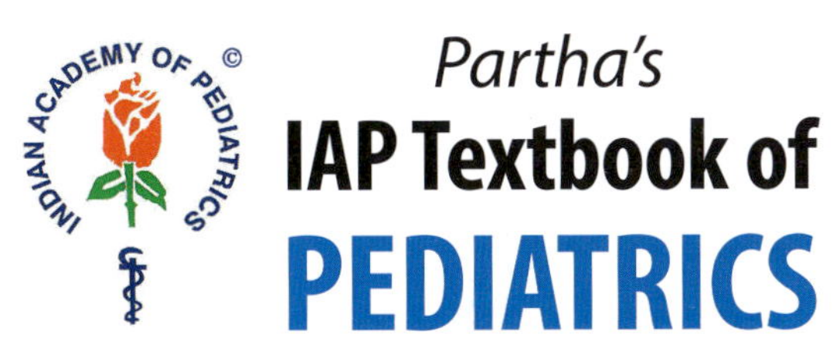

Eighth Edition

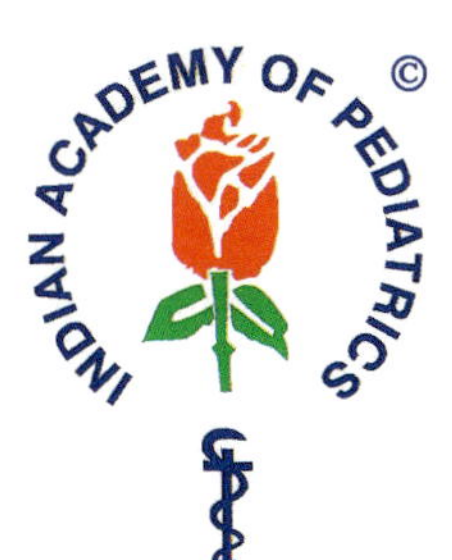

Partha's IAP Textbook of PEDIATRICS

Eighth Edition

Volume 1

Founder Editors

(Late) A Parthasarathy, PSN Menon, MKC Nair

Editor-in-Chief

PSN Menon MD MNAMS
Former Professor
Department of Pediatrics
Sub-Dean, Consultant-In-Charge
Pediatric Endocrinology and Genetics
All India Institute of Medical Sciences
New Delhi, India

Academic Editors

MKC Nair MD PhD DSc FIACAM FAMS
Director, NIMS-Spectrum
Child Development Research Centre (CDRC)
Thiruvananthapuram, Kerala, India
Formerly Vice Chancellor, KUHS
Formerly Director, CDC Kerala (Adolescent Health)

Piyush Gupta MD FRCPCH FAMS
Former Principal, Professor and Head
Department of Pediatrics
University College of Medical Sciences
and Guru Teg Bahadur Hospital
New Delhi, India

Ramachandran Padmanabhan MD DNB
Professor of Eminence, Department of Pediatrics
Head, Division of Clinical Research and Head, Bioethics Unit
Sri Ramachandra Institute of Higher Education and Research
Chennai, Tamil Nadu, India

Ritabrata Kundu MD
Professor
Department of Pediatric Medicine
Institute of Child Health
Kolkata, West Bengal, India

Executive Editor

Alok Gupta MD
Pediatrician, Counselor and Environmentalist
Pediatric Specialities Clinic, Jaipur
Former Assistant Professor of Pediatrics
MGM University
Jaipur, Rajasthan, India

Ex-Officio Editorial Advisers

GV Basavaraja MD DNB
Professor Department of Pediatrics
Indira Gandhi Institute of Child Health
Bengaluru, Karnataka, India
IAP National President 2024

Vasant M Khalatkar MD PGDID FICMCH
Consultant Pediatrician and Neonatologist
Khalatkar Hospital
Nagpur, Maharashtra, India
IAP National President, 2025

Yogesh N Parikh MD
Associate Professor
Department of Pediatrics
Government Medical College
Surat, Gujarat, India
Secretary General, IAP (2024–2025)

Atanu Bhadra DCH
Medical Superintendent
ESI Hospital
Asansol, West Bengal, India
National Treasurer, IAP (2024–2025)

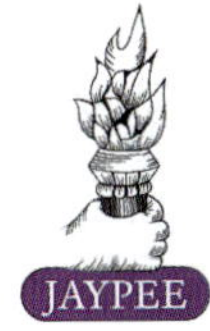

JAYPEE BROTHERS MEDICAL PUBLISHERS

The Health Sciences Publisher

New Delhi | London

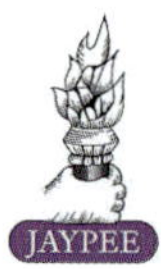

Jaypee Brothers Medical Publishers (P) Ltd

Headquarters

Jaypee Brothers Medical Publishers (P) Ltd
EMCA House, 23/23-B
Ansari Road, Daryaganj
New Delhi 110 002, India
Landline: +91-11-23272143, +91-11-23272703
+91-11-23282021, +91-11-23245672
Email: jaypee@jaypeebrothers.com

Corporate Office

Jaypee Brothers Medical Publishers (P) Ltd
4838/24, Ansari Road, Daryaganj
New Delhi 110 002, India
Phone: +91-11-43574357
Fax: +91-11-43574314
Email: jaypee@jaypeebrothers.com

Overseas Office

JP Medical Ltd
83 Victoria Street, London
SW1H 0HW (UK)
Phone: +44 20 3170 8910
Fax: +44 (0)20 3008 6180
Email: info@jpmedpub.com

Website: www.jaypeebrothers.com
Website: www.jaypeedigital.com

Inquiries for bulk sales may be solicited at: jaypee@jaypeebrothers.com

Partha's IAP Textbook of Pediatrics (3 Vols)

First Edition: 1999, 2000; Second Edition: 2002, 2003; Third Edition: 2006; Revised Reprint: 2007; Fourth Edition: 2009; Fifth Edition: 2013; Sixth Edition: 2016; Seventh Edition: 2019

Eighth Edition: **2025**

ISBN: 978-93-5696-806-6

Printed at: Samrat Offset Pvt. Ltd.

In dedication and fond memories

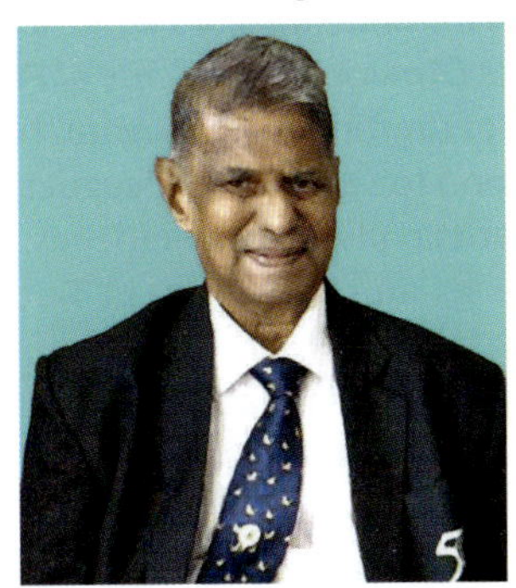

Professor Alagirisamy Parthasarathy MD DCH FIAP
DSc (Honoris Causa): The Tamil Nadu Dr MGR Medical University, Chennai, India
Emeritus Professor of Pediatrics
The Tamil Nadu Dr MGR Medical University
Chennai, Tamil Nadu, India
National President 1997, Indian Academy of Pediatrics
(August 08, 1938 – May 15, 2021)

Professor Alagirisamy Parthasarathy, National President 1997, Indian Academy of Pediatrics (IAP) was a multi-faceted person. Fondly called '*Partha Sir*' by both his contemporaries and juniors and just '*Dear Partha*' by his seniors, he had an endearing quality that made him lovable to all. Like the '*PARTHASARATHY*' (Lord Krishna) to Arjuna, he motivated and helped many academicians to come up and shine in their chosen fields.

Professor Parthasarathy graduated from the prestigious Madras Medical College, Chennai, Tamil Nadu in the year 1964. He completed his postgraduate diploma (DCH) course in the year 1973 and MD (Pediatrics) in 1976 from Madras Medical College and Institute of Child Health, Chennai. He was also trained in Clinical Epidemiology, Christian Medical College, Vellore, Tamil Nadu.

He occupied various important positions to serve the organization and was awarded the fellowship of IAP (FIAP) in 1989 for carrying out many flagship programs. He gained all-India recognition in IAP by his visionary ideas and successful implementation of many projects. He was elected as National President, IAP in the year 1997. He took up many path-breaking programs during his tenure and beyond in the field of vaccines and immunization. He served as the Regional Adviser, Association of Pediatric Societies of South-East Asia Region for three years (1997–1999).

Professor Parthasarathy worked in Tamil Nadu Health Services in various positions. He retired as Senior Clinical Professor of Pediatrics, Madras Medical College, Chennai, and Deputy Superintendent, Institute of Child Health and Hospital for Children, Chennai, Tamil Nadu. His seminal contribution was in the field of immunization services, and he was a pioneer in many successful programs in collaboration with the state health services and international organizations including UNICEF. He brought out many manuals for the healthcare workers involved in immunization activities.

Starting from the early 1990s, Professor Parthasarathy found his passion for bringing out textbooks. He was the Founder and Editor-in-Chief of Indian Journal of Practical Pediatrics which was launched under the banner of IAP in 1993. He held this post for two years and nurtured the journal from gestation to its toddlerhood. During his presidentship, he conceptualized the *IAP Textbook of Pediatrics* which proved a boon for pediatric students and practitioners. The next three decades saw a flurry of publications from IAP under his editorship in the form of *IAP Guidebook on Immunizations, IAP Immunization Card, IAP Color Atlas of Pediatrics (2011), Atlas of Pediatric Infectious Diseases (2012), Textbook of Pediatric Infectious Diseases (2012), IAP Textbook of Vaccines (2014), IAP Algorithms for Common Pediatric Illnesses (2015)* and many more. It was his brainchild to bring out a biennial treatise on *Recent Advances in Pediatrics* under IAP and two volumes have already been published in the years 2020 and 2022.

In the past 20 years, under the banner of *Partha's Series of Books for Pediatric and Adolescent Practitioners*, he brought out eight books—*Case Scenarios, Frequently Asked Questions, Management Protocols, 101 Clinical Pearls, Management Algorithms, Investigations and Interpretations, Comprehensive Manual, and Current Trends in Diagnosis and Management*—all these titles related to pediatric and adolescent practice.

He was the Founder and Editor-in-Chief of *Partha's Immunization Digest (First Edition, 2005 to 4th Edition, 2020), Handbook on Adolescent and Adult Immunization (2014), Fundamentals of Pediatrics, Selected Topics in Pediatrics for Practitioners, and* an Associate Editor in *Atlas of Tropical Pediatrics (American Academy of Pediatrics, 2009).*

Professor Parthasarathy had the unique gift of drafting in an elegant, but simple language, was prompt in communication and meticulous in detail. He showed great affection towards his colleagues, junior and senior alike. He always appreciated and encouraged the initiative by any colleague towards child health activities. He had a great command of Tamil as well and had written many beautiful Tamil poems. He wrote his autobiography in Tamil titled "*Kanne Pappa*" (Dear Child) and this was released in the Chennai Book Exhibition, 2020.

Professor Parthasarathy has a lovely family. Mrs Nirmala Parthasarathy, his wife, is a gentle and kind lady. Partha sir's children Mr Balaji and Mrs (Dr) Prathiba were extremely helpful in all his academic endeavors. He is blessed with four grandchildren.

Professor Parthasarathy was honored with numerous awards and orations. Indian Academy of Pediatrics proudly conferred him Lifetime Achievement Award of IAP in 2021.

IAP Textbook of Pediatrics was first published in 1999–2000 for which Dr Parthasarathy was the Founder and Editor-in-Chief, which he continued till the 6th edition. He continued to guide the publication of the 7th edition also. IAP considers it a great honor to name this 8th edition as *Partha's IAP Textbook of Pediatrics* as a mark of respect and affection to this great academician. Dr Parthasarathy was a very pious person, and we are sure he is blessing all of us to continue his good work in the service of children.

Section Editors

SECTION 1: Basic Concepts of Child Care

Piyush Gupta
MD FRCPCH FAMS
Former Principal, Professor and Head
Department of Pediatrics
University College of Medical Sciences
and Guru Teg Bahadur Hospital
New Delhi, India

SECTION 2: Care of the Newborn

Rhishikesh P Thakre
DM MD DNB DCH
Neonatologist
Department of Pediatrics
Neo Clinic
Aurangabad, Maharashtra, India

SECTION 3: Growth

Anju Seth MD
Director Professor and Head
Department of Pediatrics
Lady Hardinge Medical College and
Kalawati Saran Children's Hospital
New Delhi, India

SECTION 4: Development and Developmental Disorders

Samir Hasan Dalwai
MD DNB FCPS DCH LLB
Developmental Behavioral Pediatrician
New Horizons Child Development
Centre and Research Foundation
Mumbai, Maharashtra, India

SECTION 5: Nutrition and Nutritional Disorders

Praveen Kumar MD
Director Professor
Department of Pediatrics
Lady Hardinge Medical College and
Kalawati Saran Children's Hospital
New Delhi, India

SECTION 6: Immunity and Immunization

Srinivas G Kasi MD DCH
Consultant Pediatrician
Department of Pediatrics
Kasi Clinic, Bengaluru, Karnataka, India

SECTION 7: Infectious Diseases

Ritabrata Kundu MD
Professor
Department of Pediatric Medicine
Institute of Child Health
Kolkata, West Bengal, India

SECTION 8: Disorders of Central Nervous System

Sheffali Gulati MD
Professor, Child Neurology Division
Department of Pediatrics
All India Institute of Medical Sciences
New Delhi, India

SECTION 9: Diseases of Cardiovascular System

S Srinivasan DCH MD
Former Director-Professor of Pediatrics
Jawaharlal Institute of Postgraduate
Medical Education and Research
Puducherry
Professor of Pediatrics
Mahatma Gandhi Medical College and
Research Institute, Puducherry
Adjunct Professor
Department of Pediatrics
Mehta Multispecialty Hospital
Chennai, Tamil Nadu, India

SECTION 10: Disorders of Respiratory System

Sushil K Kabra MD
Former Professor and Head
Department of Pediatrics
All India Institute of Medical Sciences
New Delhi, India

SECTION 11: Disorders of Gastrointestinal Tract and Liver

Riyaz Arakkal
MD DCH DNB DM (Gastroenterology) FRCP
Professor and Head
Department of Pediatrics
KMCT Medical College
Kozhikode, Kerala, India

SECTION 12: Disorders of Hepatobiliary System and Pancreas

John Matthai
DCH MD FAB (Ped Gastro) FRCPCH
Professor
Department of Pediatric
Gastroenterology
Masonic Medical Centre for Children
Coimbatore, Tamil Nadu, India

SECTION 13: Disorders of Kidney and Urinary Tract

Arvind Bagga
MD DSc FAMS FISN
Emeritus Professor
Department of Pediatrics
All India Institute of Medical Sciences
New Delhi, India
Director of Pediatrics and Senior
Consultant (Pediatric Nephrology)
Department of Pediatrics
Indraprastha Apollo Hospitals
New Delhi, India

SECTION 14: Disorders of Hemopoietic System

Ved Prakash Choudhry
MD FIMSA FISHTM
Senior Consultant (Hematology)
Batra Hospital and Medical Research
Centre
Pushpanjali Singhania Hospital
and Research Centre
New Delhi, India

SECTION 15: Pediatric Malignancies

Purna A Kurkure MD
Head, Division of Pediatric
Hemato-oncology and BMT
Narayana Health SRCC Children's
Hospital, Mumbai
Joint Managing Trustee and Trustee
In-charge
Survivorship and Rehabilitation Division
Indian Cancer Society
Mumbai, Maharashtra, India

SECTION 16: Disorders of Endocrine System and Diabetes Mellitus

Vijayalakshmi Bhatia MD
Professor
Department of Pediatric Endocrinology
Sanjay Gandhi Postgraduate Institute
of Medical Sciences
Lucknow, Uttar Pradesh, India

PSN Menon MD MNAMS
Former Professor
Department of Pediatrics
Sub-Dean, Consultant, In-Charge
Pediatric Endocrinology and Genetics
All India Institute of Medical Sciences
New Delhi, India

SECTION 17: Genetics and Genetic Disorders

Madhulika Kabra MD
Professor and Head (Retd)
Department of Pediatrics
All India Institute of Medical Sciences
New Delhi, India

SECTION 18: Rheumatological Disorders and Allergy

Sathish Kumar
MD DCH Fellowship in Pediatric Rheumatology, Canada
Senior Professor
Division of Pediatric Rheumatology
Department of Pediatrics
Christian Medical College
Vellore, Tamil Nadu, India

SECTION 19: Adolescent Health

MKC Nair
MD PhD DSc FIACAM FAMS
Director, NIMS-Spectrum
Child Development Research Centre
(CDRC)
Thiruvananthapuram, Kerala, India
Formerly Vice Chancellor, KUHS
Formerly Director, CDC Kerala
(Adolescent Health)

SECTION 20: Intensive Care and Emergencies

Jayashree Muralidharan
MD DNB FICCM
Professor and Chief
Pediatric Critical Care Unit
Department of Pediatrics
Advanced Pediatrics Centre
Postgraduate Institute of Medical
Education and Research
Chandigarh, India

SECTION 21: Pediatric Subspecialties

Ramachandran Padmanabhan
MD DNB
Professor of Eminence
Department of Pediatrics
Head, Division of Clinical Research and
Head, Bioethics Unit
Sri Ramachandra Institute of Higher
Education and Research
Chennai, Tamil Nadu, India

SECTION 22: Community Pediatrics

Alok Gupta MD
Pediatrician, Counselor and
Environmentalist
Pediatric Specialties Clinic, Jaipur
Former Assistant Professor of Pediatrics
MGM University
Jaipur, Rajasthan, India

SECTION 23: Pediatric Procedures

Baldev S Prajapati MD DPed
Professor and Head
Department of Pediatrics
Gujarat Cancer Society Medical College,
Hospital and Research Centre
Ahmedabad, Gujarat, India

SECTION 24: Pediatric Therapeutics

Jeeson C Unni MD DCH
Senior Consultant
Department of Pediatrics and
Neonatology
Aster Medcity
Kochi, Kerala, India

Contributors

A Balachandran MD DCH PHD
Associate Head (Retd)
Division of Pulmonology
Dr Mehta's Children Hospital
Chennai, Tamil Nadu, India

Aakash Mahesan
DM (Pediatric Neurology)
Senior Resident
Department of Pediatrics
All India Institute of Medical Sciences
New Delhi, India

Aashay Abhay Shah MD FISPGHAN
Consultant
Pediatric Gastroenterologist
Director, Prism Pediatric Gastro Centre
Ahmedabad, Gujarat, India

Aashika Maria Naidu MD
Senior Resident
Department of Pediatrics
St John's Medical College and Hospital
Bengaluru, Karnataka, India

Aashima Dabas MD
Professor
Department of Pediatrics
Maulana Azad Medical College and Lok Nayak Hospital
New Delhi, India

Aathira Ravindranath
MD DM (Ped Gastro)
Consultant
Department of Pediatric Gastroenterology
Apollo BGS Hospitals
Mysuru, Karnataka, India

Abhay K Shah MD DPed
Senior Pediatrician
Consultant in Pediatric Infectious Diseases
Children Hospital
Ahmedabad, Gujarat, India

Abraham K Paul
MD DCH
Senior Consultant Pediatrician
Department of Pediatrics
Indira Gandhi Co-operative Hospital
Kochi, Kerala, India

Abraham Paulose
MD MRCPCH PDCC
Consultant Pediatrician and Pediatric Endocrinologist
Department of Pediatrics JPMC
Adjunct Senior Assistant Professor
UBD PAPRSB Institute of Health Sciences
Brunei Darussalam

Aditi Sinha MD PhD
Additional Professor
Division of Pediatric Nephrology
Department of Pediatrics
All India Institute of Medical Sciences
New Delhi, India

Akila Ganesh MDS PhD
Professor and Head
Department of Public Health Dentistry
Sri Ramachandra Dental College and Hospital
Sri Ramachandra Institute of Higher Education and Research
Chennai, Tamil Nadu, India

Alok Gupta MD
Pediatrician, Counselor and Environmentalist
Pediatric Specialties Clinic, Jaipur
Former Assistant Professor of Pediatrics
MGM University
Jaipur, Rajasthan, India

Amar Jeet Chitkara MD DNB
Senior Director
Department of Pediatrics
Max Superspecialty Hospital
New Delhi, India

Amar M Taksande
MD PhD FIAE Fellowship in Ped Cardiology
Professor and Head
Department of Pediatrics
Jawaharlal Nehru Medical College
Dutta Meghe Institute of Higher Education and Research
Wardha, Maharashtra, India

Amita Aggarwal MD DM
Professor and Head
Department of Clinical Immunology and Rheumatology
Sanjay Gandhi Postgraduate Institute of Medical Sciences
Lucknow, Uttar Pradesh, India

Amita Mahajan
MD MRCPCH CCST
Senior Consultant
Department of Pediatric Hematology/Oncology
Indraprastha Apollo Hospitals
New Delhi, India

Amita Trehan MD
Professor
Department of Pediatrics
Postgraduate Institute of Medical Education and Research
Chandigarh, India

Anika Bhandari MBBS
Resident Medical Officer
Department of Pediatrics
Sarojini Naidu Medical College
Agra, Uttar Pradesh, India

Anil Sachdev MD DCH
Director
Division of Pediatric Emergency, Criticare
Pulmonology and Allergic Disorders
Sir Ganga Ram Hospital
New Delhi, India

Aniruddha Ghosh MD DNB MNAMS
Assistant Professor
Department of Pediatric Medicine
Institute of Child Health
Kolkata, West Bengal, India

Anita Saxena MD DM (Card)
Vice Chancellor
Pt BD Sharma University of Health Sciences
Rohtak, Haryana, India

Anjali Tomar MD
FNB Trainee
Department of Pediatric Nephrology
Sir Ganga Ram Hospital
New Delhi, India

Anju Gupta MD
Professor
Department of Pediatrics
Advanced Pediatric Center
Postgraduate Institute of Medical Education and Research
Chandigarh, India

Anju Seth MD
Director Professor and Head
Department of Pediatrics
Lady Hardinge Medical College and Kalawati Saran Children's Hospital
New Delhi, India

Anju Virmani
MD DNB (Endocrinology)
Director, Pediatric Endocrinology
Pediatric Diabetes and Endocrinology
Department of Pediatrics
Max Smart Super Specialty Hospital
New Delhi, India

Anu Kiruba Devi Gunasekaran
MD DVL
Post-doctoral Fellow in Pediatric Dermatology
Department of Dermatology, Venereology and Leprosy
Christian Medical College and Hospital
Vellore, Tamil Nadu, India

Anupam Sachdeva MD
Senior Consultant and Head
Department of Pediatrics
Sir Ganga Ram Hospital
New Delhi, India

Anupama S Borker MD
Professor and Head
Department of Medical Oncology
Goa Medical College and Hospital
Panjim, Goa, India

Anupama Singh
MD (Community Medicine)
Assistant Professor
Department of Community Medicine
Santosh Medical College
Ghaziabad, Uttar Pradesh, India

Anuradha Khadilkar MD DCH (London)
Deputy Director
Department of Growth and Pediatric Endocrine Unit
Hirabai Cowasji Jehangir Medical Research Institute and Jehangir Hospital
Pune, Maharashtra, India

Anand Prakash Dubey MD
Former Director Professor
Department of Pediatrics
Maulana Azad Medical College
New Delhi, India

(Col) Aparajita Gupta
MD DM (Pediatric Neurology)
Associate Professor
Department of Pediatrics
Army Hospital (R&R)
New Delhi, India

Aparna Chandrasekaran MD DM (Neo)
Senior Consultant and Head
Department of Neonatology
KIMS Cuddles
Hyderabad, Telangana, India

Aparna Mukherjee MD PhD
Scientist E
Clinical Studies and Trial Unit
Indian Council of Medical Research
New Delhi, India, India

Aradhana Rohil MD
Senior Resident
Centre of Excellence and Advanced Research for Childhood Neurodevelopmental Disorders
Child Neurology Division
Department of Pediatrics
All India Institute of Medical Sciences
New Delhi, India

Archana S Kher MD
Former Professor
Department of Pediatrics
Seth GS Medical College and King Edward Memorial Hospital
Mumbai, Maharashtra, India

Arpana Iyengar MD DNB FRCP PhD
Professor
Department of Pediatric Nephrology
St John's Medical College Hospital
Bengaluru, Karnataka, India

Arun Bansal MD FRCPCH FCCM FAMS
Professor
Department of Pediatrics
Advanced Pediatric Centre
Postgraduate Institute of Medical Education and Research
Chandigarh, India

Arun Kumar Gupta MD
Professor and Head
Department of Imaging
Saran Ashram Hospital
Agra, Uttar Pradesh, India

Arun Kumar L MS MCh (Ped Surgery) MRCS
Associate Professor
Department of Pediatric Surgery
Christian Medical College and Hospital
Vellore, Tamil Nadu, India

Arun Phatak MD DPed
Former Professor of Pediatrics
Department of Pediatrics
Medical College, Vadodara
Government Medical College, Surat
Kashiben Gordhandas Patel Children Hospital
Vadodara, Gujarat, India

Arun Wadhwa MD
Visiting Consultant
Department of Pediatrics
Rainbow Children's Hospital
New Delhi, India

Arushi G Saini MD DM MNAMS
Associate Professor
Department of Pediatrics
Advanced Pediatrics Center
Postgraduate Institute of Medical Education and Research
Chandigarh, India

Arvind Bagga MD DSc FAMS FISN
Emeritus Professor
Department of Pediatrics
All India Institute of Medical Sciences
New Delhi, India
Director of Pediatrics and Senior Consultant (Pediatric Nephrology)
Department of Pediatrics
Indraprastha Apollo Hospitals
New Delhi, India

Asha Benakappa MD
Head
Department of Pediatrics
Dr Chandramma Dayananda Sagar Institute of Medical Education and Research (CDSIMER)
Ramanagara, Karnataka, India

Ashish R Bavdekar DCH DNB
Director of Pediatrics and Pediatric Gastroenterologist
Department of Pediatric Gastroenterology
KEM Hospital
Pune, Maharashtra, India

Ashok K Patwari MD DCH MNAMS FAMS
Former Professor
Department of Pediatrics
Lady Hardinge Medical College
New Delhi, India
Research Professor (International Health)
Boston University School of Public Health
Boston, USA

Ashok Kumar Dutta MD
Former Director Professor and Head
Department of Pediatrics
Lady Hardinge Medical College
New Delhi, India

Atul Bhaskar
MS (Orth) FRCS (Surg) FRCS (Tr & Orth) DNB (Orth) MCH (Orth) Fellowship in Pediatric Ortho (SICKKIDS, Toronto)
Consultant
Department of Pediatric Orthopedics
Bombay Hospital Institute of Medical Sciences
Apollo Hospital, Belapur, Navi Mumbai
Sir HN Reliance Hospital
Mumbai, Maharashtra, India

B Vishnu Bhat MD DHA DDE
Adviser, Medical Research and Publications
Pediatrics and Neonatology
Aarupadai Veedu Medical College and Hospital
Puducherry, India

Badira C Parambil MD DM
Professor
Department of Pediatric Oncology
Tata Memorial Hospital
Homi Bhabha National Institute
Mumbai, Maharashtra, India

Baker Ninan Fenn
MD DM (Infectious Diseases)
Senior Resident
Department of Infectious Diseases
Government Medical College
Kottayam, Kerala, India

Balasubramanian S MD DCH
Senior Consultant
Department of Pediatrics
Kanchi Kamakoti CHILDS Trust Hospital
Chennai, Tamil Nadu, India

Baldev S Prajapati MD DPed
Professor and Head
Department of Pediatrics
Gujarat Cancer Society Medical College, Hospital and Research Centre
Ahmedabad, Gujarat, India

Banani Poddar MD DNB
Professor and Head
Department of Critical Care Medicine
Sanjay Gandhi Postgraduate Institute of Medical Sciences
Lucknow, Uttar Pradesh, India

Bandlamudi Lakshmi Parvathi MD
Senior Resident
Department of Neonatology
St John's Medical College Hospital
Bengaluru, Karnataka, India

BD Gupta MD
Former Professor and Head
Department of Pediatrics
Former Superintendent and Additional Principal
Dr Sampurnanand Medical College
Jodhpur, Rajasthan, India

Bharat Mehra MD FPEM IFPCCM DPAA
Assistant Professor
Department of Pediatrics
Sri Guru Ram Das Institute of Medical Sciences
Amritsar, Punjab, India

Bharat R Agarwal MD DCH DNB MNAMS
Professor Emeritus and Former Head
Department of Pediatric Hematology and Oncology
Bai Jerbai Wadia Hospital for Children
Mumbai, Maharashtra, India

Bhaskar Raju
MD DCH MNAMS DM (Gastro)
Professor and Head (Retd)
Department of Pediatric Gastroenterology
Institute of Child Health and Hospital for Children
Chennai, Tamil Nadu, India

Bhavna Dhingra
MD DNB DBT Fellowship Genetic Diagnostics
Professor
Department of Pediatrics
All India Institute of Medical Sciences
Bhopal, Madhya Pradesh, India

Bhoomika Sharma MBBS
Registrar
Department of Pediatric Neurosciences
Rainbow Children's Hospital
Hyderabad, Telangana, India

Bikrant Bihari Lal MD PDCC
Associate Professor
Department of Pediatric Hepatology
Institute of Liver and Biliary Sciences
New Delhi, India

Biswaroop Chakrabarty
MD DNB MNAMS DM (Pediatric Neurology)
Additional Professor
Child Neurology Division
Department of Pediatrics
All India Institute of Medical Sciences
New Delhi, India

BR Nammalwar
MD DCH MNAMS DM (Nephrology)
Director
Department of Pediatric Nephrology
Mehta Multispecialty Hospitals India Pvt Ltd, Chennai, Tamil Nadu, India

C Thangadorai MD DCH MNAMS
Senior Clinical Professor (Retd)
Department of Pediatrics
Madras Medical College
Chennai, Tamil Nadu, India

Chandra Mohan Kumar MD
Professor and Head
Department of Pediatrics
All India Institute of Medical Sciences
Patna, Bihar, India

Chandrika Rao MD
Professor, Department of Pediatrics
Convener
Department of Medical Education Unit
MS Ramaiah Medical College
Bengaluru, Karnataka, India

Chandrika S Bhat
MD Fellowship in Pediatric Rheumatology (UK)
Consultant
Pediatric Rheumatology Services
Rainbow Children's Hospital
Bengaluru, Karnataka, India

Chhaya Akshay Divecha
MD DCH Fellowship in Pediatric Intensive Care (MUHS) Fellowship in Neonatal Intensive Care (IAP)
Associate Professor
Department of Pediatrics
College of Medicine and Health Sciences
National University of Science and Technology, Sohar, Sultanate of Oman

D Balachandar DCH DNB MNAMS
Senior Consultant
General Hospital
Pathanamthitta, Kerala, India

D Vijayasekaran MD DCH PhD
Consultant Pediatric Pulmonologist
Pediatric Respiratory Medicine
Apollo Children's Hospital and Kanchi Kamakoti CHILDS Trust Hospital
Chennai, Tamil Nadu, India

Deepa Bhaskaran
MD PG Diploma in Adolescent Pediatrics
PG Diploma in Developmental Neurology
Associate Professor
Department of Developmental Pediatrics
Child Development Centre
Thiruvananthapuram, Kerala, India

Deepak Bansal
MD DNB FAMS
Professor
Pediatric Hematology-Oncology Unit
Department of Pediatrics
Advanced Pediatrics Center
Postgraduate Institute of Medical Education and Research
Chandigarh, India

Deepak Ugra MD FRCPCH (London)
Senior Honorary Consultant
Pediatrics and Pediatric Pulmonology
Lilavati Hospital and Research Centre
PD Hinduja Hospital, Apollo Hospitals
Mumbai, Maharashtra, India

Dhanya Dharmapalan
MD PG Dip in PID (Oxford) FPIDS
Consultant in Pediatric Infectious Diseases
Department of Pediatrics
Apollo Children's Hospital
Navi Mumbai, Maharashtra, India

Dharshini Sathishkumar
MD (DVL) DDVL International Fellowship in Pediatric Dermatology, UK
Professor
Department of Dermatology, Venereology and Leprosy
Christian Medical College and Hospital
Vellore, Tamil Nadu, India

Dheeraj Shah MD DNB FAMS
Principal
Department of Pediatrics
University College of Medical Sciences
New Delhi, India

Dhiren Gupta MD
Deputy Director
Division of Pediatric Emergency, Critical Care, Pulmonology and Allergic Disorders
Sir Ganga Ram Hospital
New Delhi, India

Digant D Shastri
MD PGDHHM
Senior Consultant Pediatrician and CEO
Department of Pediatrics, NICU and Vaccination Center
Killol Children Hospital
Surat, Gujarat, India

Dipty L Jain
MD MSc Medicine (McMaster, Canada)
Adjunct Professor
Department of Pediatrics
Shalinitai Meghe Hospital and Research Center
Nagpur, Maharashtra, India

Divij Sachdeva MD
Associate Consultant
Department of Pediatrics
Sir Ganga Ram Hospital
New Delhi, India

Divya Nandakumar DNB
Post-doctoral Fellowship in Infectious Diseases
Department of Pediatric Infectious Diseases
Christian Medical College
Vellore, Tamil Nadu, India

Divya Prabhat MS DORL DNB FICS
Head
Department of Ear, Nose and Throat
Bai Jerbai Wadia Hospital for Children
Mumbai, Maharashtra, India

Divya Selvaraj MD
Resident, DNB Pediatric Critical Care
Pediatric Intensive Care Unit
Dr Mehta's Multispecialty Hospital
Chennai, Tamil Nadu, India

Ebor Jacob G James
DNB DCH FICCM FCCMDM
Senior Professor (Pediatric Critical Care)
Department of Pediatrics
Christian Medical College
Vellore, Tamil Nadu, India

Gargi Ajinkya Bangar
MD PGDip in Pediatric Infectious Diseases
Consultant
Department of Pediatrics
Kharghar Medicity Hospital
Navi Mumbai, Maharashtra, India

Gauri Kapoor MD PhD
Director and Head
Department of Pediatric Hematology and Oncology
Rajiv Gandhi Cancer Institute and Research Centre
New Delhi, India

Gautam Kamila
MD DNB DM (Pediatric Neurology)
Senior Research Associate
Centre of Excellence and
Advanced Research for Childhood
Neurodevelopmental Disorders
Child Neurology Division
Department of Pediatrics
All India Institute of Medical Sciences
New Delhi, India

Geetha Chanda
MD IAP PDF (Pediatric Neurology)
Consultant
Department of Pediatric Neurology
Rainbow Children's Hospital
Hyderabad, Telangana, India

Geetha Mammayil
MD DNB DM (Gastro)
Senior Consultant
Department of Pediatric
Gastroenterology
Aster Medcity
Kochi, Kerala, India

George F Moolayil DCH PGDMLE
Pediatrician and Consultant
in Medical Law (Retd)
Kottayam, Kerala, India
President IAP, Kerala 2008
Executive Board Member
CIAP 2009, 2010
CIAP, Election Commissioner 2011
2012, 2013

Gnanamurthy Narasimha DCH
Consultant Pediatrician
Department of Pediatrics
Mother and Child Care Centre
Bengaluru, Karnataka, India

Gurmeet Kaur MD
Professor
Department of Pediatrics
Christian Medical College and Hospital
Ludhiana, Punjab, India

H Paramesh
MD FAAP FIAMS FIAA FICAAI FICS FICCP
Visiting Physician Scientist
Divecha Centre for Climate Change
Indian Institute of Science
Bengaluru, Karnataka, India

Indira Agarwal MD FISN
Professor of Pediatrics
Christian Medical College
Vellore, Tamil Nadu, India

Indra Shekhar Rao M
MD DCH NEO (USA)
Director, Professor and Head
Department of Pediatrics and
Neonatology
Navodaya Hospital
Secunderabad, Telangana, India

Jagadeesh Menon VR MD DM
Consultant
Pediatric Gastroenterology, Hepatology
and Nutrition
Dr Rela Institute and Medical Centre
Chennai, Tamil Nadu, India

Jagdish Chandra MD
Professor and Head
Department of Pediatrics
ESIC Medical College and Hospital
Faridabad, Haryana, India

Jagdish Chinnappa MD
Chairman
Department of Pediatrics
Manipal Hospital
Bengaluru, Karnataka

Jagdish Prasad Goyal
MD ERS Diplomat in Pediatric Respiratory
Medicine
Professor
Department of Pediatrics
All India Institute of Medical Sciences
Jodhpur, Rajasthan, India

Jaya Agarwal MD
Senior Consultant
Department of Gastroenterology
Regency Health
Kanpur, Uttar Pradesh, India

Jayakar Thomas
MD DD MNAMS PhD FAAD FIAD FRCP (Edin)
FRCP (Glasgow) FRCP (London) FRCP (Ireland)
FRCPCH (London) DSc
Director–Research
Department of Dermatology
Chettinad Academy of Research
and Education
Chennai, Tamil Nadu, India

Jayashree Muralidharan
MD DNB FICCM
Professor and Chief
Pediatric Critical Care Unit
Department of Pediatrics
Advanced Pediatrics Centre
Postgraduate Institute of Medical
Education and Research
Chandigarh, India

Jaydeep Choudhury
DNB MNAMS
Professor
Department of Pediatric Medicine
Institute of Child Health
Kolkata, West Bengal, India

Jeeson C Unni MD DCH
Senior Consultant
Department of Pediatrics
and Neonatology
Aster Medcity
Kochi, Kerala, India

Jitendra Meena MD DM
Assistant Professor
Division of Pediatric Nephrology
Department of Pediatrics
All India Institute of Medical Sciences
New Delhi, India

John Matthai
DCH MD FAB (Ped Gastro) FRCPCH
Professor
Department of Pediatric
Gastroenterology
Masonic Medical Centre for Children
Coimbatore, Tamil Nadu, India

Joseph L Mathew MD PhD
Professor (Pediatric Pulmonology)
Department of Pediatrics
Advanced Pediatrics Centre
Postgraduate Institute of Medical
Education and Research
Chandigarh, India

JP Dadhich MD PGDDN
Director
Department of Pediatrics and
Neonatology
CK Birla Hospitals—Rukmani Birla
Hospital (RBH)
Jaipur, Rajasthan, India

Jugesh Chhatwal DCH MD FAIMER Fellow
Professor
Department of Pediatrics
School of Medical Sciences and Research
Sharda University
Greater Noida, Uttar Pradesh, India

Jyothi Janardhanan MD
Fellow
Division of Pediatric Immunology and Rheumatology
Department of Pediatrics
Aster CMI Hospital
Bengaluru, Karnataka, India

Jyothi Jayaram DM (Pediatric Critical Care)
Senior Resident
Pediatric Critical Care Unit
Department of Pediatrics
Advanced Pediatrics Centre
Postgraduate Institute of Medical Education and Research
Chandigarh, India

(Col) Jyoti Kotwal
MD (Pathology) FAMS PDF (Hemat) FRCP (Edin)
Chairperson and Professor
Department of Hematology
Sir Ganga Ram Hospital and Ganga Ram Institute of Postgraduate Medical Education and Research
New Delhi, India

Jyoti Sharma
MD DNB ISN and ISPN Fellowships in Ped Nephrology
Consultant
Renal Unit, Department of Medicine
King Edward Memorial Hospital
Pune, Maharashtra, India

Jyotindra Narayan Goswami
MD DNB DM (Ped Neurology)
Professor
Department of Pediatrics
Command Hospital
Kolkata, West Bengal, India

K Nedunchelian MD DCH
Senior Consultant Pediatrician
Head (Research and Academics)
Department of Pediatrics
Mehta Multispecialty Hospitals India Pvt Ltd
Chennai, Tamil Nadu, India

Kailash Sarathy
MS (Orthopedics)
Consultant Pediatric Orthopedic Surgeon
Department of Orthopedics
Kanchi Kamakoti CHILDS Trust Hospital
Chennai, Tamil Nadu, India

Kakali Roy MD
Clinical Tutor of Pediatrics
Department of Pediatric Medicine and Infectious Disease
Beliaghata General Hospital
Kolkata, West Bengal, India

Kamran Afzal MD
Professor
Department of Pediatrics
Jawaharlal Nehru Medical College
Aligarh Muslim University
Aligarh, Uttar Pradesh, India

Kanishka Das
MS DNB (Gen Surg) MCh DNB MNAMS (Ped Surg)
Professor
Department of Pediatric Surgery
All India Institute of Medical Sciences
Bhubaneswar, Odisha, India

Karthi Nallasamy
MD DM (Pediatric Critical Care)
Additional Professor
Department of Pediatrics
Advanced Pediatrics Centre
Postgraduate Institute of Medical Education and Research
Chandigarh, India

Kaushik Ragunathan
MD DNB DM (Pediatric Neurology)
Senior Resident
Department of Pediatrics
All India Institute of Medical Sciences
New Delhi, India

(Gp Capt) Kanwaljit S Multani MD
Associate Professor and Head
Department of Pediatrics
Maharishi Markandeshwar College of Medical Science and Research (MMCMSR)
Ambala, Haryana, India

KE Elizabeth
MD DCH PhD FRCPCH
Professor and Head
Department of Pediatrics
Sree Mookambika Institute of Medical Sciences
Kanyakumari, Tamil Nadu, India

Ketan H Shah MD
CEO
Department of Pediatrics
Ketan Children Hospital and Saachi Hospital
Surat, Gujarat, India

Ketan Parikh
MS MCh (Ped Surgery)
Senior Consultant
Department of Pediatric Surgery
Narayana Health–SRCC Children's Hospital
Mumbai, Maharashtra, India

Kiran Aggarwal
DCH FAMS (Vienna)
Former Senior Pediatrician and Unit Head
Department of Pediatrics and Neonatology
Hindu Rao Hospital
Municipal Corporation of Delhi
New Delhi, India

Komalavalli Subbiah
MD (Radiodiagnosis) PDF (HPB&GI Imaging)
Senior Consultant and Clinical Lead (HPB and Transplant Imaging)
Department of Radiology
Dr Rela Institute and Medical Centre
Chennai, Tamil Nadu, India

Krishna Mohan R
DNB Dip (Allergy & Asthma) MNAMS
Consultant Pediatrician
Kerala Government Health Services
Government Taluk Hospital
Malappuram, Kerala, India

Kriti Mohan MD
Additional Professor
Department of Pediatrics
All India Institute of Medical Sciences
Gorakhpur, Uttar Pradesh, India

Kul Bhushan MD
Assistant Professor
Department of Pediatrics
Jaipur National University Institute for Medical Sciences and Research Centre
Jaipur, Rajasthan, India

Kusum Kalla
DNB PGDAP
Senior Honorary Consultant
Department of Pediatrics
Santokba Durlabhji Memorial Hospital and Medical Research Institute
Jaipur, Rajasthan, India

L Subramanyam MD DCH
Pediatric Pulmonologist
Division of Pediatric Pulmonology
Mehta Multispecialty Hospitals
Chennai, Tamil Nadu, India

Lakshminarayanan Kannan MD DM
Senior Consultant Pediatric Neurologist and Epileptologist
Department of Neurology
Gleneagles Health City
Chennai, Tamil Nadu, India

Lalit Bharadia
MD DNB PDCC Fellowship Pediatric Gastroenterology
Consultant
Department of Pediatrics
Neo Clinic Children Hospital
Jaipur, Rajasthan, India

Lalit Takia MD DM (Pediatric Critical Care)
Assistant Professor
Department of Pediatrics (NCI)
All India Institute of Medical Sciences
New Delhi, India

Lalitha Kailas MD DCH
Professor
Department of Pediatrics
Sree Gokulam Medical College and Research Foundation
Thiruvananthapuram, Kerala, India

Lalitha Rajalakshmi S
DCH DNB MRCPCH Fellow in Neonatology
Department of Neonatology
Lancashire Teaching Hospitals
NHS Foundation Trust, UK

Leena Srivastava
DCH PGD-DN Fellowship in Pediatric Neurology-Epilepsy MA (Psychology)
Head
Division of Developmental and Behavioral Pediatrics
Department of Pediatrics
Bharati Vidyapeeth (Deemed to be) University Medical College and Hospital
Pune, Maharashtra, India

Lokesh Lingappa
MD DM (Neurology) MRCPCH (UK) Fellowship in Pediatric Neurology (UK)
Consultant, Pediatrician and Neurologist
Head, Pediatric Neurology
Department of Pediatric Neurosciences
Rainbow Children's Hospital
Hyderabad, Telangana, India

Lokesh Saini MD DM (Pediatric Neurology)
Assistant Professor
Department of Pediatrics
All India Institute of Medical Sciences
Jodhpur, Rajasthan, India

Lulu Mathews
MD PG Diploma in Palliative Medicine (Cardiff) National Fellowship in Palliative Medicine
Medical Officer
Director (Academics Programs)
Department of Palliative Medicine
Institute of Palliative Medicine (IPM)
Kozhikode, Kerala, India

M Vijayakumar MD DCH DNB FRCPCh
Professor and Head
Department of Pediatrics
Institute of Maternal and Child Health
Government Medical College
Kozhikode, Kerala, India

Madhu Nayak MD
Associate Professor
Department of Pediatrics
Sarojini Naidu Medical College
Agra, Uttar Pradesh, India

(Lt Gen) Madhuri Kanitkar
MD DNB Fellowship in Pediatric Nephrology
Vice Chancellor
Department of Pediatric Nephrology
Maharashtra University of Health Sciences
Nashik, Maharashtra, India

Madhukar R Lokeshwar MD DCH
Consultant Pediatrics, Pediatric Hematology and Oncology (Retd)
Department of Pediatrics
Lilavati Hospital and Research Center
Mumbai, Maharashtra, India

Madhulika Kabra MD
Professor and Head (Retd)
Department of Pediatrics
All India Institute of Medical Sciences
New Delhi, India

Madhusudan Samprathi
MD DM (Pediatric Critical Care)
Associate Professor
Department of Pediatrics
All India Institute of Medical Sciences
Hyderabad, Telangana, India

Mahesh A Mohite MD DCH
Medical Director
Sai Child Care Hospital
Bai Jerbai Wadia Children's Hospital
Mumbai, Maharashtra, India

Mahesh Kamate
MD DNB DM (Ped Neurology)
Professor and Head
Department of Pediatric Neurology
Jawaharlal Nehru Medical College
KAHER University
Belagavi, Karnataka, India

Malathi Sathiyasekaran
MD DCH MNAMS DM (Gastro)
Senior Consultant
Department of Gastroenterology
MGM Health Care and Rainbow Children's Hospital
Chennai, Tamil Nadu, India

Manas Kalra MD DNB FNB
Senior Consultant
Department of Pediatrics
Sir Ganga Ram Hospital
New Delhi, India

Manisha Jana
MD DNB FRCR
Professor
Department of Radiodiagnosis and Interventional Radiology
All India Institute of Medical Sciences
New Delhi, India

Manju Mehta PhD
Consultant Psychologist
Former Professor of Clinical Psychology
Department of Psychiatry
All India Institute of Medical Sciences
New Delhi, India

Maya Prasad
MD Fellowship Pediatric Oncology
Professor
Division of Pediatric Oncology
Department of Medical Oncology
Tata Memorial Hospital
Homi Bhabha National Institute
Mumbai, Maharashtra, India

Medha Mittal MD
Associate Professor
Department of Pediatrics
Chacha Nehru Bal Chikitsalaya
New Delhi, India

Menka Yadav
MD DM
Assistant Professor
Division of Pediatric Nephrology
Department of Pediatrics
All India Institute of Medical Sciences
New Delhi, India

Mihir Sarkar MD
Professor
Department of Pediatrics
Government Medical College
Kolkata, West Bengal, India

Milind S Tullu
MD DCH DNB FCPS MNAMS
Professor
Department of Pediatrics
Seth GS Medical College and KEM Hospital
Mumbai, Maharashtra, India

MKC Nair
MD PhD DSc FIACAM FAMS
Director, NIMS-Spectrum
Child Development Research Centre (CDRC)
Thiruvananthapuram, Kerala, India
Formerly Vice Chancellor, KUHS
Formerly Director, CDC Kerala (Adolescent Health)

Moinak Sen Sarma MD DM
Additional Professor
Department of Pediatric Gastroenterology
Sanjay Gandhi Postgraduate Institute of Medical Sciences
Lucknow, Uttar Pradesh, India

Monica Juneja MD
Director-Professor and Head
Department of Pediatrics
Maulana Azad Medical College and Lok Nayak Hospital
New Delhi, India

Monjori Mitra DCH DNB
Professor
Department of Pediatrics
Institute of Child Health
Kolkata, West Bengal, India

Mounika Endrakanti
MD DNB DM (Medical Genetics)
Scientist (C)
Division of Genetics
Department of Pediatrics
All India Institute of Medical Sciences
New Delhi, India

Mounika Reddy
MD DM (Pediatric Critical Care)
Assistant Professor
Department of Pediatrics
All India Institute of Medical Sciences
Hyderabad, Telangana, India

Mukul Vij MD PDCC
Senior Consultant
Department of Pathology
Dr Rela Institute and Medical Center
Chennai, Tamil Nadu, India

Muralidhar L Kulkarni
MD FRCPCH (UK) FICPCC (London) FIMSA FIANS
Former Professor and Head
Department of Pediatrics
Jagadguru Jayadeva Murugarajendra Medical College
Davangere, Karnataka, India

N Prasanna Kumar
MD DM (Child and Adolescent Psychiatry)
Professor and Head
Child and Adolescent Psychiatry
Andhra Medical College
Visakhapatnam, Andhra Pradesh, India

Namita Ravikumar
DM (Pediatric Critical Care)
Assistant Professor and Intensivist
Department of Pediatrics
MS Ramaiah Medical College
Bengaluru, Karnataka, India

Nandkishor S Kabra
MD DNB MSc (Clinical Epidemiology) DM (Neo)
Consultant Neonatologist and Director of NICU
Department of Neonatology
Surya Hospitals
Mumbai, Maharashtra, India

Narendra Kumar Bagri
MD Fellowship Pediatric Rheumatology (Bristol, UK)
Additional Professor
Division of Pediatric Rheumatology
Department of Pediatrics
All India Institute of Medical Sciences
New Delhi, India

Narendra B Rathi MD DNB
Founder, CEO, Chief Consultant Pediatrician
Smile Children Clinic
Smile Institute of Child Health
Mumbai, Maharashtra, India

Naresh Shanmugam
DCH DNB FRCPCH Dip Nutr Med
Consultant Pediatric Hepatologist and Gastroenterologist
Dr Rela Institute and Medical Centre
Chennai, Tamil Nadu, India

Naveen Parkash Gupta
MD DNB (Neonatology) Fellowship in Neonatology (BC Children's Hospital, Vancouver, Canada)
Senior Consultant
Department of Neonatology
Madhukar Rainbow Children's Hospital
New Delhi, India

Naveen Sankhyan
MD DM (Pediatric Neurology)
Professor and Head
Pediatrics Neurology Unit
Department of Pediatrics
Advanced Pediatrics Center
Postgraduate Institute of Medical Education and Research
Chandigarh, India

NC Gowrishankar MD DCH DNB FIPP
Head
Department of Pediatrics and
Pediatric Pulmonologist
Division of Pediatric Pulmonology
Mehta Multispecialty Hospitals
Chennai, Tamil Nadu, India

Neelam Mohan
DNB FPGH (UK) FIMSA FACG (USA) FRCPCH
Senior Director
Department of Pediatric
Gastroenterology, Hepatology,
and Liver Transplantation
Medanta—The Medicity
Gurugram, Haryana, India

Nidhi Dhariwal MD DM
Assistant Professor
Department of Pediatric Oncology
Homi Bhabha Cancer Hospital and
Research Centre
New Chandigarh, Punjab, India

Nigam Prakash Narain
MD DCH PhD MRCP (UK) FRCPCH
Professor and Head (Retd)
Department of Pediatrics
Patna Medical College
Patna, Bihar, India

Niranjan G Shendurnikar MD
Child Health Consultant
Ankur Children Clinic
Vadodara, Gujarat, India

Nirmala Dheivamani
DCH MD DM (Gastro)
Professor and Head
Department of Pediatric
Gastroenterology
Institute of Child Health and Hospital
for Children
Chennai, Tamil Nadu, India

Nisanth Selvam MD DM
Senior Resident
Department of Pediatric Cardiology
Amrita Institute of Medical Sciences
Kochi, Kerala, India

Nitin K Shah MD DCH
Section Coordinator and Consultant
Department of Pediatrics
PD Hinduja Hospital
Mumbai, Maharashtra, India

Nupur Ganguly
DCh DNB
Professor
Department of Pediatric Medicine
Institute of Child Health
Kolkata, West Bengal, India

P Leela Kumari
DCH DNB MPhil (Clinical Epidemiology)
PhD (Medicine)
Additional Professor
Department of Pediatrics
SAT Hospital, Government Medical
College
Thiruvananthapuram, Kerala, India

Padmaja A Marathe
MD (Pharmacology)
Additional Professor
Department of Pharmacology and
Therapeutics
Seth GS Medical College and KEM
Hospital
Mumbai, Maharashtra, India

Pallavi Prasad MD
Associate Professor
Department of Pathology
Sanjay Gandhi Postgraduate Institute
of Medical Sciences
Lucknow, Uttar Pradesh, India

Pankaj Hari MD
Professor and Head
Department of Pediatrics
All India Institute of Medical Sciences
New Delhi, India

Parang N Mehta MD
Consultant
Department of Pediatrics
Mehta Hospital
Surat, Gujarat, India

Parimalam Kumar
MD DD DNB MNAMS FIAD FAAD
FRCP (Glasgow)
Professor and Head
Department of Dermatology
Madha Medical College and Research
Institute
The Tamil Nadu Dr MGR Medical
University
Chennai, Tamil Nadu, India

Paul SS Russell MD DSc
Senior Professor of Psychiatry
Child and Adolescent Psychiatry Unit
Christian Medical College and Hospital
Vellore, Tamil Nadu, India

Payal Gupta DNB FCO FPOS (SNC)
Associate Consultant
Department of Ophthalmology
Fortis Hospital
Greater Noida, Uttar Pradesh, India

Payal Malhotra DNB FNB
Consultant
Department of Pediatric Oncology
Rajiv Gandhi Cancer Institute
New Delhi, India

Piyush Gupta MD FRCPCH FAMS
Former Principal, Professor and Head
Department of Pediatrics
University College of Medical Sciences
and Guru Teg Bahadur Hospital
New Delhi, India

Pooja Dewan MD
Director-Professor
Department of Pediatrics
University College of Medical Sciences
New Delhi, India

Pooja Soni MD
Senior Resident
Department of Pediatrics
ESIC Medical College and Hospital
Faridabad, Haryana, India

PP Maiya MD DCH
Retired Professor of Pediatrics
Senior Pediatric Consultant
Department of Pediatrics
Sagar Hospital
Bengaluru, Karnataka, India

Pranitha Reddy
DCh Fellowship in Neonatology
Consultant Neonatologist
KIMS Cuddles
Hyderabad, Telangana, India

Prasanth KS DCh DNB DM (Gastro)
Associate Professor
Division of Pediatric Gastroenterology
Department of Pediatrics
SAT Hospital
Government Medical College
Thiruvananthapuram, Kerala, India

Prashant Jauhari MD DM
Additional Professor
Child Neurology Division
Department of Pediatrics
All India Institute of Medical Sciences
New Delhi, India

Pratiksha Khatua MD
Fellow in Infectious Disease (IAP)
Department of Pediatric Medicine
Institute of Child Health
Kolkata, West Bengal, India

Pratima Anand MD DM (Neonatology)
Neonatologist
Department of Neonatology
Lady Hardinge Medical College and
Kalawati Saran Children's Hospital
New Delhi, India

Pratima R Shah MD DPed
Consulting Pediatrician
Department of Pediatrics
Ankur Institute of Child Health
Ahmedabad, Gujarat, India

Pravas Mishra
MD (Medicine) DM (Clinical Hematology)
Professor
Department of Hematology/Oncology
and Bone Marrow Transplant
Amrita Institute of Medical Sciences
Faridabad, Haryana, India

(Late) Praveen Sobti MD DCH FIMSA
Former Director
Guru Teg Bahadur Charitable Hospital
Ludhiana
Former Professor of Pediatric Hemato-oncology
Christian Medical College and Hospital
Ludhiana, Punjab, India

Praveen Kumar MD
Director Professor
Department of Pediatrics
Lady Hardinge Medical College and
Kalawati Saran Children's Hospital
New Delhi, India

Prawin Kumar MD DAA DPSM
Additional Professor
Department of Pediatrics
All India Institute of Medical Sciences
Jodhpur, Rajasthan, India

Preeti Dabadghao MD DM (Endo)
Professor and Head
Department of Endocrinology
Sanjay Gandhi Postgraduate Institute
of Medical Sciences
Lucknow, Uttar Pradesh, India

Preeti Singh MD
Professor
Department of Pediatrics
Lady Hardinge Medical College and
Kalawati Saran Children's Hospital
New Delhi, India

Prisca Colaco MD DCH
Hon Visiting Consultant in Pediatric
Endocrinology
Department of Pediatric Endocrinology
Bai Jerbai Wadia Hospital for Children
Mumbai, Maharashtra, India

Priyanka Madaan MD DM
Associate Professor
Department of Pediatrics
Amrita School of Medicine
Faridabad, Haryana, India

PSN Menon MD MNAMS
Former Professor
Department of Pediatrics
Sub-Dean, Consultant, In-Charge
Pediatric Endocrinology and Genetics
All India Institute of Medical Sciences
New Delhi, India

Pukhraj Bafna MD
Pediatrician and Adolescent Health
Consultant
United Hospital, Chhattisgarh Dental
College and Research Institute
Rajnandgaon, Chhattisgarh, India

Puneet Jain MD DM CSCN (EEG)
Assistant Professor
Division of Neurology
Department of Pediatrics
The Hospital for Sick Children
University of Toronto
Toronto, Ontario, Canada

Purna A Kurkure MD
Head, Division of Pediatric
Hemato-oncology and BMT
Narayana Health SRCC Children's
Hospital, Mumbai
Joint Managing Trustee and Trustee
In-charge
Survivorship and Rehabilitation Division
Indian Cancer Society
Mumbai, Maharashtra, India

R Bhanu Vikraman Pillai
MD FAAP Diplomate of the American Board
of Pediatrics in Pediatrics
Consultant and Head
Department of Pediatric
Gastroenterology
Amrita Institute of Medical Sciences
and Research Center
Kochi, Kerala, India

R Krishna Kumar MD DM FAHA
Professor and Head
Department of Pediatric Cardiology
Amrita Institute of Medical Sciences
Kochi, Kerala, India

Rachana Dubey
MD DNB MNAMS DM (Pediatric Neurology)
Consultant
Department of Neurology
Medanta Superspecialty Hospital
Indore, Madhya Pradesh, India

Rachna Pasi DCH DNB MNAMS
Assistant Professor
Department of Pediatrics
All India Institute of Medical Sciences
New Delhi, India

Rachna Sehgal
MD DNB DM (Pediatric Neurology) ACME
Professor
Department of Pediatrics
Vardhman Mahavir Medical College
and Safdarjung Hospital
New Delhi, India

Raghupathy Palany MD DCH FRCP
Senior Consultant
Department of Pediatric Endocrinology
Sagar Hospital
Bengaluru, Karnataka, India

Rahul Naithani
MD DM FRCP Fellowship in Pediatric
Hematology Oncology (University of Toronto)
Director and Head
Department of Hematology and Bone
Marrow Transplant
Paras Hospital
Gurugram, Haryana, India

Rajalakshmi Iyer
MD DM (Pediatric Critical Care)
PICU Fellow
Department of Pediatric Intensive Care Unit
Birmingham Children's Hospital
Birmingham, UK

Rajeev Seth MD FAAP
Medical Director and Developmental Pediatrician
Department of Child Health and Development Center
Rainbow Children's Hospital and Max Hospital
New Delhi, India

Rajesh Kumar MD DM (Neonatology)
Director and Chief Neonatologist
Department of Neonatology
Rani Hospital
Ranchi, Jharkhand, India

Rajesh Kumar MD
Assistant Professor
Department of Pediatrics
Nalanda Medical College and Hospital
Patna, Bihar, India

Rajeshwar Dayal MD DNB DCH (London)
Professor
Department of Pediatrics
Sarojini Naidu Medical College
Agra, Uttar Pradesh, India

Rajni Sharma MD
Additional Professor
Division of Pediatric Endocrinology
Department of Pediatrics
All India Institute of Medical Sciences
New Delhi, India

Rajniti Prasad MD FAMS
Professor
Department of Pediatrics
Institute of Medical Sciences
Banaras Hindu University
Varanasi, Uttar Pradesh, India

Raju C Shah MD DPed FRCPCH
Consulting Pediatrician
Department of Pediatrics
Ankur Institute of Child Health
Ahmedabad, Gujarat, India

Rakesh Lodha MD
Professor
Department of Pediatrics
All India Institute of Medical Sciences
New Delhi, India

Ramachandran Padmanabhan
MD DNB
Professor of Eminence
Department of Pediatrics
Head, Division of Clinical Research and Head, Bioethics Unit
Sri Ramachandra Institute of Higher Education and Research
Chennai, Tamil Nadu, India

Ramandeep Singh Arora
DCH MRCPCH MD
Consultant
Department of Pediatric Oncology
Disease Management Group
Max Super Specialty Hospital
New Delhi, India

Ramesh Agarwal MD DM (Neonatology)
Professor
Division of Neonatology
Department of Pediatrics
All India Institute of Medical Sciences
New Delhi, India

Ramesh Bajania
MD Diplomat-Environment and Child Health (IPA) FIPA
Consultant
Department of Pediatrics
Vitrag Children Hospital
Dhrangadhra, Gujarat, India

Ramesh Konanki
MD DM (Pediatric Neurology)
Consultant
Department of Pediatric Neurologist
Rainbow Hospital for Women and Children, Hyderabad, Telangana, India

Ramesh D Potdar MD
Consultant Pediatrician
Jeevak Children Hospital
Mumbai, Maharashtra, India

Ramesh S MD DCh
Consultant Pediatrician
Department of Pediatrics
BRS Hospital
Chennai, Tamil Nadu, India

Ranjan Kumar Pejaver
FRCP FRCPCH
Chief Neonatologist
Department of Neonatology
People Tree—Meenakshi Hospitals
Bengaluru, Karnataka, India

Ranjith Kumar Manokaran MD DM
Associate Professor
Division of Pediatric Neurology
Department of Neurology
Sri Ramachandra Institute of Higher Education and Research
Chennai, Tamil Nadu, India

Rashid H Merchant MD
Consulting Pediatrician
Apollo Hospitals, Navi Mumbai
Nanavati Max Superspecialty Hospital
Mumbai, Maharashtra, India

Rashmi Dalvi MD
Professor and Head
Department of Pediatrics
Senior Consultant Pediatric Hematology and Oncology
Bombay Hospital Institute of Medical Sciences
Narayana Health—SRCC Children's Hospital
Mumbai, Maharashtra, India

Rashna Dass Hazarika MD
Professor
Department of Pediatrics
PA Sangma International Medical College and Hospital
Ri Bhoi, Meghalaya, India

Reetha Gopinath
MD DCH Fellowship in Pediatric and Adolescent Endocrinology
Professor
Department of Pediatrics
Government Medical College
Kannur, Kerala, India

Rehna K Rahman
MD DM (Pediatric Nephrology)
Consultant Pediatric Nephrologist
Department of Pediatrics and Neonatology
Aster MIMS Hospital
Calicut, Kerala, India

Rekha Hans MD
Additional Professor
Department of Transfusion Medicine
Postgraduate Institute of Medical Education and Research
Chandigarh, India

Remesh Kumar R
MD FRCPCH
Director (Medical Services)
Senior Consultant and Head
Department of Pediatrics
Apollo Adlux Hospital
Kochi, Kerala, India

Renu Saxena
MD (Pathology) FNAMS
Director and Head
Department of Pathology and Lab Medicine
Medanta—The Medicity
Gurugram, Haryana, India

Rhishikesh P Thakre
DM MD DNB DCH
Neonatologist
Department of Pediatrics
Neo Clinic
Aurangabad, Maharashtra, India

Richa Jain MD DM
Associate Professor
Department of Pediatrics
Postgraduate Institute of Medical Education and Research
Chandigarh, India

Ridhimaa Jain
DNB DCH IAP Fellowship in Pediatric Neurology
Specialist Pediatrician
Department of Pediatrics
Lok Nayak Hospital and Maulana Azad Medical College
New Delhi, India

Rimjhim Shrivastava
PGDMCH DNB
Consultant, Pediatric Gastroenterology and Hepatology
Department of Pediatric Gastroenterology
Ekta Institute of Child Health
Swapnil Nursing Home
Petals Children's Hospital
Raipur, Chhattisgarh, India

Ritabrata Kundu MD
Professor of Pediatrics
Department of Pediatric Medicine
Institute of Child Health
Kolkata, West Bengal, India

Riyaz Arakkal
MD DCH DNB DM (Gastroenterology) FRCP
Professor and Head
Department of Pediatrics
KMCT Medical College
Kozhikode, Kerala, India

RK Agarwal MD MNAMS
Consultant Pediatrician
Department of Pediatrics
RK Hospital
Udaipur, Rajasthan, India

RK Anand MD
Emeritus Director
Department of Pediatrics and Neonatology
Jaslok Hospital and Research Centre
Mumbai, Maharashtra, India

RN Srivastava Dip Am Board FRCP FAMS
Emeritus Consultant
Pediatric Nephrologist
Indraprastha Apollo Hospital
New Delhi, India

Rohit C Agrawal MD DCH FRCP
Consultant
Department of Pediatrics
Kohinoor Hospital and Chandrajyoti Children Hospital
Mumbai, Maharashtra, India

Ruchi N Nanavati MD IBCLC (2010-2015)
Professor
Department of Neonatology
Seth GS Medical College and KEM Hospital, Mumbai, Maharashtra, India

Ruchi Rai MD
Professor
Department of Neonatology
Postgraduate Institute of Child Health
Noida, Uttar Pradesh, India

Ruchika Jha MD DNB MRCPCH
Assistant Professor
Department of Pediatrics
Armed Forces Medical College
Pune, Maharashtra, India

Ruchira Misra
DCH DNB Fellowship in Pediatric Hematology Oncology and BMT (Australia)
Senior Consultant and Head
Department of Pediatric Hematology/Oncology and BMT
MRR Children's Hospital
Thane, Maharashtra, India

S Narmada Ashok
DNB MRCPCH FRCPCH Dip Allergy & Asthma PGDDN MBA
Consultant and Director
Department of Pediatrics
Nalam Medical Center and Hospital
Vellore, Tamil Nadu, India

S Ram Sundar MD DNB (PICU)
DNB Trainee
Department of Pediatric Intensive Care
Sir Ganga Ram Hospital
New Delhi, India

S Srinivasan DCH MD
Former Director-Professor of Pediatrics
Jawaharlal Institute of Postgraduate Medical Education and Research
Puducherry
Professor of Pediatrics
Mahatma Gandhi Medical College and Research Institute, Puducherry
Adjunct Professor
Department of Pediatrics
Mehta Multispecialty Hospital
Chennai, Tamil Nadu, India

S Yamuna CCH DNB PGDAP
Consultant Pediatrician and Adolescent Physician
Department of Pediatrics
Child and Adolescent Clinic
Chennai, Tamil Nadu, India

S Sachidananda Kamath
MBBS DCH MD DHHM PGDAP
Director of Medical Affairs
Senior Consultant Pediatrician
Department of Pediatrics
Indira Gandhi Co-operative Hospital
Kochi, Kerala, India

Sachit Anand MCh (Pediatric Surgery)
Assistant Professor
Department of Pediatric Surgery
All India Institute of Medical Sciences
New Delhi, India

Sagar Bhattad
MD DM (Pediatric Clinical Immunology and Rheumatology)
Consultant
Division of Pediatric Immunology and Rheumatology
Department of Pediatrics
Aster CMI Hospital
Bengaluru, Karnataka, India

Sahana Shankar
MD Fellowship in Pediatric Gastroenterology, Hepatology, and Clinical Nutrition
Consultant
Department of Pediatrics
Mazumdar Shaw Medical Center
Bengaluru, Karnataka, India

Samir Hasan Dalwai
MD DNB FCPS DCH LLB
Developmental Behavioral Pediatrician
New Horizons Child Development Centre and Research Foundation
Mumbai, Maharashtra, India

Sandeep Agarwala
MCh (Pediatric Surgery)
Professor and Head
Department of Pediatric Surgery
All India Institute of Medical Sciences
New Delhi, India

Sandeep B Bavdekar
MD DCH DIT
Consultant and Chief (Academics)
Department of Pediatrics
Surya Children's Hospital, Surya Children's Medicare Pvt Ltd
Mumbai, Maharashtra, India

Sandeep S Kadam
MD DM
Consultant Neonatologist
Department of Pediatrics
KEM Hospital
Pune, Maharashtra, India

Sangeetha Yoganathan
MD DNB DM
Professor
Pediatric Neurology Unit
Department of Neurological Sciences
Christian Medical College
Vellore, Tamil Nadu, India

Sanjay Srirampur MD FRCPCH
Academic Head
Department of Pediatrics
Rainbow Children's Hospital
Hyderabad, Telangana, India

Sankar VH
MD DNB MNAMS DM (Medical Genetics)
Professor of Medical Genetics
Department of Medical Genetics
SAT Hospital, Government Medical College
Thiruvananthapuram, Kerala, India

Sapna Nayak
MD PDCC (Paediatric Endocrinology)
Assistant Professor
Division of Pediatric Endocrinology
Department of Pediatrics
Christian Medical College
Vellore, Tamil Nadu, India

Sasidaran Kandasamy
MD DM FIPNA European Diploma in BMT PG Diploma in Bioethics
Group Head and Senior Consultant
Pediatric Critical Care Services
Advanced Pediatric Critical Care Center
Mehta Multispecialty Hospitals
Chennai, Tamil Nadu, India

Satvik C Bansal MD
Associate Professor
Department of Pediatrics
Gajra Raja Medical College
Gwalior, Madhya Pradesh, India

Satyen K Hemrajani
MD DNB (Neonatology)
Additional Director
Department of Neonatology and Pediatrics
Dr Manjeet Institute of Critical Care
Jaipur, Rajasthan, India

Savneet Kaur MD
Assistant Professor
Department of Pediatrics
Lady Harding Medical College and Kalawati Saran Children's Hospital
New Delhi, India

Seema Alam MD
Professor
Department of Pediatric Hepatology
Institute of Liver and Biliary Sciences
New Delhi, India

Shakuntala Prabhu
MD DCH FRCPCH (London)
Medical Director and Professor
Department of Pediatrics and Pediatric Cardiology
BJ Wadia Hospital for Children
Mumbai, Maharashtra, India

Shambhavi Seth
DNB PG Diploma in Developmental Neurology
Senior Consultant
Department of Developmental Pediatrics
Max Superspecialty Hospital
New Delhi, India

Shashi N Vani
MD DPed
Emeritus Professor of Pediatrics including Neonatology
Department of Pediatrics including Neonatology
Pramukhswami Medical College and Sri Krishna Hospital
Anand, Gujarat, India

Sheffali Gulati MD
Professor
Child Neurology Division
Department of Pediatrics
All India Institute of Medical Sciences
New Delhi, India

Sheikh Minhaj Ahmed
MD DNB MNAMS Fellowship Pediatric Critical Care
Consultant PICU and NICU
Lilavati Hospital and Research Centre
Mumbai, Maharashtra, India

Sheila Samanta Mathai
DM (Neonatology)
Professor and Head
Department of Neonatology
Kasturba Medical College
Manipal, Karnataka, India

Shekhar Seshadri
MD DPM
Advisor, Samvad
Department of Child and Adolescent Psychiatry
National Institute of Mental Health and Neurosciences
Bengaluru, Karnataka, India

Shrish Bhatnagar MD
Professor and Head
Department of Pediatrics
Era's Lucknow Medical College and Hospital
Lucknow, Uttar Pradesh, India

Shruthi NM MD DM (Pediatric Neurology)
Consultant
Department of Pediatric Neurology
First Neuro Hospital
Mangaluru, Karnataka, India

Shruti Kakkar
MD Fellowship in Comprehensive Hematology-oncology
Professor of Pediatrics
Consultant, Clinical Hematology and Stem Cell Transplant Unit
Christian Medical College and Hospital
Ludhiana, Punjab, India
Visiting Consultant
(Pediatric Hematology)
Sri Guri Ram Dass University of Health Sciences
Amritsar, Punjab, India

Shubha R Phadke
MD DM (Medical Genetics)
Professor and Head
Department of Medical Genetics
Sanjay Gandhi Postgraduate Institute of Medical Sciences
Lucknow, Uttar Pradesh, India

Siddhnath Sudhanshu
MD PDCC (Pediatric Endocrinology)
Additional Professor of Pediatrics
Department of Pediatrics
All India Institute of Medical Sciences
Patna, Bihar, India

Sindhu Sivanandan MD DM
Chief Neonatologist
Department of Neonatology
Kauvery Hospital
Chennai, Tamil Nadu, India

Snehavardhan R Pandey
DM (Pediatric Hepatology)
Consultant
Department of Pediatric Hepatology
Sahyadri Superspecialty Hospital and KEM Hospital
Pune, Maharashtra, India

Somashekara HR
DCH DNB FPGHN Fellowship in Pediatric Hepatology
Consultant
Department of Pediatric Hepatology
Gleneagles Health City
Chennai, Tamil Nadu, India

Somu Sivabalan
MD DNB MNAMS FCCP (USA) FAPSR FRCP (Edin)
Consultant Pediatrician and Pulmonologist
Department of Pediatrics
Rainbow Children's Hospital
Chennai, Tamil Nadu, India

Sonali Singh
MD DNB DM
Clinical Fellow in Epilepsy
Department of Neurology, SickKids
The Hospital for Sick Children
Toronto, Ontario, Canada

Soumya Reddy MD DM (Ped Nephro)
Senior Resident
Department of Pediatric Nephrology
St John's Medical College Hospital
Bengaluru, Karnataka, India

Srikanta Basu MD MNAMS
Director Professor
Department of Pediatrics
Lady Hardinge Medical College
New Delhi, India

Srinivas G Kasi MD DCH
Consultant Pediatrician
Department of Pediatrics
Kasi Clinic
Bengaluru, Karnataka, India

Srinivas Kalyani MD
Professor
Department of Pediatrics
Osmania Medical College, Niloufer Hospital
Hyderabad, Telangana, India

Sriram Krishnamurthy
MD Fellowship (Pediatric Nephrology)
Professor
Department of Pediatrics
Jawaharlal Institute of Postgraduate Medical Education and Research
Puducherry, India

Sudha Ekambaram
DNB FPN FISPN (NUH-Singapore)
Senior Consultant
Department of Pediatric Nephrology
Apollo Children's Hospital
Chennai, Tamil Nadu, India

Sukanta Chatterjee MD
Professor
Department of Pediatrics
Government Medical College
Kolkata, West Bengal, India

Sukanya Priyadarshini MD
Senior Resident (Pediatric Endocrinology)
Department of Pediatrics
All India Institute of Medical Sciences
New Delhi, India

Suma Balan
MD MRCP CCT (UK)
Professor and Head
Department of Rheumatology and Clinical Immunology
Amrita Institute of Medical Sciences
Kochi, Kerala, India

Suman Rao PN MD DM
Professor and Head
Department of Neonatology
St John's Medical College Hospital
Bengaluru, Karnataka, India

Sumantra Kumar Raut
MD DM (Pediatric Nephrology)
Assistant Professor
Department of Nephrology
North Bengal Medical College
Siliguri, West Bengal, India

Sumathi Bavanandam
MD DCH DM (Gastro)
Professor and Head
Department of Gastroenterology
Stanley Medical College and Hospital
Chennai, Tamil Nadu, India

Sumitha Nayak
MD DNB Adv Cert in Vaccinology (IVI, S Korea & CMC, Vellore) PGDMLS PGDGC
Consultant Pediatrician
Department of Pediatrics
Shishu–The Children's Clinic
Bengaluru, Karnataka, India

Suneeta Mittal
MD FRCOG (ae) FICOG FAMS FICMCH FIMSA FICLS
Senior Director and Head
Department of Obstetrics and Gynecology
Fortis Memorial Research Institute
Gurugram, Haryana, India

Sunil Karande MD DCH
Professor of Pediatrics and Head
Department of Pediatrics
Seth GS Medical College and KEM Hospital
Mumbai, Maharashtra, India

Sunil Reddy KG
DCH DNB FISPN FNB (Ped Nephro)
Senior Resident
Department of Pediatric Nephrology
Mehta Multispecialty Hospitals India Pvt Ltd
Chennai, Tamil Nadu, India

Suravi Mohanty
DNB (Path) PDCC (Ped Path)
Professor
Department of Pathology
Kalinga Institute of Medical Sciences
Bhubaneswar, Odisha, India

Surbhi Dahiya
MD (Pathology) FIDH (Fellowship in Diagnostic Hematology)
Senior Resident
Department of Hematology
Sir Ganga Ram Hospital and Ganga Ram Institute of Postgraduate Medical Education and Research
New Delhi, India

Suresh Kumar Angurana MD DM
Associate Professor
Department of Pediatrics
Postgraduate Institute of Medical Education and Research
Chandigarh, India

Sureshkumar S
BPT MSc PhD Fellowship in Neuromuscular Rehabilitation (USA & UK)
Senior Consultant Physiotherapy and Rehabilitation
Department of Physiotherapy
Vijaya Medical and Educational Trust
Chennai, Tamil Nadu, India

Susan Uthup
MD DNB DM (Nephrology) DNB (Nephrology)
Professor
Department of Pediatric Nephrology
SAT Hospital
Government Medical College
Thiruvananthapuram, Kerala, India

Sushil K Kabra MD
Former Professor and Head
Department of Pediatrics
All India Institute of Medical Sciences
New Delhi, India

Sushila Russell
MPhil in Clinical Psychology
Senior Reader in Clinical Psychology
Department of Child and Adolescent Psychiatry Unit
Department of Psychiatry
Christian Medical College
Vellore, Tamil Nadu, India

Sushmita Banerjee
DCH MRCPI MSc in Clinical Pediatrics FRCPCH
Consultant
Department of Pediatrics
Calcutta Medical Research Institute
Kolkata, India, India

Swathi Chacham
MD DM (Neonatology) MNAMS
Former Professor
Department of Pediatrics
All India Institute of Medical Sciences, Rishikesh
Consultant Neonatologist
Nice Hospital
Hyderabad, Telangana, India

Swati Ghate
DCH PGDAP MA (Clinical Psychology)
Joint Director
Department of Pediatrics
Babylon's Newton Institute of Child and Adolescent Development
Jaipur, Rajasthan, India

Swati R Kanakia
MD DCH PhD
Consultant Pediatric Hematologist and Oncologist
Department of Pediatric Hematology
Lilavati Hospital and Research Centre
Mumbai, Maharashtra, India

Swati Y Bhave
MD DCH FCPS FAAP
Professor Emeritus Adolescent Medicine
Department of Pediatrics
Dr DY Patil Medical College, Pimpri
Dr DY Patil Vidyapeeth, Pune
Senior Consultant in Adolescent Pediatrics
Head
Family Guidance and Adolescent Wellness Clinic
Jehangir Hospital and Research Center
Pune, Maharashtra, India

Thangavelu S
MD DCH DNB MRCP
Senior Consultant and Director
Department of Pediatrics and Pediatric Critical Care
Mehta Multispecialty Hospitals India Pvt Ltd
Chennai, Tamil Nadu, India

T Jacob John
DCH MSc PhD FRCP (Edin) DSc
Retired Professor and Head
Department of Clinical Virology
Christian Medical College
Vellore, Tamil Nadu, India

T Ravikumar MD
Senior Consultant
Department of Pediatrics
Kanchi Kamakoti CHILDS Trust Hospital
Chennai, Tamil Nadu, India

Tanu Singhal
MD MSc
Consultant
Pediatrics and Infectious Diseases
Kokilaben Dhirubhai Ambani Hospital and Medical Research Institute
Mumbai, Maharashtra, India

Tanya Singla MD
Senior Resident
Department of Pediatrics
All India Institute of Medical Sciences
New Delhi, India

Tarun Patni MD
Senior Consultant
Department of Pediatrics
Lifecare Hospital
Jaipur, Rajasthan, India

Tejo Pratap Oleti
MD DM (Neo)
Consultant and Head
Department of Neonatology
Fernandez Hospital
Hyderabad, Telangana, India

TU Sukumaran
MD MPhil PhD
Professor
Department of Pediatrics
Caritas Hospital
Kottayam, Kerala, India

Tulika Seth MD ABP
Professor
Department of Hematology
All India Institute of Medical Sciences
New Delhi, India

Tushar P Shah MD LLB
Director
Department of Clinical Research and Professor of Pediatrics
Department of Pediatrics
Kashiben Gordhandas Patel Children Hospital
Vadodara, Gujarat, India

Udayakumar DS
MD (Pathology) DM (Hematopathology)
Consultant
Department of Pathology and Lab Medicine
Medanta—The Medicity
Gurugram, Haryana, India

Ujjal Poddar
MD DNB DM (Gastroenterology)
Professor and Head
Department of Pediatric Gastroenterology
Sanjay Gandhi Postgraduate Institute of Medical Sciences
Lucknow, Uttar Pradesh, India

Vaishakh Anand
MD DM (Pediatric Neurology)
Associate Professor
Department of Pediatric Neurology
Amrita Institute of Medical Sciences
Kochi, Kerala, India

Vaman Khadilkar
MD DNB MRCP DCH (London)
Senior Pediatric Endocrinologist
Department of Growth and Pediatric Endocrine Unit
Jehangir Hospital
Hirabai Cowasji Jehangir Medical Institute and Bharati Vidyapeeth
Pune, Maharashtra, India

Vandana Dhamankar MD
Deputy Director General
Department of Survivorship and Rehabilitation
Indian Cancer Society
Mumbai, Maharashtra, India

Vandana Jain MD
Professor
Pediatric Endocrinology Division
Department of Pediatrics
All India Institute of Medical Sciences
New Delhi, India

Varinder Singh MD
Director Professor
Pediatrics, Pulmonology
Department of Pediatrics
Lady Harding Medical College and Kalawati Saran Children's Hospital
New Delhi, India

Ved Prakash Choudhry
MD FIMSA FISHTM
Senior Consultant (Hematology)
Batra Hospital and Medical Research Centre
Pushpanjali Singhania Hospital and Research Centre
New Delhi, India

Vibhawari S Dani
MD DCH
Head
Research Division
(Tribal Health and Nutrition)
MAHAN
(Meditation, de-Addiction, Health, AIDS, Nutrition)
Amravati, Maharashtra, India

Vignesh Subramani MD DM
Assistant Professor
Department of Medical Oncology (Pediatrics)
Homi Bhabha Cancer Hospital
Visakhapatnam, Andhra Pradesh, India

Vijay Sriram MS (Orthopedics)
Consultant and Pediatric Orthopedic Surgeon
Department of Orthopedics
Kanchi Kamakoti CHILDS Trust Hospital
Chennai, Tamil Nadu, India

Vijayalakshmi Bhatia MD
Professor
Department of Pediatric Endocrinology
Sanjay Gandhi Postgraduate Institute of Medical Sciences
Lucknow, Uttar Pradesh, India

Vikrant Sood MD DM (Ped Hepatology)
Associate Professor
Department of Pediatric Hepatology
Institute of Liver and Biliary Sciences
New Delhi, India

Vinayan KP MD DNB DM
Professor and Head
Department of Pediatric Neurology
Amrita Institute of Medical Sciences
Kochi, Kerala, India

Vishal Sondhi
MD DM (Pediatric Neurology)
Professor
Department of Pediatrics
Armed Forces Medical College
Pune, Maharashtra, India

Vivek Kumar MD DM (Neonatology)
Research Consultant
Division of Neonatology
Department of Pediatrics
All India Institute of Medical Sciences
New Delhi, India

VR Ravikumar MS MCh
Retired Professor of Pediatric Surgery
Department of Pediatric Surgery
Coimbatore Medical College Hospital
Coimbatore, Tamil Nadu, India

VS Sankaranarayanan
MD DCH MNAMS DM (Gastro)
Former Professor and Head
Department of Pediatric Gastroenterology
Madras Medical College and Institute of Child Health and Hospital for Children
Senior Consultant and Head
Department of Pediatric Gastroenterology
Kanchi Kamakoti CHILDS Trust Hospital
Chennai, Tamil Nadu, India

Vykuntaraju KN Gowda DCH DNB DM
Professor
Department of Pediatric Neurology
Indira Gandhi Institute of Child Health
Bengaluru, Karnataka, India

YK Amdekar MD DCH
Medical Director
BJ Wadia Hospital for Children
Mumbai, Maharashtra, India

Zafar Mahmood Meenai
FRCPCH (UK) MSc Paediatric Neurodisability (UK)
Director
Child Development and Early Intervention
Ummeid Group of Child Development Centre
Bhopal, Madhya Pradesh, India

Foreword

It is with immense pride and reverence that we present the 8th edition of *Partha's IAP Textbook of Pediatrics*. This edition marks a significant milestone in the history of pediatric education in India, as it commemorates the unparalleled contributions of (Late) Professor A Parthasarathy, a visionary leader and one of the founding Editors of this esteemed textbook.

Professor Parthasarathy's dedication to advancing pediatric education and his tireless efforts to improve child health care have left an indelible mark on the medical community. His legacy continues to inspire us as we carry forward his vision through this thoroughly revised and restructured edition.

In line with the National Medical Council of India's new competency-based curriculum, this edition is designed to meet the evolving needs of undergraduate students, practicing physicians, and trainees in pediatrics. With contributions from 377 authors and 15 new Section Editors, we have endeavored to provide comprehensive and up-to-date content across 24 sections and 272 chapters. We thank Editor-in-Chief and Founder Editor, Professor PSN Menon, Founder Editor, Professor MKC Nair, Executive Editor, Dr Alok Gupta, Academic Editors, Professor Piyush Gupta, Professor Ramachandran Padmanabhan, and Professor Ritabrata Kundu, for painstaking job for bringing out the new edition.

We extend our heartfelt gratitude to M/s Jaypee Brothers Medical Publishers (P) Ltd, New Delhi, India, for their unwavering support and commitment to excellence. We are confident that this edition will serve as an invaluable resource for pediatricians and medical students in South-East Asia and other developing countries, upholding the high standards set by Professor Parthasarathy.

GV Basavaraja
MBBS MD (Pediatrics) DNB (Paediatrics) NBE
Professor (Pediatrics) and In-charge (Pediatric Intensive Care Unit)
Indira Gandhi Institute of Child Health
Bengaluru, Karnataka, India
President, Indian Academy of Pediatrics (IAP) (2024)

Foreword

With great pleasure and humility, we introduce the 8th edition of *Partha's IAP Textbook of Pediatrics*, a testament to the enduring legacy of (Late) Professor A Parthasarathy. As a past National President of the Indian Academy of Pediatrics and a Founding Editor of this textbook, Professor Parthasarathy's visionary guidance was instrumental in shaping pediatric education in India. Since its inception in 1999, this textbook has been a cornerstone of pediatric education, consistently updated to reflect the latest advancements in the field.

The 8th edition continues this tradition, offering a thoroughly revised and restructured content that aligns with the new competency-based curriculum for undergraduates prescribed by the National Medical Council of India. We are proud to present this edition, which features 140 new chapters written by esteemed experts, under the leadership of 15 new Section Editors. Highlights include the revamped sections on Care of the Newborn, Growth, Development, Immunity and Immunization, Gastrointestinal System, Hepatobiliary System and Pancreas, Nervous System, Endocrine System, Critical Care and Emergencies, Rheumatology and Allergy, and Pediatric Therapeutics. Each section has been meticulously updated to provide the most relevant and cutting-edge knowledge.

Our sincere appreciation goes to all the contributors for sharing their brilliant insight in respective topics, and the editorial team of Professor PSN Menon, Dr Alok Gupta, Professor MKC Nair, Professor Piyush Gupta, Professor Ramachandran Padmanabhan and Professor Ritabrata Kundu, and to M/s Jaypee Brothers Medical Publishers (P) Ltd, New Delhi, India, for their support in bringing this comprehensive resource to fruition.

We are confident that this edition will be an indispensable guide for undergraduate students, practicing physicians, and pediatric trainees, not only in India but also in South-East Asia and other developing regions. We hope that this textbook will continue to inspire and educate future generations of pediatricians, and help to serve children, colleagues, and country along with honoring the legacy of Professor Parthasarathy.

Vasant M Khalatkar
MD (Ped) FIAP FICMCH PG Dip Ped Inf Diseases (UNSW)
Consultant Pediatrician and Neonatologist
Khalatkar Hospital
Nagpur, Maharashtra, India
President
Indian Academy of Pediatrics (IAP) (2025)

Foreword

It is with great honor and privilege that I write the foreword for the revised 8th edition of *Partha's IAP Textbook of Pediatrics*, a cornerstone in pediatric education. This latest edition has been meticulously restructured and updated to align with the National Medical Council (NMC) syllabus for undergraduate students. It is crafted to cater to the evolving needs of medical education in India, ensuring it serves as a trusted resource for undergraduate students, diploma trainees, and private practitioners alike. Each of the 24 sections has been peer-reviewed by Section Editors, distinguished experts in their respective fields. Their dedication to ensuring accuracy, comprehensiveness, and clinical relevance makes this textbook an essential companion for learning and practice. With contributions from 377 authors, covering a total of 272 chapters, this edition embodies the collaborative spirit of academic excellence.

This textbook strikes a fine balance between theory and practical application, making it equally relevant for students preparing for their medical careers and practitioners striving to deliver evidence-based care. The inclusion of updated guidelines, clinical algorithms, and practical insights will ensure its utility across various clinical settings.

As a Pediatrician deeply committed to advancing child health and medical education, I believe this edition will empower the next generation of pediatricians with the knowledge, confidence, and skills to address the challenges of modern pediatrics. It also pays tribute to the legacy of visionary leader (Late) Professor A Parthasarathy, whose contribution continues to inspire us all.

I extend my heartfelt appreciation to the Editorial Board for their leadership and dedication: PSN Menon (Founder Editor and Editor-in-Chief), MKC Nair (Founder Editor), Alok Gupta (Executive Editor), and Academic Editors of great repute, Professor Piyush Gupta, Professor Ritabrata Kundu, and Professor Ramachandran Padmanabhan. Their collective efforts have ensured that this edition maintains the highest standards of academic excellence and clinical relevance.

I also wish to convey my sincere gratitude to M/s Jaypee Brothers Medical Publishers (P) Ltd, New Delhi, India, for their unwavering support and commitment to publishing this esteemed textbook. Their efforts have made this resource accessible to medical students and pediatricians, not only in India but across South-East Asia and other developing regions.

I recommend this textbook for all undergraduate students, diploma students, undergraduate faculty and pediatric practitioners, being confident that this revised edition will serve as an invaluable tool for them in their pursuit of knowledge and excellence.

Neelam Mohan
DNB FPGH FIMSA FACG FRCPCH
Senior Director
Department of Pediatric Gastroenterology
Hepatology and Liver Transplantation
Medanta—The Medicity
Gurugram, Haryana, India
President Elect, IAP 2025
President, Commonwealth Association of
Paediatric Gastroenterology and Nutrition

Preface to the Eighth Edition

The Executive Council of Indian Academy of Pediatrics (IAP) during the tenure of Professor Piyush Gupta as President in 2021 decided to rename the *IAP Textbook of Pediatrics* to commemorate the unparalleled contributions of (Late) Professor A Parthasarathy, a visionary leader, past President and Founder Editor of this esteemed textbook. It is with immense pride and reverence that we present this 8th edition retitled as *Partha's IAP Textbook of Pediatrics*. This edition marks a significant milestone in the history of pediatric education in India.

The new revised and updated Eighth edition of *Partha's IAP Textbook of Pediatrics (PIAPTBP)* is devoted to newborns, children and adolescents—the future citizens of India whose nurture and care are our goal, concern and commitment. It is our humble tribute to the IAP, which is at the vanguard of the care of children of all hues and colors, at all ages and without barriers; that trained and fostered us as responsible professionals to care for children with love and compassion.

The discipline of pediatrics has made substantial advances in the last decade in preventive and therapeutic care. New perspectives for the care of children have been opened and many thrust areas requiring immediate or continued attention to decrease morbidity and mortality have been demarcated. These have provided fresh impetus to improve knowledge, harvest new information and continue the process of learning. The Government of India also has embarked on new initiatives for the welfare of newborns, children and adolescents. These developments have necessitated the need for publication of an updated 8th edition of the book after a gap of six years. This was also inspired by the enthusiastic response to the previous editions from practicing pediatricians, postgraduates, undergraduates as well as faculty of departments of pediatrics throughout India and SAARC countries.

It has been our endeavor to present the subject in a simplified and practical manner to provide adequate clinical guidance to pediatricians so that children derive the benefits of early diagnosis and optimal treatment. The basic simple and practical outline of the book is retained. We have tried our best to oversee that the "art and science" of clinical pediatrics maintains its central position without being dwarfed by newer technical advances.

The book represents a substantial revision and reorganization of the text based on a complete review of the field of pediatrics. This is not a watered-down version; efforts have also been made to keep a balance with incorporation of the curricular needs of the undergraduates, postgraduates and teachers in pediatrics. This edition has 272 chapters crafted by 377 national and international experts and arranged in 24 major sections brought out in three volumes. Each section is reviewed and edited by subject experts as section editors. The text has been revised and updated by adopting three-tier review and edit system, keeping in view of the present needs and possible future requirements of practitioners and students of pediatrics. The entire contents of the textbook are reorganized to provide relevant clinical information and national priorities at one site, in line with the National Medical Council of India's new competency-based curriculum of perinatology, neonatology, pediatrics and adolescent medicine. We have made every effort to provide up-to-date content in a simplified, practical step-by-step manner in a crisp, concise and yet comprehensive text.

Some of the thrust areas in the edition refer to the felt needs of our country. It is our constant endeavor to inform, educate and update the reader about the current status of national community-oriented initiatives for children. The textbook includes details of IAP and WHO recommended Growth Charts, National Immunization Schedule (Government of India) updated in 2024 and IAP Immunization Timetable 2023 as recommended by the IAP– Advisory Committee on Vaccines and Immunization Practices (IAP–ACVIP). It provides current protocols for management of various infectious and non-infectious diseases, as recommended by various chapters and groups of the IAP.

We are justifiably proud of our achievements in preventive care with attainment of the status of polio-free nation among others, for more than 10 years. Strategies for incorporating newer technology and better coverage of immunization to contain communicable diseases and further reduction in disease burden, especially in the underprivileged areas of our society, hence, find a better thrust in this book. The book highlights the use of simple strategies to improve health status such as uniform growth charts and low-cost food supplements. More complex issues such as the increasing disease burden of new epidemics of non-infectious chronic diseases such as obesity, especially in the urban India and screening for congenital disorders in the newborns thus find adequate mention in this book, keeping in mind the changing concepts of pediatric care in the global scenario and meeting the various SDG goals related to improved child health.

The editorial board would like to place on record its appreciation to all the authors and editors who have taken great pains to contribute and/or edit reader-friendly sections with practical guidelines amidst their busy professional and academic schedules. We welcome the new team of authors, section editors and the editorial board and gratefully acknowledge their efforts, devoting a great deal of time to reviewing and editing the manuscripts. We do sincerely believe that their efforts have made the book more concise and precise.

It is our earnest hope that this book will help with early diagnosis and efficient management leading to optimal outcome and improved quality of pediatric care. Your valuable suggestions and comments are most welcome for improving the content and quality of future editions.

PSN Menon
Alok Gupta
MKC Nair
Piyush Gupta
Ramachandran Padmanabhan
Ritabrata Kundu

Preface to the First Edition

Pediatrics has grown and developed with significant milestones in preventive and therapeutic care over the past few decades. The WHO and UNICEF in their Primary Health Care (PHC) approach, have given due importance for effective child survival programs. So, the medical students need to be well oriented towards these approaches in pediatrics as the future middle level managers in primary health care.

Several luminaries in the Indian pediatric scenario have contributed their might in bringing out books for the undergraduate medical students. However, the rapid advances made in the various pediatric subspecialties have necessitated the updating of these books from time to time. Nevertheless, the need for a full-fledged textbook was felt for long. The Indian Academy of Pediatrics thought it fit to shoulder the responsibility of bringing out such a need-based textbook in pediatrics for medical students. Our erudite and enthusiastic editors and contributors made it possible at a record time. The Indian Academy of Pediatrics (IAP) owes its gratitude to all these experts for their worthy contribution.

The book has been divided into several sections. A few chapters included in this book are entirely newer concepts, which are not usually found in the conventional pediatric textbooks. It has also worthy annexures to the main contents. However, editing the text to suit the needs of medical students was a Himalayan task. The idea is to equip the medical students with adequate knowledge in pediatrics in order to make them confident to shoulder the responsibilities concerned with preventive and curative pediatrics. Thus, it is hoped that the practitioners of pediatric medicine will benefit from this book.

We are confident that the book will serve the needs of medical students, especially at a time when the Medical Council of India (MCI) has made pediatrics as a major examination. Thus, the publication of the book is not only timely but also out of necessity.

The Indian Academy of Pediatrics would like to place on record its appreciation to the senior editors, chapter editors, contributors and staff members of Indian Academy of Pediatrics (IAP), Central Secretariat, for help rendered in the creation of this book and M/s Jaypee Brothers Medical Publishers (P) Ltd, New Delhi, India, for their excellent cooperation in bringing out the 1st edition at record time.

A Parthasarathy
PSN Menon
MKC Nair

Acknowledgments

We, the members of the editorial board, are indebted to the President and Members of the Executive Boards (2024–2025) of the Indian Academy of Pediatrics (IAP) for the initiation and completion of the project of bringing out the 8th edition of *IAP Textbook of Pediatrics* for the medical students and practitioners titled *Partha's IAP Textbook of Pediatrics*. We are also grateful to the successive Presidents and Members of the previous Executive Boards from 1998–2024 for their encouragement in sustaining the project towards the publication of all the seven editions.

Our sincere appreciations go to the various contributors, section editors, and editors, past and present teachers of pediatrics who have contributed to the 8th edition and made the task of production of the current edition a reality by their precise and updated texts. The Academy is indebted to all the contributors, and members of the Production Department of M/s Jaypee Brothers Medical Publishers (P) Ltd, New Delhi, India, for their dedication, devotion and hard work.

The editorial board acknowledges the help of the new team of 24 section editors who helped in the execution of the various sections by selecting appropriate experts for contributions. Their details are provided in the list of Section Editors. This edition also marks the selection of a new team of authors, a judicious mix of both old and new for each section. Their contributions are gratefully acknowledged.

The secretarial and organizational support of the staff at the Central Office of Indian Academy of Pediatrics, Mumbai and the guidance, cooperation and coordination provided by past presidents are gratefully acknowledged.

Our grateful thanks are due to Shri Shaji Jacob Ninan for the assistance rendered to Dr PSN Menon (Editor-in-Chief) in editing, scrutinizing and proofreading of the chapters. Our special thanks are due to the staff members of the editorial board and for their assistance.

We would like to make a special mention of Ms Pragati Singh (Senior Development Editor), M/s Jaypee Brothers Medical Publishers (P) Ltd, New Delhi, India, for her untiring efforts in coordinating with more than 377 authors, 24 Section Editors and members of the editorial board. But for her outstanding harmonization, it would not have been possible to publish this edition on schedule. Our sincere and grateful thanks go to Shri Jitendar P Vij (Group Chairman), Shri Ankit Vij (Managing Director), Shri MS Mani (Group President), Ms Pooja Bhandari [Director—Production (Books and Journals)], and other members of M/s Jaypee Brothers Medical Publishers (P) Ltd, New Delhi, India, for their untiring coordination efforts in the production of the 8th edition.

All attempts have been made to acknowledge the sources of information and illustrations. Inadvertent omission, if any, is regretted.

Editorial Board

Contents

Volume 1

SECTION 1: Basic Concepts of Child Care

Section Editor: Piyush Gupta

SECTION 2: Care of the Newborn

Section Editor: Rhishikesh P Thakre

SECTION 3: Growth

***Section Editor:* Anju Seth**

SECTION 4: Development and Developmental Disorders

***Section Editor:* Samir Hasan Dalwai**

SECTION 5: Nutrition and Nutritional Disorders

***Section Editor:* Praveen Kumar**

SECTION 6: Immunity and Immunization

Section Editor: Srinivas G Kasi

SECTION 7: Infectious Diseases

Section Editor: Ritabrata Kundu

SECTION 8: Diseases of Central Nervous System

***Section Editor:* Sheffali Gulati**

Volume 2

SECTION 9: Diseases of Cardiovascular System

Section Editor: S Srinivasan

SECTION 10: Disorders of Respiratory System

Section Editor: Sushil K Kabra

SECTION 11: Disorders of Gastrointestinal System and Liver

Section Editor: Riyaz Arakkal

SECTION 12: Disorders of Hepatobiliary System and Pancreas

Section Editor: John Matthai

SECTION 13: Disorders of Kidney and Urinary Tract

Section Editor: Arvind Bagga

SECTION 14: Disorders of Hemopoietic System

***Section Editor:* Ved Prakash Choudhry**

SECTION 15: Pediatric Malignancies

Section Editor: Purna A Kurkure

SECTION 16: Disorders of Endocrine System and Diabetes Mellitus

Section Editors: Vijayalakshmi Bhatia, PSN Menon

Volume 3

SECTION 17: Genetics and Genetic Disorders

Section Editor: Madhulika Kabra

SECTION 18: Rheumatological Disorders and Allergy

Section Editor: Sathish Kumar

SECTION 19: Adolescent Health

Section Editor: MKC Nair

SECTION 20: Intensive Care and Emergencies

Section Editor: Jayashree Muralidharan

SECTION 21: Pediatric Subspecialties

Section Editor: **Ramachandran Padmanabhan**

SECTION 22: Community Pediatrics

Section Editor: **Alok Gupta**

SECTION 23: Pediatric Procedures

Section Editor: **Baldev S Prajapati**

SECTION 24: Pediatric Therapeutics

Section Editor: **Jeeson C Unni**

SECTION

Basic Concepts of Child Care

Section Editor: **Piyush Gupta**

1.1 Pediatrics: Yesterday, Today, and Tomorrow

YK Amdekar

INTRODUCTION

Care, survival, and development of children have always been our concern. The Government of India and the Indian Academy of Pediatrics (IAP) have undertaken several projects over the last few decades to improve the health of children, and it is time to introspect their impact on the ultimate goal.

DEMOGRAPHY

Due to a rapid rise in the population of India, which stands at 1.43 billion at present, there exists a shortage of health personnel and facilities. Though there has been a steady decline in infant mortality rate to 35/1,000 live births [National Family Health Survey (NFHS)-5, 2019–2021] as compared to 41 (NFHS-4), and under NFHS-5, mortality rate to 40/1,000 live births as compared to 51 (NFHS-4), it is still high and neonatal mortality rate has changed very little from 28 to 25/1,000 live births.[1] It means that the reduction in infant mortality is largely contributed by better performance in infants beyond the neonatal age of 28 days.

Breastfeeding initiation within the first hour and exclusive breastfeeding in the first 6 months have remained nearly the same—around 40% and 60%, respectively, between NFHS-4 and NFHS-5. It suggests that there is a steady improvement in some of the abovementioned indicators, but there is still along way before we achieve our goals. Only 50% of infants are on timely introduction of complementary feeds. Children <5 years of age are 35% stunted, 20% wasted, 30% underweight, and 60% anemic, and these parameters have not significantly changed. About 2–3% of children under 3 years of age suffer from acute severe malnutrition with 20–30% mortality in this group.

There is an increase in the number of children receiving primary vaccination up to 85%, though the rotavirus vaccine and second dose of measles vaccine uptake is only 30%. There is some improvement in the use of oral rehydration solution (ORS) during diarrhea episodes as it stands at around 60% in NFHS-5 (50% in NFHS-4), but the use of zinc has been low at 30%. Thus, health indices were better over the last decade *but still need much more improvement*. It suggests that medical and paramedical personnel do not follow standard simple, cost-effective preventive measures, despite contact opportunity with the community.

DISEASE PROFILE

In the 1960s and 1970s, antibiotics and vaccines appeared to have controlled infectious diseases. However, infectious diseases have returned with a vengeance. Tripartite interaction between environment, microbes, and host status decides the outcome of infectious disease. There is a complex struggle for survival between humans and microbes, and microbes are exploiting human behavior. Early and frequent exposures to infections, varying nutritional and immune status, lifestyle changes, global travel, and misuse of antibiotics have contributed to the resurgence of old infections. Microbes have an inherent ability to mutate, change virulence, and acquire resistance to antibiotics. This has made the battle against infections more difficult.

In addition, new organisms are being recognized. Forty new microbes have been recognized over the last 30 years. They include viruses such as rotavirus, Ebola virus, hantavirus, parvovirus B19, human T-lymphotropic viruses types 1 and 2, hepatitis C and E, H5N1 avian strain of influenza, severe acute respiratory syndrome (SARS), human metapneumovirus, and H1N1 swine reassortant influenza; bacteria such as *Legionella, Campylobacter jejuni*, toxin-producing staphylococci and streptococci, *Borrelia*, and *Helicobacter pylori*; and parasites such as *Cryptosporidium* and *Cyclospora*. Changing epidemiology has been observed in dengue fever, leptospirosis, brucellosis, and rickettsial fever. Due to a breakdown in public health measures, there is a resurgence of malaria and tuberculosis (TB). Coinfection with the human immunodeficiency virus (HIV) has worsened the scenario of TB. Many malignant conditions are now being attributed to an infectious agent. Hepatocellular carcinoma induced by hepatitis B and C infections and cervical cancer due to human papillomavirus are some of the examples of infection-related malignancy. Many diseases of unknown etiology (Kawasaki syndrome, sarcoidosis, and diabetes) are suspected to be induced by infections.

Infections caused by antibiotic-resistant organisms are on the increase. Multidrug-resistant *Staphylococcus aureus*, first detected in 1961 in the United Kingdom, is now known in both nosocomial and community settings. *Streptococcus pneumoniae* has become resistant to penicillin almost all over the world; surprisingly, penicillin sensitivity is still maintained in India.[2] The problem of resistance is mainly due to the misuse of antibiotics in human as well as veterinary medicine and also due to genetic mutation by bacteria. Empirical use of antibiotics, nonadherence to standard protocols by physicians, and noncompliant therapy by patients resulted in multidrug-resistant TB (MDRTB), malaria, and typhoid in the community. "ESKAPE" pathogens are problem pathogens—*Enterococcus*, *S. aureus*, *Klebsiella*, *Acinetobacter*, *Pseudomonas*, and *Enterobacteriaceae* species—and are difficult to eradicate. In addition, methicillin and vancomycin-resistant *S. aureus*, coagulase-negative *staphylococci*, penicillin-resistant *pneumococci*, macrolide-resistant *streptococci*, multidrug-resistant *Salmonella* and *Shigella*, and extended-spectrum beta-lactamase-producing *enterococci* and *Acinetobacter* are also being reported more frequently.

The recent pandemic of COVID-19 viral infection has affected global health and the economy. It has exposed scientific ignorance though it did offer opportunities to strengthen cost-effective simple measures in the community such as social distancing, masking, and sanitization (SMS) and also used the technology to invent vaccines against the COVID-19 virus. This pandemic also taught us how unpredictable is the behavior of the human immune system which may lead to multisystem inflammatory syndrome (MIS) and endanger life, a few weeks after the successful clearance of the virus. We also learned how the mental health of children is affected because of being confined to homes through this period and the further impact of online training.

Noninfective illnesses such as lifestyle diseases leading to metabolic syndrome (consisting of hypertension, coronary heart disease, and diabetes), asthma, malignancy, autism spectrum disorders, metabolic disorders, and immune deficiency disorders are being increasingly recognized. With the threat of an epidemic of obesity, the dual burden of malnutrition poses a stiff challenge.

It has been realized that vitamin D deficiency exists in significant proportion in all age groups despite the abundance of sunlight. This is because most children and adults are not exposed to sunlight due to changes in lifestyle. Vitamin D deficiency has been attributed to recurrent infections, along with many other ailments being ascribed to it. Vitamin B_{12} deficiency is being reported, especially in vegetarian families. Iron deficiency is universal in most of the children and women.

TECHNOLOGICAL ADVANCES

Etiological diagnosis of infections is possible today with modern culture techniques, such as BACTEC and polymerase chain reaction (PCR). Reverse transcription PCR for amplification of ribonucleic acid (RNA) and real-time PCR allow quantitative measurement of deoxyribonucleic acid (DNA) or RNA. Southern blot is a method of probing a specific DNA sequence in a DNA sample. Western blot measures the antibodies against a specific protein for HIV diagnosis. Gene therapy introducing a functional gene into a host genome, replacing an abnormal gene, has been successful in cystic fibrosis, hemophilia, sickle-cell disease, muscular dystrophy, and many other diseases.[3] Transfer of genes in the brain using liposomes may prove to be useful for degenerative brain disorders. Inborn errors of metabolism can be diagnosed with certainty at birth, and cost-effective umbilical cord screening of common metabolic disorders is now feasible.

The availability of several immunological tests has opened a new vista to diagnose otherwise fatal immune deficiency disorders. Imaging modalities have improved tremendously. Ultrasonography (USG) has undergone great advances over the last five decades. Color Doppler, digital subtraction angiography, and transesophageal USG are some of the newer modalities. Computed tomography and magnetic resonance imaging (MRI) give an anatomical diagnosis, while positron-emission tomography scan offers a metabolic or functional profile. Many advances have taken place for better resolution and clarity, such as diffusion MRI scans, fluid-attenuated inversion recovery (FLAIR) images, MR angiography, and MR spectroscopy. Molecular diagnosis is increasingly available for many diseases though mutations are being recognized. Thus, a negative molecular test may not completely rule out a specific disease as not all mutations have been known to science.

Advances such as computers, smartphones, apps, satellites and space technology, and telemedicine have expanded our reach to offer better health services to the community. The human genome project is capable of finding out what 23,000 genes are doing in an individual. Artificial intelligence—ChatGPT, machine learning, and neural networks are likely to dominate our lives in the near future.[4] However, we must be alert to make sure that none of these advances prove to be harmful, contrary to our expectations.

ADVANCES IN CURATIVE AND PREVENTIVE MANAGEMENT

Following a 40-year hiatus in discovering new classes of antibacterial compounds, three new classes of antibiotics have been brought into clinical use: (1) Cyclic lipopeptides (daptomycin), (2) glycylcyclines (tigecycline), and (3) oxazolidinones (linezolid). Bedaquiline and delamanid have been recently included in the treatment of MDRTB, and few other compounds are being researched. Other "new" antibiotics are merely chemically modified old molecules. With increasing antibiotic resistance, "phage" therapy needs to be revived.

Targeted therapy with better drugs and an improved understanding of their usage have modified the outcome of malignant diseases. While minimally invasive laparoscopy surgery is fast replacing conventional open surgery, interventional radiology and cardiology provide better alternatives to open surgery in many conditions. Liver or kidney transplants are now available for such end-stage diseases, in addition to bone marrow transplants and heart transplants. Stem cell therapy is yet in infancy though many centers have come up with a facility to bank stem cells collected right at birth. However, stem cells are required to be stored for decades, and it is not sure whether such centers have adequate infrastructure for the same.

The 20th century saw the development of many new vaccines. One-third of infectious disease mortality can be prevented by vaccination. The Indian Expanded Program on Immunization (EPI) covers only 7 diseases unlike 12 or more diseases covered in national programs of many developed countries. Though a greater number of vaccines are being made available by the government in selective states, such as the rotavirus vaccine, many newer vaccines are available in the open market. Combination vaccines contain six antigens in one injection. Poor coverage of susceptible populations and nonaffordability of non-EPI vaccines are the major hurdles. It is heartening that polio eradication efforts are successful though continued surveillance is needed. The time has come to phase out the oral polio vaccine (OPV) slowly over the next few years and replace it with inactivated polio vaccine (IPV). After the eradication of smallpox from the world and polio from most of the countries of the world—including India—the focus now has shifted to the eradication of measles. It may take several years before it is achieved mainly due to the logistic issues that are even more challenging than what we faced in polio eradication. However, we are on the right path with the ongoing campaign against measles.

CHANGE IN CLINICAL PRACTICE

Before the advent of modern science, physicians healed their patients with commitment, concern, and compassion. They treated the child and family, not just the disease. As science developed, physicians started treating disease and not the child. Subsequently, they started to treat diagnostic tests and not disease. Thus, modern clinical practice revolves around diagnostic tests, often without clinical correlation. Unfortunately, scientific advances have not translated into better health indices or quality of life for children at large. This is mainly because the majority of children need a simple approach to their common problems. Modern science cannot replace basic clinical bedside methods. For example, Kangaroo care and exclusive breastfeeding will save far more neonates than mechanical ventilation and modern facilities. ORS has saved many lives. Nutritional advice, growth monitoring, and immunization will contribute to a better quality of life. SMS has helped the most in the control of the recent COVID-19 pandemic. Hence, the priority in clinical practice should be the implementation of basic care, and modern advances should be reserved only for most indicated situations.

CHANGE IN EDUCATIONAL REFORMS

Before the era of superspecialization and technological advances, pediatricians were well trained in the basics of clinical medicine. While superspecialization is a boon, it is expected that superspecialist is an excellent generalist. The new generation of pediatricians has the challenging task of keeping abreast of scientific advances, but it should not be at the expense of basics. The National Board of Examination has modified the examination pattern that tests the candidates more thoroughly in actual life situations, and hence training has also been suitably modified. This has been a better step forward in pediatric education.

PEDIATRICIANS MUST CHANGE

We need to change the focus from disease to health. We must combine the traditional wisdom with modern science. The IAP has formulated guidelines for standard management of many common diseases that should be followed meticulously. Constant updating is necessary to keep up with scientific advances, and they should be used selectively. Science will undergo frequent changes as nothing is constant, and ignorance is far more than knowledge. Hence, we need to learn, unlearn, and relearn. At the same time, we must not forget the holistic approach while treating patients. While science treats the body, the art of medical practice (ethics, communication, counseling, documentation, honesty, transparency, accountability, and responsibility) treats the mind. The mind plays an important role in the ultimate recovery from disease. It is the strong, calm, and satisfied mind that stimulates the immune system which leads to divine healing. Detailed history taking is the first step toward communication, appropriate physical touch during physical examination sets up the tone of bonding, and counseling results in confidence and faith in the doctor. We must remember not to put knowledge before wisdom, science before art, cleverness before common sense, and zeal for the new before mastering the basics.

REFERENCES

1. National Family Health Survey. (2022). National Family Health Survey-5 (2019–21). [online] Available from https://www.data.gov.in/catalog/national-family-health-survey-nfhs-5 [Last accessed October, 2024].
2. Dharmapalan D, Shet A, Yewale V, Sharland M. High reported rates of antimicrobial resistance in Indian neonatal and pediatric blood stream infections. J Pediatric Infect Dis Soc. 2017;6(3):e62-8.
3. Syed N, Allawadhi P, Khurana A, Singh V, Navik U, Pasumathi SK, et al. Gene therapy: comprehensive overview and therapeutic applications. Life Sci. 2022;294:120375.
4. Kumar RR. Future of pediatric practice – Artificial intelligence beckoning? Indian Pediatr. 2021;59(6):443-4.

1.2 History Elicitation

T Ravikumar

INTRODUCTION

The clinical interview and history elicitation are very important tools in the field of pediatric medicine. Though it is mainly of diagnostic value, the process of interaction with the parents and the child during history taking has a therapeutic value as well. A pleasant and patient interaction is what any parent and the child desire. There should be fewer distractions during the interview. It is good to use lay terms when talking to the parents and avoid medical terminologies as far as possible. While interviewing, the pediatrician should also observe the child to look for any clinical clues.[1,2]

In pediatrics, the most important and distinct aspect is the fact that the person giving the history is usually not the patient (unless the child is about 4 or 5 years old). The parents are the usual source of information, and, in certain cases, when caretakers (other than the parents) are bringing up the children, then they will be the source of information.

DEMOGRAPHY

Make a note of the name of the child, his or her age in years (with months and days), parents' names, address, date, and time of the interview, the informant's name and relationship to the child, and their reliability (regarding the consistency of the information they provide).[3]

PRESENTING COMPLAINTS

The main problem or complaint for which the child has been brought for medical attention should be recorded in the informant's own terms and should be recorded in a chronological order with the duration of each complaint as shown below:[1-3]

- Fever, 5 days
- Vomiting, 4 days
- Loose motions, 4 days
- Decreased urine output, 2 days
- Lethargy, 1 day
- Fast breathing, 1 day

HISTORY OF PRESENT ILLNESS

It is important to gather more information and elaborate on the specific presenting complaints. Find out the onset of the complaints (the time up to which the child was apparently well). The evolution of the problems should then flow in a clear, concise, temporal sequence, leading up to the present moment. They should be recorded in order of occurrence, and an account of any repeated episodes of symptoms (such as seizures or respiratory infections) should be given. Symptoms pertaining to complications expected for the presenting complaint and other symptoms that will help in detecting associated conditions and in differential diagnosis should be enquired. The details of treatment given so far and the response should be noted.[1-3]

PAST HISTORY

Ask for the details of relevant past illnesses, the knowledge of which will help you in diagnosis or management. History of the occurrence of similar complaints in the past should be noted. For example, in a child with chronic suppurative lung disease or malnutrition, a history of previous exanthematous illness or whooping cough will help; in failure to thrive, a history of recurrent diarrhea; and in a child with fever and seizures, a history of febrile fits will be supportive. Past medication history will also be helpful, e.g., history of antiepileptic drugs or antituberculous drugs (history of red urine while on treatment with rifampicin). Information on previous significant hospitalizations, accidents, or surgeries may also be helpful.[1-3]

CONTACT HISTORY

History of contact with communicable diseases (e.g., tuberculosis and chickenpox) must be elicited with tact and patience. It is often denied, and repeated probing with leading questions may be necessary.

ANTENATAL HISTORY

As many illnesses in children have their origin in the womb, it is important to get a good history about the period of pregnancy of the index child. A good guide for history elicitation would be the mnemonic of the three "Is" for the mother during pregnancy—illness, irradiation, and injections (i.e., drugs). Maternal illnesses such as syphilis, toxoplasmosis, acquired immune deficiency syndrome, rubella, cytomegalovirus, and herpes virus infections are associated with specific syndromes in the child. Folic acid supplementation during early pregnancy (the first trimester) prevents neural tube defects such as meningomyelocele.[4]

BIRTH HISTORY

The actual events occurring during delivery must be enquired. The period of gestation, duration of labor, nature of delivery, drugs administered during labor, and any complications during delivery (such as cord around neck and low Apgar score) should be noted. The duration of every stage of labor (especially the second stage) is important as prolonged labor may result in fetal hypoxia. The normal first stage of labor, from the onset of labor pains to the rupture of membranes, is about 12–24 and 6–12 hours in a primigravida and multigravida, respectively. The second stage of labor, from the rupture of membranes to the delivery of the child, is about 1–2 hours in a primigravida and 0.5–1 hour in a multigravida. The third stage, which is the delivery of the placenta, lasts about 15 minutes.[4]

POSTNATAL HISTORY

The neonate and its state after birth should be enquired. The term of the child, birth weight, cry, activity, and color immediately after birth should be noted. The presence of jaundice or cyanosis, resuscitation steps used (if any), and whether hospitalized after birth must be detailed. Poor cry and lethargy suggest perinatal depression. Paucity of movements of one side or a limb may suggest a stroke or birth injury. The sucking effort of a child after delivery usually gives a clue to the neurological status of the child. All infants pass meconium within the first 24 hours; any delay would suggest cystic fibrosis, while the absence of passage would indicate intentional obstruction or anal atresia. Most infants void urine on the first day, while all will void within 48 hours; any delay would point toward an obstruction or agenesis of the renal system.[4]

DEVELOPMENT HISTORY

Development is one aspect of pediatrics that makes it unique as compared to adult medicine. The developmental milestones that a child attains are a good reflection of its physical and neurological maturity. They may be divided into gross motor (head control, rolling over, crawling, sitting, standing, walking, etc.), fine motor or adaptive (grasping, reaching and transferring objects, scribbling, etc.), social (smile, recognition, response to calls, etc.), and language (cooing, babbling, saying syllables, vocabulary, etc.). Tailor the development history to the child's age. In the case of more than one child in the family, and if the other siblings are normal, the parents may be asked if the index child's development mirrored that of the other siblings. The pace of development differs from child to child. As the child grows older, the age range of attainment of specific developmental milestones usually widens. For example, a normal child may begin to sit without support between 5 and 8 months as compared to a normal young infant developing a social smile between 6 and 8 weeks. Notice the range of normality becoming more in the older child. Always tabulate the attained milestones against the normal age for the attainment of that milestone **(Table 1.2.1)**.[1]

DIETETIC HISTORY

Dietetic history is highly problem-oriented and age-dependent. Details of the food and dietary patterns help in diagnosing protein-energy malnutrition and failure to thrive. In addition, it helps us to formulate a diet plan for nutritional rehabilitation of the child for a specific disease. The calculation of the dietary values of the food consumed should provide the actual value of proteins, calories, and fats and must mention whether it is sufficient in vitamins, minerals, and other micronutrients. Always state the approximate number of calories and protein the child is getting for that age as compared to what is recommended **(Table 1.2.2)**, which will help us to calculate the calorie and protein gap. Any problem such as feeding difficulty, regurgitation, or vomiting should be noted. Any possible natural toxins in the food consumed (fungal aflatoxins, copper, etc.) and feeding patterns during times of illness should also be mentioned. In young children, the complete breastfeeding history, including whether colostrum was given, duration of exclusive breastfeeding, weaning pattern, etc., must be elucidated. In children fed with other milk, it is important to note its dilution, mode of feeding (bottle-fed or cup and spoon-fed), frequency, and the amount consumed during each feeding.[2]

FAMILY HISTORY

The health details of all the family members must be obtained. This includes their gender, present and past health status, treatment taken, and their proximity to the child. History of similar illnesses in the family must be looked for. History of stillbirths or abortions in the family should be noted (habitual abortions occur in maternal syphilis). The birth of abnormal children or children with illness in the family and the reasons for death, if any, of children or young adults in the family should be specifically enquired into. The consanguinity pattern with the degree of relationship may be helpful for genetic disorders. The pedigree chart will help record the family history in a pictorial manner helping us to derive the inheritance pattern of an illness. Usually, three full generations should be recorded. Individuals of the same generations should be recorded in the same horizontal line and numbered from left to right using Arabic numerals. Males are usually placed on the left side of the pedigree and sibship

TABLE 1.2.1: Normal developmental milestones.

Milestones	Gross motor	Fine motor	Social	Language
First month	Grasp reflex	Starts to smile		
Second month		Hands closed	Social smile	Cooing
Third month	Head mostly held up but still bobs forward	Hands open most often	Sustained social smile	Says "Aah"
Fourth month	Head held steady	Reaches for objects, grasps objects, and brings to mouth, hands in midline	Excited at the sight of food	Laughs out loud
Seventh month	Rolls over, creeping–crawling, sits with hands leaning forward	Reaches out and grasps larger objects, palmar grasp, transfers objects from hand to hand	Smiles at mirror	Babbling
Tenth month	Sits without support, cruises	Pincer grasp	Waves bye-bye	Says "Baba, mama"
1 year	Walks with one hand held	Releases objects to other person on request/gesture	Plays a simple ball game	Says two to three words with meaning
1 year 3 months	Walks alone, crawls upstairs	Makes a tower of three cubes	Asks for objects by pointing	Follows simple commands
1 year 6 months	Runs stiff, goes upstairs by holding the rails	Makes a tower of four cubes, initiates vertical stroke scribbles	Feeds self. Dry by day	Speaks 10 words, identifies parts of the body
2 years	Runs well, walks upstairs and downstairs one foot at a time, jumps	Makes tower of seven cubes, initiates horizontal stoke	Handless spoon well and helps to undress	Puts a sentence of three words
2½ years	Goes upstairs with alternating feet	Makes a tower of nine cubes	Helps put things away	Knows full name
3 years	Rides tricycle, stands momentarily on one foot	Draws a circle, makes a tower of 10 cubes, constructs bridge or three cubes	Dresses and undresses fully when helped with buttons, joins in play	Knows age and gender
4 years	Hops on one foot, throws the ball overhead, climbs well	Draws cross and square, copies a bridge, and constructs a gate of five cubes	Plays with several children with the beginning of social interaction, goes to the toilet alone	Tells story
5 years	Skips	Draws triangle	Dresses and undresses self. Asks questions about the meaning of words	Names four colors, repeats a sentence of 10 syllables

listed in both orders. The maternal age at the time of child delivery is also important. Young mothers (<18 years) have more chances of preterm, intrauterine growth restriction babies, while older mothers (>32 years) have more chances of having children with Down syndrome and Klinefelter syndrome. In children with disease showing hereditary traits, an inquiry of a much wider circle of relatives must be made.[1-3]

SOCIOECONOMIC HISTORY

Socioeconomic history has a bearing on the type of disease the child might be suffering from, and it also helps in planning rehabilitation and treatment options, in addition to helping in giving preventive advice. The following points are worth noting:

- *Type of family:* Joint or nuclear
- Occupation and employment history
- Per capita income (total income divided by the number of dependent family members)
- Type of housing, ventilation, toilet, and potable water facilities
- Psychiatric illness and substance abuse (alcoholism and drugs) in the family
- Marital stability
- Traditional beliefs and child-rearing practices

IMMUNIZATION HISTORY

It is important to record the details of vaccines given to the child in a chronological order. The vaccination schedule of the Indian Academy of Pediatrics or the Universal Immunization Program should be followed. Special vaccines (e.g., pulse polio vaccine) must also be inquired. Look for a Bacillus Calmette-Guérin (BCG) scar at the outer aspect of the left

TABLE 1.2.2: Recommended caloric and protein requirements.

Age	Calories required/day	Protein/day
1 month to 1 year	100–110 kcal/kg/day	2 g/day
1 year	1,000 kcal/day	20 g/day
2 years	1,100 kcal/day	20 g/day
3 years	1,200 kcal/day	20 g/day
4 years	1,300 kcal/day	30 g/day
5 years	1,400 kcal/day	30 g/day
6 years	1,500 kcal/day	30 g/day
7 years	1,600 kcal/day	40 g/day
8 years	1,700 kcal/day	40 g/day
9 years	1,800 kcal/day	40 g/day
10 years	1,900 kcal/day	40 g/day
11 years	2,000 kcal/day	50 g/day
12 years	2,100 kcal/day	50 g/day
Adolescent boy	2,500–3,000 kcal/day	70 g/day
Adolescent girl	2,200–2,400 kcal/day	65 g/day

arm at the insertion of the deltoid. If any vaccine has not been given, note the reason for not doing so.[1-4]

HISTORY OF ALLERGIES

It is important to note down any known, specific drug or food allergies in the child.

CONCLUSION

A detailed history obtained by the student and/or physician from the child and parent/s or caregivers is essential in arriving at an appropriate diagnosis and to plan subsequent clinical examination and diagnostic tests. In case of newborn infants, toddlers and young children appropriate details of birth, antenatal and postnatal events, diet, and growth and development are crucial. It is important to note the immunization details. As for older children and adults, details of presenting complaints, past events, details of family with pedigree, and socioeconomic background are necessary in all children brought for medical evaluation.

REFERENCES

1. Barness LA. Pediatric history and physical examination. In: McMillan JA, DeAngelis CD, Feigin RD (Eds). Oski's Pediatrics: Principles and Practice, 3rd edition. Philadelphia, PA: JB Lippincott Williams and Wilkins; 1999. pp. 39-52.
2. Gupta P. Clinical Methods in Pediatrics, 4th edition. New Delhi: CBS Publishers; 2017.
3. Harris R. The examination of children. In: Swash M (Ed). Hutchison's Clinical Methods, 20th edition. London: ELBS-WB Saunders Co.; 1995. pp. 365-86.
4. Rees PE. Evaluating the newborn infant: diagnostic approach. In: Pediatric Clinical Skills, 2nd edition. Philadelphia, PA: Churchill Livingstone; 1997. pp. 47-76.

1.3 Physical Examination

C Thangadorai, PSN Menon

INTRODUCTION

The physical examination in a child is distinct in certain areas from that of an adult and requires a good knowledge of the variations in anatomy and physiology with growth and development. As far as possible, no child should cry or get irritated while you are examining. *"If a child cries when you examine it, then it is probably your fault"*—this statement by John Apley sums up the care one should take while handling the child. Physical examination starts as the child and the parents walk into the consultation room. Even while eliciting history, an observant eye needs to be kept on the child to watch for clinical clues. There is no definite order to be followed while examining a child. Individualize the examination for every child. Do the invasive and potentially discomforting examinations at the end. Allow the child to be in her/his most comfortable position—whether in the mother's lap, in a chair, or on a couch. Always maintain a pleasing and soothing approach and tone in your communication while examining the child. Both the child and the mother must feel secure and confident about the examining doctor.

GENERAL EXAMINATION

Before starting the physical examination, analyze the history, and based on that, look for the specific features that would be relevant, which will help you to give a probable diagnosis.[1] Examining aimlessly is unhelpful, time-consuming, and irritating to both the child and parents. In general, examination must be thorough from head to foot. Try to collect as much information as possible by general observation first. Examination of an infant or a toddler is often performed in the lap of the mother or in the presence of the parents. With an adolescent patient, privacy should be ensured; sometimes it may not be appropriate to have the parents in the examination room, as it may not allow the patient to be more forthright in expressing his/her problems. Ensure that a female staff member is present in the examination room if a male physician is examining a girl. Awareness of the legal provisions and confidentiality rules of the country is helpful to avoid uncomfortable situations.[2]

Observe the preferred position of the child, whether in the lap of the mother or on the examination table. The physician should be at the level of the child rather than at a towering position. The order of examination should be the least distressing first, followed by the most stressful last. Try your best to gain a good rapport with the child and explain as far as possible to the child at his/her level (and to the anxious parents too) what you are going to perform. Do not forget that distraction is a valuable tool for a fearful or anguished child.

In general, the examination must be as thorough as possible within a reasonable time. The golden rule is *head to foot and back, but forget not the ear, throat, genitalia, and urine.*[1,2] The sensorium (e.g., stupor or unconsciousness in intracranial pathology), posture and attitude (e.g., frog-like position in a floppy infant and limp), activity (e.g., apathy in malnutrition), expression (e.g., acutely or chronically ill-looking), and nutrition (e.g., marasmus or obesity) need special mention.

VITAL SIGNS

An important aspect of initial assessment includes triage and recognizing children who show signs that require prompt care in an intensive care facility to prevent fatality or referral to a specialist quickly.[3] A general examination should be done for important features such as the state of consciousness, toxic or distressed appearance, level of cooperation, hydration status, and cyanosis. These should be noted before starting a detailed examination.

Temperature

Digital thermometers have replaced conventional mercury thermometers and make taking a baby's temperature simple and quick. Temporal artery thermometry measures the temperature of the blood flowing through the temporal artery on the forehead. Tympanic (ear) thermometers are preferred in children more than 6 months of age, as infants have narrow ear canals. Mercury thermometers are best avoided in children as far as possible. Oral temperature should be taken in children older than 5 years, while in infants and younger children, the thermometer may be placed in the axilla. The groin or the rectum can also be used.

The temperature in the axilla or the groin is about 0.5°C lower and the rectal temperature is about 0.5°C higher than the oral temperature. The normal temperature in children is between 36.5 and 37.5°C. Temperature above 41°C is hyperpyrexia. In conditions such as malnutrition, where hypothermia is a problem, special low-reading thermometers (30–40°C) must be used.[1]

Respiratory Rate

The rate of respiration in children is important for diagnosing respiratory disease and certain other nonrespiratory conditions such as acidosis and congestive cardiac failure. The respiratory rate should be counted for a full minute since many infants normally have periodic breathing, so observing for only 15 seconds will result in a skewed number.[2] The rate varies in different age groups **(Table 1.3.1)**. However, for practical purposes, the guidelines offered in the Reproductive and Child Health (RCH) Program serve as a good guide to clinically suspect respiratory disease **(Table 1.3.2)**. It should be counted when the child is quiet. The pattern of respiration must also be noted, whether regular, irregular, Cheyne–Stokes respiration (the oscillation of breathing between apnea and hyperpnea with a crescendo–decrescendo pattern usually seen in congestive cardiac failure, stages 1 and 2, and rapid eye movement sleep), acidotic, etc. In children, the respiration is predominantly abdominothoracic.

Pulse or Heart Rate

The pulse is felt mainly over the radial artery at the wrist or brachial artery in the antecubital fossa; however, it is better to

TABLE 1.3.1: Normal respiratory rate in children of different age groups.

Age groups	*Normal respiratory rate (per minute)*
Newborn	40
1 year	30
5 years	20
10 years	18

TABLE 1.3.2: Tachypnea indicating significant respiratory disease (from the Reproductive and Child Health Program).

Age groups	*Normal respiratory rate (per minute)*
Below 2 months	60 or more
2–12 months	50 or more
12 months to 5 years	40 or more

TABLE 1.3.3: Normal heart rates in children of different age groups.

Age groups	*Normal heart rate (per minute)*
Newborn	140
1 year	110
3 years	100
8 years	90
10 years	80

auscultate or palpate the apical pulse or palpate the femoral pulse in an infant. The character, regularity, and volume must be observed. All the peripheral palpable vessels must be examined.[2] The superficial temporal, carotid, brachial, radial, femoral, popliteal, posterior tibial, and dorsalis pedis arteries are easily palpable. In infants and very young children, it may not be possible to palpate the peripheral vessels, and in such situations, the heart rate must be counted by auscultation. The normal heart/pulse rates in the different age groups in children are given in **Table 1.3.3**. For practical purposes, a heart rate of >200/min in newborns, >150/min in infants, and >120/min in older children can be taken as significant tachycardia. The radial and femoral pulses must be palpated simultaneously to look for any radio-femoral delay.

An elevated heart rate is common in infections, hypovolemia, hyperthyroidism, and anxiety. A rule of thumb is that the pulse rate increases by 10/min for an increase of each 1°C of temperature. Bradycardia is associated with hypertension, raised intracranial pressure, some intoxications, and hypometabolic states. Remember that the heart rate in a struggling or crying child will be higher.

The *pulse-oximetry test* can help identify infants with low levels of oxygen in their blood and may help diagnose critical congenital heart disease (CHD) before an infant becomes sick.

Blood Pressure

Recording the blood pressure (BP) is one of the most important aspects in a pediatric examination. It is surprising how often it is neglected. The correct size of the cuff must be used; that is, the cuff should be two-thirds of the size of the arm. A large cuff will give an erroneously low reading, while a small cuff will give a high reading.[4] In infants, the "flush method" may be used to check the BP. Here, the child's arm is raised, and a tight bandage is applied up to the level of the cuff so as to empty the blood from the upper limb. Now, the cuff is inflated, and the bandage is removed so that the limb will be pale and bloodless. Deflate the cuff slowly and note the reading at which the skin flushes and the limb becomes red again. This corresponds approximately to the systolic BP. The Doppler technique of measuring BP is more accurate and can be used in children, if available.

For every pediatric examination, both the upper limb and lower limb BP must be recorded to detect the coarctation of the aorta, while in any child with a suspected cardiac illness, the BP must be recorded in all four limbs.[4] Normally, the BP recorded in the lower limbs is about 10 mm Hg higher than in the upper limbs. Reserve recording the BP to the last in order not to irritate or scare the child.

In children <13 years of age, the definition of hypertension remains ≥95th percentile for age, sex, and height on three or more occasions. However, for adolescents ≥13 years of age, hypertension is now defined as BP ≥130/80, regardless of age, sex, or height.[5] Normal BP readings in children in the different age groups are given in Chapter 13.14: Hypertension. An observed fall of 10 mm Hg in systolic BP suggests a shock.

HEAD-TO-FOOT AND BACK EXAMINATION

Examination of Head

Note the *shape of the head* **(Fig. 1.3.1)** for microcephaly, macrocephaly, plagiocephaly (asymmetrical due to lying of the normal infants with their heads persistently on one side known as "deformational" or due to premature closure of lambdoid or coronal suture known as "synostotic"), scaphocephaly [boat-shaped with increased anteroposterior (AP) diameter due to premature closure of the sagittal suture], brachycephaly (decreased AP diameter), and oxycephaly (tower-shaped skull).

The size of the *anterior fontanel (AF)* (normal of about 2.5 cm × 2.5 cm) must be measured across the borders as shown in **Figure 1.3.2**. It normally closes in 9–18 months. Delayed closure is seen in rickets, hypothyroidism, hydrocephalus, Down syndrome, achondroplasia, and mucopolysaccharidosis. The AF in a quiet child usually shows a very slight depression from the surface and may pulsate. It is bulging when the child cries and in hydrocephalus, intracranial hypertension, and pseudotumor cerebri. A sunken fontanel is a sign of dehydration.

The *posterior fontanel* can be felt by running the finger along the sagittal suture to its junction with the lambdoid suture. It normally closes by 2–4 months of age. Ridging and overriding of *sutures* may normally be seen in the first few hours after birth, due to molding of the skull during delivery. It may also be seen in craniosynostosis due to premature fusion of the sutures. Sutures normally get ossified by 6 months of age **(Fig. 1.3.3)**.

The *Macewen's sign* is useful in clinically detecting raised intracranial tension after the sutures have closed. It is the crackpot sound elicited by the percussion of the skull. *Transillumination of the skull* in a dark room is useful in children below 1 year to detect subdural effusion or hematoma if the translucency extends beyond 2 cm in the frontal and 1 cm in the occipital region.

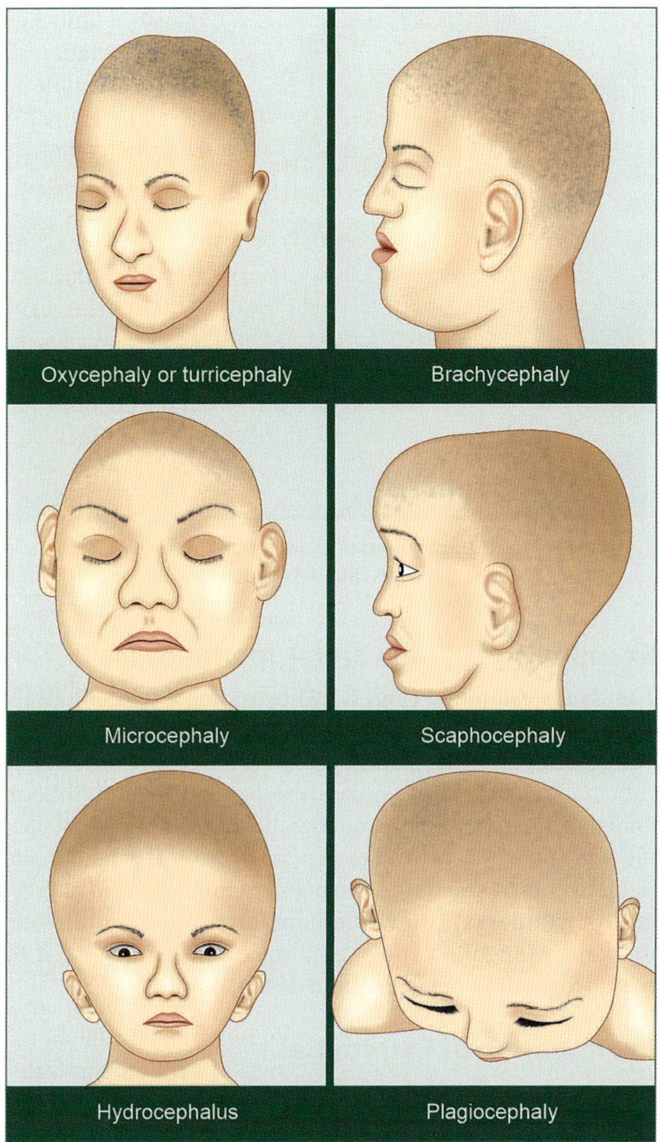

Fig. 1.3.1: Different shapes of the head.

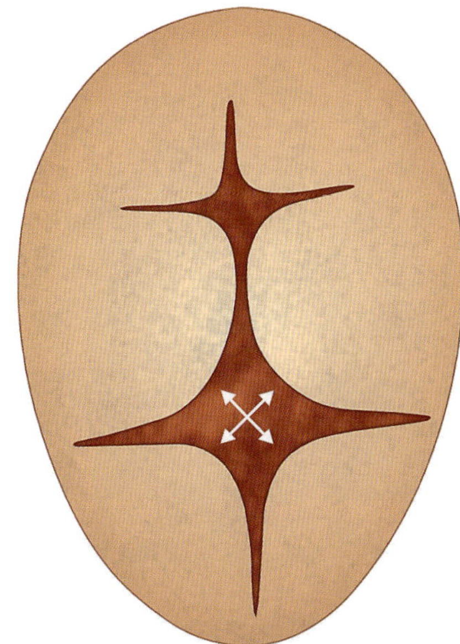

Fig. 1.3.2: Method of measuring the anterior fontanel size.

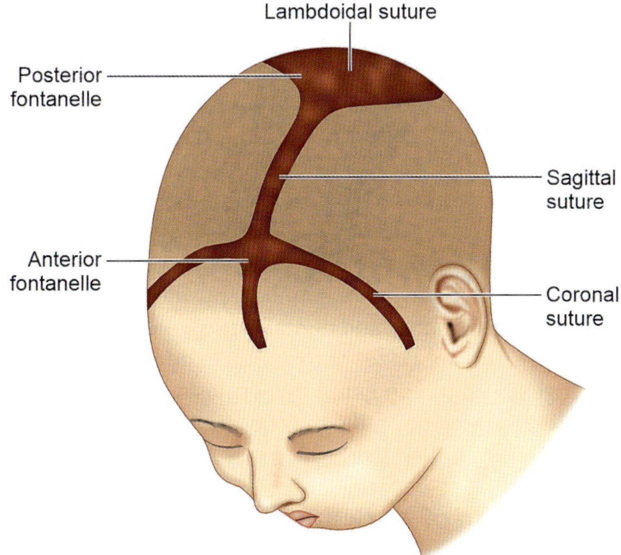

Fig. 1.3.3: Different cranial sutures at birth.

Examination of Face, Eyes, Ears, Nose, and Throat

The *face* must be observed for any dysmorphic features that may suggest chromosomal or developmental anomalies.

Eyes should be examined for signs of vitamin A deficiency, infection, icterus, pallor, strabismus, slant of palpebral fissures, hypertelorism, or telecanthus. It is important to observe the pupil size, plugging of nasolacrimal ducts, and red or fundus reflex (the coloration of the pupil from light reflecting off the back inner surface of the eye) and assess the field of vision (as best as possible). Fundus examination is important to confirm papilledema, optic atrophy, or retinitis pigmentosa. Try to be familiar with the use of a pediatric ophthalmoscope.

Examine the *ears* using a pediatric otoscope, starting with the tympanic membrane for acute otitis media or chronic suppurative otitis media. Observe the position of ears and make an assessment of hearing. The correct position for doing the ear, nose, and throat examination is shown in **Figure 1.3.4**, but this should be done preferably at the last. The interpalpebral line of the eyes, when continued horizontally backward, normally divides the ears into the upper one-third and the lower two-thirds. If the line passes above the ears, it is suggestive of low-set ears associated with genetic disorders.

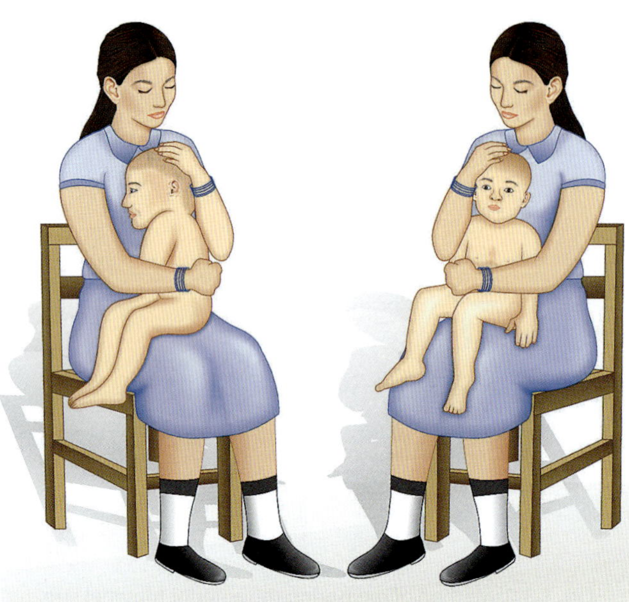

Fig. 1.3.4: Method of restraining a child for ENT examination. (ENT: ears, nose, and throat)

The *nose* examination with a torch or otoscope should include symmetry, septum, swelling, malformations, discharge, and tenderness.

The *mouth and throat* are examined with a torch and tongue depressor for the state of the lips (color and fissures), gums, buccal mucosa (color, vesicles, dry or moist, and Koplik spots), tongue (color, papillae, position, tremors, and thrush), teeth (number and dental caries), palate (intactness and arch), tonsils (size, color, and exudates), posterior pharyngeal wall (color, lymph hyperplasia, and bulge), and gag reflex. Delayed dentition may be familial or due to rickets or osteogenesis imperfecta.

Examination of Neck and Lymph Nodes

The *neck* should be examined for thyroid, position of the trachea, mass (cyst or nodes), evidence of nuchal rigidity, and torticollis. Check whether the neck is short (normal neck length:height ratio is 1:13) and has a low hairline (below C5). "Bull neck" is a feature of diphtheria.

While examining *lymph nodes,* note the site, size, consistency, tenderness, warmth, matting, and scarring. Always remember to examine the draining areas for the focus of sepsis if there is any significant lymph node enlargement. In older children, discrete and nontender lymph node enlargement of up to 1.5 cm in the cervical and inguinal regions may not be significant. Do not forget to palpate the salivary glands (parotid glands), especially with a history of fever as in mumps.

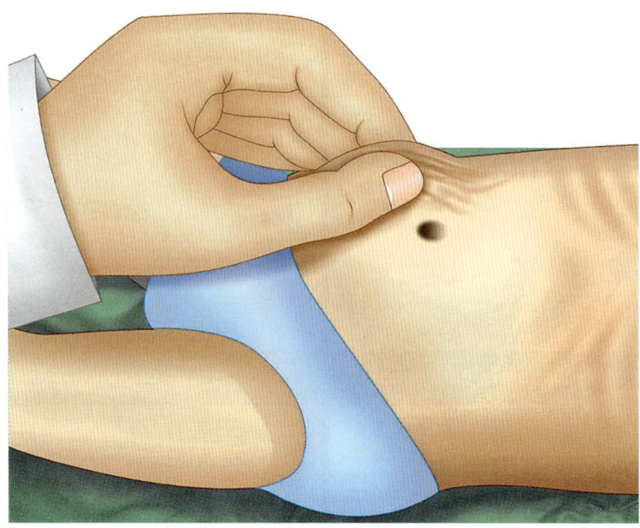

Fig. 1.3.5: Method of examining skin turgor in a child with dehydration.

Examination of Skin and Appendages

The skin is examined **(Fig. 1.3.5)** by rolling a fold of loosely adherent skin on the abdominal wall between the thumb and forefinger to determine its consistency, the amount of subcutaneous tissue present, and the degree of hydration. Look for pallor, icterus, scabies, impetigo, acanthosis nigricans, etc.; *the hair* (pale hair with "flag sign" in kwashiorkor) and nails (koilonychia in anemia). Note pigmentation, signs of allergy, and "birthmarks"—nevi, hemangioma, neurocutaneous markers, Mongolian spots, etc. Make it a regular habit to search for rashes, petechiae, and desquamation.

Examination of Extremities

Examination of the hips should always be carried out in younger children and infants to look for dislocation. The Ortolani or Barlow procedure is done, and the typical clunk of the hip moving in and out of its socket is looked for. Examine the extremities for limb deformities (seen in skeletal dysplasia), widened wrists (rickets), and nails. Infants and younger children do not exhibit classical pedal edema, as they are confined to bed; hence, sacral edema should be looked for in them.

Table 1.3.4 shows some common abnormal features and a few conditions where they are seen.

ANTHROPOMETRY

Measuring of various anthropometric data is essential for assessing the growth of the child and the nutritional status. It is also important for planning the diet and following up with the child, especially while recuperating from an illness or during nutritional rehabilitation.

TABLE 1.3.4: Some features to be looked for in the head and their associated conditions.

Features	*Important associated conditions*
Microcephaly	Familial, craniosynostosis, intrauterine infections, trisomy 13 and 21 (Down syndrome)
Macrocephaly	Hydrocephalus, hydranencephaly, porencephaly, some neurodegenerative disorders such as metachromatic leukodystrophy, Alexander disease, Canavan disease, certain intrauterine infections
Frontal bossing	Rickets, congenital syphilis, mucopolysaccharidoses
Craniotabes (ping-pong skull)	Physiological (in preterm), rickets, congenital syphilis
Increased interpupillary distance (hypertelorism)	Genetic (racial), Down syndrome, Cri-du-chat syndrome, hypothyroidism
Proptosis (sclera is visible above and below the cornea)	Thyrotoxicosis, orbital leukemic deposits, orbital cellulites, arteriovenous aneurysm (pulsatile), cavernous sinus thrombosis, neurofibromatosis, Crouzon disease
Cataract	Idiopathic, traumatic, intrauterine infections, galactosemia, diabetes mellitus, Down syndrome
Mongoloid eyes (upward slant)	Down syndrome, racial, Prader–Willi syndrome
Antimongoloid slant (downward slant)	Turner syndrome, Cri-du-chat syndrome, Treacher–Collins syndrome
Depressed nasal bridges	Down syndrome, mucopolysaccharidoses, hypothyroidism, familial
Low-set ears	Down syndrome, mucopolysaccharidoses, Turner syndrome, Potter facies (renal agenesis)
Facial puffiness	Renal disorder, kwashiorkor, congestive cardiac failures, angioneurotic edema, cavernous sinus thrombosis
Large tongue	Hypothyroidism, mucopolysaccharidoses, glycogen storage disorders, Down syndrome (relative)
Small mandible	Pierre Robin syndrome
Short neck	Turner syndrome, Down syndrome, mucopolysaccharidoses, hypothyroidism

Weight

The child must be weighed during every examination. Weight is recorded on a weighing scale, which should be frequently checked with standard weights, and zero error must be adjusted before weighing. Make it a practice to record weight on an appropriate growth chart for the corresponding ethnic population along with other anthropometric measurements (e.g., height, head circumference, body mass index) on the first visit and follow-up visits. The weight of the child is also useful for calculating the right dosage of the drugs to be given. The newborn loses up to 10% of its weight during the first week but regains it in the next few days. The child doubles its birth weight by 4 months, triples it by 1 year, and increases it four times by 2 years. While interpreting the weight of the child, the present weight must be compared to the expected weight for age, and the percentage must be calculated to find out which grade of nutrition the child falls under. Refer to Chapter 3.3 for details of growth measurements for different ages.

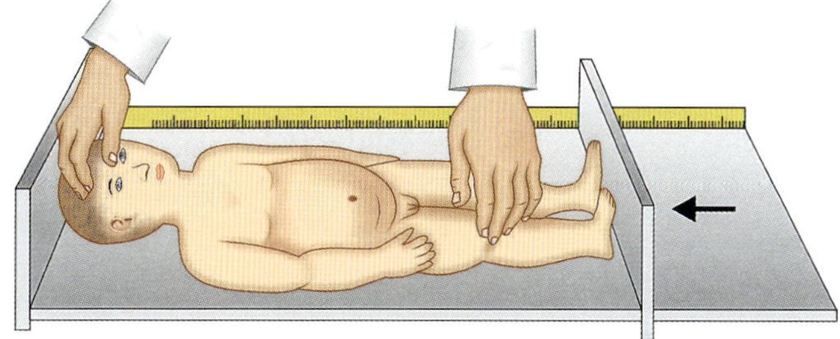

Fig. 1.3.6: Infantometer method of measuring the length of a child.

Height or Length

The height of the child is a good indicator of the chronicity of any debilitating illness. Height in an older child is ideally measured using a Harpenden stadiometer. The child should stand against a wall with her/his bare feet touching each other, the heel, calf, buttock, upper back, and occiput touching the wall, and the child looking straight ahead. A firm scale is pressed to the head to mark the point indicating height. The standing height can be measured for children more than 2 years old, while for younger children, the recumbent length should be measured using the infantometer **(Fig. 1.3.6)**. The height should be recorded on a growth chart designed for the population.

In exceptions, such as a child with quadriplegic cerebral palsy where the height or length could not be measured, the length of various segments of the body is measured separately and added together to get the length. The increase in height as shown in **Table 1.3.5** may be used for calculating the expected height.

Body Proportions

While measuring the height, it is also important to measure the upper segment (from the vertex to the pubic symphysis) and the lower segment (from the pubic symphysis to the sole of the foot). The rate of growth of upper and lower segments varies with age, as shown in **Table 1.3.6**. Hence, any difference in the proportion expected for that age may suggest the presence of specific growth disorders **(Table 1.3.7)**.

TABLE 1.3.5: Rate of increase in height in children.

Age	Height
At birth	50 cm
6 months	+12 cm (62 cm)
1 year	75 cm
2 years	85 cm (86–87 cm)
2–5 years	6–8 cm/yr
5 years and above	5 cm/yr

TABLE 1.3.6: Normal upper segment/lower segment ratio in children.

Age	Upper segment/lower segment
At birth	1.8/1
3–4 years	1.3/1
9 years	1/1
18 years	0.9/1

TABLE 1.3.7: Conditions with characteristic upper segment/lower segment ratio.

Upper segment/lower segment ratio	Probable disorder
Proportionate (normal ratio for age)	Delayed adolescence, hypopituitarism, constitutional delay in growth and puberty, undernutrition
High ratio (upper segment > lower segment)	Hypothyroidism, chondrodystrophy, achondroplasia, Ellis–van Creveld syndrome, Turner syndrome
Low ratio (upper segment < lower segment)	Mucopolysaccharidoses (Hurler syndrome, Morquio syndrome), hypogonadism

Midparental or Target Height

Stature should also be defined with the parent's height being considered, referred to as the midparental height, and the target height can be calculated using the formula given below:

For girls: Approximate projected adult height (in cm)

$$= \frac{\text{Mother's height} + (\text{Father's height} - 13)}{2}$$

For boys: Approximate projected adult height (in cm)

$$= \frac{(\text{Mother's height} + 13) + \text{Father's height}}{2}$$

This target height can be marked in the growth chart at 18 years of age and projected back to check if the child's present height falls in the target height centiles.

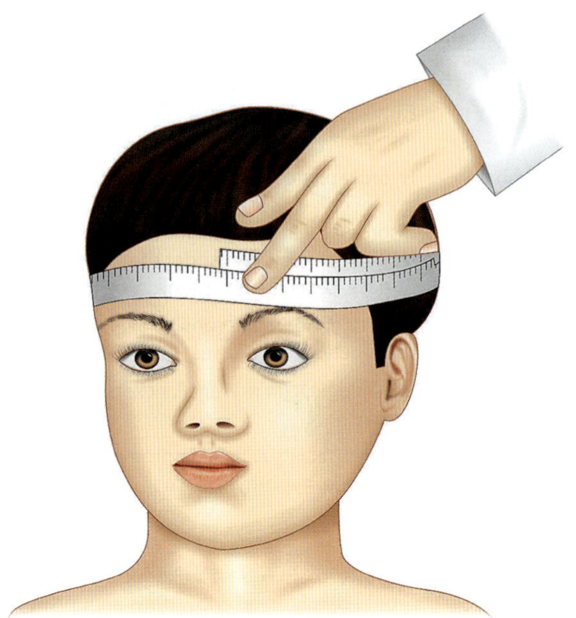

Fig. 1.3.7: Method of measuring the head circumference.

Head Circumference

The size of the head is a good indicator of the size of its contents, namely the brain and the ventricles. Any abnormality in the head circumference should alert the physician toward any problem with the brain or its related structures. Head circumference is measured with a nonstretchable tape passing through the maximum point of the external occupational protuberance posteriorly and a point just above the glabella anteriorly **(Fig. 1.3.7)**. It varies from 32 to 35 cm at birth, from 43 to 46 cm at 1 year, and from 48 to 51 cm at 5 years. Head circumference should be recorded at each visit on the growth chart of the child and checked whether it is in the normal range. The expected head circumference for the age may be calculated from **Table 1.3.8**. The adult head size is reached between 5 and 6 years. Microcephaly is defined as a head circumference of more than 3 standard deviations (SD) below the mean for the age and sex and may be a part of the disorders like Rett syndrome, congenital infection like cytomegalovirus, or abnormal brain growth as in schizencephaly. A head size of >2 SD suggests macrocephaly.[6] It may be familial in some children or part of a pathological state, as in hydrocephalus, arachnoid cyst, Canavan disease, or arteriovenous malformations of the brain.

Chest Circumference

Chest circumference is measured at the level of the nipples **(Fig. 1.3.8)**. In the infant, the chest circumference is less

TABLE 1.3.8: Expected increase in head circumference.

Age	Increase in head circumference
Till 3 months	2 cm/month
3 months to 1 year	2 cm/3 months (1/3rd of initial velocity)
1–3 years	1 cm/6 months (1/12th of initial velocity)
3–5 years	1 cm/year (1/24th of initial velocity)

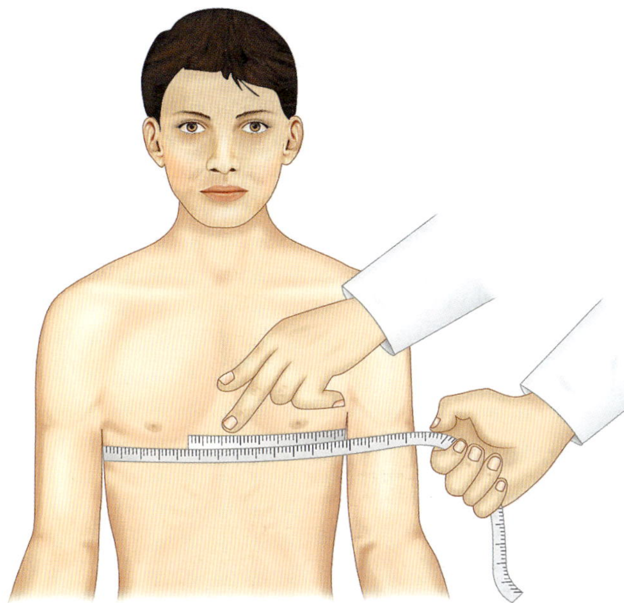

Fig. 1.3.8: Method of measuring the chest circumference.

than the head circumference by about 2.5 cm, and the two become equal by 1 year after which the chest circumference exceeds the head circumference. In undernutrition, the chest circumference remains lower than the head circumference even beyond 1.5 years, whereas in well-nourished children, the chest circumference may exceed the head circumference even before 1 year.

Midarm Circumference

The midarm circumference (MAC) is taken, as the name suggests, at the midpoint between the acromion and the olecranon, with the arm hanging by the side of the body **(Fig. 1.3.9)**. It is useful to detect malnutrition in young children (1–4 years). Values >13.5 cm may be considered normal, while values <12.5 cm indicate significant wasting and undernutrition. Shakir tape is used for measuring MAC in the community and has color bands—green color indicates a MAC >13.5 cm, yellow color a MAC between 13.5 and 12.5 cm, and red color a MAC <12.5 cm. MAC of <11.5 cm in children 6–60 months of age is also used as a diagnostic criterion for severe acute malnutrition (SAM).

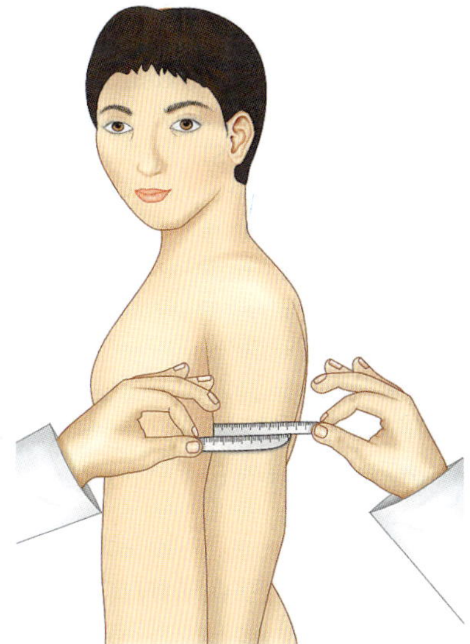

Fig. 1.3.9: Method of measuring the midarm circumference.

Arm Span

Arm span is the distance between the tips of the middle fingers with both arms held wide open, i.e., spread apart. Normally, in young children, it is 1–2 cm less than the length or height. It equals the height at 10 years, and after 10 years, it is from 1 to 2 cm more than the height. The increased arm span is seen in Marfan syndrome and homocystinuria.

Weight for Height/Length

This is calculated using the formula:

Weight for height (WFH) or length (WFL)

$$= \left(\frac{\text{Weight of child}}{\text{Weight corresponding to height of child}} \right) \times 100$$

The child's weight can be plotted against the length (up to 2 years) or height (beyond 2 years) in the Indian Academy of Pediatrics/World Health Organization (IAP/WHO) growth charts: Normal –2 to + 2 Z-score; moderate wasting <–2 to –3 Z-score; severe wasting <–3 Z-score; overweight >+2 Z-score. In children <5 years of age, obesity is defined in terms of weight for length/height. The IAP recommends using WHO weight for length/height charts as there are no under-5 IAP growth charts. The definitions in this age group for *overweight* are weight for height >2 SD but <3 SD and obesity as weight for height >3 SD for the population.[7]

Body Mass Index

Body mass index (BMI) is calculated using the formula:

$$\text{BMI} = \left(\frac{\text{Weight of kg}}{(\text{Height in meter})^2} \right)$$

For adults, the WHO defines overweight as a BMI ≥25 kg/m^2 and obesity as a BMI ≥30 kg/m^2. For children, age needs to be considered when defining overweight and obesity. Overweight for children aged between 5 and 19 years is defined as BMI-for-age >1 SD above the WHO Growth Reference median and obesity as >2 SD above the WHO Growth Reference median.[8] Please refer to Chapter 3.6: Obesity and Overweight for more details of measurements and appropriate growth charts. The BMI should be recorded on the growth charts of all children.

Growth Patterns

The common growth patterns observed during age periods are shown in **Table 1.3.9**.

TABLE 1.3.9: Growth patterns.

Age	*Approximate daily weight gain (g)*	*Growth in length (cm/month)*	*Growth in head circumference (cm/month)*
0–3 months	30	3.5	2
3–6 months	20	2	1
6–9 months	15	1.5	0.5
9–12 months	12	1.5	0.5
1–3 years	8	1	0.25
4–6 years	8	6 cm/year	1 cm/year

DEVELOPMENTAL EXAMINATION

Here, the developmental history obtained must be confirmed by examining the child for the milestones attained or lost. Many accepted methods are available for assessing development. The Gesell and Bayley Developmental Scales are commonly used. The Vadodara Developmental Screening Tests and the Thiruvananthapuram Developmental Screening Chart are useful for field assessment of children's development. The development quotient (DQ) must be calculated separately for motor and mental development using the formula:

$$DQ = \frac{\text{Developmental age}}{\text{Chronological age}} \times 100$$

Developmental evaluation is of special value in children with neurological diseases (such as neurodegenerative disorders) and chromosomal anomalies (such as Down syndrome). It is also useful for following up on children with birth asphyxia or established cerebral palsy and neurocognitive disability. The common developmental/primitive reflexes to be examined are shown in **Table 1.3.10**. The absence of appearance of the primitive reflexes at the expected time or their persistence beyond the time that they should normally disappear should lead to a suspicion of significant brain damage.

TABLE 1.3.10: Primitive reflexes to be examined during developmental assessment.

Reflexes	*Age of appearance*	*Age of disappearance*
Stepping	Birth	6 weeks
Placing	Birth	6 weeks
Moro	Birth	3 months
Sucking and rooting	Birth	4 months while awake
Palmar grasp	Birth	6 months
Plantar grasp	Birth	10 months
Tonic neck	2 months	4–6 months
Landau	3 months	24 months
Neck righting	4 months	24 months
Parachute	9 months	Persists

Puberty and Sexual Maturity Rating

The sexual maturity rating in boys and girls is shown in **Table 1.3.11**. For more details, please refer to Chapter 3.2. An appropriate psychosocial assessment appropriate to pubertal development is also necessary.

SYSTEMIC EXAMINATION

It is beyond the scope of this chapter to cover the examination of every system in detail; it can be obtained from any standard textbook of clinical examination. Here we have attempted to give salient points in clinical examination, which are different in children when compared to adults. In addition to diagnosing the underlying disease, assessment of children should involve identification of malnutrition, immunization status, level of development, screening for "4 Ds" (Defects at birth, Deficiencies, Diseases, and Developmental Delay including Disability) along with assessment of hearing and vision and detection of child abuse.[3]

Respiratory System and Thorax

Inspect the chest wall for any deformities, such as pectus excavatum or pectus carinatum. Costochondral beading is seen in rickets (broad and dome-shaped, rachitic rosary), in scurvy (sharp due to posterior subluxation of the sternum), and in chondrodystrophy. Observe the pattern of breathing, whether abdominal (which is normal in infants) or periodic (may be normal in infants with a pause of <15 seconds). Count the respiratory rate for a full minute. Look for working of the accessory muscles of respiration, i.e., flaring of alae

TABLE 1.3.11: Sexual maturity rating (SMR) in boys/girls.

SMR stage	Pubic hair (boys/girls)	Breasts (girls)	Penis	Testes
1	Preadolescent	Preadolescent	Preadolescent	Preadolescent
2	Sparse, slightly pigmented	Breast and papilla elevated, areolar diameter increased	Slight enlargement	Enlarged scrotum, pink
3	Darker, beginning to curl	Breast and areola enlarged, no contour separation	Longer	Larger
4	Coarse, curly, abundant but less than adult	Areola and papilla form secondary mound	Larger	Larger, scrotum dark
5	Adult distribution, spreads to the medial surface of thighs	Mature, nipple projects	Adult size	Adult size

nasi, sternomastoid contraction, suprasternal and subcostal and intercostal retractions, which would indicate dyspnea. Observe for indrawing of the lower ribs (Harrison's sulcus), which indicates chronic obstructive airway disease such as bronchial asthma. Vocal fremitus is rarely of value in young children. The grunting respiration in a child indicates severe respiratory disease. Percuss lightly in infants and small children; tap the chest wall directly rather than using another pleximeter finger. Due to the thin chest wall, the chest is more resonant than in adults. Before starting to auscultate, allow the child to play with your stethoscope to allay its fears. Often, it is less threatening to examine the back of the chest first. Due to the thin chest wall, breath sound is louder in children than in adults, and their character is more like the bronchial breathing of adults. This is called puerile breathing. Do not be disheartened with a crying child, as breath sounds can be auscultated better in them. Be careful to distinguish the conducted sounds from the upper respiratory tract, as in laryngomalacia, upper respiratory tract infection, etc.

Cardiovascular System

In a neonate, the apical impulse is located slightly outside the midclavicular line in the fourth intercostal space. By 2 years, it comes to the midclavicular line in the fourth intercostal space and comes to the adult position, i.e., 5th intercostal space 1 cm medial to the midclavicular line between 4 and 7 years. In infants, the right ventricles are dominant as compared to adults (where the left ventricle is dominant). Due to the short neck of infants and young children, it is difficult to see the jugular venous pulse and pressure. Use a pediatric stethoscope with a small diaphragm to auscultate, as the intercostal spaces are narrow. It is preferable to auscultate the heart while the infant is comfortably sleeping or feeding from the mother. It is easier to hear the normal splitting of the heart sounds, and the P2 is louder in young children, i.e., less than 5 years. The functional systolic flow murmurs and venous hum are often heard in normal children.

Abdomen—Liver, Spleen, Pancreas, Kidneys, and Urinary Tract

The best place to examine the child's abdomen is the mother's lap, preferably while the child is feeding. Even if the child is struggling, it may be put on the mother's shoulder, and the abdomen is palpated from behind by "ballottement," i.e., palpation just when the child breathes and the abdomen relaxes. Unlike adults, it is not necessary to fold the legs of the child while palpating the abdomen. Young children normally have a protuberant abdomen. Look for umbilical (which may be normally seen in infants) and inguinal hernia. The liver is normally palpable in children till the age of 4 years, i.e., up to 2 cm below the costal margin. In view of this, it is necessary to measure the span of the liver to figure out the actual enlargement. It is carried out by percussing the upper margin of dullness and by palpating the lower edge of the liver in the midclavicular line. The liver span ranges from about 4.5 to 5 cm at 1 week of age to approximately 7–8 cm in males and from 6 to 6.5 cm in females by 12 years of age. The spleen may be normally palpable in infants, up to 2–3 months of age. Examine the genitalia and scrotum for hydrocele/hernia, intersex, phimosis, undescended testis, hypospadias, or epispadias. The anus is examined for anal excoriation and pinworms.

Nervous System

Neurological examination of a young child is quite difficult, especially sensory examination, and requires ingenuity on the part of the doctor to get the child's cooperation. Developmental screening and assessment of the primitive reflexes should be carried out as already mentioned. Much information regarding the neurological status of the child can be learned by just observing the child, as the history is being elicited. Coordination is best tested by watching the child play. Orientation is best tested only in children above 4–5 years. Handedness becomes apparent at about 3 years of age. The signs of meningeal irritation, i.e., neck stiffness

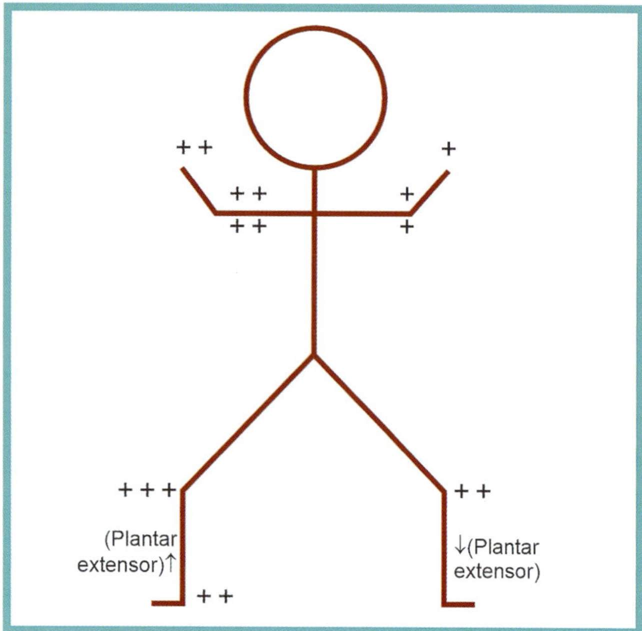

Fig. 1.3.10: Model diagrammatic representation of recording deep tendon reflexes.
(0: absent, +: sluggish, ++: normal, +++: brisk, ++++: exaggerated)

(Kernig's sign and Brudzinski's sign), must be looked for. They may not be present in infants and in the presence of severe undernutrition or overwhelming sepsis. Fundus may normally be pale in infants. Lifting the child gives a good idea about the muscle tone. If it is hypotonic, the child will slip through the hands. The plantar reflex may be extensor up to 1 year of age; however, the persistence of an extensor plantar beyond 2 years is pathological. Tendon reflexes in young infants tend to be brisk. The deep tendon reflexes may be diagrammatically represented as shown in **Figure 1.3.10**.

Musculoskeletal System

It is important to examine the back for sacral dimple, kyphosis, lordosis, or scoliosis. Examine all joints for motion, stability, swelling, and tenderness. Examine the muscles and joints for deformities, symmetry, edema, and clubbing, and note the gait or limp of the child and the presence of bow legs and knock knees. In young infants, it is important to check the hip by Ortolani's and Barlow's signs.

Genitourinary System

It is often forgotten to examine the genitalia, especially in a girl. The external genitalia should be examined in boys for hernia and hydrocele. Most hernias are indirect in infancy and childhood. Check for the presence of descended testes in the scrotum and whether they are retractile. However, it is not recommended to do a rectal examination unless there is a specific indication.

PRACTICE OF DIFFERENTIAL DIAGNOSIS

During situations when the diagnosis of the child is not very clear (which may be the case quite often), it becomes necessary to make a set of most probable diagnoses. This is called differential diagnosis. This should be based on the history, clinical symptoms, and clinical signs that have been elicited. The differential diagnoses thus made will help us to plan out investigations toward proving or disproving each probable cause. Hence, to be of practical value, the list should be as short as possible and should only include the conditions that could reasonably explain most of the child's history, symptoms, and signs. The list should be given in a descending order of probability of the various likely diagnoses, based on the positive and negative points toward each.

CONCLUSION

History taking and clinical skill development in pediatrics are learned through repeated exposure to case interviews and hands-on training in physical examination. The more a student gets this type of exposure, the more she/he can engage herself/himself in self-analysis, which will help her/him carry out the clinical examination thoroughly.

REFERENCES

1. Gupta P. Clinical Methods in Pediatrics, 5th edition. New Delhi: CBS Publishers; 2021.
2. Drutz JE, White-Satcher D'J. (2024). The pediatric physical examination: general principles and standard measurements. UpToDate. Wolters Kluwer. [online] Available from https://www.uptodate.com/contents/the-pediatric-physical-examination-general-principles-and-standard-measurements. [Last accessed October, 2024].
3. Makhija S, Tiwari P. How to proceed with examination of a child? Indian J Pediatr. 2018;85(9):738-45.
4. University of North Dakota. Outline for pediatric history and physical exam. [online] Available from https://med.und.edu>pediatrics>pediatrichp. [Last accessed October, 2024].
5. Lande MB, Batisky DL. New American Academy of Pediatrics hypertension guideline. Who is up and who is down. Hypertension. 2019;73:31-2.
6. Hanslik E, Gigante J. Microcephaly. Children (Basel). 2017;4(6):47.
7. Khadilkar VV, Shah N, Harish R, Ayyavoo A, Bang A, Basu S, et al. Indian Academy of Pediatrics Revised (2023) Guidelines on evaluation, prevention and management of childhood obesity. Indian Pediatr. 2023;60(12):1013-31.
8. World Health Organization. Obesity and overweight. [online] Available from https://www.who.int/news-room/fact-sheets/detail/obesity-and-overweight. [Last accessed October, 2024].

1.4 Communication and Counseling

Parang N Mehta

INTRODUCTION

Communication skills are a core competence for clinicians. Good communication enhances patients' understanding and adherence to therapy and improves outcomes. Poor understanding of the disease and treatment issues by parents is associated with poor outcomes.[1] Good communication and shared decision-making are essential for a positive patient experience. Poor communication puts patients at risk due to caregivers' lack of accurate information about the disease and treatment.

Communication is an important determinant of both patient satisfaction and complaints. It is everyone's responsibility to improve communication skills and provide the time and place for it. In the current climate of suspicion and even hostile doctor–patient relationships, good communication can do a lot to establish and restore trust.

COMMUNICATION SKILLS

Communication skills are, quite simply, the skills that allow human beings to communicate effectively. For pediatricians, communication skills consist of the following:

- The ability to talk with parents. Not to parents, not at parents, but with them. Listening is an essential part; communication must be a two-way process.[2] Good listening skills help not only in diagnosis but also in judging what the family expects from the medical visit and what treatment will be acceptable to them.
- The ability to communicate well enough with patients and parents to understand their concerns, problems, and beliefs and to elicit relevant information.[3]
- The ability to explain the child's illness plainly in language that the parents can easily understand. The treatment options should be explained clearly and completely so that they can make informed decisions about treatment. Health literacy is low in the general population and is associated with poor health outcomes.[1]
- The ability to convince parents to follow a treatment plan. This is especially important when embarking on prolonged, expensive, difficult, or culturally unacceptable treatment for a child.
- The ability to establish a relationship with the parents and child based on mutual respect and trust
- The ability to let parents and older children understand that they have a say in their treatment decisions.[4,5] Many people would like to participate in shared decision-making but need to be encouraged to do so.
- "Soft skills" such as being able to put all classes of parents at ease and being able to generate confidence. These components of a "good bedside manner" were once considered an important attribute of a successful practitioner.

IMPORTANCE OF COMMUNICATION AND COUNSELING SKILLS

The chief goals of communication are as follows:

- Creation of a good interpersonal relationship
- Facilitating the exchange of information
- Including patients and parents in decision-making[2]

Communication skills contribute to a doctor's respect, a patient's belief, and adherence to treatment, among other advantages **(Box 1.4.1)**.[6] A doctor with these skills is more likely to have happy, satisfied patients than an equally technically competent doctor who does not bother about communication. Even if a pediatrician's diagnosis and treatment are accurate, thoroughly rational, and successful, poor communication leaves the parents unhappy and resentful. This is especially so with chronic or incurable diseases, which are associated with anxiety, stress, and uncertainty for the whole family.[4,7]

Patients and parents do not have the knowledge to judge the quality of a doctor's examination, diagnosis, or prescription. Most complaints in healthcare systems, both public and private, arise from poor communication. Parents

BOX 1.4.1: Advantages of good communication.

- Facilitation of comprehension of medical information
- Better identification of patients' needs, perceptions, and expectations
- Patient satisfaction, leading to regular visits and referrals
- Feeling of empowerment and control
- Adherence to treatment plans
- Loyalty, even if treatment is not immediately effective
- Less chances of complaints and legal action in the event of a mistake
- Doctors with good communication skills have better clinical and commercial success, less stress, and more job satisfaction

are angered by the doctor's refusal to spend time with them, refusal to give explanations, and lack of courtesy and care.[5] When these are followed by poor treatment outcomes, complaints, quarrels, and legal action are likely.[6]

Good communication can play a significant part in avoiding complaints and malpractice claims.

BARRIERS TO GOOD COMMUNICATION

The two most important barriers are not knowing what patients want from us **(Box 1.4.2)** and not realizing the importance of good communication. Some other barriers are as follows:

- *Lack of time:* History taking, physical examination, and prescription writing are seen as essential parts of a clinical encounter. When time is short, it is the communication with parents that is sacrificed.[3]
- *Arrogance:* Doctors expect patients and their parents to follow commands unquestioningly. Explanations are considered unnecessary.
- *Shyness:* Shyness, from the patient or the doctor, stands in the way of adequate information being exchanged.[2]
- *Language and jargon:* Communication with people speaking different languages can be problematic and may need special effort.[4] If an interpreter is used, he should be given small bits of information to translate at a time, especially when the prescription is dealt with.
- Speaking in technical/medical language leaves the parents confused and uninformed and defeats the purpose of communication.[4] It is important to talk in language that a nonmedical person can understand.[5]
- *Deafness:* Speaking loudly, slowly, and distinctly helps parents with hearing impairment. Other useful measures are voice amplification devices, a quiet room, and the use of written communication.
- *Phones:* Phones are ubiquitous now, and calls can interrupt and hinder communication terribly.

BOX 1.4.2: What patients and parents want.

- Clarity and directness
- Listening
- Honesty
- More and better information about their illness, treatment plan, and expected outcome
- More openness about the hazards and side effects of treatment
- More information about the relief of symptoms and other concerns
- Advice on what they can do to help themselves
- Information on other treatments available
- A supportive, nonjudgmental, and empathetic doctor

ROLE OF COMMUNICATION IN TREATMENT ADHERENCE

The importance of adherence is often underestimated. The best diagnostic efforts and treatment plans do not yield results unless patients follow the recommended treatment, rehabilitation therapy, lifestyle changes, and other required measures. Inadequate adherence is associated with poor outcomes such as increased morbidity and disability, higher drug usage, and enhanced mortality.[8,9]

Good communication allows the detection of poor adherence. It also improves outcomes by informing parents about the disease and its dangers, the necessity of treatment, and the safety of the treatment.[9,10] Parents also cherish appreciation for the care they provide their child.

INFORMATION NEEDS

When faced with a chronic or permanent condition, most parents want to know:

- What treatment can be achieved for their child—relief of symptoms, prolongation of life, shortening of the course of the disease, etc.
- Expected progress of the child during treatment
- What to expect by way of improvement, side effects, fresh problems, etc.[10]
- Chances of a complete cure
- Treatment options

Parents also often want to know about advertised alternative medicine. They have often invested time and effort in collecting such information and do not appreciate it being brushed off as nonsense. It is necessary to explain the unscientific and unproven nature of such "magic remedies."

In the private sector, information about the likely costs of investigation and treatment should also be given. This preempts one of the major sources of conflict.

STRATEGIES FOR IMPROVING COMMUNICATION AND COUNSELING

- *Check what the parents know:* Many parents have faulty knowledge acquired from magazines, lay books, and the internet.[3]
- *Assess what the parents want to know:* Some parents want to know every little fact and detail about their child's condition. Others simply want a prescription and assurance.
- *Assess understanding:* Emotional distress, poor comprehension skills, language problems, etc., can hinder parents' comprehension. Understanding can be improved by giving time to absorb and by repetition.

TABLE 1.4.1: Do's and don'ts of communication.

Do's	*Don'ts*
• Greet the child and parent by name • Smile • Sit down when talking • Try to talk in the patient's language • Direct the conversation to relevant directions • At the end of the consultation, ask if the parents have any questions • Engage the parents in a dialog • Give time for the parents to absorb and understand the content of your explanations and then to ask questions	• Look at your watch frequently • Appear to be in a hurry • Use too many medical terms • Talk with your hand on the door handle or foot outside the door • Interrupt all the time • Start examination and then write out a prescription before the main problem has been identified • Give long lectures as explanation • Ignore concerns mentioned by parents • Be dismissive of information the parents have come with from other sources

- *Listening skills:* Listening well is an essential part of communication. This requires the provision of adequate time and patience and the willingness to listen to parents' concerns. A quiet room, lack of interruptions, provision of chairs for the parents, sitting at an appropriate distance, good eye contact, etc., are helpful.[3]
- *Build confidence:* The parents' efforts and views deserve respect. A little specific praise for the parents' efforts helps significantly in building confidence and helping parents to cope. Some suggestions for future care improve their confidence that they will be able to manage the situation. Giving false hope is wrong, but information can be given in a positive manner.
- *Truth:* Parents deserve the truth, but the bald truth can be harsh and shocking. Disclosure must be tempered with common sense and empathy. Sometimes, the whole picture may need to be delivered in small parts spread out over two or more visits. However, withholding information leads to distrust.
- *Simplicity and clarity:* Many people do not comprehend words such as "growth" and "tumor." "Cancer" sounds shocking but may be necessary to drive home the problem to parents.
- *Be tolerant:* Blame, anger, a sudden outpouring of grief—these are common reactions. They should be met with understanding and support.
- *Empathy:* Parents of sick children are going through a difficult experience. They appreciate the fact that their doctor understands their situation and their difficulties.

Many other factors affect communication positively or negatively **(Table 1.4.1)**.

CONCLUSION

Good communication and counseling is an art that is acquired, developed, and improved by experience. Efforts in this direction will lead to better patient/parent satisfaction and perhaps better clinical outcomes.[6] It is well to remember that compassion, explanation, and reassurance are valued by patients and their families as much as a diagnosis, treatment, and cure.

REFERENCES

1. Zaeh SE, Ramsey R, Bender B, Hommel K, Mosnaim G, Rand C. The impact of adherence and health literacy on difficult-to-control asthma. J Allergy Clin Immunol Pract. 2022;10(2):386-94.
2. Fong Ha J, Longnecker N. Doctor-patient communication: a review. Ochsner J. 2010;10(1):38-43.
3. Ranjan P, Kumari A, Chakrawarty A. How can doctors improve their communication skills? J Clin Diagn Res. 2015;9(3):JE01-4.
4. Crellin E, Martyn M, McClaren B, Gaff C. What matters to parents? A scoping review of parents' service experiences and needs regarding genetic testing for rare diseases. Eur J Hum Genet. 2023;31(8):869-78.
5. Grocott A, McSherry W. The patient experience: informing practice through identification of meaningful communication from the patient's perspective. Healthcare (Basel). 2018;6(1):26.
6. Moore PJ, Adler NE, Robertson PA. Medical malpractice: the effect of doctor-patient relations on medical patient perceptions and malpractice intentions. West J Med. 2000;173(4):244-50.
7. Yoo EJ, Cho SH, Park SJ, Kim TI, Kim WH, Cheon JH. Characteristics and treatment outcomes of transition among patients with inflammatory bowel disease. Yonsei Med J. 2023;64(9):541-48.
8. Ralph JE, Sezgin E, Stanek CJ, Landier W, Pai ALH, Gerhardt CA, et al. Improving medication adherence monitoring and clinical outcomes through mHealth: a randomized controlled trial protocol in pediatric stem cell transplant. PLoS ONE. 2023;18(8):e0289987.
9. Gemechu GB, Hebo H, Kura Z. Children's adherence to antiretroviral therapy and associated factors: multicenter cross-sectional study. HIV/AIDS (Auckl). 2023;15:423-34.
10. Brinkman WB, Sucharew H, Majcher JH, Epstein JN. Predictors of medication continuity in children with ADHD. Pediatrics. 2018;141(6):e20172580.

1.5 Legal and Ethical Issues in Pediatric Practice

George F Moolayil

INTRODUCTION

The doctor-patient relationship has undergone a sea of change from the olden times. Decades back, medical professionals were never questioned in their actions. If any death or other mishaps used to occur, it was attributed to the act of God, and the public used to accept it without any adverse reactions. As the times have gone by, medical professionals are being viewed with suspicion and are being dragged into the court for genuine or frivolous reasons. Deterioration in moral values, increased value for materialistic things, commercialization of the profession, higher expectation of the patients, awareness of rights and privileges of the patients, increasing consumer activism, media sensationalism, undue interference by the politicians, etc., contribute to worsening of the doctor–patient relationship. It is prudent on the part of the doctor to understand what constitutes medical negligence and how to prevent it, along with improvement in the doctor–patient relationship through good ethical practice.

MEDICAL NEGLIGENCE

Medical negligence has been divided into civil negligence and criminal negligence. In civil negligence, the affected party takes the doctor to the court for monetary compensation, whereas in criminal negligence, the prosecution is done by the State, and the punishment is usually a fine or imprisonment.

Civil Negligence

A doctor can be found guilty under civil negligence by an act of omission or commission in a situation where he/she has failed to act in a manner which an ordinary professional of his/her standing would have been expected to act or acted in a manner which an ordinary professional of his/her standing would not have been expected to act. The essential components of the modern tort of negligence propounded by Percy and Charlesworth are as follows:[1]

- The existence of a duty to take care, which is owed by the defendant to the complainant
- The failure to attain that standard of care, prescribed by the law, thereby committing a breach of such duty
- Damage, which is both causally connected with such breach and recognized by the law, has been suffered by the complainant.

Standard of care is the standard of the ordinary skilled man exercising and professing to have that special skill at that time. A man need not possess the highest expert skill. It is a well-established law that it is sufficient if he/she exercises the ordinary skill of an ordinary competent person exercising that particular art. He/she is not negligent if he/she has acted in accordance with the practice accepted as proper by a responsible body of medical practitioners skilled in that art. Failure in attaining that average standard leads to a claim for civil negligence. Compensation can be claimed under the law of contract, the law of tort, or under the Consumer Protection Act.

Criminal Negligence

The jurisprudential concept of negligence differs in civil and criminal law. In Jacob Mathew vs. State of Punjab, differentiation has been laid down, which has been followed by subsequent decisions of various courts over the country.[2] What may be negligence in civil law may not necessarily be negligence in criminal law. For an act to amount to criminal negligence, the degree of negligence should be much higher, i.e., gross or of a very high degree. Negligence that is neither gross nor of a higher degree may provide ground for action in civil law but cannot form the basis for prosecution. To prosecute a medical professional for negligence under criminal law, it must be shown that the accused did something or failed to do something that in the given facts and circumstances no medical professional in his/her ordinary senses and prudence would have done or failed to do. The hazard taken by the accused doctor should be of such a nature that the injury that resulted was most likely imminent.

OTHER PENAL PROVISIONS

Action can be taken against the medical professionals under the National Medical Commission Act for failure to follow the provisions of the Code of Medical Ethics or under infamous conduct. Penal action can also be taken against the doctors for failing to follow various other rules concerning medical professionals, such as the Prenatal Diagnostic Techniques Act, Drugs and Cosmetics Act, Transplantation of Human Organs Act, Biomedical Waste Act, Medical Termination of Pregnancy Act, etc.

PRECAUTIONS TO BE TAKEN DURING TREATMENT

In the practice of the medical profession, some precautions must be taken to make the defense strong in cases of litigations. A doctor may be treating the patient in the correct manner. However, many cases have been lost due to failure to prove the same in the judicial forums.

Documentation

A physician should document the following facts:

- Name, age, gender, religion, and address of the patient
- Date, month, and year along with the time of examination
- All relevant history, including details of previous illness along with any history of drug allergy, should be noted. If there is no history of drug allergy, it must be noted. If the patient develops an allergy to a drug subsequently, the date of occurrence
- The complete examination details, including the positive and relevant negative findings
- A record of investigations advised with reports
- A provisional diagnosis and a working diagnosis should be there before starting a line of management
- Final diagnosis
- Proper follow-up advice with review dates

Informed Consent

Currently, the courts unanimously treat lack of informed consent as a matter of negligence of the doctor to disclose necessary information. Therefore, the doctor is duty-bound to disclose the information as to the risk that can arise from the treatment of the patient. Risk is defined as exposure to a chance of an injury or loss. Most of the courts require the doctor to disclose information that other physicians possessing the same skills or practicing in the same community would disclose in the same situation. Any person of sound mind who has attained the age of 18 years may give a legally valid consent. A consent given by a child under 12 years is invalid; that given by a child between 12 and 18 years is valid if the court feels that the patient has understood the implication of the consent. In a situation where there was no proper informed consent, and if some medically acceptable complication occurs as a treatment outcome, the doctor can be punished under medical negligence, as it can always be claimed that if there was an awareness of the complications, the consent would not have been given, and hence, the doctor will be held responsible for the complications. However, in emergency or life-threatening situations, a doctor can proceed with treatment to save the life of a patient without waiting for the consent.

In a situation where the parents are not giving consent for a procedure that is essential for their ward, the doctor can proceed with the treatment in an emergency and, in other situations, can approach the court to override the decision of the parents.

Life Support: Starting, Withholding, and Stopping

When a patient is brought in a condition requiring life support, it must be started even if the condition of the patient seems to be hopeless, as not giving life support is an irreversible decision, whereas a decision to stop can be taken later also. In situations, where:

- The relatives want to stop life support, but the doctor wants to continue;
- The doctor feels that there is no use in continuing life support, but relatives want to continue; and
- If both the treating doctor and relatives want to discontinue life support.

The inability to pay should not be a criterion for withholding or stopping life support. The Supreme Court has given a judgment concerning passive euthanasia where an adult patient of sound mind can give advance directions, refusing life support when required.[3] The direction must be witnessed by two independent witnesses, preferably in the presence of a Judicial Authority. In the case of a child, a decision can be taken by parents or close relatives in consultation with the doctor.[4]

Refusal of Treatment

A patient has a right to refuse the treatment. In situations where there is a refusal of treatment, the consequences should be explained to the patients or parents in front of a witness, and it is better to get the refusal signed by them. The doctor has also got the right to refer the patients elsewhere if the treatment is refused. If the refusal involves the welfare of a minor or an unborn baby, the courts or even the Child Rights Commission can override the objections of the parents. When a medical professional advances a plea that the patient did not give his/her consent to the treatment suggested by him/her, the burden is on him/her to prove that nonadministration of the treatment was because of the refusal to give consent thereto.

ETHICS IN PRACTICE AND GOOD DOCTOR–PATIENT RELATIONSHIP

A good ethical practice should have the following elements:

- *Standard:* A doctor should keep up a high standard of behavior as prescribed in the Code of Medical Ethics, 2002 of the Indian Medical Council.

- *Choice:* The patient should be given the choice of treatment and doctor. If there is a request for reference, a proper reference letter should be given.
- *Accessibility:* The patient should have access to the best treatment in the hospital or be referred to a higher center for better care, if necessary. The doctor will earn the respect of the patient and the relatives by doing so.
- *Nondiscrimination:* No discrimination should be shown to the patients based on religion, caste, or social standing.
- *Transparency:* The doctor should be transparent with the patients and their relatives on all possible matters. All matters regarding the bill, etc., should be explained, and there should not be any practice of dichotomy (receiving commission from scan centers, laboratories, etc., for sending the patient for investigations and referrals).
- *Accountability:* The doctor should be accountable to the patient for the treatment.
- *Imparting information:* The parents and relatives should be made aware of the condition of the patient. Proper communication can avoid misunderstandings later. Imparting of information should be done in a sensitive manner.
- *Quality of service:* Expectations on the part of patients and relatives regarding the quality of medical service are quite high. Therefore, a medical professional should update his/her medical knowledge through regular attendance at continuing medical education programs.
- *Dealing with complaints:* A medical professional should give serious consideration to complaints brought by patients and their relatives and do a proper investigation on the complaints. If the complaint is genuine, an apology to pacify them is necessary; if the complaint is due to some misunderstanding, the matter should be explained.

CONCLUSION

A good doctor-patient relationship will decrease adverse incidents in the practice of the medical profession. A good understanding of the laws involving the medical profession and taking proper precautions will help the medical professional in dealing with litigations.

REFERENCES

1. Bag RK. Medical Negligence and Compensation, 3rd edition. Eastern Law House, Kolkata. 2021.
2. Lahoti RC. Jacob Mathew vs. State of Punjab. KLT. 2005;3:967.
3. Common Cause vs. Union of India. 2018;5:SCC1.
4. Supreme Court of India. Aruna Ramchandra Shanbaug vs Union of India & Ors. SC. March 7, 2011.

1.6 Media and Child Health: Handling Parents and Public

Remesh Kumar R, Krishna Mohan R

IMPACT OF MEDIA

In the present era of digital dominance, media is undoubtedly having a profound influence on our younger generation. Of course, children spend a good amount of their quality time with some form of media, television (TV), mobile, or social media. Media has got both positive and negative impacts during childhood.

Positive Effects

The educational programs on TV and the internet help students in learning. Programs such as news and quizzes help to update knowledge of current affairs. Social media platforms such as Facebook and WhatsApp help in group studies and project work.[1] They also provide an excellent opportunity for children to showcase their creative works and ideas. Social media marketing campaigns like prevention and control of substance abuse, encouraging physical activities, maintaining a healthy diet, and prevention of sexually transmitted diseases have helped to promote behavior change.[2]

Negative Effects[1]

Obesity

Increased TV viewing may lead to obesity, both directly and indirectly. More hours spent on TV viewing means less hours spent on exercise and other physical activities. Also, the various commercials on different unhealthy food products may lead to increased food consumption and overweight. Eating meals while watching TV is also a habit that should be discouraged.

Detrimental Effects on Academic Performance

Increased usage of TV and internet takes time away from reading and homework. Unsupervised TV viewing by children will have a deleterious effect on academic performance. Exposure to violence in films, TV programs, and video games can negatively affect the mental and physical health of children. This increases the likelihood of aggressive and violent behavior in both short- and long-term contexts. Violence, substance abuse, and sex in media can have a harmful influence on the behavior and personality of the developing child.

The poor posture while using cell phones and TV (head tilted forward and shoulders stooping forward) may lead to increased stress around the cervical spine with early wear and tear, followed by degeneration. Refractive errors, astigmatism, and ocular discomfort are some of the most common eye problems.

Sleep disturbance is yet another harmful effect. The blue light emitted by electronic media suppresses and disrupts melatonin secretion. The violent or sexual contents seen in the media may lead to excitement, fear, or stress in children causing a delayed onset of sleep. Sometimes, this can lead to nightmares and night awakenings, again affecting sleep quality adversely. Excess screen time in children can also lead to delayed language development, learning problems, and reading problems.

ROLE OF PARENTS AND SCHOOLS

- Children below the age of 2 years should not be exposed to any type of screen with the exception of occasional video calls with relatives. Screen time for children between the ages of 2 and 5 years should not exceed 1 hour; the lesser, the better. For older children and adolescents, it is important to balance screen time with other activities that are required for overall development. These activities include an hour of physical activity, adequate duration of sleep, and time for schoolwork, meals, hobbies, and family time.[1,3]
- Keep the TV set and internet-connected electronic devices out of the child's bedroom.
- Monitor what media the children are using and accessing, including any websites they are visiting and social media sites they may be using.
- Co-view TV, movies, and videos with children and teenagers, and use this as a way of discussing important family values.
- Model active parenting by establishing a family home use plan for all media. As part of the plan, enforce a mealtime and bedtime "curfew" for media devices, including cell phones. Establish reasonable but firm rules about cell phones, texting, internet, and social media use.
- In schools, assignments and homework that require the use of screen should be minimized, especially for children up to 10 years of age. During the COVID-19 pandemic, when online education became inevitable, PRAGYATA guidelines were issued by the Ministry of Information and Broadcasting in association with the National Council for Educational Research and Training (NCERT). Preprimary children should not be made to sit in front of screens for more than 30 minutes while children of classes 1–8 should limit online classes to two sessions (30–45 minutes duration each) and four sessions (30–45 minutes duration each) for classes 9–12.[4]

HANDLING PARENTS AND PUBLIC IN PEDIATRIC PRACTICE

Globally, media whether it is electronic, print, or internet plays a pivotal role in disseminating information to the public. The reporting by media can be biased at times and can either calm down or flare up the aggrieved parents and public alike, especially in situations such as a public health emergency. This may bring the credibility of the media information at stake, and the medical practitioner must dissect the parental perceptions on these news items and give them the best available opinion at the right time.

Types of Health News in Media

It is a known fact that media plays a tremendously influential role in public responses to health issues. It is usually during public health emergencies that demand for health information rapidly increases. On many occasions, public health officials often have the challenging task of both using the media to positively influence health practices and at the same time negating the rapid wildfire-like spread of untrue information.

Some of the positive impacts of both conventional and present-day social media include the following:

- Access to more health information, especially in developing countries
- Mass dissemination of healthy practices effectively, such as advantages of hand washing, proper immunization schedule, etc.
- Updated knowledge on innovations and openings to newer frontiers in preventive health
- More data easily available to health researchers
- Helps patients in communicating effectively with others with similar health conditions
- Helps in supporting health-related causes, such as donations toward treating poor patients and signing petitions against harmful medical practices

- Patients can broadcast their experiences about a particular healthcare provider, which makes them more accountable for the services they provide.

Despite all the virtues that media offers on the health front, policymakers and child health professionals always gauge the impact of negative information, many a time not evidence-based, as quite ominous:

- Media, especially social media, often creates problems by spreading rumors during normal health events as well as health crisis situations.
- Knowingly or unknowingly, nonexperts can share health-related information which often creates confusion and panic. This leads to active dissemination of misinformation and medical myths.
- Media field is highly competitive. Often to attain the commercial goals of the media, even health news is twisted and converted into sensationalized stories. This act of fear mongering may turn dreadful in critical situations, such as epidemics and adverse events following immunization.
- Extensive use of social media in health-related issues may lead to the breach of privacy, both for the patients and for the treating doctors.
- News columns on health care and health policies are usually overwhelmingly negative, despite measurable improvement in both. Ultimately, this may tend the public to be skeptical about national health programs.
- The tendency of the parents to find fault within the system even for trivial unanticipated sufferings of their wards in a medical care setting is often exploited by the media. Even before the authenticity of the incident could be verified by the appropriate authority, the media, who themselves always compete to flash any sensational breaking news, jump into the scene and make it viral. Further damage control is a herculean task.

"Googling" Parents

In this digital era, all information related to health is literally available at our fingertips. It is not unusual for parents to have a preliminary web browsing of their child's symptoms before presenting to the doctor's cabin. But all our net browsing tools and apps are limited by their inability to reason and think. Though there is enormous health literature in the internet, most parents will not be able to filter it properly. Ultimately, the majority of them plunge into unnecessary worry and anxiety. For such parents, the consultant in the chamber naturally becomes only a tool to either confirm or refute the diagnosis provided by the "Google" doctor. It calls for much patience and skill from the pediatrician to reassure such "fussy" parents. Moreover, this internet-driven interpretation of symptoms can negatively affect the trust between the doctor and patients.

Pitfalls in Media Usage in Child Health Issues

- The conversion of complex medical data into easily understandable public health messages continues to be an obstacle, even for most knowledgeable experts in the field.
- The media's tendency to overemphasize negative news creates unnecessary panic and confusion in society.
- There is no system to regularly censor health-related messages before being circulated through media.
- Even in the issues having overwhelming scientific consensus, the media at times fails to give clear positive messages. In the antivaccine propaganda against even expanded programs on immunization vaccines, the media often enjoys creating a verbal feud between public health officials and antivaccine campaigners rather than conveying definite positive messages supporting vaccines.
- The practitioner in their busy routines many a time tends to overlook the body language of the parents when certain newer modalities of investigations/treatment or new immunization schedules are advised.
- Lack of training of public health authorities to deal with media.

APPROACH FOR PROPER HANDLING OF IMPACT OF MEDIA[5,6]

At the Pediatrician's Desk

- The pediatrician should always be apprised about the happening in the society, especially the controversies and public dialogs on child health-related issues. This is sure to augment his/her preparedness to combat aggressive parents and calm them down with the scientific knowledge that is hitherto beyond the scope of a parent.
- Always listen to the parents' perceptions about the disease/treatment protocols and their apprehensions about it, which they might have acquired through the media. May look absurd or silly, but this is of prime importance for providing an appropriate reply. Listening to the views of one parent is sure to help us to have a better preparedness when counseling yet another family with similar complaints.
- Whenever a newer modality of treatment or investigation is advised, especially the ones that have captured public attention through media, the practitioner should be extra vigilant to convince the parents about the need for the same. The doctor needs to anticipate the allied confusions that might have already cropped into their thoughts from the messages spread through media and be prepared to clear them with available quotes from scientific updates of any sort.

Role of Indian Medical Association and Indian Academy of Pediatrics

- Professional and academic organizations, such as the Indian Medical Association (IMA) and Indian Academy of Pediatrics (IAP), should have a media cell at national, state, and district levels. An official spokesperson who is well trained in media interaction should be assigned to all these teams. At the earliest hint of any untoward public health issue, the media cell should go on a war footing to collect all evidence and information on the same. At the same time, the official spokesperson should go on air with updated scientific knowledge on that sensitive issue which can be strengthened later with the information passed by his/her team.
- It is ideal to have well-maintained websites for all professional medical organizations, with links to related websites.
- The academic bodies should identify troublemakers in the society and media. Equally important is to locate troubleshooters who can deliver the goods with maximum results in such precarious situations.

Central and State Government Initiatives

- Public health authorities need to meet the media on a regular basis and communicate to ensure a balanced scientific reporting, especially with regard to national health programs.
- Managing misinformation during health crisis situations such as an adverse effect following immunization and epidemics is very important. Ideally, all public health agencies should be well equipped before a crisis with adequate strategies, educational material, and appropriate staff to counter misinformation and myths.
- A censoring system to regularly monitor the contents of health news dealt with by mainstream as well as social media will be appropriate. Quacks and nonexperts without adequate scientific knowledge should be prevented from interacting with the public on topics related to health.

REFERENCES

1. Gupta P, Shah D, Bedi N, Galagali P, Dalwai S, Agrawal S, et al. Indian Academy of Pediatrics Guidelines on screen time and digital wellness in infants, children and adolescents. Indian Pediatr. 2022;59(3):235-44.
2. O'Keeffe GS, Clarke-Pearson K. The impact of social media on children, adolescents, and families. Pediatrics. 2011;127:800-4.
3. Ashton JJ, Beattie RM. Screen time in children and adolescents: is there evidence to guide parents and policy? Lancet Child Adolesc Health. 2019;3:292-4.
4. PRAGYATA: Guidelines for digital education. (2021). Department of School Education and Literacy. Ministry of Human Resource Development Government of India 2021. [online] Available from: https://ncert.nic.in/pdf/announcement/PRAGYATAGuidelinesEnglish.pdf [Last accessed October, 2024].
5. Leask J, Hooker C, King C. Media coverage of health issues and how to work more effectively with journalists: a qualitative study. BMC Public Health. 2010;10:535.
6. World Health Organization. Effective media communication during public health emergencies. In: WHO Handbook and Field Guide. Geneva: World Health Organization; 2005.

SECTION

2

Care of the Newborn

Section Editor: Rhishikesh P Thakre

2.1 Neonatal Nomenclature

Satvik C Bansal

INTRODUCTION

There are several terms that are used about newborn infants and their care. This section will briefly summarize the commonly used terms in reference to newborn infants.

- *Newborn/neonate:* Any infant who is up to 28 days of life is termed a newborn or neonate.
- *Early neonatal period:* The period from birth up to 7 days of life is the early neonatal period.
- *Late neonatal period:* The period from day 7 up to day 28 of life is the late neonatal period.

GESTATIONAL AGE-RELATED TERMS

- *Perinatal period:* The period from 28 weeks of fetal life up to the first 7 days after birth is the perinatal period.
- *Fetal period*
  - *Early fetal period:* This refers to a period of gestation up to 22 weeks. Usually, the fetus at this period weighs < 500 g and has a crown–rump length (CRL) of <25 cm.
  - *Intermediate fetal period:* This refers to the period of gestation from 22 to 27 weeks of fetal life. The fetus usually weighs 500–999 g and has a CRL from 25 up to 35 cm.
  - *Late fetal period:* This refers to gestations greater than 27 weeks, and the fetus usually weighs 1,000 g or more and has a CRL of at least 35 cm.

NEONATE

- *Term neonate:* A neonate born between 37 and 41 weeks of completed gestation is a term neonate.
- *Preterm neonate:* A neonate who is born before 37 weeks of completed gestation is a preterm neonate.
  - Extremely preterm (<28 weeks)
  - Very preterm (28 to <32 weeks)
  - Moderate to late preterm (32–37 weeks)
- *Post-term neonate:* A neonate who is born after 41 weeks of completed gestation is a post-term neonate.

BIRTH WEIGHT-RELATED TERMS

- *Low birth weight:* Any neonate who at birth has a weight of <2,500 g, irrespective of gestation, is a low-birth-weight (LBW) neonate.
- *Very low birth weight:* A neonate with a birth weight of <1,500 g is a very LBW neonate.
- *Extremely low birth weight:* A neonate with a birth weight of <1,000 g is an extremely LBW neonate.
- *Small for dates/small for gestation age/intrauterine growth restriction:* These are synonymous terms often used interchangeably and refer to a neonate whose birth weight is less than 10th centile or less than –2 standard deviation (SD) of the reference standard for a given gestational age.
- *Appropriate for dates/appropriate for gestation age:* It refers to a neonate whose birth weight is between the 10th and 90th centiles or between –2 and +2 SD of the reference standard for a given gestational age.
- *Large for dates/large for gestation age:* It refers to a neonate whose birth weight is greater than 90th centiles or greater than +2 SD of the reference standard for a given gestational age.

NEWBORN HEALTH STATISTICS

- *Fetal death:* It is the death that occurs before the complete expulsion or extraction of the product of conception, regardless of the duration of pregnancy.
  - *Early fetal death or abortion*—expulsion or extraction of a fetus or embryo with a gestational age under 22 weeks or a weight under 500 g
  - *Late fetal death or stillbirth*—death before expulsion or delivery of a fetus with a gestational age over 22 complete weeks or a weight of 500 g or over
- *Live birth:* This corresponds to complete expulsion and extraction of a product of conception, regardless of the duration of pregnancy, which breathes or shows evidence of life after expulsion or extraction.
- *Neonatal mortality:* It refers to the death of a newborn within the first 28 days of life.
  - *Early neonatal mortality*—death before the first 7 days of life
  - *Late neonatal mortality*—death between day 7 and day 28 of life
- *Perinatal mortality:* It is the combination of early neonatal and late fetal mortality.

2.2 Neonatal Resuscitation

Satvik C Bansal

INTRODUCTION

The transition from fetus to neonate is smooth in most cases. Approximately 10% of the babies born require some assistance, and only 1–2 babies/1,000 live births require the need for chest compressions with or without medications.

PERINATAL PHYSIOLOGY

Basic knowledge of fetal to extrauterine neonatal transition is essential in understanding the rationale behind resuscitation practices.[1]

Changes in Thermoregulation

In fetal life, the body's core temperature is just slightly higher than the surroundings (0.5°C). This situation dramatically changes after birth, when the temperature gradient between the newborn baby's core temperature and surroundings is much greater. The result is greater heat loss and a high risk for the development of hypothermia in the baby. So, in order to maintain body temperature, the newborn starts to generate heat from various metabolic processes and by the lipolysis of brown adipose tissue. Moreover, preterm infants are at an increased risk of hypothermia as they have immature skin, a greater surface area to body weight ratio, and low brown adipose tissue stores.

Changes in Respiration

The physiological adjustments in respiration are the most important. Before birth, the lungs of the fetus are filled with fluid. After birth, this fluid is cleared, and the lungs expand for effective air exchange. All these physiological adjustments generally require some time. As the infant takes the first few breaths, it causes expansion of the chest wall. This, in turn, generates negative intrathoracic pressure (around 50 mm Hg), which leads to the inflow of air into the alveoli and lung expansion. Now, there are several important circulatory transitions that occur secondary to the development of effective air exchange in the lungs. The pulmonary vascular pressures start to decrease, which reduces right-to-left shunting through the foramen ovale and ductus arteriosus. It also increases the venous return to the left atrium, leading to a rise in left atrial pressure and a further decrease in right-to-left shunting from the foramen ovale.

Changes in Circulation

Fetal circulation is unique because gas exchange takes place in the placenta. In the fetal heart, the oxygenated blood returning via the umbilical vein is mixed with deoxygenated blood from the superior and inferior vena cavae, and it is distributed differentially throughout the body. The blood returning from the placenta to the right atrium is channeled via the foramen ovale to the left atrium and ventricle and then to the ascending aorta, providing the brain with the most oxygenated blood. In fetal life, the lungs are fluid-filled, have intrinsically high vascular resistance, and do not participate in gas exchange **(Fig. 2.2.1)**.

After birth, the low-resistance placental circulation is removed, which increases the overall systemic vascular resistance. Along with this, the pulmonary vascular resistance begins to fall as a result of pulmonary expansion, increased arterial and alveolar oxygen tension, and local vasodilators. These changes result in a dramatic increase in pulmonary blood flow **(Fig. 2.2.2)**. The result is a rise in oxyhemoglobin saturation gradually over the first 5–15 minutes of life to 90% or greater, as the air spaces are cleared of fluid.

PRIMARY AND SECONDARY APNEA

The baby has to make a lot of transitions at the time of delivery and in a very short span of time, as discussed earlier. Any adverse situation compromising fetal tissue perfusion and oxygenation may affect its ability to make these necessary transitions during and immediately after birth. A newborn responds to this hypoxia (lack of oxygenation) initially by cessation of respiration, which ultimately leads to depression of cardiac function.

So, any perinatal stress will result in an initial period of rapid breathing, followed by a period of *primary apnea* (no breathing or gasping). Usually, just proper stimulation and oxygenation are sufficient to recover from this state. If the period of hypoxia continues, the fetus will have an additional brief period of irregular gasps and then will lapse into secondary apnea **(Fig. 2.2.3)**. During *secondary apnea*, stimulation will not restart the baby's breathing. Resuscitation with assisted ventilation and oxygen is required.

The basic resuscitation steps include anticipation and preparation, initial steps, ventilation followed by advanced

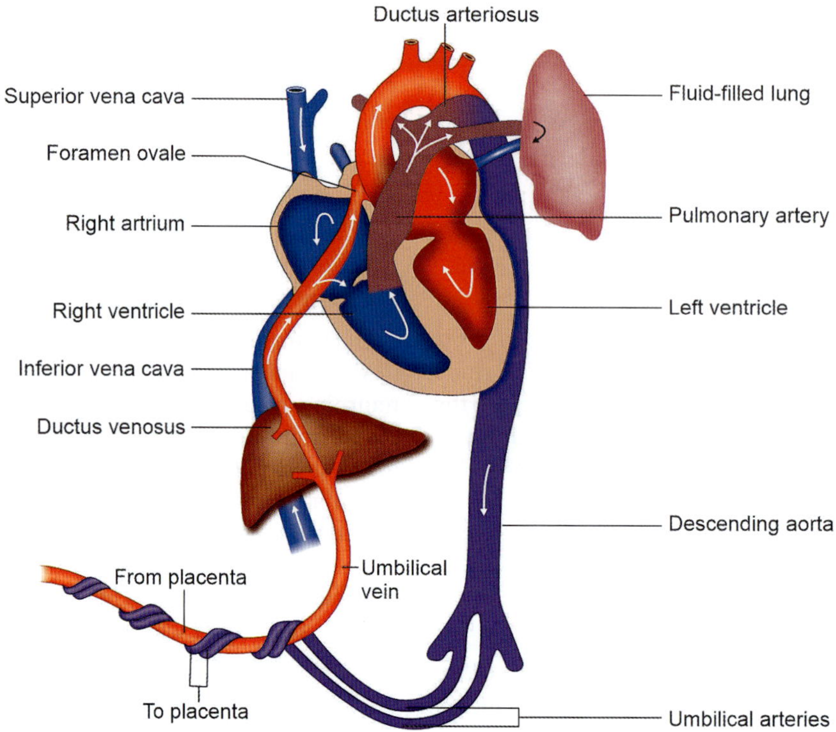

Fig. 2.2.1: Fetal circulation.

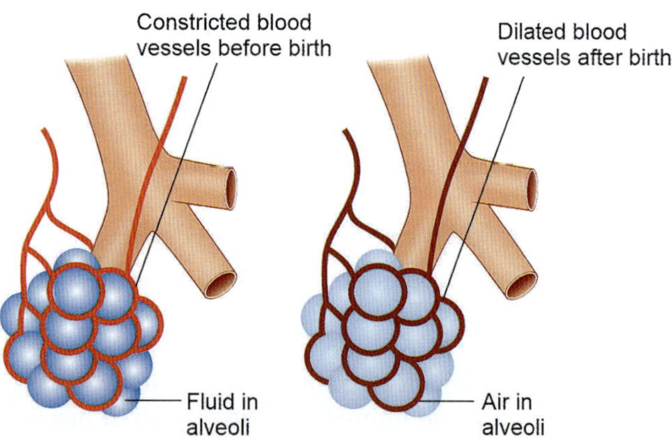

Fig. 2.2.2: Changes in pulmonary blood vessels after birth.

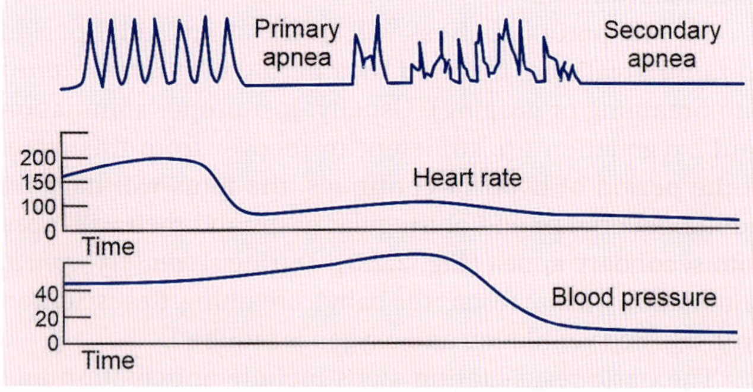

Fig. 2.2.3: Primary and secondary apnea.

steps including intubation, chest compression, medications, and dealing with difficult scenarios.[1,2]

ANTICIPATION AND PREPARATION FOR RESUSCITATION (FIG. 2.2.4)

Risk Factors

Ensuring a thorough prenatal and intrapartum history is essential, along with understanding relevant risk factors that may impact the newborn. This preparation enables the resuscitation team to be more effective and well equipped. A complete list of significant risk factors is mentioned in **Box 2.2.1**.

In up to half the cases, the requirement for resuscitation may arise even in the absence of identifiable risk factors. It is advised that each delivery be overseen by at least one individual with basic neonatal resuscitation training, and, if necessary, access to an advanced neonatal resuscitator should be readily available.

Team Briefing

The objective of team briefing is to plan a management response during resuscitation based on maternal-perinatal risk factors, resources, and expertise available at the hospital.

A team leader should be identified, and available personnel (clinical and paraclinical staff) should be assigned

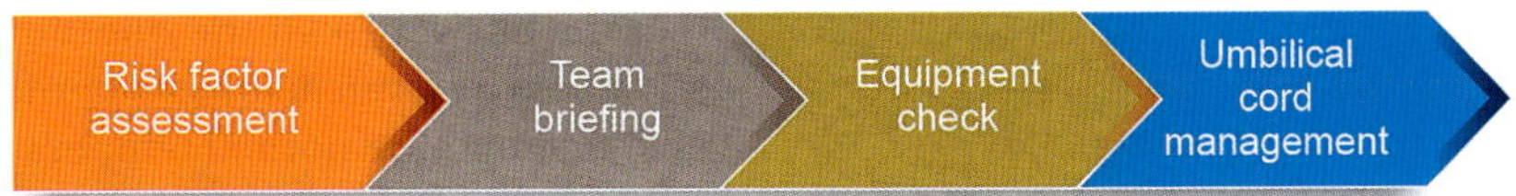

Fig. 2.2.4: Anticipation and preparation of birth.

BOX 2.2.1: Risk factors associated with the need for neonatal resuscitation.

Prenatal risk factors
- Gestational age <36 0/7 weeks or ≥41 0/7 weeks
- Pre-eclampsia or eclampsia
- Intrauterine growth restriction
- Multiple gestations
- Fetal anemia
- Polyhydramnios
- Oligohydramnios
- Fetal hydrops
- Fetal macrosomia
- Significant fetal malformations or anomalies
- No antenatal visits

Intrapartum risk factors
- Emergency cesarean delivery
- Forceps or vacuum-assisted delivery
- Breech or other abnormal presentation
- Fetal distress (Category II or III fetal heart rate pattern)
- Acute perinatal event (e.g., placental abruption, cord prolapse, abnormal fetal testing, or a scalp pH of 7.20 or less)
- Maternal general anesthesia
- Maternal magnesium therapy
- Intrapartum bleeding
- Chorioamnionitis
- Shoulder dystocia
- Meconium-stained amniotic fluid

Source: Adapted from Weiner GM, Zaichkin J. Textbook of Neonatal Resuscitation, 8th edition. Itasca, IL: American Academy of Pediatrics; 2021.

tasks during resuscitation, such as taking care of airway, supporting breathing, assisting in chest compressions, medication and auscultation, timekeeping, and documentation of resuscitative efforts. It is important to have a plan in place in case any additional help is needed.

Equipment Check

All the necessary equipment **(Table 2.2.1)** must be available and operating properly. The self-inflating bag is one of the most important equipment, and the resuscitator should be well versed with its parts and functioning **(Box 2.2.2; Fig. 2.2.5)**. It is important to have the temperature of the delivery room optimized. The entire checklist of preparation for resuscitation is given in **Box 2.2.3**.

Umbilical Cord Management

In most cases, the recommended practice is to delay the clamping of the umbilical cord by 30–60 seconds. The evidence suggests that this leads to improved survival. However, there are certain cases where early clamping of the cord may be considered, such as abruptio placenta, bleeding placenta previa, abnormal umbilical artery Dopplers, intrauterine growth restriction, and in newborns requiring active resuscitation. It is essential to have a good rapport with the obstetrician, and details of steps for cord clamping should be predecided.

TABLE 2.2.1: Equipment checklist for neonatal resuscitation.

Temperature	• Radiant warmer • Warm linen, shoulder roll • Cap • Plastic bag or plastic wrap (<32 weeks' gestation) • Thermal mattress (<32 weeks' gestation)
Airway	• Bulb syringe • 10 or 12 F suction catheter attached to wall suction • Meconium aspirator
Breathing	• Oxygen blender with flowmeter • Positive-pressure ventilation (PPV) device • Term- and preterm-sized masks • 5, 6, and 8 F feeding tubes • Equipment to give free-flow oxygen with tubing • Pulse oximeter • Laryngoscope with size-0 and size-1 straight blades (size 00, optional) • Stylet (optional) • Endotracheal tubes (sizes 2.5, 3.0, and 3.5) • CO_2 (carbon dioxide) detector • Waterproof tape or tube-securing device • Scissors • Laryngeal mask (size 1) (optional)
Circulation	• Stethoscope • Electrocardiogram (ECG) monitor leads and ECG monitor • Epinephrine (1:10,000) • Normal saline • Supplies for placing emergency umbilical venous catheter (umbilical catheters, syringes, three-way stopcocks, and a blade)

BOX 2.2.2: Checking of the self-inflating bag.

Watch for any leak or crack in the bag and replace the bag if the answer to any of the following questions is a "No"

First occlude the patient's outlet, squeeze the bag, and then assess:
- Are you able to feel pressure on your palm?
- On squeezing hard, does the pressure-release valve open?
- Is the bag able to reinflate quickly on releasing the grip?

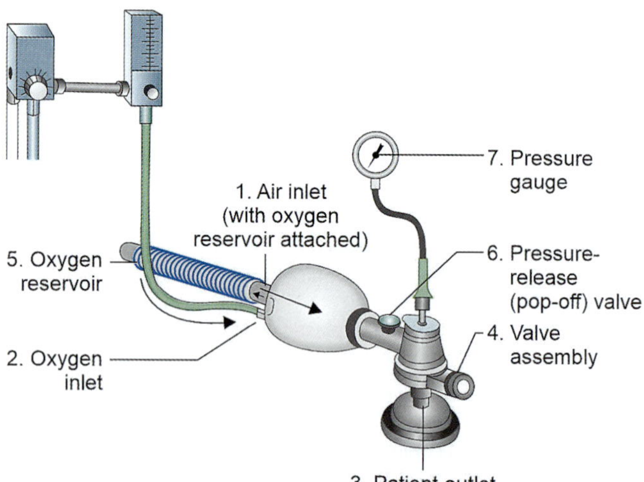

Fig. 2.2.5: Parts of self-inflating bag.

BOX 2.2.3: Preparation for resuscitation.

- The radiant warmer should be switched on 20 minutes before and put on manual mode
- Delivery room temperature should be 26°C
- Dry, warm blankets should be available
- Turn on the oxygen source or air–oxygen blend and adjust the flow to 5–8 L/min. Adjust the oxygen concentration to the desired initial level
- Test the self-inflating bag (if used) for pop-off control and leak
- Check that a proper-sized mask is present
- Make sure that the laryngoscope light is bright
- Check the availability of an appropriately sized laryngoscope blade:
  - No. 1 for full-term neonates
  - No. 0 for premature neonates
  - No. 00 for extremely low-birth-weight neonates
- Check the availability of an appropriate endotracheal (ET) tube for the expected birth weight:
  - 3.5 mm for late preterm and full-term infants (>2,000 g)
  - 3.0 mm for premature infants (>1,000 to 2,000 g)
  - 2.5 mm for smaller infants
- An intubation stylet may be used (the tip is kept at least 0.5 cm from the distal end of the tube)
- If there is any suggestion that extensive resuscitation may be needed, the following additional preparations are required:
  - Set up an umbilical catheterization tray for venous catheterization
  - Draw up 1:10,000 epinephrine and isotonic saline for catheter flush solution and volume replacement
  - Check that other potentially necessary drugs are present and ready for administration

ASSESSMENT AT BIRTH

The resuscitator should assess the answers to the following three questions:[2]

1. Is the baby of term gestation?
2. Does the baby have a good tone?
3. Is the baby breathing regularly or crying?

If the answer to all the questions is "yes," then *routine care* should be given to the newborn. This includes drying the baby, maintaining normal temperature by placing the baby in skin-to-skin contact with the mother, and maintaining the airway, that is, clearing the secretions if required and appropriate positioning. Cord clamping should be delayed by a minimum of 30–60 seconds.

"Zero separation" is preferred care where the newborn is not separated from the mother during routine care. Breastfeeding should be initiated as soon as possible. The breathing pattern and rate, activity of the baby, and color of the baby should be watched.

However, if the answer to any of the questions is "no," then the baby should be moved under a radiant warmer. Now, the baby should be managed according to the resuscitation algorithm **(Flowchart 2.2.1)**.

INITIAL STEPS OF RESUSCITATION

Warm and Maintain Normal Temperature

It is important to ensure that the infant remains warm (36.5–37.5°C). Evidence suggests that "admission temperature of newly born nonasphyxiated infants is a strong predictor of mortality at all gestational ages." The following strategies can be used in the delivery room—radiant warmer, exothermic mattresses, the use of plastic wrap, warm humidified gases, and increased room temperature. Preterm infants may require a combination of the above-mentioned techniques.

Position

The infant should be placed supine with head in midline position and slight neck extension **(Figs. 2.2.6A to C)**. This permits unrestricted air entry to the lungs. A rolled blanket or towel may be kept under the shoulders for very preterm infants and those with large caput.

Clear Airway

Whenever required [in the cases of obvious obstruction or requirement of positive-pressure ventilation (PPV)], suctioning should always be done gently. Vigorous suctioning is harmful as apart from causing injury to the tissues, it may cause bradycardia or apnea. This happens because stimulation of the posterior pharynx can generate a vagal response. Also, as a rule, the mouth should be suctioned first, followed by the nose.

Meconium-stained Amniotic Fluid

The recent guidelines suggest that resuscitation be performed irrespective of meconium-stained liquor (thick or thin) and should proceed with basic steps (initial steps and ventilation) followed by advanced steps (intubation, chest compression, medications, and difficult scenarios), if required.

Flowchart 2.2.1: Neonatal resuscitation algorithm.

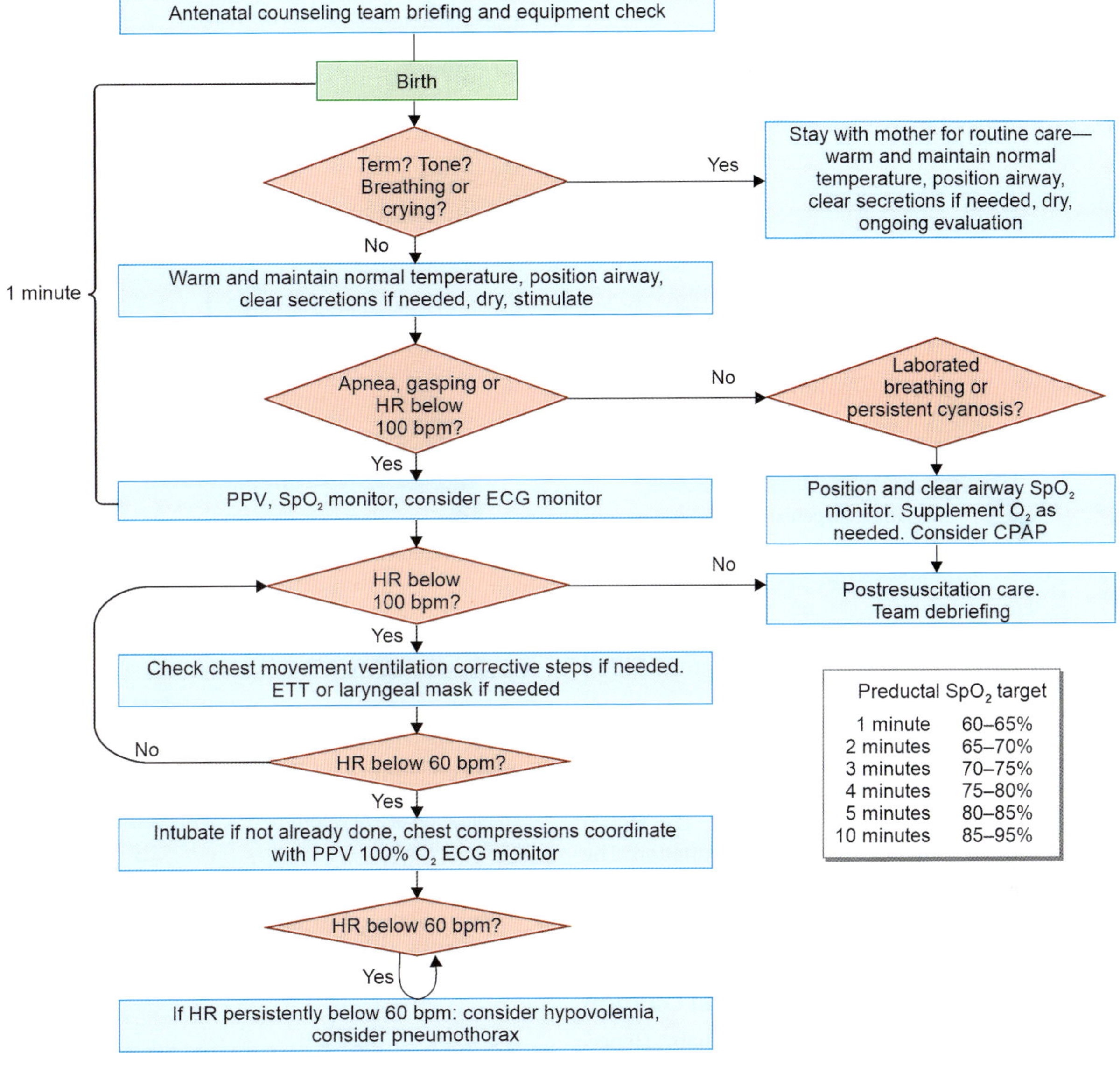

Dry and Stimulate

The baby should be gently dried using prewarmed sheets, and wet sheets should be removed immediately. Remember not to remove the vernix. In cases of preterm babies who are <32 weeks of gestation, it is recommended that they are covered in plastic wraps below the neck without drying to prevent heat loss.

Some babies may require additional tactile stimulation to improve their breathing pattern or cry. Baby's trunk, back, or extremities can be rubbed gently. It is important to remember that overly vigorous stimulation is harmful as it may cause injury to the baby. Also, if the baby remains apneic despite gentle stimulation for a few seconds, further time should not be wasted, and initiate PPV considering the possibility of secondary apnea.

ASSESSMENT OF NEWBORN AFTER INITIAL STEPS

The initial steps of resuscitation and re-evaluation of the baby should be completed within the first 60 seconds of life. The objective is that if the baby is depressed, PPV should be initiated not later than 1 minute of birth. This is termed the *"first golden minute.*

The re-evaluation after the initial steps is based on heart rate and respiratory efforts. The indications for starting PPV include apnea, gasping, or a heart rate of <100 bpm. If there

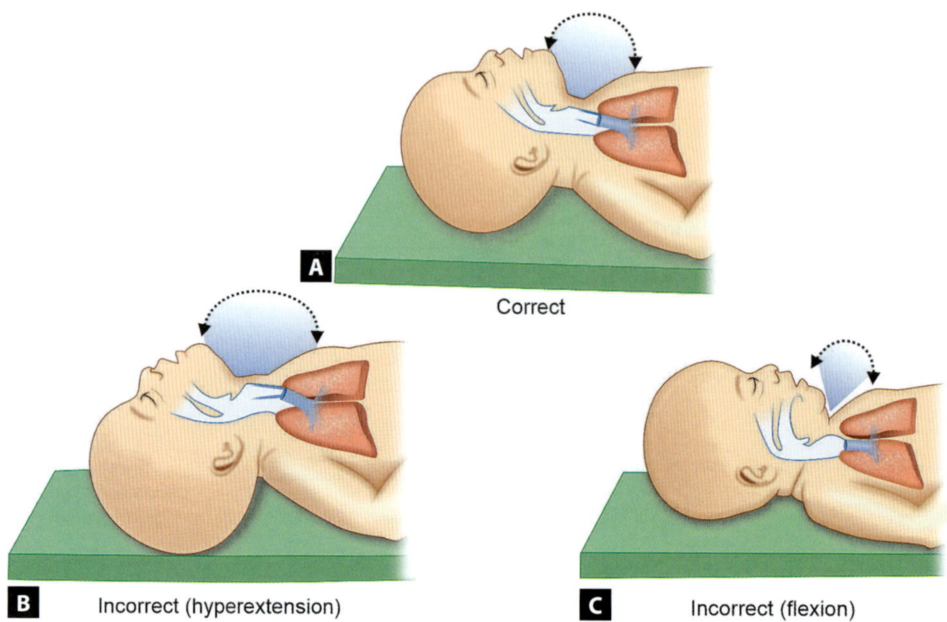

Figs. 2.2.6A to C: Correct position of head and neck to keep the airway open.

is labored breathing or persistent cyanosis, supplemental oxygen and continuous positive airway pressure (CPAP) should be considered.

Assessment of Heart Rate

An improvement in heart rate is considered the most sensitive indicator of successful resuscitation. The fastest and quickest way to assess heart rate is by auscultation. The more reliable way to assess heart rate is by a pulse oximeter. The gold standard for heart rate detection is a three-lead electrocardiogram.

Assessment for Need of Supplemental Oxygen

Both hypoxia and hyperoxia are harmful for the baby. Hence, a pulse oximeter should guide oxygen supplementation.

- *Term infants:* The resuscitation should be started with room air (21%). The supplemental oxygen may be administered, and concentration titrated, keeping the preductal oxygen saturation in the minute-specific reference range **(Flowchart 2.2.1)**.
- *Preterm infants:* The resuscitation of newborns below 35 weeks of gestation should be initiated with low oxygen (<30%). The concentration of oxygen should be titrated as per preductal saturation. In situations where blended oxygen is not available, the use of room air is recommended to initiate resuscitation.

In both term and preterm infants, 100% oxygen is used only if the heart rate remains <60 bpm with an ongoing need for chest compressions.

TABLE 2.2.2: Indications for the use of alternate airways during neonatal resuscitation.

Endotracheal tube	*Laryngeal mask airway*
• Ineffective or prolonged face-mask ventilation • Chest compressions • Stabilization of a newborn with a suspected diaphragmatic hernia • Surfactant administration • Direct tracheal suction if the airway is obstructed by thick secretions	• Ineffective or prolonged face-mask ventilation • Tracheal intubation is unsuccessful

POSITIVE-PRESSURE VENTILATION

The single-most effective and priority step for resuscitation is PPV.

Indications: The indications of starting PPV are (1) inadequate respiratory efforts—apnea or gasping respiration, (2) bradycardia—heart rate <100 bpm, and (3) newborns with respiratory distress who are unable to maintain oxygenation in the minute-specific range despite the use of free-flow oxygen or CPAP. Indications for the use of alternate airways during neonatal resuscitation are listed in **Table 2.2.2**.

Mechanism: The rationale behind the use of PPV is to force the gas into the lungs with some additional pressure, which will open up the collapsed alveoli and hence improve oxygenation. PPV should be started with higher peak

TABLE 2.2.3: Ventilation corrective algorithm.

M	Mask adjustment	Reapply the mask **(Figs. 2.2.7A to C)**
R	Reposition airway	Place the head in "sniffing position" or slightly extended
S	Suction	Use a bulb syringe or suction catheter
O	Open airway	Open the mouth and lift the jaw forward
P	Pressure increase	Increase pressure in 5–10 cmH_2O increments, maximum 40 cmH_2O
A	Alternate airway	Place an endotracheal tube or a laryngeal mask airway

pressures in the first few breaths. Once the lungs are inflated and functional residual capacity has been established, further ventilation can be continued at a lower peak pressure. There should not be excessive chest rise. This is essential so as to prevent damage to the lungs by PPV. In preterm babies, initial peak pressures of 20–25 cmH_2O are required, while full-term babies may require 30–40 cmH_2O in the first few breaths.

Devices available to ventilate a newborn are a flow-inflating bag, self-inflating bag, or T-piece resuscitator. The choice of device is based on availability, familiarity, and expertise.

Self-inflating bag (200–750 mL) is the most commonly used device. It is easier to use, does not require a compressed gas source, and is portable. The bag has a site for attaching an oxygen reservoir. It also has a pressure release "*pop-off*" valve, which prevents barotrauma to the baby's lungs **(Fig. 2.2.5)**.

If the heart rate is not rising with ventilation, chest rise should be seen, followed by breath sounds. Ventilation corrective measures should be initiated if ventilation does not yield chest rise **(Table 2.2.3)**.

Once the effective ventilation is confirmed, PPV is continued at a rate of 40–60 breaths/min to maintain minute ventilation **(Fig. 2.2.8)**. On PPV, the heart rate should be assessed after every 30 seconds. In general, before any betterment of respiratory efforts, there is improvement first in the heart rate, oxygen saturation, and tone of the baby.

The PPV should be continued till there are regular, adequate spontaneous respiratory efforts with a heart rate of >100 bpm.

Administering PEEP (5 cmH_2O) is desirable for all infants, especially preterm, during ventilation.

Continuous Positive Airway Pressure

The use of CPAP is indicated for spontaneously breathing newborns with respiratory distress. There is large evidence supporting the use of CPAP when compared with routine intubation and ventilation in such babies. The advantages include the reduction of the combined outcome of death

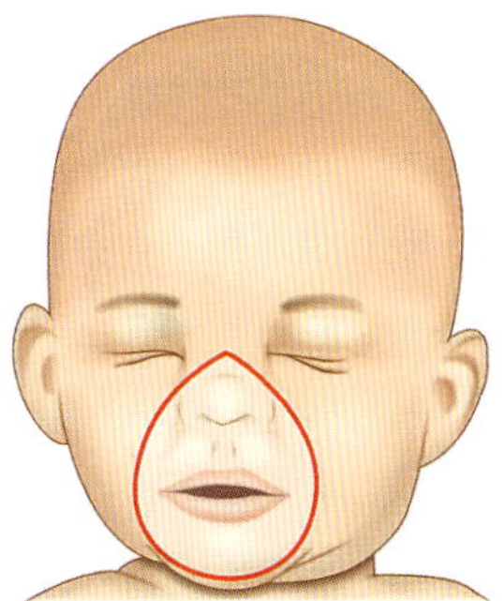

Correct
A Covers mouth, nose, and chin but not eyes

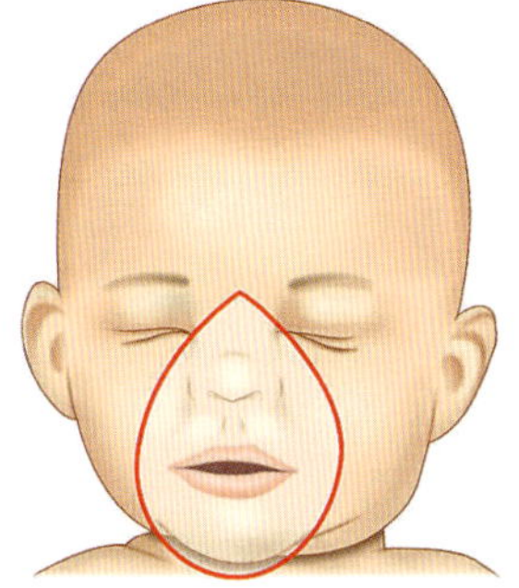

Incorrect
B *Too large:* Covers eyes and extends over chin

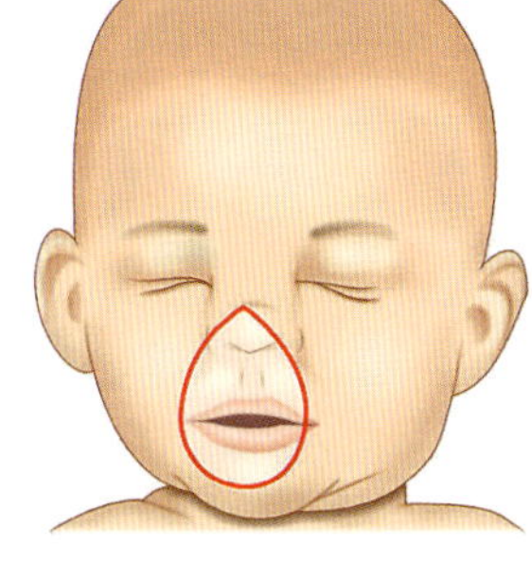

Incorrect
C *Too small:* Does not cover nose and mouth well

Figs. 2.2.7A to C: Appropriately sized mask. The mask should cover the mouth and nose but not the eyes.

and/or bronchopulmonary dysplasia in preterm babies and reduced duration of mechanical ventilation.

CHEST COMPRESSION

Indication: The chest compressions should be started if the heart rate remains below 60 bpm after 30 seconds of effective ventilation.

Prerequisite: It is advised to intubate the baby and administer 100% oxygen to the baby when starting chest compressions.

Site: The site for chest compressions is the lower third of the sternum.

Depth: The depth of compression should be at least one-third of the anteroposterior diameter of the chest **(Figs. 2.2.9A and B)**.

Technique: The chest should be compressed by two thumbs with the hands encircling the chest. There should be proper coordination between compressions and ventilation to prevent their simultaneous delivery. It is essential to allow re-expansion of the chest, but the thumbs should not rise up from the chest wall.

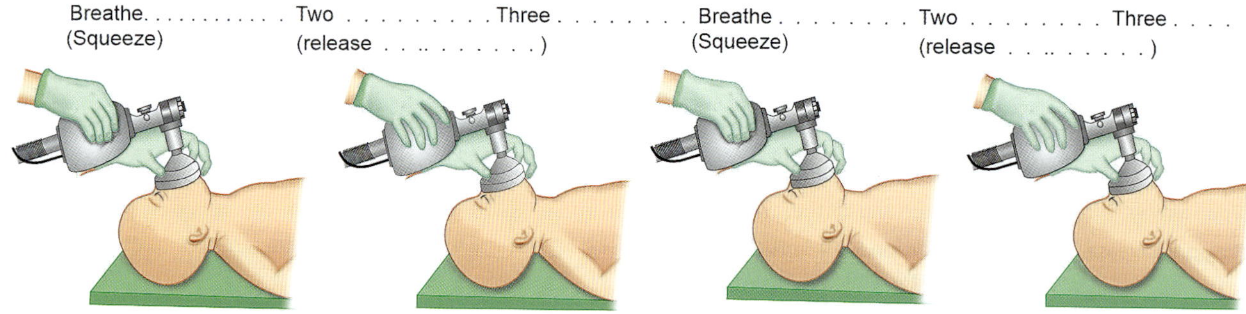

Fig. 2.2.8: Maintain the correct rate while giving positive-pressure ventilation.

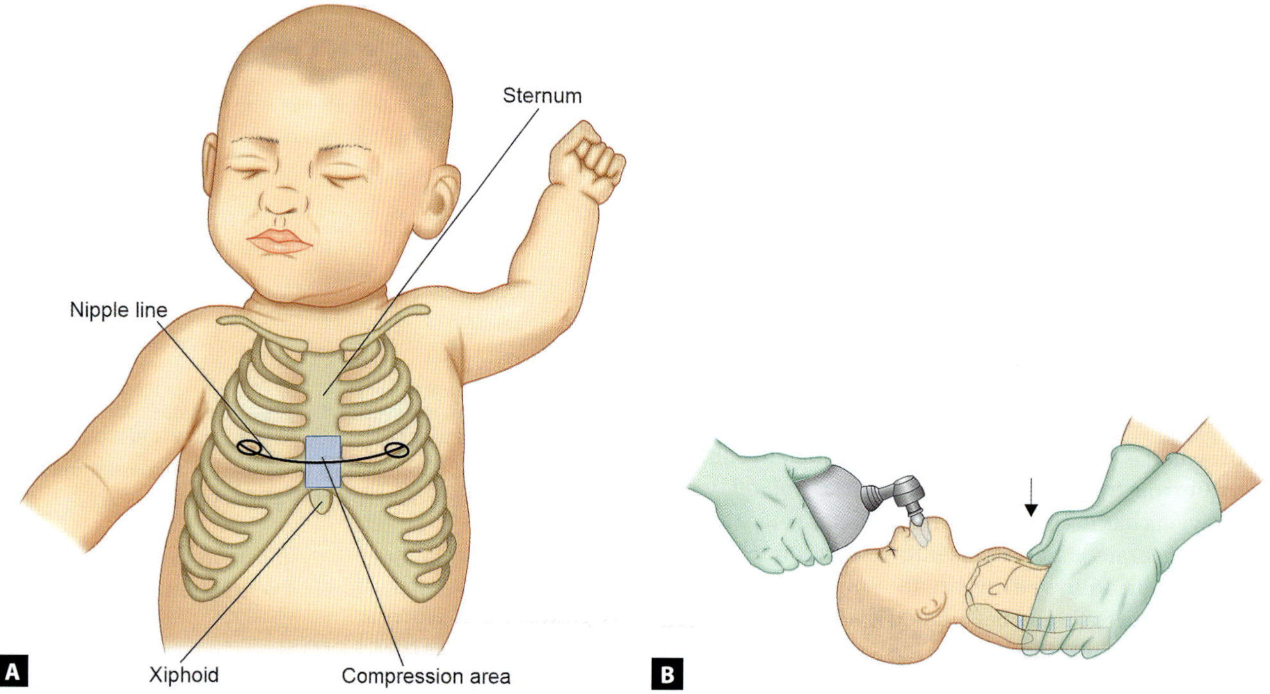

Figs. 2.2.9A and B: (A) Landmarks for chest compression; (B) Correct technique for chest compression.

The neonatal resuscitation guidelines recommend a 3:1 ratio of chest compressions to ventilation. There should be a total of 120 events each minute (90 compressions and 30 ventilations). So, each event is given around half a second.

Once chest compressions have begun, the heart rate should be checked after every 60 seconds. Once the heart rate becomes higher than 60 bpm, the chest compressions can be stopped.

MEDICATIONS

In conditions where there is no improvement in heart rate and it remains below 60 bpm despite chest compressions, the role of drugs should be considered **(Table 2.2.4)**. The following drugs are used in neonatal resuscitation.

TABLE 2.2.4: Medications used in neonatal resuscitation.

Drug	*Route*	*Dose (mL/kg)*	*Administration*
Epinephrine (1:10,000)	Intravenous or intra-osseous	0.1–0.3	Flush with 0.5–1 mL normal saline
	Endotracheal	0.5–1	PPV breaths to distribute into lungs
Normal saline or O-negative packed red cells (in suspected anemia)	Intravenous or intraosseous	10	Over 5–10 minutes. Caution in preterm newborns <30 weeks of gestation

(PPV: positive-pressure ventilation)

Epinephrine Hydrochloride

Epinephrine hydrochloride is a powerful adrenergic agent that increases the strength and the rate of cardiac contractions and causes peripheral vasoconstriction. The preferred route of administration is intravenous; however, it can be delivered through the intraosseous route or endotracheally (a higher dose is required when given endotracheally). However, as there is a lack of supportive data for endotracheal epinephrine, this route may only be considered while establishing intravenous access. The heart rate should be checked about 1 minute after giving epinephrine (longer if given endotracheally). The dose of epinephrine can be repeated after 3–5 minutes. If there is no response after two doses, while additional doses can be given, other causes of depression should be sought out. There is no benefit of using higher doses.

Volume Expansion

Volume expansion is important in conditions of known or suspected blood loss. It can also be considered when the baby is not responding to any other resuscitative measures. An isotonic crystalloid solution or blood should be administered. The recommended dose is 10 mL/kg to be given over 5–10 minutes. The dose may be repeated. It is important to remember that volume expansion should not be done rapidly in preterm newborns for the risk of intraventricular hemorrhage.

The easiest way to secure intravenous access in a baby undergoing resuscitation is the *catheterization of the umbilical vein*. There are certain points to be kept in mind while catheterizing the umbilical vein:

- Advance the catheter only up to 2–3 cm past the abdominal wall; this would be around 4–5 cm in total.
- There should be an easy backflow of blood.
- Remember to flush the medications that are administered, because there will not be any flow in the vein subsequent to cord separation.

POSTRESUSCITATIVE CARE

Once adequate ventilation and circulation are established, the infant should be transferred to an intensive care unit and kept under close monitoring of vital parameters, such as oxygen, blood glucose, and organ dysfunction.

Therapeutic hypothermia (33.5–34.5°C) is indicated for term or near-term infants (more than 36 weeks' gestation) with evolving moderate-to-severe hypoxic–ischemic encephalopathy.[3] Both whole-body cooling and selective head cooling are recommended. Cooling should be initiated and conducted under clearly defined protocols with advanced facilities in an intensive care setting. It should be commenced within 6 hours of birth and continued for 72 hours of birth. The infants are slowly rewarmed over at least 4 hours.

WITHHOLDING AND DISCONTINUING RESUSCITATION

As per medical ethics, not initiating resuscitation of a baby is equivalent to discontinuation of life-sustaining treatment during or after resuscitation.

At Border of Viability

In general, in babies <25 weeks' gestation, the appropriateness of resuscitation should be determined by region-specific guidelines. Opinions may vary regarding using aggressive therapies. Variables affecting newborn survival should be kept in mind, such as the accuracy of gestational age assigned, chorioamnionitis, and the level of care available for the newborn at the delivery center.

Withdrawal of Care

Nonimproving Apgar score **(Table 2.2.5)** of 0 at 10 minutes is a strong predictor of neonatal mortality and morbidity. It is considered reasonable to stop resuscitative efforts if, even after 10 minutes, the heart rate remains undetectable despite ongoing complete resuscitation. The variables such as optimal resuscitation, availability of advanced neonatal, special circumstances before delivery, and wishes expressed by the family should be considered.

POSTRESUSCITATION TEAM DEBRIEFING

Postresuscitation team debriefing is a method of providing constructive feedback to the team members and to promote reflective learning. The debriefing can be *quick*, which can be done immediately after the resuscitation, or can be *comprehensive*, which can be done later at a convenient time. Apart from skills, the important aspects of resuscitation, such as teamwork, communication, and documentation, are discussed.

TABLE 2.2.5: Apgar score.

Sign	*0*	*1*	*2*
Respiratory effort	Absent	Gasping	Good cry
Heart rate (bpm)	Absent	<100	>100
Color	Blue/pale	Pink body; blue extremities	Completely pink
Muscle tone	Limp	Some flexion of extremities	Active motion
Reflex*	No response	Grimace	Cry or active withdrawal

*Assessed by inserting a catheter into the nose.

QUALITY IMPROVEMENT OPPORTUNITIES

The team members should try to look out for ways and means to improve resuscitation practices and outcomes in the hospital without burdening the available limited resources. A very common quality improvement (QI) tool is the use of a PDSA (Plan-Do-Study-Act) cycle.

REFERENCES

1. Gupta P, Ramji S. IAP NNF Textbook of Neonatal Resuscitation, 1st edition. Jaypee Brothers Medical Publishers (P) Ltd; 2023.
2. Wyckoff MH, Singletary EM, Soar J, Olasveengen TM, Greif R, Liley HG, et al. 2021 International consensus on cardiopulmonary resuscitation and emergency cardiovascular care science with treatment recommendations: summary from the Basic Life Support; Advanced Life Support; Neonatal Life Support; Education, Implementation, and Teams; First Aid Task Forces; and the COVID-19 Working Group. Circulation. 2022;145(9):e645-e721.
3. National Neonatology Forum, India. (2021). Position statement and guidelines for use of therapeutic hypothermia to treat neonatal hypoxic ischemic encephalopathy in India. [online] Available from https://www.nnfi.org/assests/pdf/NNF_Position_statement_and_Guidelines_for_TH%20_Final_(10112021)-converted.pdf. [Last accessed October, 2024].

2.3 Assessment and Care of the Normal Newborn, Perinatal Care, and Follow-up

B Vishnu Bhat

INTRODUCTION

A normal newborn is an infant born at term with a birth weight >2,500 g, without any asphyxia, major congenital malformations, or birth injuries. It is important that all newborns receive essential newborn care in order to reduce morbidity and mortality.[1,2]

NORMAL FEATURES IN NEWBORN[1-3]

Anthropometry

The average birth weight of babies in India is 2,900 g. The length may vary from 47 to 52 cm and the head circumference is 33–35 cm. Generally, the head circumference is 2-3 cm more than the chest circumference at birth, and they become equal by 1 year after which the chest circumference exceeds that of the head.

Respiration, Heart Rate, and Blood Pressure

A newborn may have periodic breathing, and the normal rate may vary from 40/minute to 60/minute. The heart rate is usually 120–160 beats/min. The systolic blood pressure will vary from 40 to 60 mm Hg and the diastolic blood pressure from 25 to 40 mm Hg.

Skin Changes

Mongolian spots are bluish patches seen over the buttocks and back due to deposition of melanin pigment and disappear in 6 months to 2 years' time. Milia are tiny cream papules, which are inclusion cysts containing trapped keratinized stratum corneum and usually resolve without treatment in 2–3 weeks. Erythema toxicum is erythematous papular, macular, or rarely pustular lesions present over the body surface because of eosinophilic infiltration into the dermis. They usually appear 2 days after birth and disappear during the first week. Epstein's pearls are whitish papular lesions usually seen over the palate and sometimes over the prepuce and disappear after a few days. Small hemangiomas may be seen over the body surface, which disappear within 2 years of life.

Physiologic Events

Physiologic jaundice usually appears after 2–3 days and disappears by 7–10 days of life and does not stain the palms and soles. Enlargement of the breast during the first 3-7 days of life is known as mastitis neonatorum and does not require any treatment. This enlargement is related to the maternal transfer of hormones. A female baby may have vaginal discharge and bleeding during that period, which is also hormone related and disappears within a few days. There may be molding of the head and caput succedaneum over the presenting part, which disappears within 2–3 days. Caput should be differentiated from cephalohematoma. The latter is due to the collection of blood under the periosteum and hence does not cross the suture lines. It is usually noticed after 2 days of birth and disappears after 6–8 weeks. It usually does not require treatment.

Urine and Stool Passage

A newborn usually passes urine within 48 hours and meconium during the first 24 hours of life. If there is no distension of the abdomen, delayed passage of urine usually indicates inadequate feeding. Distension of the bladder in a male baby suggests a posterior urethral valve. When there is a delay in the passage of meconium, a soft lubricated rubber catheter should be passed into the rectum to confirm patency. The fingertip or thermometer should not be used for checking patency, since these may result in rectal injury. Prematurity, meconium plug, congenital megacolon, meconium ileus, and hypothyroidism may result in delayed passage of meconium. A baby may pass frequent yellow-colored watery to semisolid stools during the first 3–7 days of life known as transitional stools. Some babies may pass stools once in 2–3 days. Hypothyroidism should be excluded in babies with constipation.

IMPORTANT EXAMINATION FINDINGS IN NEWBORN[1-3]

Anterior and posterior fontanels are open at birth. Anterior fontanel can measure up to 3 × 3 cm at its widest points, though the size is very variable, and posterior fontanel is often open at this age. Large posterior fontanel or both anterior and posterior communicating is usually abnormal. In such cases, hypothyroidism, hydrocephalus, congenital rickets, etc., need to be excluded. Similarly, if the anterior fontanel is very small, and there is ridging of suture lines, it may indicate craniosynostosis. Natal teeth may rarely be present. They may be loose and sometimes may result in injuries to the mother's nipple; in that case, they may need to be extracted. Phimosis is normal during this period, but the meatus is visible when prepuce is retracted in more than 85% of the babies. Mucosal tags may be seen at the introitus in female babies.

Palpable liver 2–3 cm below the costal margin and palpable spleen tip are normal. Usually, both testes are at the bottom of the scrotum in term male babies. If the testes are not palpable or abnormally placed, they should be recorded and investigated. 60% of normal newborns have a systolic murmur (innocent murmur) at the age of 2 hours, but the incidence falls to around 1% by 24 hours of age. Healthy term infants move between behavioral states, spending most time in quiet and active sleep. The undisturbed normal neonate lies predominantly in a flexed position with no lateral preference.

IMPORTANT NEONATAL REFLEXES[2]

Rooting Reflex

Rooting reflex helps the baby to locate the mother's nipple without her directing the baby's mouth. The infant turns toward the point where the cheek is touched. When the corner of the mouth is touched, the lower lip is lowered, and the tongue is brought forward toward the contact **(Fig. 2.3.1)**. If the finger is moved away, the head turns to follow it.

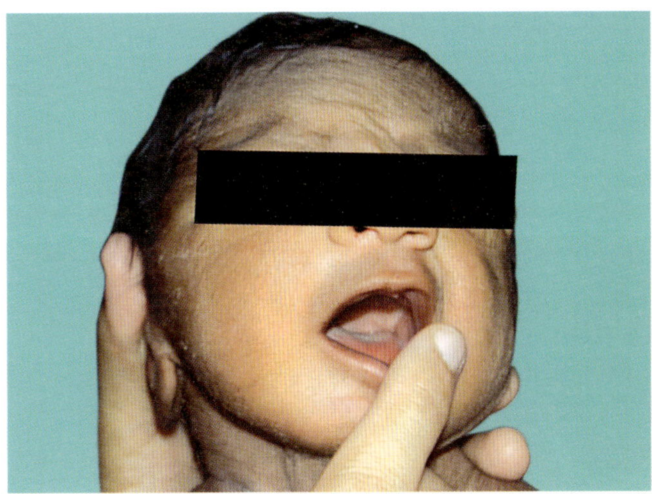

Fig. 2.3.1: Rooting reflex.

Sucking and Swallowing Reflexes

Sucking and swallowing reflexes are elicited by introducing a clean finger or mother's teat in the mouth. They disappear when voluntary control of feeding is achieved. They are decreased or absent when there is neurological depression, hypotonia, or immaturity. A baby would have usually crossed 34 weeks of gestation when he/she can feed directly from the breast.

Moro Reflex

Moro reflex is a vestibular reflex, which disappears by 3–5 months of age. It can be elicited by raising the shoulder for 45° from ground and then dropping by 30°. There will be abduction and extension of arms with opening of fingers. This is followed by flexion and adduction of arms **(Fig. 2.3.2)**. The reflex may be accompanied by crying and extension of trunk and neck with movements of legs. It is exaggerated when there is a cerebral irritation caused by hypoxia, infection, hyperbilirubinemia, etc. It is decreased with sedation, central nervous system depression, or prematurity. Asymmetrical response is seen with Erb's palsy, clavicle or humerus fracture, or shoulder dislocation.

Palmar Grasp Reflex

Palmar grasp reflex is elicited by touching the baby's palm from the ulnar side with a finger or any other suitable object **(Fig. 2.3.3)**. The fingers close and grasp the object. When the dorsum of the hand is touched, the fingers open. The grasp becomes stronger, if the head is turned to the opposite side,

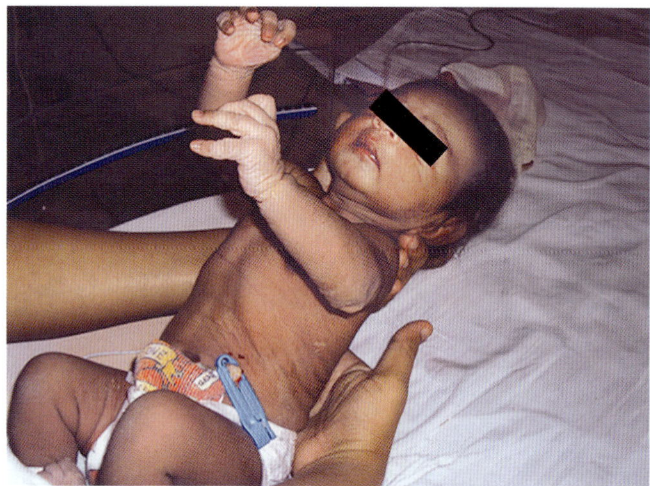

Fig. 2.3.2: Moro reflex.

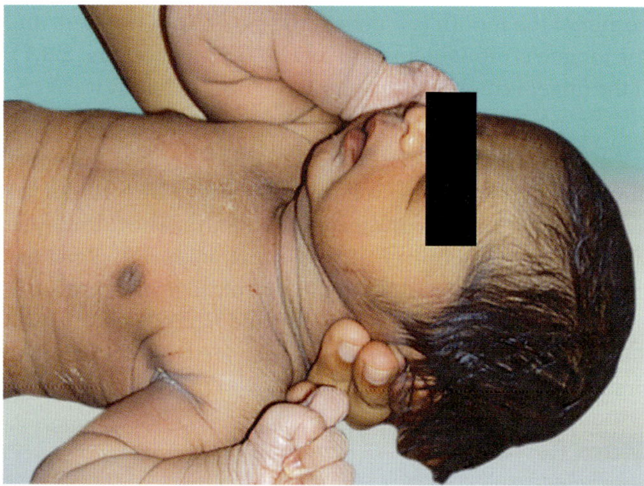

Fig. 2.3.3: Palmar grasp reflex.

and the stimulating finger is moved toward the fingers. Similar reflex can be elicited in the lower limb by stimulating the sole. Persistence of grasp after 3 months of age may indicate cerebral palsy.

MANAGEMENT[1-3]

Temperature Maintenance and Monitoring

The normal body temperature of the newborn ranges from 36.5 to 37.5°C. Newborns are uniquely susceptible to hypothermia because they have a large body surface area, which causes heat loss, and have reduced subcutaneous insulation. They are dependent on caregivers to keep them warm and dry. The temperature of the delivery room should be at least 26 ± 2°C and free from the draft of air.[3] The infant should be received over the mother's abdomen or in prewarmed sterile linen and should be dried thoroughly from head to foot. The wet linen should be removed and replaced with a dry cloth. The baby should be made to wear cap and socks. Kangaroo care position is the most ideal. Skin-to-skin contact with the mother not only prevents hypothermia but also promotes breastfeeding and bonding. A bath is delayed until the temperature is stabilized. It is better if the baby bath is not given in the hospital for fear of cross infection. Mother can be taught the simple technique of monitoring the baby's temperature by touching the periphery and observing for color change. Cold extremities with blue or pale color indicate inadequate warmth.[4]

Cord and Eye Care

The umbilical stump should be cleaned with spirit and kept dry. The local application of antiseptics is not required. Usually, the stump will fall in 7–10 days' time. The eyes should be cleaned with sterile wet cotton. There is no need to instill antibiotic drops into the eye except in areas with a high incidence of vertically acquired conjunctivitis.

Feeding

Breastfeeding should be initiated soon after birth, and exclusive breastfeeding is advised till 6 months of age in normal term babies. A baby should receive seven to eight feeds a day during the first few weeks. The mother should be explained about the benefits of breastfeeding, and the family members are encouraged to support her. It is important not to separate the newborn from the mother without a justifiable reason. The initial alert period after birth is utilized to start breastfeeding, as babies tend to sleep a lot after that. Health workers caring for newborns should learn the signs of good attachment, which include mouth wide open, more areola seen above than below, chin touching the breast, and lower lip everted. Excessive weight loss of more than 8–10% in the first 3–4 days in a term infant indicates inadequate breastfeeding or illness in the baby.

Vitamin K

All babies should receive vitamin K prophylaxis of 0.5 mg (for <1,000 g) to 1 mg (for >1,000 g) intramuscularly after birth to prevent hemorrhagic disease of the newborn.

Danger Signs

Mother should be informed about danger signs and the need to get medical advice as and when they are observed. Some of the danger signs are given in **Box 2.3.1**.

PERINATAL CARE

Essential perinatal care encompasses a holistic set of services and interventions aimed at enhancing the health and welfare

BOX 2.3.1: Danger signs in newborns.

- Poor sucking/excessive crying
- Fever/hypothermia
- Respiratory distress
- Persistent vomiting
- Blood- or bile-stained vomitus
- Abdominal distension
- Pallor
- Jaundice involving extremities
- Bleeding
- Convulsions
- Central cyanosis

BOX 2.3.2: Harmful neonatal practices.

- One should not instill oil in the nose or mouth of newborn
- Not to apply *kajal* to the eye
- Cow dung, ash, etc., not to be applied on the umbilicus
- *Vasambu*, gripe water, and native medications are not be fed to babies
- No prelacteal feeds to be given
- Squeezing of the neonate's breast to remove witch's milk
- Camphor, *neem* leaves, etc., application over the chest or body

A

POSTNATAL CARE

Date of delivery ☐☐☐☐☐☐ Place of delivery ____________ Type of delivery: N. ☐ Assisted ☐ CS ☐

Term/Preterm/Spontaneous abortion ____________

If at institution period of stay postdelivery ____________

Complications, if any (Specify) ____________

Sex of baby | M | F | *Weight of baby ☐ kg. ☐☐☐ gms

Cried immediately after birth | Y | N |

Initiated exclusive breastfeeding within 1 hour of birth | Y | N |

*(Three extra visits if birth weight <2.5 kg)

Injection vitamin K | Y | N |

B

POSTPARTUM CARE

	1st Day	3rd Day	7th Day	6th Week
Any complaints				
Pallor				
Pulse rate				
Blood pressure				
Temperature				
Breasts soft/engorged				
Nipples cracked/normal				
Uterus tenderness present/absent				
Bleeding P/V excessive/normal				
Lochia Healthy/foul smelling				
Episiotomy/Tear healthy/injected				
Family planning counseling				
Any other complications and referral				

C

CARE OF BABY

	1st Day	3rd Day	7th Day	6th Week
Urine passed				
Stool passed				
Diarrhea				
Vomiting				
Convulsions				
Activity (good/lethargic)				
Sucking (good/poor)				
Breathing (fast/difficult)				
Chest indrawing present/absent				
Temperature				
Jaundice				
Condition of umbilical stump				
Skin pustules present/absent				
Any other complications				

Figs. 2.3.4A to C: Mother and child protection card, Ministry of Health and Family Welfare (MOHFW): (A) Postnatal care; (B) Postpartum care; (C) Care of baby.

of both the mother and the newborn throughout the perinatal period, spanning pregnancy, childbirth, and the postpartum phase.[5,6] The primary objective of essential perinatal care is to guarantee a secure and favorable outcome for both the mother and the infant.

- *Antenatal care (ANC):* Regular health checkups and medical supervision for pregnant women to monitor the progress of the pregnancy, identify and manage any potential complications, and provide health education
- *Skilled attendance at birth:* Ensuring that childbirth is attended by skilled health professionals, such as midwives, nurses, or doctors, to manage and respond to any complications that may arise during labor and delivery
- *Postnatal care (PNC):* Monitoring the health of the mother and newborn in the immediate postpartum period, providing support for breastfeeding, and addressing any complications or concerns that may arise after childbirth[5,6]
- *Family planning services:* Providing information and services to help couples plan and space their pregnancies, promoting the health of the mother and the family as a whole
- *Education and counseling:* Offering health education and counseling on topics such as nutrition, hygiene, and general maternal and child health to empower expectant mothers to make informed decisions
- *Nutritional support:* Ensuring proper nutrition for pregnant women and promoting healthy eating habits to support the health and development of the fetus
- *Immunization:* Administering vaccinations to protect both the mother and the newborn from preventable diseases
- *Screening and management of complications:* Identifying and managing any complications that may arise during pregnancy, childbirth, or the postpartum period, such as infections, hypertension, or other medical conditions

DISCHARGE PLANNING

It is ideal to discharge a normal newborn after 48–72 hours of life. Parents should be told about harmful traditional neonatal practices **(Box 2.3.2)**.[5,6] The baby should be free of illness and significant jaundice, and the mother should be confident about breastfeeding. All newborns should have undergone hearing screening at discharge or during the postnatal visit. The baby should have received initial immunization with Bacillus Calmette-Guérin (BCG), oral polio, and hepatitis B vaccines and have passed meconium and urine. If the baby is discharged early, he or she should be reviewed at home or hospital after 48 hours. Babies should be followed up and anthropometry recorded in a growth chart. The growth and development should be evaluated monthly during the first few months and 3 monthly thereafter. All findings should be documented **(Figs. 2.3.4A to C)**.

REFERENCES

1. World Health Organization. (2022). World Health Organization (WHO) recommendations on maternal and newborn care for a positive post-natal experience. [online] Available from https://www.who.in/Publications/i/item/9789240045989 [Last accessed October, 2024].
2. Bhat BV. Care of normal newborn. In: Parthasarathy A, Menon PSN, Nair MKC (Eds). IAP Textbook of Pediatrics, 7th edition. New Delhi : Jaypee Brothers Medical Publishers; 2019. pp. 46-9.
3. Marshall S, Lang AM, Perez M, Saugstad OD. Delivery room handling of the newborn. J Perinat Med. 2019;48(1):1-10.
4. Tran HT, Mannava P, Murray JCS, Nguyen PTT, Tuyen LTM, Hoang Anh T, et al. Early essential newborn care is associated with reduced adverse neonatal outcomes in a tertiary hospital in Da Nang, Vietnam: a pre/post intervention study. EClinicalMedicine. 2019;6:51-8.
5. Memon J, Holakouie-Naieni K, Majdzadeh R, Yekaninejad MS, Garmaroudi G, Raza O, et al. Knowledge, attitude, and practice among mothers about newborn care in Sindh, Pakistan. BMC Pregnancy Childbirth. 2019;19(1):329.
6. Leta M. Level of knowledge toward essential newborn care practices among postnatal mothers in governmental hospitals of Harar Town, Eastern Ethiopia. SAGE Open Med. 2022;10:20503121221076364.

2.4 Kangaroo Mother Care

Shashi N Vani

INTRODUCTION

Kangaroo mother care (KMC) is a simple, low-cost, evidence-based, and holistic method of caring for newborns. It is an important component of core interventions of essential newborn care (ENBC). It is of particular importance for the care of highly vulnerable groups of newborn babies including preterm (PT) and low birth weight infants (LBWI), including even the very small and sick babies (SSB).[1,2]

Kangaroo mother care involves continuous, direct skin-to-skin contact between a mother and her baby, with both their chests in contact without any intervening clothing. This practice includes exclusive breastfeeding whenever feasible, coupled with planned early discharge and regular scheduled follow-ups for monitoring growth, administering immunizations, and assessing neurodevelopment.[3]

The concept of this care approach originated in the South American city of Bogota, Colombia, initially devised as an alternative to prevent hypothermia in infants unable to receive admission to a neonatal intensive care unit (NICU) for incubator care. Over time, numerous advantages were discovered, leading to its incorporation as a crucial component of newborn care.[4]

DEFINITION

Kangaroo mother care involves continuous and extended skin-to-skin (chest-to-chest) contact between a mother and her newborn, initiated promptly after birth, ideally as soon as possible, and administered as frequently and for as long as feasible. In instances of prolonged KMC or when the mother is unavailable, an *alternative KMC provider* (AKP), such as the father, grandmother, or another responsible and willing adult family member or friend, can offer assistance in providing KMC to the baby.[5]

Kangaroo mother care should be distinguished from the standard practice of brief skin-to-skin contact provided to every newborn soon after birth. This routine procedure, lasting only a few minutes, is administered to all infants regardless of birth weight and maturity, excluding those necessitating immediate advanced resuscitation or other urgent life-saving interventions. The primary objectives of this standard practice are to facilitate the early stabilization of physiological parameters such as heart rate and respirations, prevent hypothermia, promote the prompt initiation of breastfeeding, and yield other associated benefits.

Just skin-to-skin contact on a mother's chest by itself is not KMC.

COMPONENTS

Kangaroo mother care has three major components:[3,4]

1. Kangaroo position
2. Kangaroo nutrition
3. Kangaroo discharge and regular scheduled follow-up

Kangaroo Position

In this practice, a newborn, often a PT or LBWI, is dressed solely in a diaper, headcap, socks, mittens, and, if available, a front-open garment (Zabla). The baby, bare-chested, is placed directly on the mother's bare chest between her breasts, without any intervening layers of clothing. This positioning is preferably as vertical as possible, with the mother in a reclining posture. The baby is positioned so that their chest and epigastrium rest on the mother's chest, hands extended above the mother's breasts, and legs positioned below the mother's breasts in a frog-like posture **(Fig. 2.4.1)**. The baby's head is slightly extended in a sniffing position and turned to one side to facilitate direct eye-to-eye contact between the mother and baby. This arrangement ensures that the baby's

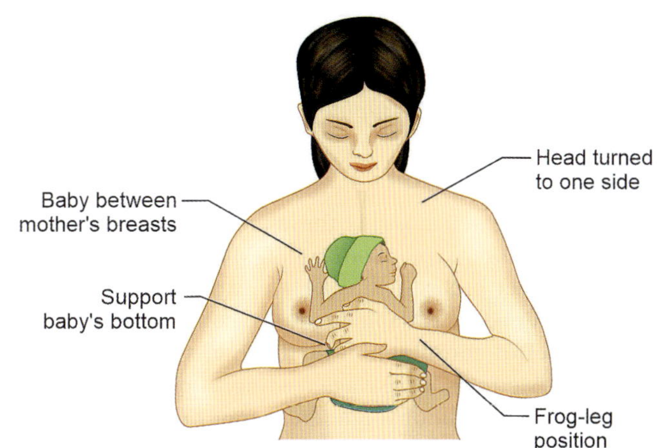

Fig. 2.4.1: Kangaroo mother care positioning.

nose is not excessively pressed against the mother's chest, preventing interference with breathing.[6]

This direct skin-to-skin contact on the mother's chest is better described as an affectionate loving body hug between the mother (or AKP) and her baby than mere superficial skin-to-skin touch.

Good-quality Kangaroo Mother Care Practice

Duration

Each cycle should not be less than at least 1–1½ hours. That enables babies to have one good sleep cycle on the mother's chest and also helps in neurosensory and behavioral development of the newborn. The duration of KMC can be gradually increased as much as possible by the mother with comfort. The total duration in 1 day should not be <8 hours and can be as prolonged in a day as much as possible, even for full 24 hours with the support of AKPs, if available. The infant in KMC needs to be removed from skin-to-skin contact only for changing diapers and clinical assessment or for the mother's personal needs.

Monitoring

Nursing personnel must ensure that the baby's neck is positioned neither excessively flexed nor overextended. They should also verify that the airway is unobstructed, breathing is consistent, the color of the neonate is pink, and the baby is maintaining an appropriate temperature. Additionally, it is important for the mother to actively participate in observing the neonate during KMC.

Precautions

Minimize handling the baby excessively. Delay bathing the baby until their weight reaches approximately 2,500 g; sponge baths are permissible. Avoid providing bottle feeds. Prevent the baby from coming into contact with individuals who have infections or illnesses.

Whenever KMC needs to be interrupted, the baby should be kept in a warm, safe, and supine position.

Kangaroo Nutrition

To the greatest extent possible, the infant should be nourished with the *mother's own milk* (MOM), delivered either through direct breastfeeding or via expressed breastmilk (EBM) obtained by suitable methods, contingent upon the baby's level of coordination in sucking, swallowing, and breathing. Methods like gavage feeding, cup feeding, spoon feeding, or the traditional *paladai* feeder may be employed depending on the baby's developmental stage. Initially, very small infants might necessitate intravenous (IV) fluids for nutrition, transitioning gradually to oral feeds. Micronutrient supplements, including iron, vitamin D, calcium, and phosphorus, are crucial for PT infants and LBWI fed with MOM, adjusting based on the baby's maturity. In some cases, human milk fortifiers may be necessary in the early stages if the anticipated weight gain is not achieved despite diligent efforts in administering MOM.

Kangaroo Discharge

Infants undergoing KMC achieve prompt physiological stability and thermal control, initiating early and successful breastfeeding. Throughout the hospital stay, with guidance and supervision from healthcare professionals, the mother, in collaboration with other involved family members through *family participatory care*, acquires the skills for caring for the tiny baby. This learning process instills confidence in the mother and family members to seamlessly continue similar care practices at home post discharge. In essence, they evolve into the primary caregivers, while physicians and nurses transition into the role of healthcare facilitators.

This facilitates the ongoing practice of KMC and home-based care. This strategically planned early discharge should be complemented by consistent follow-up appointments, preferably conducted in a hospital setting or during scheduled home visits by community health workers (CHWs).

The following criteria if met indicate that the baby is ready for discharge:

- The infant is stable in terms of respirations, heart rate, and color
- Not on any parenteral medications
- Maintaining body temperature on mother's bed for at least 3 consecutive days without any extra gadgets
- Gaining 15–20 g/kg for at least 3 consecutive days (preferable)
- Accepting direct breastfeeding or EBM by spoon, cup, or *paladai*
- Mother confident to take care of the baby at home including KMC
- Family support is assured for allowing mothers to use KMC facilities at home and even help by giving KMC by AKP

Regular follow-up is a fundamental requisite for KMC. Regular visits for growth, immunizations, and common problems must be combined with special follow-up for PT infants and LBWI for assessment for neurodevelopment and screening for retinopathy of prematurity (ROP) and hearing in PT small babies.

BENEFITS

The benefits of KMC are summarized in **Box 2.4.1**.[1,3,4,7]

BOX 2.4.1: Benefits of kangaroo mother care.

Benefits to the baby
- Prevents hypothermia
- Facilitates early physiological stability
- Reduces the risk of severe infections
- Improves neurodevelopment
- Enables better quality of quiet sleep
- Reduces stress, improves security, and less cry
- Reduces pain following painful procedures like heel puncture

Benefits to mother
- Active involvement in the care of small baby
- Increased baby bonding
- Empowered, relaxed, and confident to take care of the small baby
- Less chances of postpartum depression and psychosis
- Early initiation and longer duration of breastfeeding
- Earlier involution of uterus following delivery
- Early return to home setting

Benefits to family
- Better family support and involvement in the care of baby
- Improved breastfeeding and less chances of illness for the baby
- Less costs due to less hospital stay, less medications and other costs
- Early return to work and routine family life
- Better compliance for regular follow-up visits
- Reduced incidences of child abandonment and abuse

Benefits to the hospital
- Saves money on healthcare costs by saving on use of equipment, nursing staff, hospital stay, medications, oxygen, formula milk, etc.
- Better use of manpower and infrastructure
- Less chances of hospital-acquired infections
- Less burden on nursing staff due to more involvement of mother/parents/family in the baby care

Benefits to community and the nation
- Reduction in neonatal morbidity and mortality rates
- Better quality of survival among the LBWI and PT babies
- Reduction in harmful traditional practices
- Reduction in costs due to multiple modalities
- Optimal utilization of available resources
- Better quality of future citizens

(LBWI: low birth weight infants; PT: preterm)

SCOPE

Depending on the experience and expertise of the available staff and other support systems, each unit can decide their policy for KMC in healthcare facilities.

- KMC should be provided routinely to all the LBWI < 2,500 g of birthweight irrespective of gestational age for a minimum of 8–24 hours in a day.[2]
- It can be given to term babies also. The term babies will not continue to accept KMC for many days. But whatever few days the KMC can be given, it provides many benefits including early promotion of breastfeeding, infection prevention, and laying a strong foundation for early child development.[3,4]
- Most of the time, KMC is given to stable babies or even stabilized babies with minimal oxygen, IV fluids, antibiotics, phototherapy, etc.
- It can be given to very SSB in special newborn care units (SNCUs) or NICUs by having a mother or another willing, healthy person as an AKP to help the mother and relieve her for some time.[8,9]
- During neonatal transport of intramural and extramural neonates
- Home-based KMC as a continuum of care after planned early discharge or in rural/tribal blocks as a part of home-based newborn care[10]
- In recent years, home-based KMC is being offered to LBWI in resource-restricted areas under the guidance of a trained CHW, when no other better alternative is available.
- Soon after delivery by cesarean section or any other assisted deliveries
- In some advanced tertiary care centers, KMC is given for babies on mechanical ventilation, continuous positive airway pressure (CPAP), etc.
- KMC is recommended as a pain-relieving measure for mild-to-moderate painful procedures in SNCUs/NICUs.
- In breastmilk-collection centers of human milk banks

WEANING OFF

The hints will come from the baby. Once the infant reaches a gestational age or weight of approximately 2,500 g, signs may include squirming and discomfort, accompanied by the baby pulling limbs out of the KMC wrap. Additionally, crying and fussiness may occur whenever the mother attempts to return the baby to the kangaroo position or skin-to-skin contact on her chest. This signals that it is time to transition the baby away from KMC.

REFERENCES

1. Child Health Division, Ministry of Health and Family Welfare, Government of India. Kangaroo mother care and optimal feeding of low birthweight infants. Operational guidelines, September 2014. For program managers and service providers. 1-49. [online] Available from https://nhm.gov.in/images/pdf/programmes/child-health/guidelines/Operational_Guidelines-KMC_&_Optimal_feeding_of_Low_Birth_Weight_Infants.pdf. [Last accessed October, 2024]
2. World Health Organization. (2023). Kangaroo mother care: a transformative innovation in health care, Global Position Paper. [online] Available from https://www.who.int/publications/i/item/9789240072657 [Last accessed October, 2024]
3. Cattaneo A, Davanzo R, Bergman N, Charpak N. Kangaroo mother care in low-income countries. International Network in Kangaroo Mother Care. J Trop Pediatr. 1998;44(5):279-82.
4. Cattaneo A, Davanzo R, Worku B, Surjono A, Echeverria M, Bedri A, et al. Kangaroo mother care for low birthweight infants: a randomized controlled trial in different settings. Acta Paediatr. 1998;87(9):976-85.
5. World Health Organization. (2003). Kangaroo mother care: a practical guide. [online] Available from https://www.who.int/publications/i/item/9241590351 [Last accessed October, 2024].

6. Department of Pediatrics, WHO Collaborating Centre for Training and Research in Newborn Care, All India Institute of Medical Sciences, New Delhi. Newborn nursing for facility based care: level II units (3rd edition Jan 2014–15) Module 3 (P1 to 12). [online] Available from https://www.newbornwhocc.org/pdf/3-Ed-2014-FBNC-Nursing.pdf [Last accessed October, 2024]
7. Conde-Agudelo A, Díaz-Rossello JL. Kangaroo mother care to reduce morbidity and mortality in low birthweight infants. Cochrane Database Syst Rev. 2016;2016(8):CD002771.
8. Chellani H, Arya S, Mittal P, Bahl R. Mother-newborn care unit (MNCU) experience in India: a paradigm shift in care of small and sick newborns. Indian J Pediatr. 2022;89(5):484-9.
9. WHO Immediate KMC Study Group; Arya S, Naburi H, Kawaza K, Newton S, Anyabolu CH, Bergman N et al. Immediate "Kangaroo mother care" and survival of infants with low birth weight. N Engl J Med. 2021;384(21):2028-38.
10. Rasaily R, Ganguly KK, Roy M, Vani SN, Kharood N, Kulkarni R, et al. Community based kangaroo mother care for low birth weight babies: a pilot study. Indian J Med Res. 2017;145(1):51-7.

2.5 Identification and Approach to a Sick Newborn

Rajesh Kumar

INTRODUCTION

Early identification of a sick newborn is important because it can improve newborn survival. Early interventions in these sick newborns also reduce the risk of long-term problems. Newborn babies have very little reserve as compared to older children and adults, so it is very important to identify a sick newborn early. Early identification of the sick newborn in the emergency room or outpatient department and a proper approach to management is the key to the successful management of newborn babies. Apart from recognizing a sick newborn in the emergency room (ER), it is also very important to recognize the at-risk newborn in the labor room (LR). These at-risk newborns, if not recognized early, can become very sick very fast. Thus, early identification of life-threatening signs (emergency signs), proper triaging of a sick newborn, and proper emergency management are the keys to improved survival and also decreased morbidity.

WHO IS A SICK NEWBORN?

A sick newborn may be described as one who has one or more of the following features—cold or hot to touch; breathing fast or having difficulty in breathing; bluish lips, tongue, or face; having abnormal body movement; not feeding well; dull or cries excessively; floppy; and pale and mottled.

These are the newborn babies who require proper evaluation and many of them will require admission and lifesaving supports (oxygen, intravenous (IV) fluids, respiratory support, inotropes, close monitoring, etc.). As mentioned above, at-risk newborns are also considered "sick newborns" as they require additional support and monitoring.

EVALUATING A SICK NEWBORN IN LABOR ROOM (JUST AFTER BIRTH)

There are many newborns that cannot be shifted to the mother's side after birth because they are sick at birth or likely to get sick after some time. These newborns fall into the high-risk category and should be assessed by the attending physician for potential admission to the special newborn care unit (SNCU) or neonatal intensive care unit (NICU). The Ministry of Health and Family Welfare (MOHFW), Government of India (GOI) facility-based newborn care operational guide has defined it for inborn **(Box 2.5.1)**.[1] Newborns should not be admitted to the SNCU/NICU just for monitoring hypoglycemia, IV antibiotics, or phototherapy.

BOX 2.5.1: Criteria for admission in neonatal intensive care unit/special newborn care unit (NICU/SNCU) from the labor room (inborn babies).

- Newborns who are born at <34 weeks gestation
- Newborns weighing <1,800 g at birth (regardless of gestational age)
- Newborns with an APGAR score of <6 at 1 minute and evidence of birth asphyxia or delayed cry after 5 minutes
- Newborn requiring prolonged resuscitation, that is, after using bag and mask
- Persistent respiratory distress
- Shock or capillary refill time (CRT) >3 seconds
- Central cyanosis
- *Vomiting:* Especially bile stained
- Small for date especially; weight less than third centile for the corresponding gestational age
- Neonates with surgical problems
- Any infant who is felt to be at risk by the nursing staff or doctor

They can be managed in the ward, keeping them with the mothers.

EVALUATING A SICK NEWBORN IN THE EMERGENCY ROOM OR OUTPATIENT DEPARTMENT

History

If a newborn is seen before the 72–96 hours of life, assessment of antenatal and intrapartum risk factors is very important **(Table 2.5.1)**.[2] The history should include the details of the following:

- Age and gestation of the newborn
- Antenatal history to identify any risk factors
- Intrapartum history to identify the risk factors
- Mode of delivery
- Need for resuscitation and details of resuscitation

The postnatal history should include the history suggestive of significant illness. These are called danger signs for a newborn **(Box 2.5.2)**.

TABLE 2.5.1: Antenatal and intrapartum risk factors.

Antenatal risk factors	*Intrapartum risk factors*
• Maternal diabetes mellitus • Pregnancy-induced hypertension (PIH) • Eclampsia • Urinary tract infection (UTI) • Any medical illness • Rh-negative mother • Oligo- or polyhydramnios • Intrauterine growth retardation (IUGR) • Abnormal sonogram • Abnormal Doppler study • Premature rupture of membrane • Prolonged rupture of membrane • Abnormal nonstress test (NST) • Twins • Preterm delivery	• Malpresentation (nonvertex) • Meconium-stained amniotic fluid (MSAF) • Fetal bradycardia • Prolonged labor • Antepartum hemorrhage (APH) • Chorioamnionitis • Difficult delivery • Operative delivery

BOX 2.5.2: Features of significant illness in history.

Danger signs
- Lethargy
- Breathing difficulty
- Apnea
- Failure to pass urine/meconium in the first 24–48 hours
- Persistent vomiting
- Bilious vomiting
- Bleeding
- Excessive weight loss
- Diarrhea
- Cyanosis
- Jaundice
- Abdominal distension
- Convulsion

Examination

Examination of the sick newborn will provide important information about the etiology and severity of the illness. It can help us in triaging and formulating a management plan. Important signs and their importance are summarized below.

Temperature Instability

If a newborn is cold to touch both centrally and peripherally, the newborn is probably having hypothermia. There are two common methods to record temperature in newborns: Rectal and axillary. Axillary temperature is recorded by placing the bulb of a thermometer against the roof of the dry axilla for 5 minutes. Rectal temperature is recorded by inserting the greased bulb of the thermometer backward and downward to a depth of 3 cm in a term baby (2 cm in a preterm baby), and it is kept for at least 2 minutes. Axillary temperature is recorded as a routine monitoring of temperature. Axillary temperature is as good as rectal and probably safer. Rectal temperature is recommended for only sick and hypothermic newborns. Hypothermia (<36°C) may be due to environmental factors or because of sepsis. Severe hypothermia (<32°C) is an emergency sign. Hyperthermia is less common and can be due to environmental factors or sepsis.

Apnea

Apnea is an emergency sign. It should be differentiated with periodic breathing. Periodic breathing is a regular sequence of respiratory pauses of 10–20 seconds and it is not associated with cyanosis or bradycardia. Usually, the cessation of breathing is <10 seconds in the periodic breathing. It is common in preterm babies. Apnea is defined as cessation of breathing for >20 seconds or cessation of breathing for <20 seconds and associated with bradycardia or desaturation.

Respiratory Distress

Respiratory difficulty in newborns can be tachypnea (respiratory rate >60/min), retraction (chest indrawing), grunting, or stridor. The severity of the respiratory distress can be assessed and monitored by using Downe's score **(Table 2.5.2)**.

Cyanosis

Peripheral cyanosis of hands and feet (acrocyanosis) is common in newborns. But central cyanosis is an emergency sign. It is present throughout the body and can be assessed

TABLE 2.5.2: Evaluation of respiratory distress using Downe's score.

Features	*0*	*1*	*2*
Respiratory rate/min	<60	60–80	>80
Cyanosis	Nil	Nil on 40% O_2	Requires >40% O_2
Retraction	Nil	Mild	Moderated to severe
Grunting	Nil	Audible with stethoscope	Audible without stethoscope
Air entry	Normal	Decreased	Barely audible

Notes: Downe's score interpretation: Total of all the rows.
0–3: No/mild respiratory distress.
4–7: Moderate respiratory distress.
8–10: Severe respiratory distress with impending respiratory failure.

by looking at the mucus membrane and tongue. Respiratory illness and congenital cyanotic heart disease are the two serious causes of central cyanosis.

Shock

Shock is an emergency sign. It can be assessed using the appearance of skin (mottled or grey color of the skin), pulse (weak and fast pulse), blood pressure, and capillary refill time (CRT; >3 seconds). The preferred site for assessment of pulse is the brachial pulse. CRT is measured by pressing the index finger over the midsternum for 5 seconds and observing the complete return of skin color after the removal of the finger. CRT gives an idea about the status of peripheral circulation. CRT < 3 seconds is considered normal.

Convulsion

Convulsion is an emergency sign. Any abnormal movements should be assessed carefully. Convulsion should be differentiated from jitteriness and sleep myoclonus. Convulsion can be a pointer for serious illnesses such as meningitis, hypoxic ischemic encephalopathy, intracranial bleed, metabolic problems, etc. It is always better to look at the video of the abnormal movement, if the parents have made it. Always inquire about it from the parents.

Lethargy, Poor Feeding, and Unresponsiveness

These are very subjective and need careful assessment. A sleeping newborn may appear lethargic. If a newborn is not responsive to stimulation and does not change the state of arousal during examination or handing, it indicates that the sensorium is not normal. The six states of arousal are deep sleep, light sleep, drowsy, quiet alert, active alert, and crying. The etiology can be varied, from simpler causes, such as hypoglycemia and polycythemia to more severe ones including sepsis, meningitis, intracranial bleed, and hypoxic ischemic brain injury.

Excessive Crying, Irritability, and Restlessness

Inconsolable, excessive, and incessant crying may indicate a serious disease. It can be irritation in the brain, such as meningitis, hypoxic ischemic encephalopathy, and intracranial bleed Pain in arthritis, myocarditis, and hypoxia can all present as excessive crying.

Inadequate Weight Gain, Dehydration

Poor milk intake is the most likely cause of inadequate weight gain. However, serious problems like systemic illness and inborn error of metabolism (IEM) can present with poor weight gain. If a newborn has diarrhea, it can present with signs of dehydration such as loss of weight, sunken eyes, and depressed anterior fontanel.

Vomiting

Vomiting can be something as physiological as regurgitation, or it could be due to intestinal pathology such as intestinal obstruction. Bilious vomiting and persistent vomiting associated with abdominal distention or lethargy indicate a need for further evaluation for intestinal pathology.

Abdominal Distension

Abdominal distension usually indicates a serious underlying pathology such as sepsis, paralytic ileus, intestinal obstruction, intestinal perforation, or Hirschsprung disease.

Bleeding

Skin bleeds are usually due to thrombocytopenia. In sick newborn, skin bleeds can be due to sepsis and disseminated intravascular coagulation (DIC). In well newborn, it could be isolated thrombocytopenia or thrombocytopenia associated with some systemic disease. Bleeding per rectum could be a simpler cause due to hemorrhagic disease of newborns or serious problems like necrotizing enterocolitis and intestinal volvulus.

Pallor

Pallor may indicate anemia but may also indicate hypothermia, hypoxia, hypotension, and sepsis. It can be assessed by looking at the newborn's palm. Compare the pinkness of the palm of the newborn with your palm.

Jaundice

High levels of bilirubin can damage the brain. It is often physiological in the newborns. If icterus is present in the palms and soles, it is pathological and needs to be investigated immediately. If jaundice persists beyond 14 days of life, always check for the color of urine and stool. Pale-colored stool and high-colored urine can indicate cholestasis jaundice. The presence of cholestasis always requires detailed investigation to find out the cause.

ASSESSMENT OF ILLNESS SEVERITY

The severity of the illness can be assessed at admission by assessing the physiological alteration in the newborns.[3] Modified sick neonatal score (MSNS) is a simple scoring system that can be used to predict survival **(Table 2.5.3)**. It is very helpful in counseling the family at the time of admission. A score of >10 predicts better survival.

It is very important to decide whether a newborn requires admission to the NICU/SNCU or not. MOHFW, GOI FBNC operational guide has clearly defined it for outborn babies **(Box 2.5.3)**.[1]

TABLE 2.5.3: Scoring system for newborn sickness (modified sick neonatal score).[3]

Parameter	*Score 0*	*Score 1*	*Score 2*
Gestational age	<32 weeks	32–36 weeks + 6/7 days	≥37 weeks
Birth weight (kg)	<1.5	1.5–2.49	≥2.5
Axillary temperature (°C)	<36	36–36.5	36.5–37.5
Respiratory effort	Apnea or grunt	Respiratory rate >60/min with or without retraction	Normal
SpO_2 (in room air)	<85	85–92	>92
Heart rate (per minute)	Bradycardia (<100) or asystole	Tachycardia (>160)	Normal
Capillary refill time (seconds)	>5	3–5	<3
Blood glucose (mg/dL)	<40	40–60	>60
Total			

TRIAGING SICK NEWBORNS AND GIVING EMERGENCY TREATMENT

All newborns at admission should be immediately assessed for triage purposes. The signs have been categorized into emergency sign, priority sign, and nonurgent sign. If emergency sign is present, immediate measures should be taken. The Indian Council for Medical Research (ICMR) has developed a standard treatment workflow (STW) for neonatal emergency triage assessment and management, and it is very helpful for triaging and initial management (**Flowchart 2.5.1 and Table 2.5.4**).[2,4,5]

BOX 2.5.3: Criteria for admission in neonatal intensive care unit/special newborn care unit (NICU/SNCU) from community/referral (outborn/readmission babies).

- Delayed cry after 5 minutes
- Respiratory distress with tachypnea, grunt, chest indrawing, or central cyanosis
- Central cyanosis or spells
- Vomiting, especially bile stained
- Abdominal distension
- Suspected sepsis but child unstable
- Unstable babies with congenital abnormality requiring investigation
- Jaundice requiring exchange transfusion
- Neonates in shock (CRT >3 seconds, poor skin color, cold extremities, weak pulses, and mottled skin)
- Fits including subtle signs
- Low birth weight <1,800 g or unstable baby

Managing Hypothermia

A radiant warmer is used to treat hypothermia. Mild hypothermia can be managed by placing the baby in skin-to-skin contact [kangaroo mother care (KMC)]. For the management of moderate hypothermia, a radiant warmer is required, but skin-to-skin contact may be used till a warmer is arranged. Severe hypothermia is very dangerous and has high mortality. Apart from rewarming by a radiant warmer, the baby will require intravenous fluid and vitamin K injection.

Maintaining Airway

Place the newborn in sniffing position. Place a shoulder roll under the shoulder to position the newborn. Clear the airway of secretion by suctioning the mouth first and then the nose.

Assisting Breathing

Support the newborn's respiration if there is respiratory distress. Provide oxygen by nasal prongs; the initial flow rate should be 1 L/min which can be increased to 2 L/min if required. If oxygen requirement is >2 L/min, a newborn will require higher respiratory support [high-flow oxygen or continuous positive airway pressure (CPAP)]. The target oxygen saturation is 91–95%. Endotracheal intubation may be required in more severe distress.

Supporting Circulation

If a newborn is having shock, give IV bolus of normal saline 10 mL/kg over 20–30 minutes. Repeat 10 mL/kg normal saline if the features of shock persist. Even after that, if shock persists inotrope can be started.

Flowchart 2.5.1: ICMR standard treatment workflow for triaging a sick newborn.[2]

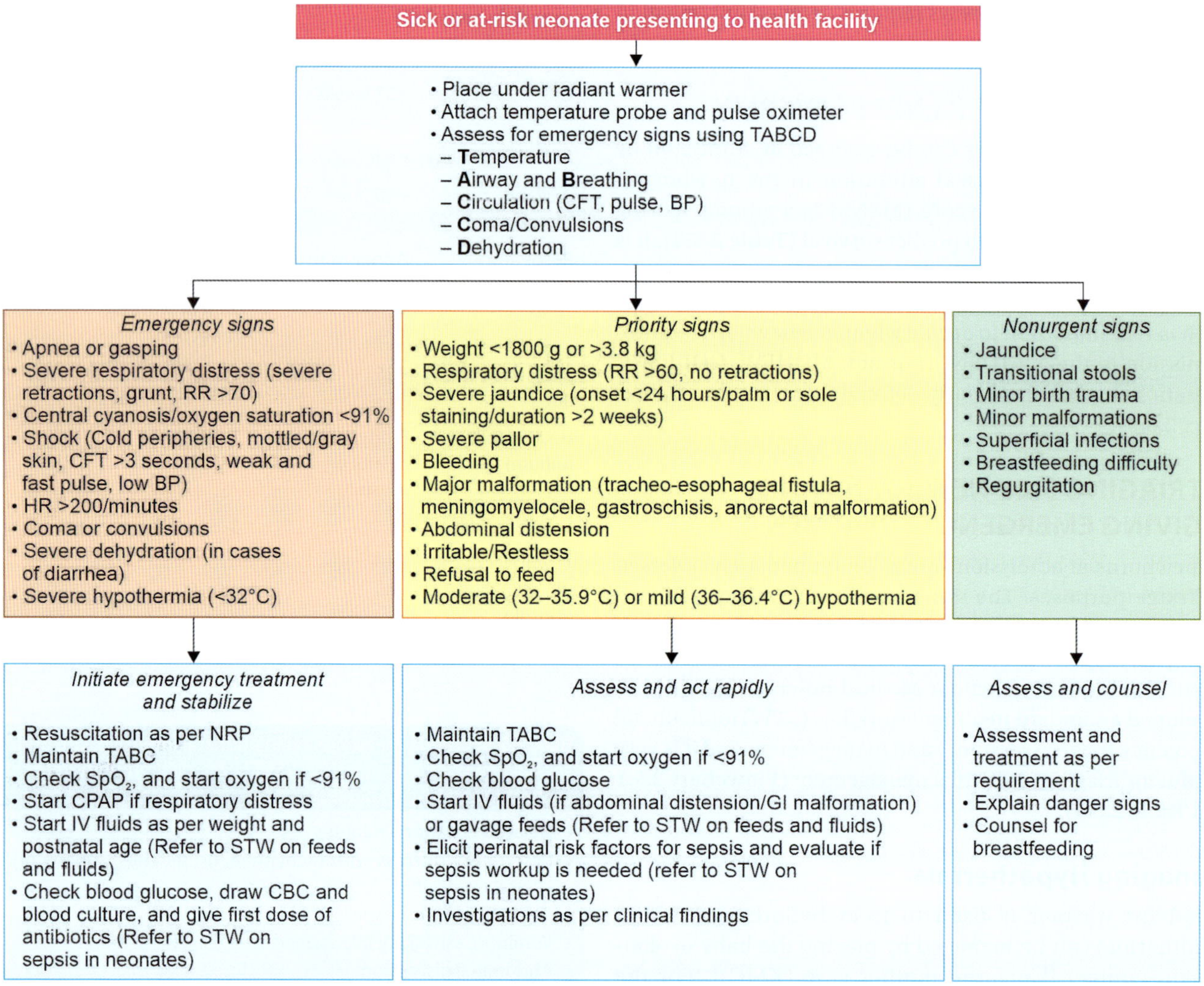

Sick or at-risk neonate presenting to health facility

↓

- Place under radiant warmer
- Attach temperature probe and pulse oximeter
- Assess for emergency signs using TABCD
  - **T**emperature
  - **A**irway and **B**reathing
  - **C**irculation (CFT, pulse, BP)
  - **C**oma/Convulsions
  - **D**ehydration

↓

Emergency signs
- Apnea or gasping
- Severe respiratory distress (severe retractions, grunt, RR >70)
- Central cyanosis/oxygen saturation <91%
- Shock (Cold peripheries, mottled/gray skin, CFT >3 seconds, weak and fast pulse, low BP)
- HR >200/minutes
- Coma or convulsions
- Severe dehydration (in cases of diarrhea)
- Severe hypothermia (<32°C)

↓

Initiate emergency treatment and stabilize
- Resuscitation as per NRP
- Maintain TABC
- Check SpO_2, and start oxygen if <91%
- Start CPAP if respiratory distress
- Start IV fluids as per weight and postnatal age (Refer to STW on feeds and fluids)
- Check blood glucose, draw CBC and blood culture, and give first dose of antibiotics (Refer to STW on sepsis in neonates)

Priority signs
- Weight <1800 g or >3.8 kg
- Respiratory distress (RR >60, no retractions)
- Severe jaundice (onset <24 hours/palm or sole staining/duration >2 weeks)
- Severe pallor
- Bleeding
- Major malformation (tracheo-esophageal fistula, meningomyelocele, gastroschisis, anorectal malformation)
- Abdominal distension
- Irritable/Restless
- Refusal to feed
- Moderate (32–35.9°C) or mild (36–36.4°C) hypothermia

↓

Assess and act rapidly
- Maintain TABC
- Check SpO_2, and start oxygen if <91%
- Check blood glucose
- Start IV fluids (if abdominal distension/GI malformation) or gavage feeds (Refer to STW on feeds and fluids)
- Elicit perinatal risk factors for sepsis and evaluate if sepsis workup is needed (refer to STW on sepsis in neonates)
- Investigations as per clinical findings

Nonurgent signs
- Jaundice
- Transitional stools
- Minor birth trauma
- Minor malformations
- Superficial infections
- Breastfeeding difficulty
- Regurgitation

↓

Assess and counsel
- Assessment and treatment as per requirement
- Explain danger signs
- Counsel for breastfeeding

(CBC: complete blood count; CFT: capillary filling time; CPAP: continuous positive airway pressure; GI: gastrointestinal; HR: heart rate; ICMR: Indian Council of Medical Research; NRP: Neonatal Resuscitation Program; RR: respiratory rate; STW: Standard Treatment Workflow)

Treating Hypoglycemia

In a sick newborn, if blood glucose (BG) is <45 mg/dL, IV dextrose is required. Give 10% dextrose bolus 2 mL/kg slowly. If the newborn is having convulsion, give 5 mL/kg of 10% dextrose. Start dextrose infusion at the rate of 6 mg/kg/min. Check BG after 30 minutes. If repeat BG is <20 mg/dL, repeat the bolus of dextrose (2 mL/kg; 10% dextrose). If repeat BG is >25 mg/dL and <45 mg/dL, increase the glucose infusion rate by 2 mg/kg/min.

Treating Convulsions

If the baby is having active convulsion, first check BG; if it is <45 mg/dL, give IV dextrose. If seizure is not controlled, give IV calcium gluconate 2 mL/kg diluted with 1:1 with 5% dextrose over 10 minutes under cardiac monitoring. If the seizure is still not controlled, give IV phenobarbitone 20 mg/kg over 15 minutes.

TABLE 2.5.4: Specific management of a sick newborn (ICMR, standard treatment workflow).[2]

Problem	***Management***
Shock	• Provide warmth • IV NS 10 mL/kg bolus over 30–60 minutes • May repeat bolus if evidence of volume deficit • Consider inotropes
HR >200/min	• Urgent ECG—look for p waves • If SVT, consider ice-pack and IV adenosine • Check for and correct hyperthermia if present
Severe dehydration	• Provide warmth • IV 30 mL/kg of RL or NS in 1 hour followed by 70 mL/kg in the next 5 hours • If IV not possible, give ORS at 20 mL/kg/h for 6 hours • Assess 1–2 hourly and titrate the volume of fluid
Hypothermia	• *Mild (36–36.4°C):* Warm environment, skin-to-skin contact, and breastfeeding • *Moderate (32–35.9°C):* Place under servo-controlled warmer; skin-to-skin contact till arranged • *Severe (<32°C):* As for moderate hypothermia plus IV fluids and injection vitamin K
Hypoglycemia	• *Blood glucose <45 mg/d and asymptomatic:* Supervised breastfeeding or EBM • *Blood glucose <20 mg/dL OR symptomatic:* 2 mL/kg 10% dextrose IV followed by infusion @ 6 mg/kg/min
Jaundice	• *Serious jaundice (onset at <24 hours of age, palm or sole staining, or signs of acute bilirubin encephalopathy):* Intensive phototherapy, consider IV fluids if suspicion of dehydration, prepare for exchange blood transfusion
Seizure	• Maintain TABC • *Check blood glucose by glucometer:* If <45 mg/dL, 5 mL/kg 10% dextrose IV followed by infusion @ 6 mg/kg/min • If not controlled, 2 mL/kg 10% calcium gluconate IV, diluted 1:1 with D5, D10 or DW, over 10 minutes under cardiac monitoring • If not controlled, Inj. Phenobarbitone 20 mg/kg IV over 15 minutes. If seizures persist after 15 minutes, consider another bolus of 10 mg/kg phenobarbitone over 10 minutes
Surgical	• Cover any skin defects with warm saline sterile gauze • Maintain hydration • Consult surgeon
Breastfeeding difficulty	• Observe and look for proper positioning and attachment of the baby during breastfeeding • Counsel mother

(EBM: expressed breast milk; ICMR: Indian Council of Medical Research; NS: nasal saline; ORS: oral rehydration salt; RL: Ringer's lactate; SVT: supraventricular tachycardia; TABC: temperature, airway, breathing, circulation)

REFERENCES

1. Facility Based Newborn Care Operational Guide, Ministry of Health and Family Welfare, Government of India. (2011). [online] Available from https://nhm.gov.in/images/pdf/programmes/CH-Programmes/FBNC/Operational-Guide-(FBNC).pdf [Last accessed October, 2024].
2. Indian Council of Medical Research (ICMR). Standard Treatment Workflow (STW) Neonatal emergency triage assessment and management. [online] Available from https://main.icmr.nic.in/sites/default/files/STWsDownload/Neonatology/NEONATAL_EMERGENCY_TRIAGE.pdf [Last accessed October, 2024].
3. Mansoor KP, Ravikiran SR, Kulkarni V, Baliga K, Rao S, Bhat KG, et al. Modified Sick Neonatal Score (MSNS): a novel neonatal disease severity scoring system for resource-limited settings. Crit Care Res Pract. 2019;2019:9059073.
4. Neogi SB, Khanna R, Chauhan M, Sharma J, Gupta G, Srivastava R, et al. Inpatient care of small and sick newborns in healthcare facilities. J Perinatol. 2016;36(s3):S18-S23.
5. Brousseau T, Sharieff GQ. Newborn emergencies: the first 30 days of life. Pediatr Clin North Am. 2006;53(1):69-84.

2.6 Birth Injuries

Satyen K Hemrajani, Naveen Parkash Gupta

INTRODUCTION

The term birth injury or birth trauma implies "any impairment of a newborn's body part or its function that are sustained during labor and delivery." This definition excludes fetal injuries due to intrauterine procedures [amniocentesis, chorion villus sampling (CVS), etc.] and neonatal injuries after resuscitation. Birth trauma often occurs in typical areas such as the head, neck, and shoulders, with less frequent incidents affecting regions like the face, abdomen, and lower limbs. The range of birth injuries is broad, extending from minor and self-limiting issues like lacerations to more critical injuries that can even cause death or irreversible disfigurement or disability, such as brachial plexus injury, intracranial injury, etc. Birth injury data serves as a quality assessment tool for the safety of maternity units.

EPIDEMIOLOGY

There has been a steady decline in birth injuries due to improved obstetric practices. The incidence of neonatal birth injuries is 0.06–0.08% of live births in developed countries.[1] Studies from India show an incidence of 3.2–15.4 per 1,000 live births.[2,3] The incidence is directly proportional to the increase in fetal weight. It is more frequent with instrumental delivery and occurs more commonly in cesarean delivery compared to vaginal delivery (3 vs. 0.6%).

RISK FACTORS OF BIRTH INJURIES

Typically, the fetus gets injured due to the manipulation used to facilitate the passage through the birth canal during the second stage of labor.[3] There are many identifiable risk factors that predispose a fetus to birth trauma **(Table 2.6.1)**.

TABLE 2.6.1: Risk factors for birth injuries.

Fetal	*Maternal*	*Delivery*
• Macrosomia • Prematurity • Abnormal presentation • Male	• Primigravida • Age (<16 years, >35 years) • Cephalopelvic disproportion • Short stature • Diabetes • Obesity	• Precipitous delivery • Instrumental delivery

SOFT-TISSUE INJURIES

Soft-tissue injuries are the most common forms of neonatal birth injuries.[4]

Bruising and Petechiae

Bruising and petechiae are most commonly seen on the presenting part of the neonate, and these are usually self-resolving. Babies with significant bruising are at an increased risk for early and severe hyperbilirubinemia.

Subcutaneous Fat Necrosis

Subcutaneous fat necrosis (SCFN) is a self-limiting panniculitis that commonly affects term neonates with a history of birth asphyxia, perinatal stress, or babies who require therapeutic hypothermia. Other risk factors include maternal diabetes, hypothyroidism, hypertension, and placental abruption. The exact pathogenesis of SCFN in the newborn remains unclear. SCFN can result from the combination of local tissue hypoxia and mechanical pressure. Another possible mechanism may be due to the crystallization of the adipose tissue, which may occur at low temperatures (in a setting of hypoxia or therapeutic hypothermia) as the neonatal adipose tissue contains stearic acids and saturated palmitic acids.

A neonate presents typically with indurated, erythematous to violaceous red to purple nodules and plaques on the cheeks, back, buttocks, or proximal extremities. Lesions on the scalp may be associated with localized alopecia. Hypercalcemia is the most common complication of SCFN and needs close calcium monitoring.[5]

Subcutaneous fat necrosis is usually diagnosed by clinical examination. Skin biopsy is the gold standard to confirm the diagnosis. Fine needle aspiration also aids in diagnosis by cytologic examination, which shows refractile, needle-shaped crystals in radial arrays within the fat cells, with necrosis, accompanied by macrophages, multinucleated giant cells, neutrophils, and lymphocytes. SCFN needs to be differentiated from cold panniculitis, sclerema neonatorum, and scleroderma.

Subcutaneous fat necrosis nodules and plaques generally resolve without scarring within several weeks, and no specific treatment is generally needed.

Lacerations

Lacerations are the most common birth injuries that occur following cesarean delivery. They are commonly seen on the face and scalp, as these parts are the presenting part during delivery **(Fig. 2.6.1)**. Most of the lacerations are usually mild and may not require any intervention.

EXTRACRANIAL INJURIES

Extracranial injuries occur due to either bleeding or edema within the scalp or skull **(Fig. 2.6.2)**.[4]

Caput Succedaneum

Caput succedaneum is a benign condition, and in this, a boggy, widespread edematous, nonfluctuant swelling of soft tissues of the scalp above the periosteum is seen mostly over the presenting part of the fetus. It can be felt immediately after birth and happens due to the prolonged compression on the engaged fetal head in the birth canal or after ventouse extraction. This swelling crosses the suture lines, gets resolved within a few days, and needs no special treatment.

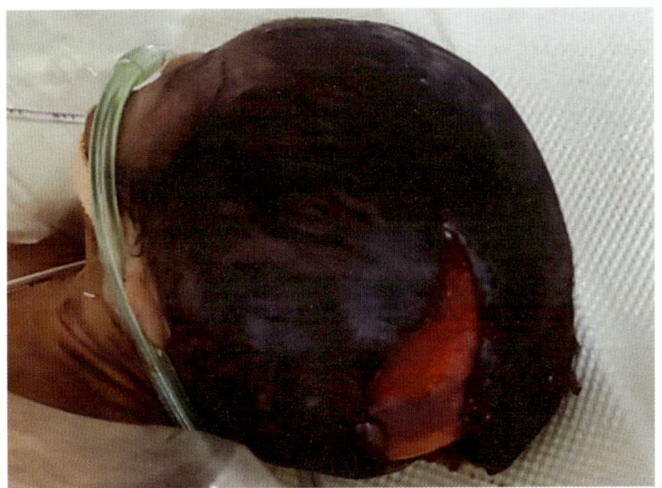

Fig. 2.6.1: Laceration of the scalp in a baby.

Cephalhematoma

Cephalhematoma is a swelling due to the collection of blood beneath the periosteum, which happens due to the rupture of vessels crossing the periosteum. It is seen commonly over the parietal or occipital bone and usually presents 2–3 days after birth and does not cross the suture line **(Fig. 2.6.3)**. Cephalhematomas usually resolve spontaneously over a few weeks without any intervention. Early and severe hyperbilirubinemia has been observed in neonates with cephalhematoma; hence, close monitoring for jaundice after discharge is advised. **Table 2.6.2** highlights the difference between cephalhematoma and caput succedaneum.

Subgaleal Hemorrhage

Subgaleal hemorrhage (SGH) is an uncommon but potentially life-threatening condition.[6] It occurs due to the accumulation of blood in the loose areolar tissue between the periosteum of the skull and the aponeurosis. Hemorrhage occurs as the emissary veins between the scalp and dural sinuses get disrupted due to the forces of traction on the scalp during delivery. This subgaleal space extends from the orbital ridges in the front to the nape of the neck in the back and to the level of the ears on both sides. SGH is more commonly associated with instrumental deliveries but can also occur spontaneously.

Subgaleal hemorrhage is similar to cephalhematoma, but it is more diffuse and more boggy depending on the amount

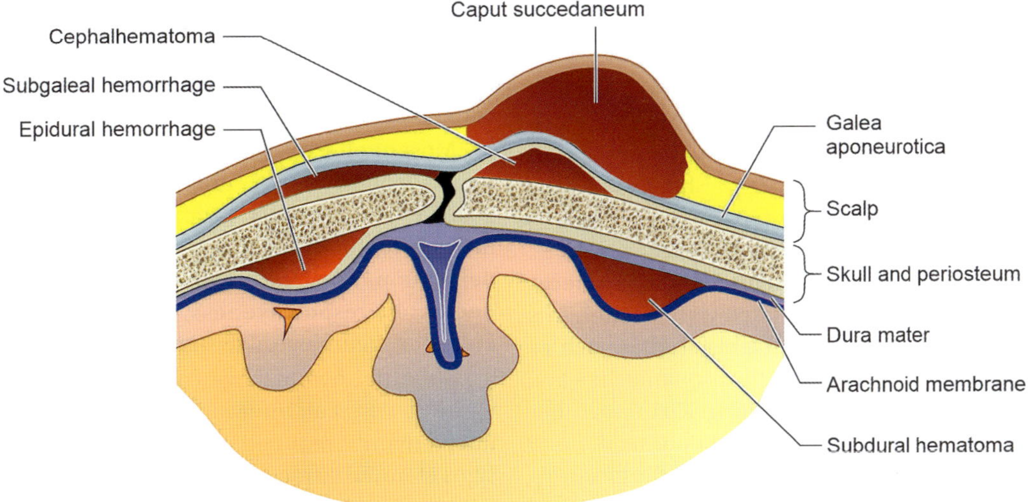

Fig. 2.6.2: Extracranial injuries in neonates.

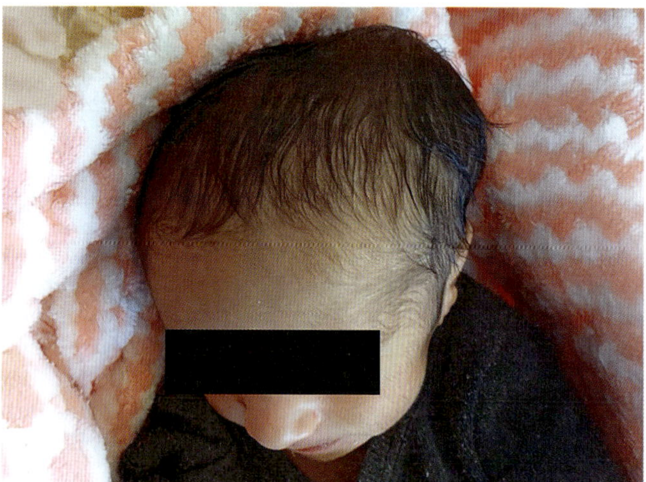

Fig. 2.6.3: Cephalhematoma.

TABLE 2.6.2: Difference between cephalhematoma and caput succedaneum.

	Caput succedaneum	*Cephalhematoma*
Manifestation	At birth	After 2–3 days
Swelling	Localized soft tissue swelling with a poorly defined outline	Soft, fluctuant, and localized swelling with a well-defined outline
Mechanism	Caused by pressure of the fetal head against the cervix during labor	Caused by rupture of vessels below the periosteum
Relation with suture line	Swelling crosses suture lines	Swelling is limited to the suture lines
Risk to the baby	None, in majority	Risk of underlying skull fracture or intracranial bleeding and increased severity of jaundice

of blood collection. Swelling may increase gradually because of continuous bleeding, which may occur for some days also after delivery. Affected neonates present with shock and pallor due to blood loss or coagulopathy. Shock is usually associated with massive blood loss (50–100 mL, which is 20–40% of blood volume) into the subgaleal space.

Serial measurements of head circumference are necessary as every 1 cm increase is associated with a 40 mL loss of blood into the subgaleal space. Imaging studies such as computed tomography (CT) or magnetic resonance imaging (MRI) brain can be useful for differentiating SGH from other causes of bleeding. A coagulation profile should be done to detect coagulopathy that may be associated with the bleeding.

Treatment includes volume resuscitation with packed red blood cells, fresh frozen plasma, and normal saline for ongoing bleeding and correction of coagulopathy. Surgical evacuation is rarely required.

Subgaleal hemorrhage may be associated with high mortality pertaining to massive blood loss into the subgaleal space.

FACIAL INJURIES

Nasal Septal Injury

Nasal septal dislocation is a common type of injury, which occurs as a result of pressure on the nose from the sacral promontory or symphysis pubis of the mother during vaginal delivery. A neonate may present with respiratory distress if the injury is severe, leading to airway obstruction. On examination, nasal septal deviation with inequal-sized nares and flattening of one side is seen. The confirmation of the diagnosis is done with the help of rhinoscopy. Treatment is possible by manual reduction, which gives satisfactory results if performed within 3 days.

Ocular Injuries

Retinal hemorrhages, subconjunctival hemorrhages, and lid edema are common ocular injuries. They resolve spontaneously without any intervention. Some other ocular injuries are hyphema (blood in the anterior chamber), vitreous hemorrhage, injury to the lacrimal duct, and disruption of Descemet's membrane of the cornea, which can result in astigmatism and amblyopia. Intervention of an ophthalmologist is required in these babies with significant ocular injuries.

INTRACRANIAL INJURIES[7]

Subdural Hemorrhage

Subdural hemorrhage (SDH) is the most frequently observed intracranial hemorrhage seen in neonates. SDH is the blood collection between the dura mater and arachnoid mater, most commonly in the tentorial and/or interhemispheric region.

Most often babies are asymptomatic, and SDH is picked up incidentally when neuroimaging (ultrasound or CT scan) is done for some other indications. Symptomatic newborns usually present within the first 48 hours of life with respiratory depression, seizures, and apnea. Other symptoms include decreased responsiveness, irritability, or altered tone, indicating neurological dysfunction.

Subdural hemorrhage can be managed conservatively without surgical intervention in the majority. Surgical intervention is required if an infant with SDH has associated signs of raised intracranial pressure or if the SDH is located in the posterior fossa, causing brainstem compression requiring emergency surgical evacuation.

Subarachnoid Hemorrhage

Subarachnoid hemorrhage (SAH) occurs as a result of damage to the bridging veins in the subarachnoid space or small leptomeningeal vessels. Neonates with SAH commonly present on the first or second day of life with apnea, respiratory depression, and seizures. A CT scan/MRI brain can easily diagnose SAH, and the treatment is usually expectant management with good recovery.

Epidural Hemorrhage

Epidural hemorrhage (EDH) is a less common type of intracranial hemorrhage in neonates. In EDH, there is a collection of blood between the dura and the inner table of the skull. EDH happens when the middle meningeal artery gets injured during delivery. EDH is commonly associated with a linear skull fracture, mostly in the parietotemporal area, and is more common with operative deliveries.

Neonates present with seizures, decreased tone, and bulging anterior fontanelle, and a decreased level of consciousness can also be seen.

Epidural hemorrhage is diagnosed by neuroimaging (CT or MRI brain). Neurosurgical follow-up is essential as EDH can progress rapidly (arterial source of bleeding), resulting in deterioration. In small EDH, neonates have a stable clinical course that can be managed conservatively. Surgical intervention is needed in cases with increased intracranial pressure and/or large EDH.

Intraventricular Hemorrhage

Although more common in preterm infants, intraventricular hemorrhage (IVH) has also been seen in term babies as a result of birth injury. The prognosis depends on the cause of the IVH. In clotting disorder or severe asphyxia, most IVH will have a poor outcome. In cases of birth trauma leading to IVH, head circumference monitoring and ultrasonogram (USG) cranial monitoring are required due to the risk of posthemorrhagic hydrocephalus as a complication of progressive IVH.

BONE INJURIES

Clavicular Fracture

Clavicular fracture is the most common bone fracture in newborns. Most of the fractures are undiagnosed at discharge, and the majority are of the greenstick type.

Majority of the fractures occur during normal, spontaneous vaginal delivery. The incidence is increased in the presence of breech with extended arms and macrosomia with shoulder dystocia.

Many times, due to the greenstick fracture, this birth injury does not present with any signs or symptoms. At times it is first detected after a callus is formed after the fourth week of life, which happens usually after discharge during routine neonatal follow-up. When any baby presents with decreased movement of the upper extremity, crepitation, swelling, and/or bruising over the affected shoulder, the examiner must try and rule out a clavicular fracture. Passive movement of the affected arm may be painful, and Moro's reflex may be absent on the affected side.

The diagnosis is confirmed with an X-ray, where a clear fracture is usually apparent at the junction between the middle and outer third of the clavicle.

Sometimes, there may be a painless swelling on the clavicle without any tenderness or limitation of movement of the shoulder and arm. This suggests the possibility of congenital pseudoarthrosis of the clavicle. In pseudoarthrosis, the radiography reveals disruption of the affected clavicle with enlargement of the end of the bone.

To treat, the affected arm is immobilized with the arm abducted and the elbow flexed. After callus formation, the immobilization may be discontinued. The prognosis is usually excellent.

Fracture of the Ribs

Fracture of the ribs is a much less common fracture. It happens when the anterior shoulder is impacted behind the symphysis pubis and the compression forces on the fetal arms and thorax, leading to spontaneous rib fractures on the same side as the posterior shoulder. Typical symptoms include discoloration, swelling, or crepitus of the chest. It is also a benign entity, and no specific treatment is required.

Fracture of the Humerus

Fracture of the humerus is the most common long bone that gets fractured during the process of birth. The fracture is usually in the diaphysis **(Fig. 2.6.4)**. It has a similar

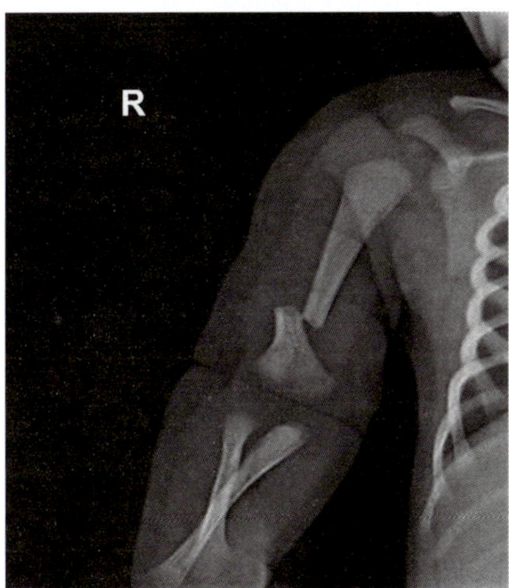

Fig. 2.6.4: X-ray of the fracture of the humerus.

presentation to that of a clavicular fracture. For treatment, immobilization is advised for 2–4 weeks by strapping the arm to the chest. Because of the excellent remodeling power of infants, the moderate overriding and angulation disappear. This fracture results in epiphyseal stimulation and leads to subsequent overgrowth.

Fracture of the Femur

Fracture of the femur is the most common long bone of the lower limb in the newborn that gets fractured. It commonly occurs in breech presentation when the leg is pulled down after the breech is partially fixed in the pelvic inlet. Babies with congenital hypotonia suffer this injury more due to decreased muscle bulk that acts as a cushion against the pressure on the femur. Most often, the bone breaks transversely in the upper half or third where it is relatively thin.

Here, the obvious deformity is noticed in the affected limb. Sometimes, an associated swelling is noted in the thigh that leads to the confirmation of this fracture. Radiographs show overriding of the fracture fragments.

Treatment is traction suspension of both lower legs and immobilization in a spica cast. This immobilization is needed for 3–4 weeks until callus is formed. Here also the complete union and restoration without shortening are expected. Extensive calcification may develop in the areas of surrounding hemorrhage but is resorbed subsequently.

Dislocation of Radius

Only radial head dislocation is a true dislocation, which is due to birth trauma and is associated with breech delivery. The head of radius can easily be reduced by supination and extension, which gives excellent results. Following this reduction, immobilization must be done for 2–3 weeks. Delayed recognition and treatment for this may result in deformity and the need for osteotomy.

Skull Fractures

Mostly, these are linear fractures that are accompanied by cephalhematoma, and usually, the infant's behavior is normal. Some fractures of the skull are however depressed fractures.

The clinical manifestation depends on the site of the fracture. The base of the skull fracture leads to separation of the basal and squamous portions of the occipital bone and it also results in severe hemorrhage due to disruption of the underlying venous sinuses. These infants will present with shock, pallor, neurologic abnormalities and cerebrospinal fluid (CSF) otorrhea or rhinorrhea. These fractures are also associated with neurologic sequelae and even death.

In X-rays of the skull, the linear fractures appear as lines of low density, whereas the depressed fractures are picked up as lines of high density. If neurological symptoms are present, consider a possible intracranial bleed, and a CT of the head should be advised.

Treatment of a complicated fracture at the base of skull needs blood transfusion, saline bolus, and broad-spectrum antibiotic cover to protect against meningitis, especially with CSF rhinorrhea or otorrhea. A small (<2 cm) depressed fracture may need only a conservative approach of treatment, but neurosurgical consultation is recommended for any neonatal skull fracture.

INJURIES TO INTRA-ABDOMINAL ORGANS

Any neonate presenting with pallor, abdominal distension, or unexplained anemia should be suspected of having a hidden injury of abdominal organs.[8]

Rupture of Liver

The liver is the most frequently injured abdominal organ during the birth process. Any trauma of liver usually results in subcapsular hematoma, which enlarges and ruptures, resulting in a massive peritoneal hemorrhage. Currently, hepatic injury is encountered most frequently in a critically ill, low-birth-weight infant, especially with sepsis and hypoxia.

In the first 3 days, the infant appears normal. Poor feeding, pallor, jaundice, tachypnea, and tachycardia may appear once the hematoma is formed and blood loss is occurring. A mass is usually palpable in the right upper quadrant of the abdomen. Serial determination of hematocrit may suggest a drop. Once the hematoma ruptures, abdominal distension and rigidity, severe anemia, and shock may develop. There may be distinct bluish discoloration of the abdomen, which at times extends into the scrotum.

An X-ray may suggest hepatomegaly, but the diagnosis can be clinched by a USG of the abdomen or CT (subcapsular hematoma without rupture). Treatment of liver trauma must focus on fluid resuscitation, transfusion of packed red blood cells, and correction of coagulopathies. Surgical treatment has a high mortality rate, but it may be unavoidable in cases of uncontrolled hemorrhage and deteriorating clinical status despite medical treatment.

Rupture of the Spleen

Although spleen is the best protected organ of the abdomen, being just below the diaphragm, it does face chances of injury during birth. When an injury occurs, there are usually mild symptoms like unexplained anemia, and there may be an associated left upper quadrant mass. The deterioration is rapid after rupture of the hematoma, leading to shock and death due to extensive blood loss.

A mass effect due to the hematoma displaces the stomach and intestine medially, which may be seen on a flat plate abdomen radiograph. Ultrasound may show intra-abdominal fluid, and CT and MRI may help in the final diagnosis of splenic rupture.

For small hemorrhages, conservative treatment is justified, but intensive monitoring of vitals and perfusion must be continued. If the bleeding is uncontrolled or if the infant is unstable clinically, then surgical exploration and repair of the spleen, partial splenectomy, or selective ligation of the blood supply of the spleen need to be performed. Along with this, aggressive resuscitation with fluid and blood products to enhance clotting must be integrated with supportive management for achieving an optimal outcome.

Adrenal Hemorrhage

The classic findings are fever, tachypnea out of proportion to the degree of fever, jaundice, pallor, and cyanosis of the lips and fingertips. There may be a mass palpable in the flanks and purpura. Also, due to leakage of blood through a patent processus vaginalis, there may be painless swelling and/or discoloration of the scrotum that may mimic testicular torsion. As a result of damage to adrenals, there can be a problem of adrenal insufficiency, which presents as seizures, hypoglycemia, hypotension, and hyponatremia.

Initially, an X-ray of the abdomen may show only the increased width of the retroperitoneal space and forward displacement of the stomach and duodenum. Later, there may be a rim-like calcification observed in the second week of life. USG in the initial phase suggests a solid lesion at the location of adrenals, which changes to cystic character.

Mild cases need only observation and packed red blood cell transfusion. More severe hemorrhages need adrenalectomy. In cases of adrenal insufficiency, replacement therapy is needed.

A late complication of adrenal hemorrhage is hypertension. Complete recovery of this hemorrhage is expected in 3 months and must be closely followed with serial ultrasound scans. Adrenal functions must also be assessed in follow-up by adrenocorticotropic hormone (ACTH) stimulation.

PERIPHERAL NERVE INJURY[9]

Facial Nerve Palsy

Facial nerve palsy is the most common neonatal traumatic nerve injury. This nerve palsy usually occurs due to compression of the peripheral portion of the nerve near the stylomastoid foramen or where the nerve traverses the ramus of the mandible. It usually happens due to the prolonged pressure applied by maternal sacral promontory, use of forceps, or in utero compression of the nerve by a tumor or mandibular deformity.

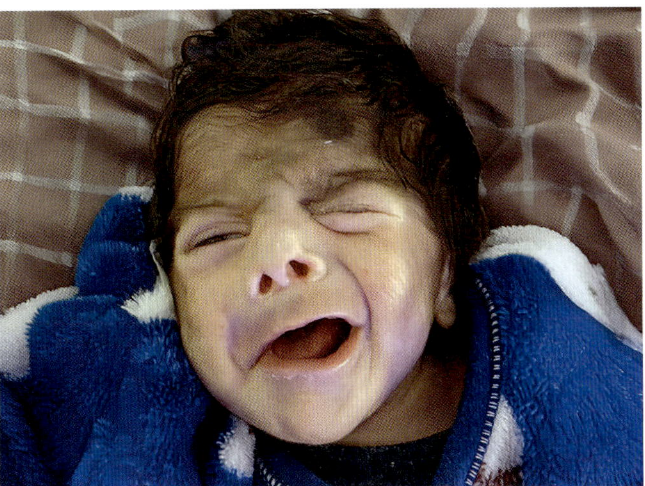

Fig. 2.6.5: Facial nerve injury.

The diagnosis of facial palsy is easily done by physical examination only and can be done on day 1 itself. Obliterated nasolabial fold, a drooping mouth, a persistently open eyelid of the affected side, and the absence of a smooth forehead on the involved side on crying are the hallmark features **(Fig. 2.6.5)**. Infants may also have ineffective sucking and swallowing and persistent drooling.

Treatment involves protecting the open eyes with patches and lubricating them with artificial tear drops (methylcellulose 1%). Full recovery may take weeks to years, depending on its severity.

Phrenic Nerve Injury

Phrenic nerve injury results in diaphragmatic paralysis and rarely occurs in isolation. This most commonly results due to lateral hyperextension of the neck during difficult breech delivery, causing injury to the third, fourth, and fifth cervical roots.

The signs of symptoms of this are episodes of cyanosis, irregular and labored breathing with the affected side having thoracic breathing and no abdominal bulging during inspiration. On chest radiography, an elevated diaphragm may be noted. A definitive diagnosis is by fluoroscopy or real-time ultrasound examination of the diaphragm.

For mild cases, conservative treatment is advised with frequent pulmonary toilet and adequate respiratory support. If there is severe respiratory distress, prolonged ventilation, recurrent pneumonia, or atelectasis, or if there is a poor response to conservative treatment after 1 month, then plication of the diaphragm or diaphragmatic pacing is needed.

Laryngeal Nerve Injury

After suffering from this injury, the neonate presents with stridor, cyanosis, airway obstruction, dysphonia, dysphagia, and aspiration. The mean age of presentation is 5.6 days. Investigations should include a modified barium swallow. Unilateral paralysis may be asymptomatic at rest and can be followed clinically, whereas bilateral paralysis usually requires tracheotomy. If no treatment happens, a funnel deformity may develop in the lower sternal area.

Obstetric Brachial Plexus Palsy

It is defined as a flaccid paresis of an arm at birth, with the passive range of motion being greater than the active range of motion.[10] Majority of these brachial plexus injuries involve C5–C6 nerve roots (Erb–Duchenne palsy). The injuries that involve the C8–T1 roots (Klumpke palsy) are more likely to persist, with only 40% resolving within a year.

In Erb's palsy, the arm is adducted, internally rotated with extended elbow, pronated forearm, and flexed wrist (waiter's tip position) **(Fig. 2.6.6)**. The deep tendon reflexes of the affected arm, (Moro's, biceps, etc.) are absent. Sensory deficit may happen on the radial side of the arm. Lower arm paralysis affects the intrinsic muscles of the hand and the long flexors of the wrist. The hand is paralyzed, and voluntary movements of the wrist are not possible. Grasp reflex is absent, and deep tendon reflexes are intact. In Horner syndrome, the features such as ptosis, miosis, and enophthalmos are present on the ipsilateral side and this may result in delayed pigmentation of the iris in later stages.

Magnetic resonance imaging of the cervical spine may reveal pseudomeningoceles suggesting nerve root avulsion, and electromyogram (EMG) and nerve conduction velocity (NCV) test after 3 months of age help identify the presence of regenerating motor units and conducting action potentials.

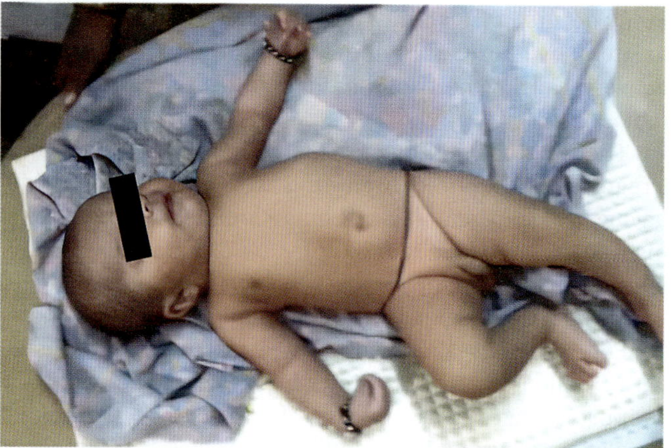

Fig. 2.6.6: Erb's palsy or brachial plexus palsy of the left hand.

Nonsurgical management with initial evaluation of the patient within 2 weeks of delivery helps in establishing a neurological baseline. The next follow-up appointment should occur at 3 months of age for assessment of spontaneous neural regeneration. Splinting and passive exercises are done to prevent contracture. Inadequate recovery in the function of shoulder abduction or external rotation, flexion of elbow, and/or hand movement by the age of 3 months prompts surgical correction before 6 months of age. Surgery is also indicated when there are nerve root avulsions in the presence of Horner syndrome. Surgical options include microsurgical repair, tendon transfers, or humeral osteotomy.

REFERENCES

1. Leung WC, Chan BC, Ma G, Lam KW, Leung KY, Pun TC, et al. Continued reduction in the incidence of birth trauma and birth asphyxia related to instrumental deliveries after the study period: was this the Hawthorne effect? Eur J Obstet Gynecol Reprod Biol. 2007,130(2):165-8.
2. Warke C, Malik S, Chokhandre M, Saboo A. Birth injuries—a review of incidence, perinatal risk factors and outcome. Bombay Hosp J 2012;54(2):202-8.
3. Ray S, Mondal R, Samanta M, Hazra A, Sabui TK, Debnath A, et al. Prospective study of neonatal birth trauma: Indian perspective. J Clin Neonatol 2016;5(2):91-5.
4. Rosenberg A. Traumatic birth injury. NeoReviews 2003;4 (10):e270-76.
5. Rodd C, Schwieger-Briel A, Hagmann C; Newborn Brain Society Guidelines and Publications Committee. Subcutaneous fat necrosis associated with hypercalcemia in neonates with neonatal encephalopathy treated with therapeutic hypothermia. Semin Fetal Neonatal Med. 2021;26(4):101269.
6. Uchil D, Arulkumaran S. Neonatal subgaleal hemorrhage and its relationship to delivery by vacuum extraction. Obstet Gynecol Surv 2003;58(10):687-93.
7. Pollina J, Dias MS, Li V, Kachurek D, Arbesman M. Cranial birth injuries in term newborn infants. Pediatr Neurosurg 2001;35(3):113-9.
8. Fuloria M, Kreiter S. The newborn examination: part 1. Emergencies and common abnormalities involving the skin, head, neck, chest and respiratory and cardiovascular systems. Am Fam Physician 2003;65(1):61-8.
9. Hughes CA, Harle EH, Milmor G, Bala R, Martorell A. Birth trauma on the head and neck. Arch Otolaryngol Head Neck Surg. 1999;125(2):193-9.
10. Evans-Jones G, Kay SP, Weindling AM, Cranny G, Ward A, Bradshaw A, et al. Congenital brachial palsy: incidence, causes, and outcome in the United Kingdom and Republic of Ireland. Arch Dis Child Fetal Neonatal Ed. 2003,88(3):185-9.

2.7 Low Birth Weight

Suman Rao PN, Bandlamudi Lakshmi Parvathi

INTRODUCTION

Low birth weight (LBW) is defined as weight at birth below 2.5 kg. LBW comprises two categories of babies—preterm infants and infants who are small for gestational age (SGA; growth-restricted) **(Table 2.7.1)**. LBW infants have a 20-fold higher risk of mortality compared to normal-weight neonates. They also have a higher incidence of neonatal morbidities, childhood growth failure, and adult health problems. Despite substantial progress in the last decade, the survival, growth, and neurodevelopment of LBW infants remain concerning in many countries. The care of preterm and LBW infants is a global priority.[1]

EPIDEMIOLOGY

"*Small vulnerable newborns*" is a term introduced in The Lancet in 2023 to encompass all newborns "*born too soon*" (<37 weeks' gestation), "*born too small*" (SGA, LBW babies, or both), and "*born too small and soon*" **(Fig. 2.7.1)**.[2] Babies born with these vulnerabilities are at an increased risk for a multitude of adverse health conditions throughout their lifespan. These vulnerabilities account for 55.3% of all neonatal deaths.

The global incidence of LBW was 14.7% in the year 2020, whereas the incidence in India has decreased from 22% (NFHS-3) to 17.29% (NFHS-4). While LBW infants constitute <20% of the births, 60–80% of newborns who die are premature and/or LBW.[3]

TABLE 2.7.1: Classification based on birth weight and gestational age.

Birth weight	***Group***
<2.5 kg	Low birth weight (LBW)
<1.5 kg	Very low birth weight (VLBW)
<1 kg	Extremely low birth weight (ELBW)
Gestation age	***Group***
Born at 37 0/7–41 6/7 weeks	Term gestation
Born before 37 0/7 weeks	Preterm
Born before 32 0/7 weeks	Very preterm
Born before 28 0/7 weeks	Extremely preterm
Born at or after 42 0/7 weeks	Post-term
Birth weight and gestation age	***Group***
Birth weight is 10–90th percentile for that gestation age	Appropriate for gestational age
Birth weight is <10th percentile for that gestation age	Small for gestational age
Birth weight is ≥90th percentile for that gestation age	Large for gestational age

ETIOLOGY

Low birth weight is caused by fetal growth restriction (FGR), prematurity, or both. FGR results in SGA babies, that is, birth weight <10th percentile for the corresponding gestational age. Most of the postnatal complications are largely dependent on the etiology of LBW. The common causes for LBW are mentioned in **Table 2.7.2**.

DIAGNOSIS

Assessment of Gestation

The best assessment of gestational age is by a first-trimester ultrasound (US; dating scan). In the absence of a dating scan, a reliable last menstrual period (LMP) or a later scan including a trimester scan can help determine gestational age. A postnatal examination can aid in the assessment of gestational age, for example, New Ballard Score **(Fig. 2.7.2)**; however, all have low accuracy of ±2.5 to 4 weeks. New Ballard Score is based on signs of neuromuscular maturity and physical maturity. Determination of gestational age is the first step to classify a baby as appropriate or small or large for gestational age.

The general appearance of an LBW preterm infant varies from an LBW growth-restricted infant and is detailed below **(Table 2.7.3)**:

- *General appearance:* Growth-restricted and SGA babies generally have an emaciated look and loose skin folds due to a lack of subcutaneous fat, which are prominent over the buttocks and thighs. They also appear plethoric in comparison to appropriately grown preterm babies.
- *Anthropometry:* Brain growth is normal in both preterm and FGR babies unless severely growth-restricted; hence, head circumference may be normal for gestational age in both groups, whereas chest circumference, length, and

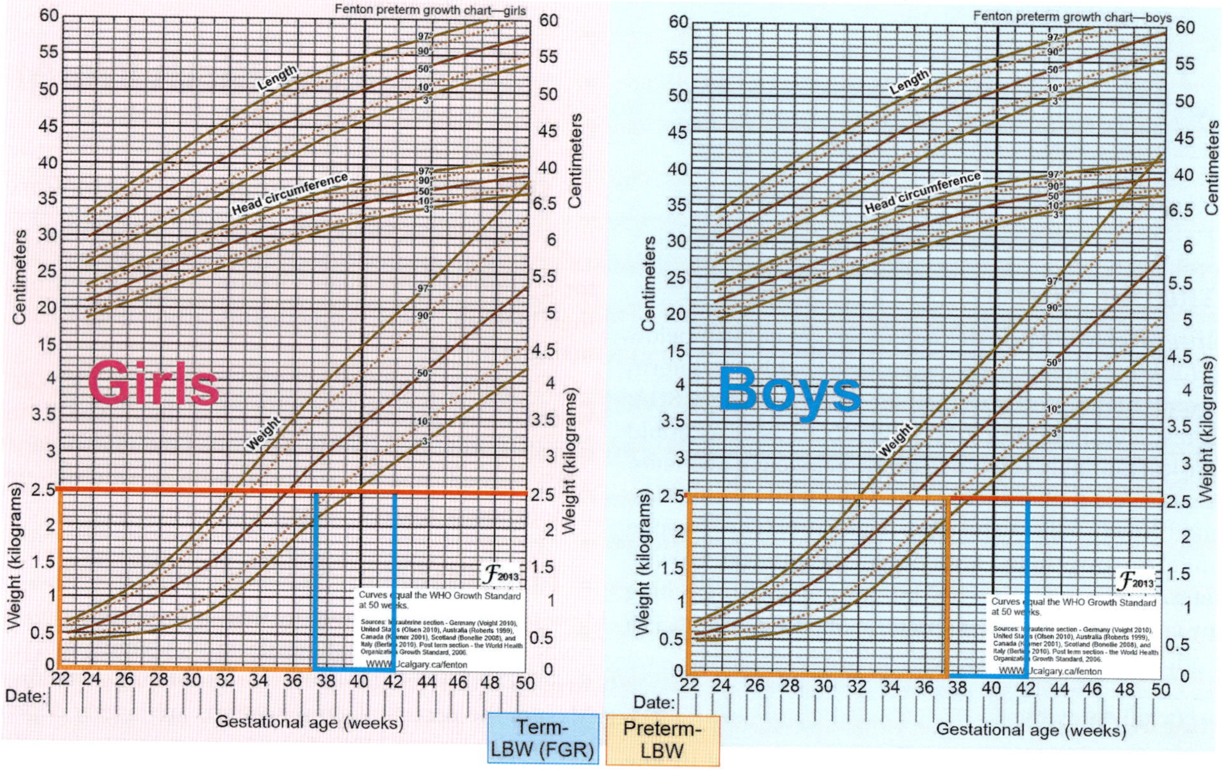

Fig. 2.7.1: Depiction of LBW on the growth chart. (FGR: fetal growth restriction; LBW: low birth weight)

TABLE 2.7.2: Etiology of low birth weight.

Fetal growth restriction	***Prematurity***
Maternal causes: • Maternal constitution—low pre-pregnancy weight, low pregnancy weight gain, short stature, and malnutrition • Chronic hypertension • Pre-eclampsia • Anemia • Substance abuse—tobacco, alcohol • High altitude	*Maternal causes:* • Short stature • Pre-eclampsia, gestational diabetes • Chronic malnutrition, anemia • Substance abuse • Infection • Teenage pregnancy, multiparity • Trauma • Iatrogenic
Placental causes: • Abnormal uterine anatomy, uterine fibroid • Incorrect cord insertion • Placental tumor • Chronic abruption • Placenta previa • Vasculitis • Cord anomalies (e.g., *single umbilical artery*)	*Uterine, placental causes:* • Cervical incompetence • Bicornuate uterus • Polyhydramnios • Placenta previa • Placental dysfunction • Placental abruption
Fetal causes: • Intrauterine infections • Chromosomal anomalies • Congenital malformations • Fetal anemia • Multiple gestation • Genetic causes	*Fetal causes:* • Fetal distress • Intrauterine infection • Chromosomal anomalies • Multiple gestation • Iatrogenic

abdominal circumference are severely compromised in growth-restricted babies.

- *Skin:* The skin is thin, edematous, and transparent with abundant lanugo in preterm babies whereas it is thick and keratinized with either sparse or lack of lanugo in term babies.
- *Ear cartilage:* The external ear or the pinna is soft and devoid of cartilage with poor re-coiling in preterm neonates. In a term baby, there is instant recoil.
- *Sole creases:* In preterm neonates, the sole creases range from barely perceptible to covering only anterior one-third of the sole, and in term neonates they extend over the anterior two-thirds or the entire sole.
- *External genitalia:* In males, the scrotum does not have rugae, and testes are not descended into the scrotum. In female infants, the labia are widely separated, not covering the labia minora, resulting in the prominent appearance of the clitoris in preterm neonates.
- *Neurological maturity:* Growth-restricted term neonates are more alert and have more neuromuscular maturity compared to preterm neonates.

CLINICAL FEATURES

Majority of LBW babies at birth are asymptomatic (**Table 2.7.4**). However, LBW is a high risk for several

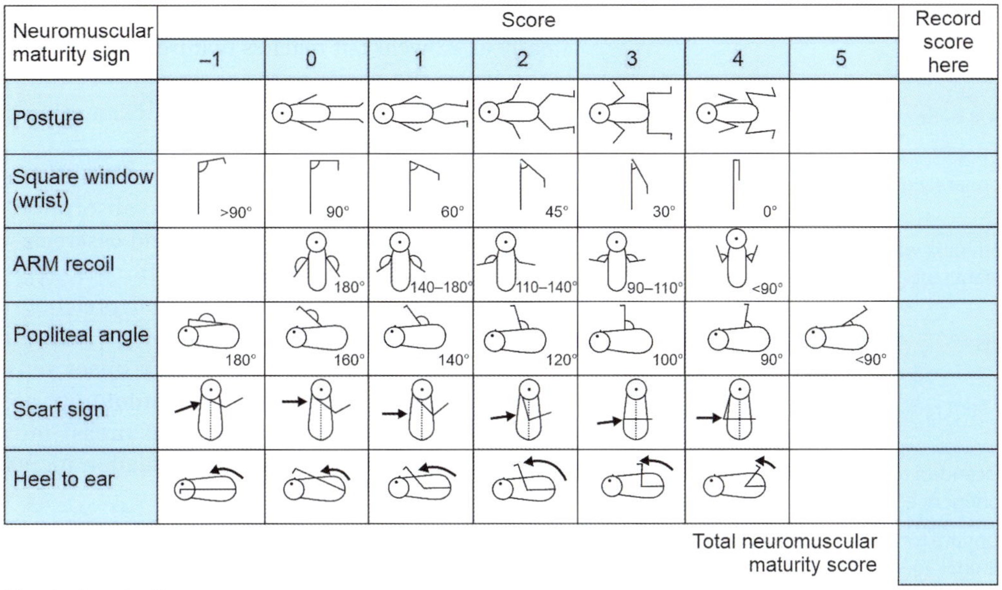

Neuromuscular maturity sign	Score							Record score here
	−1	0	1	2	3	4	5	
Posture								
Square window (wrist)	>90°	90°	60°	45°	30°	0°		
ARM recoil		180°	140–180°	110–140°	90–110°	<90°		
Popliteal angle	180°	160°	140°	120°	100°	90°	<90°	
Scarf sign								
Heel to ear								
							Total neuromuscular maturity score	

Physical maturity

Physical maturity sign	Score							Record score here
	−1	0	1	2	3	4	5	
Skin	Sticky friable transparent	Gelatinous red translucent	Smooth pink visible veins	Superficial peeling and/or rash, few veins	Cracking pale areas rare veins	Parchment deep cracking no vessels	Leathery cracked wrinkled	
Lanugo	None	Sparse	Abundant	Thinning	Bald areas	Mostly bald		
Plantar surface	Heel-toe 40–50 mm: −1 <40 mm: −2	>50 mm no crease	Faint red marks	Anterior transverse crease only	Creases ant. 2/3	Creases over entire sole		
Breast	Imperceptible	Barely perceptible	Flat areola no bud	Stippled areola 1–2 mm bud	Raised areola 3–4 mm bud	Full areola 5–10 mm bud		
Eye/Ear	Lids fused loosely: −1 Tightly: −2	Lids open pinna flat stays folded	Sl. curved pinna; soft slow recoil	Well-curved pina; soft but ready recoil	Formed and firm instant recoil	Thick cartilage ear stiff		
Genitals (male)	Scrotum flat smooth	Scrotum empty faint rugae	Testes in upper canal rare rugae	Testes descending few rugae	Testes down good rugae	Testes pendulous deep rugae		
Genitals (female)	Clitoris prominent and labia flat	Prominent clitoris and small labia minora	Prominent clitoris and enlarging minora	Majora and minora equally prominent	Majora large minora small	Majora cover clitoris and minora		
							Total physical maturity score	

Score
Neuromuscular_
Physical ____
Total_________

Maturity rating

Score	Weeks
−10	20
−5	22
0	24
5	26
10	28
15	30
20	32
25	34
30	36
35	38
40	40
45	42
50	44

Gestational age (weeks)
By dates_______
By ultrasound___
By exam_______

Fig. 2.7.2: New Ballard Score.
Source: Ballard JL, Khoury JC, Wedig K, et al. New Ballard score, expanded to include extremely premature infants. J Pediatr. 1991;119:417-423. Reprinted by permission of Dr Ballard and Mosby—Year Book. Inc.

problems at birth, during the neonatal, in infancy, and even into adulthood.

Hypothermia

Low birth weight babies irrespective of etiology are more prone to developing hypothermia due to the following deficient heat regulatory mechanisms:

- Immature skin and increased insensible water losses
- Increased surface area with a large head
- Poor subcutaneous fat and less brown fat
- Deficiency of catecholamine in the body
- Extended posture
- Increased number of interventions

The highest risk is immediately after birth and during transport to the neonatal intensive care unit (NICU). Each degree drop in admission temperature is associated with increased odds of mortality by 28% and late-onset sepsis by 11%.

TABLE 2.7.3: Comparison of the preterm LBW and the term growth-restricted LBW.

Characteristics	*Preterm neonates*	*Growth-restricted neonates*
General appearance	Small but appropriately grown	Emaciated look with loose skin fold and plethoric
Skin	Smooth pink with abundant lanugo	Thick keratinized with lack of subcutaneous fat
Ear cartilage	Deficient	Stiff, well-formed cartilage
Sole creases	No or faint red marks	Creases present over entire sole
External genitalia	Undescended testes or prominent clitoris	Testes in scrotum or majora cover minora
Anthropometry	Appropriate for gestational age	Less than expected for the gestational age
Neurological maturity	Lag as per maturity	Alert and mature

(LBW: low birth weight)

TABLE 2.7.4: Problems of low birth weight (LBW) infants.

Problems due to prematurity	*Problems due to fetal growth restriction*
• Hypothermia • Respiratory distress—respiratory distress syndrome (RDS), bronchopulmonary dysplasia (BPD) • Feeding problems—feed intolerance, necrotizing enterocolitis (NEC) • Jaundice • Metabolic—hypoglycemia, hypocalcemia, hyponatremia, hypernatremia, hyperkaliemia, hypomagnesemia • Increased susceptibility to infections • Patent ductus arteriosus (PDA) • Intraventricular hemorrhage (IVH) • Retinopathy of prematurity (ROP)	• Asphyxia • Meconium aspiration • Hypothermia • Metabolic—hypoglycemia, hypocalcemia • Hematological—polycythemia, thrombocytopenia, leukopenia • Intracranial hemorrhage (ICH) • NEC • Jaundice

Respiratory Distress

The main causes of respiratory distress at birth in the LBW neonate are:

- *Respiratory distress syndrome (RDS)* due to surfactant deficiency. The surfactant coats the alveoli and prevents them from collapsing. Though it is produced from as early as 22 weeks, it reaches mature levels only at term. The lower the gestational age, the greater the risk for RDS. Antenatal corticosteroids (dexamethasone or betamethasone) reduce the risk of RDS.
- *Transient tachypnea of the newborn (TTNB)* is due to delayed adaptation and delay in the absorption of the fluid from the alveoli. Prematurity and cesarean section without labor increase the risk of TTNB.
- *Pneumonia:* Prematurity due to preterm prelabor rupture of membranes (PPROM) or unexplained preterm labor are at risk of pneumonia and early onset sepsis. All LBW neonates are also at risk of community-acquired pneumonia. Bottle feeding, lack of breast milk, and traditional practices such as oil instillation increase the risk.
- *Meconium aspiration syndrome:* Intrauterine hypoxia and FGR increase the risk of meconium-stained amniotic fluid (MSAF) and MAS. Asphyxia also results in secondary surfactant deficiency and respiratory distress.

A careful history, examination, laboratory tests, and X-ray help in differentiating the different causes of respiratory distress. In addition, very preterm and extremely preterm infants are also at risk of needing prolonged respiratory support or oxygen beyond 36 weeks of postmenstrual age leading to chronic lung disease called *bronchopulmonary dysplasia (BPD).*

Asphyxia

Low birth weight due to FGR may not tolerate the normal stress of labor. Often, they pass meconium in utero, do not cry at birth, and may need resuscitation.

Hypoglycemia

Hypoglycemia is a common problem in LBW infants. Low stores, poor feeding, increased energy expenditure for maintaining temperature, respiratory distress, infection, and other problems predispose the LBW infant to hypoglycemia. Antenatal corticosteroids in the late preterm period also increase the risk of hypoglycemia. All LBW infants should be screened for hypoglycemia in the first 48 hours.

Jaundice

Jaundice is higher in preterm infants due to immaturity of the liver. While the activity of the enzyme uridine diphosphoglucuronyl transferase (UDP-GT) which is needed for conjugation of bilirubin is only 1% of adult value in a neonate, it is even lower in preterm infants. Preterm LBW infants are also prone to prolonged jaundice. Polycythemia in FGR infants also contributes to hyperbilirubinemia. All infants should be screened for neonatal hyperbilirubinemia.

Feeding Problems

Feeding problems are common in preterm LBW infants. Though swallowing is well established and sucking is present even at 28 weeks, the sucking, swallowing, and breathing coordination is well established only by term. Preterm infants may need alternative methods of feeding for the first few days of birth. While feed intolerance is common, the dreaded complication in preterm neonates is necrotizing enterocolitis (NEC). NEC, a disease of multifactorial etiology due to immature gut, dysbiosis, hypoxic injury, infection, and hyperosmolar feeds, presents with abdominal distension, vomiting, altered aspirates, blood in stools, and systemically with apnea, poor perfusion, and the metabolic triad of refractory hyponatremia, thrombocytopenia, and thrombocytopenia.

Infections

The risk of infections and succumbing to infections is highest in preterm infants. Many factors contribute to the risk of infections including immaturity of the skin, mucosa, and immune function, limited enteral feedings and less exposure to breast milk, and increased interventions. They are at risk of both early and late-onset sepsis. PPROM and unexplained preterm labor both predispose the preterm infant to early onset sepsis. Healthcare-associated infections are also more common in preterm infants due to the increased number of interventions such as lines, intravenous fluids, respiratory support, and prolonged stay in the NICU.

Other Complications of Prematurity

Intraventricular hemorrhage (IVH), patent ductus arteriosus (PDA), retinopathy of prematurity (ROP), and periventricular leukomalacia (PVL) are common problems of preterm LBW infants. The smaller the gestational age, the greater the risk of IVH. It typically starts in the germinal matrix which is the highly vascularized area adjacent to the ventricles, but may extend into the ventricles and also into the parenchyma. The risk is highest in the first 3 days of life. The presence of IVH is an additional risk factor for abnormal neurodevelopmental outcomes.

The immature ductus arteriosus may not close immediately after birth in the preterm infant, resulting in left-to-right shunting of blood, contributing to respiratory distress and cardiopulmonary instability.

Retinopathy of prematurity is the most common preventable cause of blindness in children. The retinal vascularization is immature in the preterm infant, and ROP screening should be done in all preterm infants <34 weeks or <2,000 g if the gestation is not known.

MANAGEMENT[4-6]

Antenatal Interventions

Women with a high likelihood of preterm birth within 7 days from 24 to 34 weeks of gestation should receive a course of antenatal corticosteroids (ACS), 4 doses of dexamethasone 12 hours apart, or 2 doses of betamethasone 24 hours apart. ACS improves survival and reduces the risk of common morbidities such as RDS, IVH, BPD, NEC, PVL, and neonatal sepsis.[7] Magnesium sulfate has also been shown to provide neuroprotection to the fetus when administered during active labor to women at <32 weeks of gestation. Antibiotics are indicated in PPROM.

Antenatal counseling, especially for the periviable fetus, is helpful for shared decision-making. It is crucial to communicate with the obstetric team about administering antenatal steroids and intravenous (IV) magnesium sulfate infusion for neuroprotection in cases of preterm delivery. Finally, preparations including organizing a team with the roles and responsibilities of each team member prior to being assigned and the arrangement of resuscitation equipment are required.

Care at Birth

The first hour of birth, called the "golden hour", is the period during which the newly born infant is resuscitated and stabilized. Interventions include strategies for thermal protection, establishment of the functional residual capacity (FRC) of the lung in the least-invasive manner, and early initiation of feeding. An organized team with well-defined roles of each team member is crucial for successful resuscitation.

Delayed Cord Clamping

For all LBW and preterm infants, delayed cord clamping (>30 seconds) is recommended to ensure placental transfusion. In infants >28 weeks who require resuscitation, intact cord milking three times before clamping the cord is an alternate method for rapidly achieving placental transfusion.

Thermoregulation

Maintaining normal temperature at birth is a key aspect of LBW resuscitation. All infants including LBW infants should be placed in skin-to-skin contact for at least 60–90 minutes after birth. In infants requiring resuscitation, the baby is placed under a servo-controlled radiant warmer with the temperature probe attached to the skin, or if <32 weeks, the infant is placed inside a plastic bag to reduce evaporative heat losses. In all LBW infants, kangaroo mother care (KMC) should be initiated immediately after birth by placing the baby in between the breasts of the mother in a skin-to-skin contact position with the head covered. The temperature of the neonate at the end of the golden hour in the delivery room is a quality indicator of care at birth.

Respiratory Support in the Delivery Room

The goal of respiratory support is to help establish FRC in the lung to ensure adequate gas exchange. This is facilitated by assisting ventilation in the least invasive manner and providing just the right amount of oxygen. Positive pressure ventilation (PPV) should be delivered if the neonate is apneic or gasping or if the heart rate is <100 bpm. T-piece is preferred over a bag and mask for delivering PPV in preterm neonates. Spontaneously breathing preterm infants who have a high risk of RDS should be supported with continuous positive airway pressure (CPAP) with a T-piece resuscitator. An oxygen blender is essential for the preterm infant to initiate resuscitation with FiO_2 between 21 and 30% and a pulse oximeter to target the Neonatal Resuscitation Program (NRP) saturation target and prevent oxygen toxicity.

Management in Special Newborn Care Unit and Neonatal Intensive Care Unit[8-10]

Low birth weight neonates who need admission to the special care unit as per National Health Mission (NHM) guidelines include those with birth weight <1,800 g, gestation <34 weeks, and any sick neonate.

Kangaroo Mother Care

Kangaroo mother care for preterm and LBW infants is the foundation of small and sick newborn care (*see* Chapter 2.4).[6] It includes continuous and prolonged (8–24 h/day, for as many hours as possible) skin-to-skin contact with support for exclusive breastfeeding or breastmilk feeding. It should be started immediately after birth and it facilitates early planned discharge from the facility with adequate follow-up. The baby is placed in between the breasts of the mother with the baby's head turned to one side with slight extension maintaining the airway open and allowing eye-to-eye contact between mother and baby. The hips should be abducted in a frog position and arms should be flexed. The baby's abdomen should be at the level of the mother's abdomen in a skin-to-skin contact position with the head and feet covered.

When not in KMC, the baby should be covered with at least two to three layers of clothes, socks, mittens, and cap. KMC not only maintains physiologic stability and euthermia but also reduces episodes of hypothermia, hypoglycemia, apnea, infection, and associated mortality in LBW neonates. In addition to a high-impact intervention to reduce mortality, it is also the best form of providing developmentally supportive care.

Skin-to-skin contact is best provided by the mother; the father and other family members also can provide KMC to support the mother to provide continuous KMC. To provide early and continuous KMC for the sick baby, the intensive care unit needs to be transformed into a mother–newborn ICU with a bed for the mother to enable her to stay with her baby on a 24/7 basis. Once the baby is stable and no longer requires intensive care, the baby and mother may be shifted to the KMC ward **(Figs. 2.7.3A and B)**. Thermal care for the sick neonate in the SNCU is provided with either a radiant warmer or an incubator **(Figs. 2.7.4A and B)**.

Regular monitoring of axillary temperature at least once every 15 minutes during the first hour and later every 6–8 hours should be carried out in all hospitalized LBW infants.

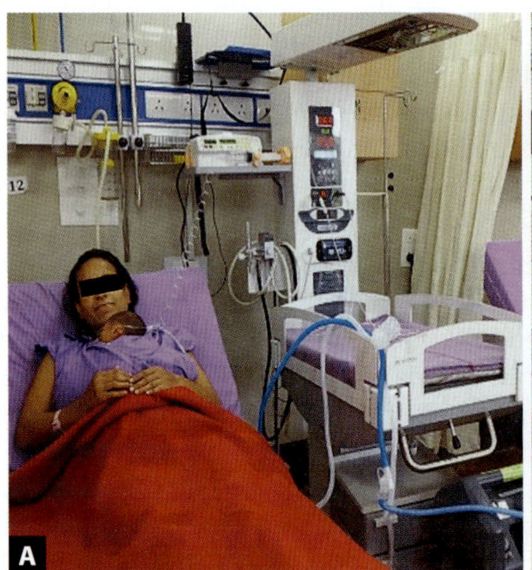

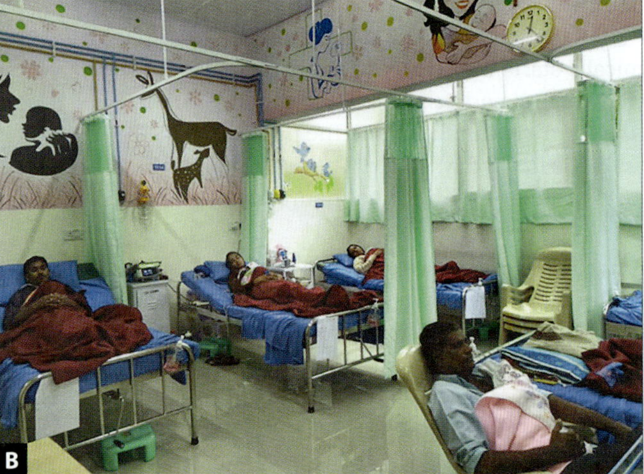

Figs. 2.7.3A and B: (A) Mother–newborn intensive care unit (Safdarjung Hospital, New Delhi); (B) Kangaroo mother care (KMC) ward (St. John's Medical College Hospital, Bengaluru).

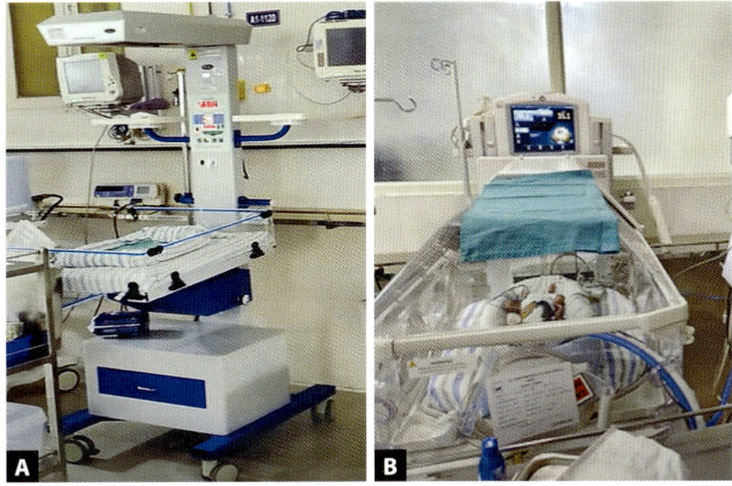

Figs. 2.7.4A and B: Thermal care for LBW in a (A) radiant warmer or (B) incubator. (LBW: low birth weight)

Respiratory Support and Safe Oxygen Use

Continuous positive airway pressure is the cornerstone of respiratory support for the preterm infant **(Fig. 2.7.5)**. Starting CPAP early establishes effective FRC and avoids the need for intubation and mechanical ventilation. Spontaneously breathing preterm neonates with respiratory distress are most effectively treated with CPAP. Bubble CPAP is preferred to ventilator CPAP. If the need for oxygen is high (FiO_2 >30%), surfactant administration is indicated. Surfactant is administered either via LISA (less invasive surfactant administration) or "InSurE" (intubate, surfactant administration, and extubate) approach. Infants on respiratory support should be monitored by a pulse oximeter and saturations are maintained between 90% and 95%.

Caffeine is recommended for the treatment of apnea or can be considered for prophylaxis in preterm infants <34 weeks. It is also indicated for extubation of preterm infants.

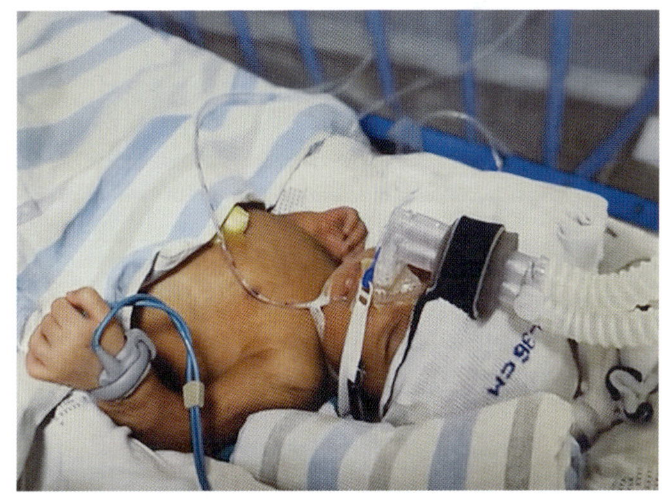

Fig. 2.7.5: Continuous positive airway pressure.

Intravenous Fluids and Enteral Feeding

Intravenous fluids are not a routine mode of fluid intake in either preterm or growth-restricted but are only considered in specific conditions where babies are sick, unable to accept or tolerate enteral feeds, and for hypoglycemia requiring IV fluid for correction. The fluid requirements volumes are given in **Table 2.7.5**. Sodium and potassium supplementation should be considered only after 48 hours of birth if unable to give enteral feeds.

The goal of nutritional management of the LBW neonate should be to achieve full enteral nutrition as soon as possible **(Figs. 2.7.6A and B)**. Mother's own milk (MOM) is the best milk for all infants including the preterm infant and the mother should be adequately counseled and supported to provide exclusive breastmilk feeding for her LBW infant. When MOM is not available, the next choice is donor human milk (DHM). When both MOM and DHM are not available, nutrient-enriched preterm formula may be considered.

Breastmilk should be started as soon as possible after birth. The preterm infant should be put to the breast as soon as possible after birth. Scheduled feeding may be considered rather than responsive feeding for preterm infants <34 weeks' gestation till discharge. Feed volumes can be increased by up to 30 mL/kg/day. The guidelines for providing enteral feeds to LBW neonates are given in **Table 2.7.6**.

Neonates can undergo a gradual transition from gastric feeding to spoon feeding and then on to breastfeeding. In infants <34 weeks, the transition from tube to breast can be facilitated by allowing the infant to suck on the empty breast of the mother (nonnutritive sucking).

TABLE 2.7.5: Fluid therapy for the LBW infant.

Fluids (mL/kg/day)	*Day 1*	*Day 2*	*Day 3–5*	*Day 6–7*	*> Day 7*
<1,000 g	80–100	100–120	120–140	140–160	160
1,000–1,500 g	80	100	120–140	140–150	150
>1,500 g	60	80	100–120	140	150

(LBW: low birth weight)

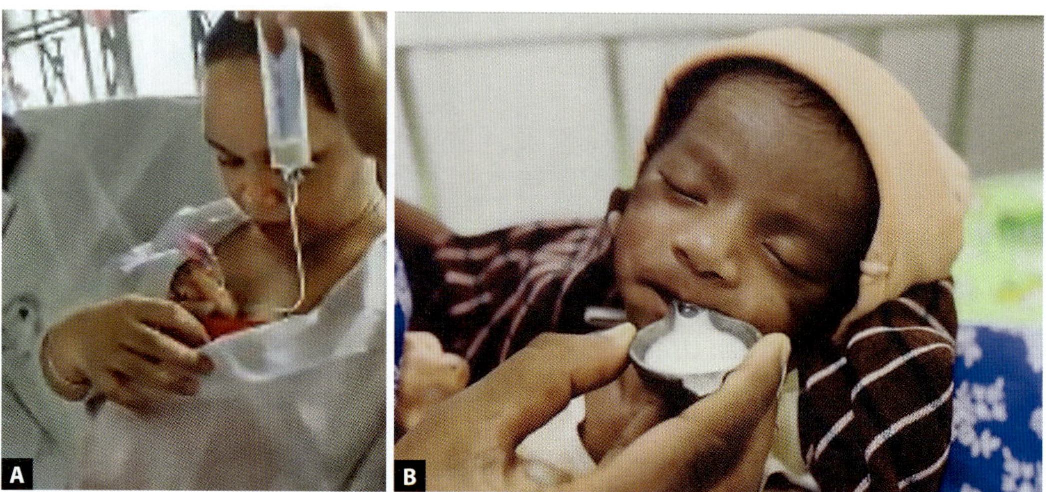

Figs. 2.7.6A and B: Alternate methods of feeding LBW. (A) Gavage feeding; (B) Paladai feeding. (LBW: low birth weight)

TABLE 2.7.6: Enteral feeding of the LBW.

Birth weight (g)	*<1,200*	*1,200–1,800*	*>1,800*
Gestation (weeks)	<30	30–34	>34
Initial feeding	IVF, try gavage feeds, if not sick	Gavage, try *katori*-spoon/*palladai* if not sick	Breastfeeding, if unsatisfactory, give *katori*-spoon/*palladai* feeds
After 1–3 days	Gavage	*Katori*-spoon/*palladai*	Breastfeeding
Later (1–3 weeks)	*Katori*-spoon/*palladai*	Breastfeeding	Breastfeeding
After some more time (4–6 weeks)	Breastfeeding	Breastfeeding	Breastfeeding

(IVF: in vitro fertilization; LBW: low birth weight)

Daily assessment of the sucking efforts of the neonate will provide an indication of when and how fast the transition from one mode to another mode of feeding should be undertaken. Also, the baby should be daily assessed for any signs of feed intolerance like abdominal distension, bilious vomiting, blood in stools, and new-onset systemic symptoms. The presence of such signs in the baby may prompt cessation of feeding and initiating investigations to rule out necrotizing enterocolitis—a multifactorial disease of the gastrointestinal tract affecting very preterm infants.

Supplementation and Fortification

Supplementation should be started as soon as the infants receive at least 120-150 mL/kg/day of enteral feeds with exclusive breast milk **(Table 2.7.7)**. The use of human milk fortifiers (HMF) can be considered in preterm LBW infants with birth weight <1,800 g and receiving enteral feeds of at least 50-80 mL/kg/day. However, in resource-limited settings, it is used only for those infants who fail to gain weight despite adequate breast milk feeding. Weight gain at the rate of about 15-20 g/day is considered adequate. Excessive weight loss or inadequate weight gain indicates inadequate feeding, cold stress, excessive insensible water loss, or systemic illness.

Monitoring

All LBW infants should be monitored frequently—at least 6-8 hourly. Sick infants may need continuous monitoring. In addition to temperature, vital parameters such as heart rate,

TABLE 2.7.7: Supplements for the LBW.

Vitamin D	400–1,000 IU/day until 1 year of age
Calcium	120–200 mg/kg/day
Phosphorus	60–100 mg/kg/day
Iron	• 2–3 mg/kg/day • Start from 2 to 4 weeks of life and given until 1 year of age
Multivitamin	1 mL/day until 6 months to 1 year of age

(LBW: low birth weight)

respiratory rate, saturations, and sugar monitoring to detect hypoglycemia are essential. They are also more prone to hypocalcemia.

Prevention of Infections

Low birth weight infants, especially preterm infants, are more at risk for infection. In addition to antenatal risk factors such as PPROM, multiple interventions, respiratory support, immaturity of the immune system and skin, delayed feeding, and separation from the mother are risk factors. Early enteral breast milk feeding, colostrum swabbing, KMC, strict adherence to hand hygiene and infection-control protocols, probiotics, avoidance and care of central lines, noninvasive respiratory support, and antibiotic stewardship all contribute to reducing infections in the very preterm infant.

Developmentally Supportive Care

At every opportunity, efforts should focus on minimizing pain and stress and promoting optimal brain growth by providing developmentally supportive care. These include noise reduction, gentle handling, clustering of procedures, attention to skincare, KMC, and early parental participation. Stimulation and early intervention harness the plasticity of the preterm brain and improve outcomes. Promoting family involvement and support to care for their infants includes education, counseling, and discharge preparation. Postdischarge, home visits by trained healthcare workers are recommended.

Discharge and Follow-up

Low birth weight neonates can be considered for discharge, if the infant has had a smooth transition to breastfeeding or breast and spoon/*paladai* feeds, is gaining weight consistently for at least 3 days, maintains temperature when being cared for by the mother in KMC, there is no active illness, and mother is confident. Assessment of the home environment prior to discharge should be done for optimal neurodevelopmental support. Regular follow-up after discharge is essential for monitoring growth, development, screen for ROP, and hearing. After discharge from the hospital, babies should be regularly followed up until 2–3 years of age in a high-risk developmental follow-up clinic.

Thrifty Phenotype (Barker Hypothesis) and Developmental Origin of Health and Disease

Early-life environment has long-term effects on the latter life and the LBW infant is at risk for developing the metabolic syndrome of diabetes, hypercholesterolemia, coronary artery disease, and diabetes mellitus which gave birth to the concept of "developmental origin of health and disease (DOHaD)."

PROGNOSIS

The mortality of LBW babies is directly related to their birth weight and gestational maturity. The lesser the weight and gestation, the poorer will be the prognosis. In general, with optimal care, most LBW babies have no major neurodevelopmental handicaps.

REFERENCES

1. World Health Organization. (2022). WHO recommendations for care of the preterm or low birth weight infant. [online] Available from https://www.who.int/publications/i/item/9789240058262 [Last accessed October, 2024].
2. Ashorn P, Black RE, Lawn JE, Ashorn U, Klein N, Hofmeyr J, et al. The Lancet small vulnerable newborn series: science for a healthy start. Lancet. 2020;396(10253):743-45.
3. Girotra S, Mohan N, Malik M, Roy S, Basu S. Prevalence and determinants of low birth weight in India: findings from a nationally representative cross-sectional survey (2019-21). Cureus. 2023;15(3):e36717.
4. Embleton ND, Moltu SJ, Lapillonne A, van den Akker CHP, Carnielli V, Fusch C, et al. Enteral nutrition in preterm infants (2022): a position paper from the ESPGHAN committee on nutrition and invited experts. J Pediatr Gastroenterol Nutr. 2023;76(2):248-68.
5. Sharma D, Shastri S, Sharma P. Intrauterine growth restriction: antenatal and postnatal aspects. Clin Med Insights Pediatr. 2016;10:67-83.
6. World Health Organization. (2023). Kangaroo mother care: a transformative innovation in health care. Global position paper. [online] Available from https://www.who.int/publications/i/item/9789240072657. [Last accessed October, 2024].
7. World Health Organization. (2023). World health statistics 2023: monitoring health for the SDGs, sustainable development goals. [online] Available from https://www.who.int/publications/i/item/9789240074323 [Last accessed October, 2024].
8. World Health Organization. (2022). WHO recommendations on antenatal corticosteroids for improving preterm birth outcomes. [online] Available from https://www.who.int/publications/i/item/9789240057296 [Last accessed October, 2024].
9. National Neonatology Forum India. Clinical practice guidelines NNF India; Feeding of low birth weight, January 2020. [online] Available from https://www.nnfi.org/assests/pdf/cpg-guidelines/Feeding%20of%20LBW-Key%20Recommendations.pdf [Last accessed October, 2024].
10. Operational guide for facility based care of sick neonate at referral. New Delhi: Ministry of Health and Family Welfare, Government of India; 2023.

2.8 Parent Counseling

Ranjan Kumar Pejaver

INTRODUCTION

Parent counseling is the process of providing assistance and guidance by giving information to the parents at various points during the perinatal period. It is the art of presenting facts enabling the parents to make the decisions. The counseling should be nondirective and nonjudgmental.[1]

WHICH PARENTS NEED COUNSELING?

Preconception

There is a history of recurrent pregnancy loss, stillbirths, or neonatal deaths. Parents would want to know why that has happened and if is there a way of preventing it in the next pregnancy.

Health of Previous Child

A previous child of the parents or any members of the immediate family of either of the spouses may be suffering from an inherited disorder, congenital abnormalities, and/or developmental delay and may have dysmorphic features. Parents would like to know information like what are the chances of the next pregnancy resulting in the same.

Age and Health of Parents

Parents are elderly and may be suffering from conditions such as severe diabetes mellitus, hypertension, and systemic diseases. They would like to know how these diseases would affect the next pregnancy and baby.

Abnormal Prenatal Ultrasound Scan

Prenatal ultrasound has revealed some congenital abnormalities or findings such as growth restriction, oligo or polyhydramnios, and the need of prospective parents for information regarding the seriousness of the same and the fate of the current pregnancy and the fetus.[2]

At Delivery

The baby is receiving extensive resuscitation and does not seem to be responding. They may need counseling regarding the continuation or stopping of resuscitation measures.[1]

Immediately After Delivery

The baby needed extensive resuscitation, has survived, and what are the repercussions? The baby is extremely low birth weight (LBW) or premature, or in case of prenatally undiagnosed abnormalities, parents may need information regarding the management and prognosis.

Neonatal Period

A preterm infant has had a stormy stay in the intensive care unit (ICU), resulting in severe damage to various organ systems. Intact survival is unlikely.[3] Parents may need information regarding possible sequelae, further continuation of care, or withdrawal of care.[1]

Predischarge Counseling

Parents of neonatal ICU graduates would need information regarding danger signs to watch out for, follow-up plans, and other instructions such as feeding, medications, immunizations, etc., or in a case of postoperative state.[4] They need information regarding home care and any follow-up procedures—timing, cost, and prognosis.

Bereavement Counseling

If a baby has expired or stillbirth has occurred, counseling is needed. Appropriate support for the grieving process and post-death arrangements should also be provided. The development of uniform clinical guidelines on "End of life Decisions (EoLDs)" would alleviate some subjectivity and enforce clarity, consistency, and transparency, enhancing parental trust.[5]

GENERAL PRINCIPLES OF PARENT COUNSELING

A counseling should be conducted in a quiet and comfortable room. It should be conducted by a senior member of the team. It is preferable that the session is conducted in a language the parents understand. If necessary, a reliable interpreter may be used.

It should be done in strict privacy, preferably with both parents being present. Some key decision-makers in the family or supportive elders may be allowed to be present with the permission of the parents. It is good to involve nurses and other specialists who are involved or likely to be involved in the care of the infant.

A counseling should be nondirective and nonjudgmental. Be careful not to hurt the local, traditional, family, cultural, and religious sentiments of the parents. Counseling provides information in simple and nontechnical language. The depth of the information should commensurate with the educational level and the understanding ability of the listeners.

Be patient; be ready to repeat the advice; and give time to the parents to understand, think, and then convey the decisions. Calmly answer the queries and be sympathetic. As they are overwhelmed by the situation, they are confused, less receptive, and may not be able to quickly process the information given. If there is any written material relevant to the discussion, it is helpful and may be given to the parents.

Physicians' and parents' shared decision-making should be based on direct and open communication sensitive to their culture and appropriate for their level of understanding complex issues regarding medical conditions, prognosis, and treatment options.

It is a good habit to summarize the discussion and decisions arrived at; write it down and take the signatures of the parents after they have read it. Signatures of the counselor and witness are also important. Many centers have started video recording the counseling sessions, informing the parents about the same.

COUNSELING: SPECIFIC TECHNICAL ASPECTS

Diagnosis

Wherever applicable, diagnosis should be known as far as possible. Where it is not known, the same should be conveyed to the parents. If a visit to a higher center would be helpful, then sufficient information about that should be supplied.

Counseling on Genetic Aspects

Family history, pedigree construction, knowledge of the prevalence of the disorder, modes of inheritance, and recurrence chances should be ascertained.

Statistical Data Supports

It should be known and quoted where necessary, for example, the survival percentage of very LBW infants and premature infants. It will guide the parents to decide roughly on the outcome and whether to seek transfer to higher centers, if available.

Resuscitation

Resuscitation is not successful all the time. Discontinuation is justified, if there are no signs of life (no heartbeat and no spontaneous respirations) after 10 minutes of full resuscitation. Parents should be informed, if possible, about the progress and status of the baby at various steps. In major congenital abnormalities incompatible with life, discussion with parents is essential before taking the decision to discontinue resuscitation. A concurrence of another colleague is ideal.

Withdrawal of Care

For babies with poor prognosis, decisions about treatment should be made jointly by the healthcare team and the infant's family with the best interests of the baby, on the basis of the infant's clinical condition including antenatal risk factors, the risks, discomforts, side effects, potential benefits, and the probabilities of death and severe disability based on the best available evidence.[3] Clinical indicators, laboratory investigations, and imaging studies showing bad prognostic signs should be documented and shown to parents. Decisions such as "do not resuscitate," "withdrawal of care," and "discharge against medical advice by parents" warrant due deliberation, proper documentation, and concurrence of authorized personnel and parents in black and white.[6] Legal sanction for any of the above does not exist at the present time!

Pregnancy Loss, Stillbirth, and Death of a Neonate

This is devastating to the family. There is a feeling of loss, guilt, shame, inadequacy, and anger in the parents. Compassionate counseling is required stressing on the point that neither of the parents is responsible for it. It may be essential that a diagnosis be arrived at in view of future pregnancies, even though it may not help in the current one. Especially, if genetic disorders or metabolic defects are suspected, investigations such as chromosomal analysis, autopsy, infantogram, clinical photographs, tissue biopsy, blood, and other body fluid analyses should be done. Informed consent of parents is needed for this. In cases of neonatal deaths, a meeting with the parents should be arranged after a few weeks when they would be more receptive having gone through the stages of bereavement, and the results of all investigations are available to have more fruitful counseling. Future reproductive options, perinatal preventive strategies such as folic acid consumption, investigations, prenatal management as high-risk pregnancy, planning of delivery, and neonatal care could be discussed.

Visits by a social worker to the abode of the unfortunate couple at least during the first few months after the tragedy to counsel will be very beneficial.

Parental counseling is an important aspect of perinatal care. It should be given its due priority. It is ideal that every unit has a person who has had some formal training in counseling.

REFERENCES

1. American Academy of Pediatrics Committee on Fetus and Newborn. The initiation or withdrawal of treatment for high-risk newborns. Pediatrics. 1995;96(2):362-3.
2. Lemos A, Soares H, Guimarães H. Decision-making at the limit of viability. Minerva Pediatr (Torino). 2021;73(4):348-62.
3. Freer Y, Lyon A, Stenson B, Russell C. BabyLink—improving communication among clinicians and with parents with babies in intensive care. Br J Healthcare Comput Inform Manag. 2005;22(2):34-6.
4. Baker K, Kuhlman T, Magliaro B. Home ward bound: discharge teaching for parents of newborns with special needs. Nursing Clin North Am. 1989;24(3):655-64.
5. Leslie L, Harris LL, Douma C. End-of-life care in the NICU: a family-centered approach. NeoReviews. 2010;11(4):e194-9.
6. Munson D. Withdrawal of mechanical ventilation in pediatric and neonatal intensive care units. Pediatr Clin North Am. 2007;54(5):773-85.

2.9 Thermoregulation in Newborn

Sindhu Sivanandan

INTRODUCTION

Thermoregulation is the ability to balance heat production and heat loss to maintain an optimal body temperature. Preterm, low birth weight (LBW), sick neonates, and those with intrauterine growth restriction (IUGR) are at a higher risk of thermal fluctuations, hypothermia, and/or hyperthermia due to poor thermoregulatory responses. There is presently inadequate awareness among healthcare professionals (HCP) regarding thermal instability as a risk to newborns. Health providers can prevent adverse conditions and provide a thermoneutral neonatal environment by understanding the physiological mechanisms of heat loss and thermogenesis in neonates.

DEFINITION

The World Health Organization (WHO) defines normal body temperature as between 36.5°C and 37.5°C and hypothermia as body temperature below 36.5°C.[1] Hypothermia is further categorized as mild (36.0-36.4°C), moderate (32.0-35.9°C), or severe (<32°C). Hyperthermia, defined as body temperature > 37.5°C, is uncommon in newborns.

EPIDEMIOLOGY

Neonatal hypothermia is a significant contributor to morbidity and mortality. The incidence varies widely based on the definition of hypothermia used and institutional thermoregulatory practices (32–85%). Nearly 1 in 5 infants born in health facilities experience hypothermia and 1 in 20 infants experience moderate-to-severe hypothermia. Infants with lower birth weight and gestational age, along with mothers of Black and Asian racial and ethnic backgrounds, exhibit the highest likelihood across all hypothermia classifications. This implies that, beyond inherent biological risk factors for hypothermia, potentially adjustable structural and social determinants may also exert significant influences.[2] Preterm, LBW, and sick neonates are at a higher risk of hypothermia. In preterm neonates, hypothermia has a dose-response relationship and is associated with a higher risk of death, intraventricular hemorrhage (IVH), bronchopulmonary dysplasia (BPD), and retinopathy of prematurity (ROP).[3] Mortality increases by 28% per 1°C decrease in temperature below the normal temperature.

ETIOPATHOGENESIS

A thermoneutral environment (TNE) is an environment in which a neonate maintains a normal body temperature while minimizing energy expenditure and oxygen consumption. Neonates maintained in TNE demonstrate better growth, respiratory stability, decreased oxygen requirements, glucose stability, and lower mortality. Thermoneutral zone temperatures vary based on the gestation, birth weight, and age of the neonate. It is 32–35°C for term infants and as high as 35°C for extremely preterm infants.

In utero, the fetal temperature is well maintained by maternal homeostasis. After birth, the baby is exposed to a cold environment, and heat exchange occurs between the neonate and the surrounding environment through four mechanisms—evaporation, conduction, convection, and radiation **(Fig. 2.9.1)**.

1. *Conduction:* Heat loss from the infant to the surface in direct contact with the body. Examples include cold mattresses, a cold weighing scale, and wet linen.
2. *Convection:* Heat loss from the infant to the surrounding area due to moving air that is cold and dry. Examples include air currents due to a fan, air conditioning, open door, or window.
3. *Evaporation:* Heat loss from the infant's skin by evaporation of water (amniotic fluid). This is the most significant source of heat loss at birth. Examples include a baby lying on a wet cloth.
4. *Radiation:* Heat loss from the infant to cooler objects without being in direct contact.

Heat loss occurs rapidly at birth. During the first 10–20 minutes, the neonate may lose enough heat for the body temperature to fall by 2–4°C if appropriate measures are not taken.

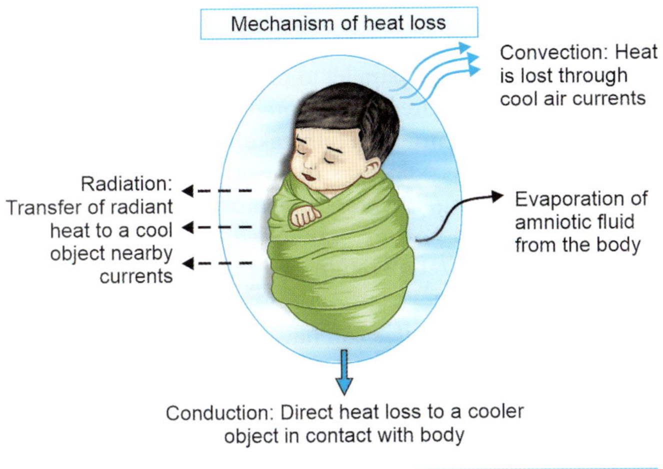

Mechanism of heat production—nonshivering thermogenesis

Anterior hypothalamus → Sympathetic nerves—norepinephrine → Brown fat: Triglycerides → Glycerol + fatty acids → Oxidation → Heat production

Skin → Afferent → Anterior hypothalamus

Fig. 2.9.1: Mechanism of heat loss and heat production in the neonate.

Preterm and LBW neonates are at a higher risk of heat loss and hypothermia due to the following risk factors:[4]

- Large body surface area compared to weight resulting in higher insensible water loss
- Immature skin characterized by the absence of a competent stratum corneum leading to higher transepidermal water loss
- Decreased subcutaneous fat offering less insulation
- Greater body water content and poorly developed metabolic mechanisms for responding to thermal stress

Risk Factors for Hypothermia

These are listed in **Table 2.9.1**.

Mechanism of Heat Production in Newborn

Heat production usually occurs by two mechanisms in neonates:

1. Muscular activity (shivering) is not a significant source of heat production in neonates as muscular activity is less.
2. Nonshivering or metabolic thermogenesis

Nonshivering or metabolic thermogenesis is the major mechanism of metabolic heat production in neonates wherein

TABLE 2.9.1: Risk factors for hypothermia in a newborn.

Infant	*Environment*	*Caretaker*	*Equipment*	*Iatrogenic*
• Preterm • Low birth weight (LBW) • Sick newborn • IUGR • Asphyxia • Congenital abdominal wall defects (e.g., exomphalos)	• Cold area (open door or window, fan, A/C) • Cold weather • Distance between the delivery room and NICU	• Limited personnel • Ignorance • Lack of training • Lack of protocol	• Lack, missing, nonfunctioning equipment/supplies • Power failure or fluctuation	• Bathing in the delivery room • Not removing wet linen • Mother–child separation • Delayed initiation of breastfeeding • During procedure, e.g., blood sampling, cannulation, exchange transfusion, X-ray, transport, etc. • Probe displacement under warmer

(IUGR: intrauterine growth restriction; NICU: neonatal intensive care unit)

heat production is not associated with muscle activity.[5] Brown fat tissue is the main site of nonshivering thermogenesis. Brown fat contributes to 2–6% of an infant's body weight and differentiates in the fetus around 20 and 30 weeks of gestational age. It is located between the scapulae, around neck blood vessels, in the mediastinum, axilla, and around the adrenal glands and kidneys. Unlike white fat, brown fat tissue is multinucleated and has an abundance of mitochondria in the cytoplasm. Cold stress increases sympathetic activity with the release of norepinephrine that activates the brown fat mitochondria and heat is generated by the uncoupling of oxidative phosphorylation. The triglycerides in fat are hydrolyzed to free fatty acids (FFA) but instead of adenosine triphosphate (ATP), the energy is released in the form of heat **(Fig. 2.9.1)**. Although both term and preterm infants are capable of thermogenesis using brown fat, their sustainability is limited when heat loss is excessive.

Consequences of Neonatal Hypothermia

Hypothermia is associated with increased mortality. While there is no direct causal link with death, hypothermia alters normal metabolic functions as listed below resulting in hypoxia, impaired fluid balance, hypoglycemia, hyperkalemia, and risk for sepsis:

- Increased oxygen consumption leads to hypoxia. Hypothermia affects surfactant function resulting in respiratory distress and causes pulmonary vasoconstriction leading to pulmonary hypertension and hemorrhage.
- Metabolic acidosis and hypoxia lead to myocardial dysfunction and hypotension.
- Affects oxidative metabolism leading to hypoglycemia and lactic acidosis
- Risk of sepsis
- Chronic hypothermia can result in poor growth.
- In preterm infants <33 weeks' gestation, hypothermia at admission to the neonatal intensive care unit (NICU) is associated with IVH, ROP, BPD, necrotizing enterocolitis (NEC), and late-onset sepsis.

CLINICAL FEATURES

Signs and symptoms of hypothermia include one or more of the following: Cold feet and trunk, lethargy, poor feeding, apnea, respiratory distress, hypoxia, tachypnea, grunting, central cyanosis, bradycardia, shock, decreased urine output, hypoglycemia, coagulopathy, bleeding tendencies, weight loss, or poor weight gain. As the clinical features are nonspecific, a high index of suspicion is needed to diagnose hypothermia.

DIAGNOSIS

The temperature in a neonate can be easily measured using a digital thermometer placed in the axilla. The thermometer is cleaned with an alcohol swab and the tip is placed in the roof of the axilla, keeping it parallel to the body. Once the beep is heard, the temperature can be noted. Rectal and tympanic measurements are not generally taken for routine practice as they are invasive. Noninvasive measurements of neonatal temperature using infrared thermometers or infrared thermography are not recommended as they are not yet reliable. The lowest temperature recordable in a conventional thermometer is 35°C.

TABLE 2.9.2: Screening by touch for thermal well-being.

Trunk	*Extremity*	*Impression*
Warm	Warm	Normal
Warm	Cold	Cold stress
Cold	Cold	Hypothermia

In the NICU, neonates can have their skin temperatures monitored continuously using the skin probe of the radiant warmer supplemented with intermittent measurement of axillary temperatures. Temperatures should be documented hourly in a seriously ill baby, two to four times per day in a small or very small baby, and once daily in a well infant. In community settings or at home where thermometers are not available, mothers can use the hand touch method. The back of the hand can be used to feel the baby's feet and compare them with the abdomen and chest **(Table 2.9.2)**.[6]

As LBW and preterm neonates are at a high risk of hypothermia at home, simple wearable devices have been tested for continuous temperature monitoring. These include the ThermoSpot, neonatal temperature monitor (NTM), and BEMPU TempWatch. The BEMPU watch creates a beeping sound and an orange light when the infant's temperature drops below 36.5°C alerting the parents to take adequate measures.[7]

TREATMENT OF HYPOTHERMIA

Treatment of hypothermia depends on the severity of the condition **(Table 2.9.3)**. For babies with cold stress, skin-to-skin contact with mothers will suffice. For moderate or severe hypothermia, the baby should be rewarmed using additional sources of heat.

Monitoring

The temperature should be monitored continuously and rewarming continued till normal body temperature is attained. Monitoring of blood glucose and electrolytes should be done and metabolic complications such as hypoglycemia should be corrected in the NICU. Consider antibiotics, intravenous (IV) glucose infusion, and oxygen administration based on clinical status.

TABLE 2.9.3: Management of hypothermia.

	Mild hypothermia	*Moderate hypothermia*	*Severe hypothermia*
Temperature	36–36.5°C	32–36°C	<32°C
Place of care	Mother	Mother or nursery	NICU or SCNU
Interventions	• Kangaroo care • Remove from source • Warm the room • Cover head, body • Breastfeed	• Kangaroo care • Warmth—bulb (200W), room heater, warm towel • Warmer, if available • Consider IV fluids, if unable to breastfeed	• Rapid rewarming till 34°C under a warmer • Slow rewarming, thereafter • Oxygen • IV fluids • Check blood glucose • Antibiotics

(NICU: neonatal intensive care unit; SCNU: special care newborn unit)

Core axillary gap measurement is considered abnormal when there is a temperature difference exceeding 2–3°C between the core and peripheral temperatures. This provides an early indication of conditions such as cold stress, hypovolemia, infection, and iatrogenic overheating.

PREVENTION

Since hypothermia can have severe consequences, it is better to prevent it than to treat it. The "warm chain" concept summarizes the salient steps in the prevention of hypothermia in newborns. It is a set of 10 interlinked procedures carried out at birth and afterward to maintain a normal temperature. The components of the warm chain are as follows:

1. *Warm delivery room:* The delivery room should be warm (25–28°C) and free from droughts from open doors, windows, or fan.
2. *Warm resuscitation:* Use at least two prewarmed linens, large enough to cover the entire baby. The radiant warmer should be set to 100% heater output in the manual mode at least 10 minutes prior to receiving the baby. Preterm babies <32 weeks' gestation need additional equipment like plastic bags or wraps and/or exothermic heat mattresses.[8] The preterm baby should be received in a plastic bag without drying and the entire resuscitation should be carried out while inside the bag. This bag is removed only after stabilizing the temperature in the NICU **(Figs. 2.9.2A to D)**.
3. *Immediate drying:* Babies who do not require resuscitation at birth should be received onto their mother's abdomen and dried while the umbilical cord is still attached. After drying, wet linen should be removed.
4. *Skin-to-skin contact between baby and mother:* Babies requiring only routine care at birth should not be separated from their mother (zero separation policy) **(Fig. 2.9.3)**. Skin-to-skin care should be initiated by placing the baby naked in between the mother's breast and continued for 1 hour. The mother–baby dyad should be covered with a warm linen and the baby's temperature, breathing, and color should be monitored every 15 minutes.
5. *Breastfeeding:* It should begin as soon as possible after delivery and preferably within the first hour of birth.
6. *Postpone bathing:* Bathing should be postponed until after the second or third day of birth and even longer in LBW babies. Bathing at home should be done quickly in warm water with drying and clothing performed immediately.
7. *Appropriate clothing and bedding:* Newborns should be dressed in two or more layers of clothing and also wear cap, socks, and mittens. The warm air trapped between two layers of clothing is an effective insulator of heat.
8. *Mother and baby nursed together:* The mother and the baby should be together 24 hours a day in the same bed, and it is easier to keep the baby warm and to breastfeed on demand.
9. *Warm transportation:* This is the weakest link in the warm chain. The baby's temperature should be recorded and stabilized before transport. The safest and most effective way to transport stable neonates is skin-to-skin contact with the mother. Sick neonates can be transported in transport incubators or low-cost equipment like Embrace warmer (which uses a phase-changing material that retains a temperature of 37°C) for 4 hours.
10. *Training of HCPs:* HCPs should be trained adequately in the principles and procedures of warm chain, early recognition, and management of hypothermia. They should also be trained in measuring temperature and operating and maintaining equipment like radiant warmers and incubators.

Preventing Hypothermia in the Community

Kangaroo mother care (KMC) is a simple and cost-effective intervention recommended for all preterm and LBW

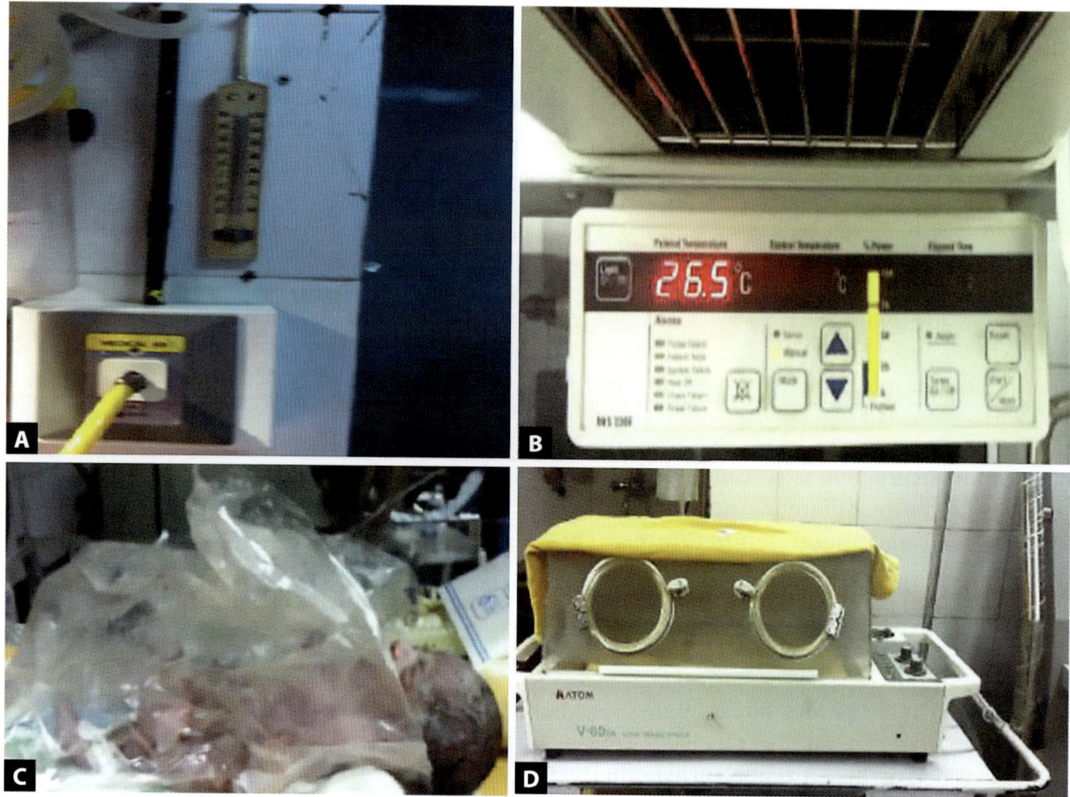

Figs. 2.9.2A to D: Components of heat loss prevention at birth: (A) Warm delivery room maintained between 25 and 26°C; (B) Radiant warmer; (C) Plastic bags for preterm neonates; and (D) Transport incubators for neonatal transport.

"Zero separation"

Benefits to mother:
- Increased rate and duration of breastfeeding
- Less stress
- Reduced postpartum hemorrhage
- Improves bonding

Benefits to baby:
- Thermal stability
- Glucose stability
- Reduced apnea
- Lesser risk of infection

Fig. 2.9.3: Skin-to-skin contact at birth.

neonates (*see* Chapter 2.4). It consists of skin-to-skin contact for prolonged periods and exclusive breastfeeding. KMC decreases the incidence of hypothermia, neonatal infections, and mortality in both facility and community settings while promoting weight gain and parent–infant bonding.[9]

HYPERTHERMIA

Hyperthermia is usually caused by raised environmental temperature (e.g., room heater and summer), dehydration, infection, or inadvertent overwarming in a radiant warmer due to temperature probe displacement. In LBW babies, infection produces hypothermia rather than fever. Management of hyperthermia involves taking the baby away from a hot environment, undressing the baby, giving a bath if needed (>39°C), frequent breastfeeding, and evaluating for infection or cause of fever. Antipyretics are generally not needed. Febrile neonates should be hospitalized and given IV antibiotics till infection is ruled out.

REFERENCES

1. World Health Organization. Thermal Protection of the Newborn: A Practical Guide. Geneva: World Health Organization; 1997.
2. Dang R, Patel AI, Weng Y, Schroeder AR, Lee NC, Aby J, et al. Incidence of neonatal hypothermia in the newborn nursery and associated factors. JAMA Netw Open. 2023;6(8):e2331011.

3. Lyu Y, Shah PS, Ye XY, Warre R, Piedboeuf B, Deshpandey A, et al. Association between admission temperature and mortality and major morbidity in preterm infants born at fewer than 33 weeks' gestation. JAMA Pediatr. 2015;169(4):e150277.
4. Trevisanuto D, Testoni D, de Almeida MFB. Maintaining normothermia: why and how? Semin Fetal Neonatal Med. 2018;23(5):333-39.
5. Cannon B, Nedergaard J. Brown adipose tissue: function and physiological significance. Physiol Rev. 2004;84(1):277-359.
6. Tuitui RL, Suwal SN, Shrestha S. Hand-touch method for detection of neonatal hypothermia in Nepal. J Trop Pediatr. 2011;57(3):236-8.
7. Nimbalkar SM, Patel VT, Patel DV, Phatak AG. Impact of hypothermia alert device (BEMPU) on improvement of duration of Kangaroo mother care (KMC) provided at home: parallel-group randomized control trial. Sci Rep. 2023;13(1):4368.
8. McCall EM, Alderdice F, Halliday HL, Vohra S, Johnston L. Interventions to prevent hypothermia at birth in preterm and/or low birth weight infants. Cochrane Database Syst Rev. 2018;2(2):CD004210.
9. Conde-Agudelo A, Díaz-Rossello JL. Kangaroo mother care to reduce morbidity and mortality in low birthweight infants. Cochrane Database Syst Rev. 2016;2016(8):CD002771.

2.10 Neonatal Hyperbilirubinemia

Rhishikesh P Thakre

INTRODUCTION

Hyperbilirubinemia is a common neonatal problem which merits medical attention. It is defined as an increased level of bilirubin in the circulation. It manifests as jaundice or icterus. Elevated levels of unconjugated bilirubin are most common and lead to indirect jaundice. In the majority, it is transient and self-limiting and manifests as "physiological jaundice," but in few instances, the indirect bilirubin may cross the blood–brain barrier to cause irreversible brain damage. Elevated levels of conjugated bilirubin lead to direct jaundice which is always pathological. A systematic approach in the form of clinical evaluation, assessment of risk factors, and timely intervention paves the way to rational management.

EPIDEMIOLOGY

Approximately 60% of the term and 80% of the preterm babies develop jaundice during the first week of life. About 5% develop severe jaundice. The incidence of jaundice, its severity, and the need for phototherapy among healthy neonates from population-based studies are scarce. There are regional, racial, and genetic differences among the population. In countries with highest neonatal mortality rates, the Global Burden of Disease Study places severe jaundice among the leading 5–10 causes of neonatal deaths. As per the National Neonatal-Perinatal Database (NNPD), neonatal hyperbilirubinemia occurs in 3.3% of in-house live-births, whereas for extramural admissions, morbidity attributed to hyperbilirubinemia constitutes 22.1%.[1]

ETIOPATHOGENESIS

Hyperbilirubinemia is the result of an imbalance between bilirubin production and its elimination. Bilirubin metabolism is described in **Table 2.10.1**. Serum bilirubin levels must reach 4–6 mg/dL to be visually detected. Unconjugated bilirubin which is unbound has the potential to cross the blood–brain barrier leading to bilirubin-induced neurological damage. Bilirubin-induced neurotoxicity leads to inflammation, oxidative stress, and damage to the cells in affected brain regions. Neuronal cells, glial cells, and other structures within the brain may be affected, causing irreversible damage.

The etiological basis for progressive hyperbilirubinemia is usually multifactorial. **Box 2.10.1** summarizes the important causes of unconjugated hyperbilirubinemia.

Physiological Jaundice

The most common cause of neonatal hyperbilirubinemia is physiological jaundice, which is a diagnosis of exclusion. The functional immaturity in bilirubin metabolism, namely increased enterohepatic circulation, increased fetal erythrocyte breakdown, decreased hepatic excretion, and immature hepatic conjugation, predisposes to early jaundice which is transient, requiring no treatment. It usually appears after 24 hours, peaks between 3 and 5 days in term and 5–7 days in preterm, and disappears by 2 weeks of life. The peak bilirubin is under 15 mg/dL.

TABLE 2.10.1: Bilirubin metabolism.

Stage	Production	Transport	Conjugation	Excretion
Organ	Reticuloendothelial system	Blood	Liver	Bowel, kidneys
Key features	• Daily bilirubin production is 2–6 mg/kg/day • 80–85% of bilirubin is derived from RBC breakdown • 1 g of Hb produces 35 mg of bilirubin • Biliverdin is reduced to bilirubin to enter circulation	• Bilirubin is bound to albumin in plasma • Unbound form deposits in fatty tissue (skin and brain) • 1 g of albumin binds to 0.8–1.2 mg of bilirubin	Hepatocyte uptake assisted by ligandin, conjugates insoluble, unconjugated bilirubin with glucuronic acid to form water-soluble, conjugated bilirubin	• Conjugated bilirubin is excreted into the biliary tract • In terminal ileum and colon, bacterial enzymes convert to urobilinogen • Majority is excreted into stools as stercobilinogen and into urine via the kidneys (1%) • 10–20% reabsorbed from intestine to portal circulation
Key enzyme	Heme oxygenase	Biliverdin reductase	Glucoronyl transferase	Beta-glucuronidase

BOX 2.10.1: Causes of indirect (unconjugated) hyperbilirubinemia.

- Physiological jaundice
- Breastfeeding jaundice, breast milk jaundice
- *Increased production:*
  - Blood group incompatibility (Rh, ABO, and minor blood group)
  - RBC membrane defects (hereditary spherocytosis and elliptocytosis)
  - RBC enzyme defects (G6PD deficiency and pyruvate kinase deficiency)
- *Disorders of bilirubin uptake:* Gilbert syndrome
- *Disorders of conjugation:*
  - Crigler–Najjar types I and II
  - Hypothyroidism
  - Pyloric stenosis
- *Enhanced enterohepatic circulation:* Small- or large-bowel obstruction or ileus
- Idiopathic
- *Others:*
  - Prematurity
  - Sepsis
  - Polycythemia
  - Infant of diabetic mother
  - Extravascular blood (cephalohematoma and bruising)

(G6PD: glucose-6-phosphate dehydrogenase; RBC: red blood cell; Rh: rhesus)

Nonphysiologic Jaundice and Risk of Bilirubin Toxicity

Jaundice within 24 hours of life, peak bilirubin >15 mg/dL, and persistence beyond 2 weeks are not physiologic and need to be investigated **(Box 2.10.2)**. The rate of rise of bilirubin >0.5 mg/dL/h or bilirubin level >25 mg/dL increases the risk of bilirubin toxicity in neonates. Bilirubin is a potential neurotoxin. Areas of the brain most commonly affected are the basal ganglia and brainstem nuclei for oculomotor and auditory functions. Studies suggest the possible impact of genetic polymorphisms on ethnic variation in the incidence and severity of jaundice. Bilirubin toxicity or kernicterus can cause permanent sequelae, characterized by a tetrad of choreoathetoid cerebral palsy, high-frequency central hearing loss, vertical gaze palsy, and dental enamel hypoplasia.

BOX 2.10.2: Nonphysiologic jaundice.

- Sick newborn
- Prematurity
- Jaundice in the first 24 hours of birth
- Jaundice beyond 14 days of birth
- Rate of rise of bilirubin >0.2 mg/dL/h
- Transcutaneous bilirubin >95th percentile on nomogram
- Total serum bilirubin >75th percentile on nomogram
- Urine staining the diapers and/or pale, clay-colored stools

CLINICAL FEATURES

Majority of infants with jaundice are asymptomatic. Jaundice appears over the face first and spreads in a cephalocaudal direction to involve the body. The presence of bruising, cephalohematoma, lethargy, vomiting, excessive weight loss, pallor, plethora, and hepatosplenomegaly are clinical clues to pathological jaundice. Abnormality in tone, cry, or sensorium should alert to the possibility of bilirubin neurotoxicity. In infants presenting with jaundice extending beyond 2 weeks, one must inquire for urine staining the diaper for cholestasis and pale or white stools, which may indicate obstructive jaundice such as biliary atresia. One must be alert to the presence of ascites, bleeding tendency, and encephalopathy in infants with direct jaundice which suggest worsening.

DIAGNOSIS

All newborns should be examined for jaundice at least once a day during the first 72 hours. Jaundice is assessed by inspecting the baby's skin, sclera, or mucous membranes,

TABLE 2.10.2: Risk factors for jaundice at the time of discharge.

Risk factors for significant hyperbilirubinemia	***Neurotoxic risk factors***
• Primipara mother • Visible jaundice at discharge • Gestation <38 weeks • Infant of diabetic mother • History of jaundice requiring treatment in previous sibling • ABO/Rh incompatibility • Geographic prevalence for G6PD deficiency • Weight loss at discharge >3%/day or >7% cumulative weight loss	• Preterm • Hemolysis • Sepsis • Unstable course over the last 24 hours • Serum albumin <3 g/dL

(G6PD: glucose-6-phosphate dehydrogenase, Rh: rhesus)

preferably in natural light.[1] The skin is blanched by digital pressure over bony parts to reveal underlying yellowing. Visual estimates are error prone; hence, the use of a transcutaneous bilirubinometer serves as an objective screening tool. All newborns should be assessed for the presence of risk factors for jaundice at the time of discharge **(Table 2.10.2)**. The more risk factors present, the greater the risk of severe hyperbilirubinemia, and the risk is extremely low, if risk factors are absent. If neonates are discharged within 24 hours, those with risk factors should be seen within 24–48 hours and those without risk factors within 72 hours of discharge.

INVESTIGATIONS

In all neonates with jaundice that is not considered physiologic, investigations need to be done to assess the severity of jaundice (for planning treatment) and the etiology of the jaundice.[2] **Box 2.10.3** summarizes the important investigations that need to be done. Cord blood is collected for typing the baby's blood group, if the mother's blood group is rhesus (Rh)-negative or O Rh-positive, or the blood group is not known. If an Rh-negative mother has an Rh-positive baby, the cord blood is subjected to a direct Coombs test, total serum bilirubin (TSB), reticulocyte count, peripheral smear, and hemoglobin. End-tidal carbon monoxide measurement in exhaled air may serve as an indirect marker of ongoing hemolysis as equimolar concentrations of CO and bilirubin are formed following the breakdown of red blood cells.

DIFFERENTIAL DIAGNOSIS

Carotenemia due to ingestion of fruits and vegetables mimics jaundice but is not seen in newborns. An acute bilirubin encephalopathy-like picture may be seen with sepsis, meningitis, or asphyxia.

BOX 2.10.3: Investigations for significant hyperbilirubinemia.

- Total and direct bilirubin
- Mother and baby blood groups
- Hemoglobin or PCV
- Peripheral blood smear (for RBC shape and evidence of hemolysis)
- Reticulocyte count
- Direct Coombs test (if the mother is O or Rh-negative)
- G6PD assay

Sick infant with jaundice or prolonged jaundice (>3 weeks):
- Complete blood count, blood culture
- Urine examination and culture
- Evaluate for infection as indicated
- Urine for reducing substances
- Thyroid profile (T4, TSH)
- Evaluate for cholestasis (if direct bilirubin is elevated)

(G6PD: glucose-6-phosphate dehydrogenase, PCV: packed cell volume, RBC: red blood cell, Rh: rhesus, T4: thyroxine, TSH: thyroid-stimulating hormone)

MANAGEMENT

Treatment of Indirect Hyperbilirubinemia

The decision-making in jaundice management is based on gestation, weight, well-being, and age of the infant. **Table 2.10.3** provides guidelines on how to decide if an infant needs treatment—phototherapy (PT) or exchange transfusion (ET) by the World Health Organization (WHO).[3] Guidelines by the American Academy of Pediatrics for >35 weeks' gestation or the National Institute for Health and Care Excellence (NICE), UK, for infants <35 weeks' gestation are widely used.[2,4]

Supportive Care

For all stable infants, mother–infant dyad should be nursed together. Breastfeeding is continued frequently. Close attention is paid to the infant's temperature, daily weight, and intake output. There is no role for routine supplementation of IV fluids or formula feeds.

Phototherapy

Phototherapy (PT) is the mainstay of treatment. When bilirubin is exposed to blue light (in the range of 420–480 nm), it undergoes a change in structure to a product called lumirubin, which can be excreted in the urine without undergoing conjugation in the liver. The efficacy of PT depends on the spectrum of light (460–480 nm), irradiance (8–30 $\mu W/cm^2/nm$), and surface area of the infant's skin exposed to light. The choice of device depends upon the severity of jaundice. For majority of infants, standard PT (six special blue lights of Philips TL 52, 20 W each) is effective. When the bilirubin is rapidly rising or nearing the ET range, intensive PT (using high-intensity light-emitting diodes) lights or double-surface standard PT tubes are provided.

TABLE 2.10.3: Treatment of indirect hyperbilirubinemia.[3]

Age	Phototherapy		Exchange transfusion	
	Healthy newborns >35 weeks' gestation (mg/dL)	Newborns <35 weeks' gestation (mg/dL)	Healthy newborns >35 weeks' gestation (mg/dL)	Newborns <35 weeks' gestation (mg/dL)
Day 1	Any visible jaundice		15	10
Day 2	15	10	25	15
Day 3	18	15	25	20

Administering PT

Phototherapy is administered continuously and interrupted only for nursing and feeding purposes. The infant is placed naked with genitalia and eyes covered. Hypoxia, hypothermia, hypoglycemia, acidosis, and sepsis need to be prevented, and if present, treated aggressively. Intravenous fluids are given only to infants who have inadequate oral intake, have significant weight loss (>10%), or are dehydrated.

Monitoring

Total serum bilirubin is monitored every 4–12 hours, depending on the patient's age and bilirubin level. PT should be stopped once serum bilirubin is 50 mmol/L or below the PT threshold. It should not be used to treat infants with conjugated hyperbilirubinemia because of the risk of bronze baby syndrome.

Exchange Transfusion

Exchange transfusion is indicated for infants whose bilirubin levels cross the threshold indicated in **Table 2.10.3** or those who have clinical features of bilirubin encephalopathy **(Fig. 2.10.1)**. During ET, twice the infant's blood volume (160 mL/kg) is exchanged; this procedure can decrease the bilirubin level by approximately 50%. The procedure is invasive and carries a small risk of complications (1–5%)—fluid overload, infection, electrolyte imbalance, hypoglycemia, thrombocytopenia, thrombosis, and death.

Drugs

The use of intravenous immunoglobulin (IVIG) and phenobarbitone is not advisable, either as a preventive measure or for treatment, in neonates experiencing hyperbilirubinemia due to alloimmune hemolytic disease.[1] Synthetic heme analogs and metalloporphyrins are competitive inhibitors of heme oxygenase, and their use has been proposed as an attractive alternative strategy for preventing or treating severe hyperbilirubinemia.

Treatment of Direct Hyperbilirubinemia

Direct hyperbilirubinemia should be suspected if the conjugated bilirubin level is >1 mg/dL.[2] A direct bilirubin

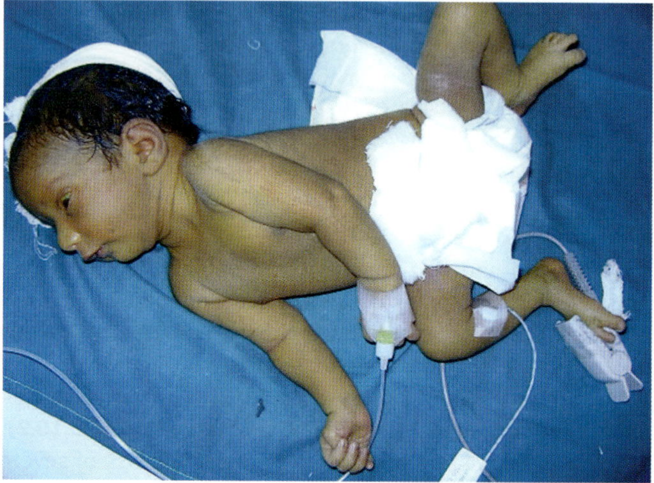

Fig. 2.10.1: Acute bilirubin encephalopathy. Note the arching of the back, tonic posture, setting sun sign, and yellowish staining of the baby.

BOX 2.10.4: Causes of conjugated (direct) hyperbilirubinemia.

- Bacterial sepsis
- Neonatal hepatitis:
  - Toxoplasmosis
  - Cytomegalovirus
  - Rubella
  - Herpes
  - Syphilis
  - Parvovirus B19
- *Biliary obstruction:*
  - Biliary atresia
  - Choledochal cyst
  - Inspissated bile plug
- *Metabolic disease:*
  - Hypothyroidism
  - Galactosemia
  - Alpha-1-antitrypsin deficiency
- *Genetic disease:*
  - Dubin–Johnson syndrome
  - Rotor syndrome
  - Cystic fibrosis
  - Alagille syndrome
- *Others:*
  - Drugs
  - Cholestasis associated with total parenteral nutrition
- *Idiopathic*

concentration exceeding 20% of the total is no longer considered essential for diagnosing cholestasis. It is an uncommon but potentially serious condition that indicates hepatobiliary dysfunction **(Box 2.10.4)**.

Evaluation should include total and direct bilirubin, urine examination and urine culture, evaluation for infection (as indicated), and thyroid profile.[2,5] Further evaluation should be tailored with expert consultation to rule out surgical causes. Treatment is directed at the specific underlying cause, if any, and remains largely supportive with a diet rich in calories, medium-chain triglycerides, adequate proteins, and supplementation of fat and water-soluble vitamins. Early detection and diagnosis are important for successful treatment for a favorable prognosis.

REFERENCES

1. Clinical Practice Guidelines, National Neonatology Forum of India. Screening, prevention and management of neonatal hyperbilirubinemia. [online] Available from https://www.nnfi.org/assests/pdf/cpg-guidelines/Jaundice.pdf [Last accessed October, 2024].
2. Kemper AR, Newman TB, Slaughter JL, Maisels MJ, Watchko JF, Downs SM, et al. Clinical practice guideline revision: management of hyperbilirubinemia in the newborn infant 35 or more weeks of gestation. Pediatrics. 2022;150(3):e2022058859.
3. World Health Organization. WHO recommendations on newborn health: guidelines approved by the WHO Guidelines Review Committee. Geneva: World Health Organization; 2017.
4. National Institute for Health and Care Excellence (NICE). (2023). Jaundice in newborn babies under 28 days. [online] Available from https://www.nice.org.uk/guidance/cg98 [Last accessed October, 2024].
5. Bhatia V, Bavdekar A, Matthai J, Waikar Y, Sibal A. Management of neonatal cholestasis: consensus statement of the Pediatric Gastroenterology Chapter of Indian Academy of Pediatrics. Indian Pediatr. 2014;51(3):203-10.

2.11 Neonatal Sepsis

Sheila Samanta Mathai

INTRODUCTION

Acquired neonatal infections are those contracted immediately before, during, or soon after birth. They are usually bacterial and are among the most common causes of neonatal morbidity. In low-resource settings, they account for almost 20% of neonatal deaths. They are distinct from congenital infections, which are typically more chronic and are transmitted from the infected mother through the placenta (vertical transmission) or rarely at the time of birth (horizontal transmission). These are usually viral [rubella, cytomegalovirus, hepatitis B, and human immunodeficiency virus (HIV)] or parasitic (malaria and toxoplasmosis).

Neonatal infections cover a wide range from superficial infections of the eyes (conjunctivitis), skin (impetigo), umbilicus (omphalitis), and mouth (oral thrush) to localized, deep-seated infections such as pneumonia, meningitis, septic arthritis, osteomyelitis, endocarditis, urinary tract infection (UTI), and otitis media. The most life-threatening form of infection in the newborn is *neonatal sepsis,* which is associated with bloodstream invasion of organisms, usually bacterial. Not all infections cause sepsis and not all cases of sepsis have an obvious focus of infection. In this chapter, we will discuss the clinical and laboratory diagnosis of neonatal sepsis and ways to treat and prevent it.

DEFINITION

The definition of sepsis has come a long way since the initial definition of the systemic inflammatory response syndrome over 20 years ago. Unfortunately, there is still no universal consensus in the definition of neonatal sepsis, and this varies in different countries and situations. Neonatal sepsis typically implies an invasive bloodstream infection, usually bacterial, leading to a dysregulated immune response, which can progress to vascular involvement and capillary leak, leading to insufficiency and multisystem organ dysfunction. The terms "septicemia," "septic," and "toxic" are obsolete and ambiguous and are not to be used.[1]

TYPES OF NEONATAL SEPSIS

Classically, neonatal sepsis is differentiated into "early-onset neonatal sepsis" (EOS) and "late-onset neonatal sepsis" (LOS) based on the time of onset being either before or after 72 hours of life.

Though sepsis is associated with bacteremia and a positive blood culture is the gold standard to confirm the diagnosis, this may not be seen in up to two-thirds of clinically suspected cases of neonatal sepsis, leading to use of the term "culture-negative sepsis," "clinical sepsis," or "presumed sepsis." Though there is controversy in the universal acceptability of these terms, they are widely used the world over and indicate situations suggestive of sepsis and unexplained by other diagnoses, with positive laboratory markers like biomarkers and blood counts but negative blood cultures. They serve as the basis for the commencement or continuation of antibiotics in many cases.[2,3]

RISK FACTORS FOR NEONATAL SEPSIS

The risk factors for EOS and LOS are different, and there have been attempts to classify them accordingly **(Table 2.11.1)**. Neonatal sepsis has been found to be inversely proportional to the period of gestation at birth, with lower gestation age being one of the highest risk factors. Male sex has also been found to be a risk factor.[4]

EPIDEMIOLOGY

The incidence of neonatal sepsis varies significantly in different countries, being highest in the low- and middle-income countries (LMICs), where it is up to 5–10 times higher as compared with high-income countries (HICs). In the United States and United Kingdom, the incidence varies from 0.5 to 2/1,000 term live births, but even in these countries it is 6–10 times higher in preterm babies. In LMICs, the incidence of clinical and laboratory-supported sepsis in neonates has been found to be as high as 47/1,000 live births. However, almost 10 times this number are treated for clinically suspected, presumed, or culture-negative sepsis. The Global Burden of Disease Study 2106/2017 estimated approximately 1.3 million annual cases of neonatal sepsis worldwide with an overall incidence of 28/1,000 live births. In India, the incidence ranges from 10 to 39/1,000 live births.[2]

TABLE 2.11.1: Risk factors for neonatal sepsis.

Risk factors for early-onset neonatal sepsis	*Risk factors for late-onset neonatal sepsis*
• Maternal fever (>37.8°C just prior to or during labor) • Prolonged rupture of membranes (PROM) for more than 24 hours • Preterm premature rupture of membranes (PPROM) of any duration • Spontaneous, unexplained onset of preterm (<37 weeks) labor with or without PPROM • Maternal urinary tract infection (UTI) within 7 days of the date of delivery • Clinical chorioamnionitis (high fever, uterine tenderness, and foul-smelling liquor) in mother	• Low birth weight (LBW) • Prematurity (<37 weeks' gestation) • Babies admitted to neonatal intensive care units for a prolonged period of time • Babies undergoing invasive ventilation • Babies on central catheters • Babies on urinary catheters • Babies on prolonged broad-spectrum antibiotics • Postsurgical cases • Male sex

ETIOPATHOGENESIS

Bacteria are the primary cause of neonatal sepsis. The adaptive immune response of newborns is essentially naïve, and the neonatal response to infection is mainly dependent on the innate immune responses and passive antibody transfer from the mother. Most of the transfer of antibodies occurs in the third trimester. Preterm neonates are more vulnerable as compared to terms, as their innate immune barriers are less robust and they have little or no transplacentally acquired maternal antibodies. In addition, other illnesses of prematurity like respiratory, cardiac, metabolic, and nutritional issues make them more likely to be subject to invasive procedures after birth, increasing their vulnerability to sepsis. The type or degree of the adaptive immune response will decide the extent of the systemic inflammatory response, which is the hallmark of severe sepsis. A dysregulated response results in a combination of immune paralysis and hyperinflammatory cytokines, which affect the stability of the vascular system and may eventually lead to shock. Circulating bacteria can also cause the production of acute-phase reactants like C-reactive protein (CRP) and procalcitonin (PCT), which serve as markers for neonatal sepsis.[5]

Several pathogenic bacteria normally colonize the maternal genital and gastrointestinal tracts but cause no symptoms in the mother. However, they can cause EOS in the baby. The most common organisms are *Escherichia coli* and group B streptococci in the West and *Klebsiella*, *Staphylococcus*, and *E. coli* in our country. The pathogenesis of EOS usually starts before birth with the invasion of the amniotic sac with these pathogenic bacteria. Environmental bacteria can also be responsible for EOS in some cases. Rarely, maternal bloodstream infections can invade the placenta and amniotic fluid, a typical example being *Listeria monocytogenes*. Most manifestations of early-onset infections in the neonate occur within the first 48 hours.

Late-onset neonatal sepsis can be either community- or hospital-acquired. The latter is often seen in babies admitted to the neonatal intensive care unit (NICU) and may involve multidrug-resistant organisms of the Enterobacteriaceae group, such as *Klebsiella pneumonia, E. coli, Acinetobacter baumani*, and *Enterobacter* species, or multidrug-resistant *Staphylococcus aureus* (MRSA). However, community-acquired LOS is not uncommon in our country and may be related to unhygienic child-rearing practices and aggravated by poor breast-feeding. Fungal sepsis is also seen in this group of babies.

Mortality in neonatal sepsis is high and worldwide is about 17–20%. Among the survivors, the incidence of adverse neurodevelopmental outcomes, including cerebral palsy, hearing loss, visual impairment, and cognitive delays, is often seen.[6]

CLINICAL FEATURES

Clinical features of sepsis can be nonspecific and mimic many other neonatal diseases. Almost two-thirds of cases of EOS are symptomatic at birth. In preterm babies, these signs and symptoms may be confused with other conditions associated with prematurity as well.

Clinical features include lethargy, feed refusal, unexplained apneic episodes, temperature instability, tachypnea, tachycardia, low blood pressure, prolonged capillary refill time (CRT), feed intolerance, abdominal distension, and hypoglycemia or hyperglycemia. The presence of convulsions, neck retraction, or bulging fontanel suggests the possibility of meningitis, though this may be present, especially in LOS, without these typical clinical features as well. Neonates with septic arthritis or osteomyelitis may not have local symptoms and present with painful limb movements and localized swelling with signs of inflammation.

The respiratory system can be involved in neonatal sepsis and may present with respiratory distress with patchy opacities on the chest X-ray. However, tachypnea can also be seen as a compensatory mechanism to shock or acidosis. Persistent pulmonary hypertension of the newborn (PPHN) is commonly seen in neonatal sepsis and can present as a progressively increasing oxygen requirement despite adequate ventilation.[3]

Due to the dysregulated immune response, vasoactive substances are produced, which affect vascular permeability and can lead to shock. This is characterized by features of circulatory insufficiency, cardiac dysfunction, and hypotension. Blood gas analysis may show acidosis with progressively rising lactate levels. If not treated aggressively in the early stages, it can lead to multisystem organ dysfunction and eventually death.

The World Health Organization (WHO) has opined that danger signs in the newborn that suggest severe infection like neonatal sepsis include lethargy, poor feeding, thermal imbalance, seizures, fast breathing, chest indrawing, yellow discoloration of palms and soles, multiple skin pustules (>10 in number), or definite evidence of significant pus collection or inflammation. These signs should be known by all healthcare workers (HCW) dealing with newborns, even at the grassroots level. In all such cases, the baby should be immediately started on antibiotics at the peripheral level and transferred to a larger healthcare facility at the earliest.[7]

INVESTIGATIONS

The working diagnosis of neonatal sepsis is based on a combination of risk factors, clinical symptoms/signs, blood counts, nonspecific markers of an inflammatory response, and response to treatment.[3,8] As many bodily fluid cultures as possible, depending on the clinical situation, should be sent for cultures. Though blood culture is the gold standard to make a definite diagnosis of sepsis, this may not be available immediately, and treatment may have to commence empirically. A diagnosis of clinical sepsis is made in a suspected case with low blood count parameters and/or inflammatory biomarkers, even if blood cultures are negative. However, other conditions may need to be reasonably ruled out in such cases.

Blood Culture

Confirmed sepsis is defined by a positive blood culture in a symptomatic baby. But even with the best of facilities, only two-thirds of cases of suspected sepsis have a positive blood culture, and in LMICs, this yield may be as low as 10–20%. Negative cultures in infected neonates can be due to many reasons, including the prior use of antibiotics, sampling issues, and poor laboratory techniques.

Collection of blood for culture should be done correctly and preferably before starting antibiotics. Skin should be cleaned with an appropriate antiseptic and at least 1 mL of blood taken by sterile techniques in a pediatric culture bottle. The sample should be transported to the laboratory as soon as possible after collection, for processing. Automated culture techniques are preferable. In an automated system, 68% of positive bacterial cultures will show up within 24 hours, 94% will give a positive signal by 36 hours, and 98% by 48 hours.

Biomarkers of Sepsis

Culture-negative sepsis has prompted the search for appropriate and available biomarkers of inflammation as surrogate evidence of sepsis in neonates. CRP is the most used marker of the available tests. It is a nonspecific marker of inflammation produced in the liver. It has been observed that it "rules out" rather than "rules in" sepsis and is often used as a guide to stop antibiotics in culture-negative suspected cases. A CRP test done at the time of taking blood culture has been found to be positive in 30–40% of culture-proven sepsis. Serum PCT has shown promise in guiding antibiotic decisions as it rises earlier than CRP and has a higher positive predictive value. However, the test is more expensive and is not as easily available in LMICs. Other biomarkers like interleukin-6 (IL6) and tumor necrosis factor (TNF) have also been seen to be useful but are not commonly used primarily because of high costs and lack of availability.

Blood Counts in Sepsis

Multiple studies have shown that total white blood cell (WBC) count, absolute neutrophil count (ANC), and immature to total neutrophil (IT) ratio are good surrogate markers of neonatal bacterial sepsis. Values obtained after 4 hours of age have been found to be more predictive of EOS than those done immediately at birth. Extreme values (WBC <5,000/cumm, ANC <2,000/cumm, and IT >0.3) are together associated with higher likelihood ratios (LRs) of sepsis. However, the sensitivity of individual parameters for detection of sepsis is low. Platelet counts may be low in specific infections like *Acinetobacter, Klebsiella,* and fungal infections or as part of disseminated intravascular coagulation (DIC) and are likely to be seen more in LOS.

Molecular Methods

Molecular diagnostic techniques in neonatal sepsis center around the detection of trace evidence of bacteria by polymerase chain reaction (PCR) amplification. These PCR-based tests have a rapid turnaround time for both detection of microbes (<3–4 hours) and antibiotic resistance patterns. Detection of microbes is much higher than with cultures and is not affected by antibiotic use. The current limitations are high cost, availability only in advanced laboratories, and false positives.

Cerebrospinal Fluid Examination

All cases of LOS, irrespective of specific symptoms pertaining to the central nervous system (CNS), warrant a cerebrospinal fluid (CSF) examination. The sample should be sent for cytology, biochemistry, and culture. In EOS, a CSF study may be indicated in symptomatic cases suggestive of meningitis or in culture-proven cases to decide the duration of antibiotics. CSF cytology of >30 cells (>50% polymorphs), with raised protein (>100 mg/dL), and/or glucose of <30 mg/dL may suggest meningitis. Meningitis requires modifications in the choice, dose, and duration of antibiotics.

Urine Culture

Urine culture is not routinely sent in the workup for neonatal sepsis but should be done in infants with failure to thrive, prolonged jaundice, and fever and those in whom there is a poor response to previous antibiotics, as these could be features of persistent UTI. All infants with congenital anomalies of the kidney and urinary tract (CAKUT) with or without obstructive uropathy should have urinary cultures sent if suspected to have sepsis. Samples for cultures should preferably be collected by suprapubic puncture or by sterile, single catheter insertion, collection, and removal.

DIFFERENTIAL DIAGNOSIS

Sepsis in neonates can mimic other diseases specifically seen at this time of life. In particular, disturbances like hypoglycemia, hypocalcemia, dyselectrolytemia, hypothermia, and necrotizing enterocolitis (NEC) can mimic sepsis. When present, inborn errors of metabolism (IEM) can also mimic sepsis.

TREATMENT[8-10]

Antibiotics

Antibiotics are the mainstay of treatment in neonatal sepsis. Most antibiotics are started empirically, as culture reports take time. The choice of antibiotics should be guided by the antimicrobial spectrum seen in that area. The Treatment Guidelines for Antimicrobial Use in Infectious Diseases 2019 of the Indian Council for Medical Research recommends the combination of ampicillin and gentamicin as the first line and piperacillin–tazobactam and amikacin as the second line if there is no improvement in 48–72 hours.[9] In neonatal meningitis, cefotaxime and gentamicin are suggested as the first line. Some evidence suggests that the use of amikacin and piperacillin–tazobactam may have low failure rates. Piperacillin–tazobactam should be avoided if the CNS is involved, as it does not penetrate the CSF barrier. A third-generation cephalosporine can be used in such cases. There may be a justification in using cloxacillin if the incidence of *Staphylococcus* is high in a given setup. Antibiotics such as carbapenems and vancomycin should be treated as reserve drugs to be used only if the primary treatment plan fails.[9]

Since EOS is likely if there are risk factors in the pregnancy and labor, certain recommendations for starting empirical antibiotics at birth, even if the baby is asymptomatic, have been made by the National Neonatology Forum (NNF) of India.[8] If a baby is <35 weeks of gestation and has risk factors for EOS but is asymptomatic, antibiotics could be considered immediately after birth. Ampicillin and gentamicin should be adequate to cover most likely organisms. In such cases, if the baby remains stable and both laboratory markers and cultures are negative at 36 hours, they can be stopped **(Flowchart 2.11.1)**. It is not recommended to start empirical antibiotics in asymptomatic babies >35 weeks of gestation with risk factors alone, and laboratory markers (biomarkers or counts) need to be positive as well. In such cases, the baby is considered to have probable sepsis, and antibiotics are to be continued for at least 7–10 days, even if the blood culture report remains negative and laboratory markers turn negative later.

Antibiotics should be started in all symptomatic neonates, irrespective of gestational age, having one or more risk factors for early onset sepsis. They should be continued

Flowchart 2.11.1: Starting antibiotics in neonates with risk factors for early-onset neonatal septicemia (EONS).

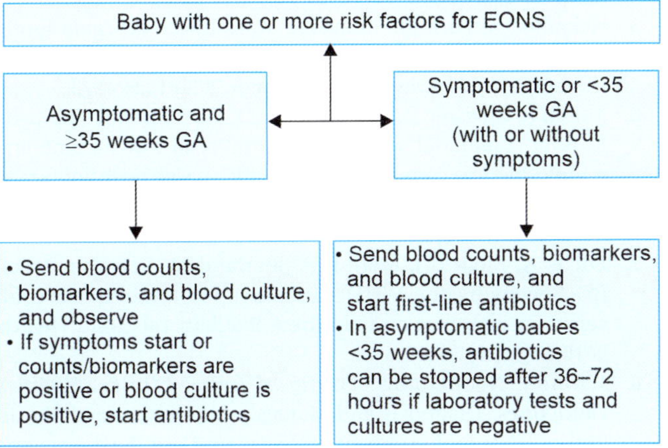

(GA: gestational age)

if biomarkers or blood counts are suggestive of sepsis, even if blood cultures are negative. The recommended duration of antibiotic therapy for uncomplicated (no meningitis, bone and joint, or staphylococcal infections), culture-positive neonatal sepsis is 10–14 days. At least one negative blood culture report should be available before stopping antibiotics. In babies in whom blood cultures are repeatedly negative, antibiotics are continued if the baby was symptomatic or had positive biomarkers or low blood counts for at least 7–10 days. In neonates with meningitis or in blood culture-proven staphylococcal sepsis, the duration of treatment is 3 weeks. In bone or joint infections, ventriculitis, endocarditis, and other deep-seated infections, antibiotics are continued for at least 4–6 weeks.

Responsible use of antibiotics is mandatory by all HCWs to decrease the incidence of multidrug-resistant organisms. Antibiotics should be stopped as soon as possible in asymptomatic preterm neonates with risk factors who had been started empirically on antibiotics. De-escalation of antibiotics should be done based on culture sensitivity. Other aspects of responsible antibiotic usage (antibiotic stewardship) are given in **Box 2.11.1**.[9]

Supportive Management

The supportive management of neonatal sepsis involves maintaining temperature, adequate ventilation, oxygenation, circulation, nutrition, and glucose homeostasis. This should preferably be in a NICU. The use of inotropes, blood products, and adequate nutrition is mandatory for good outcomes.

Adjunct treatments such as intravenous (IV) immunoglobulin, granulocyte colony stimulating factors, exchange transfusion, pentoxifylline, and activated protein C, among others, have all been tried and discarded due to a lack of scientific evidence of effectivity.

BOX 2.11.1: Antibiotic stewardship and responsible antibiotic use in neonates.

- Use appropriate drug doses and schedules based on clinical situation and culture
- Choose antibiotics based on sensitivity patterns and the antibiotic policy of your hospital
- Give antibiotic "drug holidays" as per Hospital Infection Control Committee policy
- Stop empirical antibiotics as early as possible
- De-escalate (i.e., change from a broad-spectrum antibiotics to a more specific one) based on culture sensitivity
- Refer to an appropriate drug formulary (e.g., Neofax) for the right dose, frequency, diluent, storage, interactions, and adverse events
- Do not combine antibiotics with similar toxicities, for example, vancomycin and gentamicin, or those with a similar spectrum of action
- Avoid reusing the antibiotic vial after one dose unless indicated and stored properly. Some antibiotics, such as meropenem and teicoplanin, have a short shelf life of less than 48 hours after reconstitution and should not be stored for longer periods
- Audit the use of antibiotics regularly

COMPLICATIONS

Sepsis remains the leading cause of neonatal mortality the world over. In the acute phase, hypoglycemia, coagulopathy, seizures, shock, and organ failure are common. Pneumonia, PPHN, myocardial dysfunction, renal failure, coagulation problems, and hepatic dysfunction are common, particularly with gram-negative sepsis. Meningitis can result in complications such as hydrocephalus and developmental delay.

PREVENTION OF SEPSIS[3,7]

Though not completely preventable, the incidence of neonatal sepsis can be decreased by promoting exclusive breastfeeding and skin-to-skin contact in the delivery room, rooming in with the mother, and following simple hygiene measures. Cord hygiene entails keeping the cord clean, dry, and exposed to air. The application of antiseptics and antibiotics to the cord should be avoided unless there is frank omphalitis. Hospital-acquired infections can be minimized by practicing good hand hygiene, promoting breast milk for sick low birth weight (LBW) neonates, good adherence to asepsis protocols, and following a strict antibiotic policy.

The WHO has issued recommendations to decrease infections in newborns in both the community and hospital setting and to improve early recognition and timely and appropriate treatment of neonatal sepsis. These include exclusive breastfeeding, skin-to-skin contact with the mother from birth, the empirical antibiotic treatment of neonates with risk factors or danger signs suggestive of severe infection/sepsis, and education of families and community health workers of these danger signs.

In a hospital setting, the implementation and practice of asepsis protocols are mandatory. Rapid culture techniques, antibiotic stewardship, and bundled approaches to prevent central line-associated bloodstream infections (CLABSIs) and ventilator-associated pneumonia in the neonate are now considered standard of care in NICUs and can significantly reduce morbidity and mortality from neonatal sepsis.

REFERENCES

1. Wynn JL, Polin RA. Progress in the management of neonatal sepsis: the importance of a consensus definition. Pediatr Res. 2018;83(1):13-5.
2. Fleischmann C, Reichert F, Cassini A, Horner R, Harder T, Markwart R, et al. Global incidence, and mortality of neonatal sepsis: a systematic review and meta-analysis Arch Dis Child. 2021;106(8):745-52.
3. Mukherjee T, Wazir S. Recent advances in diagnosis, prevention and treatment of neonatal sepsis. Pediatr Inf Dis. 2019;1(3):108-13.
4. Murthy S, Godinho MA, Guddattu V, Lewis LES, Nair NS. Risk factors of neonatal sepsis in India: a systematic review and meta-analysis. PLoS One. 2021;14(4):e0215683.
5. Nakamori Y, Park EJ, Shimaoka M. Immune deregulation in sepsis and septic shock: reversing immune paralysis by targeting PD-1/PD-L1 pathway. Front Immunol. 2020;11:624279.
6. Milton R, Gillespie D, Dyer C, Taiyari K, Carvalho MJ, Thomson K, et al. Neonatal sepsis and mortality in low-income and middle-income countries from a facility-based birth cohort: an international multisite prospective observational study Lancet Glob Health. 2022; 10(5):e661-72.
7. Fuchs A, Bielicki J, Mathur S, Sharland M, Van Den Anker JN. Reviewing the WHO guidelines for antibiotic use for sepsis in neonates and children. Paediatr Int Child Health. 2018;38(sup1):S3-15.
8. National Neonatology Forum of India. Clinical Practice Guidelines: Diagnosis and Management of Neonatal Sepsis. [online] Available from http://www.nnfi.org [Last accessed October, 2024].
9. Treatment Guidelines for Antimicrobial Use in Common Syndromes, 2nd edition. New Delhi: Indian Council of Medical Research; 2019.
10. Fleiss N, Schwabenbauer K, Randis TM, Polin RA. What's new in the management of neonatal early onset sepsis? Arch Dis Child Fetal Neonatal Ed. 2023;108(1):10-4.

2.12 Respiratory Distress in Newborn

Pranitha Reddy, Aparna Chandrasekaran

INTRODUCTION

Respiratory distress (RD) is the most common problem seen in neonatal intensive care units (NICUs), most often posing a diagnostic dilemma for the treating doctor. In a newborn, RD can be caused by either parenchymal lung diseases, pulmonary vascular diseases, neurological problems, metabolic issues, or congenital heart defects. In this chapter, we will discuss the most common respiratory causes of distress in newborns.

DEFINITION

According to the National Neonatal Perinatal Database (NNPD) of India, RD in newborns is defined as the presence of *any two* of the following:

- Tachypnea with respiratory rate >60/min
- Retractions—subcostal/intercostal
- Grunt

In the extremely preterm infant, the only clinical symptom of RD may be apnea. Late signs include cyanosis, gasping, apnea, and stridor.

CLASSIFICATION OF RESPIRATORY DISTRESS

Respiratory distress can be classified by assessing the appearance, breathing pattern, and circulation **(Fig. 2.12.1)**.

Grading of Severity

The grading of RD can be made relatively objective by using scores like Downes–Vidysagar score **(Table 2.12.1)** and the Silverman–Anderson (SA) score **(Table 2.12.2)**. Despite an earlier concept of using an RD score of 3–4 for deciding the initial mode of respiratory support, it has been realized that it

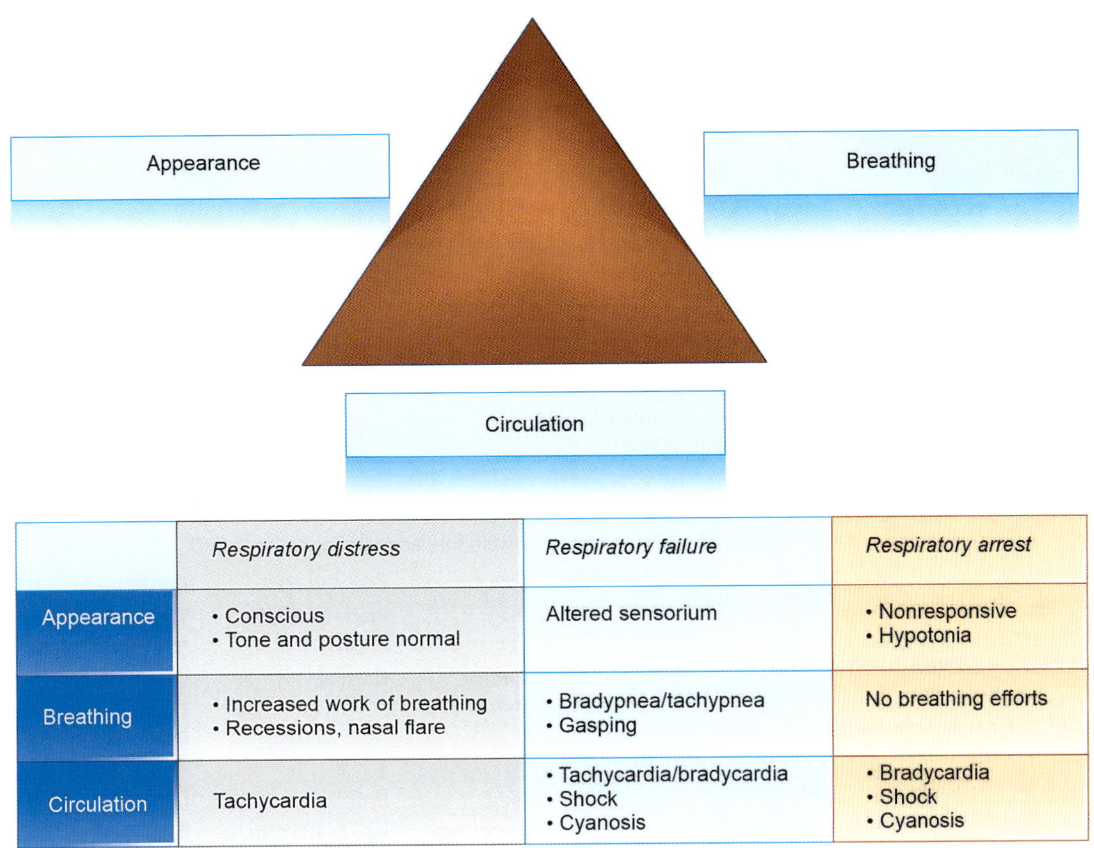

	Respiratory distress	Respiratory failure	Respiratory arrest
Appearance	• Conscious • Tone and posture normal	Altered sensorium	• Nonresponsive • Hypotonia
Breathing	• Increased work of breathing • Recessions, nasal flare	• Bradypnea/tachypnea • Gasping	No breathing efforts
Circulation	Tachycardia	• Tachycardia/bradycardia • Shock • Cyanosis	• Bradycardia • Shock • Cyanosis

Fig. 2.12.1: Classification of respiratory distress.

TABLE 2.12.1: Downes–Vidyasagar score.

Score	*Respiratory rate*	*Air entry*	*Cyanosis*	*Grunt*	*Retractions*
0	<60/min	Normal	Nil	None	None
1	60–80/min	Mildly reduced	In <40% FiO_2	On auscultation	Mild
2	>80/min	Markedly reduced or absent	In >40% FiO_2	To naked ear	Moderate

TABLE 2.12.2: Silverman–Anderson score for preterm infants.

Score[‡]	*Upper chest retractions**	*Lower chest retractions*[†]	*Xiphoid retractions*	*Nasal flare*	*Grunt*
0	Synchronized	None	None	None	None
1	Lag on inspiration	Just visible	Mild	Mild	Audible with a stethoscope
2	See-saw breathing	Marked	Marked	Marked	Audible to naked ear

*Upper chest—part of chest anterior to mid axillary line; Upper chest retractions—assess by synchrony of movement of upper chest with abdomen.
[†]Lower chest retractions—observe retractions below mid-axillary line, in between the ribs.
[‡]A score of 7 or more suggests impending respiratory failure—may need intubation and ventilation.

is better to initiate early continuous positive airway pressure (CPAP) at the appearance of even one or two signs of RD in preterm neonates below 32 weeks, such as the appearance of isolated retractions or episodes of hypoxemia without waiting for the score to go up to 3–4.

ETIOLOGY OF RESPIRATORY DISTRESS IN NEONATES

Table 2.12.3 summarizes the various etiological causes of RD in neonates.[1] Some other common causes of RD include the following:

TABLE 2.12.3: Etiology of respiratory distress in neonates.

Pulmonary	*Cardiac*	*Neurological*	*Surgical*	*Miscellaneous*
Respiratory distress syndrome (RDS)	Congenital heart disease (CHD)	Asphyxia	Tracheo-esophageal fistula (TEF)	Hypoglycemia
Meconium aspiration syndrome	Patent ductus arteriosus (PDA)	Intracranial hemorrhage (ICH)	Congenital diaphragmatic hernia (CDH)	Anemia
Transient tachypnea of newborns (TTNB)	Arrhythmia	Cerebral edema	Lung anomalies	Polycythemia
Pneumonia	Cardiomyopathy		Choanal atresia	Metabolic acidosis
Pneumothorax	Congestive heart failure (CHF)		Pierre Robin sequence	Sepsis
Pulmonary hypoplasia	High output failure			Hypo- and hyperthermia
Persistent pulmonary hypertension of newborn (PPHN)	Pneumo-pericardium/ cardiac tamponade			

- *Upper airway obstruction:* Choanal atresia, nasal stenosis, Pierre–Robin sequence, laryngeal stenosis or atresia, hemangioma, vocal cord paralysis, vascular rings, tracheobronchial stenosis, masses, cleft palate, and nasal stuffiness.
- *Pulmonary causes:* Pulmonary hemorrhage, pulmonary hypoplasia, pulmonary agenesis, cystic disease, pleural effusion, chylothorax, neoplasm, bronchopulmonary sequestration, pulmonary arteriovenous malformation, pulmonary interstitial emphysema, pulmonary edema, congenital alveolar proteinosis, and congenital lobar emphysema.
- *Thoracic causes:* Chest wall deformity.
- *Diaphragmatic causes:* Congenital diaphragmatic hernia and diaphragmatic paralysis.
- *Neuromuscular diseases:* Central nervous system damage (birth trauma and hemorrhage), medication (maternal sedation and narcotic withdrawal), muscular disease (myasthenia gravis), intraventricular hemorrhage, meningitis, hypoxic–ischemic encephalopathy, seizure disorder, obstructed hydrocephalus, infantile botulism, and spinal cord injury.

It may be often difficult to differentiate cardiac from pulmonary causes of RD. **Table 2.12.4** describes the key clinical and laboratory indicators to differentiate the two.

INCIDENCE

Respiratory distress syndrome (RDS) is the most common cause of RD in premature babies (45%). Transient tachypnea of newborns (TTNB) is the most common cause of RD in term babies.

HISTORY AND CLINICAL EXAMINATION

History and Physical Assessment

History is very helpful in guiding the cause of RD in newborns as discussed in **Table 2.12.5**.

TABLE 2.12.4: Clinical and laboratory markers to differentiate respiratory and cardiac causes of RD.

	Respiratory	*Cardiac*
RD	Predominantly retractions	Tachypnea predominant, retractions minimal or absent
Cardiac examination	Normal	Severe cyanosis, murmur, weak pulses, hepatomegaly, poor pulse volume, and differential cyanosis
pCO_2	High	Low or normal
Hyperoxia test	PaO_2 >300 mm Hg	PaO_2 does not exceed 150 mm Hg
Chest X-ray	Parenchymal infiltrates	• Cardiomegaly • Increased pulmonary vascular markings

(pCO_2: partial pressure of carbon dioxide; PaO_2: partial pressure of arterial oxygen; RD: respiratory distress)

Table 2.12.6 describes the localization of area involved and pathology based on physical findings.

Pulse Oximetry

Rightly termed the sixth vital sign, pulse oximetry plays a significant role in monitoring a neonate with RD and also provides some important clues to the diagnosis. Always check both preductal and postductal saturations. **Table 2.12.7** highlights some important observations with pulse oximetry.

Response to Oxygen Therapy

A marked response in oxygenation with supplemental oxygen delivered in the form of endotracheal ventilation or any other form of high inspired oxygen concentration is seen in respiratory causes. If PaO_2 >300 mm Hg, it usually indicates a pulmonary parenchymal cause, while PaO_2 does not exceed 150 mm Hg in congenital critical cardiac conditions. Intermediate levels can be seen in admixture lesions like hypoplastic left heart syndrome.

TABLE 2.12.5: History and clinical evaluation in determining the cause of respiratory distress (RD).

History	*Pattern of RD*	*Most probable cause*
• Preterm delivery <34 weeks • Infant of diabetic mother • Lack of antenatal steroids • Maternal abruption • Asphyxia	• Onset at/soon after birth • Progresses till 48 hours, static for 48 hours and improves later • FiO_2 requirement may be >40% • Surfactant therapy modifies the typical course	RDS
• Term/late preterm • Born by elective lower segment cesarean section • Maternal diabetes	• Onset at or soon after birth • Maximum severity at birth and improves gradually • FiO_2 requirement seldom >40% (except malignant TTNB)	TTNB
• Maternal fever • Foul-smelling liquor • Other features of chorioamnionitis	• RD with clinical features of sepsis • Onset at birth or delayed • Fails to improve with oxygen/CPAP	Congenital pneumonia/sepsis
• History of meconium-stained liquor • Prolonged labor • Oligohydramnios	• RD worsening after 6 hours of life, RR > 80/min • Barrel shaped chest • Skin and cord staining with meconium • Hyperinflated chest • Features of PPHN	MAS
• Use of PPV in delivery room	• Acute worsening of RD, especially with PPV • Shock • Chest asymmetry • Reduced air entry • Shift of mediastinum • Transillumination positive	Pneumothorax
• Obstructed labor • Fetal distress • Birth trauma • Delayed cry • Requirement of resuscitation	• Acidotic breathing	Asphyxial lung injury
• Chronic PPROM • Oligohydramnios • History of renal anomalies in antenatal scans	• Severe RD requiring high pressures and multiple doses of surfactant • Potter facies	Pulmonary hypoplasia
• Polyhydramnios • Scaphoid abdomen at birth	• Worsening of distress with bag and tube ventilation • Gurgling sounds in chest • Reduced air entry left lung • Apex beat shifted to right	CDH
• Stridor • Weak cry	• Suprasternal retractions >> intercostal recessions • Chest in-drawing • Improves after ventilation with minimal settings/pressures • Weak cry	Airway anomalies, laryngomalacia
• Polyhydramnios • OG tube cannot be passed and coils in esophagus	• Increased salivation • Excess frothing from mouth • Choking during feeds	TEF with esophageal atresia
• Polyhydramnios • NG tube cannot be passed from nose into nasopharynx	• Cyclic RD more during feeding and disappears on crying	Choanal atresia

(CDH: congenital diaphragmatic hernia; CPAP: continuous positive airway pressure; FiO_2: fraction of inspired oxygen; MAS: meconium aspiration syndrome; NG: nasogastric; OG: orogastric; PPHN: persistent pulmonary hypertension of newborn; PPROM: preterm premature rupture of membranes; PPV: positive-pressure ventilation; RDS: respiratory distress syndrome; RR: respiratory rate; TEF: tracheo-esophageal fistula; TTB: transient tachypnea of newborns)

TABLE 2.12.6: Localization of area involved and pathology based on physical findings.

Physical findings	*Localization*
Severe retractions, grunt, and nasal flaring	Pulmonary parenchymal involvement
Stridor	• Upper airway obstruction • Laryngomalacia, subglottic stenosis, and Pierre Robin sequence
Wheeze	Narrowing of bronchioles
Silent tachypnea	CHD, anemia, and metabolic acidosis
Cyanosis	CHD, severe lung disease, polycythemia, methemoglobinemia, and neurological dysfunction

(CHD: congenital heart disease)

TABLE 2.12.7: Interpretations of pulse oximetry findings.

Pulse oximetry findings	*Diagnosis*
SpO_2 <90%	Hypoxia
• Preductal greater than postductal saturations by 5–10% • Lability of saturations	PPHN
Lower limb SpO_2 > Upper limb SpO_2	TGA with pulmonary hypertension

(PPHN: persistent pulmonary hyperextension of newborn; TGA: transposition of the great arteries)

Role of Chest X-ray in Evaluation of Respiratory Distress

Chest X-ray is the most important investigation in the evaluation of RD as it helps in the diagnosis of distress in most of the cases **(Table 2.12.8; Figs. 2.12.2 to 2.12.8)**.

Role of Other Investigations in Evaluation of Respiratory Distress

- *Gastric shake test:* Mix 0.5 mL of gastric aspirate with an equal volume of 95% ethyl alcohol in a test tube, shake for 15 seconds, and let it stand for 15 minutes. The presence of a rim of bubbles is considered positive and indicates the presence of surfactant. Absence of bubbles indicates deficient surfactant and presence of RDS.
- *Transillumination:* A fiberoptic light source can be applied to the chest to diagnose pneumothorax and also for the administration of surfactant before a chest X-ray is available. It is a simple bedside test useful in severe RD and acute deterioration on respiratory support.
- *Oxygenation indices:* Oxygenation index (OI) is a sensitive indicator of oxygenation. It is calculated as OI = Mean airway pressure (MAP) × FiO_2/PaO_2 × 100. OI > 15 indicates ventilation-perfusion mismatch. OI > 20 is an indication for the initiation of inhaled nitric oxide. OI > 40 is an indication for extracorporeal membrane oxygenation (ECMO) and is associated with poor prognosis.
- *Alveolar to arterial oxygen pressure difference ($A - a\ DO_2$)* represents PAO_2 (alveolar oxygen) minus PaO_2 (arterial oxygen)

$$A - a\ DO_2 = (\text{Atmospheric} - \text{alveolar water pressure gradient} \times FiO_2) - (PaCO_2/\text{Respiratory quotient}) - PaO_2$$

- $(760 - 47) \times FiO_2 - PaCO_2/RQ$ is alveolar oxygen
- PaO_2 is arterial or capillary oxygen
- $Aa - DO_2$ is $(760 - 47) \times FiO_2 - PaCO_2/RQ - PaO_2$
- Respiratory quotient = 0.8
- Atmospheric pressure at sea level – alveolar water pressure = 760 – 47 = 713
- In healthy neonates, $A - aDO_2$ is <20

TABLE 2.12.8: X-ray findings in some of the important causes of RD in newborn.

Condition	*X-ray findings*
RDS **(Figs. 2.12.2A and B)**	• Air bronchograms • Fine reticulogranular pattern • Low volume lungs • Ground-glass appearance • White-out lung
MAS **(Fig. 2.12.3)**	• Heterogeneous parenchymal disease, fluffy infiltrates, coarse nodular opacities, hyperinflation, or patchy atelectasis • Air trapping • Features of RDS
Pneumonia **(Fig. 2.12.4)**	• Diffuse parenchymal infiltrates • Air bronchograms • Reticulogranular pattern
TTNB **(Fig. 2.12.5)**	• Prominent hilar markings • Fluid in the minor fissure • Sun burst appearance • Hyperinflation
CDH **(Fig. 2.12.6)**	Bowel loops in chest, absent gastric bubble, and mediastinal shift
Pneumothorax **(Fig. 2.12.7)**	• Area of lucency without pulmonary markings is seen • Mediastinal shift to opposite side
Congenital heart disease or PPHN	Hypoxemia disproportionate to lung findings
Pulmonary hypoplasia **(Fig. 2.12.8)**	Low volume lung

(CDH: congenital diaphragmatic hernia; MAS: meconium aspiration syndrome; PPHN: persistent pulmonary hypertension in newborn; RD: respiratory distress; RDS: respiratory distress syndrome; TTNB: transient tachypnea of newborns)

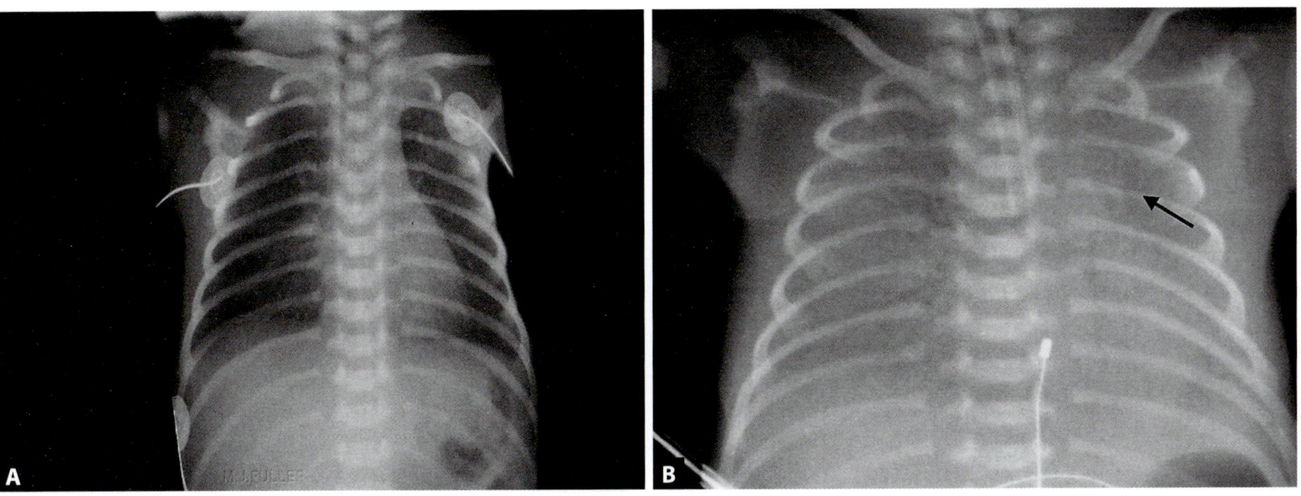

Figs. 2.12.2A and B: Respiratory distress syndrome.

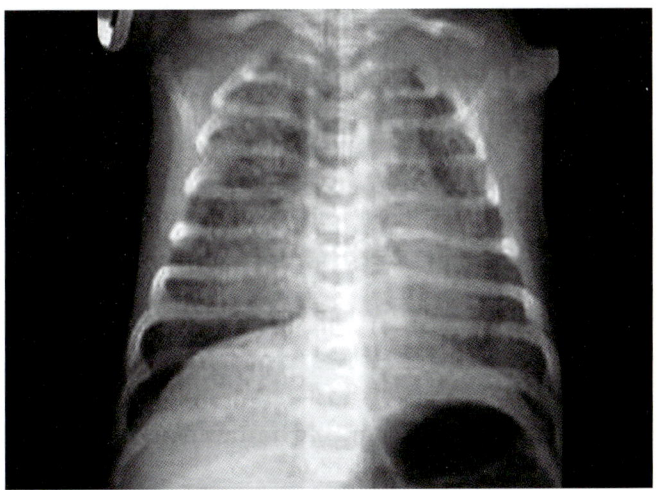

Fig. 2.12.3: Typical findings in meconium aspiration syndrome (MAS).

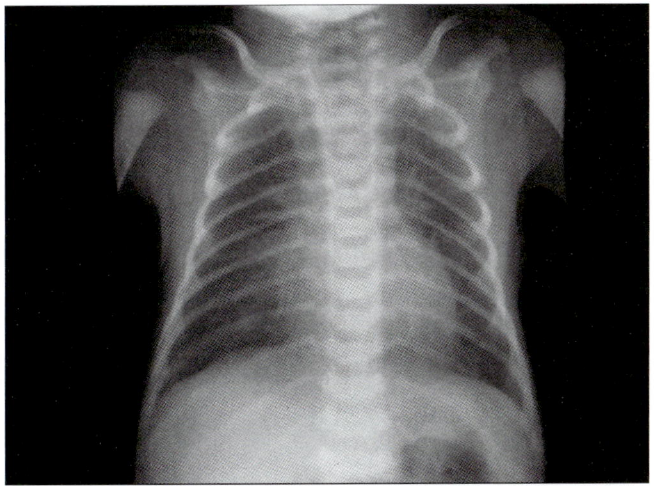

Fig. 2.12.5: Typical findings in TTNB. (TTNB: transient tachypnea of newborns)

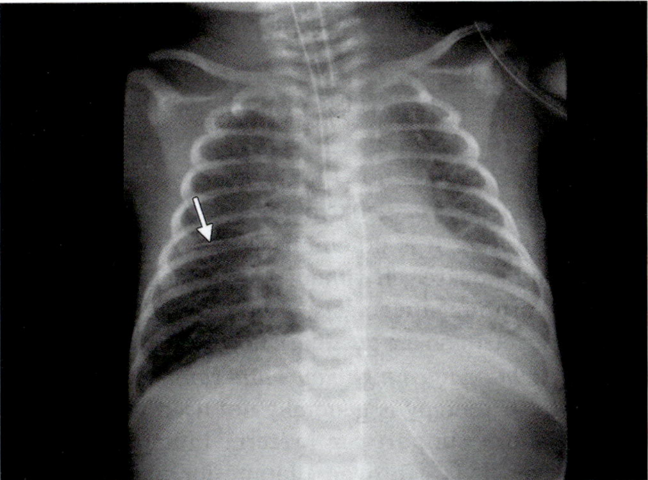

Fig. 2.12.4: Typical findings in pneumonia (arrow showing fluid in fissure).

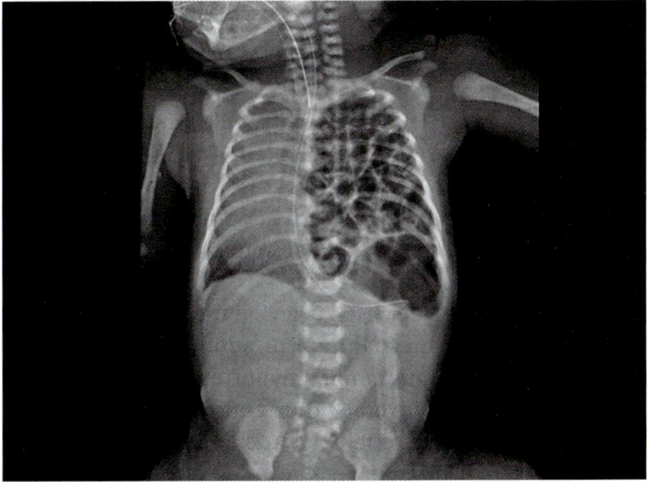

Fig. 2.12.6: Congenital diaphragmatic hernia.

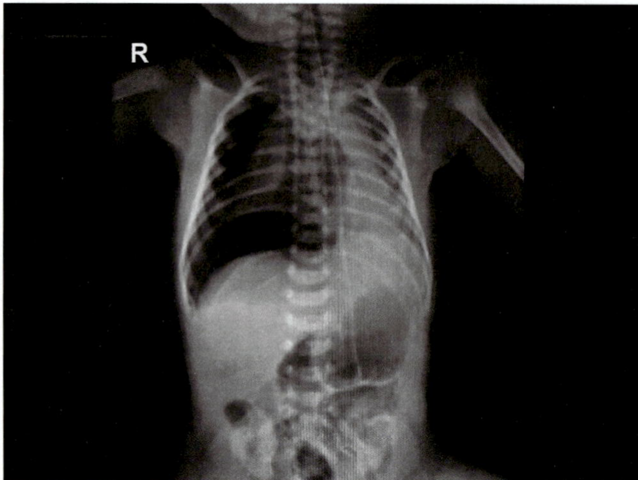

Fig. 2.12.7: Pneumothorax.

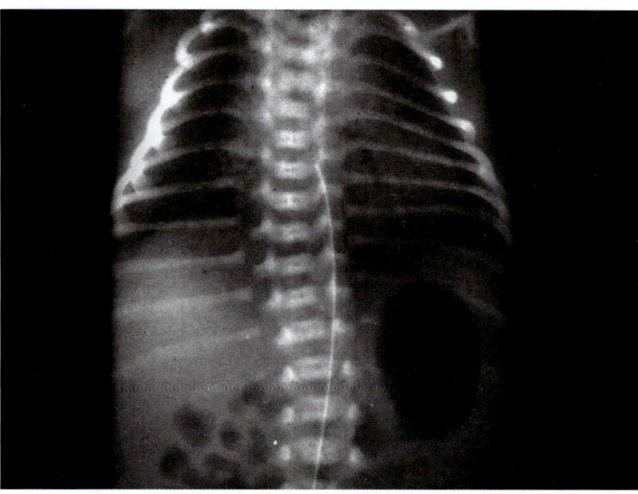

Fig. 2.12.8: Pulmonary hypoplasia.

Interpretations of some of the other investigations in RD are listed in **Table 2.12.9**.

Role of Echocardiography

Echocardiography is important in the following conditions:

- Sudden unexplained clinical deterioration
- Shock
- To rule out congenital cardiac conditions with duct-dependent pulmonary and systemic blood flow lesions and anomalous venous return
- Inhaled nitric oxide (INO) is a vital therapy in improving oxygenation in meconium aspiration syndrome (MAS) and persistent pulmonary hypertension of newborn (PPHN) due to several other causes. INO therapy is contraindicated in certain duct-dependent lesions, and it is important to do a prior echocardiogram prior to starting INO.

TABLE 2.12.9: Other investigations in respiratory distress.

Investigation	*Interpretation*
CBC	• Sepsis—leukocytosis or leukopenia, shift to left, neutropenia • Polycythemia • Anemia
Blood glucose	Hypoglycemia
CRP, PCT	• Sepsis • Pneumonia
Blood culture	• Sepsis • Pneumonia • Always obtain prior culture before initiating antibiotics
Arterial blood gases	• Assess ventilation, oxygenation, acidemia • Hypoxemia (PaO_2 <60 mm Hg, hypercarbia >60 mm Hg with falling pH. <7.2 indicates respiratory failure)
USG chest	• Pleural effusion • Diaphragmatic movements (eventration)
CT thorax	Suspected mediastinal mass, vascular ring
MRI chest/CT angiogram	To assess vascular supply in pulmonary sequestration

(CBC: complete blood counts; CRP: C-reactive protein; CT: computed tomography; PCT: procalcitonin; MRI: magnetic resonance imaging; USG: ultrasonogram)

MANAGEMENT OF RESPIRATORY DISTRESS

General Principles of Management

Supportive care includes maintenance of normal temperature, blood glucose, nutrition, and intravenous (IV) fluids (**Table 2.12.10; Flowchart 2.12.1**).

Recommendations for Respiratory Support for Neonates with Respiratory Distress

Modalities for Oxygen Therapy

- Nasal cannula
  - In babies born >34 weeks with mild RD
  - Use at 0.5–1 L/min
  - If the baby requires >1 L/min flow, warm, humidified, and blended oxygen to be given
- *Hood oxygen:* It is de-emphasized as it delivers high concentration oxygen without pressure delivery, resulting in absorption atelectasis.[2] Rebreathing and carbon dioxide retention are possible if flow rates are <4 L/min.
- *Heated, humidified high-flow nasal cannula (HHHFNC):* HHHFNC therapy is generally not used for the initial respiratory support for preterm infants with RDS. However, it is a proven therapy for postextubation support in preterm infants. HHHFNC prongs are usually

TABLE 2.12.10: Principles of supportive care in respiratory distress.

	Do's	*Don'ts*
Thermal care	Maintain normothermia by a radiant warmer/ incubator	Avoid hypo- and hyperthermia
Oxygen	• Use humidified oxygen • Strict pulse oximetry monitoring for any baby on oxygen support to target 90–95%	Avoid hypoxia <90% and hyperoxia >95%
Fluids	• Ensure proper hydration • Total volume 60–80 mL/kg/day	Avoid fluid restriction and overhydration
Circulation	• Maintain hemoglobin within acceptable limits • Monitor blood pressure • Maintain normal tissue perfusion	Do not aim for numbers
Nutrition	• Feeding as per protocol • Orogastric feeds can be given for baby on CPAP/ ventilator	• Respiratory distress is not contraindication for enteral feeding • Consider TPN if feeds cannot be started
Antibiotics	Start antibiotics as per protocol for suspected sepsis, clinical sepsis/ pneumonia	Do not give prophylactic antibiotics
Nursing	• Maintain clear airway • Suction secretions • Comfort baby • Clustering of care	

(CPAP: continuous positive airway pressure; TPN: total parenteral nutrition)

smaller in length and diameter than those used for CPAP and do not require a seal. As a result, HHHFNC may be associated with less nasal trauma and would be easier to apply than CPAP. In addition, HHHFNC enhances carbon dioxide elimination because of its ability to "washout" the posterior pharyngeal dead space with fresh inspiratory gas.

Continuous Positive Airway Pressure

Continuous positive airway pressure refers to the application of continuous pressure to the airways during both inspiration and expiration. The presence of spontaneous efforts is an essential prerequisite before starting CPAP. **Table 2.12.11** describes the mechanism of action of CPAP and **Table 2.12.12** on the initial settings on CPAP.

Flowchart 2.12.1: Approach to a case of respiratory distress.

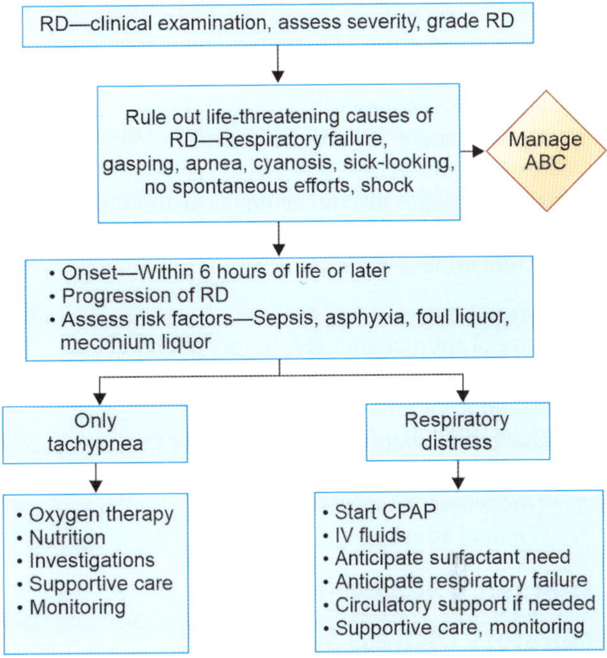

(CPAP: continuous positive airway pressure; IV: intravenous; RD: respiratory distress)

TABLE 2.12.11: Mechanisms of action of CPAP.

Continuous positive airway pressure to airways and keeps alveoli open	Increases FRC
Splints the airway by dilating lower airways and reduces airway resistance	• Helpful in airway anomalies • Prevents obstructive apnea
Better gas exchange	Reduces lung injury

(CPAP: continuous positive airway pressure; FRC: functional residual capacity)

TABLE 2.12.12: CPAP settings.

Pressure (PEEP)	4–7 cm H_2O	Start with PEEP of 5 cmH_2O for mild retractions and slowly increase PEEP in steps of 1 cm if there are persistent retractions up to 7–8 cmH_2O
Flow	4–7 L/min	• Start with flow of 4–5 L/min • Titration flow based on bubbling in pressure chamber • Preferably continuous bubbling to be present throughout the respiratory cycle
FiO_2	21–100%	Start with FiO_2 of 30%, titrate FiO_2 targeting saturations 91–95%
• Temperature • Relative humidity	37°C 100% RH	–

(CPAP: continuous positive airway pressure; PEEP: positive end-expiratory pressure; RH: relative humidity)

Indications:

- *RD:*
    - RD with SA score ≥3 in preterm neonates
    - RD due to any cause like TTNB, MAS, or pneumonia with an SA score ≥5
    - Downes score >5 in term neonates
- Postextubation
- Airway anomalies like tracheomalacia and phrenic nerve palsy
- Recurrent apneas

Contraindications:

- Absence of spontaneous respiratory efforts
- Shock
- Lung malformations like
    - Congenital diaphragmatic hernia
    - Cleft palate
    - Tracheo-esophageal fistula
    - Choanal atresia

SPECIFIC TREATMENT

Respiratory Distress Syndrome

Surfactant is essential for the reduction of surface tension. Alveoli deficient in surfactant collapse. Hence, neonates with RDS present with atelectasis, and ventilation-perfusion mismatch, leading to hypoxia and respiratory failure.

Surfactant Therapy[3-6]

Surfactant therapy is the greatest innovation contributing to the survival of preterm babies. The Laplace law states that pressure within a sphere is proportional to its surface tension and inversely proportional to its radius. Surface tension generated by a thin film of alveolar fluid prevents lung inflation and promotes alveolar collapse. So, in RDS, the pressure required to open up small alveoli is much higher owing to the high surface tension. The surfactant lowers surface tension. In alveoli lined with a surfactant, surface tension falls to zero, preventing collapse and maintaining functional residual capacity.

- *Composition:* Pulmonary surfactant is secreted by type II alveolar cells. It is a mixture of phospholipids, lipids, and surfactant proteins stored in a lamellar body. The predominant phospholipid is dipalmitoylphosphatidylcholine (DPPC).
- *Type of surfactants:* These surfactant preparations can be classified into one of five groups **(Table 2.12.13)**. Various forms of surfactant therapy used in neonatal practice are shown in **Table 2.12.14 and Flowchart 2.12.2**.
- *Indications of surfactant therapy:* The need for FiO_2 of 0.3–0.4 and/or positive end-expiratory pressure (PEEP) of >6–7 cm warrants surfactant therapy for infants with RDS. The dose of surfactant is 100 mg/kg of phospholipid.

TABLE 2.12.13: Surfactant types.

Natural	Minced lung extracts	• Surfactant TA (Surfacten) • Beractant (Survanta) • Poractant alfa (Curosurf)
	Lung lavage extracts	• CLSE/Neosurf (bLES) • Calfactant (Infasurf) • SF-RI1 (Alveofact)
	Amniotic fluid extract	• Human surfactant
Synthetic	Old synthetic (protein-free)	• Pumactant (ALEC) • Colfosceril palmitate (Exosurf) • Turfsurf (Belfast surfactant)
	New synthetic (protein analogs)	• Lucinactant (Surfaxin) • rSP-C surfactant (Venticute)

(ALEC: artificial lung expanding compound; bLES: bovine lipid extract surfactant; CLSE: calf lung surfactant extract or calfactant; rSP-C: recombinant surfactant protein C; SF-RI1: surfactant fatty acid ratio index 1; TA: therapeutic aerosol)

TABLE 2.12.14: Surfactant administration based on clinical indication and timing.

	Timing	*Clinical indication*
Prophylactic	Administration of surfactant before the onset of RD	• Not recommended routinely • May be given to preterm neonates <28 weeks' gestation requiring intubation in the delivery room
Early rescue	Giving surfactant at early signs of RDS within 2 hours of life with FiO_2 ≥30%, PEEP ≥6 cm to maintain SpO_2 ≥91%	Recommended <34 weeks' gestation
Late rescue	Administration of surfactant with clinical signs of RD at 2–4 hours of life	

(PEEP: positive end-expiratory pressure; RD: respiratory distress; RDS: respiratory distress syndrome)

- *Repeat dose of surfactant:* Repeat doses of surfactant may be required in an infant if the administered surfactant is inhibited by edema fluid, proteins, and inflammatory mediators that are present in the alveoli after lung injury due to mechanical ventilation, delayed surfactant administration, or sepsis. Infants may require repeat doses of surfactant if they require FiO_2 >0.35 and MAP >7 cmH_2O to maintain a PaO_2 50–70 mm Hg and $PaCO_2$ <50 mm Hg. The use of repetitive dosing has decreased in clinical practice, probably because more attention is being paid to avoiding lung injury prior to the first dose. Other indications of surfactant in term neonates are:

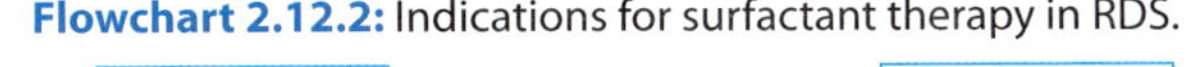

Flowchart 2.12.2: Indications for surfactant therapy in RDS.

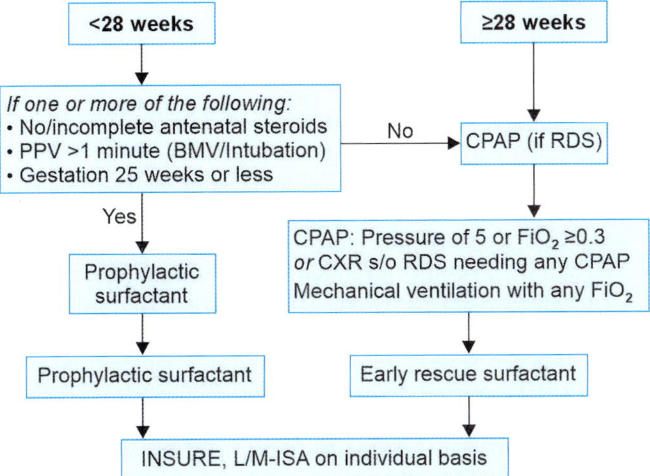

(BMV: bag-mask ventilation; CPAP: continuous positive airway pressure; CXR: chest X-ray; INSURE: intubate, surfactant, and extubate; L/M-ISA: less/minimally invasive surfactant administration; PPV: positive pressure ventilation; RDS: respiratory distress syndrome)

- Severe MAS requiring invasive ventilation with OI >15
- Severe bacterial pneumonia requiring invasive ventilation with OI >15
- Severe PPHN with OI >5

Pneumonia

Despite the lack of specific clinical signs, pneumonia accounts to be the third most common cause of RD in newborns. Clinical history of chorioamnionitis (prolonged rupture of membranes, foul-smelling liquor, maternal and fetal tachycardia, maternal fever) can serve as supportive evidence.

Etiology

Group B *Streptococcus* is the most common cause of sepsis and pneumonia in developed countries. In India, gram-negative pathogens like *E. coli* and *Klebsiella* are the most common causes of pneumonia. Other causes are Streptococci, *Staphylococcus aureus, Haemophilus influenzae, Enterococcus, Listeria monocytogenes,* fungi, viruses like respiratory syncytial virus, adenovirus, rhinovirus, cytomegalovirus, and herpes simplex virus.

Clinical Features

A newborn with pneumonia usually presents with nonspecific signs of sepsis due to the nonconfinement of infection to the lungs. Signs like lethargy, RD, hypothermia, lethargy, poor perfusion, hypotension, and in severe cases, shock and respiratory failure are seen.

Laboratory Signs

Leukopenia, increased immature granulocytes, and raised inflammatory markers such as C-reactive protein (CRP) and procalcitonin (PCT) increase the likelihood of pneumonia. Gastric aspirate for polymorphonuclear lymphocytes taken immediately after birth may be helpful in newborns with suspected congenital pneumonia. Endotracheal aspirate for culture is useful in ventilated newborns with suspected pneumonia. Blood culture is positive in only 10% of cases due to prior administration of maternal antibiotics.

Treatment

Antibiotics should be aimed toward targeted organisms. Since gram-negative organisms are commonly isolated, aminoglycoside with piperacillin/tazobactum is commonly employed. If blood culture is negative and clinical course is strongly suggestive of pneumonia, antibiotics are usually given for 5–7 days.

Transient Tachypnea of Newborns

Fetal lung epithelium produces alveolar fluid, which helps in lung growth. During the time of birth, lung epithelium transitions from secretory to resorptive type under the influence of parturition hormones. Endothelial sodium channels (ENaC) present on type II epithelial cells help in the transport of sodium and water from alveolar cells into type II cells. Sodium-potassium ATPase pumps transport sodium from type II cells into the interstitial, causing resorption of lung fluid into pulmonary circulation and lymphatics.

Meconium Aspiration Syndrome

Up to 5% of babies with meconium-stained amniotic fluid develop MAS. Fetal acidemia increases intestinal peristalsis, leading to meconium passage in utero. Perinatal hypoxia results in fetal gasping and meconium aspiration.

Pathophysiology

Respiratory distress develops in MAS by mechanisms shown in **Flowchart 2.12.3**.

Complications of MAS

- Severe RD resulting in respiratory failure in 50% of cases
- Metabolic acidosis leading to shock, cardiac dysfunction, and PPHN
- Pneumothorax is seen in 10–25% of cases

Treatment

Routine oropharyngeal and endotracheal suctioning is not recommended for babies in the delivery room born through meconium-stained liquor. MAS leads to the requirement

Flowchart 2.12.3: Pathophysiology of MAS.

Distal airways are obstructed by meconium leading to ball valve obstruction worsening hyperinflation and atelectasis
↓
Meconium causes secondary surfactant deficiency
↓
Hypoxia leads to distal pulmonary muscularization and aggravates persistent pulmonary hypertension
↓
Meconium leads to activation of inflammatory cascades

(MAS: meconium aspiration syndrome)

of mechanical ventilation in 50% of cases. The ventilator strategy involves using slower rates with long inspiratory and expiratory times. Surfactant administration is helpful in babies requiring higher FiO_2 (40–50%). PPHN is seen in 50% cases of MAS. INO is indicated, especially when the OI exceeds 20. Some babies may go on to require high-frequency oscillatory ventilation. Babies not responding to medical therapy with OI >40 should be referred to a facility with availability of ECMO.

REFERENCES

1. Dyess NF, Kinsella JP, Parker TA. Acute neonatal respiratory disorders. In: Gleason CA, Sawyer T (Eds). Avery's Diseases of Newborn, 11th edition; Philadelphia: Elsevier; 2023. pp. 594-613.
2. National Neonatology Forum, India. Oxygen therapy in neonates. NNF Clinical Practice guidelines 2021. [online] Available from https://www.nnfi.org/assests/upload/usefull-links-pdf/Oxygen_therapy_in_neonates_NNFI_CPG_Dec2021.pdf. [Last accessed October, 2024].
3. National Neonatology Forum, India. Surfactant replacement therapy in neonates. NNF Clinical Practice Guidelines 2021. [online] Available from https://www.nnfi.org/assests/upload/usefull-links-pdf/Surfactant_replacement_therapy_in_neonates-NNFI_CPG_Dec2021.pdf. [Last accessed October, 2024].
4. SUPPORT Study Group of the Eunice Kennedy Shriver NICHD Neonatal Research Network; Finer NN, Carlo WA, Walsh MC, Rich W, Gantz MG, Laptook AR, et al. Early CPAP versus surfactant in extremely preterm infants. N Engl J Med. 2010;362(21):1970-9.
5. Sweet DG, Carnielli VP, Greason G, Hallman M, Klabermass-Schrehof K, Ozek E, et al. European consensus guidelines on the management of respiratory distress syndrome: 2022 update. Neonatology. 2023;120(1):3-23.
6. Sandri F, Plavka R, Ancora G, Simeoni U, Stranak Z, Martinelli S, et al; CURPAP Study Group. Prophylactic or early selective surfactant combined with nCPAP in very preterm infants. Pediatrics. 2010;125(6):e1402-9.

2.13 Neonatal Seizures

Ruchi N Nanavati

INTRODUCTION

Seizures represent the most distinctive manifestation of neurological disease in the neonatal period. The tendency toward recurrent seizures and status epilepticus is far greater in the newborn period than at any other time of life. It is critical to recognize neonatal seizures (NS), determine their etiology, and treat them, as they usually relate to significant illness, and seizures themselves may be a cause of brain injury and potential long-term neurological sequelae.

DEFINITION

A seizure is defined as a transient occurrence of signs and/or symptoms due to abnormal excessive or synchronous neuronal activity in the brain as per the International League Against Epilepsy (ILAE) 2017 classification.[1] Seizure is a paroxysmal alteration in neurological function, including behavioral, motor, or autonomic. Neonatal status epilepticus is relatively common with poor outcome, but no widely accepted definition exists.

EPIDEMIOLOGY

Seizures, the most common neurological emergency in the neonatal period, occur in 1–5 per 1,000 live births.[2] Population-based studies of NS have revealed that the risk varies inversely with birth weight and gestational age. Hypoxic ischemic encephalopathy (HIE), intracranial hemorrhage (ICH), intracranial infections, and developmental defects account for 80–85% of all cases of NS. Indian data is limited.

ETIOPATHOGENESIS

A seizure results from excessive synchronous electrical discharge of neurons produced by the inward migration of

TABLE 2.13.1: Etiology of probable mechanisms for excessive depolarization.

Probable mechanism	Causes
Failure of Na^{+}–K^{+} pump secondary to reduced energy production	Hypoxemia, ischemia, and hypoglycemia
Excess of excitatory neurotransmitter (GABA acts as an excitatory neurotransmitter due to elevated chloride levels in perinatal neurons)	Hypoxemia, ischemia, and hypoglycemia
Relative deficiency of inhibitory neurotransmitter	Pyridoxine dependency
Membrane alteration with increased Na^{+} influx	Hypocalcemia and hypomagnesemia

(GABA: gamma-aminobutyric acid)

sodium ions (i.e., depolarization). The probable mechanisms for excessive depolarization are shown in **Table 2.13.1**.[3] Perinatal neuroanatomical and neurophysiological unique features determine NS phenomena termed *seizure semiology*. The more advanced development within the limbic system with connections to the midbrain and brainstem explains the higher frequency of subtle features, while the balance of excitatory and inhibitory processes in the immature brain is weighed toward excitation with an excess of glutamatergic synapses over inhibitory synapses with gamma-aminobutyric acid (GABA) acting as an excitatory neurotransmitter.

The threshold for seizure generation is lower in the developing brain than in the mature brain, but developing neurons are less vulnerable to injury from single prolonged seizures than mature neurons. The electrical discharges readily generated in the neonatal brain do not propagate sufficiently due to inadequate myelination and thus lead to fragmentary seizures whose electrical activity may not spread to surface electroencephalography (EEG) electrodes.

The best-documented mechanisms for the occurrence of brain injury with repeated seizures are accompanied by serious hypoventilation causing hypoxemia and hypercapnia, elevations of arterial blood pressure, disturbances of cerebral blood flow, decreased brain adenosine triphosphate (ATP) and phosphocreatine concentrations, and increased release of excitatory amino acids. Dramatic fall in brain glucose within 5 minutes of the onset of seizures with a concomitant rise in brain lactate may interfere with deoxyribonucleic acid (DNA) synthesis, glial proliferation, differentiation, and myelination. Evidence suggests that seizures may predispose to impaired cognitive and behavioral functions, or to susceptibility to epilepsy later in life.

The most common etiologies are mentioned in **Table 2.13.2**.

TABLE 2.13.2: Neonatal seizures and time of onset.

Time of onset	*Etiology*
<24 hours	HIE, severe birth trauma, congenital CNS anomalies, pyridoxine dependency, hypoglycemia, hypocalcemia, polycythemia, drug withdrawal, ICH
1–3 days	All above + Intracranial infections, ICH, IEMs, benign familial neonatal seizures
>3 days	Late hypocalcemia, sepsis, meningitis, ICH, epileptic syndromes, herpes encephalitis, IEMs

(CNS: central nervous system; HIE: hypoxic ischemic encephalopathy; ICH: intracranial hemorrhage; IEMs: inborn errors of metabolisms)

NEONATAL EPILEPTIC SYNDROMES

- *Benign familial NS:* It is an autosomal-dominant disorder with primary generalized seizures on day 2 or 3 of life without any obvious risk factor. Seizures may recur and gradually resolve over weeks. Later, epilepsy is seen in <10%.
- *Benign idiopathic NS (fifth day fits):* These are seizures that are usually multifocal clonic, often associated with apnea, and onset between days 4 and 6 of life in term infants with normal neurological state and diagnostic testing, often leading to status epilepticus. Most seizures cease after 24 hours and in all patients within 2 weeks. These are probably related to transient zinc deficiency. Long-term outcome is favorable.
- *Early myoclonic encephalopathy:* It starts as focal motor fragmentary seizures and later evolves into typical infantile spasms. It is usually associated with nonketotic hyperglycinemia. EEG reveals a burst suppression pattern with poor long-term outcomes.
- *Early infantile epileptic encephalopathy (Ohtahara syndrome):* It comprises brief tonic spasms presenting between days 10 and 90 of life. It is usually associated with structural disorders. EEG reveals a burst suppression pattern with poor long-term outcomes.

SEIZURE CLASSIFICATION

The American Clinical Neurophysiology Society had described three types of NS:

1. *Clinical only:* No simultaneous EEG seizure
2. *Electroclinical:* Clinical seizure coupled with simultaneous EEG seizure
3. *Electrographic only:* Not associated with clinical seizure

Subsequently, numerous studies have indicated that about 80–90% of electrographical seizures do not have associated clinical correlates and therefore would not be identified without continuous EEG (cEEG) monitoring.[1] In addition, treatment with anticonvulsant medication may terminate clinical seizures but not necessarily electrical seizures, thereby further highlighting the importance of cEEG monitoring.

In situations when and where full EEG is not readily available, ambulatory EEG (aEEG) may be used with coregistration of raw channels. If cEEG or aEEG is not available, observation by experienced personnel is mandatory for diagnostic certainty.

CLINICAL MANIFESTATIONS

Seizures can have a motor (automatisms, clonic, epileptic spasms, myoclonic, and tonic), nonmotor (autonomic and behavior arrest), or sequential presentation. NS are difficult to recognize because they are brief, fragmentary, and asymmetrical, and lack organization and possible association with nonmotor phenomena. NS are considered focal at onset, and thus a division into focal and generalized is unnecessary.

Motor Manifestations

Automatism: It is more or less coordinated motor activity usually occurring when cognition is impaired. It often resembles a voluntary movement and is typically oral in neonates. EEG/aEEG is mandatory. It is seen in HIE and preterm infants and is often part of sequential seizures.

Clonic: These are well-localized stereotypic and repetitive biphasic movements. These may be unifocal, multifocal (progression from one part to another in a nonordered fashion), or bilateral, usually not associated with loss of consciousness. Primary bilateral clonic seizures are extremely rare and provoked by metabolic disturbances, focal traumatic injury, subarachnoid hemorrhage (SAH), and focal infarct. The most common cause of clonic seizures that remain unifocal is neonatal stroke. An EEG reveals unifocal or multifocal abnormality, and the prognosis is good.

Epileptic spasms: A sudden flexion, extension, or mixed extension–flexion of predominantly proximal and truncal muscles that are usually more sustained than a myoclonic movement but not as sustained as a tonic seizure. Limited forms may occur: Grimacing, head nodding, or subtle eye movements. These are brief in neonates, may occur in clusters, and are difficult to differentiate from myoclonic seizures without electromyography (EMG) channel. They are rare and may be seen in inborn errors of metabolism (IEM) or early infantile developmental and epileptic encephalopathy (DEE).

Myoclonic: They are characterized by synchronous single or multiple jerks (<100 ms) and are associated with diffuse central nervous system (CNS) pathology. Focal and multifocal myoclonic seizures are most commonly unassociated with while bilateral myoclonic seizures are more likely to be associated with time-synchronized EEG discharges. An EEG may reveal a burst suppression or hypsarrhythmia pattern, and the prognosis is poor. This is a typical seizure type in IEM and preterm infants and may also be early-infantile DEE.

Tonic: Sustained extension or flexion of the axial or appendicular muscle group and resembles decerebrate or decorticate posture. These may be focal or bilateral asymmetric or symmetric, often associated with eye deviation or apnea, and are most common in preterm with ICH or diffuse CNS disease. Generalized tonic seizures may not be associated with time-synchronized EEG discharges. An EEG may depict a burst suppression pattern, and the prognosis is poor. This is a typical seizure type in early-infantile DEE and neonatal genetic epilepsies.

Nonmotor Manifestations

Autonomic: A distinct alteration of autonomic nervous system function involving cardiovascular, pupillary, gastrointestinal, sudomotor, vasomotor, respiratory (apnea), and thermoregulatory functions. EEG/aEEG is mandatory. Autonomic seizures are rare in isolation and are seen in intraventricular hemorrhage (IVH) as well as in temporal or occipital lobe lesions. They are also described in early infantile DEE.

Behavioral arrest: Arrest or pause of activities, freezing, and immobilization. EEG/aEEG is mandatory. It is rare as an isolated seizure type and is more commonly seen as part of sequential seizures.

Sequential Manifestations

Sequential: Events with a sequence of signs, symptoms, and EEG changes at different times. No predominant feature can be determined; instead, the seizure presents with a variety of clinical signs. Several features typically occur in a sequence, often with changing lateralization within or between seizures. It is often seen in self-limited neonatal epilepsy or KCNQ2 encephalopathy.

Unclassified

These comprise unusual clinical features with an inability to place in other categories. EEG/aEEG is mandatory. The research has revealed that electrographic-only seizure burden has an effect on long-term neurological outcomes comparable to that of electroclinical seizures.[4]

DIFFERENTIAL DIAGNOSIS

Certain behavioral phenomena may be confused with NS.

Jitteriness is characterized by tremulous movements (5–6 per second), is stimulus-sensitive, and is not associated with abnormal autonomic changes or eye movements. It is terminated by passive flexion of extremity, and the EEG is normal.

Tremors may be misidentified as clonic seizures. They are reported in 50% of the healthy newborns and are hypothesized due to the immaturity of inhibitory neurons. High-amplitude tremors are more likely to be secondary to brain disorders.

Benign sleep neonatal myoclonus usually presents in the first week and resolves spontaneously over weeks. It occurs during nonrapid eye movement sleep, abolishes on arousal, and never occurs during wakefulness. Neurological examination and EEG are normal. Transient dysmaturity of the brainstem reticular activating system is postulated. Anticonvulsants are not indicated. Long-term outcome is normal. Later, epilepsy does not develop.

Apnea: In a preterm, apnea associated with tachycardia suggests seizure. Associated features like automatisms, ocular events, etc., favor the diagnosis of seizure than apnea of prematurity.

Hyperekplexia: It is a rare autosomal dominant disorder characterized by hypertonia, hyperreflexia, and an exaggerated startle response. The mutation of the inhibitory glycine receptor is described. Therapy with clonazepam or diazepam causes marked improvement.

DIAGNOSIS

Table 2.13.3 lists the investigations that are required with the first seizure episode.

Continuous EEG, defined as >3 hours' monitoring, is considered the gold standard for the diagnosis of NS. Ictal EEG is useful for the diagnosis of suspected seizures, while interictal EEG is useful for predicting long-term prognosis. Abnormal background activity indicates a high risk for long-term neurological sequelae. Amplitude-integrated EEG, a bedside technique, is a useful initial complementary tool and is being increasingly used in neonatal intensive care units for neuromonitoring.

Neuroimaging: A computed tomography (CT) scan is advisable when etiology is undetermined after first-line investigations and is especially good for hemorrhages and calcifications. Magnetic resonance imaging (MRI) provides better resolution of anatomy and details of function and perfusion with diffusion-weighted MRI, spectroscopy, and angiography. Neuroimaging has more value in prognostication.

Metabolic workup: IEM should be suspected with a family history of unexplained fetal/neonatal deaths, intellectual retardation, seizures occurring after introduction of feeds, or those associated with unexplained lethargy, coma, and vomiting. Initial workup includes arterial blood gases, blood ammonia, serum and urinary amino acids, serum lactate and pyruvate, and urinary reducing substances.

TABLE 2.13.3: Investigations required with the first seizure episode.

First line	***Second line****
• Blood glucose • Serum calcium, phosphorus, and magnesium • Serum electrolytes • Cerebrospinal fluid (CSF) analysis • Cranial ultrasonography (USG) • Electroencephalography (EEG)	• Sepsis workup • Real-time PCR for bacterial, viral, and nonviral infections • MRI or CT brain scan • Inborn errors of metabolism (IEM) workup • Genetic workup • Toxic drug screen

*Based on clinical suspicion.
(CT: computed tomography; MRI: magnetic resonance imaging; PCR: polymerase chain reaction)

MANAGEMENT

Neonatal seizure is a medical emergency and mandates prompt treatment. All clinical and electrographic seizures should be promptly treated. A stepwise approach is shown in **Table 2.13.4**. With the advent of EEG monitoring, it is

TABLE 2.13.4: Approach to managing neonatal seizures.

On admission	• Assess, support, and maintain warmth, airway, breathing, and circulation • Attach multichannel monitor, EEG monitor, secure IV line, draw sample • If blood glucose <40 mg/dL, administer 2 mL/kg of 10% dextrose bolus followed by continuous infusion with GIR of 8 mg/kg/min
First-line drug	Phenobarbitone 20 mg/kg IV over 10–15 minutes; repeat 10 mg/kg IV every 5 minutes till the convulsions stop or a total dose of 40 mg/kg is reached (except in severe asphyxia)
Second-line drug	• Phenytoin (20 mg/kg, IV, over 20 minutes) OR • Fosphenytoin (30 mg/kg IV) (preferred over phenytoin) OR • Levetiracetam 50 mg/kg IV over 15 minutes
	Administer levetiracetam or phenytoin/fosphenytoin whichever is not used, if seizure continues
Seizure stops	• Start maintenance doses 12 hours after loading dose • Start weaning anticonvulsants if seizure-free for 24 hours • Continue on maintenance dose of levetiracetam (10 mg/kg, once daily) or phenobarbitone (5 mg/kg/day, BD)
Refractory seizures	• Administer lorazepam 0.05–0.1 mg/kg IV over 2–5 minutes • If seizures persist, midazolam: 0.2 mg/kg IV bolus, then 0.1–0.4 mg/kg/h • Consider other antiepileptics
Seizure continues	Investigate for neurostructural, neurometabolic, and neurofunctional disorders

(BD: twice a day; EEG: electroencephalography; GIR: glucose infusion rate; IV: intravenous)

Flowchart 2.13.1: Long-term management of neonatal seizures.

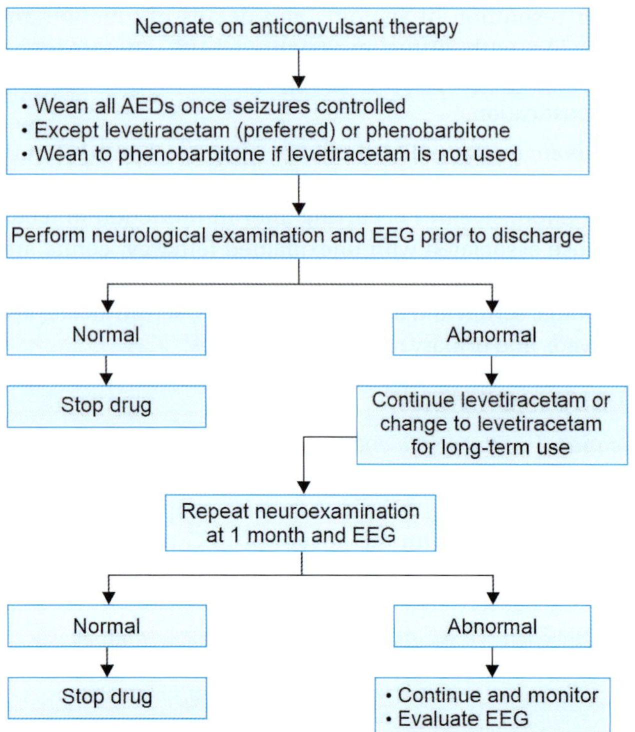

(AEDs: antiepileptic drugs; EEG: electroencephalography)

generally agreed that rare, brief seizures may not require treatment but should initiate EEG monitoring to evaluate seizure burden. A seizure burden of >30–60 s/ho should be considered as an indication to start treatment.[5]

Resistant Seizures

The following drugs can be used on a case-by-case basis for resistant seizures: Lidocaine, valproic acid, topiramate, primidone, carbamazepine, lamotrigine, vigabatrin, and pyridoxine.

Detection and Treatment of Underlying Cause

The importance of history and physical examination to detect the cause of seizures cannot be overemphasized. Treatment of the underlying cause is essential.

Hypocalcemia: Administer 10% calcium gluconate intravenous (IV) 2 mL/kg (200 mg/kg) over 10–15 minutes. The electrocardiogram or at least cardiac rhythm by auscultation should be monitored during administration. Phenobarbitone can sometimes suppress the seizures of hypocalcemia; thus, a decrease in seizures after phenobarbitone administration does not rule out hypocalcemia as the cause.

TABLE 2.13.5: Prognosis of neonatal seizures according to etiology.

Neurologic disease	***% Normal***
HIE	50
ICH with hemorrhagic infarct	<10
Primary SAH	90
Hypocalcemia—early	50
Hypocalcemia—late	100
Hypoglycemia	50
Bacterial meningitis	50
CNS malformation	0
Background EEG	***Neurosequelae***
Normal	<10
Severe abnormalities	≥90
Moderate abnormalities	~50

(CNS: central nervous system; EEG: electroencephalography; HIE: hypoxic ischemic encephalopathy; ICH: intracranial hemorrhage; SAH: subarachnoid hemorrhage)

Hypomagnesemia: Administer 50% magnesium sulfate intramuscularly at a dose of 0.2 mL/kg before treating hypocalcemia.

Long-term Therapy

The possible adverse effects on developing CNS of continuing antiepileptic drugs (AEDs) for several months have raised concerns (increased rate of apoptotic neuronal cell death). Attempts should be made to stop all AEDs and wean to only phenobarbitone or levetiracetam. Monotherapy is most appropriate. Levetiracetam has shown promising results for long-term maintenance therapy as it does not increase apoptosis.[6] Neonatal neurological examination, etiology of NS, and EEG findings are the main determinants of the duration of antiseizure medication **(Flowchart 2.13.1)**.

PROGNOSIS

Prognosis mainly depends upon gestational age, nature and cause of seizures, neurological examination, EEG background activity, and neuroimaging findings. The incidence of sequelae is different as per the etiology **(Table 2.13.5)**.

REFERENCES

1. Pressler RM, Cilio MR, Mizrahi EM, Moshe SL, Numez ML, Plouin P, et al. The ILAE classification of seizures and the epilepsies: modification for seizures in the neonate. Position paper by the ILAE Task Force on Neonatal Seizures. Epilepsia. 2021;62(3):615-28.
2. Pellegrin S, Munoz FM, Padula M, Heath PT, Meller L, Top K, et al. Neonatal seizures: case definition & guidelines for data collection, analysis, and presentation of immunization safety data. Vaccine. 2019;37(52):7596-609.

3. Volpe JJ. Neonatal seizures. In: Volpe JJ (Ed). Neurology of the Newborn, 6th edition. Philadelphia, PA: Saunders Elsevier; 2017. pp. 273-318.
4. Kharoshankaya L, Stevenson NJ, Livingstone V, Murray DM, Murphy BP, Ahearne CE, et al. Seizure burden and neurodevelopmental outcome in neonates with hypoxic-ischemic encephalopathy. Dev Med Child Neurol. 2016;58(12):1242-8.
5. Soul JS, Pressler R, Allen M, Boylan G, Rabe H, Portman R, et al. Recommendations for the design of therapeutic trials for neonatal seizures. Pediatr Res. 2019;85(7):943-54.
6. Sansevere AJ, Bergin AM. Neonatal seizures. In: Eichenwald EC, Hansen AR, Martin CR, Stark AR, (Eds). Jain N. (Ed SAE) Cloherty and Stark's Manual of Neonatal Care, South Asian edition. Gurugram: Wolters Kluwer Health (India); 2021. pp. 842-58.

2.14 Neonatal Hypoglycemia

Sandeep S Kadam

INTRODUCTION

Neonatal hypoglycemia is a common metabolic problem during the transition from the fetal to the neonatal period. It remains a risk factor for adverse neurodevelopmental outcomes, epilepsy, and cortical visual impairment. Screening of high-risk babies, prompt diagnosis, and aggressive management are indicated to help reduce long-term morbidities.

EPIDEMIOLOGY

The prevalence of neonatal hypoglycemia varies due to factors such as the infant population studied, the frequency and timing of glucose testing, the testing method employed, and the definition of hypoglycemia applied. In infants with a gestational age >35 weeks who are at risk of hypoglycemia according to the American Academy of Pediatrics (AAP) guidelines, a study revealed that 25% of all deliveries fell into the category of being at risk for hypoglycemia. Among these at-risk infants, 51% encountered at least one episode of hypoglycemia within the first 48 hours of life, as defined by a blood glucose level <47 mg/dL.[1]

DEFINITION

There is no clear definition of hypoglycemia in neonates, as different researchers have defined it in different ways.[2,3] Epidemiologists have defined it as blood glucose <2 standard deviations for that age. Clinicians have defined hypoglycemia as signs and symptoms of hypoglycemia, low serum glucose level, and the resolution of signs and symptoms with the provision of glucose (Whipple's triad). Endocrinologists recommend blood glucose >50 mg/dL within 48 hours and >70 mg/dL after 72 hours. The generally accepted definition for the diagnosis of hypoglycemia is blood glucose <47 mg/dL, severe hypoglycemia as <36 mg/dL, and adverse hypoglycemia as <27 mg/dL; however, this may lack rigorous justification.[1]

ETIOPATHOGENESIS

After birth, as the cord is cut, the steady supply of glucose in the baby ceases, and there is a fall in the blood glucose with the nadir at 2–4 hours of life, where the glucose may fall up to 25–30 mg/dL. The glucose then stabilizes in the next 4–6 hours, where the baby may be asymptomatic. The blood glucose then increases due to glycogenolysis and gluconeogenesis. This physiological nadir is seen in all babies. At-risk neonates should be screened for hypoglycemia in the first few days of life **(Box 2.14.1)**.[4]

There is a physiological basis where there is mobilization of glucagon to glucose, gluconeogenesis from the protein

BOX 2.14.1: Risk factors for neonatal hypoglycemia.

- Birth weight <2 kg
- Gestation <35 weeks
- Large for gestational age (birth weight >90th centile) (LGA)
- Small for gestational age (birth weight <10th centile) (SGA)
- Late preterm babies exposed to antenatal steroids
- Features of growth retardation
- Infants of diabetic mothers
- Rh isoimmunization
- *Mother on drugs:* Propranolol, labetalol, terbutaline, and oral hypoglycemic agents
- *Any sick neonate:* Asphyxia, polycythemia, sepsis, and shock
- Neonate receiving parenteral nutrition
- Family history suggesting inborn error of metabolism
- *Syndromic baby:* Beckwith–Weidmann syndrome, features suggesting hypopituitarism such as micropenis and midline defects

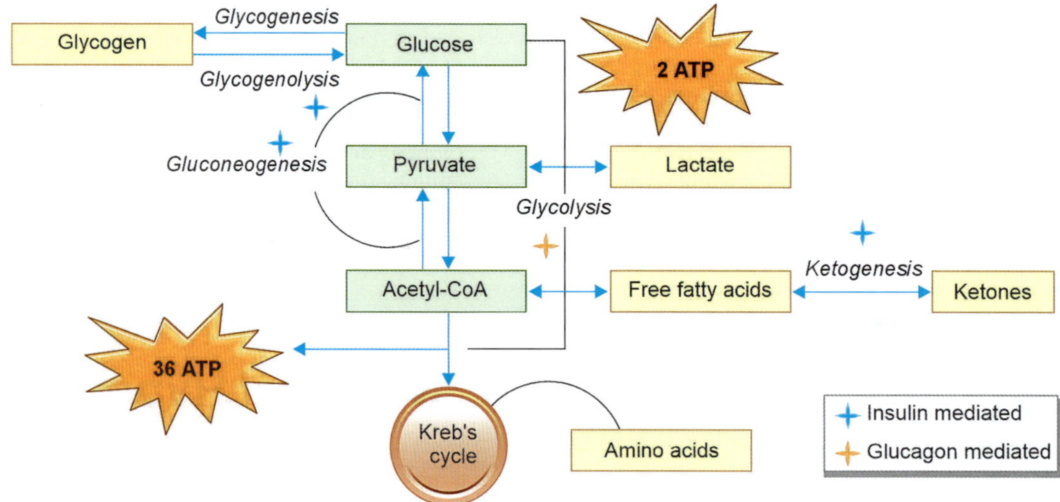

Fig. 2.14.1: Homeostasis of glucose concentration mediated by insulin and glucagon. (ATP: adenosine triphosphate; CoA: coenzyme A)

substrate, and generation of ketone bodies from the lipid tissues, which may act as glucose sparer by the neonatal brain in neonatal hypoglycemic situations **(Fig. 2.14.1)**.

CAUSES OF HYPOGLYCEMIA

Neonates may develop hypoglycemia due to decreased production/stores of glucose or due to increased glucose demands.

- *Decreased production/stores:* Prematurity, intrauterine growth restriction, delayed feeding, growth hormone or cortisol deficiency, and inborn errors of metabolism
- *Increased utilization:* Sepsis, asphyxia, hypothermia, polycythemia, infant of diabetic mothers, and hyperinsulinemia

CLINICAL FEATURES

Hypoglycemia occurs in clinical settings with comorbid conditions and rarely in isolation. Infants may exhibit certain symptoms and signs; however, majority of babies may remain asymptomatic. Hence, screening "at-risk" babies is important to diagnose and treat timely to prevent long-term sequelae **(Box 2.14.2)**. No single sign is pathognomonic of hypoglycemia. Hypoglycemia is not a clinical diagnosis but a biochemical one.[5]

BOX 2.14.2: Symptoms and signs of neonatal hypoglycemia.

Symptoms
- Abnormal cry
- Feeding difficulty
- Irritability
- Seizures
- Jitteriness
- Apnea

Signs
- Lethargy
- Hypothermia
- Tachycardia
- Tachypnea
- Cyanosis

DIAGNOSIS

The gold standard for glucose measurement involves various enzymatic methods, including the glucose oxidase (calorimetric method), glucose electrodes (used in blood gas and electrolyte analyzers), as well as the hexokinase and glucose dehydrogenase methods. Glucometers (point-of-care) are often unreliable in extremes of values (too low or too high). Laboratory assessment using the glucose oxidase method is the most accurate method of estimation.

Point-of-care measurements of blood glucose (glucometers) are often unreliable in situations where the blood glucose is too high or low. One needs to confirm the blood sugars in the laboratory for an accurate diagnosis.

It is important to understand the variation of blood glucose between plasma and whole blood glucose, as the whole blood values are 15% less than plasma levels. The glucose levels fall 15–18% per hour, and hence the time of analysis and sampling is also important.

Time Schedule for Screening

There is very little data to recommend the time to screen neonates at risk for hypoglycemia. The best time to diagnose hypoglycemia is 2 hours. Infants of diabetic mothers show hypoglycemia early. Small for gestational age (SGA) babies may show low sugar within 24–36 hours of life. High-risk babies may be screened at 2, 6, 12, 24, 36, and 48 hours of age.

Thereafter, one can screen two times a day until full feeds and as per the clinical discretion of the attending neonatologist.

Persistent Hypoglycemia

A diagnosis of resistant hypoglycemia is established if a newborn continues to require parenteral therapy for more than 7 days or requires a glucose infusion rate (GIR) of 12–14 mg/kg/min to maintain euglycemia.

Resistant hypoglycemia is always pathological, and an active search into various inborn errors of metabolism and endocrine disorders must be ensued. The diagnosis can be established by measuring the "critical sample," which includes measurement of insulin, cortisol, and growth hormone at the time of hypoglycemia. The presence of detectable insulin (>2 mIU/L), with reduced free fatty acids and ketones, establishes the diagnosis of hyperinsulinism.

DIFFERENTIAL DIAGNOSIS

Hypoglycemia manifests with nonspecific features that mimic sepsis, meningitis, electrolyte imbalance, postasphyxia encephalopathy, and inborn errors of metabolism.

MANAGEMENT

The threshold to treat hypoglycemia depends on the postnatal age and the blood glucose levels.[6] Different organizations have proposed different levels for the treatment; however, most recommendations tell us to maintain the blood glucose levels above 50 mg/dL.[7] The most important thing to remember is that one should not wait to treat hypoglycemia depending on the laboratory value, but in babies with low blood glucose on glucometer values, treatment should be started without any delay **(Table 2.14.1)**.

TABLE 2.14.1: Operational threshold for hypoglycemia.

*Glucose concentration**	*Treatment*	*Monitoring of blood glucose*
>40 mg/dL	None	• Not required • Ensure frequent feedings and adequacy of feeding and milk output
20–40 mg/dL	Oral feeds (preferably breast milk)	• Recheck blood glucose level after 60 minutes • *>40 mg/dL:* Continue oral feeds, monitor glucose 6–8 hourly for 48 hours • *<40 mg/dL:* Start IV glucose
<20 mg/dL	IV glucose infusion	• Start GIR @ 6–8 mg/kg/min • Treat as "symptomatic hypoglycemia"

*Glucose values obtained on reagent strips must be confirmed by laboratory estimation.
(GIR: glucose infusion rate; IV: intravenous)

Asymptomatic Hypoglycemia

Asymptomatic neonates at risk of hypoglycemia should be fed by 1 hour of age and screened 30 minutes later.

For asymptomatic newborns at risk, the AAP suggests a treatment plan that is divided into two time periods depending on the age of the baby.[8]

1. *In neonates with age <4 hours,* with low sugars, give an initial feed to all neonates within the 1st hour of age, and repeat blood glucose should be performed 30 minutes after the first feed. If the blood glucose is >25 mg/dL, another feeding-checking blood glucose in a 1-hour cycle is recommended, and if the blood glucose remains <25 mg/dL, then start with an intravenous (IV) glucose infusion. If the blood glucose is between 25 and 40 mg/dL, another attempt to feed may be made before progressing with IV glucose administration.
2. *In babies aged 4–24 hours,* feeding every 2–3 hours (after the initial feed) and blood glucose measurements prior to each feed are recommended. If blood glucose is <35 mg/dL in one sample, it is suggested to refeed and recheck plasma glucose (PG) concentration within 1 hour. If blood glucose remains <35 mg/dL, IV glucose should be administered. However, if blood glucose is between 35 and 45 mg/dL, active support of feeding should be continued before the initiation of treatment with an IV dextrose infusion.

Symptomatic Hypoglycemia

For any baby with symptoms and low sugars, one needs to start with a dextrose infusion.

Initiation of IV dextrose therapy should be considered if blood glucose levels remain below the operational threshold after enteral feed and dextrose gel, or if the infant is unable to tolerate oral intake or any baby with symptomatic hypoglycemia.

A continuous glucose infusion should be administered at 6–8 mg/kg/min and titrated up by 1–2 mg/kg/min every 4–6 hours to maintain euglycemia, which is desirable. A bolus of 2 mL/kg of 10% dextrose (200 mg of glucose/kg) followed by a continuous infusion rate of 6–8 mg/kg/min may be considered for infants with *serious clinical signs* (seizures, coma, or marked hypotonia with apnea) and *severe hypoglycemia* (persistently <25 mg/dL).

Intravenous glucose is indicated for a blood glucose level (1) <40 mg/dL at the time of symptoms consistent with hypoglycemia, (2) <25 mg/dL within 4 hours of life and *after* the first feeding, and (3) low values despite feeding below the operational threshold for that age.

The various formulae used for calculation while prescribing glucose infusion at the bedside are given in **Box 2.14.3**.

BOX 2.14.3: Formulae used for calculation while prescribing glucose infusion at the bedside.

- Glucose infusion rate (mg/kg/min) = (% of dextrose × Infusion rate in mL/h) ÷ (6 × Weight)
- Total concentration of dextrose (%) = (Amount of glucose in grams) × 100 ÷ (Total fluid for glucose in milliliters)
- To prepare a particular concentration (C%) of dextrose solution from D5 and D25, add "x" mL of D25 to "100 – x" mL of D5, where "x" is: 5C – 25 = "x" mL

Pharmacotherapy for Neonatal Hypoglycemia

In cases of severe and persistent hypoglycemia, the following medications can be used on a case-by-case basis—glucagon (stimulates hepatic glycogenolysis); hydrocortisone and dexamethasone (promote gluconeogenesis and decrease insulin sensitivity), and diazoxide or octreotide (suppresses insulin secretion).

PREVENTION

All high-risk babies should be monitored for blood glucose during the first 48 hours for early diagnosis and management. Common clinical practices used to prevent asymptomatic hypoglycemia include ensuring warmth by skin-to-skin contact, early initiation of breastfeeding, lactational support, supplemental feeds with breast milk or banked milk in case of inadequate breastmilk or a breast milk substitute, and applying intrabuccal dextrose gel.

REFERENCES

1. Adamkin DH. Neonatal hypoglycemia. Semin Fetal Neonatal Med. 2017;22(1):36-41.
2. Thompson-Branch A, Havranek T. Neonatal hypoglycemia. Pediatr Rev. 2017;38(4):147-57.
3. Cornblath M, Hawdon JM, Williams AF, Aynsley-Green A, Ward-Platt MP, Schwartz R, et al. Controversies regarding definition of neonatal hypoglycemia: suggested operational thresholds. Pediatrics. 2000;105(5):1141-5.
4. Hubbard EM, Hay WW Jr. The term newborn: hypoglycemia. Clin Perinatol. 2021;48(3):665-79.
5. Narvey MR, Marks SD. The screening and management of newborns at risk for low blood glucose. Paediatr Child Health. 2019;24(8):536-54.
6. Rozance PJ, Wolfsdorf JI. Hypoglycemia in the newborn. Pediatr Clin North Am. 2019;66(2):333-42.
7. Luo K, Tang J, Zhang M, He Y. Systematic review of guidelines on neonatal hypoglycemia. Clin Endocrinol (Oxf). 2024;100(1):36-49.
8. Committee on Fetus and Newborn; Adamkin DH. Postnatal glucose homeostasis in late-preterm and term infants. Pediatrics. 2011;127(3):575-9.

2.15 Neonatal Hypocalcemia

Nandkishor S Kabra

INTRODUCTION

Hypocalcemia is one of the most common metabolic problems in neonates. Ionized calcium is essential for several physiological processes in the human body, including the integrity of cell membranes, neuromuscular functioning, coagulation process, cellular secretory, and numerous other cellular enzymatic functions.

DEFINITION

For a population of preterm neonates, hypocalcemia is defined as ionized serum calcium <1 mmol/L or total serum calcium (TSC) <1.75 mmol/L. For a population of full-term neonates, hypocalcemia is defined as ionized serum calcium <1.2 mmol/L or TSC <2.0 mmol/L (for calcium, 1 mmol/L = 2 mEq/L = 4 mg/dL).[1]

Hypocalcemia in newborns is categorized into two types based on the age of onset. (1) *Early-onset neonatal hypocalcemia (EONH)* presents within the first 72–96 hours of birth, and generally, it requires short-term calcium supplementation. EONH occurs because of the insufficient release of parathyroid hormone (PTH) from immature parathyroid glands and/or the suboptimal responsiveness of the renal tubule to PTH. (2) *Late-onset neonatal hypocalcemia (LONH)* presents 96 hours after birth, and it requires long-term therapy. LONH is considered to be a manifestation of the relative unresponsiveness of the immature kidney to PTH.

EPIDEMIOLOGY

Early-onset neonatal hypocalcemia occurs earlier in premature infants as compared to at-risk full-term infants. EONH is reported to occur in 7% and 32% of infants born to mothers with gestational diabetes mellitus and pregestational diabetes, respectively.[2] It is also likely to occur more frequently in neonates who have suffered perinatal asphyxia. The severity of hypocalcemia is likely to be higher among neonates who additionally also have hyperphosphatemia, hypomagnesemia, and vitamin D deficiency. LONH is more likely to occur in infants who are fed cow's milk or formulas containing higher amounts of phosphate.[3]

ETIOPATHOGENESIS

Various causes of EONH and LONH are summarized in **Table 2.15.1**.[4-6] Body calcium exists in two main compartments: Skeletal system (99%) and extracellular fluid (1%). Calcium in the extracellular fluid is present in three different forms—bound to albumin (40%), bound to anions like phosphate, citrate, sulfate, and lactate (10%), and as a free ionic calcium (50%).

Measurement of the TSC concentration alone without considering the ionic serum calcium (ISC) component can be misrepresentative because the relationship between these two is not always directly linear. On every occasion when serum albumin concentration is low and there are disturbances in the acid–base status (which happens frequently in preterm and sick neonates), the correlation between TSC and ISC is poor. In neonates with hypoalbuminemia, TSC is low while ISC is normal. Misleadingly low ISC can occur in alkalosis and contamination with heparin. In general, the TSC decreases by a factor of 0.2 mmol/L for every 1 g/dL fall in the plasma albumin concentration. For every 0.1 unit increase in pH, there is a reduction in ISC by 0.04 mmol/L.

Mother-to-fetus transfer of calcium actively occurs during the last trimester of pregnancy. PTH-related peptide (PTHrP) is the foremost regulator of the positive calcium balance in the fetus. PTH and calcitonin do not cross the placenta. After birth, there is an abrupt termination of transplacental transfer of calcium; this leads to a drop in TSC and ISC at 24 hours after delivery. TSC and ISC concentrations subsequently rise, reaching levels comparable to adults by 2 weeks of age.

In neonates, the serum calcium levels are reliant on PTH, calcium intake, renal calcium retention, skeletal calcium, and vitamin D status.

TABLE 2.15.1: Causes of hypocalcemia.

Early-onset hypocalcemia	*Late-onset hypocalcemia*
• Prematurity • Maternal preeclampsia • Infant of diabetic mother (gestational and insulin-dependent) • Perinatal asphyxia • Maternal intake of anticonvulsants • Maternal hyperparathyroidism	• Increased phosphate load—due to cow milk, renal insufficiency • Hypomagnesemia • Vitamin D deficiency • Maternal vitamin D deficiency • Malabsorption • PTH resistance • Hepatobiliary disease • Transient neonatal pseudohypoparathyroidism • Primary hypothyroidism—DiGeorge syndrome, CATCH 22 syndrome • Secondary hypothyroidism—maternal hyperparathyroidism, metabolic disorders (long-chain fatty acyl CoA dehydrogenase deficiency) • Iatrogenic—citrated blood products, loop diuretics, sodium bicarbonate intake, intralipid infusions, phosphate therapy, glucocorticoids, aminoglycosides, and gastroenteritis

(CATCH 22: cardiac defects, abnormal facies, thymic hypoplasia, cleft palate, and hypocalcemia caused by chromosome 22q11.2 deletion; PTH: parathyroid hormone)

CLINICAL FEATURES

Asymptomatic: Most cases of EONH in neonates are asymptomatic in nature.

Symptomatic: Most cases of LONH in neonates are symptomatic in nature. The symptoms are dependent on the level of ionized calcium and usually appear when ISC drops under 0.9 mmol/L. A clinician needs to suspect hypocalcemia in a neonate who suddenly develops one or more of the following: Jitteriness, neuromuscular irritability, myoclonic jerks, clonus, focal and multifocal seizures, tetany, tonic posturing, and an exaggerated startle response. Some neonates who have cardiac involvement may present with tachycardia, prolonged QT interval, decreased cardiac contractility, and heart failure. In some cases, apnea, tachypnea, desaturations, cyanosis, vomiting, laryngospasm, and stridor (especially after crying) may also be observed.

DIFFERENTIAL DIAGNOSIS

If a seizure is the first presenting feature in neonates, other causes of seizures, such as hypoglycemia, electrolyte disturbances, sepsis, meningitis, and intracranial hemorrhage, ought to be ruled out in the beginning. Having a history of prematurity, maternal gestational or insulin-dependent diabetes, the requirement of resuscitation at birth and the age of onset of symptoms may provide a clue to a probable cause. A history of cow's milk intake could suggest a possibility of hyperphosphatemia. A general physical examination should be performed to look for dysmorphic features, cataracts, neurological abnormalities, congenital heart disease, and renal system involvement to determine the likely cause.

DIAGNOSIS

The diagnosis of hypocalcemia is made based on history, clinical examination, and supportive investigations.

Measuring total and ionic calcium levels is the most appropriate policy in case of a diagnosis of hypocalcemia. Some of the examples of the approach are summarized in **Table 2.15.2**. A suitable diagnostic approach is illustrated in **Flowchart 2.15.1**.

TABLE 2.15.2: Etiological approach based on history and clinical examination.

History and clinical examination	*Explanation*	*Action*
Prematurity	Low stores and decreased intake of calcium	Recheck amount of calcium supplementation and Ca:P ratio
LGA and hypoglycemia	Suggestive of an infant of a diabetic mother (gestational or insulin-dependent)	Recheck maternal glucose values and HbA1C
Potter facies and edema	Renal insufficiency with possible hyperphosphatemia	Antenatal USG suggestive of fetal renal abnormality and oligohydramnios
Abnormal facies, skeletal shortness, and congenital heart disease	DiGeorge, CATCH 22, other genetic causes of hypoparathyroidism	Chest X-ray and echocardiography

(LGA: large for gestational age; USG: ultrasonography)
(CATCH 22: cardiac defects, abnormal facies, thymic hypoplasia, cleft palate, and hypocalcemia caused by chromosome 22q11.2 deletion)
Source: Modified from Thakre R, Murki S (Eds). Protocols in Neonatology, 2nd edition. New Delhi: Jaypee Brothers Medical Publishers; 2020.

Flowchart 2.15.1: Diagnostic approach to hypocalcemia in newborn.

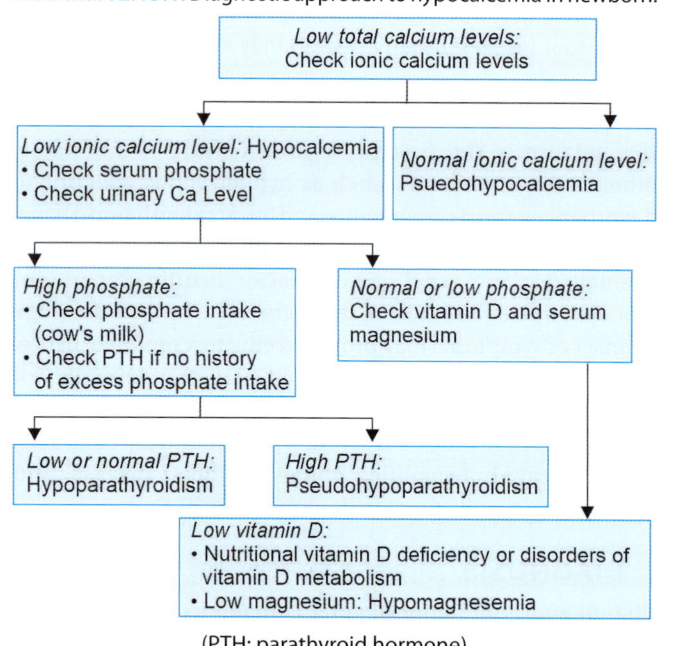

(PTH: parathyroid hormone)

Most cases of EONH in neonates are responsive to adequate calcium supplementation. If neonates with EONH linger to remain symptomatic and unresponsive notwithstanding adequate calcium supplementation beyond 72 hours of age or persistence of hypocalcemia at the end of the first week of life, it is labeled as prolonged (or persistent or resistant) hypocalcemia. These infants must be investigated as in LONH to find the particular cause.

A comprehensive list of investigations to be carried out in the case of LONH is summarized in **Table 2.15.3**. They should be carried out in the framework of history and clinical examination as appropriate.[7,8] General recommendations for interpreting these test results are summarized in **Table 2.15.4**.

MANAGEMENT

General Measures

An infant should be provided with general supportive care that helps in maintaining his/her temperature, glucose, blood pressure, and oxygenation in the normal range.

The monitoring of at-risk neonates for serum calcium levels is recommended as follows:

- Asymptomatic preterm neonates with a birth weight of ≤1 kg at 12, 24, and 48 hours
- Asymptomatic preterm neonates with a birth weight of >1 kg at 24 and 48 hours
- Sick or stressed or symptomatic neonates as indicated, usually every 24–48 hours during the acute phase of the disease

All neonates who are at risk of developing hypocalcemia have to get their daily recommended allowance of elemental calcium (60–120 mg/kg/day), preferably through the enteral route. If enteral intake is not achievable, calcium should be administered parenterally with a preference for continuous infusion over intermittent bolus administration.

TABLE 2.15.3: List of investigations required in cases of LONH, prolonged, and resistant hypocalcemia.

First line	*Second line*
• Total and ionic calcium • Serum albumin • ECG for QTc (>0.44 seconds) • USG brain if seizures • Serum phosphate • Serum alkaline phosphatase • RFT • LFT • X-ray chest and wrist • ABG for pH	• Serum magnesium • Serum PTH • 25-Hydroxyvitamin D levels • Urinary calcium:creatinine ratio • Maternal calcium, phosphorous, and alkaline phosphatase

(ABG: arterial blood gas; ECG: electrocardiogram; LFT: liver function tests LONH: late-onset neonatal hypocalcemia; PTH: parathyroid hormone; RFT: renal function tests; USG: ultrasonography)

TABLE 2.15.4: Interpreting test results in neonates with hypocalcemia.

Disorder	*Laboratory abnormality*	*Causes*	*Comments*
Vitamin D deficiency	Vitamin D level <30 mmol/L	Maternal vitamin D deficiency	Seen often in India
Chronic renal insufficiency	*High:* Phosphate, SAP, PTH *Low:* Low 25-OH D	Congenital renal problems	Additional renal workup—deranged RFT and acidotic pH
Hypoparathyroidism	*High:* Phosphate *Low:* SAP, PTH, 25-OH D	Secondary to maternal hyperparathyroidism or genetic causes	Look for the skeletal defect in mother (short fourth metacarpal)
Pseudohypoparathyroidism	*High:* SAP, PTH, phosphate *Low:* 25-OH D		
Hypomagnesemia	*High:* PTH *Low:* Phosphate, 25-OH D, Mg	May be secondary to a deficiency in mother	Magnesium level < 0.8 mmol/L (1.94 mg/dL) (1 mmol/L = 2.43 mg/dL)
High phosphate load	*High:* Serum phosphate >4.5 mg/dL with near-normal calcium levels	Cow's and other animal milk ingestion with high phosphate content	Switch to human breast milk
CATCH 22 or DiGeorge syndrome	Absence of thymic shadows on chest X-ray and presence of conotruncal anomalies	A genetic defect in chromosome 22 leading to hypoparathyroidism and arch anomalies	Genetic studies required for confirmation
Hypercalciuria	Urinary calcium excretion >4 mg/kg/day or 24-hour urinary calcium creatinine ratio >0.2	May be primary or part of renal tube defect or parathyroid defect	Seen rarely
Vitamin D-dependent rickets Type I	*High:* SAP, PTH *Low:* Phosphate, 25-OH D	Autosomal recessive disorder	Hypotonia, muscle weakness, growth failure, hypocalcemic seizures in early infancy, and radiographic findings of rickets
Vitamin D-dependent rickets Type II	*High:* SAP, PTH, 25-OH D *Low:* Phosphate	A rare autosomal recessive disorder caused by a mutation in the vitamin D receptor gene leading to end-organ resistance to $1,25(OH)_2$ vitamin D3	• Presents with refractory rickets and growth retardation in the first year of life. Alopecia is seen frequently • Will need higher doses of $1,25(OH)_2$ vitamin D3 and calcium

(25-OH D: 25 hydroxy vitamin D; CATCH 22: cardiac defects, abnormal facies, thymic hypoplasia, cleft palate, and hypocalcemia caused by chromosome 22q11.2 deletion; PTH: parathyroid hormone; RFT: renal function tests; SAP: serum alkaline phosphatase)

Source: Modified from Thakre R, Murki S (Eds). Protocols in Neonatology, 2nd edition. New Delhi: Jaypee Brothers Medical Publishers; 2020

Specific Measures[9,10]

In asymptomatic neonates, it is preferable to start with an intravenous (IV) 4–8 mL/kg/day of 10% calcium gluconate (1 mL = 9.3 mg of elemental calcium) for the initial 48 hours. After 48 hours, it can be switched to oral supplementation. It is extremely important to ensure that elemental calcium intake is targeted at 60–120 mg/kg/day.

In symptomatic neonates, calcium must be given at a bolus dose of 2 mL/kg/dose of 10% calcium gluconate, 1:1 diluted with 5% dextrose, slowly IV over 10 minutes, with continuous heart rate monitoring. It is important to ensure that the heart rate does not decrease below 100/min or >20 beats from baseline. A bolus dose may be repeated in neonates if symptoms persist. A clinical symptomatic response to this treatment confirms the diagnosis even before the results of blood reports become available. This ought to be followed by a continuous IV infusion of 6–8 mL/kg/day of 10% calcium gluconate for the next 24–48 hours. Later, this can be followed up by switching to oral calcium supplementation at normal maintenance doses. It is also important to provide adequate intake of vitamin D.

Intravenous infusion of calcium gluconate is associated with some risks. Bradycardia and cardiac bradyarrhythmia are well-known side effects of bolus IV calcium administration. Meticulous care must be taken to ensure that the IV line is secure. Prevention of extravasation of calcium-containing fluid is extremely important, as extravasation of calcium can lead to tissue necrosis. IV sites through which calcium-containing fluid is administered as an infusion must be monitored every 2–4 hours for early recognition of extravasation, if any.

Close attention also needs to be paid to the choice of calcium salt while initiating oral calcium supplementation **(Table 2.15.5)**.

TABLE 2.15.5: Elemental calcium contents of various calcium salts.

Calcium preparation	*Elemental calcium content (%)*
Calcium carbonate	40%
Calcium phosphate	38.7%
Calcium chloride	27.3%
Calcium acetate	25.3%
Calcium citrate	21.1%
Calcium lactate	13%
Calcium ascorbate	10%
Calcium gluconate	9.3%
Calcium gluceptate	8.2%
Calcium glubionate	6.6%

In symptomatic hypocalcemia, if it is not responsive to calcium supplementation, one needs to check magnesium levels. Correction of hypomagnesemia is undertaken with 0.2 mL/kg/dose of 50% magnesium sulfate injection administered deep intramuscularly (IM), two doses, 12 hours apart. If necessary, later neonates may be provided with a maintenance dose of 0.2 mL/kg/day of 50% magnesium sulfate, administered orally for 3 days.

If hypocalcemia persists for >1 week (prolonged) or remains nonresponsive despite adequate calcium, vitamin D, and magnesium sulfate administration, it is likely to be due to hypoparathyroidism, syndromic cause, and severe hyperphosphatemia. These infants may require higher doses of calcium, 1,25-dihydroxy vitamin D3 (a biologically active form of vitamin D), and in some cases phosphate binders.

Natural History and Prognosis

Most neonates with EONH resolution occur within 48–72 hours without any long-term adverse effects. LONH, which is secondary to exogenous phosphate load, responds to the restriction of phosphate. LONH, secondary to magnesium deficiency, responds to magnesium supplementation. Neonates who have hypoparathyroidism-induced hypocalcemia would need continued supplements with adequate amounts of calcium and vitamin D. The duration of therapy is directly reliant on the nature of the hypoparathyroidism, which can be transient or permanent.

Neonates with syndromes and those who have had prolonged seizures with hypoxemia would likely have unfavorable long-term neurodevelopmental outcomes.

REFERENCES

1. Mathai SS. Hypocalcemia. In: Thakre R, Murki S (Eds). Protocols in Neonatology, 2nd edition. New Delhi: Jaypee Brothers Medical Publishers; 2020. pp. 84-7.
2. Venkataraman PS, Tsang RC, Steichen JJ, Grey I, Neylan M, Fleischman AR. Early neonatal hypocalcemia in extremely preterm infants. High incidence, early onset, and refractoriness to supraphysiologic doses of calcitriol. Am J Dis Child. 1986;140(10):1004-8.
3. Smilie C, Shah D, Batra P, Ahmed RS, Gupta P. Prevalence and predictors of hypocalcaemia in severe acute malnutrition. Public Health Nutr. 2020;23(17):3181-6.
4. Kovacs CS. Calcium, phosphorus, and bone metabolism in the fetus and newborn. Early Hum Dev. 2015;91(11):623-8.
5. Hsu SC, Levine MA. Perinatal calcium metabolism: physiology and pathophysiology. Semin Neonatol. 2004;9(1):23-36.
6. Thomas TC, Smith JM, White PC, Adhikari S. Transient neonatal hypocalcemia: presentation and outcomes. Pediatrics. 2012;129(6):e1461-7.
7. Zhou P, Markowitz M. Hypocalcemia in infants and children. Pediatr Rev. 2009;30(5):190-2.
8. Singh J, Moghal N, Pearce SH, Cheetham T. The investigation of hypocalcaemia and rickets. Arch Dis Child. 2003;88(5):403-7.
9. Dhir H, Kumar D, Shah D, Batra P, Ahmed RS, Gupta P. Efficacy of oral vs. intravenous calcium supplementation for continuation therapy in hypocalcemic seizures: a randomized, controlled trial. Indian J Pediatr. 2023;90(5):433-7.
10. Mimouni F, Tsang RC. Neonatal hypocalcemia: to treat or not to treat? (A review). J Am Coll Nutr. 1994;13(5):408-15.

2.16 Hypoxic–Ischemic Encephalopathy and Intracranial Hemorrhage

Swathi Chacham, Rachna Pasi, Kriti Mohan

HYPOXIC–ISCHEMIC ENCEPHALOPATHY

INTRODUCTION

Perinatal asphyxia is a common neonatal emergency responsible for neuromorbidity and neonatal mortality. Hypoxic-ischemic encephalopathy (HIE) is the third important cause (23%) of neonatal deaths in India.[1] All the asphyxia-related deaths (97.8%) occur in the first week of life, of which most of them (70%) die in the first 24 hours.

DEFINITIONS

The World Health Organization defined asphyxia as failure to initiate or sustain respiration after birth.[2]

- *Moderate asphyxia:* It is defined as slow gasping breathing or an Apgar score of 4–6 at 5 minutes of age.
- *Severe asphyxia:* It is considered when there is no breathing or an Apgar score of 0–3 at 5 minutes of age. Essentially, it is a state of diminished gas exchange resulting in hypoxemia, hypercarbia, and fetal acidosis during the intranatal period.
- *Fetal acidosis:* It is defined as umbilical arterial blood pH <7.0.
- *Hypoxic–ischemic encephalopathy:* It refers to the altered neurobehavioral response of the neonate along with manifestations of brainstem dysfunction with objective evidence of hypoxic–ischemic etiology.

EPIDEMIOLOGY

The HIE incidence all over the world varies from 1 to 8/1,000 live births. Around four million babies succumb in the newborn period globally, and perinatal asphyxia is one of the prime causes. Furthermore, HIE is a significant concern at the individual, family, and society level. It accounts for 15–28% of children having cerebral palsy and 25% of developmental delay cases.[3]

Hypoxic-ischemic injury can occur during antenatal (5–20%), intrapartum (56%), and postnatal (5–10%) causes of the cases. Intrapartum hypoxic-ischemia is more common in developing countries than in developed countries. The incidence is inversely proportional to gestational age (GA) and birth weight (BW). It is high in pregnancies complicated with diabetes, pregnancy-induced hypertension, and abruptio placentae.

ETIOPATHOGENESIS

Asphyxia results from inefficient gas exchange through the placenta, resulting in impaired oxygenation and reduced elimination of carbon dioxide (CO_2) and hydrogen (H^+). Structural abnormalities of the respiratory, cardiovascular, and central nervous system (CNS) can result in postpartum asphyxia. Broadly, asphyxia is multifactorial resulting from maternal, placental, fetal, and neonatal causes **(Table 2.16.1)**. The clinical manifestations of neonatal encephalopathy due to different etiologies can coexist, and thus it is challenging to detect the etiology with neurological examination alone. In the absence of clear-cut perinatal risk factors, other causes of neonatal encephalopathy should be considered and excluded.[4,5]

Transient hypoxemia and limited oxygen (O_2) reserve may occur during normal labor due to uterine contractions, cord compression, and maternal dehydration. Hypoxia-ischemia results in varied physiologic and biochemical changes. Following transient asphyxia, heart rate (HR) initially increases and decreases later, while blood pressure (BP) and central venous pressure (CVP) increase. However,

TABLE 2.16.1: Etiological factors for perinatal asphyxia.

Maternal factors	Pregnancy-induced hypertension, essential hypertension, renal failure (acute or chronic), shock, hypotension, infection (including chorioamnionitis), bronchial asthma, congenital or acquired heart disease, diabetes, maternal vascular disease, and cocaine abuse
Placental factors	Abruptio placentae, placenta previa, infarction, fibrosis or hydrops fetalis, and ruptured uterus
Umbilical cord factors	Entanglement, true knot, compression, prolapse, and vasa previa
Fetal factors	Fetal anemia (fetomaternal hemorrhage), infection, cardiomyopathy, hydrops fetalis, and cardiovascular insufficiency
Neonatal factors	PPHN, cyanotic congenital heart disease, cardiomyopathy, cardiogenic shock/septic shock, respiratory failure occurring from meconium aspiration syndrome, neonatal pneumonia, and pneumothorax

(PPHN: persistent pulmonary hypertension of the newborn)

cardiac output (CO) remains unaltered. Subsequently, there is redistribution of CO, resulting in enhanced blood flow to the brain, heart, and adrenal glands (diving reflex). This phenomenon does not occur when there is complete cessation of blood flow, as in placental abruption, resulting in characteristic ischemic lesions in subcortical white matter and brainstem nuclei. When asphyxia is prolonged, cerebral autoregulation and CO_2 responsiveness are lost, leading to impaired cerebral perfusion. As cerebral blood flow (CBF) is decreased, glucose production is impaired. This is coupled with enhanced glucose utilization by the brain, depleted glycogen stores, phosphocreatine, and adenosine triphosphate (ATP). Thus, prolonged asphyxia leads to diffuse injury involving both cortical and subcortical structures, with specific predilection to neuronal populations susceptible to HI injury.[3]

The pathognomonic feature of HIE is cellular dysfunction due to impaired oxidative phosphorylation and ATP production. These events occur in two phases: (1) Primary energy failure and (2) secondary energy failure. In primary energy failure ion pump function diminishes, causing intracellular accumulation of ions, such as Na^+, Cl^-, H_2O, and Ca^{2+}, and buildup of extracellular K^+ along with excitatory neurotransmitters, such as glutamate. Secondary energy failure sets in 6–48 hours after the triggering insult. Similarly, cell death can be both necrotic and apoptotic occurring either instantly or later.

- *Immediate neuronal death (necrosis):* This is a result of ion pump failure and intracellular osmotic overload.
- *Delayed neuronal death (apoptosis):* This is due to uninhibited enzyme and secondary mediator activation within the cell (e.g., proteases, lipases, and caspases), impairment of the electron transport system in mitochondria, leukotrienes, free radicals, and nitric oxide production.
- *Reperfusion injury:* Not only the ischemic insult causes neuronal dysfunction but also the reperfusion of ischemic tissue results in neuronal injury by releasing oxygen-free radicals, such as hydroxyl, hydrogen peroxide, and superoxide, which can damage deoxyribonucleic acid, ribonucleic acid, lipids, proteins, and the blood-brain barrier. Moreover, this may lead to the activation of an inflammatory cascade with the release of tumor necrosis factor-alpha and interleukin-1 release.

CLINICAL FEATURES

Hypoxic-ischemic encephalopathy can affect any major organ, leading to multisystem involvement **(Table 2.16.2)**. It is classified as mild, moderate, or severe, according to Levene's classification **(Table 2.16.3)**, and staging of 1, 2, and 3 is given by Sarnat and Sarnat. All the three categories of HIE—mild, moderate, and severe—have altered consciousness. Differential hypotonia is seen in the early stages of HIE. Upper limbs and proximal muscles are more affected. (Abnormal scarf sign and poor flexor muscle tone during traction response). Fifty percent of the neonates with HIE manifest seizures usually within 24 hours after the HI insult in moderate or severe encephalopathy (subtle seizures followed by tonic or clonic). They need to be distinguished from jitteriness or clonus with electrographic changes. Similarly, the features of raised intracranial pressure (ICP), due to extensive cortical necrosis, can also occur, suggesting poor prognosis.

TABLE 2.16.2: Possible impacts of perinatal asphyxia.

CNS	HIE, intracranial hemorrhage (ICH), seizures, and long-term neurological sequelae
Cardiac	Myocardial dysfunction, valvular dysfunction, rhythm abnormalities, and CCF
Renal	Hematuria, acute tubular necrosis, and renal vein thrombosis
Gastrointestinal	Necrotizing enterocolitis and hepatic dysfunction
Hematological	Thrombocytopenia and DIC/coagulation abnormalities
Pulmonary	Respiratory failure, apnea, meconium aspiration, surfactant depletion, and pulmonary hypertension
Metabolic	Hypoglycemia, acidosis, hypocalcemia, and hyponatremia (SIADH or renal involvement)

(CCF: congestive cardiac failure; CNS: central nervous system; DIC: disseminated intravascular coagulation; HIE: hypoxic–ischemic encephalopathy; SIADH: syndrome of inappropriate antidiuretic hormone secretion)

TABLE 2.16.3: Levene's classification of hypoxic–ischemic encephalopathy.

Feature	*Mild grade I*	*Moderate grade II*	*Severe grade III*
Consciousness	Irritable	Lethargy	Comatose
Tone	Normal	Hypotonia	Flaccid
Seizures	No	Yes	Prolonged
Sucking	Weak suck	Weak suck/unable to suck	Unable to suck
Heart rate	Tachycardia	Bradycardia	Variable

DIAGNOSIS

A history of maternal, placental, and fetal morbidities that contribute to asphyxia needs to be identified. Additionally, one should document the fetal assessment conducted through antenatal ultrasound, biophysical profile, and nonstress test.

TABLE 2.16.4: Laboratory evaluation of asphyxia.

Metabolic	• *Blood glucose:* (2, 6, 12, 24, 48, and 72 hours of age) • Hematocrit, calcium, sodium, and potassium (daily)
CNS	Serum CK-BB, S-100, and NSE
CVS	CK-MB, CTNI, and CTNT
Renal	Blood urea nitrogen (BUN) and serum creatinine, fractional excretion of Na^+ (FeNa), and urine levels of β2-microglobulin
Brain imaging	Cranial ultrasound, CT, MRI brain, conventional T1- and T2-weighted MRI sequences, diffusion-weighted imaging (DWI), proton magnetic resonance spectroscopy (*proton-MRS* or *H-MRS*), susceptibility-weighted imaging, and magnetic resonance (MR) angiography or venography
EEG	EEG and integrated aEEG

(aEEG: amplitude EEG; CK-MB: creatine kinase-myocardial band; CNS: central nervous system; CT: computed tomography; CTNI: cardiac troponin I; CTNT: cardiac troponin T; CVS: cardiovascular system; EEG: electroencephalogram; MRI: magnetic resonance imaging; MRS: magnetic resonance spectroscopy; NSE: neuron-specific enolase)

Fetal bradycardia (HR <60/min), delivery details, and need for positive-pressure ventilation for >1 minute or delayed first cry for >5 minutes and a low Apgar score should be evaluated. Apgar score >6 at 5 minutes rules out perinatal asphyxia to a major extent.

DIFFERENTIAL DIAGNOSIS

Maternal anesthesia, birth trauma, systemic infection, CNS infection-hemorrhage or malformation or cardiac malformations, and inborn error of metabolism can mimic HIE.

INVESTIGATIONS

The evaluation of the cardiovascular system, CNS, and renal injury is an essential part of the management of asphyxiated neonates **(Table 2.16.4)**.[6]

Neuroimaging

The following neuroimaging modalities are recommended in evaluating neonates with asphyxia **(Table 2.16.4)**.

Cranial ultrasound (CUS): It is a simple, noninvasive, nonionizing bedside tool that demonstrates diminished gray-white matter differentiation and shrunken ventricles. It can demonstrate intraventricular hemorrhage (IVH) in preterm neonates associated with asphyxia.

Computed tomography (CT): CT scan in term neonates with an acute stage of HIE shows generalized low attenuation of brain parenchyma. It can depict hemorrhage and cerebral edema. It poses the risk of ionizing radiation.

BOX 2.16.1: Neuropathology seen in asphyxia.

- Selective neuronal necrosis
- Periventricular white matter injury
- Bilateral parasagittal cortical and subcortical white matter injury
- Focal or multifocal cortical necrosis/cystic encephalomalacia/ulegyria
- Diffuse cerebral cortical necrosis
- Injury of brainstem, thalamus, and basal ganglia

Magnetic resonance imaging (MRI) brain: It is the ideal investigation to delineate the degree of brain injury and various neuropathological changes **(Box 2.16.1)**. It is time-consuming, with the problem of sedation in neonates, and is costly. However, MRI brain can reveal that occurs in HIE.

Electroencephalogram

Electroencephalogram (EEG) can demonstrate seizures, differentiate seizures from seizure mimics, and help to assess the efficacy of antiepileptic drugs. Various types of EEG that are seen in asphyxia include burst suppression, discontinuous, low-voltage, or isoelectric patterns. These carry a poor prognosis. Amplitude EEG (aEEG) can also be used as a bedside tool. EEG aids in monitoring newer therapies, such as therapeutic hypothermia (TH).

MANAGEMENT

The management of HIE is multidimensional **(Box 2.16.2)**.

Treatment of Seizures

Phenobarbitone is the drug of choice for seizures [loading dose: 20 mg/kg, intravenous (IV), over 20 minutes]. If seizures persist, additional doses (5–10 mg/kg) can be given; if there is no response, phenytoin sodium (15–20 mg/kg IV over 20 minutes) can be given. If available, fosphenytoin can be used. Maintenance therapy is started 12–24 hours later (3–5 mg/kg/day, BD for phenobarbitone and 4–8 mg/kg, TID for phenytoin). Although seizures are often refractory in HIE, either of these anticonvulsants is effective in most of the cases. Infrequent, transient, mild seizures not compromising cardiopulmonary status need no treatment. For uncontrolled seizures, give lorazepam (0.05–0.1 mg/kg/dose IV). Newer anticonvulsants, such as levetiracetam, can be used. However, neonates should be investigated for other metabolic causes, such as hypocalcemia, hypomagnesemia, hypoglycemia, hyponatremia, hypernatremia, and polycythemia, which may also coexist.

Newer Modalities of Therapy

Therapeutic hypothermia is useful in term and late preterm neonates with moderate-to-severe encephalopathy. It should be initiated within 6 hours of life and continued till 72 hours of life, guided by EEG. It acts by reducing neuronal metabolism, has been shown to improve neurodevelopmental outcomes, and has become the standard of care in developed nations. It is recommended that TH should be initiated with definite protocols (used in published literature) with facilities for multidisciplinary care and longitudinal follow-up.[3]

Erythropoietin is considered to have neuroprotective effects in neonates with HIE.[7] However, its effects on neurodevelopmental outcomes when provided along with TH are still inconclusive, with some studies reporting higher adverse effects.

Other experimental treatments include allopurinol and melatonin.

OUTCOME AND PREVENTION

Neurodevelopmental sequelae correspond closely with the staging or severity of HIE. Moreover, the neonate's diagnosis is based on its worst HIE grade during the course of management. It has been noted that HIE Grade I has no long-term impairments, and 20% of HIE Grade II have long-term neurological morbidities. On the other hand, 50–70% of HIE Grade III neonates may die or have severe long-term motor, cognitive, and sensory impairments. Optimum antenatal, intrapartum, and postnatal monitoring can aid in the prevention of HIE.

BOX 2.16.2: Management of neonatal asphyxia.

- Assess, support, and maintain temperature, airway, breathing, and circulation
- Blood sugar, hematocrit, acid–base balance, and metabolic monitoring
- Management of shock/hypotension and renal impairment
- Management of seizures
- Oxygenation and ventilation
- Therapeutic hypothermia

INTRACRANIAL HEMORRHAGE

INTRODUCTION

Intracranial hemorrhage (ICH) is an important cause of morbidity and mortality in neonates. As the neonatal brain is at risk of potential damage by maternal, fetal, and neonatal factors, ICH can have a devastating effect on the developing brain with its long-term neurological sequelae. ICH can manifest as either intraparenchymal bleed or extra-parenchymal bleed. It can be classified as subdural, epidural, subarachnoid, intraventricular, and intraparenchymal hemorrhage (IPH), as shown in **Table 2.16.5**. They have varying etiopathologies, clinical manifestations, and prognoses as per the severity and GA, with an overlap among the various types.[8]

EPIDEMIOLOGY

The incidence ranges from 2% to >30% in neonates depending on the type of ICH and GA at birth. Instrumental deliveries carry a higher risk than cesarean sections.

ETIOPATHOLOGY

Subdural Hemorrhage and Epidural Hemorrhage

The basic pathology in subdural hemorrhage (SDH) is bleeding into the subdural space due to rupture of the draining veins and sinuses in it. This results in blood accumulation below the dura and above the subarachnoid villi. The process of delivery like vertical molding, torsional forces on the head during labor, and fronto-occipital elongation can precipitate SDH by laceration of the dural sinuses in the falx cerebri or the tentorium cerebelli, and hence, these are the common sites of SDH. Small clinically trivial parturition SDH can occur in uncomplicated labors. Posterior fossa SDH can

TABLE 2.16.5: Classification of intracranial hemorrhage and their determinants in neonates.

Type of hemorrhage	*Location*	*Predisposing factors*
SDH	Intracranial and below dura Amidst dura and arachnoid	Unfavorable pelvis, abnormal presentations, prolonged or precipitous delivery, bleeding disorders, clotting disorders, instrumental delivery, and difficult labor
SAH	Underneath the arachnoid mater	Bleeding disorders, clotting disorders, instrumental delivery, and difficult labor
GMH/IVH	Germinal matrix in the caudothalamic groove	Prematurity, RDS, PDA, shock, acidosis, reperfusion injury, rapid administration of hyperosmolar fluids, pneumothorax, ET suctioning, frequent intubations, and hypo-/hypercapnia
IPH	Cerebral hemorrhage and cerebellar hemorrhage	Arteriovenous malformation, aneurysm, coagulation disorders: Hemophilia, thrombocytopenia, and reperfusion injury in HIE

(ET: endotracheal intubation; GMH/IVH: germinal matrix hemorrhage/intraventricular hemorrhage; HIE: hypoxic-ischemic encephalopathy; IPH: intraparenchymal hemorrhage; PDA: patent ductus arteriosus; RDS: respiratory distress syndrome; SAH: subarachnoid hemorrhage; SDH: subdural hemorrhage)

occur due to ripping of the transverse sinus, inferior sagittal sinus, straight sinus, or vein of Galen. A severe form of SDH can result from rupture of the occipital sinus during breech presentation due to occipital osteodiastasis. Supratentorial space SDH is a manifestation of tearing off the superficial bridging veins in the cerebral cortex.

The incidence is higher in vaginal deliveries when compared to cesarean deliveries, with 2.9/10,000 spontaneous deliveries in contrast to 8–9.8/10,000 in vacuum and forceps deliveries, respectively. Recent studies report a higher prevalence of asymptomatic, small SDH (up to 45%).

Subarachnoid Hemorrhage

Subarachnoid hemorrhage (SAH) manifests frequently in the neonatal period. It has been described as primary and secondary to IVH. Primary SAH is often unnoticed and clinically asymptomatic. As with SDH, the usual process of normal labor can result in a small SAH due to the tearing of veins of subarachnoid villi. The prevalence of SAH is 1.3/10,000 spontaneous vaginal deliveries, and instrumental deliveries, such as vacuum or forceps, have a higher prevalence rate.

Subarachnoid hemorrhage can also occur due to the spreading of germinal matrix hemorrhage (GMH) or IVH into subarachnoid space in premature neonates. Similarly, SAH can develop as a progression of SDH, IPH, or rarely in term neonates manifest as subpial hemorrhage due to birth injury.

Intraparenchymal Hemorrhage

Cerebellar hemorrhage (CH) is the most common form of IPH, and primary cerebral hemorrhage is rarely due to tearing of arteriovenous malformation, aneurysm, bleeding, or coagulation disorder. It is mostly due to the expansion of GMH/IVH, SAH, SDH, reperfusion injury in HIE, hemorrhagic venous infarction, or venous sinus thrombosis **(Figs. 2.16.1 to 2.16.3)**. It can be a complication of extracorporeal membrane oxygenation therapy. CH in preterm neonates goes unnoticed by CUS, and MRI is the best tool.[8]

Intraventricular Hemorrhage

Intraventricular hemorrhage is the most frequently manifesting ICH in preterm neonates. The incidence is 25–30% in very low birth weight (VLBW) neonates and <25 weeks GA. In the preterm, IVH arises from delicate, vulnerable involuting vessels in the caudothalamic groove, which occupy the subependymal germinal matrix. The germinal matrix is situated near the ventricles and produces neurons and glial cells in the growing fetus. The blood vessels of this germinal matrix are deficient in the basement membrane, which predisposes them for rupture in the face of abnormal CBF autoregulation. The ependymal germinal matrix is extremely vascularized, receiving its blood supply from anterior choroidal vessels and anterior and middle cerebral arteries. Hence, hemorrhage can be localized to the germinal matrix or may spread into the lateral ventricles, and IVH can become unilateral or bilateral. These risk factors are enlisted in **Table 2.16.6**.

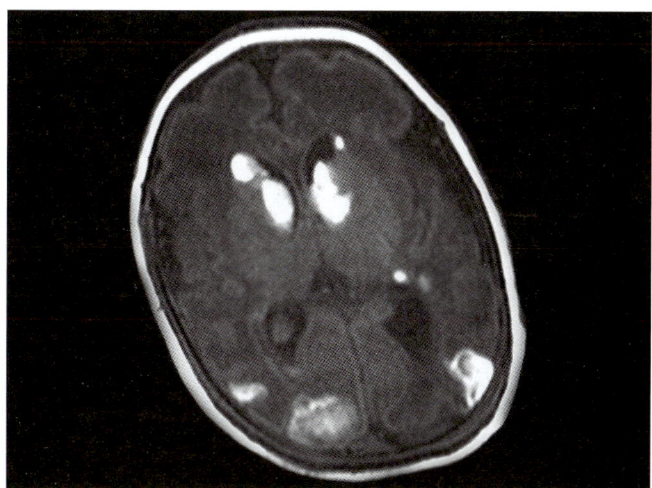

Fig. 2.16.1: MRI axial T1W image along the body of lateral ventricle, demonstrating bilateral intraventricular hemorrhage and parenchymal hemorrhages in bilateral (B/L) temporal, right occipital, and in the deep white matter associated with subacute hemorrhagic foci in (B/L) basal ganglia, thalamus, and cerebral hemispheres (abnormal T1 hyperintensities) mildly increased enhancement along the basal cisterns. (MRI: magnetic resonance imaging; T1W: T1-weighted)

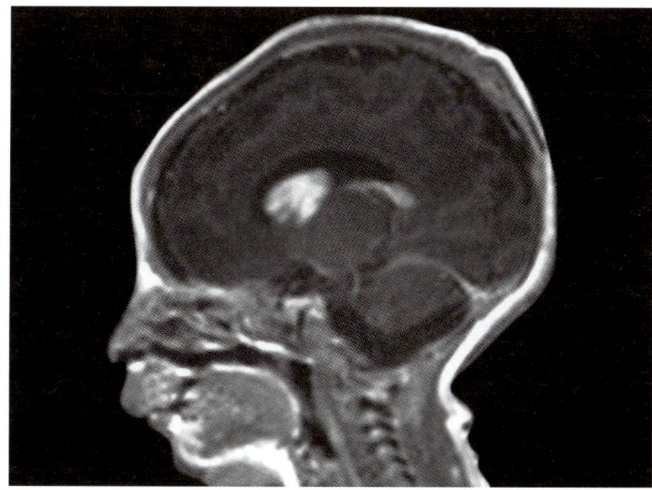

Fig. 2.16.2: MRI sagittal view revealing intraventricular hemorrhage. (MRI: magnetic resonance imaging)

Grading of IVH is given by Papile and Volpe. As per severity, Grade 1 is small, Grade 2 is moderate, and Grade 3 is severe.[8]

Intraventricular hemorrhage is less frequent in term neonates as germinal matrix involutes by >34 weeks of GA

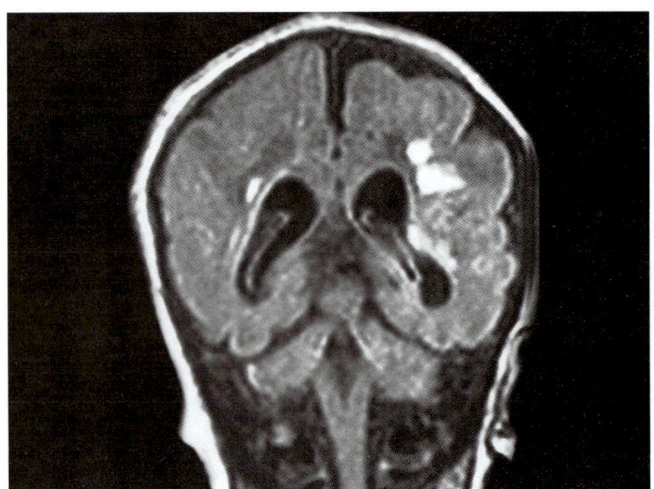

Fig. 2.16.3: MRI coronal view depicting intraparenchymal hemorrhages. (MRI: magnetic resonance imaging)

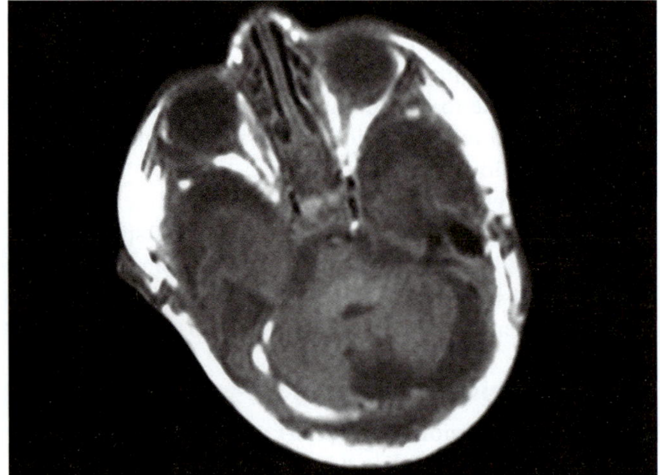

Fig. 2.16.4: MRI image axial T1W along the posterior fossa, showing distended right transverse sinus with hyperintense luminal signal, suggestive of subacute thrombus: Right transverse sinus thrombosis. (MRI: magnetic resonance imaging; T1W: T1-weighted)

TABLE 2.16.6: Causes of IVH in premature neonates.

Prenatal factors	Failure to administer antenatal steroids, chorioamnionitis, inflammation of the amniotic sac, and abruption
Intrapartum factors	Prolonged labor, obstructed labor, and instrumental delivery
Postnatal factors	Fast infusion of colloids, hyperosmolar solutions (sodium bicarbonate), normal saline in preterm, hypertension, transportation, genetic factors, acidosis, respiratory distress with hypo- or hypercapnia rapid alterations in CBF and cerebral venous pressure, patent ductus arteriosus, asynchrony on ventilator, high PEEP, tracheal suctioning, pneumothorax, anemia, and hypoglycemia
Systemic factors	Bleeding and clotting disorders

(CBF: cerebral blood flow; IVH: intraventricular hemorrhage; PEEP: positive end-expiratory pressure)

(complete involution by 36 weeks of GA). Primary IVH in term neonates arises from choroid plexus, hemorrhagic thalamic infarction, venous sinus thrombosis **(Fig. 2.16.4)**, or from subependymal germinal matrix remnants. It is predominantly due to traumatic delivery and perinatal asphyxia.[9,10]

Periventricular leukomalacia (PVL) is a neuropathological finding in premature neonates due to hypoxia, ischemia, and the inherent susceptibility of white matter of the cerebral cortex in preterm neonates enhanced by inflammation or infection. This leads to significant motor, sensory, and cognitive disturbances in childhood.

CLINICAL FEATURES

A major proportion of ICH can be small, asymptomatic, and resolve without sequelae. Depending on the location and severity of the injury, it can manifest soon after birth or within 24–48 hours of life with features of ICP and compression of the underlying brain parenchyma. Frequent clinical features consist of altered sensorium, apnea, irregular respirations, opisthotonus posture, and seizures. Bulging of fontanel and sutural separation can also be there. Hemodynamic instability, shock, and anemia can occur due to large hemorrhage.

DIAGNOSIS

Intracranial hemorrhage can be diagnosed based on history and clinical manifestations and confirmed by neuroimaging. MRI brain is the diagnostic modality for ICH. Although CUS is easy to perform in sick newborns at bedside, its utility in diagnosis is often insufficient for the majority of hemorrhages. MRI is sensitive to small hemorrhage and to detect the timing and extent of ICH. MRI is also a valuable tool for detecting other lesions like HI injury, contusion, thromboembolic infarction. Lumber puncture is contraindicated when a large ICH is suspected or ICH in the posterior fossa or supratentorial compartment is suspected. CT can be used for acute situations, where MRI is not feasible, like in an unstable neonate with raised ICP requiring neurosurgical treatment. CT head will aid both in early diagnosis and in follow-up for the evolution of hydrocephalus or subdural effusion and requires less time to perform the procedure. Along with neuroimaging, other investigations necessary to diagnose bleeding/clotting disorder and sepsis are required.

The mainstay of diagnosis of IVH is CUS. The American Academy of Neurology (AAN) recommends CUS between 7 and 14 days to all neonates <30 weeks GA and repeat CUS between 36 and 40 weeks' postmenstrual age.

MANAGEMENT

The mainstay of treatment is supportive and symptomatic. Large ICH mandates immediate stabilization with fluids, blood, inotropes, and ventilatory support as per the requirement. In all the neonates with suspected ICH, an immediate CT head should be performed, followed by the opinion of the neurosurgery team. The neonate needs close follow-up for subsequent complications, such as chronic subdural effusion and hydrocephalus. Periventricular hemorrhagic infarction (PVHI) and posthemorrhagic ventricular dilation (PVD) are the two principal complications of IVH. Larger and severe IVH have a higher predisposition to these complications and need periodic monitoring and follow-up.

REFERENCES

1. McIntyre S, Nelson KB, Mulkey SB, Lechpammer M, Molloy E, Badawi N; Newborn Brain Society Guidelines and Publications Committee. Neonatal encephalopathy: Focus on epidemiology and underexplored aspects of etiology. Semin Fetal Neonatal Med. 2021;26(4):101265.
2. Aggarwal R, Deorari A, Paul VK. Post-Resuscitation Management of Asphyxiated Neonates. New Delhi: WHO Collaboration Centre/All India Institute of Medical Sciences; 2007.
3. Victor S, Rocha-Ferreira E, Rahim A, Hagberg H, Edwards D. New possibilities for neuroprotection in neonatal hypoxic-ischemic encephalopathy. Eur J Pediatr. 2022;181(3):875-87.
4. Molloy EJ, Branagan A, Hurley T, Quirke F, Devane D, Taneri PE, et al.; Steering Group for DEFiNE (Definition of Neonatal Encephalopathy). Neonatal encephalopathy and hypoxic-ischemic encephalopathy: moving from controversy to consensus definitions and subclassification. Pediatr Res. 2023;94(6):1860-63
5. Aslam S, Strickland T, Molloy EJ. Neonatal encephalopathy: need for recognition of multiple etiologies for optimal management. Front Pediatr. 2019;7:142.
6. Chacham S, Nagasravani J, Reddy UN. Acute renal failure in neonates with perinatal asphyxia and its correlation with HIE staging: a prospective case control study. J Neurol Neurobiol. 2016;2(2). doi http://dx.doi. org/10.16966/2379-7150.119
7. Wu YW, Comstock BA, Gonzalez FF, Mayock DE, Goodman AM, Maitre NL, et al.; HEAL Consortium. Trial of erythropoietin for hypoxic-ischemic encephalopathy in newborns. N Engl J Med. 2022;387(2):148-59.
8. Volpe JJ. Intracranial hemorrhage: subdural, primary subarachnoid, cerebellar, intraventricular (term infant), and miscellaneous. In: Volpe JJ, Darras BT, du Plessis AJ, Perlman JM, Inder TE, de Vries LS, et al. (Eds). Volpe's Neurology of the Newborn, 6th edition. New York: Elsevier; 2017. pp. 665-75.
9. Bruschettini M, Romantsik O, Zappettini S, Banzi R, Ramenghi LA, Calevo MG. Heparin for the prevention of intraventricular haemorrhage in preterm infants. Cochrane Database Syst Rev. 2016;(5):CD011718.
10. Tsao PC. Pathogenesis and prevention of intraventricular hemorrhage in preterm infants. J Korean Neurosurg Soc. 2023;66(3):228-38.

2.17 Bleeding Neonate

Tejo Pratap Oleti

INTRODUCTION

Bleeding neonate is a medical emergency that poses diagnostic and therapeutic challenges in the neonatal intensive care unit (NICU). Neonates have physiological handicaps for mounting effective hemostasis and hence are at risk of bleeding. Diagnosing bleeding disorders in infants, whether congenital or acquired, necessitates comprehension of developmental hemostasis and its impact on laboratory assessments. A methodical approach to neonatal bleeding is essential for clinicians to accurately diagnose and treat conditions, given the diverse range of potential underlying diseases.[1]

EPIDEMIOLOGY

The frequency of bleeding disorders in newborns may vary depending on geographic location, healthcare accessibility, and genetic factors. While certain bleeding episodes may spontaneously resolve, others might signal underlying congenital or acquired conditions. Although the prevalence of noteworthy bleeding disorders among newborns is generally low, failure to promptly diagnose and address them can lead to considerable morbidity and mortality.[2]

ETIOPATHOGENESIS

Hemostasis consists of three steps:

1. *Primary—near the site of vessel injury:* Platelets adhere, get activated, and aggregate to form a platelet plug and will try to seal the vessel injury.
2. *Secondary*—after the platelet plug is formed, coagulation factors get activated and form crosslinking fibers to stabilize the platelet plug. **Figure 2.17.1** depicts the coagulation pathway.
3. *Tertiary*—this process involves fibrinolysis to restore the circulation in the blood flow. This step is assisted by the fibrinolytic pathway.

   Figure 2.17.1 shows the coagulation pathway.

There are several hemostatic-related handicaps in neonates:

- *Platelet:* The mean platelet count rises by 2,089 cells/cumm/week from 22 to 42 weeks of gestations.[3] The concentration of these proteins in neonates is different compared to that in children and adults. The levels match by 6 months of life after the maturation of different pathways in the organs. Neonatal platelets exhibit significant differences in function compared to adult platelets.[4] These differences impact clot formation and hemostasis.
- *Bleeding time:* Neonates have shorter bleeding time due to increased activity of von Willebrand factor (vWF). vWF plays a crucial role in platelet adhesion and aggregation at the site of vessel injury.
- *Procoagulant and inhibitor levels:* Many procoagulant levels in neonates are gestationally dependent. Inhibitors like α2-macroglobulin are elevated while antithrombin III, heparin cofactor II, protein C, and protein S are lower than the adult levels. Reduced procoagulant and inhibitor reserve affect clotting dynamics. The dynamics will elevate both prothrombin time (PT) and activated prothrombin time (APTT) values in the neonates **(Tables 2.17.1 and 2.17.2)**.
- *Fibrinolysis:* Neonates exhibit relatively impaired fibrinolysis. Tissue plasminogen activator and plasminogen activator inhibitor are elevated compared to adults while plasminogen and α2-antiplasmin are at lower levels.

Causes of Bleeding

The etiology of bleeding in the neonates is very varied. They can be broadly classified as causes related to platelets, factor

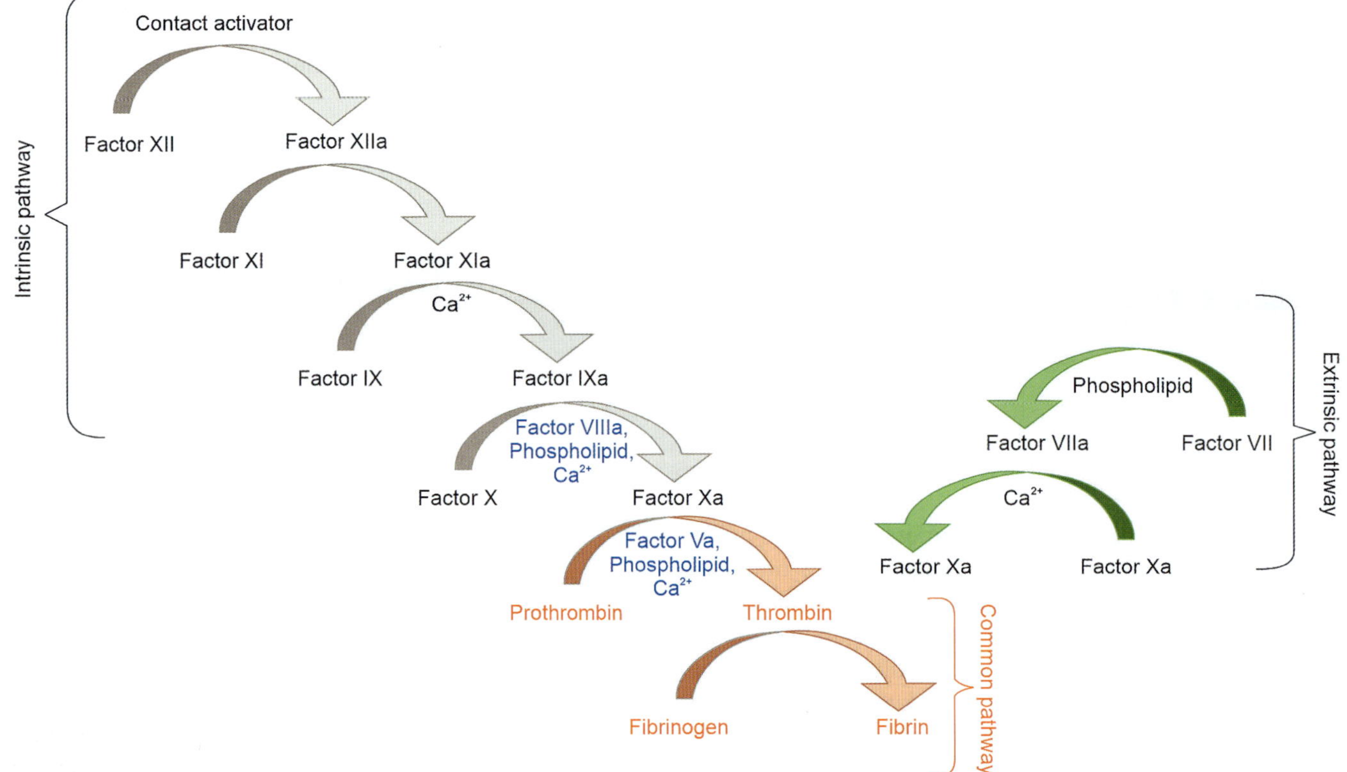

Fig. 2.17.1: Coagulation pathway.

TABLE 2.17.1: Comparison of performance of coagulation tests at different ages.

Parameters	*Preterm*	*Term*	*Infant*
Prothrombin time (PT)	Normal to ↑	Normal to ↑	<12 seconds
Activated prothrombin time (APTT)	Normal to ↑↑	Normal to ↑	<22 seconds
Fibrinogen	250 (100)	240 (150)	251 (160)
Platelet function analysis (PFA-100*)	Normal to ↓	↓	Normal

*PFA-100 will look at the qualitative aspects of platelet functioning.

TABLE 2.17.2: Coagulation factor levels at birth.

Factor levels elevated compared to adult	*Factor levels lower compared to adult*
• Fibrinogen • Factor V* • Factor VIII • von Willebrand factor (vWF)	• Factors II, VII, IX, X, XI, XII, and XIII[†] • Prekallikrein (PreK) • High-molecular-weight kininogen (HMWK)

*Reach to adult levels by day 3 of life.
[†]Levels will be 50% of the adult.

deficiencies, and others. **Table 2.17.3** depicts the common causes of the bleeding in the neonates.

CLINICAL FEATURES

The infant may be well or sick, symptomatic or asymptomatic. The symptoms and signs depend on the site and amount of bleeding. They are also influenced by prior hemodynamic status and the cause of bleeding. One or more of the following signs may be present in bleeding newborn, namely pallor, petechiae, purpura, ecchymoses, bleeding or excessive oozing from the umbilical stump, sampling sites, or cannula sites lethargy, and seizures or shock. Depending on the site, intracranial signs (seizures, altered sensorium, and breathing irregularities), extracranial signs (subgaleal hematoma or cephalhematoma), gastrointestinal signs (blood in the stools or gastric aspirates, and tense abdomen), lung signs (bloody tracheal aspirates or pulmonary hemorrhage), or renal signs (hematuria) may predominate.

DIAGNOSIS

Diagnosis is reached by focused history and physical examination **(Box 2.17.1)**.

A thorough antenatal, natal, and postnatal history will give the clues. Factor deficiencies and platelet functional disorders run in the families through different Mendelian inheritance. Hemophilia A and B are inherited as X-linked recessive inheritance patterns whereas von Willebrand disease (vWD) (types 1 and 2) is predominantly inherited as an autosomal dominant pattern (type 3: autosomal recessive).

TABLE 2.17.3: Etiology of neonatal bleeding.

Thrombocytopenia	*Factor deficiencies*
Congenital causes: • Platelet function—normal or slightly deranged • Fanconi anemia • Thrombocytopenia with absent radii syndrome (TAR) • Congenital amegakaryocytic thrombocytopenia • von Willebrand disease type 2B • Thrombotic thrombocytopenic purpura (ADAMTS13 deficiency) • Aneuploidy (trisomies- 18, 13, 21, or triploidy) • Platelet function—deranged • Wiskott–Aldrich syndrome • X-linked macrothrombocytopenia • Chediak–Higashi syndrome	*Congenital causes:* • Hemophilia (A and B) • Afibrinogenemia • von Willebrand disease • Alpha2-antiplasmin deficiency • Other individual deficiencies • Factors II, V, VII, X, and XIII • Combined factor deficiencies
Acquired causes: • TORCH [toxoplasmosis, others (syphilis, hepatitis B), rubella, cytomegalovirus, herpes simplex] group of infections • *Sepsis:* Early and late • Disseminated intravascular coagulation (DIC) • Immune thrombocytopenia: Autoimmune and alloimmune • Hypersplenism • Necrotizing enterocolitis (NEC) • *Localized:* Thrombosis, hemangioma • Intrauterine growth restriction (IUGR) • Mother having pregnancy-induced hypertension	*Acquired causes:* • DIC • Liver disease • Vitamin K-dependent bleeding disorders

BOX 2.17.1: Clues to diagnosis.

History:
- Maternal illness (e.g., infection and HELLP syndrome)
- Maternal drugs (e.g., anticonvulsants, aspirin, and coumadin)
- Difficult delivery (e.g., instrumental delivery)
- Multiple pregnancies (e.g., twin-to-twin transfusion)
- Antepartum hemorrhage (e.g., placenta previa, abruption, and vasa previa)
- Family history (e.g., unexplained deaths, frequent blood transfusions, and hemophilia)

Physical examination:
- Well or sick baby
- Single- or multiple-site bleeding
- Symptomatic or asymptomatic
- Organomegaly (e.g., sepsis and intrauterine infections)
- Dysmorphism (e.g., genetic, storage, or collagen vascular disorder)

(HELLP: hemolysis, elevated liver enzymes, and low platelets)

Knowing the site of bleeding is crucial. Petechiae are common in platelet-related disorders while hematomas are common in other coagulopathies. Mucocutaneous bleeding is more common with platelet disorders while bleeding in the visceral or deep organs is more common with coagulopathies related to factor deficiencies.

DIFFERENTIAL DIAGNOSIS

Bleeding in newborns can be due to platelet, coagulation, vascular, or iatrogenic disorder.

INVESTIGATIONS

Laboratory evaluation must focus on identifying the problems in hemostasis and to look at the underlying condition. The *first line of tests* in evaluation is listed in **Table 2.17.4**.

A routine complete blood count helps identify if it is a red blood cell (RBC), white blood cell (WBC), platelet, or combined disorder. A platelet count of <150,000 indicates thrombocytopenia. PT evaluates the extrinsic pathway, while APTT evaluates the intrinsic pathway. Both PT and APTT abnormalities might be due to factor deficiency in the common pathways or due to consumptive coagulopathies like disseminated intravascular coagulation (DIC).

The error during sample collection or incomplete dilution in citrate/ethylenediaminetetraacetic acid (EDTA) bottle can falsely lead to platelet clumping and cause erroneously low platelet counts on the measurement. Sampling obtained through the heparinized central lines or excessive heparin in the syringes can prolong the APTT and sometimes even PT also.

A careful peripheral smear examination will help us in studying the platelet morphology and can identify disorders like giant platelet disorders. Large-sized platelets are seen in giant platelet syndrome, Bernard-Soulier syndrome, and Wiskott-Aldrich syndrome. A septic screen which includes the inflammatory markers and blood cultures can help us to identify the underlying infection and inflammation. A liver function test to rule out an existing acute or chronic liver disorder which is associated with elevated PT needs to be done. The elevated D-dimer level and low fibrinogen level in a bleeding neonate indicate the presence of DIC.

TABLE 2.17.4: First-tier tests in a bleeding neonate.

Test	*Purpose*
Complete blood count (CBC)	Identifies anemia and its severity, infection, and one or more cell line affection
Peripheral smear	Red blood cell (RBC), white blood cell (WBC), and platelet morphology
Platelet count	Thrombocytopenia
Prothrombin time (PT)	Abnormal PT alone indicates vitamin K-dependent factor deficiency
Activated prothrombin time (APTT)	Abnormal APTT alone indicates VIII, IX, and XI deficiencies
Both PT and APTT abnormal	Factors V, X, prothrombin, and fibrinogen abnormalities

Second-line investigations include looking at individual factor levels and platelet functions. The individual factor assay will help in further evaluation of the disorders. Factor XIII deficiency can spuriously have normal PT and APTT and can be diagnosed only on individual factor assay. Platelet function analysis (PFA-100) will help in looking at the inherited varieties of thrombocytopenia. Genetic studies will help in confirming the familial disorders.

Flowchart 2.17.1 provides a stepwise approach to the diagnosis in a bleeding neonate.

MANAGEMENT

The management of a bleeding newborn is supportive and specific. The initial supportive management should concentrate on assessing, supporting, and maintaining temperature, airway, breathing, and circulation. Treatment should be directed toward the underlying cause.

The specific management involves providing the component therapies and also treating the underlying causes. The component therapies involve providing platelets, plasma concentrates like fresh frozen plasma (FFP) and cryoprecipitate, and also specific factor concentrates.

Platelet Transfusions

With the increasing evidence on the harmful effects of liberal strategy for platelet transfusions, we need to rationalize the unit policies for the same. Studies show that the neonates had higher mortality and bleeding tendencies in the higher threshold (<50,000/cumm) compared to the lower threshold group (<25,000/cumm).[5] The National Neonatology Forum (NNF) recommends that prophylactic transfusions be given to neonates when platelet counts fall below 25,000 (strong recommendation).[6] **Table 2.17.5** elaborates on the indications of platelet transfusions, while **Table 2.17.6** depicts the choice of platelet concentrates and their performances.

Plasma Derivatives/Concentrates

Plasma contains about 1 unit/mL of each of the coagulation factors as well as normal concentrations of other plasma proteins. Labile coagulation factors, like factors V and VIII, are not stable in plasma stored for prolonged periods at 1–6°C; therefore, plasma is usually stored frozen at –18°C or lower.

Fresh Frozen Plasma

Fresh frozen plasma is stored within 8 hours of collection. It contains about 87% of factor VIII at the time of collection and must contain at least 0.70 IU/mL of factor VIII.

Flowchart 2.17.1: Approach to a bleeding neonate.

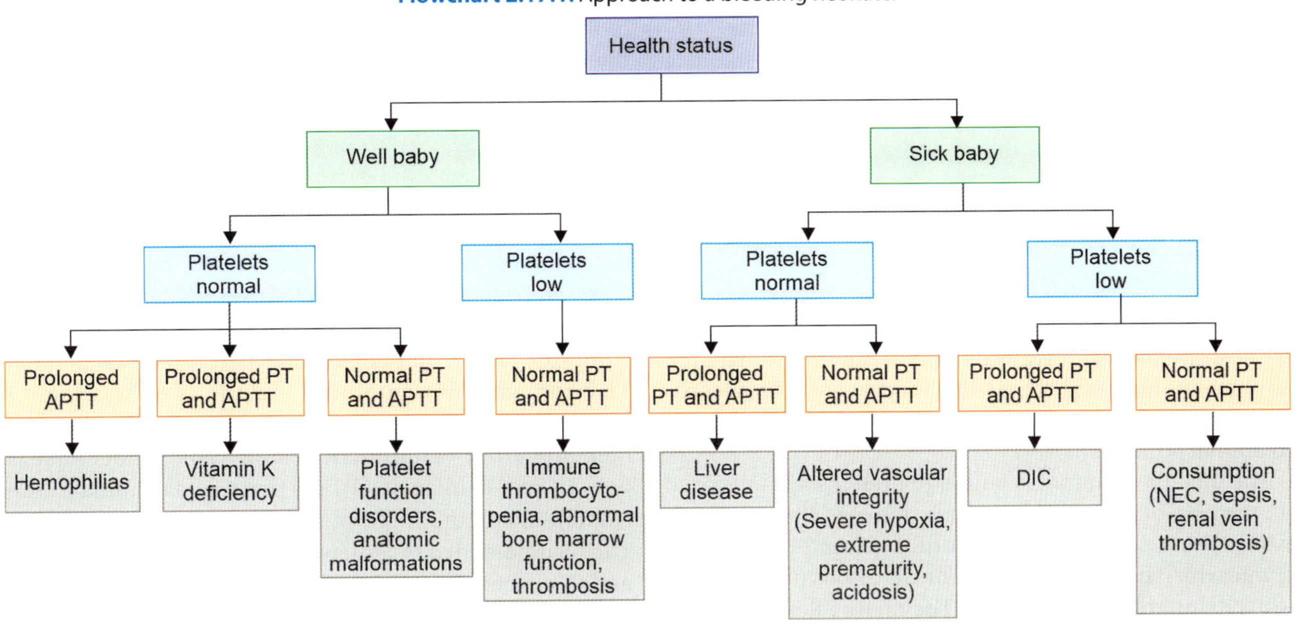

(APTT: activated prothrombin time; DIC: disseminated intravascular coagulation; PT: prothrombin time)

TABLE 2.17.5: Indications for platelet transfusion in nonimmune thrombocytopenia.

Platelet count	*Symptoms*
<30,000	None
30,000–50,000	• Sick or bleeding • <1,000 g* • <7 days old* • Concurrent coagulopathy • Major intraventricular hemorrhage (IVH) grade 3 or 4 • Requiring surgery or exchange transfusion
50,000–100,000	Actively bleeding

*Consider transfusion as the conditions are more prone to bleeding and functional studies will guide in decision.

Indications for Transfusing Fresh Frozen Plasma

- Disseminated intravascular coagulopathy
- Vitamin K-deficiency bleeding
- Inherited deficiencies of coagulation factors
- Hepatic failure
- Prophylaxis of bleeding for an invasive procedure in the presence of coagulopathy
- Exchange transfusion for hyperbilirubinemia with packed red blood cells (PRBCs)

Dosing: 10–20 mL/kg is usually adequate dose. A dose of 10 mL/kg should increase clotting factors and inhibitor levels by approximately 10 IU/dL (10%). FFP should be group AB or compatible with the recipient's ABO red cell antigens.

TABLE 2.17.6: Random donor platelets (RDPs) versus single donor platelets (SDPs).

	RDP	*SDP*
Preparation	From multiple whole blood units by pooling	From single donor by plateletpheresis
Platelet density	0.5×10^{11}/unit	3×10^{11}/unit
Dosage	15 mL/kg	15 mL/kg
Predicted improvement	20,000/cumm	60,000/cumm
Duration of administration	Over 30 minutes	Over 30 minutes
Storage period	5 days*	7 days*
Advantage	Less cost	Avoids multiple donor exposure

*Needs constant agitation.

Notes:
- Infant and donor should be ABO identical or compatible.
- Never use a *filter* during platelet transfusion.
- Platelets should be stored at 22–24°C with continuous gentle agitation in the platelet incubator and agitator.
- "Washed platelets" can be used in patients with anaphylactic reactions to the plasma component.

Cryoprecipitate

Cryoprecipitate contains about 80–100 U of factor VIII in 10–25 mL of plasma, 300 mg of fibrinogen, and varying amounts of factor XIII. It is stored at a temperature of –20°C or below. Indications for use of cryoprecipitate include the following:

- Congenital factor VIII deficiency
- Congenital factor XIII deficiency
- Afibrinogenemia and dysfibrinogenemia
- von Willebrand disease

The cryoprecipitate's suggested dose is 5 mL/kg.

Table 2.17.7 provides the shelf life of commonly used blood and blood products.

Specific Important Conditions

Vitamin K-dependent Bleeding

Vitamin K is a fat-soluble vitamin and gets stored in the body after absorption. There are two forms of vitamin K—vitamin K1 (phylloquinone, found in plant foods, e.g., leafy greens) and vitamin K2 (menaquinones found in fermented foods and animal products).

The dietary vitamin K is bound to proteins, gets released with the help of pancreatic enzymes, and gets absorbed with chylomicrons. It acts as a cofactor for gamma-carboxylase enzyme which helps in the activation of various proteins with carboxy glutamic acid residues. The factors dependent on vitamin K in the coagulation pathway are II, VII, IX, and X. The anticoagulant proteins, proteins C and S, also require the same.

The vitamin K-dependent bleeding (VKDB) has been divided into three varieties based on the time of onset:

- *Early VKDB*: It occurs in the first 24 hours and manifests as cephalhematoma, intracranial hemorrhage, or excess bleeding from the umbilical stump. It is due to maternal malabsorption or due to maternal intake of hepatotoxic medications.
- *Classic VKDB*: It occurs between 1 and 7 days and manifests as mucocutaneous bleeding, intracranial hemorrhage, gastrointestinal bleeding, bleeding from the circumcision site, or umbilical stump bleeding. It occurs due to a combination of physiological deficiency at birth, exclusive breastfeeding, or missed prophylaxis at birth.
- *Late VKDB*: It usually manifests after 2 weeks and is caused by either malabsorption or cholestasis conditions like cystic fibrosis, α1 antitrypsin deficiency, biliary atresia, and other hepatic/gastrointestinal tract (GIT) causes.

TABLE 2.17.7: Storage and shelf life of blood and blood products.

Product	Storage temperature	Shelf life	Transport temperature
Platelets' constant agitation	22°C	3–5 days	20–24°C
FFP	–20°C	1 year	1–10°C once thawed
Cryoprecipitate	–18°C	1 year	20–24°C once thawed

(FFP: fresh frozen plasma)

The incidence of late VKDB was 4–10 per 100,000 births in the absence of universal prophylaxis of vitamin K.[7] After the introduction of intramuscular (IM) vitamin K prophylaxis, the incidence of late VKDB decreased to 0.24–3.2 per 100,000 live births.[8]

Hemophilia

Hemophilia A and B are caused by factor VIII and IX deficiencies, respectively. The severity of the disease is assessed by factor activity level. In severe disease, the factor activity level will be <1%. Factor VIII deficiency is the most common factor deficiency that can occur in neonates. The common presentations include bleeding from the circumcision site, intracranial bleeding, and excessive bleeding from venipuncture sites. The milder diseases present later in infancy. APTT is prolonged in both disorders. Hemophilia is inherited by an X-linked recessive pattern. The recommended treatment for both disorders is factor VIII and IX concentrates, respectively. If the concentrates are not available, we can use FFP or cryoprecipitate in emergency situations.

von Willebrand Disease

von Willebrand disease rarely presents in the neonatal period as neonates have higher activity and more high-molecular-weight vWF multimers compared to adults. There are three types (1–3). Type 3 is the most severe form with near-complete absence of the factor, while type 1 neonates will have partial deficiency. Type 2 is caused by abnormal vWF morphology and function. It is characterized by prolonged bleeding time, decreased vWF antigen levels, reduced vWF activity (ristocetin cofactor activity), and low FVIII levels.

It can be managed by desmopressin (DDAVP) which increases vWF release from endothelial cells and is effective in type 1 vWD and some type 2 subtypes. vWF/FVIII concentrates are required for type 2 and type 3 vWD.

REFERENCES

1. McMillan D, Wu J. Approach to the bleeding newborn. Paediatr Child Health. 1998;3(6):399-401.
2. Bora K. Gaps in the coverage of vitamin K1 prophylaxis among newborns in India: insights from secondary analysis of data from the Health Management Information System. Public Health Nutr. 2021;24(17):5589-97.
3. Wiedmeier SE, Henry E, Sola-Visner MC, Christensen RD. Platelet reference ranges for neonates, defined using data from over 47,000 patients in a multihospital healthcare system. J Perinatol Off J Calif Perinat Assoc. 2009;29(2):130-6.
4. Saracco P, Rivers RPA. Pathophysiology of coagulation and deficiencies of coagulation factors in newborn. In: Buonocore G, Bracci R, Weindling M (Eds). Neonatology: A Practical Approach to Neonatal Diseases. Cham: Springer International Publishing; 2018. pp. 1431-53.

5. Curley A, Stanworth SJ, Willoughby K, Fustolo-Gunnink SF, Venkatesh V, Hudson C, et al. Randomized trial of platelet-transfusion thresholds in neonates. N Engl J Med. 2019;380(3):242-51.
6. Pandita A, Kumar A, Gupta (Chairperson) G, Taligasalam V, Tewari VV. Use of blood components in newborns. J Neonatol. 2020;34(4):199-217.
7. Sutor AH. Vitamin K deficiency bleeding in infants and children. Semin Thromb Hemost. 1995;21(3):317-29.
8. Schulte R, Jordan LC, Morad A, Naftel RP, Wellons JC, Sidonio R. Rise in late onset vitamin K deficiency bleeding in young infants because of omission or refusal of prophylaxis at birth. Pediatr Neurol. 2014;50(6):564-8.

2.18 Necrotizing Enterocolitis

Ruchi Rai

INTRODUCTION

Necrotizing enterocolitis (NEC) is the most common gastrointestinal (GI) emergency in newborns characterized by acute bowel inflammation leading to necrosis and bowel injury. It primarily affects preterm babies, although it can also be less commonly seen in term neonates. A high index of suspicion is needed to diagnose NEC as the signs and symptoms are often nonspecific.[1]

EPIDEMIOLOGY

The incidence of NEC varies from center to center with an overall incidence of 1–5% of all neonatal intensive care unit (NICU) admissions. The incidence varies inversely with the birth weight and the gestation, so the smallest and the most premature babies are at the highest risk. 7 out of 100 of all very low birth weight (VLBW) infants in the NICU are likely to develop NEC.[2] Around 10% of infants with NEC are born at term. Despite the advances in the field of neonatology, there has not been a decline in the incidence of NEC and the mortality has also remained almost constant.[3] The mortality is high, between 15% and 30%.

ETIOPATHOGENESIS

The pathogenesis of NEC is complex and multifactorial.[3-5] All factors lead to oxidative stress, inflammation, and bowel necrosis. The etiology of the disease is not very clear, but various factors seem to be involved and play a role in pathogenesis.

The risk factors associated with NEC are as follows:

- *Prematurity:* The most strongly associated factor is prematurity. The incidence of NEC is inversely proportional to the birth weight and gestation of the baby. The age of onset of NEC is inversely proportional to the weight and gestation of the baby at birth. So, the term babies have onset of symptoms much earlier than the preterm babies. Babies weighing 1,000–1,500 g at birth have an incidence of <5%; this incidence increases to >10% in babies <1,000 g at birth. The mortality also increases with decreasing gestational age.
- *Enteral feeding:* Almost universally, all the babies who develop NEC have been fed. It is hypothesized that osmolar stress due to feeds may act as a potential stress. The rapid advancement of feeds may also lead to abnormal vascular regulation of the gut. The activation of gut hormones may play a role. Feeding with human milk seems to have a protective role for NEC, whereas feeding with bovine milk increases the risk of NEC.
- *Blood transfusion:* Blood transfusion is increasingly being seen as a risk factor, with more and more evidence coming up lately. But a causal relationship has not been confirmed yet.
- *Congenital heart disease:* Critical congenital heart diseases like hypoplastic left heart syndrome and coarctation of aorta have also been found to increase the risk of NEC.
- *Infections:* Sepsis which is common in preterm babies may also lead to NEC. Organisms associated with NEC are *Klebsiella pneumonia, Escherichia coli, Clostridium perfringes*, rotavirus, etc.
- *Genetic predisposition*
- *Others:* Other risk factors are fetal growth restriction, maternal chorioamnionitis, prolonged use of antibiotics, perinatal asphyxia, polycythemia, umbilical catheterization, rapid increase in feeds, shock, and administration of indomethacin.
- *Protective factors:* Use of breast milk and antenatal corticosteroids has a protective role and decrease the incidence of NEC.

PATHOGENESIS

- *Intestinal immaturity:* In preterm babies, the GI system is immature in terms of motility, digestion, absorption, immune defenses, barrier functions, and circulatory regulation as well as microvascular tone. This makes the gut of preemies vulnerable to ischemia and necrosis.
- *Bowel ischemia:* Blood flow in splanchnic circulation is compromised in situations of stress in newborns to maintain blood flow to the vital organs, such as brain and heart. As a result, bowel ischemia and tissue necrosis ensue.
- *Dysbiosis:* The gut microflora plays a definite role in pathogenesis. When there is an overgrowth of potential pathologic bacteria (dysbiosis), they are likely to cross the compromised gut barrier and release endotoxins and cytokines, leading to inflammation.
- *Proinflammatory responses:* Excessive and inappropriate inflammatory response triggers the release of mediators, such as platelet-activating factor, lipopolysaccharides, and tumor necrosis factor (TNF), which have been suspected to play a significant role.

CLINICAL FEATURES

Like most other diseases in neonates, NEC does not have specific signs and symptoms.[3] A close observation of early signs and symptoms is crucial to suspect the disease in high-risk babies. Premature infants develop NEC around the second week of life, whereas the term babies manifest earlier. A baby with NEC may present with the following signs:

- *Systemic:* Lethargy, temperature instability, apnea, shock, irritability, and respiratory distress.
- *Abdominal:* Distention, gastric residuals, vomiting, blood in stools, abdominal wall erythema, and bilious aspirates. **Figure 2.18.1** shows a neonate with NEC having abdominal distention.
- *Course of disease:* This is also very variable, it may present with a rapidly progressive, fulminant course with tense abdominal distention or slow gradually progressing distention and feed intolerance.

Evidence suggests that routine monitoring of gastric residual has little or no effect on the incidence of NEC.[6] There is a dose-response relationship between milk intake and NEC. Overall, when the human milk accounts for at least 20% of the total enteral intake, it significantly improves outcomes. If the intake of human milk reaches 50%, the incidence and severity of NEC, as well as the time to reach enteral feeds, are reduced.[7]

DIAGNOSIS

Modified Bell staging has been used for diagnosing and staging the disease **(Table 2.18.1)**.

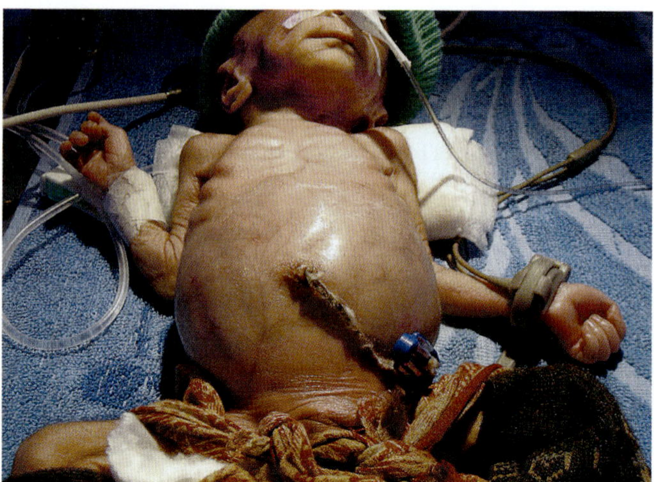

Fig. 2.18.1: Necrotizing enterocolitis with abdominal distention.

DIFFERENTIAL DIAGNOSIS

Infection (e.g., sepsis, gastroenteritis, urinary tract infection), GI anomalies (e.g., malrotation, volvulus, pyloric stenosis, duodenal atresia), and intussusception may manifest with similar clinical features.

INVESTIGATIONS

A high level of suspicion in a clinically high-risk setting is the mainstay for diagnosing NEC. However, certain supportive laboratory investigations may be of help.

Blood investigations: Clinical biomarkers have been unsuccessful in predicting as well as diagnosing NEC. The typical triad of persistent acidosis, thrombocytopenia, and refractory hyponatremia is characteristic of babies with NEC but does not aid in diagnosis.

Blood culture: It may be positive in cases of sepsis.

Stool: It may sometimes show occult blood but is not used for diagnosis.

Imaging: X-ray of the abdomen may show features of ileus, such as dilated bowel loops **(Fig. 2.18.2)**. There may be bowel wall edema, pneumatosis intestinalis (gas in bowel wall) **(Fig. 2.18.3)**, the presence of hepatobiliary gas, or if the disease has advanced to intestinal perforation, there is pneumoperitoneum **(Fig. 2.18.4)**. Pneumatosis intestinalis or portal venous gas is considered diagnostic of NEC but is seen in only some babies.

Ultrasound of the abdomen is a good tool to diagnose bowel necrosis. It has the benefit that it does not expose the baby to harmful radiation due to repeated X-rays, and it is easily available at the bedside. Ultrasound can detect pneumatosis intestinalis and portal venous gas earlier than

TABLE 2.18.1: Modified Bell staging for NEC.

Stage		Systemic signs	Intestinal signs	Radiological signs	Treatment
I Suspected NEC	A	Temperature instability, apnea, lethargy, bradycardia	Increased prefeed residue, mild abdominal distention, emesis, stool positive for blood	Normal or mild dilation of intestinal loops	NPO antibiotics × 3 days
	B	Same as I A	Same as I A + bleeding per rectum	Same as I A	Same as I A
II Definite NEC	A Mildly ill	Same as above	Same as above + absent bowel sounds, abdominal tenderness	Ileus, pneumatosis intestinalis	NPO, antibiotics × 7–10 days
	B Moderately ill	Same as above + acidosis, thrombocytopenia	Same as above + definite abdominal tenderness, ascites, abdominal cellulitis, or right lower quadrant mass	Same as above + portal venous gas, ascites	NPO, antibiotics × 14 days
III Advanced NEC	A Severely ill, bowel intact	Same as above + hypotension, bradycardia, apnea needing ventilatory support, acidosis, DIC, neutropenia	Same as above	Same as above + definite ascites	NPO, antibiotics × 14 days Inotropes, ventilator support, fluid resuscitation, paracentesis
	B Severely ill, bowel perforated	Same as III A	Same as III A	Same as III A + pneumoperitoneum	Same as III A + surgery

(DIC: disseminated intravascular coagulation; NEC: necrotizing enterocolitis; NPO: nil per oral)

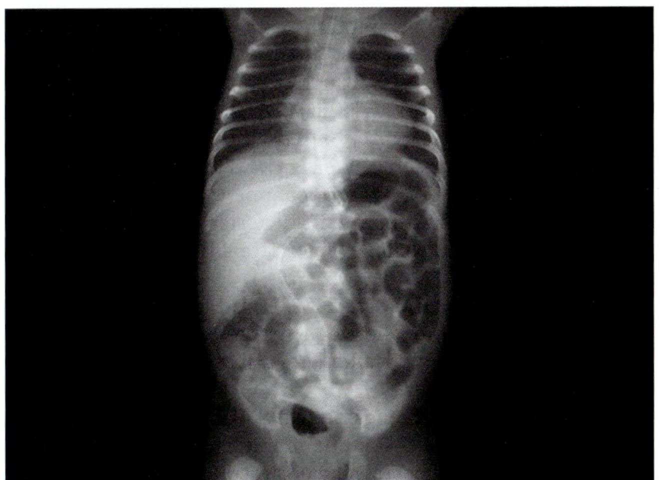

Fig. 2.18.2: X-ray of the abdomen showing dilated bowel loops (Bell stage I).

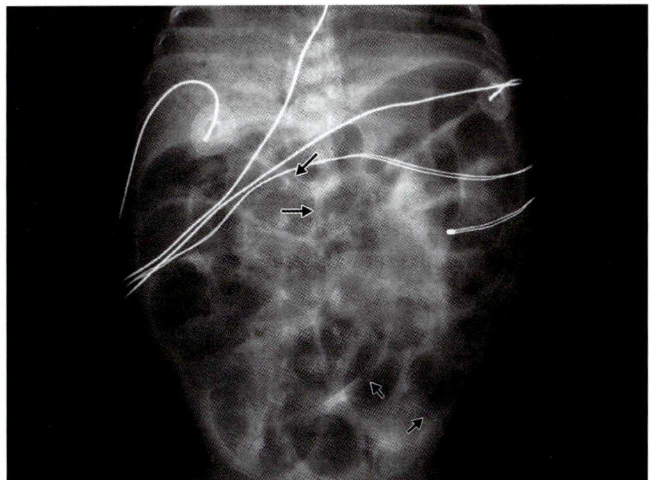

Fig. 2.18.3: Bell stage II showing pneumatosis intestinalis (arrows).

X-ray. Color Doppler is very sensitive in detecting bowel necrosis.

MANAGEMENT

No specific treatment approach is well defined.

Supportive: Supportive care during the disease can make a significant difference in morbidity and mortality, and it remains the mainstay of the management of the disease, while the disease is evolving. This includes maintenance of temperature, circulation, fluid and electrolyte balance, acid-base status, treatment of anemia, and thrombocytopenia along with close monitoring of the vitals.

Nutrition: The baby should be kept nil per oral and should be started on parenteral nutrition if possible, especially in babies with stages II and III. This will take care of the nutrition till the baby can be fed enterally.

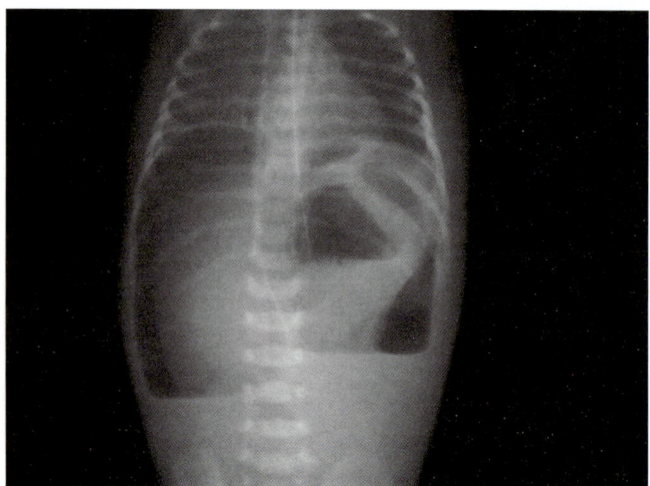

Fig. 2.18.4: Bell stage III showing pneumoperitoneum.

Decompression of the bowel: The bowel must be given rest; an orogastric tube should be kept in situ for regular decompression of the bowel and abdominal girth should be monitored.

Antimicrobials: As sepsis is one of the hypothesized factors leading to NEC, the babies must be started on broad-spectrum antibiotics after a blood culture sample has been withdrawn. Clindamycin or metronidazole should be added for anaerobic coverage.

Surgical intervention: This may be needed in 30–50% of the babies. It may be in the form of open laparotomy or insertion of a peritoneal drain. The choice and the timing of the surgical intervention remain controversial. Many recent studies have shown no definite difference in the outcomes in babies who had undergone laparotomy compared to those in whom a drain was inserted.

PREVENTION

Prevention is the most effective method to reduce NEC. The following bundle of interventions has been shown to reduce the incidence and severity of NEC.[8]

- *Feeding with human milk:* Human milk has immune-protective and anti-inflammatory factors, such as immunoglobulins, lactoferrin, and lysozyme.
- *Infection-control practices:* These should be strictly adhered to, in the NICU, to prevent any hospital-acquired infection. Prolonged empirical use of antibiotics should also be strongly discouraged.
- *Standardized feeding policy:* A consistent unit policy for feeding prevents the risk of growth failure and NEC.
- *Pre/probiotics:* Many studies show varying results regarding the protective role against NEC with no consensus on the timing, dose, duration, and type of strain.
- *Antenatal steroids:* Administration of prenatal steroids to pregnant mothers has been found to have a protective role in the development of NEC in preterm babies by enhancing gut maturity.

OUTCOME

Despite the advancement in neonatal care and diagnostic modalities, the etiology of NEC is still poorly understood; specific treatment strategies are lacking, and morbidity and mortality remain high. The mortality in babies developing NEC may be around 30%. The survivors have a high risk of developing dreaded complications, such as short bowel syndrome, intestinal strictures, and partial bowel obstruction. The neurodevelopmental outcomes in the survivors of NEC are also worse than their matched controls.

REFERENCES

1. Cuna A, George L, Sampath V. Genetic predisposition to necrotizing enterocolitis in premature infants: current knowledge, challenges, and future directions. Semin Fetal Neonatal Med. 2018;23(6):387-93.
2. Alsaied A, Islam N, Thalib L. Global incidence of necrotizing enterocolitis: a systematic review and meta-analysis. BMC Pediatr. 2020;20(1):344.
3. Afzal B, Elberson V, McLaughlin C, Kumar VH. Early onset necrotizing enterocolitis (NEC) in premature twins. J Neonatal Perinatal Med. 2017;10(1):109-12.
4. Gephart SM, Hanson C, Wetzel CM, Fleiner M, Umberger E, Martin L, et al. NEC-zero recommendations from scoping review of evidence to prevent and foster timely recognition of necrotizing enterocolitis. Matern Health Neonatol Perinatol. 2017;3:23.
5. Singh DK, Miller CM, Orgel KA, Dave M, Mackay S, Good M. Necrotizing enterocolitis: bench to bedside approaches and advancing our understanding of disease pathogenesis. Front Pediatr. 2023;10:1107404.
6. Abiramalatha T, Thanigainathan S, Ramaswamy VV, Rajaiah B, Ramakrishnan S. Routine monitoring of gastric residual for prevention of necrotising enterocolitis in preterm infants. Cochrane Database Syst Rev. 2023;6(6):CD012937.
7. Liu K, Guo J, Yang J, Su Y. The association of different proportions of human milk of the total enteral intake on health outcomes in preterm infants: a systematic review. Breastfeed Med. 2023;18(9):666-77.
8. Campos-Martinez AM, Expósito-Herrera J, Gonzalez-Bolívar M, Fernández-Marin E, Uberos J. Evaluation of risk and preventive factors for necrotizing enterocolitis in premature newborns. A systematic review of the literature. Front Pediatr. 2022;10:874976.

2.19 Common Congenital Malformations in the Newborn

Pratima Anand

INTRODUCTION

The term "congenital" means existing from birth. Therefore, congenital malformations or anomalies have their genesis in the intrauterine period. These malformations may occur as an isolated defect or they may be present in a pattern or combination involving one or more organ systems. The pattern may be a characteristic one, which is commonly known as "syndrome."

EPIDEMIOLOGY

The true incidence of malformations is still not known considering that the reported data exclude terminated pregnancies and stillbirths. Nevertheless, the reported global incidence is between 6 and 8%. In India, 1–3 out of 100 babies are born with congenital malformations; approximately 27 million babies are estimated to be born with birth defects each year.[1,2] The incidence per 1,000 live births in India of some common malformations is as follows:[1-4]

- *Central nervous system (CNS) malformations:* 0.5%
- *Cardiovascular system (CVS) malformations:* 0.5%
- *Orofacial defects:* 0.7%
- *Gastrointestinal malformations:* 0.4%
- *Musculoskeletal malformations like congenital diaphragmatic hernia (CDH), omphalocele:* 0.7%
- *Chromosomal defects:* 0.4%

COMMON TYPES OF CONGENITAL MALFORMATIONS

The malformations can be of medical, surgical, or cosmetic relevance. To note, different terms have been used in the literature to describe specific patterns of malformations. Classically, *malformations* are defects that occur due to internal abnormalities in the developmental process of the respective organ during the embryological period.[5-7] The structure is either not formed at all, partially formed, or formed in an abnormal fashion. The malformations can be classified as major or minor malformations. *Major malformations* are those which have social or surgical implications and can be life-threatening. Examples include neural tube defects and congenital heart disease. *Minor malformations,* on the other hand, are more of cosmetic importance. They may rarely require any intervention and sometimes can be a part of normal variation in the general population. Examples include ear tags and clinodactyly. As per some reports, infants with three or more minor anomalies are at an increased risk of having a major anomaly or a syndrome, and a thorough evaluation may be necessary in such cases. More than one malformation can be further classified into one of the following recognizable patterns **(Table 2.19.1)**.

TABLE 2.19.1: Pattern of multiple anomalies.[5-7]

Pattern	*Description*
Syndrome	A recognizable pattern of anomalies that occur together and have a set of clinical signs and symptoms *Example:* Down syndrome, and Edward syndrome
Association	The presence of two or more malformations that are not linked pathogenetically is known as an association *Example:* VACTERL (vertebral, anal, cardiac, tracheoesophageal, renal, and limb defects)
Sequence	The presence of a single defect that leads to a sequence of abnormalities *Example:* Potters sequence (oligohydramnios leading to renal anomalies)
Developmental field defect	An abnormality in the development of a contiguous physical space is known as developmental field defect *Example:* Holoprosencephaly, bladder exstrophy, and cloacal exstrophy. The manifestations can vary from mild to severe clinical features

As discussed above, malformations can be major or minor depending on the organ system involved, severity of clinical symptoms, and intervention needed. **Table 2.19.2** enumerates the common congenital malformations in the newborn.

ETIOPATHOGENESIS

The etiology that can be unknown is as far as 40–45% of cases of congenital malformations. However, few etiological factors have been found to be associated with some malformations as described below.[8,9]

Genetic Factors

Many genes and proteins are postulated to be associated with developmental malformations. The interference with

TABLE 2.19.2: Common congenital malformations in the newborn.

Major system	*Common malformations*
Congenital anomalies of the nervous system	• Neural tube defects **(Fig. 2.19.1)** • Anencephaly • Craniorachischisis • Iniencephaly • Encephalocele • Spina bifida • Microcephaly
Congenital anomalies of the eye and ear	• Congenital cataracts, congenital glaucoma • Microtia/anotia **(Fig. 2.19.2)**
Congenital heart defects	• Common truncus • Transposition of great arteries • Tetralogy of Fallot • Pulmonary valve atresia • Tricuspid valve atresia • Hypoplastic left heart syndrome • Interrupted aortic arch
Orofacial clefts **(Fig. 2.19.3)**	• Cleft palate • Cleft lip only • Cleft palate with cleft lip
Congenital anomalies of the digestive system	• Esophageal atresia/tracheo-esophageal fistula • Large intestinal atresia/stenosis • Anorectal atresia/stenosis
Congenital anomalies of genital and urinary organs	• Hypospadias **(Figs. 2.19.4A and B)** • Renal agenesis/hypoplasia
Congenital anomalies and deformations of the musculoskeletal system	Talipes equinovarus
Congenital anomalies and deformations of the musculoskeletal system: Limb reduction defects/ limb deficiencies	• *Limb deficiency:* Amelia, transverse terminal, transverse intercalary • *Longitudinal preaxial, longitudinal axial defects:* Split hand and foot, longitudinal postaxial
Abdominal wall defects and genitourinary defects	• Omphalocele **(Figs. 2.19.4A and B)** • Gastroschisis • Genitourinary abnormalities
Chromosomal abnormalities	Trisomy 21 (Down syndrome)
Congenital infectious syndromes	• Congenital rubella syndrome • Congenital syphilis • Congenital cytomegalovirus • Congenital Zika syndrome

any of the normal processes like apoptosis of cells, migration of neural cell crest derivatives, remodeling, etc., has the potential to cause abnormal formation of organs during the embryological period. Some of the genes implied in the genesis include the Homeobox gene (Holoprosencephaly),

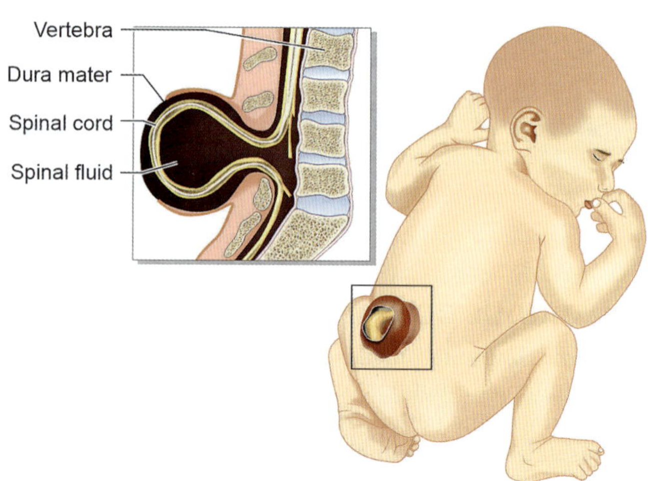

Fig. 2.19.1: Neural tube defects.[1]

transcription factors (congenital heart defects), and enzyme defects like mitochondrial myopathies. Some of the genetic mutations can be sporadic, whereas few others are known to be the result of autosomal, X-linked, or mitochondrial inheritance. For example, inborn errors of metabolism are mostly inherited as autosomal recessives.

Socioeconomic and Demographic Factors Including Nutritional Deficiencies

Nutritional deficiencies, especially folic acid deficiency, are strongly associated with neural tube defects. Periconceptional folic acid supplementation has been shown to reduce the risk of neural tube defects by 70%.

Environmental Factors Including Teratogens, Toxins, Maternal Illnesses, and Infections

Environmental toxins and teratogens [radiation exposure, maternal medications like antiepileptics (such as phenytoin and sodium valproate), and warfarin] are known to be associated with malformations like fetal hydantoin syndrome and warfarin-associated chondrodysplasias. The risk is greater if the exposure occurs during the organogenesis phase of the first trimester. Maternal infections such as cytomegalovirus, rubella, toxoplasmosis, and varicella can cause organ-specific malformations **(Table 2.19.3)**. Maternal illnesses such as insulin-dependent and pregestational diabetes mellitus, maternal phenylketonuria, and maternal antibodies like myasthenia gravis may lead to congenital malformations.

Multifactorial Etiology

These include nonsyndromic cleft lip/palate and nonsyndromic congenital heart disease.

Normal infant ear

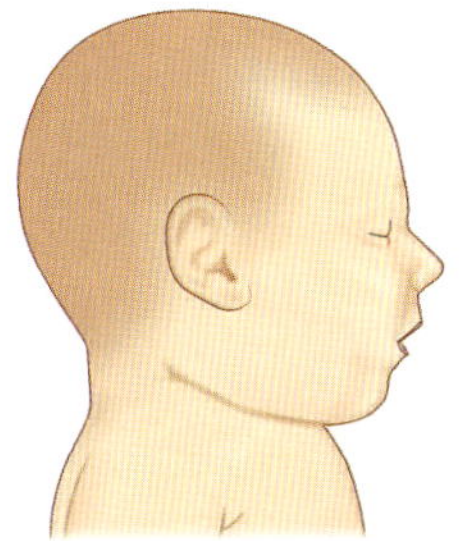

Microtia I

- Ear is small
- Ear canal may be narrowed
- Structures and ear shape are otherwise normal

Microtia II

- Ear is small
- Some components are missing
- Shape is markedly abnormal
- Ear is still recognizable

Microtia III

- Ear consists of a vertical mass of soft tissue and cartilage
- Typically associated with atresia of the external canal

Microtia IIV an Anotia

- Most extreme and rarest form
- All external ear structures are absent

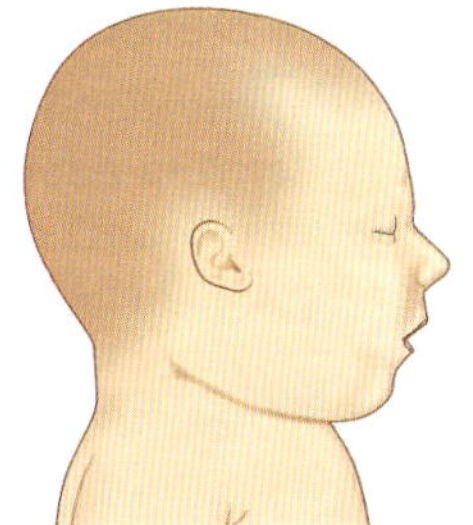

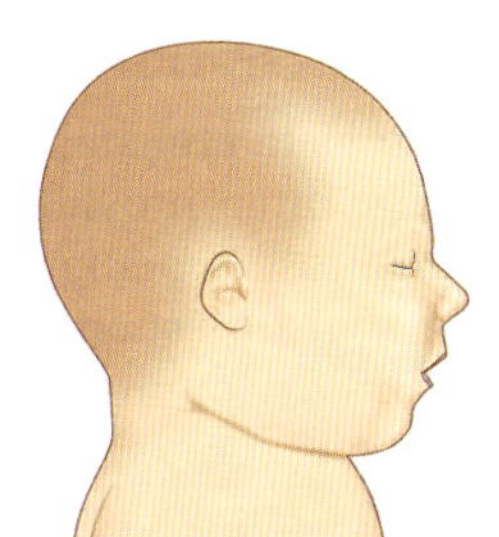

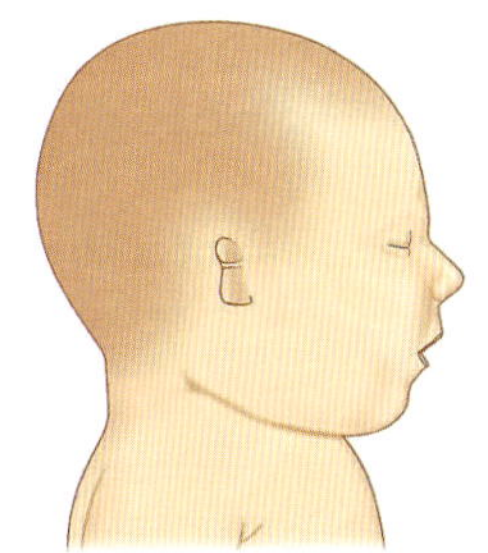

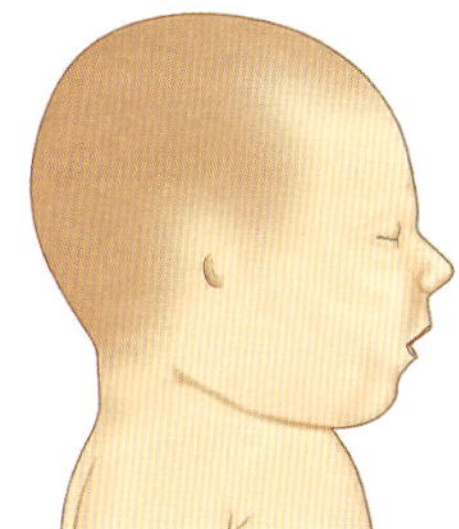

Fig. 2.19.2: Ear anomalies.[1]

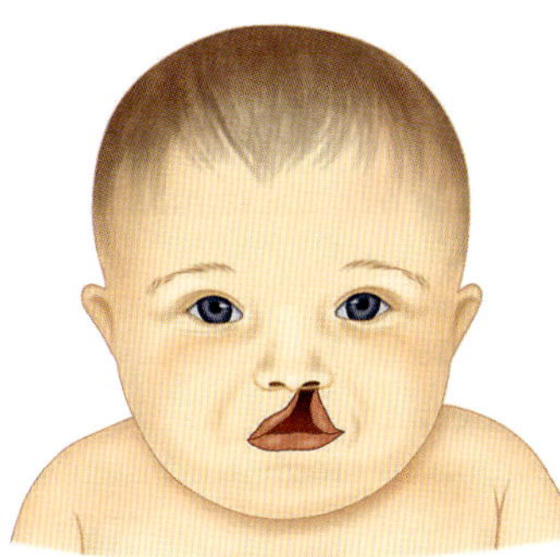

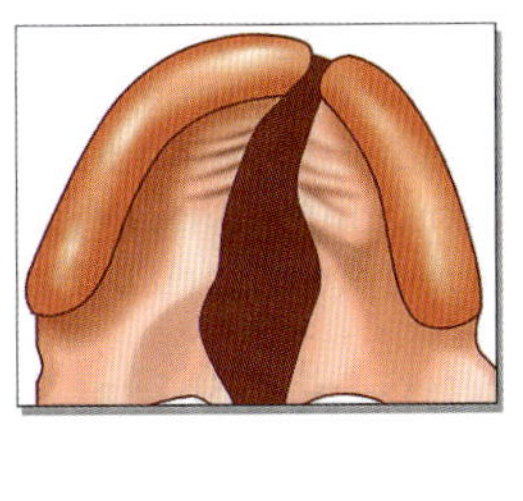

Fig. 2.19.3: Orofacial clefts—cleft lip and cleft palate.[1]

CLINICAL FEATURES

The visible birth defects are identifiable by thorough examination in the delivery room. Many others which are internal organ anomalies can be suspected at birth, based on the antenatal sonograms. Few malformations and congenital anomalies, which are not detected during the antenatal period or are not visible, may manifest with clinical symptoms in the postnatal period.

- Abnormal head size (<32 cm/too large >38 cm in full-term)
- *Gastrointestinal malformations:* Vomiting, abdominal distension and inability to pass stools
- *Cardiovascular malformations:* Failed pulse oximeter screening, shock and cyanosis
- *Neurological symptoms:* Intractable seizures, unexplained lethargy, and encephalopathy
- *Metabolic complications:* Refractory hypoglycemia and acidosis

Besides the above-presenting clinical features, if not intervened timely, many defects can also present with long-term sequelae like speech difficulty in cleft lip and palate, hearing defects in ear anomalies, limb deformities and contractures in cases of digital anomalies, lower limb paralysis in spinal cord defects, poor growth in renal anomalies, and superimposed infections in congenital skin lesions.

DIFFERENTIAL DIAGNOSIS

Unlike malformations, which may have chances of recurrence, and a graver prognosis, the deformations, disruptions, and

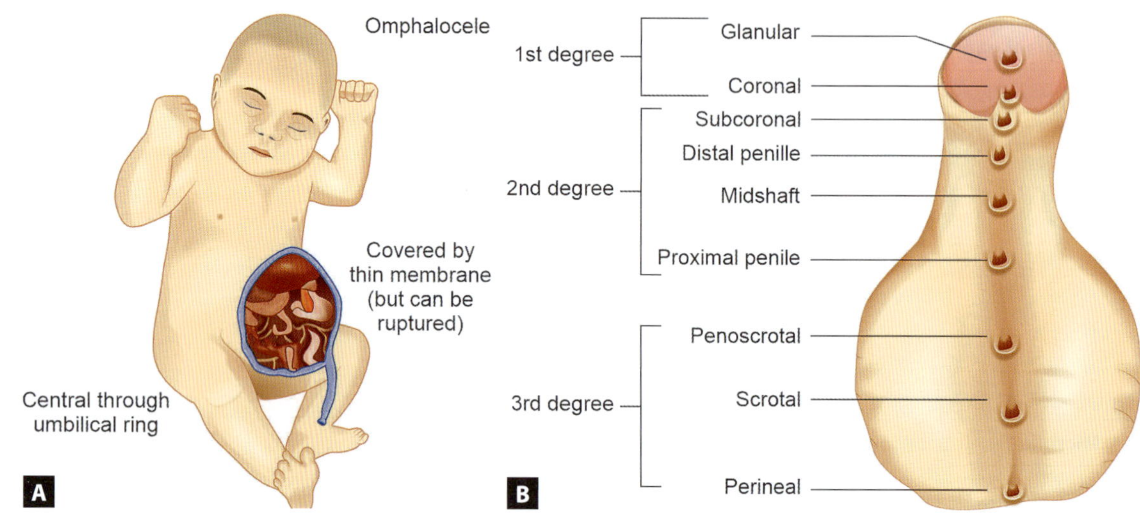

Figs. 2.19.4A and B: Genitourinary anomalies: (A) Omphalocele; (B) Hypospadias showing different sites for urethral opening.[1]

TABLE 2.19.3: Impact of maternal infections on fetus.

Viral infection	*Fetal malformation*
Cytomegalovirus	Intraventricular calcifications, microcephaly, ventriculomegaly
Rubella	• Congenital heart defects (patent ductus arteriosus, peripheral pulmonary artery stenosis, ventricular septal defects, atrial septal defects) • Auditory (sensorineural hearing impairment) • Ophthalmologic (cataracts, pigmentary retinopathy, microphthalmos, chorioretinitis) • Neurologic (microcephaly, cerebral calcifications, meningoencephalitis, behavioral disorders, mental retardation)
Toxoplasma	Intracranial calcifications, hydrocephalus, spinal cord anomalies
Varicella	Limb defects
Zika virus	Microcephaly

dysplasia may be a result of sudden and transient intrauterine events. These can sometimes present as congenital defects, and a careful evaluation is needed to differentiate these from the true congenital anomalies.

- *Deformations* are because of intrauterine mechanical forces that can alter the normally developed structure of the body. Classic examples are amniotic bands.
- *Disruptions* are defects that develop due to interference with normal development. They can be a result of vascular or mechanical processes. An example is amniotic band sequence.
- *Dysplasias* are a result of abnormal organization of cells into tissues. Examples include skeletal dysplasia.

DIAGNOSIS

Preconceptional and Antenatal Detection

A complete prenatal history and past medical and obstetric history often provide clue to the underlying etiology and exposures. A pedigree (four generations) and complete family history should be obtained. Maternal age, illnesses, and history of previous pregnancy losses and unexplained stillbirths can uncover the susceptibility of the developing fetus to anomalies. In couples with a family history of congenital defects or inherited disorders, preconceptional counseling and genetic testing can identify the specific mutations and thus aid in assessing the recurrence risk in the current pregnancy. Further, antenatal detection by noninvasive prenatal testing and sonograms can help in early identification and diagnosis of defects. This ensures that an appropriate decision is taken by the family, in cases of affected pregnancies **(Figs. 2.19.5A to C)**.

Postnatal Clinical Examination

The ideal complete postnatal examination begins with the placental and cord examination. A single umbilical artery can be associated with renal and structural heart diseases. A thorough first examination from head to toe is crucial for the identification of defects in the delivery room. A systematic approach from head to toe would minimize the chances of missing any visible defect on clinical examination **(Fig. 2.19.6)**. Additionally, complete clinical examination of the parents for any markers of inherited disorders should be done.[2,5,8,9]

Postnatal Laboratory Investigations

The laboratory tests are guided by the history and clinical examination. Targeted investigations based on clinical

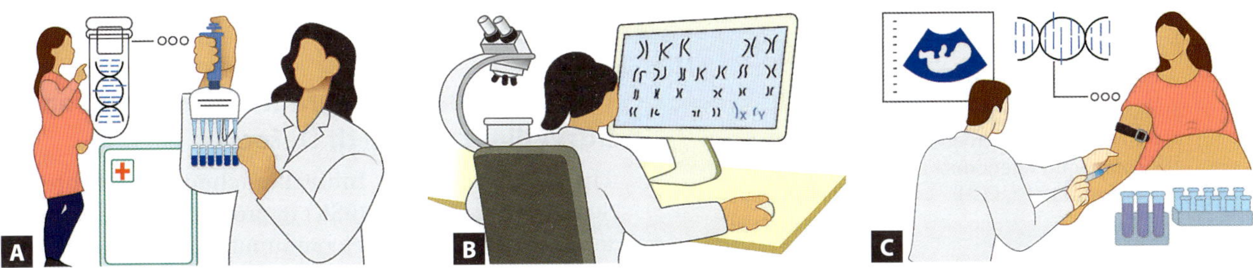

Figs. 2.19.5A to C: Diagnosis of congenital defects: (A) Preconceptional screening; (B) Testing; (C) Antenatal detection.

Mouth and oral cavity
Cleft lip, palate, high arched palate, and abnormal dentition
Tongue: Protruded tongue and macroglossia

Neck: Wide neck, short neck, and webbing of neck

Chest: Pectus excavatum, carinatum, and wide-spaced nipples
CVS: Arrythmias and deviated heartbeat (CDH)

Extremities, hands, and feet
Contractures, arthrogryposis, polydactyly, syndactyly, brachydactyly, and club foot

Head circumference, weight, and length
Head shape: Brachycephaly and plagiocephaly

Craniofacial profile
Midface hypoplasia, prognathism and asymmetry
Ears: Low set ears, shape of ear, and microtia
Eyes: Hypo- or hypertelorism, telecanthus, eso- or exotropia, and ptosis
Nose: Prominent, flat nasal bridge smooth philtrum

Spine, abdomen, and genitourinary
Spine: Tuft of hair, swelling, spina bifida, neural tube defects, and sacral dimple
Abdomen: Scaphoid abdomen, and distended abdomen
Genitourinary: Ambiguous genitalia, urethral opening, anal opening, micropenis, and cryptorchidism

Skin, hair, and nails
Light hair color (albinism), sparse hair (ectodermal dysplasias), skin pigmentation, and nail dystrophy

Fig. 2.19.6: Complete head-to-toe examination. (CDH: congenital diaphragmatic hernia; CVS: cardiovascular system)

phenotype have more yield in terms of diagnosis of precise genetic mutations **(Table 2.19.4)**. It is essential to collaborate with the geneticist to decide the most cost-effective test to identify the etiology of the particular clinical phenotype.[10,11]

MANAGEMENT

The principles of management of congenital malformations are broadly divided into the following categories:

- *Surgical:* Disorders like CDH, intestinal atresia, anorectal malformations, and tracheo-esophageal fistulas need definitive surgical management.
- *Medical (combined with surgical):* Anomalies like congenital heart diseases need preoperative, operative, and postoperative medical management for disease-free survival.
- *Multidisciplinary (special vocational and occupational therapist):* Some chromosomal disorders, neurological anomalies, and other postsurgical cases need long-term multidisciplinary management to ensure disability-free survival and improve the quality of life.
- *Prenatal counseling for next pregnancy:* It is essential that depending upon the cause and etiology and recurrence

TABLE 2.19.4: Choice of laboratory testing.

Tests	Specific modality	Remarks
Genetic testing	*Chromosome studies* Molecular-based chromosome microarray comparative genomic hybridization (aCGH)	• Identifies microdeletions • Helpful in cases of multiple anomalies and intellectual disabilities
	FISH (fluorescent in situ hybridization)	• Once aCGH detects an abnormality • Mostly for amniotic fluid samples
	Specialized metabolic genetics studies	Indicated based on clinical phenotype
	Whole exome and whole genome sequencing	Indicated in cases of multiple anomalies, intellectual disability, and/or seizures
Radiological testing	Imaging	CT/MRI brain and spine as indicated by clinical phenotype (holoprosencephaly, abnormal head shape and size, seizures, spinal defects)
	Echocardiogram	In cases of suspected congenital heart diseases

(CT: computed tomography; MRI: magnetic resonance imaging)

risk, the family is counseled appropriately for prevention, early identification, and intervention of the anomalies in net pregnancies.

PREVENTION

Individual Prevention: Early Screening and Intervention

- Appropriate vaccines should be taken regularly by adolescent females (rubella vaccine).
- Prevention and timely management of sexually transmitted diseases before conceiving
- Genetic counseling in cases of positive family history or previous pregnancies with congenital anomalies
- Avoid all possible exposure to teratogens and over-the-counter medications during the antenatal period, especially during the first trimester.

Mass Preventive Strategies

- Education and awareness programs for a nutritious diet and healthy lifestyle
- Awareness against substance abuse (alcohol and smoking)
- Promotional health activities like regular antenatal checkup

National Health Programs for Prevention and Surveillance of Birth Defects

The Government of India launched the Rashtriya Bal Swasthya Karyakram (RBSK) to provide comprehensive care to all the children in the community. This program involves screening of children from birth to 18 years of age for four "D" s—Defects at birth, Diseases, Deficiencies, and Developmental delays, spanning 32 common health conditions for early detection and free treatment and management, including surgeries at the tertiary level. The newborns are screened at the community level by health workers [Accredited Social Health Activist (ASHA)] and referred to the nearest District Early Intervention Centers (DEIC) for early intervention. All these services are provided free of cost to the families. Approximately 800 million children have benefited through 11,200 mobile health teams since 2014 under this initiative.

Another initiative in collaboration with the World Health Organization (WHO) is an online integrated newborn-birth defects [South-East Asia Region Newborn-Birth Defects Database (SEAR-NBBD)] database, to support data management for birth defects detected at birth, stillbirths, and newborns in hospital settings. The hospital staff is trained for early detection, surveillance, and reporting of birth defect data at high-load institutes across the country.

ACKNOWLEDGMENTS

Figures 2.19.1, 2.19.2, 2.19.3, and 2.19.4A and B have been accessed from reference 1 from the Centers for Disease Control and Prevention (CDC) site. The pictures are in the public domain and can be used by citing the source.

REFERENCES

1. CDC. (2024). CDC birth defects. [online] Available from https://www.cdc.gov/birth-defects/hcp/conversation-tips/resources-for-healthcare-providers.html [Last accessed October, 2024].
2. World Health Organization. (2023). Congenital disorders. [online] Available from https://www.who.int/news-room/fact-sheets/detail/birth-defects [Last accessed October, 2024].
3. Ministry of Health and Family Welfare, Government of India. Comprehensive newborn screening. Handbook for screening visible defects at all delivery points. Rashtriya Bal Swasthya Karyakram, September 2016. [online] Available from https://nhm.gov.in/images/pdf/programmes/RBSK/Resource_Documents/Birth_Defects_Handbook.pdf [Last accessed October, 2024].
4. Bellad RM, Sahni M, Venkatagiri P, Sivanandan S. Indian Academy of Pediatrics, Guidelines for Parents: Birth defects. [online] Available from https://iapindia.org/pdf/Ch-054BirthDefectsIAPParentalGuidelines.pdf [Last accessed October, 2024].

5. Graham JM, Sanchez-Lara PA. Smith's Recognizable Patterns of Human Deformation, 4th edition. Philadelphia: Elsevier; 2016.
6. Holmes LB, Westgate MN, Nasri H, Toufaily MH. Malformations attributed to the process of vascular disruption. Birth Defects Res. 2018;110(2):98-107.
7. Mai CT, Isenburg JL, Canfield MA, Meyer RE, Correa A, Alverson CJ, et al. National population-based estimates for major birth defects, 2010–2014. Birth Defects Res. 2019;111:1420-35.
8. Feldkamp ML, Carey JC, Byrne JLB, Krikov S, Botto LD. Etiology and clinical presentation of birth defects: population-based study. BMJ. 2017;357:j2249.
9. Hall J, Froster-Iskenius UG, Allanson JE. Handbook of Normal Physical Measurements, 1st edition. London: Oxford University Press; 1989.
10. Taylor CM, Smith R, Lehman C, Mitchel MW, Singer K, Weaver WC, et al. 16p11.2 recurrent microdeletion. GeneReviews. Seattle; 2015. [online] http://www.ncbi.nlm.nih.gov/books/NBK11167/ [Last accessed October, 2024).
11. McDonald-McGinn DM, Emanuel BS, Zackai EH. 22q11.2 deletion syndrome. GeneReviews. Seattle; 2013. [online] http://www.ncbi.nlm.nih.gov/books/NBK1523/ [Last accessed October, 2024].

SECTION

3 Growth

Section Editor: Anju Seth

3.1 Growth: Basic Concepts

Preeti Singh, Anju Seth

INTRODUCTION

Growth is the process of an increase in the size or mass of a living being. It occurs because of an increase in the size or number of cells, and an increase in the intracellular matrix. Growth is an integral component of childhood. It proceeds in an orderly and organized manner from the time of conception until adulthood. Normal growth represents the orderly interaction of genetic, hormonal, nutritional, and other environmental factors. Growth is also a reflection of nutritional status during childhood and an indicator of the health and well-being of an individual and populations.

Development, on the other hand, refers to maturation of function that results in acquisition of various skills for optimal functioning of the individual. It is related to maturation and myelination of nervous system. Growth and development usually proceed concurrently but may not always be inter-related.

The terms used for different phases of childhood growth are presented in **Box 3.1.1**.

BOX 3.1.1: Terms used for different age groups in a child's life.

- *Ovum:* 0–14 days
- *Embryo:*14 days to 9 weeks
- *Fetus:* 9 weeks to birth
- *Neonate:* Birth till 28 days of life
- *Infant:* Birth to 12 months of life
- *Toddler:* 1 year to 3 years of life
- *Preschooler:* 3 years to 5 years of age
- *Adolescent:* 10 years to 19 years of life

FACTORS REGULATING GROWTH

Fetal Growth

Fetal growth is the end result of a series of dynamic interactions between genetic, maternal, placental, and fetal factors **(Box 3.1.2)**. The initial 8 weeks of life in utero represent a critical phase of cell division, cell differentiation, and morphogenesis. The cells divide and differentiate to form tissues and organs. The growth of the embryo and fetus is mediated through various locally synthesized growth factors such as placental insulin-like growth factors-1 and 2 (IGF-1 and IGF-2), epidermal growth factor, nerve growth factor, fibroblast growth factor (FGF), transforming growth factor-beta, and platelet derived growth factor.[1] The primary determinant is IGF-1, which is regulated by human placental lactogen and insulin. The structural and functional integrity of the placenta facilitates nutrient transport across the placenta to the growing fetus. Factors such as growth hormone (GH), thyroid and sex hormones that are important for postnatal growth, have only a limited role in fetal growth.

Maternal health and nutrition play an important role in determining fetal growth. Mother's own childhood growth and her nutrient intake and body composition at the time of conception and during pregnancy, play an important role in determining fetal size. Teenage or advanced age at conception, high parity, undernutrition, and anemia negatively influence fetal size and health. Maternal intake of tobacco (smoked or chewed) and drug or alcohol abuse also retard fetal growth. Chronic maternal illnesses (such as diabetes mellitus, cardiovascular disease, hypertension, homozygous sickle hemoglobinopathy, and thrombophilia) or obstetric complications such as preeclampsia, smoking, alcohol can adversely affect fetal growth. Zinc and vitamin B_{12} deficiency in mothers can also result in fetal and early

BOX 3.1.2: Determinants of fetal growth.

- *Fetal:* Genetic and chromosomal defects (e.g., trisomy 13, 18, and 21; Turner syndrome), syndromic defects (e.g., Beckwith–Wiedemann, Seckel, and Russell–Silver syndromes)
- *Intrauterine infection:* Rubella, cytomegalovirus (CMV), herpes simplex virus (HSV), HIV, syphilis, and toxoplasmosis
- *Maternal health and nutrition:* Age, ethnicity, parity, preconception weight, nutrition, and weight gain during pregnancy; chronic diseases such as diabetes mellitus, cardiovascular disease, and obstetric complications such as preeclampsia and antepartum hemorrhage
- *Drug:* Alcohol, smoking, heroin, lysergic acid diethylamide (LSD), antibiotics such as streptomycin and tetracycline, anticonvulsants, and psychotropics
- *Ionizing radiations and heavy metals:* Lead, cadmium, manganese, mercury, and bisphenol A
- *Psychological and social factors:* Healthcare availability or utilization, stress, and social factors (educational status, family size, and financial condition)
- *Environmental:* Altitude and air pollution
- *Placental:* Defective placentation, chorioangiomas, IGF-1 and 2, IGFBPs, and IGF receptors

(IGF: insulin-like growth factor; IGFBPs: insulin-like growth factor-binding proteins)

infantile growth failure. On the contrary, excessive gestational weight gain is associated with increased risk of overweight and obesity during the latter part of childhood. Folic acid plays a critical role in fetal growth and development.[2] Maternal periconceptional folic acid supplementation prevents neural tube defects and decreases the risk of low birth weight and small for gestational age in the offspring.[3]

Fetal organs and tissues are extremely sensitive to teratogens, the environmental agents that impair the fetal growth and development. The exposure to teratogens during this critical period of organogenesis can result in malformations and/or functional disturbances in varying severity depending on the timing and the dose of teratogen.

Postnatal Growth

The infancy-childhood-puberty (ICP) growth model, proposed by Karlberg, divides postnatal growth into three successive and partly overlapping phases—infancy, childhood, and puberty—reflecting the major determinants of the growth process.[4] The infancy phase of the ICP model has been assumed to begin mid-gestation and tails off at approximately 3–4 years of age, representing the postnatal extension of fetal growth. It is primarily nutrition dependent, closely linked to the action of IGFs. Childhood phase of growth begins between 6 and 15 months of age. This phase is predominantly regulated by the GH–IGF-1 axis and thyroid hormones in combination with nutrition. The growth in this phase is influenced by gender, prior length/growth velocity, socioeconomic factors, systemic disease, and serum IGF-1 level. Puberty is the final phase of growth which is regulated mainly by sex hormones along with GH and thyroid hormone. However, the final height of an individual also depends on his/her genetic potential.

Growth in children and adolescents is a dynamic process that is determined by the interaction of several genetic and environmental factors. An understanding of the factors that affect growth will allow us to timely identify growth faltering and intervene. The factors affecting growth in children are summarized further **(Fig. 3.1.1)**.

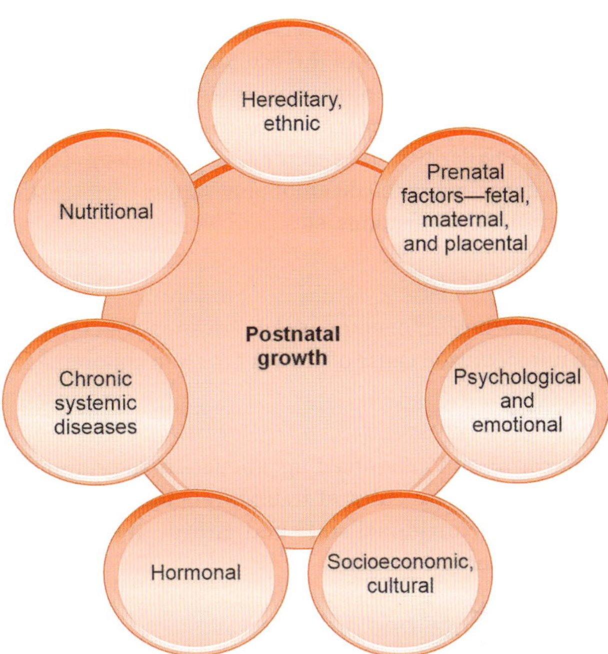

Fig. 3.1.1: Factors affecting postnatal growth in children.

Heredity and Genetics

The genetic potential of a child's linear growth is determined by the mid-parental height (MPH), which is calculated by the average of parental height corrected for sex. The age of onset of puberty is sex dependent and influenced by the genetic factors; for example, girls attain menarche at a similar age as their mothers. At the tissue level, cell growth and proliferation is determined by numerous genes and growth/transcription factors.[5] Aberrations and mutation in genes coding these pathways can also affect the child's growth. Chromosomal abnormalities can result in distinct syndromes that can be associated with growth abnormalities, e.g., Down syndrome and Turner syndrome. However, the ability of a child to achieve his or her optimum genetic potential depends on the availability of a conducive environment and nutrition.

Gender

During puberty, the growth spurt occurs earlier in girls than boys. However, the height and weight in girls are usually less than those in boys of corresponding ages and same genetic potential.

Ethnicity and Race

It was earlier thought that different ethnic groups show different patterns of growth, beginning from birth. However, the recent World Health Organization (WHO) led multicenter growth reference study demonstrated that the effect of ethnicity is minimal if the environmental and socioeconomic conditions are similar; particularly under 5 years of age. Ethnicity influences the growth during the later part of childhood and adolescence resulting in different adult size and body proportions, e.g., Chinese population groups are considered to be lighter and shorter compared to Caucasians and African Caribbean groups who are taller and heavier.[6] Population groups from African and Australian origin have the longest leg length for a given height, and Asians the shortest.

Socioeconomic Factors

The growth of a child is influenced by the socioeconomic class of the family, and the environmental conditions under which child has been reared. The educational status of parents, family size, and the economic conditions of the family determine the nurturing environment and child-rearing practices. They influence food security, feeding practices, regularity in meal timing, sleep hygiene, physical activity, capacity to provide emotional support during stress, predisposition to infections, etc.

Emotional Factors

Child abuse/neglect or emotional deprivation is an important often unrecognized cause of growth failure in children.

Cultural Factors

Child-rearing and infant-feeding practices in the community are determined by cultural habits, religious beliefs, and conventions. Nutritional state and growth of children are variably influenced by them.

Season, Climate, and Altitude

Season and climate influence the growth of children, attributed to the changes in hormone secretion.[5] At high altitudes, the growth of children gets affected due to numerous biochemical, physiological, and microanatomical changes in response to low partial pressure of oxygen. Mothers living at high altitude give birth to newborns with low birth weight due to relative intrauterine hypoxemia.

Nutrition

Nutrition exerts its effects on growth throughout childhood. The energy and nutrient requirements for infants, toddlers, preschool, and school-age children varies with age, sex, physiological state of health, and the degree of physical activity. Poor nutrition in infants and children has immediate consequences on systemic health, growth, and puberty and can lead to long-term and even intergenerational effects on reproduction, cognition, and overall well-being. Undernutrition is an important cause of stunting and wasting in children under 5 years of age. Micronutrient deficiency in children and adolescents can result in anemia, short stature, and even delayed puberty. On the other hand, overweight/obesity in children can accelerate somatic growth and lead to poor health outcomes such as hypertension, dyslipidemia, type 2 diabetes and steatohepatitis. A balanced diet that is a blend of diverse food groups to provide sufficient energy, protein, fats, micronutrients, and vitamins in adequate proportions promotes optimal growth and development.

Chronic Systemic Diseases

Growth failure is one of the earliest manifestation of chronic systemic diseases. It is secondary to an interplay of multiple factors that disturbs the balance between nutrient requirement, intake, absorption, and utilization:

- *Poor intake* (mechanical feeding problems, pain, and anorexia)
- *Poor absorption* (celiac disease, cystic fibrosis, hepatobiliary disease, enzymatic deficiencies, inflammatory bowel disease, bacterial gastroenteritis, and short bowel syndrome)
- *Increased demand* [in chronic infections viz. tuberculosis/HIV/urinary tract infections (UTIs), malignancy, chronic anemia, congenital heart diseases, interstitial lung disease, bronchopulmonary dysplasia, hyperthyroidism, and hyperaldosteronism] and
- *Poor utilization of calories* (chronic vomiting, pyloric stenosis, genetic trisomies, congenital infections, inborn errors of metabolism, renal tubular acidosis, chronic kidney disease, and chronic hypoxemia)

In most cases, more than one mechanism is responsible for growth failure. In systemic disorders, weight is more severely affected than height. In long-standing disorders, this leads to a low height velocity, ultimately leading to short stature. Serial growth monitoring with plotting of anthropometric parameters on appropriate growth chart can help in early identification of underlying disorder.

Hormones

Growth hormone and IGF-1 are the primary hormonal regulators of postnatal linear growth. GH promotes growth both directly as well as through the production of IGF-1. At the growth plate, GH stimulates the differentiation of undifferentiated cells into chondrocytes, whereas IGF-1 activates their clonal proliferation. Thyroxine (and via its conversion to triiodothyronine, T3) stimulates bone growth by its direct action on the growth plate as well as through its GH mediated IGF-1 synthesis, secretion, and action. During adolescence, the pubertal growth spurt is mediated by estrogen and androgen through their direct action on the growth plate and permissive effect on GH pulse and the amplitude. Adrenal glucocorticoids are essential for normal growth as it regulates the metabolism, salt and water homeostasis, and optimize the functioning of other organ systems.

Minor Growth Factors

Somatic growth is regulated by various peptides and their receptors, e.g., FGF and their receptors. Mutations in *FGFR3* and *FGFR2* genes cause achondroplasia and craniosynostosis, respectively. Specific tissue growth is promoted by certain peptides such as hepatocyte growth factor, endothelin, and nerve growth factor.

Secular Trend

Secular trend represents an upward shift in the height of successive generations by 1–2 cm per decade and early age of onset of puberty. This phenomena has been observed as a result of good nutrition and optimal environmental conditions for children to achieve their genetic potential. Further, in response to improved nutrition and under the effect of various environmental endocrine disruptors, children are now experiencing early puberty.[7]

IMPACT OF EARLY CHILDHOOD GROWTH TRAJECTORY ON LONG-TERM HEALTH OUTCOMES

The first year of life is characterized by rapid physical growth, development, and maturation. Malnutrition in infants under 6 months may result from multiple factors such as low birth weight, preterm birth, small for gestational age, suboptimal feeding practices, poor maternal nutrition, maternal illness, adverse maternal psychosocial status, and lack of responsive care. Early growth failure among infants can result in wasting, stunting, and is an important determinant of infant and under-5 mortality. Malnourished infants have higher risk of infections and impaired motor, cognitive, and psychosocial development. This reiterates the importance of optimizing health and nutrition in first 1,000 days (fetal and postnatal period up to 2 years age) of life to prevent adverse health outcomes later. On the other hand, rapid weight gain and obesity during infancy is associated with higher risk of overweight and/or obesity later in childhood and adolescence. Term small for gestational age subjects who have greater catch up growth in the first 2 years have an increased body fat mass and more central fat compared to children born appropriate for gestational age. Low birth weight and intrauterine growth restriction predisposes infants to noncommunicable diseases such as hypertension, type 2 diabetes, dyslipidemias, and poor cardiovascular health in adulthood. Preconceptional maternal health and nutrition has a vital role in influencing the growth and development of fetus, infant, and child across the life course, through genetic and epigenetic programming.

REFERENCES

1. Moore KL, Persaud TVN, Torchia MG (Eds). The Developing Human: Clinically Oriented Embryology, 10th edition. Philadelphia, PA: Saunders; 2015.
2. Hofman P, Mathai S, Cutfield W. Intrauterine programming, and metabolic consequences of children born preterm and small for gestational age. In: Desai M, Menon PSN, Bhatia V, Seth A (Eds). Pediatric Endocrine Disorders, 4th edition. Hyderabad: Orient Black Swan Publishers (P) Ltd.; 2022.
3. Jonker H, Capelle N, Lanes A, Wen SW, Walker M, Corsi DJ. Maternal folic acid supplementation and infant birthweight in low- and middle-income countries: A systematic review. Matern Child Nutr. 2020;16(1):e12895.
4. Benyi E, Sävendahl L. The physiology of childhood growth: Hormonal Regulation. Horm Res Paediatr. 2017;88(1):6-14.
5. Lewis R. Human genetics: Concepts and Applications, 9th edition. New York, NY: McGraw Hill; 2009.
6. Bharati S, Mukherji D, Pal M, Som S, Adak DK, Vasulu TS, et al. Influence of ethnicity, geography and climate on the variation of stature among Indian populations. Coll Antropol. 2010;34:1207-13.
7. Robert M. Secular trends in growth, maturation, and physical performance: A review. Anthropol Rev. 2004;67:3-31.

3.2 Growth during Infancy, Childhood, and Adolescence

M Vijayakumar

INTRODUCTION

Despite being influenced by many factors, normal childhood growth follows a typical pattern. Thus, even though growth pattern of every individual is unique; deviation from the expected pattern of growth may be the first warning sign of an underlying illness. Healthcare workers should be aware of the normal growth patterns in children and know how to identify the deviation from the normal. This will help to plan effective intervention before the changes become irreversible.

GROWTH DURING INTRAUTERINE PERIOD

Growth starts from intrauterine period itself. Many factors affect in utero growth, and continue to affect it during infancy and childhood. A healthy intrauterine milieu is essential for optimal growth in infancy and childhood.[1]

By the end of first week of gestation, implantation of the fertilized ovum occurs, and this event marks the beginning of embryonic period (blastocyst). By the second week, the embryo has two layers, ectoderm and endoderm (bilaminar embryo), and by third week, the mesoderm appears (trilaminar embryo). This is the time usually the mother will come to know about her missed menstrual cycle. From the fourth week onward fusion of neural folds, folding of embryo and development of organs begins. By the end of embryonic period (8 weeks) all the major organ systems are developed.[2]

Fetal period begins from the ninth week onward. During this period, rapid body growth occurs along with differentiation of various organs and other tissues. Organs start functioning and the glands secrete hormones and other secretions. During third trimester (25 weeks onward), the body starts storing proteins, fat, iron, calcium, and vitamins. During this period, weight and length rise exponentially. By the end of 37th week onward baby is termed as "full term".[2]

Though fetal life is the period of maximum growth, the organs and others structures (e.g., brain) continue to grow after birth.

During the earlier part of fetal period, increase in cell number occurs, whereas in later part (after 32 weeks of gestation) increase in cell size becomes prominent.[3]

PHASES OF GROWTH

Growth can be divided into four major phases: (1) Fetal, (2) infantile, (3) childhood, and (4) adolescence **(Table 3.2.1)**. Growth rate varies in each phase and contributing factors are different. Final adult growth parameters (height, weight, and head circumference) will be affected, if growth is restricted in any one these phases. This underscores the importance of early identification of growth faltering in each period.[4]

Fetal Period

Fetal period is the fastest phase of growth, and children with intrauterine growth restriction (IUGR) have a long period of growth impairment. If the cause of IUGR is maternal malnutrition or systemic illnesses, child may catch up her/his growth finally, but if the cause is due to fetal problems (chromosomal anomalies or intrauterine infections), child may be growth restricted in the later life too.[1]

Neonatal Period

Neonatal period comprises the first 28 days after birth. A neonate loses 10% of its birth weight following vaginal delivery and 12% after cesarean delivery during the initial days following birth. This is due to loss of extravascular fluid and limited nutrition. As the colostrum is replaced by breastmilk with higher fat content, and the baby has learnt the correct way of latching and sucking, the lost birth weight is regained. This happens by 10th day of life in a full-term baby, while a preterm baby takes 14–15 days for the same. Subsequently, the neonate puts on approximately 30 g of weight per day. Head circumference of a full term neonate is 1–2 cm, more than chest circumference.[3]

TABLE 3.2.1: Different age groups—nomenclature.[2]

Neonate	Birth to 28 days
Infant	Birth to 12 completed months of age
Toddler	1–2 years
Preschool	3–5 years
School age	6–9 years
Adolescent age	10–19 years

Infancy

The infant grows rapidly during infancy, though the growth rate declines during its later part. Thus, the baby increases his or her weight by 30 g/day during the first 3 months, about 20 g/day in next 3 months, 12 g/day in next 3 months, and 8–10 g/day in the last 3 months of infancy. By the age of 4 months, birthweight is doubled and by the end of first year, it is tripled **(Table 3.2.2)**.

The gain in length also shows a similar pattern. The average birth length of a neonate is 50 cm. It increases by 3.5 cm/month in the first 3 months, 2 cm/month in the next 3 months, 1.5 cm in the next 3 months, and 1.2 cm in the final months of infancy. The length is approximately 75 cm by the end of infancy **(Table 3.2.2)**.[1]

Head circumference indirectly denotes the brain growth of the child. At birth, the head circumference is 33-35 cm. It increases by 2 cm/month for the first 3 months, 1 cm/month for the next 3 months, and 0.5 cm/month for the last 6 months. The head circumference reaches 45 cm by the age of 1 year. By this time, the chest circumference exceeds the head circumference **(Table 3.2.2)**.[3]

Children born small for gestational age (SGA) usually show "catch up" growth and cross the growth percentiles upward during first 2–3 years of life. On the other hand, those born large for gestational age (e.g., infant of diabetic mother) demonstrate a slower growth rate during this period—they "catch down" to their genetic potential. Infants with congenital

TABLE 3.2.2: Growth in various parameters during childhood.[3]

Age	*Weight increment*	*Height increment (cm/month)*	*Head circumference increment (cm/month)*
0–3 months	30 g/day	3.5	2.0
4–6 months	20 g/day	2.0	1.0
7–9 months	0.5 kg/month	1.5	0.5
10–12 months	0.5 kg/month	1.2	0.5
1–3 years	2 kg/year	1.0	0.25
4–6 years	2 kg/year	5 cm/year	1 cm/year

anomalies (congenital heart diseases, malabsorption, and liver diseases) and genetic diseases (Turner syndrome and Down syndrome) also show slowing of growth even though their birth weight may be normal and they receive an optimal nutrition.[4]

The most important factor affecting growth during infancy is nutrition. Both macronutrient (protein, fat, and carbohydrate) and micronutrient (vitamins and minerals) deficiencies affect growth. Excessive weight gain during infancy is likely to be associated with overweight and obesity, and insufficient weight gain with underweight later in childhood.[1]

Toddler Age Group (1–2 Years)

After first year, rate of growth continues to slow down, weight gain during this period is 2–3 kg only. Increment in length also slows down, gaining about 10 cm in second year. Head circumferences increases by 2–3 cm. By 2 years, children achieve half of their adult height and 90% of adult head circumference. They start walking, initially toddle with a wide-based gait, hence the name toddler. They have a mild physiological bow leg and lordosis. The growth potentials will correspond to genetic trend by the end of 2 years as a result of continuing of catch up or catch down of growth as mentioned earlier. Height Z-score correlates with height of parents by the end of this period. Their physical activity increases and appetite decreases during this period, often causing concern in the parents **(Table 3.2.2)**.[1]

Preschool Years (3–5 Years)

The growth velocity further slows down. Weight increment of 2–3 kg/year and height increment of 6–7 cm/year is expected during this period. Head circumference increases much slowly. A higher weight increment during this time (referred to as "adiposity rebound") is seen to be associated with overweight/obesity later in childhood/adolescence **(Table 3.2.2)**. Mild genu valgus (knock knee) and pes planus (flat foot) are expected during this period. Both macro- and micronutrient intake should be ensured in this age group since protein-energy malnutrition (PEM) and micronutrient deficiencies (iron deficiency anemia, rickets, and vitamin A deficiency) are very common in this period.[1-3]

School Years (5–9 Years)

During this time, the linear growth velocity is stable at around 5–6 cm/year and the weight increases by 2 kg/year. The head circumference increases by 2 cm during the entire period since most of the brain growth is completed during first 3 years of life.

Growth in the childhood phase is usually slow and steady. Hormones such as growth hormone (GH) and thyroid hormones have tremendous influence on linear growth during this period. Deficiency of these hormones will become clinically apparent during this period. This will manifest as down-crossing of child's growth trajectory toward lower centiles.

A slight reduction of growth velocity, observed more prominently in boys, occurs toward the end of this phase, immediately before the pubertal growth spurt commences.[1-3]

Growth and Development during Pubertal Period (10–19 years)

Puberty is a period of transition from childhood to adulthood. During this period, tremendous changes occur in the physical, physiological, psychological, and social domains. These changes are primarily caused by alterations in the hormonal milieu and modified by environmental factors. This period of development, named as adolescence, is divided into three phases, namely early, mid, and late adolescence. These changes usually follow a common pattern, but with individual variations.

Three major physical changes happening in puberty are advancement in height velocity, alterations in body shape, and development of sexual organs with attainment of reproductive capacity. The onset of puberty coincides with maturation of hypothalamic–pituitary–gonadal (HPG) axis. With the activation of gonadotropin-releasing hormone (GnRH) pulse generator from hypothalamus, pituitary gland secretes luteinizing hormone (LH) and follicle-stimulating hormone (FSH), which in turn stimulate the secretion of gonadal sex steroids (testosterone and estrogen). Almost during the same time, adrenal glands start producing increasing amount of androgens, mainly dehydroepiandrosterone sulfate (DHEAS), which results in pubic hair development and under-arm odor.

Pubertal growth spurt is controlled by sex hormones (testosterone and estrogen). They act by their direct effect on growth plate and indirectly by their influence on GH secretion. The sex hormones, particularly estrogen, lead to acceleration of pulsatile secretion of GH. There is increased secretion of insulin-like growth factor-1 (IGF-1) from liver and chondrocytes, resulting in enhanced growth at epiphyseal plate. Finally, epiphyseal maturation occurs resulting eventually in bony fusion and attainment of adult stature.

Development of Secondary Sexual Characters

Tanner GM in 1962 described the progression of pubertal development in five stages known as sexual maturity rating (SMR) stages or Tanner stages. Stage 1 denotes prepuberty. Stage 2 denotes the initial changes in puberty. Stage 5 represents complete maturation or an adult pattern of development.[5]

In boys, the first sign of puberty and hence the beginning of SMR 2 is increase in testicular size measured as longitudinal measurement 2.5 cm or more or testicular volume 4 mL or more (measured by Prader's orchidometer) (**Fig. 3.2.1 and Table 3.2.3**). The testicular volume progressively increases during subsequent stages, owing to the enlargement of seminiferous tubules, epididymis, and seminal vesicles. Development of pubic hair soon follows during the same period (SMR 2). Enlargement and maturation of penis also begins during this stage and is also under the control of adrenal androgens. Sperm production, leading to nocturnal emission, happens in SMR 3. First conscious ejaculation occurs at the mean age of 13.5 years. Mild breast enlargement (gynecomastia) occurring in early pubertal period as a result of relative excess production of estrogen in some boys create anxiety in these children. Breast size decreases as puberty advances.[5,6]

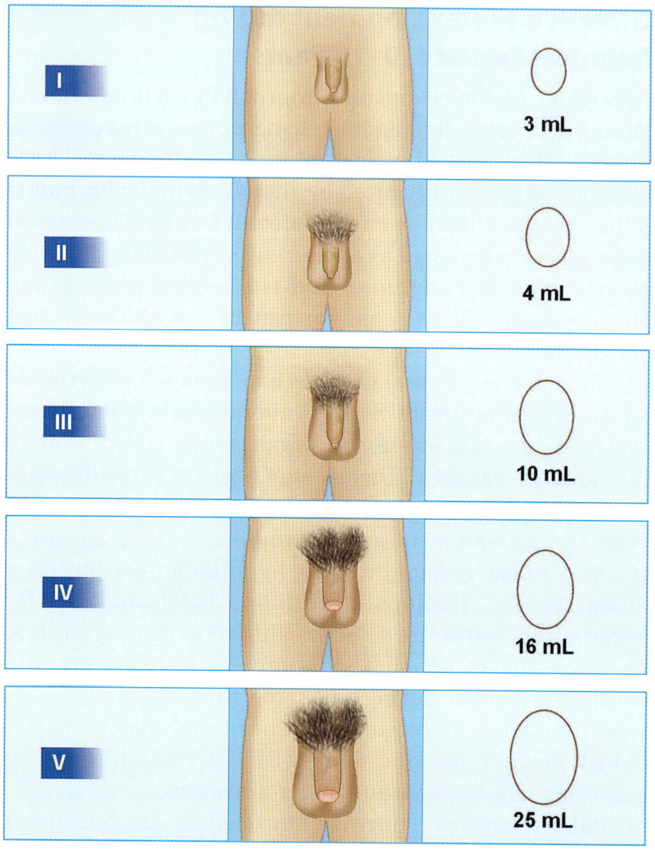

Fig. 3.2.1: Sexual maturity rating in boys.

In girls, the first sign of puberty is the appearance of breast bud (thelarche) **(Fig. 3.2.2 and Table 3.2.4)**. This denotes the beginning of SMR 2, which usually occurs around 8–9 years of age and is closely followed by appearance of pubic hair (pubarche). Internal genital organs also start developing from this period. Clear vaginal discharge (physiological leucorrhea) and change of color of vaginal mucosa (from bright red to pale pink) due to estrogenic effect, happens before menarche. Vaginal pH decreases near menarche, due to increase in lactic acid secreted by lactobacilli in the vaginal mucosa. Ovaries show multicystic appearance (more than six follicles with each one having at least 4 mm diameter) under the effect of pulsatile gonadotropins. Uterus grows in size from 2–3 cm in the pubertal age to 5–8 cm and changes its contour from tubular to a pear like structure by late puberty and is under the influence of estradiol, progesterone, GH, and IGF-1. Menarche appear 2½ to 3 years after thelarche, at SMR stage 3 or 4, usually around 12–13 years of age. Initial menstrual cycles are often irregular, and typically anovulatory. Many parameters influence pubertal development in girls which include genetic, nutritional and psychogenic factors. Increased adiposity favors early puberty and poor nutritional status leads to delayed pubertal changes. There is a secular trend toward early puberty, probably due to better nutritional status.[5-7]

Physical Development

Linear growth velocity accelerates during puberty, which contributes almost 20% of adult height. Peak height

TABLE 3.2.3: Sexual maturity rating (SMR) or Tanner staging in boys.

Pubertal stage	*Genital development (G)*	*Pubic hair development (P)*	*Axillary hair development (A)*
1	Prepubertal	Nil	Nil
2	• Testes size ≥4 mL in volume or ≥2.5 cm length • Early penile growth • Scrotal skin thin and pink	Minimally pigmented hair on base of penis	Few axillary hair
3	• Testes enlarge to 10–15 mL in volume or ≥3.3–4 cm length • Penis grows in length • Scrotal thickening and pigmentation	Darker, coarser, and curled hair extending to mons pubis	Adult pattern
4	• Testes enlarge to 15–20 mL in volume or ≥4–4.5 cm length • Penis grows in breadth; glans increases in size	Thicker adult pattern of hair not yet extending to medial surface of thighs	
5	Adult genitalia; testes 25 mL in volume or >4.5 cm length	Adult distribution spreading to medial side of thighs	

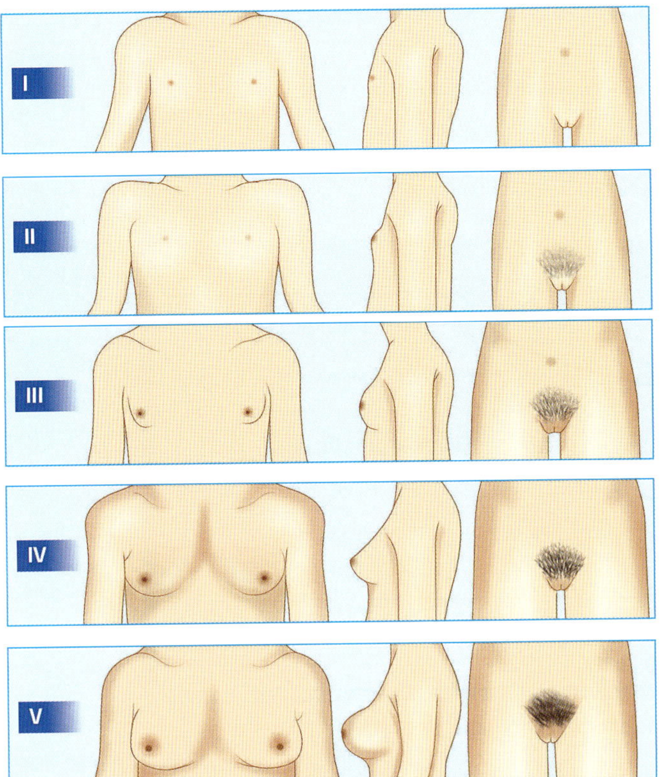

Fig. 3.2.2: Sexual maturity rating in girls.

TABLE 3.2.4: Sexual maturity rating (SMR) or Tanner staging in girls.

Pubertal stage	Breast development (B)	Pubic hair development (P)	Axillary hair development (A)
1	Prepubertal	Nil	Nil
2	Appearance of breast buds and slight areolar enlargement	Minimally pigmented hair on labia	Few axillary hair
3	Further enlargement of breast and areola	Darker, coarser, and curled hair extending to mons pubis	Adult pattern
4	Areola and nipple (papilla) form a secondary mound above the level of the breast	Thicker but not yet adult pattern	
5	Areola part of breast contour, projection of nipple only	Adult distribution extending to medial surface of thighs	

velocity (PHV) appears early in girls (SMR stages 2–3) and is about 8–9 cm/year. Increment in height after onset of menarche is only 7–8 cm.[5]

In boys, PHV starts later (SMR stages 3–4) and is about 9–10 cm/year. Boys continue their growth spurt for 2–3 years more, compared to girls. Growth spurt begins at extremities and gradually involve trunk and chest, producing a eunuchoid appearance during early puberty. In boys, lean body mass and in girls, adiposity increases toward later stages. Deposition of calcium (bone mineral accrual) and increase in bone mineral density during this period give better strength to the bones, and lack of bone mineral accrual in this period produces early osteoporosis.[5,6]

Development of sebaceous and sweat glands results in typical body odor and acne. Maturation of larynx, pharynx, and lungs produce voice changes in male (voice cracking), which occurs at around the age of 13 years and typical adult voice at 15 years. Enlargement of larynx, cricothyroid cartilage, and laryngeal muscles lead to the development of a prominence in the neck called as Adam's apple.[6,7]

In boys, facial hair first appears on the corners of upper lip during pubic hair stage 3 (14–15 years). Typical adult pattern of facial hair is attained by around SMR stage 5. Axillary hair develops by 12 years in girls and 14 years in boys. Altered sleep patterns produce delay in sleep onset at night and late awakenings in the morning.[5,6]

Early development of secondary sexual characters before 8 years in girls (thelarche) and 9 years in boys (increased testicular volume) is called precocious puberty. Delayed development of secondary sexual characters after 13 years in girls and 14 years in boys is called delayed puberty. Absence of menarche after 16 years is defined as late (primary amenorrhea).[6,7]

GROWTH PATTERNS OF DIFFERENT ORGANS

Somatic Growth

As discussed above, somatic growth (both weight and height) follows an "S"-shaped curve during childhood. Growth is maximum in intrauterine period, gradually decelerates during childhood and exponentially increases during pubertal period.[1,3]

Brain Growth

Brain growth is maximum during fetal life and infancy. At birth head size is 70% of that in adult life and at 2 years almost 90%. Brain growth slows down during childhood, but many areas will mature gradually and further differentiation (acquiring cognitive ability) occurs during this period also (**Fig. 3.2.3**).[1,2]

Gonadal Growth

Gonadal development occurs in utero. But it remains dormant during childhood. During adolescent period

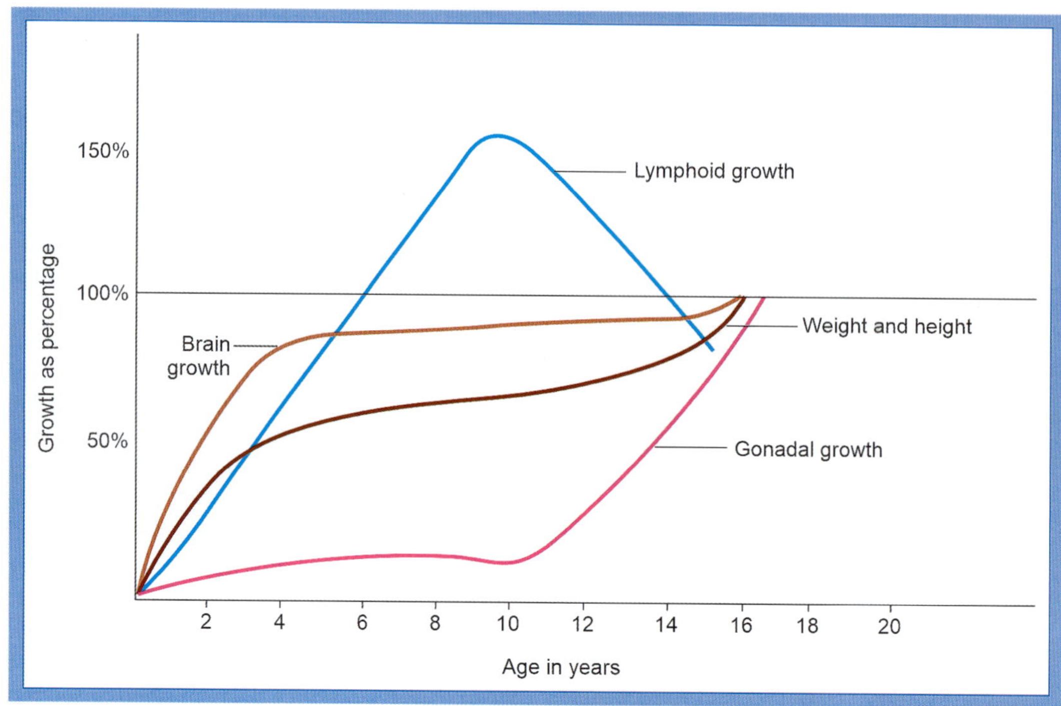

Fig. 3.2.3: Growth patterns of different organs.

further development of gonads and their function occur. The reproductive capacity begins during this phase and becomes fully mature by the end of the adolescent period **(Fig. 3.2.3)**.

Lymphoid Growth

Lymphoid tissue overgrows during childhood, and is often noted as enlarged tonsils and lymph nodes during preadolescent years (8–10 years); thereafter, their growth decelerates during puberty (**Fig. 3.2.3**).[2,3]

INFANT–CHILDHOOD–PUBERTY MODEL

The concept of infant-childhood-puberty (ICP) model of growth was put forward by Karlberg et al. According to this model, growth is the summative function of various biological processes. Rapid growth in first 2–3 years (infancy phase) is primarily nutrition dependent. Second phase, called as childhood phase, is mainly hormone dependent. Both GH and thyroid hormones play a vital role during this period. The third phase of growth is during puberty where sex hormones have a great effect on final growth spurt along with GH. Magnitude of growth spurt in adolescents is inversely related to age at PHV.[1,8]

GROWTH VELOCITY

Assessment of growth parameters over a period of time, thus enabling assessment of growth velocity (height gain per year, calculated from serial height records over a period of at least 4–6 months) yields a better idea of a child's growth compared to interpreting growth parameters at a single point. This is based on the fact that growth increment occurs in a pulsatile manner. Height velocity is higher in initial years but gradually decreases and reaches a nadir just before puberty. Height velocity increases during pubertal growth spurt reaching as high as 9 cm/year in girls and 10 cm/year in boys. A child should be evaluated for short stature if height velocity is <25th centile and for precocious puberty if height velocity is >75th percentile.[3,4]

BODY PROPORTIONS

Different parts of body grow at different paces as growth advances. The upper part of body (from highest point of head to upper end of pubic symphysis) is larger in a neonate compared to lower part (from pubic symphysis to legs), resulting in upper segment to lower segment ratio of 1.7:1. As age advances, the rate of growth of extremities is more, resulting in gradual reduction of upper segment to lower segment ratio. The ratio is 1.6:1 at 6 months and 1.5:1 at 1 year. Thereafter the ratio decreases further and reaches 1:1 at 7–10 years. During adolescent growth spurt, the ratio decreases to 0.9:1 before stabilizing. Assessment of body proportions is important in evaluation of short stature, to assess whether the abnormal stature is proportionate or disproportionate.[2,3]

Like-wise, arm span is less than the length in a neonate by about 2.5 cm, but as the age advances, it grows at a faster pace than the trunk. By the age of 10–11 years, arm span equalizes with height and thereafter exceeds height during adulthood by 5 cm in males and 2 cm in females. Pubertal growth spurt starts at distal parts of extremities (hands and feet) followed by arms and legs. Trunk and chest are involved last. This process gives a eunuchoid appearance to the body during early puberty.[1]

Body composition also alters as a child grows. In boys, lean body mass (that includes muscles, skeleton, and internal organs) increases in later adolescence, whereas in girls, higher proportion of fat accumulation occurs mainly around breasts, buttocks, and thighs.[1]

SKELETAL GROWTH AND MATURATION

Skeletal growth begins during the intrauterine period. Most of the primary centers of bones are well developed into diaphysis by 13 weeks of intrauterine period. By 6 months in utero, epiphyses of calcaneus and talus appear. By 38 weeks, distal femoral epiphysis and by 40th week, cuboid and proximal femoral epiphysis develop. After birth, diaphysis and epiphysis gradually mature and by the end of pubertal period, epiphysis fuses with diaphysis. Skeletal growth ceases thereafter. Fusion of growth plate to diaphysis occurs by 17–18 years in girls and 20–22 years in boys. Bone mineral accrual is maximum during this period. Estrogen is the prime hormone influencing epiphyseal fusion. By assessing the appearance and degree of maturation of bones, skeletal age can be assessed. Usually, an X-ray of the left hand (including distal end of radius and ulna, carpal bones, metacarpals, and phalanges) is used to assess bone age. Various methods such as Greulich and Pyle atlas and Tanner Whitehouse method are used to assess bone age in children.[3,8]

DENTAL MATURATION

Eruption of deciduous teeth begins by the age of 6 months and completed by 2½ years. Usually, teeth in the upper jaw erupts earlier than lower jaw, except central incisors and second molar. Central incisors are usually the first teeth to erupt (7 months) followed by lateral incisors (8 months). First molar erupts in the first half of second year (12–18 months) and canines in the second half (18–20 months). Second molars are the last teeth to erupt, and this occurs 21–30 months. By the end of 2½ years, all 20 primary teeth erupt.[3,8]

Permanent dentition eruption starts at 6 years of age. First molar is the first permanent dentition to erupt (6 years). This is closely followed by eruption of central incisors (7–8 years), lateral incisors (8–9 years), canines, first and second premolars (10–12 years), second molars (12–13 years), and third molars (17–21 years). The period by which first permanent molar erupts distal to second deciduous molars to the shedding down of all deciduous teeth is called mixed dentition period.[1,3]

REFERENCES

1. Carter RG, Feigelman S. Growth, Development and behavior. In: Kliegman RM, St Geme JW, Blum NJ, Shah SS, Tasker RC, Wilson KM (Eds). Nelson Text Book of Pediatrics, 21st edition. Philadelphia: Elsevier; 2020. pp. 1074-81.
2. Agarwal R, Sankhyan N, Jain V. Growth. In: Paul V, Bagga A (Eds) Ghai Essential Pediatrics, 9th edition. New Delhi: CBS Publishers & Distributors; 2019. pp. 7-37.
3. Mishra R, Jain V. Normal growth. In: Gupta P, Menon PSN, Ramji S, Lodha R (Eds). PG Textbook of Pediatrics, 3rd edition. New Delhi: Jaypee Brothers Medical Publishers; 2022. pp. 795-9.
4. Jorge AAL, Grimberg A, Dattani MT, Baron J. Disorders of child growth. In: Sperling MA, Majzoub JA, Menon RK, Stratakis CA (Eds). Sperling Pediatric Endocrinology, 5th edition. Philadelphia: Elsevier; 2022. pp. 299-356.
5. Styne DM. Physiology and disorders of puberty. In: Medmed S, Auchus RJ (Eds).Williams Textbook of Endocrinology, 14th edition. Philadelphia: Elsevier; 2020. pp. 1023-164.
6. Sharma R. Pubertal development. In: Desai MP, Menon PSN, Bhatia V, Seth A (Eds). Pediatric Endocrine Disorders, 4th edition. Hyderabad: Universities Press; 2022. pp. 130-8.
7. Holland-Hall CM. Adolescent physical and social development. In: Kliegman RM, St Geme JW, Blum NJ, Shah SS, Tasker RC, Wilson KM (Eds). Nelson Textbook of Pediatrics, 21st edition. Philadelphia: Elsevier; 2020.
8. Lifshitz F, Cervantes CD. Short stature. In: Lifshitz F (Ed). Pediatric Endocrinology, 3rd edition. New York: Marcel Dekker; 1996. pp. 3-18.

3.3 Growth Assessment and Monitoring

Vaman Khadilkar, Anuradha Khadilkar

INTRODUCTION

Human growth is a well-orchestrated highly complex process that leads to transformation of the newborn into a fully mature adult.[1] Knowledge of normal growth is of paramount importance for a pediatrician, as it is an indicator of health and disease. Regular growth monitoring is essential to detect the deviation from a normal growth pattern and diagnose nutritional, chronic systemic, and endocrine disease at the earliest so that timely intervention may be instituted. Timely management of the underlying disorder may help in achieving optimal growth as per the child's genetic potential. Growth monitoring has a positive impact on morbidity and mortality even in the absence of nutrition supplementation or education.

GROWTH MONITORING

Anthropometry

Anthropometry is the study of body measurements and proportions and forms the mainstay of growth monitoring in infants, children, and adolescents. Measurements need to be taken accurately by a trained observer using well-calibrated and maintained equipment preferably at the same time of the day and by the same observer during follow-up. Commonly used equipment for anthropometry are *stadiometer* (for measurement of height), *infantometer* (for measuring recumbent length), *nonstretchable tape* (for circumferences), *sitting height stool,* and *skinfold calipers* (for measurement of skinfold thickness). After measurement of growth parameters, it is essential to plot them on appropriate growth charts, preferably longitudinally. Following are the parameters that need to be assessed.

Height and Length

Length/height is a very critical parameter in growth assessment. Conventionally, supine length is measured in children under the age of 2 years and also in case of children who cannot stand due to a disease state or in very sick children. Under the age of 2 years, it is measured using an infantometer by two people, one to hold the head against an immovable vertical plate board while the other person extends the hips and knees to place the soles of feet along a movable footboard **(Figs. 3.3.1A to C)**.

For the measurement of height, a stadiometer is used wherein the horizontal headboard moves up and down a vertical support fixed to the wall. Footwear and socks are removed and the child is made to stand erect with heels, buttocks, back, and occiput touching the vertical support. The child's head is positioned such that the Frankfurt plane (the line joining the inferior margin of the orbit to the external auditory meatus) is parallel to the ground **(Fig. 3.3.2)**.

Height measured in the morning is usually about 8 mm more than the afternoon value because of the fatigue of the spinal muscles.

Growth in children is also accompanied by changes in body proportions and measurement of the body segments is essential for diagnosing disproportionate short stature. An *upper segment (US) to lower segment (LS) ratio* can be calculated by measuring the lower segment or by measuring the sitting height. It is important to use the correct reference values for ratios based on the method used, as US/LS ratio computed by measuring LS from symphysis pubis to the floor is not the same as *subischeal length* calculated by measuring the sitting height. The LS of the body can be measured from top of symphysis pubis to the floor. US is then calculated by subtracting the LS from height.[2] Sitting height is measured by placing a seat/stool of known height with a horizontal top under a height measuring device. Leg (subischeal limb) length is then calculated by subtracting sitting height from standing height.

Weight

This is an indicator of the nutritional status of a child. Infants must be weighed without clothes and children in minimal clothing. Electronic/mechanical beam balance type weighing scales checked for zero error each time should be used. Serial weights need to be plotted on appropriate growth charts to understand weight trajectory of the child.

Head Circumference

Growth of the head (occipital-frontal circumference) depends on the growth of the brain and is thus an estimate of the brain size. The measurement of the head circumference is performed with a nonstretchable tape which is wrapped snugly around the widest part of the head (about 1–2 fingers above the eyebrow and widest part of back of the head) **(Fig. 3.3.3)**.

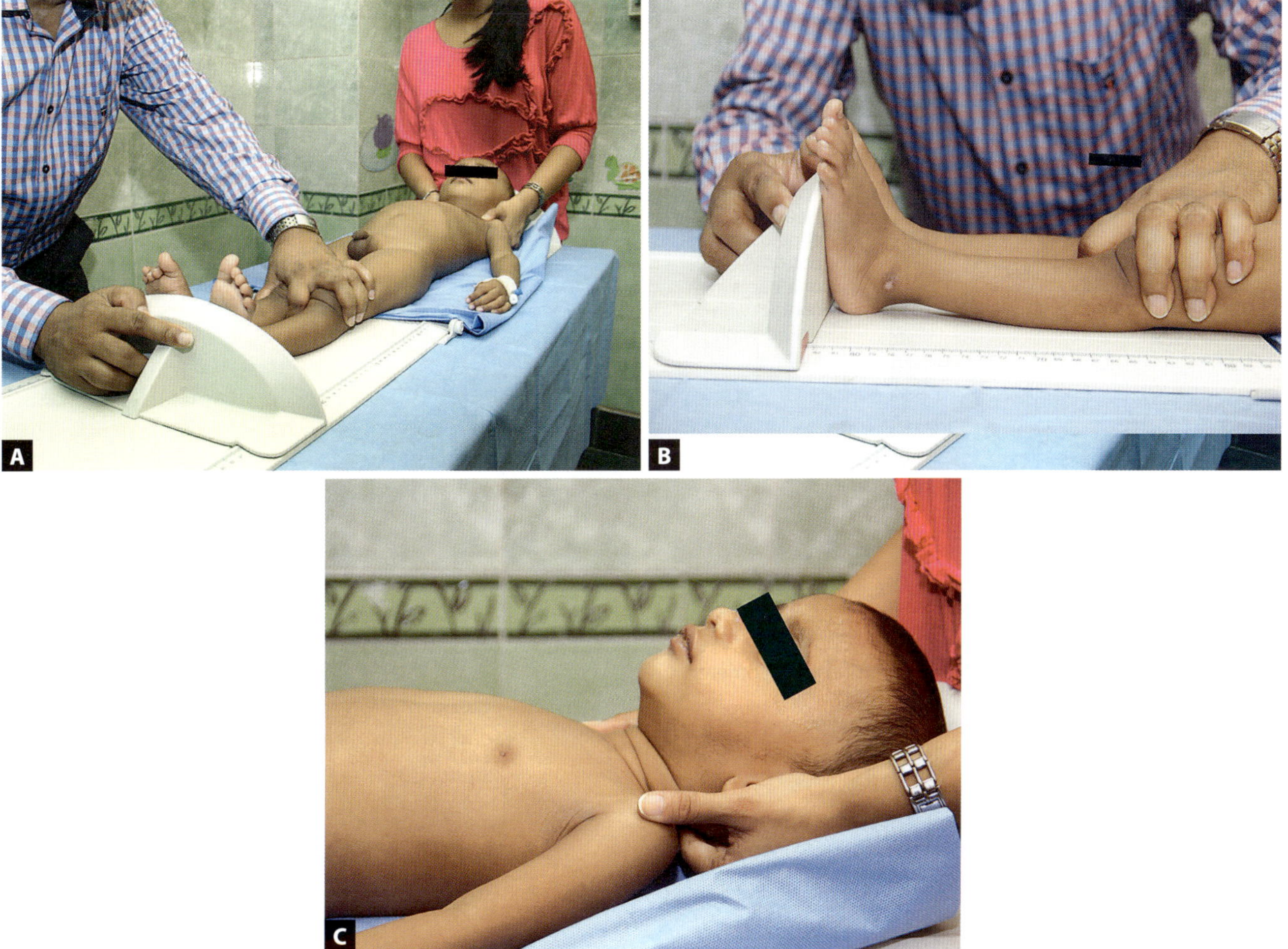

Figs. 3.3.1A to C: Baby's length being measured on an infantometer: (A) The positioning of the child on the infantometer with the help of two assistants; (B) How to place the soles of feet along a movable footboard; (C) How to hold the head against an immovable vertical plate board.

Midarm Circumference

Midarm circumference is used to assess nutritional status of a child in the community as it is an age-independent criterion and hence is useful for mass or community wide screening. The midarm circumference is measured midway between the acromion and the olecranon of the left upper arm **(Fig. 3.3.4)**. It is fairly constant between 1 and 5 years (14.8–16.2 cm), thus, for young children (1–5 years) a circumference >13.5 cm is normal, 12.5–13 cm mild to moderate, and <12.5 cm indicates severe undernutrition. The measurement varies with age in older children and thus the cutoffs are different in the older age groups.[3]

Body Mass Index

It is an estimate of adiposity in comparison to age related standards. It is the ratio of weight in kg to the square of height in meters. According to the recommendations of the World Health Organization (WHO), body mass index (BMI) cutoff value for adult Asian Indians is a BMI of 23 kg/m^2 as overweight and 27 kg/m^2 as obesity. Similar cutoffs should be used to screen Indian boys and girls. Indian Academy of Pediatrics (IAP) 2015 growth charts are designed to depict these values on the BMI charts with orange and red lines showing 23 and 27 equivalent cutoffs, respectively (available from https://iapindia.org/iap-growth-charts/).[4] In younger children under 5 years of age, WHO recommends weight for length rather than BMI to assess nutritional status. Various cutoffs as suggested by WHO are given below in **Table 3.3.1**.

Arm Span

While not measured routinely, this is an important measurement in suspected cases of short-limbed dwarfism. The arm span is measured as the distance between right and left index fingertips, with the arms held horizontally.

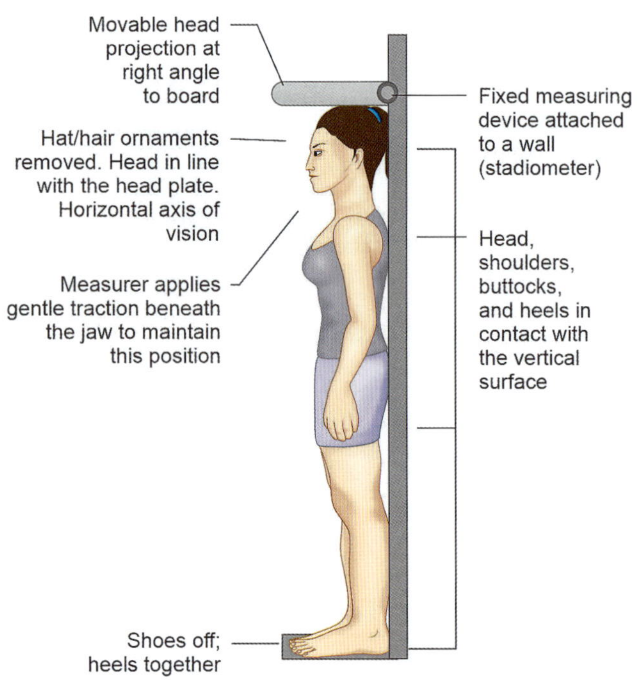

Fig. 3.3.2: Technique of recording height using a stadiometer.

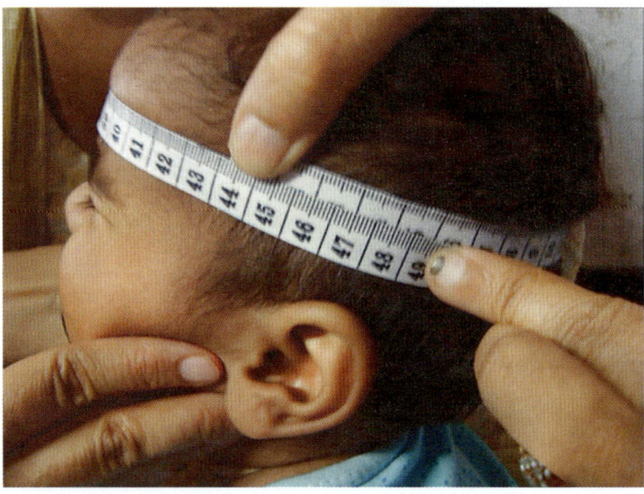

Fig. 3.3.3: Technique of measurement of head circumference.

It is almost equal to the height and exceeds the height by up to 4 cm after puberty. It may bear an abnormal relationship to height (less or more than the height) in some skeletal dysplasias or Marfan syndrome.

Skin Fold Thickness

Skin fold thickness (SFT) gives an estimate of body fat. Peripheral fat is measured on the triceps while central fat is measured by subscapular and suprailiac skinfold thickness. The skinfold thickness is measured by picking up a skin fold with one hand and measuring with a caliper held in the other hand. SFT is also usually measured in community surveys/research purposes.

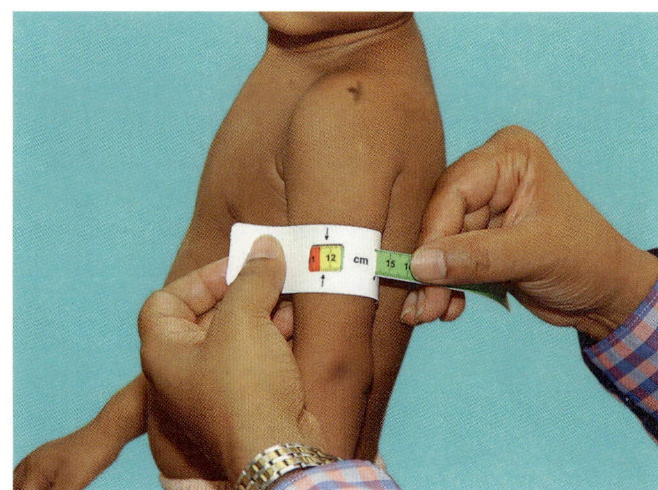

Fig. 3.3.4: Technique of measurement of midarm circumference.

TABLE 3.3.1: Interpretation of anthropometric parameters.

Age	*Growth status*	*Indicator*	*Percentile*	*Z-score*
0–5 years	Underweight	Weight for age	<3rd	<–2
WHO	Severe underweight	Weight for age	<0.1st	<–3
	Stunting	Length/height for age	<3rd	<–2
	Severe stunting	Length/height for age	<0.1st	<–3
	Wasting	Weight for height	<3rd	<–2
	Severe wasting	Weight for height	<0.1st	<–3
5–18 years	Underweight	BMI for age	<3rd	
(Revised IAP)	Short stature	Height for age	<3rd	
	Overweight	BMI for age	>23rd adult equivalent	
	Obese	BMI for age	>27th adult equivalent	

Waist Circumference

As obesity tracks from childhood to adulthood, a specific anthropometric parameter is required to correctly measure truncal obesity and thus metabolic risk. Waist circumference

(WC) provides a simple and effective measure of truncal obesity in children and adolescents.[5] Greater WC correlates better with adverse metabolic profile and health risks than the BMI. Waist circumference is measured in a standing position above the iliac crest in a horizontal plane. The median WC percentiles (5th, 10th, 15th, 25th, 50th, 70th, 85th, 90th, and 95th) are presented in a study on Indian children by Khadilkar, et al. In this study, age and sex specific reference curves for WC for Indian children and cutoff values of 70th WC percentile for screening for metabolic syndrome risk are provided **(Table 3.3.2)**.[6]

BONE AGE OR SKELETAL MATURITY

Measurement of bone age adds an important dimension to the assessment of growth in a healthy as well as diseased child. It is measured by assessing the degree of development of a large number of bones available on a radiograph of the left hand and wrist. In the Gruelich and Pyle method, bone age is estimated by comparing the maturity of ossification centers with the standard radiographs in the atlas while in the Tanner–Whitehouse method, bone age is calculated by assigning a score to either 13 or 20 individual bones.[7,8] In recent times, Gilsanz and Ratib have published an atlas of idealized digital images for the assessment of bone age.[9]

Predicted adult height is estimated by using current height and bone age. The classic method of height prediction based on Greulich and Pyle's Radiographic Atlas of Skeletal Development, was developed by Bayley and Pinneau. Tanner and colleagues introduced a system that employs height, bone age, and chronological age. The more advanced the

TABLE 3.3.2: Waist circumference reference tables for boys and girls.

Boys							
Age	***3rd***	***10th***	***25th***	***50th***	***70th***	***85th***	***95th***
5	46.9	48.2	50.5	53.5	56.1	59.1	63.1
6	48.8	50.2	52.8	56.1	59	62.2	66.7
7	50.7	52.2	55.1	58.7	61.9	65.5	70.5
8	52.6	54.3	57.4	61.3	64.9	68.8	74.3
9	54.7	56.5	59.9	64.2	68	72.3	78.2
10	57	59	62.6	67.3	71.4	76	82.3
11	59.3	61.5	65.4	70.4	74.9	79.7	86.4
12	61.5	63.8	68	73.3	78	83.1	90.1
13	63.4	65.8	70.3	75.8	80.7	86	93.2
14	64.9	67.5	72.2	78	83	88.4	95.6
15	66.2	68.9	73.8	79.8	84.9	90.4	97.6
16	67.4	70.2	75.2	81.3	86.5	92.1	99.2
17	68.4	71.3	76.5	82.7	87.9	93.5	100.6
Girls							
5	46.8	48.1	50.4	53.5	56.4	59.8	64.7
6	48.8	50.1	52.7	56.1	59.3	62.9	68.3
7	50.6	52.1	55	58.7	62.1	66	71.7
8	52.4	54.1	57.2	61.2	64.9	69	74.9
9	54.5	56.3	59.7	64	67.9	72.3	78.4
10	56.8	58.8	62.5	67.2	71.3	75.9	82.2
11	59.3	61.5	65.5	70.5	74.8	79.6	86
12	61.7	64	68.3	73.5	78.1	83	89.5
13	63.6	66.1	70.6	76.1	80.8	85.7	92.2
14	65	67.6	72.3	78	82.7	87.8	94.2
15	66	68.7	73.5	79.3	84.1	89.1	95.4
16	66.6	69.5	74.4	80.3	85.1	90.1	96.3
17	67.1	70.1	75.2	81.1	85.9	90.9	96.9

bone age, the greater the accuracy of adult height prediction, as it places the child closer to adult height.

Normally, the bone age is around 10% or one standard deviation around the chronological age. In practical terms the gap between the chronological age and bone age is usually within 1 year in younger children and 2 years in older children. When the discrepancy between the chronological age and bone age is >2 years, then the chance of an endocrine disorder increases.

GROWTH CHARTS

A growth chart is the most important objective tool for a pediatrician to monitor childhood growth, to identify growth failure, to assess nutritional status (undernutrition, overweight, and obesity) and to diagnose endocrine and nonendocrine conditions causing growth failure in a timely manner. The IAP recommends the use of IAP 2015 growth charts for growth monitoring in children from 5 to 18 years of age and IAP modified WHO charts for children under 5 years of age.

Growth charts are also useful for community health workers to diagnose and classify malnutrition as stunting, wasting or stunting, and wasting or severe and moderate acute malnutrition (MAM and SAM) at the community level.

Growth charts can be classified as growth standards and growth references. Growth standards are constructed from a population of healthy children living in ideal conditions for optimal growth (e.g., exclusive breastfeeding for 6 months, adequate nutrition, favorable psychological environment, and good living conditions). Growth standards are *prescriptive* and define how the population should grow ideally while reference charts are *descriptive*, and they are constructed from a set of children growing in a state of best possible nutrition and health in a given community. Use of growth standards such as the WHO growth standards published in 2006 presents an opportunity to compare a child of any country, race or ethnicity against a single standard with an objective assessment, however, it is likely to overdiagnose underweight and stunting in developing part of the world such as India. Ethnic specific growth reference charts are representative of existing growth patterns in children and indicate the secular trends in terms of height, weight, and obesity, but they need to be updated at least once in a decade.

Basics of Growth Charts

A growth chart consists of an X-axis on which age in years or months is plotted and a Y-axis on which various anthropometric parameters such as height, weight, head circumference, or BMI are plotted.

Growth charts for monitoring height and weight usually have 7 percentile lines that include 3rd, 10th, 25th, 50th, 75th, and 97th percentiles. Any child whose anthropometric parameters fall within the 3rd centile and 97th centile is considered as having normal growth parameters. In addition, in a child growing normally, serial recording of growth parameters on a growth chart would typically reveal a trajectory parallel to the percentile lines, indicating a normal growth velocity.

Growth velocity can also be assessed on a growth velocity chart, on which the 25th percentile is considered as the cutoff to determine low height velocity. On IAP BMI charts 23rd and 27th adult equivalent lines are considered as cutoffs for overweight and obesity, while on the WHO 2007 growth references, the 85th and 95th percentile lines are considered as cutoffs for overweight and obesity, respectively.

How to Use Growth Charts?

- At the first visit; the child's name, date of birth, and parent's heights should be entered on the growth chart and the chart should be explained to the parents to ensure their active participation.
- Calculate the child's target height by using the formula:
  - For a boy, target height = (Father's height + mother's height + 13)/2
  - For a girl, target height = (Father's height + mother's height – 13)/2
- Target height should be plotted at 18 years and marked with an arrow on the growth chart. The target range is produced by plotting two points 6–8 cm above and below the target height.
- All the points on the growth chart should be marked only as dots and not as circles.
- The height, weight, and head circumference (till 3 years) should be recorded and plotted on the chart.
- As described in earlier text, by joining the serially plotted dots, a trend line can be created which gives an idea of the growth trajectory.

GROWTH CHARTS CURRENTLY IN USE

WHO Multicentre Growth Reference Study (MGRS) Growth Charts (2006)

This is a "growth standard" for children from birth to 5 years. These charts were constructed using data from 6 countries (Brazil, Ghana, India, Norway, Oman, and USA) wherein longitudinal data for the initial 2 years of life and cross-sectional from 2 to 5 years have been used to construct percentiles and Z score lines. WHO growth standards are available from 0 to 5 years [Child growth standards (who.int)]. WHO growth charts may overdiagnose stunting, wasting, and underweight in developing countries of the world.

Indian Academy of Pediatrics Growth Charts

The revised Indian Academy of Pediatrics (IAP) growth charts are references which were published in 2015 and were derived from data collated from 9 different studies in apparently healthy children belonging to healthy families from across India. These charts are constructed from >87,000 children and depict the most modern Indian data. These charts are prescriptive for BMI as they depict 23rd and 27th adult equivalent lines for defining overweight and obesity based on the guidelines given by WHO and International Obesity Task Force (IOTF). Thus, they do not "normalize" obesity **(Figs. 3.3.5 to 3.3.10)**.

Indian Academy of Pediatrics Pediatrician-friendly Growth Charts

To make the IAP growth charts user-friendly, the IAP published pediatrician-friendly growth charts in 2020 **(Figs. 3.3.9 and 3.3.10)**. A combined WHO–IAP height and weight chart that allows monitoring of growth from birth to 18 years (using statistical smoothing procedure) on a single chart was produced. On these charts correlation between child's height and midparental height (MPH) can be readily assessed on the same chart even for children younger than 5 years which is not possible on the split chart (separate charts for under 5 and older children). A quick BMI assessment tool as well as a MPH calculation tool has also been added to the IAP–WHO combined charts eliminating all calculations that a busy pediatrician finds difficult to perform in everyday practice **(Figs. 3.3.11 and 3.3.12)**.

Disease-specific Growth Charts

Other than these standard growth charts, there are disease-specific growth charts for specific disorders like Turner syndrome, achondroplasia, and Down syndrome.[10] The advantage of these charts is that they can help in earlier detection of other associated conditions if growth faltering is observed on disease-specific charts.

GROWTH MONITORING GUIDELINES FOR CHILDREN FROM BIRTH TO 18 YEARS

Aims and Rationale

Primary Aim

To identify children with undernutrition and overnutrition and children with diseases and conditions that manifest through abnormal growth.

Secondary Aims

- To discuss health promotion related to feeding, hygiene, immunization, and other aspects of the child's health and behavior; education of parents to allay their anxiety about their child's growth.
- To sensitize pediatricians to use growth charts.

Recommended Intervals and Parameters for Growth Monitoring

- Immunization contacts at birth, 6, 10 and 14 weeks, 9 months, 15–18 months should be used for growth monitoring. An additional monitoring at 6 months with opportunistic monitoring at illnesses is recommended.
- Height, weight, and head circumference should be measured up to 3 years of age. Penile length (PL) and testicular descent should be determined in the newborn period.
- *4–8 years:* Height and weight should be measured 6 monthly and BMI, along with sexual maturity rating (SMR) should be assessed yearly from 6 years of age.
- *9–18 years:* Height, weight, BMI, and SMR should be assessed yearly.

Criteria for Referral

- Length/height, weight below 3rd percentile or above 97th percentile on a growth chart at any age from birth to 18 years.
- Head circumference below 3rd or above 97th percentile during the first 3 years.
- Crossing of two major percentile lines (above 75th or below 50th percentile) on height or weight charts at any age.
- A child below or above midparental range for height.
- Absence of weight gain for 2–3 months from 6 to 12 months.
- BMI over 23rd adult equivalent line of IAP 2015 growth charts.
- Rate of growth <5 cm/year between 3 and 9 years.
- Girls with axillary and/or pubic hair growth or breast budding before 8 years and boys with axillary and/or pubic hair growth, or genital growth, or testicular enlargement before 9 years.
- Delayed puberty—girls with absence of breast budding by 14 years or no menarche by 15 years and boys with no signs of puberty by 16 years.
- Arrest of puberty at the same stage of puberty for >2 years.

The IAP has given comprehensive guidelines for growth monitoring in children.[4]

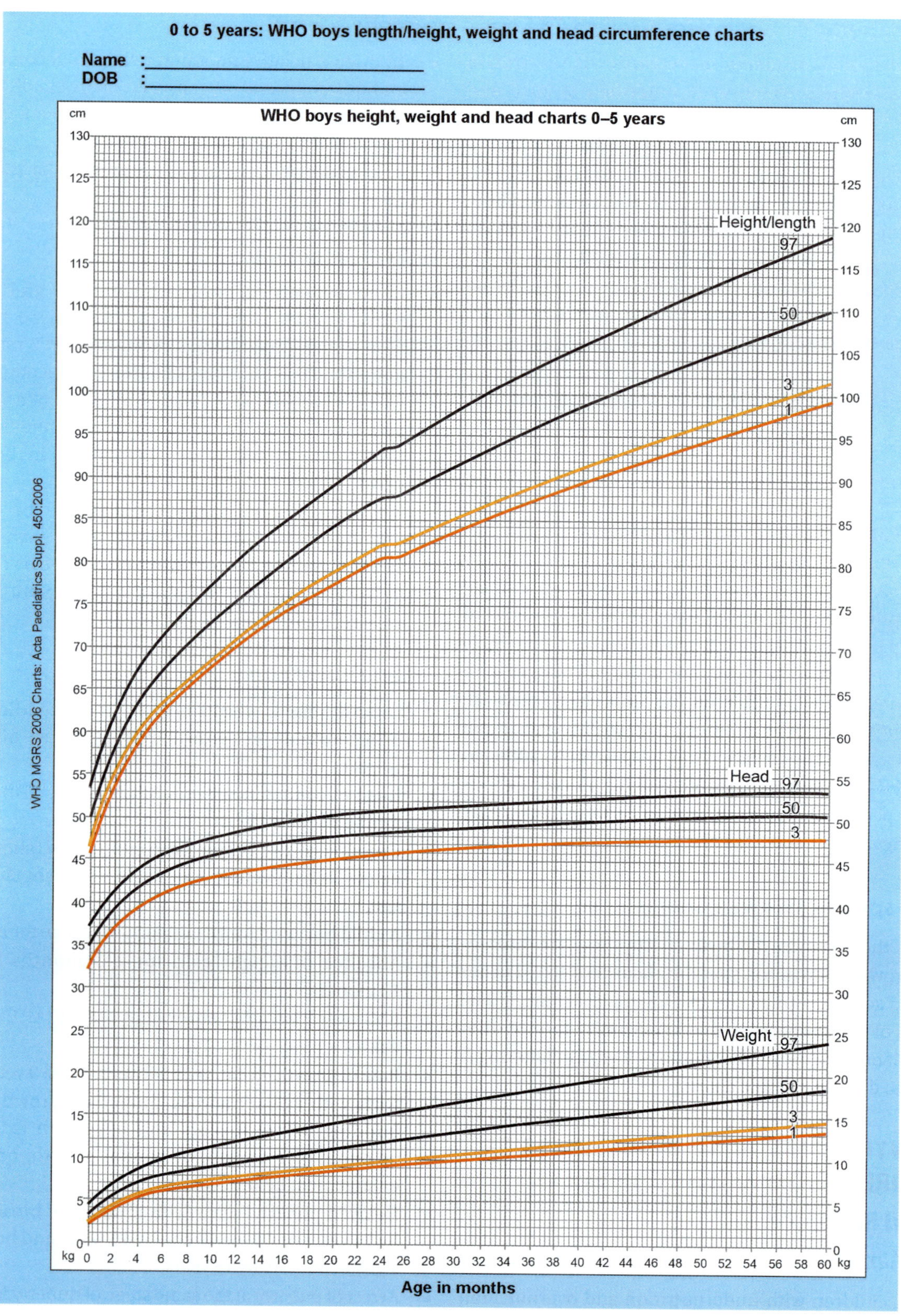

Fig. 3.3.5: Indian Academy of Pediatrics (IAP) simplified World Health Organization (WHO) height, weight, and head circumference charts for boys.

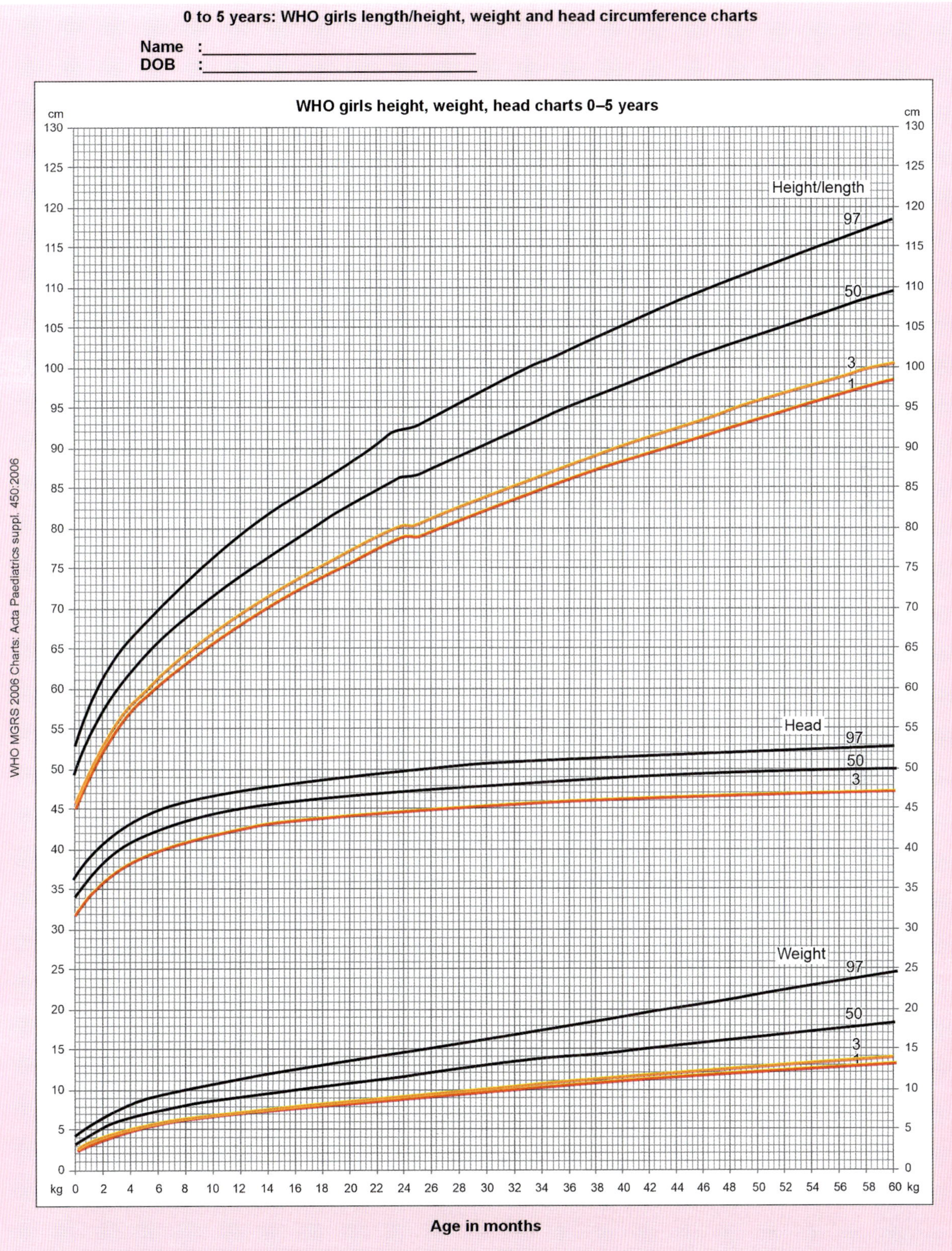

Fig. 3.3.6: Indian Academy of Pediatrics (IAP) simplified World Health Organization (WHO) height, weight, and head circumference charts for girls.

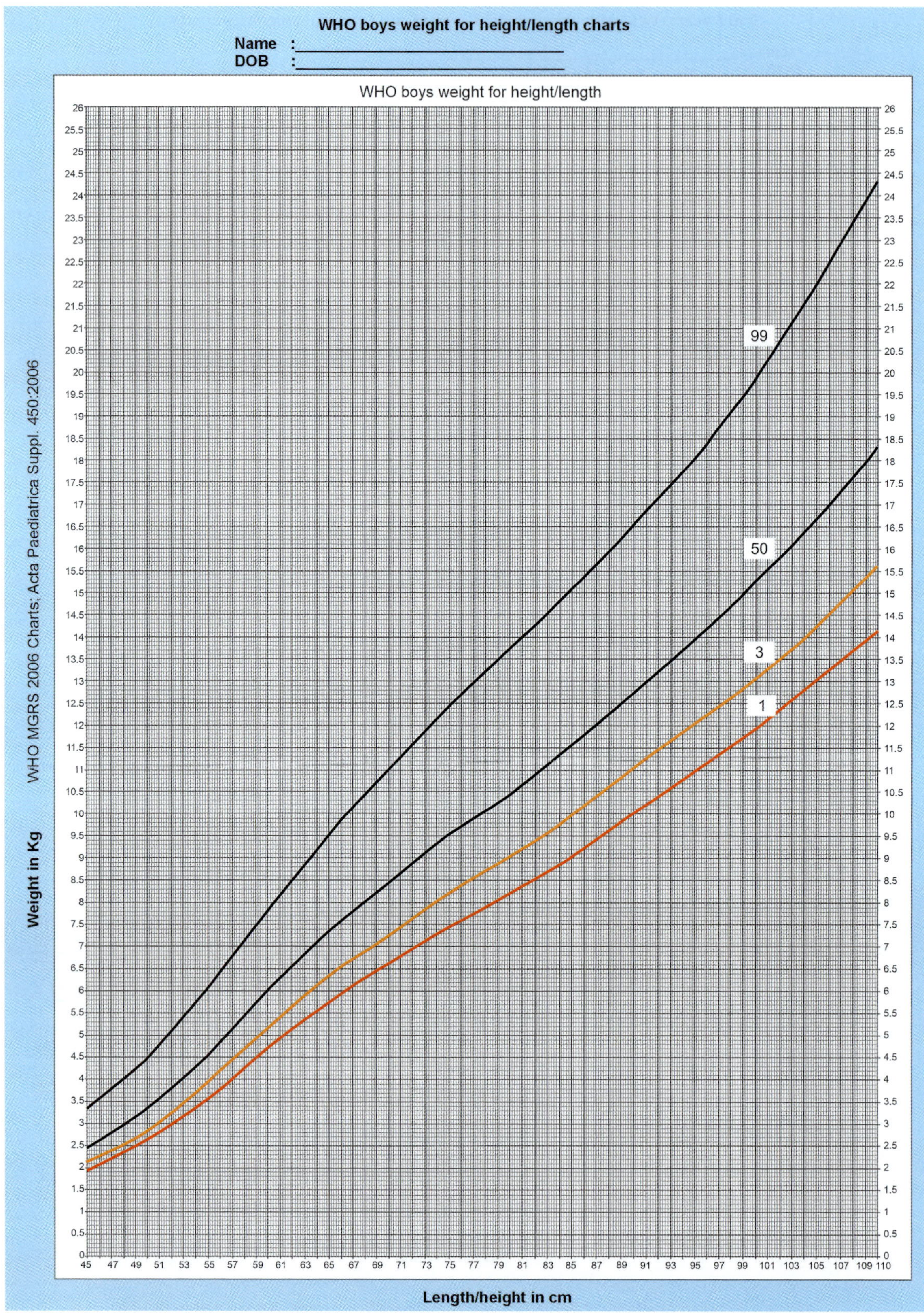

Fig. 3.3.7: Indian Academy of Pediatrics (IAP) simplified World Health Organization (WHO) weight for height charts for boys.

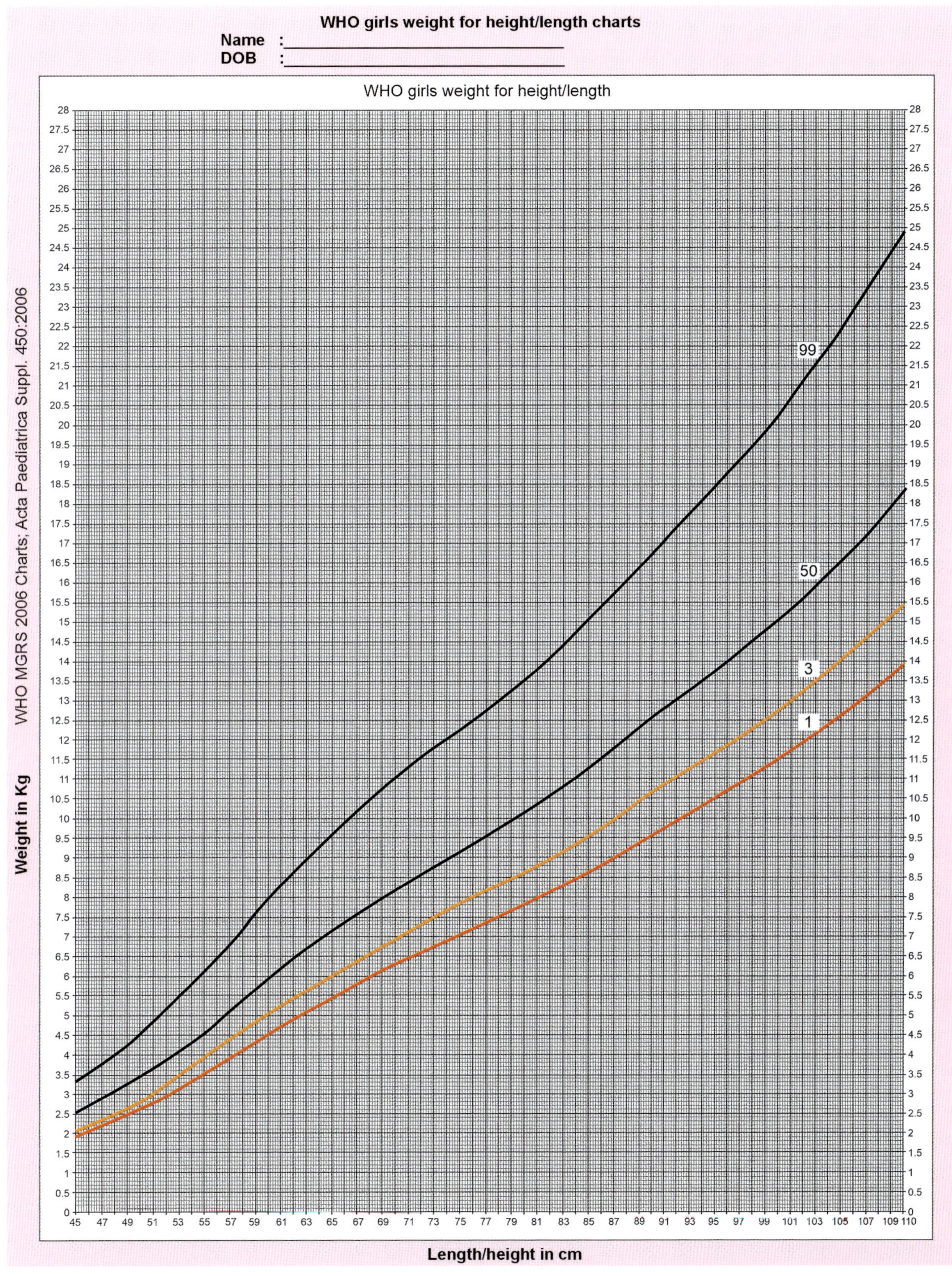

Fig. 3.3.8: Indian Academy of Pediatrics (IAP) simplified World Health Organization (WHO) weight for height charts for girls.

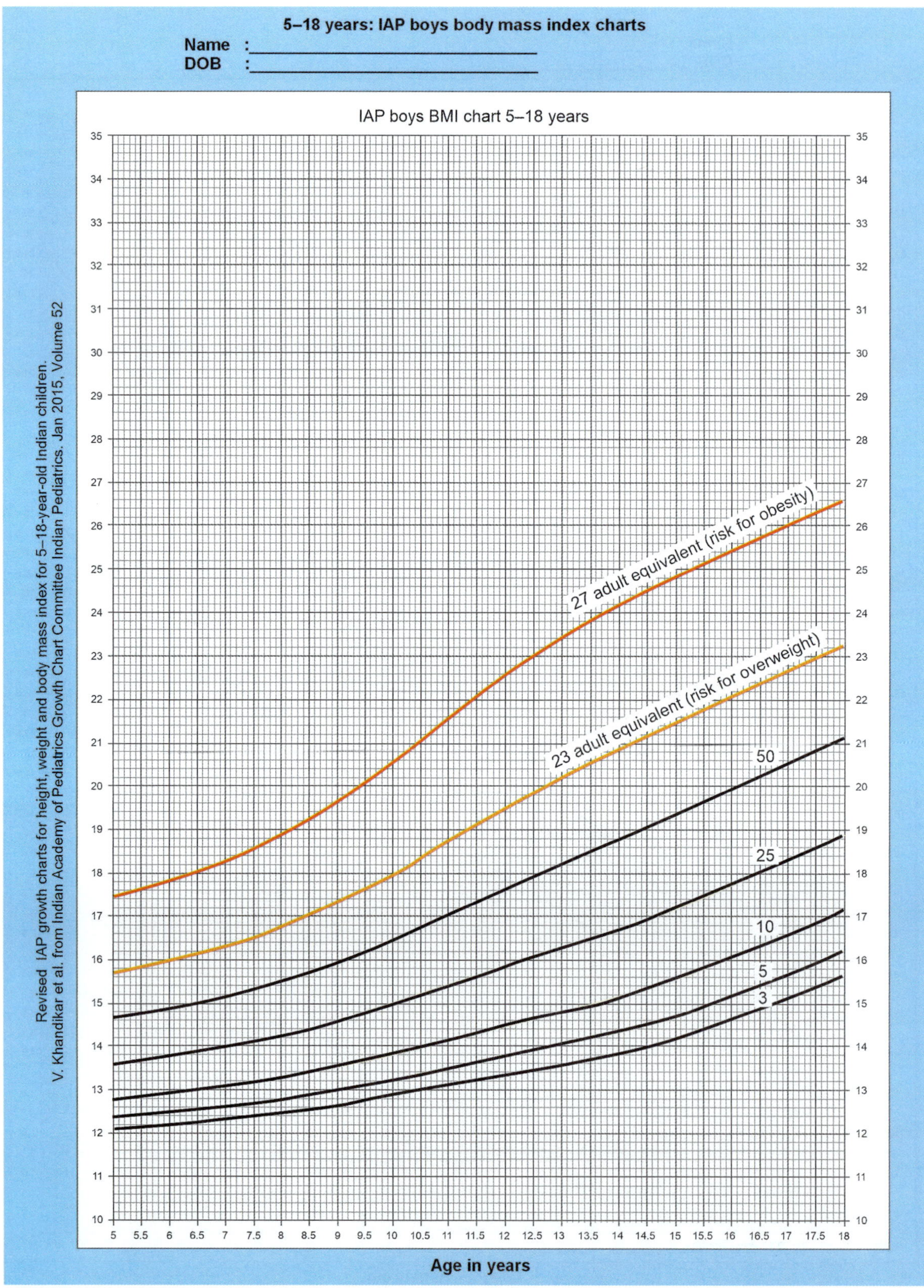

Fig. 3.3.9: Indian Academy of Pediatrics (IAP) body mass index (BMI) charts for boys 5–18 years: IAP BMI charts for boys 5–18 years.

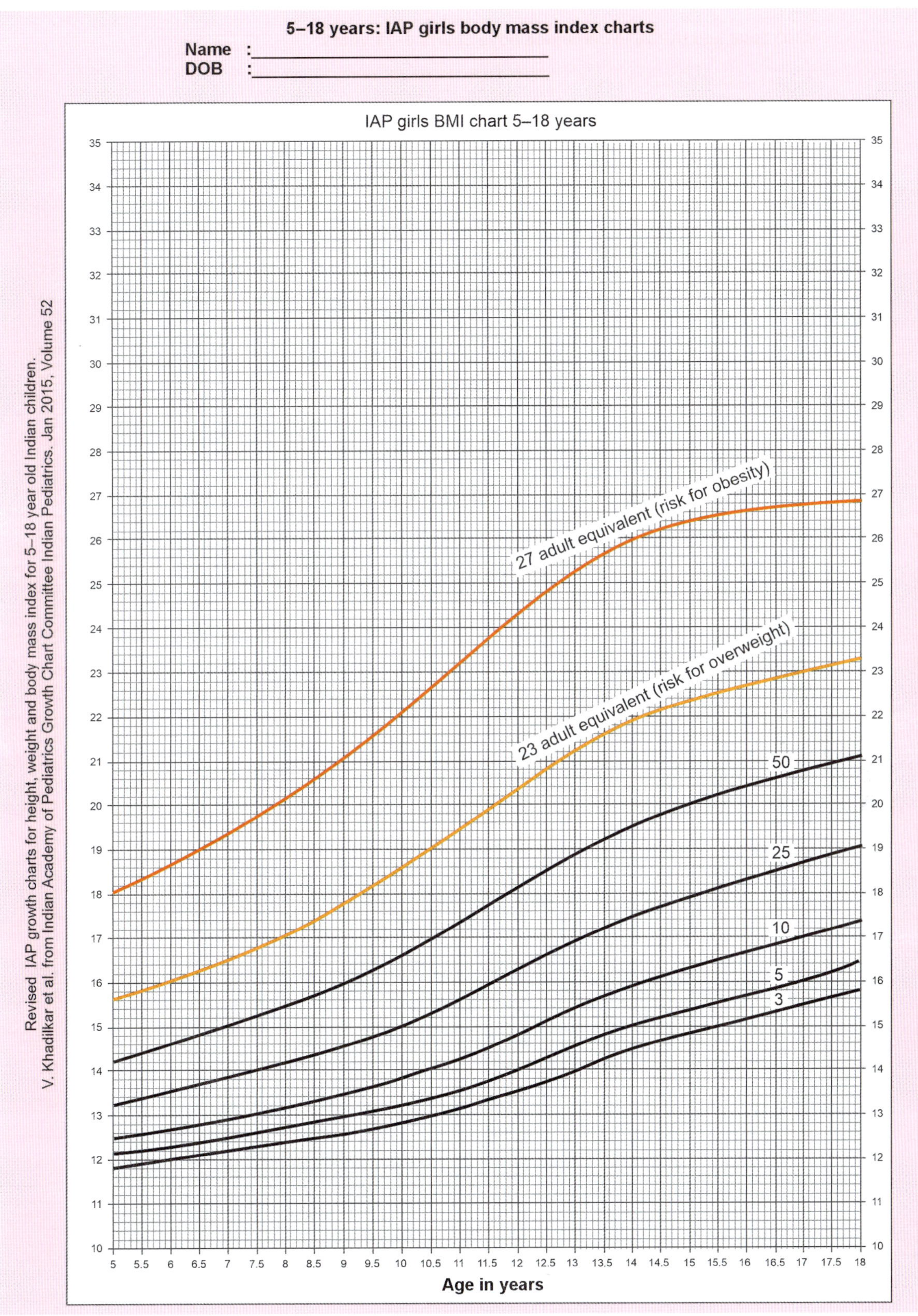

Fig. 3.3.10: Indian Academy of Pediatrics (IAP) body mass index (BMI) charts for girls 5–18 years.

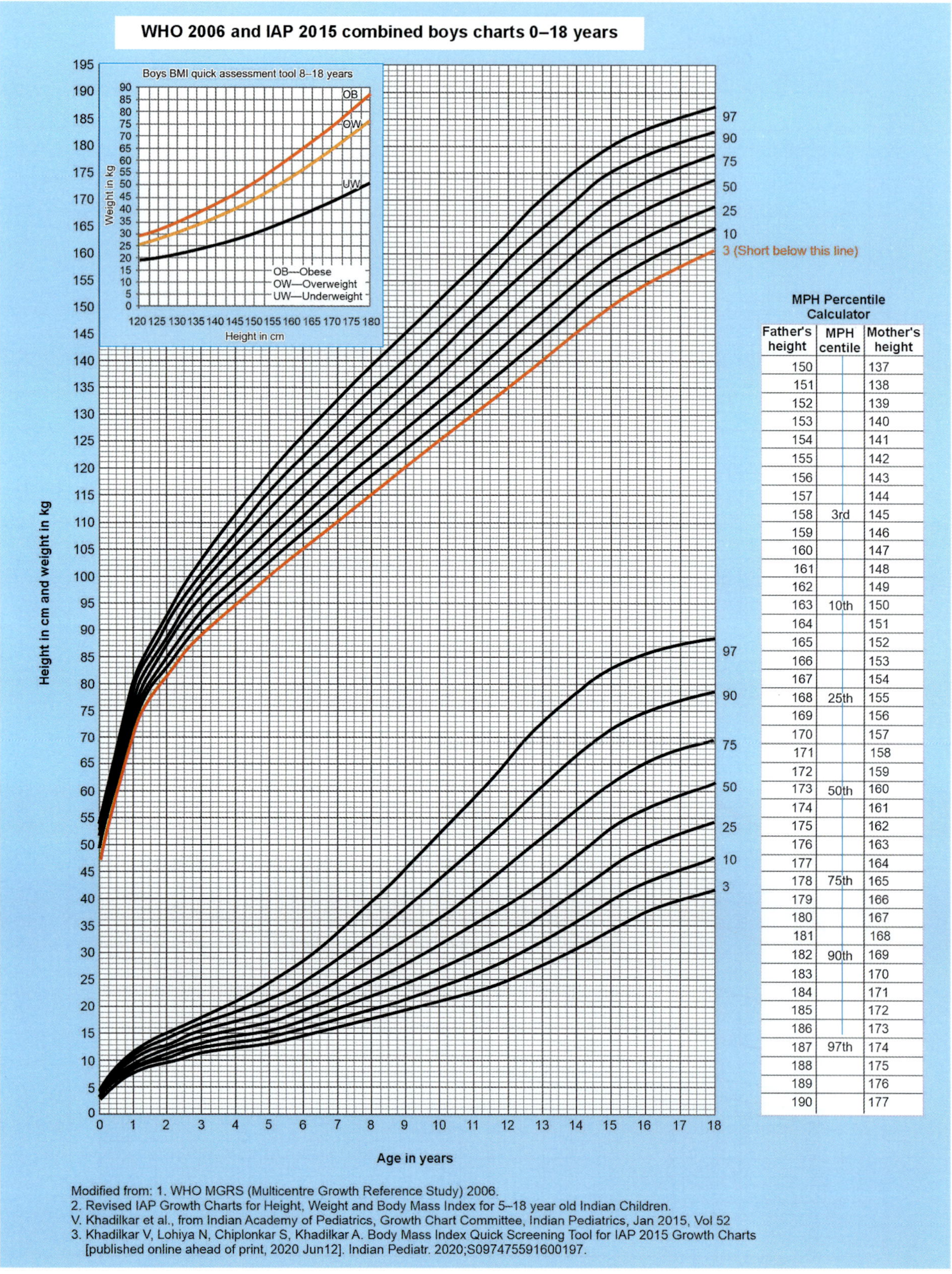

MPH Percentile Calculator

Father's height	MPH centile	Mother's height
150		137
151		138
152		139
153		140
154		141
155		142
156		143
157		144
158	3rd	145
159		146
160		147
161		148
162		149
163	10th	150
164		151
165		152
166		153
167		154
168	25th	155
169		156
170		157
171		158
172		159
173	50th	160
174		161
175		162
176		163
177		164
178	75th	165
179		166
180		167
181		168
182	90th	169
183		170
184		171
185		172
186		173
187	97th	174
188		175
189		176
190		177

Fig. 3.3.11: Indian Academy of Pediatrics (IAP) pediatrician friendly growth chart for boys.

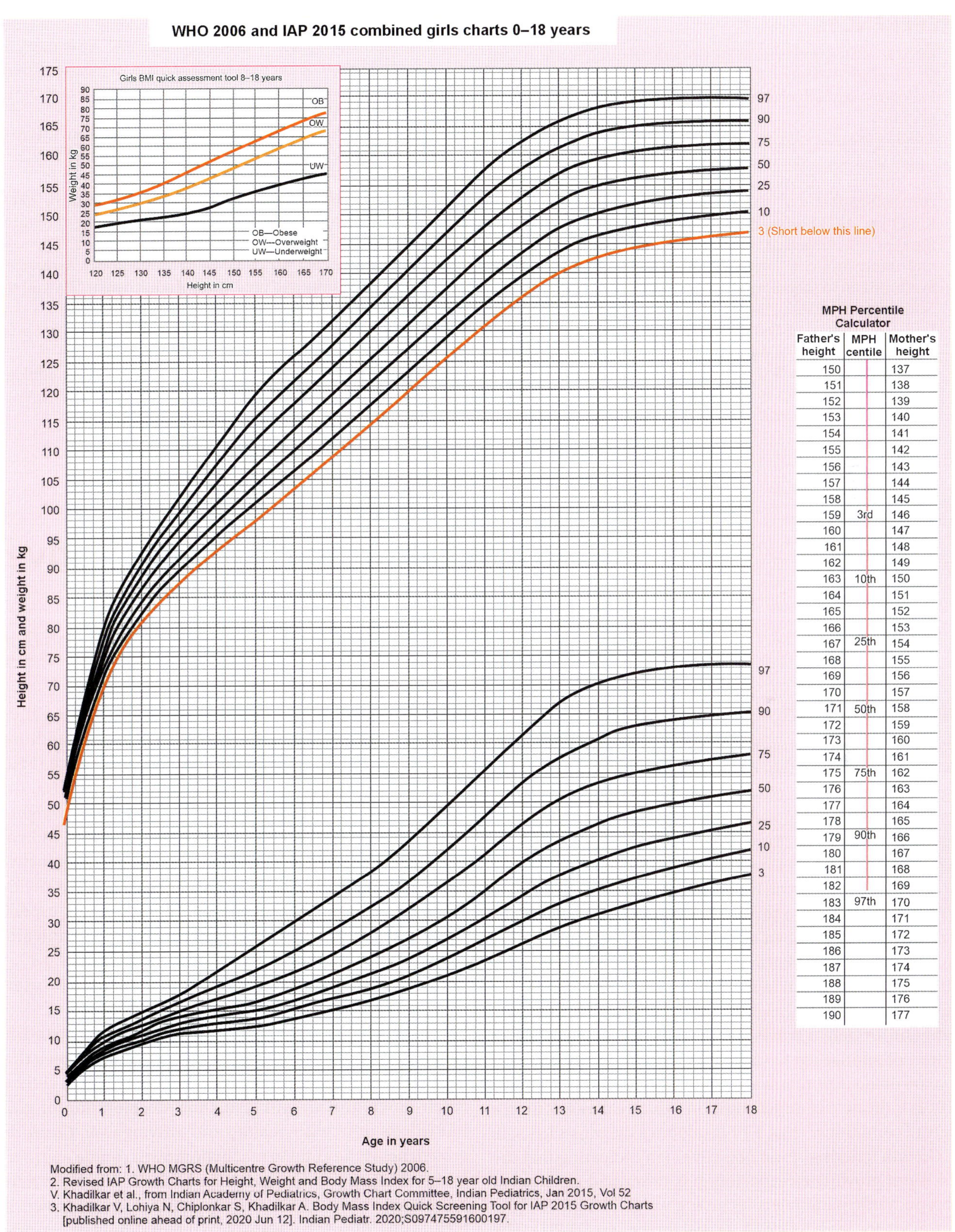

Father's height	MPH centile	Mother's height
150		137
151		138
152		139
153		140
154		141
155		142
156		143
157		144
158		145
159	3rd	146
160		147
161		148
162		149
163	10th	150
164		151
165		152
166		153
167	25th	154
168		155
169		156
170		157
171	50th	158
172		159
173		160
174		161
175	75th	162
176		163
177		164
178		165
179	90th	166
180		167
181		168
182		169
183	97th	170
184		171
185		172
186		173
187		174
188		175
189		176
190		177

Fig. 3.3.12: Indian Academy of Pediatrics (IAP) pediatrician friendly growth chart for girls.

REFERENCES

1. Jerry k. Wales. Evaluation of Growth Disorders. In: Brook C, Clayton P, Brown R (Eds). Brook's Clinical Pediatric Endocrinology, 6th edition. New Jersey: Wiley-Blackwell; 2009. pp. 126-7.
2. Kondpalle S, Lote-Oke R, Patel P, Khadilkar V, Khadilkar AV. Upper and lower body segment ratios from birth to 18 years in children from Western Maharashtra. Indian J Pediatr. 2019;86(6):503-7.
3. Khadilkar AV, Khadilkar VV, Gondhalekar KM, Kajale NA, Karkera PH, Prasad M, et al. Reference centile curves for mid-upper arm circumference for assessment of under- and overnutrition in school-aged Indian children and adolescents. Nutrition. 2021;91-92:111401.
4. Indian Academy of Pediatrics Growth Charts Committee; Khadilkar V, Yadav S, Agrawal KK, Tamboli S, Banerjee M, Cherian A, et al. Revised IAP growth charts for height, weight and body mass index for 5- to 18-year-old Indian children. Indian Pediatr. 2015;52(1):47-55.
5. Taylor RW, Jones IE, Williams SM, Goulding A. Evaluation of waist circumference, waist-to-hip ratio, and the conicity index as screening tools for high trunk fat mass, as measured by dual-energy X-ray absorptiometry, in children aged 3-19 y. Am J Clin Nutr. 2000;72(2):490-5.
6. Khadilkar A, Ekbote V, Chiplonkar S, Khadilkar V, Kajale N, Kulkarni S, et al. Waist circumference percentiles in 2-18 year old Indian children. J Pediatr. 2014;164(6):1358-62.e2.
7. Greulich WW, Pyle SI. Radiographic atlas of skeletal development of the hand and wrist, 2nd edition. Stanford: Stanford University Press; 1959.
8. Tanner JM, Healy MJR, Goldstein H, Cameron N. Assessment of skeletal maturity and prediction of adult height (TW3 method). London, UK: Saunders; 2001.
9. Gilsanz V, Ratib O. Hand Bone Age. Los Angeles, CA: Springer; 2005.
10. Khadilkar VV, Karguppikar MB, Ekbote VH, Khadilkar AV. Turner Syndrome Growth Charts: A Western India Experience. Indian J Endocrinol Metab. 2020;24(4):333-7.

3.4 Growth Faltering (Failure to Thrive)

Anju Seth, Aashima Dabas

INTRODUCTION

Assessment of growth is an essential component of evaluation of a child during childhood. On longitudinal tracking, the weight and height of a child are expected to follow the centile lines indicated on the growth chart, representing the normal weight and height trajectories for a child of that gender. This has been discussed in Chapter 3.3. A deviation from this expected pattern of growth is identified as "growth faltering."

The term "failure to thrive" (FTT) indicates a *perceived* poor growth, usually seen during the first few years of life. Infants or children that fail to thrive seem to be visibly smaller or shorter than other children of the same age. They have a low weight and often a low height; or, they have a rate of gaining weight and/or height that is significantly below that of other children of similar age and sex. As growth during the first 2–3 years of life is primarily driven by nutrition, the presence of FTT is indicative of undernutrition, which can result from a variety of conditions. Thus, FTT is seldom a diagnosis in itself.

"Growth faltering" is an objective sign indicating that the child is not growing as expected. It is described in terms of anthropometric parameters including weight, length/height, and weight-for length (WFL), or weight/height (WFH). The term "growth faltering" indicates absence or slower rate of growth than expected for the child's age and sex and is a preferred term to use over "failure to thrive". In addition to weight and length, mid-upper arm circumference (MUAC) is useful for screening for growth failure in children under 5 years of age. In children below 6 months of age, weight-for-age Z-score (WAZ) and MUAC are the preferred indicators over WFL.[1] The anthropometric parameters suggestive of *growth faltering* are summarized in **Box 3.4.1.**[2,3] A review of serial recordings of anthropometric parameters especially when plotted on a growth chart, are a better indicator of growth faltering than a single recording **(Fig. 3.4.1)**. The World Health Organization (WHO) charts should be used for monitoring growth in children 0–5 years of age.[3]

Growth faltering/FTT needs to be differentiated from *catch-down growth* that is a physiological process seen during the postnatal life in children born large-for-date. A child with catch-down growth will also show deceleration of growth but will be otherwise healthy and thriving well. *Catch-down growth* helps the child to reach the growth centile appropriate for her/his genetic potential after birth. On the other hand, a baby born small-for-date usually shows catch-up growth after birth. Thus, the birth weight of an infant should be considered when assessing for growth faltering.

BOX 3.4.1: Anthropometric parameters suggestive of growth faltering.[2,3]

Infants <6 months age

Attained growth:

- Weight-for-age Z-score (WAZ) ≤2 SD; or
- Weight-for-length Z-score (WLZ) ≤2 SD; or
- Nutritional edema; or
- Mid-upper arm circumference (MUAC) <110 mm for infants between 6 weeks to <6 months of age

Rate of growth:

- No weight gain or weight loss from one measurement to the next; or
- Downward crossing of weight-for-age centile lines*; or
- Insufficient weight gain (g/per specific time period**)

*≥1 growth centile space if birth weight <9th centile; ≥2 centile spaces if birth weight 9th–91st centile; ≥3 centile spaces if birth weight >91st centile

**Approximately <500 g/month, or if weekly measurements: Birth to 3 months, approximately <150–200 g/week and 3–6 months approximately <100–150 g per week

Children 6–59 months age

Attained growth:

- WHZ or WLZ ≤2 SD; or
- MUAC <125 mm as an alternative field measure

Rate of growth:

- No weight gain or weight loss from one measurement to the next; or
- Downward crossing of major centile lines

SIGNIFICANCE OF GROWTH FALTERING

Presence of growth faltering signifies a nonanabolic state that results in poor growth during the phase otherwise characterized by a high growth velocity. Similar risk factors underlie both wasting and stunting, the latter becoming manifest when the insult is sustained over a period. Height deficit incurred during this time cannot be compensated subsequently, leading to attainment of suboptimal adult stature. In addition, growth faltering also adversely impacts the attainment of normal developmental milestones and function of the immune system. The risk of morbidity and mortality are higher in children with growth faltering than those with normal growth. The risk of death is especially high in severely underweight infants <6 months of age, infants who have persistent wasting under 6 months (defined as >50% of measurements showing wasting), or have concurrent wasting and stunting.[4]

ETIOLOGY

Three main mechanisms contribute toward development of growth faltering, viz., increased energy consumption, decreased energy intake, or loss of nutrients. The result is an insufficient reserve of calories to ensure optimum growth.

Weight-for-age GIRLS

Birth to 5 years (percentiles)

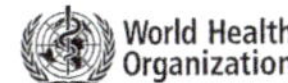

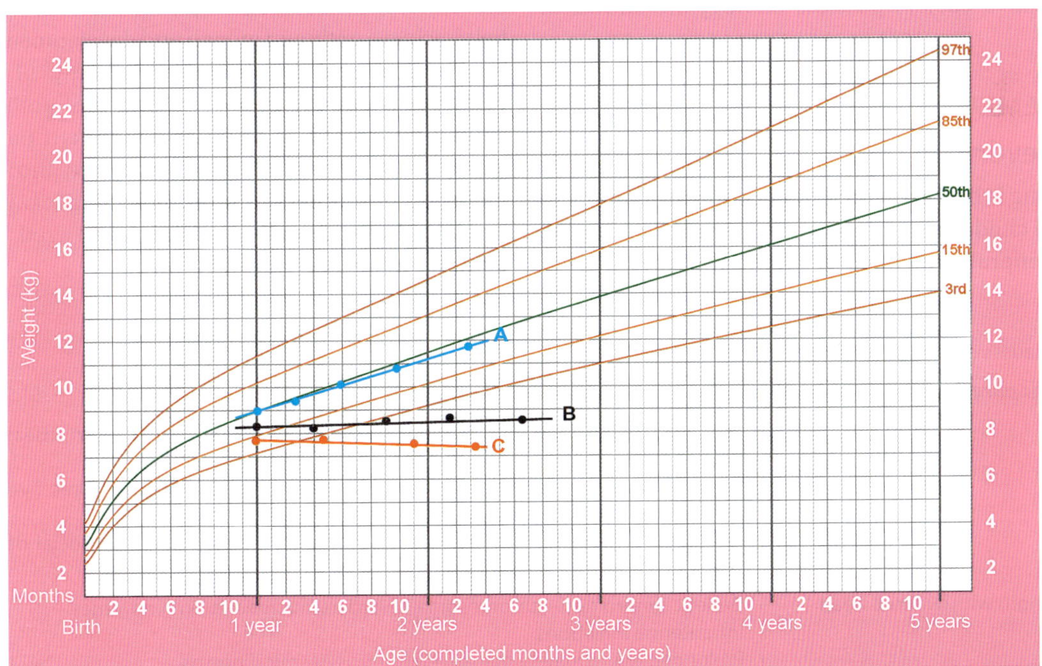

WHO Child Growth Standards

Fig. 3.4.1: Diagrammatic representation of serial weight recording in three children on World Health Organization (WHO) growth chart: (A) Slowing in weight gain; (B) Static weight; and (C) Loss of weight. All three children qualify as failure to thrive.

Broadly, etiology of growth faltering depends on whether the cause is organic, i.e., associated with an underlying disease, or nonorganic, that results from scarcity or deprivation of food. Parental risk factors such as poor education, poverty, and psychosocial stressors are associated with nonorganic causes of growth faltering. Often, there may be more than one operating factor in affected children like food insecurity and an underlying systemic disorder.

The organic causes of growth faltering can be further classified into those that first affect the weight, length/height, or the head circumference as shown in **Table 3.4.1**. Some children may only present with low length/height for age due to specific disorders/pathological conditions without deceleration in weight. These children have adequate nutrition and calories and should not be considered to have growth faltering even when height velocity is poor. Examples include children with skeletal dysplasias, genetic syndromes, and endocrine disorders such as hypothyroidism and growth hormone (GH) deficiency.

DIAGNOSTIC APPROACH TO A CHILD WITH GROWTH FALTERING INCLUDING HISTORY, EXAMINATION, AND LAB TESTS

The diagnosis of growth faltering is largely clinical. It is essential to differentiate nutritional causes from non-nutritional causes as the management of both would differ. Important clinical cues to possible etiology are shown in **Table 3.4.2**.[5]

MANAGEMENT

Primary Prevention

Growth faltering is best prevented by encouraging parents to follow optimal child rearing practices and regular monitoring of growth. General principles of infant and young child feeding should be followed to ensure adequate nutrition during the growing years. Exclusive breastfeeding should be encouraged for 6 months with timely introduction of complementary feeding. Breastfeeding packages can serve as "primary prevention" interventions for all infants under 6 months in low-middle-income countries. These include a clear policy on promotion of breastfeeding, information-education-counseling material for mothers during antenatal and postnatal visits on benefits of breastfeeding, support of breastfeeding in postpartum period, training hospital staff to support breastfeeding practices, and providing education, care, and nutrition to mothers to sustain breastfeeding and manage breastfeeding-related problems.

Mothers should be counseled to follow healthy infant practices and practice *active feeding*. Active feeding means encouraging the child to eat. The child should have her/his own serving and until the child can feed herself/himself, the mother or another caregiver should sit with the child during meals and help her/him feed. Mothers should also be counseled to continue feeding the child during illness. All children should have a longitudinal record of weight and preferably also of length/height. This is even more important for children with underlying systemic conditions (organic causes) in whom regular growth monitoring should be performed at follow-up visits with addressing their medical concerns. Optimum nutrition given as a component of overall nurturing care, comprising good practices in health, nutrition, safety and security, responsive caregiving, and early learning opportunities helps achieve optimum growth and development of children.[6]

Physical and emotional well-being of the mother/caregiver is equally important and the mother and infant should be treated as an inter-dependent pair for both to survive and thrive. Current evidence indicates greater inclusion of mothers in more holistic packages of care for small and nutritionally at-risk infants aged <6 months to optimize infant survival and growth.

TABLE 3.4.1: Causes of growth faltering.[5]

Anthropometric parameter first affected	*Etiology*
Weight	• Increased metabolism—sepsis, urinary tract infection, congenital heart disease, malignancy, CKD, and RTA • Increased loss—malabsorption, chronic diarrhea, cholestasis, chronic liver disease, and parasitic infestations (giardiasis) • Decreased intake—preterm/SGA, neuromuscular disorders, psychosocial deprivation, and GERD
Weight with length with/without head circumference	• Genetic syndromes—chromosomal disorders, microdeletion syndromes • Intrauterine infections • Prolonged inadequately managed chronic systemic illnesses • Cerebral malformations

(CKD: chronic kidney disease; GERD: gastroesophageal reflux disease; RTA: renal tubular acidosis; SGA: small-for-gestational age)
Source: Adapted from reference Franceschi et al., 2021.

TABLE 3.4.2: Clinical approach to a child with growth faltering.

History	*Pointers*	*Inference/significance*
Present illness	Ask current complaints, if any	New onset infection may predispose to systemic complications in growth faltering, will influence feeding and rehabilitation plan
Antenatal history	Maternal prepregnancy health status and any comorbidities, medical complications during pregnancy (preeclampsia, anemia, intrauterine infections)	Poor intrauterine growth leading to low birth weight, poor postnatal growth±
	Maternal substance abuse	Predisposition to low birth weight and poor postnatal growth
Birth details	Birth weight, gestation, and perinatal details	• Growth parameters to be corrected for gestation in preterm babies • Perinatal complications like birth asphyxia, sepsis, etc., may impact growth and feeding in early infancy or may be associated with a systemic condition for growth faltering
Feeding history	Breastfeeding	• Lack of exclusive breastfeeding increases risk of growth faltering • Replacement/mixed feeding is associated with higher risk of gastrointestinal infections and inadequate nutrition
	Complementary feeding	• Adequacy in terms of quality and quantity to be ascertained • Responsive feeding practices
	Feeding during current illness	Presence of "poor feeding" and "vomiting everything" are danger signs and indicate need for admission
Developmental history	Attainment of age-appropriate milestones	• Delayed or failure to gain new milestones may be seen in growth faltering, intrauterine infections, or certain syndromes • Regression of motor milestones may occur with associated muscle weakness • Regression in two or more domains should alert toward neurological disorders
Family history	Birth order, status of parents and siblings, any unexplained deaths, and history of communicable diseases in family	• Birth order and family size to identify socio-demographic risk factors • Parental health and occupation (access to resources), parental affection or neglect • Status of siblings to check for inherited disorders
Growth pattern	Growth pattern and trajectory by review of available previous weight and length records	• Growth failure since early infancy may suggest organic cause • Onset around 6–8 months of age may suggest poor complementary feeding. Recent onset of growth failure prompts the need to investigate systemic disorders
Systemic history	History of any systemic complaints, previous hospitalizations, and prolonged administration of drugs	• Recurrent infections indicate possible immunodeficiency • Recurrent loose stools indicate possible malabsorption • Recurrent lower respiratory infections indicate possibility of congenital heart diseases, airway or lung malformations • Recurrent vomiting is a pointer to likely inborn errors of metabolism/uremia • Rash may indicate immunodeficiency or inflammatory conditions • History of blood transfusions, abdominal distension (organomegaly) indicate storage disorders/bone marrow failure • Seizures and delayed milestones are a pointer to neurological disorders
Examination		
Vitals	Check temperature, heart rate, respiratory rate, and perfusion, look for presence of danger signs	• Identify hypothermia or shock in infection/sepsis/SIRS • Identify disturbance in heart rhythm if associated dyselectrolytemia • Presence of lethargy indicates serious sickness
Anthropometry	Measure weight, length, head circumference, mid-upper arm circumference	Interpretation of serial trends of weight and length on standard growth charts help understand nature, duration and possible cause of growth faltering
General and systemic examination	Cues toward specific disease	Specific and detailed examination to check systemic disease/congenital malformations/ specific syndromes. Loss of subcutaneous fat, micronutrient deficiencies to be checked in all children with growth faltering
Laboratory		
Laboratory tests	Check for nutritional deficiency and electrolyte disturbances in all, other investigations as clinically indicated	• Total protein, serum albumin, hemoglobin, blood sugar, serum sodium, potassium, calcium, renal and liver function tests • In the presence of fever/suspected infection, sepsis screen (leukocyte count, C-reactive protein, and blood culture) to be sent

Treatment of Growth Faltering

The management of growth faltering is primarily to identify and treat the underlying cause. The organic causes should be appropriately treated as required.

The most important step in management of growth faltering is nutritional rehabilitation. The family unit should be assessed for food safety, procurement, and choices. Faulty feeding practices should be identified and addressed in these children. The amount of intake and practice of feeding (responsive or coercive) should be noted. Parents should be encouraged to provide culturally acceptable home-based foods with high nutritive value to children.[7]

Once the etiology of growth faltering has been ascertained, most of the affected children can be managed at home with nutritional interventions along with management of comorbidities and underlying illness.

Inpatient management is indicated for children who are severely undernourished, in whom etiology cannot be ascertained on outpatient evaluation, and those exhibiting danger signs. Some of them may need a trial of assisted feeding using cup and spoon or tube feeding. A feeding gastrostomy tube may be required in those with persistent feeding issues (difficulty swallowing, or tongue thrust), those who fail to show catch-up in weight on cup-spoon feeds, those where cup-spoon feeding is not feasible (cleft palate, or respiratory distress), and in children with neurological conditions (global developmental delay, or cerebral palsy). All affected children need love and support for which parents and caregivers should be counseled and encouraged.

Breastfeeding support is an effective intervention in young infants. The diet plan should focus on adequate supplementation of micronutrients such as iron, calcium, zinc, and vitamins to ensure wholesome growth. These can be provided through home-based diet, but may need supplements for a brief duration. The WHO recommendations for management of acute malnutrition are discussed in Chapter 5.4.

CONCLUSION

Growth faltering during early childhood is associated with a high morbidity and mortality as well as long-term impact on development and stature. Growth monitoring is an essential tool to detect early growth faltering. The causes of growth faltering are usually multifactorial. The treatment is primarily nutritional rehabilitation with treatment of any underlying medical illness. Both mother and infant should be nurtured together as an interdependent unit with provision of nutritional package and health promotion services such as breastfeeding under the overall umbrella of nurturing care practices.

REFERENCES

1. Sinha RK, Singh RD, Verma P, Basu S, Seth A, Kumar P. Mid upper arm circumference cutoffs for identifying underweight and severe underweight among infants less than six months: a hospital based cross-sectional study. J Prev Soc Med. 2023;54(1):29-35.
2. National Institute for Heath and Care Excellence (NICE) Guideline, UK. (2017). Faltering Growth - recognition and management. National Guideline Alliance, UK. London. [online] Available from https://pubmed.ncbi.nlm.nih.gov/28991420/ [Last accessed December, 2024].
3. World Health Organization. Child Growth Standards. [online] Available from https://www.who.int/tools/child-growth-standards/standards [Last accessed December, 2024].
4. Kumar P, Meiyappan Y, Rogers E, Daniel A, Sinha R, Basu S, et al. Outcomes of hospitalized infants aged one to six months in relation to different anthropometric indices—An observational cohort study. Indian J Pediatr. 2020;87(9):699-705.
5. Franceschi R, Rizzardi C, Maines, E, Liguori A, Soffiati M, Tornese G. Failure to thrive in infant and toddlers: a practical flowchart-based approach in a hospital setting. Ital J Pediatr. 2021;47(1):62.
6. von Salmuth V, Brennan E, Kerac M, McGrath M, Frison S, Lelijveld N. Maternal-focused interventions to improve infant growth and nutritional status in low-middle income countries: A systematic review of reviews. PLoS One. 2021;16(8):e0256188.
7. World Health Organization. (2023). WHO guideline on the prevention and management of wasting and nutritional oedema (acute malnutrition) in infants and children under 5 years. [online] Available from https://www.childwasting.org/normative-guidance [Last accessed December, 2024].

3.5 Abnormalities of Stature

Rajni Sharma, Sukanya Priyadarshini

INTRODUCTION

Stature abnormalities, usually short stature, are a common presenting complaint in pediatrics. On the other hand, tall stature is seldom a presenting complaint. Both short and tall stature may also be picked up during routine anthropometric measurements in a well or a sick child. This chapter presents the etiology and approach to a child with abnormalities of stature.

SHORT STATURE

DEFINITION

Short stature is defined as a height below 2 SD (standard deviation) or less than 3rd percentile for age and gender as per standard growth charts. One must use ethnic specific growth charts to diagnose short stature.[1] For Indian children, the World Health Organization (WHO) growth charts are recommended for ages 0–5 years and the Indian Academy of Pediatrics (IAP) 2015 growth charts are recommended for ages 5–18 years (refer to Chapter 3.3 for details). Children generally follow their genetic potential for stature. This can be determined by calculating the mid-parental height (MPH) or target height. The MPH for boys is calculated by taking an average of father's height and mother's height plus 6.5 cm and for girls; the average of mother's and father's heights minus 6.5 cm. The target height range (expected adult height) for a child is MPH ± 8 cm in boys and MPH ± 6 cm in girls. MPH must be checked in all cases of short stature and compared with the child's current height.

CHILDREN WHO REQUIRE EVALUATION FOR SHORT STATURE

Apart from those who fulfill the definition of short stature, certain children who are not growing as per expectation may also require evaluation.[2]

- Ideally, the height SD score of a child should lie within ±1.5 SD of the MPH SD score. If the child is deviating too much from his/her genetic potential, he/she too warrants an evaluation for short stature.
- The rate of height gain or growth velocity is also an important consideration and growth velocity charts for Indian children are available. If the growth velocity (monitored over 6–12 months) is less than the 3rd percentile for age and gender between the age of 2 years and the onset of puberty, it is considered abnormal and needs further evaluation even if the current height is in the normal range. A short child with height <–2 SD scores (SDS) with a height velocity <25th percentile (monitored over a 6–12-month period on the height velocity chart between the age of 2 years and the onset of puberty) also merits complete evaluation.
- Children normally grow predictably along their height percentile lines between the age of 2 years until the onset of puberty. Crossing of height percentile lines between birth to 2 years of age or during puberty may be a normal phenomenon. However, deviation from the previously followed percentile line between the age of 2 years up until puberty is not normal and points to a pathological cause of growth faltering.

ASSESSMENT OF GROWTH

Anthropometric Measurements

Supine length is measured by an infantometer in infants and children <2 years and standing height by a stadiometer in older children. The techniques for measuring height are detailed in Chapter 3.3. Measurements of weight, body mass index (BMI), waist circumference, mid upper arm circumference, and head circumference are often helpful in diagnosis.

The height and weight can be expressed as SDS or *Z*-score. This is calculated using the formula (The child's height minus mean height for age) divided by 1 SD of height for that age.

Body Proportions

Measurement of body proportions is essential in a child with short stature to know if he/she has proportionate or disproportionate form of shortness. For this purpose, upper segment to lower segment ratio (US:LS ratio) and arm-span to height ratio are measured and compared to age-appropriate values. The US:LS ratio is approximately 1.7 at birth, 1.3 at 3 years, 1.1 at 6 years, and 1.0 by 10 years. Arm span is less than length at birth by 2.5 cm and equals height at about 11 years. Thereafter, it is greater than height. An abnormal US:LS ratio or arm-span to height ratio indicates disproportionate short stature, possibly a skeletal disease or dysplasia. Children with achondroplasia have a normal-sized trunk with short limbs (increased US:LS for age), while those with spinal vertebral pathology (Pott's spine, spondyloepiphyseal dysplasia, etc.) have short trunk and normal limbs (decreased US:LS for age).

Growth Charts

The growth pattern of a child should be recorded both numerically as well as graphically using appropriate growth charts (refer to Chapter 3.3 for details). MPH should be plotted at the adult equivalent (18 years) on the growth chart. The child's current height can be extrapolated using his/her current height percentile line to predicted adult height **(Fig. 3.5.1)** which should ideally lie within the target height range. As mentioned, any deviation from the genetic potential for height requires further evaluation.

Pubertal Assessment

Pubertal assessment should be performed and the stage of puberty or sexual maturity rating recorded (*See* details in Chapter 3.2). The onset of puberty is associated with a growth spurt due to gonadal hormones and increased growth hormone (GH) levels. Thus, early (precocious) or delayed puberty will be associated with corresponding changes in height spurt, ultimately impacting the child's stature.

Bone Age Assessment

Assessment of bone age or the maturity of the bones is an important investigation in the evaluation of short stature and can give important clues regarding the diagnosis. A radiograph of the left hand and wrist is done for this purpose and the appearance of epiphyseal centers of phalanges, wrist, and carpal bones is compared with standard bone atlases (Greulich-Pyle atlas) or computed using Tanner Whitehouse method (TW2 or TW3) in which bones are assigned a score according to their maturity level. Alternately, computer applications such as BoneXpert can be used for digitally calculating the bone age.

ETIOLOGY OF SHORT STATURE

Short stature can result from a variety of physiological (normal variant) or pathological causes **(Box 3.5.1)**. Majority of children presenting with short stature are physiologically short; however, it is essential to rule out any pathology in all short children by proper clinical evaluation before labeling them as normal.[3]

Physiological Short Stature

Familial Short Stature

It is one of the most common causes of short stature. Both the child and the parents are short, and the child would have a height corresponding to the MPH centile or SD score (within ±1.5 SD). The child would have a normal growth velocity, appropriate skeletal maturation (bone age), and normal age at onset of puberty, ultimately achieving a final adult height corresponding to his/her MPH.

Constitutional Delay of Growth and Puberty

Some children physiologically lag behind in growth and skeletal maturation. They are short for their MPH with a delayed bone age and delayed onset of puberty (late bloomer). However, they demonstrate a normal growth velocity in childhood and no pathology is identified on clinical evaluation. There is often a similar family history in either parent being short height in childhood or attaining puberty late. These children are said to have constitutional delay of growth and puberty (CDGP). Children with CDGP normally catch up in growth after puberty and ultimately achieve a height appropriate for their MPH.

Pathological Short Stature

Chronic Malnutrition

Some of the most common pathological causes of short stature in Indian children are protein energy malnutrition and chronic diseases.[4-6] A calorie-deficient diet can affect growth adversely. While short-term (acute) undernutrition leads to deficits in weight, long-term or chronic undernutrition leads to deficits in both height and weight. Dietary assessment for calorie and other macronutrient intake is an important part of clinical evaluation of short stature.

Chronic Systemic Disease

A child with a chronic illness or infection may suffer from ongoing systemic inflammation and undernutrition that could affect growth. Usually, both height and weight would be affected resulting in short stature and wasting. In chronic undernutrition or chronic systemic illness, weight may be more adversely affected than height, and weight percentile may be lower than the height percentile **(Fig. 3.5.2)**. This would also be reflected as low weight for height/BMI. The systemic pathology can involve any organ system including respiratory (e.g., chronic asthma, bronchiectasis, cystic fibrosis, and tuberculosis), cardiac, renal (e.g., chronic renal failure and renal tubular acidosis), gastrointestinal (e.g., celiac disease and inflammatory bowel disease), or rheumatological

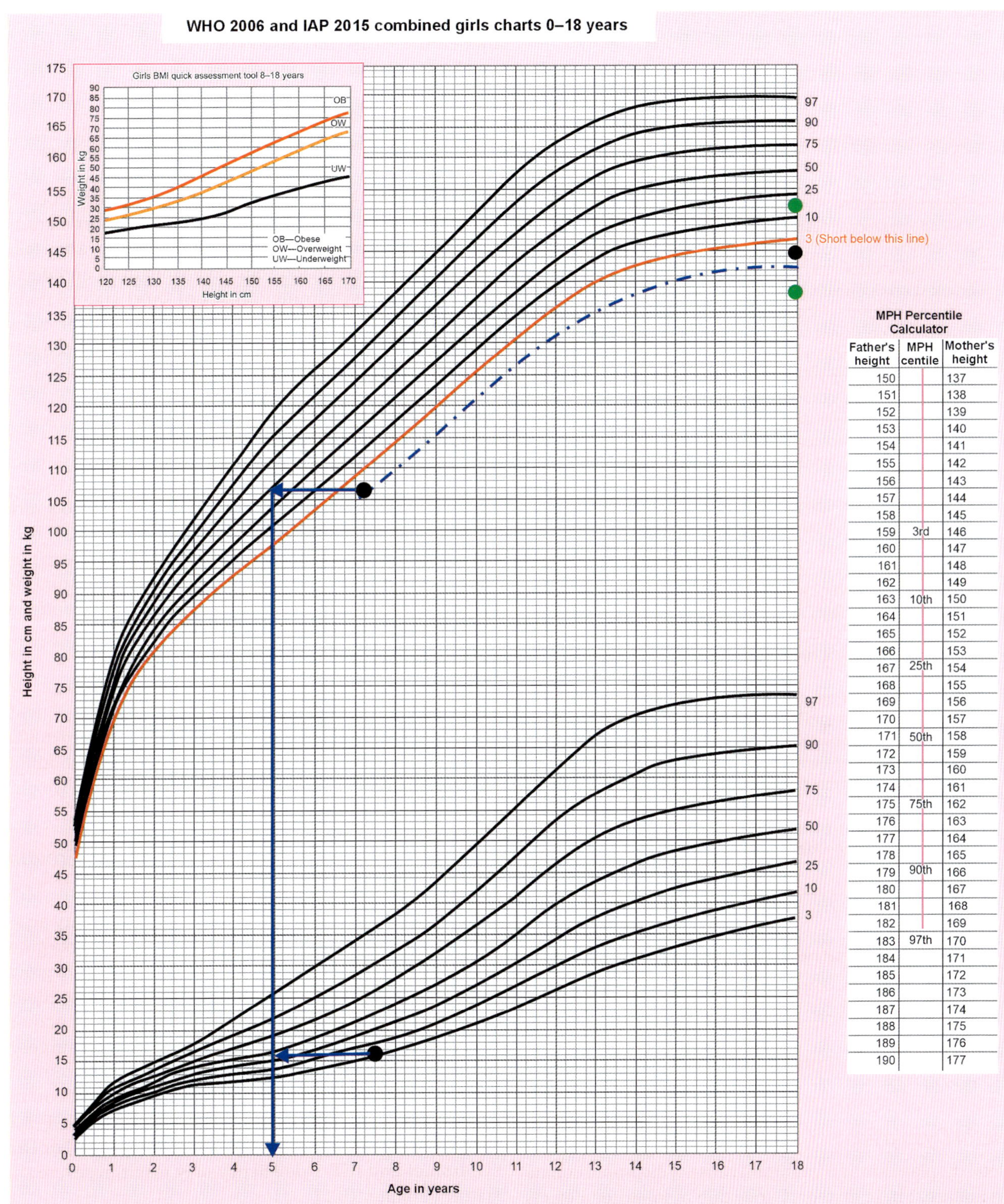

Father's height	MPH centile	Mother's height
150		137
151		138
152		139
153		140
154		141
155		142
156		143
157		144
158		145
159	3rd	146
160		147
161		148
162		149
163	10th	150
164		151
165		152
166		153
167	25th	154
168		155
169		156
170		157
171	50th	158
172		159
173		160
174		161
175	75th	162
176		163
177		164
178		165
179	90th	166
180		167
181		168
182		169
183	97th	170
184		171
185		172
186		173
187		174
188		175
189		176
190		177

Fig. 3.5.1: Growth chart of a 7-year 6-month-old girl presenting with short stature (height 106 cm; weight 16.6 kg). The mid-parental height (MPH) (145 cm) is plotted at adult height (18 years) and target height range is indicated by MPH ± 6 cm in girls. When the girl's height is extrapolated parallel to the centile lines, it lies within the target height range. She also has a bone age corresponding to her chronological age and normal growth velocity on follow-up indicating a familial cause of short stature.

BOX 3.5.1: Etiology of short stature.

- *Physiological (normal variants):*
  - Familial short stature (FGSS)
  - Constitutional delay in growth and puberty (CDGP)
- *Pathological:*
  - *Disproportionate short stature:*
    - *Skeletal dysplasia:* Achondroplasia, hypochondroplasia, and spondyloepiphyseal dysplasia
    - *Rickets:* Nutritional, metabolic
    - Mucopolysaccharidosis
  - *Nutritional causes:*
    - Nutritional disorders
  - *Chronic systemic disease:*
    - *Chronic infections:* Tuberculosis, chronic malaria, giardiasis, persistent worm infestations, and human immunodeficiency virus (HIV) infection
    - *Gastrointestinal disorders:* Celiac disease, chronic diarrhea, malabsorption syndromes, chronic liver disease, and inflammatory bowel disease
    - *Hematological disorders:* Hemolytic anemia
    - *Renal disorders:* Chronic kidney disease and renal tubular disorders
    - *Cardiac disorders:* Congenital cyanotic heart disease and chronic congestive cardiac failure
    - *Pulmonary disorders:* Cystic fibrosis, chronic asthma, and bronchiectasis
  - *Small for gestational age with poor catch-up growth:*
    - *Placental insufficiency disorders:* Gestational hypertension
    - *Intrauterine infections:* TORCH* complex
    - *Teratogens:* Alcohol, nicotine, and drugs
  - *Syndromic causes:*
    - *Dysmorphic syndromes:* Russell-Silver syndrome (RSS), Seckel syndrome, and 3-M syndrome
    - *Chromosomal anomalies:* Down syndrome, Turner syndrome, Noonan syndrome, Prader-Willi syndrome, DiGeorge syndrome, and Aarskog syndrome
  - *Endocrine disorders:* Hypothyroidism, Cushing syndrome, pseudohypoparathyroidism, and diabetes mellitus
  - *Defects in growth hormone-insulin-like growth factor 1 (GH-IGF-1) axis:*
    - GH deficiency
    - *GH insensitivity:* GH receptor defect (Laron syndrome)
    - IGF-1 deficiency
  - Psychosocial short stature

Note: *TORCH: Toxoplasma, Others (syphilis, mumps, HIV), Rubella, CMV and Herpes virus

(idiopathic juvenile arthritis) which would be apparent on clinical evaluation.

Skeletal Dysplasia

Skeletal dysplasias are an important cause of disproportionate short stature. These disorders arise due to inherited defects in cartilage or bone formation (osteochondrodysplasia). The most common among these is achondroplasia which results from an autosomal dominant defect in the fibroblast growth factor 3 receptor (*FGFR3*) which results in impaired endochondral bone growth. It is characterized by short-limbed dwarfism (increased US: LS ratio), lumbar lordosis and large head size.

Syndromic Short Stature

Various chromosomal disorders or genetic syndromes result in short stature. The most common among girls is Turner syndrome (45,X karyotype). The haploinsufficiency of *SHOX* gene located on X chromosome results in short stature in these girls, and they also manifest with primary ovarian failure resulting in hypergonadotropic hypogonadism and delayed puberty. Other syndromic causes of short stature include Down syndrome, Prader–Willi syndrome, Silver–Russell syndrome, and Noonan syndrome which can be recognized by their unique dysmorphology and associated problems.

Small for Gestational Age with Poor Catch-up Growth

Babies can be born small for gestational age (SGA) (weight or length < –2 SD for gestational age and gender) due to a variety of maternal, placental, or fetus related factors. SGA babies usually achieve catch up growth postnatally and reach their genetic potential by the age of 2 years. However, some SGA babies fail to have adequate catch-up growth and continue to remain short.

Endocrine Disorders

Endocrine problems such as hypothyroidism, Cushing syndrome, hypopituitarism, and pseudohypoparathyroidism (syndromic) may manifest with short stature in childhood. Usually, the height is more severely affected than weight in endocrine conditions **(Fig. 3.5.3)**.

Disorders of Growth Hormone-Insulin-like Growth Factor 1 Axis

Growth hormone produced by the anterior pituitary acts on the liver and bones to elicit production of insulin-like growth factor 1 (IGF-1) which is key for cartilage and bone growth. A deficiency of GH may result from developmental defects of the pituitary gland (aplasia or hypoplasia) or acquired causes (pituitary or suprasellar tumors, trauma, surgery or radiation). Craniopharyngioma, a benign developmental tumor of suprasellar/sellar origin is one of the most common causes of panhypopituitarism. Defects in the GH-IGF-1 axis such as GH receptor defect [GH insensitivity (GHI) or Laron syndrome] and IGF-1 deficiency may result in severe short stature (Chapter 16.1).

Psychosocial Causes

Physical growth in children requires not only proper nutrition and good health, but also a loving and nurturing environment.

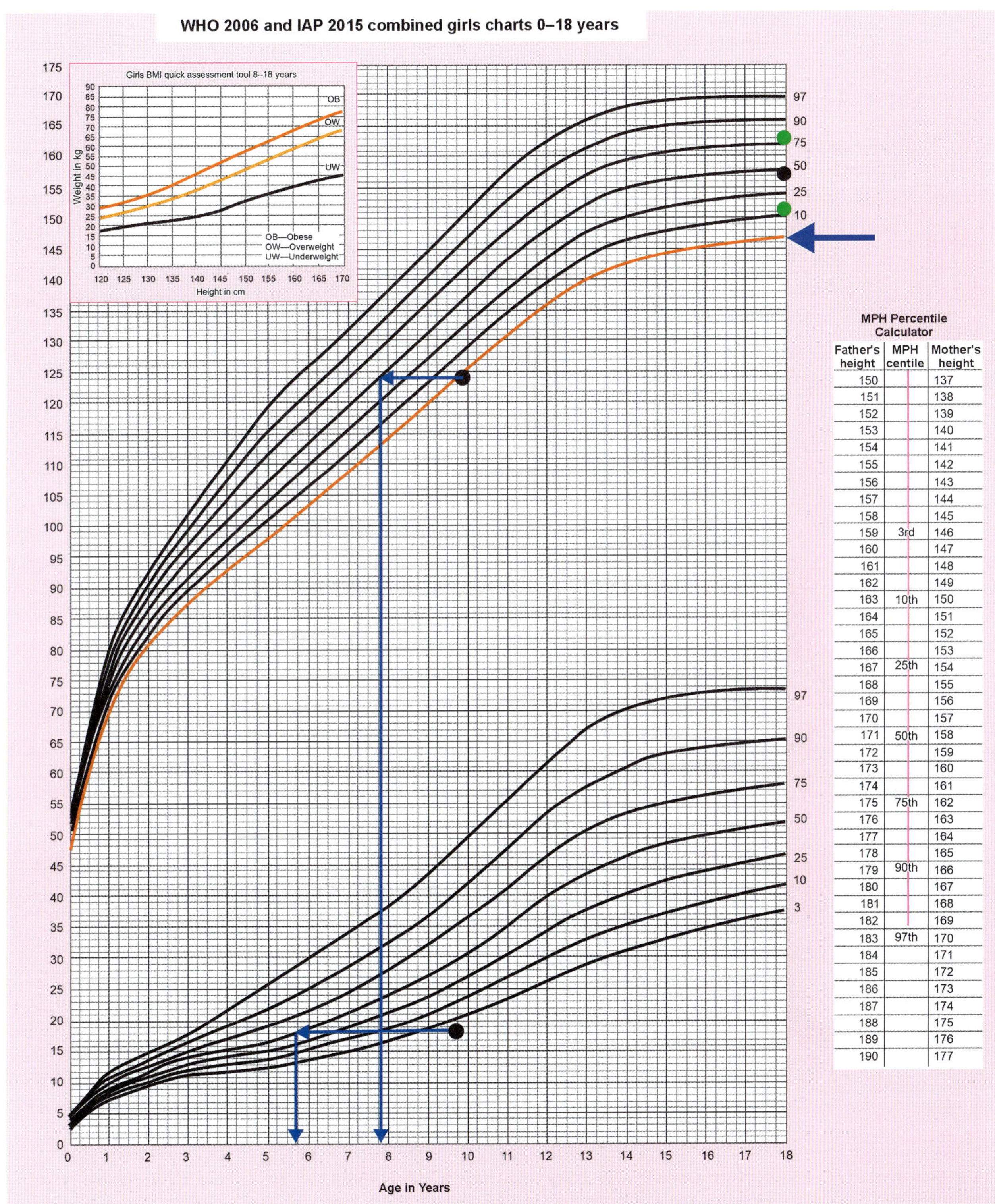

Father's height	MPH centile	Mother's height
150		137
151		138
152		139
153		140
154		141
155		142
156		143
157		144
158		145
159	3rd	146
160		147
161		148
162		149
163	10th	150
164		151
165		152
166		153
167	25th	154
168		155
169		156
170		157
171	50th	158
172		159
173		160
174		161
175	75th	162
176		163
177		164
178		165
179	90th	166
180		167
181		168
182		169
183	97th	170
184		171
185		172
186		173
187		174
188		175
189		176
190		177

Fig. 3.5.2: Growth chart of a 9-year 9-month-old girl presenting with short stature (height 124 cm; weight 18 kg). Her height is on the 3rd percentile and weight is less than the 3rd percentile. The mid-parental height (MPH) (157 cm) is plotted at adult height (18 years) and target height range is indicated by MPH ± 6 cm in girls. When the girl's height is extrapolated parallel to the centile lines, it lies below the target height range. It indicates a pathological cause of short stature. Since weight age is more affected than height age, it could be due to undernutrition or chronic disease.

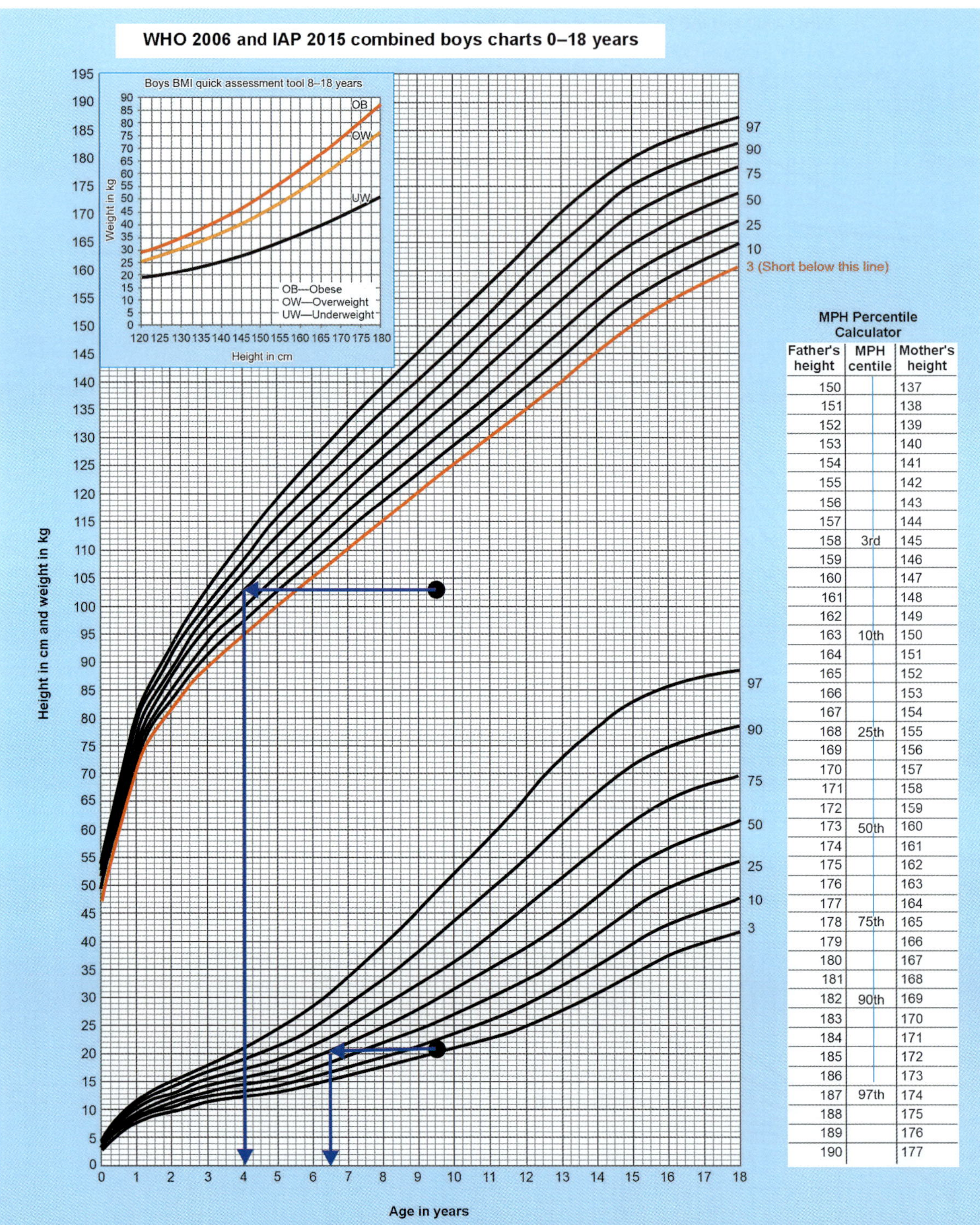

Father's height	MPH centile	Mother's height
150		137
151		138
152		139
153		140
154		141
155		142
156		143
157		144
158	3rd	145
159		146
160		147
161		148
162		149
163	10th	150
164		151
165		152
166		153
167		154
168	25th	155
169		156
170		157
171		158
172		159
173	50th	160
174		161
175		162
176		163
177		164
178	75th	165
179		166
180		167
181		168
182	90th	169
183		170
184		171
185		172
186		173
187	97th	174
188		175
189		176
190		177

Fig. 3.5.3: Growth chart of a 9.5-year boy presenting with short stature (height 104 cm; weight 20 kg). His height is way below 3rd percentile and weight is at 3rd percentile (height age more affected than weight age). He had a history of breech delivery, neonatal jaundice, and hypoglycemic seizures. He was diagnosed to have growth hormone (GH) deficiency on GH stimulation test.

A child staying in a threatening or abusive environment may suffer from psychological morbidities that could cause neurosecretory defects in pituitary GH secretion resulting in poor growth and short stature.

CLINICAL AND LABORATORY EVALUATION

An algorithmic approach to diagnosis of short stature is given in **Flowchart 3.5.1**.

Clinical History[7,8]

One needs to elicit the age at which the poor growth was first noticed and whether it affected the height, weight, or both. A detailed history needs to be taken for any systemic complaints including recurrent or chronic fever or features of systemic involvement: respiratory (cough, breathing difficulty, or chest pain), cardiac (palpitations, cyanosis, or edema), renal (dysuria, polyuria, or polydipsia), gastrointestinal (chronic diarrhea, pain abdomen, constipation, blood/mucus in stools, or jaundice), rheumatological (arthralgia, rash, or alopecia), hematological (anemia, recurrent blood transfusions, or bleeding for any site), and neurological (headache, seizures, projectile vomiting, or vision problems). Neurological problems may suggest an intracranial tumor. A history of lethargy, constipation, and cold intolerance would suggest hypothyroidism. The past history should include details of previous illnesses/hospitalizations, any history of head trauma or radiation, and a detailed drug history (including use of corticosteroids).

The antenatal history including infections, exposure to drugs/teratogens, and fetal growth is important. Birth details including gestation, birth weight, mode of delivery (breech delivery predisposes to GH deficiency), occurrence of pronged jaundice, and seizures or hypoglycemia in the neonatal period would suggest hypopituitarism. Congenital hypothyroidism is another cause of prolonged neonatal jaundice. Delayed developmental milestones may point to congenital hypothyroidism or syndromic short stature.

A detailed family history including the presence of short stature in parents, relatives, or siblings; and details of puberty in the parents (age at attainment of menarche in mother and age of shaving in father) should be recorded. If either parent had a delayed onset of puberty and/or history of short stature

Flowchart 3.5.1: Algorithmic approach to evaluation of short stature.

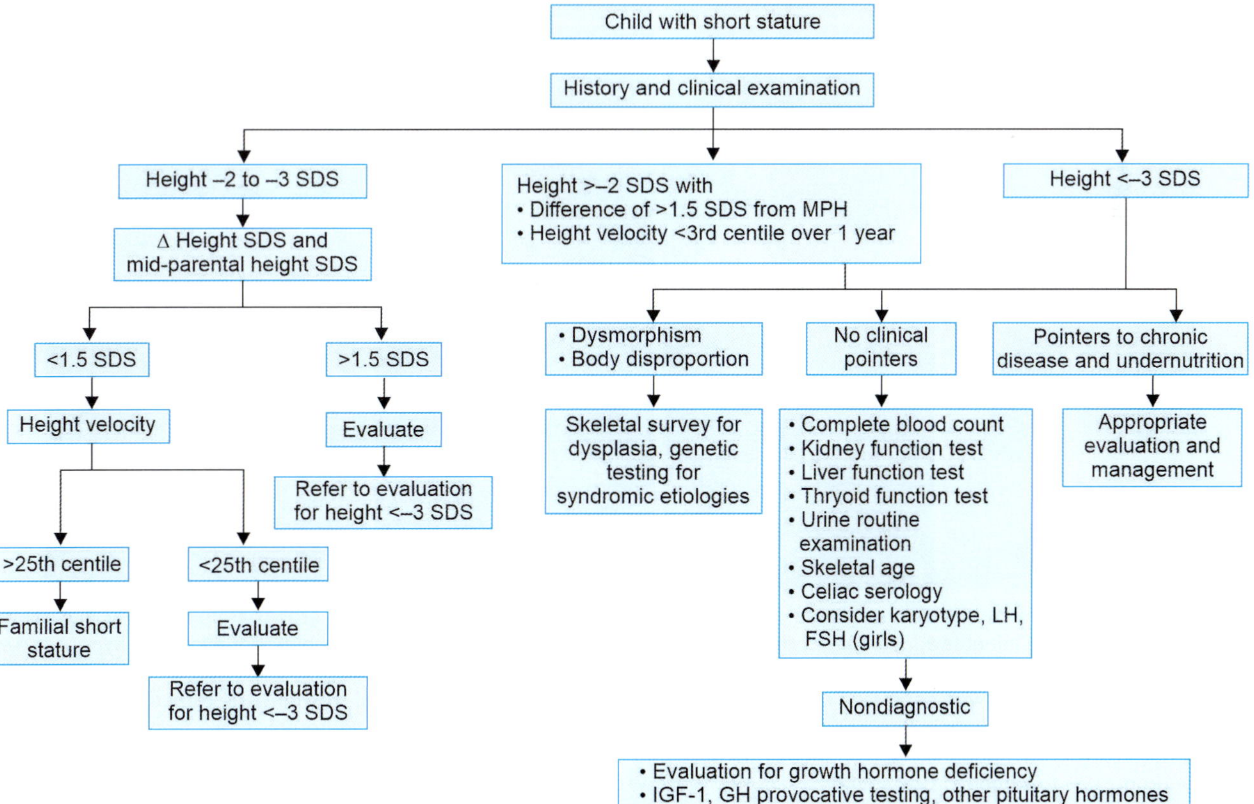

(FSH: follicle-stimulating hormone; GH: growth hormone; IGF-1: insulin-like growth factor-1; LH: luteinizing hormone; SDS: standard deviation score)

in childhood with normal adult height, it points to a diagnosis of CDGP.

Details of dietary history including energy and protein intakes are essential to rule out nutritional causes.

Examination

The assessed anthropometric parameters including height, weight, BMI and head circumference should be recorded on appropriate growth charts along with MPH. A low BMI or weight-for-height indicates undernutrition or chronic disease. Weight for height is generally normal in skeletal dysplasias and endocrine disorders. The child may even be slightly overweight/obese in endocrine disorders such as hypothyroidism, GH deficiency, and pseudohypoparathyroidism. Body proportions including US:LS ratio and arm span should be recorded. Disproportionate short stature is seen in skeletal dysplasia, rickets, congenital hypothyroidism, and some syndromes. Sexual maturity rating or Tanner staging is done in peripubertal children. Vitals including blood pressure should be measured. General physical examination can yield several clues regarding the underlying diagnosis. One should specifically look for anemia and signs of vitamin deficiencies which point to undernutrition, malabsorption, or celiac disease. The presence of goiter, signs of chronic diseases (icterus, cyanosis, clubbing, lymphadenopathy, and edema), facial dysmorphism, and neurocutaneous markers (neurofibromatosis 1) should also be carefully assessed.

The facies should be closely observed and may give important clues to diagnosis **(Figs. 3.5.4 and 3.5.5)**. Specific findings on systemic examination include the following:

- Children with *congenital GHD* are short and have a cherubic appearance, doll-like face, and micropenis. The presence of midline anomalies, such as cleft lip, cleft palate, or single central incisor tooth, crowding of midfacial structures, and abdominal adiposity, suggests the possibility of hypopituitarism. Visual field defects, optic atrophy, optic nerve hypoplasia, and papilledema are often associated with septo-optic dysplasia and

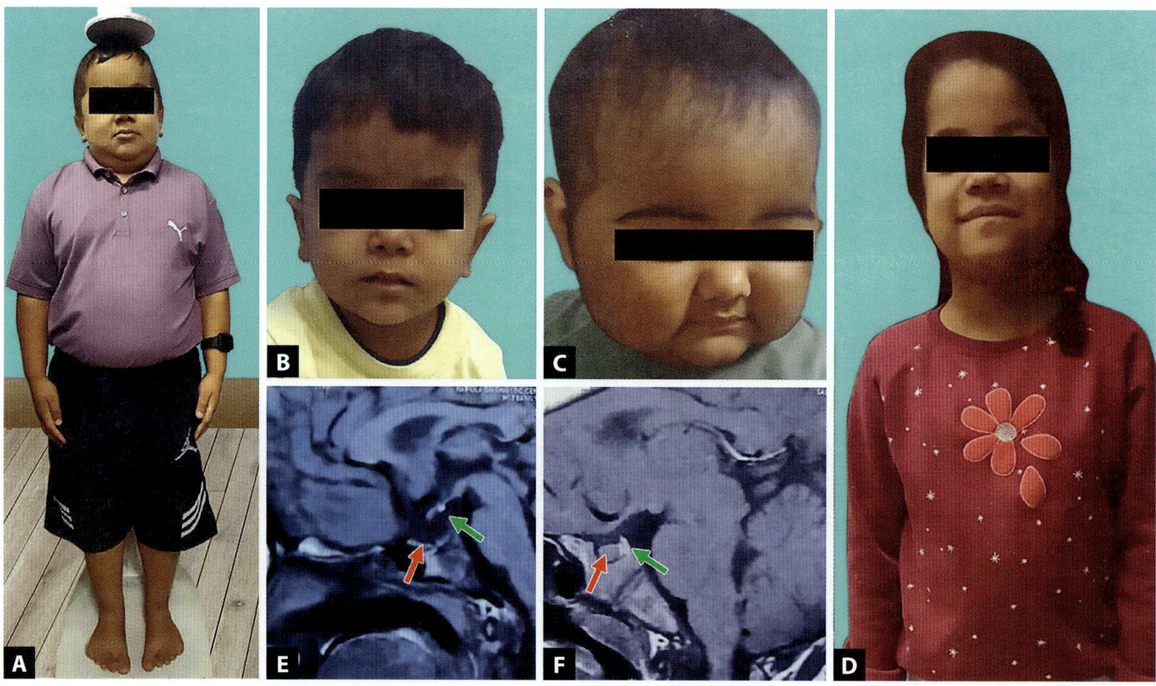

Figs. 3.5.4A to F: Endocrine causes of short stature. (A) A 16-year-old boy with short stature due to growth hormone deficiency. Note the short stature, cherubic and infantile appearance of the face, and truncal adiposity. The child also has hypogonadotropic hypogonadism as evidenced by the absence of secondary sexual characteristics; (B) A 4-year-old boy with stigmata of growth hormone deficiency. Clinical features are more pronounced with depressed nasal bridge, maxillary hypoplasia, and mid-facial crowding. He turned out to have growth hormone resistance due to a variant in the gene encoding the growth hormone receptor (Laron syndrome); (C) A 1.5-year-old girl presented with short stature. Note the moon like appearance of the face and the excessive hair growth over the forehead. The child has a case of Cushing syndrome due to adrenocortical adenoma; (D) A 13-year-old girl presented with short stature, a sallow complexion, and coarse and dull appearance. She was diagnosed to have primary hypothyroidism; (E) Pituitary magnetic resonance imaging of a patient with multiple pituitary hormone deficiency [note the empty sella (red arrow) and the ectopic posterior pituitary gland (green arrow). Compare it with the image in a normal patient with a well-formed anterior pituitary (red arrow) and normally located posterior pituitary (green arrow) (F).

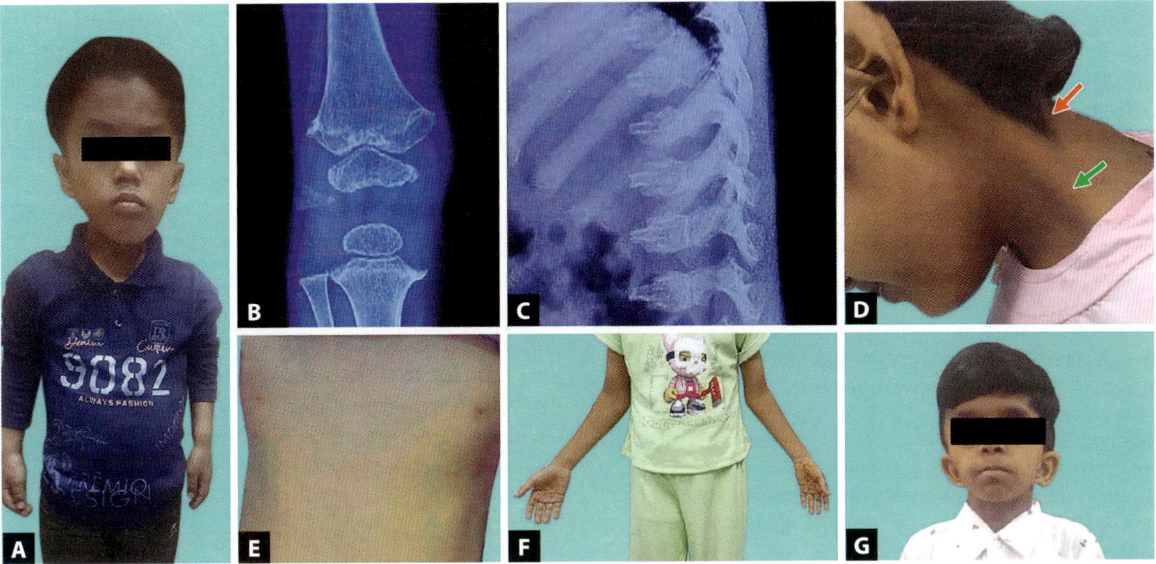

Figs. 3.5.5A to F: *Genetic and syndromic causes of short stature.* (A) Achondroplasia: Note the large head, midface hypoplasia, and extremely short limbs in a patient with achondroplasia; (B and C) Plain radiographs of the knee in a patient with skeletal dysplasia—note the small and ragged epiphyses and flared metaphyses of distal femur and proximal tibia. Vertebrae appear flattened (platyspondyly) with anterior protrusion; (D to F) Stigmata of Turner syndrome—low posterior hairline (red arrow), webbed neck (green arrow), shield chest, widely spaced nipples, and bilateral cubitus valgus; (G) Characteristic facial appearance of a child with Noonan syndrome. Note the triangular appearance of the face, the pointed chin, and low set ears. Not obvious on the image are ptosis and downward slanting palpebral fissures.

tumors of the pituitary-hypothalamic region. Children with *GHI* have almost all the features of GHD with more pronounced short stature and features of GHD (Chapter 16.1).

- *Acquired hypothyroidism* often manifests as short stature. Coarse facies, myxedema, dry rough skin, lethargy, bradycardia, constipation, and cold intolerance with delayed relaxation of deep tendon reflexes characterize hypothyroidism. Macroglossia, umbilical hernia, hoarse cry, and developmental delay may be observed in *congenital hypothyroidism* (Chapter 16.4).
- Cushing syndrome is characterized by central obesity, striae, hypertension, and proximal muscle weakness. Sometimes, growth retardation may be its only presenting feature in childhood (Chapter 16.7).
- *Pseudohypoparathyroidism* manifests with short stature, round facies, central obesity, short fourth metacarpals and mental subnormality, hypocalcemic tetany or seizures, cataract, and calcification of the basal ganglia.
- *Turner syndrome* may present in girls as isolated short stature. It is characterized by the presence of short stature, webbed neck, shield chest, wide carrying angle, widely spaced nipples, and lymphedema with characteristic cardiac, renal, and skeletal defects. Girls with Turner syndrome have primary ovarian failure resulting in delayed puberty.
- *Down syndrome,* a common cause of neurocognitive disability, is characterized by short stature with characteristic facies including mongoloid slant of the eyes.
- *Russell–Silver syndrome (RSS)* is characterized by intrauterine growth restriction (IUGR), small triangular facies, comparatively large head size, feeding difficulties in infancy, hemihypertrophy, and clinodactyly.

Investigations

If the clinical evaluation suggests a cause for short stature, the appropriate confirmatory test should be performed. Many a times, children with short stature present with no other abnormality on history and examination. Thus, in all cases of significant short stature with a low growth velocity and/or delayed bone age, it is advisable to perform a battery of screening investigations to diagnose some of the important causes **(Box 3.5.2)**.

Estimation of bone age is the first vital step in the diagnosis of short stature. Most children with CDGP, nutritional disorders, and chronic diseases have mild delay, whereas children with endocrinopathies such as GHD and hypothyroidism have significantly delayed bone age. Bone age is appropriate for chronological age in skeletal dysplasia and Turner syndrome. Additional findings that may be picked up on hand radiographs include 4th or 5th metacarpal shortening, a feature of Turner syndrome and pseudohypoparathyroidism. Madelung deformity (dorsal and radial bowing of the radius) may be present in some

BOX 3.5.2: Laboratory evaluation for short stature.

Level 1 tests:

- *Hematological tests:* Hemoglobin, hematocrit, red cell indices, total and differential leukocyte counts, peripheral blood cell morphology, and ESR
- *Blood chemistry:* Fasting blood glucose, renal function (urea, creatinine, sodium, potassium, and chloride), bone profile (calcium, phosphorus, and alkaline phosphatase), liver function (total protein, albumin, and transaminases), iron profile, and venous blood gas
- *Urinalysis:* pH, specific gravity, osmolality, microscopy, protein, and glucose
- *Stool examination:* Microscopy for parasitic infections, occult blood/mucus (inflammatory bowel disease), and fat globules for malabsorption
- *Radiology:*
  - X-ray left hand and wrist AP for bone age
  - X-ray chest, if tuberculosis or cardiorespiratory disease is suspected.
- *Thyroid hormones—T3, T4, and TSH*
- *Celiac disease screen (antiendomysial and tissue transglutaminase antibodies, IgA levels)*

Level 2 tests (For specific diagnosis):

- *Skeletal survey* (for skeletal dysplasia)
- *Karyotype in females (*for Turner syndrome)
- *Tests for hypothalamic-pituitary axis:* IGF-1, IGFBP-3, and dynamic GH testing, X-ray skull for sellar abnormalities and suprasellar calcification, CT/MRI brain, tests for other pituitary hormones

(CT: computed tomography; ESR: erythrocyte sedimentation rate; FSH: follicle-stimulating hormone; GH: growth hormone; IgA: immunoglobulin A; IGFBP-3: insulin-like growth factor-binding protein 3; IGF-1: insulin-like growth factor-1; MRI: magnetic resonance imaging; TSH: thyroid-stimulating hormone)

cases of short stature associated with homeobox gene (*SHOX*) variation and Turner syndrome.

First-line screening tests in short stature include complete blood counts with erythrocyte sedimentation rate (ESR), renal function tests (blood urea, creatinine, and electrolytes), liver function tests, and urine and stool analysis. Other tests include thyroid function tests, celiac screen, and venous blood gas (for renal tubular disorders).

Second-line tests are undertaken if the clinical suspicion points to an etiology and include karyotype in girls (for Turner syndrome) and skeletal survey for evaluation of skeletal dysplasia. For suspicion of GHD, measurement of IGF-1 is useful as a screening test. In case IGF-1 levels are low, GH levels should be checked. Since GH is secreted in a pulsatile manner from the pituitary, measurement of GH in a random blood sample is not reliable and stimulated GH levels should be checked. Various agents can stimulate GH production from the pituitary and include insulin, clonidine, arginine, etc. A GH level <7–10 ng/mL following stimulation indicates impaired pituitary secretion. Details of GHD and insufficiency are given in Chapter 16.1. Other investigations for hypopituitarism include thyroid functions, basal gonadotropins (especially in older children), prolactin, and morning cortisol along with pituitary magnetic resonance imaging. Specialized genetic testing should be considered if a genetic cause is suspected.

MANAGEMENT

After the initial visit, the family should be counseled regarding the importance of a balanced diet with adequate calories and proteins including macro- and micronutrients, coupled with regular physical exercise and adequate sleep. Children with malnutrition should receive appropriate dietary therapy. Supplemental iron and vitamins are prescribed if indicated. Height and weight should be recorded and height gain assessed every 2–3 months. The importance of regular follow-up and monitoring of therapy should be stressed. The child should receive all immunizations as recommended.

Treatment of short stature essentially depends on the cause. He/she should receive the optimal treatment for the underlying systemic disorder. Specific therapy for chronic systemic disorders includes bicarbonate supplementation for RTA and gluten free diet in celiac disease. For most skeletal dysplasias, there is no medical treatment, even though GH has been shown to benefit some selected groups. Limb lengthening surgery is an option for some skeletal dysplasias.

There is no specific treatment for familial short stature (FSS) and parents can be counseled regarding the height prognosis. Children with CDGP may experience enormous anxiety and psychological distress due to short stature and delayed puberty in adolescent years, especially during peer group interactions. In such a situation, induction of puberty should be considered as a treatment option. Boys beyond 14 years of age may benefit from a short course of low-dose testosterone (50 mg testosterone intramuscularly every 3–4 weeks) and girls >13 years may be given low dose estrogen (ethinyl estradiol/estradiol valerate) daily for 3–6 months followed by reevaluation. This will trigger the development of secondary sexual characteristics and pubertal growth spurt. Hypothyroidism should be managed with replacement by levothyroxine.

Growth hormone is indicated in children with GHD. Recombinant GH is given in a dose of 0.16–0.24 mg/kg/week (1 mg = 3 IU) given daily subcutaneously, preferably at night, till adult height is reached. Side effects of GH are rare and include edema, benign intracranial hypertension, scoliosis, and slipped capital femoral epiphysis.[9] Children gain on an average 10–12 cm in the first year of therapy and 6–8 cm/year thereafter and can attain normal adult height.

Growth hormone is also approved to treat short stature in other conditions such as Turner syndrome, *SHOX* haploinsufficiency, end-stage chronic kidney disease, and children born SGA with poor catch-up growth.[10] Additionally, it can be used in children with Prader–Willi syndrome and RSS. It has been shown to be effective in some groups of children with CDGP and idiopathic short stature. The dose of GH used in these disorders is higher than that used in GHD.

In Turner syndrome, a combination of GH with low-dose estrogen (for pubertal induction) and/or oxandrolone (synthetic anabolic steroid) has been shown to produce excellent height gain.[10] Primary IGF-1 deficiency and GHI (Laron syndrome) may be treated with daily injectable recombinant IGF-1 therapy.

TALL STATURE

INTRODUCTION

Children who have a height above 97th percentile or >2 SD above the population mean for age and gender using country-specific growth references and/or above their parental target height percentile are considered to be exceptionally tall for the reference population.[11] Compared to short stature, referrals for tall stature are uncommon.

ETIOLOGY AND CLINICAL FEATURES

A list of common causes for tall stature is given in **Box 3.5.3.**[11]

- Tall stature can be either physiological or pathological. *Physiological tall stature* includes familial and constitutional tallness. These are usually evident early in childhood. Children with familial tall stature have tall parents and their height is appropriate for MPH. Children with constitutional tallness have slightly high growth velocity and often an advanced bone age. The management of physiological tall stature mainly includes reassurance to alleviate anxiety. Medical intervention is usually not necessary. Rarely, if the tall stature is a matter of psychological concern or predicted adult height is >2.5 SD, sex steroids appropriate for the gender may be given at the onset of puberty to achieve early epiphyseal fusion.
- Children with *exogenous obesity* may be taller for age, often with an advanced skeletal age and earlier onset of puberty, but the adult height is normal.
- Children with *precocious puberty* appear to be taller than peers due to the growth enhancing action of sex steroids. However, advanced bone age and early bony epiphyseal fusion result in final short adult height, unless treated early. Precocious puberty may be central or peripheral (congenital adrenal hyperplasia and McCune Albright syndrome) (*See* Chapter 16.3 for details).
- *Hyperthyroidism* is associated with tall stature, neurobehavioral changes, and rarely eye signs (*See* Chapter 16.4 for details).
- *GH excess:* Excessive production of GH by an acidophil adenoma of the pituitary gland or a hypothalamic tumor can lead to gigantism. It is characterized by tall stature with prognathism, increased soft tissue of hands and feet, broad root of nose, profuse sweating, hypertension, and glucose intolerance. The diagnosis is confirmed by detection of raised serum IGF-1 levels and lack of suppression of GH (levels <1 ng/mL) following administration of oral glucose, 1.75 g/kg. Treatment is done by transsphenoidal pituitary surgery.
- Some *overgrowth syndromes* such as Sotos syndrome, Beckwith–Wiedemann syndrome, and Weaver syndrome can lead to tall stature. *Sotos syndrome (cerebral gigantism)* is characterized by increased birth weight and length, macrocephaly and dolichocephaly, hypertelorism, and intellectual disability. It is caused by variation in *NSD1* gene.
- *Beckwith–Wiedemann syndrome* is an overgrowth syndrome characterized by macrosomia, macroglossia, visceromegaly, renal abnormalities, and embryonal tumors.
- *Marfan syndrome* is characterized by tall stature, arachnodactyly (long thin fingers), and long thin limbs with an abnormally long LS, resulting in arm span more than height. In addition, there may be hypotonia, hyperextensible joints, scoliosis, flexion contractures, dislocation of lens, and cardiac anomalies. It is caused by variation in the fibrillin gene (*FBN1*).
- *Homocystinuria* is an inborn error of metabolism of the amino acid methionine caused by the deficiency of cystathionine-synthase and characterized by developmental delay, ectopia lentis, skeletal abnormalities, and clinical features of Marfan syndrome.
- *Klinefelter syndrome* is associated with tall stature, abnormally long legs, gynecomastia, mental subnormality, and behavioral abnormalities with a karyotype of 47,

BOX 3.5.3: Etiology of tall stature in children.

- Constitutional tall stature
- Exogenous obesity
- Precocious puberty (at initial manifestation*)
- Hyperthyroidism
- Growth hormone excess—gigantism
- *Adrenal:* Adrenal tumor, congenital adrenal hyperplasia (poorly controlled*)
- *Overgrowth syndromes:* Sotos syndrome, Weaver syndrome, Beckwith–Wiedemann syndrome
- *Genetic syndromes with tall stature:* Marfan syndrome, multiple endocrine neoplasia 2B
- *Metabolic:* Homocystinuria
- *Sex chromosome abnormalities:* Klinefelter syndrome, Fragile X-syndrome

Note: *These disorders may initially present with tall stature, but ultimately lead to a short final stature due to bone age advancement

XXY. Other sex chromosome variants associated with tall stature include 47, XYY, 47, XXX, 48, XXXY, and 48, XXYY.

- *Fragile X-syndrome* has characteristic physical features such as long and narrow face, large ears, prominent jaw, hyperflexible fingers, enlarged testicles along with delayed development, mild-to-moderate intellectual disability, and hyperactive behavior. It is due to variation in the *FMR1* gene.

CONCLUSION

The effective management of growth disorders hinges on the diligent identification of affected children through an accurate anthropometric assessment. A meticulous history and thorough examination are crucial in guiding appropriate investigations. Utilizing growth charts, and assessment of body proportions, pubertal status, and skeletal age play essential roles. It is essential not to overlook readily treatable causes such as nutritional deficiencies, chronic systemic diseases, and endocrinopathies like hypothyroidism. Even in the absence of overt indicators, first-line investigations are indispensable to rule out potential causes.

REFERENCES

1. Cheetham T, Davies JH. Investigation and management of short stature. Arch Dis Child. 2014;99(8):767-71.
2. Polidori N, Castorani V, Mohn A, Chiarelli F. Deciphering short stature in children. Ann Pediatr Endocrinol Metab. 2020;25(2):69-79.
3. Badada SK, Bhansali A, Ravikumar P, Kochhar R, Nain CK, Dutta P, et al. Changing scenario in aetiological profile of short stature in India—growing importance of celiac disease: a study from tertiary care centre. Indian J Pediatr. 2011;78 (1):41-4.
4. Velayutham K, Selvan SSA, Jeyabalaji RV, Balaji S. Prevalence and etiological profile of short stature among school children in a South Indian Population. Indian J Endocrinol Metab. 2017;21(6):820-2.
5. Chowdhury SP, Sarkar TK, Haldar D, Taraphdar P, Naskar TK, Sarkar GN. Short stature in children: experience from a tertiary care hospital in Kolkata, India. Health. 2011;2(4):139-42.
6. Garg P. Short stature in Indian children: experience from a community level hospital. Sri Lanka J Child Health. 2004;34(3): 84-8.
7. Oostdijk W, Grote FK, de Muinck Keizer-Schrama SM, Wit JM. Diagnostic approach in children with short stature. Horm Res. 2009;72(4):206-17.
8. Patel R, Bajpai A. Evaluation of Short Stature in Children and Adolescents. Indian J Pediatr. 2021;88(12):1196-202.
9. Grimberg A, Divall SA, Polychronokos C, Allen DB, Cohen LE, Quintos JB, et al. Drug and Therapeutics Committee and Ethics Committee of the Pediatric Endocrine Society. Guidelines for growth hormone and insulin-like growth factor-I treatment in children and adolescents: growth hormone deficiency, idiopathic short stature, and primary insulin-like growth factor-I deficiency. Horm Res. 2017;86(6):361-97.
10. Vyas V, Menon RK. Management of short stature: Use of growth hormone in GH-deficient and non-GH-deficient conditions. Indian J Pediatr. 2012;88(12):1203-8.
11. Corredor B, Dattani M, Gertosio C, Bozzola M. Tall stature: a challenge for clinicians. Curr Pediatr Rev. 2019;15(1):10-21.

3.6 Obesity and Overweight

Anju Virmani

INTRODUCTION

Obesity is assuming epidemic proportions worldwide, and becoming a public health problem requiring urgent and sustained attention.[1] It is now not just a cosmetic issue, but a disease that causes impaired mobility and interference with daily living activities, serious morbidity, and premature mortality. Almost 50% of obese children become obese adolescents, and nearly 80% become obese adults. Onset in childhood increases the health burden of obesity and its consequences, with severe economic implications for individuals as well as societies. Since 2008, the plateauing prevalence in high-income countries (e.g., the United States, France, Switzerland, and Australia), perhaps due to aggressive preventive measures, has given hope it can be controlled if tackled at the societal, environmental, and individual levels. On the other hand, the rapidly rising prevalence in low socioeconomic status groups, in urban and rural areas, and in low- and middle-income countries like India is worrying. In India, the National Family Health Survey (NFHS) 2019–21 found that 4% of children under 5 years old are already overweight.[2]

BOX 3.6.1: Comorbidities of obesity.

- Hypertension
- Type 2 diabetes mellitus (T2DM)
- Dyslipidemia
- *Hepatic dysfunction:* Raised transaminases, fatty liver, gallstones
- *Polycystic ovarian syndrome*: With hyperandrogenemia and hyperinsulinism
- Sleep apnea
- *Mechanical problems:* Slipped capital femoral epiphysis, genu valgum, tibia vara, Legg–Calvé–Perthes disease, low back pain, scoliosis, and osteoarthritis
- Vitamin D deficiency
- *Psychological problems and eating disorders:* Feelings of inadequacy and being different; being stereotyped as greedy, clumsy, lazy, or worthless
- *Skin:* Acanthosis nigricans, intertriginous infections
- Renal dysfunction

Obesity contributes to several noncommunicable diseases (NCDs), especially hypertension, fatty liver disease, type 2 diabetes mellitus (T2DM), dyslipidemia, musculoskeletal disorders, and sleep apnea **(Box 3.6.1)**. These conditions have a more aggressive course than in adults. In Asians, they develop at a lower body mass index (BMI), requiring active screening and management. Much of the morbidity is related to visceral rather than peripheral fat and can be reversed with weight loss. However, managing established obesity is frustrating, as weight loss is difficult to achieve and to sustain; prevention is crucial. Whether managing or preventing obesity, the entire family *must* be involved, since it is impractical to single out the child to make drastic changes in diet and lifestyle. The goal of management is *not* the attainment of ideal body weight, which may be near impossible, but achieving and maintaining steady weight loss to the extent possible. Even 5% weight loss improves metabolic parameters significantly.

Clinicians can play a key role in preventing obesity and in reducing its health impact. Measuring and plotting sequentially the length/height and weight (and BMI) of *all* children during school annual checkups/medical consultations, and taking any upcrossing of centiles seriously, enables early preventive advice.

In almost all children and adolescents, obesity is "exogenous," mainly due to an imbalance between energy intake and expenditure. In 5–10%, it is 'endogenous'. It is important to distinguish the two conditions, as management differs.

DEFINITIONS

Body mass index = weight (kg) divided by height $(m)^2$ is the most commonly used parameter to quantify obesity for diagnosis, prevention, and follow-up, as it is easy to measure and correlates well with body fat and health outcomes. However, sometimes BMI may be misleading, e.g., in persons with high muscle mass, early or delayed puberty.

The traditional definitions in adults by the World Health Organization (WHO) and the International Obesity Task Force (IOTF), were *overweight* if BMI > 25 kg/m^2; *obesity* if BMI > 30 kg/m^2, *morbid obesity* if BMI > 40 kg/m^2, and *superobesity* if BMI > 60 kg/m^2. However, South Asians tend to be "thin fat," i.e., they have more body fat for the same BMI, more adverse body fat patterning, including abdominal adiposity, and higher cardiometabolic risk. So, their recommended cutoffs are *overweight* if >23 kg/m^2; and *obesity* if >27 kg/m^2.

In children, normal BMI changes with age. For Indian children and adolescents (5–18 years), the Indian Academy of Pediatrics (IAP) recommends using the *IAP BMI charts* devised in 2015 to follow the BMI 23 and 27 kg/m^2 adult-equivalents, to diagnose overweight and obesity, as they are more appropriate for our population than WHO charts. *Extended IAP BMI charts* have since been devised to include class 2 and 3 obesity, based on 120 and 140% of the IAP obesity cut-off values, and await further validation. BMI calculation is cumbersome; to obviate this, IAP has devised *pediatrician-friendly growth charts* containing a *quick-screening BMI tool* for 8–18-year-old children (*See* Chapter 3.3.3).

Definitions of overweight/obesity in children are:

- *Overweight:* BMI > 85% [>1 SD (standard deviation)] or weight for height (WFH) up to 120% of ideal for age and gender.
- *Obese:* BMI > 95% (> 2 SD), or WFH > 120% of ideal for age and gender.

Instead of using the term "morbid obesity," obesity has been further divided into:

- *Class 2:* ≥120 to <140% of 95% based on age and gender, or BMI ≥ 35 kg/m^2 to < 40 kg/m^2
- *Class 3:* ≥140% of 95% based on age and gender or BMI ≥40 kg/m^2.

In children <5 years of age obesity is defined in terms of weight for length/height (WFL/H). IAP recommends using WHO WFL/H charts, as there are no under-5-year IAP growth charts. The definitions in this age group are:

- *Overweight:* WFL/H ≥ + 2 SD (≥97%), but < + 3 SD (<99.9%)
- *Obesity:* WFL/H ≥ 3 SD, i.e., ≥ 99.9%.

Because BMI cannot distinguish fat from muscle mass, or visceral from peripheral fat, several other parameters have been suggested. The most widely studied are *waist circumference (WC)*, or *waist-hip ratio (WHR)*, interpreted according to age, gender, and ethnicity. These parameters emphasize visceral obesity, which correlates better with insulin resistance, hypertension, dyslipidemia, and cardiovascular risk.[3] For research purposes, dual-energy X-ray absorptiometry (DXA) is a sensitive and specific measure of body fat. Bioelectrical impedance analysis is less accurate and reliable.

PATHOGENESIS

The basic reason for obesity and its metabolic consequences is *disordered energy balance,* i.e., energy intake chronically exceeds energy expenditure. The excess is stored in adipose tissue. Several hormones (e.g., insulin and leptin) and nutrients (glucose and fatty acids) link the brain and gastrointestinal (GI) tract with the adipose tissue, influencing appetite, energy expenditure, and growth. A number of hormones stimulating appetite (e.g., ghrelin, cortisol, and endocannabinoids) and suppressing it (e.g., leptin, α-melanocyte-stimulating hormone, proopiomelanocortin [POMC]), insulin, serotonin, dopamine, glucagon-like peptide-1 (GLP-1) and glucose-dependent insulinotropic peptide (GIP)] are involved in the complex processes of energy intake and expenditure and maintenance of body weight. Many of them act via the melanocortin-4 receptor (MC4R) in the arcuate nucleus of the hypothalamus. Loss-of-function mutations of the *MC4R* gene cause severe obesity by disrupting hypothalamic appetite control centers and promoting binge eating. GLP-1 and GIP ("incretin" hormones) are secreted in the intestine and brain in response to the consumption of sugary foods or beverages and stimulate beta cells to secrete insulin. Their agonists (including liraglutide, semaglutide, tirzepatide, and similar compounds) are revolutionizing therapeutic options.

ETIOLOGY

While most obesity is due to an imbalance of energy intake and output, *endogenous obesity* could be due to several conditions, including genetic, endocrine, and medications. *Infantile obesity* is usually caused by *genetic causes,* which may be syndromic, monogenic, or polygenic. Monogenic disorders include mutations in the leptin-melanocortin pathway, e.g., MC4R or leptin receptor abnormalities, or leptin or POMC deficiency. Satiety pathways are disrupted, so hyperphagia is marked, and obesity starts early (usually in infancy) and is severe. There may be other clinical features like red hair or pale skin (POMC deficiency), retinal dystrophy, frequent infections, developmental delay, other endocrine abnormalities, such as adrenocorticotropic hormone (ACTH) deficiency, hypogonadotropic hypogonadism, and diabetes insipidus.

Obesity is a feature of several rare *syndromes* including Alström, Bardet-Biedl, Carpenter, and Cohen syndromes, recognizable by dysmorphia and other features. Prader–Willi syndrome (PWS) may present as small, floppy infants, who become increasingly obese with age due to polyphagia.

Endocrine causes, marked by decreased growth velocity, include hypothyroidism, Cushing syndrome **(Fig. 3.6.1)**, and pseudohypoparathyroidism. In craniopharyngioma, obesity is multifactorial and tends to worsen after surgery.

Other disorders that alter the finely tuned satiety mechanisms include *neurological causes* (intracranial tumors, inflammation, or trauma), depression and eating disorders, and drugs (e.g., glucocorticoids, antiepileptics, and antipsychotics).

Over 90% of obese children have *exogenous obesity,* growing in an obesogenic environment, worsened by their families' unhealthy lifestyle decisions.[4] Children born small for date (SFD) or large for date (LFD) are at higher risk of obesity later.

Increasing calorie intake, especially empty calories, is a major part of the problem. An expanding food industry, supported by aggressive advertising, is altering food choices. Use of JUNCS [*J*unk foods, *U*ltra-processed foods, *N*utritionally inappropriate foods, *C*affeinated/colored/carbonated foods/beverages, and *S*ugar-sweetened beverages (SSB)] is increasing. These hyperpalatable, convenient, ultraprocessed foods consist of simple carbohydrates (fructose, sucrose, and refined cereals), laced with high fat (often trans-fat), high salt, preservatives, and additives, and low in fiber and micronutrients.[5-7] Consistently strong correlations of obesity are seen with the consumption of SSB. Low awareness of what is good nutrition, with parents consuming unbalanced diets themselves, means children get poor nutrition (in utero onward) and poor role models. Food labels are often inadequate and/or misleading.

Increasing urbanization, poor town planning, and thoughtless building architecture are reducing safe areas to play, walk, run, or cycle; and longer distances to commute. Increasing obsession with academic achievements reduces

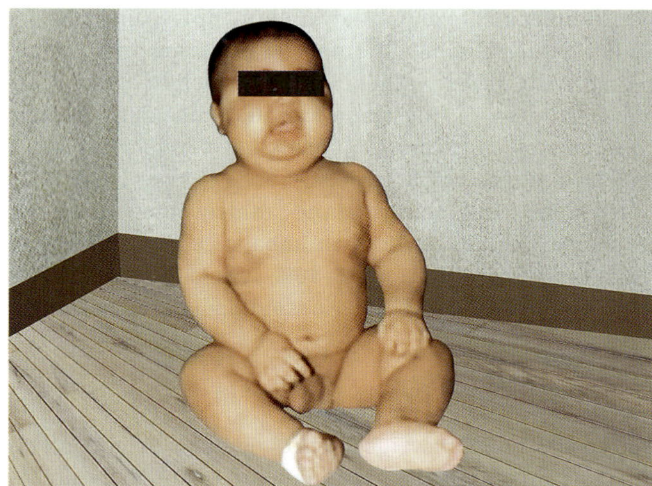

Fig. 3.6.1: An infant with Cushing syndrome. Please note that in infants, obesity may be generalized, unlike in children.

unstructured active playing time during and after school. *Increasing industrialization* is reducing the need for manual labor. The result: Sharply reducing physical activity for children and adults.

Increasing screen time is further reducing activity, while pushing wrong messages about food, thereby encouraging the intake of JUNCS. This is addicting and causes decreased physical fitness, poorer mental health, decreased self-esteem, lower school performance, and increased cardiovascular risk.

Genetic influences, seen in studies on adopted children and twins, do contribute. In general, obesity runs in families, as they share both genes and environment: 80% of children of both obese parents and 40% of one obese parent are obese/overweight. Important predictors include maternal obesity, excessive weight gain during pregnancy, prepregnancy/gestational diabetes and small or large for gestational age (SGA or LGA), especially with rapid weight gain. The "developmental origins of adult disease" concept links periconceptual, fetal, and early infant phases of life with a higher risk of obesity and metabolic consequences in adulthood.

CLINICAL EVALUATION

Ideally, rapid weight gain at any age should alert the pediatrician to advise preventive measures. Parents may present with concerns about weight gain, appearance, easy fatigability, darkening of skin (acanthosis), prominent breasts in young children or adolescent boys, or small penile size. Detailed history is important, as outlined in **Box 3.6.2**. Systemic symptoms such as breathing and vision difficulties should be asked for. Snoring indicates a need for sleep studies.

The examination should include *accurate* auxology **(Box 3.6.3)**, including *measuring* parents' heights and taking midparental height (MPH) into account. Acanthosis suggests hyperinsulinemia **(Fig. 3.6.2)**. Pinkish striae which appear with rapid weight gain should not be confused with the red striae of Cushing syndrome. Rashes in skinfolds and orthopedic problems often exist and can interfere with exercise programs. Careful genital examination is needed: the "small" penis misinterpreted as "hypogonadism," may be normal and buried in abdominal fat, not to be confused with true micropenis (stretched penile length <2 SD for age) seen in GH deficiency and some syndromes. Large breasts in an adolescent boy may be due to gynecomastia, lipomastia, or both. Assessment of the child's behavior and mental status is important. The obese child who is embarrassed, withdrawn, or has low self-esteem is less likely to exercise and more prone to binge eating. Clinical depression can interfere with management unless recognized and treated.

The *most important clinical feature,* distinguishing pathological from exogenous obesity, is *height and height velocity*. Children with exogenous obesity are taller than expected for age and MPH. Obese children who are shorter than expected, or have other red flags, should be carefully worked up for etiology, including endocrine causes. Fat distribution is truncal in Cushing syndrome but can be generalized in infants **(Fig. 3.6.1)**. Syndromic causes may have dysmorphism or other clinical findings discussed above. Children with hypothalamic satiety center abnormalities causing calorie overconsumption may be tall, but the onset of obesity would be early.

BOX 3.6.2: History.

Early influences:
- *Family history* (especially parents, grandparents, and others in joint families) of obesity, diabetes, hypertension, dyslipidemia, heart disease
- *Maternal diseases:* Diabetes, gestational diabetes, or hypertension; excess weight gain during pregnancy
- Birth weight, length, subsequent growth pattern
- Duration of breastfeeding

Diseases:
- *Central nervous system disease:* Headache, vomiting, visual disturbances, abnormal movements and school performance
- *Drug intake/topical application:* Most commonly steroids, anti-epileptics, antipsychotics, some alternative therapy medications
- Polyuria, nocturia, polyphagia
- Menstrual history, acne, hirsutism

Environment:
- *Diet details:* Recall of daily intake, frequency of junk food intake, total cooking fat intake by entire family per month
- Attitudes toward food, any eating disorder
- Details of daily activity patterns
- Availability of safe play areas
- *Duration of screen time:* TV, mobile phone, computer-including academic and nonacademic work
- Sleep duration, timing, regularity; snoring
- Intellectual development, school performance, any abnormalities
- Past attempts at dieting

BOX 3.6.3: Examination.

- Height, weight, and BMI
- Waist circumference and WHR
- Pattern of fat distribution
- Parents' heights, weights, and calculation of midparental height
- Blood pressure
- *Skin*: Striae, acanthosis, skin tags, acne, hirsutism, rashes in skin folds
- Dysmorphism, features of any syndromes, including detailed eye examination, including the retina, if indicated
- Features of endocrine disease (Hypothyroidism, Cushing syndrome, hypothalamic defects)
- Pubertal staging, including SPL and testicular volume in boys
- Distinguishing lipomastia from true breast buds in girls
- Orthopedic problems, including. Genu valgus or varus, deformities and rickets (pseudohypoparathyroidism)
- Self-esteem, behavior, and mental development

(BMI: body mass index; SPL: stretched penile length; WHR: waist-hip ratio)

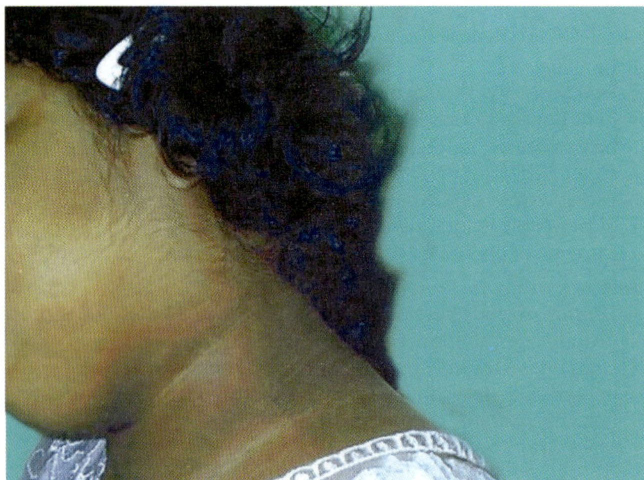

Fig. 3.6.2: Acanthosis nigricans seen as dark velvety areas at the folds of the neck in an obese girl.

LABORATORY EVALUATION

Investigations are guided by clinical presentation. The tall obese child, with normal height velocity and blood pressure (BP) (or mild hypertension), no dysmorphism or other red flags, somewhat advanced bone age (usually close to height age), is likely to have exogenous obesity. In such children, the Endocrine Society and IAP guidelines recommend *against* routine testing for causes of obesity (e.g., endocrinopathies), while testing *for* comorbidities, especially if >10 years of age.[8,9] This includes a fasting blood sample for lipids, transaminases, and blood glucose (BG), with or without a glucose tolerance test (BG 2 hours after an oral glucose load of 1.75 g/kg, up to a maximum of 75 g). Ultrasound for fatty liver or ovarian morphology may be needed. Sleep studies may reveal sleep apnea (obstructive, central, or combined). Vitamin D level may be useful, as deficiency is common; with definitely deleterious impact on the musculoskeletal system.

Needless tests can be misleading and should be avoided. Current IAP Guidelines do not recommend testing glycosylated hemoglobin (HbA1c), serum insulin, or cortisol. In the tall obese child, thyroid function and GH studies are not needed.[9]

On the other hand, the short/slowly growing obese child, often with retarded bone age, needs work up for etiology, including thyroid and adrenal function, and other tests as guided by the clinical examination. Features of any genetic syndrome mandate evaluation by a geneticist and appropriate genetic tests for prognosis and counseling. Children with steady weight gain from early infancy may have *MC4R* mutations, but the test is positive in <5% of obese children; a negative test does not alter the lifestyle aspects of management.

BOX 3.6.4: Prevention of obesity.

Family:
- Adequate breastfeeding, no force-feeding
- Ensure adequate low-fat milk and products; advise adequate, not excessive cooking fat, with saturated fat <10%, no trans fats
- Avoid processed/junk food, sweetened foods and beverages, fried foods
- Encourage fruits, salads, whole *dals*, and grilled/steamed animal products
- Encourage water as a drink, and homemade healthy drinks (*buttermilk, nimbupani, jal jeera*)
- Avoid missing meals
- Look for the calorie and carbohydrate content of packaged foods
- Encourage regular physical activity, at least 60 minutes daily
- *Controlled screen time*: Mobiles, TV, computers, and video games
- Do not use food for reward or punishment
- Express affection or approval in nonfood ways
- Avoid shaming behavior

Schools:
- No sugary or sports drinks, juices, or fried snacks available in or near school
- No high-calorie foods or snacks in school meals
- Offer fruits, low-fat dairy drinks
- Make daily exercise mandatory, ensure all children participate
- Identify, and counsel those at risk
- Specific counseling for those already obese
- Avoid shaming behavior
- Early referral if there is rapid weight gain

Community:
- Provide adequate, safe spaces for play
- Ensure cycle tracks on roads

PREVENTION

Given the protean damage caused by obesity, and the poor response to management, it is crucial to aim for prevention by guiding families and improving the environment to enable healthy lifestyles. Pediatricians should advise parents, and lobby actively with schools and society, to encourage space and time to play outdoors, reduce screen exposure, and minimize unhealthy foods and eating patterns. These messages must be started early, given consistently, and reinforced frequently, as they run counter to misleading advertising which influences societal attitudes. At the individual level, all children and adolescents should have weight and height measured and plotted at least annually. Those showing rapid weight gain (crossing percentile lines), especially in high-risk groups (SFD, obese parent/s or sibling/s, or taking certain medications), need family attention. The three windows of opportunity for obesity prevention are the first year of life, the period of adiposity rebound (age 3–7 years), and puberty, especially menarche. Diet control by the entire family (discussed further in "Management"), not "dieting" along with regular physical activity, is needed on a sustained basis **(Box 3.6.4)**. Diet changes alone, or exercise alone, are usually not adequate to prevent or manage obesity. *Consistency is critical.*

Important messages to parents include encouraging preconception normalization of the weight of obese parents, by increasing activity and reducing calorie intake themselves; encouraging parents to want children of normal weight rather than "chubby;" promoting breastfeeding; discouraging force feeding especially of SFD babies; and educating about balanced, healthy diet containing all necessary macro- and micronutrients. Each meal should contain protein (lentils, low-fat dairy products, eggs, and fish/poultry/meat) and fiber (vegetables and fruits). Central to these efforts is encouraging home-cooked food, and discouraging the use of packaged foods, i.e., JUNCS.

Parents and schools must encourage activity and discourage screen exposure. Under 5 years of age children need at least 180 minutes of physical activity daily; older children (and adults) at least 60 minutes of moderate to vigorous physical activity, preferably outdoors, including resistance exercises at least 3 days a week to strengthen muscles and bones. Activities should be safe, enjoyable, and sustainable; physical household chores can be encouraged. Understanding that exercise reduces fat, increases muscle mass, strengthens bone, and improves motor and cognitive development and psychosocial well-being, parents must follow this dictum for children and themselves.

In 2019, in its "Ending Childhood Obesity" plan, WHO recommended *nil* screen time for children below the age of 1 year, and *under 1 hour* for 1–5-year-old children. IAP Guidelines on Screen Time recommend the lesser the better: *nil* up to 2 years, *under 1 hour* for 2–5-year old, *under 2 hours* for 5–10-year-olds, with advice to the 10–18-year age group to balance recreational and educational screen time.[9]

Adequate sleep is necessary for weight control, proper physical growth and cognitive development. IAP recommends sleep of 11 hours (0–5 years), 10 hours (5–10 years), and 9 hours (>10 years). The American Academy of Pediatrics (AAP) Clinical Decision Support chart recommends "5-2-1-0" for the prevention of childhood/adolescent obesity: daily consumption of at least five servings of fruits and vegetables, screen time < 2 hours, moderate to vigorous physical activity (MVPA) at least 1 hour, and 0 intake of SSB.[10]

MANAGEMENT

Endogenous obesity needs treatment of the underlying cause: thyroxine replacement in hypothyroidism, GH in GHD, treatment of Cushing syndrome, etc. In syndromes and satiety center abnormalities, the management is as for exogenous obesity, though some new agents show promise. Setmelanotide, an MC4R agonist is being tried in POMC or LEPR deficiency; Alström and Bardet-Biedl syndrome.

Lifestyle modification remains the bedrock of managing exogenous obesity, aiming to lose weight in class 2 and 3 obesity and maintaining loss. Comorbidities must be looked for and adequately managed. Loss should be gradual (0.5 kg/month for toddlers, to a maximum of 0.5–1 kg/week for adolescents). The *entire family* has to be motivated to make *long-term* changes in diet and activity: treatment aimed only at the child/adolescent is unlikely to succeed. Small, permanent changes are more useful than drastic, short-lived ones.[7] Dietary measures, increased physical activity, reduced screen time, and sleep hygiene, supported by motivational interviewing and behavioral modification techniques, should be advised in detail, setting small, achievable goals. Considerable psychological support may be needed for the child and family. E-health methods often work with adolescents for awareness, motivation, recording, goal setting, and other behavior changes.

If basic lifestyle measures prove unsuccessful after over 6 months, referral is needed to a multidisciplinary team, consisting of pediatrician and pediatric specialists (endocrinologist, pulmonologist, dietician, and/or psychologist), working with the child, family, and school. Drug therapy is less frequently advised, but the advent of incretin mimetics and other effective drugs is changing the situation. Bariatric surgery was earlier the fallback option in class 3 obesity but may no longer be needed as often.

Dietary Advice

Diet advice should ensure healthy balanced intake, without extreme measures, for the entire family. Fat intake of <25% of total calories, protein of at least 15–20%, with 50–55% as complex carbohydrates, with adequate fiber, micronutrients, and plenty of water, should be encouraged. Carbohydrate quality is important: sucrose, high fructose corn syrup, and refined grains should be replaced by whole grains.[9,10] Nutritional deficiencies (iron, calcium, vitamin D, etc.) should be corrected and ongoing minimal supplementation given as required. Even with severe obesity, calorie restriction should be moderate, with adequate protein (0.8–1 g/kg/day), fiber and taking care to avoid eating disorders. Very-low-calorie diets (VLCD) (400–800 calories/day for 2–6 weeks) result in rapid weight loss and marked improvement in BP, BG, insulin, leptin, and lipid levels. However, they can be risky without close monitoring and adequate supplementation with minerals and vitamins, so they should be planned with careful supervision only in lifesaving situations, i.e., class 3 obesity, severe sleep apnea, or cardiopulmonary manifestations (Pickwickian syndrome). Stringent diets can hamper height gain, pubertal development, and bone health; cause irritability and behavioral problems, and often a weight loss plateau because of reduced metabolic rate. Long-term results are poor, with weight gain recurring within 1–5 years. In syndromes with abnormal satiety control, very careful attention is needed towards portion control and ensuring food is not easily accessible. This is often emotionally distressing for the family.

Principles of prevention **(Box 3.6.4)** should be strongly advocated, including encouraging intake of foods with low glycemic index (GI)—whole fruits, salads, unpolished rice, whole wheat, other coarse grains (e.g., millets), whole legumes, low-fat unsweetened milk and dairy products, variety of nuts and seeds in small quantities; plenty of plain water; and discouraging undesirable and "diet foods" or "health foods." Cooking and food purchase patterns should be discussed in detail and small changes made initially. Strategies such as "MyPlate" *(USDA choosemyplate.gov/ICMR-NIN My plate)* and "Traffic Light" can be helpful in making the family understand how to plan and consume a balanced diet. It is important to involve children in food purchases, cooking, and choices, maintain the joy of eating, and ensure food is not only healthy but also attractive and palatable. Family mealtimes (without screens) are helpful. Frequent eating should be avoided, as should large meals with long gaps, and missed meals—neither "grazing" nor "gorging." It is best to discourage sweetened drinks, juices, sugar-free desserts, chocolates, baked chips, etc. which usually have very high-calorie content; artificial sweeteners used in diet drinks and other products are also potentially harmful. While processed foods and excess cooking fat are restricted, fat must not be over-restricted: low-fat, high-carb foods have high GI (e.g., polished rice, potatoes, packaged cereals, bread, and other *maida* products, and zero-fat milk) and cause sharp BG and insulin spikes, which actually promote weight gain. At no time should diet restrictions be viewed as punishments.

Exercise

All physical activity increases energy expenditure and helps maintain good health and healthy weight loss; psychological well-being, better academic performance, lesser acne and hirsutism, regular menses, better lipid, BP, and insulin levels, reduced appetite, and increased metabolic rate (calorie restriction alone causes decreased metabolic rate).

Structured activity is important but can be challenging. A basically sedentary lifestyle, emphasis on studying, poor muscle strength and balance, deformities such as genu valgus, and even rashes caused by rubbing of thighs can impede exercise. Such factors should be identified and corrected. Compliance improves if an activity is incorporated into daily life (e.g., walking to school, and classes on different floors), is in groups, and is fun (walking with friends, swimming, dancing, and sports). Initially low impact (e.g., walking, swimming, and stationary cycling), moderate-intensity exercise (30 minutes × 5 days/week) can be advised, with a gradual increase in time and intensity to an hour or more daily of aerobics and strength training. Setting SMART (specific, measurable, achievable, realistic, and timed) goals helps.

Screen Time, Sleep, Behavior Modification and Social Support

As discussed for "prevention," reduction of *screen time* is recommended. Screen time increases weight directly by reducing time for physical activity and sleep; it also affects food choices, mental development, and mental health. Recreational screen time should be minimized.

Adequate, good quality *sleep,* at consistent timings, is essential while avoiding inadequate (and excessive) sleep. Parents, teachers, and the child must understand that adequate play and sleep are not time wasted, but crucial for growth, and physical, mental, and academic well-being.

Family-centered *behavior modification* strategies, such as maintaining diaries of food intake, activity, and screen time; motivational interviewing; and group activities ensure efforts are successful and sustained. Adolescents may be more enthusiastic about technology, e.g., mobile apps for diet or exercise monitoring, or motivational messaging.[11] Such devices can also be used for tracking behaviors and providing personalized feedback. Reasonable, clear goals must be set by the family and health personnel working together.

Occasional treats are useful to prevent frustration and dysfunctional behavior. Unhealthy family habits and disparagement of the child should be strongly discouraged. Initially, monthly reviews with reinforcement may be necessary. Yo-yo weight patterns are undesirable because each weight loss or gain cycle causes metabolic and psychological changes that make subsequent weight loss more difficult.

Treatment of Comorbidities

Associated problems **(Box 3.6.1)** should be carefully looked for and meticulously managed; including hypertension, liver dysfunction, dyslipidemia, T2DM, obstructive sleep apnea (OSA), polycystic ovary syndrome (PCOS), psychological, orthopedic, and skin problems.

Drug Therapy

Medication is considered if significant efforts at diet, exercise, and behavior control have failed over 6 months, as an add-on to these efforts, in severe grades of obesity and/or the presence of comorbidities, after age 12 years. Long-term safety is important and in children, safety data is limited.

Orlistat inhibits gastrointestinal lipases. Given at mealtimes, it decreases fat absorption by 30%, causing modest weight loss, and improving lipid and glycemic profiles; a benefit is not marked in severe obesity. Side effects include oil spotting, flatulence, frequent stools, and deficiency of fat-soluble vitamins, such as vitamins A and D.

Metformin, an insulin sensitizer, is not approved for weight loss but is indicated if the child has associated PCOS, T2DM, or prediabetes.

In children with POMC pathway defects, MC4R agonists are approved; in those with leptin deficiency, leptin therapy can be offered. Drugs such as sibutramine, topiramate, and octreotide have lesser safety profiles, lesser efficacy, little pediatric data; and are not approved. Recently, GLP-1 analogs (e.g., liraglutide, semaglutide, tirzepatide, etc.) have proved useful in adults and are being used in adolescents (above age 12 years) having received US Food and Drug Administration (FDA) approval.

Surgery

Surgical treatment should be considered only after significant efforts at diet, exercise, behavior control, and medical management have failed over at least 6 months, only as an add-on to these efforts, only in severe grades of obesity and/or the presence of significant comorbidities (OSA, liver dysfunction, slipped capital femoral epiphyses, hypertension, dyslipidemia, and T2DM), only after suitable psychological preparation, in children >13 years of age. Up to one-third of patients regain lost weight within 1–5 years.

SUMMARY

Pediatric and adolescent obesity is increasing worldwide, due to lifestyle alterations, with major health and economic implications. Endogenous obesity, marked by short stature and/or other diagnostic clues, needs to be distinguished from the far more common exogenous obesity. Efforts at prevention at all levels are crucial. Healthcare givers should push for societal changes at the community level while actively educating all parents about healthy lifestyles. The entire family should have a balanced healthy diet, aim for 60 min/day of physical activity, minimal screen time, and adequate sleep. Special focus on high-risk groups is needed—SFD/LFD babies, obese parents, single parents, only or precious children, chronic illnesses, and drug intake. Weight loss may be difficult to achieve and sustain, but a loss of even 5–10% results in substantial metabolic improvement, so high relapse rates should not discourage intensive attempts at weight loss by every family, provided by a multidisciplinary team. Comorbidities—including hypertension, T2DM, dyslipidemia, liver dysfunction, and sleep apnea—should be actively looked for and adequately treated.

REFERENCES

1. Betts SS, Adise S, Rezvan HP, Marshall AT, Kan E, Johnson DL, et al. Socioeconomic adversity and weight gain during the Covid-19 pandemic. JAMA Pediatr. 2023;177(10):1102-5.
2. GBD 2015 Obesity Collaborators; Afshin A, Forouzanfar MH, Reitsma MB, Sur P, Estep K, et al. Global Burden of Disease Obesity Collaborators Health Effects of Overweight and Obesity in 195 Countries over 25 Years. N Engl J Med. 2017;377(10):13-27.
3. Khan I, Chong M, Le A, Mohammadi-Shemirani P, Morton R, Brinza C, et al. Surrogate Adiposity Markers and Mortality. JAMA Netw Open. 2023;6(9):e2334836.
4. Bhattacharya S, Saleem SM, Bera OP. Prevention of childhood obesity through appropriate food labeling. Clin Nutr ESPEN. 2022;47:418-21.
5. Jardim MZ, de Lima Costa BV, Pessoa MC, Duarte CK. Ultra-processed foods increase noncommunicable chronic disease risk. Nutr Res. 2021;95:19-34.
6. Jakobsen DD, Brader L, Bruun JM. Association between Food, Beverages and Overweight/Obesity in Children and Adolescents - A Systematic Review and Meta-Analysis of Observational Studies. Nutrients. 2023;15(3):764.
7. Gupta P, Shah D, Kumar P, Bedi N, Mittal HG, Mishra K, et al. Indian Academy of Pediatrics Guidelines on the Fast and Junk Foods, Sugar Sweetened Beverages, Fruit Juices, and Energy Drinks. Indian Pediatr. 2019;56(10):849-63.
8. Styne DM, Arslanian SA, Connor EL, Farooqi IS, Murad MH, Silverstein JH, et al. Pediatric Obesity-Assessment, Treatment, and Prevention: An Endocrine Society Clinical Practice Guideline. J Clin Endocrinol Metab. 2017;102(3):709-57.
9. Khadilkar VV, Shah N, Harish R, Ayyavoo A, Bang A, Basu S, et al. Indian Academy of Pediatrics Revised (2023) Guidelines on evaluation, prevention and management of childhood obesity. Indian Pediatr. 2023;60(12):1013-31.
10. Hampl SE, Hassink SG, Skinner AC, Armstrong SC, Barlow SE, Bolling CF, et al. Clinical Practice Guidelines for the Evaluation and Treatment of Children and Adolescents with Obesity. Pediatrics. 2023;151(2):e2022060640.
11. Ek A, Brissman M, Nordin K, Eli K, Nowicka P. A long-term follow-up of treatment for young children with obesity: a randomized controlled trial. Int J Obes (Lond). 2023;47(11):1152-60.

SECTION

Development and Developmental Disorders

Section Editor: Samir Hasan Dalwai

4.1 Normal Development

(Gp Capt) Kanwaljit S Multani, S Sachidananda Kamath

INTRODUCTION

Growth and development are two important aspects of a child's journey after birth, with each having its own significance. *Growth* encompasses a physical increase in body size and is easily measured by changes in weight, length/height, head circumference, etc. *Development,* on the contrary, is the sequential acquisition of new skills and functions and is measured by the attainment of skills by the child that are age-specific. Both growth and development occur at a very rapid pace in infancy and early childhood; the growth rate slows thereafter till puberty, while development continues with the acquisition of more complex physical and mental skills.

The development of the child (attainment of skills) is closely related to the processes of synaptogenesis and myelination of the central nervous system (CNS) **(Fig. 4.1.1)**. Hence, an intact nervous system with functional sensory organs is an important prerequisite for normal development.[1,2] As CNS maturation is an orderly process, the child's development too is an orderly and predictable process. Along with synaptogenesis and myelination of the CNS, the development of the child occurs based on social experiences that drive the rearrangement of neural synapses (neuroplasticity). The early years of the child's development are very crucial for the achievement of the optimal developmental potential of the child, giving rise to the importance of the concept of "*Early Childhood Development*." Any insult to the developing brain or poor environmental exposure in the early years of life may result in developmental delay. Thus, nurturing care by caregivers in the early years is of vital importance.

THEORIES OF CHILD DEVELOPMENT

Historically, most theorists considered that all characteristics and behavior of a person are a result of inheritance from parents, while some favored the role of environmental influences on child development and behavior and believed that all learning and behavior was a result of conditioning. The last century saw great progress in the field of child development and behavior, like the pioneering work of Arnold Gessel. Gessel studied a set of children from birth till adolescence and quantified their physical, social, and emotional achievements based on age.[3] Gessel's maturational theory states that there is a predetermined biological timetable of development—the *Gessel Developmental Schedules* consisting of milestones achieved at particular ages.

However, this theory did not give any importance to the role of environment in child development and was

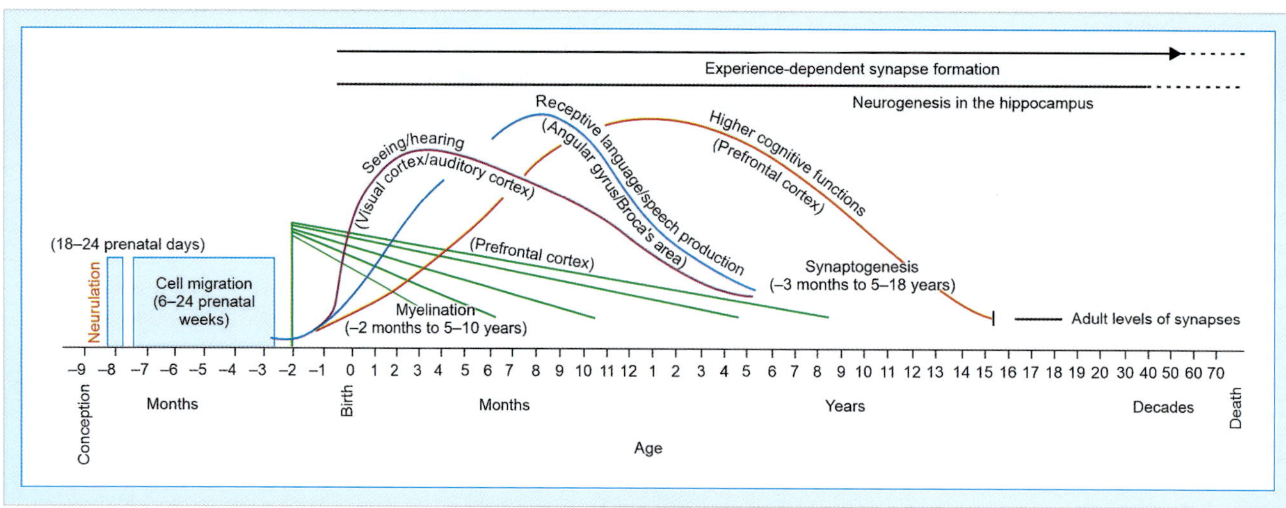

Fig. 4.1.1: Human brain development.
Source: Thompson RA, Nelson CA. Developmental science and the media: early brain development. Am Psychol. 2001;56:5-15.

considered oversimplified. This furthered the development of other theories, the most prominent of which are Jean Piaget's theory of cognitive learning, Sigmund Freud's psychosexual theory, Lev Vygotsky's sociocultural theory, Bronfenbrenner's theory of bioecological systems, and Howard Gardener's theory of multiple intelligences. All these theories explain different aspects of child development and factors involved.

The work done in the field of understanding child development over the last century clearly shows the role of interaction between nature (genes and biology) and nurture (family, society, and culture), thus laying the framework of the biopsychosocial model of child development, which looks at the child as an active participant in development. This has also led to the concept of a child achieving optimal developmental potential using an ecological life course approach, wherein the child's development is affected by complex relationships with the environment **(Fig. 4.1.2)** and the *"Nurturing Care for Early Childhood Development" (NC-ECD)*, which states the practices that support optimal development.[4]

PRINCIPLES OF DEVELOPMENT

Although the child is developing as a whole unit, the development is classified into different domains, which makes it easier to assess and understand a child's developmental status. The five domains of development commonly used are gross motor, fine motor, communication and language, personal social, and cognitive. The development process of a child is an orderly process and is guided by a set of principles elucidated by Illingworth, which are given as follows:[5]

- Development of a child is a continuous process starting from conception to maturity.
- The general sequence of development is the same for all children, though the rate of development may vary from child to child.

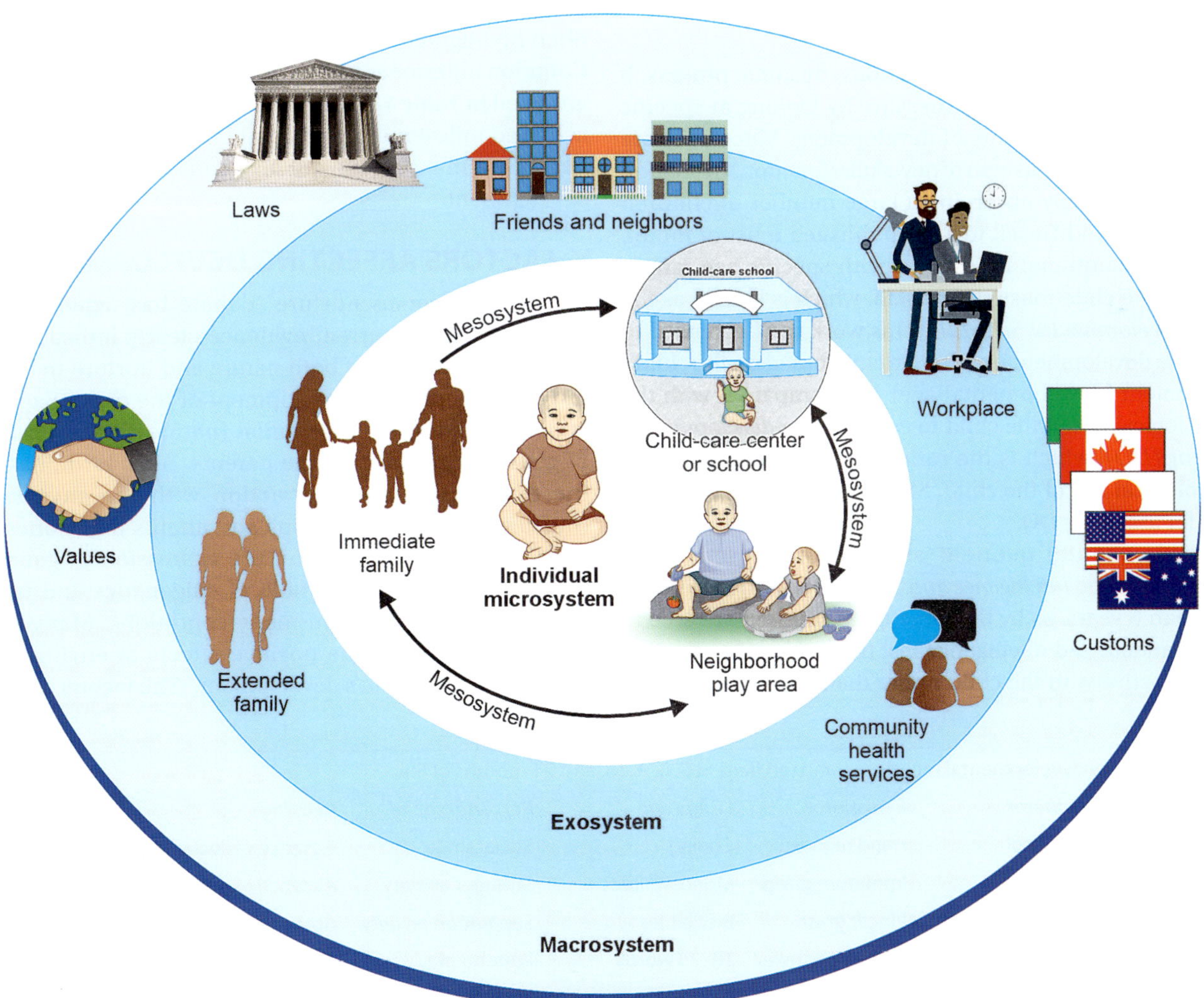

Fig. 4.1.2: Environment in ecological systems theory.

- The development should ideally run parallel in all domains of development, but there may be a difference in the different domains of development of the same child. If the differences between different domains of development in a child are marked, it is termed *"dissociation"* and the child is considered delayed in that particular domain. If two or more domains are affected, it is termed *"global developmental delay."*
- The development of the child is closely linked to the development and maturation of the CNS.
- Primitive reflexes, such as the grasp reflex, must be lost before the normal milestone corresponding to it is acquired by the child.
- Generalized mass activity of infancy is gradually replaced by specific responses in the child.
- Development occurs in a cephalo-caudal direction and proximo-distal pattern in limbs. This highlights the orderly process of myelination and maturation of the CNS.

DEVELOPMENTAL MILESTONES

Although development is a continuous, dynamic process, it is easier to understand and measure by looking at specific functions or achievements of development. Milestones are stages of a child's acquisition of new skills/functions in relation to postnatal age. By observing a large number of children over time, Arnold Gesell in 1925 published a list of motor, social, and emotional milestones with specific age ranges by which the child masters that skill, which is known as the *Gesell Developmental Schedule*. This work has been used to assess the developmental age of the child based on the child's achievement (developmental age) and compare it with the chronological age of the child to estimate the *developmental quotient (DQ)*, which is the ratio of developmental age to chronological age of the child. Many other scales have been made for assessing DQ.

Developmental quotient assessment is used up to 6 years of age, and *intelligence quotient (IQ)* is used in children older than 6 years, as by this time most children are able to take a standardized intelligence test that is far more detailed and interactive with the child rather than DQ, which merely measures easily observable milestones. Thus, the knowledge of these milestones is crucial for the assessment of a child's development. Based on the age, development can be divided into stages—infancy (<1 year), toddlerhood/preschooler (1–5 years), childhood (5–11 years), adolescence (11–18 years), and adulthood (>18 years).

DOMAINS OF DEVELOPMENT

Similar to growth, rate of development is different in different children and hence needs to be measured against a known standard. Although the child is developing as a whole unit, the development is divided into different domains—gross motor, fine motor, communication and language, personal social, and cognitive—with each domain having specific milestones, which makes it easier to assess and understand a child's developmental status. Consistent milestones are those that are always present in all children and are further quantified in detail so as to correctly identify the age at which they are present. The absence or delay of these milestones is often highlighted as *"Red flags"* in the child's development. Common milestones and red flags at 3, 6, 9, 18, and 24 months are listed in **Table 4.1.1**.[5,6] Any strong parental concern, loss of achieved milestones, early hand preference, and increased/decreased muscle tone are also considered as red flags in development.

FACTORS AFFECTING DEVELOPMENT

The "nature versus nurture" debate has raged for many decades, but the current evidence clearly indicates that it is an amalgamation of both nature and nurture that results in the final outcome/development of the child. Each child is born with a genetic potential (nature) based on the set of genes inherited from the parents. After birth, based on the experiences and interaction with the environment (nurture), the child develops and attains milestones. This effect of external factors on the expression of genes and the final outcome is the field of epigenetics and is being increasingly identified in many conditions. Many studies have demonstrated the positive effects of environmental enrichment in a child's development.[4] The factors associated

TABLE 4.1.1: Key developmental milestones and red flags at 3, 6, 9, 18, and 24 months of life.

Age	*Gross motor*	*Fine motor*	*Language*	*Personal social*	*Red flags*
3 months	Neck control	Hand regard	Cooing	Social smile	Absence of social smile
6 months	Rolls over	Immature grasp	Monosyllables	Stranger anxiety	Absence of head control and vocalization
9 months	Sits without support	Pincer grasp	Bisyllables	Separation anxiety	Absence of sitting and babbling
18 months	Walks independently	Four-cube tower	10–25 words	Pretend play	Absence of pointing and walking
24 months	Climbs stairs	Train of cubes	Two- to three-word sentences	Parallel play	Absence of two-word phrases and steady walking

with child development can be broadly grouped into three groups: (1) Genetic, (2) biological, and (3) psychosocial factors.

DEVELOPMENTAL ASSESSMENT

The two terms—developmental surveillance and developmental screening—are often used interchangeably but are very different. Developmental surveillance is the longitudinal (over time) process of following up children for early identification of any delay. *Developmental screening* is the process of using a standardized screening tool to assess the development of a child and should be carried out for all children and should be part of a complete examination of the child. All preterm newborns should be assessed after correcting age until 2 years of life (considering the postgestational age, not the chronological age). A normal vision and hearing are essential prerequisites for the normal development of a child and hence should be part of the developmental assessment. Any significant family history, dysmorphic features, or significant findings during general and systemic examination should entail a detailed developmental assessment to identify any delays.

TOOLS FOR DEVELOPMENTAL ASSESSMENT

A good screening test should be cheap, easy to use, standardized, and have acceptable sensitivity and specificity. It should be administered fairly quickly (<15 minutes). There are many screening tools available—some are parent-based questionnaires while others are clinician-administered.[7] **Table 4.1.2** compares some selected developmental tools available. Screening tools can be divided into the following:

- *General screening tools* evaluate multiple domains simultaneously, e.g., the Ages and Stages Questionnaire (ASQ), Parents' Evaluation of Developmental Status (PEDS), Bayley's Infant Neurodevelopmental Screen (BINDS), Denver Developmental Screening Test (DDST), Baroda Developmental Screening Test (BDST), and Trivandrum Development Screening Chart (TDSC).
- *Domain-specific tools* evaluate one domain of development, e.g., the Language Evaluation Scale Trivandrum (LEST) and the Early Motor Pattern Profile (EMPP).
- *Disorder-specific tools* identify a specific developmental disorder, e.g., the Modified Checklist for Autism in Toddlers (M-CHAT-R/F) and the Social Communication Questionnaire (SCQ).

Trivandrum Development Screening Chart is a simple screening tool developed by Nair et al. at the Child Development Centre, Trivandrum, for use at the community level.[8] The tool was initially developed for children up to 2 years but has been expanded to include children up to 6 years now. The tool has 51 items and has been validated against the DDST with a sensitivity and specificity of 84% and 90%, respectively. It is a simple visual tool with horizontal bars placed on the graph with age represented on the *x*-axis. Each bar represents a milestone, with the left end of the bar representing the age at which 3% of children will achieve that milestone and the right end of the bar representing the age at which 97% of the children will achieve that milestone **(Fig. 4.1.3)**.[8] A vertical line is drawn on the TDSC at the chronological age of the child being assessed, and the child should have completed all milestones that lie on the left side of the line. Any abnormality or asymmetry is considered abnormal and requires a detailed assessment using a comprehensive developmental assessment tool.

TABLE 4.1.2: Comparison of different tools for developmental assessment.

	TDSC	*BDST*	*DDST*	*PEDS*	*ASQ*
Age range	0–6 years	0–30 months	0–6 years	0–8 years	0–66 months
Method	Clinician-administered	Clinician-administered	Clinician-administered	Parent-based questionnaire	Parent-based questionnaire
Time taken	5 minutes	10 minutes	10–20 minutes	10 minutes	10–15 minutes
Sensitivity/ specificity (%)	84/90	65–93/77–94	56–83/43–80	74–79/70–80	70–90/74–91
Cost	Inexpensive	Inexpensive	$111	$30	$249
Validated in India	Yes	Yes	No	No	No
Language	English and Malayalam	English and Hindi	English	English	English and Hindi

(ASQ: Ages and Stages Questionnaire; BDST: Baroda Development Screening Test; DDST: Denver Development Screening Test; PEDS: Parents Evaluation of Developmental Status; TDSC: Trivandrum Development Screening Checklist)

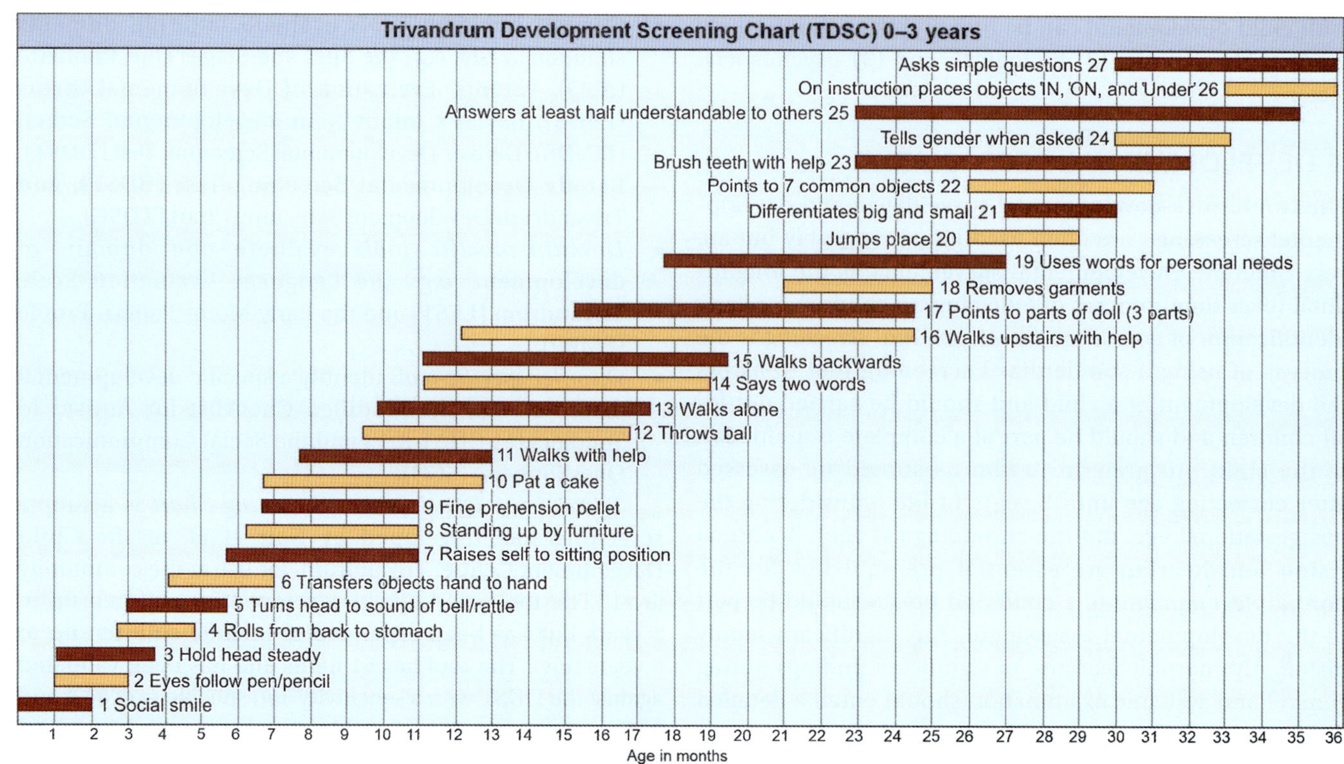

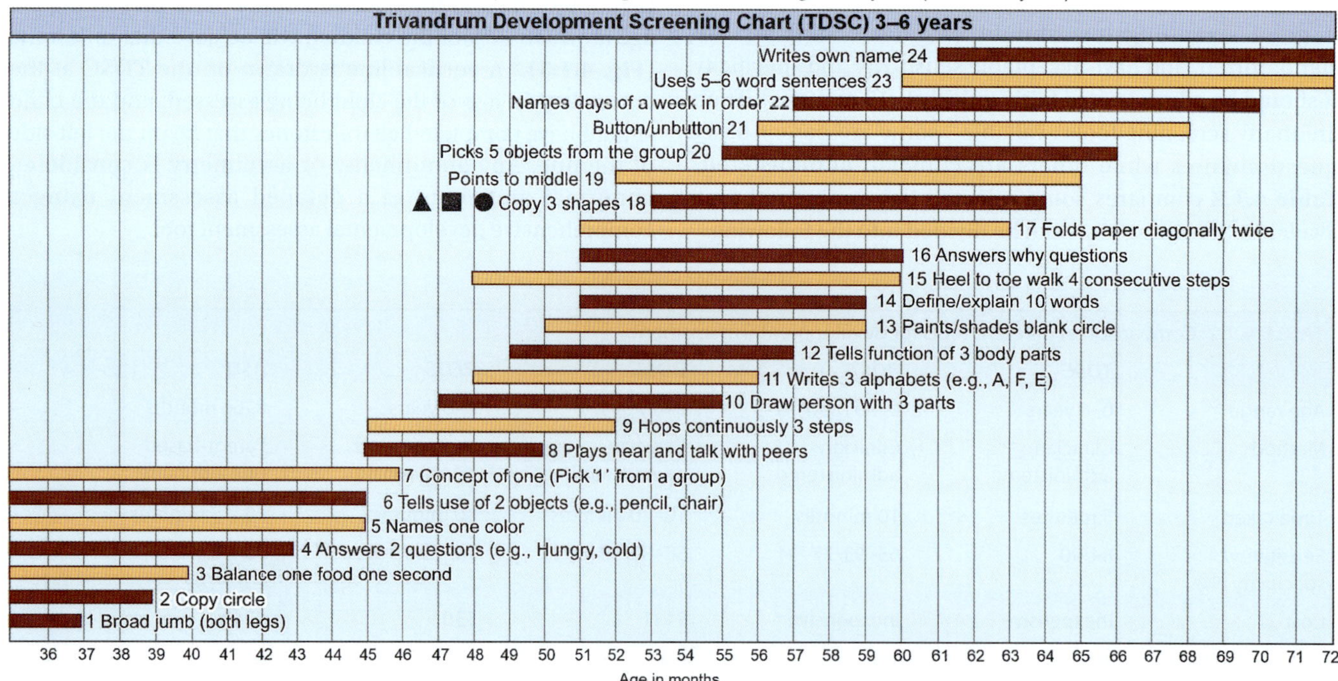

Fig. 4.1.3: Trivandrum Development Screening.[8]

Source: Nair MK, Nair GSH, George B, Suma N, Neethu C, Leena ML, et al. Development and validation of Trivandrum Development Screening Chart for children aged 0–6 years. Indian J Pediatr. 2013;80(Suppl 2):S248-55.

INTERPRETATION OF DEVELOPMENTAL ASSESSMENT

Children up to 6 years are tested using the DQ, which is derived using the formula: [developmental age (DA)/ chronological age (CA)] × 100. For children above 6 years of age, multiple tests of intelligence are available, and the results of intelligence testing are labeled as intelligence quotient. A score of 70 or less in DQ or IQ is taken as abnormal and requires further evaluation.

CRITICAL/SENSITIVE PERIOD OF DEVELOPMENT AND THE IMPORTANCE OF EARLY YEARS

After birth, the child is exposed to a large number of stimuli from the environment, and these interactions with the environment result in the formation of multiple synapses, which are essential for the development of the child. The first few months after birth are critical for vision and hearing development in children, and a delay in recognition of visual/ hearing problems will result in poor outcomes—hence the need for vision and hearing screening in the early infantile period **(Fig. 4.1.1)**. Hearing problems in the early months result in speech and language problems in the first few years. Early identification and environmental enrichment can help reduce the severity and improve the productivity of the child.

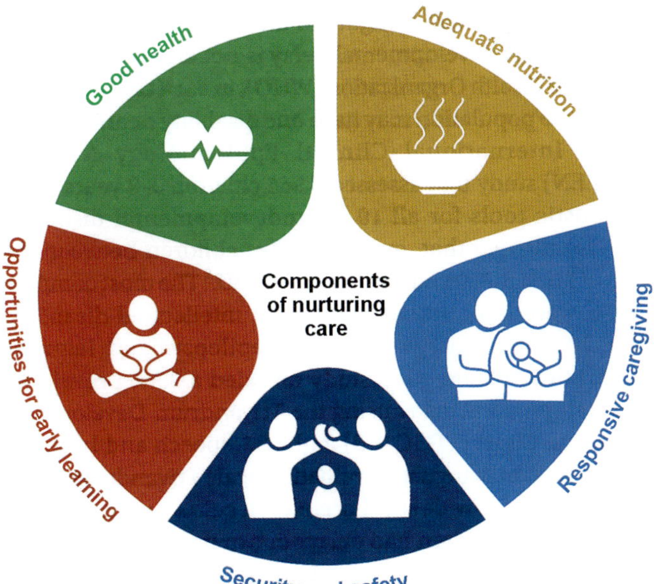

Fig. 4.1.4: Components of the NC-ECD. (NC-ECD: Nurturing Care for Early Childhood Development)

This highlights both the vulnerability and resilient nature of the child's development in the early years. The World Health Organization (WHO) has recommended a nurturing care framework in which a key principle is providing enabling environments to promote child development in the early years.[9] The NC-ECD program was started by the Indian Academy of Pediatrics (IAP) in collaboration with the Government of India, WHO, and the United Nations International Children's Emergency Fund (UNICEF) to promote awareness about the importance of development during early years in a child's life and the factors associated with it.[10] The program supports the use of five pillars to support the child's early development—good health, nutrition, responsive caregiving, safety and security, and opportunities for early learning **(Fig. 4.1.4)**. The NC-ECD framework utilizes a holistic approach to help children to survive, thrive, and learn in an enriched environment so as to achieve one's maximum human potential.

REFERENCES

1. Berk LE. Child Development, 9th edition. Boston, MA: Pearson; 2017.
2. Hagan JF, Shaw JS, Duncan PM (Eds). Bright Futures: Guidelines for Health Supervision of Infants, Children, and Adolescents, 4th edition. Elk Grove Village, IL: American Academy of Pediatrics; 2017.
3. Gesell A, Ilg FL. Child Development: An Introduction to the Study of Human Growth. New York: Harper; 1949.
4. Tomlinson M, Hunt X, Daelmans B, Rollins N, Ross D, Oberklaid F. Optimising child and adolescent health and development through an integrated ecological life course approach. BMJ. 2021;372:m4784.
5. Illingworth RS. The Development of Infant and Young Child: Normal and Abnormal, 10th edition. London: Churchill Livingstone; 2013.
6. Scharf RJ, Scharf GJ, Stroustrup A. Developmental milestones. Pediatr Rev. 2016;37(1):25-37.
7. Mukherjee SB, Aneja S, Krishnamurthy V, Srinivasan R. Incorporating development screening and surveillance of young children in office practice. Indian Pediatr. 2014;51(8): 627-35.
8. Nair MK, Nair GS, George B, Suma N, Neethu C, Leena ML, et al. Development and validation of Trivandrum Development Screening Chart for children aged 0-6 years. Indian J Pediatr. 2013;80(Suppl 2):S248-55.
9. World Health Organization. Nurturing Care for Early Childhood Development: A Framework for Helping Children Survive and Thrive to Transform Health and Human Potential. Geneva, Switzerland: WHO; 2018.
10. Mukherjee SB, Agrawal D, Mishra D, Shastri D, Dalwai, SH, Chattopadhyay N, et al. Indian Academy of Pediatrics Position Paper on nurturing care for early childhood development. Indian Pediatr. 2021;58(10):962-9.

4.2 Developmental Delay: Screening and Assessment

MKC Nair, Deepa Bhaskaran

INTRODUCTION

For too long, we have been concentrating on the developmental milestones to be achieved at each age. But from a clinical point of view, it is more important to know the major milestones that are to be reached by fixed ages like 2, 4, 8, 12, 18, and 24 months and every year after that till 6 years of age.

DEFINITION

A delay in development happens when a child does not reach milestones of development at the likely age (with acceptable allowance for the broad variation among normal children).[1] Developmental delays may occur in all the major areas of child development—gross motor, fine motor, communication, language, cognition, and social. Documentation of developmental delay is useful for introducing early intervention programs to reduce childhood disability.[2]

Developmental prediction is not always feasible, as we may be mistaken often. By doing the developmental assessment, we can only opine on present status in relation to the average performance of other children of the same age. We cannot exactly predict future intelligence, the effect of delayed maturation, and the long-term effects of emotional deprivation.

Surveillance: This is to find children who may have developmental problems. Here information is gathered and synthesized from history, observations of parents or caretakers, and healthcare professionals. This is done during periodic visits on a longitudinal basis over time.

Screening: It is done in children who are at risk for developmental delays using simple screening tools that have been validated.

Evaluation: This aims to detect a particular developmental disorder and its cause if known. This may encompass laboratory, genetic, or metabolic testing, apart from neuroimaging studies and psychological testing.

Developmental assessment: This means fundamentally looking for atypical development, which includes delay, deviation, dissociation, or regression.

- *Delay:* Significant delay in the attainment of milestones in one or more domains, but the sequence is not altered as compared to that of typically developing children.
- *Deviation:* Developmental skills are attained out of order in a given domain. For example, an infant rolls from supine to prone before prone to supine.
- *Dissociation:* When developmental skills are attained at different rates between two or more domains of development. For example, when there is a delay in motor milestones in relation to other domains of cerebral palsy.
- *Regression:* Loss of previous developmental milestones or skills or failure to acquire new skills.

EPIDEMIOLOGY

According to global statistics in 2016, about 52.9 million children reportedly had recognizable developmental problems. 95% of the population lives in low- and middle-income countries (LMICs); the risk for developmental delays and disorders is higher in these countries.[3] The exact prevalence of developmental delay is not known, but as per the World Health Organization (WHO), in each country, about 10% of the population may have one disability or another.[4]

An International Clinical Epidemiology Network (INCLEN) study that assessed 3,964 children 0–9 years using diagnostic tools for all 10 neurodevelopmental disorders (NDDs) showed that, overall, 12% of children between the ages of 2 and 9 years had at least one NDD.[5] The most common NDDs were impairment in hearing, intellectual disability, speech and language disorders, epilepsy, and learning disabilities. A state-wide study revealed a 2.5% prevalence of developmental delay using the Trivandrum Development Screening Chart (TDSC 0–3) and 2.8% speech and language delay using the Language Evaluation Scale Trivandrum (LEST 0–3).[6,7] A district-wide study of children below 6 years revealed that 3.08% of children had delays in two or more items using TDSC 0–6.[7,8] Among the screen positives (item delay cases) evaluated in detail using appropriate tools, majority had developmental delay alone (50%), speech and language delay (25%), multiple disabilities (23%), intellectual disability (17%), cerebral palsy (8%), hearing impairment (5%), seizure disorders (4%), visual impairment (3%), neuromuscular disorders (1%), and autism (1%) in that order.

The occurrence of biological risk factors for developmental delay, such as low birth weight, birth asphyxia, poor home environment, and alternate child-care services, has highlighted the need for a simple cost-effective community model for promoting early child development, like *Rashtriya Bal Swasthya Karyakram (RBSK)*.

ETIOPATHOGENESIS

Something that intensifies the likelihood of getting a disease or condition is called a risk factor. Risk can be categorized as follows:[1,2]

- *Established risk:* These include medical disorders that can lead to developmental delay. It includes Down syndrome, hydrocephalus, cerebral palsy, hearing impairment, visual impairment, and other congenital anomalies.
- *Environmental risk:* This includes limited environmental factors, which put a child at risk for developmental delay. The various factors are a very young mother, extreme poverty, low socioeconomic status, single parent, etc.
- *Biological risk:* It includes factors such as prematurity, low birth weight, neonatal hypothermia, asphyxia, hypoglycemia, hyperbilirubinemia, and convulsions. These issues happen in the prenatal, natal, and postnatal periods.
- *No apparent risk:* Developmental delays also occur in infants without any apparent risks.

The improvements in perinatal care have bettered the chances of low birth weight/preterm babies surviving more and more. This has added to the burden of developmental delay. It has been shown that 40% reduction in poor performance could be achieved among neonatal nursery graduates by the Child Development Center (CDC) model of early stimulation. UNICEF is promoting the concept of concentrating on the first 1,000 days (270 + 365 + 365) as part of the habilitation process, meaning prevention of impairment going on to disability with appropriate early stimulation. Which "high-risk" newborns require periodic screening ideally needs to be determined locally. It must also be remembered that many babies not considered "high risk" may also manifest developmental problems as they grow. These babies would not have been seen during "high-risk" focused follow-up screening.

DEVELOPMENTAL SCREENING

Developmental screening, vision, and hearing screening of all babies, especially those who have been in the neonatal intensive care unit (NICU), are important to detect potentially handicapping conditions that may be prevented or ameliorated if addressed early. A screening test helps to identify children who might have a delay and who need further developmental evaluation.[9]

Birth to 1 Year

Developmental Observation Card

This is a simple developmental card for parents to identify delay:

- *Completed 2 months:* Social smile—baby smiling back in response to smile
- *Completed 4 months:* Holds head steady—keeping head steady when the baby is held upright
- *Completed 8 months:* Sits alone—baby can sit alone with back straight, no support
- *Completed 12 months:* Stands alone—baby can stand bearing weight on both legs with minimal support
- *Completed 18 months*: Adequate communication and socialization skills and "child not in his/her own world" rule out possible autism spectrum disorder (ASD).

Child Development Center Grading for Motor Milestones

A. *Head holding grading (assessed at completed 4 months):*
   - *Grade 0:* No head holding at all
   - *Grade I:* Head erect and steady momentarily **(Fig. 4.2.1)**
   - *Grade II:* Dorsal suspension—lifts head along with body **(Fig. 4.2.2)**
   - *Grade III:* Prone position—elevates on arms, lifting chest **(Fig. 4.2.3)**
   - *Grade IV:* Holds head steady while mother moves around **(Fig. 4.2.4)**
   - *Grade V:* Head balanced always **(Fig. 4.2.5)**

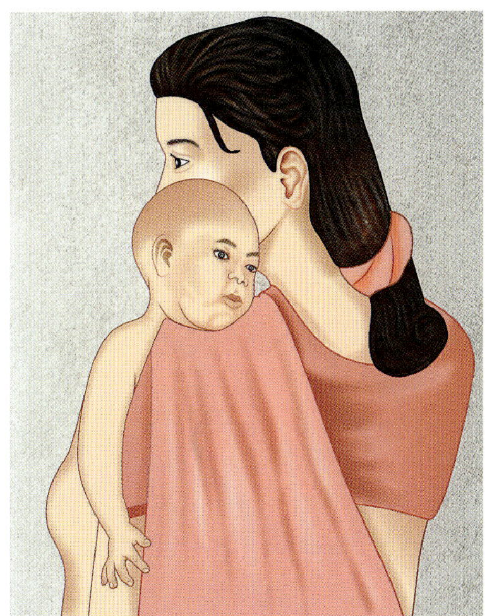

Fig. 4.2.1: Head holding Grade I.

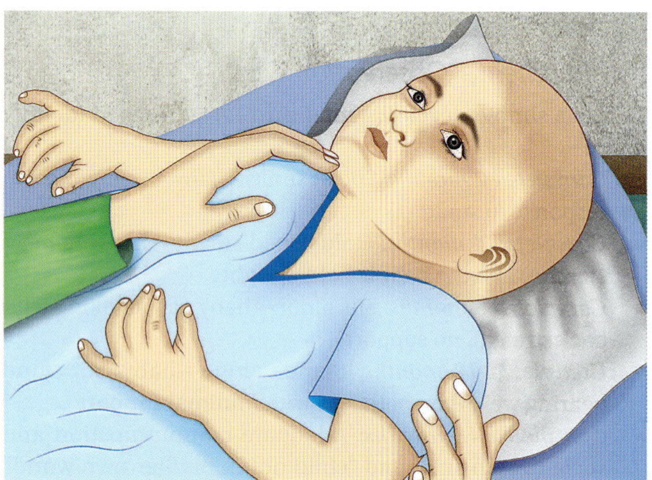

Fig. 4.2.2: Head holding Grade II.

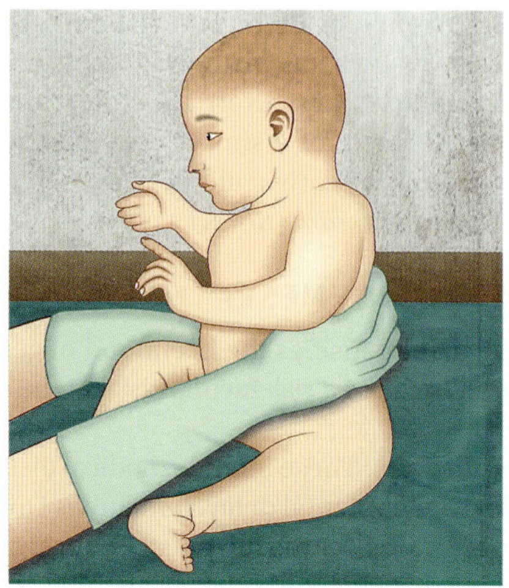

Fig. 4.2.5: Head holding Grade V.

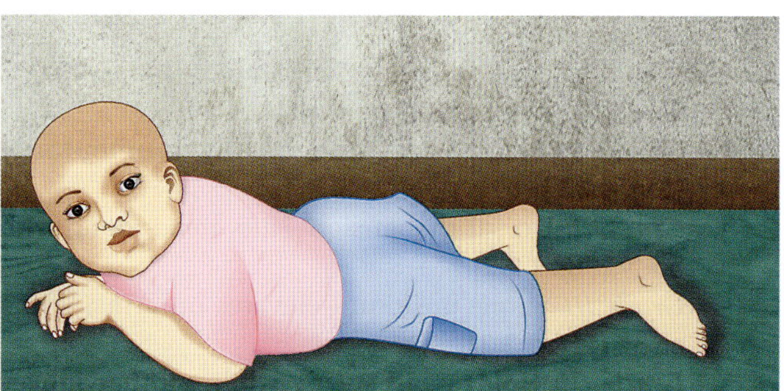

Fig. 4.2.3: Head holding Grade III.

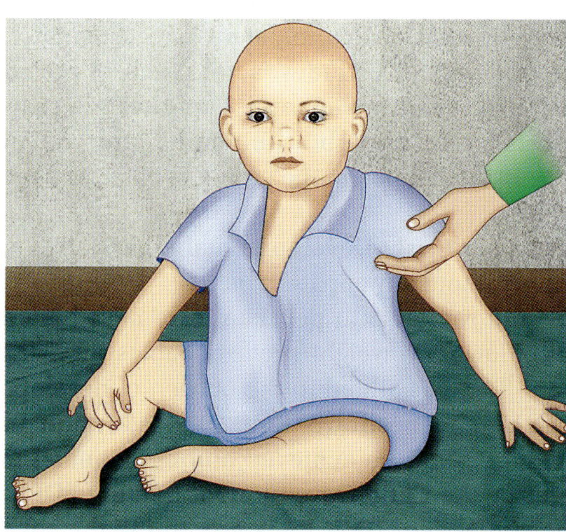

Fig. 4.2.6: Sitting Grade I.

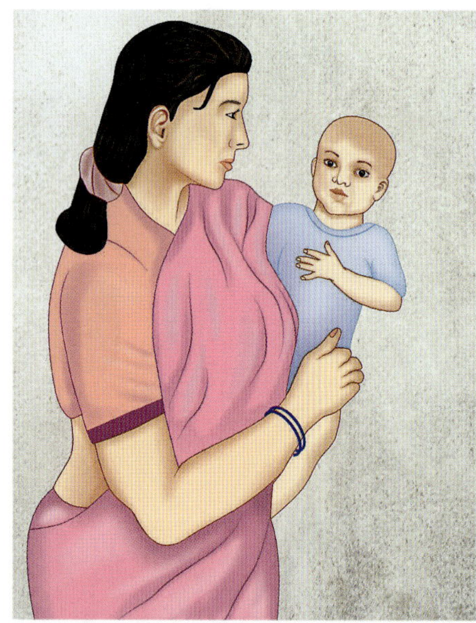

Fig. 4.2.4: Head holding Grade IV.

B. *Sitting grading (assessed at completed 8 months):*
   - *Grade 0:* No sitting at all
   - *Grade I:* Sits momentarily **(Fig. 4.2.6)**
   - *Grade II:* Sits 30 seconds or more leaning forward **(Fig. 4.2.7)**
   - *Grade III:* Sits with the child's back straight **(Fig. 4.2.8)**
   - *Grade IV:* While sitting, can turn around and manipulate a toy **(Fig. 4.2.9)**
   - *Grade V:* Raises self to sitting position **(Fig. 4.2.10)**

C. *Standing grading (assessed at completed 12 months):*
   - *Grade 0:* Not standing well
   - *Grade I:* Stands holding on to furniture momentarily **(Fig. 4.2.11)**
   - *Grade II:* Takes few steps with both hands supported **(Fig. 4.2.12)**
   - *Grade III:* Can stand alone with legs apart **(Fig. 4.2.13)**

- *Grade IV:* Comes to standing position by throwing weight on arms **(Fig. 4.2.14)**
- *Grade V:* Without support takes few steps **(Fig. 4.2.15)**

(Interpretation of CDC grading—grades III, IV, and V are normal for that age.)

Birth to 6 Years

TDSC (0–3 and 3–6 Years) (Figs. 4.2.16 and 4.2.17; Table 4.2.1)

This is a simple test to screen the development of babies below the age of 6 years that can be used in the community.[6-8] Developmental screening programs can be done in the community by "anganwadi" workers and other health workers using TDSC. The left end of each horizontal dark line is the age at which 3% of children passed the item, and the right end

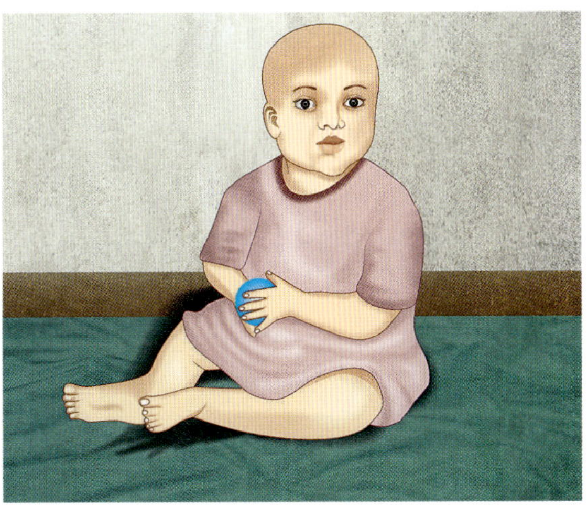

Fig. 4.2.9: Sitting Grade IV.

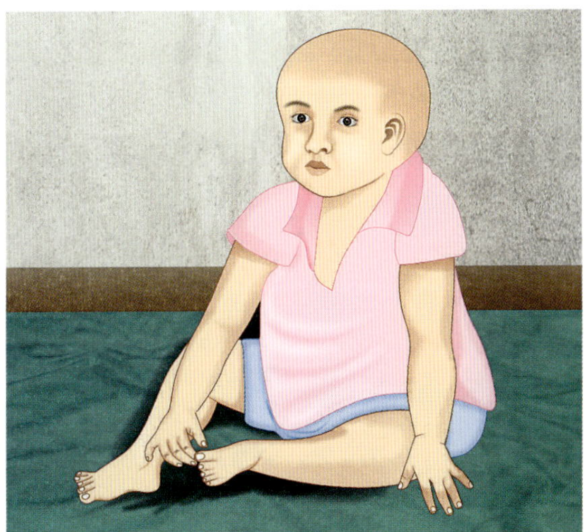

Fig. 4.2.7: Sitting Grade II.

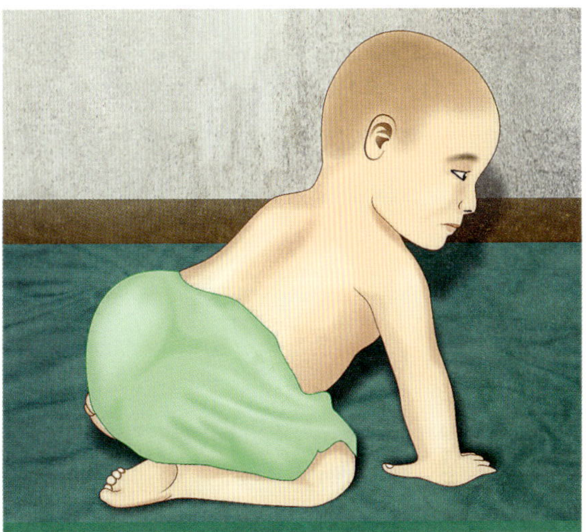

Fig. 4.2.10: Sitting Grade V.

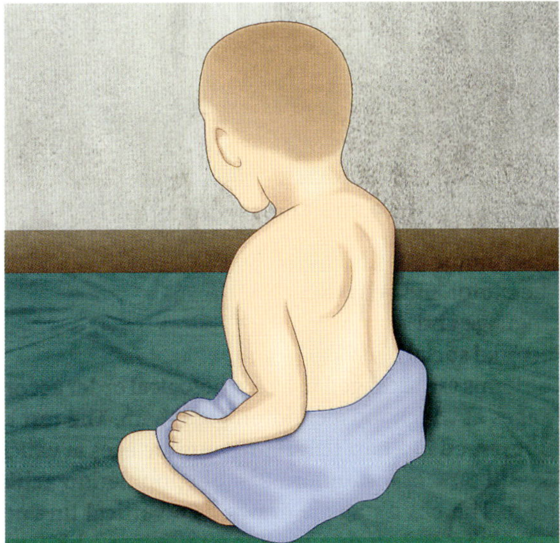

Fig. 4.2.8: Sitting Grade III.

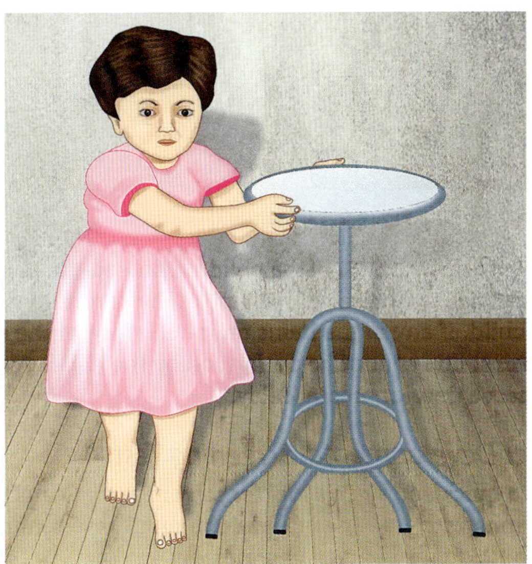

Fig. 4.2.11: Standing Grade I.

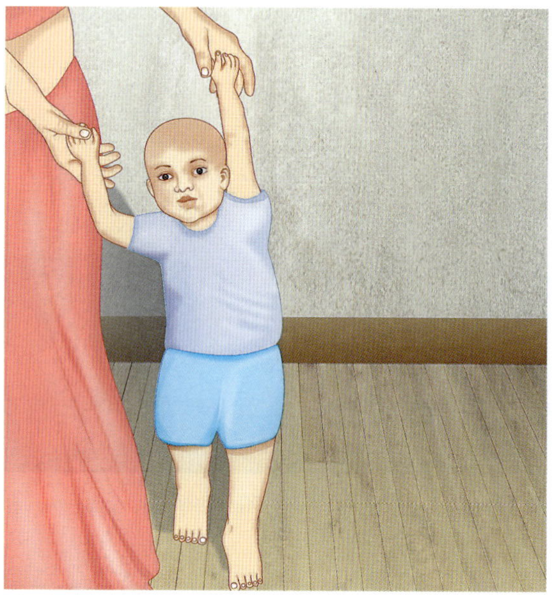

Fig. 4.2.12: Standing Grade II.

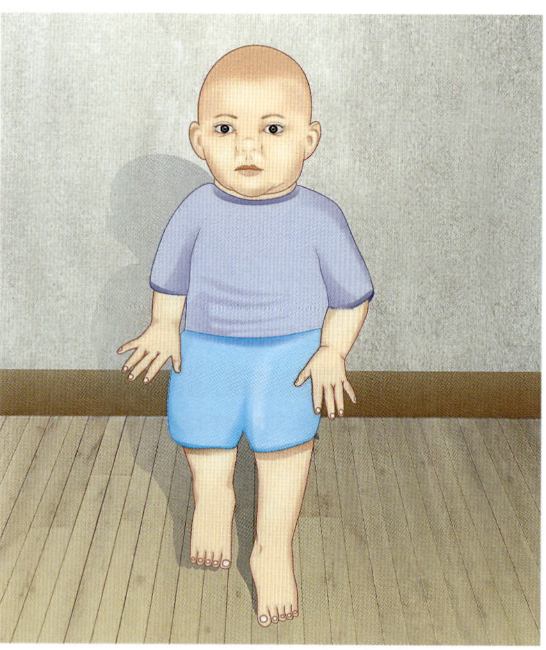

Fig. 4.2.13: Standing Grade III.

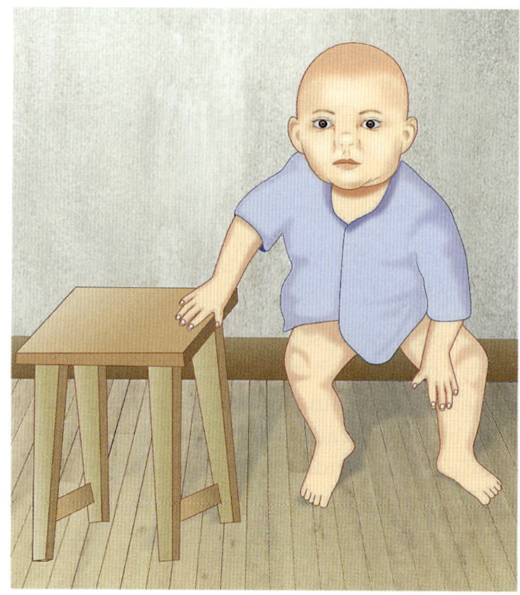

Fig. 4.2.14: Standing Grade IV.

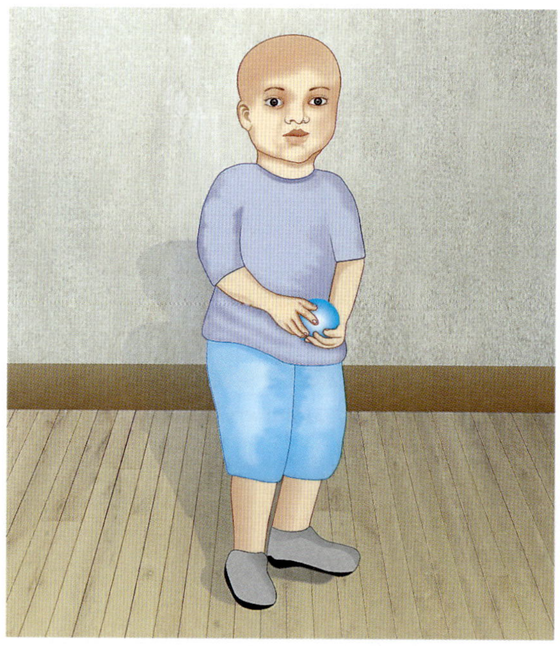

Fig. 4.2.15: Standing Grade V.

is the age at which 97% of the children passed the item. The examiner has to draw a vertical line at the chronological age of the child. If any of the items on the left side of the side of the vertical line cannot be performed by the child, you have to suspect a developmental delay.

Denver Developmental Screening Test II

This is a quick and simple tool for screening that can be used by persons with training in developmental assessment. The test has 125 items in four categories:

1. Gross motor
2. Fine motor and adaptive
3. Language and
4. Personal social

The items are arranged in a chronological order according to the ages at which most children pass them. The test items are represented in a bar. This represents the ages at which 25, 50, 75, and 90% of a standard sample population achieved that item. The child's age is drawn as a vertical line on the chart, and the examiner administers the items bisected by

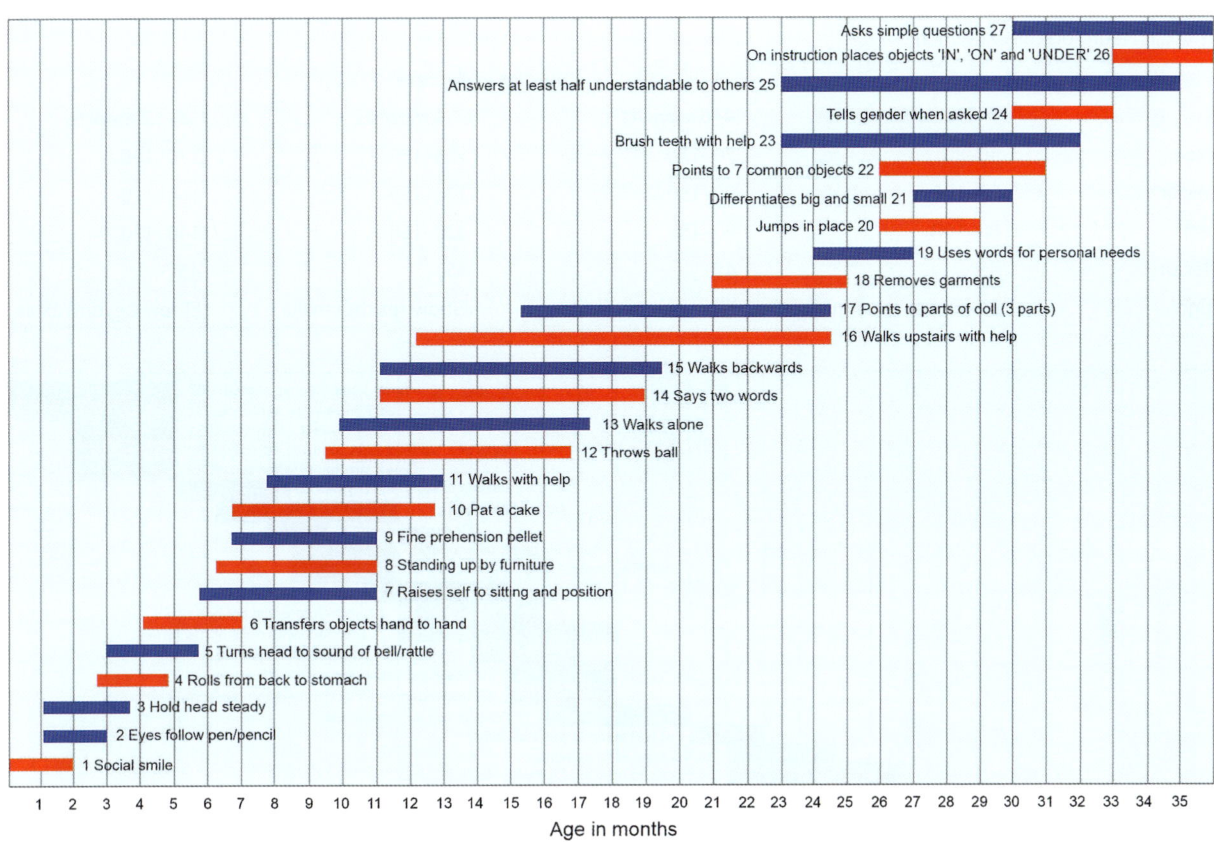

Fig. 4.2.16: Trivandrum Development Screening Chart (TDSC: 0–3 years).[7]

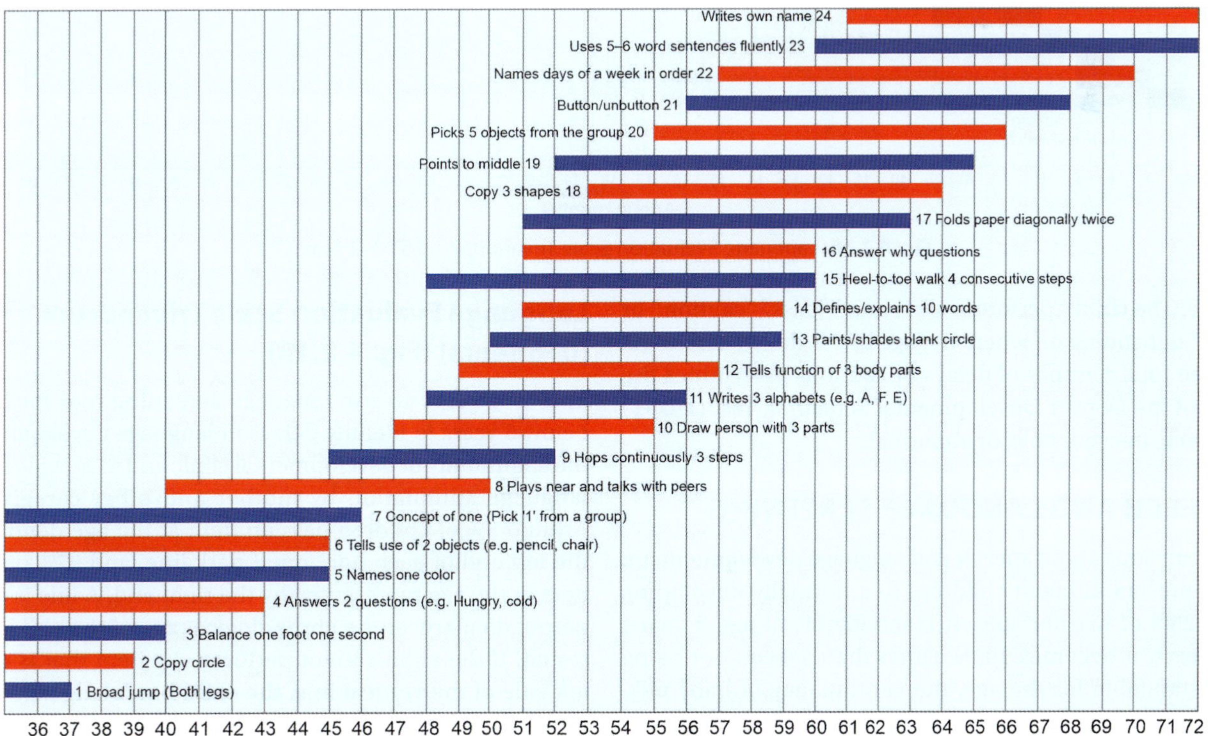

Fig. 4.2.17: Trivandrum Development Screening Chart (TDSC: 3–6 years).[6]

TABLE 4.2.1: Neurological assessment.

	Angles in degrees			
Angle	***1–3 months***	***4–6 months***	***7–9 months***	***10–12 months***
Adductor	40–80	70–110	100–150	130–150
Heel-to-ear	80–100	90–130	120–150	140–170
Popliteal	80–100	90–130	120–150	140–170
Dorsiflexion	45	45	45	45
Scarf sign	Elbow not cross midline	Elbow cross midline	Elbow reaches axilla	Elbow beyond axilla

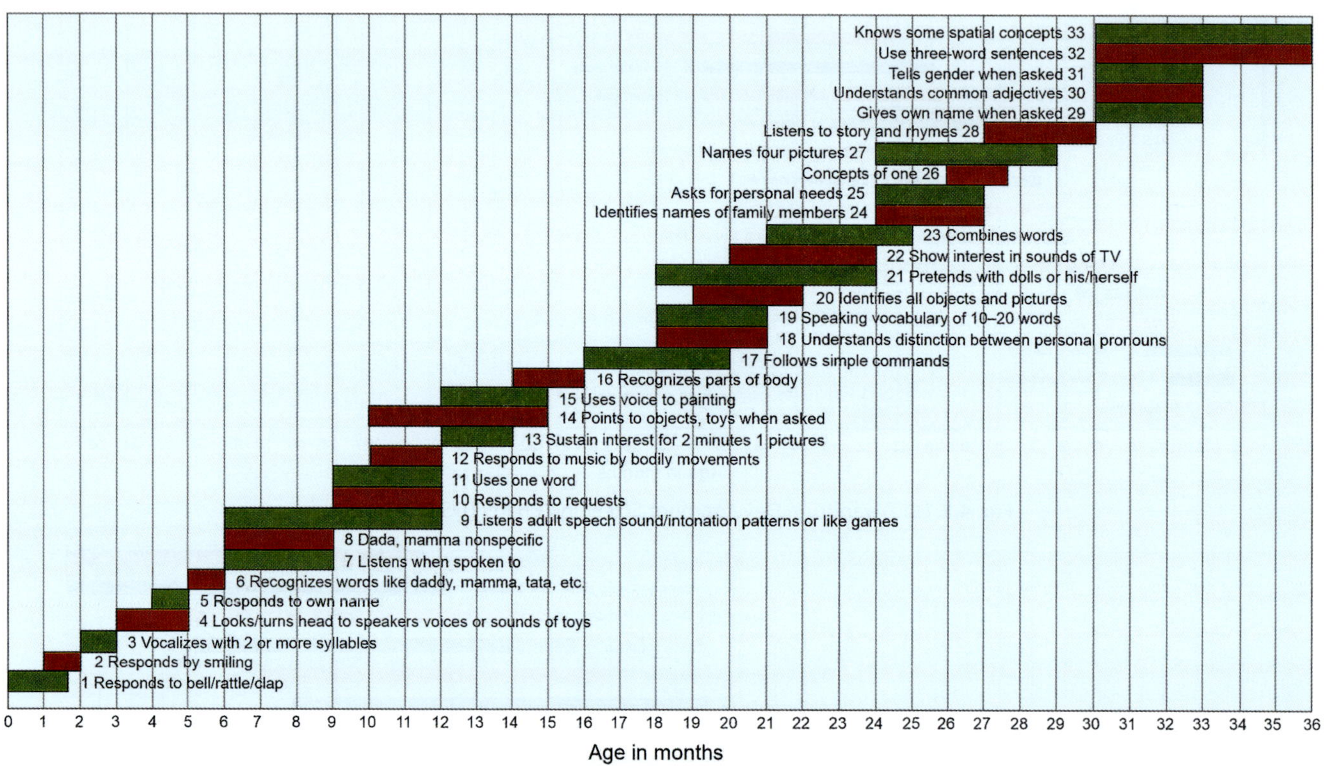

Fig. 4.2.18: Language Evaluation Scale Trivandrum (LEST 0–3 years).[6]

the line. The child's performance is rated "pass," "caution," or "delay" depending on where the age line is drawn across the bar. The total number of delays or cautions determines the rating of the Denver Developmental Screening Test (DDST) as normal, questionable, or abnormal.

SPEECH AND LANGUAGE SCREENING

Apprehensions about speech and language development are major presentations in children. In a normally developing child, 25% of his/her speech is intelligible at age 2 years. By 4 years, it becomes 100%. Other than speech not being understandable for the age, the continuance of baby talk, wrong pronunciation of words, and poor unprompted speech suggest speech and language delay.

Language Evaluation Scale Trivandrum (0–6 Years) (Fig. 4.2.18)

This is an easy-to-use language screening tool for babies below 6 years to identify delays in language development in the community or developmental clinic and to provide simple language stimulation by mother and other caregivers.[6-8] Around 3% of children pass an item at the age denoted by the left end of each horizontal dark line, and 97% pass the item at the age represented by the right end. A line is drawn perpendicularly at the chronological age of the child being tested. If the child cannot perform any item that is on the left side of the vertical line, the child has a language delay. Ideally, regular developmental assessments should be done in an "anganwadi" every year from 3 years to facilitate referral

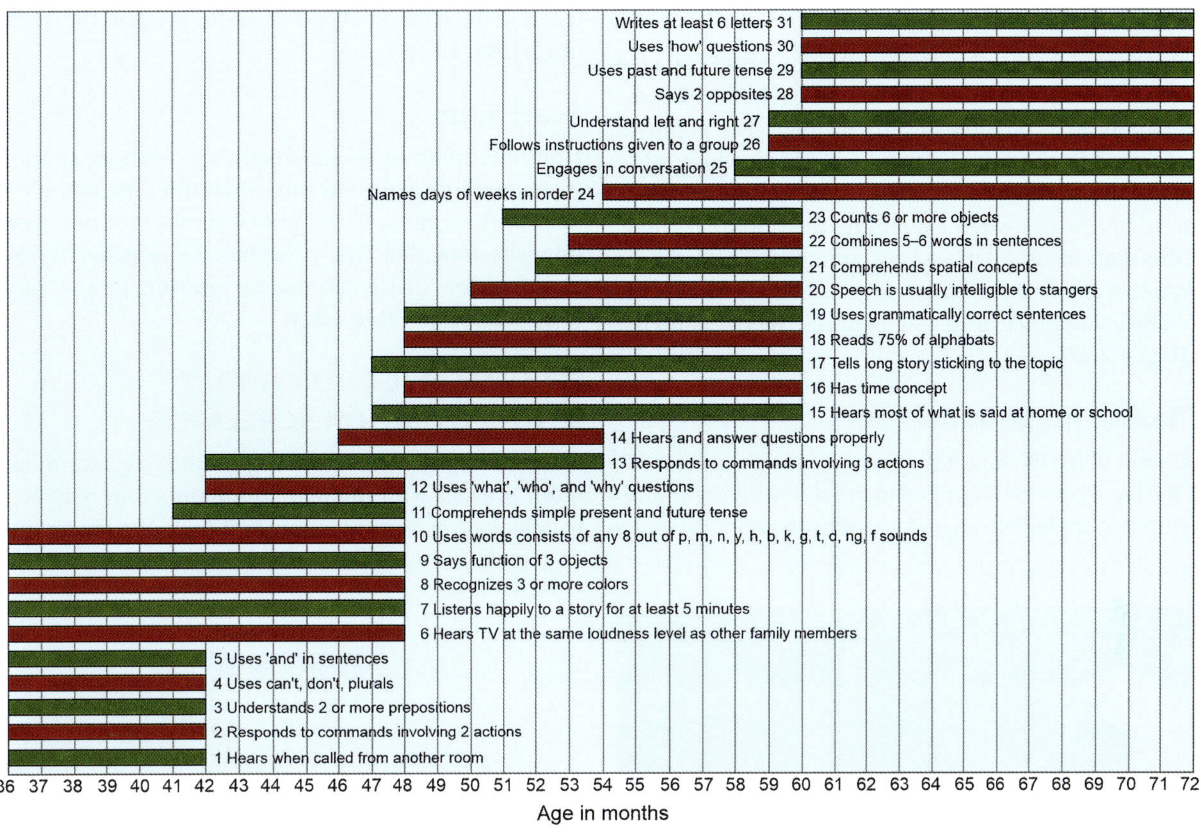

Fig. 4.2.19: Language Evaluation Scale Thiruvananthapuram (LEST 3–6 years).[7]

to District Early Intervention Centers (DEICs) under RBSK **(Fig. 4.2.19)**.

NEUROLOGICAL SCREENING (HYPOTONIA/HYPERTONIA/DYSTONIA)

Although it is easy to diagnose a given case of cerebral palsy, when it comes to follow-up of high-risk babies, a system of neurological examination that allows detection and recording of subtle neurological abnormalities that may disappear at the end of the first year (called transient abnormalities) or persist even beyond that (persistent abnormalities) is needed. Amiel-Tison has devised an all-inclusive method for neurological evaluation in the first 5 years of life. This gives us a framework for instituting a physical therapy program. In this method of neurological assessment, the presence of tone abnormalities is identified by measuring the following angles **(Table 4.2.1)**.

Adductor Angle

The infant is made to lie supine. The legs are extended and gently pulled as far apart as possible. The angle formed by the legs at this point is called the adductor angle. One should always look out for a lack of symmetry between the two sides **(Fig. 4.2.20)**.

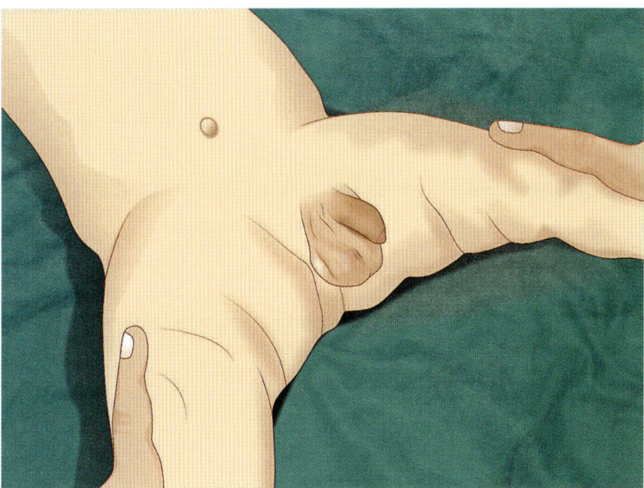

Fig. 4.2.20: Adductor angle.

Heel to Ear

Make the infant lie supine. The legs are held together and pressed as far as possible, toward the ear. Make sure not to lift the pelvis from the table. The angle is characterized by the arc formed from the infant's heel to the table. The increased resistance on one side is an indication of asymmetry, but it might be difficult to apply equal pressure to both sides **(Fig. 4.2.21)**.

Popliteal Angle

At the hip, the thighs are flexed laterally along both sides of the abdomen. Retaining this position, the examiner presses the lower leg as far as possible toward the thigh. The popliteal angle is formed by the calf and the thigh. This is assessed in both legs at the same time. It is easier to apply equivalent pressure to both sides when examining the popliteal angle. Hence, this angle is useful to assess asymmetry. The estimate of asymmetry is more unbiased. Significant asymmetry is indicated by a difference of 10°–20° between the right and left angles **(Fig. 4.2.22)**.

Dorsiflexion Angle of the Foot

The examiner holds the infant's leg straight and flexes the foot toward the leg. Pressure is applied to the sole with the thumb to measure this angle. The angle formed by the dorsum of the foot and the anterior aspect of the leg is called the dorsiflexion angle **(Fig. 4.2.23)**.

Scarf Sign

Hold the infant in a semi-reclining position, supported by the examiner's palm. At the same time, the infant's hand is held by the examiner and pulled across the chest toward the opposite shoulder. Four positions are possible in describing the position of the elbow in relation to the umbilicus **(Fig. 4.2.24; *see* Table 4.2.3)**.

COMMUNICATION AND SOCIALIZATION SCREENING

Numerous children attending a child development clinic often present with unclear complaints that may be related to a lack of communication and lack of socialization. The

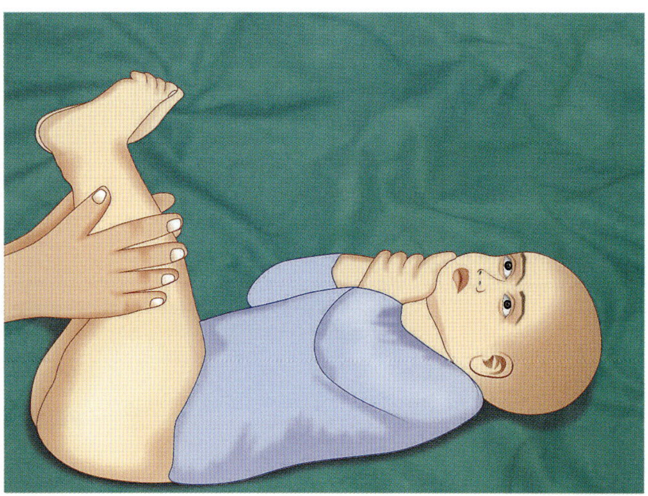

Fig. 4.2.21: Heel-to-ear angle.

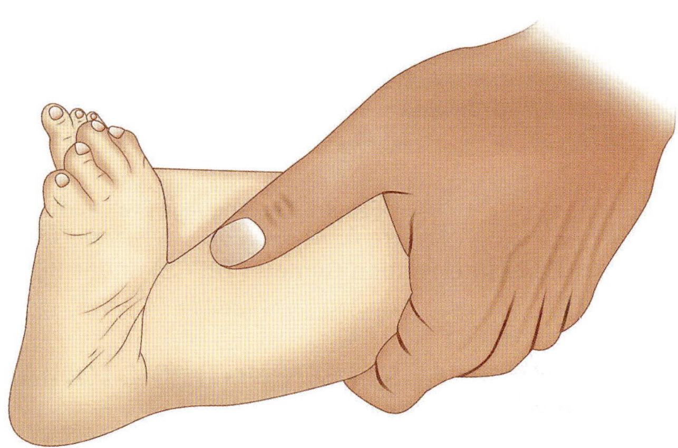

Fig. 4.2.23: Dorsiflexion angle.

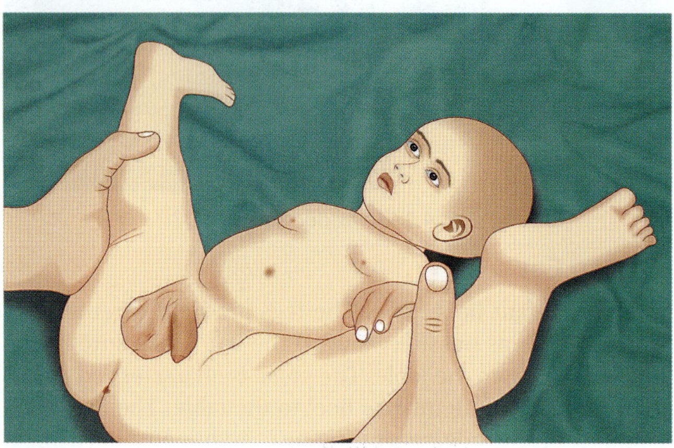

Fig. 4.2.22: Popliteal angle.

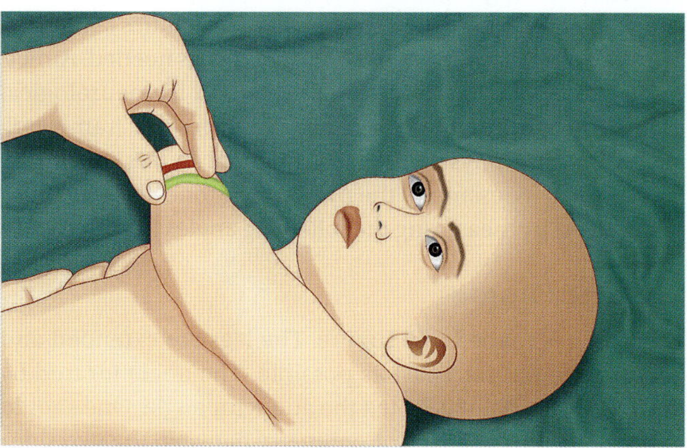

Fig. 4.2.24: Scarf sign.

parents may highlight only the speech delay. Unfortunately, the focus is often given to the speech and language delay. The more important communication and socialization delay may not be given significance, and this in turn may delay a diagnosis of possible ASD. In this setting, the accessibility of the Trivandrum Autism Behavioral Checklist (TABC) with 20 questions under four domains—(1) social interaction, (2) communication, (3) behavioral characteristics, and sensory integration—becomes more relevant as a simple screening tool for children 2–6 years **(Table 4.2.2)**. TABC has been validated against the Childhood Autism Rating Scale (CARS). CARS is a diagnostic tool for ASD and has good psychometric properties [sensitivity (96.3%), specificity (81.6%), positive predictive value (78.8%), negative predictive value (96.8%), accuracy (87.7%), positive likelihood ratio (5.2), and negative likelihood ratio (0.05)].[10]

SCHOOL READINESS SCREENING

Nursery Evaluation Scale Trivandrum—Abridged (Table 4.2.3)

When DDST II is used to assess a preschool child, we can identify children with developmental delay. However, in a borderline case, what is more important is to understand

TABLE 4.2.2: Trivandrum Autism Behavioral Checklist (TABC).[10]

		Never (1)	*Sometimes (2)*	*Often (3)*	*Always (4)*
Social interaction (five items)					
a.	Inability to establish/maintain eye contact				
b.	Child does not respond when called, sometimes appears to be deaf				
c.	Difficulty in mixing and playing with other children of the same age				
d.	Lack of appropriate emotional response				
e.	Can do certain tasks well, but not the tasks involving social understanding				
Communication (four items)					
a.	Difficulty in comprehension/communication				
b.	May indicate wants by gestures or leading adults by the hand				
c.	Echolalia/using nonsensical words and muttering to self				
d.	Lack of pretend play				
Behavioral characteristics (five items)					
a.	Like sameness in everyday routine				
b.	Inappropriate attachments to objects				
c.	Unusual body movements such as flapping hands or rocking and jumping				
d.	Extreme restlessness, hyperactivity/overpassivity or prefers to be alone all the time				
e.	Not responsive to normal teaching methods				
Sensory integration (six items)					
a.	Does not like to be hugged or touch/apparent insensitivity to pain				
b.	Intolerance/addiction to certain sounds, tastes, odors, and visuals				
c.	No understanding of fear of real dangers/excessive fear of heights and change in position				
d.	Enjoys spinning or rotating objects				
e.	Inappropriate laughing and giggling/crying spells with extreme distress for no apparent reasons				
f.	Difficulty in fine motor skills. A tendency to fall/clumsiness/resistance to new motor movement activities				

Note: Scoring: 20–35: nonautistic; 36–43: mild-to-moderately autistic; 44 and above: severely autistic.

TABLE 4.2.3: Nursery Evaluation Scale Trivandrum—abridged.[10]

	3rd, 50th, and 97th percentile age placements in months		
Items	***3rd percentile***	***50th percentile***	***97th percentile***
Gross motor development			
1. Heel-to-toe walk eight steps	61	68	72
2. Stands on one foot for 10 seconds	48	57	66
3. Walk on a 20-cm elevated balanced beam	64	69	72
4. Catches a soft ball with one hand	53	64	68
Fine motor development			
5. Paints shape	50	56	59
6. Tears simple shape	53	64	68
7. Copies diamond shape	63	66	72
8. Prints A E F	48	53	56
9. Threads 10 beads in 1 minute	50	57	65
10. Draws a picture with three parts (excluding drawing a man)	56	61	66
Cognitive development			
11. Picks a specific number of objects (5)	55	64	66
12. Builds a pyramid of 10 blocks	54	66	71
13. Arranges objects according to width and length	53	63	69
14. Puts numbers 1–10 in a sequence	48	54	59
15. Names positions of objects	46	52	65
16. Completes a simple maze	50	56	60
17. Names days of a week in order	57	65	70
18. Reads 10 printed words	61	68	72
Personal social development			
19. Buttons and unbuttons dress	56	63	68
20. Washes hands and mouth when directed	42	45	48
Expressive language development			
21. Names function associated with three body parts	49	52	57
22. Tells materials out of which objects are made of	53	60	66
Receptive language development			
23. Points to hard/soft/rough/smooth	51	59	63
24. Points to middle	52	60	65
25. Points to absurdities in a picture	51	57	62
26. Puts together five parts picture	58	68	72

the level of skill development in the child in comparison with other children of the same age (percentile position). This helps to start item-based interventions in these children with delays. Nursery Evaluation Scale Trivandrum (NEST)—Abridged is a simple tool that has skill-based items in the areas of gross motor, fine motor, cognitive, personal social, expressive language, and receptive language. NEST provides a general assessment of the child.[11]

DEVELOPMENTAL STIMULATION AND THERAPY

Therapy Based on Passive Exercises

Out of the items assessed in the Amiel-Tison method, the angles give an important clue for the therapy and stimulation part of the intervention. A restriction in angles specifies hypertonia, and a wide angle suggests hypotonia in most cases.

In such situations, the effectiveness of stimulation appears only after the muscle tone becomes normal. Passive therapy by the mother in a playful way helps to reduce these tone abnormalities. Based on Amiel-Tison passive angles, home-based therapy has been designed. This simple concept is not aimed at hastening developmental milestones but aims to prevent:

- Mental subnormality by better mother–infant interaction
- Joint stiffening by repeated passive movements
- Contractures by repetitive passive movements
- Muscle wasting and fibrosis
- Helplessness in parents

Therapy Based on Motor Milestones

Head Holding/Neck Control

- Stimulating the child to hold the head by carrying the child in an upright position by supporting the infant's head, as and when possible.
- While playing and talking with the child, lift the child by supporting his upper arm and chest, thereby stimulating him to lift and hold his head.
- The child must lie on his stomach and be guided on his elbow (a roll or round pillow can be used if necessary). Stimulate the child to lift his head and hold it up by showing a colorful toy.
- Stimulate the child in the prone position so that he lifts and holds his head. Boost him to rotate laterally by showing a colorful toy.

Sitting

- Encourage the child to sit by putting him in an armchair with the support of pillows, when possible.
- While playing and talking with the child, encourage the child to sit with his thighs apart, thereby creating a wide base and giving support at the pelvis with a downward force.
- During play, the child can be encouraged to sit in a side-sitting position on either side with support on the hand on the side toward which he is sitting.
- Guide the child to support on his hands and knees (four-point kneeling/quadruped position) during play. A roll or pillow can be used, if necessary. Then gradually guide him to sit on either side by supporting him with the hand on the same side. Help the child to stay in this position for a while. Then lead him again on to his hands and knees and then gradually to side sitting on the other side.
- A baby walker can also be used to stimulate and improve sitting.

Standing

- Guide the child on to both his knees during play. Finally, support him at the pelvis. If necessary, give support to the upper part of his body. Gradually, the support can be withdrawn, and the child can be made to support himself by holding on to a low stool. This position can be maintained by directing the child's attention to any play activity.
- From lying on the back position (supine position), stimulate the child to sit and gradually to the standing position during playtime.
- First, guide the child to both his knees while he supports himself on a low stool with his hands. Playfully, point him to a colorful toy. Gradually help on to the half-standing position-raise one leg so as to stand on one foot with the leg straight and the other on the knee. The therapist should play and talk with the child, helping him to sustain this position. Repeat on the other side. Meanwhile, depending on the child's ability, stimulate him to pull to a standing position by himself, supporting on the stool.
- Encourage the child to stand whenever possible, initially with support and then slowly diminishing the support as per the child's ability. A baby walker will also serve the purpose of developing standing and walking skills.

DEVELOPMENTAL ASSESSMENT (CONFIRMATIVE TESTS)

Formal developmental assessment is done in the developmental evaluation clinics of CDCs. Based on the experience of conducting developmental evaluation clinics for 5 years in CDC, Kerala (2,111 children), it has been seen that approximately 50% of babies attending the clinic had developmental delay without a specific clinical diagnosis; speech problems were seen in 13.9%, neurological problems in 9.5%, and chromosomal anomalies in 5.2%.[12,13]

Developmental Assessment Scale for Indian Infants

This tool developed by Ms Pramila Phatak is the gold standard test used for developmental evaluation. This is built on Bayley Scales of Infant Development (BSID). The Developmental Assessment Scale for Indian infants consists of two scales, namely mental scale and motor scale. The result is expressed as the mental developmental index and psychomotor developmental index.

Bayley Scales of Infant and Toddler Development

Bayley Scales of Infant and Toddler Development is an elaborate and formal developmental assessment tool for identifying developmental delays in early childhood years. The scores have been obtained from a norm-referenced assessment of early childhood development. BSID was first published by Nancy Bayley in 1969. The version of BSID in use now is BSID 4. It was published in 2019. This version saves time and has better clinical sensitivity and accuracy when compared to BSID 3. It takes around 30–70 minutes to complete the test.

GLOBAL DEVELOPMENTAL DELAY

As per the Diagnostic and Statistical Manual of Mental Disorders, Fifth Edition (DSM-5), global developmental delay (GDD) is to be diagnosed when a child younger than 5 years of age fails to meet expected developmental milestones in several areas of intellectual functioning and is unable to undergo standardized testing for the same.

As per Indian Academy of Pediatrics (IAP) consensus guidelines, GDD is defined as significant delay (at least 2 standard deviations below the mean with standardized developmental tests) in at least two developmental domains in children under 5 years of age. Children in whom the delay is due to a primary motor issue or severe uncorrected visual/hearing impairment are excluded.[11] Based on severity, GDD can be categorized as mild, moderate, severe, and profound based on adaptive functioning.

EARLY MARKERS OF NEURODEVELOPMENTAL DISORDERS

An early diagnosis of NDDs is possible using the INCLEN Neuro-Development Screening Tool (NDST-Research Form) and confirmed by DSM-5 criteria and INCLEN diagnostic tools like INCLEN Diagnostic Tool for autism spectrum disorder (INDT-ASD).[14] However, clinically, NDDs can be suspected early by atypical development of milestones **(Flowchart 4.2.1)**.

Flowchart 4.2.1: Evaluation of a child with suspected developmental delay.

A child suspected to have developmental delay

↓

Clinical history: Chief complaints, onset, progression, variation, precipitating and relieving factors of symptoms, if any
Developmental history: Gross motor, fine motor, speech, language and communication, personal–social, cognitive, play
Family history: With three-generation pedigree chart
Birth history: Antenatal, perinatal, and postnatal history
Family's socioeconomic condition, parenting style, family dynamics
Scholastic and academic history

↓

Clinical examination: General and head-to-foot examination focusing on dysmorphic features, neurocutaneous stigmata, clinical developmental examination, clinical neurological examination, anthropometric measurements, and systemic examination

↓

Use of clinical tools for assessment:
- Newborn and infant screening and assessment: HNNE, HINE, Prechtl's GMA, AIMS
- Developmental delay: TDSC, DDST II, DST, ASQ-3, SDQ, PEDS-DM, BSID IV, DASII
- Language and communication delay: LEST, CSBS-DP, REEL-4
- Autism screening and evaluation: M-CHAT R/F, TABC, INCLEN- ASD, CARS-2, GARS, ADOS, ADIR
- ADHD screening and evaluation: VADPRS, Conners, INCLEN-ADHD
- Behavioral assessment: ABC, CBCL, BP-2, BASC-2
- Adaptive function assessment: VABS III, VSMS
- IQ estimation: BKT, MISIC, WISC IV
- SLD assessment: NIMHANS battery for SLD, DALI, GLAD

↓

Investigation planning if necessary USG cranium, MRI brain, thyroid profile, serum iron/vitamin B_{12}, metabolic panel, genetic screening, skeletal survey

↓

Individualized intervention plan based on delays identified, early stimulation or early intervention, center- or home-based approach, bio-psychosocial model

(ABC: Aberrant Behavior Checklist; ADHD: attention-deficit/hyperactivity disorder; ADIR: Autism Diagnostic Interview Revised; ADOS: Autism Diagnostic Observation Schedule; AIMS: Alberta Infant Motor Scale; ASQ: Ages and Stages Questionnaire; BASC-2: Behavior Assessment System for Children; BKT: Binet Kamat Test; BP-2: Behavioral Profile-2; BSID: Bayley Scale of Infant Development; CARS-2: Childhood Autism Rating Scale, Second Edition; CBCL: Child Behavior Checklist; CSBS-DP: Communication and Symbolic Behaviour Scale-Developmental Profile; DALI: Dyslexia Assessment for Languages in India; DASII: Developmental Scale for Indian Infants; DDST II: Denver Developmental Screening Test II; DST: Developmental Screening Test; GARS: Gillian Autism Rating Scale; GLAD: Grade Level Assessment Device; GMA: General Movement Assessment; HNNE: Hammersmith Neonatal Neurological Examination; HINE: Hammersmith Infant Neurological Examination; INCLEN-ADHD: International Clinical Epidemiology Network attention-deficit/hyperactivity disorder; INCLEN-ASD: International Clinical Epidemiology Network Diagnostic Tool for autism spectrum disorder; LEST: Language Evaluation Scale Trivandrum; M-CHAT R/F: Modified Checklist for Autism in Toddlers, Revised with Follow-up; MISIC: Malin's Intelligence Scale for Indian Children; NIMHANS: National Institute of Mental Health and Neurosciences; PEDS-DM: Parental evaluation of Developmental Status-Developmental milestones; REEL: Receptive Expressive Emergent Language Scales; SDQ: Strengths and Difficulties Questionnaire; SLD: specific learning disability; TABC: Toddler Autism Behavior Checklist; TDSC: Total Developmental Screening Checklist; VABS: Vineland Adaptive Behavior Scale; VADPRS: Vanderbilt ADHD Diagnostic Parent Rating Scale; VSMS: Vineland Social Maturity Scale; WISC IV: Weschler's Intelligence Scale for children)

Atypical motor development/delay: Parents may notice a delay in the infant compared to other infants of the same age in acquiring motor milestones. There is always an age range for milestones to develop. Hence, a normal variation should always be kept in mind. The possibility of maturational lag or cerebral palsy, the most important cause of motor delay in infancy, should also be kept in mind.

Atypical cognitive development/delay: A child with a predominant cognitive deficit or intellectual disability generally will have normal progression of motor development, and his or her behaviors correspond with mental age. They may also have adaptive functional deficits, language delay, poor problem-solving, and poor awareness of the consequences of their actions.

Atypical social and language development/delay: Atypical development in social, cognitive, and language domains necessitates complete evaluation, particularly in infants or toddlers with the following signs: (1) No babbling, (2) no pointing (joint attention) or gestures by 12 months of age, (3) no single words by 16 months, and (4) no two-word spontaneous phrases by 24 months.

The chief recommendations of the Indian Academy of Pediatrics-Neurodevelopmental Pediatrics (IAP-NDP) chapter consensus statement on the NDD habilitation process: strategic plan for prevention, early detection, and early intervention, are as follows:

- Preconception counseling as part of focusing on the first 1,000 days
- Promoting efforts to organize systematic training programs in the Newborn Resuscitation Program (NRP)
- Lactation management
- Developmental follow-up and early stimulation for special newborn care unit (SNCU)/NICU graduates
- Risk stratification of NICU graduates
- Newborn screening
- Counseling parents
- Screening for developmental delay by trained professionals using simple validated Indian screening tools at 4, 8, 12, 18, and 24 months
- Holistic assessment of 10 NDDs at CDCs or DEICs
- Need to promote ongoing academic programs in clinical child development for capacity building of community-based therapies.[15]

REFERENCES

1. de Fátima Dornelas L, de Castro Duarte NM, de Castro Magalhães L. Neuropsychomotor developmental delay: conceptual map, term definitions, uses and limitations. Rev Paul Pediatr. 2015;33(1):88-103.
2. Brown KA, Parikh S, Patel DR. Understanding basic concepts of developmental diagnosis in children. Transl Pediatr. 2020;9(Suppl 1):S9-22.
3. Hirai AH, Kogan MD, Kandasamy V, Reuland C, Bethell C. Prevalence and variation of developmental screening and surveillance in early childhood. JAMA Pediatr. 2018;172(9): 857-66.
4. Salomone E, Pacione L, Shire S, Brown FL, Reichow B, Servili C. Development of the WHO caregiver skills training program for developmental disorders or delays. Front Psychiatry. 2019;10:769.
5. Arora NK, Nair MKC, Gulati S, Deshmukh V, Mohapatra A, Mishra D, et al. Neurodevelopmental disorders in children aged 2–9 years: population-based burden estimates across five regions in India. PLoS Med. 2018;15(7):e1002615.
6. Nair MKC, Nair GH, Mini AO, Indulekha S, Letha S, Russell PS. Development and validation of Language Evaluation Scale Trivandrum for children aged 0–3 years—LEST (0–3). Indian Pediatr. 2013;50(5):463-7.
7. Nair MKC, Nair GS, George B, Suma N, Neethu C, Leena ML, et al. Development and validation of Trivandrum Development Screening Chart for children aged 0–6 years. Indian J Pediatr. 2013;80(Suppl 2):S248-55.
8. Nair MKC, Nair GH, George B, Mini AO. Language Evaluation Scale Trivandrum (LEST 3–6 years) development and validation. Indian Pediatr. 2016;53(3):257-8.
9. Vitrikas K, Savard D, Bucaj M. Developmental delay: when and how to screen. Am Fam Physician. 2017;96(1):36-43.
10. Nair MKC, Kumar S, Lukose R, Aswathy LA, Kumar A. Diagnostic validation of Trivandrum Autism Behavior Checklist (TABC) a screening checklist for autism spectrum disorder (ASD) against Childhood Autism Rating Scale-2-Standard Version (CARS-2-ST). Int J Pharmaceut Clin Res. 2023;15(4):7-19.
11. Nair MKC, George B, Rekha R, Meenu VS, Swapna S, Sajitha J. Nursery Evaluation Scale Trivandrum (NEST)—abridged. Pediatric Compan. 2020;16(1):7-9.
12. Nair MKC, George B, Padma K, Potti N, Elizabeth KE, Jeyaseelan L. Developmental evaluation clinic—CDC experience. Indian Pediatr. 2009;46(Suppl):s63-6.
13. Juneja M, Gupta A, Sairam S, Jain R, Sharma M, Thadani A, et al. Diagnosis and management of global development delay: consensus guidelines of growth, development and behavioral pediatrics chapter, neurology chapter and neurodevelopment pediatrics chapter of the Indian Academy of Pediatrics. Indian Pediatr. 2022;59(5):401-15.
14. Juneja M, Mishra D, Russell PS, Gulati S, Deshmukh V, Poma T, et al; INCLEN Study Group. INCLEN Diagnostic Tool for autism spectrum disorder (INDT-ASD): development and validation. Indian Peditr. 2014;51(5):359-65.
15. Nair MKC, Ahmed S, Multani KS, Mohamed Ismail PM, Kamath SS, Dalwai SH, et al. Consensus statement of the IAP—neurodevelopmental chapter on neurodevelopmental disorders habilitation process: strategic plan for prevention, early detection and early intervention. Indian Pediatr. 2024; 61(1):10-23.

4.3 Cerebral Palsy

Atul Bhaskar, Shambhavi Seth

DEFINITION

Cerebral palsy (CP), as the name implies, is paresis (palsy) due to brain (cerebral) involvement. It is a broad term for a group of conditions with disturbance in the movement or posture (motor) due to a lesion in the developing brain parenchyma.

The brain lesion or damage is static but its effects on the musculoskeletal and visceral systems are progressive. Cognition, speech, and vision may also be affected based on the severity and site of the lesion.

EPIDEMIOLOGY

While the developed world predominantly deals with prematurity and extremely low birth weight (LBW)-related morbidities as causative factors for CP, developing countries are still coping with prenatal rubella, intranatal asphyxia, and postnatal hyperbilirubinemia as causes of CP. In India, environmental factors such as social attitudes, sociocultural beliefs, lack of knowledge among parents, limited availability of skilled healthcare professionals (HCPs), and resources, as well as infrastructural, transport, and financial barriers, have been found to affect treatment and participation among children with CP.[1] The incidence of CP is approximately 1–3 per 1,000 live births, and the frequency varies based on the available antenatal and postnatal care.

COMMON CAUSES AND ETIOPATHOGENESIS OF CEREBRAL PALSY

The most proximate cause of CP is damage to the brain that can occur in utero (prenatal), during birth (natal), or after birth (postnatal). High-risk maternal factors at conception such as smoking, malnutrition, systemic illnesses, and drug abuse can potentially impact the immature brain **(Table 4.3.1)**. Postnatal CP is more common in India due to a lack of experienced neonatal care in mofussil areas and sometimes because of poor healthcare infrastructure.

The exact etiology of CP is unclear, but any event that causes injury to the developing brain can lead to CP. The central nervous system (CNS), unlike visceral organs, continues to mature and form new synaptic connections after birth. The most sensitive period of CNS development occurs antenatally and in the first 2 years after birth. Undue injury or impact in any part of the developing brain can lead to various types of CP.

TABLE 4.3.1: Causes of cerebral palsy (CP).

Prenatal	First trimester	• Intrauterine maternal infection • Genetic causes • Drugs and medications • Radiation exposure
	Second trimester	• Intrapartum hemorrhage • Disorders of placenta • Oligohydramnios
	Third trimester	• Amniotic fluid infection • Placental hemorrhage • Pre-eclampsia • Rh incompatibility
Natal or birth complications leading to CP		• Prematurity • Low birth weight (LBW) • Birth hypoxia/asphyxia • Hypoglycemia • Hypocalcemia • Seizures • Prolonged labor • Meconium aspiration • Birth injury—forceps, vacuum-assisted delivery
Postnatal CP		• Infection in neonatal period • Infantile epilepsy • Head injuries • Respiratory distress syndrome • Hyperbilirubinemia • Blood dyscrasias • Hypothermia • Intracranial bleed

The incidence of CP has remained unchanged despite improvements in maternal and child health in the developed world. In the modern era, LBW (<2,500 g) and ultra-LBW (<1,500 g) babies born prematurely live to survive. There is a 70% increase in CP in children with LBW. In the past, CP was believed to have been caused during birth or after birth, but studies show that 70% of CP is caused due to prenatal factors, many of which are beyond the control of any intervention.

CLINICAL TYPES OF CEREBRAL PALSY

Cerebral palsy is commonly classified based on the part of the body segment involvement (topographic classification) or on the type of motor or muscle stiffness seen that impacts posture and function (tone-based classification).

The human body is represented in an inverted fashion in the cerebral cortex with the lower limbs at the summit and the trunk, upper limbs, and facial parts defined sequentially in the deeper cortex. Based on the area of cerebral involvement, five different types of impairments are seen.

Topographic Classification of Cerebral Palsy

The type of CP can be classified based on the body segment involved as follows **(Fig. 4.3.1)**:

- *Hemiplegia:* One-half of the body is involved—right- or left-side involvement. The arm is more severely affected than the lower limb. There may be associated sensory or speech deficits if the right or left cortex is affected.
- *Monoplegia:* Only one limb segment is involved—right or left upper or lower limb. Rare type.
- *Diplegia:* Lower limb segments are more involved than upper limb. Typically seen in children who are born premature or with LBW.
- *Triplegia:* Both legs and only one upper limb (three limb segments) are affected. Rare type.
- *Quadriplegia:* All four limb segments, trunk, and cervical spine muscles are involved. The most severe type is seen with birth asphyxia, meconium aspiration, and uncontrolled epilepsy. It can be genetic or syndromic. Significant cognitive, sensory, and visual impairment.

Motor or Muscle Tone-based Classification of Cerebral Palsy

Figure 4.3.2 provides a schematic diagram of the etio-pathogenesis of CP from abnormal tone to contracture and deformity.

- *Hypotonia*—reduced or flaccid muscle tone with poor posturing and flexible joints
- *Hypertonia:*
  - Spastic or increased tone or tension in the muscles
  - *Dyskinetic:* Dyskinetic CP is associated with abnormal and involuntary movement
    - Dystonia—the awkward and tortuous posturing is seen when the child attempts voluntary movements or even at rest. Often, these children exhibit low tone if the body is relaxed. The body segments move fast and uncontrollably impacting any useful function.
    - Athetoid—this exhibits jerky and sudden uncontrollable movements. Often, these children have good cognition and intelligence. However, speech may be impaired.
  - *Mixed tone:* This is a combination of spastic and dyskinetic movements, and management can be challenging.

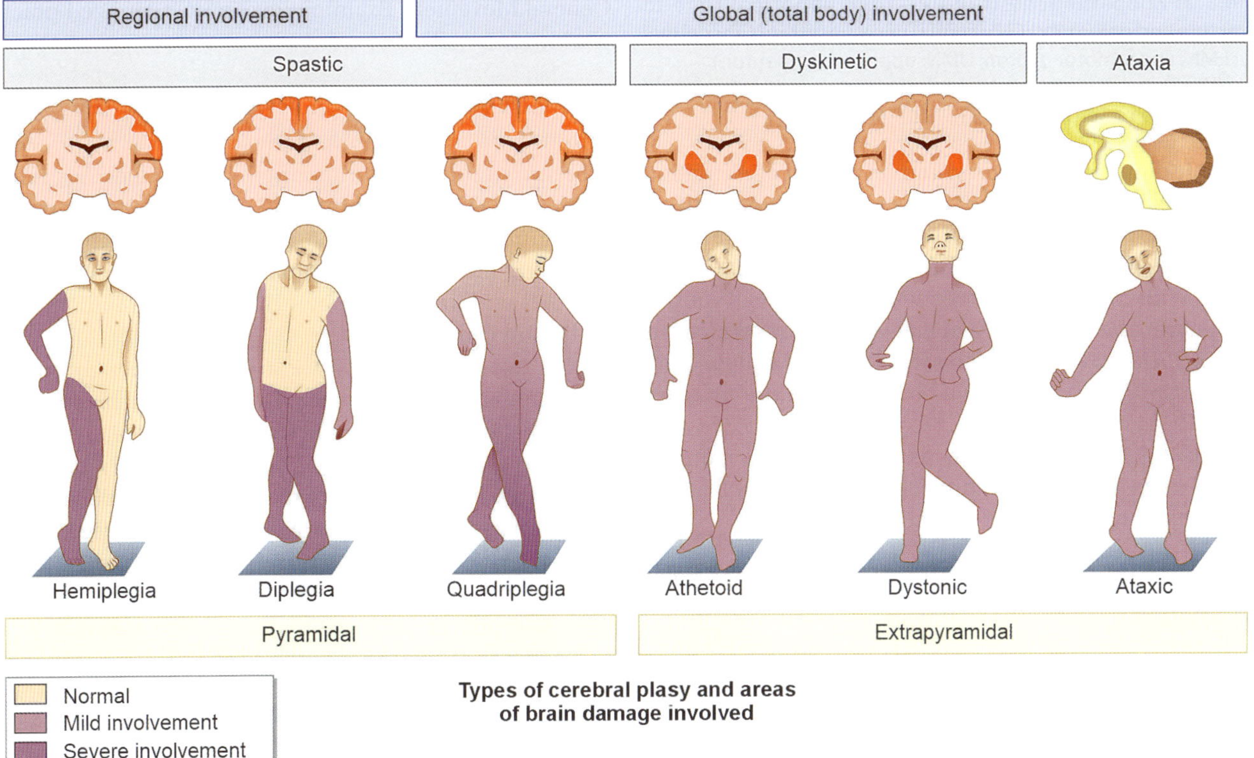

Fig. 4.3.1: Topographic classification of cerebral palsy.

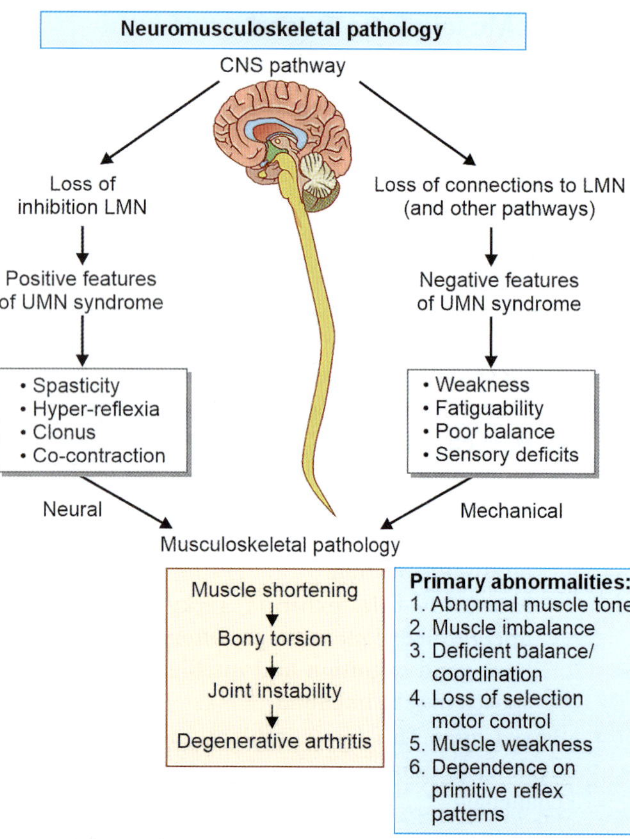

Fig. 4.3.2: Etiopathogenesis of CP—from abnormal tone to contracture and deformity. (CNS: central nervous system CP: cerebral palsy; LMN: lower motor neuron; UMN: upper motor neuron)
Source: Graham HK, Selber P. Musculoskeletal aspects of cerebral palsy. J Bone Joint Surg Br. 2003;85(2):157-66.

Spastic diplegia is the most common clinical presentation of CP with the classic finding of periventricular leukomalacia on magnetic resonance imaging (MRI) brain. Often, the tone abnormality is related to the site of brain parenchymal damage. With dystonic and dyskinetic CP, the basal ganglia and pallidum are damaged. Neonatal jaundice or kernicterus is often associated with this type of CP. Postnatal epilepsy and epileptic syndromes are often associated with the dystonic type of CP.

Often, "CP mimics" such as metabolic or genetic syndromes are associated with specific neurological features and may have mixed types of tone abnormalities.

CLINICAL FEATURES OF CEREBRAL PALSY

Early Diagnosis

The specific CP syndromes are best recognized after 3–5 years of age, although suggestive signs and symptoms may be present in infancy.[2] Picking CP early changes the management outcome. Early signs of CP on clinical examination in a young infant are listed in the following text.

Features in Neonates and Infants

Neurobehavioral Signs

Neurobehavioral signs include excessive irritability, lethargy, sleeping poorly, vomiting frequently, being difficult to handle and cuddle, and poor visual attention. Early signs may appear soon after birth. Poor cry, paucity of limb movements, abnormal posturing, difficulty sucking and feeding, and decreased response to external stimuli may be evident before 3 months.

Developmental Reflexes

Delay in disappearance of primitive reflexes such as tonic neck reflex, Moro reflex, and grasp reflex and the appearance of protective reflexes like parachute and lateral propping reactions may be an early indicator of motor disability. Also, exaggerated reflexes like exaggerated tonic labyrinthine reflex may lead to abnormal posturing in the form of opisthotonus.

Motor Examination

Motor examination, including tone and posture, should pick up any asymmetry or abnormal tone patterns like increased neck extensor tone which may lead to a false impression of improved head control, persisting hand fisting, and abnormal oromotor patterns like tongue thrust. Hammersmith Infant Neurological Examination (HINE) and more recently Prechtl's General Movement Examination are standardized practices worldwide.

Motor Milestones

Monitoring motor milestones using a standardized screening tool is recommended. The Indian Academy of Pediatrics (IAP) recommends complete developmental screening at 9, 18, and 30 months' follow-up visits. For screening of neuromotor impairments, tools developed by INCLEN and improvised by AIIMS (AIIMS Modified INDT-NMI Tool) can be used.

No two children with CP are alike although the brain damage may appear similar. The clinical signs are diverse and depend on the extent of brain damage. Many signs and symptoms overlap during infancy and childhood; the key is to watch for the red flags that depict early diagnosis and initiate investigation for early treatment and rehabilitation (**Box 4.3.1**).

Clinicians are advised to have a handy chart regarding age-appropriate milestones in their clinic and should be able to diagnose CP before 6 months.

Signs in Early Childhood

Inability to stand without support, supported sitting and toe walking either unilateral or bilateral, and brisk reflexes in

BOX 4.3.1: Red flags for early identification of CP.

Motor:
- Delay in neck holding by 6 months
- Inability to roll and sit by 1 year of age
- Persistence of primitive reflexes

Social:
- Lack of social smile by 3 months
- Poor response to tactile stimulation
- Absent visual tracking

(CP: cerebral palsy)

lower and upper limbs after 2 years could indicate CP. Early handedness before 2 years indicating that the contralateral side is weak, painless limp, and dragging of feet may be the earliest finding in hemiplegia.

The pathogenesis of muscle contracture in early and late childhood is directly related to the lack of normal physiological muscle activity. The loss of selective motor control and the inability of muscles to stretch due to increased tone lead to degeneration and fibrosis of the muscles. The skeletal growth continues unabated and with progressive muscle shortening, secondary joint contractures occur that can lead to joint subluxation or dislocation.

Flexion contractures are more common than extension attitude, with biarticular muscles more affected than monoarticular ones. Hence, in late childhood, untreated CP can lead to typical posturing in the upper and lower limbs. The attitude of the upper limb is that of shoulder adduction, elbow flexion and pronation, wrist palmar-flexion, and finger flexion due to predominant flexor contracture. The characteristic findings in the lower limb include ankle equinus, knee flexion, hip adduction and flexion (jump posture), and trunk flexion.

Secondary torsional deformities can lead to internal rotation of the femur and external rotation of the tibia.

Features during Adolescence

In children with diplegia, muscle contracture coupled with weakness causes the child to crouch with hip and knee flexion and ankle in dorsiflexion causing a labored gait. In hemiplegia, torsional deformities of the femur and muscle weakness cause the classical circumduction gait.

Scoliosis, hip joint migration and subluxation, and pelvic obliquity occur during early to later childhood and must be diagnosed early.

Scales to Measure Motor Function in Cerebral Palsy

Gross Motor Function Classification System

Gross Motor Function Classification System (GMFCS) is perhaps the best way to assess the ambulatory status of a

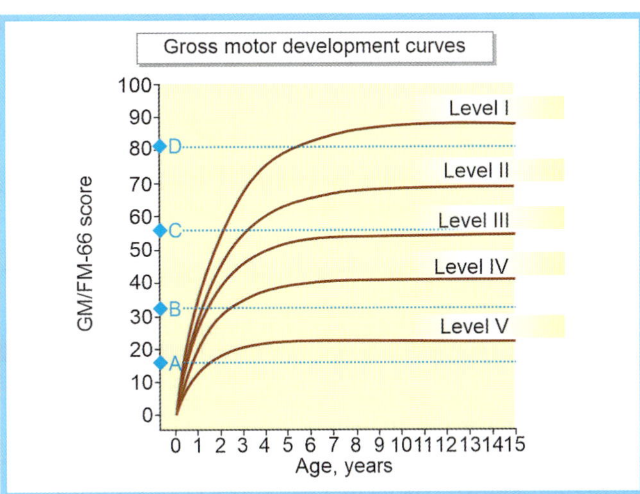

Fig. 4.3.3: GMFCS (gross motor functional classification system)—a useful tool to grade the severity of motor involvement in cerebral palsy.
Source: Rosenbaum PL, Walter SD, Hanna SE, Palisano RJ, Russell DJ, Raina P, et al. Prognosis for gross motor function in cerebral palsy: creation of motor development curves. JAMA. 2002;288(11):1357-63.

child **(Fig. 4.3.3)**. Most GMFCS curves stabilize by the age of 6–7 years, and the potential for independent ambulation is apparent around the same age.[3,4]

Associated Features in Cerebral Palsy

These include the following:
- Epilepsy
- Problems with communication and cognition
- Speech disorders
- Drooling, feeding, and swallowing issues
- Visual and hearing impairments
- Gastrointestinal difficulties
- Dental and hygiene problems

IMAGING IN CEREBRAL PALSY

Magnetic Resonance Imaging

Magnetic resonance imaging, especially of the brain, remains the cornerstone in the diagnosis of CP. Various MRI classifications exist depending on the site of involvement of the brain. *X-rays* are required to diagnose metabolic deficiencies, rule out stress fractures, and for screening of hip migration and scoliosis, especially in nonambulatory forms of CP. The salient features seen in MRI of brain in CP with respect to gestation and clinical manifestations are as follows:
- Periventricular hyperintensities are seen in premature babies and present as spastic diplegia.
- Watershed lesions with cystic encephalomalacia are seen commonly in term infants with ischemia or asphyxia and manifest clinically with spastic quadriplegia.

- Hyperintensities in the posterior putamen and thalami bilaterally are seen in infants with term hypoxic-ischemic encephalopathy (HIE) and manifest as dyskinetic CP.
- Occipital lobe involvement is characteristic of neonatal hypoglycemic insult.
- Hyperintensity involving bilateral globus pallidi is a sequelae of kernicterus.

PREVENTION

The major basic principles in the prevention of CP include the following:

- Premature babies constitute 43% of all CP, and it becomes pertinent to avoid premature birth.
- Effective preventive strategies have been developed for certain known risk factors like rhesus isoimmunization, maternal iodine deficiency, hypothyroidism, and hyperbilirubinemia.
- The role of antenatal magnesium sulfate before delivery in <30 weeks of gestation and of antenatal steroids in <34 weeks of gestation has been standard practices of care.
- For babies at term with asphyxia, therapeutic hypothermia within 6 hours of delivery is recommended.[5]

MANAGEMENT OF CEREBRAL PALSY

Management of CP is always a combination of therapies—motor interventions, tone management, medical management, surgical procedures, and newer interventions.[6] More recently, the approach has changed to improve functional outcomes based on the International Classification of Functioning, Disability and Health (ICF) framework rather than target traditional approaches of promoting normal motor tone and patterns.

Motor Interventions

Motor interventions include bimanual training, task-specific skill training to improve motor coordination and performance, constraint-induced movement therapy (restraining unaffected limb to encourage the use of the affected limb), and physical training to target underlying muscle weakness which may be provided by physiotherapy and occupational therapy. Active engagement of the child in training brings out more successful results than passive limb handling. Monitoring the acquisition of milestones is as important as the therapy—failure to acquire milestones within a reasonable period of time mandates search for comorbidities rather than continuing with the same therapies.

Tone Management

Spasticity is seen in 85% of children with CP and dyskinesia in 7% and few may have mixed tone patterns. Commonly used muscle relaxants include oral baclofen, tizanidine, and diazepam. Antidystonic medications used are trihexyphenidyl and tetrabenazine. Most of the antispasmodic agents are easy to administer but may have systemic effects with a range of side effects.

Botulinum toxin type A (BTX-A) acts by chemodenervation. When injected into the affected muscles, it blocks the presynaptic release of acetylcholine and decreases tone by limiting muscle contraction. It is more effective in dynamic contractures and ideally not more than two to three muscles should require treatment at a time.

Intrathecal baclofen with pump for children with persistent severe spasticity can be tried but significant complications may outweigh the potential benefits.

Medical Management of Associated Conditions

Medical management of associated conditions such as drooling (oral exercises and glycopyrrolate), constipation, sleep disturbances, care of feeding, and nutrition forms an integral part of the management of any child with CP.

Surgical Management

W J Little, in his classic treatise on treatment of CP (1843), had recommended surgical division of tendons to improve posture and ambulation. Prolonged casting and repeat tendon surgeries were common in the 1900s. Terhune, in the 1950s, had advocated for the first time ever "the role of teamwork in the treatment of CP." The hierarchal model of treatment, where the patient would be seen by individual specialists without any communication, has now evolved into a well-defined multidisciplinary model.

A dedicated CP clinic has development pediatricians, neurologists, physiotherapists, orthotics, nutritionists, counselors, and orthopedic surgeons all under one roof and more important as part of a documented plan. The treatment should be tailored to an individual child and the family.

Diagnostic Matrix for Management of a Child with Cerebral Palsy

Every child with CP should undergo a thorough physical examination, followed by appropriate imaging, visual or 3D gait analysis, examination under anesthesia, and pain management counseling before embarking on surgery. The appropriate classification scheme is applied based on the pattern of deformities in limbs.[7]

Orthopedic Management

Broadly, orthopedic management can be divided into four groups as described next.

Tone Management

In the past four decades, chemodenervation using botulinum toxin has revolutionized the management of spasticity. A high safety profile, locally deliverable with simple intramuscular (IM) injection and reversible effect, has the potential to control spasticity in children <7 years. The botulinum toxin works at the synaptic junction by blocking the release of acetylcholine at the neuromuscular junction, thus reducing the reflex stimulation of muscle.

Chemodenervation, coupled with splintage and physiotherapy, is the mainstay in younger children before the development of muscle fibrosis and contracture.

Muscle Contracture Management

The natural history of untreated CP is progressive contracture across joints with abnormal posture and loss of function.[8] The goal of orthopedic surgery in ambulatory CP is to improve ease of walking by optimizing gait biomechanics, improve or preserve physical function, prevent fatigue, and enhance activity participation and quality of life **(Fig. 4.3.4)**.

For nonambulatory children with CP, the chief aims of surgery are to prevent and alleviate pain due to joint deformities and to preserve or improve function and quality of life.

Early contractures occur in the flexor groups of muscles and typically ankle equinus, knee flexion, and hip flexion produce classical circumduction gait. This labored gait causes considerable energy consumption and fatigue in the child.

A single-event multilevel surgery (SEMLS) is now the gold standard of orthopedic treatment in CP—a specialized team of surgeon, anesthesiologist, and assistants perform soft-tissue releases or bony correction at each affected level in the limb, on both sides in one sitting to prevent repeat surgeries in the same child.[9] Robust pain management and nutritional and medical support with early rehabilitation have considerably improved outcomes after such major surgeries. Most surgeries involve guarded muscle recessions where only the aponeurotic covering over the muscle belly is cut circumferentially. This causes the muscles to elongate at the musculotendinous junction, thereby alleviating the contracture.

Postoperative casting and orthotics are integral to the treatment to maintain the correct weight-bearing position of the joint.

Joint and Torsional Deformity Management of Limbs and Feet

Joint deformities are seen around adolescence when the dynamics of skeletal growth, progressive muscle contracture, weight gain, and poor antigravity muscle power all contribute to angular deformities around the hip, knee, ankle, and foot joints.

Various patterns of joint and foot deformities are seen in the lower limbs and are different for diplegics and hemiplegics. Although the deformities may appear similar in this age group, treatment must be individually tailored as often some spasticity also contributes to the strength of the muscle.

Foot deformities take two or more shapes—either the foot is bent inward (equinovarus) or the heel is rotated

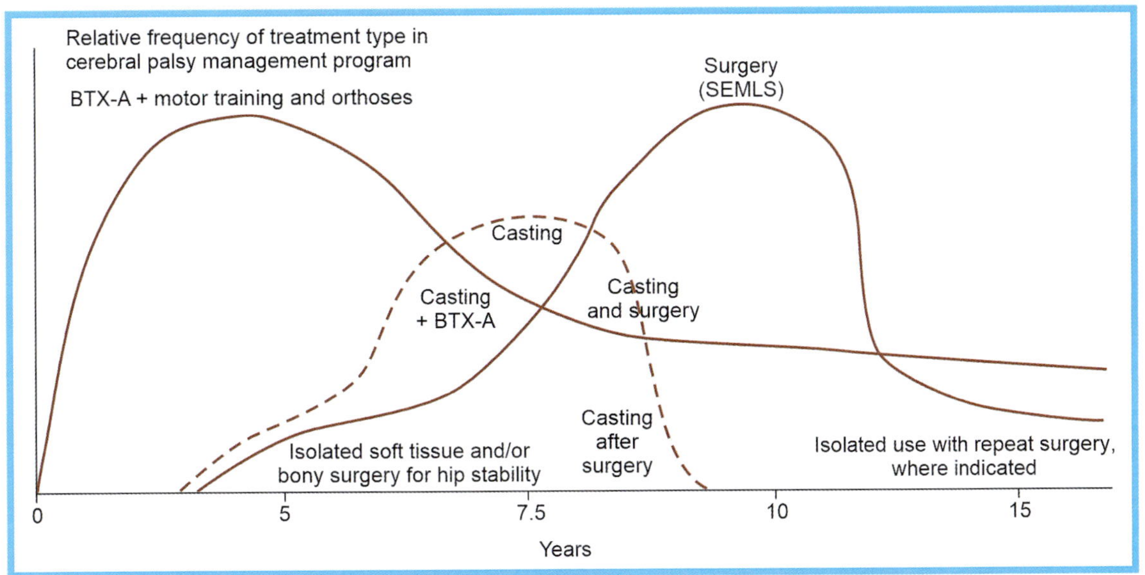

Fig. 4.3.4: Time frame of "Tone management by Casting, Botulinum Toxin, Single event multilevel surgery" from birth to adolescence. (BTX-A: botulinum toxin type A; SEMLS: single-event multilevel surgery)

outward with the forefoot in pronation with midfoot breech (planovalgus deformity). If the feet are braceable, then orthotics are applied or else the child needs corrective surgery to improve foot and overall balance.

Spine and Hip Management

Hip and spine screening is extremely important in nonambulators or functional walkers. The incidence of hip dislocation in GMFCS V is almost 60%. Hip screening, with serial pelvic radiographs, is required after the age of 2 years in nonwalkers.[10] If the hip migration is more than 40%, then chemodenervation, soft-tissue release, or bony surgery is required to maintain the joint in position. Adductor and medial hamstring release, followed by broom-stick plaster, suffices in most cases, and femoral and pelvic osteotomy for older children with greater than 50% migration.

Proposed newer interventions, including craniosacral therapy, hyperbaric oxygen, neurodevelopmental therapy in the original passive format, and sensory integration, have no proven role and are not recommended. Adjunct therapies when combined with task-specific motor training such as electrical stimulation, hydrotherapy, taping, transcranial direct current stimulation, and virtual reality serious gaming warrant more research. Literature evidence regarding the role of stem cell therapy is mixed and clinical data scarce. These are not recommended for routine clinical use as of now.

Rehabilitation

Specific goals are identified for each child, and planned sessions of rehabilitation are discussed with family and caregivers to optimize function. Assistive technology, external orthotics, physiotherapy, and rehabilitation equipment that aid the physical and mental improvement of the child are integral at every stage in the growing child.

Rehabilitation goals are tailored for each child based on their GMFCS grade. Children undergoing physiotherapy and neuromedication for tone management often need orthotic support to prevent contractures and joint deformities. Also, orthotic support is required in children who undergo multilevel surgery for correction of deformities.

CONCLUSION

The assessment and management of CP have undergone a major overhaul in terms of both diagnosis and intervention. All aspects of medical, neurological, orthopedic, and rehabilitative treatments are individualized for the child.

REFERENCES

1. Jindal P, Macdermid JC, Rosenbaum P, Direzze B, Narayan A, Nayak SL. Treatment and re/habilitation of children with cerebral palsy in India: a scoping review. Dev Med Child Neurol. 2019;61(9):1050-60.
2. Gulati S, Sondhi V. Cerebral palsy: an overview. Indian J Pediatr. 2018;85(11):1006-16.
3. Palisano R, Rosenbaum P, Walter S, Russell D, Wood E, Galuppi B. Development and reliability of a system to classify gross motor function in children with cerebral palsy. Dev Med Child Neurol. 1997;39(4):214-23.
4. Palisano RJ, Rosenbaum P, Bartlett D, Livingston MH. Content validity of the expanded and revised gross motor function classification system. Dev Med Child Neurol. 2008;50(10):744-50.
5. Graham H, Rosenbaum P, Paneth N, Dan B, Lin JP, Damiano DL, et al. Cerebral palsy. Nat Rev Dis Primers. 2016;2:15082.
6. Novak I, Morgan C, Fahey M, Finch-Edmondson M, Galea C, Hines A, et al. State of the evidence traffic lights 2019: systematic review of interventions for preventing and treating children with cerebral palsy. Curr Neurol Neurosci Rep. 2020;20(2):3.
7. Graham HK. Classifying cerebral palsy. J Pediatr Orthop. 2005; 25(1):127-8.
8. Bell KJ, Ounpuu S, DeLuca PA, Romness MJ. Natural progression of gait in children with cerebral palsy. J Pediatr Orthop. 2002;22(5):677-82.
9. Thomason P, Selber P, Graham HK. Single event multilevel surgery in children with bilateral spastic cerebral palsy: a 5-year prospective cohort study. Gait Posture. 2013;37(1):23-8.
10. Hagglund G, Andersson S, Duppe H, Lauge-Pederson H, Nordmark E, Westbom L. Prevention of dislocation of the hip in children with cerebral palsy. The first ten years of a population-based prevention programme. J Bone Joint Surg Br. 2005;87(1):95-101.

4.4 Intellectual Disability

Leena Srivastava

INTRODUCTION

The World Health Organization (WHO) defines disability as impairment, limitation, or restriction in activity caused mainly by health issues and environmental factors. The International Classification of Functioning Disability and Health (ICF), the WHO framework for health and disability, defines disability in reference to functioning in multiple life areas. Disability is seen as a result of an interaction between a person (with a health condition) and that person's contextual factors (environmental and personal factors). In this concept, disability is not seen as an individual's intrinsic feature but as a result of interaction in an environment.

Disability covers various levels of functioning at the body, person, and societal levels. Disability denotes all of the following:[1]

- Impairments in body functions and structures
- Limitations in activity
- Restriction in participation

Intellectual disability (ID) (intellectual developmental disorder), as described in the Diagnostic and Statistical Manual of Mental Disorders, Fifth Edition (DSM-5), is a neurodevelopmental disorder that begins in the early developmental period with limitations in intellectual and adaptive skills.[2] It functionally affects three adaptive domains (conceptual, social, and practical) with varying severity. The extent of adaptive impairment is key to defining ID and its severity.

The following three criteria must be met according to DSM-5:

1. *Deficits in intellectual functions*, such as reasoning, problem-solving, planning, abstract thinking, judgment, academic learning, and learning from experience, confirmed by clinical assessment and individualized, standardized intelligence testing.
2. *Deficits in adaptive functioning* that fail to meet developmental and sociocultural standards for personal independence and social responsibility. Without ongoing support, the adaptive deficits limit functioning in one or more activities of daily life, such as communication, social participation, and independent living, across multiple environments, such as home, school, work, and community
3. The *onset* of intellectual and adaptive deficits during the developmental period.

Global developmental delay (GDD) is the term used to describe intellectual impairment in children younger than 5 years. This term, also defined as developmental delay in two or more domains of development, is used to offer early intervention goals for the child until a more accurate assessment of cognition can be carried out. Not all children with GDD will continue to fulfill the diagnostic criteria for ID as they grow up. However, almost two-thirds of children with GDD will fit into an ID diagnosis later.[3]

EPIDEMIOLOGY

The prevalence of ID is stated at around 1–3% of the population.[3]

ETIOLOGY

There are varied etiologies for ID. Genetic causes account for the majority of the causes of ID. However, a significant proportion of persons with ID may have no identifiable cause.[3-6]

Genetic Causes

Genetic causes are being increasingly identified as an etiology for ID with technological advances **(Table 4.4.1)**.[5]

Chromosomal Abnormalities

The common chromosomal disorders associated with ID include the following:[3-5]

- *Down syndrome or trisomy 21*: One of the most common genetic causes with a prevalence of 1 in 800
- *Syndromes with deletions and duplications*: Another frequent cause of ID is genomic disorders resulting from deletions, microdeletions, or duplications of chromosomal material. Common examples are DiGeorge syndrome (22q11 deletion), Williams syndrome (7q11.23 deletion), Smith–Magenis syndrome (17p11.2 deletion), Angelman syndrome (15q11–13 maternal deletion), and Prader–Willi syndrome (15q11–13 paternal deletion).

TABLE 4.4.1: Common syndromes associated with intellectual disability (ID).

Syndrome	*Clinical stigmata*	*Neurodevelopmental signs*	*Genetic abnormality*
Down syndrome	• Typical facies • Hypothyroidism • Congenital heart disease	• Hypotonia • Global developmental delay (GDD) • Mild-to-moderate ID	• Trisomy 21 (95%) • Translocation (4%) • Mosaicism (1%)
Fragile X syndrome	• Elongated face • Prominent ears • Enlarged testis (postpubertal)	• Mild-to-moderate ID • Autism spectrum disorder (ASD)	CGG trinucleotide repeats (>200)
Rett syndrome	• Acquired microcephaly • Gait abnormalities • Seizures	• The initial period of normal development till 6–18 months, followed by developmental regression • Moderate-to-severe ID • Autistic features • Hand-wringing movements • Loss of purposeful hand function	Mutation in *MECP2* gene
Williams syndrome	• Typical elfin-like facies • Cardiac (e.g., supravalvular aortic stenosis) • Hypertension • Renal abnormalities	• Developmental delay • Mild-to-moderate ID	7q11 deletion
Prader–Willi syndrome	• Neonatal period-hypotonia • Lethargy • Poor feeding • Distinct faces with almond eyes • Obesity	GDD—varying levels of ID	Paternally derived deletion 15q
Angelman syndrome	• Microcephaly • Happy disposition • Ataxia • Seizures	• Developmental delay • ID/learning disabilities	Maternally derived deletion 15q

Single-Gene Disorders

These are monogenic causes of ID with autosomal dominant, autosomal recessive, or X-linked inheritance:[3-5]

- *Autosomal recessive disorders* include inborn errors of metabolism (IEMs). IEMs may account for a small percentage of patients with unexplained ID. Consanguinity, failure to thrive, episodic decompensation, developmental regression, and/or organomegaly may point to a metabolic cause. Newborn screening has increased early identification, and advances in treatment have enabled specific management in a few of these disorders.
- *Autosomal dominant ID* causality is common, and de novo variants may be responsible. Tuberous sclerosis, neurofibromatosis, and myotonic dystrophy are autosomal dominant disorders linked with ID.
- *X-linked:* Around 10–12% of X chromosome genes have been linked to ID. Fragile X syndrome is the most common X-linked cause found in males with ID. It is seen twice as commonly in males than in females. Females may manifest with milder ID. Rett syndrome, caused by mutations in the *MECP2* gene, occurs in females.

Environmental Causes

These nongenetic causes of IDs may be classified into prenatal, perinatal, and/or postnatal etiologies.[6-8]

- *Prenatal causes:*
  - Exposure to teratogens/toxins such as alcohol, tobacco, lead, and mercury; antiepileptic medications such as phenytoin and valproate; and radiation exposure
  - Congenital infections such as toxoplasmosis, syphilis, varicella zoster, parvovirus 19, rubella, cytomegalovirus, and herpes (TORCH)
- *Perinatal causes:*
  - Intrapartum asphyxia
  - Birth trauma
  - Prematurity
  - Intracranial hemorrhage
  - Congenital hypothyroidism
- *Postnatal causes:*
  - Intracranial infections (meningitis and encephalitis)
  - Head trauma
  - Malnutrition, child abuse or neglect, and extreme poverty

- Chronic iron deficiency anemia and vitamin B_{12} deficiency
- Lead poisoning
- Hypothyroidism

In many children, the etiology may be multifactorial at different phases of the early developmental period.

Diagnosis of ID will include delving into the presenting concerns, providing a detailed history, conducting a thorough general and neurological examination, and performing functional developmental assessments with targeted investigations for the etiological workup.

CLINICAL FEATURES AND HISTORY

Parental concerns that are usually present to the pediatrician are:

- Speech or language delay
- Poor understanding for the age
- Academic or learning difficulties
- Immature behavior for age

History

Personal History

- Present concerns with details of timelines and progression
- Birth history with details on the prenatal and perinatal periods with consideration of the contributory risk factors. Birth details include history of infections like chorioamnionitis, duration of labor, mode of delivery, gestation, birth weight, Apgar score, and any significant neonatal history needing special care.
- Developmental history with a chronological review of attainment of milestones in all domains with a summary of present developmental age in each domain based on history
- Social interaction and play skills, along with observation of the same
- Developmental regression or seizures
- Details of behavior, sleep, and feeding

Family History

- Obtain a three-generation pedigree of the proband with details of any developmental, genetic, metabolic, or psychiatric disorders in the family
- History of consanguinity, miscarriages, abortions, or neonatal deaths

Physical Examination

General Examination

It should focus on:

- Anthropometry—height, weight, and details of head circumference (microcephaly or macrocephaly)
- Skin—any significant neurocutaneous markers
- Dysmorphic features

Systemic Examination

A detailed neurological examination and systemic examination for organomegaly and other systemic involvement.

DIAGNOSTIC EVALUATION

Please see **Flowchart 4.4.1** for the steps in diagnostic evaluation.[6] Following a detailed history and examination, there should preferably be a referral to a developmental pediatrician or pediatric neurologist with a team for a detailed neurodevelopmental evaluation, including the following:

- Vision and hearing evaluation should be done as indicated to rule out sensory impairments. Persons with ID may have vision-related problems; around 15–20% may have hearing impairment. Thus, formal ophthalmic evaluation and hearing evaluation with audiometry are advisable.
- Routine screening for iron and vitamin B_{12} deficiency and hypothyroidism should be offered.
- Formal functional speech and language evaluation
- Intelligence and adaptive functioning assessments—a diagnosis of ID requires limitations in intellectual and adaptive functioning; thus, both need to be assessed.

Intelligence or Intelligent Quotient Testing

Intelligent quotient tests gauge impairments in intelligence or mental capacity (learning, problem-solving, reasoning, judgment, and abstract thinking). An IQ score of 2 standard deviations (SD) below the mean (i.e., <70) corresponds to intellectual impairment. Standardized tests that are commonly used for IQ testing include the following:

- Weschler Intelligence Scale for children, WISC 4
- Malin's Intelligence Scale for Indian children—an Indian adaptation of WISC
- Binet Kamat test
- Stanford Binet test

For nonverbal intelligence testing, the following are used:

- Colored/standard progressive matrices
- Bhatia's battery of tests of intelligence

Adaptive Functioning

It is essential to document impairment in a child's adaptive functioning to diagnose ID as it affects participation in settings like home, community, and school. It reflects affection in at least one conceptual, social, or practical domain. Limitations in adaptive functioning are more easily perceived in daily life functioning. They are essential in gauging the severity of ID and the extent of support that a child will need.

Flowchart 4.4.1: Multidisciplinary team evaluation of intellectual disability.

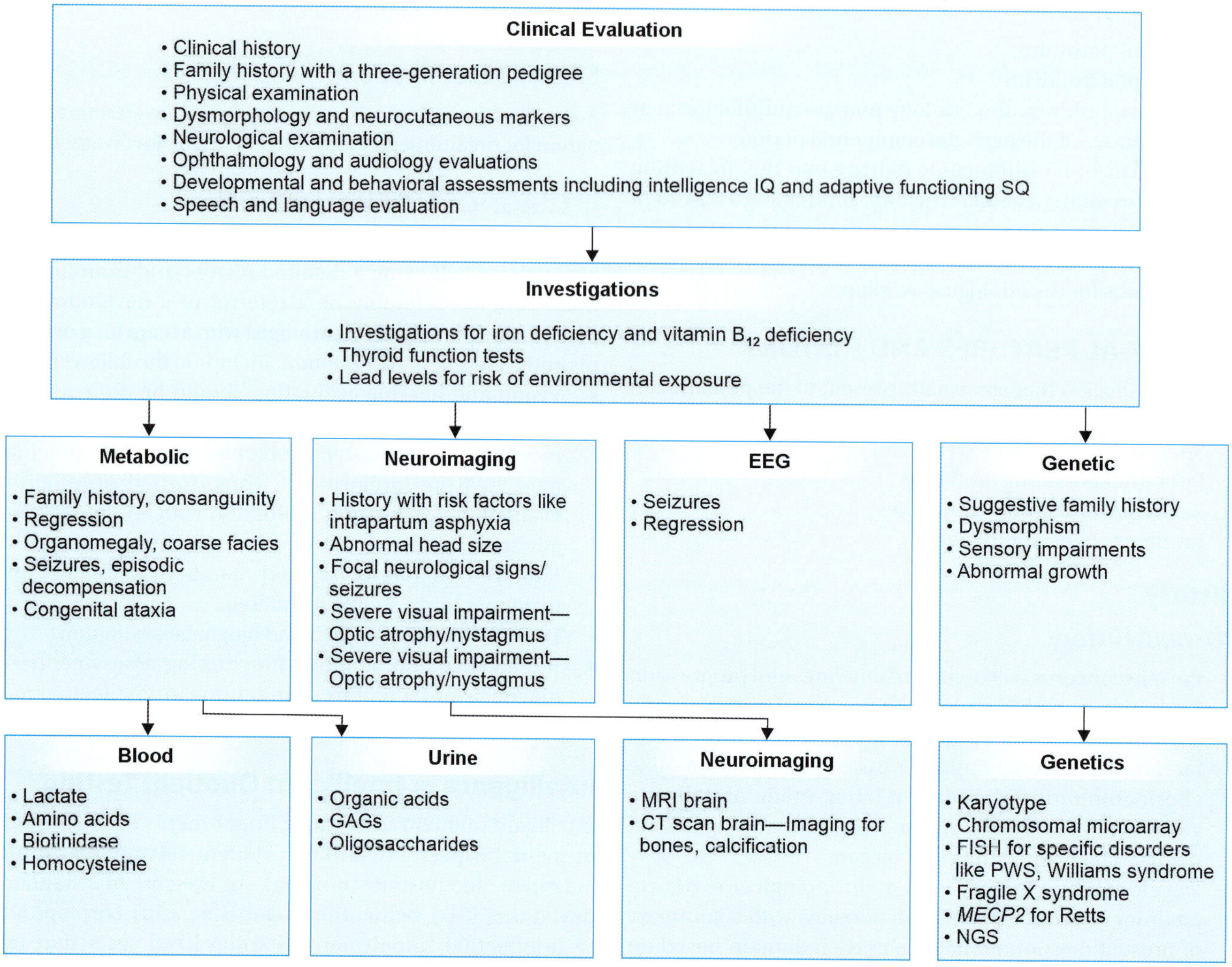

Clinical Evaluation
- Clinical history
- Family history with a three-generation pedigree
- Physical examination
- Dysmorphology and neurocutaneous markers
- Neurological examination
- Ophthalmology and audiology evaluations
- Developmental and behavioral assessments including intelligence IQ and adaptive functioning SQ
- Speech and language evaluation

↓

Investigations
- Investigations for iron deficiency and vitamin B_{12} deficiency
- Thyroid function tests
- Lead levels for risk of environmental exposure

↓

Metabolic
- Family history, consanguinity
- Regression
- Organomegaly, coarse facies
- Seizures, episodic decompensation
- Congenital ataxia

→ **Blood**
- Lactate
- Amino acids
- Biotinidase
- Homocysteine

→ **Urine**
- Organic acids
- GAGs
- Oligosaccharides

Neuroimaging
- History with risk factors like intrapartum asphyxia
- Abnormal head size
- Focal neurological signs/ seizures
- Severe visual impairment—Optic atrophy/nystagmus
- Severe visual impairment—Optic atrophy/nystagmus

→ **Neuroimaging**
- MRI brain
- CT scan brain—Imaging for bones, calcification

EEG
- Seizures
- Regression

Genetic
- Suggestive family history
- Dysmorphism
- Sensory impairments
- Abnormal growth

→ **Genetics**
- Karyotype
- Chromosomal microarray
- FISH for specific disorders like PWS, Williams syndrome
- Fragile X syndrome
- *MECP2* for Retts
- NGS

(CT: computed tomography; EEG: electroencephalogram; FISH: fluorescence in situ hybridization; GAGs: glycosaminoglycans; IQ: intelligent quotient; MECP2: methyl-CpG binding protein 2; MRI: magnetic resonance imaging; NGS: next-generation sequencing; PWS: Prader–Willi syndrome; SQ: social quotient)

Source: Adapted from: Shevell M, Ashwal S, Donley D, Flint J, Gingold, M, Hirtz D, et al. Practice parameter: evaluation of the child with global developmental delay. Neurology. 2003;60(3):367-80.

They may be interpreted as the child's social quotient (SQ). The commonly used tests are:
- Vineland Social Maturity Scale (VSMS)
- Vineland Adaptive Behavior Scale (VABS)

Grading of Severity

The presentation of children with ID is varied, but severity grading helps decide on needs, support, and interventions. Severity is now better classified based on adaptive functioning, as opposed to only IQ scores as in previous years.

Historical Classification Based only on IQ Scores

- Mild—IQ between 50–55 and 70
- Moderate—IQ between 35–40 and 50–55
- Severe—IQ between 20–25 and 35–40
- Profound—IQ <20–25

The DSM-5 now grades ID severity based on adaptive functioning as mild, moderate, severe, and profound **(Table 4.4.2)**.

Academic Achievement Tests

These are gauged using standardized academic achievement tests like the NIMHANS battery, Wide Range or Woodcock-Johnson achievement tests, or curriculum-based assessments to gauge academic functioning. It is supplemented with additional evaluation reports and observations from the school as required.

TABLE 4.4.2: Grades of severity of ID with typical adaptive skills and support needed (DSM-5).

DSM-5 categories	Conceptual	Social	Practical
Mild	• For school-aged children, there is difficulty learning academic skills like reading, writing, arithmetic, and concepts of time and money, and they require academic support to learn the age-expected skills • In adults, impairment in abstract thinking, executive functioning, and functional use of academic skills such as reading and money management	• Immaturity in social interactions compared to typical peers • Difficulties in perceiving social cues and regulating emotions and behavior as expected for age • Social judgment is also less for age	• May manage to function in personal care • Usually, they need some support in complex daily living tasks compared to peers • In adulthood, supports usually in shopping, transportation, organization, money management, health care decisions, raising a family, and learning a skilled vocation
Moderate	• Throughout developmental life, there is a lag in conceptual skills • In preschool age, language delays with weak preacademic skills • School years—reading, writing, math, and time/money concepts are limited for age • Adulthood—academic skills are at the elementary level, and assistance is needed in tasks involving conceptual understanding in daily life	• Social behavior and communication lag behind peers • Using simple spoken language and relationships with family and friends may be possible throughout life and adulthood • However, social limitations, such as difficulty interpreting social cues, social judgment, and decision-making, need assistance in friendships and work settings	• Most can become independent in personal care activities like eating, dressing, and participating in household tasks, which may be possible with extensive training, ongoing support, and reminders • Adults may be employable in jobs but with considerable support
Severe	• Limited understanding of conceptual skills and written language and minimal understanding of numbers, money, and time concepts • Extensive support for problem-solving is needed throughout their lifetime	• Limited speech abilities with single word/phrases can be augmented by other means • They may understand simple speech and communication through gestures and be able to maintain relationships with family and other familiar persons	• Require support and supervision for all activities of daily living, like eating, dressing, and bathing • Adults may achieve participation in home tasks and skills with prolonged teaching and ongoing support
Profound	• May be able to work towards self-care, recreation, and work with goal-directed use of objects • Few visuospatial skills like matching and sorting may be achieved • Comorbid motor and sensory impairments may hinder the functional use of objects	• They may display a limited understanding of speech and comprehend some simple instructions • Expression in relationships with close family and other familiar persons is mainly through nonverbal communication and gestures	• Depends mostly on others, with some participation in all self-care, health, and safety aspects • Can assist in simple daily home tasks • Recreational activities also require support • Physical and sensory impairments frequently occur, causing barriers to participation

(DSM-5: Diagnostic and Statistical Manual of Mental Disorders, fifth edition, ID: intellectual disability)
Source: Adapted from American Psychiatric Association. Intellectual disability (Intellectual developmental disorder). In: Diagnostic and Statistical Manual of Mental Disorders, 5th edition. Virginia: American Psychiatric Association.

Screening and Evaluation for Comorbidities

The assessments should include observing the child's behavior, attention, mood, social skills, and child-family interactions. Other neurodevelopmental and mental health disorders accompany ID.[9] These may additionally affect functioning in learning, daily living, behavior, and social skills.

- *Autism spectrum disorder* (ASD)*:* Children with ID may have ASD; it is more commonly seen in syndromic ID. Social and communication deficits are disproportionately more than the cognitive level, and repetitive or stereotypic behaviors are characteristic of a comorbid ASD.
- *Attention-deficit hyperactivity disorder* (ADHD) is commonly seen with ID. The hyperactivity/impulsivity and inattention levels are far more than expected with ID. It must be differentiated from situational behavior, like in situations with demands beyond their level, such as academics, and anxiety.

- *Learning difficulty* should be considered if the academic level is lower than expected for the child's intellectual ability and not explained by sensory-vision or hearing impairments or lack of exposure.
- *Anxiety and depression* may be seen in older children or adolescents. They may be challenging to recognize, given the limited communication skills of most children, but one must keep a high level of suspicion.
- *Feeding or eating disorders:* Food selectivity, lack of proper chewing, pica, or rumination disorders may be seen with ID.

Associated medical conditions such as dental caries, constipation, sleep disorders, seizures, and obesity should also be screened for in children with ID.[3]

Etiological Evaluation

Evaluation for the underlying cause helps guide the family on specific needs, a follow-up plan for the child, and a prognosis. Based on the etiology, recurrence risk and screening other at-risk persons in the family can also be discussed. In a few disorders, options for specific treatment may also be available. The findings from the thorough history and clinical examination are used as a guide for investigations.

Syndromic

A genetic cause can be identified in many children with ID.[3-6] The initial commonly used test was karyotyping, which detected only large deletions or insertions due to low resolution. *Fluorescence in situ hybridization* (FISH) is used to detect structural abnormalities and numerical changes on chromosomes with specific probes to analyze chromosomal aberration. Children with ID suspected of a known syndromic etiology can have specific tests, like karyotype for Down syndrome and FISH for Williams, Prader–Willi syndrome (PWS), and Angelman syndrome. A genetic reference may be needed for further evaluation of dysmorphic features.

Unexplained Etiology

- *Chromosomal microarray (CMA)* is the first line recommended for investigating the etiology. It has a diagnostic yield at least twice that of standard karyotype. CMA may not diagnose balanced translocations, point mutations in single-gene disorders, or triplet repeats, as in Fragile X syndrome.
- *Fragile X testing with CGG triplet repeats* in the *FMR1* gene may be recommended for patients with ID with specific features or a family history of ID.
- *Metabolic testing* may be considered, especially if there is a suggestive history of episodic decompensation, developmental regression, failure to thrive, seizures, or abnormal neurologic examination. Though the yield is relatively low, the possibility of missing a treatable metabolic etiology should be considered.
- *Whole-exome sequencing (WES)* is next-generation sequencing (NGS) used when CMA and other techniques have not found a cause. This modality has recently gained popularity, but genetic parental counseling regarding the results and yield should be accompanied to better understand the results.

Neuroimaging

Magnetic resonance imaging (MRI brain) has a better yield and is recommended when abnormal neurological findings like microcephaly, macrocephaly, focal findings, or seizures are present. Abnormalities on MRI may often not lead to a specific diagnosis but may indicate the need for more specific genetic testing.

DIFFERENTIAL DIAGNOSIS

It is essential to rule out sensory impairments like vision and hearing loss, specific language impairments, communication disorders like autism spectrum disorder, and learning disorders before making a final impression of ID. The course of ID is nonprogressive and should be differentiated from regression in cognition due to progressive neurological disorders.[6-8]

MANAGEMENT

The principles of management focus on:

- Minimize the impact of the disability
- Optimize and improve the child's daily functioning at home, school, vocation, and the environment
- Manage the comorbidities that interfere with functioning

It can be accomplished by various evidence-based interventions in a multidisciplinary and individualized plan to highlight the child's strengths and work on the weaknesses under the guidance of a developmental pediatrician.[3,6-8]

- They may include strategies to improve vision, hearing, communication, learning, behavior, activities of daily living, and social skills.
- Family support, including guidance on realistic expectations and advocacy for the child's needs, should be an integral part of the management plan.
- Treatable causes like hypothyroidism should be managed early to reduce the impact.
- Specific surveillance and follow-up should be adhered to in ID with disorders like Down syndrome, William syndrome, and neurofifromatosis-1 (NF1), among others.
- School and vocational guidance help habilitate the child based on their abilities.

Advocacy

The ID certification based on the inclusion of ID in the Persons with Disability (PWD) Act of the Indian legislation grants the child the right to be eligible for inclusive education and provisions for government schemes listed under the National Trust.[10] Various school boards also allow provisions for these children.

PREVENTION

Preconception genetic counseling with screening in those with a family history of ID or an earlier affected child coupled with newborn screening for early detection and management of treatable causes like hypothyroidism and newborn hearing screening for the early habilitation of the same are recommended. These measures and regular developmental screening for early identification and intervention for developmental concerns or delays will help reduce the impact and improve outcomes in global or cognitive delays.

REFERENCES

1. International Classification of Functioning, Disability, and Health: Children & Youth Version: ICF-CY. (2007). World Health Organization. [online] Available from https://www.who.int/classifications/international-classification-of-functioning-disability-and-health [Last accessed October, 2024].
2. American Psychiatric Association. Diagnostic and Statistical Manual of Mental Disorders. 5th edition. Washington, DC: APA Press; 2013.
3. Purugganan O. Intellectual disabilities. Pediatr Rev. 2018;39(6):299-309.
4. Ilyas M, Mir A, Efthymiou S, Houlden H. The genetics of intellectual disability: advancing technology and gene editing. F1000Res. 2020 Jan 16:9:F1000 Faculty Rev-22.
5. Moeschler JB, Shevell M; Committee on Genetics. Comprehensive evaluation of the child with intellectual disability or global developmental delays. Pediatrics. 2014;134(3):e903-18.
6. Shevell M, Ashwal S, Donley D, Flint J, Gingold M, Hirtz D, et al. Practice parameter: evaluation of the child with global developmental delay. Neurology 2003;60(3):367-80.
7. Srivastava L. Cognitive impairment. In: Ramachandran P, Thangavelu S, Nedunchelian K, Gowrishankar NC (Eds). Differential Diagnosis in Pediatrics, 1st edition. New Delhi: Jaypee Brothers; 2020. pp. 6-10.
8. Dalwai S, Rohil A. Intellectual disability. In: Dalwai S (Ed). IAP Handbook of Developmental and Behavioral Pediatrics, 1st edition. New Delhi: Jaypee Brothers Medical Publishers; 2021. pp. 54-8.
9. Siegel M, McGuire K, Veenstra-Vander Weele J, Stratigos K, King B; American Academy of Child and Adolescent Psychiatry (AACAP) Committee on Quality Issues (CQI); Bellonci C, Hayek M, Keable H, Rockhill C, Bukstein OG, Walter HJ. Practice parameter for the assessment and treatment of psychiatric disorders in children and adolescents with intellectual disability (Intellectual developmental disorder). J Am Acad Child Adolesc Psy. 2020;59(4):468-96.
10. Disability Rights (Rights of Persons with Disabilities Act & National Trust Act) and Mental Healthcare Act. 2021, National Human Rights Commission, India. [online] Available from https://nhrc.nic.in/sites/default/files/DisabilityRights.pdf [Last accessed October, 2024].

4.5 Specific Learning Disabilities

Sunil Karande

INTRODUCTION

Specific learning disabilities (SpLDs) are common neurodevelopmental disorders that occur in up to 5–10% of children.[1,2]

DEFINITION

Specific learning disabilities are a group of neurodevelopmental disorders that manifest in childhood as persistent difficulties in learning to efficiently read (dyslexia), write (dysgraphia), or do mathematical calculations (dyscalculia) despite normal intelligence, conventional schooling, intact hearing and vision, adequate motivation, and sociocultural opportunities.[1,2]

ETIOPATHOGENESIS

Specific learning disabilities are believed to be a result of functional disruption in neural systems and are genetically inherited. Dyslexia or "specific reading disability" is the most common and most carefully studied, affecting 80% of all those identified as learning-disabled. Children with dyslexia have deficits in "phonologic awareness," namely they have difficulty developing an awareness that words, both written and spoken, can be broken down into smaller units of sound and that, in fact, the letters constituting the printed word represent the sounds heard in the spoken word.[1,2]

CLINICAL FEATURES

A history of language delay or of not attending to the sounds of words (trouble playing rhyming games with words or confusing words that sound alike), along with a family history, is an important red flag for dyslexia. Children with SpLD present with persistent "academic problems" such as reading slowly and incorrectly, skipping lines while reading aloud, making repeated spelling mistakes, untidy or illegible handwriting with poor sequencing, and the inability to perform even simple additions and subtractions. These children invariably fail to achieve school grades that are commensurate with their intelligence.[1,2]

DIAGNOSIS

A conclusive diagnosis of SpLD cannot be made until the child is about 7–8 years old. Unlike children having SpLD, some of the children are "normal late developers" who by the age of 7–8 years on their own outgrow their learning problems. An evaluation for SpLD should be considered for all children presenting with learning problems in preschool or school. A multidisciplinary team comprising a developmental pediatrician or pediatric neurologist or child psychiatrist, counselor, clinical psychologist, and special educator is needed to assess each child referred for poor school performance. The sequence of evaluations done is as follows:

- *Audiometric and ophthalmic examinations* are done to rule out hearing and visual deficits, as they are common causes of poor school performance. Also, children with uncorrectable hearing and visual deficits (of >40% disability) do not qualify for a diagnosis of SpLD but are diagnosed as having "hearing impairment" and "visual impairment," respectively.
- The developmental pediatrician or pediatric neurologist or child psychiatrist then takes a detailed *clinical history* and does a detailed *clinical examination* to exclude medical causes (e.g., hypothyroidism and chronic lead poisoning) and neurological causes (e.g., cerebral palsy and Wilson disease) and to identify behavioral causes, e.g., attention-deficit hyperactivity disorder (ADHD), depression, conduct disorder (CD), or oppositional defiant disorder (ODD) of poor school performance.
- The counselor takes a detailed *interview of the parents/ family members* to rule out that emotional problem due to stress at home or school is not primarily responsible for the child's poor school performance.
- The clinical psychologist conducts the standard Wechsler Intelligence Scale for Children (WISC) test to determine that the child's *global intelligence quotient (IQ) score* is average or above average (≥85). This helps to exclude children having "borderline intellectual functioning" (IQ scores of 71–84), also known as "slow learners," who also present with poor school performance.
- The fifth edition of the Diagnostic and Statistical Manual of Mental Disorders (DSM-5) has recommended adopting *intellectual disability* as a rule-out criterion rather than using average IQ as a rule-in criterion for diagnosing learning disability (LD).[3] The DSM-5 recommendation effectively eliminates the slow learners' category.[3] However, this recommendation has raised a controversy, and till date in India, it has not been accepted.[4]
- The special educator assesses the child's *academic achievement* by administering a standard educational test (e.g., Curriculum-Based Test or Woodcock-Johnson Test of Achievement) to assess the child's performance in areas such as reading, spelling, written language, and mathematics. An academic achievement of up to 2 years below the child's actual school grade placement or chronological age is considered diagnostic of SpLD.
- The developmental pediatrician or pediatric neurologist or child psychiatrist plays an important role in confirming the diagnosis of attention deficit hyperactivity disorder (ADHD), a comorbid condition found in 12–24% of children with SpLD.[2]

TREATMENT

The cornerstone of treatment for SpLD is *remedial education,* and it should begin early when the child is in primary school. Using specific teaching strategies and teaching materials, the special educator formulates an *Individual Educational Program* to reduce or eliminate the child's deficiencies in specific learning areas of reading, writing, and mathematics identified during the child's educational assessment. The child has to undergo remedial education sessions twice or thrice weekly for a few years to achieve academic competence. However, even after adequate remedial education, subtle deficiencies in reading, writing, and mathematical abilities persist.

The management of SpLD in the more time-demanding setting of secondary school is based more on providing *provisions (accommodations).* These provisions, e.g., exemption from spelling mistakes, availing extra time for all written tests, dropping a language and substituting it with work experience, dropping algebra and geometry and substituting them with a lower grade of mathematics and work experience, are meant to help the child cope in a regular mainstream school.

The Government of India (GoI) has implemented the "Rights of Persons with Disabilities (RPwD) Act, 2016," which has recognized SpLD as a disability at the national level.[4] The GoI has also implemented the "Unique ID for Persons with Disabilities (UDID)" project in 2018. On confirmation of the diagnosis of SpLD, the student will receive the disability certificate and UDID card. This card will enable the student to avail provisions in school and board examinations. A primary school student (older than 8 years) who is diagnosed with SpLD will have to undergo revaluation first at the age of 14 years and again at the age of 18 years. Only a UDID card issued after evaluation on completion of 18 years of age states that the disability is permanent and entitles the student to get reservation in higher educational seats and government jobs.[4]

COMPLICATIONS

The "academic problems" of children with SpLD also have an adverse impact on their self-image, peer and family relationships, and social interactions.[5]

PROGNOSIS

It is well known that a favorable outcome of SpLD is dependent on early diagnosis, regular remedial education for a few years, availing of the necessary provisions, and a supportive home and school environment.

PRACTICE GUIDELINES

Every pediatrician can facilitate early detection of SpLD by enquiring about every child's school performance during a consultation and guiding the parents to get their child's psycho-educational assessment done when SpLD is suspected.

KEY MESSAGE

With appropriate remedial education and provisions, children with SpLD achieve academic competence in regular mainstream schools.

REFERENCES

1. Willcutt EG, McGrath LM, Pennington BF, Keenan JM, DeFries JC, Olson RK, et al. Understanding comorbidity between specific learning disabilities. New Dir Child Adolesc Dev. 2019;2019(165):91-109.
2. Habib M. Developmental dyslexia: A new look at clinical features and brain mechanisms. Handb Clin Neurol. 2020;174:47-59.
3. Sharma N, Mishra R, Mishra D. The fifth edition of Diagnostic and Statistical Manual of Mental Disorders (DSM-5): what is new for the pediatrician? Indian Pediatr. 2015;52(2):141-3.
4. Karande S. Specific learning disabilities in India: current situation and the path ahead. Indian Pediatr. 2022;59(5):367-70.
5. Karande S, Venkataraman R. Self-perceived health-related quality of life of Indian children with specific learning disability. J Postgrad Med. 2012;58(4):246-54.

4.6 Attention-deficit Hyperactivity Disorder

Zafar Mahmood Meenai

"Attention deficit hyperactivity disorder is not a problem with knowing what to do; it is a problem of doing what you know."

—Barkley, 2006[1]

INTRODUCTION

Attention-deficit hyperactivity disorder (ADHD) is a changing and evolving concept that refers to children and young persons whose behavior appears impulsive, overactive, and/or inattentive to an extent that is unwarranted for their developmental age and is a significant hindrance to their social and educational success. It is the most common neurodevelopmental disorder. It is a disorder of inhibition and self-regulation. Hyperactivity and inattention in childhood significantly increase the risk of academic failure later.

The gold standard for defining and diagnosing mental disorders is the Diagnostic and Statistical Manual of Mental Disorders–fifth edition-Text revision (DSM-5-TR) by the American Psychiatric Association, and it classifies ADHD into:[2]

- *Predominantly hyperactive/impulsive*—8–10% cases; typically observed by the time the child reaches 4 years of age
- *Predominantly inattentive*—25–30% cases; typically identified late and inapparent till the child is 8–9 years of age
- *Combined type*—60–70% cases

Hyperactivity is said to have a "driven" quality to it; it can be described as:

- *Exploratory*—walking, running, particularly in a new environment
- *Akathisia*—restless and fidgety
- *Stereotype*—high-frequency, repetitive movements. It manifests itself differently at different ages—preschool children with rushing around, jumping, climbing, and noisiness; school-age children being fidgety, squirming, and having difficulty remaining in their seats; and adolescents with foot-tapping, and not sitting quietly.

Impulsivity means not thinking before acting; it is often demonstrated by getting into trouble for seeming cheeky or reckless.

Poor attention span: The normal attention span is approximately 3–5 minutes per year of age. The attention gets poorly regulated and manifests particularly in difficult, imposed tasks that are not immediately rewarding. Thus, a child may be able to attend a game or watch a TV program of their choice but not a school lesson. These difficulties may give rise to other problems such as poor self-esteem, poor peer relationships, poor relationships with parents, sleep/wake problems, dietary problems (difficulty settling to eat and frequent snacking), increased risks, and repeated injuries and behavior problems.

EPIDEMIOLOGY

There is considerable variation in estimates of how common ADHD is, although recognition has increased all over the world and continues to do so. The worldwide prevalence of ADHD is 5%, with 3–16% of the children displaying symptoms of ADHD.[3] The male:female ratio varies from 2–9 boys to 1 girl, depending on the type of ADHD and the prevalence in the representative population—whether clinical or epidemiological. In India, reported prevalence varies from 11.3% (a 2013 study from southern India in primary school children) to 32.4% (2009–2012 from Mumbai).

ETIOPATHOGENESIS

It is claimed that several factors contribute to the onset and maintenance of ADHD symptoms, including genetic factors, neuroanatomical abnormalities, psychosocial factors, pregnancy and delivery complications, and environmental factors such as prenatal consumption of cigarettes, alcohol, and artificial food coloring. The most significant factor associated with ADHD is heritability, which contributes approximately 74% to the etiology of ADHD.

The neurotransmitter dopamine may be implicated in the pathogenesis of ADHD. Stimulant drugs that are used in the management of ADHD symptoms increase the availability of dopamine in the brain, and several genes related to the dopamine pathway have been implicated in ADHD.

Genetics: It is likely that we are not dealing with a single gene disorder for ADHD but a heterogeneous group of disorders with different etiologies. There is perhaps a susceptibility gene or genes that increase the risk, but other factors are necessary. The dopamine transporter gene *DAT1* is more closely associated with the ADHD combined subtype than with the inattentive subtype.

Psychologically, it has been thought of as an executive function deficit. Executive functions are believed to be located in the frontal cortex and its striatal connections. Executive functions include self-regulation, sequencing of behavior, flexibility in response, response inhibition, planning, and organization.

There may be a failure of processing between incoming information and the response generated, or a failure to inhibit responding until all the information has been considered. A key deficit that has been demonstrated in ADHD is difficulty in inhibiting a response. Another suggestion of an underlying problem in ADHD is an altered reinforcement process; reinforcement has to be immediate to be effective.

Pathologically, the development of the frontal lobes is relatively late, and myelination is not complete until into adolescence. Studies of pathology (primarily neuroimaging) have given inconsistent results, but the frontal cortex and the connections from this, as well as intracerebral connections via the corpus callosum, have shown abnormal activity. The cerebellum is also implicated.

Neurochemically, it seems likely that there is a problem with the noradrenaline/dopamine/serotonin systems in the brain. This is suggested by the response to treatment with drugs affecting this system and has some confirmation from functional imaging studies.

Medical conditions where ADHD is known to be more frequent include antenatal insults like substance abuse, smoking, and frequent alcoholism by the mother; perinatal insults like prematurity; childhood conditions like head injury resulting in frontal lobe damage, encephalitis, and meningitis; near-drowning and strangulation resulting in hypoxic episodes; cerebrovascular accidents; chronic neurological conditions like epilepsy; metabolic disorders like phenylketonuria (PKU); and medical treatment with cranial irradiation, anticonvulsants, and certain conditions like tuberous sclerosis, hyperthyroidism, Fragile X syndrome, and William syndrome.

Visual and hearing impairments, metabolic abnormalities, and nutritional deficiencies should be considered as possible influences on ADHD symptoms. ADHD is more likely in individuals with idiopathic epilepsy. ADHD is a risk factor for suicidal ideation and behavior in children and in adulthood. Sleep problems including sleep apnea and restless legs syndrome are more commonly seen.

CLINICAL FEATURES

Attention-deficit hyperactivity disorder begins in childhood but cannot be diagnosed in the absence of any symptoms before 12 years of age. One has to consider alternate mental disorders if the symptoms of what appears to be ADHD first occur after the age of 13 years. The manifestations of the disorder must be present in more than one setting (e.g., home and school, or home and work), and the essential feature of ADHD, i.e., a persistent pattern of inattention and/or hyperactivity impulsivity, should interfere with functioning or development.

Inattention typically manifests as failing to finish chores/work or follow through on instructions, wandering of task, inability to sustain focus, and being disorganized, which cannot be attributed to defiance or lack of understanding.

Hyperactivity, which often makes the disorder obvious, shows out as excessive motor activity like excessive running when socially inappropriate or as excessive talkativeness, tapping, or fidgeting. Though hyperactivity quite often reduces as age advances toward 10 years of age, quite often in adults it may also manifest as extreme restlessness or wearing others out due to their activity.

Impulsivity appears as a sudden hasty action without forethought that may harm the individual, like darting into the street without looking. Often, it looks like a desire for immediate reward or may reflect an inability to delay gratification. This often presents as social intrusiveness, like interrupting others' conversations and/or taking crucial decisions without considering the long-term consequences of it (accepting a task or a job without adequate information).

Symptoms may vary depending on the context within a given setting; hence, one has to confirm substantial symptoms across the settings by consulting with informants who have witnessed them. While evaluating, one has to be vigilant about situations when the symptoms may be minimal. Such situations include situations when a child is receiving frequent rewards for good behavior, when under close supervision, or when in a novel situation. One may also see minimal to absent symptoms when the child is engaged in interesting activities, in conditions where there is one-to-one interaction, like in a clinician's office, or when the child has a consistent external stimulus, like viewing screens or TV.

COMORBIDITIES

Comorbidity appears to be the rule rather than the exception. ADHD may coexist with oppositional defiant disorder (ODD), conduct disorder (CD), depression, and anxiety. About 50–60% of children with ADHD meet the criteria for ODD, even in the preschool period. CD may be present in 20–25%. Up to 60% of ADHD children demonstrate problems with motor coordination or deficits, and symptoms may be severe enough to meet the criteria for developmental coordination disorder (DCD).

Sleep problems and bedwetting (enuresis) occur twice as often in ADHD as in control groups. The problems are mainly more behavioral and include settling difficulties, a longer time to fall asleep, instability of sleep duration, tiredness at awakening, or frequent night waking.

Children with ADHD are usually at an educational disadvantage upon school entry, especially those with specific learning difficulties (particularly dyslexia). ADHD children are more likely than their non-ADHD peers to have basic mathematics difficulties and deficient prereading skills in their first year at school. ADHD children referred from clinics had lower intelligence scores than their controls, especially in verbal intelligence with 7–10 standard score point differences.

They appear to be at a greater risk for physical injury and accidental poisoning.

It is important to identify these other conditions because they have a bearing on the treatment. The prognosis is worsened by comorbidities.

DIFFERENTIAL DIAGNOSIS

Hyperactivity may be present in physical illness, drugs (either prescribed or abused), attachment difficulties, social issues (family break-up), child abuse (especially if change in behavior), depression/anxiety, or hearing problems. It may also manifest due to unrealistic expectations by parents or teachers, poor parenting, bullying, a bored bright child, sleep problems, or amblyopia.

- *ODD:* These are children who may resist work or school tasks requiring self-application since they resist conforming to others' demands. Negativity, hostility, and defiance are characteristic of their behavior.
- *Specific learning disorder:* These children may appear inattentive either due to a lack of interest or frustration or due to their decreased neurocognitive processing, which typically manifests as poor working memory and processing speed. However, they will have significantly lower inattention when doing tasks that do not require a cognitive process.
- *Intellectual disability:* When children with lower intellectual ability are placed in inappropriate academic settings, symptoms of ADHD are more commonly seen; during a nonacademic activity, the ADHD symptoms become nonexistent. Hence, to make a diagnosis of ADHD with intellectual disability, one should be satisfied that the hyperactivity or inattention clearly is excessive for the mental age.

- *Autism spectrum disorder:* Individuals with ADHD and those with autism spectrum disorder exhibit inattention, social dysfunction, and difficult-to-manage behavior. In ADHD, children face social dysfunction and peer rejection, whereas in autism, isolation, social disengagement, and indifference to tonal and facial cues are the hallmarks. Temper tantrums in autism are due to the inability to tolerate change from their expected course of events, but children with ADHD misbehave or throw a temper tantrum during a major transition due to impulsivity or poor self-control.
- *Anxiety disorders:* ADHD shares symptoms of inattention with anxiety disorders. Individuals with ADHD are inattentive because of their preferential engagement with novel and stimulating activities or preoccupation with enjoyable activities. This is distinguished from the inattention attributable to worry and rumination seen in anxiety disorders. Restlessness might be seen in anxiety disorders. However, in ADHD, the symptom is not associated with worry and rumination.
- *Other neurodevelopmental disorders:* The increased motor activity that may occur in ADHD must be distinguished from the repetitive motor behavior that characterizes stereotypic movement disorder and some cases of autism spectrum disorder. In stereotypic movement disorder, the motoric behavior is generally fixed and repetitive (e.g., body rocking, self-biting), whereas the fidgetiness and restlessness in ADHD are typically generalized and not characterized by repetitive stereotypic movements. In Tourette disorder, frequent multiple tics can be mistaken for the generalized fidgetiness of ADHD. Prolonged observation may be needed to differentiate fidgetiness from bouts of multiple tics.
- *Depressive disorders:* Depressive disorders in children may present with poor ability to concentrate. But in mood disorders, the inability to concentrate becomes evident only during an episode of depression.
- *Post-traumatic stress disorder:* Children following a traumatic episode may experience post-traumatic stress disorder (PTSD), which manifests as poor concentration and may be misdiagnosed as ADHD. Those who are <6 years old with PTSD may present with nonspecific symptoms like irritability, restlessness, inattention, and poor concentration—all mimicking ADHD symptoms. Furthermore, parents are likely to belittle their trauma-related symptoms, and teachers and other caregivers may be unaware of traumatic events, making the diagnosis of PTSD difficult. Hence, a comprehensive assessment of traumatic events should be done to rule out PTSD.
- *Substance-use disorders:* Differentiating ADHD from substance-use disorders may be problematic if the first presentation of ADHD symptoms follows the onset of abuse. A history of substance abuse is present.
- *Personality disorders:* ADHD is not characterized by fear of abandonment, self-injury, extreme ambivalence, or other features of personality disorder. It may take extended clinical observation and an informant interview.
- *Psychotic disorders:* ADHD is not diagnosed if the symptoms of inattention and hyperactivity occur exclusively during the course of a psychotic disorder.
- *Medications-induced symptoms of ADHD:* Symptoms of inattention, hyperactivity, or impulsivity attributable to the use of medication (e.g., bronchodilators, isoniazid, etc.).

DIAGNOSIS

Any child aged 4–18 years who presents with behavioral or academic problems and symptoms of hyperactivity, inattention, or impulsivity should be evaluated for ADHD.

A detailed history of ADHD and general evaluation should clarify presenting complaints, make a systematic evaluation of psychopathological symptoms, and describe how problems developed.

One needs to reach an adequate account of affected family members (relevant to a genetic etiology), pregnancy, and birth history (fetal growth, toxemia, bleeding or severe infections in pregnancy, maternal diabetes or epilepsy, other maternal illnesses or traumas, poor nutritional state of the mother, use of medication, nicotine, alcohol or drugs, gestational age, birth complications, birth weight, and neonatal complications).

Developmental history is important (milestones for psychomotor development, language, attachment, sleep and feeding problems, growth, and early temperament); medical history, especially tics and epilepsy; and medication (especially anticonvulsants, antihistamines, sympathomimetics, and steroids).

Diagnosis should be based on a timely, comprehensive assessment conducted by a developmental pediatrician and child/adolescent psychiatrist with expertise in ADHD. It should also involve children, parents and caregivers, and the child's school and take into account cultural factors in the child's environment. Multidisciplinary assessment, which may include educational or clinical psychologists and social workers, is advisable for children who present with indications of significant comorbidity.

As there is a modest correlation between ADHD symptoms and impaired functioning, assessment of ADHD must include evaluation of the child's functioning in the key domains of peer and sibling and parent and teacher relationships, academic progress, and the classroom and family.

No biological marker or radiological study is diagnostic for ADHD. Diagnosis is made by standardized psychological checklists. The most widely used checklist of ADHD is as per the DSM-5-TR, which includes a persistent pattern of inattention and/or hyperactivity-impulsivity that interferes with functioning or development, as characterized by (1) and/or (2) stated in the following text.

A1: Inattention

Before the age of 12 years, if 6 (or more) of the following symptoms have persisted for at least 6 months in two different settings, e.g., home/school/social gathering, to a degree that is inconsistent with developmental level and that negatively impacts directly social and academic/occupational activities, it is labeled as inattention. For older adolescents and adults (age 17 years and older), at least five symptoms are required.

1. Often fails to give close attention to details or makes careless mistakes in schoolwork, at work, or during other activities (e.g., overlooks or misses details, or work is inaccurate)
2. Often has difficulty sustaining attention in tasks or play activities (e.g., has difficulty remaining focused during lectures, conversations, or lengthy reading)
3. Often does not seem to listen when spoken to directly (e.g., mind seems elsewhere, even in the absence of any obvious distraction)
4. Often does not follow through on instructions and fails to finish schoolwork, chores, or duties in the workplace (e.g., starts tasks but quickly loses focus and is easily sidetracked)
5. Often has difficulty organizing tasks and activities (e.g., difficulty managing sequential tasks; difficulty keeping materials and belongings in order; messy, disorganized work; has poor time management; fails to meet deadlines)
6. Often avoids, dislikes, or is reluctant to engage in tasks that require sustained mental effort (e.g., schoolwork or homework; for older adolescents and adults, preparing reports, completing forms, reviewing lengthy papers)
7. Often loses things necessary for tasks or activities (e.g., school materials, pencils, books, tools, wallets, keys, paperwork, eyeglasses, mobile telephones)
8. Is often easily distracted by extraneous stimuli (for older adolescents and adults, may include unrelated thoughts)
9. Is often forgetful in daily activities (e.g., doing chores, running errands; for older adolescents and adults, returning calls, paying bills, keeping appointments).

A2: Hyperactivity and Impulsivity

Before the age of 12 years, if 6 (or more) of the following symptoms have persisted for at least 6 months in two different settings, it is termed hyperactivity and impulsivity. For older adolescents and adults (age 17 years and older), at least five symptoms are required:

1. Often fidgets with or taps hands or feet or squirms in seat
2. Often leaves seat in situations when remaining seated is expected (e.g., leaves his or her place in the classroom, in the office or other workplace, or in other situations that require remaining in place)
3. Often runs about or climbs in situations where it is inappropriate (*Note*: In adolescents or adults, may be limited to feeling restless)
4. Often unable to play or engage in leisure activities quietly
5. Is often "on the go," acting as if "driven by a motor" (e.g., is unable to be or uncomfortable being still for extended time, as in restaurants or meetings; may be experienced by others as being restless or difficult to keep up with)
6. Often talks excessively
7. Often blurts out an answer before a question has been completed (e.g., completes people's sentences; cannot wait for turn-in conversation)
8. Often has difficulty waiting his or her turn (e.g., while waiting in line)
9. Often interrupts or intrudes on others (e.g., butts into conversations, games, or activities; may start using other people's things without asking or receiving permission; for adolescents and adults, may intrude into or take over what others are doing).

Notes:

- Several inattentive or hyperactive-impulsive symptoms were present prior to the age of 12 years.
- Several inattentive or hyperactive-impulsive symptoms are present in two or more settings (e.g., at home, school, or work; with friends or relatives; in other activities).
- There is clear evidence that the symptoms interfere with, or reduce the quality of, social, academic, or occupational functioning.

Types of Attention-deficit Hyperactivity Disorders

- *Combined presentation:* If both Criterion A1 (inattention) and Criterion A2 (hyperactivity-impulsivity) are met for the past 6 months
- *Predominantly inattentive presentation:* If Criterion A1 (inattention) is met but Criterion A2 (hyperactivity-impulsivity) is not met for the past 6 months
- *Predominantly hyperactive/impulsive presentation:* If Criterion A2 (hyperactivity-impulsivity) is met and Criterion A1 (inattention) is not met for the past 6 months

Other standardized psychometric scales used to identify ADHD, its severity, and comorbidities are:

- *Child Behavior Checklist (CBCL):* This is completed by parents. The other two components are the Teacher's

Report Form (TRF) (completed by teachers) and the Youth Self-Report (YSR) (completed by the child or adolescent himself or herself). The 2001 revision of the CBCL, the CBCL/6–18, is used with children 6–18 years of age. The CBCL consists of 113 questions, scored on a three-point Likert scale.

- *Conners Scale:* The Conners 4 (2022) is a reporting measure used for evaluating children and adolescents for ADHD. The Conners 4 has forms for parents and teachers that show how a child presents in the home and the classroom. Children aged 8 years and above can also complete a self-report form that provides information about their experience of their symptoms. It is also for the 6–18 years age group and has three report forms. It is available in an online format only.
- *Vanderbilt Scale:* The Vanderbilt ADHD Diagnostic Rating Scale (VADRS) is a psychological assessment tool for ADHD symptoms and their effects on behavior and academic performance in children aged 6–12 years. It includes items related to ODD, CD, anxiety, and depression, disorders often comorbid with ADHD. There are two versions available: A parent form that contains 55 questions and a teacher form that contains 43 questions.
- *International Clinical Epidemiology Network (INCLEN):* The Development and Validation of DSM-5-Based AIIMS-Modified INDT ADHD (Indian Diagnostic Tool for Attention-deficit Hyperactivity Disorder) by Gulati et al. is an Indian tool freely available for the diagnosis of ADHD.[4]

MANAGEMENT

Information is an important aspect of management. Making the early diagnosis (and any comorbidities) and making this known to all involved may, in itself, help the child, parent, and teachers to cope with ADHD. Planning individualized early multidisciplinary intervention helps to prevent academic and functional underachievement. The focus needs to be on correcting the surroundings, which need to be made conducive, and working on the child's strengths for functional integration.[5] Building an island of excellence for the child based on his/her core strengths should be the focus of a multidisciplinary team. Management of comorbid conditions is essential. It is also important to plan and discuss safety and injury prevention.

- For ADHD preschool children (<6 years), behavioral intervention is the first line of treatment.
- For ADHD school-age children (>6 years) and adolescents, medication with or without behavioral intervention is the first line of treatment.

Educational Measures

Children with ADHD often have major difficulties in school, and help and support are needed both in the classroom and in other school activities. Simple measures can be really helpful, e.g., sitting near the teacher in the first middle row, removing distractions where possible, working alone or in groups of only two or three, providing support between lessons and at break times, addressing learning difficulties, and correcting any visual acuity defect by eyeglasses.

Behavior Management

Frequent, immediate, positive reinforcement helps children with ADHD. Children with ADHD often have low self-esteem. They usually respond best to a well-structured, predictable environment where expectations and rules are clear and consistent and consequences set down ahead of time and delivered immediately. A few effective behavior modification techniques are positive reinforcement (immediately rewarding good behavior), time out (removing any factor reinforcing problem behavior), and response cost (withdrawing privilege for unwanted behavior).

Medicinal Management

There is a lot of experience of benefit from stimulant medication in ADHD, but medication should usually be given only if certain criteria are met:

- There is a well-founded diagnosis causing significant educational and social difficulties.
- Impairment is severe or moderate, and other forms of management have been tried and failed or only partially effective.
- Attention has been given to comorbidities.
- Start medication with a low dose and increase slowly till symptoms improve.
- Medication can be carefully monitored and should never be given at night-time.

Methylphenidate

Methylphenidate is the stimulant recommended for use as part of a comprehensive treatment program for children with a diagnosis of severe ADHD. It is not currently licensed for children under the age of 6 years or for children with marked anxiety, agitation, or tension; symptoms or family history of tics or Tourette syndrome; hyperthyroidism; severe angina or cardiac arrhythmia; glaucoma; or thyrotoxicosis. The manufacturers recommend that treatment should be initiated at 5 mg once or twice daily and increased up to a maximum of 60 mg/day. Now, sustained-release once-a-day stimulant is available.

Stimulants are associated with side effects such as decreased appetite, weight loss, insomnia, stomach ache, headache, and irritability, although most will dissipate with time. There are also concerns that stimulants may cause longer-term adverse effects such as decreased growth, increased risk of substance abuse, and worsening of comorbid symptoms such as tics.

Atomoxetine

Atomoxetine is a nonstimulant selective nor-adrenergic reuptake inhibiter. Research suggests that it has a significant effect on around 70% of individuals with ADHD. The dose is 0.5–1.2 mg/kg/day (maximum 100 mg/day or 1.4 mg/kg, whichever is less). It is used as a once- or twice-daily medication (and therefore does not need giving in school). It does not have abuse potential.

Side effects include some that are similar to stimulants, including appetite suppression and consequent poor growth. Some children are sleepier on atomoxetine, but this can be beneficial if sleep is difficult for the child.

Multimodal Approach

This usually means combining some or all educational interventions, counseling, behavioral methods, family work, and medication. Much has been said about the necessity of continuing behavioral management while children are on medication, and this instinctively feels right. Additional problems are often present, and if so, they may need treatment whether or not the core symptoms of hyperactivity have been reduced by specific treatments. Training of social competence is often needed.

PROGNOSIS

Outcome studies suggest that most children with ADHD become adults with ADHD.[6] Various groups have reported similar findings with approximately:

- 30% within the normal range as adults
- About 50–60% in partial remission, continuing to have problems with concentration, impulsivity, and social interaction
- About 10–15% having significant psychiatric or antisocial problems (depression, drug and alcohol abuse, self-harm, criminal activity, etc.)

The prognosis is best for those children with "pure" ADHD. The prognosis is worse for those with severe symptoms and comorbidities, especially CD.

REFERENCES

1. Barkley RA. Attention-Deficit Hyperactivity Disorder: A Handbook for Diagnosis and Treatment, 3rd edition. New York: The Guilford Press; 2006.
2. American Psychiatric Association. (2022). Diagnostic and Statistical Manual of Mental Disorders, 5th edition, text revision. 2022. [online] Available from https://doi.org/10.1176/appi.books.9780890425787. [Last accessed October, 2024].
3. American Academy of Pediatrics. [online] Available from https://www.aap.org/en/patient-care/attention-deficit-hyperactivity-disorder-adhd/2022 [Last accessed October, 2024].
4. Gulati S, Saini L, Kaushik JS, Chakrabarty B, Arora NK, Pandey RM, The development and validation of DSM 5-based AIIMS-modified INDT ADHD tool for diagnosis of ADHD: a diagnostic test evaluation study. Neurol India. 2020;68(2):352-7.
5. National Consultation Meeting for Developing IAP Guidelines on Neuro Developmental Disorders under the aegis of IAP Childhood Disability Group and the Committee on Child Development and Neurodevelopmental Disorders; Dalwai S, Unni J, Kalra V, Singhi P, Shrivastava L, Nair MKC. Consensus statement of the Indian Academy of Pediatrics on evaluation and management of attention deficit hyperactivity disorder. Indian Pediatr. 2017;54(6):481-8.
6. Faraone SV, Biederman J, Mick E. The age-dependent decline of attention deficit hyperactivity disorder: a meta-analysis of follow-up studies. Psychol Med. 2006:36(2):159-65.

4.7 Global Developmental Delay

Monica Juneja, Ridhimaa Jain

INTRODUCTION

Developmental delay refers to a delay in attaining milestones as compared to other children of the same age. There are five main developmental domains, namely:

1. Gross and fine motor
2. Speech and language
3. Cognition
4. Social personal
5. Activities of daily living or adaptive

The delay is measured as developmental quotient (DQ), and if it is 2 or more standard deviations (SDs) below the mean for a domain, it is considered a significant delay.

The term *global developmental delay* (GDD) came into usage to describe children under the age of 5 years with suspected intellectual impairment in whom testing of intellectual function may be difficult, unreliable, and inaccurate.

Traditionally, GDD was defined as a significant delay in attaining milestones in at least two developmental domains from the following: Gross and fine motor, speech and language, cognition, social-personal, and activities of daily living in children under the age of 5 years. This definition was based on the observation that children diagnosed with intellectual disability later in life would manifest with delays across multiple developmental domains in early childhood.[1]

However, a child with isolated visual impairment can have a delay in motor milestones, delay in achieving certain sociopersonal milestones, and difficulties in activities of daily living, owing to his/her visual deficits per se without any intellectual impairment. Similarly, children with isolated neuromotor impairments (e.g., spinal muscular atrophy) or isolated severe to profound hearing impairment who have normal cognition may be misdiagnosed as GDD as they may fail to achieve milestones in multiple domains. Thus, the definition of GDD was recently modified to exclude children whose delay in two or more domains could be explained primarily by motor delay or severe uncorrected visual/hearing impairment from the diagnostic label of GDD.[2]

EPIDEMIOLOGY

The GDD is estimated to affect 1–3% of children worldwide. Various studies from India report a prevalence ranging from 3 to 13%.[1,3]

ETIOLOGY

The etiology of GDD is diverse and may be genetic or environmental. The causes are categorized as prenatal, perinatal, or postnatal based on the timing of exposure **(Table 4.7.1)**.[4]

Genetic defects are the most common etiology of GDD in India as well as globally, accounting for 30–50% of cases. Potentially preventable causes such as hypoxic-ischemic encephalopathy (HIE), intrauterine infections, congenital hypothyroidism, and toxin exposure are responsible for a significant proportion of children with GDD in developing countries. In many children, multiple risk factors may

TABLE 4.7.1: Etiology of GDD.

Timing of exposure	*Type of risk factor*	*Causes*
Prenatal	Genetic	• *Genetic syndromes:* Down syndrome, Prader–Willi syndrome, Angelman syndrome, Fragile X syndrome, Cornelia de Lange syndrome, Williams syndrome, and 22q11.2 deletion syndrome • *Neurocutaneous syndromes:* Tuberous sclerosis, Von Hippel–Lindau syndrome, and Sturge–Weber syndrome
		Metabolic/Inborn error of metabolism: Urea cycle defect, aminoaciduria, organic acidemia, and mitochondriopathy
		Cortical malformations
	Nongenetic (Environmental)	• *Intrauterine infection:* Toxoplasma, rubella, cytomegalovirus, and HIV • *Toxins/teratogen:* Alcohol, valproate, and cocaine
Perinatal	Acquired/environmental	• *Hypoxic-ischemic encephalopathy (HIE)* • *Neonatal complications:* Bilirubin encephalopathy and hypoglycemia • Birth trauma, intracranial hemorrhage
Postnatal	Acquired/environmental	• Hypothyroidism* • Nutritional deficiencies (e.g., iodine, vitamin B_{12}, and thiamine) • Toxins (e.g., lead) • Meningitis, encephalitis, stroke • Posthead injury
Common risk factors predisposing to GDD (usually in combination)		• Prematurity • Intrauterine growth restriction • *Psychosocial factors:* Poverty, parental depression or psychiatric illness, domestic violence, child abuse or neglect

*Hypothyroidism may be found overlapping with other causes such as Down syndrome, other genetic syndromes, some inborn errors of metabolism, and secondary to maternal antithyroid antibodies.
(GDD: global developmental delay; HIV: human immunodeficiency virus)

be involved such as prematurity and intrauterine growth restriction.[2,4-6]

CLINICAL FEATURES

A child not attaining age-appropriate milestones or if the parents have developmental concerns warrants an evaluation for GDD. Often, caregivers miss developmental delay in infancy if the motor milestones are normal. The children, however, may be brought with complaints of comorbid conditions such as behavioral problems (e.g., pica, temper tantrums, and hyperactivity), seizures, feeding difficulties, sleep problems (e.g., excessive sleepiness and difficulty falling asleep), or dysmorphism and congenital anomalies. Thus, a high index of suspicion should be kept in children presenting with these complaints. Also, high-risk newborns and children with risk factors **(Table 4.7.1)** should be closely monitored for development.[2]

CLINICAL EVALUATION

The diagnosis of a child with developmental delay begins with a comprehensive clinical assessment including a detailed history and examination; this itself can lead to an etiological diagnosis in 12–40% of cases.[6]

Salient points to be noted in history include:

- Documentation of major milestones in all developmental domains along with the ages at which these milestones were achieved
- History of antenatal, perinatal, and postnatal risk factors **(Table 4.7.1)**
- Family history of consanguinity, recurrent abortions, unexplained infant deaths, birth defects, GDD/intellectual disability, neurologic diseases, or genetic disorders. The presence of these points toward a genetic etiology for the GDD
- History of medical, neurological, and behavioral comorbidities **(Box 4.7.1)**

BOX 4.7.1: Common comorbidities of global developmental delay (GDD).

Medical comorbidities:

- Visual deficits
- Hearing impairment
- Epilepsy
- Cerebral palsy
- Feeding difficulties
- Sleep problems
- Protein-energy malnutrition
- Drooling
- Constipation
- Nutritional anemia
- Recurrent infections

Behavioral comorbidities:

- Behavioral problems*—pica, tantrums
- Attention-deficit hyperactivity disorder
- Autism spectrum disorder
- Aggression and disruptive behaviors

*These are more common in GDD than in typically developing children.

General physical examination must include:

- *Anthropometry, especially head circumference*. It is important to review the previous anthropometric records as microcephaly present from birth is indicative of an antenatal etiology, and low birth weight and malnutrition can be risk factors for GDD. Short or tall stature can be pointers toward some genetic syndromes.
- *Assessment of dysmorphisms* such as abnormal head shape, low set ears, mongoloid, or antimongoloid slant of eyes, hypertelorism, cataract, flat nasal bridge, short neck, limb deformities, polydactyly, and simian crease. Certain syndromes such as Down syndrome have characteristic dysmorphic features and can be easily recognized on clinical examination. Even when a specific genetic syndrome cannot be diagnosed, dysmorphic features must be documented.
- *Presence of neurocutaneous markers* such as café-au-lait spots (seen in tuberous sclerosis, neurofibromatosis, etc.), port wine stain (seen in Sturge–Weber syndrome and Klippel–Trenaunay syndrome), facial angiofibromas, ash leaf macules, and shagreen patches (tuberous sclerosis, see **Fig. 4.7.1**)

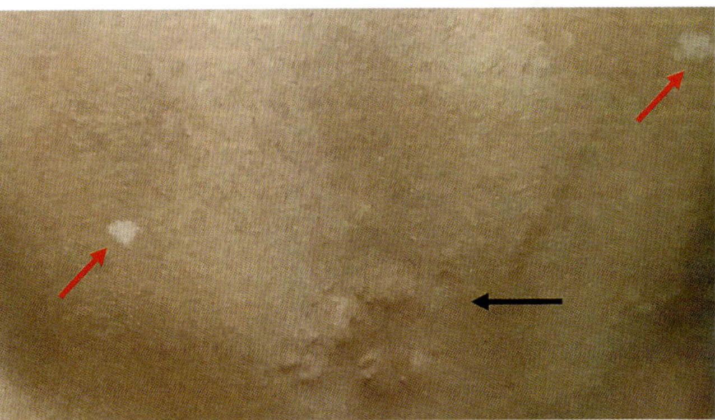

Fig. 4.7.1: Ash leaf macule (red arrows) and shagreen patch (black arrow) in a child with tuberous sclerosis.

Detailed neurological examination, developmental examination, and vision and hearing assessment must be conducted.

The definite diagnosis of GDD is made on the basis of standardized tests of development which include Development Assessment Scale for Indian Infants (DASII) and Bayley Scales of Infant Development—IV (BSID-IV). A DQ of <70 (corresponding to 2 or more SDs below the mean) on these tests is considered a significant delay.[1,2]

INVESTIGATIONS

The role of investigations is to identify the cause and recurrence risk and manage comorbidities. Investigations are prioritized to identify treatable causes such as hypothyroidism, lead toxicity, phenylketonuria, and few other metabolic disorders.[2,6,7]

Formal Testing of Vision and Hearing

These should be done in all children with developmental delay. A hearing screen is recommended as part of routine newborn screening.[2]

Neuroimaging

Indications of neuroimaging in a child with GDD are an abnormal head size, seizures, history of loss of milestones, or abnormal findings on neurological examination. The modality of choice is magnetic resonance imaging (MRI) **(Figs. 4.7.2 and 4.7.3)**.[2,8]

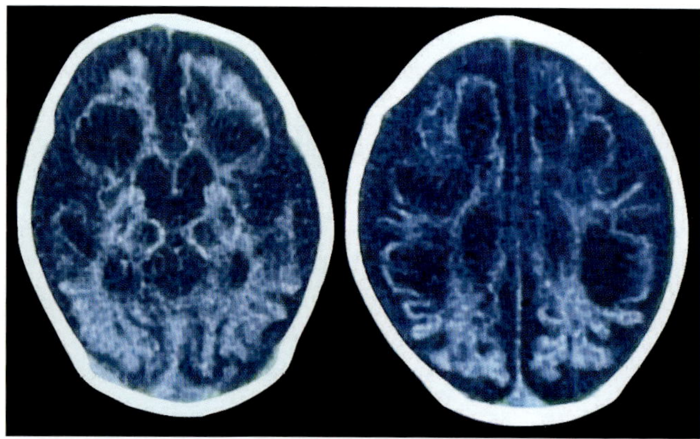

Fig. 4.7.2: Brain MRI of a 4-year-old child with global developmental delay, spastic quadriparesis, and epilepsy showing cystic encephalomalacia and cerebral atrophy. He had a history of delayed cry at birth, neonatal seizures on day 1, and required mechanical ventilation for 2 days.

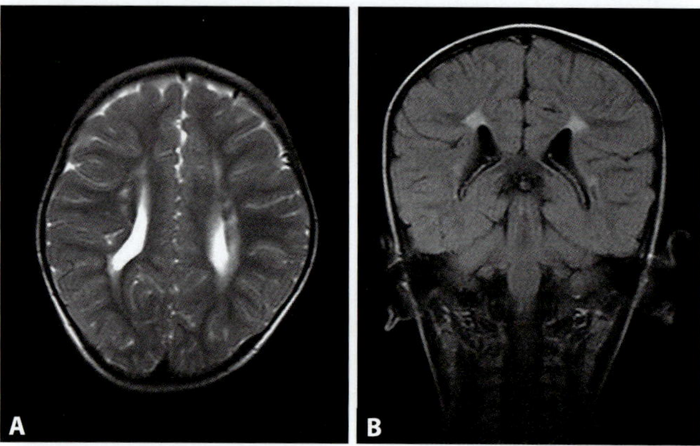

Figs. 4.7.3A and B: Brain MRI of a 2.5-year-old child with global developmental delay showing periventricular leukomalacia.

Blood Investigations

There are no serum markers for diagnosing GDD, but blood investigations may be helpful to identify etiology. They are individualized based on clinical features.

- *Thyroid function tests:* These are recommended in all cases of GDD. Children exhibiting symptoms of hypothyroidism or those at high risk (e.g., Down syndrome) require periodic retesting.[2]
- *Serum iron studies and serum lead levels* are recommended in children with a history of pica, environmental exposure to lead, or having a restricted diet.[2,7,8]
- *Metabolic testing:* It is indicated only in specific circumstances, e.g., family history of similar illness/early neonatal/infant deaths, history of loss of developmental milestones, or episodic decompensation.

Genetic Testing

Genetic conditions account for 30–50% of children with GDD. Karyotype is a simple and easily available test and should be done in children with conditions such as Down syndrome and other trisomies. Other genetic tests such as exome sequencing and chromosomal microarray should be ordered only after evaluation by specialists trained in genetics.[2,5]

TREATMENT

Management of a child with GDD entails routine medical care, treatment of the underlying cause, management of comorbidities, and developmental interventions.

Medical Care

Routine care in children with GDD is similar to typically developing children and includes growth monitoring, nutritional counseling, immunization, dental care, care during illness, and safety counseling. If a treatable condition such as hypothyroidism or certain inborn errors of metabolism is identified, specific therapies should be initiated as early as possible to improve developmental outcomes.[2]

Children with GDD should be screened for comorbidities carefully because timely management of these conditions is important for ensuring the effectiveness of developmental interventions.

Developmental Interventions

Early stimulation during the critical period of brain development (i.e., birth to 6 years) optimizes the child's development and functioning and minimizes disability. A child with suspected delay should be referred to a *child development unit* for early intervention as soon as developmental delay is detected, without waiting for a formal confirmation of diagnosis.[2,9,10]

The child development unit comprises a team of trained professionals from different disciplines under one roof. This team consists of pediatricians, clinical psychologists, speech therapists, special educators/early interventionists, and occupational therapists/physiotherapists. The pediatrician acts as the team leader who makes the diagnosis, identifies and treats comorbidities, counsels the family, ensures coordination between team members, and makes required referrals.

The team at a child development unit evaluates the functional level of the child in different developmental domains. Based on this, an individualized therapy plan is made including speech therapy, physical therapy, general stimulation, behavioral counseling, etc. Active learning of the target skills by the child is best if these interventions are delivered through play. Parents also play a core role in continuing the play-based activities all through the child's routine, thus improving the prognosis.[2]

COUNSELING

Family counseling is another core area of management. It is imperative to discuss compassionately but clearly the diagnosis, management options, and anticipated prognosis. The importance of timely interventions and compliance with therapy should be emphasized. The use of nonevidence-based complementary and alternative medicine should be firmly discouraged. The family should also be referred to an expert in genetics for genetic counseling when warranted.[2]

REFERENCES

1. Shevell M, Ashwal S, Donley D, Flint J, Gingold M, Hirtz D, et al. Quality Standards Subcommittee of the American Academy of Neurology; Practice Committee of the Child Neurology Society. Practice parameter: evaluation of the child with global developmental delay: report of the Quality Standards Subcommittee of the American Academy of Neurology and the Practice Committee of the Child Neurology Society. Neurology. 2003;60:367-80.
2. Juneja M, Gupta A, Sairam S, Jain R, Sharma M, Thadani A, et al. Diagnosis and management of global development delay: consensus guidelines of growth, development and behavioral pediatrics chapter, neurology chapter and neurodevelopment pediatrics chapter of the Indian Academy of Pediatrics. Indian Pediatr. 202;59:401-15.
3. Sharma N, Masood J, Singh SN, Ahmad N, Mishra P, Singh S, et al. Assessment of risk factors for developmental delays among children in a rural community of North India: a cross-sectional study. J Educ Health Promot. 2019;8:112.
4. Jimenez-Gomez A, Standridge SM. A refined approach to evaluating global developmental delay for the international medical community. Pediatr Neurol. 2014;51:198-206.
5. Tikaria A, Kabra M, Gupta N, Sapra S, Balakrishnan P, Gulati S, et al. Etiology of global developmental delay in young children: experience from a tertiary care centre in India. Natl Med J India. 2010;23:324-9.
6. Srour M, Mazer B, Shevell MI. Analysis of clinical features predicting etiologic yield in the assessment of global developmental delay. Pediatrics. 2006;118:139-45.
7. McDonald L, Rennie A, Tolmie J, Galloway P, McWilliam R. Investigation of global developmental delay. Arch Dis Child. 2006;91:701-5.
8. Mithyantha R, Kneen R, McCann E, Gladstone M. Current evidence-based recommendations on investigating children with global developmental delay. Arch Dis Child. 2017;102:1071-6.
9. Hwang AW, Chao MY, Liu SW. A randomized controlled trial of routines-based early intervention for children with or at risk for developmental delay. Res Dev Disabil. 2013;34:3112-23.
10. Cameron RJ. Early intervention for young children with developmental delay: the Portage approach. Child Care Health Dev. 1997;23:11-27.

4.8 Autism Spectrum Disorder

Samir Hasan Dalwai

INTRODUCTION

Autism is a condition where the child fails to connect, interact, or engage meaningfully and purposefully with others since birth. Hence, a child with autism fails to learn interaction, meaningfulness, and purpose (IMP) of social human behavior (eye contact, response to name call, behavior with others, brushing teeth, taking a shower, or dressing appropriately) as well as communication (the meaning and purposeful use of symbols—both nonverbal and verbal) while being excessively drawn to objects and patterns.

DEFINITION

Autism spectrum disorder (ASD) is defined as a biologically based neurodevelopmental disorder characterized by impairments in:

- Social communication and social interaction
- Restricted, repetitive patterns of behavior, interests, or activities[1]

The severity of presentation varies in different individuals based on these impairments and symptoms, hence the term "spectrum." The manner in which ASD affects a person's functioning depends on the severity and combination of symptoms, the presence or absence of associated conditions (e.g., intellectual impairment, epilepsy), and the quality of intervention received.

The term ASD includes disorders previously known as autistic disorder, Kanner's autism (after Dr Leo Kanner, who was the first to describe 11 cases with the disorder in 1943), childhood disintegrative disorder, pervasive developmental disorder-not otherwise specified (PDD-NOS), and Asperger's disorder (after Dr Hans Asperger, 1944).

EPIDEMIOLOGY

The prevalence estimates of ASD have increased markedly from 1 in 150 in 2000 to 1 in 44 in 2018 [Centers for Disease Control and Prevention (CDC), USA]. In 2020, 1 in 36 children aged 8 years (approximately 4% of boys and 1% of girls) was estimated to have ASD.[2] The prevalence in India was 1 in 65 [International Clinical Epidemiology Network (INCLEN), India].[3]

ETIOPATHOGENESIS

Autism spectrum disorder has a genetic etiology, which alters brain development, affecting social and communication development. Children who have a sibling with ASD have an increased risk (3–20%) of developing the condition.[4] The impact of environmental factors like nurturing or gadget and screen exposure at early ages indicates that epigenetics plays a major role. Epidemiologic evidence does not support an association between immunizations and ASD.

CLINICAL FEATURES

The earliest symptoms are the absence of normal behavior (rather than the presence of abnormal ones), i.e., the baby resists cuddling, avoids eye contact, or fails to spread her/his arms in anticipation of being picked up, or to-and-fro babbling and jargoning; similarly, a "very good" baby, i.e., quiet and undemanding.[5]

Though present since birth, symptoms of ASD like social behavior or speech impairment may not be apparent until later when the child reaches the age at which behavior or speech is expected to develop. Parents commonly notice these in the second year of life, when there is a delay in speaking meaningful words and sentences as well as in following oral instructions.

Failure in Development of Social Interaction and Communication (Flowchart 4.8.1)

- Lack of joint attention and meaningful pointing
- Failure to develop and maintain relationships
- Lack of understanding of what behavior is appropriate in a particular situation, nor the needs and emotions of others
- Involving others in activities only to reach the desired object—neglecting the person as soon as that aim is achieved
- Prefer solitary play with objects or parts of their body

Stereotyped Behaviors (Flowchart 4.8.1)

- Motor mannerisms or complex whole-body movements (e.g., hand or finger flapping or twisting, toe walking, rocking, and swaying)
- Echolalia and memorized phrases (nursery rhymes and audio jingles)
- Behaviors like lining up toys in the same manner in a stereotyped ritual without apparent understanding of what the toys represent
- Inflexible adherence to specific, nonfunctional routines or rituals that the child is used to and difficulty with change

Flowchart 4.8.1: Clinical features of ASD.

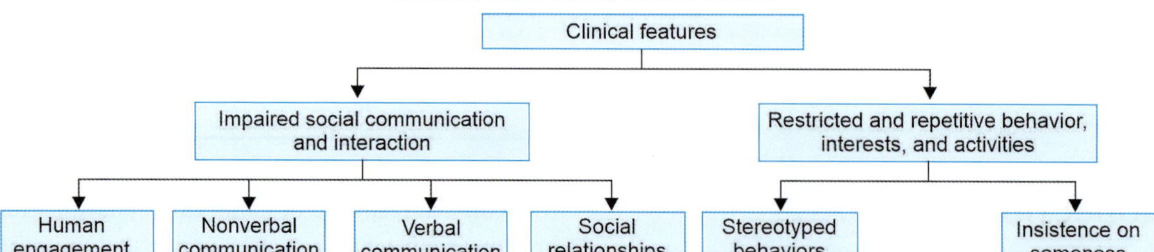

(ASD: autism spectrum disorder)

Source: Dalwai S, Ahmed S, Udani V, Mundkur N, Kamath SS, Nair MKC. Consensus statement of the Indian Academy of Pediatrics on evaluation and management of autism spectrum disorder. Indian Pediatr. 2017;54(5):385-93.

- Anxiety and distress at small changes in such routines
- Repetitive interests of older children may include phone numbers, dates, schedules, license plates, popular animation characters, or subtypes of any groups (e.g., cars, dinosaurs, planes—regarded as "higher functioning," but these may not contribute to significant functioning in daily life).

Restricted Interests

- Preoccupation or focused interests only on certain objects or part of an object
- Peculiar sensory stimuli like rubbing or rocking movements
- Preference to/for patterns of certain sensory stimuli may present as preference to particular tactile, vestibular, proprioceptive, auditory, olfactory, and visual stimuli and resistance to others.

Some children with ASD achieve early language milestones but have regression of language, communication, and/or social skills between 15 and 24 months of age. However, it is important to rule out that those "early milestones" were not merely echolalia or repetitive behaviors. For a verbal sound to be considered a word and not echolalia, it needs to be qualified by checking whether it is "interactive, meaningful, and purposeful" (IMP) for the same. If a child is reported to have achieved the milestone of saying a word at a particular age, we need to examine in detail whether it was done interactively, meaningfully, and purposefully; if not, it is doubtful if it can be considered a true milestone; rather, it is more likely to be echolalia.[6]

Associated Conditions to be Assessed for all Children with Autism Spectrum Disorder[5]

- Intellectual disability
- Medical disorders (e.g., seizures, genetic disorders, and lead poisoning in children with pica)
- Language impairment
- Developmental and mental health comorbidities (e.g., hyperactivity, anxiety, depression, or behavioral regulation)
- Sleep, feeding, and nutrition problems (e.g., constipation and restricted diet)
- Delays in acquisition of activities of daily living (ADLs) or self-help skills (e.g., toileting, dressing, and hygiene)

DIFFERENTIAL DIAGNOSIS

The common differential diagnoses include:

- Global developmental delay/intellectual disability
- Hearing impairment
- Developmental language disorder/language-based learning disability
- Landau-Kleffner syndrome
- Rett disorder (caused by mutations in *MECP2* gene)
- Severe early deprivation/reactive attachment disorder
- Anxiety disorder
- Obsessive-compulsive disorder

A comprehensive history is the best tool for distinguishing these disorders from ASD, although sometimes ancillary tests are necessary **(Box 4.8.1)**.[4,6] Comorbid global developmental delay/intellectual disability and seizures may be associated with tuberous sclerosis complex, Fragile X syndrome, Angelman syndrome, etc.

Evaluation for genetic testing and metabolic testing, neuroimaging, and/or electroencephalography (EEG) may be considered, only if the history and clinical presentation indicate associated conditions.

SCREENING

All children should be screened by a standardized autism screening tool at 18 and 24 months of age.[5]

- *18 months:* Administer the ASD-specific screening tool [Modified Checklist for Autism in Toddlers (M-CHAT)].
- *<18 months:*
  - Evaluate social communication skills.
  - Commence parental education.
  - Reschedule the next visit after 3 months (age <12 months) or after 1 month (age >12 months).
- If screening results are positive or concerning, then:
  - Continue parental education.
  - Refer the child for comprehensive ASD evaluation.
  - Initiate an early intervention program.
  - Evaluate hearing status.
  - Schedule the next follow-up visit after a month.

The M-CHAT is a freely available online questionnaire (in multiple languages) to be completed by parents, which takes about 10 minutes to complete.[7] The Social Communication Questionnaire is another tool that is also available in many Indian languages.

BOX 4.8.1: General concepts that help in differential diagnosis.

- A detailed and complete history is the most important tool for differential diagnosis.
- Additional tests are necessary only sometimes.
- Different features of social communication become obvious or are seen at different ages in the same child. This may complicate the process of differential diagnosis. Remember two groups:
  1. Young children (may need to be followed over time as symptoms evolve for a final diagnosis)
  2. Older children (information about early development may not be readily available)

Source: Dalwai S. Autism spectrum disorders. In: Gowrishankar NC, Nedunchelian K, Ramachandran P, Thangavelu S (Eds). Differential Diagnosis in Pediatrics. New Delhi: Jaypee Brothers Medical Publishers; 2020. pp. 35-8.

DIAGNOSIS

The diagnosis of ASD is clinical, based on the history, examination, and observations of behavior. There are no specific tests or investigations warranted for diagnosis **(Table 4.8.1)**. Diagnosis optimally requires a team led by a developmental pediatrician who is experienced in the diagnosis and treatment of ASD. It should include documentation of whether the child's symptoms meet the Diagnostic and Statistical Manual of Mental Disorders, Fifth Edition (DSM-5) criteria for ASD or the International Classification of Diseases, Tenth Revision (ICD-10).[5,8,9]

Key Questions to Ask

- How was your child's human engagement and social interaction as an infant and a toddler?
- How is the child's behavior and speech at home?
- Does your child use nonverbal language meaningfully?
- When did your child begin using meaningful words?
- How is the behavior and speech at school and other community and social settings?

MANAGEMENT

General Principles of Management of ASD[4,5]

- Intervention should begin as early as possible. A definitive diagnosis is not necessary for commencing intervention.
- Intervention should target core features of autism, i.e., deficits in social communication and interaction, and restricted repetitive patterns of behavior, activities, and/or interests rather than symptoms such as "delayed speech" and "hyperactivity."
- No single therapy has proven to be effective; robust evidence for treatment programs in children younger than 2 years and in adolescents is still emerging.
- Intervention should be evidence-based, structured, and appropriate to the developmental and functional needs of the child in association with the parents and family. Intervention should have a larger component of home and community-based interventions rather than merely clinic-based.
- Management of comorbidities such as intellectual disability, attention-deficit hyperactivity disorder (ADHD), anxiety, and depression is critical to the effectiveness of treatment.
- Correct, appropriate intervention is as important as early intervention. Management of ASD should target the child's milestones and enable the child toward human engagement, social behaviors, nonverbal and verbal communication, and not just rote or pattern learning of speech or solving puzzles or reading and writing.
- Pharmacologic interventions may be used to address comorbidities or provide symptom control but do not treat the core deficits.
- Intervention should be outcome-based and monitored by the physician.
- Management of children should be provided through interdisciplinary teams, coordinated by the developmental pediatrician, and documented. This team should include a pediatrician, pediatric neurologist, psychiatrist, clinical psychologist, occupational therapist, speech and language therapist, special educator, nutritionist, and social worker.

TABLE 4.8.1: Assessment for autism spectrum disorders using tools based on DSM-5.

Screening tools	
1	M-CHAT-R
2	Social Communications Questionnaire (SCQ)
3	Gilliam Autism Rating Scale (GARS)
4	Trivandrum Autism Behavioral Checklist (TABC)
Diagnostic tools	
1	Autism Diagnostic Interview-Revised (ADI-R)
2	Autism Diagnostic Observation Schedule (ADOS)
3	Childhood Autism Rating Scale (CARS)
4	INCLEN tool (INDT-ASD)[8]
5	Indian Scale for Autism Assessment (ISAA)[9]

(DSM-5: Diagnostic and Statistical Manual of Mental Disorders, Fifth Edition; INCLEN: International Clinical Epidemiology Network; INDT-ASD: Indian National Database for autism spectrum disorders; M-CHAT-R: Modified Checklist for Autism in Toddlers-Revised)

Source: Dalwai S, Ahmed S, Udani V, Mundkur N, Kamath SS, Nair MKC. Consensus statement of the Indian Academy of Paediatrics on evaluation and management of autism spectrum disorder. Indian Pediatr. 2017;54:385-93.

Domains of Management

Domains of management have been summarized in **Flowchart 4.8.2.**[5] Involving the child's family is of paramount importance in intervention and outcomes. A good autism intervention program is based on the child's developmental level (milestones attained), specific strengths and weaknesses, the goals and needs as per the child's family, and most importantly regular monitoring of the child's milestones on intervention **(Flowchart 4.8.3)**.

Interventional Models

The following interventional models are being used for ASD with limited outcomes:

- An eclectic approach using elements of different therapies as well as parent- and community-based programs
- Behavioral [e.g., Applied Behavior Analysis (ABA)], structured teaching [e.g., The Treatment and Education

Flowchart 4.8.2: Domains of management of autism.

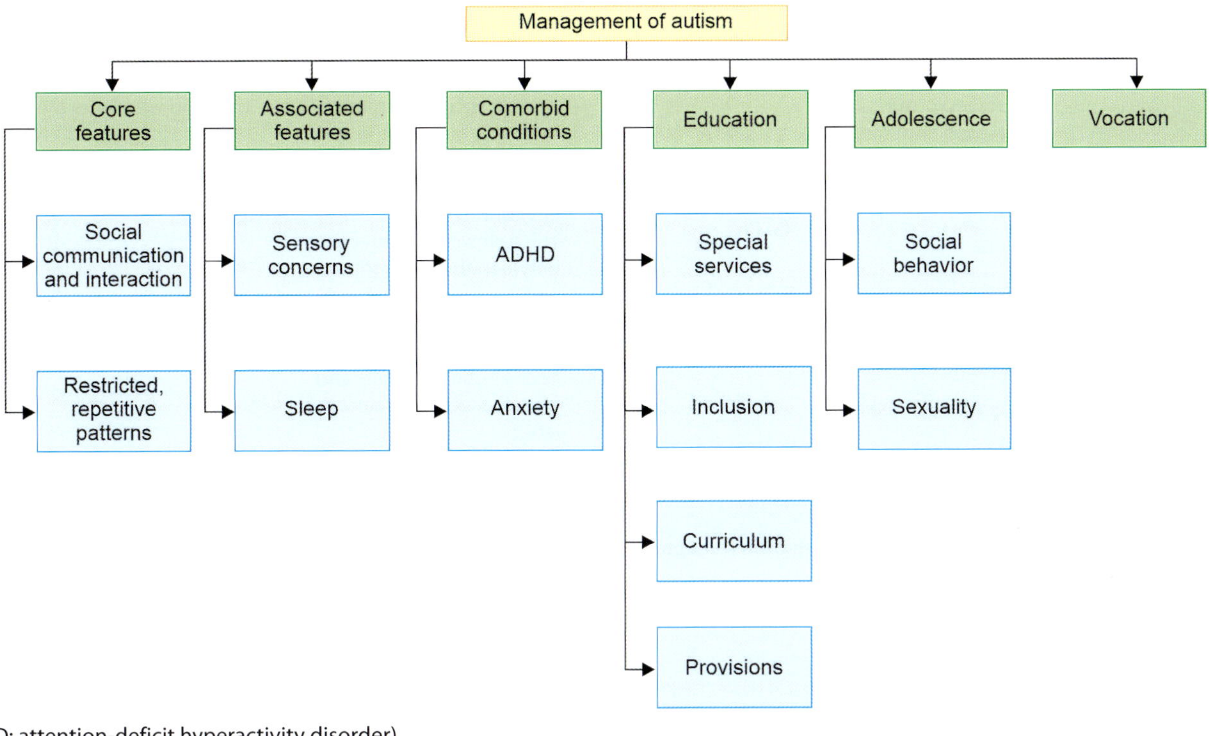

(ADHD: attention-deficit hyperactivity disorder)

Source: Dalwai S, Ahmed S, Udani V, Mundkur N, Kamath SS, Nair MKC. Consensus statement of the Indian Academy of Paediatrics on evaluation and management of autism spectrum disorder. Indian Pediatr. 2017;54(5):385-93.

Flowchart 4.8.3: Components of an ideal intervention program for autism.

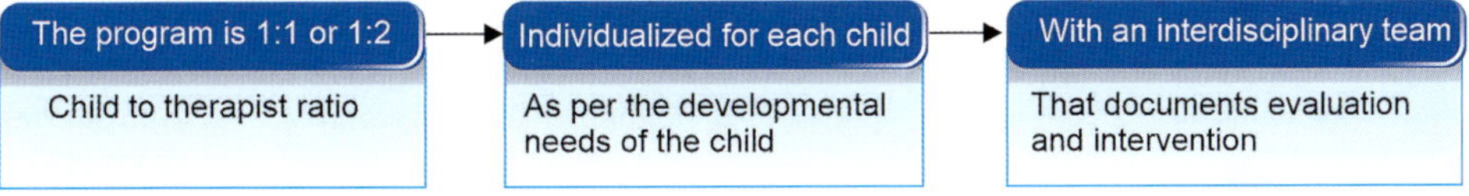

Source: Dalwai S, Ahmed S, Udani V, Mundkur N, Kamath SS, Nair MKC. Consensus statement of the Indian Academy of Paediatrics on evaluation and management of autism spectrum disorder. Indian Pediatr. 2017;54(5):385-93.

of Autistic and related Communication-handicapped Children (TEACCH)], developmental/relationship-based (e.g., "Floor Time"), and Early Start Denver Model (ESDM) Educational management of children with ASD emphasizes the following:

- Inclusion of every child in the classroom
- Curriculum adaptation
- Special needs support
- State support with certification

Pharmacologic Intervention

Pharmacologic interventions should be used in conjunction with appropriate behavioral and environmental interventions and target specific comorbid symptoms **(Table 4.8.2)**.[4,5] Though complementary therapies and stem cells have no evidence to support their use, they should be discussed with parents and explained, as parents are likely to be influenced by the same.

AUTISM—AN ALTERNATE HYPOTHESIS

The belief that autism is a disorder of speech and should be tackled by educational services in school needs re-examination. Autism should be managed appropriately as a developmental disorder by facilitating achievement of developmental milestones in a sequential manner—the New Horizons Social Behavioral and Communication Sequence **(Fig. 4.8.1)**—rather than tackling autism as a neurological regressive disorder.[10]

Autism is not the presence of a disease, but the absence of normal social communication milestones and the presence of pattern learning **(Table 4.8.3)**. In autism, the child fails to learn IMP of human behaviors and thereafter communication

TABLE 4.8.2: Pharmacologic intervention for ASD.

Symptoms	*Drug*	*Option*
Inattention and hyperactivity	Methylphenidate (S/E: Sleep disturbances, decreased appetite, irritability, tics, dullness)	Atomoxetine
Maladaptive behaviors including aggression and self-injury	Risperidone	Stimulants (SSRIs)
Repetitive behaviors	Fluoxetine (SSRI)	
Anxiety	Fluoxetine (SSRI)	
Dysregulated mood	Risperidone or SSRI	
Depressive symptoms	SSRI or serotonin norepinephrine reuptake inhibitor	

(ASD: autism spectrum disorder; SSRI: selective serotonin reuptake inhibitors)

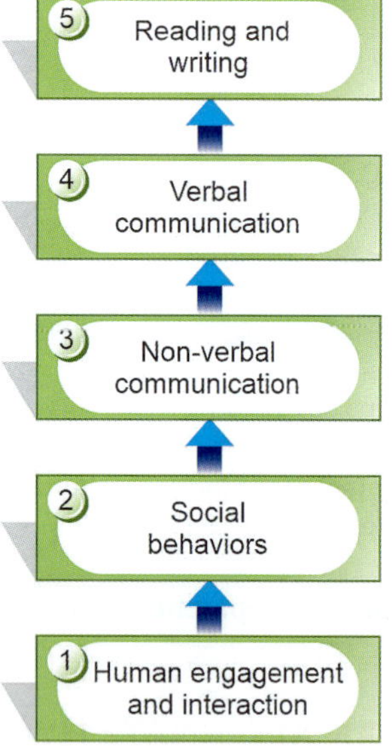

Fig. 4.8.1: The New Horizons Social Behavior Communication Sequence of milestones in the social and communication domain of child development. ©New Horizons Child Development Centre.

TABLE 4.8.3: Social behavior and communication milestones as per the theory of human engagement and interaction of autism.

Normal social communication	*Autism spectrum disorders*
• Normal social communication begins at birth, as the child learns that his needs are met by living beings in the environment • This helps it to differentiate between the living (human) and the nonliving (object) world; it can interact with the former for its needs—meaningfully and purposefully, as against the latter	The child who lacks the ability to interact fails to engage—meaningfully and purposefully—with humans for its needs
This interaction drives the child to observe, learn, and then master meaningful and purposive (1) social interaction, (2) social behavior, (3) nonverbal communication, and (4) verbal communication in a sequential manner (the "Social Communication Sequence")	This prevents the child from observing, learning, and (especially) mastering meaningful and purposive: • Social interaction • Social behavior • Nonverbal communication • Verbal communication
Finding profit in the above, the child gravitates toward learning the nuances of human social behavior and communication—a sly smile, a happy face and an angry word, and a heated conversation—and comparatively ignores the nonhuman (object) world	With the overwhelming presence of objects in the environment, the child gravitates toward learning the patterns of object "behavior" rather than the nuances of human social behavior and communication. Thus, a child with autism can master the use of a mobile gadget or patterns of movement or alphabets and numbers or musical melodies or the façade of a building to recreate it in a painting but fails to understand a sly smile, a happy face and an angry word, or a warm conversation

Source: Dalwai S. Autism spectrum disorders. In: Gowrishankar NC, Nedunchelian K, Ramachandran P, Thangavelu S (Eds). Differential Diagnosis in Pediatrics. New Delhi: Jaypee Brothers Medical Publishers; 2020.

(i.e., the meaning of symbols—nonverbal as well as verbal) **(Flowchart 4.8.4)**. This concept helps in early suspicion as well as pediatrician-guided intervention by parents. Parents are guided to increase human engagement with their child directly, avoiding articles and objects as far as possible as well as to eliminate screen time. Parents are advised to avoid rote or pattern teaching, as this may enhance echolalia. They are advised to make a schedule for the child that includes ADLs as well as include the child in household chores—this ensures that human interaction continues throughout the day even as the parent has to manage household duties. Greater use of nonverbal communication enhances the child's understanding of communication leading to easier acquisition of verbal communication and avoidance of echolalia.

Flowchart 4.8.4: Road to autism: Development of normal social behavior and communication vs. autism spectrum disorders.

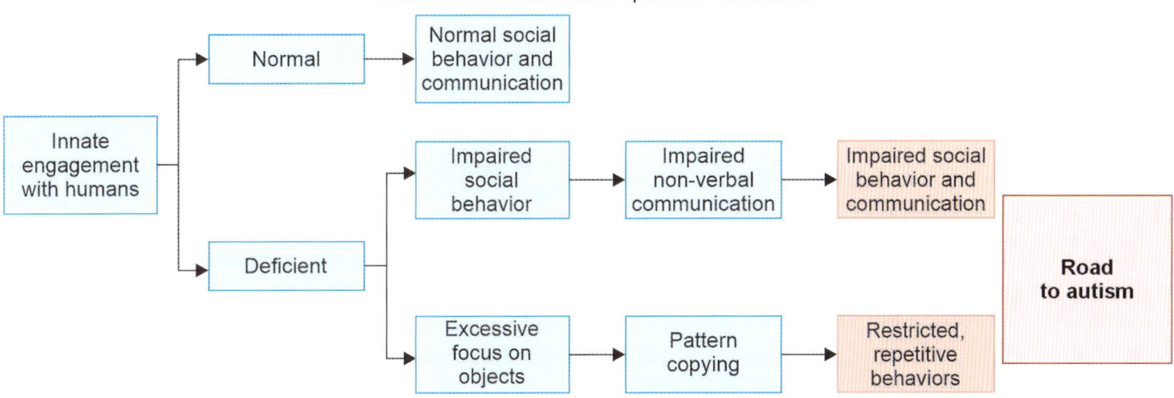

Source: ©New Horizons Child Development Centre.

REFERENCES

1. American Psychiatric Association. Diagnostic and Statistical Manual of Mental Disorders, 5th edition. Arlington, VA: American Psychiatric Association; 2013.
2. Maenner MJ, Warren Z, Williams AR, Amoakohene E, Bakian AV, Bildre DA, et al. Prevalence and characteristics of autism spectrum disorder among children aged 8 years—Autism and Developmental Disabilities Monitoring Network, 11 Sites, United States, 2020. MMWR Surveill Summ. 2023;72(2):1-14.
3. INCLEN survey findings. [online] Available from http://indiatoday.intoday.in/story/autism-autisitic-mind-western-syndrome-myths-about-autism-autistic-children/1/322242.html. [Last accessed October, 2024].
4. Dalwai SH, Ahmed S, Ravikumar CP. Autism spectrum disorders. In: Unni JC, Dalwai S, Ahmed S, Multani KS, Deshpande L, Srivastava L (Eds). IAP Standard Treatment Guidelines 2022, 1st edition. New Delhi: Jaypee Brothers Medical Publishers; 2023. pp. 592-7.
5. Dalwai S, Ahmed S, Udani V, Mundkur N, Kamath SS, Nair MKC. Consensus statement of the Indian Academy of Paediatrics on evaluation and management of autism spectrum disorder. Indian Pediatr. 2017;54(5):385-93.
6. Dalwai S. Autism spectrum disorders. In: Gowrishankar NC, Nedunchelian K, Ramachandran P, Thangavelu S (Eds). Differential Diagnosis in Pediatrics. New Delhi: Jaypee Brothers Medical Publishers; 2020. pp. 35-8.
7. Robins DL, Casagrande K, Barton M, Chen CMA, Dumont-Mathieu T, Fein D. Validation of the modified checklist for autism in toddlers, revised with follow-up (MCHAT-R/F). Pediatrics. 2014;133(1):37-45.
8. Juneja M, Mishra D, Russell PS, Gulati S, Deshmukh V, Tudu P, et al. INCLEN diagnostic tool for autism spectrum disorder (INDT-ASD): development and validation. Indian Pediatr. 2014;51(5):359-65.
9. Mukherjee SB, Malhotra MK, Aneja S, Chakraborty S, Deshpande S. Diagnostic accuracy of Indian Scale for Assessment of Autism (ISAA) in children aged 2–9 years. Indian Pediatr. 2015;52(3):212-16.
10. Dalwai S. Autism spectrum disorders. In: Unni JC, Dalwai S, Ahmed S, Multani KS, Deshpande L, Srivastava L (Eds). IAP Handbook of Developmental Behavioural Pediatrics, 1st edition. New Delhi: Jaypee Brothers Medical Publishers; 2022.

4.9 Early Interventions to Prevent Developmental Delay

Rashid H Merchant, Samir Hasan Dalwai

EARLY CHILDHOOD DEVELOPMENT

Early childhood is a critical period of rapid growth and development, laying the foundation for a child's future health and well-being. Neural circuits, which create the foundation for learning, behavior, and health, are most flexible or "plastic" during the first 3 years of life.[1] Over time, they become increasingly difficult to change. Extensive research spanning decades demonstrates that the initial experiences of children significantly influence brain development. Positive early experiences are essential prerequisites for later success in school, the workplace, and the community. The foundations of lifelong health are built in early childhood. Poor nutrition, poor nurturing and parenting practices, recurrent infections, and neurodevelopmental disorders impact child development negatively; early childhood development encompasses all aspects of a child's life holistically and includes, but not limited to, neurodevelopment.[2]

FACTORS AFFECTING OUTCOMES

- The brain is strengthened by positive early experiences, especially stable relationships with caring and responsive adults, safe and supportive environments, and appropriate nutrition.[3]
- The development of cognitive and language skills is built upon the early establishment of social/emotional skills and physical well-being.
- Positive parenting, along with child rearing and nurturing, has a high impact on the final outcomes **(Table 4.9.1)**.
- Prolonged exposure to "toxic" stress, such as extreme poverty, abuse, neglect, or severe maternal depression, can detrimentally impact brain development, resulting in long-lasting challenges in learning, behavior, and both physical and mental health.
- High-quality early intervention (EI) services have the potential to change a child's developmental trajectory, leading to improved outcomes for children, families, and communities.
- Intervening at an early stage in life is likely to yield greater effectiveness and lower costs compared to later intervention.

DEVELOPMENTAL DELAY

Developmental delay is a significant concern in pediatric practice, affecting a substantial proportion of children worldwide. Early childhood is a critical period marked by rapid physical, cognitive, and socioemotional development, and thus any disruptions during this period can have profound and long-lasting effects on a child's overall well-being.

Developmental delay refers to a significant lag in achieving developmental milestones across multiple domains, including motor skills, language and communication, cognitive abilities, and social–emotional development. It may manifest as delays in reaching developmental milestones or as atypical development compared to peers. Developmental delay can result from various factors, including genetic predispositions, prenatal exposure to toxins or infections, perinatal complications, environmental factors, and social determinants of health.

Developmental delay can have long-term consequences on a child's overall development and quality of life. However, with universal nurturing care, early identification, and appropriate EIs, many developmental delays can be prevented or minimized, allowing children to reach their full potential.

NURTURING CARE FRAMEWORK FOR EARLY CHILDHOOD DEVELOPMENT

"Nurturing Care Framework," developed by the World Health Organization (WHO) and United Nations Children's Fund (UNICEF), provides a comprehensive approach to promoting the early childhood development of children from birth to 5 years of age. It is prescribed for *all children* and not just for those with neurodevelopmental delays or disorders. It is promotive rather than therapeutic and emphasizes the critical role of nurturing care environments, which encompass responsive caregiving, opportunities for early learning, safety and security, good health, and nutrition **(Figs. 4.9.1 to 4.9.3)**.[4] By addressing these essential components, the framework aims to support children's holistic development and lay the

TABLE 4.9.1: Factors impacting child development outcomes.

Positive outcomes	*Negative outcomes*
• Positive early experiences • Stable relationships with caring and responsive adults • Positive parenting and child nurturing • Early social/emotional development–for cognitive and language skills development • Good physical health • Appropriate nutrition • Normal neurodevelopment • High-quality intervention services • Intervention provided early	• Persistent "toxic" stress • Extreme poverty • Abuse and neglect • Severe maternal depression • Poor health, multiple recurrent infections • Inadequate nutrition • Neurodevelopmental delay/ disorders • None or poor-quality interventions • Intervention provided late

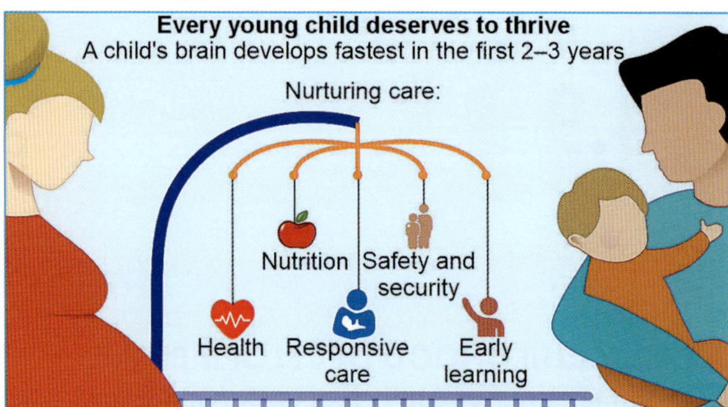

Fig. 4.9.1: The foundation for children's development.
Source: Adapted from The Lancet Early Childhood Development Series.

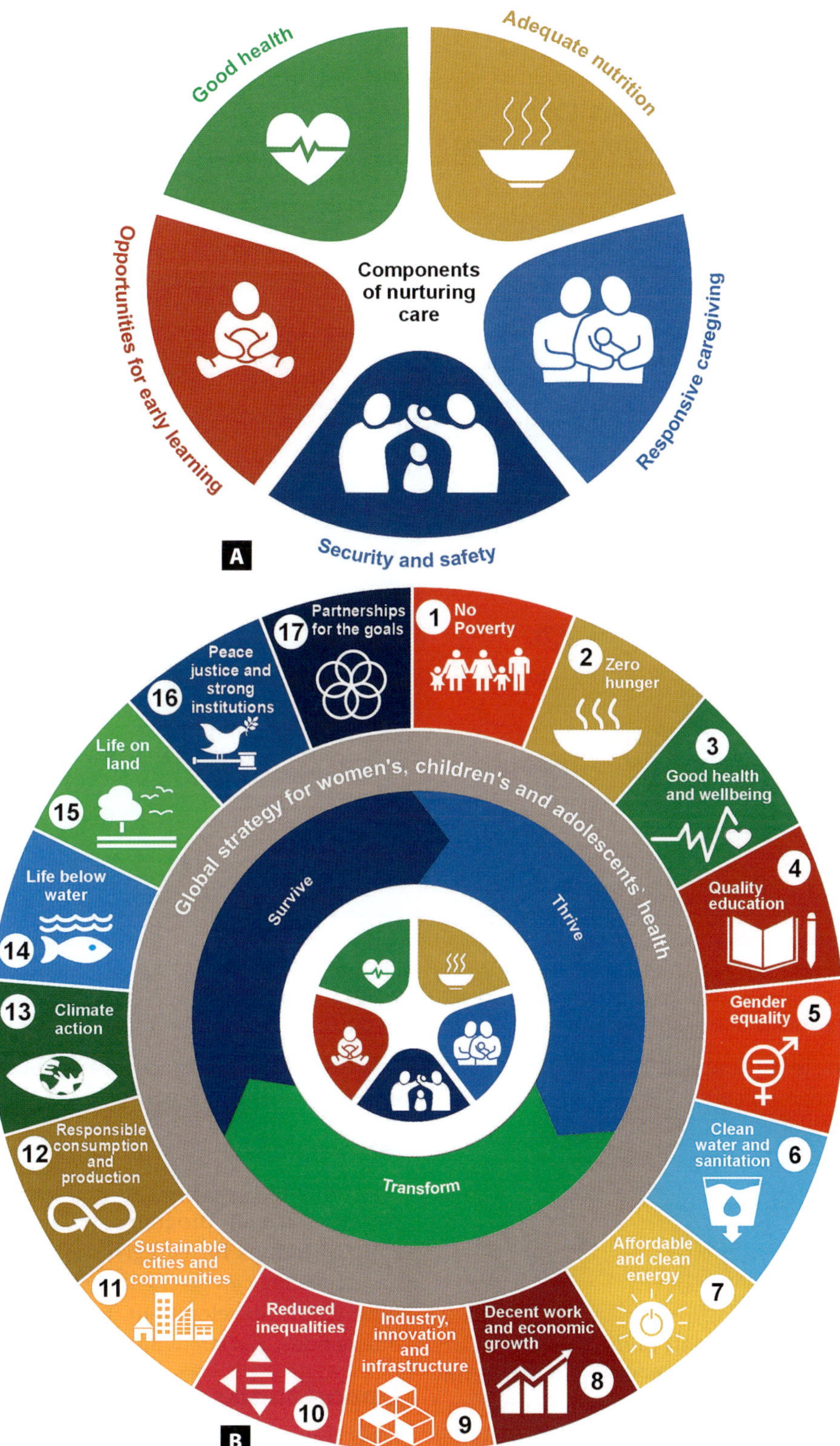

Figs. 4.9.2A and B: Care for early childhood development: A framework for helping children survive and thrive to transform health and human potential, World Health Organization, Geneva.

Source: Adapted from Scheidecker G, Chaudhary N, Keller H, Mezzenzana, F, Lancy D. "Poor brain development" in the global South? Challenging the science of early childhood interventions. Ethos. 2023;51:1-24.

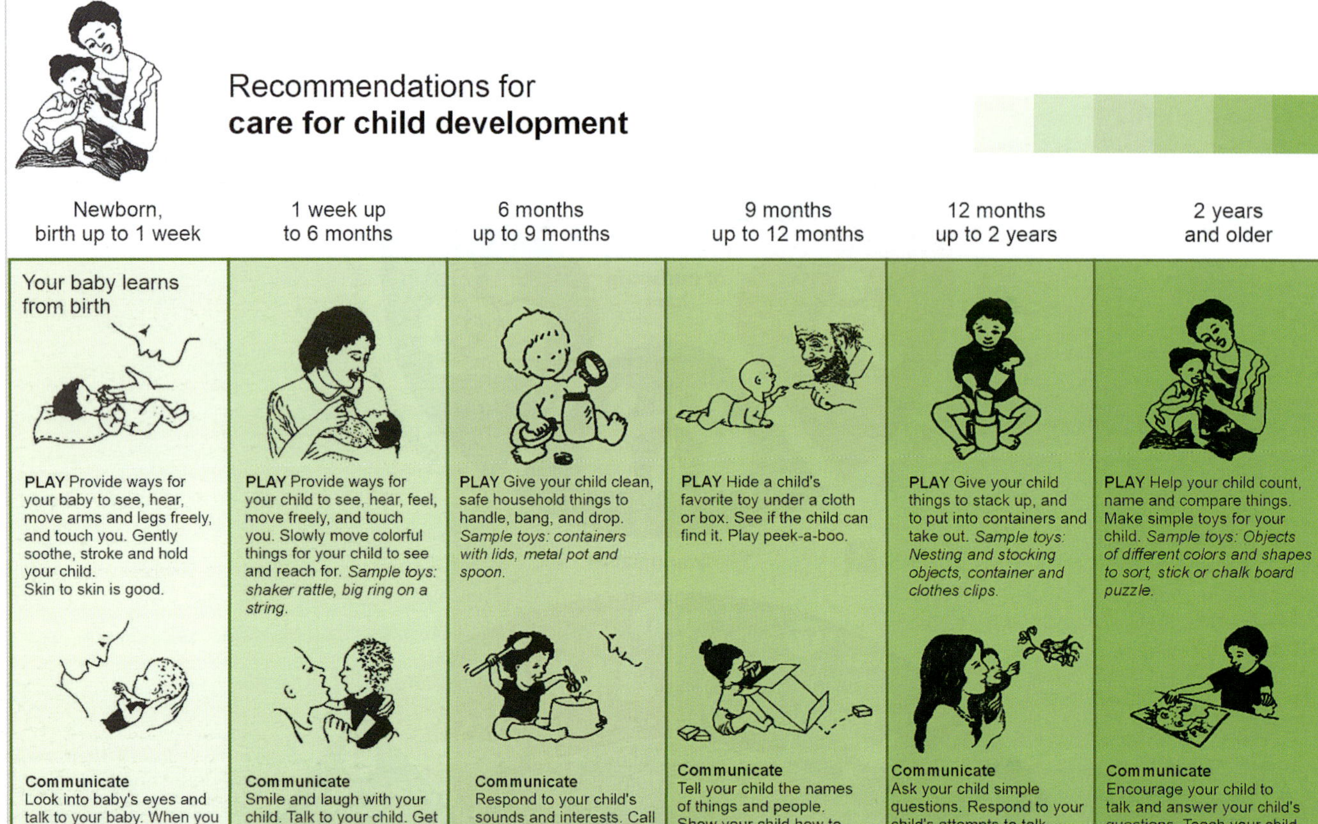

Fig. 4.9.3: Care for child development: improving the care of young children, World Health Organization, Geneva.
Source: Adapted from Scheidecker G, Chaudhary N, Keller H, Mezzenzana, F, Lancy D. "Poor brain development" in the global South? Challenging the science of early childhood interventions. Ethos. 2023;51:1-24.

foundation for lifelong health and well-being.[5] The five major components of this framework are:

1. Responsive caregiving
2. Opportunities for early learning
3. Safety and security
4. Good health
5. Adequate nutrition

Responsive Caregiving

Responsive caregiving is at the heart of the Nurturing Care Framework. It involves caregivers, whether parents, family members, or other caregivers, providing sensitive and consistent responses to children's needs. This includes responding promptly to a child's cues for feeding, comfort, and stimulation, fostering a secure attachment relationship between the child and caregiver. Secure attachments have been associated with better cognitive, social, and emotional outcomes in children and serve as a buffer against the adverse effects of stress and adversity.

Interventions

Interventions to promote responsive caregiving may include parent education programs, home visitation services, and support groups for caregivers. These interventions focus on enhancing caregivers' knowledge and skills in nurturing their child's development, fostering positive parent-child interactions, and strengthening parent-child relationships.

Opportunities for Early Learning

Early childhood is a period of rapid brain development, with neural connections forming at an astonishing pace. Providing young children with opportunities for early learning is essential for driving this cognitive development and promoting school readiness. This includes engaging children in stimulating activities that promote language development, cognitive skills, and social interaction.

Interventions

Evidence-based interventions to support early learning include high-quality early childhood education programs, such as preschools and daycare centers, that offer age-appropriate curricula and activities. Additionally, promoting early literacy through activities like reading aloud to children and providing access to books can foster a love of learning and language development from an early age.

Safety and Security

Creating safe and secure environments is crucial for promoting children's healthy development. Children who feel safe and protected are better able to explore their surroundings, form positive relationships, and develop self-confidence. Ensuring physical safety, emotional security, and protection from harm are fundamental components of nurturing care environments.

Interventions

Interventions to promote safety and security may include childproofing the home environment, providing supervision and guidance to prevent accidents and injuries, and implementing policies and programs to prevent child maltreatment and abuse. Additionally, addressing social determinants of health, such as poverty, housing instability, and community violence, is essential for creating supportive environments where children can thrive. Some measures that can be implemented are as follows:

- *Childproofing and home safety:* Offering guidance and resources to parents and caregivers on childproofing their homes, including securing hazardous items, installing safety gates, and ensuring proper supervision
- *Preventing child maltreatment and abuse:* Implementing policies and programs aimed at preventing child maltreatment and abuse, such as public awareness campaigns, mandatory reporting laws, and training for professionals working with children and families
- *Social determinants of health:* Tackling underlying social and economic factors that contribute to unsafe environments, such as poverty, housing instability, and community violence, through targeted interventions and support services.

Good Health and Adequate Nutrition

Good health and nutrition are cornerstones of early childhood development, providing the foundation for physical growth, cognitive development, and overall well-being. Adequate nutrition, access to healthcare services, and preventive care are essential for promoting children's health and reducing the risk of developmental delays.

Interventions

Interventions to promote good health and nutrition may include breastfeeding support, access to nutritious foods, immunizations, regular health screenings, and EI services for developmental concerns. Additionally, promoting maternal health and well-being during pregnancy and the postnatal period can have long-term benefits for both mother and child. Some programs that can be implemented are:

- *Breastfeeding support:* Providing education, counseling, and lactation support to mothers to promote and support breastfeeding, which offers numerous health benefits for both mother and child.
- *Nutrition programs:* Implementing programs that ensure access to nutritious foods for young children, such as subsidized food programs, school meal programs, and community food banks.
- *Early childhood health screenings:* Conducting regular health screenings and assessments to identify and address potential health concerns or developmental delays early on, enabling timely intervention and support.

IMPORTANCE OF EARLY INTERVENTION

In children who have neurodevelopmental concerns, manifesting as developmental delay or deviancies, early and appropriate intervention plays a crucial role in addressing developmental delays and promoting optimal development in young children. Timely and appropriate interventions can mitigate the risk of developmental delays and actually promote optimal development. Research has consistently shown that the earlier the interventions are initiated, the better the outcomes for children with developmental concerns—EI can help minimize the impact of developmental delays, enhance developmental trajectories, and improve children's functional outcomes. Additionally, early identification and EI can prevent secondary complications and reduce the need for more intensive interventions later in life.

Benefits of Early Intervention

Support services provided to young children experiencing or at risk of developmental delays have demonstrated significant positive effects across various developmental areas, encompassing health, language, communication, cognitive abilities, and social/emotional growth. EI benefits families by empowering them to address their children's unique requirements from an early stage and throughout their lifetime. Societal advantages include a reduction in economic strain due to a diminished demand for special education.

Challenges to Early Intervention

There is a need to serve children earlier than what is currently practiced. Only a small segment of children up to the age of

3 years who have delays actually receive services. Sociocultural and economic disparities worsen service delivery. Young children experiencing homelessness are more likely to have lower birth weights than other children, learning disabilities, developmental delays, emotional problems, and behavior issues, yet they are greatly underrepresented in early childhood programs. Almost all newborns with prenatal substance exposure, a risk factor for poor developmental outcomes, and those who have experienced substantiated abuse or neglect do not receive EI. These children often have high rates of physical, cognitive, social-emotional, relational, and psychological problems.

How does Early Intervention Work?

Nature and nurture contribute equally toward recovery in neurodevelopmental disorders in children. EI is a part of the latter that provides a wide variety of medical, educational, and psychological treatments for at-risk babies as well as socioeconomically disadvantaged children.

The goals of EI are to empower the families, facilitate service provision and coordination by developmental physicians?/pediatricians, and, when required, provide direct services by therapists. The target is to be family-centered and individualized to meet the specific needs of each infant, covering gross motor, fine motor, language, social, and self-help skills. The emphasis is on the initial 3 years of life, which is the critical period of brain development, as this is the period of effective synaptogenesis.

Early Identification

Identifying the "at-risk" or "red flags" or absent building blocks of a particular milestone is the first step in planning EI services. This requires detailed family, antenatal, and perinatal history as well as developmental history covering all domains of development. This is followed by detailed screening and assessment in relevant areas as given in the following text.

Newborn Screening

- Abnormal tone, weak suck, and lethargy for more than 24 hours indicate a 12–15-fold increased risk of developmental delay.
- Decreased spontaneous movements for more than 1 day increase the risk 19-fold.
- Poor response to touch and poor cry for more than 24 hours indicate a 21-fold increased risk of developmental delay.

Vision Screening

Fundoscopy for screening retinopathy of prematurity (ROP), retinoscopy, and visual evoked potential (VEP) is recommended.

Hearing Screening

Universal hearing screening by otoacoustic emission (OAE) and brainstem-evoked response audiometry (BERA) is recommended.

Red Flag Signs at 9 Months (American Academy of Pediatrics)

Please see **Box 4.9.1** for details.

Red Flag Signs at 18 Months (American Academy of Pediatrics)

Please refer to **Box 4.9.2** for details.

Community-based Screening and Identification—Direct Observation Card (Table 4.9.2)

Red Flags for Communication, Behavior, and Socialization

If at 2 years, the mother is:

- The mother is not satisfied with the child's speech or if there is regression in speech
- The mother is not satisfied with the child's behavior or he/she looks lost in his/her own world
- If the child is not following more than two to three single-step commands or is hyperactive
- If the child is having sensory issues like hyperacusis, chewing difficulties, and difficulty holding crayons

If any of these are present, individualized direct services should be started.

The Modified Checklist for Autism in Toddlers (M-CHAT) is an appropriate screening tool for autism.[6] Besides the above, the Denver Developmental Screening Tool (DDST) and Gross Motor Function Classification (GMFC) can be used to identify the delay in specific domains.

BOX 4.9.1: Red flag signs at 9 months (American Academy of Pediatrics).

Inability to:
- Sit well with support
- Motor symmetry without established handedness
- Grasp objects
- Transfer objects from hand to hand
- Roll over to both sides

BOX 4.9.2: Red flag signs at 18 months (American Academy of Pediatrics).

Inability to:
- Stand and walk independently
- Grasp and manipulate small objects
- Any sign of regression in gross motor (GM)/fine motor (FM) skills
- Drool

TABLE 4.9.2: Community-based screening and identification that can be carried out by the use of the Direct Observation Card.

Confirm that child can see and hear	
2-month-old infant	Social smile
4-month-old infant	Head holding
8-month-old infant	Sitting independently
12-month-old infant	Standing without support
15-month-old toddler	Should speak Mama, Papa (specifically) in his/her native language
18 months	Follow one-line command with no regression in communication, social, or play
If any of them is not achieved, it is an indication for early intervention (EI).	

Irrespective of the scale used, it is crucial to recognize issues within developmental domains and address each one individually as soon as possible, rather than delaying until a definitive diagnosis is made.[7]

MANAGEMENT

Preventive strategies should focus on adolescent girls; maternal nutrition and management of anemia and deficiencies of iron, folate, iodine, and zinc; infection prevention; rubella vaccine; treating chronic medical illnesses and gynecological issues; and better obstetric care. Antenatal steroids should be administered in premature deliveries. Adequate transport services for in utero and neonatal care should be accessible. Low birth weight and the girl child should be provided better neonatal care, literacy, and life skills.

Early Intervention Strategies should Start in the Neonatal Intensive Care Unit[7]

- Unnecessary noises of alarms should be reduced.
- Promote bonding through the Kangaroo method.
- Passive exercises of the joints and gentle massage should be given to neonates.
- Individual lighting units should be dimmed at night to simulate cycles of day and night.
- Recording of mother's voice or music (hum) can be recorded and played near the baby but not constantly.

Early Intervention for Head Control

- Carry the child in an upright position.
- Slowly lift the child from the lying-down position, holding the axilla, to the sitting position, and then slowly put him/her back to the lying position, thereby stimulating to lift and hold the head (5 minutes × 4 times/day).
- If the child does not lift his/her head, gently stroke downward over the neck muscle.

Early Intervention for Sitting

- Make the child come to a sitting position, hold her/him in this position, and then make her/him lie down (5 minutes × 4 times a day).
- Make the child sit across his/her mother's knee and then tilt the child forward and sideways so that he/she outstretches the hand. This helps in the development of righting reflex.
- Make the child sit, provide support and toys, and then slowly reduce support.

Early Intervention for Standing

- Help him/her come to a sitting position on its own.
- Make him/her come to a standing position holding a stool and put toys.
- Help him/her to balance on an inclined surface.
- Help him/her to walk with support holding both hands and later with one.
- Outdoor playing with children will help holistic development.

Early Intervention for Vision

- Hang brightly colored objects 12–15 inches above the crib.
- The mother, while maintaining eye-to-eye contact, performs singing or talking while keeping face 6–8 inches away.
- To promote visual following, use a multicolored small bulb series; this is to be hung on the wall at the foot end of the child.

Early Intervention in Speech and Communication

- No electronic gadgets before 2 years of life should be introduced.
- Speak clearly and with eye-to-eye contact with the child; do not use motherese.
- Talk to the child whenever possible and encourage him/her to ask questions.
- Encourage him/her to share his/her experiences and to tell stories.

Early Intervention for Hand Function

- For opening of hand, pull the thumb or fingers from base.
- Place an object in his/her hand and bend his/her fingers around it to promote hand grasp.
- Apply dough or colored clay to the thumb and index finger to promote pincer grasp.[8]

Early Intervention in Autism

In EI for autism spectrum disorder (ASD) in children, screening and prevention play vital roles in optimizing outcomes. Early screening allows for the timely identification of developmental concerns, facilitating prompt intervention. Prevention strategies focus on fostering a nurturing environment, promoting healthy development, and addressing risk factors proactively. By integrating screening into routine care and implementing preventive measures, healthcare providers can support children's optimal growth and development, mitigating the impact of ASD.

Screening of Autism Spectrum Disorder

The M-CHAT and its subsequent versions can be administered and scored as part of a well-child care visit and can also be used by professionals to assess risk for ASD. They were designed to screen children aged 16–30 months. For "screen-positive" children, immediate action is crucial. Parents should promptly seek a comprehensive diagnostic evaluation by a qualified healthcare professional specializing in ASD. This evaluation aims to confirm an ASD diagnosis and may involve further assessments, such as developmental evaluations and medical screenings. Additionally, EI services should be considered, as they play a vital role in supporting the child's development and addressing their unique needs. Time is of the essence in ensuring timely access to appropriate interventions and support for the child and their family.

Strategies for Early Intervention

The EI approach for children with ASD integrates a multidisciplinary approach with nurturing care principles. ASD should be appropriately managed, with emphasis being placed on coaching parents and caregivers. Through guidance, parents are empowered to support their child's functional independence by navigating sequential developmental milestones—the New Horizons Social Behavioral and Communication Sequence. Strategies are tailored for home implementation, encouraging increased social interaction and reduced object focus through enjoyable human activities like play and establishing routines. Parents are advised against rote teaching to minimize echolalia and are encouraged to involve their child in meaningful and purposeful daily living activities and household chores. This ensures sustained human interaction throughout the day. Nonverbal communication is emphasized to enhance the child's understanding and acquisition of verbal communication while discouraging screen use to promote communication and social skills. This comprehensive approach aims to maximize the child's developmental progress and overall well-being within the family context.[9]

Prevention of Autism Spectrum Disorder

Autism often results from a combination of genetic susceptibility and environmental triggers. Implementing strategies to limit screen time in children is crucial for their development and well-being. Research suggests that excessive screen time can exacerbate symptoms and hinder social and communication skills in children with autism. Parents and caregivers should be encouraged to establish clear guidelines and boundaries regarding screen use, opting for alternative activities that promote interaction and engagement, such as outdoor play, creative pursuits, and social interactions.[10] By minimizing screen exposure and promoting healthier alternatives, we can contribute to preventing autism and supporting the holistic development of children, thus enhancing their overall quality of life.

CONCLUSION

Early interventions play a crucial role in preventing developmental delays and promoting healthy development in young children. By embracing the principles of the Nurturing Care Framework for Early Childhood Development, we can create environments that support children's holistic development and lay the foundation for lifelong health and well-being. Through responsive caregiving, opportunities for early learning, safety and security, and good health and nutrition, we can ensure that every child has the opportunity to reach their full potential.

It is crucial to promptly identify infants and toddlers requiring services to intervene when the developing brain is most adaptable. Offering high-quality EI programs for vulnerable infants and toddlers can decrease the likelihood of future issues in their learning, behavior, and health. EI is likely to yield greater effectiveness and cost savings compared to later intervention.

Developmental trajectories can potentially be changed during the early years, and the development of secondary disabilities can be prevented by the provision of EI services when the child is very young. We need to incorporate EI services in our daily practice, which should be family-centered, individualized for the child, and culturally appropriate, with prompt direct services as and when indicated. One important benefit of EI is helping families be hopeful about their child's future.

REFERENCES

1. Inbrief: The Science of Early Childhood Development. (2020). Center on the developing child at Harvard University. [online] Available from https://developingchild.harvard.edu/resources/inbrief-science-of-ecd/. [Last accessed October, 2024].

2. John CC, Black MM, Nelson CA 3rd. Neurodevelopment: the impact of nutrition and inflammation during early to middle childhood in low-resource settings. Pediatrics. 2017;139(Suppl 1):S59-71.
3. Likhar A, Baghel P, Patil M. Early childhood development and social determinants. Cureus. 2022;14(9):e29500.
4. Scheidecker G, Chaudhary N, Keller H, Mezzenzana F, Lancy D. “Poor brain development” in the global South? Challenging the science of early childhood interventions. Ethos. 2023;51:1-24.
5. Nurturing Care Practice Guide: Strengthening Nurturing Care Through Health and Nutrition Services. United Nations Children’s Fund, New York and World Health Organization, Geneva; 2022.
6. Wiggins LD, Baio J, Schieve L, Lee LC, Nicholas J, Rice CE. Retention of autism spectrum diagnoses by community professionals: findings from the autism and developmental disabilities monitoring network, 2000 and 2006. J Dev Behav Pediatr. 2012;33(5):387-95.
7. Meenai Z. Early intervention. In: IAP Handbook of Developmental Behavioural Pediatrics, 1st edition. New Delhi: Jaypee Brothers Medical Publishers; 2022.
8. Meenai ZM, Nair MKC, Bhattacharya A. Standard Treatment Guidelines 2022.. India: Indian Academy of Pediatrics; 2022. [online] Available from https://iapindia.org/pdf/Ch-123-Early-Detection-and-Early-Intervention-of-a-High-risk-Neonate.pdf. [Last accessed October, 2024].
9. Dalwai S. Autism spectrum disorders. In: IAP Handbook of Developmental Behavioural Pediatrics, 1st edition. New Delhi: Jaypee Brothers Medical Publishers; 2022.
10. Gupta P, Shah D, Bedi N, Galagali P, Dalwai S, Agarwal S, et al. Indian Academy of Pediatrics guidelines on screen time and digital wellness in infants, children and adolescents. Indian Pediatr. 2022;59(3):235-44.

4.10 Digital Advances in Neurodevelopmental Disorders

Aradhana Rohil, Gautam Kamila, Sheffali Gulati

INTRODUCTION

Diagnostic and Statistical Manual of Mental Disorders, Fifth Edition (DSM-5) defines neurodevelopmental disorders (NDDs) as a group of conditions with onset in the developmental period, inducing deficits that produce impairments of personal, social, academic, or occupational functioning.[1] These chronic conditions impose significant health and cost burdens on families and society. The International Clinical Epidemiology Network (INCLEN) study of 3,964 Indian children from five different regions of India estimated the overall prevalence of NDD to be around 12% in children between 2 and 9 years of age, with a prevalence of autism spectrum disorders (ASD) around 1 in 89 overall, and 20% of children with NDD had more than one associated comorbid condition, among which autism was the most common.[2] Due to this co-occurrence, the assessment and diagnosis of NDD is a complex and lengthy procedure, and their management requires multidisciplinary care. All these factors lead to substantial delay in receiving a diagnosis and initiation of intervention, especially in resource-limited settings, further hampering the early and appropriate development in these children. Digital advances offer the opportunity to deliver automated, personalized, and self-directed interventions with improved access to therapy and the potential for better clinical effectiveness.

SPECTRUM OF DIGITAL ADVANCES

Digital advances for NDD cover a wide spectrum for their role in:

- Preventive strategies (both primordial and primary prevention)
- Assessment (for diagnosis and monitoring, which encompass secondary prevention)
- Treatment (which encompasses tertiary prevention)

They lead to the empowerment of parents of children with disabilities through education and increasing awareness via mobile applications and other computer software. They reduce the anxiety and stress among caregivers by bridging the physical distance between primary care physicians and parents. For example, by using hospital-based mobile applications, parents can put up their queries or patient-related concerns, which can be answered by the physicians. Similarly, the patient can be monitored more judiciously via telemedicine-based approaches. Doctors of different specialties, nurses, therapists, and parents can all share the same platform on a web or mobile-based application with less need to travel physically, providing ease of care. The spectrum is broad and includes:

- Artificial intelligence (AI)-based models for:
    - Detection of obstetric complications and fetal anomalies (primordial and primary prevention)

  - Screening diseases for early intervention (primary and secondary prevention)
  - Making a diagnosis (secondary prevention)
  - Management (secondary and tertiary prevention)
- Use of *assistive* technologies for management (tertiary prevention)
- Use of *adaptive* technologies for management (tertiary prevention)
- Virtual reality (VR)-based models for management (tertiary prevention)
- Robotics (tertiary prevention)
- Neurorestoration—brain-computer interfaces (BCI) and exoskeletons (tertiary prevention)
- Biofeedbacks (tertiary prevention)
- Neuromodulation—noninvasive brain stimulation (NIBS) through transcranial magnetic stimulation (TMS) (tertiary prevention)
- Telemedicine/telerehabilitation for:
  - Screening and diagnosis (primary and secondary prevention)
  - Management (secondary and tertiary prevention)
- Postimplantation genetic diagnosis (primordial and primary prevention)

DIGITAL ADVANCES IN CEREBRAL PALSY

Digital Advances Targeting Primordial Prevention in Cerebral Palsy

Preimplantation Genetic Diagnosis

Preimplantation genetic diagnosis (PGD or PIGD) is the genetic profiling of embryos prior to implantation and sometimes even of oocytes prior to fertilization. It is used primarily for genetic disease prevention by selecting only those embryos that do not have a known genetic disorder and may also be used to increase the chances of successful pregnancy. This technology has become an integral part of assisted reproductive technology (ART) procedures. There has been advancement in genetic testing of embryos from traditionally used conventional polymerase chain reaction (PCR) methods to fluorescence in situ hybridization (FISH) to comparative genomic hybridization (CGH) to next-generation sequencing (NGS).[3]

Digital Advances Targeting Primary Prevention in Cerebral Palsy

Artificial Intelligence

Artificial intelligence is a spectrum of technologies that enable machines to perform tasks traditionally requiring human-like intelligence, such as pattern recognition, language comprehension, and decision-making using logic, rules, and decision trees. AI-based predictive and classification models have been developed for use in obstetric practice based on fetal heart rate monitoring and radiology that have the potential to reduce the duration of image acquisition, enable optimization of personnel requirements, and lead to diagnostic and economic benefits with cost-saving. A recent meta-analysis showed a 50% reduction in neonatal seizures with continuous fetal cardiotocographic (CTG) monitoring; however, there are certain limitations, such as difficulty ensuring objectivity between interpretations and the need for regular observations to avoid a long gap between the detection of suspicious patterns and intervention. To overcome limitations in the interpretation of CTG by humans, AI-based models have been developed for the early detection of compromised fetuses and for predicting the risk of a pH of 7.15 or less in umbilical cord blood. Studies have also reported the efficacy of using AI in the identification of fetal structures and organs to find congenital abnormalities through fetal biometry and gross fetal ultrasound imaging. AI-based programs for predicting labor progression and prediction of prematurity are in development as well which could reduce the risk of CP. The use of AI-based models for predicting the outcomes of abnormal fetal brain magnetic resonance imaging (MRI) could reduce the probability of postnatal interventions and provide optimal advice on the continuation of pregnancy in such situations.[4]

Digital Advances Targeting Secondary Prevention in Cerebral Palsy

Artificial intelligence-based models have been developed for the prediction of CP in newborns using blood-based deoxyribonucleic acid (DNA) epigenomic data with sensitivity and specificity of 95% and 94.4%, respectively, which can be used in the future for the same.[5] Similarly, AI-based prediction models for the detection of CP based on early brain MRI findings have been developed as well, with a sensitivity of 70%, specificity of 74%, and accuracy of 73%.[6]

Digital Advances Targeting Tertiary Prevention

Assistive Technology

Assistive technology (AT) refers to any item, system, or product used to increase, maintain, or improve the functional capabilities of a child with a disability (according to IDEA, 1997). It can only improve the basic skills but does not replace the skill. It helps individuals to participate in daily life activities with greater ease and more independence. These can be of two types:

1. Low-tech gadgets such as crutches, modified pen grips, and spectacles
2. High-tech gadgets such as computers and specialized software

Adaptive Equipment

Adaptive equipment are a subcategory of AT that is modified or enhanced from its original purpose to specifically meet the needs of a person with special needs, e.g., power or electric wheelchairs customized for comfort and to support the limited upper limb function of a person with CP or neuromuscular disorder. There is an expanding list of assistive and adaptive devices for children with CP to support in their activities of daily living (ADL) and educational training **(Table 4.10.1)**.

Alternative and Augmentative Communication

Alternative and augmentative communication (AAC) is a type of AT that includes interpersonal communication techniques other than natural speech, such as manual sign language, picture exchange communications systems (PECS), communication boards, and high-tech devices like speech-generating devices. AAC systems have been used to improve communication abilities in speech-impaired children to set communication patterns between individuals with CP and their family members.

TABLE 4.10.1: Assistive devices for children with cerebral palsy (CP).

Purpose	***Devices***
Mobility	• Walkers • Nonelectric wheelchairs • Scooters • Electric wheelchairs (with a joystick) • Lifts • Functional electrical stimulation
Communication	• Electronic communication boards • Low-tech communication boards • Speech-generating devices • Eye-tracking devices • Low-technology grips or specially designed writing devices, such as a weighted pencil • Desk with adjustable height and angle • Pointer attached by Velcro to the hand or wrist, allowing an individual to press small buttons on keyboards, tablets, or phones
Assisting activities of daily life (ADL)	• Specialized toilet seats, safety bars, and bathing benches • Sponges and brushes with longer handle • Eating utensils with grips or weighted • Plates and bowls with nonslip bottoms • Nonskid rugs • Dressing aides • Tables that can be moved up and down • Adaptive scissors and art supplies • Key turners • Aids for positioning in bed or on couches and chairs
Education	• Adaptive writing and typing aids • Mobile applications • Computer software

Virtual Reality and Augmented Reality

Virtual reality is an artificial simulation or a reproduction of a real-life environment using immersive projection of virtual objects produced by computer hardware and software. It allows users to participate in virtual settings that resemble real-world objects and events in appearance, sound, and sensation. Augmented reality (AR) is a technology that projects layers of computer-generated graphics in real-world space. Mixed reality allows for the physical interaction of virtual and real elements. VR/AR systems for neurorehabilitation offer significant results to the therapy due to the feedback they provide to the patient related to performance and guidance information. They can increase cortical reorganization and cause neuroplasticity changes and are entertaining, interesting, and motivating at the same time. However, for the use of VR, there should be certain prerequisites, such as absence of hearing or vision impairment, adequate cognitive function, cooperative and motivated patients, and no significant contractures and spasticity. Studies on VR therapy (VRT) have also shown improvement in arm function, walking, and postural control as well as improvement in functional scores of gross and fine motor [bimanual motor function (BFMF), gross motor function classification system (GMFCS)] of individuals.[6,7]

Biofeedback

Biofeedback refers to extrinsic feedback where data about an individual motor performance is gathered and relayed back, e.g., using electromyography systems that give information about muscle activity during a task. This data can be combined with VR systems or with gait training to help train children more effectively. Gait training and VRT using biofeedback systems led to substantial and meaningful improvement in gait kinematics and spatiotemporal characteristics. For example, the use of avatars to visualize biomechanical inputs during rehabilitation could improve whole-body awareness. Biofeedback-related relaxation exercises could be used to target pain and spasticity.[6,7]

Robotics

Robotics is a novel technique that works on computerized control systems and assists in activities as well as helps in motor and other cognitive learning to improve the person's functional capacity. Human–robot control interfaces (both invasive and noninvasive) are technologies that acquire, decode, and commute the intentions of a human user to a device via control commands. *Robot-assisted gait training (RAGT)* has been shown to improve gait speed, walking distance, and walking, jumping, and running as compared to conventional therapy alone, and these effects were maintained for prolonged periods. However, the intensity, duration, and frequency are not yet standardized. Examples of RAGT include Honda Walking Assist (a battery-operated device for hip flexion and extension during gait cycle that fits in the lumbar and thigh area), Lokomat (training for 12 weeks with two sessions per week has shown an increase in lower limb muscle strength, speed, and step length), Innowalk, Robogait, and Waltbox-K.[6,7] Self-care robots, also called ADL robots, and social robots can help in assisting individuals with CP with physical tasks associated with ADL, hence promoting independence and increasing social interactions.[6,7]

Exoskeletons

Exoskeletons are devices that aim to interfere with the human and assist with the recovery of motor function that is compromised due to neuromuscular, sensory, or cognitive deficits. Their repetitive training assists the human nervous system in creating alternative neuronal pathways to replace the damaged ones. They also act as both active and passive support solutions to assist persons with disabilities to perform ADLs. Upper and lower limb wearable exoskeletons help in improving motor outcomes by providing high doses of guided movements, resistance, assistance, and real-time feedback. Angel Legs is a wearable torque-assisting exoskeleton robot that has been shown to improve walking abilities and gross motor skills.[6,7]

Brain–computer Interface Systems

Brain–computer interface systems interfere with the brain to acquire, decode, and translate the brain activity of the user into control commands for various devices. BCI systems are controlled by the user thinking about specific tasks, and with repetitive use, BCI learns the precise brain pattern required to perform a task (e.g., to play a game or play music). They can also be used to enhance neuroplasticity in combination with brain stimulation, VR, and assistive robotics for motor and skill relearning. BCI systems have helped children with CP regain motor function by causing activity-dependent neuroplasticity. BCI-based hand exoskeletons have been used in quadriplegic nonverbal CPs who could be trained to create artwork, operate remote cars, play computer games, and gradually select words from communication boards with their repetitive use.[6,7]

Noninvasive Brain Stimulation or Noninvasive Neuromodulation

Noninvasive brain stimulation actively and noninvasively interferes with brain function in humans. It can be used to find out the functional relevance of specific brain regions and their functional network interactions for particular cognitive tasks and to modify behavior and skills, improve certain cognitive and motor functions, and assist training. The two most widely applied NIBS methods are *TMS* and *transcranial direct current stimulation (tDCS).* TMS uses a strong, relatively focal, and rapidly changing magnetic field that induces brief electrical high-current pulses in the brain tissue under the coil and thus elicits action potentials in axons of the cortex and in subcortical white matter, which leads to the release of neurotransmitters at terminal synapses and hence modulates brain activity, which produces temporary changes in cortical excitability in a specifically targeted brain region. Neuromodulation using TMS has been used to activate corticospinal tracts and motor neurons, leading to a positive effect on gross motor, fine motor, and language as well. Studies have evaluated different protocols of TMS in spastic diplegic CP, hemiparetic CP, and dystonic CP targeting motor function, spasticity, and dystonia.

Mobile Applications

A variety of mobile applications have been developed for patients, families, and healthcare providers to guide motor, linguistic, and cognitive abilities and for empowering parents of children with disabilities.

Telemedicine is defined by the World Health Organization (WHO) as the delivery of healthcare services where distance is a critical factor, by all healthcare professionals using information and communication technologies for the exchange of valid information for diagnosis, treatment, or prevention of a disease and injury, research, and evaluation and for continuing education of healthcare providers.

Telerehabilitation is a branch of telemedicine that focuses on the delivery of rehabilitation exercises remotely with the use of information and communication technologies, either by real-time (synchronous) methods like telephone and videoconferencing or via asynchronous methods like computer software and smartphone device applications. Telerehabilitation has been used in the delivery of early intervention therapies via family coaching strategies and has been shown to have a positive impact on family social outcomes such as infant positive behavior, parent positive behavior, and maternal postpartum depression. Further, telehealth has been successfully used to deliver a highly protocolled constraint-induced movement therapy program to improve upper extremity function in infants with asymmetric CP as well as to improve fine motor and visual motor skills in children. Studies comparing telehealth-based speech and language intervention targeting speech sounds, receptive and expressive language, pragmatics, and phonological awareness in a group of children aged 3–12 years with in-person service also found equivalent responses to therapy for multiple diagnoses and diverse outcome measures.[8]

DIGITAL ADVANCES IN AUTISM SPECTRUM DISORDER

Digital Advances Targeting Primary and Secondary Prevention in Autism Spectrum Disorder

Web-based screening tools using Modified Checklist for Autism in Toddlers (M-CHAT) have been shown to be easily accessible, effective, and more feasible for screening young children with autism, even by parents.[9] Many AI-based diagnostic tools have been developed to reduce the time for lengthy evaluations and the need for trained psychologists to classify children with ASD from those who are typically developing with high sensitivity, specificity, and accuracy.[9] These include:

- Diagnostic tools based on established diagnostic scales like the Autism Diagnostic Interview (ADI-R), Autism Diagnostic Observation Schedule (ADOS), Vineland Adaptive Behavior Scales (VABS), and Mullen's Scales of Early Learning
- Mobile applications based on parent-reported symptoms
- Behavioral imaging via Behavioral Observation and Intervention System for Evaluation (BOISE), where parents upload videos of children for observation—based on naturalistic observation diagnostic assessment
- Eye tracking information can catch differences in social attention as early as 2–6 months (reduced attention to social stimuli and deficits in coordinating gaze with speech sounds are seen in children with ASD)
- Software based on multimodal behavioral analysis, which extracts the speech (pragmatic and semantic features) and facial expressions and behavior to identify atypical characteristics in language, emotional perception, and expression
- AI-based algorithms based on data from various sources such as gamified tasks, eye gaze, facial expressions, electroencephalogram (EEG), MRI, and functional MRIs individually or in combinations.

Digital Advances Targeting Tertiary Prevention in Autism Spectrum Disorder

Behavioral interventions and social skill and language training are provided through various mobile and web-based applications based on conversational agent technologies and behavioral activation therapies.

Serious games are video games with a purpose greater than pure entertainment. These gamified tasks are used to teach skills such as social skill training. AI-based gamified platforms like GOLIAH (Gaming Open Library for Intervention in Autism at Home) have shown to increase the child-therapist interaction.

Artificial intelligence-based wearable digital interventions like the Superpower glasses intervention (deployed by Google Glass and a smartphone app) can recognize emotions and their relevance and display them to the child with emoticons or colors in the peripheral vision to improve social interactions.

Video modeling, i.e., a visual teaching method where individuals watch a video of a person modeling a target behavior or skill with the aim that the individual watching it will imitate the target behavior, has been used to increase empathy and improve social behaviors and social skill accuracy.

TABLE 4.10.2: Assistive devices for children with autism spectrum disorder (ASD).

	Low-Tech	*High-Tech*
Communication	Picture boards and picture cards, including picture exchange communication system (PECS)	• Mobile apps for communication • Software—text-to-speech and speech-to-text • Speech-generating devices
Learning and executive functioning	Ordinary written planners, color-coded schedules, and visual reminders	• Watches with alarms • Visual timers • Sound-blocking headphones
Social skills training	Social stories, social skill cards, and games	• Video modeling • Social assist robots like Kiwi, QTrobot, and human-shaped robots
Sensory challenges	• Sand, slime, or putty • Rainmaker toys • Fidget spinners • Vibrating cushion or gadget	Applications like Brainworks Miracle Modus Heatpad
Safety	ID bracelets	• Tracking devices like • Alert Me Bands • AWAARE: Autism Wandering Awareness Alerts Response and Education Collaboration Project Lifesaver International

Assistive technology tools are also used in ASD for various purposes, especially for supporting basic communication with caregivers and surroundings, education, tracking times and managing schedules, learning social skills, and assistance in ADLs for tackling sensory issues **(Table 4.10.2)**.

Social skills training through VR-based gadgets like Floreo can record the learner's in-VR activity and performance and can help identify areas of improvement or of deficit. VR-based therapies have also been shown to reduce stereotypies and improve functional outcomes.

Social skill training through robotic behavioral intervention systems has been shown to have a positive impact on eye contact, facial expression, and emotion recognition.[9] A semiautonomous parrot-inspired robot called KiliRo, based on an application program interface (API) called Oxford emotion API, has been trained for analyzing facial expressions and has shown good interaction results with individuals with ASD. Humanoid robots like NAO have also been used in conjunction with LEGO therapy and cognitive behavioral therapy based on rational emotive behavior therapy (REBT). They look like science-fiction-style androids and are capable of expressing emotions by changing the color of their eyes, moving their arms, and changing the tone of their voice. Children with autism often respond more positively to NAO than to a human therapist. Also, the unlimited patience and ability to repeat the same cues in the same way repeatedly without variation have shown to help develop social skills and empathy in children with ASD. Another example is that QTrobot uses AI to record and measure the effectiveness of lessons, increasing or decreasing difficulty based on the responses of the child, and gathering information to improve its efficacy and allows for an individualized approach and is intended to increase children's willingness to interact with human therapists and decrease discomfort during therapy sessions. Kiwi, a "socially assistive robot," also intends to teach autistic children how to do math and socialize.

Telemedicine-based interventions focusing on sensory processing and speech and language therapy have also shown efficacy in children with ASD, showing improvement in their initiation and responses.[8]

Neuromodulation with TMS (theta burst TMS) has been evaluated in children with ASD, leading to a reduction of repetitive behaviors and improved quality of life.

DIGITAL ADVANCES IN SPECIFIC LEARNING DISABILITY

Digital Advances Targeting Secondary Prevention in Specific Learning Disability

Various AI-based computational models have been developed for screening and diagnosis of SLD based on various types of datasets—behavioral symptoms (working memory, phonological awareness, and facial reactions throughout the learning process), text (reading, writing, typing, handwriting, and web-based games), eye movement, infrared corneal reflection system, MRI scans, quantitative EEG (qEEG) scans, and images. There are both web-based and mobile-based applications. They have shown to be less time-consuming and achieve high accuracy in predicting SLD, reaching >90%. EEG, infrared corneal reflection system, MRI scanner, and eye tracker, although achieve higher accuracy, are expensive. Smartphone device-based applications are becoming popular due to the broader user base for an app-based data collection technique.[10]

Digital Advances Targeting Tertiary Prevention in Specific Learning Disability

There are various AT tools available for children with SLD to assist in reading, writing, mathematics, and effective communication **(Table 4.10.3)**. They range from low-tech to high-tech, with many AI-enabled applications and software now available. The tool should be chosen based on the individual's needs, taking into consideration his/her strengths and weaknesses and affordability and availability.

There are many AI-based software for remedial education, especially focusing on improving reading skills and based on concepts of phonological awareness, both mobile application-based and web-based, with some using serious games.

The Centre of Excellence and Advanced Research for Neurodevelopmental Disorders at the Child Neurology Division, Department of Pediatrics, AIIMS, New Delhi, in collaboration with IIT, Delhi, has also developed a novel AI-based model for therapeutic intervention for children with dyslexia, in the form of a web application-based phonological training program. It is a cloud-based application design that uses a bottom-up strategic learning approach, consisting

TABLE 4.10.3: Assistive technology in specific learning disability (SLD).

Purpose	*Devices*
Reading	Electronic books, single-word scanners, predictable texts, tablets, reading pens, talking electronic devices/software, text-to-speech software, digital recorders, and visual search engines
Writing	Pencil grips, templates, word processors, word cards, spelling and grammar checkers, adapted papers, voice recognition software, and literacy-specific software
Mathematics	Scientific calculators, talking clocks, and enlarged worksheets
Computer access	Word predictions, alternative keyboards, pointing options, and voice recognition software

of eight modules staggered in increasing difficulty levels, which will increase the subject's phonemic awareness and word–sound association so that he/she can better identify, categorize, blend, and segment phonemes from words. There was an improvement in phonological awareness and phonological memory in children pre- and post-intervention using this application.

Noninvasive brain stimulation using tDCS and TMS has also been evaluated in adults and children with SLD, particularly dyslexia, and is in research mode.

DIGITAL ADVANCES IN OTHER NEURODEVELOPMENTAL DISORDERS

In other neuromuscular diseases such as Duchenne muscular dystrophy (DMD), spinal muscular atrophy (SMA), limb-girdle muscular dystrophy (LGMD), and peripheral neuropathies, gait analysis systems (3D quantitative gait analysis) have been developed for a personalized approach. Customized electric/power wheelchairs and robot-based orthoses are being used, tailored to an individual's needs, strengths, and weaknesses. Also, robotic rehabilitation, BCI/exoskeletons, and VRT are being tried in these scenarios as well. AI-based models have also been developed to predict attention-deficit hyperactivity disorder (ADHD) based on gameplay data and data from MRI and EEG characteristics.

LIMITATIONS OF VARIOUS DIGITAL ADVANCES

There is currently a lack of evidence-based guidelines for the use of digital advances, and due to limited studies, there may be poor generalizability. Further, cost and availability in resource-limited settings at present are a concern that may lead to disparity in care. Their use may itself be a challenge for parents with less understanding. There is also a lack of large, high-resolution datasets from children, hindering the development of AI-based models for predictions. Further, ethical and medicolegal issues can also not be ignored.

CONCLUSION

The use of technology in NDD diagnosis and treatment is rapidly expanding. With early diagnosis through digital interventions, early intervention could be started for these children with disability, leading to better outcomes. However, with multitudes of options being available, it might be confusing for the families to choose, and hence the unbiased guidance of healthcare professionals would become necessary.

REFERENCES

1. American Psychiatric Association. Diagnostic and Statistical Manual of Mental Disorders. Arlington, VA: American Psychiatric Association Publishing; 2013.
2. Arora NK, Nair MK, Gulati S, Deshmukh V, Mohapatra A, Mishra D, et al. Neurodevelopmental disorders in children aged 2–9 years: population-based burden estimates across five regions in India. PLoS Med. 2018;15(7):e1002615.
3. Burks C, Van Heertum K, Weinerman R. The technological advances in embryo selection and genetic testing: a look back at the evolution of aneuploidy screening and the prospects of non-invasive PGT. Reprod Med. 2021;2(1):26-34.
4. Kim HY, Cho GJ, Kwon HS. Applications of artificial intelligence in obstetrics. Ultrasonography. 2023;42(1):2.
5. Bahado-Singh RO, Vishweswaraiah S, Aydas B, Mishra NK, Guda C, Radhakrishna U. Deep learning/artificial intelligence and blood-based DNA epigenomic prediction of cerebral palsy. Int J Mol Sci. 2019;20(9):2075.
6. Paul S, Nahar A, Bhagawati M, Kunwar AJ. A review on recent advances of cerebral palsy. Oxid Med Cell Longev. 2022;2022:2622310.
7. Cortés-Pérez I, González-González N, Peinado-Rubia AB, Nieto-Escamez FA, Obrero-Gaitán E, García-López H. Efficacy of robot-assisted gait therapy compared to conventional therapy or treadmill training in children with cerebral palsy: a systematic review with meta-analysis. Sensors (Basel). 2022;22(24):9910.
8. Hsu N, Monasterio E, Rolin O. Telehealth in pediatric rehabilitation. Phys Med Rehabil Clin. 2021;32(2):307-17.
9. Valentine AZ, Brown BJ, Groom MJ, Young E, Hollis C, Hall CL. A systematic review evaluating the implementation of technologies to assess, monitor and treat neurodevelopmental disorders: a map of the current evidence. Clin Psychol Rev. 2020;80:101870.
10. Kaisar S. Developmental dyslexia detection using machine learning techniques: a survey. ICT Express. 2020;6(3):181-4.

SECTION

5

Nutrition and Nutritional Disorders

Section Editor: Praveen Kumar

5.1 Infant and Young Child Feeding

RK Anand

We know that shamefully large numbers of children in both wealthy and poverty-stricken regions suffer malnutrition: the malnutrition of excess amounts of inappropriate foods and the malnutrition of insufficient nutritious foods. As adults, we should feel embarrassed that so many small children are so poorly fed. We can change this situation, if we want to and many people are already working to this end. Good nutrition for children harmonizes with good nutrition for adults... and it would be good for the world if we worked to this end.

—Gabrielle Palmer

INTRODUCTION

While adequate nutrition is important throughout childhood, it is crucial during the first 5 years of a child's life, particularly in the first 2 years when rapid growth occurs and when the child is entirely dependent on the mother and the family for food.

OPTIMAL INFANT AND YOUNG CHILD FEEDING

Optimal infant and young child feeding (IYCF) is an evidence-based measure for improving child nutrition and child survival. The "World Health Organization (WHO)/ United Nations Children's Fund (UNICEF) Global Strategy for Infant and Young Child Feeding and the National Guidelines on Infant and Young Child Feeding 2010" recommended by the IYCF Subspecialty Chapter of the Indian Academy of Pediatrics (IAP) stress that for proper growth and development, infants should be exclusively breastfed with no other food or drink—not even water—in the first 6 months of life (*See* Chapter 5.2). This must be followed by the sequential addition of nutritionally adequate, preferably home-made semisolid and solid foods to complement (not replace) breastmilk, till the child is gradually able to eat normal family food after 1 year while breastfeeding is continued up to 24 months of age or beyond **(Fig. 5.1.1)**.[1] Adequate nutrition for adolescent girls and pregnant and lactating mothers is also important for child nutrition.

The period after 6 months, when other foods are added, is also referred to as weaning, which is not preferred these days as some people wrongly interpret it as weaning the baby away from the breast. Complementary feeding is a better term than weaning.

COMPLEMENTARY FEEDING

Complementary feeding is the process of giving a child other food while continuing breastfeeding when her or his nutritional demands can no longer be fulfilled by breastfeeding alone. Appropriate complementary feeding should be timely, culturally acceptable, nutritionally adequate, safe, and responsive.[2]

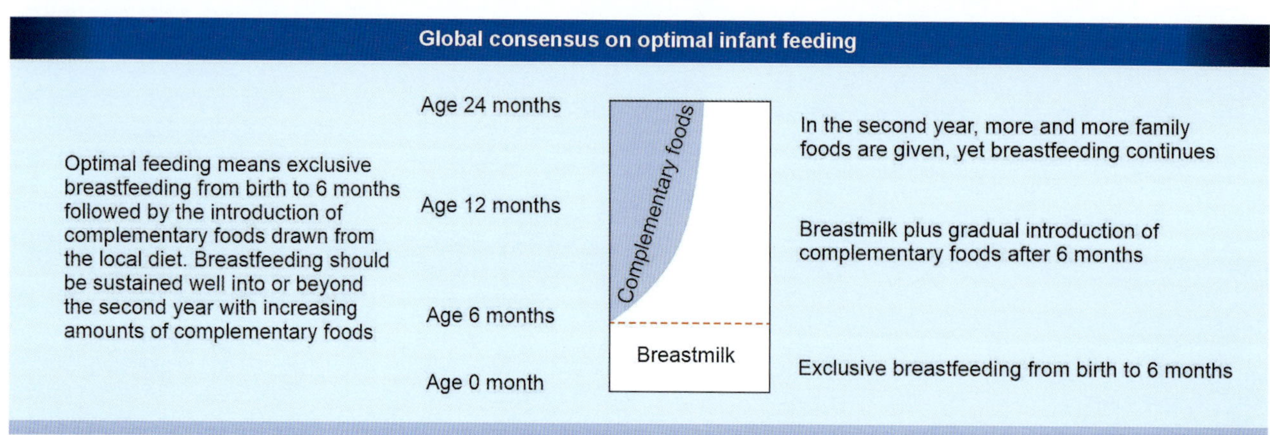

Fig. 5.1.1: Optimal infant and young child feeding.

Timely Feeding

It is recommended that infants must be exclusively breastfed for 6 months, and adequate complementary foods should be added after that **(Fig. 5.1.2)**.[3] Complementary feeding indicators in India are far from satisfactory. According to the National Family Health Survey 5 (NFHS 5), the introduction of complementary feeding along with continued breastfeeding in children of 6–8 months is only 45.9%.[4]

Addition of anything other than breastmilk before 6 months is fraught with danger for the following reasons:

- Addition of foods and other liquids (including water, soup, juice, rice water, *dal* water, etc.) interferes with optimal breastfeeding. They may fill up the child's stomach and quench the thirst and, consequently, may lead to less suckling at the breast with reduced milk production.
- Increased risk of allergic disorders due to allergens passing through the not-yet-fully mature gut of the infant. It takes about 6 months after birth for the intestine to become reasonably mature.
- The tongue-thrust reflex is active before 6 months. Infants tend to push out with the tongue anything other than liquids.
- Breastfeeding has a significant impact on cognitive growth.
- Foods other than breastmilk may result in more gastrointestinal (GI) and other infections and malnutrition. They may put an unnecessary load on the kidney and lead to obesity, hypertension, and coronary artery disease later in life.
- Breastfed children have less risk of sudden infant death syndrome (SIDS), type 1 and 2 diabetes, high cholesterol, and inflammatory bowel disease (IBD). It has also been seen that there is an increased risk of the development of Crohn's disease and ulcerative colitis in children who have not been breastfed.
- Less frequent suckling also increases the possibility of the mother becoming pregnant again.
- Breastfeeding also protects mothers against stress, postpartum depression, and breast and ovarian cancer.

Nutritionally Adequate Complementary Feeding

To be nutritionally adequate, complementary foods should contain all food groups—the staple, proteins, vitamins, and minerals **(Fig. 5.1.3; Tables 5.1.1 and 5.1.2)**.[5]

After 6 months, add homemade porridge or a fruit, such as a ripe banana. Porridge can be made with the staple cereal used by the family, such as whole-wheat flour (*atta*), rice, semolina (*suji* or *rawa*), broken wheat, *ragi* (*nachni*), or millet. Breastmilk or any other milk can be used to make the porridge. Pieces of *chapatti* could also be soaked in milk, mashed properly, and passed through a sieve to provide a soft semisolid food for the infant. Sugar and cream (*malai*) can be added to make it energy-dense.

Boiled or well-cooked mashed vegetables (pumpkin, peas, cauliflower, carrots, leafy vegetables, sweet and other potatoes, beets, and tomatoes) should be added to provide vitamins and iron. Also, offer other seasonal fruits. Gradually, introduce *khichdi* with ghee, butter, or oil, *seera* or *halwa, upma, poha, dhokla, idli, dosa, pongal,* and *missi roti* (*paratha* made with a batter of wheat flour, gram flour, spices, and *dal*). If foods of animal origin are acceptable to the family, the same may be given to the child.

Start with only one food at a time. Wait for a week before introducing another food so that we know whether the child

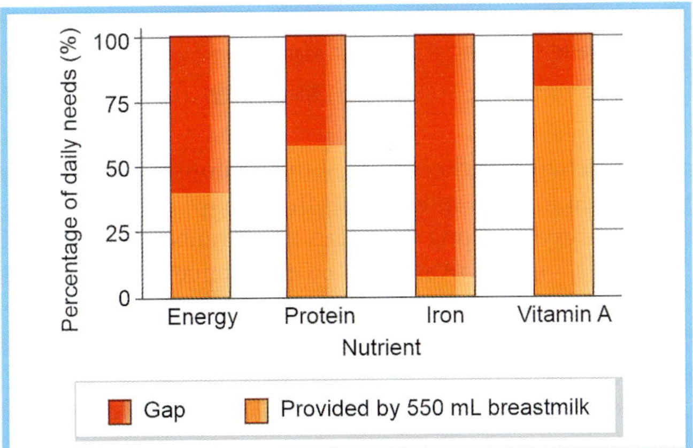

Fig. 5.1.2: Gaps to be filled by complementary foods in a breastfed child 12–23 months.[3]

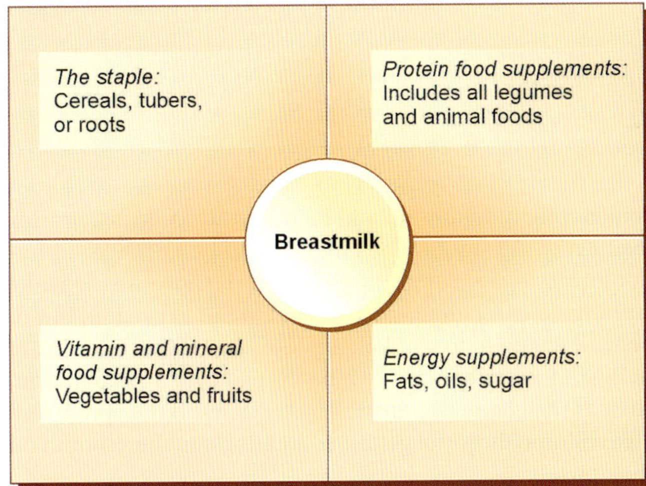

Fig. 5.1.3: Food square for the young child.
Source: Elizabeth KE. Current concepts on nutritional requirements of infants and children. Indian J Pract Pediatr. 2011;13(1):5-11.

TABLE 5.1.1: Examples of iron-rich food items (iron in mg/100 g of edible portion).

Vegetables		**Cereals**	
Cauliflower leaves	40	Ragi	3.9
Chaulai	22.9	Maize flour	2.3
Muli leaves	18	Barley	1.67
Suvani bhaji	17.4	Rawa	1.6
Pudina	15.6	**Dry fruits**	
Arvi pangreen	10	Black sesame seeds	56.7
Carrot leaves	8.8	Sesame seeds	9.3
Green onion	7.43	Coconut (dry)	7.8
Kothmir	1.42	Cashew nuts (*kaju*)	5.81
Spinach	1.14	Almonds	5.09
Arvi panblack	0.98	Walnut	2.64
Sargavapan	0.85	*Singdana*	2.5
Milk and its products		**Pulses**	
Mawa-khoa	5.8	Soybean	10.4
Cheese	2.1	Moth bean (Turkish gram)	9.5
Sugars		Black-eyed beans (*chauli*)	8.6
Jaggery	2.64	Red lentils (*masoor*)	7.86
Sago	1.3	Dried green peas	7.05
Meat		Bengal gram (*channadal*)	5.3
Liver (sheep)	6.3	Red kidney beans (*rajma*)	5.1
Egg (hen)	2.1	Green gram dal (*mung*)	4.4
Cereals		Mung bean	3.9
Rice flakes (*poha*)	20	Black gram (*urad* dal)	3.8
Pearl millet (*bajra*)	8	Pigeon peas (*tuvar* dal)	2.7
Rice puffed (*mamra*)	6.6		
Wheat flour	4.9	Poppy seeds	15.9
Sorghum bicolor (*jowar*)	4.1		
Vermicelli-sev (wheat sev)	2		

TABLE 5.1.2: Examples of foods rich in calcium and zinc.

Calcium (mg/100 g of edible portion)		***Zinc (mg/100 g of edible portion)***	
Milk products and dry fruits		Gingelly seeds	12.2
Sesame seeds	1,450	Bengal gram (*desi*)	6.1
Cheese	790	Cashew nut	5.99
Khoya	650	Safflower seeds	5.2
Coconut (dry)	400	Mustard seeds	4.8
Black sesame seeds	300	Cowpea	4.6
Almond	230	Omum seeds	4.52
Milk (buffalo)	210	Red kidney bean (*rajma*)	4.5
Curd	149	Soybean black	4.4
Pistachios	140	Poppy seeds	4.34
Milk (cow)	120	Groundnut	3.9
Watermelon seeds	100	*Samai* almond	3.7
Walnut	100	Betel leaves	3.44
Cereal and pulses		Soybean white	3.4
Finger millet (ragi)	344	Black gram (whole)	3.3
Red kidney beans (*rajma*)	260	Coriander seeds	3.26
Soybean	240	Sorghum bicolor (*bajra*)	3.1
Turkish gram (*moth*)	202	Lentil dal	3.1
Chickpeas	202	Red gram (whole)	3.1
Black gram (*urad* dal)	154	Fenugreek seeds	3.08
Vlung	124	Black gram (dal)	3
Pigeon peas (*tuvar* dal)	73	Green gram (whole)	3
Bengal gram (*channa* dal)	56	*Sanwa* millet	3
Cashew nuts	50	Garbanzo beans (*kabuli*)	2.9
Poppy seeds	1,584	Cardamom	2.81
Almond	230	Maize (dry)	2.8

is tolerating it. Infants should be offered food, fruits, or milk feed every 2–3 hours. The child should be encouraged but not forced to eat. Some children tend to choke a little while learning to eat. Parents may be told not to get scared but to be with the child to ward off any trouble. When children are helped to use a spoon, let it be dipped into a preparation, such as *shrikhand* or *phirni.* A bit will stick to the spoon and give children the joy of getting something into their mouth on their own.

A child eating well around 7 months or so may suddenly become disinterested in eating. The parents should be told not to panic but to try some new preparations. In any case, children should never be forced to eat more than what they want. Even if half a spoon is left in the bowl and the child is not interested in eating any more, the parents should respect the child's appetite. Water can be given once the child starts taking foods other than breastmilk and fruits. It should be offered from an ordinary glass. Children learn to sip from the glass within a few days.

A few general guidelines about the nutritive value of foods are as follows:

- To retain the nutrients, vegetables, including potatoes, should be scraped instead of peeled. The water in which rice or vegetables have been boiled for cooking should be used and not thrown away. The vegetables should not be overcooked. Children should be encouraged to get used to the taste of properly washed raw vegetables from an early age. In general, some amounts of spices are good for health. Most children can tolerate a moderate amount of spices used for cooking in most homes.

- Dry fruits are good, but they must also be rationed, partly because they are expensive and more so because some of these, such as dates, figs, and raisins, can remain stuck between the teeth, leading to caries. Foods that may lead to choking in children should be avoided in those below 3 years. Examples of these foods are raw carrots, roasted grams, peanuts, other nuts, popcorn, hard candies, berries, and whole grapes.
- Foods, such as *idli* and *parathas*, made from whole-wheat flour should be preferred to white bread.

Avoidable Foods

In families with a strong history of allergy, peanuts and other nuts should be avoided. If any member of the family is known to react adversely to a particular food, avoid that as well. Also, fried foods, foods containing too much sugar, artificial sweeteners, monosodium glutamate (MSG, *ajinomoto*), and a high intake of salt should be avoided.

As recommended by the National Institute of Nutrition, the following points need to be kept in mind:

- The recipes for complementary foods should be based on locally available foodstuffs.
- The cooking methods must be simple.
- The cost should be minimal.
- The recipes should be acceptable in taste and consistency.
- Gradually, the child should be introduced to healthy foods eaten by the rest of the family.

Consistency of Complementary Foods (Fig. 5.1.4)[3]

- To provide more calories from smaller volumes, food must be thick in consistency—thick enough to stay on the spoon without running off when the spoon is tilted.
- Foods, such as nuts, which can pose a choking hazard, should be avoided. Introduce lumpy or granular foods and new tastes by about 9–10 months. Missing this age may lead to fussy eating later. Avoid using mixers to make the food too smooth.
- Three to four teaspoons of roasted groundnut powder can be added to the daily diet of the infant. The meal can also be made energy-dense by adding ghee, butter, oil, and sugar or jaggery.

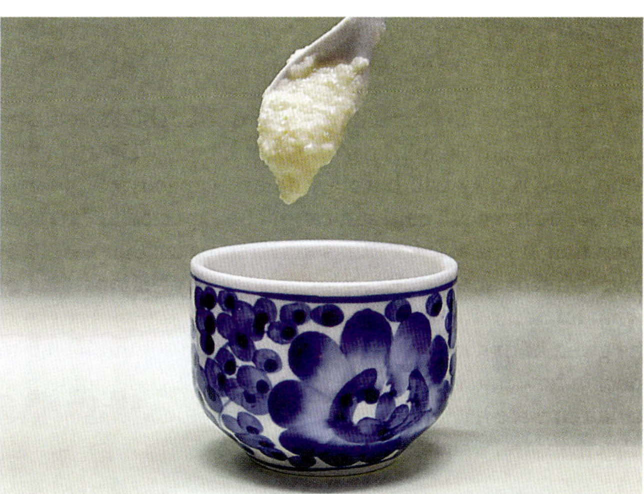

Fig. 5.1.4: Consistency of complementary food.

TABLE 5.1.3: Ready-to-use infant weaning foods.

Food	*Amount*
Pearl millet (*bajra*), (dehusked, roasted)	3 tablespoons
Roasted green gram dal (or any other dal)	1.5 tablespoon
Roasted groundnut	3/4th tablespoon
Roasted decorticated sesame (gingelly) seeds	1 tablespoon
Sugar	2 tablespoons

Ready-to-use Infant Weaning Foods

Table 5.1.3 gives the different ingredients from which weaning foods can be prepared in bulk and kept ready at hand for feeding infants. For that, powder the ingredients individually, mix them in the proportion suggested, and store them in airtight containers.

Finger Millet (Ragi, Nachni) Infant Food

Use 45 g of finger millet (*ragi*) prepared as given here instead of bajra in the earlier formula. Soak finger millet (*ragi*) in water overnight. Drain the water, spread the grains on a plate, and allow them to germinate by covering them with a damp cloth for 1 day. Dry the germinated finger millet (*ragi*) under the sun and roast till it develops a malted flavor. Powder and store in an airtight tin.

Methods of Feeding

When required, take suitable amounts (say three tablespoons) of any one of the above ready-to-use infant foods and mix with a small amount of hot water. Add more sugar or jaggery, if required, before feeding.

Amount and Frequency of Food to be Offered (Table 5.1.4)[3]

This depends on the capacity or the size of the child's stomach, which is usually 30 mL/kg of the child's body weight. A child who weighs 8 kg will have a stomach capacity of 240 mL, about one large full cup, and cannot be expected to eat more than that at one meal. Parents may not realize that a child of 1 year needs about 1,000 calories each day—almost half of what an adult may take. So, some guidance to parents may be given in this respect. After that, children should be left to decide how much they want to consume. A good guide that children were having optimum quantity of food is their level of activity and weight gain.

Safe Complementary Feeding

All utensils used for feeding must be washed thoroughly. There is no need to sterilize the utensils. Eating by hand need not be discouraged. Finger foods, which the child can hold and chew, may be given. However, the hands of the caregiver and the child must be washed thoroughly with soap and water before and after eating. Microbial contamination of complementary foods is more common in hot weather. It is slower if the food is refrigerated. When that is not possible, the food should be eaten within 2 hours of its preparation. Even if the food is kept in the refrigerator, it should be consumed within a day or two.

RESPONSIVE FEEDING (FIG. 5.1.5)[6]

While feeding young children, the caregivers should provide psychosocial stimulation to the child through age-appropriate play and praise. Children sitting on the lap of a caregiver or eating with loved ones learn to enjoy eating. Self-feeding must be encouraged even if the child makes a mess **(Figs. 5.1.6A and B)**. Forced feeding, threatening, and punishment interfere with the development of proper feeding habits. Distractions during meals and feeding in front of the television or smartphone, etc., should be avoided.

FEEDING DURING AND AFTER ILLNESS[7]

The appetite during an illness may go down. However, even sick babies continue to breastfeed quite often. They should

TABLE 5.1.4: Amount of food to be offered.

Age	*Texture*	*Frequency*	*Average amount of each meal*
6–8 months	Start with thick porridge and well-mashed foods	2–3 meals per day plus frequent breastfeeding	Start with 2–3 tablespoons full
9–11 months	Finely chopped or mashed foods and foods that the baby can pick up	3–4 meals along with breastfeeding. Depending on appetite, offer 1–2 snacks	1/2 of a 250 mL cup or bowl
12–23 months	Family food chopped or mashed, if necessary. As per appetite, offer 1–2 snacks	3–4 meals plus breastfeeding. Depending on appetite, offer 1–2 snacks	3/4 to 1 of a 250 mL cup or bowl

Note: If the baby is not breastfed, give in addition 1–2 cups of milk per day and 1–2 extra meals per day.

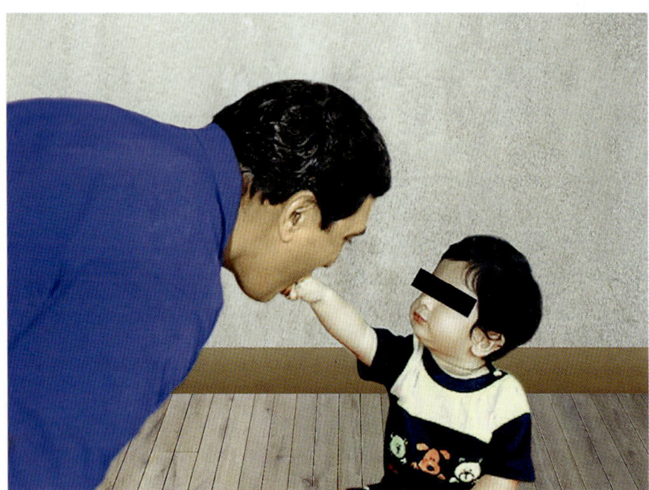

Fig. 5.1.5: Responsive feeding.

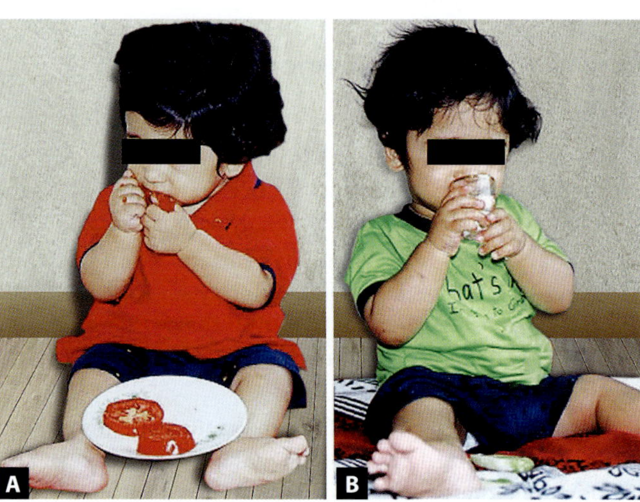

Figs. 5.1.6A and B: Self-feeding.

be encouraged to take enough liquids and small quantities of nutrient-rich food that they like to eat. After the illness, the nutrient intake can be increased by adding one or two extra meals in the daily diet for about a month by offering nutritious snacks between meals, by giving an extra amount at each meal, and by continuing breastfeeding.

JUNK AND COMMERCIAL NUTRITION SUPPLEMENTS

Commercial ready-made cereals, though convenient to use, are not preferred over homemade foods. In addition to the high cost, the smooth consistency of such products may make the children get so used to them that they may not accept homemade foods. Families must be equipped with means and knowledge to feed their children without the need for processed foods. All efforts must be made to ensure that government policies protect public health before private profits.

Unhealthy foods and beverages like foods high in sugar, salt, and trans fats and sugar-sweetened beverages should not be consumed.[6] Tinned food, juices, cold drinks, packaged drinks and packaged wafers, health drinks, nutrition supplements promoted for "picky eaters," bakery products, and drinks with low nutrient value, such as tea and coffee, should be avoided.

PICKY EATERS

Of late, a nutritional supplement is being aggressively promoted for so-called picky eaters for better growth and height. Before the parents start using such a product, they should be given the following information:[5,8]

- An infant grows rapidly in the early months of life. In the second year, the growth will be slower; the appetite may decrease and vary from day to day. Between 15 months and 3 years, the child often passes through a phase of negativism and does the opposite of what the parents want. If the child is unwell, the appetite may suffer even more, though the mother's milk is often not refused.
- Keeping the earlier point in mind, the child should not be forced to eat. Of course, various healthy food options must be offered at frequent intervals. Allow children to eat with their hands even if it turns out to be a messy affair. Then let them learn to use the spoon. The parents may fill the spoon off and on or may offer the child some food with a separate spoon, while gradually encouraging the child to eat independently.
- Parents need not get upset if the child does not eat "nourishing" foods for a few days. Children have their moods; for some days, they may eat less of certain foods, but if left to themselves, they may start eating the same again after a gap of a few days.
- Children who are small at birth may not weigh as much as their peers. The parents should be told that so long as the child follows the growth curve, they should be happy. In fact, if these children are given food or products too high in calories and become obese, they become potential candidates for developing diabetes and cardiovascular diseases.
- Make sure that the child is not anemic and does not have urinary or any other infection responsible for anorexia.
- Convey to the parents that the product promoted for "picky eaters" is expensive, not wholesome, and comes in the way of the child developing healthy food habits. Moreover, one may get a false sense of security while the underlying causes for fussy eating mentioned earlier are missed.

KEY MESSAGES FOR OPTIMUM INFANT AND YOUNG CHILD FEEDING

- Initiate breastfeeding as early as possible after birth, preferably within 1 hour.
- Except for any essential medicine or supplements, practice exclusive breastfeeding from birth to 6 months of age, and introduce complementary foods at 6 months (180 days).
- Continue frequent on-demand breastfeeding until 2 years of age or beyond.
- Start complementary foods at 6 months of age with a small amount. Increase the quantity and frequency as the child gets older while maintaining frequent breastfeeding.
- Gradually, increase food consistency and ensure that all nutrient needs of the child are met.
- Practice responsive feeding by applying the principles of psychosocial care.
- Practice good hygiene by handwashing with soap and water before preparing food and feeding the child and after using the toilet.
- Increase fluid intake during illness, including more frequent breastfeeding, and encourage the child to eat soft favorite foods. After illness, encourage the child to eat more often.
- Ensure adequate nutrition, including control of anemia in infants, young children, adolescent girls, and pregnant and lactating mothers. Vitamin and mineral supplements must be given, if required.
- Support the implementation and monitoring of the Infant Milk Substitutes Act.

REFERENCES

1. World Health Organization/United Nation Children's Fund. Global Strategy for Infant and Young Child Feeding. Geneva: WHO Press; 2003. [online] Available from https://www.who.int/publications/i/item/9241562218. [Last accessed October, 2024].

2. Bellad R. Complementary feeding. In: Bharadva K, Tiwari S, Chaturvedi P, Bang A, Agarwal RK (Eds). Feeding Fundamentals: Handbook on Infant and Young Child Nutrition. Jaipur: PEDICON; 2011. pp. 141-8.
3. World Health Organization. Infant and Young Child Feeding: Model Chapter for Textbooks for Medical Students and Allied Health Professionals. Geneva: WHO Press; 2009. [online] Available from https://iris.who.int/bitstream/handle/10665/44117/9789241597494_eng.pdf?sequence=1. [Last accessed October, 2024].
4. National Family Health Survey—5, 2019-21; India report. [online] Available from https://dhsprogram.com/pubs/pdf/FR375/FR375.pdf. [Last accessed October, 2024].
5. Kushwaha KP. Complementary feeding of breastfed children. In: Anand RK, Kumta NB, Kushwaha KP, Gupta A (Eds). The Science of Infant Feeding. New Delhi: Jaypee Brothers Medical Publishers (P) Ltd; 2002. pp. 117-34.
6. World Health Organization. (2023). Guideline for complementary feeding of infants and young children 6–23 months of age. [online] Available from https://www.who.int/publications/i/item/9789240081864. [Last accessed October, 2024].
7. Lutter CK, Grummer-Strawn L, Rogers L. Complementary feeding of infants and young children 6 to 23 months of age. Nutr Rev. 2021;79(8):825-46.
8. Emmett PM, Hays NP, Taylor CM. Antecedents of picky eating behaviour in young children. Appetite. 2018;130:163-73.

5.2 Breastfeeding

JP Dadhich

The provision has been made for infants to be fed upon their mother's milk. They find their food and their mother at the same time. It is complete nourishment for them, body and soul. It is their first introduction to the great truth that man's true relationship with the world is that of personal love and not that of the mechanical law of causation.

—Rabindranath Tagore

INTRODUCTION

Optimal *infant and young child feeding (IYCF)* practices are critical for a child's nutrition, growth, development, and survival. Breastfeeding is a vital component of IYCF. The "global strategy for IYCF" states that "breastfeeding is an unequalled way of providing ideal food for the healthy growth and development of infants; it is also an integral part of the reproductive process with important implications for the health of mothers. As a global public health recommendation, infants should be *exclusively breastfed for the first 6 months of life* to achieve optimal growth, development, and health. Thereafter, to meet their evolving nutritional requirements, infants should receive nutritionally adequate and safe *complementary foods* while breastfeeding continues for up to 2 years of age or beyond."[1] Presently, when global efforts are on to achieve better nutritional status and survival for children enshrined in the sustainable development goals (SDGs), breastfeeding emerges as a very effective intervention to achieve these targets.

DEFINITIONS RELATED TO BREASTFEEDING

Various definitions used in the context of breastfeeding are summarized in **Box 5.2.1**.

RECOMMENDATIONS FOR BREASTFEEDING

Child health and nutrition programs across the world (including India) conform to these guidelines based on global recommendations. These recommendations are based on the available scientific evidence, some of which are defined in the following text.[2-4]

Initiation of Breastfeeding Immediately after Birth, Preferably within 1 hour

Early initiation has been documented to improve neonatal survival and be protective against infection-specific mortality among newborn infants. Early initiation of breastfeeding helps to develop a bond between a mother and her baby. Early initiation is extremely important to establish successful and sustained lactation. It stimulates uterine contractions and the expulsion of the placenta. The practice of delaying breastfeeding after birth and giving something else, i.e., prelacteal feeds, exposes the infant to infections and leads to problems in establishing a successful lactation. Scientific evidence suggests that the earlier the initiation

BOX 5.2.1: Definitions related to infant feeding.

- *Exclusive breastfeeding:* Giving a baby only breastmilk/breastfeeding and no other food or drink, including water (syrup/drops of vitamins, minerals, and medicines are permitted)
- *Predominant breastfeeding:* Giving small amounts of water in addition to breastfeeding
- *Partial breastfeeding:* Giving a baby some breastfeeds and some artificial feeds, either milk, cereal, or other food
- *Bottle feeding:* Feeding a baby from a bottle, whatever is in the bottle, including expressed breastmilk
- *Cup feeding:* Feeding a baby from a cup (*katori*, *paladai*, etc.) whatever is in the cup, including breastmilk
- *Artificial feeding:* Feeding a baby on any kind of artificial milk, such as animal milk, and tinned milk, and not breastfeeding at all
- *Complementary feeding:* The process of providing foods in addition to milk when breastmilk or milk formula alone are no longer adequate to meet nutritional requirements
- *Replacement feeding:* Process of feeding a child who is receiving no breastmilk with a diet that provides all nutrients the infants need until the age at which they can be fully fed on family foods

Source: Adapted from Infant and Young Child Feeding Counseling: A Training Course, the "4 in 1 Course" (Integrated Course on Breastfeeding, Complementary Feeding and Infant Feeding and HIV); Breastfeeding Promotion Network of India (BPNI); New Delhi: 2015; and WHO Guideline for Complementary Feeding of Infants and Young Children 6–23 Months of Age. Geneva: World Health Organization; 2023.

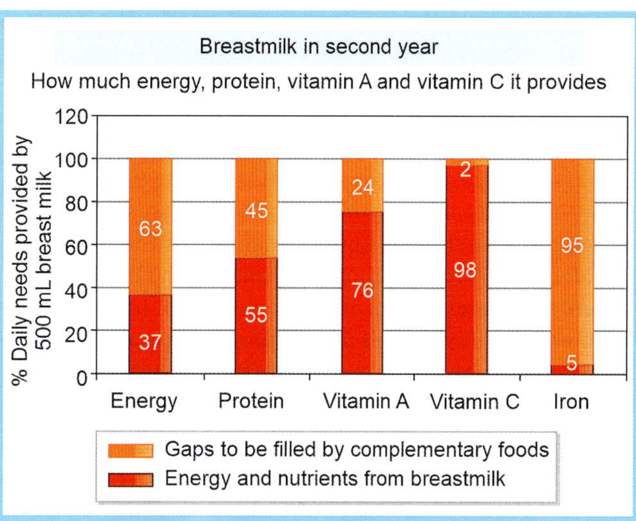

Fig. 5.2.1: Nutrition provided by breastmilk in the second year of life.
Source: Reproduced with permission from Infant and Young Child Feeding Counseling—A Training Course, the "4 in 1 Course" (Integrated Course on Breastfeeding, Complementary Feeding and Infant Feeding and HIV). New Delhi: Breastfeeding Promotion Network of India (BPNI); 2015.

of breastfeeding, the higher the chances of survival of the neonate.

After a cesarean section, some delay in the initiation of breastfeeding may be unavoidable due to the condition of the mother or infant. After a cesarean section with spinal anesthesia, breastfeeding can often be initiated immediately. With general anesthesia, breastfeeding can be initiated within a few hours as soon as the mother regains consciousness.

Exclusive Breastfeeding for the First 6 Months

Exclusive breastfeeding is recommended for the first 6 months of life, as breastmilk contains all the necessary nutrients, which are sufficient to sustain the appropriate growth and development of a healthy term infant. There is sufficient evidence that a significant number of under-6-month deaths in resource-poor countries could be prevented through the achievement of 90% coverage with exclusive breastfeeding for 6 months. Any supplementation during the first 6 months will expose infants to infections and decrease breastmilk output.

Appropriate and Adequate Complementary Feeding after 6 Months of Age while Continuing Breastfeeding

Additional foods are needed at this stage to complement the breastmilk and sustain the growth and development of the infant. Along with breastfeeding, children aged 6–24 months should be fed from three/four or more different food groups, two to three times a day (see more details in Chapter 5.1).[5]

Continued Breastfeeding up to the Age of 2 Years or Beyond

Breastfeeding along with other foods remains an important and safe source of high-quality protein, energy, and other nutrients, such as vitamins A and C, between 6 and 24 months of life. It is, therefore, crucial in preventing undernutrition and morbidities. It can provide about one-third of energy needs, half of protein, and 75% of the vitamin A requirements of a child of this age **(Fig. 5.2.1)**. Thus, breastmilk helps a child to get enough energy and high-quality nutrients from breastfeeding during the second year of life. These nutrients may not be easily available from the family diet. Continuing to breastfeed during the second year can help to prevent malnutrition and vitamin deficiencies.

STATUS OF BREASTFEEDING PRACTICES IN INDIA

The status of breastfeeding and complementary feeding practices is very dismal in India. According to the National Family Health Survey-5 (NFHS-5), only 41.4% of children are breastfed within the first hour of birth and about 86.8% initiate breastfeeding within the first day of life.[6] Approximately

15.5% of newborn infants receive prelacteal feeds, such as milk other than breastmilk, honey, sugar or glucose water, and plain water. The exclusive breastfeeding rate up to the age of 6 months is only 63.7%. Exclusive breastfeeding rapidly declines from the first month to the sixth month.

Possible reasons for suboptimal breastfeeding are primarily due to the lack of proper information to mothers, inadequate healthcare support, inability of the healthcare providers (HCP) to help mothers experiencing breastfeeding difficulty, aggressive promotion of baby foods by the commercial industry, and lack of proper support structures at the community and at the workplace, which include maternity entitlements and crèches. Cultural beliefs also appear to be important; for example, breastfeeding initiation is delayed because of the belief that mother's milk does not "come" at the time of childbirth but flows 2–3 days later.

NUTRITIONAL COMPOSITION OF BREASTMILK

The breastmilk contains all the macronutrients (carbohydrates, proteins, and fats), micronutrients, such as vitamins and minerals, and adequate water to meet the requirements of a healthy term infant for the first 6 months of life.[7] Apart from these, breastmilk provides a variety of bioactive factors, which protect the infant against infection and modulate the composition of the indigenous intestinal microbiota. Breastmilk also contains some factors to help in digestion and absorption of nutrients.

Fats

The mature human breastmilk contains 3.2–3.8 g/dL of fats. Fats provide 50% of the total energy content of the breastmilk. Breastmilk fat in the immediate postpartum period contains fat needed for gray matter development and in later months, fat, which is needed for myelination. Breastmilk fat has a steady higher level of cholesterol than animal milk and formula. Breastfed babies have significantly higher total cholesterol and low-density lipoprotein (LDL) cholesterol compared to mixed-fed babies in the first 6 months of life, with an improving high-density lipoprotein (HDL) cholesterol/LDL cholesterol ratio at 6 months. High-cholesterol intake in infancy may have a beneficial long-term programming effect on the synthesis of cholesterol by downregulation of hepatic enzymes.

Human milk contains essential fatty acids and *n*-3 fatty acids (docosahexaenoic acid and eicosapentaenoic acid), which are needed for a baby's growing brain and eyes and for healthy blood vessels. Human milk contains the enzyme lipase, which helps to digest fat. Thus, the fat in breastmilk is more completely digested and more efficiently used by a baby's body than the fat in cow's milk or formula. The lipase in breastmilk is called bile salt-stimulated lipase because it starts working in the intestine in the presence of bile salts. The lipase is not active in the breast or in the stomach before the milk mixes with bile.

Carbohydrates

Lactose is the main carbohydrate in human breastmilk and provides about 50% of its energy content. Breastmilk also contains oligosaccharides, such as glucose, galactose, *N*-acetylglucosamine, and sialic acid. These oligosaccharides attach to the epithelial cell surface in the intestines and prevent adhesion of microorganisms, thereby preventing their growth.

Proteins

Proteins in breastmilk provide amino acids for growth and anti-infective factors. Mature breastmilk contains 0.9 g/dL of protein, while colostrum contains 2.3 g/dL. The breastmilk protein contains more whey protein and less casein. Due to the high whey-to-casein ratio, the breastmilk forms softer curds, which are easier to digest.

In human milk, much of the whey protein consists of anti-infective proteins, which help to protect a baby against infection. The anti-infective proteins in human milk include lactoferrin (which binds iron and prevents the growth of bacteria that need iron) and lysozyme (which kills bacteria), as well as antibodies [immunoglobulin (Ig), mostly IgA]. Animal milk and formula may lack the amino acid cystine, and formula may lack taurine, which newborns need especially for brain growth. A human infant is ill-equipped to handle phenylalanine and tyrosine, two amino acids that are in high concentration in animal milk in comparison to breastmilk.

DYNAMIC COMPOSITION OF BREASTMILK

The composition of breastmilk is not always the same. It varies according to the age of the baby and from the beginning to the end of a feed. It also varies between feeds and may be different at different times of the day.

Colostrum

The milk produced during the first few days after the delivery is known as colostrum, which is a special, thick, sticky, bright lemony yellowish fluid. It is secreted in small quantities for the first 3–4 days of life. Although it is in small quantities, it is sufficient to meet the needs of the newborn baby. Colostrum contains more protein than later milk. Colostrum is considered the first immunization for newborns, as it is rich in anti-infective factors that help protect the baby against diarrhea, respiratory, and other infections. Colostrum contains more epidermal growth factors (EGFs) in comparison to mature breastmilk, which help a baby's immature intestine to develop after birth. This helps to prevent the baby from developing allergies and intolerances to other foods. Colostrum helps to clean the baby's intestine, which is important to prevent jaundice in the newborn. Colostrum is also rich in vitamin A.

Transitional Milk

During the transition from colostrum to mature milk, the amount of Ig, proteins, vitamins A and E decreases, and the amount of lactose, fats, energy, and water-soluble vitamins increases.

Mature Milk

After a few days, colostrum changes into mature milk. Mature milk is in large amounts, and the breasts feel full, hard, and heavy. Some people call this the milk "coming in."

Foremilk is the bluish milk that is produced early in a feed. It is produced in larger amounts and provides plenty of protein, lactose, and other nutrients. Because a baby gets large amounts of foremilk, he or she gets all the water that he or she needs from it. *Hindmilk* is the whiter milk that is produced later in a feed. It contains more fat than foremilk. This fat provides much of the energy of a breastfeed. Therefore, it is important not to take a baby off a breast too quickly, not until he or she leaves the breast on her/his own.

BENEFITS OF BREASTFEEDING

The benefits of breastfeeding for infant, mother, and community include the following:[8,9]

- Breastfeeding provides all the nutrients a baby needs for the first 6 months of life, after which it continues to provide a major portion of the infant's nutrition along with appropriate family foods. It provides almost half of the nutritional requirements between 6 and 12 months of age and up to one-third between 12 and 24 months of age.
- Breastmilk is easily digested by the baby.
- Breastmilk contains antibodies and other factors, which protect the baby against diarrhea and other infections.
- It contains enough water, which is sufficient even for very dry and hot climates.
- It is clean, safe, and cheap.
- Breastfeeding provides a perfect opportunity for building a close bond between mother and baby.
- It helps the mother by reducing the postdelivery bleeding and thus preventing anemia.
- Breastfed babies are less prone to diabetes, heart disease, eczema, asthma, rheumatoid arthritis, and other allergic disorders later in life.
- Breastfeeding enhances brain development, visual development, and visual acuity, leading to learning readiness.
- Breastfeeding has a contraceptive effect for the mother if she exclusively breastfeeds her infant for the first 6 months.
- Mothers have a lower risk of breast and ovarian cancers.
- Breastfeeding costs less in terms of healthcare expenses as breastfed infants get ill less often.
- Breastfeeding protects the environment.

RISKS OF FORMULA FEEDING

Infant formula, which is generally used as an artificial substitute for human breastmilk, is time-consuming, less nutritious, and expensive. It is also fraught with innumerable risks for infants and children in comparison with breastfeeding.[10] Some of these risks are depicted in **Box 5.2.2.**

SCIENCE OF MILK TRANSFER

Understanding the structure of the breast and the process of breastmilk production and transfer to the infant is useful to provide effective skilled help to the lactating mother.

Anatomy of the Breast

The human breast consists of the nipple and areola, mammary tissue, soft tissue, including supporting connective tissue and fat, blood and lymphatic vessels, and nerves **(Fig. 5.2.2).**[11] The nipple is the area from which the milk comes out of the breast through multiple small openings. This area of the breast is very richly supplied with nerves. The nerve endings in the nipple are important to provide a stimulus for the hormonal reflexes important for the production and release of milk from the breast. The areola is the dark skin surrounding the nipple. The milk ducts beneath the areola are filled with milk and become wider during a feed. Areola is an important anatomical landmark as it is important to ensure that the majority of areola is in the baby's mouth during the feed to achieve an effective suckling. The mammary tissue is composed of alveoli, which are small sacs made up of millions of milk-secreting cells.

BOX 5.2.2: Risks of formula feeding.

- Increased risk for infection from inherent and subsequent contamination of formula with microbes, such as *Enterobacter sakazakii* and *Salmonella*
- Increased risk of acute respiratory infections, diarrhea, otitis media, and ear infections
- Increased risk of necrotizing enterocolitis
- Increased risk of asthma and other allergies
- Increased risk of chronic diseases, such as type 1 diabetes, ulcerative colitis, and Crohn's disease
- Increased risk of cardiovascular disease, increased blood pressure, obesity, altered blood cholesterol levels, and atherosclerosis in later adulthood
- Increased risk of side effects of environmental contaminants and harmful chemicals such as melamine and bisphenol A

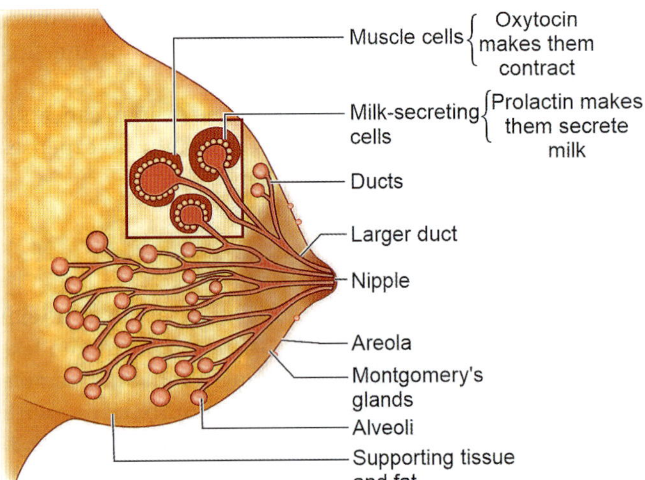

Fig. 5.2.2: Anatomy of the breast.
Source: Reproduced with permission from World Health Organization. Infant and Young Child Feeding: Model Chapter for Textbooks for Medical Students and Allied Health Professionals. Geneva: WHO Press; 2009.

Milk produced in the alveoli is carried toward the nipple via tubular structures called ducts. These ducts open outside at the nipple area. The alveoli are surrounded by myoepithelial tissue, which helps in pushing the milk present in the alveoli toward the nipple.

PHYSIOLOGY OF LACTATION

Production of Breastmilk

Production of the breastmilk is controlled by the hormone prolactin.[11,12] When a baby suckles at the breast, sensory impulses go from the nipple to the brain. In response, the anterior part of the pituitary gland at the base of the brain secretes prolactin. Prolactin goes in the blood to the breast and makes the milk-secreting cells produce milk. This process is known as the prolactin reflex **(Fig. 5.2.3)**. From this, it is evident that milk production is dependent on the suckling stimulus. If the baby suckles more, the breast will produce more milk. For the same reason, if a mother has two babies, breastmilk production increases accordingly. Prolactin is present in the blood for about 30 minutes after the baby finishes the feed. It makes the breast produce milk for the next feed. More prolactin is produced at night due to the inhibition of dopaminergic drive during sleep, so breastfeeding at night is especially helpful for keeping up the milk supply. Prolactin also suppresses ovulation, so breastfeeding can help to delay a new pregnancy.

Flow of Breastmilk

When a baby suckles, sensory impulses go from the nipple to the brain. In response, the posterior part of the pituitary gland at the base of the brain secretes the hormone oxytocin.

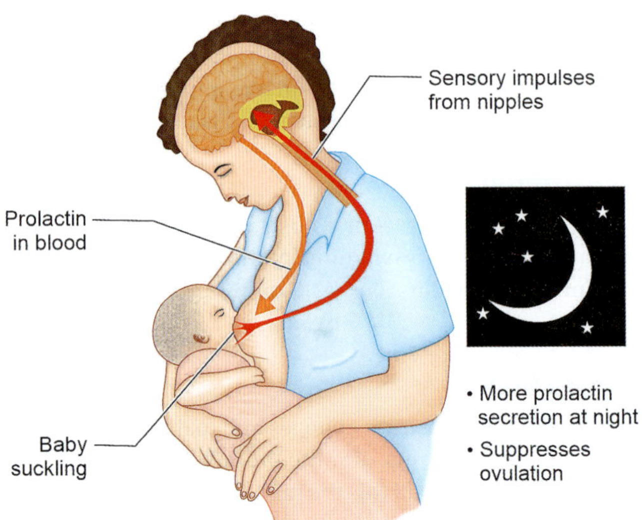

Fig. 5.2.3: Prolactin reflex.
Source: Reproduced with permission from World Health Organization. Infant and Young Child Feeding: Model Chapter for Textbooks for Medical Students and Allied Health Professionals. Geneva: WHO Press; 2009.

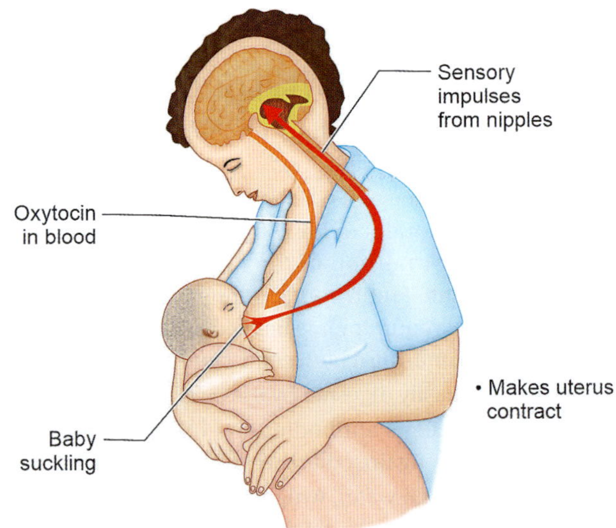

Fig. 5.2.4: Oxytocin reflex.
Source: Reproduced with permission from World Health Organization (WHO). Infant and Young Child Feeding (IYCF); Model Chapter for Textbooks for Medical Students and Allied Health Professionals. Geneva: WHO Press; 2009.

Oxytocin goes in the blood to the breast and makes the muscle cells around the alveoli contract. This makes the milk, which has collected in the alveoli, flow along the ducts toward the nipple. It makes the milk in the breast flow for this feed **(Fig. 5.2.4)**. Sometimes, the milk is ejected in fine streams.

This is the oxytocin reflex or the milk ejection reflex. Oxytocin can start working before a baby suckles, when a mother expects a feed. The oxytocin reflex is positively affected by a mother's sensations and feelings, such as thinking lovingly about the baby; touching, smelling, or seeing the baby; or hearing the baby cry. If the oxytocin reflex does not work well, the baby may have difficulty getting the milk. This may happen if the mother is emotionally disturbed or experiencing pain and discomfort. In such a condition, the mother needs support to make her physically and/or emotionally comfortable to make the oxytocin reflex work again and let the milk flow.

Signs of an active oxytocin reflex are a tingling sensation in the breast before or during a feed, milk flowing from breasts when the mother thinks of the baby or hears him/her crying, milk flowing from the other breast when the baby is suckling, milk flowing from the breast in streams if suckling is interrupted, and uterine pain or a flow of blood from the uterus during the feed. However, the absence of these signs does not indicate an inadequate oxytocin reflex.

Breastmilk Inhibitor

Breastmilk production is also controlled within the breast itself. Sometimes one breast stops making milk, while the other breast continues to make milk, although oxytocin and prolactin go equally to both breasts. There is a substance in breastmilk that can reduce or inhibit milk production. If a lot of milk is left in a breast, the inhibitor stops the cells from secreting any more. If suckling or expression removes breastmilk, the inhibitor is also removed, and the breast makes more milk.

Positioning and Attaching the Baby at the Breast

For effective milk transfer from mother to infant, good breastfeeding skills, including proper positioning of the baby and good attachment at the breast, are required.[11]

Positioning

A woman can feed her baby in any comfortable position, such as sitting, lying, or even standing. If the baby suckles properly from the breast, he or she will get sufficient milk. However, for a good attachment on the breast, some basic principles need to be observed for the relative positioning of the baby while breastfeeding. These are as follows:

- Baby turned toward the mother, and his or her ears, shoulder, and buttock are in a straight line.
- His face should face the breast with the nose opposite the nipple.
- The mother should hold the baby close to her.
- In a newborn, she should support his bottom with her hand and not just his head and shoulders.

The mother should be explained how to support the breast with her hand while offering it to the baby:

- With her fingers and palm placed on her chest wall below the breast so that her first finger forms a support at the base of the breast.
- With her thumb placed on the top of the breast so that it is easier for her baby to attach well.
- She should not hold her breast too near to the nipple.

The mother should be explained how to bring the baby to the breast:

- Touch baby's lips with her nipple;
- Wait until the baby's mouth is wide open;
- Move the baby quickly onto the breast from below.

Attachment

This is important how the baby's mouth is attached to the mother's breast for a successful suckling **(Figs. 5.2.5 and 5.2.6)**. In a good suckling position, the baby is suckling with nipple and a larger breast tissue being in his or her mouth. In a poor suckling position, the baby is suckling with nipple only or nipple with a small breast tissue in his or her mouth.

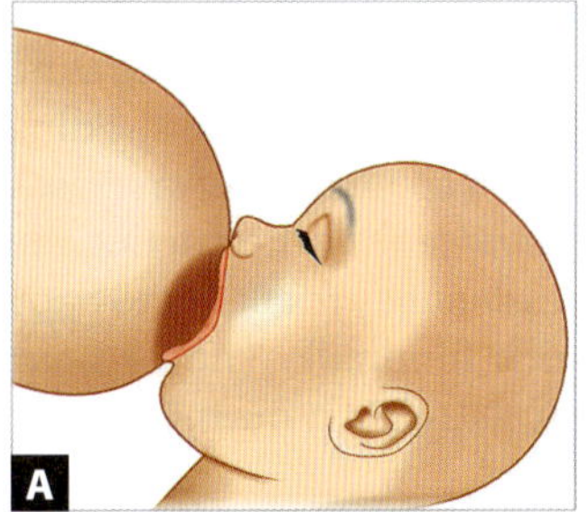

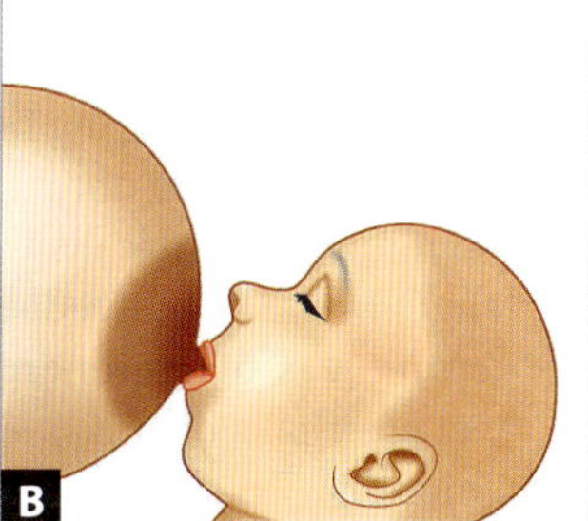

Figs. 5.2.5A and B: (A) Good and (B) Poor attachment. External signs.
Source: Reproduced with permission from World Health Organization (WHO). Infant and Young Child Feeding (IYCF); Model Chapter for Textbooks for Medical Students and Allied Health Professionals. Geneva: WHO Press; 2009.

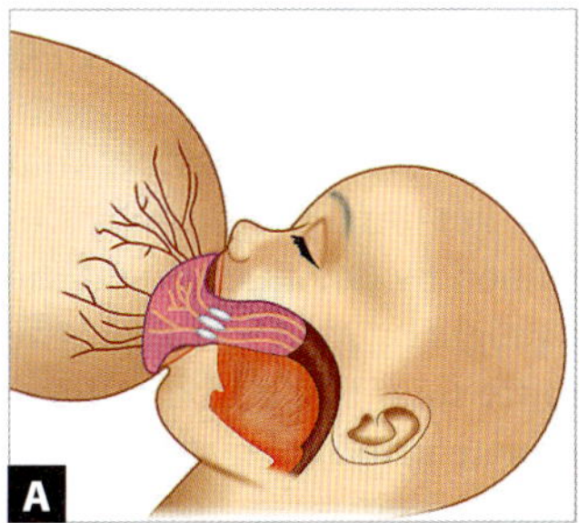

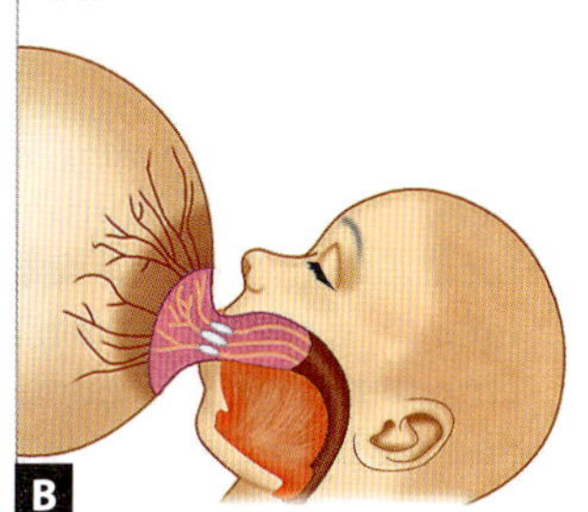

Figs. 5.2.6A and B: (A) Good and (B) Poor attachment inside the infant's mouth.
Source: Reproduced with permission from World Health Organization. Infant and young child feeding: Model chapter for textbooks for medical students and allied health professionals. Geneva: WHO Press; 2009.

The signs of good suckling attachment are as follows:

- The baby's chin touches the breast.
- His/her mouth is wide open.
- His/her lower lip is turned outward.
- One can see more of the areola above his or her mouth and less below. This shows that he or she is reaching with his/her tongue under the lactiferous sinuses to press out the milk.

Poor attachment may lead to pain and damage to the mother's nipple, and she may develop sores or fissures in the nipple. It may also lead to engorgement of the breast due to improper milk removal. The baby remains hungry and frustrated, which leads to refusal to suck. Ultimately, it leads to the production of less milk in the breast; the baby is not able to feed properly, leading to weight loss. Common causes of poor attachment are use of a feeding bottle, inexperience of the mother, and lack of skilled support.

PRACTICES FOR SUCCESSFUL BREASTFEEDING

To ensure adequate milk production and flow for 6 months of exclusive breastfeeding and thereafter continued breastfeeding, certain practices are very important.

- The infant should be fed as frequently and for as long as he or she wants to, during both day and night. The suckling should be allowed until the infant spontaneously releases the nipple. This is called *demand feeding*. Restricting the length of the breastfeeding session may result in the baby getting less of the energy-rich hindmilk. The 24-hour average intake of milk is about 800 mL/day during the first 6 months.
- At the time of delivery, before breastfeeding is initiated, no prelacteal feed should be given to the infant. Apart from having harmful effects on the infant, such as risk of infection, such a practice may interfere with the establishment of breastfeeding. Later, in the first 6 months of life, no supplementary feed, such as other milks, should be given to the infant. This may lead to a decreased supply of breastmilk.
- Sometimes, a mother may have the perception that her milk is not sufficient for her infant. Adequacy of breastfeeding may be ascertained by documenting if the infant has regained the birth weight by 2 weeks of age, the cumulative weight gain is more than 500 g in a month, and the infant is passing adequate urine at least six times a day, while on exclusive breastfeeding.

HOSPITAL PRACTICES AND BREASTFEEDING

Maternity homes and healthcare practices should support exclusive breastfeeding during the first 6 months of life and continued breastfeeding along with appropriate complementary feeds thereafter.[4] To motivate maternity facilities to practice 10 steps to successful breastfeeding, the World Health Organization (WHO) and the United Nations Children's Fund (UNICEF) launched the *baby-friendly hospital initiative (BFHI)* in 1991. The initiative is a global effort for improving the role of maternity services to enable mothers to breastfeed babies for the best start in life. It aims at improving the care of pregnant women, mothers, and newborns at health facilities that provide maternity services for protecting, promoting, and supporting breastfeeding. The BFHI package was relaunched in 2009 with an updated version that included new evidence and specifically addressed infant feeding by women living with human immunodeficiency virus (HIV). In 2018, the BFHI package was further revised, which is based on the 2017 WHO guideline on protecting, promoting, and supporting breastfeeding in facilities providing maternity and newborn services, and an implementation guidance has been published. The key to successful breastfeeding lies in the prenatal priming of the expectant mother about the undisputed facts of the benefits of breastfeeding the newborn child within 1 hour of birth and addressing all the issues that may delay or prevent the initiation of breastfeeding the newborn. The elders in the family should also be taken into confidence about breastfeeding soon after the birth.

Components of Baby-friendly Hospital Initiative

Ten steps to successful breastfeeding have been regrouped under two headings, critical management procedures and key clinical practices, which are given in **Table 5.2.1**.

BREASTFEEDING THE PRETERM BABIES

Nutritional management plays a large role in the immediate survival and subsequent growth and development of preterm infants. The optimal diet for premature infants should support growth at intrauterine rates without imposing stress on the infant's immature metabolic and excretory functions and ensure healthy short-term and long-term outcomes. Breastmilk produced during the early postpartum period offers nutritional advantages because of its higher protein and electrolyte concentrations.[13,14] Preterm infants fed preterm milk demonstrate an increase in weight, length, and head circumference as well as retention rates of various nutrients comparable to those for the fetus of similar postconception age. Fat absorption in preterm babies fed their own mother's milk is significantly higher in comparison to infants fed cow's milk formula. Long-chain polyunsaturated fatty acids, which are important for mental and visual development, are also higher in human milk.

TABLE 5.2.1: Ten steps of baby-friendly hospital initiative (revised 2018).

Step no.	Description
Critical management procedures	
1a	Comply fully with the International Code of Marketing of Breastmilk Substitutes and relevant World Health Assembly resolutions
1b	Have a written infant feeding policy that is routinely communicated to staff and parents
1c	Establish ongoing monitoring and data management systems
2	Ensure that the members of the staff have sufficient knowledge, competence, and skills to support breastfeeding
Key clinical practices	
3	Discuss the importance and management of breastfeeding with pregnant women and their families
4	Facilitate immediate and uninterrupted skin-to-skin contact and support mothers to initiate breastfeeding as soon as possible after birth
5	Support mothers to initiate and maintain breastfeeding and manage common difficulties
6	Do not provide breastfed newborns any food or fluids other than breastmilk, unless medically indicated
7	Enable mothers and their infants to remain together and to practice rooming in 24 hours a day
8	Support mothers to recognize and respond to their infants' cues for feeding
9	Counsel mothers on the use and risks of feeding bottles, teats, and pacifiers
10	Coordinate discharge so that parents and their infants have timely access to ongoing support and care

Preterm infants fed breastmilk have a lesser incidence of necrotizing enterocolitis compared to those fed with formula milk. Even if the disease occurs in infants fed with breastmilk, the course of the disease is less severe, and the prevalence of intestinal perforation is lower. This is due to various protective factors in breastmilk, such as secretory IgA, IgM, IgG erythropoietin, interleukin-10, platelet-activating factor—acetylhydrolase enzyme, lactoferrin, lactadherin, and oligosaccharides, which are in greater quantity than in term milk. These factors may prevent intestinal attachment of enteropathogens by acting as receptor homologs, resulting in the suppression of enteral colonization with harmful microorganisms. EGF in preterm milk leads to enhanced proliferation and differentiation of epithelial cells and healing of damaged gastrointestinal (GI) mucosa. Breastmilk also provides protection against retinopathy of prematurity and helps in preventing a host of neonatal infections. Breastfed infants have preferred intestine microbiota; that is, beneficial bifidobacteria predominate over the potentially harmful bacteria, while in formula-fed infants disease-causing microbiota coliforms, enterococci, and bacteroides predominate.

The use of human milk can be adopted as an important healthcare intervention in neonatal units.

BREAST CONDITIONS AND DIFFICULTIES IN BREASTFEEDING

There are several common breast conditions that sometimes cause difficulties with breastfeeding.[12] Management of these conditions is important both to relieve the mother and to enable successful breastfeeding. The difficulties in breastfeeding can be overcome by careful guidance, reassurance, and encouragement to the mother during the prenatal period to prepare for breastfeeding and by providing skilled counseling after birth.

Flat Nipple

Many times, a mother becomes apprehensive that a flat nipple is a hindrance to successful breastfeeding. However, in a good suckling attachment, the infant takes the nipple and the breast tissue underlying the areola into his mouth to form a "teat." The anatomical nipple only forms about one-third of the "teat" of breast tissue in the baby's mouth. This is therefore evident that the shape of the nipple is immaterial for successful suckling. The nipple is just a guide to show where the baby must take the breast. A woman with flat nipples should be reassured that she has normal nipples, even if they look short, provided her nipples protract easily.

Inverted Nipple

Sometimes, a nipple does not protract, and on attempting to pull out the nipple, it goes deeper into the breast. The condition is known as inverted nipple **(Figs. 5.2.7A and B)**. The mother needs support in such a situation. She should be reassured that with some help, she will be able to breastfeed her infant successfully. Help is most important soon after delivery when the baby starts breastfeeding.

A mother with inverted nipple may be helped with the syringe method as follows **(Fig. 5.2.8)**:

- Cut the nozzle end of a disposable syringe (10–20 mL).
- Introduce the piston from the ragged cut end side.
- Ask the mother to apply the smooth side of the syringe on the nipple, gently pull out the piston, and let her wait for a minute.
- The nipple would then protrude into the syringe. Ask the mother to slowly release the suction and put the baby to the breast; at this time, it helps the nipple to erect out, and the baby is able to suckle in the proper position.

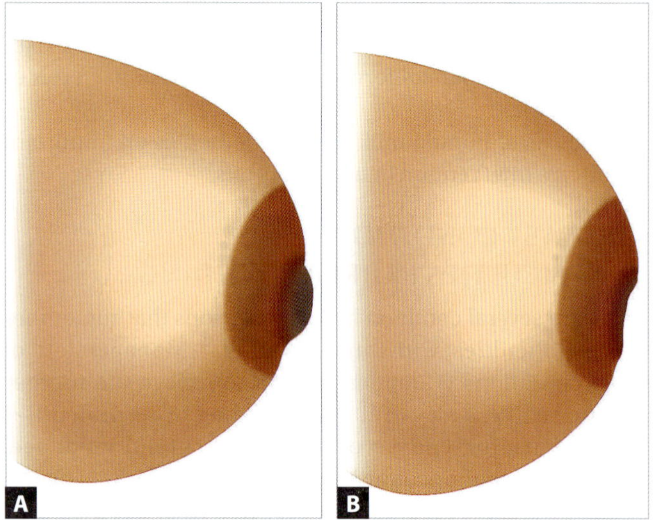

Figs. 5.2.7A and B: (A) Flat and (B) Inverted nipple.
Source: Adapted with permission from Gupta A, Kushwaha KP, Sobti JC, Jindal T. Breastfeeding and complementary feeding. New Delhi: Breastfeeding Promotion Network of India (BPNI); 2001.

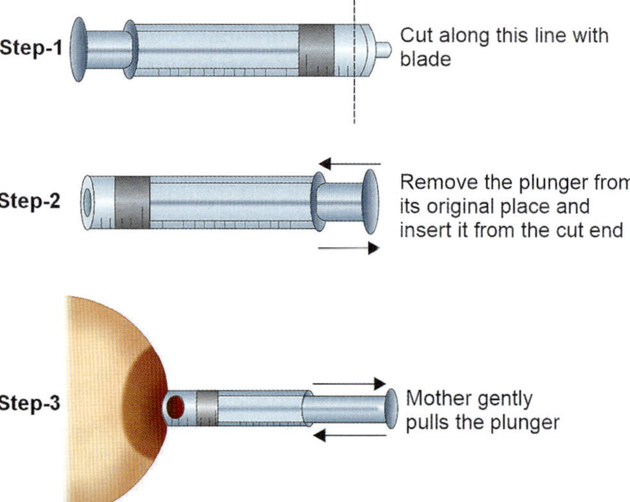

Fig. 5.2.8: Syringe method for correction of inverted nipple.
Source: Adapted from Infant and Young Child Feeding Counseling—A Training Course, the "4 in 1 Course" (Integrated Course on Breastfeeding, Complementary Feeding and Infant Feeding and HIV). New Delhi: Breastfeeding Promotion Network of India (BPNI); 2015.

- After feeding, the nipple may retract back, but doing it each time before feeding over a period of few days will help to solve the problem.

Engorgement of Breasts

If breasts are not emptied, the milk gets collected in the breast, leading to engorgement. The engorged breast is tight, shiny (because of edema), and painful. Moreover, the milk may stop flowing. The factors that cause engorgement of breasts are as follows:

- Giving prelacteal feeds to the baby
- Delayed initiation of breastfeeds
- Long intervals between feeds
- Early removal of the baby from the breast
- Bottle-feeding and any other restrictions on breastfeeding

Engorgement of the breast can be prevented by avoiding the factors mentioned earlier. If the baby can suckle, he or she should feed frequently. If pain and tightness of the breast do not allow suckling, expressed milk may be given to the infant with a cup/spoon. Once the mother feels comfortable, she should be advised again to breastfeed the infant on demand. Applying a cold compress may reduce edema of the breasts. Engorged breasts may cause mild fever, which subsides spontaneously within a day or two.

Mastitis and Abscess

Mastitis is an inflammation of the breast, which makes it red, hot, tender, and swollen. The mother feels sick and has fever and severe pain in the breast. Mastitis usually affects a part of the breast and is usually unilateral. Mastitis may develop in an engorged breast or may follow a condition called blocked duct. It must be treated promptly and adequately. If treatment is delayed or incomplete, there is an increased risk of developing breast abscess. An abscess is when a collection of pus forms in part of the breast. The most important part of treatment is supportive counseling and improved drainage of milk from the affected part of the breast.

The mother needs clear information and guidance about all measures needed for treatment and how to continue breastfeeding or expressing milk from the affected breast. This is important to help the mother improve the infant's attachment at the breast with frequent, unrestricted breastfeeding. If necessary, express breastmilk by hand or with a pump until suckling is resumed. Antibiotics should be given if laboratory tests indicate infection, symptoms are severe, or symptoms do not improve after 12–24 hours of improved milk removal. Pain should be treated with an analgesic and warm packs to the breast. Incision and drainage should be done if an abscess develops.

Sore and Cracked Nipples

The most common cause of sore nipples is poor attachment in which the infant pulls the nipple in and out as he or she sucks and rubs the skin of the breast against his or her mouth. If the baby continues to suckle in this way, it damages the nipple skin and causes a crack or fissure. Oral thrush in the infant's mouth is another important cause of sore nipple, but it usually develops when a baby is few weeks old. The situation is very painful for the mother. If a mother has sore or cracked nipples, improving the infant's attachment to the breast relieves the pain. Medicated creams are best avoided as they may worsen the soreness. Hindmilk, which is rich in fat, should be applied on the nipple after feeding. For oral thrush, 1% gentian violet or 1% clotrimazole mouth paint should be applied over the nipple as well as inside the baby's mouth every 4–6 hours for 5–7 days.

BREASTFEEDING AND MATERNAL ILLNESS

Maternal illnesses can have adverse effects on lactation.[8,15] A sick woman may perceive that her milk supply has gone down because of illness. She may also believe that her milk will make the baby ill. These factors may lead to the discontinuation of breastfeeding. Minor illnesses, such as cold and other mild viral infections, which are self-limiting, should not prevent a mother from continuing breastfeeding. However, major illness requires a more careful approach. The potential role of breastfeeding in the transmission of infections must also be acknowledged, and appropriate precautions should be taken.

Breastfeeding should be temporarily avoided in a maternal herpes simplex virus type 1 (HSV-1) infection when lesions on the breast lead to direct contact with the baby's mouth. If the mother has tuberculosis, the mother–infant dyad should be treated together, and breastfeeding should be continued.

In maternal hepatitis B infection, hepatitis B immunoglobulin should be given to the infant at delivery along with the hepatitis B vaccine, and breastfeeding should be practiced. Similarly, in the case of hepatitis A and C, breastfeeding can continue normally as the risk of transmission by breastfeeding is very low.

In an HIV-positive mother, the mother should be provided with counseling and support for appropriate infant feeding practices. With adequate and appropriate antiretroviral drugs for mother and infant, exclusive breastfeeding for the first 6 months of life is now the preferred recommendation in India.

Certain maternal drugs may affect the breastfed infant adversely as they are secreted in the breastmilk. Breastfeeding should be avoided if the mother is consuming cytotoxic drugs, such as cyclophosphamide, methotrexate, and doxorubicin, and radioactive compounds, such as gallium 67, indium 111, iodine 131, and technetium-99m.

INFANT FEEDING DURING EMERGENCIES

In disasters and emergencies, such as earthquakes, floods, typhoons, and tsunamis, breastfeeding is the safest, often the only reliable choice for infants and young children.[16] It provides adequate and appropriate nutrition to the affected infants in a situation where child survival is a key issue. In disasters, infants are more likely to become ill and die from malnutrition. Uncontrolled distribution of breastmilk substitutes during disasters may lead to early and unnecessary cessation of breastfeeding. For the vast majority of infants, the emphasis should be on protecting, promoting, and supporting breastfeeding and ensuring timely, safe, and appropriate complementary feeding.

PROTECTING BREASTFEEDING FROM COMMERCIAL INFLUENCE

During the last many decades, extensive promotion by infant food manufacturing companies through advertisements, free samples, gifts to mothers, and health workers has led to convince them that formula feeding is as good as breastfeeding. This has also made a dent in the confidence of lactating women in their capacity to optimally breastfeed and has contributed to the decline of breastfeeding rates.[17] Recognizing this trend, the Indian Parliament enacted the "infant milk substitutes (IMSs), feeding bottles and infant foods (regulation of production, supply and distribution) Act 1992 (IMS Act)." The IMS Act was further amended in the year 2003. The IMS Act controls the marketing and promotion of IMSs, infant foods, and feeding bottles. Some salient features of the IMS Act include the following:

- It bans any kind of promotion or advertisement of IMSs, infant foods, and feeding bottles to the public, including electronic and print media.
- It prohibits providing free samples of IMSs, infant foods, feeding bottles, and gifts to anyone including pregnant women, mothers of infants, and members of the families.
- It prohibits the donation of free or subsidized supplies of IMSs, infant foods, and feeding bottles for healthcare institutions except donations to the orphanages.
- It prohibits the display of posters of IMSs, infant foods, and feeding bottles at healthcare facilities, hospitals, and health centers.
- It prescribes rules for information on the containers and labels of IMSs and infant foods, including a specific statement in English and local languages that "mother's milk is best for the baby" in capital letters.
- It prohibits having pictures of infants or women or phrases designed to increase the sale of the product on the labels of the products.
- It prohibits any contact of employers of manufacturing and distributing companies with pregnant women, even for providing educational material to them.
- It prohibits direct or indirect financial inducement or gift to a health worker or to any members of his family by the producer, supplier, or distributor of the IMSs, infant foods, and feeding bottles.

- The IMS Act also prohibits offering or giving any contribution or pecuniary benefit to a health worker or any association thereof, including funding of seminar, meeting, conference, educational course, contests, fellowship, research work, sponsorship, etc., by the manufacturers, supplier, or distributors of the products mentioned earlier.
- It prescribes standards for the IMSs, infant foods, and feeding bottles.

REFERENCES

1. World Health Organization. United Nations Children's Fund. (2003). Global strategy for infant and young child feeding. [online] Available from https://www.who.int/publications/i/item/9241562218. [Last accessed October, 2024].
2. Ministry of Women and Child Development, Food and Nutrition Board, Government of India. National Guidelines on Infant and Young Child Feeding, 2nd edition. New Delhi: Food and Nutrition Board; 2006.
3. Tiwari S, Bharadva K, Yadav B, Malik S, Gangal P, Banapurmath CR, et al. Infant and young child feeding guidelines, 2016. Indian Pediatr. 2016;53(8):703-13.
4. World Health Organization. (2018). Implementation guidance: protecting, promoting and supporting breastfeeding in facilities providing maternity and newborn services—the revised baby-friendly hospital initiative. [online] Available from https://www.who.int/publications/i/item/9789241513807. [Last accessed October, 2024].
5. World Health Organization. (2023). Guideline for complementary feeding of infants and young children 6–23 months of age. [online] Available from https://www.who.int/publications/i/item/9789240081864. [Last accessed October, 2024].
6. National Family Health Survey-5, 2019-21; India report. [online] Available from https://dhsprogram.com/pubs/pdf/FR375/FR375.pdf. [Last accessed October, 2024].
7. Anand RK, Kumta NB, Kushwaha KP, Gupta A (Eds). The Science of Infant Feeding. New Delhi: Jaypee Brothers Medical Publishers; 2002.
8. Meek JY, Noble L; Section on Breastfeeding. Policy statement: breastfeeding and the use of human milk. Pediatrics. 2022;150(1):e2022057988.
9. World Health Organization. Long-term effects of breastfeeding: a systematic review (Horta BL, Victora CG). 2013. [online] Available from http://apps.who.int/iris/bitstream/10665/79198/1/9789241505307.eng.pdf. [Last accessed October, 2024].
10. INFACT Canada/IBFAN North America. (2006). Risks of formula feeding—a brief annotated bibliography. [online] Available from http://www.infactcanada.ca/risksofformulafeeding.pdf. [Last accessed October, 2024].
11. Infant and Young Child Feeding: Model Chapter for Textbooks for Medical Students and Allied Health Professionals. Geneva: World Health Organization; 2009.
12. Breastfeeding Promotion Network of India. Infant and Young Child Feeding Counseling—A Training Course, the "4 in 1 Course" (Integrated Course on Breastfeeding, Complementary Feeding and Infant Feeding and HIV). New Delhi: Breastfeeding Promotion Network of India; 2015.
13. Altobelli E, Angeletti PM, Verrotti A, Petrocelli R. The impact of human milk on necrotizing enterocolitis: a systematic review and meta-analysis. Nutrients. 2020;12(5):1322.
14. Underwood MA. Human milk for the premature infant. Pediatr Clin North Am. 2013;60(1):189-207.
15. World Health Organization. (2009). Acceptable medical reasons for use of breastmilk substitutes. [online] Available from https://iris.who.int/bitstream/handle/10665/69938/WHO_FCH_CAH_09.01_eng.pdf?sequence=1. [Last accessed October, 2024].
16. Infant and young child feeding in emergencies—operational guidance for emergency relief staff and programme managers, version 3.0—October 2017; Developed by the IFE Core Group. [online] Available from https://www.ennonline.net/resources/operationalguidancev32017. [Last accessed October, 2024].
17. Ministry of Women and Child Development, Government of India. The infant milk substitutes, feeding bottles and infant foods (regulation of production, supply and distribution) Amendment Act, 2003. [online] Available from https://www.indiacode.nic.in/handle/123456789/1958?view_type=browse. [Last accessed October, 2024].

5.3 Human Milk Banking

RK Agarwal, Asha Benakappa

INTRODUCTION

Breastfeeding is the best method of infant feeding because human milk is uniquely suited to the human infant. All mothers should be encouraged to breastfeed their infants. Early initiation of breastfeeding (EIBF) is recommended by the World Health Organization (WHO), where all mothers are supported to initiate breastfeeding as soon as possible after birth, within the first hour after delivery.[1] When a mother, for some reason, is unable to feed her infant directly, her breastmilk should be expressed and fed to her infant.[2] If the mother's own milk is unavailable or insufficient, the next best option is to use pasteurized donor human milk (PDHM). The WHO and the United Nations Children's Fund (UNICEF) made a joint statement in 1980 that "where it is not possible for the biological mother to breastfeed, the first alternative, if available, should be the use of human milk from other sources." Human milk banks should be made available in appropriate situations.

Though "wet nursing" has been in practice since mythological ages, modern human milk banking is in its infancy in India. The first human milk bank in Asia was established by Armida Fernandez in 1989 in Mumbai. Currently, the number of human milk banks has grown to nearly 118 in India, and Rajasthan leads with 27 banks.[3] Brazil has the largest network of 210 banks in the world. Its strategy includes innovative measures, such as training postmen to provide information on breastfeeding to pregnant women and using firefighters to collect surplus milk for donation from lactating women. One of the major reasons for the slow growth and loss of interest in human milk banking was the promotion of milk formula by the industry.

LOCATION OF HUMAN MILK BANK

Human milk banks are primarily focused on providing donor milk to high-risk newborns.[4] Thus, a location near or even inside the boundaries of the neonatal unit is desirable. Postnatal wards are most suited for the purpose as the number of donors is likely to be in large number, where lactation counselors can encourage them to donate milk. Certain nongovernmental organizations (NGOs) that take care of abandoned babies should have a human milk bank in their facility. The presence of human milk banks in the neonatal intensive care units (NICUs) is associated with increased rates of exclusive breastfeeding rates in very low birth weight (VLBW) babies with better survival.

National guidelines suggest establishing comprehensive lactation management centers (CLMCs) and lactation management centers (LMCs) at various medical colleges and district hospitals which provide milk collection, screening, storage, and dispensing facilities to the mothers.[3,4]

THE RECIPIENTS

Pasteurized donor human milk can be prescribed on priority for:[4]

- Preterm and sick babies[5]
- Babies of mothers with postpartum illnesses
- Babies whose mothers have difficult lactation till their milk output improves.

Therapeutic benefits of PDHM are noted in short gut syndrome, sepsis, and postsurgical gut healing in omphalocele, gastroschisis, bowel obstruction, and intestinal fistula. In extremely preterm infants given only preterm formula versus human milk, there was a significantly greater duration of parenteral nutrition and a higher rate of surgical necrotizing enterocolitis (NEC) in infants receiving preterm formula.[5] It is possible to do gut priming exclusively with human milk.

If there is an adequate supply of PDHM, donor milk can be provided for the following purposes:[4]

- Infants born prematurely and with a low birth weight (LBW). Preterm newborns, particularly in the initial days, are the primary beneficiaries of donated human milk until their mothers can produce sufficient milk[5]
- Preterm neonates who are ill with conditions such as NEC and gastrointestinal (GI) procedures and are in the process of healing
- Severe fetal growth restriction within the uterus [intrauterine growth restriction (IUGR)]
- Infants who do not have the opportunity to consume their mother's breastmilk or when the mother is unable to nurse or express milk due to a medical condition
- Infants born to women experiencing conditions such as eclampsia, postpartum hemorrhage (PPH), and febrile diseases
- Infants admitted to the facility whose moms are unavailable (due to physical absence or decease)
- Infants born to mothers with lactation insufficiency
- Extraordinary circumstances, supported by medical rationale
- Delivery of several babies, if necessary
- Infants delivered through surrogacy

INFRASTRUCTURE

There are recommendations laid down by the Government of India for the establishment of CLMCs and LMCs.[3] The average requirement is a room of 250 sq. ft., which can accommodate the equipment required for milk banking, a work area for the technician, some storage space for records and administration, an area for counseling donors, etc. Privacy is of paramount importance for the area of breastmilk expression. Provision of music or television and crèche for her baby helps in reducing the stress of donors. Teaching videos of Kangaroo mother care (KMC), expression of breastmilk, and advantages of breastmilk feeding can be shown.

EQUIPMENT[3]

Pasteurizer (Shaker Water Bath)

It is essential to have a device to carry out heat treatment of donor milk at the recommended temperature of 62.5°C for 30 minutes (Holder pasteurization). A conventional pasteurizer is extremely expensive and of dairy-industry size and is not suitable for a human milk bank. A well-accepted alternative is the use of a shaker water bath with a microprocessor-controlled temperature regulator, an electronic timer device, and a shaker speed controller. The milk in the container is boiled through the steam and hot water in the water-shaker bath. To avoid coagulation of the milk and to distribute heat evenly, the tray on which the stainless-steel containers are placed is shaken and wobbled. This shaker water bath should be double-walled and made of steel. The size of the shaker water bath varies according to the need of the milk bank with the tray capacity varying from 9 to 24 flasks or stainless-steel containers of 200–400 mL capacity.

Effect of Pasteurization on Human Milk

Pasteurization at a temperature of 62.5°C for a duration of 30 minutes does have an impact on some nutritional, immunological, and other constituents of human milk. This heat therapy effectively eradicates all functional white blood cells and bacteria; deactivates human immunodeficiency virus (HIV), human T-lymphotropic virus (HTLV), and cytomegalovirus; and reduces or substantially lowers the levels of most other viruses.[6] Heat treatment has diverse effects on immunologic variables. The majority of secretory immunoglobulin A (IgA), bifid growth factor, and lysozymes is eliminated, while lipids remain untouched. However, 57% of lactoferrin and 34% of IgG are destroyed. Holder pasteurization did not seem to have an impact on the absorption or retention of nitrogen in LBW infants. The majority of enzymes, growth hormones, vitamins, and minerals remain unaltered or experience only modest reduction. The process of subjecting donor milk to heat treatment seems to promote faster growth of intestinal epithelial cells by deactivating heat-sensitive inhibitory cytokines, thus enabling heat-resistant epidermal growth factor to function. Cryopreservation renders milk cells and most viruses inert, while leaving the nutritious and anti-infective properties of the milk unaffected.

Deep Freezer

It is necessary to have a deep freezer to keep the milk at –20°C. Ordering a deep freezer with an alarm feature and a digital temperature display is preferable.

- Milk awaiting culture is stored in the first deep freezer; it is kept there until the postpasteurization milk culture reports are available. In order to prevent milk from being unintentionally used before the culture results are available, this freezer should always be locked.
- Once the culture reports are negative and the milk is deemed safe for distribution, the pasteurized milk is stored in the second deep freezer.

Refrigerators

Refrigerators are required to store the milk till the whole day's collection is over and the milk is ready to be mixed and pooled for further processing. They are also required for thawing the milk before being dispatched.

Hot Air Oven or Autoclave

A hot air oven or autoclave in the milk bank is essential for sterilizing the containers used for collection from donors, containers for pasteurizing and storing the milk, and test tubes needed for sending milk culture samples to the microbiology laboratory.

Breastmilk Pumps

When it comes to milk banking, it is preferable to use medical-grade electric pumps because they yield higher quantities of expressed milk and are generally painless and comfortable to operate. There is negligible disparity among the various models of electrical breast pumps. If there are limitations on expenses, one might utilize manually operated devices for extracting milk from lactating animals.[7] They can be reused through chemical sterilization. Simultaneous breast expression in lactating mothers is more effective than sequential breast expression. Breast pumps have the potential to cause infection. They should be well cleaned. Detachables should undergo sterilization according to the guidelines provided by the manufacturer.

Containers

For collection and storing the collected milk, single-use hard plastic containers of polycarbonates, Pyrex, or propylene are used; however, cylindrical, wide-mouthed stainless-steel containers of 200 mL capacities with tight-fitting or screwed caps are equally effective. They are easily available, durable, easy to clean, and autoclave. There is no significant decrease in nutrient composition on storage; however, cellular components are reduced. Polythene milk bags are not suitable as they are fragile, associated with loss of lipids and vitamins, and there is a risk of contamination.

Generator or Uninterrupted Power Supply

Every milk bank should have a centralized source of uninterrupted power supply in the form of a generator, UPS, or inverter, to run the deep freezers and refrigerators in case of electricity failure.

Milk Analyzer

It is desirable to have a macronutrient analysis of breastmilk to estimate the calorie, protein, and fat of a milk sample, using infrared spectroscopy technology, in teaching hospitals as a step toward lacto-engineering.

ADMINISTRATIVE STAFF

Milk banks should have a panel from pediatrics, neonatology, microbiology, nutrition, lactation management, public health and food technology, milk bank officer (usually a doctor), lactation support staff, full time (for counseling mothers and assisting expression of breastmilk), technician (for pasteurization of breastmilk and microbiological surveillance), attendant/hygiene helper (for collecting, sterilization of the containers, and maintaining hygiene), receptionist (for record keeping and public relations), and a microbiologist (for microbiology testing and infection-control policies).[3]

General Guidelines for Staff[3]

Maintaining hygienic measures, such as thorough handwashing, wearing gowns, masks, and gloves, keeping nails trimmed, and securing long hair, is essential.

- It is necessary to use gloves when handling raw and heat-treated milk, and they should be changed between these two tasks.
- The bank's standard operating procedures, which should be prominently stated, must be followed.
- It is necessary for the staff to regularly undergo health checks and receive immunization against the hepatitis B virus (HBV).
- Banks should aim to provide complete traceability from the donor to the beneficiary and keep a record of all storage and processing conditions.

DONOR POPULATION

The donor population consists of nursing moms who are in good health and have healthy infants. These mothers willingly donate their surplus breast milk to other infants, while ensuring that their own baby's nutritional needs are not compromised. In India, donors do not receive any remuneration for their contributions. The individuals who may be included are moms who attend well-baby clinics, mothers with babies in the NICU, women who have experienced the loss of their kids but are willing to donate breast milk, lactating working personnel inside the hospital, and motivated mothers from the community.

The maximum number of potential donors should be achieved through the dissemination of information and widespread communication. NGOs, social groups, and senior female students can contribute significantly to this endeavor.

Who can Donate?[3]

A donor is deemed ineligible if she:

- Engages in the use of illicit drugs or consumes tobacco products or nicotine replacement therapy
- Consistently consumes more than two ounces of alcohol or its equivalent, or three caffeinated beverages per day
- Tests positive for HIV, HTLV, hepatitis B or C, or syphilis in a blood test[6]
- Has engaged in sexual activity with a partner who has engaged in high-risk behavior or has been diagnosed with HBV, HIV, hepatitis C virus, or venereal illnesses during the past 12 months[6]
- Has undergone an organ or tissue transplant, received a blood transfusion, or received a blood product in the past 12 months
- Is currently taking drugs that are radioactive or have chemical environmental exposure, or is taking over-the-counter prescriptions or high doses of vitamins that are known to be harmful to the newborn and are excreted in breastmilk
- Has mastitis or fungal infections of the nipple or areola, or has reactivated herpes simplex or varicella-zoster infections in the breast or chest area.

COLLECTION OF BREASTMILK

Once the suitability for donation has been assessed, written informed consent obtained, medical history taken, physical examination conducted, and samples collected for laboratory tests, the donor mother is directed to the designated place for breastmilk collection. Trained personnel collect the breastmilk once the donor has selected a method for expressing it. While home collection of breastmilk is being implemented in certain countries, experts advise against it in our country owing to the risk of contamination and tracking difficulties. However, milk-collecting camps can be conducted under adequate supervision. Washing the breast with plain water prior to expression is equally effective as washing with a disinfectant. There is no logical reason to reject the initial few milliliters of foremilk in order to decrease the likelihood of infection. Breast milk can be obtained using either electric or manual breast pumps. Donations should be gathered in appropriately labeled sterile receptacles.

Processing

It is important to refrigerate all batches of collected raw breastmilk immediately in a refrigerator before processing until the serological analysis shows a negative result.[3] It is not advisable to mix fresh raw milk with frozen milk, as this can cause the frozen milk to thaw and result in the breakdown of triglycerides by hydrolysis.[8] When combining recently expressed raw breastmilk with previously frozen raw breastmilk from the same donor, it is important to cool the fresh milk before adding it to the frozen milk. However, it is recommended to utilize a fresh container for each pumping session when dealing with ill or premature infants.[5]

Microbiological analysis of donated milk is conducted before and immediately following pasteurization, assuming cost is not a limiting factor.[7] In certain situations, prepasteurization microbiology might lead to a loss of approximately 30% of milk. Although pasteurization is performed, residual toxins from organisms may still be present in the milk in certain instances. However, these toxins have not been observed to have any clinical impact on the newborn. A bacterial count of 105 CFU/mL or higher in raw breastmilk can be regarded as an indication of the milk's substandard quality. The expert panel chose threshold values of 105 CFU/mL for total bacterial count and 104 CFU/mL for *Enterobacteriaceae* and *Staphylococcus aureus*, based on the concern that heavily contaminated milk may still contain enterotoxins and thermostable enzymes even after pasteurization. These values are consistent with those used by milk banks in other countries.

Zero growth is deemed unacceptable in postpasteurization microbiological cultures. The entire batch of pasteurized milk that tested positive for contamination should be disposed of. Prior to pasteurization, the act of combining and blending may be performed, including numerous contributors, in order to facilitate the procedures of processing and storage.

Storage

Pasteurized milk that is awaiting the culture report should be stored in a designated freezer location, ensuring that it is not disturbed until the culture test results are confirmed as negative. It is important to store culture-negative processed milk at a temperature of –20°C in a tightly sealed container. The container should include a label that clearly states the expiry date and other necessary information. It has a shelf life of 4–6 months. Predistributing random samples of preserved milk can help ensure quality control.

Disbursal

Pasteurized donor human milk should be distributed to the NICU upon request, following the recipient's parents' informed consent. The task should be completed based on the "first-in-first-out" principle from the storage. Frozen PDHM should be thawed by either fast defrosting the milk in a water bath at a temperature that does not exceed 37°C or by placing it under running lukewarm water. Thawing the milk in the microwave should be avoided, as it leads to a decrease in the IgA content of the milk. Refreezing milk should be avoided as it accelerates the hydrolysis of the triglycerides present in the milk.[8] Prior to use, the substance should be gently stirred while allowing it to reach room temperature in order to achieve a uniform combination. It is recommended to utilize the substance within 3–4 hours to avoid any potential contamination. It is preferable for preterm babies to receive PDHM from donors who were also preterm.[5] **Flowchart 5.3.1** illustrates the procedure of a human breastmilk bank.

Labeling and Record Keeping

Proper labeling at all levels is mandatory, from the sterile container for the collection of milk during donation, pooling vessel, and pasteurization container to storage containers. Labels should be water resistant and read clearly names and identification number of donors and dates of pasteurization batch numbers. Record keeping at all levels should be meticulous for the donor record file containing the consent form, donor's data and screening reports, and pasteurization batch files and for the PDHM disbursal record file, containing relevant data including the recipient consent form.

As the incubation period for most infections varies from a few weeks to 6 months and the appearance of symptoms is faster in infants and children, there seems to be no rationale

Flowchart 5.3.1: Summary of the process for a human milk bank.

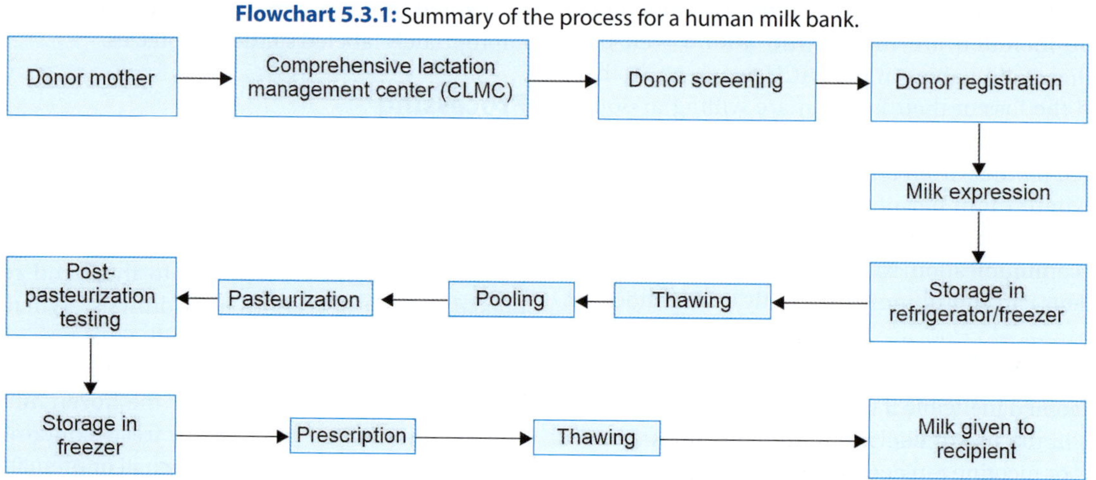

for keeping records beyond 5 years, unless one is working in an area where the milk kinship issue is of paramount importance. In India, the milk refrigeration record, milk pooling record, milk pasteurization record, dispensing record, and culture report records are preserved for a minimum period of 5 years.

ECONOMIC IMPLICATIONS

There has been a definite cost effectiveness of using banked human milk in NICUs observed in western countries largely by a reduction in the rate of NEC.[7] In a country, such as ours, the cost of running a milk bank with potential cost savings due to the reduction in NEC and sepsis rate and, ultimately, the duration of hospital stay has not been adequately evaluated, but given the high incidence of sepsis and a large burden of premature births, this intervention is likely to result in substantial saving for the nation.[9]

CONCLUSION

Artificial formula will never provide the broad range of benefits of human milk.[2] Given the high rate of preterm births in the country and the level of malnutrition that ensues in the postnatal growth of such babies after birth, there is an urgent need for establishing milk banks across the country, especially in the large NICUs of all hospitals. The authors are of the opinion that human milk banks be opened in all 707 (2018) districts of India to help in reducing neonatal mortality rate, infant mortality rate (IMR), and under-five mortality rate (U5MR). It only requires a pediatrician and microbiologist and very little budget.

ACKNOWLEDGMENTS

Dr Nida Asif, Senior Resident, Department of Pediatrics, CDSIMER, Dayananda Sagar University, Harohalli, Karnataka.

REFERENCES

1. Shrimpton R. (2017). Early initiation of breastfeeding, World Health Organization. [online] Available from https://www.who.int/tools/elena/commentary/early-breastfeeding [Last accessed October, 2024].
2. Duale A, Singh P, Al Khodor S. Breast milk: a meal worth having. Front Nutr. 2022;8:800927.
3. Child Health Division. (2017). National Guidelines on Lactation Management Centers in Public Health Facilities. Ministry of Health and Family Welfare, Government of India. [online] Available from https://nhm.gov.in/images/pdf/programmes/child-health/guidelines/Enhancing-optimal-IYCF-practices.pdf [Last accessed October, 2024].
4. Infant and Young Child Feeding Chapter, Indian Academy of Pediatric; Bharadva K, Tiwari S, Mishra S, Mukhopadhyay K, Yadav B, Agarwal RK, et al. Human milk banking guidelines. Indian Pediatr. 2014;51(6):469-74.
5. Wight NE. Donor human milk for preterm infants. J Perinatol. 2001;21(4):249-54.
6. Israel-Ballard K, Chantry C, Dewey K, Lönnerdal B, Sheppard H, Donovan R, et al. Viral, nutritional, and bacterial safety of flash-heated and pretoria-pasteurized breast milk to prevent mother-to-child transmission of HIV in resource-poor countries: a pilot study. J Acquir Immune Defic Syndr. 2005;40(2):175-81.
7. Arnold LD. The cost-effectiveness of using banked donor milk in the neonatal intensive care unit: prevention of necrotizing enterocolitis. J Hum Lact. 2002;18(2):172-7.
8. Morera Pons S, Castellote Bargallo AI, Lopez Sabater MC. Evaluation by high-performance liquid chromatography of the hydrolysis of human milk triacylglycerides during storage at low temperatures. J Chromatogr A. 1998;823(1-2):467-74.
9. Simmer K, Hartmann B. The known and unknowns of human milk banking. Early Hum Dev. 2009;85(11):701-4.

5.4 Malnutrition

Praveen Kumar

INTRODUCTION

Nutrition is important for ensuring growth, development, and immunity. *Malnutrition* is a generic term that includes abnormal nutritional status, that is, both *undernutrition* and *overnutrition*. However, in children, malnutrition is interchangeably used for undernutrition, as this is more common than overnutrition or obesity. Malnutrition remains one of the most common causes of morbidity and mortality among children. Strong evidence exists on the synergism between undernutrition and child mortality due to common childhood illnesses, including diarrhea, acute respiratory infections, malaria, and measles.

CLASSIFICATION

For several decades, the term *protein-energy malnutrition (PEM)* was being used to describe undernutrition and was broadly divided into two types—*Kwashiorkor*, which occurs due to a gross deficiency of proteins with reasonable intake of calories and is characterized by edema, and *marasmus,* which occurs due to inadequate intake of protein and calories and is characterized by emaciation.

Malnutrition in children <5 years of age is most commonly identified by the measurement of weight and length/height and then plotting it on a growth chart and determining the standard deviation (SD) as compared to the World Health Organization (WHO) growth standard median for age and gender. It is the most commonly used method for determining nutritional status. In a normally growing child, serial recordings of these parameters on a growth chart over time should yield a curve parallel to one of the standard growth curves of their growth trajectory. When the child's growth parameters falter, serial recordings on a growth chart will no longer be parallel to the standard growth curves.

By using anthropometric indices [weight-for-age (WFA), length or height-for-age (HFA), and weight-for-length/height], nutritional status may be graded into four categories that are being used internationally to classify malnutrition, as summarized in **Table 5.4.1**:[1]

1. Normal
2. Underweight
3. Wasted
4. Stunted

Underweight is defined as WFA <2 SD below the median for age and gender as compared to WHO growth standards 2006. When it is <–3 SD for age and gender, it is known as severely underweight. Underweight can result from acute or chronic malnutrition.

If weight for length/height is <–2 SD, then it is known as *wasted*, while <–3 SD is known as *severely wasted*. Wasting/severe wasting indicates acute malnutrition, that is, nutritional deficiencies of short duration, and has the highest risk of mortality among all forms of malnutrition.

Stunting, an indicator of linear growth retardation, results from failure to receive adequate nutrition over a long period and is defined as HFA <–2 SD.

The WHO has recommended the use of combined criteria for the identification of children with acute malnutrition as summarized in **Table 5.4.2.**[2]

Measuring mid-upper arm circumference (MUAC) and looking for bilateral pitting pedal edema are other methods

TABLE 5.4.1: World Health Organization classification of nutritional status based on the combined use of growth indicators.

	Growth indicator		
Standard deviation (SD) score	***Height/length for age***	***Weight for age***	***Weight for height/length***
+2 SD to –2 SD	Normal	Normal	Normal
<–2 SD to –3 SD	Stunted	Moderate underweight	Wasted or moderate acute malnutrition
<–3 SD	Severely stunted	Severely underweight	Severely wasted or severe acute malnutrition (SAM)

Source: World Health Organization Child Growth Standards and the Identification of Severe Acute Malnutrition in Infants and Children: Joint Statement by the World Health Organization and the United Nations Children's Fund. Geneva: World Health Organization; 2009.

TABLE 5.4.2: Criteria for identification of children with acute malnutrition (wasting/severe wasting).

Age in completed months	***Nutritional status***	***Criteria***
0–5 months (infants under 6 months)	Wasting/moderate acute malnutrition	Weight for length <–2 SD and no edema
	Severe wasting/severe acute malnutrition (SAM)	Weight for length <–3 SD* and/or bilateral pitting pedal edema†
6–59 months	Wasting/moderate acute malnutrition	Weight for length < –2 SD to –3 SD and/or mid-upper arm circumference 11.5 –12.4 cm and no edema
	Severe wasting/severe acute malnutrition (SAM)	Weight for length/height <–3 SD* and/or mid-upper arm circumference 11.5 –12.4 cm and/or bilateral pitting pedal edema*

*In emergency settings when length/height measurement is not possible, very severe wasting may be used as one of the criteria. Very severe wasting is also used to identify severe wasting in infants with length <45 cm.
†Edema without a known cause of edema like congestive heart failure, nephrotic syndrome, etc.
(SD: standard deviation)
Source: Guideline: Updates on the Management of Severe Acute Malnutrition in Infants and Children. Geneva: World Health Organization; 2013.

of identifying children with acute malnutrition. MUAC measurement is very useful in community settings where length/height measurements are not feasible.

PREVALENCE OF WASTING AND SEVERE WASTING IN INDIA

As per the National Family Health Survey-5 (NFHS-5), the prevalence of underweight, stunting, and wasting is 32.1%, 35.5%, and 19.3%, respectively, among under-5 children, while 7.7% of children are severely wasted [severe acute malnutrition (SAM)].[3] Wasting and severe wasting are highest in the first 6 months of life **(Fig. 5.4.1)**.

MANAGEMENT OF CHILDREN WITH WASTING OR UNDERWEIGHT

All children with wasting/moderate acute malnutrition or who are underweight should be assessed for their feeding practices and underlying medical conditions. If any underlying medical condition is identified (e.g., tuberculosis, cleft palate, congenital heart disease, infections), they should be treated appropriately along with nutritional rehabilitation. Mothers and caregivers should be counseled to give feeds in an adequate amount and frequency that have adequate energy density and are hygienic. They should also be counseled for improving food diversity and feeding actively. They should be followed up after 15 days for ensuring improvement.

MANAGEMENT OF SEVERE WASTING OR SEVERE ACUTE MALNUTRITION

As described earlier, children with SAM usually have a significantly higher risk of mortality if they develop medical complications such as pneumonia, diarrhea, malaria, and measles. Malnutrition and infections make a vicious cycle; that is, malnutrition predisposes the child to infection and infection makes the child more malnourished. To break this vicious cycle, it is important to prevent, identify, and treat malnutrition early.

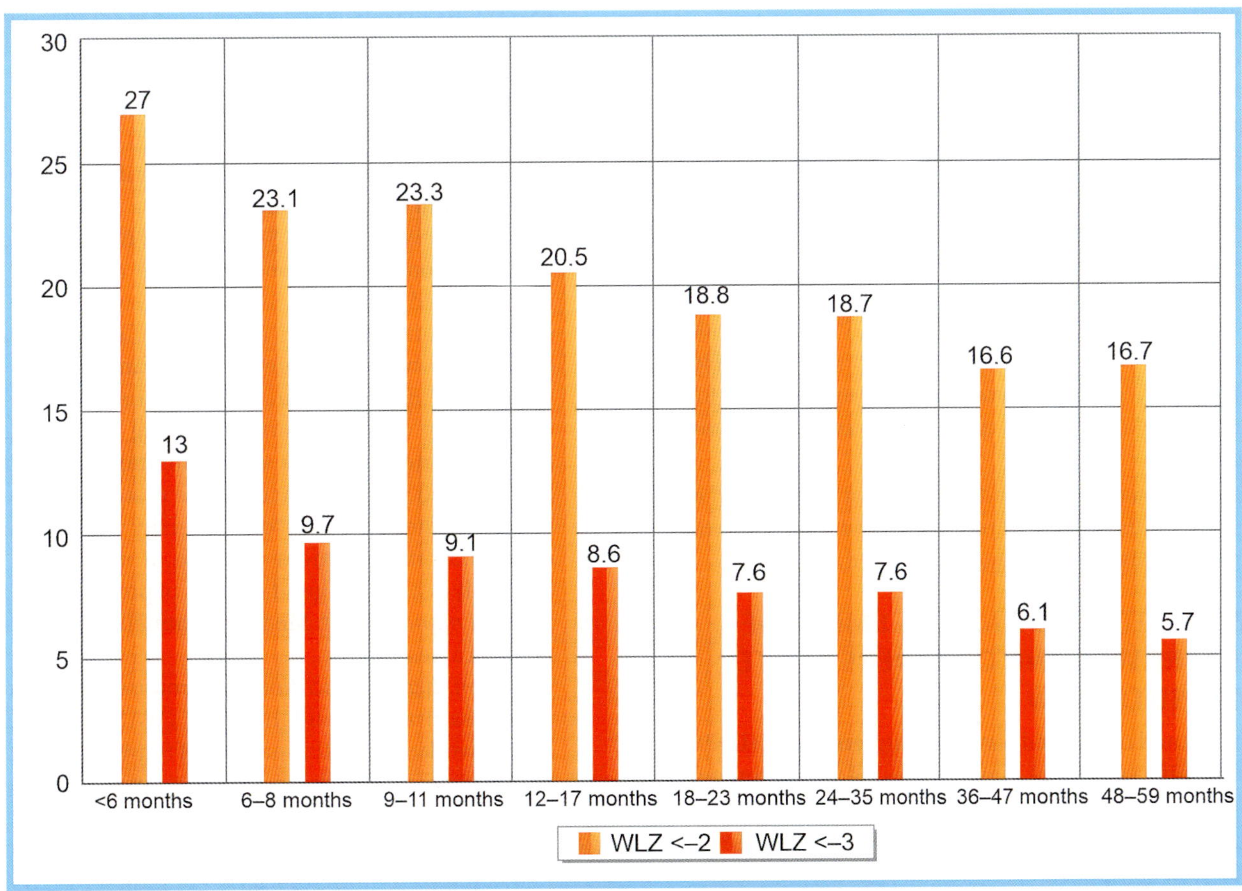

Fig. 5.4.1: Prevalence of wasting/severe wasting in different age group children. (WLZ: weight for length standard deviation score)
Source: National Family Health Survey (NFHS-5) 2019–2021. Government of India: Ministry of Health and Family Welfare; 2022.

METABOLIC AND PHYSIOLOGICAL CHANGES IN SEVERE MALNUTRITION (REDUCTIVE ADAPTATION)

Children with SAM have several metabolic and physiological changes that happen due to nutritional deficiencies, which is known as *reductive adaptation*.[4] In a severely malnourished child, as the vital systems of the body begin to slow down, energy is conserved by reducing basal metabolism by slowing protein turnover, slowing the sodium and potassium pumps in cell membranes and reducing their number. The functional reservoir of organs is also reduced. Important changes are summarized as follows:

- The liver has less reserve and is less able to make glucose, which increases the risk of *hypoglycemia and hypothermia* if they are not fed for a long duration.
- The kidneys are not able to handle excess fluid and sodium. So, excess fluid can quickly build up in the circulation with the *risk of fluid overload and congestive heart failure*.
- The heart is smaller and weaker and has reduced output. If children with SAM are given the fluid volume recommended for normal children, they are not able to handle, causing excess fluid in the circulation, stress to the heart, and risk of *heart failure*.
- The gut produces less acid and smaller amounts of enzymes, so they are not able to digest food fully. *Villi become flattened and motility is reduced* and bacteria may colonize the stomach and small bowel, damaging the mucosa and deconjugating bile acids.
- The *sodium-potassium pump is slow*, which leads to leak of sodium, causing excess body sodium. Potassium leaks out of cells and is lost in urine, contributing to *hypokalemia*.
- *Reduction of muscle mass* is accompanied by loss of intracellular nutrients and smaller reserves of muscle glycogen.
- Red cell mass is also reduced, liberating iron. *Free iron promotes the growth of pathogens* and the production of free radicals, which damage cell membranes.

MODALITIES FOR MANAGEMENT OF SEVERE WASTING OR SEVERE ACUTE MALNUTRITION

The WHO and the United Nations Children's Fund (UNICEF), in their joint statement, have suggested the following two modalities for the management of children with SAM:

1. *Community-based care* for children with SAM without medical complications and good appetite
2. *Facility/hospital-based care* for SAM children with medical complications and/or poor appetite.

Community-based Management

About 85–90% of children with SAM do not have medical complications and can be treated in their communities without being admitted to a health facility. Therefore, it is essential to categorize children with SAM into "complicated" and "uncomplicated" cases based on the presence or absence of medical complications and appetite.

Community-based Management of SAM

The Ministry of Women and Child Development and the Ministry of Health have jointly launched a protocol for the community-based management of malnourished children on October 10, 2023.[5] Management has been divided into the following 10 steps:

1. *Growth monitoring:* To identify children with SAM by measuring weight and length/height and determining their nutritional status by entering measurements in the Pradhan Mantri Overarching Scheme for Holistic Nutrition (POSHAN) Tracker
2. *Appetite test for children with SAM:* Identified SAM children are given food items by anganwadi workers (AWW) to check whether the child is accepting food or has a poor appetite. If the child is not accepting food, the child has a poor appetite.
3. *Medical assessment:* Auxiliary nurse midwife (ANM) during Village Health, Sanitation, and Nutrition days performs a medical assessment to identify SAM children with medical complications.
4. *Deciding level of care:* SAM children with medical complications and/or poor appetite are referred to facility-based care, while SAM children without medical complications and good appetite are enrolled in the community-based management program.
5. *Nutritional management:* Nutritional management is by ensuring adequate nutrition using a combination of take-home rations as supplementary foods and a home-based culturally acceptable diet. The guideline also advocates ensuring food diversity while planning nutritional management and use of milk, eggs, and culturally acceptable good sources of protein.
6. *Medical management:* Medical treatment is done as per medical assessment.
7. *Nutrition, health education, and counseling,* including water, sanitation, and hygiene (WASH) practices: Health workers sensitize parents of SAM children about appropriate diet, including the importance of dietary diversity, safe drinking water, and hygiene.
8. *Visit by AWW and referral:* Each SAM child enrolled in a community-based program is visited by AWW for monitoring their progress weekly during the first month of enrolment and then fortnightly.

9. *Duration of monitoring:* As per the guideline, all SAM children will be monitored till 6 years of their age.
10. *Follow-up care:* During each follow-up, the weight and length/height of enrolled children will be measured and entered in the POSHAN Tracker.

Ready-to-use Therapeutic Food

The WHO and the UNICEF have recommended ready-to-use therapeutic food (RUTF) for the management of children with SAM.[6] Conventionally, the ingredients used are milk powder, vegetable oil, peanuts, sugar, minerals, and vitamins. The absence of water in RUTF gives them protection against bacterial contamination and ease of storage.

However, RUTF is not approved in India, as the evidence on the efficacy of RUTF comes from studies done in Africa. Pilot studies from India did not show much benefit over augmented local food items. There is also better sustained recovery when children are managed on locally available food items.

Facility-based Management of Severe Acute Malnutrition

Indications for inpatient care are summarized in **Box 5.4.1**.

BOX 5.4.1: Indications for inpatient treatment in children with SAM.

If children with SAM have any of the following medical complications:
- Presence of any emergency signs (severe respiratory distress, coma, convulsion, and shock)
- Poor feeding or loss of appetite
- Presence of edema
- Severe pneumonia
- Pneumonia (fast breathing and/or chest indrawing) and oxygen saturation <94% on room air
- Very severe febrile disease
- Diarrhea with some or severe dehydration
- Dysentery
- Severe persistent diarrhea (diarrhea for 14 days or more and dehydration)
- Severe anemia (hemoglobin <4 g/dL or hemoglobin 4–6 g/dL with signs of cardio-pulmonary decompensation)
- Hypothermia (axillary temperature <35°C or <95°F)
- High-grade fever (axillary temperature ≥38.5°C or ≥101.3°F)
- Hypoglycemia
- Severe complicated measles or postmeasles state
- Mastoiditis
- Extensive skin lesions or eye lesions
- All children with history or clinical signs suggesting secondary causes like recurrent pneumonia, hemoglobinopathies (thalassemia and sickle cell anemia), tuberculosis, HIV, congenital anomalies like cleft palate or congenital heart disease, abnormal tone, history of recurrent seizures, jaundice, or abnormally protruded abdomen

(HIV: human immunodeficiency virus; SAM: severe acute malnutrition)
Source: Facility Based Care of Severe Acute Malnutrition. India: National Health Mission. Ministry of Health and Family Welfare; 2013.

Sick children with SAM are predisposed to metabolic derangements and infections and due to reductive adaptation, they do not manifest typical signs and symptoms of infections. Hence, all admitted children should undergo basic investigations to rule out common complications and infections **(Table 5.4.3)**.

The WHO has recommended 10 steps of management for children with SAM and medical complications that take care of their metabolic and physiological changes.[8] Management is broadly divided into two phases—stabilization and rehabilitation **(Table 5.4.4)**.

Step 1: Treat or Prevent Hypoglycemia

Children with SAM are at risk of hypoglycemia. Hypoglycemia in a child with SAM is defined as blood glucose <3 mmol/L (<54 mg/dL). If hypoglycemia is not prevented or detected early, these children may become lethargic, unconscious, or develop convulsion. Treatment is as follows:

- *Hypoglycemia without convulsion/unconsciousness:* Give 50 mL of 10% glucose or sucrose orally or by a nasogastric (NG) tube immediately, followed by a starter diet (F-75) (1/4th of 2 hourly feed volume) every 30 minutes for the first 2 hours and thereafter 2-hourly feeds. More details about F-75/starter diet are given in Step 7.
- *Hypoglycemia with unconsciousness, lethargy, or convulsions:* Give 5 mL/kg of 10% glucose intravenously (IV), followed by 10% glucose or sucrose 50 mL orally. Start feeding F-75 diet (one-fourth of the 2-hourly feed volume) every 30 minutes for the first 2 hours and thereafter 2-hourly feeds to prevent further episodes of hypoglycemia.

Step 2: Treat or Prevent Hypothermia

Hypothermia in a child with SAM is defined as axillary temperature below 35°C or rectal temperature below 35.5°C. In children with SAM, less heat is generated due to a low-basal metabolic rate and they are at high risk of losing heat due to a lack of insulating fat and a higher surface area per kg body weight.

If the child is hypothermic, rewarm using one of the following techniques:

- *Kangaroo technique:* Skin-to-skin contact
- Overhead warmer or radiant heater

In case of severe hypothermia (rectal temperature < 32°C), give warm humidified oxygen, 10% glucose bolus (5 mL/kg), and IV maintenance fluid till the child's general condition is stabilized.

Hypothermia and hypoglycemia often occur together. Always look for hypoglycemia in a child with hypothermia and vice versa.

TABLE 5.4.3: Investigations for children with SAM requiring inpatient care.

Laboratory investigations	*Details*
Blood glucose (BG)	At admission, during the stabilization phase, if the child becomes hypothermic or lethargic during the rehabilitation phase
Hemoglobin (Hb) or packed cell volume (PCV) in all children	• Hb with total and differential leukocyte counts (TLC, DLC) in all cases • Peripheral smear if the child has anemia/palmar pallor
Serum electrolytes	Sodium, potassium, and calcium (whenever possible)
Screening for infections	• TLC, DLC, and blood culture (wherever available) • Urine routine and microscopy, and culture (wherever indicated and available) • Stool examination for ova/cysts • Chest X-ray

Additional investigations to identify secondary causes:
- Screening for HIV (recurrent infections, presence of oral thrush, lymphadenopathy, unexplained death of parents, persistent diarrhea, parotid enlargement, etc.)
- Rapid diagnostic tests (RDT) or peripheral smear for malaria, if admitted with fever and malaria is a possibility
- Screening for tuberculosis: Gastric aspirate for acid-fast bacillus (AFB) and nucleic acid amplification test (NAAT) as per National Tuberculosis Elimination Program (NTEP) guidelines
- Neuroimaging in children with neurological diseases
- Workup for thalassemia and sickle cell anemia when clinically indicated.
  Workup for celiac disease in high-prevalence areas, particularly if the child has recurrent/chronic diarrhea, abdominal distension, and family history of celiac disease

(HIV: human immunodeficiency virus; SAM: severe acute malnutrition)

TABLE 5.4.4: Ten steps of facility-based management of children with SAM.

		Stabilization phase		*Rehabilitation*
Steps		*1–3 days*	*3–7 days*	*2–6 weeks*
1	Treat/prevent hypoglycemia	——→		
2	Treat/prevent hypothermia	——→		
3	Treat/prevent dehydration	——→		
4	Correct electrolyte imbalance	————	——→	
5	Treat infections	————	——→	
6	Correct micronutrient deficiencies Iron supplementation	———— No iron	————	——→ With iron
7	Start cautious feeding	————	——→	
8	Achieve catch-up growth	——→		
9	Provide sensory stimulation and structured play therapy	————	————	——→
10	Prepare for discharge and follow-up	————	——→	

(SAM: severe acute malnutrition)

Source: Ashworth A, Khanum, S, Jackson A, Schofield EC. Guidelines for the Inpatient Treatment of Severely Malnourished Children. Geneva: World Health Organization; 2003.

Step 3: Treat or Prevent Dehydration

Diarrhea is a common morbidity with which children with SAM are admitted. It is difficult to determine dehydration status correctly in a child with SAM, as the usual signs of dehydration (such as lethargy and sunken eyes) are unreliable in these children. Hence, all children with SAM, whether they have some or severe dehydration, should be rehydrated orally and slowly over 10–12 hours unless they present with shock. During rehydration, all children should be closely monitored with weight, pulse rate, respiratory rate, and signs of overhydration. They should be rehydrated with oral rehydration solution (ORS) 5 mL/kg every 30 minutes during the first 2 hours and then 5–10 mL/kg every alternate hour with a starter (F-75) diet for 10–12 hours. The amount offered in this range is based on the child's willingness to drink and the amount of ongoing losses.

The WHO-recommended commercial ORS for children with SAM (ReSoMal) is not available in India. Wherever hygienic preparation is possible, modified ORS for SAM may be prepared by dissolving one sachet (1 L) of low-osmolarity oral rehydration salt, 50 g of glucose/sugar, and 45 mL of potassium chloride syrup in additional water to make a total volume of 2 L in place of 1 L. Modified ORS will have a composition closer to ReSoMal. In case modified ORS preparation is not possible or the child has profuse watery diarrhea or cholera is suspected, use low osmolarity ORS without any modification.

Management of children with SAM who present with diarrhea and shock is summarized in **Flowchart 5.4.1**.

Step 4: Correct Electrolyte Imbalance

All children with SAM who are managed with locally prepared starter and catch-up diets should be given potassium supplements (3–4 mEq/kg/day) and intramuscular (IM) magnesium sulfate 50% once (0.3 mL/kg) up to a maximum of 2 mL on day 1 followed by 0.2–0.3 mL/kg/day orally with feeds till discharge or up to 14 days.

Step 5: Give Antibiotics

Majority of children with SAM have an underlying infection and in spite of infection, the usual signs of infection, such as fever, are often absent. Hence, all children with SAM should be given broad-spectrum antibiotics. Uncomplicated children should receive oral amoxicillin while admitted children should receive a combination of ampicillin or third-generation cephalosporin with aminoglycosides.

Step 6: Give Micronutrients

Micronutrient deficiency is common in children with SAM. Commercial F-75/F-100 and RUTF have these micronutrients premixed. Most children with SAM in India are managed with locally prepared starter and catch-up diets, which are not able to meet their micronutrient requirements. Hence, they should be given a dose of vitamin A on admission unless they have received it during the previous month. Children with clinical signs of vitamin A deficiency should be given three doses of vitamin A on days 1, 2, and 14. These children should also be supplemented with multivitamins (containing vitamins A, C, D, E, and B_{12}) for at least 2 weeks at twice the recommended dietary allowances (RDA); folic acid 5 mg on day 1, then 1 mg/day; elemental zinc 2 mg/kg/day; and copper 0.3 mg/kg/day. Iron should be added only in the rehabilitative phase after 2 days of the child being on a

Flowchart 5.4.1: Fluid therapy in a child with severe acute malnutrition and shock.[9]

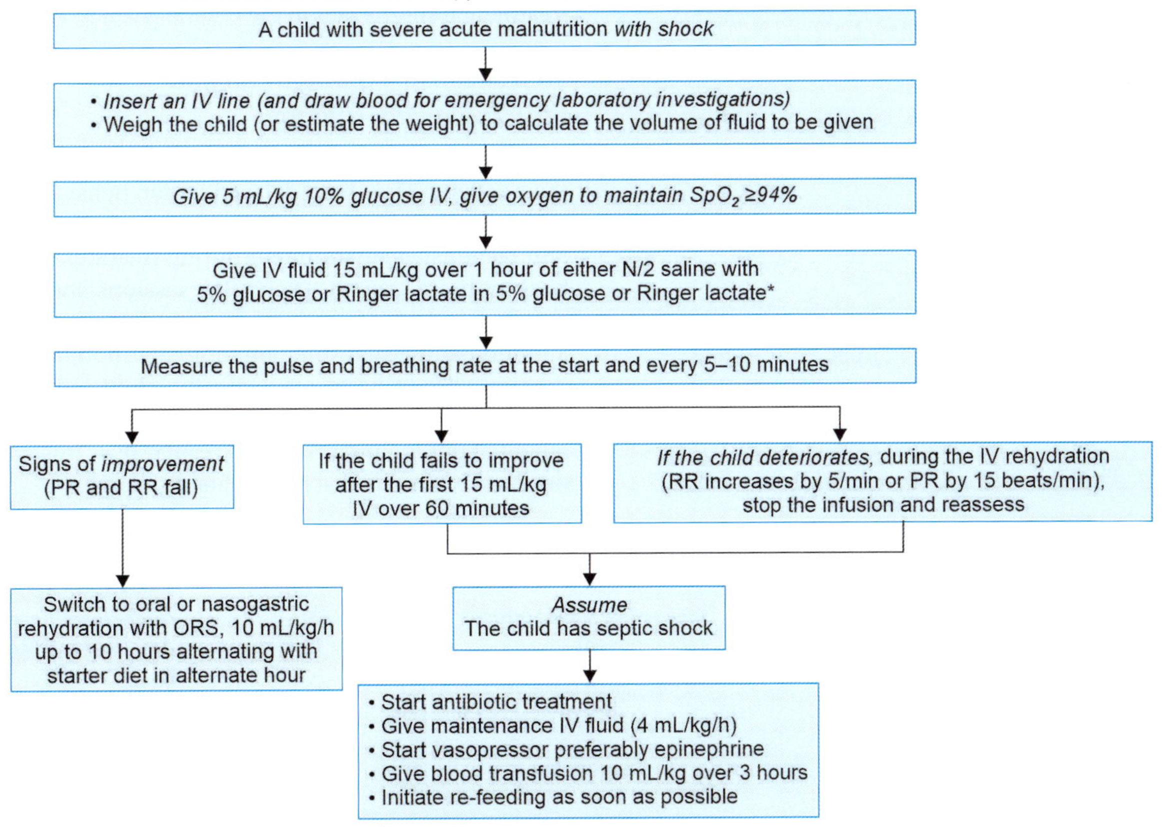

(IV: intravenously; ORS: oral rehydration solution; PR: pulse rate; RR: respiratory rate)
*If profuse diarrhea or suspected cholera, repeat 15 mL/kg of IV fluid.

catch-up diet. Emerging evidence also indicates that a large number of these children are also vitamin B_{12} deficient and need therapeutic supplementation.[10]

Blood transfusion, preferably packed cell transfusion, is indicated in children with SAM if hemoglobin (Hb) is <4 g/dL or 4–6 g/dL with cardiorespiratory distress.

Step 7: Start Cautious Feeding

Children with SAM cannot tolerate usual amounts of protein, sodium, or high amounts of fat initially. The WHO recommends F-75 therapeutic diet to be used during the stabilization phase, which provides 75 calories per 100 mL, has low protein (0.9 g/100 mL), and provides the required micronutrients **(Table 5.4.5)**. During stabilization, give 130 mL/kg (100 mL/kg in children with SAM with +++ edema) divided into 12 feeds (i.e., give every 2 hours).

When commercial F-75 therapeutic is not available, locally prepared therapeutic feed starter diet may be prepared **(Table 5.4.6)** and given. However, these children need electrolytes and micronutrient supplementation as described in Steps 4 and 6. The child is gradually shifted to larger, less frequent feeds (every 3 or 4 hours). In case the child is very weak, has mouth ulcers that prevent drinking, or is not able to finish 80% of the feeds, an NG tube should be used for feeding.

TABLE 5.4.5: Composition of World Health Organization recommended F-75 and F-100 diets.

Constituents per 100 mL	*F-75*	*F-100*
Energy (calories)	75	100
Protein (g)	0.9	2.9
Lactose (g)	1.3	3.0
Potassium (mmol)	3.6	5.9
Sodium (mmol)	0.6	1.9
Magnesium (mmol)	0.43	0.73
Zinc (mg)	2.0	2.3
Copper (mg)	0.25	0.25
Osmolality (mOsm)	333	419

Step 8: Achieve Catch-up Growth

F-100 diet is the recommended feed to be used during rehabilitation, which provides 100 kcal of energy and 2.9 g of protein per 100 mL **(Table 5.4.5)**. When commercial F-100 is not available, a locally prepared catch-up diet **(Table 5.4.6)** is used along with electrolyte and micronutrient supplementation as described in Steps 4 and 6.

The following signs indicate readiness to move from F-75/starter diet to F-100/catch-up diet:

- Return of appetite (finishes >80% of the 4-hourly F-75 diet)
- No episodes of hypoglycemia or hypothermia
- Edema starts disappearing

Transition usually takes 3 days, during which catch-up/F-100 diet should be given according to the schedule given in **Box 5.4.2**. The goal is to achieve a calorie intake of 150–220 kcal/kg/day and protein of 3.5–5.5 g/kg/day.

Weight should be recorded daily to monitor the progress:

- *Good weight gain:* 10 g/kg/day or more
- *Moderate weight gain:* 5–10 g/kg/day
- *Poor weight gain:* <5 g/kg/day

A child with SAM is said to be nonresponder to the treatment if she/he falls in the criteria given in **Table 5.4.7**.

Step 9: Sensory Stimulation and Structured Play Therapy

As children become malnourished, they gradually reduce their activity. They have delayed motor, behavioral, mental, and emotional development. A cheerful, cordial, stimulating, and responsive environment during treatment encourages healthy brain growth. Daily play sessions should include social, emotional, language, cognitive, motor development, auditory, and visual stimulation. In addition to group play, the aim should be to play with the child individually for 30 minutes, two sessions each day. Also, mothers should be taught about the importance of regular play sessions, which need to be continued at home after discharge.

TABLE 5.4.6: Constituents of locally prepared starter and catch-up diet.[7]

Contents	*Starter (F-75 diet) (cereal-based)*	*Starter (F-75 diet) (non-cereal-based)*	*Catch-up (F-100) diet (cereal-based) Amount for 100 mL*	*Catch-up (F-100) diet (non-cereal-based) Amount for 100 mL*
Cow's milk or full-cream dairy milk	30 mL	30 mL	75 mL	90 mL
Sugar	7 g	10 g	2.5 g	7.5 g
Vegetable oil	2 g	2 g	2 g	2 g
Puffed rice	3.5 g	–	7 g	–
Water to make	100 mL	100 mL	100 mL	100 mL

BOX 5.4.2: Schedule of transition from F-75/starter diet to F-100/catch-up diet.

- *First 48 hours (2 days):* Give catch-up (F-100) diet every 4 hours in the same amount as last given F-75 diet
- *On the third day:* Increase each feed by 10 mL if the child is finishing feeds up to a maximum of 220 mL/kg. If the child does not finish a feed, offer the same amount at the next feed
- Encourage the mother to breastfeed between feeds
- After the transition, F-100 diet is given in the range of 150–220 mL/kg according to the current weight of the child

TABLE 5.4.7: Failure to respond [nutritional rehabilitation center (NRC)/pediatric facility].

Criteria	*Approximate time after admission*
Failure to regain appetite	Day 4
Failure to start losing edema	Day 4
Edema still present	Day 10
Failure to gain at least an average of 5 g/kg/day for 3 successive days after feeding freely on a catch-up diet even after treatment of 4 weeks	

TABLE 5.4.8: Discharge criteria for children with SAM requiring inpatient care.

Child	*Mother/caregiver*
• Edema has resolved • Child has average weight gain of ≥5 g/kg/day over the last 3 consecutive days • All infections and other medical complications have been treated • Immunization is updated • Child is eating an adequate amount of food	• Knows how to prepare energy-dense foods and how to feed the child • Knows how to give prescribed medications, vitamins, folic acid, and iron at home • Knows how to make appropriate toys and play with the child • Knows how to give home treatment for diarrhea, fever, and acute respiratory infections and how to recognize danger signs for which medical assistance must be sought • Follow-up plan is discussed and understood

(SAM: severe acute malnutrition)

Step 10: Prepare for Discharge and Follow-up

Mothers/caregivers should be involved in all aspects of the management of children with SAM. It is very important to teach mothers/caregivers the preparation of energy-dense food; feed children hygienically and actively; bathe and change clothes; and play with children, supervise play sessions, and make toys. Food items demonstrated should be culturally acceptable and made of locally available items that mothers can afford and prepare at home.

Children should be discharged from inpatient care when they fulfill discharge criteria **(Table 5.4.8)**.

Before discharge, immunization should be updated and treatment for helminthic infections should be given as 200 mg albendazole for children aged 12–23 months and 400 mg for older children.

Follow-up plan: Follow-up should be done periodically to document sustained recovery and identify cases with relapse.

PREVENTION

Key interventions to prevent the development of acute malnutrition include nutritional care of adolescent girls and pregnant mothers so that babies are born with a normal birth weight. Appropriate breastfeeding and complementary feeding practices, timely immunization, adherence to WASH practices, care during illnesses, and improving food security at household levels are needed to prevent malnutrition.

REFERENCES

1. World Health Organization. WHO Child Growth Standards and the Identification of Severe Acute Malnutrition in Infants and Children: Joint Statement by the World Health Organization and the United Nations Children's Fund. Geneva: World Health Organization; 2009. [online] Available from https://www.ncbi.nlm.nih.gov/books/NBK200775. [Last accessed October, 2024].
2. World Health Organization. Guideline: Updates on the Management of Severe Acute Malnutrition in Infants and Children. Geneva: World Health Organization; 2013.
3. National Family Health Survey (NFHS-5) 2019–21. Government of India: Ministry of Health and Family Welfare. [online] Available from https://mohfw.gov.in/sites/default/files/NFHS-5_Phase-II_0.pdf [Last accessed October, 2024].
4. World Health Organization. Management of Severe Malnutrition: A Manual for Physicians and Other Senior Health Workers. Geneva: World Health Organization; 1999.
5. Ministry of Women and Child Development: Protocol for Management of Malnutrition in Children. Ministry of Women and Child Development, Government of India; 2023.
6. Community-Based Management of Severe Acute Malnutrition. A Joint Statement by the World Health Organization, World Food Programme, United Nations Standing Committee on Nutrition, United Nations Children's Fund. Geneva: World Health Organization/World Food Programme/United Nations Standing Committee on Nutrition/United Nations Children's Fund; 2007.
7. Facility Based Care of Severe Acute Malnutrition. India: National Health Mission, Ministry of Health and Family Welfare; 2013. [online] Available from https://www.nhm.gov.in/images/pdf/programmes/child-health/IEC-materials/PARTICIPANT-MANUAL_FBCSA-Malnutrition.pdf. [Last accessed October, 2023].
8. Ashworth A, Khanum, S, Jackson A, Schofield EC. Guidelines for the Inpatient Treatment of Severely Malnourished Children. Geneva: World Health Organization; 2003. [online] Available from https://apps.who.int/iris/handle/10665/42724. [Last accessed October,2024].
9. World Health Organization. Updated Guideline: Pediatric Emergency Triage, Assessment and Treatment. Geneva: World Health Organization; 2016.
10. Chandra J, Kumar P. Anemia in severe acute malnutrition: ten steps of management need to be fine-tuned. Indian J Pediatr. 2023;90(11):1061-4.

5.5 Water-soluble Vitamins

Dheeraj Shah

INTRODUCTION

Water-soluble vitamins include all vitamins in the B-complex group [thiamine (vitamin B_1), riboflavin (vitamin B_2), niacin (vitamin B_3), pyridoxine (vitamin B_6), cobalamin (vitamin B_{12}), folate, biotin, pantothenic acid, choline, and inositol] and ascorbic acid (vitamin C). These vitamins act as coenzymes in many interrelated metabolic pathways. As these vitamins are water-soluble and heat-labile, large amounts are lost from the ingredients, if they are repeatedly washed, and when the cooking water is discarded. These vitamins are not stored for prolonged periods in the body; significant toxicities at therapeutic doses are uncommon.[1]

VITAMIN B COMPLEX

Thiamine

The active form of this vitamin acts as a cofactor for enzymes involved in carbohydrate catabolism, nucleic acid synthesis, and nerve conduction.

Dietary Sources

Rice, wheat, legumes, fortified flours, fish, lean meat, and poultry are good sources of thiamine. Polished rice is depleted of thiamine. It can be retained in rice by steaming the rice in the husk before milling (parboiling).[2]

Deficiency State

Malnutrition, gastrointestinal (GI) disorders (such as malabsorption, blind loops, and short bowel), and chronic debilitating conditions (such as malignancies) are common causes of deficiency. Fatigue, irritability, poor mental concentration, anorexia, and nausea are the early manifestations of deficiency. A full-fledged deficiency state *(beriberi)* manifests as peripheral neuropathy, resulting in tingling, paresthesia, leg cramps, hyporeflexia, ataxia, and lack of coordination. Cardiac manifestations include cardiomegaly and congestive heart failure (CHF). Central nervous system (CNS) involvement occurs late in the disease and is characterized by psychic disturbances, optic atrophy, hoarseness, raised intracranial pressure, and coma. Thiamine-responsive megaloblastic anemia and biotin-thiamine-responsive basal ganglia disease are genetic disorders of thiamine metabolism where high doses of thiamine provide therapeutic benefit.[3]

Treatment

Oral administration of thiamine is sufficient in mild-to-moderate deficiency states. Children with cardiac and CNS manifestations should be given 10–50 mg of thiamine intramuscularly (IM) or intravenously (IV) daily for the first week, followed by 3–5 mg/day orally for 6–12 weeks. Most children show dramatic improvement to oral or parenteral thiamine.[2,4]

Riboflavin

Majority of this vitamin in tissues is found in the form of coenzymes flavin adenine dinucleotide and flavin mononucleotide, which participate in oxidation–reduction reactions in numerous metabolic pathways and in energy production via the respiratory chain.

Dietary Sources

Dietary sources include milk and its products, eggs, fortified cereals and grains, and liver. Vegan diets are poor sources.

Deficiency State

Ariboflavinosis is characterized by glossitis, angular cheilosis, keratitis, conjunctivitis, photophobia, corneal vascularization, and seborrheic dermatitis. Malnutrition, malabsorption, and GI infections commonly precipitate the deficiency.

Treatment

Oral administration of riboflavin (3–10 mg/day) as a part of vitamin B-complex mix rapidly corrects the deficiency and controls the associated symptoms.[4]

Niacin

Niacin is a component of the coenzymes nicotinamide adenine dinucleotide (NAD) and nicotinamide adenine dinucleotide phosphate (NADP), which are important for many redox reactions involved in carbohydrate metabolism, fatty acid synthesis, and steroid synthesis.

Dietary Sources

Niacin is rapidly absorbed from the stomach or the intestine. Good sources are fish, meat, cereals, legumes, milk, and green leafy vegetables. Predominantly, maize-eating populations suffer from niacin deficiency as maize is a poor source of tryptophan, a precursor of niacin.

Deficiency State

The classical triad of niacin deficiency (*pellagra*) is diarrhea, dermatitis, and dementia. Certain inborn errors of tryptophan metabolism (carcinoid syndrome and Hartnup disease) are also associated with niacin deficiency. Skin lesions of pellagra start as symmetric erythematous areas, resembling sunburn. These lesions are distributed on hands and feet in a "glove-and-stocking" pattern and are sometimes present over the neck (Casal necklace). Infants and young children often do not develop classical deficiency signs and present with irritability, fatigue, anorexia, and scaly skin.

Treatment

Oral administration of niacin (50–200 mg/day) as a part of vitamin B-complex mix is indicated for pellagra. Severe cases may require IV administration. Sun exposure should be avoided during active skin lesions, and soothing agents should be applied.[2,4]

Pyridoxine

Pyridoxine (vitamin B_6) is a component of pyridoxine hydrochloride, pyridoxal, and pyridoxamine cofactors in the metabolism of carbohydrates, amino acids, steroids, and nucleic acids.

Dietary Sources

Poultry, meat, fish, fortified cereals, and bananas are good sources of pyridoxine. Drugs inhibiting pyridoxine activity (e.g., isoniazid, oral contraceptives, penicillamine, phenytoin, and carbamazepine) may precipitate the deficiency.

Deficiency State

Early symptoms or signs are listlessness, irritability, and vomiting. Seizures, failure to thrive, skin lesions, and microcytic anemia may occur in severe deficiency states. Pyridoxine-dependent epilepsy is a genetic defect of pyridoxine metabolism, which needs high doses of pyridoxine for its treatment.

Treatment

Oral administration of 10–100 mg/day is sufficient for correcting the deficiency and dependency. Pyridoxine 100 mg IM or IV is administered in the case of seizures. Treatment should be followed by ensuring adequate dietary consumption.[2,4]

Folate and Vitamin B_{12}

Folate is involved in a variety of reactions involved in amino acid and nucleotide metabolism. Vitamin B_{12} (cobalamin) is required as a cofactor for methyl group transfer from a folic acid cofactor to form methionine. The unmethylated folate cofactor then participates in single-carbon reactions for nucleic acid synthesis. Thus, some B_{12} and folic deficiency symptoms are similar. The risk of folate and vitamin B_{12} deficiency increases during periods of rapid growth such as infancy and adolescence. Severe malnutrition and malabsorptive states also predispose to deficiency of both nutrients.

Dietary Sources

Legumes, fortified cereals, citrus fruits, and leafy vegetables are good sources of folate. On the other hand, vitamin B_{12} is found only in foods from animal sources. Organ meats, sea foods, egg yolk, fish, and poultry are rich sources of vitamin B_{12}. Vegetarians get their requirements mainly from fortified cereals and milk.

Deficiency State

Megaloblastic anemia results from either (or combined) folate or vitamin B_{12} deficiency.[5] Maternal folate deficiency increases the risk of neural tube defects in the fetus. Vitamin B_{12} also results in neurological manifestations, such as irritability, poor attention span, hypotonia, abnormal movements, and peripheral neuropathy progressing to subacute combined degeneration. Hyperpigmentation of knuckles is a commonly observed sign of vitamin B_{12} deficiency. Hereditary folate malabsorption and cerebral folate deficiency are genetic disorders resulting in symptoms of severe folate deficiency. Hereditary intrinsic factor deficiency and Imerslund–Grasbeck disease are genetic disorders of B_{12} absorption, leading to its continued deficiency.[5,6]

Treatment

Megaloblastic anemia due to folate deficiency requires oral administration of 0.5–1 mg/day of folic acid for 3–4 months or until a definite hematologic response has occurred. Parenteral (IM or deep SC or IV) vitamin B_{12} (25 μg daily for initial 2–3 days, 50–100 μg daily for next 7 days, 100 μg on alternate days for next 7 days, and thereafter 1,000 μg every week over the next 1 month) is administered for achieving hematological response in vitamin B_{12} deficiency. Alternatively, vitamin B_{12} (500 μg daily in infants, 1,000 μg daily in older children) can be given orally for 3 months, especially when there is no neurological involvement. A combined treatment is required, if the blood levels for both are not available. In case vitamin B_{12} deficiency has not been excluded, treatment with only folic acid should not be instituted as it can precipitate vitamin B_{12} deficiency and worsen the neurological symptoms.[4,5,7]

Other Vitamin B Complex Vitamins

Biotin

Biotin (found in a variety of vegetarian and nonvegetarian foodstuffs) deficiency causes scaly periorificial dermatitis, alopecia, hypotonia, and apathy. The deficiency state can be treated using 1–10 mg/day of oral biotin.

Pantothenic Acid

Pantothenic acid (found in seafood, organ meats, egg yolk, legumes, and milk) deficiency causes muscle cramps and burning feet syndrome; clinical deficiency is extremely rare.

Choline and Inositol

Although important for normal body functions, choline and inositol are not known to be associated with any specific deficiency syndromes.

VITAMIN C (ASCORBIC ACID)

Vitamin C has an important role in collagen synthesis and the synthesis of steroid hormones, neurotransmitters, and bile acids. It increases the GI absorption of iron and has an important antioxidant activity.[8]

Dietary Sources

Citrus fruits, guava, tomato, capsicum, cauliflower, and green leafy vegetables are good sources of vitamin C. Breast milk is a good source of vitamin C, but children consuming animal milk are at risk of deficiency.

Deficiency State

Scurvy, resulting from severe vitamin C deficiency, manifests as gum bleeding, petechial hemorrhages, painful and swollen bones, and poor wound healing. Children with scurvy often have other nutrient deficiencies including severe malnutrition, anemia, and vitamin B-complex deficiency. The diagnosis of scurvy is usually made by radiographs, the changes being most prominent at the knee **(Fig. 5.5.1)**. The shafts of the long bones have a typical ground-glass appearance with a thin and dense cortex (pencil thinning). Metaphyseal changes are characterized by thickened bands (white line of Frankel) with a zone of destruction underneath (Trummerfeld zone). Ends of the white lines often end abruptly into a spur (Pelkan's spur). Epiphyses are also outlined by dense lines giving the appearance of a ring (Wimberger's ring). Subperiosteal hemorrhages may complicate the disease causing periosteal elevation and underlying calcifications.[8,9]

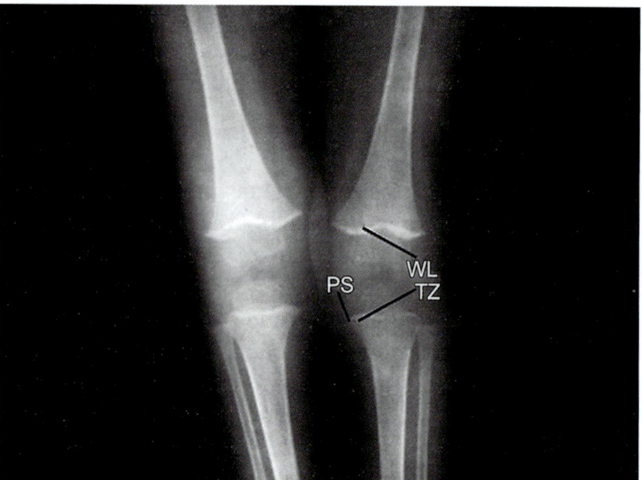

Fig. 5.5.1: Bony changes of scurvy at knee. (PS: Pelkan's spur; TZ: Trümmerfeld zone; WL: white line)

Treatment

Oral administration of vitamin C (100–200 mg/day) results in complete recovery. The resolution of clinical symptoms is rapid, whereas bony changes and subperiosteal hemorrhages take more time to recover. Treatment should be continued for 3 months and must be followed by ensuring adequate dietary vitamin C to prevent recurrence.[7,9,10]

REFERENCES

1. Yue T, Zhang Q, Li G, Qin H. Global burden of nutritional deficiencies among children under 5 years of age from 2010 to 2019. Nutrients. 2022;14(13):2685.
2. Martini L, Pecoraro L, Salvottini C, Piacentini G, Atkinson R, Pietrobelli A. Appropriate and inappropriate vitamin supplementation in children. J Nutr Sci. 2020;9:e20.
3. Nazir M, Lone R, Charoo BA. Infantile thiamine deficiency: new insights into an old disease. Indian Pediatr. 2019;56(8):673-681.
4. Sachdev HPS, Shah D. Vitamin B complex deficiencies and excess. In: Kliegman RM, St Geme JW, Blum NJ, Shah S, Tasker RC, Wilson KM (Eds). Nelson Textbook of Pediatrics, 21st edition. Philadelphia: Elsevier; 2020.
5. Socha DS, DeSouza SI, Flagg A, Sekeres M, Rogers HJ. Severe megaloblastic anemia: vitamin deficiency and other causes. Cleve Clin J Med. 2020;87(3):153-164.
6. Ali MA, Hafez HA, Kamel MA, Ghamry HI, Shukry M, Farag MA. Dietary vitamin B complex: orchestration in human nutrition throughout life with sex differences. Nutrients. 2022;14(19):3940.
7. Chandra J, Dewan P, Kumar P, Mahajan A, Singh P, Dhingra B, et al. Diagnosis, treatment and prevention of nutritional anemia in children: recommendations of the Joint Committee of Pediatric Hematology-Oncology chapter and Pediatric and Adolescent Nutrition Society of the Indian Academy of Pediatrics. Indian Pediatr. 2022;59(10):782-801.
8. Shah D, Sachdev HPS. Vitamin C (ascorbic acid) deficiency and excess. In: Kliegman RM, St Geme JW, Blum NJ, Shah S, Tasker RC, Wilson KM (Eds). Nelson Textbook of Pediatrics, 21st edition. Philadelphia: Elsevier; 2020.
9. Gandhi M, Elfeky O, Ertugrul H, Chela HK, Daglilar E. Scurvy: rediscovering a forgotten disease. Diseases. 2023;11(2):78.
10. Kinlin LM, Weinstein M. Scurvy: old disease, new lessons. Paediatr Int Child Health. 2023;43(4):83-94.

5.6 Fat-soluble Vitamins

Pooja Soni, Bhavna Dhingra

INTRODUCTION

Vitamins are vital micronutrients for the human body that neither can be synthesized endogenously nor synthesized in sufficient amounts, thus requiring an outside source for replenishment of the required amount of necessary vitamin, which is mostly obtained through the diet. Vitamins are classified into two categories: Water-soluble and fat-soluble vitamins. Fat-soluble vitamins play a crucial role in various physiological processes of the body and include four vitamins—vitamins A, D, E, and K. These fat-soluble vitamins are soluble in organic solvents and are absorbed in the micelle forms in the small intestine, packaged and transported in chylomicrons, and then get entered into the bloodstream through the lymphatic system, where chylomicrons are metabolized by lipoprotein lipase (LPL), releasing these vitamins into the tissues for their use and storage. Since fat-soluble vitamins can be stored in the tissues, these are retained in the body for a longer duration and may precipitate their toxicity too.[1,2]

VITAMIN A

Vitamin A is a subgroup of retinoids showing the biological activity of retinol and includes retinyl palmitate (vitamin A ester), retinal (vitamin A aldehyde), retinoic acid (vitamin A acid), and retinol (vitamin A alcohol). Hepatic stellate cells can store up to 80% of vitamin A in the form of retinyl palmitate, which is present in lipid droplets and is available for body supply. The recommended daily allowance (RDA) of vitamin A is 300–400 μg or retinol activity equivalents (RAE) in infants, 400–600 μg in children, and 750 μg in adolescents. 1 RAE is equal to 1 μg of retinol, 3.33 international unit (IU) of vitamin A activity from retinol, 10 IU of vitamin A activity from β-carotene, 6 μg of β-carotene, or 12 μg of other provitamin-A carotenoids.[3]

Sources

Vitamin A can be obtained through both plant and animal sources. Animal sources include eggs, milk, butter, yolk, cheese, and liver and contain the retinol form of vitamin A. Plant sources are dark green, leafy vegetables, yellow and orange vegetables, and fruits containing carotenoids, especially β-carotene, which is converted to vitamin A (retinol) in the body. Retinol is further converted to active forms of vitamin A—retinal and retinoic acid.[2,4]

Functions

Vitamin A is required for the proliferation and differentiation of epithelial cells in the salivary glands, eyes, and genitourinary tract. It also stimulates T-lymphocyte differentiation and activation of B-lymphocytes in response to immune stimuli, thus aiding in vision, especially in low light settings, immune function, growth and development of the embryo, and also maintains a normal mucous membrane. In the retina, vitamin A is converted to retinal (11-cis-retinal) and binds to the protein opsin, forming rhodopsin. When light enters the retina, 11-cis-retinal gets converted to all-trans-retinal and detaches from opsin. Opsin also changes shape to generate an electrical impulse in the retina cells, which transfers the signal to nerve cells and then to the brain. The brain interprets the signal as light. Subsequently, all-trans-retinal is reconverted into 11-cis-retinal, while some retinal is lost during every cycle. Therefore, vitamin A must be replenished through diet. Retinoic acid assists with the levels of natural killer cells, which can provide antitumor and antiviral activity in the body; it helps to increase the phagocytic activity in macrophages and increases the interleukin (IL)-1 and other cytokines to serve as mediators of inflammation. Vitamin A is a precursor for a nuclear hormone, all-trans retinoic acid (ATRA), which heterodimerizes with retinoic acid receptors in the nucleus and mediates the formation of structural proteins, extracellular matrix proteins, and enzymes.[5]

Deficiency

Vitamin A deficiency is responsible for more than 500,000 cases of corneal defects in children every year in India, Bangladesh, Indonesia, and the Philippines, and half of these cases are likely to result in blindness. The common causes of vitamin A deficiency are severe acute malnutrition, persistent diarrhea, poor dietary intake, fat malabsorption syndrome, liver disease, pancreatic insufficiency, inflammatory bowel disease, and iron deficiency in children. Mild vitamin A deficiency causes follicular hyperkeratosis of skin, causing roughness of skin with raised hyperkeratotic patches like goosebumps. Deficiency leads to night blindness (nyctalopia)

TABLE 5.6.1: WHO classification of xerophthalmia.

Primary signs		***Secondary signs***	
X1A	Conjunctival xerosis	XN	Night blindness
X1B	Bitot's spots	XF	Fundus changes
X2	Corneal xerosis	XS	Corneal scarring
X3A	Corneal ulceration (less than one-third of the cornea)		
X3B	Corneal ulceration (more than one-third of the cornea)		

(WHO: World Health Organization)

due to defective dark adaptation (inhibition of reformation of rhodopsin) and xerophthalmia due to dryness of the ocular epithelium. Keratin accumulation in the conjunctiva labeled as Bitot's spots is a pathognomonic feature of vitamin A deficiency. The classification of eye manifestations of vitamin A deficiency is shown in **Table 5.6.1**. Vitamin A has a role in the protection of the skin and mucosal barrier involving the gastrointestinal and respiratory tracts and the proliferation and differentiation of T-lymphocytes; therefore, its deficiency also increases the risk of infections and also leads to squamous metaplasia of the renal pelvis, ureter, vaginal epithelium, and pancreatic and salivary ducts. Vitamin A deficiency also may interfere with neutrophil development and cytokine release, causing poor physical growth, intellectual impairment, and apathy.[3]

Investigation

The dark adaptation test is used to diagnose early stages of vitamin A deficiency; other tests to diagnose less severe deficiency are relative dose-response, modified relative dose-response, and conjunctival impression cytology tests. A serum retinol test is done for assessment of vitamin A levels in the body, and levels below 15 µg/dL or 0.7 µmol/L suggest deficiency (normal 20–80 g/dL).[6]

Treatment

Oral vitamin A on days 0, 1, and 28 with a dose of 50,000 IU for infants <6 months, 1,00,000 IU for infants 6–12 months of age, and 2,00,000 IU for children >1 year of age is given for the treatment of vitamin A deficiency. Alternatively, parenteral water-soluble preparations can be given to children having persistent vomiting or severe malabsorption (doses are half of the oral dose for children >6 month-old and 75% for <6 month-old children).

Prevention

The National Vitamin A Prophylaxis Programme by the Ministry of Health and Family Welfare (MoHFW) provides oral vitamin A supplementation of 1,00,000 IU at 9 months of age with the measles vaccine; 2,00,000 IU at 15–18 months with the diphtheria, pertussis, and tetanus (DPT) booster; and then every 6 months to children below 3 years of age.

Toxicity

Vitamin A toxicity results from oversupplementation (>50,000 IU/day for several months) and taking excessive isotretinoin therapy. Acute manifestations of toxicity include pseudotumor cerebri (headache, vomiting, irritability, diplopia, papilledema, and seizures). Other chronic manifestations include anorexia, arthralgia, alopecia, dryness of mucosa, skin desquamation, hypercalcemia, and liver damage. Radiographs may show hyperostosis affecting long bones, particularly the middle of the bony shafts. Symptoms subside rapidly after withdrawing the vitamin intake, but the rate of clinical improvement is dependent on the amount of vitamin A stored in the body tissues. Vitamin A is teratogenic if consumed in high doses in early pregnancy, and its intake should not exceed 3,000 µg daily or 7,500 µg weekly.[3]

Carotenodermia, which is a state of yellowishness of the skin due to high doses of carotenoids, is not associated with severe outcomes and also resolves slowly when carotene intake is reduced. Individuals with food faddism, liver disease, hypothyroidism, and diabetes mellitus are more susceptible to developing carotenemia.

VITAMIN D

Sources

Vitamin D is found in two forms, D_2 (ergocalciferol) and D_3 (cholecalciferol). Vitamin D_2 is present in salmon, tuna, mackerel, and fortified milk, and in small quantities in egg yolk, cheese, butter, and beef liver. Vitamin D_3 gets synthesized in the skin after exposure to sunlight of wavelength 290–315 nm on the precursor 7-dehydroxycholesterol, and thus is also known as "sunshine vitamin." The amount of formation of vitamin D depends upon the length of ultraviolet (UV) radiation, intensity, and skin pigmentation. The RDA for vitamin D is 10 µg (400 IU) per day in infants and 15 µg (600 IU) per day in children >1 year of age.[2,4]

Functions

Vitamin D helps in maintaining calcium and phosphorus homeostasis and effective bone mineralization. A normal calcium level is required for the proper functioning of the neuromuscular junction, nerve transmission, secretion, and actions of various hormones. Prohormones, vitamin D_3 (from skin), and vitamin D_2 (from diet) undergo hydroxylation to form 25-hydroxycholecalciferol [25(OH)D or cholecalcidiol] in the liver via action of enzyme 25-hydroxylase, and then

25(OH)D further hydroxylates into the biologically most active form 1,25-dihydroxycholecalciferol [1,25$(OH)_2$D or cholecalcitriol] in the kidneys via the 1α-hydroxylase enzyme. The synthesis pathway of the active form of vitamin D is shown in **Flowchart 5.6.1.** Vitamin D stimulates an active calcium transport system that increases absorption of calcium and phosphorus from duodenum, reabsorbs calcium from distal convoluted tubules in the kidneys by upregulating calcium transporters, and acts for effective bone mineralization by maintaining adequate plasma concentrations of calcium and phosphorus and by bone remodeling. Parathyroid hormone (PTH) and low serum phosphate levels increase the activity of the 1α-hydroxylase enzyme, while fibroblast growth factor (FGF) decreases its activity.[1,5]

Deficiency

Common risk factors for vitamin D deficiency are exclusively breastfeeding with no vitamin D supplementation in infants, immobility, deranged renal function, chronic liver disease, malabsorption syndrome, use of antiseizure medicines, dark skin complexion, less sunlight exposure, full body clothing, living at high latitudes, and obesity. Vitamin D deficiency presents with muscle aches, weakness, bone pain, growth faltering, bony deformities like bow leg deformity, knock knees, spinal curvature defects, craniotabes, frontal bossing, frequent fractures, rachitic rosary, dental deformities, and hypocalcemic seizures.[7]

Flowchart 5.6.1: Synthesis pathway of the active form of vitamin D [1,25$(OH)_2$D].

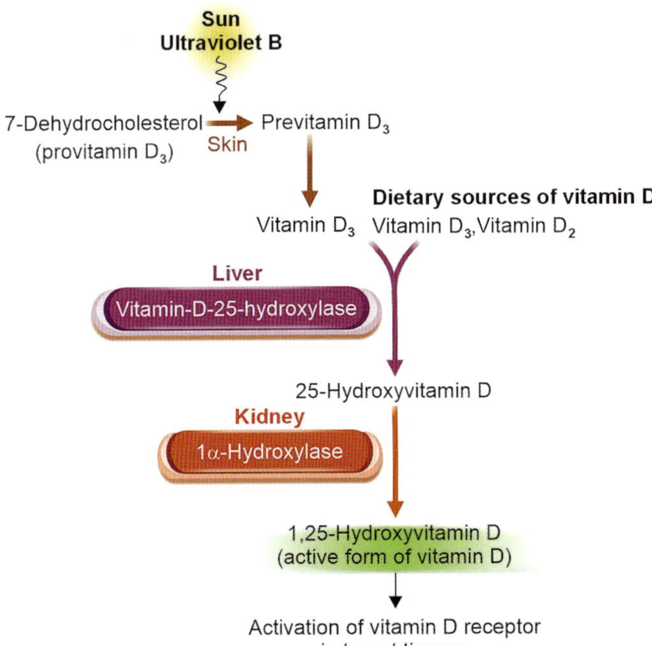

Investigation

Vitamin D level may be measured in serum using 25(OH) D and 1,25$(OH)_2$D. 25(OH)D has a half-life of ~3 weeks and is the preferred form for measurement. 25(OH)D levels <20 ng/mL are considered insufficient, <10 ng/mL are indicative of deficiency, and >100 ng/mL are considered as toxic. 1,25$(OH)_2$D levels are indicated in patients with renal failure, suspected hypercalcemia in sarcoidosis, and suspected hyperparathyroidism. 1,25$(OH)_2$D level is reduced in early renal failure while increased in sarcoidosis and primary hyperparathyroidism. Other markers of vitamin D deficiency are hypocalcemia, hypophosphatemia, raised alkaline phosphatase, radiographic evidence like loss of normal zone of calcification at the metaphysis, and osteopenia. X-ray reveals poor mineralization and widening of growth plate cartilage, cupping, fraying, and splaying of metaphysis.

Treatment

Lower daily doses of 2,000, 2000, and 3000 IU are advised for infants <6 months, children between 6 and 12 months, and those >12 months of age, respectively, for a duration of 12 weeks for the treatment of vitamin D deficiency, followed by a maintenance dose of 400–600 IU/day [as per Indian Academy of Pediatrics revised guidelines (2021) (Please refer to Chapter 16.6]. Higher doses or Stoss therapy (oral 60,000 IU daily or alternate day to reach a maximum total dose of 6,00,000 IU) can be given to patients with poor compliance to daily therapy. This should be associated with oral calcium supplementation (30–75 mg/kg/day) for 2 months. Patients show radiological healing within 4 weeks of therapy. Reduction of alkaline phosphatase level and resolution of clinical signs occur slowly. Bony malformations also improve with treatment, although patients with severe disease may have permanent short stature and deformities requiring orthopedic intervention.[1]

Prevention

Most of the cases of vitamin D deficiency rickets can be prevented by providing 400 IU/day of vitamin D from birth until 1 year of age. After 1 year of age, all children and adults should meet their nutritional requirements for vitamin D through diet and/or supplements.

Toxicity

Vitamin D toxicity is rare but can occur in individuals receiving higher doses of vitamin D supplementation, excess intake of fortified foods, or excessive intake of synthetic vitamin D analogs (25-D, 1,25-D). The upper limit for long-term vitamin D intake is 1,000 IU for infants and 2,000 IU for children >1 year. Manifestations occur due to hypercalcemia because of excessive absorption of calcium in the duodenum and nephrons and predominantly excessive bone resorption, causing reduced appetite, diarrhea, nausea, vomiting, dehydration, constipation, pancreatitis, polyuria, polydipsia, pruritus, calcium deposition in soft tissues and vessels, renal stones, acute renal failure, muscle or bony pain due to increased bone resorption, hypertension, arrhythmias, hypotonia, disorientation, confusion, depression, psychosis, hallucinations, and coma. Laboratory findings are hypercalcemia, high 25(OH)D (>100 ng/mL), hypercalciuria, decreased PTH, and hyperphosphatemia. $1,25(OH)_2D$ levels are usually normal, resulting from downregulation of renal 1α-hydroxylase because of low PTH, hyperphosphatemia, and $1,25(OH)_2D$. Management of vitamin D toxicity consists of elimination of the source of excess vitamin D, control of hypercalcemia, aggressive rehydration, loop diuretic therapy, glucocorticoids, bisphosphonates, and hemodialysis in refractory cases.[7]

VITAMIN E

Predominantly, vitamin E is found in alpha-tocopherol form, although other tocopherols and tocotrienols are also found in the circulation like alpha, beta, gamma, and delta forms. Alpha-tocopherol is transported into lipoprotein by specific tocopherol transfer protein (TTP) in the liver, and mutation of this protein leads to vitamin E deficiency. For premature infants, 15–20 µg/day vitamin E is required. For term infants, RDA increases from 3 to 6 mg tocopherol from birth to 2 years of age.[2]

Sources

Natural sources of vitamin E include vegetable oils (the richest source), seeds, nuts, wheat germ, milk, leafy vegetables, and whole grains. The vitamin E content of animal foods is generally low.[4]

Functions

Vitamin E is an important antioxidant and anti-inflammatory micronutrient and inhibits the generation of reactive oxygen species during fat oxidation. It also protects polyunsaturated fatty acids (PUFAs) in cell membranes from oxidative destruction, thus maintaining fluidity and stability of the cell membrane. It has a role in the growth of erythrocytes and is associated with impacting the aging process. Vitamin E inhibits protein kinase activity, resulting in halting platelet aggregation, which may decrease atherosclerosis.[5]

Deficiency

Deficiency of vitamin E is extremely rare and majorly occurs in individuals with fat malabsorption, cholestasis, chronic hepatitis, short bowel syndrome, pancreatic disorders, cystic fibrosis, Crohn's disease, and hypo- or abetalipoproteinemia. Premature infants are more susceptible to deficiency owning to significant transplacental transfer of vitamin E occurring during the last trimester and high content of PUFAs in premature formula milks. Deficiency leads to breakdown of cell membranes and tissue damage due to oxidative stress. Manifestations of vitamin E deficiency include peripheral neuropathy, axonal degeneration, limb and truncal ataxia, hyporeflexia, decreased proprioception (Romberg sign positive), decreased vibratory sensation, dysarthria, ophthalmoplegia, nystagmus, muscle weakness, hemolysis, visual field abnormalities, pigmentary retinopathy, blindness, memory impairment, and arrhythmias. Premature infants with vitamin E deficiency develop hemolysis (which may precipitate with iron supplementation) during the second month of life.

Ataxia with isolated vitamin E deficiency (AVED) is a rare autosomal recessive disorder with mutation in the α-tocopherol transfer protein (*TTPA*) gene, making the patient unable to incorporate the vitamin E into lipoproteins and thus leading to reduced levels of serum vitamin E with normal intestinal vitamin E absorption. Ataxia, dysarthria, and clumsiness usually manifest in late childhood.

Investigation

Alpha-tocopherol is measured in serum, and 3–5 µg/mL is considered a normal level in children. The ratio of vitamin E to serum lipids is preferred, and ratio < 0.6 mg/g in infants and <0.8 mg/g in older children is considered deficient. Premature infants with hemolysis may also have a raised platelet count.

Treatment

Treatment of vitamin E deficiency consists of providing large doses of oral vitamin E (15–20 mg/kg/day). Hemolysis resolves with correction of the deficiency, but neurological manifestations may have little or no improvement.

Prevention

Premature infants should get adequate vitamin E through formula milk (without high PUFA content) or fortified breastmilk to prevent the development of vitamin E deficiency. High-risk patients for vitamin E deficiency should be screened for deficiency and receive sufficient supplementation.

Toxicity

Oversupplementation is the main cause of toxicity of vitamin E, and this inhibits platelet aggregation and thus causes bleeding.

VITAMIN K

Vitamin K is responsible for the formation of clotting factors. The RDA for vitamin K in newborns is 3–5 µg/day, which increases to 10 μg/day at 2 years of age and 10–30 μg/day in older children.[2]

Sources

Two primary forms of vitamin K are K_1 and K_2. Vitamin K_1 or phylloquinone is present in green leafy vegetables, cauliflower, cabbage, cereals, dairy products, fish, meat, and some fruits, whereas vitamin K_2 or menaquinone is synthesized by gut microflora, though its contribution to overall vitamin K status is unknown.[4]

Functions

Vitamin K activates clotting factors II, VII, IX, X, and proteins C and S in the liver by vitamin K-dependent gamma-carboxylation and thus helps in coagulation function. Vitamin K acts as a cofactor for the enzyme gamma-glutamyl carboxylase and catalyzes post-translational synthesis of gamma-carboxy-glutamyl residues.

Deficiency

The risk factors for the deficiency of vitamin K are prolonged antibiotic use interfering with gut microbiota, nutritional deficiency, newborns (more predisposition in preterm babies as vitamin K does not cross placenta well), maternal ingestion of antiseizure medicines, high ingestion of vitamins A and E, cystic fibrosis, biliary obstruction, short bowel syndrome, celiac disease, and patients receiving total parental nutrition (TPN) without vitamin K supplementation. Vitamin K has limited body stores and high turnover with short half-lives of vitamin K-dependent clotting factors, predisposing to the development of deficiency symptoms early within weeks of inadequate supply. Deficiency of vitamin K leads to poor clot formation and hence manifests as systemic bleeding like gastrointestinal, genitourinary, pulmonary, and central nervous system (CNS) bleed. Hemorrhagic disease of newborns or vitamin K deficiency bleeding (VKDB) is a vitamin K deficiency manifestation in newborns that consists of severe systemic bleeding and ecchymosis appearing in the first week of life.

Investigation

Prolonged prothrombin time (PT) is a marker of vitamin K deficiency and should be confirmed by normalization of prothrombin time/international normalized ratio (PT/INR) in response to vitamin K supplementation. Activated partial thromboplastin time (APTT) is usually prolonged, but it may be normal in the early stages of deficiency. In situations of mild vitamin K deficiency, PT may be normal, but there are increased levels of undercarboxylated forms of protein, also known as "proteins induced by vitamin K absence (PIVKA)." Thus, measurement of undercarboxylated factor II (PIVKA-II) can be used in cases of mild deficiency of vitamin K.[1]

Treatment

Infants with VKDB should receive parenteral 1 mg vitamin K, after which the PT should decrease within 6 hours and normalize within 24 hours. In adolescents, parenteral 2.5–10 mg vitamin K is recommended for rapid correction of vitamin K deficiency. Apart from vitamin K, patients with severe life-threatening bleeding should also receive fresh frozen plasma (FFP) transfusion for rapid correction of coagulopathy. At-risk children should receive supplemental vitamin K with periodic PT level assessments.

Prevention

Routine administration of intramuscular vitamin K (0.5–1 mg) at birth to all healthy newborns is useful for the prevention of hemorrhagic disease in newborns. Maternal intake of medications predisposing to hemorrhagic disease of newborns should be stopped before delivery.

Toxicity

Hypervitaminosis K is uncommon but may occur in infants on formula feeds and those who receive menadione (water-soluble) form of vitamin K, which causes excessive lipid peroxidation in liver, leading to hepatocyte damage. Symptoms of vitamin K toxicity include hemolytic anemia, jaundice, and liver damage.

REFERENCES

1. Sharma R. Micronutrients in health and disease. In: Paul VK, Bagga A (Eds). Ghai Essential Pediatrics, 9th edition. Delhi: CBS Publishers; 2023. pp. 100-10.
2. Johnson EJ, Mohn ES. Fat-soluble vitamins. World Rev Nutr Diet. 2015;111:38-44.
3. Ross AC. Vitamin A deficiencies and excess. In: Kliegman RM, ST Geme JW, Blum NJ, Shah SS, Tasker RC, Wilson KM, Behrman RE (Eds). Nelson Textbook of Pediatrics, 21st edition. Philadelphia, PA: Elsevier; 2020. pp. 360-5.
4. Stevens SL. Fat-soluble vitamins. Nurs Clin North Am. 2021;56:33-45.
5. Reddy P, Jialal I. (2023). Biochemistry, fat soluble vitamins. In: StatPearls [Internet]. Treasure Island, FL: StatPearls Publishing. [online] Available from https://www.ncbi.nlm.nih.gov/books/NBK534869/. [Last accessed October, 2024].
6. de Pee S, Dary O. Biochemical indicators of vitamin A deficiency: serum retinol and serum retinol binding protein. J Nutr. 2002;132(9 Suppl):2895S-901S.
7. Greenbaum LA. Vitamin D deficiency (rickets) and excess, vitamin E deficiency, vitamin K deficiency. In: Kliegman RM, St Geme JW, Blum NJ, Shah SS, Tasker RC, Wilson KM, Behrman RE (Eds). Nelson Textbook of Pediatrics, 21st edition. Philadelphia, PA: Elsevier; 2020. pp. 375-87.

5.7 Trace Elements

KE Elizabeth, P Leela Kumari

INTRODUCTION

Trace elements are minerals required only in minute amounts for living organisms for normal body function and growth. They are present in concentrations <0.01% of body dry weight. The World Health Organization (WHO) Expert Consultation has categorized nutritionally significant trace elements into three groups:[1]

1. *Essential trace elements:* Iron, iodine, zinc, selenium, copper, molybdenum, and chromium
2. *Elements that are probably essential:* Manganese, silicon, nickel, boron, and vanadium
3. *Potentially toxic elements:* Fluorine, lead, cadmium, mercury, arsenic, aluminum, lithium, and tin

EPIDEMIOLOGY

Trace element deficiencies are common in growing children and pregnant women because of the increased requirement. A balanced diet that includes all the food groups can supply all the trace elements. *Infant and young child feeding* (IYCF) practices, especially in the minus nine to plus 24 months that correspond to the first 1,000 days of life, are crucial in preventing deficiency and ensuring enough stores of trace elements. Trace element deficiencies occur usually in those with childhood undernutrition, picky eaters, and low birth weight (LBW) babies and in those on exclusion diets and total parenteral nutrition (TPN).[2] Excess intake of dietary fiber, phytates, and oxalates reduces trace element absorption. Both deficiency or excess of trace elements can affect normal body functions. So the trace elements should be present in the human body at optimum levels. Recent epidemiological surveys and animal studies have revealed the significant role of trace elements in human health and highlighted the association of trace element deficiency state with reduced antioxidant potential leading to accelerated aging, onset of cancer, atherosclerosis and lifestyle diseases, growth retardation in children, and immunological abnormalities.[2]

The various aspects related to trace elements are summarized in **Table 5.7.1**.

DIAGNOSIS

Except in a few items like iron, iodine, zinc, and selenium, specific features of deficiency may not occur. So, clinical diagnosis may be difficult. Recent advances in analytical technologies like atomic absorption spectrometry have made it possible to measure these elements precisely and to determine their deficiency and excess state. A high index of suspicion and therapeutic response to supplementation help in clinching the diagnosis. Methods currently used for diagnosis include the following:[3-5]

- *Measurement of trace elements in samples:* Serum, erythrocytes, leukocytes, hair, and urine
- *Measurement of activity of enzymes containing trace elements:* 5'nucleotidase (zinc), thyroid hormones (iodine), and glutathione peroxidase (selenium)
- *Function tests:* Taste test (zinc) and electroretinogram (zinc)
- *Analysis of daily intake:* Not practical
- Observing for the response to supplementation

IRON

Iron deficiency is the most common micronutrient deficiency worldwide. Iron is needed in the human body for hemoglobin and myoglobin synthesis. Moreover, it is a cofactor for many enzymes in the human body and for many metabolic processes. It is needed for brain growth and maturation and for neurotransmitter synthesis and metabolism. Literature evidence reveals that early iron deficiency can lead to irreversible changes in the growing brain. It is needed for immunity and cell maturation and differentiation. The stages of iron deficiency are prelatent stage, latent stage, and frank iron deficiency.[3]

Iron Deficiency

Iron insufficiency leads to iron depletion, iron deficiency anemia (IDA) with microcytic hypochromic red blood cells (RBCs) with increased red cell distribution width (RDW), reduced physical stamina, lack of concentration and learning ability, pica, and koilonychia. Pica includes eating disorders like geophagia (mud), amylophagia (eating raw rice), pagophagia (ice cubes), and other nonedible things. Even mild-to-moderate anemia in infancy and childhood may lead to permanent changes in the brain. IDA is an added risk factor for breath-holding spells, febrile fits, and hypercyanotic blue spells.[4]

TABLE 5.7.1: Sources, functions, deficiencies, clinical features, requirements, and toxicity of the various trace elements.

TE	*Sources*	*Functions*	*Deficiency*	*Clinical features*	*Requirement*	*Remarks and toxicity*
Iron	• *Heme:* 7–35% and nonheme: 2–20% • Fish, meat, liver, and 3 Gs (grams, grains, and greens) • Jaggery/ molasses, asafetida, turmeric, dates, and watermelon • Cooking in iron vessels	• Constituent of myoglobin and enzymes • Role in oxygen transport learning ability and myelination • Also known as the "energy mineral"	• LBW • Excess cow's mIlk • *Blood loss:* Hookworm and whipworm • Malabsorption • Poor intake • Increased demands	• Pallor • Dyspnea • CCF • Irritability • Lack of concentration • Pica • Koilonychia ***Investigation:*** • Hb low • Serum iron (50–150 µg/dL), • Iron-binding capacity (100–400 µg/dL) • Serum ferritin (50–250 ng/mL) • Transferrin saturation <15%, • *Blood smear:* Hypochromic microcytic anemia • *MCV, MCH, MCHC:* Reduced • *RDW:* Increased	***Prophylaxis:*** • 2–3 mg/kg/day • *Children:* 10–20 mg/day • *Pregnancy and lactation:* 30–40 mg/day ***Treatment:*** • *Oral:* 4–6 mg/ kg/day for 3–4 months • *Parenteral:* Weight in kg × deficit in g/ dL × 2.5 + 25% • Iron sucrose IV/IM • *Packed red cell transfusion:* 5–10 mL/kg • Always treat the cause	• Oxalate, phytates, Zn, and coffee/tea inhibit absorption • Vitamin C, cobalt, lime juice, and acid medium increase absorption ***Toxicity:*** • *Chronic:* Hemosiderosis and hemochromatosis • *Acute:* GI upset, stages of the quiescent phase, metabolic derangement, hepatic failure, and strictures • Gastric lavage with soda bicarbonate and desferrioxamine • IV Desferal 50 mg/kg followed by 10 mg/ kg/h × 24 h • Serum iron >1,800 µg/dL is fatal
Iodine	• Seafoods • Drinking water (two-thirds requirement) • Iodized salts	Constituent of thyroxine for metabolic control, modulation of estrogen, and fetal health	• Low content in water, especially in mountainous areas • Excessive intake of Brassica species, cabbage, and cauliflower	• Endemic goiter • Hypothyroidism • Stillbirth • CNS defect ***Investigation:*** • Urinary iodine • PBI • T3, T4, and TSH • Iodine uptake study	50–150 µg/day	• Iodized salt to contain 15 µg/g (15 ppm); up to 30 ppm added to tackle loss • Excess can cause iodism, reversible dermatitis, and cobalt deficiency/ excess iron deficiency • Manganese excess and fluorine excess may aggravate goiter
Copper	• Liver • Fish • Meat • Oyster • Legumes • Competes with Zn and Mo for absorption	• Constituents of enzymes, ceruloplasmin, and hormone function • Role in hemopoiesis • Essential for Zn, iron and vitamin C function, and bone • Also called twin mineral of iron	• LBW • Preterm • TPN • Childhood undernutrition • Nephrotic syndrome • *Menke's kinky hair syndrome* is an X-linked metabolic disturbance of copper metabolism characterized by intellectual deficits, abnormal hair texture, hypocupremia (<65 µg/dL), and low circulating ceruloplasmin (<20 mg/dL)	• Hypochromic anemia • Neutropenia • Hypopigmented hair • Bony defects ***Investigation:*** • Serum copper 75–150 µg/dL • Serum ceruloplasmin 10–50 µg/dL	1–2 mg/day	***Toxicity:*** • Indian childhood cirrhosis hepatitis (ICC) • Cirrhosis • Coomb's negative • hemolytic anemia • Zn deficiency • Cu deposition occurs in Wilson disease

Contd...

Contd...

TE	Sources	Functions	Deficiency	Clinical features	Requirement	Remarks and toxicity
Zinc	• Liver • Beef • Oyster • Cereals • Nuts • Grapes	• Constituents of enzymes • Role in protein and nucleic acid synthesis, epithelial repair, fluid electrolyte transport, taste function, and immunity	• Childhood undernutrition • TPN • Hepatitis • Nephrotic syndrome • Acrodermatitis enteropathica, especially as a genetic defect	• Growth retardation • Anorexia • Gonadal atrophy • Alopecia • Dermatitis • Diarrhea • Reduced taste sensation ***Investigation:*** • Serum Zn 60–150 μg/dL • Zn in hair	• 5–15 mg/day ***Treatment:*** • Diarrhea; ORS and Zn: 2–6 months: 10 mg/day • >6 months: 20 mg/day × 2 weeks • Dose 1–2 mg/kg/day up to 150 mg elemental zinc	• Phytates reduce absorption • Excess reduces iron and copper levels • Used as adjuvant in Wilson disease ***Toxicity:*** • GI upset • Cu deficiency
Chromium	• Yeast • Liver • Cereals • Nuts • Cocoa • Pepper	• Facilitates insulin action and weight loss • Help to prevent diabetes	• Childhood undernutrition • TPN	• Hyperglycemia • Encephalopathy ***Investigation:*** • Serum Cr 0.02 μg/dL	10 μg/day ***Treatment:*** Single dose 180 μg in hyperglycemia	*Toxicity:* Renal failure and Dermatitis
Fluorine	• Drinking water • Seafoods • Tea • Cheese	Constituent of bone and teeth	Poor water content	Dental caries	1–5 mg/day Drinking water up to 1 ppm	***Excess:*** • Dental and skeletal fluorosis • Genu valgum with excess in drinking water and sorghum intake • >2–3 ppm in drinking water needs defluoridation by alum and/or by reverse osmosis (OS)
Selenium	• Meat groups • Green • Garlic	• Antioxidant • Cofactor of enzyme function • Maintains liver integrity	• Childhood undernutrition • TPN • Poor soil content	• *Keshan cardiomyopathy* • Arthritis • Myalgia • Growth retardation • Liver necrosis • Risk of liver cancer • *Kashin–Beck disease:* Endemic osteoarthropathy ***Investigation:*** • Serum Se 13 μg/dL	100 μg/day	• Dental caries • Alopecia • Garlic odor in breath
Manganese	• Cereals • Legumes • Greens • Tea	• Component of superoxide • Dismutase • Role in oxidative phosphorylation	TPN	• Growth retardation • Reddening of hair • Increased • prothrombin time ***Investigation:*** • Serum Mn 0.06 μg/dL	1–5 mg/day	• Iron decreases Mn absorption ***Toxicity:*** • Encephalitis • Goiter • Cardiomyopathy • Cholestasis

Contd...

Contd...

TE	Sources	Functions	Deficiency	Clinical features	Requirement	Remarks and toxicity
Nickel	Chocolate	• Component of urease • Nickel plasmin stabilizes membranes	TPN	***Investigation:*** S. nickel 0.02 µg/dL	Not known	***Excess:*** • Dermatitis • Liver necrosis • Nasal and lung cancers
Silicon	–	• Cross-linkage of collagen • Helps in bone formation	TPN	• Growth retardation • Defective bone growth	Not known	***Excess:*** • Granuloma and fibrosis of lung • Silicosis • Urolithiasis
Vanadium	Protein-rich food	Regulation of enzymes Na^+/K^+-ATPase, adenylate cyclase, and protein kinase	PEM	Deficiency associated with nutritional edema	Not known	–

(CCF: congestive cardiac failure; CNS: central nervous system; GI: gastrointestinal; IM: intramuscular; IV: intravenous; LBW: low-birth weight; MCH: mean corpuscular hemoglobin; MCHC: mean corpuscular hemoglobin concentration; MCV: mean corpuscular volume; ORS: oral rehydration salts; PBI: protein-bound iodide; PEM: protein-energy malnutrition; RDW: red cell distribution of width; TE: trace element; TPN: total parenteral number; TSH: thyroid-stimulating hormone)

TABLE 5.7.2: Hemoglobin levels and grade of anemia.

Population	Anemia (hemoglobin g/dL)		
	Mild	Moderate	Severe
Children 6–59 months of age	10–10.9	7–9.9	<7
Children 5–11 years of age	11–11.4	8–10.9	<8
Children 12–14 years of age	11–11.9	8–10.9	<8
Nonpregnant women (15 years of age and above)	11–11.9	8–10.9	<8
Pregnant women	10–10.9	7–9.9	<7
Men (15 years of age and above)	11–12.9	8–10.9	<8

Source: World Health Organization. Nutritional Anemia: Tools for Effective Prevention and Control. Geneva: World Health Organization-; 2017.[6]

The prevalence of anemia among six groups, as per the National Family Health Survey-5 (2019–2021), is: 25.0% in men (15–49 years), 57.0% in women (15–49 years), 31.1% in adolescent boys (15–19 years), 59.1% in adolescent girls, 52.2% in pregnant women (15–49 years), and 67.1% in children (6–59 months).

Table 5.7.2 lists the hemoglobin levels and the grade of anemia.

In 2018, the Government of India launched the Anemia Mukt Bharat (AMB) strategy with the target to reduce anemia in vulnerable age groups such as women, children, and adolescents in a life cycle approach, providing preventive and curative mechanisms through a "6 × 6 × 6" strategy including six target beneficiaries, six interventions, and six institutional mechanisms. The six beneficiaries include children of 6–59 months, children of 5–9 years, adolescent boys and girls (10–19 years), women of reproductive age group, and pregnant and lactating women. The six interventions include prophylactic iron and folic acid supplementation, deworming, testing of anemia using digital methods and point-of-care treatment, intensified year-round behavioral change communication campaigns, mandatory provision of iron and folic acid fortified foods in public health programs, and addressing non-nutritional causes of anemia.[5]

Prophylactic iron and folic acid supplementation for children aged 6–59 months includes 1 mL of iron and folic acid syrup given biweekly [20 mg of elemental iron (Fe) and 100 µg of folic acid]. For children aged 5–9 years, the dose is a weekly 1 Fe and folic acid tablet (45 mg of elemental Fe + 400 µg of folic acid, sugar-coated pink tablet). The recommended dose for adolescent boys and girls is a weekly 1 Fe and folic acid tablet (60 mg of elemental Fe + 500 µg of folic acid, sugar-coated blue tablet); for women of reproductive age (20–49 years, nonpregnant, nonlactating) a weekly 1 Fe and folic acid tablet (60 mg of elemental Fe + 500 µg of folic acid, sugar-coated red tablet); for pregnant and lactating mother, daily one iron and folic acid tablet starting from the fourth month of pregnancy and continued throughout pregnancy and continued for 180 days postpartum (60 mg of elemental Fe + 500 µg of folic acid, sugar-coated red tablet).[5]

Regarding deworming, for children of 1–2 years, tablet albendazole 200 mg biannually and for children of 2 years and above, tablet albendazole 400 mg biannually are recommended.

IODINE

Iodine is one of the essential trace elements needed for normal human growth and development. It is needed for the synthesis of thyroid hormones. About two-thirds of this is generally derived from drinking water and one-third from diet. The daily requirement is 150 µg.[3]

Iodine Deficiency Disorders

Iodine deficiency is a preventable cause of intellectual deficiency. Iodine deficiency disorders (IDDs) can affect children's mental health and survival. Severe iodine deficiency during pregnancy can lead to stillbirths, abortions, and cretinism. Universal iodization of salt, ensuring potassium iodate 15 ppm (15 µg/g), is recommended in India. Salt testing kits are made available to ensure optimum iodization. In commercial iodized salt, up to 30–50 ppm is added to cover losses. Double-fortified salt contains potassium iodate and ferrous sulfate to tackle IDA and IDD. Urinary iodine excretion is reduced in deficiency. Urinary iodine can be tested using a dipstick or laboratory method. The daily requirement is 150 µg/L; excretion <100 µg/L indicates iodine deficiency, 50–100 µg/L mild, 20–50 µg/L moderate, and <20 µg/L severe deficiency. Goiter is an indication of a previous deficiency state, and rates >5% in prepubertal children indicate endemic goiter: 5–20% mild, 20–30% moderate, and >30% severe. Goiter is graded as follows: *Grade 0*: Goiter not visible or palpable; *Grade 1*: Goiter palpable; and *Grade 2*: Both visible and palpable.[4,5]

ZINC

Zinc (Zn) is an essential trace element, is a component of many proteins and metalloproteins, and is needed for many biological functions in the human body. The initial cases of zinc deficiency in humans were reported in the early 1960s in male adolescents from the middle east characterized by delayed sexual development and short stature. Subclinical zinc deficiency is not uncommon. It is useful in the treatment of Wilson disease. Zinc supplementation results in better catch-up growth in LBW and protein-energy malnutrition (PEM). In field settings, oral rehydration salts (ORS) and zinc are promoted in diarrhea for diarrhea control program and also for prevention of diarrhea, as zinc results in the repair of mucosa, replenishment of brush border enzymes, and fluid regulation.[3]

About 20 mg zinc sulfate tablets are made available in the reproductive and child health (RCH) kit, 1/2 tablet in 2–6 months old and 1 tablet in >6 months old for 14 days. In those <2-month-old, it is not given as a routine medication but can be prescribed, whenever indicated. Skin changes induced by zinc deficiency in acrodermatitis enteropathica are symmetrical and periorificial **(Fig. 5.7.1)** compared to more extensive lesions in nutritional dermatosis of severe malnutrition, which is also associated with growth failure.[4]

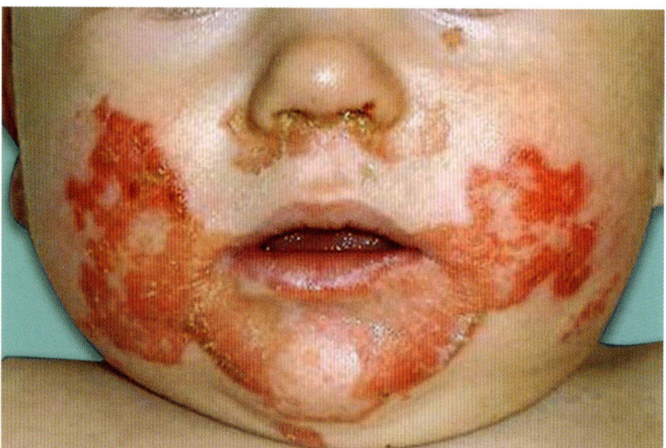

Fig. 5.7.1: Symmetrical periorificial lesions in zinc deficiency due to acrodermatitis enteropathica (note that overall growth is normal).

COPPER

Copper is widely distributed in biological tissues as organic complexes, many of which are metalloproteins. The adult human body contains 80 mg of copper with an arrangement of 50–120 mg. The tissue copper level ranges from <1 µg/g (dry weight) in many tissues to >10 µg/g (dry weight) in the liver and brain. The concentration of copper may be 6–10-fold greater in the liver of infants during the first 2 months of postnatal life. Copper in human blood is mainly distributed between erythrocytes and plasma. In the erythrocytes, 60% of copper occurs as metalloenzymes (superoxide dismutase, cytochrome C oxidase, and tyrosine oxidase) and the remaining 40% is loosely bound to other proteins and amino acids. Total erythrocyte copper is 0.9–1 µg/mL of packed red cells. In the plasma, 93% of copper is firmly bound to the enzyme ceruloplasmin, and the remaining 7% is less firmly bound to albumin and amino acids.[3]

Normal serum copper level is 0.8–1.2 µg/mL, and hypocupremia is defined as a serum copper level of 0.8 µg/mL or less (WHO) and is usually accompanied by hypoceruloplasminemia.[7]

Recent investigations have increased the understanding of the physiologic roles of copper in the human body, copper homeostasis, and copper needs throughout the lifecycle.

Biological Functions

Copper is an essential element in the human body. It is the cofactor for many enzymes, needed for hemoglobin synthesis, essential for zinc, iron, and vitamin C functions, melanin synthesis, neurotransmitter synthesis, cross-linkage and synthesis of elastin and collagen, and central nervous system (CNS) functions. It is needed for the formation of neuroactive compounds like catecholamines and enkephalins.

Dietary Sources

Good dietary sources (>2 μg/g) include liver, fish, oysters, organ meat, legumes, nuts, and seafood. The upper limit of the safe range of population mean intake is 12 mg/day for males, 10 mg/day for females, and 150 μg/kg for infants (WHO).[7] Toxicity leads to hepatic cirrhosis, hemolytic anemia, zinc deficiency, and gastritis. Absorption occurs in the small intestine. Absorption varies from 25 to 60%.[5]

Deficiency

Copper deficiency occurs in LBW and preterm babies, PEM, malabsorption, high intake of zinc and vitamin C, and during TPN. Clinical features of deficiency include hypochromic anemia refractory to iron therapy, neutropenia, hypopigmented hair, abnormal bone formation with skeletal fragility, osteoporosis, and neurological manifestations. Metabolism of copper is deranged in Wilson disease. Menkes kinky hair syndrome is an X-linked metabolic disturbance of copper metabolism characterized by intellectual retardation, abnormal hair texture, hypocupremia (<65 μg/dL), and low-circulating ceruloplasmin (<20 mg/dL). Toxicity can result from contamination of water from copper pipes, cooking in copper vessels, exposure to chemicals containing high levels of copper, etc.[4]

CHROMIUM

Chromium is an essential micronutrient that potentiates the action of insulin and thus influences carbohydrate, lipid, and protein metabolism. It reduces the oxidative stress and inflammation. It facilitates weight loss and prevents diabetes. Chromium exists in two forms: Trivalent (3+) and hexavalent (6+). Trivalent form is naturally present in many foods and is safe for humans. Hexavalent form is a toxic byproduct of stainless steel and other manufacturing processes. Dietary sources include yeast, liver, cereals, nuts, eggs, butter, and cheese. The average basal requirement of chromium is <20 μg/day, and the mean population intake to meet basal needs may be 25 μg/day.[7] The upper limit of the safe range of population mean intake is 250 μg/day (WHO).

Deficiency and Excess

Deficiency may occur in PEM and during TPN. Deficiency leads to impaired growth, elevated serum cholesterol and triglycerides, hyperglycemia, increased incidence of aortic plaques, corneal lesions, and decreased fertility. Tissue chromium status may not be actually reflected by fasting plasma or serum chromium status. Serum chromium levels <0.14–0.15 ng/mL may indicate severe chromium deficiency.[8,9]

Chromium toxicity due to oral intake is rare. Toxicity usually occurs in an industrial environment where concentration in the air is high or contact with skin is frequent. Toxicity leads to renal failure and dermatitis. Elevated serum chromium (>0.15 ng/mL) is a useful indicator of excessive exposure to chromium. Another indicator is the high urinary chromium level.

SELENIUM

Selenium is a trace element that is naturally present in many foods, added to others, and available as a dietary supplement. Selenium, which is nutritionally essential for humans, is a constituent of selenoproteins that play critical roles in reproduction, thyroid hormone metabolism, deoxyribonucleic acid (DNA) synthesis, and protection from oxidative damage and infection.[10]

Selenium is a component of the enzymes superoxide dismutase, glutathione peroxidase, deiodinase, and glycine reductase and plays an important role in the antioxidant defense system. It maintains liver integrity and helps in thyroid hormone synthesis.

Because of its effects on DNA repair, apoptosis, and the endocrine and immune systems as well as other mechanisms, including its antioxidant properties, selenium might play a role in the prevention of cancer. Epidemiological studies have suggested an inverse association between selenium status and the risk of colorectal, prostate, lung, bladder, skin, esophageal, and gastric cancer.

Selenium can protect against heart disease by influencing platelet aggregation.

Grains, garlic, green leafy vegetables, mushrooms, nuts, cereals, fish, eggs, and meat are good dietary sources of selenium. Selenium compounds are well absorbed in humans. The rate-limiting step in the overall bioavailability of dietary selenium is its conversion within the tissues to its metabolically active form (e.g., its incorporation into glutathione peroxidase). A level of 40 μg/day is considered the acceptable intake of selenium for Indians and is necessary to maintain glutathione peroxidase, an enzyme containing selenium. The selenium content of cereals and pulses ranges between 30 and 400 μg/g. The safe upper limit of population mean intake of selenium for adults is 400 μg/day.[3,10]

The most commonly used measures of selenium status are plasma and serum selenium concentrations. Concentrations in blood and urine reflect recent selenium intake. Analyses of hair or nail selenium content can be used to monitor longer-term intakes over months or years. Quantification of one or more selenoproteins (such as glutathione peroxidase and selenoprotein P) is also used as a functional measure of selenium status.

Deficiency and Toxicity

Deficiency is common in childhood undernutrition and TPN. Clinical features include myalgia, cardiomyopathy, arthritis, and liver necrosis. The endemic cardiomyopathy associated with selenium deficiency is known as *Keshan disease*. It is seen in certain areas of China where the lowest selenium content of soil exists, and the selenium deficiency was first reported in the human population in 1979. It can be clinically categorized into four types: Acute, subacute, chronic, and insidious. Once the disease is established, selenium supplementation does not help. The major histopathological picture of the disease is multifocal myocardial necrosis. The coronary arteries are essentially unaffected. *Kashin-Beck disease* is an endemic osteoarthropathy associated with low selenium status. It occurs in children aged 5–13 years, endemic in certain regions of China. Degeneration and necrosis of hyaline cartilage lead to joint swelling and deformity.[10]

It is absorbed from the upper part of the small intestine. Selenium status can be assessed by measuring selenium or glutathione peroxidase in serum, platelets, or erythrocytes.

Early indicators of toxicity are a garlic odor in the breath and a metallic taste in the mouth. The most common clinical signs of chronically high selenium intakes or selenosis are hair and nail loss or brittleness. Other symptoms include lesions of the skin and nervous system, nausea, diarrhea, skin rashes, mottled teeth, fatigue, irritability, and nervous system abnormalities.

Acute selenium toxicity can cause severe gastrointestinal and neurological symptoms, acute respiratory distress syndrome, myocardial infarction, hair loss, muscle tenderness, tremors, lightheadedness, facial flushing, kidney failure, and cardiac failure.

OTHERS TRACE ELEMENTS[3-5]

Boron is recognized as essential for healthy bones and utilization of vitamin D and calcium in the body.

Cobalt is an essential component of vitamin B_{12}; it increases iron absorption and iodine utilization. Deficiency produces anemia and goiter and excess can lead to goiter and cardiomyopathy.

Germanium is said to be the secret behind the health benefits of garlic, ginseng, and mushrooms.

Fluorine is not considered an essential mineral by some, as humans do not require it for growth or to sustain life. However, it prevents dental caries, and primary action occurs topically.

Strontium is involved in the utilization of calcium. It promotes calcium uptake into bone at moderate dietary levels but has rachitogenic action at higher dietary levels.

Arsenic, bromine, cadmium, silicon, tungsten, and vanadium have biochemical roles as structural or functional cofactors in other organisms. Arsenic is thought to promote nail and hair growth. Excess residue found in cow's milk may be toxic to the skin, CNS, and respiratory tract.

Mercury is toxic to enzymes and ribonucleic acid (RNA). Excess leads to Minamata disease in fetus and acrodynia in others.

KEY MESSAGES

- Most of the trace elements are essential or probably essential, but a few are potentially toxic.
- Trace elements are required only in minute quantities and are present in selected food items.
- Deficiency of these micronutrients causes various pathologic effects in the human body.
- Excess can also cause serious adverse reactions in the body. So optimum trace element balance in the body is essential.
- An optimum trace element balance should be considered in TPN and food fortification.
- Trace element deficiencies should be diagnosed in the early phase and corrected.
- Along with optimum dietary intake recommendations, factors influencing the absorption and bioavailability should be considered.

REFERENCES

1. World Health Organization. Trace Elements in Human Nutrition and Health. Report of a WHO Expert Committee. Geneva: World IIealth Organization.; 1996.
2. Bailey RL, West KP, Black RE. The epidemiology of global micronutrient deficiencies. Ann Nutr Metab. 2015;66(Suppl 2):22-33.
3. Elizabeth KE (Ed). Vitamins, minerals and micronutrients. In: Nutrition and Child Development, 6th edition. Hyderabad: Paras Medical Publishers; 2022. pp. 205-19.
4. Williams AF. Pediatric nutrition. In: Gibney MJ, Elia M, Ljungqvist O, Dowsett J (Eds). Clinical Nutrition. Oxford: Blackwell Science; 2006. pp. 379-427.
5. Sharma R. Micronutrients in health and disease. In: Paul VK, Bagga A (Eds). Ghai Essential Pediatrics, 10th edition, Reprint. New Delhi: CBS Publishers; 2024. pp. 100-17.
6. World Health Organization. Nutritional Anemia: Tools for Effective Prevention and Control. Geneva: World Health Organization; 2017.
7. World Health Organization. Vitamin and Mineral Requirements in Human Nutrition, 2nd edition. Geneva: World Health Organization.; 2005.
8. Vincent JB, Lukaski AC. Chromium. Adv Nutr. 2018;9(4):505-6.
9. Hsu C-W, Weng C-H, Lee C-C, Yen T-H, Huang W-H. Association between serum chromium levels with malnutrition in hemodialysis patients. BMC Nephrol. 2019; 2(1):302.
10. Terry EN, Diamond AM. Selenium. In: Erdman JW, Macdonald IA, Zeisel SH (Eds). Present Knowledge in Nutrition, 10th edition. Washington, DC: Wiley-Blackwell; 2012. pp. 568-87.

SECTION

6 Immunity and Immunization

Section Editor: Srinivas G Kasi

6.1 Basics of Immune System

Abhay K Shah, Aashay Abhay Shah

INTRODUCTION

The immune system is an extremely important defense mechanism that can identify an invading organism, from outside the body (e.g., viruses, bacteria, parasites, allergens) or within the body (e.g., malignant cells), and destroy it. Our environment contains a huge range of pathogenic microbes and toxic substances that challenge the host by various pathogenic mechanisms. It requires a vigorous and vigilant immune system to keep the body free from such pathogens. Immunity is the ability of an individual to resist and/or fight a particular infection or toxin by the action of specific antibodies or sensitized white blood cells (WBCs). This immune system consists of major lymphoid organs such as the spleen and lymph nodes, as well as smaller lymphoid tissues lining the mucosal entry points of the body like the airway (adenoids and tonsils) and gut-associated lymphoid tissue. The immune cells are found in the reticuloendothelial system of many organs and in circulation. There is a constant traffic of these cells from one point to the other in the body, which helps disseminate immune messages throughout the body.

TYPES OF IMMUNE SYSTEMS

Immune system is broadly classified as innate and adaptive immunity **(Fig. 6.1.1)**.[1,2]

Innate immunity is inherent and comes into play within hours of the entry of an infective agent. The components of the innate immune system comprise epithelial and mucosal barriers, the antibacterial chemicals present in these barriers, phagocytes [neutrophils, macrophages, and natural killer (NK) cells], as well as complement. It is not very specific as it is triggered by structures shared by different microbes instead of specific microbial antigens. There is no immune memory. It plays a very important role as it is the first line of defense. It is the effector pathway of adaptive immunity.

Adaptive immunity is triggered by antigen presentation by the cells of the innate immune system. It takes time to

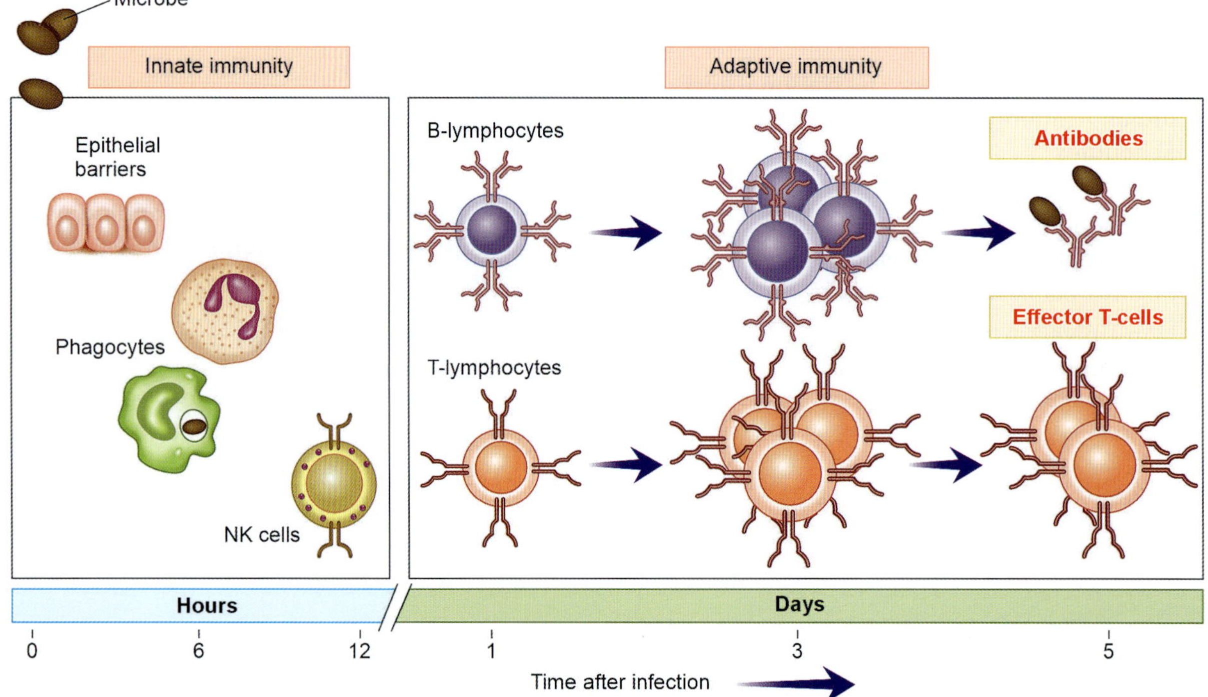

Fig. 6.1.1: Innate and adaptive immunity. (NK: natural killer)

develop. The two arms of adaptive immunity are *humoral immunity* and *cell-mediated immunity* **(Fig. 6.1.2)**. It has intense diversity, can respond to millions of antigens, and possesses immune memory. **Table 6.1.1** describes the comparison between the two types of immunity.

- *Humoral immunity* is mediated by *B-lymphocytes* by the production of immunoglobulins (antibodies) in the blood. Humoral immunity is the major defense system against bacterial infections and extracellular microbes.
- *Cellular immunity* is mediated by *T-lymphocytes*. It is responsible for delayed allergic reactions and rejection of foreign tissue transplants. It constitutes a major defense against infections due to viruses, fungi, and a few bacteria, such as the tubercle bacilli. It also plays an important role in protection against tumors. It mainly protects against intracellular pathogens.

COMPONENTS OF THE IMMUNE SYSTEM

The immune system consists of T-lymphocytes, B-lymphocytes, antigen-presenting cells (APCs), NK cells, phagocytic cells, and complement proteins **(Fig. 6.1.3)**.[1,2]

T-lymphocytes

Cellular immunity is mediated by T-lymphocytes which are derived from the thymus. In the blood, T-cells constitute 60–70% of the peripheral lymphocytes. Each T-cell can recognize a specific cell-bound antigen by an antigen-specific

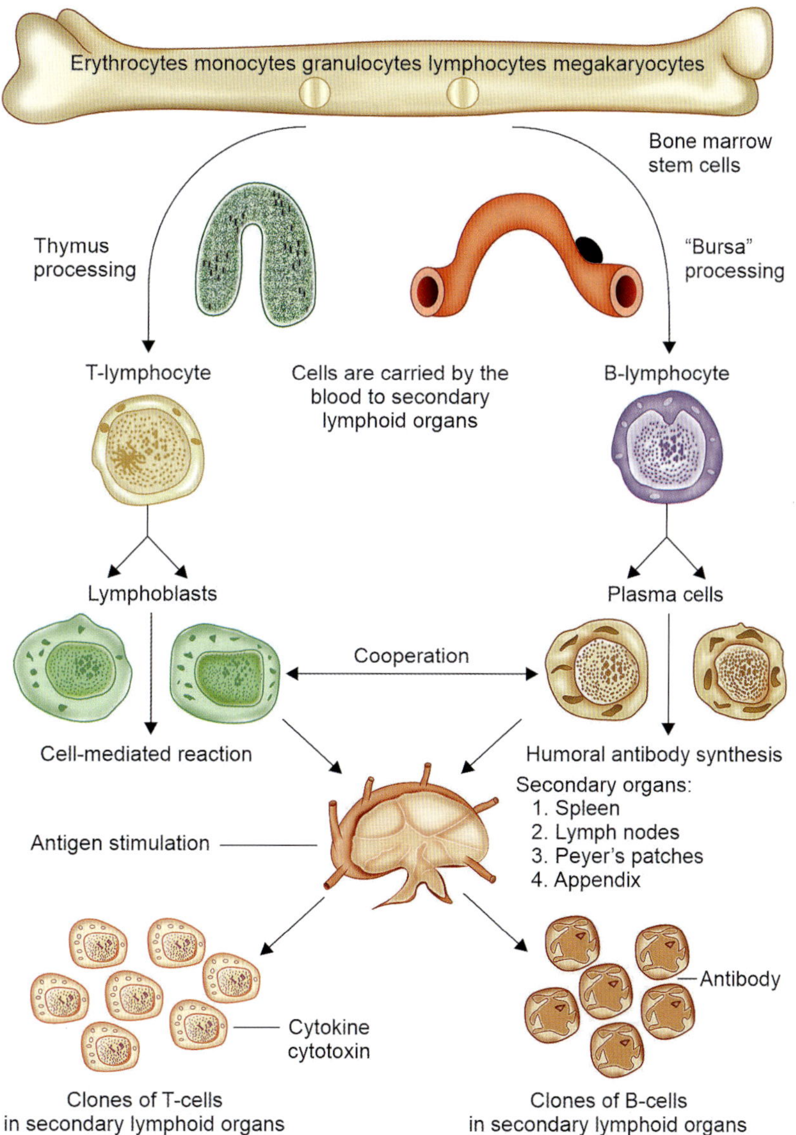

Fig. 6.1.2: Cellular and humoral immunity.

TABLE 6.1.1: Comparison of innate and adaptive immunity.

Innate immunity	*Adaptive immunity*
Its response is *antigen-independent*	Its response is *antigen-dependent*
There is *immediate* response	There is a *lag time* between exposure and maximal response
It is *not antigen-specific*	It is *antigen-specific*
Exposure does *not* result in induction of *memory* cells	Exposure results in induction of *memory* cells
Some of its cellular components or their products *may aid* innate immunity	Some of its products *may aid* adaptive immunity

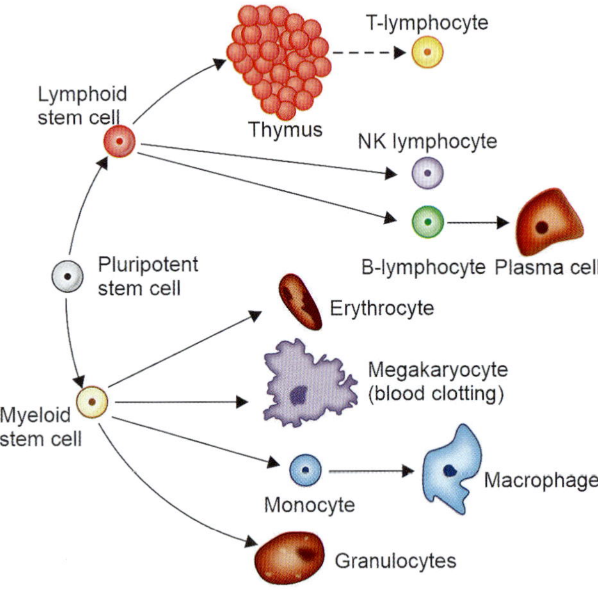

Fig. 6.1.3: Components of the immune system. (NK: natural killer).

T-cell receptor (TCR). Subpopulations of lymphocytes may be identified by surface markers as well as by functional abilities. Markers on the surface of the lymphocytes are assigned CD (clusters of differentiation) numbers on the basis of their reactions to a panel of monoclonal antibodies. Most *cytotoxic T-cells* display the glycoprotein CD8, and the *helper T-cells* display the glycoprotein CD4. These proteins are closely associated with the TCRs and may function as coreceptors. CD4 is expressed on approximately 60% of the mature T-cells, whereas CD8 is expressed on about 30% of the T-cells. In a normal healthy person, the CD4 to CD8 ratio is about 2:1.[1]

There are three types of T-lymphocytes.

CD4+ Helper Cells

CD4+ helper cells help in the maturation of B-cells into plasma cells and memory B-cells. They also help activate cytotoxic T-cells and macrophages. They become activated when they are presented with peptide antigens by major histocompatibility (MHC) class II molecules, which are expressed on the surface of APCs. Once activated, they divide rapidly and secrete small proteins called cytokines that regulate or assist in the active immune response.[1]

There are two subtypes of helper T-cells depending on the cytokines they produce on activation. *T-helper 1 (TH1) cells* secrete interleukin (IL)-2 and gamma interferon, which promote cytotoxic T-cell or delayed hypersensitivity types of responses. *T-helper 2 (TH2) cells* secrete IL-4 and IL-5 and interact primarily with B-cells in relation to humoral immunity and allergic sensitization. Cytotoxic T-cells recognize foreign or self-altered antigens on the surface and destroy them. This mechanism may play a role in the rejection of transplanted tissues, detection of virus-infected cells, and surveillance against malignancy.

CD8+ Cytotoxic Cells

CD8+ cytotoxic cells cause lysis of virus-infected and tumor cells. They are also involved in transplant rejection. These cells recognize their targets by binding to antigens associated with MHC class I molecules, which are present on the surface of all nucleated cells. Cytotoxic cells secrete hole-forming proteins called perforins for their cytolytic action.[1]

NK T-cells

Approximately 10–15% of the peripheral blood lymphocytes do not bear TCR or cell-surface immunoglobulins. These cells are endowed with an innate ability to lyse a variety of tumor cells and virally infected cells without prior sensitization. Hence, they are called NK cells. Two cell-surface molecules, CD16 and CD56, are widely used to identify NK cells. They bridge the adaptive immune system with the innate immune system. Whilst most T-cells function based on recognition of MHC class molecules, NK T-cells are able to recognize other antigen classes. Once activated, they are also able to perform the same functions as CD4+ and CD8+ cells.[1,2]

Clinical Significance of T-cell Responses

- The T-cell responses are more robust, long-lasting, and more cross protective than humoral responses.
- Normal newborn infants are also capable of mounting antigen-specific T-cell responses at birth, as evidenced by the vigorous tuberculin reactivity a few weeks after Bacillus Calmette-Guérin (BCG) vaccination even on the first day of life.[3]
- Patients with severe defects of T-lymphocyte number and/or function, such as severe combined immune deficiency and thymic aplasia (DiGeorge syndrome), show an increased susceptibility to infections due to

Candida, cytomegalovirus, and *Pneumocystis carinii*. They also have a higher incidence of malignancies, if they survive infections.

- Human immunodeficiency virus (HIV) selectively binds to the cells expressing CD4 molecules on their surface, primarily helper T-cells (CD4 cells), leading to the progressive depletion of these cells.

B-lymphocytes

B-cells are derived from *bursa of Fabricius* in birds (hence, the name B-cells). But in mammals, as there is no bursa, the transformation occurs in bursal equivalents, i.e., the fetal liver and, after birth, the bone marrow. B-lymphocytes constitute 10–20% of the circulating peripheral lymphocyte population. B-cells can bind to antigens directly, but they must contact helper T-cells to produce full activation and antibody production. It is the TH2 subtype that is mainly involved. The activated B-cells proliferate and transform into plasma cells. Plasma cells secrete large quantities of antibodies into the general circulation. Circulating antibodies protect their host by binding to and neutralizing some protein toxins, by blocking the attachment of some viruses and bacteria to cells, by opsonizing bacteria, and by activating complement.

As with T-cells, each B-cell receptor has unique antigen specificity, derived in part from the somatic rearrangements of immunoglobulin genes. Thus, the presence of rearranged immunoglobulin genes in a lymphoid cell is used as a molecular marker of B-lineage cells. B-cells also possess several other molecules that are essential for their function. These include complement receptors, Fc receptors, and CD19.[2]

B-lymphocytes produce five different classes of immunoglobulins called IgG, IgA, IgM, IgE, and IgD.[1]

1. *Immunoglobulin G (IgG)* is the most abundant of all immunoglobulins found in plasma and plays a major role in the prevention of infections. It crosses the placenta and thus is the primary defense against infections in the first few weeks of life in the neonate.
2. *Immunoglobulin M (IgM)* is the first antibody to be produced after an antigenic stimulation and is especially important in the initial period of the primary immune response. The fetus can synthesize IgM in utero starting from 20 weeks of gestation.
3. *Immunoglobulin A (IgA)* is the secretory immunoglobulin that is secreted by the B-cells and protects the mucosal surfaces of the gastrointestinal, respiratory, and genitourinary tracts and the breast. IgA guards the entrance to the body. It concentrates in body fluids such as tears, saliva, and secretions of the respiratory and gastrointestinal tracts. IgA response depends upon the route and the type of infection. Serum IgA is seen in organisms that invade from the mucosa, whereas surface IgA is classically seen with localized mucosal infections such as in cholera, respiratory syncytial virus infection, etc.
4. *Immunoglobulin E (IgE)* is found in low concentrations in the serum. The normal biological role of the IgE antibody is not clear. It is probably important in defense against parasitic infestations. Generally, an elevated level of IgE is found in patients suffering from atopic diseases.
5. *Immunoglobulin D (IgD)* is found in small amounts in serum and also on the surface of the lymphocytes.

Clinical Significance of B-cell Responses

- Patients with immune deficiency syndromes involving B-lymphocytes, namely, X-linked agammaglobulinemia, suffer from recurrent pyogenic infections primarily involving the sinopulmonary tract. These defects usually manifest after 6 months of life when the passively transferred maternal IgG antibody level begins to decline.
- The capacity to produce specific antibodies to protein antigens is intact at the time of birth. However, normal infants cannot produce antibodies to polysaccharide (PS) antigens until usually after 2 years of life. But if the PS antigen is conjugated to a protein carrier, as in the conjugate *Haemophilus influenzae* type b (Hib) and *Streptococcus pneumoniae* vaccines, the child <2 years of age can produce the immune response.[3,4]

Antigen-presenting Cells and Dendritic Cells

Antigen-presenting cells are a heterogeneous group of immune cells that mediate the cellular immune response by processing and presenting antigens for recognition by certain lymphocytes, such as T-cells. Classical APCs include dendritic cells (DCs), macrophages, Langerhans cells, and B-cells. T-cells do not interact directly unless presented by APCs. B-cells directly interact with antigens to produce humoral response. APCs are the cells that capture antigens by endocytosis or phagocytosis, process them into small peptides, display them at their surface through MHC molecules, and provide costimulation signals that act synergistically to activate antigen-specific T-cells. APCs include B-cells, macrophages, and DCs, although only the DCs are capable of activating naïve T-cells.

The major role of these cells is to identify danger signals, which is done by the special receptors on the APC named toll-like receptors (TLRs).

Antigens are taken up by immature DCs activated by the local inflammation, which provides the signals required for their migration to draining lymph nodes. During this migration, DCs mature and their surface expression of molecules changes. DCs sense "danger signals" through their TLRs and respond by a modulation of their surface or secreted molecules. Simultaneously, antigens are processed into small fragments and displayed at the cell surface in the grooves of *MHC–human leukocyte antigen (HLA)* molecules in humans. As a rule, MHC class I molecules present peptides from antigens that are produced within infected cells, whereas phagocytosed antigens are displayed on MHC class II molecules. Thus, mature DCs reaching the T-cell zone of lymph nodes display MHC–peptide complexes and high levels of costimulation molecules at their surface. CD4+ T-cells recognize antigenic peptides displayed by class II MHC molecules, whereas CD8+ T-cells bind to class I MHC–peptide complexes.

Antigen-specific TCRs may only bind to specific MHC molecules (e.g., HLA-A2), which differ among individuals and populations. Consequently, T-cell responses are highly variable within a population.

Macrophages

Macrophages are a part of the mononuclear phagocyte system. The functions carried out by macrophages in the immune response are as follows:

- They are required to process and present antigens to immunocompetent T-cells.
- They produce a variety of cytokines, such as IL-1 and tumor necrosis factor, and thus exert a modulatory effect on the inflammatory response.
- They are the effector cells of some forms of cell-mediated immunity, e.g., delayed hypersensitivity reaction.

The enzymes in macrophages include lysozymes, cathepsins, acid hydrolases, and neutral proteases. They can secrete digestive enzymes, complement components, arachidonic acid metabolites, enzyme inhibitors, interferons, and chemotactic factors in their environment.

Clinically, the deficiency of phagocyte function is acquired secondary to systemic illnesses, namely diabetes mellitus, malnutrition, and neoplasia, in which the defects of chemotaxis may contribute to susceptibility to infections. The most common congenital deficiency is chronic granulomatous disease. *Staphylococcus*, gram-negative rods, and fungi are troublesome for these individuals who suffer from skin, periorificial, and deep organ infections.

Cytokines

Cytokines are substances that regulate the immunologic, inflammatory, and reparative host responses and comprise previously designated lymphokines (lymphocyte-derived), monokines (monocyte-derived), and several other polypeptides.

Complement System

The cell-killing effects of innate and acquired immunity are mediated in part by a system of plasma enzymes, originally named the complement system. Complement activation occurs in two phases, namely the activation of the C3 component followed by the activation of the attack or lytic sequence. The critical event is the cleavage of C3 by complement-derived enzymes termed *C3 convertases*. The major fragment (C3b) of activated C3 mediates a number of vital biological activities.

Two different pathways or enzyme cascades activate the system: (1) The *classic pathway*, triggered by immune complexes, and (2) the *alternative or properdin pathway*, triggered by contact with various viruses, bacteria, fungi, and tumor cells. These proteins have two functions:

1. They help kill invading organisms by opsonization, chemotaxis, and eventual lysis of the cells.
2. They serve in part as a bridge between innate and acquired immunity by activating B-cells.

IMMUNE RESPONSE

Antigens and Antibodies

Antigen is a protein, toxin, or other substance of high molecular weight to which the body reacts by producing antibodies and stimulating an immune response.

Antibodies (immunoglobulins; Ig) are protein molecules that bind specifically to a particular part of an antigen, called antigenic site or epitope. There are multiple epitopes on the same antigen, and there are multiple antigens on the same organism. The immune system mounts multiple antibodies to the same organism. Only some of these antibodies are protective in nature and the rest are not useful in this sense. In general, viruses contain a lesser number of antigens than bacteria, fungi, or parasites. Humoral immunity is mediated through B-lymphocytes by secreting antibodies (immunoglobulins) that act by neutralization, by complement activation, or by promoting opsonophagocytosis, which results in an early reduction of pathogen load and clearance of extracellular pathogens and their toxins. Some humoral antibodies prevent colonization, which is the first step in pathogenesis by encapsulated organisms like Hib, pneumococcal, meningococcal, and organisms like diphtheria and pertussis.

During acute infection, IgM antibodies appear within a few days, peak at around 7–10 days, and disappear in the next few months to undetected levels. Hence, the presence of IgM indicates a recent infection. Similarly, IgM, being a large molecule, is not transferred transplacentally in a newborn. The IgM response is usually seen in the primary response. It is short-lived, and the titers of the antibodies are lower.

Immunoglobulin G response usually picks up along with IgM, or after a few days, peaks it around 2–3 weeks, and lasts for a very long time. It is usually seen best during the secondary response, classically seen on re-exposure, and the titers are very high.

SEQUENCE OF EVENTS AFTER VACCINATION

The ability to recognize the antigen is innate and develops without exposure to the antigen. Stem cells differentiate into many million different T- and B-lymphocytes, each with the ability to respond to a particular antigen.

The first and crucial step following the intramuscular administration of a vaccine is the recognition of the vaccine antigen or adjuvant as foreign and as a "danger." This is accomplished by the interaction between the pathogen-associated molecular patterns (PAMPs) on the pathogen and the pattern recognition receptors (PRRs), which are present in the APCs.[3,4] This interaction results in intracellular messaging within the APCs, gene transcription, and production of proinflammatory cytokines, which creates a proinflammatory environment and recruits more and more APCs at the site of vaccine administration. This step is crucial because the type of APCs involved in this process skews the immune response toward either a TH1 or TH2 pathway. During this phase, APCs undergo molecular changes, which induce them to migrate toward the regional lymph nodes. In the primary immune response, native antigen is carried to a lymph node and taken up by specialized cells called follicular DCs. Virgin B-cells, bearing surface Ig, specific for that antigen, then bind to this antigen. This antigenic adherence stimulates the B-cells to differentiate into antibody-producing plasma cells. Initially, these plasma cells produce IgM. Later, a switchover in the production of immunoglobulins takes place, and plasma cells start producing the IgG class of immunoglobulins. When the stimulus is removed, the B-cell division and differentiation stop, but the circulating pool of B-lymphocytes still contains a large population of memory cells. During re-exposure to the same antigen (secondary immune response), immediate and extensive divisions of the B-cells with IgG receptors take place, and a large quantity of IgG antibodies are produced. These antibodies combine with the antigen. The type of response elicited will depend upon the antigenic type, its content, and the immune status of an individual.[5,6]

Activation of the follicle germinal center (GC) is the key to a robust and long-lasting immune response. In the case of a protein antigen, in an extrafollicular reaction, B-cells rapidly differentiate into plasma cells that produce low-affinity antibodies (of the IgM +/– IgG/IgA isotypes) that appear at low levels in the serum within a few days after immunization. Some antigen-specific helper T-cells that have been activated by antigen-bearing DCs trigger some antigen-specific B cells to migrate toward follicular dendritic cells (FDCs), initiating the GC reaction. In GCs, B cells receive additional signals from follicular T-cells and undergo massive clonal proliferation. This intense proliferation is associated with two major events: Ig class switch from IgM toward IgG, IgA, or IgE and affinity maturation of B cells for their specific antigen, which differentiate into plasma cells secreting large amounts of antigen-specific antibodies.

T-cell-dependent Immune Response

Certain antigens, mainly proteins, induce both B-cell and T-cell stimulations, leading to what is called a T-cell-dependent immune response, whereas large molecular antigens like PS induce only a B-cell response as they are incapable of inducing a T-cell response on their own.

The *T-cell-dependent response* is usually prompt with higher titers, IgG type, and longer lasting. It also shows booster effects with repeated exposure. Infants of 6 weeks of age onward are capable of T-cell-dependent responses. Finally, IgA antibodies are also produced in such a response, which probably helps in providing mucosal protection and eradicating the carrier state. As compared to this, the T-cell-independent response is only B-cell-mediated. It is predominantly IgM type with low titers. The response is short-lived and does not lead to boosting, and such vaccines are actually revaccination rather than boosters when given repeatedly, which produces the same type of response every time the antigen is introduced. Lastly, IgA is not produced, and hence, there is no local mucosal protection with this type of antigen.[5,6]

A T-cell-independent antigen like PS can be converted to a T-cell-dependent antigen by the technique of conjugation, where a carrier protein is conjugated with the PS. When this conjugated moiety is presented to the T-cell, it recognizes the protein carrier as an antigen and leads to internalization of the whole complex, which leads to the T-cell now responding even to the carbohydrate antigen of the complex, producing T-cell response to the PS. This technique is very useful in producing vaccines such as conjugated Hib, pneumococcal, typhoid, and meningococcal vaccines.[6]

T-cell-independent Immune Response

It is elicited by B-cells only and has the following characteristics:

- Only B-cell response, T-cell independent
- Poorly immunogenic below 2 years due to immaturity of the marginal zones
- Do not trigger GC activity
- Weaker and shorter immune response
- No induction of immune memory, hence no booster responses
- There is no local immunity, as IgA is not produced
- Repeated doses lead to hyporesponsiveness

Bacterial (*S. pneumoniae, Neisseria meningitidis, H. influenzae,* and *Salmonella typhi)* PS antigens are T-cell-independent antigens.

Primary versus Secondary Immune Response

When an antigen is introduced for the first time, the immune response starts after a lag of 10 days or so. This is called primary response. Such a response is short-lived and has a lag period, mainly IgM type with low titers of antibodies. In the primary immune response, the antigen exposure elicits an extrafollicular response that results in the rapid appearance of low IgG antibody titers.

Secondary immune responses start on subsequent exposure (booster) to the same antigen. There is no lag phase; response starts in <7 days and persists for a long time, mainly IgG type with high antibody titers.

Active and Passive Immunity

Active immunity is acquired through natural infection/immunization and is long-lasting. Passive immunity is conferred by transplacental passage of maternal antibodies or immunoglobulin/antitoxin sera preparations and is short-lasting.

Immunoglobulins are transferred predominantly in the last trimester and are mainly of IgG type. This protects the child for the first few months till the time she/he develops her/his own immunity after repeated exposure to various antigens after birth. The protection offered by transplacental passive immunity depends on the half-life of the specific antibody; for example, the antibody against poliomyelitis does not protect the child for more than 4–6 weeks (the time of starting the polio vaccination in the baby), whereas the antimeasles antibody protects the child until 6–9 months (the reason for delaying the measles vaccine until 9 months). Not only does passive immunity protect the child against specific diseases, but it also interferes with the immune response to the concerned vaccine, if given in the presence of maternal antibody, such as for measles, as discussed earlier.[5]

Limitations of Early Life Immune Response[5,6]

- Maternal antibodies inhibit antibody responses.
- Do not affect T-cell response.
- Antibody responses elicited in early life are short-lasting.
- BCG can be given as maternal antibodies actually enhance T-cell responses.
- Oral polio vaccine may be given as there is no maternal IgA in the gut to neutralize the virus (maternal Ab are only IgG).
- Measles at 6 months in an outbreak situation may protect by inducing T-cell immunity.

REFERENCES

1. Chaplin DD. Overview of the immune response. J Allergy Clin Immunol. 2010;125(Suppl 2):S3-23.
2. Lahiri KR, Taori RN. Basics of immune system in children. In: Parthasarathy A, Menon PSN, Nair MKC (Eds). IAP Textbook of Pediatrics, 4th edition. New Delhi: Jaypee Brothers Medical Publishers (P) Ltd; 2009. pp. 1080-4.
3. Paul Y, Vashishtha VM. Immunology of vaccines: basics and beyond. In: Vashishtha VM, Kalra A, Thacker N (Eds). FAQs on Immunization, 1st edition. New Delhi: Jaypee Brothers Medical Publishers; 2011. pp. 3-23.
4. Shah NK, Thacker N. General principles of vaccination. In: Thacker N, Shah NK (Eds). Immunization in Clinical Practice. New Delhi: Jaypee Brothers Medical Publishers; 2005. pp. 1-5.
5. Paul Y, Vashishtha V. Vaccine immunology—basics and beyond. In: FAQs on Vaccines and Immunization Practices, 3rd edition. New Delhi: Jaypee Brothers Medical Publishers; 2021. pp. 1-27.
6. Shah AK. Basic Immunology in IAP Q&A on Vaccines and Vaccinology, 1st edition. New Delhi: Jaypee Brothers Medical Publishers; 2021.

6.2 Inborn Errors of Immunity

Tanu Singhal

INTRODUCTION

Inborn errors of immunity (IEI), previously termed primary immunodeficiency disorders (PIDs), are a group of approximately 500 inherited genetic disorders that result in defects in normal immune development and function.[1] They occur at a prevalence ranging from 1 in 1,000 to 5 in 1,000 and are often underdiagnosed or diagnosed late. The clinical presentation is variable and includes recurrent, severe, and unusual infections, autoimmunity, autoinflammatory diseases, and malignancies. This section gives a bird's-eye view of the common IEIs. The new classification of IEI by the International Union of Immunological Societies (IUIS) is listed in **Table 6.2.1**.[2,3]

TABLE 6.2.1: International Union of Immunological Societies (IUIS) classification of inborn errors of immunity (IEI).

Group	*IEI disease category*	*Characteristics*	*Examples*
I	Cellular and humoral IDs	• Recurrent viral, fungal, and bacterial infections • Autoimmunity	• SCID • DOCK8 deficiency
II	Syndromic combined IDs	• Recurrent viral, fungal, and bacterial infections • Autoimmunity • Nonimmune features • Dysmorphology	• HIES • Wiskott–Aldrich syndrome • DiGeorge syndrome
III	Antibody deficiencies	Recurrent bacterial sinopulmonary infections	• Agammaglobulinemia • AR hyper-IgM syndrome • Selective IgA deficiency
IV	Immune dysregulatory diseases	• Autoimmunity • Hemophagocytic lymphohistiocytosis (HLH) • Lymphoproliferation	• Familial HLH • Chédiak–Higashi syndrome • Autoimmune lymphoproliferative syndrome (ALPS)
V	Phagocytic diseases	• Severe bacterial infections of the skin, lungs, and lymph nodes • Inflammatory bowel disease	• Chronic granulomatous disease • Leukocyte adhesion deficiency • Congenital neutropenias
VI	Innate IDs	• Invasive bacterial infections (sepsis and meningitis) often in the absence of fever • Recurrent fungal, mycobacterial, and viral infections	• Mendelian susceptibility to mycobacterial disease (MSMD) • STAT1, STAT2 deficiencies • TLR3, CARD9 deficiency
VII	Autoinflammatory diseases	• Recurrent fever, rash, and arthritis/arthralgia • Amyloidosis • Inflammatory bowel disease	• Familial Mediterranean fever • Mevalonate kinase deficiency • TRAPS
VIII	Complement deficiencies	• Disseminated Neisseria infections • Recurrent pyogenic infections • SLE • Atypical hemolytic uremic syndrome	• Deficiency of complement components • Properdin deficiency
IX	Bone marrow failure	• Macrocytic anemia and other cytopenias • Skeletal, nail, hair, and/or skin abnormalities	• Fanconi anemia • Dyskeratosis congenita
X	Phenocopies of PIDs	Multiple phenotypes	• Chronic mucocutaneous candidiasis • Recurrent staphylococcal infections

(AR: autosomal recessive; CARD9: caspase recruitment domain-containing protein 9; DOCK8: dedicator of cytokinesis 8; HIES: hyperimmunoglobulin E syndrome; ID: immunodeficiency; IgA: immunoglobulin A; IgM: immunoglobulin M; PID: primary immunodeficiency; SCID: severe combined immunodeficiency; SLE: systemic lupus erythematosus; STAT: signal transducer and activator of transcription; TLR3: toll-like receptor 3; TRAPS: tumor necrosis factor receptor-associated periodic fever syndrome)

OVERVIEW OF SOME COMMON INBORN ERRORS OF IMMUNITY

Severe Combined Immunodeficiency

Severe combined immunodeficiency (SCID) is a group of syndromes of differing genetic mutations that impair the development and function of T- and B-cells and sometimes natural killer (NK) cells. Inheritance is either X-linked dominant or autosomal recessive (AR). The CD3 (T-cell count) in SCID is generally <300/μL and there is panhypogammaglobulinemia. In some cases in early life, the lymphocyte count and immunoglobulins may be near normal due to the transplacental passage of maternal cells and immunoglobulins. There is an absence of lymphoid tissue and no thymic shadow on the radiograph.

These children present in the first few months of life with recurrent infections, diarrhea, and severe failure to thrive. Common manifestations include mucocutaneous candidiasis, severe and often fatal viral infections [cytomegalovirus (CMV), respiratory syncytial virus (RSV), influenza, parainfluenza, rotavirus, norovirus, Epstein–Barr virus (EBV), measles, herpes zoster virus (HSV), and varicella zoster virus (VZV)], pneumocystis pneumonia, and complications from live vaccines including Bacillus Calmette-Guérin (BCG) vaccine, oral polio vaccine (OPV), mumps–measles–rubella (MMR) vaccine, and varicella vaccine. SCID is almost uniformly fatal in the first year of life.

It is a medical emergency, and patients need to be referred for hemopoietic stem cell transplantation (HSCT) as soon as possible. Till HSCT, antimicrobial, antifungal, antiviral, antimycobacterial (if BCG was given), and immunoglobulin therapy should be initiated.

DiGeorge Syndrome

DiGeorge syndrome, also known as velocardiofacial syndrome, is caused by heterozygous deletion at chromosomal 22q11.2 leading to errors in the development of the pharyngeal pouch system. It is characterized by a triad of conotruncal heart defects, immunodeficiency, and hypocalcemia (due to parathyroid aplasia). Other manifestations include craniofacial and palatal abnormalities, developmental delay, allergic disease, and autoimmunity. The phenotype is very variable. The immunologic defects can range from mild to profound immunodeficiency with complete thymic aplasia.

Wiskott–Aldrich Syndrome

Wiskott–Aldrich syndrome is an X-linked syndrome of variable phenotype due to mutation in the gene coding for the Wiskott–Aldrich syndrome protein (WASP). The classic WASP phenotype is characterized by early onset thrombocytopenia with bleeding manifestations, eczema, and recurrent bacterial, viral sinopulmonary and gastrointestinal infections. There is a tendency for the development of autoimmunity and malignancy in later life. The characteristic laboratory finding is thrombocytopenia with levels between 20,000 and 50,000/mm^3 and small platelet volumes. Treatment options include prophylactic antibiotics, antivirals, platelet transfusions, thrombopoietin receptor agonist therapy, gammaglobulin replacement, splenectomy, and eventually HSCT. Gene therapy trials are ongoing.

Hyperimmunoglobulin E Syndrome

Hyperimmunoglobulin E syndromes (HIES) are a group of disorders caused by multiple genetic mutations with common features of recurrent eczema, skin infections, pneumonia, eosinophilia, and high immunoglobulin E (IgE) levels. An unusual feature of HIES is a lack of local inflammation at sites of infection leading to cold abscesses and severe pneumonia with few systemic features. The autosomal dominant variant due to the signal transducer and activator of transcription-3 (STAT3) deficiency (Job syndrome) has additional craniofacial abnormalities, hyperextensibility of joints, recurrent fractures, and retention of primary teeth. The AR variant due to the dedicator of cytokinesis 8 (*DOCK8*) gene deficiency is more severe and has an increased tendency for severe viral infections (HSV, VZV, HPV, and molluscum contagiosum), pneumocystis, and cryptosporidia and allergies. Treatment of HIES includes antibiotic/antifungal and antiviral prophylaxis and skin and bone care. HSCT is recommended for *DOCK8* deficiency.

Antibody Deficiencies

Antibody deficiencies account for half of the IEIs.

Bruton's Agammaglobulinemia

The most dramatic is Bruton's agammaglobulinemia (X-linked inheritance) due to a defect in the *BTK* gene. It is characterized by the absence of tonsils and adenoid tissues, near absence of CD19+ B cells, and very low levels of immunoglobulin G (IgG), IgM, and IgA. Most children present beyond the age of 3–6 months once the maternal immunoglobulins have decayed with severe and recurrent bacterial ear, nose, and throat (ENT) infections, pulmonary infections, and gastroenteritis. The other salient feature is susceptibility to severe enteroviral meningitis or encephalitis and OPV-induced paralytic poliomyelitis. Bronchiectasis and pulmonary insufficiency are seen as age advances. Treatment consists of lifelong immunoglobulin replacement therapy and antibiotic prophylaxis. Live vaccines, especially OPV, are contraindicated in these children and their close contacts. Gene therapy and HSCT are investigational.

Class-switch Immunoglobulin Deficiencies

These are due to the inability of B cells to switch from IgM to IgG/IgA production characterized by low levels of IgG and IgA and normal or high levels of IgM. The X-linked hyper-IgM syndrome due to mutations in the *CD40* ligand gene is distinct from the other class-switch disorders as it is also associated with neutropenia and T-cell defects. It is associated with a propensity for severe pneumocystis infections in addition to respiratory bacterial infections.

Common Variable Immunodeficiency

This is a heterogeneous group of disorders that are characterized by the inability of B cells to differentiate into plasma cells. It is characterized by low levels of IgG/IgA and IgM (<2 standard deviations of age-related cutoff), impaired response to immunization, absence of profound T-cell deficiency, and exclusion of other causes of hypogammaglobulinemia. The disease usually presents in late childhood or young adulthood with recurrent bacterial ENT and pulmonary infections and bronchiectasis. Gastrointestinal manifestations including chronic diarrhea, malabsorption, and giardiasis are also common. Patients often have lymphadenopathy, splenomegaly, and granuloma formation. Autoimmune disease with cytopenias, hypothyroidism, arthritis, and increased risk of malignancies are other manifestations. Treatment includes antibiotic prophylaxis, immunoglobulin replacement, and immunomodulatory drugs in those with autoimmune disease.

Transient Hypogammaglobulinemia of Infancy

This is a condition where there is a delay in the production of immunoglobulins after the disappearance of maternal immunoglobulins. Many cases are asymptomatic; others may have recurrent airway infections, severe sepsis, meningitis, recurrent diarrhea, oral candidiasis, and severe varicella infection. Antibody levels generally normalize by 2–3 years but in some children remain depressed for years. Treatment consisting mainly of antibiotic prophylaxis and immunoglobulin replacement is indicated only in those with severe infections.

Other Humoral Immunodeficiencies

Other humoral immunodeficiencies include selective IgA deficiency (most common IEI and defined as an IgA level <7 mg/dL in children 4 years or older), immunoglobulin G2 subclass deficiency, and specific polysaccharide antibody deficiency (SPAD; where there is impaired response to pneumococcal polysaccharide vaccine). These disorders may be asymptomatic or present with recurrent airway infections or chronic diarrhea. IgA deficiency is associated with chronic giardiasis and anaphylaxis or allergic reactions when blood products are administered.

Familial Hemophagocytic Lymphohistiocytosis

These syndromes result from defects in perforin/syntaxin genes among others that lead to defective NK cells and cytotoxic T-cell activity. Patients can present at any age with life-threatening HLH characterized by fever, cytopenias, jaundice, splenomegaly, hyperferritinemia, hypofibrinogenemia, and hypertriglyceridemia. Treatment involves immunosuppressive therapy with steroids, cyclosporine, and etoposide followed by HSCT.

Chédiak–Higashi Syndrome

Chédiak–Higashi syndrome is an AR disorder in which a gene mutation results in abnormal lysosomal transport. The peripheral smear shows giant cytoplasmic granules in leukocytes and platelets. The presentation is with recurrent bacterial infections of skin, respiratory tract with oculocutaneous albinism, progressive neurologic defects, and coagulation abnormalities and, at later stages, HLH. Definitive treatment is HSCT.

Chronic Granulomatous Disease

The most prominent defect of phagocyte function is chronic granulomatous disease (CGD), inherited mostly as X-linked recessive inheritance and less commonly as AR. It is due to the defect in the phagocyte NADPH oxidase complex which prevents the oxidative burst killing of microbes. It is characterized by recurrent skin, soft tissue, lymph node, liver infections, granulomatous abscesses in internal organs, and inflammatory bowel disease. Commonly implicated organisms are *Staphylococcus aureus*, *Aspergillus*, *Serratia*, *Nocardia*, *Candida*, and *Burkholderia*. In India, it is often misdiagnosed as tuberculosis due to the presence of granulomas on histopathology. Diagnosis is by the estimation of neutrophil oxidase activity by the nitroblue tetrazolium or dihydrorhodamine (NBT/DHR) test. Treatment includes cotrimoxazole prophylaxis, itraconazole prophylaxis, use of interferon-gamma (IFN-γ), and, in severe cases, HSCT. Gene therapy is investigational. Female carriers can also exhibit an increased rate of inflammatory diseases and rarely develop typical CGD infections due to skewed X chromosome lyonization.

Leukocyte Adhesion Deficiency

Leukocyte adhesion deficiency (LAD I, II, and III) is due to the inability of the leukocytes to migrate from the vasculature to tissues during infection or inflammation. LAD presents in the newborn period with delayed separation of the umbilical cord and later recurrent cellulitis and abscesses with the absence of pus formation, severe periodontitis, marked neutrophilia (up to 100,000/mm^3), and delayed wound healing. LAD I is the most severe; LAD II has less severe infections but neurologic disabilities, short stature, and abnormal facies. LAD III has associated bleeding due to platelet dysfunction. Treatment involves oral and dental care, prompt treatment of infections, antimicrobial prophylaxis, fucose supplementation (LAD II), and HSCT (LAD I and III).

Congenital Neutropenia

Congenital neutropenias (CNs) are due to the failure of bone marrow in producing neutrophils with an absolute neutrophil count of <500/mm^3. CN includes severe congenital neutropenia (SCN, Kostmann syndrome), cyclic neutropenia, and Diamond–Schwachman syndrome (associated pancreatic insufficiency and bony abnormalities). The nadir in cyclic neutropenia is usually 21 days but may range from 14 to 36 days. Manifestations include recurrent skin, soft tissue, respiratory, rectal infections, and gingivitis/oral ulcerations. Treatment is with granulocyte-macrophage colony-stimulating factor (GM-GCF) and HSCT in unresponsive cases.

Mendelian Susceptibility to Mycobacterial Disease

Mendelian susceptibility to mycobacterial disease (MSMD) is a group of disorders arising from defects in the IFN-γ or interleukin-12 axis. These patients present in early life with disseminated infections due to the BCG vaccine (BCGiosis) and later with environmental nontuberculous mycobacteria (NTM) and *Mycobacterium tuberculosis*. The common manifestations of these include fever, failure to thrive, adenopathy, hepatosplenomegaly, diarrhea, osteomyelitis, and central nervous system (CNS) disease. BCGiosis is also characterized by abscesses or lymphadenitis at the BCG injection site. Patients are also at risk for other intracellular pathogens such as *Salmonella typhi* and nontyphoidal *Salmonella*. Diagnosis is best established by genetic sequencing. Treatment involves regular administration of subcutaneous IFN-γ or, in some cases, HSCT.

Autoinflammatory Disorders

These groups of disorders are characterized by overactivation of the innate inflammatory pathways leading to excess of proinflammatory cytokines. The common autoinflammatory disorders include familial Mediterranean fever, hyperimmunoglobulin D syndrome, tumor necrosis factor-associated periodic fever syndrome (TRAPS), and chronic recurrent multifocal osteomyelitis (CRMO). The clinical manifestations include recurrent fever, rash, serositis, uveitis, meningitis, arthritis, enteritis, vasculitis with a rise in neutrophil count, and C-reactive protein (CRP). These disorders are important differentials for the recurrent fever phenotype. Diagnosis is by genetic sequencing. Treatment involves the use of anti-inflammatory drugs, steroids, colchicine, and biologicals.

Complement Defects

The complement arm of the immune system protects the body from bacterial pathogens by opsonizing bacteria and also forming a membrane attack complex to cause lysis of bacteria. Complement proteins also play a role in the clearance of apoptotic cell debris, which can cause autoimmune inflammation. There are three main complement protein pathways: Classical complement, alternative complement, and lectin pathway. Early classical complement component deficiencies (C1q, C1r, C1s, C2, C4, and C3) present with systemic lupus erythematosus (SLE) and susceptibility to infections from encapsulated bacteria. Terminal classical complement component deficiencies (C5, C6, C7, C8, and C9) and alternative complement pathway defects present with a unique susceptibility to recurrent *Neisseria* meningitis. A deficiency of factor H and factor I (both complement regulatory proteins) can cause a phenotype of recurrent atypical hemolytic uremic syndrome or susceptibility to Neisseria, depending upon the mutation. Initial screening tests for complement deficiency include CH50 (total hemolytic complement) and AH50 (measures total functional activity of the alternative pathway). Treatment consists of antibiotic prophylaxis and immunization (especially meningococcal vaccine).

Bone Marrow Failure Syndromes

The classical disorder here is Fanconi's anemia, a chromosomal breakage syndrome that is characterized by insidious loss of bone marrow function. They have associated short stature and organ abnormalities. Most cases present late in the first decade with pancytopenia. There is a higher tendency for the development of hematologic malignancies and acute myeloid leukemia (AML) in later life. Treatment strategies include androgens, transfusions, growth factors, and HSCT. Gene therapy is investigational.

Phenocopies of Inborn Errors of Immunity

Phenocopies of IEI are noninherited disorders that occur due to the formation of autoantibodies against various components of the immune system. These include chronic mucocutaneous candidiasis due to autoantibodies to IL-17 and/or IL-22, adult-onset MSMD with autoantibodies to IFN-γ, recurrent staphylococcal skin infections due to autoantibodies to IL-6, autoantibodies to GM-CSF that can cause pulmonary alveolar proteinosis, acquired angioedema with autoantibodies to C1 inhibitor, and many others.

APPROACH TO DIAGNOSIS OF A CHILD WITH A SUSPECTED INBORN ERRORS OF IMMUNITY

Fortunately, the most common causes of recurrent infections in a child are due to increased exposure, atopy, or anatomic defect rather than IEI. IEI should be suspected in the setting of infections that are:

- Recurrent [defined as two or more severe infections in 1 year, three or more respiratory infections (e.g., sinusitis, otitis, and bronchitis) in 1 year, or the need for antibiotics for 2 months/year]
- Of unusual severity [persistent evidence of inflammation (e.g., fever) or confinement to bed for a week or more (e.g., missing school or other activities), failure to respond to oral antibiotics, and/or the need for intravenous antibiotics or hospitalization]
- Due to uncommon organisms
- At unusual sites

The warning signs of PIDs are listed in **Box 6.2.1**. The approach to diagnosis of IEI and type of IEI begins with a detailed history and physical examination keeping in mind the various manifestations detailed previously.[1,4,5] The age of onset, site of infections, underlying organisms, and associated physical abnormalities give a clue to the type of immunodeficiency.[6]

BOX 6.2.1: The warning signs of primary immunodeficiency disorder (PID) (the first 10 are from the Jeffrey Modell Foundation).

1. Four or more new ear infections within 1 year
2. Two or more serious sinus infections within 1 year
3. Two or more months on antibiotics with little effect
4. Two or more pneumonias within 1 year
5. Failure of an infant to gain weight or grow normally
6. Recurrent deep skin or organ abscesses
7. Persistent thrush in mouth or fungal infection on skin
8. Need for intravenous antibiotics to clear infections
9. Two or more deep-seated infections including septicemia
10. A family history of primary immunodeficiency
11. Infection caused by an unusual microbial organism and/or in an unusual location
12. Complications from a live vaccine [e.g., rotavirus, varicella, and Bacillus Calmette-Guérin (BCG) vaccines]
13. Chronic diarrhea
14. Nonhealing wounds
15. Extensive skin lesions
16. Persistent lymphopenia
17. Unexplained autoimmunity or fevers
18. Granulomas
19. Hemophagocytic lymphohistiocytosis (HLH)
20. Lymphoma in childhood
21. Features typical of syndromic PIDs (e.g., cartilage-hair hypoplasia, Chédiak–Higashi syndrome, and ataxia-telangiectasia)
22. Absent thymus on chest X-ray, cardiac abnormalities, and hypocalcemia

APPROACH TO LABORATORY DIAGNOSIS OF A CHILD WITH SUSPECTED INBORN ERRORS OF IMMUNITY

Please refer to **Table 6.2.2**.

MANAGEMENT OF INBORN ERRORS OF IMMUNITY

Patients with IEI should be referred to specialist centers for care. Infections should be identified and treated promptly.[6-8] Effort should be made to find the etiologic agent even if it involves invasive testing as the differential diagnosis is very wide. Nutritional and micronutrient support is crucial. Prophylactic strategies include isolation, antimicrobial prophylaxis with cotrimoxazole, antifungal prophylaxis (fluconazole/itraconazole), antiviral prophylaxis (acyclovir and ganciclovir), antimycobacterial prophylaxis (isoniazid), gamma interferon, and replacement immunoglobulin therapy.[3,9] Blood products should be irradiated and leukocytes depleted.

Immunizations should be given carefully as live vaccines are often not safe and killed vaccines are poorly effective.[10] The immunization strategy depends on the type of IEI. Children with major antibody deficiencies and combined

TABLE 6.2.2: Approach to laboratory diagnosis of a child with suspected inborn errors of immunity (IEI).

Test	***Comments***
Complete blood count with peripheral smear	• Attention to absolute lymphocyte count (lymphopenia if <1,500 in children >5 years and <2,500 for younger children) • Low platelets in Wiskott–Aldrich syndrome • Attention to absolute neutrophil count (ANC) • Eosinophilia in hyper-IgE syndrome • Howell–Jolly bodies in asplenia • Acanthocytes in ataxia telangiectasia • Cytoplasmic granules in Chédiak–Higashi syndrome
Imaging: Chest X-ray, ECHO, CT, and MRI	Look for thymic shadow, heart defects, and signature infections/abnormalities
Biochemistry, ESR, and CRP	Look for low globulins, low calcium (DiGeorge syndrome), high acute phase reactants in infection
HIV serology	To exclude HIV infection
Serum IgG, IgM, IgA, and IgE levels	• Correlate with age-related cutoffs • A serum IgG level of <300 mg/dL or serum IgG + IgA + IgM <500 or complete absence of IgM or IgA above the age of 6 months is suggestive of antibody deficiency • Very high IgE levels indicate hyper-IgE syndrome
Flow cytometry	Enumeration of T, B, and NK cell subsets (may be falsely low during an acute infection)
NBT and DHR tests	For diagnosis of CGD
CH50, AH50	For diagnosis of complement deficiencies
Clinical or whole exome sequencing or whole genome sequencing	• The molecular bases for many of the common PIDs have been identified • Diagnosis at the genetic or molecular level by clinical/whole exome sequencing is always desirable to establish unequivocal diagnosis, to permit accurate genetic counseling, to define better the genotype–phenotype associations, and for the best therapy of specific disorders now and in the future

(CGD: chronic granulomatous disease; CRP: C-reactive protein; CT: computed tomography; DHR: dihydrorhodamine; ESR: erythrocyte sedimentation rate; HIV: human immunodeficiency virus; IgA: immunoglobulin A; IgE: immunoglobulin E; IgG: immunoglobulin G; IgM: immunoglobulin M; NBT: nitroblue tetrazolium; NK: natural killer; PIDs: primary immunodeficiency disorders)

immunodeficiencies on immunoglobulin replacement therapy should only be given influenza inactivated vaccines; other inactivated vaccines are not recommended and all live vaccines, especially OPV, are contraindicated. Patients with MSMD should be given all age-appropriate inactivated vaccines including pneumococcal vaccines; live vaccines including BCG are contraindicated. Children with CGD should be given all inactivated and live vaccines except BCG. Children with complement deficiencies should be given all inactivated and live vaccines; the meningococcal vaccine is especially recommended. Family members should be vaccinated completely with the exception of OPV to protect the index case.

Psychosocial support is paramount.

Definitive therapy for serious IEI is by HSCT. Gene therapy is emerging.

CONCLUSION

Inborn errors of immunity are rare but often missed serious disorders. Diagnosis and treatment are complicated, expensive, and not readily available. It is crucial to increase awareness among practitioners about these diseases and develop regional referral centers that can evaluate and treat children with IEI.

REFERENCES

1. Notarangelo LD, Fischer A, Geha RS, Casanova JL, Chapel H, Conley ME, et al. Primary immunodeficiencies: 2009 update. J Allergy Clin Immunol. 2009;124(6):1161-78.
2. Tangye SG, Al-Herz W, Bousfiha A, Cunningham-Rundles C, Franco JL, Holland SM, et al. Human inborn errors of immunity: 2022 update on the classification from the International Union of Immunological Societies Expert Committee. J Clin Immunol. 2022;42(7):1473-507.
3. UpToDate. [online] Available from www.uptodate.com [Last accessed November, 2024].
4. Bonilla FA, Bernstein IL, Khan DA, Ballas ZK, Chinen J, Frank MM, et al. Practice parameter for the diagnosis and management of primary immunodeficiency. Ann Allergy Asthma Immunol. 2005;94(5 Suppl 1):S1-63.
5. Hernandez-Trujillo VP. Approach to children with recurrent infections. Immunol Allergy Clin North Am. 2015;35(4):625-36.
6. Buckley RH (Ed). (2006). Diagnostic and clinical care guidelines for primary immunodeficiency diseases: Immune Deficiency Foundation. [online] Available from www.primaryimmune.org [Last accessed October, 2024].
7. Wood P, Stanworth S, Burton J, Jones A, Peckham DG, Green T, et al. Recognition, clinical diagnosis and management of patients with primary antibody deficiencies: a systematic review. Clin Exp Immunol. 2007;149(3):410-23.
8. Marciano BE, Holland SM. Primary immunodeficiency diseases: current and emerging therapeutics. Front Immunol. 2017;8:937.
9. Perez EE, Orange JS, Bonilla F, Chinen J, Chinn IK, Dorsey M, et al. Update on the use of immunoglobulin in human disease: a review of evidence. J Allergy Clin Immunol. 2017;139(3S):S1-46.
10. Rubin LG, Levin MJ, Ljungman P, Davies EG, Avery R, Tomblyn M, et al. 2013 IDSA clinical practice guideline for vaccination of the immunocompromised host. Clin Infect Dis. 2014;58(3):e44-100.

6.3 Principles and Practice of Immunization

T Jacob John

INTRODUCTION

Immunization against vaccine-preventable diseases (VPDs) is an integral part of both individual medical care (as preventive medicine) and community-level disease control (a public health function of governments). While national immunization programs in low-income countries use vaccines selected by their governments using epidemiologic and economic criteria against diseases identified for control, in pediatrics, we use vaccines against other locally prevalent diseases also, as per individualized choice, based on risk assessment.

Since disease episodes disrupt daily life's routine, may necessitate medical care (involving expenditure), and may cause "disability" (retarded brain development and scholastic performance, muscle paralysis, immunodeficiency, stunting, and wasting),[1] even death, disease prevention by immunization is a fundamental right of the child.[2]

In the absence of overarching public health infrastructure in India, the national "Universal Immunization Programme" (UIP) is "vertical"—designed or funded by the central government and implemented by state governments, through their respective Ministries of Health and Family Welfare.

UIP policies regarding old vaccines were inherited from the World Health Organization's (WHO) Expanded Program on Immunization (EPI), but for the choice of newer vaccines and their schedules, we rely on a National Technical Advisory Group on Immunization (NTAGI).[3] Organizationally, UIP is a silo, managed through dedicated immunization officers at state and district levels and field staff under them—typical of all vertical programs. Unfortunately, disease control remains incomplete without validated "outcome monitoring."[4,5]

Immunization coverage is monitored regularly but it is a measure of "inputs efficiency" as a tool of management. UIP's input achievements are excellent, reaching about 90% coverage with the set of vaccine doses given during infancy. In districts lagging behind in coverage, well-planned multivaccine campaigns are conducted under *"Project Indradhanush"* and *"Intensified Project Indradhanush."*

Outcome monitoring requires systematic case-based disease surveillance.[4,5] In its absence, we have a highly efficient UIP and, side by side, large numbers of VPDs. When polio was targeted for elimination, India had to create a polio-specific "acute flaccid paralysis" (AFP) surveillance with laboratory support for confirming polio. Currently, India is striving for the elimination of measles and rubella and has established a fever and rash surveillance with laboratory support for confirming diagnosis. The legacy of smallpox eradication was a fever and rash surveillance, which was discontinued in the early 1980s after EPI was adopted.

The Indian Academy of Pediatrics (IAP) has its own immunization schedule and Advisory Committee on Immunization. IAP has a web-based disease reporting modality, IDsurv, illustrating what can be done for filling the gaps in disease surveillance (see www.idsurv.org). The guiding principle of pediatric immunization is the best interests of children, to mitigate risks of diseases, while UIP's goal is community-level disease control—in the best interests of the majority—what can be accomplished within the government's budget.

Thankfully, the government's regulatory agency [Drugs Controller General of India (DCGI)] licenses other vaccines on merit, if target diseases are prevalent. The IAP schedule covers all UIP vaccines and includes more vaccines and improved schedules.

BROAD BIOLOGICAL PRINCIPLES

During infection by pathogens, the host-pathogen interaction in the body has three dimensions:

1. Pathogen amplification and spread within the body, with or without pathogen shedding
2. Cell/tissue/organ damage, hence physical/biochemical pathology, causing symptoms/signs of disease
3. Immune responses irrespective of the presence/severity of symptoms[6]

The concurrently developing immunity is essential for recovery processes, curtailing the first two dimensions.

If exposed again to the same pathogen, the host-pathogen interactions are drastically modified compared to those in the first instance in the immunity-naïve. Immunity denotes, conceptually, this new physiological state. Immunity can also be induced by immunization, avoiding risks of disease. This is a unique contribution of scientific medicine, absent in other traditional systems of medicine or health care.

Pathogen shedding has epidemiological implications. Transmission (pathways and dynamics) of pathogens is a critical element in epidemiology, relevant for understanding the principles of both disease prevention (individual level) and control (community level). If shedding leads to transmission to other human hosts, humans become the pathogen's reservoir and the infectious disease is "anthroponosis." In many (not all) anthroponoses, shedding and transmission are reduced in magnitude and/or duration due to immunity induced by immunization. This is the basis of the "herd effect" of immunization, elaborated in the following text.

WHAT ARE VACCINES?

Substances introduced into the body (inoculated) in order to stimulate the immune system and elicit adaptive immune response(s) are together called vaccines. As a biomedical product for use in humans, only the ones approved by DCGI are to be inoculated. Vaccine may be inoculated through injection (intradermal, subcutaneous, or intramuscular), by mouth, or by nostril. Skin as an absorptive organ was a teaching of Ayurveda, and scientific medicine has adopted it in modern times. Interestingly, even an antigen can be applied on skin under a skin patch and the immune system will respond. We can look forward to its increasing use for injection-free vaccination in the future.

Generations of vaccines were made with the pathogen's antigens: either as whole pathogen—live attenuated to make it nonvirulent or as inactivated, noninfectious; or toxin converted to toxoid, or the pathogen's best structural subunits as antigens. Additive substances, called "adjuvants", were found to enhance immune response.

The time taken to develop such vaccines through the investigational and evaluation processes used to be several years. Faced with the COVID-19 pandemic, two approaches were applied. One was to grow the virus and inactivate it. One Indian vaccine manufacturer (Bharat Biotech) made such a vaccine with a novel adjuvant Alhydroxiquim-II that enhanced both antibody production and cell-mediated immunity (CMI). Its safety record is excellent. It is highly immunogenic too.

The other approach was innovative. If the genes for the microbial antigens in the form of deoxyribonucleic acid (DNA) could be injected, they would be internalized, transcribed to messenger ribonucleic acid (RNA), and translated as antigen that would provoke an immune response. For the sake of simplicity, it was called DNA vaccine. It did not work out well since its immunogenic capacity was rather limited. But the idea remained alive and was applied effectively in 2020 in the face of the COVID-19 pandemic.

COVID-19 is caused by infection with severe acute respiratory syndrome coronavirus 2 (SARS-CoV-2)—a coronavirus with a single-stranded positive-sense *RNA* gene. Positive sense means that it functions directly as messenger RNA (mRNA). The ligand recognized by the host cell virus receptors is the spike (S) protein. A particular segment of viral RNA codes for S protein. If that piece of RNA is injected, it will soon be broken down and removed by the body. Two clever ways were used to deliver RNA without getting rapidly destroyed. One was to package its DNA within a genetically disabled adenovirus—the nonreplicating adenovirus will gain cell entry and then deliver its cargo, the DNA, which in turn will be transcribed as mRNA. This adenovirus-vectored vaccine was developed in the UK and Europe, and the Serum Institute of India was given a license to manufacture it in India.

The 2023 Nobel Prize for Physiology/Medicine was awarded to Katalin Kariko of Hungary and Drew Weissman of the United States for their discovery of nucleotide base modifications so that mRNA remains functionally active when injected into the host, protected within a lipid cover (liposome) until it is internalized in body cells. This method has been in use to create immunity to cancer cells—by synthesizing and modifying the mRNA of the chosen cancer cell antigen. That was for an individualized mRNA vaccine. Synthesizing SARS-CoV-2 spike protein mRNA was a rapid process, and a few companies manufactured mRNA vaccines against COVID-19 in record time, and they were available within several months from the beginning of the pandemic, after completing safety and immunogenicity/efficacy studies.

Both adenovirus-vectored and mRNA vaccines direct host cells to synthesize large amounts of S protein, a portion of which functions as the immunogenic vaccine. However, both vaccines cause very rare serious adverse events following immunization (AEFI). Synthesizing S protein by host cells is an integral step in SARS-CoV-2 infection itself; presumably for that reason (only as speculation), both these vaccines appear to be associated with, or rather mimicking, some of the inflammatory and other pathology-eliciting reactions associated with blood clotting and/or bleeding. During the pandemic, the benefit–risk balance was highly favorable, on account of the high frequencies of severe disease and case fatality. We need a careful reassessment of the benefit–risk balance now that the target disease is endemic and the currently prevalent variant Omicron has very low case fatality.

VACCINOLOGY

As the number of vaccines increased, including in the case of polio where two vaccines with contrasting qualities—inactivated and live-attenuated vaccines—were developed and as the manufacturing processes became increasingly complex, there was a need to understand and apply stringent quality control, in addition to evaluation of efficacy and safety. In 1977, Jonas Salk coined the term "vaccinology" to cover all such aspects as an integrative discipline.

Currently, there are about 30 vaccines in regular use in various countries. A few more vaccines are available against geographically restricted diseases like typhoid fever and cholera prevalent in several countries across the globe and Ebola virus disease that occurs in just a few countries in Africa. Vaccinology is an important part of the specialties/subspecialties of pediatrics, infectious diseases, laboratory immunology, community health, epidemiology, and public health. There are several national-level and international-level courses on vaccinology for interested clinicians, epidemiologists, immunization officers, and industry scientists.

All vaccines are necessarily commercially manufactured and are marketed at a range of prices. Some individuals suspect that some companies may hide safety issues or exaggerate efficacy evaluations. Some ask if the purpose of promoting immunization is for the financial profit of manufacturers and doctors. In this manner, explicitly expressed mistrust and sentiments against some or many vaccines are often encountered in social media. Such "antivaccine" propaganda is detrimental to the honest practice of immunization. As pediatricians, we need to understand all sides of such issues and go by scientific evidence and ethical standards. We need to teach and learn vaccinology. Since the prevention of diseases is the right of children, vaccines should be considered an essential commodity. However, opportunities for unethical promotion and use of vaccines do exist, and thorough knowledge of vaccinology and wise choices are essential for promoting the health of children and regaining trust.

One major aspect of vaccinology is regarding vaccine safety. Unlike therapeutic drugs to mitigate pathology, symptoms, and signs, vaccination is given to persons without the target diseases but who are at risk of contracting them at a later time. Safety is assessed on the basis of the severity of AEFI. Causality assessment must be properly done so that we can separate coincidental diseases from true vaccine-induced AEFI. Trivial, short-term, self-limited, and inconsequential

AEFI do not render a vaccine unsafe. Injection site pain, swelling, systemic unease, or fever of very short duration and the like are common after injected vaccines.

Serious AEFI is one that leads to illness necessitating hospitalization for management, to chronicity of symptoms, to disability, and to death—all only if causally associated. Such vaccines are not safe for routine use unless the benefit-risk balance is highly favorable. In many Western countries, oral poliovirus vaccine (OPV) was used to prevent and control poliomyelitis when its incidence was high but was later replaced by the inactivated polio vaccine (IPV) when the benefit-risk balance of OPV turned unfavorable as vaccine viruses can cause "vaccine-associated paralytic polio" (VAPP).

VACCINATION AND IMMUNIZATION

Although often used synonymously, they actually mean different but overlapping processes. The inoculation of a vaccine is vaccination. Eliciting the desired immune response through vaccination is immunization. For various reasons, vaccination may fail to immunize, which is "vaccine failure."

Immunization against diphtheria, pertussis, and tetanus requires vaccination with three doses (priming/primary immunization) plus one or more booster doses. Parents should understand that the entire course is required for immunization. Incomplete course is partial immunization, not partial vaccination. Such nuances are important also in teaching immunization to various health professionals, including vaccinators.

Reporting of vaccine failure to the government functionaries is important. In the early 1990s, several vaccine-failure cases of neonatal tetanus were reported in Bangladesh. Investigation showed that in-country manufacture of tetanus toxoid had developed a snag and its efficacy was very low. Errors in manufacture were corrected, and thereafter there was no more vaccine failure.

ADVANTAGES AND ATTRIBUTES OF IMMUNIZATION

Immunity, as a function of the body's immune system, has two arms—innate and adaptive. Immunization can induce or modify adaptive immunity. For immune responses and their protective functions, innate and adaptive immunity act in tandem, the former in "recognizing" the infecting pathogens and "informing" the latter to respond. Innate immunity, along with other barriers, is often called the first line of defense.

Innate means inborn; evolutionarily, we have inherited an innate ability to protect against invasion by pathogenic microbes but within limits. Dendritic cells and macrophages, both derived from monocytes in circulation, have two intrinsic properties—phagocytosis and migration to draining lymph nodes carrying the antigen components of the pathogen's structure or secretions. They express major histocompatibility complex (MHC), and the pathogen's antigen is displayed juxtaposed to MHC. Since all dendritic cells and macrophages have all pathogen-associated molecular patterns, their function is called "nonspecific" in contrast to the specificity of antigen recognition of T and B cells. But their function is specific for invading infectious agents, particularly pathogens.

Innate immunity, to an extent, discriminates between virulent and harmless microbes.[7] Repeatedly alerted innate immunity due to many infections may explain why live-attenuated OPV is often ignored by the body in countries with low standards of hygiene/sanitation. However, wild poliovirus (WPV) infects infants and children, seemingly with ease. The inoculum dose in OPV is quite high (1 million infectious particles of type 1 and 6 lakhs of type 3) but likely to be very small in natural exposure to wild virus. Yet, vaccine failure is very common.[8] In countries with high standards of sanitation/hygiene, vaccine virus infection occurs nearly every time when OPV is inoculated. Two phenomena are involved:

1. The potential of innate immunity in discriminating between virulent and attenuated polioviruses
2. Influence of environmental conditions on the efficacy of OPV

These are common to other oral live vaccines also: Ty21a *Salmonella typhi* and Rotavirus vaccines.

In infections in which pathogen load is not much affected by immunity, vaccines tend to not be successful; acquired immunodeficiency syndrome (AIDS), malaria, and, to a certain extent, tuberculosis (TB) are examples. However, there is a malaria vaccine with low/moderate protective efficacy. Bacillus Calmette-Guérin (BCG) offers good protection against progressive primary TB but not against reactivation TB or reinfection TB.

When immune individuals are exposed to infection, in most cases, "breakthrough" infection will occur, but pathogen amplification will be drastically curtailed. Immunity induced by the human papillomavirus (HPV) vaccine is effective enough to abort breakthrough infection. The HPV vaccine [nonreplicating virus-like particles (VLPs), a superb immunogen] induces unnaturally high antibody levels. Passively transduced antibodies on the cervix mucosa neutralize the infectivity of any deposited virus. Vaccine immunity surpasses natural immunity, which is low and not capable of preventing infection when exposed.

Human papillomavirus immunization protects against cancer of the cervix caused by the genotypes in the vaccine. Similarly, hepatitis B immunization protects against infection, its chronicity, and the development of adenocarcinoma of the liver.

Transmucosally transduced antibodies inhibiting infection and/or shedding frequency (the basis of the herd effect) occur after immunization with many live infectious (replicating) vaccines. Children immunized with the measles vaccine do not become a link in the transmission chain, whereas children immunized with OPV may continue to act as links in chains of WPV transmission. Several nonreplicating vaccines also induce immunity with high herd effect—protein-conjugated *Haemophilus influenzae* b and pneumococcal, aluminum-salt adjuvanted diphtheria and pertussis vaccines, and IPV. The "success factor" seems to be unnaturally high antibody levels.

In a measles-immunized child, exposure does not result in disease, but unrecognized "reinfection" may occur without tissue invasion/viremia. Coryza and copious nasal virus shedding, occurring after the incubation period, are the consequences of viremia—once it is blocked, the child does not shed virus.

In diphtheria, antitoxin immunity prevents disease but not asymptomatic (subclinical) reinfection. Reinfection has a very low bacterial load on the pharyngeal mucosa. Heavy bacterial load requires the action of toxins on the pharyngeal epithelium. Immunization reduces bacterial shedding, sufficient to prevent transmission. In polio, breakthrough infection results in virus shedding and transmission. Importation of virulent poliovirus from endemic to nonendemic countries is mostly through immune adults, who themselves are protected from disease. Because of the unnaturally high antibody level induced by IPV (three or more doses), the transmission frequency is reduced, providing an excellent herd effect.[9]

In common parlance, immunity is taken as protection from disease. For the professional, immunity is the presence of any desired parameter of the immune response.

HUMORAL AND CELL-MEDIATED IMMUNITY

Adaptive immunity has two pathways: humoral (antibody-mediated) and cellular (cell-mediated). The "humor" (extracellular body fluids) distributed widely in the body are blood, lymph, intercellular fluids, transduced fluids across the mucosa, cerebrospinal fluid, etc. Hence, the antibody has to be soluble. Gammaglobulin—"adapted" (structurally modified at the Fab terminals), functioning as an immunity-mediator, is denoted immunoglobulin (Ig).

Antibody binds to the virus at the structural site that would normally attach to the host-cell receptor. That blocks cell attachment of the virus, thereby preventing host-cell infection. The virus is "neutralized" (from infection). If the Ig is chemically dissociated from the virus in the laboratory test tube, the virus regains infectivity, showing that antibody attachment does not chemically modify it. When the antibody binds to a bacterial toxin, the toxicity is similarly neutralized irreversibly.

The antibody can be transferred by injection into tissues or infused intravenously, thereby passively rendering the person immune, just for the occasion. This process is "passive immunization." When pathology is mediated by bacterial toxins (e.g., diphtheria and tetanus), the antiserum that binds and neutralizes it is used as therapy.

The Ig molecule is Y-shaped, with two Fab (fragment antigen binding) limbs and the single Fc (fragment crystallizable) limb. Antisera raised in animals can be made safe from hypersensitivity reactions by cleaving off Fc limbs; Fab is the functional portion.

When rabies virus is introduced via dog or cat bite into tissue, the immediate treatment has three steps:

1. Flush the wound with water and toilet soap for detergent and lipid solvent actions to dislodge virus and disrupt virus envelope for drastically reducing tissue virus load.
2. Passive immunization by injecting rabies-specific Ig around the wound to neutralize the infectivity of residual virus.
3. Commence rabies vaccination to induce acquired immunity to be ready as passive immunity wanes.

The vaccination schedule is "peculiar" in that multiple doses are given at short intervals in order to force the immune system to start synthesizing antibodies very early and to reach high levels. This mimics replicating antigen, as if it is persisting over many days.

Viviparous mammals with placenta have two physiological processes of transferring maternal Igs into the offspring. Transplacental transfer occurs in humans and primates. In bovines, there is no such transfer; instead, colostrum is rich in Igs—calves ingest and absorb them. Milk (animal and human) contains Igs but in lower concentration. Babies, unlike calves, do not absorb Igs from ingestion.

The half-life of Ig is about 28 days. The antibody level halves in 4 weeks and the process repeats. The higher the mother's antibody levels, the longer the persistence in the infant. Normally, the poliovirus antibody wanes to a functionally insignificant level in about 4–5 months, whereas the measles antibody may survive for 6–12 months. This duration has implications for immunization. Injected measles vaccine virus will be neutralized by maternal antibody, rendering it ineffective to stimulate immunity induction. Inactivated poliovirus in IPV may be bound by maternal antibodies, thus inhibiting immunogenicity. However, live virus infection by wild or vaccine poliovirus in the nasopharynx and intestine is not prevented by humoral passive immunity. As long as the maternal antibody level is adequate in body fluids, mucosal infection cannot invade body tissues; hence, the infant is protected from polio (natural or vaccine-virus-induced VAPP).

Cell-mediated immunity is collectively the function of immune-adapted T cells. Instead of Ig, CMI involves a set of immune system cells that have been programmed to encounter infected cells. Both humoral immunity and CMI are involved in all infections by pathogens. Immune response to some pathogens is predominantly CMI and to many others predominantly humoral. In general, bacteria that invade cells (intracellular pathogens) and viruses that are always intracellular pathogens elicit CMI, and the immune functions are fulfilled by both CMI and antibodies. The major role of CMI is played by immune-adapted cytotoxic T cells, particularly CD8 cells.

SELF AND NONSELF-RECOGNITION BY IMMUNE SYSTEM CELLS

The fundamental principle of the immune system is the recognition of microbes and microbial subunits/molecules as "non-self" so that the system can respond to defend against the ill effects of infection. During infection, the "foreign" proteins, lipoproteins, carbohydrates, and nucleic acids, generally called "antigens" or "immunogens," sourced from microbes, are recognized by the cells of the immune system, primarily by physical contact between the foreign molecules and antigen-recognizing cells. This physiological process is utilized/imitated by immunization using vaccines.

The antigen-recognizing cells (dendritic cells and macrophages) physically carry the antigens into the germinal centers of lymph nodes, where they inform T cells and B cells about their cargo, again by physical contact. While antigens may be displayed on the surfaces of infected cells, they are not important in the immune response. The antigen has to be presented to T-cells alongside the MHC, and that is what dendritic cells and macrophages do. So, they are called "professional" antigen-presenting cells (APCs). MHC-II helps in identifying T4 cells and MHC-I helps in identifying T8 cells.

T and B lymphocytes recognize "nonself", but individual cells recognize specific "nonself" molecules, one T or B cell recognizing one antigen epitope of one pathogen. Such recognition does not activate T and B cells sufficient for robust immune responses. There are literally tens of thousands of antigens that T and B cells have to recognize. Since pathogen inoculation can occur at any location in the body, it is impossible to locate T and B cells of all specificities all over the body—their sheer numbers will not have space in tissues. So, they are packed in lymph nodes. APCs carry antigens into lymph nodes and meet with T and B cells that have receptor specificity to the antigens. In the lymph node germinal centers, T helper (Th) cells and B cells interact via cytokines, and together they continue the complex processes of immunity—antibody production and formation of memory cells and CMI.

Carbohydrate antigens are not directly recognized by APC—they lack receptors. They are recognized by B cells that are specific for the antigen, but that process does not involve T cells. Immune response is "T-independent", hence without generating memory cells that are necessary for booster response. If conjugated with a microbial peptide like a nontoxic mutant of diphtheria toxin called "cross-reacting material no. 197" (CRM197) or tetanus toxoid, the pattern-recognizing receptors on APC will pick up the "carrier" protein, internalize the entire complex, and then present the carbohydrate antigen to Th cells in conjunction with MHC-II. Immunization is more than simply mimicking nature; we can also "surpass" the natural limits of infection-induced immunity.

The cells of the immune system have to communicate with other cells at distances within the network of the system. That is achieved through cytokines. The effector functions of CMI are fulfilled by direct contact of cytotoxic cells with infected cells or by calling them to the site through cytokines.

Immunity protects through the "effector functions" of immune system cells and their secretory products—activated T cells, assisted in some specific situations by complement activation, plasma cells derived from activated B cells, Igs, and cytokines. These are the main mediators of immunity.

T cells have several functions and have been likened to the conductor of an orchestra. Regulatory functions over B cells are achieved by Th and T regulatory (reg) cells. Evolutionarily, the more ancient arm of immunity is CMI; T helper 1 (Th1) cells promote CMI, while T helper 2 (Th2) cells promote the induction of humoral immunity. Most adjuvants in vaccines promote the Th2 pathway and enhance antibody levels. The novel adjuvant (used in the Indian COVID-19 vaccine made by inactivating SARS-CoV-2), namely Alhydroxiquim-ll [a toll-like receptor (TLR) 7/8 agonist molecule chemisorbed on aluminum hydroxide], enhances both humoral and cellular immunity.

Cytokines are another set of mediators of immune functions—peptides that "communicate" between cells of the immune system. Many cytokines are involved in immune responses to infection, while others are involved in regulatory functions for the growth and integrity of the immune system itself. Thus, there are different kinds of cytokines, such as chemokines, interleukins, interferons, colony-stimulating factors (CSFs), and tumor necrosis factor (TNF). In the immune system and in its responses, cytokines play crucial roles: To activate cells, to direct cell differentiation, and cell proliferation.

IMMUNIZATION FOR DISEASE CONTROL

All "developed" countries have had public health and universal primary/secondary healthcare as two separate divisions in health management, even from the 19th century. The immunization program was an integral part of public health and healthcare. Low-income countries had no public health infrastructure or universal healthcare and hence no immunization program. The WHO launched the EPI in 1974, to popularize the application of BCG, OPV, DPT (diphtheria, pertussis, and tetanus), and the measles vaccines in infants, and tetanus toxoid in antenatal immunization was included in the EPI. Neonatal tetanus has been virtually eliminated in many low-income countries.

India adopted EPI in 1978 without the measles vaccine, which remained unlicensed. In 1979, a state-wide measles immunization program was begun in Tamil Nadu with special permission from the central government. The vaccine was gifted by Rotary International. Its success led to the inclusion of the measles vaccine in EPI in 1984/1985 and expanded to cover all states in 1990—when EPI was renamed the UIP. Today, measles and rubella are targeted for elimination.

Disease control is defined as the deliberate reduction of incidence by immunization, bringing incidence down to a preset target level within a planned time frame. Bringing incidence to zero in a country is elimination, and elimination in all countries is global eradication. A sufficiently high herd immunity induced by immunization is necessary for control and elimination. Only anthroponoses can be eliminated and eradicated. All other VPDs (such as zoonoses) can be controlled by sustained high herd immunity.

The terms herd immunity and herd effect are obviously borrowed from veterinary usage. In the human health sciences, the term herd immunity has been defined as the proportion in the community that is immune.[10] In vaccinology, we are concerned with vaccination-induced herd immunity.

The proportions of immune and nonimmune in the community influence the dynamics of transmission of pathogens that are human-to-human transmitted anthroponoses. In most of them, such as measles, disease cases are the source of transmission. In endemic (steady state) one case results in one secondary case and case reproduction number $R = 1$. In an outbreak, R is >1 and as it ends, R is <1, and endemicity is regained with $R = 1$. If a case occurs in a group of nonimmune children, one case results in many cases. If all contacts are nonimmune, the number infected by one case is called "basic reproduction number" R_0, which would be about 15 for measles. With high herd immunity, R can be sustained <1, progressively, until it reaches $R = 0$ and transmission ceases. If immunization "pressure" is kept up over sufficient time, we can eliminate transmission. The reduction of incidence in the unvaccinated segment of children is denoted as the "herd effect" of immunization.[9]

Immunization is a common component of primary healthcare and public health, often cited as the most cost-effective medical intervention.

REFERENCES

1. Khandaker G, Muhit M, Rashid H, Khan A, Islam J, Jones C, et al. Infectious causes of childhood disability: results from a pilot study in rural Bangladesh. J Trop Pediatr. 2014;50(5):363-9.
2. Srivastava RN. Right to health for children. Indian Pediatr. 2015;52(1):15-8.
3. John TJ. India's National Technical Advisory Group on Immunisation. Vaccine 2010;28(Suppl 1):A88-90.
4. John TJ, Samuel R, Balraj V, John R. Disease surveillance at district level: a model for developing countries. Lancet. 1998;352(9121):58-61.
5. John TJ, Plotkin SA, Orenstein WA. Building on the success of the Expanded Programme on Immunization: enhancing the focus on disease prevention and control. Vaccine. 2011;29(48):8835-7.
6. John TJ, Kompithra RZ. Eco-epidemiology triad to explain infectious diseases. Indian J Med Res. 2023;158(2):107-12.
7. Alberts B, Johnson A, Lewis J, Raff M, Roberts K, Walter P.. Innate immunity. In: Molecular Biology of the Cell, 4th edition. New York: Garland Science; 2002. [online] Available from: https://www.ncbi.nlm.nih.gov/books/NBK26846/. [Last accessed October, 2024].
8. Patriarca PA, Wright PF, John TJ. Factors affecting the immunogenicity of oral poliovirus vaccine in developing countries: review. Rev Infect Dis. 1991;13(5):926-39.
9. Stickle G. Observed and expected poliomyelitis in the United States, 1958-61. Am J Pub Health. 1964;54(8):222-9.
10. John TJ, Samuel R. Herd immunity and herd effect: new insights and definitions. Eur J Epidemiol. 2000;16(7):601-6.

6.4 Scheduling of Vaccines; the National and Indian Academy of Pediatrics Immunization Schedules

Srinivas G Kasi

INTRODUCTION

A vaccination schedule is a timetable of vaccines that every child should receive to prevent commonly encountered infectious diseases. The schedules are formulated or recommended by national or professional bodies. Catch-up vaccinations and vaccination of high-risk individuals are also mentioned. Every schedule mentions the following factors:

- *Name of the vaccine:* Product name, e.g., pneumococcal conjugate vaccines (PCVs); brand names are not mentioned
- *The age range* at which the vaccine needs to be administered
- *The interval between doses* where applicable
- *The age for booster doses* as required
- *Age range for catch-up vaccination*
- *The footnotes* which provide some additional information about the vaccines to be administered

The main objectives of scheduling vaccines are to achieve maximum coverage and minimize the number of healthcare system interactions to achieve this goal.

REQUIREMENTS OF A VACCINATION SCHEDULE

An ideal vaccination schedule should be immunologically acceptable, epidemiologically appropriate, and programmatically feasible.

Immunologically Acceptable

The schedule has to balance early life immunological immaturity, maternal antibodies inhibiting the vaccine responses, with the need for initiating the schedule early enough to provide protection before exposure to disease. Early life immunological immaturity is multifactorial and involves innate and adaptive immune responses.

Neonatal responses to pathogen-associated molecular patterns (PAMPs) are reduced compared to adults, leading to reduced production of chemokines and cytokines and inflammatory mediators, e.g., interleukin-12 (IL-12) and interferon-α (IFNα).[1] B-cell immaturity is caused by limited germinal center (GC) responses caused by delayed development of follicular dendritic cells (FDCs) and the limited induction of T follicular helper (Tfh) cells. This results in a limited magnitude of antibody responses to proteins.[1]

Antibody responses tend to wane earlier due to the limited survival of antigen-specific long-lived plasma cells in the bone marrow.[1] A suboptimal antigen-presenting cell/T-cell interaction is observed, probably resulting from reduced levels of IL-12 and IFN-α.[1]

The neonatal immune system exhibits a preferential differentiation of early life GC B-cells toward memory rather than immunoglobulin (Ig)-producing plasma cells. This explains the usefulness of neonatal priming doses, e.g., oral polio vaccine (OPV) and hepatitis B vaccine.[1] The neonatal and infant T-cell responses are skewed toward the T helper 2 (Th2) response with reduced production of IL-12 and IFNα production, which in turn adversely affects antibody production.[1]

Maternal Antibodies

Maternal antibodies transferred from mother to offspring have a major role in protecting the newborn, with an immature immune system, against infectious diseases. B-cell inhibition is mediated through a cross-link between the B-cell receptor (BCR) with the Fcγ-receptor IIB by a vaccine–antibody complex. Most maternal antibodies are of the IgG isotype. Maternal antibodies inhibit B-cell function and the production of antibodies. This can result in suboptimal responses to all types of vaccines (live attenuated, inactivated, and subunit), although the effect is most marked with live-attenuated vaccines.[2]

Most maternal antibody titles tend to decline over a period of time. In humans, maternal antibodies wane over a period of 6–12 months **(Fig. 6.4.1)**. The rate of decline of maternal antibodies is related to the initial titers in the newborn, with the highest titers showing a more gradual decline. However, even very low titers of persisting maternal antibodies can interfere with the immune response to live-attenuated vaccines. This is best exemplified by the measles vaccine wherein the measles vaccine administered at 6 months of age elicits poor antibody responses; when administered at 9 months of age, responses are acceptable; and when administered after 12 months of age, the responses are optimal **(Fig. 6.4.2)**.[2]

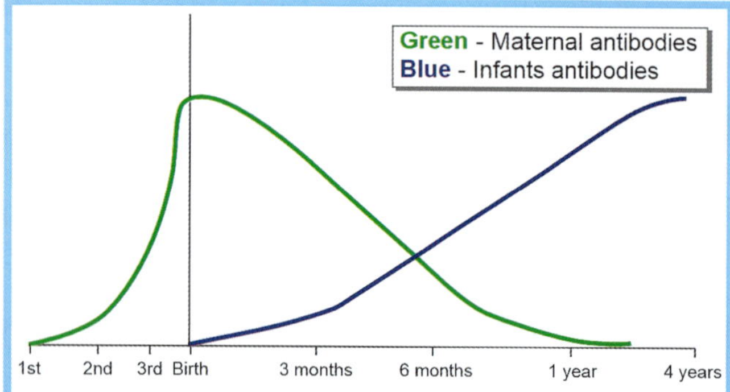

Fig. 6.4.1: Maternal antibody persistence in infants.

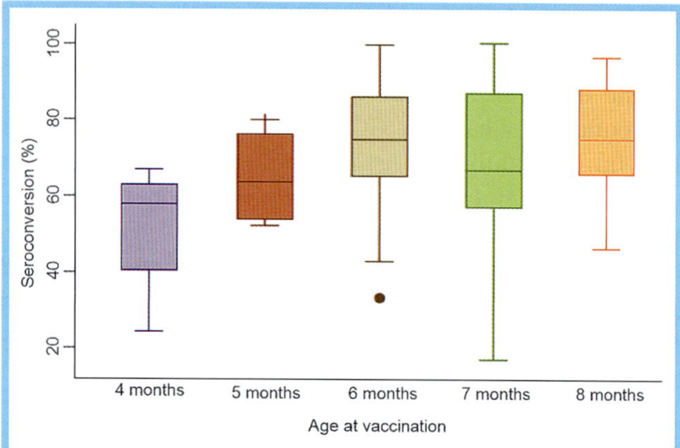

Fig. 6.4.2: Seroconversion (%) by age of first dose of the measles vaccine.

Maternal antibodies do not significantly affect the T-cell function. Hence, Bacillus Calmette-Guérin (BCG) can be administered at birth, and the measles vaccine administered at 6 months may not elicit good antibody responses, but induction of measles-specific T-cells can offer protection against measles complications.[3]

Epidemiologically Appropriate

It is essential that the vaccine should induce protective immune responses prior to the most vulnerable age and prior to exposure to natural infection. In countries with a high disease burden, the most vulnerable age is earlier and vice versa.

Programmatically Feasible

New vaccine introduction should be piggybacked on to existing programs to minimize the number of contacts with the healthcare system. The widely accepted schedule for the hepatitis B vaccine is the 0-1m-6m schedule. This schedule implies the creation of additional healthcare encounters, which is not programmatically feasible. The seroconversion rates following a 0-6w-10w-14w schedule have been found to be noninferior to the 0-1m-6m schedule. Hence, the hepatitis B vaccine is given in combination with a pentavalent/hexavalent vaccine as it is programmatically feasible.[4]

MINIMUM AGE OF INITIATION OF SCHEDULE

Most inactivated vaccines need priming doses to induce immune memory. These priming doses generate a GC reaction that results in the production of memory B-cells, antibody-producing plasma cells, and long-lived plasma cells that sustain antibody production for long periods.

The age of the first dose depends on:

- Age-specific risk for disease and of disease complications
- Age-specific immunogenicity of the vaccine
- Potential interference with maternal antibodies
- Interaction with other vaccines in the schedule

In low-income countries (LICs) and low-middle-income countries (LMICs), most infectious diseases occur at an earlier age.

In the PNEUMONET study, the estimated incidence rate (per 100,000 children) of invasive pneumococcal disease (IPD) was highest in the first 12 months of life [28d–6m: 36.7 (13.5, 79.8) and 7–12m: 49.9 (26.5, 85.2)]. The incidence of clinical pneumonia, X-ray-confirmed pneumonia, and X-ray-confirmed pneumonia with a C-reactive protein (CRP) value ≥40 mg/L was highest in the 28d–6m cohort.[5]

In a longitudinal study of 464 newborns from a rural area in South India, 54% were colonized with *Streptococcus pneumoniae* by 2 months of age, 64.1% at 4 months, and 70.2% at 6 months.[6] In a follow-up of 452 children, from birth till 3 years of age, 56% were infected with rotavirus by 6 months of age and 20% of all diarrheal episodes occurred within 6 months of age.[7]

The minimum age for any vaccine schedule is the youngest age group at risk for a disease for whom the efficacy and safety of a vaccine have been demonstrated. For most antigens, immunization before 6 weeks of age results in a weaker response and poorer immune persistence, mainly because of the immaturity of the immune system.

For LICs, the expanded program on immunization (EPI) schedule of 6-10-14 weeks is followed, whereas the developed countries employ the 2-4-6 month schedule. While the 2-4-6 month schedule elicits higher antibody levels, the 6-10-14-week schedule, along with the addition of a booster dose, generates equivalent immune memory compared with schedules that start at or after 2 months of age and is more appropriate depending on the local epidemiology of the disease. Delaying the first dose in countries with a high and early burden of disease may result in inadequate protection for the most vulnerable age group.[8]

NUMBER OF DOSES IN THE PRIMARY SCHEDULE

Most inactivated vaccines, when administered in early infancy, require multiple doses in the priming schedule. An increased number of doses is necessary to overcome the effects of immune immaturity and the effects of maternal antibodies. Generally, three priming doses are necessary when the schedule begins before 6 months of age, two priming doses between 6 and 12 months, and one priming dose beyond the age of 1 year. This is applicable to diphtheria-pertussis-tetanus (DPT), inactivated polio vaccine (IPV), PCV, *Haemophilus influenzae* type b (Hib), and hepatitis B vaccines. **Table 6.4.1** is an example of the primary schedule of PCV.

In contrast, live-attenuated vaccines [except measles, mumps, and rubella (MMR) and BCG] are not administered before the age of 1 year. By 1 year of age, all maternal antibodies will have completely disappeared from the infant's blood, and there will be no interference to the take of live-attenuated vaccines. Generally, only one dose of live-attenuated vaccines is sufficient to induce good antibody titers and a memory cell response. However, a small percentage of vaccinees do not respond to the first dose. This is known as primary vaccine failure, and to overcome this, a second dose is administered 4–12 weeks later. A second dose of some live-attenuated vaccines is also administered for programmatic reasons, for those who missed the first dose, during immunization sessions.

SPACING OF VACCINE DOSES

Primary Schedule

A minimum of 4 weeks between primary doses prevents interference of primary waves of immune response. This is because a primary response self-terminates in 3–6 weeks. Vaccines are spaced out at 4- to 8-week intervals to avoid competing immune responses between primary waves of GC reaction.[1]

As can be seen in **Figure 6.4.3**, the antibody titers following a previous dose are highest after 4 weeks, intermediate after 6 weeks, and least after 8 weeks. The longer the interval between doses, the more robust the antibody response. Thus, an interval of 8 weeks between doses elicits much higher antibody levels than an interval of 4 or 6 weeks. Irrespective of the interval between doses in the primary schedule, all schedules generate immune memory.

TABLE 6.4.1: Example of a primary schedule for PCV.

Age at first dose	***Primary series PCV 13***	***Primary series PCV 10***	***Primary series 10vPCV 10***
6 weeks to 6 months	3 doses	3 doses	3 doses
7–11 months	2 doses	2 doses	2 doses
12–23 months	1 dose	1 dose	1 dose

(PCV: pneumococcal conjugate vaccine)

Booster Doses

High-affinity antibodies and memory cells capable of producing antibodies with the highest affinity are produced during the GC reaction. This process takes approximately 4–6 months. An interval of at least 6 months between the last primary dose and the first booster dose allows completion of the affinity maturation process and development of highly specific memory B-cells. The longer the gap between the primary and booster doses, the better the immune persistence.[1]

For pathogens with a short incubation period (e.g., Hib and *S. pneumoniae*), the incubation period is much shorter than the time taken for a booster dose (anamnestic reaction) to raise protective antibody levels. Hence, periodic boosters are necessary.[9]

For pathogens with a long incubation period [e.g., hepatitis B, human papilloma virus (HPV), and hepatitis A], the incubation period is longer than the time taken for a booster dose (anamnestic reaction) to raise protective antibody levels. Hence, periodic boosters are not necessary.

For most live-attenuated vaccines, protective antibody titers persist almost lifelong. Periodic boosters are not necessary.

SPACING OF DIFFERENT VACCINES

Generally, all vaccines can be administered simultaneously. In order to attain protection against multiple pathogens that pose a threat in infancy, multiple vaccines are administered at each healthcare encounter in early infancy. Multiple injections are avoided by the use of licensed combination

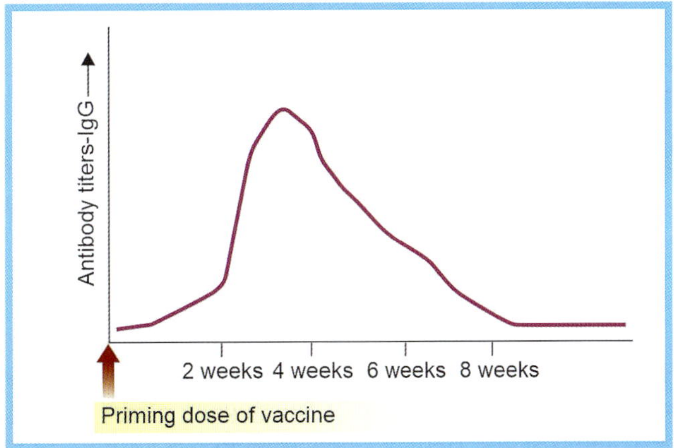

Fig. 6.4.3: Primary immune response. (IgG: immunoglobulin G)

vaccines. Combination vaccines make the immunization process more acceptable to the caregiver and child. In addition, combination vaccines have programmatic benefits in terms of lesser costs, need for lesser cold storage space, and lesser use of syringes, needles, etc.

Live vaccines are best administered after 12 months of age. Epidemiologic needs dictate the necessity of measles-containing vaccine at 9 months. Since the seroconversion rates of the measles vaccine given at 9 months are suboptimal, additional doses are given in the second year of life.

NATIONAL IMMUNIZATION PROGRAM AND INDIAN ACADEMY OF PEDIATRICS SCHEDULES

The immunization schedule in the government sector [National Immunization Program (NIP)] differs from that in the private sector [Indian Academy of Pediatrics (IAP)], in terms of both the number of vaccines and the schedules of vaccines. The selection of vaccine for possible introduction in the NIP is a complex process. It includes:

- Disease burden (incidence/prevalence, absolute number of morbidity/mortality, epidemic/pandemic potential)
- Safety and efficacy of the vaccine under consideration
- Affordability and financial sustainability of the vaccination program, even if the initial introduction is supported by the external funding agency
- Program capacity to introduce a new antigen, including cold chain capacity
- Availability of a domestic or external vaccine-production capacity
- The cost effectiveness of the vaccination program and also of the alternatives other than vaccination

The aim is to maximize the benefit of the vaccine to the largest population possible in the most cost-effective manner. The aim is to control a disease and induce herd immunity. Cost comes first, efficacy next, and safety last. The vaccines are provided free to all the beneficiaries. It is for this reason that the Universal Immunization Program (UIP) recommends bivalent oral polio vaccine (bOPV) as the primary vaccine for protection against polio; inactivated polio vaccine (IPV) is used in fractional doses; and PCV is recommended in a 2+1 schedule **(Table 6.4.2)**. Mumps-rubella (MR) vaccine is used instead of the MMR vaccine, as this is more cost-effective and mumps is not considered as a major public health issue.

In the IAP schedule, the probability of risk to an individual child is the determining factor for the inclusion of a vaccine in the schedule **(Table 6.4.3)**. Safety comes first, efficacy next, and cost last. Here, the beneficiaries pay for the cost of the vaccine and administration. Vaccines against pathogens that are not considered as major public health issues are also included in the IAP schedule (hepatitis A and varicella). The schedule recommended is the one that elicits the best possible immunological response (6w-10w-14w schedule for PCV, full dose IM-IPV in a 6w-10w-14w schedule, with boosters at 4–6 years).

Catch-up Schedules

Delayed or missed doses of any vaccine in a schedule do not necessitate restarting of the series. The remaining doses should be administered as per the schedule. The World Health Organization (WHO) has published tables for catch-up schedules.[8]

Adolescent Schedules

Adolescent immunization is the most neglected aspect of the immunization scenario in India. Waning immunity following the earlier childhood vaccinations given, availability of vaccines for specific use in adolescents [tetanus, diphtheria, and pertussis (Tdap), HPV], and catch-up vaccinations underline the need for exclusive adolescent immunization schedules. The Centers for Disease Control and Prevention (CDC) of the United States regularly updates its adolescent schedule. The IAP has an adolescent immunization schedule that has been updated by the Adolescent Health Academy.

Revision of Schedules

Vaccination schedules need to be revised/updated periodically. The CDC and the American Academy of Pediatrics (CDC/AAP) updates schedule every year, while the IAP and the Advisory Committee on Vaccines and Immunization Practices (IAP/ACVIP) revises them every 1–2 years.

Revision of schedules is necessary in certain situations. These include:

- Availability of a new vaccine (e.g., HPV vaccine)
- New indication for an available vaccine (e.g., HPV vaccine for boys)
- Availability of improved vaccines (conjugate typhoid vaccine)
- Availability of combination vaccines (e.g., HB vaccine)
- New data about available vaccines (e.g., varicella second dose, PCV (2+1), HPV 1 dose)
- Changing disease patterns (e.g., JE for adults)
- Changes to the group of people most susceptible to the disease (e.g., hepatitis A vaccine)
- Discontinuation of vaccine (e.g., smallpox, type 2 OPV).

TABLE 6.4.2: NIP schedule.[9]

Age	Vaccines	Route	Site
Birth	BCG	Intradermal (ID)	Left upper arm at insertion of deltoid
	bOPV-0 dose	Oral	Oral
	Hepatitis B birth dose	Intramuscular (IM)	Anterolateral side of mid-thigh
6 weeks	bOPV-1	Oral	Oral
	Pentavalent-1	IM	Anterolateral side of mid-thigh
	Rotavirus vaccine (RVV)-1	Oral	Oral
	Fractional dose of inactivated polio vaccine (fIPV)-1	ID	Right upper arm
	Pneumococcal conjugate vaccine (PCV)-1	PCV-2: IM	Anterolateral midthigh
10 weeks	bOPV-2	Oral	Oral
	Pentavalent-2	IM	Anterolateral midthigh
	RVV-2	Oral	Oral
14 weeks	bOPV-3	Oral	Oral
	Pentavalent-3	IM	Anterolateral side of mid-thigh
	fIPV-2	ID	Right upper arm
	RVV-3	Oral	Oral
	PCV-2	IM	Anterolateral midthigh
9–12 months	Measles and rubella (MR)-1	Subcutaneous (SC)	Right upper arm
	Japanese encephalitis (JE)-1	SC	Left upper arm
	PCV-booster	*PCV-booster:* IM	Anterolateral midthigh
	fIPV-3	ID	Right upper arm
16–24 months	MR-2	SC	Right upper arm
	JE-2	SC	Left upper arm
	Diphtheria, pertussis, and tetanus (DPT)-booster-1	IM	Anterolateral midthigh
	bOPV–booster	Oral	Oral
5–6 years	DPT-booster-2	IM	Upper arm
10 years	Tetanus and adult diphtheria (Td)	IM	Upper arm
16 years	Td	IM	Upper arm
Pregnant women	TT-1, TT-2, or TT-booster	IM	Upper arm

(BCG: Bacillus Calmette-Guérin; bOPV: bivalent oral polio vaccine; NIP: National Immunization Program; TT: tetanus toxoid)

TABLE 6.4.3: IAP immunization schedule.[10]

Vaccine	*Age in completed weeks/months/years*																
	Birth	***6 weeks***	***10 weeks***	***14 weeks***	***6 months***	***7 months***	***9 months***	***12 months***	***13 months***	***15 months***	***16–18 months***	***18–24 months***	***2–3 years***	***4–6 years***	***9–14 years***	***15–16 years***	***17–18 years***
BCG																	
Hepatitis B	HB 1	HB 2	HB 3	HB 4													
Polio	OPV	IPV 1	IPV 2	IPV 3							IPV B1			IPV B2			
DTwP/DTaP		DPT 1	DPT 2	DPT 3							DPT B1			DPT B2			
Hib		Hib 1	Hib 2	Hib 3							Hib B1						
PCV		PCV 1	PCV 2	PCV 3				PCV B									
Rotavirus		RV 1	RV 2	RV 3													
Influenza					Dose 1	Dose 2	Annual vaccination										
MMR							Dose 1			Dose 2				Dose 3			
TCV																	
Hepatitis A								Dose 1				Dose 2					
Varicella										Dose 1		Dose 2					
Tdap																	
Td																	
HPV															1 and 2	1, 2, and 3	
Meningococcal							Dose 1	Dose 2									
JE								Dose 1	Dose 2								
Cholera								Dose 1	Dose 2								
PPSV 23																	
Rabies																	
Yellow fever																	

(BCG: Bacillus Calmette-Guérin; DTaP: diphtheria, tetanus, and acellular pertussis; DPT: diphtheria, pertussis, and tetanus; DTwP: diphtheria, tetanus, and whole-cell pertussis; HB: hepatitis B; Hib: *Haemophilus influenzae* type b; HPV: human papillomavirus; IAP: Indian Academy of Pediatrics; IPV: inactivated polio vaccine; JE: Japanese encephalitis; MMR: measles, mumps, and rubella; OPV: oral polio vaccine; PCV: pneumococcal conjugate vaccine; PPSV: pneumococcal polysaccharide vaccine; RV: rotavirus vaccine; TCV: tetanus conjugate vaccine; Td: tetanus and diphtheria; Tdap: tetanus, diphtheria, and pertussis)

Recommended age | **Catch-up age range** | **Vaccination in special situations**

REFERENCES

1. Siegrist CA. Vaccine immunology. In: Plotkin SA, Orenstein WA, Offit PA, Edwards KM (Eds). Plotkin's Vaccines, 7th edition. Philadelphia: Elsevier; 2018.
2. Zimmermann P, Curtis N. Factors that influence the immune response to vaccination. Clin Microbiol Rev. 2019;32(2):e00084-18.
3. National Institute for Public Health and the Environment. (2015). Measles vaccination below 9 months of age: systematic literature review and meta-analyses of effects and safety. [online] Available from https://terrance.who.int/mediacentre/data/sage/SAGE_Docs_Ppt_Oct2015/5_session_measles_and_rubella/Oct2015_session5_MCV_use_at_9months.pdf. [Last accessed October, 2024].
4. World Health Organization. Optimizing the hepatitis B vaccination schedules. [online] Available from https://terrance.who.int/mediacentre/data/sage/SAGE_Docs_Ppt_Oct2016/9_session_HepB/Oct2016_session9_review_hepB_vax_childhood.pdf. [Last accessed October, 2024].
5. Nisarga R, Premalatha R, Shivananda, Ravikumar KL, Shivappa U, Gopi A, et al. Hospital-based surveillance of invasive pneumococcal disease and pneumonia in South Bangalore, India. Indian Pediatr. 2015;52(3):205-11.
6. Jebaraj R, Thomas C, Raghupathy P, Brahmadathan K, Lalitha M, Kurien T, et al. Nasopharyngeal colonization of infants in southern India with *Streptococcus pneumoniae*. Epidemiol Infect. 2000;123(3):383-8.
7. Gladstone BP, Ramani S, Mukhopadhya M, Muliyil J, Sarkar R, Rehman AM, et al. Protective effect of natural rotavirus infection in an Indian birth cohort. N Engl J Med. 2011;365(4):337-46.
8. World Health Organization. WHO recommendations for routine immunization—summary tables. [online] Available from https://www.who.int/teams/immunization-vaccines-and-biologicals/policies/who-recommendations-for-routine-immunization---summary-tables. [Last accessed October, 2024].
9. Ministry of Health and Family Welfare. Universal immunization program. [online] Available from https://mohfw.gov.in/sites/default/files/41016395871489662752.pdf. [Last accessed October, 2024].
10. Kasi SG, Shivananda S, Marathe M, Chatterjee K, Agarwalla S, Dhir SK, et al. Indian Academy of Pediatrics (IAP) Advisory Committee on Vaccines and Immunization Practices (ACVIP): recommended immunization schedule (2020-21) and update on immunization for children aged 0 through 18 years. Indian Pediatr. 2021;58(1):44-53.

6.5 Polio Eradication Endgame: Global and National Perspectives

Dhanya Dharmapalan, T Jacob John

INTRODUCTION

Global polio eradication efforts were initiated by the World Health Organization (WHO), enabled by a World Health Assembly Resolution passed in 1988, stipulating the time target of the year 2000. As the target was missed, the WHO uses the term "Endgame" for continued efforts for completing the project, as announced in a symposium titled "Progress in polio eradication: Vaccine strategies for the Endgame" in Institute Pasteur, Paris, during June 28–30, 2000.[1] Endgame literally means the final stage of an organized program.

The goals of the first polio Endgame were:[2]

- To achieve eradication of wild poliovirus (WPV) types 1 and 3 infection in all remaining endemic countries by 2002
- To minimize the risk of WPV reintroduction from laboratory stock
- To block transmission of vaccine-derived polioviruses (VDPVs) and circulating VDPVs (cVDPVs)
- To obtain certification of global WPV eradication by 2005

In 2001, there were 10 countries in South Asia and sub-Saharan Africa with endemic polio due to WPV transmission, and the 2002 target was also missed. Emergence and transmission of VDPVs types 1, 2, and 3 and consequent iatrogenic polio were observed from 2000, and their frequency increased substantially from 2006 with polio outbreaks due to cVDPV type 2 (cVDPV-2) **(Table 6.5.1)**.

Announcing further extensions of Endgame became an iterative process. The latest Endgame plan is for 2022–2026.[3] The two pending endpoints, namely (1) interrupting WPV transmission in Afghanistan and Pakistan and (2) interrupting transmission of VDPVs, were the targets to be achieved by 2023, so that eradication could be certified 3 years later, in 2026. However, WPV-1 polio continues to occur in those two countries in 2023, heralding the failure of even the latest Endgame. In 2022, WPV-1 was imported from Pakistan to Malawi and Mozambique. Also in 2022, cVDPV-2 was imported from an unknown source country into Israel, UK, and USA, illustrating the emergence of new lineages and the persistence of previously emerged lineages.[4] In 2023, polio

TABLE 6.5.1: Shifting goalposts of the Polio Eradication Programme from 2000 onward.[2,3]

Polio Endgame plan	*Reasons for missing target*	*Added challenges with cVDPV polio*
2001–2005	*10 countries reported WPV:* Afghanistan, Angola, Egypt, Ethiopia, India, Pakistan, Niger, Nigeria, Somalia and Sudan	China, the Dominican Republic, Haiti, Indonesia, Madagascar, and the Philippines
2005–2009	WPV transmission in India, Nigeria, Pakistan, and Afghanistan	Afghanistan, Angola, Benin, Cambodia, Cameroon, Central African Republic, Chad, DR Conga, Dominican Republic, Ethiopia, Ghana, Guinea, Haiti, India, Indonesia, Israel, Kenya, Pakistan, Laos, Madagascar, Niger, Malawi, Mozambique, Myanmar, Nigeria, Papua New Guinea, Philippines, Somalia, South Sudan, Syria, USA, Ukraine, and Yemen
2009–2013	WPV transmission in India, Nigeria, Pakistan, and Afghanistan	
2013–2018	WPV transmission in Nigeria, Pakistan, and Afghanistan	
2018–2022	WPV transmission in Pakistan and Afghanistan	
2022–2026	WPV transmission continues in Pakistan and Afghanistan in 2023	

(cVDPV: circulating vaccine-derived poliovirus; WPV: wild poliovirus)

due to cVDPV-1 was detected in three African countries and due to cVDPV-2 in 15 African and 2 Asian countries.[5]

The proposed budget for the 2022–2026 Endgame is in US dollars: 0.932 billion in 2022, 1.005 billion in 2023, 1 billion in 2024, 0.935 billion in 2005, and 0.888 billion in 2026, totaling 4.76 billion.[3] The global partners supporting the Global Polio Eradication Initiative (GPEI) are the Rotary International, Centers for Disease Control and Prevention (USA), Gates Foundation, and GAVI, the Vaccine Alliance.

GLOBAL PERSPECTIVE

The original global polio eradication project was for 12 years (1988–2000), but its six Endgames have lasted 23 years until now, without any hope that the project will be concluded in 2026. Any project delayed beyond plan will entail extra expenditure. Thus, the Endgames have so far consumed 22 billion US dollars and have budgeted for nearly 5 billion more until 2026.

By 1988, when the WHO launched the project, all rich countries in North America and Europe had controlled polio.

Two factors hindered the successful outcome of the polio Endgames.[6] They were:

1. Exclusive reliance on trivalent oral polio vaccine (tOPV), which showed very low vaccine efficacy for types 1 and 3 in countries such as India, Pakistan, and Afghanistan in Asia and Nigeria, the Democratic Republic of Congo, and their neighboring countries in sub-Saharan Africa
2. Not factoring the risk–benefit balance of oral polio vaccine (OPV) as the years passed by

The risks from OPV include vaccine-associated paralytic polio (VAPP) in vaccinated children and their contacts; chronic vaccine virus infection in children and adults with any B-cell function deficiencies; genetic reversion of vaccine polioviruses toward wild-like properties, the emergence of VDPVs, their wide circulation as cVDPVs and exportation to non-OPV-using countries; and polio outbreaks caused by cVDPVs.

When the incidence of natural, wild virus-induced polio, was high, these risks were small in comparison, but after the incidence of natural polio declined under vaccination pressure, their risks surpassed benefits. Once WPV-2 was eradicated (in 1999), the type 2 vaccine virus in OPV had to be removed, because it made no scientific sense to immunize against a nonexistent pathogen. The unfortunate consequences of persisting with tOPV are described in the following text.

The two factors that hindered progress were compounded by the failure to enunciate a time-bound plan to replace OPV with an inactivated polio vaccine (IPV). Scientifically, it appears that any use of OPV is incompatible with polio eradication; a polio-eradicated world can use only IPV. IPV can shorten the duration of eradication Endgame.[6]

The polio Endgames till 2014 used tOPV exclusively as its tool for meeting the target of polio eradication. However, as early as the 1970s, studies from India had reported the low efficacy of the tOPV and failure to protect from polio despite three doses of tOPV.[7] A paralytic case from Vellore was the first global report of failure of tOPV in the world.[7] Repeated doses of tOPV had to be administered in tropical countries, especially in campaign mode (called pulse immunization), to overcome the challenge of the low efficacy of the vaccine. However, many children developed polio despite receiving over 15 doses of tOPV. In 2023, in Afghanistan, four children had developed polio due to WPV-1 despite 21–28 doses of bivalent OPV (bOPV containing types 1 and 3) and one case despite 16 doses.

While type 2 could be eradicated before 2000 as the vaccine efficacy of tOPV was satisfactory against WPV-2, tOPV containing type 2 vaccine virus was continued to be administered until the global switch from tOPV to bOPV without type 2 in 2016.[8] By then, the type 2 vaccine virus had already led to the emergence of VDPVs and cVDPV-2 and had caused many outbreaks in many countries. To control the cVDPV type 2 outbreaks, at first, tOPV and later monovalent OPV type 2 (mOPV-2) were used in campaign mode, adding fuel to the fire. That resulted in more cVDPV lineages.

The rare adverse event following immunization with tOPV and bOPV is VAPP, more frequently associated with type 3 vaccine virus than the other two. This clearly shows that an attenuated vaccine virus can regain neurovirulence like WPV and invade the spinal cord to cause paralysis in the recipient of the vaccine. When genetic reversion results in regained neurovirulence and transmission efficiency, in other words, losing both attenuating properties, the result is the emergence of cVDPV.

Both VDPV polio and VAPP are clinically indistinguishable from WPV polio and therefore the suffering endured by the victim and family is also no different when paralysis is induced by WPV, OPV, or VDPV. VAPP is never reported as such by the GPEI, but is classified as "nonpolio acute flaccid paralysis." Our estimate has been 400–800 VAPP cases annually, globally.

The continued use of OPV was untenable, when the number of paralytic polio cases caused by VAPP exceeded the number caused by the WPV. The alternate polio vaccine was the IPV, which was licensed in western countries even before the OPV came into use. IPV had no serious adverse effects and is highly efficacious against all three serotypes with three doses plus a booster dose. Many rich countries of North America, the Western Pacific, and Europe had abandoned the use of OPV due to safety concerns by or before 2000 and have been free of polio caused by WPV or vaccine viruses. Roughly, the efficacy of three doses of IPV surpasses that of about 30 doses of OPV in many tropical low-income countries.

A major problem for the Endgames beyond 2005 was the increasing number of outbreaks of cVDPV-2. To overcome this problem, recently a novel OPV type 2 (nOPV-2) was created in the laboratory, which does not revert genetically to neurovirulence and easy transmissibility. This genetically engineered vaccine is safer than Sabin OPV-2. Unfortunately, the wide use of nOPV-2 in African countries has also resulted in its evolution as cVDPV-2, causing polio outbreaks in Africa.[9]

The exclusive dependence on live-attenuated oral polio vaccines was justified until 1999 as OPV was less expensive than IPV and easy to administer in campaigns. The belief that it would be more efficient in interrupting WPV transmission than IPV was based on the erroneous assumption of the route of transmission. Polio epidemiology—such as all cases by age 5 years and a low median age of <18 months, polio in exclusively breastfed infants, no waterborne outbreaks, and polio having affected countries irrespective of high or low standards of sanitation/hygiene—points to the respiratory route of transmission rather than a fecal-oral route. The real route of transmission was not scientifically investigated.

The fact that fecal excretion of the vaccine virus by the large numbers of OPV recipients would laterally spread by fecal-oral transmission and induce immunity in most if not all the unvaccinated children (herd effect) was a concept every Endgame greatly relied on.

When cVDPV-2 polio was detected in USA in 2022 in an unvaccinated adult, it was found that the virus had spread widely in New York where the local immunization coverage by IPV had dipped during the pandemic. In 2000, USA had switched from OPV to IPV. In 2022, as coverage was improved, the circulation of cVDPV-2 stopped. There, and in UK, which had also experienced importation and circulation of cVDPV-2 in 2022, the transmission route was clearly respiratory and could not have been fecal-oral as there was no fecal/sewage contamination of water supplies.[4] In India, we know that it is very uncommon (except in urban slums) for infant feeds to have fecal contamination.

NATIONAL PERSPECTIVE

During the first, second, and third Endgame periods, India continued to have polio caused by WPV types 1 and 3.

The world's last case of WPV-2 polio was in India in October 1999. Several studies in India had shown that the vaccine efficacy was higher for type 2 than for types 1 and 3. When sufficient OPV coverage was reached to interrupt WPV-2 transmission in 1999, it became obvious that interrupting WPV-1 and -3 would be a formidable task, on account of the very low efficacy of tOPV against them. India could not have succeeded in interrupting transmission of WPV-1 and -3 in 2010/2011 by persisting with tOPV.

Given that the vaccine efficacy of mOPV-1 and mOPV-3 was two-and-a-half times higher than that of tOPV against types 1 and 3, respectively, as early Indian research had demonstrated, India introduced mOPV-1 and mOPV-3 in 2006 and succeeded in interrupting WPV-3 and -1 (in 2010 and 2011, respectively). India was then declared polio-free in 2014. Studies in India also showed that the vaccine efficacies of the two mOPVs given separately or together as bOPV were very similar.

India's success story of WPV elimination was largely due to the huge efforts by the Ministry of Health and full support from the community, together achieving nearly 100% coverage of mOPVs through repeated pulse polio campaigns.

In 2016, India complied with the WHO recommendation of two fractional intradermal doses of IPV at 6 and 14 weeks of age (for vaccine efficacy equivalent to one intramuscular dose at 14 weeks) before switching to bOPV. More recently, another fractional intradermal IPV dose has been included at 9 months of age.

The Indian Academy of Pediatrics (IAP) advocates the use of IPV-containing pentavalent or hexavalent vaccines to complete three doses of IPV in the primary series in infancy and booster doses between 15 and 18 months and between 4 and 5 years. The National Immunization Schedule of India uses fractional doses of IPV at 6 and 14 weeks in the primary series, with one booster dose at 9 months. However, there are the following risks:

- There is a long interval of several months between the second fractional dose and the booster dose. Therefore, there is a certain vulnerability to the cVDPV-2 outbreak in the event of importation into the country.
- Continued use of type 3 in OPV has only risk for continued cases of VAPP with no benefit in protection against type 3 after its global eradication in 2012 (last case in 2012 in Nigeria).
- There is a persistent risk of immunodeficiency-related VDPVs (iVDPVs) until OPV use is stopped.[10]

For these reasons, India ought to use only mOPV-1 and also increase the IPV coverage in its full-dose primary series with one booster, preferably as a combination vaccine. India will then be able to safely withdraw OPV completely. India must also count and record VAPP cases and place the data in the public domain.

These steps by India will ensure equity and justice for all children to remain polio-free from both wild and vaccine viruses.

CONCLUSION

To summarize, the polio Endgames should not continue with shifting goalposts and without their endpoint in sight. It is the responsibility of all stakeholders to revisit the failed Endgames and change the old strategies in a way that could assure a definite victory in the shortest time possible. India can very well emerge as a nation to script its own final polio Endgame with an improved schedule and sustained coverage with IPV.

REFERENCES

1. Global Polio Eradication Initiative. [online] Available from https://polioeradication.org/wp-content/uploads/2019/06/english-polio-endgame-strategy.pdf. [Last accessed October, 2024].
2. Progress in polio eradication: vaccine strategies for the End Game. Paris, France, 28–30 June 2000. Proceedings. Dev Biol (Basel). 2001;105:1-244.
3. Global Polio Eradication Initiative (GPEI) strategy 2022–2026. [online] Available from http://polioeradication.org/gpei-strategy-2022-2026/. [Last accessed October, 2024].
4. John TJ, Dharmapalan D. Lessons from vaccine-related poliovirus in Israel, UK and USA. Vaccines (Basel). 2022;10(11):1969.
5. Global Polio Eradication Initiative. [online] Available from https://polioeradication.org/wp-content/uploads/2023/11/weekly-polio-analyses-cVDPV-20231121.pdf. [Last accessed October, 2024].
6. John TJ, Dharmapalan D. Challenges en route to polio eradication. Lancet. 2022;400(10350):428-9.
7. John TJ. Problems with oral polio vaccine in India. Indian Pediatr. 1972;9:252-6.
8. Garon J, Seib K, Orenstein WA, Ramirez Gonzalez A, Chang Blanc D, Zaffran M, et al. Polio endgame: the global switch from tOPV to bOPV. Expert Rev Vaccines. 2016;15(6):693-708.
9. Global Polio Eradication Initiative. cVDPV2 outbreaks and the type 2 novel oral polio vaccine (nOPV2). [online] Available from: https://polioeradication.org/wp-content/uploads/2024/08/GPEI_nOPV2_Factsheet_5-January-2024.pdf. [Last accessed October, 2024].
10. Mohanty MC, Desai M, Mohammad A, Aggarwal A, Govindaraj G, Bhattad S, et al. Assessment of enterovirus excretion and identification of VDPVs in patients with primary immunodeficiency in India: outcome of ICMR-WHO collaborative study phase-I. Vaccines (Basel). 2023;11(7):1211.

6.6 Non-Universal Immunization Programme Vaccines in India

Chandra Mohan Kumar

INTRODUCTION

Vaccines are included in the immunization schedule of a country based on recommendations of the World Health Organization (WHO) as well as the National Immunization Technical Advisory Group of that country. This organization is known as the National Technical Advisory Group on Immunization (NTAGI) in India. Their recommendations take into consideration the epidemiology, cost-effectiveness, and availability of the vaccines in the country, along with the scientific evidence of the efficacy, immunogenicity, and safety of a particular vaccine in the country. In the last decade, several new vaccines have been developed and licensed and are available in India, in addition to the vaccines delivered under the *National Immunization Schedule (NIS)*. Some vaccines against vaccine-preventable diseases (VPD), which are not considered as a public health burden, are not included in the NIS but are available in the private sector. These are called *non-Universal Immunization Programme (UIP) vaccines*. In addition, some vaccines common to both the NIS and the private sector [e.g., pneumococcal conjugate vaccine (PCV) and inactivated polio vaccine (IPV)] have different schedules in the NIS and the schedule followed by the private practitioners.

The Indian Academy of Pediatrics-Advisory Committee on Vaccination and Immunization Practices (IAP-ACVIP) periodically reviews the need for these vaccines and recommends their use **(*See* Table 6.4.3)**. Physicians should be able to counsel the parents regarding the efficacy and importance of these vaccines in the present health situation.[1]

This chapter includes a brief description of these vaccines. Almost all these vaccines are included in the Expanded Program on Immunization (EPI) national schedules of several developed countries. In India, almost all these vaccines find a place in the *IAP-ACVIP immunization timetable 2023* **(*See* Table 6.4.3)** for routine use.[2]

PNEUMOCOCCAL VACCINES

Currently, two types of pneumococcal vaccines are marketed in India:

1. Polysaccharide pneumococcal vaccines [23-valent capsular polysaccharide vaccine (PPSV23)]
2. Conjugate vaccines:
   - 13-valent PCV (PCV-13)
   - 10-valent PCV (PCV-10)
   - 14-valent PCV (PCV-14)

PCV-10 and PCV-14 (both developed in India) are now included in the National Immunization Program (NIP) of India.[3]

23-Valent Capsular Polysaccharide Vaccine

The 23-valent capsular polysaccharide vaccine is available for use in children above 2 years of age who belong to the "high-risk group" and for use in older children, adolescents, and adults, routinely. This vaccine covers most of the prevalent strains (over 80%) of *Pneumococci*-causing disease. Being a polysaccharide vaccine, it is T-cell independent and has poor immunogenicity in children below 2 years of age. It has poor immune memory, does not reduce nasopharyngeal carriage, and does not provide herd immunity.

Indications

This vaccine is recommended in children with sickle cell disease, functional and anatomic asplenia, nephrotic syndrome, patients with cerebrospinal fluid leak, and children with malignancies and human immunodeficiency virus infection. *It is not recommended for immunocompetent and normal children.*

Schedule

It is given as a single dose of 0.5 mL subcutaneously (SC) or intramuscularly (IM) in children, above 2 years of age. A second dose is recommended in immunosuppressed children, at least 5 years after the first dose.

Given the limitations mentioned above, conjugated vaccines are preferred.

Pneumococcal Conjugate Vaccines

Four brands of PCVs are available in India. Their serotype composition and Indian Academy of Pediatrics (IAP) schedules are mentioned in **Tables 6.6.1 and 6.6.2**. PCVs are used in the NIS as a 2P + 1 schedule (6w–14w–9m), with the 9-month dose considered as a booster dose.

TETANUS TOXOID WITH LOW DOSE OF DIPHTHERIA AND ACELLULAR PERTUSSIS VACCINE (TDAP VACCINE)

Immunity following primary/booster diphtheria, tetanus, and pertussis (DTP)/diphtheria, tetanus, and acellular pertussis (DTaP) vaccination wanes over 5–10 years. Standard-strength DTP and DTaP vaccines cannot be used in children above 7 years of age due to increased reactogenicity. Tetanus toxoid with reduced quantity diphtheria and acellular pertussis [tetanus, diphtheria, and pertussis (Tdap)] vaccine contains lower doses of diphtheria and acellular pertussis components and hence can be used in children above 7 years. While DTP

TABLE 6.6.1: PCVs available in India and their serotype composition.

Brand	*Serotypes present*														
PCV-10 GSK	1		4	5		6B	7F	9V	14	18C		19F		23F	
PCV-10 SII	1			5	6A	6B	7F	9V	14		19A	19F		23F	
PCV-13	1	3	4	5	6A	6B	7F	9V	14	18C	19A	19F		23F	
PCV14 (BE)	1	3	4	5		6B	7F	9V	14	18C	19A	19F	22F	23F	33F

(PCVs: pneumococcal conjugate vaccines)

TABLE 6.6.2: PCV immunization schedules (IAP).

Age at 1st dose	Primary series				Booster dose			
	PCV 13	PCV 10 (GSK)	PCV 10 (SII)	PCV 14	PCV 13	PCV 10 (GSK)	PCV 10 (SII)	PCV 14
6 weeks to 6 months	3 doses	3 doses	3 doses	3 doses	1 dose at 12–15 months*	1 dose at 12–15 months*	1 dose at 12–15 months*	NR‡
7–11 months	2 doses	2 doses	2 doses	NR‡	1 dose during 2nd year	1 dose during 2nd year	1 dose during 2nd year	NR‡
12–23 months	2 doses†	2 doses†	2 doses†	NR‡				NR‡
24–59 months	1 dose	2 doses†	NR‡	NR‡				NR‡

*At least 6 months after the 3rd dose.
†At least 8 weeks apart.
‡No recommendations (NR).
(IAP: Indian Academy of Pediatrics; PCV: pneumococcal conjugate vaccine)

and Tdap contain 5 Lf units of tetanus toxoid, diphtheria, pertussis, and tetanus (DPT) contains 15–25 Lf of diphtheria toxoid versus 2–2.5 Lf units in Tdap and 10–25 mg of pertussis toxin versus 2.5–5 mg in Tdap.[4]

Schedule

A dose of this vaccine should be given at 10–11 years of age as an adolescent booster. For those who have never received this vaccine, one dose is recommended at any interval after the last tetanus and diphtheria (Td) dose. In unimmunized children, a schedule of 0–1m–6m is recommended; of this, any one dose should be Tdap, e.g., Tdap-Td-Td. This vaccine is recommended after 7 years. Systemic side effects are rarely seen. The IAP-ACVIP and Federation of Obstetric and Gynaecological Societies of India (FOGSI) now recommend a single dose of Tdap in pregnancy during the third trimester (preferred 26–27 weeks) regardless of previous immunization with Tdap. This protects the young infant from pertussis till ~3 months of age. It should be given during every pregnancy.

TYPHOID VACCINE

Although with improved sanitation and increased access to safe drinking water, the enteric fever disease burden has reduced significantly in the last three decades, it is still a public health problem in India. Now typhoid is occurring in younger age groups, and there is emergence of multiple drug resistance. Hence, there is a need for typhoid vaccines. Two types of typhoid vaccines are now available.[5]

Vi-Polysaccharide Typhoid Vaccine

The Vi antigen of *Salmonella typhi* is a capsular antigen with known virulence property of the organism and is available as an injectable vaccine containing 25 mg of purified Vi-capsular polysaccharide (Vi-PS) per dose. The dose is 0.5 mL IM in the deltoid region above the age of 2 years, with revaccination every 3 years beginning at the age of 2 years. The efficacy of the vaccine varies from 64% to 72% in various studies. Adverse reactions include pain, erythema, and induration at the local site and rarely fever. All the reactions are of mild nature and self-limiting.

Conjugated Typhoid Vaccines

The limitations of the polysaccharide typhoid vaccine include the following:

- Noneffectiveness below the age of 2 years
- Limited efficacy (of around 60%)
- T-cell-independent response, which lacks immune memory
- It is not boostable

Conjugation of the Vi antigen with a protein carrier is hence desirable, as it would induce a T-cell-dependent immune response.

Vi-Polysaccharide Vaccines Conjugated with Tetanus Toxoid (Vi-CPS)

There are different typhoid conjugate vaccines (TCVs) available in India using tetanus toxoid or CRM197 as the carrier protein. All are developed in India and contain 25 µg/0.5 mL of purified Vi-PS antigen.

Recommendations for Use

The Indian Academy of Pediatrics-Advisory Committee on Vaccination (IAP-ACV) recommends vaccination with Vi capsular polysaccharide (Vi-CPS) between 6 and 9 months of age. The current evidence suggests persistence of robust antibody levels up to 7 years postvaccination and based on this data, the IAP-ACVIP recommends a single dose of TCV and no boosters.[6]

INACTIVATED POLIO VACCINE

Inactivated polio vaccine is a formaldehyde killed (Salk) poliovirus vaccine made from wild poliovirus strain types 1, 2, and 3. It is grown in monkey kidney, Vero cell culture, or human diploid cells. Each 0.5 mL dose contains 40, 8, and 32 D antigen units of types I, II, and III polioviruses, respectively. IPV induces primarily a humoral immune response compared to oral polio vaccine (OPV), which induces mucosal immunity.

Following two doses of IPV at 2 and 4 months, seroprotection rates ranged from 89% to 100% for poliovirus type 1, from 92% to 100% for poliovirus type 2, and from 70% to 100% for poliovirus type 3. The 2–4–6-month schedule gives the highest seroprotection rates and geometric mean titers (GMT).[7]

Studies in developing countries have shown that IPV is immunogenic in an EPI schedule, although the titers achieved and the seroconversion rates may be lower compared with vaccination of infants at 2–4–6 months. Since IPV does not cause vaccine-associated paralytic poliomyelitis (VAPP) or circulating vaccine-derived poliovirus (cVDPV), it is the mainstay vaccine for the eradication of polio.

This vaccine is a part of UIP in which fractional IPV (fIPV) is given 0.1 mL intradermal (ID) at 6 weeks, 14 weeks, and 9 months.

Dosage and Schedule

IAP Schedule

Three doses of 0.5 mL IM at 6–10–14 weeks, followed by boosters at 16–18 months and 4–6 years. IPV is administered along with DPT-containing vaccines.

Catch-up Immunization

Three doses at 0, 2, and 6 months up to 5 years of age.

Fractional Dose IPV

Fractional IPV has been recommended by the Global Polio Eradication Initiative (GPEI) and the WHO for use in developing countries, after the switch from trivalent oral polio vaccine (tOPV) to bivalent oral polio vaccine (bOPV). fIPV is a dose-sparing strategy to reduce cost and stretch supply to a larger number of children in situations of limited supply of IPV. fIPV is immunogenic but slightly less immunogenic than the administration of the regular IM dose. fIPV elicited significantly lower seroconversion rates and GMT than IM IPV for all three poliovirus types when administered at 6, 10, and 14 weeks of age.

Seroprotection rates, following two doses of fIPV or IPV given at 14 and 36 weeks, were noninferior to three doses given at 10, 14, and 36 weeks. The GMTs were higher at 40 weeks for the three-dose IPV groups versus two or three doses of fIPV for all three serotypes.

NIP Schedule (fIPV)

Three doses at 6 weeks, 14 weeks, and 9 months.

Adverse Effects

Inactivated polio vaccine is one of the safest vaccines. Local minor adverse reactions include pain, swelling, and erythema, which are self-limiting.

HEPATITIS A VACCINE

Two types of hepatitis A vaccines are available: Inactivated and live-attenuated formulations.

Inactivated Hepatitis A Vaccine

This contains formaldehyde inactivated hepatitis A virus derived from the HM175, GBM strain, or TZ84 strain, adsorbed onto aluminum hydroxide.[8]

Immunogenicity

Following the first dose, 95% of healthy children, adolescents, and adults seroconvert and 99% following the second dose.

Dose and Schedule

Hepatitis A vaccine is given in a prime-boost schedule, namely the priming dose on the elected date "0," followed by a single booster at a 6-month interval. The IAP-ACVIP recommends the vaccine to be given at 12 months of age routinely for optimal protection in view of waning maternal antibodies in infants. The dose is 0.5 mL IM and a booster between 18 and 24 months of age, for children till 18 years of age.

Adverse Effects

Adverse reactions are minimal and include self-limiting local reactions at the injection site. It can be given after 1 year in children as a routine vaccine.

Live-attenuated Hepatitis A Vaccine

The vaccine is derived from the H2 strain of the virus attenuated after serial passage in human diploid cells. It has been in use in China since the 1990s in mass vaccination programs. The vaccine meets the requirements of the Chinese Drug Authority and WHO. It is also licensed and available in India. Immunogenicity studies with a single dose show seroconversion rates of >98%, 2 months after vaccination, and persistence of protective antibodies in >80% of vaccines at 10-year follow-up. Two immunogenicity studies from India in 143 and 505 children, respectively, have demonstrated >95% seroconversion with a single dose of the live-attenuated vaccine with persistence of antibodies on follow-up.[8]

Schedule

The IAP-ACVIP recommends a single dose of 0.5 mL given SC after the age of 12 months.[4]

VARICELLA VACCINE

Varicella vaccines are live-attenuated vaccines, derived from the original Oka strain, with the virus contents varying from one manufacturer to another. The recommended dose is 0.5 mL by the subcutaneous route, and the minimum infectious virus content should be at least 1,000 plaque-forming units. It is available as a lyophilized vaccine. It should be protected from light and needs to be used within 30 minutes of its reconstitution. It may be given with all other childhood vaccines.

Immunogenicity

After a single dose of the varicella vaccine, in children older than 12 months, 76–85% develop a protective immune response. After two doses, seroprotection rates and cell-mediated immune responses approach 100%.[9]

IAP/ACVIP Recommendations

The first dose of varicella vaccine is at ≥15 months of age and the second dose is at 18–24 months. For catch-up vaccination, children below the age of 13 years should receive two doses 3 months apart, and those aged 13 years or more should receive two doses at an interval of 4–8 weeks.

A combined measles, mumps, rubella, and varicella (MMRV) vaccine is also licensed in India. It has an efficacy of 95–100%. It is recommended in the 4–6-years age group, as there is a chance of increased incidence of febrile seizure if it is used below 2 years.

HUMAN PAPILLOMAVIRUS VACCINE

Human papillomavirus (HPV) serotypes 16 and 18 are implicated in 70% of cervical cancers globally. Types 6 and 11 are known to cause 90% of anogenital warts. HPV has also been implicated in the causation of oropharyngeal, anal, and penile carcinomas.

Four HPV vaccines are licensed in India: Two quadrivalent, a nonavalent, and a bivalent vaccine, which is no longer marketed. HPV vaccines are manufactured by recombinant deoxyribonucleic acid (RNA) technology that produces noninfectious virus-like particles comprising the HPV L1 protein, the major capsid protein of HPV. The quadrivalent vaccine available in India is a mixture of L1 proteins of HPV serotypes 16, 18, 6, and 11 with an aluminum-containing adjuvant. The bivalent vaccine is a mixture of L1 proteins of HPV serotypes 16 and 18 with ASO_4 as an adjuvant. The nonavalent (9-valent) vaccine contains 31, 33, 45, 52, and 58 HPV serotypes in addition to 6, 11, 16, and 18 that are present in the quadrivalent HPV vaccines.[10]

The IAP-ACVIP recommends routine vaccination with the HPV vaccine to all girls and boys in a two-dose schedule between 9 and 14 years as a gender-neutral vaccine. Since protection is seen only when the vaccine is given before infection with HPV, the vaccine should be given prior to sexual debut. Both the quadrivalent and nonavalent vaccines are equally efficacious and safe for protection against cervical cancer and percutaneous lesions, including anogenital warts.[11]

The vaccines should be stored at 2–8°C and must not be frozen. The dose is 0.5 mL by the intramuscular route in deltoid. The vaccine can be given to females above 15 years of age. Three doses of either vaccine are recommended at 0, 2, and 6 months in the 15–26-year-old age group. Both vaccine formulations are now recommended in women up to 45 years of age after a one-to-one discussion. Pregnancy is a contraindication.

ROTAVIRUS VACCINES

Four rotavirus vaccines are marketed in India. These are the monovalent vaccine (RV1-GSK), the pentavalent human bovine reassortant vaccine (RV 5-MSD), the Indian neonatal rotavirus live vaccine, 116 E (BBIL), and the bovine rotavirus pentavalent vaccine (BRVPV-SII). Of these, the latter two are used in the NIP.

Schedules

- *NIS:* Three doses at 4-week interval, 6 weeks of age onward. The first dose can be given latest by one completed year and the last dose by two completed years.
- *IAP:* Three doses at 4-week intervals, 6 weeks of age onward. The first dose should be given not later than 14 completed weeks and the final dose not later than 32 completed weeks.[12]

MEASLES, MUMPS, AND RUBELLA VACCINE

This is a live-attenuated vaccine containing the attenuated strains of measles, mumps, and rubella. The vaccine is available as a combined vaccine with the measles, mumps, and rubella (MMR) vaccine **(Table 6.6.3)**.

Schedule

- The NIS recommends MR (measles, rubella) vaccine in two doses at 9–12 months and 16–24 months.

TABLE 6.6.3: Characteristics of MMR vaccines available in India.

	MMR-SII	***MMR-GSK***	***MMR-Zydus***
Measles strain	Edmonston-Zagreb (EZ)	Schwartz	Edmonston-Zagreb (EZ)
Dose	Not <1,000 $CCID_{50}$	Not <$10^{3.3}$ $CCID_{50}$	Not <1,000 $CCID_{50}$
Mumps strain	Leningrad—Zagreb	RIT 4385 (Jeryl Lynn)	Hoshino
Dose	Not <5,000 $CCID_{50}$	Not <$10^{3.7}$ $CCID_{50}$	Not <5,000 $CCID_{50}$
Rubella strain	Wistar RA 27/3	Wistar RA 27/3	Wistar RA 27/3
Dose	Not <1,000 $CCID_{50}$	Not <$10^{3.0}$ $CCID_{50}$	Not <1,000 $CCID_{50}$

(CCID: cell culture infectious dose; MMR: measles, mumps, and rubella vaccine)

- The IAP-ACVIP recommends three doses of MMR vaccine at 9 months, 12–15 months, and 4–6 years.

It is a safe vaccine. Minor allergic reactions, febrile seizure, rash, pruritus, and encephalopathy have been reported. Rarely, the vaccine may cause thrombocytopenia. Being a live vaccine, it cannot be used in immunocompromised individuals or in pregnancy.[13]

INFLUENZA VACCINE

Currently, there are three types of vaccines used worldwide: Inactivated influenza vaccine (IIV), live-attenuated influenza vaccine (LAIV), and recombinant HA vaccine. Each type of vaccine has its advantages and disadvantages.

Inactivated Influenza Vaccine

The inactivated virus vaccine is the most common worldwide approach due to its high safety and relatively low production costs. As a result, it has the highest percentage in the flu vaccine global market. The IIV can be given for children 6 months and older. The virus is generally grown in embryonated chicken eggs or cultured cells of mammalian origin for this type of vaccine. IIV has three types: Whole-virus inactivated vaccines, split-virus inactivated vaccines, and subunit inactivated vaccines.

Live-attenuated Influenza Vaccines

The LAIV was developed to mimic natural infection and immunity without causing severe illness and consequently induces humoral and cellular immunity. It has some superiority over IIV because it induces mainly local mucosal immunity and local immunoglobulin A (IgA) production as well as IgG, in contrast to only systemic IgA and IgG antibodies with IIV. However, it is not recommended in immunocompromised children or individuals who are in close contact with them. In India, a quadrivalent intranasal LAIV is licensed to be used safely in children and adults, ages 2–49 years.

Recombinant HA Vaccine

Recombinant HA vaccine can be produced using recombinant protein expression technology by insect cells and baculovirus due to their high yield and cost effectiveness. The recombinant HA vaccine has its suitability for an influenza pandemic because it might take a shorter time to manufacture, and it would be much safer than other influenza vaccines due to the absence of highly pathogenic viruses. However, due to its lack of efficacy in children, the recombinant HA vaccine is limited to adults.

Dose and Schedule

Two doses, 1 month apart, are given for the first time for children from 6 months to <9 years, with revaccination every year. The dose is 0.5 mL. After 9 years, only a single dose of 0.5 mL is given, followed by a single revaccination every year. It is recommended in high-risk groups, e.g., immunocompromised children and children with cardiopulmonary diseases. It should also be given to children whose parents ask for the vaccine.[14]

MENINGOCOCCAL VACCINE

There are two types of vaccines: Polysaccharide vaccines and polysaccharide protein conjugate vaccines. As with other PSVs, the polysaccharide meningococcal vaccine is composed of serogroup-specific capsular polysaccharides that elicit humoral responses independent of T-cells; thus, it does not provide immunological memory, and additionally, it exhibits low immunogenicity in children under 2 years of age. Therefore, it is recommended for adults and children older than 2 years old. It is available as bivalent (serogroups A and C) and tetravalent (serogroups A, C, Y, and W135) vaccines. These vaccines are currently not marketed in India. In contrast, the polysaccharide protein conjugate vaccine has higher immunogenicity, longer efficacy, and the potential for herd immunity; moreover, it is even effective for children below 2 years old. Therefore, it is preferred over polysaccharide vaccines, particularly in children. There are two types of polysaccharide protein conjugate vaccines available in India.

1. *Quadrivalent conjugate vaccine (serogroups A, C, Y, and W135):* It includes Menactra and Menveo vaccines; Menactra vaccine uses diphtheria toxin as a carrier protein, while Menveo uses a nontoxic mutant of diphtheria toxin known as cross-reactive material 197 (CRM197) as a carrier protein.
2. *Monovalent (serogroup A or C):* It includes MenAfriVac and PsA-TT for serogroup A and uses tetanus toxoid as a carrier protein, while the MenC vaccine protects against serogroup C and uses CRM197 as a carrier protein.

The quadrivalent conjugated vaccine is preferred in India, whereas the monovalent conjugated vaccine is primarily used in Africa (MenAfriVac/PsA-TT) and Europe (MenC). Quadrivalent meningococcal conjugate vaccine (Menactra™) has been licensed for use of individuals aged 9 months onward in India. Two doses at 9 months to 2 years at a 6-month interval and a single dose of 0.5 mL IM above 2 years is recommended. Menveo™ is licensed as a single dose above 2 years of age. For those at high risk of invasive meningococcal disease, boosters are recommended every 5 years.[15]

The IAP-ACVIP recommends the use of meningococcal vaccines, especially in certain high-risk situations in children:

- During outbreaks, if caused by serogroups included in the vaccine
- Children with complement deficiency
- Children with asplenia
- Travelers to the Kingdom of Saudi Arabia for Haj (mandatory)
- Travelers to the African meningitis belt
- Students going abroad (mandatory in the United States of America)[9]

CONCLUSION

Non-UIP vaccines are very important components of immunization strategy in childhood for prevention of VPDs. The government cannot include all vaccines in the UIP, as resources are limited; and not all vaccines are absolutely essential for all children as some vaccines are essential in some specific groups or geographies. IAP-ACVIP reviews the scientific evidences available and comes up with recommendations regarding these non-UIP vaccines from time to time. Depending on changing priorities and availability of resources the vaccines which are currently non-UIP may be included in UIP in future.

REFERENCES

1. Rao MIS, Kasi SG, Dhir SK, Wadhwa A, Rajsekhar B, Kumar CM, et al. Indian Academy of Pediatrics (IAP) Advisory Committee on Vaccines and Immunization Practices (ACVIP): Recommended Immunization Schedule (2023) and update on immunization for children aged 0 through 18 years. Indian Pediatr. 2024;61(2):113-25.
2. World Health Organization. Strategic Advisory Group of Exports on Immunization (SAGE)- October 2017. [online] Available from https://www.who.int/news-room/events/detail/2017/10/17/default-calendar/strategic-advisory-group-of-experts-on-immunization-(sage)---october-2017 [Last accessed, February 2024].
3. Khadke R, Abhay Shah A. Pneumococcal vaccines. In: Shekhar Rao MI, Kasi SG (Eds). Purple Book: IAP Guidebook on Immunization 2022, 4th edition. New Delhi: Indian Academy of Pediatrics; 2022. pp. 193-220.
4. Kasi SG, Shah A. Diphtheria, tetanus, and pertussis vaccines. In: Shekhar Rao MI, Kasi SG (Eds). Purple Book: IAP Guidebook on Immunization 2022, 4th edition. New Delhi: Indian Academy of Pediatrics; 2022. pp. 171-3.
5. Kumar CM, Vashishtha VM, Kalra A. Typhoid vaccines. In: Vashishtha VM (Ed). FAQs on Vaccines and Immunization Practices. New Delhi: Jaypee Brothers Medical Publishers; 2021. pp. 333-55.
6. Chatterjee K, Kasi SG. Typhoid vaccines. In: Shekhar Rao MI, Kasi SG (Eds). Purple Book: IAP Guidebook on Immunization 2022, 4th edition. New Delhi: Indian Academy of Pediatrics; 2022. pp. 289-99.
7. Shenoy B, Agarwalla SK. Polio vaccines. In: Shekhar Rao MI, Kasi SG (Eds). Purple Book: IAP Guidebook on Immunization 2022, 4th edition. New Delhi: Indian Academy of Pediatrics; 2022. pp. 118-38.
8. Kumar CM, Marathe S. Hepatitis A vaccines. In: IAP Guidebook on Immunization, 4th edition. New Delhi: Indian Academy of Pediatrics; 2022. pp. 270-84.
9. Khadke R, Sanjay S. Varicella vaccines. In: Shekhar Rao MI, Kasi SG (Eds). Purple Book: IAP Guidebook on Immunization 2022, 4th edition. New Delhi: Indian Academy of Pediatrics; 2022. pp. 253-69.
10. Human papillomavirus vaccines: WHO position paper, December 2022 Weekly Epidemiological Record No 50, 2022, 97, 645–672. [online] Available from https://www.who.int/publications/i/item/who-wer9750-645-672. [Last accessed October, 2024].
11. Kalyani S, Kasi SG. Human papilloma virus vaccines. In: Shekhar Rao MI, Kasi SG (Eds). Purple Book: IAP Guidebook on Immunization 2022, 4th edition. New Delhi: Indian Academy of Pediatrics; 2022. pp. 305-21.
12. Dhir SK, Kasi SG. Rotavirus vaccines. Shekhar Rao MI, Kasi SG (Eds). IAP Guidebook on Immunization, 4th edition. New Delhi: Indian Academy of Pediatrics; 2022. pp. 221-39.
13. Rajsekhar B, Verma S. Measles, mumps and rubella vaccines. In: Shekhar Rao MI, Kasi SG (Eds). Purple Book: IAP Guidebook on Immunization 2022, 4th edition. New Delhi: Indian Academy of Pediatrics; 2022. pp. 240-52.
14. Rajsekhar B, Agarwalla SK. Influenza vaccines. In: Purple Book: Shekhar Rao MI, Kasi SG (Eds). IAP Guidebook on Immunization 2022, 4th edition. New Delhi: Indian Academy of Pediatrics; 2022. pp. 323-39.
15. Ananda Kesavan TM, Pemde HK. Meningococcal vaccines. In: Shekhar Rao MI, Kasi SG (Eds). Purple Book: IAP Guidebook on Immunization 2022, 4th edition. New Delhi: Indian Academy of Pediatrics; 2022. pp. 357-72.

6.7 Vaccines for SARS-CoV-2

Sumitha Nayak

INTRODUCTION

The severe acute respiratory syndrome coronavirus-2 (SARS-CoV-2) pandemic attacked all regions of the globe with an enormous intensity. The morbidity and mortality were unparalleled. The rapid replication and mutation of the virus needed vaccines to be prepared at an extremely rapid pace. Several existing platforms were used, and many newer platforms were explored as the world realized that it was a race against time. As the virus genome was unraveled, the spike protein was found to be the most natural target to be selected by vaccine makers across the world. Currently, several vaccines are in clinical usage, while many more are in various stages of clinical trials and awaiting approvals.

SARS-COV-2 VIRUS

The SARS-CoV-2 virus belongs to the family *Coronaviridae*, subfamily *Coronavirinae*. This subfamily contains four genera: *Alphacoronavirus, betacoronavirus, gammacoronavirus,* and *deltacoronavirus*.[1] SARS-CoV-2 virus belongs to the betacoronavirus 2B lineage, a new betacoronavirus that infected humans. This virus was first reported from a cluster of supposedly viral pneumonia cases in Wuhan, China.[2]

Structure of the SARS-CoV-2 Virus

The genome of the coronavirus is a single-stranded ribonucleic acid (RNA), 27–32 kb in size, and is larger than other RNA viruses.[1] The genome is packed inside an envelope surrounded by the capsid **(Fig. 6.7.1)**. This capsid contains the nucleocapsid protein (N). The envelope packing of the genome contains three structural proteins: Membrane protein (M), spike protein (S), and envelope protein (E). There are 4 structural proteins—S, E, M, and N—and 16 nonstructural proteins (NSPs 1-16). Each NSP has a distinct function.

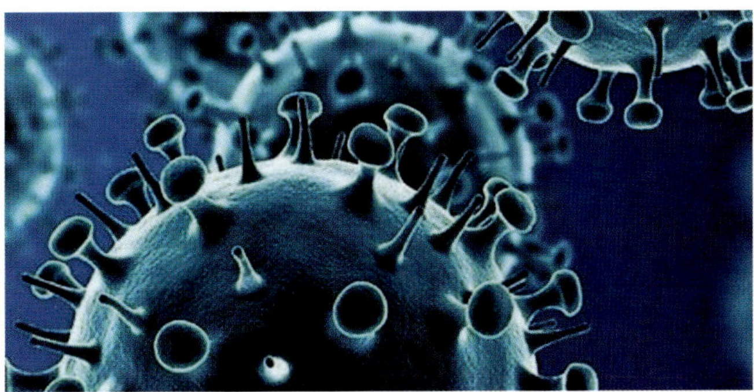

Fig. 6.7.1: Structure of SARS-CoV-2 virus.[1] (SARS-CoV-2: severe acute respiratory syndrome coronavirus-2)

Spike Glycoprotein

The spike protein (S-protein), which is crucial for viral entry into the host cell, is a transmembrane protein and has two subunits: S1 and S2, each with differing functions. The S1 subunit consists of an N-terminal domain (NTD) and a receptor-binding domain (RBD) **(Fig. 6.7.2)**. The S1 subunit functions to bind the receptor on the host cell, while the S2 subunit fuses the membranes of the virus and host cells.

The S-protein contains an RBD, which has a specific affinity to the acetylcholinesterase receptors (ACE2).[1] This RBD has two domains—the core and the external subdomains. This core subdomain contains most of the binding sites for SARS-CoV-2 and the ACE2 receptors.[1]

VACCINES AGAINST COVID-19 VIRUS

Challenges

Most RNA viruses are known to mutate and result in variants with increased or decreased transmission, increased or decreased pathogenicity, and attack rates. In keeping with this pattern, the SARS-CoV-2 virus has shown a high mutation rate with numerous mutant strains.[2] The major challenges include:

- Rapid virus mutation rate
- Lack of correlates of protection

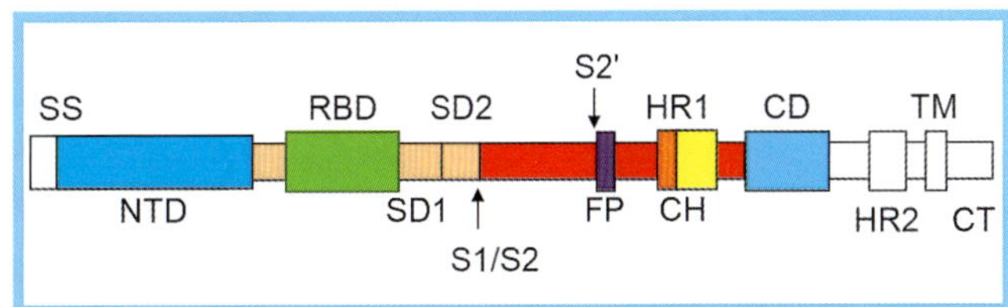

Fig. 6.7.2: Structure of the spike glycoprotein of SARS-CoV-2 virus.[1] (CD: codon deoptimization; NTD: N-terminal domain; RBD: receptor-binding domain; SARS CoV-2: severe acute respiratory syndrome coronavirus-2)

- Poor mucosal immunity of the vaccines under development
- For vaccines developed later, lack of SARS-CoV-2 naive populations for testing vaccines

According to the data from the World Health Organization (WHO), as of March 30, 2023, there are 183 candidate vaccines in clinical development and 199 in preclinical development.[3]

Vaccine Platforms

Several vaccine platforms have been employed in the manufacture of COVID-19 vaccines.[2] Some are tried and tested platforms [live-attenuated vaccines, inactivated vaccines, protein-based subunit vaccines, and protein-based virus-like particle (VLP)-containing vaccines], while some are novel platforms [deoxyribonucleic acid (DNA) vaccines, RNA vaccines, and viral vector vaccines] **(Fig. 6.7.3)**.[2]

VIRUS-BASED VACCINES

Live-attenuated Virus Vaccines

These vaccines utilize the attenuated form of the SARS-CoV-2 virus.[2] They are classically produced by serial passages in cell cultures until the pathogenicity is attenuated.[4] Codon deoptimization (CD) techniques are utilized to attenuate the virus. CD represents a potential strategy to modify the expression efficiency of a gene, thereby altering the amount of its protein product. This strategy involves synthetic recoding of viral genomes, such that synonymous codons are suppressed and nonsynonymous codons are retained, resulting in suboptimal production of proteins.

The live-attenuated vaccines are advantageous, as they are capable of providing mucosal and robust cellular immunity for protection against the virus.

Inactivated Virus Vaccines

As a time-tested and proven method of vaccine design, the use of inactivated vaccines against viral infections has stood the test of time. The inactivated virus is injected into the host, and a strong and wide range of immune responses occur in the body.[2,4] Chemicals like psoralen, ascorbic acid, hydrogen peroxidase, formaldehyde, and ultraviolet (UV) treatment are used to inactivate the virus.[2] Multiple inoculations and powerful adjuvants are required to ensure the optimal immune response.[2]

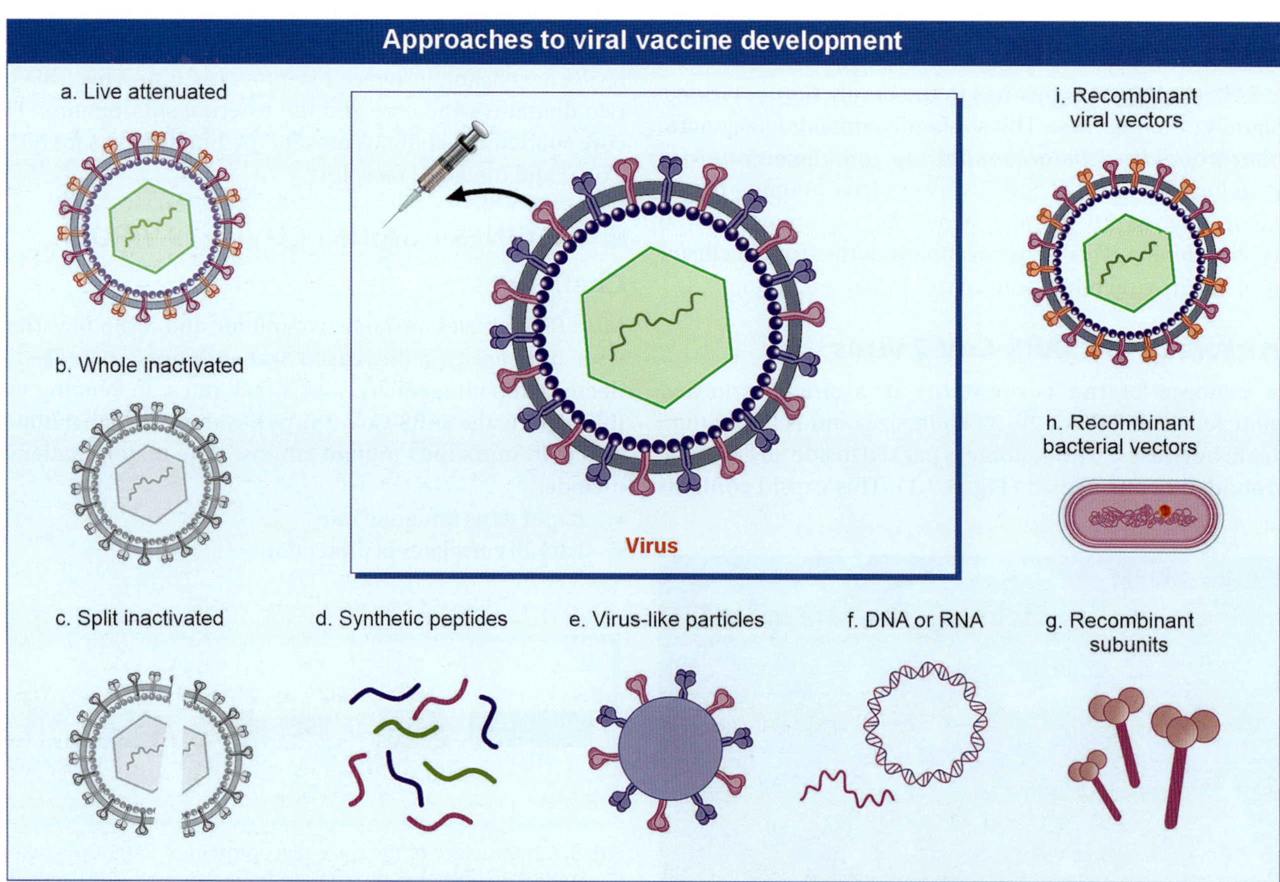

Fig. 6.7.3: Newer vaccine platforms. (DNA: deoxyribonucleic acid; RNA: ribonucleic acid)
Source: https://app.biorender.com/illustrations/6537c4eafa52c12370ad3719.

Protein-based Vaccines

These are of two types—the subunit vaccines and the VLP-containing vaccines.[2,4] The subunit vaccines consist of viral antigenic fragments produced by recombinant techniques along with adjuvants that improve the immunogenicity.[2,4]

The RBD domain of the SARS-CoV-2 virus contains the spike protein and is the highly immunogenic region of the virus.[2] As per studies done, the S1 and S2 subunits as well as the RBD proteins are critical for generating neutralizing antibodies.[2] Hence, the protein subunit vaccines comprise the virus components that activate the human immune system without the remaining portion of the viral particles.[2,4] However, these recombinant vaccines generally trigger a humoral response that may provide partial protection against the virus.[4] Hence, repeated doses may be required to produce immune memory.[4] Adjuvants are necessary to enhance the immunogenicity of subunit vaccines.[4] Around 33 protein subunit vaccines against SARS-CoV-2 are in various stages of clinical development.[4] The RBD-based vaccines may be more prone to changes that arise with antigenic drift, compared to vaccines that contain the entire length of the spike protein.[5]

Viral Vector Vaccines

These are produced by using an attenuated recombinant virus that encodes the sequence of the desired antigen. This is introduced into the host and induces elevated levels of humoral and cellular immune responses.[2] These can be nonreplicating or replicating viral vector vaccines.

Nonreplicating Viral Vector Vaccines

These are attenuated recombinant vaccines, which encode the antigen sequence for high-level endogenous production of that antigen, resulting in elevated endogenous cellular and humoral immune responses.[2] Some viruses are commonly used as vectors on this platform and include lentivirus, retrovirus, adenovirus, and adeno-associated virus (AAV).[4] Due to the safety and immunogenicity, usually no adjuvants are required, and a single dose may be sufficient to produce robust immunity.[4] The Ad5-nCoV and Ad.26.CoV2.S vaccines have been tested for safety and immunogenicity. The ChAdOx-1 nCoV-19 vaccine (AZD1222) has been studied at Oxford University together with Astra Zeneca and received emergency use licensing, following which the phase IV clinical trial is ongoing since February 2021.[2,4] The Gamaleya Institute in Russia uses two adenoviruses, Ad5 and Ad26, with the spike protein inserted.[2] The additional recombinant vector has been shown to boost the RBD-specific antibody titers.[2]

Replicating Viral Vector Vaccines

These vaccines use different viral vectors compared to the nonreplicating vector vaccines. The various vectors that have been used include the flu virus, measles virus, and vesicular stomatitis virus (VSV).[2] Several replicating vaccines that have been produced and are undergoing various stages of trials include the intranasal flu-factored Del NS1-2019-nCoV-RBD-OPTI1 vaccine, the rVSV-SARS-CoV-2-S/IIBR-100 vaccine, and the measles vector-based TMV-083 vaccine. Besides these, the live recombinant Newcastle disease virus-vectored COVID-19 vaccine is in the early stages of trials. These vaccines are based on the sequence of the antigenic viral protein and do not mandate the presence of the viral particles.[2]

Gene-based Vaccines

DNA Vaccines

These vaccines do not use the live virus and are constructed with a plasmid vector that encodes a target vaccine molecule.[2] The plasmids replicate the main chromosomal DNA including the inserted material.[2] The immune system responds to this genetically engineered DNA with both humoral and cell-mediated responses. DNA vaccines are safe and advantageous, as they can be produced in large amounts in a very short period of time.[6-8] Upon injection, the plasmid encoded genes are processed by class I and II major histocompatibility cells (MHCs), resulting in a complete and adequate immunization.[2]

RNA Vaccines

The antigen of interest is encoded in the messenger RNA (mRNA) or in a self-amplifying RNA, which acts as a template to produce the proteins.[2,4] The vaccine must be available in the host's cytoplasm for translation into the antigenic proteins. BNT 162b2 was the first mRNA vaccine candidate against SARS-CoV-2 that received authorization. It utilizes the protein RBD trimer in the lipid-soluble nanoparticle formulation.[2]

Virus-like Particles-containing Vaccines

These vaccines are created using 10–200 nm nanoparticles assembling viral proteins, which have been recombinantly generated and are referred to as VLPs. The VLPs of the S protein of SARS-CoV-2 have the capability of host cell fusion via the ACE2 receptors.[2]

Table 6.7.1 provides a detailed list of various platforms to prepare SARS-CoV-2 vaccines.

VACCINES LICENSED FOR USE IN PEDIATRIC AND ADOLESCENT AGES

According to the current 2023 guidelines released by the American Academy of Pediatrics (AAP), children above the age of 6 months should be protected with the SARS-CoV-2 vaccine. Healthy children and adolescents aged 6 months to 17 years are classified in the low-priority group by WHO. Some of the vaccines licensed for use in children are discussed in the following text.

Pfizer BioNTech COVID-19 Vaccine

This vaccine contains the latest 2023–2024 formula. The vaccine contains 3 msg of nucleoside-modified mRNA encoding the viral spike S glycoprotein of the SARS-CoV-2 Omicron variant of the XBB.1.5 lineage. This vaccine is licensed for use above 6 months of age.[7]

Route of administration: The vaccine is administered intramuscularly (IM).

- *For children between 6 months and 4 years of age:* A three-dose schedule is recommended as follows:[8]
  - *For naive children, not previously vaccinated:* Administer dose 1 now; dose 2 at least 3–8 weeks after dose 1; dose 3 at least 8 weeks after dose 2.
  - *For children who have previously taken one dose of vaccine:* Administer dose 2 to be given at least 3–8 weeks after the previous dose; dose 3 to be given at least 8 weeks after dose 2.
  - *For those who have taken two or more doses of the vaccine:* Complete the series; administer dose 3 to be given 8 weeks after the last dose.

  The single dose is 0.3 mL of vaccine; the color code of the label border and vial cap is yellow.
- *For children from age 5 years through 11 years, irrespective of previous COVID-19 vaccine status,* give a single dose of vaccine. If previously vaccinated, give the dose at least 2 months since the last dose. Single dose: 0.3 mL. The color code of the vial cap and label border is blue.
- *For immunocompromised children aged 6 months to 11 years,* a three-dose schedule of a COVID-19 vaccine is recommended. At least one dose must be of the latest 2023–2024 formulation.

It is not licensed for use in those below 6 months of age or those aged 12 years or more.

Contraindications to this vaccine include history of severe allergic reaction or anaphylaxis to the previous dose or to any component of the vaccine.

Adverse reactions include injection site pain, redness, and swelling at all ages. Below 24 months of age, there could be decreased appetite, drowsiness, fever, or irritability. Above 2 years of age, chills, diarrhea, fatigue, worsening joint pains, or vomiting may occur as adverse effects. All serious adverse events, cases of myocarditis, multisystem inflammatory syndrome (MISC), cases of pericarditis, hospitalization, or death that may occur after vaccine administration must be reported to the Vaccine Adverse Events Reporting System.

For those above the age of 12 years, Comirnaty is the vaccine indicated for active immunization. It is administered as a single dose of 0.3 mL given IM, at least 2 months after any previous dose of the COVID-19 vaccine given.

TABLE 6.7.1: List of platforms and SARS-CoV-2 vaccines.

Vaccine platforms	*Types of vaccines*	*Developers*
Inactivated viruses	Vero cell	Sinopharm
	VLA 2001	Valneva, National Institute for Health Research, UK
	BBIBP-CorV	Sinovac
	Covaxin, inactivated vero cell	Bharat Biotech India
Live-attenuated	COVI-VAC	Codagenix/Serum Institute of India
	MV-014-212	Meissa Vaccines, Inc.
DNA-based	Covigen	Univ of Sydney, Bionet Co. Ltd., Technovalia
	INO4800+Electroporation	Invio Pharma + IVI + Advaccine
	AG0301-COVID-19	AnGes + Takara Bio + Osaka Univ
	Zycov-D	Zydus Cadila, India
	GX-19N	Genexine Consortium
RNA-based	mRNA-1273, mRNA-1273.351	Moderna
	BNT162b2b	Pfizer/BioNTech + Fosun Pharma
	ARCT-021	Arcturus Therapeutics
	ARCoV	Academy of Military Science, Walvax Biotechnology, Suzhou Abogen Biosciences
	LNP-nCoVsaRNA	Imperial College, London
	Gemcovac-19 (m-RNA is adsorbed on the surface)	Gennova, India

Contd...

Contd...

Vaccine platforms	Types of vaccines	Developers
Protein subunit	VAT 00008	Sanofi Pasteur + GSK
	Recombinant SARS-CoV-2 Fusion Protein vaccine (V-01)	Livzon Pharmaceuticals
	Nancovax	Nanogen Pharmaceutical Biotechnology
	CIGB-66	Center for Genetic Engineering and Biotechnology
	Covovax (Recombinant nanoparticle vaccine)	Serum Institute of India
	Novovax	
	Corbevax	Biological E
Viral vector (nonreplicating)	Recombinant novel coronavirus vaccine (Adenovirus type 5 vector)	CanSino Biological Inc./Beijing Institute of Biotechnology
	Sputnik V (rAd26-S+rAd5-S)	Gamaleya Research Institute
	Cov2373/Nuvaxovid/Covovax (Recombinant nanoparticle vaccine)	Novavax
	Ad26.CoV2.S	Janssen Pharma
	VXA-CoV2-1Ad5 adjuvanted Oral Vaccine platform	Vaxart
	AZD1222 Vaxzevria	Astra Zeneca
	COVISHIELD (ChAdOx1_nCoV-19)	Serum Institute of India
Viral vector (replicating)	DeINS 1-2019-nCoV-RBDOPT1(Intranasal flu-based RBD)	University of Hong Kong, Xiamen University, and Beijing Wantal Biological Pharmacy
	rVSV-SARS-CoV-2-S Vaccine	Israel Institute of Biological Research
Virus-like particle	RBD SARS-CoV2 HBsAg VLP Vaccine	Serum Institute of India + AccelagenPty +SpyBiotech
	VBI-2902a	VBI Vaccines Inc.
	SARS-CoV-2 VLP Vaccine	The Scientific and Technological Research Council of Turkey
	ABNCoV2 Capsid VLP ± adjuvant MF59	Radboud University

(DNA: deoxyribonucleic acid; mRNA: messenger RNA; RBD: receptor-binding domain; RNA: ribonucleic acid; SARS-CoV-2: severe acute respiratory syndrome coronavirus-2; VLP: virus-like particle)

Sources:

1. Beni-Suef Univ J Basic App Sci. 2022;11:35.
2. Status of COVID-19 Vaccines within WHO EUL/PQ evaluation process. [online] Available from https://extranet.who.int/prequal/sites/default/files document_files/Status_COVID_VAX_08AUgust2023.pdf [Last accessed November, 2024].

Moderna COVID-19 Vaccine

This vaccine includes a single component corresponding to the Omicron variant XBB.1.5 of SARS-CoV-2 and has received emergency use authorization (EUA) from the US Food and Drug Administration (FDA) for use in individuals 6 months through 11 years of age.[8]

Route of administration: IM. *Dose:* 0.25 mL.

- *For children 6 months through 4 years of age,* the doses given depend on the number of previous doses received:
    - *In case of children who have not received any previous doses:* Two-dose schedules at 0 and 1 months are given.
    - *In case of one dose received previously:* A single dose is to be given 1 month after the last dose of the Moderna vaccine received.
    - *In case of two or more doses received previously:* A single dose is to be given 2 or more months after the previous dose of the Moderna vaccine.
- *For children 5 years through 11 years of age, irrespective of previous immunization status:* Give a single dose, 2 or more months after the last dose of the previous COVID-19 vaccine given.
- *For immunocompromised individuals from 6 months through 11 years:* Complete a three-dose series, each given 1 month apart at 0, 1, and 2 months.

Contraindications: History of a severe allergic reaction like anaphylaxis to any component of the vaccine or anaphylaxis after a previous dose of the Moderna vaccine is a contraindication for using this vaccine.

Spikevax is the vaccine that is indicated for use in *those above the age of 12 years*. It is administered as a single dose of 0.5 mL, given at least 2 months after the last dose of any COVID-19 vaccine that had been given.

Novavax COVID-19 Adjuvanted Vaccine

This vaccine is given EUA for those aged 12 years and above.[6] The vaccine is a protein subunit vaccine, given at a dose of 0.5 mL IM.

- *For those above the age of 12 years who have previously been vaccinated with any COVID-19 vaccine,* administer a single dose at least 2 months after the last dose.
- *For those above the age of 12 years who have not been previously immunized with any COVID-19 vaccine,* administer two doses of 0.5 mL each 3 weeks apart.
- *For those with immunocompromised,* an additional dose of Novavax COVID-19 vaccine adjusted (2023–2024) may be administered at least 2 months following the last dose of the COVID-19 vaccine.

Contraindications to use of this vaccine include any history of anaphylaxis or severe allergic reactions to any components of Novavax COVID-19 or history of anaphylaxis following any previous dose of a Novavax COVID-19 vaccine.

Adverse reactions include local site redness and pain, fatigue or malaise, muscle pain, headache, joint pain, nausea, vomiting, and fever. Any serious adverse reactions, including myocarditis, pericarditis, MISC, etc., must be reported to the Vaccine Adverse Event Reporting System.

Covaxin COVID-19 Vaccine

This vaccine is the first in the world to generate data in the 2–18-year age group.[9] This vaccine has received approval for use in ages 6–12 years in the year 2022. With this, the vaccine is licensed for use above the age of 6 years. The Drugs Controller General of India (DCGI) has issued EUA for use in all age groups above 6 years.[10]

This is a whole virion-inactivated vaccine (BBV152) that is safe and immunogenic. The vaccine is administered IM in a two-dose schedule, given 28 days apart. The vaccine can be safely used in immunocompromised individuals also.

The only *contraindications* to the use of Covaxin are severe allergic reactions or anaphylaxis to any component of the vaccine or to any previous dose of the vaccine.

The *adverse effects* include injection site pain, redness and swelling, fever, body ache, malaise, vomiting, nausea, or rashes.

Corbevax COVID-19 Vaccine

This is India's indigenously developed protein subunit vaccine. This vaccine has received EUA for children in the 12–18-year age group.[10] The vaccine has been shown to be safe and immunogenic following trials in this age group. The vaccine is administered IM. It is administered in a two-dose regimen.

ZYCOV-D COVID-19 Vaccine

This is the world's first DNA vaccine that was developed in India.[10] This vaccine received EUA for use in humans for protection against SARS-CoV-2. Developed using the plasmid DNA platform, this vaccine can be easily adapted to deal with mutations. As early as August 2021, this vaccine has received EUA for use in all individuals above the age of 12 years.

The vaccine is administered using a needle-free injector into the intradermal space. The schedule consists of three doses administered 28 days apart—days 0, 28, and 56. A dose of 2 mg of the vaccine must be given at each visit. The vaccine is administered as two shots given at different sites, preferably the deltoid region, at each visit.

IMPACT OF COVID-19 VACCINATION

The COVID-19 vaccines have a substantial impact on mitigating the disease severity. However, disease transmission and outbreaks are not affected by the vaccination. Reports from large efficacy trials in the USA have shown an efficacy of over 90% against symptomatic and severe disease.[9] Indian data gathered from 21 states have shown that the vaccine has been effective in curbing disease spread in 16 of these states.[10] Vaccines are the key measures to reduce the disease burden, mitigate outbreaks in the future, and decrease disease incidence, hospitalizations, and deaths due to the COVID-19 infection.[10]

REFERENCES

1. Wang M-Y, Zhao R, Gao L-J, Gao X-F, Wang D-P, Cao J-M, et al. SARS-CoV-2: structure, biology, and structure-based therapeutics development. Front Cell Infect Microbiol. 2020;10:587269.
2. Savina K, Sreekumar R, Soonu VK, Variyar EJ. Various vaccine platforms in the field of COVID-19. Beni Suef Univ J Basic App Sci. 2022;11:35.
3. World Health Organisation. (2023). COVID-19 vaccine tracker and landscape. [online] Available from https://www.who.int/publications/m/item/draft-landscape-of-COVID-19-candidate-vaccines. [Last accessed October, 2024].
4. Jafari A, Pouya FD, Niknam Z, Abdollahpour-Alitappeh M, Rezaei-Tavirani M, Rasmi Y. Current advances and challenges in COVID-19 vaccine development: from conventional vaccines to next-generation vaccine platforms. Mol Biol Rep 2022;49(6):4943-57.

5. Krammer F. SARS-CoV-2 vaccines in development. Nature. 2020;586(7830):516-27.
6. US Food and Drugs Administration. Fact sheet for healthcare providers administering vaccine: emergency use authorization of Novavax covid-19 vaccine, adjuvanted (2023–2024 formula), for individuals 12 years of age and older. [Last accessed October, 2024].
7. US Food and Drugs Administration. Fact sheet for healthcare providers administering vaccine: emergency use authorization of Pfizer-BioNTech COVID-19 vaccine (2023–2024 formula), for 6 months through 11 years of age. [Last accessed October, 2024].
8. US Food and Drugs Administration. Fact sheet for healthcare providers administering vaccine: emergency use authorization of Moderna COVID-19 vaccine (2023–2024 formula), for individuals 6 months through 11 years of age. [Last accessed October, 2024].
9. Moghadas SM, Vilches TN, Zhang K, Wells CR, Shoukat A, Singer BH, et al. The Impact of Vaccination on Coronavirus Disease 2019 (COVID-19) Outbreaks in the United States. Clin Infect Dis. 2021;73(12):2257-64.
10. Vikaspedia. COVID-19 vaccines in India. [online] Available from https://vikaspedia.in/health/health-campaigns/all-about-covid-vaccines/COVID-19-vaccines-in-india. [Last accessed October, 2024].

6.8 Vaccine Storage and Handling

Sanjay Srirampur

INTRODUCTION

Immunization programs have significantly reduced infectious diseases worldwide. This has improved child morbidity and morbidity significantly. These programs rely heavily on correctly storing and handling vaccines, which is a responsibility that involves everyone, from the manufacturers to those who administer the vaccines, as well as on the logistics and administration of the vaccines. Most mistakes in storing and handling vaccines can be avoided. Even with good systems, problems related to keeping vaccines cold can still happen, often due to technical issues. But if there are good procedures in place, these issues can be quickly found and fixed, ensuring that the vaccines work well and reducing waste. Therefore, taking care of how vaccines are stored is a very important part of ensuring quality in healthcare services that provide vaccinations.

COLD CHAIN

The concept of the "cold chain" refers to a crucial process in vaccine logistics. This involves the transportation and storage of vaccines from their production site to the point of use, while strictly maintaining them within a specified temperature range. This system comprises three key elements:[1]

1. *Personnel:* The trained individuals responsible for handling vaccines throughout the supply chain
2. *Equipment:* The specialized tools and storage units used for preserving vaccines at the correct temperatures
3. *Procedures:* The established guidelines and methods (outlined in a flowchart) that ensure the safe and efficient handling of vaccines

The ideal storage temperatures are +2 to +8°C for refrigerated vaccines and –15 to –25°C for frozen ones. Additionally, certain vaccines require protection from light as part of their storage conditions. This comprehensive approach ensures the integrity and efficacy of vaccines until they reach the recipients.

IMPORTANCE OF COLD CHAIN

Maintaining the cold chain is critical for vaccine efficacy. Vaccines, composed of proteins, nucleic acids, lipids, and carbohydrates, lose effectiveness or degrade when exposed to inappropriate temperatures. Cold-sensitive vaccines immediately lose potency if frozen. When vaccines are exposed to high temperatures, they gradually lose potency with each episode of exposure. This loss, especially when repeated, is irreversible.[1,2] The importance of maintaining vaccine potency is multifaceted:

- It prevents vaccine-preventable diseases (VPDs) from re-emerging.
- It avoids resource wastage due to vaccine loss.
- It prevents vaccine supply shortages from impacting immunization schedules.
- It safeguards public trust in vaccines and healthcare systems.

EQUIPMENT

Vaccine storage equipment is divided into:[3]

- *Electrical:* Walk-in freezers and coolers, deep freezers, ice-lined refrigerators (ILRs), and domestic refrigerators
- *Nonelectrical:* Cold boxes and vaccine carriers

ELECTRICAL EQUIPMENT

Walk-in Freezers

Walk-in freezers are used for bulk storage of vaccines like oral polio vaccine (OPV) and for ice pack preparation, maintaining temperatures around -18 to -20°C.

Walk-in Coolers

Walk-in coolers, typically controlled between 2 and 8°C, have digital temperature displays and alarms and are used for bulk vaccine storage at state and regional stores.[3,4]

Deep Freezers

Deep freezers, maintaining -18 to -20°C, are used for storing OPV at districts and for ice pack freezing.

Ice-lined Refrigerators

Ice-lined refrigerators are suitable for areas with irregular power supply. They can keep vaccines safe with minimal electricity. They have specific storage recommendations based on vaccine heat sensitivity.[1]

Ice-lined refrigerators are designed with either a top-opening or front-opening configuration. These refrigerators feature an internal lining composed of water containers—in the form of either ice packs or tubes—strategically fitted along the walls and secured by a supporting frame. When the ILR is operational, the water within these containers freezes. In events where the electricity supply is disrupted, this ice lining plays a crucial role in maintaining a safe internal temperature for vaccine storage. Remarkably, the ILR can ensure the safety of vaccines with a minimal requirement of continuous electricity supply: Only 8 hours within a 24-hour cycle.

Due to its ability to maintain temperature stability with limited electricity, the ILR is particularly advantageous in regions plagued by irregular power supplies. To optimize the storage of vaccines within these refrigerators, it is recommended to use baskets. This precaution prevents the vaccines from directly contacting the sides and bottom of the ILR. The coldest area in an ILR is at the bottom, necessitating a strategic placement of vaccines based on their heat sensitivity: The most heat-sensitive vaccines are stored at the bottom, while the more heat-resistant ones are kept in the top compartment. This arrangement is the opposite of what is typically seen in domestic refrigerators.

Vaccine Storage Guidelines for Ice-lined Refrigerators[3,5]

- *Bottom compartment:* Ideal for the storage of highly heat-sensitive vaccines such as measles, measles-rubella (MR), measles-mumps-rubella (MMR), Bacillus Calmette-Guérin (BCG), OPV, yellow fever (YF), live Japanese encephalitis (JE), varicella, rotavirus, and live-attenuated hepatitis A vaccines.
- *Middle and upper compartments:* Suitable for storing vaccines with a higher tolerance to temperature variations. This includes all pertussis-containing combination vaccines, inactivated hepatitis A vaccines, typhoid conjugate vaccine (TCV), pneumococcal conjugate vaccine (PCV), meningococcal vaccine (MCV), inactivated influenza vaccine, human papillomavirus (HPV) vaccine, rabies, and inactivated JE vaccines.

This structured approach to vaccine storage in ILRs ensures optimal preservation of vaccine efficacy, especially crucial in settings with unreliable electricity.[3,4]

Domestic Refrigerators

Most private vaccination providers store vaccines in domestic refrigerators. However, these fridges are meant for food and drinks and do not meet the specific temperature needs for vaccines, which poses risks.[1]

Risks of a Domestic Refrigerator

- Temperature fluctuates every time the door is opened.
- Temperature increases during defrosting in cyclic defrost and frost-free refrigerators.
- Ambient temperature easily affects the cabinet temperature.
- Temperature setting is crude and often inaccurate.

If a domestic refrigerator is the only option, it can be used to store vaccines only if the fridge and freezer have separate external doors. There are two types of domestic fridges: Frost-free and manual/cyclic defrost. Frost-free is better for vaccines as it maintains more uniform temperatures.

For safe vaccine storage in domestic fridges:[3]

- Use a dedicated fridge for vaccines without food, water, or other medications.
- Maintain the fridge compartment between 2 and 8°C and the freezer at or below -15°C.
- Ensure that door seals are tight and the door closes automatically.
- The fridge should have a separate freezer compartment, a quiet compressor, and no coolant or water leaks.
- Staff should be trained in vaccine storage.

If these conditions cannot be met, a purpose-built refrigerator should be used for storing vaccines.

Some simplified tips for better vaccine storage in domestic refrigerators are given in the following text.[3]

Refrigerator Placement

- Keep it away from direct sunlight, doors, and windows.
- Ensure 10 cm of space around it for air circulation.
- Place it on a stand at least 5 cm high.
- Use a switchless electric socket or tape the switch to prevent accidental off-switching.

Restricted Access

Only vaccination staff should access the fridge to minimize door opening and prevent power shut-off.

Temperature Stabilization

- Set the thermostat to +2 and +5°C when first installed.
- Use it for vaccines only after consistent temperature readings within +2 to +8°C have been recorded for 2 consecutive days.

Minimize Door Opening

Limit opening the fridge door to reduce temperature fluctuations.

Monitoring Temperatures

Regularly check the internal temperature with a digital thermometer placed in the center of the storage compartment.

Power Source Safeguard

Clearly mark the power source to prevent accidental unplugging or switching off.

Increase Cool Mass

Place water bottles or gel packs in the fridge and freezer to help stabilize temperature.

Ideal Storage Method

- Use labeled containers for vaccines for easy identification and minimal door opening.
- Store vaccines in their original packing and avoid overfilling.
- Never store vaccines in the fridge door.

Vaccine Placement

- Store freeze-resistant vaccines such as measles and YF on the top shelf.
- Place freeze-sensitive vaccines such as diphtheria, tetanus, and pertussis (DTP) and Hepatitis B on the middle shelf.
- Keep diluents next to their respective vaccines or on the bottom shelf if space is limited.

Staff Training

- Train staff in proper vaccine storage and handling.
- Assign specific responsibilities for fridge management and cold chain.

Maintenance

- Report breakdowns immediately and arrange alternative storage.
- Defrost the fridge regularly for efficient functioning.

Power Failure Protocol

- Keep the fridge closed during power failures of 4 hours or less.
- If there is no backup generator, find an alternate storage site nearby.
- Remember to keep a chart or map on the fridge door showing vaccine locations, and train staff on these guidelines to ensure effective vaccine storage.

Purpose-built Vaccine Refrigerator

The purpose-built vaccine refrigerator is the preferred choice for vaccine storage in hospitals, pharmacies, and larger medical practices.[3] This specialized refrigerator offers several advantages over standard domestic refrigerators:[1]

- It is specifically designed for vaccine storage, eliminating the need for modifications.
- It maintains a consistent internal temperature between 2 and 8°C.
- The cabinet temperature remains stable and uniform, unaffected by external ambient temperatures.
- It features an evaporator that operates at 2–8°C, preventing the freezing of vaccines.
- It includes a defrost cycle that allows for defrosting without increasing cabinet temperature.
- It ensures even temperature distribution through continuous air circulation.
- It is equipped with an external temperature display, a continuous maximum/minimum temperature display, and an alarm for out-of-range temperatures.
- It demonstrates excellent temperature recovery following door openings to access vaccines

NONELECTRICAL EQUIPMENT

Cold Boxes

Cold boxes, used for vaccine transport, can maintain vaccine efficacy for extended periods under specific conditions. In emergencies, cold boxes can be used to keep vaccines and ice packs frozen. To prepare the cold box, conditioned ice packs are placed at the bottom and sides. Vaccines like DPT (diphtheria, pertussis, and tetanus), DT (diphtheria and tetanus), hepatitis B, and TT (tetanus toxoid) should not touch the ice packs directly. Instead, they should be put in a cardboard or plastic bag. A 5-L cold box can keep vaccines for 90 hours and a 20-L box for 6 days if the outside temperature is 43°C. This works as long as the boxes are in good condition and remain closed during this time.

Vaccine Carriers

Vaccine carriers are used by health workers to transport 16–20 vials of vaccines to smaller health centers or community programs. They keep vaccines cold for 1 day during transport from primary health centers, maintaining a temperature between +2 and –8°C using four conditioned ice packs, provided they're not opened too often.[1]

Icepacks are leak-proof plastic containers filled to 80% capacity with tap water and frozen in deep freezers at –25°C. When taken out, they are at –20°C, which can harm vaccines sensitive to freezing. To prepare them for use, they undergo "sweating." This involves placing the icepacks on a table and shaking them periodically until the ice inside starts moving, which can take a few minutes to an hour. Once this is done, the icepacks are ready to be used in vaccine carriers and cold boxes.

Automatic Voltage Stabilizers

An automatic voltage stabilizer functions to regulate voltage fluctuations, maintaining the main voltage at 220 V with a tolerance of ±10 V.

COLD CHAIN TEMPERATURE MONITORING

Monitoring temperature is very important in a cold chain system.[1] Without accurate temperature records, even the best equipment might not be useful. The temperature in vaccine storage should be checked and recorded at least twice a day. This helps to identify any major temperature changes.[3,4] There are different thermometers for this, like the minimum/maximum thermometer.

Minimum/Maximum Thermometer

It shows the current, lowest, and highest temperatures reached. It helps spot temperature changes outside the safe range. It comes in two types: Fluid-filled and digital. The digital one with a probe is the most effective. Place the probe against a vaccine vial or package for accurate readings. The thermometer needs to be reset regularly, and its battery should be checked and changed when needed.

Digital Thermometer

It is very accurate and can alert you if the fridge malfunctions. For correct readings, place the probe in the right spot.

Data Loggers

They record temperatures over time and can give visual and audio alarms. They work like chart recorders but store data electronically. Their purpose is to create a "temperature map" of the fridge to identify safe and risky areas for storing vaccines, especially to avoid freezing. Each logger is a small computer. Once set up, it is placed in the fridge near the temperature probe and works on its battery until the data is downloaded.

Recording Temperatures

The temperature in vaccine fridges/freezers should be recorded twice daily, at 10 AM and 4 PM, and noted in a logbook. All temperature monitoring devices in the cold chain should be calibrated every 6 months or sooner if needed.

Vaccine Vial Monitor

This is a label with heat-sensitive material on vaccine vials, showing cumulative heat exposure over time. It helps health workers know if a vaccine has been damaged by heat. The vaccine vial monitor (VVM) has a square inside a circle. The square changes color with heat exposure; it gets darker with more heat over time. This color change is permanent. The rate of color change depends on the temperature: Slower at lower temperatures and faster at higher ones.

VACCINE-HANDLING PERSONNEL

Designated Vaccine Coordinators

Each vaccination clinic should have a primary vaccine coordinator and a backup. Their job is to make sure that all vaccines are handled properly, procedures are recorded, and everyone gets training on how to maintain the cold chain. They should be well trained in both routine and urgent vaccine storage and handling.[1,4]

Other Staff

All staff, including those who are not directly handling vaccines, like receptionists who receive vaccine shipments, should know the vaccine storage and handling policies and procedures.[3]

Training Personnel

Every staff member who handles or administers vaccines needs training in correct vaccine storage and handling.[3] They should all understand how important it is to maintain the cold chain and know the basic practices. This way, they are aware of their role in keeping the vaccines safe. If staff members who check and log the temperatures of vaccine storage units notice any problems, like wrong temperatures or exposure to light, they should quickly tell the vaccine coordinator.[3,4]

EFFICIENT VACCINE MANAGEMENT PROTOCOLS

Ordering and Accepting Vaccine Deliveries[1]

- Keep about a month's supply of vaccines in stock.
- Make sure that vaccines are delivered when the vaccination unit is open and staff is there to store them right away at 2–8°C.
- Keep a record of each vaccine's details such as name, quantity, arrival date, condition, manufacturer, lot number, and expiration date.

Storing and Handling Vaccines[6]

- Use vaccines and diluents with the nearest expiration date first.
- Organize vaccines by expiry dates, putting those with longer expiry dates behind those with shorter ones.
- Remove expired vaccines and diluents from the usable stock.
- Keep an organized stock and a map of vaccine locations outside the fridge for easy access.
- Check the storage unit every day to ensure that vaccines and thermometers are placed correctly.
- Dispose of vaccine materials as medical waste.
- Managing potentially compromised vaccines:
    - Separate and label any vaccines and diluents that might be compromised as "DO NOT USE."
    - Store them at the right temperature but away from other vaccines.
    - Contact vaccine manufacturers or the state immunization program for guidance on what to do with these vaccines.[2]

EMERGENCY VACCINE RETRIEVAL AND STORAGE

Planning for Emergencies

Staff should be trained for situations like equipment failures, power outages, or natural disasters that can affect vaccine storage. Have an emergency plan that includes:[6]

- A backup storage site with proper storage units, temperature monitoring, and a generator
- Ready-to-use packing materials like gel packs and bubble wrap
- Clear instructions for packing and transporting vaccines and diluents with a calibrated thermometer in each pack
- Procedures for dealing with potentially compromised vaccines
- Contact details for vaccine manufacturers and immunization programs
- Electronic Vaccine Intelligence Network (eVIN):[7]
    - eVIN is a digital system started in 2015 to improve vaccine supply chain management in India.
    - It allows real-time monitoring of vaccine stocks and temperatures at multiple locations.
    - Cold chain handlers use smartphones with an app to manage vaccine inventory, monitor stocks and temperatures, manage emergencies, plan routes, and reallocate stock.
    - Temperature loggers attached to cold chain equipment record temperature every 10 minutes and update it hourly via GPRS. Alerts for temperature breaches are sent via email and SMS.
    - It has been implemented across all 36 states and 733 districts in India, covering over 29,000 storage centers. It has significantly improved vaccine availability and reduced instances of vaccine shortages.

REFERENCES

1. Gupta SK, Shastri DD. Cold chain and vaccine storage. In: Shah NK, Agrawal R, Sukumaran TU, Vashishtha VM (Eds). IAP Textbook of Vaccines, 1st edition. New Delhi: Jaypee Brothers Medical Publishers; 2014. pp. 89-99.
2. Rao MIS, Kasi SG. Purple Book: IAP Guidebook on Immunization 2022 By Advisory Committee on Vaccines and Immunization Practices (ACVIP). 2023. pp. 49-72.
3. Centers for Disease Control and Prevention. (2023). Vaccine storage and handling toolkit. [online] Available from https://www.cdc.gov/vaccines/hcp/admin/storage/toolkit/storage-handling-toolkit.pdf. [Last accessed October, 2024].
4. Department of Health and Ageing, Australian Government. (2013). National vaccine storage guidelines, "Strive for 5". [online] Available from https://www.health.gov.au/resources/publications/national-vaccine-storage-guidelines-strive-for-5. [Last accessed October, 2024].
5. Galazka A, Milstien J, Zaffran M. (1998). Thermostability of vaccines: global programme for vaccines and immunization. [online] Available from https://apps.who.int/iris/bitstream/handle/10665/64980/WHO_GPV_98.07.pdf?sequence=1&isAllowed=y. [Last accessed October, 2024].
6. Ketan B, Jariwala V, Kirit S. Target-5: Guide to Vaccine Storage and Handling, 1st edition. Gujarat: IAP Surat Publication; 2006.
7. National Health Portal. Ministry of Health and Family Welfare. Electronic Vaccine Intelligence Network (EVIN). [online] Available from https://pib.gov.in/PressReleasePage.aspx?PRID=1643172. [Last accessed October, 2024].

6.9 Adverse Events Following Immunization

Indra Shekhar Rao M

INTRODUCTION

Immunization is a major contributor to the success story of child health in the last century, which has enhanced and improved the child survival all over the world. Vaccines used in National Immunization Programs (NIPs) are safe and effective. Several scientific, ethical, and statutory obligations are fulfilled by the manufacturers and elaborate field trials regarding safety and protection offered by individual vaccines are established before they are recommended for routine use. However, no vaccine is perfectly safe and adverse events can occur following immunization.

The adverse event following immunization (AEFI) is defined as *a medical incident that takes place after immunization, causes concern, and is believed to be caused by the immunization.*[1] Any untoward medical occurrence which follows immunization and which does not necessarily have a causal relationship with the use of the vaccine is clubbed under AEFI. Coincidental occurrence of any ill health events during postvaccination stage are falsely incriminated to vaccines by most of the vaccinees.

The vaccines are foreign for human bodies, given to healthy infants and children. In the natural process of developing immunity, a vaccine may cause fever, erythema, local pain, etc. In addition, there is a slight risk of foreign body reaction to the components in the vaccines. These factors are likely to cause some concerns in the caregivers and parents.

Vaccines are given to healthy individuals and their tolerance for AEFI is lower than that of medication; safety has therefore always been a key concern. Whatever the cause, an AEFI may upset people to an extent that they may refuse further vaccination for their children. This makes it more likely for the children to get a vaccine preventable disease (VPD), become seriously ill, disabled, and risk death. This contributes significantly to the vaccine hesitancy by parents resulting in vaccine undercoverage.

The AEFI surveillance, therefore, helps to preserve public confidence in the immunization program. A reported adverse event can be true adverse event or an event coincidental to the immunization. Most of the vaccine safety data available is based on the postvaccination data, i.e., AEFI rather than an estimate of attributable risk.

CLASSIFICATION OF ADVERSE EVENT FOLLOWING IMMUNIZATION

The AEFIs are classified into five categories **(Table 6.9.1)**.[2] Immunization can cause adverse events from the inherent properties of vaccine (*vaccine reaction*), which comprises vaccine product-related reactions and vaccine quality defect-related reactions. It may be due to some error in immunization process (*program error*) such as contaminated vaccine or diluent, reuse of disposable syringe or needle, and reuse of reconstituted vaccine. The event may be unrelated to the immunization but have temporal association (*coincidental event*). Anxiety-related reactions can arise from fear or pain of the injection rather than the vaccine itself, e.g., fainting, hyperventilation, vomiting, and convulsions. In some cases, the cause of AEFI remains unknown.

Vaccine reactions can be classified into two groups:

1. *Minor reactions* usually occur within a few hours of injection; resolve after short period of time and pose little danger. They are mostly local reactions (pain, swelling, or redness at the site of injection) and occasionally systemic (fever, malaise, muscle pain, headache, or loss of appetite).

TABLE 6.9.1: Classification of adverse events following immunization (AEFI).[3]

Types of AEFI	*Definition and characteristics*
Vaccine product related	Event caused by inherent properties of the vaccine
Vaccine quality related	Event caused by a vaccine due to one or more quality defects of the vaccine product, including its administration device as provided by the manufacturer
Immunization error related	Event caused by an error in vaccine preparation, handling, storage, or administration
Immunization anxiety related	Event from anxiety about or pain from the injection itself rather than the vaccine
Co-incidental event	Event that happens after immunization but not caused by the vaccine or its administration. Caused by something other than the vaccine product or quality, immunization error, or immunization anxiety

2. *Severe reactions* usually do not result in long-term problems; but can be disabling and include seizures and allergic reactions caused by the body's reaction to a particular component in a vaccine.

The AEFI may be anticipated and may not be severe enough to cause discomfort for a long duration of time [e.g., pain or fever after diphtheria, tetanus, and pertussis (DTP) vaccination], whereas a severe or a rare event following the vaccine may be in the form of unexpected anaphylactic shock or induction of active disease following measles or oral polio vaccine (OPV), respectively. Hypothetical type of reaction may be related to vaccine scares, which have causal relationship relating to the issues which are of controversial nature occurring in vaccinated children. The common vaccine reactions are due to the immune response of the host and sometimes due to vaccine components (e.g., aluminum adjuvant and preservatives). A successful vaccine reduces these reactions to a minimum while inducing the best possible immunity. These anticipated reactions occur within a day or two of immunization and are listed in **Table 6.9.2.**[3]

TABLE 6.9.2: Anticipated reactions after immunization.[3]

Vaccine	Local reaction (pain, swelling, and redness)	Fever >38°C	Irritability, malaise, systemic symptoms
BCG	90–95%	–	–
Hib	5–15%	2–10%	–
Hepatitis B	Adults: 15% Children: 5%	1–6%	–
Measles/ MMR/MR	10%	5–15%	5% (Rash)
Oral polio vaccine	–	<1%	<1%
Tetanus/DT/Td	10%	10%	25%
Pneumococcal conjugate	~20%	~20%	~20%
Pertussis (DTwP)	Up to 50%	Up to 50%	Up to 55%
HPV[4]	20%	10–13%	<5%
COVID-19[5]	30%	16%	60%
Treatment	• Cold sponging at injection site • Oral paracetamol	• Give extra fluids • Wear cool clothing • Tepid sponge or bath • Oral paracetamol	Give extraoral fluids

(BCG: Bacillus Calmette–Guérin; DT/Td: tetanus-diphtheria vaccine; DTP/DTwP: diphtheria, tetanus, and pertussis; Hib: *Haemophilus influenzae* type b; HPV: human papilloma virus; MMR: measles, mumps, and rubella; MR: measles and rubella virus vaccine)

Another notable component of AEFI is due to program errors that would result from errors and accidents in vaccine preparation, handling, or administration **(Table 6.9.3)**.[3] The identification and correction of these errors are of great importance which would otherwise lead to a cluster of other events associated with immunization. The most common program error is iatrogenic infection as a result of nonsterile injection, e.g., sterile abscess, which may have a systemic effect or blood-borne infection (e.g., human immunodeficiency virus and hepatitis B).

VACCINATION COMPLICATIONS AND THEIR MANAGEMENT

Bacillus Calmette–Guérin Vaccine

- *Local adverse reactions:*
  - Persistent discharging sinus at the site of vaccination
    - Regional axillary lymphadenitis
    - Below 2 cm—no treatment
  - Fluctuant, >2 cm—treatment with isoniazid for 3–6 months and/or excision

TABLE 6.9.3: Program errors leading to adverse events.[3]

Nonsterile injections: • Reuse of disposable syringe or needles • Improperly sterilized syringe or needles • Contaminated vaccine or diluents • Reuse of reconstituted vaccine at subsequent session	• Local injection site reactions (e.g., abscess, swelling, cellulitis, induration) • Toxic shock syndrome • Blood-borne transmission of disease, e.g., hepatitis B, HIV • Sepsis, death
Vaccine prepared incorrectly: • Vaccine reconstituted with incorrect diluent • Drugs substituted for vaccine or diluent	• Vaccine ineffective • Effect of drug, e.g., insulin, oxytocin, etc.
Immunization injected at wrong site: • Subcutaneous instead of intradermal for BCG • Too superficial for toxoid vaccine (DTP, DT, and TT) • Buttocks	• Local reaction or injection site abscess • Local reaction or injection site abscess • Sciatic nerve damage
Vaccine transported/stored incorrectly: • Freezing vaccine during transport • Failure to keep vaccine in cold chain	• Increased local reaction from frozen vaccine • Ineffective vaccine
Contraindications ignored	Avoidable severe reaction

(BCG: Bacillus Calmette–Guérin; DT: diphtheria-tetanus vaccine; DTP: diphtheria, tetanus, and pertussis; HIV: human immunodeficiency virus; TT: tetanus toxoid)

- BCG complex (local lymphadenitis + positive Mantoux reaction + paratracheal lymph node): Treat with rifampicin (R), pyrazinamide (Z), and isoniazid (H) [RHZ (2 months)] plus R + H [RH (4 months)]

- *Systemic reactions:* Disseminated infection, tuberculous osteomyelitis, and scrofuloderma—treat these like tuberculosis.

Diphtheria, Tetanus, and (Whole-cell) Pertussis Vaccine

Adverse reactions:

- Incessant cry (>3 hours)
- Febrile convulsions
- Hyperpyrexia
- Hypotonic hyporesponsive episode (HHE, shock-like state)
- Acute encephalopathy
- Anaphylactic shock.

Diphtheria, Tetanus, and (Acellular) Pertussis Vaccine

Adverse events such as pain or swelling are minimal with above vaccine.

Clinical features of anaphylaxis:

- These involve multiple body systems (skin, respiration, and circulation)
- Itchy, urticarial rash, and facial flushing
- Progressive edema involving face, mouth, and body parts
- *Respiratory symptoms:* Sneezing, coughing, wheezing, and airway obstruction
- Hypotension and shock

Oral Polio Vaccine

- Adverse event following immunization almost none
- Very rarely vaccine-associated paralytic poliomyelitis (VAPP).

Inactivated Polio Vaccine

- *Local reactions:* Erythema and induration if the patient is sensitive to streptomycin/neomycin. She/he might develop hypersensitive reactions as inactivated polio vaccine (IPV) contains these as preservatives.
- *Systemic reactions:* Transient arthralgia, rarely agitation, somnolence, and convulsions.

Measles

Reaction anticipated: 7–12 days following immunization, localized discomfort, soreness, and sickness resembling measles. Paracetamol is used as treatment.

Adverse reactions:

- *Toxic shock syndrome (TSS):*
  - Measles vaccine does not contain any preservatives. When measles vaccine cap is punctured, it allows bacterial growth, especially staphylococci which can cause TSS due to the exotoxins liberated by it. This can happen due to usage of unsterile syringes, needles, and using a vaccine vial beyond 4 hours after reconstitution. It can occur after 30 minutes to few hours after vaccination and the child presents with fever, vomiting, diarrhea, and shock.
  - *Treatment:* It should be treated as medical emergency. Child should be resuscitated with intravenous (IV) fluids (Ringer's lactate and normal saline), and treated with antibiotics (cloxacillin 100–200 mg/kg/day in divided doses), steroids, antipyretics, and supportive therapy.
- Thrombocytopenic purpura may occur at 1 per 30,000 vaccines.

Measles, Mumps, and Rubella Vaccine

- *Anticipated reactions:* Mild fever, rash, and febrile seizures.
- *Adverse reactions:*
  - *Mumps component:* Fever, rarely encephalopathy, seizures, Guillain-Barré syndrome (GBS), parotid swelling, hemolytic uremic syndrome (HUS), and aseptic meningitis.
  - *Rubella component:* Arthralgia, lymphadenopathy, fever, and sore throat; rarely thrombocytopenia and peripheral neuropathy.

Hepatitis B Vaccine and Hepatitis A Vaccine

- *Local reactions:* Soreness at the site of injection
- *Systemic reactions:* Mild fever, myalgia, arthralgia, and rarely anaphylaxis

Typhoid Vi Antigen Vaccine

- *Local reaction:* Mild pain and swelling for 1 day.
- *Vi-polysaccharide conjugate vaccine conjugated with tetanus toxoid (TT):* No major local or systemic side effects are seen.
- *Adverse effects:* Pain at injection site and fever

Tetanus Toxoid

Systemic reactions: Frequent TT injections can lead on to increased severity of local and systemic reactions due to binding of the toxoid with the preformed antitoxin leading on to immune complex-mediated reactions (swollen limbs and Arthus type 2 reactions).

Haemophilus influenzae Type B Vaccine

Local reactions: Mild redness, pain, and swelling.

Varicella Vaccine

- *Local reactions:* Pain, redness, and swelling at injection site
- *Systemic reactions:* Varicella-like rash in around 5% of the vaccines

Rabies Tissue Culture Vaccine

- *Local reactions:* Soreness
- *Systemic reactions:* Headache and fever

Meningococcal Vaccine (Quadrivalent)

- *Local reactions:* Pain and swelling at injection site
- *Systemic reactions:* GBS is possible but unproven risk in adolescents.

Pneumococcal Vaccine

- *Local reactions:* Swelling, redness, and pain
- *Systemic reactions:* Fever, vomiting and diarrhea, convulsion, and HHE rarely

Japanese Encephalitis Vaccines

Vaccination against SA 14-14-2 Obtained from Live-attenuated Cell Culture

- *Local effects* include pain, irritation, and swelling.
- *Systemic effects* include rash and fever.

SA 14-14-2 Japanese Encephalitis Vaccine, Developed from Inactivated Vero Cell Culture

No significant negative occurrence.

Influenza Vaccine (Trivalent Influenza Vaccines)

- *Local responses:* Swelling and pain.
- *Systemic effects* include myalgia, fever, and malaise. A statistically significant rise in hospitalizations due to GBS has not been linked to the trivalent influenza vaccine's marginally elevated risk of GBS. If the advantages of the vaccination outweigh the risks of side effects, it should be avoided in people with a history of GBS and given cautiously to people who are allergic to eggs.

Rotavirus Vaccine

Systemic reactions: Mild undesirable side effects such as fever, vomiting, irritability, and rash may occur. The risk of intussusception with rotavirus is not increased as with placebo group.

Human Papillomavirus Vaccine

Common side effects:[4]

- Pain, redness, or swelling in the arm where the shot was given.
- Fever
- Headache or feeling tired
- Nausea
- Muscle or joint pain
- Brief fainting spells and related symptoms (such as jerking movements) can happen after any medical procedure, including vaccination. Sitting or lying down for about 15 minutes after a vaccination can help prevent fainting and injuries caused by falls.
- Severe (anaphylactic) allergic responses can very rarely happen following vaccination. Vaccines should not be administered to anyone who have severe allergies to any of their ingredients.

COVID-19 Vaccine[5]

- There are reports of cutaneous adverse effects similar to acute generalized exanthematous pustulosis and drug reaction with urticarial, petechial eruptions after COVID-19 vaccine.
- Several cases of facial nerve palsy have been reported post-COVID-19 vaccination. This is most likely caused by additive adjuvants that elicit an immunomodulatory response.[6]
- The incidence of nonhemorrhagic stroke, acute myocardial infarction, and deep vein thrombosis were common in people above 85+ years of age. The incidence of acute myocardial infarction range from 1/10 to 1/100.[7]
- Allergic individuals cannot be excluded from vaccination. As AEFI with major case fatalities are very rare, vaccination should be encouraged since it helps prevent a potentially deadly illness. Moreover, healthcare personnel should clear up misconceptions regarding COVID-19 vaccines among the recipients.

GUILLAIN-BARRÉ SYNDROME AS ADVERSE EVENT FOLLOWING IMMUNIZATION

Clinical Features

The GBS is a severe neurological disease with limb pain and muscle weakness as cardinal symptoms.[8] Vaccines with risk of GBS as AEFI include:

- Influenza vaccine
- Meningococcal vaccine
- Measles, mumps, and rubella (MMR) vaccine
- Polio vaccine
- Human papillomavirus (HPV) vaccine
- Hepatitis A and B vaccines
- Varicella vaccine

The time window between prior infection and vaccination was considered as 6 weeks based on a literature review and expert survey.

RISK OF SEIZURES AS ADVERSE EVENT FOLLOWING IMMUNIZATION[9]

- Concomitant administration of vaccines causes seizures due to synergistic effect of those vaccines. When these vaccines are given separately, the risk of seizures is decreased, e.g., MMR + varicella (MMRV).
- Diphtheria, tetanus, and whole-cell pertussis (DTwP) associated risk of seizures is attributed to whole cell pertussis component of vaccine affecting acellular signaling by decreasing release of inhibitory neurotransmitters [gamma-aminobutyric acid (GABA)] via interleukin 1-alpha (IL-1α) production. Acellular pertussis vaccine does not induce the IL-1α production. Whole cell pertussis vaccines contain 3,000 different proteins, whereas acellular pertussis vaccine [diphtheria, tetanus and acellular pertussis (DTaP)] contains 2–5 proteins.[10]
- Febrile seizures post-MMR vaccination is common after 8–14 days but not in the 0–7 and 15–30 days.[11] Children who had febrile seizures within 15 days postimmunization showed only a slight elevated risk of recurrent febrile seizures.
- Pneumococcal conjugate vaccine 7 (PCV 7) increases the risk of febrile seizures in the 2 days postvaccination. There is no difference in febrile seizures between PCV 13 and PCV 7.[12]
- Vaccine-induced encephalopathy may be due to inherent genetic condition with no causal relationship with vaccination. It is possible that vaccinations cause fever, which precipitates the manifestations genetic defects (seizures and encephalopathy).[13]

ADVERSE EVENT FOLLOWING IMMUNIZATION SURVEILLANCE SYSTEMS FOR PREGNANT WOMEN AND THEIR INFANTS

- The World Health Organization (WHO) has made it a priority to strengthen prenatal care as a platform for maternal immunization.
- Pregnancy-related vaccinations can shield both the mother and the unborn child from the consequences of serious infection.
- A number of vaccinations, such as the TT, seasonal influenza, and the tetanus-diphtheria-acellular pertussis vaccine (Tdap), are currently advised during pregnancy.[14]
- Patients' and healthcare professionals' vaccination reluctance, which is occasionally linked to worries about vaccine safety, is one possible obstacle to immunization.

MEASURES TO IMPROVE ADVERSE EVENT FOLLOWING IMMUNIZATION SURVEILLANCE IN MATERNAL AND CHILD IMMUNIZATION PROGRAMS

- Existing health systems can be expanded to include active surveillance capabilities, especially in nations with integrated electronic health information systems.
- Countries with passive surveillance systems should think about including a question regarding pregnancy status in their standard AEFI surveillance reporting forms in order to better capture AEFI in pregnant women.
- Every nation should receive assistance in setting up a procedure for determining the causation of serious AEFI during pregnancy and disclosing the results. An essential component of AEFI surveillance is the determination of causality.
- To enable uniform reporting and data sharing on vaccine safety in expectant mothers and their children worldwide, a system and procedure are required.
- To confirm whether progress has been made, active and passive surveillance surveys for AEFI in expectant mothers and their unborn children should be conducted on a regular basis.

MANAGEMENT OF AN ANAPHYLAXIS AFTER A VACCINE

Anaphylaxis Emergency Management

- In the anterolateral thigh, inject 0.01 mL/kg of epinephrine (1:1,000 solution) at a maximum dose of 0.5 mL.
- Establish IV access.
- If tolerated, lay the patient flat and raise their legs. If necessary, administer high flow oxygen and ventilation.
- If hypotensive, arrange for a second wide-bore access and administer 20 mL/kg of IV normal saline under pressure for 1–2 minutes.
- If necessary, IM adrenaline can be administered again in 3–5 minutes.
- While IV antihistaminic are not advised, oral antihistaminic may be administered to relieve skin problems.
- Although the benefit has not yet been established, oral or injectable corticosteroids that are equivalent to prednisone 1–2 mg/kg may be used.
- Emergency medications and resuscitation should be available to all medical professionals.

VACCINES AND CONTRAINDICATIONS

It is often difficult to prove definite cause-effect relationship between the act of vaccination and subsequent complication. The following guidelines as well as the list of contraindications

TABLE 6.9.4: Vaccines and contraindications.

Avoid: Live vaccine	• Immunodeficient individuals • Immunosuppressant therapy • Chronic debilitating illness (till recovery)
Avoid: DTP (first dose)	• Progressive neurological disease • Uncontrolled seizure disorder (postpone till control)
Avoid: Rubella vaccine	During pregnancy
Avoid: Measles vaccine/should not be given	If person is sensitive to egg protein
Delay: Live vaccine	• Measles/MMR for 6 weeks following immunoglobulin therapy • Severe febrile illness
Do not stop vaccination in	• Malnutrition • Moderate fever • Respiratory infections • Mild diarrhea • Any benign ailment

(DTP: diphtheria, tetanus, and pertussis; MMR: measles, mumps, and rubella)
Source: Bhatia R, Ichhpujani RL. Immunization against infectious disease. New Delhi: Jaypee Brothers Medical Publishers Pvt Ltd.; 1994. pp. 20-60.

for vaccinations will help in deciding vaccine administration **(Table 6.9.4)**.

GUIDELINES FOR SAFE VACCINATION

- Always ensure safe injection practices for safe health by using disposable syringes.
- Select proper vaccine and follow manufacturer's instructions (dose/route/administration).
- Maintain cold chain.
- Inform the parents regarding vaccine benefits and their anticipated reactions.
- Obtain written or at least oral consent before vaccination.
- Keep the child under observation for 30 minutes after vaccination. Be equipped and geared up to treat any untoward reactions.
- Have always resuscitation kit ready.
- Use desired injection procedure, i.e., load the vaccine into appropriate syringe size.
- Do not mix vaccines in single syringe unless approved for such use. Use different syringes for different vaccines. Use different sites for injection.
- Always use anterolateral aspect of thigh in young children and deltoid area for older children for injections. Never use gluteal region in children.
- Avoid fomentation/vigorous rubbing after vaccination. Firm pressure for a few minutes is sufficient.
- Document every vaccination procedure in the immunization card and keep a copy of it.
- Complete the vaccination schedule as per immunization calendar. Remind the parents regarding next date.
- There is no need to restart immunization of multidose vaccine, e.g., *Haemophilus influenzae* type B (Hib), DTP, etc. If the child is not brought for immunization on suggested date. Instead just continue and complete the schedule.

PREVENTION AND TREATMENT OF VACCINE REACTION

It is mandatory for the person administering the vaccine to have sufficient knowledge regarding vaccines and expected side effects and to inform parents thoroughly regarding such adverse effects, which may however occur very rarely. It is also essential to be prepared and to always have a "kit" with lifesaving drugs and equipment at each place of vaccination. Advice on managing the common reactions as well as the instructions to return to the clinic if there are more serious symptoms should be given to parents. This will help to reassure parents about immunization and prepare them for common reactions. Program errors are easily preventable. Identification and correction of these errors are of great importance. WHO guidelines to avoid program errors are as follows:

- Vaccines must be reconstituted only with the diluents supplied by the manufacturer.
- Reconstituted vaccines must be discarded at the end of each immunization session and never retained.
- No other drugs or substances should be stored in the refrigerator of the immunization center.
- Immunization workers must be adequately trained and closely supervised to ensure that proper procedures being followed.
- Careful epidemiological investigation of an AEFI is needed to pinpoint the cause and to correct immunization practices.

REPORTING ADVERSE EVENT FOLLOWING IMMUNIZATION

The reportable AEFI must include any death or serious event believed by the public or health worker to be caused by immunization **(Table 6.9.5)**.[3]

The minor common reactions such as local reactions, fever, and self-limiting systemic symptoms need not be reported. It is important for the persons administering the vaccine to advise the parent/patient at the time of immunization that these reactions are expected and advise them how to manage these common reactions (e.g., paracetamol to treat fever).

TABLE 6.9.5: List of reportable adverse event following immunization (AEFI).[3]

Time period	*Type of adverse effects*
Occurring within 24 hours of immunization	• Anaphylactoid reaction (acute hypersensitivity reaction) • Anaphylaxis • Persistent (>3 hours) inconsolable screaming and crying • Hypotonic hyporesponsive episode (HHE)
Occurring within 5 days of immunization	• Toxic shock syndrome (TSS) • Severe local reaction • Sepsis • Injection site abscess (bacterial/sterile)
Occurring within 15 days of immunization	• Seizures, including febrile seizures (6–12 days for measles/MMR; 0–2 days for DTP) • Encephalopathy (6–12 days for measles/MMR; 0–2 days for DTP)
Occurring within 3 months of immunization	• Acute flaccid paralysis (4–30 days for OPV recipient; 4–75 days for contact) • Brachial neuritis (2–28 days after tetanus containing vaccine)
Occurring within 1 month and 12 months	• Thrombocytopenia (15–35 days after measles/MMR) • Lymphadenitis and disseminated BCG infection after BCG immunization • Osteitis/osteomyelitis
No time limit	Any death, hospitalization, or other severe and unusual events that are thought by health workers or the public to be related to immunization

(BCG: Bacillus Calmette–Guérin; DTP: diphtheria, tetanus, and pertussis; MMR: measles, mumps, and rubella vaccine; OPV: oral polio vaccine)

For more serious problems, the patient should be advised to return or to seek medical attention and to allow detection of AEFI. More importantly, they should be advised not to delay treatment of a coincidental illness falsely attributed as vaccine reaction.

Severe local reactions, especially if occurring in clusters, should be reported, as they can be markers for program errors or for problems with specific vaccine lots.

Channels and Timeline for Reporting Serious Adverse Event Following Immunization (Private)

Private sectors contribute to about 20% of total immunization and also provide vaccines not available in government sector. Hence, AEFI from this sector is also reported and investigated as per the laid down national guidelines.[2] Also the AEFI reporting from private sector will provide vital information on the safety of new and underutilized vaccines in India. Once, a serious AEFI happens in the private sector at a clinic of pediatricians in the rural area, she/he should immediately inform medical officer (MO) in-charge of nearest primary health center (PHC) or other health facility. In the urban area, either she/he can inform MO in-charge of nearest urban health center (UHC) or to the District Immunization Officer (DIO). By all channels, the information should reach DIO as soon as possible.

The private practitioners (including pediatricians) should use the "first information report (FIR)" form for reporting serious AEFI cases to the district officials. Once an AEFI is reported from private sector, the DIO, and district AEFI committee members would then investigate the reported AEFI case. The pediatricians should help the investigation team in collection of all the related information.

Indian Academy of Pediatrics (IAP) through its IAP Advisory Committee on Vaccines and Immunization Practices (IAP ACVIP) has resolved to collaborate with the national AEFI program by suggesting the following measures—Integrate IAP Disease Surveillance Project (IDSURV) with AEFI reporting for a web-based and integrated voice recording reporting (already incorporated: *www.idsurv.org*). The IDSURV program is fine-tuned to automatically send information to the concerned DIO/state immunization officer (SIO) for prompt action.

Serious Adverse Event Following Immunization Cases (Government)

When to report? Who should report?[2]

- Minor AEFI are to be reported by the village health nurse (VHN) to the MO of PHC in the monthly reports who will include the report from all VHNs in the monthly report to the district headquarters authority.
- Pediatricians can report any AEFI case to the PHC/community health center MOs (in rural area) or may directly report to DIO **(Flowcharts 6.9.1 and 6.9.2)**.
- The DIO reports this in the monthly report to the state and the state to the Government of India (GOI) as per the timeline for monthly report.
- The report should contain the following details at a minimum as per standard operating procedure:
  - Description of the event
  - Timing of the event in relation to immunization
  - Vaccine/s given
  - Patients identifying details

This is called FIR. The routine vaccination program should continue while awaiting the completion of the reporting and investigation.

Flowchart 6.9.1: Channels and timeline for reporting serious AEFI cases.[2]

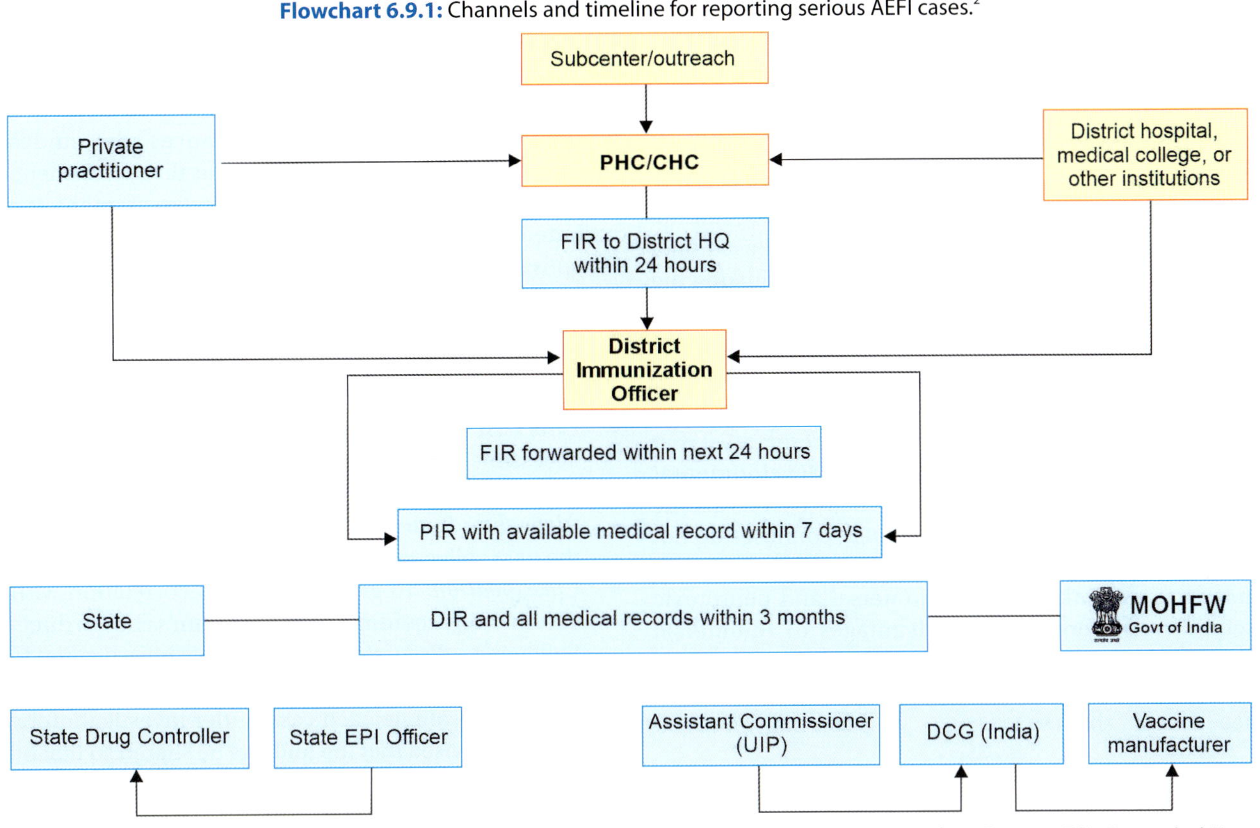

(AEFI: adverse event following immunization; DCG: Drug Controller General; DIR: Domestic Incident Report; EPI: Expanded Program Immunization; FIR: First Information Report; HQ: Headquarter; MOHFW: Ministry of Health and Family Welfare; PHC/CHC: Primary Health Center/Community Health Center; PIR: Program Information Report; UIP: Universal Immunization Program)

COMMUNICATING WITH THE MEDIA

The media plays an important role in public perception. The media is more interested in stories that will attract attention; hence, there is tendency to dramatize and personalize the event. It is easy for the media to create sense of panic and outrage about the events which are unrelated to immunization (coincidental). The guiding principle while dealing with media must be that one should show empathy and caring, honesty and openness, and dedication and commitment; whenever possible, positive terms like immunization safety or vaccine safety should be used. Key messages have to be prepared before media contact, and they should include some of these facts:

- Benefit of immunization in preventing disease is well proven.
- It is very risky not to immunize (risk of disease and complications).
- Vaccine preventable diseases caused millions of deaths and/or disability before the introduction of vaccines and that situation would return without continued use of vaccines.

Flowchart 6.9.2: Where to send samples for testing.[2]

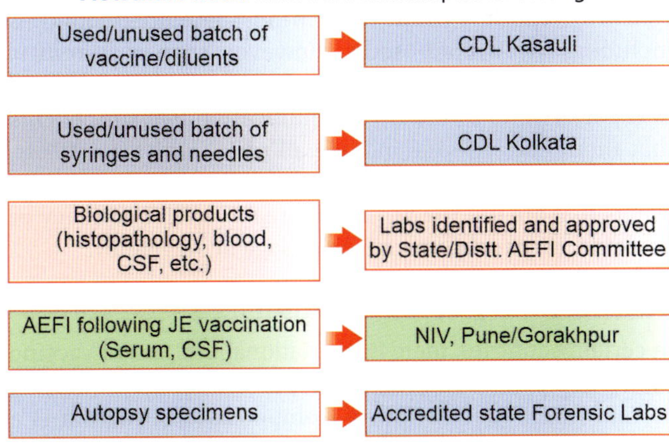

- Vaccines do cause reactions, but these are rarely serious and hardly ever cause long-term problems.
- Immunization safety is of paramount importance, and any suspicion of a problem is investigated (advantage of well-established immunization safety surveillance).
- The AEFI is currently being investigated but is likely to be coincidental due to a local problem (depending on type of

event), and the immunization program must continue to keep the population safe from diseases.

CONTROVERSIES IN VACCINE SAFETY

Autism and Vaccines

The link between immunizations, namely the MMR vaccine, and autism/autistic spectrum disorder (ASD) has been the subject of intense debate over the last 10 years. Based on a review of all available data, there is no evidence linking the MMR vaccine to autism.

Safety of Thiomersal

Inactivated vaccinations, especially those in multidose vials, include thiomersal (50% ethylmercury), a preservative that has previously been connected to neurodevelopmental problems and ASD. As a result, the majority of vaccine formulations that are accessible in affluent countries do not contain thiomersal. However, a thorough analysis of the data has not proven a link between thiomersal and neurotoxic consequences. Therefore, the advantages of thiomersal greatly exceed any potential hazards in developing countries where multidose vials drastically reduce vaccine prices and the need for cold chain space.

VACCINE-ASSOCIATED ADVERSE EVENT REPORTING SYSTEM

A system for reporting vaccine-associated adverse event reporting system (VAERS) is crucial in any immunization program, so as to pick up previously unrecognized adverse effects and generate further data on vaccine safety. A robust system for reporting VAERS exists in most developed countries including the United States. However, such a system is currently not available in India. Pediatricians are encouraged to report VAERS to the IAP immunization website. Events that should be reported include all serious adverse effects, irrespective of causal association, and nonserious adverse events that are unexpected in nature, severity, frequency or outcome, vaccine failures, and all usage in pregnancy.

Vaccine Injury Compensation

In certain countries, there is the National Childhood Vaccine Injury Compensation Program to provide compensation for certain AEFI. Vaccine Injury Compensation Program is a "no-fault" system to compensate individuals whose injuries may have been caused by any routinely recommended childhood vaccines. Vaccine Injury Compensation Program is separate from VAERS.

Causality Assessment[2]

The process of systematically analyzing the data gathered regarding an AEFI in order to ascertain the probability that the event was brought on by the vaccine or vaccines received is known as causation assessment. It boosts trust in the NIP and is an essential component of AEFI monitoring. The updated WHO/CIOMS Causality (2014) is used in the updated guidelines. For reported AEFI instances, the guidelines recommend the state to perform a causality assessment. For the AEFI report to qualify for causality assessment, it must include investigative formats, pertinent documents, and a diagnosis. There are four steps in the causality assessment process:

- *Eligibility:* To ascertain whether the reported AEFI case meets the previously stated minimal requirements for causality evaluation.
- *Checklist:* To thoroughly examine the pertinent and accessible data in order to address any potential causative elements of the AEFI.
- *Algorithm:* To determine the causal relationship between the data collected in the checklist.
- *Classification:* To group the AEFI's correlation with the vaccination according to the algorithm's chosen direction.

Following a discussion of all available investigation forms and reports, the state AEFI committee's causality assessment experts shall evaluate each case under investigation by the district. It is advised that the findings be shared so that others might benefit from the experience. Errors in immunizations will need to be fixed, and communication is required to preserve trust in cases that happen by accident.

ADVERSE EVENT FOLLOWING IMMUNIZATION COMMITTEES

Along with the members' terms of reference, the updated standards also provide comprehensive details about the district, state, and national AEFI committees. AEFI committees offer technical assistance in examining the causes of adverse events and in enhancing the system to ensure safe and efficient vaccination. A pediatrician, microbiologist, pathologist, epidemiologist, neurologist, forensic specialist, cold chain officer, IDSP, drug authority, Municipal Corporation, and partner agencies should all be represented on the committee.

Adverse Event Following Immunization Surveillance Monitoring

The AEFI surveillance system's performance monitoring is emphasized in the recommendation. The following are the defined key indicators:

For routine AEFI:

- The proportion of routine reports that are received on time (zero reports)
- A list of the percentage of AEFI cases.
- The proportion of cases of severe AEFI.

For severe AEFI:

- The proportion of instances that are promptly reported.
- The proportion of AEFI cases when the case reporting form (CRF) was promptly communicated with the state and center.
- How many serious AEFI cases were promptly investigated
- The proportion of significant AEFI cases with a full investigation
- The proportion of significant AEFI cases promptly designated as causative by the state AEFI committee.

ASPECTS OF ADVERSE EVENT FOLLOWING IMMUNIZATION SURVEILLANCE OPERATIONS

The AEFI surveillance's overarching objective is to reduce AEFI-related morbidity and mortality as well as the disease's detrimental effects on public health. The roles and responsibilities of the key players in the AEFI surveillance system are outlined in the updated rules. It is stressed how crucial it is that ASHA, anganwadi workers, and health supervisors participate in the surveillance system at all levels (community, subcenter). In addition to identifying and reporting the incident, the MO is also in charge of case management. Professional organizations such as IAP and IMA can help improve AEFI surveillance.

One option for reporting AEFI is to use internet software (IDsurv) for infectious illness reporting. The district authorities' roles and responsibilities are described, including reporting, investigating, keeping track of reported AEFIs, and liaising with the ADR monitoring center and private and public medical colleges. At the state level, the SIO is responsible for keeping track of AEFI documentation, assisting with case investigations as needed, and collaborating with the state drug controller and other partner organizations. The causality assessment of reported instances should be carried out by the state.

An essential part of the National Regulatory Authority's (NRA) operations is AEFI. The NRA is crucial for vaccine prequalification as well as for ensuring the nation's vaccinations are of high quality.

To improve AEFI surveillance across the nation, the AEFI Secretariat was founded in 2012 inside the Ministry of Health and Family Welfare (MOHFW), GoI. The Immunization Technical Support Unit (ITSU), established by the MOHFW (GoI), serves as its host. At the state and district levels, four Zonal AEFI Consultants have been assigned to communicate with the managers of immunization programs and other vaccine safety stakeholders.

In addition to receiving ongoing direction and assistance from the National AEFI Committee, the AEFI Secretariat has partnered with Lady Hardinge Medical College in New Delhi, which is known as the National AEFI Technical Collaborating Centre (NATCC), to offer supervision and assistance. The Guidelines also outline how the District Committee must coordinate with the police in order to investigate the reported AEFI.

THE CONVERGENCE OF THE AEFI SURVEILLANCE PROGRAM WITH THE NATIONAL REGULATORY AUTHORITY AND ITS AFFILIATED INSTITUTIONS

The recommendations outline the functions of the Pharmacovigilance Program of India (PVPI) and the National Drug Regulatory Authority (NDRA), as well as the significance of collaboration between the Immunization Division of MOHFW and the CDSCO. The CDSCO receives the results of the causality assessment that has been approved by the National AEFI Committee. It evaluates the findings and takes any additional regulatory action that may be required (such as inspections, manufacturer reporting, or changes to product inserts). To guarantee consistency in vaccine safety reports and their sufficient investigations, the Indian Pharmacopoeia Commission (IPC) and the AEFI secretariat have formed a data exchange agreement.

CONCLUSION

The immunization focus as established by the WHO has the objective to eliminate sickness and death caused by VPDs through the development of strong, sustainable NIP, capable of delivering high-quality vaccines in a safe and effective way to all children. Safe and efficient immunization practices with thorough knowledge of the vaccines, well-maintained cold chain, proper parent education, and efficient resuscitation equipment are vital components essential to make immunization most cost-effective public health tool in child survival programs.

REFERENCES

1. Indian Academy of Pediatrics. IAP GuideBook on Immunization. Mumbai: Indian Academy of Pediatrics; 2011. pp. 43-6.
2. Ministry Health & Family Welfare, Government of India. (2015). AEFI (Adverse Events Following Immunization). Surveillance and Response Guidelines. [online] Available at https://nhm.gov.in/New_Updates_2018/NHM_Components/Immunization/Guildelines_for_immunization/AEFI_Surveillance_and_Response_Operational_Guidelines_2015.pdf [Last accessed December, 2024].
3. World Health Organization. Immunization Safety Surveillance: Guidelines for managers of immunization programmes on reporting and investigation adverse events following immunization. Manila: World Health Organization; 1999.
4. Meites E, Szilagyi PG, Chesson HW, Unger ER, Romero JR, Markowitz LE. Human Papillomavirus Vaccination for Adults:

Updated Recommendations of the Advisory Committee on Immunization Practices. MMWR Morb Mortal Wkly Rep. 2019;68(32):698-702.

5. Kanizsai A, Molnar T, Varnai R, Zavori L, Tőkés-Füzesi M, Szalai Z, et al. Fever after Vaccination against SARS-CoV-2 with mRNA-Based Vaccine Associated with Higher Antibody Levels during 6 Months Follow-Up. Vaccines (Basel). 2022;10(3):447.
6. Shemer A, Pras E, Hecht I. Peripheral facial nerve palsy following BNT162b2 (COVID-19) vaccination. Isr J Med Sci. 2021;23(3):143-4.
7. Li X, Ostropolets A, Makadia R, Shoaibi A, Rao G, Sena AG, et al. Characterizing the incidence of adverse events of special interest for COVID-19 vaccines across eight countries: a multinational network cohort study. BMJ. 2021;373:n1435.
8. Lee H, Kang HY, Cho S, Park S, Kim AY, Jung SY, et al. Causality Assessment Guidelines for Adverse Events Following Immunization with a Focus on Guillain-Barré Syndrome. Vaccines (Basel). 2020;8(1):101.
9. Rahman MM, Fatema K. Risk of seizures after immunization with vaccine in children. Bangladesh J Child Health. 2020;44(1):40-7.
10. Geier DA, Geier MR. An evaluation of serious neurological disorders following immunization: A comparison of whole-cell pertussis and acellular pertussis vaccines. Brain Dev. 2004;26(5):296-300.
11. Barlow WE, Davis RL, Glasser JW, Rhodes PH, Thompson RS, Mulloly JP, et al. Centers for Disease Control, Prevention Vaccine Safety Datalink Working Group. The risk of seizures after receipt of whole cell pertussis or measles, mumps, and rubella vaccine. N Engl J Med. 2001;345:656-61.
12. Tseng HF, Sy LS, Liu IL, Qian L, Marcy SM, Weintraub E, et al. Postlicensure surveillance for prespecified adverse events following the 13-valent pneumococcal conjugate vaccine in children. Vaccine. 2013;31(22):2578-83.
13. Cendes F, Sankar R. Vaccinations and febrile seizures. Epilepsia. 2011;52(Suppl 3):23-5.
14. Centers for Disease Control and Prevention (CDC). Updated recommendations for use of tetanus toxoid, reduced diphtheria toxoid, and acellular pertussis vaccine (Tdap) in pregnant women ¡ Advisory Committee on Immunization Practices (ACIP). 2012. MMWR Morb Mortal Wkly Rep. 2013;62:131-5.

6.10 Vaccination in Special Situations

Arun Wadhwa

INTRODUCTION

A "special situation" is a situation in which the administration of a vaccine may result in suboptimal efficacy or increase the chances of adverse effects following immunization (AEFI). In such circumstances, vaccination procedures and schedules must be modified, either to maintain the expected efficacy of the vaccine or to prevent AEFI.

ALTERED IMMUNOCOMPETENCE

The terms immunosuppression, immunodeficiency, and immunocompromise are now collectively referred to as "*altered immunocompetence*." This altered immunocompetence can be primary or secondary. Primary immunodeficiencies are usually inherited and can be because of total absence or quantitative deficiency of cellular component, humoral component, or both. Examples can be congenital immunodeficiency diseases, severe combined immunodeficiency (SCID), and chronic granulomatous disease (CGD). Secondary immunodeficiencies are acquired and are loss or qualitative reduction in cellular or humoral immune components. These can occur because of the disease itself or because of its therapy. Some examples of secondary immunodeficiency are human immunodeficiency virus (HIV) infection and hematopoietic malignancies, which also result from treatment with radiotherapy and immunosuppressive drugs. The degree to which immunosuppressive drugs cause immunodeficiency is dose-related and also varies from drug to drug. Medical conditions like asplenia (congenital or acquired) and chronic kidney disease can also cause altered immunocompetence.

Knowing the patient's immunocompetence is important because the incidence or severity of some diseases may be higher in these persons, and they may need to be vaccinated on a priority basis. Non-live vaccines may also be less effective during the period of altered immunocompetence and thus might be deferred for a later date. Here, the concern is with effectiveness and not safety. Also, if a non-live vaccine is administered during the period of altered immunocompetence, it might need to be repeated after the immune function has improved. Similarly, administration of live vaccines to immunocompromised patients might need to be deferred. This is primarily because patients who have altered immune function and receive live vaccines might be at an increased risk of adverse reactions because of uninhibited growth of the bacteria or live-attenuated virus. Certain situations that may be associated with altered immunocompetence.

CORTICOSTEROID THERAPY

Corticosteroids are probably the most common drugs used in children which may cause immunosuppression. The recommendations for vaccination of children on steroid therapy are:[1]

- *Dose of <2 mg/kg (if <10 kg), <20 mg/day (if >10 kg):* No immunosuppression, can receive live vaccines
- *Dose of >2 mg/kg (if <10 kg), >20 mg/day (if >10 kg), for a duration of <2 weeks:* Can receive live vaccines immediately after stopping steroids
- *Dose of >2 mg/kg (if <10 kg), >20 mg/day (if >10 kg), for a duration of >2 weeks:* No live vaccines until 1 month after stopping steroids

Killed vaccines are safe but may be less efficacious.

Patients on alternate-day steroid therapy, inhalation formulations, topical steroids, maintenance physiologic doses (replacement therapy), intra-articular, bursal, or tendon injection are not immunosuppressed and can receive all vaccines.[1]

When initiating immunosuppressive therapy after a live vaccine, if possible, we should wait for 4 weeks after a live vaccine and 2 weeks after a non-live vaccine. However, if a patient requires urgent corticosteroid therapy for any condition, it should not be delayed because of past administration of vaccines.[2]

OTHER IMMUNOSUPPRESSIVE DRUGS

Whenever feasible, all vaccines indicated should be administered before the initiation of chemotherapy, treatment with immunosuppressive drugs, radiotherapy, or before undergoing splenectomy. Persons receiving chemotherapy or radiation for hematopoietic malignancies or solid tumors should be assumed to have altered immunocompetence. Live, attenuated vaccines should not be administered for at least 3 months after cessation of immunosuppressive therapy **(Table 6.10.1)**.[3,4] Non-live vaccines administered during chemotherapy should be readministered after immune competence is regained **(Table 6.10.2)**.[5] Children vaccinated before receiving chemotherapy for leukemia, lymphoma, other malignancies, or radiation generally are thought to retain immune memory after treatment, although single-dose revaccination with the common childhood vaccines after chemotherapy for acute lymphoblastic leukemia might be indicated.[5] In general, revaccination of a person after chemotherapy or radiation therapy is considered unnecessary if the previous vaccination occurred before therapy and not during therapy, except for recipients of hematopoietic stem cell transplantation (HSCT), who should be revaccinated. In solid organ transplant recipients, immunosuppressive medications are administered to prevent organ rejection. In these children, live vaccines should be withheld for 2 months following discontinuation of antirejection therapy.[3] Determination of the level of immune memory and the need for revaccination has to be made by the treating physician, as there are no perfect laboratory tests to do so.

The Bacillus Calmette-Guérin (BCG) vaccine, if not received earlier, is contraindicated during ongoing chemotherapy and can only be given after 6 months of completion of chemotherapy. In children previously immunized with a visible scar, no further doses are recommended.

Oral polio vaccine (OPV) is contraindicated during and up to 6 months after chemotherapy, including pulse polio immunization days. After 6 months of stopping chemotherapy, it is recommended to vaccinate children with

TABLE 6.10.1: Recommendations for live vaccines after chemotherapy.[4]

		After the end of chemotherapy	
Vaccine	***During chemotherapy***	***Previously unimmunized***	***Completely immunized***
BCG	Not recommended	Single dose after 6 months of completion of chemotherapy	Not recommended if scar is present
OPV	Not recommended	IPV preferred; otherwise three doses of bOPV—1 month apart	IPV preferred; otherwise two doses of bOPV—1 month apart
MMR and varicella	Not recommended	Two doses 1–3 months apart, 6 months after completion of chemo	Single dose, 6 months after completion of chemo
Live HAV	Not recommended	Single dose, 6 months after completion of chemo	
Rotavirus	Not recommended	Child generally outgrows the maximum permissible age limit	

(BCG: Bacillus Calmette-Guérin; bOPV: bivalent oral polio vaccine; HAV: hepatitis A virus; IPV: inactivated polio vaccine; MMR: measles, mumps, and rubella; OPV: oral polio vaccine)

TABLE 6.10.2: Recommendations of non-live vaccines after chemotherapy.[5]

		After the end of chemotherapy	
Vaccine	***During chemotherapy***	***Previously unimmunized***	***Completely immunized***
DPT, DTaP, Tdap, and Td	Not recommended	Three doses at 0, 1, and 6 months after stopping chemo	Single dose, 6 months after stopping chemo
Hib	Not recommended	Age-appropriate doses, 6 months after stopping chemo	Single dose 6 months after stopping chemo
IPV	Not recommended	Three doses of IPV at 0, 2, and 6 months after stopping chemo	Single dose 6 months after stopping chemo. Two doses if primary vaccination was OPV
HBV	Four doses—0, 1, 2, and 12 months in double dose in unimmunized child. No extra dose if completely immunized child	Three doses—0, 1, and 6 months after stopping chemo	One booster 6 months after stopping chemotherapy
HAV	Not recommended	Two doses—0, and 6 months after stopping chemotherapy	One dose, 6 months after stopping chemotherapy
Pneumococcal vaccine		Age-appropriate PCV doses 6 months after stopping chemotherapy. PPSV booster not recommended	Single dose 6 months after stopping chemotherapy
Inactivated flu vaccine	Single dose annually	Not recommended beyond 1 year of stopping chemotherapy	
Typhoid vaccine	Not recommended	Single TCV dose 6 months after stopping chemotherapy	
HPV	Not recommended	Age-appropriate doses 6 months after stopping chemotherapy	Insufficient data. Single booster may be given

(DPT: diphtheria, pertussis, and tetanus; DTaP: diphtheria, tetanus, and acellular pertussis; HAV: hepatitis A virus; HBV: hepatitis B virus; Hib: *Haemophilus influenzae B*; HPV: human papillomavirus; IPV: inactivated polio vaccine; OPV: oral polio vaccine; PCV: pneumococcal conjugate vaccine; PPSV: pneumococcal polysaccharide vaccine; TCV: typhoid vaccine; Tdap: tetanus with lower doses of diphtheria and acellular pertussis vaccine)

the inactivated polio vaccine (IPV). When IPV is unavailable, bivalent OPV (bOPV) as three doses 1 month apart are recommended for unimmunized children. In children with previously completed immunization, two doses of bOPV, 1 month apart, are recommended if IPV is not available. After 6 months of stopping treatment, children should be actively encouraged for pulse polio immunization days.

After 6 months of stopping treatment, a single dose of hepatitis B virus (HBV), diphtheria, pertussis, and tetanus (DPT), tetanus with lower doses of diphtheria and acellular pertussis (Tdap), tetanus and diphtheria (Td), *Haemophilus influenzae B* (Hib), pneumococcal conjugate vaccine (PCV), measles, mumps, and rubella (MMR), chickenpox, hepatitis A virus (HAV), and typhoid vaccine (TCV) may also be given. Influenza vaccine is given annually during chemotherapy but not recommended beyond 1 year of stopping treatment.

If there is a risk of suboptimal blood transfusion practices in a child diagnosed with cancer who is unimmunized and who is HBV surface antigen negative, then it is recommended to administer four doses of HBV vaccine at 0, 1, 2, and 12 months at double dosage as well as an age-appropriate dose of HBV immunoglobulin every 3 months until there is no risk of exposure to blood products.

If a child on chemotherapy gets a wound, it can be assumed that the antibody levels are inadequate. Therefore, in a clean, minor wound, Td/Tdap booster regardless of immunization status is recommended; for all other wounds, Td/Tdap + tetanus immunoglobulin is advised. For the human papilloma virus vaccine (HPV), in children with previously completed immunization, there is no data to make any recommendation, but a single dose may be considered.

Other immunosuppressive medications in use now are immune mediators like interleukins (IL) and colony-stimulating factors, immune modulators, tumor necrosis factor-alpha (TNFα) inhibitors, and anti-B-cell agents. Non-live vaccines should be administered at least 2 weeks before initiating any of these therapies, and live vaccines should be given at least 4 weeks before their initiation. Also, live vaccines should not be given for 3 months following these treatments.

After therapy with anti-B-cell agents, both non-live and live vaccines should be withheld for 6 months or more, as these agents suppress antibody-producing cells for a prolonged duration.[3] Zoster vaccine is an exception here and should be withheld for just 1 month following anti-B-cell agents. After vaccination, anti-B-cell agents can be resumed 1 month later.[3]

RECIPIENTS OF HEMATOPOIETIC CELL TRANSPLANT

A HSCT involves ablation of the bone marrow followed by reimplantation of the person's own stem cells or stem cells derived from a donor. The process results in immunosuppression not only because of the hematopoietic ablative therapy but also because of the drugs used to prevent or treat graft-versus-host disease (GVHD) and, in some cases, also from the underlying disease itself, which led to transplantation. The ablation reduces or removes the immune memory acquired from previous vaccinations. Antibody titers to tetanus, poliovirus, MMR, and encapsulated bacteria decrease 1–4 years after autologous or allogeneic HSCT if the recipient is not revaccinated.

Hematopoietic stem cell transplantation recipients of all ages are at an increased risk for diseases caused by encapsulated bacteria (e.g., pneumococcal and Hib infections). As a result, HSCT recipients who received vaccines prior to their HSCT should receive repeat doses routinely after HSCT, regardless of the source of the transplanted stem cells.[6] Revaccination doses following HSCT are indicated with pneumococcal vaccines, diphtheria, tetanus, and acellular pertussis (DTaP)/Tdap vaccines, Hib vaccine, HAV vaccine, HBV vaccine, IPV, inactivated influenza vaccines (IIV), meningococcal conjugate vaccines (MCV) (for individuals at high risk), and HPV vaccine.[6]

Most non-live vaccines should be reinitiated 6 months after the HSCT.[1] IIV should be administered 6 months after HSCT and annually thereafter for the life of the patient. If a dose of IIV is given at 4 months after HSCT, a second dose should be given after 4 weeks.[1] As with other children, a second dose is recommended routinely for all children younger than 9 years receiving the influenza vaccine for the first time.

Hematopoietic stem cell transplantation patients must be given pneumococcal vaccine irrespective of their pretransplant vaccine status. Starting after 3–6 months of the transplant, the first three doses of PCV should be given at a minimum 4-week interval and then the fourth dose should be administered 6 months after the third dose or 1 year after the HSCT, whichever is later. It should be followed by the pneumococcal polysaccharide vaccine (PPSV23) 1 year after the last dose of PCV.

A three-dose regimen of Hib vaccine should be administered beginning 6 months after transplant; at least 1 month should separate the doses.[1]

The revaccination schedule for pertussis-containing vaccines: For patients <7 years old, three doses of DTaP at least 4 weeks apart. For patients ≥7 years, we have three options for revaccination:

1. Three doses of DTaP
2. One dose of Tdap and two doses of diphtheria and tetanus (DT) or
3. One dose of Tdap and two doses of Td[2]

Varicella and MMR vaccines may be readministered after HSCT if 24 months have passed since HSCT, the patient does *not* have GVHD, and is considered immunocompetent. Recombinant zoster vaccine may be readministered 6–12 months after an allogeneic HSCT and 3–12 months after an autologous HSCT. As the yellow fever, rabies, tick-borne encephalitis, and Japanese encephalitis vaccines are not routinely administered, their use post HSCT will be determined by the disease-specific risk such as exposure or travel. BCG, live-attenuated influenza vaccine (LAIV), and rotavirus vaccine are not recommended after HSCT.[4] A single dose of the typhoid conjugate vaccine may be given in disease-endemic countries.

We need to make a clinical judgment on whether to follow the revaccination schedules described above in circumstances where particular vaccines were *not* administered prior to the HSCT. In this circumstance, we may just vaccinate according to routine recommendations for that appropriate age. There are specific recommendations for Hib and pertussis-containing vaccines. Use of the three-dose Hib schedule following HSCT is supported for both patients who received Hib prior to HSCT and those who did not receive Hib prior to HSCT.[7]

ANATOMIC OR FUNCTIONAL ASPLENIA

Patients with anatomic asplenia (surgical removal or congenital absence) or functional asplenia (e.g., children with sickle cell disease) are at an increased risk for infection by encapsulated bacteria like *Streptococcus pneumoniae* (*Pneumococcus*), *Neisseria meningitidis* (*Meningococcus*), and Hib. Children should receive an age-appropriate series of PCV. Unvaccinated children between 2 and 5 years of age should receive two doses of PCV13. Children aged 6 years and above should receive a dose of PCV13 if they have not previously received any dose. Children above 2 years of age should receive two doses of PPSV23 separated by 5 years, beginning 8 or more weeks after completion of recommended doses of PCV13. In circumstances where both PCV13 and PPSV23 are indicated, doses of PCV13 should be administered first, followed by PPSV23, 8 weeks after the last dose of PCV13 **(Table 6.10.3)**.[7]

Both quadrivalent MCV4 and meningococcal serogroup B (MenB) vaccines are recommended for patients with anatomic or functional asplenia. For children 2–23 months of age, two doses, 3 months apart, of MenACWY-D should be administered. For persons ≥2 years of age, a two-dose primary series, 8 weeks apart, of either MenACWY-CRM or MenACWY-D should be administered. The required doses of

TABLE 6.10.3: Vaccination of persons with primary and secondary immunodeficiencies.[4]

Basic deficiency	*Specific disease*	*Contraindications*	*Risk-specific vaccine required*	*Comments*
Primary B-cell deficiency (humoral)	Severe Ab deficiency	BCG, OPV, MMR, chickenpox, LAIV, and other live vaccines	Pneumococcal, Hib (12–59 months),* recombinant zoster vaccine	Effectiveness may be less for pure polysaccharide vaccines
	Less severe deficiency	BCG, OPV, and yellow fever Other live vaccines are safe	Pneumococcal, Hib (12–59 months), recombinant zoster vaccine	All vaccines are likely effective; the immune response might be attenuated
Primary T-cell deficiency (humoral + cell-mediated)	Complete defects like SCID	All live vaccines	Pneumococcal, Hib (12–59 months), recombinant zoster vaccine	Vaccines unlikely to be effective
	Partial like DiGeorge, Wiskott–Aldrich, ataxia telangiectasia	All live vaccines	Pneumococcal, meningococcal, Hib, recombinant zoster vaccine	Effectiveness will depend on the degree of immune suppression
	Interferon (IF-α and IF-γ) deficiencies	All live vaccines	Recombinant zoster vaccine	
	IF-γ, interleukin-12 axis deficiencies	Live bacterial vaccines	Recombinant zoster vaccine	
Phagocytic deficiency	Chronic granulomatous disease	Live bacterial vaccines	Recombinant zoster vaccine	Live viral vaccines are safe and effective
	Phagocytic deficiencies accompanied by defects in T-cell and NK cell dysfunction like Chédiak–Higashi, leukocyte adhesion deficiency, and myeloperoxidase deficiency	All live vaccines	Pneumococcal and recombinant zoster	All non-live vaccines safe and likely effective
Primary: Compliment	Persistent complement, properdin, or factor B deficiency	None	Pneumococcal, meningo-coccal, Hib (12–59 months)	All routine vaccines are likely to be effective
Secondary	HIV/AIDS	OPV, BCG, LAIV Withhold MMR and varicella in severely immunosuppressed (CD4 count <15%)	Pneumococcal, Hib, HBV, MenACWY, recombinant zoster	MMR and varicella vaccine in those with mild immunosuppression, rotavirus, and all non-live vaccines, including inactivated influenza as per routine vaccination schedule, might be effective
	Generalized malignant neoplasm, transplantation, immuno-suppressive or radiation therapy	Live viral and bacterial, depending on immune status	Pneumococcal, Hib, recombinant zoster	The effectiveness of any vaccine depends on the degree of immune suppression
	Taking eculizumab or ravulizumab	None	Meningococcal	
	Asplenia	LAIV	Pneumococcal, mening-ococcal, Hib, typhoid	Discussed above
	Chronic kidney disease	None	Pneumococcal, hepatitis B	All routine vaccines are likely effective

*Hib in children 12–59 months: If a child is unimmunized or received only one dose, and that dose was administered before 12 months of age, they should receive two Hib doses, 8 weeks apart; if they received two or more doses before age 12 months, and none after 12 months, they should receive one Hib dose 8 weeks after the last dose; if they completed a primary series and received a booster dose at age 12 months or older, no additional Hib doses are recommended. Patients who have not received a primary series and booster dose or at least one dose of the Hib vaccine after 14 months of age are considered unimmunized.

(AIDS: acquired immunodeficiency syndrome; BCG: Bacillus Calmette-Guérin; CD: clusters of differentiation; DPT: diphtheria, pertussis, and tetanus; DTaP: diphtheria, tetanus, and acellular pertussis; HAV: hepatitis A virus; HBV: hepatitis B virus; Hib: *Haemophilus influenzae B*; HIV: human immunodeficiency virus; HPV: human papillomavirus; IPV: inactivated polio vaccine; LAIV: live-attenuated influenza vaccine; MMR: measles, mumps, and rubella; NK: natural killer; OPV: oral polio vaccine; PCV: pneumococcal conjugate vaccine; PPSV: pneumococcal polysaccharide vaccine; SCID: severe combined immunodeficiency; TCV: typhoid vaccine; Tdap: tetanus with lower doses of diphtheria and acellular pertussis vaccine)

PCV should be completed first and then MenACWY should be given 4 weeks after the PCV13 series is completed. For children <7 years of age, after the primary series of MCV-4 vaccine, another dose is recommended after 3 years. A 5-year interval is recommended for persons who received their last MCV4 dose at age 7 years or older.[4] Meningococcal B (MenB) vaccine (not available in India) should be administered as either a two-dose series of MenB-4C (Bexsero) or a three-dose series of MenB-FHbp (Trumenba). Either of the MenB vaccines may be administered concomitantly with MenACWY vaccines, but at a different anatomic site. Unlike MCV4, there are at present no recommendations for booster doses of the MenB vaccines.[3]

Hib vaccine is recommended routinely for all children below 5 years of age. Patients between 12 and 59 months old with functional or anatomic asplenia and who are unvaccinated or who received only a single dose of Hib before their first birthday should receive two additional doses of Hib vaccine. Those who received two or more doses of Hib before 12 months of age should receive one additional dose. Unimmunized asplenic patients older than 59 months of age should also receive one dose of the Hib vaccine.[3]

Pneumococcal, meningococcal, and Hib vaccinations should be administered at least 14 days before elective splenectomy, if possible. If the vaccinations are not administered before surgery, they should be administered after the procedure as soon as the patient's condition is stable.

The TCV can be given to those children who are living in endemic countries, although there is no published data related to this.

PRIMARY IMMUNODEFICIENCIES

Children with primary immunodeficiencies are rare and present a challenging situation. The summary of the conditions along with the vaccines that may be specifically required and those that are contraindicated is given in **Table 6.10.3**.

PATIENTS WITH BLEEDING DISORDERS

Physicians tend to avoid giving intramuscular (IM) injections to patients with bleeding disorders, fearing the risk of hematoma formation. In one study, the HBV vaccine was administered intramuscularly to 153 persons with hemophilia, using a 23-gauge needle, followed by the application of steady pressure on the site for 1–2 minutes. The bruising rate was low (4%), and no patients required factor supplementation.[8] Antigens that produce more local reactions (e.g., pertussis) will produce an equally low rate of bruising is not known.

When any IM vaccine is indicated for a patient with a bleeding disorder, the vaccine should be administered intramuscularly by a physician familiar with the patient's bleeding risk. If the patient receives antihemophilia or similar therapy, vaccinations can be scheduled shortly after such therapy is given. A fine-gauge needle (23-G or smaller) should be used for the vaccination, followed by firm pressure on the site, without rubbing, for at least 2 minutes. The patient or family should be given information about the risk of hematoma formation. Patients receiving any anticoagulation therapy should also follow the same guidelines for IM administration. If possible, vaccination can be scheduled prior to the use of these medications, so that the patients' risk of bleeding is not increased after their administration.[8]

VACCINATION OF PREGNANT WOMEN

There is no evidence of risk to the fetus from vaccinating pregnant women with non-live virus or bacterial vaccines.[9] HPV vaccine, although a non-live vaccine, is not recommended during pregnancy.[9] Live vaccines given to pregnant women do pose a theoretical risk to the fetus; therefore, live-attenuated virus and live bacterial vaccines are generally contraindicated during pregnancy. Also, women should avoid conception for 4 weeks after getting vaccinated with live vaccines. However, the benefits of vaccinating pregnant women may outweigh the potential risks if the likelihood of disease exposure is high and if the infection poses a serious risk to the mother or fetus.[10]

Women who are pregnant should receive a dose of Tdap in each pregnancy, irrespective of whether they have previously received Tdap or not. Vaccination of the mother produces antibodies that pass transplacentally and protect the infant in the initial months. Additionally, preventing pertussis in the mother reduces the risk that the infant is exposed to pertussis after birth.[9] Mothers should receive Tdap during the third trimester, preferably between 27 and 36 weeks. If Tdap is not administered during pregnancy, it should be given immediately postpartum.

BREASTFEEDING AND VACCINATION

Except for yellow fever and smallpox vaccines, no live or killed vaccines administered to a lactating woman affect the safety of breastfed infants. Yellow fever vaccine is avoided because two cases (one confirmed, one probable) of vaccine-associated acute neurotropic disease have been reported in infants.[9] Although live viruses in vaccines replicate in the mother, most of these viruses have been demonstrated not to be excreted in human milk. Although the rubella vaccine virus has been excreted in human milk, the virus usually does not infect the infant. If infection does occur, it is well tolerated because the virus is attenuated.[9]

VACCINATION OF PRETERM INFANTS

Children born before 37 weeks' gestation should be vaccinated at the same chronological age, according to the same schedule, and using the same precautions as for full-term infants and children, irrespective of their birth weight. Weight at birth and gestation are not the factors that decide whether to vaccinate or not vaccinate a clinically stable preterm infant.[9] The full recommended dose of each vaccine should be used; reduced doses are not recommended.

HOUSEHOLD CONTACTS OF IMMUNOCOMPROMISED PATIENTS

Administering vaccines to household contacts of patients with altered immunocompetence prevents the potential transmission of a potential contagious disease. All close contacts of persons with altered immunocompetence should receive all age- and exposure-appropriate vaccines, *except* for the smallpox vaccine. MMR, varicella, and rotavirus vaccines should be given to unvaccinated, eligible close contacts. No specific precautions are needed unless the varicella vaccine recipient has a rash after vaccination, in which case direct contact with the immunocompromised patient should be avoided till the rash resolves.[3] Also, all members of the household should wash their hands after changing the diaper of an infant who received the rotavirus vaccine for up to 1 month after the last dose.[3] Household and other close contacts of persons with altered immunocompetence should receive annual influenza vaccination. LAIV can also be administered to healthy household and other close contacts of persons with altered immunocompetence unless the person is in a protective environment, typically defined as a specialized patient-care area with a positive airflow relative to the corridor, high-efficiency particulate air filtration, and frequent air changes.[10] There is no recommendation of influenza vaccine use by healthcare workers or other persons who have close contact with persons with lesser degrees of immunosuppression, like patients with diabetes, asthma patients on high-dose corticosteroids, or HIV patients.

CONCLUSION

The degree of altered immunocompetence in a patient should be determined by a physician. The challenge for clinicians and other healthcare providers is assessing the safety and effectiveness of vaccines for conditions associated with primary or secondary immunodeficiency, especially when new therapeutic modalities are being used and information about the safety and effectiveness of vaccines has not been characterized fully in persons receiving these immunomodulatory drugs. Tests useful to assess humoral immunity include immunoglobulins and their subset levels and specific antibody levels (e.g., Td). Tests that demonstrate the status of cellular immunity include flow cytometry, a test that delineates concentrations and proportions of lymphocyte subsets, and tests that measure T-cell proliferation or function in response to specific or nonspecific stimuli (e.g., lymphocyte proliferation assays). The ability to characterize a drug or disease condition as affecting cellular or humoral immunity is only the first step; using this information to draw inferences about whether particular vaccines are indicated or whether caution is advised with the use of live or non-live vaccines is more complicated and might require consultation with an infectious diseases or immunology specialist.

REFERENCES

1. American Academy of Pediatrics. Immunization in special clinical circumstances. In: Pickering L, Baker C, Kimberlin D, Long S (Eds). Red Book: 2009 Report of the Committee on Infectious Diseases, 28th edition. Elk Grove Village, IL: American Academy of Pediatrics; 2009.
2. Rubin L, Levin M, Ljungman P, Davies EG, Avery R, Tomblyn M, et al. 2013 IDSA clinical practice guideline for vaccination of the immunocompromised host. Clin Infect Dis. 2014;58(3):e44-100.
3. Centers for Disease Control and Prevention (CDC). (2023). General best practice guidelines for immunization. Altered immunocompetence. [online] Available from https://www.cdc.gov/vaccines/hcp/acip-recs/general-recs/immunocompetence.html#ref-37. [Last accessed November, 2024].
4. Moulik NR, Mandal P, Chandra J, Jog P, Sanjay S, Shah N, et al. Immunization of children with cancer in India treated with chemotherapy—consensus guideline from the Pediatric Hematology Oncology Chapter and the Advisory Committee on Vaccination and Immunization Practices of the Indian Academy of Pediatrics. Indian Pediatr. 2019;56(12):1041-8.
5. Brodtman DH, Rosenthal DW, Redner A, Lanzkowsky P, Bonagura VR. Immunodeficiency in children with acute lymphoblastic leukemia after completion of modern aggressive chemotherapeutic regimens. J Pediatr. 2005;146(5):654-61.
6. Tomblyn M, Chiller T, Einsele H, Gress R, Sepkowitz K, Storek J, et al. Guidelines for preventing infectious complications among hematopoietic cell transplantation recipients: a global perspective. Biol Blood Marrow Transplant. 2009;15(10):1143-238.
7. Strikas RA; Centers for Disease Control and Prevention (CDC); Advisory Committee on Immunization Practices (ACIP); ACIP Child/Adolescent Immunization Work Group. Advisory committee on immunization practices recommended immunization schedules for persons aged 0 through 18 years—United States, 2015. MMWR Morb Mortal Wkly Rep. 2015;64(4):93-4.
8. Centers for Disease Control and Prevention (CDC). General best practice guidelines for immunization. Special situations. [online] Available from https://www.cdc.gov/vaccines/hcp/acip-recs/general-recs/special-situations.html#ref-11. [Last accessed November, 2024].
9. Centers for Disease Control and Prevention (CDC). Guiding principles for development of ACIP recommendations for vaccination during pregnancy and breastfeeding. MMWR Morb Mortal Wkly Rep. 2008;57(21):580
10. Grohskopf LA, Olsen SJ, Sokolow LZ, Bresee JS, Cox NJ, Broder KR, et al. Prevention and control of seasonal influenza with vaccines: recommendations of the Advisory Committee on Immunization Practices (ACIP)—United States, 2014-15 influenza season. MMWR Morb Mortal Wkly Rep. 2014;63(32):691-7.

6.11 Future Vaccines, Vaccine Technologies, Adjuvants, and Immunization Techniques

Bharat Mehra, Amar Jeet Chitkara

INTRODUCTION

Anecdotal evidence of vaccination has existed since the 11th century, but it was the landmark observation of Edward Jenner and Louis Pasteur about 200 years ago that started the success story of vaccination.[1] Over the last two centuries, modern vaccinology has evolved into a complex and multidisciplinary science encompassing the fields of microbiology, immunology, molecular biology, epidemiology, and public health. Advancements in the fields of immunology, structural biology, systems biology, and bioinformatics have led to the development of newer, effective, and highly safe vaccines. The synthetic microbial antigens, expression of protective antigens in live vectors and plants, antigen-sparing adjuvants that manipulate the desired immune response in the host, alternate modes of delivery, high productivity, and thermostability are some of the exciting developments that shall not only revolutionize the prevention of infectious diseases but also target noninfectious ailments like malignancy and degenerative diseases. The advances in vaccinology with its innumerable applications have led all the stakeholders to adopt the "call to action for the new decade of vaccines," emphasizing the need of intensified research, funding, and advocacy at all levels for not only equity in distribution and access to vaccines but also to ensure their consumption. The argument that vaccines create wealth and prevent unnecessary deaths has to be percolated at all levels to ensure global health.

TARGETING NEW DISEASES

Recent Advances Affecting Vaccine Development

The empirical approach of selecting a vaccine antigen had an inherent problem of a longer gestation period till it could be available for mass usage and was associated with a high failure rate as well as safety concerns. *Genomics* has changed the concept of antigen selection by reverse vaccinology. This technique of *reverse vaccinology* was developed by the Italian researchers Rino Rappuoli and Maria Grazia Pizza. This technique elucidates the entire genetic framework of the microorganism by genome sequencing and thus helps to identify those molecules that have the capacity to function as potential antigens. Meningococcal B protection, which had eluded researchers till now, became a reality, thanks to this novel technology. The rapid development of the influenza vaccine is another example of reverse vaccinology.

Nanovaccinology is another rapidly evolving science that comprises technology to identify and produce nanoparticles and nanomaterials as potential antigens.[1] Also, nanoparticles are being developed to be used as delivery vehicles and/or immune potentiators. These nanoparticles can improve not only antigen uptake from antigen-presenting cells (APCs) but also immunogenicity and the slow release of antigens. Moreover, most nanoparticles are biodegradable and biocompatible and have minimal toxicity; therefore, they can offer a safe and effective alternative to traditional vaccines. Hepatitis B vaccine (HBV) and human papillomavirus vaccine (HPV) are some examples of vaccines based on nanoparticles.

The detailed atomic configuration of an antigen by *structural biology* shall further help to identify the specific epitopes determining viral entry into the cell or the virulence and can be used as a vaccine antigen. Such efforts are being made for a new measles vaccine.

Systems biology is another emerging discipline, which is based on cytokine and immunological responses and can identify markers that can predict the safety and efficacy of a vaccine using modeling techniques. These developments have helped to identify numerous potential vaccine antigens but have complicated the issue of selecting the best.

The antigens being targeted today are not only the virulence factors but also those having a crucial role in the pathogenesis of disease and the survival of bacteria and viruses in the host. Pneumococcal adhesin antigen is being looked upon as a potential candidate for multiserotype protection with a high herd effect. Glyco-conjugation of polysaccharide antigen has already revolutionized protection against *Haemophilus influenzae* type b (Hib), meningococcal, and pneumococcal organisms and is being further exploited for group A and B *Streptococcus* and *Staphylococcus aureus*.

The first marvel of genetic engineering in vaccinology has been the HBV made from yeast carrying the surface antigen gene. Subsequently, recombinant proteins as effective immunizing agents have been enabled by gene insertion in yeast, *Escherichia coli*, and Chinese hamster ovary cells for Lyme disease, cytomegalovirus (CMV), and pertussis. Vectored vaccines are live recombinants using pathogenic viruses or bacteria to deliver vaccine antigens, which have met with reasonable success for diseases such as Japanese encephalitis, dengue (yellow fever virus vector), and respiratory syncytial virus (RSV) (human parainfluenza virus-3). The vectors serve as a carrier for the pathogenic gene and have the advantage of simulating a natural infection and stimulating both humoral and cell-mediated immunity (CMI) effectively. The vectored approach also has the potential for therapeutic vaccines for cancer, e.g., fowl poxvirus encoding prostate-specific antigen for prostatic cancer. The preferred vector candidates are poxviruses, adenoviruses, yellow fever, and the Bacillus Calmette–Guérin (BCG) vaccine. The strategy is being used for much work on human immunodeficiency virus (HIV) and malaria vaccines. Virus-like particles produced in vitro by the assembly of viral proteins are highly immunogenic and the basis for the HPV vaccines available today. A severe acute respiratory syndrome vaccine is being developed on the same premise. Cell culture techniques in use since 1950 are being further refined and offer the advantages of attenuation (many live viral vaccines), cold adaptation live-attenuated influenza vaccine (LAIV), single clone selection with the highest efficacy and lowest virulence, rapid and high productivity, and reassortment, i.e., mixing ribonucleic acid (RNA) segments of the attenuated strain with the protective antigen from the wild strain (pandemic influenza and rotavirus vaccines).

Deoxyribonucleic Acid and Ribonucleic Acid Vaccines

Deoxyribonucleic acid (DNA) vaccines are bacterial plasmids containing viral or nonviral genes that get integrated with the host-cell DNA and encode for the surface proteins of the pathogen, which are carried to the cell surface and incite an immune response in the body.[2] The first-generation DNA vaccines, though safe and well tolerated, failed miserably because of erratic immunogenicity. The second-generation DNA vaccines formulated with plasmids encoded with carefully designed antigens, delivered effectively by needle-free approaches, such as electroporation, particle bombardment, dermal patches, and simultaneous incorporation of genes encoding for molecular adjuvants, such as cytokines, chemokines, or costimulatory factors, such as granulocyte–macrophage colony-stimulating factor, have renewed interest in this platform. The second-generation DNA vaccines lead to a high antigen expression and a directed and predictable immune response.

Currently, there are 43 ongoing clinical trials, the majority being for HIV and cancer. The other targets being evaluated are influenza, HBV, hepatitis C virus (HCV), malaria, and HPV. Safe, stable, cheaper, and unaffected by maternal antibodies, there are concerns about genomic integration and anti-DNA immune responses, but these have not been substantiated in many nonhuman primate studies till now. The DNA vaccines undergoing trials, at present, are targeted for cancers (breast, ovarian, cervical, and lymphoma), HIV treatment, malaria (*Plasmodium falciparum*), hepatitis B, and influenza.

Due to rapid advancements in mRNA technology over the last few decades, compounded by the mRNA-based COVID-19 vaccine success during the COVID-19 pandemic, the current vaccinology world is focusing on utilizing mRNA-based vaccines. The mRNA-based vaccines offer several theoretical and logistical advantages to the traditional vaccines (live and attenuated pathogens, subunit-based, and DNA-based vaccines). These include:

- *Safety,* as mRNA is noninfectious and does not integrate with the host DNA.
- *Efficacy,* as rapid modifications in the mRNA structure can make the vaccine more stable and effective, with reduced immunogenicity.
- *Manufacturing and scale-up efficiency,* as mRNA vaccines are produced in a cell-free environment, hence allowing rapid, scalable, and cost-effective production.
- Moreover, mRNA vaccines have the provision to code for multiple antigens, thus *strengthening the immune response* against some resilient pathogens.

Currently, there is a wide variety of mRNA vaccines in clinical trials intended for infectious diseases (COVID-19, influenza, Zika virus, Nipah virus, RSV, and others), genetic disorders, and cancers due to the ability of the mRNA vaccine to balance both adaptive and innate immune responses. Majority of these vaccines are liposome-based and are in Phase 1 and 2 clinical trials. Moreover, around 60–70% of the ongoing clinical studies are being conducted with mRNA-based COVID-19 vaccines.

Transgenic Approaches

The euphoria of developing edible vaccines in the form of locally available fruits or other plant parts for oral use, providing mucosal immunity about two decades back was short-lived. The difficulties of standardization, regulatory affairs, and the potential risk of contaminating the food chain halted further progress. However, there has been a renewed interest in plant-made vaccines utilizing plants like tobacco, which are not staple foods, and using recombinant protein synthesis as used in yeast, bacteria, and mammalian cells. The proteins are highly purified and used as vaccine antigens. The two closest products have been a veterinary vaccine for Newcastle disease virus and the most recent attempts to express the protective antigens of various influenza viruses, including H5N1, in the tobacco plant *Nicotiana benthamiana* using an agrobacterium-mediated transient expression system, yielding a purified vaccine within 3 weeks of viral sequence release, and have completed phase II human trials in the United States of America. However, regulatory permissions would be delayed for such novel products.

NEWER ADJUVANTS

Live vaccines mimic a natural infection and induce a strong immunological response without unacceptable adverse events. However, the inactivated vaccines, be it subunits, peptides, polysaccharides, or DNA plasmids, need adjuvants to enhance immunogenicity. The conventional alum adjuvant, though safe, had its limitations of reactogenicity, incompatibility with certain antigens, and a narrow spectrum of only TH2 stimulation (humoral). Newer adjuvants, such as MF59, ASO_4, lipidated peptides, and the most recent lecithin nanoparticles, appear to be promising to overcome these limitations. Molecular adjuvants, which are plasmid-encoded vectors, are another novel approach to target specific regional APCs and are being tried for DNA vaccines **(Table 6.11.1)**.[3]

ADVANCES IN IMMUNOLOGY AND VACCINOLOGY

Immunology and vaccinology have a long, intertwined relationship. Both have had a different pace of development, and often vaccinology has lagged behind. The success of vaccines till now has rested on high avidity, long-lasting protective antibodies. The role of CMI, especially for chronic diseases, such as HIV, tuberculosis, HCV, HBV, malaria, and cancer, as well as mucosal immunity and the interaction between mucosal and systemic immunity (many respiratory and enteric pathogens), has given the necessary fillip to the development of vaccines regulating these pathways for higher efficacy. RSV disease can worsen with a vaccine that only enhances humoral response without adequately stimulating T-cell responses. The most recent studies on toll-like receptors (TLR)-mediated stimulation of innate immunity and neuroregulation of host defenses, newer adjuvants capable of inducing CMI, availability of laboratory assessment of CMI by enzyme-linked immunosorbent spot tests and tetramer staining, and systems biology techniques to study innate immunity have further opened exciting opportunities in vaccinology. The impact of T-regulatory cells on pathogens evading immune response has been another recent development. One can foresee vectored DNA and RNA vaccines and synthetic peptides using adjuvants, such as lecithin nanoparticles, lipid-in-water emulsions, TLR agonists, liposomes, and cytokines, to selectively guide host TH1 and/or TH2 for effective protection against many infectious and noninfectious diseases. Therapeutic vaccines for chronic infections by CMI viral load for HCV, HPV (E6, E7 oncogenes), and HIV (gag and tat genes) appear feasible in the future.

VACCINES IN THE PIPELINE

Though vaccines against 35 infectious diseases have been licensed, the future vaccine list is gradually expanding. A few recently approved vaccines against dengue, malaria, and RSV are mentioned here.

TABLE 6.11.1: Newer adjuvants and the immunological characteristics.[3]

Adjuvant	*Immunological characteristics*	*Usage in vaccines*
Alum (aluminum salt)	Depot and proinflammatory effects	Many vaccines (e.g., DTaP-hepatitis B)
MF59 oil-in-water emulsion	Local proinflammatory effects and immune-cell activation	Influenza and pandemic influenza
AS03 oil-in-water emulsion	Local proinflammatory effects and immune-cell activation	Influenza and pandemic influenza
AS02 oil-in-water emulsion containing MPL and Q-21	Induces antibody and cell-mediated immune response	Malaria vaccine candidate
AS04 (combination of aluminum salts and MPL)	Strong antibody and cell-mediated immune response, and toll-like receptor 4-dependent	Hepatitis B and HPV vaccine
CG sites	Toll-like receptor 9 agonist	Hepatitis B, cancer, and malaria
IC31 (oligonucleotides plus KLKL5 bacterial peptide)	Toll-like receptor 9 agonist	Influenza and tuberculosis
GLA synthetic lipid A	Activates toll-like receptor 4 receptors and induces Th1 CD4 helper cells with broad humoral response	Tuberculosis, leishmaniasis, and malaria
ISA51 (water-in-oil emulsion)	Enhances antigen-specific antibody titers and cytotoxic T-lymphocyte (CTL) responses	Therapeutic vaccine against lung cancer, HIV, and malaria

(CD4: cluster of differentiation 4; DTaP: diphtheria, tetanus, and acellular pertussis; GLA: glucopyranosyl lipid adjuvant; HPV: human papilloma virus; KLKL5: kallikrein-like protein 5; MPL: monophosphoryl lipid A)

Dengue Vaccines[4]

Dengvaxia® (CYD-TDV by Sanofi) is a recombinant, live, attenuated tetravalent dengue vaccine licensed for clinical use in 2015 and recently approved by the United States Food and Drug Administration (US FDA) in individuals aged 9–45 years with previously laboratory-confirmed dengue and residing in endemic areas. This vaccine did not perform well in younger children (aged 2–5 years), as there was a risk of severe disease and hospitalization in participants who were previously seronegative.

Denvax (TAK-003) by Takeda is a live-attenuated tetravalent dengue vaccine that showed efficacy at 80% and 56% against DENV2 and DENV1, respectively, in virologically confirmed dengue.[5] Even in seronegative patients, it showed efficacy of 88% and 45% against DENV2 and DENV1, respectively. TAK-003 vaccine has been approved in multiple countries, namely the European Union, the UK, Brazil, Argentina, Indonesia, and Thailand.

Dengusiil, another tetravalent live-attenuated vaccine, is under trial and showing promising results.

RSV Vaccines

Arexvy® (by GSK) is a recombinant subunit vaccine using prefusion RSV F glycoprotein antigen (RSVPreF3) combined with $AS01_E$ adjuvant. It was approved by the US FDA in May 2023 on the basis of "pivotal AReSVi-006" phase III clinical-trial data for clinical use as a single dose in adults aged 60 years and older.[6]

ABRYSVO® (by Pfizer Inc.), a bivalent vaccine, has been approved by the US FDA for use in both adults above 60 years and pregnant women (32–36 weeks of gestation) as a single dose to prevent severe RSV disease in infants <6 months.[6]

Malaria Vaccines

RTS,S/AS01 (RTS,S) is the world's first malaria vaccine recommended by the World Health Organization (WHO) against the deadly *Plasmodium falciparum*. The vaccine efficacy was 51% against clinical malaria and 45% against severe malaria. *R21/Matrix-M* Malaria Vaccine (by the University of Oxford) is the second vaccine recommended by WHO for the prevention of malaria in children.[7] With 77% efficacy, it is the first malaria vaccine that meets the WHO's goal of a malaria vaccine with at least 75% efficacy. In April 2023, Ghana's Food and Drugs Authority approved the use of the R21 vaccine for use in children aged between 5 months and 3 years old.

Other Vaccines

The world's first chikungunya vaccine, IXCHIQ (manufactured by Valneva), is a live-attenuated single-dose vaccine, approved by the US FDA in November 2023 for use in adults aged 18 years and older.

Many novel antigens from cancer cells and autoimmune disorders are being targeted for specific immune responses to prevent or treat disease and improve survival **(Table 6.11.2)**.[8]

TABLE 6.11.2: Vaccines in the pipeline showing technology and disease targeted.[9]

Vaccine/technology	*Targeted disease/pathogen*
Live vaccines: • Virus variant • Recombinant virus • Recombinant viral vector • Bacterial using recombinant bacterial vector	 • Rotavirus, RSV • HSV, polio, HIV using vaccinia/adenovirus, Ebola, allergy, and CMV using alphavirus • *Salmonella typhi, Vibrio cholerae, Shigella flexneri, Streptococcus gordonii, Listeria monocytogenes*, BCG
Inactivated vaccines: • Recombinant polypeptide-based • B-cell epitope-based • T-cell epitope-based • Conjugated polysaccharide-based • DNA-based • Nucleic acid-based viral vector	 • HIV and HSV, Group-A *Streptococcus* • Malaria • HBV and HIV • Group-B *Streptococcus*, *Shigella* • Influenza, HBV, and HIV • *Flavivirus*
Vaccines for noninfections	Glioblastoma, autoimmunity, multiple myeloma, diabetes, allergy, Alzheimer, hypercholesterolemia, fertility, pancreatic cancer, nonsmall cell lung cancer, HIV, melanoma, and prostate cancer

(BCG: Bacillus Calmette–Guérin; CMV: cytomegalovirus; DNA: deoxyribonucleic acid; HBV: hepatitis B virus; HIV: human immunodeficiency virus; HSV: herpes simplex virus; ROTA: rotavirus; RSV: respiratory syncytial virus)

TARGETING NEW AGE GROUPS

Conventionally, vaccines have been primarily used for infants and children, but the future needs demand universal immunization of adolescents and adult populations, especially targeted for diphtheria, tetanus toxoids, and pertussis because of the changing epidemiology of the herpes simplex virus, HPV, CMV, and influenza. A structured vaccination schedule may be desirable. The concerns of an aging population will merit a similar program for the elderly, e.g., zoster, influenza, pneumococcal, cancer, and degenerative diseases, such as Alzheimer's disease. Vaccination during pregnancy is done to prevent vertical transmission of infections (Guillain–Barré syndrome and HIV), ensure high levels of protective antibodies in neonates, especially for RSV, pneumococcal infection, and pertussis, and protect pregnant women against diseases, such as influenza, compounded by various ethical issues that merit consideration in the future. Protection against nosocomial infections and bioterrorism are areas where lots of new vaccines are being targeted.

COMBINATION VACCINES

The ever-increasing list of not only available but also desirable vaccines for children will result in babies becoming pin cushions. The introduction of new vaccines shall become challenging in such a scenario. To simplify the immunization schedule, it is imperative that age-appropriate combination vaccines are made available to simplify the schedule and provide better compliance and coverage with feasible costs and logistics. However, there are multiple technical challenges in maintaining the immunogenicity and safety of different antigens in combination vaccines. The need to combine pneumococcal and meningococcal vaccines with existing diphtheria–tetanus–pertussis combinations is being explored. To address these immunogenicity and safety issues, different carrier proteins, such as protein D, diphtheria toxin, CRM197, peptides containing T-helper cell epitopes, novel adjuvants, and developing in vitro assays for potency, are being researched. Several types of combination vaccines are currently under development, such as severe acute respiratory syndrome coronavirus 2 (SARS-CoV-2) + influenza and human metapneumovirus + parainfluenza virus 3.

TARGETING NEWER ROUTES OF ADMINISTRATION

Since most pathogens invade through the epithelia (skin, mucosa) or blood (cuts and abrasions, insect bites), the same routes have been conventionally used for vaccination, guided by the fact that most of the immune system is within or close to these entry portals. Because of the physical and chemical barriers posed by the skin and mucosa, the mainstay has been the parenteral route, which is painful and poses a big challenge to mass vaccination. It is now an established fact that mucosal immunity is highly important for protection against many pathogens. Recent developments in immunology, biotechnology, pharmacology, microbiology, and biomedical engineering have opened new vistas in alternative routes of immunization, chiefly the nasal and painless cutaneous administration.

Nasal administration has been found effective for LAIV, RSV, group-B meningococcal, Ebola, and human parainfluenza virus-3 (HPIV-3).[10] The nasal-associated lymphoid tissue elicits a strong mucosal secretory immunoglobulin A (IgA) and systemic immunoglobulin G (IgG) response. The secretory IgA can also be detected in other mucosal sites following nasal administration. Attempts are in progress to develop highly safe and immunogenic nasal vaccines by optimizing antigenic formulations and novel adjuvants and mass administration by inhalational devices.

Painless cutaneous administration by microneedles containing transdermal patches shall soon revolutionize vaccination practices. The microneedles just pierce the stratum corneum without reaching the pain receptors in the dermis. The breach in skin helps deliver antigen and/or the adjuvant to the abundant dendritic cells and Langerhans cells in the dermis.[11] Several studies using various formulations of influenza vaccine have demonstrated a dose-sparing, stable formulation and an early and directed immune response better than the intramuscular administration. Electroporation, jet propulsion, and ultrasonic (sonophoresis) are other methods being evaluated but are cost-intensive. Oral administration of inactivated vaccines and rectal or vaginal administration are other areas of future research (**Figs. 6.11.1 and 6.11.2**; www.path.org**)**.

TARGETING SAFETY AND EFFICACY CONCERNS

New vaccine development is highly cost-intensive and has a long gestation period until licensing. The stringent regulatory approach to guard against the remotest adverse event puts the industry on the back foot. Translational studies can help identify the early predictors of success by the assessment of early events after vaccination, such as inflammatory biomarkers and innate immunity activation within 1–5 days of vaccination. The safety concerns in the preclinical stage can be addressed using bioinformatics and systems biology to avoid vaccine antigens that can mimic human antigens (proteins

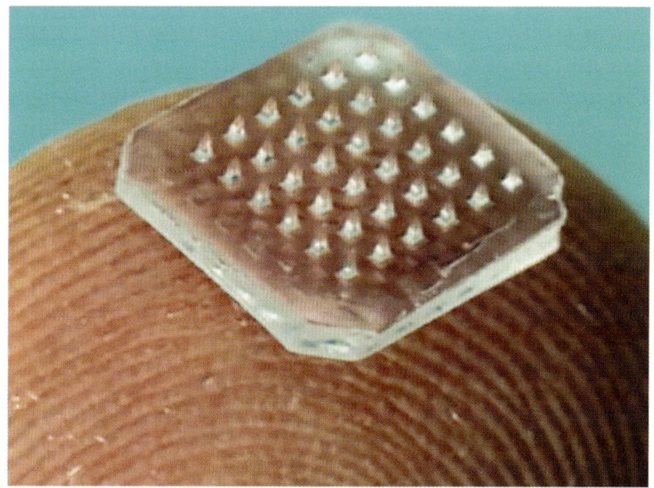

Fig. 6.11.1: Microneedle patch.
Source: www.path.org.

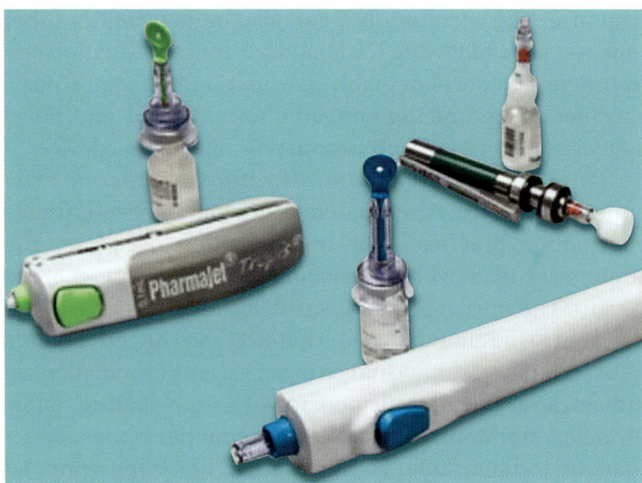

Fig. 6.11.2: Needle-free devices.
Source: www.path.org.

and polysaccharides) and cause autoimmunity. Microarray technology can effectively demonstrate immune stimulation at the site of injection within hours of administration. The vaccine formulations with extensive nonspecific immune stimulation are best avoided. Identification of specific genetic risk factors for adverse events is being studied to further ensure safety. This "bench-to-bedside" methodology can expedite the rapid development of safe and effective vaccines in the near future. The challenges of postlicensure assessment of vaccine safety and effectiveness are also likely to be addressed by the availability of large computer databases, comprehensive surveillance networks, and genomic information of the population.

TARGETING CHALLENGES

Vaccines are perfect interventions that prevent morbidity and mortality, yet their introduction into public health is a herculean task, especially in a developing country. The availability, cost, its sustainability, safety and efficacy concerns, regulatory constraints, logistics of access, and political will are the major impediments. In countries with a high disease burden, some trade-off for safety may be acceptable, but it may erode the already meager public confidence in the vaccination program. This decade shall clearly witness unprecedented development in vaccines, and a highly consistent advocacy by all the stakeholders is necessary to promote the simple idea that "vaccines save lives, prevent suffering, and create wealth."

REFERENCES

1. Facciolà A, Visalli G. Past and future of vaccinations: from Jenner to nanovaccinology. Vaccines (Basel). 2023;11(2):384.
2. Ferraro B, Morrow MP, Hutnick NA, Shin TH, Lucke CE, Weiner DB. Clinical applications of DNA vaccines: current progress. Clin Infect Dis. 2011;53(3):296-302.
3. Rappudi R, Black S, Lambert PH. Vaccine delivery and translation of new vaccine technology. Lancet. 2011;378(9788):360-8.
4. World Health Organization. WHO position paper on dengue vaccines - May 2024. Weekly epidemiological record. [online] Available from https://www.who.int/publications/i/item/who-wer-9918-203-224 [Last accessed November, 2024].
5. Rivera L, Biswal S, Sáez-Llorens X, Reynales H, Lopez-Medina E, Borja-Tabora C, et al. Three-year efficacy and safety of Takeda's dengue vaccine candidate (TAK-003). Clin Infect Dis. 2022;75(1):107-17.
6. CDC Newsroom. CDC recommends RSV vaccine for older adults. Centers for Disease Control and Prevention. [online] Available from https://www.cdc.gov/media/releases/2023/s0629-rsv.html. [Last accessed November, 2024].
7. World Health Organization. R21/Matrix-M malaria vaccine: Evidence to recommendations framework, 2023. [online] Available from https://www.who.int/publications/m/item/r21-matrix-m-malaria-vaccine--evidence-to-recommendations-framework—2023 [Last accessed December, 2024].
8. Plotkin SA. Vaccines: past, present and future. Nat Med. 2005;11(4 Suppl.):S5-11.
9. Plotkin SA, Orenstein WA, Offit PA. Vaccines, 6th edition. Philadelphia, PA: Elsevier; 2015.
10. Bitter C, Zimmermann KS, Surber C. Nasal drug delivery in humans. Curr Probl Dermatol. 2011;40:20-35.
11. Hegde NR, Kaveri SV, Bayry J. Recent advances in administration of vaccine for infectious diseases: microneedles as painless delivery device for mass vaccination. Drug Discov Today. 2011;16(23-4):1061-8.

6.12 Vaccine Hesitancy

Srinivas Kalyani

INTRODUCTION

Vaccine hesitancy, the reluctance or refusal to vaccinate despite the availability of vaccines, threatens to reverse the progress made in tackling vaccine-preventable diseases (VPD). Vaccine hesitancy has been recognized as an important emerging risk factor for nonvaccination, and was listed as one of the World Health Organization (WHO)'s "Ten Threats to Global Health" in 2019.[1] The WHO's Strategic Advisory Group of Experts (SAGE) on Immunization defines vaccine hesitancy as an individual's behavior that is influenced by the three Cs, i.e., issues of:

1. *Confidence* (no trust in the vaccine or provider)
2. *Complacency* (does not perceive a need for the vaccine, does not value the vaccine)
3. *Convenience* (ease or difficulty of access)[2]

India has a large number of unvaccinated and undervaccinated children. As of 2019, India is home to the world's second largest population of infants without the first dose of the diphtheria–pertussis–tetanus (DPT) vaccine.[3] A 2018 Wellcome Trust study found that over 95% of Indian parents surveyed believed vaccines to be safe, effective, and important. In Chandigarh, those with a high school education had 0.10 times the odds of vaccine hesitancy compared to those with less education. Those having more antenatal care visits were less vaccine-hesitant.[4] During Mission Indradhanush, the awareness gap was responsible for 48% of missed vaccine sessions, fear of adverse event following immunization (AEFI) was noted in 24%, and vaccine resistance in 11%.[5]

During the COVID-19 pandemic, fear of getting the infection, social distancing norms, and other infection-prevention control practices have adversely affected health-seeking behavior and routine visits. Primary healthcare services, including immunization, were disrupted, putting women and children at risk for VPD.[3]

As vaccine uptake peaks, the disease incidence declines and the adverse effects of the vaccine become more noticeable. Extensive media coverage of these adverse effects leads to a loss of confidence in the vaccine, as the public perceives the risk of vaccination to outweigh the risk of disease ("loss of confidence" phase). This, in turn, may increase vaccine refusal and ultimately lead to disease resurgence. Then, after a disease resurgence or an outbreak, as the public again appreciates the increasing burden of disease, vaccine acceptance is restored and vaccination rates increase ("resumption of confidence" phase).[6]

Determinants of vaccine hesitancy are grouped into three categories:[2]

1. *Contextual influences:* Influences arising due to historic, sociocultural, environmental, health system/institutional, economic, or political factors
2. *Individual and group influences:* Influences arising from personal perception of the vaccine or influences of the social/peer environment
3. *Vaccine/vaccination*: Specific issues directly related to vaccine or vaccination

Individual decision about vaccination is related to beliefs about disease etiology, safety and efficacy of vaccines, and views on the need for preventive measures. Previous experience with local health services and vaccination settings is another important determinant of the individual decision about vaccination. Moreover, the demand by parents for an active involvement in the decision-making process about health-related issues for their child has given rise to the practice of "shared decision-making" between health professionals and parents, which may hinder vaccination uptake.

Vaccine-related issues revolve around perceived risks of vaccines themselves or preservatives and adjuvants in vaccines. Classical examples include the measles–mumps–rubella (MMR) vaccine and autism, hepatitis B virus (HBV) vaccines and multiple sclerosis, meningococcal vaccines and Guillain-Barré syndrome, and human papillomavirus (HPV) vaccines and primary ovarian failure.

APPROACH TO MANAGEMENT OF VACCINE HESITANCY

Vaccine hesitancy is a continuum, from a parent who accepts all vaccines to a parent who refuses all vaccines **(Fig. 6.12.1)**. The aim of any vaccine hesitancy intervention is to move the caregiver from a state of hesitancy to acceptance of vaccinations.[2]

Motivational Interviewing

Motivational interviewing (MI) is an effective counseling method, in which the autonomy of the patient is respected.

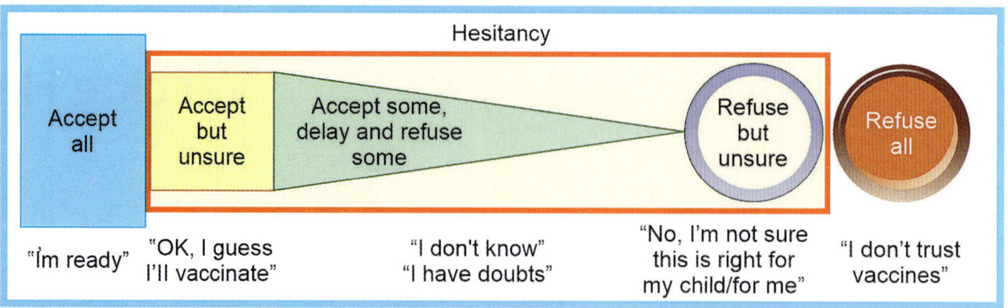

Fig. 6.12.1: Vaccine hesitancy continuum.

The approach is nonconfrontational and guides the caregiver toward change.[7] The process of MI includes the following:

- *Ask open-ended questions*: Every question should create opportunities for more discussion. "Do you think MMR vaccines cause autism?" is a close-ended question. The response could be yes or no. If the answer is yes, the conversation ends. On the other hand, "What is your opinion about the link between the MMR vaccine and autism?" is an open-ended question. There is scope for discussion.
- *Reflective listening*: Pay respectful attention to the content and feeling expressed in another person's communication. This lets the opposite person know that his/her views are being heard, respected, and analyzed.
- *Eliciting pros and cons of change*: Risk of disease versus the risk of vaccination. Discuss the indirect benefits of vaccination.
- *Establish a positive dialogue*: Listen to parental views, seek sources of information, discuss about what vaccines have achieved in reducing mortality and suffering, and emphasize the process by which vaccine safety is assured at all stages of development and after use in the population.
- *Discuss information* from authentic sources and explain in simple language without medical jargon.
- *Discuss specific concerns*: Autism, adjuvants, preservatives, overload of the immune system, injection pain, etc.

In observational studies, a presumptive approach (e.g., "He is due for three shots today") was associated with less parental resistance to immunizations than a participatory approach (e.g., "What would you like to do about shots?").

Maintain a relationship whenever possible—encourage providers to make continuous and strident efforts toward educating parents who are vaccine-hesitant, maintaining the relationship whenever possible.[8]

Healthcare providers (HCPs) have a unique opportunity to counsel women of reproductive age, including pregnant and postpartum patients, about the importance of receiving COVID-19, influenza, and tetanus toxoid, reduced diphtheria toxoid, and acellular pertussis (Tdap) vaccines.

Communication Strategies

The goal is to maintain public trust in vaccines and immunization safety and achieve a high level of immunization coverage. Healthcare workers (HCWs) must communicate the importance and benefits of vaccination, as well as restore confidence in the National Immunization Program (NIP) should an AEFI occur.

Vaccine hesitancy is increasing now because of the "crowded" vaccination schedule along with "greater access to vaccine-critical messages via digital networks."[9] Lack of awareness of the need to vaccinate is one key factor in people not getting vaccinations.

Selecting Proper Media

New digital technologies have "disrupted" traditional vaccine information communication. The challenge for NIPs is to proactively apply innovative and participatory communication approaches with evidence-based messages.[10]

Mobile applications that are helpful in reminding parents of their children's next vaccination appointments while providing information on child development, growth, nutrition, and vaccines would prove to be popular. As technology is highly dynamic, mobile apps should be rapidly produced, introduced, evaluated, and then reiterated to incorporate new findings.

Building partnerships with the media and social media influencers is key to keeping the public regularly informed about and engaged with the benefits of immunization and to timely information sharing on vaccine safety issues.

PRE-EMPTING VACCINE HESITANCY

Discussions and dissemination of information about vaccines should be initiated with the prospective parents before the delivery and during the first few postnatal appointments. Parents can be provided with the *"IAP Q&A on vaccines"* leaflets and credible web sources of information about vaccines, and opportunities should be provided to ask questions. One-on-one discussion with a trusted pediatrician is the most likely avenue for changing a parent's stance on vaccines. An observational study found that 47% of parents eventually consented to vaccines after initial refusal when their physicians continued to engage with them on the issue.[11]

REFERENCES

1. World Health Organization. Ten threats to global health in 2019. [online] Available from https://www.who.int/news-room/spotlight/ten-threats-to-global-health-in-2019. [Last accessed November, 2024].
2. MacDonald NE; the SAGE Working Group on Vaccine Hesitancy. Vaccine hesitancy: definition, scope and determinants. Vaccine. 2015;32(34):4161-4.
3. Chard AN, Gacic-Dobo M, Diallo MS, Sodha SV, Wallace AS. Routine vaccination coverage worldwide, 2019. MMWR Morb Mortal Wkly Rep. 2020;69(45):1706-10.
4. Wagner AL, Shotwell A, Boulton ML, Carlson BF, Mathew JL. Vaccine hesitancy in Chandigarh, India. Front Med (Lausanne). 2021;7:585579.
5. Gurnani V, Haldar P, Aggarwal MK, Das M, Chauhan A, Murray J, et al. Improving vaccination coverage in India: lessons from intensified mission Indradhanush, a cross-sectoral systems strengthening strategy. BMJ. 2018;363:k4782.
6. World Health Organization (WHO). Vaccine Safety Communication: Guide for Immunization Programme Managers and National Regulatory Authorities. Manila: WHO Regional Office for the Western Pacific; 2016. p. 76.
7. Gagneur A. Motivational interviewing: a powerful tool to address vaccine hesitancy. Can Commun Dis Rep. 2020;46(4): 93-7.
8. Navin MC, Wasserman JA, Opel DJ. Reasons to accept vaccine refusers in primary care. Pediatrics. 2020;146(6):e20201801.
9. Leask J, Willaby HW, Kaufman J. The big picture in addressing vaccine hesitancy. Hum Vaccin Immunother. 2014;10(9): 2600-2.
10. Penţa MA, Băban A. Message framing in vaccine communication: a systematic review of published literature. Health Commun. 2018;33(3):299-314.
11. Edwards KM, Hackell JM; Committee on Infectious Diseases, the Committee on Practice and Ambulatory Medicine. Countering vaccine hesitancy. Pediatrics. August 2016;138(3):e20162146.

SECTION

7 Infectious Diseases

Section Editor: Ritabrata Kundu

7.1 Fever and Fever of Unknown Origin

PP Maiya

INTRODUCTION

Fever in children is one of the most common manifestations of an illness, which makes the parents seek medical attention early. Fever occurs when various infectious and noninfectious processes interact with the host's defense mechanism. It is important that all children with fever are carefully assessed to find the cause. Nevertheless, the reason remains undetermined in a significant percentage of cases, leading to the designations of fever without focus (FWF) and fever of unknown origin (FUO). Even when the etiology is determined, fever remains the overriding source of anxiety.

DEFINITION

Fever may be defined in both physiological and clinical terms. Physiologically, fever is an interleukin-1 (IL-1)-mediated elevation of the thermoregulatory set point of the hypothalamic center.

Clinically, fever is a body temperature of 1°C (1.8°F) or greater above the mean at the site of temperature recording as follows:

- Rectal temperature >38.0°C
- Oral temperature >37.6°C
- Axillary temperature >37.4°C

Body temperature measurement sites are as follows:

- *From birth until 2 years of age:* Rectal, tympanic, and axillary areas
- *2–5 years of age:* Rectal, tympanic, and axillary areas
- *>5 years of age:* Oral and axillary areas

The ranges and means of temperature according to body site are listed in **Table 7.1.1.**[1]

TABLE 7.1.1: The ranges and means of temperature according to body site.

Body site	*Type of thermometer*	*Range (mean) Celsius*	*Fever in Celsius*
Axilla	Hg in glass, electronic	34.7–37.3 (36.4)	37.4
Sublingual	Hg in glass, electronic	35.5–37.5 (36.6)	37.6
Rectal	Hg in glass, electronic	36.6–37.9 (37)	38
Ear	Infrared emission	35.7–37.5 (36.6)	37.6

PHASES OF FEVER

Fever is characterized by three phases:[2]

1. *Phase of temperature rise* is often characterized by discomfort and is the result of decreased heat loss through vasoconstriction and increased heat production through shivering. The patient feels cold and the skin also feels cold to the touch.
2. *Phase of temperature stabilization (fastigium)* occurs at the new level of the thermoregulatory set point. Heat production and heat loss are balanced as in normal health, but at the higher hypothalamic set point. A flushed or pink appearance signifies that the fever has peaked. Once this phase is reached, the child usually feels comfortable without shivering.
3. *Phase of falling temperature or defervescence* occurs either by lysis (falling gradually within 2–3 days to a normal level) or by crisis (falling within a few hours to a normal level).

MECHANISM OF FEVER

The fever reaction is a series of cellular events that begins peripherally and ends centrally with a resetting of the body's temperature set point. Unlike hyperthermia, fever does not represent a failure of temperature control but rather an upward shift of the regulated temperature as a result of the body's exposure to infecting microorganisms, immune complexes, and other sources of inflammation. Various mediators like cytokines, tumor necrosis factor (TNF), IL-1, and IL-6 stimulate prostaglandin E2 (PGE2) production in the anterior hypothalamus, which brings about a rise in the temperature set point by a variety of physiological mechanisms, including activation of cyclic adenosine monophosphate (cAMP). When this happens, signals are sent to various efferent nerves innervating peripheral blood vessels to conserve heat. The vasoconstriction causes the feeling of chills, which may lead to rigors with sudden elevation of body temperature. Also, the thermoregulatory center sends signals to the cerebral cortex to initiate behavioral changes like seeking a warm environment, extra clothing, and flexed posture. All these mechanisms act to elevate the core body temperature so that the blood-bathing neurons in the anterior hypothalamus are warm and match the new temperature set point. **Flowchart 7.1.1** summarizes the pathogenesis of fever.

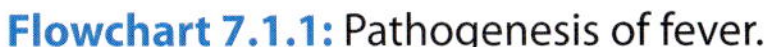
Flowchart 7.1.1: Pathogenesis of fever.

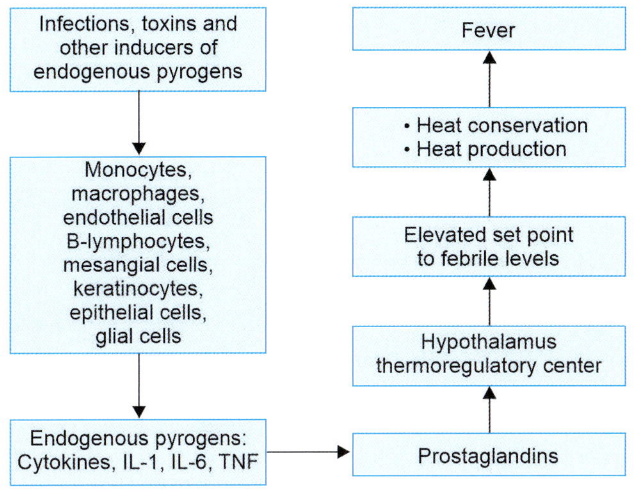

(IL: interleukin; TNF: tumor necrosis factor)

PATTERNS OF FEVER

Patterns of fever include the type of onset (insidious or abrupt), variation in temperature degree during a 24-hour period and during the entire episode of illness, cycle of fever, and response to therapy.[2]

- *Continuous or sustained fever* is characterized by a persistent elevation of body temperature with a maximal fluctuation of 0.4°C during a 24-hour period. Normal diurnal fluctuation temperature is usually absent or insignificant, e.g., enteric fever and malignant falciparum malaria **(Fig. 7.1.1)**.
- *Remittent fever* is characterized by a fall in temperature each day or recurring fever spikes daily or more than once per day with a variation of >1°C but not returning to a normal level. This is the most common type of fever in pediatric practice and is not specific to any disease. Diurnal variation is usually present, particularly if the fever is infectious in origin, e.g., most viral or bacterial diseases and pyelonephritis **(Fig. 7.1.2)**.
- *Intermittent fever:* The temperature returns to normal each day, usually in the morning, and peaks in the afternoon. This is the second most common type of fever encountered in clinical practice, e.g., malaria, lymphoma, and endocarditis **(Fig. 7.1.3)**.
- *Hectic or septic fever* occurs when remittent or intermittent fever shows a very large difference between the peak and the nadir, e.g., Kawasaki disease and pyogenic infection **(Fig. 7.1.4)**.
- *Undulant fever* describes a gradual increase in temperature that remains high for a few days and then gradually decreases to a normal level like a wave **(Fig. 7.1.5)**.
- *Prolonged fever* describes a single illness in which the duration of the fever exceeds that expected for this illness, for example, >10 days for a viral upper respiratory tract infection.
- *Recurrent fever* is an illness involving the same organ (e.g., urinary tract) or multiple-organ systems in which fever recurs at irregular intervals, e.g., familial Mediterranean fever **(Fig. 7.1.6)**.

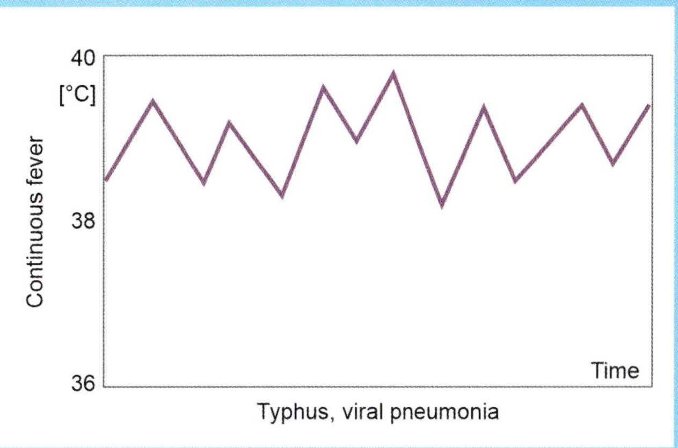

Fig. 7.1.1: Continuous or sustained fever.

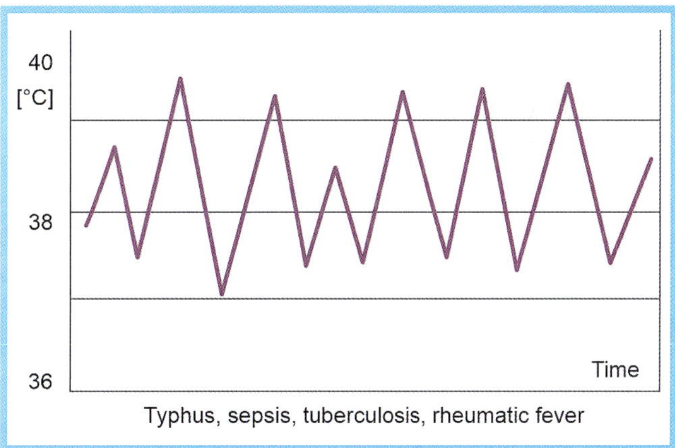

Fig. 7.1.2: Remittent fever.

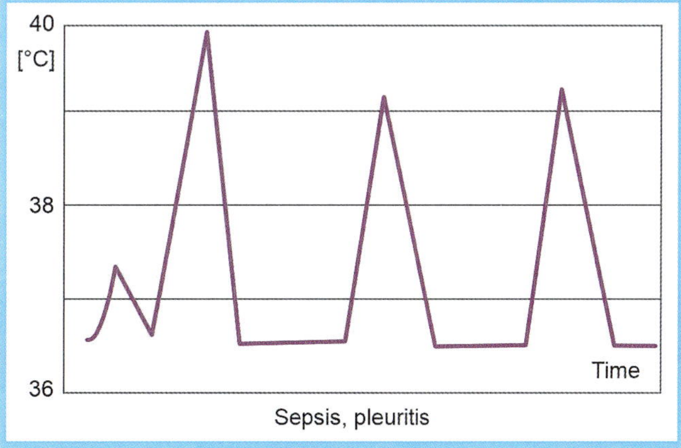

Fig. 7.1.3: Intermittent fever.

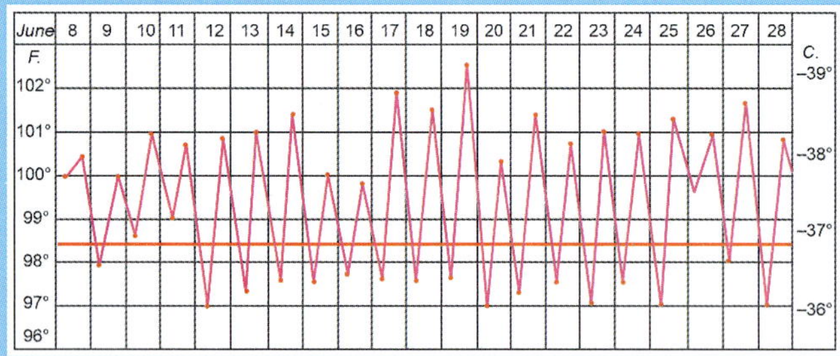

Fig. 7.1.4: Hectic or septic fever.

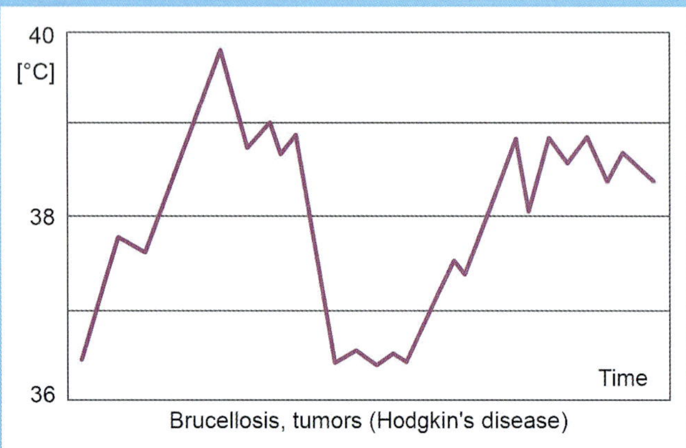

Fig. 7.1.5: Undulant fever.

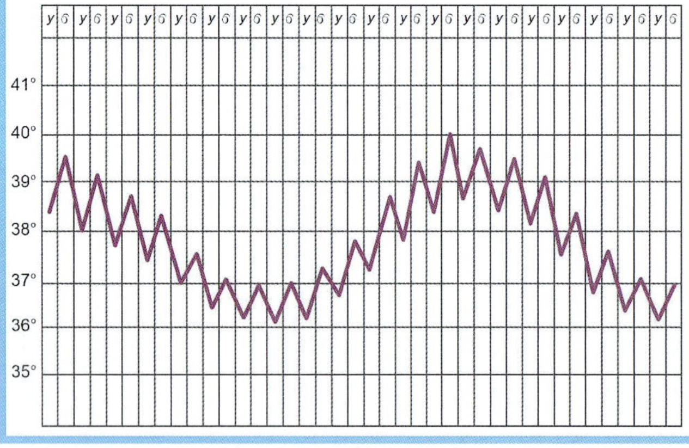

Fig. 7.1.6: Periodic fever.

- *Periodic fever* is characterized by episodes of fever recurring at regular or irregular intervals. Each episode is followed by one to several days and weeks or months of normal temperature. Examples are seen in malaria (termed tertian when the febrile spike occurs every third day and quartan when the spike occurs every fourth day) and brucellosis **(Fig. 7.1.7)**.
- *Relapsing fever (RF)* is the term usually applied to recurrent fevers caused by numerous species of Borrelia and transmitted by lice (louse-borne RF) or ticks (tick-borne RF) **(Fig. 7.1.8)**.

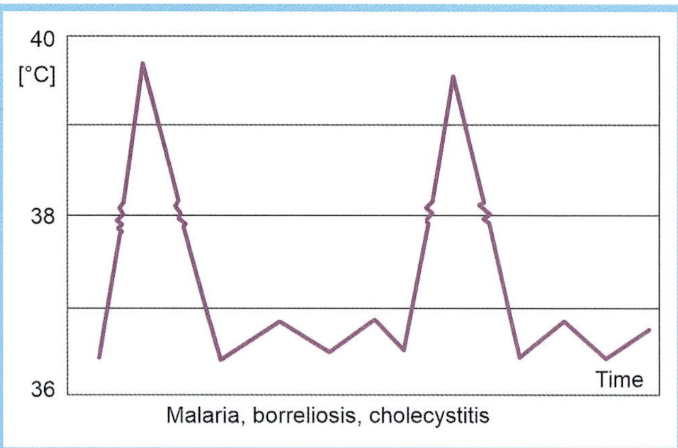

Fig. 7.1.7: Recurrent fever.

- *Pel-Ebstein fever* was originally thought to be characteristic of Hodgkin lymphoma (HL). The pattern consists of recurrent episodes of fever lasting 3–10 days, followed by an afebrile period of similar duration **(Fig. 7.1.9)**.

CLASSIFICATION OF FEVER SYNDROMES

The majority of febrile episodes in children is associated with infections. The diagnosis is made by identifying the focus, e.g., ear discharge and otalgia in otitis media, cough and respiratory distress in respiratory infections, vomiting and diarrhea in gastrointestinal (GI) infections, convulsions and focal neurological deficit in central nervous system (CNS) infections, and joint swelling in collagen vascular diseases.[3]

Majority of the children presenting with acute fever are due to viral infections. Many a time, one may find difficulty in differentiating between viral and bacterial infections. **Table 7.1.2** gives clues to differentiate between viral and bacterial infections.

Fever Without Focus

This term refers to fever of acute onset and short duration (<1 week) without any localizing symptoms or any clinical signs on physical examination. The following conditions are important causes of FUO:

- Acute viral fever
- Septicemia or bacteremia
- Vaccine-associated fever
- Urinary tract infection
- Sinusitis
- Occult bacteremia
- Prodrome of conditions like infectious mononucleosis, Kawasaki's disease, etc.

Fever with Nonspecific Signs

When the duration of fever is <2 weeks at presentation and the child manifests with hepatomegaly, splenomegaly, rash, jaundice, or lymphadenopathy, specific investigations

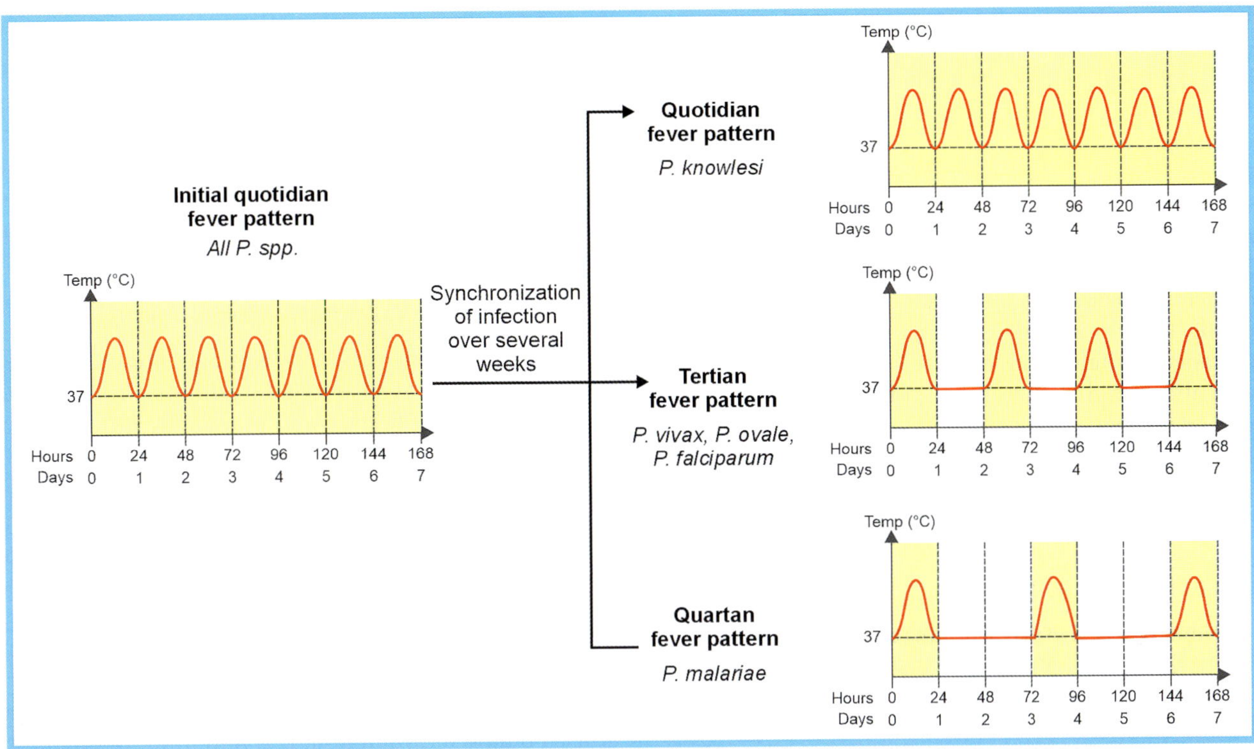

Fig. 7.1.8: Relapsing fever.

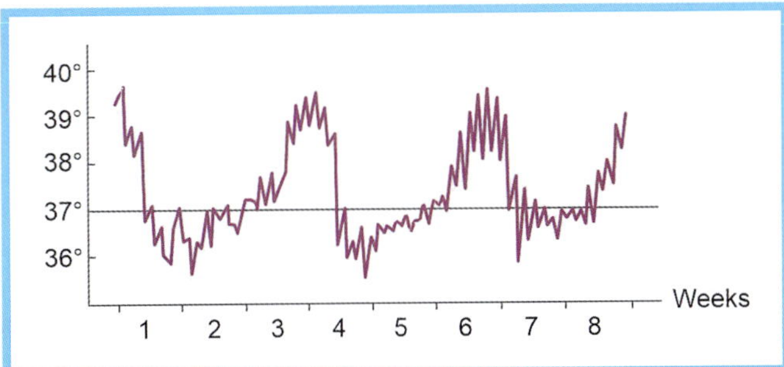

Fig. 7.1.9: Pel–Ebstein fever.

TABLE 7.1.2: Clinical differentiation between viral and bacterial infections.

Viral infections	*Bacterial infections*
Abrupt onset	Insidious onset
Duration 3–5 days	May last for more than 7 days
Prodrome usually present	No prodrome
Rash is very common	Rash is less common
Seasonal variations	No seasonal variation
Investigations are usually normal	Elevated WBC counts, CRP positive and culture positivity
No localizing findings	May have systemic localization and organomegaly
Mostly self-limiting	Require antibiotic therapy

(CRP: C-reactive protein; WBC: white blood cell)

for anicteric or icteric hepatitis, enteric fever, malaria, and infectious mononucleosis may provide clues to diagnosis. Assess the epidemiological details suggestive of dengue fever, leptospirosis, and malaria. COVID-19 and dengue infection are important examples of fever with nonspecific signs.[3]

Fever Complicating Chronic Illness

A child who has fever persisting for over 2 weeks may have a chronic disease to be investigated for lymphoma or leukemia. Childhood tuberculosis may present in a similar way.

TREATMENT OF FEVER

Whether or not to treat elevated temperature is a common question. To decide an answer, one must first identify the cause of fever and the degree of fever and then establish the goals of therapy. In patients with a fever of <40°C, there is no benefit of antipyretic therapy. The use of antipyretics will alter the pattern of fever, which may mask the diagnosis. The goal of the treatment is to correct the fluid deficit and ensure that the child's fluid intake is adequate. The knowledge that fever is an important immunologic defense mechanism has always been used to support the arguments against treating fever. There is enough evidence to support this view that uncomplicated fever is relatively harmless.

Fever has physiological benefits to the human body, which include the following:

- Increases immune response by increased production of interferons, B-cell proliferation, and increased bactericidal effect of polymorphonuclear cells
- Improves the nutrition of cells with a protective influence on their activity
- Growth and virulence of several bacteria like malaria and syphilis are impaired
- Augments hepatic synthesis of acute-phase reactants

There are situations where fever can be harmful in young children if not treated, e.g., debilitated children with systemic infections. It is a common experience that fever often makes a child uncomfortable and increases metabolic rate, oxygen consumption, and carbon monoxide production. It also increases demands on the cardiopulmonary system. Therefore, administration of antipyretics becomes necessary in children.

Indications for antipyretic therapy for fever >101°F include:

- Children known to have febrile convulsions
- Shivering
- Children with heart disease

The characteristics of an ideal antipyretic are as follows:

- Give a rapid result and be effective in reducing fever by at least 1°C (1.8°F)
- Be available in liquid and suppository forms
- To have a low rate of side effects in therapeutic doses and low toxicity when taken in overdose
- To have a low incidence of interaction with other medications and rarely contraindication in pediatric doses

Drug Therapy for Fever

Table 7.1.3 lists commonly used medications for fever in children.[2,4,5]

SUPPORTIVE THERAPY

Physical therapy is often used to promote loss of heat in high grades of fever, which includes the following:

- Remove excess clothing or blankets and keep the child in a well-ventilated room.
- Encourage to take extra fluids to compensate for increased insensible fluid loss and to maintain blood flow necessary for heat dissipation.
- Discourage vigorous activities.

TABLE 7.1.3: Drug therapy for fever.

Drug	Preparations	Dosing	Frequency
Paracetamol	Oral	15 mg/kg	4–6 hourly
	Intravenous	10 mg/kg	4–6 hourly
	Suppository	15 mg/kg	4–6 hourly
Ibuprofen	Oral	5–10 mg/kg	6–8 hourly
Mefenamic acid	Oral	4–8 mg/kg	8–12 hourly

Tepid Sponging

Tepid sponging is a cheap, easy, and safe physical measure to reduce body temperature. Studies have found that tepid sponging is effective in the first 30 minutes. Some studies have found that tepid sponging for 20 minutes is ineffective and recommended 2–4 hours of therapy. Rapid cooling methods such as ice baths, alcohol rub down, and cool water enemas should be avoided.

FEVER OF UNKNOWN ORIGIN

Fever of unknown origin is a diagnostic dilemma for pediatricians because it is often difficult to distinguish clinically between benign and potentially life-threatening causes. Pediatricians face the important challenge of not missing the diagnosis of a serious illness or an easily treatable condition that can result in increased morbidity. Fortunately, FUO is usually an uncommon presentation of a common disease, with most of these common diseases being easily treatable.

The term FUO is best reserved for children with a temperature >38°C (100.4°F) documented by a healthcare provider and for which the cause could not be identified after at least 8 days of evaluation. It is important to differentiate FUO from fever without a source (FWS). FWS is fever where the source has not yet been identified and is differentiated from FUO by the duration of the fever. FWS can progress to FUO if no cause is elicited after 7 days of evaluation.[6]

MAJOR SUBTYPES OF FEVER OF UNKNOWN ORIGIN

- *Classic FUO:* This is defined as a fever of 38°C (100.4°F) lasting for >3 weeks with more than two visits within this period or 1 week in hospital. The possible etiologies of classic FUO infections are inflammatory conditions, undiagnosed malignant hyperthermia, and malignancy.
- *Healthcare-associated FUO:* It is defined as a fever of ≥38°C (100.4°F) persisting for >1 week that was not present or incubating on admission to the hospital. The causes include healthcare-associated infections, postoperative complications, and drug fever.
- *Immune-deficient FUO:* It is defined as a fever of ≥38°C (100.4°F) lasting for >1 week, with negative cultures even after 48 hours. Etiology is infectious in 40–60% of cases, but in 30–50% of cases, no cause is documentable.
- *Human immunodeficiency virus (HIV)-related FUO:* It is defined as a fever of ≥38°C (100.4°F) lasting for >3 weeks for outpatients and >1 week for inpatients in an HIV infection-confirmed patient.

ETIOLOGY OF FEVER OF UNKNOWN ORIGIN

Table 7.1.4 lists the common etiological agents of FUO.

TABLE 7.1.4: Etiology of FUO.

Abscesses	***Bacterial diseases***	***Localized infections***	***Spirochetes***
• Abdominal • Brain • Dental • Hepatic • Paraspinal • Pelvic • Perinephric • Rectal • Subphrenic • Psoas	• Actinomycosis • *Bartonella henselae* (cat-scratch disease) • Brucellosis • *Campylobacter* • *Chlamydia* • *Francisella tularensis* (tularemia) • *Listeria monocytogenes* (listeriosis) • Meningococcemia (chronic) • *Mycoplasma pneumoniae* • Rat-bite fever (*Streptobacillus moniliformis*; streptobacillary form of rat-bite fever) • *Salmonella* • Tuberculosis • Whipple disease • Yersiniosis	• Cholangitis • Infective endocarditis • Lymphogranuloma venereum • Mastoiditis • Osteomyelitis • Pneumonia • Pyelonephritis • Psittacosis • Sinusitis	• *Borrelia burgdorferi* (Lyme disease) • Relapsing fever (*Borrelia recurrentis*) • Leptospirosis • Rat-bite fever (*Spirillum minus*; spirillary form of rat-bite fever) • Syphilis
Fungal diseases	***Rickettsiae***	***Viruses***	***Parasitic diseases***
• Blastomycosis (extrapulmonary) • Coccidioidomycosis (disseminated) • Histoplasmosis (disseminated)	• African tick-bite fever • Ehrlichia canis • Q fever • Rocky Mountain spotted fever • Tick-borne typhus	• Cytomegalovirus • Hepatitis viruses • HIV • Epstein–Barr virus • COVID-19 infection	• Amebiasis • Babesiosis • Giardiasis • Malaria • Toxoplasmosis • Trichinosis • Trypanosomiasis • Visceral larva migrans (Toxocara)
Rheumatologic/inflammatory diseases	***Hypersensitivity diseases***	***Neoplasms***	***Granulomatous diseases***
• Behçet disease • Juvenile dermatomyositis • Juvenile idiopathic arthritis • Rheumatic fever • Systemic lupus erythematosus • Kawasaki disease • Kikuchi–Fujimoto disease • Metal fume fever • Pancreatitis • MIS-C	• Drug fever • Hypersensitivity pneumonitis • Serum sickness • Weber–Christian disease	• Atrial myxoma • Cholesterol granuloma • Hodgkin disease • Inflammatory pseudotumor • Leukemia • Lymphoma • Pheochromocytoma • Neuroblastoma • Wilms tumor	• Granulomatosis with polyangiitis • Crohn disease • Granulomatous hepatitis • Sarcoidosis • Familial Mediterranean fever, many other autoinflammatory diseases

(FUO: fever of unknown origin; HIV: human immunodeficiency virus; MIS-C: multisystem inflammatory syndrome in children)

DIAGNOSTIC APPROACH TO FEVER OF UNKNOWN ORIGIN

The diagnostic approach for each child has to be individualized. It has to be kept in mind that in most cases, the cause of FUO is a familiar disease with an uncommon presentation rather than a rare disease. For most patients, diagnostic evaluation may be initiated on an outpatient basis. However, young infants, children who appear toxic or chronically ill, and children who have been febrile for a prolonged period should be hospitalized for evaluation. Hospitalization helps in documenting the fever, exploring the history further, repeating the physical examination, and maintaining constant observation along with laboratory evaluation.[7,8]

History

Carefully taken and detailed history is the most important tool in the diagnosis of FUO.

- *Age:* Neonates and young children are susceptible to specific organisms like *Listeria monocytogenes* and group *B Streptococcus*. Connective tissue disorders are four times more common in children who are >6 years old.

- *Sex:* Chronic granulomatous disease and Bruton's agammaglobulinemia are restricted to boys. Pelvic inflammatory disease occurs more often in females.
- *History of fever in family members or neighbors* may point toward an infectious cause of fever.
- *Contact with tuberculosis* may suggest the possibility of tuberculosis.
- *Pets in the house* raise the possibility of toxoplasmosis, visceral larva migrans, and cat scratch disease.
- *History of pica and ingestion of dirt* provide clues for toxocara or toxoplasma infection.
- Note should be made about the *presence of epidemics in the community* like dengue, enteroviral, and leptospira infections for considering appropriate diagnosis.
- Take details regarding *travel* to areas with endemic illnesses.
- *Recent history of surgery* suggests the possibility of occult infection.
- *Medication history* should be looked into and should include over-the-counter preparation and topical agents, including atropine (atropine-induced fever).
- *Genetic background of the patient* is important for conditions like Riley–Day syndrome.

Physical Examination and Clues to the Diagnosis of Fever of Unknown Origin

Careful and meticulous physical examination is mandatory in all children with FUO. Repetitive examinations, preferably daily, are important to pick up subtle or new signs that appear during the course of illness and help in identifying the etiology. Following are the clinical parameters, which give clues to the diagnosis:[7,8]

- *Pulse rate:* Relative bradycardia in enteric fever, meningitis, dengue, and Weil's disease
- *Anemia:* Malaria, kala-azar, subacute bacterial endocarditis (SABE), and acute lymphoblastic leukemia (ALL)
- *Lymph node:* All lymph nodes should be described and recorded
  - *Generalized lymphadenopathy* is seen in Hodgkin's disease, ALL, and secondary syphilis
  - *Localized lymphadenopathy:* Glandular fever, Kawasaki disease, and Kikuchi–Fujimoto disease
- *Jaundice:* Infectious hepatitis, Weil's disease, malaria and liver abscess, and infectious mononucleosis
- *Skin rash:* Viral exanthematous illnesses like measles and varicella, meningococcemia, dengue fever, septicemia, SABE, and rickettsial illness
- *Clubbing:* Lung abscess, bronchiectasis, SABE, and liver abscess
- *Arthritis:* Rheumatic fever, SABE, meningococcemia, and leukemia
- *Bony tenderness:* Arthritis and leukemia
- *Eye examination:*
  - *Uveitis:* Sarcoidosis, juvenile idiopathic arthritis (JIA), systemic lupus erythematosus, Kawasaki disease, Behçet disease, and vasculitis
  - *Chorioretinitis:* Cytomegalovirus (CMV), toxoplasmosis, and syphilis
  - *Proptosis:* Orbital tumor, thyrotoxicosis, metastasis neuroblastoma, orbital infection, Wegener granulomatosis, or pseudotumor
  - *Fundus:* Choroid tubercles in tuberculosis
- *Cardiovascular system* should be examined for murmurs daily.
- *Musculoskeletal system:*
  - *Point tenderness* over a bone can suggest occult osteomyelitis or bone marrow invasion from neoplastic disease
  - *Generalized muscle tenderness* suggests dermatomyositis, Kawasaki disease, or mycoplasma or arboviral infection

LABORATORY EVALUATION OF A CHILD WITH FEVER OF UNKNOWN ORIGIN

Investigations should be appropriate and based on clinical history and physical findings. Additional investigations depend upon the child's presentation, which is listed as advanced investigations in **Box 7.1.1**.[9,10] Routine investigations should include total and differential blood counts, peripheral smear, erythrocyte sedimentation rate (ESR), urine analysis, and blood culture.

A total white blood cell (WBC) count >11,000/mm has a high likelihood of bacterial infection. Peripheral eosinophilia provides clues to parasitic infestation, immunodeficiency disorder, or occult malignancies. Direct smear examination with Giemsa or Wright stain reveals organisms of malaria, toxoplasma, relapsing fever, etc.

Erythrocyte sedimentation rate exceeding 30 mm/h indicates inflammation and needs further evaluation. ESR >100 mm/h may suggest tuberculosis, Kawasaki disease, autoimmune, or malignant diseases. *Procalcitonin (PCT)*, a precursor to the hormone calcitonin, is a biomarker for bacterial infection. Levels >2.0 ng/mL are highly suggestive of systemic bacterial infection.

Blood culture should include aerobic and anaerobic cultures.

The chest X-ray should be an initial investigation. An X-ray of the sinuses, mastoids, or GI tract may be indicated by a specific history or physical findings. Other investigations like ultrasonography, computed tomography (CT) scan, and bone marrow examination must precede stepwise. Lumbar puncture is necessary in a young infant or child with meningeal signs and altered mental status.

Isotope scans with technetium-99 m, gallium citrate, and indium-111 labeled leukocytes help in localizing

BOX 7.1.1: Laboratory evaluation of a child with FUO.

Routine workup:
- Complete blood count with differential count; peripheral blood swear C-reactive protein; ESR; ferritin; procalcitonin
- Blood cultures
- Renal and hepatic function tests; LDH
- *Urine:* Routine and microscopy examination with culture
- Throat swab culture
- Mantoux test (PPD, 2 TU)
- Cardiologic evaluation with echocardiography
- Abdominal ultrasound
- Chest X-ray (to rule out infiltrates, effusions, or enlarged hilar lymph nodes)
- HIV serology

Categorical workup:
- Infectious diseases
  - Specific antibody or molecular test for EBV, CMV, *Toxoplasma*, Parvovirus, HIV, *Salmonella*, *Brucella*, *Bartonella*, *Yersinia*, *Borrelia*, and *Leishmania*
  - Blood culture-aerobic and anaerobic
  - Cerebrospinal fluid culture if indicated
  - Thick and thin blood smears for malaria FDG-PET/CT whole-body scanning to diagnose infectious and noninfectious inflammatory foci
  - Whole-body Tc-99m MDP bone scan for suspected bone infection; head MRI for suspected central nervous system infections

Oncologic diseases:
- Bone marrow biopsy and aspiration
- *Lymph node biopsy:* Uric acid for suspected leukemia and lymphoma (consider tumor lysis syndrome)
- Chest-abdomen-pelvic CT scan for suspected masses (or pyogenic collections) and related enlarged lymph nodes
- Positron emission tomography/computed tomography (PET/CT) in order to detect neoplasms, infections and inflammation
- Lymphangiography to localize retroperitoneal, aortic, and iliac lymph nodes
- 24-hour urine collection for total catecholamines, vanillylmandelic acid, and metanephrines, monitoring for suspected pheochromocytoma

Autoimmune/rheumatological:
- Autoimmune workup (RA factor and ANA factors)
- Thyroid function tests

Immunodeficiency:
- Immunoglobulins and lymphocyte surface marker analysis for humoral and cellular immunodeficiencies
- Assessment of neutrophil function

Gastrointestinal:
- Upper GI series and barium enema to detect changes or abnormalities in esophagus, stomach, duodenum, and colon
- ASCA, ANCA, LKM, and ASMA antibodies for suspected inflammatory GI disorders
- Exploratory laparotomy

(2 TU: 2 tuberculin unit; ANCA: anti-neutrophil cytoplasmic antibodies; ASCA: antisaccharomyces cerevisiae antibody; ASMA: anti-smooth muscle antibody; CT: computed tomography; CMV: cytomegalovirus; ESR: erythrocyte sedimentation rate; EBV: Epstein–Barr virus; FDG-PET/CT: fluorodeoxyglucose-positron emission tomography/computed tomography; FUO: fever of unknown origin; GI: gastrointestinal; HIV: human immunodeficiency virus; LDH: lactate dehydrogenase; LKM: kidney microsomal antibodies; MDP: methylene diphosphonate; MRI: magnetic resonance imaging; PPD: purified protein derivative; RA: rheumatoid arthritis)

inflammatory processes. 18F-fluorodeoxyglucose positron emission tomography (18-FDG-PET), in which radiolabeled glucose marks foci of increased glucose metabolism, has been used successfully in oncology diagnostics and can also be used to diagnose infectious and noninfectious inflammatory foci. Bronchoscopy, laparoscopy, GI endoscopy, and mediastinoscopy may be warranted on the individual merits of the case. Lymphangiography is resorted to localize aortic, iliac, and retroperitoneal lymph nodes.

Exploratory laparotomy is performed when all the other diagnostic procedures fail.

TREATMENT OF FEVER OF UNKNOWN ORIGIN

As far as possible, any treatment for FUO should be started only when sufficient grounds for diagnosis are available. Mild antipyretics are given for patient comfort. An empirical trial with antibiotics may mask the diagnosis of infective endocarditis, osteomyelitis, or meningitis. In general, observation of the temperature pattern, repeated clinical examination, careful laboratory evaluation, and interpretation of the results might throw a light on the diagnosis. Specific treatment depends on the diagnosis.

REFERENCES

1. National Institute for Health and Care Excellence. (2019). Fever in under 5s: assessment and initial management. NICE guidelines [NG143]. [online] Available from https://www.nice.org.uk/guidance/ng143 [Last accessed November, 2024].
2. Ashwath D. Fever: pathophysiology and types. Indian J Pract Pediatr. 2021;23(3):225-8.
3. Long SS. Distinguishing among prolonged recurrent and periodic fever syndromes. Pediatr Clin North Am. 2005;52(3):811-35.
4. El-Radhi AS, Carroll J, Klein N, Abbas A. Fever. In: El-Radhi AS, Carroll J, Klein N (Eds). Clinical Manual of Fever in Children. Berlin: Springer-Verlag. 2009. pp. 1-25.
5. Chandra J, Bhatnagar SK. Antipyretics in children. Indian J Pediatr. 2002;69(1):69-74.
6. Arora R, Mahajan P. Evaluation of child with fever without source: review of literature and update. Pediatr Clin North Am. 2013;60(5):1049-62.
7. Lorin MI. Fever of unknown origin. In: McMillan JA, Feigin RD, DeAngelis C, Jones DM (Eds). Oski's Principles and Practice of Pediatrics. Philadelphia: Lippincott Williams & Wilkins; 1999. pp. 848-50.
8. Powell KR, Behrman RE, Kliegman RM, Nelson WE, Vaughan VC. Fever of unknown origin. In: Kliegman RM, Stanton BM, St. Geme J, Schor NF, Behrman RE (Eds). Nelson Textbook of Pediatrics, 19th edition. Philadelphia: Saunders; 2011. pp. 896-902.
9. Attard L. Overview of fever of unknown origin in adult and paediatric patients. Clin Exp Rheumatol. 2018;36(Suppl. 110):S10-24.
10. Steenhoff AP. Fever of unknown origin. In: Kliegman RM, Stanton BM, St. Geme J, Schor NF, Behrman RE (Eds). Nelson Textbook of Pediatrics, 21st edition; Philadelphia: Saunders; 2020.

7.2 Approach to a Child with Fever and Rash

Baker Ninan Fenn, Ebor Jacob G James

INTRODUCTION

A child with fever and rash frequently poses a diagnostic dilemma. Healthcare providers must be able to distinguish between benign and more serious conditions of this common clinical scenario. Making an appropriate diagnosis and formulating a suitable course of treatment are achievable with a systematic review of history and physical examination. Hence, an understanding of the common differentials of exanthematous fever in children would aid in appropriate evaluation and management.

Various causes of fever with rash in children seen in India are summarized in **Table 7.2.1**.

TABLE 7.2.1: Common causes of fever with rash in children.[1]

Infectious etiology	*Noninfectious etiology*
Viral infections: • Dengue • Measles • Varicella • Herpes simplex viruses (HSV) 1 and 2 • Human herpes viruses 6 and 7 (HHV6 and HHV7) • Parvovirus B19 • Epstein–Barr virus (EBV) • Chikungunya • Rubella • Influenza A and B • Adenovirus • Hepatitis B	*Drug rash:* • Stevens–Johnson syndrome (SJS) • Toxic epidermal necrolysis (TEN) • Drug reaction with eosinophilia and systemic symptoms (DRESS)
Bacterial infections: • Group A *Streptococcus* • *Staphylococcus aureus* • *Neisseria meningitidis* • *Salmonella typhi* • *Leptospira* *Rickettsial infections:* • *Rickettsia tsutsugamushi* (Scrub typhus) • *Rickettsia conorii* (Indian tick typhus) • *Rickettsia akari* (rickettsial pox)	*Collagen vascular diseases:* • Kawasaki disease • Systemic onset juvenile rheumatoid arthritis (SOJIA) • Juvenile dermatomyositis • Henoch–Schönlein purpura (HSP) • Systemic lupus erythematosus (SLE)

HISTORY TAKING

Most cases can be diagnosed based on a thorough history. It also helps to identify the day of illness, thus enabling the clinician to have a clear idea regarding expected complications, period of infectivity, etc. History should include the following points:

- Age
- Onset
- Duration of fever
- Type of fever
- Presence of prodromal symptoms
- Temporal association between fever and rash
- Sequence of distribution of rash
- Blanching or nonblanching
- Change in the appearance of the rash
- Treatment modalities for the rash
- Associated systemic symptoms
- Close contact with other people who have fever and rash
- History of travel
- Immunization history
- Recent medication
- Exposure to allergens and pets

The age of a child can help determine possible etiologies as summarized in **Table 7.2.2.**

TABLE 7.2.2: Age-based differential diagnoses.[2]

Age	*Differential diagnoses*
Infectious etiology	
<3 years	Measles, roseola infantum (sixth disease), Epstein–Barr virus (EBV), enterovirus
<5 years	Kawasaki disease, staphylococcal scalded skin syndrome, meningococcemia (second peak 15–24 years)
3–10 years	Varicella, rubella, erythema infectiosum
Noninfectious etiology	
<1 year	Systemic onset juvenile rheumatoid arthritis (SOJIA)
2–8 years	Henoch–Schönlein purpura (HSP)
>6 years	Systemic lupus erythematosus (SLE), juvenile dermatomyositis, rheumatic fever, polyarteritis nodosa (PAN)

The timing of the onset of rash after fever is also typical of various viral exanthematous illnesses. This can be remembered by the mnemonic "Very Sick Patients Must Take Double Tablets," where the letters stand for the following:

- *V*aricella: First day of fever
- *S*carlet fever: Second day of fever

- Small *P*ox: Third day of fever
- *M*easles: Fourth day of fever
- *T*yphus: Fifth day of fever
- *D*engue: Sixth day of fever
- *T*yphoid: Seventh day of fever

The associated clinical features, along with the rash, can help one come to a reasonable conclusion on the diagnosis, thus preventing unnecessary investigations and treatment. An etiological approach based on systemic features is elaborated in **Box 7.2.1**.

EXAMINATION

A meticulous examination helps corroborate the information obtained from the history and allows, most often, to arrive at a clinical diagnosis or helps in narrowing down the differentials. Care should be taken in accurately describing the rash based on its morphology and distribution. Examination should also include careful documentation of lymph nodes, involvement of the palms and soles, genitalia, oral mucosa, and hair. Targeted examination should be done to look for hepatosplenomegaly [Epstein–Barr virus (EBV)] and murmurs of the heart (infective endocarditis and rheumatic fever).

Rash can be described as primary features and secondary features of the rash, as elucidated in **Table 7.2.3**.

The morphology of the rash would also be characteristic of different infections. Macular or maculopapular rash tends to be due to a viral exanthem. Examples of different infective agents with their rash morphology are described in **Table 7.2.4**.

BOX 7.2.1: Differential diagnosis based on associated clinical features.

- *Prodrome of an upper respiratory tract infection:* Measles, rubella, erythema infectiosum, exanthem subitem, varicella, adenovirus, coxsackie, Epstein–Barr virus, and scarlet fever
- *Acute onset of fever:* Measles, rubella, erythema infectiosum, exanthem subitum, varicella, adenovirus, scarlet fever, infectious mononucleosis, infective endocarditis, Kawasaki disease, systemic-onset juvenile rheumatoid arthritis (SOJIA), and rheumatic fever
- *Insidious onset of fever:* Systemic lupus erythematosus (SLE), juvenile dermatomyositis (JDM), polyarteritis nodosa (PAN), and Wegener's granulomatosis
- *Small joint arthritis:* Chikungunya, dengue, leptospira, SOJIA, SLE, PAN, and JDM
- *Large joint arthritis:* Acute rheumatic fever and Henoch–Schönlein purpura (HSP)
- *Hepatosplenomegaly with lymphadenopathy:* Infectious mononucleosis, brucellosis, leptospirosis, and *Borrelia*
- *Shock with multiorgan dysfunction:* Meningococcemia, toxic shock syndrome, dengue, leptospirosis, and chikungunya

CLINICAL FEATURES

Viral Infections

Measles

Measles has a typical prodromal phase with fever and the 3 Cs—cough, coryza, and conjunctivitis. Koplik spots, which are gray-white sand-like lesions with surrounding erythema, opposite the lower second molar tooth are pathognomonic. An erythematous, confluent maculopapular rash (as seen in **Fig. 7.2.1**) develops on the fourth day of fever, starting behind the ears and forehead, which progresses downward (centrifugally and inferiorly). The person is usually infective

TABLE 7.2.3: Terms to describe a rash.

Primary features	
Macule	Nonpalpable lesion <1 cm in diameter
Papule	Palpable lesion <0.5 cm in diameter
Patch	Nonpalpable lesion >1 cm in diameter
Nodule	Palpable lump >0.5 cm in diameter
Vesicle	Blister <0.5 cm containing clear fluid
Bulla	Blister >0.5 cm
Pustule	Vesicle-containing pus
Secondary features	
Excoriation	Scratch mark
Lichenification	Thickening of skin caused by rubbing
Erosion	Partial loss of epidermis
Ulcer	Full-thickness loss of epidermis
Necrosis	
Scarring	

TABLE 7.2.4: Morphology of rash and etiology.

Type of rash	***Etiology***
Maculopapular rash	Measles, rubella, roseola infantum (sixth disease), erythema infectiosum (fifth disease), EBV, chikungunya, adenovirus, enterovirus, *Brucella*, *Rickettsia*, SLE, SOJIA, and drug rash
Vesicular rash	Varicella zoster, HSV, and enterovirus
Petechiae or purpura	Meningococcemia, dengue, chikungunya, *Rickettsia*, HSP, and cutaneous vasculitis
Urticaria	Coxsackie, *Yersinia enterocolitica*, and *Coxiella burnetti*
Nodular rash	Erythema nodosum (in tuberculosis), fungal infections, *Yersinia enterocolitica*, sarcoidosis, and IBD

(EBV: Epstein–Barr virus; HSP: Henoch–Schönlein purpura; HSV: herpes simplex virus; IBD: inflammatory bowel disease; SLE: systemic lupus erythematosus; SOJIA: systemic-onset juvenile rheumatoid arthritis)

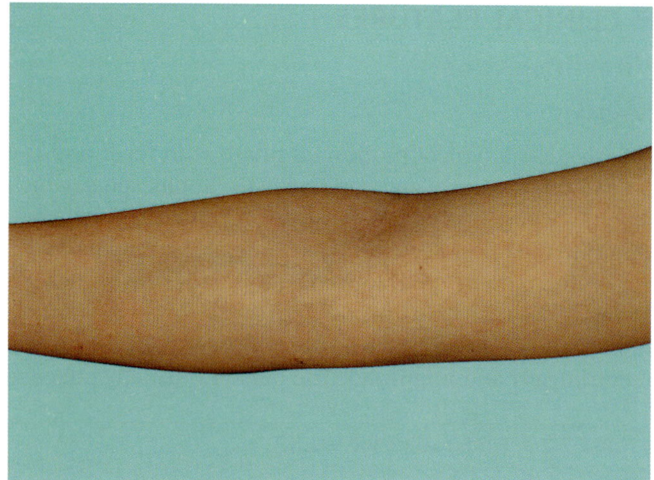

Fig. 7.2.1: Confluent maculopapular rash of measles.

4 days before and 4 days after the rash. It resolves in the same order with residual brownish discoloration and desquamation and fades over 10 days. Stimson line is a transverse line of inflammation along the eyelid margin seen in measles.

Rubella

Rubella characteristically has small, discrete macules, which are different from the confluent measles rash. Here the rash appears within 24 hours of fever and spreads from the face to the trunk and limbs rapidly and disappears by day 3. Even though the rash looks like measles, the patient does not look toxic. Another common observation is postauricular, suboccipital, and posterior cervical lymphadenopathy. Forschheimer spots are petechiae seen on the soft palate. The rubella immunoglobulin M (IgM) becomes detectable only 1–2 weeks after the onset of rash.

Varicella

The rash seen in varicella appears in crops and is typically polymorphic, as different stages of evolution from macule, papule, vesicle, and crusts can be seen at the same time. The rash usually occurs on day 1 of fever and disappears 3–7 days later. The vesicle is fluid-filled, surrounded by erythema, and described as "dewdrops on a rose petal." The child is infective till no new lesions appear or the last lesions have crusted.

Infectious Mononucleosis

Infectious mononucleosis, caused by EBV, has symptoms such as fever, throat inflammation, generalized lymphadenopathy, and hepatosplenomegaly accompanied by skin rash, which may appear as either erythema multiforme (EM) or urticaria. This rash occurs in 3–13% of cases but increases to 50% when treated with ampicillin or amoxicillin. Diagnosis can be made with antiviral capsid antigen (anti-VCA) IgM.

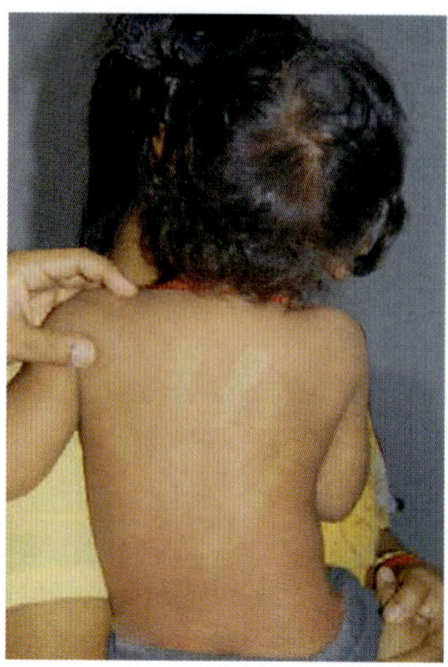

Fig. 7.2.2: Febrile rash and convalescent rash of dengue fever.
Source: With permission from Vijayalakshmi AM, Jayavardhana A. An infant with skin rash. Indian Pediatr. 2012;49(10):853-4.

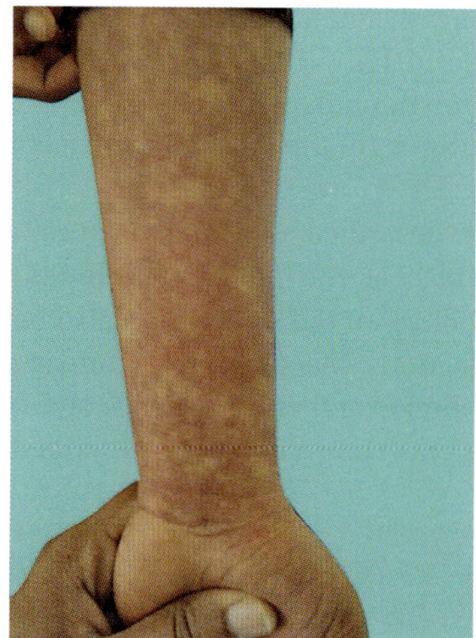

Fig. 7.2.3: Dengue recovery rash (white islands in the red sea).

Dengue Fever

Children with dengue fever experience a sudden onset of high fever along with facial redness, headache, muscle and joint pain, and abdominal discomfort. Within 48 hours of fever onset, they develop a transient generalized, blanching macular rash giving the child a flushed appearance **(Fig. 7.2.2)**. The fever may subside after 2–7 days, only to return after 1–2 days, following a typical biphasic pattern. The critical phase begins when the fever subsides and is marked by warning signs such as severe abdominal pain, persistent vomiting, bleeding from mucous membranes, accumulation of fluid, lethargy, and tender hepatomegaly. In the convalescent phase, a widespread rash resembling measles appears, sparing the palms and soles, described as "isles of white in a sea of red" **(Fig. 7.2.3)**.

Chikungunya

Chikungunya fever is marked by high fever with chills, along with severe joint pain, headache, myalgia, and a rash. The arthritis is polyarticular and migratory, typically affecting small joints. The most common presentation is a maculopapular rash occurring over the trunk, face, and extremities and associated with severe pruritus. It occurs 2–3 days after the onset of fever. Rarer manifestations include vesicles and bullae **(Fig. 7.2.4)**. Erythema and edema of post-traumatic scars and striae have also been described. Skin lesions usually subside without sequelae in the majority; however, many children can have hyperpigmentation, the most common site being the nose, followed by the face, trunk, neck, and palms **(Fig. 7.2.5)**. Some children can also have desquamation and xerosis. There are also reports of aphthous ulcers and purpuric lesion.[3]

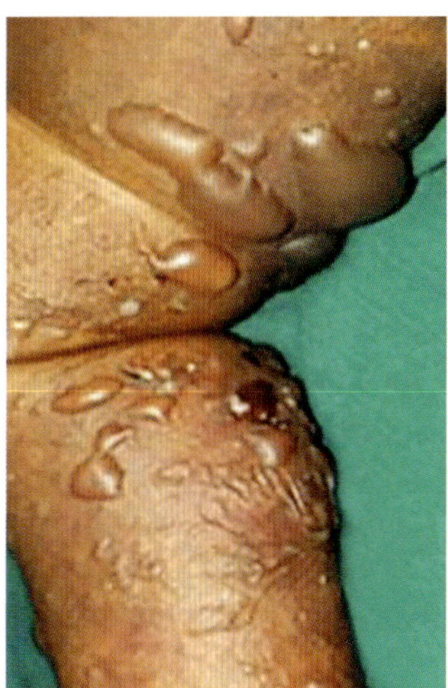

Fig. 7.2.4: Vesiculobullous rash.

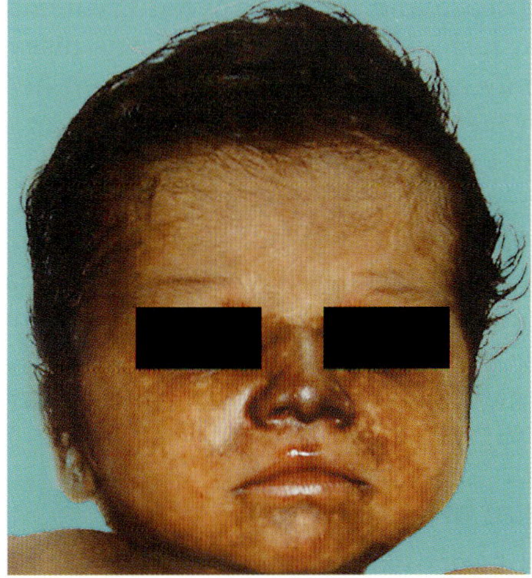

Fig. 7.2.5: Hyperpigmentation seen in chikungunya.

Herpes Simplex Virus 1 and 2

The lesions of *herpes simplex virus (HSV)* types appear as single or clustered vesicles ranging from 2 to 10 mm in size on an erythematous base. Recurrent HSV-1 infections commonly manifest as fever blisters, primarily on the lips, chin, nose, cheek, or oral mucosa.

Human Herpes Virus Types 6 and 7

Children infected with human herpes virus types 6 and 7 (HHV6 and 7) develop a rash known as exanthem subitum (roseola infantum or sixth disease), usually between 6 months and 2 years. The nonpruritic pink papular rash begins on the trunk and can involve the neck as well. HHV6 is known to be associated with a 10% risk of febrile convulsions. Pityriasis rosea, which mainly affects adolescents and young adults, has been linked to HHV6 and HHV7. It starts with a primary "herald patch" after a prodromal period. Within 1–2 weeks, smaller lesions with similar characteristics appear on the trunk and proximal extremities, distributed along skin lines and surrounded by scales.

Parvovirus B19

Erythema infectiosum caused by Parvovirus B19 presents as redness on the cheeks, resembling a "slapped cheek," along with a rash on the extremities and trunk **(Fig. 7.2.6)**. The rash fades and reappears due to triggers like local irritants, high temperature, and emotional stress. Parvovirus B19 also causes papular-purpuric gloves and socks syndrome (PPGS), characterized by edema and redness of the hands and feet with associated petechiae and purpura. The rash may extend to the dorsal surfaces but stops abruptly at the wrists and ankles, often causing burning and itching. Oral erosions, vesicles, lip swelling, and petechiae on the hard palate, pharynx, and tongue may also occur.

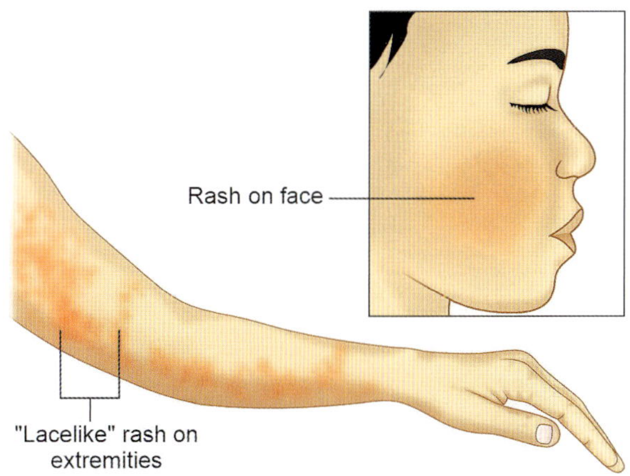

Fig. 7.2.6: Slapped cheek appearance and rash on extremities seen in Parvovirus B19.

Enteroviruses

Enteroviruses cause various exanthems, with hand-foot-and-mouth (HFM) disease being the most common. After a 2-4-day prodrome, large oval gray blisters with a red base develop on the hands, feet, and buttocks, accompanied by painful mouth ulcers. The rash resolves in 5-7 days.

Gianotti–Crosti Syndrome

This syndrome is also called papular acrodermatitis of childhood. This affects children aged 1-6 years and is linked to viruses such as hepatitis B, EBV, cytomegalovirus, and coxsackie virus. It presents with symmetric, flat-topped pink-brown papules on the cheeks, extensor extremities, and buttocks, often accompanied by hemorrhagic or moist eczematous papules. The rash lasts for about 15-20 days or longer.

Bacterial Infections

Staphylococcal Infections

In children, *Staphylococcus* can cause infections ranging from furuncles, carbuncles, and folliculitis to bullous impetigo, which may or may not be associated with fever, as well as toxic shock syndrome (TSS) and staphylococcal scalded skin syndrome (SSSS), both of which are associated with high temperatures. TSS is characterized by high fever, vomiting, diarrhea, conjunctival congestion, a "sunburn-like" rash, altered consciousness, disseminated intravascular coagulation, and low blood pressure. Symptoms resolve within 7-10 days, with desquamation of the palms and soles. SSSS predominantly affects children under 5 years old and is characterized by a scarlatiniform rash that becomes wrinkled with peeling of large sheets of skin **(Fig. 7.2.7)**, healing within 10-15 days without scarring.

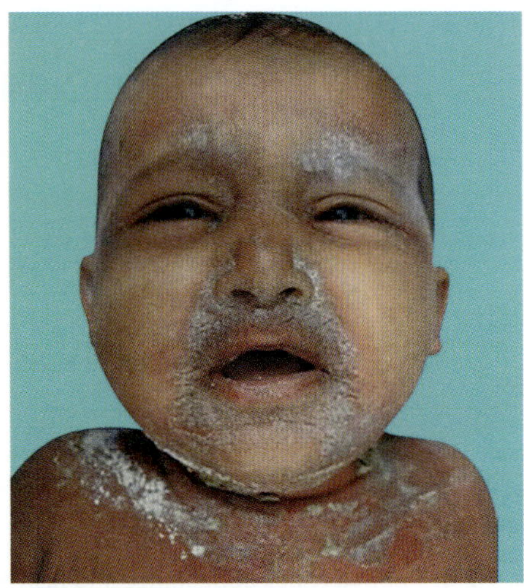

Fig. 7.2.7: Staphylococcal scalded skin syndrome.

Streptococcal Infection

Scarlet fever (SF) caused by group A *Streptococcus* (GAS) is characterized by a rash and strawberry tongue appearing 1-2 days after an upper respiratory tract infection. The rash is typically diffuse, red, and finely papular (like sandpaper), starting around the neck and spreading over the trunk and extremities but sparing the face. The rash fades with desquamation after 3-4 days. SF is noted to have the Koebner phenomenon characterized by skin lesions appearing along lines of trauma or pressure.

Erysipelas, also caused by GAS, is a well-defined, hardened, tender rash that appears suddenly with a high fever. Erythema marginatum is a major diagnostic criterion of acute rheumatic fever (RF), a nonsuppurative complication of prior GAS infection. The rash consists of red, serpiginous, nonitchy macules with central pallor, primarily occurring on the trunk and extremities but sparing the face. Enterococci and Viridans group streptococci can cause bacterial endocarditis, with cutaneous manifestations including petechiae, splinter hemorrhages, Osler's nodes, and Janeway's spots **(Figs. 7.2.8A and B).**

Meningococcus

Meningococcemia is mainly characterized by fever with petechiae. The petechiae are often raised with a "smudged" appearance, involving the trunk and extremities. Fulminant meningococcemia is associated with gangrenous hemorrhagic areas resembling purpura fulminans **(Fig. 7.2.9)**, as well as adrenal hemorrhage, low blood pressure, and multiorgan failure, with or without meningitis.

Borrelia

Borrelia infections can cause fever with rash, particularly in Lyme disease and relapsing fever. Erythema migrans, an annular rash, is characteristic of Lyme disease. It may be uniformly red or resemble a target with necrosis and vesicles in the center. The rash enlarges to an average of 15 cm with a sharply defined reddish border about 1-2 cm wide and resolves without treatment in 4 weeks. Relapsing fever consists of recurrent febrile and afebrile periods, each lasting 2-7 days. Usually, the end of the primary febrile episode is associated with a diffuse, red, macular, or petechial rash on the trunk and shoulders lasting 1-2 days. Jaundice, splenomegaly, lymphadenopathy, and central nervous system (CNS) symptoms may also occur.

Rickettsial Infections

Rickettsial fevers typically present with fever, headache, myalgia, hepatosplenomegaly, and lymphadenopathy, along with a rash that may be macular, maculopapular, or

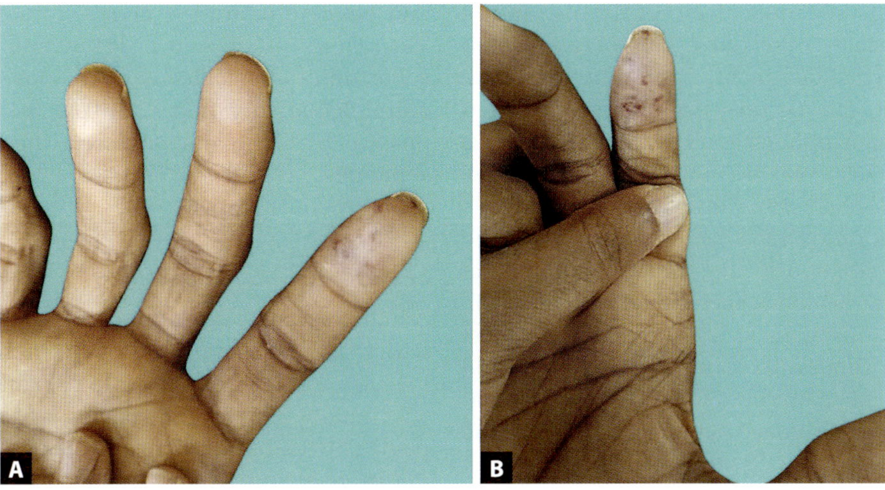

Figs. 7.2.8A and B: Janeway lesions in a child with infective endocarditis.

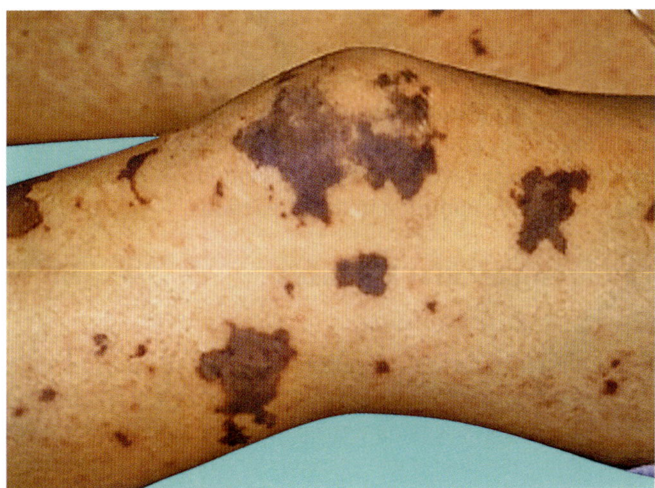

Fig. 7.2.9: Purpura fulminans seen in meningococcemia.

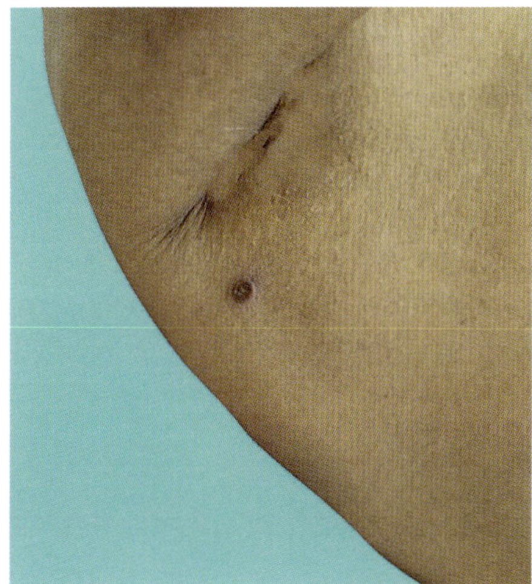

Fig. 7.2.10: Eschar in a child with scrub typhus.

occasionally petechial. Scrub typhus is usually associated with a painless eschar with an erythematous rim at the site of the vector bite resembling a skin burn of a cigarette butt **(Fig. 7.2.10)**. The rash involves the palms and soles in Rickettsial spotted fever. Thrombocytopenia is seen in Rickettsial fever due to clumping of platelets; the Weil-Felix test may be positive, and specific serology for anti-scrub typhus IgM and antispotted fever IgM is available. Doxycycline is the drug of choice.

Drug Eruptions

Acute Generalized Exanthematous Pustulosis

It is characterized by a sudden onset of fever accompanied by widespread scarlatiniform erythema and numerous small, sterile, nonfollicular pustules. The main cause is antibiotics, although mercury exposure or ultraviolet (UV) radiation can also trigger it. Acute generalized exanthematous pustulosis (AGEP) typically resolves spontaneously within 7–10 days, followed by desquamation over a few days.

DRESS Syndrome

Drug rash with eosinophilia and systemic symptoms (DRESS) syndrome is a severe idiosyncratic drug reaction characterized by a prolonged latency period. It typically appears anywhere from 2 to 8 weeks after starting the offending drug. Common drugs implicated are lamotrigine, abacavir, allopurinol, and minocycline. The clinical manifestations often include fever, rash, lymphadenopathy, eosinophilia, and various systemic presentations ranging from mild to severe. A wide range of cutaneous findings have been observed, including diffuse maculopapular inflammatory reactions (most common), erythroderma, Stevens-Johnson syndrome (SJS) or toxic epidermal necrolysis (TEN), EM, and pruritic eruptions.

Eosinophilia is the most frequently occurring hematological abnormality, observed in >50% of cases. Other hematological abnormalities include thrombocytopenia, anemia, neutropenia, and the presence of large, activated lymphocytes (atypical lymphocytes). Lymphadenopathy is present in a majority (80%) of cases involving minocycline, but it is rare in cases where other drugs are used. Hepatic involvement in the form of hepatocellular necrosis is the most common visceral abnormality, although abdominal pain, nausea, and diarrhea have been noted with abacavir. Renal dysfunction, mostly in the form of proteinuria, is most often observed with allopurinol. Minocycline (associated with eosinophilic pneumopathy in 33% of cases) and abacavir (associated with tachypnea, cough, and pharyngitis) are the drugs most frequently associated with lung involvement.[4]

The Japanese group criteria (J-SCAR) for diagnosing DRESS/DIHS (drug-induced hypersensitivity) include the following:

- Maculopapular rash developing >3 weeks after starting the suspected drug
- Prolonged clinical symptoms persisting 2 weeks after discontinuation of the suspected drug
- Fever above 38°C
- Liver abnormalities (alanine aminotransferase >100 U/L)
- Leukocyte abnormalities, including leukocytosis ($>11 \times 10^9$/L), atypical lymphocytosis (>5%), and eosinophilia ($>1.5 \times 10^9$/L)
- Lymphadenopathy
- HHV6 reactivation

A score of 7: Typical DRESS, 5: Atypical DRESS, <5: Consider alternate diagnosis.

Prompt recognition of DRESS syndrome is crucial, and the causative drug should be withdrawn immediately. Early withdrawal of the drug has been associated with better prognosis. Treatment is mainly supportive and symptomatic, and corticosteroids are often used, although the evidence regarding their effectiveness is limited. Other immunosuppressants, such as cyclosporin, may also be necessary in some cases.

SJS and TEN

Stevens–Johnson syndrome is a severe mucocutaneous illness with systemic symptoms. It is characterized by flat, atypical target lesions, epidermal detachment involving <10% of the total body surface area (BSA), and involvement of two or more mucosal sites. TEN is a life-threatening condition characterized by high fever, widespread (involving >30% of BSA) confluent erythema, and subsequent necrolysis. SJS–TEN overlap refers to epidermal involvement between 10 and 30% of BSA. Anticonvulsants, especially carbamazepine and phenytoin, are the most common causes of SJS and TEN. Other implicated drugs include antibiotics such as sulfonamides, penicillins, fluoroquinolones, and nonsteroidal anti-inflammatory drugs (NSAIDs). Nikolsky's sign is usually positive in these conditions, seen when the outer epidermis separates easily from the basal layer on exertion of firm sliding manual pressure.

Leukocytoclastic Vasculitis

Another severe drug eruption is leukocytoclastic vasculitis, which is characterized by blanching erythematous macules that later develop into palpable purpura. It may be accompanied by fever, myalgias, arthritis, and abdominal pain. This condition typically appears 7–21 days after the initiation of drug therapy.

Serum Sickness

Antibiotics have also been reported to cause serum sickness and serum sickness-like cutaneous eruptions. These reactions start with erythema on the sides of the fingers, hands, and toes and progress to a widespread morbilliform or urticarial eruption. Multiorgan involvement, fever, arthralgia, and arthritis are common in these reactions.

Collagen Vascular Diseases

Kawasaki Disease

Children with Kawasaki disease (KD) typically present with a remittent or continuous fever lasting about 1–2 weeks. The acute phase of KD is characterized by erythema and/or edema of the hands and feet, polymorphous erythema over the body and extremities, bilateral nonexudative bulbar conjunctivitis, redness, dryness, and fissuring of the lips, a strawberry tongue, and nonsuppurative cervical lymphadenopathy. During this phase, fever and all acute signs subside, except for conjunctivitis. The subacute phase, lasting about 2 weeks, is associated with desquamation **(Figs. 7.2.11A and B)**, thrombocytosis, and coronary aneurysms. The convalescent phase begins with the disappearance of all clinical features and lasts for the next 2–4 weeks until erythrocyte sedimentation rate (ESR) and C-reactive protein (CRP) levels normalize.

Systemic Lupus Erythematosus

Childhood-onset systemic lupus erythematosus (cSLE) is a serious, chronic, and systemic autoimmune disorder. The cutaneous manifestations include malar rash, oral ulcers, vasculitis, photosensitivity, alopecia, and discoid lupus erythematosus. Periungual erythema, Raynaud's phenomenon, periungual gangrene, nail involvement, and subacute discoid lupus erythematosus are rare.

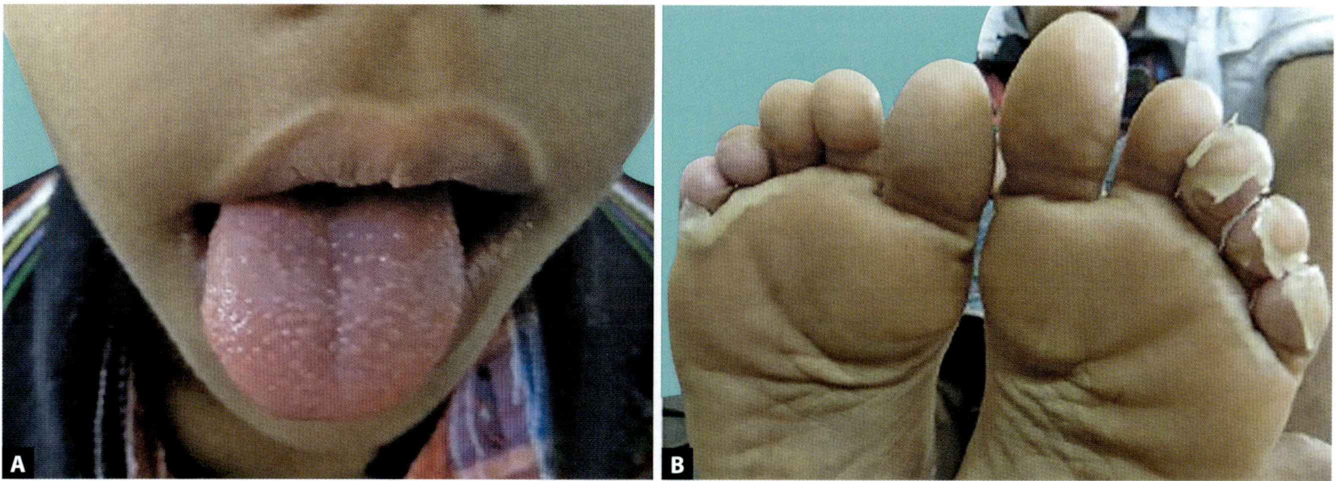

Figs. 7.2.11A and B: Strawberry tongue (prominent papillae) and peripheral desquamation.

Juvenile Dermatomyositis

Juvenile dermatomyositis (JDM) is a rare yet severe systemic autoimmune disease that primarily affects the proximal muscles and skin in children. The skin manifestations of JDM can be severe and challenging to manage, potentially leading to ulcerative disease or subcutaneous calcification, significantly impacting long-term quality of life. The clinical examination should include a formal assessment of muscle strength using a validated tool, such as the Childhood Myositis Assessment Scale (CMAS). Additionally, a thorough assessment of the skin is essential, including examination of the nail fold capillaries.

Myositis-specific autoantibodies are likely to be associated with distinct cutaneous manifestations. In the case of anti-MDA5 antibody-associated DM, cutaneous ulceration due to vascular injuries was related to rapidly progressive interstitial lung disease (ILD) and palmar violaceous macules/papules.

Severe cutaneous manifestations, including V-neck sign, shawl sign, heliotrope rash, Gottron's papules/sign, and flagellate erythema, are often observed in patients with anti-TIF1γ antibody-associated DM.

Mechanic's hands, characterized by keratotic erythema on the sides of the thumbs and forefingers, are generally specific to patients with antisynthetase syndrome, including those with anti-ARS antibody-associated DM.

Juvenile and adult myopathy patients positive for the anti-NXP2 antibody have a high risk of calcinosis. In contrast, anti-SAE antibody-positive patients with DM demonstrated extensive rash, including erythroderma with an "angel wings" sign, with pink, atrophic plaques on the back in an "angel wing" distribution.[5]

IgA Vasculitis

Immunoglobulin A (IgA) vasculitis, formerly known as Henoch-Schönlein purpura (HSP), is a complex immune-mediated vasculitis characterized by the involvement of small blood vessels in various organ systems. It primarily affects the small vessels of the joints, kidneys, gastrointestinal tract, and skin. As a result, patients often present with a diverse range of clinical manifestations, including gastrointestinal complaints, palpable purpura, arthralgias, and renal involvement. The purpura is typically painless and palpable, manifesting over the dependent areas of the body, such as lower limbs, buttocks, and back.

Systemic-onset Juvenile Idiopathic Arthritis

Systemic-onset juvenile idiopathic arthritis (SoJIA) is a subtype of juvenile idiopathic arthritis (JIA) characterized by at least 6 weeks of arthritis accompanied by intermittent fever, occurring daily or twice daily for at least 2 weeks, in children aged <16 years, in the absence of an identifiable underlying etiology. According to the newer International League of Associations for Rheumatology (ILAR) criteria, SoJIA is now more strictly defined as having a daily fever of ≥39°C and requiring the presence of at least one of the following clinical features of systemic inflammation—characteristic evanescent erythematous skin rash, generalized lymphadenopathy, hepatosplenomegaly, and serositis. The fever is classically quotidian, which means that it occurs once or twice a day, and with the spike of fever, an evanescent salmon pink rash appears over the body, which later fades with defervescence.

Polyarteritis Nodosa

Polyarteritis nodosa (PAN) is a rare systemic vasculitis characterized by necrotizing arteritis of predominantly medium-sized vessels, leading to microaneurysms, ruptures, and hemorrhages. It manifests with multisystem involvement of the skin, kidney, peripheral nerves, muscles, and gastrointestinal tract. Skin signs include purpura, Raynaud's phenomenon, skin gangrene, skin infarct, subcutaneous nodules, and livedo reticularis.

Flowchart 7.2.1: NHS fever and rash pathway.

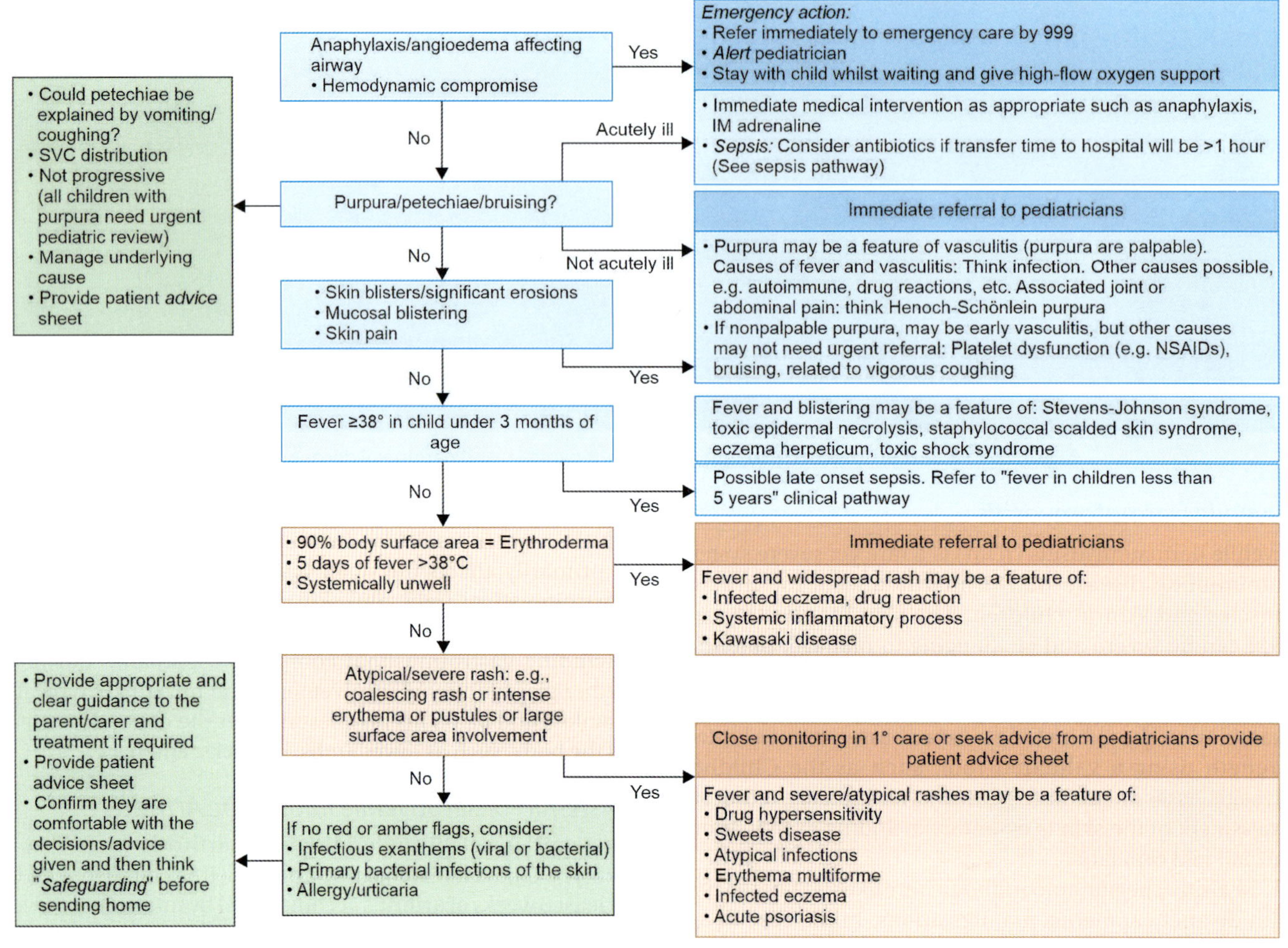

(NHS: National Health Service; NSAIDs: nonsteroidal anti-inflammatory drugs)
Source: https://abbhealthiertogether.cymru.nhs.uk/application/files/9815/2846/5539/CS45385_NHS_Rash_Pathway_Acute_Hospital_Setting_Mar_18_final.pdf

INVESTIGATIONS

Initial investigations could include a complete blood count (CBC), urinalysis, blood cultures, and specific serologies as indicated. Fluid from the vesicular lesions can be examined, the base of unroofed vesicles can be swabbed for cultures and sent for polymerase chain reaction (PCR), and a skin biopsy can be carried out.[6]

MANAGEMENT

Management plans should be carried out by determining the most possible etiology clinically. It is also imperative that clinicians be aware of life-threatening conditions presenting with fever and rash, and such cases be managed immediately or referred at the earliest. The National Health Service (NHS) fever and rash pathway, given in **Flowchart 7.2.1**, gives an example of a treatment algorithm from the primary care level.[7]

ACKNOWLEDGMENT

We thank Dr Winsley Rose, Professor of Pediatrics, Pediatric ID, CMC, Vellore, for guidance on the topic and permission to use clinical pictures in his custody.

REFERENCES

1. Sarkar R, Mishra K, Garg VK. Fever with rash in a child in India. Indian J Dermatol Venereol Leprol. 2012;78:251-62.
2. Manoharan KS, Ramasamy K, Heinz P. Rash with fever in children: a clinical approach. Paediatr Child Health. 2017;27(4):196-201.
3. Kumar R, Sharma MK, Jain SK, Yadav SK, Singhal AK. Cutaneous manifestations of chikungunya fever: observations from an outbreak at a tertiary care hospital in Southeast Rajasthan, India. Indian Dermatol Online J. 2017;8(5):336-42.

4. Choudhary S, McLeod M, Torchia D, Romanelli P. Drug reaction with eosinophilia and systemic symptoms (DRESS) syndrome. J Clin Aesthet Dermatol. 2013;6(6):31-7.
5. Okiyama N, Fujimoto M. Cutaneous manifestations of dermatomyositis characterized by myositis-specific autoantibodies. F1000Res. 2019;8:F1000
6. Kang JH. Febrile illness with skin rashes. Infect Chemother. 2015;47(3):155-66.
7. The NHS fever and rash pathway. [online] Available from https://abbhealthiertogether.cymru.nhs.uk/application/files/9815/2846/5539/CS45385_NHS_Rash_Pathway_Acute_Hospital_Setting_Mar_18_final.pdf

7.3 Healthcare-associated Infections

Digant D Shastri

INTRODUCTION

Healthcare-associated infections (HCAIs) are defined as infections that patients acquire while receiving health care. Previously, HCAIs were referred to those infections that were linked with hospital admission (called nosocomial infections), but now they also include infections developed in different types of healthcare settings where patients obtain healthcare (e.g., ambulatory care, home care, long-term care, family medicine clinics, etc.). They refer to infections that were not present in a patient at the time of approach to a healthcare setting, and there was no evidence of incubation of such infections at the time of hospitalization. The HCAIs are infections that first appear 48 hours or more after hospitalization or within 30 days after having received health care. These occur worldwide and affect both developed and resource-poor countries. Hospital-acquired infections increase the use of antibiotics, increase the cost of treatment, extend hospitalization duration, and result in elevated morbidity and mortality. They are a significant burden for both the patient and public health. Increased incidence of HCAIs reflects a poor quality of health service delivery.

EPIDEMIOLOGY

Magnitude

The prevalence of HCAIs at a given time in developed countries varies between 3.5% and 12%. The European Centre for Disease Prevention and Control reports an average prevalence of 7.1% in European countries. The estimated incidence in the USA was 4.5% in 2002, corresponding to 9.3 infections per 1,000 patient-days and 1.7 million affected patients. The prevalence of HCAI varies between 5.7% and 19.1% in low- and middle-income countries. The proportion of patients with intensive care unit (ICU)-acquired infections ranged from 4.4% to 88.9%, with a frequency of overall infections as high as 42.7 episodes per 1,000 patient-days.[1,2]

Sources

The source of infectious agents for causing HCAI may be endogenous or exogenous:

- *Endogenous sources:* Normal flora present in one site can cause infection in any other site when antibiotics are given inappropriately or if there is a breach in the skin or mucosa, e.g., wounds and catheters, which allows the overgrowth of *Clostridium difficile* and *Candida;* gram-negative organisms in the gastrointestinal tract can invade the surgical site or the urinary tract.
- *Exogenous sources:* Bacteria are transmitted between the patients through direct contact, e.g., hands, saliva, droplets, or by staff via contaminated hands or by contaminated equipment, visitors, water, or food.

Risk Factors for Healthcare-associated Infection

A hospitalized patient is usually in a "poor state of health," impairing his/her defense. Advanced age or premature birth, malnutrition, and immunodeficiency (congenital or acquired) present a general risk, while other diseases can present specific risks; for instance, chronic obstructive pulmonary disease can increase the chances of respiratory tract infection. Invasive devices, such as intubation tubes, central lines, catheters, surgical drains, and tracheostomy tubes, all bypass the body's natural lines of defense against pathogens and provide an easy route for infection.[3,4] Patients already colonized at the time of admission are instantly put at a greater risk when they undergo invasive procedures. Treatment modality in patients may leave him/her vulnerable to infections: Immunosuppression and antacid treatment

BOX 7.3.1: Risk factors for healthcare-associated infections.

- Prior antibiotic therapy
- Immunodeficiency
- Immunosuppression
- H_2 blocker administration
- Prior intralipid use (in newborn babies causing *Candida* infection)
- Parenteral nutrition, central venous line placement (in newborn babies causing *Candida* infection)
- *Extremes of age:* Gestational age of less than 32-week-old people
- *Associated comorbidities:* Diabetes and obesity
- Hospital stay longer than 7 days
- Cerebral palsy (urinary tract infections in pediatric patients)
- Reintubation (ventilator-associated pneumonia)

undermine the body's defenses, while antimicrobial therapy (removing competitive flora and only leaving resistant organisms) and recurrent blood transfusions have also been identified as risk factors (**Box 7.3.1**).

Contributory Factors

- *Reuse of disposable material:* Lack of affordability due to financial constraints in private healthcare facilities or inadequate supply of disposable material in public sector hospitals
- *Inadequate infrastructure* leading to overcrowding of patients and sharing of equipment (due to insufficient equipment)
- *Inadequate staff* leading to increased workload and increased chances of cross-infections
- *Lack of knowledge and application of basic infection-control measures*
- *Lack of well-written protocols*
- *Lack of local and national guidelines and policies*

CAUSATIVE AGENTS FOR HEALTHCARE-ASSOCIATED INFECTION

Healthcare-associated infections are caused by bacteria, fungi, viruses, and protozoa. About 90% of nosocomial infections are due to bacteria, whereas protozoans, viruses, and fungi account for the rest of 10%. The agents that are usually involved in hospital-acquired infections include *Streptococcus* spp., *Acinetobacter* spp., enterococci, *Pseudomonas aeruginosa*, coagulase-negative staphylococci (CoNS), *Staphylococcus aureus, Bacillus cereus, Legionella*, and *Enterobacteriaceae* family members including *Proteus mirabilis, Klebsiella pneumoniae, Escherichia coli*, and *Serratia marcescens.* Out of these enterococci, *P. aeruginosa, S. aureus*, and *E. coli* have a major role. Urinary tract infections (UTIs) usually contain *E. coli*, while it is uncommon in other infection sites. Contrarily, *S. aureus* is frequent at other body sites and rarely causes UTI. In blood-borne infections, coagulase-negative *S. aureus* is the main causative agent. Surgical-site infections

TABLE 7.3.1: Facility types and HCAIs.

Acute care hospitals (ACHs)	*Inpatient rehabilitation facilities (IRFs)*	*Long-term acute care hospitals (LTACHs)*
• CLABSI • CAUTI • VAE • SSI • *Clostridium difficile* • MRSA bacteremia	• CLABSI • CAUTI • *Clostridium difficile* • MRSA bacteremia	• CLABSI • CAUTI • VAE • *Clostridium difficile* • MRSA bacteremia

(CLABSI: central-line-associated bloodstream infection; CAUTI: catheter-associated urinary tract infection; HCAIs: healthcare-associated infections; MRSA: methicillin-resistant *Staphylococcus aureus* infection; SSI: surgical-site infection; VAE: ventilator-associated event; VAP: ventilator-associated pneumonia)

(SSIs) contain *Enterococcus* spp., which is less prevalent in the respiratory tract. One-tenth of all infections are caused by *P. aeruginosa*, which is evenly distributed to the entire body sites.[5]

The distribution of bacteria in nosocomial infections is changing over time. For example, *Proteus* spp., *Klebsiella* spp., and *Escherichia* spp. were responsible for HCAI in the 1960s, but from 1975 to the 1980s, *Acinetobacter* spp. with *P. aeruginosa* created clinical difficulties. As per a multicentric-multistate survey on HCAI involving 11,282 patients from 183 US hospitals conducted by the Centers for Disease Control and Prevention (CDC) and published in 2014, *C. difficile* (12.1%) was the leading pathogen for HCAIs, closely followed by *S. aureus* (10.7%), *K. pneumoniae* (9.9%), and *E. coli* (9.3%). As per the 2021 National and State Healthcare-Associated Infections Progress Report of the CDC, for different types of healthcare facilities, the HCAIs prevalence varies (**Table 7.3.1**).[5,6]

TYPES OF HEALTHCARE-ASSOCIATED INFECTIONS

The National Healthcare Safety Network with the CDC for surveillance has classified HCAI sites into 13 types, with 50 infection sites, which are specific and based on biological and clinical criteria.[6] The most common types are (**Table 7.3.2**):[7]

- Bloodstream infection (BSI)
- Central-line-associated bloodstream infections (CLABSIs)
- Pneumonia [e.g., ventilator-associated pneumonia (VAP)]
- Catheter-associated urinary tract infection (CAUTI)
- Surgical-site infection (SSI)

Catheter-related Bloodstream Infections

In ICUs, longline insertions and vascular accesses are the important factors for catheter-related bloodstream infections (CRBSIs). In CLABSI, the possible mechanisms for infection are colonization, biofilm formation, and

TABLE 7.3.2: Types of healthcare-associated infections (HCAIs).

Healthcare-associated infections	***Common organisms***
Central-line-associated bloodstream infections	*Candida* species, coagulase-negative *staphylococci*, *Staphylococcus aureus*, *Enterococcus* species, *Escherichia coli*
Catheter-associated urinary tract	*Escherichia coli*, *Klebsiella pneumoniae/K. oxytoca*, *Enterococcus* species
Ventilator-associated pneumonia	*S. aureus*, *K. pneumoniae/K. oxytoca*, *Pseudomonas aeruginosa*, *Streptococcus* species
Surgical-site infections	*S. aureus*, *Enterococcus* species, *E. coli*, *K. pneumoniae/K. oxytoca*, *Streptococcus* species

extraluminal migration.[3] The femoral site is associated with an increased risk of infections and should preferably be avoided. CoNS, commonly found in skin flora, is a common cause of colonization and thereby CLABSI.[3] *S. aureus* and *Staphylococcus epidermidis* are common organisms associated with biofilm formation on catheters.[5,7]

The incidence of CRBSI varies widely among different healthcare institutions, ranging from 1.12 to 4.2 per 1,000 catheter days, with the risk being higher in central lines than peripheral lines in the pediatric ICUs (PICUs).[3]

Risk Factors

- Settings such as PICUs
- Site of catheterization
- Type of catheter
- Frequency of dressing
- Duration
- Length of hospital stay
- Type of antiseptic solutions
- Local and systemic antibiotics

Common Organisms

The likely organisms are *Staph.* group 10–50%, *Enterococcus* 15–20%, methicillin-resistant *S. aureus* (MRSA) 20–25%, and extended-spectrum beta-lactamase-producing bacteria 15–20%.

Management

Empirical antibiotics with coverage against gram-positive and gram-negative organisms, including *Pseudomonas*, should be started and then modified based on the susceptibility pattern of isolated organisms. Antifungal therapy is added to empiric antibiotic coverage in some cases, particularly those who are immunocompromised patients, those who have prolonged ICU stay, and those who had exposure to antibiotics in the last 90 days. In cases where disseminated viral infection is suspected, antiviral therapy (e.g., ganciclovir and acyclovir) may be added. The duration of therapy depends on the isolated pathogen, retention of the catheter, or the presence of complications, such as endocarditis and sepsis. For most bacterial organisms, the duration of therapy is 10–14 days after blood cultures become negative. The removal of the central line should be considered, if:[3]

- The line is no longer needed.
- The infection is caused by *S. aureus*, *Candida* species, or mycobacteria.
- The patient is critically ill.
- The patient fails to clear bacteremia in 48–72 hours.
- The symptoms of BSI persist beyond 48–72 hours.

Catheter-associated Urinary Tract Infections

Urinary tract infection is the most common HCAI associated with the least morbidity. Occasionally it can lead to bacteremia, septicemia, and rarely death. Majority of the time, it is due to an indwelling catheter. The World Health Organization (WHO) defines a positive culture as more than 1 lakh count with a maximum of two isolated organisms.[1,7]

Common Organisms

The bacteria responsible are *E. coli* and multiresistant *Klebsiella*.[8]

Management

To avoid the persistence and recurrence of infection, as far as possible, the indwelling catheters should be removed. In some instances, the removal of the catheter may result in spontaneous resolution of bacteriuria or asymptomatic cystitis. Consider empiric antibiotic and antifungal therapy (immunocompromised individuals) to avoid complications, such as pyelonephritis, renal scarring, and generalized septicemia. For CAUTIs, typically 7 days of antibiotics is recommended. However, in case of a delayed response or bacteremia, in children with sepsis, pyelonephritis, or urinary tract abnormalities, antibiotics of 10–14 days have been recommended by most of the experts.

Ventilator-associated Pneumonia

Ventilator-associated pneumonia occurs in ICU settings associated with high morbidity and mortality and enormous cost to health care. Microorganisms colonize the stomach, upper airway, and bronchi and cause infection in the lungs (pneumonia); they are often endogenous (digestive system or nose and throat) but may be exogenous, often from contaminated respiratory equipment.[5]

World Health Organization definitions of pneumonia include clinical and radiological criteria that are readily available but nonspecific: Recent and progressive radiological opacities of the pulmonary parenchyma, purulent sputum, and recent onset of fever.[1]

Diagnosis is more specific when quantitative microbiological samples are obtained using specialized protected bronchoscopy methods.

Risk Factors

Known risk factors for infection include:

- The type and duration of ventilation
- The quality of respiratory care
- Severity of the patient's condition (organ failure)
- Previous use of antibiotics

Management

For the management of VAP, one should initially start with broad-spectrum empirical antibiotic therapy, and the regimen should be modified based on the culture results of sputum/endotracheal suction material/bronchial lavage wash. The choice of empiric antibiotic coverage should take into consideration the risk for multidrug-resistant (MDR) pathogens.[8] The regimens typically include antibiotics having activity against *S. aureus* and *P. aeruginosa*. In hospital-acquired pneumonia (HAP) or VAP, the usual duration of the antibiotic regimen is 7 days.

Surgical-site Infections

The WHO defines SSI clinically as: "A purulent discharge around the wound or the insertion site of the drain, or spreading cellulitis from the wound."[1] The CDC classifies SSI as being either incisional or organ/space, occurring within 30 days after the operation, and may be deep involving the organs or superficial involving the shin and soft tissues, which are manipulated during the procedure.[6,7]

The incidence depends on the place, hospitals, invasive procedures, elective or emergency surgery, persons, quality of care, immune status of the individuals, age, and surgical site. The incidence varies from 1% to 20%.[9]

Risk Factors

- Type of surgery—more in cardiothoracic orthopedic, gastrointestinal (GI) surgeries
- In implanted surgeries and less in pinhole surgeries
- *Wound type:* Clean or contaminated
- Experience of the surgical team
- Duration of stay in the hospital
- Immune status of the child
- Emergency or elective surgery
- Duration of surgery and age
- Infection-control policy of the hospital contributes greatly.

Common Organisms

Organisms involved in SSI depend upon the site of surgery; that is, if surgery is close to the perineum and hollow viscous organs, the organisms may be endogenous, such as fecal flora, e.g., *E. coli*, and sometimes anaerobes, such as *Bacillus fragilis*.

Staphylococcus aureus continues to be at the top in the list of pathogens isolated from SSI, followed by CoNS, *Enterococcus* spp., *E. coli*, *P. aeruginosa*, and *Enterobacter* spp. Other pathogens involved include *P. mirabilis*, *K. pneumoniae*, *Candida albicans*, and other *Streptococcus* spp.[9]

Management

Management of SSIs must be a dual-prong approach—combination of surgical care and antibiotic therapy. After starting empirical antibiotic therapy, the regimen should be modified based on the culture results. Aggressive surgical interventions are needed for severe infections, such as streptococcal gangrene and extensive tissue necrosis, as antibiotics alone may not work.[7,9]

PREVENTION OF HEALTHCARE-ASSOCIATED INFECTIONS

Standard precautions are to be applied to the care of all patients in all healthcare settings, regardless of the suspected or confirmed presence of an infectious agent. This is the primary strategy in preventing the transmission of infectious agents among patients and healthcare personnel. Transmission-based precautions are used in addition to standard precautions when caring for patients who are infected or colonized with pathogens transmitted by airborne, droplet, or contact routes.

- Preventive precautions to prevent transmission of airborne droplet infections include the use of single-patient rooms, negative air-pressure ventilation, and N95 respirator masks.
- Preventive precautions to prevent transmission of microorganisms via direct or indirect contact with infected or colonized persons include the use of a single-patient room (if not feasible, cohort patients infected with the same organism), use of gowns and gloves, and hand hygiene after glove removal.

- Preventive precautions to prevent intravascular catheter-associated infections include avoidance of unnecessary catheter placement, removal of catheter as soon as possible, aseptic technique during catheter insertion, and minimal manipulation of catheter. Scrubbing the catheter hub with devices containing isopropyl alcohol has been found to reduce these infections.[4,10]
- Preventive precautions to prevent healthcare-associated bacterial pneumonia include education of healthcare workers (HCWs) about infection-control procedures, thorough cleaning of devices for sterilization or disinfection, changing the breathing circuit only when it is visibly soiled, hand hygiene, and change of soiled gloves.[4,11,12]

Other General Measures

Handwashing

Poor hand hygiene is responsible for 40% of infections transmitted in hospitals. Surveys have shown that the improvement in compliance with handwashing reduces HCAIs. Accessibility to the handwashing stations and the use of alcohol gels improves compliance with handwashing. It is recommended to use a hand scrub after the examination of each patient, either by handwashing or by using an alcohol-based hand rub. Hands should also be washed before and after aseptic procedures and after the removal of gloves. When washing hands with soap and water, wet hands first with water, apply an amount of product recommended by the manufacturer to hands, rub hands together vigorously for at least 15 seconds, covering all surfaces of the hands and fingers, and then rinse hands with water and dry thoroughly with a disposable towel. While using an alcohol-based hand rub, apply the recommended quantity of product to the palm of one hand and rub hands together, covering all surfaces of hands and fingers, until the hands are dry. It is advisable to use a handwash formulation containing 60–95% alcohol alone or 50–95% alcohol in combination with a quaternary ammonium compound or 50–95% alcohol in combination with hexachlorophene or 50–95% alcohol in combination with chlorhexidine gluconate **(Fig. 7.3.1)**.

Environmental Sanitation

Environmental surfaces could potentially contribute to cross-transmission through hand contact with contaminated surfaces, medical equipment, or patients. Daily wet mopping of floors and surfaces close to patient care is a must. Particular attention is to be paid for surfaces, such as door-knobs, which are most commonly handled by patients in the clinic. It is preferable to use a disinfectant over plain soap and water with a contact time of at least 30–60 seconds. Spills of blood on surfaces should be promptly cleaned with detergent, followed by bleach (1:100) using gloves.

Disinfection of Hospital Rooms

Disinfection of hospital rooms with hydrogen peroxide vapor in addition to standard cleaning reduces environmental contamination and the risk of infection with MDR organisms.[8,11]

Safe Practices During Procedures

The use of invasive procedures increases the risk of nosocomial infections. For insertion of intravascular catheters and other invasive procedures and for obtaining blood cultures, 2% chlorhexidine, chlorhexidine in 70%

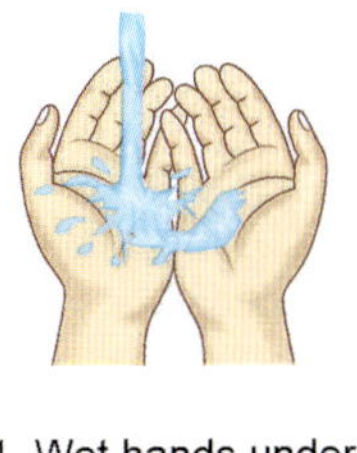

1. Wet hands under running water

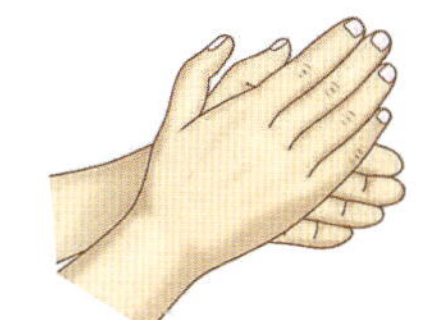

2. Apply soaps and rub palms together to ensure complete coverage

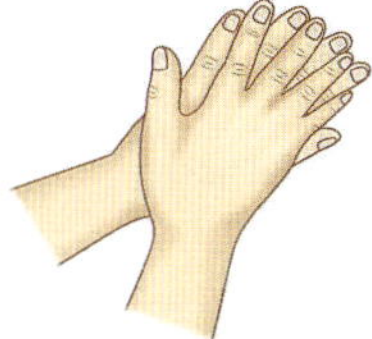

3. Spread the lather over the backs of the hands

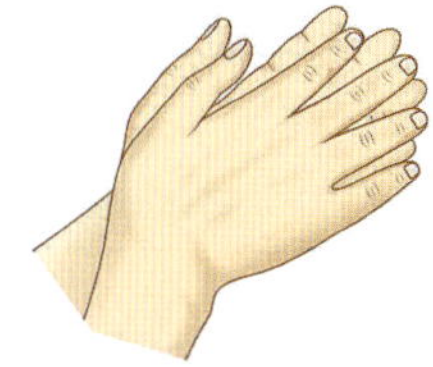

4. Make sure the soap gets in between the fingers

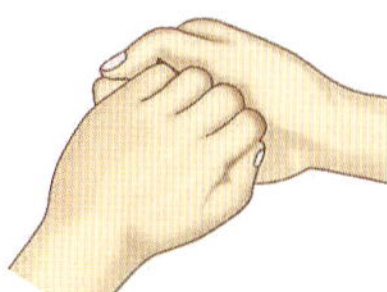

5. Grip the fingers on each hands

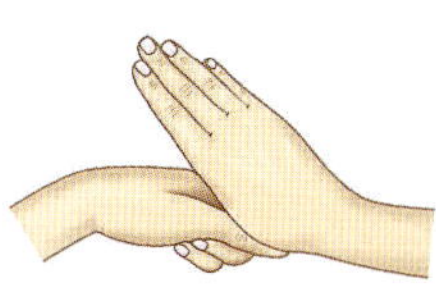

6. Pay particular attention to the thumbs

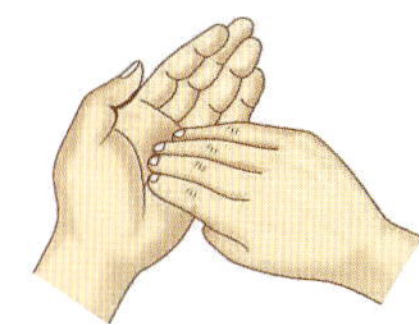

7. Press fingertips into the palms of each hand

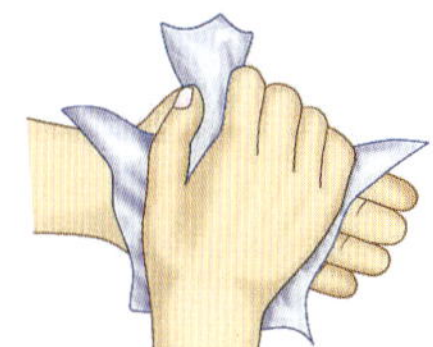

8.Dry thoroughly with a clean towel

Fig. 7.3.1: Steps of handwashing.

alcohol, 10% povidone-iodine, or alcoholic tincture of iodine should be used. Povidone-iodine should be left to dry for 2 minutes. Tunneling the catheter reduces the risk of nosocomial infection. Antimicrobially impregnated catheters can reduce catheter-related infections. The use of a strict, aseptic technique is paramount in the insertion of intravascular catheters. By using isolation rooms for patients with MRSA, *C. difficile*, vancomycin-resistant enterococci (VRE), and resistant gram-negative infections, the spread of infection can be reduced owing to improved awareness of the implementation of appropriate infection-control precautions.[8]

Biowaste Management

As per the Infection Management and Environment Plan Policy Framework, March 2007, by the Indian Ministry of Health, it is the duty of every occupier of a clinic, dispensary, nursing home, or hospital to take all steps to ensure handling and disposal of biowaste generated without any adverse effect on human health and the environment. Waste should be segregated as per the color coding provided by the Bio-Medical Waste Management Rules, 1998 and disposed of through biowaste management protocols **(Flowchart 7.3.1)**.

INFECTION-CONTROL PROGRAM

The important components of the infection-control program are:

- Basic measures for infection control, i.e., standard and additional precautions
- Education and training of HCWs

Flowchart 7.3.1: Treatment of hazardous and nonhazardous waste.

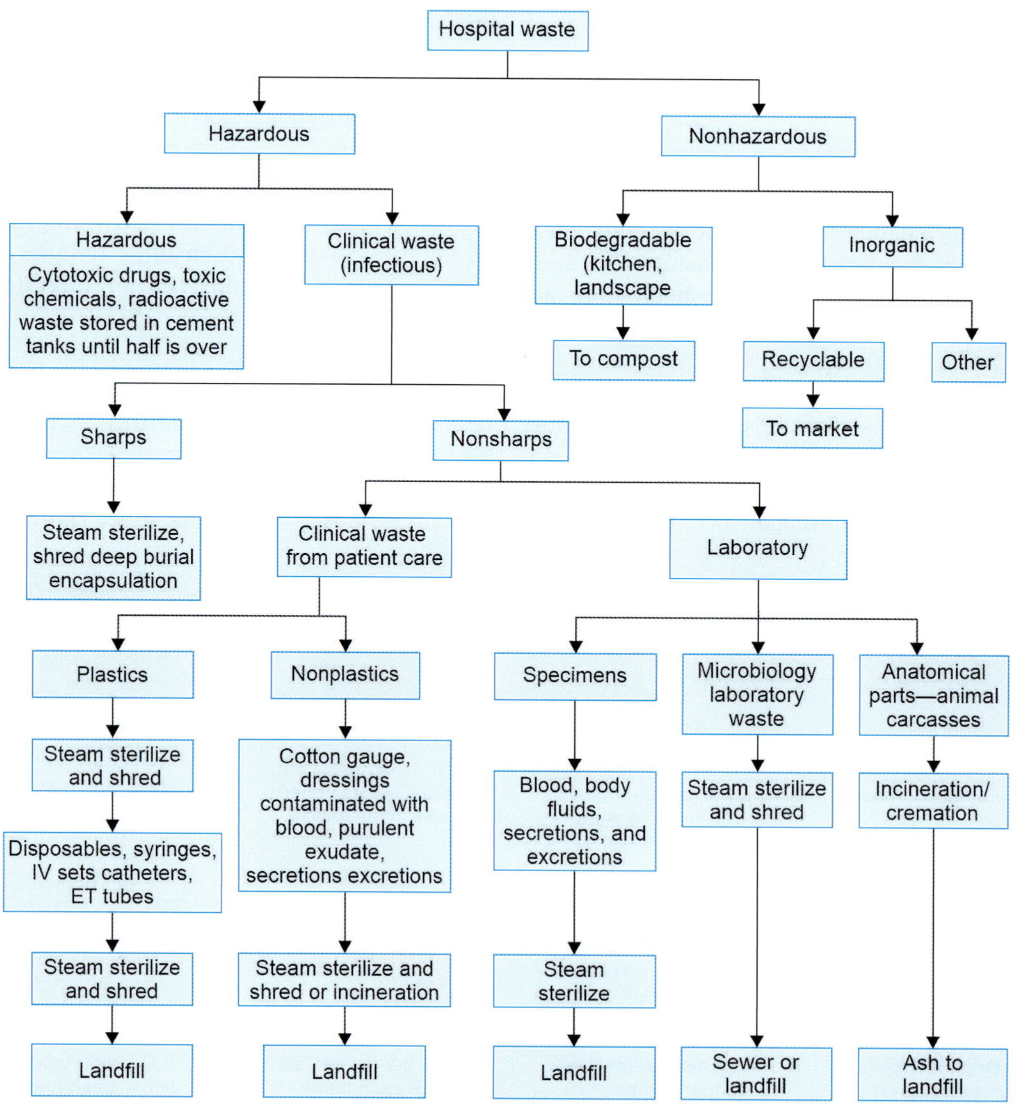

(ET: endotracheal; IV: intravenous)

- Protection of HCWs, e.g., immunization
- Identification of hazards and minimizing risks
- Routine practices essential to infection control, such as aseptic techniques, use of single-use devices, reprocessing of instruments and equipment, antibiotic usage, management of blood/body fluid exposure, handling and use of blood and blood products, and sound management of medical waste[4]
- Effective work practices and procedures, such as environmental management practices, including management of hospital/clinical waste, support services (e.g., food and linen), and use of therapeutic devices
- Surveillance
- Incident monitoring
- Outbreak investigation

Recommendations for Infection Control in Waiting Area

- The waiting room should be adequately ventilated. Ideally, it should provide at least six air exchanges per hour. A facility for handwash or alcoholic hand rub should be available.
- In office practice, the waiting time may be minimized by consultation on appointment, thereby minimizing the risk of exposure.[13]
- Healthcare professionals should try for early pickup and triage of patients with obvious communicable diseases such as chickenpox, measles, and conjunctivitis while they are waiting in the waiting area, and they should then provide consultation on priority. These will minimize exposure to other patients waiting for their turn.
- Prioritize the consultation for immunocompromised patients so as to minimize the chances of exposure to patients with communicable diseases.
- Regular cleaning of floors and surfaces in the waiting area through wet mopping is recommended as they can easily get contaminated with settling of droplets or contact with shoes. Any visible soiling by vomitus/urine/feces is to be promptly cleaned, followed by disinfection.[11]
- Toys are easily mouthed by children and can act as fomites. They should be washed with soap and water daily or when soiled by secretions. The risks of sharing toys or books should not outweigh the advantages of entertaining children, and toys should be removed, if supervised and regular cleaning is not feasible.
- Educational posters for respiratory etiquette and emphasis on hand hygiene displayed in the waiting area can help in dissemination of information.

Maintenance of Reusable Medical Equipment[10]

- The bell and diaphragm of a stethoscope, ear curettes of an otoscope, infantometer, and blood pressure cuffs are noncritical equipment that encounters intact skin, and therefore they are at low risk of infection transmission and require low disinfection, such as washing with plain water and soap.
- Infant weighing scales can be washed with soap and water. Separate clean paper (clean newspaper, if sterile paper is not economically feasible) should be used for every baby to prevent the risk of hypothermia and cross-contamination.
- The clinical thermometer should preferably be used in contact with intact skin, such as in the axillary fold, rather than mucous membrane, such as rectal mucosa. It can be washed with soap water or wiped with 70–90% ethyl or isopropyl alcohol with a contact time of at least 30 seconds and air-dried.
- Metallic tongue depressors come in contact with mucous membrane and saliva and require sterilization after washing by either boiling or autoclave. Disposable sterile tongue depressors are recommended but are expensive.[12]
- The nebulizer machine should be maintained as per the manufacturer's instructions. In general, the mask and T-shaped part of the nebulizer machine should be washed with mild soap and water and air-dried on a clean cloth.
- Instruments required for suturing should be placed inside a clean-folded cloth, and the tray should be autoclaved.

Prevention of Occupational Infections of the Healthcare Workers

- *Equipment for personal safety:*
    - Gloves should be worn by the HCW just before any invasive procedure, or contact with sterile sites and nonintact skin or mucous membrane, or where there is a risk of exposure to body fluids or blood, or while handling sharps and contaminated devices. The gloves should be removed soon after the procedure and disposed of appropriately. Hands should be washed after the removal of gloves.
    - A surgical mask should be worn, if there is a high risk of the procedure being exposed to respiratory secretions, splash of blood, and body fluids. For example, for procedures such as nebulization-induced sputum collection for acid-fast bacilli. Mask should be appropriately disposed of soon after use. Also, it should be used only once and changed, if wet or soiled. For severe acute respiratory syndrome, coronavirus, or avian influenza, the current recommendations are for personnel to wear an N95 mask for pandemic influenza; an N95 mask is recommended only for personnel performing certain aerosol-generating procedures.
    - Gloves and facemask should be worn when handling biowaste.

- *Immunization:* All HCWs should be vaccinated against hepatitis B. They are recommended to be immunized against vaccine-preventable diseases such as measles, mumps, varicella, influenza, diphtheria, and tetanus.
- *Education and training of staff:* The rationale behind infection-control practices should be taught to the staff. The correct methods of disinfection should be explained and supervised. Repeated discussions and training can help in maintaining high standards of compliance.
- *Personal hygiene:* The staff should maintain high standards of hand hygiene, keep nails short and free of false nails, and wear short sleeves.
- *Postexposure prophylaxis* should be promptly undertaken on exposure to needle-stick injury or exposure to contagious material.

REFERENCES

1. World Health Organization. Prevention of Hospital-Acquired Infections: A Practical Guide, 2nd edition. WHO/CDS/CSR/EPH/2002. Geneva: WHO; 2002.
2. Magill SS, Edwards JR, Bamberg W, Bedavs ZG, Dumyati G, Kainer MA, et al; Emerging Infections Program Healthcare-Associated Infections and Antimicrobial Use Prevalence Survey Team. Multistate point-prevalence survey of health care-associated infections. N Engl J Med. 2014;370(13):1198-208.
3. Novosad SA, Fike L, Dudeck MA, Allen-Bridson K, Edwads JR, Edens C, et al. Pathogens causing central-line-associated bloodstream infections in acute-care hospitals-United States, 2011–2017. Infect Control Hosp Epidemiol. 2020;41(3):313-9.
4. Zaoutis TE, Coffin SE. Clinical syndromes of device-associated infections. In: Long SS, Pickering LK, Prober CG (Eds). Principles and Practice of Pediatric Infectious Diseases, 3rd edition. Philadelphia, PA: Churchill Livingstone; 2008. (Chapter 102).
5. Coffin SE, Zaoutis TE. Healthcare-associated infections. In: Long SS, Pickering LK, Prober CG (Eds). Principles and Practice of Pediatric Infectious Diseases, 3rd edition. Philadelphia, PA: Churchill Livingstone; 2008. (Chapter 101).
6. 2022 National and State Healthcare-Associated Infections Progress Report of CDC. [online] Available from https://www.cdc.gov/hai/data/portal/progress-report.html. [Last accessed November, 2024].
7. Horan TC, Andrus M, Dudeck MA. CDC/NHSN surveillance definition of health care-associated infection and criteria for specific types of infections in the acute care setting. Am J Infect Control. 2008;36(5):309-32.
8. Serra-Burriel M, Keys M, Campillo-Artero C, Agodi A, Barchitta M, Gikas A, et al. Impact of multi-drug resistant bacteria on economic and clinical outcomes of healthcare-associated infections in adults: systematic review and meta-analysis. PLoS One. 2020;15(1):e0227139.
9. Rosenthal VD, Richtmann R, Singh S, Apisarnathanarak A, Kubler A, Viet-Hung N, et al. Surgical site infections, International Nosocomial Infection Control Consortium (INICC) report, data summary of 30 countries, 2005–2010. Infect Control Hosp Epidemiol. 2013;34(6):597-604.
10. Mehta A, Rosenthal VD, Mehta Y, Chakravarthy M, Todi SK, Sen N, et al. Device-associated nosocomial infection rates in intensive care units of seven Indian cities: findings of the International Nosocomial Infection Control Consortium (INICC). J Hosp Infect. 2007;67(2):168-74.
11. Healthcare Infection Control Practices Advisory Committee (HICPAC); Rutala WA, Weber DJ. (2008). Guideline for disinfection and sterilization in healthcare facilities. [online] Available from http://www.cdc.gov/hicpac/Disinfection_Sterilization/3_4surfaceDisinfection.html. [Last accessed November, 2024].
12. Patwardhan N, Kelkar U. Disinfection, sterilization and operation theater guidelines for dermatosurgical practitioners in India. Indian J Dermatol Venereol Leprol. 2011;77(1):83-93.
13. Canadian Pediatric Society. Infection control in paediatric office settings. Paediatr Child Health. 2008;13(5):408-19.

7.4 Diphtheria

Monjori Mitra

INTRODUCTION

Diphtheria is a potentially acute, respiratory infectious disease caused by the exotoxin-producing *Corynebacterium* genus, mostly *Corynebacterium diphtheriae* and occasionally other closely related species, including *Corynebacterium ulcerans* and *Corynebacterium pseudotuberculosis.*[1,2] Morbidity and mortality result from the bacterial toxin (*tox*-encoding diphtheria toxin, i.e., DT) that may cause obstructive pseudomembranes in the upper respiratory tract (croup) or damage myocardium and other tissues.

Diphtheria predominantly affects children of ≤15 years of age with a high case-fatality rate (5–17%) among the unvaccinated population. Diphtheria was a major cause of childhood morbidity and mortality during the prevaccine era. Numerous major diphtheria outbreaks (respiratory/pharyngeal/cutaneous/ocular) have been recorded across all global regions, and it is still prevalent as per recent reports. A trivalent vaccine for diphtheria, tetanus, and pertussis (DTP) and booster doses of toxoid (i.e., inactivated toxin) are available against diphtheria for childhood and adults, respectively. Also, many immunological and molecular detection tools, administration of diphtheria antitoxin (DAT), and antibiotic therapy are effective in patients with typical disease symptoms.[3,4]

EPIDEMIOLOGY

Humans are the only natural reservoir of *C. diphtheriae*, although occasionally it has been isolated from a variety of domestic animals. Spread occurs in close-contact settings through respiratory droplets or direct contact with respiratory secretions or skin lesions. The majority of nasopharyngeal *C. diphtheriae* infections result in asymptomatic carriage, with clinical disease developing in only about one in seven individuals.

Diphtheria immunization protects against disease but does not prevent carriage. Vaccination with diphtheria toxoid (formalin-treated inactivated toxin) was introduced in the 1920s. Immunization of children in an era when the majority of older individuals had natural immunity resulted in a dramatic drop in the incidence of diphtheria and an even more rapid decline in the proportion of toxigenic strains isolated, presumably because the selective advantage of the *tox* gene promotion of greater replication and spread of the organism is lost in an immune host. In most Western countries, toxigenic *C. diphtheriae* has virtually been eliminated.

Vaccine-induced immunity to diphtheria wanes with time, and there is a growing cohort of individuals with no natural diphtheria immunity. Serosurveys indicate that 20–60% of adults in industrialized countries have DAT levels below minimal protective levels. As long as a high proportion of the population remains susceptible, the danger of reintroduction or re-emergence of toxigenic strains exists. Since 1990, there has been a major resurgence of diphtheria in several countries of the former Soviet Union.

According to the latest estimates of the World Health Organization (WHO), about 84% of children globally received the recommended three doses of diphtheria-containing vaccine during infancy, leaving 16% with no or incomplete coverage. There is a wide coverage variation between and within countries.[5] In 2005, India contributed 5,826 (71%) of the 8,229 diphtheria cases reported globally. According to new numbers released by the Central Bureau of Health Intelligence, under the Union Ministry of Health and Family Welfare in 2010, a total of 3,129 cases of diphtheria were reported out of which 731 were found to be from Delhi and a huge 90% of reported diphtheria deaths (163 out of 177) recorded in 2010 were also in Delhi. In the recent July 2015 update from WHO global monitoring system data, India contributed 6,094 cases out of the total number of 7,382 reported cases. The data about diphtheria cases reported to WHO indicate that India accounts for 52.8% of the 16,648 diphtheria cases reported globally in 2018. Thus, despite the introduction of the diphtheria vaccine four decades ago, the persistence or re-emergence of diphtheria in India still remains a concern.[6]

PATHOGENESIS

Corynebacterium diphtheriae is a member of a group of aerobic, nonmotile, unencapsulated, nonsporulating, and pleomorphic organisms. Both nontoxigenic and toxigenic *C. diphtheriae* strains exist. Toxigenicity is conferred when a nontoxigenic organism is infected with a beta-phage carrying the gene for the toxin (*tox*). *C. diphtheriae* has three biotypes: (1) Gravis, (2) mitis, and (3) intermedius, which are distinguished by colonial morphology and varying biochemical and hemolytic reactions. Strains may be distinguished for epidemiologic purposes by molecular techniques. *Corynebacterium ulcerans* can also produce classic diphtheria, including local respiratory tract and distal toxic complications.

Corynebacterium diphtheriae colonizes the mucosal surface of the nasopharynx and multiplies locally without bloodstream invasion. Released toxin causes local tissue necrosis with the formation of a tough, adherent pseudomembrane composed of a mixture of fibrin, dead cells, and bacteria. The membrane usually begins on the tonsils or posterior of the pharynx. In more severe cases, it spreads over the pharyngeal wall, fauces, and soft palate and into the larynx, resulting in respiratory obstruction. Toxin entering the bloodstream causes tissue damage at distant sites, particularly the heart (myocarditis), nerves (demyelination), and kidneys (tubular necrosis).

Nontoxigenic tox-bearing *C. diphtheriae* (NTTB) strains may cause mild local respiratory disease, sometimes including a membrane. The pathogenesis of NTTB infections is largely unclear; the most common entry routes are skin lesions or dental caries and the possible virulence factors are biofilm formation and pilus proteins (SpaD and SpaH). Moreover, as an emerging zoonotic agent of diphtheria, the genome of *C. ulcerans* presents a higher similarity to the genome of *C. pseudotuberculosis* as compared with *C. diphtheriae.*[7]

CLINICAL MANIFESTATIONS

Anterior Nasal Diphtheria

Anterior nares colonization leads to chronic serosanguineous or seropurulent discharge and erosive rhinitis without fever or significant toxicity. A whitish membrane may be observed on the septum. Mild clinical features are usually observed due to apparently poor systemic absorption of toxin from this location, and rapid termination is possible by DAT and/or antibiotic therapy.[8]

Pharyngeal and Tonsillar Diphtheria

The faucial (pharyngeal) form is the most common. It is manifested with sore throat, malaise, and mild-to-moderate fever. Initially, there is mild pharyngeal erythema, usually followed by progressive formation of whitish tonsillar exudates, which over a period of 24–48 hours changes into a grayish membrane that is tightly adherent and bleeds on attempted removal. Cervical adenopathy and soft-tissue edema result in the typical bull neck appearance and stridor.

Laryngeal Diphtheria

Laryngeal involvement is manifested as hoarseness, stridor, and dyspnea. Most laryngeal lesions exist with a deep layer of lymphocytes. The acute inflammatory reaction often goes beyond the mucous glands of the respiratory tract.

Cutaneous Diphtheria

Classic cutaneous diphtheria is an indolent, nonprogressive infection characterized by a superficial, erythemic, nonhealing ulcer with a gray-brown membrane. Diphtheritic skin infections cannot always be differentiated from streptococcal or staphylococcal impetigo, and these conditions frequently coexist. In most cases, a primary process, such as dermatosis, laceration, burns, bite, or impetigo, becomes secondarily infected with *C. diphtheriae*. Extremities are more often affected than the trunk or head. Pain, tenderness, erythema, and exudate are typical. Local hyperesthesia or hypoesthesia is unusual.

COMPLICATIONS

Most complications of diphtheria, including death, are attributable to the effects of the toxin. Myocarditis typically occurs in the first week or second week after the onset of respiratory symptoms and develops either suddenly or insidiously with signs of low cardiac output and congestive failure. Conduction disturbances, such as ST-T wave abnormalities, arrhythmias, and heart block, may occur without myocarditis.

Neurologic impairment is manifested as cranial nerve palsies and polyneuritis. Palatal or pharyngeal paralysis (or both) occurs during the acute phase; peripheral neuritis, symmetrical and predominantly motor, occurs 2–12 weeks after the onset of the disease. Motor deficit may range from minor proximal weakness to complete paralysis. Complete recovery is the rule.

Other complications include otitis media and respiratory insufficiency due to airway obstruction, especially in infants.

DIAGNOSIS

The specimen should be collected immediately after clinical diagnosis with the swab from the inflamed tissue, and one is sent for staining and the other for the culture. It is obtained from the nose and throat and any other mucocutaneous lesion. A portion of the membrane should be removed for culture. Evaluation of a direct smear using Gram stain is used to accurately identify the organism and subsequently with the special stain, such as Albert's stain and Ponder's stain; the metachromatic granular structure is identified.

Alert the laboratory to the suspicion of diphtheria because isolation of *C. diphtheriae* requires special culture media. *C. diphtheriae* may be grown on various selective media, including Tellurite agar or specially enriched Loeffler, Hoyle, Mueller, or Tinsdale medium.

Culture isolates of coryneform organisms should be identified to the species level, and toxigenicity and antimicrobial susceptibility tests should be performed for *C. diphtheriae* isolates. Elek's test is used for toxigenicity to determine whether the organism can produce the DT or not. While chest X-ray and echocardiogram are the preferred imaging studies, other laboratory practices include CBC and/or troponin levels.[3,5]

DIFFERENTIAL DIAGNOSIS

The differential diagnosis includes streptococcal and viral tonsillopharyngitis, infectious mononucleosis (often characterized by fatigue, malaise, sore throat, fever, nausea, anorexia, pharyngitis, lymphadenopathy, and cough.), Vincent's angina (i.e., gum infection with pain and bleeding and ulcerative gingiva necrosis), candidiasis (grayish pseudomembrane presented in diphtheria vs. whitish appearance observed in oral candidiasis), and acute epiglottitis (typically characterized by acute inflammation of the epiglottis and associated structures).[9]

MANAGEMENT

The goals of treatment are to neutralize the toxin rapidly, eliminate the infecting organism, provide supportive care, and prevent further transmission. The mainstay of therapy is equine DAT and should be administered based on clinical grounds. A single dose ranging in quantity from 20,000 U for localized tonsillar diphtheria up to 100,000 U is given for extensive disease with severe toxicity. Antitoxin may be administered intramuscularly or intravenously; particularly for more severe cases, the intravenous route is preferred. Tests for sensitivity to antitoxin should be performed before administering it and desensitization carried out if necessary.

Antibiotic therapy should be started simultaneously. Parenteral penicillin (4–6 million units/day) or macrolides, such as erythromycin, clarithromycin, and azithromycin, are the drugs of choice. The antibiotic is given for 10–14 days.

General supportive care includes ensuring a secure airway, electrocardiographic monitoring for evidence of myocarditis, treating heart failure and arrhythmias, and preventing secondary complications of neurologic impairment, such as aspiration pneumonia. The patient should be in strict isolation until follow-up cultures are negative. Convalescing patients should receive diphtheria toxoid.

The local health department must be notified. Close contacts should have cultures performed and be administered prophylactic antibiotics. All contacts without full primary immunization and a booster within the preceding 5 years should receive diphtheria toxoid.

Antibiotic therapy is not a substitute for antitoxin therapy. Some patients with cutaneous diphtheria have been treated for 7–10 days. Elimination of the organism should be documented by negative results of at least two successive cultures of specimens from the nose and throat (or skin) obtained 24 hours apart after completion of therapy. Treatment with erythromycin is repeated if either culture yields *C. diphtheriae.*

Active immunization against diphtheria is recommended during convalescence from diphtheria, as the disease does not necessarily confer immunity. Moreover, apart from standard prevention measures, droplet precautions should be undertaken for patients and carriers with respiratory diphtheria until two cultures from both the nose and throat collected 24 hours after completing antimicrobial treatment are negative for *C. diphtheriae.*[10]

PREVENTION

Immunization with diphtheria toxoid is the only effective means of primary prevention. The primary series is four doses of diphtheria toxoid (given with tetanus toxoid and pertussis vaccine) at 6, 10, and 14 weeks, and 15–18 months, and a preschool booster dose is given at 4–6 years of age. Thereafter, boosters [tetanus and diphtheria (Td) or tetanus-diphtheria-acellular pertussis (Tdap)] should be given as part of the adolescent immunization visit (i.e., at 10 and 16 years of age), followed by doses administered every 10 years. Since 2005, the Centers for Disease Control and Prevention (CDC) recommends the routine use of tetanus toxoid, reduced diphtheria toxoid, and acellular pertussis vaccine (Tdap) in adolescents 11–18 years of age in place of Td toxoid vaccines. In addition, the CDC recommends routine use of a single dose of Tdap for adults 19–64 years of age to replace the next booster dose of Td.

In countries that are rendered nonendemic through high immunization coverage, the primary vaccination series of the three doses should be extended by at least one booster dose. Revaccination of adults against diphtheria (and tetanus) every 10 years may be necessary to sustain immunity in some epidemiological settings. Particular attention should be given to the revaccination of healthcare workers. To further promote immunity against diphtheria, combined diphtheria toxoid and tetanus toxoid rather than tetanus toxoid alone should be used when tetanus prophylaxis is needed following injuries.

PROGNOSIS

Although most infections with *C. diphtheriae* are asymptomatic or run a relatively mild clinical course, high case-fatality rates (>10%) have been reported even in recent outbreaks. In the prevaccination era, diphtheria had a very high case-fatality rate in preschool children. With the widespread vaccination in both developed and developing countries, the incidence of diphtheria has decreased, but there is also a decrease in the circulating toxigenic *C. diphtheriae* organisms, resulting in less natural boosting of antibody levels. Hence, if an adequate booster dose is not given, the chances of outbreaks will be there, leading to increased case-fatality rates.

Diphtheria is still, in many developing countries, a preventable health issue with the urgent requirement of early detection, effective treatment through improved vaccine and booster coverage, and intensive care interventions in severe to rare cases. Diphtheria must be recognized as another important vaccine-preventable disease of the modern age. As the robust and prioritized preventive immunization protocols along with booster doses demand special attention for countries like India, the manufacturing and supply chain of the DTP vaccine and DAT should be strengthened, expedited, and made readily available globally at all scales. Another issue is the periodic assessment and call-to-action specific to the antigen units of the vaccines and boosters, as well as the molecular characterization of *C. diphtheriae.*[11,12] Hence, the ideal public health policy should put efforts into reaching at least 90% coverage with the three doses of diphtheria toxoid in children <1 year of age.[13] In countries where diphtheria has been successfully controlled, immunity levels should be maintained by booster doses to achieve immediate reduction in diphtheria-associated mortality.

REFERENCES

1. Bitragunta S, Murhekar MV, Hutin YJ, Penumur PP, Gupte MD. Persistence of diphtheria, Hyderabad, India, 2003-2006. Emer Infec Dis. 2008;14(7):1144-7.
2. Sharma NC, Efstratiou A, Mokrousov I, Mutreja A, Das B, Ramamurthy T. Diphtheria. Nat Rev Dis Primers. 2019;5(1):81.
3. Buescher ES. *Corynebacterium diphtheria.* In: Kliegman RM, Stanton BF, Behrman RE (Eds). Nelson Textbook of Pediatrics, 18th edition. Philadelphia, PA: WB Saunders; 2009. pp. 1153-7.

4. Centers for Disease Control and Prevention. Respiratory diphtheria-like illness caused by toxigenic *Corynebacterium ulcerans*-Idaho, 2010. MMWR. 2011;60(3):77.
5. Clarridge JE, Popovic T, Inzana TJ. Diphtheria and other corynebacterial and coryneform infections. In: Hausler WJ, Sussman M (Eds). Topley and Wilson's Microbiology and Microbial Infections. New York: Oxford University Press; 1998. p. 347.
6. Murhekar MV. Resurgence of diphtheria in India. J Infect. 2020;80(2):232-54.
7. Fauzi IS, Nuraini N, Sari AM, Wardani IB, Taurustiati D, Simanullang PM, et al. Assessing the impact of booster vaccination on diphtheria transmission: mathematical modeling and risk zone mapping. Infect Dis Model. 2024;9(1):245-62.
8. Galazka AM, Robertson SE. Diphtheria: changing patterns in the developing world and the industrialized world. Eur J Epidemiol. 1995;11(1):107-17.
9. Philip AM. *Corynebacterium diphtheria*. In: Mandell GL, Bennette JE, Dolin R (Eds). Mandell, Douglas and Bennett's principles and practice of infectious diseases, 7th edition. Philadelphia, PA: Churchill Livingstone; 2009. pp. 2678-93.
10. Sharma NC, Banavaliker JN, Ranjan R, Kumar R. Bacteriological and epidemiological characteristics of diphtheria cases in and around Delhi—a retrospective study. Indian J Med Res. 2007;126(6):545-52.
11. World Health Organization. Diphtheria vaccine-WHO position paper. Wkly Epidemiol Rec. 2006;81:24-31.
12. Nicholson L, Adkins E, Karyanti MR, Ong-Lim A, Shenoy B, Huoi C, et al. What is the true burden of diphtheria, tetanus, pertussis and poliovirus in children aged 3–18 years in Asia? A systematic literature review. Int J Infect Dis. 2022;117:116-29.
13. Berger A, Badell E, Åhman J, Matuschek E, Zidane N, Kahlmeter G, et al. *Corynebacterium diphtheriae* and *Corynebacterium ulcerans*: development of EUCAST methods and generation of data on which to determine breakpoints. J Antimicrob Chemother. 2024;79(5):968-76.

7.5 Pertussis

Aniruddha Ghosh

INTRODUCTION

Pertussis or whooping cough, also known as 100-day cough, is a respiratory tract infection caused by the bacteria *Bordetella pertussis*. *Bordetella parapertussis* and other rare *Bordetella* sp. also contribute to a small number of cases of pertussis. It can affect any age group of the population, but affected infants and young children mostly contribute to the high mortality and morbidity due to pertussis globally. After the development of the pertussis vaccine in the 1940s, the incidence came down significantly. According to reports from all over the world, pertussis cases are again on the rise and pose a real threat to healthcare professionals.[1,2]

EPIDEMIOLOGY

Bordetella pertussis only infects men. Mild, missed, or unrecognized infected persons act as reservoirs of the infection. There is no subclinical infection or chronic carrier state in this disease. The bacteria do not survive long outside the human body. Infection spreads via nasopharyngeal secretions of an infected person as droplets or aerosol. The incubation period is 7–10 days with a range of 4–21 days. The period of transmission starts after 5–7 days of contact, persisting for 3 weeks if left untreated. With appropriate antibiotic therapy, the transmission period may be blocked after 5 7 days. The infant death rate is ~2% due to pertussis. A secondary attack rate of up to 90% has been described in susceptible family members.[1,2]

Global Perspective

Pertussis is an endemic disease globally and has epidemic peaks every 2–5 years. As per the World Health Organization (WHO) database, worldwide over 24 million cases are reported every year with mortality estimated to be over 160,000.[3] The incidence has been increasing lately in infants and young children as well as in adolescents and adults who contract the infection and contribute to the further spread of the contagion.[1,2,4]

India Outlook

Around 4,362 cases of pertussis have been reported in 2022 from India, with an incidence of 3.1 per 1,000,000 total population. There might be under-reporting due to the lack of availability of definitive diagnostic modalities. As per the National Family Health Survey-4 (NFHS-4), the national coverage for full immunization is around 62% and the third primary dose of diphtheria, tetanus, and pertussis (DPT)/

pentavalent vaccine has been received in 78.4% of the targeted population of infants countrywide.

The re-emergence of pertussis in the last two decades is poorly understood and several factors including genetic modifications in the *B. pertussis* contributing to greater virulence, strains not recognized by vaccines, waning vaccination immunity, adolescents and adults being affected more than before and working as reservoirs, less long-lasting immune response by the acellular vaccines, introduction of diagnostic modalities which are more sensitive than traditional cultures and thereby giving higher positivity than previous years, etc., have been implicated as the cause of this re-emergence.

ETIOPATHOGENESIS

Bordetella pertussis is a gram-negative bacillus that primarily causes the disease by numerous toxins/antigens, namely pertussis toxin (PT), filamentous hemagglutinin (FHA), pertactin (PRN), several fimbrial agglutinogens, heat-labile toxin, adenylate cyclase toxin, and tracheal cytotoxin, *Bordetella* resistance to killing protein (BrkA), and endotoxin.[5] The toxins bind to the cilia of the respiratory tract epithelial cells. These toxins paralyze the ciliary movements hampering mucociliary clearance and cause severe inflammation and destruction of epithelial cells. Pertussis antigens induce lymphocytosis in the host immune system but impair chemotaxis thereby evading the host defense. Previously, it was thought that pertussis bacilli cannot invade tissues directly, but recent studies have demonstrated the bacteria inside alveolar macrophages.[1,2,6]

Host factors like age, immunological status, vaccination status, time passed since the last dose of vaccination against pertussis, virulence of the strain of pertussis, etc., are factors that influence the clinical presentation.[7] Immunized children and adolescents may present with chronic cough-mimicking bronchitis. On the other hand, newborn babies may only have cyanosis, apneic spells, and mild cough. Maternal antibody does not provide any immunity to the newborns. Immunity acquired by natural infection or vaccinations is not lifelong and wanes with time. Also, there is no cross immunity against *B. parapertussis*.

CLINICAL FEATURES

Classically, the disease course of pertussis follows three stages as mentioned in the following text:

Catarrhal Stage

During this phase, the patient has a running nose, low-grade fever, mild occasional cough, etc. This is a highly contagious stage with a very high secondary attack rate. This phase lasts for 1–2 weeks.

Paroxysmal Stage

This phase lasts for 1–6 weeks, sometimes as long as 10 weeks. During this stage, the patient develops debilitating bouts of numerous successive coughs followed by the "whoop" sound produced by inspiration through the swollen glottis. Vomiting and exhaustion often ensue after paroxysms of cough.

Convalescent/Recovery Stage

Recovery is slow with the intermittent return of paroxysms. Often during this phase, which lasts for around 1–2 weeks, the patient may acquire secondary infections, and there might be sudden clinical deterioration. Coinfections and superadded infections by other bacterial or viral respiratory pathogens are quite common as PTs suppress the respiratory tract defense mechanisms of the host. This might again lead to diagnostic difficulty and delay in treatment. The most common bacterial pathogens causing the superadded infection are *Streptococcus pneumoniae, Streptococcus pyogenes, Haemophilus influenzae*, and *Staphylococcus aureus*. Respiratory syncytial virus, cytomegalovirus, and adenovirus superinfections have also been reported frequently.

Usually, these stages are evident in unimmunized older children or adolescents. Pertussis affects all ages but it is most severe in infants. In them, the classical stages of pertussis are not followed and may start as a mild upper respiratory tract infection. An occasional cough proceeds to paroxysms within 1–2 weeks increasing in both severity and frequency. Often a series of vigorous coughing occurs without taking a breath leaving the baby breathless and cyanosed. Apneic spells are often the sole presentation along with mild upper respiratory tract symptoms. Post-tussive vomiting may be present. Cough increases during feeding and crying and is often worse at night. Usually, the baby is well in between the paroxysm. Fever is not a very common presentation in this age group of patients. The classical "whoop" is not witnessed in smaller infants and is commonly seen in patients of the age group of 6 months to 5 years.

Several pulmonary complications are reported in infants and smaller children. Interstitial and alveolar pneumonia along with respiratory failure may occur. As a result of leukostasis in pulmonary microcirculation, pulmonary hypertension, impaired gaseous exchange, cardiogenic shock, or cerebrovascular thrombosis may develop which again increases mortality. Cough paroxysms and associated hypoxia may give rise to encephalopathy, intracerebral bleeding, cerebral infarcts, hypoxic seizure, etc. Prolonged difficulty in feeding due to paroxysms may lead to nutritional deficiencies. Other complications reported include subconjunctival hemorrhage, pneumothorax and pneumomediastinum, epistaxis, subcutaneous emphysema, edema of face, rib fractures, syncope, rectal prolapse, etc.

DIFFERENTIAL DIAGNOSIS

Pertussis mimics any other respiratory tract infection initially. Viral upper respiratory tract infection, bronchiolitis, bacterial pneumonia, etc., should be kept in the differential diagnosis in this phase. When bouts of cough start and persist, then foreign body aspiration (especially in toddlers), tuberculosis, acute exacerbation of reactive airway disease, or bronchial asthma, bronchitis, etc., should be excluded as alternative diagnoses. Sometimes, very high leukocytosis with lymphocytic leukemoid reaction may be confused with leukemia.

DIAGNOSIS

Pertussis usually has *leukocytosis* with a rise in absolute lymphocyte counts during the catarrhal stage. In infants, these two markers are directly linked to disease severity. Very high leukocyte counts (>60,000/μL) *with lymphocytic preponderance* often lead to severe pneumonia and pulmonary hypertension. Neutrophilic counts may indicate toward alternate diagnosis or secondary bacterial infection.

Chest radiograph findings are nonspecific and may show infiltrates, peribronchial thickening, atelectasis, and, rarely, lobar consolidation. A "shaggy" right heart border, although not pathogenomic, has been associated with pertussis in many literature.

Modalities for definitive diagnosis of pertussis have evolved over time. *Culture* was traditionally the gold standard. Nasopharyngeal samples collected by swab or aspiration were traditionally cultured in specialized culture media like Regan–Lowe or freshly prepared Bordet–Gengou medium. However, this process was difficult as the organism is fastidious (starting from proper sample collection and effective transport in a medium to finally culture it in the specialized media), and it took almost 2 weeks to culture the organism. Often the clinical suspicion of pertussis is made later in the disease course and samples collected at that time were often associated with poor yield.

A standardized polymerase chain reaction (PCR) for *B. pertussis* is now the preferred mode for definitive diagnosis in clinical fields. It has the following advantages over cultures:

- It is a rapid diagnostic procedure, helping in early diagnosis of the disease.
- It will remain positive even in the later part of the disease course.
- Despite antibiotic therapy, it may give a positive result even as late as 21 days.
- It has got higher specificity and sensitivity in comparison with traditional cultures.

Serological tests traditionally being used [direct fluorescent antibody assay, anti-PT immunoglobulin G (IgG) assay, anti-PT immunoglobulin A (IgA) and immunoglobulin M (IgM) assay, etc.], mostly for epidemiological studies, lack sensitivity and specificity and some have problems with standardization. Currently, the use of enzyme-linked immunosorbent assay (ELISA) is increasing day by day for higher sensitivity and specificity and it is vital for seroepidemiological studies.

MANAGEMENT

Early case detection, timely intervention with appropriate antibiotic therapy, and supportive care are the mainstay of treatment. Supportive therapy includes proper care for airway and breathing, adequate hydration, and, if required, supplemental oxygen therapy.

Strict isolation is necessary throughout the catarrhal stage and 3 weeks after the onset of the paroxysmal stage. In patients treated with antibiotics, the isolation period is shorter (5 days after starting the antibiotic).

During the earlier stage of the disease, antibiotics can significantly reduce the course of the disease and also prevent severe outcomes. But later on, when toxin-mediated damage has already set in, the role of antibiotic therapy is limited for curative purpose. Although, even at this stage, the period of contagiousness gets reduced as almost within 5 days of initiation of antibiotic therapy, bacteria get rapidly cleared off the nasopharynx of an infected person. As per the American Academy of Pediatrics (AAP) and Centers for Disease Control and Prevention (CDC), macrolides (erythromycin, azithromycin, and clarithromycin), and cotrimoxazole [trimethoprim-sulfamethoxazole (TMP-SMX)] are the antibiotics of choice for both cases and chemoprophylaxis of close and high-risk household, daycare, or school contacts and healthcare workers (HCWs).[8]

Macrolides

Erythromycin

In infants <1 month of age, erythromycin should be avoided. If at all prescribed, then they are to be closely monitored for the development of pyloric stenosis. Infants >1 month and older children can be prescribed erythromycin.

Dosage: Infants and children—40–50 mg/kg/day in four divided doses for 14 days. Maximum daily dose 2 g/day.

Adults—dose is 2 g/day in four divided doses for 14 days.

Azithromycin

Dosage: Infants <6 months of age—10 mg/kg for 5 days.

Infants >6 months and older children—10 mg/kg on day 1 (maximum 500 mg) followed by 5 mg/kg/day (maximum 250 mg) on days 2–5.

Adults—500 mg on day 1 followed by 250 mg/day on days 2–5.

Clarithromycin

Not recommended for infants < 1 month age.

Dosage: Pediatric patients—15 mg/kg/day (maximum 1 g/day) in two divided doses for 7 days.

Adults—1 g/day in two divided doses each day for 7 days.

Cotrimoxazole (Trimethoprim–Sulfamethoxazole)

Cotrimoxazole is contraindicated in children <2 months of age. Dosages for all other pediatric and adult patients are as follows:

Pediatric—TMP 8 mg/kg/day, SMX 40 mg/kg/day in two divided doses for 14 days

Adults—TMP 320 mg/day, SMX 1600 mg/day in two divided doses for 14 days

Sick infants often require intensive care unit admission, mechanical ventilation, and if in shock, inotropes and vasopressor medications. Exchange transfusion and leukapheresis may be helpful for the management of pertussis-related respiratory or cardiac failure and pulmonary hypertension, but have to be initiated before distress becomes severe or multiorgan failure sets in.

There is no proven role of corticosteroids, bronchodilators, pertussis immune globulin, cough suppressants, or antihistamines.

PREVENTION

As a preventive measure, the Indian Academy of Pediatrics (IAP) has recommended whole-cell or acellular pertussis-containing vaccines at 6, 10, and 14 weeks, 16–18 months, and 4–6 years. Adolescents should also receive a single dose of the Tdap vaccine at 10–12 years of age. During 27–36 weeks of pregnancy, pregnant women should receive 1 dose of Tdap/Td.[9,10]

REFERENCES

1. Decker MD, Edwards KM. Pertussis (Whooping cough). J Infect Dis. 2021;224(4):S310-S320.
2. Machado MB, Passos SD. Severe pertussis in childhood: update and controversy—systemic review. Rev Paul Pediatr. 2019;37(3):351-62.
3. World Health Organization. WHO SAGE pertussis working group. Background paper. [online] Available from https://terrance.who.int/mediacentre/data/sage/SAGE_Docs_Ppt_Apr2014/8_session_pertussis/Apr2014_session8_pertussis.pdf [Last accessed November, 2024].
4. Boulet SL, Chamberlain AT, Biswas HH, Jamieson DJ. Trends in infant pertussis hospitalizations in the United States, 2009–2017. JAMA. 2019;322(21):2134-6.
5. Kilgore PE, Salim AM, Zervos MJ, Schmitt HJ. Pertussis: microbiology, disease, treatment, and prevention. Clin Microbiol Rev. 2016;29:449-86.
6. Paddock CD, Sanden GN, Cherry JD, Gal AA, Langston C, Tatti KM. Pathology and pathogenesis of fatal *Bordetella pertussis* infection in infants. Clin Infect Dis. 2008;47:328-38.
7. Muloiwa R, Dube FS, Nicol MP, Hussey GD, Zar HJ. Risk factors for *Bordetella pertussis* disease in hospitalized children. PLoS One. 2020;15:e0240717.
8. American Academy of Pediatrics. Pertussis (Whooping cough). In: Kimberlin DW, Brady MT, Jackson MA, Long SS (Eds). Red Book: 2018 Report of the Committee on Infectious Diseases, 31st edition. Itasca, IL: American Academy of Pediatrics; 2018. p. 620.
9. Tiwari T, Murphy TV, Moran J. National Immunization Program CDC recommended antimicrobial agents for the treatment and postexposure prophylaxis of pertussis. 2005 CDC Guidelines. MMWR Recomm Rep. 2005;54:1-16.
10. Vashishtha VM. Adolescent immunization schedule: need for a relook. Indian Pediatr. 2019;56(2):101-4.

7.6 Enteric Fever (Typhoid and Paratyphoid Fever)

Baldev S Prajapati

INTRODUCTION

Enteric fever (also known as typhoid fever) is a major public health problem, especially in countries with poor sanitation and limited access to safe drinking water. It is the disease of developing countries. In developed countries, it mainly occurs in travelers returning from the developing country.

ETIOLOGY

Typhoid fever is caused by *Salmonella typhi*. Paratyphoid fever is due to *Salmonella paratyphi* A, B, and C. Enteric fever includes both typhoid and paratyphoid and cannot be differentiated clinically. They can be differentiated only by blood culture. Currently, paratyphoid fever is on the rise and reported as 10–20% of total cases of enteric fever from different centers in India. *Salmonella* organisms are gram-negative, rod-shaped bacilli. All *Salmonella* organisms are closely related and are considered as a single species, *Salmonella enterica*. The organism has three major antigens: somatic (S), flagellate (H), and virulence factor (Vi).[1]

EPIDEMIOLOGY

There are about 50–60 million cases with 600,000 deaths per year due to enteric fever worldwide.[2] Enteric fever is endemic in Asia (especially the Indian subcontinent), Africa, Latin America, the Caribbean, and Oceania. Children aged 5–19 years are at the highest risk of infection. However, there is an increasing trend of enteric fever in infants and young children. They are also at the highest risk of morbidity and mortality.

The infection is transmitted through the fecal–oral route. Food or water contaminated by excreta or urine from patients or chronic carriers or food handled by infected persons or carriers act as a primary source of infection. Secondary sources of infection include contaminated fingers and flies.

Humans are the only reservoir and only known host to get infected. Carriers are asymptomatic who shed typhoid bacilli after the disease. The bacilli are shed from the gall bladder through feces or urine. The convalescent carrier sheds bacilli for about 3 months following the disease, whereas the chronic carrier sheds for more than a year. Fortunately, the carrier state is not common in children.[2]

PATHOGENESIS

The infecting dose of typhoid fever is 10^3–10^6 bacilli. Those bacilli surviving the acidic environment of the stomach will pass through the intestinal mucosa to invade Peyer's patches, where macrophages engulf them but cannot kill them. Subsequently, via mesenteric lymph nodes and lymphatics, they reach the bloodstream. This primary bacteremia is usually asymptomatic. Then, they multiply within the reticuloendothelial tissues of the liver, spleen, bone marrow, lymph node, and Peyer's patches. After a critical concentration is reached, it induces macrophage apoptosis and gets released into the bloodstream again. This results in secondary bacteremia, which causes clinical symptoms. The gall bladder can get infected via either bacteremia or direct extension of infected bile. Organisms via bile re-enters the gut and are shed in stool. Gut epithelium overlying hyperplastic Peyer's patches may get sloughed out and result in ulceration, which can bleed or progress to cause perforation. In neonates, vertical transmission from the mother is known.[1]

CLINICAL FEATURES

The *incubation period* is 7–21 days, depending upon the inoculum size and immunity status of the host.[1]

The usual initial manifestations include fever, malaise, abdominal discomfort, and headache. The fever may have an insidious onset and begins as a low-grade fever rising in a stepladder pattern, but a stepladder pattern of fever is not seen these days due to frequent use of antipyretics and antibiotics. Untreated children demonstrate the following manifestations.[1,3]

First Week

The child may have a sick or toxic look. They may have gastrointestinal symptoms such as anorexia, pain in the abdomen, nausea, vomiting and diarrhea, followed by constipation. Physical findings of coated tongue, abdominal tenderness, splenomegaly or hepatosplenomegaly, relative bradycardia, and chest signs like wheezing and crepitations may be present. Spleen is usually palpable at the end of the first week. Relative bradycardia is not seen in children and may be found in older children and adolescents.

Second Week

Persistent high-grade fever and hepatosplenomegaly are common manifestations in the second week. Salmon-colored blanching truncal maculopapular rose spots may develop but are not commonly appreciated in Indian complexion.

Third Week

Manifestations referable to complications are noted in the third week. These include jaundice, altered sensorium, encephalopathy, encephalitis, meningitis, cholecystitis, osteomyelitis, etc. Malena or hematochezia due to intestinal hemorrhage and acute abdomen related to intestinal perforation are hardly seen nowadays because of effective and early antibiotic therapy. However, Guillain–Barré syndrome following enteric fever has been reported.

COMPLICATIONS

Complications occur in 10–15% of patients and are usually seen in the second and third weeks of the infection. They are not commonly encountered with the institution of effective antimicrobial therapy. The known complications of enteric fever are as follows:[4]

- Intestinal hemorrhage
- Intestinal perforation
- Myocarditis
- Cardiac arrythmias
- Venous thrombosis
- Encephalopathy
- Meningitis
- Hepatitis
- Cholecystitis
- Osteomyelitis

- Guillain-Barré syndrome
- Arthritis
- Cerebellar ataxia
- Transverse myelitis
- Pancreatitis

RELAPSE

Relapse occurs in 5–10% of patients. It presents with a recurrence of fever 2–3 weeks after the initial fever has subsided. The relapse rate of enteric fever is found more in patients treated with cephalosporins compared to patients treated with azithromycin and fluoroquinolones. Azithromycin and fluoroquinolones have better action with intracellular organisms.[1]

DIAGNOSIS

The clinical presentation of enteric fever is nonspecific, most common as "fever without focus." No laboratory test is diagnostic except positive blood culture.

Complete Blood Count

Complete blood count (CBC) shows nonspecific changes. Mild anemia may be due to a nutritional cause or chronic illness. Leukopenia is seen in 20–25% of cases, whereas leukocytosis is also seen in a few cases. White blood cell (WBC) count is normal in most patients. Eosinopenia favors enteric fever. Thrombocytopenia may develop in the second week of illness. Severe anemia may follow complications like intestinal hemorrhage.

Biochemical Tests

Mild elevation of serum glutamic pyruvic transaminase (SGPT) and serum glutamic oxaloacetic transaminase (SGOT) may occur. Serum bilirubin may be raised in a case of enteric hepatitis.

Cultures

Blood culture: This is the gold standard for the diagnosis of enteric fever. It is positive in >75% of patients during the first week of illness. The sensitivity is greatest in the first week at around 90% but drops to 40% by the fourth week. Its overall sensitivity is 60%, which reduces to 20–40% after antibiotics; its specificity is 100%. *Salmonella* is an easy organism to culture. At least 5 mL of blood should be collected for a ratio of 1:5–1:10 of blood to broth to neutralize the bactericidal effect of serum. Prior treatment with antibiotics is a very common factor for failure to obtain a positive culture.

BACTEC, an automated blood culture system, certainly increases the isolation rate. Blood culture should be done in all suspected cases of enteric fever, as a positive culture not only establishes the diagnosis but also gives an antibiotic sensitivity pattern, which is important in this era of multidrug-resistant enteric fever.

Bone marrow culture: Median bacteremia in bone marrow is high compared to blood. The bone marrow to peripheral blood ratio of an organism is around 4.8 in the first week, which increases to 158 during the third week due to a decrease in bacteria in peripheral blood. It is not a preferred investigation routinely being invasive, but sensitivity is 80–95% and leads to good yield even in late disease treated with antibiotics. It is, however, a very useful and valid investigation in the evaluation of pyrexia of unknown origin, where the marrow should be inoculated in the culture bottle at the bedside.

Stool and urine culture: The organisms can be isolated in the third week if untreated. A stool specimen of adequate amount should be processed within 2 hours or should be kept at 4°C. For the detection of a carrier, several samples should be examined because of irregular shedding of the organism. The sensitivity of urine culture is very poor. Duodenal string and skin snip culture of rose spot is of academic interest only.

Serological Tests

No tests are enough sensitive or specific to replace culture-based diagnosis. The *Widal test* has been in use for 100 years for serological diagnosis of enteric fever. It detects the presence of immunoglobulin M (IgM) and immunoglobulin G (IgG) antibodies to H (flagellar antigen) of *S. enterica var typhi* and *paratyphi* A and B and O (somatic antigen) common to typhi and paratyphi A and B. Anti-O titers are both IgG and IgM that rise and decline early, while anti-H are primarily IgG that rise and decline late in the course of the disease. The conventional method of interpretation of the Widal test has been to demonstrate a fourfold rise in antibody titers in two samples; since this is often not practical, a single titer of at least 1:160 for both O and H is considered positive. Even with this compromise, the Widal test has several limitations. Sensitivity is low in the first week of illness and in patients treated with prior antibiotics. Specificity is low owing to anamnestic reactions, cross-reactivity with other enterobacteriaceae, and subclinical infection in endemic areas.[1]

Other tests, such as Tubex and Typhidot, that detect IgM antibodies against typhoid have not proven to be superior to the Widal test. Serological tests are losing their utility in practice.

Antigen Detection Tests

To detect serum or urinary O, H or Vi antigens have suboptimal with variable sensitivity and specificity.

Molecular Methods

Polymerase chain reaction (PCR) is not used in day-to-day practice as it is not evaluated extensively in field practice.

DIFFERENTIAL DIAGNOSIS

During the first week, enteric fever needs to be differentiated from common febrile illnesses that present as fever without focus, such as viral fever, malaria, dengue fever, and urinary tract infection. Once the spleen becomes palpable, other differential diagnoses that need consideration include malaria, hepatitis, infectious mononucleosis, brucellosis, etc. Undiagnosed enteric fever beyond 2 weeks needs to be differentiated from tuberculosis, leukemia, and collagen vascular diseases.

MANAGEMENT

Indications for Inpatient Treatment

Most cases of enteric fever can be managed at home with oral antibiotics and advice to seek medical follow-up in case of failure to respond to therapy or development of complications. Children with persistent vomiting, inability to take orally, severe diarrhea, or abdominal distention require intravenous (IV) antibiotic therapy and IV fluids, necessitating hospitalization.

Antimicrobial Sensitivity

The antimicrobial sensitivity of *S. typhi* and *S. paratyphi* has shown changes over decades.[3,5] Though resistance to chloramphenicol was first reported in the 1940s, it was not until 1972 that chloramphenicol-resistant enteric fever became a major problem. Multidrug-resistant typhoid fever (MDRTF) became a major issue by the end of the 1990s, with the emergence of *S. typhi* resistant to all the primary drugs such as chloramphenicol, cotrimoxazole, and ampicillin. Fluoroquinolones were introduced in the 1990s and had good results initially, but the past decade has been progressive resistant. Recently, several studies showed return of sensitivity to first-line drugs like chloramphenicol, cotrimoxazole, and ampicillin.[6]

Currently, third-generation cephalosporins such as ceftriaxone and cefixime are the first-line antibiotics for the treatment of enteric fever. Azithromycin is another molecule that is being used as a second line of medicine. However, there are recent reports of the emergence of plasmid-borne ceftriaxone resistance in *Salmonella* that is of serious concern. Cephalosporin-resistant *Salmonella* outbreaks have been reported from some centers in India recently.[3,5,6]

Choice of Empirical Therapy

Where enteric fever is clinically diagnosed and a blood culture report is awaited or the culture is sterile, empirical therapy is started. The choice of empirical antibiotics is decided with consideration of various factors such as known local sensitivity pattern, severity of disease, indoor or outdoor therapy, and presence of complications.[3,5] The current choice of empirical antibiotic therapy is summarized in **Table 7.6.1**.

TABLE 7.6.1: Empirical choice of antimicrobial therapy for enteric fever.

Type of fever	*First line*	*Alternative*
Uncomplicated enteric fever	Cefixime 20 mg/kg/day in two divided doses Maximum 1,200 mg	Azithromycin 20 mg/kg/day once a day Maximum 1,000 mg
Severe enteric fever	Ceftriaxone 100 mg/kg/day in two divided doses as IV infusion therapy Maximum 4 g	Aztreonam 150 mg/kg/day in three divided doses Maximum 6 g/day

Once a blood culture report is available, antibiotics can be modified. Cefixime should be completed for a period of 14 days; a shorter duration of therapy is associated with relapse. Azithromycin should be continued for 7–10 days. An indoor patient who is on injection ceftriaxone can switch to oral cefixime once he is afebrile and showing recovery, to complete 14 days of treatment. There is no data at present to support combination therapy in enteric fever. Recently, extensively drug-resistant *S. typhi* infections have been reported from Pakistan and Iraq. The use of azithromycin or carbapenems may be indicated in this situation. Some of the centers in India also have reported outbreaks of ceftriaxone-resistant enteric fever recently. Many of the patients from these outbreaks responded to cephalosporins (ceftriaxone or cefixime) on continuation of therapy, in spite of their blood culture results showing ceftriaxone and/or cefixime-resistant *Salmonella*.[3,5,6]

Some patients with culture-proven enteric fever do not defervesce up to a week of treatment despite being on a susceptible antimicrobial agent. In such situations, thrombophlebitis, coinfection, drug fever, and development of complications should be considered. If all of these are excluded, continue the same medicine; it may respond late. In blood culture-negative nonresponders, a thorough search for alternative etiology for fever should be made.

Steroids in Enteric Fever

Use of steroids may decrease mortality in children with complications like encephalopathy, toxic shock, etc. Dexamethasone is used in an initial dose of 3 mg/kg IV over 30 minutes, followed by 1 mg/kg every 6 hours for 48 hours.

Therapy of Relapse

Relapse rates vary with the type of drug and are most common with cephalosporins (ceftriaxone and cefixime), especially if a shorter duration of therapy is used. Relapse may be satisfactorily treated with the same drug used as for primary therapy but for an appropriate dose and duration. Azithromycin may be used, if not used earlier.

Treatment of Complications

Complications such as intestinal perforation and intestinal hemorrhage may require surgical intervention besides appropriate antimicrobials and blood transfusion therapy.

PREVENTION

The most effective and desirable measures for the prevention of enteric fever are improving hygiene and sanitation. It will also reduce the burden of other water-borne diseases. Vaccination is a proven strategy for the prevention of enteric fever at present. Chronic carrier is defined as >1 year of fecal shedding and is of public health importance and treated effectively by 4–6 weeks of fluoroquinolones.

REFERENCES

1. Jeffrey SM. Enteric Fever (Typhoid and Paratyphoid Fever). In: Kliegman RM, Geme III JE, Blum NJ, Tasker RC, Wilson KM (Eds.). Nelson Textbook of Pediatrics, 22nd edition. Philadelphia; Elsevier. 2025. pp. 1771-6.
2. Bhan MK, Bahl R, Bhatnagar S. Typhoid and paratyphoid fever. Lancet. 2005;366:749-62.
3. Crump JA. Progress in typhoid fever epidemiology. Clin Infect Dis. 2019;68(Suppl 1):54-9.
4. Khatun H, Islam SB, Naila NN, Islam SA, Nahar B, Alam NH, et al. Clinical profile, antibiotic susceptibility pattern of bacterial isolates and factors associated with complications in culture-proven typhoid patients admitted to an urban hospital in Bangladesh. Trop Med Int Health. 2018;23(4):359-66.
5. Espinoza LMC, McCreedy E, Holm M, Im J, Mogeni OD, Parajulee P, et al. Occurrence of typhoid fever complications and their relation to duration of illness preceding hospitalization: a systematic literature review and meta-analysis. Clin Infect Dis. 2019;69(Suppl 6): S435-8.
6. Kumar Y, Sharma A, Mani KR. Antibiogram profile of *Salmonella enterica* serovar Typhi in India—a two-year study. Trop Life Sci Res. 2013;24(1):45-54.

7.7 Tuberculosis

Aparna Mukherjee, Rakesh Lodha

INTRODUCTION

Tuberculosis (TB) is one of the most common causes of mortality worldwide. Globally, in 2022, an estimated 10.6 million people fell ill with TB and there were an estimated 1.3 million deaths. Children represent about 11% of all TB cases. The overall case notification is about 70% in adults and about 50% in children. Approximately 67 million children are infected with TB (latent TB) and are therefore at risk of developing disease in the future. Despite the best of efforts, childhood TB is still under-reported in most of the countries.[1]

EPIDEMIOLOGY

The incidence of TB cases varies among different populations and regions, from under 10 per 100,000 population in most high-income countries to 150–300 in most of the 30 high-burden countries. The World Health Organization (WHO) South-East Asia Region (WHO-SEAR) accounted for 45% of the incident cases. TB is the ninth leading cause of death worldwide; it is the main cause from a single infectious agent. More than 80% of TB deaths occurred in the WHO African Region and the WHO-SEAR in 2022. In 2022, the estimated incidence of TB in India was 199 per 1,00,000; the estimated human immunodeficiency virus (HIV)-negative TB mortality rate was 23 per 100,000 population.[1,2]

The incidence of drug-resistant TB has increased over the past few years and is a challenge for the whole world due to diagnostic and therapeutic challenges. In 2022, worldwide estimates for the proportions of multidrug-resistant (MDR)/rifampicin-resistant TB in new and previously treated cases were 4.1% and 19%, respectively.

PATHOGENESIS

Mycobacterium tuberculosis bacilli (MTB) are acid-fast, nonspore-forming, nonmotile, pleomorphic, weakly gram-positive curved rods, 1–5 µm long, typically slender and slightly bent. They may appear beaded or clumped under microscopy. They are obligate aerobes that grow in synthetic media containing glycerol as the carbon source and ammonium salts as the nitrogen source. Other closely related mycobacteria, such as *Mycobacterium bovis*, *Mycobacterium africanum*, and *Mycobacterium microti*, along with *M. tuberculosis*, form the *M. tuberculosis* complex. The characteristic property is acid fastness, which is imparted by the ability to form stable mycolate complexes with arylmethane dyes that resist discoloration with ethanol.

The spectrum of affliction by MTB includes exposure, infection, and disease.

- *Exposure* means that the child had significant contact with a person with infectious TB but lacks proof of infection.
- *Infection* occurs when an individual inhales droplets, which contain mycobacteria, which survive intracellularly in lung and lymphoid tissue. In this stage, the child is *asymptomatic* and has a normal physical examination.
- *Disease* occurs when the symptoms, signs, or radiographic manifestations become apparent.

Not all infected individuals have the same risk of developing the disease. An immunocompetent adult with untreated TB infection has approximately a 5–10% lifetime risk of developing disease. In contrast, an infected infant has a 40% chance of developing the disease within 9–12 months.

Lung is the portal of entry in the majority of cases. Bacilli enter alveolar passage in an aerosol droplet, interact with macrophages or type II pneumocytes, and are phagocytosed in a process initiated by bacterial contact with macrophage mannose and/or complement receptors. On entry into a host macrophage, *M. tuberculosis* initially resides in an endocytic vacuole called the phagosome. If the normal phagosomal maturation cycle occurs, i.e., phagosome–lysosome fusion, these bacteria may encounter a hostile environment that includes acid pH, reactive oxygen intermediates, lysosomal enzymes, and toxic peptides. Interferon-gamma (IFN-γ) plays a key role for a protective immune response. IFN-γ, produced mainly by cluster of differentiation 4 ($CD4^+$), $CD8^+$ T cells, and the natural killer (NK) cells, synergizes with tumor necrosis factor-alpha (TNF-α) and activates macrophages to kill intracellular bacilli. Bacteria may evade destruction by preventing phagosome–lysosome fusion and causing macrophage necrosis. These bacilli, which survive within macrophages, are carried to regional lymph nodes. The *primary complex (Ghon complex)* of TB includes local infection at the portal of entry and the regional lymph nodes that drain the area.

There is tissue reaction at initial foci over the next 2–12 weeks and hypersensitivity develops, which heals by calcification or fibrosis. Occasionally, this portion may continue to enlarge and lead to focal pneumonitis and pleuritis, and if caseation is intense then it may lead to cavitation. During the development of the primary complex, tubercle bacilli are carried to most tissues of the body through the blood and lymphatic vessels.

Disseminated TB occurs if host cellular immunity is inadequate. Bacterial replication is more likely to occur in organs with conditions that favor their growth, such as lung apices, brain, kidneys, and bones. The time between initial infection and apparent disease is variable. Pulmonary TB that occurs after 1 year of primary infection is due to endogenous growth of bacilli. This reactivation of TB is rare in children but common in adults and adolescents. Occasionally, reinfection can occur in immunocompromised individuals or those living in highly endemic areas.

DIFFERENCES BETWEEN TUBERCULOSIS IN ADULTS AND CHILDREN

Childhood TB is not simply a reflection of the adult spectrum of disease. Characteristics of TB in children include the paucibacillary nature; preponderance of primary focus and lymph node disease; a higher chance of dissemination into serious manifestations such as miliary TB, tuberculosis meningitis (TBM), and spinal TB; a higher burden of extrapulmonary TB (EPTB); challenges in diagnosis due to the inability to expectorate sputum; and a difference in pharmacokinetic or pharmacodynamic characteristics of antitubercular drugs.[2]

PULMONARY TUBERCULOSIS

Intrathoracic involvement in children is varied and may include the following:

- *Primary focus:* Primary focus, or Ghon focus, results from primary infection and is usually a single focus of parenchymal involvement with or without pleural component. The primary focus, along with the draining regional lymph node, is called the primary or Ghon complex. This may get complicated and result in cavitation or intrabronchial spread.
- *Lymph node disease:* As a result of primary infection, parahilar and paratracheal nodes may be involved; complications may include airway involvement leading to alveolar collapse or pneumonia.
- *Pleural or pericardial effusion:* This represents a hypersensitivity reaction resulting in straw-colored fluid with a high lymphocyte count. If *Mycobacterium bacillus* grows in pleural space, localized empyema is formed. Pericardial effusion may lead to constrictive pericarditis.
- *Miliary disease:* This results from hematogenous dissemination of bacilli; <2 mm nodules are seen on chest X-ray extending up to the periphery.
- *Adult-type cavitary lesion:* This is usually seen around 8–10 years of age and beyond.

Clinical Features

Pulmonary TB can present with cough and/or fever for >2 weeks, not responding to a course of antibiotic for 7–10 days, weight loss (>5% of the highest recorded weight in the past 3 months) or not gaining weight, poor appetite, lethargy or easy fatigability, and night sweats. There may be a history of contact with an open case of TB within the last few years.[2,3]

Diagnosis (Flowchart 7.7.1)

Microbiological Confirmation

In spite of the fact that approximately 50% of intrathoracic TB in children is diagnosed clinicoradiologically, every attempt should be made to document a microbiological confirmation in each case.

- *Sample collection:* A major challenge in the microbiological diagnosis of childhood TB is the difficulty in obtaining an appropriate sample, as children usually cannot expectorate sputum. Gastric aspirate/lavage and induced sputum are feasible options for collecting respiratory samples even in ambulatory, nonhospitalized children. Recently, stool specimens have also been used to diagnose TB.
- *Examination of smears from respiratory samples under light microscopy after Ziehl–Neelsen (ZN) staining:* It is still the most widely accessible investigation in the majority of high-burden areas. In spite of a high specificity, the sensitivity of smear examination remains variable (5–10%).
- *Culture:* Löwenstein–Jensen culture media (LJ medium) is the most widely used solid media for the determination of characteristic features of colonial morphology, growth rate, and pigment production. The yield of culture varies from 30% to 50%. The excessively long period required for the isolation of MTB by conventional culture techniques has led to the development of other techniques for

Flowchart 7.7.1: Diagnostic algorithm for childhood intrathoracic tuberculosis.

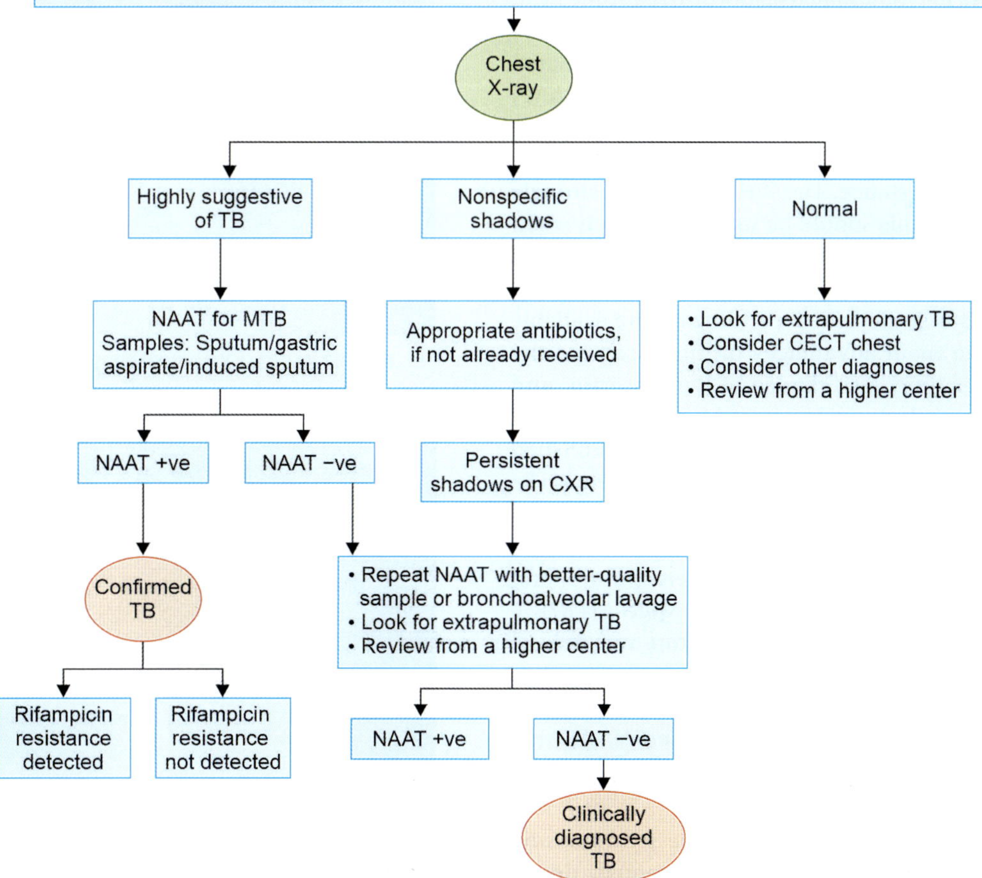

(CECT: contrast-enhanced computed tomography; CXR: chest X-ray; MTB: *Mycobacterium tuberculosis*; NAAT: nucleic acid amplification test; TB: tuberculosis)

culture—BACTEC radiometric assay, Septi-Chek acid-fast bacilli (AFB) system, and mycobacterial growth indicator tube (MGIT) culture. Liquid systems are more sensitive for detecting mycobacteria and may increase the case yield by 10% over solid media as well as reduce the time to result from weeks to days. For drug susceptibility testing (DST), the delay may be reduced to as little as 10 days, compared with 28–42 days with conventional solid media.

- *Microscopic observation drug susceptibility (MODS) assay:* MODS assay is an inexpensive, rapid, and sensitive diagnostic method utilizing the manual liquid culture method (Middlebrook 7H9 broth culture) and an inverted light microscope to detect the growth of MTB in the form of "tangles or cords." In a study from Peru, where the assay was developed, MODS detected 94% of 1,908 positive sputum cultures, whereas conventional LJ culture detected only 87%. This assay is not yet available widely and has some problems as it is operator-dependent and labor-intensive, and more studies in nonresearch settings are needed to validate its use.
- *Nucleic acid amplification test (NAAT):* Polymerase chain reaction (PCR), fully automated platform of real-time PCR, and loop-mediated isothermal amplification (LAMP) platform are the available variations of NAAT. Automated cartridge-based nucleic acid amplification test (CBNAAT) such as Xpert MTB/RIF test is a fully automated real-time PCR-based assay that detects not only *M. tuberculosis* but also rifampicin resistance. The WHO as of now strongly recommends that this should be used in children when there is strong suspicion of MDR-TB or in the case of HIV-TB coinfection. It may also be used in any case where pulmonary TB is suspected, depending on the available resources. The main advantages of this assay are the rapid turnover time, less chance of human error, and the ability to simultaneously detect *M. tuberculosis* and resistance to rifampicin. In the meta-analysis published by the WHO, the overall pooled sensitivity of Xpert MTB/RIF compared against culture as a reference standard in children presumed to have TB was 66%; the samples used were induced sputum, expectorated sputum, and gastric lavage. The pooled specificity of Xpert MTB/RIF compared against the gold standard culture was at least 98%. The sensitivity of Xpert MTB/RIF to detect rifampicin resistance in specimens from children was 86%. *Truenat* is an indigenously developed chip-based NAAT that sequentially detects the presence of *M. tuberculosis* and rifampicin resistance.
- *Molecular drug resistance testing—line probe assays (LPAs):* LPAs are strip tests that simultaneously detect MTB as well as genetic mutations that indicate isoniazid (INH) and/or rifampicin resistance.

Tuberculin Skin Test (Mantoux Test)

Tuberculin skin test (TST) is an intradermal skin test with 5 TU of PPD-S or 2 TU of PPD RT 23 or equivalent, read after 48–72 hours. An induration of 10 mm or more is considered positive. In immunocompromised individuals, an induration of 5 mm or more is considered positive. A positive TST merely indicates the presence of tubercular infection and not disease; hence, it can only *aid in the diagnosis* of TB disease and not *confirm* it.

Imaging

- *Chest X-ray:* Radiological features highly suggestive of TB include hilar or paratracheal lymph nodes with or without parenchymal involvement, miliary pattern, and fibrocavitary lesion. Some examples are given in **Figures 7.7.1 to 7.7.4.** If left untreated, miliary nodules

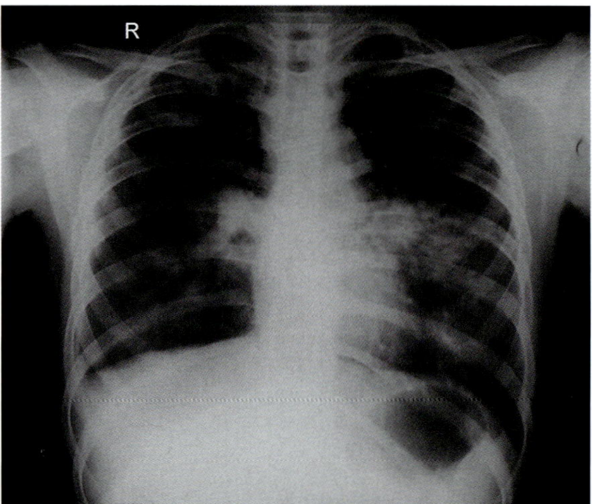

Fig. 7.7.1: Chest X-ray showing bilateral infiltrates.

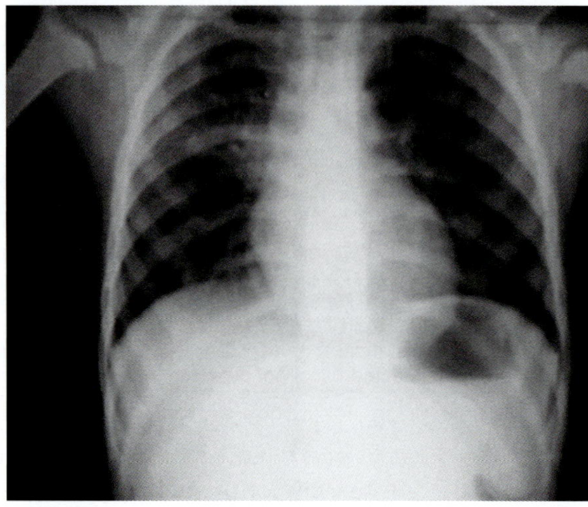

Fig. 7.7.2: Chest X-ray of a 5-year-old with collapse consolidation of the right middle lobe.

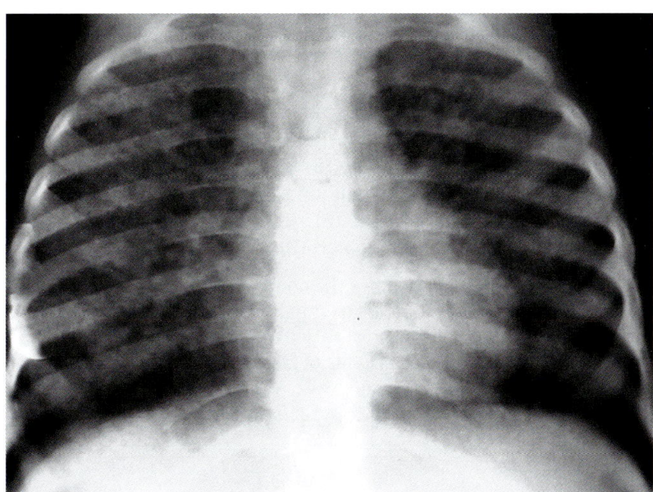

Fig. 7.7.3: Chest X-ray of a 2½-year-old girl with miliary tuberculosis.

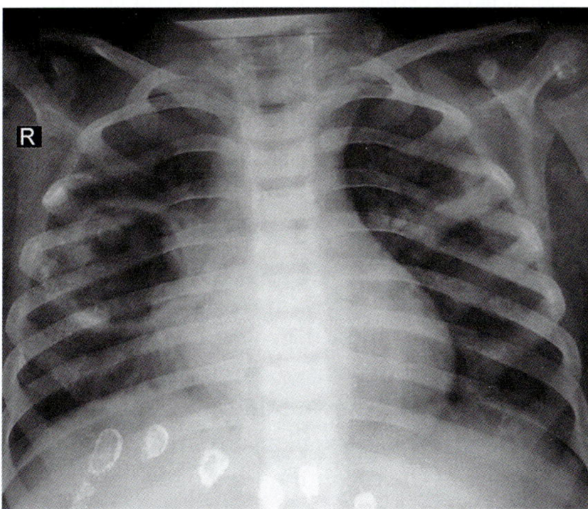

Fig. 7.7.4: Chest X-ray showing a cavitary lesion.

may coalesce and may reach 3–5 mm in size, radiologically described as a "snow-storm" appearance.

- *Contrast-enhanced computed tomography (CECT) chest:* CT chest may be done in cases where the chest X-ray is not conclusive. CECT chest enables evaluation of parenchymal lesion, identification of necrosis in lymph nodes, description of pleural, airway, and diaphragmatic pathologies, and evaluation of visualized bones. CECT features suggestive of TB include a necrotic lymph node with a low-density center surrounded by rim enhancement (rim sign), 2–4 mm centrilobular nodules, and tree-in-bud appearances (sharply marginated linear branching opacities around the terminal and respiratory bronchioles) indicating endobronchial spread, thick-walled cavity surrounded by parenchymal lesion indicating active disease. CT may also be useful in undertaking guided aspiration/biopsy from mediastinal nodes for cyto/histopathology and microbiological diagnosis.
- *Endobronchial ultrasound (EBUS):* EBUS is a newer modality of diagnosis that is feasible and useful in older children. In case of older children with large hilar or subcarinal lymph nodes, EBUS-transbronchial needle aspiration (TBNA) may be tried to obtain a sample for cytological and microbiological diagnosis. Studies have documented a definitive diagnosis of 57% using TBNA in cases of mediastinal lymphadenopathy in children. However, this is a technique that is yet to be available widely for the diagnosis of TB in children. Also, EBUS may reveal a pattern of multiple hyperechoic foci without an acoustic shadow over a hypoechoic background. This is called the "starry sky sign" and is about 51.6% and 100% sensitive and specific in the diagnosis of tubercular mediastinal nodes. This mode of diagnosis can be employed for follow-up of mediastinal nodal disease instead of CT chest to reduce radiation exposure. The presence of diffusion restriction in lymph nodes along with peripheral enhancement suggests active disease.

T-cell-based Interferon-gamma Release Assays

Interferon-gamma release assays (IGRA) are in vitro tests of cell-mediated immune response, which are mostly helpful in detecting latent TB infection, not disease. The two common commercially available IGRAs are the QuantiFERON-TB Gold In-Tube (QFT-GIT) assay (Cellestis Ltd., Carnegie, Australia) and the T-SPOT.TB assay (Oxford Immunotec, Oxford, UK). The QFT-GIT assay is an enzyme-linked immunosorbent assay (ELISA)-based whole-blood test that quantitates IFN-γ released in response to antigenic stimulation from three TB specific peptides, namely ESAT-6, CFP-10, and TB7.7, in a simple in-tube format. T-SPOT.TB is an enzyme-linked immunospot (ELISPOT) assay designed to measure the number of IFN-γ-producing T-cells in response to ESAT-6 and CFP-10 peptides. The advantage of these assays lies in the fact that they are not affected by previous Bacille Calmette-Guérin (BCG) vaccination, do not cross-react with most of the nontubercular mycobacterium (except *Mycobacterium kansasii*, *Mycobacterium szulgai*, and *Mycobacterium marinum*), are not affected by observer bias, and require only one visit for testing. The sensitivity of QFT assay and T-SPOT.TB assay is 75–85% and 90–95%, respectively. The sensitivity is lower in high-incidence regions. The shortcoming of these assays includes the inability to distinguish between latent and active TB and high cost. The immune response leading to the release of IFN-γ is inconsistent in children below 4 years of age, and hence interpretation of IGRA may be difficult in this age group. The sensitivity of QFT-GIT is variable in children below 4 years of age, with a higher number of indeterminate results. These tests are recommended for use in the country.

C-Tb (Statens Serum Institut, Copenhagen, Denmark)

C-Tb is an intradermal skin test that utilizes ESAT-6 and CFP-10 as the antigen; 5 mm induration is considered as a positive indication of tubercular infection. C-Tb findings have high concordance with those of IGRA, such as QFT. It is yet to be included in the programmatic setting in India.

Antigen Detection Tests

Lipoarabinomannans (LAM) are phosphorylated lipopolysaccharides, which are a major cell wall component of bacteria of the genus *Mycobacterium*. Antigen detection assays based on capture ELISA format to detect LAM in urine hold promise as an easy, point-of-care, noninvasive tool for diagnosing active TB. However, the low sensitivity of urinary LAM (17–50%) as compared with the gold standard of culture offsets the advantages. The specificity is acceptable (88–95%). This diagnostic tool may be particularly helpful in the selected subset of patients with HIV/TB coinfection, where the sensitivity increases.

Antibody Detection Tests

There is no role of any serological diagnosis in the form of antibodies against tubercular antigens in the diagnosis of any type of TB—pulmonary or extrapulmonary. Such tests are currently banned by the Government of India.

Treatment

Treatment of TB comprises two phases—intensive phase (IP) and continuation phase (CP).[2,3] The IP is administered at the beginning of therapy when the bacterial load is expected to be higher and rapid killing of bacteria is required, whereas the CP refers to the later phase where the residual disease is being treated.

The current treatment plan has changed in the following aspects:

- Drug sensitivity is tested upfront with the widespread availability of NAAT.
- Category-based treatment has been abolished.
- There is no provision of extension of IP even if there is an unsatisfactory response; the patient is to be investigated for drug resistance.

All rifampicin-sensitive new or previously treated cases are prescribed 6 months of antitubercular therapy (ATT), which includes 2 months of IP consisting of daily isoniazid, rifampicin, pyrazinamide, and ethambutol, followed by 4 months of CP of daily isoniazid, rifampicin, and ethambutol. Fixed-dose combinations are preferred as they are easier to administer to the children. **Table 7.7.1** shows the ATT for children.

TABLE 7.7.1: Treatment for tuberculosis in children.

Type of cases	***Regimen***
• Newly diagnosed microbiologically confirmed rifampicin-sensitive (RS) pulmonary or extrapulmonary TB • Newly clinically diagnosed pulmonary or extrapulmonary TB (probable TB) • Drug-sensitive previously treated TB	2HRZE + 4HRE

Notes: The prefix number denotes the number of months.
Newly diagnosed TB case refers to situations where the child is either treatment naïve or has received anti-TB treatment for <4 weeks.
Previously treated TB includes cases of failure, relapse, or lost to follow-up.
(H: isoniazid; R: rifampicin; Z: pyrazinamide, E: ethambutol; TB: tuberculosis)

TABLE 7.7.2: Daily dose and maximum doses of isoniazid, rifampicin, ethambutol, and pyrazinamide in children.

Drug	***Dose (range) (mg/kg body weight/day)***	***Maximum dose (mg/day)***
Rifampicin	15 (10–20)	600
Isoniazid	10 (7–15)	300
Ethambutol	15–25	1,500
Pyrazinamide	35 (30–40)	2,000

The medications should preferably be given daily on a mg/kg body weight basis. A meta-analysis conducted on studies in children showed that intermittent therapy of antitubercular drugs was less likely to cure than daily therapy. **Table 7.7.2** details the recommended daily doses of the four first-line antitubercular drugs according to the latest WHO guidelines. The dose of the antitubercular drugs should be adjusted according to the current weight of the child in each follow-up visit during therapy. For children, the current program uses a daily regimen and weight-band-based dosing using fixed-dose combinations (FDCs).

Monitoring

Any child on ATT should be regularly monitored for the following:

Response to Treatment

Monthly follow-up while on therapy and 6-monthly visits after completion of treatment for a total of 2 years are advised. In each visit, symptomatic improvement, as well as reduction in clinical signs like abnormal breath sounds, size of lymph nodes, etc., along with a change in weight, should be noted. If the child is not responding at the end of 4 weeks, a radiological assessment and MGIT culture should be performed.

Adverse Events

Any feature suggestive of hepatitis, rash, and/or peripheral neuropathy should be promptly investigated. The antitubercular drugs should be modified if the child is symptomatic with pain in the abdomen, vomiting, or yellowish discoloration of sclera and urine, or if the liver enzymes [aspartate aminotransferase (AST)/alanine aminotransferase (ALT)] are deranged more than five times the upper limit, or if the total bilirubin is raised. Isoniazid, rifampicin, and pyrazinamide should be stopped, and the modified regimen should contain ethambutol and fluoroquinolone such as levofloxacin. Injectable streptomycin may be added if the disease severity warrants. Once the symptoms are relieved and liver parameters are normalized, the first-line antitubercular drugs should be restarted sequentially, increasing every 5–7 days after checking the liver functions. Once the full dose of conventional antitubercular drugs is reached, the modified regimen may be stopped.

Role of Corticosteroids in Tuberculosis

Routinely, there is no role of corticosteroids in the management of intrathoracic TB in children. However, in the case of superior mediastinal compression syndrome due to mediastinal nodes or in miliary disease with alveolocapillary block, oral corticosteroids may be used. Other definite indications for concomitant steroid therapy in TB include TBM, pericarditis, and TB uveitis.

TUBERCULAR LYMPHADENITIS

Tuberculosis in any organ other than the lung is considered as EPTB. Lymph node TB is the most common form of EPTB, especially in children. Approximately 35% of EPTB cases are lymph node TB. Deep-seated nodes of the mediastinum (mediastinal TB) or abdomen (abdominal lymph node TB) may also be affected.

A child with lymph node TB presents with matted, usually nontender lymph nodes >2 cm size at one or more sites, not responding to antibiotic treatment and persisting for >1 month. The child may also have fever, poor appetite, and weight loss/inability to gain weight. The lymph node may become fluctuant and burst forming a sinus or ulcer with undermined edges **(Fig. 7.7.5.)**.

Diagnosis

Tuberculin skin test: Positive TST ≥ 10 mm suggests tubercular infection, but does not confirm disease. An X-ray of the chest should be done to evaluate pulmonary involvement.

Fine needle aspiration of the nodes: The antigravity Z technique should be applied for aspiration. Deep-seated nodes can be accessed by ultrasound guidance. Samples should be sent for cytopathology, AFB, MGIT culture, and CBNAAT assay. The cytopathological characteristics of tubercular lymphadenitis include epithelioid cell granuloma with or without Langhans cell with or without necrosis. Staining for AFB is a must in all cases suspected to be lymph node TB.

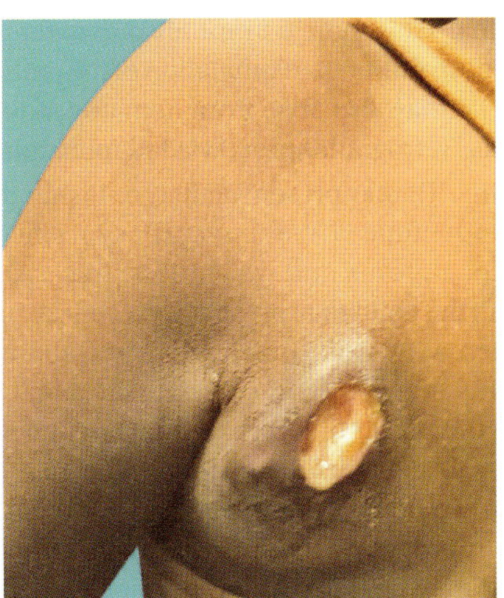

Fig. 7.7.5: Tubercular axillary lymph nodes with overlying ulcer formation.

Excision biopsy: It may be needed if cytopathology from aspiration is inconclusive and there is a high index of suspicion of malignancy.

Treatment

Treatment of tubercular lymphadenitis follows the same principle of ATT as pulmonary TB.[2,3] Newly diagnosed, microbiologically confirmed, or clinically diagnosed TB lymphadenitis is treated by a 6-month course of ATT (2HRZE + 4HRE). There is no role of surgery in the treatment of tubercular lymphadenitis.

ABDOMINAL TUBERCULOSIS

Abdominal TB occurs in approximately 3.5% of patients with extrapulmonary TB. Approximately 30% of patients with intra-abdominal TB have evidence of pulmonary TB at the time of diagnosis. Miliary TB cases will have abdominal involvement in about one-third of cases.

Abdominal TB may involve the various regions of the gastrointestinal (GI) tract, the peritoneum, or both. The most common site of involvement in the GI tract is the ileocecal region, followed by the ascending colon, jejunum, appendix, duodenum, stomach, esophagus, sigmoid colon, and rectum. In case of peritoneal involvement, it may be wet type with the development of ascites, dry type with adhesions, and fibrotic type along with pockets of ascites.

Abdominal TB is more commonly due to the ingestion of infected sputum rather than inhalation of the pathogen. Intra-abdominal TB may also arise from hematogenous spread or, in some cases, retrograde spread via fallopian tubes.

Abdominal TB may present acutely or insidiously. Clinical features of abdominal TB may be very nonspecific and include abdominal pain, fever, and weight loss. In case of intestinal involvement, the child may present with colicky pain, chronic diarrhea alternating with constipation, and abdominal mass. Ascites is frequently present; subacute intestinal obstruction can also be the presenting complaint. Omental involvement may give rise to a characteristic doughy feel to the abdomen. Isolated involvement of the hepatobiliary system by MTB is rare; it usually is part of a more disseminated process. Hepatic involvement may be miliary with multiple miliary tubercles, granulomatous with tuberculomas, nodular with abscess formation, ductal, or nodal where nodes cause obstruction at the porta leading to jaundice.

Diagnosis

Diagnosis of abdominal TB requires the following:

- *Chest X-ray:* An X-ray should be done in all cases of presumptive abdominal TB to look for pulmonary involvement.
- *Ascitic fluid analysis:* Ascitic fluid is usually straw-colored, exudative in nature, with majority of lymphocytes. Protein concentration is higher than 2.5 g/dL; serum albumin to ascitic ratio (SAAG) > 1.1.
- *Microbiological confirmation* should be attempted in all cases. Samples that can be sent for Z-N staining, MGIT culture, and CBNAAT assay include ascitic fluid, ultrasonography (USG), or CT-guided fine-needle aspirate or biopsy from the mesenteric/retroperitoneal nodes or peritoneum.
- *Imaging:* Imaging for abdominal TB includes USG and CECT or CT enterography. The most common imaging features detected in abdominal TB include a conglomerate of lymph nodes with central necrosis, mesenteric thickening (>15 mm), peritoneal thickening, ascites, lesions in the spleen or liver, etc. Characteristically, a pulled-up and contracted caecum, distorted ileocecal angle, and short strictures (<3 cm) can be seen on CT enterography.

Treatment

- 6 months of ATT (2HRZE + 4HRE) is the mainstay of therapy.
- Supportive treatment should be provided for ascites.
- Subacute intestinal obstruction is to be managed conservatively.

OSTEOARTICULAR TUBERCULOSIS

Bones and joints account for approximately 10% of extrapulmonary TB. Spinal TB, or Pott's spine, is the most common type of bone TB, the thoracic spine being the most common site. Spinal TB results from hematogenous spread from either a pulmonary site or an extrapulmonary site like a lymph node.

Tuberculosis of the spine may present with localized back pain for more than 6 weeks, fever, weight loss, or failure to gain weight. There may be localized tenderness with gibbus formation, with or without spinal cord involvement and neurological manifestations.

All suspected cases of spinal TB should undergo an X-ray of the spine followed by MRI of the spine. MRI of the spine demonstrates characteristic features of bone destruction earlier than X-ray and can also give important information regarding spinal cord involvement. A chest X-ray should also be done in all cases to look for pulmonary involvement. Samples should be taken (guided by radiology from any paravertebral collection and joint effusion) for MGIT culture and CBNAAT assay along with cytopathology.

The treatment option for bone TB is 2 months of HRZE followed by 10 months of HRE. The development and progression of a neurological deficit may need surgical intervention.

The other forms of osteoarticular TB include TB dactylitis, usually involving the short tubular bones of the hand and feet.

CENTRAL NERVOUS SYSTEM TUBERCULOSIS

Central nervous system (CNS) TB includes an array of conditions—meningitis (TBM), cerebral and spinal tuberculoma, myelitis, and arachnoiditis.[4] Approximately 1% of total TB cases are due to CNS TB. CNS TB can lead to considerable mortality and morbidity, especially in younger children <3 years of age.

Tuberculosis Meningitis

Tuberculosis meningitis may present as acute, subacute, or chronic meningitis. According to the Wallgren timeline, TBM develops within approximately 3 months of primary infection, if not contained. TBM may initially present with nonspecific symptoms like fever, listlessness or apathy, poor appetite, failure to thrive, neck stiffness, and headache if the child is old enough to complain. Later, it may progress to altered sensorium, seizures, and focal neurological deficits. Because of the nonspecific nature of the symptoms, any meningitis-like presentation before 1 year of age should be investigated for TBM. Also, there is a close association with miliary TB and immunocompromised states.

The disease begins with the development of small tuberculous foci (Rich foci) in the brain, spinal cord, or meninges caseating into the subarachnoid space.

There are various clinical classifications of the severity of TBM. The British Medical Council Research criteria classify TBM into the following stages:

- *Mild:* Fully conscious with no focal neurological deficit
- *Moderate:* Conscious but with altered sensorium, confusion, lethargy, and moderate neurological signs like single nerve palsy, hemiparesis, and paraparesis
- *Severe:* Comatose, multiple cranial nerve palsies, hemiplegia, and/or paraplegia

Effort should be made for early diagnosis and treatment of TBM to avoid an unfavorable outcome and lasting disability.

Diagnosis

- *Lumbar puncture and cerebrospinal fluid (CSF) analysis*—clear appearance, pleocytosis with lymphocytic predominance, raised protein (0.5–2.5 g/L, and low CSF: Plasma glucose ratio <0.5). CSF should also be sent for AFB, MGIT culture, and CBNAAT assay. Samples should also be sent for ruling out bacterial and fungal pathology.
- *Imaging*—noncontrast CT brain shows basal hyperdense exudates; contrast studies may demonstrate basal meningeal enhancement, infarcts, or hydrocephalus. MRI brain is a better imaging option for determining the features of TBM, especially brainstem lesions and early infarcts. Contrast-enhanced MRI can help in the visualization of leptomeningeal tubercles and vascular involvement (most commonly affecting the terminal portions of the internal carotid arteries and proximal parts of the middle and anterior cerebral arteries).
- *Adenosine deaminase (ADA) assay* in CSF does not have any role in diagnosing TBM.
- Like any other extrapulmonary TB, a *chest X-ray* should always be done to look for pulmonary involvement.
- *HIV infection* should also be ruled out.
- *Other risk factors for TBM*, e.g., severe acute malnutrition or history of contact with active pulmonary TB cases, should be considered.

The main complications of TBM are hydrocephalus (communicating variety in 70–80% of cases), vasculitis, stroke, and opticochiasmatic arachnoiditis leading to loss of vision.

Tuberculoma

Tuberculomas are granulomas in solid organs. CNS tuberculoma can occur anywhere in the brain or spinal cord and may be present along with TBM. Clinical features of CNS tuberculoma are mainly seizures and/or focal neurological deficit; fever and headache may also be present.

TABLE 7.7.3: Differences between CNS tuberculoma and neurocysticercosis.

CNS tuberculoma	***Neurocysticercosis***
May present at any age	Rare before 3 years of age
Progressive neurological deficit	Usually, no neurological deficit
Lesion size is usually >20 mm; an irregular outline with marked cerebral edema; it may be conglomerate	Usually smaller; a regular rounded outline with less cerebral edema
May be supra- or infratentorial	Usually, supratentorial
Likely to cause midline shift	Usually, no midline shift
Magnetic resonance spectroscopy shows lipid peak	No lipid peak

(CNS: central nervous system)

Diagnosis

Important differential diagnoses include neurocysticercosis, pyogenic abscess, and malignancy. The differentiating features between CNS tuberculoma and neurocysticercosis are outlined in **Table 7.7.3**. MRI brain is the main modality of diagnosis of CNS tuberculomas. Tuberculomas may occasionally increase in size or number in the first 3 months after starting ATT; this is due to paradoxical reaction or immune reconstitution syndrome.

Treatment of CNS TB

Treatment of any form of CNS TB entails 12 months of ATT (2HRZE + 10HRE) for new cases.[3] Adjunctive steroid therapy in the form of prednisolone (1–2 mg/kg/day) or dexamethasone (0.6 mg/kg/day) for 4 weeks followed by tapering over the next 2 weeks improves the outcome. Mannitol may be used for emergency management of cerebral edema. In more subacute cases and in hydrocephalus, acetazolamide or furosemide may be used. Surgical intervention may be needed for hydrocephalus in the form of ventriculoperitoneal shunting if there is no response to medical management or if there is noncommunicating hydrocephalus. In case of seizures, an appropriate antiepileptic drug should be added.

TUBERCULOSIS AND HUMAN IMMUNODEFICIENCY VIRUS

With the spread of the HIV infection, there has been a resurgence in TB. The two infections have significantly detrimental interactions. Coexistent TB and HIV infections accelerate the progression of both diseases. HIV-infected children are more likely to have extrapulmonary and disseminated TB; the course is also likely to be more rapid. An HIV-infected child with latent tubercular infection is more likely to develop the disease than a seronegative child.

Diagnosis

In the absence of significant immunosuppression due to HIV infection, the clinical manifestations of TB are not much different from those in seronegative children. The diagnosis of TB in HIV-infected children poses greater challenges than in other children. Even with the use of a lower cutoff of 5 mm, the tuberculin test is often negative, particularly in children with severe immunosuppression. In extensive disease, the bacteriological confirmation rates are likely to be greater. All attempts should be made to isolate *M. tuberculosis*. Other than providing a definitive diagnosis, it offers the opportunity to do drug sensitivity analysis. The incidence of MDR-TB is higher in HIV-infected patients.

Management

Most current international guidelines recommend that TB in HIV-infected children should be treated according to the same treatment plan as in non-HIV-infected children. A close follow-up is essential to diagnose nonresponse/drug resistance early. In an HIV-positive child, starting ATT takes precedence over antiretroviral therapy (ART).

There is no clear-cut consensus for the *optimal timing of commencing ART* when a child is on ATT, but all HIV-infected children who have developed TB have to be started on ART irrespective of the CD4 count. The decision has to be taken weighing the possibilities of drug interaction, immune reconstitution syndrome, and overlapping toxicities against the possibility of worsening immune status. However, it is advisable to start ART as soon as possible within 8 weeks of the initiation of ATT. Earlier initiation of ART is more crucial in HIV-TB coinfected children with low CD4 values.

After timing, the next important concern in the treatment of HIV-TB coinfected children is the *drug interaction between rifampicin and antiretroviral drugs,* particularly nevirapine, efavirenz, lopinavir/ritonavir, and dolutegravir. Rifampicin is known to be a potent inducer of the hepatic microsomal CYP 450 enzyme system. Nevirapine and efavirenz are no longer used in the ART regimens. For a regimen containing lopinavir/ritonavir, ritonavir boosting is recommended. In the presence of coadministration of rifampicin, lopinavir needs to be super-boosted with ritonavir (1:1 ratio). In children where dolutegravir is used, the weight band dosing frequency is increased to twice a day from once a day. All children diagnosed with TB-HIV coinfection should receive cotrimoxazole prophylaxis.

Isoniazid preventive therapy is to be offered to all children living with HIV, whether on ART or not.

Please refer to Chapter 7.23 "Pediatric Human Immunodeficiency Virus Infection and Acquired Immunodeficiency Syndrome" for more specific details.

MULTIDRUG-RESISTANT TUBERCULOSIS

Multidrug-resistant TB is defined as a case of TB with confirmed resistance to isoniazid and rifampicin with or without resistance to other first-line ATT. Other forms of drug-resistant TB are as follows:

- *Monoresistant TB* where resistance is conformed to only one first-line antitubercular drug
- *Isoniazid-resistant TB (Hr-TB)* where resistance is conformed only to isoniazid and not rifampicin or any other ATT.
- *Pre-extensively drug-resistant TB:* TB caused by *M. tuberculosis* strains that are resistant to rifampicin and isoniazid, along with resistance to any fluoroquinolone (levofloxacin or moxifloxacin)
- *Extensively drug-resistant TB (XDR-TB):* TB caused by *M. tuberculosis* strains that are resistant to rifampicin and isoniazid, along with resistance to any fluoroquinolone (levofloxacin or moxifloxacin) and bedaquiline (Bdq) and/or linezolid

As per the report of the First National Anti-Tuberculosis Drug Resistance Survey India 2014–2016, an estimated 2.8% (2.3–3.5) among new TB cases and 14% (12–17) among previously treated cases have been diagnosed with MDR-TB.

In children, the drug resistance can be confirmed by either CBNAAT/LPA or culture and sensitivity using MGIT. In the absence of a microbiological confirmation either due to the paucibacillary nature of the disease or inadequate biological sample, probable MDR-TB can be diagnosed based on the following criteria:

- Signs of symptoms of active TB and history of close contact with a known case of MDR-TB or
- Close contact with a person who died while on TB treatment or
- Close contact with a person who failed TB treatment, nonresponse or failure of a first-line regimen, or
- Previous treatment with second-line medications.
- The treatment of MDR-TB follows the same principles as those of an adult.
- Children above 5 years of age and weighing at least 15 kg are eligible for both the shorter (Lfx, Cfz, Z, E, Hh, Eto, Bdq, followed by Lfx, Cfz, Z, E) or longer oral MDR/RR-TB regimens (Lfx, Cfz, Lzd, Cs, Bdq).
- For age below 5 years, Bdq is to be replaced by injectable second-line drugs like kanamycin or amikacin. A child on this therapy should be very carefully monitored for clinical improvement and adverse events of the drugs prescribed.

PREVENTION

Prophylaxis

Isoniazid is prescribed for chemoprophylaxis at a dose of 10 mg/kg of body weight/day, for 6 months.[5]

Tuberculosis preventive therapy or chemoprophylaxis should be provided to:

- All asymptomatic contacts <5 years of age of a bacteriologically confirmed case of pulmonary TB, after ruling out active disease. The status of BCG vaccination or TST reading does not preclude one from receiving this chemoprophylaxis.
- In children above 5 years of age who are household contacts of an active TB case, tuberculosis preventive treatment (TPT) may be prescribed if they are IGRA positive or IGRA is not available and active TB has been ruled out.
- All HIV-infected children with no active TB disease.
- All TST-positive children who are receiving immunosuppressive therapy.
- A child born to a mother who was diagnosed to have TB in pregnancy after ruling out congenital TB. BCG vaccination can be given at birth even if chemoprophylaxis is planned.

Vaccination

Bacille Calmette-Guérin is the only vaccine for TB disease used at present. The protection it provides against pulmonary TB is variable; however, it has 60–80% protective efficacy against more serious, disseminated diseases in children like CNS TB.

REFERENCES

1. Marais BJ, Schaaf HS. Tuberculosis in children. Cold Spring Harb Perspect Med. 2014;4(9):a017855.
2. World Health Organization. WHO Operational Handbook on Tuberculosis: Module 5: Management of Tuberculosis in Children and Adolescents. Geneva: WHO; 2022.
3. World Health Organization. Guidance for National Tuberculosis Programmes on the Management of Tuberculosis in Children. Geneva: WHO; 2014.
4. Thwaites GE, van Toorn R, Schoeman J. Tuberculous meningitis: more questions, still too few answers. Lancet Neurol. 2013;12: 999-1010.
5. National Tuberculosis Elimination Program. (2022). Paediatric TB management guideline. [online] Available from https://tbcindia.mohfw.gov.in/pediatric-tb/ [Last accessed November, 2024].

7.8 Leprosy

Rajeshwar Dayal, Madhu Nayak, Anika Bhandari

INTRODUCTION

Leprosy, also known as Hansen's disease, is a chronic granulomatous disease caused by *Mycobacterium leprae*. It particularly affects the skin and nerves, along with affecting all the organs.

EPIDEMIOLOGY

According to the World Health Organization (WHO), a total of 174,056 new cases of leprosy were detected in 2022. India accounted for 59.6% (103,819) of the total new cases detected.[1] The global prevalence of leprosy at the end of 2021 was 16.3 per million population, which is a reduction from the 2019 prevalence of 22.9 per million population. The prevalence rate of leprosy in India has come down from 0.69/10,000 population (2014–2015) to 0.45 (2021–2022), and the annual new case detection rate per 100,000 population has come down from 9.73 (2014–2015) to 5.52 (2021–2022).[1] Leprosy in children is a marker for ongoing transmission in the community. As of 2022, 5.9% (10,300 cases) of the total new cases detected were <15 years old. India accounts for 54.2% (5586 cases) of the total new pediatric leprosy burden.[1] Grade II disability rates, an indicator of late detection and treatment of disease, saw a fall between 2019 and 2022 worldwide. As of 2022, the grade II disability detection rate in India stands at 1.67 per million population.[1]

Achieving eradication of the disease from the elimination stage is a giant task. It requires the cases to be identified at an early stage and treated promptly so that deformity and spread of infection can be prevented. For the diagnosis of early and suspicious cases of leprosy, newer diagnostic concepts of molecular biological approaches, such as polymerase chain reaction (PCR), in situ PCR, *and in situ* hybridization, have evolved and are the need of the time.

ETIOLOGY

Leprosy is caused by *M. leprae*, which is an acid-fast, nonsporing bacillus and occurs both intracellularly and extracellularly. In a stained smear, it lies singly, as rods, or in clumps called globi. They have an affinity for the Schwann cells and cells of the reticuloendothelial system. Till date, it cannot be grown in any artificial media. *M. leprae* does not produce any toxin and is well adapted to reside within macrophages, yet it may survive outside the body for months.

Source of Infection and Mode of Transmission

The only source of infection is the infected human being. The capacity of multibacillary (MB) leprosy patients to infect is 4–11 times that of patients with paucibacillary (PB) leprosy.

Direct Transmission

For direct transmission, prolonged and close contact is required. An "intrafamilial" contact with a patient is more risky than an "extrafamilial" one.

Untreated lepromatous patients discharge as many as 100 million bacilli from their nasal secretions every day. These bacilli remain viable outside the human body for several days. Inhalation of these bacilli, via droplets, is now regarded as the most common mode of entry of leprosy bacilli into the contact person. After inhalation, these inhaled leprosy bacilli enter the respiratory system, from where they are disseminated by blood to skin and peripheral nerves where, depending on the host immune response, the disease may manifest either as tuberculoid leprosy (where there is a good cell-mediated immune response to *M. leprae*) or as lepromatous leprosy (LL) (where there is anergy to *M. leprae*).

Other portals of entry include scratched, abraded, or insect-bitten skin, which facilitates the passage of organisms via the droplets laden with leprosy bacilli through the epidermis into the dermis. Case reports of leprosy in young infants suggest a vertical mode of transmission from mothers to fetus via placenta or via breastfeeding. However, it is uncommon. In infants, the most likely routes of transmission are skin-to-skin contact with the mother and through nasal droplets if the mother is untreated.

Indirect Transmission

Mycobacterium leprae remains viable for several days outside the human body. Occasionally, leprosy may spread by fomites being used by a patient suffering from MB leprosy. Localized infections via infected syringes and tattooing needles have been reported.

CLINICAL MANIFESTATIONS

Incubation Period

The incubation period varies from a few months to as long as 20 years, with an average between 5 and 7 years. The onset of this disease is usually gradual but may be sudden in highly susceptible people.

Early Signs of the Disease

- A hypopigmented patch in the skin, present for a long duration, nonirritating with loss of sensation to touch, pain, and temperature
- Thickening of the skin, more red and shiny in appearance than the surrounding parts, more prominent on the face and hands
- Loss of sensation, numbness, feeling of "pins and needles" or "crawling of ants," tingling sensation in any part of the body, especially in hands and feet. There may be paresis in hands and feet or difficulty in fine movements of fingers.
- Appearance of spontaneous blisters and ulcers, especially in fingers.

CLASSIFICATION

According to the classification laid down by the Indian Association of Leprologists, the cases have been divided into five broad groups:

1. Indeterminate
2. Borderline
3. Tuberculoid
4. Lepromatous
5. Polyneuritic

The borderline group is further subdivided into mid-borderline (BB), borderline lepromatous (BL), and borderline tuberculoid (BT) types.

Indeterminate Leprosy

This type of leprosy is seen in only 10–20% of infected individuals and is the earliest detectable form of leprosy.

This is characterized by the presence of a single hypopigmented macule measuring 2–4 cm in diameter, with a poorly defined border, without any erythema or induration. Anesthesia may be minimal or even absent. A biopsy may show a granuloma, but bacilli are rarely seen in the section. In 50–75% of patients, this lesion heals spontaneously, and in the remaining cases, it gradually progresses to one of the classic forms.

Tuberculoid Leprosy

Tuberculoid leprosy is characterized by the presence of single or few asymmetrical, well-defined, hypopigmented, erythematous, or copper-colored patches with sensory impairment. The entire patch or only its margins are raised above the level of the surrounding skin. Initially, a single nerve trunk related to the lesions is affected. The nerve trunk becomes enlarged, hard, and tender and later may form a nerve abscess.

In this form of leprosy, the lepromin test is positive, and there is an absence of bacilli in the skin smear. On biopsy, foci of lymphocytes, epithelioid cells, and Langhans giant cells are seen.

This form of leprosy is the most common, especially in children, and is relatively benign and stable with a good prognosis.

Borderline Leprosy

Borderline leprosy is further classified into three subtypes based on clinical and histological criteria.

1. *Borderline tuberculoid leprosy:* Here the lesions are greater in number but smaller in size than in tuberculoid leprosy. There may be small satellite lesions around older lesions, and the margins of the BT lesions are less distinct and the center is less atrophic and anesthetic. This form usually involves the thickening of two or more superficial nerves.
2. *Mid-borderline leprosy:* In the BB subtype, the lesions are more numerous and heterogeneous. The lesions may become confluent, or even plaques may be present. The borders are poorly defined, and the erythematous rim fades into the surrounding skin. Hyperesthesia is more common than anesthesia.
3. *Borderline lepromatous leprosy:* In BL leprosy, there are a large number of asymmetrically distributed lesions, which are heterogeneous in appearance. Macules, papules, plaques, and nodules may all coexist. Usually, the individual lesions are small unless confluent. Anesthesia is mild and superficial nerve trunks are spared.

Lepromatous Leprosy

Most cases of LL develop from borderline leprosy (BB or BL). This form of leprosy is relatively uncommon in the pediatric age group. There are two symptoms, which may precede the classical skin lesions by months or years and serve to alert the physician to a possible early diagnosis. They are:

1. Nasal symptoms, which constitute stuffiness, crust formation, and bloodstained discharge
2. Edema of legs and ankles is always bilateral, usually prominent late in the evening, and disappears after overnight rest

Skin lesions may take the form of macules, papules, nodules, or a combination of them. Numerous symmetrically distributed erythematous or coppery, shiny macules with ill-defined margins are usually the first ones to appear. Patients may have a leonine facies due to the loss of eyebrows and eyelashes. There is no sensory impairment in these lesions, but as the disease progresses, many peripheral nerves get symmetrically affected. Due to enormous bacillary infiltration, nerves are initially softer, larger than normal, and tender. In advanced cases, nerves become thin and hard due to fibrosis and result in extreme anesthesia. The skin smear is almost always positive, and the lepromin test is negative.

This form of LL is the most infectious, prone to lepra reactions, and if left untreated, the prognosis is poor.

The features of these varieties of leprosy are summarized in **Table 7.8.1**. As age advances, the disease moves from the tuberculoid end of the spectrum toward the lepromatous end.

TABLE 7.8.1: Clinical aspects of tuberculoid, borderline, and lepromatous leprosy.

	Types of leprosy				
Features	***TT***	***BT***	***BB***	***BL***	***LL***
Number of lesions	Single usually	Single or few	Several	Many	Very many
Size of lesions	Variable	Variable	Variable	Variable	Small
Surface of lesions	Very dry and sometimes scaly	Dry	Slightly shiny	Shiny	Shiny
Sensation in lesions	Absent	Markedly diminished	Moderately diminished	Slightly diminished	Not affected
Hair growth	Absent	Markedly diminished	Moderately diminished	Slightly diminished	Not affected
AFB in lesions	Nil	Nil or scanty	Moderate numbers	Many	Very many (plus globi)
AFB in nasal scrapings/ in nose blows	Nil	Nil	Nil	Usually nil	Very many (plus globi)
Lepromin test	Strongly positive (+++)	Weakly positive (+ or ++)	Negative	Negative	Negative

(AFB: acid–fast bacilli; BB: mid-borderline; BL: borderline lepromatous; BT: borderline tuberculoid; LL: lepromatous leprosy; TT: tuberculoid)

Polyneuritic Leprosy

These cases show nerve involvement but do not have any skin lesion. This may be of primary or secondary variety. In the former, the nerves are directly infected without any skin lesion, while in the latter, infection spreads up the nerves from leprous skin lesions. The affected nerves become thickened and tender, producing sensory motor and trophic changes in their areas of distribution. This dysfunction leads to deformities, neuropathic ulcers, and lagophthalmos, which may result in serious eye complications.

Neuritic leprosy most commonly involves the ulnar, median, lateral popliteal, tibial, great auricular, and rarely radial nerves. It also affects the V and VII cranial nerves.

Reactions

Reactions are acute exacerbations due to changes in the host–parasite immune relationship. They are common during the initial years of treatment. The types are noted in the following subsections.

Type 1 Reversal Reaction

This is seen in borderline cases and consists of acute tenderness and swelling at the site of the lesion. Irreversible nerve injury can occur if this reaction is not treated immediately.

Type 2 Erythema Nodosum Leprosum Reaction

This occurs in lepromatous and BL cases as a systemic inflammatory response. There is high fever, migrating polyarthralgia, orchitis, iridocyclitis, and lymphadenitis. Tender red papules or nodules resembling erythema nodosum are seen characteristically.

DIAGNOSIS

The diagnosis of leprosy is based on the presence of at least one of the following three cardinal signs:[1]

1. A definite loss of sensation in a pale (hypopigmented) or reddish skin patch
2. Thickened or enlarged peripheral nerve with loss of sensation and/or weakness of the muscles supplied by that nerve
3. Presence of acid-fast bacilli in a slit-skin smear

Smear Examination

Sites of bacteriological examination are usually from the most affected parts of the body. If no definite patches or areas of thickened skin are visible, a smear should be taken from ear lobules and buttocks. Smears should be made by the "slit and scrape" method and stained by Ziehl–Neelsen (ZN) or by Fite-Faraco staining. Smears are positive in LL, BL, and some BB and BT cases. It is of limited help in tuberculoid and indeterminate lesions and in patients with early atypical clinical presentation.

Histopathology

In some cases of indeterminate lesions, it becomes necessary to carry out a histological examination for the purpose of diagnosis and classification of the lesion.

Bacillary Index

Bacillary index is a semiquantitative estimation of the density of bacilli present in the skin smears and biopsies and is measured on two scales, namely (1) Dharmendra scale and (2) Ridley scale. It measures the total acid-fast bacilli in the microscopic field, which includes both live and dead bacilli.

Patients are labeled as having PB infection when there are less than or equal to *five* skin lesions and no bacilli on skin smears. They are labeled as having MB infection when there are more than or equal to *six* skin lesions and bacilli are present on skin smears. The bacterial index can range from 0 (no bacilli in 100 oil immersion fields) to 6 (>1,000 bacilli per field).

Footpad Culture

Inoculation of material into the mouse footpad is the only certain way to demonstrate the multiplication of bacilli. This method is 10 times more sensitive at detecting *M. leprae* than slit skin smear examination.

Immunological Methods

Test for Cell-mediated Immunity

Lepromin test: This is a test using intradermal injection of 0.1 mL of lepromin (Dharmendra or Mitsuda antigen) into the inner aspect of the forearm of the individual. The reaction is read at 48 hours (Fernandez reaction) and 21 days (Mitsuda reaction) to classify the stage of leprosy. The lepromin test is not a diagnostic test for leprosy, but it has been found to be useful for classifying the disease. This test is positive in the cases of tuberculoid and BT, negative in LL and BL, and weakly positive and variable in BB leprosy. The lepromin-negative contacts have been found to be at a much higher risk of developing disease than the lepromin-positive contacts. This test signifies the cell-mediated immunity of a person. Two kinds of lepromin are commonly used:

1. Crude antigen of Mitsuda
2. Refined antigen of Dharmendra

Serological Assays

Specific serological tests can detect subclinical infection. The major serological assays include the following:

- *Fluorescent leprosy antibody absorption test (FLA-ABS):* This technique is highly sensitive in detecting the antibodies against *M. leprae* antigen by the immune-fluorescent technique and is useful in identifying healthy contacts of patients who are at risk of developing disease. This test is 92% sensitive and 100% specific in detecting *M. leprae*-specific antibody.
- *Radioimmunoassay:* It detects antibodies to the cell wall antigen of *M. leprae*. An antibody competition test, the serum antibody competition test (SCAT), based on this approach has been found to be sensitive for the detection of *M. leprae* antibody.
- *Enzyme-linked immunosorbent assay (ELISA):* Phenolic glycolipid (PGL)-ELISA was found highly positive in MB cases, but positivity in PB and subclinical cases was quite low. Further simplified dot ELISA and dipstick ELISA using a monoclonal antibody targeting PGL-1 have also been studied.

Molecular Biological Approaches

Identification of organisms can be done in a more rapid and specific way, both from culture and directly from clinical specimen, by recombinant deoxyribonucleic acid (DNA) technology. Based on the gene sequences of *M. leprae*, several probes have been designed in recent years. In recent years, several gene amplification techniques, such as PCR, for amplifying *M. leprae*-specific sequences from a variety of specimens have been published. These have been reported to be highly sensitive and specific.

In Situ PCR

In situ PCR is a method to run PCR directly on small tissue samples, tissue microarrays, or other small cell samples rather than extracting DNA or ribonucleic acid (RNA) first and then performing PCR, real-time PCR, or quantitative PCR from the extracted material. In our studies, in situ PCR on a slit-skin smear has an average positivity of 72%, which is better than that on skin biopsy (60%).[2] In addition, it has the added advantages of being minimally invasive and less cumbersome and can be performed even at sites where skin biopsy is difficult.

Other series have shown similar results.[3] Hence, it can be concluded that in situ PCR, with the added advantages of providing structural correlates and concomitant study of tissue pathology, improves diagnostic yield in early doubtful cases of leprosy and when histopathology is nonspecific.

In Situ Hybridization

In situ hybridization uses a labeled complementary DNA/RNA strand to localize specific DNA/RNA in a portion or section of tissue. In situ hybridization significantly enhances the diagnosis in early cases. In our series, it showed a positivity of about 42.8% in the early I/BT and 46.7% in the BB/BL group, thus enhancing the diagnosis by 18.1%.[2]

M. leprae-specific Genes

Many specific genomic regions, such as 16S ribosomal RNA (rRNA), *rpoT, soda*, 36-kDa antigen, complex 85, and the repetitive sequences (LEPRPT, LEPREP, REPLEP, and RLEP), have been targeted to detect *M. leprae* using PCR or quantitative PCR (qPCR) techniques. The RLEP region was found to be the most sensitive and specific sequence among the above genes.[4]

In our series, we showed that *M. leprae*-specific repetitive element (RLEP)-based PCR on slit-skin smears is a useful tool to confirm early cases of leprosy, where skin smears are negative. In this series, it was found positive in 72% of cases, while skin smears were positive in only 18% of cases.[5]

Other genes that have been used include 16srRNA, esxA, Ag85B, soda, pra, rpoT, ML2179, ML1545, ML0098, ML0024, MntH, AT repeats, AGT repeats, and TTC repeats.

Loop-mediated Isothermal Amplification Assay

Isothermal amplification is a process that rapidly amplifies nucleic acid sequences at constant temperature. It uses four to six primers to identify specific regions in the DNA, which can be multiplied at a constant temperature. Gene amplification and detection are achieved in one step within less time and with a high specificity. Commonly used DNA targets for loop-mediated isothermal amplification (LAMP) include 16srRNA, RLEP, 18-kDa, SodA, rpoT, and Pra.[6]

MANAGEMENT

Leprosy patients should be treated with patience, perseverance, and understanding. Along with the medical treatment, the patients and their parents need moral support and reassurance. Parents should be explained hygienic measures, proper diet, and the importance of taking treatment completely and regularly.

Multidrug Therapy

The WHO Guideline Development Group (GDG) recommends the same three-drug regimen with rifampicin, dapsone, and clofazimine for all leprosy patients, with a duration of treatment of 6 months for PB leprosy and of 12 months for MB leprosy (conditional recommendation, very-low-quality evidence) **(Table 7.8.2)**.

Parents should be advised to give rifampicin on an empty stomach and clofazimine with meals or with a glass of milk. Red staining of skin and lesions is very common with clofazimine.

TABLE 7.8.2: World Health Organization (WHO) multidrug therapy regimens.

Age group	*Drugs*	*Dose and frequency*	*MB*	*PB*
Children (10–14 years)	• Rifampicin • Clofazimine • Dapsone	450 mg once a month 150 mg once a month, 50 mg on alternate days 50 mg daily	12 months	6 months
Children <10 years or <40 kg	• Rifampicin • Clofazimine • Dapsone	10 mg/kg once a month 100 mg once a month, 50 mg twice weekly 2 mg/kg daily	12 months	6 months

(MB: multibacillary leprosy; PB: paucibacillary leprosy)

Treatment of Drug-resistant Leprosy

The treatment schedule is given in **Table 7.8.3**.

TABLE 7.8.3: Treatment of drug-resistant leprosy.

	Treatment	
Resistance type	*First 6 months (daily)*	*Next 18 months (daily)*
Rifampicin resistance	Ofloxacin 400 mg + Minocycline 100 mg + Clofazimine 50 mg	Ofloxacin 400 mg *or* Minocycline 100 mg + Clofazimine 50 mg
	Ofloxacin 400 mg + Clarithromycin 500 mg + Clofazimine 50 mg	Ofloxacin 400 mg + Clofazimine 50 mg
Rifampicin and ofloxacin resistance	Clarithromycin 500 mg + Minocycline 100 mg + Clofazimine 50 mg	Clarithromycin 500 mg *or* Minocycline 100 mg + Clofazimine 50 mg

Treatment of Reactions

Drugs commonly used in these conditions are antimalarials, such as chloroquine (given orally), antimonials, e.g., potassium antimony tartrate intravenously (IV), clofazimine, corticosteroids, and thalidomide (all the three given orally). Symptoms, such as iritis and neuritis, occurring during reactions (or occurring independently) should be properly treated in order to avoid irreversible sequelae, i.e., deformities and neuropathic ulcers.

PROPHYLAXIS

Chemoprophylaxis

In high-risk contacts of MB patients like children (>2 years of age), the WHO recommends single-dose rifampicin (SDR) to be given at a dose of 600 mg in adults, 450 mg for children 10–14 years of age, 300 mg for children 6–9 years (or >20 kg), and 10–15 mg/kg for children <20 kg (>2 years) as a chemoprophylactic agent. The National Leprosy Eradication Programme (NLEP) also recommends SDR for "a person who has been living/working/having social activities for >3 months and 20 hours a week with a newly detected case of leprosy in the last 1 year."

Vaccines

Bacille Calmette-Guérin

In 2018, the WHO recommended one dose of the Bacille Calmette-Guérin (BCG) vaccine for healthy neonates at the earliest opportunity to reduce the risk of leprosy in countries or settings where it is common. However, meta-data analyses of clinical trials found that the BCG vaccine has variable protection ranging from 18 to 90% against leprosy.[7]

Recombinant BCG

Recombinant BCG is a mixed vaccine with the addition of killed *M. leprae* or killed *M. vaccae* (an environmental mycobacterium) and recombinant BCG (rBCG) for enhanced immunogenicity. Clinical trials have been equivocal about its efficacy in offering protection against leprosy.

Mycobacterium indicus pranii

Mycobacterium w (Mw) or *Mycobacterium indicus pranii* (MIP) is a vaccine that has been indigenously developed in India for use in leprosy. The MIP vaccine has received approval from the Drugs Controller General of India and the US Food and Drug Administration.[8] After various trials suggesting enhanced bacterial clearance, reduction in duration of multidrug therapy (MDT), and reduction in bacillary load with the use of MIP in leprosy, the NLEP has introduced the vaccine in a project mode in India from the year 2016.[9]

LepVax

LepVax is a subunit vaccine whose phase 1a trial was completed in 2019, which showed that the vaccine was safe with no serious adverse effects.[10] It is currently in its 1b/2a trial.

Use of Artificial Intelligence in Leprosy

An artificial intelligence (AI)-enabled diagnostic assistant called *AI4leprosy* was developed by Microsoft's AI for Health team and the Novartis Foundation that can help identify suspected patients by assessing skin lesion images in combination with patient symptoms. According to a study published in The Lancet, the diagnostic assistant indicates the disease likelihood in more than 90% of the cases.[11]

REFERENCES

1. World Health Organization. (2023). The Global Health Observatory Leprosy (Hansen's disease). [online] Available from https://www.who.int/data/gho/data/themes/topics/leprosy-hansens-disease. [Last accessed November, 2024].
2. Dayal R, Agarwal M, Natrajan M, Katoch VM, Katoch K, Singh K, et al. PCR and in-situ hybridization for diagnosis of leprosy. Indian J Pediatr. 2007;74(7):645-8.
3. Dayal R, Singh SP, Mathur PP, Katoch VM, Katoch K, Natarajan M. Diagnostic value of in situ polymerase chain reaction in leprosy. Indian J Pediatr. 2005;72(12):1043-6.
4. Sharma M, Singh P. Advances in the diagnosis of leprosy. Front Trop Dis. 2022;3:893653.
5. Kamal R, Dayal R, Gaidhankar K, Biswas S, Gupta Sb, Kumar N, et al. RLEP PCR as a definitive diagnostic test for leprosy from skin smear samples in childhood and adolescent leprosy. Indian J Lepr. 2016;88:193-7.
6. Jiang H, Tsang L, Wang H, Liu C. Loop-mediated isothermal amplification (LAMP) assay targeting RLEP for detection of *Mycobacterium leprae* in leprosy patients. Int J Infect Dis. 2021;107:145-52.
7. Setia MS, Steinmaus C, Ho CS, Rutherford GW. The role of BCG in prevention of leprosy: a meta-analysis. Lancet Infect Dis. 2006;6(3):162-70.
8. Talwar GP, Gupta JC, Mustafa AS, Kar HK, Katoch K, Parida SK, et al. Development of a potent invigorator of immune responses endowed with both preventive and therapeutic properties. Biologics. 2017;11:55-63.
9. Talwar GP, Singh P, Atrey N, Gupta JC. Making of a highly useful multipurpose vaccine. J Transl Sci. 2016;2(1):69-73.
10. Duthie MS, Frevol A, Day T, Coler RN, Vergara J, Rolf T, et al. A phase 1 antigen dose escalation trial to evaluate safety, tolerability and immunogenicity of the leprosy vaccine candidate LepVax (LEP-F1 + GLA-SE) in healthy adults. Vaccine. 2020;38(7):1700-7.
11. Barbieri RR, Xu Y, Setian L, Souza-Santos PT, Trivedi A, Cristofono J, et al. Reimagining leprosy elimination with AI analysis of a combination of skin lesion images with demographic and clinical data. Lancet Reg Health Am. 2022;9:100192.

7.9 Tetanus

Raju C Shah, Pratima R Shah

INTRODUCTION

Tetanus, historically called "*lockjaw*," is an acute, often fatal, severe exotoxin-mediated infection caused by *Clostridium tetani*. Rosenbach in 1886 demonstrated for the first time these slender bacilli. The disease first described by Carlie and Rattone is characterized by severe muscular spasms or acute spastic paralysis and is caused by the action of a potent neurotoxin produced during the growth of the bacteria in dead tissues.

EPIDEMIOLOGY

Tetanus occurs worldwide and is an important cause of neonatal death in the developing world. The causative organism *C. tetani* is part of the normal flora in human and animal intestines and is disseminated through the excreta and found in soil and dust. In the spore form, they are hard and long-lasting in soil and dust. As the spores of *C. tetani* are ubiquitous, wound contamination is unavoidable. The contamination of wound, unhygienic and improper handling of the umbilical cord in newborns, lack of hygienic habits, and aseptic care during and after delivery in women are the main risk factors for infection.[1] Tetanus can occur in a child having chronic ear discharge.

Tetanus is the only vaccine-preventable disease (VPD) that is infectious but not contagious from person to person. Among the burden of VPDs world over, tetanus ranks fourth with 13% disease burden. The incidence is high in tropical countries with humid climate. According to the World Health Organization (WHO) in 2015, global reported cases of tetanus were 10,301, which include 3,551 cases of neonatal tetanus. In 2019, global mortality due to tetanus was reported as 34,684 cases and in under 5 years the number of cases was 18,293. The reported cases of tetanus from India in 2018 were 7,000, of which 129 cases were of neonatal tetanus. In 2022, reported cases were 65 and all of them were of neonatal tetanus. More cases were reported from rural than urban areas. In April 2015, the WHO included India in the list of countries that have eliminated neonatal tetanus.[2] It means that India has

BOX 7.9.1: Global magnitude of tetanus.

- 6,554 reported cases in 2022
- *Total deaths:* 34,684 while those of <5 years were 18,293 in 2019

less than 1 case of neonatal tetanus per 1,000 live births in every district.

Worldwide, all countries are committed to "elimination" of maternal and neonatal tetanus (MNT), i.e., a reduction in the incidence of neonatal tetanus to below one case per 1,000 live births per year in every district. As of March 2018, 14 countries remain that have not eliminated MNT **(Box 7.9.1)**.[2]

ETIOLOGY

The causative organism *C. tetani* is a gram-positive, anaerobic, and spore-forming organism. It forms terminal spores resembling drumsticks. The spores are resistant to boiling, usual antiseptics, and chemical agents like phenol. They can survive autoclaving at 121°C for 10–15 minutes.

Clostridium tetani usually enters the body through a wound. The bacilli themselves are noninvasive. The spores germinate in anaerobic conditions. They produce two types of toxins—tetanospasmin and tetanolysin. Of these, tetanospasmin is a neurotoxin and is responsible for the clinical signs and symptoms of the disease. Toxins act at several sites within the nervous system.

CLINICAL MANIFESTATIONS

The incubation period of tetanus is around 10 days (range 3–30 days). Based on clinical findings, three different forms of tetanus have been described:[3]

1. The most common type (80%) is "generalized tetanus."
2. "Localized tetanus" produces pain and spasm of the muscles in proximity to the site of injury. Occasionally, this form of disease may precede a generalized form.
3. "Cephalic tetanus" is a rare form of the disease seen in children with otitis media.

Generalized Tetanus

Generalized tetanus is usually present with a descending pattern. The first sign most of the time is trismus or lockjaw due to spasm of masseter muscle. Headache, restlessness, and irritability may be the early symptoms followed by stiffness of the neck, difficulty in swallowing, and rigidity of abdominal muscles. The spasms can be precipitated by bright light, noise, and even touch. The rigidity of facial muscles leads to the sardonic smile of tetanus or risus sardonicus, a typical grinning appearance. Rigidity and spasm of back and abdominal muscles cause arching (opisthotonos). Laryngeal and respiratory muscle spasm can lead to airway obstruction and asphyxia. Constipation and retention of urine may also occur. Hyperpyrexia, hypertension, excessive sweating, tachycardia, and cardiac arrhythmia can occur due to sympathetic nerve involvement. Paralysis is evident in the first week, stabilizes in the second week, and ameliorates in the next 1–4 weeks.

Neonatal Tetanus

Neonatal tetanus typically occurs when the umbilical cord is cut with an unsterilized instrument or some unhygienic materials are applied to the stump of the cord. It manifests within 3–12 days of birth. It is generalized tetanus, a serious condition and often fatal. Progressive difficulty in feeding (sucking and swallowing) with associated hunger and crying is generally seen. Paralysis and diminished movement, stiffness to touch, and spasms with or without opisthotonos are the clinical features. Opisthotonos may be extreme or sometimes absent.

Localized Tetanus

Localized tetanus is painful spasm to the site of infection preceding generalized tetanus. Cephalic tetanus with bulbar muscle involvement is seen with wounds of the head, face, and nostrils or with chronic otitis media. Retracted eyelids, deviated gaze, trismus, risus sardonicus, spastic paralysis of the tongue, and pharyngeal muscles are the presenting features.

DIAGNOSIS

The diagnosis is mainly clinical. The typical setting is an injured unimmunized patient or baby born to an unimmunized mother presenting within 2 weeks with trismus, rigid muscles, and clear sensorium. The organism can be isolated from the wound or ear discharge.

MANAGEMENT

Management comprises wound debridement, immunoglobulin administration, antibiotics, and supportive care. The aim of therapy is to neutralize all toxins, eradicate *C. tetani*, ensure an environment not conducive for multiplication of anaerobic organisms and provide supportive care.

Human tetanus immunoglobulin (TIG), 3,000–6,000 U intramuscular (IM), is recommended to be given immediately. TIG has no effect on toxin, which is already fixed to the neural tissue and does not penetrate the blood–cerebrospinal fluid (CSF) barrier. It can neutralize circulating tetanospasmin. If TIG is not available, human intravenous immunoglobulin (IVIg) can be used. Antitetanus serum (ATS) is recommended only when TIG is not available. It can be given in a single dose of 50,000–1,00,000 U, half the dose IM, and the rest intravenously (IV) after a skin test.

TABLE 7.9.1: Wound management.

History of tetanus toxoid doses	Clean minor wounds		All other wounds*	
	TT/Td/Tdap	TIG	TT/Td/Tdap	TIG†
Unknown, less than three doses, immunocompromised	Yes	No	Yes	Yes
More than three doses	No‡	No	No§	No

*Including, but not limited to, wounds contaminated with dirt, feces, soil, and saliva; puncture wounds; avulsions; and wounds resulting from missiles, crushing, burns, and frostbite.
†TIG: 250–500 U IM.
‡Yes, if it has been >10 years since the last dose.
§Yes, if it has been >5 years since the last dose.
(IM: intramuscular; Td: tetanus and diphtheria; Tdap: tetanus-diphtheria-acellular pertussis; TIG: tetanus immunoglobulin; TT: tetanus toxoid)

Penicillin is the antibiotic of choice for *C. tetani.* Penicillin G 2,00,000 U/kg body weight can be given IV in four divided doses for 10–14 days. Local wound, discharging ears, and umbilical cord should be cleaned and debrided if needed.

All patients with generalized tetanus require muscle relaxants. Diazepam is preferred as it causes both muscle relaxation and seizure control. The initial dose is 0.1–0.2 mg/kg every 3–6 hours given IV. Midazolam and baclofen can also be used. The best survival rates with generalized tetanus are achieved with neuromuscular blocking agents, such as vecuronium and pancuronium. These drugs produce general flaccid paralysis, which can be managed by mechanical ventilation.

Meticulous nursing care is imperative. The patient should be kept in a quiet, dark environment with minimum auditory or visual stimuli. Maintenance of nutrition, fluid and electrolyte balance, suctioning of secretions, and cardiorespiratory monitoring should be done. Provision for tracheostomy should be kept ready.

Wound Management

All wounds should be cleaned; necrotic tissue and foreign material should be removed. As shown in **Table 7.9.1**, wounds, which are not minor, require human TIG except those in fully immunized patients. In patients with a history of unknown or incomplete immunization, crush, puncture, or bone-projecting wounds, wounds contaminated with soil, saliva, or feces, avulsion injuries, and compound fractures, 250 U of TIG should be given IM. In cases where the wound could not be properly debrided or wound >24 hours old, 500 U of TIG should be given. Tetanus toxoid may be administered immediately depending on the immunization status of the child.[3,4]

COMPLICATIONS

Aspiration of secretions leading to pneumonia is one of the major complications. Autonomic system irregularities in the form of cardiac arrhythmias, asystole, and labile blood pressure may be noted. Few children may get seizure-related injuries, rhabdomyolysis, myoglobinuria, bone fractures, and renal failure.

PROGNOSIS

The average mortality of tetanus is 45–55%. For neonatal tetanus, the mortality is 60–70%. The most important factor influencing outcome is supportive care. Recovery from tetanus does not confer immunity; therefore, active immunization of the patients following recovery is imperative.

PREVENTION

Tetanus is an entirely preventable disease. Active immunization is the best method to prevent tetanus. The WHO recommends a three-dose primary vaccination series with diphtheria-containing vaccine, followed by three booster doses. The three-dose primary series should begin as early as 6 weeks of age, with subsequent doses given with a minimum interval of 4 weeks between doses. The three booster doses should preferably be given during the second year of life (12–23 months), at 4–7 years, and at 9–15 years of age. Ideally, there should be at least 4 years between booster doses. After 7 years of age, Tdap (tetanus-diphtheria-acellular pertussis) (low-dose diphtheria and acellular pertussis) should be used as a booster dose.

Neonatal tetanus could be prevented by immunizing the pregnant women with two doses of tetanus toxoid or tetanus and diphtheria (Td) (preferably one-dose Tdap) between 16 and 36 weeks of pregnancy and with only one dose of Tdap or Td in the subsequent pregnancies.[5]

REFERENCES

1. Arnon SS. Tetanus. In: Kliegman RM, Jenson HB, Behrman RE, Stanton BF (Eds). Nelson Textbook of Pediatrics, 18th edition. Philadelphia, PA: Elsevier; 2007. pp. 1228-30.
2. World Health Organization. Weekly epidemiological record, 1st May 2020, 95th Year, No. 18. 2020;95(18):173-84. [online] Available from http://www.who.int/wcr. [Last accessed November, 2024].
3. Centers for Disease Control and Prevention. Diphtheria, tetanus and pertussis: recommendations for vaccine use and other preventive measures. Recommendations of the Immunization Practices Advisory Committee (ACIP). MMWR Recomm Rep. 1991;40(RR-10):1-28.
4. Centers for Disease Control and Prevention. Epidemiology and Prevention of Vaccine-Preventable Diseases, 10th edition. Atlanta: Department of Health and Human Services, CDC; 2007.
5. World Health Organization. The "high risk" approach: the WHO—recommended strategy to accelerate elimination of neonatal tetanus. Wkly Epidemiol Rec. 1996;71:33-6.

7.10 Leptospirosis

Ramesh S

INTRODUCTION

Leptospirosis is an acute febrile generalized disease whose manifestations can range from mild self-limiting illness to fatal multiorgan involvement. Leptospirosis, an infectious disease that affects humans and animals, is considered the most common zoonosis in the world. Leptospirosis is caused by pathogenic (spirochetes) bacteria that belong to the genus *Leptospira*. By genomic studies, 64 species of *Leptospira* have been identified which include pathogenic and nonpathogenic *Leptospira*. Pathogenic *Leptospira* are highly diversified spirochetes currently composed of 10 identified species.

There is an older classification of pathogenic *Leptospira* based on its antigenic structure, with 300 serovars grouped into 32 serogroups. The same serovars can exist across species. As a result, by convention, isolates are identified by both species and serovar (e.g., *L. interrogans serovar Copenhageni*).[1]

EPIDEMIOLOGY

The rat is the principal source and a reservoir of infection. In rats, the *Leptospira* exists as a commensal in the kidney. Other important reservoirs include wild mammals and domestic and farm animals. The infected animals excrete spirochetes in urine for an extended period of time. Human infection occurs due to exposure to water or soil contaminated with rat urine. It can also occur through direct contact with blood, tissues, organs, urine, or reproductive secretions of infected animals.[2]

Leptospirosis occurs as an epidemic in India during the monsoon and immediate postmonsoon period. It can also be endemic in areas that result from exposure to leptospire contamination of stagnant water with sewerage. Recreational activities such as swimming, canoeing, and water skiing in contaminated water are other reasons to acquire leptospirosis.

PATHOPHYSIOLOGY

Leptospirosis gains access to the human body through cuts and abrasions in the skin and intact mucous membranes. The primary lesion caused by leptospire is damage to the endothelial lining of small blood vessels and vasculitis with leakage with resultant ischemic damage to the liver, kidneys, meninges, and muscles.[2]

CLINICAL FEATURES OF LEPTOSPIROSIS

Leptospirosis usually presents with an abrupt onset of fever, associated with rigors, myalgia, and headache. Conjunctival suffusion, if present, is considered an important finding in Leptospirosis. Leptospirosis should be included in the differential diagnosis of undifferentiated fevers, especially during or after the monsoon season. The clinical spectrum of leptospirosis varies widely confounding the clinical diagnosis; it can range from mild and self-limiting to a life-threatening illness.

The following approaches are useful to make a presumptive clinical diagnosis of leptospirosis.

- *According to the World Health Organization (WHO)*, which adopts a syndromic approach, the disease can present in one of the four ways:[3]
  1. As a nonspecific febrile illness
  2. As Weil's syndrome with jaundice, renal failure, hemorrhage, and myocarditis
  3. As meningitis or meningoencephalitis
  4. As pulmonary hemorrhage with respiratory failure
- *Diagnosis based on the Indian Leptospirosis Society.* This illness should be suspected when a child presents with a history of abrupt-onset fever and body ache/headache and with any one or more of the following features:
  - Jaundice
  - Oliguria
  - Cough and breathlessness
  - Hemorrhagic tendency
  - Signs of meningeal irritation, or altered sensorium, or convulsions
- *Conventional approach.* It is conventional to describe the clinical presentation of leptospirosis which can occur as *anicteric disease* which is more common with less severe manifestation or as a rare *icteric form* which is more severe.

Anicteric Leptospirosis

Anicteric leptospirosis occurs as a biphasic illness with a septicemic phase followed by the immune phase. The septicemic phase is associated with the multiplication of *Leptospira* in the bloodstream, cerebrospinal fluid (CSF), and other tissues, and the immune phase that follows is characterized by the development of antibodies to *Leptospira* and disappearance of the organisms. The distinction between the first and second phases may not be clinically apparent.

Septicemic Phase

The child may present with fever of abrupt onset, associated with muscle pain, headache, nausea, vomiting, abdominal pain, and conjunctival suffusion. Less common findings include a transient skin rash, photophobia, and mild signs of meningism. The septicemic phase lasts 4–7 days.

Immune Phase

The immune phase is characterized by circulating antibodies. There is a brief asymptomatic interlude between the septicemic and immune phases. The important clinical features in the immune phase are as follows:

- Fever which is less pronounced than in the early phase
- Aseptic meningitis with abnormal CSF pleocytosis is seen occasionally among children.
- Hepatitis is characterized by enlargement of the liver and elevation of bilirubin with a modest increase in liver enzymes.
- Renal involvement is characterized by abnormal findings in the urine analysis (hematuria, proteinuria, and casts), azotemia with oliguria or anuria. Renal failure is the principal cause of death in fatal cases.

Icteric Leptospirosis (Weil's Syndrome)

Weil's syndrome is characterized by liver, kidney, and vascular dysfunction in addition to the other symptoms of anicteric leptospirosis. Individuals with Weil's syndrome will usually develop jaundice without hepatocyte destruction and azotemia by the third to the seventh day of illness. The liver may be enlarged and there may be right upper quadrant tenderness. With an increasing severity of jaundice, the individual is at a greater risk of developing renal failure, hemorrhage, and cardiovascular collapse. Uremia, oliguria, and anuria may occur with the onset of kidney failure unless dialysis is provided. Fatalities due to icteric leptospirosis are typically because of renal failure, cardiopulmonary failure, and fatal hemorrhages.

LABORATORY DIAGNOSIS

Culture of *Leptospira*

Leptospira can be cultured from blood or CSF during the first 10 days of illness and from the urine for several weeks beginning in the second week. However, results take up to 3 months; hence, its use is limited in routine clinical practice.

Dark-field Microscopy

Dark-field microscopy (DFM) is used to detect leptospires in blood within the first 10 days of illness and from the urine from the second week onward. False-positive results are common due to the extrusion of fibrillar material from red blood cells (RBCs) which mimics leptospirosis. Urine samples must be examined within half an hour of collection. This investigation has low specificity and sensitivity. Hence, it has fallen out of favor with clinicians.

Serology—Detection of Antibodies to Leptospirosis

Serologic tests form the mainstay in the diagnosis of leptospirosis. Antibodies to leptospirosis start appearing 5–10 days after the onset of fever. Therefore, the timing of tests is important.

Immunoglobulin M Enzyme-linked Immunosorbent Assay

These tests detect genus-specific leptospiral immunoglobulin M (IgM) antibodies which tend to become positive early in the disease from around the fifth day of illness. Detection of IgM antibodies indicates current infection. The performance of commercial enzyme-linked immunosorbent assay (ELISA) tests varies by geographical setting, with the sensitivity of the *Leptospira* IgM-ELISA being 35–76% and specificity being 76–98% in different endemic settings. The IgM ELISA test does not differentiate between pathogenic and saprophytic *Leptospira*, and the infecting serovar cannot be identified.

Immunoglobulin G ELISA

Immunoglobulin G (IgG) ELISA detects genus-specific antibodies and indicates past infection, though in a reinfection, the IgM and IgG can be positive. In a clinical setting, IgM ELISA is the most commonly ordered test for the detection of leptospiral antibody.

Microscopic Agglutination Test

Microscopic agglutination test (MAT) is a serovar-specific test and is considered the gold standard in serological tests to detect leptospirosis due to its high specificity. It detects serovar-specific antibodies. It detects both IgG and IgM antibodies. The MAT is usually positive 10–12 days after symptom onset and reaches a peak by the third week. It involves the use of a battery of live leptospiral cultures to be used as antigens, done in specialized laboratories. Available antisera may not identify all *Leptospira* serotypes. Serotypes commonly seen in the community are usually identified including the virulent and serious types. Initial high titers of 1:800 or rising titers (fourfold increase) obtained 2 weeks apart are diagnostic.

Other Serological Tests

Other serological tests include slide agglutination test, indirect immunofluorescence test, and indirect hemagglutination tests.

Polymerase Chain Reaction

Polymerase chain reaction (PCR) can be used to detect leptospiral DNA in blood, urine, and CSF. Loop-mediated isothermal amplification (LAMP) of the *Leptospira* rrs (165) gene has been developed for the diagnosis of leptospirosis.

Next-generation Sequencing

Next-generation sequencing (NGS) is a technology for sequencing an exponentially greater number of genes than conventional DNA sequencing. Currently, these investigations are not readily available. These tests when readily available would increase the sensitivity and specificity of the diagnosis.

The WHO suggests that the gold standard laboratory method for confirming leptospirosis diagnosis should be:[3]

- Isolation of *Leptospira* by the culture method
- Detection of organism DNA by PCR
- Detection of antibodies by MAT

As these investigations are not readily available, the detection of *Leptospira* IgM and IgG antibodies by ELISA remains a cost-effective investigation to make the laboratory diagnosis of leptospirosis.

TREATMENT

Initiation of treatment early in the disease before the seventh day shortens the clinical course.[3,4]

For Children with Less Severe Illness who can be Managed as Outpatients

Oral doxycycline 2 mg/kg in two divided doses not to exceed 200 mg/day for a total of 7 days can be given. Doxycycline can be used in children across all age groups. Other drugs include oral azithromycin 10 mg/kg on day 1 and 5 mg/kg for 3 days, oral amoxycillin 25–50 mg/kg in three divided doses, or cefixime 10 mg/kg/day in two divided doses for 7 days.

For Hospitalized Children with Severe Leptospirosis

IV crystalline penicillin is the drug of choice and the dose is 250,000 units/kg/24 h in four divided doses (maximum dose: 6–12 million units per day). Alternative drugs include Inj. ceftriaxone 75–100 mg/kg in a single dose or two divided doses and doxycycline IV 4 mg/kg/day in two divided doses; the maximum dose is 200 mg/day. The duration of treatment is for at least 7 days.

Jarisch Herxheimer Reaction

Jarisch Herxheimer reaction (JHR) is a transient clinical phenomenon that occurs in patients with spirochetal infections undergoing antibiotic treatment. It occurs within 24 hours of starting antibiotic treatment. It manifests as fever, rigors, chills, headache, nausea, vomiting, hyperventilation, tachycardia, and hypotension. The breakdown of spirochetes after initiation of antibiotics leads to the release of toxins and inflammatory cytokines which is responsible for this phenomenon. Most cases are mild and resolve without treatment. For severe JHR, treatment includes IV crystalloid fluids, steroids, vasopressors, and inotropic agents.

PREVENTION

Rodent control and avoidance of contact with contaminated water and soil will prevent infection. Parents should instruct children not to wade through flood waters or play in stagnant water.

REFERENCES

1. Vincent AT, Schiettekatte O, Goarant C, Neela VK, Bernet E, Thibeaux R, et al. Revisiting the taxonomy and evolution of pathogenicity of the genus *Leptospira* through the prism of genomics. PLoS Negl Trop Dis. 2019;13:e0007270.
2. Davies HD, Simonsen KA. Leptospira. In: Kliegman RM, St Geme II JW, Blum NJ, Tasker RC, Shah SS, Wilson KM (Eds). Nelson Textbook of Pediatrics, 21st edition. Philadelphia: Saunders; 2020. pp. 1601-2.
3. World Health Organization. Human leptospirosis: guidance for diagnosis, surveillance and control. WHO/CDS/CSR/EPH 2002.23.
4. Choudhury J, Shah T, Kewal Kishore Arora KK. Leptospirosis/ Standard Treatment Guidelines 2022. Indian Academy of Pediatrics. [online] Available from https://iapindia.org/pdf/Ch-021-STG-leptospirosis.pdf [Last accessed November, 2024].

7.11 Rickettsial Diseases

Narendra B Rathi

INTRODUCTION

Family *Rickettsiae* comprises a group of micro-organisms that phylogenetically occupy a position between bacteria and viruses. The order rickettsiae contains six genera, i.e., *Rickettsia*, *Orientia*, *Anaplasma*, *Ehrlichia*, *Neoehrlichia*, and *Neorickettsia*. *Rickettsia* are small, nonflagellate, gram-negative pleomorphic coccobacilli adapted to obligate intracellular parasitism and transmitted by arthropod vectors such as fleas, ticks, mites, and lice. *Rickettsia* spp. are subdivided into two types, i.e., spotted fever group and typhus group, while *Orientia* spp. comprise the scrub typhus group.[1,2]

EPIDEMIOLOGY

Rickettsial diseases have a global distribution (except Antarctica), and recent reports suggest their continuing presence and re-emergence in India. The presence of rickettsial disease in India has been documented in Jammu and Kashmir, Himachal Pradesh, Uttarakhand, Rajasthan, Assam, West Bengal, Maharashtra, Kerala, and Tamil Nadu.[3] Recent studies from western Maharashtra and central India have documented that rickettsial diseases are important re-emerging infections in India.[1]

ETIOPATHOGENESIS

Family *Rickettsiae* comprises three genera, namely *Rickettsia*, *Orientia*, and *Ehrlichia*. Former members of this family, *Coxiella burnetii*, which causes Q fever, and *Rochalimaea quintana*, causing trench fever, have been excluded because the former is not primarily arthropod-borne and the latter is not an obligate intracellular parasite. Various members of this family can be grouped into four biogroups, as shown in **Table 7.11.1**, based on the lipopolysaccharide group antigen.[1,2]

Man is an accidental host except for louse-borne epidemic typhus caused by *Rickettsia prowazekii*. Transmission to humans occurs by infected arthropod vector or exposure to an infected animal reservoir host. Vector-to-human transmission occurs as vector defecate while feeding (flea feeding reflex) so that feces contaminate pruritic bite wounds (seen with typhus fever group) or primarily by bite, where the regurgitation of infected saliva occurs during feeding (seen with the spotted fever group and scrub typhus).

TABLE 7.11.1: Biogroups of rickettsia.

Biogroup	*Disease*	*Vector*	*Organism*
Spotted fever	RMSF	Tick	*Rickettsia rickettsii*
	Rickettsialpox	Mite	*Rickettsia akari*
	Indian tick typhus, boutonneuse fever, and MSF	Tick	*Rickettsia conorii*
Typhus	Epidemic louse-borne typhus	Louse	*Rickettsia prowazekii*
	Brill–Zinsser disease (recrudescent typhus)	Louse	*R. prowazekii*
	Endemic or murine flea-borne typhus	Flea	*Rickettsia typhi*
Scrub typhus	Scrub typhus	Chigger	*Orientia tsutsugamushi*
Miscellaneous	Ehrlichiosis and anaplasmosis	Tick	*Ehrlichia, Anaplasma*
	TIBOLA	Tick	*Rickettsia slovaca*
	DEBONEL	Tick	*R. slovaca*

(DEBONEL: Dermacentor-borne necrosis-eschar-lymphadenopathy; MSF: Mediterranean spotted fever; RMSF: Rocky Mountain spotted fever; TIBOLA: tick-borne lymphadenopathy)

The risk of transmission of rickettsial diseases is directly proportional to the time spent in outdoor activities, more so during seasons of peak feeding and lifecycle activity for the corresponding vector.

Skin rash, capillary leak leading to edema, and organ ischemic injury are secondary to vasculitis, which is the basic pathogenetic mechanism of rickettsial diseases.

CLINICAL FEATURES

A high index of suspicion is key to early diagnosis because of nonspecific signs and symptoms in the early stages of the disease. Various clinical features of rickettsial infections are shown in the following sections.[1,2]

Fever

Fever of undetermined origin is the most frequent presentation of rickettsial disease. Fever is usually abrupt onset, high grade, sometimes with chills, occasionally with morning remissions, and associated with headache and myalgia. In fact, the diagnosis of rickettsial disease should always be considered in patients with acute febrile illness accompanied by headache and myalgia, particularly in endemic areas with a history of tick exposure or contact with dogs.

Headache and Myalgia

Severe frontal headache and generalized myalgia, especially in muscles of the lumbar region, thigh, and calf, are seen in a variable proportion of cases.

Rash

Rash is the major clinical feature, though not universally seen. Thus, spotted fever is a misnomer. 3-5 days after the onset of fever, rash usually becomes apparent. Typical rash is evolving, i.e., from macular to popular to ecchymotic to gangrenous; rash evolves without treatment. Palpable purpura is the hallmark of vasculitis **(Fig. 7.11.1)**. Vasculitis and thrombosis can progress to gangrene of digits **(Fig. 7.11.2)**, earlobes, scrotum, nose, or limbs. There is a centripetal spread of rash from extremities near ankles, lower legs, and wrists to the trunk. Rash on palms and soles, considered so typical of rickettsial disease, can be seen in various diseases like infective endocarditis, syphilis, meningococcemia, enteroviral diseases, adverse drug reactions, and rickettsial diseases.

Eschar

An eschar is a necrotic tissue seen at the point of entry of organisms that looks like a burn from a cigarette butt and is seen in Indian tick typhus, scrub typhus, and rickettsialpox **(Fig. 7.11.3)**. There is an erythematous rim around eschar, and regional lymph nodes are enlarged.

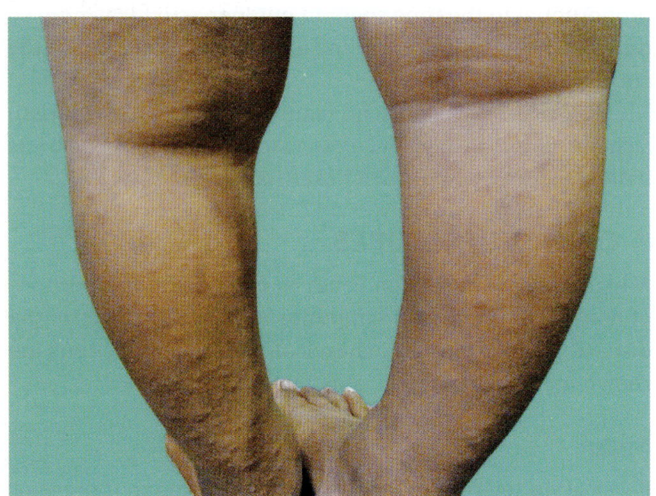

Fig. 7.11.1: Palpable purpuric rash.

Generalized Lymphadenopathy and Hepatosplenomegaly

It is found in the majority of scrub typhus patients.

Systemic Features

Clinical features referable to various systems are sometimes seen in rickettsial infections. Gastrointestinal symptoms, such as nausea, vomiting, abdominal pain, and diarrhea, are seen with varying frequencies. Constipation is seen particularly in epidemic typhus. Respiratory symptoms, such as cough and distress, are sometimes seen. Neurological manifestations, such as dizziness, drowsiness, disorientation, tinnitus, photophobia, delirium, meningismus, and visual disturbances, are seen more commonly with typhus group infections.

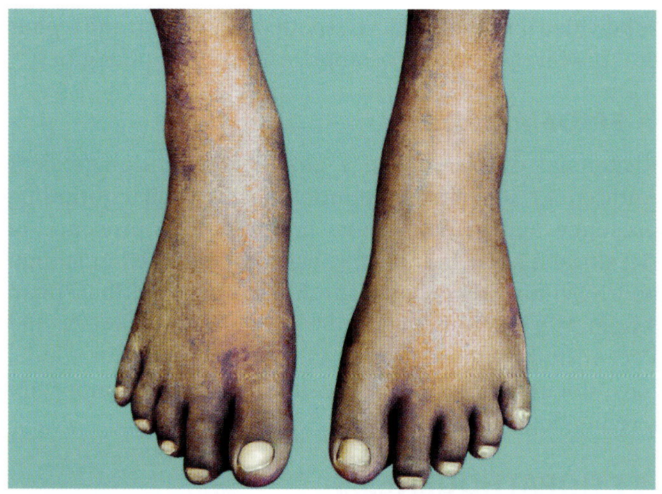

Fig. 7.11.2: Pedal edema with gangrenous changes in toes.

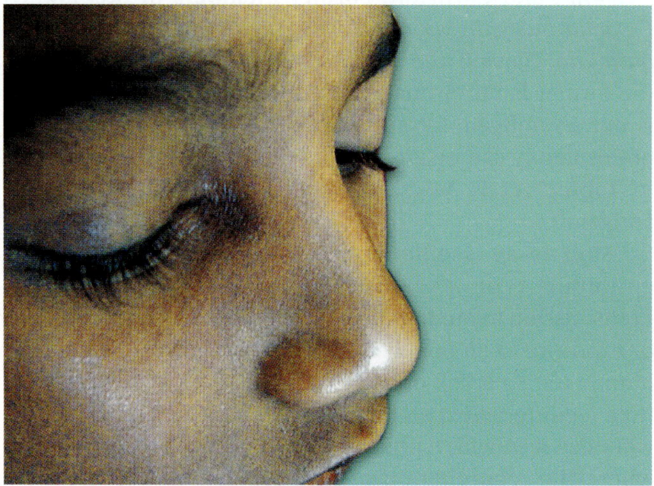

Fig. 7.11.3: Eschar near medial canthus of right eye.

Miscellaneous

Periorbital edema, conjunctival hyperemia, epistaxis, acute reversible hearing loss, and arthralgia are sometimes reported.

MODALITIES OF DIAGNOSIS

Clinical laboratory findings include a normal-to-low total leukocyte count during the early course of the disease with a marked shift to the left, low platelet counts, and a high erythrocyte sedimentation rate.[3] There may be hyponatremia, hypoalbuminemia, and raised hepatic transaminases. The RGA (Rathi Goodman Aghai) scoring system can be used for early detection, treatment, and prevention of mortality and morbidity in the spotted fever group **(Table 7.11.2)**. The RGA scoring system has a total score of 35 (25 clinical and 10 laboratory findings).[4] A cutoff score of 14 has a sensitivity and specificity of 96.15% and 98.84%, respectively, in making a diagnosis of the spotted fever group. This scoring system was validated for the diagnosis of scrub typhus by a study to compare the effectiveness of RGA scoring with respect to polymerase chain reaction (PCR), which found that an RGA score of >14 shows a sensitivity of 92% and a specificity of 83.3% when compared with the PCR. An RGA score of >14 showed a sensitivity of 93.8% in those who were both immunoglobulin M enzyme-linked immunosorbent assay (IgM) ELISA and PCR positive for scrub typhus.[5]

TABLE 7.11.2: RGA scoring system to diagnose spotted fever group (total score = 35).[4]

Clinical features	*Score*	*Laboratory features*	*Score*
Rural	1	Hemoglobin <9 g/dL	1
Pets	1	Platelets <1,50,000 cells/L	1
Tick exposure	2	C-reactive protein >50 mg/dL	2
Tick bite	3	Serum albumin <3 g/dL	1
Conjunctival congestion (nonexudative)	2	Urine albumin >2 +	1
Maculopapular rash	1	SGPT >100 U/L	2
Purpura	2	Serum sodium <130 mEq/L	2
Palpable purpura/ ecchymosis/necrotic rash	3		
Rash appearing 48–96 hours after fever	2		
Pedal edema	2		
Rash on palms and soles	3		
Hepatomegaly	2		
Lymphadenopathy	1		
Total	*25*	*Total*	*10*

(RGA: Rathi Goodman Aghai; SGPT: serum glutamate pyruvate transaminase)

Serological diagnosis is difficult during the acute stage of the disease as a definite diagnosis usually requires examination of paired serum samples after convalescence. The most common serological test for confirmed diagnosis is the indirect immunofluorescence assay, but a diagnostic titer is not detectable until the second week of the disease.

Blood or tissue samples can be tested for rickettsial nucleic acid by PCR, but it is relatively insensitive as the level of rickettsemia is very low.

As no clinical or laboratory clues are specific for early diagnosis, diagnosis should be made with a combination of compatible clinical presentation, history of tick exposure, epidemiological data, suggestive laboratory parameters, and rapid defervescence with appropriate antibiotics.

The Indian Academy of Pediatrics (IAP) has formulated guidelines for rickettsial diseases in children and has elaborated an algorithm of case definitions **(Flowchart 7.11.1)**, various clinical scenarios in which rickettsial disease should be considered **(Box 7.11.1)**, epidemiological features that suggest these infections **(Box 7.11.2)**, differential diagnosis **(Box 7.11.3)**, and laboratory features that suggest diagnosis of these infections **(Box 7.11.4)**.[6]

TREATMENT

Definitive treatment should be instituted based on clinical and epidemiological clues as early as possible to avoid severe disease and fatal outcome. Various antibiotics useful for treating different rickettsial diseases include tetracycline (preferably doxycycline), chloramphenicol, macrolides (especially azithromycin, clarithromycin, and roxithromycin), and fluoroquinolones (especially ciprofloxacin, ofloxacin, pefloxacin, and levofloxacin).[1,2]

Doxycycline is the drug of choice. The dose is 5 mg/kg/day in two divided doses for children below 45 kg and 200 mg/day in two divided doses for children above 45 kg. The duration of therapy should be minimum 5–7 days or at least 3 days after defervescence. It can be used for treatment of rickettsial diseases in children below 8 years of age as tooth discoloration is dose-dependent.

Chloramphenicol should be used in case of doxycycline allergy (50–100 mg/kg/day every 6 hours intravenously, maximum 3 g/day).

COMPLICATIONS

Respiratory (interstitial pneumonitis and *acute respiratory distress syndrome*), neurologic (meningoencephalitis), renal (acute renal failure), disseminated intravascular coagulation, hepatic failure, gangrene, and myocarditis are various complications seen in rickettsial infections.

Flowchart 7.11.1: Indian Academy of Pediatrics (IAP) guidelines for diagnosis and management of rickettsial diseases.[6]

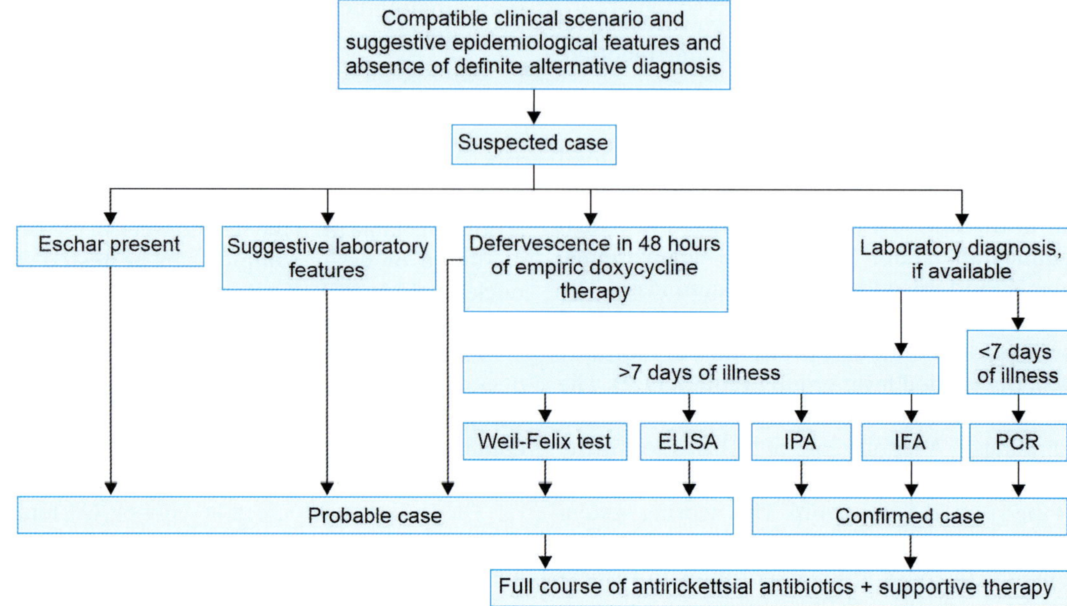

(ELISA: enzyme-linked immunosorbent assay; IFA: indirect immunofluorescence assay; IPA: immunoperoxidase assay; PCR: polymerase chain reaction)

BOX 7.11.1: Compatible clinical scenario for rickettsial infection.[6]

One or more of the following:
- Undifferentiated fever of >5 days' duration
- Sepsis of undetermined etiology
- Fever with a skin rash
- Fever with edema
- Dengue-like febrile disease
- Fever with headache and myalgia
- Fever with hepatosplenomegaly and/or lymphadenopathy
- Features of aseptic meningitis/meningoencephalitis/acute encephalitic syndrome
- Fever with cough and pulmonary infiltrates or community-acquired pneumonia
- Fever with acute kidney injury (AKI)
- Fever with acute gastrointestinal or hepatic involvement

BOX 7.11.2: Suggestive epidemiological features for rickettsial infections.[6]

One or more of the following within 14 days of illness onset:
- Tick bite
- Ticks seen on clothes or in and around homes or in areas where children play
- Visit to areas that are common habitats of vectors, like high uncut grass or weeds or bushes or rice fields or woodlands (where rodents share habitats with animals) or grassy lawns or river banks or poorly maintained kitchen gardens
- Animal sheds in proximity of homes
- Contact with pet or stray dog infested with ticks
- Living in or traveling to areas endemic for rickettsial diseases
- Occurrence of similar clinical cases simultaneously or sequentially in family members, coworkers, neighborhood, or pets
- Exposure to rodents

BOX 7.11.3: Differential diagnoses for rickettsial infections.[6]

- *Viral diseases:* Enteroviral diseases, measles, dengue fever, chikungunya, and infectious mononucleosis
- *Bacterial diseases:* Meningococcemia, leptospirosis, typhoid fever, scarlet fever, secondary syphilis, and infective endocarditis
- *Protozoal diseases:* Malaria
- *Vasculitis:* Kawasaki disease and thrombotic thrombocytopenic purpura
- Adverse drug reactions
- Differential diagnoses pertaining to each systemic presentation

BOX 7.11.4: Suggestive laboratory features for rickettsial infections.[6]

- *Complete blood counts:* Normal-to-low total white blood cell count with a shift to the left in early stages and leukocytosis later
- *Platelets:* Thrombocytopenia
- *Acute phase reactants:* Raised ESR and CRP
- *Serum electrolytes:* Hyponatremia
- *Serum proteins:* Hypoalbuminemia
- *Liver function tests:* Elevated hepatic transaminases

(CRP: C-reactive protein; ESR: erythrocyte sedimentation rate)

PROGNOSIS

Untreated cases can have fatality rates as high as 30–35%, but when diagnosed early, they are often easily treated and carry an extremely good prognosis.

PREVENTION

Effective prevention warrants minimizing exposure to vectors (fleas, lice, mites, and ticks) and avoiding animal reservoirs (mainly dogs and rats). Avoiding tick bites, limiting exposure to tick habitats, inspecting the body carefully for ticks after being in a tick habitat, and removing attached ticks immediately by grasping with tweezers close to skin and pulling gently with steady pressure are various means of prevention. Antibiotic prophylaxis after tick bite given to asymptomatic people is usually not beneficial. No vaccine is available for rickettsial infections.

REFERENCES

1. Edwards MS, Feigin RD. Rickettsial and ehrlichial diseases. In: Feigin RD, Cherry JD, Demmler-Harrison GJ, Kaplan SL, Steinbach WJ (Eds). Textbook of Pediatric Infectious Diseases, 6th edition. Philadelphia, PA: Saunders Elsevier; 2009. pp. 2669-83.
2. Nicholson W, Paddock C. (2024). Rickettsial Diseases, CDC Yellow Book. [online] Available from https://wwwnc.cdc.gov/travel/yellowbook/2024/infections-diseases/rickettsial-diseases [Last accessed November, 2024].
3. Rathi N, Rathi A. Rickettsial infections—Indian perspective. Indian Pediatr. 2010;47(2):157-64.
4. Rathi NB, Rathi AN, Goodman MH, Aghai Z. Rickettsial diseases in Central India: proposed clinical scoring system for early detection of spotted fever. Indian Pediatr. 2011;48(11):867-72.
5. Naik IB, Sailaja A, Anusha T, Kumar A, Priya P, Prasanna S. A prospective study of the effectiveness of clinical RGA (Rathi Goodman Aghai) score in relation with PCR in the diagnosis of scrub typhus. In J Paediatr Geriatr. 2019;2(2):1-5.
6. Rathi NB, Kulkarni A, Yewale V. IAP guidelines on rickettsial diseases in children. Indian Pediatr. 2017;54(3):223-9.

7.12 Measles

Anand Prakash Dubey

INTRODUCTION

Measles is a contagious disease characterized by catarrhal symptoms, followed by the appearance of a typical rash. The incidence of measles has come down world over with effective immunization, but still it is a major cause of preventable blindness and the leading vaccine-preventable killer in children.

EPIDEMIOLOGY

India contributes 27% of the global measles deaths. The World Health Organization (WHO) has started the Measles Surveillance Project in India from 2007. Measles vaccination resulted in an 84% drop in measles deaths between 2000 and 2016 worldwide. In 2016, about 85% of the world's children received one dose of the measles vaccine by their first birthday through routine health services—up from 72% in 2000. During 2000–2016, measles vaccination prevented an estimated 20.4 million deaths, making the measles vaccine one of the best buys in public health. In 2016, there were 89,780 measles deaths globally—marking the first year that measles deaths had fallen below 1,00,000 per year.[1]

The 11 member states of the WHO South-East Asia Region committed to eliminate measles by 2030. In a phased manner, the Government of India is working on this goal and has introduced a two-dose strategy for the measles vaccine in routine immunization.

Molecular epidemiology of measles in India has been considerably growing and would be useful for understanding the circulation of wild-type measles in the pre- and postelimination period. However, recently, due to the COVID-19 pandemic, a drop in the measles vaccine coverage has been noticed resulting in more measles cases being reported now. India reported a total of 6,967 measles cases in 2022. To overcome this, mass campaigns of measles–rubella (MR) vaccination have been undertaken.

ETIOLOGY

Measles is caused by a ribonucleic acid (RNA) virus of the genus *Morbillivirus*, of the family *Paramyxoviridae.* Only one serotype of measles is known.

Measles is seen in early childhood in the developing countries. The disease usually occurs in infants below 3 years of age. Infants are usually protected until the age of 4–6 months due to immunity acquired transplacentally from the mother. Usually, these antibodies are undetectable by the age of 9 months, but antibodies may persist up to 12 months of age. The disease runs a mild course in healthy children, whereas the disease is severe in malnourished children. Transmission occurs either by direct contact or by droplet spray. The period of infectivity is 4 days before and 4 days after the appearance of rash. It is rarely subclinical. It is highly contagious, and the secondary attack rate is approximately 90% in susceptible household contacts.[2]

PATHOGENESIS

The measles virus enters the human body through the respiratory epithelium of the nasopharynx. The virus replicates initially in these cells, including the epithelial cells lining the buccal mucosa and conjunctiva. Later, it spreads to the regional lymph nodes. Further replication of the virus leads to primary viremia with seeding of the cells of the reticuloendothelial system. Infection of these cells leads to secondary viremia, whereby the measles virus is disseminated throughout the body, coincident with the clinical manifestations of the disease. Measles causes immunosuppression, which may persist for weeks to months and predisposes individuals to severe bacterial infection.[2]

CLINICAL MANIFESTATIONS

The clinical course of measles can be divided into four stages:

1. Incubation period
2. Prodromal stage
3. Catarrhal stage
4. Postmeasles stage of complications

The *incubation period* ranges from 10 to 12 days. In the later part of the incubation period, the child shows prodromal symptoms, which last for 2–4 days and consist of fever, malaise, coryza, and tracheobronchitis.

At the end of the *prodromal phase*, the child gets a fever, which may be high grade. Koplik spots, which are pathognomonic signs of measles, are seen on days 2–3 of fever. These are grayish-white or bluish-white dots with reddish areola. Occasionally, they are hemorrhagic, mostly seen on buccal mucosa opposite lower molars but may be seen all over the buccal mucosa. Conjunctival congestion and photophobia are also classical of measles, which occur before Koplik spots appear. The temperature rises abruptly as rash appears and often reaches 40°C or higher.

Rash appears on the fourth to the sixth day of fever. It starts as a faint erythematous maculopapular rash on the upper lateral aspect of the neck and typically behind the ears and increasingly involves the face, then spreading on to trunks, and then to legs and arms over the next 3–4 days. By the time rash appears on the feet, it starts disappearing from the face and fades down in the same pattern. Temperature also suddenly normalizes once rash starts fading and the child suddenly looks well from the sick look. The severity of the disease is directly related to the extent and confluence of rash. In severe cases, rash may become hemorrhagic. The rash fades in the next 3–4 days. As the rash disappears, it leaves behind the brownish desquamation and brownish discoloration characteristic of the postmeasles state and disappears in 7–10 days.

COMPLICATIONS

Measles can affect various systems in the body, resulting in the following complications:

- *Respiratory system:* Postmeasles bronchopneumonia, empyema, mediastinal and subcutaneous (SC) emphysema, and flaring of pulmonary tuberculosis
- *Gastrointestinal tract:* Diarrheal episodes are quite common after measles
- *Ear–nose–throat:* Otitis media
- *Central nervous system:* Measles encephalitis and encephalopathy
  - *Subacute sclerosing panencephalitis:* It is a degenerative disease of the brain caused by a persistent infection with the measles virus. It can manifest several years (usually 7 years) after measles infection. The patient develops progressive personality changes, developmental delay, myoclonic seizures, and motor disability. The measles virus has been isolated from the brain tissue of such patients. Their sera and cerebrospinal fluid show a high titer of measles-specific antibodies
- *Eye:* Keratitis
- Cancrum oris (Noma) and stomatitis
- *Systemic:* Acute malnutrition, secondary bacterial infections, such as septicemia with *Streptococcus*, etc.

PROGNOSIS

In developing countries, measles has a devastating course with a mortality of 1–3% and may go up during epidemics up to 5–15% with a high rate of complications.

MANAGEMENT

Management is mainly supportive. The child may be given antipyretics, fluids, and antihistamines during the acute phase. No antiviral therapy is available. The child may be isolated for the period of infectivity. There is an inverse correlation between serum retinol concentration and measles severity. A single dose of vitamin A, 1,00,000 U orally for children 6–12 months of age and 2,00,000 U orally for children >1 year of age, reduces mortality. Antibiotics may be indicated if there is evidence of otitis media or bacterial pneumonia.[2]

PREVENTION

Isolation of the patient from the seventh day of exposure to 5 days after rash appearance is recommended.

Measles Vaccine

Measles can be effectively prevented by the *measles vaccine.* The newborn baby is protected by transplacentally acquired maternal antibodies. The antibody gradually wanes, and the infant becomes susceptible to measles starting at 6 months of age. By 9–12 months of age, most infants become susceptible. At this age, the live-attenuated measles vaccine offers good protection. The vaccine that is not reconstituted remains viable for 2 years at 2–8°C, but once reconstituted, it should be used within 4 hours, as the vaccine does not contain any preservative or antibiotic.

Measles vaccine is a potent and effective vaccine with a seroconversion rate of 95–98%. As per the National Immunization Program in India and Expanded Program of Immunization (EPI) policy, the first dose of the measles vaccine is given as *measles and the rubella* vaccine at 9 months of age as a 0.5 mL SC injection, followed by a second dose at 15–18 months of age. The highly infectious nature of the measles virus requires the maintenance of very high levels of population immunity through high routine coverage. Measles remains widespread in India because of the delayed implementation of mass vaccination campaigns.

MMR vaccine is a combination of vaccines against measles, mumps and rubella. The global recommendation now is two doses for the MMR vaccine—the first dose at 15 months and the second at 4–6 years. It will be ideal to administer the second dose at 5th year along with diphtheria, tetanus, pertussis booster, and oral polio vaccines. The Indian Academy of Pediatrics (IAP) Advisory Committee on Vaccination and Immunization Practices (ACVIP) recommends three-dose MMR vaccines at 9 months, 15 months, and 4–6 years, respectively.[3]

The measles vaccine is contraindicated in pregnancy, children with primary immunodeficiency, untreated tuberculosis, cancer, organ transplantation, those receiving long-term immunosuppressive therapy, or severely immunocompromised human immunodeficiency virus (HIV)-infected children.

Postexposure Prophylaxis

For a child <6 months of age (the mother is usually immune in India), there is no need for prophylaxis as the child is already protected from passively transferred maternal antibodies.

- For a child of 6–12 months of age, if unimmunized, vaccinate with the measles vaccine within 72 hours.
- For a child >12 months of age, if unimmunized, vaccinate with measles or the MMR vaccine within 72 hours of exposure.
- For an immunocompromised child, give 0.5 mL/kg immunoglobulin (maximum 15 mL) intramuscularly, irrespective of immunity status.

REFERENCES

1. Center for Disease Control and Prevention. Epidemiology and Prevention of Vaccine-preventable Diseases, 10th edition. Georgia: Department of Health and Human Services, CDC; 2007.
2. WHO SEARO. India EPI Fact Sheets, 2023, Country Fact Sheet. Geneva: WHO SEARO; 2023.
3. National Operational Guidelines for Introduction of Measles-Rubella Vaccine. New Delhi: Ministry of Health and Family Welfare, Government of India; 2017.

7.13 Rubella

Nupur Ganguly, Pratiksha Khatua

INTRODUCTION

Rubella, also known as "German measles" or the 3-day measles, is derived from the Latin, meaning little red. The disease was first described by German physicians in the mid-18th century; hence, it is also known as German measles. This disease is often mild, and attacks pass unnoticed as trivial infection. The rash may last 3 days, with children recovering faster than adults. Its importance lies in its teratogenic effects on the fetus. Infection during early pregnancy may cause fetal death or congenital rubella syndrome (CRS), causing various congenital abnormalities, the most common being hearing loss, cardiac defects, and eye anomalies, with development and growth delay leading to considerable morbidity and mortality. There is no treatment for rubella, but it can be prevented by vaccination. By vaccinating all children in the age group of 9 months to 15 years, India aims to eliminate rubella by 2023.

EPIDEMIOLOGY

Humans are the only natural host of the rubella virus. The virus is transmitted by aerosol droplets from person to person and transplacentally causing CRS. Volunteer studies have shown that the virus remains in the nasopharynx from 7 days before to 14 days after the onset of rash. It replicates in the mucosal cells of the upper respiratory tract and spreads to the regional lymph nodes, especially the posterior auricular and the suboccipital group. A small number of infants with congenital rubella can continue to shed the virus in nasopharyngeal secretions and urine and can transmit infection to susceptible contacts.

The secondary attack rate is 50–60% in family contacts and almost 100% in closed populations, such as institutions or military barracks.

Reliable statistics on CRS are rare in developing countries. The World Health Organization (WHO) estimates that worldwide, >1,00,000 children are born with CRS each year, and most of them are in developing countries. Data regarding the prevalence of rubella in India is scarce. Serosurveys have shown that 8–47% of women are susceptible to rubella infection.[1]

ETIOLOGY

The rubella virus is a cubical, medium-sized (70 nm) virus. It is a ribonucleic acid (RNA) virus of the genus *Rubivirus* in the family *Togaviridae*. A capsid protein surrounds the viral RNA. The virus has two transmembrane proteins, E1 and E2. Only one serotype has been identified.

CLINICAL MANIFESTATIONS

The *incubation period* is 14–21 days.

Initial *prodromal symptoms* include malaise, headache, mild catarrhal symptoms, and low-grade fever. The most characteristic features are retroauricular, posterior cervical, and suboccipital lymphadenopathy. Discrete rose-colored spots on the soft palate (Forchheimer spots) may be seen in approximately 20% of patients before the onset of skin rash. Skin rash is mostly discrete maculopapular but quite variable in size and confluence. It starts on the face and spreads rapidly over the trunk. Progression is so fast that by the third day, it usually clears up without significant desquamation. Occasionally, conjunctivitis is seen. In women and young girls, arthralgia and polyarthritis may occur. Any joint can be involved, but small joints of the hand are affected most frequently, lasting for a few days to a few weeks and leaving no sequelae.

Congenital Rubella Syndrome

In pregnant women, the rubella virus can cross the placenta and infect the developing embryo or the fetus, resulting in various congenital malformations. The exact nature and extent of these malformations depend on the gestational age of the affected fetus. The risk for congenital defects is greatest with primary maternal infection. Congenital defects occur in about 90% infants if maternal infection occurs before 11 weeks of pregnancy and about 10–20% by the end of the first trimester. CRS may result in spontaneous abortion or birth of a severely malformed baby. Maternal infection after the 16th week is associated with a low risk of congenital defects.[2]

BOX 7.13.1: Main clinical manifestations of congenital rubella syndrome.

General:
- Fetal loss (spontaneous abortion and stillbirths)
- Low birth weight
- Micrognathia

Ears and central nervous system:
- *Sensorineural deafness:* Unilateral or bilateral
- Central auditory deafness
- Intellectual deficits
- Speech defects

Cardiovascular system:
- Patent ductus arteriosus
- Pulmonary arterial stenosis
- Ventricular septal defect

Eyes:
- Retinopathy
- *Cataracts:* Pearly, dense, nuclear; 50% bilateral; always accompanied by retinopathy
- Microphthalmos

Transient neonatal manifestations:
- Thrombocytopenia, which may manifest as purpura
- Hepatosplenomegaly
- Meningoencephalitis
- Bony radiolucencies

Late emerging or developmental:
- Late-onset interstitial pneumonitis, at age 3–12 months
- Chronic diarrhea
- Insulin-dependent diabetes mellitus

Thyroid dysfunction

Classically, the CRS includes a triad of malformations: Cataract, sensorineural hearing loss, and congenital heart disease. It may also be a disease with multisystemic involvement and a wide spectrum of clinical expression. It can also lead to intrauterine growth retardation, microphthalmia, microcephaly, and neurocognitive and motor retardation **(Box 7.13.1)**. In the postnatal period, infants with congenital rubella should be isolated, particularly from pregnant women, as they can shed the virus through urine and nasopharyngeal secretion and infect others.

Though the exact burden of CRS in India is not known, it is one of the most important causes of vaccine-preventable blindness and deafness in the country.

DIAGNOSIS

Confirmation is by serology or viral culture. Virus can be isolated from throat and urine from 1 week before to 2 weeks after the onset of rash. Congenital rubella is associated with low platelet counts, abnormal liver function tests, hemolytic anemia, pleocytosis, and very high immunoglobulin M (IgM) antibody titer. X-ray shows pneumonitis and bone metaphyseal longitudinal lucencies in CRS.[3,4]

DIFFERENTIAL DIAGNOSIS

Rubella is often confused with a mild variety of scarlet fever or rubeola. Other viral illnesses, such as roseola infantum, infectious mononucleosis, enteroviral infection, and drug rash, often closely resemble rubella.

PROGNOSIS

The prognosis of childhood rubella is better than that of congenital rubella, which varies with the gestational age at the time of infection and the organ involved.

TREATMENT

No specific antiviral therapy is available for rubella. Antipyretics are used for symptomatic relief.

PREVENTION

Congenital rubella syndrome is a significant public health problem and is entirely preventable by ensuring the vaccination of children with a rubella-containing vaccine (RCV).[5] Rubella vaccination induces seroconversion rates of 95% or higher after the administration of a single dose. Hence, it is an excellent vaccine for the prevention of CRS. The WHO rubella vaccine position paper recommends that countries take advantage of the measles platform to introduce RCV as either measles and rubella (MR) or measles–mumps–rubella (MMR) vaccine. Countries should give RCV in the routine schedule at the same age as they currently give the first dose of the measles-containing vaccine (MCV). WHO global recommendations for rubella also recommend regular follow-up campaigns with MR-containing vaccines in the countries with MCV1 coverage <90–95%, efforts to reach women of childbearing age, and surveillance for rubella and CRS. Special care should be taken in reproductive females to avoid pregnancy for 3 months after MMR vaccination. However, inadvertent vaccination during pregnancy is not an indication for termination of pregnancy.

The first step taken by the Government of India was Mission Indradhanush to incorporate the MR vaccine from 9 months until the age of 2 years, from 2017 in Universal Immunization Program (UIP), along with routine immunization (RI), for rubella and measles elimination by 2023. However, the achievements were hindered during the COVID pandemic with limited resources and population migration. As a result, many cohorts remained unvaccinated, giving rise to the measles outbreak. As India moved toward the last mile for MR elimination, catch-up campaigns were conducted across the country.

Intensified Mission Indradhanush 5.0 (IMI 5.0) was planned to catch up the gaps between unvaccinated and reach the unreached child from the age of 9 months to 5 years (previously it was up to 2 years), covering all the districts of the country.

Three rounds of *IMI 5.0* were conducted with MR along with RI.

1st round: August 7–12, 2023

2nd round: September 11–16, 2023

3rd round: October 9–14, 2023

Each round was spread over 6 working days. Vaccination sessions were flexible for better turnout of the beneficiaries. This was undertaken along with RI. The U-Win portal was used for registering, data collection, and reporting of the number of beneficiaries. This was a big leap toward MR elimination.

Further with a goal of rubella elimination by 2023, a nationwide MR vaccine introduction campaign was done targeting children from 9 months to 15 years, irrespective of their previous vaccination status with the measles/MR/MMR vaccine. The campaign was being carried out in schools, health care, health facility, or a private clinic.

Both girls and boys are at an equal risk of getting infected as well as transmitting the rubella virus, if not already protected against the disease. Therefore, both boys and girls were immunized with the MR vaccine during the MR vaccination campaign.

Further roadmaps to MR elimination in India by 2023 are made by the India Expert Advisory Group for surveillance of measles and rubella (IEAG-MR), where the focus has also shifted from surveillance of measles to "fever and rash" surveillance.[6] Every child reporting with fever and rash (irrespective of age) is to be notified to the District Medical Officer (DMO), the District Immunization Officer (DIO), or the District Surveillance Officer (DSO). For reported cases, nasopharyngeal or throat swab and/or urine specimen within 7 days of the onset of rash and one blood sample for a virological/serological study for measles/rubella or nonmeasles/nonrubella within 28 days of the onset of rash are to be sent.

REFERENCES

1. Cutts FT, Robertson SE, Diaz-Ortega JL, Samuel R. Control of rubella and congenital rubella syndrome (CRS) in developing countries, Part 1: Burden of disease from CRS. Bull World Health Organ. 1997;75(1):55-68.
2. Dewan P, Gupta P. Burden of congenital rubella syndrome (CRS) in India: a systematic review. Indian Pediatr. 2012;49(5):377-99.
3. Levin MJ, Weinberg A. Infections: viral and rickettsial. In: Hay WW, Levin MJ, Sondheimer JM, Deterding DR (Eds). Current Diagnosis and Treatment: Pediatrics, 20th edition. New York: McGraw-Hill Medical; 2009. pp. 1107-47.

4. Mason WH. Rubella. In: Kliegman RM, Jenson HB, Behrman RE, Stanton BF (Eds). Nelson Textbook of Pediatrics, 18th edition. Philadelphia: Elsevier; 2007. pp. 1337-41.
5. Sharma H, Chowdhari S, Raina TR, Bhardwaj S, Namjoshi G, Parekh S. Sero-surveillance to assess immunity to rubella and assessment of immunogenicity and safety of a single dose of rubella vaccine in school girls. Indian J Community Med. 2010;35(1):134-7.
6. Ministry of Health and Family Welfare, GOI. Roadmap to Measles and Rubella Elimination in India by 2023. New Delhi, India; 2022.

7.14 Mumps

Jaydeep Choudhury

INTRODUCTION

Mumps is an acute viral infection that is characterized by swelling of one or more of the salivary glands, most commonly the parotid glands. It generally occurs in children and young adults. The salivary glands, the pancreas, the testes or ovary, the brain, the breast, the liver, the joints, and the heart are the organs that are usually affected by the virus. About one-third of infections do not cause clinically apparent gland swelling and manifest only as respiratory infection.[1]

ETIOLOGY

Mumps virus is a ribonucleic acid virus of the genus *Paramyxovirus* in the family *Paramyxoviridae*. Only one serotype of the mumps virus is known.

EPIDEMIOLOGY

The mumps virus is endemic worldwide; it also occurs in small epidemics. The only known host is the human. In unimmunized populations, epidemics tend to occur every 2–5 years, throughout the year but often with a peak in late winter or early spring.[2]

ETIOPATHOGENESIS

The mumps virus is transmitted by infected respiratory tract secretions such as saliva, through airborne droplets, by direct contact, through fomites contaminated by saliva, and possibly by urine. The secondary infection rates in susceptible populations have been as high as 80%.[1] The period of maximum communicability extends from 1 to 2 days before the onset of symptoms to 5 days thereafter. The incubation period is 2–4 weeks, average 16–18 days. The virus proliferates in the upper respiratory tract epithelium and then enters circulation. Viremia occurs after 12–25 days and lasts for 3–5 days.[2] During viremia, the virus spreads to multiple tissues. It then localizes in glandular and neural tissue. Infection with the virus or immunization is thought to confer lifelong immunity.

CLINICAL FEATURES

Symptoms begin acutely with fever, malaise, and headache to be followed by parotitis, which is the most common manifestation and occurs in 30–40% of infected persons.[1] It may involve one or both glands. Earache, jaw tenderness with chewing, and dry mouth are among the presenting complaints that worsen over the next several days. Sucking a sour stimulus produces significant worsening of the pain. The swelling is at the angle of the jaw and obliterates the angle, often extending to the lower portion of the ear, which may be lifted upward and outward. Defervescence and resolution of parotid tenderness take about a week.[3] The orifice of Stensen's duct is commonly red and swollen.

The submaxillary and sublingual glands are involved less often and may be without parotid swelling.[3] Presternal pitting edema has been described due to lymphatic obstruction.

Other than parotitis, orchitis is the second most common feature in adolescent and postpubertal males but uncommon in prepubescent males.[4] Epididymo-orchitis, bilateral in 30%, usually occurs 1–2 weeks after parotitis, but it may occur without parotitis. Symptoms begin abruptly with testicular swelling and tenderness and associated nausea, vomiting, and headache. The testicle may enlarge three or four times and become very tender. Some degree of atrophy develops in nearly half of the affected organs, but sterility is uncommon. Oophoritis in girls is much uncommon and may cause lower abdominal pain but does not lead to sterility.[2]

The central nervous system (CNS) involvement, in both children and adults, is characterized by aseptic meningitis that occurs in 1–10% of patients.[4] Meningeal symptoms may develop anytime between a week before and several weeks after the parotitis. Pleocytosis of cerebrospinal fluid (CSF) with a lymphocytic predominance of about 500 cells is usual, but total white cell counts may rise to over 2,000 in the spinal fluid. CSF glucose is usually normal but may be low at times, and the protein is normal or slightly elevated. These findings revert to normal after about a week, and sequels are uncommon.

Encephalitis is rare, but it can be very serious with seizures and cortical blindness.[3] Recovery is usually complete. Occasionally, meningitis or encephalitis may occur without manifest parotitis. Aqueductal stenosis and hydrocephalus have been associated with mumps infection. Other CNS problems include transverse myelitis, cerebellar ataxia, facial palsy, and Guillain-Barré syndrome (GBS).

Mumps pancreatitis may be present with pain in the abdomen, but diagnosis is difficult as serum amylase is elevated in both parotitis and pancreatitis, but serum lipase is normal in the former and elevated in the latter.[1]

WORLD HEALTH ORGANIZATION (2016) MUMPS CASE DEFINITION

Clinical Case Definition

Acute onset of unilateral or bilateral tender, self-limited swelling of the parotid or other salivary gland, lasting 2 or more days, and without other apparent cause is the clinical case definition of mumps.[4]

Laboratory Criteria for Diagnosis

- Isolation of mumps virus from a clinical specimen *OR*
- Seroconversion or significant (at least fourfold) rise in serum mumps immunoglobulin G *OR*
- Positive serological test for mumps-specific immunoglobulin M antibodies

Case Definition

- *Clinical case:* A case that meets the clinical case definition
- *Laboratory confirmed:* A case that meets the clinical case definition and is laboratory confirmed
- *Epidemiologically confirmed:* A case that meets the clinical case definition and is linked epidemiologically to a laboratory-confirmed case

COMPLICATIONS

The CNS is commonly affected by mumps infection, and it is also the most common site of mumps affection after the salivary glands. Usually, it presents as benign aseptic meningitis, seen in about 10% of cases. But it may also present as meningoencephalitis. Other manifestations include ataxia, acute disseminated encephalomyelitis, auditory nerve involvement, and GBS.

Pancreatitis is a manifestation of mumps and occurs in approximately 5% of the patients. Infection with the mumps virus has been implicated as a possible cause of juvenile onset of diabetes, but the causal link has not been proven.[1]

There is no evidence of impairment of fertility in postpubertal girls with oophoritis. Other complications including myocarditis, deafness—unilateral or bilateral (transient or permanent), arthritis, optic neuritis, and thyroiditis have been reported.[2]

Deafness caused by the mumps virus may be unilateral in about 80%. It may be associated with vestibular reactions. Onset is usually sudden and results in permanent hearing impairment.

Electrocardiogram changes typical of myocarditis are seen in 3–15% of patients with mumps. Usually, there is complete recovery.

Arthralgia, arthritis, and nephritis are other less common complications.

DIAGNOSIS

Virus Isolation

Mumps virus can be isolated in cell culture inoculated with buccal swab, throat washing, saliva, or CSF.

Serologic Tests

Serologic tests are rarely done, but it is possible to identify infection acutely by detecting antibodies to the "S" antigen by complement fixation antibody titers, which rise in the first week of illness, and the "V" antigen by complement fixation antibody titers that follow with a rise several weeks later and may persist at low levels for years. Neutralizing and hemagglutination-inhibiting antibodies appear during convalescence.[1]

MANAGEMENT

There is no specific treatment. The majority of cases resolve within 2 weeks.[3] Symptomatic and supportive treatment includes simple analgesics, such as paracetamol. Mumps immunoglobulin treatment is of no value.

PROGNOSIS

Mumps is a self-limited disease, and the prognosis is generally good in children.

PREVENTION

Immunization is necessary to protect children against mumps and its complications. Live-attenuated mumps virus vaccine strains include Leningrad-Zagreb, Leningrad-3, Jeryl-Lynn, RIT 4385, or Urabe AM9 strains and are grown in chick embryo or human diploid cell cultures.[5] The measles, mumps, and rubella (MMR) vaccines are supplied in lyophilized form and should be frozen for long-term storage. In the clinic, these vaccines can be stored at 2–8°C. The vaccines should be protected from light. Reconstituted vaccine should be stored at 2–8°C, protected from light, and used within 4–6 hours. The Indian Academy of Pediatrics (IAP) Advisory Committee on Immunization Practices (ACVIP) has recommended MMR vaccines indicated at 9 months, 15 months, and 4–6 years of age in combination with measles and rubella vaccination.[5,6] The dose is 0.5 mL subcutaneously. The vaccine can be given along with all other childhood vaccines except the bacillus Calmette-Guérin (BCG) vaccine. The virus does not spread from the vaccinee to contacts. Mumps-containing vaccines should be given at least 2 weeks before or 3 months after administration of immunoglobulins or blood transfusion. There is a theoretical possibility that antibodies will neutralize the vaccine virus and interfere with seroconversion.

In patients who have received a high dose of corticosteroid (>2 mg/kg/day or >20 mg/day of prednisolone or equivalent) for 14 days or more and who are otherwise not immunocompromised, mumps-containing vaccines should be given at least 1 month after the discontinuation of corticosteroid.[5]

The seroconversion rate against mumps is >90%, but clinical efficacy and long-term protection are 60–90%. with single dose. Outbreaks have been reported in the previously vaccinated population. Hence, two dosages are needed for adequate protection. Waning of immunity and poor B-cell memory responses induced by mumps strain can be the reason for outbreaks. The third dose of MMR is indicated as time since vaccination is crucial for protection.[6] High population density and antigenic differences between vaccine strain and wild-type strain could be other reasons for outbreaks. Recently, outbreaks of mumps have been reported from different places in India. Surveillance of mumps should also be started in India and make it a notifiable disease.

CONCLUSION

Mumps is usually a benign disease characterized by fever, malaise, and headache, followed parotitis. Orchitis is the second common feature in adolescent and postpubertal males. Mumps is a self-limited disease and there is no specific treatment. However it can be prevented by vaccination. MMR vaccines, which also contains mumps is indicated at 9 months and 15 months and 4–6 years of age.

REFERENCES

1. Cherry JD, Quinn KK. Mumps. In: Cherry JD, Harrison GJ, Kaplan SL, Steinbach WJ, Hotez PJ (Eds). Feigin and Cherry's Textbook of Pediatric Infectious Diseases, 8th edition. Philadelphia: Elsevier; 2019. pp. 1771-9.
2. Arora SK, Gupta P. Mumps. In: Gupta P, Menon PSN, Ramji S, Lodha R (Eds). PG Textbook of Pediatrics, 2nd edition. New Delhi: Jaypee Brothers Medical Publishers; 2018. pp. 1377-80.
3. Rai A. Mumps. In: Choudhury J, Shastri DD, Kundu R, Yewale V (Eds). Textbook of Pediatric Infectious Diseases, 3rd edition. New Delhi: Jaypee Brothers; 2023. pp. 411-3.
4. American Academy of Pediatrics. Mumps. In: Red Book 2015: Report of the Committee on Infectious Diseases, 30th edition. New Delhi: Jaypee Brothers Medical Publishers; 2015. pp. 566-8.
5. Purple book. In: Rao MIS, Kasi SG (Eds). IAP Guidebook on Immunization 2022, 4th edition. New Delhi: Jaypee Brothers Medical Publishers; 2024.
6. Marlow MA, Marin M, Moore K, Patel M. CDC guidance for use of a third dose of MMR vaccine during outbreaks. J Public Health Manag Pract. 2020;26:109-15.

7.15 Poliomyelitis

Ashok Kumar Dutta

INTRODUCTION

Poliomyelitis is a highly infectious, crippling, and often-fatal disease caused by any of the three serotypes—types 1, 2, and 3—that mainly affects children under 5 years of age. It is most often recognized by acute-onset flaccid paralysis of the limbs. The condition was considered in the past as one of the most feared infectious diseases because of permanent residual paralysis and disability. However, with the intelligent use of the available polio vaccines, the disease by wild poliovirus has become a rarity, with only two countries in the world—Pakistan and Afghanistan—as the only endemic countries in the world. The wild type 3 and 2 poliovirus has been eradicated from the world. In addition, there is always the threat of the spread of the disease from the endemic countries to the neighboring countries if the immunity level of the population declines. At present, vaccine-associated paralytic poliomyelitis (VAPP) and vaccine-derived poliovirus (VDPV) are occurring in many countries. The World Health Organization (WHO) aims at eradicating both wild and vaccine viruses causing poliomyelitis.[1,2]

EPIDEMIOLOGY

Poliovirus is a highly communicable disease for which human is the only reservoir. It multiplies in the intestine and is spread via the fecal-oral route. The average incubation period is 7-10 days (range 4-35 days). The maximum excretion of the virus occurs just before the onset of paralysis and during the first 2 weeks after the onset of paralysis. However, the virus is excreted intermittently for up to 2 months after infection.

Polio cases have decreased by over 99% since 1988, from an estimated 350,000 cases to only 12 cases in 2023 globally. There is an increase in the number of cases of paralytic poliomyelitis in 2024. Till 16th December, 2024, the data from WHO shows a total of 88 cases of paralytic poliomyelitis, 25 from Pakistan and 63 cases from Afghanistan. The number of cVDPV cases reported are as follows: cVDPV1 - 10, cVDPV2 - 225 and cVDPV3 - 3. There are four categories of countries in relation to poliomyelitis disease:[1,2]

1. *Endemic countries*, which have never stopped the transmission of indigenous wild poliovirus, can also be affected by outbreaks of circulating VDPV (cVDPV). Only two countries—Pakistan and Afghanistan—fall into this category, where six cases each of paralytic poliomyelitis due to the type 1 virus have been reported from both countries.
2. *Outbreak countries* are those that have stopped indigenous wild poliovirus but are experiencing reinfection either through the importation of wild or VDPV from another country or through the emergence and circulation of VDPV. There are at present 35 countries in the world that are in this group. The following countries belong to this group:
   a. *African region:* Algeria, Benin, Botswana, Burkina Faso, Burundi, Cameroon, Central African Republic, Chad, Cote d'Ivoire, Congo, Democratic Republic of Congo, Ghana, Guinea, Kenya, Madagascar, Malawi, Mali, Mauritania, Mozambique, Niger, Nigeria, Tanzania, Togo, Zambia, and Zimbabwe
   b. *American region:* The United States of America and Canada
   c. *Eastern Mediterranean:* Djibouti, Egypt, Somalia, Sudan, and Yemen
   d. *Europe:* Israel, Ukraine, and the United Kingdom
   e. *Southeast Asia:* Indonesia

   To stop these outbreaks, it is necessary to fully implement international outbreak response guidelines.
3. *Key at-risk countries:* Low levels of immunity and surveillance leave countries at risk of polio returning. To ensure that every country stays free from polio, it is essential to reach every child with polio vaccines and to strengthen disease surveillance. There are the following eight countries that belong to this category, e.g., Indonesia, Mozambique, Myanmar, Papua New Guinea and Philippines.
4. *At-risk countries:* All countries remain at risk of polio until the disease has been completely eradicated from the world. Until then, the best way for countries to minimize the risk and consequences of polio infection is to maintain strong population immunity levels through high vaccination coverage and strong disease surveillance in order to rapidly detect and respond to polio.

However, cases of cVDPV are still occurring in many countries of the world with poor immunization coverage. Almost all cVDPV cases are occurring with the type 2 oral polio vaccine (OPV) virus. In 2023, a total of 491 cases of cVDPV have been reported from around the world.

ETIOPATHOGENESIS

Poliomyelitis is caused by three antigenically distinct serotypes (types 1, 2, and 3) of polioviruses. The polioviruses are nonenveloped, positive-stranded ribonucleic acid (RNA) viruses and belong to the genus *Enterovirus* in the family *Picornaviridae*. These viruses can remain active for several days at room temperature and can be stored indefinitely frozen at a temperature of -20°C. It is rapidly inactivated by heat, chlorine, and ultraviolet light. Wild-type 2 and 3 polioviruses have been eradicated from the world, and only type 1 wild poliovirus is causing disease. However, cVDPV in almost all the cases and 60% of VAPP cases are caused by type 2 poliovirus. Polioviruses enter the intestine by the fecal-oral route of transmission through contaminated water and food. The primary site of replication is the small intestine and regional lymph nodes. Poliovirus probably accesses the central nervous system (CNS) through peripheral nerves and primarily infects motor neuron cells in the spinal cord (anterior horn cells) and the medulla oblongata.

CLINICAL MANIFESTATIONS

In 90-95% of infected individuals, poliovirus infection is unapparent. In the remaining 5-10% of individuals infected by poliovirus, one of the following three syndromes may occur:[1]

1. *Abortive polio:* This occurs in 4-8% of infections and is characterized by a minor illness with low-grade fever, sore throat, vomiting, abdominal pain, loss of appetite, and malaise. Recovery is rapid and complete; there is no paralysis.
2. *Nonparalytic polio:* It occurs in 1-2% of infections and is characterized by headache and neck, back, and leg stiffness, which occurs several days after the prodrome (fever, malaise, etc.). Presentation resembles other causes of aseptic meningitis and recovers within 2-10 days.
3. *Paralytic polio:* This form occurs in 0.5-1% of infections (i.e., one case of paralysis in every 100-200 infected children). Symptoms often occur in two phases, minor and major, and are often separated by several days without symptoms. The minor phase consists of symptoms similar

to those of abortive poliomyelitis. The major phase of the illness begins with muscle pain, spasms, and fever. This is followed by the rapid onset of flaccid paralysis that is usually complete within 72 hours.

There are four types of paralytic poliomyelitis:[1]

1. *Spinal paralytic poliomyelitis* is the most common form of paralytic poliomyelitis, seen in approximately 80% of paralytic cases. It results from a lower motor neuron lesion of the anterior horn of the spinal cord and affects the muscles of the legs, arms, and/or trunk. The affected muscles are flaccid (lower motor neuron type), and reflexes are diminished. There is no sensory involvement. Paralysis is often asymmetrical, affecting legs more often than arms. Paralytic manifestation in extremities begins proximally and progresses to involve distal muscle groups (i.e., descending paralysis). Severe cases may develop quadriplegia and paralysis of the trunk, abdominal, and thoracic muscles. Residual flaccid paralysis is usually present after 60 days.
2. *Bulbar polio* accounts for up to 2% of paralytic cases and results from a cranial nerve lesion, resulting in respiratory insufficiency, difficulty in swallowing, nasal regurgitation, and difficulty in phonation.
3. *Bulbospinal polio* accounts for approximately up to 20% of paralytic cases, which is a combination of both the spinal and bulbar components.
4. In rare cases, an *encephalitic type of poliomyelitis* has been reported.

Residual Paralysis

As the acute phase of illness (0–4 weeks) subsides, the recovery begins in paralyzed muscles. The extent of recovery is variable depending upon the extent of damage caused to the neurons by the virus. Maximum neurological recovery of the paralyzed muscle takes place in the first 6 months of the illness, but slow recovery continues for up to 2 years. After 2 years, no more recovery is expected, and the child is said to have "postpolio residual paralysis," which remains as such throughout life.

Vaccine-associated Paralytic Poliomyelitis

In some of the recipients of OPV (in <1%), genetic changes in the *VP1* gene of the vaccine virus take place, and the vaccine virus becomes virulent and causes paralysis in the same recipient or among close contacts who are not immune. Approximately one case of VAPP occurs after 2.3 million first doses and after 12 million subsequent doses. According to the WHO, approximately 500 cases per year occur in the world, out of which 75 cases are from India. VAPP is clinically indistinguishable from paralysis due to wild poliovirus.[2]

Vaccine-derived Poliovirus

Vaccine-derived poliovirus is a derivative of the Sabin strain from OPV, which exhibits about 1–15% genetic changes in the *VP1* gene and usually transmits disease to nonimmune individuals. The strain has the potential for human infection and paralysis, including sustained circulation and spreading disease in other countries through human travel, and is a serious threat to the spread of the disease in various countries of the world. In the last 5 years, more than 500 cases of cVDPV type 2 disease have occurred in various countries, which were declared polio-free. This mutant strain is of three types, as described in the following subsections.

Circulating Vaccine-derived Poliovirus

This emerges in areas with poor OPV coverage and chances of sustained person-to-person spread. WHO considers cVDPV a serious threat to the polio eradication process. In 2018, until the end of April 2018, a total of 35 cases of cVDPV have been reported from the Democratic Republic of the Congo and the Syrian Arab Republic, where no case of wild poliovirus has been reported. Somalia and Kenya are the other two outbreak countries for cVDPV, as per the WHO. Several other countries in Africa and the Middle East are at risk for cVDPV.[2]

Immunodeficient-associated Vaccine-derived Poliovirus

This strain is isolated from persons with primary immune deficiency states who exhibit prolonged infection after OPV exposure. These strains can persist for over 20 years.

Ambiguous Vaccine-derived Poliovirus

This strain is a clinical isolate from a nonimmunocompromised individual or environmental isolation from an unidentified source.

DIFFERENTIAL DIAGNOSIS

The differential diagnosis of abortive and nonparalytic polio includes other viral fevers. Paralytic poliomyelitis needs differentiation from other causes of acute flaccid paralysis (AFP). Paralytic poliomyelitis, Guillain–Barré syndrome, traumatic neuritis, and transverse myelitis represent the most common causes of AFP, but the complete differential diagnosis includes numerous etiologies (hypokalemia, encephalitis, meningitis and other enterovirus infections, polymyositis, peripheral neuritis, myasthenia and other myopathies, etc.). Distinguishing characteristics of paralytic polio are asymmetric, AFP, mostly involving proximal muscles with fever and muscular pain at onset, rapid progression from onset to maximum paralysis (usually <4 days), intact sensory nerve function, and most often, residual paralysis or weakness after 60 days.

TABLE 7.15.1: Differential diagnosis of paralytic poliomyelitis.

Signs and symptoms	*Polio*	*GBS*	*Transverse myelitis*	*Traumatic neuritis*
Fever at onset	High, present	Not common	Rarely present	Present
Flaccidity	Asymmetrical and proximal	Symmetrical and distal	Symmetrical lower limbs	Asymmetrical limb
DTR	Decreased or absent	Absent	Absent in LL early, hyperreflexia late	Decreased or absent
Sensation	Myalgia, no sensory loss	Cramps, tingling, and hypo-esthesia of palms and soles	Loss of sensation with sensory level	Pain in gluteal region
Cranial nerves involvement	Only in bulbar and bulbospinal	Often present VII, IV, X, XI, and XII	Absent	Absent
CSF: WBCs, protein	• High WBCs • Normal or slight increase in protein	<10 WBCs High protein	Normal or slight increase in protein	Normal protein
Bladder dysfunction	Absent	Transient	Present	Never
NCV—3rd week	• Abnormal • Anterior horn cell disease	Abnormal demyelination	No diagnostic value	Abnormal in sciatic nerve
EMG—3rd week	Abnormal	Normal	Normal	Normal

(CSF: cerebrospinal fluid; DTR: deep tendon reflexes; EMG: electromyography; GBS: Guillain–Barré syndrome; LL: lower limbs; NCV: nerve conduction velocity; WBCs: white blood cells)

Salient features of differentiation are summarized in **Table 7.15.1**.

DIAGNOSIS

The characteristic clinical presentation of acute lower motor neuron type of asymmetrical paralysis of proximal limb muscles without any sensory involvement is highly suggestive of poliomyelitis. However, all cases of AFP should be investigated by sending a stool sample for isolation of the virus.

Stool for Virus Isolation

It is recommended in every case of AFP. The virus usually can be found in the feces from onset to up to 8 or more weeks after paralysis, with the highest probability of detection during the first 2 weeks after onset. Isolation of wild poliovirus from stool is the recommended method for laboratory confirmation of paralytic poliomyelitis. Two stool specimens are collected from each case for laboratory confirmation.

An adequate stool specimen is defined as two specimens collected at least 24 hours apart within 14 days of the onset of paralysis. Each sample should have volume (8–10 g or thumb size) and sent to a WHO-accredited laboratory in good condition with no desiccation, leakage, and maintaining cold chain.

TREATMENT

The aim of treatment is to promote recovery to minimize residual muscle paralysis and disability. Treatment of the child with paralytic poliomyelitis varies with the stage of illness and the severity of paralysis. Children with bulbospinal polio and respiratory paralysis would require hospitalization. In the acute stage, children with isolated limb/limb paralysis should be advised complete rest, proper positioning of the affected limb, and passive range of movement at the joints. Massage and intramuscular (IM) injections should be avoided during the acute phase of illness. The child should be made to lie on a firm bed and maintain limbs in a neutral position. The child should lie with trunk and hip straight with slight flexion (5–10°) at knees and feet at the right angle at the ankle joint. This position can be maintained with pillows, rolled towels, or sandbags. The support should also be given on the lateral sides of limb/limbs to prevent external rotation. Warm moist fomentations and passive range of movements of all the joints of the affected limb/limbs should be given.

As the acute phase of illness subsides, recovery in muscle power is helped by giving physiotherapy in the form of active exercises aimed at strengthening weak muscle groups, improvement of functional skills of the child, helping ambulation, and prevention of deformities. Physiotherapy plays an important role in the management of children during recovery and the postpolio residual paralysis stage. Some children with fixed deformities and contractures may require orthopedic surgery.

STRATEGIES FOR POLIO ERADICATION INCLUDING ENDGAME STRATEGY

In May 1988, the World Health Assembly committed the member nations of the WHO to achieving the goal of global eradication of poliomyelitis. Since most of the countries in the world have been declared as polio-free, the endgame strategy has been defined now by the WHO Strategic Advisory Group on Polio Eradication as complete eradication and containment of all wild, vaccine, and Sabin poliovirus diseases from the world.[2] For the eradication of poliomyelitis from the world, the strategies include the following:

- Continuation of mass polio vaccination with bivalent (bOPV1 and 3) to susceptible individuals in national immunization days (NID) and sub-NID (SNID)
- Maximum coverage of infants in routine immunization
- Excellent clinical and virological surveillance of AFP
- Environmental surveillance of wild as well as vaccine-derived poliovirus
- Inclusion of fractional dose of inactivated polio vaccine (IPV) along with the bOPV at 6 weeks, 14 weeks, and 9 months
- Use of safe novel type 2 OPV in countries to contain outbreaks of cVDPV

In the country, this strategy would prevent cVDPV type 2 responsible for almost all cVDPV and also most of the VAPP cases (caused by type 2 virus). Please refer to Chapter 6.5, Polio Eradication Endgame: Global and National Perspectives for more details.

PREVENTION OF POLIOMYELITIS

Polio Vaccines

There are currently two effective polio vaccines—the IPV, which was the first vaccine to become available in 1955, and the live-attenuated OPV, which was licensed in 1959.[3,4]

Oral Polio Vaccine

Oral polio vaccine induces both circulating antibodies and intestinal immunity, and by secondary spread, probably protects susceptible contacts. The seroconversion after three doses of OPV has been reported to be more than 95% in the developed countries, but data from the developing countries has shown wide variation in seroconversion and protective efficacy, with rates varying from 70% against types 1 and 3 and approximately 90% for type 2 strains. Presently, only bOPV (containing types 1 and 3 Sabin live-attenuated strain) is available in the world. Type 2 OPV is no longer used anywhere in the world.

Dosage, Administration, and Formulation

The oral polio vaccine is formulated as a bivalent vaccine, containing antigens for poliovirus serotypes (1–3). The bivalent vaccine is used for both routine immunizations and NID and SNID.

Oral polio vaccine should be administered orally, that is, directly into the mouth. Each single dose consists of two drops of live OPV. OPV is given at birth, followed by three more doses at 6, 10, and 14 weeks and at 16–18 months as per the National Immunization Schedule of India. In addition, bOPV doses are recommended as per recommendations regarding NID or SNID from time to time.

Oral polio vaccine is one of the most heat-sensitive vaccines in common use. The vaccine should be stored at 2–8°C at all times. Unopened vials of OPV may be stored for up to 6 months at –20°C. The potency is monitored with color changes in the vaccine vial monitor.

Trivalent OPV (tOPV) has been discontinued in 2016, and there has been a switch to bOPV (types 1 and 3). This strategy was adopted to prevent cVDPV by augmenting the immunity induced by earlier doses of tOPV. By 2019, it is expected that if there is no case of poliomyelitis in the world, there shall be complete cessation of OPV, and at least one dose of IPV will be given to each child until 2024.

Inactivated Polio Vaccine

Inactivated polio vaccine, also known as Salk vaccine, is a mixture of the three polioviruses made by harvesting cell culture supernatants and submitting them to inactivation by formalin. When used as primary vaccination of infants, the vaccine produces seroconversion in 90–95% of children. IPV is relatively heat stable. The risk of vaccine-associated paralysis is nonexistent with IPV and can be safely used in immunocompromised individuals. Three doses are recommended as the primary schedule at 6, 10, and 14 weeks, followed by booster doses at 18 months and 5 years by the Indian Academy of Pediatrics (IAP).[5] However, in the National Immunization Schedule, three fractional doses of IPV (one-fifth) of the IM dose at 6 weeks, 14 weeks, and 9 months, along with pentavalent vaccine and bOPV, are used for routine immunization. Studies have shown that three doses of intradermal IPV are not inferior to IM doses.

REFERENCES

1. World Health Organization. Poliomyelitis (Polio). [online] Available from https://www.who.int/health-topics/poliomyelitis#tab=tab_1 [Last accessed November, 2024].
2. World Health Organization. Polio vaccines. WHO Position Paper. June 2022 Weekly epidemiological Report No 25. [online] Available from https://www.who.int/publications/i/item/WHO-WER9725-277-300. [Last accessed November, 2024].
3. Sutter RW, Kew OM, Cochi SL. Poliovirus vaccine-live. In: Plotkin SA, Orenstein WA, Offit PA (Eds). Vaccine, 6th edition. Philadelphia: Elsevier Saunders; 2013. pp. 598-645.
4. John TJ, Koirala A. Poliovirus vaccine-inactivated and live. In: IAP Textbook of Vaccines, 2nd edition. New Delhi: Jaypee Brothers Medical Publishers; 2020. pp. 198-213.
5. Shenoy B, Agarwalla S. Polio vaccine. In: Purple Book, 4th edition. Mumbai: Indian Academy of Pediatrics; 2022–2023. pp. 119-39.

7.16 Hand, Foot, and Mouth Disease

Tarun Patni

INTRODUCTION

Robinson described an outbreak of a highly infectious disease with skin rash in Toronto, Canada, in the last century. This disease had characteristic vesicles in the oral cavity, lips, hands, feet, and around the buttocks.[1] After investigations, it was concluded that it is caused by the coxsackievirus (CV) A16. The hand, foot, and mouth disease (HFMD) is a highly transmissible disease that mainly infects children below 10–12 years of age; occasionally, adults too may suffer.[2,3] It normally recovers on its own and, in a few cases, may lead to very severe and catastrophic complications.

ETIOLOGY

The causative agent of HFMD is CV, of the *Enterovirus* family, and is a single-stranded ribonucleic acid (RNA) virus of around 28 nm in size. These are from the *Picornaviridae* family. Human enteroviruses have many subgroups, like poliovirus, CV A and B, echovirus, and other enteroviruses. These viruses can attack various organs of the body and manifest with symptoms and signs in the skin, neurological organs, and other visceral organs.[4]

EPIDEMIOLOGY

Hand, foot, and mouth disease occurs in all areas of the world; young infants and toddlers suffer mostly and also children up to 10–12 years of age. Adults get infected rarely, which may be due to immunity because of the disease being acquired in childhood. Those living in congested places, camps, schools, or hostels and close contacts in the family suffer the infection most. In close contacts, the virus gets transferred through various body secretions like saliva, or throat and upper respiratory tract discharges. The vesical fluids in the perioral area, hands, or feet and even stool of an infected child are potential sources of transmission. The presence of the virus in feces and oral secretions before the onset of symptoms and even after the recovery makes the transmission of the disease easier.

The most implicated HFMD-associated serotypes are enterovirus (EV) A71 and CVA16; however, increasing cases of HFMD due to CVA10 and CVA6 were reported recently.[5-7] CVA10 has been implicated in severe disease, and atypical cases were found to be associated with CVA6 and A16.[5-7]

SIGNS AND SYMPTOMS

The disease has a short incubation period of around 3–6 days. The disease course starts with low-grade fever and upper respiratory symptoms like mild cough and pain in the throat. Slowly, it may lead to malaise, body pain, and anorexia. These general symptoms are usually followed by a maculopapular rash, small in size, and surrounded by erythema. This maculopapular rash turns into vesicles in exposed skin areas and small ulcers in the oral cavity, often in the peritonsillar area and end of the hard palate **(Fig. 7.16.1)**. These ulcers can cause a lot of discomfort and pain and lead to difficulty in feeding. The rash and vesicles develop over the hands and feet and perianal area **(Fig. 7.16.2)**. The disease in fingers may involve the nails leading to shedding of nails too **(Figs. 7.16.3 and 7.16.4)**. Thus, in a suspected case of HFMD, a thorough search for rash in the oral cavity, perianal area, hands, nails, and feet should be done.[8]

The clinical signs and symptoms are usually the same in HFMD caused by various types of causative virus, but still a little difference is there depending upon the causative virus. CVA16 is associated with large vesicles. Petechial rash on trunks and limbs is present when the HFMS is caused by EVA71. Many atypical presentations occur when the disease is caused by CVA6. Usually in CV-caused disease, nail shedding is present in the convalescent phase.[6-8] Central nervous

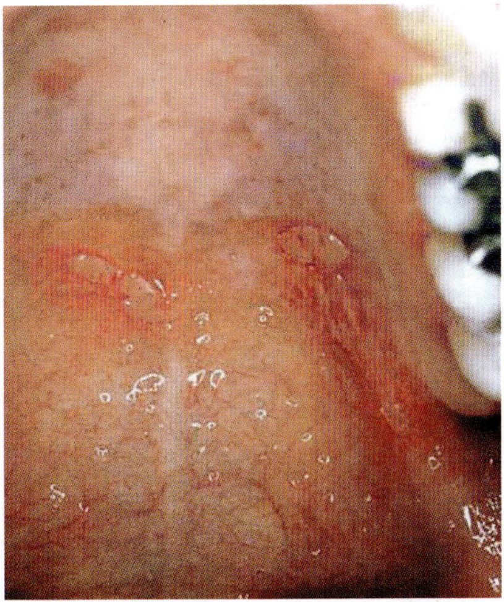

Fig. 7.16.1: Oral lesions in HFMD.
(HFMD: hand, foot, and mouth disease)

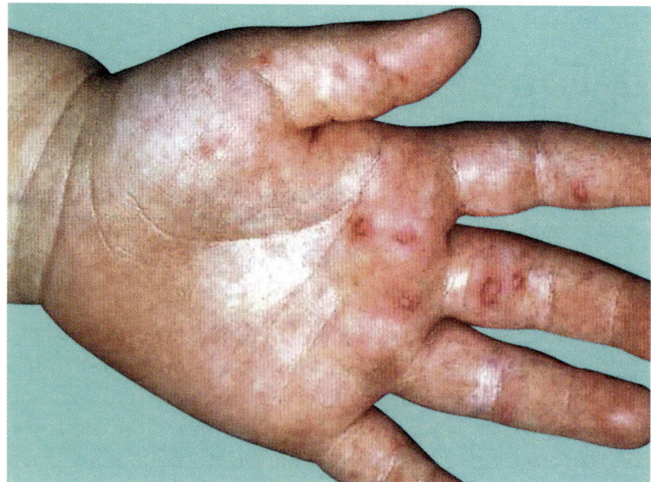

Fig. 7.16.2: Papular rash over palms in HFMD. (HFMD: hand, foot, and mouth disease)

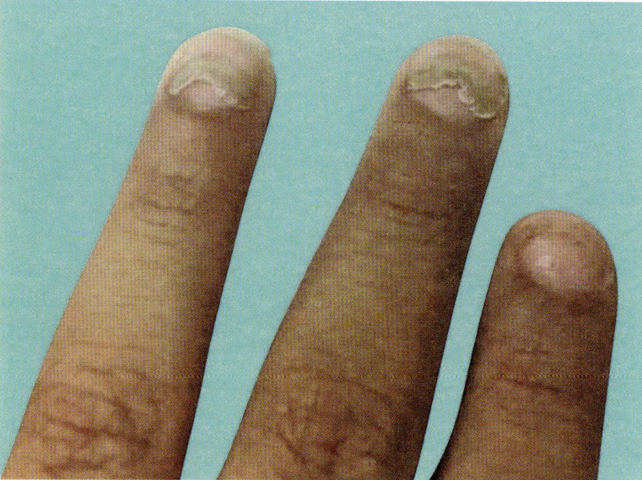

Fig. 7.16.3: HFMD leading to nail changes. (HFMD: hand, foot, and mouth disease)

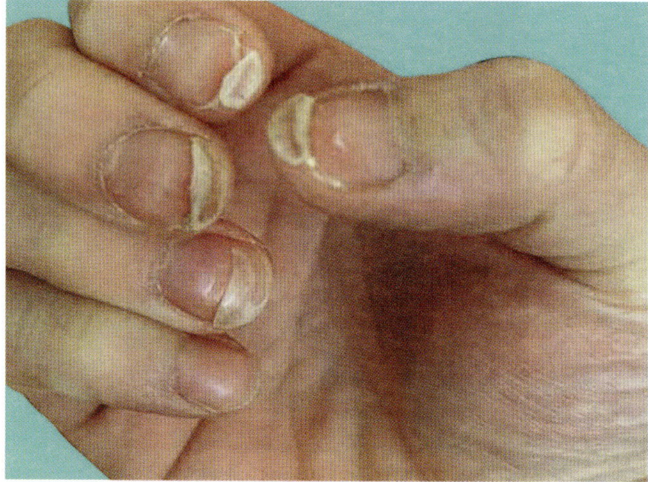

Fig. 7.16.4: Nail shedding after HFMD. (HFMD: hand, foot, and mouth disease)

system (CNS) manifestations of HFMD can be varied and very severe. Complications, including myoclonic seizures, tremors, nystagmus, brainstem encephalitis, and polio-like paralytic disease are a part. Severe cardiovascular (CVS) manifestations, including tachycardia, and even potentially lethal manifestations like congestive heart failure (CHF) and pulmonary edema are rarely encountered.[9]

DIAGNOSIS

In the majority of cases, the disease is diagnosed based on clinical signs and symptoms only. The various diseases that may have a similar picture, like herpes simplex, herpangina, and erythema multiforme, should be ruled out in atypical cases. Epidemiological history has a major role in diagnosing the disease, as it usually spreads in a local area, school, or camps. In atypical cases, the need for sophisticated diagnostic tools like polymerase chain reaction (PCR), etc., is needed. Vesical scraping may be used to differentiate the disease from herpes.

TREATMENT AND PREVENTION

Hand, foot, and mouth disease is usually a self-limiting viral disease. The disease usually needs symptomatic treatment of pain and fever, along with reassurance. Hydration and care of vesicles and general hygiene are always to be stressed upon. As the disease involves a huge number and even small atypical cases can be observed in large volumes, there is a need for a specific vaccine against HFMD. Few vaccines are being developed at the laboratory level, but it might take a long time to have a regular vaccine for prevention.[10] As the disease leads to a lot of loss to the quality of life of children with the disease and society, the need for preventive measures in the form of vaccines is there. Most of the vaccines are in the developmental stage and currently being developed against single strains of EVA71 and CVA16.[10]

REFERENCES

1. Robinson CR, Doane FW, Rhodes AJ. Report of an outbreak of febrile illness with pharyngeal lesions and exanthema: Toronto, summer 1957; isolation of group A Coxsackie virus. Can Med Assoc J. 1958:79(8):615-21.
2. Wang Y, Feng Z, Yang Y, Seif S, Gao Y, Longini IM, et al. Hand, foot and mouth disease in China: patterns of spread and transmissibility. Epidemiology. 2011;22(6):781-92.
3. Zhang X, Yan H-p, Huang C, Tan Y-f, Ma D-m, Zhang H-p, et al. The etiology and clinical manifestations of 70 patients in hand-foot-mouth disease. Zhonghua Yu Fang Yi Xue Za Zhi. 2009;43(10):872-4.
4. Wang J-f, Guo Y-S, Christakos G, Yang W-Z, Liao Y-L, Li Z-J, et al. Hand, foot and mouth disease: spatiotemporal transmission and climate. Int J Health Geogr. 2011;10:25.
5. Mirand A, Henquell C, Archimbaud C, Ughetto S, Antona D, Bailly J-L, et al. Outbreak of hand, foot and mouth disease/

herpangina associated with coxsackievirus A6 and A 10 infections in 2010, France: a large citywide, prospective observational study. Clin Microbiol Infect. 2012;18(5):E110-8.
6. Chen K-T, Lee T-C, Chang H-L, Yu M-C, Tang L-H. Human enterovirus 71 disease. Clinical features, Epidemiology, Virology, and Management. Open Epidemiol J. 2008;1:10-6.
7. Feder HM, Bennet N, Modlin JF. Atypical hand, foot and mouth disease: a vesicobullous eruption caused by Coxsackie virus A6. Lancet Infect Dis. 2014;14(1):83-6.
8. Keawcharoen J. Hand, foot and mouth disease. Thai J Vet Med. 2012;42:255-7.
9. Chang L-Y, Lin T-y, Hsu KH, Huang YC, Lin KL, Hsueh C, et al. Clinical features and risk factors of pulmonary oedema after enterovirus-71 related hand, foot, and mouth disease. Lancet. 1999;354(9191):1682-6.
10. Liu C-C, Chow Y-H, Chong P, Klein M. Prospect and challenges for development of multivalent vaccines against hand, foot, and mouth disease. Vaccine. 2014;32(47):6177-82.

7.17 Chickenpox (Varicella) and Monkeypox

Lalitha Kailas

CHICKENPOX (VARICELLA)

INTRODUCTION

Chickenpox is a common childhood disease, caused by the *Varicella zoster* virus (VZV). Though generally considered as a benign, self-limited infection, this may cause severe illnesses, especially in newborns, immunocompromised children, and elderly patients. The incidence of the disease has now markedly decreased as the varicella vaccine has become more widely used.

EPIDEMIOLOGY

Chickenpox is worldwide in distribution; epidemics do not have any definite periodicity. The age of peak varicella incidence has shifted from children younger than 10 years to children 10–14 years of age. Immunity to wild-type varicella generally is lifelong.[1,2]

ETIOLOGY

Varicella zoster virus is a double-stranded deoxyribonucleic acid (DNA) virus, a member of the herpesvirus family. Humans are the only reservoir for VZV and cause primary, latent, and recurrent infections. Primary infection causes chickenpox and results in a lifelong latent infection of sensory ganglion neurons. Reactivation of latent infection causes a localized form of the disease known as herpes zoster (HZ) (shingles), which is not common in children.[1,2]

Recovery from primary varicella infection usually results in lifetime immunity. In otherwise healthy persons, a second occurrence of varicella is uncommon; it is more common in immunocompromised persons.

PATHOGENESIS

The virus presents in the respiratory secretions and in the fluid of skin lesions of an affected child is transmitted either by airborne or by direct contact. Viral replication occurs initially in the respiratory tract, followed by subclinical viremia. Host immune responses limit viral replication and facilitate recovery from infection. In immunocompromised children, however, viral replication continues with resultant injury to the lungs, brain, and other organs. The virus is transported in a retrograde manner through sensory axons to the dorsal route ganglia through the spinal cord and establishes as a latent infection; subsequent reactivation of this lesion results in HZ. The maximum period of infectivity is from 2 days prior to the onset of rash until all the lesions have crusted, which is usually 5 days after the onset of rash. Chickenpox is highly contagious, with a secondary household attack rate of >90% in susceptible individuals.[1,2]

CLINICAL FEATURES

The illness usually begins 14–16 days after exposure, although the incubation period can range from 10 to 21 days. The prodromal period starts as mild fever, headache, generalized body ache, and tiredness. Fever is usually moderate ranging from 38 to 39°C After 2–3 days the rash appears initially as maculopapular, which evolves into vesicles filled with clear fluid, which becomes cloudy and umbilicated, described as "dew drops on rose petals" **(Fig. 7.17.1)**. The rash is intensely pruritic, and distribution is typically central or centripetal. Lesions also occur in the oral mucosa, pharynx, conjunctiva, and genitalia. New lesions appear for 1–7 days. While the initial lesions are crusting, new crops form on the trunk and then extremities. *Simultaneous presence of lesions in various*

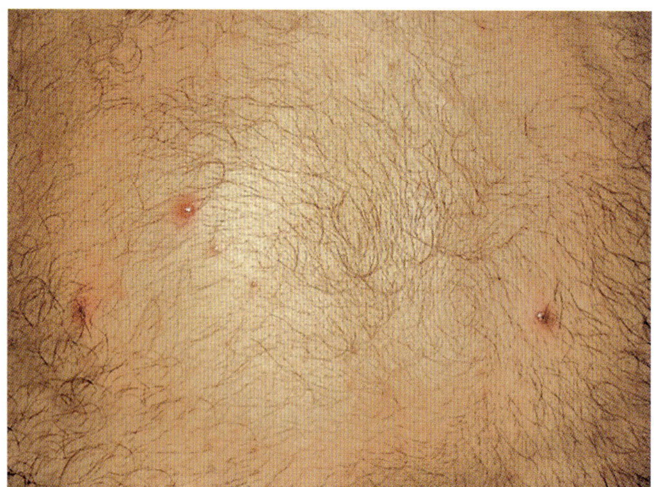

Fig. 7.17.1: Varicella rashes as "dewdrops on rose petals."

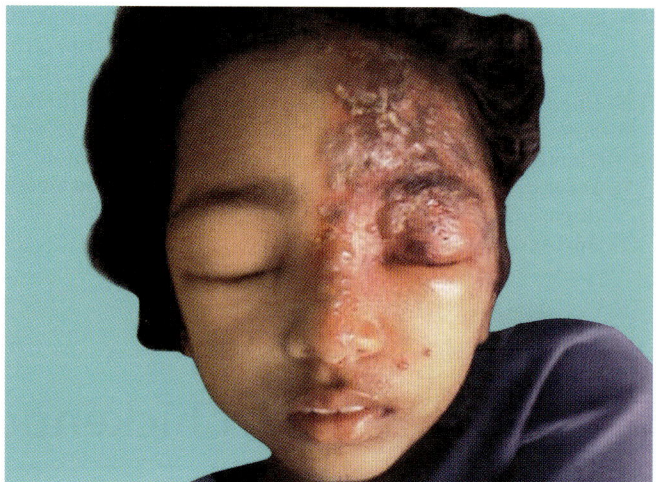

Fig. 7.17.2: Herpes zoster.

stages of evolution is characteristic of varicella.[3] New vesicle formation generally stops within 4 days, and most lesions have fully crested by day 6 in normal children. The lesions vary in number, from 10 to 1,500 and the crusts completely fall off within 1–2 weeks leaving behind hypo- or hyperpigmented marks that persist for days to weeks. Scarring is unusual unless the lesions are secondarily infected or scabs are removed prematurely.[1,2]

Herpes Zoster

Herpes zoster is caused by the reactivation of latent VZV and is not common in childhood. Zoster is not caused by exposure to a patient with varicella; in fact, exposures to varicella boost the cell-mediated immune response to VZV in individuals with prior infection, decreasing the likelihood of reactivation of latent virus. The lifetime risk for HZ for individuals with a history of varicella is at least 30%, with 75% of cases occurring after 45 years of age. HZ is characterized by clustered vesicular lesions on the erythematous base, distributed over one or two dermatomes. Unlike in adults, severity is less except in immunocompromised children **(Fig. 7.17.2)**.[4]

Breakthrough Varicella

Breakthrough varicella is defined as varicella developing >42 days after immunization and usually occurs 2–5 years following vaccination. It occurs in about 1–4% of vaccinees per year. Generally, it is mild with <50 skin lesions, predominantly maculopapular rather than vesicular rash, low or no fever, shorter (4–6 days) duration of illness, and less contagious.

COMPLICATIONS

Complications of varicella are not common; uneventful recovery is the rule except in immunocompromised persons. The specific types of complications in patients with varicella vary with age; bacterial complications are common in children, whereas respiratory complications are more seen in adults.[5]

Bacterial Infections

Secondary bacterial infections of skin (cellulitis and abscess) occur most commonly due to *Staphylococcus aureus* and *Streptococcus pyogenes*, which can lead to complications such as necrotizing fasciitis, septicemia, septic arthritis, and even toxic shock syndrome occasionally.

Neurologic Complications

Encephalitis and cerebellar ataxia are the common neurologic complications encountered, usually manifest 2–6 days after the onset of rash but may occur in the incubation period also. Cerebellar ataxia can appear as late as 21 days. This is benign and with complete recovery within 2–4 weeks. Encephalitis is more serious and occurs in 0.1–0.25% of persons with the disease, with the mortality established between 5 and 20%. Other complications include transverse myelitis, Guillain-Barré syndrome, and optic neuritis.

Respiratory Complications

Varicella pneumonia is a severe complication, which is more common among immunocompromised children, and it sets in during the first 6 days after the onset of rash.

Other Complications

Other complications include purpura fulminans, central nervous system vasculitis, autoimmune thrombocytopenia, and Reye syndrome.

Progressive Varicella

Progressive varicella is a dreaded complication that follows primary varicella infection in children with congenital cellular immune deficiency, malignancy, human immunodeficiency virus (HIV), after-organ transplantation, or on chronic steroid therapy. It is characterized by severe visceral organ involvement, coagulopathy, and hemorrhage, and lesions will continue to develop for a longer time. Severe and even fatal varicella has been reported in otherwise healthy children on high-dose corticosteroids (>2 mg/kg/day of prednisone or equivalent) for treatment of asthma and other illnesses.[5]

Varicella Embryopathy

Chickenpox in pregnancy is associated with an increased risk of fetal malformations, especially if infection occurs in the first or second trimester. The incidence of congenital varicella syndrome following gestational varicella in the first 20 weeks is approximately 2% and is characterized by cicatricial skin scarring in a dermatomal fashion, limb hypoplasia, and ocular and brain abnormalities (microcephaly, seizures, neurocognitive deficits, etc.). Children infected with VZV in utero may develop zoster early in life without having had extrauterine varicella.

Neonatal Varicella

Varicella is associated with high mortality in newborn. The risk in newborn is dependent on the amount of maternal antibody that the fetus has acquired transplacentally before birth. If there is 1 week or more of interval between maternal chickenpox and delivery, it is likely that the newborn received sufficient antibody to VZV to ameliorate neonatal infection. Alternatively, if the interval was <1 week, the newborn is unlikely to have enough VZV antibodies, and neonatal chickenpox may be exceptionally severe.[5]

DIFFERENTIAL DIAGNOSIS

The differential diagnosis of varicella includes vesicular rashes caused by other infectious agents, such as herpes simplex virus, enterovirus, monkeypox, rickettsialpox, and *S. aureus;* drug reactions; disseminated HZ; contact dermatitis; and insect bites (especially for breakthrough varicella).[3]

DIAGNOSIS

Diagnosis is clinical and not usually difficult in a typical case. Often, a history of exposure to the disease is helpful in reaching the diagnosis. Laboratory abnormalities include leukopenia in the initial 72 hours, followed by relative lymphocytosis. Although multinucleated giant cells can be detected with nonspecific stains (Tzanck smear), they have poor sensitivity and do not differentiate VZV from herpes simplex viral infections. Vesicular fluid or a scab can be used to identify VZV using a polymerase chain reaction (PCR) test, which is currently the diagnostic method of choice. VZV immunoglobulin G (IgG) antibodies can be detected by several methods, and a four-fold increase in IgG antibodies is also confirmatory of acute infections. Testing for VZV immunoglobulin M (IgM) antibodies is not useful for clinical diagnosis as the kits available are generally unreliable.[1,2,5]

MANAGEMENT

Management is symptomatic and includes antipyretics, antipruritic agents, and good hygiene. Antiviral treatment modifies the course of both varicella and HZ. There is controversy in treating uncomplicated varicella in a healthy child.

Oral acyclovir and valacyclovir are not recommended for routine use in otherwise healthy younger children with varicella because their use results in only a modest decrease in symptoms. For healthy children <12 years old, varicella is typically self-limited, and most of the viral replication stops by 72 hours after the onset of rash. The American Academy of Pediatrics (AAP) recommends treatment only in high-risk individuals such as unvaccinated children >13 years, those with chronic cutaneous/pulmonary diseases, secondary cases in household contacts, and children on oral/inhaled steroids. Acyclovir is the drug of choice; 20 mg/kg/dose four times a day for 5 days. Valacyclovir, 20 mg/kg/dose three times daily for 5 days, is also licensed for the treatment of varicella in children aged 2–18 years. Treatment should be initiated within 24 hours of the onset of the disease to get maximum effectiveness. Intravenous (IV) acyclovir is indicated in severe varicella, neonates, and immunocompromised individuals in a dose of 10 mg/kg 8 hourly for 7–10 days.[1,2]

Acyclovir-resistant VZV has been identified primarily in children infected with HIV. These children may be treated with IV foscarnet (120 mg/kg/day divided every 8 hours for up to 3 weeks).

PREVENTION

Active Immunization

Varicella is a vaccine-preventable disease. Vaccines are available either as monovalent (V)-varicella only or as quadrivalent measles-mumps-rubella-varicella (MMRV) vaccines. Varicella vaccine, a live-attenuated vaccine, is recommended as a two-dose regimen at all ages. For primary immunization, the first dose should be given at the age of 15 months, *and the second dose should be preferably administered 3–6 months after the first dose (ACVIP recommendation 2021)*. A short interval between two doses of the varicella vaccine might be preferable to reduce breakthrough varicella, especially in countries with poor coverage and where the wild-type virus circulates predominantly, like in our country. Also, 2–3 years is the usual entry age for preschool in India, which may result in breakthrough varicella before the receipt of a delayed second dose. In India, the varicella vaccine is not in the National Immunization Program (NIP) and is recommended only by the Indian Academy of Pediatrics (IAP), and the overall uptake is low, and exposure to varicella following the first dose may give rise to breakthrough varicella.[6] Since the aim of varicella vaccination, in office practice, is the best possible protection for the individual child, an earlier second dose will be beneficial over a delayed second dose.

For catch-up vaccination, children below the age of 13 years should receive two doses at 3 months apart and, above 13 years of age, two doses at a 4–8-week interval. No booster is recommended.

Herpes Zoster Vaccines

Two vaccines, Zostavax™ (live attenuated) and Shingrix™ (recombinant), are available in the global market for protection against HZ.[1] Presently, they are not available in India.

Postexposure Prophylaxis

A *vaccine* given within 3–5 days of exposure (as soon as possible preferably) is effective in preventing or modifying varicella, especially in a household setting. *Antivirals like oral acyclovir/valacyclovir* administered late in the incubation period, beginning 7 days after exposure and continuing for 7 days, may prevent or modify subsequent varicella in a healthy child.

Varicella Zoster Immunoglobulin

Varicella zoster immunoglobulin (VZIG) is recommended for postexposure prophylaxis for susceptible individuals with significant contact with varicella or HZ. Immunocompromised children and newborns of mothers with varicella within 5 days before delivery and 2 days after delivery should be protected with passive immunization. VZIG should be given as soon as possible within 96 hours after exposure; it can be given up to 10 days. The dose is 125 U/10 kg body weight [maximum 625 international units (IU)]; the minimum is 62.5 IU in a neonate, administered intramuscularly (IM). The currently available VZIG is for IV use (Varitect) and administered at a dose of 0.2–1 mL/kg. If VZIG is not available, IVIG can be considered as an alternative in the dose of 400 mg/kg once.

CONCLUSION

Chickenpox in children differs from the disease in adults, with usually a milder clinical presentation and relatively less complications. Early diagnosis and prompt treatment are recommended to alleviate symptoms and prevent potential complications. Countries where varicella vaccine was introduced have witnessed a fall in the incidence of varicella infection in pediatric population.

MONKEYPOX

INTRODUCTION

Monkeypox (Mpox) is a zoonotic viral infectious disease caused by the monkeypox virus that has been endemic in Central and West Africa for many decades. A global outbreak occurred in May 2022, involving more than 70 nonendemic countries.[7]

ETIOLOGY

Mpox is caused by the monkeypox virus, a member of the *Orthopoxvirus* genus, which also includes the smallpox (variola) and vaccinia viruses. Two different Clades exist: Clade I and Clade II, and the 22 global outbreak is caused mostly by the Clade IIb virus.[7,8]

EPIDEMIOLOGY

The monkeypox virus was first isolated in Denmark in 1958 from a laboratory for monkeys in Singapore and was identified as a cause of disease in humans in the 1970s in the Democratic Republic of the Congo. Ever since, the disease has been endemic in nearly 11 countries of the Central and Western African regions, with thousands of cases being reported annually. In the period between January 1, 2022, and July 22, 2022, 16,016 laboratory-confirmed cases of monkeypox and five deaths have been reported to the World Health Organization (WHO) from 75 countries. The five countries that have reported the highest cumulative number of cases globally are Spain, the United States of America, Germany, the United Kingdom of Great Britain, and Northern Ireland. In India, as on July 24, 2022, four cases of Mpox were reported; the first case was reported on July 14, 2022. All four were men. The first three were from Kerala with a history of foreign travel, but the last case from Delhi had no history of foreign travel.[8-10]

CLINICAL FEATURES

The incubation period of monkeypox is usually 7–14 days, but it can be longer (5–21 days). The prodromal features include fever, myalgia, headache, backache, sore throat, and swollen lymph nodes. The lymphadenopathy appears with the onset of fever and may be unilateral/bilateral, cervical, axillary, or inguinal. This is followed by the appearance of rash generally within 1-3 days (sometimes longer) after the patient develops fever. Rashes evolve over sequential stages—macules, papules, vesicles, pustules, and umbilication—prior to crusting and desquamating over a period of 2–3 weeks. Eruption tends to be centrifugal, starting on the face and progressing toward the hands and feet, and can involve the oral mucous membranes, conjunctiva, cornea, and/or genitalia. Rashes are similar to smallpox in appearance, distribution, and pathological progression, but often less severe. In Mpox, all lesions in the person are similar in nature, unlike chickenpox, where multiple phases can be found at the same time and also the distribution is centripetal. The commonly involved sites in order of frequency are face (98%), palms and soles (95%), oral mucous membranes (70%), genitalia (28%), and conjunctiva (20%). Involvement of palms and soles is the hallmark of Mpox.[8-11]

Mpox is transmitted through close contact with an infected person or animal or with material contaminated with the virus. A person is considered infectious from the onset of clinical manifestations until all skin lesions have crusted.

Mpox is mostly self-limiting, and most patients recover spontaneously within 2–4 weeks. However, some children may develop complications, especially immunocompromised ones, and those who have certain skin conditions, such as eczema.[7]

COMPLICATIONS

Secondary bacterial infection is the most common complication and may include furuncle, carbuncle, cellulitis, abscess, necrotizing soft-tissue infection, suppurative lymphadenitis, and posterior pharyngeal abscess. Sepsis and septic shock can also occur. Other complications are bronchopneumonia, vomiting, and/or diarrhea, which can lead to severe dehydration, electrolyte disturbances, and encephalitis.[8,10]

Eye infection and corneal scarring, which can lead to permanent vision loss, can also occur. Complications observed in the current outbreak include proctitis/ulcerative pharyngitis or tonsillitis and genital, perianal, or facial lesions that evolve into large plaques, ulcers, or crusts and cellulitis requiring antibiotic treatment.

The transplacental transmission of monkeypox has resulted in miscarriages and fetal deaths. However, the association between the severity of maternal illness and these outcomes is unclear.[7]

DIFFERENTIAL DIAGNOSIS

Differential diagnosis includes varicella (chickenpox), varicella zoster (shingles), hand, foot, and mouth disease (HFMD), measles, scabies, molluscum contagiosum, herpes, allergic skin rashes, and drug eruptions. **Table 7.17.1** lists the differentiating features between Mpox and varicella.

TABLE 7.17.1: Differentiating features between Mpox and varicella.

Features	Monkeypox	Chickenpox
Rash	Single-stage lesions	Often in multiple stages
Evolution of rash	Slow	Rapid
Distribution of rash	• More dense on face • Palms and soles commonly affected	• More on trunk • Not common on palms and soles
Lymphadenopathy	Common	Rare
Secondary attack rate in household contacts	Less (10%)	High (90%)

DIAGNOSIS

The diagnosis of monkeypox should consider the epidemiological, clinical, and (if available) laboratory findings. Clinical cases may be classified as suspected, probable, or confirmed, guided by any history of exposure to monkeypox within the last 21 days.[12]

Laboratory Tests

Multiple nonspecific laboratory findings seen in patients with Mpox include abnormal aminotransferases, leukocytosis, thrombocytopenia, and hypoalbuminemia.

Viral Testing

Detection of viral DNA by reverse transcription-polymerase chain reaction (RT-PCR) from specimens obtained from skin rash, fluid or crusts (collected by vigorous swabbing), blood, oropharyngeal, anal, or rectal swabs is confirmatory.[8]

Serological Testing

Serological testing includes estimation of levels of antiorthopox IgM antibody 4–56 days after rash onset or a four-fold rise in IgG antibody titer between acute and convalescent (day 21 onward) samples.[7]

MANAGEMENT

Treatment of Mpox is symptomatic therapy with antipyretics/analgesics, early identification of secondary infections, and prompt treatment with appropriate antimicrobial agents.[12]

Antiviral Drugs

Tecovirimat is currently the first-line treatment for Mpox virus infection in people with severe disease or who are at risk for severe disease, including children and adolescents. The other antivirals include Brincidofovir and Cidofovir, which were approved for the treatment of smallpox in humans based on in vitro and animal studies. Antivirals can be considered in severe disease, immunocompromised individuals, children, pregnant and breastfeeding women, those with complicated lesions, and when lesions appear in proximity to the mouth, eyes, and genitals.[7]

PREVENTION AND VACCINES

The smallpox vaccine may provide some protection against Mpox. ACAM2000, (a live-attenuated) second-generation smallpox vaccine, is considered as the best choice for postexposure prevention of monkeypox and smallpox. A third-generation smallpox vaccine, MVA-BN (modified vaccinia Ankara-Bavarian Nordic strain), was approved against monkeypox in 2019.[11,12]

To prevent the spread of Mpox to others, persons with Mpox should be kept in isolation for the duration of the infectious period.

CONCLUSION

Mpox is a viral infection transmitted primarily through close skin contact that typically causes a self-resolving illness but may result in severe illness and death in immunocompromised individuals. First-line therapy is supportive care, although patients with severe Mpox infection may be treated with advanced therapeutic agents. It is an evolving global health threat, and clinicians must be aware of the characteristic signs and symptoms of Mpox to ensure timely diagnosis and appropriate management.

REFERENCES

1. American Academy of Pediatrics. Varicella-zoster virus infections. In: Kimberlin DW, Lynfield R, Sawyer MH (Eds). Red Book: 2021 Report of the Committee on Infectious Diseases, 32nd edition. Illinois: American Academy of Pediatrics; 2021. pp. 831-43.
2. LaRussa PS, Marin M. Varicella zoster virus. In: Kliegman RM, Jenson HB, Behrman RE, Stanton BF (Eds). Nelson Textbook of Pediatrics, 21st edition. Philadelphia: Elsevier; 2020. pp. 1708-15.
3. Albrecht MA, Hirsch MS, Kaplan SL. (2023). Clinical features of varicella-zoster virus infection: chickenpox. UpToDate. https://www.uptodate.com/contents/clinical-features-of-varicella-zoster-virus-infection-chickenpox, (Last accessed November 2024)
4. Whitely R. Chickenpox and herpes zoster. In: Bennett JE, Dolin R, Blaser MJ (Eds). Mandell, Douglas and Bennett's Principle and Practice of Infectious Diseases, 8th edition. Philadelphia: Elsevier, Saunders; 2014. pp. 1731-3.
5. Blair RJ. Varicella zoster virus. Pediatr Rev. 2019;40(7):375-7.
6. Kasi SG, Shivananda S, Marathe S, Chatterjee K, Agarwala S, Dhir SK, et al. Indian Academy of Pediatrics (IAP) Advisory Committee on Vaccines and Immunization Practices (ACVIP): recommended immunization schedule (2020-21) and update on immunization for children aged 0 through 18 years: Indian Pediatr. 2021;58(1):44-53.
7. Isaacs SN, Shenoy ES, Goldfarb IT. (2024). Treatment and prevention of mpox (monkeypox) UpToDate. [online] Available from https://www.uptodate.com/contents/treatment-and-prevention-of-mpox-formerly-monkeypox [Last accessed November, 2024].
8. World Health Organization. Mpox (monkeypox), key facts, 18 April 2023. [online] Available from https://www.who.int/news-room/fact-sheets/detail/monkeypox. [Last accessed November, 2024].
9. Lahariya C, Thakur A, Dudeja N. Monkeypox disease outbreak (2022): epidemiology, challenges, and the way forward. Indian Pediatr. 2022;59(8):636-41.
10. Singhal T, Kabra SK, Lodha R. Monkeypox: a review. Indian J Pediatr. 2022;89(10):955-60.
11. World Health Organization. (2022). Clinical management and infection prevention and control for monkeypox: interim rapid response guidance, 10 June 2022. [online] Available from https://www.who.int/publications/i/item/WHO-MPX-Clinical-and-IPC-2022.1 [Last accessed November, 2024].
12. Jiang R-J, Zheng Y-J, Zhou L, Feng L-Z, Ma L, Xu B-P, et al. Diagnosis, treatment, and prevention of monkeypox in children: an experts' consensus statement. World J Pediatr. 2023;19(3):231-42.

7.18 Influenza

Nitin K Shah, Gargi Ajinkya Bangar

EPIDEMIOLOGY

In recent centuries, the influenza virus has given rise to recurrent outbreaks of acute febrile syndrome every 1–4 years. In 1173–1174, the first epidemic report of an influenza-like illness (ILI) was seen, and in 1674, the first definitive influenza epidemic was reported. During 1918–1919, the greatest H1N1 pandemic in recorded history occurred with approximately 21 million deaths.[1] Thereafter, three pandemics occurred in the 20th century: The 1957 H2N2 pandemic, the 1968 H3N2 pandemic, and the 2009 influenza A (H1N1) virus pandemic (pH1N1). As of 2023, an estimated 1 billion cases of seasonal influenza occur annually worldwide. Of these, 3–5 million are severe cases. Influenza is responsible for 2,90,000–6,50,000 respiratory deaths each year. Here, 99% of deaths occur in children <5 years of age residing in developing nations. National Influenza Centers (NICs) and other national influenza laboratories from 118 countries, areas, or territories report their data to FluNet for pandemic preparedness. Real-time statistics are available at the Global Influenza Surveillance and Response System (GISRS).

INFLUENZA STRAINS

There are four types of influenza viruses: A, B, C, and D. Influenza A and B viruses cause seasonal epidemics of disease in humans. They are from *Orthomyxoviridae* family, with negative-strand ribonucleic acid (RNA) viruses.

Influenza A viruses are divided into subtypes based on two proteins on the surface of the virus: Hemagglutinin (HA) and neuraminidase (NA). There are 18 different HA subtypes and 11 different NA subtypes. They are further broken down into different genetic "clades" and "subclades."

Influenza B viruses are not divided into subtypes but instead are further classified into two lineages: B/Yamagata and B/Victoria. Similar to influenza A viruses, influenza B viruses can be further classified into specific clades and subclades.

Influenza (flu) viruses are constantly mutating in two different ways—antigenic drift and antigenic shift.[2]

Antigenic Drift

Drift consists of small mutations in the influenza virus genes that happen continually with time as the flu virus replicates. This leads to changes in the HA or NA surface proteins. The HA and NA surface protein antigens are recognized by the human immune system, which then triggers an immune response consisting of antibodies to fight the infection. The mutated virus may still have similar antigenic properties to the previous virus, so the immune system recognizes and responds to it. This is known as cross-protection. However, small changes in HA and NA continue to accumulate, and as a result, the virus becomes antigenically different in that antibodies bind differently or do not bind at all. This results in reduced or loss of recognition and neutralization. Antigenic drift is the primary reason to administer flu vaccine annually to keep up with the evolving flu viruses.

Antigenic Shift

Antigenic shift is a sudden major change in influenza A virus which results in new HA or NA proteins giving rise to a new flu subtype. It may occur in animal populations and present as a novel virus in humans. An example is the 2009 H1N1 virus. This has the potential to cause a pandemic because most people are immunologically naïve and may have some or no immunity against the new strain of the virus.

MODE OF INFECTION

The flu virus is transmitted via the nasopharyngeal route. It spreads mainly via coughing, sneezing, hands, social contact, and medical interventions, such as suctioning, nebulization, and open ventilation, which generate respiratory mist. It can spread by infected fomites such as shared napkins and handkerchiefs. A person is infective from 1 day before to 7 days after the symptoms develop. If the illness persists beyond 7 days, the person remains infective till the resolution of symptoms.

CLINICAL MANIFESTATIONS

Influenza affects children of all ages. During an outbreak, the attack rate is 9.3% in children <17 years, 8.8% in 18–64 years, and 3.9% in those >65 years. It is twice as likely to develop in children as adults over 65 years. Around 99% of deaths are noted in children under 5 years of age.[3]

There is a wide spectrum of presentation, ranging from asymptomatic in over 50% of people to mild upper respiratory symptoms, mild-to-severe acute lower respiratory infection (ALRI) to extrapulmonary multiorgan involvement and death. Most commonly, symptoms are of ILI which include cold, cough, fever, malaise, sore throat, and headache. Symptoms last for 7–10 days and recover spontaneously. Other symptoms include cough with sputum, dyspnea, headache, myalgia, fatigue, diarrhea, nausea, and vomiting. Fatigue may take weeks to resolve. A more serious presentation includes initial bronchioalveolar pathology and cytokine storm which leads to primary viral pneumonia, acute respiratory distress syndrome (ARDS), and pulmonary edema. Secondary bacterial pneumonia may occur during resolution. In around 32% of patients with viral pneumonia, bacterial coinfection occurs, most commonly with *Streptococcus pneumoniae*.[4-6]

Acute otitis media is seen in 3–5% of children. Myositis with influenza is noted as severe myalgia in lower limbs wherein there is reluctance to walk for 2–3 days. Gastrocnemius and soleus muscles are most commonly affected. Investigations show high creatinine phosphokinase and myoglobinuria.

Sometimes, seizures can occur and imaging reveals bilateral thalamic necrosis and brainstem involvement. Gastrointestinal symptoms such as diarrhea and vomiting are common in children (7.7%). This is followed by myositis, otitis media, hepatitis, and then worsening of underlying conditions.

Moderate complications include ear and sinus infections. Serious complications include pneumonia along with bacterial coinfection.[4-6] Flu may trigger inflammation of the heart (myocarditis), brain (encephalitis), muscle tissues (myositis and rhabdomyolysis), and multiorgan failure (respiratory and kidney failure). An extreme inflammatory response in the body can occur leading to a sepsis-like picture. Hematologically, a child may have mild-to-severe leukopenia and thrombocytopenia and may land into hemophagocytic lymphohistiocytosis (HLH).

IMPLICATIONS IN PEDIATRIC POPULATION

A higher attack rate is noted in children. Unvaccinated children have considerably higher exposure risk compared to adults. During the influenza epidemic, the attack rate was 40% in preschool and 30% in school children, implying high infectivity. The incidence of influenza episodes and associated ALRI is significantly higher in developing countries when compared with developed countries. Children are a major source of transmission.[5,6]

The Japanese experience demonstrated the impact of childhood vaccination or the absence of it on overall mortality in the entire community. With increasing coverage of the influenza vaccine in school children, the excess mortality fell in the community and the trend reversed with decreasing coverage in children proving that children were the main source of spread of the influenza virus in the community.[7]

There is an increase in respiratory and other complications due to flu in children. Otitis media and pneumonia with coinfections are higher in the influenza season.[4] Outpatient visits and antibiotic prescriptions go up by 30% during flu season. A high incidence of type A in the 0–4-year age group may lead to a high incidence of type A-associated encephalopathy. Children have a higher mortality rate. In 2011, a meta-analysis estimated that 28,000–111,500 children <5 years of age die each year due to influenza-associated acute lower respiratory tract infections (LRTI) with 99% in developing nations.[8] There is a >15-fold difference in meta-estimates of influenza-associated case-fatality ratio between developing and developed regions. An increase in healthcare utilization and antibiotic use is noted due to influenza. Increased hospital admissions burden the pediatric wards. There is also an increase in children's absenteeism from daycare centers and schools. For every 100 children with influenza, 274 days of absence in <3 years, 262 in 3–6 years, and 216 days in 7-year-old children were noted.

DIAGNOSIS

Definitive diagnosis of influenza infection is made by a reverse transcriptase-polymerase chain reaction (RT-PCR) test, viral culture, or a fourfold rise in influenza-specific neutralizing antibodies. PCR is the gold standard. Various respiratory specimens can be collected including nasopharyngeal swab, nasal swab, throat swab, wash or aspirate, or tracheal aspirate (in case of an intubated child) ideally within 48 hours of the onset of illness. Bronchoalveolar lavage or tracheal aspirate should be 3–5 mL and collected in sterile screw-capped containers. The swab should be placed in a transport medium-containing tube and stored and transported at 4°C within 24 hours of collection or it should be stored at –70°C. The sensitivity and specificity in a symptomatic patient are nearly 100%. Results normally take 24–48 hours.

Serological testing is not recommended as it can only tell whether the strain is type A or type B and cannot differentiate between pH1N1 and other type A seasonal influenza strains. The Government of India guidelines recommend to reserve PCR-based tests only for severe hospitalized patients and not for outdoor patients who should be started on oseltamivir on clinical grounds. A PCR-based test is also useful to monitor drug sensitivity to oseltamivir.

MANAGEMENT

National Guidelines[9]

Patients are categorized based on clinical examination as category A, B, and C.

- *Category A* are mild, uncomplicated cases and those with mild fever and cough/sore throat with or without body aches, headache, diarrhea, and vomiting. Testing is not required and home treatment should be symptomatic including paracetamol and adequate fluid intake. They are asked to follow-up if other symptoms of ILI develop. Isolation is advised.
- *Category B* is uncomplicated but with additional severe symptoms such as high-grade fever (≥102°F) and severe sore throat or any high-risk child with high-risk conditions. Testing for influenza is not advised. However, they should receive oseltamivir (as discussed in **Box 7.18.1**) with symptomatic treatment.
- *Category C* are those with signs and symptoms of severe disease. Symptoms include breathlessness,

BOX 7.18.1: Recommended antiviral treatment regimens.[10]

Oseltamivir: For adolescents, 13–17 years of age, and for adults, the recommended oral dose is 75 mg oseltamivir twice daily for 5 days. For children, the recommended doses are as follows:	
By weight	
15 kg or less	30 mg orally twice a day for 5 days
15–23 kg	45 mg orally twice a day for 5 days
24–40 kg	60 mg orally twice a day for 5 days
>40 kg	75 mg orally twice a day for 5 days
For infants	
<3 months	12 mg orally twice a day for 5 days
3–5 months	20 mg orally twice a day for 5 days
6–11 months	25 mg orally twice a day for 5 days
For preterm infants—1–3 mg/kg/dose twice daily	
(Available as 75 mg per tablet and syrup containing 12 mg/mL)	
(Duration of treatment can be extended up to 10 days in a severe case)	
Zanamivir: Zanamivir is indicated for the treatment of influenza in adults and children (>5 years). The recommended dose for the treatment of adults and children from the age of 5 years is two inhalations (2–5 mg) twice daily for 5 days	

hemoptysis, altered mental status, poor feeding, seizures, decreased urine output, persistence, or worsening of initial symptoms beyond 72 hours or worsening of any underlying medical conditions. Signs to check are tachypnea, $SpO_2 < 90\%$, hypotension, reduced urine output, and cyanosis. Immediate hospitalization is necessary. Testing for influenza is advised. Oseltamivir should be started empirically without waiting for results.

Antiviral Therapy[10]

Three drug types are registered that specifically target the influenza virus. These are M2 proton channel antagonists (amantadine), NA inhibitors (NAI; Zanamivir, oseltamivir, peramivir, and laninamivir), and polymerase acidic endonuclease inhibitors (baloxavir marboxil). At present, oseltamivir is recommended as the first line of treatment for children. It should be started within 48 hours of the onset of illness for maximum effect. However, it should be started, even if it is delayed at any stage of active disease when ongoing viral replication is anticipated or documented. It is especially recommended in individuals at high risk of complications, such as children <5 years of age, patients with progressive respiratory disease including pneumonia, and those with high-risk medical conditions.[4] It is best administered along with food to reduce gastrointestinal side effects.

Zanamivir is approved for children >5 years to be given by inhalation, not for those with underlying airway disease. Older antivirals, amantadine, and rimantadine have not been recommended since 2006 due to increased global resistance which may cause treatment failures.

Supportive Measures

Adequate hydration, proper nutrition, use of moist oxygen, early detection of respiratory failure, timely management with moist oxygen, and ventilatory support are some of the important general supportive measures. Antibiotics are not used routinely and are reserved for cases with suspected secondary bacterial infection. *Pneumococcus* and *Staphylococcus* are important organisms involved in secondary infection in pandemic influenza in children. Routine use of corticosteroids is best avoided. Infection-control measures are of utmost importance in preventing the spread of disease to close contacts.

PREVENTION

General Infection Control Measures

At Home

Hand hygiene and cough etiquette are important measures for a patient who is managed at home. A surgical mask is not as effective and tends to clog within 2–4 hours, making it ineffective and uncomfortable. Only N95 masks are highly effective in preventing the spread of the virus but are expensive, not easily available, and are best used in hospital setups. Hand sanitizers are useful in preventing the spread of the virus to contacts. Isolation in the home for 5–10 days also helps in preventing the spread of contacts at workplaces.

At the Community Level

Availability of hand sanitizers at public places will help the spread of the virus for people touching things of common interest. Avoidance of mass gathering will also prevent the spread of the virus. Closure of schools, though practiced during peak transmission, is not found to be effective and is impractical. General awareness about how the virus spreads and messages regarding hand hygiene and cough etiquette help regulate personal behavior and the spread of the virus.

At the Healthcare Facility

Healthcare personnel are at a great risk of spread of virus from a suspected case of influenza, especially if there is an uncontrolled mist of respiratory tract secretions such as with open nebulization, suctioning, or open ventilation systems. Use of protective gears, such as an N95 mask (ideal) or surgical disposable mask, head cap and gowns, and strict hand hygiene before and after touching the patient are strongly recommended for those handling patients of influenza which include healthcare workers and caretakers. Such patients also have to be isolated in a reserved area with separate entrance and exit where no or minimum human visitors are allowed.

Influenza Vaccines

The most effective strategy for the prevention of influenza and its complications is annual vaccination against seasonal strains. The first vaccine against the novel pH1N1 strain was a monovalent vaccine and was approved for manufacturing by the US Food and Drug Administration on September 15, 2009, and was available for mass use in the United States on October 5, 2009. Now, novel pH1N1 vaccines are available as a live-attenuated quadrivalent vaccine for intranasal administration and as quadrivalent inactivated split-virus or subunit vaccines (QIV) for injection which again may be with or without adjuvant. There are several manufacturers of these vaccines. Most of the manufacturers use chicken eggs for producing these vaccines. A high-dose influenza vaccine is available abroad for use in >70 years of age.

Vaccine Compositions

As discussed before, the antigenic drifts and shifts enable the virus to evade existing immunity. The strains are selected based on the GISRS data from circulating influenza strains and new strains found globally. Accordingly, the influenza vaccine is a quadrivalent vaccine containing circulating seasonal pH1N1, H3N2, and both the type B strains. Manufacturing flu vaccines is literally a race against time. Every year, the circulating virus drifts and hence the vaccine strains change accordingly. About 4–6 months are required to manufacture and approve a new vaccine. For each season, recommendations are made in February for the next northern hemisphere vaccine and in September for the next southern hemisphere vaccine.

India is geographically diverse; hence, the surveillance data gives suggestions based on local transmission dynamics. Areas above 30° latitude (Srinagar) and those with late monsoon season (Chennai and Vellore) should have winter vaccination strategies using the Northern Hemisphere vaccine, while in other parts of the country, vaccination should take place in May–June using the Southern Hemisphere vaccine.[5,11]

The World Health Organization (WHO) recommendations of quadrivalent vaccines for the Northern Hemisphere 2023–2024 contain:[11]

- Egg-based vaccines—A/Victoria/4897/2022 (H1N1) pdm09-like virus, A/Darwin/9/2021 (H3N2)-like virus, B/Austria/1359417/2021 (B/Victoria lineage)-like virus, and B/Phuket/3073/2013 (B/Yamagata lineage)-like virus
- Cell culture or recombinant-based vaccines—A/Wisconsin/67/2022 (H1N1) pdm09-like virus, an A/Darwin/6/2021 (H3N2)-like virus, B/Austria/1359417/2021 (B/Victoria lineage)-like virus, and B/Phuket/3073/2013 (B/Yamagata lineage)-like virus

The WHO recommendations of quadrivalent vaccines for the Southern Hemisphere 2024 contain:

- Egg-based vaccines—A/Victoria/4897/2022 (H1N1) pdm09-like virus, A/Thailand/8/2022-like virus, A/Thailand/8/2022 (H3N2)-like virus, B/Austria/1359417/2021 (B/Victoria lineage)-like virus, and B/Phuket/3073/2013 (B/Yamagata lineage)-like virus
- Cell culture or recombinant-based vaccines—A/Wisconsin/67/2022 (H1N1) pdm09-like virus, A/Massachusetts/18/2022 (H3N2)-like virus, B/Austria/1359417/2021 (B/Victoria lineage)-like virus, and B/Phuket/3073/2013 (B/Yamagata lineage)-like virus

Schedule

The influenza vaccine is to be given annually as the vaccine changes every year as discussed before. Two doses are recommended at a 4-week interval in the first year for children <9 years of age. Subsequently, one dose is given annually. For children >9 years old, one dose is given in the first year and then one dose annually.[9]

Inactivated Influenza Vaccine

The inactivated influenza vaccine can be used only for children >6 months of age; for both healthy subjects and populations at risk of medical complications of influenza infection. The dose is 0.5 mL intramuscularly (IM) for all ages.

Live-attenuated Influenza Vaccine

Cold-adapted live nasal flu vaccines are recommended only for healthy nonpregnant 2–49-year-old. These are contraindicated in immune-compromised hosts as well as in those with chronic medical conditions. Children aged 2–9 years require two doses given 1 month apart in the first year. Children >9 years of age require one dose. Live-attenuated influenza vaccine (LAIV) can be used even if one has received another live injectable vaccine within the last 4 weeks. The dose is split equally between two nostrils and administered using a nasal sprayer. The Indian live nasal vaccine has been approved for a single dose even in the first year for 2–9-year-old children.

Adverse Effects

Inactivated influenza vaccines commonly cause local reactions in 30% of vaccine recipients such as soreness, swelling, and redness at the injection site, and less often fever, muscle- or joint pains, or headache. These symptoms are generally mild, do not need medical attention, and last for 1–2 days. Fever, aches, and headaches can occur more frequently in children compared to elderly people. Rarely, influenza vaccines can cause allergic reactions, such as hives, rapid swelling of deeper skin layers and tissues, asthma, or a severe multisystem allergic reaction due to hypersensitivity to certain vaccine components. Live vaccines are given via a nasal spray and can commonly cause runny nose, nasal congestion, and cough and can less frequently cause sore throat, low-grade fever, irritability and headache, and muscle aches. Wheezing and vomiting episodes have been described in children receiving live influenza vaccines. Hence, LAIV should be used with caution in 2–5-year-old children with wheezing on inhaled corticosteroids.

Immunogenicity

With the experience of using seasonal flu vaccines in the past, it has been shown that HA titers of >1:40 are considered seroprotective and known to provide at least 50% protection against seasonal H1N1 disease. Monovalent novel H1N1 vaccines have shown that >90% of children achieve seroprotection rates with one or two doses. Two doses are better in children <9 years of age for the first year. In general, the geometric mean titer achieved after one or two doses is >1,000 U/mL. Adjuvant vaccines are better immunogenic and hence need fewer antigen doses than nonadjuvant vaccines. The WHO recommends that children >6 months and <9 years of age need two doses.[11,12]

Efficacy/Effectiveness

Studies suggest that flu vaccination has prevented millions from falling sick and visiting doctors each year. Vaccination prevents the risk of severe life-threatening disease in children by 75% and reduces flu-related hospital admissions by 41% and outpatient department (OPD) visits by 50%, antibiotic prescription by 32%, parental work absenteeism by 77%, and school absenteeism in children aged 6 months to 17 years by 47%. Studies from 2014 indicated that flu vaccine reduced flu-related pediatric intensive care unit (PICU) admissions by 74% during flu seasons from 2010 to 2012. Vaccination reduces cardiac events in those with existing heart disease, worsening of chronic obstructive pulmonary disease (COPD), and worsening of other chronic illnesses due to flu. Vaccination reduces children's risk of dying from flu significantly.

Moreover, when administered to pregnant women, it reduces the risk of being hospitalized for flu by 40%. It also protects newborn babies till they are too young to receive the vaccine.

Contraindications

Flu vaccine is not indicated in children <6 months old. It is contraindicated in patients with a past history of anaphylactic reaction to egg or previous flu vaccine. Guillain–Barré syndrome within 6 weeks of the previous dose of the flu vaccine is a precaution for subsequent use of influenza vaccines. Like with any other vaccine, any severe acute illness is a temporary contraindication to use the flu vaccine till the person recovers from the illness. LAIV is contraindicated in children <2 years and adults >50 years old. It is also contraindicated, if the children have moderate-to-severe febrile illness, receive salicylates, have anaphylactic reaction to egg protein, have reactive airway disease, and in patients at risk of medical complications following influenza infections, pregnant women, and contacts of immune-compromised conditions requiring protected environment such as stem-cell transplant recipients.

CONCLUSION

Influenza remains a significant public health challenge due to its high infectivity, potential for severe complications, and capacity to cause widespread outbreaks. Its ability to undergo antigenic drift and shift necessitates continuous monitoring and annual updates to vaccines. Children, especially those under five years of age, are particularly vulnerable, with a higher risk of complications such as pneumonia, otitis media, and exacerbation of underlying conditions.

Effective prevention strategies, including annual vaccination and public health measures such as hand hygiene and respiratory etiquette, are critical in limiting the spread of the virus. Antiviral therapies like oseltamivir, combined with timely diagnosis and supportive care, remain essential tools in reducing disease severity and preventing complications.

Global efforts to improve vaccine access, enhance surveillance, and educate communities about preventive measures are crucial for minimizing the impact of influenza. Continued research and investment in healthcare infrastructure are vital to addressing the disparities in disease burden and ensuring better outcomes for all populations.

REFERENCES

1. Moghadami M. A narrative review of influenza: a seasonal and pandemic disease. Iranian J Med Sci. 2017;42(1):2-13.
2. Centers for Disease Control and Prevention. (2023). How flu viruses can change: "drift" and "shift". CDC. [online] Available from https://www.cdc.gov/flu/php/viruses/change.html. [Last accessed November, 2024].
3. Jayasundara K, Soobiah C, Thommes E, Tricco AC, Chit A. Natural attack rate of influenza in unvaccinated children and adults: a meta-regression analysis. BMC Infect Dis. 2014;14:670.
4. Van der Sluijs KF, van der Poll T, Lutter R, Juffermans NP, Schultz MJ. Bench-to-bedside review: bacterial pneumonia with influenza-pathogenesis and clinical implications. Crit Care. 2010;14(2):1-8.
5. Dharmapalan D. Influenza. Indian J Pediatr. 2020;87(10):828-32.
6. Ghosh U, Bharathy RVN, Prasad DJH, Moorthy M, Verghese VP. An eight-year profile of children with influenza A (H1N1) in a large hospital in India. J Trop Pediatr. 2021;67(4):fmab084.
7. Gu Y, Shimada T, Yasui Y, Tade Y, Kaku M, Okabe N. National surveillance of influenza-associated encephalopathy in Japan over six years, before and during the 2009–2010 influenza pandemic. PLoS One. 2013;8(1):e54786.
8. Nair H, Brooks WA. Katz M, Roca A, Berkley JA, Madhi SA, et al. Global burden of respiratory infections due to seasonal influenza in young children: a systematic review and meta-analysis. Lancet. 2011;378(9807):1917-30.
9. Ministry of Health & Family Welfare-Government of India. Technical guidelines for H1N1. National Centre for Disease Control (NCDC). [online] Available from https://ncdc.mohfw.gov.in/technical-guidelines-for-h1n1/. [Last accessed November, 2024].
10. Świerczyńska M, Mirowska-Guzel DM. Antiviral drugs in influenza. Int J Environ Res Public Health. 2022;19(5):3018.
11. World Health Organization. (2023). Influenza seasonal. [online] Available from https://www.who.int/news-room/fact-sheets/detail/influenza-(seasonal). [Last accessed November, 2024].
12. Chadha MS, Potdar VA, Saha S, Koul PA, Broor S, Dar L, et al. Dynamics of influenza seasonality at sub-regional levels in India and implications for vaccination timing. PLoS One. 2015;10(5):e0124122.

7.19 Chikungunya Fever

Rajniti Prasad

INTRODUCTION

Chikungunya fever is caused by an alphavirus and is transmitted by the bite of the *Aedes aegypti* mosquito. The name derives from the Tanzanian Kimakonde dialect "*kungunyala*," which means "to dry up" or "become contorted," that is, the "bent" posture of patients. It has caused numerous outbreaks and epidemics in both Africa and Southeast Asia, involving thousands of children.

CHIKUNGUNYA VIRUS

Chikungunya virus (CHIKV), a positive-stranded, enveloped ribonucleic acid (RNA) virus, is a member of the *Alphavirus* genus and belongs to the *Togaviridae* family. Genetic analysis based on partial *E1* envelope glycoprotein gene sequences showed the presence of three distinct phylogroups. The first contained all isolates from West Africa; the second comprised all Central, Southern, and Eastern African strains; and the third contained isolates from Asia.[1]

EPIDEMIOLOGY

Chikungunya virus is commonly transmitted to humans through the bite of infected mosquitoes of the *Aedes* genus, which usually bite during daylight hours. In Africa, CHIKV appears to be maintained in a sylvatic cycle involving wild primates such as monkeys that may serve as reservoirs of the virus. The secondary attack rate is 4–45%. *Aedes aegypti*, *Aedes albopictus*, and *Aedes polynesiensis* are commonly involved in the transmission of virus, although *Culex* has also been reported for some transmission. Vertical transmission has also been reported.[2]

Aedes aegypti, the principal vector of CHIKV in India, is anthropophilic and endophagic and bites during the daytime. It mainly breeds in man-made discarded containers where rainwater accumulates. The recent epidemic in India suggested that the Asian tiger mosquito was responsible for the spread. The mutation in the envelope protein gene (*E1-A226V*) was reported in some strains of CHIKV. This mutation is responsible for CHIKV adaptation to the Asian tiger mosquito. With global climate warming, CHIKV could expand to new geographic locations.

PATHOGENESIS

Chikungunya virus replicates primarily in fibroblasts and macrophages but can replicate in various human cells, including fibroblasts and epithelial and endothelial cells. Viral entry occurs through a power of hydrogen (pH)-dependent, endocytic pathway. It is highly cytopathic and induces apoptosis of infected cells. In CHIKV-infected fibroblasts, there are marked losses of major histocompatibility complex (MHC) class-I surface expression and antigen presentation, which result in evasion of $CD8^+$ T-cell response and persistence of infection. In humans, CHIKV produces symptoms after 48 hours of a mosquito bite.

Patients have a high viral load in their blood during the first 2 days of illness. Viremia declines around day 3 or day 4 and usually disappears by day 5. Hemagglutination inhibition and neutralizing antibodies can usually be detected after day 5. Clinical or silent infection is thought to confer lifelong immunity. A recent study has suggested CHIKV tropism for muscular satellite cells, which can act as small reservoirs for virus or virus-encoded components or both for longer periods.[3]

Pro- and anti-inflammatory cytokines, especially interleukin-6 and -8, may act in synergy to cause bleeding in patients with plasma leakage. It is postulated that these cytokines may act on the endothelium to increase vascular permeability leading to plasma leakage compromising hemodynamics and coagulopathy.[4]

CLINICAL MANIFESTATIONS

Chikungunya fever is characterized by the triad of abrupt-onset fever, rashes, and arthralgia followed by other constitutional symptoms. The incubation period is usually 2–3 days (range 1–12 days). All age groups are affected, including newborns, but full-blown disease is common in adults. *Fever* rises abruptly, often reaching 39°C accompanied by intermittent shaking chills. This acute phase lasts for 2–3 days. The temperature may remit for 1–2 days after a gap of 4–10 days, resulting in a "saddle back" fever curve.[5]

Arthralgia is polyarticular and migratory and predominantly affects the small joints of hands, wrists, ankles, and feet with lesser involvement of larger joints **(Fig. 7.19.1)**.

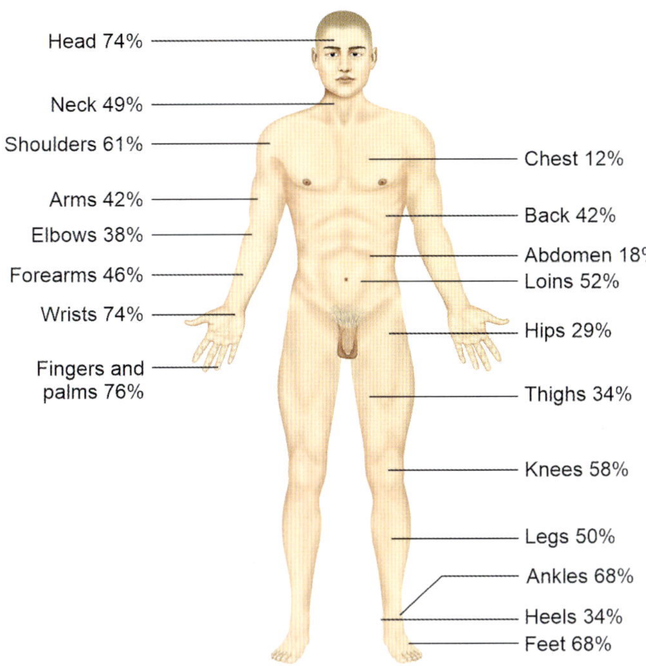

Fig. 7.19.1: Frequency of pain and arthritis by location during acute stage.

In the acute stage, patients complain bitterly of pain, when asked to move assuming an attitude of flexion. Pain on movement is worse in the morning, improved by mild exercise and exacerbated by strenuous exercise. Swelling may occur but fluid accumulation is uncommon. Patients with mild articular manifestation are usually symptom-free within a few weeks, but severe cases require months to resolve entirely.

Cutaneous manifestations include flushing of the face and trunk. This is usually followed by a maculopapular rash present usually over trunk and limbs; but face, palms, and soles also may show lesions. Rashes may simply fade or desquamate. Petechiae may occur alone or in association with rash and observed during the acute stage of illness and convalescence. Pigmentary changes have been reported to be the most common cutaneous finding (42%), followed by maculopapular eruption (33%) and intertriginous aphthous ulcers (21.37%). Exacerbation of existing psoriasis and unmasking of undiagnosed Hansen's disease may occur. The rash usually lasts for 1–7 days.[6]

Iridocyclitis and retinitis are the most common ocular manifestations associated with chikungunya fever, with a typically benign clinical course. Less frequent ocular lesions include episcleritis. Other rare manifestations include meningoencephalitis, fulminant hepatitis, and mild hemorrhagic manifestations.[7]

Most symptomatic patients (93.7%) complain of a chronic stage of the disease, which is characterized by pains in joints, bones, or both. This persisting pain may be continuous or discontinuous with alternation of clinical remission and relapses (58.7%). Some infected individuals may also have fever at this stage. The atypical manifestations reported in recent outbreaks include severe arthralgia and neurological complications, such as encephalitis, meningitis, and Guillain–Barré syndrome.[3]

LABORATORY DIAGNOSIS

Some patients show leukopenia with a mildly decreased platelet count. Elevated levels of aspartate aminotransferase [AST or serum glutamic-oxaloacetic transaminase (SGOT)] and C-reactive protein (CRP) are also seen. However, virus isolation is the most definitive test in the 1st week. Recently, the reverse transcription-polymerase chain reaction (RT-PCR) technique for diagnosis has been developed using nested primer pairs amplifying specific components of three structural gene regions. PCR results may be available within 1–2 days.[8]

A four-fold increase in antibody titer in acute and convalescent sera by ELISA is suggestive of chikungunya fever, but RT-PCR is done to confirm the diagnosis. Demonstrating immunoglobulin M (IgM) antibodies is also specific for CHIKV. A commonly used test is the IgM antibody capture enzyme-linked immunosorbent assay (MAC-ELISA). Results of MAC-ELISA may be available within 2–3 days. Cross-reaction with other flavivirus antibodies, such as O'nyongnyong and Semliki, may occur in MAC-ELISA; however, the latter viruses are relatively rare in Southeast Asia. A positive virus culture supplemented with neutralization is taken as the definitive proof of the presence of CHIKV.

MANAGEMENT

There is no specific treatment for chikungunya fever. The illness is usually self-limiting and resolves with time. Supportive care with rest is recommended during the acute joint symptoms. Movement and mild exercise tend to improve stiffness and morning arthralgia, but heavy exercise may exacerbate rheumatic symptoms.

Nonsteroidal anti-inflammatory drugs (NSAIDs) are recommended for joint pain. In debilitating arthritis refractory to NSAID, chloroquine (10 mg/kg/day) or methotrexate is recommended. Chloroquine inhibits viral replication by blocking pH-dependent endocytosis of CHIKV in host cells. Although chloroquine blocks CHIKV replication, the therapeutic index of chloroquine in cell cultures is narrow. Thus, one should be cautious when planning the use of chloroquine as an antiviral treatment in infected individuals. Methotrexate in a weekly dose of 15 mg/m^2 for 6–8 weeks may be given for disabling arthritis. Anti-CHIKV monoclonal antibodies inhibit viral fusion and release and may be given to children in the acute phase with a severe life-threatening illness.[9]

Self-resolution occurs with cutaneous lesions. Patients with hyperpigmentation may be treated with sunscreens and topical steroids. All patients with only centrofacial involvement usually show complete clearance during follow-up by 3 weeks. Patients with more diffuse involvement show a slower resolution. Aphthous ulcers usually heal over 7–10 days with local cleaning and topical antimicrobials to prevent secondary infection. Iridocyclitis and retinitis have a typically benign clinical course. All patients respond well to the treatment with preservation of good vision.

Infected persons should be protected from further mosquito exposure (staying indoors and/or under a mosquito net during the first few days of illness) so that they do not contribute to the transmission cycle.

VACCINE

The current live attenuated vaccine (Valneva) approved and recommended by the United States Food and Drug Administration (US FDA) and the Centers for Disease Control and Prevention (CDC) in the United States in endemic regions for children above the age of 6 months is safe and well tolerated and produces no severe adverse events. The efficacy of this vaccine is 99% with long-lasting immunity in human beings. The vaccine is recommended for travelers in endemic regions with active outbreaks, working or staying in an endemic region for >6 months, and laboratory workers handling this virus. Immunization of children with vaccine in an endemic area during outbreaks may prevent disease and debilitating arthritis.[3]

PREVENTION

Prevention is entirely dependent on taking steps to avoid mosquito bites, which includes wearing full-sleeve clothes and eliminating mosquito-breeding sites. The use of mosquito coils, repellents, electric vapor mats during the daytime and permethrin-treated mosquito nets during sleep prevents transmission of disease. Drainage of water from coolers, tanks, barrels, drums, buckets, and empty coolers, when not in use, prevents mosquito breeding.

Active surveillance by health workers of cases should be undertaken. This will help in identifying the affected areas so that control measures may be initiated. Vector surveillance should also be done and will help in initiating early control measures and assessing the impact of the measures taken. Education of people about the disease, mode of transmission, availability of treatment, and adoption of control measures are important for the prevention of the disease.

REFERENCES

1. Chhabra M, Mittal V, Bhattacharya D, Rana U, Lal S. Chikungunya fever: a re-emerging viral infection. Indian J Med Microbiol. 2008;26:5-12.
2. Nyamwaya DK, Thumbi SM, Bejon P, Warimwe GM, Mokaya J. The global burden of chikungunya fever among children: a systematic literature review and meta-analysis. PLOS Glob Public Health. 2022;2(12):e0000914.
3. de Lima Cavalcanti TYV, Pereira MR, de Paula SO, de Oliveira Franca RF. A review on chikungunya virus epidemiology, pathogenesis and current vaccine development. Viruses. 2022;14(5):969.
4. Imad HA, Phumratanaprapin W, Phonrat B, Chotivanich K, Charunwatthana P, Muangnoicharoen S, et al. Cytokine expression in dengue fever and dengue hemorrhagic fever patients with bleeding and severe hepatitis. Am J Trop Med Hyg. 2020;102(5):943-50.
5. Queyriaux B, Simon F, Grandadam M, Michel R, Tolou H, Boutin J-P. Clinical burden of chikungunya virus infection. Lancet Infect Dis. 2008;8(1):2-3.
6. Inamadar AC, Palit A, Sampagavi VV, Raghunath S, Deshmukh NS. Cutaneous manifestations of chikungunya fever: observations made during a recent outbreak in South India. Intern J Dermatol. 2008;47(2):154-9.
7. Mahendradas P, Ranganna SK, Shetty R, Balu R, Narayan KM, Babu RB, et al. Ocular manifestations associated with chikungunya. Ophthalmology. 2008;115(2):287-91.
8. Imad HA, Phadungsombat J, Nakayama EE, Suzuki K, Ibrahim AM, Afaa A, et al. Clinical features of acute chikungunya virus infection in children and adults during an outbreak in the Maldives. Am J Trop Med Hyg. 2021;105(4):946-54.
9. Tumkosit U, Siripanyaphinyo U, Takeda N, Tsuji M, Maeda Y, Ruchusatsawat K, et al. Anti-chikungunya virus monoclonal antibody that inhibits viral fusion and release. J Virol. 2020;94:e00252-20.

7.20 Severe Acute Respiratory Syndrome Coronavirus-2 Infection

Balasubramanian S, Divya Nandakumar

INTRODUCTION

The severe acute respiratory syndrome coronavirus-2 (SARS-CoV-2), belonging to the *Betacoronavirus* family, usually causes a disease characterized mainly by fever, cough, myalgia, and fatigue. It can also lead to severe respiratory distress and cytokine storm in some children. Acute infection with SARS-CoV-2 is usually mild in children; however, the postinfectious complications like multisystem inflammatory syndrome in children (MIS-C) can be quite complex in diagnosis and management. Although mortality and morbidity are less among children, certain children with comorbid conditions and risk factors can have severe infections, and hence, four vaccines were given emergency-use approval for the pediatric population in the early part of 2022 in India.

EPIDEMIOLOGY

A novel coronavirus was isolated in Wuhan, China, in December 2019 and was identified to be the cause of a cluster of cases of severe pneumonia and acute respiratory distress syndrome. The World Health Organization (WHO) named the virus severe acute respiratory syndrome coronavirus 2 (SARS-CoV-2), and the disease was called coronavirus disease-2019 or COVID-19 in February 2020. The virus rapidly spread globally, leading the WHO to declare a pandemic on March 11, 2020. India reported its first case of COVID-19 on January 30, 2020, in Kerala. SARS-CoV-2 infection has been reported worldwide, and there have been 771,549,718 confirmed cases of COVID-19 and 6,974,473 deaths reported to WHO so far.[1] In India, 45,001,052 confirmed cases and 5,33,291 deaths have been reported so far. Numerous reasons, like the variable expression of the angiotensin-converting enzyme-2 (ACE-2) receptor with age, lesser incidence of comorbidities, effective innate immune system, and excellent regeneration capacity of pediatric alveolar epithelium, were attributed to a lesser rate of hospitalization, intensive care unit (ICU) admission, and a lower mortality rate in children when compared to adults.

MODE OF TRANSMISSION

The most common method of transmission is mainly from person to person following close exposure (<6 feet) to respiratory droplets (>5–10 μm) when an infected person coughs, sneezes, or talks loudly. Children usually acquire infection from household contacts, but transmission from schools and healthcare settings can also occur. It can also spread by direct contact through an infected person's hands or by contact with contaminated surfaces and touching the eyes, nose, or mouth. Aerosol-generating procedures like endotracheal intubation, nebulization, bronchoscopy, etc., have also resulted in aerosol transmission of the virus, but this is not a very common mode of transmission. Neonates can get infected during delivery or in the postnatal period, but vertical transmission is reportedly rare. The possibility of fecal-oral transmission, blood-borne transmission, and nonmucous membrane contact transmission remains uncertain. Airborne transmission is not yet well established.

INCUBATION PERIOD

The median incubation period is 5 days, with a range of 2–14 days after the initial exposure. Transmission of SARS-CoV-2 starts prior to the development of symptoms and is highest early in the course of illness. Infected individuals are more likely to be contagious within the first 7–10 days of infection, and the chances of transmission decrease thereafter.

ETIOPATHOGENESIS

Virology

SARS-CoV-2 belongs to the beta subgroup of the *Coronaviridae* family. It is an enveloped virus containing a positive-sense, single-stranded ribonucleic acid (RNA). The virus is encircled with an envelope containing viral nucleocapsid (N) and together appears as a coiled tubular helix inside the bilayer lipid envelope, which anchors membrane (M), envelope (E), and spike (S) protein.[2] ACE2 is the receptor for cell entry in humans, and spike S protein binds to ACE2, resulting in membrane fusion and uptake of the virus into human cells.

New Variants

SARS-CoV-2 has constantly evolved over a period of time, and new mutations have been identified. Variants with rapid transmission, causing severe disease, decreased neutralizing antibodies generated during previous infection or vaccination, reduced effectiveness of treatments or vaccines, or diagnostic detection failures were considered as variants of concern.

The first variant—alpha variant (B.1.1.7 lineage)—was first isolated in late 2020 in the United Kingdom and had greater potential for infectivity without an increase in disease severity or impact on vaccine efficacy. Other variants identified include B.1.351 lineage (beta variant) and P.1 lineage (gamma variant).

The delta variant (B.1.617.2 lineage) was first identified in December 2020 in India and was found to be highly transmissible and was also associated with a higher risk of severe disease and hospitalization.

Omicron was first identified in Botswana and South Africa in late November 2021, and cases quickly began to occur and multiply in other countries. Even though they are associated with less severe infection, they have the ability to evade infection- and vaccine-induced humoral immunity to a greater extent than the other variants.

Life Cycle

- The spike S protein binds to the cellular receptor ACE2. The S protein is composed of two functional subunits, S1 and S2. The S1 subunit helps in binding the virus to the host cell receptor, and the S2 subunit plays a role in the fusion of viral and host cellular membranes.
- Once the receptor binding occurs, there occurs a conformational change in the S protein, which facilitates viral envelope fusion with the cell membrane through the endosomal pathway.[3]
- The viral genomic messenger RNA (mRNA) is released into the host cell cytoplasm; thereby, it is translated into viral replicase polyproteins pp1a and 1ab, which are cleaved by proteases to yield 16 nonstructural proteins that form the RNA replicase–transcriptase complex, which drives the production of negative-sense RNAs through both replication and transcription.
- The polymerase produces a series of subgenomic mRNAs which are finally translated into relevant viral proteins.
- Viral proteins and genome RNA are finally assembled into virions in the endoplasmic reticulum and Golgi apparatus.
- Virions are then released from the infected cell through exocytosis.

PATHOPHYSIOLOGY

It remains unclear why children and young adults are less severely affected than older individuals, but this might involve differences in immune system function in the elderly and/or differences in the expression/function of the cellular receptor for SARS-CoV-2—ACE2.[4]

Viral Entry and Early Infection

SARS-CoV-2 virus from respiratory droplets binds to the nasal epithelial cells in the upper respiratory tract, with ACE2 acting as the host receptor for viral entry. The virus undergoes local replication; however, the infected person remains asymptomatic initially. Later, fever and constitutional symptoms like headache, throat pain, myalgia, and dry cough develop.

Pulmonary Phase

Some progress to the second phase. In this phase, the virus reaches the lungs and predominantly involves the ACE2 receptor expressing alveolar type II pneumocytes, causing them to undergo apoptosis and thereby releasing a large number of viral particles to infect the surrounding cells. The patients manifest with pneumonia-like symptoms evidenced as lung opacities as seen in chest radiography or as glass opacities in computed tomography (CT). Depending on the severity of lung involvement, patients can improve or worsen further, requiring intubation and ventilation.

Hyperinflammatory Phase

A majority of children seem to recover after stage II or even directly after stage I. Due to the release of various cytokines and inflammatory markers, a cytokine storm ensues, which results in subsequent inflammation and lung injury.[5] Some go on to develop multiorgan dysfunction and often require intensive care treatment.

CLINICAL FEATURES

Most infections in children caused by the SARS-CoV-2 virus are asymptomatic or mildly symptomatic infections. Less severe infections in children can be attributed to the strong innate immunity in children, variable expression of the ACE2 receptor with age, and fewer comorbidities. The common symptoms associated with COVID-19 infection include fever, cough, rhinorrhea, myalgia, sore throat, headache, etc. Gastrointestinal symptoms like abdominal pain, diarrhea, and vomiting can also be the presenting complaints in children. Loss of smell or taste is very rare in children. Cutaneous manifestations like maculopapular, urticarial, and vesicular rashes; livedo reticularis; and reddish-purple nodules on the distal digits, called COVID toes, can also be seen with COVID-19 infection in children. Neurological and cardiovascular manifestations are relatively rare in children.

Majority of children with mildly symptomatic acute SARS-CoV-2 infection recover within 1–2 weeks of disease onset. Severe illness and acute respiratory distress syndrome are rare in children.

No specific clinical feature can pinpoint a definitive clinical diagnosis.

DIAGNOSIS

Guidelines on testing strategy for SARS-CoV-2 infection have been laid down by the WHO, the Infectious Diseases

Society of America (IDSA), and local government agencies. It is appropriate to follow local governmental guidelines for diagnosis. In resource-limited settings, it may be appropriate to test only those who are hospitalized and with high-risk factors when the burden of the disease is high.

Indications for Testing

Outpatient Settings

Children with clinical features suggestive of COVID-19 with comorbidities or who are at risk for severe disease need to be tested for COVID-19, and these include children with:

- Chronic systemic disease
- Neuromuscular disorder
- An immunocompromised child
- Uncontrolled type I diabetes mellitus
- Ex-preterm with prolonged preterm care
- Obesity with body mass index (BMI) ≥120% of the 95th percentile
- Exposure to a laboratory-confirmed case of COVID-19 within the previous 14 days

Inpatient Settings

Testing children at admission is beneficial when community transmission of COVID-19 is high and the children need to be cohorted to prevent nosocomial spread of infection. When children present with severe symptoms and a respiratory illness, SARS-CoV-2 can be tested as a part of a multiplex viral respiratory panel.

Laboratory Diagnosis

Blood investigations in COVID-19 may reveal:

- Lymphopenia
- Elevated C-reactive protein (CRP) >5 mg/L
- Elevated liver enzymes—serum glutamic oxaloacetic transaminase (SGOT) and serum glutamic pyruvic transaminase (SGPT)
- Severely ill children can have abnormal renal function tests

Molecular Diagnostics

- The reverse transcription polymerase chain reaction (RT-PCR) test from the nasopharyngeal swab is the diagnostic test of choice for detecting infection with the SARS-CoV-2 virus.
- The test detects the presence of viral RNA in samples. The yield of positive rates from the lower respiratory tract specimens may be higher than the upper respiratory tract specimens in view of the higher viral load.
- RT-PCR has a high specificity for SARS-CoV-2, and sensitivity varies depending on the timing of the test and the type of sample tested.
- The sensitivity varies with time as the amount of virus particles shed by an individual changes over the course of their infection. 4–5 days after infection, the RT-PCR sensitivity peaks at 92.7% and it drops to around 88% between 5 and 14 days after infection.[6]
- Children with COVID-19 can have detectable SARS-CoV-2 RNA in upper respiratory tract specimens for several weeks after the onset of symptoms. RT-PCR positivity does not necessarily mean that an individual is infectious, particularly more than 10–14 days after infection, because nonviable viral RNA may be present for some time.
- The cycle threshold (Ct) value in an RT-PCR test refers to the number of cycles needed to amplify viral RNA to reach a detectable level. The lower the value, the greater the amount of viral RNA present in the sample, and hence, the Ct value can reflect the relative viral RNA load in a specimen. Ct values are not standardized across laboratories, and their clinical application is uncertain.
- Antigen testing may be used as the initial test in resource-limited settings, but the sensitivity of antigen tests is lower than that of RT-PCR. A negative antigen test does not rule out COVID-19 and an RT-PCR test needs to be done in such circumstances for confirmation if warranted.

Serological Tests

Serology testing detects targeted antibodies that bind to SARS-CoV-2-specific antigens. In view of the greater efficacy of immunoglobulin G (IgG) antibody, serology testing to detect IgG or total antibody tests is preferred rather than immunoglobulin M (IgM) antibody, IgA antibody, or IgM/IgG differentiation tests.[7] They cannot be used to diagnose acute infection because it takes several days to weeks of infection for them to become reactive. The mere presence of IgG antibodies does not guarantee protection from future infection since data is limited regarding their protective immunity and the duration of protection offered by them.

The main application of serology testing is to identify individuals who have previously been infected with SARS-CoV-2 and thus help in epidemiology and seroprevalence studies. Serology tests may also be used to evaluate the immune response to vaccines in clinical trials; however, it is not advised routinely to check antibody titers post vaccination.

Radiological Investigations

Radiological imaging is infrequently required in children with mild COVID-19 infection. Only in severe cases are chest X-rays and CT chest indicated. Ground-glass opacities followed by patchy infiltrates and consolidation are the most frequently reported radiological findings.

MANAGEMENT

The management is focused on symptomatic care for SARS-CoV-2 infection, monitoring for clinical worsening and isolation of the patient to prevent transmission of infection.

Supportive Care

For determining the line of management, the severity of the COVID-19 illness can be classified as follows:

- *Mild or moderate disease:* No need for supplemental oxygen requirement
- *Severe disease:* Need for supplemental oxygen without the need for ventilatory support
- *Critical disease:* New or increased need for noninvasive or invasive mechanical ventilation, sepsis, and multiorgan dysfunction

Home Isolation

Children with mild disease and without risk factors for severe illness can be effectively managed at home by appropriate counseling. Home isolation is recommended for at least a duration of 10 days after the first appearance of symptoms and 24 hours without fever and until other symptoms of COVID-19 have improved. Caregivers of children who are managed at home should be counseled regarding the warning signs and to seek urgent medical care when the following warning signs are present:

- Severe respiratory distress or difficulty in breathing
- Grunting
- Cyanosis
- Lethargy
- Poor feeding or oral intake
- Decreased urine output
- Cold clammy mottled skin

Medications

For relief of fever with discomfort or pain, paracetamol can be given at a dose of 10–15 mg/kg every 4 or 6 hours once. Nonsteroidal anti-inflammatory drugs (NSAIDs) may be avoided.

Treatment of Hospitalized Children with Severe Illness

- Respiratory support consisting of supplemental oxygen or ventilatory support (noninvasive or invasive)
- Although bacterial coinfections are rare with COVID-19, antibiotics as indicated for community-acquired pneumonia can be started empirically in a sick child. De-escalation can be done once the child is stable based on cultures and other microbiological tests
- Fluid and electrolyte management
- Continued monitoring for cytokine release syndrome with blood pressure measurements, worsening hypoxemia, and biomarkers

Antiviral Therapy

Antiviral therapy can be considered if the following conditions are present, despite a lack of evidence of strong benefit:

- Documented severe or critical COVID-19
- Mild or moderate disease with an underlying condition that may increase the risk of progression to severe disease

Remdesivir

Remdesivir is the drug of choice, and it is approved by the Food and Drug Administration (FDA) for hospitalized pediatric patients aged ≥28 days and weighing ≥3 kg. The active form of remdesivir acts as a nucleoside analog and inhibits RNA-dependent RNA polymerase. For most hospitalized patients, remdesivir should be administered for 5 days. Treatment may be extended to 10 days for patients with severe disease who have not clinically improved or for children who are severely immunocompromised.

Dose of remdesivir:

- ≥3 to <40 kg—5 mg/kg intravenous (IV) loading dose on day 1, followed by 2.5 mg/kg IV every 24 hours
- ≥40 kg—200 mg IV loading dose on day 1, followed by 100 mg IV every 24 hours

Immunomodulators

Corticosteroids

Corticosteroids may modulate inflammation-mediated lung injury and thereby decrease the risk of progression to respiratory failure and death. The RECOVERY (Randomised Evaluation of COVID-19 Therapy) trial concluded that the use of dexamethasone for up to 10 days resulted in lower 28-day mortality than usual care in patients who received invasive mechanical ventilation at randomization and those who received oxygen without invasive mechanical ventilation.[8] It had eventually shown benefit from low-dose dexamethasone therapy in adults, although pediatric data is limited.

Among children with severe COVID-19 who require mechanical ventilation or those who require supplemental oxygen and have risk factors for progression to severe disease, low-dose corticosteroids may be indicated for a duration of up to 10 days or until discharge, whichever is shorter. Low-dose glucocorticoid regimens that can be used are as follows:

- Dexamethasone 0.15 mg/kg orally or IV once daily (maximum dose 6 mg)
- Prednisolone 1 mg/kg orally once daily (maximum dose 40 mg)
- Methylprednisolone 0.8 mg/kg IV once daily (maximum dose 32 mg)

Other Immunomodulatory Therapies

The National Institute of Health guidelines recommend the use of baricitinib or tocilizumab for children on mechanical ventilation or extracorporeal membrane oxygenation (ECMO) who do not have rapid improvement in oxygenation after initiation of dexamethasone. However, immunomodulators like interleukin (IL)-6 inhibitors (e.g., tocilizumab), Janus kinase inhibitors (JAK) inhibitors (e.g., baricitinib), and convalescent plasma from recovered COVID-19 patients are not routinely used in the treatment of children with COVID-19 in India.

Anticoagulants

Anticoagulation therapy is not routinely recommended in all children with COVID-19. It may be considered on a case-to-case basis, depending on the presence of risk factors. All hospitalized children should be evaluated for the risk of developing thrombosis and monitored regularly for the development of thrombosis. Prophylactic anticoagulant is indicated in the following conditions:

- Strong personal or family history of venous thrombotic event
- Presence of an indwelling central venous line
- Decreased mobility from baseline
- Morbid obesity
- Other associated medical conditions like burns and severe dehydration

Low-molecular-weight heparin is the preferred anticoagulant.

SEQUELAE OF COVID-19

Sequelae after COVID-19 are rare in children. *Pulmonary fibrosis* has been reported in some cases. However, majority of children recover completely 12 weeks after the onset of illness. *Long COVID* is defined as symptoms and signs that develop during or after an infection consistent with COVID-19 that continues for >12 weeks and is not explained by any other alternative diagnosis. Symptoms might include fatigue, dyspnea, palpitations, headache, dizziness, poor concentration, and myalgia.

MULTISYSTEM INFLAMMATORY SYNDROME IN CHILDREN

Multisystem inflammatory syndrome in children is a postinfectious complication of COVID-19 seen in children who present with clinical features similar to incomplete Kawasaki disease (KD) or toxic shock syndrome. It is also referred to as pediatric multisystem inflammatory syndrome (PMIS), pediatric inflammatory multisystem syndrome temporally associated with SARS-CoV-2 (PIMS-TS), or pediatric hyperinflammatory syndrome.

Pathogenesis

Epidemiologic data have clearly shown a temporal association between MIS-C and SARS-CoV-2 infection, with MIS-C presenting 3–6 weeks after SARS-CoV-2 infection. MIS-C is believed to be related to immune dysregulation, which leads to delayed hyperinflammatory response, resulting in immune cell activation and cytokine storm.

Cardiac manifestations noted in the acute phase of MIS-C include ventricular dysfunction, coronary artery (CA) dilation and aneurysms, arrhythmia, and conduction abnormalities. Severe cases can present in vasodilatory or cardiogenic shock, requiring fluid resuscitation and inotropic support. The causes of myocardial injury are thought to be a combination of factors like systemic inflammation, acute viral myocarditis, hypoxia, stress cardiomyopathy, and, rarely, ischemia caused by CA involvement.

Clinical Features

MIS-C usually presents with symptoms such as:

- Fever for >3 days
- Gastrointestinal symptoms (abdominal pain, vomiting, and diarrhea)
- Nonpurulent conjunctivitis and mucositis
- Neurocognitive symptoms (headache, lethargy, and confusion)
- Respiratory symptoms often caused by shock

They can also present with:

- Shock
- Myocardial dysfunction
- Acute respiratory failure requiring noninvasive or invasive ventilation
- Acute kidney injury
- Hepatitis or hepatomegaly
- Encephalopathy, seizures, coma, or meningoencephalitis

Laboratory Investigations

- Hematologic abnormalities include lymphocytopenia, neutrophilia, anemia, and thrombocytopenia
- Elevated CRP with variable increase in the erythrocyte sedimentation rate (ESR) and ferritin
- D-dimer and fibrinogen
- Hyponatremia, hypoalbuminemia, elevation in alanine transaminase (ALT), aspartate aminotransferase (AST), and lactate dehydrogenase (LDH)
- Children with suspected MIS-C should be tested for SARS-CoV-2, including both serology and RT-PCR. The baseline rate of seropositivity for SARS-CoV-2 has increased significantly in view of the widespread infection and postvaccination. Hence, a positive SARS-CoV-2 IgG antibody alone does not confirm the diagnosis of MIS-C

Echocardiography (ECHO)

Echocardiographic findings may include:

- Left ventricular (LV) dysfunction
- CA dilation or aneurysm
- Mitral regurgitation
- Pericardial effusion

World Health Organization Criteria for Diagnosis of Multisystem Inflammatory Syndrome in Children[9]

- Children and adolescents 0–19 years of age
- Fever >3 days
- Clinical signs of multisystem involvement (at least two of the following):
  - Rash or bilateral nonpurulent conjunctivitis or mucocutaneous inflammation signs (oral, hands, or feet)
  - Hypotension or shock
  - Features of myocardial dysfunction, pericarditis, valvulitis, or coronary abnormalities [including ECHO findings or elevated Troponin/N-terminal pro B-type natriuretic peptide (NT-proBNP)]
  - Evidence of coagulopathy [by prothrombin time (PT), partial thromboplastin time (PTT), and elevated D-dimers]
  - Acute gastrointestinal problems (diarrhea, vomiting, or abdominal pain)
- Elevated markers of inflammation such as ESR, CRP, or procalcitonin
- No other obvious microbial cause of inflammation, including bacterial sepsis, staphylococcal, or streptococcal shock syndromes
- Evidence of SARS-CoV-2 infection (any of the following):
  - Positive SARS-CoV-2 RT-PCR
  - Positive serology
  - Positive antigen test
- Contact with an individual with COVID-19

Treatment

A multidisciplinary approach to treatment is usually needed. Empirical antibiotics are a must in sick children until infection is ruled out because sepsis and toxic shock syndrome may present with similar clinical features. Shock often requires the use of vasoactive agents, preferably norepinephrine or epinephrine.

- Intravenous immunoglobulin (IVIG) at 2 g/kg (maximum dose—100 g) over 12–24 hours is recommended as the first line of therapy.
- Corticosteroids (methylprednisolone) are recommended in the presence of:
  - Severe or refractory shock
  - KD-like features with a risk factor for IVIG resistance [e.g., CA enlargement (Z-score ≥2.5), age ≤12 months]
  - Persistent fever and rising inflammatory markers
  - The dose may vary from 10 mg/kg OD for 3 days initially, followed by oral therapy tapered over 2–4 weeks.
- Aspirin at 3–5 mg/kg/day (maximum 75 mg/day) is indicated in all children with MIS-C for a period of 4–6 weeks or longer among those with coronary aneurysms. It is contraindicated if the platelet count is <80,000 or in the presence of bleeding manifestations.
- Anticoagulant therapy with low-molecular-weight heparin is indicated if there is either of the following:
  - Giant coronary aneurysm with absolute coronary diameter ≥8 mm or Z score ≥10
  - Documented thrombus
  - Ejection fraction (EF) <35%

Biologicals

Treatment with biological agents like IL-1 inhibitors (anakinra), IL-6 inhibitors (tocilizumab), and tumor necrosis factor (TNF) inhibitors (infliximab) can be considered among children with MIS-C who are refractory to initial therapy with IVIG and glucocorticoids.

Prevention

Prevention of pediatric COVID-19 is essentially through universal masking for all persons above 5 years of age, social distancing precautions, and maintaining hand hygiene when the disease transmission in the community is high. Even though COVID-19 is mild in children, they might be important sources of transmission to high-risk adults, and among children with comorbid conditions and risk factors, it can progress to severe infection. Four vaccines have received emergency-use authorization for the pediatric population in India. Details regarding the vaccines are outlined in **Table 7.20.1**.

Infection Prevention in Healthcare Settings

Infection-prevention measures to limit the transmission of SARS-CoV-2 include universal masking, early identification, and isolation of patients with suspected disease, use of appropriate personal protective equipment when caring for patients with COVID-19, hand hygiene, and environmental disinfection.

Isolation

- For immunocompetent children with mild-to-moderate disease, infection-prevention precautions can be discontinued when the following criteria are met:[9]
  - At least 10 days have passed since symptoms started.

TABLE 7.20.1: Vaccines for SARS-CoV-2 infection.

Type of vaccine	*Route of administration*	*Schedule*	*Age group*
Whole virion inactivated vaccine	Intramuscular	Two-dose schedule at 0 and 28 days	6–18 years
• Protein subunit vaccine • Contains the receptor binding domain of spike protein, which is produced through recombinant technology	Intramuscular	Two-dose schedule at 0 and 28 days	5–18 years
DNA-based vaccine	Intradermal route using needle-free injector	Three-dose schedule on days 0, 28, and 56	12–18 years
Recombinant nanoparticle vaccine	Intramuscular	Two-dose schedule on days 0 and 21	12–17 years

(DNA: deoxyribonucleic acid; SARS-CoV-2: severe acute respiratory syndrome coronavirus-2)

    - At least 1 day (24 hours) has passed since the resolution of fever without the use of fever-reducing medications.
    - There is improvement in symptoms.
- For children with severe infection, isolation can be discontinued when:[10]
    - At least 10 and up to 20 days have passed since symptoms first appeared.
    - At least 1 day (24 hours) has passed since the resolution of fever without the use of fever-reducing medications.
    - There is improvement in symptoms.
- For children with moderate-to-severe immunocompromise, the duration of isolation should typically be extended to at least 20 days after symptom onset (or first positive viral test for those who are asymptomatic), since such patients can shed viable virus for prolonged periods of time, regardless of disease severity.[10]

Neonatal COVID-19

Neonates can be infected by SARS-CoV-2 through vertical (via placenta or genital tract) or horizontal (through respiratory droplets) transmission following contact with family members or healthcare workers. Neonatal COVID-19 is less common; vertical transmission is infrequent and mostly asymptomatic, with most of the reported cases due to postnatal infection.

Clinical Features

Most of the neonates remain asymptomatic or may develop mild symptoms like cough, rhinorrhea, low-grade fever, and vomiting. Some may go on to develop severe symptoms like respiratory distress, lethargy, poor feeding, and hemodynamic instability.

Neonatal multisystem inflammatory syndrome (MIS-N) has been described as the result of neonatal hyper-responsiveness to the SARS-CoV-2-specific maternal IgG antibodies.[11] The diagnosis of MIS-N secondary to maternal infections remains debatable, and there are no specific criteria for the diagnosis of MIS-N.[12] The multiorgan involvement, the presence of signs of inflammation, and IgG SARS-CoV-2 antibodies are commonly seen in MIS-N. Cardiac involvement may include myocarditis, pericarditis, or coronary aneurysm. Respiratory, renal, and neurological symptoms can also be seen.

Laboratory Findings

Leukocytosis or lymphopenia, thrombocytopenia, and elevated inflammatory markers are commonly seen. In the presence of a suspected MIS-N, elevated inflammatory markers [CRP, ferritin, D-dimer, and lactate dehydrogenase (LDH)], elevated NT-proBNP, and troponin can be observed along with detectable SARS-CoV-2 IgG (in the absence of maternal immunization).

Diagnosis

Neonatal COVID-19 can be diagnosed in those with a history of exposure to a COVID-19-positive adult, mother with COVID-19 infection within 14 days before birth, and history of contact with COVID-19-positive persons in the postnatal period.

Management

Stable neonates should be roomed in with mothers, and breastfeeding should continue. Neonates who are sick and are born to a mother with suspected or proven COVID-19 infection should be managed in a separate isolation room. Supportive management and specific measures for systemic COVID-19 are similar to any other critical illness in neonates.

REFERENCES

1. World Health Organization. WHO coronavirus (COVID-19) dashboard. [online] Available from https://covid19.who.int/. [Last accessed November, 2024].
2. Kung YA, Lee KM, Chiang HJ, Huang SY, Wu CJ, Shih SR. Molecular virology of SARS-CoV-2 and related coronaviruses. Microbiol Mol Biol Rev. 2022;86(2):e00026-21.
3. V'kovski P, Kratzel A, Steiner S, Stalder H, Thiel V. Coronavirus biology and replication: implications for SARS-CoV-2. Nat Rev Microbiol. 2021;19(3):155-70.

4. Bohn MK, Hall A, Sepiashvili L, Jung B, Steele S, Adeli K. Pathophysiology of COVID-19: mechanisms underlying disease severity and progression. Physiology (Bethesda). 2020;35(5):288-301.
5. Binny RN, Priest P, French NP, Parry M, Lustig A, Hendy SC, et al. Sensitivity of reverse transcription polymerase chain reaction tests for severe acute respiratory syndrome coronavirus 2 through time. J Infect Dis. 2023;227(1):9-17.
6. Hanson KE, Caliendo AM, Arias CA, Englund JA, Lee MJ, Loeb M, et al. Infectious Diseases Society of America guidelines on the diagnosis of coronavirus disease 2019. Clin Infect Dis. 2020:ciaa760.
7. RECOVERY Collaborative Group. Dexamethasone in hospitalized patients with COVID-19. N Engl J Med. 2021; 384(8):693-704.
8. World Health Organization. (2020). Scientific brief: multisystem inflammatory syndrome in children and adolescents with COVID-19. [online] Available from https://www.who.int/news-room/commentaries/detail/multisystem-inflammatory-syndrome-in-children-and-adolescents-with-covid-19[Last accessed November, 2024].
9. United States Centers for Disease Control and Prevention. Ending isolation and precautions for people with COVID-19: interim guidance. [online] Available from https://www.cdc.gov/coronavirus/2019-ncov/hcp/duration-isolation.html. [Last accessed November, 2024].
10. Balasubramanian S, Rao NM, Goenka A, Roderick M, Ramanan AV. Coronavirus disease 2019 (COVID-19) in children—what we know so far and what we do not. Indian Pediatr. 2020;57(5): 435-42.
11. Dhanalakshmi K, Venkataraman A, Balasubramanian S, Madhusudan M, Amperayani S, Putilibai S, et al. Epidemiological and clinical profile of pediatric inflammatory multisystem syndrome—temporally associated with SARS-CoV-2 (PIMS-TS) in Indian children. Indian Pediatr. 2020; 57(11):1010-4.
12. Galderisi A, Lista G, Cavigioli F, Trevisanuto D. Clinical features of neonatal COVID-19. Semin Fetal Neonatal Med. 2023;28(2):101430.

7.21 Dengue Illnesses

Thangavelu S, Lalitha Rajalakshmi S

INTRODUCTION

Dengue illness is an acute systemic mosquito-borne viral infection that has become a global public health concern, especially in Southeast Asian countries. It is hyperendemic in the urban and semiurban areas, with more than half of the world's population at risk.

The World War II heightened the expansion of disease by shipping vessels to the coastal regions across the world. Postwar urbanization and industrialization were the primary reasons for hyperendemicity and the emergence of severe forms of the disease, especially in Southeast Asia. Dengue illness presents with a wide spectrum of clinical features ranging from nonspecific febrile illness to life-threatening dengue shock syndrome (DSS).

EPIDEMIOLOGY

Global Situation

Before 1970, only nine countries were affected by dengue illnesses, which have now spread to over 100 countries. The most severely affected continents are the Americas, Southeast Asia and Western Pacific regions, and Asia representing 70% of the global disease burden. Dengue has also now invaded new areas in Europe, with cases reported for the first time in 2010 in France and Croatia. A study conducted across 12 Southeast Asian countries showed a yearly economic burden of US$ 950 million, and nearly 52% of this is incurred from loss of productivity.

Globally, the highest reported incidence of dengue was 5.2 million cases in the year 2019, with an estimated incidence between 100 and 400 million cases per year. It is also estimated that dengue is responsible for 20,000 deaths annually. However, poor disease surveillance, under-reporting, lower case fatality rate, and difficulty in diagnosis may be some of the reasons that mask the exact incidence and impact of dengue across the globe.

Indian Scenario

Earlier, dengue was considered a benign disease with pain and fever, and since the mid-1990s, it has become a potentially fatal disease. In the following decades, dengue had spread throughout India from urban to rural areas, with the first national outbreak in 1996. A dramatic increase in the frequency of outbreaks and the disease burden followed. Currently, in India, all four serotypes are prevalent in most of the states. According to recent data, 1,93,245 cases were reported in the year 2021.

Recent studies have documented a shift in the affected age group from the adult population to children and young adults. Also, concurrent infection with multiple serotypes makes India hyperendemic for dengue infection and a major contributor to the global disease burden.

Dengue surveillance in India is conducted by the Department of Health Research through over 600 sentinel hospitals managed by the National Vector Borne Disease Control Program (NVBDCP), Integrated Disease Surveillance Program (IDSP), and 52 Virus Research and Diagnostic Laboratories (VRDL).

ETIOPATHOGENESIS

Etiology

Dengue virus belongs to the family *Flaviviridae* of the genus *Flavivirus*, which includes four serotypes—DEN-1, DEN-2, DEN-3, and DEN-4. The bite of the vector *Aedes aegypti* transmits the virus to humans, primarily in the rainy seasons. The most common serotypes are DEN-3 and DEN-4, and DEN-2 is considered as the most virulent.

Viral Factors

The dengue virus is a single-stranded ribonucleic acid (RNA) virus with a glycoprotein envelope. The envelope is involved in hemagglutination, neutralization, and host cell interaction in the early phase of infection. The soluble membrane-associated NS1 (nonstructural protein-1) antigen activates the human complement system and is expressed in the early phase of infection in blood, which is used for diagnosis in the early stages.

The dengue virus is composed of three structural and seven nonstructural proteins. These proteins determine the four serotypes, and due to mutations in the virus, the severity varies from time to time. Infection with one serotype confers lifelong immunity; however, cross-reactivity leads to severe disease with reinfection of a different serotype. There is never a complete herd immunity for all four serotypes, as periodic outbreaks happen with different serotypes, making natural elimination not achievable.

Vector Factors

The primary vector, the female *A. aegypti*, is a domestic mosquito that breeds in clean water containers, is day-biting, and the feeding episodes often go unnoticed. They frequently take multiple blood meals in a single breeding cycle; hence, the mosquito may transmit a dengue virus to several individuals within the household. The eggs can survive in dried conditions for several months, and the first contact with water initiates the cycle. This is an important vector with high affinity for human blood and is highly adapted to urban living.

The other host is *Aedes albopictus* or the tiger mosquito. They do not feed on humans as frequently as *A. aegypti* and hence have become less-efficient natural vectors. But it has the ability to transmit both the dengue and chikungunya infections, and simultaneous outbreaks of both diseases have occurred. They have a very limited flight range, maximum of 512 m, making humans the most important factor for the global spread. Globalization, travel and trade, climate, and settlement factors influence the global spread of the vector and thus the dengue illness. Thus, vector control is the most important measure in the control and prevention of outbreaks and endemicity.

The vector gets infected on taking a blood meal from patients in the febrile phase of dengue illness. After an extrinsic incubation period of 8–10 days, the infected *Aedes* transmits the virus to the host through the bite.

Host Factors

Dengue virus gains entry to the host by the infected mosquito bite and replicates in the subdermal Langerhans dendritic cells from where the virus migrates to lymph nodes. Viremia occurs and infects the solid organs and bone marrow. Humoral, cellular, and innate host responses determine the severity and progression of the illness and are not related to the viral load. A seroprevalence study in India noted seropositivity between 60% and 80%.[1]

Transmission Cycle

Dengue virus transmission is enhanced by multiple factors of urbanization like population growth, poor urban planning with overcrowding, poor sanitation, and modern transportation. These factors allow increased movement and colocation of humans, mosquitoes, and viruses. Increasing global temperatures are one of the major contributing factors for the growing vector density and prolonged infective period of mosquitoes. Viral transmission is maintained through a human–mosquito–human cycle, as represented in **Figure 7.21.1**.

Other methods of spread are nosocomial transmissions, where mosquito bites can transmit the infection to other inpatients in the hospital; transmission via blood products, needlestick injury, and vertical transmission.

PATHOGENESIS

Various mechanisms of severe dengue are antibody-dependent enhancement (ADE) in secondary dengue, T-cell and immune complex-mediated disease, complement and its pathways, and "cytokine tsunami" leading to massive concentrations of cytokines that mediate plasma leakage. Anti-NS1 antibodies behave as autoantibodies against platelets and endothelium, which trigger intracellular

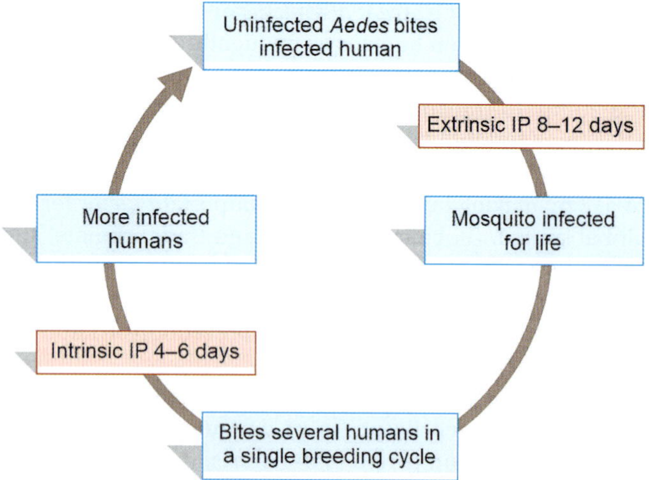

Fig. 7.21.1: Diagrammatic representation of transmission cycle of *Aedes aegypti*—dengue virus—human. (IP: incubation period)
Source: World Health Organization.

signaling resulting in increased capillary permeability. Severe dengue presents with increased capillary permeability without damage to the capillary endothelium, altered function and number of leukocytes and platelets, altered hemostasis, and liver damage. Sudden fluid shift into third space, such as serous cavities like the pleura, pericardium, and peritoneum and associated hemorrhage results in shock, *DSS*.

Coagulopathy is a consistent finding in severe dengue, while mechanisms are still unclear. Thrombocytopenia, platelet dysfunction, prothrombin complex deficiency, endothelial injury, disseminated intravascular coagulation (DIC), decreased fibrinogen and increased fibrinogen degradation products (FDP), increased D-dimers, and platelet sequestration all could be causes of bleeding in *dengue hemorrhagic fever (DHF)*.

Direct organ damage has also been reported with the dengue virus having high affinity to hepatocytes.

Dengue NS1 disrupts the endothelial glycocalyx, resulting in vascular leak, which is the hallmark of severe dengue. However, there is no concordance between the timing of NS1 antigenemia and the development of vascular leak.[2]

CLASSIFICATION OF DENGUE ILLNESSES

There are two types of severity grading classification systems in dengue according to the World Health Organization (WHO).

World Health Organization 1997 Classification and World Health Organization Guideline 2012[3]

Presentation of symptomatic dengue varies from *undifferentiated dengue fever (UDF)* to fatal DHF/DSS. Plasma leakage is important for the diagnosis of DHF and DSS.

Undifferentiated Dengue Fever

Primary dengue infection is not different from other viral febrile illnesses. There may be maculopapular rash. Signs of capillary leakage and bleeding are absent.

Clinical criteria: Acute febrile illness that lasts 2–7 days with two or more of the following—headache, retro-orbital pain, myalgia, arthralgia, and rash.

Dengue Hemorrhagic Fever

Clinical criteria: Dengue fever (DF) *plus*

- Hemorrhagic tendencies, which may be *one or more* of the following:
  - Positive torniquet test
  - Petechiae, ecchymoses, or purpura
  - Bleeding from mucosa, gastrointestinal (GI) tract, injection, and other sites
- Thrombocytopenia (<1,00,000 cells/mm^3) and
- Plasma leakage evidenced by *one or more* of the following:
  - ≥20% rise in average hematocrit (HCT) for age and sex
  - >20% drop in HCT following volume replacement compared to baseline
  - Third spacing (pleural effusion, ascites, and hypoproteinemia)

Dengue Shock Syndrome

All the above features of DHF plus evidence of circulatory failure presenting as rapid and weak pulse, narrow pulse pressure <20 mm Hg, hypotension, cold clammy skin, and restlessness comprise DSS.

Grades of DHF

- DHF I—DF *plus* positive torniquet test and evidence of plasma leakage. Platelet <1,00,000 cells/mm^3 and HCT rise >20% from baseline
- DHF II—DHF I *plus* spontaneous bleeding (melena, epistaxis, and gum bleed) and abdominal pain
- DHF III/DSS—DHF II *plus* circulatory failure (rapid and weak pulse, narrow pulse pressure <20 mm Hg, hypotension, cold clammy skin, and restlessness)
- DHF IV/DSS—profound shock with undetectable pulse or blood pressure (BP) (DHF III and IV are classified as DSS)

Expanded Dengue Syndrome

Unusual manifestation of organ system involvement can occur in both DF and DHF groups. Expanded dengue syndrome (EDS) presents as the following based on the organ system involved. This is common in patients with comorbidities or coinfections.

- Central nervous system (CNS)—encephalopathy, encephalitis, and intracranial bleed
- GI—acute hepatitis, fulminant hepatic failure, pancreatitis, cholecystitis, and cholangitis
- Renal—acute kidney injury (AKI), hemolytic uremic syndrome (HUS), and acute tubular necrosis (ATN)
- Cardiac—myocarditis, pericardial effusion, arrhythmia, and cardiomyopathy
- Respiratory—pleural effusion, pulmonary edema, adult respiratory distress syndrome (ARDS), and pulmonary hemorrhage
- Eye—conjunctival or macular hemorrhage, impaired vision, and optic neuritis

World Health Organization 2009 Classification[4]

Figure 7.21.2 provides the details of the WHO 2009 classification of dengue. The difficulty observed in the WHO 1997 classification is its overlapping and complexity. A comparison of both classifications is given in **Table 7.21.1**.

CLINICAL FEATURES

In a dengue epidemic, a significant proportion of the affected may be asymptomatic. As per a study done in schoolchildren, inapparent infections are equal to or more than those of children with symptomatic infection.[5] In another study, it was estimated that only one-fourth of dengue infections are symptomatic.[6] Clinical features depend on the phase of illness, severity, and rarely because of the presence of coinfections.

COURSE OF DENGUE ILLNESS AND THREE PHASES

Dengue illness progresses usually in three phases—febrile phase, critical phase, and recovery phase **(Fig. 7.21.3)**.[4]

Febrile Phase

Febrile phase starts with acute-onset high-grade fever, body pain, headache, eye pain, nausea, vomiting, diarrhea, flushing and erythema of palms and soles, conjunctival congestion, and hepatomegaly. Warning signs may start appearing after 2–3 days, which include GI symptoms such as abdominal pain or tenderness, persistent vomiting, hepatomegaly >2 cm, clinical fluid accumulation without respiratory distress, lethargy, and restlessness.

Features are indistinguishable from other viral infections. Dengue being a dynamic disease, features in the febrile phase will not predict the course and severity of the illness. A *tourniquet test* may be positive at this stage. It is done by inflating the BP cuff between systolic and diastolic for 5 minutes and observing for the appearance of 10 or more petechiae in 1 inch^2 area in the forearm, which is considered positive for DHF **(Fig. 7.21.4)**.

Laboratory features are increasing HCT and concurrent decrease in platelet count. C-reactive protein (CRP) may be negative; leukopenia and lymphocytosis may be seen.

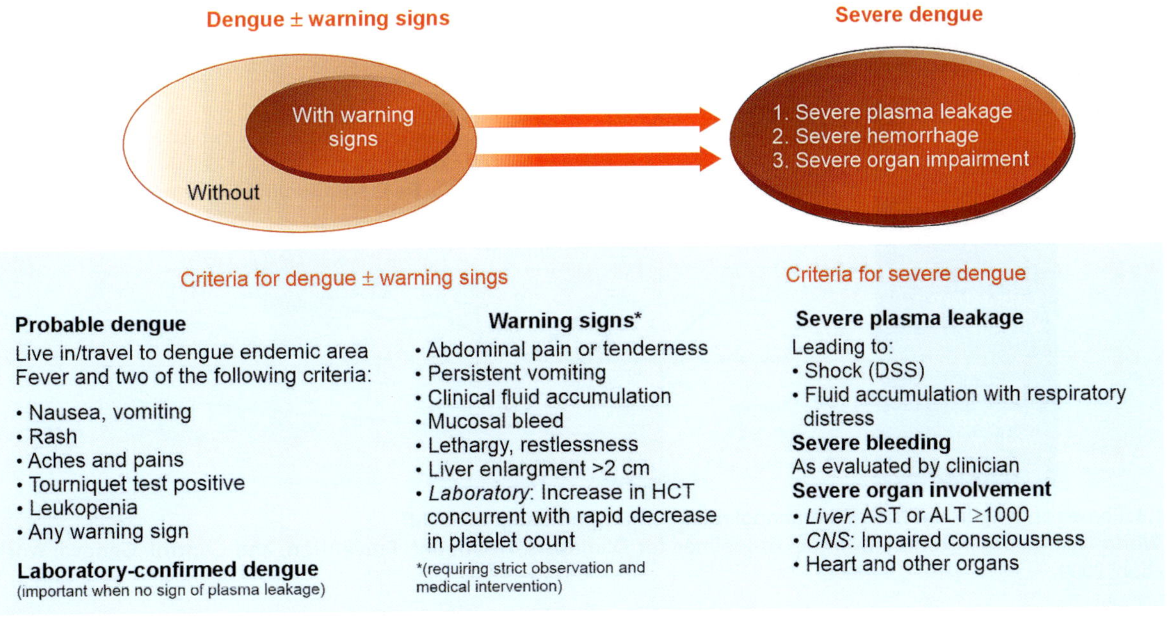

Fig. 7.21.2: WHO 2009 classification of dengue. (ALT: alanine transaminase; AST: aspartate aminotransferase; CNS: central nervous system; DSS: dengue shock syndrome; HCT: hematocrit; WHO: World Health Organization)
Source: World Health Organization. Dengue: Guidelines for Diagnosis, Treatment, Prevention, and Control. Geneva: World Health Organization; 2009.

TABLE 7.21.1: Comparison of WHO 1997 and 2009 classification systems.

	1997 WHO classification[3]	*2009 WHO classification*[4]
Basis	First one, based on data	
Categories	• Dengue fever (DF) • Dengue hemorrhagic fever (DHF I and II) • Dengue shock syndrome (DSS) (DHF III and IV)	• Dengue without warning signs (probable dengue) • Dengue with warning signs • Severe dengue
DF = D without shock	• DF (as per this classification, mild hemorrhage and skin mucosal bleeds are included here) • Features of plasma leak absent	Dengue without warning signs
DHF II and II = D with without shock	• Features of DF + GI bleeding • Features of capillary leak (rise in HCT by 20%, platelets <1,00,000, ascites, pleural effusion) are present • Without shock	• Dengue with warning signs—abdominal pain/tenderness, persistent vomiting, fluid accumulation evidenced by ascites, pleural effusion, mucosal bleeding, lethargy or restlessness, hepatomegaly >2 cm • Rise in HCT and fall in platelet count • Without shock
DHF grades III and IV = severe dengue	Rapid and weak pulse, cold, clammy skin and restlessness, narrow pulse pressure, hypotension, and severe bleeding	Severe dengue: • *Severe plasma leakage:* Shock, fluid accumulation with respiratory distress, severe bleeding (as evaluated by clinician) • *Severe organ involvement:* AST or ALT ≥ 1,000 units, impaired consciousness, and organ failure
	Expanded dengue syndrome	Severe dengue with multiorgan dysfunction syndrome (MODS), which may be due to hypotensive shock, coinfection, or hyperferritinemic HLH

(ALT: alanine transaminase; AST: aspartate aminotransferase; D: dengue; GI: gastrointestinal; HCT: hematocrit; HLH: hemophagocytic lymphohistiocytosis; WHO: World Health Organization)

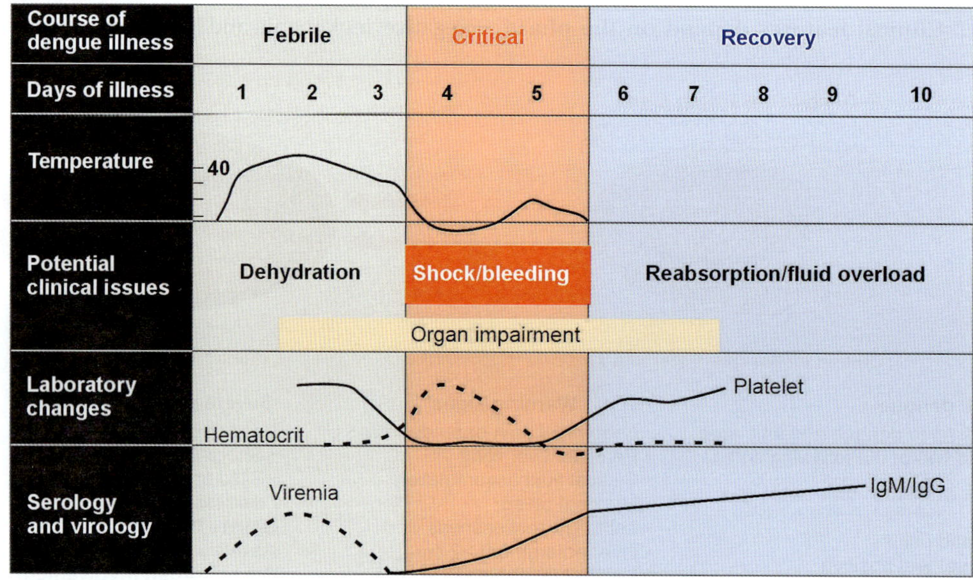

Fig. 7.21.3: Phases of dengue illness. (IgG: immunoglobulin G; IgM: immunoglobulin M)
Source: World Health Organization. Dengue: Guidelines for Diagnosis, Treatment, Prevention, and Control. Geneva: World Health Organization; 2009.

Differential Diagnosis in Febrile Phase

Other viral infections like influenza and tropical infections like enteric fever, leptospirosis, malaria, and scrub typhus may resemble the febrile phase of DF. Environmental clues like monsoon and other cases of dengue occurring in the community aid in diagnosis.

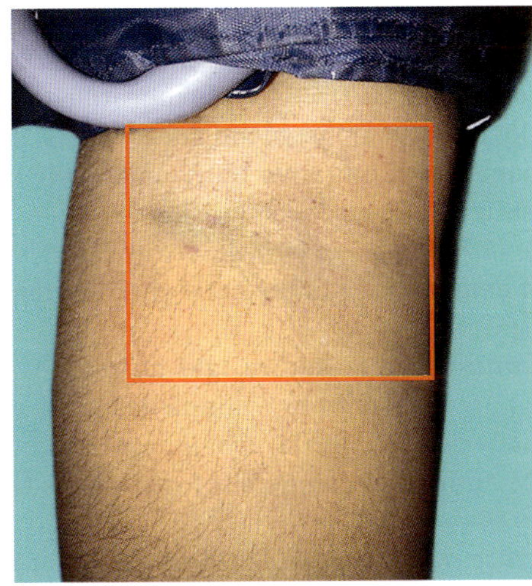

Fig. 7.21.4: Positive tourniquet test.

Critical Phase

Critical phase commences with the resolution of fever with or without warning signs. This period is characterized by:

- Serious features like shock, respiratory distress due to ascites, and pleural effusion secondary to plasma leak
- Severe hemorrhage (GI, menstrual) as assessed by the treating pediatrician
- Organ involvement resulting in encephalopathy, AKI, myocardial impairment, acute liver failure (ALF), and hyperferritinemic hemophagocytic lymphohistiocytosis (HLH)

Laboratory parameters include a 20% rise in HCT with concurrent thrombocytopenia, impaired renal parameters, raised transaminases, prolonged international normalized ratio (INR), and high inflammatory markers such as ferritin and lactate dehydrogenase (LDH).

Differential Diagnosis in Critical Phase

Septic shock is a close differential diagnosis **(Table 7.21.2)**. Tropical infections such as enteric fever, malaria, leptospirosis, and malaria may present as septic shock. Presence of eschar, splenomegaly, anemia, and thrombocytopenia and specific investigations like blood culture, typhoid immunoglobulin M (IgM), and scrub IgM may point toward the diagnosis.

Recovery Phase

Some children with nonsevere dengue do not develop critical features and improve from the febrile phase immediately to develop the recovery phase after defervescence. Others recover after 48–72 hours of critical phase, or on day 8 of illness, and the signs of recovery are improvement in appetite and well-being. Mostly, hemodynamic stability occurs and diuresis occurs in the recovery phase of dengue. *Recovery rash*, island of pallor in the sea of redness **(Fig. 7.21.5)**, and sinus bradycardia and sinus arrhythmia are common ssfeatures. In those who receive excessive fluids, fluids are absorbed into the intravascular compartment, leading to hypervolemia and respiratory distress. HCT starts falling and platelets start increasing.

TABLE 7.21.2: Differences between dengue shock and septic shock.

Features	*Dengue*	*Septic shock*
Fever	Shock develops after the fever subsides	Shock develops at the peak of fever
Hepatomegaly	Present	Usually, absent
Heart rate	Relative bradycardia	Tachycardia
Pulse pressure	Narrow	Wide
Focus of sepsis	Absent and flushing of palm, soles, and conjunctival congestion	Septic focus may be absent or involve skin and soft tissues, lungs in pneumonia, etc.
Bleeding tendency	Skin or gastrointestinal bleed	Generally, absent in early stages
Complete blood count (CBC)	Leukopenia, lymphocytosis, raised hematocrit (HCT), and thrombocytopenia	Neutrophilic leukocytosis
C-reactive protein (CRP)	Normal	Raised
Blood and urine culture	Negative	Positive

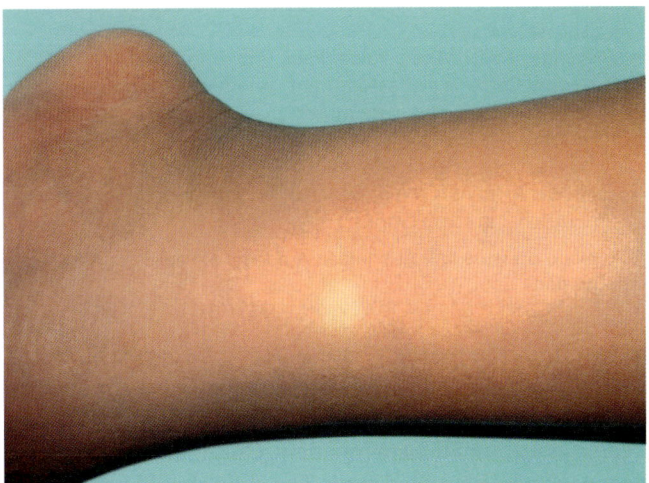

Fig. 7.21.5: Recovery rash—"Island of pallor in red sea."

MANIFESTATIONS OF SEVERE DENGUE

Severe dengue is potentially fatal and can present with features as shown in **Box 7.21.1**.

Dengue is a dynamic disease exhibiting abrupt changes in clinical features and laboratory parameters when the disease

BOX 7.21.1: Clinical features of severe dengue.

- *Severe plasma leakage* leading to hypovolemic shock; third spacing causes pleural effusion and ascites, including abdominal compartment syndrome, which results in worsening of shock and respiratory distress
- *Severe bleeding* as assessed by the treating physician, which may be hematemesis, melena, epistaxis, menstrual bleeding in adolescent girls, and very rarely pulmonary hemorrhage
- *Severe organ involvement:* Multiple organ system impairment can lead to multiorgan dysfunction syndrome (MODS), which may be due to direct invasion of the organs by DENV, secondary to hypotensive shock and hypoxia, or due to hyperferritinemic HLH. A child may have clinical signs of acute encephalitis or encephalopathy, acute kidney injury, acute hepatic failure, myocardial impairment, and cardiogenic shock

(DENV: dengue virus; HLH: hemophagocytic lymphohistiocytosis)

BOX 7.21.2: Assessment as per IAP ALS guidelines.

- *Airway:* Stable or unstable
- *Breathing:* Assess rate, increased work of breathing, breath sounds and saturation. Tachypnea and increased work of breathing will indicate the presence of fluid overload
- *Circulation:* Assess pulse rate, pulse volume, capillary refill time (CRT), BP, urine output and level of consciousness. Presents with weak pulses, hypotension, and low urine output (<0.5 mL/kg/h). Unlike in other types of shock, classical features like tachycardia will be absent
- *Disability:* AVPU (Alert, Voice, Pain, and Unresponsive) or GCS (Glasgow Coma Scale) assessment can identify depressed level of consciousness. There are multiple causes for encephalopathy, including metabolic causes like hypoglycemia, hyponatremia, hypoxia, shock, encephalitis, etc.
- *Exposure:* To identify the presence of jaundice in acute liver failure (ALF), eschar in scrub typhus

(BP: blood pressure; IAP ALS: Indian Academy of Pediatrics Advanced Life Support)

moves from the febrile phase to the critical phase. In the critical phase, the child needs to be monitored very frequently, i.e., two to four times a day, depending on whether the child is treated as an outpatient or inpatient. Only then signs of severe dengue can be identified early. The child should be assessed as per the Indian Academy of Pediatrics (IAP) Advanced Life Support (ALS) guidelines **(Box 7.21.2)**.

DIAGNOSIS

The diagnostic test depends on the duration of illness and clinical presentation. Laboratory diagnosis is done either by detecting viral antigens or by serology for antibodies.

In addition to complete blood count (CBC), CRP and dengue NS1 antigen in the first 5 days and dengue IgM after day 7 are important. Frequent monitoring of packed cell volume (PCV), platelet count, electrolyte, urea, creatinine, alanine transaminase [ALT or serum glutamic pyruvic transaminase (SGPT)], aspartate aminotransferase [AST or serum glutamic oxaloacetic transaminase (SGOT)], ferritin, LDH, electrocardiogram (ECG), and echocardiogram (ECHO) help identify complications; blood culture, CRP, scrub IgM, malarial parasite quantitative buffy coat (QBC) test, and leptospirosis IgM to identify coinfections.

- *Enzyme-linked immunosorbent assay (ELISA)-based NS1 antigen* detects cases in the early viremic stage and is a highly specific test.
- *IgM capture ELISA*—serum IgM antibodies (dengue-specific) are measured by a simple test. IgM antibodies are usually detected by day 5 of illness (range 2–8 days). The IgM antibodies can persist for >90 days but usually wane by 60 days.
- *Polymerase chain reaction (PCR)* is useful for molecular diagnosis in acute-phase serum samples and has replaced viral isolation methods from serum, plasma, or leukocytes.
- *Immunoglobulin G (IgG) ELISA* differentiates primary and secondary dengue and is simple and easy to perform.
- *Rapid detection test kits* are commercially available that give results in 15–25 minutes; however, the sensitivity and specificity vary and may give a false-negative result.

Probable Dengue Fever/Dengue Hemorrhagic Fever

This is a clinical description compatible with DF during an outbreak or non-ELISA-based NS1 antigen or IgM positive.

Confirmed Dengue Fever

Clinical description compatible with DF with at least one of the following:

- Virus isolation demonstrated by positive virus culture
- Positive IgM antibody titer by ELISA in a single serum sample
- Positive viral antigen in the serum sample by NS1-ELISA
- IgG seroconversion demonstrated by the fourfold increase in IgG titer in paired sera after 2 weeks
- Detection of viral nucleic acid by PCR

MANAGEMENT OF DENGUE

As dengue is a dynamic illness, management depends on the severity and stage of the illness.

Management in Febrile Phase

In this stage, the child needs only paracetamol to control fever, and nonsteroidal anti-inflammatory drugs (NSAIDs) are to be avoided. Parents should be instructed to ensure adequate hydration, which is evident by the voiding of urine more than five times in the day, and to watch for warning signs like abdominal pain or vomiting. A child without warning signs or without signs of severe dengue can be treated as an outpatient, provided the pediatrician can examine and assess the child twice a day and document the progress. The child needs to be hospitalized when he/she develops warning signs or features of severe dengue. Children with high-risk factors like younger age, comorbidities, or warning signs should be admitted to the hospital to be monitored at least 6 hourly, and vital signs are to be charted. **Figure 7.21.6** shows a model dengue monitoring chart.

Management of Dengue in the Critical Phase

While following up on the child in the hospital during the critical phase, one should watch for the following six serious problems:

1. Shock
2. Fluid overload (FO)
3. Hemorrhage
4. Organ systems failure (acute encephalopathy, AKI, ALF, and myocardial impairment)
5. Hyperferritinemic HLH
6. Infections (coinfections or secondary infection)

Management of Shock

After starting oxygen, administer isotonic crystalloid as a bolus of 10 mL/kg over 1 hour for compensated shock and 20 mL/kg over 30 minutes for hypotensive shock. Crystalloids can be normal saline or Ringer lactate. Close monitoring and continuing fluids are shown in **Flowchart 7.21.1**. Monitoring includes pulse rate, pulse volume, capillary refill time (CRT), BP, urine output (UO), respiratory rate (RR), oxygen saturation (SpO_2), liver span, level of consciousness, and HCT. The best method is to assess HCT, which is the capillary blood from a finger prick or venous blood, for immediate results within 5 minutes, which will help further in fluid management **(Fig. 7.21.7)**. Bladder catheterization will ensure hourly UO, ensuring at least 0.5 mL/kg/h. A child will need admission to a high-dependency unit (HDU) or pediatric intensive care unit (PICU), as shock may resurface even after the initial correction of shock. Serum electrolytes, urea, creatinine, transaminases, and ferritin need to be assessed periodically.

In case of nonresponse to 20–30 mL/kg boluses, consider massive plasma leakage, obvious or occult bleed, metabolic disturbances, or myocardial dysfunction, and the management options are given below:

- Colloid resuscitation with 5% albumin is preferred over synthetic colloids.
- Low-dose adrenaline starting from 0.05 µg/kg will help if the child has a component of myocardial impairment.
- Correction of metabolic abnormalities like hypoglycemia, hypocalcemia, and hyponatremia.
- If there is obvious blood loss, a packed red blood cell (PRBC) transfusion may be needed.
- If facilities are available, bedside echocardiography should be done to note for inferior vena cava (IVC) filling and myocardial depression.

Dengue Monitoring Chart

Name: Age/Sex: IP NO: Date of Admission:

Onset of Fever: NS1: IgM: CRP:

Date	Time	Temp	HR bpm	RR bpm	SpO_2	BP	Pulse volume	CRT	AVPU	Rashes	Warning signs	Intake	Output (mL/kg/hr)	PCV	Platelet	Sign

Fig. 7.21.6: Dengue monitoring chart, designed and used in our institution. (AVPU: Alert, Voice, Pain, and Unresponsive; BP: blood pressure; CRP: C-reactive protein; CRT: capillary refill time; HR: heart rate; IgM: immunoglobulin M; IP: in-patient; NS1: nonstructural protein-1; PCV: packed cell volume; RR: respiratory rate)

Flowchart 7.21.1: Fluid management in dengue shock.

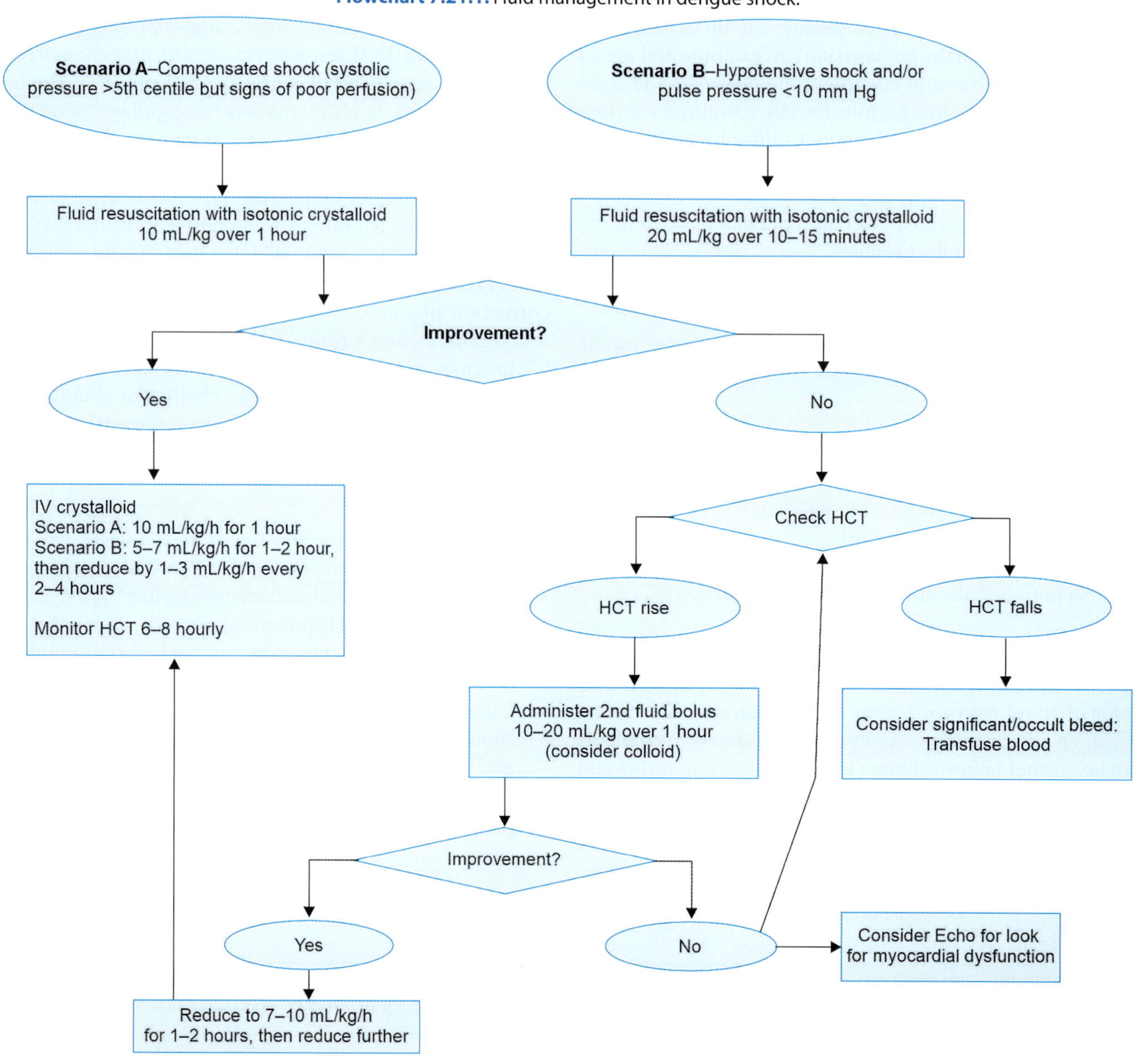

(HCT: hematocrit; IV: intravenous)

Source: Randhawa MS, Nallasamy K. Management of severe dengue. In: Pediatric Intensive Care Unit Protocols. Indian J Pract Pediatrics. IJPP Series 13.

Rethinking about the shock management charts and how restricted fluid management evolved are given in **Box 7.21.3**. The restrictive group (who received <40 mL/kg) had 53% lower mortality compared to the liberal group (who received >40 mL/kg) ($p = 0.18$).[7]

Management of FO

Capillary leak leading to puffiness of the face, pleural effusion, and pulmonary congestion, which leads to respiratory distress, and ascites results in abdominal compartment syndrome, resulting in worsening of shock and respiratory distress. FO can be calculated by the following formula:

$$FO\% = \text{Total fluid intake (L)} - \text{Total fluid output (L)/body weight (kg)} \times 100$$

Fluid overload (FO) can occur secondary to excessive intravenous fluid (IVF) administration, either as bolus or as IVF maintenance. FO should be calculated daily and also cumulative volume over the duration of the hospital stay.

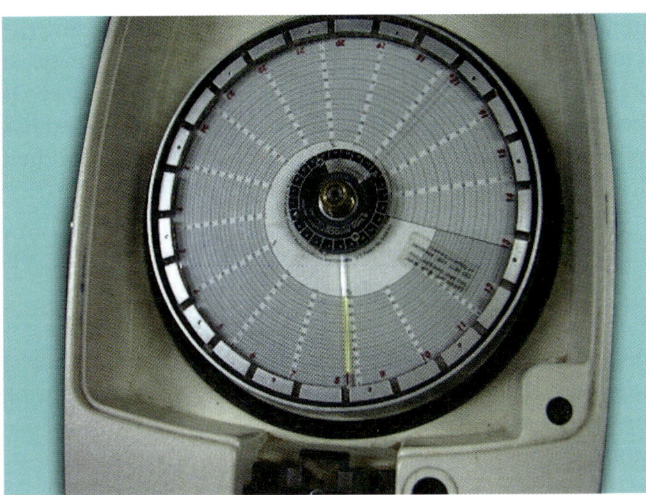

Fig. 7.21.7: Microhematocrit machine with centrifuge.

BOX 7.21.3: Restricted fluid management.[8]

Over the years, many clinicians understood the fact that fluid overload kills more children than shock, and the initial fluid volume is restricted to 20–30 mL/kg only and restricted intravenous fluids (IVF) maintenance

- Though the algorithms of shock management are very clear on paper, rechecking and tapering the fluid rate in the initial 12–24 hours do not happen in an orderly manner, unless the child is admitted to the PICU. Hence, the initial tapering rate of 7 mL/kg may be continued inadvertently for a longer period
- After a bolus of 10 mL/kg, hourly fluid administered at tapering volumes of 7, 5, 3, and 2 mL/kg means a lot. For example, if a child weighing 40 kg receives fluid in a perfect tapering method for 12 hours, the child will receive 840 + 600 + 360 + 240 mL = 2040/12 = 170 mL/h. For a 40 kg child, maintenance volume is 80 mL/h; however, with this approach, in 12 hours, the child will receive twice maintenance in 12 hours and so four times of maintenance volume in 24 hours
- This will unintentionally lead to fluid overload and related complications
- So, following a maintenance fluid calculation will be a safer one. After shock correction, the child can be started on 100%, 80%, or 70% maintenance fluid, which will be 80, 64, or 56 mL/h
- If tolerated well and the child has no abdominal symptoms, IV fluids can be stopped and oral fluids, including oral rehydration solutions (ORS), can be started

(IV: intravenous; PICU: pediatric intensive care unit)

Daily monitoring will caution against FO by restricting fluid use and early colloid or vasoactive agents. Mild FO can be managed by oxygen administration. Progressive increase in FO is managed by noninvasive (NIV) supports such as high-flow nasal cannula (HFNC) oxygen therapy, bilevel positive airway pressure (BiPAP), or invasive ventilation.

Fluid removal can be done by diuretic therapy or continuous renal replacement therapy (CRRT).

- *Diuretics:* Mainly used when the child is in the recovery phase by day 7 and not in shock by using frusemide 0.1 mg/kg as an infusion over 6 hours. Close monitoring is needed as it can precipitate shock.
- If the child is still in the critical phase or has AKI, CRRT can be used, which will remove the fluid as well as cytokines. When FO% > 10%, renal replacement therapy is warranted. CRRT is performed in only specialized centers with required skills.

Hemorrhage

In dengue, causes of hemorrhage are multiple—thrombocytopenia, platelet function disorder, coagulopathy, vasculitis, and low fibrinogen. It is more commonly seen in children with profound hypoxia and multiorgan dysfunction syndrome (MODS). It is managed by correcting hypoxia and platelet transfusion if the platelet number is <20,000, along with PRBC and fresh frozen plasma (FFP).

Organ System Impairment

Organ system impairment manifests as myocardial impairment, acute encephalopathy, AKI, and ALF.

- *Myocardial impairment:* In any child who remains in shock after 20–30 mL/kg of boluses, myocardial impairment should be suspected as obvious features of cardiogenic shock such as gallop, murmur, or hepatomegaly (which will be present in dengue) are absent. Studies do not favor the use of vasoactive agents without ECHO evaluation. Low ejection fraction (EF) and systolic and diastolic dysfunction can be identified, which are transient, and improvement will occur fast. Low-dose epinephrine intravenous (IV) infusion at doses of 0.05–0.1 µg/kg is used. In a sick child, the point of care of echocardiography will be helpful.
- *Acute encephalopathy with or without seizures:* Supportive management with antiepileptics, intracranial pressure (ICP) control measures, and mechanical ventilation are helpful strategies. As metabolic disturbances such as hypoglycemia, hyponatremia, and hypocalcemia, as well as encephalitis, intracranial bleed, and coinfection, can also cause encephalopathy, investigation and management should be extended in these lines.
- *ALF:* This can occur due to direct invasion of dengue virus, paracetamol overdose, coinfection, or hypoxic injury. ALF is managed by supportive management with *N*-acetylcysteine (NAC) infusion, ventilation, plasma exchange, ICP control, and blood products. Hyperammonemia and encephalopathy may warrant CRRT.
- *Respiratory failure (RF):* There are many reasons for a child with severe dengue to develop RF, including pleural effusion, pulmonary edema, abdominal compartment syndrome, and rarely central cause, such as acute encephalopathy. In the initial stages, standard

O_2 supplements, HFNC, or BiPAP are helpful; when they fail, invasive ventilation may be needed. A child requiring intubation is at risk of hemorrhagic complications and worsening of shock during the procedure.

- *Hyperferritinemic HLH:* Serum ferritin is found to be higher in dengue than in other febrile illnesses. Elevated ferritin levels are becoming a potential early biomarker for predicting severe dengue.[9] A typical child with dengue will go into an afebrile stage by day 5 of illness and expected to improve by day 7. If a child remains febrile and sick after day 7, there are three possible causes—coinfections, secondary sepsis, or hyperferritinemic HLH. Evolution of HLH in dengue is difficult to differentiate from uncomplicated dengue, but persistence of fever beyond day 7 of illness, fall in HCT without bleeding, persistent cytopenia, hypoalbuminemia, very high or rising ferritin levels (usually >10,000 ng/mL), and new-onset or progressive organ dysfunction may be suggestive. Coinfections are to be excluded in this situation as they are close differentials. HLH is managed by immunomodulators such as intravenous immunoglobulin (IVIg) and steroids.
- *Infections:* Coinfections such as enteric fever, malaria, leptospirosis, scrub typhus, and secondary sepsis are to be excluded, if fever persists or with a new onset of fever.

Antidengue Drug Therapy

There is no drug currently approved and at the same time, alternative medicines have to be avoided as their efficacy is unproved and safety is not established.

PREVENTION

Public health authorities are taking measures to monitor and reduce the larval density of the *Aedes* vector; source reduction of mosquito-breeding sites to control the *Aedes* mosquito population, with insecticides, indoor space spray, and fogging as well as encouraging personal protection measures such as adequate clothing and the use of mosquito repellents have benefits.[10] Several newer strategies including genetically modified male mosquitoes, sterile insect techniques, infecting mosquitoes with *Wolbachia* bacterium, and using larvivores fish and crustaceans are employed to reduce vector density. Focused surveillance with geographical information system (GIS) is one of the new strategies to identify vector foci. Using pheromones to attract and kill and insect growth regulators are also new strategies.

Vaccines Against Dengue

Vaccine development is tricky as it has to cover all four serotypes, and immune augmentation is a problem. Lack of an animal model is a major drawback in understanding the pathogenesis and development of drugs and vaccines. At present, many vaccines are under development. Dengvaxia is the only approved vaccine; however, there is an increased risk for severe dengue, especially in persons who acquired their first natural dengue infection after vaccination due to ADE.[11] So, it requires prevaccination screening for past dengue infection, and it is currently not licensed in India.

CONCLUSION

Dengue is a common arboviral infection in the South-east Asian countries and could be fatal. Meticulous monitoring and methodical treatment to stabilize the child will reduce morbidity and mortality.

REFERENCES

1. Garg S, Chakravarti A, Singh R, Masthi NRR, Goyal RC, Jammy GR, et al. Dengue serotype-specific seroprevalence among 5- to 10-year-old children in India: a community-based cross-sectional study. Int J Infect Dis. 2017;54:25-30.
2. Malavige GN, Ogg GS. Pathogenesis of vascular leak in dengue virus infection. Immunology. 2017;151(3):261-9.
3. World Health Organization. Dengue Haemorrhagic Fever: Diagnosis, Treatment, Prevention and Control, 2nd edition. Geneva: World Health Organization; 1997.
4. World Health Organization. Dengue: Guidelines for Diagnosis, Treatment, Prevention and Control. Geneva: World Health Organization; 2009.
5. Endy TP, Chunsuttiwat S, Nisalak A, Libraty DH, Green S, Rothman AL, et al. Epidemiology of inapparent and symptomatic acute dengue virus infection: a prospective study of primary school children in Kamphaeng Phet, Thailand. Am J Epidemiol. 2002;156(1):40-51.
6. Bhatt S, Gething PW, Brady OJ, Messina JP, Farlow AW, Moyes CL, et al. The global distribution and burden of dengue. Nature. 2013;496(7446):504-7.
7. Yuliarto S, Kadafi K, Anitasari D. Restrictive versus liberal fluid resuscitation in children with dengue shock syndrome: the differences in clinical outcomes and hemodynamic parameters. Int J Pediatr. 2019;7(4):9215-24.
8. Ranjit S, Ramanathan G, Ramakrishnan B, Kissoon N. Targeted interventions in critically ill children with severe dengue. Indian J Crit Care Med. 2018;22(3):154-61.
9. Soundravally R, Agieshkumar B, Daisy M, Sherin J, Cleetus CC. Ferritin levels predict severe dengue. Infection. 2015;43(1):13-9.
10. National Vector Borne Diseases Control Programme, Directorate General of Health Services, Ministry of Health & Family Welfare, Government of India, New Delhi. The National Guideline for Dengue Case Management During COVID-19 Pandemic. National Health Mission; 2020.
11. Tayal A, Kabra SK, Lodha R. Management of dengue: an updated review. Indian J Pediatr. 2023;90(2):168-77.

7.22 Rabies

Rashna Dass Hazarika

INTRODUCTION

Rabies in humans is a 100% fatal but preventable viral disease. It is spread by the bite of rabid animals but bites from a rabid dog remain the most common form of transmission. It has a variable incubation period and symptoms and signs may take months to years to develop. It is important to take preventive action as soon as animal bites occur. Wound management is important to halt the spread of the virus. Along with these effective rabies vaccines, monoclonal antibodies and immunoglobulins are available for prompt use and augmentation of therapy.[1]

EPIDEMIOLOGY

Rabies occurs in most countries except Antarctica. Worldwide estimates put the rabies deaths at 59,000–60,000 annually (most common in Asia and Africa). More than 99% of these bites are caused by dogs. In India, an estimated 20,000 deaths occur annually.[2] Children between 5 and 14 years are the most common victims. The global burden of disease study has shown a decrease in the number of rabies cases in the world from 24,744 in 1990 to 14,075 in 2019.[3] The age-standardized incidence rate (ASIR) decreased from 45.99/10,000,000 population in 1990 to 18.45/10,000,000 population in 2019. An improvement in the socio-demographic index was inversely correlated with the occurrence of rabies. The cases continue to be more in males but again with a decreasing trend in the last 30 years. Rabies has been made a notifiable disease in India in 2021.[2,4]

RABIES VIRUS

The rabies virus is a negative-stranded bullet-shaped ribonucleic acid (RNA) virus of 120 × 80 nanometer size **(Fig. 7.22.1)**. It belongs to the family *Rhabdoviridae* and the genus *Lyssavirus*. The virus is sensitive to ethanol, iodine preparations, soaps and detergents, and liquid solvents like ether, chloroform, and acetone. It is inactivated by phenol, formalin, carbon dioxide (CO_2), β-propriolactone, ultraviolet (UV), or sunlight.[4]

RESERVOIRS OF RABIES

In Africa and Asia, the reservoirs of the rabies virus are dogs, cats, jackals, wolves, foxes, and mongoose. In Latin America, rabies is mostly spread by bats, dogs, and cats. In Europe, bats and foxes are the main reservoirs, whereas in North America, bats, raccoons, shunks, and foxes spread the virus.[1]

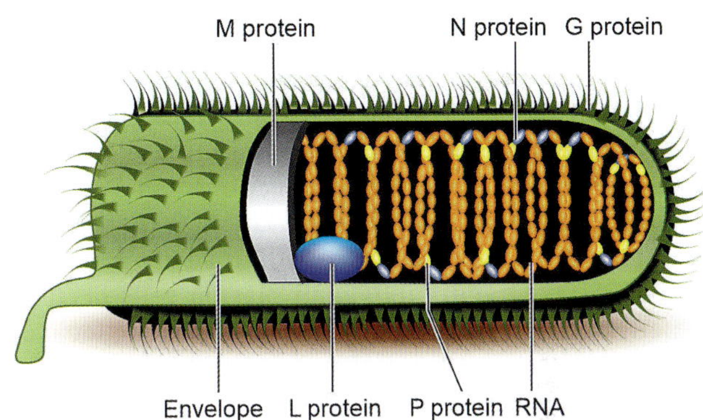

Fig. 7.22.1: Structure of the rabies virus. (G protein: glycoprotein; L protein: large RNA polymerase protein; M protein: matrix protein; N protein: nucleoprotein; P protein: phosphoprotein; RNA: ribonucleic acid)
Source: Creative—diagnostics.com.

In India, ~97% of human rabies is caused by dog bites, 2% by cats, and 1% by bites caused by mongoose, jackals, foxes, etc. Rodents, squirrels, rabbits, birds, and bats do not transmit rabies.[4]

RABIES VIRUS TRANSMISSION

The commonest mode of transmission to humans is by the bite of a rabid dog or contamination of a wound by the saliva of a rabid dog or animal. The other modes of transmission are through oral mucous membranes, conjunctiva, anus, and genitalia. The rabies virus resides in the saliva of the rabid animal. It is a neurotropic virus and after biting, the virus travels via the adjacent nerve roots to reach the spinal cord and then the brain. The multiplication of the virus then affects the function of the brainstem and causes hydrophobia, aerophobia, photophobia, and finally respiratory paralysis and death. The time (incubation period) between the bite and the onset of hydrophobia is variable depending on viral load, virulence, site, severity and route of exposure, individual host factors and host immunity, timing and standard of wound management, and rabies prophylaxis.[1,4]

PATHOGENESIS AND PATHOLOGY

After inoculation, the virus multiplies in the tissue at the site of inoculation. From here, the virus enters the peripheral nerves (both the sensory and motor nerves) through the neuromuscular junction followed by transport to the central nervous system (CNS) in the endoneurium of the Schwann cells. In the CNS, spread is rapid with the early involvement of the limbic system neurons. Rapid multiplication occurs along with centrifugal spread, especially to the salivary glands. It is during this stage of CNS multiplication and spread that the classical symptoms of rabies develop.

Occasionally, the virus may go into an eclipse phase within the host and escape detection. This phase may last for several days or months and is affected by the cell-mediated immunity generated by the virus. Pathologic changes that occur in the human host are encephalitis with myelitis. Infiltration with leucocytes, neutrophils, and plasma cells occurs in the perivascular areas. *Negri bodies* (cytoplasmic inclusion bodies suggestive of active viral replication) are typically seen in the neuronal cells, especially in the pyramidal cells of the hippocampus and Purkinje cells of the cerebellum.

CLINICAL PRESENTATION

The clinical presentation may start with a subtle tingling sensation at the site of the bite followed by nonspecific symptoms such as fever, headaches, muscle aches, loss of appetite, nausea, and fatigue. As the virus enters the CNS, the patient develops symptoms and signs of encephalitis such as irritability, agitation, confusion, hallucination, aggressiveness, and bizarre thoughts, followed by muscle spasms, abnormal posturing, seizures, and paralysis. As the spread occurs to other organs, excessive salivation and heightened sensitivity to light, sound, and touch appear. This is further followed by hydrophobia, photophobia, and aerophobia. In the last stages, the patient develops double vision, difficulty in movement of facial muscles, abnormal breathing movements, and difficulty in swallowing along with foaming at the mouth. Death can occur anytime between 2 and 10 days.[4]

The stages of rabies infection are as follows:

- *Incubation period:* 20–90 days—no clinical clue
- *Prodrome phase:* 2–10 days of nonspecific symptoms
- *Acute and late neurologic phases:* 2–7 days—features of acute encephalitis followed by hydrophobia, photophobia, etc.
- *Coma:* 0–14 days
- *Death:* Within a few days of the onset of symptoms

ASSESSMENT OF BITES

The bites need to be categorized to assess the severity of exposure and the treatment modality **(Table 7.22.1, Figs. 7.22.1 and 7.22.2)**.

TABLE 7.22.1: Categorization of bites.

Category	*Type of contact*	*Type of exposure*
I	• Touching or feeding of animals • Licks on intact skin	None (if history is reliable)
II **(Fig. 7.22.2)**	• Nibbling of uncovered skin • Minor scratches or abrasions without bleeding	Minor
III **(Fig. 7.22.3)**	• Single or multiple transdermal bites or scratches with oozing of blood, licks on broken skin • Contamination of mucous membranes with animal saliva	Severe

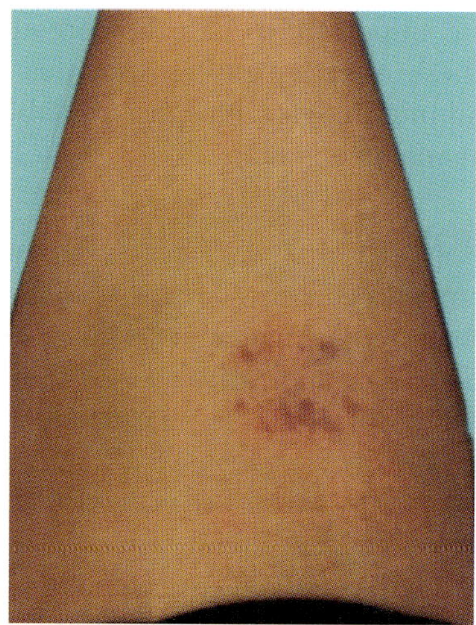

Fig. 7.22.2: Category II bite.
Courtesy: Dr MK Sudarshan, Bengaluru.

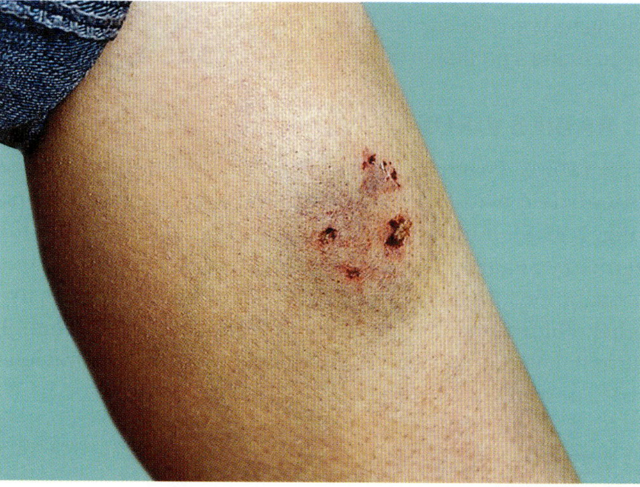

Fig. 7.22.3: Category III bite.
Courtesy: Dr MK Sudarshan, Bengaluru.

LABORATORY DIAGNOSIS

The diagnosis is mostly clinical. Laboratory tests are done to confirm the presence of the virus by the four following methods:[1]

1. *Histopathology:* Demonstration of Negri bodies in infected tissue—positive in about 71% of the cases.
2. *Virus cultivation:* This can be done by tissue culture of the infected tissue and the use of immunofluorescence (IF) to detect the rabies antigen in the tissue culture. Saliva, salivary gland tissue, and brain tissue are commonly inoculated into the laboratory mice and the infected mice's brain is examined for the presence of viruses by IF on the death of the mice.
3. *Serology:* Symptomatic patients have circulating antibodies that can be detected by enzyme-linked immunoassays. It is reported to be the most useful method for diagnosis.
4. *Rapid virus antigen detection:* This is done by incubation of infected tissue with fluorescein-labeled antibody. Usual specimens are corneal impressions, or sensory nerves from neck skin biopsy.

MANAGEMENT

Management consists of three main categories: Pre-exposure prophylaxis (PrEP), immediate postexposure treatment, and care of the rabid patient.

Pre-exposure Prophylaxis

This is done to individuals at high risk of exposure such as laboratory workers, clinicians, and other health workers attending to rabies patients, veterinarians, animal handlers, pet owners, quarantine officers, wildlife wardens, door-to-door salespersons, police and security personnel, and travelers from rabies-free areas to endemic areas. The Indian Academy of Pediatrics (IAP) recommends PrEP as an optional vaccine for children considering the large numbers of street dogs in India. The PrEP schedule includes the antirabies vaccine full dose given intramuscular (IM) or 0.1 mL intradermal (ID) on days 0, 7, and 21 or 28. Boosters are recommended only if the rabies virus-neutralizing antibody titers fall <0.5 IU/mL.[1,5]

Immediate Postexposure Treatment

This consists of two aspects—wound management and postexposure prophylaxis (PEP) with the rabies vaccine and rabies immunoglobulin (RIG) or rabies monoclonal antibody (RmAb).

1. *Wound management:* The first step is to wash the wound properly with soap and water. This reduces the viral load in the area of the bite. Local antiseptics are to be applied to prevent infection of the wound. Exposed wounds require local infiltration with RIG or RmAb. Large wounds that require suturing are infiltrated with the RIG or RmAb after a thorough cleaning. A gap of 30 minutes is allowed after wound infiltration and then the wound is sutured.
2. *PEP:* The PEP regimen depends on the exposure status of the individual. In an individual without any past exposure to the rabies vaccine, one can use the following schedule:
   - Two sites ID on days 0, 3, and 7 (Cambodia regimen)
     OR
   - One site IM on days 0, 3, 7, and between 14 and 28 days (Essen regimen)
     OR
   - Two sites IM on days 0, 1 site IM on days 7, 21 (Zagreb regimen)

   No PEP required if PEP or PrEP was received within the previous 3 months.

   In those individuals who have received the rabies vaccine before, the PEP regimens are:
   - 1 site ID on days 0 and 3
     OR
   - 4 sites ID on day 0
     OR
   - 1 site IM on days 0 and 3

   No RIG/RmAb required irrespective of category of bite.

   The treatment guidelines as per category of bite are outlined in **Table 7.22.2**.

Rabies Monoclonal Antibodies

Currently, two RmAbs are approved by the World Health Organization (WHO), Drugs Controller General of India

TABLE 7.22.2: PEP recommendations.

Category	Type of contact	Type of exposure	Recommended treatment
I	• Touching or feeding of animals • Licks on intact skin	None	No treatment if history reliable
II	• Nibbling of uncovered skin • Minor scratches or abrasions without bleeding	Minor	• Wound management • Antirabies vaccine
III	• Single or multiple transdermal bites or scratches with oozing of blood, licks on broken skin • Contamination of mucous membranes with animal saliva	Severe	• Wound management • RIG/RmAb • Antirabies vaccine

(PEP: postexposure prophylaxis; RIG: rabies immunoglobulin; RmAb: rabies monoclonal antibody)

(DCGI), as well as the IAP Advisory Committee on Vaccines and Immunization Practices (IAP ACVIP).[1,5] The first is the single RmAb (Rabishield) produced by the Serum Institute of India and the second is the cocktail RmAb (Twinrab) from Zydus vaccines. The dose of Rabishield is 3.33 IU/kg and that of Twinrab is 40 IU/kg. Both have to be administered along with the rabies vaccines.[6]

Care of the Rabid Patient

Mostly supportive care is given in the form of sedation, physical and emotional support, alleviate thirst, and intravenous sedatives such as midazolam and antipyretics.[1]

CONCLUSION

Rabies is 100% fatal but a preventable viral disease. The most common mode of transmission in India is by the bite of a rabid dog or contamination of a wound by the saliva of a rabid animal. Rapid multiplication and spread via the peripheral nerves to the central nervous system and involvement of the limbic system results in clinical signs and symptoms. Patients are usually recognized during the acute encephalitic stage, rapidly progressing to coma in a matter of 2 weeks and finally death. The clinical assessment revolves around the assessment and categorization of the bites which determines the plan of management of the cases. Management consists of pre-exposure and postexposure prophylaxis. The pre-exposure prophylaxis consists of administration of antirabies vaccine to high-risk individuals. Post-exposure prophylaxis consists of wound management by properly washing with soap and water followed by local wound infiltration with RIG or RmAb in exposed wounds. The administration of anti-rabies vaccine is done either by IM or ID route, the doses depend on the status of prior rabies vaccine exposure. For the rabid patient the only treatment available is supportive care.

REFERENCES

1. World Health Organization. WHO Expert Consultation on Rabies: Third Report; WHO Technical Report Series 1012: Geneva, Switzerland, 2018; ISBN 9789241210218.
2. Sudarshan MK, Madhusudana SN, Mahendra BJ, Rao NSN, Ashwath Narayana DH, S Abdul Rahman S, et al. Assessing the burden of human rabies in India. Results of a national multi-center epidemiological survey. Int J Infect Dis. 2007;11(1):29-35.
3. Gan H, R, Xue M, Hu H, Liu M, Cheng ZJ, Zhu Z, et al. Global burden if rabies in 204 countries and territories from 1990 to 2019: results from the Global Burden of Disease Study. Int J Infect Dis. 2023;126:136-44.
4. Sudarshan MK. Pocketbook of rabies. Kothari Medical Subscription Services Pvt. Ltd; 2020.
5. Kasi SG, Shivananda S, Marathe S, Chatterjee K, Agarwalla S, Dhir SK, et al. IAP Advisory Committee on Vaccines and Immunization (ACVIP): recommended immunization schedule (2020-21) and update in immunization for children aged 0 through 18 years. Indian Pediatr 2021;58(1):44-53.
6. Fan L, Zhang L, Li J, Zui F. Advances in the progress of monoclonal antibodies for rabies. Hum Vaccin Immunother. 2022;18(1):2026713.

7.23 Pediatric Human Immunodeficiency Virus Infection and Acquired Immunodeficiency Syndrome

Chhaya Akshay Divecha, Milind S Tullu

INTRODUCTION

Acquired immunodeficiency syndrome (AIDS) is caused by the human immunodeficiency virus (HIV), HIV-1 and 2. Children constitute 4% of the global HIV disease burden, 10% of new HIV infections, and 13% of AIDS-related deaths and have rapid progression and a high mortality. The disease has now become a chronic disorder due to the availability of antiretroviral (ARV) therapy (ART) and drugs to treat opportunistic infections (OIs). HIV infection also has social implications (especially in children, due to the demise of parents) and economic consequences.[1]

EPIDEMIOLOGY

World/Global Scenario

As per the United Nations Program on HIV/AIDS report on the global AIDS epidemic, there were 39 million adults and children living with HIV (CLHIV) or AIDS at the end of 2022, of which 1.54 million were children below 15 years of age. In 2022, an estimated 1.3 million people became newly infected, while 1,30,000 children contracted HIV (a 58% drop in the annual new infections in children globally between 2010 and 2022), mainly through transmission of the virus from their mothers during pregnancy, delivery, or while breastfeeding.

Annual AIDS-related deaths have reduced from 1.3 million in 2010 to 6,30,000 in 2022 (a decline of 51%). Childhood AIDS-related deaths have also reduced from 2,10,000 in 2010 to 84,000 in 2022 (reduction by 64%). In 2022, about 8,80,000 children under the age of 15 years (57% of infected children) received ART. In the Asia and Pacific region, there were 6.5 million people living with HIV (PLHIV) in 2022, with 3,00,000 new infections and 1,50,000 AIDS-related deaths. There were 12,000 new HIV infections in children (0–14 years).[2,3]

Indian Scenario

India has the third largest population of patients with HIV/AIDS. As of 2021, 2.4 million people in India are living with HIV, of which 65% are on ART. There were 62,970 new infections and 41,970 AIDS-related deaths in 2021 (76% decline in AIDS-related deaths since 2010). Of the total new infections, an estimated 39% are females and 8% are children. There are 70,000 CLHIV, of which 95% are on ART. New HIV infections have declined by 46% since 2010. Mizoram, Nagaland, Manipur, Andhra Pradesh, and Telangana are the states with the highest adult prevalence (%) of HIV in India. About 62% of pregnant women living with HIV received ART for prevention of mother-to-child transmission (MTCT) of HIV (2021).[4]

Modes of Human Immunodeficiency Virus Transmission

Human immunodeficiency virus infection occurs through sexual contact, parenteral exposure to infected blood or blood products, sharing of needles by drug users, or vertical transmission from the mother to child. The route of infection in the pediatric population is mostly through vertical transmission. As per 2020–2021 figures from India, heterosexual transmission accounts for 83.1% of cases (the most common), parent-to-child transmission 3.4%, infected syringe and needle use 6.3%, homosexual transmission 2.5%, blood or blood products use 0.7%, and unknown route 3.9%.[4] The final MTCT rate (including the breastfeeding period) in India in 2020 reduced to 27.4% from around 40.2% in 2010. However, it is far from the global target of 5% for breastfeeding countries. Vertical transmission can occur during intrauterine, intrapartum, or breastfeeding periods.[3,5]

The overall risk of transmission without ART and breastfeeding is about 20–25%. With breastfeeding in the absence of ART, the risk is about 30–45%. Using ART (3 ARVs) has reduced the risk of transmission to as low as 1% in nonbreastfed and 2% in breastfed children. The mechanism of intrapartum transmission is exposure to infected blood and cervicovaginal secretions during birth. Risk factors increasing the rate of vertical transmission include preterm delivery (<34 weeks), low maternal antenatal cluster of differentiation (CD4) count, high maternal viral load, symptomatic disease in mothers, >4-hour duration of ruptured membranes, intrapartum hemorrhage, and birth weight <2,500 g.

ETIOPATHOGENESIS

Etiology

Human immunodeficiency virus-1 and 2 belong to the *Retroviridae* family (genus *Lentivirus*). The HIV-1 genome contains two copies of single-stranded ribonucleic acid (RNA). At either end of the genome exist the "long terminal repeats," which contain the regulation and expression genes of HIV. The HIV genome includes three major regions:[1]

1. GAG region (encoding the viral core proteins, including p24)
2. POL region (encoding the viral enzymes, including reverse transcriptase and protease)
3. ENV region (encoding viral envelope proteins gp120 and gp41)

The gp120 glycoprotein carries the binding site for the CD4 molecule. The viral tropism for CD4+ T cells reduces the effectiveness of the host immune system. Other CD4-bearing cells include macrophages and microglial cells. After viral attachment, the gp120 and CD4 molecules undergo conformational changes, with the gp41 interacting with the fusion receptor on the cell surface. Viral fusion with the cell membrane occurs, allowing entry of viral RNA into the cell cytoplasm.[5]

Viral DNA copies are transcribed from virion RNA (viral reverse transcriptase enzyme), with duplication of the DNA copies producing double-stranded circular DNA, which is transported into the host cell nucleus and gets integrated into chromosomal DNA (referred to as "provirus," which has the advantage of latency or dormancy for a long period). The proviral DNA encodes the production of viral RNA, leading to the synthesis of viral proteins required for viral assembly. The virus-specific protease is important for HIV-1 viral assembly. The HIV-1 reverse transcriptase is error-prone leading to multiple mutations, thus creating wide genetic variation in the isolates. HIV-1 transcription is followed by translation. The RNA genome is incorporated into newly formed viral capsids with the generation of new virus particles, which then bud off from the host cell to infect other cells.[3]

Pathogenesis

Human immunodeficiency virus is lymphotropic in nature. When the mucosa serves as the portal of entry, the initial cells to be infected are the dendritic cells, which transport the virus to lymphoid tissues. In lymph nodes, the virus binds to cells expressing CD4+, primarily the helper T-lymphocytes (CD4+ T cells) and cells of the monocyte-macrophage lineage.

The infected CD4+ lymphocytes get activated in lymph nodes and proliferate (causing generalized lymphadenopathy).[1]

When HIV replication reaches a threshold (usually within a month), a burst of viremia occurs, leading to flu-like illness (fever, rash, lymphadenopathy, arthralgia, etc.). A complex immune (cellular and humoral) response is mounted by the immune system of the host, leading to control of the viremic episode in the next 2–4 months, and the patients enter a clinically silent latent phase.

The long period of clinical latency (up to 8–12 years) does not indicate viral latency but has very high virus turnover and depletion of CD4+ lymphocytes. Viral replication in infected monocytes may suggest their role as reservoirs of HIV and as effectors of tissue damage. CD8 T cells play an important role in containing the infection. During states of immunologic quiescence, a complex interaction of cytokines leads to a constant level of viral expression (especially in lymph nodes). With the progression of the disease, there is an increase in viral replication and a progressive decline in CD4 cell counts, ultimately compromising immunity and leading to OIs.[6] The progression of the disease is related to the gradual disruption of lymph nodes with loss of their ability to restrict the virus; the virus thus recirculates, producing a high level of viremia and a rapid decline of CD4+ T cells (during later stages).[5]

When compared with adults, the disease progression is more rapid in children, the immune system is more immature with higher CD4 counts, and high viremia in perinatally transmitted HIV leads to rapid progression in infants. Lymphopenia is usually only seen in older children or in those with end-stage disease. Infections such as invasive bacterial infections and *Pneumocystis carinii* (*jirovecii*) pneumonia (PCP) are more common in children, while malignancies such as Kaposi's sarcoma are more common in adults.[3]

Clinical Patterns

Three clinical patterns of HIV disease have been described in children [prior to the availability of the highly active ART (HAART)].[5]

1. *Rapid progressors or rapid disease course (15–25%):* In these, the onset of AIDS occurs within the first few months of life with a median survival time of 6–9 months (if left untreated). OIs and neurological manifestations are common. It is common in resource-poor countries.
2. *Short-term progressors or slower progression (60–80%):* The majority of those infected perinatally (intrapartum) have a median survival time of 6 years with slower progression. HIV-related illnesses develop in 3–4 years, progressing to AIDS by 6–7 years. They present clinically with recurrent bacterial infections, failure to thrive, and lymphocytic interstitial pneumonia (LIP).
3. *Long-term progressors or long-term survivors (<5%):* Few of those perinatally infected have minimal or no progression of disease with relatively normal CD4 counts and very low viral loads for longer than 8 years. Possible mechanisms for this delay in disease manifestations include effective humoral immunity and/or cytotoxic T-lymphocytic responses, host genetic factors, and infection with an attenuated or defective virus.

CLINICAL FEATURES

The HIV infection is a disease with various clinical manifestations of varying severity. Important manifestations occurring in infancy and childhood include lymphadenopathy, hepatosplenomegaly, failure to thrive, chronic or recurrent diarrhea, recurrent pneumonia, oral thrush, recurrent otitis media, tuberculosis (TB), PCP, pyrexia of unknown origin, etc. Recurrent bacterial infections, chronic parotid swelling, LIP, and early onset progressive neurologic deterioration are manifestations seen more commonly in children as compared to adults.[1,3]

World Health Organization's (2007) Clinical Staging of HIV/AIDS in Children Below 15 Years

This system is used in children proven to have HIV infection to decide the severity and to determine the need for ART. Only the common or important manifestations are mentioned below, and readers are referred to the original WHO document for a complete list:[7]

- *Clinical stage 1:* Asymptomatic or persistent generalized lymphadenopathy
- *Clinical stage 2 (mild):* Unexplained persistent hepatosplenomegaly, persistent parotid enlargement, herpes zoster, recurrent or chronic upper respiratory tract infections, etc.
- *Clinical stage 3 (advanced):* Unexplained moderate malnutrition or wasting, persistent diarrhea, persistent fever, persistent oral candidiasis, lymph node or pulmonary TB, recurrent bacterial pneumonia, bronchiectasis, etc.
- *Clinical stage 4 (severe):* Unexplained severe malnutrition or wasting, PCP, recurrent severe bacterial infections, esophageal or tracheobronchial or lung candidiasis, extrapulmonary TB, HIV encephalopathy or cardiomyopathy or nephropathy, etc.

Opportunistic Infections

With gradual deterioration of the immune system, children are at a high risk for infections from bacteria, viruses, fungi, and protozoa.[6] These OIs need to be diagnosed and treated early to prevent morbidity and mortality. Young children generally have primary infections, and owing to a lack of prior immunity, the infections often have a more fulminant course. Some important OIs are discussed here.[3,5] Some other OIs are summarized in **Table 7.23.1**.

TABLE 7.23.1: Opportunistic infections in HIV infection: Clinical manifestations, diagnosis, and treatment.

Infectious agent	*Clinical features*	*Diagnostic test(s)*	*Treatment*
Pneumocystis carinii (jirovecii)	Fever, cough, breathlessness, cyanosis, tachypnea, fine rales, etc.	• *Demonstration of trophozoite* (Wright stain) on specimen obtained by BAL or in sputum or tracheal secretion/lung biopsy • *Chest radiograph* shows interstitial infiltrates or diffuse alveolar disease • *High level of LDH*	• TMP–SMX *Alternatives:* • Pentamidine • Atovaquone • Primaquine plus Clindamycin, Dapsone + Trimethoprim (adult studies) • Steroids (adjuvant therapy)
MAC Nontuberculous, especially with low CD4 counts (*Mycobacterium avium, Mycobacterium intracellulare, Mycobacterium paratuberculosis*)	• Isolated lymphadenitis or disseminated (involvement of lungs, liver, spleen, bone marrow, and GI tract) • Recurrent fever, malaise, weight loss, night sweats, chronic diarrhea, recurrent abdominal pain, etc.	• *Isolation of organism or culture* (blood/biopsy) with typical histopathological features on biopsy of lymph node, bone marrow, or other tissues • *Associated laboratory features* such as disproportionate anemia, neutropenia, leukopenia, and raised ALP or LDH levels	• Clarithromycin or azithromycin and ethambutol • Combination of two or more drugs for at least 12 months • *Disseminated disease* needs 3–4 drugs. Third drug (rifabutin) or alternative (levofloxacin/ciprofloxacin and/or amikacin, streptomycin) given until improvement followed by two drugs
CMV (usually with severe CD4 depletion below 50 cells/mm^3) 8–10% of pediatric AIDS-defining illness	CMV retinitis, GI involvement, colitis, esophagitis, liver, lungs, pancreas, CNS, kidney, and sinuses	• *Fundoscopy:* Yellowish-white area of retinal necrosis with perivascular exudates and hemorrhage at the periphery • *GI—mucosal biopsy* and demonstration of CMV inclusion bodies • *Endoscopy:* Small confluent ulcers • *Staining* with CMV monoclonal antibodies • *Serology:* Not very useful, but negative IgG makes CMV disease unlikely CMV—antigenemia (acute or latent infection): Viral matrix protein pp65 on infected neutrophils • *Viral cultures, CMV DNA PCR* • *Congenital CMV:* Gold standard for diagnosis is a positive viral culture from saliva/urine collected within the first 21 days of life	• *Ganciclovir (6 weeks) or Valganciclovir* (6 months) for symptomatic congenital infection with neurologic involvement • *Induction with ganciclovir* followed by chronic maintenance with ganciclovir/valganciclovir for disseminated disease with retinitis and CNS involvement • *Secondary prophylaxis* is recommended following initial therapy of disseminated disease, retinitis, neurologic disease, or GI disease with relapse • *Dilated retinal check* by ophthalmologist every 6 months in children with HIV <5 years old who are CMV infected and severely immunosuppressed
Cryptococcus neoformans	• Subacute or chronic meningoencephalitis • Others—joints, bones, skin, and lungs	• In suspected first episode of meningitis—*prompt lumbar puncture* (LP) with measurement of CSF opening pressure and *rapid cryptococcal antigen assay* (or CSF India ink examination if rapid test unavailable) is recommended for diagnosis • Serum/plasma/whole-blood rapid *cryptococcal antigen assay* if LP contraindicated or not possible	• *Induction therapy:* Amphotericin B plus flucytosine • *Alternate:* Fluconazole plus flucytosine *or* amphotericin B plus fluconazole • *Consolidation therapy:* Fluconazole for 8 weeks • *Maintenance therapy:* Secondary prophylaxis with fluconazole as maintenance phase until immune reconstitution (CD4 > 200 cells/mm^3 and suppression of viral loads on ART • *Delay ART* by 4–6 weeks once treatment for cryptococcal meningitis is started; *steroids* are not recommended

Contd...

Contd...

Infectious agent	***Clinical features***	***Diagnostic test(s)***	***Treatment***
Toxoplasma gondii	• *Commonly asymptomatic*; however, congenital infections can develop visual, intellectual, or neurologic abnormalities (late sequelae) • *Symptomatic presentation* can be generalized disease (maculopapular rash, lymphadenopathy, hepatosplenomegaly, hematological abnormalities) or predominantly neurological (hydrocephalus, intracerebral calcification, microcephaly, seizures)	• *CT scan/MRI brain* (ring-enhancing lesions in basal ganglia, corticomedullary junction, intracranial granulomas, and calcification) • *IgG antibodies* in CSF, *T. gondii* PCR in CSF • *Congenital toxoplasmosis* by positive IgG with positive IgM and/or IgA, positive CSF PCR, or persistence of specific IgG beyond 12 months of age • *In suspected toxoplasmosis:* – Ophthalmologic, auditory, and neurologic examinations – Lumbar puncture – Imaging of the head	• *Pyrimethamine-sulfadiazine* (with folinic acid) • *Alternative drugs*—clindamycin plus Pyrimethamine (with folinic acid) • *Steroids* may be added in severe chorioretinitis or CNS lesions with mass effect • *Alternative:* Atovaquone, azithromycin, or TMP–SMX (studies in adults)
Recurrent bacterial infections • 20% of AIDS-defining illness in children • *Streptococcus pneumoniae, Haemophilus influenzae, Staphylococcus, Pneumococcus, Pseudomonas aeruginosa*, etc.	Bacteremia, pneumonia, meningitis, osteomyelitis, sinusitis, and skin, ear, and upper respiratory infections	• Relevant investigations are to be carried out depending upon the site of infection • All efforts should be made to isolate the causative organism	Appropriate antimicrobial therapy
Isospora belli and *Cyclospora*	• Rarer causes of chronic diarrhea • Watery (nonbloody) diarrhea, biliary disease (cholecystitis/ cholangiopathy) and reactive arthritis	• Stool examination demonstrating the acid-fast oocyst • IF • ELISA	• TMP-SMX • *Alt:* Pyrimethamine plus folinic acid • *Second-line alternatives:* Ciprofloxacin and Nitazoxanide
Cryptosporidia	• *Diarrhea* (acute/persistent) • *Other complications:* Severe malabsorption, hepatitis, pancreatitis, and cholangitis	• *Stool examination* demonstrating the acid-fast oocyst • Monoclonal antibody-based direct fluorescent assays and antigen-detection assays, PCR, and histopathology	Effective ART, Nitazoxanide, correct dehydration and electrolyte abnormalities, and nutritional support
Microsporidia	• Chronic diarrhea with weight loss • *Uncommon:* Involvement of CNS, eyes, sinus, muscle, and disseminated infection	• Stool microscopy and staining • Immunofluorescent antibody assays and PCR	• Albendazole for ocular infection • Topical fumagillin • Bicyclohexyl-ammonium (Fumidil B) ± albendazole
Giardiasis	• Acute or protracted intermittent diarrhea, fever, malabsorption, failure to thrive, malnutrition • *Extraintestinal:* Ocular, muscular, and metabolic complications; reactive arthritis	Stool specimens, duodenal fluid, or small-bowel tissue microscopy; direct fluorescent antibody (DFA) assays; soluble stool antigens using enzyme immunoassays (EIA); PCR	• Tinidazole and nitazoxanide are preferred therapies; metronidazole is the alternative • Correct dehydration and electrolyte abnormalities

(AIDS: acquired immunodeficiency syndrome; ALP: alkaline phosphatase; ART: antiretroviral therapy; BAL: bronchoalveolar lavage; CB-NAAT: cartridge-based nucleic acid amplification test; CD: cluster of differentiation; CMV: cytomegalovirus; CNS: central nervous system; CSF: cerebrospinal fluid; CT: computed tomography; DNA: deoxyribonucleic acid; ELISA: enzyme-linked immunosorbent assay; GI: gastrointestinal; HIV: human immunodeficiency virus; IF: immunofluorescence; IgG: immunoglobulin G; IgM: immunoglobulin M; IV: intravenous; LA: latex agglutination; LDH: lactate dehydrogenase; MAC: *Mycobacterium avium* complex; MRI: magnetic resonance imaging; PCR: polymerase chain reaction; TMP–SMX: trimethoprim–sulfamethoxazole)

Tuberculosis

Tuberculosis remains the leading cause of deaths among PLHIV—30% of the AIDS-related deaths reported in 2019 were due to TB.[6] CLHIV are at a higher risk for primary progressive TB, extrapulmonary TB **(Fig. 7.23.1)**, and multidrug-resistant TB. CLHIV should be regularly screened for TB during their visits for any of the following four symptoms (4S)—cough and/or fever for 2 weeks, failure to thrive/weight loss/ poor weight gain, and history of contact with a TB case. Extrapulmonary TB may present with lymphadenopathy, central nervous system (CNS) symptoms (headache and altered sensorium), joint pain/spinal deformity (bone TB), chest pain and respiratory distress (pleural/pericardial TB), or abdominal pain/swelling/discomfort (abdominal/ peritoneal TB).

Diagnosis is by X-ray chest (infiltration, hilar lymphadenopathy, pleural effusions, etc.) and rapid molecular test using cartridge-based nucleic acid amplification test (CB-NAAT) of sputum, gastric aspirate (<3 years old), gastric lavage, induced sputum, or bronchoalveolar lavage (BAL). Tuberculin skin test (TST) or Mantoux test is a useful adjunct in the diagnosis of TB—a reaction of 5 mm or more is considered positive. Extrapulmonary TB can be diagnosed using ultrasonography, fine-needle aspiration cytology (FNAC), excision/biopsy of specimen, fluid cytology, or neuroimaging (CNS TB). The interferon-gamma release assay (IGRA) is not recommended for diagnosis.

In TB-coinfected HIV children, initiation of antituberculosis treatment (ATT) is a priority and should be started first. TB preventive therapy should be offered to HIV-infected children above 12 months of age and to adolescents who are unlikely to have active TB on clinical evaluation/ national guidelines and without TB contact. However, in those below 12 months of age, only those with TB contact with a negative evaluation of TB should receive TB preventive therapy. The dose of isoniazid (INH) for preventive therapy is 10 mg/kg body weight daily for a minimum period of 6 months. INH preventive therapy should also be considered if TST is positive without active TB disease and after successful completion of ATT (6 months).

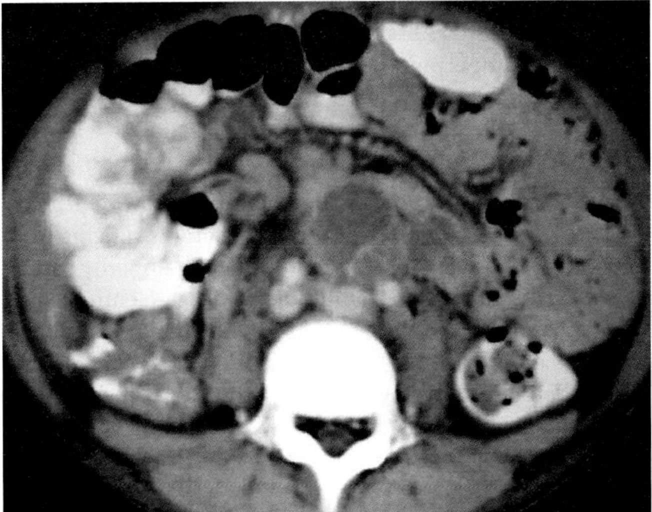

Fig. 7.23.1: *Computed tomographic scan of abdomen:* Multiple enlarged conglomerated peripherally enhancing and necrotic lymph nodes (para-aortic, peripancreatic, periportal, and mesenteric) in an HIV-infected child with abdominal tuberculosis. (HIV: human immunodeficiency virus)

Pneumocystis carinii (jirovecii) Pneumonia

This is the most common OI in infants (mortality rate up to 35%), with the highest occurrence at the age of 3–6 months (highest mortality in <1 year age).[6] The infant presents with acute-onset fever, dyspnea, tachypnea, cough, cyanosis, and marked hypoxia. The radiographic findings include interstitial infiltrates or diffuse alveolar disease (which progresses rapidly), nodular lesions, streaky or lobar infiltrates, or pleural effusions. Presumptive diagnosis is supported by clinical manifestations, radiological findings, hypoxia on arterial blood gas [partial pressure of arterial oxygen (PaO_2) typically 30 mm Hg], and high lactate dehydrogenase (LDH). Diagnosis is confirmed by demonstration of *P. carinii (jirovecii)* in induced sputum or BAL, transbronchial biopsy by fiber-optic bronchoscopy (if BAL is negative), or open lung biopsy with appropriate staining.

Treatment is with intravenous (IV) cotrimoxazole [trimethoprim (TMP)–sulfamethoxazole (SMX)] (15–20 mg/kg/day of TMP and 75–100 mg/kg/day of SMX every 6 hourly) with adjunctive corticosteroids (prednisolone or dexamethasone) if PaO_2 is <70 mm Hg (in room air). The duration of treatment is 21 days with oral TMP–SMX replacing IV drug after clinical improvement. Alternative therapy includes IV pentamidine (4 mg/kg/day). Other etiologies/coinfections or treatment failure should be considered [such as *Pneumococcus* and cytomegalovirus (CMV)] if the child fails to respond within 4–7 days of therapy.

Cotrimoxazole (TMP–SMX) prophylaxis reduces the incidence of PCP infection (6 mg/kg/day of TMP) and protects against other bacterial infections, malaria, toxoplasmosis, etc. All HIV-exposed infants should receive cotrimoxazole preventive therapy (CPT) from 6 weeks of age until HIV is reliably excluded. It is also recommended for HIV-infected children <5 years (regardless of CD4 cell count or clinical stage) and in HIV-infected children >5 years with WHO clinical stage 3 or 4 and/or CD4 <350 cells/mm^3. It may be discontinued in those ≥5 years of age with WHO stage 1 or 2 and CD4 count of >350 cells/mm^3 twice at least 6 months apart. In those HIV-infected children with TB coinfection, PCP prophylaxis should be initiated regardless of the CD4 counts and discontinued as per age-appropriate criteria. Secondary prophylaxis in children with previous infection with PCP is similar to primary prophylaxis. Cotrimoxazole is administered as a syrup or tablet at a dose of 5 mg/kg/day of TMP + 25 mg of the SMX combination once daily.

Candidiasis

Candidiasis is the most common fungal infection in HIV-infected children.[6] Oral thrush is the most common presentation, and its recurrence in infants older than 8 weeks of age is a clinical indicator for HIV. Esophageal candidiasis is an AIDS-defining condition and common in those with CD4 counts <100 cells/mm^3, neutropenia, high viral load, and coexisting oropharyngeal candidiasis. Also, extended antibiotic duration predisposes these individuals to systemic candidiasis, with severe presentations.

For oropharyngeal disease, oral fluconazole, clotrimazole troches, or nystatin suspension by mouth is recommended. Treatment for esophageal disease is oral fluconazole; amphotericin B or an echinocandin (caspofungin, micafungin, and anidulafungin) can be used if oral therapy is not tolerated. For invasive disease/critically ill patients, echinocandin such as anidulafungin/caspofungin/ micafungin is recommended treatment. For nonserious infections, IV fluconazole is recommended. *Secondary prophylaxis* is recommended for frequent or severe recurrences with fluconazole or itraconazole.

Other Opportunistic Infections

Some other OIs include *Herpes simplex* virus (HSV), *Varicella zoster* virus (VZV), Histoplasmosis, Penicilliosis (Talaromycosis), and Coccidiomycosis. Diagnosis is either by microscopy, staining, cultures, polymerase chain reaction (PCR), antigen detection, or serology. Treatment is by acyclovir (HSV and VZV) or amphotericin B and itraconazole (Histoplasmosis, Penicilliosis, and Coccidiomycosis).[6]

Organ-specific Manifestations[5]

Pulmonary or Respiratory Tract

Recurrent infections (pneumonia), complications (invasive sinusitis and mastoiditis), and bronchiectasis **(Fig. 7.23.2)** may be seen. In addition to PCP, *Streptococcus pneumoniae*, *Haemophilus influenzae*, *Pseudomonas aeruginosa*, viruses (CMV), and fungi (*Aspergillus*, *Histoplasma*, or *Cryptococcus*) can cause lung disease. Pulmonary and extrapulmonary TB are an important association.

Lymphocytic interstitial pneumonia, a noninfectious lymphoproliferative condition due to HIV-related immune deficiency, can occur in up to 25% of HIV-infected children with onset around 2–3 years of age. It is chronic with

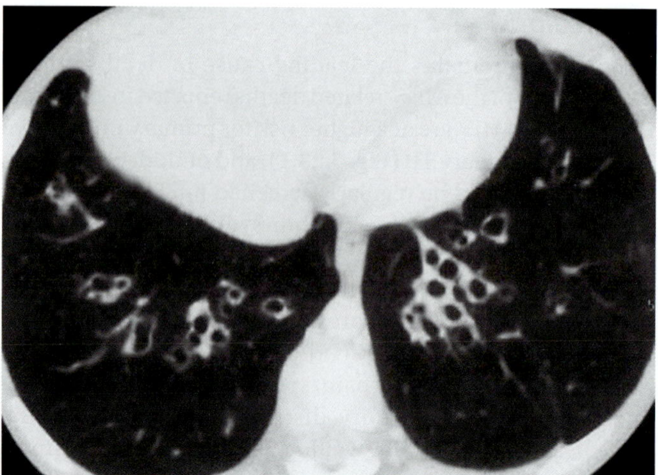

Fig. 7.23.2: *High-resolution computed tomographic scan of chest.* Note the bilateral bronchiectatic changes in an HIV-infected child (HIV: human immunodeficiency virus)

progressive alveolar capillary block due to infiltration of lymphoid cells in the lung interstitial parenchyma, alveolar septa, and lymphatics, along with pulmonary lymphoid tissue hyperplasia (PLH). It progresses with an insidious onset of cough, tachypnea, fatigue, clubbing, and hypoxia with minimal rales or normal auscultatory findings. Hepatosplenomegaly, generalized lymphadenopathy, and parotid enlargement may occur. Chest radiograph shows chronic diffuse bilateral reticulonodular infiltrates (predominantly lower zones) with hilar/mediastinal lymphadenopathy. Serum immunoglobulin (IgG) levels of >2,500 mg/dL have been observed. High-resolution computed tomography (CT) confirms interstitial involvement and monitors disease extent and severity. Severe disease is treated with systemic corticosteroids (2–4 weeks with gradual tapering); continuing at the lowest doses for 4–6 months if refractory.

Central Nervous System

Human immunodeficiency virus is neurotropic with primary CNS involvement. Neurological manifestations ranging from developmental delay to progressive encephalopathy can be caused by the virus itself, OIs, tumors, or drugs. Neuroimaging reveals cerebral atrophy, increased ventricular size, basal ganglia calcifications, leukomalacia, etc. **(Fig. 7.23.3)**. HIV encephalopathy needs early initiation of ART with drugs penetrating well in the CNS [zidovudine (ZDV) and efavirenz (EFV)]. It also helps to pick up associated CNS TB **(Fig. 7.23.4)**.

Gastrointestinal and Hepatic Manifestations

Chronic or recurrent diarrhea with malabsorption, abdominal pain, dysphagia, and failure to thrive are common

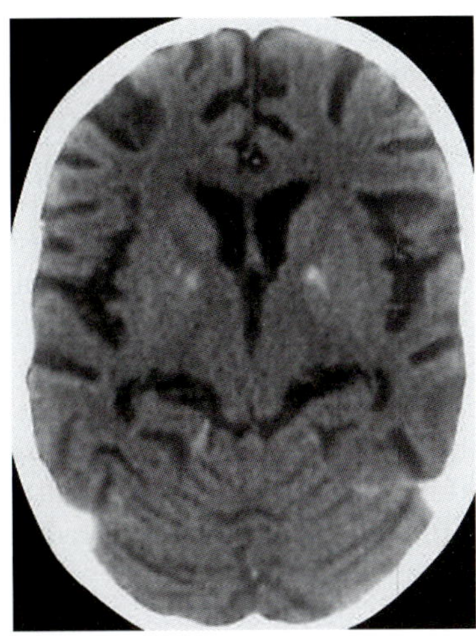

Fig. 7.23.3: *Computed tomographic scan of the brain.* Note the bilateral basal ganglia calcification, generalized cerebral atrophy, and dilatation of ventricles in a child with HIV encephalopathy. (HIV: human immunodeficiency virus)

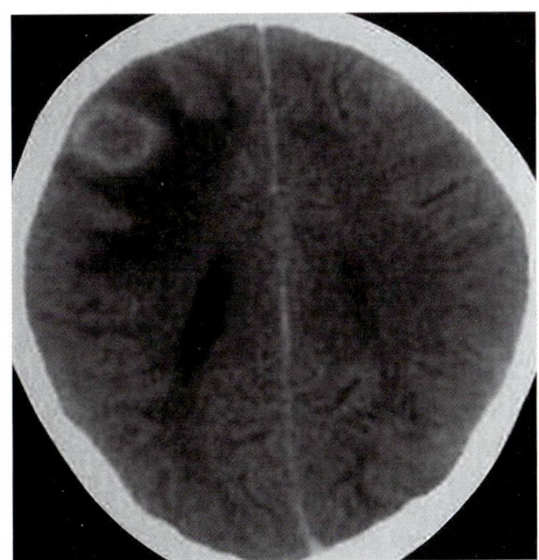

Fig. 7.23.4: *Computed tomographic scan of the brain.* Note the ring-enhancing lesion in the right frontal cortex with perilesional edema (tuberculoma) in an HIV-infected child. (HIV: human immunodeficiency virus)

gastrointestinal (GI) symptoms. Pathogens include bacteria (e.g., *Salmonella, Campylobacter*), protozoa (e.g., *Giardia, Cryptosporidium*), viruses (CMV, rotavirus), or fungi (*Candida*). Candidiasis, periodontal disease, salivary gland disease, oral hairy leukoplakia, oral ulcerations, or HIV/AIDS enteropathy can occur. Hepatitis and pancreatitis may also occur.

Cardiovascular System

Cardiac involvement can be due to prolonged immunosuppression by HIV, intercurrent infections, nutritional deficiencies, OIs, immune-mediated reactions, and drugs (ZDV). Dilated cardiomyopathy, coronary artery disease, left ventricular hypertrophy, pulmonary hypertension, arrhythmias/conduction disturbances, etc., can occur. Electrocardiography and echocardiography are helpful in assessment while treatment is supportive.

Renal Disease

Nephrotic syndrome is the most common manifestation of pediatric renal HIV disease. Renal disease can occur due to HIV infection, immune-complex-mediated, OIs, hyperviscosity, or use of nephrotoxic drugs (indinavir). Treatment consists of ART and angiotensin-converting enzyme inhibitors.

Dermatological Disorders

Cutaneous manifestations seen in HIV-infected children such as seborrheic dermatitis, severe eczema, HSV, and herpes zoster are not necessarily unique but are disseminated and less responsive to conventional therapy. HIV-related characteristic conditions include oral hairy leukoplakia, bacillary angiomatosis, and Kaposi's sarcoma.

Hematologic Disorders

Anemia (20–70%), leukopenia (one-third of untreated), and thrombocytopenia (up to 20%) are known in HIV and can be due to chronic infection, inadequate nutrition, immunologic drugs or OIs, or bone marrow suppression. ART can reverse thrombocytopenia.

Malignancies

As compared to adults, malignant diseases are uncommon in children. Non-Hodgkin lymphoma and primary CNS lymphoma are known to occur. Epstein–Barr virus is associated with most lymphomas.

Growth, Nutrition, Endocrine System, and Others

Delay in growth and puberty may be seen due to infections, abnormalities in GI and metabolic functions, drugs, ART, and malnutrition. Other metabolic abnormalities include HIV-associated lipodystrophy, lipoatrophy, hyperlipidemia, insulin resistance, hyperinsulinemia, and hyperglycemia. Other organ involvement, such as HIV arthropathy, myopathy, and rheumatologic manifestations, may be seen.

DIAGNOSIS OF HUMAN IMMUNODEFICIENCY VIRUS INFECTION

HIV Antibody Detection

Infants born to HIV-infected mothers are antibody positive (IgG) at birth (transplacental passive transfer of maternal HIV antibody), which cannot be used for definitive diagnosis until 18 months of age. Most uninfected infants lose the maternal antibody between 6 and 12 months of age (seroreverters). Rapid diagnostic tests (RDT) for HIV serology can be used to diagnose HIV infection among children older than 18 months.[5]

HIV DNA or Antigen Testing

Tests detecting HIV DNA or antigens are most useful for infant HIV diagnosis with a window period of 6 weeks post exposure. Testing for HIV-1 total nucleic acid (TNA) PCR has replaced conventional DNA PCR testing. It is a qualitative test with high sensitivity (99%) and specificity (98%) and detects viral nucleic acids from HIV RNA and proviral DNA. However, the false positivity rate increases with lower MTCT rates (<5%), which may cause wrong diagnosis and treatment.

National AIDS Control Organization Protocol for Diagnosis of HIV-1 Infection in Infants and Children

The National AIDS Control Organization's (NACO) early infant diagnosis testing protocol is applicable for *HIV-exposed infants and sick infants with clinical features of HIV infection but unknown HIV exposure status.*[7,8] HIV exposure status should be ascertained by antibody tests of the mother. The first HIV TNA PCR test for HIV-1 in dried blood spot (DBS) should be conducted at 6 weeks of age and confirmed on another DBS at the earliest if positive. If the second test is negative, another HIV-1 TNA PCR test should be done, relying on its result for a final diagnosis. If the first TNA PCR test is negative, screening for HIV antibodies is done by rapid testing at 6 months of age. Those infants testing positive on rapid testing are retested with a PCR on DBS. The TNA PCR may also be repeated earlier if the child develops symptoms. In breastfed children, retesting is done after 3 months after cessation of breastfeeding, even if initial PCR tests are negative.

Infants seen for the first time after 6 months of age are screened by HIV serology testing. If positive, PCR is performed on a DBS sample. Due to the ongoing risk of transmission by breastfeeding, HIV serology should be repeated in those with initial negative serology 3 months after cessation of breastfeeding. An age-appropriate test [TNA PCR or antibody test by enzyme-linked immunosorbent assay (ELISA)/rapid] should be performed any time a child develops symptoms.

The *final diagnosis* for all HIV-exposed children is by HIV antibody testing (all three serological tests) at 18 months of age or 3 months after breastfeeding is stopped, whichever is later. In cases of discordance (initial positive HIV TNA PCR followed by negative serology at 18 months), separate algorithms for the management of serodiscordance are applied. In symptomatic infants <6 months of age with unknown exposure, rapid testing should be performed in the mother, followed by HIV TNA PCR in the child if the mother tests positive. If the mother is unavailable for testing, the infant should be tested by HIV serology followed by HIV TNA PCR (from the same sample) if positive. Symptomatic children between 6 and 18 months of age should be tested by rapid test irrespective of the availability of the mother, simultaneously collecting a DBS sample for a nucleic acid test (NAT).

In older children >18 months, serological testing, including RDT, is used to diagnose HIV. Two consecutive positive tests in a clinically symptomatic child (suggesting HIV infection) and three consecutive positive tests in a clinically asymptomatic child are mandatory to diagnose HIV infection. In an asymptomatic child >18 months of age, two initial positive results followed by one negative result (consecutively) are reported as indeterminate HIV status requiring follow-up testing.

Presumptive Diagnosis

A presumptive diagnosis is made in patients (below 18 months) with symptoms and signs suggestive of HIV infection where virological testing is not available. A presumptive diagnosis is made when an infant is confirmed HIV antibody positive and a diagnosis of any of the AIDS-indicator conditions can be made (or if the infant is symptomatic with two or more of the following: oral thrush, severe pneumonia, or severe sepsis). Other factors supporting the diagnosis of severe HIV disease in an HIV-antibody-positive infant include recent HIV-related maternal death or advanced HIV disease in the mother and child's CD4 count below 20%. These infants can be started on ART. However, virological testing should be done to confirm the diagnosis of HIV infection as soon as possible.

MANAGEMENT OF HUMAN IMMUNODEFICIENCY VIRUS INFECTION

Though there is no cure for HIV infection, the goals of treatment are to achieve normal growth and development, prevent OIs and organ involvement, and maintain good health and an acceptable quality of life.

Antiretroviral Therapy

Antiretroviral therapy does not eradicate the virus but only suppresses the virus, thus changing the course of the disease to a chronic illness. ART should be given in consultation with an expert in pediatric HIV disease.[7,8]

Principles of Antiretroviral Therapy

It is necessary that the OIs are stabilized before initiating the ART.[6] Suppression of HIV replication to an undetectable level restricts the selection of ARV-resistant mutants. Sustainable suppression of HIV replication is best achieved by simultaneous initiation of combinations of ARV agents and adherence to complex drug regimens.

Drugs Used in Antiretroviral Therapy and Combination Therapy

The main types of ART drugs include NRTIs (nucleoside/nucleotide reverse transcriptase inhibitors), NNRTIs (non-nucleoside reverse transcriptase inhibitors), PIs (protease inhibitors), FIs (fusion inhibitors), and INSTIs (integrase inhibitors). A combination antiretroviral therapy (cART) including at least three drugs with at least two different mechanisms of action should be used initially.[7,8]

Antiretroviral agents are categorized by their mechanism of action (ability to inhibit the HIV reverse transcriptase or protease enzymes). Maximum viral suppression is possible by targeting different points in the viral life cycle and stages of cell activation and delivering drugs to all tissue sites. Thus, combination of drugs such as a thymidine analog NRTI [azidothymidine (AZT)/ZDV], a nonthymidine analog NRTI [2′,3′-dideoxy-3′-thiacytidine (3TC)-lamivudine] to suppress replication in both active and resting cells, a PI [lopinavir/ritonavir (LPV/r) or nelfinavir] or an NNRTI [EFV or nevirapine (NVP)], or an INSTI [dolutegravir (DTG) or raltegravir (RAL)] is effective. Most NNRTI and PI drugs are inducers or inhibitors of the cytochrome P450 system. There are syrup formulations of ZDV, 3TC, NVP, and EFV. Fixed-drug combinations (which help in reducing the pill burden and improving compliance) are available through the national program.

Adherence Issues

Adherence to treatment is vital to the initiation and success of ART. Compliance below 90% results in suboptimal viral load suppression. Poor adherence to ART regimens results in subtherapeutic drug concentrations and drug resistance (PIs and NNRTIs). The family or caretaker should participate in the decision to initiate ART. Education on drug administration, follow-up visits, relationship of drug adherence to viral suppression, and commitment of the family and the child are essential. Other interventions include peer counselors, mobile phone text messages and reminder devices, cognitive-behavioral therapy, behavioral skills training/medication adherence training, and once-daily and fixed-dose combinations.[7,8]

Initiation of Antiretroviral Therapy and Regimens

As per NACO guidelines, all children and adolescents living with HIV should be started on ART irrespective of their age, CD4 counts, and WHO clinical staging.[9,10] Dosing in children is dependent on body surface area/weight bands. In children <6 years and body weight <20 kg, the recommended ART is Abacavir (ABC) + 3TC + LPV/r; for those between 6 and 10 years and weight between 20 and 30 kg, the recommended regimen is ABC + 3TC + DTG; and in those >10 years and body weight >30 kg, the recommended first line is tenofovir disoproxil fumarate (TDF) + 3TC + DTG.

Children living with HIV coinfected with TB should be initiated as soon as possible on ART regardless of CD4 cell count or WHO clinical staging, within 2 weeks of starting ATT. In case of TB meningitis, ART should be delayed for at least 4 weeks but not >8 weeks of initiating management for TB meningitis (with adjuvant corticosteroids). While on ATT, children weighing >20 kg body weight and on a DTG-based regimen should continue their ART with an increased dose of DTG—50 mg twice daily for 2 weeks after the last dose of rifampicin. Those on an LPV/r-based regimen require superboosting of LPV with ritonavir (at a ratio of LPV:r as 1:1) until 2 weeks after rifampicin is stopped. No modification is required for an EFV-based regimen while using rifampicin. ART should also be initiated in all CLHIV with hepatitis B virus (HBV) coinfection regardless of CD4 cell counts, HBV viral load, or severity of liver disease. Treatment with TDF + 3TC + DTG is recommended when feasible.[9,10]

Immune Reconstitution Inflammatory Syndrome

Immune reconstitution inflammatory syndrome (IRIS) is a collection of signs and symptoms resulting from the ability to mount an immune response to antigens or organisms associated with immune recovery on ART. IRIS may present with *paradoxical* unexpected clinical deterioration in an HIV-infected patient with previously diagnosed and/or treated infection or *unmasking* of disease clinically unapparent/subclinical infections prior to ART initiation as immune function is being restored with ART. It can occur in up to 10% of all patients initiated on ART. The incidence is up to 25% in those with a CD4 count below 50 cells/mm^3. Most of these are associated with mycobacterial infections (MTB), *P. carinii*, *Toxoplasma*, *Cryptococcus*, hepatitis B and C viruses, CMV, herpes zoster, etc. It is characterized by fever and worsening of the clinical manifestations of OIs or new manifestations, typically within the first few weeks (2–12 weeks) after the initiation of ART but may also occur up to several months after initiation of ART. It is difficult to differentiate IRIS from worsening existing infection, new OI, or drug toxicity.

Immune reconstitution inflammatory syndrome may be reported for infectious, noninfectious conditions, and tumors. The most serious and life-threatening forms of paradoxical IRIS are TB, cryptococcosis, Kaposi's sarcoma, and herpes zoster. Risk factors for IRIS include lower CD4+ cell count or high HIV RNA at ART initiation and a shorter treatment duration for OIs before starting ART. IRIS is generally self-limiting, and ART should be continued in those who can tolerate it with reassurance. The unmasked OI needs to be treated, and life-threatening reactions may require a short course of corticosteroids. The incidence of IRIS may be reduced by early diagnosis of HIV and initiation of ART (before CD4 falls below 200 cells/mm^3) and screening of OIs with optimal treatment prior to ART initiation.

Changing the Antiretroviral Therapy

Antiretroviral therapy should be changed when the existing regimen is failing in an adherent child (treatment failure) as seen by an increase in plasma viral load (virological failure—persistent viral load above 1,000 RNA copies/mL seen in two consecutive viral load measurements 3 months apart after at least 6 months of initiation of ART with adherence support), deterioration of the CD4 cell count (immunological failure), or clinical failure [appearance/reappearance of WHO clinical stage 4 events (except TB) after 6 months of effective ART, progressive neurological deterioration, or growth failure]. When a decision is made to change the ARV therapy, all drugs should ideally be changed. However, in many situations (previous ART experience, intolerance, or toxicity), this may not be possible, and hence, at least two drugs should be changed based on the resistance mutation genotype or previous ART regimen. The new ART regimen should include an unused class, either DTG/ritonavir-boosted PI (LPV/r)/ NNRTI (EFV), along with one new and unused NRTI (ABC, ZDV, or TDF) along with continuation of 3TC. Failing first-line AZT-based regimen should be replaced by ABC/TDF-based regimen (TDF in children >10 years and body weight >30 kg). Children on a failing ABC/TDF-based first-line regimen should be started on an AZT-based second-line regimen (if Hb is >9 g/dL). DTG can be substituted as a third drug in second-line treatment (in >6 years and >20 kg body weight) for failing LPV/r or EFV-based first-line treatment, while LPV/r can be substituted as a third drug in a second-line regimen for EFV-based first-line treatment in children <6 years old and <20 kg weight, transitioning to DTG on reaching 6 years of age and 20 kg body weight. For children between 3 and 6 years of age and body weight between 10 and 20 kg, EFV can be substituted for failing LPV/r-based first-line regimen, while continuation of the existing regimen with monitoring may be done in children <3 years of age.[7,9]

Monitoring the Antiretroviral Therapy

People established on ART should be offered clinical visits and refills every 3–6 months, preferably 6 monthly. Clinical assessment and laboratory tests play a key role in follow-up. Serial plasma viral load monitoring is recommended in children initiated on ART at 6 and 12 months after starting ART and annually thereafter. In the case of unavailability of viral loads, CD4 counts and clinical monitoring may be used to evaluate treatment failure. Other monitoring recommended at HIV diagnosis and ART initiation includes TB symptom screening and cryptococcal antigen in children >10 years old. Optional tests are HBV and hepatitis C virus (HCV) serology, hemoglobin (if starting AZT), creatinine, and estimated glomerular filtration rate (if starting TDF).[9,10]

Toxicities of Antiretroviral Therapy

Adverse reactions to ART drugs are many and should be based on the report of the child on ART (or caregiver), history, clinical findings, or laboratory reports. Due to similar manifestations, it is necessary to rule out concurrent medications and diseases (OIs, IRIS, etc.) while considering adverse reactions to ART. Mild reaction (grade 1) requires reassurance with no change in ART; moderate reaction (grade 2) requires continuation of ART as long as possible with single-drug substitution (if no improvement occurs). Stress should be given on the need to adhere to ART despite some toxicity in both mild and moderate reactions. Severe reactions (grade 3) require substitution of the offending drug with continuation of the remaining regimen, while severe life-threatening reactions, such as Stevens–Johnson syndrome and lactic acidosis (grade 4), require immediate discontinuation of all drugs while treating the event and reintroducing a modified regimen once the patient stabilizes.

Resistance to Antiretroviral Therapy

Resistance to ART should be suspected in the case of multiple failed regimens or suboptimal viral load response to treatment. For some drugs (NNRTIs or 3TC), a single mutation is associated with resistance, while for other drugs (AZT, ABC, TDF, and most PIs), several mutations are needed to develop resistance. Testing for drug resistance is becoming the standard of care and should be done before initiating ART as well as changing ART due to failure. Treatment success is noted to be higher in patients whose ART is guided by genotype or phenotype testing.

Drug Interactions

Rifampicin reduces levels of NNRTIs and PIs. Antifungals increase levels of NVP, LPV, and saquinavir. Drug interactions of ART can also occur with oral contraceptives, lipid-lowering agents, and anticonvulsants. Amongst ART drugs, EFV is not used with NVP, NVP should not be used with atazanavir (ATV)/r, and LPV/r requires dose adjustments when used with NVP.

Monitoring

Monitoring is required in patients on ART and even those not on ART. A complete hemogram, liver functions, urine and stool examination, fundoscopy, echocardiography, and height should be done at least annually. Additional investigations may be required depending on the symptomatology, suspected OIs, and organ involved. Checking the immunization status and looking for symptoms of OIs is required at each visit. It should be ensured that the child is on cotrimoxazole prophylaxis, and concomitant medications should be noted. Assess criteria for ART initiation at every visit and reassess family situation.[9,10]

Counseling

Disclosure of HIV-positive status of self or parents or caregivers should be done in children of school age (6–12 years old). Younger children should be gradually prepared for disclosure by incremental updating of their status, adapting to their cognitive skills and emotional maturity. Counseling the parents or caretakers about the disease, course of illness, and therapy is of utmost importance in treatment. Starting ART is not an emergency, and adherence should be ensured.

Immunization, Nutrition, and Supportive Treatment

Immunization is an important mode of preventing infections. In general, HIV-exposed infants, children and adolescents with HIV should receive all routine vaccinations according to national recommendations. Live vaccines (varicella and measles–mumps–rubella) are contraindicated in severely immunocompromised HIV-infected children. Inactivated or killed vaccines should be preferred to live vaccines, and supplemental doses or revaccination may be needed after ART-induced immune reconstitution. Asymptomatic infants living with HIV may be given an inactivated polio vaccine or a bivalent oral polio vaccine.

Bacillus Calmette-Guérin (BCG) can be given to asymptomatic neonates of unknown HIV status born to HIV-infected mothers. In HIV-infected infants and children, BCG is delayed until ART is initiated and the child is clinically well and immunologically stable (CD4 <25%) while for those on ART but not received BCG earlier can be vaccinated once immunologically and clinically stable. All can receive diphtheria, tetanus, and pertussis (DTP) containing vaccines. Measles vaccination can be given to asymptomatic children with HIV and in symptomatic HIV infection, if without severe immunosuppression. Besides the national immunization schedule, additional vaccines such as Hib, inactivated influenza vaccine, pneumococcal, varicella, and inactivated hepatitis A vaccine are also recommended. Seroconversion should be confirmed after hepatitis B vaccination, with boosters if required.[8,9]

Current WHO-recommended COVID-19 vaccines are safe for PLHIV. However, immunizations may not always offer adequate protection in HIV-infected children.[7,8] Counseling and psychosocial support are the cornerstone for the management of HIV-infected children, irrespective of ART. The caretakers should be counseled about the importance of good handwashing, avoiding raw or undercooked food (to prevent *Salmonella* infection), avoiding drinking or swimming in lake or river water or being in contact with young farm animals (to prevent *Cryptosporidium* infection), and the risk of playing with pets (to prevent *Toxoplasma gondii* from cats). Simple interventions, such as good general hygiene (including food and water), dental care, adequate nutrition (including nasogastric and parenteral nutrition, if required), balanced diet, timely immunizations, vitamin A supplementation, counseling about micro- or macronutrient deficiency, using locally available nutritious foods, plotting weight and height on growth charts, provision of a safe and stimulating environment, developmental evaluation, and interventions, such as occupation therapy or speech therapy, etc., can help a child with HIV to be free of infections and grow well. Nutritional assessment and growth monitoring should be done in infants (monthly) and children (3 monthly). In asymptomatic patients, energy intake should be increased by 10% of recommended dietary allowance, while in symptomatic patients, it should be increased by 20–30%. In severely malnourished patients, 50–100% additional energy is required. The WHO recommends an average of 60 minutes of moderate to vigorous physical activity per day, vigorous and strengthening activities at least three times per week and a limitation of time spent in sedentary activities.[7,8]

PROGNOSIS

Better understanding of the pathogenesis with availability and access to healthcare and medications, including effective ART, has considerably changed the outcomes. In developed countries, the progression of HIV to AIDS and mortality rate have decreased, with improved quality of life. Even with a partial decrease in the viral load, children have significant clinical and immunologic advantages. High viral load (>1,00,000 copies/mL) or CD4 lymphocyte percentage of below 15% is associated with higher mortality and morbidity.

In developing countries with limitations of ART availability and diagnostic tests, a clinical staging system can be used to predict disease progression. Lymphadenopathy, splenomegaly, hepatomegaly, LIP, and parotitis are indicators of a comparatively better prognosis. Children with OIs [PCP or *Mycobacterium avium* complex (MAC)], encephalopathy, or severe wasting syndrome have poor prognosis (75% die before 3 years of age). Persistent fever with or without oral thrush, serious bacterial infections (meningitis, pneumonia, and sepsis), hepatitis, and persistent anemia (<8.0 g/dL) with or without thrombocytopenia (<1,00,000/mm^3) also suggest a poor prognosis.

PREVENTION

Prevention of Perinatal Transmission

Mother-to-child transmission of HIV (during pregnancy, labor or delivery, or after delivery through breastfeeding) is a significant contributor to the HIV pandemic, accounting for 10% of new infections globally. Prevention of perinatal transmission from mother to child has been achieved (to as low as 2%) by effective access to HIV testing and counseling, initiation of lifelong ART with support for adherence and retention, viral suppression for mothers living with HIV, safe delivery practices, optimal infant feeding practices, and access to postnatal ARV prophylaxis for infants. In some situations, the mother may be counseled about the potential benefit of a cesarean section to reduce the risk for vertical transmission. As the coverage of ARV medicines in pregnant HIV-infected women to prevent perinatal transmission has increased from 47% to 82% since 2010, so have the new infections in children declined by 58% during the same period.

National Guidelines for Prevention of Perinatal Transmission

The use of ARV drugs during pregnancy and breastfeeding is advocated for maternal health, prevention of infection in the exposed baby, and reduction of sexual transmission. National guidelines recommend lifelong ART to all pregnant and breastfeeding women, irrespective of WHO clinical stage or CD4 counts. The preferred first-line therapy in mothers is TDF + 3TC + DTG. Infant prophylaxis is another component of prevention of parent-to-child transmission (PPTCT). The NACO recommends that all infants born to HIV-infected mothers should receive ARV prophylaxis starting immediately after birth or at the first healthcare encounter.[9,10] In high-risk infants (born to HIV-infected mothers not receiving ART, viral loads unavailable/not suppressed in mother between 32 weeks of pregnancy and delivery, or mother newly diagnosed postpartum within 6 weeks of delivery), dual prophylaxis with AZT (twice daily) and NVP (once daily) should be given for the first 6 weeks of life in exclusive replacement feeding (ERF) and 12 weeks in exclusive breastfeeding (EBF). Low-risk infants [born to mothers with suppressed plasma viral loads (<1,000 copies/mL) assessed between 32 weeks of pregnancy and delivery] should receive NVP (once daily) or AZT (twice daily) until 6 weeks of age, irrespective of feeding practices (breastfed or formula-fed). If AZT syrup is unavailable, syrup NVP should be used for the first 14 days after birth, followed by syrup LPV/r until 6 weeks (ERF) or 12 weeks in EBF.

Human Immunodeficiency Virus and Breastfeeding

Since HIV is known to be transmitted through breastfeeding, it is necessary to balance HIV prevention (by omission of breastfeeding) with protection from other causes of childhood mortality. National guidelines recommend that HIV-infected mothers should exclusively breastfeed for the first 6 months, continue breastfeeding for at least the first 12 months of life, and may extend breastfeeding until 24 months or longer with good ART adherence. Reassurance that breastfeeding of durations <12 months is better compared to never initiating breastfeeding at all should be offered. Breastfeeding is made safe by providing ART to the mother and ARV prophylaxis to the baby. It should stop only when infants can be provided with nutritionally appropriate and safe replacement feeds. For those on replacement feeding, it is necessary to ensure safe water and good sanitation, sufficient supply for normal growth and development, adequate hygiene (to prevent diarrhea and malnutrition), family support, and access to comprehensive child healthcare. (It should follow the AFASS criteria—Acceptable, Feasible, Affordable, Safe, Sustainable). Though EBF is recommended, in a setting of mixed feeding, mothers can be reassured that breastfeeding need not be stopped if they are on ART.

Other Measures

Early identification of mothers with HIV can be ensured by recommended prenatal visits and pregnancy care followed by proper adherence counseling. In addition, screening for sexually transmitted infections, nutritional support, and counseling about infant feeding and family planning should be provided. Rapid HIV testing should be provided to women in labor/immediate postpartum with unknown HIV status to enable early ART/infant prophylaxis if tested positive. Also, mothers at a higher risk of treatment failure/perinatal transmission should be identified by conducting viral load at 34–36 weeks of gestation (latest at delivery) and in all breastfeeding women 3 months postdelivery and 6 monthly thereafter (to detect viremia during the postnatal period). Due to the high risk of acquiring HIV during pregnancy, HIV testing should be repeated in the third trimester, postpartum, and/or during labor in HIV-negative pregnant mothers.

Deliveries should be conducted in a facility with trained skilled birth attendants, avoiding unnecessary instrumentation or premature rupture of membranes and following universal precautions. In HIV-exposed infants, at birth, the baby's mouth and nostrils should be wiped as soon as the head is delivered; infants should be handled with gloves until all blood and maternal secretions are washed off; and the cord should be clamped soon after birth (avoid milking). Postdelivery, appropriate follow-ups, linkages to treatment, and postpartum care should be ensured. Infants should be provided with initial care during the first immunization visit at 4–6 weeks of age (reinforce safe feeding practices, early infant diagnosis, and ARV coverage), while mothers should be reviewed for postpartum checkup, family planning advice, and review of ARV therapy and adherence.

Indian Initiatives

The Government of India setup the National AIDS Control Program (NACP)-I in 1992 and the NACO.[9,10] Through its 36 State/Union Territory/District AIDS Prevention and Control Societies (SACS) and various nongovernmental organizations (NGOs), NACO reaches out to the population and enables preventive programs at the state, district, and village levels. Subsequent phases of NACP were introduced—NACP II in 1999, NACP III in 2007, NACP IV in 2012, NACP IV (extension phase) from 2017 to 2021, and NACP V phase (2021 to 2026, currently under implementation). NACP V aims at 95-95-95 by 2025 (i.e., 95% of estimated people with HIV know their HIV status, 95% of those who know their HIV status are on ART, and 95% of those accessing ART have suppressed viral load). These goals are directed toward global targets of achieving "End of AIDS" by 2030. The HIV and AIDS (Prevention and Control) Act, 2017 provides for safeguarding human rights, legal rights, and reinforcing constitutional rights of the PLHIV, coming into force from September 10, 2018.[4,]

REFERENCES

1. Hayes EV. Human immunodeficiency virus and acquired immunodeficiency syndrome. In: Kliegman RM, St Geme III JW, Blum NJ, Shah SS, Tasker RC, Wilson KM, Behrman RE (Eds). Nelson Textbook of Pediatrics, 21st edition, Vol. 1. Philadelphia: Elsevier; 2020. pp. 1778-805.
2. Selik RM, Mokotoff ED, Branson B, Owen SM, Whitmore S, Hall HI. Revised surveillance case definition for HIV infection—United States, 2014. MMWR. 2014;63(RR-03):1-10.
3. UNAIDS. (2023). The path that ends AIDS: 2023 UNAIDS global AIDS update. Joint United Nations Programme on HIV/AIDS 2023. [online] Available from https://www.unaids.org/en/resources/documents/2023/global-aids-update-2023. [Last accessed November, 2024].
4. Ministry of Health and Family Welfare. Training Modules (1-4) for Programme Managers and Medical Officers. New Delhi, India: Central TB Division, MoHFW, Government of India; July 2020. [online] Available from http://www.tbcindia.gov.in. [Last accessed November, 2024].
5. Divecha CA, Tullu MS. HIV and acquired immunodeficiency syndrome. In: Gupta P, Menon PSN, Ramji S, Lodha R (Eds). PG Textbook of Pediatrics, 3rd edition. New Delhi: Jaypee Brothers Medical Publishers; 2022. pp. 1544-63.
6. Panel on Opportunistic Infections in Children with and Exposed to HIV. Guidelines for the prevention and treatment of opportunistic infections in children with and exposed to HIV. Department of Health and Human Services. [online] Available from https://clinicalinfo.hiv.gov/sites/default/files/guidelines/documents/pediatric-oi/guidelines-pediatric-oi.pdf. [Last accessed November, 2024].
7. World Health Organization. Updated Recommendations on First-Line and Second-Line Antiretroviral Regimens and Post-Exposure Prophylaxis and Recommendations on Early Infant Diagnosis of HIV: Interim Guidelines. Supplement to the 2016 Consolidated Guidelines on the Use of Antiretroviral Drugs for Treating and Preventing HIV Infection. Geneva: World Health Organization; 2018. [online] Available from https://apps.who.int/iris/bitstream/handle/10665/277395/WHO-CDS-HIV-18.51-eng.pdf?sequence=1&isAllowed=y. [Last accessed November, 2024].
8. World Health Organization. Consolidated Guidelines on HIV Prevention, Testing, Treatment, Service Delivery and Monitoring: Recommendations for a Public Health Approach. Geneva: World Health Organization; 2021. Update to 2nd edition. [online] Available from https://www.who.int/publications/i/item/9789240031593. [Last accessed November, 2024].
9. National AIDS Control Organization. (2021). National Guidelines for HIV Care and Treatment, 2021. New Delhi: NACO, Ministry of Health & Family Welfare, Government of India. [online] Available from https://naco.gov.in/sites/default/files/National_Guidelines_for_HIV_Care_and_Treatment_2021.pdf. [Last accessed November, 2024].
10. National AIDS Control Organization. (2022). Sankalak: Status of National AIDS Response, 4th edition. New Delhi: NACO, Ministry of Health and Family Welfare, Government of India. [online] Available from https://naco.gov.in/sites/default/files/Sankalak_Report_1.pdf. [Last accessed November, 2024].

7.24 Malaria

Kakali Roy, Ritabrata Kundu

INTRODUCTION

Malaria is a major public health problem in developing countries. More than 1,70,000 cases of malaria are reported annually, of which >50% are due to *Plasmodium falciparum*, which has been rising in recent years. The magnitude of the problem is further enhanced by the resistance of *P. falciparum* to standard antimalarial drugs, particularly chloroquine. The important contributing factors to drug resistance are population movement, infrastructure deficiency, deforestation, unplanned development, drug pressure, and haphazard use of drugs. Drug pressure is the single most important factor in the development of resistance, followed by presumptive antimalarial treatment.

ETIOLOGY

Malaria is caused by the protozoan parasite of the genus *Plasmodium* through the bite of a female *anopheles* mosquito. The four *Plasmodium* species that infect humans are *P. falciparum*, *Plasmodium vivax*, *Plasmodium ovale*, and *Plasmodium malariae*, of which the first two are the main causative agents in our country. Malaria is not seen 2,000 m above the mean sea level and thrives in high humidity with ambient temperatures between 20 and 30°C.

CLINICAL FEATURES

Fever is the most important feature of malaria. The symptom complex is nonspecific and may mimic other diseases with fever. *P. vivax* malaria may cause a well-defined febrile paroxysm with chills and rigor every alternate day, while *P. falciparum* malaria may cause erratic fever without a definite paroxysm. Fever is often accompanied by headache, nausea, vomiting, aches and pains in muscles and joints, chills, and lassitude. In endemic areas, the diagnosis of malaria on the basis of symptoms alone invariably leads to overdiagnosis due to their nonspecificity. If not diagnosed in time, the parasite burden, particularly in falciparum malaria, may increase, leading to severe malaria often in a few hours. Severe malaria, if left untreated, has mortality of nearly 100%, but timely adequate supportive care and specific antimalarial therapy can reduce around 80% of deaths.

Severe malaria is characterized by one or more of the following clinical or laboratory features:

- Impaired consciousness or nonarousable coma
- Prostration so that the patient is unable to walk or sit up without assistance
- Failure to feed
- Multiple convulsions, more than two episodes in 24 hours
- Deep breathing, respiratory distress (acidotic breathing)
- Circulatory collapse or shock, systolic blood pressure <50 mm IIg in children
- Clinical jaundice plus evidence of another vital organ dysfunction
- Hemoglobinuria
- Abnormal spontaneous bleeding
- Pulmonary edema (radiological)

The *laboratory features* include:

- Hypoglycemia (blood glucose <40 mg/dL)
- Metabolic acidosis (plasma bicarbonate <15 mmol/L)
- Severe normocytic anemia [hemoglobin <5 g/dL, packed cell volume (PCV) <15%]
- Hyperparasitemia (>2% or 1,00,000/mL)
- Renal impairment (serum creatinine >3 mg/dL)
- Hyperlactatemia (serum lactate >5 mmol/L)

Though all manifestations of severe malaria may be seen in children, the most common are cerebral malaria, severe anemia, respiratory distress due to acidosis, and hypoglycemia. Convulsions are common in children, and symptoms preceding coma are very brief, that is, 1–2 days. Generalized seizures are the most common feature of cerebral malaria in children. Repeated seizures more than two in a 24-hour period may occur. The most common neurological feature is symmetrical upper motor neuron lesions. Severe anemia with hepatomegaly, gallop rhythm, and heart failure are common. Indrawing of the lower chest wall, without any localizing sign in the chest, suggests metabolic acidosis and is seen in malaria with severe anemia and dehydration. Hypoglycemia often presents with convulsions or coma.

Relapse of Malaria

In *P. vivax* malaria, there may be reappearance of symptoms with asexual parasitemia after resolution of primary infection, due to persistence of hypnozoites in the liver. The inert hypnozoites in the liver start a fresh cycle. Relapse may occur after weeks to years following resolution of the primary infection. As *P. falciparum* malaria does not have hypnozoites, there is no relapse in falciparum malaria.

Recrudescence of Malaria

Adequate or incomplete treatment may result in the persistence of few erythrocytic forms of parasites in the circulation. With time, they multiply and cause recurrence of asexual parasitemia of the same genotype with reappearance of symptoms; this is especially seen in falciparum malaria, which can occur within 2–3 months following treatment.

DIAGNOSIS OF MALARIA

All efforts should be made to diagnose malaria before commencing treatment. However, in complicated malaria or malaria with danger signs, presumptive treatment may be started after collecting blood for examination.

Microscopic Diagnosis

Light microscopy of well-stained thick and thin films by a skilled microscopist has remained the "gold standard" for diagnosis. Thick films are nearly 10 times more sensitive for the diagnosis of malaria as a larger amount of blood is there in a given area compared to thin films. Species identification is better with thin films as the morphology of the parasite and red blood cells (RBCs) is well preserved.

Sample collection should be done as soon as malaria is suspected. It can be collected at any time, irrespective of fever, and not necessarily only at the height of fever. Collection should be done before the administration of antimalarials, as they cause detection of parasites difficult due to their morphologic alteration.

Smear should be prepared immediately after collection or within 2 hours from anticoagulant-mixed blood, which enables better film adhesion to the slide and causes minimal distortion of parasites and RBCs.

Rapid Diagnostic Tests

Rapid diagnostic tests (RDTs) are immunochromatographic tests to detect *Plasmodium*-specific antigens in a blood sample. They employ monoclonal antibodies directed against targeted parasite antigens, namely *histidine-rich protein II (HRP-II)* and *parasite lactate dehydrogenase (pLDH),* in currently available RDTs. In our country, where falciparum and vivax malaria parasites cocirculate, typically occurring as a single species infection, an RDT that can detect both falciparum and vivax malaria and distinguish between them is warranted.

Laboratory confirmation of malaria is an essential component of disease management. The National Drug Policy of Malaria (2013) asks all fever cases suspected to have malaria go for confirmation either by RDT or by microscopy.[1] Expert microscopic diagnosis is available at central levels of the healthcare system, such as metro cities, but is often unreliable or unavailable in areas with poor health facilities. So, RDT will be useful in the following situations in our country:

- In faraway communities with poor healthcare facilities where microscopic diagnosis is not available and in areas where laboratory service is inadequate, of an unacceptable standard, or not available at odd hours.
- In places where quality microscopy is available, RDT and microscopy can run in parallel. RDT will provide rapid or screening diagnosis, whereas microscopy is reserved for resolution of confusing cases and confirmation of negative results in RDT with high clinical suspicion of malaria.
- The advantage of RDT is that it can be done in remote places by an unskilled health worker with minimal training.

Even after successful therapy, HRP-II antigen persists at detectable levels for >28 days whereas pLDH rapidly falls to an undetectable level following effective treatment but is expressed in gametocytes, which may appear after clinical infection is cleared. So RDTs are not useful for monitoring the response to treatment, for which microscopy is the investigation of choice.

Other Methods of Diagnosis

Other diagnostic methods, namely microscopy using fluorochromes on centrifuged blood specimens, molecular probes, polymerase chain reaction (PCR), and serology, are available. Unfortunately, they are not suitable for routine disease management and do not have wide field applications. Their use is currently for only research and epidemiological purposes.

MANAGEMENT OF UNCOMPLICATED MALARIA IN CHILDREN

Malaria in children has some unique features. Young children <5 years of age, whose passive immunity wanes and who have not developed sufficient immunity of their own, are most vulnerable. Falciparum malaria can be rapidly progressive, leading to rapid clinical deterioration; hence, this group needs constant monitoring. Children can tolerate antimalarial drugs better than adults, and their symptoms resolve more quickly following successful treatment.

The malaria parasite develops resistance to drugs randomly due to de novo genetic mutations. Nonimmune patients of our country are infected with a large number of parasites, and if they receive inadequate treatment, they become potent sources of de novo resistance. Here lies the importance of prescribing a highly effective treatment regimen in hyperparasitemic patients and ensuring good adherence to prescribed drugs.

It has been noted that monotherapy in the case of resistant falciparum malaria invariably results in failure. Sulfadoxine-pyrimethamine (SP) introduced following chloroquine resistance was ineffective in the early 1980s. Similarly, mefloquine (MQ) introduced as monotherapy took only 4–5 years to report resistance. So, to counter the threat of resistance of falciparum to monotherapy, the World Health Organization (WHO) recommends combinations of antimalarials for the treatment of falciparum malaria.[2]

Status of Drug Resistance in India

In India, the first reports of resistance of *P. falciparum* to chloroquine came from Diphu of Karbi Anglong district in Assam. Thereafter, it started spreading throughout the country. There are reports of resistance to SP at various levels in districts of seven northeastern states. Though few reports of the emergence of chloroquine-resistant *P. vivax* are there, the drug still retains its effectivity against vivax malaria in our country.

Antimalarial Combination Therapy

The WHO recommends a combination of antimalarials for the treatment of falciparum malaria to improve treatment outcomes and halt the threat of resistance to monotherapy.[2] Antimalarial combination therapy is the simultaneous use of two or more blood schizonticidal drugs with independent modes of action and unrelated biochemical targets in the parasite. If a mutant parasite arises de novo during the course of infection with one drug, it will be killed by the other drug. However, to reap the benefit of combination therapy, the partners in the combination should be individually effective. This mutual protection will prevent or at least delay the emergence of resistance to individual drugs. The only disadvantage of combination therapy is an increased risk of adverse effects and increased cost of therapy.

According to the WHO, one of the partners in combination therapy will be artemisinin and its derivatives, hence known as artemisinin-based combination therapy (ACT).[2] The reason for choosing artemisinin is its rapid clearance of parasitemia and resolution of symptoms. They reduce the parasite number by approximately 10,000-fold (10^4) in each asexual cycle. The second important reason is its rapid elimination from the body, so that the residual concentration of the drug does not provide a selective filter for resistant parasites. The other reasons include its lack of serious adverse effects and absence of significant resistance until date. It has also the advantage of reducing gametocyte carriage and thus transmission of malaria, which is particularly important in malaria control.

If artemisinin is combined with other rapidly eliminated antimalarials like tetracycline or clindamycin, a 7-day course of treatment is required. This long course invariably results in poor adherence, but when combined with slowly eliminated antimalarials, such as SP, MQ, or lumefantrine, shorter courses of treatment (3 days) will be effective and also ensure adherence. Slowly eliminated partner drug persists at parasiticidal concentrations until all the infecting parasites have been killed.

The following ACTs are currently available in our country:

- Artesunate (AS) + SP
- AS + MQ
- Artemether–lumefantrine

Of these, artemether–lumefantrine is available as coformulated tablets, and lumefantrine is not available as monotherapy. Other combinations are available separately.

TREATMENT REGIMEN OF UNCOMPLICATED MALARIA

Treatment regimens are to be tailored specifically according to the resistance pattern of the region under consideration. According to the National Vector Borne Disease Control Program, all falciparum cases may be treated with ACT in both public and private healthcare systems to win the war against ongoing drug resistance.[1]

Different treatment regimens in different parts of the country are shown in **Boxes 7.24.1 to 7.24.3**.

MANAGEMENT OF SEVERE MALARIA IN CHILDREN

Severe life-threatening malaria is nearly always due to *P. falciparum*. All cases with severe manifestations are to be treated in the same line of complicated malaria with

BOX 7.24.1: Recommended treatment of uncomplicated *Plasmodium vivax* malaria.

Recommended treatment

Chloroquine 10 mg base/kg stat orally followed by 5 mg/kg at 6, 24, and 48 hours (total dose 25 mg/kg)

OR

Chloroquine 10 mg base/kg stat orally, followed by 10 mg/kg at 24 hours and 5 mg/kg at 48 hours (total dose 25 mg base/kg)

Primaquine should be given in a dose of 0.25 mg/kg once daily for 14 days to prevent relapse

I. Chloroquine should not be given in an empty stomach and high fever. Temperature should be brought down first. If vomiting occurs within 45 minutes of a dose of chloroquine, that particular dose is to be repeated after taking care of vomiting by using an antiemetic (domperidone or ondansetron)
II. As primaquine can cause hemolytic anemia in children with G6PD deficiency, they should be preferably screened for the same prior to starting treatment. As infants are relatively G6PD deficient, it is not recommended in this age group, and children with a 14-day regimen should be under close supervision to detect any complications. In cases of borderline G6PD deficiency, a once-weekly dose of primaquine 0.6–0.8 mg/kg is given for 6 weeks

(G6PD: glucose-6-phosphate dehydrogenase deficiency)

BOX 7.24.2: Recommended treatment of uncomplicated *Plasmodium falciparum* malaria in all states other than the northeastern states of India.

Recommended treatment

Artesunate 4 mg/kg of body weight orally once daily for 3 days and a single administration of SP as 25 mg/kg of sulfadoxine and 1.25 mg/kg of pyrimethamine on day 1

OR

Artesunate as above and mefloquine 25 mg/kg of bodyweight in two divided doses (15 and 10 mg/kg) on days 2 and 3

OR

Coformulated tablets containing 20 mg of artemether and 120 mg of lumefantrine can be used as a six-dose regimen orally twice a day for 3 days

- For 5–14 kg body weight, one tablet at diagnosis, again after 8–12 hours, and then twice daily on days 2 and 3
- For 15–24 kg body weight, the same schedule with two tablets
- For 25–35 kg body weight and above, the same schedule with three and four tablets

I. A single dose of primaquine (0.75 mg/kg) is given for gametocytocidal action. Currently, there are insufficient safety and tolerability data on mefloquine at its recommended dosage of 25 mg/kg body weight in children. Mefloquine shares cross-resistance with quinine, which is still an effective drug in our country. Health planners in our country do not advocate the use of mefloquine

II. The advantage of the artemether–lumefantrine combination is that lumefantrine is not available as monotherapy and has never been used alone for the treatment of malaria. Lumefantrine absorption is enhanced by coadministration with fatty foods such as milk

III. Artemether–lumefantrine is not recommended in children weighing <5 kg

(SP: sulfadoxine-pyrimethamine)

BOX 7.24.3: Recommended treatment of uncomplicated *Plasmodium falciparum* malaria in northeastern states of India.

Recommended treatment

Coformulated tablets containing 20 mg of artemether and 120 mg of lumefantrine can be used as a six-dose regimen orally twice a day for 3 days

- For 5–14 kg body weight, one tablet at diagnosis, again after 8–12 hours, and then twice daily on days 2 and 3
- For 15–24 kg body weight, the same schedule with two tablets
- For 25–35 kg body weight and above, the same schedule with three and four tablets

OR

Artesunate 4 mg/kg of body weight orally once daily for 3 days and mefloquine 25 mg/kg body weight in two divided doses (15 and 10 mg/kg) on days 2 and 3

A single dose of primaquine (0.75 mg/kg) is given for gametocytocidal action:

Rest same as (I, II, III) **(Box 7.24.2)**

injectable antimalarials, irrespective of the species. A high degree of suspicion of severe malaria is of utmost importance, and any delay in the initiation of treatment can be fatal. Confirmation of the diagnosis is preferable, but one should not delay the treatment if it needs >1 hour. Further, in cases of strong clinical suspicion, prompt antimalarial therapy is needed even if parasites are not found in the initial blood examination.

Effective therapy in children with severe malaria includes antimalarial chemotherapy, supportive management, and management of complications. All these three interventions are equally important and to be taken care of simultaneously.

Antimalarial Chemotherapy of Severe and Complicated Malaria (Box 7.24.4)

Ideally, the antimalarial drug should be given initially by intravenous (IV) infusion, which should be replaced by oral administration as soon as the condition permits. After weighing the patient, antimalarials should be given according to the body weight.

According to the National Antimalarial Program, the drug policy in all cases of severe malaria, either IV AS or quinine, should be given irrespective of chloroquine-resistant status.[1] AS, 60 mg per ampoule, is dissolved in 0.6 mL of 5% sodium bicarbonate diluted to 3–5 mL with 5% dextrose and given immediately by IV bolus (push injection).

- Artemether is dispensed in a 1 mL ampoule containing 80 mg of artemether in peanut oil.
- A loading dose of quinine should not be used if the patient has received quinine, quinidine, or MQ within the preceding 12 hours. Alternatively, the loading dose can be administered as 7 mg salt/kg by IV infusion pump over 30 minutes, followed immediately by 10 mg salt/kg diluted in 10 mL isotonic fluid/kg by IV infusion over 4 hours.
- Quinine should not be given by bolus or push injection.
- Infusion rate should not exceed 5 mg salt/kg/h.
- If there is no clinical improvement after 48 hours of parenteral therapy, the maintenance dose of quinine should be reduced by one-third to one-half, that is, 5–7 mg salt/kg.
- Quinine should not be given subcutaneously as this may cause skin necrosis.

Choice of Therapy

Artemisinin is the most rapidly acting of all known antimalarial drugs; it often produces a 10,000-fold reduction of parasites per asexual cycle. It has the broadest time window of antimalarial effects from ring forms to early schizonts. Thus, it can stop parasite maturation, particularly from the less pathogenic circulating ring stages to the more pathogenic cytoadherent stages.

Artemisinin also has an excellent safety profile, and the cost of therapy as compared to quinine is almost similar. There are no reports of resistance to artemisinin at present,

BOX 7.24.4: Recommended treatment of complicated and severe malaria.

Drug dosage

Artesunate 2.4 mg/kg IV stat, then at 12 and 24 hours, then once a day

Children weighing <20 kg should receive a higher dose of artesunate (3 mg/kg bw per dose) than larger children (2.4 mg/kg bw per dose) to ensure equivalent exposure to the drug

Once the patient is able to swallow oral medication, complete the treatment by giving a course of:

- *Artemether plus lumefantrine* in northeastern states, as shown in **Box 7.24.3**
- *Artesunate plus sulfadoxine–pyrimethamine* in all states other than northeastern states of India, as shown in **Box 7.24.2**

If IV drugs are not available:

Artemether 3.2 mg/kg (loading dose) IM, followed by 1.6 mg/kg daily

Once the patient is able to swallow oral medication, complete the treatment by giving a course of:

- *Artemether plus lumefantrine* in northeastern states, as shown in **Box 7.24.3**
- In all states other than northeastern states of India, as shown in **Box 7.24.2**
- *Artesunate plus sulfadoxine–pyrimethamine*

OR

- *Quinine* salt 20 mg salt/kg (loading dose) diluted in 10 mL of isotonic fluid/kg by infusion over 4 hours
- Then give a maintenance dose of 10 mg salt/kg every 8 hours, calculated from the beginning of the previous infusion, until the patient can swallow, then quinine tablets, 10 mg salt/kg every 8 hourly, to complete a 7-day course of treatment (including both parenteral and oral)
- Tetracycline, doxycycline, or clindamycin is added to quinine as soon as the patient is able to swallow and should be continued for 7 days
- Tetracycline (>8 years) or doxycycline (>8 years) to be given for 7 days 4 mg/kg/dose four times daily or 3.5 mg/kg once a day, respectively. Clindamycin to be given 20 mg/kg/day in two divided doses for 7 days
- If controlled IV infusion cannot be administered, then quinine salt can be given in the same dosages by IM injection in the anterior thigh (not in buttock)
- The dose of quinine should be divided between two sites, half the dose in each anterior thigh. If possible, IM quinine should be diluted in normal saline to a concentration of 60–100 mg salt/mL (quinine is usually available as 300 mg salt/mL). Tetracycline, doxycycline, or clindamycin should be added as above
- Parenteral treatment in severe malaria should be continued at least for 24 hours, irrespective of the patient's ability to tolerate oral medication earlier than 24 hours
- Loading dose of quinine should not be used if the patient has received quinine, quinidine, or mefloquine within the preceding 12 hours. Alternatively, the loading dose can be administered as 7 mg salt/kg by IV infusion pump over 30 minutes, followed immediately by 10 mg salt/kg diluted in 10 mL isotonic fluid/kg by IV infusion over 4 hours
- Quinine should not be given by bolus or push injection. Infusion rate should not exceed 5 mg salt/kg/h
- If there is no clinical improvement after 48 hours of parenteral therapy, the maintenance dose of quinine should be reduced by one-third to one-half, that is, 5–7 mg salt/kg
- Quinine should not be given subcutaneously as this may cause skin necrosis
- Artesunate, 60 mg per ampoule, is dissolved in 0.6 mL of 5% sodium bicarbonate diluted to 3–5 mL with 5% dextrose and given immediately by IV bolus (push injection)
- Artemether is dispensed in a 1 mL ampoule containing 80 mg of artemether in peanut oil
- Mefloquine should be avoided in cerebral malaria due to neuropsychiatric complications associated with it

(bw: bodyweight; IM: intramuscular; IV: intravenous)

but declining sensitivity to quinine has been reported from some Southeast Asian countries like Thailand. Randomized trials comparing AS and quinine from Southeast Asia show clear evidence of benefit with AS. However, artemisinin should be used when rate-controlled IV infusion of quinine is not possible; patients have contraindications to quinine use and evidence of inadequate response or resistance to quinine noted. Simultaneous use of quinine and artemisinin is not indicated as it may be harmful, and there is no added advantage. In limited studies available, AS has been found to be better than artemether.

Supportive Management

- Rapid clinical assessment with respect to the level of consciousness (use Blantyre coma scale), blood pressure, rate and depth of respiration, anemia, state of hydration, and temperature
- Good nursing care with proper positioning and meticulous attention to airways, eyes, mucosa, and skin should be done.
- For an unconscious child, a nasogastric tube is to be inserted to reduce the risk of aspiration.
- Oxygen therapy and respiratory support should be given if necessary.
- In case of shock, resuscitate with normal saline or Ringer lactate by bolus infusion; avoid under- or overhydration.
- Hyperpyrexia should be treated with tepid sponging, fanning, and paracetamol.
- Close monitoring of the vital signs, preferably every 4 hours, to be done until the patient is out of danger.

Also, maintain an intake-output chart and watch for hemoglobinuria.

- Monitoring of the response to treatment is essential. A blood smear examination every 6–12 hours for parasitemia for the first 48 hours is needed.
- In case of artemisinin derivatives, the parasite count usually comes down within 5–6 hours of starting therapy. Asexual parasitemia generally disappears after 72 hours of therapy.
- In case of quinine, the parasite count may remain unchanged or even rise in the first 18–24 hours, which should not be taken as an indicator of quinine resistance. However, the parasite count should fall after 24 hours of quinine therapy and should disappear within 5 days.

MANAGEMENT OF COMPLICATIONS OF MALARIA

Of the various complications of falciparum malaria, the common and important ones in children are as follows:

- Cerebral malaria
- Severe anemia
- Respiratory distress (acidosis)
- Hypoglycemia

Cerebral Malaria

The initial presentation is usually fever followed by inability to eat or drink. Progression to coma or convulsion is usually very rapid within 1 or 2 days. Convulsions may be very subtle with nystagmus, salivation, or twitching of an isolated part of the body. Effort should be given to exclude other treatable causes of coma (e.g., bacterial meningitis or hypoglycemia). Patients should be given good nursing care, convulsions should be treated with diazepam/midazolam, and harmful adjuvant treatments such as corticosteroids, mannitol, adrenaline, and phenobarbitone should be avoided.

Severe Anemia

Children with hyperparasitemia due to acute destruction of red cells may develop severe anemia. Packed red cell transfusion should be given cautiously when PCV is 12% or less or hemoglobin is <4 g/dL. Transfusion should also be considered in patients with less severe anemia in the presence of respiratory distress (acidosis), impaired consciousness, or hyperparasitemia (>20% of RBCs infected).

Lactic Acidosis

Deep breathing with indrawing of the lower chest wall without any localizing chest signs suggests lactic acidosis. It usually accompanies cerebral malaria, anemia, or dehydration. Correct hypovolemia, treat anemia, and prevent seizures. Monitor acid-base status, blood glucose, and urea and electrolyte levels.

Hypoglycemia

Hypoglycemia is common in children <3 years, especially with hyperparasitemia or convulsion. It also occurs in patients treated with quinine. Manifestations are similar to those of cerebral malaria, so it can be easily overlooked. Monitor blood sugar every 4–6 hours. If facilities to monitor blood glucose are not available, assume hypoglycemia in the symptomatic patient and treat accordingly. Correct hypoglycemia with IV dextrose (25% dextrose 2–4 mL/kg by bolus), and it should be followed by a slow infusion of 5% dextrose-containing fluid to prevent recurrence.

PREVENTION OF MALARIA

- Awareness
- Avoid being bitten by mosquitoes with effective vector control:
  - Insecticide-treated nets
  - Long sleeves and pants
  - Insect repellents
- *Chemoprophylaxis:* It is indicated in high *P. falciparum*-endemic areas
  - *Short-term chemoprophylaxis (until 6 weeks): Doxycycline 1.5 mg/kg once daily for children >8 years (maximum 100 mg once daily).* It should start 2 days before coming and should be continued 4 weeks after leaving the endemic area.
  - *Long-term chemoprophylaxis (>6 weeks):* MQ 5 mg/kg weekly (up to 250 mg) to be administered 2 weeks before coming and should be continued 4 weeks after leaving the endemic area.

REFERENCES

1. Directorate of National Vector Borne Diseases Control Program; Directorate General of Health Services. National Drug Policy on Malaria. New Delhi: Ministry of Health and Family Welfare, Government of India; 2013.
2. World Health Organization. Guidelines for the Treatment of Malaria, 2nd edition. Geneva: World Health Organization; 2010.

7.25 Kala-Azar (Visceral Leishmaniasis)

Nigam Prakash Narain, Rajesh Kumar

INTRODUCTION

Leishmaniasis, also known as kala-azar (KA), is a vector-borne protozoan disease[1] caused by parasites belonging to the *Leishmania* genus within the Trypanosomatidae family.[2] This disease is predominantly prevalent in tropical and subtropical areas. The main causative agent differs by region, with *Leishmania donovani* being prominent in the Indian subcontinent, Middle East, and Africa, and *Leishmania infantum* causing the disease in the Mediterranean, Central Asia, and China.[3] Leishmaniasis can manifest in one of three distinct forms: (1) Visceral leishmaniasis (VL), also known as KA, (2) mucocutaneous leishmaniasis (MCL), and (3) cutaneous leishmaniasis (CL).

EPIDEMIOLOGY

Visceral leishmaniasis is one of the 20 neglected tropical infectious diseases (NTDs) recognized by the World Health Organization (WHO).[4] Annually, there are 0.7–1.0 million new cases of leishmaniasis worldwide.[5] Although there has been a global decline in VL cases in recent years, with an annual occurrence of 50–90 thousand cases,[6] the disease continues to be prevalent in approximately 83 countries. Over 95% of new VL cases are concentrated in 10 countries, including Brazil, China, Ethiopia, India, Iraq, Kenya, Nepal, Somalia, South Sudan, and Sudan.[5] In the Southeast Asia Region (SEAR), India, Bangladesh, and Nepal are the most affected countries. In India, VL is endemic in 54 districts across four states: Bihar, West Bengal, Jharkhand, and Eastern Uttar Pradesh, contributing to over 70% of the nationwide total cases.[7] Sporadic cases are reported in Assam, Himachal Pradesh, Kerala, Madhya Pradesh, Sikkim, and Uttarakhand. Nearly half of the new VL cases are seen in children, with the most commonly affected age group being 5–9 years.[8] Overall, VL remains a significant global health challenge, particularly in specific endemic regions, necessitating ongoing efforts for control and elimination.

ETIOPATHOGENESIS

The protozoan parasite *L. donovani* exhibits two distinct developmental stages. The aflagellar *amastigote* form is characterized by small, round to oval-shaped cells, measuring around 3–5 µm. These obligate intracellular parasites reside within host reticuloendothelial cells, including macrophages, neutrophils, and endothelial cells in organs such as the liver, spleen, and bone marrow of vertebrate hosts like men, dogs, rodents, etc. Their nucleus, typically <1 µm in size, can be centrally or laterally located, and they possess a kinetoplast with mitochondrial deoxyribonucleic acid (DNA) copies, positioned at a right angle to the nucleus, along with an axoneme and an adjacent vacuole. In contrast, the flagellar *promastigote* form is larger, measuring 8–15 µm, and exhibits a pear-shaped appearance. These motile, single-flagellated cells are found extracellularly, within sandflies and laboratory cultures. Promastigotes are the infective stage for humans and feature a centrally located nucleus, a transversely placed kinetoplast near the anterior end, and include a parabasal body and blepharoplast, but they lack an undulating membrane.

Leishmania donovani is transmitted to humans through the bites of certain species of female sandflies, specifically those belonging to the genus *Phlebotomus* in Asia, Africa, and Europe, and *Lutzomyia* sandflies in the Americas. These sandflies can have various hosts, including canids, rodents, marsupials, hyraxes, and humans. Human leishmaniasis can be transmitted in two primary ways. First, it can have a *zoonotic transmission* pattern, where the disease is initially present in an animal reservoir and then transmitted to humans through a vector. Alternatively, it can follow an *anthroponotic transmission* pattern, where the disease is directly transmitted between humans through a vector. In the case of Indian KA, caused by *L. donovani*, it has a unique epidemiological characteristic. It is exclusively anthroponotic, meaning that humans are the sole known reservoir of infection. In India, the sandflies of the genus *Phlebotomus argentipes* are the only known vectors responsible for transmitting KA. Transmission can also occur through needles among intravenous drug abusers, and there is also the possibility of in utero transmission from an infected mother to her fetus.

The life cycle of *Leishmania* is intricately linked to two primary hosts: A vertebrate host, such as humans, dogs, or rodents, and a female sandfly vector. Sandflies are diminutive insects, approximately one-fourth the size of mosquitoes, characterized by a body length ranging from 1.5 to 3.5 mm. These adult sandflies feature erect large wings and are covered in long hairs. *Leishmania*'s life cycle encompasses multiple stages, including eggs, four larval instars, pupa, and the adult stage.[6] The complete life cycle spans over a month, with the duration influenced by factors like temperature and ecological conditions. Sandflies thrive in environments characterized by high relative humidity, warm temperatures, abundant subsoil water, and vegetation rich in organic matter, which serves as a food source for their larvae. The transmission of *Leishmania* commences when a female sandfly feeds on the blood of an infected individual, ingesting amastigotes. Inside the sandfly's midgut, these amastigotes undergo transformation into promastigotes, which proliferate through longitudinal fission, eventually giving rise to metacyclic promastigotes. These metacyclic promastigotes multiply within the midgut and subsequently migrate to the foregut (proboscis) of the sandfly. *Leishmania*'s life cycle in sandflies varies in duration, typically ranging from 4 to 18 days. After taking an infected blood meal, the female sandfly requires another meal, often fruit juice, before becoming capable of transmitting the parasite. Promastigotes obstructing the sandfly's buccal cavity are released into the bite wound created by the sandfly's proboscis during its subsequent blood meal. Once in the host, promastigotes are phagocytosed by skin macrophages and, within 12–24 hours, transform into amastigote forms. These amastigote forms replicate within macrophages, causing their rupture and the release of amastigotes into the bloodstream. Through the circulatory system, amastigotes are transported to various organs, including the liver, spleen, and bone marrow, where they invade reticuloendothelial cells like macrophages and endothelial cells. It is essential to note that Indian KA is classified as a nonzoonotic disease, with humans serving as the exclusive reservoir of infection in this context. Comprehending this intricate life cycle is pivotal for initiatives aimed at controlling and preventing the transmission of *Leishmania* parasites.

Leishmaniasis is a disease that can affect individuals of all ages, including infants, but it is most commonly observed in the pediatric age group of 5–9 years in India. There is a notable gender discrepancy, with males being twice as susceptible as females (a 2:1 ratio). The movement of people, such as migrants, laborers, and tourists, from areas where the disease is prevalent (endemic) to nonendemic regions can contribute to its spread. Individuals with lower socioeconomic status are frequently affected by KA. Additionally, those engaged in occupations such as farming, forestry, mining, and fishing are at an elevated risk of contracting the disease. These various host factors play a significant role in the prevalence of leishmaniasis.

Environmental factors also play a crucial role in the distribution of KA. The disease is predominantly found in the alluvial plains along the Ganges River, where conditions are favorable, including adequate monsoon rains, temperatures ranging from 15 to 38°C, high humidity, lush vegetation, and subsoil water availability. The disease is rarely encountered at altitudes exceeding 2,000 feet. Historical outbreaks have shown two distinct peaks, one occurring in November and the other in March–April. The sandflies, particularly *P. argentipes*, which are responsible for transmitting the disease, reproduce in a variety of habitats, including soil cracks, buildings, tree hollows, and caves. Factors like overcrowding, poor ventilation, and the accumulation of organic matter in the surroundings facilitate disease transmission. These sandflies primarily exhibit nocturnal habits, with only female sandflies being responsible for biting, predominantly during night-time hours.

INCUBATION PERIOD

The extrinsic incubation period in sandflies typically spans from 6 to 9 days. On the other hand, the intrinsic incubation period in humans varies considerably, generally lasting from 1 to 4 months, with a range that can extend from 10 days to as long as 2 years.

CLINICAL FEATURES

The clinical presentation of KA varies depending on the onset pattern.

Acute Onset

This is less common and typically occurs in individuals from nonendemic areas. Fever is the predominant symptom, which can manifest as high-intensity intermittent or remittent episodes lasting 2–6 weeks or even longer. Rapid spleen enlargement is a characteristic feature, often occurring within a few days.

Chronic Onset

This is the most common form in endemic areas, with an incubation period ranging from 2 to 32 weeks. Without proper treatment, individuals with VL may succumb within 2 years, primarily due to secondary bacterial infections, severe anemia, or hemorrhage from thrombocytopenia. Some infected individuals may remain asymptomatic for years, developing symptoms only when their immune system weakens. Infections in the reticuloendothelial system can be subclinical, with mild or noticeable symptoms.

Typically, KA presents with high fever, abdominal discomfort, emaciation, and pallor. The fever is usually high grade and intermittent, featuring a double rise in temperature within a day (double quotidian fever), a characteristic rarely seen nowadays. Children with KA often remain relatively well and ambulant, with a reasonably preserved appetite. Almost all cases exhibit splenic enlargement, with the spleen becoming palpable within the first month and gradually increasing in size by about an inch per month, eventually becoming massively enlarged and firm. The liver is also enlarged but not to the same extent. Marked splenomegaly and moderate hepatomegaly become evident around 6 months after onset. Hepatic functions are generally unaffected, and jaundice is rare. Skin hyperpigmentation, particularly on the face, hands, feet, and abdomen, may occur due to cytokine-induced enhanced adrenocorticotropic hormone (ACTH) production, giving rise to the Hindi name "kala-azar" or black fever,[9] although this feature is less common in children nowadays.

At-risk populations include preschool children, immunocompromised individuals, and the malnourished. The incidence of Leishmaniasis has been increasing in individuals with acquired immunodeficiency syndrome (AIDS), intravenous drug users, or both, suggesting potential transmission through contaminated syringes. Late-presenting patients may exhibit hypergammaglobulinemia with nonprotective antileishmanial antibodies, leading to chronic diarrhea and growth retardation. In the absence of treatment, cachexia and multisystem failure can occur. CD4 cell reductions may result in disease recurrence, especially in patients receiving corticosteroids, chemotherapy, transplants, or those with human immunodeficiency virus (HIV) infection.

COMPLICATIONS

In certain cases, an extreme degree of anemia is evident, usually of a normocytic and normochromic nature. Multiple factors contribute to this anemia, including autoimmune hemolysis, replacement of bone marrow by *Leishmania*-infected macrophages, ineffective erythropoiesis, hypersplenism, hemodilution, the suppressive impact of cytokines on bone marrow function, nutritional deficiencies, and gastrointestinal bleeding.

Most patients also experience leukopenia, with some having very low total white blood cell counts, some as low as 1,000/mm^3. Several factors contribute to this leukopenia, such as increased margination of white blood cells, splenic sequestration, or even an autoimmune process. Secondary infections are a common complication, with tuberculosis being the most frequently associated infection. Frequently observed additional infections comprise pneumonia, measles, otitis media, and cancrum oris. Patients may also experience symptoms like cough and diarrhea. Eosinopenia, characterized by the absence of eosinophils, is frequently observed.

Thrombocytopenia and hypergammaglobulinemia are also commonly present. Severe thrombocytopenia can occasionally result in bleeding from mucous membranes, leading to epistaxis and hematemesis, as well as the development of petechiae and purpura. However, this presentation is less common in the endemic regions of Bihar.

DIFFERENTIAL DIAGNOSIS

Visceral leishmaniasis should be considered in individuals experiencing persistent fever, weakness, weight loss, marked enlargement of the spleen and liver, cytopenias, and elevated gamma globulin levels, especially if they have had potential exposure in an endemic region. Distinguishing VL from other illnesses can be challenging due to its similarity to various febrile conditions. Notably, it can be mistaken for malaria, typhoid fever, disseminated tuberculosis, brucellosis, schistosomiasis, histoplasmosis, amebic liver abscess, and infectious mononucleosis. Furthermore, conditions such as portal hypertension, chronic myeloid leukemia, and tropical splenomegaly syndrome, presenting with splenomegaly, may be mistaken for VL.

In malaria-endemic areas, suspicion of VL should arise when a fever persists for >2 weeks and does not respond to antimalarial treatment (assuming that drug-resistant malaria has been considered as a possibility).

Case Classification (By WHO Operational Definition)

- *Suspected case of KA:* A patient with a history of fever lasting >2 weeks and an enlarged spleen and liver that do not respond to antimalarial treatment, particularly in an individual from an endemic area
- *Confirmed case of KA:* A person residing in an endemic area who has been having fever for over 2 weeks along with splenomegaly and diagnosis has been confirmed through either a rapid diagnostic test (RDT) or a biopsy

Laboratory Criteria for Diagnosis

- *Confirmation through parasitology:* Positive findings in stained smears from bone marrow, spleen, liver, lymph nodes, blood, or culture of the organism from biopsied or aspirated material.
- *Confirmation through serology:* Positive results in serological tests such as IFAT (indirect fluorescent antibody test), ELISA (enzyme-linked immunosorbent assay), rK39 test, and direct agglutination test (DAT).
- *Confirmation through polymerase chain reaction (PCR) and related techniques:* Positive results in PCR and other related molecular techniques for detecting the presence of the parasite.

Laboratory Diagnosis of Visceral Leishmaniasis (Box 7.25.1)

Nonspecific Tests

- *Blood analysis:*
  - A complete blood count (CBC) often reveals normocytic normochromic anemia, thrombocytopenia,

BOX 7.25.1: Diagnosis of visceral leishmaniasis.

Laboratory investigations:

Nonspecific tests

- *CBC:* Anemia, leucopenia, thrombocytopenia
- Raised ESR, mildly elevated liver enzymes
- *Napier's aldehyde or Formogel test, Chopra's antimony test:* Due to hypergammaglobulinemia
- *Leishmanin skin test/Montenegro test:* Delayed hypersensitivity test

Direct evidence (demonstration of *Leishmania donovani)*

- *Microscopy: Gold standard.* Demonstration of amastigotes in smears prepared with tissue aspirates from bone marrow, spleen, or lymph node
- *Culture:* Demonstration of promastigote forms. Uses special media like NNN medium, Schneider's liquid medium with 20% calf serum, bactoagar biphasic medium
- *Animal inoculation:* Not routinely used

Indirect evidence

- *Detection of antigen:* ELISA and PCR
  - *KAtex test* is a latex agglutination test, which detects leishmanial antigen in urine
- *Detection of antibodies:* rK39 rapid test, ELISA, complement fixation test, IFA, and DAT
  - rK39 rapid test is *method of choice* for VL
- *PCR:* DNA detection

(CBC: complete blood count; DAT: direct agglutination test; DNA: deoxyribonucleic acid; ELISA: enzyme-linked immunosorbent assay; ESR: erythrocyte sedimentation rate; IFA: indirect immunofluorescence; NNN: Novy–McNeal–Nicolle; PCR: polymerase chain reaction; VL: visceral leishmaniasis)

and leukopenia. Neutropenia is common, along with relative lymphocytosis and monocytosis. The leukocyte-to-erythrocyte ratio is significantly altered and may be around 1:2,000 (normal: 1:750).

- Liver function tests may show mild elevations in liver enzymes.
- Elevated erythrocyte sedimentation rate (ESR) is typically observed.

- *Hypergammaglobulinemia:*
  - Increased levels of gamma globulins with a reversal of the albumin-to-globulin ratio are common. This hypergammaglobulinemia was the basis for *Napier's aldehyde or Formogel test* and Chopra's *antimony test,* which are no longer used now.
  - *Montenegro test*: The leishmanin skin test, also known as the *Montenegro test,* is a delayed hypersensitivity test. It involves injecting 0.01 mL of a killed promastigote suspension intradermally on the forearm. Induration of 5 mm or more after 48–72 hours suggests a positive result, indicating prior exposure to the leishmanial parasite. In active KA, this test is negative and becomes positive usually 6–8 weeks after cure from the disease.

Direct Evidence

- *Microscopy:* The *gold standard* for VL diagnosis involves identifying amastigotes in smears of tissue aspirates. These samples can be obtained from the bone marrow, splenic aspirate, or rarely enlarged lymph nodes. Smears are stained by Leishman, Giemsa, or Wright's stains and examined under an oil immersion microscope, revealing the presence of amastigote parasites within macrophages.
- *Culture:* Aspirates from the spleen, bone marrow, or other tissues are cultured in specialized media. This includes Novy–McNeal–Nicolle (NNN) medium, Schneider's liquid medium with 20% calf serum, bactoagar biphasic medium, and others.
  Both techniques (microscopic exam and culture) have a sensitivity of 85%.
- *Animal inoculation:* It is not routinely used for diagnosis.

Indirect Evidence

- *Serodiagnosis:*
  - *Detection of antigen:* Antigen concentration in serum or other body fluids is very low. ELISA and PCR tests have been developed for detecting leishmanial antigen. The *KAtex* test, a latex agglutination test, detects leishmanial antigen in urine and is especially useful in VL-HIV coinfection cases.
  - *Detection of antibodies:* VL patients often have high parasite-specific antibody titers. Various serological tests are available, including ELISA, complement fixation test, indirect immunofluorescence (IFA), and DAT. However, serologic tests alone are neither sufficiently sensitive nor specific to definitively confirm or exclude leishmaniasis. Serology may be positive in individuals from endemic areas because of past exposure and may not be indicative of current active disease.
    - *rK 39 rapid test for VL:* This rapid bedside test, using a recombinant leishmanial antigen rK 39, has become the mainstay for VL diagnosis. This immune-chromatographic dipstick test is developed using a recombinant leishmanial antigen *rK 39* consisting of 39 amino acids conserved in the kinesin region of *Leishmania chagasi.* It is highly specific and sensitive (98% sensitivity and 97% specificity). False positives may occur in hepatitis and tuberculosis cases, while false negatives can be seen in HIV patients with a depressed immune response. The RDT can remain positive for months or years after treatment of VL. For this reason, this test is not useful in the diagnosis of relapse cases. In post-kala-azar dermal leishmaniasis (PKDL), it can be used only to rule out the disease if negative but not for confirmation.

- *PCR*: This is a highly sensitive and specific DNA detection method. It can detect even a single parasite in a specimen, making it a valuable diagnostic tool for VL.

TREATMENT OPTIONS FOR VISCERAL LEISHMANIASIS (BOX 7.25.2)

Treatment options for VL include several approaches:

- *Antimony compounds:* Sodium stibogluconate (SSG) and meglumine antimonate have been used for decades. However, starting in the early 1980s, there was a significant rise in the prevalence of SSG resistance on a large scale in North Bihar. As a result, only 35–38% of patients in Bihar responded positively to SSG treatment, leading to its decreased popularity. It is administered at 20 mg/kg body weight via intramuscular injection or intravenous infusion over the course of 28–30 days. Side effects may include pain at the injection site, arthralgia, myalgia, metallic taste, elevated levels of serum transaminases, lipase, and amylase, bone marrow suppression, cardiac toxicity manifested as cardiac arrhythmias, prolonged QTc interval, ventricular premature beats, ventricular tachycardia, ventricular fibrillation, and torsades de pointes. SSG therapy demonstrates reduced effectiveness and a higher occurrence of adverse effects, including increased mortality, in individuals coinfected with HIV.
- *Amphotericin-B:* Amphotericin-B deoxycholate, a potent polyene antifungal drug, is highly effective, approximately 400 times more so than SSG. It is administered at a dose of 0.75–1 mg/kg through slow intravenous infusion over 15–20 doses on alternate days. Major side effects include infusion-related reactions, nephrotoxicity, hypokalemia, and myocarditis.

BOX 7.25.2: Treatment options for kala-azar (visceral leishmaniasis).

Drugs, dosage, route of administration, and duration:

- *Sodium stibogluconate (SSG):* 20 mg/kg/day, OD, IM/IV for 28–30 days
- *Amphotericin-B deoxycholate:* 0.75–1 mg/kg/dose, alternate days, slow IV infusion for 28 days
- *Liposomal amphotericin-B (first-line treatment):* 10 mg/kg (*for all age groups*) IV, dissolved in 5% dextrose, *single dose*
- *Miltefosine*
  - 2–11 years, 2.5 mg/kg, OD orally, after meals for 28 days
  - >12 years and weight <25 kg, one capsule of 50 mg, daily for 28 days
  - >12 years and weight 25–50 kg, two doses of 50 mg each (total 100 mg), daily for 28 days
  - >50 kg body weight, 150 mg/day, in divided doses for 28 days
- *Paromomycin:* 15 mg of paromomycin sulfate (11 mg/kg base), IM for 21 days
- *Pentamidine:* 4 mg/kg, on alternate days, IM/IV for 15–30 doses

- *Lipid formulations of amphotericin-B:* Liposomal amphotericin-B (AmBisome), amphotericin-B lipid complex (ABLC; Abelcet), and amphotericin-B colloidal suspension (Amphomul/Amphocil) are advanced options with a cure rate of approximately 94%. They require shorter hospital stays and have fewer side effects. Liposomal amphotericin-B (AmBisome) is recommended by the WHO and is designated as the primary treatment option in the National Vector Borne Disease Control Program's (NVBDCP) Accelerated Plan for Kala-azar Elimination-2017. This recommendation is due to its ease of administration, effectiveness, and high compliance rate. In comparison to conventional amphotericin-B, it is considerably safer; however, its widespread use is hampered by its elevated cost. The recommended dosage for all age groups is a single intravenous dose of 10 mg/kg, dissolved in 5% dextrose, and administered over a 2-hour period.
- *Miltefosine:* Miltefosine, the first orally active drug proven effective in managing leishmaniasis, eliminates the need for parenteral therapy and hospitalization. This alkyl phospholipid, specifically hexadecylphosphocholine, has an impressive cure rate of 95–100%. It was officially registered in India in 2002 and was adopted as the first-line regimen by the Asian elimination initiative in 2005. The recommended dosing for miltefosine is as follows: Children aged 2–11 years: 2.5 mg/kg once daily after meals for 28 days; Children >12 years and weighing <25 kg: One 50 mg capsule daily for 28 days, Children >12 years and weighing 25–50 kg: 100 mg daily, split into two 50 mg doses after meals, for 28 days; and for individuals weighing >50 kg: 150 mg/day orally, divided into doses, for 28 days. However, miltefosine does come with certain side effects, including gastrointestinal symptoms like vomiting and diarrhea, occasional asymptomatic elevation of hepatic enzymes, and rare cases of nephrotoxicity. It is crucial to note that miltefosine is a teratogenic drug and should not be used during pregnancy or in females of childbearing age. Due to its relatively long half-life of approximately one week, contraception should be continued for an additional 3 months after discontinuing the drug. Its extended half-life also makes it susceptible to the rapid development of drug resistance. While miltefosine is utilized as a first-line drug for treating adults on an outpatient basis in North Bihar, it has not been as successful in children due to gastrointestinal intolerance. Nonetheless, it represents a significant advancement in the management of VL, offering an alternative to parenteral therapy and hospitalization for affected adults.
- *Injectable paromomycin:* Paromomycin, a globally marketed aminoglycoside-aminocyclitol antibiotic with a history spanning over two decades, has proven its clinical

efficacy in treating VL through well-established clinical trials conducted in Africa and India. This drug boasts high overall cure rates, with a remarkable success rate of 94.2%. In 2006, it gained approval from the Indian government for VL treatment, and the recommended dosage involves a 15 mg dose of paromomycin sulfate (equivalent to 11 mg/kg base) administered intramuscularly for a 21-day period. Paromomycin stands out for its affordability and safety, making it a viable option.

Common adverse events associated with its use include pain at the injection site, a transient rise in hepatic transaminases, and reversible ototoxicity. Importantly, paromomycin has demonstrated effectiveness in treating resistant cases of VL in North Bihar.

- *Pentamidine:* Pentamidine, an aromatic diamidine, was once employed in the early 1980s as a treatment for antimony-resistant VL in India. However, it fell out of favor due to a combination of reduced effectiveness and the emergence of severe toxicities, including pancreatitis that could lead to insulin-dependent diabetes, as well as issues such as hypoglycemia, hypotension, QT prolongation, and hyperkalemia. In contemporary medical practice, pentamidine has found a role in secondary prophylaxis, primarily to prevent VL relapses in patients coinfected with HIV and VL, provided their CD4 count is ≤200 cells/μL. This prophylactic regimen involves a monthly dose of 4 mg/kg for 12 months, with the possibility of a 6-month extension.
- *Combination therapy:* It has garnered significant attention in the context of diseases like HIV, tuberculosis, and malaria, and due to increasing drug resistance in the Indian subcontinent, researchers have turned their focus to its potential in treating VL. The rationale behind this approach lies in the amplification of treatment effectiveness by using compounds with synergistic or additive activities that target different sites of the disease. Combination therapy offers several advantages, including the reduction of treatment duration, lowered dose requirements, decreased risk of toxic side effects and cost, and the prevention of drug resistance emergence. Various combination therapies have been recommended for the treatment of KA, including antimonial with interferon-gamma, AmBisome with paromomycin, AmBisome with miltefosine, miltefosine with paromomycin, and SSG with paromomycin.
- *Supportive care:* Transfusions of packed red blood cells and platelets for severe anemia and thrombocytopenia. Antibiotics for secondary bacterial infections.

TREATMENT OUTCOMES IN VISCERAL LEISHMANIASIS

Treatment outcomes in VL are assessed at two points: At the end of drug treatment and 6 months after the last dose, with four main outcomes identified: Cure, nonresponse, relapse, and treatment failure.

1. *Cure:* A patient is considered clinically cured when they have successfully completed the entire treatment regimen and there are no remaining signs or symptoms of KA.
2. *Nonresponse:* Nonresponse is characterized by the persistence or recurrence of signs and symptoms despite receiving appropriate treatment for a duration exceeding 2 weeks.
3. *Relapse:* The term "relapse" is defined as the reappearance of KA signs and symptoms within a 6-month period following the conclusion of treatment.
4. *Treatment failure:* Treatment failure encompasses cases of nonresponse and relapse, where the initial treatment proves ineffective or where signs and symptoms recur despite initial treatment.

Response to treatment: Following effective treatment, the majority of patients typically experience a resolution of fever within 1 week, and a reduction in spleen size becomes evident within 2 weeks. Over the course of 6 months to a year, the spleen usually fully regresses. Patients' overall health and well-being improve, and within 2 weeks, there is a noticeable increase in both their total blood count and hemoglobin levels.

POST-KALA-AZAR DERMAL LEISHMANIASIS

Post-kala-azar dermal leishmaniasis is observed in approximately 3–10% of patients recovering from VL in endemic regions, typically appearing about a year or two after systemic illness recovery, primarily in India and East Africa. PKDL manifests as nonulcerative skin lesions, and most cases occur after the cure of VL, lacking the typical KA symptoms like fever, splenomegaly, or anemia. However, some PKDL cases, around 5–6%, occur without any prior history of KA, presenting only with diverse skin lesions. Importantly, sensation over the lesions is preserved, unlike leprosy, where similar lesions lack sensation. PKDL lesions can be classified into three types: *Depigmented or hypopigmented macules*, commonly found on the face, trunk, and extremities, resembling tuberculoid leprosy; *erythematous patches* distributed on the face in a "butterfly distribution"; and *nodular lesions* that may evolve from the previous two categories.

Case definitions for PKDL include *probable PKDL* for patients with multiple hypopigmented macules, papules, plaques, or nodules who test positive in an RDT and *confirmed PKDL* for patients from VL-endemic areas with similar lesions who test positive for the parasite in a slit-skin smear (SSS) or biopsy.

Diagnosis involves biopsying the nodular lesions and demonstrating amastigote forms in stained sections with treatment options including miltefosine, SSG, amphotericin "B" deoxycholate injection, and liposomal amphotericin-B (AmBisome). Treatment outcomes are assessed in two stages: *Initial cure*, characterized by clinical improvement at the end of treatment, and *final cure*, confirmed 12 months after the end of treatment, indicating complete resolution of skin lesions.

COINFECTION WITH HUMAN IMMUNODEFICIENCY VIRUS

Visceral leishmaniasis has emerged as an opportunistic infection in HIV patients, and the atypical clinical presentations in these individuals can pose diagnostic challenges. Approximately 2,000 cases of coinfection with HIV and VL have been reported across 35 countries.[10] Notably, coinfected patients may lack the typical VL symptom of hepatosplenomegaly. Diagnosis in such cases often relies on bone marrow examination due to the lower sensitivity of immunodiagnostic tests based on antibodies. Screening and diagnosis may also involve demonstrating amastigotes in buffy coat smears or analyzing whole blood or its buffy coat using PCR.

Treatment for coinfected patients entails the use of liposomal amphotericin-B at a dose of 3–5 mg/kg daily or intermittently for 10 doses, administered on days 1–5, 10, 17, 24, 31, and 38, with a total cumulative dose of 40 mg/kg. Additionally, the initiation of antiretroviral therapy is recommended, and secondary prophylaxis should be administered until the CD4 count exceeds 200/μL. The recommended secondary prophylaxis options, in order of priority, include liposomal amphotericin-B (3–5 mg/kg/dose every 3 weeks), SSG at 20 mg/kg every 2 weeks, or amphotericin-B at 1 mg/kg/dose every 2 weeks, for all patients with a CD4 T-cell count <350/μL. This comprehensive approach is crucial for the management and prevention of VL recurrence in HIV-positive individuals.[10]

PREVENTION

Controlling leishmaniasis poses significant challenges, given its prevalence in sylvatic and rural areas. Timely detection and swift treatment of all cases remain paramount. Integrated insecticidal spraying programs can be effective in reducing sandfly populations. Bed net usage, proper clothing, and other personal protective measures can mitigate the risk of infection.

In 2005, the World Health Assembly established a goal to reduce VL incidence in the Indian subcontinent to less than 1 case per 10,000 people by 2015. This initiative, called the kala-azar Elimination Program, has made substantial progress in many endemic countries. Control strategies focus on early detection and rapid treatment of cases, vector control through indoor residual spraying, use of insecticide-treated bed nets, and health education. These efforts have resulted in a significant reduction in VL cases in the region, with some areas successfully achieving elimination status. Currently, there is no available vaccine for preventing leishmaniasis, but there are several trials, including both killed and live-attenuated vaccines, in progress to develop one.

CONCLUSION

Over the past two decades, the burden of VL in the Indian subcontinent—comprising India, Nepal, and Bangladesh—has significantly decreased. This remarkable progress is largely attributed to national health programs in the region, which have adopted the use of single-dose liposomal amphotericin B (L-AmB) therapy, with multidrug therapy added when necessary. The single-dose L-AmB treatment is highly effective, safe, and ensures maximum patient compliance. Its ability to reduce hospital stays has not only made it convenient for patients but also one of the most cost-effective options for treatment of VL. This approach has played a key role in reducing the impact of the disease across the region.

REFERENCES

1. Torres-Guerrero E, Quintanilla-Cedillo MR, Ruiz-Esmenjaud J, Arenas R. Leishmaniasis: a review. F1000Research. 2017;6:750.
2. Karimi A, Alborzi A, Amanati A. Visceral leishmaniasis: an update and literature review. Arch Pediatr Infect Dis. 2016;4(3):e31612.
3. Ghosh S. Paniker's Textbook of Medical Parasitology, 8th edition. New Delhi: Jaypee Brothers Medical Publishers (P) Ltd; 2017. pp. 52-65.
4. World Health Organization. The NTD road map: together towards 2030. [online] Available from https://www.who.int/neglected_diseases/diseases/en/. [Last accessed November, 2024].
5. World Health Organization. Leishmaniasis. [online] Available from https://www.who.int/news-room/fact-sheets/detail/leishmaniasis. [Last accessed November, 2024].
6. Burza S, Croft SL, Boelaert M. Leishmaniasis. Lancet. 2018;392(10151):951-70.
7. National Vector Borne Disease Control Programme. Accelerated Plan for Kala-Azar Elimination 2017. [online] Available from https://ncvbdc.mohfw.gov.in/WriteReadData/l892s/Accelerated-Plan-Kala-azar1-Feb2017.pdf [Last accessed November, 2025].
8. https://ncvbdc.mohfw.gov.in/Doc/opertional-guideline-KA-2015.pdf
9. Chatterjee KD. Parasitology: Protozoology and Helminthology in Relation to Clinical Medicine, 12th edition. New Delhi: CBS Publishers; 1980. pp. 54-65.
10. Chakravarty J, Sundar S. Current and emerging medications for the treatment of leishmaniasis. Expert Opin Pharmacother. 2019;20(10):1251-65.

SECTION

8

Diseases of Central Nervous System

Section Editor: **Sheffali Gulati**

8.1 Neuroanatomical Localization in Children

Aradhana Rohil, Prashant Jauhari

INTRODUCTION

One of the most important aspects of approaching a neurological case is the localization of the possible lesion within the nervous system. This is a process of precisely identifying the site of abnormality within the nervous system that best explains the occurrence of a particular sign or symptom. It is undoubtedly the most interesting part of neurology and can be compared to solving a crossword or sudoku. The science of neuroanatomical localization can be easily mastered; however, two important prerequisites must be fulfilled: A basic knowledge of the physiological function of each part of the nervous system and a detailed history along with a vigilant neurological examination, to identify and characterize the clinical presentation of the patient. History is the most important component of neurological assessment and provides an introduction to neuroanatomical localization. In this chapter on localization of the lesion, a detailed discussion on neurologic history-taking and examination is beyond the scope. In simple terms, the history should be able to define the presenting complaint(s) and provide a detailed description of the temporal evolution of the complaint. The examination should be able to confirm the findings from the history and pick up minor deficits or soft signs.

In clinical neurology practice, localization of the lesion(s) often follows the completion of the history and examination, preceding consideration of a set of differential diagnoses. Some disorders will have a predilection to involve a particular region of the neuraxis, while others may be unlikely to do so, thus making the formulation of an etiological diagnosis easier. **Flowchart 8.1.1** provides a simple, stepwise algorithm used in neurology to arrive at a diagnosis.

NEURAXIS

Neuraxis consists of the central nervous system (CNS) and peripheral nervous system (PNS), which can be further subdivided into segments for precise localization of the disease process **(Table 8.1.1)**.

BASIC PRINCIPLES GOVERNING LOCALIZATION ALONG THE NEURAXIS

- *"KISS" principle and Occam's razor*: KISS stands for "keep it super simple," meaning that while attempting to localize a particular symptom, one should try to explain the findings by simple concepts rather than by a complex approach. The simplest explanation is often the correct one. Thus, when a finding can be explained by two competing reasonings, one should prefer the simpler one.

Flowchart 8.1.1: Algorithmic approach to a neurological case.

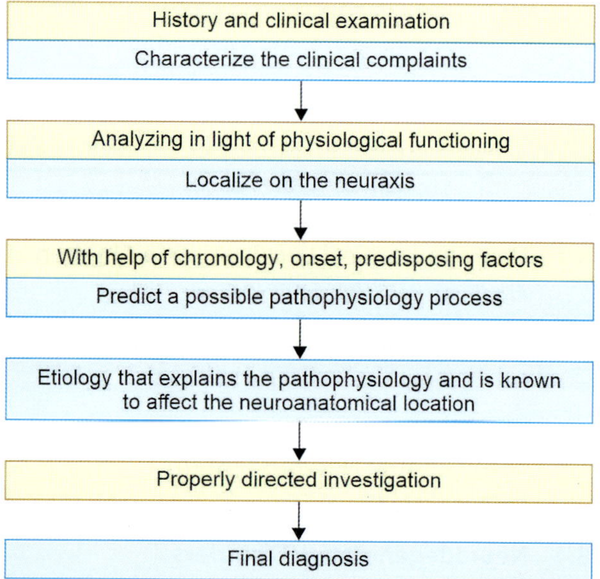

TABLE 8.1.1: Parts of the neuraxis.

CNS	Cerebral hemispheres	Cerebral cortex (gray matter)
		Subcortical white matter
	Basal ganglia	
	Brainstem	
	Cerebellum	
	Spinal cord (tracts)	
PNS	Spinal cord (AHCs)	
	Peripheral nerves	
	NMJ	
	Muscle	

(AHCs: anterior horn cells; CNS: central nervous system; NMJ: neuromuscular junction; PNS: peripheral nervous system)

This problem-solving approach is known as "Occam's razor," an age-old principle applicable in many disciplines of science.

- We must understand that brain regions are not strict compartments. Disorders may initially have a predilection for a specific CNS region but may progress and eventually involve other brain structures. For example, a gray matter degenerative brain disease affecting the cerebral cortex may later also affect the basal ganglia and the pyramidal tracts. In such scenarios, the clinical findings at the onset of the illness should be used to localize the disease process on the neuraxis.[1]
- The clinician is not required to match the signs and symptoms of a particular child with all possible sites of localization on the neuraxis. Instead, one should consider broader categories of localization. Thus, the first step is to localize a particular neurological finding or disease to the CNS or PNS. Once this is successfully done, the clinician can then be more precise by attempting to localize the set of complaints to a particular region within the CNS or PNS. CNS affection is hallmarked by the presence of cognitive and/or behavioral changes, alteration of sensorium, seizures, movement disorders, upper motor neuron (UMN) type of motor weakness, ataxia, etc., either in isolation or in various combinations depending upon the exact site of affection within the CNS **(Table 8.1.1)**. PNS affection is characterized by involvement of the lower motor neuron (LMN) and presents with motor and/or sensory abnormality without any affection of higher cortical functions.
- At times, a particular neurological sign/symptom may be explained by different sites on the neuraxis, for example, unilateral weakness which may have its origin in the cortex or can be distally localized even to muscle groups. What leads a clinician to prefer a particular site is the presence of other clinical features characteristic of that site. It might be necessary to re-elicit relevant history or perform a detailed neurological examination to identify these features. Thus, unilateral weakness with the presence of focal seizures clearly localizes it to the cerebral cortex.[2]
- The clinician should ideally take each sign and symptom and try to consider all potential sites of localization on the neuraxis. Then, using the KISS principle, choose a common region that explains the majority or all of the clinical findings.
- Cortical lesions produce a less pronounced neurological deficit in comparison to a similar lesion in the internal capsule or brainstem because a large number of neurons and axons are widely spaced out within the cortex, while they are compactly packed within the internal capsule and brainstem.[2]
- In case the clinical signs and symptoms are not congruent with any specific neuraxial site, consider the possibility of a multifocal (demyelinating) or diffuse disease process (toxic-metabolic). A high index of suspicion for a nonorganic etiology (malingering) should be kept in older children and adolescents in such a scenario.
- It must be remembered that although localization is the initial step toward identifying the neurological diagnosis, it may not always tell us the etiology. History, specifically the temporal evolution of deficits is important in identifying the precise etiology.[1] For example, a spinal cord dysfunction over seconds to minutes is more likely due to trauma or vascular insult, as compared to a demyelinating pathology such as transverse myelitis, which could take a few days to develop. However, an infiltrating tumor might take months to present.

LOCALIZATION OF A FOCAL NEUROLOGICAL SIGN ON THE NEURAXIS

The most common neurological finding on history and examination that requires precise localization on the neuraxis is focal weakness or motor deficit. The child could present with:

- Monoplegia/monoparesis (weakness in a single limb)
- Hemiplegia/hemiparesis (weakness on one side of the body)
- Paraplegia/paraparesis (weakness in both lower limbs)
- Quadriplegia (involvement of all four extremities)
- Diplegia (involvement of all four extremities, with legs more affected than arms)
- Double hemiplegia (involvement of all four extremities, with arms more affected than legs)[1]

A motor deficit can be explained by two broad sites on the neuroaxis: The pyramidal tract or the UMN and the LMN. However, a lesion within the deep gray matter (basal ganglia) and the cerebellum might also lead to motor abnormalities by primarily affecting muscle tone. UMN lesions could be anywhere from the motor cortex to the end of the corticospinal tract in the spinal cord, while LMN lesions span from the anterior horn cells (AHCs) to the muscle **(Fig. 8.1.1)**.[3] A UMN lesion above the level of pyramidal decussations will lead to a deficit on the contralateral side, whereas a UMN lesion after pyramidal decussation and an LMN lesion will lead to ipsilateral manifestations. UMN and LMN lesions can be differentiated as described in **Table 8.1.2**.[3]

After ascertaining the UMN pathology, for further localization, one should consider the involvement of cranial nerves, whether the upper and lower extremity weakness is proportionate or disproportionate, and the presence of additional signs and symptoms such as seizures, altered sensorium, aphasia, hemianopia, sensory deficits, and

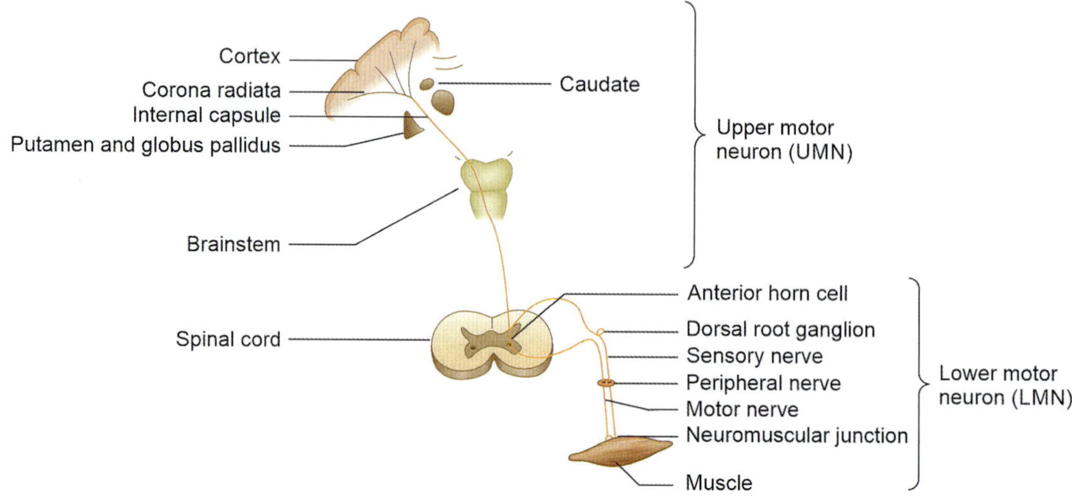

Fig. 8.1.1: Upper and lower motor neuron.

TABLE 8.1.2: UMN versus LMN lesion.

	UMN	*LMN*
Extent	Cortex, coronal radiata, internal capsule, descending corticospinal tract in cerebral peduncles, pons, medulla, spinal cord tracts	AHC, peripheral nerve, NMJ, muscle
Primary function	Inhibitory effect on muscle stretch reflex	Motor component of muscle stretch reflex
Type of paralysis	Spastic (involves antigravity muscles—upper limb flexors and lower limb extensors)	Flaccid
Tone	Increased (spasticity)	Hypotonia
Bulk	No/later disuse atrophy	Early wasting
Power	Weakness involves extensors and supinators of upper limb (deltoid, triceps, wrist, and finger extensors) and lower limb (hip and knee flexors, foot dorsiflexors, and evertors)	• Proximal weakness—myopathy • Distal weakness—neuropathy
Extent of involvement	Diffuse	Mostly localized if it involves a single nerve/ plexus lesion or a group of muscles
DTRs	Brisk	Normal/hyporeflexia/absent
Superficial reflexes	Absent	Present
Plantar reflex	Extensor (Babinski positive)	Flexor
Clonus	Present	Absent

(AHC: anterior horn cell; DTRs: deep tendon reflexes; LMN: lower motor neuron; NMJ: neuromuscular junction; UMN: upper motor neuron)

abnormal movements **(Table 8.1.3)**. If a cranial nerve palsy, such as facial nerve palsy, is seen on the side of the hemiplegia ("uncrossed hemiplegia"), then the lesion is above the brainstem. If the weakness is disproportionate, the lesion is often cortical or subcortical in location, whereas internal capsular lesions often involve both upper and lower extremities proportionately. A "crossed hemiplegia," that is, cranial nerve involvement on the ipsilateral side of the lesion and contralateral hemiparesis, often points to a brainstem lesion, with the level depending on the cranial nerves involved.[3]

WHEN TO SUSPECT A CEREBRAL LESION?

Affection of the cerebral hemispheres is well noted on examination of higher mental function, with the child presenting with altered sensorium, disturbances in attention, memory, and emotions, as well as disturbances in somatosensory perceptions leading to agraphia, acalculia, agnosia, right-left disorientation, disturbances in sensorimotor integration, and movement executions leading to apraxia, aphasias, hallucinations, and the presence of primitive reflexes.

Lesions affecting the cortex (gray matter) primarily present with seizures, cognitive affection, and aphasia, whereas subcortical white matter lesions lead to weakness, spasticity, hemisensory, and visual field deficits.[4]

Within the cortex, especially in older children and adolescents, an attempt should be made to localize the findings to a particular lobe **(Table 8.1.4)**.

TABLE 8.1.3: Localizing upper motor neuron lesions.

Site	*Symptoms/signs*
Cortex	• Differential weakness of limbs and face • Associated cognitive dysfunction, attentional alterations • Seizures • *Sensory symptoms:* Aphasia, hemianopia, and hemineglect • Language deficits
Corona radiata	Differential weakness of limbs and face with primary sensory loss
Internal capsule	Equally and densely affected face, arms, and legs
Brainstem	• Unilateral or bilateral weakness with involvement of cranial nerves (ocular/oropharyngeal involvement, vertigo, diplopia, dysarthria) • Crossed hemiplegia
Spinal cord	• Face spared • Sensory level • Bladder/bowel incontinence

A focal weakness of hyperacute or acute onset localizing to the cerebral cortex may result from a vascular insult, either in the form of arterial ischemic stroke or hemorrhage. In such cases, the clinical findings, instead of localizing to a specific lobe, get localized to the area supplied or vascular territory of the affected artery. For localizing stroke, a basic knowledge of the vascular supply of the CNS should be kept in mind, as depicted in **Figures 8.1.2 and 8.1.3**.

- Anterior cerebral artery (ACA) supplies the medial and superior parts of the frontal lobe as well as the anterior parietal lobe, which covers the supplementary motor cortex as well as parts of the primary motor and sensory cortex supplying the leg area. Hence, a stroke in the ACA territory would manifest as behavioral change and contralateral leg weakness.[4]
- Middle cerebral artery (MCA), however, supplies the majority of the lateral surface of the cerebral hemispheres,

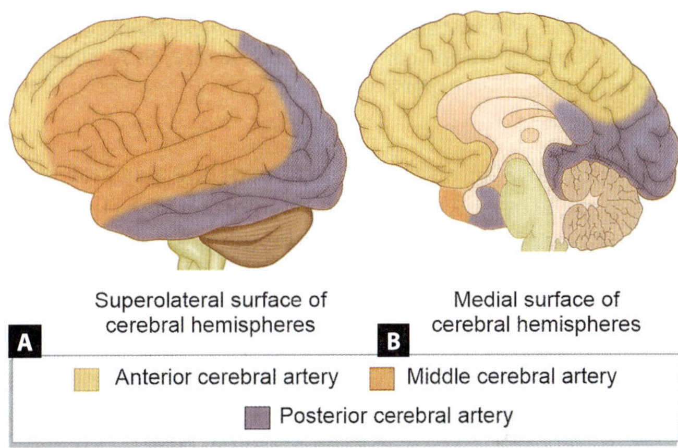

Figs. 8.1.2A and B: Vascular supply of cerebral hemispheres.

TABLE 8.1.4: Major localizing signs/symptoms of various cerebral lobes.

Frontal lobe	***Parietal lobe***
• Disinhibition • Antisocial behavior • Defective executive functioning • Impaired memory • Urinary incontinence • Appearance of primitive reflexes • Akinesia/akinetic mutism • Motor aphasia	• Contralateral sensory loss and pain, paresthesia (postcentral gyrus) • Homonymous hemianopia *Dominant hemisphere* • Dyscalculia • Dyslexia • Apraxia • Finger agnosia • Right–left disorientation *Nondominant hemisphere* • Neglect of nondominant side • Spatial disorientation • Constructional apraxia • Dressing apraxia
Temporal lobe	***Occipital lobe***
• Amnesia • Complex hallucinations • Auditory agnosia (bilateral lesion) *Dominant hemisphere* • Sensory aphasia • Dyslexia • Agitated delirium *Nondominant hemisphere* • Poor nonverbal memory • Loss of musical skills • Impaired recognition of facial emotions	• Homonymous hemianopia • Visual agnosia • Impaired face recognition (prosopagnosia) • Visual hallucination

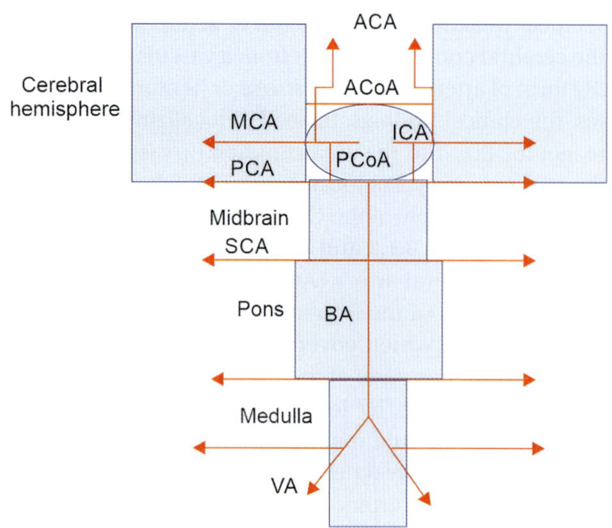

Fig. 8.1.3: Circle of Willis. (ACA: anterior cerebral artery; ACoA: anterior communicating artery; BA: basilar artery; ICA: internal carotid artery; MCA: middle cerebral artery; PCA: posterior cerebellar artery; PCoA: posterior communicating artery; SCA: superior cerebellar artery; VA: vertebral artery)

except for the superior portion of the parietal lobe (supplied by ACA) and the inferior portion of the temporal and occipital lobes [supplied by the posterior cerebral artery (PCA)]. Hence, an MCA territory infarct presents as contralateral face and arm predominant weakness with sensory deficits, hemineglect, and speech disturbances.[4]

- PCA supplies the occipital lobe, inferomedial surface of the temporal lobe, and thalamus. Hence, a PCA territory infarct would present with visual field defects and sensory deficits.[4]
- Posterior circulation infarction refers to the affection of vertebrobasilar vasculature supplying the brainstem, cerebellum, and thalamus along with areas of the temporal and occipital lobes. It presents with vertigo, ataxia, dizziness, and impaired balance along with cranial nerve involvement causing pupil and eye movement abnormalities, changes in voice and swallowing, decreased levels of consciousness, and occasionally motor and sensory findings.

WHEN TO SUSPECT INVOLVEMENT OF DEEP GRAY MATTER (BASAL GANGLIA)?

Lesions of the basal ganglia or the extrapyramidal system can present with either a change in tone (increase or decrease in tone) or abnormal movements (hypokinetic or hyperkinetic involuntary movements). The findings can be either bilateral or contralateral. Tone abnormalities can be classified as rigidity or variable tone (a feature of dystonia).

TABLE 8.1.5: Differences between spasticity and rigidity.

Spasticity	***Rigidity***
More resistance in the initial part followed by release—"clasp knife"	• *Lead pipe:* Uniform increase in tone • *Cogwheel:* Tremor superimposed on this hypertonia that results in intermittent increase in tone during the movement
Velocity-dependent (i.e., more noticeable with fast movements)	*Not velocity-dependent:* Does not vary with the speed of movement of muscle groups involved
More resistance in one direction than the other direction	Same resistance in all directions
Caused by pyramidal tract lesions	Caused by basal ganglia lesions

It is important to distinguish between hypertonia (spasticity) caused by pyramidal tract involvement and hypertonia (rigidity) originating from extrapyramidal involvement. The differences between spasticity and rigidity are discussed in **Table 8.1.5**. Further, due to superimposed abnormal movements (described below), there can be variable tone on repeated neurological examinations.

The abnormal involuntary movements resulting from extrapyramidal involvement can be classified as either hyperkinetic or hypokinetic movements. Hyperkinetic movements include chorea, athetosis, and hemiballismus.

- *Chorea* is described as involuntary, forcible, rapid, arrhythmic, and flowing "dance-like" movements and leads to distortion of voluntary movements, with preserved muscle power, but due to the inability to maintain muscular contractions, may give the impression of diminished power (which has traditionally been described as milkmaids' grip).[1]
- *Athetosis* is comparatively slower movements than chorea, traditionally described as slow, sinuous, writhing movements seen over distal extremities (hands), face, and tongue and seem to flow into one another. Chorea and athetosis are poorly localized and can be caused by lesions involving the striatum, pallidum, thalamus, or subthalamus.[1]
- *Ballismus or hemiballismus* is described as violent, flinging movements involving the proximal joints, resulting from lesions of the contralateral subthalamic nucleus.[1]
- *Dystonias* are characterized by slow, sustained, involuntary twisting movements or postures, which can involve axial as well as appendicular muscles, and are caused by lesions of the globus pallidus.[1]
- *Hypokinetic movement disorders* are relatively rare in children and are traditionally described as features of parkinsonism, which include bradykinesia or hypokinesia,

that is, slowness of movements with reduced arm swing, shuffled walk, lack of facial expressions (masked facies or hypomimia), along with slow, monotonous speech with reduced volume, associated rigidity, and resting tremors. These are seen in lesions of the substantia nigra and globus pallidus.

WHEN TO SUSPECT BRAINSTEM LESION?

The brainstem is subdivided into the midbrain, pons, and medulla. Affection of the brainstem causes a constellation of motor and sensory deficits with involvement of cranial nerves with crossed signs (as described above) due to the transection of major pathways at various levels **(Table 8.1.6)**.

WHEN TO SUSPECT A CEREBELLAR LESION?

The cerebellum is predominantly involved in coordinating movements and balance. Hence, a cerebellar lesion will manifest as a wobbly or clumsy child with truncal imbalances, gait difficulties, and head titubations, that is, constant to-and-fro nodding movement of the head in an upright position. Truncal instability will be manifested during walking with a tendency to fall, and even while sitting, the child may lean to one side (mostly toward the side of the lesion). Ataxia is the term used for the lack of muscle coordination and control. Ataxic gait involves a wide-based stance and a gait with increased trunk sway, irregular stepping with a tendency to stagger as if intoxicated, with inappropriate timing of foot placement.[1] Ataxia secondary to cerebellar injury characteristically persists despite visual cues (unlike sensory ataxia, which is more pronounced with eyes closed).[5] Hence, there will be an inability to do tandem walking and an inability to perform Romberg's test even with eyes open. The dysfunction is ipsilateral, with ipsilateral hypotonia and accompanying asynergia, dysmetria (finger-nose and heel-shin tests), and dysdiadochokinesia.[5] Accompanying cerebellar dysarthria has labored speech with occasional excessive facial grimacing with intact comprehension. Cerebellar dysarthria is described as scanning, slurred, staccato, explosive, hesitant, slow altered accent, and garbled speech. Nystagmus is also associated with a cerebellar lesion and could be gaze-evoked upbeat, rebound, and abnormal optokinetic nystagmus. The midline lesions affecting the cerebellar vermis will typically cause truncal ataxia and titubations, whereas the lesions involving the cerebellar hemispheres will present with appendicular predominant symptoms.

TABLE 8.1.6: Brainstem localization.

Site	*Signs/symptoms*
Midbrain	• Ipsilateral cranial nerve 3 and 4 palsy • Contralateral hemiplegia including lower facial weakness (corticospinal and corticobulbar tracts)
Pons	• Contralateral hemiplegia • Ipsilateral facial paresis • Ipsilateral 6th cranial nerve palsy • Ipsilateral gaze palsy • Contralateral pan-sensory loss • Locked-in syndrome
Lateral medulla	• Ipsilateral face and contralateral trunk and extremity pain and temperature: Sensory involvement • No motor weakness as pyramidal tract spared
Medial medulla	Contralateral hemiplegia with hemisensory loss with ipsilateral hypoglossal palsy

LOCALIZING LOWER MOTOR NEURON LESION

The LMN lesion presents predominantly with flaccid weakness, with or without sensory deficit. The higher mental functions stay intact. LMN lesions can be further localized to the AHC in the spinal cord or could involve the nerve, neuromuscular junction (NMJ), or muscle, as described in **Flowchart 8.1.1**. The differentiating features are tabulated in **Table 8.1.7**.

Anterior Horn Cell

Involvement of AHC, as in spinal muscular atrophy, will cause a pure motor deficit in the form of flaccid weakness, paucity of antigravity movements, more prominently proximal with areflexia and preserved sensations, along with associated fibrillations and fasciculations (twitching and flickering movements) evident in tongue muscles and hands. Muscles supplied by cranial nerves such as facial and ocular muscles are spared.[6]

Peripheral Nerve

Disorders of the peripheral nerves such as hereditary or acquired neuropathies may present with accompanying sensory loss, as the nerve consists of both motor and sensory components and has predominant distal involvement manifesting as foot or wrist drop.[6]

Neuromuscular Junction

Disorders involving the NMJ such as myasthenia gravis will have a predilection for highly active small muscles of the body such as ocular and oropharyngeal muscles. Another characteristic of NMJ involvement is easy fatigability and diurnal variation.

Muscle

Involvement of muscle will generally present with proximal weakness, except in a few rare conditions such as myotonic

TABLE 8.1.7: Localizing LMN lesion.

	AHC	*Nerve*	*NMJ*	*Muscle*
Distribution: Arms, legs, and face	Arms, legs, and late involvement of face	Arms and legs	Face, arms, and legs	Variable
Pattern of weakness	Proximal	Distal	Small muscles (extraocular)	Proximal
DTRs	Absent	Hyporeflexia	Normal	Hyporeflexia
Fluctuating/diurnal	No	No	Yes	No
Sensory deficits	No	Yes	No	No
Fasciculations and fibrillations	Present	May be present	Absent	Absent
EMG	Fasciculations/ fibrillations	Fibrillations	Decremental (myasthenia gravis) or incremental (botulism) response on RNST	Short duration, small amplitude, and polyphasic motor unit potentials
Muscle biopsy	Denervation pattern	Denervation pattern	Normal	Myopathic pattern
CPK	Normal	Normal	Normal	Elevated

(AHC: anterior horn cell; CPK: creatinine phosphokinase; DTRs: deep tendon reflexes; EMG: electromyography; NMJ: neuromuscular junction; RNST: repetitive nerve stimulation test)

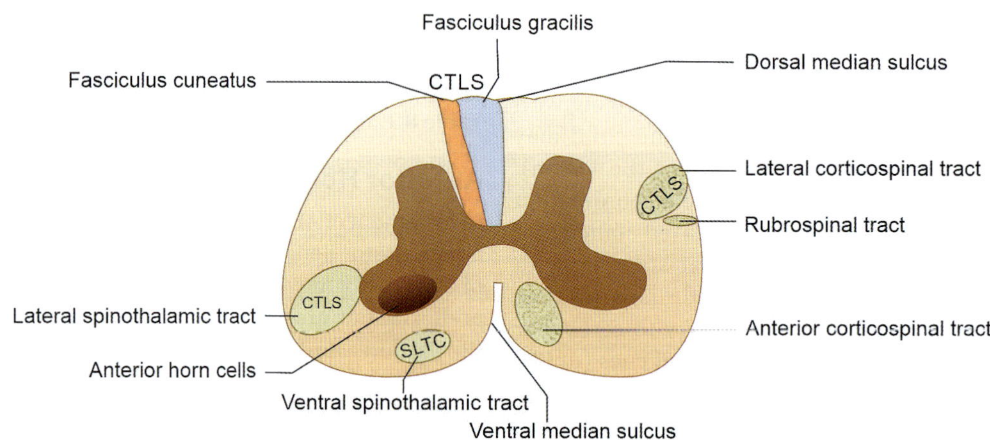

Fig. 8.1.4: Transverse section of the spinal cord.

dystrophy. Myopathies and muscular dystrophies often have a predilection to involve certain muscle groups, while other muscles are spared. Thus, hypertrophy and atrophy of different muscle groups may be seen. Face and extraocular muscles may get involved.

LOCALIZING THE LESION IN THE SPINAL CORD

The spinal cord is a tubular structure running from the foramen magnum to the lower lumbar vertebrae, and the organization of gray and white matter is opposite to that in the brain, with white matter lying in the periphery and gray matter lying in the center. The various tracts running in the white matter are either ascending tracts, which carry sensory information from receptors to the CNS, or descending tracts carrying signals from the CNS to various body parts. The location of the various tracts in the spinal cord is depicted in **Figure 8.1.4**, an understanding of which is essential for localizing lesions in the spinal cord. The most important descending tract is the corticospinal tract (or pyramidal tract), which comprises anterior and lateral corticospinal tracts. Almost 90% of the fibers in the tract cross to the opposite side in the medullary pyramids.[7] The two important ascending tracts include the anterior and lateral spinothalamic tracts, which carry pain and temperature sensation and cross to the contralateral side one to two segments above the origin in the spinal cord. The other ascending tract that runs in the posterior column carries proprioception and vibration sensation and crosses in the lower medulla.[7]

The clinician should consider spinal cord localization when:

- Motor/sensory symptoms (bilateral > unilateral) are associated with bladder/bowel dysfunction.

- Neck or back pain is present.
- A sensory level across the trunk or a tight band around the trunk or torso is evident.
- Presence of dissociative sensory loss, that is, the presence of loss of proprioception on one side and loss of pain and temperature sensation on the other side.[8]
- The presence of certain signs must alert a novice examiner against spinal cord localization, such as the presence of cranial nerve deficits, a pure LMN presentation, monoparesis of a limb, or proximal muscle weakness, especially with normal sensation and reflexes.

Localization in the spinal cord is both horizontal and longitudinal.

Horizontal Localization

- The spinal cord is surrounded by a meningeal cover called the dura mater. Any pathology affecting the cord may originate outside the dura mater and compress the cord (extradural lesion) or may originate inside the dura (intradural lesion). These intradural lesions can originate from within the spinal cord parenchyma (intramedullary) or outside the spinal cord but within the dural covering (extramedullary). While localizing a cord lesion, the clinician is required to identify the same **(Table 8.1.8)**.[8]
- Intramedullary lesions affect the central gray matter first. The UMN motor signs come late. They tend to have symmetric involvement with early bladder affection. These lesions involve the centrally placed spinothalamic tract and spare the posterior columns (hence cause dissociation of sensation) and cause a descending type of sensory loss (due to the somatotopic organization of spinothalamic tracts with cervical and upper limb represented medially).[8]

TABLE 8.1.8: Extramedullary versus intramedullary spinal cord lesion.

Signs and symptoms	*Extramedullary*	*Intramedullary*
Spontaneous pain	Radicular type	Dysesthesia/burning type, poorly localized
Sensory deficit	Contralateral loss of pain and temperature and ipsilateral loss of proprioception	Pain and temperature affected, proprioception intact
Saddle anesthesia	Yes	No
LMN signs	Segmental	More marked
UMN signs	Early	Late
DTRs	Increased	Late changes
Trophic changes	Less marked	More marked

(DTRs: deep tendon reflexes; LMN: lower motor neuron; UMN: upper motor neuron)

- Extramedullary lesions involve the white matter first. These involve the posterior columns (causing Lhermitte's sign), the corticospinal tracts (depicting UMN signs), and cause an ascending sensory loss, that is, sacral involvement first due to the somatotopic organization of spinothalamic tracts, with sacral segments represented more laterally.[8]

Longitudinal Localization

- A lesion at a specific level will cause LMN signs at the level of the lesion and UMN signs below the level of the lesion. Further, sensory and local tenderness/back pain and vertebral level can also help to localize the level.
- A lesion at the cervical level—LMN signs in arms with spastic legs and involvement of the diaphragm.[8]
- A lesion at the thoracic level—presence of Beevor's sign (abnormal upward movement of the umbilicus on attempting to raise the head from supine position due to a rectus abdominis muscle weakness), Horner's syndrome (C8–T1 lesion), and intercostal neuralgia. There would be no arm deficits in lesions below T1.[8]
- A lesion at the lumbar level—may present as a conus medullaris or cauda equina syndrome (as described in **Table 8.1.9**).

TABLE 8.1.9: Conus medullaris versus cauda equina lesions.

	Conus medullaris	*Cauda equina*
Distribution	Spinal cord tip containing sacral and coccygeal segments (S1 and below): UMN (+LMN because of AHCs)	Lumbar 2 (L2) spinal nerve roots and below: LMN type involvement
Onset	Sudden/bilateral	Gradual/unilateral
Pain	Uncommon	*Common:* Radicular, severe, asymmetric over perineum and thigh
Sensory deficit	*Saddle:* Symmetric and dissociation	*Saddle:* Asymmetric, not dissociation
Motor loss	Symmetric, less severe, fasciculation present	Asymmetric, severe, atrophy
DTRs	Ankle jerk absent (lesion below S1)	Knee and ankle jerks absent
Bowel/ bladder	Early/marked	Late/less marked
Trophic changes	Common	Less common

(AHCs: anterior horn cells; DTRs: deep tendon reflexes; LMN: lower motor neuron; UMN: upper motor neuron)

CONCLUSION

Localization on the neuroanatomical axis, coupled with a comprehensive history and examination, constitutes the initial stride toward identifying an etiology. Accurate localization significantly narrows down the differentials. Once the lesion's location is pinpointed, consideration turns to the pathophysiologic causes. Nearly all neurologic lesions fall into one of seven pathophysiologic processes:

1. Traumatic
2. Vascular
3. Inflammatory (infective/parainfective/noninfective)
4. Toxic–metabolic
5. Degenerative
6. Neoplastic
7. Congenital/genetic

A detailed history outlining the onset and temporal evolution of symptoms aids in identifying the underlying pathophysiology. A hyperacute presentation suggests a vascular or traumatic etiology, while an acute presentation evolving over days may indicate an inflammatory pathology. Conversely, a subacute to chronic presentation aligns more closely with a neoplastic etiology. The final step entails identifying the specific etiology, which, through one of the aforementioned pathophysiologic processes, has generated a lesion at the identified site, resulting in the observed clinical manifestations in the patient.

When applied appropriately, such a structured, stepwise approach empowers clinicians to arrive at a correct diagnosis with a minimal set of investigations. This method significantly reduces the likelihood of being misled by atypical or complex presentations.

REFERENCES

1. Brazis PW, Masdeu JC, Biller J. Localization in Clinical Neurology. Philadelphia: Lippincott Williams & Wilkins; 2012.
2. Ranganathan LN. Localization of Clinical Neurology. Gurugram: Wolters Kluwer India Pvt. Ltd.; 2020.
3. Assir MZ, Das JM. How to Localize Neurologic Lesions by Physical Examination. StatPearls. St. Petersburg: StatPearls Publishing; 2022.
4. Berkowitz AL. Clinical Neurology and Neuroanatomy: A Localization-Based Approach. Boston: McGraw Hill Professional; 2022.
5. D'Arrigo S, Loiacono C, Ciaccio C, Pantaleoni C, Faccio F, Taddei M, et al. Clinical, cognitive and behavioural assessment in children with cerebellar disorder. Appl Sci. 2021;11(2):544.
6. Leung R, Yiu EM. Practical approach to the child presenting with acute generalised weakness. J Paediatr Child Health. 2024;60(2-3):41-6.
7. Cho TA. Spinal cord functional anatomy. Continuum (Minneap Minn). 2015;21(1):13-35.
8. Gruener G, Biller J. Spinal cord anatomy, localization, and overview of spinal cord syndromes. Continuum Lifelong Learning Neurol. 2008;14(3):11-35.

8.2 Investigations in Pediatric Neurology

Lokesh Lingappa, Bhoomika Sharma

INTRODUCTION

Developmental stages of children are distinctive, and physiology of the pediatric population is dynamic, due to which timely and specific investigations are crucial for effective management and intervention of pediatric neurological disorders. This requires a multidisciplinary approach that combines clinical assessments, neuroimaging, electrophysiological studies, and laboratory analyses. This chapter discusses the different diagnostic tools and methodologies employed in pediatric neurology, highlighting their applications and benefits. The investigations that need to be performed in children with neurological illnesses are dependent on:

- *State of the illness:* Acute, subacute, or chronic
- *Age of child:* Newborn, infant, toddler, childhood, or adolescence
- *Etiology of the illness:* Acquired versus genetic or metabolic

Thus, no single investigation plan suits every child with a neurological illness. It is essential to have a general awareness of the range of available tests for any given condition.

TESTING IN ACUTE CARE NEUROLOGY IN CASES WITH ENCEPHALOPATHY OR FOCAL WEAKNESS

Complete Blood Counts

Red Blood Cell Profile

- *Low mean corpuscular volume (MCV) or low mean corpuscular hemoglobin concentration (MCHC)* is indicative of iron deficiency anemia, which puts the child at an increased risk for stroke.

- *Sickling* is associated with stroke and sickle cell crises.
- *Increased rouleaux formation* is seen in mycoplasma-associated stroke or encephalopathy.

Low Platelet Count

Low platelet count is considered an indicator of central nervous system (CNS) bleed.

White Blood Cell Count

- *Low white blood cell (WBC) count (especially lymphocytes):*
  - Consider immunodeficiency—T-cell deficiency associated with CNS manifestations
  - In children on chemotherapy—absolute lymphocyte count of <500 could be indicative of febrile neutropenia due to an uncommon organism affecting the brain
- *High WBC count:*
  - Evidence of *neutrophilic leukocytosis* may be indicative of bacterial infection.
  - Elevated *absolute lymphocyte count* is suggestive of tuberculous or fungal infections.
  - *Eosinophilia* (specifically, eosinophils >1,000/μL) in the context of an acute illness is suggestive of a noninfectious (e.g., autoimmune), parasitic (e.g., acute schistosomiasis), or fungal (e.g., coccidiomycosis, etc.) cause for the illness.[1]

Erythrocyte Sedimentation Rate

High erythrocyte sedimentation rate (ESR; specifically toward 100 mm/1st hour) is seen in tubercular meningitis or other chronic infections, systemic vasculitis, and systemic malignancy.

Coagulation Profile

- In infants or newborns with prolonged *prothrombin time (PT) or activated partial thromboplastin time (aPTT)*, with or without mucosal bleeds or prolonged ooze from venipuncture sites, consider hemorrhagic disease of newborn (HDN).
- CNS bleeds with normal coagulation profile are seen in arteriovenous (AV) malformations or aneurysmal bleeds.
- In cases other than AV malformations and aneurysmal bleeds, factor 13 assay with platelet function studies should be done.
- Stroke or sinovenous thrombosis in children may be associated with low protein C, protein S, factor V Leiden deficiency, or antithrombin III deficiency in small percentage of population.

Cardiology evaluation is important for children with stroke, and infections are one of the high-risk factors for stroke in children.

Biochemistry Tests

Serum Sodium

Sudden drop in sodium levels is associated with acute encephalopathy, symptomatic seizures, and pontine or extrapontine myelinolysis.

Serum Potassium

- Low levels are more likely to be associated with acute weakness.
- In case of hypokalemic periodic paralysis, investigate for renal tubular acidosis

Blood Urea and Serum Creatinine

While sudden high levels are seen in acute uremic encephalopathy, low creatinine levels are generally indicative of low muscle mass.

Serum Uric Acid

- In case of significantly *low serum uric acid* in infants with recurrent unexplained CNS presentation or spastic diplegia, a variant of purine nucleoside phosphorylase (PNP) deficiency may be considered.
- *Elevated serum uric acid levels* in children with developmental delay, self-mutilation, and movement abnormality help in diagnosis of Lesch–Nyhan syndrome.

Liver Function Tests

- Significantly elevated liver enzymes in acute encephalopathy is indicative of hepatic encephalopathy.
- In case of acute liver failure with Coombs negative hemolysis, moderate aminotransferase elevation, low alkaline phosphatase levels, and alkaline phosphatase/bilirubin ratio of <2, Wilson's disease should be considered.
- Chronic unconjugated hyperbilirubinemia with chronic encephalopathy—consider Crigler–Najjar syndrome

C-reactive Protein

- Significantly elevated C-reactive protein (CRP) levels are seen in infections (e.g., bacterial infections including subdural empyema or brain abscess).
- CRP levels can also be elevated in inflammatory or vasculitic conditions.

Procalcitonin

Procalcitonin is predominantly a marker of bacterial infections.

Microbiology

Blood Cultures

- Blood cultures are essential investigations in all pediatric cases presenting with acute encephalopathy, with or without seizures.
- Bactec cultures are sent for diagnosis of tuberculosis.

Serological Tests

They are most commonly done in suspected rickettsial infections, mycoplasma, dengue with acute encephalopathy, and brucellosis, which may present with chronic meningitis.

Serum Myelin Oligodendrocyte Glycoprotein and Neuromyelitis Optica Antibodies

These are investigated when there is evidence of demyelination on magnetic resonance imaging (MRI) brain, optic neuritis, myelitis, and diffuse encephalopathy with or without fever and minimal cerebrospinal fluid (CSF) pleocytosis with raised proteins.

Metabolic Investigations

Blood Lactate

There are various reasons for the elevation of blood lactate levels. Some examples include:

- In acutely unwell children with shock, lactate levels are elevated but get rapidly corrected during resuscitation.
- In children with inherited metabolic disorders—mitochondrial, organic acidurias, fatty acid oxidation disorders, carbohydrate metabolism disorders, etc.—lactate remains elevated for longer periods of time.
- Mitochondrial deoxyribonucleic acid (DNA) disorders such as MELAS (mitochondrial encephalomyopathy, lactic acidosis, and stroke-like episodes), MERRF (myoclonic epilepsy with ragged red fibers), etc., have more consistently elevated lactate levels compared to nuclear DNA-associated mitochondrial disorders. In nuclear DNA-associated mitochondrial disorders, it is important to check lactate levels a few times, especially during acute decompensation, to demonstrate lactic acidosis.
- Lactic acidosis is usually suspected when acidosis is persistently >5 mmol/L.
- Lactate levels alone do not provide definitive confirmation of disease presence, its severity, or prognosis.

Serum Ammonia

This is one investigation that is prone to most erroneous reports if not performed well. For accurate results, the sample tube must be filled completely, mixed well, and kept tightly stoppered at all times. The sample must be placed on ice immediately, and plasma from cells has to be separated within 15 minutes of collection. Patients should *not* clench their fists during the collection of samples. Transfer the specimen to a plastic transport tube before freezing.

Even at 4°C, ammonia levels in whole blood samples are only stable for about 1 hour before they start to rise. In as few as 2 hours at room temperature (which may be how long a phlebotomy sample stays on a collection tray), serum ammonia levels can double. The levels stay stable in plasma samples when compared to whole blood.

- Elevated ammonia is seen in synthetic liver dysfunction, but there is no exclusive correlation between the two.
- High ammonia levels are also noted in urea cycle disorders, and moderate elevation is seen in organic acidurias.

Serum Homocysteine

- Hyperhomocystinemia is associated with a higher incidence of stroke and intellectual disabilities. The reason for elevation can be genetic disorders of homocysteine or methionine metabolism or cobalamin pathway disorders.
- It is one of the most preferred investigations in children with intellectual delay associated with features such as marfanoid habitus, ectopia lentis, and in infants with developmental delay and nonfamilial hypopigmented hair.
- Acquired vitamin B12 deficiency due to a strictly vegetarian diet is a common cause of elevated homocysteine levels.

Tandem Mass Spectrometry

- Tandem mass spectrometry (TMS) is a very cost-effective method of screening for multiple small-molecule diseases such as amino acidurias, organic acidurias, and fatty acid oxidation defects.
- The best time to use this investigation as a screening tool is during the newborn period, after the baby has been fully fed for at least 48 hours.

Miscellaneous

- Abnormal liver function tests (LFT), renal function tests (RFT), leukopenia, low platelets, and low hemoglobin levels are all seen together in an encephalopathic child with a normal MRI and are generally attributed to sepsis-associated encephalopathy.
- In cases of secondary hemophagocytic lymphohistiocytosis (HLH), elevated levels of serum ferritin and lactate dehydrogenase (LDH) are seen.

NEUROIMAGING

Computed Tomography and Computed Axial Tomography

- Computed tomography (CT) scan is the imaging of choice in unstable cases of acute-onset encephalopathy due to a traumatic brain injury or if an intracranial (IC) bleed is suspected.
- CT brain with 3D reconstruction bone window is done in suspected primary craniosynostosis or plagiocephaly.
- CT brain with coronal and sagittal reconstruction to visualize lenticulostriate vessel calcification is done in infants with minor trauma and stroke **(Figs. 8.2.1A to C)**.

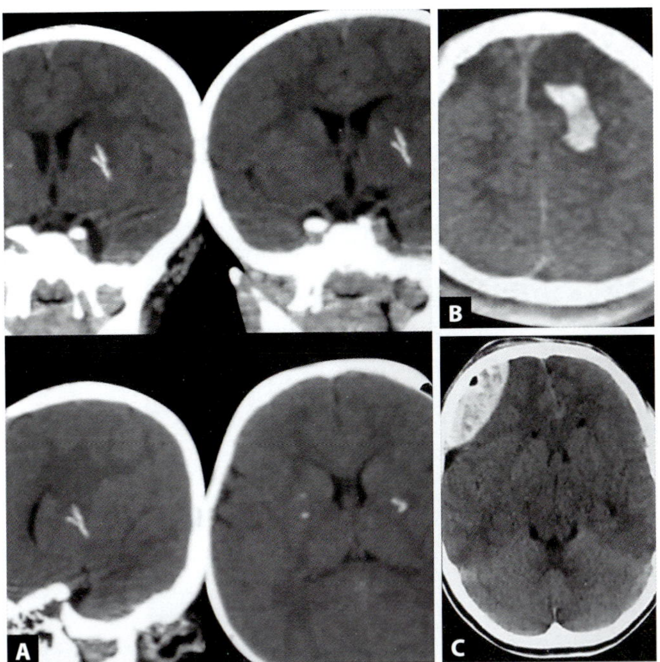

Figs. 8.2.1A to C: (A) Top: Coronal; Bottom left: Sagittal; Bottom right: Axial images demonstrating mineralizing angiopathy of lenticulostriate arteries with left lentiform nucleus infarct; (B) Right frontal epidural hematoma; and (C) Left high frontal intraparenchymal hematoma with L > R contusion, along with subgaleal collection.

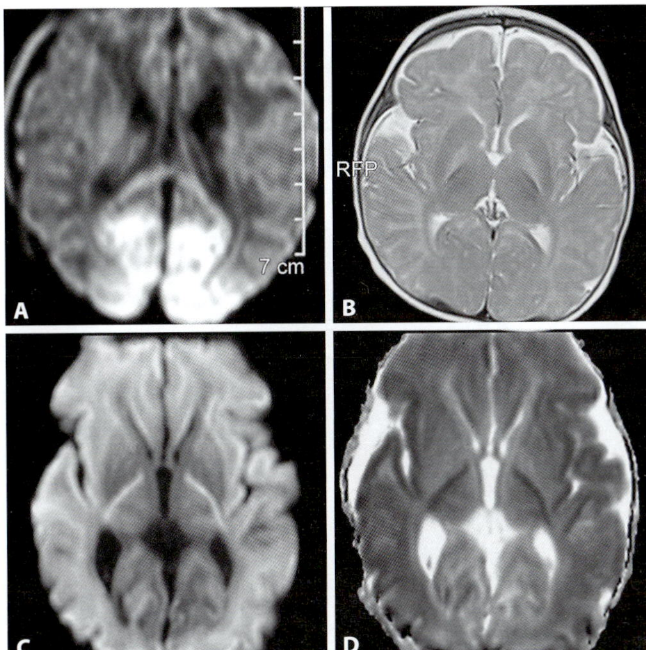

Figs. 8.2.2A to D: (A) Bilateral medial occipital gliosis in NHBI; (B) T2WI globus pallidus hyperintensities in BIND or kernicterus; (C and D) DWI and ADC images of a global devastating brain injury demonstrating restricted diffusion in the cortical region and posterior limb of the internal capsule. (ADC: apparent diffusion coefficient; BIND: bilirubin-induced neurological dysfunction; DWI: diffusion-weighted image; NHBI: neonatal hypoglycemic brain injury; T2WI: T2-weighted imaging)

Magnetic Resonance Imaging

- MRI is the imaging of choice in all acute encephalopathies, pediatric stroke, optic neuritis, degenerative brain disorders, focal epilepsies, and refractory epilepsy **(Figs. 8.2.2 and 8.2.3)**.
- MRI should always be done in liaison with pediatric neuroradiologists to choose appropriate imaging sequences.
- In cases of suspected demyelination, an early MRI brain done within 24–48 hours of onset of neurological symptoms might be normal or nonspecific. In cases of high suspicion, imaging needs to be repeated after 5–7 days of onset of symptoms.
- *Magnetic resonance spectroscopy* (MRS) is usually done to differentiate between tumors, abscesses, and demyelination. It is also the investigation of choice in suspected Canavan's disease and creatine deficiency disorders.
- *Magnetic resonance angiogram (MRA)* is the preferred imaging method in cases of stroke. It helps in the differentiation of focal cerebral arteriopathy, Moyamoya syndrome, and dissection. MRA is also done in cases of IC bleed to look for aneurysms or AV malformations. In such cases, the appropriate timing for imaging, since the onset of symptoms, should be discussed with a neuroradiologist **(Figs. 8.2.4A and B)**.
- *Magnetic resonance venogram (MRV)* is the optimal imaging technique in suspected venous strokes.

CEREBROSPINAL FLUID EVALUATION

Lumbar puncture and/or spinal tap is done in cases of suspected meningitis, meningoencephalitis, unexplained encephalopathy, demyelination, and autoimmune disorders. Rarely, it is used as a diagnostic tool in cases of malignancy. Always preserve an extra ethylenediaminetetraacetic acid (EDTA) sample for any further analysis. CSF glucose is done in the fluoride tube. Contraindications for lumbar puncture include:

- Acute raised IC pressure
- Intracranial space-occupying lesion
- Local site infection
- Coagulopathy
- Platelet count <50,000/mm^3

Opening pressure during lumbar puncture should always be measured, preferably without ketamine sedation, and should ensure that the child is not flexed excessively. The normal range of opening pressure in children is 5–15 cmH_2O.

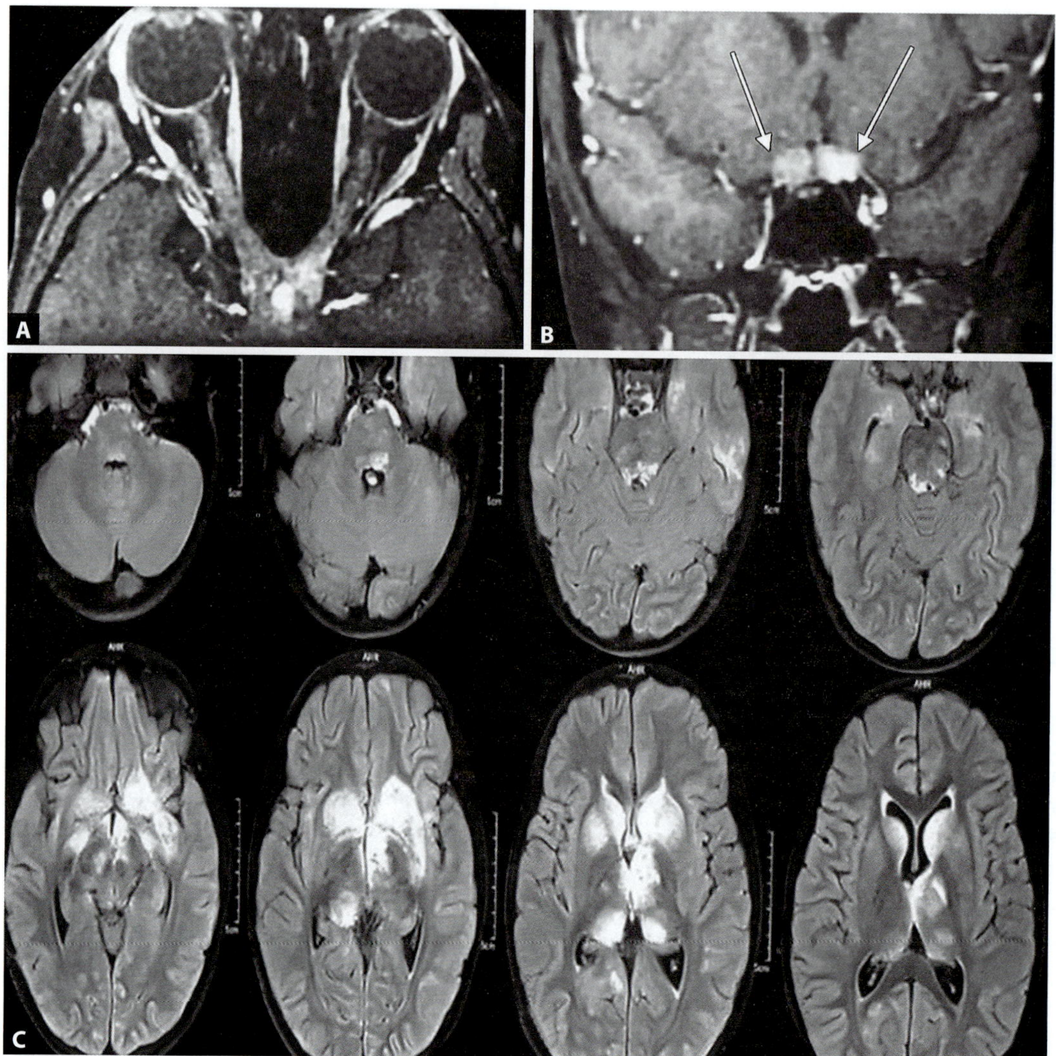

Figs. 8.2.3A to C: (A and B) Postcontrast, bilateral enlarged optic nerves (R > L) with chiasm and infundibulum involvement in case of optic neuritis; (C) Axial FLAIR images demonstrating bilateral asymmetric basal ganglia and thalamic involvement along with left dorsal pons involvement noted in children with MOG antibody disease. (FLAIR: fluid-attenuated inversion recovery; MOG: myelin oligodendrocyte glycoprotein)

Elevated opening pressure with normal cell count, normal glucose, and protein levels in CSF is seen in idiopathic IC hypertension. All acute infections and sinovenous thrombosis may have raised ICP.

Cerebrospinal Fluid Cell Count

- Normal number of cells is ≤5, all mononuclear WBCs, and no red blood cells (RBCs)
- Raised cell count with neutrophilic response could point toward a bacterial or early stages of viral infection.
- Cell counts higher than 2,000 is indicative of ventriculitis or a ruptured brain abscess.
- Lymphocytic predominance in cells is seen with viral, tubercular, and fungal infections; to a certain extent, it is also evident in partially treated pyogenic meningitis.
- Eosinophils are elevated in fungal and protozoan infections.

Cerebrospinal Fluid Protein

- Normal range of protein in CSF is 20–40 mg/dL.
- Protein levels up to 100 mg/dL are commonly seen in viral meningitis or encephalitis.
- Bacterial infection can have protein elevated up to 1,000 mg/dL or even higher.
- Rarely, tubercular meningitis can have protein levels elevated to 2–3 g/dL as well.
- Elevation of protein up to 100–200 mg/dL with a minimal increase in the number of cells is usually indicative of a peripheral or central demyelination process.

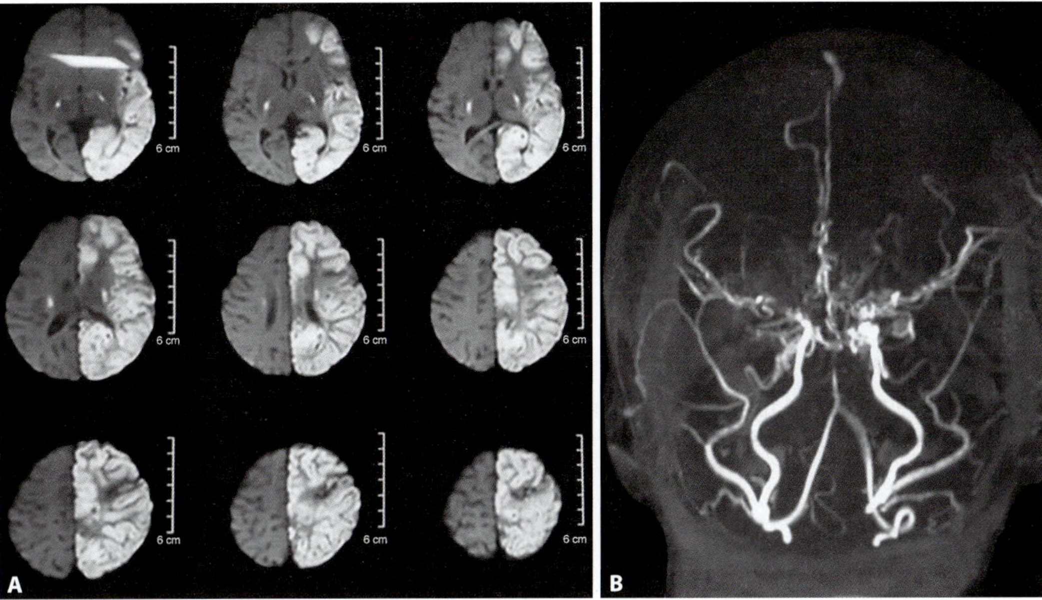

Figs. 8.2.4A and B: (A) DWI demonstrating middle cerebral artery, posterior cerebral artery, and patchy anterior cerebral artery infarcts on the left side, along with patchy restricted diffusion in the right posterior limb of the internal capsule; (B) MRA demonstrating severe narrowing of the supraclinoid internal carotid artery, along with collaterals and irregularity of the middle cerebral artery in Moyamoya disease. (DWI: diffusion-weighted image; MRA: magnetic resonance angiogram)

- When CSF proteins are very high, the cell count might be too low or zero (as cells can get trapped in the protein debris). In such instances, the possibility of Froin's syndrome should also be considered due to spinal blockade.
- In the presence of significantly elevated protein with a normal cell count, spinal cord imaging should be done.

Cerebrospinal Fluid Glucose

- Normal level of CSF glucose is usually >50% of blood glucose levels.
- Blood glucose levels should always be checked for before the lumbar puncture, as the stress of the procedure might increase blood glucose levels.
- Hypoglycorrhachia is when the CSF glucose level is <45 mg/dL or a CSF-to-serum glucose ratio ≤0.5 is seen, and it is commonly noticed in bacterial, tubercular, and fungal infections of the meninges and brain. Hypoglycorrhachia in the absence of an infection marker in a child with epilepsy and developmental delay may point toward glucose transporter-1 (GLUT1) deficiency.
- Mumps meningitis can also have low CSF glucose.

Cerebrospinal Fluid Autoimmune Antibodies

- *N*-methyl-D-aspartate receptor (NMDAR) antibody is the most common antibody-associated disease seen in children and as an investigation has higher sensitivity and specificity as compared to serum antibodies.
- Anti-glutamic acid decarboxylase (GAD) antibodies are elevated to 100–1,000 times the normal levels in acquired stiff-person syndrome.
- Voltage-gated potassium channel (VGKC) antibodies are elevated in faciobrachial seizures. They should also be looked at in cases of other refractory focal epilepsies that are nonstructural.
- CSF oligoclonal bands are done in the setting of demyelination to assess the risk of the development of multiple sclerosis.

ELECTROENCEPHALOGRAM

Electroencephalograms (EEGs) are ordered when there is a possibility of an event being epileptic in nature. Normal EEGs do not help in differentiation of epileptic and nonepileptic events. In most situations, the distinction between epileptic and nonepileptic events is made clinically based on history and home videos. EEG done within the first 12–16 hours following epileptiform seizure has the best yield, provided no intravenous benzodiazepine injections are given.[2]

The EEG has to include a record of electrical activity during sleep and awake periods, along with all activation procedures such as hyperventilation and photic stimulation (possible only in cooperative children). When necessary, sleep-deprived EEG can be done to increase the yield in cases of focal epilepsies. While the sensitivity of a standard 1-hour recording of the EEG is good for diagnostic confirmation of epileptic spasms, Lennox–Gastaut syndrome, absence epilepsy, and benign focal epilepsies of childhood, it is low for most other conditions, including focal epilepsies.[3]

The sensitivity of EEG is also age- and syndrome-dependent. Drugs that can be safely used to induce sedation for EEG include chlordiazepoxide and melatonin.

Figures 8.2.5 and 8.2.6 show normal patterns seen during normal wake and sleep periods, whereas **Figures 8.2.7 to 8.2.12** show a spectrum of abnormal EEG patterns seen in various disorders.

VISUAL EVOKED POTENTIAL

Visual evoked potential (VEP) is used to investigate anterior visual pathway abnormalities. The presence of waveforms should be established first.

Latency Measurements

- Absolute/peak latency is the duration in milliseconds from the start of click to the appearance of a wave.
- Interpeak latency or interval is the duration in milliseconds between peaks of two waves.
- Peak-to-peak amplitude is calculated most often. This is the difference in voltage between two successive peaks.
- The procedure involves independent stimulation of each eye. Multiple stimuli are given and then the latencies are averaged. Primarily, P100 latencies along with amplitudes are measured. Usually, the maximum latencies in children are around 107 ms. Anything above 113 ms latency for boys and 109 ms for girls is considered abnormal and is predominantly seen in demyelinating disorders.
- Flash VEP is done in children who are unable to cooperate and fixate well.
- Pattern reversal VEP has much better reliability but can be performed only in cooperative children.

BRAINSTEM EVOKED RESPONSE AUDIOMETRY

Brainstem evoked response audiometry (BERA) is also known as brainstem auditory evoked potential (BAEP). It is the first 10 ms of response produced in the brainstem after an auditory stimulus.

- Amplitude of a wave is measured in microvolts (μV) from the peak of a wave to the peak of next trough.
- Absolute peak latency is the duration in milliseconds from the start of click to the appearance of a wave; interpeak latency or interval is the duration in milliseconds between peaks of two waves.
- Interaural peak latency is the difference in milliseconds of a particular wave between two ears. This is useful in unilateral ear disease, for example, acoustic neuroma (interaural wave V latencies).
- Up to 20% of newborns may not have reproducible BERA at birth, and only 1–5% of them will have persistent abnormalities at 3 months.[4]

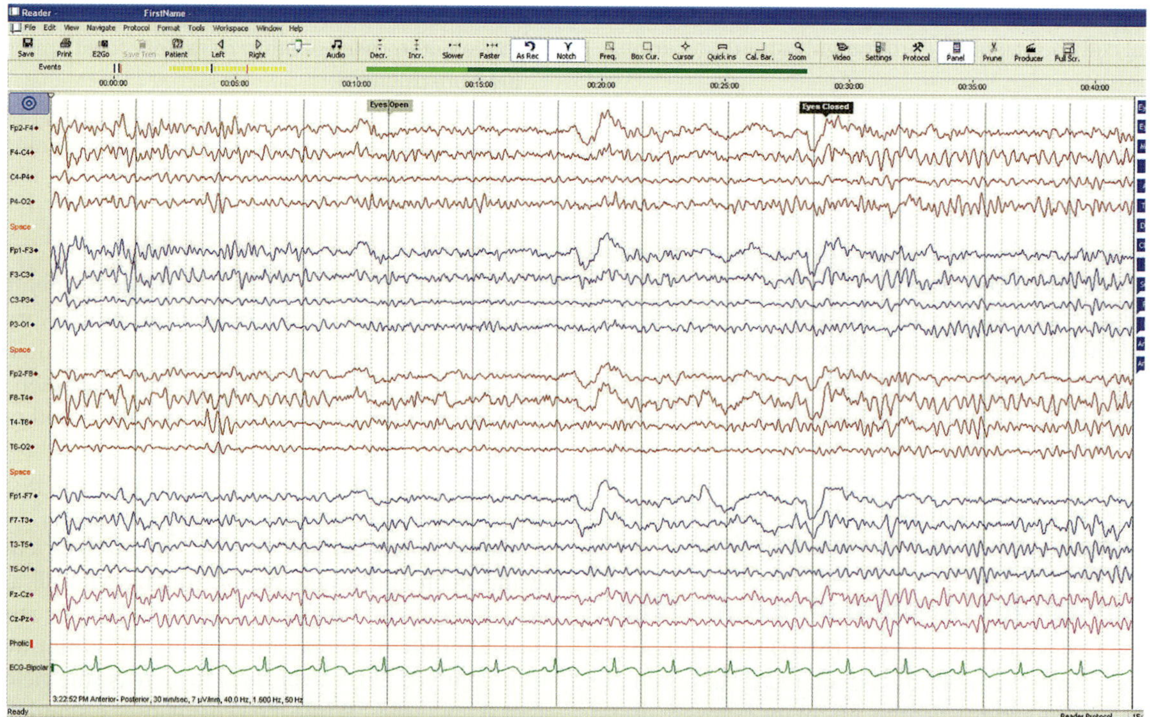

Fig. 8.2.5: Normal awake EEG with good posterior dominant alpha rhythm. (EEG: electroencephalogram)

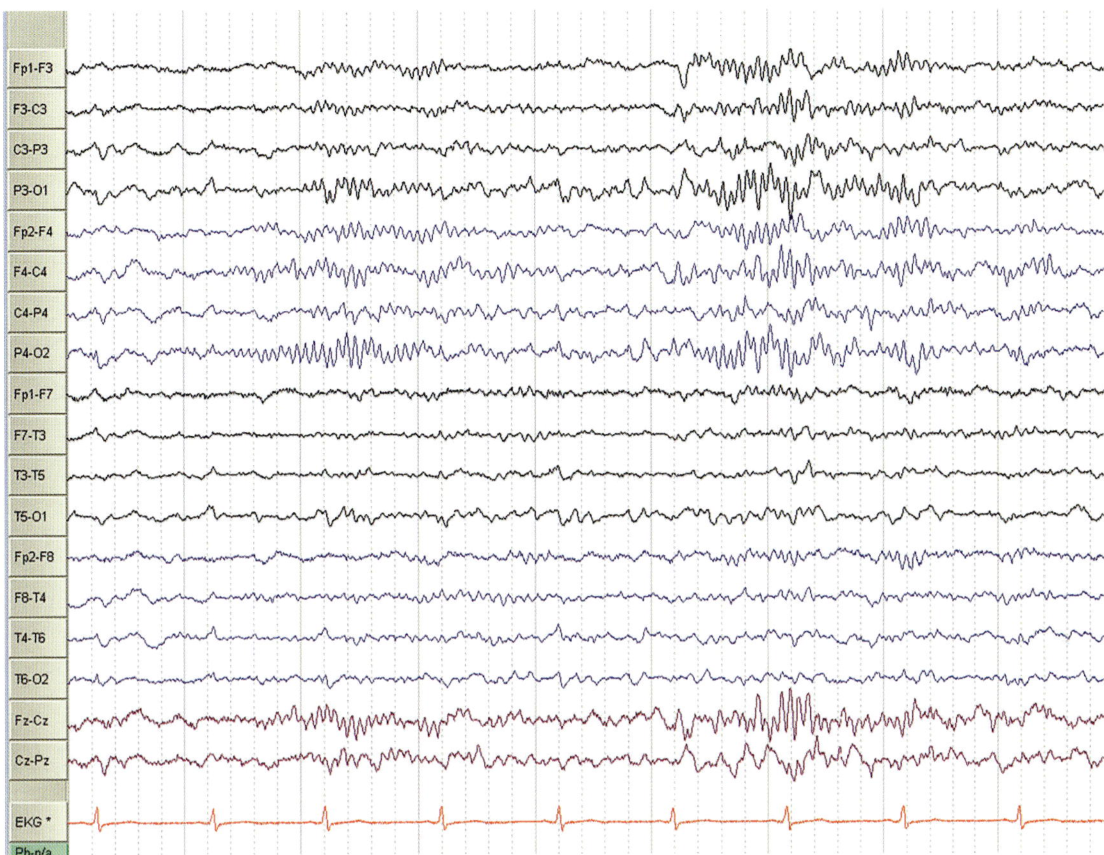

Fig. 8.2.6: Normal sleep record with sleep spindles.

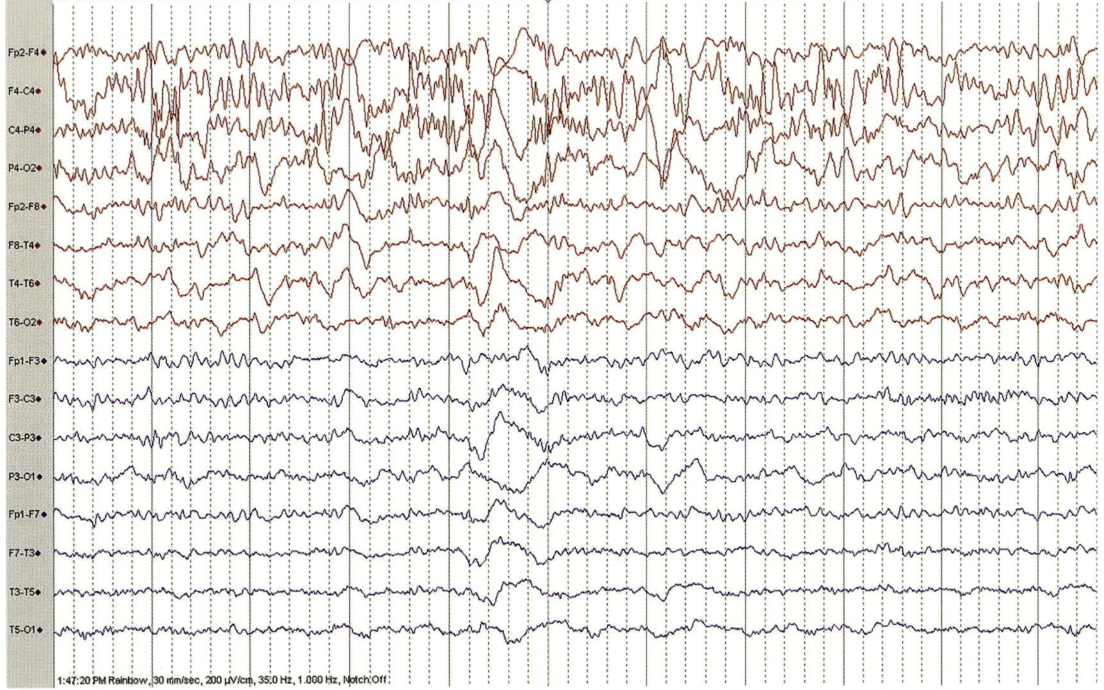

Fig. 8.2.7: Right hemispheric discharges noted in an infant with right hemimegalencephaly.

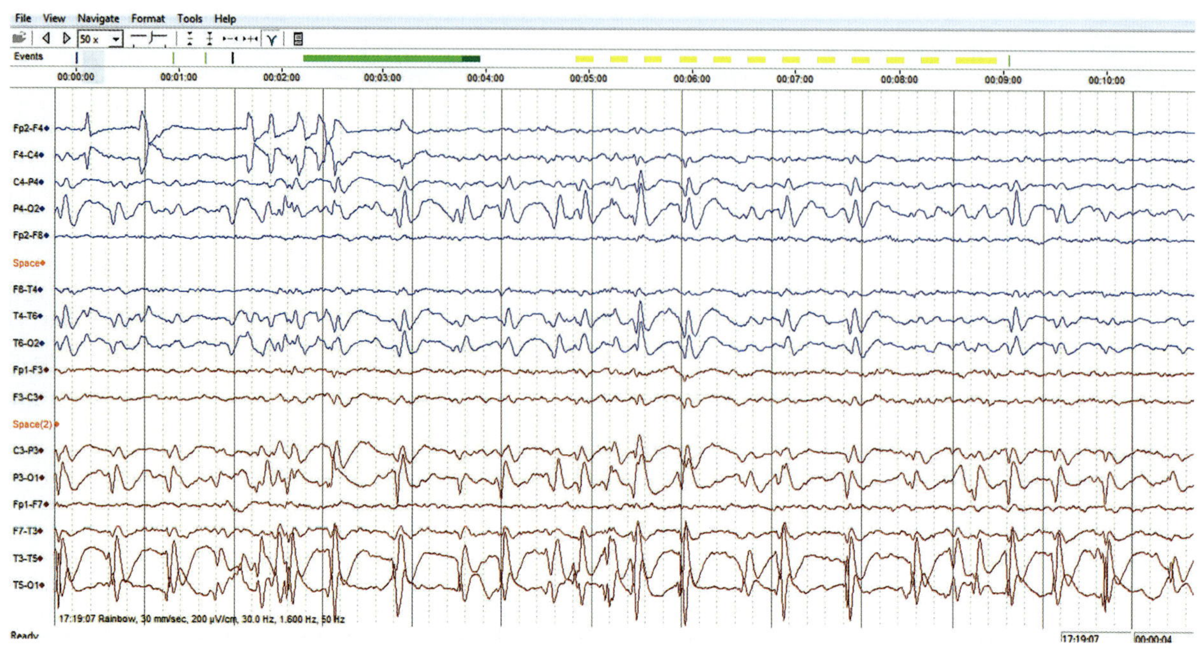

Fig. 8.2.8: Benign occipital lobe epilepsy of Gastaut type (COVE) with frequent occipital lobe discharges. (COVE: childhood-onset visual epilepsy)

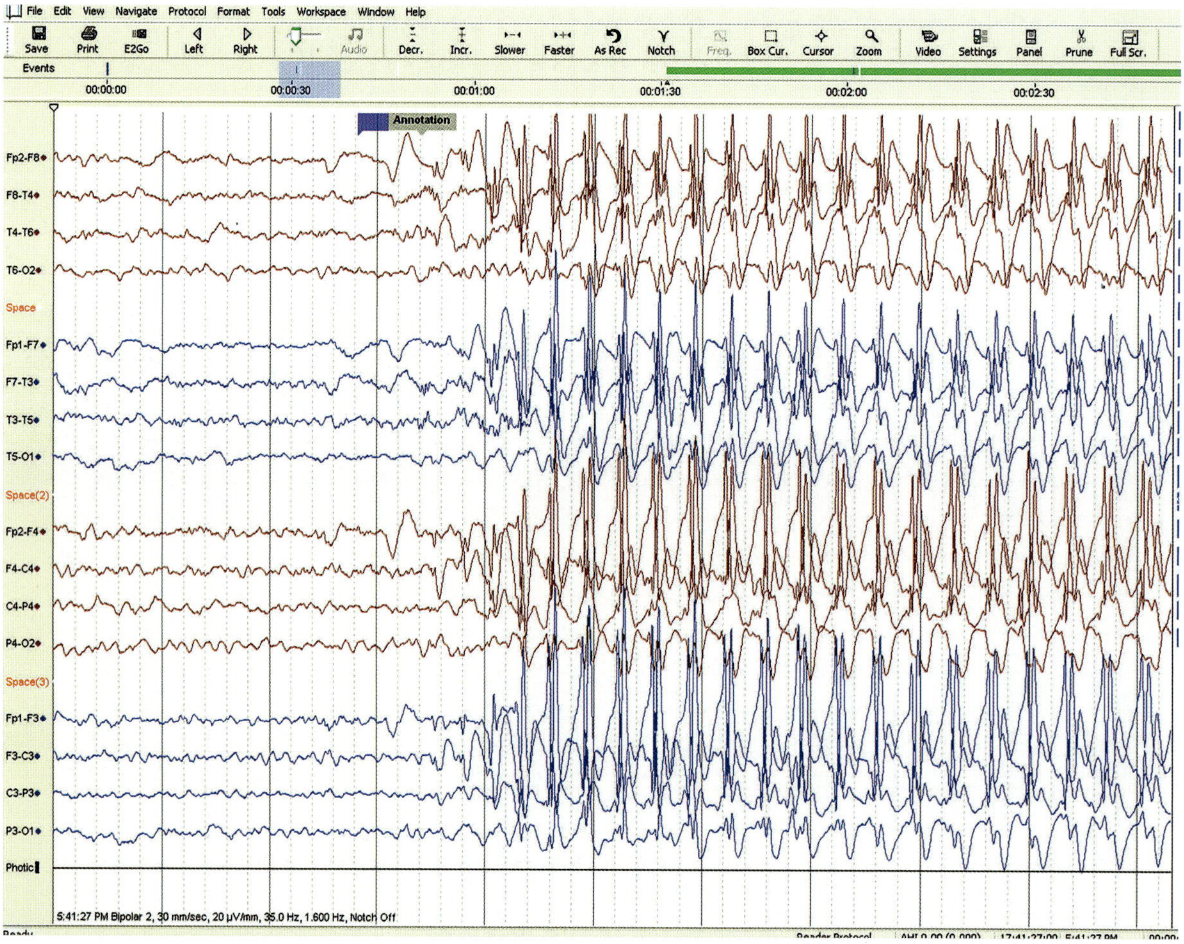

Fig. 8.2.9: Abrupt onset of generalized 3 Hz spike and slow wave discharges on hyperventilation in absence epilepsy.

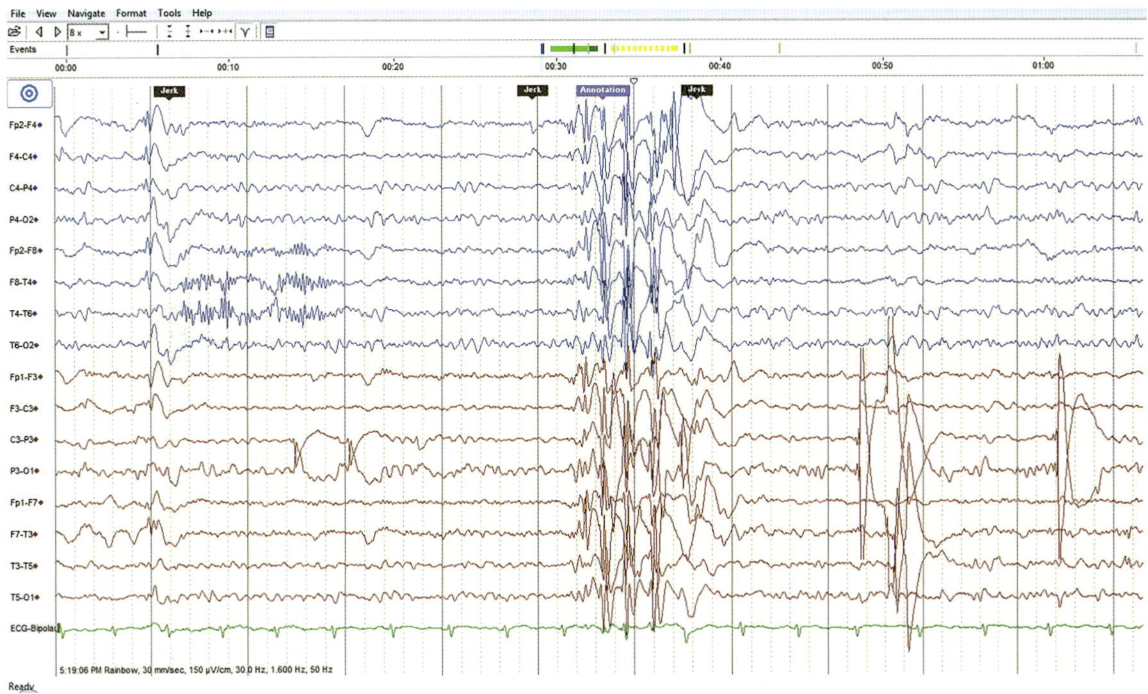

Fig. 8.2.10: Intermittent burst of generalized spike and poly-spike wave discharges with myoclonic jerks noted on normal background in JME. (JME: juvenile myoclonic epilepsy)

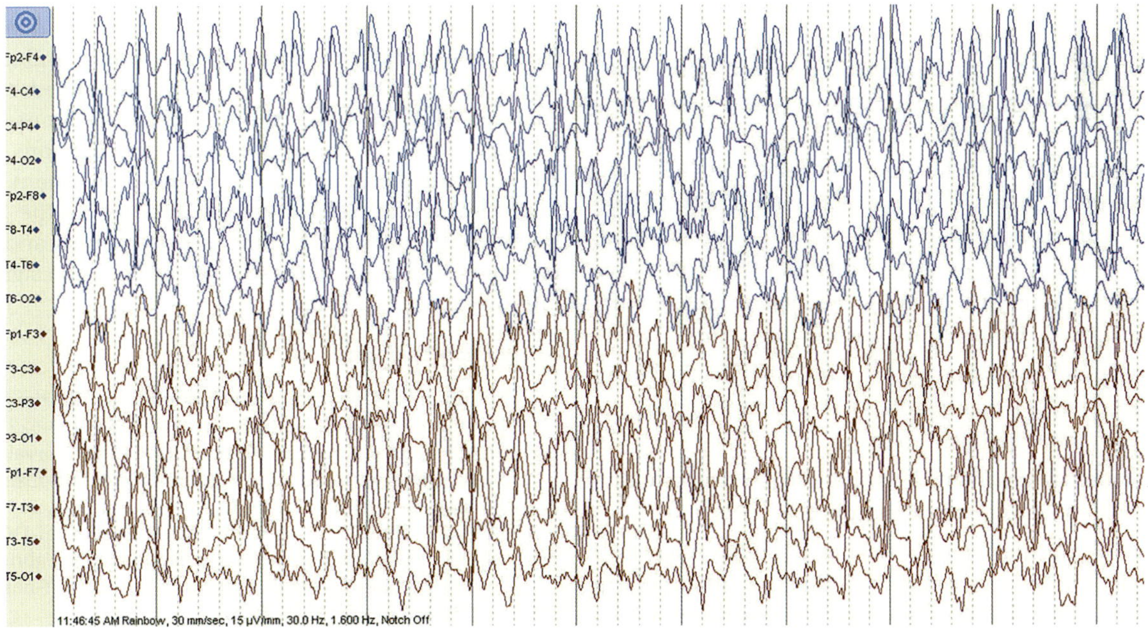

Fig. 8.2.11: EEG in pediatric ICU to look at nonconvulsive status and for monitoring of SRSE. (EEG: electroencephalogram; ICU: intensive care unit; SRSE: super refractory status epilepticus)e

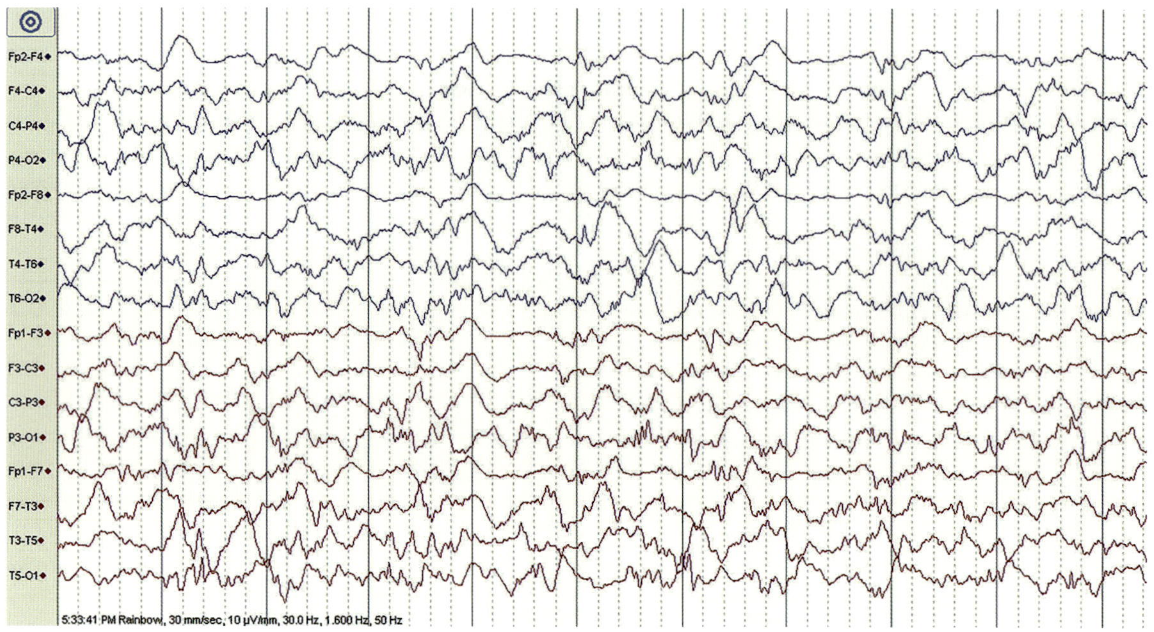

Fig. 8.2.12: EEG of the same child while on midazolam infusion with clearance of NCSE. (EEG: electroencephalogram; NCSE: nonconvulsive status epilepticus)

NERVE CONDUCTION STUDIES

Nerve conduction studies (NCS) are a useful tool to study the functioning of both motor and sensory nerves. The procedure requires cooperation of the patients, and in young children, it is performed after administering oral sedation. NCS requires small electrical stimulation to be administered to the motor and sensory nerves. This electrical stimulation produces an electrical response, which in turn is recorded and then tabulated. The distal motor latencies, velocities, and amplitudes are all recorded. The sensory testing is done with small electrical currents, and the response is documented. Only large, and to a certain extent, medium-sized fibers are tested during routine NCS. We can also look at the proximal part of the nerve by performing F wave testing.

- The pattern of abnormalities helps to distinguish between length-dependent neuropathies and acquired nonlength-dependent neuropathies
- This procedure also helps in elicitation of sensory-motor, only sensory, or only motor neuropathies.
- *Caveat*—Acute abnormalities of nerve function may take a few days to be reflected in the NCS. In Guillain-Barré syndrome (GBS), the abnormalities may take a few days before we find clear abnormalities in NCS. In this situation, an MRI of the lumbosacral spine with contrast will provide a necessary clue to diagnoses of GBS.

CONCLUSION

Investigations in pediatric neurology are essential for diagnosing a wide range of CNS disorders in children. A comprehensive approach, including clinical assessment, neuroimaging, electrophysiological studies, and laboratory tests, is crucial for accurate diagnosis and effective management. The choice of tests is influenced by factors such as the child's age, the nature of the illness, and its etiology. Selecting the appropriate investigations not only aids in accurate diagnosis and timely treatment but also helps reduce unnecessary cost, minimizing the financial burden on families and healthcare system. Early and targeted interventions based on these investigations can significantly improve patient outcomes.

REFERENCES

1. O'Connell EM, Nutman TB. Eosinophilia in infectious diseases. Immunol Allergy Clin North Am. 2015;35(3):493-522.
2. Sofat P, Teter B, Kavak KS, Gupta R, Li P. Time interval providing highest yield for initial EEG in patients with new onset seizures. Epilepsy Res. 2016:127:229-32.
3. Baldin E, Hauser WA, Buchhalter JR, Hesdorffer DC, Ottman R. Yield of epileptiform electroencephalogram abnormalities in incident unprovoked seizures: a population-based study. Epilepsia. 2014;55(9):1389-98.
4. Singh R, Vates E. Brainstem auditory evoked response test. In: StatPearls. Treasure Island, FL: StatPearls Publishing; 2024. [online] Available from https://www.ncbi.nlm.nih.gov/books/NBK597358/. [Last accessed November, 2024].

8.3 Prenatal Development and Malformations of the Central Nervous System

Rachna Sehgal

INTRODUCTION

Central nervous system (CNS) malformations arise in earlier stages of embryogenesis. They have a multifactorial etiopathogenesis with a developmental genetic basis and environmental risk factors. The presentation can be myriad.

EPIDEMIOLOGY

The global incidence is 3.2 per 1,000 live births and the global prevalence is 2.2 per 1,000 live births. However, in a cerebral palsy cohort, the prevalence was found to be as high as 88 per 1,000 live births.[1,2] In a recent study on prenatally detected CNS abnormalities, ventriculomegaly and cortical or complex brain malformations were found to be the most common diagnoses. A genetic diagnosis was positive in only 5%. A longitudinal follow-up of these infants demonstrated neurological deficits and therapy requirements in 14–54% of the children.[3] Another study of 110 patients reported the common CNS malformations in order of prevalence as neuronal migration defects, congenital hydrocephalus, neural tube defects (NTDs), and posterior fossa malformations.[4]

PRENATAL DEVELOPMENT OF CNS AND EMBRYOLOGIC BASIS OF CNS MALFORMATIONS[5]

The CNS evolves from a specialized ectoderm called neural ectoderm. Between weeks 2 and 8 of embryogenesis, within the trilaminar germ disc, a primitive streak emerges from a thickened area of the caudal ectoderm. This structure grows in a caudocranial direction to form *primitive node* at its cranial end. Migration of mesenchymal cells from the primitive node leads to the formation of the *notochordal process*. At the same time, the ectodermal tissue thickens and flattens cranial to the primitive node to form *neural plates*. Neural plate infolds to form *neural groove* whose lateral margins move closer and fuse to form *neural tube*. This process is known as *neurulation* and is induced by the notochord. The elevation, juxtaposition, and fusion of neural tube in the midline of the axis of body is known as *primary neurulation* (16–26 days of gestation). The closure of anterior neuropore occurs on day 25 (fourth week) and the posterior neuropore closes on day 27 (4 weeks).

The neural tube then separates from the overlying ectoderm by a process of *dysjunction*. Thereafter, *secondary neurulation* (45–53 days of gestation) occurs at the caudal region by steps of cellular condensation and epithelial transition to mesenchymal tissue. Mesodermal cells migrate into the space between the neural tube and ectoderm, forming *somites*. These somites develop into the posterior components of the vertebral bodies and the paraspinal muscles. *Notochord* ultimately forms nucleus pulposus of the intervertebral discs.

Neural tube defects occur due to failed neurulation. When the anterior neuropore does not close, NTD develops at the cranial end, such as anencephaly. Similarly, failure of closure of the posterior neuropore leads to NTD at the caudal end, like spina bifida with myeloschisis.

The brain forms from the cranial two-thirds of the neural plate, while the spinal cord originates from the caudal one-third. During brain development, three primary brain vesicles give rise to five secondary brain vesicles. These include the prosencephalon, mesencephalon, and rhombencephalon.

The *prosencephalon (forebrain)*, later, differentiates into the cerebral hemispheres, epithalamus, thalamus, and hypothalamus. The cleavage of the prosencephalon occurs from the posterior to the anterior end of the neural tube, between fifth and sixth week of gestation. The horizontal cleavage gives rise to a pair, each of optic vesicles, olfactory bulbs, and tracts. The telencephalon is separated from the diencephalon by transverse cleavage, whereas sagittal cleavage results in separation of cerebral hemispheres, basal nuclei, and ventricles. By the end of the second month, the commissural, chiasmatic, and hypothalamic plates are formed, which are crucial for the development of the corpus callosum, septum pellucidum, optic chiasma, and hypothalamic structures, respectively.

Mesencephalon gives rise to the midbrain. The *rhombencephalon*, which forms the hindbrain, is divided into three segments: Metencephalon, caudal myelencephalon, and rostral myelencephalon. The metencephalon includes the cerebellum, the caudal myelencephalon corresponds to the central canal of the medulla that is closed, and the rostral myelencephalon is the open component of the medulla where cerebrospinal fluid (CSF) is produced by the choroid plexus.

Normally, aprosencephaly or atelencephaly results from nonseparation into prosencephalon, mesencephalon, and telencephalon. *Holoprosencephaly (HPE)* results from failure of prosencephalic cleavage to different degrees.

Disorders of midline prosencephalic development in areas of commissural plate, chiasmatic plate, and hypothalamic plates are responsible for *agenesis of corpus callosum (ACC), septo-optic dysplasia (SOD)*, and *septo-optic-hypothalamic dysplasia.*

During normal brain development, the cerebral cortex develops seven layers of cells. The subplate neurons in layer 7 migrate to layer 1, i.e., marginal zone. Abnormal migration can cause *lissencephaly*.

The *hypophysis*, the precursor to the pituitary gland, has two developmental origins. The anterior pituitary arises from an ectodermal growth in the mouth, while the posterior pituitary develops from an outgrowth of the hypothalamus.

The spinal cord has three layers: Ventricular layer, which lines the central canal; mantle layer, containing neuronal cell bodies; and marginal layer, containing axons.

Neural crest cells give rise to the pia and arachnoid mater, dorsal root ganglia, and connective tissue in the head and neck. The dura mater originates from the surrounding mesenchyme.

Myelination of peripheral axons is carried out by the neurolemma, formed by Schwann cells, which are derived from neural crest cells. Myelination of CNS axons occurs through oligodendrocytes, which are derived from neuroepithelium.

ETIOPATHOGENESIS

There is a complex relationship of brain malformations with environmental, genetic, and epigenetic factors, molecular signaling, and neurometabolic disorders which are believed to act in concert to produce malformations.

Genetics

Neurulation is a complex process governed by over 300 genes, influenced by specific molecular signals such as bone morphogenetic protein (BMP), wingless signaling pathway (Wnt), and transcription factors like Grhl2/3, Pax3, Cdx2, and Zic2. When neural tube closure (NTC) fails, it often results in defects in the surrounding bony structures, including the cranial vault and neural arches. The most common chromosomal abnormalities associated with NTDs and HPE are trisomy 13, trisomy 18, and triploidy.

Holoprosencephaly is also seen in association with many malformation syndromes with the normal karyotype like Pallister–Hall syndrome, Rubinstein–Tayebi syndrome, Smith–Lemli–Opitz syndrome. Nonsyndromic and nonchromosomal HPE is seen with autosomal dominant and autosomal recessive inheritance patterns with mutations in genes including Sonic Hedgehog (*SHH*), *TGIF, BATCHED-1, NODAL, fox H1, PTCH-1*, and *GL12.*

Most cases of *ACC* are associated with chromosomal causes like aneuploidies, translocations, deletions, and duplications. ACC has also been found to be associated with genetic syndromes like Andermann syndrome *(KCC3), XLAG (ARX)*, pyridoxine-dependent epilepsy *(ALDH7A1)*, pyruvate dehydrogenase deficiency *(PDHA1, PDH8, PDHX)*, ACC with fatal lactic acidosis *(MRPS 16)*, etc. ACC is seen consistently with syndromes like acrocallosal syndrome and Aicardi syndrome although the gene has not yet been identified. It may also be seen occasionally with orofaciodigital syndrome, SOD, Meckel–Gruber syndrome, etc. Genes implicated in SOD include *SOX2, SHH, ARID1A*, and filamin A gene.

Around 40% of children with hydrocephalus also have an underlying genetic etiology with at least 43 known gene mutations. *L1CAM* gene at XQ28 is a common underlying cause of X-linked hydrocephalus.

Megalencephaly may be associated with somatic overgrowth syndromes, germline mutations in Ras/mitogen-activated protein kinase pathway, *PTEN*, a tumor suppressor gene, mammalian target of rapamycin (mTOR) pathway, and loss-of-function mutations in genes that regulate programmed cell death, such as caspase-3 and caspase-9.

There is no genetic mutation consistently associated with focal cortical dysplasia (FCD) 1A. FCD 2B may be associated with somatic mutation of the mTOR pathway. The classical lissencephaly is usually due to mutations of tubulin and *MAP* genes, whereas variant lissencephaly has been found to have mutations in *ARX*, Aristaless-related homeobox gene and *RELN*, reelin signaling pathways.

Heterotopias may be linked to mutations in *FLNA* and *ARFGEF2*, which are thought to play a role in vesicle trafficking and neuroependymal repair.

Among neurometabolic factors, ACC may be seen in nonketotic hyperglycemia, cerebellar hypoplasia or heterotopias have been seen with multiple acyl-CoA dehydrogenase deficiency (MADD), cobblestone malformation and cerebellar hypoplasia with congenital disorders of glycosylation, and pachygyria is associated with Zellweger syndrome.

Environmental Factors

Several environmental factors are also associated with brain malformations. Major teratogens include alcohol, tobacco, certain prescription medications, and illicit drugs, particularly during the critical 3–8-week period of embryogenesis.

The established risk factors for spina bifida include history of previous affected pregnancy with the same partner (RR 30), inadequate maternal intake of folic acid, pregestational maternal diabetes, and intake of valproic acid, carbamazepine, topiramate. Suspected risk factors

TABLE 8.3.1: Risk factors for central nervous system (CNS) malformations.

Risk factor	*Associated CNS malformation*
Intraventricular hemorrhage in preterm, hypoxic ischemic encephalopathy, CNS infections	Microcephaly or hydrocephalus
Gestational diabetes	Holoprosencephaly (HPE)
Ionizing radiation	Periventricular nodular heterotopia
Intrauterine cytomegalovirus (CMV) infection and vascular disruption in second trimester	Schizencephaly, polymicrogyria

include low maternal vitamin B_{12}, maternal obesity, maternal hyperthermia, chlorination, electromagnetic fields, and pesticides.

The environmental factors implicated in HPE are maternal illnesses like diabetes, drugs like salicylates, and contraceptives; alcohol; low calorie diets, hypocholesterolemia, viral infections; and even artificial reproductive therapy.

Nongenetic causes of ACC include fetal alcohol syndrome, intrauterine infections notably cytomegalovirus (CMV) and *herpes simplex* virus (HSV), and heavy metal toxicity. Environmental factors like chronic maternal illness and exposure to drug and toxin exposure are implicated in SOD. Some of the factors are summarized in **Table 8.3.1**.

CLINICAL FEATURES

In a recent retrospective chart review of 110 cases of CNS congenital malformations, the most common presenting features were developmental delay, seizures, microcephaly, and dysmorphism. Nearly 1% of children had a history of birth asphyxia too.[4] Moreover, autism or infantile spasms may be presentations associated with hypoplasia of cerebellum or ACC. They can have associated comorbidities of sleep, feeding, mood, and hormonal and autonomic dysregulation.

CLASSIFICATION

The classification is complicated as there is a tendency for malformations to co-occur. These disorders can be classified on the basis of underlying genetic disorders, embryology, brain imaging, or clinical features. The chapter would cover the CNS malformations under these subheads:

- NTDs
- Disorders of development of forebrain: Cleavage or midline development
- Disorders of development of cerebellum and brainstem
- Disorders of development of cortex:
  - *Group 1: Malformations due to abnormal cell proliferation or apoptosis*
    - Primary microcephaly
    - Megalencephaly
    - Dysplastic malformations (FCD)
  - *Group 2: Malformations due to abnormal neuronal migration*
    - Heterotopias
    - Cobblestone malformations
    - Lissencephaly
  - *Group 3: Malformations due to abnormal development after neuronal migration*
    - Polymicrogyria (PMG)
    - Schizencephaly
- Hydrocephalus

SECTION 1: NEURAL TUBE DEFECTS[5]

Neural tube defects are the most common CNS malformations, with around 300,000 cases occurring globally each year. In India, the incidence is reportedly higher in the northern regions compared to the south. Any disruption in the complex process of neural tube formation during embryogenesis can result in NTDs, with the severity depending on the timing and extent of the disruption. The defects can be broadly subdivided into open and closed defects as shown in **Table 8.3.2.**[6]

Embryologically, NTDs may arise due to a defect of neural folding and formation, disordered postneurulation development, incomplete dysjunction, disordered gastrulation, disordered secondary neurulation, and failure of caudal neuraxial development. The types of defects based on stage and their clinical features are depicted in **Table 8.3.3** and encephalocele is shown in **Figures 8.3.1A to C**.

Spina bifida occulta is the mildest type of spina bifida. It is characterized by a tuft of hair, a small dimple, vascular nevus, lipoma, and dermal sinus in the lumbosacral region. It may indicate the presence of underlying malformation like diastematomyelia (split cord malformations) or lipoma, or tethered cord syndrome. The term *spina bifida multiplex* is used when there is tethering of the spinal cord at more than two locations, along with a myelomeningocele (MMC).

Diagnosis

Diagnosis is done with the help of clinical features and characteristic MRI findings.

Management

Elective LSCS has been found to reduce the chance of rupture of the defect during delivery in cases of antenatally diagnosed MMC. Children born with MMC often require multiple surgeries, including defect repair and placement of a ventriculoperitoneal (VP) shunt for associated hydrocephalus. Surgery to repair an open defect is needed within 24–48 hours after birth to reduce the risk of meningitis.

TABLE 8.3.2: Types of neural tube defects.[6]

	Open	*Closed*
Cause	Due to disruption of primary neurulation	Due to disruption of secondary neurulation
Covering	May not be covered by skin	Covered with skin
Biochemical	Increased levels of a-fetoprotein and acetylcholinesterase in amniotic fluid.	Normal levels
Clinical features	Below the lesion level, there is a loss of neurological function.	• Generally asymptomatic, may have paraparesis or bladder dysfunction in case of tethering • May have sinus, lipoma, or tuft of hair overlying the defect
Outcome	Poor	Better
Examples	Exencephaly–anencephaly, myelomeningocele (MMC, open spina bifida), lipomyelomeningocele, and craniorachischisis	Spina bifida occulta, encephalocele, split cord malformation, dermal sinus, or dermal nevus to extreme spinal cord tethering

TABLE 8.3.3: Embryologic basis of neural tube defects (NTDs).

Stage of defect	*Type*	*Clinical features*
Defect of neural folding and formation	Anencephaly	• Both cerebral hemispheres and calvaria are absent, incompatible with life • Craniorachischisis occurs when this is associated with thin and flattened spinal cord • Iniencephaly has associated retroflexed neck • Meroanencephaly has malformed cranial bones and midline cranial defect
	Myelomeningocele (MMC)	• Mortality rate is 50% in untreated MMC • Neurological deficit is based on the site of lesion • Associated neurogenic bladder and renal complications, clubfeet, hip dislocation, bowel dysfunction, hydrocephalus, and epilepsy are common
Disordered postneurulation development	Encephalocele	Herniation of intracranial contents through a midline defect in occipital, frontal, and basal transsphenoidal regions. Severe intellectual delay, spasticity, and microcephaly results. Associated malformations may be present
Incomplete dysjunction	Dermal sinus and associated dermoid and epidermoid tumors	• It may be a cause of recurrent meningitis • Presence of glucose in the fluid helps to distinguish CSF from other body fluids
Disordered gastrulation	Split cord malformation	A midline septum divides the spinal cord longitudinally by a bony or fibrous septum into equal or unequal parts. Presents with scoliosis, hydrocephalus, and progressive myelopathy
	Neurenteric cyst	• Due to incomplete resorption of neurenteric canal • Intradural extramedullary cysts can cause obstruction to CSF flow
Disordered secondary neurulation	Thickened filum terminale (>2 mm thick)	It may be associated with low conus, bladder dysfunction, leg numbness, weakness, and scoliosis
	Myelocystocele	• Large ependyma-lined cystic dilatation of the caudal end of central canal of spinal cord • May be associated with cloacal exstrophy • Can progress to lower extremity paresis unless repaired
Failure of caudal neuraxial development	Sacral agenesis	• Congenital absence of whole or part of sacrum • May be autosomal dominant or in mothers with insulin dependent diabetes mellitus • Maybe associated with neurogenic bladder, bowel impairment, paraparesis, clubfeet, renal anomalies, flattened buttocks, anterior meningocele, presacral teratoma

Without this procedure, only 20% of affected infants survive beyond 2 years of age.

Management of seizures is challenging in these children and intermittently shunt malfunction or ventriculitis may even cause further exacerbation of seizures. Neurogenic bladder necessitates ongoing monitoring for hydronephrosis and vesicoureteric reflux. Treatment entails clean intermittent catheterization, anticholinergics, ureteric reimplantation, ileal conduits, and resection of external sphincter. Constipation and fecal incontinence are usually

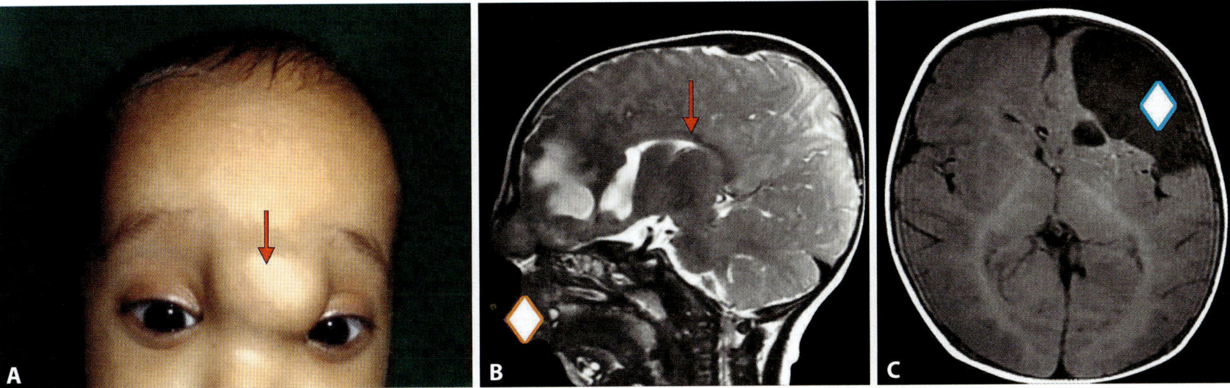

Figs. 8.3.1A to C: (A) Frontal encephalocele in a child; (B) MRI brain T2 sagittal section showing dysgenesis of genu of corpus callosum with preserved body and splenium (red arrow) and encephalocele (orange diamond); (C) Left frontal porencephalic cyst (blue diamond).

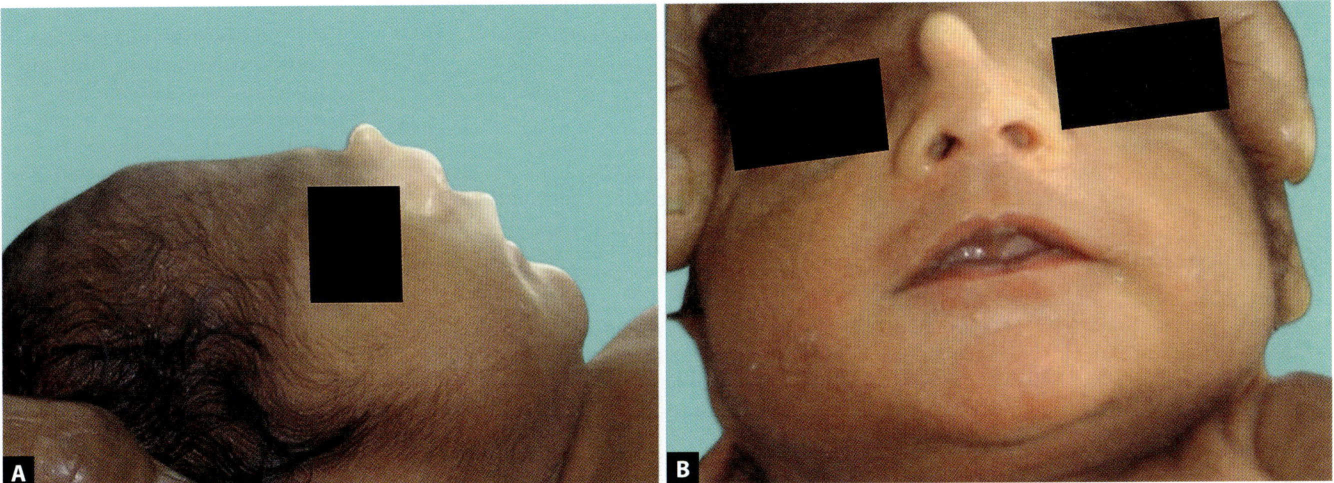

Figs. 8.3.2A and B: Sagittal and frontal views of a newborn showing proboscis.

managed with dietary manipulation, laxatives, and manual evacuation or enemas. Splinting or casting may be needed for orthopedic deformities.

Prevention[6]

Around 70% of NTDs can be prevented through prenatal folic acid supplementation, with a recommended daily dose of 0.4 mg for all prospective mothers. For high-risk pregnancies, a dose of 4 mg/day should be started 1 month before conception and continued until the 12th week of pregnancy as secondary prevention. Maintaining an adequate body mass index (BMI) before conception is also advised. Literature suggests the role of inositol and zinc also for NTC.

SECTION 2: DISORDERS OF FOREBRAIN DEVELOPMENT

The prosencephalic development occurs by ventral inductive influence of the prechordal mesoderm that results in the formation of face and forebrain. Therefore, severe disorders of forebrain development are associated with striking facial anomalies resulting in the common adage "The face predicts the brain" with the presence of cyclopia, proboscis **(Figs. 8.3.2A and B)**, and microform as shown in **Table 8.3.4**. This table also shows features of disorders of forebrain cleavage or midline development, namely HPE, ACC, and SOD. ACC has an incidence of 1:3000 live births and is the second most common anomaly after spina bifida. "SOD plus" syndrome is when there are associated brain anomalies like cortical malformations hydrocephalus or hippocampal malformations.

Diagnosis

MRI Brain Findings

- Alobar HPE is characterized by a single midline mass of forebrain parenchyma, fused thalami and basal ganglia, and a primitive monoventricle that frequently communicates with a large cyst situated dorsally. There is absence of interhemispheric fissure and corpus callosum.

TABLE 8.3.4: Forebrain malformations.

	Holoprosencephaly (HPE)	
Types	***Clinical features***	***Outcome***
• Aprosencephaly • Alobar HPE • Semilobar HPE • Lobar HPE • Middle interhemispheric variant (MIH)	*Severe varieties have:* • Cleft lip and palate • Cyclopia (single central eye) • Coloboma • Retinal dysplasia • Proboscis (rudimentary nose with single nostril above the eye) *Milder variants have:* • *Microform:* Anosmia • Solitary maxillary median incisor • Choanal atresia • Pyriform aperture stenosis • Hypotelorism	• *More severe forms* like alobar, are associated with early demise in utero or in the first 6 months • Usually, microcephaly but normo- or macrocephaly if associated with hydrocephalus • Developmental and motor delay epilepsy, oromotor dysfunction, hypothalamic dysfunction particularly diabetes insipidus
Agenesis of corpus callosum		
• Isolated or with associated brain anomalies • Complete or partial • Associated with other system anomalies	• *Isolated may be normal or may have* Behavioral anomalies • Epilepsy • Developmental delay • Autism • Cerebral palsy • Attention-deficit hyperactivity disorder (ADHD) • Associated cardiac, renal, musculoskeletal, and gastrointestinal anomalies	• If associated malformations like cortical malformations, cysts and posterior fossa abnormalities neurological deficits are usually present • IQ may be normal if detected incidentally or may have social or behavioral deficits
Septo-optic dysplasia (SOD) or de Morsier syndrome		
Diagnostic criteria • Any two features from the classic clinical triad of optic nerve hypoplasia • Agenesis of brain midline structures (e.g., corpus callosum, septum pellucidum) • Hypoplasia of the hypothalamic–pituitary axis	*Neonatal period* • Maybe normal at birth or may present within the first week of life with abnormalities related to hypothalamic dysfunction, such as hypoglycemia and hyperbilirubinemia, nystagmus, apnea, and hypotonia. Also, microphthalmia or anophthalmia, cleft lip and palate and microphallus *After the newborn period* • Progressive visual impairment due to optic nerve hypoplasia • Endocrine abnormalities due to insufficient interaction between the hypothalamus and pituitary gland like growth hormone abnormalities • Neurological dysfunction, developmental delay, and epilepsy • Facial abnormalities (e.g., hypertelorism) that have been associated with a worse prognosis	• SOD patients may have sudden death due to endocrine abnormalities that can lead to hypoglycemia, diabetes insipidus, and poor thermoregulation. • The survivors need multidisciplinary management

- In the semilobar HPE, anterior hemispheres fail to separate and there is absence of genu and body of corpus callosum and frontal horns of the lateral ventricle. However, posterior hemispheres, splenium, and posterior horns are partially separated. There is often partial fusion of the thalami.
- In the lobar HPE, only the most rostral aspect of the frontal lobes (<50%) is incompletely cleaved. The septum pellucidum is absent, but the ventricular system and basal ganglia appear near-normal with mildly dysplastic callosal genu.
- In the middle interhemispheric (MIH) variant, the midsection of the cerebral hemispheres is fused across the midline, with the corpus callosum absent in the body region. The anterior frontal lobes, basal forebrain, and occipital lobes are separated. There may be incomplete cleavage of the thalami and caudate nuclei.
- In the mildest variety of septo-preoptic HPE, there is cortical fusion limited to preoptic suprachiasmatic region and anterior hypothalamus and/or septal region.

Management of Forebrain Malformations

The mainstay of management is symptomatic targeting neurological concerns like epilepsy, speech delay, tone and behavior abnormalities, and endocrine abnormalities. The medical armamentarium includes antiseizure, antispasticity, and dystonia medications like trihexyphenidyl, physical therapy, occupational therapy, speech therapy, and behavioral therapy.

For children with HPE, screening electrolyte needs to be performed to look for subacute development of diabetes insipidus. Comprehensive hormonal analysis also includes cortisol, thyroid stimulating hormone (TSH), free thyroxine (FT4), and insulin-like growth factor-1 (IGF1) assays.

Surgical options include gastrostomy tube placement for severe feeding issues and VP shunt placement for hydrocephalus even in children with severe HPE to facilitate caring of the child.

SECTION 3: DISORDERS OF CEREBELLAR AND BRAINSTEM DEVELOPMENT[7,8]

These disorders are being characterized with greater accuracy due to advances in MRI that have better resolving power for posterior fossa and the use of genetic testing. These disorders may be further delineated as Chiari malformations, posterior fossa cystic malformations **(Table 8.3.5)**, pontocerebellar hypoplasias **(Tables 8.3.6 and 8.3.7)**, and isolated cerebellar atrophy (CA) **(Figs. 8.3.3A to C)**.

Clinical Features

The affected children usually present with signs of cerebellar dysfunction, like nystagmus, head stereotypies, hypotonia, and delayed motor development. There may sometimes be features of raised intracranial tension if associated with hydrocephalus, like Dandy-Walker malformation or Chiari II malformation.

Chiari Malformations

Chiari malformations are subclassified on the basis of their morphology and severity.

- *Chiari I malformation* is the least severe and has herniation of one or both cerebellar tonsils 3–5 mm below the McRae line, an imaginary line drawn from the basion to the opisthion. It can cause syringomyelia.
- *Chiari II or Arnold-Chiari malformation* consists of brainstem herniation in addition to the herniated cerebellar tonsils and vermis due to an open distal spinal dysraphism or MMC.
- *Chiari III malformation* is characterized by herniation of the cerebellum with or without the brainstem into a low occipital or high cervical meningoencephalocele.
- *Chiari IV malformation* is now considered to be obsolete. Earlier, it was synonymous with severe cerebellar hypoplasia. These present with occipital headache exacerbated by Valsalva maneuver with or without features of myelopathy.

Cerebellar Hypoplasia

Cerebellar hypoplasia consists of reduced volume, while dysplasia is characterized by abnormal cerebellar architecture. Unlike atrophy, this term excludes conditions where cerebellar development was initially normal but later followed by progressive degeneration, as in Friedreich ataxia. With physical rehabilitation and nervous system maturation, children usually improve with age.

Rhombencephalosynapsis

Rhombencephalosynapsis is characterized by complete or partial absence of vermis, fusion of cerebellar hemispheres, and absence of primary fissure of vermis on midsagittal MRI with keyhole-shaped fourth ventricle.

TABLE 8.3.5: Cystic malformations of posterior fossa.

	MRI features						
Malformation	***Vermis***	***Cerebellar hemispheres***	***Fourth ventricle***	***Posterior fossa***	***Hydrocephalus***	***Displaced torcula heterophily***	***Occipital scalloping***
Dandy–Walker malformation	Hypoplastic, rotated	Normal	Enlarged	Enlarged	Frequent	Yes	Yes
Blake pouch cyst	Normal, maybe upward rotated	Normal	Enlarged	Normal	Frequent	No	No
Mega cisterna magna	Normal	Normal	Normal	Normal or slightly enlarged	Absent	No	Possible
• Posterior fossa • Arachnoid cyst	Normal, maybe compressed, not rotated		Normal or reduced	Normal or slightly enlarged	Rare	No	Yes
• Isolated vermian • Hypoplasia	Hypoplastic inferior portion, occasionally slightly rotated	Normal	Normal or slightly enlarged	Normal	Absent	No	No

TABLE 8.3.6: Pontocerebellar hypoplasia.

Predominant associated feature	Course and outcome	MRI brain	PCH type
• Motor neuron degeneration • Peripheral neuropathy	Prolonged survival	Sparing of pons	PCH1A/1B/1C
	Lethal		PCH1D
	Turkish descent	Mild cerebellar atrophy	PCH10
	Respiratory failure, congenital contractures		PCH4
	• Lactic acidosis • Rapid progression		PCH6
Chorea, dystonia	• Neonatal jitteriness • No gain in milestones • Swallowing impairment	Dragonfly cerebellum	• PCH2A • Rarely PCH2B-F
	• Stable, developmental gain	Dragonfly cerebellum	PCH8
Disorder of sex differentiation			PCH7
		Figure of 8 brainstem	PCH9
Optic Nerve atrophy			PCH3
	Associated neocortical malformations		RELN, VLDR, CASK mutations
	Associated ataxia	Sparing pons	PCH2D
Ataxia	Delayed myelination, multiorgan failure, facial dysmorphism		CDG1a
	Non degenerative		PCH11
			Spinocerebellar ataxia

TABLE 8.3.7: Genetic basis of cerebellar hypodysplasias.

Cerebellar phenotype	Associated features	Possible genetic basis
Cysts	Cobblestone, brainstem kinking, increased CPK	Alpha dystroglycanopathies *(DGP)*
	Cobblestone, associated eye, muscle abnormalities	*LAMB1*
	Frontoparietal polymicrogyria	*GPR56/COL3A!*
	Myopia, retinal abnormalities (Poretti–Bolthauser syndrome)	*LAMA1*
Hypoplasia	Simplified gyration	*CASK*
	Lissencephaly/pachygyria	*VLDR/REELIN*
Dysplasia	• Diagonal folia across cerebellar vermis • Basal ganglia, corpus callosum, cortical anomalies	Tubulins
	• Abnormal foliation, fissuration inferior cerebellar hemispheres • Agenesis of corpus callosum, cingulate and frontal polymicrogyria, hearing loss (Chudley–McCollough syndrome)	*GPSM2*
Hypodysplastic	Hypoplastic superior vermis and dysplastic inferior vermis and cerebellar hemispheres (molar tooth sign- Joubert syndrome) **(Figs. 8.3.4A to C)**	Ciliopathy (>30 genes)

Pontocerebellar Hypoplasia

Pontocerebellar hypoplasia is a heterogenous group of disorders of prenatal onset having genetic basis (*CASK, RELN,* and *VLDLR* genes) or metabolic (like congenital disorder of glycosylation 1a), or environmental origin like disruption due to extreme prematurity characterized by reduction in the volume of both pons and cerebellum with variable supratentorial abnormalities. **Figures 8.3.3A to C** show Joubert syndrome.

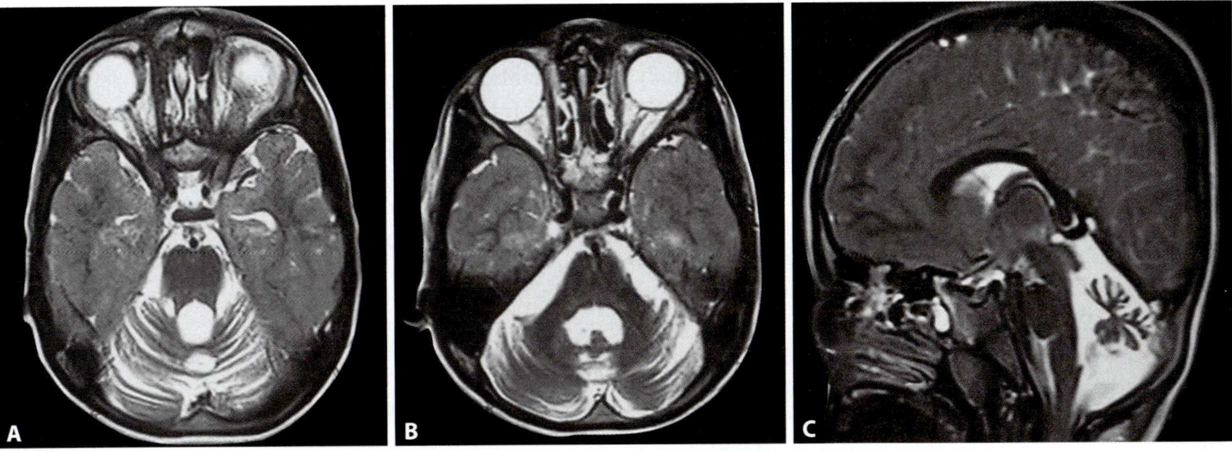

Figs. 8.3.3A to C: MRI brain T2 axial (A and B) and sagittal (C) showing cerebellar atrophy.

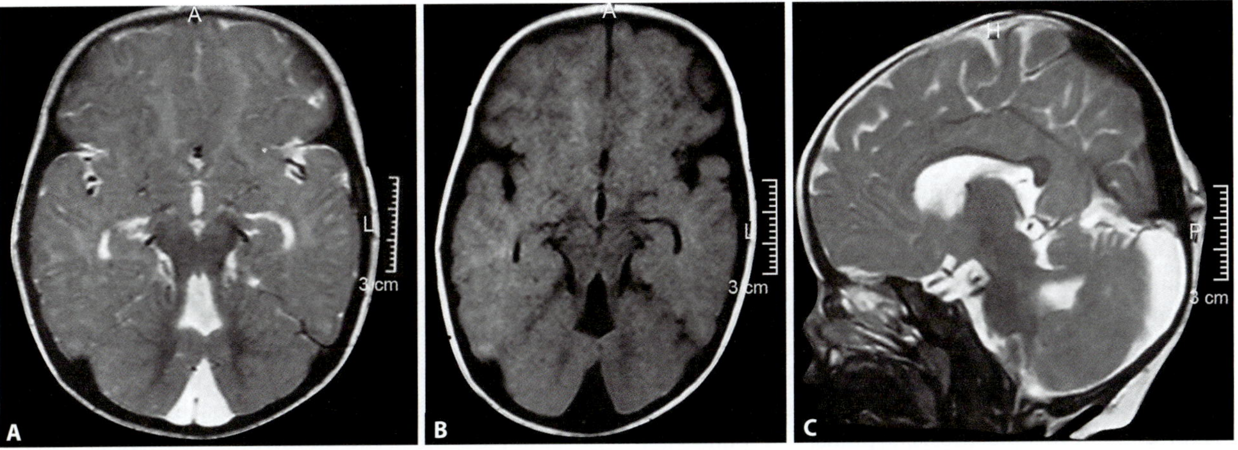

Figs. 8.3.4A to C: Joubert syndrome showing molar tooth appearance (A and B) and elongated superior cerebellar peduncle with vermian atrophy on sagittal section (C).

Cerebellar Atrophy

Cerebellar atrophy **(Figs. 8.3.4A to C)** refers to progressive attenuation of cerebellar parenchyma preceded by normal development. Pure CA may be seen with ataxia telangiectasia; with associated hypomyelination, one can consider Pelizaeus–Merzbacher disease or Salla disease; with progressive demyelination, neuronal ceroid lipofuscinosis and Nieman–Pick type C should be considered. Associated basal ganglia involvement is seen in Kearns-Sayre, Wilson, and Cockayne syndromes, and associated cerebellar cortex hyperintensities are seen with infantile neuroaxonal dystrophy.

Management

Depending on the type of Chiari malformation, this can include duraplasty to facilitate surgical decompression of posterior fossa and repair of neural tube and shunt for hydrocephalus. Children with cerebellar hypoplasias improve with rehabilitation and age. Vitamin E and mitochondrial cocktail may be useful if there is suggestive etiology.

SECTION 4: MALFORMATIONS OF CORTICAL DEVELOPMENT[9]

Malformations of cortical development are a diverse group of disorders that frequently cause neurodevelopmental delay and epilepsy, arising from disruptions in the normal development of the human cerebral cortex. These disorders can be subclassified into three groups.

Group 1: Malformations due to Abnormal Cell Proliferation or Apoptosis

These result in brain size alteration and may manifest with microcephaly or macrocephaly.

Microcephaly

Severe microcephaly is characterized by an occipitofrontal circumference (OFC) >3 standard deviations (SD) below the mean, while mild microcephaly has an OFC between –2 and –3 SD. It is considered a neurological sign rather than a disorder, as it can result from any developmental defect or brain injury affecting prenatal or early postnatal brain growth.

Primary microcephaly refers to congenital microcephaly that occurs without other significant brain or somatic malformations. In severe cases of congenital microcephaly, brain imaging and pathology show disproportionately small frontal lobes, along with reduced number, complexity, and depth of gyri and sulci.

Other types of microcephaly may have associated CNS malformations. Some of the representative causes of microcephaly are depicted in **Table 8.3.8**.

Clinical features: Severe microcephaly may be associated with variable degrees of cognitive impairment, epilepsy, poor feeding, and recurrent vomiting. Several syndromes with microcephaly have variable ocular malformations like coloboma, microphthalmia, cataracts, etc. (e.g., mitochondrial depletion syndrome, mucolipidosis IV) or ear or hearing impairment (e.g., Allan-Herndon-Dudley syndrome, Coffin-Lowry syndrome) or proportionate growth deficiency (Seckel syndrome, etc.). Familial microcephaly tends to have milder phenotype.

Diagnosis:[10] The diagnostic evaluation is complex. If the clinical features, other organ involvement, vision/hearing impairment or eye/ear anomalies or antenatal or birth or family history suggest a specific disease or syndrome, specific testing should be done for that condition.

If the microcephaly is disproportionate to weight and height, MRI brain should be done first. If it shows a specific pattern of injury, diagnostic strategy should be directed to it. However, if MRI brain shows nonspecific changes, laboratory studies for titers of toxoplasmosis, syphilis, CMV, and HSV and genetic testing including karyotype for chromosome analysis and fluorescent in situ hybridization (FISH) with subtelomeric probes may be done. One can consider testing for metabolic, endocrine, and toxic causes as per the case. Testing for Rett syndrome should be considered in girls.

If the microcephaly is proportionate to weight and height, a similar algorithm may be adopted if the child has or develops neurologic signs or symptoms or severe or worsening microcephaly.

Megalencephaly

Megalencephaly refers to an increased brain mass that exceeds the mean by 2 SD for age and gender. Anatomic megalencephalies are disorders of neuronal development caused by either excessive cell production or a failure in programmed cell death. While megalencephaly can be diagnosed through pathological and radiological means, due to the challenges in accurately measuring brain volume, it is considered the cause of macrocephaly after hydrocephalus or an enlarged extra-axial space has been excluded.

Types of megalencephaly: Familial (nonsyndromic) megalencephaly: These children have normal intracranial pressure, development, facial, cutaneous and neurological examination with large OFC in parents or siblings. Follow-up visits show leveling off of OFC and normality of a patient's development course. An approach to syndromic megalencephaly is depicted in **Flowchart 8.3.1**.

Focal cortical dysplasias: These are diverse disorders with more localized dysplastic neurons that are responsible for epilepsy. These are subdivided into types 1A, 1B, 2A, and 2B. They can be differentiated microscopically by the

TABLE 8.3.8: Causes of microcephaly.

	Congenital	***Postnatal onset***
Genetic		
Isolated/inborn errors of metabolism	Autosomal recessive/dominant/ X-linked/chromosomal	Aminoacidopathies, congenital disorders of glycosylation, glucose transporter defect, mitochondrial, peroxisomal, organic acidemia
• Syndromic • Chromosomal • Contiguous gene deletion	• Trisomy 21, 18, 13 • 4p deletion, 5p deletion, 7q deletion, 22q deletion	17p13.3 deletion (Miller–Dieker syndrome)
Single-gene defects	Cornelia de Lange, holoprosencephaly (HPE), Seckel syndrome	Rett syndrome, Cockayne syndrome
Acquired		
Disruptive injuries	Stroke, fetal death of a twin	Trauma, hypoxic-ischemic encephalopathy (HIE), stroke
Infections	TORCH, HIV	Meningitis, encephalitis
Teratogens	Alcohol, hydantoin, uncontrolled diabetes	Lead, chronic renal failure
Deprivation	Maternal hypothyroidism, folate deficiency, malnutrition, placental insufficiency	Hypothyroidism, anemia, malnutrition, congenital heart disease

Flowchart 8.3.1: Approach to syndromic megalencephaly.

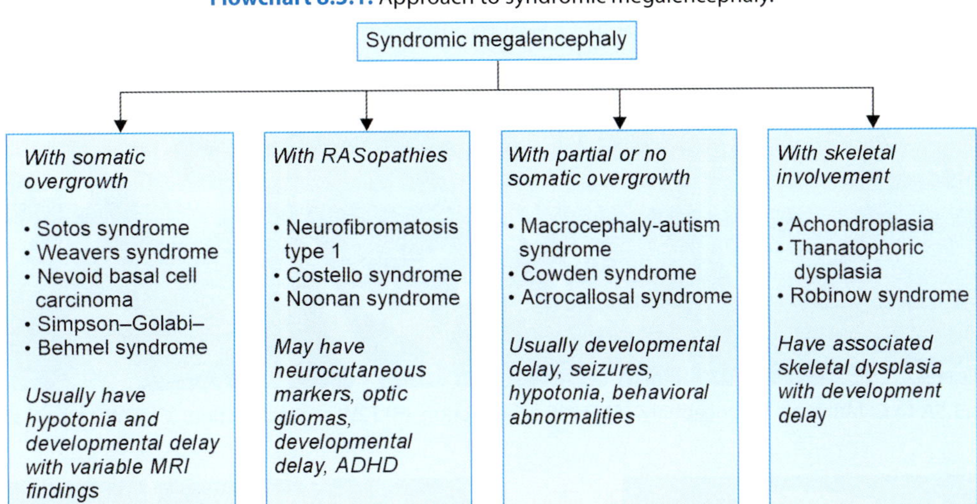

way cortical neurons are placed. FCD 1A may involve the entire frontal lobe, parietal lobe, and temporal lobe and is associated with delayed myelination. FCD type 2A has a localized dyslamination with blurring of gray-white matter boundary and cortical thickening. FCD type 2B appears as a funnel-shaped T2/FLAIR hyperintensity from the superolateral margin of the lateral ventricle to dysplastic cortex (transmantle sign).

Group 2: Malformations Due to Abnormal Neuronal Migration

Migration disorders are usually the result of mutations in genes for tubulin or microtubule-associated protein. These proteins are crucial prerequisite for migration of neurons. Therefore, disorders of microtubule formation or function can result in lissencephaly, band heterotopias, and malformations of midbrain and hindbrain.

Lissencephaly

Lissencephaly, or "smooth brain", is a malformation resulting from insufficient neuronal migration from layer 7 to layer 1 of the cerebral cortex. It is characterized by a thick cortex, with either no sulci (complete lissencephaly) or unusually broad gyri separated by shallow sulci (incomplete lissencephaly) **(Figs. 8.3.5A to C)**.

Subcortical Band Heterotopia

Subcortical band heterotopia, also called "double cortex", is a related malformation where only some neurons carry a harmful mutation in the tubulin or *DCX* gene. On MRI, band heterotopia appears as an undulating band of subcortical gray matter made up of incompletely migrated neurons. The band can vary in thickness and may or may not run parallel to the overlying cortex **(Fig. 8.3.6)**.

Gray Matter Heterotopias

They are neuronal accumulations in abnormal locations. These can be periventricular nodular heterotopia or subcortical or subpial based on location **(Figs. 8.3.7A and B)**.

Group 3: Malformations Due to Abnormal Development after Neuronal Migration

Polymicrogyria

Polymicrogyria is a common malformation characterized by an excessive number of small convolutions, which can be observed both grossly and on imaging. Its histological correlate is overfolding and abnormal cortical lamination. Clinically, it may present as developmental delay, epilepsy, or behavioral issues in childhood. PMG has a multifactorial origin and can result from genetic factors or prenatal brain injury due to ischemia, teratogens, or infections. Cobblestone appearance can masquerade as PMG before myelination is completed. Location wise, it can be bilateral perisylvian, unilateral perisylvian, generalized, frontal only, or parasagittal parieto-occipital type.

Schizencephaly

Schizencephaly is less common than PMG and is linked to maternal factors such as young age or alcohol use or inadequate prenatal care. It commonly presents with delayed development or epilepsy. MRI of the brain reveals a cleft lined by gray matter from the cortex to the ventricle, often containing CSF and, in some cases, blood vessels.

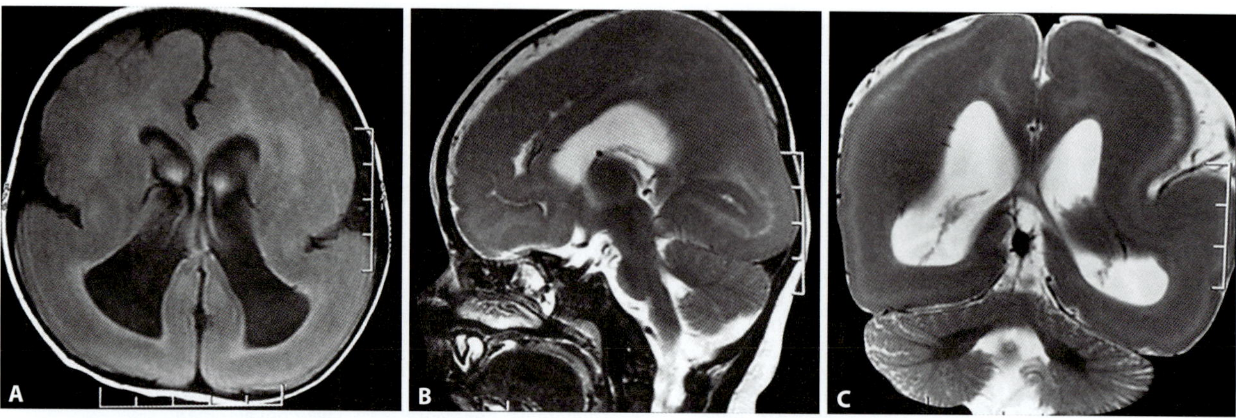

Figs. 8.3.5A to C: MRI brain lissencephaly. (A) FLAIR axial section; (B) T2W sagittal section; (C) T2W coronal section.

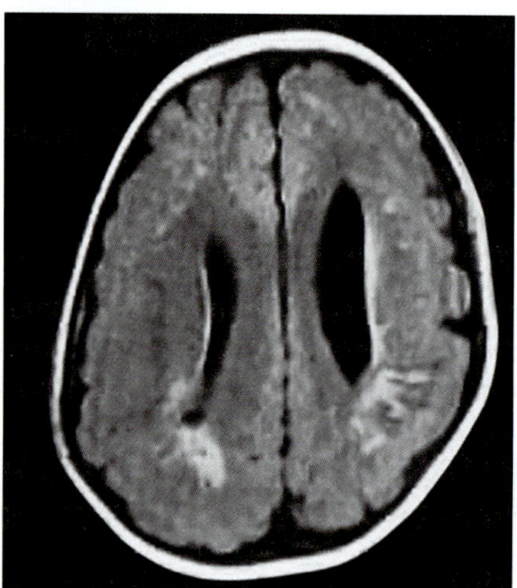

Fig. 8.3.6: MRI brain axial FLAIR: Pachygyria with double cortex suggestive of band heterotopia with cysts.

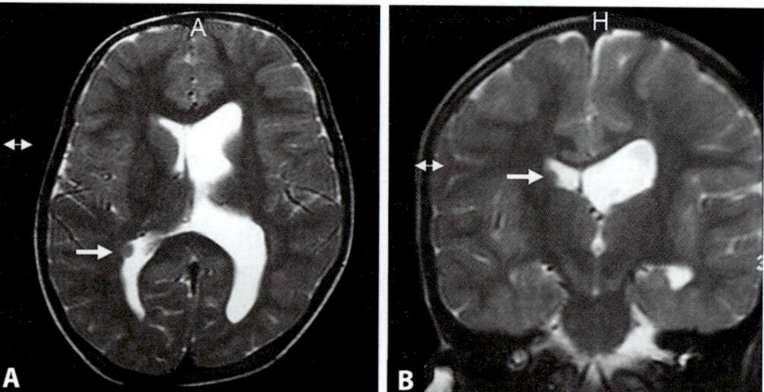

Figs. 8.3.7A and B: MRI brain T2W images. (A) *Axial section:* Right occipital subependymal gray matter heterotopia; (B) *Coronal section:* Right frontal subependymal gray matter heterotopia.

HYDROCEPHALUS[11]

Hydrocephalus is defined as a net accumulation of CSF due to an imbalance between production and absorption characterized by an increase in the size of cerebral ventricles and elevation of intracranial pressure. Thus, the disturbance may be in any of the steps of formation, flow, or absorption of CSF.

Classification

Hydrocephalus can be classified in the following ways:

- *Obstructive or communicating* based on whether the flow of CSF from the ventricles to the subarachnoid space is obstructed or there is inadequate resorption by arachnoid granulations
- *Acquired or congenital* based on presence at birth or later
- *Arrested/compensated* or *progressive/uncompensated* based on if the ventricular size has stabilized after reaching a new equilibrium and absence of features of raised intracranial pressure
- *Ventricular or extraventricular obstructive hydrocephalus.* Extraventricular hydrocephalus is equivalent to benign extra-axial collection of infancy. This is usually familial. It resolves by 18–24 months and does not require any treatment.

Cerebrospinal fluid is produced by choroid plexus within the cerebral ventricles and by transependymal subarachnoid secretion. The CSF flows from the lateral ventricles to the foramen of Monro and then to the third ventricle. From there, it travels via aqueduct of Sylvius to fourth ventricle. Then it traverses into the subarachnoid space through the foramina of Luschka and Magendie. The CSF formation requires active transport of sodium, but resorption is not an energy-dependent process. The hydrostatic force behind the absorption is the pressure difference of 5–7 mm Hg between subarachnoid space and dural venous sinuses.

Causes

The causes can be congenital malformations like Arnold-Chiari malformation, autosomal recessive aqueductal stenosis, basilar impression, and Dandy-Walker malformation. The acquired etiologies can be because of infectious, neoplastic, traumatic, or vascular causes. The infectious subgroup includes TORCH group of infections, meningitis, and encephalitis. The neoplasms include brainstem gliomas, medulloblastoma, ependymoma, and leukemia. The traumatic causes can be hemorrhage, hypoxic ischemic encephalopathy (HIE), and posterior fossa surgery and the vascular causes include arteriovenous malformations, jugular venous catheterization, vein of Gallen malformation, and cerebral sinus venous thrombosis. Certain syndromes that are associated with hydrocephalus include achondroplasia, Cockayne syndrome, Crouzon syndrome, Hurler syndrome, Krabbe disease, muscle eye-brain disease, neurofibromatosis, osteopetrosis, etc.

Clinical Features

- *Infants:* Delayed development, irritability, poor feeding and vomiting, bulging tense anterior fontanelle, large head, distended scalp veins, cracked pot (McEwen's sign), seizures, papilledema (rare) setting sun sign, and spasticity at more than 6 months of age
- *Older children:* Headache, cognitive deterioration, gait changes, papilledema, Parinaud syndrome [light-near dissociation, convergence-retraction nystagmus, and eyelid retraction (Collier sign)], and abnormal hypothalamic function

Diagnosis

Cranial USG in fetus, neonates, and infants and CT or MRI brain in older children are done to demonstrate ventricular size, periventricular ooze, and underlying pathology and is also useful in follow-up of patient after shunt surgery. Ewan's ratio is the ratio of largest width of the frontal horns to the maximal biparietal diameter. A ratio >30% is suggestive of hydrostatic hydrocephalus.

Management

The management can be conservative by careful follow-up with neurological examination, neuropsychological assessment, and reassessment of the ventricular size and medical management (acetazolamide, glycerol, and frusemide) in patients with mild and slowly progressive hydrocephalus, and in arrested hydrocephalus where CSF pressure is normal.

Surgery

- In obstructive hydrocephalus secondary to a surgically resectable mass, the lesionectomy may be curative.
- Rapid-onset hydrocephalus with increased intracranial pressure has to be treated on an emergency basis with either ventricular tap (in infants) or extraventricular drainage or placement of a VP or ventricular-pleural or ventricular-atrial or (vascular) shunt, lumbar puncture may be done in posthemorrhagic and postmeningitic hydrocephalus.

GENETIC COUNSELING[11]

An important component is prediction of recurrence risk. For HPE, the recurrence risk has been found to vary between 6 and 13%. There is a 25% recurrence risk with pontocerebellar hypoplasia, molar tooth malformation, and congenital microcephaly as they all have autosomal recessive inheritance. On the other hand, ACC, PMG, and Dandy-Walker malformation have been found to have a very low recurrence risk. Moreover, there are no reported recurrences with FCD and rhombencephalosynapsis.

CONCLUSION

- Central nervous system (CNS) malformations arise between 2 and 8 weeks of embryogenesis.
- Several environmental, genetic, and epigenetic factors, molecular signaling, and metabolic factors act in concert to produce CNS malformations.
- The presentation can be myriad.
- Medical management focuses on epilepsy, tone and behavior abnormalities, and endocrine abnormalities associated with some of the malformations.
- Bladder, bowel care, physical therapy, occupational therapy, speech therapy, oromotor training and behavioral therapy are cornerstones of management.
- Surgical options include gastrostomy tube placement, ventriculoperitoneal shunt placement or third ventriculostomy for hydrocephalus and repair of neural tube defects.
- The prognosis is variable based on severity of deficit.
- Preventive strategies involve folic acid, zinc supplementation, control of obesity for neural tube defects and prenatal diagnosis for the malformations with identified genetic locus.

REFERENCES

1. von Wendt L, Rantakallio P. Congenital malformations of the central nervous system in a 1-year birth cohort followed to the age of 14 years. Childs Nerv Syst. 1986;2(2):80-2.
2. Rankin J, Cans C, Garne E, Colver A, Dolk H, Uldall P, et al. Congenital anomalies in children with cerebral palsy: a population-based record linkage study. Dev Med Child Neurol. 2010;52(4):345-51.
3. Siddesh A, Gupta G, Sharan R, Agarwal M, Phadke SR. Spectrum of prenatally detected central nervous system

malformations: neural tube defects continue to be the leading foetal malformation. Indian J Med Res. 2017;145(4):471-8.
4. Gowda VK, Sugumar K, Vamyanmane DK, Shivappa KS. Profile of central nervous system malformations in children from a tertiary care center in southern India. J Pediatr Neurosci. 2022. DOI: 10.4103/jpn.jpn_181_21.
5. Elshazzly M, Lopez MJ, Reddy V, Caban O. Embryology, Central Nervous System. StatPearls [Internet]. Treasure Island (FL): StatPearls Publishing; 2023.
6. Ravi KS, Divasha, Hassan SB, Pasi R, Mittra S, Kumar R. Neural tube defects: different types and brief review of neurulation process and its clinical implication. J Family Med Prim Care. 2021;10(12):4383-90.
7. Severino M, Huisman TAGM. Posterior Fossa Malformations. Neuroimaging Clin N Am. 2019;29(3):367-83.
8. van Dijk T, Baas F, Barth PG. What's new in pontocerebellar hypoplasia? An update on genes and subtypes. Orphanet J Rare Dis. 2018;13(1):92.
9. Desikan RS, Barkovich AJ. Malformations of cortical development. Ann Neurol. 2016;80(6):797-810.
10. Ashwal S, Michelson D, Plawner L, Dobyns WB; Quality Standards Subcommittee of the American Academy of Neurology and the Practice Committee of the Child Neurology Society. Practice parameter: Evaluation of the child with microcephaly (an evidence-based review): report of the Quality Standards Subcommittee of the American Academy of Neurology and the Practice Committee of the Child Neurology Society. Neurology. 2009;73(11):887-97.
11. Swaiman KF, Ashwal S, Ferriero MD, Schor NF, Finkel RS, Gropman AL, et al. Swaiman's Pediatric Neurology Principles and Practice, 6th edition. China: Elsevier; 2017.

8.4 Neurodegenerative Disorders

Naveen Sankhyan, Arushi G Saini

INTRODUCTION

Neurodegenerative disorders (NDDs) are characterized by neuroregression. They are genetic disorders causing progressive intellectual and neurological deterioration, which results from a progressive loss of neurons. Neuroregression in children is associated with loss of memory, ability to think, understand, and recognize and is frequently associated with personality changes or distressing behavior. Additionally, vision loss, hearing loss, tone abnormalities, and epilepsy are other common symptoms in NDDs. Although most of the childhood NDDs are fatal, an accurate diagnosis is crucial for genetic counseling, prognostication, initiating prevention strategies, and prenatal diagnosis. Also, with advancing research and new drug development, treatment of certain disorders is now possible.

Neuroregression may result from NDD, neurometabolic problems, or may be acquired **(Flowchart 8.4.1)**.

EPIDEMIOLOGY

The true burden of NDD in India remains unknown. However, most of the common NDDs have been reported from India. The prevalence varies as per settings in which research is conducted. A clinic-based study of 117 children in North India reported that the three most common gray matter NDDs were

Flowchart 8.4.1: Causes of neuroregression.

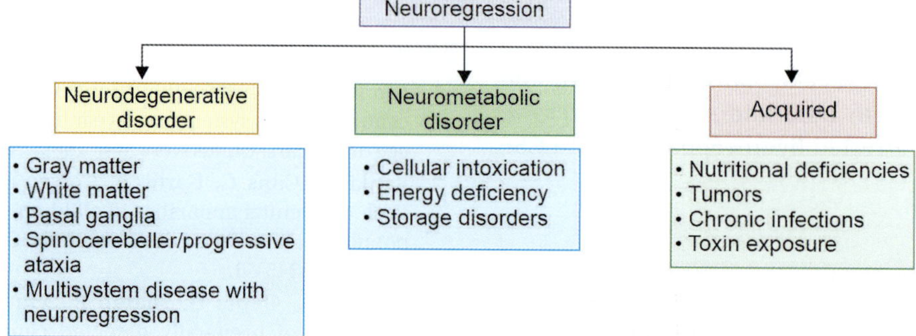

Wilson disease (18%), neuronal ceroid lipofuscinosis (NCL) (17%), and neurodegeneration with brain iron accumulation (NBIA) (16%). On the other hand, a single-center laboratory-based study of 464 patients from Hyderabad reported 23 different lysosomal storage disorders. Sphingolipidosis was the most frequent lysosomal storage disorder in this report followed by mucopolysaccharidosis (MPS). Neurometabolic diseases likely contribute to a significant proportion of neuroregression secondary to a genetic cause, although exact estimates are not available from India. Among the white-matter degenerations, megalencephalic leukodystrophy with subcortical cysts is particularly common in India, especially in the Agarwal community.

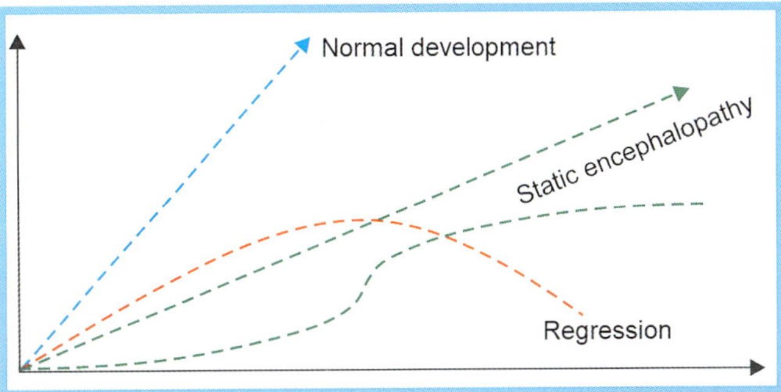

Fig. 8.4.1: Developmental trajectory in static encephalopathy versus neuroregression.

PATHOGENESIS

Both intrinsic and extrinsic factors are involved in pathogenesis. The underlying gene defect may affect the whole population of neurons or a functionally related group of neurons. The nerve cells may be affected as a whole, or certain components may be preferentially involved (e.g., axon and myelin). Some disease processes may affect synaptic connections, neurotransmitter synthesis or action, or neuromodulators. In some diseases, certain cellular proteins become structurally abnormal, accumulate, and disrupt functions in the nervous system (proteopathies). Further, a dysfunction of the elimination pathways for damaged cellular components, such as ubiquitin-proteasome system (UPS), lysosomal-autophagy, and apoptosis pathways, contributes to the pathogenesis of NDDs. For most disorders, the precise process by which the abnormal enzyme activity or abnormal metabolite accumulation causes brain damage is being extensively studied but is yet to be defined. In some disorders, the culprit metabolite has been identified (e.g., psychosine in Krabbe leukodystrophy, polyglutamine in Huntington's disease, and abnormal sterol in defects of cholesterol synthesis). Extrinsic factors, such as fasting, high protein load, fever, and hypoglycemia, may contribute to worsening the underlying condition, especially metabolic and mitochondrial disorders. Although the central nervous system (CNS) has been considered as an immune-privileged organ, increasing evidence supports the role of chronic inflammation in various neurodegenerative diseases, such as Aicardi-Goutières syndrome, neuronal ceroid lipofuscinoses, and several leukodystrophies and gangliosidoses. Metals, such as iron, copper, and manganese, have an important role in NDD and alterations in their homeostasis in the body can result in metal accumulation, free radical damage, and progressive neurodegeneration.[1,2]

APPROACH TO DIAGNOSIS

The first question we need to ask is "whether the development is delayed but improving or regressing?" **(Fig. 8.4.1)**.[3] There are certain red-flag signs in children with a diagnosis of static encephalopathy **(Box 8.4.1)** that should make us think about an underlying NDD. Once an NDD is suspected, the objective of a careful initial evaluation is to ascertain the age of onset, extent, and evolution of the disease [white matter, gray matter, cerebellum, etc. **(Table 8.4.1)**].

BOX 8.4.1: Red-flag signs in children with encephalopathy suggestive of NDD.

- Excessive delay or arrest in psychomotor development
- No definite history of a preceding brain injury
- Family history of neurological symptoms
- Parental consanguinity or family history of neurodegenerative disorders
- Inadequately explained oculomotor abnormalities, muscle atrophy, or sensory loss
- Recurrent episodic altered mentation, vomiting, or abnormal movements (IEM)
- Progressive difficulty in walking
- Unsteady gait, ataxia, or involuntary movements
- Intentional myoclonus (polymyoclonus)
- Skeletal and visceral abnormalities
- Recent unexplained behavioral problems or memory loss

(IEM: inborn errors of metabolism; NDD: neurodegenerative disorder)

As a first step in clinical evaluation, pseudoregression should be excluded in all children with neuroregression. Regression can occur without an underlying neurodegenerative process due to poorly controlled seizures, overmedication with anticonvulsants or antipsychotics, intercurrent systemic illness, raised intracranial pressure caused by brain tumor, hydrocephalus, chronic CNS infections, vitamin B_{12} deficiency, chronic lead poisoning, hypothyroidism, autistic regression, or recurrent strokes. Secondary neurological problems in a child with static encephalopathy (e.g., loss of mobility due to the development of joint contractures, seizures, and movement disorder) or depression or other emotional problems, especially in older children, are also not uncommon.

TABLE 8.4.1: Clinical features of gray- and white-matter diseases.

Features	Gray matter	White matter
Dementia	Early	Late
Seizures	Early and prominent	Late
Psychological symptoms	May be present	Uncommon
Basal ganglia signs and symptoms	Often present	Absent
Retinitis pigmentosa	May be present	Absent
Primary optic atrophy	Rare	May be seen
Primary neuropathy	Rare	May be seen
MRI	Cortical atrophy, abnormalities in basal ganglia, cerebellum	Clearly identifies abnormalities in white matter
ERG	May be abnormal	Normal
Visual-evoked response	May be abnormal	Normal
Brainstem auditory-evoked responses	Usually normal	Abnormal

(ERG: electroretinogram; MRI: magnetic resonance imaging)

History and Examination[2,4]

A detailed history is aimed at ascertaining the age of onset, and the spheres of development affected motor, cognitive, vision, and hearing. A family history of three generations obtained by pedigree charting is important to identify the possible modes of transmission. There are certain specific clues in general physical and systemic examinations, which give an indication of the nature of the disorder **(Table 8.4.2)**. After a careful history and examination, one is able to decide about the range of pathology within the nervous system and whether other organ systems are involved or not. Broadly, if one can assign the patient to one of the following groups, further evaluation is easier:

- *Gray-matter degenerations:* Poliodystrophies
- *White-matter degeneration:* Leukodystrophies
- Progressive ataxias
- Basal ganglia disorders
- Multisystem disorders with neuroregression

Regression in a Child Below 2 Years (Flowcharts 8.4.2 and 8.4.3)[1,2,4]

During infancy, delayed milestones are a common manifestation of NDDs. Many infants have not gained many distinctive abilities, so the loss of abilities is difficult to quantify or localize. Commonly, the affected infant lacks visual interest or socialization and has poor head control or inability to use hands. Other common symptoms are developmental retardation with severe hypotonia, especially with feeding difficulties and/or vomiting and failure to thrive.

Many disorders that present in the second year of life are frequently recognizable by the obvious loss of motor abilities. This may result from corticospinal, cerebellar, extrapyramidal, or peripheral nerve involvement. The second year of life is also the age for disorders with gradually increasing dysmorphism, skeletal abnormalities, and cognitive decline (MPS and mucolipidosis) to manifest. Some children may present with progressive mental deterioration, seizures, and vision loss. Yet, another group of children presents with recurrent neurological deterioration interspersed with apparent recovery (organic aciduria, mitochondrial disorders, urea cycle disorders, etc.).

- In girls with regression in cognitive spheres starting in infancy and microcephaly and associated with loss of purposeful hand movements, a possibility of Rett syndrome should be considered.
- In addition, the possibility of human immunodeficiency virus (HIV) encephalopathy should always be kept in mind and a systematic evaluation for risk factors should be undertaken.

Neuroregression in Later Childhood and Adolescence (Flowcharts 8.4.4 and 8.4.5)[1,2,4]

In older children, NDDs result in neuroregression after a considerable period of normal development. Hence, the onset and course of the disorder can be clinically more accurately determined.

It is much easier to view individual patients as having the predominant involvement of a particular area of the nervous system. The major clinical problem one faces is the varied ways in which the same disorder can present. This is particularly true for autosomal dominant disorders.

Subacute sclerosing panencephalitis (SSPE), though not a hereditary NDD, is a common cause of neuroregression in our country. It should be considered in all children with behavioral changes and cognitive deterioration with or without myoclonic jerks.

An extrapyramidal syndrome, developmental delay, and self-mutilation behavior are seen in boys with Lesch–Nyhan syndrome **(Fig. 8.4.4A)**. Chilblains-like distal red rash is seen in Aicardi–Goutières syndrome **(Fig. 8.4.4B)**.

Investigations

Investigations help in excluding differentials and making the diagnosis and are guided by history and examination.

Imaging

A high-resolution magnetic resonance imaging (MRI) with spectroscopy would be the best to pick up abnormalities.

TABLE 8.4.2: Some clinical pointers in hereditary neurodegenerative disorders.

Organs or features	***Abnormality***	***Disorders***
Head	Microcephaly	NCL, Krabbe disease, Rett syndrome
	Macrocephaly	MPS, Alexander disease, Canavan disease, GM1 gangliosidosis, Tay–Sachs disease, MLSC
Hair	Alopecia	Biotinidase deficiency
	Pigmentary changes	PKU, Menkes disease
	Wooly, kinky hair	Menkes disease **(Fig. 8.4.2)**
Skin	Rash	Biotinidase, holocarboxylase deficiency
	Subcutaneous nodules	Farber disease
	Angiokeratomas	Fabry disease
	Fat pads, focal atrophy	Congenital disorders of glycosylation
	Hyperpigmentation	Adrenoleukodystrophy
Eyes	Cataract	Galactosemia, Zellweger disease, Wilson disease
	Retinitis pigmentosa	Peroxisomal disorders, NCL, mitochondrial encephalomyopathies, MPS, PKAN, ABLP
	Cherry red spot	Tay–Sachs disease, Niemann–Pick disease, GM1 gangliosidosis, sialidosis
	Optic atrophy	NCL, MLD, Krabbe disease, Canavan disease, GM2 gangliosidosis
	Chorioretinitis	MPS, SSPE, Lowe syndrome
	Dislocated lens	Homocystinuria, sulfite oxidase deficiency
Ears	Deafness	MPS, ALD, mitochondrial disorders, peroxisomal disorders
	Hyperacusis	Krabbe disease, Tay–Sachs disease
Abdomen	Hepatosplenomegaly	MPS, GM1 gangliosidosis, Gaucher disease, Niemann–Pick disease
	Hernia	GM1 gangliosidosis, MPS
Nervous system	Peripheral neuropathy	MLD, Krabbe disease, mitochondrial disorders
	Hydrocephalus or raised intracranial pressure	MPS, infantile Alexander disease
Cardiac	Cardiomyopathy	FAOD, mitochondrial disorders, Friedreich ataxia, AVED, Pompe disease
	Valvular defects	MPS, Zellweger syndrome, Fabry disease

(ABLP: abetalipoproteinemia; ALD: adrenoleukodystrophy; AVED: ataxia with vitamin E deficiency; FAOD: fatty acid oxidation defects; MLD: metachromatic leukodystrophy; MLSC: megalencephalic leukodystrophy with subcortical cysts; MPS: mucopolysaccharidosis; NCL: neuronal ceroid lipofuscinosis; PKAN: pantothenate kinase-associated neurodegeneration; PKU: phenylketonuria; SSPE: subacute sclerosing panencephalitis)

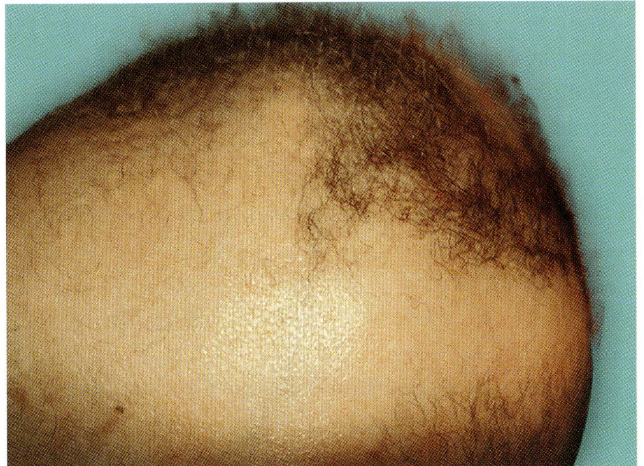

Fig. 8.4.2: Note the sparse, hypopigmented curly, stubby hair in a child with Menkes disease.

MRI in certain patients may provide a diagnostic clue, e.g., pantothenate kinase-associated neurodegeneration with "Eye of Tiger" sign in globus pallidi **(Fig. 8.4.5)**, megalencephalic leukodystrophy with subcortical cysts **(Figs. 8.4.6A to C)**, SSPE **(Fig. 8.4.7)**, metachromatic leukodystrophy (MLD) **(Fig. 8.4.8)**, adrenoleukodystrophy (ALD) **(Fig. 8.4.9)**, Wilson disease **(Fig. 8.4.10)**, mitochondrial encephalopathies, and creatine deficiency disorders. MRI with spectroscopy helps in the diagnosis of certain disorders, such as Canavan disease **(Figs. 8.4.11A and B)**.

Radiographs

A skeletal survey is important to look for abnormalities in certain storage disorders, such as MPS **(Figs. 8.4.12A and B)** and infantile GM1 gangliosidosis.

Flowchart 8.4.2: A simplified approach to a child <2 years with suspected degenerative brain disorder.

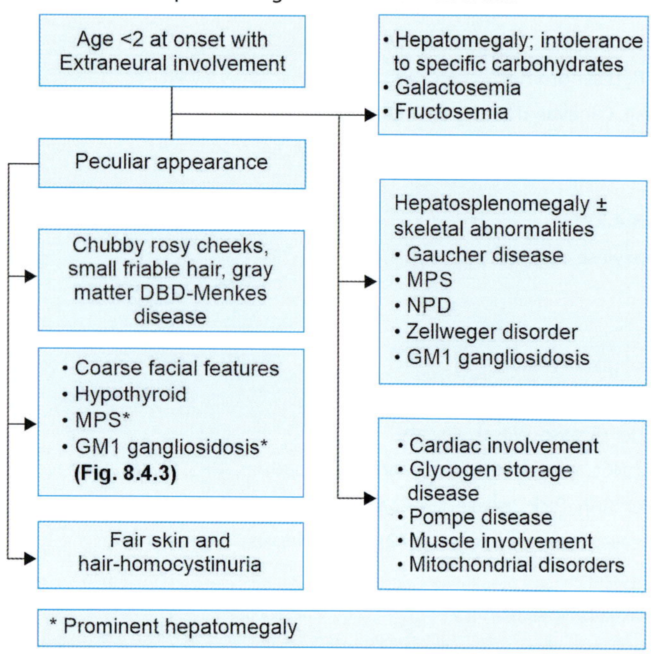

(DBD: degenerative brain disorder; MPS: mucopolysaccharidosis; NPD: Niemann–Pick disease)

Flowchart 8.4.3: A simplified approach to a child <2 years with suspected degenerative brain disorder with no extraneural abnormalities.

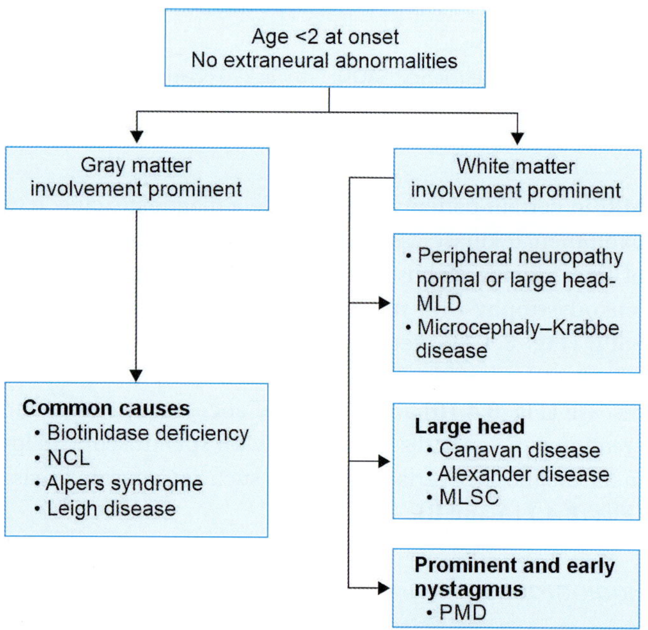

(MLD: metachromatic leukodystrophy; MLSC: megalencephalic leukodystrophy with subcortical cysts; NCL: neuronal ceroid lipofuscinosis; PMD: Pelizaeus–Merzbacher disease)

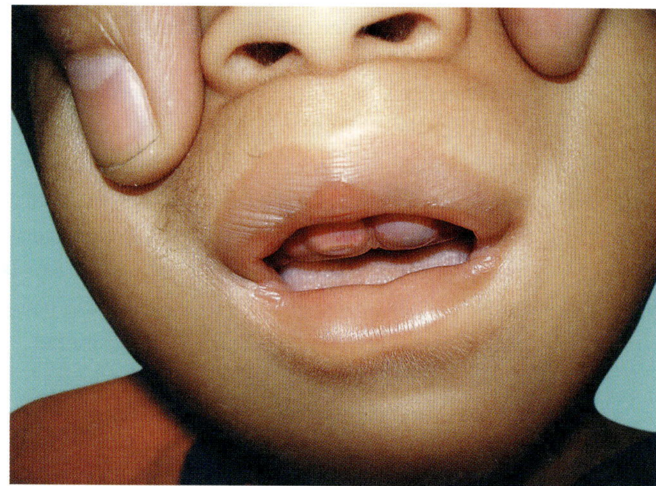

Fig. 8.4.3: Gum hypertrophy and coarsening in an 18-month-old child with infantile GM1 gangliosidosis.

Urine and Blood Assay for Plasma Ammonia, Blood Lactate and Pyruvate, Plasma Amino Acids

These tests guide the course of further investigations in a suspected neurometabolic disorder to arrive at the diagnosis.

Electrophysiological Tests

Electrophysiological tests include "visual evoked potentials," brainstem auditory-evoked responses, "nerve conduction studies," electroencephalography, electromyography, and somatosensory-evoked potentials. These help to delineate the extent of central and peripheral nervous system involvement in the patient.

Other Tests

- *Histopathological and ultrastructural information from selected biopsies*
- *Bone marrow:* Storage cells are seen in Niemann–Pick disease, Gaucher disease
- *Conjunctival, skin, rectal biopsy:* NCL
- *Muscle:* Mitochondrial disorders
- *Hair microscopy:* Menkes disease

Specific investigations are done based on clues obtained from preceding investigations:

- *Serology:* HIV, SSPE
- *Urine copper, serum ceruloplasmin:* Wilson disease
- *Urine MPS*: MPS
- *Enzyme analysis:* Lysosomal storage disorders, biotinidase deficiency
- *Urine organic acids:* Organic acidemias
- *Very long-chain fatty acids (VLCFA) and plasmalogen levels:* Peroxisomal disorders

Flowchart 8.4.4: Approach to progressive neurological deterioration in the 2–5 years age group.

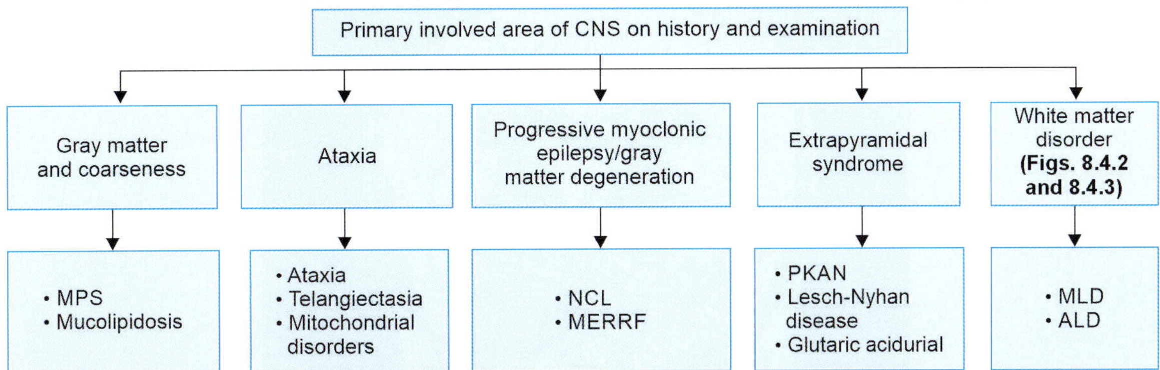

(ALD: adrenoleukodystrophy; CNS: central nervous system; MERRF: myoclonic epilepsy with ragged red fibers; MLD: metachromatic leukodystrophy; MPS: mucopolysaccharidosis; NCL: neuronal ceroid lipofuscinosis; PKAN: pantothenate kinase-associated neurodegeneration)

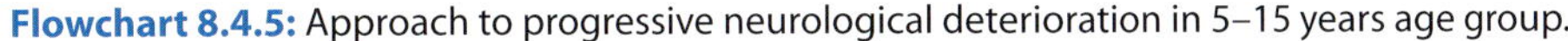

Flowchart 8.4.5: Approach to progressive neurological deterioration in 5–15 years age group.

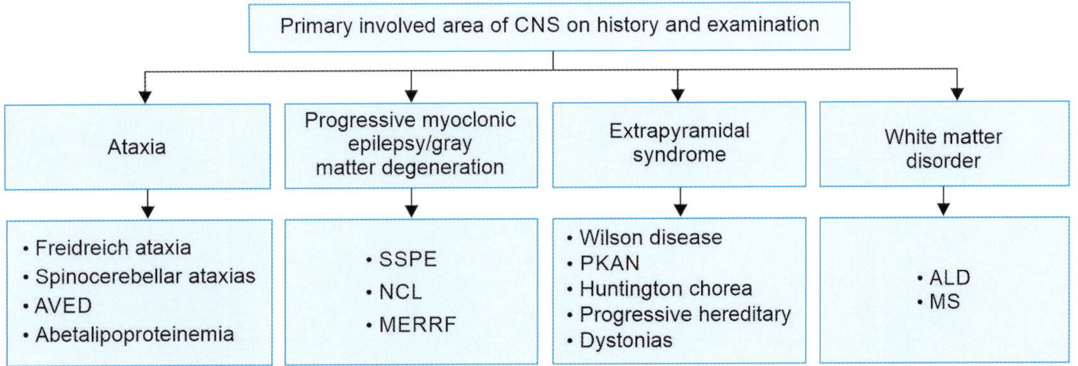

(ALD: adrenoleukodystrophy; AVED: ataxia with vitamin E deficiency; CNS: central nervous system; MERRF: myoclonic epilepsy with ragged red fibers; MS: multiple sclerosis; NCL: neuronal ceroid lipofuscinosis; PKAN: pantothenate kinase-associated neurodegeneration; SSPE: subacute sclerosing panencephalitis)

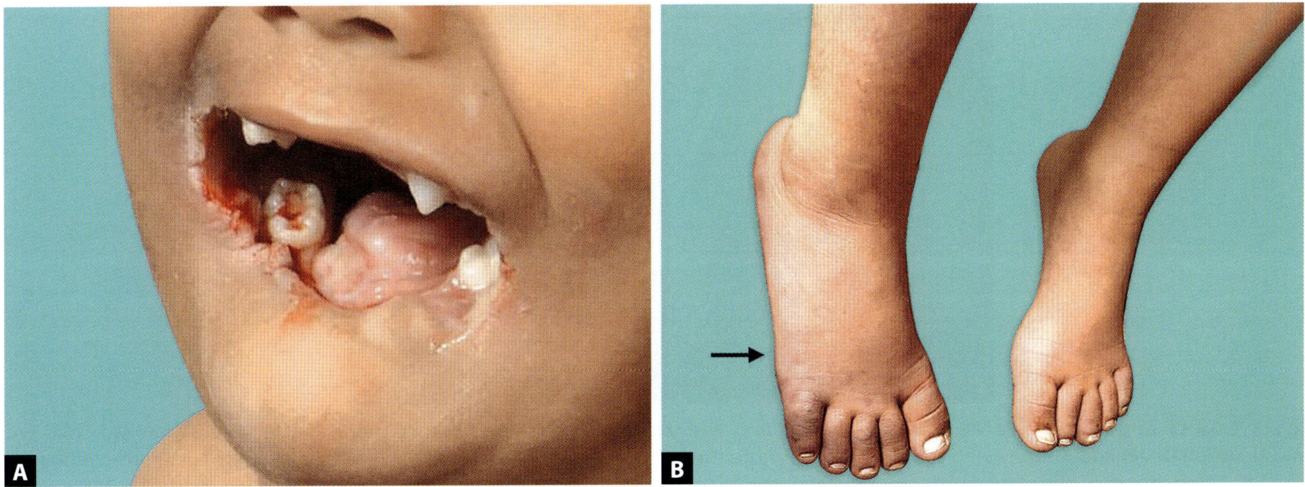

Figs. 8.4.4A and B: (A) Severe self-mutilation in a 3-year-old boy with Lesch–Nyhan disease; (B) Chilblains-like distal red rash in a child with Aicardi–Goutières syndrome.

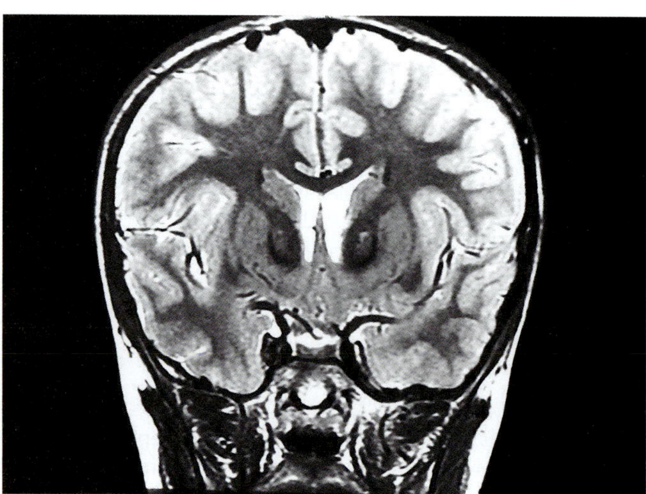

Fig. 8.4.5: Coronal T2W MRI in a child with pantothenate kinase-associated neurodegeneration showing the bilaterally hypointense globus pallidi with an area of central hyperintensity. (MRI: magnetic resonance imaging; T2W: T2 weight)

A

B

C

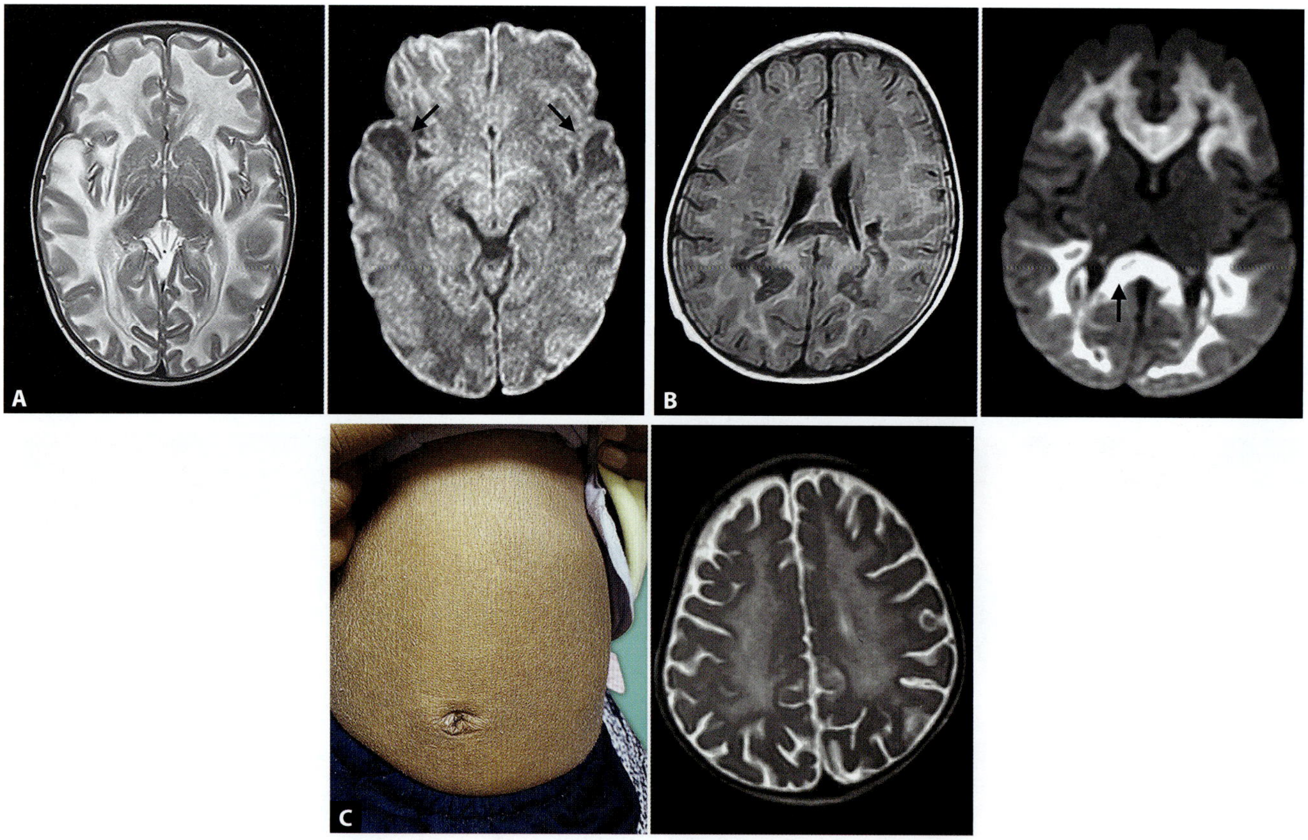

Figs. 8.4.6A to C: (A) Axial T2W MRI of the brain showing abnormal diffusely hyperintense white matter in a 3-year-old child with "megalencephalic leukodystrophy with subcortical cysts", note the temporal cysts (black arrows); (B) MRI brain in an 11-month-old boy with complex-1 mitochondrial disease with extensive white matter changes with cystic degeneration and intense diffusion restriction (black arrow); and (C) Extensive ichthyosis and progressive spasticity in a child with multiple sulfatase deficiency. MRI showing periventricular white matter changes similar to those seen in metachromatic leukodystrophy. (MRI: magnetic resonance imaging; T2W: T2 weight)

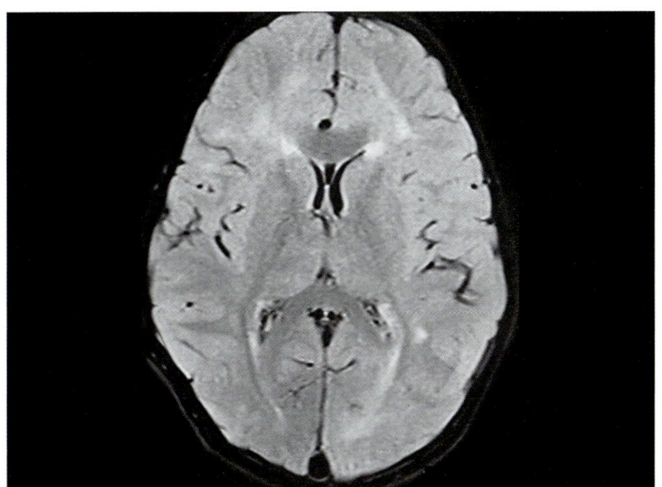

Fig. 8.4.7: Axial FLAIR-MRI of the brain showing ill-defined, bilateral, asymmetrical, patchy hyperintensities in the periventricular and subcortical white matter of frontal and parieto-occipital regions in a child with SSPE. (FLAIR-MRI: fluid-attenuated inversion recovery-magnetic resonance imaging; SSPE: subacute sclerosing panencephalitis)

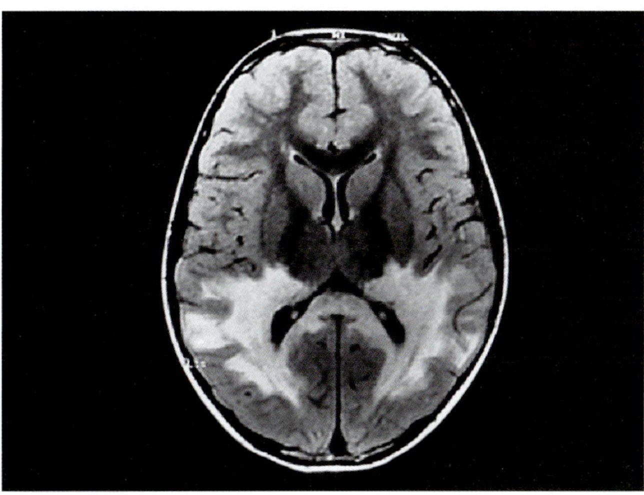

Fig. 8.4.9: Axial FLAIR-MRI of the brain showing posterior dominant abnormal hyperintense white matter in a child with adrenoleukodystrophy. The splenium of the corpus callosum is also prominently involved. (FLAIR-MRI: fluid-attenuated inversion recovery-magnetic resonance imaging)

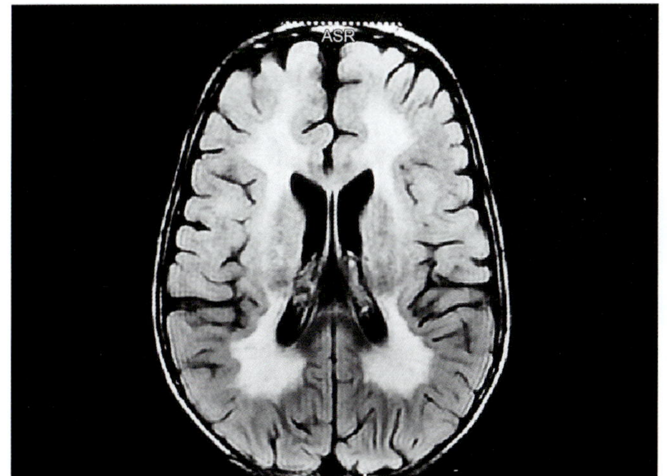

Fig. 8.4.8: Axial FLAIR-MRI of the brain showing bilateral periventricular abnormal hyperintense white matter in a child with metachromatic leukodystrophy. (FLAIR-MRI: fluid-attenuated inversion recovery-magnetic resonance imaging)

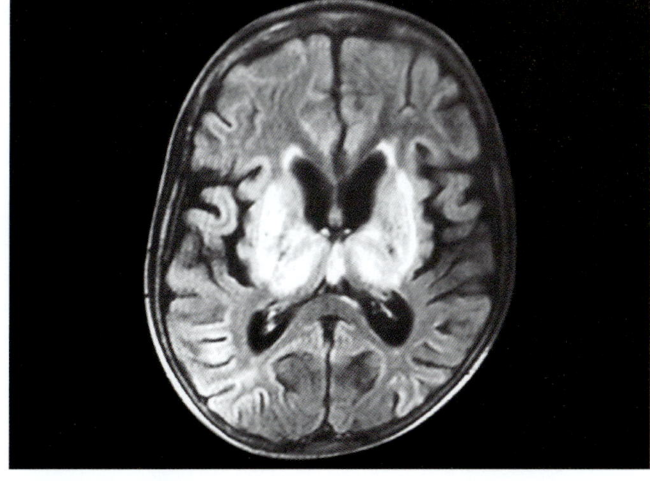

Fig. 8.4.10: MRI in a child with Wilson disease showing the involvement of bilateral basal ganglia. (MRI: magnetic resonance imaging)

- *Genetic testing*: This is now one of the first-line tests in degenerative disorders. The next-generation sequencing of the exome offers an easy and quick way to establish the diagnosis of these disorders. However, it is important to make a clinical diagnosis of these disorders before genetic testing to inform proper bioinformatics interpretations and avoid wrong diagnoses. Parental and family testing is often needed to clearly define the genetic defect.

MANAGEMENT

First, never miss out on a treatable cause of neuroregression, such as hydrocephalus, HIV infection, hypothyroidism **(Fig. 8.4.13)**, and lead toxicity. It must be remembered that many NDDs are amenable to treatment **(Table 8.4.3)**. Therapies under research include mitochondrial genome manipulation of heteroplasmic mitochondrial deoxyribonucleic acid mutations; defective mitochondrial

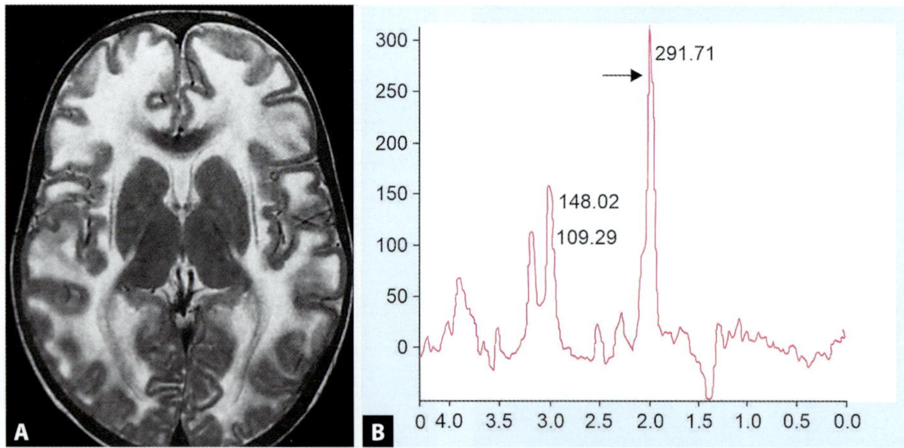

Figs. 8.4.11A and B: T2-weighted MRI image showing (A) diffuse, symmetrical white-matter hyperintensities involving the periventricular and subcortical white matter and (B) NAA peak on MR spectroscopy in a 2-year-old boy with progressively increasing head size and developmental delay suggestive of Canavan disease. (MR: magnetic resonance; NAA: *N*-acetyl aspartate)

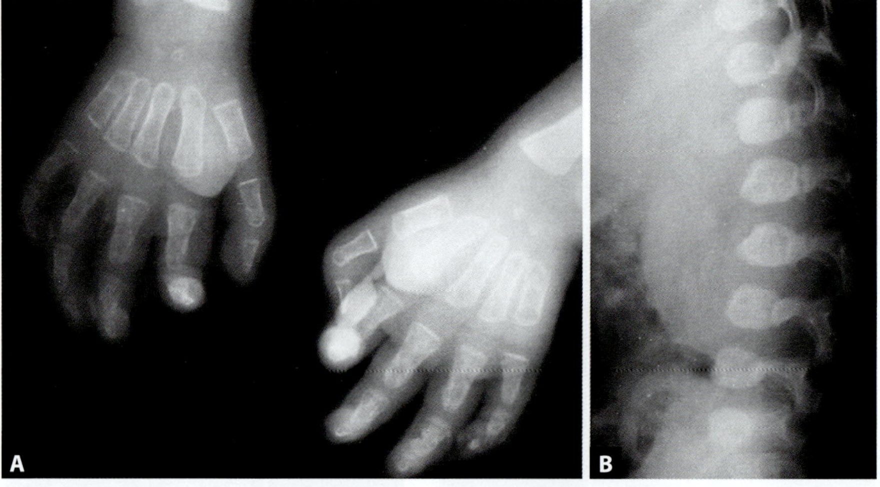

Figs. 8.4.12A and B: (A) X-ray of hands of a child with infantile GM1 gangliosidosis showing mild changes of dysostosis multiplex with early conical shape of proximal bases of 2–5 metacarpals with tapering of the proximal phalanges; (B) Lateral radiograph of the spine in child.

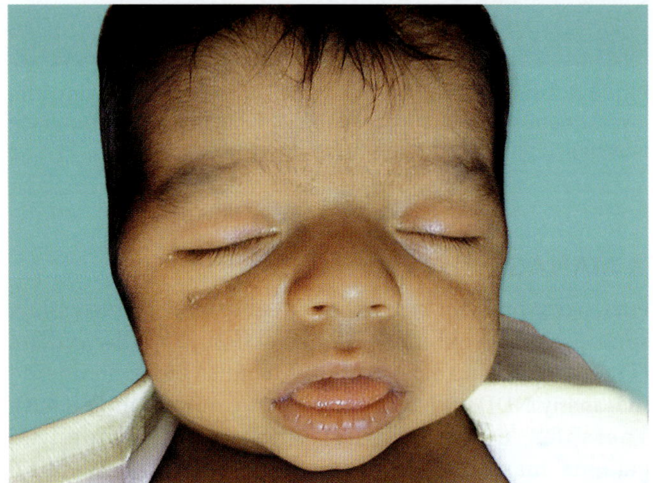

Fig. 8.4.13: Note the coarsening of facial features, and large tongue in an infant with hypothyroidism.

replacement by genome editing, gene-editing tools, such as zinc finger nucleases, meganucleases, and transcription activator-like effector nucleases; CRISPR (clustered regulatory interspaced short palindromic repeats)-Cas9 (CRISPR-associated protein 9); and antiapoptotic drugs, such as minocycline, rasagiline, melatonin, resveratrol, and lithium.

Supportive Measures

It is never wise or correct to say that the disease is "untreatable." Such statements only result in parents feeling a profound sense of anguish, abandonment, and loneliness. Something can almost always be done to help the child. Supportive treatment may add significantly to the quality of life of a child with NDD. Measures to reduce spasticity, dystonia, drooling, swallowing problems, control seizures, control pain, improve nutrition, prevent constipation, prevent bed sores, and enhance mobility all contribute to the quality of life

TABLE 8.4.3: A few examples of treatment in neurodegenerative disorders.

Disease	*Therapeutic agent*
Gaucher disease	Enzyme replacement, miglustat
Fabry disease	Enzyme replacement
MPS I, MPS II, MPS IVA, MPS VI, MPS VII	Enzyme replacement
Pompe disease	Enzyme replacement
Neuronal ceroid lipofuscinosis-2	Enzyme replacement
Ataxia (Co-Q deficiency)	Coenzyme Q10
Ataxia with vitamin E deficiency	Vitamin E
Minimally symptomatic X-linked adrenoleukodystrophy, Krabbe disease	Bone marrow transplant
MPS 1H-Hurler disease	Bone marrow transplant
Glycogen storage disease	Liver transplant
Glutaric aciduria-II, biotinidase deficiency	Cofactor replacement
Wilson disease	D-Penicillamine, trientine, zinc acetate, liver transplantation
Menkes disease	Copper sulfate
Creatine-deficiency disorders	Creatine supplements
Hypermanganesemia	Chelation
Glucose transporter disorder, pyruvate dehydrogenase deficiency, Refsum disease	Special diet
Neurotransmitter disorder	Specific cofactors or drugs
Lesch–Nyhan disease	Allopurinol
Rett syndrome	Trofinetide
Metachromatic leukodystrophy	Gene therapy
Cerebral adrenoleukodystrophy	Gene therapy

(Co-Q: coenzyme Q10; MPS 1: mucopolysaccharidosis type 1)

of the patient and indirectly to the quality of life of the parents and any unaffected siblings. The use of a mitochondrial cocktail (a mixture of oral vitamins and supplements, such as L-carnitine, coenzyme Q, riboflavin, thiamine, and vitamins C and E) in disorders with impaired mitochondrial function has been shown to produce modest improvements in broad patient outcomes in small-scale clinical trials. Formulating a chronic care and follow-up plan and communicating this to all professionals involved are of immense benefit to the child and the family.

PREVENTION

One of the very important aspects of the management of a child with NDD is to accurately establish the diagnosis. This becomes important not only for proper care and prognostication but also for accurate prenatal diagnosis to prevent children from further being affected by the same disease. The diagnosis may also help identify pauci- or presymptomatic siblings or other family members who may benefit from early therapy (e.g., zinc therapy in Wilson disease). It would be wise to refer parents for prenatal diagnosis to an equipped center before they plan any future pregnancies.

PROGNOSIS

It is sensible to first confirm the diagnosis and then prognosticate. The prognosis in NDD depends on the underlying disorder. In general, an earlier onset of disease predicts a poorer outcome. However, several late-onset diseases can also rapidly progress (e.g., ALD).

CONCLUSION

- A thorough clinical evaluation that includes a detailed history, family history, and general physical and systemic evaluation forms an important starting point for further evaluation. If the history and examination are strongly indicative, more specific diagnostic testing can be undertaken (e.g., HIV testing, urine MPS, and VLCFA).
- Based on the clinical presentation, always keep the treatable causes in mind and exclude them systematically.
- Second-line investigations including genetic testing are best undertaken at referral centers or by qualified experts with expertise in proper interpretations of these tests.
- While managing these children, always focus on issues that make the child's and caregiver's life comfortable (e.g., control of seizures, spasticity, adequate nutrition, and skin care).

REFERENCES

1. Lyon G, Kolodny EH, Pastores GM. Neurology of Hereditary Metabolic Diseases in Children, 3rd edition. New York: McGraw-Hill; 2006.
2. Neurologic syndrome. In: Clarke JTR (Ed). A Clinical Guide to Inherited Metabolic Diseases, 3rd edition. Cambridge: Cambridge University Press; 2006. p. 2889.
3. Fenichel GM. Clinical Pediatric Neurology: A Signs and Symptoms Approach, 5th edition. Philadelphia: Elsevier; 2005.
4. Swaiman KF, Ashwal S, Ferriero DM, Schor NF, Finkel RS, Gropman AL, et al. (Eds). Swaiman's Pediatric Neurology: Principles and Practice, 6th edition. Philadelphia: Elsevier; 2017.

8.5 Neurocutaneous Disorders

Lokesh Saini

INTRODUCTION

Neurocutaneous syndromes, also referred to as *phakomatoses* (from the Greek "*Phakos*" meaning birthmark), represent a diverse group of disorders characterized by the simultaneous involvement of the central and peripheral nervous systems, skin, and internal organs.[1,2] The term *phakomatoses* was introduced by a Dutch ophthalmologist, Jan van der Hoeve, in 1932. Among the neurocutaneous syndromes, neurofibromatosis (NF), tuberous sclerosis complex (TSC), Sturge–Weber syndrome (SWS), and ataxia telangiectasia (AT) are considered as prototypes of the disease. Additionally, pediatric practitioners may encounter other syndromes such as linear nevus sebaceous syndrome (LNSS), incontinentia pigmenti (IP), McCune-Albright syndrome (MAS), Von Hippel-Lindau syndrome (VHLS), megalencephaly-capillary malformation-polymicrogyria syndrome (MCAP), and PHACE syndrome (posterior fossa malformations, hemangioma of the cervicofacial region, arterial anomalies, cardiac anomalies, eye anomalies, and sternal or abdominal clefting or ectopia cordis). The significant comorbidities of neurocutaneous syndromes are drug-resistant epilepsy, neurodevelopmental disorders including autism spectrum disorder (ASD), intellectual disability (ID), attention deficit hyperactivity disorder (ADHD), and sleep disturbances.

EPIDEMIOLOGY

The estimated birth prevalence of neurocutaneous syndromes is 1 in 2,000–3,500 for NF1, 1 in 6,000–10,000 for TSC, and 1 in 25,000–40,000 for NF2.[2-4]

PATHOPHYSIOLOGY

Neurocutaneous syndromes are predominantly inherited in an autosomal dominant mode. The genetic mutations with defective proteins and gene mapping for the common neurocutaneous syndromes are summarized in **Table 8.5.1**. While the mechanisms leading to epileptogenesis vary across neurocutaneous disorders, there is a shared involvement in molecular pathways, particularly the mammalian target of rapamycin (mTOR) signaling pathways.[3,4]

Common neurocutaneous syndromes are described in the following text.

TABLE 8.5.1: Genetic mutations of common neurocutaneous syndromes.

Syndrome	Gene	Protein	Chromosome
Neurofibromatosis 1 (von Recklinghausen disease)	*NF1*	Neurofibromin	17q11
Neurofibromatosis 2 (NF2-related schwannomatosis)	*NF2*	Schwannomin/ Merlin	22q12
Tuberous sclerosis complex (Bourneville disease)	*TSC1/ TSC2*	Hamartin/Tuberin	9q34/16p13
Sturge–Weber syndrome (Encephalotrigeminal angiomatosis)	*GNAQ*	Guanine nucleotide-binding protein, Q polypeptide protein	9q21
Von Hippel–Lindau disease	*VHL*	Von Hippel–Lindau protein	3p35
Ataxia telangiectasia	*ATM*	Ataxia telangiectasia mutated protein	11q22

NEUROFIBROMATOSIS

Neurofibromatosis-1

Among the neurocutaneous syndromes, neurofibromatosis type 1 (NF1), also known as von Recklinghausen disease, is the most prevalent, exhibiting autosomal dominant inheritance. NF1 is classified as a RASopathy, arising from pathogenic variations in the *NF1* gene, a tumor-suppressor gene responsible for encoding the neurofibromin protein.[3] NF1 displays considerable variability both within and between families and shares some features with other RASopathies.[5] This loss of neurofibromin causes dysregulation of the RAS/MAPK, RAF, PI3K, AKT, and mTOR pathways.

Cutaneous manifestations of NF1 encompass café-au-lait macules, freckling, and juvenile xanthogranulomas. Ophthalmological signs include Lisch nodules (iris hamartomas) and choroidal anomalies. NF1 is linked to a higher likelihood of benign and malignant tumors forming in both neural and nonneural tissues. Tumors commonly associated with NF1 are optic pathway gliomas,

BOX 8.5.1: Revised diagnostic criteria for NF1.*

A: For an individual who does not have a parent diagnosed with NF1 if two or more of the following are present:
- Six or more café-au-lait macules over 5 mm in greatest diameter in prepubertal individuals and over 15 mm in greatest diameter in postpubertal individuals
- Freckling in the axillary or inguinal region
- Two or more neurofibromas of any type or one plexiform neurofibroma
- Optic pathway glioma
- Two or more iris Lisch nodules identified by slit-lamp examination or two or more choroidal abnormalities (CAs)—defined as bright, patchy nodules imaged by optical coherence tomography (OCT)/near-infrared reflectance (NIR) imaging
- A distinctive osseous lesion such as sphenoid dysplasia, anterolateral bowing of the tibia, or pseudarthrosis of a long bone
- A heterozygous pathogenic NF1 variant with a variant allele fraction of 50% in apparently normal tissue such as white blood cells

B: A child of a parent who meets the diagnostic criteria specified in *A* merits a diagnosis of NF1 if one or more of the criteria in *A* are present

*Revised diagnostic criteria for NF1—2021.

BOX 8.5.2: Revised diagnostic criteria for NF2.*

A diagnosis of NF2-related schwannomatosis (previously termed neurofibromatosis 2, NF2) can be made when an individual has one of the following:
- Bilateral vestibular schwannomas (VS)
- An identical NF2 pathogenic variant in at least two anatomically distinct NF2-related tumors (schwannoma, meningioma, and/or ependymoma)
- Either two major or one major and two minor criteria as described in the following:
  - *Major criteria:*
    - Unilateral vestibular schwannomas
    - First-degree relative other than sibling with NF2-related schwannomatosis
    - Two or more meningiomas (*Note:* Single meningioma qualifies as minor criteria)
    - NF2 pathogenic variant in an unaffected tissue such as blood
  - *Minor criteria:*
    - Can count >1 of a type (e.g., two distinct schwannomas would count as two minor criteria)
    - Ependymoma, meningioma (*Note:* Multiple meningiomas qualify as major criteria), schwannoma (*Note:* If the major criterion is unilateral VS, at least one schwannoma must be dermal in location)
    - Can count only once (e.g., bilateral cortical cataracts count as a single minor criterion)
    - Juvenile subcapsular or cortical cataract, retinal hamartoma, epiretinal membrane in a person aged <40 years, meningioma

*Updated diagnostic criteria and nomenclature for NF2—2022.

medulloblastomas, ependymomas, and spinal neoplasms, including malignant peripheral nerve sheath tumors (MPNST), neurofibromas, gangliogliomas, and astrocytomas. Other associated manifestations are precocious puberty, excess/deficiency of growth hormone, epilepsy, neurodevelopmental disorders, bone dysplasias, scoliosis, and moyamoya vasculopathy.

The revised diagnostic criteria for NF1 are summarized in **Box 8.5.1**.

The proposed targeted therapies for NF1 plexiform neurofibroma include sirolimus, imatinib, and trametinib, and for optic pathway glioma is everolimus.

Neurofibromatosis-2

Neurofibromatosis type 2 (NF2) (NF2-related schwannomatosis) follows an autosomal dominant pattern of Mendelian inheritance and arises from mutations in the *NF2* gene.[3] *NF2*, a tumor-suppressor gene, encodes the Merlin protein that regulates the PI3kinase/Akt, Raf/MEK/ERK, and mTOR pathways.[6]

NF2 typically manifests with sensorineural hearing loss, tinnitus, headaches, and balance issues. Additionally, NF2 is linked with seizures, cataracts, and sensations of numbness or tingling (paresthesias). In children, the most common symptoms and signs of NF2 are associated with skin or spinal tumors. Tumors commonly associated with NF2 include vestibular schwannomas, intracranial meningiomas, ependymomas, and spinal intramedullary and extramedullary tumors. Additionally, individuals with NF2 may develop schwannomas affecting cranial, spinal, and peripheral nerves and astrocytomas. Ocular abnormalities seen in NF2 are cataracts and retinal hamartomas.

The revised diagnostic criteria for NF2 are summarized in **Box 8.5.2**. The proposed targeted therapies for NF2 vestibular schwannoma are erlotinib, everolimus, and bevacizumab.

TUBEROUS SCLEROSIS COMPLEX

Tuberous sclerosis complex (Bourneville disease) is a multisystemic disorder with an autosomal dominant pattern of Mendelian inheritance due to mutations in *TSC1* or *TSC2* genes encoding the hamartin and tuberin proteins, respectively.[3] This causes the loss of the mTOR signaling cascade, leading to disordered regulation of cell division, growth, and differentiation, and altered neuronal migration, resulting in the development of hamartomas.[7]

The dermatological features in TSC are facial angiofibromas (adenoma sebaceum), shagreen patches, hypomelanotic (ash-leaf) macules, and fibrous plaques.[5] Hypomelanotic macules are the primary skin signs seen in TSC; although they

TABLE 8.5.2: Revised diagnostic criteria for tuberous sclerosis complex (TSC).*

Genetic criteria: A pathogenic variant in TSC1 or TSC2 is diagnostic for TSC	
Clinical criteria:	
Major features: • Hypomelanotic macules (≥3; at least 5 mm diameter) • Angiofibroma (≥3 or fibrous cephalic plaque • Ungual fibromas (≥2) • Shagreen patch • Multiple retinal hamartomas • Cortical dysplasias (tubers and cerebral white matter radial migration lines) • Subependymal nodule (≥2) • Subependymal giant cell astrocytoma • Cardiac rhabdomyoma • Lymphangioleiomyomatosis • Angiomyolipomas (≥2)	*Minor features:* • "Confetti" skin lesions • Dental enamel pits (≥3) • Intraoral fibromas (≥2) • Retinal achromic patch • Multiple renal cysts • Nonrenal hamartomas
Definite TSC: Two major features or one major feature with ≥2 minor features *Possible TSC*: Either one major feature or ≥2 minor features	

*Updated tuberous sclerosis complex diagnostic criteria—2021.

are very sensitive indicators, they lack specificity. Shagreen patches typically form on the lower back and have a texture resembling orange peel. Facial angiofibromas, the most noticeable sign, start as erythematous macules and evolve into fibrous growths. Ophthalmological features in TSC are lid angiofibromas, hypopigmented choroidal lesions, and retinal hamartomas. The revised diagnostic criteria for TSC are summarized in **Table 8.5.2**.

Tuberous sclerosis complex is associated with significant comorbidities, including drug-refractory epilepsy, sleep disturbances, and TSC-associated neuropsychiatric disorders (TAND).[8] In childhood, the primary seizure types observed in TSC are epileptic spasms and focal seizures. The central nervous system tumors in TSC include hamartomas, cortical tubers, subependymal nodules (SENs), and subependymal giant cell astrocytomas (SEGAs). Other lesions include cardiac rhabdomyomas, retinal hamartomas, neuroendocrine tumors (NETs), renal angiomyolipoma, renal cell carcinoma, lymphangioleiomyomatosis (LAMs), and multifocal micronodular pneumocyte hyperplasia (MMPH).[9]

Computed tomography (CT) of the brain is valuable for detecting calcifications. Electroencephalography (EEG) abnormalities precede clinical seizures, and periodic EEG monitoring is advocated in infancy. Magnetic resonance imaging (MRI) of the brain helps in identifying and monitoring the growth of SENs and SEGAs.[9] MRI and fluorine-18 fluorodeoxyglucose (^{18}F-FDG) positron emission tomography (PET) can be used to locate the tubers. Epileptogenic cortical tubers are only identified using the α-[^{11}C]-methyl-L-tryptophan (AMT)-PET scan.[9,10]

The management involves a multidisciplinary approach combining medical and surgical interventions. It is recommended that all children diagnosed with TSC undergo neuroimaging at diagnosis and every 1–3 years for surveillance, even if they are asymptomatic. mTOR inhibitors such as sirolimus and everolimus are utilized to manage conditions such as LAM, renal angiomyolipoma, SEGAs, and drug-resistant epilepsy. Vigabatrin is the FDA-approved first-line monotherapy for treating epileptic spasms in TSC. Surgically removing SEGAs is an option if they are clinically symptomatic. Supportive therapies, including occupational therapy, physiotherapy, and speech therapy, are provided for neurodevelopmental disorders.

STURGE–WEBER SYNDROME

Sturge–Weber syndrome (encephalotrigeminal angiomatosis) is a neurocutaneous syndrome with sporadic inheritance and presents with angiomas involving the face, choroid, and leptomeninges. SWS is a triad of capillary–venous malformations of the skin (port-wine stain/nevus flammeus), leptomeningeal angiomatosis, and glaucoma.[2,4] The port-wine stain is seen in the ophthalmic division of trigeminal nerve distribution of forehead and cheeks, and the leptomeningeal angiomatosis is usually seen in the occipital and posterior parietal lobes. Glaucoma occurs almost always in the ipsilateral side of the port-wine stain. The reduction of intraocular fluid decreases intraocular pressure, subsequently lowering the risk of vision loss associated with glaucoma. The facial and pial angiomas are due to persistent primordial sinusoidal vascular channels.

Common presentations in SWS are stroke-like events, focal motor seizures, headache, migraine, learning and behavioral problems, and mood disorders. Stroke-like events involve transient episodes of hemiparesis caused by focal seizures, ischemia, and vascular leakage from blood vessels.

Neuroimaging typically reveals unilateral hemispheric atrophy, leptomeningeal angiomatosis, and tram-track (gyriform) calcifications.[10] Aspirin at 3–5 mg/kg/day may reduce the frequency and also the severity of stroke-like episodes. Laser photocoagulation is used for treating port-wine stains. Topical medications and surgical procedures such as trabeculotomy or goniotomy are used for the management of glaucoma. For cases of drug-resistant epilepsy, surgical interventions such as hemispherectomy or resection of the epileptogenic focus may be performed.

VON HIPPEL–LINDAU SYNDROME

Von Hippel–Lindau syndrome is an autosomal dominant syndrome with multisystemic neoplasms and has an estimated incidence of 1 in 27,000–43,000 live births. The *VHL* gene that encodes the VHL protein (pVHL) is located on chromosome 3p35.[3] The lack of VHL protein results in tumorigenesis due to increased expression of platelet-derived growth factor (PDGF) peptide, vascular endothelial growth factor (VEGF), and transforming growth factor-alpha (TGF-α).

Von Hippel–Lindau syndrome is divided into two subtypes (type I and II) based on the absence and presence of pheochromocytomas, respectively.[2,4] The common tumors of VHL are central nervous system hemangioblastoma, retinal hemangioblastoma, pheochromocytoma, and renal clear cell carcinoma. Other tumors seen in VHL are endolymphatic sac tumors, paragangliomas, cystadenomas of the epididymis, and pancreatic neuroendocrine tumors (PNETs).

Plasma-free metanephrines are used for diagnosing pheochromocytomas.[9] CT and MRI of the brain and abdomen are used to assess lesions at various sites. Hearing assessment should be done as endolymphatic sac tumors can cause unilateral or bilateral hearing loss. Targeted therapies for advanced renal cell carcinoma in VHL are pazopanib, and belzutifan has been approved for renal cell carcinoma, CNS hemangioblastomas, and PNETs. Surgical removal is required for large tumors in VHL with adjuvant chemotherapy.

ATAXIA TELANGIECTASIA

Ataxia telangiectasia (Louis-Bar syndrome) is a chromosomal instability syndrome with autosomal recessive inheritance and has an estimated incidence of 1 in 40,000–100,000 live births. It is due to mutations in the *ATM* gene, a tumor-suppressor gene located in chromosome 11q22–23.[3] This results in a nonfunctional ATM protein that is involved in DNA repair, cellular response to ionizing radiation, oxidative damage, and immunoglobulin production. Unrepaired breaks in double-strand DNA elevate radiosensitivity and the likelihood of cancer.

The clinical spectrum of AT includes cerebellar ataxia, telangiectasias, heightened sensitivity to radiation, increased susceptibility to malignancies, immunodeficiencies, and recurrent respiratory infections.[2,4] Telangiectasias are frequently observed on the conjunctiva, brain, and bladder. Immunological changes in AT involve reduced levels of IgA and IgG, variable IgM, decreased total CD4 cell count, and elevated alpha-fetoprotein. Leukemia and lymphoma often manifest in early life, while solid tumors become more common in later stages of life.

No curative treatment is available at present. Avoidance of ionizing radiations, regular tumor surveillance, and periodic intravenous immunoglobulin (IVIg) infusions for immunodeficiency are recommended.

INVESTIGATIONS

The common cutaneous findings are shown in **Figures 8.5.1A to D**. Investigations should be individualized for specific syndromes:

- *Routine investigations:* Hemogram, renal and liver function tests
- *Dermatological examination*: Wood's lamp
- *Ophthalmological examination:* Slit-lamp examination, fundoscopy, visual acuity
- *Radiology:* X-rays of skull, chest, limbs, and spine
- Ultrasonogram of abdomen and pelvis
- Brainstem evoked response audiometry (BERA)
- 2D echocardiography
- MRI of abdomen and pelvis
- *Neuroimaging:* CT or MRI with contrast and PET of brain and/or spine
- Electroencephalogram
- Neurodevelopmental assessment

MANAGEMENT

Although neurocutaneous syndromes lack a cure, the management primarily revolves around managing symptoms and addressing accompanying comorbidities. Due to the complexity of managing affected children, comprehensive care is typically delivered by a multidisciplinary team

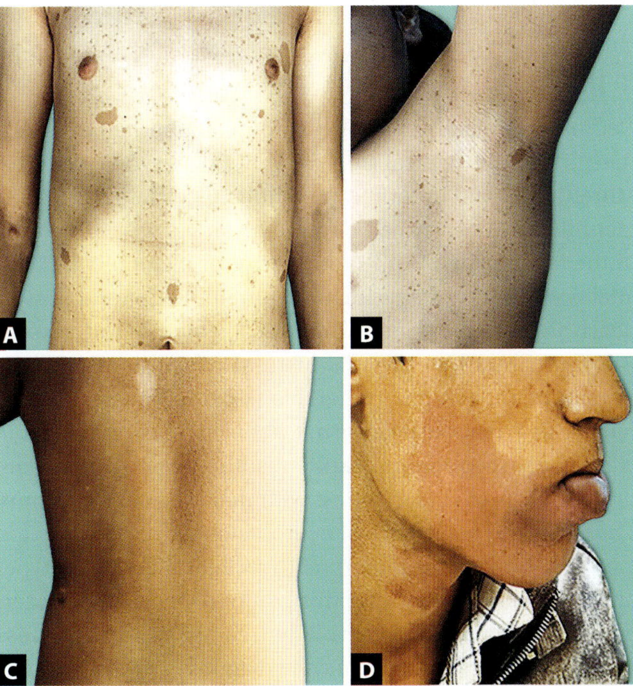

Figs. 8.5.1A to D: Café-au-lait macules over the (A) Body and (B) Axilla; (C) Hypomelanotic macules; (D) Hemangioma over face and neck.

comprising pediatric neurologist, ophthalmologist, surgical specialist, geneticist, dermatologist, physiotherapist, and occupational and speech therapist. Supportive treatment involves educating both children and parents, offering psychological and genetic counseling, and providing social support. Regular surveillance using neuroimaging is recommended to monitor the disease progression in all neurocutaneous syndromes.

REFERENCES

1. Kliegman RM, St. Geme III JW (Eds). Nelson Textbook of Pediatrics, 22nd edition. Amsterdam: Elsevier; 2022.
2. Klar N, Cohen B, Lin DDM. Neurocutaneous syndromes. Handb Clin Neurol. 2016;135:565-89.
3. Gürsoy S, Erçal D. Genetic evaluation of common neurocutaneous syndromes. Pediatr Neurol. 2018;89:3-10.
4. Kioutchoukova I, Foster D, Thakkar R, Ciesla C, Cabassa JS, Strouse J, et al. Neurocutaneous diseases: diagnosis, management, and treatment. J Clin Med. 2024;13(6):1648.
5. Legius E, Messiaen L, Wolkenstein P, Pancza P, Avery RA, Blakeley J, et al. Revised diagnostic criteria for neurofibromatosis type 1 and Legius syndrome: an international consensus recommendation. Genet Med. 2021;23(8):1506-13.
6. Plotkin SR, Messiaen L, Legius E, Pancza P, Avery RA, Blakeley JO, et al. Updated diagnostic criteria and nomenclature for neurofibromatosis type 2 and schwannomatosis: an international consensus recommendation. Genet Med. 2022;24(9):1967-77.
7. Northrup H, Aronow ME, Bebin EM, Bissler J, Darling TN, de Vries PJ, et al. Updated international tuberous sclerosis complex diagnostic criteria and surveillance and management recommendations. Pediatr Neurol. 2021;123:50-66.
8. de Vries PJ, Belousova E, Benedik MP, Carter T, Cottin V, Curatolo P, et al. TSC-associated neuropsychiatric disorders (TAND): findings from the TOSCA natural history study. Orphanet J Rare Dis. 2018;13(1):157.
9. Ullrich NJ. Neurocutaneous syndromes and brain tumors. J Child Neurol. 2016;31(12):1399-411.
10. Nandigam K, Mechtler LL, Smirniotopoulos JG. Neuroimaging of neurocutaneous diseases. Neurol Clin. 2014;32(1):159-92.

8.6 Neurometabolic Disorders

Sangeetha Yoganathan

INTRODUCTION

Neurometabolic disorders are a group of inherited disorders that affect the central and peripheral nervous systems. More than 1,400 inherited metabolic disorders have been identified and nearly half of these disorders were described in the last two decades.[1] Inborn error of metabolism (IEM) affects multiple systems including brain, peripheral nerves, heart, liver, kidney, lungs, blood cells, and blood vessels. Brain attributes to 25–30% of total oxygen and glucose consumption, and it is vulnerable to oxidative stress due to relative deficiency of defense mechanisms.[2] The human brain is highly susceptible to insults resulting from IEM. About three-fourths of IEM manifest with neurological symptoms. The estimated prevalence of neurometabolic disorders is 1 in 1,000 live births.[3] It is important to recognize the phenotypes and diagnostic methods for this group of inherited disorders as many of them are potentially treatable. Many of these neurometabolic disorders may be diagnosed in the neonatal period by newborn screening tests. Establishing a diagnosis of IEM helps to offer prenatal diagnosis to prevent subsequent affected live births.

CLASSIFICATION OF INBORN ERRORS OF METABOLISM

Defects of enzymes, proteins, receptors, or transporters involved in metabolic pathways result in IEM. Broadly, IEM may be classified into categories I and II.[4] Disorders under category I predominantly affect one functional system, such as the endocrine or immunological or a single anatomic system, such as intestine, renal tubules, or erythrocytes. The clinical symptoms of these disorders are uniform and are easy to diagnose. Category II disorders occur due to defects in the metabolic pathways common to many cells or organs or restricted to one organ but give rise to systemic manifestations. Category II disorders can be divided into:[4]

- *Group 1:* Disorders of metabolism affecting small molecules
- *Group 2:* Disorders involving energy metabolism
- *Group 3:* Disorders involving complex molecules

Group 1 Disorders

Group 1 disorders include intermediary metabolism affecting small molecules **(Box 8.6.1)** and there is an acute

BOX 8.6.1: Disorders of metabolism affecting small molecules.

- Amino acidopathies (e.g., phenylketonuria, maple syrup urine disease)
- Urea cycle disorders (e.g., *N*-acetyl glutamate synthetase deficiency, carbamoyl-phosphate synthetase I deficiency, ornithine transcarbamylase deficiency, argininosuccinic acid synthetase deficiency, arginase deficiency, argininosuccinic acid lyase deficiency)
- Organic acidurias (e.g., methylmalonic acidemia, propionic acidemia, isovaleric acidemia, glutaric acidemia type 1)
- Porphyrias
- Galactose and fructose metabolism defects
- Disorders involving the synthesis of amino acids (serine, asparagine, proline, glutamine)

or progressive intoxication due to accumulation of normal or unusual metabolites or compounds proximal to the block in the metabolic pathway.[4]

In addition to the disorders affecting small molecules, disorders of metal metabolism and neurotransmitter disorders are also categorized under group 1 disorders. The disorders of metal metabolism include accumulation of copper (Wilson disease) or deficiency of copper (Menkes disease), accumulation of iron (neurodegeneration with brain iron accumulation, hemochromatosis), and accumulation of manganese (*SLC30A10* or *SLC39A14* gene mutations) or deficiency of manganese (*SLC39A8* gene mutation). Neurotransmitter disorders result from defects in the synthesis, transport, release, or reuptake of neurotransmitters (e.g., monoamines, glycine, and gamma aminobutyric acid).

In children with group 1 disorders, the presentation is usually acute though few of these disorders may have a chronic progressive or nonprogressive course. Children with group 1 disorders such as amino acidopathies, organic aciduria, or urea cycle disorders may have a symptom-free period and the symptoms are usually precipitated by an intercurrent illness, fever, prolonged fasting, or inappropriate food intake.

Group 2 Disorders

Group 2 disorders involve primary energy metabolism, and these disorders occur due to the deficiency in energy production or utilization in the brain, muscle, heart, or other tissues.[4] Group 2 disorders may be classified into cytoplasmic energy defects **(Box 8.6.2)** and mitochondrial energy defects **(Box 8.6.3)**. Cytoplasmic energy defects are usually less severe and several of them are treatable, while mitochondrial energy defects are severe and generally partially treatable or not treatable.

Few of the mitochondrial energy defects are partially treatable and the mitochondrial energy defects are enlisted in **Box 8.6.3**.

BOX 8.6.2: Group 2 disorders—cytoplasmic energy defects.

- Disorders of glycolysis
- Disorders of glycogen metabolism and gluconeogenesis
- Glucose transporter defects
- Disorders of creatine metabolism (cerebral creatine deficiency syndrome)
- Disorders of pentose phosphate pathways
- Hyperinsulinism

BOX 8.6.3: Group 2 disorders—mitochondrial energy defects.

- *Aerobic glucose oxidation defects:* Congenital lactic acidemias (pyruvate transporter defect, pyruvate carboxylase deficiency, pyruvate dehydrogenase deficiency, Krebs cycle defects)
- Mitochondrial respiratory chain disorders
- Fatty acid oxidation defects and ketone body defects

BOX 8.6.4: Disorders involving complex molecules.

- Lysosomal storage disorders (defects in the catabolism of sphingolipids, mucopolysaccharides, and oligosaccharides)
- Carbohydrate-deficient glycoprotein (CDG) syndrome
- Peroxisomal disorders
- Purine and pyrimidine metabolism disorders
- Inborn errors of cholesterol and bile acid synthesis
- Inborn errors of intracellular triglycerides, phospholipids, and glycosphingolipids synthesis and remodeling

Group 3 Disorders

Disorders involving complex molecules are categorized under group 3 disorders and they result from the defect in synthesis, remodeling, recycling, intracellular trafficking, and catabolism of complex molecules. It involves one or more cellular organelles such as peroxisomes, lysosomes, endoplasmic reticulum, Golgi apparatus, and mitochondria.[4] Children with group 3 disorders usually manifest with a chronic progressive course without episodic decompensation following catabolic stress. The list of disorders involving defects in the metabolism of complex molecules is given in **Box 8.6.4**. Lysosomal storage disorders are one of the commonly encountered group 3 disorders in clinical practice and include sphingolipidosis, mucopolysaccharidosis, oligosaccharidosis, and neuronal ceroid lipofuscinoses. Sphingolipidosis includes GM1 gangliosidosis, GM2 gangliosidosis, Gaucher disease, Niemann-Pick disease, Farber disease, Fabry disease, Krabbe disease, and metachromatic leukodystrophy. Mucopolysaccharidosis encompasses Hurler syndrome (type I), Hunter syndrome (type II), Sanfilippo disease (type III), Morquio disease (type IV), Maroteaux-Lamy disease (type VI), Sly disease (type VII), and Natowicz disease (type IX). Oligosaccharidosis includes mannosidosis, fucosidosis, sialidosis, and aspartylglucosaminuria.

CLINICAL MANIFESTATIONS

The age at onset of symptoms is often variable depending upon the underlying etiology.

Fetal Period

A few of the metabolic disorders may have onset of symptoms in the intrauterine period and might result in major malformations, dysplasias, and functional signs. Major malformations in the affected fetus include skeletal malformations, cardiac anomalies, and neural tube defects. Dysplasias include cortical dysplasias, posterior fossa malformations, cortical cysts, liver cysts, and polycystic kidney disease. Functional signs in an affected fetus are hydrops fetalis, intrauterine growth restriction, visceromegaly, microcephaly, coarse facies, and facial dysmorphism.[5] The list of disorders that interfere with the embryofetal development is summarized in **Box 8.6.5**.

Neonatal and Early Infantile Period

Most disorders of intermediary metabolism affecting small molecules may manifest in the neonatal or early infantile period. The affected neonates usually become symptomatic after a symptom-free period of hours to weeks. The neonates and infants usually develop poor feeding, lethargy, vomiting, fast breathing, seizures, altered sensorium, hiccups, involuntary movements, hypothermia, and hypotonia. The neonates may have poor repertoire of symptoms and inherited metabolic disorders closely mimic sepsis, but these neonates deteriorate rapidly and do not respond to symptomatic therapy.[5] However, history of consanguinity, positive family history, abnormal urine odor, and negative sepsis screening test should alert the clinician to think of an underlying metabolic disorder.

Seizures refractory to antiseizure medications occur in pyridoxine-dependent epilepsy, folinic acid-responsive epilepsy, pyridox(am)ine-5-phosphate oxidase deficiency, biotinidase deficiency, serine biosynthesis defect, pyrimidine biosynthesis defects, and glucose 1 transporter deficiency. These disorders are potentially treatable, and early diagnosis and treatment often result in a better neurodevelopmental outcome. Other inherited metabolic disorders that manifest with refractory seizures in the neonatal or early infantile period are nonketotic hyperglycinemia, sulfite oxidase deficiency, Menkes disease, peroxisomal biogenesis defects, carbohydrate-deficient glycoprotein (CDG) disorders, and respiratory chain disorders. The latter group of disorders is only partially treatable or not treatable and the long-term neurodevelopmental outcome remains poor.

BOX 8.6.5: Disorders with onset of symptoms in the embryofetal period.

- Amino acid synthesis disorders (glutamine and asparagine synthetase deficiency)
- Glutaric aciduria type II
- Respiratory chain disorders
- Mitochondrial thiamine pyrophosphate carrier defect
- Manganese transporter defect
- Omega 2 fatty acid transporter defect
- Carbohydrate-deficient glycoprotein syndrome

Hepatomegaly without liver cell failure, hypoglycemia, and seizures occur in infants with glycogen storage disorders types I and III. Hepatomegaly with liver cell failure occurs in fructosemia, tyrosinemia, respiratory chain disorders, and transaldolase deficiency.

Neonates with disorders of energy metabolism may exhibit hypotonia, progressive neurological deterioration, malformations, and cardiac and hepatic involvement. Hypoglycemia and lactic acidosis may be observed.

Disorders of complex molecules rarely have onset of symptoms in the neonatal period with the exception of a few lysosomal storage disorders, peroxisomal biogenesis defects, and CDG disorders. They manifest with progressive neurological deterioration, seizures, facial dysmorphism, malformations, skeletal dysplasias, and visceromegaly.

Late Infantile and Early Juvenile Period (1–5 Years of Age)

Group 1 disorders, as discussed earlier, have acute episodic presentation characterized by encephalopathy, seizures, fast breathing, hypoglycemia, metabolic acidosis, hyperammonemia, or elevated lactate. The symptoms are precipitated by fasting, excessive protein intake, infection, stress, or surgical procedures. A few of the amino acidopathies such as classic homocystinuria and methylene tetrahydrofolate reductase deficiency may have a chronic progressive course. Neurotransmitter disorders manifest with unexplained developmental delay, tone abnormalities, dystonia with or without diurnal variation, oculogyric crisis, and behavioral and sleep disturbances. As neurotransmitter disorders may mimic dyskinetic cerebral palsy, the absence of a history of perinatal insult should alert the clinician to consider the possibility of neurotransmitter disorders.

Treatable cytoplasmic energy defects should be considered in children with unexplained developmental delays, behavioral symptoms, autistic features, and seizures. Magnetic resonance imaging (MRI) with spectroscopy reveals absent creatine peaks in patients with cerebral creatine deficiency syndromes. Mitochondrial energy defects may occur due to mutations in nuclear genes or mitochondrial genes. These disorders have a myriad of presentations ranging from acute encephalopathy, intellectual disability, status epilepticus, stroke, movement disorders, myopathy, and neuropathy with or without systemic involvement.

Many of the complex molecule disorders typically have onset of symptoms in the late infantile or early juvenile period. The usual presentations in disorders predominantly involving white matter in this age group are developmental delay, regression of motor skills, hypotonia, progressive spasticity, and ataxia with or without peripheral neuropathy. On the contrary, gray matter disorders manifest with psychomotor retardation, regression of cognitive skills, vision impairment, refractory seizures, and movement disorders.

Late Childhood and Adolescence (5–15 Years of Age)

Children and adolescents with neurometabolic disorders manifest with a constellation of neurological and systemic symptoms, such as psychomotor retardation, psychiatric manifestations, behavioral disturbances, seizures, spasticity, extrapyramidal symptoms (dystonia, chorea, and athetosis), cerebellar symptoms, peripheral neuropathy, skeletal dysplasias, and organomegaly, depending upon the underlying etiology.

CLINICAL EXAMINATION

As the symptoms and signs of neurometabolic disorders are diverse, a systematic clinical and laboratory approach is needed to establish an early diagnosis. The following key points are to be analyzed to arrive at a clinical diagnosis:[6]

- Positive family history/consanguinity/pattern of inheritance
- Age at onset of symptoms
- Course of illness (acute episodic, chronic progressive, nonprogressive)
- Precipitating factors
- Sites of neuroaxis involvement (cerebral cortex, pyramidal, extrapyramidal, cerebellar, cord involvement, peripheral neuropathy, myopathy)
- Systemic involvement (hepatic, cardiac, skeletal, renal)

The constellation of clinical symptoms and signs helps to narrow down the list of differentials. The head-to-toe findings that need to be focused on the general examination are summarized in **Table 8.6.1**. Most metabolic disorders have an autosomal recessive inheritance, while few metabolic disorders have autosomal dominant, X-linked, or mitochondrial inheritance.

A systematic neurological examination helps to identify the anatomical sites of neuroaxis involvement and pattern recognition. Neurologic findings in IEM are encephalopathic crisis, developmental delay, regression of milestones, behavioral disturbances, psychiatric disturbances, epilepsy, ocular movement abnormalities, vision impairment, hearing loss, hypotonia/myopathy, spasticity, ataxia, dystonia, choreoathetosis, neuropathy, stroke, and neuroimaging abnormalities involving one or more sites such as cerebrum, white matter, basal ganglia, cerebellum, cysts/dysgenesis, or mixed are observed.[7] An overlap of these symptoms and signs is not an uncommon finding in children with untreated neurometabolic disorders at a later stage.

TABLE 8.6.1: Head-to-toe clinical findings in children with neurometabolic disorders.[6]

Diagnostic clues	*Possible neurometabolic disorders*
Coarse facies	Mucopolysaccharidoses, mannosidosis, mucolipidosis, GM1 gangliosidosis, fucosidosis
Facial dysmorphism	Peroxisomal biogenesis defect
Marfanoid habitus, arachnodactyly	Classic homocystinuria
Flexural dermatitis, seborrheic dermatitis, sparse scalp hair	Biotinidase deficiency
Hypopigmented sparse scalp hair, fair skin complexion, kinky hair, joint hyperlaxity	Menkes disease
Persistent Mongolian spots	GM1 gangliosidosis
Ichthyosis	Refsum disease, Sjogren–Larsson syndrome
Angiokeratomas	Fabry disease
Diffuse skin hyperpigmentation, hyperpigmentation of oral mucosa	Adrenoleukodystrophy
Hypertrichosis	Mitochondrial disorders
Macrocephaly	Glutaric aciduria type I, l-hydroxy glutaric aciduria, GM2 gangliosidosis, Canavan disease, Alexander disease
Microcephaly	• Most neurometabolic disorders • Krabbe disease, neuronal ceroid lipofuscinoses
Eye examination findings:	
• Keyser–Fleischer ring	• Wilson disease
• External ophthalmoparesis	• Mitochondrial disorders
• Corneal clouding	• Mucopolysaccharidosis
• Cataract	• Wilson disease, galactosemia, mitochondrial disorders
• Lens dislocation	• Sulfite oxidase deficiency, molybdenum cofactor deficiency, homocystinuria
• Pigmentary retinopathy	• Neuronal ceroid lipofuscinoses, mitochondrial disorders, peroxisomal biogenesis disorders
• Cherry red spot	• GM2 gangliosidosis, metachromatic leukodystrophy, sialidosis, Niemann–Pick disease
Hepatomegaly ± splenomegaly	• Glycogen storage disorder • Gaucher disease • Niemann–Pick disease • Mucolipidosis • Mannosidosis

INVESTIGATIONS

A structured diagnostic approach is needed to plan appropriate investigations to establish an early diagnosis. The basic investigations for the diagnosis of IEM include complete blood count; estimation of blood glucose, electrolytes, lactate, arterial blood gas, ammonia, and ketosis (GELAK); renal function tests; liver function tests; and estimation of uric acid, homocysteine, creatine phosphokinase (CPK), fasting lipid profile, and serum copper levels.[8] Urine analysis includes the examination of color, odor, and urine multistix tests. Urine odor abnormalities are listed in **Table 8.6.2.**[8]

Advanced testing includes tandem mass spectrometry, serum amino acids levels estimation by high-performance liquid chromatography (HPLC), urine organic acid analysis by gas chromatography–mass spectrometry (GC–MS), enzyme assays, urine screening tests for porphyria, mucopolysaccharides and oligosaccharides, and estimation of serum copper and ceruloplasmin.[8] Neuroimaging including brain MRI with magnetic resonance spectroscopy (MRS) plays a key role in the pattern recognition and diagnosis of many of these neurometabolic disorders. Brain MRI acquisition should include diffusion-weighted images (DWI) and apparent diffusion coefficient (ADC) images. MRI spine screening will be needed in children with few neurometabolic disorders to look for the other sites of neuroaxis involvement.

A tier-based approach has been created recently to diagnose all treatable metabolic disorders in clinical practice. The first-tier investigations are easily accessible and affordable and have the potential to diagnose 60% of all treatable IEMs.[7] The second-tier investigations are planned based on the identification of specific clinical signs and symptoms of the patient. The tier-based approach to diagnose neurometabolic disorders is summarized in **Table 8.6.3**. Normal blood and urine biochemistry test reports may be obtained if done during the interim period of normalcy in children with IEM. This is one of the major pitfalls of biochemical testing, and repeat testing during acute metabolic crisis may improve the yield of testing.

TABLE 8.6.2: Urine odor abnormalities in children with neurometabolic disorders.

Neurometabolic disorder	*Urine odor*
Phenylketonuria	Musty or mousy odor due to phenylacetic acid
Maple syrup urine disease	Burnt sugar odor due to 2-oxoisocaproic acid
• Tyrosinemia • Hypermethioninemia	Boiled cabbage odor due to 2-hydroxybutyric acid, 2-keto-4-methiolbutryric acid
Multiple carboxylase deficiency	Tom cat urine odor due to 3-hydroxyisovaleric acid
Isovaleric acidemia, glutaric acidemia type II	Sweaty feet odor due to isovaleric acid

Other investigations such as electrocardiography (ECG), echocardiography, and ultrasound abdomen and pelvis are used in children with inherited metabolic disorders with systemic involvement. Electroencephalography (EEG) has to be considered in all children with suspected IEM and seizures. A detailed ophthalmology assessment should be considered in the evaluation of all children with neurometabolic disorders. Nerve conduction studies and electromyography are recommended in the evaluation of children with metabolic myopathies or neuropathies. Visual evoked potential (VEP) and brainstem auditory evoked responses (BAER) must be included in the evaluation of children with neurometabolic disorders to identify vision or hearing disturbances.

The recent advances in genetic testing have facilitated a rapid diagnosis of neurometabolic disorders in children. Whole exome sequencing helps in the confirmation of the diagnosis of monogenic inherited neurometabolic disorders. Mitochondrial disorders are caused by mutations in the nuclear or mitochondrial genes. Nuclear gene-mediated mitochondrial disorders can be diagnosed by whole exome sequencing, while mitochondrial gene mutations can be identified only by mitochondrial genome sequencing.

MANAGEMENT

Group 1 Disorders

Ensure airway, breathing, and circulation in an acutely ill child. The emergent measures are to be initiated to decrease the production and facilitate the excretion of toxic metabolites. Maintain adequate hydration and good urine output. Reverse the catabolic state as early as possible and

TABLE 8.6.3: Tier-based approach for diagnosis of treatable metabolic disorders.[7]

Tier-1 investigations	*Tier-2 investigations*
Blood investigations: • Ammonia • Lactate • Homocysteine • Plasma amino acid • Acylcarnitine profile • Copper • Ceruloplasmin *Urine investigations:* • Organic acids • Creatine metabolites (Guanidinoacetate, creatine: Creatinine ratio) • Oligosaccharides • Mucopolysaccharides • Pyrimidines • Purines	• Plasma vitamin B_{12}, folate • CSF/plasma glucose ratio • Blood and CSF lactate/pyruvate ratio • CSF amino acids • CSF neurotransmitters • Plasma cholesterol • Plasma 7-dehydrocholesterol: cholesterol ratio • Plasma very long chain fatty acids • Plasma pipecolic acid • Urine AASA • Blood manganese • Urine deoxypyridinoline • Measurement of CoQ • Molecular studies (genetic testing)

(AASA: α-Aminoadipic semialdehyde; CoQ: coenzyme Q; CSF: cerebrospinal fluid)

maintain euglycemia. Remove and treat the precipitating factors such as infections and exposure to a high protein diet. Acidosis may be corrected by the administration of bicarbonate. High-calorie and protein-restricted diet should be initiated to provide 100 kcal/kg/day.[7] If gastric intolerance is observed, parenteral nutrition should be considered initially, with a switch to enteral nutrition as soon as possible.

Special formula preparations are available for specific amino acidopathies, organic aciduria, and urea cycle disorders. Hyperammonemia may be managed with the administration of a protein-restricted diet, sodium benzoate, or sodium phenylbutyrate. Children with urea cycle disorders need long-term administration of L-citrulline, L-arginine, or *N*-carbamylglutamate depending on the defect in the biochemical pathway. Arginine has to be restricted in children with arginase deficiency. Peritoneal dialysis and hemodialysis are to be considered in children with refractory metabolic acidosis and hyperammonemia. Supplementation of cofactors is an important step in the management of amino acidopathies. Carnitine should be initiated in all children with organic acidurias. Liver transplantation may be considered in children with urea cycle disorders and few organic acidemias.

Vitamin-responsive neurological disorders include pyridoxine-dependent epilepsy, folinic acid-responsive epilepsy, biotinidase deficiency, biotin thiamine-responsive basal ganglia disease, hereditary folate malabsorption, and riboflavinopathies. Children with suspected neurotransmitter disorders should be given a therapeutic trial with the administration of oral levodopa and carbidopa to exclude dopa-responsive dystonias. Other treatment options in children with neurotransmitter disorders are supplementation of folinic acid, trihexyphenidyl, dopa agonists, and monoamine oxidase (MAO) inhibitors.

Wilson disease may be treated with copper-restricted diet and administration of chelators such as D-penicillamine or triethylenetetramine.[4] The treatment of Menkes disease includes subcutaneous administration of copper histidine injections. Children with manganese transporter defects are treated with manganese-restricted diet and intravenous administration of calcium disodium ethylenediaminetetraacetic acid (EDTA).

Group 2 Disorders

Glycogen storage disorders are managed with frequent feeding, avoidance of fasting, and administration of uncooked cornstarch to maintain euglycemia. Liver transplantation remains an option in children with glycogen storage disorders. Children with glucose transporter defects are managed with ketogenic diet, carnitine supplementation, and avoidance of valproate. Cerebral creatine deficiency syndromes (CCDS) are managed with the administration of creatine monohydrate. Depending on the enzyme defects, supplementation or restriction of arginine, supplementation of ornithine and glycine has to be decided. Mitochondrial disorders are managed with avoidance of mitochondrial toxic drugs and administration of vitamins and cofactors cocktail including carnitine, thiamine, riboflavin, coenzyme Q10, vitamin C, folinic acid, and vitamin E.

Group 3 Disorders

Hematopoietic stem cell transplantation can be considered in selected patients with adrenoleukodystrophy, metachromatic leukodystrophy, and Krabbe disease. Enzyme replacement therapy is an option in neuronal ceroid lipofuscinoses, mucopolysaccharidosis, Pompe disease, Fabry disease, and Gaucher disease. Pharmacological chaperones have been tried in children with Gaucher disease.[6] Gene therapy seems to be evolving as a potentially promising treatment option in few of the neurometabolic disorders.

Multidisciplinary team care, comprising pediatrician, pediatric neurologist, neuroradiologist, geneticist, physical therapist, and dietitian, plays a key role in the management of children with neurometabolic disorders. In addition to the targeted treatment in each of these neurometabolic disorders, other medications such as antiseizure medications, antispasticity drugs, and antidystonic medications are administered to manage seizures, spasticity, and movement disorders. A structured clinical evaluation, diagnostic tests, and tailored therapeutic modalities will facilitate early diagnosis and management and reduce the morbidity and mortality in these children. Prenatal diagnostic tests should be offered in families with previously affected children not only to prevent subsequent births with neurodegenerative disorders but also to facilitate early diagnosis and management of treatable neurometabolic disorders. Also, nationwide policies should be considered to include extended newborn screening tests as mandatory in both public and private hospitals.

CONCLUSION

Neurometabolic disorders may have overlapping clinical symptoms and hence, establishing an accurate clinical diagnosis may be challenging. However, meticulous history taking, and careful clinical examination combined with the utility of appropriate laboratory diagnostic methods and inclusion of newborn screening tests will improve the ability of clinicians to establish an early diagnosis and initiate timely management. Timely therapeutic interventions will improve the long-term neurodevelopmental outcomes in children with neurometabolic disorders.

REFERENCES

1. Tabarki B, Ortigoza-Escobar JD, Lee WT, Alfadhel M. Editorial: pediatric neurometabolic disorders. Front Neurol. 2021;12:737398.

2. Panagariya A, Agarwal V. Neurometabolic disorders. Indian J Clin Biochem. 2007;22:1-2.
3. Karimzadeh P, Ghofrani M, Nasiri S. Approach to patients with neurometabolic diseases who show characteristic signs and symptoms. Iran J Child Neurol. 2020;14:19-32.
4. Saudubray JM, Sedel F, Walter JH. Clinical approach to treatable inborn metabolic diseases: an introduction. J Inherit Metab Dis. 2006;29:261-74.
5. Saudubray JM, Garcia-Cazorla À. Inborn errors of metabolism overview: pathophysiology, manifestations, evaluation, and management. Pediatr Clin North Am. 2018;65:179-208.
6. Bindu PS, Tally AB. Pediatric neurology neurometabolic disorders: a diagnostic approach. Indian J Pract Pediatr. 2016;18:158-70.
7. van Karnebeek CD, Shevell M, Zschocke J, Moeschler JB, Stockler S. The metabolic evaluation of the child with an intellectual developmental disorder: diagnostic algorithm for identification of treatable causes and new digital resource. Mol Genet Metab. 2014;111:428-38.
8. Bijarnia-Mahay S, Kapoor S. Testing modalities for inborn errors of metabolism – what a clinician needs to know? Indian Pediatr. 2019;56:757-66.

8.7 Seizures, Epilepsy, and Nonepileptic Events

Lakshminarayanan Kannan, Puneet Jain

INTRODUCTION

Epilepsy is one of the most prevalent chronic neurological disorders in childhood, and it denotes an endurable propensity to have chronic and repeated unprovoked seizures. In patients with epilepsy, recurrent seizures are the primary concern and, in many instances, the only symptom. Seizures manifest when there are abnormally excessive and synchronized neuronal discharges that occur due to any reason. Depending on the anatomical site of onset and its spread in the brain regions, the ensuing manifestations vary in seizures. Thus, childhood epilepsy has a diverse spectrum of clinical manifestations, from subtle to overt. However, many neurological and other conditions may mimic epilepsy. Thus, the diagnosis of epilepsy is clinical, and the same may not be straightforward in many instances.

EPIDEMIOLOGY

Epilepsy affects approximately 50–70 million individuals worldwide, with a significant burden falling on low- and middle-income countries. Estimates suggest that around 80% of patients with epilepsy reside in developing nations. Several factors contribute to this disparity, including a higher incidence of perinatal complications, limited access to quality healthcare services in rural areas, a high incidence of central nervous system (CNS) infections such as neurocysticercosis, traumatic brain injuries, and a lack of awareness leading to delayed diagnosis and treatment. The incidence of epilepsy follows a bimodal distribution, with peaks occurring during childhood (typically between 5 and 9 years of age) and in the elderly population.

DEFINITION

As per the International League Against Epilepsy (ILAE) 2005 definition, an epileptic seizure is a transient occurrence of signs and/or symptoms due to abnormal excessive or synchronous neuronal activity in the brain. Operationally, these signs or symptoms may include sudden and transitory abnormal phenomena such as alterations of consciousness, or involuntary motor, sensory, autonomic, or psychic events perceived by the patient or an observer.

CLASSIFICATION

A critical first step in the diagnosis of epilepsy is to differentiate between seizures and seizure mimics. This distinction is done clinically by way of a detailed history of reported symptoms by the patients and first-hand witnesses. As epilepsy is not a single disease, the precise diagnosis of the seizure type, epilepsy type, and epilepsy syndrome guides the individualization of the precision treatments.

Seizure Type

A comprehensive clinical history is essential for distinguishing epileptic seizures from seizure mimics. It is crucial to gather detailed information when a paroxysmal event is witnessed, including the time, duration, frequency, seizure triggers, aura, initial signs, sequential progression, and postictal manifestations. Caregivers or healthcare providers may simulate common seizure types to assist in event descriptions, and home videos, if available, can provide valuable insight. A structured approach for documenting seizure history is outlined in **Box 8.7.1**.

BOX 8.7.1: Sample history-taking for description of a suspected seizure.

- Age at first seizure:
- History of status epilepticus: Yes/no (if yes, details)
- Longest seizure-free interval:
- Triggers (if any): Usual triggers—fever, missed dose of medicine, sleep deprivation
- Frequency (e.g., daily/weekly/monthly):
- Duration (seconds/minutes):
- Timing (specific time of day, awake or asleep):
- Detailed description of the seizure phenomenology
  - Aura:
  - Ictus:
  - Postictal:
- Review home video (if available) to corroborate the seizure description
- Evolves to bilateral tonic–clonic seizure: Yes/no
- Last episode:
- Current medications:
- Past medications:

Epilepsy Type

Once nonepileptic events have been reasonably ruled out, the next step is to categorize the seizure as either "focal onset" or "generalized onset" based on the initial manifestations during the seizure episodes.[1] Focal seizures originate in a localized site or neural network in the brain before spreading to other regions, whereas generalized seizures simultaneously engage bilateral widespread neural networks. Focal seizures may exhibit a sequence of symptoms, and they can later progress to involve both hemispheres, termed focal to bilateral tonic–clonic seizures.

Epilepsy Syndrome

Epilepsy syndrome is a distinctive disorder defined by characteristic seizure types, typical age at onset and remission, comorbidities, characteristic electroencephalography (EEG) features, and neuroimaging findings. Epilepsy syndromes are usually heterogeneous concerning etiology. The diagnosis of epilepsy syndrome usually has therapeutic and prognostic implications.[2] Common epilepsy syndromes have been summarized in **Table 8.7.1**.

FIRST UNPROVOKED SEIZURE

Unprovoked seizures are characterized by their occurrence without a discernible underlying clinical condition or beyond the expected timeframe for acute symptomatic seizures. Typically, multiple seizures within 24 hours are regarded as a single-seizure event. These unprovoked seizures differ from acute symptomatic seizures in terms of their risk of recurrence and mortality across various etiologies. The incidence of single unprovoked seizures ranges from 23 to 61 per 100,000 person-years, with a higher prevalence observed in infants under the age of 1 year. Approximately 10–12% of children experiencing their first unprovoked seizure will have a seizure lasting >30 minutes [status epilepticus (SE)]. A structured approach to managing a child with a first unprovoked seizure is depicted in **Flowchart 8.7.1**.

Electroencephalography and neuroimaging play a pivotal role to evaluate the risk of recurrence and determine the need for treatment. In general, the risk of seizure recurrence at 2 years after one unprovoked seizure is around 42%, escalating to 70–80% with two or more unprovoked seizures. This risk tends to be higher in cases of "remote symptomatic" etiology (e.g., prior underlying brain lesion or insult), the presence of global developmental delay/intellectual disability, focal neurological deficits, focal seizures, and seizures occurring during sleep.

On the other hand, provoked seizures, also known as acute symptomatic seizures, occur either during or shortly after a systemic insult or documented brain injury. Common scenarios include seizures within 1 week of events such as stroke, traumatic brain injury, ischemia–hypoxia, or intracranial surgery. They may also manifest at the time of first identification of subdural hemorrhage, during active CNS infections, in conjunction with autoimmune diseases such as multiple sclerosis, during episodes of severe metabolic derangement, drug or alcohol intoxication and withdrawal, or following exposure to known epileptogenic drugs. Hyponatremia, hypocalcemia, and hypoglycemia are the common metabolic derangements that can cause seizures.

FEBRILE SEIZURES

Febrile seizures are the most common provoked seizures in children under the age of 5 years, occurring in approximately 2–5% of all children within this age group. These seizures typically occur in response to a febrile illness, characterized by a body temperature of 100.4°F or 38°C or higher. The American Academy of Pediatrics (AAP) sets the lower cutoff age for febrile seizures at 6 months, excluding neonatal seizures and unprovoked seizures from the criteria. Febrile seizures are distinct from other acute symptomatic seizures and are further classified into simple and complex febrile seizures.

Simple febrile seizures involve generalized seizures with or without convulsions lasting <15 minutes and occurring only once within 24 hours. Sudden unresponsiveness with up-rolled eyes, with or without stiffening of the body and limbs, is a common manifestation. On the other hand, complex febrile seizures are prolonged (lasting >15 minutes), exhibit focal manifestations during seizures or cause postictal focal deficits, and may recur within 24 hours of the first

TABLE 8.7.1: International League Against Epilepsy (ILAE) "three-tier" approach to classification of seizures and epilepsies.

Seizure types						
Focal onset (aware or impaired awareness)		***Generalized onset***		***Unknown onset***		
Motor onset	***Nonmotor onset***	***Motor onset***	***Nonmotor onset***	***Motor onset***	***Nonmotor onset***	
• Automatisms • Tonic • Clonic • Epileptic spasms • Hyperkinetic • Myoclonic • Tonic	• Autonomic • Behavioral arrest • Cognitive • Emotional • Sensory	• Tonic–clonic • Clonic • Tonic • Myoclonic • Myoclonic–tonic–clonic • Myoclonic–atonic • Atonic • Epileptic spasms	• Typical • Atypical • Myoclonic • Eyelid myoclonia	• Tonic–clonic • Epileptic spasms	Behavioral arrest	
Epilepsy types						
Focal	***Generalized***		***Combined generalized and focal***		***Unknown***	
Epilepsy syndromes						
Neonatal/infantile	***Childhood***		***Adolescent/adult***		***Any age***	***Comorbidities***
• Self-limited familial neonatal epilepsy • Early infantile-developmental/epileptic • Encephalopathy • Epilepsy of infancy with migrating focal seizures • Infantile epileptic spasm syndrome • Myoclonic epilepsy in infancy • Self-limited familial infantile epilepsy • Dravet syndrome • Genetic epilepsy with febrile seizure plus (GEFS+)	• Self-limited epilepsy with centrotemporal spikes (SeLECTS) • Atypical childhood epilepsy with centrotemporal spikes • Self-limited epilepsy with autonomic seizures (SeLEAS) • Childhood occipital visual epilepsy (COVE) • Epileptic encephalopathy with spike wave activation in sleep • Landau–Kleffner syndrome (LKS) • Childhood absence epilepsy (CAE) • Epilepsy with myoclonic absences • Epilepsy with myoclonic atonic seizures • Sleep-related hypermotor epilepsy (SHE) • Lennox–Gastaut syndrome		• Juvenile absence epilepsy (JAE) • Juvenile myoclonic epilepsy (JME) • Epilepsy with generalized tonic–clonic seizures alone • Autosomal dominant epilepsy with auditory features (ADEAF) • Other familial temporal lobe epilepsies		• Familial focal epilepsy with variable foci • Reflex epilepsies • Progressive myoclonic epilepsies	
Etiology						
Structural	Genetic	Infectious	Metabolic	Immune	Unknown	

episode. The peak incidence of febrile seizures is typically observed around 18 months of age, with over 80% occurring before the age of 3 years.

Various viral and bacterial infections, including human herpesvirus type 6 (HHV-6), have been associated with febrile seizures, as well as certain vaccinations such as mumps–measles–rubella (MMR), diphtheria–pertussis–tetanus (DPT), influenza, and pneumococcal vaccines. Genetic epilepsy with febrile seizure plus (GEFS+) is a syndrome characterized by febrile seizures and other seizure types, including focal and generalized seizures. Major genes associated with GEFS+ include *SCN1A*, *GABRG2*, and *SCN1B*. Dravet syndrome, which involves mutations in the *SCN1A* gene, may also present with a history of febrile seizures, particularly if the onset of febrile seizures is before 7 months of age.

Management of febrile seizures involves acute measures, as outlined in **Box 8.7.2**. Most children with febrile seizures have a favorable prognosis, but there is a risk of recurrence (17–42%) and a risk of future epilepsy (2–8%). Certain factors increase the risk of recurrent febrile seizures, including age younger than 18 months, fever duration <1 hour before seizure onset, and a family history of febrile seizures. Conversely, risk factors for future epilepsy include age over 3 years at the time

Flowchart 8.7.1: An approach to the management of a child with a first unprovoked seizure.

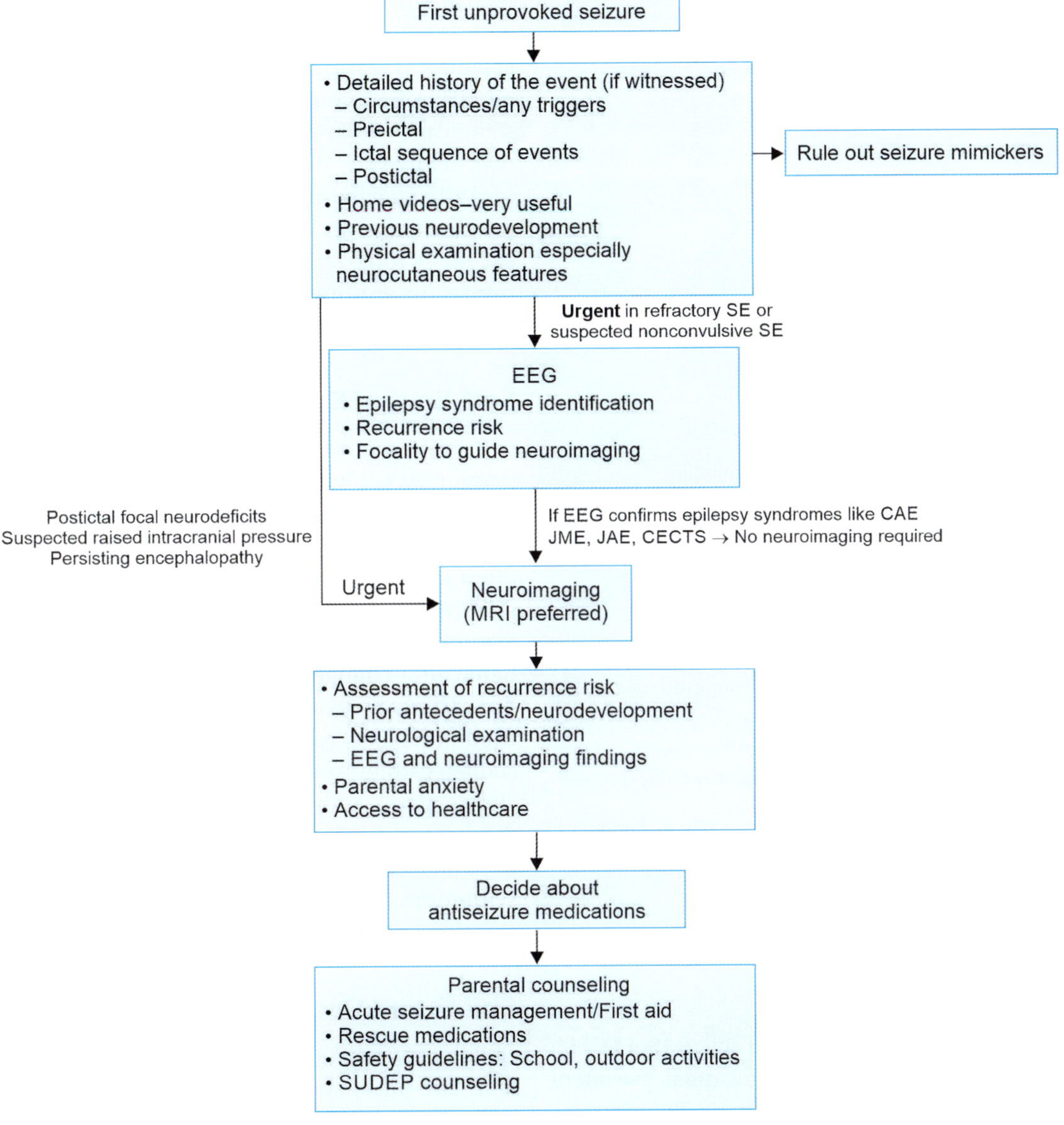

(CAE: childhood absence epilepsy; CECTS: childhood epilepsy with centrotemporal spikes; EEG: electroencephalography; JAE: juvenile absence epilepsy; JME: juvenile myoclonic epilepsy; MRI: magnetic resonance imaging; SE: status epilepticus; SUDEP: sudden unexpected death in epilepsy)

of the first febrile seizure, complex febrile seizures, multiple febrile seizure episodes, and underlying neurodevelopmental abnormalities.

Intermittent clobazam prophylaxis is not to be used routinely in all patients. This is reserved for children with frequent recurrent febrile seizures, recurrent febrile SE, significant parental anxiety, and limited access to healthcare. However, it is important to note that fever may not always be recognized before a febrile seizure, and recurrence can still occur despite prophylaxis.

SELF-LIMITED CHILDHOOD FOCAL EPILEPSIES

Self-limited childhood focal epilepsies (previously called benign focal epilepsies) are the most prevalent epilepsies encountered in childhood, including in children with neurodevelopmental disabilities. They are characterized by age-related pharmacoresponsive focal seizures (usually nocturnal), sleep-activated focal epileptiform abnormalities on EEG, and spontaneous resolution with age.[3]

BOX 8.7.2: Management of FS.

- Most FS are self-limited and end before patients reach the hospital
- If seizure is ongoing → follow institutional SE protocol
- Focus on acute stabilization (airway, breathing, circulation, etc.) of the child
- History and examination
  - Focus of infection
  - Recent immunization/immunization status
  - Past history of febrile or afebrile seizures
  - Birth history, neurodevelopment
  - Prior antibiotic use
  - Daycare attendance
  - Family history of FS/epilepsy
- *Examination:* Signs of meningitis, persisting encephalopathy, focal deficits
- Individualize investigations
- Infection workup
- *Lumbar puncture, indicated if:**
  - History/exam suggests the presence of meningitis
  - Patient pretreated with antibiotics
  - In infants between 6 and 12 months of age, if the immunization (Hib or pneumococcal) is deficient or unknown
  - Focal neurological findings
- *Neuroimaging, indicted if:*
  - Abnormal neurological examination
  - First episode of febrile SE
- *EEG:* Only indicated if epilepsy or fever-triggered seizure is suspected
- Treatment of fever and infection, as appropriate

*Local meningitis rates and immunization coverage may guide the need for lumbar puncture.
(EEG: electroencephalography; FS: febrile seizures; Hib: haemophilus influenzae type b; SE: status epilepticus)

Self-limited Epilepsy with Centrotemporal Spikes

Self-limited epilepsy with centrotemporal spikes (SeLECTS), also known as Rolandic epilepsy, is the most prevalent age-related focal epilepsy in childhood, typically occurring between 5 and 10 years of age. Seizures are characterized by their infrequent incidence, with approximately 15% of children encountering just one seizure, and their short duration, although they may progress to bilateral tonic–clonic seizures in certain instances, often occurring during sleep. Rolandic seizures are characterized by hemifacial clonic movements, laryngeal symptoms, speech interruption, swallowing/chewing automatisms, and excessive salivation. While most children with SeLECTS demonstrate typical development, some may encounter challenges affecting language and executive functioning. EEG typically exhibits classical sleep-induced bilateral (or unilateral) centrotemporal spikes with their characteristic polarity. Neuroimaging is generally deemed unnecessary for classical presentations.

Children presenting with the first or second episode of typical Rolandic seizure of SeLECTS are usually not treated with medications as these are infrequent nocturnal sleep seizures. Treatment is required only for those children enduring frequent, prolonged, or daytime seizures or with significant scholastic worsening and behavior abnormalities due to epilepsy. Preferred antiseizure medications (ASMs) include carbamazepine, oxcarbazepine, valproate, levetiracetam, and clobazam. Patients with SeLECTS show excellent long-term prognosis with spontaneous seizure remission around the age of puberty, irrespective of the treatment received.

Self-limited Epilepsy with Autonomic Seizures

Self-limited epilepsy with autonomic seizures (SeLEAS), previously known as Panayiotopoulos syndrome, typically presents between 3 and 6 years of age, though onset can range from 1 to 14 years. Seizures are infrequent but often prolonged, with two-thirds of children experiencing seizures during sleep. They are characterized by autonomic features, including vomiting, sweating, and pallor, along with behavioral changes, eye deviation, or "strange" coughing. Approximately two-thirds of patients exhibit the full emetic triad of nausea, retching, and vomiting. Ictal syncope and sudden cardiorespiratory arrest may also occur. EEG typically shows sleep-activated stereotypic occipital spike-wave discharges. Carbamazepine and valproate are commonly used medications, though carbamazepine may rarely worsen symptoms. The prognosis is excellent, with most children achieving complete seizure remission within a few years.

Childhood Occipital Visual Epilepsy

Childhood occipital visual epilepsy (COVE), formerly referred to as late-onset childhood occipital epilepsy (Gastaut type), typically manifests around 8 years of age, with onset ranging from 3 to 15 years. Approximately 20% of patients may have a family history of migraine. Seizures are predominantly diurnal, frequent but brief, and often commence with visual symptoms such as elementary or formed visual hallucinations, transient amaurosis, or visual illusions. These may be followed by hemisensory or motor signs, or unresponsiveness. Postictal symptoms may mimic migraine, with severe headache, nausea, or vomiting. EEG typically reveals bilateral occipital spike/sharp waves, activated by sleep and eye-closed states, with characteristic fixation-off sensitivity and photosensitivity. Seizures are generally responsive to pharmacotherapy, with a favorable prognosis, as more than half of patients achieve remission within 2–4 years of onset.

GENETIC (IDIOPATHIC) GENERALIZED EPILEPSIES

Genetic generalized epilepsy (GGE) as a group is one of the common epilepsy syndromes encountered in childhood. GGEs represent a cluster of epilepsy syndromes characterized by normal neurodevelopment, the presence of generalized seizures such as absences, generalized tonic–clonic seizures (GTCS), or myoclonus, typically responsive to medication(s), normal neurological examination, characteristic EEG pattern, normal brain imaging findings, and a favorable long-term prognosis.[3] However, subtle behavioral abnormalities such as inattention, hyperactivity, or learning disabilities may be observed. The definitive diagnosis of GGEs heavily relies on EEG findings, with neuroimaging generally deemed unnecessary if clinical and EEG features suggest GGEs. Though the terminology suggests "genetic" etiology, routine genetic testing is not warranted in typical GGE cases. Most patients do not have a monogenetic cause, and polygenic inheritance is the underlying mechanism in most. Some common GGEs are detailed in the following text.

Childhood Absence Epilepsy

Childhood absence epilepsy (CAE) usually manifests between the ages of 4 and 12 years, with multiple daily episodes of brief staring spells or behavioral arrest.[4] These episodes are often accompanied by subtle twitching of the eyelids or face and hand automatisms. Other seizure types are infrequent, and EEG typically reveals characteristic 3 Hz generalized spike-wave discharges, often triggered by hyperventilation. Patients with CAE are typically responsive to treatment. Ethosuximide is the drug of choice for CAE. Sodium valproate and lamotrigine are other alternatives.

Juvenile Absence Epilepsy

Juvenile absence epilepsy (JAE) is similar to CAE, but onset occurs between ages 8 and 20 years. Besides absence seizures, patients may also experience myoclonic seizures and GTCS. EEG findings are typically diagnostic and show generalized 3–3.5 Hz polyspike-wave discharges. While most cases are responsive to medication(s) and remit over time, some patients may require long-term treatment to mitigate the risk of GTCS. The drugs of first choice for the treatment include sodium valproate in boys and levetiracetam in girls.

Juvenile Myoclonic Epilepsy

Juvenile myoclonic epilepsy (JME) presents between ages 8 and 25 years with myoclonic jerks upon waking, GTCS, and absence seizures. Similar to JAE, JME may necessitate lifelong treatment, with a high proportion (80%) of patients developing recurrence of seizures, including GTCS, on medication withdrawal.

Other Genetic Generalized Epilepsies

Other GGEs include epilepsy with GTCS alone, epilepsy with eyelid myoclonia (Jeavon syndrome), and epilepsy with myoclonic absences. Treatment usually involves broad-spectrum antiseizure medications such as valproate, levetiracetam, lamotrigine, and benzodiazepines. Ethosuximide is particularly effective for absence seizures, but it is a narrow-spectrum drug that is ineffective against GTCS or myoclonus. However, drugs such as carbamazepine, oxcarbazepine, phenytoin, vigabatrin, tiagabine, and gabapentin should be avoided as they may exacerbate absence or myoclonic seizures.

DEVELOPMENTAL AND EPILEPTIC ENCEPHALOPATHIES

Epileptic encephalopathy, first introduced as a term in 2006 and later incorporated into the 2010 ILAE classification, refers to a group of disorders where the epileptic activity itself exacerbates severe cognitive and behavioral impairments beyond what would be expected from the underlying pathology alone, such as cortical malformation.[4] These disorders often present with developmental concerns that may be independent of ongoing seizures and may be associated with the underlying etiology.

Developmental delay may manifest before the onset of seizures, exacerbating with the emergence of epileptic encephalopathy, or persisting despite seizure management postresolution of epileptic encephalopathy. Distinguishing between the contributions of the underlying cause and the epileptic activity to the developmental aspects of encephalopathy can pose challenges. In 2017, to tackle these complexities, the term "developmental and epileptic encephalopathies" (DEEs) was introduced, allowing for the inclusion of either or both descriptors, "epileptic" and "developmental."[5] Isolated developmental encephalopathy denotes developmental delay or intellectual disability without epileptic encephalopathy, representing a static impairment that may become more noticeable with age. These individuals face a heightened risk of epilepsy, although not necessarily epileptic encephalopathy. Infantile epileptic spasms syndrome, Dravet syndrome, epilepsy of infancy with migrating focal seizures, Lennox-Gastaut syndrome, and epileptic encephalopathy with continuous spike and wave during sleep (CSWS) are some of the examples of DEEs **(Fig. 8.7.1)**.

Managing DEEs proves challenging owing to the resistance of seizures to medications. Judicious use of multiple ASMs in combination (polypharmacy) to mitigate seizures is beneficial. The ketogenic diet might offer benefits and should be contemplated early in treatment. Structural causes amenable to epilepsy surgery warrant prompt referral

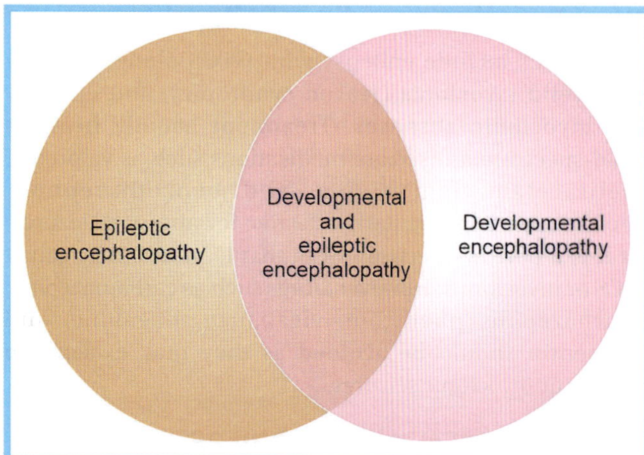

Fig. 8.7.1: Concept of developmental and epileptic encephalopathy.

to an epilepsy surgery center. Neuromodulation techniques, such as vagal nerve stimulation or deep brain stimulation, may be considered in specific cases following a thorough evaluation.

Precision therapies are also emerging for certain genetic etiologies.[6] For example, memantine may be used in *GRIN2A*-related DEEs with gain-of-function variants, quinidine in *KCNT1*-related DEE, and mammalian target of rapamycin (mTOR) inhibitors in tuberous sclerosis complex (TSC)-related epilepsy/DEE. These precision therapies offer targeted approaches to management, potentially improving outcomes in specific genetic subtypes of DEEs.

INVESTIGATIONS

Role of Electroencephalography

Electroencephalography is one of the most useful investigations in patients with epilepsy/suspected epilepsy if used appropriately.[7] It is an important aid in the clinical diagnosis of epilepsy, but it cannot rule in or out the diagnosis of epilepsy. EEG is a supportive investigation and is not a confirmatory test. Up to 50% of children with epilepsy can have a normal EEG, especially in the first instance when the EEG is taken. Sleep deprivation, sleeping during the EEG test, and activation procedures such as hyperventilation and photic stimulation increase the diagnostic yield of the EEG. On the contrary, 1–2% of normal children can show epileptiform abnormalities on EEG.

The common indications for performing an EEG are listed in **Box 8.7.3**.

Ordering EEG is not recommended in cases of febrile seizures, autism without seizures, evident nonepileptic events during infancy such as breath-holding spells (BHS) and self-gratification, as well as other paroxysmal events such as syncope, headache, dizziness, and vertigo, and for monitoring the "progress" of epilepsy. It is highly advisable to conduct synchronized video recording for all EEG recordings.[8]

BOX 8.7.3: Common indications for performing EEG.

- *Non-ICU setting*
  - *First unprovoked seizure**
    - Diagnosis of an epilepsy syndrome
    - To classify epilepsy into generalized versus focal
    - To prognosticate the risk of seizure recurrence
  - *Diagnosed cases of epilepsy*
    - Clarification of epilepsy syndrome
    - Clinical change, regression
    - Monitoring treatment (only in certain epilepsy syndromes, not routinely)
    - Infantile spasms, EE-CSWS, absence epilepsy
    - Before weaning off antiseizure medications (risk of seizure recurrence)
    - Presurgical evaluation
  - *Others*
    - Febrile status epilepticus
    - Apparent life-threatening event/brief resolved unexplained event (BRUE)
    - Unexplained global development delay
    - Neuroregression (cognitive/language) even in the absence of seizures
    - Paroxysmal events (detailed history is a prerequisite)
- *ICU setting*
  - Refractory status epilepticus, to guide treatments
  - Encephalopathy with suspicion of electrographic seizures
  - Characterize paroxysmal events suspected to be seizures

(EE-CSWS: epileptic encephalopathy with continuous spike and wave during sleep; EEG: electroencephalography; ICU: intensive care unit)

Role of Neuroimaging

Magnetic resonance imaging (MRI) is the preferred imaging method for children with epilepsy, and computed tomography (CT) scan has a limited role.[9] However, in areas where inflammatory granulomas are a significant cause of epilepsy, CT may serve as a reasonable initial imaging modality. It may also be considered when MRI is inaccessible or contraindicated (e.g., the presence of metal implants or an unstable patient condition). Due to radiation hazards, CT scanning should be avoided whenever possible.

Neuroimaging is generally beneficial in most epilepsy cases, except in certain epilepsy syndromes such as childhood epilepsy with centrotemporal spikes and typical genetic generalized epilepsies (e.g., childhood absence or juvenile myoclonic epilepsies), where it may not be necessary. Urgent neuroimaging may be warranted in children experiencing prolonged seizures/SE, clusters of seizures, focal neurological deficits, persistent encephalopathy, or systemic symptoms/signs (e.g., fever, new-onset behavioral concerns, meningeal signs). Lesions detected on MRI should be correlated with clinical seizure characteristics and EEG findings. Sometimes, MRI "lesions" may be incidental and may not necessarily be responsible for the ongoing seizures (e.g., incidental neurocysticercosis or arachnoid cyst).

Role of Genetic Testing

Approximately two-thirds of individuals with epilepsy may have a genetic basis. The genetic landscape of epilepsy is diverse, encompassing single-gene disorders, epilepsies with complex inheritance, and susceptibility genes/modifiers.

Common indications for genetic testing in epilepsy include epileptic encephalopathy, unexplained drug-resistant epilepsy, associated neurological comorbidities, multisystem involvement, dysmorphic features, and family history of affected individuals or sibling death. Well-controlled epilepsy, idiopathic generalized epilepsies (e.g., childhood absence, juvenile absence, or JME), self-limited (benign) focal epilepsies, and acquired epilepsies typically do not necessitate genetic testing.

Available genetic tests range from karyotype and chromosomal microarray to epilepsy gene panels, whole exome, or genome sequencing. These tests should be ordered following a thorough evaluation of the epilepsy phenotype and initial investigations by a childhood epilepsy expert.

TREATMENT

Antiseizure medications are the mainstay of treatment in epilepsy.[10] The choice of ASM depends primarily on the precise epilepsy type (or epilepsy syndrome) diagnosis. Determining when to initiate medication presents a common therapeutic dilemma following a first unprovoked seizure. The primary consideration in such cases typically revolves around the risk of seizure recurrence. Generally, if the likelihood of recurrence is deemed significant (typically >60%), initiating ASMs may be considered appropriate. Factors such as a "remote symptomatic" etiology, focal seizures in the context of developmental delay, abnormal neuroimaging or EEG findings, and nocturnal seizures elevate the risk of recurrence. The decision to commence ASM therapy becomes more straightforward in children experiencing very frequent (often daily) new-onset seizures, such as absence seizures or infantile spasms.

Both the advantages and disadvantages must be carefully weighed and discussed with the patient's family. Initiating an ASM implies a potential decrease in the risk of seizure recurrence, consequently reducing the likelihood of injuries and even sudden unexpected death in epilepsy (SUDEP). Additionally, it may offer psychological and social benefits. Considerations such as the impact on schooling in younger children or employment/driving for older adolescents should also be taken into account. Conversely, commencing ASMs may lead to potential adverse effects (both short- and long-term), drug interactions, or financial burdens (in terms of cost/insurance).

BOX 8.7.4: The commonly used antiseizure medications (ASMs), classified based on mechanism of action.

- *Drugs acting on extra-synaptic membrane*
  - Voltage-gated sodium channel blockers (mainly fast inactivation): Carbamazepine, oxcarbazepine, phenytoin, lamotrigine, topiramate, zonisamide, rufinamide, felbamate, valproate, lacosamide (slow inactivation)
- *Drugs acting on inhibitory synapse*
  - GABAA receptor modulators: Benzodiazepines, barbiturates, stiripentol, felbamate, topiramate
  - GABA-transaminase inhibitor: Vigabatrin
- *Drugs acting on excitatory synapse*
  - α-Amino-3-hydroxy-5-methyl-4-isoxazolepropionic acid (AMPA) receptor blockers: Perampanel, topiramate, lamotrigine, phenobarbital
  - *N*-methyl-D-aspartate (NMDA) receptor blockers: Felbamate, valproate, ketamine
- *Voltage-gated calcium channel inhibitors: Gabapentin*
- *Miscellaneous*
  - Low voltage-activated (T-type) calcium channel blocker: Ethosuximide
  - Synaptic vesicle protein 2A (SV2A) blocker: Levetiracetam, brivaracetam
  - Carbonic anhydrase inhibitor: Sulthiame, acetazolamide
  - Diverse mechanisms: Ketogenic diet, cannabidiol

(GABA: gamma-aminobutyric acid; GABAA: gamma-aminobutyric acid type A)

The commonly used ASMs, classified based on their mechanism of action, are listed in **Box 8.7.4**.

The choice of any ASM is usually governed by variables related to seizure type/epilepsy syndrome, underlying etiology, properties of the ASMs (efficacy spectrum, adverse effect profile, dosing intervals, drug interactions, cost, and availability), and various patient characteristics (age, sex, allergies, comorbidities, lifestyle, occupation, and past ASM trials). Treatment should be individualized based on the child's specific needs and response to therapy. Close monitoring for efficacy and adverse effects is essential, and dosage adjustments may be necessary over time. Additionally, nonpharmacological treatments such as the ketogenic diet, vagus nerve stimulation (VNS), and epilepsy surgery may be considered in certain cases, especially when medications fail to adequately control seizures.

When to Stop Medications?

Based on both evidence-based practices and expert consensus, most physicians typically consider tapering ASMs after a minimum of 2 years of seizure freedom. The likelihood of seizure recurrence is influenced by factors such as the specific epilepsy syndrome, underlying etiology,

TABLE 8.7.2: Nonepileptic paroxysmal disorders.

Neonates	Infancy	Childhood
• Jitteriness • Benign neonatal sleep myoclonus • Hyperekplexia	• Benign upgaze of infancy • Benign paroxysmal torticollis • Shuddering attacks • Infantile self-stimulation behavior • Breath-holding spells • Benign myoclonus of infancy	• Alternating hemiplegia of infancy and childhood • Paroxysmal dyskinesias • Parasomnias • Tics—motor and vocal • Benign paroxysmal vertigo • Cyclical vomiting syndrome • Episodic ataxia • Transient ischemic attacks • Psychogenic nonepileptic seizure • Syncope

comorbidities, EEG and neuroimaging findings, and past history of seizure recurrence on medication withdrawal. For certain age-dependent epilepsy syndromes such as self-limited childhood epilepsy with centrotemporal spikes or Panayiotopoulos syndrome, the risk of recurrence may be relatively low. Conversely, children with genetic/metabolic epilepsies, epileptic encephalopathies, or significant structural malformations (particularly if bilateral and unsuitable for surgery) may face a higher risk of recurrence.

The greatest risk of seizure recurrence typically occurs within the initial 1–2 years following ASM discontinuation. Once the decision to taper off medication has been made, it is usually accomplished over a period of 2–3 months to minimize potential risks.

Status Epilepticus

Status epilepticus is a neurological emergency characterized by prolonged seizures or a series of recurrent seizures without recovery of consciousness between episodes. While SE can occur in individuals of all ages, its incidence is higher in children. Febrile SE, infections such as meningitis or encephalitis, traumatic brain injury, and electrolyte imbalances are some of the common causes of SE in children. Children with known epilepsy are at increased risk of developing SE, especially if their seizures are poorly controlled or if they miss their antiepileptic medications.

Prompt and effective management of SE is crucial to prevent neurological damage and reduce morbidity and mortality. Initial treatment is to administer emergency rescue medications such as benzodiazepines (e.g., lorazepam, midazolam) intravenously to terminate ongoing seizures. Intranasal or buccal midazolam is administered in out-of-hospital settings. Home use of emergency rescue nasal midazolam is routinely advised for patients with recurrent prolonged seizures. Midazolam can be administered intramuscularly if immediate intravenous access is difficult.

If seizures persist despite initial treatment, second-line medications such as phenytoin, fosphenytoin, levetiracetam, or phenobarbitone may be administered as an intravenous loading dose over 20 minutes. In refractory cases, other interventions such as intravenous anesthetics or ketamine may be considered. Close monitoring of vital signs, continuous EEG, and supportive measures to maintain adequate oxygenation and cardiovascular function are essential during the management of SE.

NONEPILEPTIC PAROXYSMAL DISORDERS

Nonepileptic paroxysmal disorders in children encompass a range of conditions characterized by sudden, transient episodes of altered behavior or consciousness, without the characteristic electrographic abnormalities seen in epilepsy. These episodes may mimic epileptic seizures but are caused by nonepileptic mechanisms. Paroxysmal disorders are diagnosed primarily based on characteristic phenomenology, detailed history, and clinical examination. Home video recordings of typical episodes often clinch the diagnosis. Common nonepileptic paroxysmal disorders encountered in children are listed in **Table 8.7.2** according to the age groups. BHS, syncope, and psychogenic nonepileptic seizures (PNES) are the most commonly encountered nonepileptic events in children.

Breath-holding Spells

Breath-holding spells typically occur in infants and young children during moments of frustration, anger, or pain. They are characterized by a sudden, involuntary cessation of breathing, leading to cyanosis (or pallor) and loss of consciousness. BHS are classified into cyanotic or pallid spells depending on the lips' color change. Although frightening for caregivers, BHS are benign and resolve spontaneously without long-term consequences.

Syncope

Syncope is characterized by a temporary loss of consciousness due to a brief reduction in blood flow to the brain. Various contributory factors include the vasovagal reflex, orthostatic hypotension, cardiac arrhythmias, or neurological issues. The primary objective of evaluation is to pinpoint the underlying cause and implement measures to prevent future occurrences.

Psychogenic Nonepileptic Seizures

Psychogenic nonepileptic seizures are characterized by altered behavior or consciousness, resembling epileptic seizures but lacking abnormal brain electrical activity. These episodes are believed to stem from psychological triggers, such as stress, trauma, or emotional turmoil. Diagnosing and managing PNES in children often necessitates a collaborative approach involving pediatric neurology, psychiatry, and psychology.

CONCLUSION

The diagnoses of seizures and epilepsy are clinical; the EEG is only a supportive investigation. Correct clinical diagnosis ensures precise treatments apart from avoiding unnecessary investigations. Normal EEG does not rule out epilepsy and an abnormal EEG per se is not diagnostic of epilepsy. Diagnosis and management of children with epilepsy warrant a systematic approach.

REFERENCES

1. Fisher RS, Cross JH, French JA, Higurashi N, Hirsch E, Jansen FE, et al. Operational classification of seizure types by the International League Against Epilepsy: position paper of the ILAE Commission for Classification and Terminology. Epilepsia. 2017;58(4):522-30.
2. Scheffer IE, Berkovic S, Capovilla G, Connolly MB, French J, Guilhoto L, et al. ILAE classification of the epilepsies: position paper of the ILAE Commission for Classification and Terminology. Epilepsia. 2017;58(4):512-21.
3. Specchio N, Wirrell EC, Scheffer IE, Nabbout R, Riney K, Samia P, et al. International League Against Epilepsy classification and definition of epilepsy syndromes with onset in childhood: position paper by the ILAE Task Force on Nosology and Definitions. Epilepsia. 2022;63(6):1398-442.
4. Jain P. Absence seizures in children: usual and the unusual. Indian J Pediatr. 2020;87(12):1047-56.
5. Scheffer IE, Liao J. Deciphering the concepts behind "epileptic encephalopathy" and "developmental and epileptic encephalopathy". Eur J Paediatr Neurol. 2020;24:11-4.
6. Byrne S, Enright N, Delanty N. Precision therapy in the genetic epilepsies of childhood. Dev Med Child Neurol. 2021;63(11):1276-82.
7. Benbadis SR, Beniczky S, Bertram E, MacIver S, Moshé SL. The role of EEG in patients with suspected epilepsy. Epileptic Disord. 2020;22(2):143-55.
8. Kannan L, Jain P, Nayak D. Role of video-EEG in children. Indian J Pediatr. 2021;88(10):1007-16.
9. Lee YJ. Advanced neuroimaging techniques for evaluating pediatric epilepsy. Clin Exp Pediatr. 2020;63(3):88-95.
10. Perucca E. The pharmacological treatment of epilepsy: recent advances and future perspectives. Acta Epileptol. 2021;3(1):22.

8.8 Headache and Migraine

Shruthi NM

INTRODUCTION

Headache is one of the most common pediatric neurologic disorders and affects about 80–85% of the pediatric population. Headaches can be primary like migraine or tension-type headaches (TTH), or secondary to an underlying systemic cause. Primary headache disorders are more commonly seen in children than secondary headache disorders. Migraine headaches affect 5–10% of children in the adolescent age group and lead to significant disability in some children, affecting school and extracurricular activities. It is also one of the leading causes of emergency visits among children. This chapter elucidates the nature of migraine in children.

EPIDEMIOLOGY

Migraine is seen in 1–3% of children between 5 and 7 years and in 4–10% in the adolescent age group. Up to 18% of pediatric emergency visits are found to be related to the same. The prevalence increases with increasing age. About 1 in 10 children experience recurring and disabling headaches due to migraine. It is seen equally in prepubertal boys and girls and two to three times more frequently in postpubertal girls.[1]

PATHOPHYSIOLOGY

The pathophysiology of primary headache disorders is unclear but is probably the complex interaction of genetic and environmental factors. There are different theories explaining the pathophysiology of migraine. The vascular theory of migraine headache has raised controversies during recent times, and it is now considered to be a disease of the brain. Cortical spreading depression leading to alteration in the neurotransmitter systems and trigeminal vascular system activation releasing vasoactive peptides such as calcitonin gene-related peptide (CGRP), substance P, and nitric oxide triggering the nociceptive receptors are among the few mechanisms. The insula, hypothalamic–pituitary–adrenal axis, and the serotoninergic system are also involved. Children have reduced cholinergic function, and the neurotransmitter balance differs compared to adults. Hence, children have different clinical manifestations with respect to their adult counterparts.[2]

The secondary headaches are usually due to an underlying cause and are not uncommon in children. Systemic infections, intracranial infections, trauma, intracranial space-occupying lesions, idiopathic intracranial hypertension (IIH), rhinosinusitis, cerebral venous sinus thrombosis (CVST), and subarachnoid hemorrhage are some of the causes of secondary headaches. **Box 8.8.1** outlines the brief classification of headache disorders in children.[3]

CLINICAL FEATURES

Children with migraine do not usually have the classical unilateral throbbing headache seen in adults. Instead, it is characterized by recurrent episodes of moderate to severe intensity of throbbing or pulsating pain, which increases with head movements and other activities and lasts for 1–72 hours. It may be unilateral or bilateral, unlike in adults where it is usually unilateral. It is associated with nausea, vomiting, photophobia, phonophobia, aversion to certain smells, cutaneous allodynia (pain due to a stimulus that does not normally provoke pain), and heightened sensitivity to environmental stimuli adding to the disability. There are specific triggers such as lack of sleep, sunlight, inadequate food habits, or excessive screen exposure. Rarely, when migraine is with aura (as in one-third of children), it is additionally associated with sensory, visual (most commonly fortification spectra), motor, or speech disturbances preceding the onset of headache for less than an hour. Brainstem phenomena like vertigo/giddiness or abdominal pain/cyclical vomiting are also seen in children with migraine headaches. It is frequently associated with a positive family history. Fatigue, depression, yawning, and food cravings may be premonitory symptoms.[1]

Tension-type headaches are like migraine headaches but without any associated nausea or vomiting or sensitivity to environmental stimuli. It is a band-like or constricting type of pain of mild-to-moderate intensity. These attacks are more frequent compared to migraine headaches.

BOX 8.8.1: Classification of headache disorders (derived from ICHD-3).[3]

Primary headache
- *Migraine headache*
  - Migraine with aura
  - Migraine without aura
  - Chronic migraine
  - Complications of migraine
  - Probable migraine
  - Episodic syndromes
- *TTH*
  - Infrequent episodic TTH
  - Frequent episodic TTH
  - Chronic TTH
  - Probable TTH
- *Trigeminal autonomic cephalalgias*
  - Cluster headache
  - Paroxysmal hemicrania
  - Short-lasting unilateral neuralgiform headaches
  - Hemicrania continua
- *Other primary headache disorders*
  - Primary cough headache
  - Primary exercise headache
  - Primary thunderclap headache and others
- *Secondary headache disorders*
  - Post-traumatic headache
  - Cranial or cervical vascular disorder-related headache
  - Headache attributed to nonvascular intracranial disorder
  - Headache attributed to substance abuse or its withdrawal
  - Headache related to infections
  - Headache attributed to disorders of homeostasis
  - Headache related to disorders of the cranium/eye/neck/ears/nose/sinus/teeth/mouth or other facial or cervical structures
  - Headache due to psychiatric disorder
  - Painful lesions of cranial nerve and other facial pain

(ICHD-3: International Classification of Headache Disorders, 3rd edition; TTH: tension-type headaches)

APPROACH TO A CHILD WITH HEADACHE

Diagnosis of headache is primarily based on history and examination. **Table 8.8.1** details the important aspects of history taking, and **Table 8.8.2** details the important aspects of examination. Investigations are needed only in the presence of red flag signs **(Box 8.8.2)**.

DIAGNOSTIC TESTING

In children with headaches, diagnostic testing is warranted only in the presence of red flag signs as detailed in **Box 8.8.2**. There is no role of routine blood work, imaging, and lumbar puncture in a child with normal neurological examination and in the absence of red flags as per the current guidelines. Headache is a clinical diagnosis, and the diagnostic criteria for primary headache disorders are detailed in **Box 8.8.3**.[1]

Magnetic resonance imaging (MRI) of the brain is very sensitive in identifying intracranial pathologies and considered as the investigation of choice in routine cases.

TABLE 8.8.1: Important aspects of clinical history in a child with headache.

History	*Comments*
Onset of headache	• Acute/explosive onset in patients with hemorrhage or trauma • Acute intermittent headaches in infections/secondary headaches/primary headache disorders • Chronic recurrent as in migraines or tension headaches
Temporal pattern	• Acute recurrent headaches seen in pediatric migraine and other primary headache disorders • Acute headaches in infections or systemic causes • Chronic progressive headaches as in tumors or intracranial pathologies • Chronic nonprogressive headaches in medication overuse
Triggers	• Sun exposure, lack of sleep, disturbance in daily routine, diet pattern, trauma
Frequency and duration of headache	• To characterize the headache type as in primary headaches • To classify as acute/recurrent/chronic headaches • Migraine headaches are usually infrequent whereas cluster headaches and tension headaches can occur more frequently
Aura/prodrome	• Migraine/epilepsy with postictal headaches
Distribution of pain	• Bifrontal in migraine/rhinosinusitis headache • More diffuse in tension headaches/intracranial pathologies
Nature of the pain	• Throbbing in migraine • Band-like in tension headaches • Dull aching in raised intracranial pressure
Associated symptoms	• Nausea/vomiting/photophobia or phonophobia are common associations with migraine • Fever is a sign of infection • Associated dental pain or earache are causes of secondary headaches
Disability associated with pain	• Restriction of daily activities can help quantify the severity of pain and guide the management • Younger children are unable to express pain, and identifying the restrictions of daily activities may be useful for diagnosing the severity of pain
Relieving factors	• Rest/sleep or medications
History of other comorbidities	• Learning disability, attention deficits, cognitive decline, regression of behavior may point to secondary causes
Associated medical conditions	• Systemic illness leads to hypertension and secondary headaches, or due to stress associated with chronic illness, primary headaches may be triggered • Preexisting malignancy/neurocutaneous disorders give a clue for etiological diagnosis
Medication intake	• As adverse reaction to certain drugs/chronic headaches due to analgesic overuse
Family history	• A positive history of migraine is usually seen among family members • Family dynamics may be altered leading to stress headaches/functional headaches

Computed tomography (CT) of the head is preferred in case of emergencies and when bleeding or trauma is suspected, as it has a shorter acquisition time. Incidental MRI brain abnormalities may be found in up to 20% of patients routinely imaged for headaches and may wrongfully be attributed as a causative factor. Lumbar puncture is diagnostic in cases of intracranial infections and can be therapeutic in children with IIH syndrome.

Primary headache disorders can coexist in the same patient. It is important to identify them individually because the treatment varies. Maintaining headache diaries will greatly help to distinguish the coexisting conditions and help in avoiding medication overuse and its adverse consequences.

TREATMENT

Flowchart 8.8.1 provides an algorithm for the management of a child with headache. The goal of treatment is to reduce disability associated with recurrent headaches and improve the quality of life. In children with secondary headache disorders, the underlying etiology should be rightly identified and treated. The goal of treatment of migraine headaches is to reduce the duration, frequency, and intensity of the headaches, thereby reducing the disability and improving the quality of life.[4] There are two aspects of the treatment of primary headache disorders—preventive and abortive therapy.

TABLE 8.8.2: Important aspects of clinical examination in a child with headache.

Hypertension	Seen in systemic disorders like chronic kidney disease, malignancies, drug intake, raised intracranial pressure-related conditions
Fever	Infections
Macrocephaly	Hydrocephalus, neurocutaneous disorders
Head and neck examination	Look for signs of meningeal irritation, cranial bruit, trauma, evidence of sinusitis, dental caries
Skin examination	• Pallor, icterus, or cyanosis indicative of systemic illness • Petechiae and purpura indicating bleeding tendencies
Fundus and refraction/eye movements	• Papilledema and paralytic squint may be associated with raised ICP • Decrease in visual acuity is seen in IIH
Detailed neurologic examination	Look for alteration in mental status, behavioral issues, cranial nerve deficits, focal deficits, reflexes, sensory deficits, coordination, and gait
Other system examination	• Look for cardiac murmurs • Organomegaly • Crepitations and wheeze on respiratory examination indicating fluid overload

(ICP: intracranial pressure; IIH: idiopathic intracranial hypertension)

Preventive Therapy of Migraine Headache/ Tension-type Headache

Lifestyle changes and biobehavioral therapy are the most important strategies to prevent recurrent headaches in children. Nonpharmacological therapy is the first-line treatment.[5] Maintaining a headache diary and noting the triggers is the initial step, followed by measures to avoid those triggers.

An effective way to reduce triggers is by adapting the "SMART" action plan:

- S—*S*leep hygiene; *S*tress reduction
- M—stop *M*edication overuse
- A—regular physical *A*ctivity
- R—*R*egular diet, avoiding caffeine, cheese, fast foods, irregular food intake, and skipping meals; relaxation exercises and biofeedback techniques/cognitive behavioral therapy (CBT)
- T—reduce *T*elevision exposure and screen time

Pharmacological treatment for preventing migraine headaches is not routinely recommended in children. They are only used if there are very frequent (1–2 attacks/ week) disabling headaches [Pediatric Migraine Disability Assessment (PedMIDAS) questionnaire score > 30] and

BOX 8.8.2: Red flag signs for considering further evaluation in children with headache.

Red flags in history
- Acute explosive headache
- New onset severe headache of <1-month duration
- Progressive headaches—acute/chronic
- Change in nature of the headache
- Age <6 years
- Occipital headaches
- Associated symptoms such as fever/recurrent projectile vomiting/ vision issues/loss of consciousness or altered mental status/ seizures/headache disturbing sleep in the night/vertigo
- No family history of headache
- Associated systemic conditions like immunosuppression

Red flags in examination
- Fever
- Hypertension
- Pallor/cyanosis/icterus/clubbing/edema
- Papilledema in fundus examination
- Squint
- Altered mental status
- Focal neurological deficits
- Abnormal other system examination

BOX 8.8.3: ICHD-3 criteria for diagnosis of migraine without aura and episodic TTH.[3]

Criteria for pediatric migraine without aura

A. At least five attacks fulfilling criteria B–D

B. Headache attacks lasting 2–72 hours (untreated or unsuccessfully treated)

C. Headache has at least two of the following four characteristics:
  1. Unilateral location
  2. Pulsating quality
  3. Moderate or severe pain intensity
  4. Aggravation by or causing avoidance of routine physical activity

D. During headache at least one of the following:
  1. Nausea and/or vomiting
  2. Photophobia or phonophobia

E. Not better accounted by any other ICHD-3 diagnosis

Criteria for frequent episodic TTH

A. At least 10 episodes of headache occurring on 1–14 days/month on average for >3 months (≥12 and <180 days/year) and fulfilling criteria B–D

B. Lasting from 30 minutes to 7 days

C. At least two of the following four characteristics:
  1. Bilateral location
  2. Pressing or tightening quality (nonpulsatile)
  3. Mild to moderate intensity
  4. Not aggravated by routine physical activity

D. Both of the following:
  - No nausea or vomiting
  - No more than one of photophobia or phonophobia

E. Not better accounted for by another ICHD-3 diagnosis

(ICHD-3: International Classification of Headache Disorders, 3rd edition; TTH: tension-type headache)

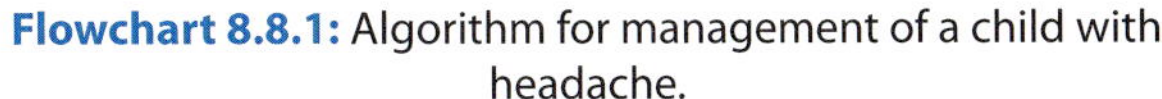

Flowchart 8.8.1: Algorithm for management of a child with headache.

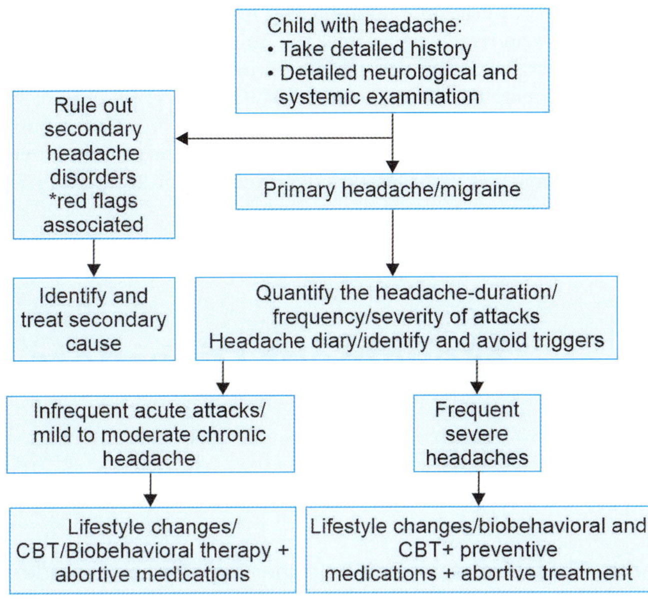

*Frequency of headaches that warrant initiation of preventive medications is not defined and should be tailored according to the patient's presenting symptoms and severity.
(CBT: cognitive behavioral therapy)

frequent school absenteeism, for a period of 3–4 months. A recent randomized controlled study [CHAMP (Childhood and Adolescent Migraine Prevention) trial done in 2017, in 8–17-year-old children] comparing topiramate and amitriptyline to placebo has shown no added benefits. The available quality of evidence on the use of drugs in the pediatric population is low. Some of the commonly used medications are:

- *Propranolol*: 2–4 mg/kg/day
- *Flunarizine*: 5–10 mg/day
- *Valproate*: 20–40 mg/kg/day
- *Topiramate*: 1–10 mg/kg/day
- *Cyproheptadine*: 0.25–1.25 mg/kg/day
- *Amitriptyline*: 1 mg/kg/day
- *Nutraceuticals*: Magnesium/riboflavin/coenzyme Q10

Early preventive treatment is advocated by some studies to reduce the risk of migraine chronification during adulthood.

Abortive Therapy for Migraine Headache

Abortive therapy is commonly used in case of acute severe attacks or in status migranosus.[1] Frequently used drugs are analgesics (acetaminophen 15 mg/kg), nonsteroidal anti-inflammatory drugs (NSAIDs; ibuprofen 10 mg/kg and naproxen 5–10 mg/kg), and triptans (5-hydroxytryptamine receptor agonists, oral rizatriptan 5–10 mg/day). The focus should be to use them early and in optimal doses to abort the headache. Triptans are exclusively effective for migraine, and their effectiveness is thought to be diagnostic of migraine. For vomiting associated with headaches, metoclopramide, domperidone or ketorolac may be used. Intravenous ketorolac and prochlorperazine combination, sodium valproate infusions, and fluid boluses have been used in severe attacks. During an acute attack, the child should be allowed to rest in a dark and quiet room. Parents should be educated to use the drugs judiciously to avoid medication overuse headache (occurs with use of >15 days/month for 3 months with NSAIDs and >10 days/month for 3 months with triptans).

PROGNOSIS

Most of the children (approximately 50%) continue to have persistent headaches in adulthood. There are studies to indicate that children can have different types of primary headaches over time. Headache frequency increases during menstruation and childbearing age, and women are two to three times more likely to experience migraine compared to men.

Studies have shown that children with recurrent migraine headaches have reduced academic performance compared to their healthy peers. They are also more prone to anxiety, depression, mood and behavioral disorders, Tourette syndrome, and attention-deficit hyperactivity disorder. Other systemic comorbidities known to be associated with headache are epilepsy, obesity, asthma, atopic dermatitis, restless leg syndrome, and sleep disorders.

RECENT ADVANCES

Newer medications such as lasmiditan, a serotonin antagonist, and gepants, CGRP receptor antagonists/anti-CGRP monoclonal antibodies, have recently been approved in adults for chronic migraine and as an abortive treatment. Further studies are needed in children for the same. The pathophysiology of primary headaches is still evolving, and new developments may help us manage the headaches better. Several pain and severity assessment scales such as PedMIDAS tool have been approved and proven to be beneficial in quantifying pediatric headaches.

CONCLUSION

- Pediatric headache is very common and is not to be overlooked.
- Prompt identification of red flags helps us to treat secondary headaches timely and adequately.
- Nonpharmacological treatment is always preferred over medications; healthy lifestyle is the key to managing primary headache disorders.
- Early and optimal doses of abortive medications are to be used to reduce the disabling pain in acute attacks.

REFERENCES

1. Langdon R, DiSabella MT. Pediatric headache: an overview. Curr Probl Pediatr Adolesc Health Care. 2017;47(3):44-65.
2. Førland-Schill A, Berring-Uldum A, Debes NM. Migraine pathophysiology in children and adolescents: a review of the literature. J Child Neurol. 2022;37(7):642-51.
3. Headache Classification Committee of the International Headache Society (IHS). The International Classification of Headache Disorders, 3rd edition. Cephalalgia. 2018;38(1): 1-211.
4. Ailani J, Burch RC, Robbins MS, Board of Directors of the American Headache Society. The American Headache Society Consensus Statement: update on integrating new migraine treatments into clinical practice. Headache. 2021;61(7):1021-39.
5. Papetti L, Ursitti F, Moavero R, Ferilli MA, Sforza G, Tarantino S, et al. Prophylactic treatment of pediatric migraine: is there anything new in the last decade? Front Neurol. 2019;10:771.

8.9 Movement Disorders

Priyanka Madaan, Rachana Dubey

INTRODUCTION

Movement and posture are functions of the central and peripheral nervous systems. The motor system controls voluntary movements (directed by the motor cortex), subconscious movements, and involuntary reflexes and prevents abnormal involuntary movements (movement disorders). The nervous system integrates sensory inputs (from different senses including proprioception) with volitional control to elicit a movement. The motor cortex is involved in planning and voluntary control of movement. The basal ganglia and cerebellum are involved in fine-tuning of these movements. The spinal cord, on the other hand, carries the motor tracts (both pyramidal and extrapyramidal tracts) and the anterior horn cells, which constitute the lower motor neurons (i.e., the final common pathway to the muscle fibers through peripheral nerves and neuromuscular junction), generating movement.

Motor control develops with maturation of the motor system with age. The maturation of the motor system goes hand in hand with maturation of the nervous system, occurring as a result of innervation remodeling, synaptic pruning, and myelination. The initial fetal movements are very simple and patterned. With maturation of the motor system, these simple fetal movements evolve into relatively complex general movements in fetal life and early infancy and subsequent goal-directed voluntary and habitual movements. Achievement of selective motor control contributes to better control of isolated movements by preventing coactivation of undesired muscle groups, based on the demands of a voluntary motion or posture.

Movement disorders occur as a result of abnormalities in motor control. They include either an impairment of voluntary movements or the presence of involuntary movements or both. Therefore, these can be either hypokinetic disorders (e.g., parkinsonism) or hyperkinetic disorders (e.g., dystonia).

TYPES OF ABNORMAL MOVEMENTS

Movement disorders in children can be classified as hyperkinetic or hypokinetic disorders **(Box 8.9.1)**.[1-4] Hyperkinetic disorders are more common in children than hypokinetic disorders. Many times, a variety of abnormal movements coexist. The different abnormal movements are as follows:

- *Dystonia:* It refers to abnormal twisting posture occurring as a result of cocontraction of agonist and antagonist muscles. Dystonia is often worsened by attempted movement or posture, excitement, crying, etc., and is task-specific (occurs with specific tasks such as writing dystonia). It reduces with rest and sleep.
- *Chorea/Ballism:* Chorea is chaotic, randomly triggered, rapid, flowing movements involving proximal muscle groups. When very large in amplitude, choreic limb movements are often called ballism. Motor impersistence is an important feature associated with chorea. Chorea is worsened by attempted movement or posture, excitement, crying, etc., and reduces with rest and sleep.
- *Athetosis:* It refers to slow, writhing movements of distal body parts, especially the fingers and hands. These often occur in combination with chorea.
- *Myoclonus:* It refers to sudden, brief, shock-like movements that may be repetitive or rhythmic. It is more rapid than chorea. It may be epileptic (cortical myoclonus) or nonepileptic (subcortical myoclonus).
- *Tremor:* It is a rhythmic oscillation (to and fro movement) about a central point or position, involving one or more body parts. It is classified based on the time of greatest severity such as rest, postural, action, or intention tremor.

BOX 8.9.1: Common movement disorders in children.

Hyperkinetic
- Dystonia
- Chorea
- Athetosis
- Myoclonus
- Tremors
- Stereotypes

Hypokinetic: Rigid/akinetic (parkinsonism)

- *Tics:* These refer to sudden, rapid, abrupt, repetitive, recurrent, and nonrhythmic movements or vocalizations mostly involving the face, neck, and upper trunk. These are associated with premonitory urge and voluntary suppressibility. These are exacerbated by emotions such as stress and excitement and improve with concentration and sleep.[5]
- *Parkinsonism:* It is a hypokinetic syndrome characterized by a triad of resting tremor, slow movement (bradykinesia), and rigidity.

In comparison with dystonia, it is important to understand the concept of spasticity and rigidity, which are abnormalities of tone (resistance to passive stretch). Spasticity refers to a velocity-dependent increase in muscle tone (clasp-knife effect), while rigidity refers to constant resistance throughout the range of motion, irrespective of velocity. Ataxia is another disorder of motor control that affects balance and coordination.

PATHOPHYSIOLOGY AND LOCALIZATION

Different abnormalities of tone, movement, and posture have different underlying pathophysiology and localization. There is an intricate balance and complex interplay between different parts of the motor system that, if altered, leads to movement disorders.[2-4]

Spasticity occurs as a result of damage to cortico-reticulospinal (pyramidal) tracts, while rigidity occurs due to problems with the extrapyramidal system. Ataxia occurs due to cerebellar dysfunction. Dystonia has been associated with disorders of the thalamus and basal ganglia, especially the lentiform nucleus; chorea localizes to the caudate nucleus; and ballism to the subthalamic nucleus. Myoclonus may be of epileptic (cortical myoclonus) or nonepileptic (subcortical myoclonus—brainstem, spinal) origin. Localization of tremor depends on its type; for example, intention tremor localizes to the cerebellum. Tic disorders localize to basal ganglia and cortical mechanisms.[5]

ETIOLOGY

The etiology of movement disorders can be multifactorial. It depends on the types of abnormal movements. To simplify, the etiology can be acquired or congenital.[3,4]

Acquired causes include a variety of brain injuries such as hypoxic–ischemic brain injuries, traumatic brain injuries, stroke, and infections [such as meningoencephalitis, central nervous system (CNS) tuberculosis, and viral encephalitis, e.g., Japanese B encephalitis]. Other causes include autoimmune causes (such as autoimmune encephalitis, Sydenham chorea, and systemic lupus erythematosus), nutritional causes (such as infantile tremor syndrome), tumors, drugs and toxins, and endocrine disorders (such as hyperthyroidism).[2-4]

Congenital causes include congenital malformations of the brain, congenital infections such as TORCH (toxoplasmosis, rubella, cytomegalovirus, and herpes simplex), genetic disorders including metabolic disorders such as organic acidemias, neurotransmitter disorders, neurodegenerative disorders such as neurodegeneration with brain iron accumulation (NBIA), gray matter and white matter disorders, and primary movement disorders.

Neurological disorders with abnormalities of movement and posture in children are listed in **Table 8.9.1**.[3,4] Some important disorders are discussed in the following text.

Cerebral Palsy

Cerebral palsy (CP) refers to a heterogenous group of permanent disorders of movement and posture, causing activity limitation, occurring as a result of static insult to the developing fetal or immature brain. The motor disorders of CP are often associated with problems of cognition and communication, epilepsy, and secondary musculoskeletal issues. CP is the most common cause of motor disability in children. Common clinical syndromes include spastic CP and extrapyramidal CP [dyskinetic (choreoathetotic, dystonic), ataxic–hypotonic, or mixed (dyskinetic and spastic)]. Based on the extent of involvement, CP is further classified as: (1) quadriplegic (all four limbs involved), (2) hemiplegic (unilateral involvement), (3) diplegic (predominant lower limb involvement), and (4) other monoplegic or triplegic limb distribution. Dyskinetic CP occurs due to sequelae of kernicterus. Please refer to Chapter 4.3: Cerebral Palsy for more details.

Sydenham Chorea

Sydenham chorea is one of the common causes of chorea in children. It occurs after a group A beta-hemolytic streptococcus infection and is one of the major Jones criteria for the diagnosis of rheumatic fever. It has been described as "St Vitus dance" in the initial reports. Antibasal ganglia antibodies have been reported in some cases and are believed to occur as a result of molecular mimicry. Sodium valproate, neuroleptics, etc., have been used for symptomatic benefit. Immunotherapy in the form of corticosteroids and intravenous immunoglobulin hastens recovery. The prognosis is usually excellent.

TABLE 8.9.1: Neurological disorders with abnormalities of movement and posture in children.

Broad causes	
Static insult	• Cerebral palsy • Stroke • Tumors • Malformations • Demyelination
Autoimmune	• Sydenham chorea • Systemic lupus erythematosus • Autoimmune encephalitis
Infections	Encephalitis
Drugs/toxins	• Neuroleptic medications • Tricyclic antidepressants • Calcium channel blockers • Levodopa
Genetic—metabolic	• Organic acidemias • Wilson's disease • Lesch–Nyhan disease • Mitochondrial disorders, including Leigh's syndrome • Neurotransmitter disorders
Genetic—degenerative	• NBIA such as PKAN • Ataxia telangiectasia • Juvenile Parkinson's disease • Huntington's disease • Spinocerebellar ataxia • Progressive myoclonic epilepsies
Genetic—paroxysmal movement disorders	• Complex migraine • Paroxysmal dyskinesias
Other genetic disorders	Rett syndrome
Functional movement disorders	

(NBIA: neurodegeneration with brain iron accumulation; PKAN: pantothenate kinase-associated neurodegeneration)

Primary or Genetic Dystonias

These include dystonias of genetic origin with normal neuroimaging. A variety of genetic dystonias (DYT-1, DYT-2, DYT-5, DYT-11, etc.) have been described due to different genes. All have different clinical features. DYT-5 dystonia is associated with diurnal variation and is dopa-responsive.

Pantothenate Kinase-associated Neurodegeneration

Pantothenate kinase-associated neurodegeneration (PKAN) is categorized under a broad group of disorders with NBIA. This occurs as a result of pathogenic variations of *PANK-2* gene. Clinical features include progressive dystonia, dysarthria, rigidity, dementia, and pigmentary retinal degeneration. Brain magnetic resonance imaging (MRI) reveals a characteristic "eye of the tiger" sign. Treatment is symptomatic. Prognosis is poor.

TABLE 8.9.2: Analysis of abnormal movements.

Parameter	
Movement description • Rhythmicity	 • Rhythmic (e.g., tremor), nonrhythmic (e.g., dystonia)
• Amplitude	• Low (e.g., athetosis), high (e.g., chorea)
• Velocity	• Slow (e.g., athetosis), rapid (e.g., chorea)
• Character	• Flowing (e.g., chorea), writhing (e.g., athetosis), flinging (e.g., ballismus), twisting (e.g., dystonia)
• Joints and muscle groups involved	• Proximal (e.g., chorea), distal (e.g., athetosis)
Temporal repetition	Paroxysmal (sudden onset and offset), continual (repeated again and again), or continuous (without stop)
Any premonitory sensation or urge	Present in tics
Voluntary suppressibility	Present in tics
Effect of voluntary movement and posture	Resting, postural, and intention tremors

Tourette Syndrome

Tourette syndrome is a movement disorder characterized by multiple motor tics and at least one vocal tic. The tics would be frequent (many times a day or intermittently) for a period of 1 year.[5,6]

CLINICAL FEATURES AND DIAGNOSIS

The identification and characterization of abnormal movements are very important clinically as it guides the diagnosis and management. Clinically, abnormal movements can be characterized based on a variety of parameters such as rhythmicity (to and fro nature), amplitude, velocity, character, muscle groups involved, temporal repetition, etc. These parameters have been discussed in **Table 8.9.2**.[2-4]

Based on history, clinical examination, phenomenology of movements, age of onset, progression, and extent of involvement, further etiological evaluation is considered.[3,4,7] Neuroimaging (brain MRI) gives clues to the underlying etiology such as bilateral globus pallidus involvement in kernicterus and metabolic disorders, eye of the tiger sign in PKAN, panda sign in Wilson's disease, etc. Brain MRI is usually normal in genetic dystonias and Sydenham chorea. Depending on differential diagnosis, specific testing is considered such as serum ceruloplasmin for Wilson's disease, antistreptolysin titers in Sydenham chorea, autoantibody testing in autoimmune encephalitis, and metabolic testing (e.g., arterial lactate and mass spectrometry) for metabolic disorders. Lastly, genetic testing such as whole exome sequencing, triple repeat testing (e.g., spinocerebellar ataxias), etc., is considered in cases with suspected genetic etiology.[3,4,7]

MANAGEMENT

Treatment of movement disorders in children is based primarily on the phenomenology of the movement and sometimes on underlying etiology (such as in dopa-responsive dystonia). The treatment is usually specific for phenomenology.[2-4]

- *Dystonia:* For dopa-responsive dystonia, levodopa is the drug of choice. Levodopa may help in secondary dystonias also. Other medications for dystonia include anticholinergics (such as trihexyphenidyl), baclofen, gabapentin, and benzodiazepines. Deep brain stimulation may be helpful in some disorders.
- *Chorea:* Except for Sydenham chorea, which responds to symptomatic treatment with neuroleptics, valproic acid, etc., other choreas are difficult to treat. Benzodiazepines or dopamine depletors (tetrabenazine, reserpine) may be helpful in some cases. Deep brain stimulation may help in severe cases.
- *Parkinsonism:* Bradykinesia responds to L-dopa and dopamine agonists.
- *Tremor:* Drugs for essential tremor include propranolol, primidone, benzodiazepines, etc.
- *Myoclonus:* Cortical myoclonus is usually treated with benzodiazepines such as clonazepam.
- *Tics:* Behavioral intervention, clonidine, neuroleptic drugs such as pimozide, and atypical neuroleptics such as risperidone might be useful.[5,6]

CONCLUSION

To conclude, movement disorders in children include a broad spectrum of conditions with different etiologies. Phenomenological analysis aids in diagnosis. Early recognition and accurate diagnosis are important for management, which may include pharmacological interventions, physical therapy, and rarely surgical options. A multidisciplinary approach involving neurologists, pediatricians, and therapists is essential for providing comprehensive care.

REFERENCES

1. Nardocci N, Fernandez-Alvarez E (Eds). Movement Disorders in Children: A Clinical Update with Video Recordings. Montgrue: John Libbey Eurotext; 2007. [online] Available from https://www.researchgate.net/publication/332769109_Movement_Disorders_in_Children_A_Clinical_Update_with_Video_Recordings_2007_Edited_by_Nardo_Nardocci_Emilio_Fernandez-Alvarez_Published_by_John_Libbey_Eurotext_192_pages_Price_C86 [Last accessed January, 2025]
2. Jain R, Pandey S, Raghav S. Movement disorders in children. Indian Pediatr. 2021;58(9):861-70.
3. Singer HS, Mink JW, Gilbert DL, Jankovic J. Movement Disorders in Childhood, 2nd edition. London: Academic Press; 2016.
4. Swaiman KF, Ashwal S, Ferriero DM, Schor NF, Finkel RS, Gropman AL, Pearl PL, Shevell ML (Eds). Movement Disorders, 6th edition. Amsterdam: Elsevier; 2018.
5. Nilles C, Hartmann A, Roze E, Martino D, Pringsheim T. Tourette syndrome and other tic disorders of childhood. Handb Clin Neurol. 2023;196:457-74.
6. Ramsey KA, McGuire JF. Advancements in the phenomenology, assessment, and treatment of Tourette syndrome. Curr Opin Psychiatry. 2024;37(2):57-64.
7. O'Malley JA. Diagnosing common movement disorders in children. Continuum (Minneap Minn). 2022;28(5):1476-519.

8.10 Sleep Disorders in Children

Biswaroop Chakrabarty

INTRODUCTION

Pediatric sleep disorders are prevalent yet frequently underreported due to a lack of awareness among both physicians and caregivers.[1] Sleep disturbances can have significant consequences, such as poor school performance, lower intelligence quotient (IQ) scores, excessive daytime sleepiness, and socioemotional problems.[2] Unrecognized sleep disorders result in hypertension, growth retardation, cognitive impairment, and right heart failure.[3] Poor quality of sleep in children and adolescents impairs parental sleep and quality of life.

Children's sleep patterns vary, evolving from the immature patterns of preterm babies to adult sleep patterns, making identification and diagnosis more challenging. Additionally, efforts to screen for these problems have led to the development of numerous questionnaires over the years.

Using appropriate questionnaires can facilitate focused referrals to sleep experts, which are essential for the optimal evaluation and management of sleep-related problems in children and adolescents. This, in turn, translates into improved sleep hygiene and better academic, behavioral, and socioemotional performance.

EPIDEMIOLOGY

Across various age groups, the prevalence of sleep disorders varies from 30–50% in infancy, 15–30% in pre-schoolers and toddlers, to 20–40% in school-going children and adolescents. In infants and toddlers, insomnia and sleep-related movement disorders predominate. In school-going children and adolescents, along with these, parasomnia, sleep-related breathing disorders, hypersomnolence, circadian rhythm disorders, and enuresis are also reported.[4]

Epilepsy and sleep share a reciprocal relationship; sleep activates interictal and ictal discharges, and epilepsy has a significant detrimental effect on sleep duration, quality, and restorative functions, in both generalized and focal seizures.[5] More than half of children with attention deficit hyperactivity disorder and three-fourths with Down syndrome and autism are reported to have sleep problems.[6] Sleep disturbances are also frequent in boys with Duchenne muscular dystrophy (DMD) and spinal muscular atrophy and are strongly associated with immobility.

SLEEP ONTOGENY

The organization of sleep initiates around 26 weeks of gestation. A discontinuous record with an interburst interval (IBI) of fewer than 30 seconds evolves to an IBI of fewer than 20 seconds beyond 30 weeks. The predominant sleep stage at this point is rapid eye movement (REM). At term, 60% of sleep is nonrapid eye movement (NREM). The first 3 months postnatally show further maturation with the emergence of sleep spindles and the development of circadian rhythm. The adult sleep pattern is achieved in the second year of life, characterized by 75–80% NREM and 15–25% REM sleep. A sleep cycle of 90 minutes passes through stages N1 to N3 of NREM followed by REM, occurring approximately five to six times during sleep.[7] The salient features of sleep ontogeny and mature sleep stages have been enumerated in **Box 8.10.1**.

CLASSIFICATION OF SLEEP DISORDERS

The diagnostic classification of sleep disorders is crucial for standardizing definitions and enabling a systematic diagnostic approach. The International Classification of Sleep Disorders (ICSD) is used for categorizing sleep disorders. The third edition, ICSD-3, encompasses seven major categories of sleep disorders **(Box 8.10.2)**. It is worth noting that pediatric diagnoses align with adult diagnoses across most categories, except for sleep-related breathing disorders (SRBD).[1]

BOX 8.10.1: Landmark events in sleep ontogeny.

- *EEG patterns*:
  - <30 weeks PMA: Discontinuous, IBI <30 seconds, hypersynchronous background
  - >30 weeks PMA: IBI <20 seconds, asynchrony
- *Maturational rhythms*: STOP (<28 weeks), temporal theta (28–32 weeks)
- *REM*: 31 weeks
  - 0–3 months postnatally: Sleep spindles
  - 2–3 months postnatally: Circadian rhythm
  - 4–6 months postnatally: NREM differentiated into three stages
  - 1–2 years postnatally: Adult pattern of sleep, NREM 75–80%

(EEG: electroencephalogram; IBI: interburst interval; NREM: nonrapid eye movement; PMA: postmenstrual age; REM: rapid eye movement; STOP: spontaneous occipital theta activity)

BOX 8.10.2: Major categories of ICSD-3.

- Insomnia
- Sleep-related breathing disorders (SRBD)
- Central disorders of hypersomnolence
- Circadian rhythm sleep–wake disorders (CRSWD)
- Parasomnias
- Sleep-related movement disorders (SRMD)
- Other sleep disorders

(ICSD-3: International Classification of Sleep Disorders, third edition)

DIAGNOSIS OF SLEEP DISORDERS

The gold standard method for diagnosing pediatric sleep disorders is clinical assessment and polysomnography (PSG). PSG involves the continuous and simultaneous recording of multiple physiological parameters throughout a sleep period to characterize sleep and identify sleep disorders. The components assessed on PSG and the various sleep stages depicted have been enumerated in **Box 8.10.3** and **Table 8.10.1**. While PSG is considered a relatively painless, noninvasive procedure, it can be challenging and frightening for children. The first-night effect may result in sleep records not being fully representative of the usual sleep pattern. Moreover, PSG requires a laboratory setup and may not be available in all centers.[8,9]

In children, alternative methods to screen for sleep disorders include questionnaires, sleep logs, and sleep diaries. Components of a sleep log/diary are depicted in **Box 8.10.4**. Newer methods, such as actigraphy, have evolved for diagnosing and assessing treatment responses in pediatric sleep disorders.

Questionnaires Used in Assessing Pediatric Sleep Disorders

The gold standard for evaluating sleep disorders is overnight PSG. However, this procedure is technically challenging,

BOX 8.10.3: Components of polysomnography.

- Pressure transducer and thermistor for nasal flow
- Chest and abdominal belts
- Pulse oximetry
- Extended electroencephalogram (EEG)
- Chin electromyogram (EMG)
- Two leg channels
- An electrocardiogram (ECG)
- Simultaneous video monitoring

TABLE 8.10.1: Polysomnographic characteristics of sleep stages.

Stages	*EEG*	*EOG*	*Chin EMG*
Awake	Posterior dominant α rhythm	nonspecific	Muscle activity of variable amplitude, more than sleep stages
N1	θ (theta) activity	Sinusoidal conjugate slow eye movements	Reduced activity
N2	Sleep spindles, vertex waves, K complexes	Reduced eye movements	Further reduced activity
N3	δ (delta) activity	Further reduced eye movements	Further reduced activity
REM	Mixed frequency, predominant θ	Sinusoidal eye movements Conjugate rapid eye movements	No muscle activity

(EEG: electroencephalogram; EMG: electromyogram; EOG: electrooculogram; REM: rapid eye movement)

BOX 8.10.4: Essential components of a sleep log.

- Time to go to bed and time to get out of bed
- How long taken to fall asleep
- Number of hours slept
- Number of awakenings and their times, durations, and causes (e.g., nightmare, noise)
- Feelings before and after sleep
- Activities before going to sleep
- Presence during the day of a nap, exercise, medication, caffeine, or alcohol

and expertise is limited. Therefore, simple questionnaires for screening children and adolescents for sleep problems can help identify those who need expert evaluation and focused assessment using overnight PSG. Commonly used questionnaires are described below.

The *BEARS* questionnaire (the acronym stands for *B*edtime problems, *E*xcessive daytime sleepiness, *A*wakenings during night, *R*egularity of evening sleep time and morning awakening, and *S*noring) is a brief screening tool for ages 2–18 years.

The *Children's Sleep Habits Questionnaire (CSHQ)* is a parent-rated 33-item questionnaire for children aged 4–10 years, rated on a three-point scale. CSHQ yields a total score and eight sleep domain scale scores: Bedtime resistance, sleep duration, parasomnias, sleep-disordered breathing (SDB), night awakenings, daytime sleepiness, sleep anxiety, and sleep onset delay.

The *Pediatric Sleep Questionnaire (PSQ)* is a parent-rated, 22-item questionnaire for children aged 2–18 years. All items except for inattention/hyperactivity, which are rated on a four-point Likert scale, are rated on a three-point scale. PSQ provides a total score and describes five subscales, namely SRBD, snoring, sleepiness, behavior, and periodic limb movement disorder (PLMD).

The latest addition to the list of questionnaires is the *Childhood and Adolescent Sleep Evaluation Questionnaire (CASEQ)*, the first questionnaire developed and validated based on ICSD-3. It is a bilingual questionnaire (Hindi and English) comprising 27 primary and 9 secondary questions validated in 2–18-year-olds. All the primary and secondary questions have binary responses (yes/no), except one secondary question, which mentions the frequency and duration of symptoms. The presence or absence of a sleep problem is decided by the response to the primary questions. It covers all major subtypes of disorders under ICSD-3 and has questions related to insomnia, hypersomnolence, sleep-related breathing and movement disorder, circadian rhythm sleep–wake disorder (CRSWD), and parasomnias, including nocturnal enuresis. The response to secondary questions provides information on sleep hygiene, the frequency and duration of the symptoms mentioned in response to primary questions, and associated medical and psychological comorbidities.[10] The salient properties of the questionnaires are enumerated in **Table 8.10.2**.

Role of Actigraphy in Diagnosing Sleep Disorders

Actigraphy, utilizing ambulatory devices to estimate sleep–wake patterns from activity levels, has become common in pediatric research and practice. It provides a more objective measure than parent report and is advantageous for studying sleep–wake patterns over extended periods in a child's natural environment. Actigraphy involves using small wristwatch-sized activity monitors with internal accelerometers, translating collected data into sleep or awake epochs. While it is sensitive to sleep changes associated with interventions, its low specificity in detecting wakefulness within sleep periods is a limitation. Despite this, actigraphy is particularly applicable to field-based studies, offering more objectivity

TABLE 8.10.2: Characteristics of commonly used sleep questionnaires.

Questionnaire	*Age*	*Characteristic properties*
BEARS	2–18 years	Screens for *b*edtime problems, *e*xcessive daytime sleepiness, *a*wakenings during night, *r*egularity of evening sleep time and morning awakening, and *s*noring
CSHQ	4–10 years	• Based on ICSD-1 • 33-items questionnaire reporting bedtime resistance, sleep duration, parasomnias, SDB, night awakenings, daytime sleepiness, sleep anxiety, and sleep onset delay
PSQ	2–18 years	• Based on ICSD-1 • 22-items screening primarily for SDB, daytime sleepiness, and behavioral problems
CASEQ	2–18 years	• Based on ICSD-3 • 36-items questionnaire screening for symptoms of insomnia, SDB, hypersomnolence, SRMD, CRSWD, parasomnia, and nocturnal enuresis

(CASEQ: Childhood and Adolescent Sleep Evaluation Questionnaire; CRSWD: circadian rhythm sleep–wake disorder; CSHQ: Children's Sleep Habits Questionnaire; ICSD: International Classification of Sleep Disorders; PSQ: Pediatric Sleep Questionnaire; SDB: sleep-disordered breathing; SRMD: sleep-related movement disorder)

than questionnaires or sleep diaries. The American Academy of Sleep Medicine recommends the use of actigraphy in children with insomnia, CRSWD, and SRBD, but not in place of electromyogram (EMG) for the diagnosis of PLMD.[11]

MANAGEMENT OF PEDIATRIC SLEEP DISORDERS

The clinical and polysomnographic gold standard criteria for diagnosing pediatric sleep disorders are mentioned in the ICSD-3 manual.[12] The salient clinical characteristics and steps in management of these disorders are mentioned in the following text.[4,12,13]

Insomnia

Insomnia refers to persistent difficulty in sleep initiation despite adequate opportunity associated with daytime impairment. The prevalence of insomnia is up to 40% in children and 10% in adolescents. It comes in three types: Behavioral, psychophysiological, and transient. The behavioral subtype, more common in younger children, is treated with appropriate sleep hygiene, behavioral therapy, gradual withdrawal of parental involvement, and training children to self-soothe. The psychophysiological variety, more common in older children and adolescents, is treated with teaching appropriate relaxation techniques. Pharmacotherapy, specifically melatonin along with behavioral therapy, is considered when nonpharmacological measures are ineffective.

Sleep-related Breathing Disorders

Sleep-related breathing disorders encompass OSA syndrome, central sleep apnea syndromes, sleep-related hypoventilation disorders, and sleep-related hypoxemia disorder. Clinical features include snoring, witnessed apneas, daytime sleepiness, and associated behavioral and academic complaints. Treatment considerations for OSA are based on specific clinical and PSG criteria, with adenotonsillectomy (AT) considered the treatment of choice for moderate-to-severe cases. AT combined with weight loss is the first-line treatment in pediatric SRBD. Other options include intranasal corticosteroids, leukotriene-receptor antagonists for milder forms, and nasal continuous positive airway pressure (CPAP) for more severe sleep apnea. Screening for SRBD in children with underlying ADHD and learning difficulties is recommended.

Central Disorders of Hypersomnolence

Central disorders of hypersomnolence are characterized by excessive daytime sleepiness not attributable to another sleep disorder. This group includes narcolepsy type 1, narcolepsy type 2, idiopathic hypersomnia, Kleine–Levin syndrome, hypersomnia due to medical disorders or substances, and insufficient sleep syndrome. Diagnosis involves PSG followed by multiple sleep latency tests (MSLT), with reduced hypocretin-1 in cerebrospinal fluid seen in narcolepsy type 1. Treatment involves an individualized plan, incorporating education, good sleep hygiene, behavioral changes, and medication. Scheduled naps and medications such as psychostimulants, modafinil, and sodium oxybate may be used.

Circadian Rhythm Sleep–Wake Disorder

This group includes delayed sleep–wake phase disorder (DSPD), advanced sleep–wake phase disorder, irregular sleep–wake rhythm disorder, non-24-hour sleep–wake rhythm disorder, shift work disorder, jet lag disorder, and circadian sleep–wake disorder not otherwise specified. DSPD is the most common in adolescence, and treatment involves proper sleep hygiene practices and sometimes oral melatonin administered 3–5 hours before bedtime.

TABLE 8.10.3: Salient features of various parasomnias.

NREM parasomnias (first half of sleep)			***REM parasomnias (early morning)***	
Sleep walking	***Confusional arousals***	***Sleep terrors***	***Sleep terrors***	***REM behavioral disorder***
Simple or complex behavior with ambulation	Disorientation with slurred and incoherent speech	Terrorized, inconsolable and unresponsive child	Frightening dreams with arousal and agitation	Bizarre motor and behavioral patterns
Cloudy recollection	Complete amnesia	Associated autonomic manifestations	Complete recall	Associated narcolepsy

(NREM: nonrapid eye movement; REM: rapid eye movement)

Parasomnias

Parasomnias are undesirable physical events or experiences occurring during NREM, REM, or transitions to and from sleep. Treatment recommendations vary based on the type of parasomnia. For infrequently occurring confusional arousals, sleep terrors, and sleepwalking, reassurance and education about the self-limiting nature are often sufficient. Behavioral interventions and, if necessary, a low dose of benzodiazepine may be prescribed for persistent cases. The differentiating features between various parasomnias are enumerated in **Table 8.10.3**.

BOX 8.10.5: Components of sleep hygiene.

- Clear daytime schedule
- Parents to use positive, not negative, reinforcement for sleeping
- Avoid playing in bedroom
- Avoid heavy and stimulating food and beverages before sleep
- Promote sleeping by own and parents to avoid staying until the child falls asleep
- Consistency in schedule
- Reading for younger children and relaxation exercises for older children and adolescents
- Calm, dark room (dimmed light preferably)
- Avoid using electronic gadgets before sleep and remove them from bedroom

Sleep-related Movement Disorders

This group includes RLS, PLMD, sleep-related leg cramps, sleep-related bruxism, sleep-related rhythmic movement disorder, benign sleep myoclonus of infancy, propriospinal myoclonus at sleep onset, sleep-related movement disorder (SRMD) due to a medical disorder, SRMD due to a medication or substance, and SRMD unspecified. For RLS/PLMD, behavioral interventions and iron supplementation are recommended based on subjective data and objective findings from PSG.

The various components of sleep hygiene, which are integral to management of all types of sleep disorders, are listed in **Box 8.10.5**.

SYSTEMIC DISORDERS AND SLEEP[13]

Craniofacial Syndromes

Within this group of disorders, sleep morbidity often presents as SDB, encompassing conditions such as OSA, upper airway resistance syndrome, and snoring. Examples of craniofacial syndromes include CHARGE, Crouzon, Apert, Pfeiffer, Pierre Robin, and Treacher Collins syndromes.

Medical Conditions

Children and adolescents with asthma may exhibit features of SRBD and insomnia, such as nocturnal awakenings and decreased sleep duration. Additionally, individuals with gastroesophageal reflux disease may experience delayed sleep onset.

Neurological and Behavioral Disorders

In cerebral palsy, the most common sleep morbidity is OSA. Various sleep disorders, including parasomnia, insomnia, hypersomnia, circadian rhythm sleep disorders (CRSD), and OSA, are observed in intellectual disability and autism spectrum disorders. Patients with epilepsy often experience fragmented sleep and frequent nocturnal awakenings. ADHD may present with various sleep morbidities such as OSA, RLS/PLMD, and narcolepsy. Neuromuscular disorders, Down syndrome, Arnold–Chiari malformation, mitochondrial disorders, and Joubert syndrome may exhibit both obstructive and central sleep apnea. Rett syndrome cases typically show CRSD and parasomnias. Narcolepsy is associated with Prader–Willi syndrome and Niemann–Pick disease. Mucopolysaccharidoses like Hurler syndrome can present with isolated OSA.

Medications and Sleep

Various medications, including antidepressants, antipsychotics, anticonvulsants, antiemetics, and antihistamines, can adversely affect sleep and lead to a range of sleep disorders.

Salient steps in evaluation of a child with sleep disorder are enumerated in **Box 8.10.6**.

BOX 8.10.6: Salient components of clinical evaluation for sleep disorders.

History
- The sleep environment
- Need for sleep aids
- Time of going to bed, sleep onset, and final morning awakening
- Snoring, mouth breathing, cessation of breathing
- Paroxysmal motor and behavioral events during sleep
- Daytime behavior and need for naps
- Medications

Examination
- Body mass index
- Craniofacial abnormalities (micrognathia, macroglossia, dental malocclusion, myopathic facies, midface hypoplasia)
- Deviated nasal septum, tonsillar hypertrophy, mouth breathing
- Brainstem involvement
- Features of neuromuscular disorders
- Parent–child interaction
- Home videos

Indications for PSG
- Obstructive sleep apnea
- Hypersomnia, including narcolepsy (along with multiple sleep latency test)
- Suspected parasomnia and sleep-related movement disorder (after ruling out epilepsy in both the scenarios)
- Repeat PSG to be considered if no REM record obtained, technically inadequate record, or sleep differs from home

(PSG: polysomnography; REM: rapid eye movement)

CONCLUSION

Adequate sleep holds paramount significance for optimal health, well-being, and cognitive functioning. Research indicates that insufficient sleep is associated with adverse physical, behavioral, and cognitive outcomes. Questionnaire-based tools have revealed sleep morbidities in up to 50% of normal school-going children and adolescents, rising to 80% among those with underlying medical and developmental disorders.

Currently, awareness regarding sleep and its morbidities among caregivers and healthcare professionals is suboptimal.[14] Moreover, there is a shortage of sleep experts. The gold standard for evaluating sleep disorders, PSG, is a cumbersome and technically demanding procedure, necessitating a specific laboratory setup and an overnight hospital stay. Simple, holistic, easy-to-apply, and scientifically sound questionnaires have been designed to screen children for the entire spectrum of sleep disorders. This approach can enhance awareness, leading to better and optimal referrals to sleep experts and the judicious use of resources such as PSG.

REFERENCES

1. Sateja MJ. International classification of sleep disorders-third edition: highlights and modifications. Chest. 2014;146:1387-94.
2. Lewandowski AS, Toliver-Sokol M, Palermo TM. Evidence-based review of subjective pediatric sleep measures. J Pediatr Psychol. 2011;36:780-93.
3. Luginbuehl M, Kohler WC. Screening and Evaluation of Sleep Disorders in Children and Adolescents. Child Adolesc Psychiatric Clin N Am. 2009;18:825-38.
4. Ophoff D, Slaats MA, Boudewyns A, Glazemakers I, Van Hoorenbeeck K, Verhulst SL. Sleep disorders during childhood: a practical review. Eur J Pediatr. 2018;177:641-8.
5. Manokaran RK, Tripathi M, Chakrabarty B, Pandey RM, Gulati S. Sleep abnormalities and polysomnographic profile in children with drug-resistant epilepsy. Seizure. 2020;82:59-64.
6. Aathira R, Gulati S, Tripathi M, Shukla G, Chakrabarty B, Sapra S, et al. Prevalence of Sleep Abnormalities in Indian Children With Autism Spectrum Disorder: A Cross-Sectional Study. Pediatr Neurol. 2017;74:62-7.
7. Scher MS. Ontogeny of EEG-sleep from neonatal through infancy periods. Sleep Med. 2008;9:615-36.
8. Boss EF, Benke JR, Tunkel DE, Ishman SL, Bridges JFP, Kim JM. Public insurance and timing of polysomnography and surgical care for children with sleep-disordered breathing. JAMA Otolaryngol Head Neck Surg. 2015;141:106-11.
9. Konka A, Weedon J, Goldstein NA. Cost-benefit analysis of polysomnography versus Clinical Assessment Score-15 (CAS-15) for treatment of pediatric sleep-disordered breathing. Otolaryngol Head Neck Surg Off J Am Acad Otolaryngol Head Neck Surg. 2014;151:484-8.
10. Zulfiqar L, Chakrabarty B, Gulati S, Jauhari P, Pandey RM, Tripathi M, et al. The Childhood and Adolescent Sleep Evaluation Questionnaire (CASEQ): Development and validation of an ICSD-3-based screening instrument, a community and hospital-based study. J Sleep Res. 2022;31: e13479.
11. Smith MT, McCrae CS, Cheung J, Martin JL, Harrod CG, Heald JL, et al. Use of Actigraphy for the Evaluation of Sleep Disorders and Circadian Rhythm Sleep-Wake Disorders: An American Academy of Sleep Medicine Systematic Review, Meta-Analysis, and GRADE Assessment. J Clin Sleep Med. 2018;14:1209-30.
12. American Academy of Sleep Medicine. International classification of sleep disorders, 3rd ed. Darien, IL: American Academy of Sleep Medicine; 2014.
13. Sheldon SH. Sleep in infants and children. In: Lee-Chiong TL (Ed). Sleep: A Comprehensive Handbook. Hoboken: John Wiley & Sons, Inc.; 2006.
14. Rajan A, Chakrabarty B, Gulati S, Jauhari P, Pandey RM, Tripathi M, et al. Childhood and Adolescent Sleep Awareness in Caregivers and Health Care Providers: A Community- and Hospital-Based Survey. Pediatr Neurol. 2023;147:14-23.

8.11 Autoimmune and Demyelinating Neurologic Disorders

Ruchika Jha, Vishal Sondhi

INTRODUCTION

Although individually uncommon, autoimmune causes collectively comprise a significant proportion of autoimmune neurologic disorders in children, with an acute or subacute presentation.[1] Antibody-mediated diseases of the central nervous system (CNS) are now increasingly recognized in childhood, where the antibodies directed toward ion channels, receptors, or membrane proteins bind to cell surface epitopes on neuronal or glial proteins, and the patients demonstrate either focal or more generalized clinical signs depending on the extent of brain regions targeted by the antibodies.[2] The spectrum of presentation of autoimmune neurologic disorders is broad **(Flowchart 8.11.1)**, based on the underlying immune dysregulation, mandating a high degree of suspicion. Moreover, their timely detection and appropriate management are of paramount importance due to the possible chronic sequelae and disease burden entailed.

EPIDEMIOLOGY

In a recent study on the incidence of autoimmune neurologic disorders, the mean incidence rates were 1.54 children/million [95% confidence interval (CI) 0.95–2.35] and 2.49 children/million (95% CI 1.73–3.48) for autoimmune encephalopathy (AIE) and acute disseminated encephalomyelitis (ADEM), respectively.[3] The annual incidence of all acquired demyelinating CNS disorders is estimated at 0.5–1.66 per 100,000 children.[4-7] With the advent of well-defined guidelines for diagnosis and antibody testing, a more accurate estimation of these autoimmune disorders will be more likely.

ETIOPATHOGENESIS

Different pathogenic mechanisms have been identified such as cell-mediated, antibody-mediated, infection-triggered, paraneoplastic, and genetically defined mechanisms that can occur in previously healthy children, and these can contribute to different stages of the disease **(Table 8.11.1)**.[8]

Infections

A history of a recent infection, typically a nonspecific upper respiratory or gastrointestinal illness, is commonly elicited in pediatric patients with autoimmune neurologic conditions. Selected examples of notable infectious triggers include

Flowchart 8.11.1: The spectrum of pediatric autoimmune neurologic disorders.

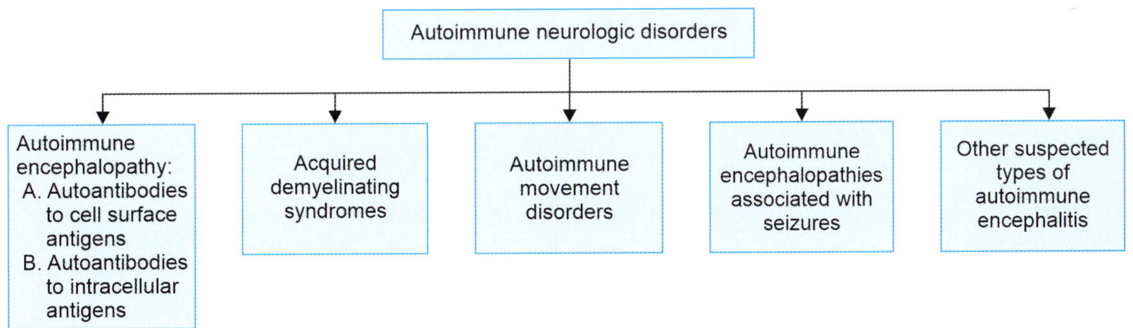

TABLE 8.11.1: Proposed triggers/agents for autoimmune disorders, including encephalopathies.

Triggers/etiological factors	
Infections • Postviral immune encephalitis • Nonviral agents	 • HSV, VZV, EBV, HHV-6, CMV, HIV, adenovirus • *Rickettsia*, *Mycoplasma*, *Streptococcus*
Postvaccination	Influenza, poliomyelitis, DPT, Japanese B encephalitis
Paraneoplastic: Tumoral antigens shared by neuronal cell antigens	Ovarian teratoma, testicular carcinoma, Hodgkin lymphoma, neuroblastoma

(CMV: cytomegalovirus; DPT: diphtheria–pertussis–tetanus; EBV: Epstein–Barr virus; HIV: human immunodeficiency virus; HHV-6: human herpes virus type 6; HSV: herpes simplex virus; VZV: varicella zoster virus)

Herpes simplex encephalitis with anti-*N*-methyl-D-aspartate receptor (NMDAR) antibody encephalitis and the range of poststreptococcal immune-mediated disorders. While some infections may trigger autoimmunity following a relatively short period, others may predispose to chronic inflammation in the CNS, such as in Epstein–Barr virus (EBV) infection and multiple sclerosis. In some instances, the infection, by increasing circulating cytokines that alter blood–brain barrier permeability, may merely serve to precipitate subclinical disease related to a preexisting antibody.

Genetics

A personal or family history of other autoimmune conditions suggests an autoimmune cause for a child's neurologic presentation. However, with the exception of human leukocyte antigen (HLA) DRB1*1501 in pediatric multiple sclerosis (MS), the other genes involved are unknown.

CLINICAL FEATURES

Autoimmune Encephalopathies

Children with AIE present with acute or subacute onset of neuropsychiatric symptoms due to an underlying abnormal immune response to the CNS.[9,10] Typically, children with AIE are previously healthy and present with rapid onset of neuropsychiatric symptoms **(Table 8.11.2)**. Prodromal symptoms, including fever, occur in over 50% of patients. Between disease onset and initiation of therapy, symptoms

TABLE 8.11.2: Clinical features of autoimmune encephalopathies.

Disease	*Antibodies/mechanisms*	*Syndrome*
A. Autoantibodies to cell surface antigens		
Anti-NMDAR encephalitis	• Antibodies against GluN1 subunit of NMDAR • Triggering factor may be HSV encephalitis or tumor; however, most cases are idiopathic	• Psychiatric symptoms • Decreased verbal output • Sleep disorder (mainly insomnia) • Seizures • Dyskinesias (orofacial, limbs) • Dystonia, rigidity, and other abnormal movements • Autonomic dysfunction • Hypoventilation
VGKC complex	The target antigens for some VGKC-complex antibodies are proteins tightly complexed with the VGKC, including the secreted synaptic protein leucine-rich glioma inactivated 1 (LGI1), the transmembrane axonal protein, contactin-associated protein 2 (CASPR2), and contactin 2	• Limbic encephalitis • Neuromyotonia • Morvan syndrome
Encephalitis associated with $GABA_AR$ antibodies	Antibodies against subunits of $GABA_AR$	• Refractory seizures • Epilepsia partialis continua • Limb or orofacial dyskinesias
Encephalitis with mGluR5 antibodies (Ophelia syndrome)	Antibodies against mGluR5	• Abnormal behavior • Seizures • Memory deficits
Other autoimmune encephalitis (infrequent in children)	Antibodies against $GABA_BR$, DPPX, GlyR, D2R	• *$GABA_BR$:* Encephalitis, seizures, cerebellar ataxia • *DPPX:* CNS hyperexcitability, PERM, cognitive dysfunction, psychiatric features, resting tremor, and myoclonus • *GlyR:* PERM, stiff person syndrome • *D2R:* Basal ganglia encephalitis
B. Autoantibodies to intracellular antigens		
Autoimmune encephalitis	Antibodies to intracellular/intraneuronal antigens (Hu, Ma2, GAD65, amphiphysin)	• *Hu:* Brainstem/limbic encephalitis • *Ma2:* Encephalitis • *GAD65:* Limbic encephalitis, epilepsy • *Amphiphysin:* Stiff person syndrome, myelopathy and myoclonus, encephalomyelitis, or sensory neuronopathy (not reported in children)

(anti-NMDR: anti-*N*-methyl-D-aspartate receptor; CNS: central nervous system; DPPX: dipeptidyl-peptidase-like protein 6; D2R: antidopamine receptor; $GABA_AR$: antibodies against the α1 subunit of the γ-aminobutyric acid A receptor; $GABA_BR$: antibodies against the β subunit of the γ-aminobutyric acid A receptor; GAD65: glutamine acid decarboxylase 65; GlyR: glycine receptor; HSV: Herpes simplex virus; mGluR5: metabotropic glutamate receptor 5 antibodies; PERM: progressive encephalomyelitis with rigidity and myoclonus; VGKC: voltage-gated potassium channel) typically persist over time.[7] Children with AIE are more likely to present with multifocal neuropsychiatric symptoms rather than isolated clinical syndromes. Pediatric AIE is less associated with tumors compared with adults.

Acquired Demyelinating Disorders

Acquired demyelinating syndrome (ADS) represents a group of different inflammatory demyelinating disorders of the CNS, characterized by immune-mediated damage to the myelin, manifesting as neurologic dysfunction.[11] These immune-mediated dysfunctions can be classified based on four different criteria. *First,* based on the localization of neurological deficits, they may be classified into monofocal and multifocal. In monofocal ADS, the child presents with neurologic signs and symptoms attributable to a single CNS location such as optic neuritis (ON). In multifocal ADS, the patient presents with signs/symptoms attributable to multiple CNS sites (as in ADEM). *Second,* ADS may be classified based on disease course into monophasic (ADEM) or relapsing disorders (MS). *Third,* ADS can be classified based on the presence of encephalopathy (ADEM) or the absence of the same (MS). *Last,* one can classify ADS depending on the presence or absence of specific antibodies such as antiaquaporin antibodies (AQP4) and myelin oligodendrocyte glycoprotein (MOG). The clinical features of ADS have been illustrated in **Table 8.11.3**.

TABLE 8.11.3: Clinical features of acquired demyelinating disorders.

Phenotype	*Clinical features*
Acute disseminated encephalomyelitis (ADEM)	*Neurological manifestations:* • Polyfocal deficits • Encephalopathy (defined as behavioral change and/or alteration in the level of consciousness) • Behavioral abnormality (aggression, irritability, psychosis, mood changes) • Seizures • Speech defects (aphasia) • Optic neuritis • Motor deficits • Cerebellar ataxia • Movement disorders • Spinal cord dysfunction (paraparesis, bladder/bowel dysfunction) *Other manifestations:* • Febrile illness in 4 weeks prior to onset of neurological symptoms • Fever at time of presentation • Headache • Vomiting • Meningismus
Clinically isolated syndrome	*Neurological manifestations:* • Optic neuritis • Transverse myelitis • Seizures • Motor deficits (paraparesis/hemiparesis) • Brainstem syndrome (internuclear ophthalmoplegia/diplopia/dysarthria) *Other manifestations:* • No fever • No encephalopathy
Optic neuritis	• Reduced visual acuity • Unilateral/bilateral • Pain with ocular movement • Increased central scotoma • ±Papillitis • Red color desaturation
Transverse myelitis	• Paraparesis • Sensory level • Bladder involvement • Initial flaccidity and hyporeflexia; evolves to spasticity and hyperreflexia
Multiple sclerosis	• Optic neuritis (usually unilateral) • Motor deficits (focal motor deficits, paraparesis, hemiparesis) • Sensory dysfunction • Cerebellar abnormalities (dysarthria, ataxia) • No encephalopathy
Neuromyelitis optica spectrum disorder	• Optic neuritis (unilateral or bilateral) • Transverse myelitis • Vomiting at the onset

Autoimmune Movement Disorders

In a prospective study of 52 children presenting with an acute-onset movement disorder, an immune etiology was identified in 42% of patients.[12] NMDAR antibody encephalitis and basal ganglia encephalitis associated with antidopamine receptor (D2R) antibodies, opsoclonus–myoclonus syndrome (OMS), Sydenham chorea (SC), and systemic lupus erythematosus (SLE) are the autoimmune etiology-based movement disorders. The clinical features of autoimmune movement disorders have been summarized in **Table 8.11.4**.

Autoimmune Encephalopathies Associated with Epilepsy and Status Epilepticus

The role of the immune system in epilepsy has been critically reviewed, particularly how neuroinflammation is integrally related to the pathogenesis of epilepsy and in sustaining seizure activity.[13] The International League Against Epilepsy (ILAE) has included "immune" as an etiology in the ILAE revised terminology for the organization of seizures and epilepsies. These patients present primarily with seizures, sometimes in the absence of other features of encephalitis

TABLE 8.11.4: Clinical features of autoimmune movement disorders.

Disease	*Antibodies/mechanisms*	*Syndrome*
Autoimmune movement disorders		
OMS	Only a small minority of pediatric patients have Hu antibodies, and most patients do not have an identifiable autoantibody	• OMS classically causes opsoclonus, nonepileptic myoclonus, ataxia, sleep disturbance, cognitive dysfunction, and behavioral disruption • Approximately 50% of pediatric patients with OMS have a neuroblastoma
SC	Despite indicators of autoimmunity and the recent identification of D2R antibodies in a proportion (10/30) of SC patients, a definitive autoimmune process or autoantibody is yet to be proven	• The onset of chorea is often acute • Orofacial involvement is often noted, alongside vocalizations due to chorea involving orolingual movements • Speech can be affected in up to 40% of patients with dysarthria, reduced fluency, and reduced prosody • Accompanying features are motor impersistence, emotional lability, obsessive–compulsive disorder, attention deficit hyperactivity disorder, and psychosis
• Autoimmune tic and neuropsychiatric disorder • Pediatric Autoimmune Neuropsychiatric Disorders associated with streptococcal (PANDAS) infections	D2R antibodies have been identified in a subgroup of patients; however, the clinical relevance and pathogenicity of these antibodies remain unclear at present	The primary movement disorder is tics, although the dominant phenotype is emotional lability with anxiety, obsessive–compulsive behaviors, irritability, and change in function

(D2R: antidopamine receptor antibodies; OMS: opsoclonus–myoclonus syndrome; SC: Sydenham chorea)

TABLE 8.11.5: Clinical features of autoimmunity in epilepsy syndromes.

Disease	*Antibodies/mechanisms*	*Syndrome*
Autoimmune encephalopathies associated with epilepsy and status epilepticus		
Rasmussen encephalitis	• Proposed etiology includes the presence of neuronal antibodies and T-cell-mediated mechanisms triggered by a viral infection • Antibodies found are against GluR3, alpha-7-nicotinic acetylcholine receptor, and Munc-18-1	Refractory encephalopathy characterized by progressive refractory focal seizures, cognitive deterioration, and focal neurological deficits occurring with gradual atrophy of one brain hemisphere
• Fever-induced refractory epileptic encephalopathy syndrome (FIRES) • Acute encephalitis with refractory repetitive partial seizures (AERPS) • Devastating epilepsy of school-aged children (DESC) • New-onset refractory status epilepticus (NORSE)	CSF oligoclonal bands, or serum antibodies to GluR-epsilon2 and VGKC-complex have been found in a few patients; however, the pathogenic significance of these antibodies in this clinical context is unclear	Devastating encephalopathies with refractory seizures that are induced by fever or an inflammatory process

(CSF: cerebrospinal fluid; GluR3: glutamate receptor 3; VGKC: voltage-gated potassium channel)

or encephalopathy, although the seizures and electrographic abnormalities might be severe enough to produce an "epileptic" encephalopathy **(Table 8.11.5)**.

Other Autoimmune Encephalopathies

The features of other autoimmune encephalopathies have been illustrated in **Table 8.11.6**.

DIFFERENTIAL DIAGNOSIS

The differential diagnosis of pediatric autoimmune neurological disorders has been summarized in **Box 8.11.1**.

DIAGNOSIS

Clues in the history that an autoimmune disorder may be present include acute to subacute onset, preceding infection

TABLE 8.11.6: Clinical features of other autoimmune encephalopathies.[7]

Disease	Antibodies/mechanisms	Syndrome
Other autoimmune encephalopathies		
Bickerstaff encephalitis	Anti-GQ1b antibodies	Ophthalmoplegia, ataxia, and decreased level of consciousness with frequent hyperreflexia
Hashimoto encephalitis	Antithyroperoxidase (TPO) antibodies	Stroke-like symptoms, tremors, myoclonus, aphasia, seizures, ataxia, sleep, and behavioral problems
Rapid onset obesity with hypothalamic dysfunction, hypoventilation, and autonomic dysregulation (ROHHAD)	An autoimmune or paraneoplastic etiology is supported by frequent association with neural crest tumors	Rapid onset obesity, hyperphagia, abnormal behavior, autonomic dysfunction, and central hypoventilation
Chronic lymphocytic inflammation with pontine perivascular enhancement responsive to steroids (CLIPPERS)	No specific antibody association	Episodic diplopia or facial paresthesias with subsequent brainstem or spinal cord dysfunction
Systemic inflammatory disorders such as SLE, antiphospholipid syndrome	• Some patients with SLE have been shown to have neuronal surface antibodies, suggesting specific autoimmune targeting of the brain • Patients with antiphospholipid syndrome presenting with movement disorders have shown elevated IgG binding to the cell surface of neuron-like cells	• Systemic autoimmune disorders may also result in CNS inflammation as a component of the same disease process • This may be mediated by a less specific mechanism, whereby systemic inflammation results in "spillover" inflammation into the CNS, or a more disease-specific mechanism, where the primary etiology, as in a vasculitis, is also present in the brain

(CNS: central nervous system; SLE: systemic lupus erythematosus)

BOX 8.11.1: Differential diagnosis of pediatric autoimmune neurological disorders.[7]

- *Infections*
  - Meningitis
  - Viral encephalitis
  - Relapsing post-HSV encephalitis
  - Intracerebral abscess
  - Systemic infections
- *Seizures/epilepsy*
  - Convulsive or nonconvulsive status epilepticus
  - Epileptic encephalopathy
- *Genetic*
  - Genetic disorders that can manifest as autoimmune encephalitis: HLH, RANBP2 mutations, interferonopathies, autoinflammatory syndromes (including cryopyrin-associated periodic syndromes), CTLA4 deficiency
  - Leukoencephalopathies
  - Mitochondrial encephalopathy
- *Metabolic:* Inborn errors of metabolism such as glutaric aciduria type I, 3-methylglutaconic aciduria, creatine transport deficiency, Leigh syndrome, Wilson syndrome, Lesch–Nyhan syndrome, Pantothenate kinase-associated neurodegeneration, porphyria, urea cycle defects
- *Psychiatric disorders*
- New-onset psychosis
- Kleine–Levin syndrome
- Childhood disintegrative disorder/late-onset autism
- *Others*
- Monoamine neurotransmitter disorder
- CNS vasculitis
- Limbic encephalitis
- Encephalitis lethargica
- Neuroleptic malignant syndrome
- *Drugs:* Drugs affecting the dopaminergic pathways such as ketamine, phencyclidine, etc.

(CNS: central nervous system; CTLA4: cytotoxic T-lymphocyte-associated protein-4; HLH: hemophagocytic lymphohistiocytosis; HSV: herpes simplex virus; RANBP2: Ran-binding protein 2)

TABLE 8.11.7: Initial investigations for suspected AIE.

Diagnostic imaging	Brain MRI with gadolinium (T1, T2, FLAIR, and DWI sequences) + MRI spine (if features suggestive of spinal cord involvement)
Blood tests	• CBC with differential, ESR, CRP, ferritin • Serum testing for antibodies associated with AIE • Vitamin B12, vitamin D levels • Free T3, TSH, and thyroid autoantibodies [antithyroperoxidase (TPO), antithyroglobulin, anti-TSH receptor antibodies] • ANA and expanded nuclear antigen panel if features suggestive of systemic autoimmunity also present • Serum complement levels, immunoglobulin levels
Lumbar puncture	• Opening pressure, CSF cytology, protein, lactate, oligoclonal bands, infectious testing based on regional epidemiology • CSF testing for antibodies associated with AIE • Save 5–10 mL for future testing
Respiratory tests	Nasopharyngeal swab for respiratory viruses, mycoplasma
EEG	Epileptiform discharges, changes in background activity
Others	PET/SPECT if indicated

(AIE: autoimmune encephalopathy; ANA: antinuclear antibodies; CBC: complete blood count; CRP: C-reactive protein; CSF: cerebrospinal fluid; DWI: diffusion-weighted imaging; EEG: electroencephalography; ESR: erythrocyte sedimentation rate; FLAIR: fluid-attenuated inversion recovery; MRI: magnetic resonance imaging; PET: positron emission tomography; SPECT: single photon emission computed tomography; T3: triiodothyronine; TSH: thyroid stimulating hormone)

or vaccination, fluctuating course, prior episodes of similar symptoms, and personal or family history of autoimmunity. A comprehensive physical examination may yield clues to the presence of a systemic autoimmune disorder. The neurologic examination should attempt to localize the symptoms and signs within the nervous system and seek pathognomonic patterns that can point toward specific autoimmune disorders.

Diagnostic Approach to a Child with Suspected Autoimmune Encephalopathy

The diagnostic approach and the relevant investigation in a child with suspected autoimmune encephalitis are outlined in **Table 8.11.7**.

Diagnostic Approach to a Child with Suspected Acquired Demyelinating Syndrome

The diagnostic approach and the relevant investigation in a child with suspected acquired demyelination have been outlined in **Box 8.11.2**.

BOX 8.11.2: Initial investigations for suspected acquired demyelination.

- *Investigations that should be considered for all cases with suspected acquired demyelination*
  - Contrast-enhanced MRI brain + spine + optic nerves
  - Serum AQP4
  - Serum MOG-Ab
  - CSF for:
    - Cells, glucose, proteins
    - IgG and albumin
    - CSF IgG index
    - Oligoclonal bands
- *Investigations that may be considered based on a case-to-case basis*
  - Evoked potentials
    - Visual evoked potentials
    - Brainstem evoked response audiometry
    - Somatosensory evoked potentials
  - Optical coherence tomography
  - Investigations for systemic autoimmunity
    - C3, C4
    - ANA, anti-ds-DNA
    - ESR
    - CRP
  - 25(OH)-vitamin D
  - Bacterial and viral studies

(ANA: antinuclear antibody; anti-ds-DNA: anti-double-stranded deoxyribonucleic acid; AQP4: aquaporin-4; CRP: C-reactive protein; CSF: cerebrospinal fluid; ESR: erythrocyte sedimentation rate; IgG: immunoglobulin G; MOG-Ab: myelin oligodendrocyte glycoprotein antibody; MRI: magnetic resonance imaging)

TABLE 8.11.8: Initial investigations for suspected autoimmune movement disorders.

Diagnostic imaging	• Brain MRI with contrast • Whole body imaging for tumor evaluation if positive antibody • Ovarian/testicular ultrasonography (USG)
Lumbar puncture	• CSF cell count, protein, glucose, IgG index, oligoclonal bands, neopterin, antibodies • Also consider CSF neurotransmitters, lactate, pyruvate, amino acids
Serum autoimmune studies	• Antinuclear antibody (ANA), thyroid autoantibodies • Serum autoimmune antibody panel
EEG	Epileptiform discharges, changes in background activity
Genetic/metabolic evaluation	To ascertain other etiologies of movement disorders

(CSF: cerebrospinal fluid; EEG: electroencephalography; IgG: immunoglobulin G; MRI: magnetic resonance imaging)

Diagnostic Approach to a Child with Suspected Autoimmune Movement Disorders

The investigations for a child with suspected autoimmune movement disorder are outlined in **Table 8.11.8**.

TABLE 8.11.9: Diagnostic criteria for autoimmune encephalopathy/encephalitis.[7]

Diagnostic criteria for possible autoimmune encephalitis	• Subacute onset (<3 months) of working memory deficits, altered mental status, or psychiatric symptoms • At least one of the following: – Reasonable exclusion of alternative causes such as CNS infection, septic encephalopathy, drug toxicity, cerebrovascular disease, neoplasm, Creutzfeldt–Jakob disease, epilepsy, rheumatologic disorders, Kleine–Levin syndrome, Reye syndrome, mitochondrial disorder, and inborn errors of metabolism
Diagnostic criteria for anti-NMDAR encephalitis	Probable anti-NMDAR encephalitis: *All three of the following* • Rapid onset (<3 months) of at least four of the six following major groups of symptoms: – Abnormal (psychiatric) behavior or cognitive dysfunction – Speech dysfunction (pressured speech, verbal reduction, mutism) – Seizures – Movement disorder, dyskinesias, or rigidity/abnormal postures – Decreased level of consciousness – Autonomic dysfunction or central hypoventilation • At least one of the following laboratory study results: – Abnormal EEG (focal or diffuse slow or disorganized activity, epileptic activity, or extreme delta brush) – CSF with pleocytosis or oligoclonal bands • Reasonable exclusion of other disorders *Definite anti-NMDAR encephalitis:* Diagnosis can be made in the presence of one or more of the six major groups of symptoms and IgG anti-GluN1 antibodies,* after reasonable exclusion of other disorders
Diagnostic criteria for Bickerstaff's brainstem encephalitis	*Probable Bickerstaff's brainstem encephalitis* Diagnosis can be made when both of the following criteria have been met: • Subacute onset (rapid progression of <4 weeks) of all the following symptoms: – Decreased level of consciousness – Bilateral external ophthalmoplegia – Ataxia • Reasonable exclusion of alternative causes *Definite Bickerstaff's brainstem encephalitis:* Diagnosis can be made in the presence of positive IgG anti-GQ1b antibodies, even if bilateral external ophthalmoplegia is not complete, ataxia cannot be assessed, or if recovery has occurred within 12 weeks after onset
Diagnostic criteria for Hashimoto's encephalopathy	*Diagnosis can be made when all six of the following criteria have been met:* • Encephalopathy with seizures, myoclonus, hallucinations, or stroke-like episodes • Subclinical or mild overt thyroid disease (usually hypothyroidism) • Brain MRI normal or with nonspecific abnormalities • Presence of serum thyroid (thyroid peroxidase, thyroglobulin) antibodies • Absence of well-characterized neuronal antibodies in serum and CSF • Reasonable exclusion of alternative causes
Criteria for autoantibody-negative but probable autoimmune encephalitis	*Diagnosis can be made when all four of the following criteria have been met:* • Rapid progression (<3 months) of working memory deficits (short-term memory loss), altered mental status, or psychiatric symptoms • Exclusion of well-defined syndromes of autoimmune encephalitis (e.g., typical limbic encephalitis, Bickerstaff's brainstem encephalitis, acute disseminated encephalomyelitis) • Absence of well-characterized autoantibodies in serum and CSF, and at least two of the following criteria: – MRI abnormalities suggestive of autoimmune encephalitis – CSF pleocytosis, CSF-specific oligoclonal bands, or elevated CSF IgG index, or both – Brain biopsy showing inflammatory infiltrates and excluding other disorders (e.g., tumor) • Reasonable exclusion of alternative causes
Diagnostic criteria for definite autoimmune limbic encephalitis	*Diagnosis can be made when all four[†] of the following criteria have been met:* • Subacute onset (rapid progression of <3 months) of working memory deficits, seizures, or psychiatric symptoms suggesting involvement of the limbic system • Bilateral brain abnormalities on T2-weighted fluid-attenuated inversion recovery MRI highly restricted to the medial temporal lobes* • At least one of the following: – CSF pleocytosis (white blood cell count of >5 cells/mm^3) – EEG with epileptic or slow-wave activity involving the temporal lobes* • Reasonable exclusion of alternative causes

*^{18}Fluorodeoxyglucose (^{18}F-FDG) positron emission tomography (PET) can be used to fulfill this criterion. Results from studies in the past 5 years suggest that ^{18}F-FDG-PET imaging might be more sensitive than MRI to show an increase in FDG uptake in normal-appearing medial temporal lobes.

†If one of the first three criteria is not met, a diagnosis of definite limbic encephalitis can be made only with the detection of antibodies against cell-surface, synaptic, or onconeural proteins.

(CNS: central nervous system; CSF: cerebrospinal fluid; EEG: electroencephalography; IgG: immunoglobulin G; MRI: magnetic resonance imaging; NMDAR: *N*-methyl-D-aspartate receptor)

Diagnostic Criteria

There are well-defined diagnostic criteria proposed for these clinical syndromes, which can be referred to while establishing a diagnosis. They have been illustrated in **Tables 8.11.9 and 8.11.10**.

MANAGEMENT

The general therapeutic approach comprises the treatment or removal of the immunologic trigger when present, such as infections or tumors, and the early start of first-line immunotherapy. First-line drugs include corticosteroids, which have a broad mechanism of action on the immune system and may modulate the blood–brain barrier. Intravenous immunoglobulin (IVIG) is often given combined with corticosteroids and may have a broad immunomodulatory potential. Plasma exchange can also be applied, preferably before IVIG.

In patients who do not respond to first-line drugs in the first 2 weeks of treatment, second-line therapy with rituximab or cyclophosphamide should be started. Rituximab has a B cell depletion mechanism of action, resulting in a significant reduction of pro-inflammatory CD4 and CD8 T-cell responses, underlining broad immunosuppressant properties. In this regard, it is effective in refractory cases, and it may reduce the risk of relapses. Cyclophosphamide is the alternative second-line drug, and it has a broad cellular immunosuppressive action. It should be given to refractory cases with severe disease, weighing its potential for long-term infertility and secondary malignancy.

A subset of patients may benefit from maintenance immunotherapy. Oral prednisone or monthly IVIG may also be prescribed after clinical remission to reduce the relapse rate. When steroid dependence is proven or a relapsing course is detected in steroid-responsive patients, steroid-sparing agents such as azathioprine and mycophenolate mofetil are commonly used. When the first- and second-line treatments fail to achieve disease remission, very limited options such as bortezomib, tocilizumab, intrathecal steroids, or methotrexate might be considered. The basic aspects of

TABLE 8.11.10: Diagnostic criteria for various acquired demyelinating syndromes.

Entity	*Definition*
ADEM	*Clinical features (all are required)* • A first polyfocal, clinical CNS event with presumed inflammatory demyelinating cause • Encephalopathy that cannot be explained by fever • No new clinical and MRI findings emerge 3 months or more after the onset • Brain MRI is abnormal during the acute (3-month) phase *Lesion characteristics on brain MRI* • Diffuse, poorly demarcated, large (>1–2 cm) lesions involving predominantly the cerebral white matter • T1 hypointense lesions in the white matter are rare • Deep gray matter lesions (e.g., thalamus or basal ganglia) can be present
Multiphasic ADEM	*Multiphasic ADEM is defined as:* • Two episodes consistent with ADEM separated by 3 months but not followed by any further events • The second ADEM event can involve either new or a reemergence of prior neurologic symptoms, signs, and MRI findings Due to its very low frequency, the category of "recurrent ADEM" has been eliminated
Clinically isolated syndrome	*All of the following are required* • A monofocal or polyfocal, clinical CNS event with presumed inflammatory demyelinating cause • Absence of a prior clinical history of CNS demyelinating disease (e.g., absence of past ON, TM, and hemispheric or brainstem-related syndromes) • No encephalopathy (i.e., no alteration in consciousness or behavior) that cannot be explained by fever • The diagnosis of MS based on baseline MRI features is not met
MS	*Can be satisfied by any of the following:* • Two or more nonencephalopathic (e.g., not ADEM-like) clinical CNS events with presumed inflammatory cause, separated by >30 days and involving more than one area of the CNS • One nonencephalopathic episode typical of MS, which is associated with MRI findings consistent with the 2010 Revised McDonald criteria for DIS, and in which a follow-up MRI shows at least one new enhancing or nonenhancing lesion consistent with DIT MS criteria • One ADEM attack followed by a nonencephalopathic clinical event, 3 or more months after symptom onset, which is associated with new MRI lesions that fulfill the 2010 Revised McDonald DIS criteria • A first, single, acute event that does not meet ADEM criteria and whose MRI findings are consistent with the 2010 Revised McDonald criteria for DIS and DIT (applies only to children ≥12 years old)

Contd...

Contd...

Entity	Definition
Neuromyelitis optica	*All of the following are required:* • ON • Acute myelitis • At least two of three supportive criteria: – Contiguous spinal cord MRI lesion extending over three vertebral segments – Brain MRI not meeting diagnostic criteria for MS – Anti-AQP4 IgG seropositive status
MOG-AD	• The presence of a core clinical demyelinating event: – ON – TM – ADEM – Cerebral monofocal or polyfocal deficits – Brainstem or cerebellar deficits – Cerebral cortical encephalitis, often with seizures • A positive MOG-IgG antibody test – *Clear positive assay:* A clear positive MOG-IgG is defined by a live cell-based assay according to the individual assay cutoffs or by fixed cell-based assay result with a titer ≥1:100 – *Low positive assay:* A low positive MOG-IgG is defined by a live cell-based assay according to the individual assay cutoffs or by fixed cell-based assay result with a titer ≥1:10 and <1:100 In cases where the serum MOG-IgG titer is low positive, positive without a reported titer, or seronegative but with clear positive cerebrospinal fluid (CSF) MOG-IgG, at least one additional supportive clinical or MRI feature is required, along with a seronegative AQP4-IgG test to fulfill this criterion • The exclusion of a better diagnosis, including multiple sclerosis *Supportive features*: One or more of the following clinical and MRI features are required for the diagnosis in the absence of a clear positive cell-based serum MOG-IgG assay: • *For ON:* – Bilateral simultaneous clinical involvement – Longitudinal optic nerve involvement (>50% length of the optic nerve) – Perineural optic nerve sheath enhancement – Optic disc edema • *For myelitis:* – Longitudinally extensive myelitis – Central cord lesion or axial H-sign on imaging – Conus lesion • *For brain, brainstem, or cerebral syndrome*: – Multiple ill-defined T2-hyperintense lesions in supratentorial and often infratentorial white matter – Deep gray matter involvement – Ill-defined T2-hyperintensity involving pons, middle cerebellar peduncle, or medulla – Cortical lesion with or without lesional and overlying meningeal enhancement

(ADEM: acute disseminated encephalomyelitis; AQP4: aquaporin-4; CNS: central nervous system; DIT: dissemination in time; IgG: immunoglobulin G; MOG-AD: myelin oligodendrocyte glycoprotein antibody disease; MOG-IgG: myelin oligodendrocyte glycoprotein immunoglobulin G; MRI: magnetic resonance imaging; MS: multiple sclerosis; ON: optic neuritis; TM: transverse myelitis)

management are initiating immunotherapy, maintenance immunotherapy, supportive therapy, and screening for tumors as indicated.

The management of patients with AIE has been outlined in **Flowchart 8.11.2**. Patients with demyelination during the acute phase may be managed with pulse steroids. The subsequent management depends on the type of demyelination:

- *Neuromyelitis optica spectrum disorder (NMOSD)*: Long-term immune suppression
- *Myelin oligodendrocyte glycoprotein antibody disease (MOG-AD)*: No long-term immune suppression if first episode; else, will need maintenance immunotherapy
- *Multiple sclerosis*: Disease-modifying therapies such as interferon, glatiramer, fingolimod, etc.

Flowchart 8.11.2: Management of patients with autoimmune encephalopathy.

Clinically suspected autoimmune encephalopathy
- Acute or subacute (<12 weeks) onset of a recognizable antibody specific syndrome (NMDAR/VGKC/Glycine receptor/Dopamine receptor
- If partial syndrome, one additional supportive criteria required:
  - Previously normal
  - Viral or fever prodrome
  - History of autoimmunity
  - Evidence of CNS inflammation (CSF or imaging)

↓

Investigations

Serum studies
- Neuronal surface antibody studies (NMDAR, VGKC) and associated proteins (LGI1, CASPR2, Contacting; AMPAR; GABA; Glycine receptor; D2R)
- Other antibodies: GAD, Thyroid antibodies
- Onconeuronal if concerned
- Exclude other infective, systemic inflammatory, and metabolic disorders

EEG

CSF studies
- Cytology
- Biochemistry
- Microscopy
- IgG index
- Oligoclonal bands
- Extra samples to be stored for antibody studies if needed
- PCR for ruling out infective etiology based on cytology and biochemistry

Imaging
- MRI with contrast
- PET (Brain ± Whole body depending on antibody and onconeuronal pattern suspected)

↓

Treatment

Exclude infections and metabolic causes

- Chest radiograph
- Mantoux

↓

Acute Treatment
- First-line immunotherapy
  - IV methylprednisolone (30 mg/kg/day) x 5 days
  - ± IVIG 0.4 g/day × 5 days
  - ± Plasmapheresis
- Second-line immunotherapy
  - Rituximab (750 mg/m^2) day 1 and day 15
  - ± Cyclophosphamide

Factors influencing decision
- Severity of acute condition
- Early in disease course and reversible disease
- Risk of permanent disability
- Relapse risk
- Favorable side effect profile of treatment

Maintenance immunotherapy
- Long-term oral steroids
- Monthly IVIG pulse
- Steroid sparing agents like mycophenolate mofetil or azathioprine or rituximab

If no response and no antibody identified evaluate diagnosis again

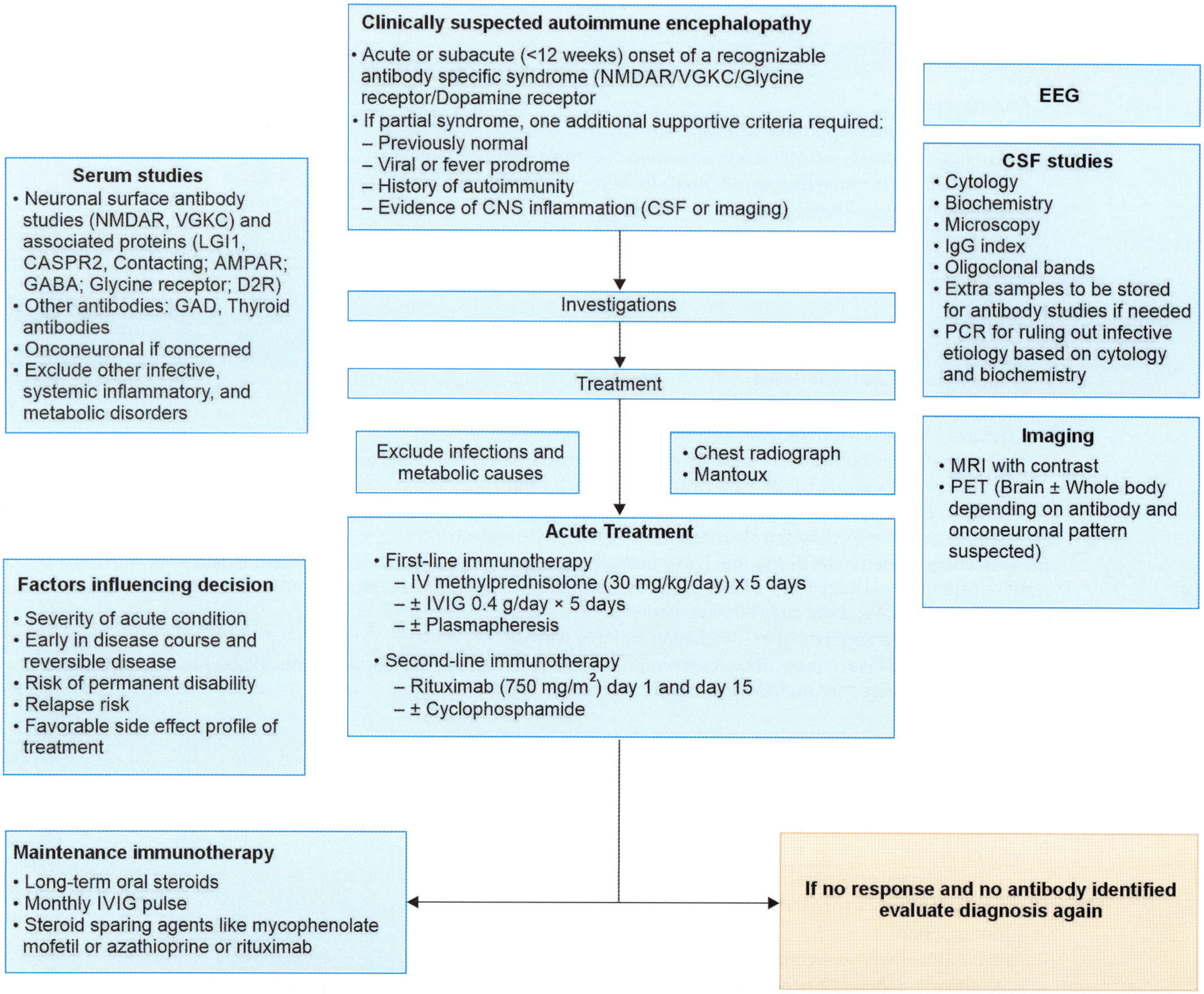

(CNS: central nervous system; CSF: cerebrospinal fluid; EEG: electroencephalography; GABA: gamma-aminobutyric acid; GAD: glutamic acid decarboxylase; IgG: immunoglobulin G; IV: intravenous; IVIG: intravenous immunoglobulin; LGI1: leucine-rich glioma inactivated 1; MRI: magnetic resonance imaging; NMDAR: *N*-methyl-D-aspartate receptor; PCR: polymerase chain reaction; PET: positron emission tomography; VGKC: voltage-gated potassium channel)

CONCLUSION

Over the past two decades, a broad range of autoimmune disorders of the central nervous system have been identified. In genetically vulnerable individuals, these disorders can be initiated by various factors. The manifestations of these disorders may vary from demyelination (MOGAD, NMOSD) to encephalitis (NMDAR, GAD). The autoimmune attacks target specific antigens that are clearly identified in disorders such as NMDAR encephalitis, MOGAD, and NMOSD; however, in conditions like multiple sclerosis, the targets are not well understood. Autoimmune attacks and their associated pathology can mainly be mediated by B cells and autoantibodies, as observed in NMOSD, or they can be primarily mediated by T cells, as seen in classic paraneoplastic disorders. Current treatment focuses on removing pathogenic autoantibodies through plasma exchange and administration of immunosuppression.

REFERENCES

1. Pillai SC, Hacohen Y, Tantsis E, Prelog K, Merheb V, Kesson A, et al. Infectious and autoantibody-associated encephalitis: clinical features and long-term outcome. Pediatrics. 2015;135(4):e974-84.

2. Lim M, Gorman M. Autoimmune neurologic disorders in children. Handb Clin Neurol. 2016;133:485-510.
3. de Bruijn M, Bruijstens AL, Bastiaansen AEM, van Sonderen A, Schreurs MWJ, Smitt PAES, et al. Pediatric autoimmune encephalitis: recognition and diagnosis. Neurol Neuroimmunol Neuroinflamm. 2020;7(3):e682.
4. Banwell B, Kennedy J, Sadovnick D, Arnold DL, Magalhaes S, Wambera K, et al. Incidence of acquired demyelination of the CNS in Canadian children. Neurology. 2009;72(3):232-9.
5. Langer-Gould A, Zhang JL, Chung J, Yeung Y, Waubant E, Yao J. Incidence of acquired CNS demyelinating syndromes in a multiethnic cohort of children. Neurology. 2011;77(12):1143-8.
6. Ketelslegers IA, Catsman-Berrevoets CE, Neuteboom RF, Boon M, van Dijk KJG, Eikelenboom MJ, et al. Incidence of acquired demyelinating syndromes of the CNS in Dutch children: a nationwide study. J Neurol. 2012;259(9):1929-35.
7. Graus F, Titulaer MJ, Balu R, Benseler S, Bien CG, Cellucci T, et al. A clinical approach to diagnosis of autoimmune encephalitis. Lancet Neurol. 2016;15(4):391-404.
8. Matricardi S, Farello G, Savasta S, Verrotti A. Understanding childhood neuroimmune diseases of the central nervous system. Front Pediatr. 2019;7:511.
9. Van Mater H. Pediatric inflammatory brain diseases: a diagnostic approach. Curr Opin Rheumatol. 2014;26(5):553-61.
10. Dalmau J, Graus F. Antibody-mediated encephalitis. N Engl J Med. 2018;378(9):840-51.
11. Neuteboom R, Wilbur C, Van Pelt D, Rodriguez M, Yeh A. The spectrum of inflammatory acquired demyelinating syndromes in children. Semin Pediatr Neurol. 2017;24(3):189-200.
12. Dale RC, Singh H, Troedson C, Pillai S, Gaikiwari S, Kozlowska K. A prospective study of acute movement disorders in children. Dev Med Child Neurol. 2010;52(8):739-48.
13. Vezzani A, French J, Bartfai T, Baram TZ. The role of inflammation in epilepsy. Nat Rev Neurol. 2011;7(1):31-40.

8.12 Infections of the Central Nervous System (including Acute Encephalitic Syndrome)

Aradhana Rohil, Gautam Kamila, Sonali Singh

INTRODUCTION

Infections of the central nervous system (CNS) are medical emergencies warranting neurointensive care. A detailed history and physical examination are necessary for localization, establishing the etiological agent, and guiding further investigations and management plans. The spectrum of CNS infections includes:

- Meningitis—acute, subacute, and chronic
- Encephalitis—acute, subacute, and chronic
- Localized infections—brain abscess, tuberculomas, and neurocysticercosis (NCC)
- Postinfectious syndromes

ACUTE BACTERIAL MENINGITIS

DEFINITION

Meningitis is characterized by inflammation of the leptomeninges surrounding the brain and spinal cord, often affecting the brain to a varying degree. It is categorized as acute, subacute, and chronic depending on the duration of illness—acute is defined as symptoms persisting for <5 days, subacute lasts 5 days to 4 weeks, and chronic persists for >4 weeks.

Acute bacterial meningitis (ABM) predominantly affects young children, with 90% of cases occurring between 1 month and 5 years of age. The incidence is highest in early infancy and decreases through childhood and adolescence.

The most common organisms causing bacterial meningitis vary by age, immune status, and other clinical conditions **(Tables 8.12.1 and 8.12.2)**. Beyond the neonatal period, *Haemophilus influenzae* type b (Hib), *Streptococcus pneumoniae,* and *Neisseria meningitidis*, are predominantly responsible for around 90% cases of ABM. In neonates, group B *streptococcus* (GBS), specifically *Streptococcus agalactiae*, and *Escherichia coli* are the primary culprits, followed by *Listeria monocytogenes.*

PATHOGENESIS

Mode of Spread

Most bacteria that cause meningitis, such as meningococcus, pneumococcus, and *H. influenzae*, are carried in the human nose and throat and are spread from person to person by respiratory droplets or throat secretions. GBS is often carried in the human gut or vagina and may infect the neonate during birth.

Predisposing Factors (Table 8.12.2)

- Younger age is associated with increased risk.
- People living in close proximity (mass gatherings, in refugee camps, in overcrowded households, or students)

TABLE 8.12.1: Etiological agents for acute bacterial meningitis.

Age	Causative bacteria
0–1 month—early onset	• *Escherichia coli* • *Klebsiella pneumoniae* • Other gram-negative bacilli • *Streptococcus agalactiae* • Group B Streptococcus • *Listeria monocytogenes*
Neonate—late onset	• *E. coli* • *K. Pneumoniae* • Enterobacter • Salmonella • *Staphylococcus aureus*
1–3 months	• *E. coli* • *K. pneumoniae* • Enterobacter • Salmonella • *S. aureus* • *Streptococcus pneumoniae* • *Neisseria meningitidis* • *Haemophilus influenzae* type B
3 months to 5 years	• *S. pneumoniae* • *H. influenzae* • *N. meningitidis* • Rarely—Pseudomonas and *Salmonella typhi*
5 years to adults	• *S. pneumoniae* • *N. meningitidis* • Rarely—*Pseudomonas* and *S. typhi*

TABLE 8.12.2: Etiological agents implicated in special scenarios.

Predisposing factors	Causative organisms
Cerebrospinal fluid (CSF) leak	*Streptococcus pneumoniae*
CSF shunt, meningomyelocele, and cranial trauma	• *Staphylococcus aureus* • *Staphylococcus epidermidis*
Splenic dysfunction—nephrotic syndrome/sickle cell anemia, etc.	• *S. pneumoniae* • *Haemophilus influenzae* • *Neisseria meningitidis*
Defects in complement system	*N. meningitidis*
T-cell defects	*Listeria monocytogenes*

- Congenital or acquired immunodeficiencies—human immunodeficiency virus (HIV) infection, complement deficiency, asplenia, autosplenectomy (sickle cell anemia), immunosuppression
- Anatomic defects of the spinal cord, brain, or inner ear (e.g., lumbosacral dermal sinus and meningocele)
- Acquired cranial defects due to basilar skull fracture or surgery
- Medical devices [cerebrospinal fluid (CSF) shunt, cochlear implant]
- Travel to endemic areas
- Parameningeal infections (sinusitis and mastoiditis)
- Recent infections (especially respiratory and ear infections)

Major Mechanisms for the Spread of Pathogen

The major mechanisms for the spread of pathogen to CNS includes colonization of the nasopharynx, with subsequent bloodstream invasion followed by CNS invasion. Another mechanism of nonhematogenous spread involves direct entry of organisms into the CNS from a contiguous infection site (e.g., sinusitis and mastoiditis), post-trauma, neurosurgery, or through direct communication of the subarachnoid space (SAS) with the skin or mucosa as in head trauma, dermal sinuses, and through infected CSF shunts, CSF leak, and cochlear implants.

The pathogens multiply in the SAS due to deficient local host defenses. It is followed by activation of the immune response, resulting in bacterial lysis, which further triggers an inflammatory response leading to disruption of the blood–brain barrier (BBB). Subsequently, leukocytes enter the CSF, leading to CSF pleocytosis, with the release of various toxic mediators adversely affecting the cerebral blood flow and metabolism. This results in the development of cerebral edema leading to decreased cerebral perfusion, raised intracranial pressure (ICP), and cerebral herniation. The inflammatory exudates cover the brain and cerebral blood vessels and cause vasculitis and thrombosis; ischemia may lead to cerebral infarction.

CLINICAL FEATURES

Diagnosis of ABM requires a high index of clinical suspicion in children. Typical symptoms of meningitis include fever along with symptoms of meningeal irritation such as headache, vomiting, stiff neck, photophobia, irritability with or without symptoms suggestive of brain involvement, or complications such as altered sensorium, confusion, seizures, or neurological deficits.

The clinical features vary depending on the age at presentation, underlying etiology, extent of involvement, and complications. In infants, symptoms suggestive of meningeal irritation such as stiff neck are less common, whereas systemic manifestations such as fever or hypothermia, lethargy, poor feeding, irritability, vomiting, diarrhea, respiratory distress, and jaundice are more common along with features such as bulging fontanel, seizures, and vomiting that could indicate complications.

Meningitis due to meningococcal infection may present with a fulminant course along with systemic features such as rash, petechiae or purpura, sepsis, shock (Waterhouse–Friderichsen syndrome), rapidly progressive cerebral edema, and raised ICP, evolving over a few hours.

Seizures occur in 20–30% of patients with meningitis, either prior to presentation or within the first 48 hours of admission, and are typically generalized but may be focal. If they occur later in the course, they are more likely a manifestation of an underlying complication.

The signs of meningeal inflammation include nuchal rigidity, Kernig sign, tripod sign, and Brudzinski sign and are present only in 60–80% of affected children at presentation. In *Kernig sign* with thighs flexed on the abdomen, passive extension of the knee produces pain in the back. In *Brudzinski sign* passive flexion of the neck produces flexion of both lower limbs. In the sitting position, child supporting himself/herself with both arms extended behind the back, is termed as *tripod sign*. Meningeal signs may be absent in children <18 months of age, those with severe malnutrition, terminal illness, immunocompromised state, or in partially treated meningitis. In conditions such as upper lobe pneumonia, typhoid fever, cervical spine disease, retropharyngeal abscess, myalgia, cervical lymphadenitis, cerebellar tonsillar herniation, and subarachnoid hemorrhage, meningeal signs may be falsely positive.

Features suggestive of raised ICP include bulging fontanel, headache, vomiting, and altered mental status. Late signs include the presence of Cushing triad (systemic hypertension, bradycardia, and respiratory depression), papilledema on funduscopic examination, and cranial nerve palsies of the 3rd, 4th, or 6th cranial nerves.

Features of parenchymal involvement include altered sensorium such as stupor, coma, obtundation, seizures, and focal neurological deficits including stroke.

Extra-CNS manifestations include rashes, petechiae, arthralgias, disseminated intravascular coagulation (DIC), shock, and pneumonia, which may be seen in some cases, depending on the etiology.

DIAGNOSIS

Diagnosis requires a high index of suspicion, especially in neonates and infants. Lack of fever or meningeal signs do not rule out meningitis in the presence of a clinical setting for the same. Blood investigations and CSF analysis should be performed preferably before initiation of therapy, on an emergency basis to confirm the diagnosis and identify the underlying etiological agent.

Cerebrospinal Fluid Analysis

Cerebrospinal fluid analysis should be performed in all suspected cases once contraindications are ruled out. Contraindications for performing a lumbar puncture (LP) include signs of raised ICP, or evidence of obstructive hydrocephalus, cerebral edema, and presence of local skin infection in needle track. Sepsis, hypotension, coagulation disorder (DIC or platelet counts <50,000/mm^3), or poor Glasgow coma scale (GCS) score <8 are relative contraindications for performing an LP. LP can be repeated after 48–72 hours in case of a traumatic tap or in case of no response to treatment.

While performing an LP, the CSF opening pressure should be checked. The CSF should be analyzed for its gross appearance (clear or turbid) and sent for biochemistry (CSF/blood glucose and proteins), cytology (total and differential counts), Gram stain for bacteria, Giemsa staining for cell differentiation, and cultures and sensitivity.

Rapid diagnostic tests detect bacterial antigens in the serum by countercurrent immune-electrophoresis, enzyme-linked immunosorbent assay (ELISA), and latex agglutination tests and multiplex polymerase chain reaction (PCR) assays can rapidly detect many organisms; however, these tests are not readily available at all centers.

The CSF picture in various scenarios is depicted in **Table 8.12.3**. CSF opening pressure is typically raised in ABM. Cloudy CSF under pressure is suggestive of ABM. The presence of polymorphonuclear leukocytosis (a few hundred to thousands), decreased glucose (<40 mg/dL or a CSF to

TABLE 8.12.3: CSF picture in meningitis caused by different etiological agents.

	Normal	*Pyogenic*	*Viral*	*Mycobacterial*	*Fungal*
Gross appearance	Clear	Turbid	Clear to turbid	Clear cobweb coagulum forms	Turbid/clear
Glucose (mg/dL)	>50	<40	Normal	<50	30–40
CSF/blood glucose	(≥2/3)	Very low ratio	Normal ratio	1/2–2/3 ratio	Low ratio
Protein	<40 mg/dL	100–500	Normal or slight increase	Up to 300 may be increased >500	100 (20–500)
Total cells	<5/mm^3	Up to several 1,000	Up to 100	25–100 (rarely >500)	Up to 50
Cell type	No polys	Neutrophils	Lymphocytes generally	Lymphocytes	Lymphocytes generally
Gram/other stains		Giemsa		Ziehl–Neelsen staining	
Other tests		Latex agglutination ELISA/PCR	PCR/ELISA viral panel	• PCR/BACTEC/ antigen-based tests • Gene Expert	Antigen-based tests PCR

(CSF: cerebrospinal fluid; ELISA: enzyme-linked immunosorbent assay; PCR: polymerase chain reaction)

serum glucose ratio of 0.4 or less in children and 0.6 or less in neonates), and increased protein concentration are common findings in ABM. An initial polymorphonuclear response may be seen in viral meningitis and an initial lymphocytic response in bacterial meningitis. The CSF glucose is normal in most cases of viral meningitis, except for a few like mumps, but is rarely below 20 mg/dL. CSF culture is the gold standard for organism identification; however, it is positive in only around 70% of cases, the detection rate being even lower in developing countries.

Blood and Other Investigations

These should include complete blood count (CBC) with differential counts, blood culture, inflammatory markers [e.g., C-reactive protein (CRP) and procalcitonin (PCT)], and tests to rule out complications such as serum electrolytes, glucose, blood urea nitrogen and creatinine, lactate levels, and coagulation studies, especially in patients with petechiae or purpuric lesions. Blood cultures are positive only in approximately 60–85% of patients with ABM.

Samples from other sites of infection, such as pleural fluid, cellulitis, otitis, aspiration of petechiae in suspected meningococcemia, and urine in young infants, should also be collected for organism identification.

Neuroimaging

Neuroimaging is not routinely indicated in ABM. Indications for neuroimaging in a case of ABM include coma or GCS < 8, papilledema or other signs of raised ICP, focal neurologic deficit, status epilepticus, CSF shunt in place, history of hydrocephalus, recent CNS trauma or neurosurgery, and poor response to treatment, to rule out complications [such as subdural empyema, focal cerebritis, evolving brain abscess, ventriculitis, vasculitis, parainfectious immune-mediated changes such as acute disseminated encephalomyelitis (ADEM), and hydrocephalus]. A normal computed tomography (CT) does not rule out raised ICP.

DIFFERENTIAL DIAGNOSIS

- Aseptic meningitis
- Tubercular meningitis (TBM)
- Fungal meningitis
- Parasitic infections—Naegleria
- Other causes of meningismus—pneumonia with right upper lobe involvement, retropharyngeal abscess, cervical lymphadenitis, and subarachnoid hemorrhage
- Other causes of coma/altered sensorium—acute encephalitis (viral, atypical bacteria, fungal, parasitic, and cerebral malaria), metabolic causes (neurometabolic disorders—acute decompensation, Reye syndrome, and hepatic encephalopathy)
- Other causes of neurological deficits—cerebral abscess, stroke, herpes encephalitis, intracranial bleeds, and space-occupying lesions

MANAGEMENT

Early antibiotic initiation, vigilant monitoring for complications, and appropriate supportive care are all pivotal in improving outcomes for children with ABM.

Antibiotic Therapy

The key principles for the antibiotic management of ABM include the following:

- *Early initiation of appropriate antibiotics in antimeningitic doses administered intravenously (IV).* Bactericidal antibiotics with good penetration into CSF are preferred. Therapeutic concentration in CSF should ideally be 10–30 times higher than the minimum bactericidal concentration (MBC) for the specific pathogen.
- *Empirical antibiotic therapy* should be started based on the likely pathogens and their resistance patterns in the community or hospital (antibiogram). A third-generation cephalosporin such as cefotaxime or ceftriaxone is recommended as initial monotherapy due to their broad spectrum of activity and ability to penetrate the BBB effectively. In neonates or infants up to 3 months of age, ampicillin should be added to the initial regimen to cover for *L. monocytogenes.*[1,2]
- *Antibiotic modification after culture and sensitivity results* are obtained from CSF or blood analysis **(Table 8.12.4)**. If there is no response after 48–72 hours, add vancomycin or a new antibiotic according to the CSF culture report. If there is still no response after addition of vancomycin after 48 hours change the third-generation cephalosporin antibiotic to meropenem. If there is a clinical response, but the culture is insensitive to the antibiotic/s being used, continue both.
- *Duration of antibiotic therapy:*
  - *Unspecified bacterial meningitis:* 10 days of antibiotic therapy
  - *N. meningitidis:* 7 days of antibiotic therapy
  - *H. influenzae:* 10–14 days of antibiotic therapy
  - *S. pneumoniae:* 10 days of antibiotic therapy
  - *Gram-negative bacillary and pseudomonal meningitis:* 21 days of antibiotic therapy
  - *Staphylococcus:* 28 days[2]
- The changes expected in CSF with antibiotic treatment are as follows:
  - CSF cultures are typically expected to become sterile within 24 hours of starting effective antibiotic therapy.
  - CSF glucose usually normalize within 48–72 hours of starting appropriate antibiotic therapy.

TABLE 8.12.4: Choice of antibacterial agents in acute bacterial meningitis.

Organism	*Empiric antibiotic of choice*	*Dose/day*	*Second-line choices*	*Minimum duration of treatment*
Unknown agent current regimen	• Ceftriaxone or • Cefotaxime	100 mg/kg/day in two divided doses 200–300 mg/kg/day (6–8 h)	–	10 days 10 days
Unknown agent conventional regimens used	• Ampicillin or • Penicillin G + chloramphenicol	• 200–300 mg/kg/day (6 h) • 250,000–400,000 U/kg/day (4–6 h) • 100 mg/kg/day (6 h)	–	10–14 days
Meningococcus	Penicillin G	250,000–400,000 U/kg/day	(% Resistance hence not recommended)	7 days
Pneumococcus	• Penicillin G; (resistance suspected) • Ceftriaxone + vancomycin	• 250,000–400,000 U/kg/day • Ceftriaxone—100 mg/kg/day in two divided doses • Vancomycin—60 mg/kg/day in three divided doses)	Meropenem ± aminoglycoside	10 days
Haemophilus influenzae	Ceftriaxone or Cefotaxime	• 100 mg/kg/day in two divided doses • 200 mg/kg/day in three divided doses	• Cefepime, 150 mg/kg (8 h) • Fluoroquinolones	10–14 days
Gram negative (except Pseudomonas)	Ceftriaxone or cefotaxime ± aminoglycosides (specific situations)	As above 200 mg/kg/day in three divided doses	Cefepime or Meropenem, 120 mg/kg/day (8 h)	21 days
Pseudomonas	Ceftazidime	150 mg/kg/day in two to three divided doses	Meropenem ± aminoglycides	14–21 days
Staphylococcus	Vancomycin + rifampicin	• 60 mg/kg/day in three divided doses • 20 mg/kg/day in two divided doses	• Linezolid • Cefepime	28 days
Enterococci	Ampicillin + gentamicin	• 150–200 mg/kg/day in four divided doses • 7.5 mg/kg/day in three divided doses	Vancomycin + gentamicin, 5 mg/kg (12 h)	21–28 days
Listeria	Ampicillin + gentamicin	• 200 mg/kg/day in four divided doses + • 7.5 mg/kg/day in three divided doses	Trimethoprim + sulfamethoxazole	21 days
Failed empiric therapy	• Meropenem • Cefepime	• 150 mg/kg/day in three divided doses • 120 mg/kg/day in two divided doses	• Linezolid, 10 mg/kg (12 h) • Fluoroquinolones, 20 mg/kg (6h)	Duration to be decided based on individual case scenarios

- Initially, there may be an increase in the total cell count in the CSF due to the influx of neutrophils. As therapy progresses and the infection begins to resolve, there is a shift toward a predominance of lymphocytes in the CSF. Persistence of neutrophils beyond 48 hours may indicate inadequate response to therapy or ongoing infection.
- Proteins in CSF take longer to normalize and may not be a reliable parameter for monitoring the adequacy of antibiotic therapy in the short term.

Role of Corticosteroids in Acute Bacterial Meningitis

Corticosteroids, particularly dexamethasone, have been studied for their role in managing ABM, primarily to mitigate inflammation-mediated damage (cytokine-mediated damage) and potentially improve outcomes. Dexamethasone use has also been associated with earlier resolution of fever and may help in reducing raised ICP, potentially improving clinical outcomes.

Guidelines for Corticosteroid Use and Dosing

- Dexamethasone should be administered 15 minutes before the first dose of antibiotics.
- The recommended dose is 0.15 mg/kg/dose every 6 hours for 3 days.
- It is specifically indicated for Hib meningitis, where its use has demonstrated efficacy in reducing neurological sequelae, especially hearing loss. The effectiveness of dexamethasone in pneumococcal or meningococcal meningitis remains uncertain and has not been consistently demonstrated and its use may potentially reduce the penetration of antibiotics into the CNS.

- Dexamethasone is not recommended for neonatal meningitis. It is also not useful if the child has already received antibiotics before steroid administration.

Supportive Care

- *Stabilization of airway, breathing, and circulation and temperature control* is important to prevent complications and maintain cerebral perfusion.
- *Intensive monitoring*
- *Seizure control with prompt antiseizure medications:* There is no role for prophylactic antiseizure medications.
- *Monitoring and optimization of metabolic parameters* (blood glucose, electrolyte balance, and arterial blood gases) *and fluid management:* Once the child's sensorium improves, oral feeds can be initiated cautiously after the first 24 hours of illness.
- *Management of raised ICP:*
    - First-line measures include head elevation, avoidance of noxious stimuli, and maintenance of normal physiological parameters (e.g., euthermia, euglycemia, and euvolemia).
    - Osmotherapy with 20% mannitol or 3% hypertonic saline
    - Mean arterial pressure should be maintained to ensure adequate cerebral perfusion.
    - Caution is exercised with fluid management to avoid hypotonic fluids that can exacerbate cerebral edema.
    - Additional medications such as acetazolamide or glycerol may be considered if ICP remains elevated beyond 48 hours.
    - In refractory cases, second-line (e.g., decompressive craniotomy) or third-line therapies (e.g., barbiturate coma) may be necessary.

COMPLICATIONS

Early Complications

- Seizures
- Subdural effusion and empyema (Hib)
- Arterial stroke
- Ventriculitis and hydrocephalus
- Venous sinus thrombosis
- Brain abscess

Late Complications

- Cognitive impairment
- Behavioral and emotional disorders
- *Hearing loss:* Common sequelae, particularly Hib
- Motor disability (including cerebral palsy)
- Vision impairment
- Seizures or epilepsy

COURSE OF ACUTE BACTERIAL MENINGITIS

If treated properly, usually defervescence occurs within 48–72 hours of starting antibiotics. Persistent fever (>10 days) may be due to thrombophlebitis, subdural effusion, empyema, brain abscess, spread of infection to extra-CNS sites (such as pneumonia, arthritis, or osteomyelitis), drug fever, and rarely resistant organisms. A repeat complete CSF examination and change of antibiotics is warranted, if fever persists >5 days.

In the case of recurrent meningitis, one should rule out CSF rhinorrhea or otorrhea or spinal dysraphism. In case of progressively increasing head size (more than the accepted normal for that age), the possibility of subdural effusion/empyema, hydrocephalus, or ventriculitis should be considered.

PROGNOSIS

- *Mortality:* Overall mortality rate is approximately 10%, with the highest rates seen in pneumococcal infections and among patients who present with shock.
- *Risk factors for adverse outcomes:* Major risk factors for adverse outcomes include the duration and/or progression of illness before effective antibiotic therapy, younger age, and etiological agent (*S. pneumoniae* is associated with the worse outcome). The presence of neurologic complications in the acute phase also predicts long-term neurologic sequelae such as prolonged seizures or seizures that begin >72 hours after admission, focal neurologic deficits, hydrocephalus, etc.
- *Neurologic sequelae:* About 20–30% of survivors of bacterial meningitis experience long-term neurologic sequelae. These include:
    - Deafness, occurring in up to 10–25% of children, often permanent and more common in infections caused by *S. pneumoniae* and *H. influenzae.*
    - Neurodevelopmental retardation, neuromotor deficits, speech and learning problems
    - Seizures, focal motor deficits, and cranial nerve deficits are also common consequences.

ADVICE AT DISCHARGE

- *Follow-up* for sequelae
- *Hearing assessment:* Before discharge and again 6 weeks postdischarge. Up to 90% of children with hearing loss due to meningitis can develop ossification of the cochlea, which complicates treatment with cochlear implants.
- Continued anticonvulsants and neurological follow-up as indicated
- Neurodevelopmental monitoring and support for children with hearing loss, intellectual disability, or other neurologic deficits
- Physiotherapy

PREVENTION

- *Immunoprophylaxis*
  - Hib vaccine reduces severe Hib disease in children under 2 years of age by >95%.
  - Meningococcal vaccine, especially during epidemics, and recommended for individuals over 2 years of age
  - Pneumococcal conjugate vaccine (PCV) prevents pneumococcal meningitis and invasive pneumococcal disease, particularly in immunocompromised individuals, those with asplenia, hemoglobinopathies, and transplant recipients.
- *Chemoprophylaxis for household contacts*
  - *Hib:* Rifampicin 20 mg/kg/day (maximum 600 mg) as a single dose for 4 days
  - *Meningococcus:* Rifampicin 20 mg/kg/day (maximum 600 mg) in two divided doses for 2 days, or ciprofloxacin 500 mg orally as a single dose

BRAIN ABSCESS

DEFINITION

Brain abscess is a localized suppurative (pus-forming) infection within the brain parenchyma, characterized by a sequence starting with cerebritis (early focal inflammation) that evolves into an encapsulated collection of pus. It typically involves pyogenic bacteria, though fungal, mycobacterial, and parasitic causes are also possible. Brain abscesses account for approximately 1–2% of intracranial space-occupying lesions in developed countries and up to 8% in developing countries, with a significant percentage occurring in children.

ETIOLOGY

The most common agents causing brain abscess in immunocompetent hosts are bacterial. Polymicrobial etiology is seen in 25–30% of cases. Common bacterial agents include:

- Streptococci (including *S. pneumoniae*)
- Anaerobic bacteria (e.g., *Bacteroides fragilis*)
- *S. aureus*
- *Pseudomonas* spp.
- Mixed infections are common, involving both aerobic and anaerobic organisms.

PATHOGENESIS

Predisposing Conditions and Associated Etiological Agents

- *Otitis media, mastoiditis:* Temporal lobe involvement with *Streptococcus* spp., including *S. pneumoniae*, and anaerobic bacteria, or microaerophilic bacteria (e.g., *B. fragilis*, *Eikenella corrodens*, *Abiotrophia*, and *Granulicatella* spp.), *Pseudomonas*, and *Staphylococcus*
- *Sinusitis:* Frontal lobe abscesses with streptococci and mixed anaerobic or microaerophilic bacteria
- *Odontogenic infections:* Frontal lobe abscesses with streptococci, gram-negative bacilli, and *B. fragilis*
- Congenital cyanotic heart disease: Multiple abscess sites with group A streptococcus
- *Infective endocarditis:* Multiple abscess sites with *Streptococcus viridans* and *S. aureus*
- *Trauma to skull:* Abscesses at the site of trauma with *S. aureus*, coagulase-negative staphylococci, or gram-negative bacilli
- *Neurosurgical procedures [e.g., ventriculoperitoneal (VP) shunt]:* Various bacteria including *S. aureus, Pseudomonas aeruginosa*
- *Neonates: Citrobacter* spp., *Cronobacter sakazakii, and Candida* spp.
- *Immunocompromised hosts:* Fungal abscesses (cryptococcus, aspergillus, etc.), mycobacterial (tubercular) abscesses, and *Nocardia* spp.
- History of contact with persons with tuberculosis (TB)—tubercular abscess

Routes of Infection

- *Contiguous spread (approximately one-half of the cases):* Often from nearby infections in sinuses, middle ear, dental infections, or inflamed meninges
- *Hematogenous spread (one-third cases):* From distant sites such as the heart (congenital cyanotic heart disease, bacterial endocarditis), lungs (empyema), skin, or intra-abdominal infections
- *Direct inoculation*: Post-trauma or postsurgical procedures

Stages of Abscess Formation

1. *Stage I:* Early cerebritis (1–3 days)—microglia and astrocyte activation, neutrophil accumulation, edema, and tissue necrosis
2. *Stage II:* Late cerebritis (4–9 days)—macrophage and lymphocyte infiltration, expansion with a central necrotic focus
3. *Stage III:* Early capsulation (10–14 days)—formation of a ring-enhancing dense collagenous and vascularized abscess capsule, peripheral gliosis, and fibrosis
4. *Stage IV:* Late capsulation (>14 days)—thickening of abscess capsule, completely walled-off suppuration, may be amenable to surgical excision

CLINICAL FEATURES

- *Classic triad* (present in 20% of cases): Fever, headache, and acute neurological deficits
- *Common symptoms:* Headache (70%), fever (50%), focal neurologic deficits (50%) such as seizures, cranial nerve

palsies, aphasia, ataxia, and visual field defects, and behavioral changes (frontal lobe or right temporal lobe)
- *Signs of raised ICP:* Headache, vomiting, papilledema, altered sensorium, and Cushing's triad (hypertension, bradycardia, and irregular respiration)
- *Specific features in infants:* Irritability, excessive crying, lethargy, fever, vomiting, bulging fontanelle, seizures, and increased head circumference
- *Location:* Supratentorial in 85%, infratentorial in 13%, combined in 2%, with frontal and parietal lobes being most common. Pontine abscess leads to compression of aqueduct of Sylvius leading to obstructive hydrocephalus
- *Features suggestive of rupture:* Sudden worsening of sensorium, high-grade fever, severe headache, and meningismus

DIAGNOSIS

Neuroimaging

Contrast-enhanced CT (CECT) or contrast-enhanced magnetic resonance imaging (CEMRI) with gadolinium enhancement is essential. MRI is superior for detecting early stages, abscess characteristics, and nearby infections. Early cerebritis is seen as a hypodense lesion on CT scan and as T2 hyperintense lesions (focal edema) on MRI. Mature abscess is seen as a ring-enhancing lesion (REL) with hypodense core (necrotic) and perilesional edema on CECT. On CEMRI, a mature abscess is seen as a hypointense lesion with ring enhancement postgadolinium contrast on T1 and a central hyperintense lesion surrounded by a hypointense capsule (fibrous capsule) and irregular hyperintense perilesional edema on T2 with diffusion restriction.

Cerebrospinal Fluid Analysis

It is not useful for etiological diagnosis due to low yield (<10%) and risk of herniation. The most common CSF findings in brain abscesses are mild mononuclear pleocytosis, mildly elevated protein, and normal to slightly low glucose with sterile cultures. CSF may show marked leukocytosis with 50,000–100,000 cells, significant hypoglycorrhachia (CSF glucose <40 mg/dL), raised protein, and elevated lactate (> 500 mg/dL) after rupture of abscess in the ventricles.

Definitive Diagnosis

Excision biopsy or stereotactic aspiration for microbiological and histopathological examination is indicated for definitive diagnosis. Specimens are assessed using Gram staining, KOH mount, acid-fast bacillus (AFB) staining, culture, and molecular tests such as nucleic acid amplification test (NAAT) for *Mycobacterium tuberculosis*, PCR for bacterial or fungal deoxyribonucleic acid (DNA)/ribonucleic acid (RNA), and 16S ribosomal DNA PCR for specific species or genera of bacteria.

Other Investigations

- *Sepsis and inflammatory markers*—leukocytosis, raised ESR, CRP, and procalcitonin
- *Blood culture*—diagnostic yield, 25–30%

MANAGEMENT

Medical Management

- *Selection of antibiotics*
  - *Empirical therapy:* Initiate treatment with broad-spectrum antibiotics:
    - Third or fourth-generation cephalosporin (e.g., ceftriaxone, cefotaxime) for coverage against gram-negative and some gram-positive organisms with good CNS penetration
    - Metronidazole for anaerobic coverage
    - Vancomycin to cover methicillin-resistant *S. aureus* (MRSA), especially in cases of penetrating trauma or neurosurgical procedures[3]
  - *Duration:* 4–6 weeks or until radiologic stabilization of the abscess is achieved.
- Adjustment based on culture and sensitivity
- *Special considerations:* In immunocompromised patients, consider potential fungal or mycobacterial etiologies, and adjust treatment accordingly. Early drainage may be necessary to obtain samples for definitive diagnosis and guide appropriate therapy.

Surgical Management

- *Indications for surgical drainage:*
  - Large abscess size (>2.5 cm in diameter)
  - *Impending rupture:* Increasing neurological deficits, or worsening symptoms despite antibiotics
  - Impending herniation
  - Abscesses involving noneloquent cortex
  - Multiloculated abscess
  - *Fungal abscess:* Due to their more indolent nature and difficulty in penetration by antibiotics
  - Traumatic abscess with foreign body[4]
- *Surgical approaches:*
  - Burr hole for superficial abscesses
  - Craniotomy for deeper or larger abscesses
  - *Stereotactic drainage:* Minimally invasive procedure

Supportive Care

- Management of raised ICP and seizures
- *Corticosteroids:*
  - Avoid use in bacterial and fungal abscesses due to its potential to worsen the infection
  - *Potential benefit:* May be considered in mycobacterial abscesses or cases with impending herniation due to perilesional edema to reduce inflammation and edema

Monitoring

Repeat neuroimaging (typically CT) after 2–4 weeks of antibiotic initiation to monitor response to treatment and assess for any changes or in case of sudden neurological deterioration to evaluate for complications such as abscess expansion, hemorrhage, or new lesions.

Prognosis

- *Complications:*
  - Raised ICP
  - Herniation
  - *Rupture into ventricular system:* Leads to ventriculitis, obstructive hydrocephalus, and further neurological complications
  - Status epilepticus
- *Mortality:*
  - *High mortality rate:* Up to 25%
- *Poor prognostic factors:*
  - Neonates and young children
  - Complications such as ventriculitis, hydrocephalus, or abscess rupture
  - Poor GCS at presentation indicating severe neurological impairment
  - Immunocompromised state, which may lead to difficulties in managing infections
  - Fungal etiology of the abscess, which is often more challenging to treat

CHRONIC MENINGITIS

Chronic meningitis is the persistence of symptoms and signs of meningitis for >4 weeks associated with CSF pleocytosis. Chronic meningitis can have either an acute or insidious onset. The causes of chronic meningitis include both infectious and noninfectious etiologies with the most common causes being TB, fungal agents, and neoplasms. Establishing the correct cause and timely targeted therapies are the major challenges in its management. A case of chronic meningitis with acute onset can be mistaken for partially treated meningitis.

Partially treated meningitis implies meningitis which has been treated with inappropriate selection of the drugs and/or inadequate doses/duration resulting in an altered clinical picture with nonclearance of the CSF.

Recurrent meningitis is defined as separate episodes of meningitis at least 1 week or more apart during which time the patient's clinical profile is essentially normal.

ETIOLOGICAL SPECTRUM OF CHRONIC MENINGITIS AND PATHOGENESIS

The etiology may be varied and difficult to identify **(Table 8.12.5)**. TBM is the most common and important cause of chronic meningitis in developing countries, especially with the advent of HIV infection and acquired immunodeficiency syndrome (AIDS). It may occur at any age but is most common between 6 and 24 months; usually within a year of primary infection or concomitantly with miliary TB.

TABLE 8.12.5: Etiology of chronic meningitis.

Infectious	*Noninfectious*
• *Bacterial*: – Spirochetal: - *Borrelia burgdorferi* - *Treponema pallidum* – *Leptospira* species – *Brucella* species – *Listeria monocytogenes* • Partially treated meningitis • *Mycobacterium tuberculosis* • Others: – *Francisella tularensis* – *Actinomyces* species – *Ehrlichia chaffeensis* – *Nocardia* species – *Tropheryma whipplei* (Whipple disease) • *Viral*: – Human immunodeficiency virus – Human T cell lymphotropic virus I and II – Herpes simplex virus – Epstein–Barr virus – Varicella-zoster virus – Enterovirus – Mumps – Cytomegalovirus • *Fungal*: – Cryptococcus – Candida – Histoplasma – Sporothrix – Blastomyces – Coccidioides – Aspergillus • *Parasitic*: – Cysticercosis – Toxoplasma – Acanthamoeba – *Balamuthia mandrillaris* • Nosocomial infections	• *Collagen vascular disease*: – Systemic lupus erythematous – Wegener's granulomatosis – Polyarteritis nodosa – Behcet's syndrome – Sarcoidosis – CNS vasculitis • *Malignancies*: – Leukemia – Lymphoma – Metastasis • *Drugs*: – Chemotherapeutic agents – Intravenous immunoglobulin – Intrathecal agents

(CNS: central nervous system)

DIAGNOSTIC APPROACH

The diagnostic approach to chronic meningitis requires a comprehensive evaluation integrating clinical history, thorough physical examination, CSF analysis, imaging studies, and targeted laboratory investigations. Early identification of the underlying etiology is crucial for initiating appropriate treatment and improving patient outcomes. Close collaboration among different specialties is often necessary to manage complex cases effectively.

Clinical History

- *Symptoms:* Patients may present with headaches (mild to severe), fever, neck stiffness, irritability, focal neurological deficits, and seizures. They may present with subtle signs and symptoms or acutely due to complications.
- *Etiological pointers:*
    - *Immune status:* Recurrent infections, known immunodeficiency (e.g., HIV), drug-induced immunosuppression (e.g., posttransplant)
    - *Immunization history:* Pertinent for vaccine-preventable diseases
    - *Travel/residence history:* Endemic areas for specific infections
    - *Drug history:* Chemotherapy, immunoglobulins
    - *Animal exposure:* Dog bites, ticks, bats
    - *Environmental toxins:* Lead exposure
    - *Exposure to TB:* Contact history
    - *Parasitic infections:* Raw or poorly cooked foods (e.g., NCC)
    - *Water exposure:* Acanthamoeba meningitis
    - *Systemic involvement:* Eye or joint symptoms suggesting rheumatological conditions
    - *Neurosurgical history:* Procedures, CSF leaks, VP shunt
    - *Shock:* Nosocomial infections, candidemia, fungal infections (especially in premature infants)

Neurological and Systemic Examination

- *Signs of raised ICP:* Altered sensorium, poor GCS, Cushing's triad (late), papilledema, and unequal dilated pupils
- *Skin findings:* Rash (erythema migrans in Lyme disease), petechiae, and purpura (meningococcal infection)
- *Meningeal signs:* Neck rigidity, Kernig sign, and Brudzinski sign
- *Cranial nerve palsies:* Seen in TB or Lyme disease
- *Focal neurological deficits:* Stroke (basilar meningitis in TB), vasculitis (TB and fungal infections)
- *Respiratory involvement:* TB, fungal infections (histoplasmosis, blastomycosis)
- *Hepatic involvement:* Jaundice, liver failure

Laboratory Investigations

The diagnostic evaluation of chronic meningitis involves a combination of blood investigations and CSF analysis tailored to the suspected etiology based on clinical history and examination findings.

Blood Investigations

- *Sepsis markers:* CBC, procalcitonin, and CRP
- *Blood culture:* Bacterial (aerobic and anaerobic) and fungal cultures
- *Serological tests*:
    - Antibodies against atypical organisms (e.g., atypical organisms—brucella, mycoplasma, legionella, leptospira, and rickettsiae)
    - Antigen detection tests (e.g., cryptococcal antigen)

Cerebrospinal Fluid Analysis

- *Centrifugation and microscopic examination:* Increases diagnostic yield for certain pathogens, particularly fungi and mycobacteria
- *Cell counts and differential:*
    - *Neutrophilic pleocytosis:* Early in TBM and certain fungal infections
    - *Lymphocytic pleocytosis:* Common in most cases of chronic meningitis
- *Glucose and protein levels:*
    - *Glucose:* Low CSF to serum glucose ratio suggestive of atypical bacteria or fungal infections, NCC, neurosarcoidosis, and carcinomatous meningitis
    - *Protein:* Elevated levels in inflammation and disruption of the BBB
- *Special findings:*
    - Eosinophilia suggestive of parasitic etiology or coccidioidomycosis
    - Stained smears occasionally reveal fungal elements or bacteria
    - *India ink microscopy:* Cryptococcus
- *CSF culture:* Use large volumes (10–25 mL) to increase sensitivity for routine bacterial and fungal cultures
- *CSF PCR testing:*
    - *M. tuberculosis*
    - Fungal agents such as aspergillus or panfungal PCR for nonspecific fungal detection
- *Serological testing:*
    - Fungal infections (e.g., histoplasmosis and sporothrix); detecting specific antibodies in CSF
- *Antigen testing:*
    - Detection of cryptococcal antigen in CSF
- *Other biomarkers:*
    - *CSF galactomannan:* Used for diagnosing aspergillosis (70% sensitivity)
    - *CSF 1,3-β-d-glucan:* Nonspecific marker for fungal infections, indicating fungal cell wall components

- *Advanced testing:* Multiplex PCR; 16S, 18S, and 28S ribosomal RNA (rRNA) PCR; and metagenomic deep sequencing—these are novel methods, especially useful in patients who have received empirical antibiotic treatment and are under development in both blood and CSF samples.

Role of Neuroimaging

Magnetic resonance imaging and CT scans are useful for assessing the parameningeal focus of infection and complications such as brain abscess, cerebral edema, hydrocephalus, stroke, vasculitis, basilar meningitis, or differentials (e.g., tumor). Contrast imaging is preferable in the absence of complications. If indicated, vascular imaging [MR angiography (MRA) or MR venography (MRV)] should be performed as in cases of stroke.

Brain or Meningeal Biopsy

Meningeal and/or brain biopsy may be valuable, especially in cases in which areas of enhancement are identified on postcontrast MRI.

Workup for Tuberculosis

Tuberculosis should be ruled in or ruled out upfront as it is a major cause of chronic meningitis. The details are explained below in the section on TBM.

MANAGEMENT OF CHRONIC MENINGITIS

Empirical Treatment

Empirical treatment with antitubercular drugs is started based on the presence of risk factors (such as contact history, in endemic areas) and clinical manifestations such as hydrocephalus, stroke, raised ICP with neuroimaging suggestive of basilar meningitis, or tuberculomas. Since TB is one of the most common causes of chronic meningitis, the threshold for starting antitubercular treatment (ATT) should be kept low in cases of chronic meningitis.[5,6] Specific treatment of tuberculous meningitis is described in the central nervous system tuberculosis.

Empirical treatment with antibacterials should be started, especially if there is suspicion of partially treated meningitis and/or setting of a CSF leak or history of neurosurgical procedure or a VP shunt in situ.

Empirical antifungal treatment should be considered in settings of immunocompromised hosts, posttransplant patients, HIV/AIDS or premature neonates, and a prolonged hospital stay. However, response to such empiric therapy may be hard to assess because patients with fungal meningitis often respond slowly to appropriate therapy. A low threshold should be kept in those who are neutropenic or have AIDS and in posttransplantation patients, given the risk for fulminant infection with significant morbidity and mortality.[2]

Empirical glucocorticoids may be useful in selected patients who fail to improve during follow-up, or in those with high suspicion of tubercular etiology. In such cases, early therapeutic response must be interpreted with caution given the temporary clinical benefit many patients may experience from steroids alone. Empirical glucocorticoids should be avoided or used with caution in patients with HIV/AIDS with suspected fungal etiologies.

Specific Treatment for Other Infective Causes of Chronic Meningitis

Specific treatment of fungal, bacterial, viral, and parasitic causes of chronic meningitis is outlined in **Table 8.12.6** for fungal meningitis, **Table 8.12.7** for specific bacterial infections, **Table 8.12.8** for viral meningitis, and **Table 8.12.9** for specific parasitic meningitis.[7]

Supportive Treatment for Chronic Meningitis

- Monitoring for neurological deterioration and hemodynamic and respiratory support and fluid and electrolyte management as required clinically
- Management of raised ICP and seizures
- Neurosurgical intervention for:
  - Decompressive craniotomy for raised ICP, which is refractory to first-line measures
  - Brain abscess drainage
  - CSF diversion procedures such as VP shunt insertion or external ventricular drainage as indicated for obstructive hydrocephalus or raised ICP not responding to treatment
- Rehabilitation

COURSE OF DISEASE AND PROGNOSIS

In approximately one-third of the cases, etiology remains unidentified in spite of extensive workup. With appropriate treatment, patient starts showing clinical improvement in 1–2 weeks, although neurological improvement may continue for as long as a year.

Repeat LP might be indicated after 1–2 weeks to assess CSF response, to review diagnosis if no clinical improvement, or in case of deterioration. CSF may take as long as 2 months to normalize.

Repeat CT scan might be needed 4 weeks later, or earlier if there is clinical progression, increasing head size, new-onset neurological signs, to evaluate need for VP shunt, or to detect sequelae of the disease.

TABLE 8.12.6: Treatment of fungal causes of chronic meningitis.

Organism	*Treatment*
Cryptococcosis	Three-step approach with induction, consolidation, and maintenance phases: • Induction phase, amphotericin B (liposomal amphotericin B 10 mg/kg/day) with flucytosine (25 mg/kg/dose q six hourly) for 2 weeks • Consolidation therapy with fluconazole for at least 8 weeks • Maintenance therapy with lower-dose fluconazole for a minimum of 1 year • Antifungal treatment for cryptococcal infection in patients who are HIV infected should be lifelong or until the immune system has recovered with ART to a $CD4^+$ T-cell count of >200 cells/mm^3 • Current recommendations do not advocate treatment with adjunctive steroids in cases of definitive cryptococcal meningitis, especially in those who are HIV positive
Histoplasmosis	• Amphotericin B for induction therapy for at least 3 months, followed by fluconazole or itraconazole • VP shunt placement in hydrocephalus to be delayed until the patient has received at least a few weeks of amphotericin B to reduce the likelihood of shunt colonization
Blastomycosis	• Amphotericin B for at least 1 month followed by an oral azole • Antifungal treatment should be continued until clinical stability is achieved and CSF parameters normalize (typically >1 year)
Coccidioidomycosis	• Lifelong azole treatment
Aspergillosis	• Voriconazole—first line • Lipid formulations of amphotericin B are reserved for those intolerant or refractory to voriconazole • Duration—continued for a minimum of 6–12 weeks
Candidiasis	• For initial treatment, liposomal amphotericin B, 5 mg/kg/day, with or without oral flucytosine, 25 mg/kg, four times daily is recommended • For step-down therapy after the patient has responded to initial treatment, fluconazole, 400–800 mg (6–12 mg/kg/day), is recommended • Treatment should be continued till complete resolution of clinical, CSF, and radiographic abnormalities • With clinical improvement, therapy can be changed to fluconazole if the isolated species is susceptible

(ART: antiretroviral therapy; CSF: cerebrospinal fluid; HIV: human immunodeficiency virus; VP shunt: ventriculoperitoneal shunt)

CENTRAL NERVOUS SYSTEM TUBERCULOSIS

Tuberculosis is a multisystem infectious disease, commonly affecting the lungs followed by CNS, lymph nodes, abdomen, and bones, caused by *M. tuberculosis,* a gram negative acid-fast bacilli. In India, approximately 3.42 lakh children are estimated to be affected by TB every year (refer to Chapter 7.7: Tuberculosis).

Neurotuberculosis or TB of the CNS (CNS-TB) is the most severe extrapulmonary complication of TB with high morbidity and mortality rates, accounting for 1–10% of all TB cases. It is most common in children between 6 months and 4 years of age. In children, TBM is associated with about 50% mortality, and most of the survivors have permanent neurologic sequelae including severe disability. *Tuberculoma* is an uncommon presentation of CNS-TB in children, occurring in 5% of children. Risk factors for TBM include age <5 years, household contact with TB, protein-energy malnutrition (PEM) grades III and IV, recent measles or pertussis infection and HIV infection, immunosuppression, high prevalence of TB in the community, and no history of Bacillus Calmette-Guérin (BCG) vaccination.

PATHOGENESIS OF CENTRAL NERVOUS SYSTEM-TUBERCULOSIS

Dissemination of Tuberculosis Bacilli to Central Nervous System

Tuberculosis bacilli primarily infect the respiratory epithelium. If it survives the initial encounter with the innate immune system, primary infection is established in the lung parenchyma. From the primary focus, TB bacilli are disseminated to CNS via hematogenous spread, where a single meningeal or subcortical granuloma called Rich focus is formed. Rupture of the Rich focus years after initial hematogenous dissemination discharges acid-fast bacilli into the SAS.

Role of Host Immune Response to Tuberculosis Infection in Central Nervous System

In response to TB bacilli, there is granulomatous inflammation affecting basal meninges. Inflammatory exudates obstructing CSF passage led to obstructive hydrocephalus and raised ICP. Furthermore, vasogenic edema that occurs due to an influx of proteins through the leaky BBB and cytotoxic edema that occurs due to cellular damage, both add to raised ICP. Cerebral infarcts may occur due to inflammation and occlusion of small and medium-sized intracerebral arteries. Local inflammation is pronounced over basal meninges in proximity to the circle

TABLE 8.12.7: Antibiotics indicated in specific bacterial infections causing chronic meningitis.

Organism	***Antibiotic recommended***
Methicillin-susceptible *Staphylococcus aureus* (MSSA)	• Nafcillin or oxacillin • If cannot tolerate lactams—desensitize or may receive vancomycin as an alternative agent • If susceptible to rifampin, may be considered but in combination • If beta-lactam agents or vancomycin cannot be used, linezolid, daptomycin or trimethoprim-sulfamethoxazole with selection of a specific agent based on in vitro susceptibility testing • *Duration:* 10–14 days
Methicillin-resistant *S. aureus* (MRSA)	• Vancomycin • *Duration:* 10–14 days or continue for another 14 days after last positive culture
Coagulase-negative *staphylococci*	• Similar to that for *S. aureus* (MRSA or MSSA based on in vitro susceptibility testing) • Duration: 10–14 days
Propionibacterium acnes	• Penicillin G • *Duration:* 10–14 days
Gram-negative bacilli	• Third-generation cephalosporins, ceftriaxone, or cefotaxime is recommended if susceptible • Extended-spectrum beta-lactamase-producing gram-negative bacilli—meropenem • Prolonged infusion of meropenem (each dose administered over 3 hours) can be given—resistant gram-negative organisms • *Duration:* 21 days or continue for another 14 days after last positive culture
Pseudomonas species	• Cefepime, ceftazidime, or meropenem • Alternative antimicrobial agents are aztreonam or a fluoroquinolone with in vitro activity
Acinetobacter	• Meropenem • For carbapenem resistance, colistimethate sodium or polymyxin B (either agent administered by the intravenous and intraventricular routes)
Bartonella bacilliformis	Chloramphenicol, ciprofloxacin, doxycycline, ampicillin, or trimethoprim-sulfamethoxazole
Bartonella henselae	Doxycycline or azithromycin, with or without rifampin
Listeria monocytogenes	• Ampicillin + gentamicin is recommended • Trimethoprim-sulfamethoxazole is an alternative in the penicillin-allergic patient
Mycoplasma pneumoniae	Azithromycin, doxycycline, or a fluoroquinolone
Borrelia burgdorferi	Ceftriaxone, cefotaxime, or penicillin G
Treponema pallidum	• Penicillin G is recommended • Ceftriaxone is an alternative
Tropheryma whipplei	Ceftriaxone followed by either trimethoprim-sulfamethoxazole or cefixime is recommended
Anaplasma	Doxycyclin
Ehrlichia chaffeensis	Doxycycline
Rickettsia rickettsii	Doxycycline Chloralmphenicol is an alternative
Coxiella burnetii	Doxycycline + a fluoroquinolone + rifampin

of Willis, predisposing to infarcts. In children with good cellular immunity, the focus gets organized into tuberculoma. Cytokine-mediated inflammatory response causes vasculitis, obstructive hydrocephalus, and cranial nerve palsies as well as late paradoxical reaction. Tumor necrosis factor alpha (TNF-α) is an important cytokine in this response. The disequilibrium of pro- and anti-inflammatory cytokines is implicated in the pathogenesis of CNS-TB and its various complications.

CLASSIFICATION OF CENTRAL NERVOUS SYSTEM-TUBERCULOSIS

- *Intracranial:*
  - TBM
  - Tubercular encephalopathy
  - Tubercular vasculopathy
  - CNS tuberculoma
  - Tubercular brain abscess

TABLE 8.12.8: Specific antiviral agents in chronic meningitis.

Agent	Antiviral	Duration
Herpes simplex virus	Acyclovir (10 mg/kg IV every 8 hours in children and adults with normal renal function; 20 mg/kg IV every 8 hours in neonates)	14–21 days
Varicella zoster virus	• Acyclovir (10–15 mg/kg IV every 8 hours) • Alternative—gancyclovir	10–14 days
Cytomegalovirus	• Combination ganciclovir (5 mg/kg IV every 12 hours) and foscarnet (60 mg/kg IV every 8 hours or 90 mg/kg IV every 12 hours) • Cidofovir is not an alternative, because its ability to penetrate the blood–brain barrier is poorly studied	3 weeks
Epstein–Barr virus	• None • Acyclovir is not recommended	
Human herpesvirus 6	Ganciclovir or Foscarnet	
Influenza	Oseltamivir	
Measles virus	Ribavirin	
Nipah virus	Ribavirin	
West Nile virus	Ribavirin is not recommended	
Japanese encephalitis virus	IFN-α is not recommended	
St. Louis encephalitis virus	IFN-2α can be considered	
HIV	HAART	
JC virus	Reversal of immunosuppression or HAART in HIV-infected patients is recommended	

(HAART: highly active antiretroviral therapy; HIV: human immunodeficiency virus; IFN: interferon; IV: intravenous; JC virus: John Cunningham virus)

TABLE 8.12.9: Treatment for specific parasitic infections.

Acanthamoeba	Trimethoprim-sulfamethoxazole + rifampin + ketoconazole or fluconazole + sulfadiazine + pyrimethamine
Balamuthia mandrillaris	Pentamidine, combined with a macrolide (azithromycin or clarithromycin), fluconazole, sulfadiazine, flucytosine, and a phenothiazine can be considered
Naegleria fowleri	Amphotericin B (intravenous and intrathecal) and rifampin, combined with other agents, can be considered
Toxoplasma gondii	Pyrimethamine + either sulfadiazine or clindamycin is recommended or Trimethoprim-sulfamethoxazole alone or Pyrimethamine + either atovaquone, clarithromycin azithromycin, or dapsone are alternatives
Trypanosoma brucei gambiense	• Eflornithine • Melarsoprol is an alternative
Trypanosoma brucei rhodesiense	Melarsoprol

- *Spinal:*
  - *Osseous spinal TB:* Pott's spine and Pott's paraplegia
  - *Nonosseous:*
    - Spinal tuberculoma
    - Arachnoiditis
    - Epidural abscess

CLINICAL PRESENTATION

These include fever >5 days duration, headache, vomiting, irritability, lethargy, coma, neck stiffness, loss of appetite, loss of weight, seizures, cranial nerve palsies, hemiparesis, paraparesis, quadriparesis, altered sensorium, and other organ system symptoms (such as cough, lymphadenopathy, and abdominal mass) as well as spinal deformities (gibbus). History of contact with TB may be present.

Modified Vellore Grading of Central Nervous System Tuberculosis with Hydrocephalus

- *Grade I:* Headache, fever, vomiting, neck stiffness, normal sensorium, and no neurological deficits
- *Grade II:* Normal sensorium with neurological deficit
- *Grade III:* Altered sensorium but arousable, dense neurological deficit may or may not be present
- *Grade IV:* Coma, decerebrate, or decorticate posturing

DIFFERENT PRESENTATIONS OF CENTRAL NERVOUS SYSTEM-TUBERCULOSIS

Tuberculous Meningitis

It constitutes 70–80% cases of CNS-TB with peak age of 2–4 years and occurs usually within 3–6 months of primary infection. It is often subacute in onset. Neurological symptoms are noted 1–4 weeks after the onset of fever, ranging from meningismus, protracted headache, vomiting, lethargy, confusion, and varying degrees of cranial nerve and long-tract signs, seizures, hemiplegia/paraplegia to stupor and coma, and decerebrate posturing. Untreated patients may die within 5–8 weeks from symptoms onset.

Cerebrospinal fluid analysis reveals lymphocytosis (50–500 white cells/mL) with elevated protein 100–4,000 mg/mL, and low CSF glucose (less than two-thirds of serum glucose, usually <45 mg/dL).

Differential diagnosis includes partially treated pyogenic meningitis, fungal meningitis (cryptococcosis, histoplasmosis, blastomycosis, and coccidioidomycosis), neoplastic meningitis, brain abscess, and viral meningitis (Herpes simplex and mumps).

Hydrocephalus

Hydrocephalus is a common complication of TBM. It may be communicating, obstructive, or mixed. Falsely, low CSF opening pressure is found on LP. A progressive dip in sensorium in a patient with TBM, signs of raised ICP, or progressive increase in head size are clues and warrants an emergency imaging.

Tuberculoma

Tuberculomas are conglomerates of tubercles within the brain parenchyma. Nearly 10% of TBM have coexisting tuberculomas, one-third of which are multiple. They commonly present as mass lesions, with or without fever, headache, focal seizures, papilledema, or other signs of increased ICP, and progressive focal neurological deficit. Tuberculomas are supratentorial in adults, while in children, it is infratentorial. Differentials to be considered are tubercular brain abscess, NCC, brain tumor, cryptococcal infection, CNS toxoplasmosis, and tumefactive ADEM. Paradoxical enlargement of tuberculomas after starting ATT is seen in 2–23% due to interaction between the host's immune response and the direct effects of mycobacterial products. It should be suspected when there is transient worsening or appearance of new signs or symptoms or radiographic manifestations of TB 2–4 weeks after starting ATT. The presentation of brain abscess is more subacute (1 week to 3 months) than tuberculoma but slower in onset than pyogenic brain abscesses.

Cerebrovascular Complications of Tubercular Meningitis

Cerebrovascular complications of TBM that occur typically as multiple or bilateral lesions in the territories of the middle cerebral artery perforating vessels are termed tuberculous vasculopathy. Vessel pathology is a consequence of its immersion in the local inflammatory exudate. Vasospasm may mediate early strokes. Luminal thrombosis due to necrotizing vasculitis, proliferative intimal disease, and infiltrative pathology leads to later strokes. Due to the development of collaterals, there may be an appearance of the moyamoya pattern in the region of basal ganglia and the base of the brain. Infarcts in TBM are multiple, bilateral, and localized to the "tuberculous zone" involving the caudate nucleus, anterior thalamus, anterior limb, and genu of the internal capsule, in contrast to the posterior location of the ischemic thromboembolic infarcts.

Optochiasmatic Arachnoiditis

It presents as vision impairment.

Immune Reconstitution Inflammatory Syndrome or Paradoxical Reaction

Two forms of immune reconstitution inflammatory syndrome (IRIS) are recognized in the case of TBM. First is paradoxical TB-IRIS occurring in patients diagnosed with TB and established on TB treatment before antiretroviral treatment (ART) for HIV infection or in patients not infected with HIV-1. The other type includes unmasking TB-IRIS occurring in patients who are not on TB treatment when they start ART (within the first 3 months of ART). Clinical features include recurrent fever, worsening pulmonary infiltrates, enlarging pleural effusions, the development of TBM, new or enlarging tuberculomas, or tuberculous lesions developing at other anatomic sites. Release of new antigen targets during mycobacterial killing, hypersensitivity to killed antigens, and exaggerated immune restoration (following TB-induced immunosuppression) occurring during TB treatment are implicated in its pathogenesis.

DIAGNOSIS

Detailed history taking (fever, weight loss, chronic cough, loss of appetite, jaundice, and evidence of TB contact) and examination (lymphadenopathy, hepatosplenomegaly, bone, joint, and skin manifestation, as well as choroid tubercles) should be done to look for clues of systemic TB.

Every attempt should be made to demonstrate the presence of bacilli (in pulmonary or extrapulmonary specimens). Culture on solid or liquid media is the gold standard for diagnosis. Other tests for supportive evidence include neuroimaging, pathogen-based tests (NAATs), antigen detection tests, advanced testing (CRISPR MTB and metagenomic next-generation sequencing], and host-based tests—cytokine or cell-stimulation-based tests [tuberculin skin test, interferon-gamma release assay test (IGRA), serological tests, adenosine deaminase (ADA) test, etc.].

Cerebrospinal Fluid Examination

Gold standard confirmation of CNS-TB is the isolation of the agent in CSF. CSF examination is recommended for all children with TBM. Typical findings include low glucose, increased proteins (100–500 mg/dL), protein concentrations (up to >1 g/dL in more advanced stages of the disease in combination with a spinal block), lymphocytic pleocytosis, with most patients presenting between 100 and 500 cells/dL.

In Ziehl–Neelsen staining for the demonstration of *M. tuberculosis*, though it has a low sensitivity of 10–25%, a higher yield can be seen by analyzing at least 10 mL of the CSF sample, centrifuging the sample for at least 20 minutes, and performing a thorough CSF examination.

Cerebrospinal fluid-NAATs, such as Gene Xpert/RIF and Xpert Ultra, are rapid tests that have high specificity (94–96%) and sensitivity (60–85%). These tests can detect >99.5% of rifampicin resistance mutations. The World Health Organization (WHO) recommends Xpert Ultra in CSF to be used as the first-line investigation for the diagnosis of TBM. Conventionally used TB-PCR, which amplifies the *MPB64* gene or the insertion element IS6110, had a sensitivity of 56% and specificity of 98%. Routine PCR testing is completely replaced by cartridge-based NAAT (CBNAAT).[6]

Conventional culture media include solid culture [Löwenstein–Jensen (LJ) medium, Dubos] and synthetic (7H10/7H11 Middle Brook) and liquid culture media (7H9/7H12 Middle Brook, Kirshner). Automation systems, such as BACTEC and mycobacterium growth Indicator tubes (MGIT), are now available, which allow earlier detection compared to LJ media. MGIT is recommended by the WHO. Novel culture-based assays include microscopic observed drug susceptibility assay (MODS), nitrate reduction assay (NRA), thin layer agar (TLA), phage-based assays, and calorimetric redox indicator (CRI media).

Neuroimaging

It is helpful both in making diagnosis and management of patients with CNS-TB. MRI brain is superior to CT scan and helpful in detecting lesions of the brainstem, mid-brain, and basal ganglia.

Computed tomography scan can be normal in 30% of cases in early stages and later hyperdense basal exudates may be visualized. Other findings include hydrocephalus, parenchymal tuberculomas, and calcifications. On MRI, apart from basilar enhancement, periventricular infarcts especially in the basal ganglia are seen. The triad of basilar enhancement, thalamic infarcts, and hydrocephalus are highly suggestive of TBM.

Tuberculoma on CT scan appears as a REL >20 mm in size, irregular margin, with marked perilesional edema and associated calcification. Large tuberculoma or abscess can be associated with midline shift. MRI shows a REL with central core on T2-weighted images hypointense or isointense in caseating granuloma and hyperintense in noncaseating granuloma. MRS shows a lipid peak.

MANAGEMENT

Objective of Antitubercular Treatment

- Rapidly reduce the number of actively growing bacilli, thereby decreasing severity of the disease, preventing death, and halting transmission of *M. tuberculosis*.
  - INH and fluoroquinolones
- Eradicate populations of persisting bacilli in order to prevent relapse.
  - Rifamycin and pyrazinamide
- Prevent acquisition of drug resistance during therapy.
  - Avoiding monotherapy, irregular drug intake

Treatment Regimen in Central Nervous System-tuberculosis (Table 8.12.10)

In general, treatment for drug-susceptible TB includes 2 months HRZE followed by 4 months HRE (refer to Chapter 7.7: Tuberculosis). In case of CNS-TB, WHO recommends 2 months HRZE in induction phase (IP) followed by 10 months HR in continuation phase (CP). Ethambutol or streptomycin could be used in CP. According to IAP RNTCP Guidelines 2019, the recommendation is treatment with HRZE for 2 months in intensive phase followed by HRE for at least 7 months in continuation phase (making total duration at least 9 months), which can be extended to 3 more months in continuation phase (making the total duration of treatment to 12 months) on a case to case basis in case of delayed response and as per the discretion of the treating physician/pediatrician.

Role of Corticosteroids in Tubercular Meningitis

Corticosteroids are potent anti-inflammatory and immunomodulatory agents and lead to reduced local inflammation, reduction in swelling, and congestion of

TABLE 8.12.10: Antitubercular drugs dosing.

Drug	*Range (mg/kg/day)*	*Average (mg/kg/day)*	*Maximum dose (mg/day)*
Isoniazid (H)	7–15	10	300
Rifampicin (R)	10–20	15	600
Pyrazinamide (Z)	10–20	15	600
Ethambutol (E)	15–25	20	1,500
Streptomycin (S)	15–20	20	1,000

the meninges, thereby reducing ICP, cerebral edema and CSF outflow resistance and promote BBB repair. WHO recommends the use of corticosteroids in TBM as an initial adjuvant therapy tapered over 6–8 weeks as they reduce the risk of death and disabling neurological deficits later on. Children should be given prednisolone 4 mg/kg/24 h (or an equivalent dose of dexamethasone: 0.6 mg/kg/24 h) for 4 weeks, followed by a tapering course over 4 weeks. In sick patients, dexamethasone is given IV until oral dexamethasone can be initiated. Pulse methylprednisolone may be given in patients with optochiasmatic arachnoiditis and spinal arachnoiditis followed by oral steroids.[6]

Drug-resistant Tuberculosis

Absence of initial response and continued worsening of symptoms, exposure to drug-resistant TB contacts, concomitant HIV infection, and previous poor treatment are the risk factors for drug-resistant TB. The second-line drugs include:

- *Group A:* Includes all three—levofloxacin (Lfx) or moxifloxacin (M), bedaquiline (Bdq), linezolid (Lzd)
- *Group B:* Includes one or both—clofazimine (Cfz), cycloserine
- *Group C:* When group A/B drugs cannot be used and to complete the regimen—ethambutol (E), delamanid (Dlm), pyrazinamide (Z), imipenem-cilastatin or meropenem (Ipm-Cln or Mpm), amikacin or streptomycin (Am) or (S), ethionamide (Eto) or prothionamine (Pto), *p*-amino salicylic acid (PAS)

Multidrug resistance: It is defined in the presence of resistance to both H and R. Shortened 6 + 5-month regimens or longer 18–20-month regimens are available. The shorter MDR regimen consists of seven second-line ATT drugs for 4–6 months of intensive phase (moxifloxacin, ethambutol, clofazimine, pyrazinamide, kanamycin, high-dose isoniazid, and ethionamide) followed by a CP of 5 months, which consists of the former four drugs only. Longer 18–20-month regimens consist of all oral drugs such as levofloxacin, bedaquiline, clofazimine, linezolid, and cycloserine.

Extensive drug resistance (XDR): It is defined as a multidrug resistance along with additional resistance to fluroquinolone or other category A drugs (levofloxacin or moxifloxacin, bedaquiline, linezolid). Here, a longer individualized 18–20-month regimen consisting of preferably only oral drugs from group A and B (levofloxacin, bedaquiline, linezolid, clofazimine and cycloserine) is recommended, with no separate IP or CP. In case if the need may arise replacements can be taken from group C drugs to complete the regimen as recommended by WHO and included in National TB Elimination Programme Guidelines for Drug Resistant TB in India, March 2021.

Monitoring

- Compliance and adherence to therapy.
- *Liver functions tests:* Withhold R and Z if AST/ALT >5 times upper limit of normal (ULN) with normal bilirubin or AST/ALT >3 times ULN with elevated bilirubin >2 times ULN or symptomatic patient; reintroduce once AST/ALT <2 times ULN one by one and if cannot be reintroduced successfully to be substituted by other category drugs such as levofloxacin and extend treatment duration
- Vision loss
- MGIT and LPA (line probe assay) for resistance to ATT

Those on drug-resistant regimens will need more monitoring including CBC, thyroid function tests, electrocardiogram (QT prolongation), electrolytes, skin discoloration, hearing loss, psychiatric symptoms, and urine routine.

Management of Paradoxical Reaction

Steroids are the mainstay of treatment. TNF-α blockers such as thalidomide, infliximab, and etanercept have been tried as well.

Management of Tubercular Vasculopathy/Stroke

- Aspirin (low dose 2–3 mg/kg) for antithrombotic action is started. Role of high-dose aspirin for anti-inflammatory action and its prophylactic role is not well-established
- Antitubercular therapy with corticosteroids
- Early physiotherapy after stabilization and supportive care

Other Aspects of Supportive Management in Tubercular Meningitis

- Stabilization of airway, breathing, and circulation and management of raised ICP and seizures if indicated
- *Early neurosurgical intervention* for CSF diversion procedures (external ventricular drainage or VP shunt in case of hydrocephalus, decompressive craniotomy in case of refractory raised ICP, and aspiration and drainage or decompressive craniotomy in case of a large tuberculoma/tubercular abscess causing midline shift)
- *Appropriate fluid and electrolyte management*—hyponatremia is the most frequently observed electrolyte abnormality in children with TBM with a prevalence of 35–65% of all cases. Hyponatremia has been identified as an independent risk factor for poor prognosis. The two common etiologies associated with hyponatremia are cerebral salt wasting (CSW) and syndrome of inappropriate secretion of antidiuretic hormone (SIADH). For SIADH, fluid restriction is recommended while CSW is treated with adequate fluid and sodium replacement.

PREVENTION OF CENTRAL NERVOUS SYSTEM-TUBERCULOSIS

- *BCG:* BCG vaccination has 60–80% efficacy in preventing TBM and the BCG-vaccinated children who develop TBM have a milder clinical course and better outcomes.
- *INH prophylaxis:* All children <5 years with a history of contact with AFB+ve pulmonary TB patients after ruling out active TB should be given 10 mg/kg isoniazid.

OUTCOME AND PROGNOSIS

Tubercular meningitis is associated with high mortality (20%) and morbidity (10–85%). The clinical outcome in TBM depends upon the extent of the disease at diagnosis, delay in initiation of ATT, number of antitubercular drugs administered, HIV coinfection, whether adequate steroid cover was given or not, and the presence of drug resistance. The late sequelae of TBM includes gait disturbances, hemiplegia, cranial nerve palsies, blindness, deafness, learning issues, dementia, and endocrine problems (pituitary and hypothalamic disturbances).

ACUTE ENCEPHALITIS SYNDROMES

DEFINITION

Encephalitis is the inflammation of the brain parenchyma, which can present as a diffuse and/or focal neurological dysfunction (mental, behavior, motor sensory, speech, movement, or personality change) with evidence of CNS inflammation (CSF picture and abnormalities in neuroimaging and EEG). If associated with meningitis it is known as meningoencephalitis. Acute encephalitis is inflammation of the brain of acute onset (<4 weeks). A case of acute encephalitis syndrome (AES) is defined as a person of any age, at any time of the year with the acute onset of fever and a change in mental status (including symptoms such as confusion, disorientation, coma, or inability to talk), and/or new onset of seizures.

ETIOLOGY

Acute encephalitis can be attributed to both infectious and noninfectious causes **(Table 8.12.11)**. The most common infectious causes implicated are viral in etiology. Herpes simplex virus-1 (HSV-1) is the leading cause of sporadic encephalitis globally. Herpes simplex virus-2 (HSV-2) causes encephalitis in the neonatal period or in immunocompromised hosts only.

PATHOGENESIS

Routes of spread to CNS: Hematogenous spread from other sites in systemic infections, antegrade spread via neuraxis as in rabies, reactivation of a latent infection as in HSV, and contiguous spread from adjacent infectious sites such as ear, nose, sinuses, and dental sites.

Predisposing factors: Young age, immunocompromised host, travel to endemic areas, animal bite or exposure, and vaccination status.

CLINICAL MANIFESTATIONS

The clinical profile is highly variable depending on the etiological agent, extent of spread, stage of illness at presentation, age of the patient, and his/her immunological status. Common signs and symptoms are fever, altered sensorium, ranging from irritability to deep coma, seizures, focal neurologic deficits, features of raised ICP, meningeal signs, behavioral changes, and systemic involvement—respiratory involvement, bleeding diathesis, hepatic involvement, and bone or joint pains.

Historical Evaluation

- Antecedent history of viral infections, flu-like symptoms, exanthem, or vaccination
- Epidemic forms—arboviral diseases
- Travel history—knowledge about endemicity of Japanese B encephalitis, leptospira
- Contact exposure or history of similar illness in family or neighborhood
- Immunization history
- History of exposure to animals—dog bite or exposure to bats in rabies, exposure to cats in bartonella, ticks
- Exposure to fresh-water bodies
- History of drug ingestion, toxins, trauma
- History of similar illness in the past

Clinical Examination

Systemic Examination

- Pallor—cerebral malaria or intracranial bleed
- Icterus—leptospirosis, hepatic encephalopathy, or cerebral malaria
- Parotitis and orchitis point-mumps
- Skin rashes—meningococcemia, dengue, measles, rickettsial diseases, varicella, arboviral diseases, and enteroviral encephalitis
- Petechiae and ecchymosis—meningococcemia, dengue, and viral hemorrhagic fevers
- Animal bite marks—rabies, insect bites, or eschar in scrub typhus
- Vitals—for features of shock or raised ICP requiring urgent management and ICU care

TABLE 8.12.11: Etiology—acute encephalitis.

Infectious		***Noninfectious***	
Viral—sporadic: • Herpes simplex virus • HHV-6 • EBV • Varicella zoster virus • Mumps • Measles • ECHO viruses • Influenza • Enterovirus • Rota virus • Polio • Rabies • HIV • Chickenpox • Cytomegalovirus	*Viral—endemic:* • JE (Japanese B encephalitis) • KFD (Kyasanur forest disease) • Chikungunya • Rabies • Chandipura • Nipah • Dengue • St. Lewis encephalitis • Western equine encephalitis • California encephalitis • West Nile	*Autoimmune—neuronal cell surface antigen:* • Anti-NMDAR • Anti-LGI1 • Anti-CASPR2 • Anti-AMPAR • Anti-GABA-A-R • Anti-GABA-B-R • Anti-GlyR • Anti-mGluR5	*Autoimmune—intracellular antigen:* • Anti-Hu • Anti-Ma/Ta • Anti-GAD65 • Anti-GFAP
Bacterial: • Mycoplasma • Rickettsia • Rocky mountain spotted fever • Scrub typhus • Leptospirosis • Enteric fever		*Systemic autoimmune disorders:* • SLE • Behcet's disease • Sarcoidosis	
Parasitic: • Cerebral malaria • Acanthamoeba • Naegleria toxoplasma		*CNS demyelinating conditions:* • ADEM • MOGAD	
Fungal: Cryptococcosis			

(ADEM: acute disseminated encephalomyelitis; EBV: Epstein–Barr virus; HHV-6: human herpesvirus 6; HIV: human immunodeficiency virus; MOGAD: myelin oligodendrocyte glycoprotein antibody-associated disease; NMDAR: *N*-methyl-D-aspartate receptor; SLE: systemic lupus erythematosus)

Neurological Examination

- Assessment of encephalopathy and its severity—GCS
- Look for signs of raised ICP—altered pupillary size and responses, Cushing's triad, abnormal posture (decorticate or decerebrate), and papilledema
- Focal neurological deficits (cranial nerve involvement, hemiparesis, and abnormal posturing)
- Movement disorders including parkinsonian features
- Seizures—tonic eye deviation, nystagmus, subtle clonic movements of face or fingers
- Specific pointers to various etiologies are enumerated in **Table 8.12.12.**[8,9]

Management of acute encephalitis syndrome (AES):

1. *Step 1:* Rapid assessment and stabilization (airway, breathing, circulation, metabolic or electrolyte abnormalities, seizures, and raised ICP)
2. *Step 2:* Detailed history and focused examination (as described above)
3. *Step 3:* Investigations
4. *Step 4:* Empirical treatment

INVESTIGATIONS

Lumbar Puncture

Lumbar puncture should be performed as soon as possible after stabilization and ruling out contraindications. CSF should be examined for cytology, biochemistry, Gram stain, Ziehl–Neelsen stain for acid-fast bacilli, bacterial culture, India ink staining or latex agglutination for cryptococcal antigen, PCR for HSV-1 and 2, and IgM antibodies for Japanese encephalitis (JE) and for dengue serology or PCR. **Table 8.12.12** also enlists the various tests to be considered for various etiologies.

Neuroimaging

Neuroimaging is of particular importance, especially when LP cannot be performed due to contraindications. It provides details regarding the sites and extent of involvement, which can point toward specific etiological agents as depicted in **Table 8.12.13**. Furthermore, it helps to look for complications such as cerebral edema, midline shift, herniation, bleed or

TABLE 8.12.12: Pointers to different etiological agents.

Cause	*Pointers to diagnosis*	*Diagnostic tests*
Herpes simplex virus 1 and 2 (HSV-1 and 2)	Periodic lateralized epileptiform discharges (PLEDS) on EEG, MRI showing temporal lobe involvement, CSF RBC	CSF HSV PCR for HSV-1 and 2
Human herpesvirus 6 (HHV6) and HHV7	• Rash • Most frequently occurs at the time of primary infection (roseola infantum) in children <2 years of age	Specific PCR in CSF
Epstein–Barr virus (EBV)	• Rash, generalized adenopathy, tonsillitis, organomegaly • Typically follows acute mononucleosis by 1–3 weeks, metamorphopsia variably present, isolated cerebellar involvement can occur	• EBV VCA IgM in blood • EBV PCR in CSF
Cytomegalovirus (CMV)	Immunocompromised host	
Varicella zoster virus (VZV)	Antecedent rash	• Varicella IgM in blood • CSF varicella PCR
Human immunodeficiency virus (HIV)	Fever, rash, lymphadenopathy	• HIV ELISA in blood • HIV PCR in blood
Japanese encephalitis (JE)	• Epidemiology, dystonic and extrapyramidal movements • MRI shows changes in thalami, basal ganglia, substantia nigra	IgM antibody in serum and CSF
Measles	• Antecedent or concurrent rash • History of vaccination	Measles IgM in blood and CSF
Mumps	Antecedent or concurrent parotitis, high amylase, low sugar in CSF	• Mumps IgM in blood • Mumps virus in CSF by PCR
Influenza	• Respiratory prodrome, ongoing outbreak • Diffuse cerebral edema or focal thalamic necrosis due to acute necrotizing encephalopathy (ANE)	Influenza PCR in throat swab
Dengue	Ongoing outbreak, rash, low WBC and platelets, biochemical hepatitis	• Dengue-specific PCR in CSF • Dengue IgM, NS1 antigen in blood
Enterovirus	Vesicular lesions in the mouth, GI symptoms, brain stem involvement	Specific PCR in CSF
Rabies	Animal bite, hydrophobia, brain stem involvement	• Specific IgM antibody in CSF • Nuchal skin biopsy/conjunctival smears for direct fluorescent antibody • Brain biopsy
Mycoplasma	Respiratory illness, skin rash, hemolytic anemia	• Mycoplasma IgM in blood • Mycoplasma PCR in throat swab
Rickettsia	Epidemiology, rash, eschar, multisystem involvement	• IgM and IgG antibodies in serum • Scrub typhus DNA in whole blood, buffy coat, eschar/skin rash
Leptospira	• Icterus, myalgia, renal failure • Occurs due to rat bite	• Leptospira PCR in blood • Specific IgM in blood
Enteric	Protracted illness, hepatosplenomegaly	Blood cultures
Cerebral malaria	Pallor, splenomegaly	Smear or rapid antigen test for malaria
Acanthamoeba and Balamuthia mandrillaris	• Occur in immunocompromised children • Granulomatous amoebic encephalitis	
Naegleria toxoplasma	Acquired by swimming in infected water	

(CSF: cerebrospinal fluid; DNA: deoxyribonucleic acid; EEG: electroencephalogram; GI: gastrointestinal; HIV ELISA: human immunodeficiency virus enzyme-linked immunosorbent assay; HIV PCR: human immunodeficiency virus polymerase chain reaction; IgG: immunoglobulin G; IgM: immunoglobulin M; MRI: magnetic resonance imaging; WBC: white blood cell)

TABLE 8.12.13: Central nervous system (CNS) sites involved in various etiologies.

Area involved	*Etiological agent*
Frontal lobe	Naegleria
Temporal lobe	• Herpes simplex virus (HSV) • Human herpesvirus 6 (HHV-6) • Autoimmune limbic encephalitis
Deep gray matter (basal ganglia, thalamus)	• Japanese encephalitis (JE) • West Nile virus
Brainstem	• Rabies • Enterovirus • Listeria
Cerebellum	• Epstein–Barr virus (EBV) • Varicella zoster virus (VZV)
White matter	• Acute demyelinating encephalomyelitis (ADEM) • Parechoviruses
Acute ischemic lesion	• VZV • Syphilis • Fungal • Rickettsia • Tuberculosis

stroke, and hydrocephalus and to rule out alternate diagnosis such as ADEM.

Electroencephalogram

Electroencephalogram is implicated in children with subtle motor seizures and those with persistently altered sensorium in postictal phase or in those with poor sensorium after ruling out or treating raised ICP to look for nonconvulsive status epilepticus. Specific findings such as periodic lateralized epileptiform discharges (PLED) point toward HSV, delta brush is seen in autoimmune encephalitis (NMDA-R), and the presence of diffuse cerebral dysfunction could predict poor prognosis.

Other Etiological Workup

- Sepsis and inflammatory markers—hemogram, CRP, erythrocyte sedimentation rate (ESR), procalcitonin
- Blood culture—bacterial, viral, fungal
- Serological testing—leptospira, legionella, Lyme disease, mycoplasma, scrub typhus
- Antigen testing
- Autoimmune antibody panel in blood and CSF (anti-NMDA, anti-GAD, anti-AMPA, anti-GABR, anti-LGI1, anti-CASPR, etc.)
- Oligoclonal antibodies in serum and CSF
- Serum myelin oligodendrocyte glycoprotein (MOG) antibodies
- Autoimmune workup—antinuclear antibody (ANA), antineutrophil cytoplasmic antibody (ANCA), C3, C4, anti-dsDNA, antithyroid peroxidase (anti-TPO), etc.

TREATMENT

Empirical Treatment

Third-generation cephalosporin ceftriaxone (100 mg/kg/day in two divided doses) or cefotaxime (150–200 mg/kg/day in two or three divided doses) should be started for antibacterial cover with or without staphylococcal cover (IV vancomycin). Acyclovir IV should be started in all suspected sporadic viral encephalitis (such as in the presence of focal seizures). In areas endemic to scrub typhus or in the presence of eschar, doxycycline or azithromycin should be started. In malaria-endemic regions, in the presence of clinical suspicion of malaria, empirical antimalarial (artemisin-based combination therapies) should be started.[8,9]

Specific Treatment of Underlying Etiology

It can be revised as soon as the results of the investigations are obtained.

Supportive Management

- *Stabilization* of airway, breathing, circulation, and treatment of raised ICP and seizures
- *Steroids:* Pulse steroids (methylprednisolone or dexamethasone) must be given to children with suspected ADEM
- *Rehabilitation:* Physiotherapy, posture change, prevent bed sores and exposure keratitis
- *Prevention of complications:* Aspiration pneumonia, nosocomial infections, coagulation disturbances
- *Nutrition:* Early feeding
- *Psychological support* to patient and family

PROGNOSIS

The main determinant of prognosis in a child with AES depends on the underlying etiology and extent of brain injury. Rapid clinical progression, duration of coma, prolonged seizures, focal deficits, and certain EEG abnormalities may indicate adverse outcomes.

NEUROCYSTICERCOSIS

Neurocysticercosis is the most common preventable cause of epilepsy in the developing world and is an important public health issue in Asia, South America, and many other countries. In India, NCC contributes to 1.2 % of all space-occupying lesions and 5.2% of late-onset epilepsies.

ETIOLOGY

Neurocysticercosis is a parasitic infection of the CNS, caused by encysted larvae of human tapeworm *Taenia solium*, characterized by a range of pathological symptoms including epileptic seizures, headaches, and hydrocephalus.

PATHOGENESIS

Neurocysticercosis is acquired through the fecal–oral route, by eating food contaminated with *T. solium* eggs. Typically, eggs or gravid proglottid are ingested by pigs and the oncospheres from these hatch in the pigs' intestine, penetrate the intestinal walls, and circulate to the pigs' muscles, developing there as cysticerci. When humans eat raw or undercooked meat, they develop intestinal teniasis and excrete the eggs of *T. solium* in feces. When humans eat these eggs, they hatch in the human intestine to release larvae that penetrate the intestinal mucosa and migrate throughout the body to produce human cysticercosis (subcutaneous tissue, eye, and brain). Cysticerci often live asymptomatically within host tissues for years as vesicular cysts, which are cystic lesions containing the larva without any perifocal edema, and excite very little host reaction. When they degenerate, colloidal or granular nodular stages occur and cause symptoms. The various stages result in different image morphology on CT and MRI.

CLINICAL MANIFESTATIONS

Neurocysticercosis is classified into parenchymal and extraparenchymal (ventricular, cisternal, ophthalmic, or spinal). The latter is uncommon in children. In India, parenchymal cysticercosis is the most common. Most children present with single degenerating parenchymal cysts, and some with multiple cysts.

Parenchymal Neurocysticercosis

Cysticercosis may be asymptomatic and identified during incidental neuroimaging. The most common presentation is seizure (occurs in 70–90% of cases), which is focal in two-thirds of cases and is more common in degenerating cysts, but rare in patients with only viable, noninflamed cysts. Almost one-third of children have headache and vomiting. Papilledema, focal neurological deficits, visual symptoms, or hydrocephalus are uncommon. Cysticercal encephalitis presents with severe acute raised ICP. It rarely occurs in children with innumerable cysts and extensive cerebral edema.

Extraparenchymal Neurocysticercosis

Extraparenchymal NCC is rare in children and may present as obstructive hydrocephalus, chronic meningitis, or spinal cysticercosis (arachnoiditis, transverse myelitis, or other spinal cord syndromes). Ophthalmic cysticercosis can cause visual deficits and limitation of eye movements.

DIAGNOSIS

Neuroimaging

Neuroimaging is the diagnostic modality of choice for NCC. Conclusive evidence is the demonstration of scolex within a cystic lesion on a CT/MRI brain. The typical NCC lesion is <20 mm with thin, well-defined wall with eccentrically placed scolex located near the grey–white matter junction. The scolex appears as a bright, high-density eccentric nodule in these cysts and is pathognomonic of NCC. Lesions of varying stages can be seen in the same patient at one point of time. "Starry sky" appearance is typical of NCC and consists of disseminated NCC with numerous cysts. MRI is useful for detecting relatively small lesions, evaluating degenerating changes, detecting edema around calcified lesions, and visualizing scolices within calcified lesions. MRI distinguishes cysticercosis from tuberculoma better **(Table 8.12.14)**.

Serologic Tests

Enzyme-linked immuno-electrotransfer blot (EITB) using parasite glycoproteins or ELISA which uses crude antigens have a low positivity (17–25%) particularly for single lesions and have no role in the diagnosis and management of NCC.

DIFFERENTIAL DIAGNOSIS

- Tuberculomas
- Chronic brain abscesses
- Tumors
- Other parasitic infestations (acanthamoeba) toxoplasma
- Fungal lesions

TABLE 8.12.14: Difference between tuberculoma and neurocysticercosis (NCC) in neuroimaging.

Features	*Tuberculoma*	*NCC*
Size	≥25 mm	Variable, generally smaller
Midline shift	Greater	Lesser
Perilesional edema	Greater	Lesser
Thickness of ring	Greater	Lesser
Scolex	Absent	Present in one-third
Intracystic space	Isodense with brain	Hypodense
Meningeal involvement	Present	Absent

TREATMENT[10]

Cysticidal Therapy

Indications

- All multiple cysts/live cysts need treatment.
- Calcified lesions do not require cysticidal therapy.
- With therapy, even in single RELs there is faster resolution of active/RELs and diminished acute symptomatic seizures. Radiologic resolution is also higher after therapy; however, the risk of calcification is not significantly altered.

Contraindications

- *Ocular cysticerci:* Always check the fundus (indirect ophthalmoscopy, USG B scan for intraocular cysts before cysticidal treatment). Treatment involves surgical management and later anticysticercal drugs.
- Encephalitis
- *Ventricular cysts, hydrocephalus, and spinal cysts:* Treatment involves surgical management and later anticysticercal drugs.

Dose

- *One to five viable NCC:* Albendazole (preferred)—15 mg/kg/day for 7 days with steroids
- *More than five viable cysts:* Cysticidal therapy is not recommended.

Other Cysticidal Therapy

Praziquantel (50 mg/kg/day) can be combined with albendazole in case of no resolution with albendazole monotherapy.

Role of Corticosteroids

Corticosteroids (oral dexamethasone 0.6 mg/kg/day) must be given for 2 days before and 5 days after starting cysticidal therapy. Initiation of cysticidal therapy alone may enhance perilesional edema and worsen symptoms; hence, steroids should be given with anticysticidal treatment. However, routine use of steroids is not recommended in patients with calcified NCC with contrast enhancement presenting as seizure, except in conditions with marked perilesional edema.[10]

Role of Repeat Neuroimaging

A repeat CT is generally done after 3–6 months to determine whether the lesions have resolved.

Supportive Care

Treatment of Seizure

The antiepileptic drugs used most commonly are carbamazepine, oxcarbazepine, phenytoin, and levetiracetam. Duration varies from 6 to 9 months (much shorter than epilepsy) or till the lesion disappearance. Longer treatment is indicated in calcified lesions and persistent or multiple cysts.

Treatment of Cysticercal Encephalitis

There is no role for cysticidal therapy. For the management of acute symptomatic edema patients can be treated with pulse methylprednisolone (30–50 mg/kg/day for 3–5 days, maximum 1,000 mg/day). Anti-raised ICP measures and osmotherapy are indicated for the management of raised ICP.

Indications of Surgery

- Ocular cysticercosis
- Obstructive hydrocephalus
- Spinal cord lesions which warrant high-dose steroids
- Epilepsy surgery in drug-refractory epilepsy

PREVENTION

Proper hygiene and sanitation, community awareness to prevent open field defecation, pork-eating precautions (inspection to look for measly meat, adequately freezing and cooking meat to destroy cysticerci) should be practiced.

PROGNOSIS

Cases with single lesions generally have a good prognosis. Cysticercus encephalitis and extraparenchymal NCC have a poor prognosis.

CONCLUSION

- Meningitis can be defined as acute, subacute, and chronic based on the duration of illness being <5 days, 5 days to 4 weeks, and >4 weeks, respectively.
- Neck rigidity may be falsely negative in infants, severe malnutrition, terminally ill patients, partially treated meningitis, and immunocompromised hosts.
- In the presence of CSF leak, VP shunt in situ or history of neurosurgical procedure antimicrobial with *Staphylococcus* cover (vancomycin) should be added along with third-generation cephalosporins in the management of ABM.
- Role of corticosteroids in the management of pyogenic meningitis is established only in infection with *H. influenzae* but is controversial in others.
- The most common agents causing brain abscess in immunocompetent hosts are aerobic and anaerobic streptococci. Polymicrobial etiology is seen in 25–30% of cases.
- Indications of surgical drainage in brain abscess include abscess >2.5 cm, impending rupture or herniation, abscess involving noneloquent cortex, abscess size

increasing despite antibiotic treatment or no decrease in size even after 3–4 weeks of antibiotics, fungal abscess, traumatic abscess with foreign body, etc.

- TB should be ruled in or ruled out upfront as it is a major cause of chronic meningitis and the threshold for starting ATT should be kept low in cases of chronic meningitis.
- Steroids in the initial intensive phase are the only treatment that has been shown to reduce mortality in TBM.
- Immune-mediated paradoxical reaction should always be considered in case of new-onset neurological worsening in children with TBM receiving adequate antitubercular therapy.
- IV acyclovir should be considered in all cases of acute febrile encephalopathy, especially with focal seizures, focal deficits, temporal involvement, or a high suspicion of HSV encephalitis.
- For multifocal CNS involvement in a young child with acute febrile encephalopathy, possibility of ADEM should be considered upfront and steroids should be started after ruling out infection.
- Differentiating NCC from tuberculoma is crucial, especially in Indian settings where both are common and endemic.
- Ocular NCC should be ruled out before initiating cysticidal therapy.
- NCC should be considered as a differential in a child presenting with unprovoked seizures, especially focal seizures.

REFERENCES

1. Tunkel AR, Hasbun R, Bhimraj A, Byers K, Kaplan SL, Scheld WM, et al. 2017 Infectious Diseases Society of America's clinical practice guidelines for healthcare-associated ventriculitis and meningitis. Clin Infect Dis. 2017;64(6):e34-65.
2. Tunkel AR, Hartman BJ, Kaplan SL, Kaufman BA, Roos KL, Scheld WM, et al. Practice guidelines for the management of bacterial meningitis. Clin Infect Dis. 2004;39(9):1267-84.
3. Bodilsen J, D'Alessandris QG, Humphreys H, Iro MA, Klein M, Last K, et al. European Society of Clinical Microbiology and Infectious Diseases guidelines on diagnosis and treatment of brain abscess in children and adults. Clin Microbiol Infect. 2024;30(1):66-89.
4. Arlotti M, Grossi P, Pea F, Tomei G, Vullo V, De Rosa FG, et al. Consensus document on controversial issues for the treatment of infections of the central nervous system: bacterial brain abscesses. Int J Infect Dis. 2010;14(Suppl 4):S79-92.
5. Thakur KT, Wilson MR. Chronic meningitis. Continuum (Minneap Minn). 2018;24(5):1298-326.
6. Dian S, Ganiem AR, van Laarhoven A. Central nervous system tuberculosis. Curr Opin Neurol. 2021:34(3):396-402.
7. Chang CC, Harrison TS, Bicanic TA, Chayakulkeeree M, Sorrell TC, Warris A, et al. Global guideline for the diagnosis and management of cryptococcosis: an initiative of the ECMM and ISHAM in cooperation with the ASM. Lancet Infect Dis. 2024:24(8):e495-512.
8. Sigfrid L, Perfect C, Rojek A, Longuere KS, Lipworth S, Hassis E, et al. A systematic review of clinical guidelines on the management of acute, community-acquired CNS infections. BMC Med. 2019;17(1):1-7.
9. Bloch KC, Glaser C, Gaston D, Venkatesan A. State of the art: acute encephalitis. Clin Infect Dis. 2023;77(5):e14-33.
10. White AC Jr, Coyle CM, Rajshekhar V, Singh G, Hauser WA, Mohanty A, et al. Diagnosis and treatment of neurocysticercosis: 2017 clinical practice guidelines by the Infectious Diseases Society of America (IDSA) and the American Society of Tropical Medicine and Hygiene (ASTMH). Clin Infect Dis. 2018;66(8):1159-63.

8.13 Disorders of Consciousness and Coma

(Col) Aparajita Gupta

INTRODUCTION

Disorders of consciousness include states such as coma, vegetative state (VS) or unresponsive wakefulness syndrome, and minimally conscious state. These are complex medical conditions caused by infection, trauma, hypoxic-ischemic brain injury, intracranial hemorrhage, and metabolic disorders. However, before jumping onto the complex terminologies in use for disorders of consciousness, it is vital to understand the meaning of the word "consciousness."

- Consciousness is defined by the state of *wakefulness* and *awareness*.
- *Wakefulness* simply means the child's state of wakefulness, that is, whether he or she opens his/her eyes spontaneously.
- *Awareness* means "awareness of our surroundings," the people around us, and of ourselves.

Together, these two elements make up our consciousness.

Disorders of consciousness may vary from clouding of consciousness to minimally conscious state to VS (unresponsive wakefulness) to coma and lastly to brain death.

Altered consciousness may be transient or permanent in nature. The outcome for transient disorders of consciousness is usually favorable when compared to those with persistent disorders of consciousness. There is no eye opening in comatose patients, and most often it is confused with conditions such as concussion and syncope. For a patient to be in coma, there should be total absence of arousal and awareness for *>1 hour duration.*[1]

Duration of altered consciousness is also used when defining VS. VS may be transient, persistent, or permanent. Transient VS lasts < 4 weeks, and persistent VS lasts > 4 weeks regardless of the etiology. VS is termed permanent if it lasts for >3 months for nontraumatic brain injury and after 12 months for traumatic brain injury (TBI).

It is best to avoid terms such as somnolence, obtundation, stupor, and lethargy because these are very subjective terms and no objective criteria are available to define them.

TERMINOLOGY

Before understanding the pathophysiology of disorders of consciousness and coma, it is important to know the defining terms for each of the following **(Table 8.13.1)**.

- *Brain death*: Irreversible state of coma with apnea, permanent absence of all brain functioning including the brainstem reflexes
- *Coma*: In simple words, it means complete absence of arousal and awareness. It is a state of unconsciousness in which the child is not arousable to external stimuli nor responsive to internal needs. The eyes are closed, and wakefulness and awareness are indistinguishable. There are no sleep-wake cycles. The patient can neither vocalize nor localize any noxious stimuli.
- *VS/unresponsive wakefulness*: It is also known as "arousal without awareness." It is a state of disordered consciousness in which the child does not respond to external stimuli consistently. There is no sustained, reproducible response to visual, auditory, tactile, or noxious stimuli. The sleep-wake cycles are present, and some spontaneous movements may be present; however, these children may lack the awareness of themselves to the external stimuli. There is no evidence of any form of language expression or comprehension. Periodic eye opening may be present, manifesting as intermittent wakefulness.
- *Minimally conscious state:* This state refers to a slightly higher level of consciousness than VS, wherein the children may show inconsistent signs of awareness, which may not be always present. In simple terms, awareness is minimal but definite. The sleep-wake cycles are maintained. There may be localization to painful stimuli, some nonreflexive movement patterns, intelligible vocalizations, inconsistent following of commands, and unreliable yes or no responses.

TABLE 8.13.1: States of wakefulness.

State	***Definition***
Coma	Complete absence of arousal and awareness
Vegetative/unresponsive wakefulness (UWS)	Arousal without awareness
Minimally conscious state– (MCS–)	Minimal reproducible but inconsistent awareness without language
Minimally conscious state+ (MCS+)	Minimal, reproducible but inconsistent awareness with language comprehension and expression (intelligible verbalization or intentional communication)
Wakefulness	Arousal and awareness both present

ETIOLOGY

The etiology of disorders of consciousness is varied. Broadly, they can be classified as traumatic or nontraumatic as shown in **Table 8.13.2**.

EVALUATION OF A CHILD WITH COMA/ DISORDERS OF CONSCIOUSNESS

Any alteration in consciousness is an emergency requiring prompt evaluation of the hemodynamic stability and etiology. While the evaluation of etiology of coma is underway, the most important step in the management is stabilization of the child.

Airway should be stabilized, and breathing should be ensured because a child with coma is prone to airway instability and aspiration due to loss of protective brainstem reflexes. Circulation should be assessed, and appropriate measures to maintain adequate circulation should be ensured at all times, including fluid bolus and initiation of vasopressor drugs if required. Electrolyte abnormalities and hypoglycemia or hyperglycemia should be promptly corrected. Hematological, biochemical, and acid-base status should be assessed and corrected promptly. Any ongoing seizure activity requires administration of intravenous antiseizure drugs. Simultaneously, there should be an ongoing evaluation of any internal or external injuries along with assessment of any intake of drugs, accidental poisoning, and toxins.[2]

EXAMINATION

Hemodynamic Stability

On admission, hemodynamic stability should be ensured by charting vital parameters such as temperature, blood

TABLE 8.13.2: Etiology of disorders of consciousness.

Traumatic	
• Accidental • Nonaccidental head injury (abusive trauma)	
Nontraumatic	
CNS infections	• Viral encephalitis • Bacterial meningoencephalitis • Brain abscess • Scrub typhus • Lyme's disease • Rock mountain spotted fever • Cerebral malaria • HIV disease • Fungal abscess • Multiple neurocysticercosis
Vascular lesions	• Stroke • Vasculitis • Moyamoya disease • Arteriovenous (AV) malformations causing intracranial bleeding • Cerebrosinous venous thrombosis
Diffuse hypoxic brain injury	• Shock • Postcardiac arrest • Drowning • Electric current
Postinfectious	• ADEM • MOG-related demyelination • NMOSD • Primary progressive multiple sclerosis • Acute necrotizing encephalopathy • Hemorrhagic shock and encephalopathy syndrome
Metabolic disturbances	• Hypoglycemia • Diabetic ketoacidosis • Uremic encephalopathy • *Hepatic failure:* Hyperammonemia • *Inborn errors of metabolism:* Organic acidemias, aminoacidopathies, urea cycle deficits, fatty acid oxidation defects • *Electrolyte disturbances:* Hyponatremia, hypernatremia
Systemic infections	• Bacterial sepsis • Enteric encephalopathy • Shigella encephalopathy
Intracranial tumors	• Brainstem glioma • Anaplastic astrocytoma
Hypertensive encephalopathy	
Postictal states	• Nonconvulsive status • *Postseizure state:* Todd's paresis • Status migrainosus
Drugs/toxin and poisoning	

(ADEM: acute disseminated encephalomyelitis; CNS: central nervous system; HIV: human immunodeficiency virus; MOG: myelin oligodendrocyte glycoprotein; NMOSD: neuromyelitis optica spectrum disorder)

pressure (BP), heart rate, respiratory rate, and oxygenation. Elevated BP may indicate underlying hypertensive encephalopathy, while a low BP may indicate shock, the etiology of which may be septic shock or myocardial dysfunction. Elevated temperature may indicate underlying infection, while tachycardia may be indicative of underlying infection or shock. Bradycardia may indicate elevated intracranial pressure (ICP). Tachypnea or bradypnea may indicate disorders of consciousness with involvement of the brainstem. Silent tachypnea is an indicator of underlying metabolic derangement, such as metabolic acidosis seen in diabetic ketoacidosis, inborn errors of metabolism, and uremia.

General Examination

This examination should include assessment of pallor, icterus, anthropometry, measurement of head size, rashes, eschar, purpura, and neurocutaneous markers. In young infants, the size of anterior fontanelles should be measured and the presence of a bruit should be looked for.

Systemic Examination

Assess for the presence of any organomegaly, size of the heart, and any evidence of myocardial dysfunction, which may lead to stroke; evidence of pneumonia, etc., should be assessed.

Focused Neurological Examination

Detailed neurological examination should include assessment of meningeal signs, size of the pupils, pupillary reaction to light, evidence of any cranial nerve (CN) palsies, presence of corneal reflexes, presence of nystagmus, ocular bobbing, ophthalmoplegia, papilledema, retinal hemorrhages, and persistent ocular deviation. Unilaterally fixed and dilated pupil is suggestive of transtentorial herniation. Persistent ocular deviation and nystagmus may indicate ongoing status epilepticus. Preserved pupillary reflexes despite abnormal brainstem reflexes indicate a metabolic or toxic cause. Nystagmus may indicate phenytoin toxicity.

Further, motor system should be assessed for reflexes, bulk, tone, and asymmetry. *Decerebrate posture* literally means "to remove the cerebrum from." It is an abnormal body posture resulting from arms being in adducted position, internally rotated and extended at elbows, wrists being flexed and the neck being stiffly extended, legs being held straight out, and the toes being pointed downward. This kind of posturing is also known as "extensor posturing." A child displaying decerebrate posturing in response to pain receives a score of 2 in the motor section of the Glasgow Coma Scale (GCS). Decerebrate posturing indicates brainstem damage, specifically below the red nucleus. Usually, there is a lesion in the midbrain and lesions in the pons and adjoining areas. Whenever a child shows signs of *decorticate posturing* that further progress to decerebrate posturing, it is always indicative of uncal (transtentorial herniation) or tonsillar brain herniation due to raised ICP. Raised ICP may be due to a variety of causes, including intracranial bleeds, metabolic encephalopathies, space-occupying lesions, TBI, and malignant strokes.

Decorticate posturing is an abnormal posture consisting of flexion at the elbows and the wrists with extension in the lower limbs and the toes being pointed outward. This posturing is also known as "arms to the core." This posturing results from damage to one or both corticospinal tracts in the internal capsule or the cerebral hemispheres and the thalamus. A child displaying decorticate posturing in response to pain gets a score of 3 in the motor section of the GCS.

There are two parts of the decorticate posturing. The first part is the disinhibition of the red nucleus with facilitation of the rubrospinal tracts which in turn facilitates the motor neurons in the upper extremities. The rubrospinal tract and medullary reticulospinal tract-based flexion outweighs the pontine reticulospinal tract-based extension in the upper extremities. The second component is the disruption of the lateral corticospinal tract, which in normal state facilitates the motor neurons of the flexor muscles in the lower limbs. Due to the interruption of the corticospinal tract, the pontine reticulospinal tract-based extension overwhelms the flexion in the lower limbs and causes extension posture of the lower limbs. Therefore, lesions above the red nucleus involving the corticospinal tract and the rubrospinal tract cause characteristic flexion of the upper limbs and extension of the lower limbs.

While decorticate posturing is still an ominous sign of severe brain damage, decerebrate posturing is indicative of more severe damage at the rubrospinal tract, and hence the red nucleus is also involved, suggesting a lesion in the brainstem. Children displaying decorticate and/or decerebrate posturing are in coma and are always at risk of sudden cardiorespiratory arrest.

Other neurological signs may be observed, including absent reflexes and flaccidity, which are indicative of a grave prognosis due to the severe brainstem involvement, while the presence of dystonia and dyskinesias is suggestive of infectious causes such as Japanese B encephalitis. Neurometabolic disorders may also present with dystonia and states of altered consciousness.[3,4]

The other most important examination is the *pattern of respiration* in a child with altered consciousness, which may also help in localization of the disease.

Abnormal Patterns of Respiration

- *Cheyne-Stokes respiration:* This is a periodic breathing pattern characterized by cyclical episodes of apnea and hyperventilation. This type of respiration is usually seen in TBI, stroke, toxic metabolic encephalopathy, congestive heart failure, and brain tumors, or involvement of the respiratory center in the brainstem.
- *Central neurogenic hyperventilation:* This is characterized by episodes of hyperventilation that persist even during sleep. It is usually seen as a result of infiltrative tumors that stimulate the pontine respiratory center and central chemoreceptors.
- *Apneustic pattern of respiration:* This is characterized by prolonged gasping inhalations followed by short and inadequate exhalations. The lesion is generally in the upper pons, usually due to infiltrative lesions, trauma, and stroke.
- *Ataxic:* It is characterized by a completely irregular breathing pattern with irregular pauses of apnea. The lesion is usually caused by damage to the medulla oblongata due to trauma or stroke.

Any form of these breathing patterns indicates severe brain injury due to trauma, toxins, vascular insults, or infiltrative lesions, and recognition of these breathing patterns requires mechanical ventilation and treatment of underlying condition.

Grading of Coma

Grading of coma may be done using a pediatric GCS for children. The grading of GCS is given in **Table 8.13.3**. The maximum score obtained is 15 and the minimum score obtained is 3. Any child with a GCS of <8 requires invasive ventilation.

Eye Findings

The eye findings in a child with coma are important localizing signs. The eye examination includes testing the size of pupils (anisocoria) along with the pupillary reflexes (both direct and consensual), the relative afferent pupillary defect, the extraocular eye movements, lid position, ophthalmoscopic findings, ocular motility including ocular bobbing, ophthalmoplegia, ocular misalignment, ocular dipping, and ocular misalignment.

- *Unilateral dilated fixed pupil* in a comatose patient is an emergency suggestive of uncal herniation. This occurs due to the compression of the third cranial nerve (CN III) at the Kernohan notch due to uncal herniation. Inadvertent pupillary dilation due to use of atropine drops should be ruled out in all cases. Administration of 1% pilocarpine will not constrict an atropinized pharmacologically dilated pupil and can be used to differentiate CN III palsy.
- *Bilateral pinpoint pupils*: Seen in dorsal pontine involvement such as pontine hemorrhage

TABLE 8.13.3: Pediatric Glasgow Coma Scale.

Eye opening	***>5 years***	***<5 years***
E4	Spontaneous	Spontaneous
E3	To voice	To voice
E2	To pain	To pain
E1	None	None
Verbal		
V5	Oriented in person or place	Alert/babbles/coos/words or sentences to usual ability
V4	Confused	Less than usual ability, irritable cry
V3	Inappropriate sounds	Cries to pain (inconsolable)
V2	Incomprehensible sounds	Moans to pain
V1	No response to pain	No response to pain
T	Intubated	Intubated
Motor		
M6	Obeys command	Normal spontaneous movements
M5	Localizes to supraorbital pain or withdraws to touch	Localizes to supraorbital pain or withdraws to touch
M4	Withdraws from pain	Withdraws from pain
M3	Flexion to pain (decorticate)	Flexion to pain (decorticate)
M2	Decerebrate to pain	Decerebrate to pain
M1	No response	No response

- *Bilateral small but reactive pupils*: Suspect injury to diencephalon and drug toxicity
- *Unilateral small but reactive pupil*: This suggests Horner syndrome due to the damage of the ipsilateral oculosympathetic pathway (hypothalamus to the posterolateral brainstem) descending caudally to the ciliospinal center (cervical C8 to thoracic T2 level). In addition to miosis, anisocoria is worse in the dark; there is presence of ipsilateral ptosis and anhidrosis.
- *Bilateral fixed and dilated pupils*: Suggestive of CN III dysfunction as seen in bilateral infarction of the dorsal midbrain
- *Papilledema on fundus examination* is suggestive of high ICP due to a space-occupying lesion or hemorrhage.
- *Ocular motility*: Ocular movements may be affected due to cranial neuropathy (CN III, IV, and VI) or skew deviation may be seen in children with coma. In CN III palsy, the eye is typically down and out (hypotropia and exotropia), and in CN VI palsy, the eye is typically deviated inward (esotropia). A lesion in the frontal eye fields will result in conjugate deviation toward the side of lesion, whereas a lesion in the paramedian reticular formation causes conjugate deviation away from the side of the lesion.

Similarly, abnormal *saccades* (eye movement toward a stationary target) may occur in a comatose patient due to the involvement either of the frontal eye fields, pons, CN III, CN VI, and the medial longitudinal fasciculus. The presence of a smooth visual pursuit describes a slow tracking movement of the eyes, which is voluntary. Therefore, the presence of smooth pursuit movements suggests that the patient is at least in a minimally conscious state rather than VS.

Similarly, the presence of an *oculocephalic reflex* (Doll's eye maneuver) is an assured sign of brainstem intactness. Oculocephalic response consists of conjugate eye movement in the opposite direction of head rotation with a gradual return to the midline position.

Other Neurological Signs

Other neurological signs in a comatose child consist of meningeal signs such as neck rigidity, Kernig's sign, and Brudzinski's sign. Neck rigidity may be present in subarachnoid hemorrhage, herniation, or trauma.

ASSESSMENT IN A CHILD WITH ALTERED CONSCIOUSNESS

The list of investigations in a child with coma may be exhaustive and therefore needs to be tailored as per the history, examination, and the differential diagnosis. The list of investigations is given in **Table 8.13.4**.

MANAGING A CHILD WITH COMA

Recognizing a child with altered consciousness is an emergency. Maintenance of airway, breathing, and circulation takes precedence. The principles of management include rapid assessment and stabilization. Once the child has been stabilized, a quick detailed history and clinical examination should be carried out to assess the depth of coma and localize the lesion.

The specific management strategies are as given in **Table 8.13.5**.

OUTCOME

A coma is a transient state usually lasting 2–4 weeks. Children recover, die, or may slip into a vegetative or minimally conscious state. VS is considered to be permanent if it lasts >12 months for TBI and longer than 3 months for non-traumatic brain injury.[4,5]

TABLE 8.13.4: List of investigations for disorders of consciousness.

Sample	*Indications*
Complete blood count	Infections such as meningitis/encephalitis/malaria/rickettsial/fungal infection
Blood sugar	• Hypoglycemia in sepsis and IEM • Hyperglycemia in diabetic ketoacidosis
Electrolytes	Metabolic encephalopathy such as hyponatremia and hypernatremia
Liver function tests	• Hepatic encephalopathy/certain IEMs • Toxins • Infections such as malaria/rickettsial infections/Reye syndrome
Renal function tests	• Uremic encephalopathy • Toxins and infections such as sepsis
Arterial blood gas	• Acidosis and lactate in sepsis • Increased anion gap in IEMs
Ammonia	Metabolic encephalopathy/drug induced
Blood culture	Bacterial sepsis
IgM for rickettsia Weil–Felix test	Rickettsial infections
Widal test	Enteric encephalopathy
Leptospira serology	Leptospirosis
• CSF for cytology, biochemistry, Gram stain, lactate, Biofire, and galactomannan • MOG antibody • Oligoclonal bands	• Viral encephalitis/bacterial meningoencephalitis • Invasive CNS fungal infections • Specific demyelination syndromes
• Urine ketones • Toxicology screen	• Metabolic and toxicology screen • Toxic encephalopathy
Neuroimaging • CT scan • MRI brain (preferred)	• Only in emergency for a traumatic brain injury, intracranial hemorrhage, and stroke • CNS infections, demyelination, acute necrotizing encephalopathy, vascular strokes, neurometabolic disorders, space-occupying lesions
MRA	Vascular strokes/Moyamoya disease and CNS vasculitis
Electroencephalogram (EEG)	Nonconvulsive status epilepticus/burst suppression in children on barbiturate coma

(CNS: central nervous system; CSF: cerebrospinal fluid; IEM: inborn errors of metabolism; IgM: immunoglobulin M; MOG: myelin oligodendrocyte glycoprotein; MRA: magnetic resonance angiography; CT: computed tomography; MRI: magnetic resonance imaging)

TABLE 8.13.5: General management principles in a child with disorders of consciousness and coma.

General management	
Raised ICP	• Head in midline position at a 30° elevation • Maintain euthermia and normoglycemia • Maintain adequate analgesia and sedation • Hyperventilation and osmolar agents such as mannitol (0.25 g/kg) or 3% hypertonic saline (0.1–1 mL/kg/h) to maintain sodium between 145 and 155 mEq/L may be instituted • *Mannitol is contraindicated in children with intracranial hemorrhage and in children with hypovolemic shock* • In children with impending herniation, emergency decompressive craniectomy should be carried out
Seizures	• Intravenous benzodiazepines (lorazepam/midazolam 0.1 mg/kg) followed by a broad-spectrum intravenous antiseizure drug such as fosphenytoin should be started to prevent recurrence of seizure • Recurrent seizures may increase the intracranial pressure, causing secondary neuronal injury • Nonconvulsive status epilepticus should be looked through continuous EEG monitoring
Hypoglycemia/hyperglycemia	• Fingerstick evaluation and estimation of blood glucose should be done as soon as the coma is recognized • Hypoglycemia should be treated with 2.5 mL/kg of 10% dextrose • In case of hyperglycemia, urine ketone bodies should be checked for diabetic ketoacidosis, and insulin drip should be started for the same
Infections	• Pending definitive diagnosis of CNS infections, empiric treatment with antibacterial medication such as ceftriaxone at 100 mg/kg/day (maximum 4 g per day) plus vancomycin 60 mg/kg per day plus acyclovir 30–60 mg/kg/day should be instituted • Therapy should not be delayed pending CSF results
Fever	• Requires aggressive management with antipyretics because hyperthermia can contribute to neuronal damage at cellular level • Hyperthermia can also worsen raised intracranial pressure • Controlled induced hypothermia is the treatment of choice for elevated intracranial pressure due to traumatic brain injury. However, this treatment is still not recommended for nontraumatic brain injury
Electrolyte imbalance	• No intervention is generally needed to manage mild to moderate hypernatremia. • Hyponatremia can increase cerebral edema and should be corrected

(CNS: central nervous system; EEG: electroencephalogram; ICP: intracranial pressure)

The outcome of a comatose child depends on the etiology. Children with drug overdose have a better outcome as compared to children with hypoxic ischemic injury. The potential for recovery is greater for TBI as compared to hypoxic brain injury. Associated hypotension or continued seizures are associated with worse outcomes. Presence of acute kidney injury, hepatic injury, and elevated lactate correlate with poor neurological outcome. In TBI, hyperglycemia, need for mechanical ventilation, and raised ICP are associated with poor outcomes. Similarly, a low GCS both at admission and at 24 hours is associated with poor prognosis. Generally, as a rule, the prognosis of TBI is better than hypoxic ischemic insult.[6-8]

Neuroimaging findings of diffuse axonal injury, brainstem injury, involvement of the basal ganglia, involvement of water-shed areas, and severe cerebral edema causing herniation are associated with poor prognosis. Electroencephalogram (EEG) findings of burst suppression pattern, periodic lateralized epileptiform discharges, and nonreactive background activity are also associated with poor prognosis.[9]

CONCLUSION

Management of a child with altered consciousness needs evaluation of etiology along with a detailed neurological assessment, to be able to prognosticate the outcome. Children with altered consciousness generally have an optimistic outcome with a possible late emergence. Therefore, it is important to provide optimal management with simultaneous care withdrawal with extreme caution. There is a growing need for standardization of neurophysiological tools in the assessment of children with disorders of consciousness.

REFERENCES

1. Taylor DA, Ashwal S. Impairment of consciousness and coma. In: Swaiman KF, Ashwal S, Ferriero DM (Eds). Pediatric Neurology: Principles and Practice, 4th edition. Philadelphia: Elsevier; 2006. pp. 1379-400.
2. Brazis PW, Masdeu JC, Biller J. Coma. In: Brazis PW, Masdeu JC, Biller J (Eds). Localization in Clinical Neurology, 4th edition. Philadelphia: Lippincott Williams and Wilkins; 2001. pp. 559-86.
3. Shewmon DA. Coma prognosis in children. Part I: definitional and methodological challenges. J Clin Neurophysiol. 2000;17(5):457-66.
4. Giacino JT, Ashwal S, Childs N, Cranford R, Jennet B, Katz DI, et al. The minimally conscious state: definition and diagnostic criteria. Neurology. 2002;58(3):349-53.
5. Multi-Society Task Force on PVS. Medical aspects of the persistent vegetative state (2). N Engl J Med. 1994;330(22): 1572-9.
6. Murthy SNK, Faden HS, Cohen ME, Bakshi R. Acute disseminated encephalomyelitis in children. Pediatrics. 2002;110(2 Pt 1):e21.
7. Prasad MR, Ewing-Cobbs L, Swank PR, Kramer L. Predictors of outcome following traumatic brain injury in young children. Pediatr Neurosurg. 2002;36(2):64-74.
8. Jacinto SJ, Gieron-Korthals M, Ferreira JA. Predicting outcome in hypoxic-ischemic brain injury. Pediatr Clin North Am. 2001;48(3):647-60.
9. Trübel HK, Novotny E, Lister G. Outcome of coma in children. Curr Opin Pediatr. 2003;15(3):283-7.

8.14 Primary Brain Tumors

Jyotindra Narayan Goswami

INTRODUCTION

Primary brain tumors are the most common solid tumors in children. After leukemia, primary brain tumors are the second most common malignancy of childhood, and they account for almost one-quarter of the total childhood neoplasms. Age-adjusted incidence varies among countries from 1.12 to 5.14 cases per 100,000/year for children and adolescents <19 years of age. The incidence is more common in boys.[1,2]

Brain tumors in childhood differ from those in adults in their sites of origin, clinical presentation, dissemination potential, histological features, and biological behaviors.[3] Astrocytoma and embryonic tumors are more common in children, whereas metastases, glioma, and meningioma are seen predominantly in adults. The incidence of infratentorial tumors and tumors with malignant behavior (medulloblastoma and ependymoma) decreases with increasing age, whereas the occurrence of supratentorial tumors and tumors with benign nature (pilocytic astrocytoma/glioma) increases with age.[2] Local dissemination is faster in young children. Manifestations and outcomes depend upon the location, behavior of the tumor, degree of surgical resection, and response to adjuvant therapy.

Though significant advances in the field of diagnosis and treatment have occurred over the years, the overall survival rate remains modest. The survivors face considerable morbidity throughout their lives due to long-term sequelae of surgical or adjuvant radio- and chemotherapy. Introduction of molecular diagnostics has helped in understanding the behavior of these neoplasms and their response to treatment. The World Health Organization (WHO) has changed the classification and grading of childhood neoplasms due to fast-evolving molecular diagnostics.[4] Aggressive surgery is the undisputable primary modality of treatment, but long-term postsurgical sequelae are still very high. Distressing cognitive/endocrine and growth-related issues are intolerable after adjuvant therapy. There is a great hope that innovative treatment modalities, such as immunotherapy and gene therapy, will improve the overall survival and quality of life of these children in coming times.[5]

ETIOLOGY

The etiology of childhood brain neoplasms remains unknown. Two strong risk factors are associated with childhood brain neoplasms, namely genetic syndromes and exposure to therapeutic ionized radiotherapy. The common genetic syndromes associated with increased risk of brain neoplasms are shown in **Table 8.14.1**. The inheritance pattern in all of these familial disorders is autosomal dominant.

Primitive embryonic tissue can also be a potential risk for the development of primitive neuroectodermal tumors.[3] Craniopharyngioma, a common midline supratentorial tumor in children, arises from persistent remnants of craniopharyngeal pouch. Intracranial germ cell tumors with the exception of mature teratoma are seen commonly during adolescence. This is probably due to hormonal drive to gonadal development, which interacts with potential tumor cells within the brain. Another potent risk factor is therapeutic ionizing radiation exposure. The common neoplasms recurring after radiation are malignant glioma and meningioma, and they can occur as late as 5–15 years. Other possible risk factors are higher birth weight, nervous system anomalies, diagnostic ionizing radiation, advanced parental age, folic acid deficiency, exposure to electromagnetic radiation (cell phones), immunosuppression, and residual pesticides. The etiology in majority of the brain tumors is probably multifactorial, where genetic instabilities and environmental factors play a role in pathogenesis. The common genetic mutations associated with childhood brain tumors are depicted in **Table 8.14.2**. These mutations help in establishing the correct diagnosis and prognostication. Some of them are useful markers for tumor prediction.

TABLE 8.14.1: Common genetic syndromes associated with primary brain tumors.

Genetic syndrome and mutations	*Brain tumors*
NF1 and *NF2*	Pilocytic astrocytoma of visual pathways
TSC1 and *TSC2*	Giant cell astrocytoma
VHL	Hemangioblastoma of cerebellum
Li–Fraumeni (germ cell line *TP53*)	Glioma medulloblastoma
Atypical teratoid/rhabdoid tumor syndrome (*SMARCB1*, *SMARCA4*)	Atypical teratoid/rhabdoid tumor
Gorlin syndrome (germline *PTCH1* mutation)	Medulloblastoma

(NF: neurofibromatosis; *TP53*: tumor protein p53; TSC: tuberous sclerosis complex; VHL: von Hippel–Lindau)

CLASSIFICATION

Brain tumors can be classified according to their location **(Table 8.14.3)**, immunohistochemical or molecular markers, and behavior of the neoplasm. The WHO has revised the classification of childhood brain neoplasms based on their molecular behaviors in 2016.[4] In brain tumors, the terms "benign" and "malignant" are often misleading. Malignant tumors, such as medulloblastoma, may be curable in up to 80%, if they occur in older children or when well localized and completely surgically resectable. On the contrary, some benign tumors, such as low-grade astrocytoma and glioma,

TABLE 8.14.2: Common childhood neoplasms with genetic mutations.

Tumor	*Genetic mutations*
Astrocytoma (diffuse and anaplastic) grades II and III	*IDH* (>80%), *TP53* (94%), *ATRX* (86%)
• Glioblastoma mutant grade IV • Glioblastoma wild-type grade IV	*IDH1* (>95%), *ATRX* (90–95%), *TP53* (62–65%), *IDH2* (2–5%), *TP53* (25–35%), *TERT* promoter (>80%), *EGFR* amplification, *CDKN2A* homogeneous deletion (35–50%)
Oligodendroglioma grades II and III	*IDH* (98%), 1p/19q codeletion (100%), *TERT* promoter (96%), *MGMT* methylation (85%)
Subependymal giant cell astrocytoma grade I	*TSC1* and *TSC2* (100%)
Pilocytic astrocytoma grade I	*BRAF-KIAA*1549 fusion (70%), *BRAF-V600E* (15%)
Diffuse midline glioma grade IV	Histone *K27M* (100%), *ATRX* (50%), *TP53* (50%)
Craniopharyngioma	*BRAF V600E* and *CTNNB1* (100%)
AT/RT grade IV	*SMARCB1* (95%), *SMARCA4* (2%)
Medulloblastoma grade IV	*TERT* promoter (21%)
Meningioma	*TRAF7/KLF4* (100%)

(AT/RT: atypical teratoid/rhabdoid tumor)

TABLE 8.14.3: Classification of brain tumors based on their anatomical localization and common ages of occurrence.

Infratentorial (43.2%)	*Supratentorial (40.9%)*	*Multiple sites and spinal cord (15.9%)*
• *Astrocytoma (40%)*: 5–15 years • *Medulloblastoma (40%)*: 1–4, 7–10 years • *Brainstem glioma (10–20%)*: 5–15 years • *Ependymoma (10–20%)*: 1–4 years • *Atypical teratoid/rhabdoid (3%)*: 1–3 years	• *Cortical glioma* – Low grade (50%): 1–15 years – High grade (20%): 10–19 years – Diencephalic (10%): 0–3 years • *Craniopharyngioma* (10%): 5–15 years • *Choroid plexus papilloma* (<1%): 0–12 years	• Astrocytoma • Glioma • Ependymoma

TABLE 8.14.4: World Health Organization grading of primary brain tumors.

Grade of the tumor	*Characteristics*	*Examples*
Grade I (benign)	• The least malignant tumors associated with long-term survival • Their growth is slow, and the appearance under a microscope is almost normal • Surgery alone may be an effective treatment	• Pilocytic astrocytoma • Subependymal giant cell astrocytoma • Craniopharyngioma • Neurofibroma • Choroid plexus papilloma • Meningioma
Grade II (semibenign)	• These tumors are slow-growing and look slightly abnormal under a microscope • Some can spread into nearby normal tissue and recur • Surgery with additional adjuvant therapy is required	• Ependymoma • Diffuse astrocytoma, IDH mutant • Neurocytoma • Atypical choroid plexus papilloma • Atypical meningioma
Grade III (semimalignant)	• By definition, these tumors are malignant • The cells of a grade III tumor are actively reproducing abnormal cells, which grow into nearby normal brain tissue • These tumors tend to recur, often as a grade IV	• Anaplastic astrocytoma, IDH mutant • Anaplastic ependymoma • Anaplastic ganglioglioma • Anaplastic meningioma
Grade IV (malignant)	• The most malignant tumors • These tumors reproduce rapidly, look bizarre when viewed under the microscope, and easily invade into nearby normal brain tissue • They form new blood vessels, so they can maintain their rapid growth • They also have areas of dead cells in their centers	• Glioblastoma, IDH mutant and wild type • Pineoblastoma • Medulloblastoma (all subtypes) • Atypical teratoid/rhabdoid tumors

(IDH: isocitrate dehydrogenase)

can disseminate to surrounding normal brain and may be quite difficult to remove completely and behave like a malignant mass.

Supratentorial tumors peak during the first year of life and after 10 years of age, whereas infratentorial tumors are more common in 1–10-year age-group children. In India, the most common childhood brain tumors are astrocytoma, medulloblastoma, and craniopharyngioma.[1]

STAGING AND GRADING OF PRIMARY BRAIN TUMORS

Staging of central nervous system (CNS) tumors depends upon the degree of surgical resectability, the residual tumor mass left after surgery, and the extent of the spread beyond the primary location of the tumor.[3] Staging of CNS tumors is usually performed based on magnetic resonance imaging (MRI) images of the brain and the spinal cord and/or by cerebrospinal fluid (CSF) analysis for tumor cells. Scans taken after surgery are used to determine the left-out tumor mass. CNS tumors that have the tendency to spread are exposed to both the scan images and CSF studies. Patients with medulloblastoma, for example, will often have their CSF examined for the presence of tumor cells. These patients also require spinal cord scans because of the tumor's tendency to spread to the spinal cord. Since embryonal and glial neoplasms rarely spread to nonneuronal sites, evaluation for disease spread outside the nervous system is not recommended.

Immunohistology and molecular diagnostics have been incorporated to determine treatment response and risk stratifications.[6] The same neoplasm at different locations and at different ages of presentation can have different underlying mutations and different behaviors. For example, the underlying genetic mutations and behavior of the midline and cortical gliomas are different.

Grading helps in deciding the benign or malignant nature of the tumor, treatment response, and outcome. The higher the grade, the more malignant the tumor. Based on the WHO grading system, there are four tumor grades—I, II, III, and IV **(Table 8.14.4)**.

CLINICAL FEATURES

Clinical features depend on location, size, evolutionary behavior of the tumor, and the age of the child. Aggressively growing tumors manifest early with severe symptoms, whereas initial signs and symptoms of slow-growing tumors are subtle.

Subtentorial tumors become symptomatic in the beginning because of the compact space. Extra-axial subtentorial tumors obstruct CSF pathways and present with early features of raised intracranial pressure, such as early morning headache, vomiting, bradycardia, hypertension, visual disturbances, papilledema, mental changes, and gait disturbances. Intra-axial masses in the subtentorial region, such as pontine glioma, present with features of multiple cranial nerve palsy and long-tract signs. Supratentorial tumors present with seizures and focal neurological deficit.

In infants and young children, presentations can be nonspecific, and there are difficulties in detection and evaluation. Before closure of skull sutures and fontanels, the only manifestations can be a progressively enlarging head size without features of raised intracranial pressure and focal neurological symptoms and signs. Slowly growing neoplasms may present with developmental delay in the beginning and regression of developmental milestones in the later part of progression. There may be disk pallor instead of papilledema, particularly in suprasellar masses. Sunsetting sign is a common feature of raised intracranial tension, manifested by impaired upward gaze with persistent downward gaze due to dilated third ventricle with pressure on tectum due to obstructive hydrocephalus.

Hypothalamic neoplasms in children may present with diencephalic syndrome, characterized by failure to thrive and emaciation in an otherwise normal child. These children may present with gelastic seizures, particularly in hypothalamic hamartoma. Such children are usually irritable with significant developmental delay, but some of them are also happy and euphoric.

Expanding neoplasms also cause secondary brain dysfunction because of herniation due to a pressure gradient in different compartments. Herniation causes overcrowding of brain matter, stretching and rupturing of blood vessels, edema, and pressure over vital structures, notably cranial nerves and vital centers in the brainstem.

DIAGNOSIS

Key features while assessing primary brain neoplasms are the site, size, type of brain tissue involved, surgical resectability, and spread within the brain and spinal cord. Neuroimaging, histopathology, immunology, and molecular diagnostics are the primary tools used in diagnostic assessment of brain tumors.

- *MRI* with gadolinium-diethylenetriamine pentaacetic acid (GD-DTPA) is a generally preferred diagnostic method **(Figs. 8.14.1 to 8.14.4)**. Most tumors enhance with contrast. MRI is better at delineating benign masses from malignant growths, inflammatory and infectious conditions, and normal brain tissue. Tumors in the posterior fossa, temporal lobe, and sellar and chiasmatic regions are also best visualized with MRI.
- *Positron emission tomography (PET) and magnetic resonance spectroscopy (MRS)* have a role in the

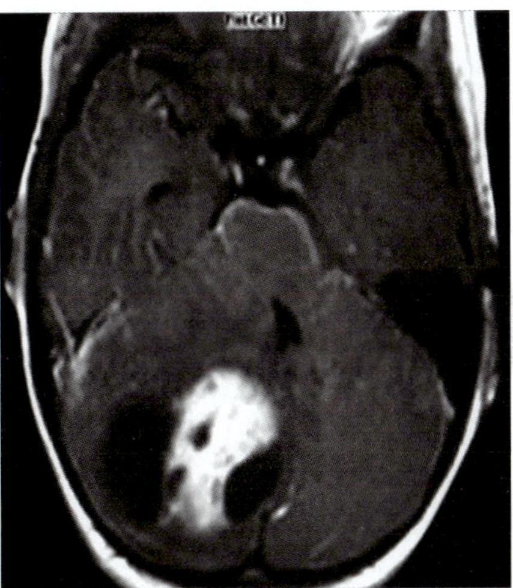

Fig. 8.14.1: Postgadolinium T1-weighted transverse MRI image of the brain showing a well-defined heterogeneously enhancing mass lesion in the right cerebellar hemisphere. Biopsy-proven case of cerebellar astrocytoma. (MRI: magnetic resonance imaging; T1: transverse 1)

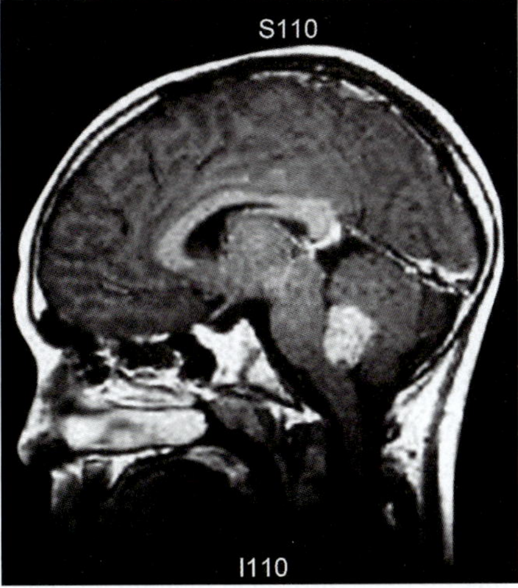

Fig. 8.14.2: Postgadolinium T1-weighted sagittal MRI image of the brain showing a well-defined intensely enhancing mass lesion expanding the fourth ventricle and displacing the brainstem anteriorly. Biopsy-proven case of medulloblastoma. (MRI: magnetic resonance imaging; T1: transverse 1)

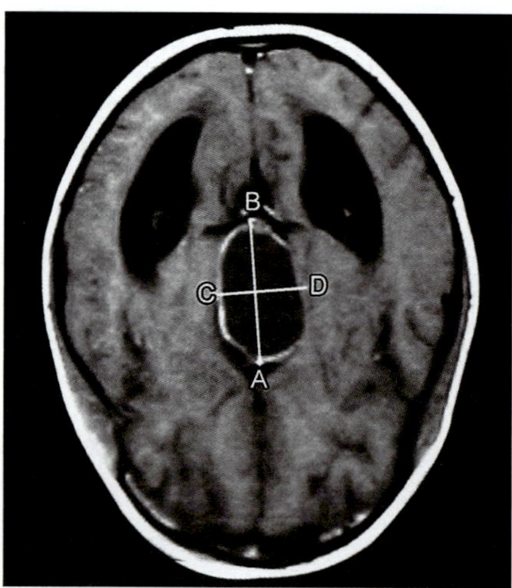

Fig. 8.14.3: Postgadolinium T1-weighted coronal MRI image of the brain showing a well-defined rim-enhancing lesion in the third ventricle. Biopsy-proven case of third ventricle ependymoma. (MRI: magnetic resonance imaging; T1: transverse 1)

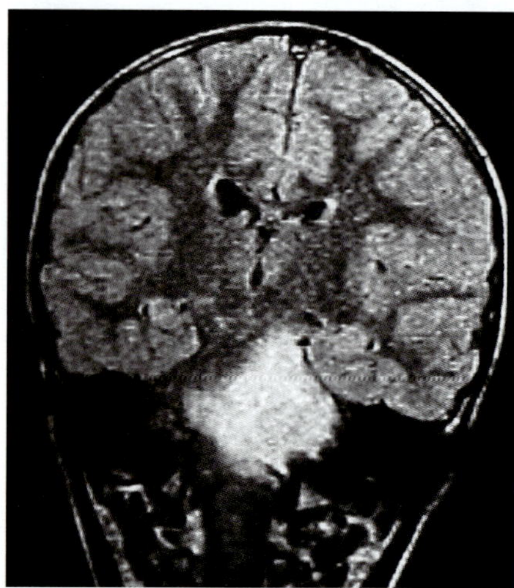

Fig. 8.14.4: FLAIR coronal MRI images of the brain showing an ill-defined mass lesion expanding the pons. Biopsy-proven case of pontine glioma. (FLAIR: fluid-attenuated inversion recovery; MRI: magnetic resonance imaging)

characterization of brain tumors, in follow-up, and in differentiation from other nonmalignant conditions.

- *Computed tomography (CT)* is the imaging modality of choice in an emergency.
- CSF studies for malignant cells are advised in tumors that have a tendency to spread.

Immunohistopathology of the resected tumor and molecular testing have improved diagnostic accuracy, better targeted therapy, and prognostication.[7]

TREATMENT

Surgery remains the mainstay and the initial step in the treatment of brain tumors.[5] Total resection may not be possible in many cases, but partial resection is useful to reduce the bulk of tumor, thus permitting destruction of the remaining malignant cells by irradiation or chemotherapy. Partial resection provides tissue for immunohistology that is essential for the specific diagnosis and characterization of tumor's behavior. Significant postsurgical sequelae are unavoidable in many situations. Hypothalamic and pituitary abnormalities are common in supratentorial midline tumors, such as craniopharyngioma. Cerebellar mutism syndrome, characterized by postoperative mutism, emotional liabilities, irritability, hypotonia, and other cerebellar deficits, is seen primarily but not exclusively after medulloblastomas resection.[8] This is thought to be secondary to disruption of cerebellar dentate nuclei or pathways between dentate nuclei and cortex. It can be permanent in 50% of cases.

Many pediatric brain tumors are radiosensitive. Newer radiotherapy techniques are more precisely targeted to the tumor with lower radiation doses and minimal or no collateral damage to the surrounding brain tissue. Newer modalities include brachytherapy, three-dimensional conformal radiation therapy, confronted proton beam radiation therapy, intensity-modulated radiation therapy, and stereotactic radiotherapy. Radiotherapy is the pillar of palliative care in most malignant and aggressive neoplasms or infiltrative benign masses not amenable to surgery.[9,10] Overall survival has improved with radiotherapy, but long-term sequelae are a concern. Common long-term effects are endocrine function, growth/development, and cognition. Long-term sequelae depend on the age of the child, dose and type of radiation, and preexisting brain injury. Secondary neoplasms after radiation exposure are another long-term concern.

The addition of chemotherapy has increased median survival rates for high-risk neoplasms.[5] The common chemotherapeutic agents used are deoxyribonucleic acid alkylators and alkaloids. Overall success remains unchanged; reasons are impairments to drug delivery across blood–brain barrier and resistance to drugs. Newer strategies have been designed to concentrate chemotherapy agents directly into the tumor with least effect on the body stem cells and regional delivery systems, such as intrathecal or intraventricular.

Recent advances in biological therapy include primarily supportive care measures, such as the use of hematopoietic growth factors and autologous stem cell harvesting and reinfusion. Identification of major targets, such as the epidermal growth factor receptor, platelet-derived growth factor receptor, vascular endothelial growth factor, and key signaling pathways, such as the mitogen-activated protein kinase and phosphatidylinositol 3-kinase (PI3K)/AKT/mammalian target of rapamycin (mTOR) pathway, has enhanced the knowledge of physicians in understanding the tumor behavior and design-tailored therapy.

Immunotherapy, a novel modality to treat deadly or incurable brain neoplasms, has a supportive role in prolonging survival and improving the quality of life of such children.[11] Adverse effects and toxicity related to conventional treatment of brain tumors significantly reduce the quality of patient's life. Although most immunotherapy approaches are not successful in solid tumors, several early phase clinical trials are beginning to reveal a potential role for immunotherapy in the treatment of brain neoplasms. Promising immunotherapy includes de novo activation of T cells through cancer vaccines, oncolytic viral therapy, or ex vivo engineered cell therapy. Monoclonal antibodies are also showing a promising role; however, the main concern is how to deliver them across the blood–brain barrier.[12]

In gene therapy, genetic material is transferred to cancer cells to either stop or slow the growth and multiplication of these cells. Genetic material in the cells also increases susceptibility to other treatment modalities. Gene transfer technology has used many viruses as delivery agents.

Endocrine dysfunctions are common before and after surgery and after craniospinal radiation or chemotherapy for supratentorial midline neoplasms. Complete endocrine workup before surgery for midline tumors is essential for better outcome. Children with tumors near the hypothalamic–pituitary axis are prone to fluid and electrolyte abnormalities during perioperative period. All children (except those having Cushing disease) with midline tumors near the pituitary–hypothalamic axis are administered hydrocortisone 100 mg every 6–8 hourly during surgery and postoperative period for 3 days. Hydrocortisone is continued if serum cortisol levels are low. Endocrine follow-up is recommended after the resection of a craniopharyngioma and other midline masses and cranial irradiation for a long time.

Prophylactic antiepileptic drugs, such as intravenous phenytoin (10 mg/kg as slow loading followed by 4–8 mg/kg/day), are recommended during the perioperative period. Psychological assessment is critical as these children are more prone to cognitive and behavioral problems **(Table 8.14.5)**.

TABLE 8.14.5: Common childhood brain tumors.

Type of tumor	*Salient features*
Glioma	• Gliomas arise from glial precursors and are differentiated along astrocytic and oligodendroglial lineage. They occur through all ages and throughout neuraxis. Histologically, these are either low-grade (WHO grade I or II) or high-grade gliomas (WHO grade III or IV) • *Low-grade gliomas* are the most common brain tumors in childhood, constituting >20% of all childhood primary brain tumors. The common sites are the cerebellum, visual pathways, and diencephalon. According to the WHO grading system, gliomas are either grade I or grade II. Common tumors in grade I are pilocytic astrocytoma, subependymal giant cell astrocytoma, and astrocytic astrocytoma. Grade II examples are oligodendroglioma, oligoastrocytoma, neurocytoma, and diffuse astrocytoma • *Common genetic abnormalities* in low-grade astrocytoma are gain in chromosomes 7, 4, 5, 6, 8, and 11, and deletions of 17p and 1q. In DIPG, the genetic aberrations are gains of chromosomes 1q, 2p, 2q, 8q, and 9q, and common deletions of 16q, 14q, 17p, and 20p. High-grade gliomas have more association with familial genetic syndromes, such as Li–Fraumeni, Turcot type-1, and CMMRD syndrome. Common tumors in this group, according to the WHO grading, are glioblastoma (IV), anaplastic oligodendroglioma (III), and anaplastic oligoastrocytoma (III) • *Clinical presentations* depend upon the location, age of the child, and behavior of the tumor. High-grade gliomas present with recent history of symptoms and progress very fast. Low-grade tumors present slowly, and presentations can be atypical. In DIPG, the median duration of symptoms is about 1 month. Signs include cranial nerve palsy and cerebellar and long-tract signs. Rarely, pathological laughter can also be the presenting symptom • *Modalities of investigations* are MRI brain with contrast and MRS • *Treatment options* are radical surgical resection, radiotherapy, and chemotherapy. In DIPG, radiotherapy is the mainstay of treatment; chemotherapy and surgery have a poor role. In glioblastoma, management is radical surgery, followed by radiation. In adults, temozolomide is considered the standard care, but in pediatric glioblastoma, its role is limited
Medulloblastoma	• *Embryonal tumor of the cerebellum* is believed to arise from the stem cells and neuronal progenitor cells in and around the cerebellum. It accounts for 20% of primary brain neoplasms and 40% of all posterior fossa tumors • It has a *bimodal incidence* peak between 3 and 4 years and 7–10 years of age. It is commonly associated with familial syndromes, such as Gorlin syndrome (germline mutation of *PATCHED*-1 gene on chromosome 9), Turcot's type-1 (mutations of the adenomatous polyposis gene), and Li–Fraumeni syndrome (germline mutation of *TP53*). Rarely, medulloblastoma has association with Rubinstein–Taybi and Fanconi syndrome. Therapeutic radiation exposure is another risk factor • *Age of onset, sex predilection, and outcome* depend upon the molecular subgrouping. They commonly present with the features of raised intracranial pressure. Macroscopic bleeding and rapid progression can lead to sudden altered sensorium and coma. The classical sunsetting sign is seen rarely • Medulloblastoma can spread along neuraxis, but there are no signs and symptoms of dissemination • Lesion is well-defined and homogenous; hypointense on T1-weighted images and hyperintense on T2. The majority of them enhance with contrast

Contd...

Contd…

Type of tumor	*Salient features*
	• *Treatment* is surgical excision, followed by radiotherapy and chemotherapy. Posterior fossa mutism syndrome is the most common complication following surgery, seen in almost 20–30% of children. With current means of treatment, most of the children are expected to survive >5 years after the diagnosis. Majority of the survivors are left with neurocognitive delay, endocrine problems (most common growth hormone deficiency). High-grade gliomas are the common recurring neoplasms after adjuvant therapy and are very resistant to treatment
Craniopharyngioma	• Craniopharyngioma is a benign tumor histologically, but its unique relationship with vital structures, such as optic pathways and hypothalamic–pituitary axis and its high recurrence rate, makes the management very challenging. It arises from the embryonic remnants of the Rathke's pouch in the parasellar region. Tumor is partially calcified and heterogeneous, having solid and cystic components • *Histologically,* it has three variants: Adamantinomatous, papillary, and rarely mixed variety. It often infiltrates the surrounding critical structures • Tumor has a *bimodal age distribution* with peaks at age 5 and 15 years and another peak in adults between 50 and 75 years of age • The *diagnosis* is delayed because of the slow growth. Headache due to raised intracranial pressure is the presenting complaint in about 75% of cases. Visual complaints due to pressure on visual pathways are observed in >50%. Hypothalamic and pituitary dysfunctions as presenting complaints are seen in 25–50% of cases. Growth hormone deficiency is seen in 75% of children with craniopharyngioma, followed by deficiency of gonadotropins (93%). Diabetes insipidus develops in two-thirds of cases • *Preoperative endocrinal workup* is essential • *MRI contrast* shows an enhancing cystic capsule and solid tumor • *Treatment*: Presently, there is no consensus on optimal management strategies. Treatment can be radical surgery, subtotal resection with radiation, and intracystic irradiation/bleomycin/interferon. Frequent follow-up with neuroimaging is essential to detect early recurrence. Hypothalamic–pituitary dysfunction is common and includes obesity, hyperphagia, memory deficit, thermoregulation instability, labile behavior, and sleep–awake cycle abnormalities
Ependymoma	• *Second most common primary malignant neoplasm* of the central nervous system, accounting for about 10% of all childhood primary brain tumors. More than 50% of intracranial ependymomas arise in children <5 years of age. In adults, spinal origin predominates. Prevalence is slightly more in males. During childhood, 75% of them originate in the fourth ventricle • *Most common presentation* is features of raised intracranial pressure. Some of the children may present with cerebellar or lower cranial nerves features. A very young child is brought with excessive irritability or lethargy • *Probable location of origin* is the ependymal lining of ventricles and central canal; however, these may arise anywhere along neuraxis not related to ependymal lining. Dissemination via cerebrospinal fluid is reported in 10–20%. In adults, the most common spinal site is filum terminale • *MRI* typically displays iso- to hypointensities on T1W and hyperintensities on T2W images. Contrast enhancement is heterogeneous. There is genetic and epigenetic heterogeneity between different spinal cord and intracranial locations. In intracranial ependymomas, there is upregulation of *RAF-1* gene, and in spinal cord, there is upregulation of PLA2GS-ITIH2 and *HOX* family of genes. In supratentorial neoplasms, EPHB-EPHRIN is overexpressed, while there is a loss of chromosomes 22q, 6q, and 17q in infratentorial tumors • *Treatment* is primarily surgical excision, followed by chemo- and radiotherapy. Recurrence is common, and the outcome becomes poor with subsequent recurrences. Prognostic features are degree of surgical resection, age (older children have a better outcome), and location (supratentorial, where the outcome is better)
AT/RT	• *Highly malignant tumor* that occurs predominantly in children younger than 3 years of age. It accounts for 3% of total childhood primary central nervous system neoplasms. About 15% of children <3 years of age with primary brain tumors have AT/RT • Due to the aggressive nature of the disease, children present with very *brief onset of symptoms.* Clinical presentations depend upon the location of the tumor and the age of the child. Infratentorial neoplasm presents with the features of raised intracranial pressure, and presentation of supratentorial masses is seizures and focal neurodeficits. Other nonspecific features can be progressively enlarging head, neuroregression, and lethargy. AT/RT can also arise in the spinal cord, and manifestations are those of spinal cord compression • *MRI* shows heterogeneous intensities on T1W and T2W images because of intralesional bleed. Contrast enhancement is also heterogeneous because of bleed in the mass lesion. MRS typically shows high choline peak and absent or reduced *N*-acetyl-aspartate peak. Histological picture is a mix of rhabdoid cells, primitive neuroectodermal cells, and epithelial and mesenchymal cells. Genetically, there is complete or partial loss of chromosome 22 (mutated genes—*SMARKB1*, *SMARKA4*) • *Treatment* is radical surgical excision. Chemotherapy is the mainstay of adjuvant therapy. Radiotherapy can also be given. Outcome is poor due to high toxicity related to adjuvant treatment

(AT/RT: atypical teratoid/rhabdoid tumor; CMMRD: constitutional mismatch repair deficiency; DIPG: diffuse intrinsic pontine glioma; MRI: magnetic resonance imaging; MRS: magnetic resonance spectroscopy; T1: transverse 1; T2: transverse 2; T1W: transverse 1 weight; T2W: transverse 2 weight; TP53: tumor protein p53; WHO: World Health Organization)

CONCLUSION

Primary brain tumors comprise of a large segment of neoplasms among children. These tumors differ from adult brain tumors in many aspects. Genetics and epigenetics play a major role in the etiopathogenesis, differentiation and prognosis of pediatric brain tumors. There is a major role of early clinical suspicion and specific investigations for establishing diagnosis. Though these entities have limited definitive treatment options and generally poor prognosis, multipronged supportive therapy, anticipation of complications and their timely management are associated with improved survival. Advances such as genetic therapy, biological therapeutic regimes, new radiotherapy protocols and evidence-based chemotherapeutic regimes with better disease control and fewer adverse effects hold promise for more effective management in the future.

REFERENCES

1. Jain A, Sharma MC, Suri V, Kale SS, Mahapatra AK, Tatke M, et al. Spectrum of pediatric brain tumors in India: a multi-institutional study. Neurol India. 2011;59:208-11.
2. Johnson KJ, Cullen J, Barnholtz-Sloan JS, Ostrom QT, Langer CE, Turner MC, et al. Childhood brain tumor epidemiology: a brain tumor epidemiology consortium review. Cancer Epidemiol Biomarkers Prev. 2014;23:2716-36.
3. Packer RJ. Pediatric neuro-oncology: an overview. In: Swaiman KF, Stephen A, Donna MF, Nima FS, Richard SF, Adrea LG, et al. (Eds). Swaiman's Pediatric Neurology: Principles and Practice, 6th edition. Edinburgh: Elsevier; 2017. pp. 957-62.
4. Louis DN, Perry A, Reifenberger G, von Deimling A, Figarella-Branger D, Cavenee WK, et al. The 2016 World Health Organization classification of tumors of the central nervous system: a summary. Acta Neuropathol. 2016;131:803-20.
5. Lutz K, Jünger ST, Messing-Jünger M. Essential management of pediatric brain tumors. Children (Basel). 2022;9(4):498.
6. Kim KE, Kim KU, Kim DC, Park JI, Han JY. Cytogenetic characterizations of central nervous system tumors: the first comprehensive report from a single institution in Korea. J Korean Med Sci. 2009;24:453-60.
7. Park SH, Won J, Kim SI, Lee Y, Park CK, Kim SK, et al. Molecular testing of brain tumor. J Pathol Transl Med. 2017;51:205-23.
8. Wibroe M, Cappelen J, Castor C, Clausen N, Grillner P, Gudrunardottir T, et al. Cerebellar mutism syndrome in children with brain tumours of the posterior fossa. BMC Cancer. 2017;17:439.
9. Ludmir EB, Grosshans DR, Woodhouse KD. Radiotherapy advances in pediatric neuro-oncology. Bioengineering. 2018;5:97.
10. Veeravagu A, Lee M, Jiang B, Chang SD. The role of radiosurgery in the treatment of craniopharyngiomas. Neurosurg Focus. 2010;28:E11.
11. Lieberman NAP, Vitanza NA, Crane CA. Immunotherapy for brain tumors: understanding early success and limitations. Expert Rev Neurother. 2018;18:251-9.
12. Cabanas R, Saurez G, Alert J, Reyes A, Valdes J, Gonzalez MC, et al. Prolonged use of nimotuzumab in children with central nervous system tumors: safety and feasibility. Cancer Biother Radiopharm. 2014;29:173-8.

8.15 Raised Intracranial Pressure

Ranjith Kumar Manokaran

INTRODUCTION

Increased intracranial pressure (ICP) is a common pediatric neurocritical care problem. An increase in brain volume, cerebral blood flow (CBF) or cerebrospinal fluid (CSF) volume or a combination of these can result in an increase in the cerebral pressure.[1] However, treatments for intracranial hypertension are not extensively researched, and recommendations are mostly based on clinical experience and studies in traumatic brain injury patients.

INTRACRANIAL PRESSURE: NORMATIVE VALUES

Intracranial pressure refers to the combined pressure exerted by the brain, blood, and CSF within the skull. According to the Monro-Kellie hypothesis, the total volume inside the skull, comprising the brain (about 80%), blood (approximately 10%), and CSF (around 10%), remains constant. Therefore, any increase in one of these components must be balanced by a decrease in another to maintain equilibrium; otherwise, pressure within the skull rises. The normal range of ICP varies with age and is not well established for children. Typically, normal values are below 10–15 mm Hg for adults and older children, 3–7 mm Hg for young children, and 1.5–6 mm Hg for term infants. ICP readings exceeding 20–25 mm Hg generally require medical intervention.[2] Sustained ICP levels surpassing 40 mm Hg indicate severe and potentially life-threatening intracranial hypertension.[3]

CEREBRAL PRESSURE DYNAMICS

Cerebral pressure dynamics involve cerebral perfusion pressure (CPP), a crucial factor influencing CBF within the brain. CPP is quantified in millimeters of mercury and is calculated by subtracting ICP from mean arterial pressure (MAP) (CPP = MAP – ICP). The CPP formula indicates that CPP can decrease due to a drop in MAP, an increase in ICP, or a combination of both. CPP measurements help assess the volume of blood in the intracranial space, serving as a vital clinical marker for CBF and ensuring adequate oxygen supply. While normal CPP values for children are not definitively established, the following thresholds are generally considered the minimum pressure needed to prevent ischemia: Adults should have a CPP > 70 mm Hg, children >50–60 mm Hg, and infants/toddlers >40–50 mm Hg.[3]

CAUSES OF RAISED INTRACRANIAL PRESSURE

Raised ICP can stem from a variety of factors, either independently or in combination, as outlined in **Box 8.15.1**. According to the Monro-Kellie hypothesis, elevated ICP may arise due to an increase in the volume of the brain, blood, or CSF. Often, it is a blend of these elements that leads to elevated ICP.[1] The causes of elevated ICP can be categorized as primary or secondary based on the primary pathology involved. In primary causes, rectifying the underlying brain disorder promptly is key to normalizing ICP. Conversely, in secondary causes of elevated ICP, managing the underlying systemic or extracranial issue is necessary.

BOX 8.15.1: Causes of raised intracranial pressure.

Increase in brain volume
- Intracranial space-occupying lesions
- Brain tumors
- Brain abscess
- Intracranial hemorrhage
- Intracranial vascular malformations
- Cerebral edema
- Encephalitis (viral, inflammatory, autoimmune)
- Meningitis
- Hypoxic–ischemic encephalopathy
- Traumatic brain injury
- Hepatic encephalopathy
- Reye's syndrome
- Stroke

Increase in CSF quantity/volume
- Hydrocephalus
- Choroids plexus tumors, such as papilloma

Increase in perfusion
- Vascular malformations
- Cerebral venous thrombosis
- CNS infections such as meningitis, encephalitis

(CNS: central nervous system; CSF: cerebrospinal fluid)

ASSESSMENT AND MONITORING

Children at an increased risk for raised ICP, as outlined in **Box 8.15.1**, include those with head trauma, suspected neuroinfections, or suspected intracranial mass lesions. Elevated pressure often presents with symptoms such as headache, vomiting, irritability, squinting, tonic posturing, or deteriorating sensorium. It is important to note that the manifestation of symptoms depends on factors such as age, underlying cause, and the progression of raised ICP.

Initial Assessment

When dealing with any sick child, the initial step is to assess and maintain the airway, breathing, and circulatory function. It is crucial to promptly identify and address potentially life-threatening signs of herniation, such as impairment of consciousness, neck rigidity, opisthotonus, decerebrate rigidity, vomiting, irregular respirations, apnea, and bradycardia. If these signs are present, immediate measures to reduce ICP should be implemented. Cushing's triad (comprising bradycardia, hypertension, and irregular breathing) is a late indicator of herniation, guiding the subsequent course of management. Additionally, abnormalities in pupillary responses and ocular movements, assessed through spontaneous, doll's eye, or cold caloric testing, provide important clues about brainstem dysfunction localization. Fundus examination is focused on detecting papilledema, although its absence does not rule out raised ICP. The motor system examination aims to identify any posturing or flaccidity.

Neurological Assessment

Following the initial assessment, a comprehensive history and clinical examination are conducted to ascertain the potential causes of raised ICP or focal deficits. The findings from a general physical and systemic examination can offer insights into the underlying cause of elevated ICP, such as jaundice or hepatomegaly indicating hepatic encephalopathy, or a rash suggesting viral encephalitis, among others.

Neuroimaging

For patients presenting to the emergency room with raised ICP, the imaging study of choice is a computed tomography (CT) scan. A contrast study can be beneficial for identifying infection-related features such as meningeal enhancement, brain abscesses, or tumors. If the CT scan results are normal but the patient exhibits clinical features of raised ICP, then a magnetic resonance imaging (MRI) with magnetic resonance venogram should be obtained after stabilizing the patient. An MRI can detect early stroke, venous thromboses, posterior fossa tumors, and demyelinating lesions that might not be visible on a CT scan.

Invasive Intracranial Pressure Monitoring

Intracranial pressure monitoring is primarily used to guide therapeutic decisions, such as determining the timing for CSF drainage, administering mannitol or sedation, and planning further management. Invasive monitoring also allows for the observation of individual and consecutive ICP waveforms, providing insights into intracranial compliance, cerebrovascular status, and cerebral perfusion. Guidelines for ICP monitoring are specifically available for traumatic brain injury cases.[4] Indications for ICP monitoring include patients with a Glasgow Coma Scale (GCS) score of 3–8 after resuscitation, along with an abnormal admission head CT or motor posturing and hypotension. However, the role and benefits of ICP monitoring in other conditions such as subarachnoid hemorrhage, hydrocephalus, intracranial infections, and Reye syndrome are not well defined, and the availability of this monitoring modality is limited in some cases. Additionally, for brain injuries such as hypoxic and ischemic injuries, there is no clear evidence that monitoring ICP improves outcomes.

MANAGEMENT OF INTRACRANIAL HYPERTENSION

The primary goal for patients with raised ICP is to identify and address the underlying cause while implementing measures to reduce ICP, as illustrated in **Box 8.15.2**. Timely treatment is crucial, especially in cases where identifying the underlying cause may require some time. In situations where elevated ICP is clinically evident, urgent action to reduce ICP is necessary. It is important to avoid factors that can worsen or trigger raised ICP, which is a critical goal for all children with intracranial hypertension. While the availability of ICP monitors may vary, it should not hinder urgent therapy and management.

BOX 8.15.2: Measures to decrease ICP.

- *Assessment and management of ABCs* (airway, breathing, circulation)
- *Early intubation if:* Glasgow Coma Scale (GCS) <8, evidence of impending herniation, bradypnea, nonmaintainable airway
- *Head elevation* of 15–30°
- *Maintain euvolemia*
- *Hyperventilation:* Target $PaCO_2$: 30–35 mm Hg (for acute increases in ICP or features of impending herniation)
- *Mannitol:* Initial bolus: 0.25–1 g/kg, then 0.25–0.5 g/kg, q2–6h, as per requirement, up to 48 hours (contraindicated for hypotension and renal failure)
- *Hypertonic saline:* Can be used in hypotension, hypovolemia, serum osmolality >320 mOsm/kg, renal failure; dose: 0.1–1 mL/kg/h infusion, target Na^+ 145–155 mEq/L
- *Steroids:* Brain tumors, multiple neurocysticercosis, ADEM, TBM
- *Acetazolamide:* Hydrocephalus, idiopathic intracranial hypertension, high-altitude illness
- *Adequate sedation and analgesia*
- *Prevention and treatment of seizures:* Use lorazepam or midazolam followed by phenytoin as initial choice
- *Avoid noxious stimuli:* Use lignocaine prior to endotracheal tube suctioning [nebulized (4% lidocaine mixed in 0.9% saline) or intravenous (1–2 mg/kg as 1% solution) given 90 seconds prior to suctioning]
- *Control fever:* Antipyretics, cooling measures
- *Maintenance IV fluids:* Only isotonic or hypertonic fluids (Ringer's lactate, 0.9% saline, 5% dextrose in 0.9% normal saline); hypotonic fluids are not preferred
- *Maintain blood glucose:* 80–120 mg/dL
- *Maintain hemoglobin:* >10 g/dL
- *Refractory raised ICP*
  - Heavy sedation and paralysis
  - Barbiturate coma
  - Hypothermia
  - Decompressive craniectomy

(ADEM: acute disseminated encephalomyelitis; ICP: intracranial pressure; IV: intravenous; $PaCO_2$: partial pressure of carbon dioxide; TBM: tuberculous meningitis)

Airway, Breathing, and Circulation

The initial step in management involves assessing and managing the airway, breathing, and circulation (ABCs). Early consideration should be given to endotracheal intubation for children with a GCS score of <8, signs of herniation, apnea, or inability to maintain the airway. Intubation should be performed with the administration of medications to reduce ICP during the procedure. Recommended medications include lidocaine, thiopental, and a short-acting nondepolarizing neuromuscular blockade agent such as vecuronium or atracurium. Adequate oxygenation must be ensured throughout the process. If there are indications of circulatory failure, a fluid bolus should be administered. Additionally, samples should be collected for investigations based on the patient's medical history and presentation.

Positioning

Raising the head of the bed by 15–30° has been proven to lower ICP without adversely affecting CPP or CBF. The child's head should be centered and elevated at this angle to promote drainage from the jugular veins. It is important to avoid sharp angles of the head and tight neck garments or taping. Before placing the child in this position, ensure they are adequately hydrated (euvolemic) and not in a state of shock.

Hyperventilation

Lowering partial pressure of carbon dioxide ($PaCO_2$) to the range of 30–35 mm Hg is a swift and effective method to reduce ICP.[5] Hyperventilation achieves this by narrowing cerebral blood vessels and reducing CBF. However, this vasoconstrictive impact on cerebral arterioles is temporary, lasting only 11–20 hours as the CSF pH quickly adjusts to the new $PaCO_2$ level. Excessive hyperventilation can significantly lower CBF, potentially leading to or worsening cerebral ischemia. Therefore, hyperventilation is most beneficial for acute, sudden increases in ICP or indications of impending herniation.

Osmotherapy

Mannitol

Mannitol has long been a key treatment for reducing elevated ICP.[6] However, the most effective dosing of mannitol remains unclear. A reasonable strategy involves an initial bolus of 0.25–1 g/kg (higher doses for more urgent ICP reduction), followed by 0.25–0.5 g/kg boluses every 2–6 hours as needed. Care must be taken to maintain fluid balance to avoid hypovolemia and shock. There is a concern about potential mannitol leakage into damaged brain tissue, which could lead to "rebound" increase in ICP. To mitigate this risk, mannitol should be tapered off and used for a limited duration, typically 48–72 hours. In addition to hypotension and rebound ICP, mannitol can also cause hypokalemia, hemolysis, and renal failure.

Hypertonic Saline

Hypertonic saline offers distinct advantages over mannitol, especially in children with hypovolemia or hypotension.[7] It is also preferable in cases of renal failure or when serum osmolality exceeds 320 mOsm/kg. Its efficacy has been noted even in patients with serum osmolality levels up to 360 mOsm/kg. However, there are concerns associated with its use, such as bleeding, rebound increase in ICP, hypokalemia, hyperchloremic acidosis, central pontine myelinosis, acute volume overload, renal failure, cardiac failure, or pulmonary edema. Despite these potential risks, current evidence indicates that hypertonic saline, as currently administered, is generally safe and does not lead to significant adverse effects.

The concentration of hypertonic saline used can vary widely, ranging from 1.7 to 30%. Similarly, the method of administration also varies, making evidence-based recommendations challenging. A reasonable approach is to administer hypertonic saline as a continuous infusion at a rate of 0.1–1.0 mL/kg/h, aiming for a target serum sodium level of 145–155 mEq/L. Close monitoring of serum sodium levels and neurological status is crucial during therapy. When hypertonic saline therapy is no longer needed, serum sodium should be gradually corrected to normal values, with an hourly decline not exceeding 0.5 mEq/L, to prevent complications related to fluid shifts. Monitoring of serum sodium and serum osmolality should be conducted every 2–4 hours until the target level is achieved, followed by 12-hourly estimations. Under careful monitoring, hypertonic saline has been safely used for up to 7 days.

Other Agents

- *Acetazolamide* is a carbonic anhydrase inhibitor that reduces the production of CSF. It is typically prescribed at a dose of 20–100 mg/kg/day, divided into three doses, with a maximum daily dose of 2 g. This medication is particularly beneficial for patients with hydrocephalus, high-altitude illness, and benign intracranial hypertension.
- *Furosemide*, a loop diuretic, is sometimes used alone or in combination with mannitol to manage raised ICP, although its success can vary. It is typically administered at a dose of 1 mg/kg/day every 8 hours.
- *Glycerol* is another osmotic agent that can be used to treat elevated ICP. It can be given orally at a dose of 1.5 g/kg/day every 4–6 hours or intravenously. When administered intravenously, glycerol reduces ICP for approximately 70 minutes without significantly affecting serum osmolality. Glycerol easily crosses the blood–brain barrier into the brain, but there is a concern, although not proven, about a potential rebound rise in ICP following its use.[8]

Steroids

Glucocorticoids are very effective in ameliorating the vasogenic edema that accompanies tumors, inflammatory conditions, infections, and other disorders associated with increased permeability of the blood–brain barrier, including surgical manipulation. Dexamethasone is the preferred agent due to its very low mineralocorticoid activity (dose: 0.4–1.5 mg/kg/day, q6h). Steroids are not routinely indicated in individuals with traumatic brain injury. Steroids have not been found to be useful and may be detrimental in ischemic lesions, cerebral malaria, and intracranial hemorrhage.[9]

Sedation and Analgesia

Raised ICP can be exacerbated by factors such as agitation, pain, and patient–ventilator asynchrony. To manage this, adequate analgesia, sedation, and sometimes neuromuscular blockade can be beneficial. However, analgesia and sedation are generally preferred over neuromuscular blockade because they are reversible and allow for neurological monitoring.

When using sedatives, it is preferable to choose agents with minimal impact on blood pressure. Short-acting benzodiazepines, such as midazolam, are commonly used for sedation in children. If these sedatives are not sufficient, a neuromuscular blocking agent such as pancuronium, atracurium, or vecuronium may be necessary.

Minimizing stimulation is also crucial. Limiting painful or overly stimulating interventions can help reduce ICP. For example, instilling lidocaine into the endotracheal tube before suctioning has been shown to prevent an increase in ICP and a reduction in CPP in adults with severe traumatic brain injury. Lidocaine can be administered endotracheally at body temperature, slowly, and through a fine tube inserted into the endotracheal tube without direct mucosal contact. Nebulized or intravenous forms of lidocaine can also be used for this purpose.

Fluids

The primary objective of fluid therapy in patients with ICP is to maintain normal fluid balance, glucose levels, and prevent hyponatremia. Fluid management aims to keep the patient in a state of euvolemia, with adequate blood volume and electrolyte levels.

Children with raised ICP should receive fluids at a rate that meets their daily maintenance requirements. Fluid boluses may be necessary in cases of hypovolemia, hypotension, or reduced urine output. Maintenance fluids typically include isotonic or hypertonic solutions such as normal saline or Ringer's lactate. Potassium chloride may also be added to maintenance fluids based on the child's weight and electrolyte needs.

It is crucial to avoid hypotonic fluids such as 0.18% saline in 5% dextrose or isolyte P, as these can contribute to hyponatremia, which must be corrected slowly if it occurs. Maintaining a careful balance of fluid intake and electrolyte levels helps support optimal cerebral perfusion and reduces the risk of complications related to fluid imbalances.

Blood Glucose

Maintaining blood glucose levels between 80 and 120 mg/dL is crucial for children with raised ICP. Hyperglycemia, with levels above this range, has been linked to poor neurological outcomes and increased mortality in children with traumatic brain injury. Conversely, hypoglycemia, with blood glucose levels below normal, can trigger a systemic stress response and disrupt CBF, potentially leading to neuronal injury.

Hypoglycemia should be managed aggressively to prevent these complications. It is essential to monitor blood glucose levels closely and intervene promptly to maintain glucose within the target range. This careful glucose management supports optimal brain function and reduces the risk of further neurological complications.

Temperature Regulation

Maintaining normothermia is crucial to prevent complications associated with temperature fluctuations in patients with raised ICP. This involves regularly monitoring body temperature and promptly addressing any deviations from the normal range. Antipyretic medications can be used to lower elevated temperatures, while assisted cooling or heating methods may be employed as needed to regulate body temperature within the optimal range. Consistent monitoring and management of body temperature contribute to better patient outcomes and reduce the risk of temperature-related complications.

Prevention and Treatment of Seizures

Children with significant head injuries and neuroinfections are prone to seizures, which can exacerbate raised ICP by increasing CBF and volume. Seizures also elevate the brain's metabolic demands, potentially leading to ischemia. Therefore, it is essential to treat seizures promptly when they occur. While evidence-based recommendations for prophylactic antiepileptic therapy in children with nontraumatic raised ICP are lacking, it is common practice to consider short-term prophylactic anticonvulsants unless contraindicated. Continuous electroencephalography (EEG) can be beneficial in identifying subclinical seizure activity in high-risk children, aiding in timely intervention.

Anemia

Anemia theoretically increases CBF and can consequently elevate ICP. There are case reports of severe anemia leading to symptoms of raised ICP and papilledema. While this aspect has not been extensively studied, it is a common clinical practice to maintain hemoglobin levels above 10 g/dL in patients with traumatic brain injury and raised ICP to mitigate these risks.

Surgical Therapy

Cerebrospinal fluid drainage using an external ventricular drainage (EVD) or ventriculoperitoneal shunt is an effective method to immediately lower ICP. EVD also allows for continuous monitoring of ICP. While CSF drainage is particularly beneficial in cases of hydrocephalus, it can also be considered in children without hydrocephalus. Studies have shown its efficacy in reducing ICP to be comparable to intravenous mannitol or hyperventilation. However, its utility is limited in cases of diffuse brain edema with collapsed ventricles.

Surgery to resect mass lesions is another crucial intervention when a lesion suitable for surgical intervention is identified as the primary cause of raised ICP. This neurosurgical approach is commonly recommended in situations such as acute epidural or subdural hematomas, brain abscesses, or brain tumors.

Target of Therapy

When facilities for ICP monitoring are available, the management is customized to ensure an adequate CPP and lower ICP to acceptable levels. For children, a CPP of >50–60 mm Hg is targeted, while for infants and toddlers, it should be maintained above 40–50 mm Hg. The target ICP levels are generally below 20 mm Hg for children older than 8 years, below 18 mm Hg for ages 1–8 years, and below 15 mm Hg for infants.

Other Therapies for Refractory Raised Intracranial Pressure

Barbiturates

Barbiturates such as thiopentone are typically reserved for cases of refractory raised ICP. Thiopentone is used with dosing adjusted based on the target ICP as monitored by an ICP monitor. The drug is titrated to achieve 90% burst suppression (2–6 bursts/min) using an EEG monitor. Monitoring a child under barbiturate-induced coma should include EEG, ICP monitoring, invasive hemodynamic monitoring [arterial blood pressure, central venous pressure, jugular venous oxygen saturation ($SjvO_2$)], and frequent assessment of oxygenation status. However, it is important to note that barbiturate therapy comes with a high complication rate, including hypotension, hypokalemia, respiratory complications, infections, hepatic dysfunction, and renal dysfunction.

Hypothermia

Evidence from carefully conducted studies in adults and children does not show any improvement in the neurologic outcome in head-injured patients with the use of therapeutic hypothermia.[10] However, studies do suggest a lowered ICP during hypothermia therapy in children. So, in children with refractory raised ICP, controlled hypothermia may be considered.

Decompressive Craniectomy

On rare occasions when all other measures fail, decompressive craniectomy with duraplasty may be a valuable procedure. Reports of its use in children with traumatic brain injury have shown benefits. It may offer an alternative treatment option in uncontrolled ICP refractory to other measures.

REFERENCES

1. Welch K. The intracranial pressure in infants. J Neurosurg. 1980;52(2):693-9.
2. Rangel-Castillo L, Gopinath S, Robertson CS. Management of intracranial hypertension. Neurol Clin. 2008;26(2):521-41.
3. Mazzola CA, Adelson PD. Critical care management of head trauma in children. Crit Care Med. 2002;30(1 Suppl.):S393-401.
4. Adelson PD, Bratton SL, Carney NA, Chesnut RM, du Coudray HEM, Goldstein B, et al. Guidelines for the acute medical management of severe traumatic brain injury in infants, children, and adolescents. Chapter 5. Indications for intracranial pressure monitoring in pediatric patients with severe traumatic brain injury. Pediatr Crit Care Med. 2003;4(3 Suppl.):S19-24.
5. Skippen P, Seear M, Poskitt K, Kestle J, Cochrane D, Annich G, et al. Effect of hyperventilation on regional cerebral blood flow in head-injured children. Crit Care Med. 1997;25(8):1275-8.
6. Marcoux KK. Management of increased intracranial pressure in critically ill child with acute neurological injury. AACN Clin Issues. 2005;16(2):212-31.
7. Ziai WC, Toung TJ, Bhardwaj A. Hypertonic saline: first-line therapy for cerebral edema? J Neurol Sci. 2007;261(1-2):157-66.
8. Berger C, Sakowitz OW, Kiening KL, Schwab S. Neurochemical monitoring of glycerol therapy in patients with ischemic brain edema. Stroke. 2005;36(2):e4-6.
9. French LA, Galicich JH. The use of steroids for control of cerebral edema. Clin Neurosurg. 1964;10:212-23.
10. Adelson PD, Ragheb J, Kanev P, Brockmeyer D, Brown SD, Cassidy LD, et al. Phase II clinical trial of moderate hypothermia after severe traumatic brain injury in children. Neurosurgery. 2005;56(4):740-54.

8.16 Stroke in Children

Ramesh Konanki, Geetha Chanda

INTRODUCTION

A cerebrovascular accident or stroke is not an uncommon emergency in children. The World Health Organization (WHO) has defined pediatric stroke as "acute onset focal dysfunction of the brain, spine, or retina lasting for >24 hours, or of any duration of symptoms if neuroimaging or autopsy shows infarction or hemorrhage consistent with clinical symptoms." A transient ischemic attack (TIA) is defined as "a focal neurological dysfunction of duration <24 hours and normal neuroimaging."

Based on the age of onset, pediatric stroke can be classified as "perinatal stroke", when the stroke occurs between 20 weeks of gestation and 28 days of life ("acute neonatal stroke" presents in first 28 days of life and "presumed perinatal stroke" presents later in life but attributed to presumed perinatal events), or "childhood stroke" when the stroke occurs beyond the neonatal period (i.e., after 28 days of life).

Based on the pathophysiological mechanism, childhood stroke can be classified as "ischemic stroke" when it occurs secondary to acute blockage of arterial blood supply [arterial ischemic stroke (AIS)] or venous thrombosis of cerebral vessels [cerebral sinovenous thrombosis (CSVT)], or "hemorrhagic stroke" when a stroke occurs due to the rupture of blood vessels with bleeding into the brain.

EPIDEMIOLOGY

Worldwide, the reported incidence of childhood stroke (stroke occurring between 1 month and 18 years of age) ranges from 1.2 to 13 cases per 100,000 population, with significant male predominance. The incidence varies widely depending on the age at stroke occurrence: 2.5 per 100,000 population per year, for strokes occurring within 1 year of life (infancy), to 1.25 per 100,000 population, for those occurring beyond 1 year of life. This may be attributed to a higher incidence of congenital heart disease (CHD) and perinatal complications in children below 1 year of age. The hospital-based data from India shows that 5–15% of all strokes in young individuals (below 40 years of age) are attributed to childhood stroke.

ETIOPATHOGENESIS

The etiological and risk factor profile in childhood stroke is comprehensive and heterogeneous, and often, identifying the precise etiology is challenging. Broadly, the causes and risk factors in pediatric ischemic stroke can be categorized into the following groups: Structural heart disease, vasculopathies (inflammatory and noninflammatory), hematological disorders, prothrombotic states (inherited and acquired), and miscellaneous conditions.

The risk factors' spectrum may vary from nation to nation and region to region within a nation. For example, moyamoya disease is one of the most common causes in Japan. In India, sickle cell disease (SCD) is an important cause in central India, while CHDs are more often reported from tertiary care centers involved in the management of children with complex CHDs.

Acute Ischemic Stroke

Acute ischemic stroke (AIS) can occur secondary to cardiac causes, intra- and extracranial arteriopathies, thrombophilia, hematologic disorders, and inflammatory, genetic, or metabolic disorders.

Cardia Causes

Cardioembolic phenomenon accounts for ~30% of all pediatric AIS. The underlying pathogenesis is predominantly thromboembolism, with a possible role of associated extracranial vascular abnormalities. Thromboembolism occurs secondary to stasis in CHD, extracorporeal membrane oxygenation (ECMO), and ventricular assist devices. The role of arrhythmias and patent foramen ovale (PFO) remains unclear.

Extracranial Arteriopathy

Extracranial arteriopathy resulting in stroke is usually secondary to craniocervical arterial dissection (CCAD) due to a tear in the intimal layer of the endothelium, which triggers platelet aggregation and coagulation cascade. With time, it can result in pseudoaneurysm formation. CCAD accounts for ~7.5% of pediatric strokes. When present in the posterior circulation, there is an increased risk of recurrent stroke. Recurrent posterior circulation CCAD should prompt evaluation of V3 segment of vertebral artery (C1–C2 segment) dissection/pseudoaneurysm using digital subtraction angiography (DSA) or computed tomographic angiography (CTA) with intraprocedural head turning to look for compression of the vertebral artery with head turning, which causes repeated trauma and dissection. CCAD can change over time, and ~50% of vessel abnormalities can progress in the first year after the first episode; hence, serial imaging over 1-year poststroke is recommended.

Intracranial Arteriopathies

Intracranial arteriopathies account for ~45% of pediatric AIS. Focal cerebral arteriopathy (FCA) is defined as unilateral, unifocal stenosis or irregularity of large intracranial arteries of the anterior circulation, including the distal internal carotid artery (ICA) or its proximal branches. FCA-d (dissection) includes dissection involving the intracranial anterior circulation. In FCA-I (inflammation), an infectious or parainfectious process results in localized vessel wall inflammation, secondary thrombus formation, and lumen occlusion, resulting in AIS. Varicella infection in the preceding 6–12 months is the most commonly associated infection and was previously known as postvaricella arteriopathy. The role of doing cerebrospinal fluid (CSF) and varicella polymerase chain reaction (PCR) or immunoglobulin G (IgG)/immunoglobulin M (IgM) is not clear in cases of postvaricella angiopathy.

Progressive diseases of distal ICA or its proximal branches with the development of collaterals are known as moyamoya disease. It is associated with the presence of a characteristic imaging pattern of "puff-of-smoke appearance" due to the extensive collaterals. It is commonly bilateral, although unilateral disease can be seen. When associated with conditions such as neurofibromatosis-1, Down syndrome, or SCD, it is known as moyamoya syndrome. Asian ancestry is a risk factor for moyamoya disease, with 30–56% of patients harboring a mutation in the *RNF126* gene, in contrast to only 3.6–29% in non-Asian patients.[1] Compared to FCA, where 1-year recurrence rate of stroke is ~19–25% (beyond which progression is uncommon), the recurrence risk of strokes in moyamoya disease is 35% for the first year.

Thrombophilia Disorders

Prothrombotic disorders result in a hypercoagulable state in the body, which, in the presence of other triggering factors such as cardiac disease or infection, may result in systemic embolic manifestations. These can be inherited or acquired. Inherited conditions of increased lipoprotein-A, PTG20210, FVLG1691A, protein C mutations, and methylenetetrahydrofolate reductase (MTHFR) polymorphisms are independently associated with increased stroke risk. Antiphospholipid antibody syndrome (lupus anticoagulant, anticardiolipin antibody, and anti-β2 microglobulin Ib antibody) is one of the major acquired prothrombotic conditions. Of note, antiphospholipid antibodies can be positive in childhood after an acute viral illness and stroke. In case positive immediately after a stroke episode, these should be rechecked after 12 weeks to ensure validity.

Systemic Disorders

Systemic disorders, both inflammatory and inherited genetic conditions, are associated with increased stroke risk. Childhood primary angiitis of the central nervous system (cPACNS)-large vessel type has some overlap with FCA-I, with the monophasic illness being the same as FCA-I. Rheumatological disorders such as systemic lupus erythematosus (SLE), ADA2 deficiency, and polyarteritis nodosa can have stroke as a manifestation. Persistent elevated inflammatory markers, such as C-reactive protein (CRP) and erythrocyte sedimentation rate (ESR)], for >1 month after acute stroke should prompt investigations for progressive inflammatory disorders of childhood.

Genetic Conditions

Genetic conditions such as MELAS (mitochondrial encephalomyopathy, lactic acidosis, and stroke-like episodes), PHACES syndrome, *ACTA2*, *COL4A1* mutations, and Fabry disease should be investigated when other clinical features are present.

Miscellaneous

Lenticulostriate artery mineralization is a new entity, causing subcortical (basal ganglia) strokes, especially in children aged 6–24 months, following a trivial head injury. The pathophysiology is mineralization/calcification of lenticulostriate arteries, which is best picked up on CT and is the investigation of choice when suspected.

Cerebral Sinovenous Thrombosis (CSVT)

The risk factors for CSVT are diverse and are listed in **Box 8.16.1**. The underlying pathogenesis pertains to poor venous blood flow or stasis, or factors resulting in the procoagulant state, which results in activation of the thrombosis cascade and thrombus formation in the cerebral venous system. Both acquired and inherited factors are known to result in CSVT; hence, a thorough search for the precipitating factor(s) is essential to initiate proper workup and prevent recurrences.

Hemorrhagic Stroke

Hemorrhagic stroke results from either structural malformation of the arteriovenous system of the brain or acquired or inherited deficiencies of procoagulant factors **(Box 8.16.1)**.

BOX 8.16.1: Etiological factors for pediatric CSVT and hemorrhagic strokes.

CSVT
- Fever
- Anemia (iron deficiency anemia)
- Dehydration
- Infections (otitis media, mastoiditis, sinusitis, orbital cellulitis, meningoencephalitis)
- *Chronic systemic inflammatory disorders:* Inflammatory bowel disease, Behcet's disease, systemic lupus erythematosus (APLA, lupus anticoagulant), protein-losing enteropathy/nephropathy
- Congenital heart diseases (vascular stasis and instrumentation)
- Thyrotoxicosis
- Childhood malignancies [e.g., acute lymphoblastic leukemia (prothrombotic state, treatment-related—l-asparaginase), brain tumors (mass effect with venous compression or invasion)]
- Prothrombotic drugs: Steroids, estrogen-containing contraceptives

Hemorrhagic stroke
- *Trauma*
- *Structural*
  - Arteriovenous malformations
  - Arteriovenous fistula
  - Aneurysm
  - Cavernous malformation
  - Bleeding into a tumor
- *Hematological causes*
  - Inherited:
    - Common: Hemophilia A (factor VIII deficiency) or B (factor VII deficiency)
    - Rare: Factor VII deficiency, factor II, factor XIII deficiency
    - Vitamin K-dependent clotting factors deficiency
  - Acquired: Idiopathic thrombocytopenic purpura
- *Others*
- Hypertension (rare)

(APLA: antiphospholipid antibody; CSVT: cerebral sinovenous thrombosis)

CLINICAL FEATURES

Neonatal Stroke

Acute Symptomatic Neonatal Stroke

Neonates with AIS or hemorrhagic stroke may present with seizures (50–70%), encephalopathy, tone abnormalities, and feeding difficulties. Acute onset focal deficits are usually not evident in the neonatal period.

Presumed Perinatal Stroke

These infants usually present later in the first 2 years of life with focal weakness, developmental delays, or seizures. Diagnosis is usually made based on neuroimaging consistent with sequelae of an acute ischemic event.

Childhood Stroke

The most common symptoms of childhood stroke are acute onset hemiparesis and hemifacial weakness (67–90%), speech or language dysfunction (20–50%), vision disturbances (10–15%), and ataxia (8–10%). Nonlocalizing symptoms such as headache (20–50%) and altered mental status (17–38%) may also be seen in children. Seizure at stroke onset can be present in 15–25% of cases, especially in children aged <6 years. A cardioembolic stroke usually presents with an abrupt onset of symptoms, whereas a staggering or fluctuating course may be more commonly present in vasculopathic strokes. Children with moyamoya disease as the diagnosis may have a history of recurrent TIAs with hemiparesis or hemisensory deficits (~72%), chronic headaches (~52%), and seizures (<10%). In infants and young children, excessive crying preceding neurological deficits is a clue to possible underlying cerebral vasculopathy.

Posterior circulation strokes are usually present in previously healthy boys, with a median age of presentation of 7–8 years. The presentation can be with localizing features such as hemiparesis, ataxia, dysarthria, visual field defects, and oculomotor deficits. Nonlocalizing features including headache, vomiting, and altered sensorium may be present in 60–70% of children.

Cerebral Sinovenous Thrombosis

The presentation of CSVT may be subtle and nonspecific. The neonates usually present with encephalopathy and seizures. Infants and children can present with signs of raised intracranial pressure (ICP) such as headache, nausea, vomiting, lethargy, seizures, sixth cranial nerve palsy, or diplopia. Cavernous sinus thrombosis usually presents with ipsilateral proptosis and palsies of cranial nerves III–VI, which course through the cavernous sinus.

Hemorrhagic Stroke

Hemorrhagic stroke usually presents with acute signs of raised ICP, focal neurological deficits, or seizures. Symptoms onset occurs more abruptly and progresses more rapidly in hemorrhagic stroke than in ischemic stroke.

DIFFERENTIAL DIAGNOSIS

Various differential diagnoses of AIS are discussed in **Table 8.16.1**. Common conditions that may mimic a stroke include demyelinating disorders (which can present with encephalopathy and focal neurological deficits), hemiplegic migraine, intracranial space-occupying lesions (ICSOLs), etc.

DIAGNOSIS AND INVESTIGATIONS

Investigations in childhood stroke aim to diagnose the type of stroke and identify the underlying risk factors.

TABLE 8.16.1: Stroke mimics and differential diagnoses.

Etiologies	*Clinical features*
Todd's palsy	Paralysis of one or more parts of the body after a seizure episode; usual duration is from 30 minutes to 36 hours. It resolves completely without any intervention
Acute demyelination syndrome of CNS	Can present with unilateral weakness, with or without other associated features such as encephalopathy, seizures, and visual symptoms. Usually preceding febrile illness/vaccination is common
ICSOL	ICSOLs such as brain infections (neurocysticercosis, tuberculoma), brain abscess, and brain tumors may present with hemiparesis
AHC	Characterized by recurrent episodic hemiplegia with onset <18 months of age, involving either side of the body and relieved by sleep. Additional features, such as paroxysmal extrapyramidal symptoms, epilepsy, and developmental delay, may be associated
Hemiplegic migraine	Typically begins with weakness in one hand, followed by spread over the entire arm and leg. This is usually associated with a headache and lasts for 20–30 minutes, although a longer duration, lasting for days, is known. Rapid onset of symptoms may mimic stroke
Stroke-like episodes in MELAS	Recurrent episodes of focal deficits may be seen in MELAS. Neuroimaging shows nonterritorial vascular area infarcts. Elevated arterial or CSF lactate and elevated lactate peak on MRS may be present
Posterior reversible encephalopathy syndrome (PRES)	PRES is a clinico-radiological syndrome associated with hypertension. Typical areas involved are parieto-occipital areas. It usually presents with seizures and encephalopathy

(AHC: alternating hemiplegia of childhood; CNS: central nervous system; CSF: cerebrospinal fluid; ICSOL: intracranial space-occupying lesions; MELAS: mitochondrial encephalomyopathy, lactic acidosis, and stroke-like episodes; MRS: magnetic resonance spectroscopy; PRESS: posterior reversible encephalopathy syndrome)

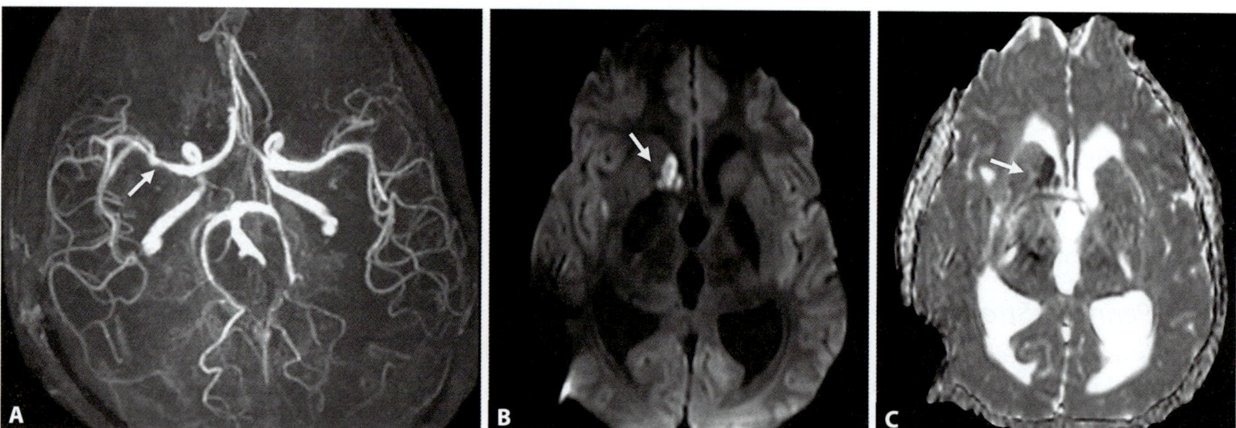

Figs. 8.16.1A to C: *Focal cerebral arteriopathy.* MRA showing right middle cerebral artery stenosis and beading (A), acute infarct in right lenticulostriate artery territory (right caudate) showing diffusion restriction (B), and GRE showing blooming (C). (GRE: gradient recalled echo; MRA: magnetic resonance angiography)

Neuroimaging

Neuroimaging is the first step in the diagnosis of stroke by confirming the vascular nature and ruling out other differential diagnoses. Neuroimaging should be done as early as possible in a child with suspected stroke. Magnetic resonance imaging (MRI) is the diagnostic modality of choice along with magnetic resonance angiography (MRA) and magnetic resonance venography (MRV) if required. Computed tomography (CT) and DSA can be considered in specific conditions, especially if intervention is planned. In those children with hemodynamic instability and posing challenges with sedation, a CT scan of the brain along with CTA is a reasonable alternative mode of imaging.

Magnetic Resonance Imaging

Brain MRI is the gold standard for the diagnosis of stroke. It should include T1-weighted (T1W), T2-weighted (T2W), T2-fluid-attenuated inversion recovery (T2-FLAIR), and diffusion-weighted imaging (DWI) sequences. The DWI is the most sensitive sequence to identify abnormalities as early as 2–6 hours and small ischemic infarcts in AIS. All children with AIS should also undergo MRA to assess the intracranial arteries and neck vessels (external carotid arteries and vertebrobasilar system). In the hyperacute setting (within 6 hours of symptom onset), imaging should include axial DWI and apparent diffusion coefficient (ADC), T2 axial/FLAIR, gradient recalled echo/susceptibility-weighted imaging (GRE/SWI), and 3D time of flight magnetic resonance angiography (TOF MRA) of the brain and neck vessels.[2] In children with suspected AIS, beyond the hyperacute period of stroke onset (>6 hours from symptom onset), neuroimaging can be tailored depending on the initial MRI sequences and likely etiology/risk factors.

Magnetic resonance imaging features of AIS include infarcts in the vascular territory [visualized as territorial area(s) of diffusion restriction and T2/FLAIR hyperintensity in the acute phase, T1 hypointensity and corresponding T2/FLAIR hyperintensity in the chronic stage]. Vessel wall thinning, stenosis, and collaterals can sometimes be visualized on T2 sequences. MRA may show vessel wall stenosis, dilation, or beading in cases of FCA **(Figs. 8.16.1A to C)**, extensive collateral formation in supraclinoid, distal ICA regions with stenosis, and vessel dropout of distal middle cerebral artery (MCA) branches in moyamoya disease in addition to multiple, chronic infarcts on MRI **(Figs. 8.16.2A to D)**. In suspected CSVT, MRI with MRV is the imaging modality. Neuroimaging

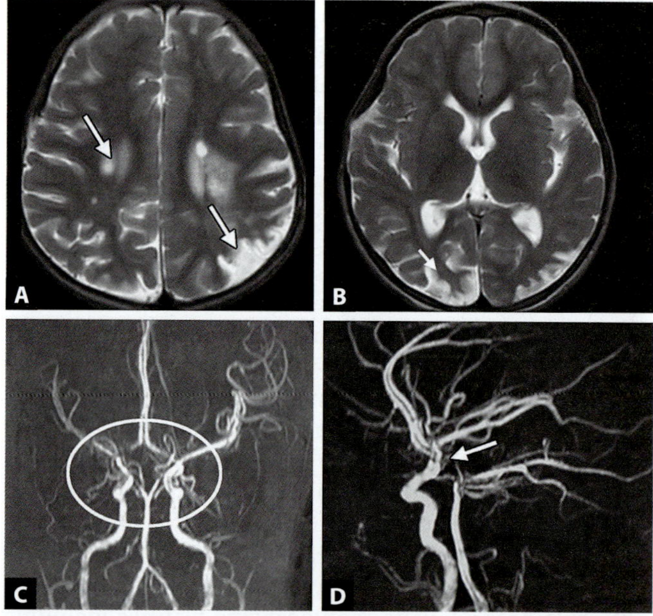

Figs. 8.16.2A to D: *Moyamoya disease*: (A) and (B) Multiple chronic infarcts in middle and posterior circulation; (C) MRA showing extensive collaterals; and (D) Bilateral internal carotid artery stenosis. (MRA: magnetic resonance angiography)

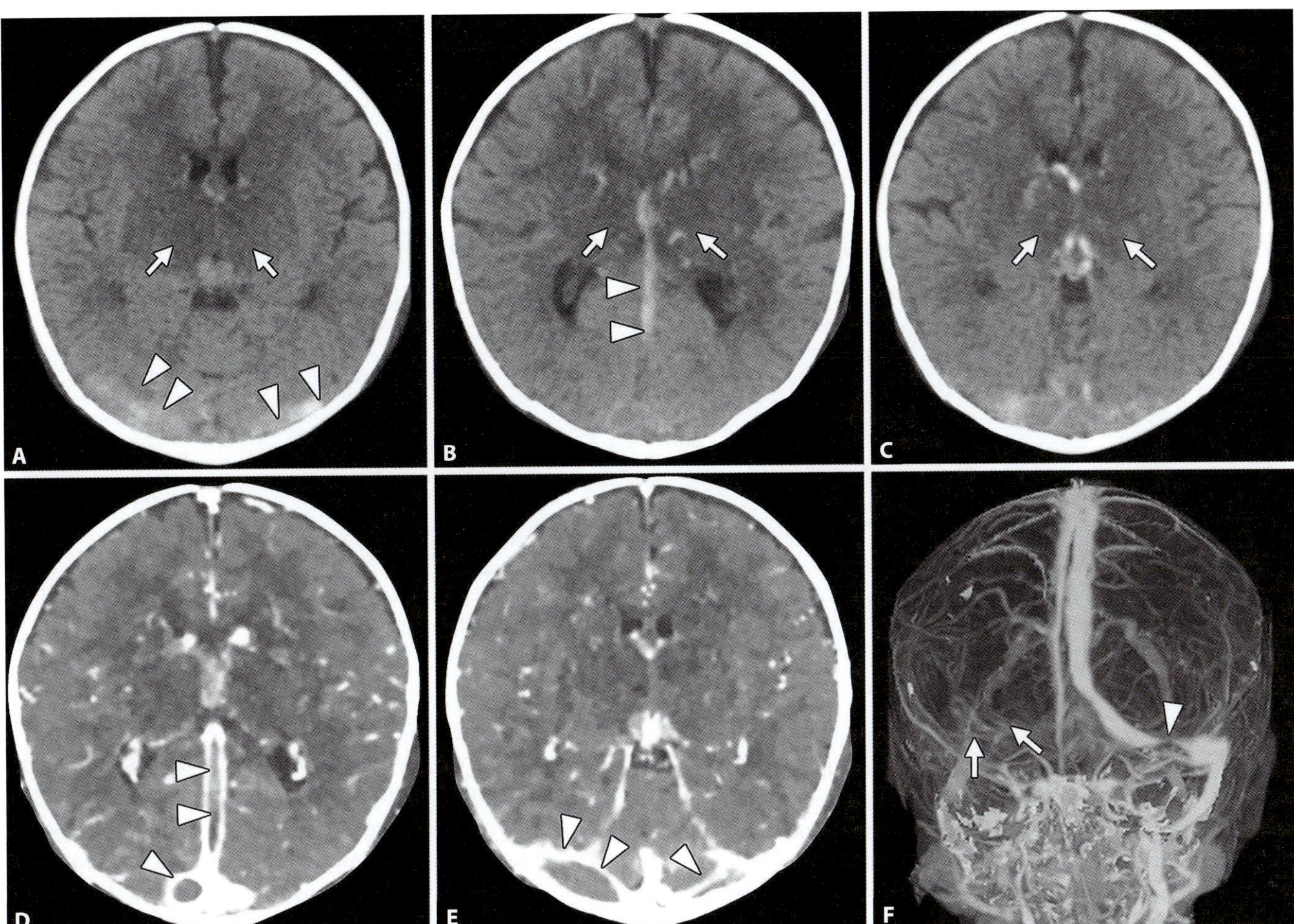

Figs. 8.16.3A to F: *Cerebral sinovenous thrombosis (CSVT)*: Dense cord sign on noncontrast CT in the bilateral transverse sinus (A) and deep cerebral vein (B) marked by arrowheads; bilateral thalami show hypodensities in the upper panel, consistent with deep venous thrombosis (C); contrast CT shows filling defect in the deep cerebral vein (D) with extension to bilateral transverse sinuses (E) (arrowheads); (F) CT venogram shows a filling defect in the left transverse sinus (arrowhead) and nonvisualization of the right transverse sinus. (CT: computed tomography)

shows hyperdense signals in areas of thrombosed sinuses known as dense cord signs, with filling defects on contrast CT and MRV **(Figs. 8.16.3A to F)**.

Computed Tomography

The CT of the brain has low sensitivity for AIS. It is commonly used in emergencies, when children are hemodynamically unstable, to rule out hemorrhagic stroke or CSVT. In such situations, CT of the brain is recommended along with CT angiography or venography, respectively.

In mineralizing angiopathy, axial CT sections show basal ganglia punctate calcifications, and sagittal and coronal reconstructed sections usually demonstrate the linear mineralization of the perforating arteries (linear hyperdensities along vessels) **(Figs. 8.16.4A and B)** along with infarcts (hypodensity).

Digital Subtraction Angiography

Digital subtraction angiography is the gold standard for diagnosis of vasculopathies and, hence, is performed in children with suspected moyamoya disease, small-vessel vasculitis, cervicocephalic arterial dissection, and arterial stenosis of other etiologies.

Transcranial Doppler

The transcranial Doppler (TCD) is used to measure blood flow velocity in major cerebral vessels. It is used in SCD. Children with a time-averaged mean velocity of >200 cm/s on TCD have a higher risk of stroke. Hence, it is recommended that, in children with SCD, periodic TCD should be done annually if the initial TCD is normal, a month later if abnormal, and 3–6 months later if borderline abnormal.

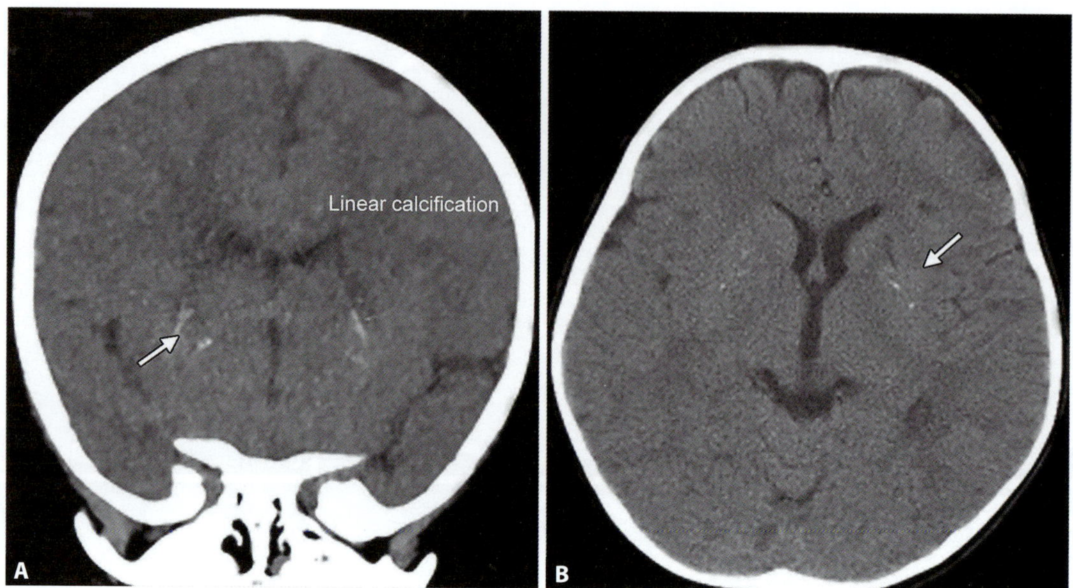

Figs. 8.16.4A and B: *Mineralizing angiopathy*: (A) Linear calcification in right basal ganglia; and (B) Punctate areas of calcification in bilateral basal ganglia.

Etiological Evaluation

Detailed birth, perinatal, and developmental history, as well as history pertaining to inflammatory and cardiac disorders in the patient or family members, and a three-generation family tree should be obtained for all patients. In addition to detailed clinical examination, focused cardiac examination and four-extremity blood pressure measurement should be recorded for all patients. Furthermore, risk factor identification for stroke recurrence has to be obtained and should answer three questions regarding the antithrombotic management plan:

1. Does the child have predisposing factors for stroke?
2. Is there an immediate trigger for thrombosis?
3. What is the risk of recurrence in the immediate and distant future?

The first-line investigations are aimed to identify the most common etiologies and should be done in all children. Second-line investigations such as evaluation for inherited prothrombotic states are desirable in all children; however, they can be individualized. Anticoagulant protein levels should preferably be done 3 months after an acute stroke to prevent falsely low values secondary to consumption of these factors. Beyond this, third-line investigations for rare etiologies can be tailored according to specific indications **(Table 8.16.2)**.

TREATMENT

Acute Ischemic Stroke

Acute symptomatic management with securing of airway, breathing, and circulation is the priority and should be managed in-hospital in the first 24 hours **(Flowchart 8.16.1)**. Practice points are detailed as follows:[3]

- *Neuroprotective and neurocritical care*, as indicated, should be provided to all patients.
- *Blood glucose*: Hyperglycemia in the first 24 hours after stroke has been associated with poor outcomes. Hence, blood glucose values should be maintained between 140 and 180 mg/dL in children with hyperglycemia, and values should not fall <60 mg/dL.
- Normal *temperature and age-appropriate blood pressure* should be maintained.
- *Pediatric National Institutes of Health Severity Scale* (PedsNIHSS) score should be recorded in all children to quantify stroke severity and for objective follow-up.
- Indications for *decompressive surgery*:
  - Prophylactic decompressive surgery should be considered in malignant MCA infarcts involving >50% of MCA territory within 24 or 72 hours with serial monitoring for worsening cerebral edema.
  - Posterior fossa masses or strokes with brainstem compression
- Children with acute stroke should be started on *antithrombotic agents*, which include either antiplatelet drugs (Aspirin) or anticoagulants such as heparin [low molecular weight heparin (LMWH) or unfractionated heparin (UFH)] or warfarin for the prevention of further strokes. Preventive therapy should be continued for at least 1 year (or more depending on the underlying etiology).

TABLE 8.16.2: Investigations for acute stroke.

Tier 1	*Tier 2*
• Complete hemogram with peripheral smear • Sickling test • Prothrombin time and international normalized ratio (PT-INR) • ESR, CRP • Fasting lipid profile • Liver and renal function tests • ECG, 2D-echocardiography, carotid doppler • Serum iron studies • Plasma homocysteine • Vitamin B_{12} levels	• Protein C, protein S • Antithrombin III • Activated protein C resistance • Factor V Leiden • Anticardiolipin antibodies (aCL-IgM, IgG) • Lupus anticoagulant • Lipoprotein(a) • MTHFR polymorphisms, prothrombin gene mutations
Tier 3: Individualized investigations	
Preceding varicella infection in the past 6–12 months	Varicella CSF PCR, IgG, and IgM antibodies
Sickle cell disease—painful abdomen/chest episodes, severe anemia, hemolytic facies, recurrent blood transfusions, endemic area	Hemoglobin electrophoresis
Recurrent infections, failure to thrive, lymphadenopathy, weight loss	Tuberculosis workup, retroviral serology
Preceding respiratory tract infections	IgM for mycoplasma
Mitochondrial cytopathies (failure to thrive, short stature, regression, stroke-like episodes, myoclonic epilepsy)	Arterial and CSF lactate, MRI with MRS, ophthalmic evaluation for retinitis pigmentosa, EEG, genetics
Systemic inflammatory diseases (recurrent pyrexia, weight loss, joint pains/swellings, rash, lymphadenopathy, cytopenia)	ANA, dsDNA, rheumatology consult
IEMs—regression, episodic symptoms, family history, consanguinity, dysmorphism, organomegaly	Blood ammonia, lactate, TMS, GC-MS, eye evaluation, genetic testing
Teenagers with possible drug abuse	Toxicology profile—urine and blood

(ANA: antinuclear antibody; CRP: C-reactive protein; CSF-PCR: cerebrospinal fluid polymerase chain reaction; dsDNA: double-stranded deoxyribonucleic acid; ECG: electrocardiography; EEG: electroencephalogram; ESR: erythrocyte sedimentation rate; GC-MS: gas-chromatography-mass spectroscopy; IEMs: inborn errors of metabolism; IgG: immunoglobulin G; IgM: immunoglobulin M; MRI: magnetic resonance imaging; MRS: magnetic resonance spectroscopy; MTHFR: methylenetetrahydrofolate reductase; TMS: tandem mass spectroscopy)

- Indications for using anticoagulants include thromboembolic stroke (cardiac and known thrombophilic disorder) and extracranial dissection for 3–6 months after stroke.[4]
- *Role of acute thrombolysis*: The safety and efficacy of acute thrombolysis are not available for children <18 years of age. Intervention with intraarterial thrombolysis [with tissue plasminogen activator (tPA)—alteplase] can be considered till 4.5 hours, and for mechanical thrombectomy till 6 hours, with possible extension up to 24 hours after acute stroke onset for basilar artery or MCA thrombosis. Mechanical thrombectomy intervention can be considered in children with:
  - Persistent neurological deficits—PedsNIHSS score >6 at the time of intervention
  - Radiographically confirmed intracranial large artery occlusion
  - Larger/older children
  - Intervention should be performed by an endovascular surgeon with expertise in treating children and performing thrombectomy in adult stroke patients.
  - *Neonatal AIS:* Supportive care in the neonatal intensive care unit (NICU) should be provided to all neonates. Long-term prophylactic treatment with antithrombotic drugs is not recommended for all neonates and should be considered for babies with thrombophilia and complex CHDs (high risk of stroke recurrence).

Cerebrovenous Sinus Thrombosis

Supportive Care

Precipitating factors such as dehydration, fever, sepsis, or ear infections should be appropriately managed. Raised ICP management is paramount and can be challenging with ongoing anticoagulation.

Anticoagulation

Evidence for *anticoagulation* in childhood CSVT has been extrapolated from adult studies, which have demonstrated a clear benefit of anticoagulation.[5] The only major exception is the presence of septic CSVT (complication of otitis media and Lemierre syndrome), where antibiotics and surgical intervention are the mainstays of management with the controversial role of anticoagulation. Intravenous UFH, subcutaneous LMWH, or oral warfarin can be used with appropriate monitoring using factor Xa, activated partial thromboplastin time (aPTT), or international normalized ratio (INR), respectively.

In conditions with concerns for bleeding or surgical intervention, treatment may initially be started on

Flowchart 8.16.1: Management of acute stroke with specific practice points.

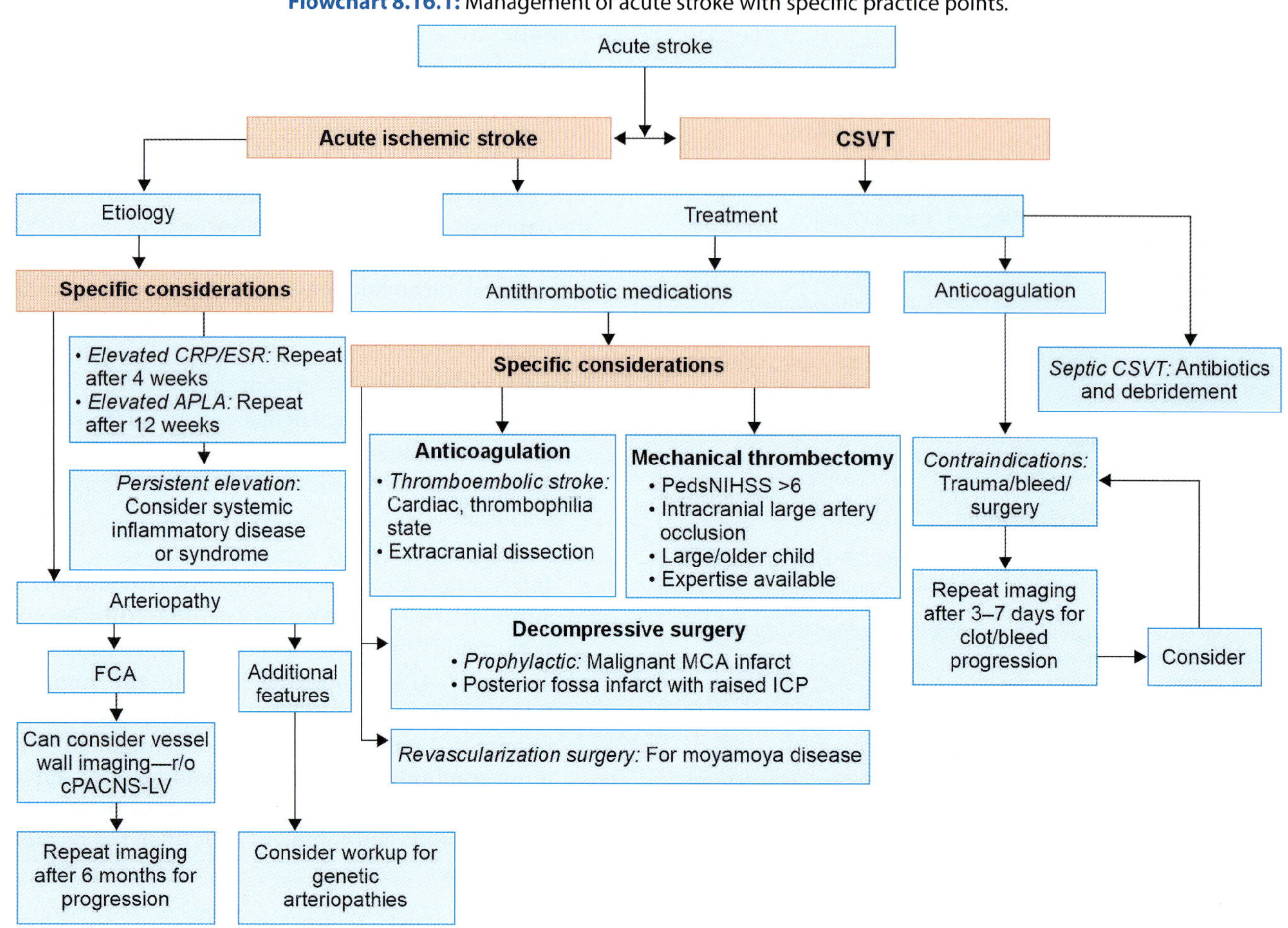

(APLA: antiphospholipid antibody; cPACNCS-LV: childhood primary angiitis of central nervous system, large vessel type; CRP: C-reactive protein; CSVT: cerebral sinovenous thrombosis; ESR: erythrocyte sedimentation rate; FCA: focal cerebral arteriopathy; ICP: intracranial pressure; MCA: middle cerebral artery; PedsNIHSS: Pediatric National Institutes of Health Severity Scale)

UFH followed by conversion to LMWH or warfarin. In case anticoagulation is deferred due to the presence of contraindications (surgery, recent head trauma, or bleeding), repeat imaging after 3–7 days should be obtained to look for clot progression. Approximately one-third of children who are not anticoagulated will have clot progression, of which 40% will have additional hemorrhage.

Anticoagulation should be considered in neonates with CSVT. Although there is a lack of strong evidence to support its use, preliminary data suggest better outcomes with anticoagulation.

Hemorrhagic Stroke

In addition to supportive care with neuroprotection and control of raised ICP, management depends on the specific underlying etiology. Surgical evacuation of the hematoma is beneficial in some cases.

PROGNOSIS

Mortality rates have been variably reported to be approximately 4–5% for acute strokes in children. In-hospital mortality of 3.6% has been recently reported in a large cohort of pediatric stroke patients. Normal neurological outcomes were recorded in 30% of children in the Canadian Pediatric Stroke Registry. Of the remaining 70%, 36% had mild deficits. This study also recorded poorer cognitive outcomes with respect to verbal memory, processing speed, working memory, and overall intelligence in children with AIS compared to normal children.

Younger age at stroke (after the neonatal period) and larger stroke volume at stroke onset are related to poorer 1-year outcomes, whereas hemorrhagic stroke was not seen to influence 1-year outcomes.

Neonatal and perinatal strokes have high long-term neurological sequelae. Although motor deficits are predominant, seizures, learning, behavioral, and language issues can also be present. Overall, prognosis depends on risk factors, causes and severity of neuronal involvement, and timely treatment given.

REFERENCES

1. Cecchi AC, Guo D, Ren Z, Flynn K, Santos-Cortez RLP, Leal SM, et al. RNF213 rare variants in an ethnically diverse population with moyamoya disease. Stroke. 2014;45(11):3200-7.
2. Mirsky DM, Beslow LA, Amlie-Lefond C, Krishnan P, Laughlin S, Lee S, et al. Pathways for neuroimaging of childhood stroke. Pediatr Neurol. 2017;69:11-23.
3. Klučka J, Klabusayová E, Musilová T, Kramplová T, Skříšovská T, Kratochvíl M, et al. Pediatric patient with ischemic stroke: initial approach and early management. Child Basel Switz. 2021;28;8(8):649.
4. Ferriero DM, Fullerton HJ, Bernard TJ, Billinghurst L, Daniels SR, DeBaun MR, et al. Management of stroke in neonates and children: a scientific statement from the American Heart Association/American Stroke Association. Stroke. 2019;50(3):e51-96.
5. Felling RJ, Hassanein SMA, Armstrong J, Aversa L, Billinghurst L, Goldenberg NA, et al. Treatment and outcome of childhood cerebral sinovenous thrombosis. Neurol Clin Pract. 2020;10(3):232-44.

8.17 Disorders of Spinal Cord

Vykuntaraju KN Gowda

INTRODUCTION

The etiology, clinical features, and treatment of spinal cord disorders in children is different from adults. Spinal cord disorders can cause permanent severe neurologic disability. For some patients, such disability can be avoided or minimized if evaluation and treatment are rapid. In children, causes of spinal cord disorders are congenital, developmental, traumatic, and rarely neoplastic disorders. In children, spinal cord disorders are present with scoliosis, pain, weakness, or numbness due to rapid growth. The surgical treatment in children must be considered carefully due to expected growth and development of the spine.[1,2]

EPIDEMIOLOGY

The most common causes of spinal cord disorders in children are meningomyelocele (MMC) and spinal cord injuries (SCIs). The incidence of neural tube defects (NTDs) in North India is 3.9–9/1,000 live births. The last few decades have demonstrated significant success in reduction of NTD by simple intervention of periconceptional folate supplementation.[1,2]

ANATOMY

The spinal cord extends cranially from the medulla at the foramen magnum and terminates at the upper lumbar vertebrae, usually between L1 and L2, where it forms the conus medullaris. In the lumbosacral region, nerve roots from lower cord segments descend within the spinal column in a nearly vertical sheaf, forming the cauda equina.[3]

The white matter at the cord's periphery contains ascending and descending tracts of myelinated sensory and motor nerve fibers. The central H-shaped gray matter is composed of cell bodies and nonmyelinated fibers. The anterior (ventral) horns of the "H" contain lower motor neurons, which receive impulses from the motor cortex via the descending corticospinal tracts and, at the local level, from internuncial neurons and afferent fibers from muscle spindles. The axons of the lower motor neurons are the efferent fibers of the spinal nerves. The posterior (dorsal) horns contain sensory fibers that originate in cell bodies in the dorsal root ganglia. The gray matter also contains many internuncial neurons that carry motor, sensory, or reflex impulses from dorsal to ventral nerve roots, from one side of the cord to the other, or from one level of the cord to another. The spinothalamic tract transmits pain and temperature sensations contralaterally in the spinal cord; most other tracts transmit information ipsilaterally. The cord is divided into functional segments (levels) corresponding approximately to the attachments of the 31 pairs of spinal nerve roots.[3]

Bony Spine and Ligaments

The bony spine provides protection to underlying spinal cord movements. The cervical spinal cord is the most common site of injuries because it is the most common mobile portion of the spinal cord.

Spinal Cord

The caudal end of the cord lies at the first lumbar level in adults and at second lumbar vertebrae at birth. This disparity should be considered with children's age during approach to spinal cord disorders.

Blood Supply

The anterior spinal artery is formed by the union of paired branches of the intracranial vertebral arteries. It is present in the entire length of the spinal cord in the anterior median fissure. The anterior spinal artery receives additional blood supply from anterior radicular arteries derived from lateral spinal arteries from C3 to L3. The posterior spinal artery is the first intracranial branch of vertebral artery, one on each side which runs along the posterolateral sulcus. The anterior spinal artery supplies anterior two-thirds while posterior spinal artery supplies posterior one-third of the spinal cord.[3]

CLINICAL FEATURES

Symptoms and Signs

The spinal cord disorders cause neurological dysfunction at the level and below the spinal cord segments **(Table 8.17.1)**, except in the central cord syndromes **(Table 8.17.2)**. In central cord syndrome, there will be a sparing of segments below. Neurological deficits depend on the location of disease in the intramedullary, extramedullary, or extradural locations. Spinal nerve injury causes motor or sensory abnormalities in the distribution of nerves affected. The clinical manifestations are paresis, loss of sensation, reflex changes, and autonomic dysfunction such as neurogenic bladder and bowel, loss of sweating. Injuries can be complete or partial. Corticospinal tract lesion causes upper neuron dysfunction. Acute SCIs

TABLE 8.17.1: Effects of spinal cord dysfunction by segmental level.

*Location of lesion**	*Possible effects*
At or above C5	Respiratory paralysis, quadriplegia
Between C and C6	Paralysis of legs, wrists, and hands; weakness of shoulder abduction and elbow flexion; loss of biceps jerk reflex; loss of brachioradialis deep tendon reflex
Between C6 and C7	Paralysis of legs, wrists, and hands, but shoulder movement and elbow flexion usually possible
Between C7 and C8	Loss of triceps jerk reflex, paralysis of legs and hands
At C8 to T1	Horner syndrome, paralysis of legs
Between T1 and conus medullaris	Paralysis of legs

*Abbreviations refer to vertebrae; the cord is shorter than the spine, so that moving down the spine, cord segments and vertebral levels are increasingly out of alignment. At all levels of cord injury, deep tendon reflexes are altered (initially decreased and later becoming brisk) below the level of the lesion, bowel and bladder control is lost, and sensation is lost below the level of injury.

TABLE 8.17.2: Spinal cord syndromes.

Syndrome	*Cause*	*Symptoms and signs*
Anterior cord syndrome	Lesions disproportionately affecting the anterior spinal cord, commonly due to infarction (e.g., caused by occlusion of the anterior spinal artery)	Malfunction of the all the tracts except posterior columns, thus sparing position and vibration sensation
Brown–Sequard syndrome	Unilateral spinal cord lesions, typically due to penetrating trauma	Ipsilateral paresis, ipsilateral loss of touch, position, and vibratory sensation. Contralateral loss of pain and temperature sensation*
Central cord syndrome affecting the cervical spinal cord	Lesions affecting the center of the cervical spinal cord, mainly central gray matter (including spinothalamic tracts, which cross), commonly due to trauma, syrinx, or tumors in the central spinal cord	• Paresis tending to be more severe in the upper extremities than in the lower extremities and sacral regions • Tendency to lose pain and temperature sensation in a cape-like distribution over the upper neck, shoulders, and upper trunk, with light touch, position, and vibratory sensation relatively preserved (dissociated sensory loss)
Conus medullaris syndrome	Lesions around L1	• Distal leg paresis, perianal and perineal loss of sensation (saddle anesthesia) • Urinary retention, frequency, or incontinence • Fecal incontinence • Hypotonic anal sphincter • Abnormal bulbocavernosus and anal wink reflexes
Transverse myelopathy	Lesions affecting all or most tracts of the spinal cord at ≥1 segmental level	Deficits in all functions mediated by the spinal cord (because all tracts are affected to some degree)

*Occasionally, only part of one side of the spinal cord malfunctions (partial Brown–Sequard syndrome)

cause spinal shock. It presents acute flaccid paresis in the form of weakness, hypotonia, hyporeflexia, and absent extensor plantar. It may last days to weeks.

The various spinal cord syndromes are transverse sensorimotor myelopathy, Brown-Séquard syndrome, central cord syndrome, anterior cord syndrome, and conus medullaris syndrome **(Table 8.17.2)**. Cauda equina syndrome is not a spinal cord syndrome as it involves nerve roots and cord is spared. However, it can masquerade as medullaris syndrome, however, in this syndrome muscle tone and deep tendon reflexes are decreased in the legs.

CLINICAL SYNDROMES

Intraspinal Intramedullary Lesions

Intraspinal intramedullary lesions can cause complete or incomplete loss of spinal cord function. With complete loss, there is absence of all motor, sensory, and reflex function below the level of injury. With incomplete loss, some motor, sensory, and reflex function persists.

Complete Spinal Cord Lesions

Complete loss of spinal cord function can be either physiologic or pathologic. In physiologic loss, there is no morphologic alteration of the spinal cord, which becomes dysfunctional after impact. This dysfunction may occur with transient compression of the spinal cord by a dislocated vertebra. Development of anatomical disruption followed by pathologic changes with long-standing compression of the spinal cord.

Table 8.17.3 shows various findings, how to differentiate intramedullary and extramedullary lesions.

DIAGNOSIS

Spinal cord disorders should be suspected in case of deficits at segmental levels. If deficits are unilateral suggests nerve root or nerve involvement. Clinical examination is helpful in localization of the lesion. MRI gives the most reliable details of spinal cord parenchyma, soft tissues lesion, and bony lesions.

MANAGEMENT

The general principles of managing children and adolescents with spinal cord disorders are significantly different when compared to adults with similar impairments. Pediatric care must be family-centered, because of the central role of parents and family in a child or adolescent's life.

The growth of the child and spine should be considered when deciding surgical treatment. The care of children and young adolescents with spinal cord disorders must be developmentally appropriate, with compatible physical and philosophic characteristics, including child-life and recreation therapy.

GENETIC AND CONGENITAL MALFORMATIONS

NEURAL TUBE DEFECTS (DYSRAPHISM)

Neural tube defects account for most congenital anomalies of the central nervous system (CNS) and result from failure of the neural tube to close spontaneously between the 3rd and 4th week of in utero development. Classifications of NTD are shown in **Box 8.17.1** and etiology of NTD are shown **Box 8.17.2**.[4]

Assessment

History including family history of NTD and risk factors should be taken. The back should be examined for the location of the defect and its skin cover (whether intact or ruptured). The examination should include checking for a cerebrospinal fluid (CSF) leak (by looking for features of meningitis if CSF leak present), transillumination (to differentiate MMC from meningocele), and presence of vertebral defect/and/or kyphoscoliosis. The most common site is lumbosacral (75%). **Figures 8.17.1A and B** show cervical swelling in a case of cervical meningocele. **Figures 8.17.2A and B** show the tail and deformity in the bilateral lower limbs due to caudal regression syndrome. **Figures 8.17.3A and B** show tuff of hair on lower back due to spinal

TABLE 8.17.3: Clinical guidelines to differentiate intramedullary and extramedullary tumors.

Symptoms/signs	*Intramedullary tumors*	*Extramedullary tumors*
Radicular pain	Unusual	Common, may occur early
Vertebral pain	Unusual	Common
Funicular pain	Common	Less common
Upper motor neuron signs	Yes, late	Yes, early
Lower motor signs	Prominent and diffuse	Unusual, if present, segmental distribution
Paresthesia's progression	Descending progression	Ascending
Sphincter abnormalities	Early with caudal lesion (conus cauda equine)	Late
Trophic changes	Common	Unusual

BOX 8.17.1: Classification of neural tube defects (NTDs).

Primary NTD (95%) (failure of closure of neural tube at 17–28 days of gestation)
- Meningomyelocele—the most common NTD, thoracic or lumbosacral. Commonly associated with hydrocephalus (90%), Arnold-Chiari II and corpus callosal agenesis
- Encephalocele—occipital or frontal
- Anencephaly

Secondary NTD (5%) (occur after neural tube closes due to defects in mesoderm)
- Meningocele—no neural elements, can be distinguished from meningomyelocele (MMC) by transillumination—80% at lumbosacral
- Lipomeningocele, intradural lipoma 1–4%. More common in girls. Cervical/thoracic
- Diastematomyelia—sagittal clefting of cord between T9 and S1 separated by fibrous or bony spur
- Dorsal dermal sinus, tethered cord

BOX 8.17.2: Etiology of neural tube defect (NTD).

- Primary NTD—multifactorial inheritance
- Maternal risk factors—alcohol, radiation, type 1 diabetes, valproate, methotrexate, aminopterin, hyperthermia, antiepileptic drugs-carbamazepine, zinc, and folate deficiency
- Genetic—*MTHFR* gene defects
- Chromosomal abnormalities—trisomy 13 and 18 and syndromes such as Meckel-Gruber, acrocallosal syndrome, amnion rupture sequence, and caudal dysplasia sequence

dysraphism. **Figures 8.17.4A and B** show scoliosis and MRI of the spine shows syringomyelia. Hydrocephalus (90%), and type II Chiari defect may be present at birth in most children with NTD or may appear later. Head size should be recorded frequently. Power in the lower limbs should be checked to look for paraparesis; bladder, and bowel examination should include assessing anal tone, perineal sensation and compressibility of bladder. Musculoskeletal examination should be done to detect developmental dysplasia of hip (DDH) and congenital talipes equinovarus (CTEV). Other malformations such as cardiac, renal, and gastrointestinal tract anomalies should also be noted.[4]

Investigations

X-ray of chest, spine, and hip tare were done to detect spina bifida, hemi-vertebrae, and hip dysplasia. Ultrasound of the sac should be done for detection of contents. Ultrasound of the head is done to detect hydrocephalus and ultrasound of hip joint for DDH. CT head should be done for hydrocephalus; MRI of spine and brain to look for other associated malformations of brain.

Management

Severe paralysis at birth with bladder, bowel involvement, and hydrocephalus predicts a poor neuromotor outcome despite

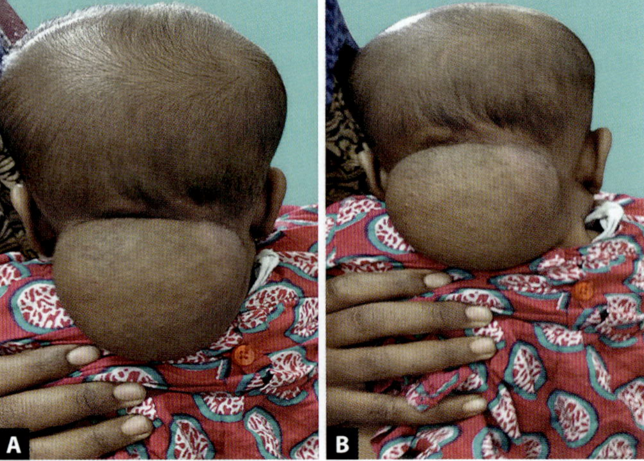

Figs. 8.17.1A and B: Cervical swelling in child with cervical meningocele.

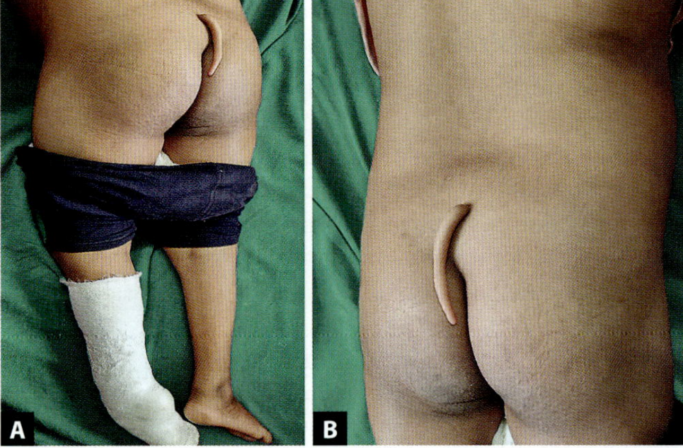

Figs. 8.17.2A and B: Tail and deformities in the lower limbs due to caudal regression syndrome.

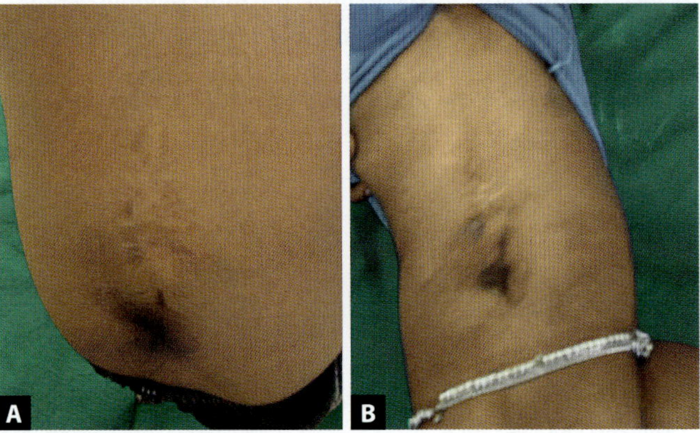

Figs. 8.17.3A and B: Tuff of hair in the lower back in children with spinal dysraphism.

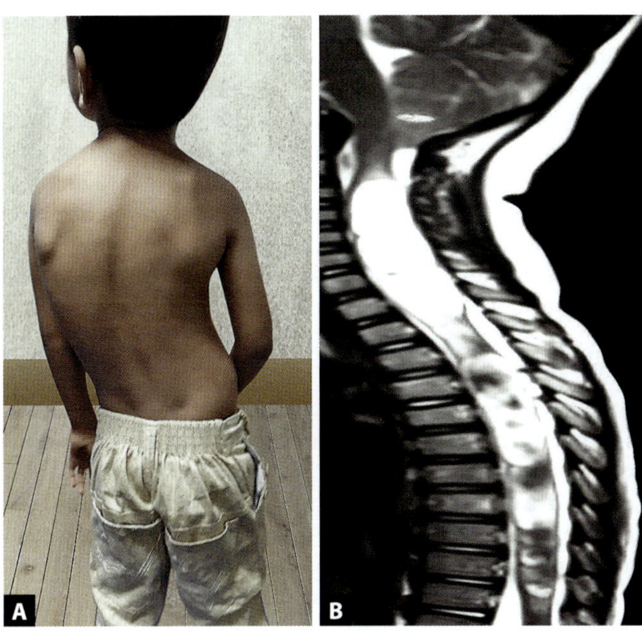

Figs. 8.17.4A and B: Clinical photograph showing scoliosis and MRI of the spine showing syringomyelia.

early surgery. It requires a multidisciplinary approach with involvement of pediatric surgeon/neurosurgeon, pediatrician, pediatric neurologist/orthopedician, physiotherapist, and social worker. Surgery should be done early, after evaluation of associated deficits. Emergency surgery is required if CSF leak is present (to avoid meningitis). Management of neurogenic bladder includes Crede's method of emptying bladder, clean intermittent catheterization, vesicostomy, and frequent urine cultures to detect and treat urinary tract infections. Bowel management includes daily evacuant enema. Correction of DDH and CTEV by orthopedic surgeon is required. Long-term multidisciplinary care includes monitoring neurological status, appropriate physiotherapy, and rehabilitation.[4]

SPINA BIFIDA OCCULTA

This common anomaly consists of a midline defect of the vertebral bodies without protrusion of spinal cord or meninges. Most individuals are asymptomatic and lack neurologic signs. In some cases, patches of hair, a lipoma, discoloration of the skin, or a dermal sinus in the midline of the low back signifies an underlying malformation of the spinal cord. A spine X-ray shows a defect in closure of the posterior vertebral arches and laminae, typically involving L5 and S1. Spinal bifida is occasionally associated with more significant developmental abnormalities of the spinal cord, including syringomyelia, diastematomyelia, and a tethered cord.

A dermoid sinus usually forms a small skin opening, which leads into a narrow duct, sometimes indicated by protruding hairs, a hairy patch, or a vascular nevus. Dermoid sinuses occur in the midline at the site of occurrence of meningocele or encephalocele (the lumbosacral region or occiput). Dermoid sinus tracts may pass through the dura, acting as a conduit for the spread of infection. This can cause recurrent meningitis.

SYRINX

Syringomyelia and syringobulbia are fluid-filled cavities in the spinal cord and brainstem, respectively. Various predisposing factors include craniocervical junction anomalies, spinal trauma, and spinal tumors. Fifty percentage of patients will have congenital abnormalities such as Chiari malformation, encephalocele, or myelomeningocele. These congenital abnormalities often expand during teenage group probably due rapid increase in the growth.

Symptoms and Signs

Syringomyelia is characterized by features of central cord syndrome **(Table 8.17.2)**. Early symptoms are pain and temperature sensory deficits, however, difficult recognize. Initially, they can present painless burn or cut. Later they develop weakness, atrophy, and fasciculations. Cape-like distribution of in the form deficit in pain and temperature sensation with café-like distribution. over the shoulders, with preserved light touch and position and vibration.

Diagnosis

An MRI of the entire spinal cord and brain shows gadolinium enhancement is useful for diagnosis and to assess associated anomalies.

Treatment

Correction of underlying abnormalities to considered. After compression of spinal cord, surgery will not reverse neurological function but prevents further worsening.

Prevention of Neural Tube Defects

Primary prevention by folate supplementation (0.4 mg/day) to all prospective mothers. Food fortification is another possible approach as food provides only half the requirement. Secondary prevention is by periconceptional folate (higher dose) 5 mg/day. It should be taken 1–2 months before and continued till 3 months after conception. Folate supplementation reduces recurrence risk by 70% and first occurrence by 50%.[4]

CRANIOCERVICAL JUNCTION ABNORMALITIES

Abnormalities of the occipital bone, foramen magnum, or first 2 cervical vertebrae due to acquired or congenital that decreased the space for the cervical spinal cord or lower brainstem are called craniocervical junction anomalies.

The unique embryological development of this region can give rise to a wide spectrum of anatomic and pathological disorders. These disorders may range from trivial, asymptomatic problems to conditions with the potential to cause devastating neurological problems, paralysis, or even death. Disorders affecting this craniovertebral junction can be reflected in the anatomic structures in the region, including the brain stem, cerebellum, cranial nerves, spinal cord, and vertebrae. **Box 8.17.3** shows craniocervical abnormalities and their clinical consequences.[5]

Etiology

Both congenital and acquired lesions can cause craniocervical junction abnormalities. Various causes are mentioned in **Box 8.17.4**. The bone that replaces all or a part of the odontoid process is called os odontoideum. Congenital fusion of the atlas and occipital bone is called atlas assimilation. Atlanto-occipital anomalies are often seen in Klippel–Feil malformation. Platybasia sometimes seen in Chiari malformation.

Achondroplasia sometimes causes the foramen magnum to narrow or fuse with the atlas and thus may compress the spinal cord or brain stem. Down syndrome, Morquio syndrome, or osteogenesis imperfecta can cause atlantoaxial subluxation or dislocation. Individuals with Down syndrome have a much higher incidence of instability at C1/C2, and at the atlanto-occipital (O-C1) junction. It is recommended that these patients should undergo routine flexion-extension X-rays to identify any significant instability, with treatment provided when indicated in order to prevent progressive deformity or neurological impairment. These problems are usually diagnosed from 6 to 12 years of age.

BOX 8.17.3: Craniocervical abnormalities and their clinical consequences.

- *Fusion of the atlas (C1) and occipital bone:* Spinal cord compression if the anteroposterior diameter of the foramen magnum behind the odontoid process is <19 mm
- *Basilar invagination (upward bulging of the occipital condyles):* A short neck and compression that can affect the cerebellum, brain stem, lower cranial nerves, and spinal cord
- *Atlantoaxial subluxation or dislocation (displacement of the atlas anteriorly in relation to the axis):* Acute or chronic spinal cord compression
- *Klippel-Feil malformation (fusion of cervical vertebrae):* Deformity and limited motion of the neck but usually no neurologic consequences
- *Platybasia* (flattening of the skull base so that the angle formed by the intersection of the clival and anterior fossa planes is >135°), seen on lateral skull imaging: No symptoms or cerebellar or spinal cord deficits or normal-pressure hydrocephalus

The common injuries caused by vehicle or bicycle accidents, fall, and driving involve bone, ligaments or both can be fatal and causes long term sequalae.

The pattern of spinal injury in children differs from that of adults. They often have isolated ligamentous injury. Atlantoaxial dislocation or subluxation, basilar invagination, or platybasia can be due to rheumatoid arthritis and Paget disease of the cervical spine. The brain stem or spinal cord compression can be seen in slowly growing craniocervical junction tumors.[5]

Symptoms and Signs

Clinical features can develop after a minor neck injury of spontaneously and vary in progression based on severity. Presentation depends on level and severity of compression. Common features are neck pain and compressive myelopathy. Compression of C2 root and the greater occipital nerve causes local pain radiating to the arms, and headache. Short neck, webbing of neck, torticollis, decreased neck movements can be seen in platybasia, basilar invagination, and Klippel–Feil malformation. Upward compression can cause brain stem, cranial nerve, and cerebellar deficits. Variation in head position can trigger vertebrobasilar ischemia.

Diagnosis

A craniocervical abnormality is suspected when patients have pain in the neck or occiput plus neurologic deficits referable to the lower brain stem, upper cervical spinal cord,

BOX 8.17.4: Etiology of craniocervical junction abnormalities.

Congenital
- Structural abnormalities
  - Os odontoideum
  - Atlas assimilation
  - Congenital Klippel–Feil malformation (e.g., with Turner or Noonan syndrome)
  - Atlas hypoplasia
  - Chiari malformations, sometimes associated with platybasia
- General or systemic disorders that affect skeletal growth and development
  - Achondroplasia
  - Down syndrome
  - Morquio syndrome
  - Osteogenesis imperfecta

Acquired: Acquired causes include injuries and disorders
- Spontaneous—C1/2, atlanto-axial rotatory subluxation
  - Traumatic ligamentous injury—atlanto-occipital dislocation (AOD), C1/2 (atlantoaxial) instability
  - Fracture—occipital condyles, C1 (burst), and C2 odontoid, hangman's
  - Infection—osteomyelitis, empyema
  - Ligamentous laxity
  - Rheumatoid arthritis
  - Paget disease of the cervical spine
  - Slowly growing craniocervical junction tumors

or cerebellum. The lower cervical spine disorders can usually be distinguished clinically and by neuroimaging.

Neuroimaging

The CT has the advantage of identification of bone structures more accurately than MRI and can be on emergency basis. Sagittal MRI of MRI brain detects associated hindbrain, cerebellar, spinal cord, and vascular anomalies, syringomyelia. Plain X-rays of both lateral and anteroposterior view identify vertebral fractures. If MRI and CT are unavailable or inclusive CT myelography can be considered. Magnetic resonance angiography (MRA) or vertebral angiography to be done if any suspicion of vascular injures.

If MRI and CT are unavailable, plain X-rays with a lateral view of the skull showing the cervical spine, an anteroposterior view, and oblique views of the cervical spine are taken. If MRI is unavailable or inconclusive and CT is inconclusive, CT myelography is done. If MRI or CT suggests vascular abnormalities, MRA or vertebral angiography is done.

Treatment

If neural structures are compressed, treatment consists of reduction (traction or changes in head position to realign the craniocervical junction and thus relieve neural compression). After reduction, the head and neck are immobilized. Acute or suddenly progressive spinal cord compression requires emergency reduction. Several different methods of instrumentation (e.g., plates or rods with screws) can be used for temporary stabilization until bones fuse and stability is permanent. In general, all unstable areas must be fused.

INFECTIONS AND INFLAMMATORY DISORDERS

SPINAL EPIDURAL ABSCESS

A spinal epidural abscess is an accumulation of pus in the epidural space that can mechanically compress the spinal cord. They usually occur in the thoracic or lumbar regions. An underlying infection is often present; it may be remote (e.g., endocarditis, furuncle, or dental abscess) or contiguous (e.g., vertebral osteomyelitis, pressure ulcer, or retroperitoneal abscess). In about one-third of cases, the cause cannot be determined. The most common causative organism is *Staphylococcus aureus*, followed by *Escherichia coli* and mixed anaerobes. Occasionally, the cause is a tuberculous abscess of the thoracic spine (Pott disease). Rarely, a similar abscess occurs in the subdural space.

Symptoms and Signs

Symptoms begin with local or radicular back pain and percussion tenderness, which become severe; pain may be worsened by recumbency. Fever is common. Spinal cord compression may develop. Deficits progress over hours to days.

Diagnosis

Because rapid treatment is necessary to prevent or minimize neurologic deficits, clinicians should consider this diagnosis if patients have significant atraumatic back pain, particularly when there is focal percussion tenderness over the spine, or if they have a fever or have had a recent infection or dental procedure. Diagnosis is by MRI; CT may be used if MRI is not available. Samples from blood and infected areas are cultured. Lumbar puncture is contraindicated because it may trigger cord herniation if the abscess completely obstructs CSF flow. Plain X-rays are not routinely indicated but show osteomyelitis in about one-third of patients. erythrocyte sedimentation rate (ESR) is elevated, but this finding is nonspecific.

Treatment

Abscesses causing neurological compromise should be surgically drained immediately. Other abscesses require antibiotics with or without needle aspiration. Antibiotics that cover *Staphylococcus* and anaerobes are given as for brain abscess. An aminoglycoside is added to cover gram-negative bacteria if abscess develops after neurosurgical procedures.

TUBERCULOUS SPINAL OSTEITIS

It is still common in India and other developing countries. Infection usually starts in the vertebral body and spreads to adjacent bodies, leading to collapse and angular deformity of the spine. Spinal cord compression is usually due to extradural TB abscess or TB meningomyelitis rather than vertebral infections. Another mechanism of injury is interference with the vascular supply of subjacent segments, either by compression of radicular arteries or by endarteritis, which causes paraplegia. Most of the patients recover with antitubercular chemotherapy, rarely require surgical intervention. **Figure 8.17.5** shows tuberculosis of the spine.

Syphilitic spinal osteitis is now a very rare cause of spinal compression and produces effects like those of tuberculous caries.

VIRAL MYELITIS

In the last century, viral myelitis is caused by poliomyelitis virus and now other nonpolio enteroviruses such as, coxsackie viruses, herpes zoster, herpes simplex, human immunodeficiency virus (HIV), Epstein-Barr virus, cytomegalovirus (CMV), and HTLV-1. Usually, these viruses commonly cause postinfectious transverse myelitis.

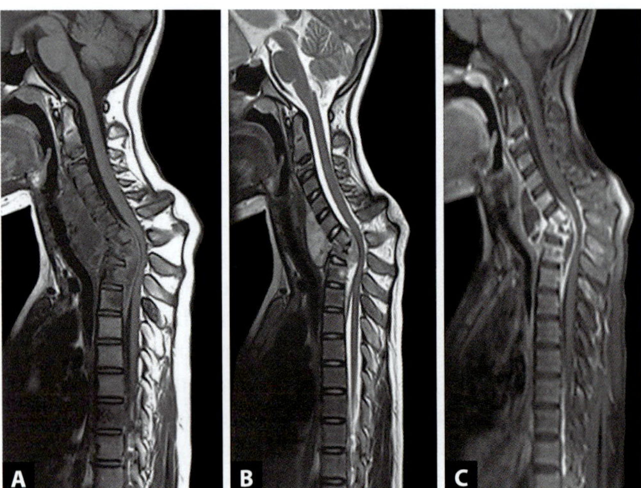

Figs. 8.17.5A to C: Tuberculosis of the spine. (A) T1 sagittal; (B) T2 sagittal; (C) Postcontrast T1. There is anterior wedge collapse with destruction of the C7 and D1 vertebrae and the intervertebral disk, causing a kyphotic deformity. A large heterogeneous mass is seen in the adjacent anterior epidural space (C7–D4 levels) and the pre- and paravertebral regions (C4–D2 levels). The epidural lesion severely compromises the spinal canal. The lesion is hyperintense on the T2-weighted image and hypointense on the T1-weighted image with evidence of diffusion restriction and peripheral enhancement.

In poliomyelitis usually anterior horn cells are involved presenting with patchy, multifocal, or sometimes extensive muscle weakness and wasting without sensory involvement. After polio eradications polio such as disorders are usually caused by coxsackie and other entero-viruses. Varicella zoster initially presents with dermatomal vesicular rash followed by sensory dermatomal deficit, marked pain, due to predominant involvement of the dorsal root ganglion. Transverse myelitis due to viral infections is likely to occur in immunocompromised states, and difficult to differentiate from demyelinating spinal cord lesions. The confirmation of diagnosis is made by including those with HIV infection. The diagnosis is confirmed by the isolation of viral in the CSF by polymerase chain reaction (PCR).

AIDS VACUOLAR MYELOPATHY

The tempo is subacute with symptoms typically evolving over several weeks. Motor, sensory, and sphincter abnormalities all appear, sometimes asymmetrical and predominantly in the legs, although the arms may also be involved. It can be delayed or prevented using effective antiretroviral therapies.

SPINAL CORD ARTERIOVENOUS MALFORMATIONS

An arteriovenous malformation (AVM) of the spinal cord consists of a collection of tortuous dilated veins. The most common malformations are extramedullary in the thoracolumbar, posterior side, and rest are intramedullary situated in the cervical or upper thoracic region. The malformation may cause neurologic symptoms by its mass effect on the cord or by the steal phenomenon, by which blood is shunted through the abnormal veins, bypassing the spinal cord, which produces transient and, in some cases, progressive loss of neurologic function. Patients occasionally present with acute paraparesis and a sensory deficit due to a subarachnoid bleed from the malformation. More commonly, gradual onset of gait abnormalities, low back pain, and bowel and bladder dysfunction are noted. In approximately one-third of cases cutaneous angioma overlies the AVMs and spinal bruit may occasionally be auscultated.

Diagnosis

X-ray of the spine may show erosion of the pedicles. MRI and MRA are the most useful tests to detect. Contrast myelography and selective spinal angiography are required to delineate the blood supply and the extent of the malformations.

Treatment

If cord function is compromised surgical intervention should be considered. In case of AVM is small and located in surgically inaccessible locations, stereotactic radio surgery may require. Embolization of artery occludes feeder arteries before surgical intervention.

SPINAL CORD INFARCTION

Spinal cord infarction usually results from ischemia originating in an extravertebral artery. Symptoms include sudden and severe back pain, followed immediately by rapidly progressive bilateral flaccid limb weakness and loss of sensation, particularly for pain and temperature. The diagnosis is by MRI. Treatment is generally supportive. Anterior spinal artery has one large feeder artery, that artery of Adamkiewicz in the lower thoracic region and only few feeder arteries in the cervical region. Spinal cord ischemia is common between the 2nd and 4th thoracic segments because of less collateral in the anterior spinal artery. Extravertebral feeder artery or aorta injury due to dissection or clamping during surgery or thrombosis causes infarctions.

Symptoms and Signs

Sudden pain in the back with tightness radiating circumferentially is followed within minutes by segmental bilateral flaccid weakness and sensory loss.

Sudden bilateral flaccid weakness and sensory loss with back pain and tightness radiating circumferentially is the most common presentation. Temperature and pain sensations are disproportionately impaired. The anterior cord syndrome is caused due to anterior spinal artery infarction **(Table 8.17.2)**. It can mimic central cord syndrome if the infarct is small and affects primarily tissue farthest away from an occluded artery. It may recover completely.

Diagnosis

An MRI of the brain and MRA is helpful in the diagnosis of infarction and excludes close differential diagnosis such as acute transverse myelitis, spinal cord compression, and demyelinating disorders. CSF analysis is also helpful to exclude infectious causes.

Treatment

Supportive care with sometimes specific treatment for the underlying etiologies such as aortic dissection and polyarteritis nodosa.

SPINAL CORD INJURY

Half of the spine injuries in children 0–3 year-old occur at the C1 to C2 level, whereas only 8% affect this level in children aged 4–12 years. The probable reason is higher fulcrum of motion in younger children and weakness of C2 due to incomplete ossification of its synchondrosis.[6-8]

The various causes of SCIs are moto vehicle accidents, including belt injuries to the lumber spine, falls, recreational, or sports activities, especially driving accidents and football injuries and penetrating injuries such as gunshot or knife. Since the 1980s, violence has increased from 10 to 30% as a cause of SCI in patients ages 16–20 years. Even though traumatic birth injury decreased it accounts for only 10–15% of all cases.[8]

The various factors that determine the severity of injury after spinal cord trauma are shown in **Box 8.17.5**. SCIs cause more mortality in children compared to adults. **Box 8.17.6** shows predisposing factors for the upper cervical spine injury. The various predisposing factors for cervical SCI in children are shown in **Box 8.17.7**.

Pathogenesis: Mechanisms of Spinal Cord Injury

The five mechanisms of SCI following trauma are—(1) forward flexion, (2) lateral flexion, (3) rotation, (4) axial compression, and (5) hyperextension. The forces generated by these movements can result in vertebral distraction, dislocation, fracture, and disk herniation. The most common cause of SCI is fracture or displacement. SCI without radiographic abnormality (SCIWORA) is common in children due to ligamentous injury. Forward flexion can lead to wedge or teardrop fractures, which usually begin at or near the intervertebral disk. These fractures are often encountered in motor vehicle accidents in passengers not wearing seat belts, but also can be seen in children wearing ill-fitting adult types of lap-sash belts (cervical seat-belt syndrome).

Clinical Assessment

History of the activity of the child at that time, and the use of restraining devices, such as seat belts, car seats, head rests, and air bags, is helpful in assessing type and mechanism of injury. Examination findings of genetic disorders (e.g., Down syndrome), congenital abnormalities of the bony spine (e.g., hemivertebrae), or blood dyscrasias (e.g., hemophilia) that may predispose a child more vulnerable to SCI. Even minor trauma predisposes to injuries. Type breathing and vitals should be examined. The entire spine should be examined with great care to prevent further SCIs.

Spinal cord injury should be suspected in cases of breech or difficult delivery, trauma, child abuse, and sports injuries, such as football, gymnastics, and ice hockey. Patients can present with any combination of the following symptoms and signs—neck or back pain, weakness, sensory loss, decrease in deep tendon reflexes, loss of bladder or bowel control, autonomic dysfunction, and meningismus.[6,7]

BOX 8.17.5: Determinants of the severity of injury after spinal cord trauma.

- Nature, direction, and degree of the traumatic insult
- Site of injury
- Presence of any preexisting spine anomaly
- Extent of tissue damage
- Degree of vascular compromise complicating the spinal trauma
- Rapidity and efficacy of treatment

BOX 8.17.6: Factors predisposing the upper cervical spine injury in the young child.

- A proportionally larger and heavier head
- Relative under development of the neck muscles and ligaments
- Incomplete ossification of the vertebral bodies with relative anterior wedging
- Incomplete development of the uncinate processes
- Smaller vertebral bodies of C1 to C2 compared with C3 to C5
- More horizontal orientation of the articular surfaces of the cervical facet joints

BOX 8.17.7: Conditions predisposing to cervical spinal cord injury in the children.

- Down syndrome (15% have atlantoaxial instability)
- Klippel–Feil syndrome
- Morquio syndrome
- Larsen's' syndrome
- Achondroplasia
- Previous spine surgery

Laboratory Studies

Approximately, 50% of children with severe SCIs show no abnormality on the spine X-ray, where CT or MRI of spine are useful. CT is useful in detecting subtle spinal fractures and clarifying findings on plain films. MRI of the spine has replaced CT and myelography as the preferred means of imaging the injured spinal cord.

Management

Medical management includes measures aimed at treating acute cord injury and more long-term management. It must include stabilization of spine to prevent further injury, in addition to maintenance of vital signs. Injection of methylprednisolone, bolus of 30 mg/kg, given intravenously after an acute SCI and followed by methylprednisolone infusion at 5.4 mg/kg/h for the next 23 hours can be considered. The role of steroids as neuroprotective agents in acute SCI remains controversial. Although the NASCIS 2 and 3 studies show some improvement in neurological function from high-dose methylprednisolone, the benefit seems to be modest at best, and against, this one needs to weigh the risk of potentially serious complications of high-dose steroid therapy.

SPINAL CORD TUMORS

Spinal cord neoplasms are less common compared to the brain. The ratio of brain to intraspinal neoplasms in adults is 5:1, whereas for children, the ratio varies from 20:1 to 5:1. The tumors commonly seen in the following frequency, thoracic spinal cord followed by cervical, thoracolumbar, and lumbosacral areas probably related to number of number of segments in the areas.

Clinical Characteristics

Usually, presents with insidious onset of vague symptoms. Changing pattern of continence, crying while micturition and straining at stools can be present. Pain is a common symptom, but further location is difficult because of poor description by children. Weakness and sensory abnormalities like Brown–Sequard syndrome are rarely encountered. Pain can be accentuated by either Valsalva's maneuvers, or by straight leg raising. Mild scoliosis, discrepancy in foot or leg length, or vasomotor changes in the lower extremities, hyperreflexia, clonus, Babinski's response, proprioceptive, vibratory loss, or a sensory level can be seen.

Diagnostic Studies

An X-ray of spine may show an increase in the interpedicular distance suggestive of long-standing intramedullary lesion. Distortion or widening of the neuroforamina is seen in extramedullary tumors such as neurofibromas. MRI is useful to differentiate intramedullary masses from the extramedullary lesions. Protein content is invariably elevated. Froin syndrome, clotting of CSF after its removal, is attributed to marked elevation of cerebrospinal protein.

Types of Tumors

Extramedullary Tumors

Spinal cord tumors can be divided into extramedullary and intramedullary locations as shown in the **Table 8.17.4**. Dumbbell lesions are rarely encountered with features of both inside and outside the foramina such as neurofibromas. Reticulum cell sarcomas, lymphomas, neuroblastomas, and other sarcomatous lesions usually occur epidurally and are present as compressive lesions. Meningiomas are rare in children, except in cases of neurofibromatosis-2 (NF-2).

Dysembryoplastic lesions are commonly seen in children. In dermoid tumors, we can see teeth, bones, or calcification on X-ray film. This can be associated with sinus tract, spina bifida, sacral dimple, port-wine nevus, and excessive clumps of coarse hair. With or without surgery, patients relatively stable.

Intramedullary Tumors

Intramedullary tumors constitute 35% of pediatric intraspinal tumors. Most intramedullary tumors in children are either astrocytomas or ependymomas. The mean duration of symptoms may vary from 1 day to 4 years. Astrocytomas can involve single or multiple segments of the cord. Surgical resection is the treatment of choice, in the presence of dissemination radiotherapy should be given.

High-grade astrocytoma has a poor prognosis with median survival of 12 months. Ependymomas are less common than astrocytoma and treated with laminectomy with decompression and total resection. Radiation is useful in case of incomplete removal of tumor. Prognosis in

TABLE 8.17.4: Tumors of the spinal cord.

Intramedullary	*Extramedullary*
• *Astrocytomas*: – Cystic – Noncystic • *Ependymomas*: – Myxopapillary – Well-differentiated • Oligodendrogliomas	• Neurofibromas • *Dysembryoplastic*: – Dermoids – Epidermoids – Teratomas – Lipomas • Meningiomas • Arachnoid cysts • *Metastatic*: – Neuroblastoma – Sarcoma – Lymphoma

ependymomas is better than astrocytoma with 5-year survival rates of 72–100%.

Management

Surgery

Surgical decompression should be considered in all cases; however, surgery will not correct irreversible damage already happened.

Adjuvant Management

Radiation should be considered in all spinal cord tumors if tumor is not able resect completely.

Chemotherapy

Chemotherapy can be considered in cases of low-grade astrocytoma's; commonly used drugs are combinations of carboplatin and vincristine.

Complications

These include radiation myelopathy, arachnoiditis, kyphoscoliosis, and limited growth of the vertebral column. Loss of sensation can cause nonhealing ulcers, fractures, and hip dislocations.

In conclusion, the prognosis for patients with spinal cord tumors is better than brain tumors. Surgical resection is the treatment of choice, in whom tumor not able resect completely radiotherapy can be considered. Long-term morbidity is high despite the above treatment.

NUTRITIONAL, METABOLIC AND OTHER DISORDERS

SUBACUTE COMBINED DEGENERATION OF THE CORD

Vitamin B_{12} deficiency produces a characteristic subacute myelopathic syndrome, although rare, it is very important to diagnose and treat promptly in order to minimize the extent of permanent neurological deficit. The clinical picture is usually due to combined features of posterior column, corticospinal tract, and peripheral nerve degeneration, but involvement of the optic nerves and brain is not uncommon. Vitamin B_{12} must be given intramuscularly, followed by oral treatment.

RADIATION MYELOPATHY

Delayed myelopathy can occur following radiation to neck or chest, where spinal cord was included in the radiation field. Three types of spinal cord syndrome have been described because of radiation. The first is a transient and benign disorder manifesting limb paresthesia and a positive Lhermitte's sign, usually appearing 2–6 months after radiotherapy. The second, most common and most serious problem is that of a steadily progressive myelopathy, which appears after a somewhat longer interval from the time of radiotherapy; the most common latent period is between 12 and 15 months, but it may range from 6 months to 5 years or even longer. The third postradiation syndrome is rare and presents as a segmental lower motor neuron disorder (with weakness, wasting, and reflex loss), suggesting that there has been damaged to anterior horn cells in the irradiated part of the cord. In patients with progressive radiation myelopathy, corticosteroids or anticoagulation has been employed although there is no proof of efficacy, some patients appeared to stabilize on steroids and trial of this therapy would seem reasonable.

COPPER DEFICIENCY

The neurological manifestations of acquired copper deficiency in humans have been recognized, the most common being a myelopathy presenting with a spastic gait and prominent sensory ataxia. The clinical features and neuroimaging findings are like the subacute combined degeneration seen in patients with vitamin B_{12} deficiency. Copper and vitamin B_{12} deficiency may coexist. The neurological syndrome may be present without the hematologic manifestations. Copper supplementation resolves anemia and neutropenia promptly and completely and may prevent the neurological deterioration. Improvement, when it occurs, is often subjective and preferentially involves sensory symptoms.

KEY POINTS

- Neural tube defects account for most of the congenital anomalies of the CNS.
- Trivial injury can cause spinal injury in Down syndrome and Morquio syndrome.
- Permanent severe neurologic disability can be avoided or minimized if evaluation and treatment are rapid.
- MRI is a sensitive test to detect spinal cord disorders.
- Spinal dermoid can cause recurrent meningitis.
- Tuberculosis of spine requires antituberculosis chemotherapy rarely requires surgery.
- In SCI without radiographic abnormality (SCIWORA), X-ray spine will be normal.
- Copper deficiency can cause myelopathy like vitamin B_{12} deficiency.
- Growth and development of the spine should be considered when planning for spinal surgical treatment.
- Neural tube defects can be prevented with simple periconceptional folic acid supplementation.

CONCLUSION

Neural tube defects are still common and one of the most common malformations. Spinal dermoid can cause recurrent meningitis. Tuberculosis of the spine still commonly exists, however, conservative treatment using antitubercular therapy can achieve good outcomes. Spinal cord injury without radiographic abnormality (SCIWORA) is a ligamentous injury causing SCI without bone disruption and is common in children. Magnetic resonance imaging is the imaging of choice for spinal cord disorders. The surgical treatment of spinal disorders in children must consider the expected growth and development of the spine. Rapid evacuation and treatment prevent permanent severe neurologic disability in spinal cord injuries.

REFERENCES

1. Rekate HL. Spinal Cord Disorders. In: Kliegman RM, Stanton BF, St. Geme III JW, Schor NF, Behrman RE (Eds). Nelson Textbook of Pediatrics, 19th edition. Philadelphia;, Elsevier; 2011. pp. 2101-8.
2. Kalra V. Practical Pediatric Neurology, 2nd edition. New Delhi: Arya Publications; 2008.
3. Brazis PW. Localization in clinical neurology, 6th edition, Philadelphia: Wolters Kluwer Lippincott Williams and Wilkins; 2011.
4. Copp AJ, Stanier P, Greene ND. Neural tube defects: recent advances, unsolved questions, and controversies. Lancet Neurol. 2013:12(8):799-810.
5. Menezes AH. Cranivertebral junction database analysis: incidence, classification, presentation, and treatment algorithms. Childs Nerv Syst. 2008:24(10):1101-8.
6. Rosman NP, Harini C. Spinal cord Injury. In: Swaiman KF, Ashwal S, Ferriero DM, Schor NF (Eds.) Pediatric Neurology Principles and Practice, 5th edition. Philadelphia: Elsevier; 2011. pp. 1198-220.
7. Garton HJ, Hammer MR. Detection of pediatric cervical spine injury. Neurosurgery. 2008;62(3):700-8.
8. Polk-Williams A, Carr BG, Blinman TA, Masaikos PT, Wiebe DJ, Nance ML. Cervical spine injury in young children: A National Trauma Data Bank review. *J Pediatr Surg. 2008;*43(9):1718-21.

8.18 Floppy Infant: Clinical Approach

Mahesh Kamate

INTRODUCTION

The term "floppy infant" refers to an infant who has hypotonia and/or weakness and presents as floppiness while handling the child. It poses an important diagnostic challenge, as it is a sign of both benign and serious conditions. The maintenance of normal tone requires an intact nervous system (central and peripheral) and the connective tissues. Hence, hypotonia is a common symptom of neurological dysfunction and occurs in diseases of the brain, spinal cord, nerves, and muscles, and also in some connective tissue disorders.

The differential diagnosis for this presentation is exhaustive and includes many rare disorders. In the last few decades, there have been overwhelming advances in the diagnosis and management of the various causes of a "floppy infant." Many conditions like spinal muscular atrophy (SMA) now have specific treatment such as gene therapy, and many novel treatments are in pipeline for other neuromuscular conditions that may present as a "floppy infant." This underlines the need for an early accurate diagnosis, so that appropriate therapy can be initiated for better final outcomes.

Recent advances in the field of neuromuscular disorders and neonatal neurology have completely changed both the diagnostic pathway and the level of intervention possible, especially with the advent of genetic testing and gene therapies. Despite the tremendous advances in imaging and in genetic diagnostic tools such as next-generation sequencing (NGS) or whole-exome sequencing (WES), there is still a need to perform a detailed clinical assessment for targeting and for the interpretation of the genetic findings.[1]

DEFINITIONS AND TERMINOLOGIES

Tone

Tone is the resistance of muscle to passive stretch. Clinicians test two kinds of tone—phasic and postural. While phasic tone is the rapid contraction in response to a high-intensity stretch, as in tendon reflex response, postural tone is the prolonged contraction of antigravity muscles in response to the low-intensity stretch of gravity. When postural tone is depressed, the trunk and limbs cannot maintain themselves against gravity, and the infant appears floppy. Muscle tone is most easily shown as movement of an extremity, but certainly includes trunk, neck, back, shoulder, and pelvic girdle.

Phasic tone is assessed by the passive resistance to movement of the limbs (appendicular structures), whereas postural tone is tested by the resistance to passive movement of the axial muscles (e.g., neck, back, and trunk). There may be a discrepancy between phasic tone and postural tone in a given patient. This is commonly appreciated in the 3- or 4-month-old infant who has had a hypoxic-ischemic insult at birth and now has poor head and trunk control (postural hypotonia) but is beginning to become stiff (hypertonic) in the extremities (phasic tone) and will eventually develop increased reflexes and tone (spasticity) in the appendicular and axial muscles.

The maintenance of normal tone needs intact central and peripheral nervous systems. While "hypotonia" is defined as reduced resistance to passive range of motion in joints, weakness is the reduction in the maximum power that can be generated by the muscle. While both can present a floppy infant, it is important to differentiate the two and also be aware that both can coexist in a given case.

Weakness is the reduction in power, which is the maximum strength that is generated by muscle contraction. While evaluating a child with floppiness, it is important to ascertain whether the patient is "hypotonic" or "hypotonic and weak" together. When a child presents later (beyond neonatal period), the pediatrician must ascertain whether the delay, when present, is just a motor delay or a combination of motor and cognitive delay. The following terms are important in the approach to diagnosis:[2]

- *Motor unit:* One anterior horn cell and all the muscle fibers that it innervates make up a motor unit. The motor unit is the unit of force. Therefore, weakness is a symptom of all motor unit disorders.
- *Neuronopathy:* A primary disorder of the anterior horn cell body
- *Neuropathy:* A primary disorder of the axon and its myelin covering
- *Myopathy:* A primary disorder of the muscle fiber

EVALUATION OF A FLOPPY INFANT[3,4]

History Taking

Weakness[2,4,5]

- *Timing of onset of complaints*: When was the floppiness first appreciated? Was it intrauterine (in the form of decreased fetal movements or polyhydramnios), at the time of birth, a few hours or days after birth, or after a few weeks to months after birth?
- *Presentation*: Acute (developing over few hours) versus subacute or chronic (floppiness developing over few days to weeks/months)
- *Distribution of weakness*:
  - Symmetrical versus asymmetrical
  - Upper limb versus lower limb
  - Proximal versus distal
  - Cry and sucking/swallowing (weak cry suggests bulbar and respiratory muscles involvement, while swallowing and sucking difficulty suggests an involvement of the facial and bulbar muscles)
  - Ptosis and extraocular muscle movements
- *Respiration:* The involvement of respiratory muscles, as both the intercostal and diaphragmatic weakness are frequent in several neuromuscular disorders with neonatal onset and can help in the differential diagnosis
  - Sphincters (bowel/bladder)
  - Deformities of limbs/contractures
- *Fatiguability and diurnal variation* in the severity of weakness suggest a neuromuscular junction disorder.
- *Severity of weakness* (just flicker of movements/antigravity movements or vigorous movements)
- *Presence of other neurological symptoms* that suggest central nervous system (CNS) involvement, such as seizures, abnormal movements, irritability, and effect on nonmotor domains of development
- *Choking episodes*—bulbar and pharyngeal muscles
- *Differentiation of bulbar versus pseudobulbar weakness*

Other Relevant History

- Any significant *family history*—affected parents or siblings, consanguinity, stillbirths, childhood deaths
- *Maternal disease*—myotonic dystrophy
- *Pregnancy and delivery history*—drug or teratogen exposure, decreased fetal movements, abnormal presentation, polyhydramnios or oligohydramnios, Apgar score, resuscitation requirements, and cord blood gases
- *Postnatal history*: Respiratory effort, ability to feed, level of alertness, level of spontaneous activity, and character of cry
- *Detailed developmental history*: Check all the domains of development and see if there is isolated motor delay and/or delay in other domains also along with motor delay (psychomotor delay)

Physical Examination

General and Systemic Physical Examination[2,4]

Detailed general physical examination, including eyes and systemic examination, should be done to look for abnormalities and clues. Look for lethargy and dysmorphism, and measure head circumference. Examine the skin and joints for hyperextensible joints and soft velvety skin, which could suggest a possibility of hypermobility syndrome due to a connective tissue disorder or can be an accompanying feature in a few congenital muscular dystrophies.

- *Resting position*: Limb position and spontaneous limb movements. The presence of antigravity movements indicates mostly a central cause of hypotonia or a milder disease.
- *Respiration*: Shape of chest, work of breathing, and pattern of breathing (thoracoabdominal, abdominothoracic, and seesaw or paradoxical)
- *Seizures and contractures*
- *Face*: Facial expression, secretions, and eyes (cataracts in Lowe syndrome, ptosis, and extraocular movements in myasthenic syndromes and myopathies). Look for myopathic facies with an open mouth, reduced facial expressions, and inverted "V" shaped upper lips. Facial weakness is invariably found in myotonic dystrophy and in several congenital myopathies or muscular dystrophies while it is never observed in SMA.
- *Cry*: High-pitched or unusual-sounding cry suggests CNS pathology; a weak cry suggests diaphragmatic weakness; and a fatigable cry indicates congenital myasthenic syndrome

Tone in all four Limbs and Central Tone (Head Lag, Ventral Suspension)

Palpate the muscles for flabbiness and look for the passive range of movements. In infants and children <2–3 years, different angles and signs are used to demonstrate hypotonia.

- *Adductor angle*: Angle between the thighs when the hips are maximally abducted at the hips with extension at the knees
- *Popliteal angle*: Hips flexed onto the abdomen by holding at the knees
- *Dorsiflexion angle of the foot*: By gentle pressure on the sole
- *Heel to ear maneuver*: Both extended legs lifted toward the ear without lifting the pelvis
- *Scarf sign*: Flexed at the elbow and pulled across the chest by holding at the wrist and hands

Weakness and Contractures

Weakness is assessed by looking for good antigravity movements of the upper and lower limbs, both proximally and distally. Even though born preterm, many babies have antigravity movements of the limbs. Absence of antigravity movements indicates significant muscle weakness. If no spontaneous movement is observed when the infant is awake and calm, it is important also to assess the presence of movements at peak of activity, such as when crying or stimulated.

Neonatal contractures are often the result of reduced motility in utero. It is important to assess the possibility of contractures, especially at the ankle, knee, hip, shoulder, and elbow levels, which can only be fully observed by performing an assessment of each joint, checking whether there is a full range of extension.

Reflexes

Look for primitive reflexes such as sucking, Moro, plantar grasp, palmar grasp, and deep tendon jerks such as biceps, knee, and ankle reflexes, as well as the presence of clonus. Deep tendon reflexes are more difficult to be elicited in term babies as opposed to preterm infants in whom tendon reflexes can even be exaggerated. Thus, not easily elicitable reflexes, when occurring in isolation, are not necessarily a negative prognostic sign in infants who do not have additional risk factors.

Eyes

Pupil size and reaction are important in infantile botulism.

Examination of the Child in Different Positions

- *180° flip examination*: Examination of the child in different positions, carefully observing the movements and postures, and developmental milestones such as social smile and tracking objects in supine position
- *Supine position*: Developmental milestones and pithed-frog posture
- *Pull-to-sit traction response*: The "pull-to-sit" maneuver is performed by holding the supine infant's hands and slowly pulling them to a sitting position. While head lag is normal in the neonatal period, by about 2 months of age, this should be minimal if still present at all. Premature infants will have lower tone than term infants, and term infants will have lower tone than post-term infants normally. This response tests both the axial tone (neck and back) and the appendicular tone (shoulder and arms) and also tests strength to some extent because the normal response from the infant being tested is to resist the pull on the arms and shoulder. Look for a straight or rounded back
- *Vertical suspension and weight-bearing*: Look for Forster's sign, slippage, and flexion of the hips and knees
- *Ventral suspension*: Jug handle or inverted U position, Landau and parachute reflex (based on age)
- *Prone position* with hands by the side: Head/chest off the couch, flexion of the knees

STEPWISE APPROACH TO FLOPPY INFANT[2,4,5]

Step 1

- Differentiate neurological from non-neurological (due to lax joints and ligaments from connective tissue disorders such as Ehlers–Danlos syndrome, which presents with hypotonia but with normal power or no weakness)
- Differentiate central hypotonia from peripheral hypotonia
- Classify hypotonia as central, mixed, or peripheral
- Central hypotonia could be due to a systemic cause, with altered sensorium due to acute brain injury, either syndromic or nonsyndromic

Central Hypotonia

Central hypotonia is due to a CNS cause, while peripheral hypotonia is due to a lower motor neuron (LMN) or peripheral nervous system cause. The central causes can be due to insults/dysfunction in the brain, brainstem, or cervical spinal junction, while peripheral hypotonia is due to a problem in the motor unit. Weakness is more common in LMN causes of floppiness. Central hypotonia can also be due to a systemic illness such as sepsis or congestive cardiac failure complicating a severe congenital heart defect that influences the nervous system (brain and brainstem). These need to be ruled out before we workup for nervous system cause for floppiness. Hypoxic-ischemic encephalopathy (HIE) and inborn errors of metabolism (IEM) are another two important causes of central hypotonia and are associated with altered sensorium. Once we have ruled out these central causes, look for dysmorphism or syndromic features. Those with these features are labeled as syndromic central hypotonia (e.g., Down syndrome, Prader–Willi syndrome, Joubert syndrome, Smith–Lemli–Opitz syndrome, and other chromosomal or genetic disorders). The other group is nonsyndromic central hypotonia. Based on neuroimaging, they can be those with cerebral dysgenesis (malformations such as lissencephaly or holoprosencephaly) or with grossly normal brain (some cases may be associated with subtle changes such as delayed myelination and macrocerebellum). Rarely, craniovertebral junction injury or anomalies can also present as central hypotonia.

The common causes of floppiness are shown in **Table 8.18.1**.

Central versus Peripheral Hypotonia

Central hypotonia usually presents as "floppy strong," that is, babies are floppy to handle, but most of them have limb movements, which can be antigravity movements also, while peripheral hypotonia presents as "floppy weak," that is, they are floppy and weak. Causes due to central hypotonia account for 60–80% of hypotonia cases and peripheral hypotonia occurs in 15–30% of cases. There is a considerable overlap of involvement and clinical manifestations between the two types. The key differences between the two groups are summarized in **Table 8.18.2**.

Step 2: Family History and Examination of Family Members, Especially Parents

Look for consanguinity and draw a three-generation pedigree chart to know if there are any similarly affected family members and the pattern of inheritance if there is a genetic disorder in the family. This helps in recognizing conditions with maternal inheritance that could suggest a possibility of mitochondriopathy and anticipation, which could suggest triplet nucleotide expansion disease. It is important, as the tests we choose to diagnose these conditions are very different, and our routine genetic tests, such as exome sequencing and microarray, can miss these disorders.[1] History of similar complaints in other family members may not be appreciated by parents. Check photographs of relatives if available and examine other family members if available. Examine the parents, especially the mother, for grip myotonia, myopathic facies, pes cavus, wasting of small muscle of hands, and areflexia. Examine siblings for any evidence of neuromuscular illness or IEM. Maternal history should be taken in detail to look for a difficult delivery that presents as central hypotonia at birth due to HIE and the presence of uterine dystonia that can suggest myotonic dystrophy in the mother.

Step 3: Recognize the Patterns of Weakness and Attempt to Localize the Origin of Hypotonia in a Child with Peripheral Hypotonia

Based on the distribution of weakness, reflexes, and other features, we can localize the disease to different parts of the neuroaxis as follows.

Anterior Horn Cell (e.g., Spinal Muscular Atrophy)

The anterior horn disorders are characterized by proximal more than distal weakness, prominent wasting and fasciculations, wasting of tongue, presence of polyminimyoclonus in fingers/toes, areflexia, sparing of social/language milestones and sensory system, flexor plantar response, and involvement of bulbar/respiratory muscle involvement.

Muscle Disease/Myopathies

Pure motor weakness (normal sensory examination), proximal more than distal involvement, normal or sluggish deep tendon jerks, less prominent wasting, absence of fasciculations, with or without involvement of the extraocular

TABLE 8.18.1: Common causes of floppiness.

Type	Key features	Localization	Examples
Central hypotonia	With preserved DTR and altered sensorium	Brain and brain stem	Hypoxic-ischemic encephalopathy, meningitis/encephalitis, inborn errors of metabolism
	With preserved DTR and normal sensorium without dysmorphism	Brain and brain stem	• Systemic causes such as sepsis, congestive cardiac failure with CHD • Cerebral dysgenesis or malformations such as lissencephaly, holoprosencephaly • With normal neuroimaging—essential or benign congenital hypotonia, or GDD/ID, or ASD • With subtle neuroimaging findings such as delayed myelination associated with GDD/ID and may have underlying chromosomal aberration
	With preserved DTR and dysmorphism	Brain and brainstem	Syndromic hypotonia such as Down syndrome, Prader–Willi syndrome, Smith–Lemli–Opitz syndrome, Angelman syndrome, Sotos syndrome, Coffin–Lowry syndrome, and other deletion syndromes
	Hypotonia or hypotonia followed by hypertonia; may have depressed, normal, or hyperreflexia	Spinal cord or craniovertebral junction anomaly	Spinal cord injury Chiari malformations
Peripheral hypotonia	Weakness with absent or sluggish DTR	Anterior horn cell	• Spinal muscular atrophy • BVVL syndrome
		Peripheral nerve	HMSN, CHN, infantile neuroaxonal dystrophy
		Muscle	Congenital myopathies, congenital muscular dystrophies, metabolic myopathies
	Weakness with normal DTR	Neuromuscular junction	• Transient-acquired myasthenia gravis • Congenital myasthenic syndromes • Botulism
Central plus peripheral or both	With normal DTR or depressed DTR	Brain, brain stem, muscle, peripheral nerves	Congenital muscular dystrophies such as muscle eye brain disease, Walker–Warburg disease, mitochondrial cytopathies, congenital disorders of glycosylation
Extraneurological	Hyperlaxity of joints	Skin and connective tissue	Ehlers–Danlos syndrome

(ASD: autism spectrum disorder; BVVL: Brown–Vialetto–Van-Laere syndrome; CHD: congenital heart disease; CHN: Charcot–Marie–Tooth neuropathy; DTR: deep tendon reflexes; GDD: global developmental delay; HMSN: hereditary motor and sensory neuropathy; ID: intellectual disability)

muscles, facial and bulbar muscles, and normal social/language milestones (can be seen in congenital muscular dystrophies) characterize the muscle disorders.

Neuromuscular Junction Disorders

Presence of ptosis, fatigable muscle weakness, diplopia/extraocular muscle involvement, generalized muscle involvement with bulbar and respiratory muscles, presence of deep tendon reflexes, flexor plantar response, and absence of fasciculations/wasting are suggestive of neuromuscular junction disorders.[2,4,5]

Peripheral Neuropathy

There is symmetrical weakness that is more distal than proximal. The sensory complaints are less pronounced. Deep tendon jerks are absent, and the plantars are flexor. There is normal cognition.

Step 4: Course of the Disease

The onset and course of the weakness in a given child can give an important clue to the underlying cause of floppiness. A term infant who is born healthy but develops floppiness after 12–24 hours suggests a possibility of an IEM. Infants suffering central injury usually develop increased tone and deep tendon reflexes. Central congenital hypotonia does not worsen with time but may become more readily apparent. Fluctuation in weakness usually suggests neuromuscular junction illness. Degenerative disorders such as SMA have progressive loss of power in muscles, while static disorders such as congenital myopathies slowly but steadily improve with age.[2,4,5]

TABLE 8.18.2: Key differences between central and peripheral hypotonia.

Finding	*Central hypotonia*	*Peripheral hypotonia*
Appearance	Lethargy/dull	Active, alert
Language and social milestones	Delayed/ affected	Normal
Power	Weakness relatively less	Weakness is prominent
Deep tendon reflexes	Normal or brisk	Sluggish or absent
Primitive reflexes	Present or exaggerated	Absent
Fisting of hand	Present	Absent
Plantar	Extensor	Flexor
Wasting and fasciculations	Absent	Present
Dysmorphism	May be present	Absent
Systemic features such as deranged liver function tests, abnormal eye movements, apneas, and shock	Present	Absent
Seizures	Present	Absent
Micro/macrocephaly	May be present	Usually absent

Step 5: Specific Clues on Examination (General Physical/Systemic Examination)

A detailed general physical examination and systemic examination can suggest the underlying disease. Coarse facies, jaundice, and constipation can be seen in congenital hypothyroidism, while facial dysmorphism can suggest chromosomal abnormalities such as Down syndrome. Large head, wide open fontanelle, and costochondral beading can be seen in rickets, which is associated with hypotonia in infancy. Hypopigmentation and undescended testes are findings seen in Prader–Willi syndrome. Abnormal odor in urine or body can suggest IEM and congenital cataracts, and glaucoma suggests oculocerebrorenal (Lowe) syndrome. The presence of hepatosplenomegaly suggests storage disorders and congenital infections, whereas renal cysts, high forehead, and wide fontanelle are seen in Zellweger syndrome. Hepatomegaly and retinitis pigmentosa are seen in neonatal adrenoleukodystrophy, while cardiomegaly and large tongue can be seen in Pompe disease.

Step 6: Investigations

If central hypotonia is suspected, then magnetic resonance imaging (MRI) of the brain is done to look for features of HIE, structural brain abnormalities, and evidence of injury to the brain. If there is associated dysmorphism along with floppiness, then genetic tests such as chromosomal microarray, karyotyping, or whole-exome/genome sequencing can be ordered depending on the clinical scenario.[1] If there is suspicion of IEM, screening tests like serum ammonia, lactate, arterial blood gases, urine ketone bodies, liver/renal function tests, glucose, and electrolytes are done, followed by other confirmatory tests like tandem mass spectrometry or gas chromatography/mass spectrometry and plasma amino acidogram. Serum creatine phosphokinase is a must in all cases of a floppy infant. It suggests muscle disease, and the levels are very much increased (in several thousands) in muscular dystrophies and levels are in few hundreds in myopathies. Electrophysiological studies such as nerve conduction studies and electromyography are also ordered to diagnose anterior horn cell diseases, neuropathies, and myopathies. When we suspect neuromuscular junction disorders, repetitive nerve stimulation (RNS) needs to be ordered. Muscle biopsy used to be done earlier in most cases of myopathies/muscular dystrophies. But because of its invasive nature, nowadays genetic tests like whole-exome/genome sequencing are done first.[1] When they are negative or inconclusive, then muscle biopsies are done. For triplet nucleotide expansion diseases like myotonic dystrophies, special genetic tests such as triplet repeat primed polymerase chain reaction (TP-PCR) needs to be ordered as other tests may not yield positive results in these disorders.[2,4,5]

CONCLUSION

Many conditions can present as a floppy neonate or infant. A careful history and physical examination can suggest the correct diagnosis in many cases. Systematic and stepwise examination and/or evaluation helps in majority of the patients. A correct clinical diagnosis is a must to choose the appropriate test for confirmation of the diagnosis and treatment.

REFERENCES

1. Prasad AN, Prasad C. Genetic evaluation of the floppy infant. Semin Fetal Neonatal Med. 2011;16(2):99-108.
2. Pitt M. Neurophysiological strategies for the diagnosis of disorders of the neuromuscular junction in children. Dev Med Child Neurol. 2008;50(5):328-33.
3. Cutrona C, Pede E, De Sanctis R, Coratti G, Tiberi E, Luciano R, et al. Assessing floppy infants: a new module. Eur J Pediatr. 2022;181(7):2771-8.
4. Bodensteiner JB. The evaluation of the hypotonic infant. Semin Pediatr Neurol. 2008;15(1):10-20.
5. Kaler J, Hussain A, Patel S, Majhi S. Neuromuscular junction disorders and floppy infant syndrome: a comprehensive review. Cureus. 2020;12(2):e6922.

8.19 Neuromuscular Disorders

Sheffali Gulati, Shruthi NM, Aakash Mahesan, Kaushik Ragunathan

INTRODUCTION

Neuromuscular disorders (NMDs) are a heterogeneous group of disorders, which result from pathology anywhere in the motor unit. The motor unit comprises a single anterior horn cell, peripheral nerve, neuromuscular junction, and all the muscle fibers that are innervated by it. NMDs comprise neuronopathy (primary disorder of anterior horn cell), neuropathy (primary disorder of axon or its myelin), neuromuscular junction disorders, and myopathy/ muscular dystrophy (primary disorder of muscle). They may be hereditary [e.g., spinal muscular atrophy (SMA) and congenital myopathies] or acquired [e.g., inflammatory myopathies and myasthenia gravis (MG)]. Many NMDs are multisystem disorders affecting multiple organ systems, e.g., myotonic muscular dystrophy (affecting brain and eye) and mitochondrial cytopathies.[1]

In recent times, inherited NMDs have witnessed a paradigm shift in their recognition from histopathology to genetic identity. Detailed history and careful physical examination are the fundamental tools in the evaluation of a child with NMDs. **Table 8.19.1** enumerates key features to differentiate between various NMDs.

CLINICAL APPROACH

Weakness and hypotonia are the two cardinal features of NMDs.

Hypotonia

The maintenance of normal tone requires intact central and peripheral nervous system. Dysfunction of either or both leads to hypotonia. *Cerebral (central) hypotonia* differs from *peripheral hypotonia* (due to motor unit disorders) by having preserved muscle stretch reflexes, extensor plantar, preserved power (hypotonia is out of proportion to weakness and predominance of axial weakness), persistence of neonatal reflexes, associated seizures, dysmorphic features, and malformations of brain or other organs. *Mixed hypotonia* occurs in both the central and peripheral nervous system involvement with relatively preserved power and areflexia or hyporeflexia. **Table 8.19.2** shows common etiologies of peripheral and central hypotonia.[2]

Weakness

Weakness is a common feature of motor unit dysfunction. Different patterns of weakness such as limb-girdle,

TABLE 8.19.1: Key features to differentiate between motor unit disorders.

Site of involvement	***Proximal (P) vs distal (D) involvement***	***Facial involvement***	***Atrophy***	***Muscle stretch reflexes***	***Sensations***	***Electrophysiological studies***	***Muscle biopsy***
Anterior horn cell	P ≥ D	Absent	Yes	Absent	Normal	Evidence of denervation and fasciculation	Type grouping
Nerve	D > P	Absent	Yes	Depressed/ absent	Decreased	Abnormal nerve conduction studies and denervation potentials on EMG	Denervation pattern
Neuromuscular junction	Variable, fatigable	Present (ptosis and ophthalmoparesis)	No	Normal	Normal	Repetitive nerve stimulation—abnormal decrement/increment	Normal
Muscle	P > D	Present variably (ptosis in congenital myopathies)	Late stages	Depressed	Normal	Low-amplitude short-duration polyphasic motor unit action potential on EMG	Usually characteristic

(EMG: electromyogram)

TABLE 8.19.2: Differential diagnosis of hypotonia.

Central hypotonia (floppy strong)	Peripheral hypotonia (floppy weak)	Mixed hypotonia
Chromosomal disorders: • Prader–Willi syndrome • Trisomy *Static encephalopathies:* • Cerebral malformations • Cerebellar disorders • Hydrocephalus • Perinatal insult *Neurometabolic:* • Acid maltase deficiency • Biotinidase deficiency • GM1/GM2 gangliosidoses • Peroxisomal disorders • Congenital disorders of glycosylation *Infections:* • Sepsis/meningitis • Intrauterine infections *Benign congenital hypotonia* *Genetic defects:* • Lowe syndrome • Familial dysautonomia	*Anterior horn cell:* • Spinal muscular atrophy • Poliomyelitis • Enteroviral infections *Neuropathies:* • Giant axonal neuropathy • Hereditary sensory autonomic neuropathies • Congenital hypomyelinating neuropathy • Charcot–Marie–Tooth disease • Guillain–Barré syndrome *Infections*: Diphtheria, HIV *Traumatic neuropathies* *Toxic neuropathies*: Lead, porphyria *Neuromuscular junction disorders:* • Myasthenia gravis • Congenital myasthenic syndromes • Botulism *Myopathies:* • Central core disease • Myotubular myopathy • Nemaline rod myopathy • Congenital fiber-type disproportion myopathy • Metabolic myopathies • Inflammatory myopathies *Muscular dystrophy:* • Dystrophinopathy • Myotonic dystrophy • Facioscapulohumeral dystrophy • Congenital muscular dystrophy • Emery–Dreifuss muscular dystrophy	• Hypothyroidism • Acid maltase deficiency • Hypoxic ischemic encephalomyelopathy • Familial dysautonomia • Infantile neuronal degeneration • Motor unit disease with superimposed asphyxia • Mitochondrial disorders • Lysosomal storage disorders • Peroxisomal disorders

(GM1: ganglioside M1; GM2: ganglioside M2; HIV: human immunodeficiency virus)

scapulo-peroneal, distal upper limbs and proximal lower limbs, facial, oculopharyngeal, and axial weakness exist. In general, muscle involvement results in proximal weakness (except myotonic dystrophy and Miyoshi myopathy), and nerve involvement leads to distal weakness. Anterior horn cell involvement leads to generalized weakness. Neuromuscular junction disorders lead to fatigable weakness with predilection to facial/ocular muscles and limb-girdle muscles. Key features to differentiate and localize motor unit disorders have been enumerated in **Table 8.19.1**.

History

Key points in history should include three-generation pedigree, consanguinity, drug or teratogen exposure (alcohol, solvents, and drugs), reduced fetal movements, history of polyhydramnios, detailed birth and perinatal history (details of resuscitation and feeding history), family history of recurrent infantile deaths, and developmental history. Detailed history of neuromuscular symptoms such as age at onset, progression, extent of involvement, pattern of involvement, positive and negative symptoms, fluctuations, precipitating factors, associated features of central nervous system, and other system involvement should be taken.[1]

Evaluation

One should perform focused general, musculoskeletal and neurologic, and systemic examinations to direct further diagnostic workup. Electrodiagnostic studies, including nerve conduction studies and electromyography (EMG), are considered extensions of physical examination and help to guide further tests, such as muscle/nerve biopsy or genetic testing. With this approach and skilled synthesis of all the available information, one can make an accurate diagnosis and anticipate complications, provide prognostic information, and guide for specific molecular therapies if available.

MUSCLE DISORDERS

Congenital Myopathy

Congenital myopathies are a heterogeneous group of muscle diseases, and they typically present with hypotonia, motor delay, and muscle weakness with variable age of onset. Majority of the patients present from birth to early infancy or childhood. Usually, they have a benign course with nonprogressive hypotonia and weakness leading to predominant motor delay. Sometimes, the severe forms present with early-onset respiratory distress and feeding difficulties. Children may have myopathic facies (long facies, temporal hollowing, dolichocephaly, high-arched palate, tented upper lip, and open mouth). There may be variable involvement of facial, extraocular, bulbar, and respiratory muscles. Intellectual function is usually preserved, and primary cardiac involvement is rare.

Four broad pathological variants are as follows:

1. *Protein inclusion myopathies*, such as nemaline rod and myosin storage myopathies
2. *Core myopathies*, such as central core and multiminicore myopathies
3. *Myopathies with internalized nuclei*, such as myotubular myopathy (MTM) and centronuclear myopathy
4. *Myopathies associated with abnormal fiber size*, such as congenital fiber-type disproportion myopathy

Histopathological review at All India Institute of Medical Sciences, New Delhi, has found core myopathies to be the most common variant.

Diagnosis

Diagnosis is based on history, clinical findings, electrophysiology, muscle biopsy, and genetic testing. In muscle biopsy, the presence of morphological and ultrastructural sarcolemmal skeletal changes and the absence of histological features of dystrophies, such as fiber necrosis, fibrosis, fatty, and inflammatory infiltration, are the defining features of congenital myopathy. Creatine phosphokinase (CPK) is usually normal. Popularly, they have been classified based on the major characteristic features seen on muscle biopsy, e.g., rods (nemaline myopathy), cores (central core disease and multiminicore disease), central nuclei (centronuclear/MTM), and selective atrophy/hypotrophy of type 1 fibers (congenital fiber-type disproportion). Genetic diagnosis is gaining importance in view of the prognostic implications and for genetic counseling.[3]

At present, *treatment* is mainly supportive with a focus on rehabilitative measures. There are no curative therapies. Therapies, such as l-tyrosine for nemaline myopathy, salbutamol in core myopathies, pyridostigmine in centronuclear myopathy and MTM, *N*-acetylcysteine in selenoprotein N1 (*SEPN1*) and ryanodine receptor 1 (RYR1)-related myopathies, gene and enzyme replacement therapies in MTM, microribonucleic acids and histone deacetylases in RYR1 myopathies, are under investigation. Care should be taken while using halogenated anesthetic agents and muscle relaxants in RYR1 myopathies due to the risk of malignant hyperthermia. Dantrolene is the treatment of choice.

Table 8.19.3 depicts common congenital myopathy subtypes with their clinical, muscle biopsy and muscle magnetic resonance imaging (MRI) features.[4]

Congenital Muscular Dystrophies

Congenital muscular dystrophies (CMDs) are early onset muscle disorders (onset within 2 years of age) that are usually progressive. Affected infants typically present as floppy infants with skeletal abnormalities and other organ involvements, such as eye and brain, to a variable extent. Early joint contractures and spinal deformities are particularly prominent. The muscle biopsy is consistent with dystrophic process (even if not fully developed, with variation in fiber size, necrosis, increased endomysial fibrosis, and regenerative changes) without histological evidence of another neuromuscular disease. CPK levels are usually elevated but can be normal.[2]

Now, it is known that there is overlap between CMDs and congenital myopathies at the clinical, morphological, and genetic levels. Recently, classification of CMDs has underwent major revision with emerging knowledge of genes causing CMDs. **Table 8.19.4** gives an outline of classification of CMDs.[2]

Laminin alpha-2-related CMDs are the most common variants with variable spectrum. Abnormalities on neuroimaging are found in laminin alpha-2 deficiency (white matter changes) and dystroglycanopathies (structural brain abnormalities). Normal cognitive abilities and neuroimaging are found in collagen VI deficiencies and SEPN1-related CMDs. Dystroglycanopathies have severe presentations with eye and brain involvement (Walker–Warburg syndrome and Fukuyama CMD, and muscle–eye–brain disease). Collagen VI-deficient CMDs (Ullrich and Bethlem myopathies) have prominent skeletal manifestations with early proximal joint contractures and distal joint laxity **(Fig. 8.19.1)**.[2] Serum CPK levels are normal or mildly increased in collagen VI-deficient CMD, SEPN1-related CMD, and lamin A/C-related CMD, whereas those with primary merosin deficiency (laminin alpha-2 deficiency) or secondary merosin deficiency (dystroglycanopathies) have raised levels (>4 times normal).[2]

No specific therapy is available for any of the variants, and treatment is mainly focused on supportive respiratory, cardiac, orthopedic, and general care.

TABLE 8.19.3: Clinical features and genetics of subtypes of congenital myopathy.[4]

Subtype (with genes and inheritance)	Clinical features and muscle biopsy	Muscle MRI features
NM		
• *ACTA1* • *NEB* • *TPM2* • *TPM3* • *TNNT1* • *CFL2* • *KBTBD13* • *KLHL40*	• *NEB* mutation is the most common cause of NM (>50%), autosomal recessive inheritance • Most common presentation is congenital • Severity may vary from mild to lethal • Significant bulbar involvement, facial weakness, neck weakness, foot drop, variable extremity weakness, chest deformity, and scoliosis are common • Ophthalmoparesis is infrequently observed, except in some specific genetic variants, such as *LMOD3* • *Muscle biopsy* shows rods in Gomori trichrome staining as dark red/purple dense bodies in the cytoplasm or as intranuclear inclusions	Relative sparing of thigh with early involvement of lower leg with sparing of tibialis anterior and gastrocnemius
Core myopathies (central core disease and multiminicore disease)		
• *RYR1* • *SEPN1* • *ACTA1* • *TTN* • *MYH7* • *KBTBD13*	• *RYR1* is the most common cause of both central (autosomal dominant *RYR1*) and multiminicore (autosomal recessive *RYR1*) myopathies • Risk of malignant hyperthermia is high in patients having *RYR1* mutations • *SEPN1* (multiminicore disease) mutation-related myopathy presents with congenital axial weakness (head drop) and thin built with reduced muscle mass • Spinal rigidity may be marked. Scoliosis and congenital dislocation of hip may be present • The presence of ptosis, ophthalmoparesis, and facial weakness is more common with *SEPN1* than *RYR1*-related disorders • *Muscle biopsy* shows regions with lack of staining on oxidative stains. Central core disease shows single central cores with well-defined borders, best appreciated on longitudinal sections. Multiminicore disease shows multiple smaller cores with less-defined boundaries	• Marked involvement of sartorius, vasti, adductor magnus, and sparing of rectus femoris, adductor longus, and hamstrings • Calf level-lateral head of gastrocnemius, soleus with sparing of peroneal, medial head of gastrocnemius, and anterior compartment
Centronuclear myopathies		
• *MTM1* • *DNM2* • *BIN1* • *RYR1* • *TTN* • *SPEG*	• *MTM1* (X-linked) and *DNM2* (autosomal dominant) are the common mutations associated • It may present with varying severity from newborn to adulthood • Diagnostic clues are facial weakness, neck flexors weakness, ptosis and external ophthalmoplegia, swallowing, and respiratory weakness along with distal predominant extremity weakness • *Muscle biopsy* shows increased fibers with internalized nuclei (>25%) in H/E staining and radial sarcoplasmic strands and central aggregates of staining material on NADH stain. Myofiber hypotrophy and type 1 fiber predominance is seen	Predominant and progressive distal lower leg involvement (soleus, peroneal, tibialis anterior) and in thigh recti and hamstrings involved with sparing of sartorius and gracilis
CFTD		
• *ACTA1* • *TPM3* • *TPM2* • *RYR1* • *SEPN1*	• Most common is due to *TPM3* mutations (autosomal dominant) • Majority has less severe phenotype and many of them can walk into adulthood • *Muscle biopsy* shows variation in fiber sizes (type 1 fibers consistently smaller than type 2 by >25%, type 1 fiber predominance of >75%) or ratios, with no cores, rods, or central nuclei	No characteristic findings

(CFTD: congenital fiber-type disproportion; H/E: hematoxylin/eosin; *LMOD3*: leiomodin-3; MRI: magnetic resonance imaging; NADH: nicotinamide adenine dinucleotide; NEB: nebulin; NM: nemaline myopathy; RYR1: ryanodine receptor 1; SEPN1: selenoprotein N1)

Muscular Dystrophies

Muscular dystrophies are heterogeneous and inherited disorders, characterized by progressive muscle degeneration and loss of strength, defined by the presence of variable dystrophic changes on muscle biopsy. These are caused by various defects of the cytoskeletal proteins or enzymes leading to the degeneration of the muscle fibers and replacement by fibrous tissue. Classically, there is involvement of facial, axial, and limb-girdle muscles, with the involvement of cardiac and smooth muscles in some subtypes. They may be X-linked (dystrophinopathies), autosomal dominant [limb-girdle muscular dystrophy (LGMD) D1-5] or recessively inherited

TABLE 8.19.4: Classification of congenital muscular dystrophy (CMD).[2]

Subtypes of CMD and associated genes	Clinical phenotypic spectrum
COL6-RD *COL6A1, COL6A2, COL6A3*	• UCMD, autosomal recessive • BM, milder disease course, ambulatory, autosomal dominant • Proximal contractures, increased distal flexibility, prominent calcaneum, keratosis pilaris, and velvety palm are few notable features
Laminin alpha-2-related dystrophy (LAMA2-RD), includes MDC1A and merosin deficient (MD) *Gene: LAMA2*	• Nonambulant LAMA2-RD (complete merosin deficiency in muscle biopsy) • Ambulant LAMA2-RD (partial merosin deficiency) • Brain MRI shows white matter T2 hyperintensities usually sparing the corpus callosum along with cortical malformations
Alpha-dystroglycan-related dystrophy (aDG-RD, also alpha dystroglycanopathy) *Common genes: FKRP, FKTN, POMT1, POMT2, POMGnT1*	• Walker–Warburg syndrome • Muscle–eye–brain disease; Fukuyama CMD; Fukuyama-like CMD • CMD with cerebellar involvement; cerebellar abnormalities may include cysts, hypoplasia, and dysplasia • CMD with mental retardation and normal brain on imaging • CMD with no mental retardation; no evidence of abnormal cognitive development • LGMD with mental retardation or without mental retardation (milder weakness, may be later onset) and a structurally normal brain on imaging
LMNA-related dystrophy (LMNA-RD, including LMNA-CMD and Emery–Dreifuss) *LMNA*	• *CMD presentation*: Dropped head syndrome, axial and scapula–peroneal involvement, and absent or early loss of ambulation • Milder presentations fuse with early-onset Emery–Dreifuss muscular dystrophy
SEPN1-related myopathy (SEPN1-RM, also rigid spine CMD) *SEPN1*	*CMD presentation:* Present with cervicoaxial weakness, scapular winging, facial and bulbar involvement, progressively developing joint contractures, spinal rigidity, and scoliosis; secondary respiratory insufficiency and cardiac involvement common

(BM: Bethlem myopathy; COL6-RD: collagen VI-related dystrophies; LGMD: limb–girdle muscular dystrophy; LMNA: lamin A/C; MDC1A: congenital muscular dystrophy type 1A; SEPN1: selenoprotein N1; UCMD: Ullrich congenital muscular dystrophy)

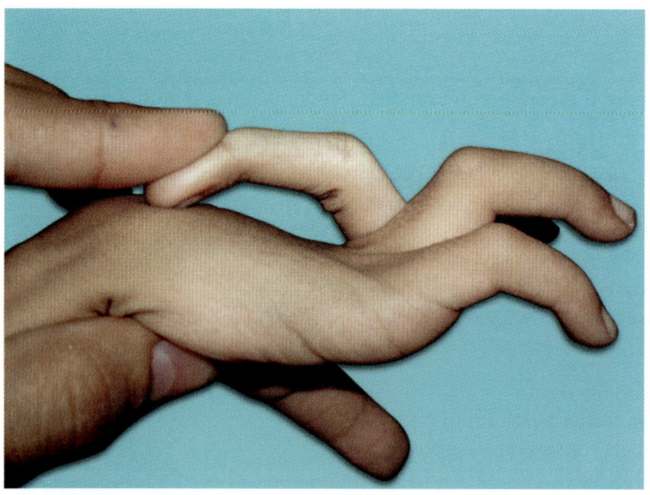

Fig. 8.19.1: Ullrich muscular dystrophy–distal hyperextensible joints.[2]

(LGMD R1-24). Dystrophinopathy [Duchenne muscular dystrophy (DMD) and Becker muscular dystrophy (BMD)] is the most common muscular dystrophy having a prevalence of 1 in 3,500 live male births. It accounts for approximately 60% of all muscular dystrophy cases.[5]

Dystrophinopathies

Dystrophinopathies are a group of disorders resulting from mutations in the *dystrophin* gene (located on the short arm of X chromosome in the *Xp21* region). Dystrophin is expressed in skeletal, cardiac, and smooth muscles and brain. These may be affected variably in dystrophinopathies. Dystrophin is located underneath the sarcolemma and is responsible for cytoskeletal stability. Decreased dystrophin will lead to membrane instability and susceptibility to mechanical stress and calcium-mediated cell injury, resulting in degeneration of muscle fibers.[1]

Duchenne Muscular Dystrophy and Becker Muscular Dystrophy

- *Duchenne muscular dystrophy:* It is the most common dystrophinopathy.
- *Becker muscular dystrophy:* Its rarer allelic variant differs from DMD by its later age of onset (usually >6 years of age), more prolonged unaided ambulation (>15 years), more incidence of myalgias, occasional rhabdomyolysis following exercise, and cardiac findings, which are "out of proportion" to limb weakness. Symptomatic cardiac involvement is more common in BMD. Cognitive impairment is not prominent, but these patients may have behavioral issues, such as impaired attention and learning difficulties. Both form the two ends of a spectrum.

Clinical features: Children with DMD often have delayed motor milestones. Gait disturbances often become apparent

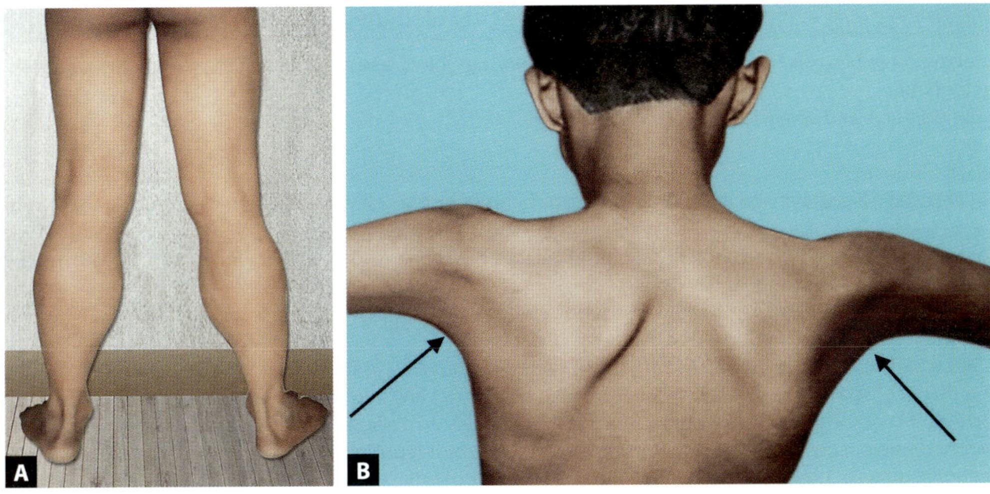

Figs. 8.19.2A and B: Duchenne muscular dystrophy: (A) Calf hypertrophy; (B) Valley sign.

at 3–4 years of age. Waddling gait, Gower sign, and calf muscle hypertrophy **(Figs. 8.19.2A and B)** are classical findings at this stage. Neck flexor muscle weakness is seen early. Other muscles may also show hypertrophy (extensor digitorum brevis, calf and tongue muscles). The progression of weakness may plateau between 3 and 6 years of age. Subsequently, there is increasing gait difficulty, contractures, and increased lumbar lordosis. Natural history studies have shown that the age of loss of independent ambulation in untreated DMD is between 8.8 and 10.5 years. After the loss of ambulation, there is worsening kyphoscoliosis, increasing upper limb weakness, and bulbar dysfunction.

Weakness of intercostal and diaphragmatic muscles with spinal deformity compromises respiratory function. Cardiomyopathy and arrhythmias are the two major cardiac manifestations in DMD. The cause of death in DMD patients is usually the combination of respiratory insufficiency and cardiomyopathy. Other clinical features of DMD may include variable degrees of intellectual disability and impaired gastric motility and smooth muscle dysfunction.

More than 90% of female carriers are asymptomatic. However, few may have variable degree of weakness with elevated CPK levels. Full DMD phenotype may be present in the case of complete inactivation of normal X chromosome. Increased risk of cardiomyopathy may be seen in female carriers.

Diagnosis:

- *Serum CPK* levels are greatly elevated (>10 times). It has no correlation with severity of the disease or response to treatment. Other muscle enzymes are also elevated. The levels decrease as the muscle mass is lost with the progression of the disease.
- *Genetics:* Multiplex polymerase chain reaction (PCR) can detect intragenic deletions (65% cases), Southern blotting and quantitative PCR detect duplications (5% cases), and multiplex ligation-dependent probe amplification (MLPA) detects the rest 30–35% (small insertion or deletion, single base changes, or splicing). In around 90% of boys with DMD, the "out-of-frame" mutation disrupts the normal dystrophin transcription, resulting in almost undetectable dystrophin. The "in-frame" mutations result in the production of some abnormal molecular weight dystrophin leading to BMD phenotype. This "reading frame rule" was proposed by Koenig and has a sensitivity of 93–96% in predicting DMD. Mutation analysis is currently preferred over invasive methods, such as biopsy. It also helps in carrier detection, prenatal, and genetic counseling.
- *Muscle biopsy* may be required in detection of negative cases to differentiate between DMD and BMD. Genetic diagnosis is mandatory in biopsy-confirmed cases as per recent recommendations.

Management: Management of a child with DMD is briefly outlined in **Box 8.19.1**.[4]

Other Common Dystrophies Apart from Dystrophinopathies

These are summarized in **Table 8.19.5 (Figs. 8.19.3A to C)**.[5]

Metabolic myopathies: These are a group of muscle disorders resulting from failed energy production related to defects in glycogen, lipid, or mitochondrial metabolism. Fatty acid oxidation is the chief source of energy for resting muscle, with glucose utilization accounting for 10–15% of total oxygen consumption. During exercise, for the initial 5–10 minutes,

BOX 8.19.1: Management of a child with Duchenne muscular dystrophy.[4]

Physical therapy: Effective stretching and appropriate positioning at various joints, assistive devices to prevent contractures, avoid high-resistance strength training

Surgery: Persistent contractures and spinal fusion

Steroids:

- Standard of care
- Usually started in children >2 years of age with static or declining functions; in <2-year-old steroids are not started in presymptomatic or plateau phase
- Most effective dose 0.75 mg/kg/day of prednisolone (increased till the child reaches 40 kg weight with a cap at 30–40 mg/day of prednisolone); daily schedule more effective than alternate day dosing
- Deflazacort (0.9 mg/kg/day; maximum 36–39 mg/day) may be preferred in children with excessive weight gain with prednisolone or with preexisting behavioral problems but has increased incidence of cataracts
- *Nonambulatory DMD children:* Low-dose (0.3–0.6 mg/kg/day) prednisolone may be started with the aim of preserving upper limb strength, reducing the progression of scoliosis and delaying the decline in respiratory and cardiac function
- *Before starting steroids:* Adequate immunization (pneumococcal/influenza/varicella); screening with chest X-ray and Mantoux test
- *Monitoring of children on steroid therapy:* Screening for side effects of steroids (cushingoid features, obesity, cataracts, hypertension, glucose intolerance, infections, growth, hirsutism, acne, behavioral changes, polyuria/polydipsia, GERD/PUD, fractures, and color of urine after exercise)
- *In the case of side effects:* Reduce steroid dose by 25–33%, reassess monthly, up to a minimum effective daily dose of steroid is reached (3 mg/kg/day); switch to alternative regimen (intermittent day regimen: 10 days on and 10 days off/10 days in a month; alternate day regimen: 0.75–1.25 mg/kg on alternate days or high-dose weekend regimen) if side effects still persist

Follow-up:

- *At each visit:* Monitor weight/height/body mass index, blood pressure, and blood sugar
- Annual SMR staging
- Annual ophthalmologic evaluation
- Pulmonary function tests (6 monthly in nonambulatory; annually in ambulatory patients)
- Echocardiography (once in 2 years <10 years of age; annually >10 years of age)
- ACE inhibitors or angiotensin-receptor blockers for symptomatic patients of asymptomatic patients >10 years of age
- Serum calcium, phosphate, 25(OH) vitamin D (biannually)
- DEXA scan annually
- Respiratory and cardiac care
- *Orthopedic management:* Surveillance for scoliosis after 5 years of age (surgery if >25% scoliosis or reduction in vital capacity >30%)
- Management of gastrointestinal problems
- Psychosocial management

Approved newer therapies:

- *Antisense oligonucleotide and exon skipping (for out-of-frame deletions):* Eteplirsen (Exondys 51), Golodirsen (Vyondys 53), Viltolarsen (Viltepso 53), and Casimersen (Amondys 45)
- *Read through stop codon strategies (for nonsense mutations)*: *PTC124* (Ataluren)
- *Histone deacetylase inhibitor:* Givinostat
- *Newer synthetic steroid:* Vamorolone
- *Gene therapy using microdystrophin:* Delandistrogene moxeparvovec (Elevidys) *AAV-rh 74*

Drugs under trial:

- *Utrophin upregulation:* SMT *C1100* (phase 1B trials on going)
- Stem cell therapy and induced pluripotent stem cell therapy used in research settings only
- Isosorbide dinitrate with ibuprofen
- SERCA1 delivery
- CRISPR editing
- Osteopontin inhibitor
- Drugs, such as oxandrolone, azathioprine, creatine monohydrate, nifedipine, leucine, selenium, vitamin E, methysergide, pizotifen, sildenafil, tadalafil, inhibitors of myostatin and idebenone, have been tried in research without much benefits and evidence for use

[DEXA: dual energy X-ray absorptiometry; DMD: Duchenne muscular dystrophy; FDA: Food and Drug Administration; GERD: gastroesophageal reflux disease; PUD: peptic ulcer disease; SMR: sexual maturity rating (Tanner staging)]

high-energy phosphates are used, followed by glycogenolysis. At around 90 minutes of exercise, glucose and free fatty acids are the major sources. During prolonged exercise, free fatty acids and triglycerides are the major fuel sources.[6]

Affected older children and adults present primarily with exercise intolerance, weakness, and myoglobinuria; newborns and infants present with severe multisystem disorders. In patients with glycolytic/glycogenolytic defects,

TABLE 8.19.5: Other muscle dystrophies.

Muscular dystrophy	*Underlying defect*	*Clinical features*
Myotonic dystrophy type 1 (AD) type 2 (AD) (less severe)	Abnormal expansion of *[CTG] n* repeats in the *DMPK* gene (chromosome 19) type 1; (CCTG) tetranucleotide repeat intron 1 of the *ZNF9* gene type 2	• *Congenital form:* Respiratory failure, poor feeding, hypotonia, facial diplegia, clubfoot and gastroparesis, decreased fetal movements, and polyhydramnios in mother • *Late-onset form* presents during adolescence; myotonia (percussion and handgrip myotonia), facial weakness, distal limb weakness (finger flexor and intrinsic hand muscles, dorsiflexors of feet), cataracts, frontal baldness, myotonic facies, palatal weakness mental retardation, endocrinopathies, cardiac arrhythmias, and disturbed gastrointestinal motility • *Diagnosis:* DNA analysis; EMG-dive bomber potentials, abnormal CPK levels • *Treatment:* Quinine, procainamide, phenytoin, mixeletine, acetazolamide; supportive treatment. *AAV.U7snRNAs* vectors targeting DMPK are promising
Facioscapulohumeral muscular dystrophy (AD)	*FSHD1 protein*: • *Type 1: D4Z4* deletion • *Type 2 (5%):* Hypomethylation of *DUX4* allele due to *SMCHD1* gene mutation	• *Age of onset variable:* The disease may start with asymptomatic facial weakness (may be asymmetric) followed sequentially by scapular fixator (chicken wing appearance), humeral, truncal, and lower extremity weakness; hearing loss; polyhill sign; Beevor sign; Popeye effect (thin arms and preserved forearms) slowly progressive; extraocular and bulbar muscles are spared; contractures are rare; side-to-side asymmetry of muscle weakness is typical; extramuscular manifestations include deafness (70–75%), Coats' disease (60–70%), atrial arrhythmias, and restrictive respiratory disease **(Figs. 8.19.3A to C)** • *Diagnosis:* CPK mildly elevated; EMG shows myopathic potentials; nonspecific dystrophic features on muscle biopsy with angulated fibers; genetic diagnosis • *Treatment:* Supportive
Emery–Dreifuss muscular dystrophy (EMDM 1-6) • X-linked (1,6) • AD (2,4,5) • AR (3)	• *EDMD 1: EMD* • *EDME 2: LMNA* • *EDMD 3: LMNA* • *EDMD 4: SYNE 1* • *EDMD 5: SYNE 2* • *EDMD 6: FHL 1*	• Variable age of onset from childhood-to-late adolescence or adulthood. Weakness initially in the pectoral and shoulder girdles, progressing to pelvic girdle and distal leg. Triad of early contractures, slowly progressive muscle weakness and cardiac conduction defects • *Diagnosis:* CPK levels elevated; EMG myopathic potentials; skin and muscle biopsy with immunostaining; DNA analysis • *Management* is supportive
Oculopharyngeal muscular dystrophy (AD)	*PABPN1* gene symbol (GCG repeats). Ch locus *14q11.2*	• *Late onset*, initial features are ptosis and dysphagia, followed by proximal lower limb weakness and external ophthalmoplegia, lower limbs are more commonly involved than upper limbs, facial and tongue muscles are also involved variably • *Diagnosis:* Elevated CPK; EMG myopathic potentials; dystrophic changes, rimmed vacuoles, and intranuclear inclusions on muscle biopsy; genetic analysis (no anticipation, as the triplet expansion is mitotically stable) • *Management* is supportive; Doxycycline is under trial to reduce intranuclear aggregates
LGMD (few notable ones)[5]		
Calpainopathy (LGMD R1)	• *Gene locus: 4p21* • *Protein:* Calpain-3	Most frequent form worldwide. Onset is variable. Mild phenotype in majority. Early onset has more severe progression. Loss of ambulation 10–30 years after onset. Pelvic girdle is more involved than shoulder girdle, relative preservation of hip abductors and scapular winging, calf hypotrophy, joint contractures seen
Dysferlinopathy (LGMD R2)	• *Gene locus: 2p12–14* • *Protein:* Dysferlin	Mean age of onset 17–20 years. Slow progression. Most walk till their fourth decade. Patchy involvement of muscle or muscle groups with the areas of atrophy and hypertrophy; may have a presentation, such as inflammatory myopathies with subacute onset pain and raised CPK levels with normal sporting ability; posterior leg and biceps brachii involvement is seen
Sarcoglycanopathy (LGMD R3-6)	• *Gene locus: 13q12, 17q21, 4q12, 5q33* • *Protein:* Gamma-sarcoglycan, alpha- sarcoglycan, beta-sarcoglycan, theta-sarcoglycan	*Age of onset* is variable. Most present in early childhood. They have moderate-to-severe progression. Patients with gamma-sarcoglycanopathy behave in similar way, such as DMD or BMD, while patients with theta-sarcoglycanopathy have rapid progression and succumb in their second decade. Markedly elevated CPK levels usually in thousands. Predominantly limb–girdle weakness. Scapular winging is present. Cardiac involvement is seen in later course. Calf hypertrophy is prominent

Contd...

Contd...

Muscular dystrophy	*Underlying defect*	*Clinical features*
Previously classified as LGMD 1 and removed in the current classification of LGMD include AD MYOT, LMNA, CAV3, DES and AR DES, GAA, LIMS2, BVES, TOR1AIP1. Bethlem and milder laminin alpha 2-related muscular dystrophy are now considered as LGMD[5]		
Myofibrillar myopathy	• *Gene locus*: *5q31* • *Protein*: Myotilin	Onset variable, usually the third to seventh decade, anticipation is seen. Slow progression. Limb–girdle weakness including facial and wrist and finger extensors involvement. Early foot drop is seen. Cardiomyopathy in up to 50%, dysarthria is seen
EDMD phenotype	• *Gene locus: 1q11–q21* • *Protein*: Lamin A/C	Age of onset is <20 years. Slow progression. Upper limbs involved by third or fourth decade. Cardiomyopathy is seen up to 62%; may result in neonatal hypotonia
Rippling muscle disease	• *Gene locus*: *3p25* • *Protein*: Caveolin-3	Onset 5 years to adulthood. Moderate severity and progression; may present as asymptomatic hyperCKemia; rippling muscle disease; calf hypertrophy seen

(AD: autosomal dominant; BMD: Becker muscular dystrophy; CPK: creatine phosphokinase; DMD: Duchenne muscular dystrophy; DMPK: dystrophia myotonica-protein kinase; DNA: deoxyribonucleic acid; EMG: electromyography; LGMD: Limb–girdle muscular dystrophy; LMNA: lamin A/C)

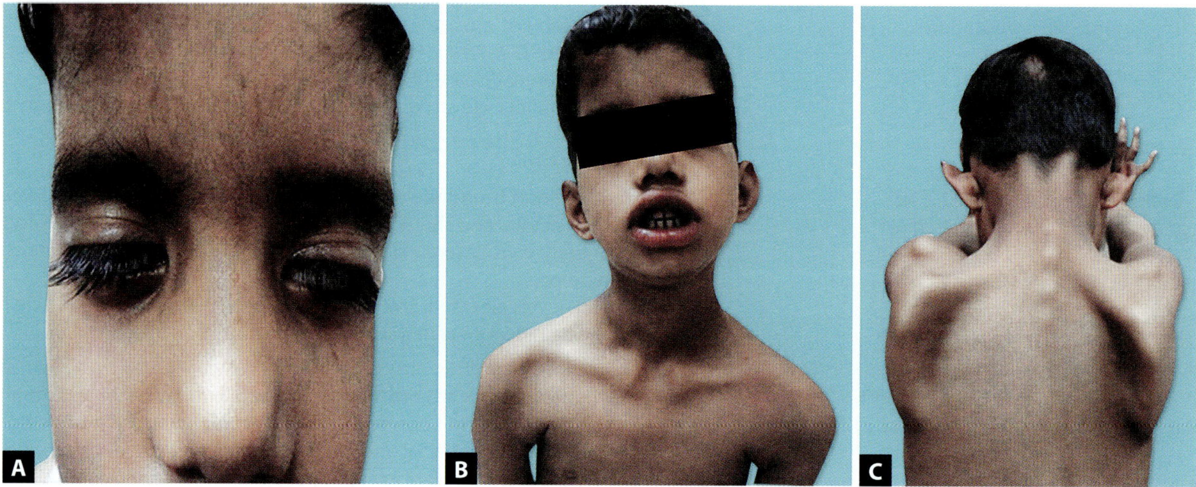

Figs. 8.19.3A to C: Facioscapulohumeral muscular dystrophy: (A) Inability to close eyes completely; (B) Forward sloping of shoulders with straight clavicles; (C) Scapular winging on attempted forward flexion.

symptoms are induced by either brief isometric exercise, such as lifting heavy weights, or by less intense but sustained dynamic exercise. With disorders of lipid metabolism, the abnormalities are usually induced by prolonged exercise and prolonged fasting. Investigations include serum CPK, urine myoglobin, serum ammonia, tandem mass spectrometry, gas chromatography–mass spectrometry (GC–MS), electrophysiological studies, forearm ischemia exercise test, muscle biopsy, and molecular studies.

NEUROMUSCULAR JUNCTION DISORDERS

Neuromuscular junction disorders comprise presynaptic, synaptic, and postsynaptic disorders. The cardinal features of these disorders are a waxing–waning course and easy fatigability, which improve after rest. In infants and children, three forms of MG are characterized:

1. Juvenile MG (JMG) (autoimmune), such as adult type
2. Congenital MG
3. Transient neonatal MG in an infant born to a myasthenic mother

Juvenile Myasthenia Gravis

Juvenile MG is an autoimmune disorder of synaptic transmission. All age-groups can be affected, with equal incidence in males and females before puberty, and in <40 years more predominant in females. Circulating acetylcholine receptor (AChR) antibodies interfere with fixation, placement, or survival of nicotinic AChR. Muscarinic receptors are not affected; therefore, pupillary and autonomic responses are spared. Other antibodies associated are antibodies to muscle-specific kinase. About 10–15% are antibody negative, designated as seronegative myasthenia.

The salient features of JMG are given in **Box 8.19.2**. It can have purely ocular/generalized presentations with variable bulbar involvement. Most of the patients with ocular presentation progress to generalized MG by 2 years.

BOX 8.19.2: Presentation of juvenile myasthenia gravis.

Clues from history:
- Slowly progressive course with relapsing-remitting tendency with variable or fatigable weakness
- *Perinatal:* Reduced fetal movements, polyhydramnios, arthrogryposis
- *Infancy:* Hypotonia, weakness, weak cry, feeding difficulties, and recurrent apneic episodes
- *Childhood:* Difficulty in chewing or swallowing, fatigability or hoarse voice, diplopia especially on sustained gaze or continuous activity, such as reading, weakness of jaw, orthopnea secondary to diaphragmatic weakness; limb-girdle weakness; ocular symptoms are the most common

Clues on neurological examination:
- *Eye signs:* Ptosis (may be asymmetric); peep sign (on attempting to tightly close eyes, after few minutes the cornea gets exposed due to inability to sustain contraction of orbicularis oculi), ophthalmoparesis, curtain sign (when examiner lifts the more affected eyelid, contralateral less affected eyelid ptosis worsens)
- *Facial weakness:* Compensatory wrinkling of forehead (due to hypercontracted frontalis to maintain eye opening), expressionless facies, snarl on trying to smile, inability to close the jaw
- *Other cranial musculature:* Bulbar weakness, tongue may show triple longitudinal furrowing
- *Skeletal musculature:* Proximal limb weakness and tachypnea/shallow respiration

Thymic hyperplasia (60–70%) is mostly observed compared to thymoma (10%). Various tests used in the diagnosis of JMG are discussed in **Box 8.19.3 (Figs. 8.19.4A and B)**.

Management

- *Chronic treatment*: The aims of treatment for MG patients should be to induce and maintain complete clinical or pharmacological remission with minimal adverse effects.
- *Nonimmune modulatory:* Pyridostigmine
- *Immune modulatory:* Steroids, steroid-sparing agents, and thymectomy **(Table 8.19.6)**

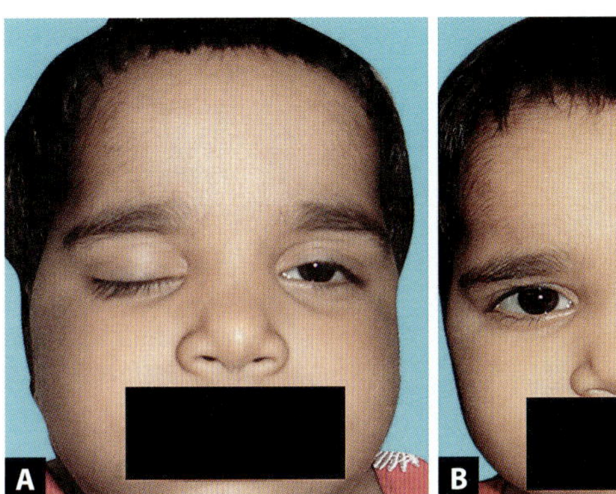

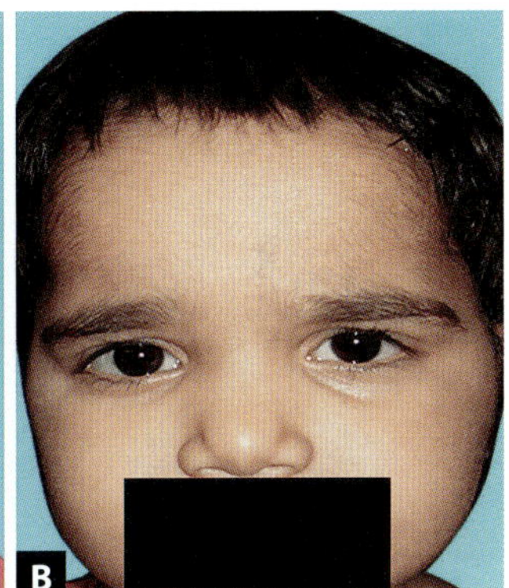

Figs. 8.19.4A and B: Juvenile myasthenia gravis; neostigmine challenge test: (A) Pre- and (B) Post-test; also note the asymmetric ptosis.

BOX 8.19.3: Diagnosis of myasthenia gravis.

- *Edrophonium testing:* A rapid acting, short duration cholinesterase inhibitor. Effects are seen within 10 seconds and persist till 120 seconds; positive: transient resolution of the clinical signs (ptosis/ophthalmoplegia/dysarthria); diagnostic dose is 0.1–0.2 mg/kg [may be repeated every minute to a total maximum dose of 5 mg (weight <34 kg) or 10 mg (weight >34 kg)]; should be done in a monitored setting with available atropine and cardiorespiratory resuscitation kit
- *Infants*: Edrophonium is not recommended for use in infants due to high risk of arrhythmias and short duration of action, which precludes objective assessment. Neostigmine (prostigmine methylsulfate) by intramuscular injection slower in action, response anticipated in 10–15 minutes and maximum in 30 minutes, a more objective assessment of response can be made; dose used is 0.125 mg/kg in an infant and 0.04 mg/kg in an older child. If the result is equivocal or negative, the dose may be repeated in 4 hours. **Figures 8.19.4A and B** demonstrate a positive response to neostigmine challenge test
- *Ice pack test:* It may be helpful for the diagnosis of ocular myasthenia; should only be interpreted as positive when there is clear and unequivocal improvement in ptosis following a 2-minute application of an ice pack to the affected eyelid
- *Electrophysiological testing:* RNST—the fatigability of neuromuscular transmission is demonstrated by a decrement of more than 10% in compound muscle action potential after repetitive nerve stimulation (2–5 Hz). SFEMG may show increased jitter or variation in contraction time in muscle fibers. RNST is positive in 80% of the generalized MG with 50–100% sensitivity and in 50% of the ocular MG with 10–20% sensitivity. SFEMG is virtually always abnormal, showing increased jitters and is the most sensitive test
- *Serum antibodies:* Acetylcholine receptor antibodies may be positive (up to 80% in the generalized MG and in up to 50% of the ocular MG patients); positivity rates are lower in peri and prepubertal children (50–60%). Specificity is up to 98%. Anti-MuSK antibodies may be demonstrable in 40% of the seronegative MG patients and is 80–90% specific
- *Muscle biopsy:* It is not indicated routinely
- X-ray chest or CT of anterior mediastinum may show thymoma/thymic hyperplasia
- Thyroid profile should always be done in suspected juvenile MG patients

(CT: computed tomography; MG: myasthenia gravis; MuSK: muscle-specific kinase; RNST: repetitive nerve stimulation test; SFEMG: single fiber electromyography)

TABLE 8.19.6: Management of juvenile myasthenia gravis.

Drugs	***Mechanism of action***	***Dose***	***Indications***	***Monitoring/precautions***
Pyridostigmine	AChE inhibitor	• 1–7 mg/kg in 5 or 6 divided doses 30 minutes before meals • *Maximum dose*: 300 mg • *Dose of IV pyridostigmine* is 1/30th of oral dose	First line for all JMG patients	May use glycopyrrolate/ atropine for muscarinic side effects
Corticosteroids	Exact mechanism unknown; immunosuppressive; reduces anti-AChR antibody level	• *In nonacute setting:* Start at low dose (@ 0.5 mg/kg/day); dose can be gradually increased as tolerated; once in remission, decrease dose gradually; effect starts within 2–3 weeks, full improvement is seen in 3 months; occasionally steroids can worsen the symptoms • *Acute setting*: Intravenous pulse steroids at 30 mg/kg/day for 3–5 days	*Cases:* Unresponsive to pyridostigmine and acute settings	Monitor for side effects
Azathioprine	Purine antimetabolite—inhibits T-cell proliferation	1–3 mg/kg/day as single dose; may be increased by 0.5–1 mg/kg/day every 4–8 weeks; takes a longer duration for the effects to appear, maximal effect is observed by 18–20 months	May be used as steroid-sparing drug; may be used alone also	CBC, hepatic function monthly Withhold treatment if counts <3,000; reduce if <4,000/mm^3
Mycophenolate mofetil	Selectively blocks purine synthesis in T and B cells by inhibiting the action of inosine-5-monoposphate dehydrogenase	1,000–1,500 mg every 12 hourly; slow onset of action with maximum benefit seen by 9–10 months	May be used as steroid-sparing drug	Monthly CBC for 1 year, then 3 monthly
IVIG	Blocks Fc receptor of antibodies	• *Acute setting:* 2 g/kg/day IV over 2 days or 5 days • *Maintenance:* 1 g/kg/day × 2 days every 4–8 weeks • Maximal benefit observed over 1–2 weeks; effect persists up to 1 month	May be used in myasthenic crises or as maintenance therapy, if child unresponsive to other immunomodulatory therapy	Monitor for side effects
Plasmapheresis	Removes AChR antibodies from circulation	• *Acute setting:* 3–5 exchanges every other day; number may depend on the severity • *Maintenance:* 3–5 exchanges/ month	May be considered in children who failed to respond to anti-AChE; and in crises	Monitor for side effects
Thymectomy	Immunomodulator	–	Necessary in thymoma; may be considered in nonthymomatous hyperplasia; thymectomy within 2 years of diagnosis results in a higher rate of remission; benefit may be delayed for years; timing of surgery is debatable	Undertaken with caution in very young children due to the occurrence of immunological abnormalities

(AChE: acetylcholinesterase; CBC; complete blood count; IVIG: intravenous immunoglobulin; JMG: juvenile myasthenia gravis)

Spontaneous remission is seen in 20% of the patients. Drugs are withdrawn if the patient remains asymptomatic up to 1 year.

Treatment of Acute Exacerbations/Crisis

- *Causes:* Disease progression, stressor/illness, withdrawal of chronic treatment, use of contraindicated medication **(Box 8.19.4)**. A close differential diagnosis is cholinergic crisis due to overdosage of acetylcholinesterase (AChE) inhibitors.
- *Short-term immunotherapy:* Intravenous immunoglobulin (IVIG) 2 g/kg over 2–5 days and plasmapheresis

BOX 8.19.4: Medications exacerbating myasthenia gravis.

- *Absolutely contraindicated:* Curare, penicillamine, Botox, and IFN-α
- *Relatively contraindicated*:
  - *Antibiotics:* Fluoroquinolones (ciprofloxacin, levofloxacin, etc.)
  - Macrolides (erythromycin, azithromycin, etc.)
  - Aminoglycosides (gentamicin, tobramycin, etc.)
  - Quinine
  - Class IA antiarrhythmic (procainamide, quinidine, lidocaine, etc.)
  - Magnesium
- *Use with caution:* Calcium-channel blockers, lithium, statins, and steroids

(IFN: interferon)

- *Supportive care:* Temporary nil per oral or nasogastric tube feeding to prevent aspiration. Close respiratory monitoring and provide ventilatory support if necessary.
- *Cholinergic crisis:* Cholinergic symptoms and signs may include diarrhea, urinary incontinence, miosis, bronchospasm, salivation, and lacrimation. If the patient is in crisis, withhold AChE inhibitor.

Congenital Myasthenia Syndromes

Congenital myasthenia syndromes (CMS) are a genetically determined heterogeneous group of neuromuscular junction disorders. Age of onset is variable, ranging from neonatal period to adulthood. Patients may present with ptosis, external ophthalmoparesis, facial weakness, general hypotonia, proximal greater than distal muscle weakness, and variable degrees of functional impairment.[7] Up to 35 CMS disease genes have been identified till date; among them, the most common cause of CMS is the gene, responsible for defects in AChR. **Table 8.19.7** gives outline of classification and therapeutics for common subtypes of CMS.

PERIPHERAL NEUROPATHIES IN CHILDHOOD

Peripheral neuropathy is a heterogeneous group of disorders affecting peripheral nerves, which can be acquired or genetic

TABLE 8.19.7: Outline of classification and therapeutics of common subtypes of congenital myasthenia syndromes (CMS).[7]

Subtypes	***Treatment***	***Caveats***
Presynaptic defects		
Choline acetyltransferase deficiency	Pyridostigmine parenteral neostigmine for acute apneic episodes	Recurrent apneas are common. They are floppy and weak with respiratory and bulbar muscle involvement. Severely affected patients may not respond to any cholinergic drugs and may require permanent respiratory support
SNAP25B deficiency	Amifampridine	
Synaptic defects		
Acetylcholinesterase deficiency	Salbutamol or ephedrine	Avoid pyridostigmine and amifampridine
Laminin-β_2 deficiency	Ephedrine	Avoid pyridostigmine
Postsynaptic defects		
Primary acetylcholine receptor deficiency	Pyridostigmine; amifampridine also helps; salbutamol may be given in refractory cases	Most common variant of CMS
Slow-channel syndrome	Quinine, quinidine, or fluoxetine	Avoid pyridostigmine and amifampridine
Fast-channel syndrome	Pyridostigmine and amifampridine	Avoid quinine, quinidine, or fluoxetine
Dok-7 deficiency	Salbutamol or ephedrine	Presents as limb–girdle myasthenia. Avoid pyridostigmine
End-plate rapsyn deficiency	Pyridostigmine, amifampridine, and salbutamol	–

(CMS: congenital myasthenia syndromes; SNAP25B: synaptosomal-associated protein 25)

in origin. Hereditary neuropathy is represented by Charcot–Marie–Tooth (CMT) disease, a heterogeneous entity, the most common inherited NMD with estimated prevalence of 40 per 100,000. Acquired neuropathies are usually due to vitamin deficiencies, drugs/toxins, immune dysfunction, and focal mononeuropathies. Among the acquired causes, Guillain–Barré syndrome (GBS) is the most common, with an annual incidence of 1.2–2.3 per 100,000. Outline of diagnostic approach to peripheral neuropathy is depicted in **Flowchart 8.19.1**.

Charcot–Marie–Tooth Disease (Hereditary Motor Sensory Neuropathy)

Charcot–Marie–Tooth disease is the most common hereditary neuropathy and comprises a heterogeneous group of inherited, nonmetabolic neuropathies. Salient features include positive family history, long slowly progressive course, and foot deformities. Individuals with CMT1 have a hypertrophic demyelinating neuropathy (onion bulbs in histopathology) and reduced nerve conduction velocities, whereas CMT2 denotes individuals with an axonal neuropathy and normal or slightly reduced nerve conduction velocities. CMT3 (Dejerine–Sottas disease) refers to individuals with a demyelinating peripheral neuropathy having a more severe phenotype presenting in infancy. CMT4 refers to autosomal recessive CMT, whereas CMT 1, 2, and 3 are historically considered autosomal dominant conditions.

Distal weakness, impaired sensation, and diminished or absent reflexes are the salient features. Individuals present with complaints of clumsiness, slippage of slippers, difficulty in running or climbing stairs, or impaired fine motor skills (such as writing, buttoning clothes, or tying shoelaces). High arches, hammertoes, pes cavus, and claw hands are useful clinical indicators for hereditary neuropathy. Sensory symptoms may include numbness, dysesthesias, or ataxia. Autonomic symptoms, such as abnormal sweating, cardiac arrhythmias, hypotension, or bowel and bladder dysfunction, may accompany peripheral neuropathy.

One should keep in mind that in large families with known hereditary neuropathies, only 20% of the affected family members seek medical attention because of its symptoms. One should inquire in detail before arriving at a conclusion regarding family history—difficulty in running; sports or military activities; high-arched feet or flat feet; hammer or

Flowchart 8.19.1: Diagnostic approach to peripheral neuropathy.

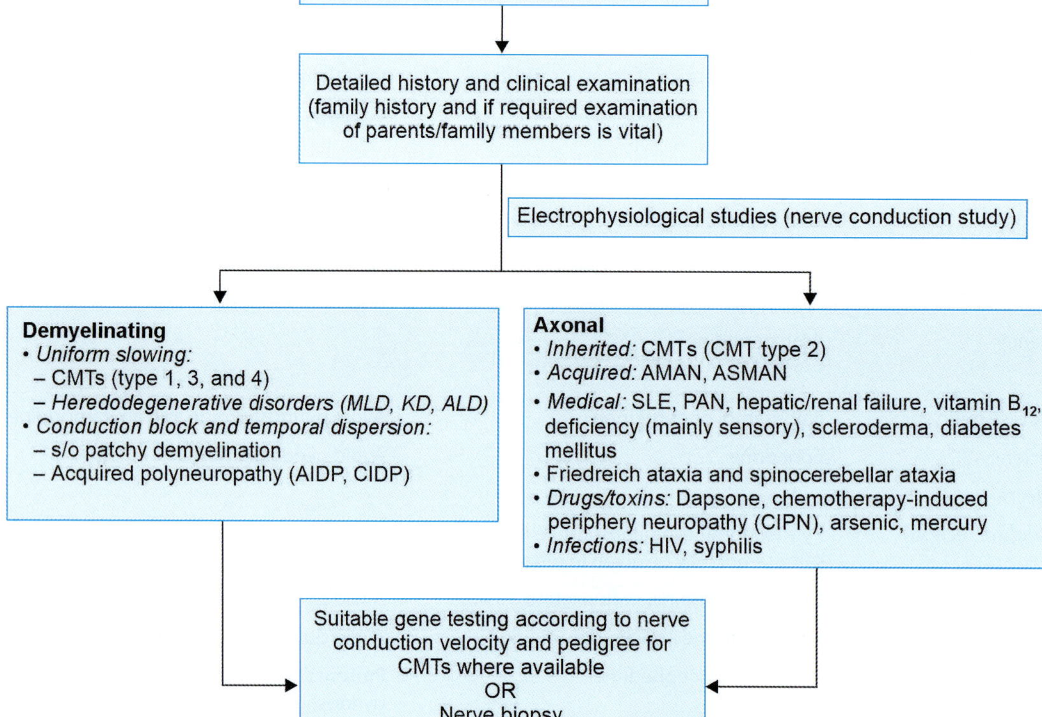

[AIDP: acute (chronic) inflammatory demyelinating polyneuropathy; ALD: adrenoleukodystrophy; AMAN: acute motor axonal neuropathy; ASMAN: acute sensory motor axonal neuropathy; CMT: Charcot–Marie–Tooth disease; KD: Krabbe disease; MLD: metachromatic leukodystrophy; PAN: polyarteritis nodosa; SLE: systemic lupus erythematosus]

curled-up toes; claw hands; wasting of muscles; foot troubles; foot ulcers; use of orthosis, arthritis, or poliomyelitis (incorrect diagnosis); and difficulty in walking on heels and toes.

There are various gene locations and known protein abnormalities associated with various forms of CMT (hereditary motor sensory neuropathy) and the clinical subtypes.

Guillain–Barré Syndrome

Guillain–Barré syndrome is a common cause of acute flaccid paralysis in children. Many subtypes have been described and include acute inflammatory demyelinating polyradiculoneuropathy (AIDP), acute motor axonal neuropathy (AMAN), acute motor and sensory axonal neuropathy, and the Miller–Fisher syndrome (MFS). There are many variants of GBS, such as acute pandysautonomia, acute sensory neuropathy, Bickerstaff brainstem encephalitis, acute paraplegic variant, acute ophthalmoparesis variant, pharyngo-cervico-brachial variant, and polyneuritis cranialis.

About two-thirds GBS cases have an antecedent infection 1–6 weeks prior to symptom onset, generally an upper respiratory tract infection or gastroenteritis. The clinical manifestations include an acute-onset symmetrical ascending weakness (both proximal and distal) with frequent facial weakness and respiratory weakness in one-fourth of the cases. Dysautonomia is also common. Pain and refusal to walk may be the initial manifestations. The axonal forms of GBS exhibit is more common in the Asian population, including India compared to western population, and is usually associated with *Campylobacter* infection. Weakness reaches its nadir by 2–4 weeks, with AMAN variants having a severe and faster progression. Areflexia is commonly seen, though AMAN variants may have preserved reflexes.

The diagnosis depends on classical clinical picture, electrophysiological findings, and cerebrospinal fluid (CSF) examination. Electrophysiology may reveal absent F-responses or H-reflexes, reduced compound muscle action potentials or sensory nerve action potentials (in axonal forms), prolonged distal latencies, reduced conduction velocities, abnormal temporal dispersion, and conduction blocks (in demyelinating types).[8] CSF analysis may reveal raised CSF protein concentration (80%) with the mononuclear cell count being either normal (albuminocytological dissociation) or <50 cells/mm^3.[9] Both electrophysiological studies and CSF analysis may be normal in the 1st week of the illness. Certain antibodies may also be detected in some subtypes, such as antiganglioside M1 and antiganglioside D1a antibodies in AMAN variant, antiganglioside Q1b in MFS variant, but they are not helpful in early establishment of diagnosis. Antigen involved in AIDP is unknown. **Boxes 8.19.5 and 8.19.6** give clinical diagnostic criteria and management principles for the patients suffering from GBS, whereas **Table 8.19.8** gives differential diagnosis of GBS.[10]

BOX 8.19.5: Clinical diagnostic features for Guillain–Barré syndrome.[9]

Features required for diagnosis:
- Progressive symmetrical weakness in more than one limb (might start with weakness only in the legs)
- Areflexia (or decreased tendon reflexes)

Features that strongly support diagnosis:
- Progression of symptoms over days to 4 weeks
- Minimal sensory symptoms
- Pain (often present) and autonomic dysfunction
- Cranial nerve involvement (may involve bilateral 7th cranial nerves)
- High concentration of protein in CSF and albumin-cytological dissociation
- Typical electrodiagnostic features

Features that should raise doubt about the diagnosis:
- High-grade fever at the onset of illness
- Severe pulmonary dysfunction with limited limb weakness at onset
- Severe sensory signs with limited weakness at onset and sharp sensory level
- Persistent and significant bowel bladder involvement
- Slow and staggered course of weakness progression (may consider subacute or chronic inflammatory demyelination)
- Marked persistent asymmetry of symptoms
- Increased CSF cell count (>50 × 10^6/L) suggesting other infections, such as HIV

(CSF: cerebrospinal fluid; HIV: human immunodeficiency virus)

ANTERIOR HORN CELL DISORDERS

Spinal muscular atrophy is the most common anterior horn cell disorder encountered in children. It will be discussed briefly further. Other disorders affecting the anterior horn cells are infective (polio, nonpolio enteroviruses, human immunodeficiency virus, West Nile virus, human T-lymphotropic virus, Lyme disease, and Japanese encephalitis); inflammatory (para/postinfectious/autoimmune, such as multifocal motor neuropathy and sarcoidosis); hereditary (amyotrophic lateral sclerosis or other motor neuron disorders that commonly manifest in adults), toxic; paraneoplastic; and vascular causes.

Spinal Muscular Atrophy

Spinal muscular atrophy is an autosomal recessive genetic disorder characterized by progressive degeneration of motor neurons of the spinal cord, which results in progressive muscle weakness and paralysis. It is one of the most common fatal autosomal recessive disorders caused by mutations in the survival motor neuron (*SMN*) gene present on *5q13*. The homozygous deletion of the *SMN1* exon 7 is observed in most of the patients and is being utilized as a reliable and sensitive SMA diagnostic test. *SMN2* produces less full-length transcript than *SMN1*; the number of *SMN2* copies has been shown to modulate the clinical phenotype; the more the number of copies, less severe the phenotype. SMA

BOX 8.19.6: Management of a patient with Guillain–Barré syndrome.[9,10]

Give good general care:
- Regularly monitor pulmonary function (initially every 2–4 hours, in stable phase every 6–12 hours)
- Regularly check for autonomic dysfunction (blood pressure, heart rate, pupils, and ileus)
- Check for swallowing dysfunction
- Recognize and treat pain and prevent decubitus ulcers and contractures
- Prevent and treat infections and pulmonary embolism
- Prevent corneal ulceration due to facial weakness

Consider specific treatment with IVIG or PE:
- *Indications to start IVIG or PE:*
  - Severely affected patients (inability to walk unaided)
  - *Start IVIG preferably within first 2 weeks from onset*: 2 g/kg over 2–5 days or 5 × PE with total exchange volume of five plasma volumes in 2 weeks (can be given up to 4 weeks from the onset of illness)
- *Indications for retreatment with IVIG:*
  - *Secondary deterioration after initial improvement or stabilization (treatment-related fluctuation)*: Treat with 2 g/kg over 2–5 days
  - No proven effect of retreatment with IVIG in patients who continue to worsen

Is there an indication for admission to an intensive care unit?
- Rapid progressive severe weakness often with impaired respiration (vital capacity <20 mL/kg)
- Respiratory failure
- Insufficient swallowing with high chance of pulmonary infection/aspiration
- Severe autonomic dysfunction

Fluctuations during the course of disease or continued slow progression:
- *Consider treatment-related fluctuation*: Repeat treatment
- Consider acute-onset CIDP (A-CIDP) and treat accordingly (intravenous steroids)

(A-CIDP: acute-onset chronic inflammatory demyelinating polyneuropathy; IVIG: intravenous immunoglobulin; PE: plasma exchange)

TABLE 8.19.8: Common differential diagnosis of Guillain–Barré syndrome.

Muscle disorders	*Neuromuscular junction disorders*	*Neuropathies*	*Central nervous system and spinal cord disorders*	*Others*
• Inflammatory myopathy • Periodic paralysis • Hypokalemia • Infections	• Myasthenia gravis • Eaton–Lambert syndrome • Botulism	• Diphtheritic neuropathy • Acute intermittent porphyria • Traumatic neuritis • Vasculitic neuropathy	• Acute myelopathy • Acute anterior poliomyelitis • Acute transverse myelitis • Brainstem stroke • Brainstem encephalitis • Acute cerebellar ataxia	*Antalgic conditions:* • Fracture • Trauma • Bone pain • Joint synovitis • Discitis • Scurvy • Leukemia

TABLE 8.19.9: Subtypes of spinal muscular atrophy.

Subtypes	*Age of onset*	*Maximum function achieved*	*SMN copy number*
Type 0 (very severe)	Neonatal with prenatal signs	Never sits	
Type 1 (severe) (Werdnig–Hoffmann disease)	0–6 months	Never sits	SMN2 ≤ 2 copies
Type 2 (intermediate)	7–18 months	Sits but never stands	SMN2: 3 copies
Type 3 (mild) (Kugelberg–Welander disease)	>18 months	Stands and walks	SMN2: 3–4 copies
Type 4 (adult)	10–30 years	Stands and walks	SMN2: 4 or more copies

(SMN: survival motor neuron)

is conventionally classified according to the age of onset and the highest motor function achieved, including SMA type 0 to describe the severe forms of prenatal onset SMA **(Table 8.19.9)**. A summary of recent advances in management of SMA is given in **Box 8.19.7**. Disease-targeted therapies such as Nusinersen, Zolgensma, and Risdiplam are approved by the US Food and Drug Administration (US-FDA) for SMA, but they have prohibitive-exorbitant costs.

BOX 8.19.7: Therapeutic approaches in spinal muscular atrophy.

- *SMN1 gene replacement*: Onasemnogene abeparvovec-xioi (Zolgensma) is an AAV9-based therapy that delivers a fully functional copy of SMN complementary (cDNA)
- *Promotion of exon 7 inclusion*:
  - Antisense oligonucleotides (Nusinersen/Spinraza is an ASO/ intrathecally-delivered splicing modifier that binds to the exon-7 silencer region on *SMN2* pre-mRNA
  - Risdiplam is an orally available, selective small molecule that modifies SMN2 pre-mRNA (pre-mRNA) splicing. It increases exon-7 inclusion in SMN2 mRNA transcripts and production of full-length SMN protein
- *SMN2 activation*: Histone deacetylase inhibitors (valproate, phenylbutyrate, and sodium butyrate) and hydroxyurea—investigational
- *Stabilization of SMN protein*: Aminoglycosides
- *Neuroprotection*: Riluzole, gabapentin, creatine, albuterol, olesoxime—investigational

(SMN: survival motor neuron)

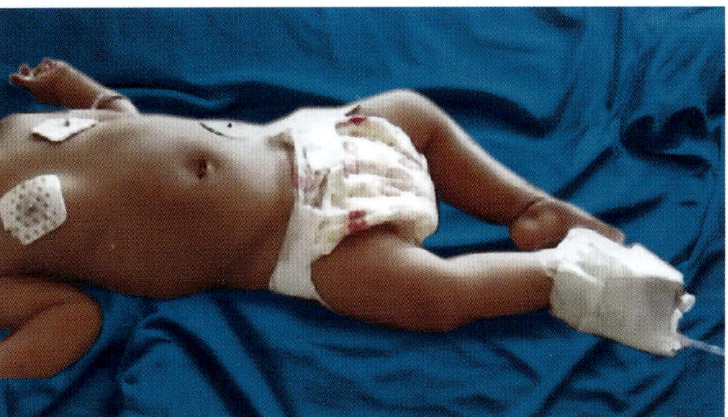

Fig. 8.19.5: Frog-like posture in a child with spinal muscular atrophy type 1.

Spinal muscular atrophy type 1 presents with profound hypotonia and flaccid weakness. Weak sucking, poor swallowing, labored breathing during feeding, frequent aspiration of food or secretions, and weak cry are commonly seen. Aspiration pneumonia is an important cause of morbidity and mortality. In the supine position, the lower extremities may be abducted and externally rotated in a "frog-leg" position, and the thorax is flattened anteroposteriorly, hence is bell-shaped because of intercostal weakness **(Fig. 8.19.5)**.[1] Children with type 2 disease are usually able to sit unassisted. They may develop kyphoscoliosis, tremors of upper limbs (polyminimyoclonus), poor swallowing, and respiratory insufficiency. Types 3 and 4 patients are usually able to walk. They may mimic LGMD or myopathy.

CONCLUSION

- Detailed history and examination, in a child with suspected neuromuscular disease, is essential to localize the lesion in the motor unit.
- Family history with pedigree drawing is imperative to reach appropriate diagnosis.
- Investigations must be planned judiciously while managing children with NMD.
- Never miss potentially treatable conditions, such as neuromuscular junction disorders, which may mimic common muscle disorders. They may also have potentially fatal complications, if unrecognized.
- Genetic counseling and prenatal diagnosis are important in selected clinical scenarios. When we come across families with multiple siblings affected by common conditions, such as SMA and DMD, the medical fraternity carries the blame for not offering appropriate genetic counseling and prenatal diagnosis.
- Early diagnosis is supported by the knowledge of the common initial clinical presentations of specific NMDs, and in many cases, the early diagnosis has potential implications for treatment and prevention of secondary conditions.
- Newer treatment options such as gene therapy, exon skipping, antisense oligonucleotide therapies give optimism for overall better outcome in the future, especially for DMD and SMA.

REFERENCES

1. McDonald MC. Clinical approach to the diagnostic evaluation of hereditary and acquired neuromuscular diseases. Phys Med Rehabil Clin N Am. 2012;23(3):495-563.
2. Bönnemann GC, Wang CH, Quijano-Roy S, Deconinck N, Bertini E, Ferreiro A, et al. Diagnostic approach to the congenital muscular dystrophies. Neuromuscul Disord. 2014;24(4):289-311.
3. North KN, Wang CH, Clarke N, Jungbluth H, Vainzof M, Dowling JJ, et al. Approach to the diagnosis of congenital myopathies. Neuromuscul Disord. 2014;24(2):97-116.
4. Birnkrant DJ, Bushby K, Bann CM, Apkon SD, Blackwell A, Brumbaugh D, et al. Diagnosis and management of Duchenne muscular dystrophy, part 1: diagnosis, and neuromuscular, rehabilitation, endocrine, and gastrointestinal and nutritional management. Lancet Neurol. 2018;17(3):251-67.
5. Straub V, Murphy A, Udd B, LGMD Workshop Study Group. 229th ENMC international workshop: Limb girdle muscular dystrophies - Nomenclature and reformed classification Naarden, the Netherlands, 17–19 March 2017. Neuromuscul Disord. 2018;28(8):702-10.
6. Lilleker JB, Keh YS, Roncaroli F, Sharma R, Roberts M. Metabolic myopathies: a practical approach. Pract Neurol. 2018;18(1):14-26.
7. Engel AG, Shen XM, Selcen D, Sine SM. Congenital myasthenic syndromes: pathogenesis, diagnosis, and treatment. Lancet Neurol. 2015;14(4):420-34.
8. England JD, Gronseth GS, Franklin G, Carter GT, Kinsella LJ, Cohen JA, et al. Evaluation of distal symmetric polyneuropathy: the role of laboratory and genetic testing (an evidence-based review). Muscle Nerve. 2009;39(1):116-25.

9. Leonhard SE, Mandarakas MR, Gondim FAA, Bateman K, Ferreira MLB, Cornblath DR, et al. Diagnosis and management of Guillain-Barré syndrome in ten steps. Nat Rev Neurol. 2019;15(11):671-83.
10. Joint Task Force of the EFNS and the PNS. European Federation of Neurological Societies/Peripheral Nerve Society Guideline on management of paraproteinemic demyelinating neuropathies. Report of a Joint Task Force of the European Federation of Neurological Societies and the Peripheral Nerve Society—first revision. J Peripher Nerv Syst. 2010;15(3):185-95.

8.20 Neurotoxicology

Vaishakh Anand, Vinayan KP

INTRODUCTION

Innumerable natural and synthetic substances are proven to be toxic to the human brain and nervous system. The clinical manifestations of these exposures vary widely depending on the route of exposure, level of exposure, coadministered substances, age of the subject, and coexisting disease conditions. Infants and young children are particularly vulnerable to the adverse effects of these substances since their brains are immature and developing. This chapter will describe common poisonings in children causing neurological manifestations; neurological toxic effects of various drugs, substances of abuse, and environmental toxins; neuroteratology; and developmental neurotoxins.

When a child arrives at the emergency department (ED) with impaired sensorium, numerous differential diagnoses could be made. Poisoning or exposure to chemicals is not uncommon cause in this situation. Some of the common etiologies that closely resemble poisonings are head trauma, metabolic disorders, psychiatric disorders, and central nervous system (CNS) infections. The neurological dysfunction may be isolated or part of the systemic derangement. The cluster of clinical features occurring together in a case of suspected poisoning is called *toxidromes* and helps identify the etiological agent. The common toxidromes and the responsive agents are listed in **Table 8.20.1**.

TABLE 8.20.1: Common toxidromes.

Toxidrome	*CNS effects*	*Vitals*	*Pupils and others*	*Examples of agents*
Sympathomimetic	Hallucination, agitation, excitement, tremors, seizures	Tachycardia, hypertension	Dilated pupils, diaphoresis	Cocaine, amphetamines, theophylline, caffeine
Cholinergic	Confusion, coma, fasciculations, seizures	Bradycardia, hypo/hypertension	Constricted pupils, salivation, lacrimation, urination, defecation, gastrointestinal distress, emesis (SLUDGE syndrome)	Organophosphates, carbamates, nicotine, physostigmine
Anticholinergic	Confusion, disorientation, agitation, hallucinations, incoordination, ataxia, and psychosis ("mad, hot, dry, and blind")	Hyperthermia, tachycardia, dry skin	Dilated pupils, urinary retention	Atropine, datura poisoning, TCA, antihistamines
Opioid	CNS depression with coma, flaccidity	Bradycardia, bradypnea	Pinpoint pupils	Heroin, morphine, oxycodone, fentanyl
Sedative-hypnotic	Confusion, stupor, coma, sedation, ataxia	Bradycardia, hypotension	Constricted pupils	Benzodiazepines, barbiturates, alcohol
Serotonin syndrome	Confusion, agitation, clonus, hyperreflexia, rigidity	Hyperthermia, tachycardia, autonomic hyperactivity	Dilated	MAO inhibitors ± SSRIs, TCAs, L-tryptophan

(CNS: central nervous system; MAO: monoamine oxidase; SSRIs: selective serotonin reuptake inhibitors; TCAs: tricyclic antidepressants)

BIOLOGICAL TOXINS

Snakebite

There are over 236 different kinds of snakes in India, 15 of which are venomous. The "Big Four species" are the group of four that are considered to be the most significant: Common krait (*Bungarus caeruleus*), common cobra (*Naja naja*), saw-scaled viper (*Echis carinatus*), and Russel's viper (*Daboia russelii*). Among these, krait and cobra are neurotoxic. The snake venom contains numerous proteins, peptides, and lipids with various biological actions that differ according to the species. The neurotoxic effects of krait and viper venom are related to the neuromuscular transmission blockade and not due to CNS effects since it cannot cross the blood–brain barrier. Krait venom contains a phospholipase A2 complex called β-bungarotoxin, which binds presynaptically at the neuromuscular junction (NMJ). It destroys the vesicles carrying acetylcholine and affects the formation of new vesicles. This results in an irreversible neuromuscular blockade and skeletal muscle paralysis. The earliest clinical manifestation is ptosis followed by external ophthalmoplegia and then descending paralysis. Often, the history of snakebite is not obtained since krait bite is notorious for being painless and often nocturnal. On the contrary, cobra toxin contains α-cobratoxin, a three-fingered complex that binds to the acetylcholine receptors (AChR) postsynaptically, preventing the attachment of acetylcholine on it. This is more often reversible with antisnake venom (ASV). The ASV available in India is not species-specific and contains pooled antibodies against the toxins present in all Big Four species. Hence, it is not the identification of the snake but the clinical features that decide the initiation of ASV. In cases of cobra envenomation, anticholinesterase drugs such as neostigmine may help in the reversal of neuromuscular blockade.

Botulism

Botulism is a syndrome of acute flaccid paralysis caused by the toxin produced by *Clostridium botulinum* bacteria. Three forms of botulism exist: (1) Infantile botulism, (2) food-borne botulism, and (3) wound botulism. Botulinum toxin attaches to the presynapse of the NMJ and cleaves the SNAP-25 protein, resulting in the inhibition of acetylcholine release from the synaptic vesicles. This produces the characteristic clinical features of botulism with or without gastrointestinal (GI) manifestations.

Infantile botulism is caused by ingestion of the spores of botulinum toxin-producing strains, with subsequent spore germination, multiplication, and production of botulinum toxin in the large intestine. A major association reported commonly is the ingestion of honey. Infants appear floppy and lethargic with head drop. Cranial nerve palsy results in bulbar dysfunction with poor sucking, drooling, and oculomotor palsy followed by descending paralysis. Constipation is commonly present rather than diarrhea. Food-borne botulism results from the ingestion of preformed botulinum toxin in improperly canned or preserved food items. Along with the classical neurological signs, GI symptoms such as vomiting and diarrhea may be present. Detection of the presence of the toxin or organism in fluid or feces confirms the diagnosis. In cases of suspected botulism, human botulism immunoglobulin along with supportive measures should be provided.

Litchi-associated Toxic Encephalopathy

Muzaffarpur district of Bihar has been witnessing seasonal outbreaks of unexplained encephalopathy and deaths during premonsoon periods in children for many decades. The typical clinical scenario is children developing acute encephalopathy mostly in the early morning along with refractory hypoglycemia and metabolic acidosis. In severe cases, cerebral edema sets in with high rates of mortality. An infectious etiology was ruled out since there was no fever, serum inflammatory markers were absent, and the cerebrospinal fluid (CSF) study was normal. Later, a case–control study detected two major epidemiological associations in cases: Litchi consumption and absence of an evening meal in the preceding 24 hours.[1] Toxins present in litchi, namely hypoglycin A and methylenecyclopropylglycine (MCPG), were implicated in the pathogenesis. These toxins act at the mitochondrial level, inhibiting the beta-oxidation of fatty acids and resulting in hypoketotic hypoglycemia with metabolic acidosis. Widespread awareness programs have reduced the incidence of such cases in later years.

Neurolathyrism

Lathyrism is a neurodegenerative condition caused by excessive and prolonged consumption of *Lathyrus sativus* (grass pea). The culprit is a neurotoxin named BOAA (beta-*n*-oxalylamino-L-alanine), an analog of glutamate that results in excitotoxicity mediated through α-amino-3-hydroxy-5-methyl-4-isoxazolepropionic acid (AMPA) receptors. It primarily affects the corticospinal tracts, resulting in progressive spastic paraparesis. Neurolathyrism was reported in impoverished communities, especially during periods of famine when other food crops were not readily available. With widespread awareness programs and the availability of other cereals and pulses, the incidence of this condition is almost nil currently. There is no curative treatment for this condition.

INSECTICIDES

Organophosphate and Carbamate Poisoning

Organophosphates (malathion, parathion, diazinon, fenthion, chlorpyrifos, and ethion) and carbamates are potent cholinesterase inhibitors capable of systemic toxicity following cutaneous exposure, inhalation, or ingestion. They cause irreversible (organophosphates) or transient (carbamates) inhibition of the acetylcholinesterase enzyme, leading to excess of acetylcholine in the NMJ or neuronal synapses, leading to cholinergic symptoms. Acute cholinergic poisoning is characterized by bradycardia, miosis, lacrimation, salivation, bronchorrhea, bronchospasm, urination, emesis, and diarrhea as the main clinical manifestations, which are related to excess muscarinic action. Due to the nicotinic action at NMJ, skeletal muscle weakness and fasciculations may be present along with CNS symptoms. With some highly fat-soluble organophosphorus agents, an intermediate syndrome with neck flexion weakness, decreased deep tendon reflexes, cranial nerve abnormalities, proximal muscle weakness, and respiratory insufficiency develops 24–96 hours after the exposure. After 1–3 weeks of acute exposure, some individuals develop organophosphorus agent-induced delayed neuropathy (OPIDN).

Decontamination, general supportive care, and the administration of certain antidotes, such as oximes and atropine, are all part of the treatment. Activated charcoal used as a single dose works best if administered within an hour of consumption. These therapies usually do not work well for delayed or intermediate exposures.

Lindane

Lindane (1,2,3,4,5,6-hexachlorocyclohexane) is used as a topical pediculicide worldwide. It can enter the CNS following excess topical application or accidental ingestion and result in significant neurological toxicity. Infants, small children, the elderly, patients with other skin conditions, and those receiving repeated treatment are at risk. Acute toxicity is associated with generalized seizures and altered mental status. Along with general supportive measures, active seizure management needs priority. Phenytoin is known to exacerbate lindane-associated seizures and should be avoided.

HEAVY METALS

Lead

Children are exposed to lead through variable sources such as chips of paint or lead dust from lead-painted surfaces; food or beverages stored or served in lead-soldered cans or lead-glazed pottery; water from lead-soldered plumbing; automobile emissions; and lead-using industries. Nervous system affection is an important feature of acute and chronic lead poisoning, along with blood and renal involvement. Although no "safe blood lead level" exists, levels >10 μg/dL have been consistently shown to be associated with neurobehavioral issues in children. Acute lead encephalopathy is associated with levels of >90 μg/dL. It is clinically characterized by persistent vomiting, altered or fluctuating state of consciousness, ataxia, seizures, or coma. Chronic lead toxicity is associated with neurocognitive deficits, behavioral issues, hearing loss, and peripheral neuropathy. Oral meso-2,3-dimercaptosuccinic acid (DMSA), dimercaprol [British anti-Lewisite (BAL)], and calcium disodium versenate ($CaNa_2EDTA$) are the chelating agents recommended for lead poisoning.

Mercury

Mercury poisoning can be due to exposure to elemental, inorganic, or organic mercury. While acute mercury poisoning is associated with GI symptoms, chronic toxicity is predominated by neurological manifestations such as coarse tremors, personality change, and peripheral neuropathy. Erethism or mad hatter disease, characterized by a change in personality, anxiety, irritability, excitability, pathologic shyness, insomnia, memory loss, etc., was historically associated with chronic mercury exposure. Acrodynia or pink disease is specifically seen in infants and young children who get exposed to mercury salts. Apart from supportive measures, dimercaprol (BAL), DMSA, and 2,3-dimercapto-propanesulfonate (DMPS) may be used for chelation, especially in acute toxicity.

Thallium

Thallium is present in rat poison, ant killer, and several herbal medications. Thallium toxicity is characterized by the triad of abdominal pain, alopecia, and mixed peripheral neuropathy. Other neurologic effects such as cranial neuropathies involving the optic and oculomotor nerves, dementia, delirium, and seizures are not uncommon. Painful distal glossitis, Mees' lines, and cardiovascular manifestations such as hypertension and shock are other clinical features. Hemodialysis is the best way to reduce blood thallium levels.

Arsenic

Chronic arsenic poisoning is associated with prominent cutaneous manifestations such as diffuse hyperpigmentation, raindrop pigmentation, and arsenic keratosis. Neurological manifestations include asymmetric sensory-motor polyneuropathy mimicking Guillain–Barré syndrome. Cardiovascular, renal, and hepatic manifestations may also be associated. Chelation is useful only in cases with acute toxicity.

DRUGS OF ABUSE

Cocaine

Cocaine is a stimulant alkaloid derived from the leaves of *Erythroxylum coca*. It inhibits the reuptake of norepinephrine, dopamine, and serotonin, which explains its CNS and systemic effects. Acute toxicity symptoms are supposedly due to norepinephrine excess, leading to hyperthermia, tremors, tachycardia, cardiac dysrhythmias, myocardial infarctions, diaphoresis, vasoconstriction, and hypertension. The behavioral effects such as a sense of well-being, excitement, and increased alertness are attributed to its dopaminergic action. It can lead to psychomotor agitation, seizures, stroke, or intracranial hemorrhage. Symptomatic management is done using benzodiazepines, alpha, and beta-blockers.

Cannabis

Cannabis is a commonly abused illicit substance taken by inhalation or ingestion. The active ingredient is tetrahydrocannabinol (THC). Clinical features postintoxication include cognitive slowing, short-term memory loss, euphoria, analgesia, appetite stimulation, conjunctival hyperemia, pupillary dilation, and tachycardia. Supportive therapy is indicated along with benzodiazepines for seizures and agitation.

Opiates

Opioids are natural and synthetic substances with morphine-like activity. Opioids used therapeutically other than morphine are hydromorphone, codeine, buprenorphine, meperidine, methadone, oxycodone, and fentanyl. Heroin is the prototypic recreationally abused opioid. Opioids exert their action on the limbic system, thalamus, and hypothalamus through three receptors: (1) mu (μ), (2) kappa (κ), and (3) delta (δ). Opioid intoxication in an adolescent may be due to recreational drug abuse, whereas in a young child, drug overdose needs to be considered. The clinical features of opioid intoxication include apnea, CNS depression, miosis, seizures, and cardiovascular collapse. Naloxone is the preferred antagonist for reversing acute opioid toxicity. It is a synthetic derivative of oxymorphone that binds opioid receptors competitively.

THERAPEUTIC DRUGS

Barbiturates

Barbiturate toxicity is usually caused by accidental drug overdose or suicidal attempts. Clinical features include confusion, sedation, and ataxia. High doses may lead to respiratory depression, miosis, areflexic paralysis, and brainstem dysfunction. Activated charcoal may be used in acute toxicities. Respiratory and cardiovascular support remains the most important step in management. Unlike benzodiazepines, no specific antidote is available for barbiturate poisoning.

Benzodiazepines

Benzodiazepine overdose can produce ataxia in children more commonly than CNS depression compared to adults. Depending on the dose, other CNS manifestations such as confusion, somnolence, and even coma with normal vitals may be seen. Benzodiazepine toxicity in isolation is not considered fatal. However, coadministration of other CNS suppressant medications may lead to respiratory depression and even death. Supportive care and the particular benzodiazepine antagonist flumazenil are the two mainstays of treatment.

Antipsychotics

First-generation antipsychotics act through the blockade of D2 dopamine receptors in the brain postsynaptically. They are associated with extrapyramidal symptoms (EPS), tardive dyskinesia, hyperprolactinemia, neuroleptic malignant syndrome (NMS), QT prolongation, and sudden death. Acute dystonic reactions are common with these drugs and are not dose-related. First-generation antihistaminic drug diphenhydramine is commonly used to revert this reaction. Atypical antipsychotics also have a similar mechanism of action with better selectivity and less affinity than first-generation antipsychotics. They have lesser extrapyramidal adverse effects.

Neuroleptic malignant syndrome is a unique and life-threatening adverse effect associated with antipsychotic use, especially first-generation ones. It is characterized by a tetrad of mental status changes, rigidity, fever, and dysautonomia. Myoglobinuria and acute renal failure may complicate the clinical condition. Treatment consists of intensive supportive care, aggressive fluid management, and dantrolene or bromocriptine administration.

Tricyclic Antidepressants

Tricyclic antidepressants (TCAs) act by the inhibition of reuptake of norepinephrine and serotonin presynaptically. TCA toxicity can cause hyperthermia, flushing, dilated pupils, delirium, ileus, urinary retention, and delirium due to its anticholinergic action. The antihistaminic action can cause sedation, and the gamma-aminobutyric acid type A ($GABA_A$) receptor antagonism can cause seizures. TCA toxicity also produces cardiac toxicity through inhibition of the fast sodium channels in the His–Purkinje system and myocardium. Management protocols include benzodiazepines for seizures, sodium bicarbonate for cardiac toxicities, and supportive measures.

Salicylates

Salicylates are present in various preparations from aspirin to herbal medicines. Their toxicity can have neurologic, pulmonary, and hepatic manifestations. The acute toxicity is characterized by the triad of hyperventilation, tinnitus, and GI manifestations. It can also cause high anion gap metabolic acidosis along with respiratory alkalosis caused by central neurogenic hyperventilation. Management considerations include fluid and electrolyte correction, serum and urine alkalinization, correction of hypoglycemia, and hemodialysis.

Reye syndrome is a type of acute toxic noninflammatory encephalopathy described in children associated with hepatic dysfunction. Clinical features include vomiting, confusion, recurrent seizures, coma, and hepatomegaly. The use of aspirin in the setting of an acute viral illness was identified as a strong risk factor for Reye syndrome. This led to a drastic decline in the use of aspirin as an antipyretic, and the incidence of Reye syndrome also reduced. It is supposed that many of the previously diagnosed cases of Reye syndrome may in fact be inborn errors of metabolism such as fatty acid oxidation defects.

Theophylline

Theophylline inhibits adenosine receptors and has indirect adrenergic activity. Toxicity can be associated with nausea, vomiting, tachycardia, and agitation. Seizures are a major neurological manifestation, especially in younger children. Cardiac arrhythmias are a major cause of mortality in theophylline toxicity. Activated charcoal and hemodialysis can be used for elimination from the GI tract and serum.

Calcineurin Inhibitors

Cyclosporine and tacrolimus are calcineurin inhibitors widely used as immunosuppressants. They bind to cyclophilin and FK-binding protein, respectively, and inhibit calcineurin, which is crucial for transcriptional activation of various cytokines such as interleukin-2 (IL-2). Subsequently, the proliferation of cytotoxic T cells is inhibited. Both these drugs are used widely for immunosuppression in solid organ transplantation. While both can cause neurological toxicity, cyclosporine has a more favorable adverse effect profile. Adverse effects may be related to direct CNS involvement or related to complications such as acute hypertension or nephrotoxicity-related metabolic disturbances. Seizures, tremors, encephalopathy, headache, and visual disturbances may be present. Posterior reversible encephalopathy syndrome (PRES) may present as encephalopathy, seizures, and focal neurological deficits. The therapeutic options are reducing the drug dosage, changing to oral formulations, or discontinuing the medicine.

Antineoplastic Drugs

Anticancer therapy-induced neurologic side effects can occur from direct toxic effects on the nervous system, or indirectly from drug-induced metabolic disturbances or cerebrovascular disturbances. Often, the neurological toxicity of chemotherapeutic agents is confused with disease relapse or metastasis.

Platinum-based Compounds

Platinum-based compounds are among the most common chemotherapeutic agents causing neurotoxicity.

Cisplatin

Peripheral neuropathy and ototoxicity are the most common neurological adverse effects associated with cisplatin. Symmetrical sensory polyneuropathy develops following the affection of the dorsal root ganglion. Clinical features are numbness, paresthesias, and pain. Examination reveals loss of vibration and proprioception with loss of deep tendon reflexes. Reducing the dose or discontinuing the drug is indicated based on the severity. In many patients, the symptoms progress even after drug discontinuation, which is called the coasting effect.

Cisplatin can cause dose-dependent high-frequency sensorineural hearing loss due to the toxic effects on the outer hair cells in the organ of Corti and the vascularized epithelium in the lateral wall of the cochlea. Most often, this condition is irreversible. Children <5 years old, subjects with CNS tumors, subjects receiving cranial irradiation, and those with renal dysfunction are particularly at risk. Sodium thiosulfate has been approved recently by the Food and Drug Administration (FDA) for reducing cisplatin-related ototoxicity in children. Other drugs tried for the same are amifostine, vitamin E, and diethyldithiocarbamate. Cisplatin has also been associated with an encephalopathy syndrome similar to PRES following infusion.

Oxaliplatin and Carboplatin

Oxaliplatin is well known to cause acute sensory neuropathy with distal limbs and perioral paresthesias, pharyngeal, and laryngeal dysesthesias shortly after an infusion and is usually reversible. Limiting the exposure to cold during the immediate postinfusion period was found to mitigate these symptoms. Oxaliplatin can also cause chronic sensory neuropathy. In contrast to cisplatin and oxaliplatin, carboplatin is less recognized to cause deleterious effects on the nervous system.

Methotrexate

Methotrexate is a dihydrofolate reductase inhibitor, widely used in childhood cancers and pediatric rheumatological conditions. It is well known to cause acute, subacute, and chronic neurological toxicities based on the dose and route of administration. The most common adverse effect associated with intrathecal (IT) methotrexate is aseptic meningitis presenting with neck and back pain and headache. Most of the time, only symptomatic management is needed. Noncompressive transverse myelopathy develops in some subjects receiving IT methotrexate, especially if cranial radiotherapy is received concurrently. Following high-dose methotrexate administration, some patients develop altered sensorium, seizures, and sleepiness within the first 24 hours. Another characteristic presentation is the development of stroke-like episodes with transient hemiparesis or hemianopia, weeks after a high dose of IT methotrexate. Diffusion-weighted images of the magnetic resonance imaging (MRI) brain show diffusion restriction in the involved white matter, which returns to baseline later. Methotrexate-related leukoencephalopathy is a dreaded long-term neurological complication of methotrexate use, especially in those who had concurrent CNS irradiation. MRI brain typically shows diffuse white matter T2/fluid-attenuated inversion recovery (FLAIR) hyperintensities without contrast enhancement, mimicking a leukoencephalopathy.

Methotrexate-induced transverse myelopathy warrants discontinuation of the drug, and further administration of the drug is contraindicated. For other manifestations, discontinuing the drug depends on the clinical severity. Therapeutic agents tried apart from leucovorin are aminophylline, dextromethorphan, cyanocobalamin, and intravenous (IV) steroids. Accidental overdose of methotrexate can be treated with IV or IT glucarpidase, a recombinant enzyme that rapidly hydrolyzes the carboxyl-terminal glutamate residue from extracellular methotrexate into inactive metabolites.

Vinca Alkaloids

Vincristine

Peripheral neuropathy is the most well-known adverse effect associated with vincristine. Almost all patients receiving vincristine will develop some degree of neuropathy. Owing to the antimicrotubule activity of vincristine, the microtubules in the axons of the neurons are disrupted. This results in sensory or mixed axonal polyneuropathy. The symptoms start as distal paresthesias, muscle cramps, and mild distal weakness resulting in foot drop. Rarely, cranial neuropathy can set in, resulting often in ophthalmoparesis. Due to the involvement of the autonomic nervous system, subjects may experience colicky abdominal pain, constipation, or even paralytic ileus. Examination reveals an absence of deep tendon reflexes most commonly. Reducing the dosage or stopping the medication altogether is advised because the severity of symptoms is dose-related. The signs and symptoms are reversible in the majority of cases, albeit taking months. Vincristine neuropathy also may be associated with the coasting effect. Oral glutamine supplementation has been tried without much evidence. Symptomatic management using gabapentin or duloxetine is indicated if pain predominates.

Vinblastine can also cause similar neuropathy features but with lesser incidence.

Other Agents

L-asparaginase is commonly used in acute lymphoblastic leukemia (ALL). Asparaginase does not directly cause neurotoxicity, but it can cause cerebral sinus venous thrombosis (CSVT) because of its prothrombotic impact. Cytarabine may be associated with acute cerebellar syndrome following high doses, hours to days after the infusion. Although it is reversible with drug discontinuation, symptoms may be permanent in some cases. Cyclophosphamide and ifosfamide are associated with encephalopathy after IV infusion, resembling PRES clinically and radiologically. Spontaneous improvement as well as improvement with steroids and methylene blue is reported.

Antimicrobials

Beta-lactam Antibiotics

Beta-lactam antibiotics with penicillin being the prototype are known to be associated with multiple neurological adverse effects. It may be characterized by seizures, myoclonus, altered sensorium, delirium, and hyperreflexia. Cefepime, the fourth-generation cephalosporin, is reported to be associated with seizures and nonconvulsive status epilepticus (NCSE), particularly in subjects with impaired renal functions. Among carbapenems, imipenem is implicated in reducing seizure threshold. It is thought that the proconvulsive action of beta-lactam antibiotics results from their blockage of GABA receptors.

Aminoglycosides

Ototoxicity and neuromuscular blockade are the most important neurotoxic effects of aminoglycosides. They are linked to vestibular and cochlear toxicity in patients who use the medication for extended periods. Neomycin, kanamycin, and amikacin are considered more ototoxic, while gentamicin and tobramycin are mostly vestibulotoxic. The neuromuscular blocking action of aminoglycosides becomes clinically significant when coadministered with another neuromuscular blocking drug such as succinylcholine. For the same reason, they are avoided in subjects with myasthenia gravis or congenital myasthenic syndromes.

Drug-induced Peripheral Neuropathy

Many antimicrobials are implicated in peripheral neuropathy. The most important one is isoniazid, which can cause a sensory polyneuropathy manifesting as numbness and paresthesias of the distal extremities. Other antimicrobials implicated in causing peripheral neuropathy include nucleoside reverse transcriptase inhibitors (NRTIs) such as didanosine, stavudine, dapsone, metronidazole, nitrofurantoin, fluoroquinolones, and ethambutol.

Ethambutol is also associated with optic neuropathy, mostly after 3–5 months of therapy. The clinical features are reduced visual acuity or red-green color blindness. Other antibiotics implicated in optic neuropathy are chloramphenicol, linezolid, isoniazid, and dapsone.

DEVELOPMENTAL NEUROTOXICITY

Developmental neurotoxicity refers to the adverse effects of toxic substances on the developing brain in utero or early postnatal years when development and maturation occur the most. About 214 industrial chemicals are known to be toxic to the adult brain. Among those, a few are established to cause developmental neurotoxicity at even lower levels. The vulnerability of the developing brain to toxic substances is related to many factors. In utero, the placenta is not an effective barrier to many toxins and even concentrates some such as alcohol, lead, and mercury. While breastfeeding, many environmental toxins are transferred to infants. The immaturity of the blood–brain barrier also plays a role in developmental toxicity. Initial studies identified lead, methylmercury, polychlorinated biphenyls, arsenic, and toluene as developmental neurotoxins.[2] Later, manganese, fluoride, chlorpyrifos, dichlorodiphenyltrichloroethane (DDT), tetrachloroethylene, and polybrominated diphenyl ethers were added to the list.[3] Lead is the most extensively studied developmental neurotoxin, and it was concluded that no safe lead levels exist. Another study revealed that the overall intelligence quotient (IQ) losses linked to lead, pesticides, and other neurotoxicants were comparable to, or even higher than, the losses brought on by medical occurrences such as congenital heart disease, traumatic brain damage, brain tumors, and premature birth.[4] Prenatal exposure to manganese, organophosphates, and phthalates has been linked to neurodevelopmental disorders such as attention-deficit hyperactivity disorder (ADHD) and autism spectrum disorder (ASD). Organochlorine compounds such as DDT and organophosphates are notorious for persisting in the environment and body. Many studies showed an inverse association between the serum levels of these compounds (which indicate accumulated exposures) and neurodevelopmental performance. Endosulfan, an organochlorine pesticide, was implicated in causing many birth defects and neurological toxicities in the Kasaragod district of Kerala, where aerial spraying of this pesticide was done for 20 years. However, the initial epidemiological studies pointing toward this association were found to be methodologically and statistically incorrect later.[5] Larger robust epidemiological studies are needed to establish the association between the higher prevalence of birth defects and endosulfan.

There is mounting evidence that links behavioral problems and neurodevelopmental delays to air pollution. The main culprits are perfluorinated chemicals, carbon monoxide, and tobacco smoke. A study reported that infants exposed prenatally to polycyclic aromatic hydrocarbons from vehicle exhausts had a lower IQ and more cognitive impairment at 5 years than infants exposed to lower concentrations of these substances.[6]

NEUROTERATOLOGY

Many neurotoxins are confirmed to have teratogenic effects depending on the timing of administration, the dose, distribution, and placental transfer. The most well-known is prenatal exposure to alcohol, which can cause a range of physical, behavioral, and cognitive effects collectively termed as *fetal alcohol spectrum disorder* (FASD). The major features include facial dysmorphism: Short palpebral fissures, midfacial hypoplasia, and thin upper lip; pre- and postnatal growth retardation, microcephaly, and intellectual disability. *Fetal hydantoin syndrome* is caused by prenatal exposure to phenytoin. It is characterized by dysmorphic features such as short neck, low-set ears, cleft lip and palate, deep nasal bridge, and hypoplastic distal phalanges of both upper and lower limbs. Microcephaly and intellectual disability also may be associated.

First-trimester exposure to sodium valproate is well known to cause neural tube defects such as spina bifida and meningomyelocele and other major malformations. Early maternal folic acid intake can ameliorate this risk. Similarly, an increased association between ASD and prenatal exposure to valproate has been proven in many studies. The Neurodevelopmental Effects of Antiepileptic Drugs (NEAD) study prospectively evaluated the cognitive effects of offspring born to mothers on antiepileptic drug monotherapy (i.e., carbamazepine, lamotrigine, phenytoin, or valproate) at 6 years.[7] Children exposed to valproate had IQ scores seven to ten points lower than those exposed to lamotrigine, phenytoin, or carbamazepine. Other identified neuroteratogens include isotretinoin, lead, mercury, cocaine, marijuana, and chemotherapeutic agents such as cisplatin, methotrexate, and 5-fluorouracil (5-FU).

CONCLUSION

Developing brain is vulnerable to the toxic effects of a variety of natural and synthetic chemicals. The clinical manifestations and prognosis might differ depending on the degree and route of administration as well as the age at exposure. Biological toxins should be considered in suspected cases especially in rural settings. Substance abuse among adolescents is rising exponentially. Hence, pediatricians should be made aware of the toxidromes associated with drugs of abuse along with those of commonly used therapeutic agents. Developmental neurotoxicity is an important domain which needs further large-scale research studies. This chapter describes the most common neurotoxic agents and their manifestations to help the pediatricians manage them appropriately in an emergency setting.

REFERENCES

1. Shrivastava A, Kumar A, Thomas JD, Laserson KF, Bhushan G, Carter MD, et al. Association of acute toxic encephalopathy with litchi consumption in an outbreak in Muzaffarpur, India, 2014: a case-control study. Lancet Glob Health. 2017;5(4):e458-66.
2. Grandjean P, Landrigan P. Developmental neurotoxicity of industrial chemicals. Lancet. 2006;368(9553):2167-78.
3. Grandjean P, Landrigan PJ. Neurobehavioural effects of developmental toxicity. Lancet Neurol. 2014;13(3):330-8.
4. Bellinger DC. A strategy for comparing the contributions of environmental chemicals and other risk factors to neurodevelopment of children. Environ Health Perspect. 2012;120(4):501-7.
5. Sreekumar KM, Prathapan KD. A critique of the epidemiological studies on health in allegedly endosulfan-affected areas in Kasaragod, Kerala. Curr Sci. 2013;104(1):16-21.
6. Perera FP, Li Z, Whyatt R, Hoepner L, Wang S, Camann D, et al. Prenatal airborne polcyclic aromatic hydrocarbon exposure and child IQ at age 5 years. Pediatrics. 2009;124(2):e195-202.
7. Meador KJ, Baker GA, Browning N, Cohen MJ, Bromley RL, Clayton-Smith J, et al. Fetal antiepileptic drug exposure and cognitive outcomes at age 6 years (NEAD study): a prospective observational study. Lancet Neurol. 2013;12(3):244-52.

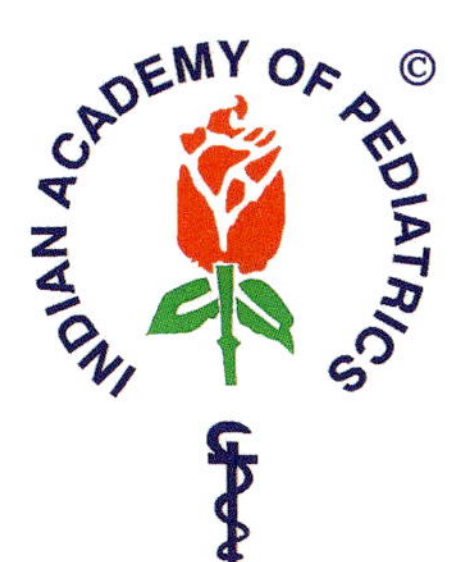

Partha's

IAP Textbook of PEDIATRICS

Eighth Edition

Volume 2

Founder Editors

(Late) A Parthasarathy, PSN Menon, MKC Nair

Editor-in-Chief

PSN Menon MD MNAMS
Former Professor
Department of Pediatrics
Sub-Dean, Consultant-In-Charge
Pediatric Endocrinology and Genetics
All India Institute of Medical Sciences
New Delhi, India

Executive Editor

Alok Gupta MD
Pediatrician, Counselor and Environmentalist
Pediatric Specialities Clinic, Jaipur
Former Assistant Professor of Pediatrics
MGM University
Jaipur, Rajasthan, India

Academic Editors

MKC Nair MD PhD DSc FIACAM FAMS
Director, NIMS-Spectrum
Child Development Research Centre (CDRC)
Thiruvananthapuram, Kerala, India
Formerly Vice Chancellor, KUHS
Formerly Director, CDC Kerala (Adolescent Health)

Piyush Gupta MD FRCPCH FAMS
Former Principal, Professor and Head
Department of Pediatrics
University College of Medical Sciences
and Guru Teg Bahadur Hospital
New Delhi, India

Ramachandran Padmanabhan MD DNB
Professor of Eminence, Department of Pediatrics
Head, Division of Clinical Research and Head, Bioethics Unit
Sri Ramachandra Institute of Higher Education and Research
Chennai, Tamil Nadu, India

Ritabrata Kundu MD
Professor
Department of Pediatric Medicine
Institute of Child Health
Kolkata, West Bengal, India

Ex-Officio Editorial Advisers

GV Basavaraja MD DNB
Professor Department of Pediatrics
Indira Gandhi Institute of Child Health
Bengaluru, Karnataka, India
IAP National President 2024

Vasant M Khalatkar MD PGDID FICMCH
Consultant Pediatrician and Neonatologist
Khalatkar Hospital
Nagpur, Maharashtra, India
IAP National President, 2025

Yogesh N Parikh MD
Associate Professor
Department of Pediatrics
Government Medical College
Surat, Gujarat, India
Secretary General, IAP (2024–2025)

Atanu Bhadra DCH
Medical Superintendent
ESI Hospital
Asansol, West Bengal, India
National Treasurer, IAP (2024–2025)

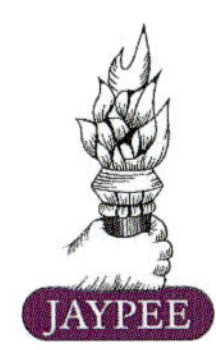

JAYPEE BROTHERS MEDICAL PUBLISHERS
The Health Sciences Publisher
New Delhi | London

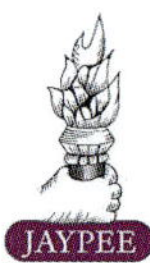

Jaypee Brothers Medical Publishers (P) Ltd

Headquarters

Jaypee Brothers Medical Publishers (P) Ltd
EMCA House, 23/23-B
Ansari Road, Daryaganj
New Delhi 110 002, India
Landline: +91-11-23272143, +91-11-23272703
+91-11-23282021, +91-11-23245672
Email: jaypee@jaypeebrothers.com

Corporate Office

Jaypee Brothers Medical Publishers (P) Ltd
4838/24, Ansari Road, Daryaganj
New Delhi 110 002, India
Phone: +91-11-43574357
Fax: +91-11-43574314
Email: jaypee@jaypeebrothers.com

Overseas Office

JP Medical Ltd
83 Victoria Street, London
SW1H 0HW (UK)
Phone: +44 20 3170 8910
Fax: +44 (0)20 3008 6180
Email: info@jpmedpub.com

Website: www.jaypeebrothers.com
Website: www.jaypeedigital.com

Inquiries for bulk sales may be solicited at: jaypee@jaypeebrothers.com

Partha's IAP Textbook of Pediatrics (3 Vols)

First Edition: 1999, 2000; Second Edition: 2002, 2003; Third Edition: 2006; Revised Reprint: 2007;
Fourth Edition: 2009; Fifth Edition: 2013; Sixth Edition: 2016; Seventh Edition: 2019

Eighth Edition: **2025**

ISBN: 978-93-5696-806-6

Printed at: Samrat Offset Pvt. Ltd.

Contents

Volume 1

SECTION 1: Basic Concepts of Child Care

Section Editor: Piyush Gupta

SECTION 2: Care of the Newborn

Section Editor: Rhishikesh P Thakre

SECTION 3: Growth

Section Editor: Anju Seth

SECTION 4: Development and Developmental Disorders

Section Editor: Samir Hasan Dalwai

SECTION 5: Nutrition and Nutritional Disorders

Section Editor: Praveen Kumar

SECTION 6: Immunity and Immunization

***Section Editor:* Srinivas G Kasi**

SECTION 7: Infectious Diseases

***Section Editor:* Ritabrata Kundu**

SECTION 8: Diseases of Central Nervous System

Section Editor: **Sheffali Gulati**

Volume 2

SECTION 9: Diseases of Cardiovascular System

Section Editor: S Srinivasan

SECTION 10: Disorders of Respiratory System

Section Editor: Sushil K Kabra

SECTION 11: Disorders of Gastrointestinal System and Liver

Section Editor: Riyaz Arakkal

SECTION 12: Disorders of Hepatobiliary System and Pancreas

Section Editor: John Matthai

SECTION 13: Disorders of Kidney and Urinary Tract

Section Editor: Arvind Bagga

SECTION 14: Disorders of Hemopoietic System

Section Editor: Ved Prakash Choudhry

SECTION 15: Pediatric Malignancies

Section Editor: **Purna A Kurkure**

SECTION 16: Disorders of Endocrine System and Diabetes Mellitus

Section Editors: **Vijayalakshmi Bhatia, PSN Menon**

Volume 3

SECTION 17: Genetics and Genetic Disorders

Section Editor: **Madhulika Kabra**

SECTION 18: Rheumatological Disorders and Allergy

Section Editor: Sathish Kumar

SECTION 19: Adolescent Health

Section Editor: MKC Nair

SECTION 20: Intensive Care and Emergencies

Section Editor: Jayashree Muralidharan

SECTION 21: Pediatric Subspecialties

Section Editor: **Ramachandran Padmanabhan**

SECTION 22: Community Pediatrics

Section Editor: **Alok Gupta**

SECTION 23: Pediatric Procedures

Section Editor: **Baldev S Prajapati**

SECTION 24: Pediatric Therapeutics

Section Editor: Jeeson C Unni

SECTION

Diseases of Cardiovascular System

Section Editor: S Srinivasan

9.1 Clinical Approach to Pediatric Cardiology

S Srinivasan

INTRODUCTION

The objectives of the clinical examination of the cardiovascular system in newborns, young infants, and older children are as follows:

- To assess rapidly *A*irway, *B*reathing, *C*irculation, *D*isability, and *E*xposure (ABCDE) without delay to institute appropriate life-saving remedial and resuscitative measures before taking a detailed history, e.g., critical ductus-dependent congenital heart disease (CHD) in neonates or other associated life-threatening complications, such as cardiogenic shock, pulmonary edema, tachyarrhythmia or bradyarrhythmia, endocarditis, cardiac tamponade, or hypertensive encephalopathy.
- To institute appropriate, immediate, and urgent resuscitative measures before resorting to detailed history-taking and physical examination
- To carry out proper history taking and clinical examination to ascertain the presence of a cardiovascular problem and identify the nature of the underlying cardiac condition in terms of structural involvement and its severity
- To ascertain its etiology—congenital/acquired, genetic, chromosomal, or dysmorphogenic syndromes
- To assess the urgency and severity of the condition and the functional limitation
- To identify the presence or absence of other related and associated complications and their impact on a child's nutritional, growth, developmental status, and functional limitation at home, play, and school activities

HISTORY TAKING

The mother must be allowed to give without unnecessary interruption her own account of the presenting symptoms, which necessitated her to bring the child to medical attention and narrate the evolution of these symptoms from the time of their onset.[1-4] Only open-ended questions must be used. The historical points of interest, of course, will vary considerably, depending upon the age of the patient and the presenting signs, symptoms, and complaints. If the child is brought in a state of breathlessness, cyanosis, or shock, precious time must not be wasted in taking elaborate history. Neonates with marked shortness of breath, cyanosis, and pallor with lethargy need immediate attention with regard to the adequacy of breathing, circulation (perfusion), and airway patency; quick clinical and investigative assessment (pulse oximetry and echocardiography) to rule out life-threatening, acute cardiac emergency states, e.g., ductus-dependent congenital cardiac lesions that restrict pulmonary or systemic blood flow. Other relevant and important details in history taking that have bearing on the diagnosis of the cardiac condition, its severity, and in planning treatment and counseling have been summarized in **Table 9.1.1**.

Moreover, while taking the history, one should take note of the evolution of symptoms according to chronology and mode of presentation, duration, progression, severity, relieving factors, aggravating factors, associated symptoms, and functional impairment.

Cardiac Symptoms

Symptoms of CHD can be very varied and subtle at times and may manifest anytime from the fetal period to adulthood **(Box 9.1.1)**.[5,6] Many of these symptoms may not be the presenting problem, and therefore, it has to be elicited by asking pertinent questions.

GENERAL PHYSICAL EXAMINATION

Examination of an infant and young child needs a lot of tact, and the general principles of examining a child should be applied. Although it is a usual routine to follow a definitive order in clinical examination, in a young child, such an orderly examination may not be always possible because of their apprehensive and anxious nature.[1-4] In a sleeping child, it is better to perform auscultation of the precordium for the nature of cardiac sounds and the presence of murmurs and other sounds. Infants and young children must be comfortably seated in the mother's lap with their dresses removed earlier before sitting in front of the examiner. The standard format of general physical examination has been summarized in **Table 9.1.2**.

It is important to remember that vital signs should be examined first before undertaking a detailed cardiac examination. The pertinent points to note are airway, breathing (rate, type, and signs of distress), circulation (capillary filling time, details of pulse, and blood pressure), and temperature.

TABLE 9.1.1: Important documentation of history relating to causative or precipitating factors.

History of abnormal facial features or minor or major congenital malformations	Many chromosomal and genetic syndromic disorders, such as Down syndrome, other trisomies, Turner syndrome, DiGeorge syndrome, Williams syndrome, Alagille syndrome, and other genetic, metabolic, and isolated malformations may indicate the presence of associated CHD
Past history	Any physical symptoms, health problems, hospital visits or admissions in the past for recurrent chest infections, bacterial endocarditis, symptoms suggestive of rheumatic fever (such as arthritis and abnormal movements), tuberculosis, delayed motor development, and rashes, skin peeling in palms, soles, tips of fingers and toes, or sore throat preceding onset of joint pains
Prenatal history	• History of acute or chronic infections in various trimesters—fever and rashes • Other maternal illnesses—metabolic disorders, such as gestational diabetes, phenylketonuria, and autoimmune disorders, such as SLE • Drugs—phenytoin, lithium, and other anticonvulsants • Substance abuse; alcohol, addictive drugs, etc. • Exposure to irradiation and pollutants • Maternal dietary history—micronutrient deficiencies like thiamine, vitamin D, and others
Birth history, immediate postnatal, and neonatal history*	Delayed crying and breath initiation, bluishness, sucking and feeding difficulty, lethargy, importance of finding out the gestational age, birth weight, need for resuscitation, need for breathing and oxygen support, prolonged stay in the neonatal unit, need for tube feeding or intravenous fluids, type of medications given during neonatal stay in the hospital and subsequent to discharge
Nutritional history	• Dietary micronutrient deficiencies in children like iron, vitamin B_1, and vitamin D—thiamine deficiency can cause wet Beri-Beri, thiamine-responsive pulmonary hypertension • Children with cardiac conditions with frequent heart failure or recurrent infections will have loss of appetite, and their nutritional intake will be greatly compromised
History of growth and developmental impairment	• Growth impairment and failure to thrive in the first few years of life are commonly noted in moderate-to-severe cardiac structural lesions • Tall stature or short stature, delayed gross motor milestones have a bearing on underlying cardiac disease • In a child with tall stature, the possibility of Marfan syndrome must be considered • In a female child with short stature, Turner syndrome and associated coarctation of the aorta must be ruled out • Moderate-to-severe CHD will be associated with delays in gross motor milestones in relation to other areas of development • Chromosomal and dysmorphogenetic syndromes with associated heart diseases may exhibit global developmental delay
Family history	• Record any of the following present in the family members: Sudden death, SIDS, rheumatic fever, structural or congenital cardiac abnormalities in siblings, genetic or dysmorphogenic syndromes in the family • The estimated recurrence risk of CHD is 2–6% when a previous sibling is affected, nearly 30% with two siblings affected, and 3% if one of the parents is affected
History of functional limitations	School attendance and absenteeism, academic performance, inability to participate in games and sports activities
Treatment history	Past and present treatment (medical and surgical) details
Personal/socioeconomic history	In a developing country with the majority of the population being below the poverty line, long-term treatment facilities, including surgical corrections at an appropriate age, may not be possible. Hence, children and adults at all ages may have CHD with or without advanced complications, such as PAH

*Preterm babies have a higher incidence of PDA. They also go into heart failure early in their first week with even moderate-sized defects with left-to-right shunts.
(CHD: congenital heart disease; PAH: pulmonary arterial hypertension; PDA: patent ductus arteriosus; SIDS: sudden infant death syndrome; SLE: systemic lupus erythematosus)

CARDIAC EXAMINATION

Precordium

The objectives of inspection of the chest are to identify chest wall asymmetry if present, in the form of precordial prominence, pectus excavatum, carinatum, kyphosis, scoliosis, and Harrison's sulcus; abnormal pulsations in the neck, suprasternal notch, parasternal region, epigastric region, and over the back; the location of apical impulse—left side or right side; and scars of previous operative procedures.[1-4]

Jugular Venous Pulse and Pressure

The jugular venous pulse waveform consists of three positive upstrokes—a, c, and v—and two negative waves—*x* descent

BOX 9.1.1: Presentation of cardiac problems.

Fetus (diagnosed by fetal echocardiography):
- Hydrops
- Arrhythmias
- Cardiomegaly

Neonate and infant:
- Heart failure (tachypnea with feeding or activities, labored breathing/dyspnea, feeding difficulties, sweating on head)
- Failure to thrive
- Cyanosis, circulatory failure, collapse
- Abnormal heart rate/rhythm, murmur, weak femoral pulses
- Noticeable excessive precordial activity or pulsations observed by parents
- Sleep disturbances
- Recurrent lower respiratory infections
- Dysmorphism
- Noncardiac congenital abnormalities

Older child:
- Heart failure (exercise intolerance, shortness of breath with activities), palpitation
- Increased precordial pulsations or prominence
- Dizzy or fainting spells, syncope
- Chest pain on activity
- Recurrent lower respiratory infections
- Failure to thrive
- Murmur
- Hypertension, as a part of multisystem disease (rheumatic fever, Kawasaki disease)
- Seizures (presenting as a complication of cyanotic heart disease)
- Cyanotic spells, squatting

after a and c waves, and *y* descent after a v wave. The abnormalities of various waveforms have been summarized in **Table 9.1.3**.[7,8]

Arterial Pulse

Pulse is the peripherally transmitted waveform of propagated arterial blood from the aortic root along the arterial tree generated by systolic contraction of the left ventricle. The travel speed of the arterial pulse wave is 10 times faster than that of the blood column. The importance of palpating the arterial pulse at various sites, e.g., both radial, femoral, brachialis, popliteal, posterior tibial, dorsalis pedis, carotid, and superficial temporal arteries, should be kept in mind at the beginning of each clinical posting and perhaps throughout life so as to ensure that one does not miss coarctation of the aorta, and thromboembolic phenomena need to be repeatedly emphasized to the students at every posting of theirs.[5,6]

The various types of abnormal pulses have been depicted in **Table 9.1.4**.

Precordial Palpation[7,8]

The learning objectives of palpation of the precordium are:
- To identify the site and type of apical impulse, whether normal or abnormal

TABLE 9.1.2: Proforma for general examination in a cardiac patient.

General appearance	Comfortable, consolable, state of distress
Posture/decubitus	Squatting by an acyanotic child—tetralogy of Fallot
General health	Failure to thrive in large left-to-right shunt in VSD
Body build and proportion	• Short stature in females—Turner syndrome • Tall stature with arachnodactyly—Marfan syndrome
Nutritional and growth status	Anthropometry
Features of chromosomal/ genetic/dysmorphogenic syndromes	Down syndrome, Turner syndrome, other trisomies, Williams syndrome, Noonan syndrome, etc.
External isolated/multiple congenital external malformations	Short neck, webbing, polydactyly, syndactyly, camptomelia
Oral cavity, teeth, and pharynx	Sore throat, caries
Skin	Rashes, erythema marginatum, nodules, desquamation
Joints	Rheumatic fever, rheumatoid arthritis
Abnormal movements	Chorea
Dependent edema	Sites—feet, legs, back, eyelids
Lymph nodes	Kawasaki disease, tuberculosis
Clubbing of fingers and toes	Cyanotic heart defects, bacterial endocarditis
Central cyanosis, differential cyanosis	

(VSD: ventricular septal defect)

- To identify the presence of abnormal pulsations, heaves, and thrills in specified precordial sites—left parasternal and epigastric regions, suprasternal notch, and second left intercostal space (LICS)
- To ascertain enlargement of right ventricle, left ventricle, or both or dilatation of great arteries—aorta and pulmonary arteries[5,6]

Apical Impulse

Apical impulse refers to the outermost and lowermost definitive palpable outward thrust of cardiac impulse in the lower precordium imparted by the anterior movement of the left ventricular (LV) apex during early systolic contraction of the left ventricle. Its location, amplitude, duration, size, character, or contour must be recorded.

In the first 3–4 years of life after birth, the normal location of the apical impulse is in the fourth LICS, 1–2 cm lateral to the

TABLE 9.1.3: Abnormal jugular venous pulse and its clinical interpretation.

"A" wave abnormalities		
Large "a" waves	Forcible contraction of right atrium against obstruction at AV valve area	Tricuspid stenosis, RA myxoma
	Increased resistance offered by noncompliant right ventricle	Severe PAH, PS (moderate-to-severe), RV cardiomyopathy, acute pulmonary embolism
Cannon or very large giant "a" waves	Contraction of the right atrium against a closed tricuspid valve	Tricuspid atresia, AV dissociation, complete heart block
	Regular cannon waves	Junctional rhythm, isorhythmic AV dissociation
	Irregular cannon waves	Complete heart block, classic AV dissociation, ventricular pacing, ventricular ectopics
Absent "a" waves	Ineffective atrial contraction	Atrial fibrillation, marked sinus tachycardia
"V" wave abnormalities		
Large "v" waves	Rapid and excessive RA filling	TR, TAPVD, ASD with MR

(ASD: atrial septal defect; AV: atrioventricular; MR: mitral regurgitation; PAH: pulmonary arterial hypertension; PS: pulmonary stenosis; RA: right atrial; RV: right ventricular; TAPVD: total anomalous pulmonary venous drainage; TR: tricuspid regurgitation)

TABLE 9.1.4: Abnormal pulses.

Pulsus parvus	Low-volume pulse with slow rise; its presence suggests the possibility of severe AS or severe low-output states, such as severe heart failure
Pulsus tardus	Slow-rising pulse with a late peaking closer to the second sound, is reported in fixed LV obstructive lesions
Hypokinetic pulse	Weakly felt, small-volume pulse felt with difficulty in the cases of low-cardiac-output states, such as shock, severe heart failure, myocarditis, cardiac tamponade, constrictive pericarditis, severe left heart obstructive lesions, such as MS and AS, and aortic outflow obstructions, such as aortic arch syndromes and coarctation of the aorta
Hyperkinetic (bounding) pulse	High-amplitude, large-volume pulse with rapidly rising ascending wave felt in augmented high cardiac output states with decreased peripheral arterial resistance and wide pulse pressure, e.g., anxiety, exercise, fever, anemia, thyrotoxicosis, arteriovenous fistulas, beriberi, moderate MR, moderate-sized ventricular septal defects, AR, PDA
Water hammer/ collapsing pulse	• Water hammer pulse is elicited by suddenly and gently elevating the child's arm above his/her shoulder, while the radial pulse is continuously felt by the palmar surface of the examiner's hand instead of the usual three fingertips. It is a large-volume pulse with sudden and rapid upstroke with equally rapid downstroke. The term "water hammer" refers to a famous Victorian era English toy • Collapsing pulse indicates rapid and reverse diastolic runoff into the left ventricle in AR and rapid runoff to the peripheral vessels due to decreased systemic peripheral vascular resistance. For example, AR, PDA, AP window, and RSOV into the right ventricle and arteriovenous fistulas • Collapsing pulse in a cyanotic child suggests truncus arteriosus with truncal regurgitation, pulmonary atresia with AP collaterals, TOF with AP collaterals, or PDA. Collapsing pulse is also felt in hyperkinetic states, such as anemia, fever, thyrotoxicosis, pregnancy, and beriberi
Bisferiens pulse	Pulse with two beats in a single systolic wave upstroke; when the examiner's palpating finger feels two positive upward peaks during systole, it is termed pulsus bisferiens, better appreciated over the carotids than radials. They indicate the presence of severe AR or AR with AS or HOCM
Corrigan's pulse	Prominently visible dancing pulsation over the carotids in AR
Brisk/jerky pulse	Pulse with a sharp, tapping upstroke with normal volume, and downstroke is characteristic of HCM
Anacrotic pulse	It is felt in severe AS and is a small-volume (low amplitude), slow-rising (ana = up, and crotos = beat) upstroke wave with late peaking. The anacrotic notch occurs during the early half of the ascent; earlier it is felt, severe is the AS. In severe MS, the notch is felt in the latter half of the ascending limb
Dicrotic pulse	It refers to pulse waveforms with two peaks in each wave, one in the systolic ascending limb and the second prominent one in the descending limb of the wave during diastole. This is seen in cardiac conditions with low stroke volume and decreased peripheral arterial resistance—typhoid fever, LV failure, dilated cardiomyopathies, and cardiac tamponade

Contd...

Contd...

Pulsus paradoxus	It occurs when there is an exaggerated decrease in pulse volume and blood pressure >10 mm Hg recorded during inspiration. In normal individuals, there is usually a normal physiological drop of systolic blood pressure during inspiratory phase ranging from 5 mm Hg to a maximum of 10 mm Hg, which may be appreciated by experienced clinicians on feeling the arterial pulse in the absence of tachycardia. Hence, the term paradox used as an adjective is not true. It is seen in cardiac tamponade, pericardial effusion, constrictive pericarditis, acute severe asthma, and in conditions that obstruct superior vena cava return to the right atrium as noted in anterior and superior mediastinal tumors
Pulsus alternans	It refers to the occurrence of an alternating pulse of high and low amplitudes or volumes in the presence of normal rhythm and is indicative of moderate-to-severe LV failure
Pulsus bigeminy, pulsus trigeminy	It refers to the coupling of two or three beats, followed by a pause with a stronger beat after the pause. It occurs in the AV block and sinoatrial block with ventricular escape

(AP: aortopulmonary; AR: aortic regurgitation; AS: aortic stenosis; AV: atrioventricular; HCM: hypertrophic cardiomyopathy; HOCM: hypertrophic obstructive cardiomyopathy; LV: left ventricular; MR: mitral regurgitation; MS: mitral stenosis; PDA: patent ductus arteriosus; RSOV: ruptured sinus of Valsalva; TOF: tetralogy of Fallot)

midclavicular line (MCL). Between 4 and 8 years, the location is in the fifth LICS on the MCL. Beyond 8 years, it lies in the fifth LICS, 1–2 cm or half an inch medial to the MCL. The apex beat is shifted to the left in cardiomegaly, scoliosis, pectus excavatum, and right-sided pneumothorax or effusion. It is shifted to the right side in the cases of congenital dextrocardia, acquired dextroposition (heart pushed or pulled to the right side as in left-sided pleural effusion or pneumothorax), and diaphragmatic hernia. **Table 9.1.5** summarizes different types of apical impulse.

Other Palpable Sounds and Pulsations

The second heart sound (S2) may be palpable in pulmonary hypertension. The third heart sound (S3) may be rarely palpable in severe mitral regurgitation (MR) or dilated cardiomyopathy. The fourth heart sound (S4) is more often palpable in adults than in children in the following conditions: Hypertrophic cardiomyopathy, severe aortic stenosis (AS), acute MR, and long-standing hypertension.[5,6] Suprasternal pulsations are seen and palpable in patent ductus arteriosus, AS, aortic regurgitation, coarctation of aorta, and aortic aneurysm. Pulsations in the parasternal area without a perceptible or palpable left parasternal lift are characteristic of right ventricular (RV) volume-overload conditions, such as atrial septal defect, tricuspid regurgitation, and moderate-to-large ventricular septal defect without pulmonary arterial hypertension, in addition to hyperdynamic high-output states. Epigastric pulsations are seen, and the impulse is felt in RV volume-overload states. Apart from these sounds, murmurs are also palpable in various areas.

Parasternal Heave

Parasternal heave is both seen and felt by the ulnar border of the examiner's hand over the left parasternal region of the precordium overlying the heart. It indicates RV enlargement.[7,8]

TABLE 9.1.5: Characteristics of apical impulse.

Tapping apical impulse	Palpable S1 noted in MS; it represents a hypokinetic, underfilled left ventricle. Tapping apical impulse is also felt in ASD
Hyperdynamic apex	Suggests LV dilatation seen in high-cardiac output states and ventricular volume overloads seen in MR and AR, VSD, or PDA. In hyperdynamic apex, the apical impulse, in addition to being shifted outward and downward, has increased amplitude with brisk upstroke and is felt in more than one ICS, usually over two or three ICSs exceeding 3 cm. It is ill sustained with the duration of impact between the one-third and half of systole
Heaving apex	It is said to be present when the systolic thrust is sustained and increased in duration, almost like a wave felt for more than the two-thirds of systole with increased amplitude and is confined to one ICS. It is indicative of pressure overload and LVH seen in AS, systemic arterial hypertension, or coarctation of the aorta
Retractile apical impulse	Indicative of constrictive pericarditis where there is systolic retraction away from the chest wall and forward or positive diastolic thrust
Double apical impulse	It suggests AS with AR, HOCM, LBBB, and in adults, LV aneurysm. Triple or quadruple impulse may be felt in HOCM
Absence of apical impulse	Dextrocardia, pericardial effusion, obesity, apex under the rib, emphysema, or large pleural effusion on the left side

(AR: aortic regurgitation; AS: aortic stenosis; ASD: atrial septal defect; HOCM: hypertrophic obstructive cardiomyopathy; ICS: intercostal space; LBBB: left bundle branch block; LV: left ventricular; LVH: left ventricular hypertrophy; MR: mitral regurgitation; MS: mitral stenosis; PDA: patent ductus arteriosus; S1: first heart sound; VSD: ventricular septal defect)

Heart Sounds

The first heart sound (S1) is produced by the closure of mitral and tricuspid valves, marking the beginning of systole.

It is best heard over the apex and in the mitral area. The S2 is produced by the closure of semilunar valves of the aorta and pulmonary arteries. The normal variable split of S2 is because the pulmonary component (P2) is normally heard 30 ms after the aortic component (A2) during inspiration (increased RV ejection time and pulmonary artery hangout interval) and within 20 ms during expiration. The S3 is low pitched, may be normally heard in early diastole, and is caused by rapid ventricular filling. It may also be heard in athletes and pregnant women. If S3 occurs in a child with cardiac symptoms, one should suspect diastolic overload conditions or LV dysfunction (dilated left ventricle, decreased ejection fraction, and constrictive pericarditis) or LV failure. The S3 gallop refers to an exaggerated sound with a cadence heard when significant tachycardia occurs with the above conditions. The S4 is often an abnormal sound, and it is a low-pitched, late diastolic sound produced by forceful atrial contraction against a certain degree of resistance and decreased ventricular compliance during late ventricular filling. The characteristics of various heart sounds have been summarized in **Table 9.1.6**.[5,6]

Other Abnormal Sounds

Clicks, opening snap, and pericardial friction rub are the other added sounds one should try to detect during auscultation.

Heart Murmurs

Heart murmurs are audible sound waves in the range of 20–2,000 Hz that occur as a result of turbulent blood flow due to functional or structural hemodynamic alterations in the pattern of blood flow in the heart chambers across the valves or the atrial or ventricular septum or in the vessels as in coarctation of the aorta, renal artery stenosis, or pulmonary arteriovenous collaterals or malformations.[7,8]

When the presence of murmur over the precordium is appreciated by the student, it becomes essential to make a clinical decision about whether the murmur is functional/innocent or organic/pathological due to an underlying cardiac disorder. When one or more of the following are present, the murmur is likely to be pathologic and requires further evaluation: Symptoms, cyanosis, systolic murmur that

TABLE 9.1.6: Characteristics of different heart sounds.

Intensity of S1	***Cardiac conditions***
Loud	Exercise, sinus tachycardia, short PR interval states, such as WPW syndrome, MS, tricuspid stenosis, atrial myxoma
Soft	Long PR interval, pericardial effusion, MR, TR, calcific MS, myocarditis and cardiomyopathy, proximal LBBB
Split S1	Ebstein anomaly, RBBB, large ASD
Intensity of S2	
Increased A2	Systemic hypertension, aortic root dilatation, L-TGA, TOF
Decreased A2	Severe AS, AR, calcific aortic valve
Increased P2	Pulmonary hypertension, ASD
Decreased P2	PS, TOF, TGA
Splitting of S2	
Wide (both A2 and P2 audible in inspiration and expiration)	*Due to early A2 closure:* VSD, MR
	Due to late P2 closure: PAH, PS, RBBB, pulmonary embolism, LV ectopic beat
	Increased hangout interval due to decreased impedance to pulmonary artery: ASD, PS, TAPVC, Ebstein, idiopathic dilatation of pulmonary artery
Wide and fixed split	ASD, severe RV failure
Paradoxical or reverse split	Delayed A2
P2, then A2 (split audible in expiration but not in inspiration)	*Mechanical:* AS, hypertension, CAD *Electrical:* Proximal LBBB; RV ectopics
	Decreased impedance to aorta: PDA, poststenotic dilatation in AS
Single S2	*Absent A2:* HLHS, aortic atresia
	Absent P2: Pulmonary atresia, truncus arteriosus, absent pulmonary valve
	Very soft/masked P2: TOF, TGA, severe PS
	Synchronous A2 and P2: Severe PAH, PPH, Eisenmenger VSD
Intensity of S3	
LV overload states	MR, VSD, PDA
RV overload states	TR, ASD
Intensity of S4	
LA S4 gallop	Aortic valvular stenosis, systemic arterial hypertension
Right atrial S4 gallop	PAH, PS, Ebstein anomaly, ASD, prolonged PR interval

(A2: aortic component of S2; AR: aortic regurgitation; AS: aortic stenosis; ASD: atrial septal defect; CAD: coronary artery disease; HLHS: hypoplastic left heart syndrome; LA: left atrial; LBBB: left bundle branch block; LV: left ventricular; L-TGA: levo-transposition of great arteries; MR: mitral regurgitation; MS: mitral stenosis; P2: pulmonary component of S2; PAH: pulmonary arterial hypertension; PDA: patent ductus arteriosus; PPH: primary pulmonary hypertension; PR: pulmonary regurgitation; PS: pulmonary stenosis; RBBB: right bundle branch block; RV: right ventricular; S1: first heart sound; S2: second heart sound; S3: third heart sound; S4: fourth heart sound; TAPVC: total anomalous pulmonary venous connection; TGA: transposition of great arteries; TOF: tetralogy of Fallot; TR: tricuspid regurgitation; VSD: ventricular septal defect; WPW: Wolff–Parkinson–White).

is loud (grade, harsh, and long in duration), diastolic murmur, abnormal heart sounds, presence of a click, and abnormally strong or weak pulses. The characteristics of organic heart murmurs have been summarized in **Table 9.1.7**.

TABLE 9.1.7: Characteristics of organic heart murmurs.

Organic systolic murmurs			
Pansystolic	*Ejection*	*Mid/late systolic*	
MR, TR, VSD	AS, PS, ASD, VSD	MVP	
Organic diastolic murmurs			
Early diastolic	*Mid-diastolic*	*Presystolic*	
AR, PR	MS TS Carey Coombs murmur of mitral valvulitis Austin flint murmur in AR	Severe MS	
	Secondary flow murmurs (ASD, VSD, PDA, MR, TR)		
Organic continuous murmurs			
Acyanotic • PDA • Aortopulmonary window, rupture of sinus of Valsalva into the right ventricle or pulmonary artery • Coronary arteriovenous fistulas • Systemic arteriovenous fistulas • Peripheral pulmonary artery branch stenosis • ALCAPA *Cyanotic* • Pulmonary arteriovenous fistulas • Truncus arteriosus Blalock-Taussig shunt		*Secondary collaterals in* • TOF • Aortic coarctation • Aberrant LCA with RCA collaterals	*Combination of defects* • VSD + AR • AR + AS • MR + AR/TR + MR + AR

(ALCAPA: anomalous left coronary artery from the pulmonary artery; AR: aortic regurgitation; AS: aortic stenosis; ASD: atrial septal defect; LCA: left coronary artery; MR: mitral regurgitation; MS: mitral stenosis; MVP: mitral valve prolapse; PDA: patent ductus arteriosus; PR: pulmonary regurgitation; PS: pulmonary stenosis; RCA: right coronary artery; TOF: tetralogy of Fallot; TR: tricuspid regurgitation; TS: tricuspid stenosis; VSD: ventricular septal defect)

Innocent Murmurs

A murmur heard in a child without a structural heart disease is termed an innocent murmur. The child has no cardiac-related symptoms or other signs on careful history and physical examination, and basic investigations, such as chest X-ray, electrocardiogram, and echocardiogram, are normal. A significantly large proportion of children have innocent murmurs beginning at 3–4 years of age.

The characteristics of innocent or functional murmurs are usually the following: They are localized to specific areas, short, often early or midsystolic, grade 1/6 or 2/6 (not associated with thrill), and vary in intensity with change in posture, decreasing in intensity when the child stands, sits up, or strains during a Valsalva maneuver.

REFERENCES

1. Allen HD, Philips JR, Chan DP. History and physical examination. In: Shaddy RE, Penny JP (Eds). Moss and Adams' Heart Disease in Infants, Children and Adolescents Including the Young Adult, 10th edition. Philadelphia, PA: Lippincott; 2021. pp. 58-66.
2. Park MK. History taking. In: Park MK, Salamat M (Eds). Pediatric Cardiology for Practitioners, 7th edition. Philadelphia, PA: Mosby Elsevier; 2023. pp. 1-5.
3. Park MK. Physical examination. In: Park MK, Salamat M (Eds). Pediatric Cardiology for Practitioners, 7th edition. Philadelphia, PA: Mosby Elsevier; 2023. pp. 6-30.
4. Roy DL. Cardiovascular assessment of infants and children. In: Goldbloom RB (Ed). Pediatric Clinical Skills, 3rd edition. Philadelphia, PA: Saunders; 2003. pp. 169-89.
5. Saadoon AQ. 4.9 Cardiovascular system examination. In. Saadoon AQ (Ed). Essential Clinical Skills in Pediatrics—A Practical Guide to History Taking and Clinical Examination. New York: Springer; 2018. pp. 166-76.
6. Srinivasan. S. Evaluation of the cardiovascular system. In: Gupta P (Ed). Piyush Gupta Clinical Methods in Pediatrics, 5th edition. New Delhi: CBS Publishers & Distributors; 2022. pp. 235-301.
7. Tandon R. Bedside diagnosis of congenital heart disease. In: Bahl VK (Ed). Cardiology Update 2008. New Delhi: Cardiological Society of India; 2008. pp. 484-90.
8. Thompson WR, Mehrotra SM. Approach to heart diseases in children: cardiac history and physical examination. In: Raid A (Ed). Heart Diseases in Children: A Pediatrician's Guide. New York: Springer; 2011. pp. 3-16.

9.2 Congenital Heart Disease

Nisanth Selvam, R Krishna Kumar

INTRODUCTION

Congenital heart disease (CHD) encompasses a broad and extremely diverse range of conditions that can manifest anytime from fetal life to late adulthood. In common parlance, CHD refers to structural heart defects that are present at birth. Conditions, such as hypertrophic cardiomyopathy and mitral valve prolapse, may have a congenital basis, but these are often discussed separately. Similarly, electrical and conduction disorders, such as prolonged "QT" syndrome, Brugada syndrome, arrhythmogenic right ventricular dysplasia, and congenital complete heart block, are not usually categorized as CHD, even though in the strictest terms they should perhaps be. In this chapter, we will be discussing common structural defects that are present at birth.

The bewildering array of CHD is intimidating to the uninitiated pediatrician. Many defects are quite complex, and a very large number of combinations often defy predictable patterns. The most significant challenge that a student faces is striking the right balance between acquiring an in-depth understanding of individual conditions and acquiring a broad overall understanding of most "commonly encountered" CHDs.[1-3]

A practical approach lies in remembering the following:

- The most important role of the pediatrician today is to ensure that, as far as possible, serious CHD should not be missed; this is especially true in the neonatal period and during infancy where maximal attrition from CHD occurs.
- History, physical examination, chest X-ray, and electrocardiogram (ECG) are the traditional tools available to the pediatrician. With this, it is usually possible to identify whether CHD is present except perhaps in the early newborn period where CHD diagnosis can be challenging.
- Despite numerous anatomic possibilities, the physiologic categories of CHD are limited and can be understood. Understanding the basic hemodynamic and physiologic concepts is important because they have an important bearing on the clinical picture, interpretation of echocardiographic reports, natural history, and decision-making on the timing of surgical or catheter intervention.
- The traditional diagnostic tools allow classification of CHD into physiologic categories in a significant proportion of babies. The limitations of the traditional tools in identifying the precise anatomy are substantial, and this is exposed by the widespread use of echocardiography.
- Numerous recent advances have dramatically changed the outlook of children with CHD. As a result, some form of palliation or correction is feasible for most CHD, provided that it is undertaken in a timely fashion.
- The improved understanding of CHD today suggests that management needs to be individualized or tailored to each patient. It is possible to identify and determine the severity of all the specific lesions through echocardiography. Recognizing the numerous combinations and specific features with each lesion, each patient needs to be approached according to the specifics of the lesion(s).
- It is increasingly evident that a substantial proportion of children with CHD have significant problems in other organ systems. A growing proportion of children with CHD are being identified to have specific chromosomal (such as CATCH 22) and single-gene disorders. The pediatrician has an important role in identifying them because they have a significant bearing on eventual outcomes and counseling of the family.
- Despite significant recent advances, long-term concerns after palliation and many forms of "correction" of CHD are significant, and many of these children need lifelong follow-up.

  This chapter will expand on the above-mentioned points. A detailed description of individual congenital heart defects is beyond the scope of this chapter, and the reader should refer to standard textbooks of pediatric cardiology.[1-3] Brief descriptions of "common" CHDs are included in a section at the end of the chapter.

EPIDEMIOLOGY OF CONGENITAL HEART DISEASE

Congenital heart disease accounts for about 10% of infant deaths and nearly half of all deaths are due to congenital malformations in developed countries. The prevalence of CHD diagnosed in the first 12 months is estimated at 6–8 per 1,000 live births. Of these, at least 25% are life-threatening CHDs that require very early intervention. A large recent prospective study was recently undertaken from Kochi, and

5,487 consecutive newborns were screened. Of these, 425 had CHD (prevalence: 7.75%) and 17 (0.31%) had major CHD (lesions that are likely to require early intervention). The rest (408 patients, 7.44%) had minor CHD [such as small muscular ventricular septal defects (VSDs), closing patent ducts, and small atrial septal defects (ASDs)/patent foramen], most of which were normalized by 6 weeks.[4] In a larger and more recent study from Delhi, involving nearly 20,000 consecutive newborns, CHD was identified in 159 (prevalence 8.36 per 1,000 live births). Of these, 70 had a major CHD (3.68 per 1,000 live births), of whom 44 had serious CHDs (requiring surgical or catheter intervention in the first year of life) and 26 had critical CHDs (requiring intervention in the first month of life).[5]

Extrapolating this data on a national scale suggests that the absolute burden of CHD in India is substantial. For a population of 1.2 billion, it can be expected that there would perhaps be approximately 1,00,000 newborns born each year with CHD requiring some form of intervention early in life.

In relative terms, CHD is of importance in those parts of the country that are showing improved human development indices (such as Kerala, Tamil Nadu, Himachal Pradesh, and Goa). In these regions, infant mortality from readily preventable conditions (such as diarrhea and respiratory infections) has declined substantially.

It is estimated that only 6–10% of newborns and infants with CHD are receiving timely surgery in India. Most newborns with CHD escape timely detection. Even after a diagnosis is made, the economic and logistic barriers to reaching a center and successfully undergoing surgery are substantial in our country. As a result, CHD has a unique profile in India (such as in other low- and middle-income countries). This is characterized by remarkable early attrition, late survival selected by natural history, and significant numbers of older children with complications, such as pulmonary hypertension and overt (brain abscess and stroke) and covert (neurodevelopmental abnormalities) neurological damage.

ETIOPATHOGENESIS

The link between the etiology and embryogenesis of CHD is often very complex. A lot of recent research has focused on the chain of events in early embryogenesis of the heart and great vessels. As a result, there have been dramatic conceptual upheavals. The details are beyond the scope of this chapter. In simplified terms, the pediatrician should recognize today that a growing proportion of patients with CHD have an identifiable genetic basis. **Table 9.2.1** summarizes common genetic conditions that are associated with CHD. The association with acquired conditions and teratogens and occurrence of CHD is summarized in **Table 9.2.2**.

PHYSIOLOGY AND PHYSIOLOGIC CLASSIFICATION OF CONGENITAL HEART DISEASE

Once the basic physiologic concepts are understood, it is relatively easy to understand clinical manifestations (history and physical examination). These concepts enable better interpretation of chest X-ray, ECG, and echocardiographic findings and allow correct management decisions (timing of surgical or catheter interventions).[1-3]

For many years, CHD has been broadly classified as cyanotic and acyanotic, with certain specific subtypes in each category **(Table 9.2.3)**. While broad classifications based on physiology work for many situations, there are several patients who cannot be classified into common physiologic categories. In addition, there are often specific issues, such as valve regurgitation that dictate the clinical presentation. The broad categories of CHD in **Table 9.2.3** have limitations, and some patients may have a combination of lesions belonging to more than one category. For example, a child may have a large VSD with moderate pulmonary stenosis (PS) and mild pulmonary hypertension.

Another way of understanding the physiology of CHD is to list the various physiological perturbations **(Table 9.2.4)** that are commonly associated with CHD. Here again, it is evident that many defects have more than one physiological perturbation. The table is, however, useful in that it illustrates various mechanisms by which CHD produces clinical manifestations. The reader is encouraged to study this table carefully. A thorough understanding of the physiology of individual forms of CHD can be acquired through a detailed study of individual lesions. This is clearly beyond the scope of this chapter.

Here, the focus will be on illustrating selected key physiological concepts that are important to understand many lesions. These include:

- Pretricuspid versus post-tricuspid shunts
- VSD–PS physiology
- Single ventricle physiology
- Duct-dependent lesions
- Unfavorable streaming and parallel circulation

Pretricuspid versus Post-tricuspid Shunts

Acyanotic heart disease with left-to-right shunts is traditionally classified as pretricuspid and post-tricuspid shunts. There are important differences in physiology that have an important bearing on clinical manifestations and natural history.

Left-to-right shunts at the level of the atria are known as pretricuspid shunts. They include ASDs and partial anomalous pulmonary venous connection. The left-to-right shunt and the consequent excessive pulmonary blood flow are dictated by the relative stiffness of the two ventricles.

TABLE 9.2.1: Common genetic conditions that are linked to the occurrence of congenital heart disease.

Specific condition	*Genetic basis*	*Cardiac lesions*	*Other manifestations*
CATCH 22 syndrome	Microdeletion on long arm of chromosome 22, 22q11 deletion; autosomal dominant inheritance	*Conotruncal defects:* Interrupted aortic arch, tetralogy of Fallot (TOF), ventricular septal defect (VSD), persistent truncus arteriosus, double outlet right ventricle	Cleft lip/palate, hypocalcemia/ hypoparathyroidism, thymic hypoplasia/T-cell abnormality, nasal regurgitation of feeds, failure to thrive, gastroesophageal reflux, facial dysmorphism, hypernasal speech, learning disabilities, behavioral disorders (ADHD), older children may have psychiatric disorders
Williams–Beuren syndrome	Microdeletion at chromosome 7q11.23 (elastin gene located in this segment); autosomal dominant inheritance	Supravalvular aortic stenosis, pulmonary arterial stenosis, aortic and mitral valve abnormalities, adult systemic hypertension/renal artery stenosis	Elfin facies (periorbital fullness, stellate iris pattern, full lips-wide mouth, short, upturned nose, flat nasal bridge) strabismus, mental retardation, cognitive disability, hyperacusis, hypersocial personality, failure to thrive, short stature, hypercalcemia, hypothyroidism, chronic urinary tract infections, nephron-calcinosis
Down syndrome/ Trisomy 21	Meiotic nondisjunction of chromosome 21 (rarely Robertsonian translocation or mosaicism), sporadic mutation	Frequent (40–50%) AV canal defect, perimembranous VSD, TOF, PDA	Characteristic flat facies, clinodactyly, single palmar crease, mental deficiency, hypotonia, hearing and visual disturbances, early-onset dementia
Turner syndrome	Chromosomal (45, XO karyotype and variants mosaicism, structurally abnormal X chromosome)	Predominantly left-sided lesions [i.e., bicuspid aortic valve (BAV), coarctation]; risk for aortic root dilation/aortic dissection in later life	*Variable phenotype:* Short stature, gonadal dysgenesis, lymphedema over the dorsum of hands and feet, renal anomalies, normal intelligence but can have a learning disability. Seen in phenotypic females
Noonan syndrome	Protein tyrosine phosphatase, nonreceptor type (PTPN11) mutations in 50%; half of cases are de novo autosomal dominant inheritance in the next generation	Pulmonic stenosis (20–50%), hypertrophic cardiomyopathy (20–30%), and atrial septal defect (ASD)	*Variable phenotype:* Short stature, webbed neck-widely placed nipples, dysmorphic facies, varying developmental delay; cryptorchidism; coagulation defects. Both males and females are affected
VATER association/ VACTERL syndrome	No specific recurring etiology, sporadic; very small risk to offspring	VSD, TOF	*V*ertebral defects, *a*nal atresia, *TE*F, *r*enal and *l*imb anomalies, normal intelligence
Holt–Oram syndrome	TBX5 mutation (70%); 15% familial, autosomal dominant inheritance	Ostium secundum ASD, VSD, conduction defects	Upper limb anomalies of varying degrees (especially radial ray and thumb anomalies) in 100% (complete penetrance)
CHARGE association	CHD7 mutation (60%) or deletion; most cases are *de novo* autosomal dominant inheritance	Commonly right-sided lesions: Branch pulmonary artery stenosis and conotruncal lesions (TOF, VSD)	Colobomas, growth failure, developmental delay, choanal atresia, genitourinary anomalies, genital hypoplasia, ear anomalies, and hearing loss
Alagille syndrome	JAG1 mutation (90%) or deletion (7%); 50–70% of cases are de novo; autosomal dominant inheritance	Pulmonary valve and branch PA—most affected; TOF in 7–15%	*Hepatic disease/chronic cholestasis, dysmorphic facies:* Triangular facies with pointed chin, hypertelorism and malformed ears, butterfly vertebrae, renal anomalies, neurovascular anomalies, posterior embryotoxon

(ADHD: attention deficit hyperactivity disorder; AV: atrioventricular; CHD7: chromodomain-helicase-DNA-binding protein 7; JAG1: jagged1; PA: pulmonary atresia; PDA: patent ductus arteriosus; TBX5: T-box transcription factor 5; TEF: tracheoesophageal fistula; VATER: vertebrae, anus, trachea, esophagus, renal)

Since the right ventricle (RV) is relatively stiff (noncompliant) at birth and during early infancy, the shunt is small. Over the years, the RV progressively enlarges to accommodate the excessive pulmonary blood flow. The pulmonary vasculature also becomes more capacious to gradually accommodate the excessive blood flow. This explains why ASDs typically do not manifest with the symptoms of pulmonary overcirculation during infancy and childhood. The clinical signs are also easily explained by the physiology of pretricuspid shunts. The diastolic flow murmur of ASD is across the much larger

TABLE 9.2.2: Etiology of congenital heart disease (CHD)—prenatal exposure to acquired factors.

Acquired condition	***Association with CHD***
Diabetes	A variety of forms of CHDs (3–5%) are now linked with maternal gestational and pregestational diabetes. The list includes transposition, atrioventricular septal defects, ventricular septal defect (VSD), hypoplastic left heart syndrome, cardiomyopathy, and patent ductus arteriosus (PDA)
Febrile illnesses in the first trimester	Any febrile illness during the first trimester of pregnancy may have a twofold increase in the risk of CHD
Maternal rubella (usually in the first trimester)	Specific cardiac manifestations of rubella embryopathy include PDA, pulmonary valve abnormalities, peripheral pulmonary stenosis, and VSD
Epilepsy	The association is perhaps because of the risk of CHD from anticonvulsant medications
Lupus (apart from typical symptoms of SLE, it may be useful to ask for a history of previous abortions)	*Neonatal lupus:* Maternal systemic lupus erythematosus (SLE) is associated with the risk of complete heart block in the offspring
Phenylketonuria	Phenylketonuria is associated with a greater than six-fold increase in the risk of CHD (specifically VSD, TOF, PDA, and single ventricle)
Vitamin deficiency	Multivitamin supplements, including folic acid derivatives, have been shown to protect against the occurrence of CHD in two studies. Multivitamins may also reduce the risk of CHD associated with febrile illnesses in the first trimester
Prenatal exposure to medications in the first trimester (teratogenic)	The list of medications known to be associated with a risk of CHD in the offspring includes anticonvulsants (valproic acid, phenytoin), nonsteroidal anti-inflammatory drugs (NSAIDs), trimethoprim–sulfonamide, lithium, ACEI, thalidomide, and vitamin A congeners
Occupational exposure	Exposure to organic solvents, herbicides, pesticides, and ionizing radiation may increase the risk of CHD in the offspring

(ACEI: angiotensin-converting enzyme inhibitor; TOF: tetralogy of Fallot)

TABLE 9.2.3: Broad physiologic categories of congenital heart disease.

Physiologic category	***Examples***
Acyanotic congenital heart disease	
Simple left-to-right shunts	
Pretricuspid	Partial anomalous pulmonary venous drainage and atrial septal defect
Post-tricuspid	
Ventricular	Ventricular septal defects (VSDs)
Great artery	Aortopulmonary window, patent arterial duct, coronary cameral fistula, and ruptured sinus of Valsalva
Combination of pre- and post-tricuspid	Atrioventricular septal defect and left ventricle to right atrial communications (Gerbode defect)
Obstructive lesions	
Inflow: Left-sided	Cor triatriatum and obstructive lesions of the mitral valve apparatus
Outflow	
Right ventricle	Infundibular stenosis, pulmonary valve stenosis, and branch pulmonary artery stenosis
Left ventricle	Subaortic membrane, valvular aortic stenosis, supravalvular aortic stenosis, and coarctation of the aorta
Miscellaneous lesions	Coronary artery abnormalities, congenital mitral, and tricuspid valve regurgitation
Cyanotic heart disease	
Reduced pulmonary blood flow	
Intact interventricular septum	Pulmonary atresia (PA) with intact ventricular septum, critical pulmonic stenosis (PS) with R-L shunt at atrial level, Ebstein anomaly, and isolated RV hypoplasia
Unrestrictive ventricular communication	All conditions listed under VSD with PS or PA physiology*

Contd...

Contd...

Physiologic category	*Examples*
Miscellaneous conditions	Pulmonary arteriovenous malformation and anomalous drainage of systemic veins to LA
Increased pulmonary blood flow	
Pretricuspid	Total anomalous pulmonary venous communication and common atrium
Post-tricuspid	All single-ventricle physiology lesions† without PS and persistent truncus arteriosus
Pulmonary hypertension	Shunt reversal after the development of pulmonary vascular obstructive disease in any of the conditions associated with increased pulmonary blood flow (Eisenmenger physiology)

**VSD with PS or PA physiology:* This includes all conditions with unrestrictive interventricular communication and pulmonary stenosis or pulmonary atresia. *Included in this list are the following:* Tetralogy of Fallot, double-outlet right ventricle, single ventricle, transposition with VSD, corrected transposition with VSD, atrioventricular septal defect, and tricuspid atresia

†Admixture lesions are all conditions with single-ventricle physiology

(LA: left atrium; R-L: right-to-left; RV: right ventricle)

TABLE 9.2.4: Physiological perturbations in congenital heart disease.

Physiological derangement	*Hemodynamic consequences*	*Clinical consequences*	*Examples*
Increased pulmonary blood flow	Inefficient circulation, pulmonary congestion, and pulmonary hypertension	Failure to thrive, heart failure symptoms, tachypnea, and frequent respiratory infections	All post-tricuspid shunts, some large pretricuspid shunts
Reduced pulmonary blood flow	Hypoxia in the presence of an atrial or ventricular septal defect (VSD); reduced cardiac output if both septa are intact	Cyanosis and fatigue on exertion	All congenital heart defects that are associated with pulmonary stenosis
Mixing of systemic and pulmonary venous return (single-ventricle physiology)	Some hypoxia will result, but the exact oxygen saturation will be dictated by pulmonary blood flow. If pulmonary blood flow is increased (shunt ratio of 2:1 or more). Saturations are usually above 85%	Cyanosis of varying severity depending on pulmonary blood flow	All forms of univentricular hearts; double-inlet left ventricle (LV) or right ventricle (RV); tricuspid atresia, primitive hearts associated with asplenia; and polysplenia
Unfavorable streaming and parallel circulation	Hypoxia tends to be severe unless pulmonary blood flow is significantly elevated	Severe cyanosis in the face of excessive pulmonary blood flow	All variations of transposition of the great arteries; double outlet RV with subpulmonic VSD (Taussig–Bing)
Pulmonary venous hypertension	Pulmonary venous congestion with pulmonary arteriolar vasoconstriction and resultant elevation in pulmonary vascular resistance	Tachypnea from pulmonary edema and severe elevation in pulmonary vascular resistance translate into reduced pulmonary blood flow and increased cyanosis	Obstructed total anomalous pulmonary venous connection, cor triatriatum, congenital mitral stenosis, mitral atresia with restrictive atrial septal defect (ASD), and pulmonary vein stenosis
Elevated pulmonary vascular resistance	Inability to increase cardiac output during exercise or stress and increased right-to-left shunting across associated defects	*Fatigue on effort:* Patients with defects in the atrial or ventricular septum will have increasing cyanosis	All conditions associated with increased pulmonary blood flow increase the risk for the development of increased pulmonary vascular resistance
Left-sided atrioventricular valve regurgitation	Left ventricular volume overload, elevation in left atrial pressures, and pulmonary venous congestion	Tachypnea, fatigue on effort, and heart failure symptoms	Atrioventricular septal defects, corrected transposition, ASDs (5–10% have associated mitral valve prolapse and MR), congenital MR, and anomalous coronary artery from pulmonary artery
Right-sided atrioventricular valve regurgitation	Right ventricular volume overload, elevated right atrial pressures, and systemic venous congestion	Fatigue and right heart failure	Ebstein anomaly and congenital anomalies of tricuspid valve
Left ventricular hypertrophy	Elevated filling pressures result in left heart failure	Tachypnea from pulmonary venous congestion	All forms of left ventricular outflow tract obstruction and hypertrophic cardiomyopathy

Contd...

Contd...

Physiological derangement	*Hemodynamic consequences*	*Clinical consequences*	*Examples*
Right ventricular hypertrophy	Elevated right-sided filling pressures with systemic venous congestion	*Right heart failure:* Liver enlargement and fluid accumulation (edema and ascites)	*Advanced forms of right ventricular outflow obstruction:* Critical pulmonary stenosis and advanced pulmonary hypertension
Reduced coronary perfusion	Left ventricular dysfunction	Tachypnea and fatigue	Anomalous left coronary artery from pulmonary artery
Pulmonary valve regurgitation	Dilation of branch pulmonary arteries with airway compression and right ventricular dilation	Respiratory symptoms in infants with tetralogy of Fallot (TOF) and absent pulmonary valve, fatigue on effort in patients with long-standing pulmonary valve incompetence	TOF with absent pulmonary valve and pulmonary hypertension (usually mild)
Aortic valve regurgitation	Left ventricular dilation	Fatigue and palpitation	Bicommissural aortic valve, in association with subpulmonic and some perimembranous defects

(MR: mitral regurgitation)

tricuspid valve and is, therefore, subtle or even inaudible. The second heart sound split is wide and fixed largely because of the prolonged "hang-out" interval resulting from increased capacitance of the pulmonary circulation. In addition, the large communication at the atrial level minimizes any differences in the impact of respiration on the right versus left heart. Pulmonary arterial hypertension (PAH) is typically absent or at most mild. The presence of moderate or severe PAH in ASD is worrisome and may suggest the onset of irreversible changes in the pulmonary vasculature.

Post-tricuspid shunts are different in that there is direct transmission of pressure from the systemic to the pulmonary circuit at the ventricular level (VSD) or great arteries [patent ductus arteriosus (PDA) and aortopulmonary (AP) window]. For patients with large post-tricuspid shunts, symptoms begin in early infancy, typically after some regression of elevated pulmonary vascular resistance (PVR) in the newborn period together with progressive development of the pulmonary vascular tree. The excessive pulmonary blood flow returns to the left atrium (LA) and flows through the mitral valve, resulting in the apical diastolic flow murmur that is a consistent marker of large post-tricuspid shunts. The LA and left ventricle (LV) are dilated because of this extra volume. Elevation in pulmonary artery (PA) pressures is an inevitable consequence of large (or unrestrictive) post-tricuspid shunts and is labeled as hyperkinetic PAH. This needs to be distinguished from the elevation of PVR that results from sustained exposure to increased pulmonary blood flow.

Ventricular Septal Defect: Pulmonary Stenosis Physiology

This situation is characterized by a large communication at the ventricular level together with varying degrees of obstruction to pulmonary blood flow. Typically, this is in the form of subvalvular (infundibular), valvular, annular (small valve annulus), and occasionally supravalvular stenosis. The free communication between the two ventricles results in the equalization of pressures. Severity of PS dictates the volume of blood flowing through PAs and, therefore, the amount of oxygenated blood returning via pulmonary veins. Severe PS results in a right-to-left shunt across the VSD with varying degrees of hypoxia and, consequently, cyanosis. Cyanosis is directly proportionate to the severity of PS. Since the RV is readily decompressed by the large VSD, heart failure is unusual. The best example of VSD–PS physiology is tetralogy of Fallot (TOF). In its least severe form, TOF is often not associated with cyanosis (pink TOF). Here, PS is significant enough to result in a large pressure gradient across the right ventricular outflow tract (RVOT) but not severe enough to result in a reduction in pulmonary blood flow. Pink TOF is typically associated with a loud ejection systolic murmur (ESM) because of the reasonable volume of blood flowing across the RVOT. As the severity of PS increases, pulmonary blood flow declines, and the intensity and duration of murmur decline progressively. Other examples of VSD–PS physiology include double-outlet RV (DORV) with subaortic VSD and PS, corrected transposition with PS, and atrioventricular (AV) septal defect with PS. These conditions are often indistinguishable from TOF at the bedside.

Single-ventricle Physiology

This refers to a group of conditions where there is complete mixing of pulmonary and systemic venous returns. In addition to single ventricle (double-inlet ventricle), a variety of conditions come under the category of single ventricular/

admixture physiology based on the level of mixing of blood. Atresia of one of the AV valves, severe hypoplasia of one of the ventricles, and severe straddling of one of the AV valves over a large VSD are all examples of situations where there is mixing of pulmonary and systemic venous returns at the ventricular level. Persistent truncus is an example of mixing at the great artery level. The clinical manifestations are dictated by whether there is PS. In the absence of PS, there is excessive pulmonary blood flow, especially in infants, because of the relatively lower PVR. As a result, the proportion of oxygenated blood from pulmonary veins that mixes with the systemic venous return is high. As a result, cyanosis is minimal and measured oxygen saturation may be in the 90s. However, the price for this preserved oxygenation is heart failure and development of permanent elevation of PVR [pulmonary vascular obstructive disease (PVOD)]. Over time, if the child survives infancy, PVR progressively increases with increasing cyanosis.

Single ventricle and its physiologic variants can be associated with varying degrees of PS. Here, the situation is quite like VSD-PS physiology except for relatively severe hypoxia because of free mixing systemic and pulmonary venous return.

Duct-dependent Lesions

An infant or a newborn with CHD that is dependent on the patency of the ductus arteriosus for survival can be termed suffering from a duct-dependent lesion. Typically, these are newborns in which either the systemic blood supply or the pulmonary blood flow is critically dependent on an open PDA termed duct-dependent systemic circulation (DDSC) or duct-dependent pulmonary circulation (DDPC), respectively.

Closure of the PDA in DDSC results in systemic hypoperfusion and shock-like presentation (often mislabeled as neonatal sepsis). Examples of DDSC include hypoplastic left heart syndrome, where the entire systemic circulation is supported by the RV through the PDA, and interrupted aortic arch, where the descending aortic flow is entirely through the PDA. Severe coarctation and critical aortic stenosis (AS) are also examples of DDSC.

Closure of PDA in DDPC results in severe hypoxia and cyanosis in the affected newborn. Examples of DDPC include all forms of pulmonary atresia (irrespective of underlying heart defect) where the PDA is the predominant source of pulmonary blood flow. There are examples of pulmonary atresia where pulmonary blood supply is from major AP collaterals. These children may survive even after the PDA closes. Critical pulmonic stenosis ("nearly atretic" pulmonary valve) can present as duct-dependent pulmonary blood flow.

Neonates with duct-dependent physiology require prostaglandin E1 (PGE1) for survival. Early recognition of a duct-dependent situation allows early initiation of PGE1 and stabilization until a definitive procedure can be accomplished. The usual dosage of PGE1 is 0.05–0.5 μg/kg/min. Adverse effects include hypotension, flushing/fever, and apnea.

Unfavorable Streaming and Parallel Circulation

Unfavorable streaming refers to a situation where oxygen-rich pulmonary blood flow is directed toward the pulmonary valve and poorly oxygenated blood toward the aortic valve. An extreme form of unfavorable streaming is the parallel circulation in transposition of the great arteries (TGA) with an intact ventricular septum. Here survival is dependent on the presence of a communication (ideally at the atrial level) that allows mixing of pulmonary and systemic venous return. The presence of a VSD may improve the saturation in TGA, but significant cyanosis is usually present unless the pulmonary blood flow is torrential.

RECOGNITION OF CONGENITAL HEART DISEASE

The manifestations of CHD are different in a neonate, an infant, or a child. It is often easy to recognize the presence of CHD in older children. In infants, and particularly in newborns, manifestations of heart disease can often be subtle. Further, several conditions that do not involve the cardiovascular system can result in clinical manifestations that overlap with those resulting from heart disease. Notwithstanding these difficulties, it is possible to identify the presence of heart disease in most infants and newborns after careful clinical evaluation. The following clinical features should alert the pediatrician regarding the presence of CHD.

Cyanosis

Cyanosis may be peripheral or central. Peripheral cyanosis (acrocyanosis) almost exclusively involves lips (perioral region) and extremities. Normal neonates may have bluish extremities that respond to warming or moving extremities. Similarly, some infants may have peripheral cyanosis following exposure to cold Saturations of 90% or lower while breathing room air beyond the first 20 minutes are considered abnormal. Central cyanosis involving the mucous membranes and trunk along with the lips and extremities strongly suggests the likelihood of CHD. Unfortunately, however, cyanosis often remains unnoticed. This is particularly true in the Indian context, where it is difficult to detect cyanosis in the presence of a dark skin complexion. The tip of the tongue is a good place to look for cyanosis as the circulation is not sluggish and its color is not affected by race/ethnicity. Further, cyanosis is often masked by anemia. When central cyanosis is suspected, its presence should be confirmed, and severity quantified by measuring oxygen saturation using a skin oximeter probe. Unfortunately, however, the availability of this instrument is limited to a few selected institutions. Differentiating cardiac versus pulmonary cyanosis is of upmost importance; a hyperoxia test helps in differentiating these conditions. Cyanosis from pulmonary disease responds to inhalation of 100% O_2 by an increase in arterial pO_2, whereas cardiac disease does not.

Difficult Feeding and Poor Growth

The parent of an infant with CHD may complain that the child has difficulty in feeding. This is usually a feature of an infant with congestive heart failure resulting from CHD. The history may be of slow feeding, small volumes consumed during each feed, tiring easily following feeds, and the requirement of periods of rest during feeds. Not infrequently, no history of feeding difficulty may be obtained, but examination of the growth charts will reveal that the child's growth rate is not appropriate for age. A steady decline in the growth rate (falling off the growth curve) or weight that is inappropriate for age (<third percentile) may result from a large left-to-right shunt. Characteristically, growth retardation affects weight significantly more than height. In cyanotic children, there may be equal retardation in weight and height.

Difficult Breathing

Tachypnea [respiratory rates consistently >60/min in infants <2 months; >50/min in older infants (2–12 months); >40/min after 1 year] is a characteristic manifestation of heart failure (preterm newborns may normally have respiratory rates of up to 60/min). For infants, subcostal or intercostal retractions/ use of accessory muscles of respiration together with flaring of nostrils (alae nasi) are frequently associated with tachypnea.

Frequent Respiratory Infections

Respiratory infections that are frequent, severe, and difficult to treat are common in infants with CHD associated with large left-to-right shunts, resulting from increased lung blood flow. Not infrequently, heart disease may be detected for the first time during an episode of respiratory tract infection.

Clinical Stigmata of Specific Syndromes

Evidence of the presence of chromosomal anomalies or other syndromes that are known to be associated with CHD should alert the clinician to the presence of specific cardiac defects that are known to be associated with these conditions. The list of such conditions is a long one. Trisomy 21 is the most common chromosomal anomaly that is associated with heart disease. Other common examples include trisomy 13, trisomy 18, Turner syndrome, Noonan syndrome, velocardiofacial, and DiGeorge syndrome **(Table 9.2.1)**.

CARDIOVASCULAR EXAMINATION

A thorough and systematic cardiovascular examination provides valuable clues to the presence of heart disease. With practice, such an examination can be accomplished in a short time. For the pediatrician, thorough familiarization with what is normal is a useful initial step. It is useful to answer the following questions that can serve as a checklist for a preliminary cardiac examination. This checklist is comprehensive and is designed primarily to answer the question: *Does the patient have heart disease?* It can also help identify the broad physiologic category of heart defect.

- *Are arterial pulsations normal?*
  Is the pulse volume normal or increased?
  Is there a discrepancy of pulsation in any of the four extremities?
  A careful evaluation of pulsations in all extremities should always be a part of physical examination. Coarctation is readily diagnosed when weak femoral artery pulsations are detected in comparison to brachial or radial arteries. When a discrepancy in pulses is suspected, four-extremity blood pressure measurements should be obtained. An automated, noninvasive blood pressure instrument is preferred over manual recording for four-extremity blood pressure measurement.
- *Does the precordium feel normal?*
  Are there visible precordial pulsations?
  Is the apex beat displaced, hyperdynamic, or heaving? Is there a thrill palpable?
- *Are the heart sounds normal?*
  Can the two components of the second heart sound be separated?
  Is there an additional heart sound in diastole (such as S3)?
  Are there any additional systolic sounds (ejection clicks)?
- *Is (or are) there a murmur (or murmurs)? If so:*
  Is it systolic or diastolic, or both systolic and diastolic (diastolic murmurs always have a structural basis)?
  Is it loud (grade 3 or louder murmurs are seldom innocent)?

DIAGNOSIS

Electrocardiogram and Chest X-ray

If there is a suspicion of heart disease based on the history or physical examination, an ECG and a chest X-ray should be obtained. The ECG should be interpreted keeping the age of the child in mind. Interpretation of the chest X-ray should involve evaluation of the cardiac silhouette and lung vasculature. The X-ray also provides information about the location of abdominal organs (for determination of the situs) and the aortic arch. Beyond the neonatal period, a normal ECG and chest X-ray make the diagnosis of a hemodynamically significant heart defect unlikely. In the newborn, however, ECG and chest X-ray change and may take a few days to evolve. For the newborn, particularly in the first few days, a "normal" ECG and a normal X-ray do not rule out serious heart disease.

Echocardiography

Echocardiography has revolutionized the diagnosis of CHD, and its high diagnostic yield makes this investigation very cost-effective in most situations. This statement is, however, only true if it is performed by an experienced individual who understands the anatomy and physiology of CHD. In many children with CHD, a very thorough evaluation is possible, and all the questions addressed in the checklist (below) can be answered. This is particularly true for infants and newborns, in which excellent images are readily obtained. Such patients can undergo a definitive procedure based on the information provided by the echocardiogram. Transesophageal echocardiography can supplement transthoracic studies. This is particularly true for patients with poor thoracic echocardiography windows that do not permit adequate imaging. Unlike adults, children undergoing transesophageal echocardiography often require general anesthesia. Echocardiography has a few inherent limitations; however, it consistently fails to define certain structures, such as the PA branches beyond the hila of the lungs. Here, cardiac computed tomography (CT) or cardiac magnetic resonance (CMR) imaging works well. Newer modalities, such as three-dimensional echocardiography, are in the evolving phase and at present do not add significance to two-dimensional echocardiography.

Checklist of Diagnosis of CHD Through Echocardiography

- What is the visceral and atrial situs (solitus, inversus, or ambiguous)?
- What is the relationship of the abdominal aorta to the inferior vena cava (IVC)?
- What are the systemic venous connections like? Is the IVC intact? Is there a separate left superior vena cava (SVC)? If so, how does it drain?
- What are the pulmonary venous connections like? Normal drainage into LA? Any anomalous drainage?
- What is the appearance of the atria like? Is the atrial septum intact? Is there an ASD or a patent foramen ovale? If so, in what direction does blood flow?
- How do the atria connect to the ventricles (concordant or discordant)?
- Is it possible to identify two separate AV valves?
- How are the AV valves in their appearance and function?
- The ventricles, their size, shape, and function?
- Are the various components of the interventricular septum intact?
- How do the ventricles connect to the great arteries?
- Is there any outflow tract obstruction?
- What is the appearance and function of the semilunar valves?
- What is the great artery relationship?
    - Are the branch PAs in continuity? Is there any branch PA stenosis?
    - What side is the aortic arch? What is its branching pattern? Is there a PDA or a coarctation?
    - What is the coronary artery anatomy?
    - How are the hemodynamics and physiology altered?

Cardiac Magnetic Resonance Imaging

Cardiac magnetic resonance imaging (MRI), a useful noninvasive imaging modality, has established itself as an important modality for the evaluation of CHD. It is especially useful in older patients and postoperative patients where imaging from echo is limited. In addition, CMR has tremendous value in defining extracardiac structures, such as branch PAs, pulmonary veins, and AP collaterals. Very useful physiologic data (especially blood flow calculations at several locations along with functional assessment) is also obtained through MRI. It is likely to replace cardiac catheterization in most situations. Limitations with CMR include limited expertise for interpretation and the requirement of general anesthesia to enable breath holding in children.

Computed Tomography

Anatomic information from CT is like that of MRI. CT overcomes some of the key limitations of MRI because it has a much lower image acquisition time. However, exposure to ionizing radiation is a major concern. In addition, unlike adults, children have faster resting heart rates that come in the way of satisfactory imaging of coronary arteries.

Diagnostic Cardiac Catheterization

The role of diagnostic cardiac catheterization for patients with CHD has declined considerably with the availability of high-quality echocardiography, MRI, and CT. Since cardiac catheterization is an invasive procedure, its performance requires careful planning so that the information desired may be obtained with the minimum risk to the patient. Simply stated, a diagnostic cardiac catheterization may be performed whenever noninvasive investigations do not provide crucial information that is required for surgical planning. Accurate estimation of filling pressures and PA pressures, determination of blood flows and vascular resistance, and definition of coronary arteries are often best performed through cardiac catheterization.

NEWBORN SCREENING FOR CONGENITAL HEART DISEASE

Notwithstanding its significant limitations, pulse oximetry offers the best prospect of detecting critical CHD among all the available tools in the newborn period. Clinical examination alone has very poor sensitivity and specificity. Systematic efforts to examine the utility of pulse oximetry for screening for newborn heart disease in Indian settings have yielded mixed results. Among the 19,009 newborns screened in the recent study from Delhi, pulse oximetry detected 39 major (sensitivity 55.7% and specificity 68.3%) and 22 critical CHDs (sensitivity 84.6% and specificity 68.3%). The addition of pulse oximetry to clinical examination significantly improved sensitivity for major CHDs (35.7–75.7%) and critical CHDs (11.5–84.6%).[6] There are important challenges in applying screening for newborn CHD on a national scale.[4] The existing numbers of centers are simply not capable of dealing with the existing volume of cases that are incidentally identified. With the introduction of widespread systematic screening, there is likely to be a substantial increase in the numbers of children that will completely overwhelm the existing programs. A nationwide screening program can only be introduced after the downstream consequences of identifying large numbers of children with CHD are fully considered. **Flowchart 9.2.1** shows the recommended protocol for newborn pulse oximeter screening.

DEFINITIVE TREATMENT AND PALLIATION FOR CONGENITAL HEART DISEASE

To ensure the best possible results of management of CHD, it is necessary to assemble a team of especially qualified individuals who should ideally be a part of a comprehensive pediatric heart program. The details are shown in **Flowchart 9.2.2**. Definitive treatment for CHD requires the collaborative (and not competitive) use of surgery and catheter-based interventions.

Surgery

Surgery is still the best option for definitive treatment or palliation of most forms of CHD. A simple scheme of classification of surgery for CHD is shown in **Flowchart 9.2.3**. This classification is a practical one and is from the point of view of follow-up issues. A detailed description of all congenital heart operations is clearly beyond the scope of the chapter. Congenital heart operations are also broadly classified as open heart [requiring the use of cardiopulmonary bypass (CPB)] and closed heart (not requiring CPB). Most corrective operations and many palliative operations fall under the category of open-heart operations. These procedures are generally a more significant and expensive undertaking because of the use of the CPB circuit and a substantially larger number of disposable items. The morbidity of open-heart operations is proportionate to the duration of exposure to

Flowchart 9.2.1: Recommended protocol for newborn pulse oximeter screening.

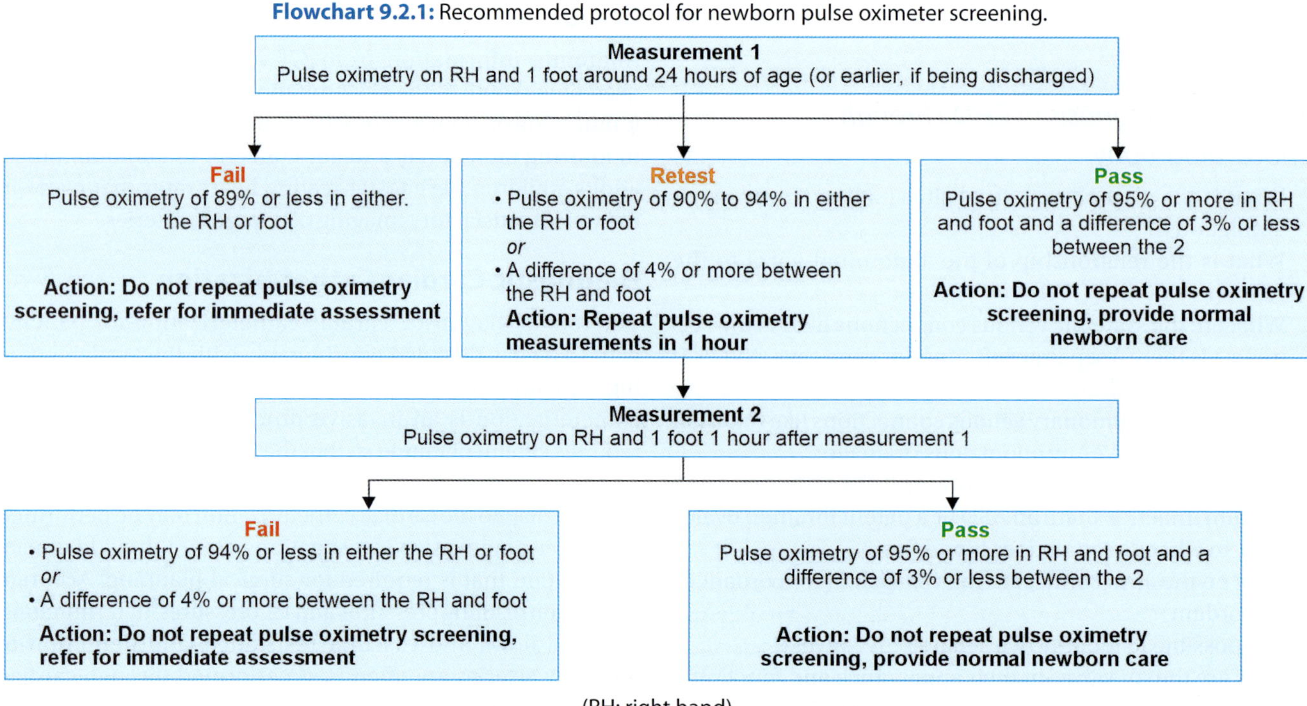

(RH: right hand)

Flowchart 9.2.2: Constituents of a comprehensive pediatric heart program for optimal care of children with congenital heart disease.

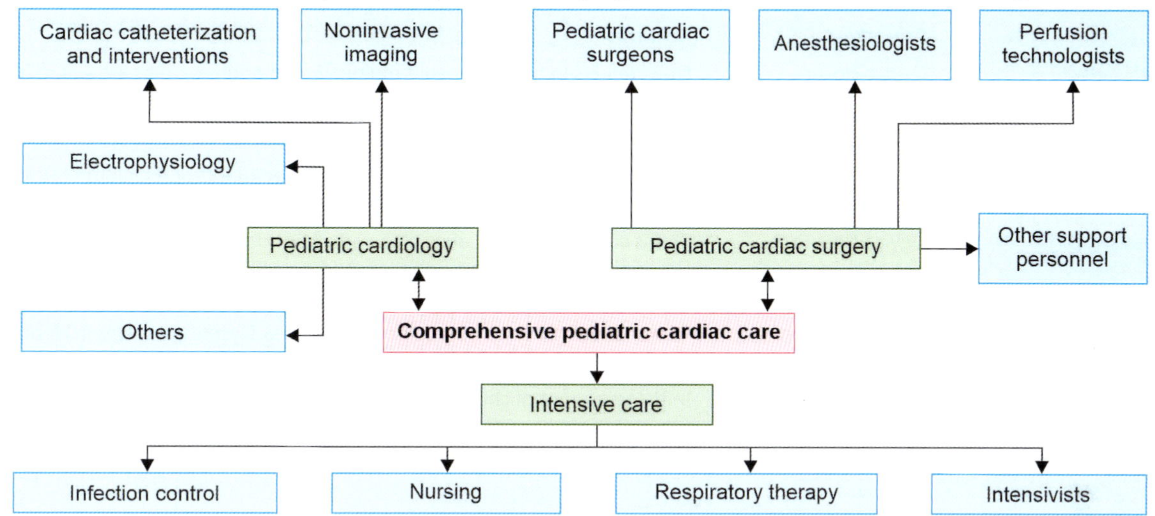

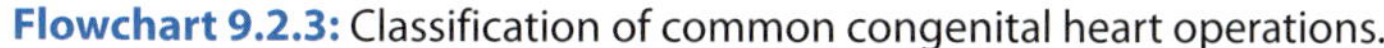

Flowchart 9.2.3: Classification of common congenital heart operations.

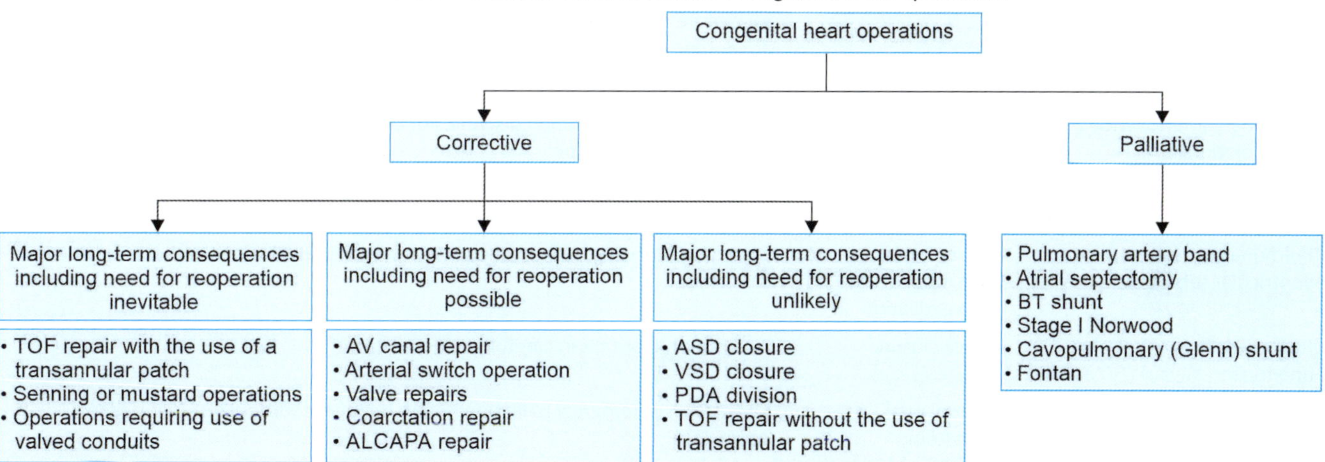

(ALCAPA: anomalous left coronary artery arising from the pulmonary artery; ASD: atrial septal defect; AV: atrioventricular; BT shunt: Blalock–Taussig shunt; PDA: patent ductus arteriosus; TOF: tetralogy of Fallot; VSD: ventricular septal defect)

CPB and the cross-clamp time (the period when heart beating is deliberately brought to a standstill using cardioplegia).[7]

Catheter Interventions for Congenital Heart Disease

The scope of catheter interventions has grown by leaps and bounds in the last two to three decades, and this treatment option has transformed the care of many children with CHD. Many simple defects, such as secundum ASD, PDA, and selected muscular VSD, can now be closed in the catheterization laboratory. In addition, balloon valvuloplasty is now the first line of treatment for congenital stenosis of the pulmonary and aortic valves. Additional details of catheter intervention procedures are shown in **Table 9.2.5**. The advantages of catheter-based interventions are obvious, and this has become an increasingly appealing option for many children. The procedures are far less traumatic than surgery, accomplished with greater ease, allow rapid recovery, and leave behind no scars.

For the best and consistently reproducible results in newborn and infant heart surgery, the presence of such a team is vital.

COMPLICATIONS OF CONGENITAL HEART DISEASE

Several adverse complications occur because of CHD (**Table 9.2.6**). For the sake of simplicity, we will focus on the selected common complications.

TABLE 9.2.5: Congenital heart defects amenable to catheter-based interventions.

Lesion	*Procedure*	*Remarks*
Atrial septal defect	Device closure	Only defects in the fossa ovalis region with enough margins are suited for device closure
Patent ductus arteriosus (PDA)	Coil or device closure	Most PDAs can be closed in the cath lab except for large PDAs in small infants
Muscular ventricular septal defect (VSD)	Device closure	Device closure is an option for relatively older infants and children (>8 kg)
Membranous VSD	Device closure	This is controversial because of the small but definite possibility of heart block. However, an increasing number of children with membranous defects are being offered closure
Pulmonary valve stenosis	Balloon pulmonary valvuloplasty (BPV)	Treatment of choice for most forms at all ages. Dysplastic valves in Noonan syndrome may not respond well to BPV
Aortic valve stenosis	Balloon aortic valvuloplasty (BAV)	Initial treatment of choice at all ages; eventually the dilated aortic valves with regurgitation may need surgical management
Branch pulmonary artery stenosis	Balloon dilation with stenting	Stenting is often preferred to surgery in branch PA stenosis
Coarctation of aorta	Balloon dilation with or without stenting	Surgery is the preferred option in the newborn period because recurrence after balloon dilation is very common. For older infants, balloon dilation is a reasonable alternative. Older children and adolescents (>10 years) may be offered stenting for a more complete relief. Neither balloon dilation nor stenting has a proven advantage over surgery
Coronary artery fistula	Coil or device closure	Treatment of choice
Pulmonary arteriovenous malformations	Coil or device closure	Treatment of choice when discrete. For diffuse malformations, coil or device closure is not an option
Duct-dependent pulmonary circulation	Stenting of the PDA	Stenting can be offered in carefully selected cases as an alternative to the Blalock–Taussig shunt
Pulmonary atresia with intact ventricular septum	Perforation of the valve followed by balloon dilation	Emerging as the procedure of choice in selected institutions with the facility and expertise
Ruptured sinus of Valsalva aneurysm	Device closure	A reasonable option in carefully selected cases
Transposition of the great arteries	Balloon atrial septostomy	Short-term emergency palliation before definitive surgery (arterial switch operation)

(cath lab: catheterization laboratory; PA: pulmonary atresia)

Pulmonary Arterial Hypertension

Pulmonary arterial hypertension occurs commonly in the context of CHD. With increasing emphasis on early correction, the magnitude of the problem is on the decline in most developed nations. Unfortunately, because most children with CHD do not receive timely attention, this is still a problem of considerable magnitude in low- and middle-income countries.

The lesions that have the greatest likelihood include cyanotic heart disease with increased pulmonary blood flow. Here irreversible changes in pulmonary vasculature develop rapidly, often during infancy itself. Therefore, it is particularly important to correct or appropriately palliate these lesions early (ideally within the first few months of life). Large acyanotic post-tricuspid shunts are also prone to early development of PAH and should be ideally corrected early, preferably within the first year. In pretricuspid shunts, PAH develops slowly and unpredictably. Most patients with ASD will have mild or no PAH throughout their lives. A small proportion of them develop accelerated changes in the pulmonary vasculature. Some of the key features responsible for the development of PAH are summarized in **Figure 9.2.1**.

Infective Endocarditis or Endarteritis

Endocarditis can complicate CHD with a suitable substrate. This includes the presence of a region of significant turbulence created by high-pressure gradients. Examples include unrepaired cyanotic CHD and repaired CHD with residual defects or use of artificial material, such as restrictive VSD and PDA, TOF (pulmonary valve), and other VSD–PS situations, and left ventricular outflow tract obstruction. Some surgical operations [palliative shunts such

TABLE 9.2.6: Common adverse consequences of congenital heart disease (CHD).

Lesion category	*Adverse consequences*
Duct-dependent systemic blood flow in the newborn: • Hypoplastic left heart syndrome • Critical coarctation • Interrupted aortic arch • Critical aortic stenosis	Systemic hypoperfusion and death with closure of the duct
Duct-dependent pulmonary blood flow in the newborn: • Pulmonary atresia intact ventricular septum • Pulmonary atresia with other CHD conditions • Critical pulmonary stenosis • Severe Ebstein anomaly	Severe hypoxia and death with the closure of the ductus
Conditions associated with increased pulmonary blood flow: • Left-to-right shunts • *Admixture lesions with increased pulmonary blood flow:* Transposition with ventricular septal defect (VSD), persistent truncus arteriosus, double outlet right ventricle, tricuspid atresia with unrestricted pulmonary blood flow, single ventricle, etc.	*Early:* • Heart failure • Lower respiratory infections that are frequent, prolonged, and difficult to treat • Growth retardation *Late:* • Pulmonary vascular obstructive disease and Eisenmenger syndrome *Development of valve dysfunction:* • Aortic regurgitation in VSD • Mitral regurgitation in atrial septal defect (ASD)
Conditions with reduced pulmonary blood flow and right-to-left shunting in the heart tetralogy of Fallot (TOF) Other conditions with TOF (VSD with pulmonic stenosis) physiology	• Cyanotic spells • Brain infarction/ cerebrovascular thrombosis • Brain abscess • Seizure disorder • A variety of adverse long-term neurodevelopmental consequences • Cognitive impairment • Lower intelligence quotient (IQ) • Learning disturbance • Problems associated with polycythemia
Obstructive lesions: • Aortic and pulmonary valve stenosis • Subaortic obstruction • Supravalvular aortic stenosis • Isolated infundibular stenosis • Coarctation • Peripheral pulmonic stenosis	• Heart failure • Sudden death • Dysrhythmias
Congenital valve regurgitation	• Heart failure • Ventricular dysfunction • Dysrhythmia

as the Blalock-Taussig (BT) shunt, use of conduits] are also associated with an increased risk of infective endocarditis or endarteritis. Lesions with little or no turbulent flows, such as ASD, are not associated with increased risk. Typically, the risk of endocarditis increases after dentition begins. Current guidelines do not routinely recommend antibiotic prophylaxis for many conditions (including some of the above lesions). However, the importance of maintaining good dental hygiene and cutaneous hygiene in all children with CHD cannot be overemphasized.

Growth and Nutrition

This is affected in all forms of CHD and is particularly striking in large left-to-right shunts. Children with CHD show a high prevalence (59% in recent Indian studies) of significant malnutrition (weight is more affected than height), and this tends to improve after correction, irrespective of the underlying lesion. However, catch-up growth is slow, especially if CHD is corrected late or there is syndromic association/noncardiac lesions.[8]

Myocardial Dysfunction and Myocardial Damage

Chronic volume overload results in ventricular enlargement and ventricular dysfunction that is typically reversed after correction. A small proportion of patients with severe hypoxia also develop severe ventricular dysfunction involving both ventricles. Heart failure is mostly the result of hemodynamic consequences of increased pulmonary blood flow, mitral or tricuspid valve regurgitation, and severe myocardial hypertrophy. Systolic dysfunction is a relatively less common cause.

Neurologic and Neurodevelopmental Consequences

These are listed in **Table 9.2.6**. Chronic hypoxia, in utero hypoxia and hypoperfusion, and open-heart surgery (especially operations performed under total circulatory arrest) contribute substantially to morbidity from the neurological consequences of CHD. Brain abscess is uniquely associated with cyanotic heart disease involving the temporal and parietal lobes predominantly (typically beyond the age of 2 years) where the right-to-left shunt bypasses the pulmonary filter.

Polycythemia and Its Adverse Consequences

Older children with cyanotic CHD are prone to complications from a chronically elevated red cell turnover. These include symptoms of hyperviscosity (mucosal bleeding, visual disturbances, and neurological complications), gout, renal failure, and gallstones.

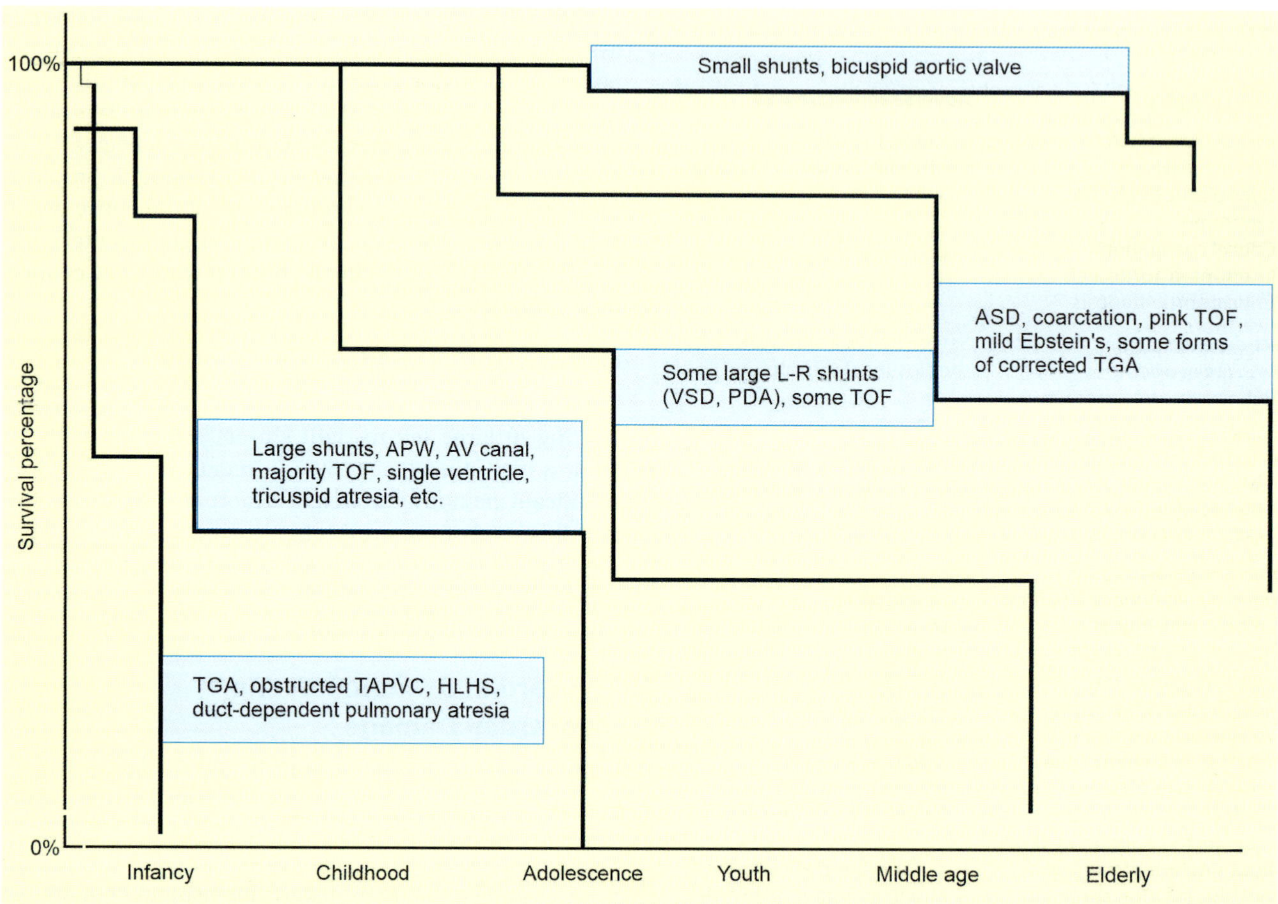

Fig. 9.2.1: Natural history of uncorrected CHD; this is a simplified representation showing the survival for most common congenital heart defects. (APW: aortopulmonary window; ASD: atrial septal defect; AV: atrioventricular; CHD: congenital heart disease; HLHS: hypoplastic left heart syndrome; L-R: left-to-right; PDA: patent ductus arteriosus; TAPVC: total anomalous pulmonary venous connection; TGA: transposition of the great arteries; TOF: tetralogy of Fallot; VSD: ventricular septal defect)

Rhythm Disorders and Sudden Death

Chronic enlargement of heart chambers predisposes to tachyarrhythmia. Chronic right atrial (RA) enlargement (such as in ASD, Ebstein, and severe tricuspid regurgitation) predisposes to atrial flutter. This can be persistent and refractory. Chronic right ventricular enlargement predisposes to malignant ventricular tachycardia (VT) and can precipitate sudden cardiac arrest in a small fraction of patients. This is starting to become a significant long-term concern after TOF repair where the pulmonary valve is rendered incompetent. Similarly, left ventricular hypertrophy (LVH) and dysfunction are associated with a higher-than-usual risk of malignant VT.

Cyanotic Spells

All patients with the VSD-PS physiology are prone to cyanotic spells. Cyanotic spells are due to an acute decrease in pulmonary blood flow, increased right-to-left shunt, and systemic desaturation, possibly due to the following reasons:

- Infundibular spasm due to increased circulating catecholamines because of the effort of feeding or crying
- Activation of mechanoreceptors in RV due to a decrease in systemic venous return or that in LV due to decreases in pulmonary blood flow, leading to peripheral vasodilation and fall in systemic vascular resistance, producing increased right-left shunt and systemic desaturation. The same mechanism can account for occasional episodes of bradycardia (Bezold-Jarisch reflex).

A cyanotic spell is a pediatric emergency that requires prompt recognition and intervention to prevent disabling cerebrovascular insults or death. A cyanotic spell needs to be taken seriously not just because of the immediate threat but also because it indicates the need for early operation. It is commonly seen below 2 years (peaks between 2 and 6 months). The onset is usually spontaneous and unpredictable and occurs more often early in the morning after waking up, although it can occur at any time of the day. The infant cries incessantly, is irritable, and is often inconsolable. Tachypnea is prominent and a cardinal feature. Typically, these infants have a pattern of deep and rapid breathing without significant subcostal recession. Cyanosis deepens as the spell progresses. Later gasping respiration and apnea ensue, which leads to limpness and ultimately anoxic seizures. Spells can last from minutes to hours. Auscultation reveals softening or disappearance of pulmonary ejection murmur. The management of cyanotic spell is summarized in **Box 9.2.1**.

BOX 9.2.1: Management of hypercyanotic spells.

Management of cyanotic spells

Immediate steps

- *Check airway and start oxygen*: If a child is uncomfortable with a mask or nasal cannula, deliver oxygen via a tube whose end is held 16–1 in away from the nose. This corresponds to delivering 80% oxygen
- Knee-chest position
- Sedate the child with subcutaneous morphine (0.2 mg/kg/dose) or intramuscular (IM) ketamine (3–5 mg/kg/dose)
- Obtain reliable intravenous (IV) access
- Soda bicarbonate 1–2 mL/kg (1–2 mEq/kg) given as 1:1 dilution or can be diluted in 10 mL/kg of isolyte "P," which is given a bolus as the initial resuscitating fluid
- Correct hypovolemia (10 mL/kg fluid bolus of isolyte "P" or dextrose normal saline)
- Keep the child warm
- Correct anemia by packed cell transfusion. Hemoglobin levels <12 g/dL merit correction through a blood transfusion in children with cyanotic spells
- Start beta-blockade. Beta-blockade is fairly safe unless a specific contraindication such as bronchial asthma or ventricular dysfunction exists. It should always be given with heart rate monitoring

Medications and dosages

Intravenous metoprolol: 0.1 mg/kg, given slowly over 5 minutes

- Can repeat every 5 minutes for a maximum of three doses
- Can be followed by infusion 1–2 µg/kg/min
- Monitor saturation, heart rates, and blood pressure (BP)
- Aim to keep heart rate below 100/min

Other options

- *IV esmolol:* 500 µg/kg over 1 minute as loading dose, 50 µg/kg/min for 4 minutes; if desaturation persists without a significant decrease in heart rate the loading dose will need to be repeated and the infusion rate can be increased in 50 µg/kg/min increments until 300 µg/kg/min; this infusion should be maintained at the rate that produces the desired result. Esmolol is relatively expensive but has the advantage of being very short acting
- *IV propranolol (0.1 mg/kg):* If desaturation persists, and there is still no significant trend toward improvement despite maximum beta-blockage
- *Start vasopressor infusion*: Methoxamine given IV at a dose of 0.1–0.2 mg/kg/dose or IM (0.1–0.4 mg/kg/dose). *Phenylephrine:* 5 µg/kg as bolus and then 1–4 µg/kg/min as infusion
- If spells are persistent, consider paralyzing the child, elective intubation, and ventilation, and plan for surgery/catheter-based intervention, which can be corrective or palliative (BT shunt) or rescue RVOT stenting/emergency BPV
- If convulsions occur—consider IV diazepam 0.2 mg/kg or IV midazolam 0.1–0.2 mg/kg/dose, as slow push

After a spell:

- After a spell is successfully managed, a careful neurological examination is mandatory. In the case of suspicion of neurologic insult during a spell, a CT scan is to be done to assess the presence and extent of cerebral infarcts
- Initiate maximally tolerated beta-blockade (propranolol 0.5–1.5 mg/kg/dose 8 hourly or 6 hourly). The dose can be titrated by the heart rate response. Beta-blockade may help improve resting saturation and can decrease the frequency of spells
- Do a detailed segmental analysis by 2D echo for a complete diagnosis
- Plan toward early corrective or palliative operation (depending on the age and anatomy)
- Continue therapeutic (if anemic) or prophylactic iron therapy (if not anemic)

Prevention:

- Parents of patients diagnosed to have a cyanotic congenital heart defect should be counseled, if the possibility of occurrence of a spell is anticipated
- Explain to them the circumstances when a spell may occur and teach them the knee-chest position for aborting a spell when there is a delay in availing medical care
- Avoid dehydration
- Rapid control of temperature whenever fever occurs
- Encourage early surgical repair
- Obtaining IV access in a cyanotic child can precipitate spells. This can be avoided by sedating the child with IM ketamine (3–5 mg/kg) and/or by using local anesthetic skin ointment (Emlap) before attempting for venous access or blood sampling

(2D echo: two-dimensional echocardiography; BPV: balloon pulmonary valvuloplasty; BT: Blalock–Taussig; CT: computed tomography; RVOT: right ventricular outflow tract)

Spontaneous Closure of Heart Defects (Table 9.2.7)

Some defects have a tendency toward spontaneous closure, and this can influence the timing of intervention. The defects known to close spontaneously are ASDs, VSDs, and PDA (during the first few months of life). The variables that influence the likelihood of spontaneous closure include age at evaluation (the likelihood of spontaneous closure declines with age, and most ASDs and many VSDs are unlikely to close after the first 3 years of age), size of the defect (smaller defects are more likely to close), and location of the defects (fossa ovalis ASDs, perimembranous, and muscular VSDs can close on their own). **Table 9.2.7** summarizes the variables that influence spontaneous closure. It is important to recognize the possibility of spontaneous closure while interpreting echocardiogram reports in infancy.

SURVIVAL OF PATIENTS WITH CONGENITAL HEART DISEASE

The natural history of common forms of CHD is shown in **Figure 9.2.1**. This figure is an approximation but serves to illustrate the fact that, without correction, many children with CHD (especially those with cyanotic CHD) will not survive beyond infancy or early childhood. This is dramatically altered by correction through surgery and, in some situations, through catheter interventions.

Following surgical correction, the natural history of many CHDs is dramatically improved. With accumulating follow-up data, however, it is becoming increasingly apparent that many "curative" operations have important long-term sequelae. The best example is surgery for TOF. For many years, it was thought that TOF repair was curative. A transannular patch that sacrifices the pulmonary valve and leaves behind severe pulmonary regurgitation was not thought to be of major importance. However, after 25–30 years of experience, most patients will develop progressive RV dilation with an increased risk of late heart failure and sudden cardiac death.

Similarly, there are growing long-term concerns after the arterial switch operation (aortic root dilation and silent coronary occlusion), AV canal repair (AV valve regurgitation), and coarctation (residual hypertension and aortic aneurysm). In addition, there are operations that involve placement of conduits (pulmonary atresia, Rastelli operations for TGA–VSD–PS). These require replacement with growth.

The Fontan operation, a final solution for all univentricular hearts (single-ventricle physiology), is best described as palliative with several significant long-term concerns.

PREVENTION OF CONGENITAL HEART DISEASE

Education of the lay public on the dangers of consanguinity, drugs, and teratogens in the first trimester of pregnancy and widespread immunization against Rubella can prevent CHDs to a limited extent. However, since most CHDs do not yet have an identifiable etiology, there is no effective strategy available for their prevention in the periconceptional period. Fetal echocardiography is emerging as a modality for CHD prevention after 14–16 weeks of gestation. Fetal echo is best suited to diagnose relatively severe forms of CHD. Conditions that involve major chamber discrepancy (such as hypoplastic left heart syndrome), single ventricles, and a common AV canal can be identified in a simple screening protocol (the four-chamber view). With some refinement (outflow tract and three vessel views), additional conditions, such as TOF, large VSD, TGA, persistent truncus arteriosus, and arch abnormalities, can be picked up as well.

The most significant challenge of fetal echocardiography lies in identifying the population at risk. The low incidence of CHD, together with the relatively small proportion of CHD that occurs in "high-risk" pregnancies, makes fetal screening of CHD an inefficient exercise. Further, the expertise and equipment required for accurate fetal echocardiography are scarce in regions with poorly developed facilities for pediatric heart care.

TABLE 9.2.7: Spontaneous closure of heart defects.

Variable	*Effect of likelihood of spontaneous closure*
Age at evaluation	Younger patients have a higher likelihood of spontaneous closure of defects. Most ASDs and VSDs that are destined to close or become very small do so before the age of 3 years. PDAs have a tendency to close in the first 2–4 weeks after which they seldom close, particularly in a preterm infant
Size of the defect	Larger defects have little likelihood of spontaneous closure. ASDs > 8 mm are unlikely to close spontaneously. Similarly, large unrestrictive VSDs are also unlikely to close
Location of the defect	Only fossa ovalis ASDs tend to close. Primum and sinus venosus types of ASDs do not close. Muscular VSDs have the highest likelihood of spontaneous closure. Perimembranous VSDs can also close spontaneously. Outlet (subpulmonic) VSDs may close by prolapse of the aortic valve, with the risk of aortic regurgitation. Inlet VSDs and misalignment types of VSDs (such as those occurring in TOF) do not close spontaneously

(ASD: atrial septal defect; PDA: patent ductus arteriosus; TOF: tetralogy of Fallot; VSD: ventricular septal defect)

Once a serious CHD is identified, it is vital to counsel the families carefully and thoroughly about the postnatal manifestations, natural history, surgical options, and their long-term outlook. Before 20 weeks of gestation, medical termination of pregnancy (MTP) is an option. After the legal period of MTP, fetal echocardiography enables directed delivery at a center with a comprehensive pediatric heart program. This overcomes the logistic challenges of transporting a newborn with CHD and allows prompt institution of treatment in the newborn period (such as PGE1 for duct-dependent lesions).

It is a common practice to recommend fetal echocardiography for future pregnancies after the diagnosis of serious CHD in a child. This practice is likely to have a low yield because only 2–8% of CHD tends to recur. The highest chance of recurrence is with obstructive lesions of the left heart.

The detection of certain specific chromosomal anomalies in a child should prompt an evaluation of parents to identify a carrier state. Examples of these conditions include partial deletion of chromosome 22 (22q11 or the CATCH 22 syndrome) and translocation variants of trisomy 21 through fluorescence in situ hybridization or karyotyping. The growing list of single-gene mutations that are known to be associated with CHD that can be detected through laboratory tests may enable precise counseling for a larger proportion of families where a child is affected by CHD.

SELECTED INDIVIDUAL CONGENITAL HEART DEFECTS

The following section has a brief description of selected individual heart defects. This is an incomplete list of conditions. It is important to recognize that many patients have one or more defects. It is, therefore, important to individualize the approach depending on the exact combination of the lesion and the overall clinical situation.

ATRIAL SEPTAL DEFECT

Incidence: ASDs occur as an isolated anomaly in 5–10% of all CHDs.

Anatomy: Based on anatomy, ASDs are classified as follows:

- *Fossa ovalis ASD:* They are in the central portion of atrial septum, in the position of foramen ovale. Only these defects are amenable to closure in the catheterization laboratory.
- *Sinus venosus ASD:* In the region of SVC—right atrium junction. These defects do not have a superior margin because the SVC straddles the defect.
- *Ostium primum ASD:* These defects are created by failure to seal the septum primum. They are in the lower part of the atrial septum, and the inferior margin of the defect is formed by the AV valve.
- *Coronary sinus ASD:* An unroofed coronary sinus is a rare communication between the coronary sinus and the LA, which produces a clinical picture like other types of ASD.
- *Physiology:* The physiology of ASD is that of a pretricuspid shunt [*see* Section on "Physiology and Physiologic Classification of Congenital Heart Disease" (page 696)]. The heart murmur in ASD originates from the pulmonary valve because of the increased blood flow through this normal-sized valve; therefore, the murmur is systolic in timing. An increased flow through the tricuspid valve may result in a diastolic rumble at the lower left sternal border. The dilated RV cavity prolongs the time required for the depolarization of RV, resulting in delayed P2. This delay also results from the prolonged "hang-out" interval because of the very low resistance in the pulmonary circulation, thereby a wide split S2.

In addition, the large ASD tends to abolish respiration-related fluctuations in systemic venous return to the right side of the heart, thereby the fixed S2.

Natural history and complications: Heart failure is exceptional in infancy. Pulmonary hypertension is also relatively rare. A small proportion of patients develop PAH. It appears that those who are destined to develop PAH do so relatively early (often in the second or third decade). ASD closure is primarily recommended to prevent complications in late adulthood. These include atrial arrhythmias and heart failure.

Treatment: Fossa ovalis defects with good margins can be closed percutaneously in the catheterization laboratory with occlusive devices. Some selected cases of sinus venosus ASDs are amenable to closure in the catheterization laboratory as well. Others require surgical closure. Closure is recommended before school entry to prevent late complications. Small defects (<8 mm) can be observed. Spontaneous closure is well recognized in small defects that are diagnosed in infancy or early childhood.

VENTRICULAR SEPTAL DEFECT

Incidence: VSD accounts for 15–20% of all CHDs. It is the most common heart defect.

Anatomy: The ventricular septum may be divided into a small membranous portion and a large muscular portion **(Fig. 9.2.2)**. The muscular septum has three components: The inlet, the trabecular, and the outlet septum. The trabecular septum is further divided into central, marginal, and apical portions. A VSD may be classified into perimembranous, inlet, outlet, central/mid muscular, marginal muscular, and apical muscular defects.

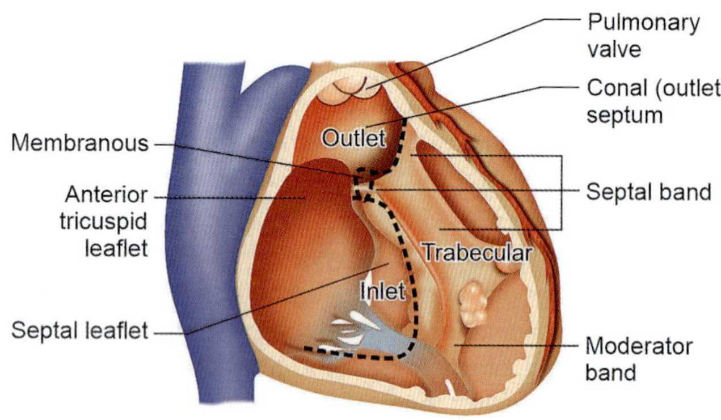

Fig. 9.2.2: En-face view of the right ventricular septal surface to show various landmarks that are used to classify ventricular septal defects.

Pathophysiology: The physiology is that of a post-tricuspid left–right shunt. The magnitude of the shunt is determined by the size of the VSD and downstream PVR. The lower the PVR, the greater the magnitude of left-to-right shunts. In VSD, the LV starts contracting before RV, and a high-pressure gradient is maintained between two ventricles throughout systole. Hence, the murmur is pansystolic. Passing through a normal mitral valve, the relatively larger volume of blood results in a mid-diastolic murmur at the apex. This is a very useful clue indicating a large, significant flow and operability of the lesion.

Since the LV has two outlets, it empties relatively early; this results in early A2. Since ejection into RV and PA is increased, P2 is delayed. Therefore, the S2 is widely split but varies with respiration. In a large VSD with increasing PVR, S2 splitting becomes less and less obvious. It is single once PVR is significantly elevated because of the reduced "hang-out" interval.

Treatment: Decisions to close a VSD are dictated by many considerations that include anatomic subtype, number and size of the defects, age at diagnosis, symptom status, comorbidity, and logistics of follow-up. Infants with large defects should be referred to a center for infant heart surgery early. The consequences of delaying surgery in the hope that the defect will close spontaneously are, sometimes, quite devastating. They include pneumonia that is severe and refractory to treatment, severe malnourishment, and premature pulmonary vascular disease. Catheter closure is usually unrealistic in early infancy because of technical challenges. The long-term results of surgical closure in infancy are excellent.

PATENT DUCTUS ARTERIOSUS

Patent ductus arteriosus is the persistence of normal fetal channel connecting the aorta and PA and accounts for 5–10% of all CHDs. Functional closure of the ductus occurs within 12–24 hours after birth due to constriction of the medial smooth muscle. Anatomic closure occurs between 2 and 3 weeks and is produced by fibrosis of the ductal tissue. Prematurity is associated with delay in the closure of the PDA.

Anatomical and Physiological Considerations

The PDA needs to be understood in two circumstances: As a source of pulmonary blood flow in cyanotic heart disease with reduced pulmonary blood flow and as a cause of left-to-right shunts. In the former situation, the PDA tends to be vertical, often from the undersurface of the aorta, while in the latter, it connects the roof of the main PA with the proximal descending thoracic aorta. In this section, we will focus on the latter only. The PDA is programmed to close early in life. In the cases where the ductus fails to close normally, blood will shunt from left to right into the PA and lungs. This occurs increasingly as the PVR drops and the pressure in the aorta exceeds that of PA. The volume of shunted blood will increase pulmonary blood flow, increase venous return to LA, and cause LA/LV volume overload. The flow in the PDA occurs throughout the cardiac cycle. This results in a murmur that starts in systole after S1, peaks at S2, and continues in diastole. This is a continuous murmur. The passage of increased blood across the mitral valve produces a mid-diastolic murmur as in any other post-tricuspid shunt. The prolonged LV systole results in delayed closure of the aortic valve and a late A2. With large PDA, S2 may be paradoxically split. The excessive diastolic backflow from the aorta results in low diastolic pressure and bounding pulses.

Clinical Circumstances

Preterm Infants

Persistent patency of ductus arteriosus in preterm infants is well recognized in the era of modern preterm care. The prevalence of PDA in babies <1,750 g is 45%, and it increases closer to 80% in very-low-birth-weight babies <1,200 g weight. PDA with a significant left-to-right shunt is associated with varied complications, such as necrotizing enterocolitis, renal dysfunction, intraventricular hemorrhage, and chronic lung disease in preterm babies. Effective and timely treatment of PDA enhances preterm survival and reduces the risk of complications. Studies showed that closure of hemodynamically significant PDA is beneficial, but the timing and the best method of closure are not clear.

A hemodynamically significant duct is identified clinically by features of heart failure, bounding pulses, and evidence of pulmonary overcirculation (tachypnea, tachycardia, and continued requirement of mechanical ventilation and higher FiO_2). An easily audible murmur often accompanies the hemodynamically significant duct, but this is typically absent if the duct is large and unrestrictive. Echocardiography aids considerably in determining the hemodynamic significance of a PDA. A size of >1 mm/kg body weight is considered the minimum for the PDA to be of significance. Additional findings that suggest an important PDA include flow reversal in the descending aorta and LA and LV enlargement.

Older Infants

Older infants with PDA present like any other post-tricuspid shunts (such as VSD).

Treatment

Three modalities of definitive treatment are available for the PDA, and they need to be tailored to anatomy and clinical circumstances. For the preterm infant, indomethacin or ibuprofen should ideally be the first line of treatment. The younger the gestational age of the infant, the lesser the likelihood of a response to indomethacin or ibuprofen (10 kg/kg/dose/day on D1 and 5 mg/kg/dose/day on D2 and D3). Recent literature has found paracetamol to be an effective alternative with minimal side effects in the treatment of preterm neonates. The standard dosing is 15 mg/kg/dose 6th hourly, for 3 consecutive days.

Beyond 10-day postnatal age, the ductus rarely responds to indomethacin. In these circumstances, surgery should be considered. Transcatheter closure of preterm PDA has gained wide attention in recent years as an effective alternative with minimal complications to surgical ligation.

Catheter closure has emerged as a very promising option for all forms of PDA. Two methods are available. They include coil occlusion and closure with occlusive devices. Today, surgery is reserved for large ducts in small infants.

ENDOCARDIAL CUSHION DEFECTS

Very commonly encountered in children with Down syndrome (50% association), the failure of normal development of the endocardial cushion to form the lower part of the atrial septum and upper part of the ventricular septum, along with mitral and tricuspid valves, results in this defect. It can be classified as partial or complete endocardial cushion defect (ECD). Partial form comprises only ostium primum ASD with/without mitral cleft; usually, presentation is like that of a fossa ovalis ASD. Complete ECD encompasses both ASD and VSD along with AV valve abnormalities. Hemodynamic changes behave like that of an ASD and VSD. They present with congestive heart failure (CHF) early in life. The ECG axis is very peculiar in these lesions—they have a superior axis deviation/left axis deviation. In partial ECD, the timing of closure around 3–4 years or earlier if there is a failure. Complete ECD needs repair in infancy, ideally within 2–4 months of age, as they are prone to early development of PVOD.

AORTOPULMONARY WINDOW

This uncommon malformation consists of communication usually nonrestrictive between the adjacent walls of the ascending aorta and pulmonary trunk. This condition results from the failure of the spiral septum to completely divide the embryonic truncus. The pathophysiology of the AP window is like that of a large PDA. In 80% of the patients, the murmur is systolic rather than continuous and is punctuated by eddy sounds. A moderately restrictive AP window (rare) can generate a continuous murmur. Apical mid-diastolic murmur represents increased flow across the mitral valve. AP window requires early surgical correction.

OBSTRUCTIVE LESIONS

These lesions can be divided into two groups:

1. *Ventricular outflow obstructive lesions:*
   - AS
   - PS
   - Coarctation of aorta
2. *Stenosis of AV valves/ventricular inflow tract:*
   - Congenital mitral stenosis (MS)
   - Supramitral ring
   - Cor triatriatum
   - Tricuspid stenosis

Features common in ventricular outflow obstruction are concentric hypertrophy of the chamber proximal to obstruction due to pressure overload and an ESM due to the turbulent flow of blood through the obstruction.

Congenital Aortic Stenosis

The most common cause of congenital AS is the bicommissural aortic valve (80–85%). The partial or complete fusion of commissures between right-left or right-noncoronary commissures results in variable degrees of severity of AS. Very severe stenosis presents early in the newborn period with left ventricular dysfunction and heart failure; less severe forms present later. Bicuspid aortic valve (BAV) should always be followed up meticulously as they are associated with incompetence later in life secondary to concomitant aortic root dilation, which is now considered a primary aortopathy.

Other forms of LV outflow tract obstruction are less common and include subaortic membrane and supravalvular AS. The latter is seen in association with the Williams-Beuren syndrome.

The symptoms of AS are related to LV outflow obstruction and include effort angina, dyspnea, syncope, and fatigue on effort. There is a significant risk of sudden death with severe AS, especially in adolescents and young adults.

The murmur of AS is loudest over the ascending aorta (i.e., upper right sternal border or aortic valve area) and characteristically radiates to the carotid arteries. Constant systolic ejections click just after the first heart sound is a consistent physical finding in bicommissural aortic valve. This is highly sensitive and specific in children and often better heard at the apex. The ECG is characterized by evidence of LV hypertrophy (voltage with strain pattern in severe cases). Severe aortic valve stenosis can be relieved by balloon dilation in the catheterization laboratory. Many of these patients require aortic valve surgery to deal with progressive aortic regurgitation. Other forms of AS require surgical relief.

Congenital Pulmonary Stenosis

Like in AS, pulmonic stenosis may involve the valve or occur above or below the valve. Subvalvular or infundibular PS (double-chambered RV) results from hypertrophied muscle bundles within the RV cavity. In the common form of pulmonary valve stenosis, the valve is thickened, with fused or absent commissures. This valve characteristically domes in systole; the resultant click is best heard during expiration when the excursion of the valve is exaggerated by a relatively underfilled RV cavity. Another form of pulmonary valve stenosis is the dysplastic valve (frequent in Noonan syndrome) that is characterized by tethering of the leaflets to the adjacent main PA with narrowing of the main PA at the sinotubular junction.

Supravalvular PS often refers to the narrowing of the main or branch PAs. Peripheral PS is usually associated with Williams syndrome, Alagille, congenital rubella, and Ehler-Danlos syndrome.

Most patients are acyanotic and well developed. Newborns with critical PS are cyanotic and tachypneic. Majority of patients are asymptomatic in infancy and childhood. Dyspnea and fatigue are mild, if the RV maintains normal stroke volume at rest and augments its stroke volume with exercise. The murmur of PS is loudest over the main PA (i.e., second left intercostal space) and is associated with systolic thrill. The intensity and length of ESM are directly proportional to the severity of PS.

Wide spitting of S2 is due to delayed closure of pulmonary valve. The pulmonary component of S2 is soft. An inconstant ejection click louder in expiration is also audible at the site of the murmur; the interval between S1 and click varies inversely with the degree of PS. The ECG shows right ventricular hypertrophy (RVH). Neonates with critical PS may show predominant LV forces because of associated hypoplasia of RV.

Balloon valvuloplasty is a relatively simple intervention that is now accepted as the standard treatment for valvular PS. While dysplastic valves have a characteristically suboptimal response, balloon dilation is still attempted in them.

Coarctation of Aorta

Isolated coarctation is more common in males (3:1) and is characterized by narrowing of the aorta, typically located near the aortic attachment of the ligamentum arteriosum or PDA (juxta-ductal).

It can be a localized or discrete narrowing or associated with long-segment tubular hypoplasia of the segment proximal to the coarctation (isthmus). There are two types of presentations described:

1. Symptomatic newborns or infants with heart failure
2. Relatively asymptomatic adolescents or young adults who may have "minor" symptoms in the form of headache, epistaxis, and claudication pain over their legs after exercise

The presentation depends on the development of good collateral circulation in fetal life.

Depending on the severity of obstruction, the femoral pulses are both weak and delayed (due to delayed upstroke of the arterial pulse in lower extremity sites) or absent. This is a valuable physical sign and an excellent screening test in newborns as well.

In older children, a systolic murmur is present over the descending aorta, distal to obstruction (in the left interscapular region). Sometimes, a continuous murmur of collaterals between vessels arising from pre- and postcoarctation segments is present over the back of the chest.

Hypertension with a significant difference in upper and lower limb systolic blood pressure (>20 mm Hg) exaggerates on exercise. It is an inevitable consequence in older children, and this accounts for most of the late morbidity. In addition, vascular complications, such as aortic dilation with aneurysm formation and berry aneurysms in the cerebral vasculature, are commonly seen. The ECG in symptomatic infants shows RVH, while LVH is present in older children and adults.

Newborns with severe coarctation require surgery for lasting relief. In older children, balloon dilation is a less invasive option, and in adolescents and adults, stenting of the coarctation segment can yield maximum reduction in gradient. Irrespective of the treatment modality chosen, all patients with coarctation should ideally be followed lifelong for hypertension and vascular complications that may occur despite relief of the obstruction.

Congenital Mitral Stenosis

Congenital MS results from a variety of mechanisms that include a membrane at the level of the annulus (supramitral ring), thickening of chordal apparatus and reduction of leaflet motion, and single papillary muscle (parachute mitral valve). The onset and severity of symptoms are related to the severity of MS. Congenital MS is often associated with other forms of left heart obstruction (LV outflow obstruction at various levels), coarctation (as a part of the Shones complex), and other CHD (such as VSD and DORV). Clinical examination is characterized by the typical mid-diastolic murmur with presystolic accentuation. However, unlike in rheumatic MS, the opening snap is unusual. Management is challenging.

Surgical relief is often the only option (balloon mitral valvuloplasty seldom works for congenital MS). However, this too is unsatisfactory in most situations.

Cor Triatriatum

This is a rare anomaly in which LA is divided into two compartments by an abnormal fibromuscular septum with a small opening, producing pulmonary venous return obstruction. Embryologically, this results from the failure of incorporation of the embryonic common pulmonary vein into LA. Therefore, the upper compartment is a dilated common pulmonary vein, and the lower compartment is the true LA. It produces pulmonary venous and PAH, as in MS. This condition is easily amenable to surgery.

Tetralogy of Fallot

Tetralogy of Fallot is the most common cyanotic CHD. Among the cyanotic CHDs, TOF has a relatively favorable natural history that allows survival beyond infancy in about 75% of cases. As a result, it is the most common CHD encountered beyond the age of 1 year. The disease has been a subject of intense study over several decades.

The physiology is that of VSD with PS and has been described earlier in this chapter.

Anatomically, it is characterized by the classic tetrad: Severe RV outflow obstruction, large VSD, aorta that overrides the VSD and RVH. Within this classic tetrad, there are numerous anatomical variations, most of which have an important bearing on treatment strategies **(Table 9.2.8)**.

Corrective operation for TOF involves closure of the VSD and relief of the RVOT obstruction. There is growing emphasis on retaining the pulmonary valve during initial repair to prevent pulmonary regurgitation and its major late consequences (RV dilation, arrhythmia, heart failure, and sudden death). However, this is not often possible if the component(s) of the RVOT are small. Cyanotic spells are a major concern in severe TOF, and their management and prevention have been elaborated upon in the section on complications.

Although corrective operation is feasible in very young infants, many centers opt for palliative options initially. Palliation is possible in the very young through the BT shunt, balloon dilation of the pulmonary valve, or stenting of the patent arterial duct (if present)/RVOT stenting.

Ebstein Anomaly

There is downward and apical displacement of the septal and the posterior leaflets of the tricuspid valve into the RV cavity.

TABLE 9.2.8: Anatomic variations in tetralogy of Fallot and their significance.

Structure	***Common variation***	***Implications***
RVOT	Degree of stenosis at various levels: Infundibulum, valve, pulmonary annulus, main PA	Severe stenosis manifests early; annular narrowing requires correction with a transannular patch with significant late sequelae; predominant stenosis of the valve may allow palliation with a balloon valvuloplasty in selected cases
Branch PAs	Stenosis of LPA, absence of either branch PA, hypoplastic PAs	Small branch PA may not allow correction at an early age; severe stenosis of LPA origin will need to be addressed at the time of surgery; the absence of one branch PA may require the placement of a conduit
Pulmonary valve	Absent pulmonary valve with aneurysmal branch PAs	This results in a dramatically different manifestation. There is severe airway compression in the worst affected and the manifestations are essentially related to respiratory consequences
VSD	Extension of the VSD to the inlet or outlet septum, restrictive VSD with severe right ventricular hypertrophy and strain, additional muscular VSD	Surgical approach needs to be tailored accordingly
Coronary arteries	Origin of left anterior descending artery from right coronary artery. This abnormal vessel may cross the RVOT	The abnormal vessel comes in the way of corrective surgery. If it is running along the pulmonary annulus, a transannular patch is not feasible, and this may require a conduit
Atrial communication	ASDs, PFO	While it is necessary to close an ASD, PFO is often helpful in the early postoperative period. Many surgeons choose to leave it behind because it helps with early postoperative recovery
Aortopulmonary collaterals	Large major aortopulmonary collaterals	These collaterals will need to be clearly defined. They will need to be closed if their supply overlaps with the native PA supply

(ASD: atrial septal defect; LPA: left pulmonary artery; PAs: pulmonary arteries; PFO: patent foramen ovale; RVOT: right ventricular outflow tract; VSD: ventricular septal defect)

A portion of RV is incorporated into the RA (i.e., atrialized RV). This contracts asynchronously with the RV, resulting either in right-to-left shunting via a patent foramen ovale (majority) or in heart failure (rare). In addition, there is also an additional leak through the severely deformed tricuspid valve. Presentation is variable and dependent on the severity of the involvement. Severe disease may manifest in the newborn period with cyanosis. Mild disease may resent for the first time in adulthood. Reentrant arrhythmias [Wolff-Parkinson-White (WPW) (pre-excitation)] are a frequent accompaniment, and this may result from accessory (bypass) tracts in the region of the displaced leaflets.

NEONATAL HEART DISEASE

Because of the fact that many heart diseases that are present in the newborn period are potentially fatal and need to be recognized early, it is important to be familiar with them. **Table 9.2.9** describes the most common CHDs that are present in the newborn period. For a detailed description of the individual conditions, the reader should refer to standard textbooks included in the reference.

SELECTED HEART DISEASES THAT PRESENT IN THE NEWBORN PERIOD

Dextrotransposition of the Great Arteries

This condition is characterized by parallel circulation resulting from aorta arising from RV and PA arising from LV. Hypoxia is inevitable, and survival is dependent upon communications at the atrial, ventricular, or great vessel level that allows mixing between the two parallel circulations. Such a communication is created at the atrial level by a balloon atrial septostomy procedure or by PGE1 that opens the closing ductus arteriosus. The neonatal arterial switch operation has dramatically transformed the outlook of transposition. This operation needs to be done early. The operation is ideally performed within 2–4 weeks for dextro-TGA (D-TGA) with an intact ventricular septum because of the regression of the LV that is connected to the low-resistance pulmonary circuit. In D-TGA with a large VSD, the concern relates to the rapid development of PVOD, and these babies often need surgery before 3 months of age.

Total Anomalous Pulmonary Venous Connection

This condition, as the name suggests, involves all pulmonary veins that typically come together in a confluence or a common chamber, which then drains into the right atrium, often via one of the systemic venous channels draining into the heart. Depending upon the site of drainage, they can be classified as supracardiac, cardiac, infracardiac, and mixed total anomalous pulmonary venous connection (TAPVC).

The critical determinant of physiology is whether pulmonary venous drainage is obstructed or not. Obstructed TAPVC presents early, often in the newborn period, with heart failure and hypoxia. Severe pulmonary hypertension is invariably present. Emergency surgery often offers the only prospect for survival. Unobstructed TAPVC presents variably,

TABLE 9.2.9: Cardiac emergencies in the newborn.

Physiologic category	*Conditions*	*Manifestation*
Duct-dependent systemic blood flow*	Hypoplastic left heart syndrome, critical coarctation, interruption of aortic arch, critical aortic stenosis	Heart failure, shock, circulatory failure, acidosis
Duct-dependent pulmonary blood flow*	Pulmonary atresia, critical pulmonary stenosis, Ebstein anomaly	Cyanosis, hypoxia
Obstruction of pulmonary venous return	Obstructed total anomalous pulmonary venous return, mitral atresia with a restrictive patent foramen ovale	Cyanosis, hypoxia, heart failure
Parallel circulation with poor mixing	Dextrotransposition with intact ventricular septum	Cyanosis, hypoxia
Valve regurgitation	Congenital mitral valve regurgitation	Heart failure
High-output state	Atrioventricular (AV) malformations (usually intracranial)	Heart failure
Myocardial dysfunction	Myocardial diseases (inflammatory and metabolic, sometimes infectious)	Heart failure
Tachyarrhythmia	Atrial flutter, neonatal atrioventricular reentrant tachycardias, ectopic atrial tachycardia	Tachycardia, heart failure
Bradyarrhythmia	Complete heart block	Bradycardia, heart failure

*Some of the duct-dependent conditions (critical PS, AS, and coarctation) manifest with varying severity. The most severe forms manifest early (in the first few days) with absolute dependence on the duct for survival. Others may manifest later in the neonatal period (first few weeks) with heart failure or cyanosis and may not be strictly "duct dependent."
(AS: aortic stenosis; PS: pulmonary stenosis)

often a little later in infancy. A small fraction of unobstructed TAPVC (~10%) remains relatively symptom-free and presents later, like an ASD.

CONCLUSION

Early detection, referral and management of critical CHD is vital. Understanding the physiological perturbations of these heart defects aids in the initial stabilization of these children before referring to a specialist. With considerable advances in management of CHD, there is a paradigm shift in the overall approach towards active screening, diagnosis and proactive intervention. Early corrections or palliations offers the best chance for children with CHD towards a near normal quality of life.

REFERENCES

1. Allen HD, Shaddy RE, Driscoll DJ, Feltes TF. Moss Adams' Heart Disease in Infants, Children and Adolescents, 7th edition. Philadelphia, PA: Kluwer/Lippincott Williams and Wilkins; 2008.
2. Kumar RK, Shrivastava S. Pediatric heart care in India. Heart. 2008;94:984-90.
3. Kumar RK, Prabhu SS, Ahamed Z. IAP Specialty Textbook of Pediatric Cardiology. New Delhi: Jaypee Brothers Medical Publishers (P) Ltd.; 2008.
4. Vaidyanathan B, Sathish G, Mohanan S, Sundaram KR, Warrier KK, Kumar RK. Clinical screening for congenital heart disease at birth: a prospective study in a community hospital in Kerala. Indian Pediatr. 2011;48:25-30.
5. Saxena A, Mehta A, Sharma M, Salhan S, Kalaivani M, Ramakrishnan S, et al. Birth prevalence of congenital heart disease: a cross sectional observational study from North India. Ann Pediatr Cardiol. 2016;9:205-9.
6. Saxena A, Mehta A, Ramakrishnan S, Sharma M, Salhan S, Kalaivani M, et al. Pulse oximetry as a screening tool for detecting major congenital heart defects in Indian newborns. Arch Dis Child Fetal Neonatal Ed. 2015;100(5):F416-21.
7. Viswanathan S, Kumar RK. Assessment of operability in congenital cardiac shunts with increased pulmonary vascular resistance. Catheter Cardiovasc Interv. 2008;71:665-70.
8. Vaidyanathan B, Radhakrishnan R, Sarala DA, Sundaram KR, Kumar RK. What determines nutritional recovery in malnourished children undergoing correction of congenital heart defects? A prospective study. Pediatrics. 2009;124:e294-9.

9.3 Acute Rheumatic Fever and Rheumatic Heart Disease

Shakuntala Prabhu, Amar M Taksande

INTRODUCTION

Acute rheumatic fever (ARF) results from a complex interaction between group A *Streptococcus* (GAS) and a susceptible host in a stage set by environmental factors. This process commonly affects the joints and heart. Cardiac involvement occurs in the form of carditis, which can be of variable severity, and results in significant morbidity. Acute rheumatic carditis may resolve completely or persist and evolve into a chronic process of rheumatic heart disease (RHD). The important predisposing factors include a family history of rheumatic fever (RF), low socioeconomic status (poverty, poor hygiene, and medical deprivation), and age between 6 and 15 years (with a peak incidence at 8 years of age). Although the sexes are nearly equally affected, mitral valve disease and chorea are more common in girls, whereas aortic valve involvement is often seen in boys.[1-3]

EPIDEMIOLOGY

Though the global burden might have declined, in India, RHD continues to be a significant public health problem. The prevalence of RHD is also not uniform in all regions of our country. Indian states with improved human development are reporting a significant decline in the incidence of RF. School-based clinical surveys conducted at Chandigarh, Kochi, Indore, and Vellore (2004–2007) indicate that the prevalence has dropped to between 0.5 and 1/1,000. Recent studies in India using echocardiography show a higher prevalence of RHD (20 per 1,000) in selected regions. The incidence of ARF following streptococcal throat infection is 0.3% in the general population and 1–3% in the presence of epidemics of streptococcal pharyngitis.[4-6]

ETIOPATHOGENESIS

The etiology of RF is unknown. ARF is believed to be an immunologic response that occurs as a delayed sequela of group A beta-hemolytic streptococcal infection of the pharynx but not of the skin. The attack rate of ARF after streptococcal infection varies with the severity of the infection, ranging from 0.3 to 3%. The streptococcal antigens, such as M protein and carbohydrate antigen (*N*-acetyl-beta-D-glucosamine), produce antibodies that cross-react with human cardiac proteins such as myosin and laminin and result in humoral-mediated injury.[7] Additionally, the involvement of GAS superantigens such as pyrogenic exotoxins in the pathogenesis of ARF has been proposed. Streptococci have never been isolated from rheumatic lesions in joints, heart, or the bloodstream. Only heart valves are permanently damaged during an episode of RF. All other affected tissues typically heal without residua: Pericarditis, chorea, and arthritis resolve completely.

Pathologically, ARF results in diffuse exudative and proliferative reactions resulting in infiltration with lymphocytes, polymorphonuclear leukocytes, histiocytes, and eosinophils. There is also T cell recruitment, leading to granulomatous inflammation and Aschoff body formation, which is the pathologic hallmark of RHD. CD4+ T cells are the major effectors of this process, which leads to the development of chronic RHD. These inflammatory changes are diffuse, affecting the heart, large joints, brain, and subcutaneous tissue. Long-term sequelae occur as a result of the involvement of the endocardium of valvular and subvalvular regions resulting in valvular heart disease. The most common involvement is of the mitral valve, followed by aortic, tricuspid, and very rarely pulmonary valves.

Microscopically, there is edema, inflammatory cell infiltration, and capillary proliferation. Inflammatory infiltrates are also frequently seen in the myocardium with scanty injury and loss of myocardial fibers. Pericardial involvement results in fibrinous pericarditis, which may result in pericardial effusion, which is serosanguinous. It usually resolves completely, never causing constrictive pericarditis. Genetic factors such as human leukocyte antigen (HLA) class II alleles (DR and DQ), specific B cell alloantigen (D8/17), genetic polymorphisms [tumor necrosis factor-alpha (TNF-α), interleukins, transforming growth factor-beta 1 (TGF-β1), etc.] have been proposed to contribute to this host susceptibility.[8,9]

CLINICAL FEATURES

The classical clinical picture of ARF consists of streptococcal sore throat followed 10 days to a few weeks later by various manifestations of ARF, although the history of acute streptococcal sore throat is available only in 50% of patients. The guidelines for the diagnosis of ARF were originally suggested by T Duckett Jones in 1944, subsequently revised by the American Heart Association (AHA) in 1965, updated in 1992, and later revised and updated by the World Health Organization (WHO) in 2003. The most recent guidelines for the diagnosis of ARF have been endorsed by the World Heart Federation (WHF). These guidelines are different for the low-risk population versus moderate- or high-risk population. The major changes in the latest 2015 update include population risk stratification based on the disease endemicity and inclusion of subclinical carditis as a major criterion. Lower thresholds for joint manifestations, fever, etc., are adopted for the high-risk population **(Table 9.3.1)**. These modifications are made to improve the sensitivity of the criteria in moderate-/high-risk populations. The guidelines consist of major, minor, and essential criteria. Two major or one major and two minor criteria are required in the presence of essential criteria to diagnose the first episode of ARF. Additionally, for ARF recurrence, three minor criteria are sufficient. It is important to emphasize that these guidelines

TABLE 9.3.1: 2015 update of Jones criteria for the diagnosis of acute rheumatic fever.

	Low-risk population	***Moderate/high-risk population***
Definition	Annual incidence of ARF ≤ 2 per 1,00,000 school-aged children or all-age prevalence of RHD ≤ 1 per 1,000	Those not fulfilling the criteria for low risk
Major manifestations		
	• Polyarthritis • Clinical and/or subclinical carditis • Chorea • Erythema marginatum • Subcutaneous nodules	• Polyarthritis and/ or polyarthralgia; monoarthritis • Clinical and/or subclinical carditis • Chorea • Erythema marginatum • Subcutaneous nodules
Minor manifestations		
	• Polyarthralgia • Fever ≥38.5°C • ESR ≥60 mm in the first hour and/or CRP ≥3.0 mg/dL • PR prolongation (age-adjusted)	• Monoarthralgia • Fever ≥38°C • ESR ≥30 mm in the first hour and/or CRP ≥3.0 mg/dL • PR prolongation (age-adjusted)
Supporting evidence of antecedent GAS infection	• Increased or rising antistreptolysin O titer or other streptococcal antibodies (anti-DNAseB) • Positive throat culture for GAS or positive rapid GAS carbohydrate antigen	
First episode of ARF: Two major or one major plus two minor (in the presence of supporting evidence)		
Recurrence: Two major or one major plus two minor or three minor (in the presence of supporting evidence)		

(ARF: acute rheumatic fever; CRP: C-reactive protein; ESR: erythrocyte sedimentation rate; GAS: group A *Streptococcus*; RHD: rheumatic heart disease)

are meant to help a physician in making a firm diagnosis of ARF and do not mean that a physician should not use his/her clinical judgment in diagnosing ARF in the absence of these criteria.

Major Criteria

Carditis

Carditis is an early manifestation, with 80% of patients developing it in the first 2 weeks of the onset of RF. Tachycardia (out of proportion to the degree of fever) is an early sign of carditis. Rheumatic carditis is a pancarditis involving the pericardium, myocardium, and endocardium, although studies indicate a limited myocardial component. Clinical carditis is diagnosed in 50–70% of cases, whereas echocardiography can diagnose an additional 12–21% of cases.[10]

- *Pericarditis:* It results in precordial pain that may be quite severe. On auscultation, a friction rub is present. Clinical pericarditis is seen in approximately 15% of those who have carditis. The electrocardiogram (ECG) may show ST and T changes consistent with pericarditis. As a rule, rheumatic pericarditis is associated with only small effusions and does not result in either cardiac tamponade or constrictive pericarditis. A patient with rheumatic pericarditis always has additional mitral or mitral and aortic regurgitation (AR) murmurs. If after the disappearance of the pericardial friction rub, there are no murmurs, it is unlikely to be due to ARF.
- *Myocarditis:* The features diagnostic of myocarditis are (1) cardiac enlargement, (2) soft S1, (3) protodiastolic (S3) gallop, (4) congestive cardiac failure, and (5) Carey Coombs murmur. Carey Coombs murmur is a low-pitched delayed diastolic mitral murmur heard during the course of ARF. It tends to disappear after the myocarditis subsides. Most likely, it is due to increased diastolic flow secondary to mitral regurgitation (MR) across the inflamed rigid mitral valve. The disappearance can be explained by the decrease in the left ventricular (LV) size following subsidence of myocarditis and better function of the mitral valve—papillary muscle complex, resulting in a decrease in MR and subsidence of inflammation, causing a decrease in turbulent flow.
- *Endocarditis:* Endocardial lesions are most important and tend to leave permanent scarring in most cases. The endocardial inflammation is most severe and common in the mitral and aortic valves, less common in the tricuspid valve, and least in the pulmonary valve. Pathologically, the mitral valve is involved in all cases of RF with carditis. The inflammation results in regurgitation murmurs. The most common finding of carditis is apical pansystolic murmur of MR occurring in 92–95% of patients. Aortic valve involvement results in early diastolic murmur of AR. Aortic valve is involved in 20–25% of cases; it is an isolated finding in only 5–8% of cases. Pathologically, tricuspid valve involvement is seen. Tricuspid valvulitis resulting in tricuspid regurgitation (TR) occurs in 10–30% of cases. Isolated tricuspid valvulitis as a manifestation of rheumatic endocarditis does not occur. Clinical evidence of pulmonary valve involvement in ARF is never seen. The acute hemodynamic overload resulting from acute MR and/or AR leads to left ventricular failure (LVF) and is the main reason for the morbidity and mortality of RF and RHD. Signs of congestive heart failure (CHF) (gallop rhythm, distant heart sounds, and cardiomegaly) are indications of severe cardiac dysfunction.
- *Subclinical carditis:* Carditis may occasionally be clinically silent and only identified by echocardiography that shows MR.

Arthritis

Rheumatic arthritis is an early manifestation, seen in 40–70% of ARF episodes. It is a "migratory polyarthritis" involving large joints (knees, ankle, elbow, and wrists). Unusually smaller joints can be involved. However, such migratory polyarthritis is becoming uncommon, and monoarthritis and arthralgias are more common, especially among patients with recurrences. The affected joints have redness, warmth, swelling, pain, and limitation of movements. The pain and swelling appear rather quickly, last 3–7 days, and subside spontaneously to appear in some other joints. There is no residual damage to the joints. Arthritis responds dramatically to salicylate therapy; if patients do not improve with salicylates in 48 hours, the diagnosis of ARF is probably incorrect.

Subcutaneous Nodules

Subcutaneous nodules appear as hard, nontender, nonpruritic, freely movable nodules varying in size from pinhead to almond on bony prominences, such as the shin, wrist, elbow, knee, ankle, spine, and occiput. They are not transient, lasting for weeks, and have a significant association with carditis. Subcutaneous nodules are not exclusive to RF. They are late manifestations occurring around 6 weeks after the onset of ARF, rarely as early as 3 weeks after the onset. They occur in about 3–20% of cases of RF in India. Usually, they disappear in a few days to a few weeks, rarely lasting even up to 1 year. Patients who have subcutaneous nodules always have carditis. They are seen in <10% of ARF episodes. They last from a few days to weeks but have been known to last for almost 3 years.

Chorea

Sydenham's chorea (St. Vitus' dance) is a neuropsychiatric disorder commonly affecting females consisting of both neurologic signs (choreic movement and hypotonia) and psychiatric signs (e.g., emotional lability, hyperactivity, separation anxiety, obsessions, and compulsions). Chorea is characterized by involuntary, purposeless, jerky movements resulting in abnormal speech, muscular incoordination, dropping of articles, awkward gait, and motor weakness. Clinical maneuvers to elicit features of chorea include (1) demonstration of *milkmaid's grip* (irregular contractions of the muscles of the hands while squeezing the examiner's fingers), (2) spooning and pronation of the hands when the patient's arms are extended, (3) wormian darting movements of the tongue upon protrusion, and (4) examination of handwriting to evaluate fine motor movements. Diagnosis is based on clinical findings with supportive evidence of GAS antibodies. It is a late manifestation occurring about 3 months after the onset of ARF. It is reported to occur in 5–36% of cases. It is usually self-limiting. The levels of the antineuronal antibody titer are positively related to the severity of choreic movements. These findings suggest that chorea may be related to dysfunction of basal ganglia and cortical neuronal components. Rarely, chorea may be the sole manifestation of ARF.

Erythema Marginatum

The maculopapular rash is painless, reddish, not raised above the skin, and nonitching, with serpiginous margins. It starts as a red spot with a pale center, increasing in size to coalesce with adjacent lesions to form a serpiginous margin. They are most prominent on the trunk and the inner proximal portions of the extremities; they are never seen on the face. It increases by applying heat. It is a rare and difficult to detect manifestation, particularly in individuals with dark skin. It occurs in <10% of patients with ARF.

Minor Criteria

They are divided into clinical and laboratory criteria.

Clinical Criteria

- *Fever:* Usually present in 90% of patients, the temperature usually goes above 39.5°C.
- *Arthralgia:* Subjective joint pains without physical signs are labeled as arthralgia, whereas arthritis means subjective symptoms and objective signs of inflammation. Figures from India indicate that arthritis and arthralgia together occur in about 90% of the patients.
- *History of previous ARF or RHD:* This criterion applies only for recurrent episodes of RF.

Laboratory Findings

- *Acute phase reactants* consist of polymorphonuclear leukocytosis, increased erythrocyte sedimentation rate (ESR), and presence of C-reactive protein (CRP). The leukocyte count usually is between 10,000 and 15,000/mm^3. The ESR is almost always elevated during ARF and remains so for 4–10 weeks in almost 80% of patients. In a small proportion of patients, it may remain elevated even beyond 12 weeks. CRP is a beta-globulin, which is increased uniformly in all ARF patients and subsides rapidly if the patient is treated with corticosteroids. Absence of raised CRP goes strongly against the diagnosis of ARF. Presence of increased CRP, however, is not diagnostic since it becomes positive in many infections. CRP and ESR are invariably elevated in ARF and help differentiate acute carditis from indolent RHD.
- *Electrocardiogram:* First-degree atrioventricular (AV) block (prolonged PR interval) is a nondiagnostic criterion since it can occur in many infections. Higher grades of block, such as second-degree AV block, especially of the Wenckebach type, may also be seen. A complete AV block is extremely rare as a manifestation of ARF. Prolongation of QTc (corrected QT interval) is suggestive of myocarditis.

Essential Criteria

The essential criteria include evidence of recent streptococcal infection.

- *Antistreptolysin-O (ASO) titer* is well standardized and therefore is the most widely used test for the presence of antibodies against streptococci. Elevated levels of ASO only indicate previous streptococcal infection and not ARF. The higher the level, the more the likelihood of a recent streptococcal infection; lower levels considered "normal" do not necessarily exclude a recent streptococcal infection. A basal ASO titer of 50 U/dL that goes up to 250 U/dL is indicative of a recent streptococcal infection. A rising titer of ASO is strong evidence of a recent streptococcal infection. If three antistreptococcal antibody tests (ASO, antideoxyribonuclease B, and antihyaluronidase tests) are obtained, a titer for at least one antibody test is elevated in over 95% of patients. Single antibody sensitivity is 70%. With two antibodies tested, it rises to 90%; with three antibodies tested, it rises to 95%.
- *Positive throat culture for streptococci* is relatively uncommon when a patient presents with ARF. Positive throat culture cannot be equated with the diagnosis of ARF. Positive throat culture means that streptococci are present in the throat. The patient may or may not have ARF. Positive throat cultures or rapid streptococcal antigen tests for group A streptococci are less reliable than antibody tests because they do not distinguish between recent infection and chronic pharyngeal carriage.

Echocardiography

After the inclusion of "subclinical carditis" as a major criterion, the role of echocardiography has become vital in the management of ARF. Echocardiography is useful not only to assess the severity of lesions but also to establish alternative etiologies.[11] World Health Federation (WHF) has elaborated echocardiographic features to identify rheumatic valves and criteria to differentiate pathologic and physiologic regurgitation.[12] Features suggestive of rheumatic carditis include annular dilatation, elongation of the chordae to the anterior leaflet of the mitral valve causing a prolapse, and lack of coaptation of the two leaflets resulting in MR. There is focal nodular thickening of the tips of the mitral leaflets; they however do not show the independent chaotic movement seen with infective endocarditis. Occasionally, the tip of the mitral valve leaflet is flail because of chordal rupture, resulting in severe MR. The left atrial (LA) and LV sizes are increased. Involvement of the aortic valve is recognized as AR. Echocardiography has improved recognition of carditis, which at times is not possible on auscultation. This has led to the recognition of subclinical carditis, characterized by no clinical but echocardiographic findings of MR.

DIFFERENTIAL DIAGNOSIS

Table 9.3.2 lists the differential diagnosis of ARF.

TREATMENT

There is no specific treatment. Management is symptomatic combined with suppressive therapy **(Box 9.3.1)**. In suppressive therapy, either aspirin or steroids can be used. The total duration of aspirin or steroid therapy is generally 12 weeks. With aspirin, the full doses are given for 10 weeks and then tapered off in the next 2 weeks. The dose of aspirin is 90–120 mg/kg/day in four divided doses (if facilities for blood salicylate level estimation are available, the dose is modified to maintain a blood salicylate level of 20–25 mg/dL for 10 weeks and later tapered off over 2 weeks). Alternatively, a full dose of steroid is given as prednisolone 2 mg/kg/day (maximum 60 mg) for 3 weeks and then tapered gradually to cover a total period of 12 weeks.

TABLE 9.3.2: Differential diagnosis of ARF.

Arthritis	• Juvenile rheumatoid arthritis • Reactive arthritis (e.g., *Shigella, Salmonella, Yersinia*) • Sickle cell disease • Other collagen vascular diseases (systemic lupus erythematosus, mixed connective tissue disease) • Serum sickness • Infectious arthritis (such as gonococcal) • Virus-associated acute arthritis (rubella, parvovirus, hepatitis B virus, herpesviruses, enteroviruses)
Carditis	• Infective endocarditis • Viral myocarditis • Viral pericarditis • Kawasaki disease • Congenital heart disease
Chorea	• Wilson disease • Huntington chorea • Hyperactivity

(ARF: acute rheumatic fever)

PREVENTION

It would be ideal to provide primary prevention of RF. Primary prevention requires the identification of streptococcal sore throat and its treatment with penicillin in the population. Its success depends on the awareness of parents regarding the dangers of sore throat. Therefore, for primary prevention **(Table 9.3.3)**, it is necessary to educate the community regarding the consequences of streptococcal sore throat. Logistically, it is difficult in our country since it requires:

- Identification of sore throat, which is dependent on the education of parents;
- Rapid laboratory confirmation of streptococcal infection of the throat; and
- Medical help and availability of penicillin.[13]

BOX 9.3.1: Treatment of acute rheumatic fever.

Bed rest
- It is advised in all patients with carditis until activity subsides
- Prolonged bed rest (>2–3 weeks) is seldom necessary unless there is clinically apparent carditis with heart failure

Diet
- Salt restriction is not necessary unless congestive cardiac failure is present
- An easily digestible nutritious diet with vitamin supplements should be given

Antimicrobial therapy

Penicillin:
- After obtaining throat cultures, the patient should receive penicillin
- A single injection of benzathine penicillin is given after sensitivity testing when the diagnosis of ARF is made

Dose: 1.2 megaunits (>27 kg) and 0.6 megaunits IM (<27 kg)
- Alternatively, oral penicillin in a dose of 250 mg four times a day for 10 days
- Patients sensitive to penicillin are advised to take oral azithromycin 12.5 mg/kg/day once daily for 5 days or cephalexin 15–20 mg/kg/dose bid for 10 days

Suppressive therapy
- Aspirin or steroids are given as suppressive therapy
- For patients having carditis with congestive cardiac failure, use steroids
- For carditis without congestive cardiac failure, one may use either steroids or aspirin, but most use steroids
- For patients without carditis, it is preferable to use aspirin

Management of chorea
- Usually, self-limiting
- Complete physical and mental rest
- Chlorpromazine, diazepam, diphenhydramine, haloperidol, or promethazine can be used

(ARF: acute rheumatic fever; IM: intramuscularly)

TABLE 9.3.3: Primary and secondary prevention of ARF.

Drugs	*Dose*	*Route of administration*	*Duration*
Primary prevention: Prophylaxis of ARF (treatment of streptococcal sore throat)			
Benzathine penicillin G (after sensitivity test)	1.2 million unit (>27 kg) 0.6 million unit (<27 kg)	Deep IM	Single dose
Penicillin V (oral)	*Children:* 250 mg twice daily	Oral	10 days
Azithromycin (oral)	12.5 mg/kg/d once daily	Oral	5 days
Secondary prevention: Chemoprophylaxis for recurrences of ARF			
Benzathine penicillin	1.2 million unit (>27 kg) 0.6 million unit (<27 kg)	Deep IM	Every 3–4 weeks Every alternate week
Penicillin V	*Children:* 250 mg qid	Oral	Twice daily

Note: In high-risk situations, administration every 3 weeks is recommended.
(ARF: acute rheumatic fever; IM: intramuscularly)

TABLE 9.3.4: Duration of prophylaxis for people who have had ARF.

Category	*Duration of prophylaxis*
• Patients without proven carditis	• 5 years after the last episode, or until they are 18 years old (whichever is longer)
• Patient with carditis (mild mitral regurgitation or healed carditis)	• 10 years or until 25 years of age, whichever is longer
• Patient with established RHD or following valvular surgery of balloon mitral valvuloplasty	• Lifelong prophylaxis, or at least until the age of 40 years

(ARF: acute rheumatic fever; RHD: rheumatic heart disease)

Secondary prevention consists in giving long-acting benzathine penicillin intramuscularly. The injection is painful, and some patients get fever for 24–36 hours following the injection. As such, it is preferable to give the injection on a Saturday afternoon to avoid loss of studies for the child.[14]

In the presence of carditis, ideally penicillin prophylaxis **(Table 9.3.4)** should continue lifelong whereas patients without proven carditis should receive prophylaxis for 5 years after the last episode or until they are 18 years old (whichever is longer).[15]

CHRONIC RHEUMATIC HEART DISEASE

In pediatric cardiac practice, roughly 20–25% of cases have RHD, with crippling valvular heart disease in many of them. RHD has a variety of clinical manifestations, including myocarditis, decompensated CHF, arrhythmias [i.e., atrial fibrillation (AF)], and valvular heart disease. Chronic RHD commonly manifests with symptomatic valvular disease, with heart failure, AF, and pulmonary hypertension (PHT) being the predominant clinical manifestations. Mitral valve is the most common valve involved in RHD. It can be regurgitant, stenotic, or may exhibit a combination of regurgitation and stenosis. Additionally, there may be cases of *combined mitral and aortic valve disease* in the next most common subset. Isolated aortic valve involvement is seen only in 2–8% of cases. Isolated rheumatic tricuspid valve disease does not occur. Tricuspid stenosis occurs rarely and mostly with mitral stenosis (MS). The utilization of screening echocardiography in various studies has revealed that the true burden of asymptomatic RHD is considerably greater than that detected clinically. Most individuals have minor valvular dysfunction, which may progress in severity or even regress. A transthoracic echocardiogram is more sensitive and specific than auscultation during the physical examination for the detection of RHD.

MITRAL REGURGITATION

Mitral regurgitation is the result of structural changes that usually include some loss of valvular substance and shortening and thickening of the chordae tendineae. The chronic lesion is most often mild or moderate in severity, and the patient is asymptomatic. More than half of patients with acute mitral insufficiency no longer have the mitral murmur 1 year later. In patients with severe chronic mitral insufficiency, pulmonary arterial pressure becomes elevated, the right ventricle and atrium become enlarged, and right-sided heart failure subsequently develops.

Clinical Manifestations

Exertional fatigue and palpitation are common features. Exertional dyspnea and features of right-sided cardiac failure are late manifestations of severe grades of MR and LVF. There is no tachycardia, tachypnea, or basal rales unless significant LV overload/LVF occurs. The pulse pressure is wide with significant MR. The cardiac size increases with increasing severity of MR, resulting in an LV hyperdynamic impulse that is downward and outward. There may be a palpable LV S3.

The S1 may be soft, normal, or loud. It may be masked by the murmur. The S2 is normal with mild MR; with severe grades of MR, it becomes a wide variable split due to early A2 as LV systole is shortened due to part of stroke volume regurgitating in the left atrium.

- *With mild disease,* signs of heart failure are not present, the precordium is quiet, and auscultation reveals a high-pitched holosystolic murmur at the apex that radiates to the axilla.
- *Moderate-to-severe degree of MR* results in a low-pitched delayed diastolic murmur at the apex, which may be palpable as a diastolic thrill. A diastolic thrill is more commonly felt with MR than a systolic thrill. Systolic thrill is uncommonly felt at the apex in MR as the blood is regurgitating in the left atrium, which is posteriorly placed.
- *With severe MR and CHF,* P2 becomes loud due to high pulmonary arterial pressures. LV S3 is generally audible with significant MR due to an increase in early diastolic filling.

The diagnostic feature of MR is a pansystolic murmur best heard at the apex and radiating to the axilla. With significant MR, a low-frequency delayed diastolic murmur is audible at the apex; the duration of murmur increases with increasing severity of MR. If MR is severe, the diastolic rumble is audible throughout the diastole but has no presystolic accentuation in the absence of MS. In patients with severe MR, there are also features of CHF, such as raised jugular venous pressure (JVP) and hepatomegaly.

Investigations

- *Electrocardiogram:* It reveals sinus rhythm and may be normal with mild MR. With increasing degree of MR, LA overload and LV volume overload are seen. LA enlargement results in bifid "P" wave (P-mitrale). LV enlargement results in tall R waves in left-sided leads (I, augmented vector left, V5, V6) with deep "Q" waves indicating volume overload of the left ventricle. In the cases of severe MR, right ventricular hypertrophy (RVH) may be seen due to the development of PHT.
- *Chest X-ray:* Significant MR results in LA and LV enlargement with the changes of pulmonary venous hypertension (PVH).
- *Echocardiogram:* It clearly shows the altered valve pathology, degree of LA and LV enlargement and function, and quantum of regurgitation **(Fig. 9.3.1)**. In addition, other common features include doming of the anterior mitral leaflet and shortening of the anterior leaflet, accompanied by varying degrees of leaflet thickening and calcification. The jet of MR is often eccentric and is due to malcoaptation and/or shortening of the anterior leaflet with an immobile or restricted posterior leaflet.

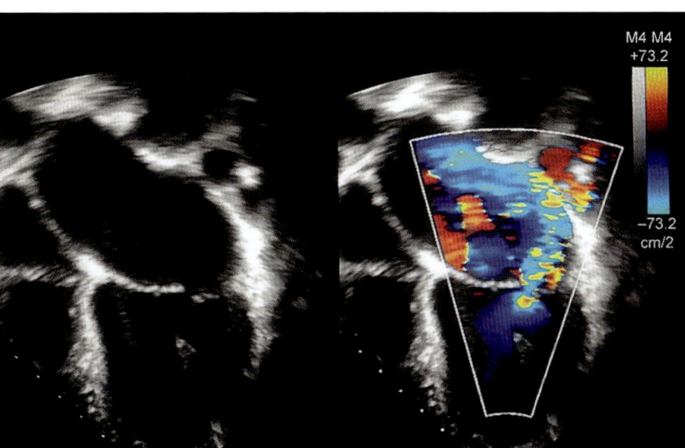

Fig. 9.3.1: Apical four-chamber view showing dilated LA and LV (2D-echo) and mitral regurgitation (color Doppler). (LA: left atrial; LV: left ventricular)

Differential Diagnosis

In a child with MR, one should keep in mind other causes, such as mitral valve prolapse, cleft mitral valve, levotransposition with regurgitant left AV valve, and connective tissue disorders.

Complications

Severe mitral insufficiency may result in cardiac failure that may be precipitated by progression of the rheumatic process, the onset of AF, or infective endocarditis.

Management

Symptomatic patients with moderate-to-severe MR will need decongestive therapy, including angiotensin-converting enzyme (ACE) inhibitors. Angiotensin receptor blockers partially lessen the physiological consequences. Beta-blockers have also been used in severe regurgitation, with little evidence favoring long-term benefits. Surgical treatment is indicated for patients who despite adequate medical therapy have persistent heart failure, dyspnea with moderate activity, and progressive cardiomegaly, often with PHT. Although annuloplasty provides good results in some children and adolescents, valve replacement may be required. The patients should be carefully evaluated to see if the mitral valve could be repaired surgically. Patients with severe MR with decreasing LV ejection fraction need early surgical intervention. If the valve cannot be repaired, they will need mitral valve replacement.

RHEUMATIC MITRAL STENOSIS

Mitral stenosis of rheumatic origin results from fibrosis of the mitral ring, commissural adhesions, and contracture of the valve leaflets, chordae, and papillary muscles over time. It usually takes 10 years or more for the lesion to become fully established, although the process may occasionally be accelerated. It is the most common isolated lesion encountered after the age of 30 years.

Clinical Manifestations

In the pediatric age group, male patients commonly have MS. The patient complains of shortness of breath on exertion initially. With increasing severity, this becomes more severe, and the child becomes breathless when walking short distances. Subsequently, the child starts getting paroxysmal nocturnal dyspnea and breathlessness at rest. In the later stages, with the development of severe PHT and TR, features of CHF develop. When PHT has developed, right ventricular (RV) dilatation may result in functional tricuspid insufficiency, hepatomegaly, ascites, and edema. The patient can also have hemoptysis or pulmonary edema due to severe PVH.

On examination, there may be tachycardia and low pulse volume. JVP is normal with mild MS. With severe MS and TR, elevated JVP with prominent "V" wave (due to regurgitation of blood into the right atrium) and rapid "Y" descent is seen (in the presence of TR without tricuspid stenosis). Enlarged and tender hepatomegaly, which may be pulsatile, is seen with severe TR. Respiratory rate with mild MS is normal; tachypnea develops with significant MS. Basal crepitations are also heard with significant MS. If the patient develops pulmonary edema, severe respiratory distress, extensive rales, and cyanosis are seen.

Precordial examination reveals normal heart size in most cases. Cardiac enlargement is seen in the presence of CHF and TR. The apex beat is tapping; parasternal heave is present with the development of PHT. At this stage, P2 may also be palpable. Mild TR does not result in RV dilatation. Therefore, there is no parasternal pulsation. Significant TR results in RV dilatation resulting in parasternal lift. If the pressure in the right ventricle is elevated, parasternal pulsations can be seen, and on palpation, parasternal heave is felt.

A systolic thrill is rarely felt along the left or right sternal border. A diastolic thrill could be felt at the apex.

- On auscultation, the S1 is loud; the S2 is normally split with a loud pulmonary component, loudness depending on the degree of PHT.
- An opening snap—hallmark for the diagnosis of MS—is audible at the apex at the beginning of diastole. The closer the opening snap is to the A2, the severe is the MS.
- A low-pitched delayed diastolic rumble is audible at the apex with presystolic accentuation immediately after the opening snap.
- In the presence of significant TR, systolic pulsations can be felt over the liver, which enlarges with the development of CHF.
- A holosystolic murmur along the left sternal border increasing with inspiration or leg raising is the hallmark for the diagnosis of TR.
- With significant regurgitation, S3 can be heard in the tricuspid area; if the quantum of regurgitation is significant, a delayed diastolic murmur across the tricuspid valve is heard.
- Rarely, an opening snap and presystolic accentuation of the diastolic murmur are heard, if tricuspid stenosis is present.

Investigations

Electrocardiogram: The rhythm is usually sinus. The most common finding is LA enlargement (p-mitrale); however, this finding disappears if the patient enters AF **(Fig. 9.3.2)**. With increasing PHT, an increasing degree of right-axis deviation, RVH (tall R wave in right-sided leads), and right atrial (RA) overload (tall peaked "P" wave) are seen.

Chest X-ray: Heart size is usually normal, with the development of TR and CHF. Cardiomegaly develops due to RA and RV enlargement. The left atrium is enlarged. Features of varying grades of pulmonary venous and arterial hypertensions are also seen.

Echocardiography shows thickening of the mitral valve and distinct narrowing of the mitral orifice during diastole and LA enlargement. Doppler can estimate the transmitral pressure gradient. 2D-echo with color flow mapping clearly shows the stenotic mitral valve; the mitral valve area can be calculated. The gradient across the mitral valve is calculated by taking the velocity of the mitral inflow on Doppler. The peak velocity of TR gives the estimate of pulmonary arterial pressures.

The key pathological feature of rheumatic MS is commissural fusion which can be detected on echocardiography by short-axis imaging of the mitral valve and inferred by the presence of doming of the anterior leaflet during diastole **(Fig. 9.3.3)**. The posterior leaflet usually has restricted leaflet motion during diastole and is not infrequently immobile. The leaflets are thickened at their tips and may have superimposed calcification. There are varying degrees of thickening and calcification of the leaflet body,

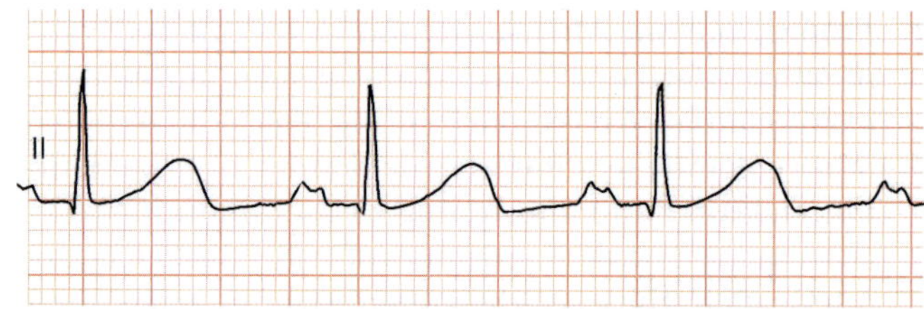

Fig. 9.3.2: Notched P wave indicating left atrial enlargement as seen in mitral stenosis.

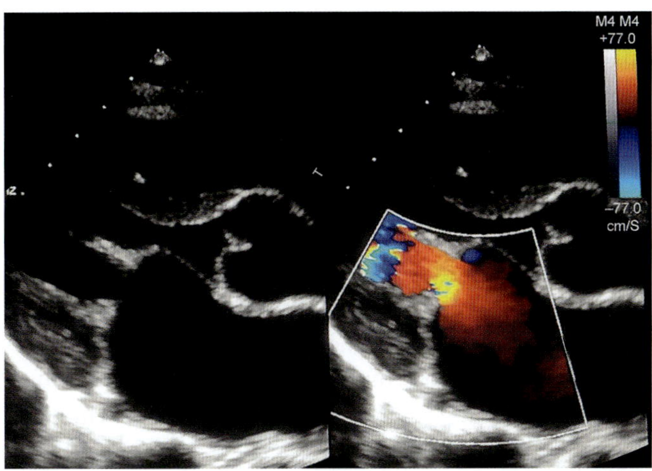

Fig. 9.3.3: Parasternal long-axis view (2D and color Doppler), showing diastolic doming (hockey-stick shape) of anterior mitral valve leaflet and thickened, restricted posterior mitral valve leaflet suggestive of mitral stenosis.

which may be accompanied by varying degrees of chordal shortening and fusion. This variability in the rheumatic process forms the basis of the Wilkins score to assess the likelihood of a valve being suitable for percutaneous mitral commissurotomy (PMC).

Differential Diagnosis

Cor triatriatum, supramitral ring, congenital MS, and LA myxoma are rare entities that can sometimes mimic MS.

Management

A salt-restricted diet and diuretics are useful to reduce pulmonary venous congestion. If there is evidence of cardiomegaly and CHF, digoxin is useful. Intervention is indicated in patients with clinical signs and hemodynamic evidence of severe obstruction but before the severe manifestations outlined earlier. Surgical valvuloplasty or balloon catheter mitral valvuloplasty generally yields good results; valve replacement is avoided unless absolutely necessary. Balloon valvuloplasty is indicated for symptomatic, stenotic, pliable, noncalcified valves of patients without atrial arrhythmias or thrombi.

AORTIC REGURGITATION

In chronic rheumatic aortic insufficiency, sclerosis of the aortic valve results in distortion and retraction of the cusps. Regurgitation of blood leads to volume overload with dilatation and LVH. Combined mitral and aortic insufficiency is more common than aortic involvement alone.

Clinical Features

Aortic regurgitation is common in male patients. The presenting symptom is usually palpitation and increased neck pulsations due to high stroke volume. The large stroke volume and forceful LV contractions may result in palpitations. Sweating and heat intolerance are related to excessive vasodilation. Dyspnea on exertion can progress to orthopnea and pulmonary edema; angina may be precipitated by heavy exercise. Nocturnal attacks with sweating, tachycardia, chest pain, and hypertension may occur.

TABLE 9.3.5: Peripheral signs of aortic regurgitation (AR).

Corrigan's pulse	Dancing carotids
de Musset's sign	Head nodding
Quincke's sign	Capillary pulsations over nail bed
Traube's sign	Pistol-shot sounds over femorals
Hill's sign	Lower extremity BP > upper extremity BP >20 mm Hg—mild AR >40 mm Hg—moderate AR >60 mm Hg—severe AR
Müller's sign	Systolic pulsation of the uvula
Rosenbach's sign	Pulsatile liver
Gerhardt's sign	Enlarged pulsatile spleen
Lighthouse sign	Blanching and flushing of the forehead
Landolfi's sign	Alternating constriction and dilatation of the pupil
Becker sign	Visible pulsations of retinal arteries seen through an ophthalmoscope

The pulse pressure is the best clinical parameter to assess the degree of AR. The wider the pulse pressure, the more severe the regurgitation. The wide pulse pressure results in several signs. It also results in prominent neck, suprasternal, peripheral, and abdominal pulsations. The pulse shows a sharp rise and fall, the so-called water hammer pulse, which becomes more evident on elevating the arm. Nodding of the head with cardiac cycle may be seen (de Musset's sign). The increased pressure difference between the systolic pressure of the upper and lower limbs is called Hill's sign **(Table 9.3.5)**. Normally, this difference is <20 mm Hg. With mild, moderate, and severe regurgitation, it is 20–40, 40–60, and >60 mm Hg, respectively. Pistol-shot sounds can be heard over large arteries with significant regurgitation. If slight pressure is applied over these arteries, a systolic murmur can be heard, and if pressure is applied distally, a diastolic murmur is heard. This is called the Duroziez sign. Palpation of the precordium may be unremarkable with mild AR; with significant regurgitation, the cardiac apex is displaced down and out and is of LV hyperdynamic type. The greater the amount of regurgitation, the bigger the heart size. Rarely, with severe regurgitation, the whole of the precordium is pulsatile.

The S3 may be felt over the LV apex. In some cases, a systolic thrill may be felt in the second left intercostal space. The S1 is soft, and the S2 is normally split with mild-to-moderate regurgitation; it may be paradoxical with severe regurgitation, particularly with LV failure. The murmur of AR is high-pitched decrescendo diastolic starting with A2. A systolic ejection murmur is commonly heard in the aortic area conducted to the neck in cases with significant AR. Delayed diastolic rumble is heard in some cases of AR (Austin Flint murmur). Some of the other signs have been listed in **Table 9.3.5**.

Doppler studies demonstrate the degree of aortic runoff into the left ventricle. Magnetic resonance angiography (MRA) can be useful in quantitating regurgitant volume. Cardiac catheterization is necessary only when the echocardiographic data are equivocal.

Investigations

- *X-ray chest:* In the cases of mild AR, there is no cardiomegaly, and aorta may be prominent. With increasing AR, heart size enlarges due to an enlarged left ventricle. Changes in PVH develop with severe regurgitation and LV failure.
- *Electrocardiogram:* The ECG may be normal with mild AR. If significant regurgitation is present, the ECG shows evidence of volume overload of left ventricles—increased LV voltage with prominent "Q" waves and tall "T" waves. In patients with severe AR, particularly in the presence of CHF, LA overload may also be seen.
- *Echocardiography:* Two-dimensional and color Doppler echocardiography can confirm the diagnosis and also estimate the severity of AR, degree of LV enlargement, and function. Doppler studies demonstrate the degree of aortic runoff into the left ventricle.

Differential Diagnosis

In the case of isolated AR, one should look for Marfan syndrome, Hurler syndrome, and nonspecific aortoarteritis. The other causes of AR, such as congenital aortic valve disease, rupture sinus of Valsalva, or ventricular septal defect with AR, should be kept in mind.

Management

Mild AR is well tolerated. Significant AR causing LV dilatation may benefit from ACE inhibitors. If the left ventricle is progressively dilating and the patient is symptomatic or there is evidence of CHF, decongestive therapy along with an ACE inhibitor should be started and the patient planned for surgery, aortic valve repair, or replacement. In most of these patients, the aortic valve repair is not possible, and they end up with valve replacement. The improvement with surgery is remarkable, but with a prosthetic valve, the child has to take lifelong anticoagulant therapy with its own inherent hazards.

TRICUSPID REGURGITATION

Tricuspid regurgitation is commonly seen in patients of rheumatic mitral valve disease (20–50%). It can be functional or organic. If TR is present in the absence of severe pulmonary arterial hypertension (PAH), it is likely to be organic, but if PAH is present, it can be either functional, organic, or both.

Clinical Features

There are no specific symptoms of TR except pain in the right hypochondria and fatigue due to low cardiac output. The symptoms will depend on the lesion with which TR is associated. The signs diagnostic of TR are a prominent "V" wave with rapid "Y" descent in JVP, systolic pulsations over the liver, and systolic murmur at the lower left or right sternal border, increasing in severity with inspiration. It may sometimes be associated with a systolic thrill, enlarged right ventricle, S3, and delayed diastolic rumble over the tricuspid area. Tricuspid stenosis results in slow Y descent in JVP, diastolic rumble with presystolic accentuation in the tricuspid area, and rarely an opening snap before the diastolic rumble. The other physical finding will be of the associated lesion; isolated tricuspid valve diseases of rheumatic etiology do not occur.

Investigations

An ECG may reveal evidence of RA and RV overload patterns in addition to other changes due to the associated lesions. Significant TR results in cardiac enlargement due to the dilatation of the right atrium and right ventricle. Two-dimensional and color Doppler evaluation easily confirms tricuspid valve disease. The degree of regurgitation is estimated by color flow mapping.

Management

The presence of significant TR results in cardiomegaly and CHF, and the patients need decongestive therapy. The complete management will depend on the associated valvular lesions. Severe grades of TR result in dilatation of the tricuspid annulus. If the tricuspid annulus is >21 mm/m^2, then it has to be repaired by annuloplasty in addition to the other valvular lesions at surgery.

REFERENCES

1. Gewitz MH, Baltimore RS, TaniL Y, Sable CA, Shulman ST, Carapetis J, et al. Revision of the Jones criteria for the diagnosis of ARF in the era of Doppler echocardiography: a scientific statement from the American Heart Association. Circulation. 2015;131(20):1806-18.
2. Jones TD. The diagnosis of rheumatic fever. JAMA. 1944;126:481-4.
3. Kumar RK, Paul M, Francis TP. RHD in India: are we ready to shift from secondary prophylaxis to vaccinating high-risk children? Curr Sci. 2009;97(3):397-404.
4. Misra M, Mittal M, Singh R, Verma A, Rai R, Chandra G, et al. Prevalence of rheumatic heart disease in school-going children of Eastern Uttar Pradesh. Indian Heart J. 2007;59(1):42-3.

5. Padmavati S. Rheumatic fever and rheumatic heart disease in India at the turn of the century. Indian Heart J. 2001;53(1):35-7.
6. Arvind B, Ramakrishnan S. Rheumatic Fever and Rheumatic Heart Disease in Children. Indian J Pediatr. 2020;87(4):305-11.
7. Azevedo PM, Pereira RR, Guilherme L. Understanding rheumatic fever. Rheumatol Int. 2012;32(5):1113-20.
8. Guilherme L, Kalil J. Rheumatic fever and rheumatic heart disease: cellular mechanisms leading autoimmune reactivity and disease. J Clin Immunol. 2010;30(1):17-23.
9. Bryant PA, Robins-Browne R, Carapetis JR, Curtis N. Some of the people, some of the time: susceptibility to ARF. Circulation. 2009;119(5):742-53.
10. Tubridy-Clark M, Carapetis JR. Subclinical carditis in rheumatic fever: a systematic review. Int J Cardiol. 2007;119(1):54-8.
11. Ramakrishnan S. Echocardiography in acute rheumatic fever. Ann Pediatr Card. 2009;2(1):61-4.
12. Reményi B, Wilson N, Steer A, Ferreira B, Kado J, Kumar K, et al. World heart federation criteria for echocardiographic diagnosis of rheumatic heart disease—an evidence-based guideline. Nat Rev Cardiol. 2012;9(5):297-309.
13. Gerber MA, Baltimore RS, Eaton CB, Gewitz M, Rowley AH, Shulman ST, et al. Prevention of rheumatic fever and diagnosis and treatment of acute Streptococcal pharyngitis: a scientific statement from the American Heart Association Rheumatic Fever, Endocarditis, and Kawasaki Disease Committee of the Council on Cardiovascular Disease in the Young, the Interdisciplinary Council on Functional Genomics and Translational Biology, and the Interdisciplinary Council on Quality of Care and Outcomes Research: endorsed by the American Academy of Pediatrics. Circulation. 2009;119(11):1541-51.
14. Peters F, Karthikeyan G, Abrams J, Muhwava L, Zühlke L. Rheumatic heart disease: current status of diagnosis and therapy. Cardiovasc Diagn Ther. 2020;10(2):305-15.
15. Watkins DA, Beaton AZ, Carapetis JR, Karthikeyan G, Mayosi BM, Wyber R, et al. Rheumatic heart disease worldwide: JACC Scientific Expert Panel. J Am Coll Cardiol. 2018;72(12):1397-416.

9.4 Congestive Heart Failure

Anita Saxena

INTRODUCTION

Congestive heart failure (CHF) is defined as an abnormality of cardiac structure or function leading to failure of the heart to deliver oxygen at a rate commensurate with the requirements of the metabolizing tissues, despite normal filling pressures (or only at the expense of increased filling pressures). In children, this requirement includes growth and development. The term CHF is increasingly being replaced by heart failure (HF), since peripheral congestion may not be present in all cases. HF is often a transient state in children that is secondary to an underlying condition, the most common being congenital heart defects (CHDs). Less common causes include cardiomyocyte dysfunction secondary to myocarditis/cardiomyopathies. Palliated CHDs leading to HF are increasingly being recognized.

EPIDEMIOLOGY OF HEART FAILURE IN CHILDREN

True global incidence and prevalence are difficult to estimate due to lack of a standard definition of HF. CHD may account for 25–75% of pediatric HF cases.[1] About one-third to one-fourth of CHDs are severe enough to warrant attention; half of these result in HF. Dilated cardiomyopathy is another important cause of HF at any age; its incidence has been reported between 0.87 and 7.4/100,000 children in a systematic literature review.[2] Rheumatic heart disease (RHD) is an important cause of HF in children in developing countries, such as India.

CAUSES OF HEART FAILURE IN INFANTS AND CHILDREN

Children can have diverse causes of HF depending on the age, geographical location, and many other factors. The prominent causes of HF or ventricular dysfunction in children are provided in **Table 9.4.1**.

Different causes of HF according to age at presentation are given in **Table 9.4.2**.

Heart failure presenting on the first day of life is commonly due to metabolic abnormalities and not CHD. Conditions producing fetal HF, such as Ebstein anomaly or abnormal heart rate/rhythm, are also causes of HF on day 1 of life.

Obstructive and duct-dependent lesions can present with HF or acute circulatory shock soon after birth. HF due to left-to-right shunts occurs later (4–6 weeks) as the pulmonary vascular resistance falls, though large ventricular septal defect

TABLE 9.4.1: Causes of HF in children by underlying pathology.

Cause	*Comment*
Volume overload (relative or absolute)	CHD with increased pulmonary blood flow (VSD, PDA, AVSD, TGA, truncus, TAPVC, etc.)* arteriovenous fistula or malformations, anemia, and thyrotoxicosis†
Obstructive lesions/atretic valves or great vessels	AS, PS, mitral valve atresia or stenosis, coarctation of aorta, and aortic interruption‡
Regurgitant lesions (MR/TR)	Congenital (e.g., as part of AVSD, Ebstein anomaly), acquired (e.g., RF/RHD), and postoperative*
Myocyte dysfunction (pump failure)	
Primary	Inborn errors of metabolism, muscular dystrophies, DCM, drug-induced, and hemoglobinopathies†
Inflammatory	Myocarditis, Chagas disease, and HIV*
Hemodynamic	Obstructive or regurgitant lesions and HT‡
Abnormal rate/ rhythms	Tachycardiomyopathy, bradycardia, and AV dyssynchrony†
Abnormal morphology	SV physiology‡ and ALCAPA
Ischemic	CAD (including premature CAD)†
Postoperative	Post-bypass, SV surgeries, and post-TGA repair‡
Abnormal homeostasis	Hypothermia, hypoxia, hypocalcemia, hypoglycemia, and sepsis† (peculiar to the neonatal period)

*Common.
†Rare (may be common in specific age groups/settings).
‡Uncommon.
(ALCAPA: anomalous left coronary artery from the pulmonary artery; AS: aortic stenosis; AV: atrioventricular; AVSD: atrioventricular septal defect; CAD: coronary artery disease; CHD: congenital heart disease; DCM: dilated cardiomyopathy; HF: heart failure; HIV: human immunodeficiency virus; HT: hypertension; MR: mitral regurgitation; PDA: patent ductus arteriosus; PS: pulmonary stenosis; RF: rheumatic fever; RHD: rheumatic heart disease; SV: single ventricle; TAPVC: total anomalous pulmonary venous connection; TGA: transposition of the great arteries; TR: tricuspid regurgitation; VSD: ventricular septal defect)

(VSD), patent ductus arteriosus (PDA), and atrioventricular septal defect (AVSD) may present earlier. Children with an isolated atrial septal defect (ASD) are mostly asymptomatic; if an infant is diagnosed to have ASD and is in failure, the likely diagnosis is the much more malignant CHD and total anomalous pulmonary venous connection (TAPVC).

Heart failure secondary to CHD is unusual after the first year of life unless complicated by infective endocarditis (IE), anemia, infections, or arrhythmias. Thus, older children (usually beyond 2 years) are likely to have other causes for HF, such as acute/chronic RHD, myocarditis, cardiomyopathies, and postoperative CHD.

TABLE 9.4.2: Common causes of HF by age at presentation.

Day 1 of life/fetal	*1–2 months*
• Asphyxia • Metabolic • Systemic arteriovenous fistula • Myocarditis • Hematological • SVT • CHB • Severe TR (Ebstein anomaly) • Severe MR	• VSD • PDA • AVSD • Aortopulmonary window • Unobstructed TAPVC • TGA and malposition complexes • ALCAPA • DCM
First week of life	***2–6 months***
• Critical AS/PS • Obstructive TAPVC • Hypoplastic left heart • Coarctation of aorta • Adrenaline sufficiency • TGA with intact septum • Other causes listed above for day 1 of life/fetal	• Coarctation of aorta • Aortic stenosis • Other causes listed above for age group 1–2 months
Second week of life	***Older children***
• Large VSD • Large PDA • AVSD • Persistent truncus arteriosus • Unobstructive TAPVC	• RF/RHD • CHD with complications • Cardiomyopathies • Severe AS/PS with ventricular dysfunction • Palliated/postoperative CHD • Tachycardiomyopathies • Severe hypertension

(ALCAPA: anomalous left coronary artery from the pulmonary artery; AS: aortic stenosis; AVSD: atrioventricular septal defect; CHB: complete heart block; CHD: congenital heart disease; DCM: dilated cardiomyopathy; HF: heart failure; MR: mitral regurgitation; PDA: patent ductus arteriosus; PS: pulmonary stenosis; RF: rheumatic fever; RHD: rheumatic heart disease; SVT: supraventricular tachycardia; TAPVC: total anomalous pulmonary venous connection; TGA: transposition of the great arteries; TR: tricuspid regurgitation; VSD: ventricular septal defect)

CLINICAL FEATURES

The initial signs and symptoms of HF may be mistaken for common diseases in children such as pneumonia and sepsis. Those presenting with nausea and vomiting due to an enlarged congested liver may be diagnosed as having acute gastroenteritis. Specific cardiac symptoms that are common include breathlessness on exertion, fatigue, palpitations, and right upper abdominal pain. Parents may notice tachypnea and respiratory distress in infants. Failure to gain weight, feeding difficulties, suck–rest–suck cycle, and excessive sweating over the head, especially during feeds, are other symptoms noted in infants.

Physical examination may not reveal classical signs of HF, such as raised jugular venous pulse (JVP) and pedal edema in infants and toddlers. A triad of tachypnea, tachycardia, and hepatomegaly may be indicative of HF in infants. A gallop rhythm may also be present. All patients must also be evaluated for arterial oxygen saturation by using a pulse oximeter. In severe cases, signs of poor perfusion, such as delayed capillary refill and cool distal extremities, may be seen. A careful precordial examination helps in making a diagnosis of underlying CHD, such as a large VSD. A murmur of mitral regurgitation (MR) may be audible in some cases of dilated cardiomyopathy. Common signs and symptoms of HF are given in **Table 9.4.3**.

The conventional New York Heart Association (NYHA) functional classification is not applicable to children under 6 years of age. For this reason, the modified Ross classification is used for the assessment of younger children.[3] A comparison of the two classifications is given in **Table 9.4.4**.

DIAGNOSTIC WORKUP

Chest Radiograph

A chest radiograph should be done in all patients with suspected HF; an echocardiogram is not a substitute for a radiograph. It enables the diagnosis of cardiomegaly, quantification of pulmonary blood flow, presence of associated chest infection, pleural effusion, etc., as well as showing pathognomonic cardiac silhouette in certain disease states. A cardiothoracic ratio of >60% in neonates and >55% in older children suggests that cardiomegaly through expiratory films should be interpreted with caution. A large thymus can also give a false impression of cardiomegaly in neonates and infants **(Fig. 9.4.1)**. Cardiomegaly with increased pulmonary blood flow (pulmonary plethora), prominent main and branch pulmonary arteries are the features of significant left-to-right shunts **(Fig. 9.4.2)**. Typical radiographs are rare but if present are diagnostic of certain CHD, e.g., egg-on-side appearance in transposition of the great arteries (TGA) **(Fig. 9.4.3)**, normal heart size with ground-glass lungs in obstructed TAPVC **(Fig. 9.4.4)**, figure-of-eight appearance in unobstructed supracardiac TAPVC **(Fig. 9.4.5)**, and so on.

TABLE 9.4.3: Common signs and symptoms of HF at different ages.

Age	Common signs and symptoms	Less common signs and symptoms
Infants	Growth failure, persistent tachypnea, tachycardia, feeding difficulties, diaphoresis, subcostal recession, and hepatomegaly	Cyanosis, palpitation, syncope, seizures, and wheeze
Toddlers	Respiratory distress, tachypnea, tachycardia, fatigue, and hepatomegaly	Poor appetite, palpitations, and edema
School age	Fatigue, effort intolerance, poor appetite, orthopnea, abdominal pain, nausea, vomiting, hepatomegaly, and raised JVP	Palpitations, chest pain, leg edema, ascites, and basal crepitations
Adolescents	Effort intolerance, poor appetite, abdominal pain, orthopnea, and hepatomegaly	Nausea, vomiting, leg edema, and ascites

(HF: heart failure; JVP: jugular venous pulse)

Electrocardiogram

An electrocardiogram (ECG) is a much-underutilized investigation in children. It is often useful for diagnosing types of CHD and tachyarrhythmia. Biventricular hypertrophy

TABLE 9.4.4: NYHA and modified Ross heart failure classifications for children.

Class	NYHA	Modified Ross
Class I	No limitations on physical activity	No limitations or symptoms
Class II	May experience fatigue, palpitations, dyspnea, or angina during moderate exercise but not during rest	*Infants:* Mild tachypnea or diaphoresis with feeding *Older children:* Mild-to-moderate dyspnea on exertion
Class III	Symptoms with minimal exertion that interfere with normal daily activity	*Infants:* Growth failure and marked tachypnea or diaphoresis with feeding *Older children:* Marked dyspnea on exertion
Class IV	Unable to carry out any physical activity because they typically have symptoms at rest that worsen with any exertion	Symptoms at rest such as tachypnea, retractions, grunting, or diaphoresis

(NYHA: New York Heart Association)

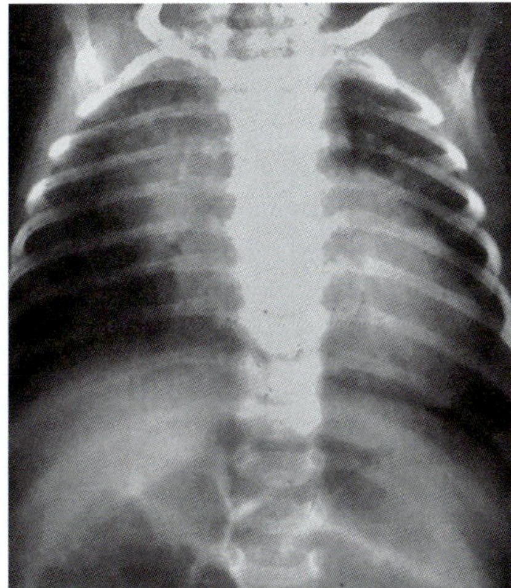

Fig. 9.4.1: A large thymus may give a false impression of cardiomegaly in neonates and infants.

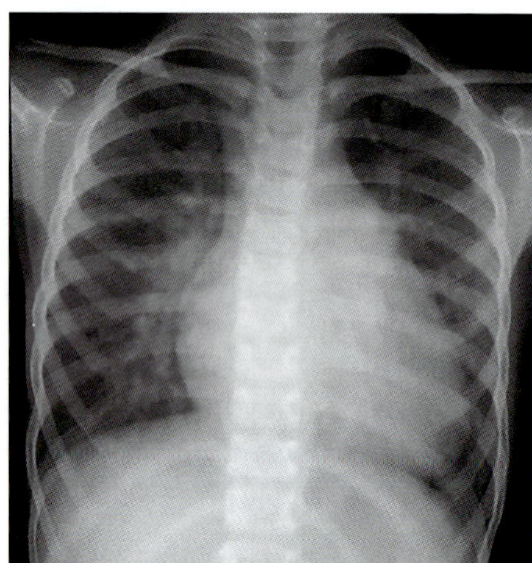

Fig. 9.4.2: Features of significant left-to-right shunts: Cardiomegaly with increased pulmonary blood flow (pulmonary plethora) and prominent main and branch pulmonary arteries.

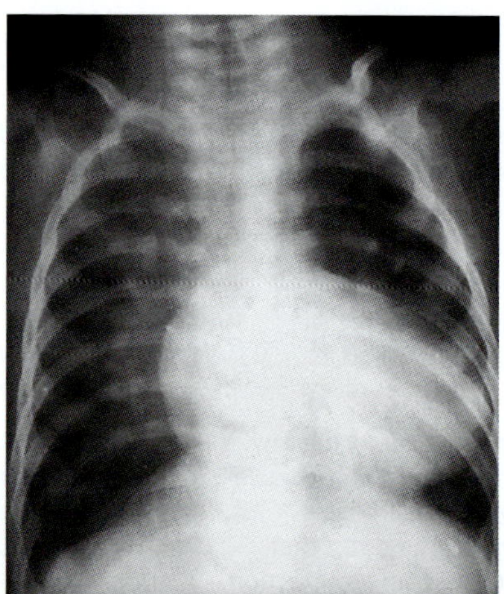

Fig. 9.4.3: Egg-on-side appearance in transposition of great arteries (TGA).

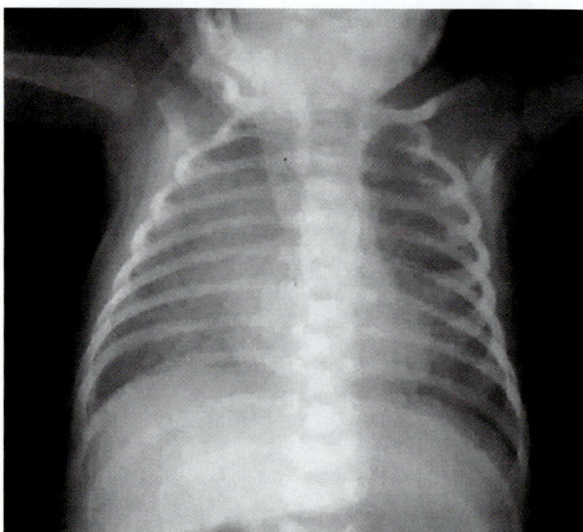

Fig. 9.4.4: Normal heart size with ground-glass lungs in obstructed total anomalous pulmonary venous connection (TAPVC).

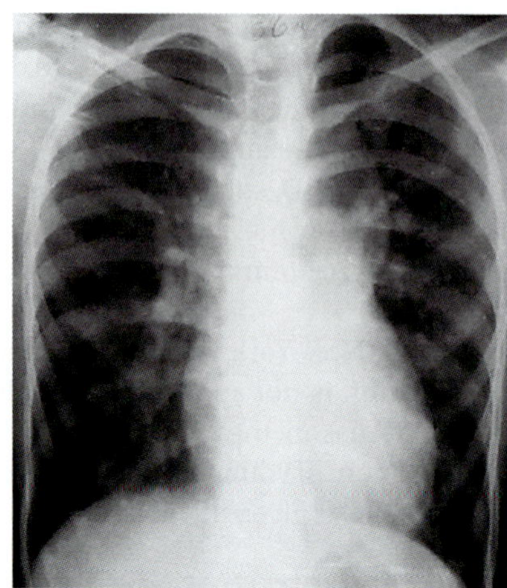

Fig. 9.4.5: Figure-of-eight appearance in unobstructed total anomalous pulmonary venous connection (TAPVC).

(Fig. 9.4.6) with volume overload of the left ventricle is seen in large VSD, the most common cause of HF in infants. Tachycardiomyopathy, a potentially reversible cause of HF, due to incessant supraventricular tachycardia (such as ectopic atrial tachycardia) can only be picked up by ECG. Similarly, bradyarrhythmias due to congenital complete heart block (CHB) are detected on ECG **(Fig. 9.4.7)**. Anomalous left coronary artery from pulmonary artery produces a very specific pattern, pathologic "q" waves in anterolateral leads **(Fig. 9.4.8)**. Left-axis deviation in a child with a large shunt lesion suggests AVSD as a cause of HF **(Fig. 9.4.9)**. Rarely, hypocalcemia may cause left ventricular dysfunction (LVEF); ECG shows prolonged corrected QT (QTc) interval with terminal "T"-wave inversion **(Fig. 9.4.10)**. Nonspecific ST- and T-wave changes may be present in the ECGs of patients with cardiomyopathy.

Echocardiogram

Echocardiography is the most useful investigation as it provides the precise diagnosis in most cases and is widely available. It provides information on the function of right and left ventricles, size of cardiac chambers, wall thickness, severity of valvular stenosis, or incompetence, if present, and associated structural abnormalities of the heart and great vessels. Pericardial effusion and intracardiac thrombi are also easily seen on echocardiography. Information obtained on echocardiography is crucial to make a correct diagnosis and also to guide appropriate management.

Biomarkers

Brain natriuretic peptide (BNP) and/or its cleavage product amino-terminal pro-brain natriuretic peptide (NT-proBNP) are often elevated in children with HF. BNP or amino terminal, NT-proBNP has been shown to be of use in differentiating HF from pulmonary causes of respiratory distress in acute

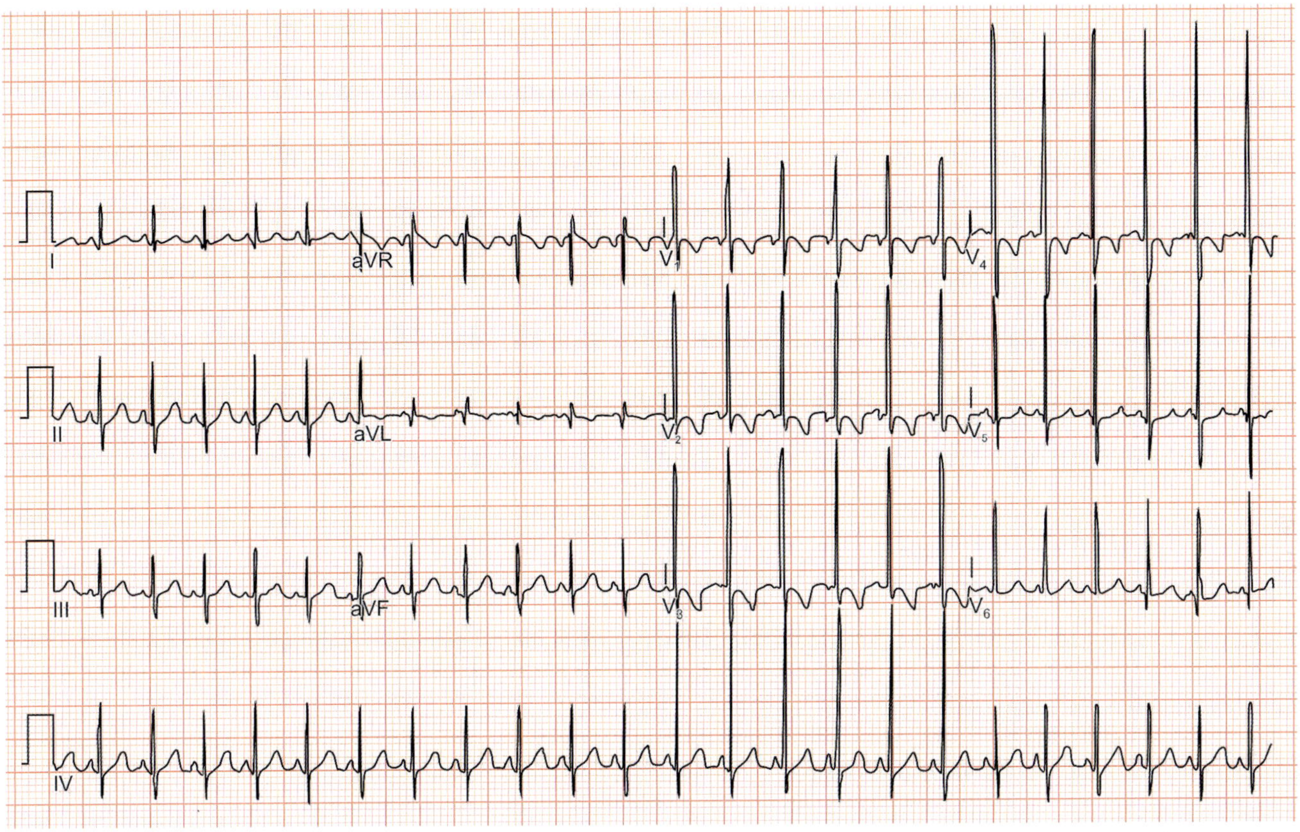

Fig. 9.4.6: Biventricular hypertrophy with volume overload of the left ventricle seen in large ventricular septal defect (VSD).

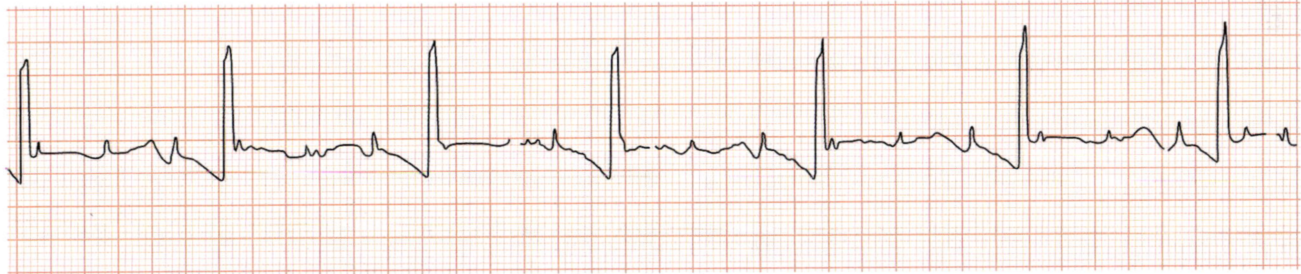

Fig. 9.4.7: Electrocardiogram detecting bradyarrhythmias due to congenital complete heart block.

settings. According to some studies, higher levels of these biomarkers may represent a poor prognosis.[4] Similarly, a strong correlation has been found between NT-proBNP and symptoms and ventricular function.[5] High levels of these biomarkers may be associated with the worst outcome in HF, high likelihood of admission to the hospital, high chances of need for mechanical circulatory support, or heart transplant. Serial BNP or NT-proBNP measurements may be useful for monitoring the progress of the patient.

Other Investigations

- *Hemoglobin* estimation is important as anemia can cause decompensation in children with an underlying heart disease but no HF.
- *Electrolytes, such as serum calcium, phosphorus, and blood glucose,* should be routinely measured in all children with HF, especially neonates, where their abnormalities are an uncommon but reversible cause of ventricular dysfunction. Serum electrolytes and renal function may be impaired, either due to HF or due to diuretic therapy, and need to be monitored.
- *Other tests:* Screening tests for hypoxia and sepsis in newborns. Antistreptolysin O and C-reactive protein if suspecting acute rheumatic fever with carditis as the cause of HF.
- *Second-line investigations:* Second-line tests may be required in some specific cases for making a diagnosis.

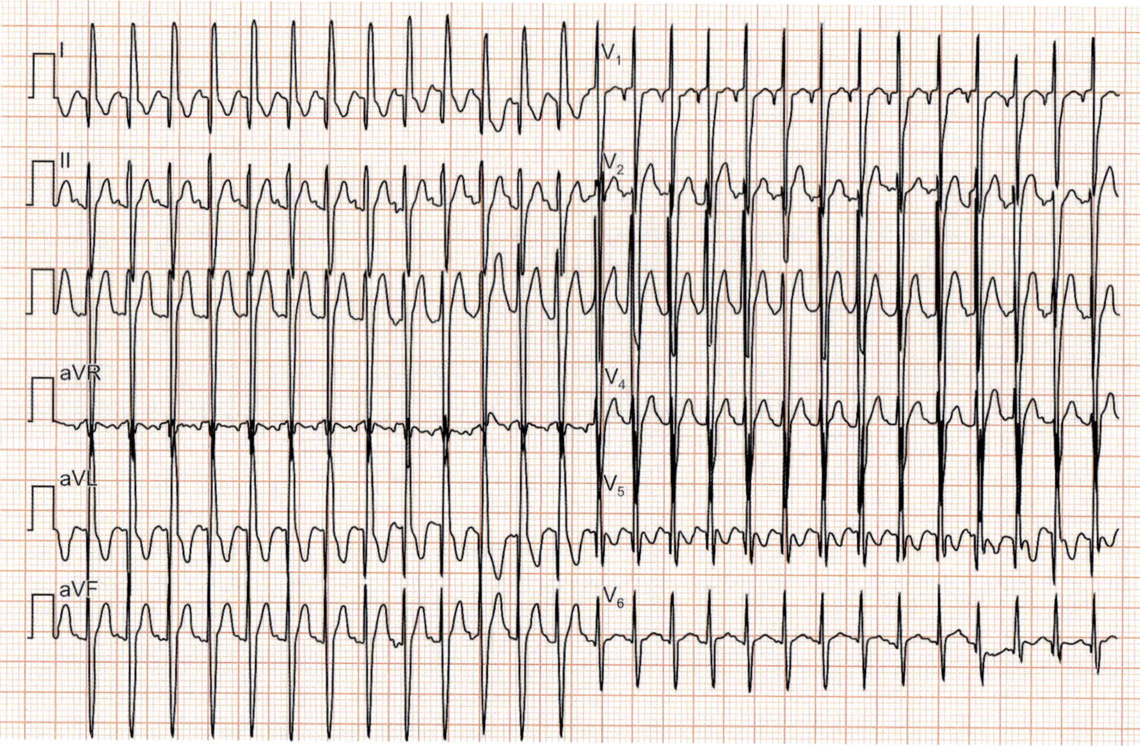

Fig. 9.4.8: Anomalous left coronary artery from pulmonary artery (ALCAPA) producing a very specific pattern, pathologic "q" waves in anterolateral leads.

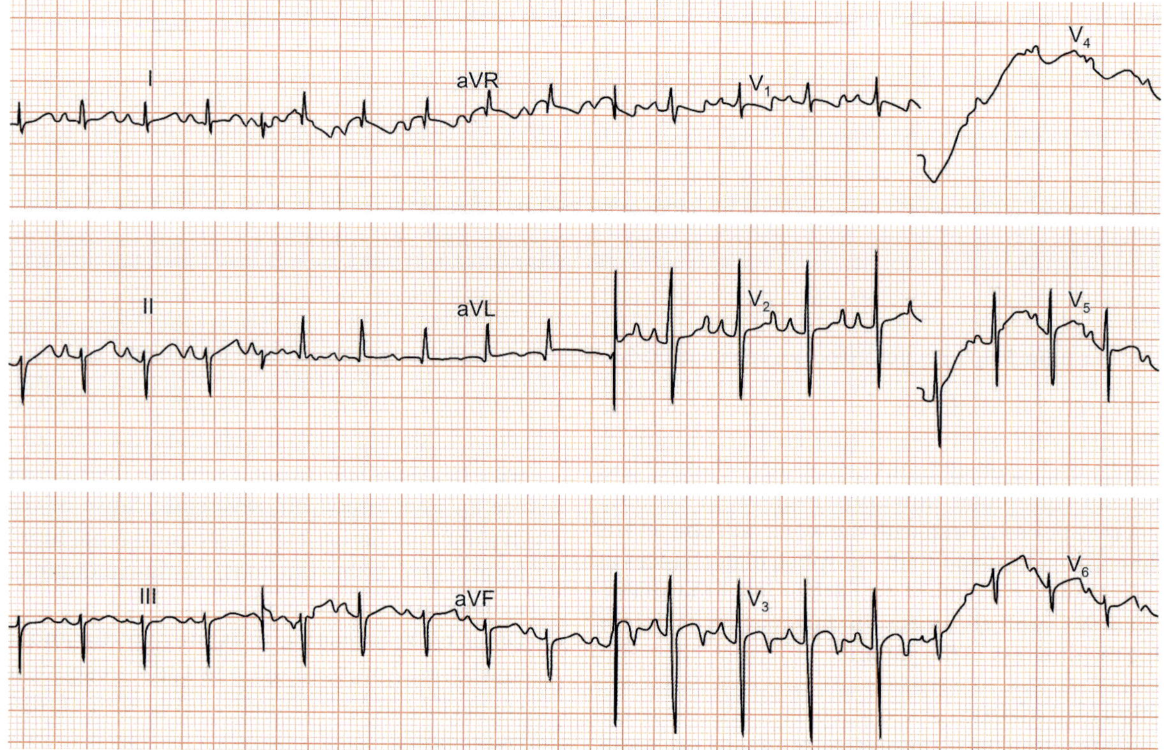

Fig. 9.4.9: Left-axis deviation in a child with a large shunt lesion suggesting atrioventricular septal defect (AVSD) as a cause of HF. (HF: heart failure)

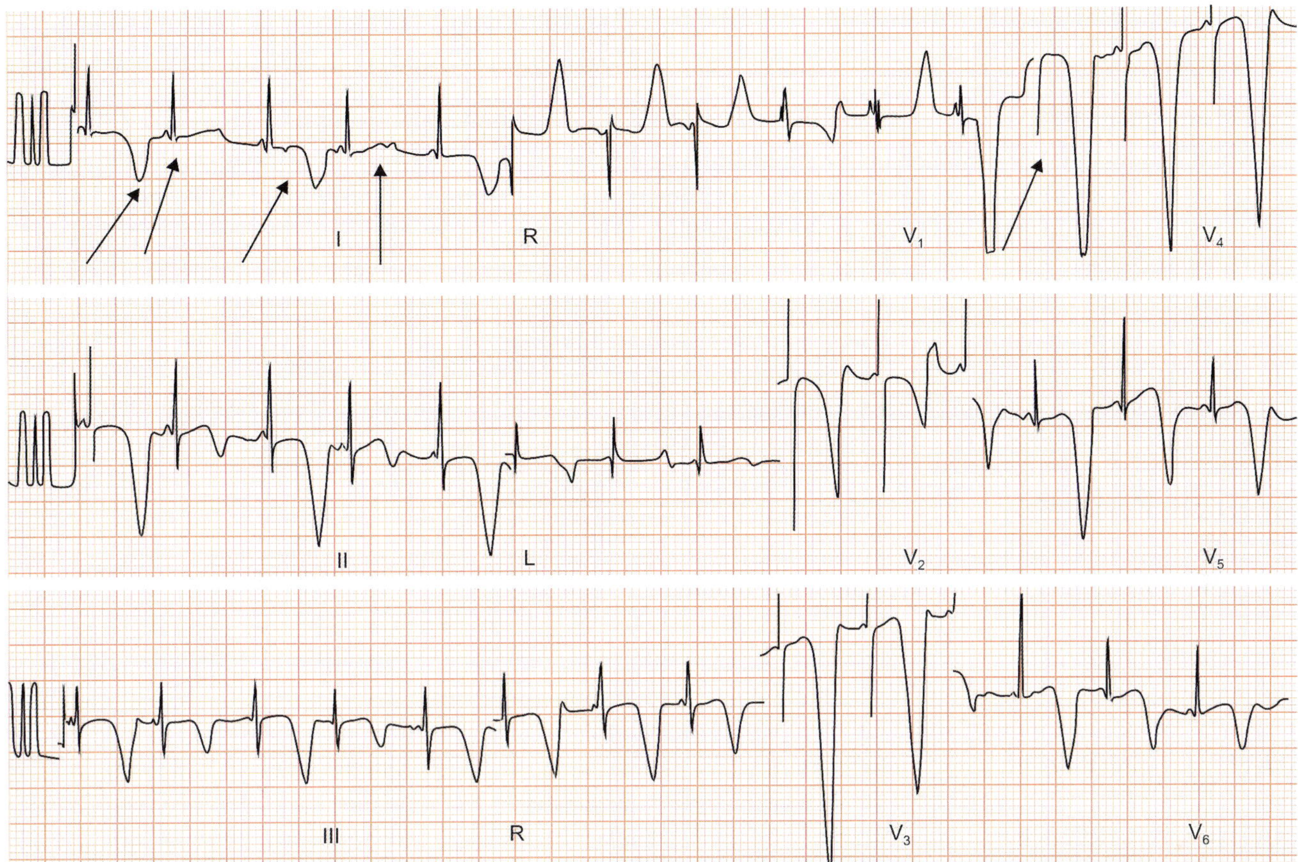

Fig. 9.4.10: Electrocardiogram showing prolonged QTc interval with terminal "T" wave inversion in hypocalcemia.

These include cardiac magnetic resonance imaging (MRI), computed tomography (CT) angiography, endomyocardial biopsy, Holter monitoring, metabolic and genetic testing, viral pathogenic screening, etc.

MANAGEMENT

In contrast to HF therapy in adults, few evidence-based data exist to guide the management of HF in children. Most of the drugs for HF are used in children based on experience in adults. Key concepts in the management of HF in children are listed below:

- Treatment of HF in children should consist of treatment of the cause, precipitating factors (anemia, IE, infections, acute rheumatic fever, electrolyte imbalance, noncompliance with drug or diet, and arrhythmias), and treatment of the congested state.
- Therapy should allow for somatic growth and development.
- Therapy should reduce congestion and improve cardiac output and end-organ perfusion.
- During early infancy, supplementation of potassium is usually not required up to 2 mg/kg of dose for furosemide or equivalent. In cases requiring higher doses and in older children, a combination of loop diuretics and spironolactone (or other potassium-sparing diuretics) may be preferred.

Management includes supplemental oxygen therapy, nutrition supplements, and fluid management. Pharmacologic agents form the backbone of treatment. Extracorporeal membrane oxygenation (ECMO), left ventricular assist devices (LVAD), and other advanced therapies may be required in cases not responding to conventional management.

Nutrition

In infants, a calorie intake of 120–150 kcal/kg/day is recommended with a fluid intake of 100 mL/kg/day. Many patients are unable to tolerate this amount of fluid. Calorie-dense food, adding fat to feeds (coconut oil or medium-chain triglyceride), frequent small feeding, and at times feeding through the nasogastric tube may achieve adequate calories. Calcium and vitamin D_3 supplements should be prescribed. Unlike in adults, dietary restriction of sodium is generally not recommended in children unless there is severe edema that is not responding to diuretic therapy. Frequent weight measurement is encouraged, especially in infants, to assess their nutritional status.

Fluid Management

Fluid intake is generally not restricted unless the child has acute HF with significant lung congestion and edema despite diuretics. Fluid restriction may also be required in cases with hyponatremia.

Bed Rest

Bed rest is generally not required. In fact, some amount of physical activity should be encouraged in children with controlled HF.

Correction of Anemia

A large proportion of these children are anemic due to various reasons, and they should receive iron and vitamin supplements. If Hb is <7 or 8 g/dL, blood transfusion is recommended.

Pharmacological Therapy

Figure 9.4.11 depicts the various sites for action of pharmacologic agents to treat HF. **Table 9.4.5** provides the most common pediatric HF drugs and doses.

Several studies in adults have shown the role of diuretics, angiotensin-converting enzyme (ACE) inhibitors,

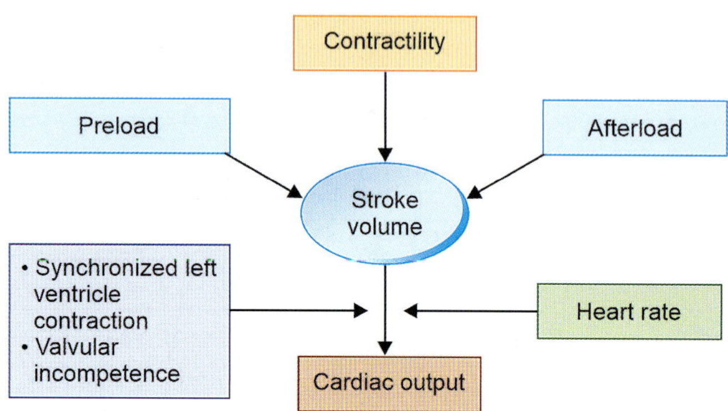

Fig. 9.4.11: Pharmacologic targets for treatment of heart failure.

TABLE 9.4.5: Dosages, mechanism of action, and side effects of common drugs used in the treatment of HF in children.

Drug	*Standard dose*	*Mechanism of action*	*Comments*
Diuretics Furosemide Torsemide Metolazone	 1 mg/kg dose BD max 6 mg/kg/day 0.4 mg/kg day 0.1 mg/kg dose BD max 20 mg/day	Relieves congestive symptoms; useful in volume overload/fluid retention states; do not change the long-term outcomes	Aggressive use can reduce preload resulting in neurohormonal activation and fluid retention; patients refractory to the usual oral dose of diuretics may need IV diuretics to relieve congestion
Spironolactone	1 mg/kg dose BD max 200 mg/day	Decreases mortality and morbidity; improves endothelial dysfunction	Should be used with caution in patients with hyponatremia, renal insufficiency, hyper-kalemia, and hepatic disease; can cause gynecomastia
Digoxin	3–5 µg/kg dose BD	Increases inotropy; decreases neurohormonal activation, results in reduced norepinephrine, improves baroreceptor function, decreases sympathetic activity	Very narrow toxic to therapeutic ratio; common side effects are conduction disturbances (AV block); useful for atrial arrhythmia; excreted by the kidney, so the dose must be reduced with renal insufficiency
ACEi Captopril Enalapril	 0.1 mg/kg dose TD max 2 mg/kg/dose 0.1 mg/kg dose BD max 0.5 mg/kg/day	Decrease mortality and morbidity; blocks the conversion of angiotensin I to II, activates bradykinin and kallidin; causes vasodilation and natriuresis; reduces afterload	Beneficial in HF patients; not recommended for asymptomatic children with mild ventricular dysfunction; side effects include chronic cough, hypotension, and renal insufficiency
ARB Losartan	 0.5–2 mg/kg/day	Action similar to that of ACEi. Less likelihood of cough	Should not be combined with ACEi. May cause hypotension
Betablockers Metoprolol Carvedilol	 0.1 mg/kg dose BD max 1 mg/kg dose 0.025 mg/kg/dose BD, max 0.5 mg/kg/dose BD	Decrease morbidity and mortality; Carvedilol has vasodilatory, antioxidant, antiproliferative, and antiapoptotic properties, reversing cardiac remodeling	Patients with compensated HF. Should not be used for NYHA class IV patients. May be beneficial in children with HF due to CHD when LV is systemic ventricle

(ACEi: angiotensin-converting enzyme inhibitor; ARB: angiotensin receptor blocker; AV: atrioventricular; CHD: congenital heart disease; HF: heart failure; IV: intravenous; LV: left ventricle; NYHA: New York Heart Association)

mineralocorticoid antagonists, angiotensin receptor antagonists (ARBs), and beta blockers in HF management to relieve symptoms and improve survival. Despite the lack of such robust data in pediatrics, drugs commonly used in adults are diuretics, ACE inhibitors, and ARBs. Aldosterone antagonists (spironolactone or eplerenone) are the current standard of care therapy for chronic HF. The addition of a β-adrenergic receptor antagonist (β-blocker) for both asymptomatic and symptomatic patients with chronic HF is less well supported in the pediatric literature, but is being increasingly used in practice. Digoxin is not routinely recommended but can be reserved for patients who remain symptomatic despite maximum doses of the above-stated drugs and in those with tachyarrhythmia such as atrial fibrillation.

New Drugs for Heart Failure

Despite conventional therapy, several children, especially those with impairment of ventricular function, continue to deteriorate. A number of new drugs have been added to the armamentarium of HF therapy for adults. Again, the evidence for these drugs in the pediatric age group is lacking. Some of the newer drugs are discussed in the following text.

Ivabradine

Ivabradine is an inhibitor of the funny channels located in the sinoatrial node that slows the rate of phase-4 depolarization, thereby reducing the heart rate. Though tachycardia is a common compensatory mechanism in HF, elevated heart rates have been shown to increase the risk of death and cardiac transplant in registry data of children with dilated cardiomyopathy.[6] A randomized, double-blind, placebo-controlled, phase II/III clinical trial of children with stable HF reported the safety of Ivabradine in children.[7] The trial showed reduction in the resting heart rate and an increase in the left ventricular ejection fraction. The recommended dose is 0.02–0.05 mg/kg twice a day for children under 40 kg and 2.5 mg twice a day for children >40 kg.

Sacubitril–Valsartan

This new drug Sacubitril–Valsartan is a combination of a neprilysin inhibitor and an angiotensin II receptor antagonist. The enzyme neprilysin degrades natriuretic peptides, which decrease the sympathetic tone and aldosterone levels. Inhibition of neprilysin prevents degradation of natriuretic peptides, thereby promoting sodium excretion and lowering blood pressure. The combination of a neprilysin inhibitor with an angiotensin II receptor antagonist provides inhibition of neprilysin as well as blockade of the renin–angiotensin–aldosterone system. This combination is available as sacubitril/valsartan. Based on the analysis of interim data in 110 pediatric subjects, the United States Food and Drug Administration (FDA) approved the use of this drug in October 2019 for children, 1 year of age or older, with symptomatic HF with left ventricular systolic dysfunction.[8] The starting dose for children <40 kg is 1.6 mg/kg of the combined amount of both valsartan and sacubitril. The dose is titrated upward every 2 weeks from 2.3 mg/kg up to a maximum dose of 3.1 mg/kg based on tolerance.

Sodium–Glucose Cotransporter 2 Inhibitors

Drugs included under this group are canagliflozin, dapagliflozin, and empagliflozin. These were initially developed for patients with diabetes mellitus. The mechanism of action is to inhibit the sodium/glucose cotransporter situated in the kidney and to promote glucose excretion and improve sugar control in a diabetic patient. The first description of the use of sodium-glucose cotransporter 2 (SGLT2) inhibitors in the pediatric age group was reported in the year 2021.[9] More data in pediatric HF is required before recommending this drug for HF. The dose in the pediatric age group is 0.1–0.2 mg/kg once daily with a maximum of 10 mg.

Investigational Supplement Drug

Recently published data suggest that coenzyme Q10 (a potent antioxidant) improves cardiac function. Its mechanism of action is to stabilize myocardial calcium-dependent ion channels and to prevent the consumption of some of the essential metabolites.[10]

WHICH DRUG FOR WHICH PATIENT: THE LOGICAL APPROACH

It seems reasonable to start with a drug in the ACE inhibitor or ARB group, except in patients having HF secondary to obstructive lesions. For patients with dilated cardiomyopathy, an aldosterone antagonist drug may also be added. There is evidence that sacubitril/valsartan is tolerated well in this setting, so this may become the preferred option in place of an ACE inhibitor in the future. It is also important to use the maximally tolerated doses of vasodilators to reap the maximum benefit of these drugs. Generally, the doses can be escalated rapidly in stable patients with chronic HF. This can be followed by a β-blocker. β-blockers can be started prior to discharge in hospitalized patients. Those treated in the outpatient department can be given a lower dose to ensure tolerability, and the dose is gradually increased. Target dosing of ACE inhibitors can be achieved within 6–7 days in most patients, but optimizing the dose of β-blockers generally takes longer. For those having high heart rate despite β-blockers or intolerant to β-blockers, additional treatments with ivabradine may be prescribed. Diuretics may be prescribed for reducing pulmonary or systemic congestion in symptomatic patients; the dosage may be given daily or as and when required. Indications for SGLT2 inhibitors are not very clear at this stage for children. Based on excellent results in adults, these drugs may be used in adolescent patients with reduced function of the left ventricle due to dilated cardiomyopathy who have persistent symptoms.

ACUTE HEART FAILURE

Acute HF may occur due to worsening of ongoing HF, either due to progression of the disease or due to suboptimal treatment of chronic HF. At times, it can occur de novo, e.g., due to a mechanical cause such as acute MR (chordal or papillary muscle rupture) or tachyarrhythmias. The treatment algorithm is given in **Table 9.4.6**.

TABLE 9.4.6: Treatment algorithm for acute heart failure in neonates and infants.

Supportive measures	
Avoid hypothermia and hypoglycemia; check for hypocalcemia	
Maintenance of adequate oxygenation	• Monitoring of blood gases if perfusion is poor • Ventilate, if required, with modest PEEP to achieve PaO_2 of 50–60 mm Hg and SaO_2 of 75–85% to avoid pulmonary congestion
Adequate hydration	Stop oral feeds if severe tachypnea
IV access	IV and CVP lines (umbilical vein cannula)
IV inotropes for shock	• Isoproterenol 0.5–2 µg/kg/min • Dopamine 5–20 µg/kg/min • Dobutamine 5–20 µg/kg/min • Avoid digoxin
Milrinone	• Inotrope and vasodilator • Load with 25–50 µg/kg/min; maintain at 0.25–1 µg/kg/min
Diuretics	Furosemide 2–4 µg/kg PO/IV
Vasodilators	• Captopril 0.1–1 mg/kg/day PO q 8 hourly • Sodium nitroprusside 0.5–4 µg/kg/min IV • Careful monitoring of blood pressure is necessary
Prostaglandin infusion for ductus-dependent lesions	Start at 0.1 µg/kg/min (up to 0.4 µg/kg/min if no response), taper to the lowest dose possible (0.005 µg/kg/min) monitor for apnea; keep the minimum required dose

(CVP: central venous pressure; IV: intravenous; PEEP: positive end-expiratory pressure; PO: per oral)

Advanced Nonpharmacologic Therapy

Cardiac Resynchronization Therapy

This device therapy is indicated in adults who have a left ventricular ejection fraction of <35%, dilated left ventricle, and NHYA classes II, III, and IV despite maximization of drug therapy and QRS duration of >120 ms. A clear benefit has been shown with cardiac resynchronization therapy (CRT) in terms of slower progression of HF due to the improvement of cardiac motion and a reduced risk of sudden death.

Implantable Cardioverter Defibrillator

This device is implanted for patients with a history of cardiac arrest or symptomatic sustained ventricular tachycardia in association with CHD. Some pediatric patients with a history of severe LVEF (<30%) with or without documented ventricular arrhythmias may benefit from a combination of CRT and implantable cardioverter defibrillator (ICD), the so-called defibrillator-associated cardiac resynchronization therapy (CRT-D).

Extracorporeal Membrane Oxygenation and Ventricular Assist Device

This approach has been widely used in acute settings of cardiopulmonary arrest, especially when the cause of HF is likely to be reversible, such as fulminant myocarditis. ECMO or ventricular assist device (VAD) is used as a temporizing measure allowing ventricular function to recover. ECMO is also often used in emergency during the perioperative period if there is ventricular pump failure. For patients who require long-term support as a bridge to cardiac transplantation, VAD is increasingly being used. VAD devices can offer isolated left or right ventricular support or biventricular circuit support. However, VADs have high complication rates, including thrombosis, bleeding, and infections, more so in infants with a body weight of <10 kg. Patients can stay on VAD till a heart becomes available for transplantation but have high morbidity and mortality.

Cardiac Transplantation

Heart transplantation is to be considered only for end-stage HF, which is refractory to surgical and medical therapy. The most common indication is cardiomyopathy; other indications are uncorrectable CHD, such as hypoplastic left heart syndrome or failed Fontan due to ventricular dysfunction. Approximately 600–700 pediatric heart transplantation procedures are performed worldwide each year. Complications include systemic viral infections (cytomegalovirus, Epstein–Barr virus, and adenovirus), acute rejection, vasculopathy with graft failure, and hypertension.

TABLE 9.4.7: Stepwise guide to the management of HF.

Step	Management
Step 1	*In acute decompensation*: Bed rest, propped-up position, humidified oxygen sodium, and, if required, volume restriction
Step 2	• Start digoxin (not in myocarditis) • Assess reversible and precipitating causes • Assess the need for surgery/interventional procedure in the case of structural heart disease
Step 3	• Add ACE inhibitor • In the case of ACE-inhibitor-induced cough, switch to ARB like losartan • Switch to nitrates if ACE inhibitor/ARB is not tolerated
Step 4	Add carvedilol in compensated HF, especially in the cases with tachycardia
Step 5	• Once or twice weekly dobutamine therapy • Consider stem-cell coronary infusion
Step 6	• Cardiac transplantation • Ventricular assist device as a bridge in the case of delays or even destination therapy

(ACE: angiotensin-converting enzyme; ARB: angiotensin receptor blocker; HF: heart failure)

Malignancies like lymphoproliferative disorders are other major complications of cardiac transplantation in children. Advances in immunosuppression have reduced episodes of rejection and have resulted in improved survival and quality of life. Survival is >70% at 5 years; a large number of children survive for over 20 years. A major limitation to cardiac transplantation is the inadequate donor supply.

Pulmonary Artery Banding

Recently, this procedure has been used in selected infants or toddlers with dilated cardiomyopathy as a bridge to recovery or to more definitive therapy such as cardiac transplantation. Band results in right ventricular pressure overload, which straightens the interventricular septum, thereby improving the filling of the left ventricle, its end-diastolic volume, and pressure. This improves left ventricular ejection fraction. A multicenter survey reported 70 patients from 15 centers in 11 countries.[11] 60% of the patients showed a clinical improvement after pulmonary artery banding, and 48% showed a functional recovery in 1 year. Right ventricular function must be normal for this modality of pulmonary artery banding to be of use. The best response is obtained in children <1 year, normal pulmonary artery pressure, and normal or mild left atrial dilatation.

A stepwise guide to the management of HF is given in **Table 9.4.7**.

CONCLUSION

Heart failure in children is a complex syndrome resulting from diverse etiologies and varied clinical presentation. Correction of an underlying heart disease can reverse HF in a large number of cases. Thus, the overall outcome with HF is better in children than that in adults. Clinical presentation of HF in younger children can be nonspecific requiring a heightened degree of suspicion. In particular, some conditions that can present with acute shock are important to recognize, as they can be effectively treated or palliated on an urgent basis. A systematic clinical approach is necessary for the exact clinical diagnosis. Treatment has evolved in the last three decades or so. However, most of the pharmacotherapy for HF in children is extrapolated from data in adults. In the future, pediatric-specific data should be developed with the goal of identifying an individualized management regimen.

REFERENCES

1. Boucek MM, Edwards LB, Keck BM, Trulock EP, Taylor DO, Mohacsi PJ, et al. The registry of the International Society for Heart and Lung Transplantation: sixth official pediatric report-2003. J Heart Lung Transplant. 2003;22(6):636-52.
2. Shaddy RE, George AT, Jaecklin T, Lochlainn EN, Thakur L, Agrawal R, et al. Systematic literature review on the incidence and prevalence of heart failure in children and adolescents. Pediatr Cardiol. 2018;39(3):415-36.
3. Ross RD. The Ross classification for heart failure in children after 25 years: a review and an age-stratified revision. Pediatr Cardiol. 2012;33(8):1295-300.
4. Auerbach SR, Richmond ME, Lamour JM, Blume ED, Addonizio LJ, Shaddy RE, et al. BNP levels predict outcome in pediatric heart failure patients post hoc analysis of the Pediatric Carvedilol Trial. Circ Heart Fail. 2010;3(5):606-11.
5. Kocharian A, Shabanian R, Rahimzadeh M, Kiani A, Hosseini A, Zanjani KS, et al. N-terminal pro-B-type natriuretic peptide and ventricular dysfunction in children and adolescents. Cardiol Young. 2009;19(6):580-8.
6. Rossano JW, Kantor PF, Shaddy RE, Shi L, Wilkinson JD, Jefferies JL, et al. Elevated heart rate and survival in children with dilated cardiomyopathy: a multicenter study from the pediatric cardiomyopathy registry. J Am Heart Assoc. 2020;9(15):e015916.
7. Bonnet D, Berger F, Jokinen E, Kantor PF, Daubeney PEF. Ivabradine in children with dilated cardiomyopathy and symptomatic chronic heart failure. J Am Coll Cardiol. 2017;70(10):1262-72.
8. Shaddy R, Canter C, Halnon N, Kochilas L, Rossano J, Bonnet D, et al. Design for the sacubitril/valsartan (LCZ696) compared with enalapril study of pediatric patients with heart failure due to systemic left ventricle systolic dysfunction (PANORAMA-HF study). Am Heart J. 2017;193:23-34.
9. Newland DM, Hong BJ, Albers EL, Friedland-Little JM, Kemna MS, Law YM. Safety of Dapagliflozin in children with heart failure. J Heart Lung Transplant. 2021;40(4):S280.
10. Al Saadi T, Assaf Y, Farwati M, Turkmani K, Al-Mouakeh A, Shebli B, et al. Coenzyme Q10 for heart failure. Cochrane Database Syst Rev. 2021;(2):CD008684.
11. Schranz D, Akintuerk H, Bailey L. Pulmonary artery banding for functional regeneration of end-stage dilated cardiomyopathy in young children: World Network Report. Circulation. 2018;137(13):1410-2.

9.5 Diseases of Endocardium, Myocardium, and Pericardium

Srikanta Basu

DISEASES OF ENDOCARDIUM

INFECTIVE ENDOCARDITIS

Infective endocarditis (IE) is defined as the "endovascular microbial infection of cardiovascular structures," which involves infection of the endocardium or of the endothelium of the great vessels. This condition usually occurs as a complication of congenital heart disease (CHD) or rheumatic heart disease (RHD) but rarely develops without a pre-existing heart disease. It is associated with 16–25% of mortality, and 20% of the patients require emergency surgery.[1]

Epidemiology

Infective endocarditis is more common in adults as compared to children and accounts for 0.8–3.3 cases for every 1,000 admissions to the hospital with a cumulative risk of 6.1 per 1,000 children up to 18 years. The incidence in children and neonates may be rising due to the increasing use of newer devices, indwelling catheters, increasing sophistication of resuscitative techniques, especially in sick babies, and overall improved survival. In India or other developing countries, RHD still forms a significant proportion of cases with IE.

In general, cardiac lesions with steep pressure gradients [ventricular septal defect (VSD), patent ductus arteriosus (PDA), and left-sided valvular regurgitation] are associated with an increased risk of IE. It is extremely rare in patients with atrial septal defects (ASDs). Tetralogy of Fallot (TOF), bicuspid aortic valve, and children who had undergone repair or palliation for cyanotic CHD are also at a higher risk of IE. In newborns, endocarditis often involves right-sided structures, and the diagnosis may be difficult with a very high mortality rate.

Etiopathogenesis

Gram-positive cocci are the most likely organisms, although gram-negative rods and fungi can cause IE. *Streptococcus viridans* is the most common causative agent, followed by *Staphylococcus aureus* in children beyond the age of 1 year. This has been reported in Indian studies as well. However, *S. aureus* and fungus are more common in children where a vascular in-dwelling catheter or prosthetic valve is used and in immunocompromised patients.

The cardiac lesions consist of vegetations of fibrin, leukocytes, platelets, and bacteria. Many clinical manifestations are related to destructive aspects of the infection or to embolization of portions of the vegetation. Endocarditis, particularly from *Staphylococcus*, may cause valvular damage, such as perforation of the aortic cusps or ruptured chordae tendineae of the mitral valve. Embolization may occur in the pulmonary or systemic circulations and cause infarction, abscess, or inflammation of various tissues. Emboli to the lungs, kidneys, spleen, or brain are reported most frequently because in each location there are major clinical or laboratory findings of the phenomenon.

Clinical Features

The clinical presentation is insidious with prolonged fever, malaise, myalgia, anorexia, weight loss, pallor, arthralgia, and headache. The classical signs, such as Janeway lesions, Osler's node, and Roth spot, are rarely seen in children. The diagnosis should be suspected in any child with a significant cardiac murmur and a prolonged fever. Congestive cardiac failure (CCF) may develop, especially if aortic or mitral valve regurgitation is created by the infection. Signs and symptoms of embolic phenomenon should be sought. Signs of recurrent pneumonia or a pleuritic type of pain may indicate embolization of infected material to the lungs. Signs of systemic embolization, such as splenomegaly, hematuria, splinter hemorrhages, and central nervous system signs, should be sought in any febrile patient with a cardiac anomaly, and rarely the children may present with these signs acutely. Acute IE has a fulminant course often requiring emergency intervention. It presents with high-grade fever, rapidly changing signs and symptoms, and shock, and *S. aureus* is the most common causative organism.

Diagnosis

The diagnosis can be confirmed by obtaining the organisms from a *blood culture*. Usually, three blood cultures should be taken aseptically within the first 12 or 24 hours, and 2–3 mL of blood may be enough. Blood culture may be negative in nearly 7% of the cases, although studies from India have shown that the percentage is much higher, which may be due to prior use of antibiotics and insufficient samples of blood for culture, especially in our setup. Nonspecific *acute-phase reactants*, such as erythrocyte sedimentation rate (ESR), C-reactive protein (CRP), and rheumatoid factor, are usually elevated; the tests may also be useful in following the progress of therapy.

Echocardiography has become an important modality for the diagnosis of IE and is taken as major criteria in the modified Duke's classification **(Table 9.5.1 and Box 9.5.1)**.

TABLE 9.5.1: Modified Duke criteria.

Major criteria
A. Positive blood culture for IE
• Typical microorganisms consistent with IE from two separate blood cultures, as noted below: – *Streptococcus viridans*, *Streptococcus bovis*, or HACEK group, or *Staphylococcus aureus* – Community-acquired enterococci in the absence of a primary focus • Microorganisms consistent with IE from persistently positive blood cultures defined as: – Two positive cultures of blood samples drawn >12 hours apart, or – All of three or a majority of four separate cultures of blood (with the first and last samples drawn 1 hour apart) – Single positive blood culture for *Coxiella burnetii* or antiphase 1 IgG antibody titer >1:800
B. Evidence of endocardial involvement
Echocardiogram positive for IE (TEE recommended for patients with prosthetic valves rated at least "possible IE" by clinical criteria, or complicated IE paravalvular abscess; TTE as the first test in other patients)
• Positive echocardiogram for IE is defined as: – Oscillating intracardiac mass on valve or supporting structures, in the path of regurgitant jets, or omni-planted material in the absence of an alternative anatomic explanation, or – Abscess, or – New partial dehiscence of prosthetic valve – New valvular regurgitation (worsening or changing of preexisting murmur not sufficient)
Minor criteria
• *Predisposition:* Predisposing heart condition or intravenous drug use • *Fever:* Temperature >38°C (100.4°F) • *Vascular phenomena:* Major arterial emboli, septic pulmonary infarcts, mycotic aneurysm, intracranial hemorrhage, conjunctival hemorrhages, and Janeway lesions • *Immunologic phenomena:* Glomerulonephritis, Osler's nodes, Roth spots, and rheumatoid factor • *Microbiological evidence:* Positive blood culture but does not meet a major criterion as noted above* or serological evidence of active infection with organism consistent with IE • Echocardiographic minor criteria eliminated

*Excludes single positive cultures for coagulase-negative staphylococci and organisms that do not cause endocarditis.
(HACEK: *Haemophilus* species, *Actinobacillus actinomycetemcomitans*, *Cardiobacterium hominis*, *Eikenella corrodens*, *Kingella* species; IE: infective endocarditis; IgG: immunoglobulin G; TEE: transesophageal echocardiography; TTE: transthoracic echocardiography)

It is important to remember that the diagnostic yield of echocardiography is influenced by the image quality, size of vegetation [vegetation <2–3 mm may not be well seen by transthoracic echocardiography (TTE)], location of vegetation, and the experience of the echocardiographer. The absence of valve changes or vegetations does not exclude endocarditis. TTE is very sensitive in children due to better acoustic window, but occasionally, transesophageal echocardiography is advised in situations when the window is poor, in patients with prosthetic valves, grafts, or conduits, and rarely in aortic valve endocarditis or aortic root abscess.[1]

Management

The aim of the management is to treat infection with antibiotics, manage complications, and surgical intervention in selected cases. If the patient is very ill, antibiotic treatment can be initiated empirically after the cultures are taken. However, in all the other cases, initiation of therapy should await the results of blood cultures. The exact treatment depends upon the organism isolated and its antibiotic sensitivities.

Usually, penicillin (or vancomycin if sensitive to penicillin) and gentamicin are the preferred antibiotics that are administered parenterally. The total duration of therapy for native valve endocarditis varies from 2 to 6 weeks. The duration of therapy depends on the type of etiological agent, site of valvular infection, and complications. Following completion of therapy, blood cultures should be obtained to verify the eradication of the infection. The American Heart Association has listed various regimens for IE in adults, and the same can be followed in children with dose modification. Fungal endocarditis may be difficult to treat and may require surgery along with antifungals, such as amphotericin B, for a duration of 6–8 weeks followed by oral antifungals, such as fluconazole, for a prolonged duration of time (may take up to a year).[1]

BOX 9.5.1: Diagnosis of infective endocarditis (IE) according to the modified Duke's criteria.

Definite IE:
- *Pathologic criteria:* Microorganism demonstrated by culture or histologic examination of vegetation, emboli, intracardiac abscess; or active endocardial lesions on pathology examination
- *Clinical criteria:* Two major criteria, or one major criterion and three minor criteria, or five minor criteria
- *Possible IE:* One major criterion and one minor criterion, or three minor criteria

Rejected:
- Firm alternative diagnosis explaining evidence of IE; or
- "IE syndrome" resolved within 4 days of antibiotic therapy; or
- No pathological evidence of IE at surgery or autopsy within 4 days of antibiotic therapy; or
- Does not meet criteria for "possible IE" as above

The indications of surgery in the acute phase are listed in **Box 9.5.2**. The aims of the surgery are to repair the cardiac defects, eradicate infection, and prevent complications. Despite the availability of antimicrobials, endocarditis can lead to major complications **(Box 9.5.3)**. Complications are more likely to occur in patients with prosthetic valves, age <2 years, left-sided IE, fungal and staphylococcal IE, symptoms continuing for >3 months, and cyanotic CHDs.[1]

Prophylaxis

Antibiotics are recommended for the prevention of IE prior to certain medical and dental procedures. The guidelines by the American Heart Association have undergone changes in 2007. The cardiac conditions for which prophylaxis is recommended have been listed in **Box 9.5.4**. Presently, it is recommended for all dental procedures that involve treatment of gingival tissue or periapical region of the teeth or oral mucosal perforation and for invasive procedures that involve incision or biopsy of respiratory mucosa, such as tonsillectomy and adenoidectomy. It is no longer recommended for genitourinary or gastrointestinal tract procedures solely for bacterial endocarditis prophylaxis. The application of these guidelines in the Indian context is debated by various pediatric cardiologists. The drugs recommended are oral amoxicillin (50 mg/kg) and intravenous ampicillin, and those allergic to penicillin can take cefazolin, ceftriaxone, clindamycin, cephalexin, azithromycin, or clarithromycin. The antibiotic should be given before the procedure and up to 2 hours after the procedure in those who did not take it earlier.[2]

BOX 9.5.2: Indications for surgery in the acute phase of infective endocarditis.

- Myocardial or periannular abscess
- Continued bacteremia after 2 weeks of antibiotic therapy
- Worsening of heart failure due to valvular regurgitation
- Embolic events
- Fungal endocarditis
- Prosthetic valve dysfunction

BOX 9.5.3: Complications of infective endocarditis.

- *Embolic events:* Cerebral, pulmonary, renal, and coronary
- Congestive heart failure
- Persistent bacteremia or fungemia
- Periannular extension of abscess
- Metastatic infection
- Glomerulonephritis/renal failure
- Mycotic aneurysm
- Mesenteric or splenic abscess or infarct
- Arrhythmia or development of new heart block

BOX 9.5.4: Cardiac conditions for which antibiotic prophylaxis is recommended for dental, respiratory tract, infected skin, skin structures, or musculoskeletal tissue procedures.

- Prosthetic cardiac valve or prosthetic material used for cardiac valve repair
- Previous IE
- Unrepaired cyanotic CHD, including palliative shunts and conduits
- Completely repaired congenital heart defect with prosthetic material or device, whether placed by surgery or by catheter intervention during the first 6 months after the procedure
- Repaired CHD with residual defects at the site or adjacent to the site of a prosthetic patch or prosthetic device (which inhibits endothelialization)
- RHD, if prosthetic valves or prosthetic materials are used for valve repair
- Cardiac transplantation recipients who develop cardiac valvulopathy

(CHD: congenital heart disease; IE: infective endocarditis; RHD: rheumatic heart disease)

DISEASES OF MYOCARDIUM

CARDIOMYOPATHY

Cardiomyopathy refers to a group of diseases of heart muscle that are not secondary to structural heart disease, hypertension, or pulmonary vascular disease. These are categorized by the World Health Organization (WHO) as dilated, hypertrophic, restrictive, and arrhythmogenic right ventricular dysplasia—cardiomyopathy. One more form of cardiomyopathy, that is, left ventricular (LV) noncompaction (spongy myocardium or fetal myocardium), is also recognized as a distinct form of cardiomyopathy by the American Heart Association.[3] This entity is not so rare as was previously believed as the incidence in various studies in children varies between 8% and 9% and mimics dilated cardiomyopathy (DCM) as far as clinical features and outcome are concerned.

Cardiomyopathy is characterized by the abnormality of systolic and/or diastolic functions. Factors identified as causes of myocardial damage are shown in **Table 9.5.2**. Broadly, cardiomyopathy can be primary or secondary (where heart muscles are affected along with the involvement of the other systems). The incidence of primary cardiomyopathy in population-based studies in the US, Australia, and Finland is around 1 case per 100,000 person-years in children <20 years of age.

Dilated Cardiomyopathy

Dilated cardiomyopathy is the most common type of heart muscle disease in children where both ventricles are dilated with reduced contractility. Most cases of DCM are idiopathic.[4,5]

Etiopathogenesis

Three major factors, namely preceding viral myocarditis, autoimmunity, and underlying genetic predisposition, have

TABLE 9.5.2: Etiology of myocardial damage.

Infections	***Metabolic, endocrinal, and nutritional***
Viral infections (myocarditis): • Coxsackievirus B • Adenovirus • Parvovirus • Human immunodeficiency virus • Echovirus • Rubella • Varicella • Mumps • Epstein–Barr virus • Cytomegalovirus • Measles • Polio *Others:* • Diphtheria • *Mycoplasma* • Tuberculosis • Lyme disease • Psittacosis • Rocky mountain-spotted fever • *Toxoplasma* • *Toxocara* • *Cysticercus* • *Histoplasma* • *Coccidioidomycosis* • *Actinomycosis*	• Pompe disease • Carnitine-deficiency syndrome • Hyperthyroidism • Carcinoid syndrome • Infant of diabetic mother • Kwashiorkor • Pellagra • Thiamine deficiency • Selenium deficiency
Familial—hereditary	***Coronary arteries***
• Mitochondrial myopathy syndrome • Hypertrophic cardiomyopathy • Duchenne or Becker muscular dystrophies • Friedreich ataxia • Kearns–Sayre syndrome • Other muscular dystrophies	• Kawasaki disease • Anomalous left coronary artery *Drugs—toxins:* • Doxorubicin • Cyclophosphamide • Chloroquine • Hemosiderosis
Connective tissue—granulomatous—infiltrative: • Systemic lupus erythematosus • Scleroderma • Rheumatoid arthritis • Sarcoidosis • Amyloidosis • Dermatomyositis • Leukemia	*Others:* • Anemia • Sickle cell disease • Endomyocardial fibroelastosis • Histiocytosis

been implicated in the pathogenesis of myocardial damage in DCM. Injury to the myocardial cells is the initiating factor that leads to cell death. If considerable cell loss occurs, the myocardium fails to generate enough contractile force to produce adequate cardiac output and leads to chronic heart failure (CHF). Overstretching of the ventricles causes myocardial thinning, cavity dilatation, secondary valvular regurgitation, and compromised myocardial perfusion. The resulting subendocardial ischemia perpetuates myocyte damage. The most common known causes of DCM are myocarditis, neuromuscular disorders, and familial.[4]

Myocardial remodeling is an important contributor to worsening heart failure (HF). Lost myocyte cells are replaced with fibrous tissue, thereby decreasing the compliance of one or more ventricles and adversely affecting performance. Aldosterone, angiotensin II, catecholamines, endothelins, and mechanical factors, such as excessive myocardial stretch and ischemia, have been identified as mediators of remodeling.

Altered gene expressions resulting in calcium-handling abnormalities, downregulation of myosin or conversion to the less-active beta isoform, and abnormal beta-receptor signal transduction have all been identified at the molecular level in the chronically failing heart.[5]

Clinical Features

Children with DCM usually present typically after HF. Cough, poor feeding, irritability, and difficulty in breathing are usually the initial presenting symptoms. Older children complain of easy fatigability, dyspnea, and palpitation and rarely may present with pulmonary edema. The clinical examination may reveal displaced apical impulses and muffled heart sounds with a prominent S3 or S4. Murmurs are usually not audible, but rarely the murmur of mitral regurgitation (MR) or tricuspid regurgitation (TR) may be heard. The liver may be enlarged, and in older children, other signs of venous congestion, such as neck vein congestion and peripheral edema, may be observed. A short duration of symptoms (2–4 weeks) may suggest myocarditis. The infant or young child with the disease is often tachypneic and tachycardic with weak peripheral pulses and has cool extremities and hepatomegaly. Blood pressure is low with a decreased pulse pressure, accentuated P2, and murmurs of MR and TR; murmurs may be inconspicuous initially if the patient presents with acute HF and cardiomegaly.[4]

Cardiomyopathy should always be suspected in cases of acute decompensated HF in emergency and primary care settings, especially if the infant presents with lethargy, weakness, abdominal pain, and unexplained tachypnea or disproportionate tachycardia. Even in the absence of cardiomegaly in the chest X-ray, myocarditis should always be considered in the differential diagnosis in cases presenting with a viral prodrome and nonspecific respiratory or abdominal symptoms associated with tachycardia, hypotension, hypertension, or cardiac rhythm abnormalities. One should rule out three important correctable causes of DCMs, that is, anomalous left coronary artery from the pulmonary artery, tachycardiomyopathy, and hypocalcemia in newborn and young infants.[5]

Diagnosis

The main aim of diagnostic evaluation for a patient with DCM is to identify the underlying etiology so that etiology-specific therapy can be planned. Even in the best of centers, the cause is usually identified in only 34% of children. An additional purpose is to determine the extent of myocardial dysfunction and its complications, such as clot formation in the heart **(Fig. 9.5.1)**. **Table 9.5.3** provides a list of useful diagnostic tests.

Screening of Family Members

Recent reports suggest a genetic cause for >50% of patients with DCM. With the advancement of molecular genetics techniques, prospective controlled studies on screening of family members have revealed a genetic transmission in up to 20–30% of cases involving more than 37 genetic mutations with DCM and a prevalent autosomal trait. Due to limited awareness about genetic predisposition, screening and echo of family members are not performed, but it is advisable in view of the above findings.

Treatment

Treatment is mainly supportive management of CHF (discussed in detail in Chapter 9.4: Congestive Heart Failure).[6] Ideally, etiology-specific treatment is recommended, but it requires clear proof of association of etiology, which is not possible always; other various treatment modalities (immunoglobulins or carnitine) are administered without good evidence. These treatment modalities have been enlisted in **Table 9.5.4**.[7,8]

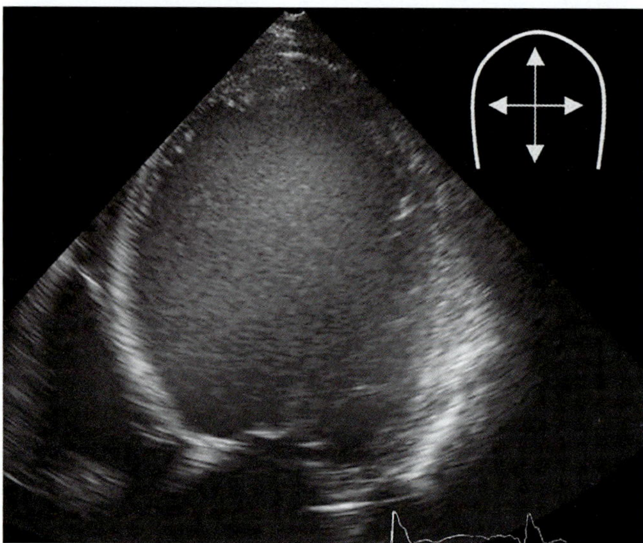

Fig. 9.5.1: Transthoracic echocardiogram of a patient with dilated cardiomyopathy (apical four-chamber view shows dilated left ventricle).

Immunoglobulins and immunosuppression: Intravenous immunoglobulin (IVIG) has been used as an immune modulator, which neutralizes pathogenic antibodies and suppresses the ongoing process and is used in cases of myocarditis. The Pediatric Cardiac Society of India, in a consensus review (2009), has recommended IVIG in cases where symptoms are preceded by viral illness, or when history is short (<3 months) or cardiac enzymes are elevated. The role of immunosuppressive agents (prednisolone, azathioprine, or cyclosporine) is debatable and is not recommended routinely due to the lack of convincing evidence.[8]

Surgical and other interventions: Reduction cardiomyoplasty or Batista operation, assist devices, extracorporeal membrane oxygenation, and artificial heart are some procedures, which

TABLE 9.5.3: List of investigations in the dilated cardiomyopathy.

Investigations	*Findings and comments*
Chest X-ray	Cardiomegaly and features of pulmonary venous congestion
Electrocardiogram	Low-voltage waves, "ST" segment depressions with "T" wave inversion in the anterolateral precordial leads, prominent "Q" wave, changes suggestive of arrhythmias
Echocardiogram **(Fig. 9.5.1)**	EF and FS. LV systolic dysfunction in children is currently defined by a fractional shortening <25% and/or an ejection fraction <55%. Quantification of MR, clots, thrombus, and coronaries; rule out any structural heart lesion
Basic laboratory tests	Hemogram, ESR, glucose, urea, creatinine, LFT, electrolytes, calcium, phosphorous, ABGs
Metabolic screening	Blood lactate, serum ammonia, urinary ketones
Muscle enzymes	CPK, CPK-MB, cardiac troponin T
Biomarkers: BNP/ NT-proBNP	Differentiates symptoms due to lung disease or heart failure, can be used as a confirmatory test in the acute evaluation of pediatric HF
Screening and echocardiogram of family members	Screening of first-degree relatives of the case
Endomyocardial biopsy and viral culture	Not advised routinely and should only be performed if confirming the clinical diagnosis of myocarditis will have a clear effect on the patient's treatment plan
CMRI with gadolinium contrast	Can detect patchy myocardial involvement and provide additional information by tissue and scar characterization

(ABGs: arterial blood gases; BNP: B-type natriuretic peptide; CMRI: cardiac magnetic resonance imaging; CPK: creatine phosphokinase; CPK-MB: creatine phosphokinase-muscle/brain; EF: ejection fraction; ESR: erythrocyte sedimentation rate; FS: fractional shortening; HF: heart failure; LFT: liver function test; LV: left ventricular; MR: mitral regurgitation; NT-proBNP: N-terminal pro-b-type natriuretic peptide)

TABLE 9.5.4: Treatment options for the dilated cardiomyopathy.

Treatment options	*Comments*
Digoxin	Can be given in myocarditis but loading dose is to be avoided
Furosemide + spironolactone	Helps in reducing systemic and pulmonary venous congestion
Intravenous inotropes and vasodilators (dobutamine, dopamine, and milrinone)	• Dobutamine is the first choice in the stage of decompensation • Milrinone is becoming the first-line treatment as it causes less mechanical stress as compared to other cardiotonics • To be used cautiously in cases of hypotension
Levosimendan	• Oral agent with similar properties to milrinone but not superior to dobutamine
ACE inhibitors (captopril and enalapril)	• Benefits by reducing systemic vascular resistance • Initiate treatment with captopril and can be changed to enalapril • Avoid during acute decompensated state • Improved survival in chronic CHF
Beta-blockers and carvedilol	Carvedilol is the most widely used and improves symptoms and LV failure. It should be considered in the absence of overt heart failure, particularly in the presence of tachycardia
Anticoagulation and aspirin	All children with DCM and severe LV dysfunction (EF <30%) should ideally be anticoagulated and in the absence of monitoring INR, aspirin can be tried. The presence of LV thrombus is a strong indication for oral anticoagulation
Carnitine	If metabolic screening suggests carnitine deficiency (elevated ammonia levels, high blood lactate, or presence of urinary ketones), carnitine can be given

(ACE: angiotensin-converting enzyme; CHF: chronic heart failure; DCM: dilated cardiomyopathy; EF: ejection fraction; INR: international normalized ratio; LV: left ventricular)

are often used as options to "bridge to transplantation procedure" and are very expensive. Cardiac transplantation is the final treatment for DCM with severe LV dysfunction and the reported survival benefit of 1 year is 90%, 5 years 75%, and 20 years 40%.[7,8]

Stem-cell therapy: This is another promising option, and several studies are going on in the adult and pediatric populations.

Prognosis: In a small proportion of pediatric patients, DCM may resolve completely. In a few pediatric case series, the mortality from DCM at 5 years after the presentation varied from 33% to 66%. In a large case series from the All India Institutes of Medical Sciences on 128 children, it was reported that 54% improved on medication and of these 24% became symptom-free without medication. Around 35% deteriorated despite therapy, and 19% died. Female sex was the only multivariate predictor of death. Another study from South India of 233 cases showed good recovery of LV function in 36% of children with a poor outcome in the infantile group.[9] Overall, the prognosis of DCM will improve only if various etiologies are understood and etiology-specific therapy is instituted.

Hypertrophic Cardiomyopathy

Hypertrophic cardiomyopathy (HCM) is a condition in which myocardial thickness is increased. In contrast to DCM, the LV cavity has a normal or decreased size. During systole, the hypertrophied myocardium bulges into the LV outflow tract and may result in subaortic obstruction.

Etiology and Genetics

The disease may be caused by one of many possible mutations of genes coding for various contractile proteins. This condition frequently occurs as autosomal dominant with a variable penetrance. Multiple generations may be involved. Manifestations can begin at any age. Siblings of the proband may not be affected as children but may show evidence of the disease as they reach adolescence and adulthood. The natural history and prognosis are variable; sudden death is not uncommon even in patients who have no important obstruction or sentinel arrhythmia. Genetic testing is advised in proband with HCM, atypical clinical features, and suspected other genetic conditions.

Clinical Features

Patients with HCM usually come to medical attention in one or more of the following ways:

- Detection of a murmur
- An angina kind of chest pain
- An abnormal electrocardiogram (ECG)
- From family screening or a positive family history
- From evaluation of syncope, palpitations, or out-of-hospital cardiac arrest

The physical findings can be variable. The peripheral pulse may be of bisferiens character with a rapid upstroke, and palpation of the apex may reveal a double impulse. A long systolic ejection murmur is present along the left sternal border and faintly radiates to the base. The murmur varies in intensity with a change in position; it is usually the loudest with the patient standing in contrast to functional flow murmurs. Third and fourth sounds may be present.

Investigations

Chest X-ray is not diagnostic, and ECG shows evidence of left and frequently biventricular hypertrophy with or without ischemic changes. Septal changes are evidenced by abnormal "q" waves in V5 and V6. The echocardiogram may reveal asymmetric septal hypertrophy. Left ventricular thickness ≥2 standard deviation above the mean (*Z*-score) for age, sex, or body size is diagnostic of HCM in children; the interventricular septum may be 2–3 cm thick compared with the normal, which is ≤1 cm. Systolic anterior motion of the mitral valve anterior leaflet is a classic two-dimensional echocardiographic finding. It results from the high-velocity flow occurring in the LV outflow tract. This creates low pressure, which "pulls" the valve leaflet toward the interventricular septum during systole. Cardiac catheterization and angiography are rarely required. Cardiac MRI is indicated when echocardiography is inconclusive.

Treatment

The greatest risk with HCM is sudden death despite medical and surgical treatments. For symptomatic patients, beta-blockers or verapamil can be tried, and for the control of arrhythmias, disopyramide and amiodarone are the drugs of choice. Digitalis, other inotropic drugs, and afterload-reducing agents, which increase the gradient, are contraindicated. It is necessary that patients with HCM should undergo a 24-hour Holter to document for arrhythmias and should be restrained from strenuous games and exercises. Implantable automatic cardioverter/defibrillator devices may abort potentially lethal arrhythmia in some patients.

For patients with significant LV outflow tract obstruction, surgical myomectomy or alcohol ablation can be done. There is increasing evidence that elimination of the obstruction prolongs life and relieves symptoms.

Prognosis

Although ultimately fatal in majority, the interval between the discovery and death often goes in decades. The risk of sudden death in recent population-based studies has shown to be nearly 1% per year. The following features may be associated with a higher risk for sudden death: Diagnosis in childhood, septal thickness exceeding 3 cm, nonsustained ventricular tachycardia, failure of normal increase of systolic blood pressure during exercise, family history of premature death associated with HCM, significant LV outflow tract obstruction, and prior cardiac arrest.

Restrictive Cardiomyopathy

This is the rarest form of cardiomyopathy characterized by poor ventricular compliance and limited filling. It may be idiopathic or may be associated with a systemic disease, such as scleroderma, amyloidosis, sarcoidosis, or inborn error of metabolism (mucopolysaccharidoses).

The two common types are endocardial fibroelastosis with normal or less than normal left ventricle and endomyocardial fibrosis. Endomyocardial fibrosis is endemic in Kerala but rare in North India.

Symptoms are nonspecific and like those of CHF seen with DCM. In contrast to DCM, the left ventricle is of normal size and may have normal systolic function. This condition alters diastolic ventricular function, so the clinical manifestations are those of elevated left and right atrial pressures.

Examination reveals hepatic and splenic enlargement and jugular venous distension. Electrocardiographic abnormalities are usually limited to atrial enlargement. Chest X-ray shows pulmonary vascular congestion with a relatively normal cardiac silhouette. The echocardiogram reveals striking dilatation of the atria and great veins but normal or small ventricles. Physiologically, the condition is like constrictive pericarditis, and differentiating the two can be difficult. Overall, the prognosis is poor in infants and children, and cardiac transplantation is advised once the diagnosis is made.

A comparison of the three variants of cardiomyopathy has been summarized in **Table 9.5.5**.

TABLE 9.5.5: Overview of myopathy.

	Dilated	*Hypertrophic*	*Restrictive*
Prevalence	50/100,000	1/500	Unknown
Inheritance	25–50% AD, AR, X-L, MT	50% AD	Unknown
Ventricular function	Systolic and diastolic dysfunction	Diastolic dysfunction	Severely reduced diastolic function
Arrhythmias	Atrial, ventricular, and conduction disturbances	Atrial and ventricular dynamic systolic outflow obstruction	Atrial fibrillation normal to reduced systolic function

Contd...

Contd...

	Dilated	*Hypertrophic*	*Restrictive*
Echocardiographic findings	Dilated LV cavity with normal to thin wall thickness	Asymmetric, concentric, or apical LV hypertrophy	Normal or small ventricular cavity size, marked biatrial enlargement
Medical management	ACE inhibitors diuretics (furosemide, spironolactone) digitalis β2-blocking agents	Propranolol pacemaker calcium antagonists (digitalis/catechols and nitrates contraindicated, and diuretics may worsen symptoms)	Antiarrhythmic agents: Careful use of diuretics, milrinone
Surgical/interventional	ICD, resynchronization biventricular pacing transplantation	ICD, septal myomectomy transplantation	ICD transplantation
Sudden death	Yes	Depends on gene 0.7–11% per year, associated with exercise	1.5% per year

(ACE: angiotensin-converting enzyme; AD: autosomal dominant; AR: autosomal recessive; ICD: implantable cardioverter defibrillator; LV: left ventricular; MT: mitochondrial; X-L: X-linked)

PERICARDIAL DISEASE

PERICARDITIS

Pericarditis is the inflammation of the visceral and parietal layers of the pericardium. The causes are variable and are listed in **Table 9.5.6**. Pericardial effusion is the accumulation of excess fluid in the pericardial sac. The symptoms that result from pericardial fluid depend upon the status of the myocardium and the volume and the speed at which the fluid accumulates. It may be exudative due to bacterial infections, serous to increased capillary pressures (e.g., CHF) or decreased plasma oncotic pressure (e.g., hypoproteinemia). Cardiac tamponade is a life-threatening, slow or rapid compression of the heart due to accumulation of fluid, blood, clots, or gas in the pericardial space leading to significant impairment of ventricular filling with reduction in stroke volume and cardiac output. It is most commonly associated with viral infections, neoplasm, uremia, and acute hemorrhage. Constrictive pericarditis is due to adherent, thick, and noncompliant pericardium that restricts ventricular filling. In children, tuberculosis is the most common cause in India.

Clinical Features

The clinical manifestations of pericarditis, which may vary from a simple inflammatory response with no cardiovascular compromise to cardiac tamponade and constrictive pericarditis, are noted in **Table 9.5.7**. The differentiation of constrictive pericarditis and restrictive myocarditis can be challenging.

TABLE 9.5.6: Causes of pericardial diseases.

Congenital:
- Absence of pericardium
- Pericardial cyst

Infectious:
- Viral (*coxsackievirus A and B, Epstein–Barr virus, hepatitis, HIV*, and *adenovirus*)
- Bacterial (*Staphylococcus, Haemophilus influenzae type B Streptococcus, Pneumococcus*)
- Tuberculosis
- Fungal (*histoplasmosis and actinomycosis*)
- Parasitic (*Toxoplasmosis and Echinococcosis*)

Connective tissue diseases:
- Rheumatic fever
- Rheumatoid arthritis
- Systemic lupus erythematosus
- Systemic sclerosis
- Kawasaki disease
- Wegener granulomatosis

Hematology-oncology:
- Bleeding diathesis
- Malignancy (primary and metastatic)
- Radiotherapy induced

Postprocedural:
- Postcardiac catheterization
- Cardiac surgery
- Central line placement

Drugs:
- Anticoagulants
- Antithrombolytics
- Hydralazine
- Phenytoin
- INH
- Rifampicin

Others:
- Renal failure
- Hypothyroidism
- Chylopericardium

(HIV: human immunodeficiency virus; INH: isonicotinylhydrazide)

Management

The management of these conditions will depend on the cause, which are listed in **Table 9.5.7**.

TABLE 9.5.7: Manifestations and management of pericarditis.

	Nonconstrictive pericarditis	*Pericardial effusion*	*Cardiac tamponade*	*Constrictive pericarditis*
Symptoms	• Retrosternal chest pain (occasionally radiating to back) • Aggravated by supine position • Relieved by leaning forward, dyspnea	• May be asymptomatic • Dull ache • Other features of cardiac tamponade	• Dyspnea • Fatigue • Anorexia • Cough • Cold extremities	• Exercise intolerance • Syncope with exertion • Dyspnea • Fatigue • Anorexia
Signs	• Fever • Tachypnea • Pericardial rub • Distant heart sound	• Muffled heart sound • Ewart sign (dullness of posterior left chest wall) • Tachycardia	• Raised JVP • Hypotension • Tachycardia • Pulsus paradoxus (decrease in systolic blood pressure >10 mm Hg with each inspiration) • Decreased capillary refill time • Silent precordium • Distant heart sound • Hepatomegaly	• Tachycardia • Pedal edema • Raised JVP • Hepatomegaly • Ascites • Pericardial knock • Signs of low cardiac output
ECG	• "ST" segment elevation in all leads • PR segment depression	• Decreased voltage "QRS" complex • Electrical alternans	• Electrical alternans • Sinus tachycardia • Low-voltage waves • Electrical alternans	• Low-voltage waves • Intraventricular conduction delay
Chest X-ray	Normal	Globular, symmetrical cardiomegaly	Globular, symmetrical cardiomegaly	• Normal • Pericardial calcification or effusion
Echocardio-graphy	Usually normal	An echo-free space (suggesting fluid) around the heart	• Global fluid collection • Compressed and collapsing chambers with hyperdynamic cardiac function	• Flattening of the left ventricular posterior wall endocardium • Abnormal septal motion • Dilated SVC, IVC, atria
Treatment	• Treat the cause; symptomatic treatment with rest • Analgesic and rarely antibiotics	• Treat the underlying condition • Pericardiocentesis if sudden accumulation of fluid • NSAIDs or steroids are required occasionally	Needle pericardiocentesis or surgical drainage, pericardial stripping or window in recurrent condition	• Analgesic, corticosteroids, and antibiotics • Pericardiectomy is definitive treatment but mostly unwarranted as many cases, including TB, resolve spontaneously

(ECG: electrocardiogram; IVC: inferior vena cava; JVP: jugular venous pressure; NSAIDs: nonsteroidal anti-inflammatory drugs; SVC: superior vena cava; TB: tuberculosis)

CONCLUSION

Infective endocarditis is a serious infection of the valves of the heart associated with significant morbidity and mortality, requiring early recognition and treatment. Modified Duke's criteria is the commonly used diagnostic criterion used in practice. Prolonged antibiotic therapy and timely surgical interventions in selected cases are the mainstay of treatment. Rigorous dental hygiene and antibiotics prophylaxis before the indicated surgical procedures should be routinely followed.

Dilated cardiomyopathy is the most common form of cardiomyopathy in children characterized by dilated ventricles and heart failure. Hypertrophic cardiomyopathy is a genetically inherited disease followed by rarer restrictive cardiomyopathy which carries a poorer prognosis. Myopathies present as heart failure and treatment entails managing failure and preventing associated complications like thromboembolic events, arrhythmias and sudden death. Heart transplant is the only therapy available for end-stage heart disease following cardiomyopathy.

Viruses are the most common cause of acute pericarditis in children. In cases of constrictive pericarditis, tuberculosis should be ruled out as it is an important cause. Connective tissue disorders (SLE, JIA, acute rheumatic fever, etc.) are the important noninfectious etiologies.

REFERENCES

1. Baddour LM, Wilson WR, Bayer AS, Fowler VG, Bolger AF, Levison ME, et al. Infective endocarditis: diagnosis, antimicrobial therapy, and management of complications: a statement for healthcare professionals from the Committee on Rheumatic Fever, Endocarditis, and Kawasaki Disease, Council on Cardiovascular Disease in the Young, and the Councils on Clinical Cardiology, Stroke, and Cardiovascular Surgery and Anesthesia, American Heart Association: endorsed by the Infectious Diseases Society of America. Circulation. 2005;111(23):e394-433.
2. Wilson W, Taubert KA, Gewitz M, Lockhart PB, Baddour LM, Levison M, et al. Prevention of infective endocarditis guidelines from the American Heart Association: a guideline from the American Heart Association Rheumatic Fever, Endocarditis, and Kawasaki Disease Committee, Council on Cardiovascular Disease in the Young, and the Council on Clinical Cardiology, Council on Cardiovascular Surgery and Anesthesia, and the Quality of Care and Outcomes Research Interdisciplinary Working Group. Circulation. 2007;116(15):1745-54.
3. Lipshultz SE, Law YM, Asante-Korang A, Austin ED, Dipchand AI, Everitt MD, et al. Cardiomyopathy in children: classification and diagnosis: a scientific statement from the American Heart Association. Circulation. 2019;140(1):e9-e68.
4. Mallavarapu A, Taksande A. Dilated cardiomyopathy in children: early detection and treatment. Cureus. 2022;14(11): e31111.
5. Jefferies JL, Towbin JA. Dilated cardiomyopathy. Lancet. 2010;375(9716):752-62.
6. Kantor PF, Lougheed J, Dancea A, McGillion M, Barbosa N, Chan C, et al. Presentation, diagnosis, and medical management of heart failure in children: Canadian Cardiovascular Society guidelines. Can J Cardiol. 2013;29(12):1535-52.
7. Working Group on Management of Congenital Heart Diseases in India. Consensus on timing of intervention for common congenital heart disease. Indian Pediatr. 2008;45(2):117-26.
8. Working Group on Management of Congenital Heart Diseases in India. Drug therapy of cardiac diseases in children (Saxena A, Ramakrishnan S, Tandon R, et al.). Indian Pediatr. 2009;46(4):310-38.
9. Mukhtar G, Sasidharan B, Krishnamoorthy KM, Kurup HKN, Gopalakrishnan A, Sasikumar D, et al. Clinical profile and outcomes of childhood dilated cardiomyopathy—A single center three-decade experience. Ann Pediatr Cardiol. 2023;16(3):175-81.

9.6 Cardiac Arrhythmias

S Srinivasan

INTRODUCTION

Cardiac arrhythmias refer to the occurrence of *irregularities in rate or rhythm or both heartbeats* due to disturbances, alterations, or dysfunction in cardiac electrical impulse generation, conduction, or excitability. Arrhythmias are often seen in hearts with abnormal conduction pathway structures or altered cardiac structural or pathological states compared to normal hearts during certain physiological states. They may occur in periodic or paroxysmal episodes or have continuous runs unless terminated by appropriate therapeutic interventions. When the heart rate slows down to <60/min, it is termed *bradycardia*, and when the same is >120/min, it is called *tachycardia*.[1]

The myocardial contraction is initiated by electrical impulses [action potentials due to phasic alteration in electrical voltage of membrane potential by the influx of ionic sodium (Na^+) and calcium (Ca^{++})], causing depolarization and efflux of potassium (K^+), resulting in repolarization generated in the sinoatrial (SA) node located at the junction of the superior vena cava and right atrium by a well-regulated sequence of electrically charged transmembrane ion exchanges through highly specialized channels. The SA node acts as an electrical impulse generator or pacemaker with its own intrinsic rate depending on the age of the child, controlled by the autonomic nervous system.

The impulses thus generated by the SA node pass through the internodal pathways in the atrium to the atrioventricular (AV) node and bundle of His, and then its right and left branches having specialized fibers for rapid transmission of electrical impulses on either side of the interventricular septum (IVS) to depolarize the atria and ventricles in sequence determined by the slower conductivity of the AV node. The right and left bundle branches terminate in millions of small Purkinje fibers projecting through the myocardium. The action potentials passing through the specialized internodal pathways in the atria depolarize the atrial myocytes. The respective right and left branches depolarize the myocytes of the corresponding right and left ventricles with the IVS. The cardiomyocytes contract by a process termed "excitation-contraction coupling."

If the sinus rate generated by the master pacemaker SA node slows down considerably, a shift in pacemaker activity occurs, and the AV node (nodal rhythm) or the myocytes of the ventricle (idioventricular rhythm) take over the function of impulse generation and propagation **(Table 9.6.1)**.

The SA node, consisting of specialized electrical impulse-generating cardiac fibers with few contractile myofibril elements and nerve terminals from the autonomic nervous system, has inherent automatic rhythmicity to generate regular electrical impulses to be conducted to the AV node, thus setting the pace for cardiac contractility to occur at a regular rate. Hence, it is also known as the primary pacemaker or generator of the heart.

The AV node is stimulated by the transmission of impulses at a specific rate per minute from the SA node and transmits them to the contractile elements, e.g., the myocardial fibers of the ventricles. The AV node is thus directed by the SA node to intensify and transmit or relay the electrical signals to the ventricular myocardium to contract at a specific rate. AV node functions mostly as a receiver and a pace transmitter or relay station and occasionally takes over as a pacesetter. The AV node is not influenced directly by the autonomic nervous system, unlike the SA node. It is governed by the SA node automaticity, rhythmicity, and conductivity.

If the SA nodal generated rate slows down considerably, a shift in pacemaker activity occurs, and the AV node (nodal rhythm) or the ventricle (idioventricular rhythm) takes over the function of impulse generation and propagation.

On the standard surface electrocardiogram (ECG) recording, the "P" wave in the PQRST represents the depolarization wave spreading from the SA node throughout the atrial musculature, causing atrial contraction ahead of ventricular depolarization and contraction. Its duration is usually 0.08–0.1 seconds. The atrial rate is calculated by determining the time interval between P waves. The brief isoelectric period after the P wave and before the inscription of QRS represents the travel time of electrical impulse within the AV node with decreased conduction velocity and the bundle of His.

TABLE 9.6.1: Cardiac cell types, their location, and their inherent electrical pacemaker potentials.

Pacemaker	*Location*	*Inherent rate (beats/min)*
Sinoatrial (SA) node	Right atrium (RA) at superior vena cava (SVC) junction	60–100
Atrioventricular (AV) node	RA at the posteroinferior area of the interatrial septum	40–60
Purkinje fibers	Throughout the ventricles	2–40
Ventricular cardiomyocytes	Throughout the ventricles	2–40

The *PR interval* duration, the distance between the onset of the P wave and the beginning of the QRS complex (normal duration: 0.12–0.20 seconds), is the time duration between the onset of atrial and ventricular depolarizations. A prolonged PR interval beyond the upper range of the normal for that age (>0.2 seconds) indicates a delay between the SA node and the AV node, termed *AV block*.

The *QRS complex* represents ventricular depolarization. The distance between two successive QRS complexes in a child with regular rhythm helps in arriving at the ventricular rate. When this time gets prolonged beyond the upper range of normal for that age (range: 0.06–0.1 seconds), it indicates slowed and impaired conduction within the ventricles occurring in bundle branch blocks or in situations where an abnormal ventricular focus acts as an abnormal ectopic pacemaker directing the rate of ventricular contractions.

The *ST segment*, the isoelectric segment that follows the QRS, is the time taken for ventricular depolarization. An elevated or depressed ST segment from the isoelectric line is of diagnostic importance in ischemic, hypoxic, or inflammatory insults to the ventricular myocardium and pericardium.

The *T wave* representing ventricular repolarization is longer in duration than its depolarization. It may be sometimes followed by a "U wave" representing the late phase of repolarization. When present, its prominence or inversion indicates abnormal physiological or pathological states affecting repolarization.

The *QT interval* is the average ventricular electrical action potential representing the total duration of ventricular depolarization and repolarization time (heart-rate-dependent range 0.2–0.4 seconds). Prolonged QT interval indicates an increased risk for the development of tachyarrhythmias, and hence, it is vital to accurately determine and interpret the duration of QT interval as normal, prolonged, or short. It is often expressed as "corrected QT interval (QTc)." Thus, heart rate-independent "QTc" is calculated by dividing the QT interval by the square root of the RR interval (interval between two successive ventricular depolarizations). Prolonged QTc interval is beyond 0.44 seconds.

SINUS RHYTHMS

Sinus Bradycardia and Sinus Tachycardia

Sinus bradycardia (heart rate less than what is mentioned in **Table 9.6.2** for that age) occurs in older children who are athletic. It also occurs following therapy with drugs, such as parasympathomimetic drugs or poisons; antisympathomimetic drugs, such as beta-blockers, digitalis, and verapamil; and pathological conditions, such as hypothyroidism, hypothermia, and raised intracranial pressure.

Sinus tachycardia (heart rate more than what is mentioned in **Table 9.6.2** for that age) occurs with sympathetic

TABLE 9.6.2: Approximate range of normal heart rate variability in neonates, infants, and children.

Age range	*Heart rate*	*Age range (years)*	*Heart rate*
Neonates	100–160	3–5	80–120
1–5 months	90–150	6–10	70–110
6–12 months	80–140	11–14	60–105
1–3 years	80–130	15–20	60–100

stimulation after exercise, fever, anxiety, anemia, pregnancy, heart failure, thyrotoxicosis, and administration of drugs that stimulate the sympathetic nervous system.

Sinus arrhythmia is a manifestation of normal automatic nervous activity with an increase in sinus heart rate during inspiration and a decrease during expiration. This is seen in young children.

TACHYARRHYTHMIAS

Supraventricular Tachycardia (Supraventricular Tachyarrhythmia, Paroxysmal Atrial Tachycardia, and Atrioventricular Nodal Reentrant Tachycardia)

Supraventricular tachyarrhythmia is the most common of the rapid rhythm abnormalities encountered in children, the greatest frequency being recorded in infancy. It is known to occur in fetus as early as in the middle fetal life.[2]

The two basic mechanisms of initiation of supraventricular tachycardia (SVT) are:[2]

1. Impulse generation abnormalities, e.g., increased automaticity resulting in ectopic impulse formation
2. Propagation abnormalities in ectopic impulse generated (re-entry loop or closed-circuit propagation), termed "reentrant tachycardia"

The sites in which these mechanisms operate determine the type of SVT:

- Re-entry of the electrical impulse back into the conducting system either through an accessory pathway (Wolff-Parkinson-White syndrome) or accessory pathway re-entry
- AV nodal re-entry
- AV junctional focus
- Ectopic localized atrial focus of enhanced automaticity

In AV reentrant tachycardia, retrograde conduction occurs from the ventricles back to the atrium by a concealed bypass tract.

In the absence of antegrade conduction by the bypass accessory pathway, re-entry through the AV node or through a concealed bypass tract is responsible for >90% of all SVTs. AV nodal reentrant tachycardia, being the most common of all SVTs, has no specific predisposing factors. It most often occurs in children who are otherwise normal. In infancy, it is more common in children below 6 months of age.

Symptoms

These children are often asymptomatic. In infants, if it persists for >24 hours, symptoms and signs of congestive heart failure (CHF) occur along with pallor, fatigue, and tachypnea. An older child may sense palpitation with sudden onset. Syncope and hypotension may be the presenting symptoms. Acute pulmonary edema can ensue.[1]

Supraventricular tachyarrhythmia occurring in the fetus, when prolonged, results in heart failure and nonimmune hydrops fetalis.

Diagnosis

The heart rate is regular and often ranges between 200/min and 320/min, and all impulses are conducted to the ventricles. The onset of the paroxysm is as sudden and abrupt as its termination.[2]

Whenever the heart rate in an infant is >200 beats/min (ranging up to 320 beats/min) and in a child >180 beats/min and often regular, and in the absence of possible causes for sinus tachycardia, SVT is strongly suspected and confirmed by immediate electrocardiographic examination. There may be symptoms or history suggestive of SVT either now or in the past.

The ECG shows marked tachycardia (>200/min) with regular narrow QRS complexes, and the P waves may be normal, absent, buried in the QRS complex, or appear as distortions at the terminal part of the QRS complexes. When QRS complexes become wider in the presence of an associated bundle branch block, it becomes difficult to differentiate from ventricular tachycardia (VT).

Treatment

In stable children with an abrupt, brief episode without symptoms:[3]

First step: Simple *vagal stimulation techniques or maneuvers*, such as carotid sinus massage, placement of ice water bags over the face, and then the child blowing through a closed straw, can effectively terminate SVT in the majority of cases. The progress must, however, be monitored by concurrent ECG recording.

Second step: Medical management—with unsuccessful vagal stimulation tactics, in a stable child with normal perfusion and with normal QRS < 0.08 seconds, immediate vascular access is established. Adenosine, with its short half-life, is the drug of choice for all ages.[4] Intravenous rapid bolus administration of 0.1 mg/kg of adenosine (maximum first dose of 6 mg and second dose of 12 mg) is resorted to. Verapamil is the next drug of choice and may be given to children above 1 year of age if adenosine is not readily available. Beta-blockers, disopyramide, and digitalis are less preferred alternatives, and digoxin is not helpful in acute cases.

Third step: Electroconversion or direct-current (DC) cardioversion—if administration of adenosine (two blouses) is not terminating the normal or narrow QRS complex SVT, electrical DC cardioversion (first dose: 0.5–1 J/kg, and second dose, if the first dose is ineffective: 2 J/kg) is performed with a trained pediatric team in an advanced life support system and resuscitation. Sedation before cardioversion is given to a conscious child.

Fourth step: Prevention of recurrences—further recurrences of SVT due to AV nodal re-entry are achieved by the use of drugs, such as digitalis, beta-blockers, or calcium channel blockers, which act primarily on the antegrade slow pathway.

- Temporary percutaneous venous, atrial, or ventricular pacing terminates the attack when drugs fail to do so or in recurrent cases
- Catheter radiofrequency ablation of the reentrant circuit is frequently being resorted to in refractory cases
- Cryoablation using cold energy is another recent, potentially safe, faster, and more effective method that is being increasingly employed and being evaluated
- Surgical ablation is rarely resorted to

Wolff–Parkinson–White Syndrome (Pre-excitation Syndrome)

An abnormal band of specialized electrically conductible atrial tissue acts as an accessory pathway bypassing the junctional tissue. This occurs in association with some congenital heart diseases and most commonly with Ebstein anomaly.

Wolff–Parkinson–White syndrome refers to antegrade conduction by the AV bypass tract resulting in a short PR interval, a slurred upstroke of the QRS complex termed a delta wave and a wide QRS complex. Differential conducting speeds of accessory and normal pathways with differing refractory periods cause the re-entry phenomenon to occur, resulting in paroxysmal SVT. Atrial flutter and atrial fibrillation also occur commonly in this condition. This, in turn, may lead to very rapid ventricular rates, even resulting in VT and ventricular fibrillation (VF) because of the lack of decremental conducting properties in the bypass tract as in the AV node.[1]

Supraventricular tachyarrhythmia is treated as mentioned earlier. Class 1A drugs (quinidine, procainamide, and disopyramide) or Class 1C drugs (flecainide) may be used to slow conduction and increase refractoriness primarily in the bypass tract. Flecainide is limited to use in an otherwise normal heart. Digitalis and verapamil can precipitate VF by shortening the refractory period of the bypass tract.

Radiofrequency ablation of an accessory pathway is another treatment option commonly used in patients with reentrant rhythm or atrial ectopic tachycardia. It is often used electively in children and teenagers, as well as in patients who require multiple agents, find drug side effects intolerable, or for whom arrhythmia control is poor. The overall initial success rate ranges approximately from 80% to 95%, depending on the location of the bypass tract. Surgical ablation of the bypass tract may also be successful in related patients **(Table 9.6.3)**.

ATRIAL TACHYARRHYTHMIAS

Atrial Ectopic Beats or Extrasystoles

Premature atrial beats are recognized by abnormally shaped premature "P" waves, followed by a near-normal PR interval with a normal QRS complex. Rarely, QRS complex may be aberrant. They may occur in normal newborns and disappear with age and do not cause symptoms. Multiple atrial premature beats may sometimes result in transient atrial fibrillation.[2]

Atrial Flutter

Atrial flutter is uncommon in children. In atrial flutter, the characteristic feature is a very rapid atrial activity (250–400 beats/min), with the ventricles responding to every second to fourth atrial beat, resulting in regular or regularly irregular tachycardia.[5]

Causes

It is rare in children and may be seen rarely in congenital heart diseases, resulting in a grossly enlarged atria, e.g., mitral or tricuspid insufficiency, atrial septal defects (ASDs), tricuspid atresia, Ebstein anomaly, acquired rheumatic mitral valvular heart disease, acute viral myocarditis, cardiomyopathy, pericarditis, hypertension, and intra-atrial surgery.[2]

Pathophysiology

An electrically active (irritable), abnormal focus in atria produces an abnormal impulse, which gets repeatedly propagated by a circus rhythm, resulting in an extremely rapid atrial rate. All of these rapid atrial beats cannot get transmitted through the AV node. Varying degrees of AV block result in anywhere from 2:1 to 8:1 atrial ventricular rate ratios.[5]

Symptoms

Symptoms depend upon the ventricular rate. No symptoms occur in atrial flutter with a reasonable ventricular rate. Prolonged episodes of atrial flutter with a very rapid ventricular rate precipitate left ventricular (LV) dysfunction

TABLE 9.6.3: Intravenous antiarrhythmic agents commonly employed in SVT, atrial, and ventricular tachyarrhythmias.

Drug (types of arrhythmia)	*Dosage*	*Comments*	*Monitoring*
Adenosine (SVT)	0.05 mg/kg through a central line; double the dose until effect is seen to a maximum of 0.4 mg/kg	Caution in asthmatics, contraindicated in preexisting types 2 and 3 AV block without pacemaker	
Verapamil (SVT)	0.05–0.2 mg/kg IV (maximum 5 mg) over 5–10 minutes	Contraindicated in children <12 months of age	For hypotension
Propranolol	0.05–0.15 mg/kg IV slowly every 5 minutes (maximum 0.3 mg/kg, 5 mg)	Contraindicated in children with asthma and congestive heart failure. Not to be given with verapamil	Pulse, BP
Esmolol (SVT, VT)	0.5 mg/kg bolus over 1 minute; maintenance: 50–300 µg/kg/min	Contraindicated in children with asthma, congestive heart failure, hypersensitivity, sick sinus syndrome, and second- and third-degree heart blocks	Pulse, BP
Procainamide (AF, AVN, and VT tachyarrhythmias)	10–20 mg/kg IV over 30–45 months; maintenance: 20–60 µg/kg/min	Continuous monitoring	Dizziness, hypotension
Lidocaine (VAs)	1–2 mg/kg IV over 15 months by continuous infusion: 30–50 µg/kg/min maintenance	Causes respiratory depression, hypotension	BP
Lignocaine (VAs)	1 mg/kg IV bolus 20–50 µg/kg/min IV		
Amiodarone (SVT, AAs, and VAs)	Ventricular fibrillation: 5 mg/kg IV load over 20 minutes, then 5–15 µg/kg/min (maximum 15 mg/kg/day) SVT: 5 mg/kg over 10 minutes × five doses	Safety and efficacy in pediatric patients have not been well established	
Phenytoin (VAs)	20 mg/kg over 30 minutes IV LD		

(AAs: atrial arrhythmias; AF: atrial fibrillation; AV: atrioventricular; AVN: atrioventricular node; BP: blood pressure; IV: intravenous; LD: loading dose; SVT: supraventricular tachycardia; VAs: ventricular arrhythmias; VT: ventricular tachycardia)

characterized by syncope, dyspnea, and other features of LV failure.

Diagnosis

The ECG is characteristic showing the rapid and regular atrial saw-toothed flutter "F" waves.

Treatment

Direct-current cardioversion is the most effective method of reverting to sinus rhythm. If the clinical status is stable, the ventricular rate is first slowed by the administration of AV node blocking drugs, such as beta-blockers, calcium channel antagonists (verapamil), or digitalis.

Once the ventricular rate is slowed, an attempt is made to convert the flutter into normal sinus rhythm by the use of Class 1A drugs (quinidine, procainamide, or disopyramide), Class 1C drugs (flecainide), or amiodarone. The same drugs also prevent recurrences of atrial flutter and fibrillation.[5]

Atrial Fibrillation

Atrial fibrillation is characterized by totally distorted, chaotic, rapid, and ineffective atrial contractions with an irregular and erratic ventricular response, resulting in the diagnostic "irregularly irregular" radial arterial pulse with a pulse deficit. It may be paroxysmal or persistent. Atrial fibrillation is extremely uncommon in neonates, infants, and young children.[1]

Causes

The causes mentioned in the preceding text in atrial flutter may also lead to atrial fibrillation. Chronic rheumatic heart disease with mitral valve disease with significant atrial dilatation in adolescents in tropical countries and chronic unoperated moderate-to-severe ASDs in older children may develop atrial fibrillation. In sick sinus syndrome, atrial fibrillation may occur in the tachycardiac phase.[5]

Symptoms

Symptoms occur with rapid ventricular rate—fatigue, palpitation, giddiness or syncope, symptoms of heart failure, and symptoms of systemic embolization in children with mitral valvular disease.

Diagnosis

The ECG is characteristic with no organized discernible "P" waves, except for irregular, fibrillatory "F" waves in the baseline with irregular but normal QRS complexes.

Treatment

The therapeutic goal is to immediately slow down the ventricular rate by using either beta-blockers (propranolol) or calcium channel antagonists (verapamil). Quinidine or other Class 1A drugs as mentioned above or Class 1C drugs, such as flecainide, may then correct the condition to sinus rhythm. If no response occurs within 24 hours, electrical DC conversion is resorted to. The causative factors have to be immediately attended. Anticoagulation 2 weeks prior and 2 weeks after any attempt at cardioversion is indicated to prevent the dreaded thromboembolic complications in situations where atrial fibrillation has been persistent for >48–72 hours.[4]

In exceptional circumstances of refractory atrial fibrillation, surgical or transvenous catheter radiofrequency ablation may be resorted to deliberately induce complete heart block (CHB) with simultaneous permanent pacemaker implantation.[5]

VENTRICULAR TACHYARRHYTHMIAS

Ventricular Tachycardia

Ventricular tachycardia is defined as a tachycardia arising below the bundle of His with at least three or more ectopic ventricular beats in sequence. Sustained VT means a run of ventricular premature contractions in succession for a period of 30 seconds or more. Nonsustained VT represents episodes <30 seconds.

Monomorphic VT has a regular rate and rhythm with the same QRS complex morphology.

Polymorphic VT has a variable rate and variable QRS morphology.

The mechanisms involved in VT are the same as mentioned above for the generation of SVT, e.g., ectopic automaticity of impulse generation, re-entry, and altered propagation in the ventricular myocardium.

Ventricular tachycardia, a potentially life-threatening arrhythmic condition in all age groups, is thankfully less common in children. It accounts for 6% of all childhood tachyarrhythmias. When it occurs, it indicates the presence of a serious underlying structural or functional cardiac problem. VT with pulses may cause high variability in heart rate, varying from normal to even 200 beats/min. It compromises stroke volume and hence the cardiac output. The prognosis is poor and carries a great risk of mortality unless corrected immediately.[2]

Causes

Electrolyte disturbances, such as hypokalemia, hypomagnesemia, severe acidosis, hypoxia, proarrhythmogenic drugs, myocarditis, ischemic myocardial damage, anomalous origin of the coronary artery, cardiomyopathy, mitral valve prolapse, prolonged QT interval (congenital or acquired), Wolff–Parkinson–White syndrome, cardiac tumors, and drug abuse with cocaine or amphetamine, are all known predisposing factors. In a significant number of children with VT, an underlying cause may not be found.

Symptoms

Symptoms vary depending upon the duration, type, and the underlying cause of initiating the VT, and these include dizziness, syncope, chest pain, palpitations, breathlessness, and cardiac arrest.

Diagnosis

Electrocardiography: VT must be differentiated from SVT, and the golden rule is that all wide QRS tachycardia should be considered and treated as VT until proved otherwise. The helpful electrocardiographic features in the diagnosis of VT are the wide or broad QRS complexes (prolonged QRS duration), usually unidentifiable P waves, and regular and fast ventricular beats, usually around 120 beats/min. Other features include T waves with opposite polarity to QRS, ventricular arrhythmias dissociation, capture fusion beats, extreme left axis deviation, and no response to carotid sinus massage, or intravenous administration of adenosine. The features that differentiate VT from SVT with wide QRS are the variation in RR intervals and the presence of fusion complexes.

Treatment

- *Acute management of VT:*[3]
    - In an "unstable" VT child, instantaneous synchronized cardioversion with 2 J/kg is the treatment of choice. The dose may be increased, if needed. It is mandatory to have an electric defibrillator in every emergency room, intensive care area, and all wards or in each floor of the hospital.
    - In a "stable" VT child, drug treatment with 5 mg/kg of amiodarone is administered intravenously over 30–60 minutes. The other drug that is employed is intravenous procainamide at a dose of 15 mg/kg over the same period.
- *Drugs:*
    - *Lignocaine:* If a defibrillator to deliver DC shock is not available or if VT is relatively well tolerated, a bolus dose of lignocaine (1 mg/kg) is intravenously administered with a continuing intravenous infusion at a rate of 10–50 mg/kg/min.
    - Bretylium is an alternative drug in lignocaine refractory cases. Mexiletine, flecainide, disopyramide, and amiodarone are suitable alternatives.
    - Phenytoin is effective in VT, especially when it occurs following the digitalis toxicity.

- *Treatment or elimination of the precipitating factors and prevention of recurrences:* All underlying precipitating factors must be identified and effectively treated or eliminated. Electrolyte disturbances, such as hypokalemia, hypomagnesemia, and others, such as drugs, have to be identified and immediately corrected or stopped. Myocardial tumor, anomalous origin of the coronary artery, and similar surgical problems are appropriately tackled.
- *Alternative treatment strategies:*
  - When the drug therapy fails to control or prevent recurrences, other modalities of treatment are contemplated and executed as mandated by the causative factors.
  - Implantation of automatic cardioverter, implantable defibrillator, or surgical resection of the diseased myocardial area

Ventricular Fibrillation

Ventricular fibrillation is a chaotic ventricular tachyarrhythmia with no effective ventricular contraction. The ECG record shows a wavy line without any discernible QRS complexes; P waves may be discernible.

Ventricular fibrillation may be a preterminal event in many conditions, disturbances, or diseases. Hypokalemia, digitalis or quinidine toxicity, myocardial inflammation or damage, catecholamines, aminophylline, anesthetic drugs, and plant toxins may precipitate VF. Uncontrolled VT, multifocal ventricular ectopic beats, or long QT interval syndromes may result in VF. If not terminated instantaneously, death ensues.

A thump in the chest may restore sinus rhythm. External cardiac massage with artificial ventilation and DC defibrillation are immediate measures to be undertaken. The precipitating factors are corrected without delay. After defibrillatory conversion to VT, VT is treated with drugs as mentioned above. Refractory cases are treated by an implantable automatic cardioverter–defibrillator.

BRADYARRHYTHMIAS

Sinus Arrest and Sinoatrial Block

Sinus arrest is failure of impulse formation within the SA node. *Sinoatrial arrest* refers to blockade of the generated sinus impulse from reaching the atrium. Though rare in children, these disturbances may occur secondary to digitalis toxicity and extensive atrial surgery.

Atrioventricular Block

Atrioventricular block occurs when interference occurs in the normal conduction of the electrical impulses from the atria to the ventricles through the AV node.[2]

First-degree Atrioventricular Block

Prolongation of *PR interval* beyond the *stipulated normal range for that age and heart rate* without conduction blockade of any of the atrial impulses to the ventricles is defined as *first-degree heart block*. No evidence of heart disease is seen in the majority of such cases. However, it may be seen in children with coronary heart disease, such as ASD, corrected transposition of the great vessels, Ebstein anomaly, primary myocardial disease, rheumatic carditis, and diphtheria and in children receiving drugs, such as digitalis and quinidine. Children with first-degree block are asymptomatic and need no treatment except for the treatment of the primary cause.

Second-degree Atrioventricular Block

Some of the atrial impulses are blocked and hence not conducted to the ventricles.

In *Mobitz type I (Wenckebach phenomenon)*, while the PP interval remains constant, a progressive increase in the PR interval occurs with successive beats until an atrial impulse seen as a P wave is not conducted to the ventricle (absent QRS complex). The PR interval is again shorter in the cycle following the dropped ventricular complex. It will then progressively increase to result in another blocked ventricular impulse.

In *Mobitz type II*, atrial conduction is blocked at constant intervals, e.g., once every three, four, or five beats with no change in the PR interval.

It is less often noticed in individuals with normal hearts. The same predisposing factors mentioned in first-degree AV block also play a role. No treatment is necessary. If Stokes–Adams syndrome occurs, although rare, pacemaker insertion is undertaken.

Complete or Type 3 (Third-degree) Atrioventricular Heart Block

Complete AV block refers to complete nonpropagation of SA nodal-generated electrical impulses to the AV nodes. There is total dissociation between the SA node and AV node, and the AV node starts generating its own electrical impulse at its inherent slow-paced rhythmicity with a rate ranging between 50/min and 100/min in neonates and infants and between 50/min and 60/min in older children and adults.

Idioventricular rhythm: Rarely when the AV node stops generating impulses or there is a failure of conduction in the bundle of His, the ventricular myocytes intrinsically generate their own action potential to be propagated to adjacent ones, causing the heart to beat at a rate of 20–40/min.

Congenital or Acquired Complete Atrioventricular Heart Block

Congenital CHB is a rare entity with a reported incidence of 1 in 20,000 live births.

Causes

Autoimmune injury of the fetal conduction tissue by immunoglobulin G antibodies transferred from the mother with active or inactive systemic lupus erythematosus is one of the well-known causes of this condition. The reported incidence of fetal CHB in women with anti-Ro/SSA (Sjögren's syndrome-related antigen A) *antibodies* is 1–5%, and in the cases of a previously affected child, it rises 6–25%. In neonates with lupus rash, the incidence of CHB may be as high as 20%. It is seen in association with congenitally corrected transposition of the great arteries.

Other autoimmune diseases, such as rheumatoid arthritis, are reported to cause congenital heart block. Myocarditis and postsurgical repair involving ventricles are other known causes of acquired CHB. In utero, it may result in hydrops fetalis. It may also result in fetal wastage. In some children, it may occur at 3–6 months of age.

Symptoms

Older children are asymptomatic. Syncope, fatigue, irritability, and night terrors may be some of the symptoms.

Diagnosis

Slow, bounding pulse <60/min not increasing by >10–20 beats/min after exercise or atropine administration; cannon A waves; and varying intensity of the S1 are clinically diagnostic of this condition. The ECG strip is diagnostic with regular P waves with the same PP interval but with varying PR intervals.

Prognosis

The prognosis of this condition is usually good. In symptomatic children with Stokes-Adams syndrome, the insertion of an artificial pacemaker is imperative to prevent sudden death. All cardiac depressants should be avoided.

Treatment

Isoproterenol, atropine, or epinephrine is temporarily employed.

Temporary transvenous ventricular pacing is often employed to increase the heart rate temporarily until pacemaker placement can be arranged.

Transthoracic epicardial pacemakers: The permanent measure is to go for permanent implantable epicardial pacemakers.

Indications for cardiac pacing:[5]

- Neonates with an extremely low ventricular rate below 50/min
- Associated with congenital cardiac malformations, such as cyanotic heart disease, single-ventricle physiology, complete AV septal defect, or significant AV valve disease
- The onset or the presence of symptoms and signs of low cardiac output or heart failure
- Life-threatening wide complex rhythms, such as prolonged QT interval, ventricular arrhythmia, or unstable escape rhythm

REFERENCES

1. Walsh EP, Saul JP, Triedman JK (Eds). Cardiac Arrhythmias in the Pediatric Patient. Philadelphia, PA: Lippincott Williams and Wilkins; 2001.
2. Sacchetti A, Moyer V, Baricella R, Cameron J, Moakes ME. Primary cardiac arrhythmias in children. Pediatr Emerg Care. 1999;15(2):95-7.
3. Ziegler VL, Gillette PC (Eds). Practical Management of Pediatric Cardiac Arrhythmias. New York: Futura Publishing Inc.; 2001.
4. Losek JD, Endom E, Dietrich A, Stewart G, Zempsky W, Smith K. Adenosine and pediatric supraventricular tachycardia in the emergency department: multicenter study and review. Ann Emerg Med. 1999;33(2):185-91.
5. Wolff G, Gelband H, Deal BJ. Arrhythmias in Infants and Children: Current Concepts in Diagnosis and Management of Atrial Arrhythmias in Infants and Children. New York, NY: Futura Publishing Inc.; 1998.

SECTION

Disorders of Respiratory System

Section Editor: Sushil K Kabra

10.1 Examination of the Respiratory System

TU Sukumaran

INTRODUCTION

Respiratory disorders are as common in children as it is in adults. A systematic history taking coupled with a physical examination is necessary for arriving at a diagnosis. In this chapter, the practical aspects of the examination of the respiratory system are discussed.

Physical examination consists of general assessment of the patient, vital signs, and examination of upper and lower respiratory tract.[1-3]

GENERAL ASSESSMENT

Look for Danger Signs

These include abnormal breathing patterns, altered sensorium, convulsions, cyanosis, inability to drink, sweating, hypotonia, repeated vomiting, dehydration, and paralysis. Altered sensorium and convulsions indicate hypoxemia.

Vital Signs

Tachypnea (Fast Breathing)

This usually occurs in pneumonia but can also occur in anxiety, asthma, collapsed lung cardiac failure, pulmonary edema, pneumothorax, and pleural effusion. The rate of breathing should be assessed by counting it for 1 minute; it should be repeated in case of any doubt. Rapid, shallow breathing denotes respiratory muscle paralysis. Metabolic acidosis of any etiology is characterized by an increased rate and depth of breathing.

Tachycardia

Sinus tachycardia may be a manifestation of respiratory tract infection. Anxiety, cardiac failure, respiratory failure, and simultaneous intake of sympathomimetic drugs should also be considered.

Temperature

Fever indicates upper (sinusitis, otitis media, tonsillopharyngitis, and mastoiditis) as well as lower respiratory tract infection. Common causes for high fever in lower respiratory illness are pneumonia, empyema, lung abscess, and bronchiectasis. Low-grade fever occurs in mycoplasma infections.

Blood Pressure

Blood pressure should always be recorded. Hypertension and pulsus paradoxus indicate serious respiratory impairment.

EXAMINATION OF THE RESPIRATORY SYSTEM[1-3]

- *Apnea,* which is cessation of breathing for >20 seconds, is associated with bradycardia or neurologic impairment. A duration of <20 seconds, which is associated with pallor, limpness, cyanosis, or convulsions, should be a cause for alarm.
- *Cheyne-stokes* breathing is characterized by rhythmic waxing and waning of the depth of respiration, with regularly recurring periods of apnea. It is seen in congestive heart failure and raised intracranial pressure with cerebral cortical impairment.
- *Biot's breathing* also called ataxic respiration is characterized by irregular periods of apnea, alternating with periods of four or five breaths of identical depth, and indicates severe brain stem damage.
- *Kussmaul breathing* is rapid deep breathing of metabolic acidosis.
- *Gasping or jaw breathing* is of slow rate with rapid inspiration, prominent jaw movement, and slow expiration. It indicates severe hypoxia due to any cause.

Work of Breathing

This includes flaring of alae nasi, head nodding (sternomastoid and scalene overactivity), and chest retractions (intercostals, subcostal, suprasternal, and infrasternal).

Chest and Abdominal Movements

Observe the chest movements from the side in supine and standing positions to confirm that both sides are moving equally and to assess the relative contributions of chest and abdomen. In normal inspirations, the lower chest flares out and the abdomen moves forward by the actions of the lower intercostal muscles and diaphragm, respectively. When the intercostals are paralyzed, as in spinal muscular atrophy, inspiration causes the lower chest to be drawn inward by the diaphragm, and the outward movement of the abdominal wall is prominent. Such movements can occur also in upper airway occlusion and are caused by the violent action of the diaphragm. The reverse movement is seen in diaphragm weakness, in which the abdomen is drawn inward during inspiration (paradoxical breathing). In unilateral phrenic nerve paralysis, the abdomen is drawn in on the paralyzed side during inspiration but is normal (i.e., moves out) on the nonparalyzed side.

Cyanosis in respiratory diseases indicates a serious degree of hypoxia and can be identified by the hyperoxia test. Associated circulatory failure or underlying cardiac lesions should be ruled out.

Clubbing in respiratory diseases is seen early in cystic fibrosis, bronchiectasis (of at least 1 year duration) lung abscess, empyema, and malignancies.

Indicators of Serious Chronic Respiratory Illness

These include persistent fever, limitation of physical activity, chronic purulent sputum, cyanosis, clubbing, persistent tachypnea, labored breathing, growth retardation, persistent chest hyperinflation, and a family history of heritable lung diseases.

EXAMINATION OF THE UPPER RESPIRATORY TRACT[1-3]

Use a bright torch to examine the nose, ears, and throat.

Signs of Allergic Problems

People with allergic rhinitis frequently develop a transverse nasal crease resulting from repeated rubbing of the nose to relieve the itching (Darier's line). Another feature of nasobronchial allergy is dark circles under the eyes (allergic shiners).

Changes in the Anatomical Structures

The nasal passages may be narrow, as in midface hypoplasia associated with various syndromes. Congenital abnormalities, like a deviated nasal septum, should be looked for. Extensive nasal polyps cause widening of the nasal bridge. Signs, such as the presence of ulceration, crusting, purulent or a blood-stained discharge, presence of foreign bodies, trauma, and tumors (vascular and nonvascular) should be noted.

Examination of Sinuses

Sinus tenderness can be elicited over the affected sinus.

Examination of the Ears

The ears should be examined for congenital anomalies, infections, foreign bodies, and impacted wax. Gently move the pinna and tragus; tragal pain suggests otitis externa. Examine the mastoids and retroauricular areas for eczema, tenderness, and lymph node enlargement. For better visualization of the external ear canal and tympanic membrane, pull the pinna up, and posteriorly with the thumb and index finger.

Otoscopic evaluation is a must for patients with fever of unknown or known origin, as well as those with ear symptoms. In the latter situation, the healthy side should be evaluated first. The otoscope should have a strong light and the speculum should be of the largest size that can fit comfortably into the ear canal. Gently place the otoscope over the external auditory meatus and inspect the external ear canal. Carefully advance it to observe the tympanic membrane. Absence of the normal light reflex, dull appearance, bulging, retraction, perforation, and so on should be noted.

Examination of the Throat

The tonsils should be examined for size (hypoplastic in X-linked agammaglobulinemia, enlarged in infections and tumors), congestion, follicles, or membranes. Other symptoms of pharyngeal infection are redness and mottling over the soft palate and uvula. In a retropharyngeal abscess, the neck is hyperextended, and respiration becomes noisy with gurgling sounds and pooling of secretions. In lateral pharyngeal abscess, the features are torticollis toward the same side, trismus, and bulging in of the lateral pharyngeal wall. Peritonsillar abscess also is characterized by trismus and torticollis. Adenoidal tissue hypertrophy on the posterior pharyngeal wall may reveal cobble stoning.

The integrity of the palate should be investigated by palpation to exclude a submucous cleft. A bifid uvula is a clue to an occult submucous cleft palate.

EXAMINATION OF THE LOWER RESPIRATORY TRACT[1-3]

Neck

The important aspects to be assessed in relation to the respiratory tract are the trachea, neck vein, and the presence of surgical emphysema.

Trachea

This is inspected and palpated for deviation (in the standing or sitting position), with the examiner facing the patient. Tracheal deviation causes the clavicular head of the sternomastoid muscle on that side to appear prominent (*Trail sign*). In severe respiratory distress, "tracheal tug" (i.e., pulling in of the trachea) occurs because of the vigorous contraction of the diaphragm pulling down the mediastinum. Gently palpate the trachea with the middle finger at the suprasternal notch. Should there be massive pleural effusion, pneumothorax, and large intrathoracic cysts and tumors, the trachea will shift to the opposite side. It is pulled to the same side in upper lobe collapse, fibrosis, and pleural adhesions.

Signs of Superior Mediastinal Obstruction

Signs of superior mediastinal obstruction are edema of the head and neck, cyanosis, proptosis, Horner syndrome, and distended nonpulsatile neck veins. The common cause is mediastinal mass, notably because of a lymphoma.

Examination of the Chest

Inspection

This should be performed with the chest as maximally exposed as the custom permits, with the eyes at the level of the chest, from head and foot ends, and from front and lateral aspects. Evaluate the overall shape and appearance of the chest. Assess the shoulders for drooping (indicates painful conditions of the chest wall on the same side, pleurisy, pneumonia, collapse, and fibrosis), position of the cardiac apical impulse, and precordial shape. The anteroposterior diameter of the chest is increased in hyperinflation. A localized bulge indicates parietal wall inflammatory swellings, hematoma, or tumors. In pleural effusion or pneumothorax, intercostal spaces (ICS) appear bulging. Look for chest movements. Localized paucity of movements occurs in trauma and in painful conditions of the chest wall and pleura, pleural effusion, pneumothorax, pneumonia, collapse, and tumors of the lung.

Palpation

This includes measurement of the expansion of the chest at the level of the nipples after deep inspiration and expiration. Expansion of identical sides of the chest should be assessed. Chest movements are assessed over supraclavicular, upper interscapular, and lower interscapular areas from the back, and infraclavicular and inframammary areas from the front. To do this, encircle the chest from both sides with four fingers and palm, with the thumbs meeting in the midline but not touching the chest wall. On inspiration, if one thumb remains closer to the midline, it indicates reduced chest movements on that side. Tactile vocal fremitus is compared for spoken words over identical areas on both sides of the chest with the medial margin of the right palm.

Percussion

The examiner should master the technique of percussion to feel, rather than hear, the normal and abnormal lung resonance. The patient should be in a comfortable position, i.e., sitting or lying down. The left middle finger (the pleximeter) is placed parallel to the long axis over the area to be percussed; back of the middle phalanx of the pleximeter finger is struck, as a tapping movement arising from the wrist. The plexor finger should immediately be raised after the tap. The terminal phalanx of the plexor finger should be at right angles to the metacarpal bone and the pleximeter finger while the blow is delivered. Proceed down the intercostal space (ICS) in mammary line, with each blow being compared with that on the other side. The upper border of liver dullness reaches the fifth ICS on the right side in the mammary line and will shift to one space lower down on deep inspiration (tidal percussion). On the left side, the normal resonance is replaced by the tympanitic note of the stomach at the same level. The cardiac dullness should be verified on the left side and will be more resonant in emphysema. To percuss the lateral side of chest, patients' limbs should be raised above the shoulders with the hands resting over the vertex—one over the other. Each ICS is percussed and compared with the opposite side, with the examiner standing or sitting on the side to be percussed. The normal resonance on the right side is replaced by liver dullness in the seventh space in the midaxillary line and on the left side by the tympanitic note of the stomach almost at the same level.

Percussion of the back should start from the supraclavicular area, i.e., from the medial to the lateral side, the pleximeter finger being placed across the area with the tip directed forward. A band of lung resonance that normally presents in the central area (Kronig isthmus) will be replaced by a dull note in massive pleural effusion, consolidation, neoplasia, or collapse of the apical part of lung. Subsequently, the upper and lower interscapular and the infrascapular spaces should be percussed. The normal resonance is replaced by the dullness at the 9th and 10th ICS in the infrascapular area on the right (liver) and left side (spleen), respectively.

Resonance is the normal feel and sound caused by air being set into vibration. Lung resonance is increased in airway obstruction and pneumothorax; in the latter situation, it reaches up to a tympanitic note. Localized obstruction occurs in congenital lobar emphysema or in partial obstruction by a foreign body in the bronchus (check valve or ball valve). Overall, hyperinflation occurs in obstructive airway disease, as in asthma pushing down the liver dullness. Percussion note is impaired or dull when the lung becomes more solid (pneumonia, consolidation, collapse, fibrosis, sequestration, abscess, and infarction), or the pleura becomes thickened or contains fluid (pleural effusion, empyema, and hemothorax) or solid (mesothelioma). A feel of resistance below the pleximeter finger is perceived in pleural effusion, as if percussed against a wall, and is described as a "stony dullness."

In hydropneumothorax, a *shifting dullness* can be identified by percussing the chest (from anterior to posterior) in the supine, lying position of the patient. As the fluid shifts to the posterior part of the chest in the lying position, the dull lower chest (in the sitting position) becomes resonant anteriorly and a definite level below which there is complete dullness can be demonstrated.

Auscultatory Percussion

It is helpful to detect mediastinal masses. The patient sits with arms resting on both thighs while the examiner sits facing the patient. With the tip of the terminal phalanx of the middle finger of the dominant side, light percussion is directly applied over the sternum from the center to either side, while the note is auscultated from behind over the corresponding areas. The area of impaired resonance reveals the size of the mediastinal mass.

Auscultation

Developing an expertise in interpreting auscultatory findings is an experimental process, and as such, there is no substitute for the experience of having listened to a large number of patients, both with and without lung disease. Follow a consistent pattern for auscultation to avoid missing any area. Start from the infraclavicular area and proceed to mammary, inframammary, axillary, and infra-axillary areas, each time comparing with the opposite side. Segmental auscultation is the technique of comparing breath sounds of homologous segments. The examiner should sit facing the patient when auscultating the anterior aspect of the chest. The lateral side of the chest can be auscultated from front as well as from behind the patient. Posteriorly, auscultation is performed in the same way as in the order of percussion, with the examiner sitting behind the child.

The parameters to be assessed are the breath sounds, added sounds, and vocal resonance. Assess the intensity and quality of the breath sounds. Intensity may be normal (when the lung tissue is inflating normally), reduced, or increased. It is reduced in airway obstruction, lung damage, pleural thickness, effusion, and pneumothorax. The normal breath sounds are vesicular. The inspiration is loud and high-pitched followed by harsh low-pitched expiration (without a pause in between), which is of short duration, i.e., almost up to half of inspiration. The cycle is followed by a pause. In bronchovesicular breathing, the expiration is prolonged up to or more than the inspiration, and there is no pause in between. This is typical of asthma.

Bronchial breathing is louder in intensity. Expiration is high-pitched, loud, and prolonged (equal to or more than the duration of inspiration). There is a pause in between. The normal vesicular breathing is replaced by bronchial breathing when the lung becomes more solid (as in consolidation, collapse consolidation, fibrosis, abscess lung, massive pleural effusion, and neoplastic growth) or contains a cavity. In these situations, the sounds generated in large airways are transmitted more efficiently and resemble those obtained by listening over the trachea. Adventitious sounds are wheezes, crackles, pleural rub, mediastinal crunch, peristaltic sounds, and crepitus.

Wheezes arise from narrowed intrathoracic airways. Monophonic wheeze is due to localized narrowing of a single bronchus, as in foreign body aspiration or bronchial adenoma. Widespread polyphonic wheezes (of differing intensity), usually heard in expiration, indicate diffuse airway obstruction as in asthma.

Crackles or crepitations are short bubbling or crackling noises arising from large airways with secretions (coarse), or from small airways (fine), and from alveoli containing exudates (fine). These sounds are produced by sudden changes in gas pressure from the rapid opening of previously closed small airways or alveoli. Crackles are heard in obstructive airway disease, pneumonia, and pulmonary edema. Localized loud and coarse crackles may indicate bronchiectasis.

The added sounds should be differentiated from conducted sounds from the throat and pharynx. Conducted sounds disappear after suction and changes in position and are heard with equal intensity over equidistant parts of the chest and better by auscultation in front of the mouth and neck.

Pleural rub has a rubbing, superficial, leathery character, and is heard during an identical phase of inspiration and expiration; unlike crackles, it does not change after coughing. The intensity increases as the chest piece is pressed firmly, it can be felt also with the palpating hand.

Mediastinal crunch (Hamman's sign) is heard in emphysema and left-sided pneumothorax. A crunching sound will be heard over the left sternal border during a systole.

Peristaltic sounds are gurgling sounds occasionally heard over the lower part of the left side. Frequent peristaltic sounds with other clinical evidences indicate diaphragmatic hernia.

In addition to peristaltic and diaphragmatic sounds, crepitus sounds may occur over the region of a broken rib or surgical emphysema. Additional false sounds arise by the movement of the stethoscope on the patient's skin and should be differentiated from the symptomatic sounds.

Vocal resonance is the sound perceived by the chest piece, as the voice is transmitted through the lungs. The child is auscultated while saying one or his name in the same order of auscultation, and both sides are compared. The intensity of resonance will be decreased in airway obstruction, collapse, pleural effusion, or pneumothorax (except when bronchial breathing is present). Intensity is increased over consolidation, cavity, infraction, and collapse consolidation. If the patient is asked to whisper the same words, they will be heard clearly in the examiners ears (*whispering pectoriloquy*) in massive consolidation and bronchopleural fistula **(Table 10.1.1)**.

TABLE 10.1.1: Salient features of common lower respiratory diseases in children.

Parameter	*Acute asthma*	*Consolidation*	*Collapse*	*Pleural effusion*	*Pneumothorax*
Respiratory rate	↑	↑	↑↑	↑↑	↑↑↑
Chest in-drawing	+++ Overall	++ Spares affected region	++ Spares affected region	++ Spares affected region	++ Spares affected region
Chest expansion	Overall reduction	Reduced over affected area	Reduced over affected area	Reduced over affected area	Reduced over affected area
Tracheal and mediastinal shift	Nil	Nil	Toward the affected side	Toward the opposite side	Toward the opposite side
Lung resonance	Hyper-resonant, liver dullness pushed down	Dull over affected area	Dull over affected area	Stony dullness over affected area	Tympanitic over affected area
Breath sound intensity	N/↓	↑	↓/– over affected area	↓/– over affected area	↓/– over affected area
Breath sound quality	Bronchovesicular	Bronchial	Vesicular/bronchial	Vesicular	Vesicular
Vocal resonance	Normal	↑↑	↓↓	Imperceptible	Imperceptible

REFERENCES

1. Empey D. The respiratory system. In: Swash M (Ed). Hutchison's Clinical Methods, 10th edition. London: WB Saunders and Company Ltd; 1995. pp. 60-8.
2. Kuruvilla VJ, Thulasi Prasad K. Clinical Evaluation of Newborns, Infants and Children, 2nd edition. New Delhi: Jaypee Brothers Medical Publishers; 2009. pp. 112-20.
3. Silverman M, Callaghan CL. Practical Pediatric Respiratory Medicine, 1st edition. New Delhi: Viva Books (P) Ltd.; 2005.

10.2 Diagnostic Procedures and Investigations in Respiratory Diseases

D Vijayasekaran

INTRODUCTION

Respiratory diseases are a major cause of mortality and morbidity in children. Methodical, detailed history taking, and clinical examination help to arrive at provisional diagnosis but to confirm, investigations are required. Children with chronic lung problems require many investigations and common investigations and procedures in those situations are discussed in the following text **(Table 10.2.1)**.

HEMATOLOGICAL INVESTIGATIONS

Complete Blood Count

Complete blood count (CBC) includes measurement of parameters such as white blood cells (WBCs), hemoglobin (Hb), platelet, and red blood cells (RBCs) which gives information about the underlying infection and inflammation. Leukocytosis (WBC >16,000/μL) and leukopenia (WBC <4,000/μL) may suggest infection. It is important to consider age-specific normal ranges. Lymphocytosis suggests viral infection and pertussis, and increased atypical lymphocytes may suggest infectious mononucleosis.

Acute Phase Markers

C-reactive protein (CRP) increases with infections, both viral and bacterial. It is useful in monitoring the disease. *Procalcitonin* (PCT) raises much earlier (4–12 hours) than CRP (24–38 hours) and is used as prognostic marker in bacterial infection. Raised *erythrocyte sedimentation rate* (ESR) suggests chronic infection and inflammatory disorders.

TABLE 10.2.1: Investigations and procedures in respiratory diseases.	
Hematological • Complete blood count (CBC) • Erythrocyte sedimentation rate (ESR) • C-reactive protein (CRP) • Procalcitonin (PCT)	*Pulmonary function tests* • Spirometry • Peak expiratory flow rate (PEFR)
Imaging studies • X-ray chest • Chest ultrasonography • Computed tomography (CT) • Magnetic resonance imaging (MRI) • Barium studies • Fluoroscopy	*Monitoring* • Arterial blood gas analysis • Pulse oximetry • Polysomnography
Skin tests • Tuberculin skin test • Skin prick test	*Endoscopy* • Flexible bronchoscopy • Bronchoalveolar lavage (BAL) • Laryngoscopy
Microbiological tests and specimens • Smear microscopy • Gastric lavage • Induced sputum • Solid and liquid culture for TB • Nucleic acid amplification test	*Miscellaneous* • Thoracentesis • Intercostal chest drainage • Sweat chloride

SKIN TESTS

Tuberculin Skin Test

In tuberculin skin test (TST) (*Mantoux test*) 1 or 2 tuberculin unit of purified protein derivative (PPD) with Tween 80 is injected intradermally and the reaction read between 48 and 72 hours. The test is considered positive if the induration is 10 mm or more which denotes tuberculosis (TB) infection and not the TB disease.

Interferon-gamma Release Assays

Interferon-gamma release assays (IGRA) uses selective antigens namely early secretion antigen target (ESAT 6) and culture filtrate protein 10 (CFP 10), and thus it is not affected by prior BCG and infection due to nontuberculous mycobacteria. IGRA also detects TB infection only and not the TB disease, similar to TST.

QuantiFERON-TB Gold In-Tube (QFT-IT) might be used in children over 2 years of age investigated for recent immigration/adoption screening and in cases of recent low risk TB contact.[1] Both TST and QFT-IT tests are recommended in cases of strong clinical suspicion or high-risk TB contact in children <5 years of age, to avoid misdiagnosis.

Skin Prick Test and Immunoassays

Type I hypersensitivity reaction is the basis of atopic (allergic) diseases with immunoglobulin E (IgE) release. It runs in families which include atopic dermatitis (occur first), food allergy, asthma, and allergic rhinitis; and the diagnosis is always clinical and tests support the diagnosis. Skin prick test is a manual test (in vivo test) considered as more sensitive with a greater selection of antigens.

Immunoassays are blood tests (in vitro test) which measure the specific IgE to a suspected allergen. Serum IgE >100 IU/mL before age 6 years and a four-fold increase of value for the age (increases during childhood and reaches adult values by 10 years (380 IU/mL) is a nonspecific test for allergy.

IMAGING STUDIES

Chest Radiography

Chest X-ray (CXR) is considered as an extension of clinical examination.[2] The standard chest radiograph is the posteroanterior view (PA), but in younger children, anteroposterior view (AP) is taken for convenience. CXR delineates only four densities namely air, fluid, soft tissue, and bone density, further delineation and minute details can be possible only with computed tomography (CT) scan.

CXR is very useful in the diagnosis of common lung problems such as:

- Pneumonia (consolidation without any shift or volume loss)
- Collapse (triangular shadow with ipsilateral shift and volume loss)
- Pleural fluid (opacity without any bronchovascular markings with contralateral shift)
- Lung abscess (cavity with air fluid level) **(Figs. 10.2.1A to D)**.

Normal mediastinum is such that it occupies one-third on the right and two-thirds on the left of midline. Conditions which push the mediastinum are pleural fluid, pneumothorax, emphysema, and space occupying lesion. Conditions which pull the mediastinum are collapse, hypoplasia, fibrosis, and pleural thickening.

The CXR gives the two-dimensional representation of a three-dimensional structure so while interpretation, the lesions should be specified to three zones. Upper zone extends from apex to lower border of anterior end of second costal cartilage, middle zone extends from the above line to lower border of fourth costal cartilage, and lower zone (from lower border of fourth costal cartilage to the bases of the lungs).

Barium Studies

Barium swallow is used in the evaluation of gastroesophageal reflux, achalasia, and hiatus hernia. Modified barium swallow (videofluoroscopic swallowing study) gives better information about the swallowing evaluations.

Barium meal gives information about stomach and upper gut and helps in the evaluation of malabsorption syndromes.

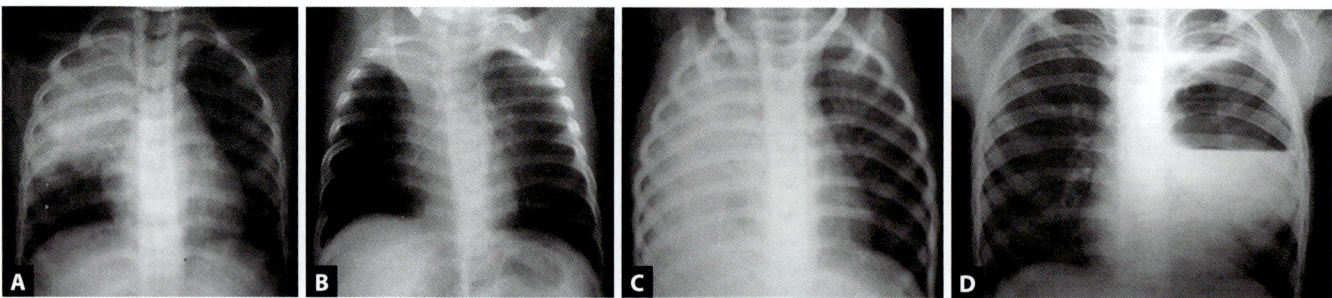

Figs. 10.2.1A to D: Chest X-ray showing four important lung lesions. (A) Pneumonia right upper zone; (B) Collapse right upper zone; (C) Pleural fluid right; and (D) Lung abscess left.

Barium follow-through gives information about the lower gut, helps in the evaluation of abdominal TB, and ileocecal problems.

Chest Ultrasonography

Chest ultrasonography (USG) is an imaging test that uses high-frequency sound waves to look at the organs.[3] Prenatal USG plays an important role in the early diagnosis of congenital lung lesions such as congenital pulmonary airway malformation (CPAM), pulmonary sequestration, congenital lobar emphysema (CLE), diaphragmatic hernia, and pleural diseases.

Computed Tomography

Computed tomography provides more information than the plain chest radiograph because of its higher resolution, cross-sectional perspective, and three-dimensional reconstructions.

Multidetector CT (MDCT) a breakthrough in CT technology uses multiple parallel rows of X-ray detectors (range from 16 to 64) and each of the rows records data independently as the gantry rotates (when the X-ray tube and X-ray detectors rotate together in a fixed geometrical orientation) thereby providing better image quality with improved spatial resolution.

Magnetic Resonance Imaging

Magnetic resonance imaging (MRI) uses magnetic properties of atoms and radio waves. Since it does not use ionizing radiation, it is safer than CT. MRI is more useful in differentiating the soft tissue shadows particularly in the evaluation of mediastinum and vessels.

MICROBIOLOGICAL TESTS AND SAMPLES

The positivity of microbiological tests depends upon good samples (specimens). The common samples used in microbiological tests are gastric lavage, induced sputum and bronchoalveolar lavage (BAL).

Gastric lavage (GL) is done in the early morning in children below 6 years who are unable to expectorate the sputum. Ambulatory GL procedure done after 4–6 hours of fasting.

Induced sputum (IS) give higher bacteriological yield in which the child is nebulized with 3% hypertonic saline to induce sputum and secretions are collected from the throat or nasopharynx. Spontaneous sputum can be collected from older children and adolescents. Sputum specimens with epithelial cells of >10 per high-power field are unsuitable because of high contamination with upper respiratory flora.

Smear Microscopy and Culture

Smear microscopy for TB bacilli with *Ziehl–Neelsen stain* is positive only if the number of bacilli is >10,000 per mL of specimen. Of late, smear positive specimens are used in linc probe assay to detect drug resistance for anti-TB drugs.

Since conventional solid *TB culture* done with Löwenstein–Jensen media takes about 8 to 12 weeks for TB detection, liquid cultures are widely used.

Mycobacteria growth indicator tube (MGIT) is an automated liquid culture system that exploits the fluorescence of an oxygen sensor to detect growth of mycobacteria in culture. The growing mycobacteria depletes oxygen which is indicated by oxygen sensitive fluorescence and the results are available by 4 weeks.

Nucleic Acid Amplification Test

Nucleic acid amplification test (NAAT) is a rapid molecular test that detects TB and rifampicin drug sensitivity, based on real-time polymerase chain reaction (PCR). Cartridge-based NAAT (CBNAAT) are available commercially as GeneXpert or Xpert MTB/RIF which detects presence of DNA of TB bacilli and rifampicin resistance in <4 hours.

Ultra Xpert MTB/RIF is the recent advance in (CBNAAT) with increased sensitivity which detects TB with minimum of 16 bacilli/mL as against GeneXpert which requires about 131 bacilli/mL and also detects few silent mutations.

TrueNat a battery-operated rapid PCR test developed in India that can be carried to the field and is a promising test especially in high-burden countries.[4]

PULMONARY FUNCTION TESTS

Spirometry Test

Spirometry by measuring lung volume and flow rates detects physiological problems of lung and broadly differentiates lung diseases into obstructive and restrictive diseases but does not give any information about the etiology.

Spirometry measures the *forced vital capacity* (FVC) and indices such as *forced expiratory volume* in one second (FEV_1), the ratio of FEV1 with FVC (FEV_1/FVC), forced expiratory flow (FEF) 25–75% of FVC (FEF 25–75%) are derived from FVC by the machine **(Figs. 10.2.2A to C)**.

Achieving a good FVC curve is the most important aspect of spirometry. The child should take a deep breath to full inhalation followed by a brief hold and then a sustained exhalation and to make the curve plateau with maximum effort to produce a good curve (flow volume curve or loop). With adequate coaching many above 6 years can do the test.

Spirometry helps to differentiate obstructive and restrictive lung diseases.[5] FVC is diminished in both obstructive and restrictive diseases. FEV_1 is decreased in obstructive diseases. FEV_1 /FVC ratio may be normal or even increased in restrictive diseases.

Peak Expiratory Flow Rate

Peak flow meter records peak expiratory flow rate (PEFR) which is the greatest flow obtained on forced expiration after full inspiration. PEFR is effort dependent and measures mostly large airway function. It plays a major role in monitoring asthma therapy (correlates with FEV_1) and sudden fall may be an indicator of an impending asthma attack.

MONITORING

Arterial Blood Gas Analysis

Arterial blood gas (ABG) analysis reveals oxygenation status, adequacy of ventilation, and acid–base balance. Many serious acid–base disturbances can coexist without significant clinical manifestations.[6]

The radial artery at the wrist is the most preferred site of ABG specimen collection as it has adequate collaterals. Heparinized syringe with 22-gauge needle should be held like a pen with a 45° angle (with the beveled edge of the tip facing downward) and the artery should be punctured just 2 cm above the wrist crease, the sample should be analyzed immediately.

While reading ABG, four parameters such as pH, HCO_3, $PaCO_2$, and partial pressure of oxygen (PaO_2) are important. The normal pH of our body is 7.4 (range 7.35–7.45) which depends upon the levels of $PaCO_2$ and HCO_3 and their disturbance results in four simple acid–base disorders namely metabolic acidosis (↓ HCO_3), metabolic alkalosis (↑ HCO_3), respiratory acidosis (↑ $PaCO_2$), and respiratory alkalosis (↓ $PaCO_2$) or mixed disorders.

Metabolic acidosis (↓ HCO_3) results due to loss of HCO_3 from the body (severe diarrhea, renal tubular acidosis) or due to the addition of acids (lactic acid accumulation after shock and asphyxia, keto acid accumulation after diabetes mellitus). The above two types of metabolic acidosis are differentiated by anion gap calculation.

Metabolic alkalosis (↑ HCO_3) results due to loss of acids (H^+ ions) from the gastrointestinal (GI) tract (e.g., vomiting) or through renal mechanisms (e.g., Bartter syndrome, rapid correction with HCO_3).

Respiratory alkalosis occurs in mild respiratory disorders due to hypoxemia following CO_2 washout (↓ $PaCO_2$).

Respiratory acidosis occurs in severe respiratory diseases and neuromuscular dysfunction due to carbon dioxide retention (↑ $PaCO_2$).

The normal PaO_2 is 80–100 mm Hg which depends upon the inspired O_2 concentration (FiO_2). When fraction of the inspired O_2 (FiO_2) concentration increases the arterial PaO_2 increases by five times ($PaO_2 = FiO_2 \times 5$).

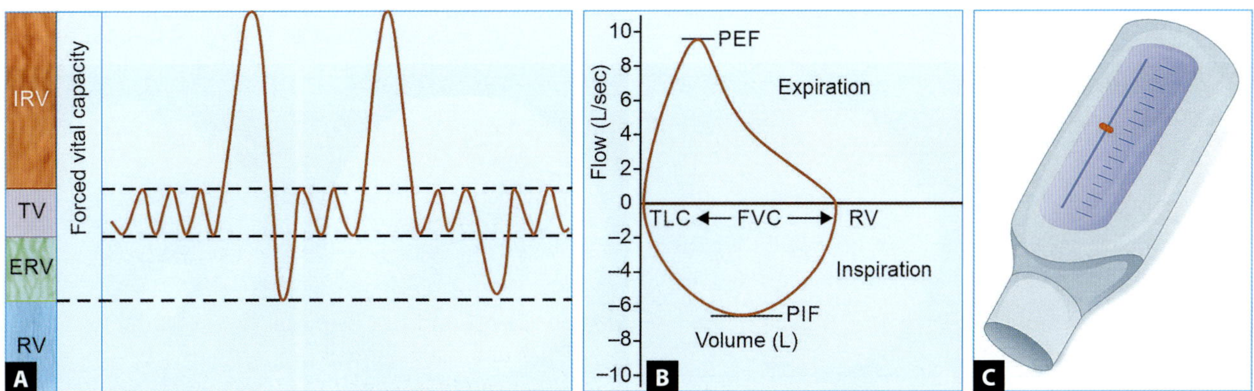

Figs. 10.2.2A to C: Spirometry recordings of: (A) Lung volumes; (B) Flow volume loop; and (C) Peak expiratory flow meter.

Pulse oximetry is a noninvasive method which denotes how much hemoglobin is saturated with oxygen (SaO_2), measures light wavelengths of oxygenated hemoglobin to deoxygenated hemoglobin. Nail polish, low cardiac output, and hypothermia may impair the value.

Polysomnography

Polysomnography is the gold standard test for the diagnosis of obstructive sleep apnea (OSA); and is used to assess apnea (A), hypopnea (H), desaturation/h, and total sleep time. Apnea-hypopnea index (AHI) >1 episode/h suggests the diagnosis of OSA; 2–5 episodes mild OSAS and >5 episodes moderate-to-severe OSA.

ENDOSCOPY

Flexible Bronchoscopy

Flexible bronchoscopy (FBS) is an important diagnostic technique, done under conscious sedation. The diagnostic and therapeutic indications are increasing after the advent of smaller size and video bronchoscopes **(Table 10.2.2)**.

After application of lignocaine gel into the nostril, lignocaine solution (1%) is instilled through the suction channel of bronchoscope as "spray and proceed technique." Dynamic lesions such as vocal cord pathology, laryngomalacia, tracheomalacia, and foreign body are better identified with flexible bronchoscopy (**Figs. 10.2.3A to D**).

TABLE 10.2.2: Flexible bronchoscopy–indications.

Diagnostic	*Therapeutic*
• Persistent pneumonia, atelectasis • Prolonged stridor and wheezing • Suspected foreign body • Endobronchial tuberculosis • Suspected airway anomaly • Evaluation of hemoptysis • Bronchoalveolar lavage	• Removal of mucous plug/ bronchial cast • Removal of retained secretions • Drug instillation • Bronchoscopy-guided endotracheal intubation • Endobronchial biopsy • Tracheostomy evaluation

Bronchoalveolar Lavage

Bronchoalveolar lavage is a diagnostic procedure that allows the recovery of both cellular and noncellular components from the epithelial lining of the alveolar and bronchial airspaces and considered as the "liquid biopsy of the lung."[7] After wedging the scope into the desired subsegmental bronchus, BAL is performed by instilling 3 mL/kg of normal saline (divided into three equal fractions).

The BAL is helpful in diagnosis of pulmonary hemorrhage (by detecting hemosiderin laden macrophages with Perls, stain or Prussian blue stain), lipoid pneumonia (by detecting lipid laden macrophages with Oil Red O stain), alveolar proteinosis (milky, with Periodic Acid Schiff stain), pulmonary eosinophilia (eosinophils >25%) and to detect infections such as *Mycobacterium tuberculosis, Aspergillus* species (Galactomannan), and *Pneumocystis jirovecii.*

INVASIVE PROCEDURES

Thoracentesis

Thoracentesis also known as thoracocentesis or pleural tap is done to diagnose pleural fluid [preferably ultrasonography (USG) guided]. Nature of the fluid and biochemistry may be useful to differentiate transudate versus exudate **(Table 10.2.3)** which decides the further management. Exudate fluid warrants surgical intervention like intercostal chest tube drainage or video-assisted thoracoscopic surgery.

Intercostal Chest Tube Drainage

Intercostal chest tube drainage (ICD) is the procedure to remove pus from the pleural cavity by inserting a chest tube. Insertion of a chest tube is done at the lower aspect of fifth intercostal space at the mid-axillary line (avoid injury to neuromuscular bundle which runs on the lower margin of ribs). The movement of air column in the ICD tube denotes whether it is functioning; if not it should be adjusted. When the drainages reduce to 50 mL/day, ICD can be removed after ensuring other parameters such as absence of fever and the general wellbeing.

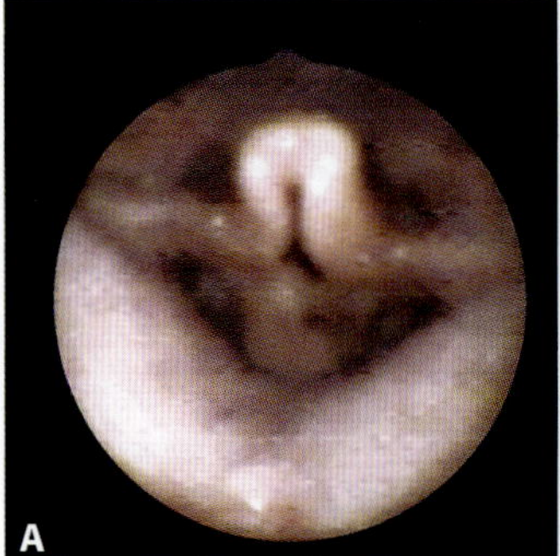

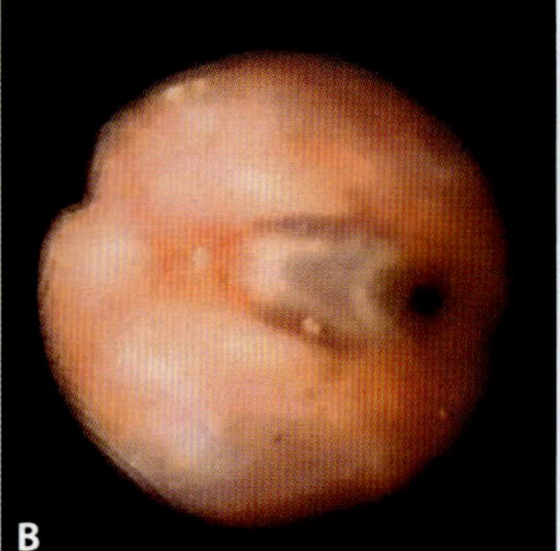

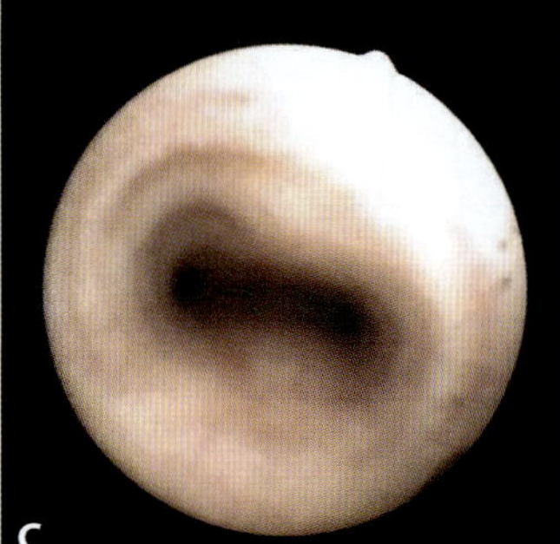

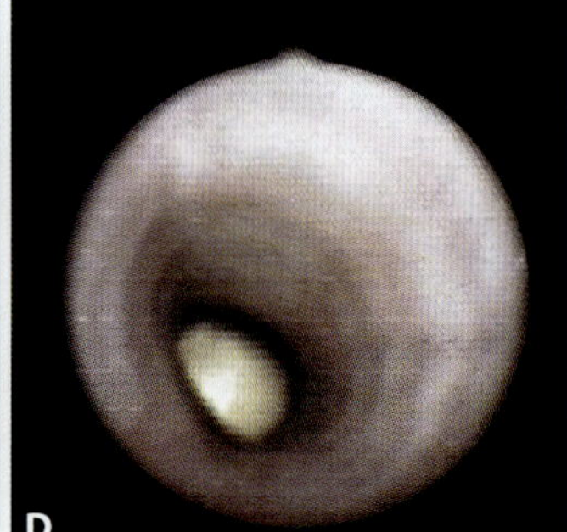

Figs. 10.2.3A to D: Bronchoscopic view of (A) Laryngomalacia; (B) Laryngeal web; (C) Tracheomalacia; and (D) Central foreign body.

TABLE 10.2.3: Distinguishing features between transudate and exudate.

	Transudate	*Exudate*
Appearance/color	Clear	Turbid, pus, straw
Protein	<3 g/dL	>3 g/dL
Lactate dehydrogenase (LDH)	<200 IU/L	>200 IU/L
pH	>7.2	<7.2
Glucose	>40 mg/dL	<40 mg/dL
Pleural fluid/ serum protein	<0.5	>0.5
Pleural fluid/ serum LDH	<0.6	>0.6
Cause	• Congestive cardiac failure • Nephrotic syndrome • Cirrhosis • Hypoproteinemia	• Complicated parapneumonic effusion • Empyema
Pathophysiology	Occurs due to ↑ hydrostatic or ↓ oncotic pressure	Occurs due to inflammation or infiltration of pleura

SWEAT CHLORIDE

Cystic fibrosis (CF) is an autosomal recessive disease due to mutational defect of *CF* gene in the long arm of chromosome (7qI3) resulting in defective chloride transport, diagnosed by elevated chloride in the sweat (>60 mEq/L), done by pilocarpine iontophoresis technique. In the normal sweat gland, chloride is absorbed out of the sweat as the sweat travels from the gland to the skin surface but in CF it is hindered and when the sweat reaches the skin surface it has higher chloride concentrations.

CONCLUSION

It is the clinical history and thorough examination that make a major part of the diagnosis. Since newer investigations are getting added day by day, while planning for investigation parents of the affected child should be counseled properly and the most appropriate investigation with minimal expenditure should be considered.

REFERENCES

1. Chiappini E, Storelli F, Tersigni C, Venturini E, de Martino M, Galli L. QuantiFERON-TB Gold In-Tube test performance in a large pediatric population investigated for suspected tuberculosis infection. Paediatr Respir Rev. 2019;32:36-47.
2. Parekh M, Balasubramanya R. Chest and mediastinal imaging. In: StatPearls [Internet]. Treasure Island (FL): StatPearls Publishing; 2023.
3. Quercia M, Panza R, Calderoni G, Di Mauro A, Laforgia N. Lung ultrasound: A new tool in the management of congenital lung malformation. Am J Perinatol. 2019;36(S 02):S99-S105.
4. Singh UB, Singh M, Sharma S, Mahajan N, Bala K, Srivastav A, et al. Expedited diagnosis of pediatric tuberculosis using Truenat MTB-Rif Dx and GeneXpert MTB/RIF. Sci Rep. 2023;28;13(1):6976.
5. Boonjindasup W, Chang AB, McElrea MS, Yerkovich ST, Marchant JM. Does the routine use of spirometry improve clinical outcomes in children? A systematic review. Pediatr Pulmonol. 2022;57(10):2390-7.
6. Sekaran DV, Subramanyam L, Balachandran A. Arterial blood gas analysis in clinical practice - Personal practice. Indian Pediatr. 2001;38(10):1116-28.
7. Vijayasekaran D. Bronchoalveolar lavage. In: D Vijayasekaran (Ed). Pediatric Respiratory Medicine - The judicious application of investigations including bronchoscopy, 3rd edition. Chennai; Kural Publications. 2019. pp.150-5.

10.3 Upper Respiratory Tract Infections

Sushil K Kabra

INTRODUCTION

Acute respiratory infections are the major causes of morbidity and mortality in children and of particular significance in the developing countries, such as India. Outpatient attendance attributed to acute respiratory infections is as high as 20–40% of all outpatients and 12–35% of inpatients. The overall incidence of acute respiratory infection in the children under the age of 5 years may be between 3 and 8 episodes/child/year. Majority of these are due to upper respiratory tract infections (URTIs).

Upper respiratory tract infection is an umbrella term that includes infection of nasal cavity, throat, nasopharynx, ears, and sinuses. They are common causes of morbidity in children.

ACUTE NASOPHARYNGITIS

Infection of nasopharynx is also called common cold. It is probably the most common infection in children. In young children, three to eight episodes of common cold may occur in a year.

Etiology

Acute nasopharyngitis is caused by viruses. The common viruses include rhinovirus and corona viruses. The other viruses include adenoviruses, influenza, parainfluenza, or respiratory syncytial viruses.[1] These are spread by droplet infection. Predisposing factors include chilling, sudden exposure to cold air, and overcrowding. Rhinitis could also be due to allergy.

Clinical Features

Clinical features of common cold are due to congestion, swelling, and increased secretion of nasopharyngeal mucosa. Clinical manifestations are more distressing in infants and young children. The common manifestations include nasal discharge (initially watery followed by thick white to yellowish), nasal block, cough, and conjunctival congestion. Nasal block causes difficulty in feeding, irritability, excessive crying, and mouth breathing. Occasionally, it may be complicated by secondary bacterial sinusitis and otitis media. Otitis media should be suspected in a child with no relief in crying, even after treatment for nasal block. If a course of common cold is prolonged beyond 7–10 days, sinusitis should be considered in a school-going child.

Treatment

Acute nasopharyngitis is usually caused by virus, and is self-limiting, and requires no specific treatment. For fever, paracetamol can be given every 4–6 hours. For nasal block, normal saline can be instilled in nostrils every 4–6 hours, especially before feeds. The child may be given plenty of warm liquids to drink. There is no role of antibiotics, antihistamines, local decongestive drops, or steroids. Home remedies for cough and cold, such as *tulsi*, ginger, or honey, may be beneficial in common cold. However, the mother should be told to bring the child to hospital immediately, if there is rapid respiration, lower chest in drawing, poor feeding, or persistent vomiting.

ACUTE PHARYNGITIS

Acute pharyngitis includes infection of pharynx and tonsils. This is also called acute tonsillopharyngitis. Most of the times, it is associated with rhinitis, sinusitis, and occasionally laryngitis.

Etiology

This is commonly caused by viruses, such as rhinovirus, coronavirus, influenza, parainfluenza, and adenoviruses.[1]

About 10–20% of sore throats are caused by bacteria. The most important bacterial pathogen is group A beta-hemolytic *Streptococcus*. Rarely, *Corynebacterium diphtheriae* may present with acute pharyngitis.

Clinical Features

Children with acute pharyngitis may have fever, sore throat, pain during deglutition, nasal discharge, conjunctival congestion, and discomfort in throat. There may be enlargement of tonsils and soreness in throat. Sore throat may lead to dysphagia and drooling of saliva. Cervical lymph nodes may be enlarged and tender. Examination may reveal grayish-white pseudomembrane specifically in infection with *diphtheria* and Epstein–Barr virus. Infection due to group A *Streptococcus* may show pus points over tonsillar surface, palate, or pharyngeal wall.

Viral pharyngitis is self-limiting and recovers in 5–7 days. Pharyngitis caused by group A beta-hemolytic *Streptococcus* may lead to suppurative complications, such as retropharyngeal and peritonsillar abscesses. Presence of these complications may be indicated by high-grade fever, severe dysphagia, and bulge in the posterior wall of pharynx or around tonsils. The nonsuppurative complications due to streptococcal pharyngitis include acute rheumatic fever and acute glomerulonephritis. These complications can be prevented by administration of antibiotics.

It is very difficult to differentiate viral from bacterial pharyngitis. Presence of exudates/pus points on pharynx with enlarged tender cervical nodes and absence of nasal discharge suggests bacterial pharyngitis.

Diagnosis

Acute pharyngitis is a clinical diagnosis. At times, it is very difficult to differentiate nasopharyngitis from pharyngitis. Diagnosis of streptococcal pharyngitis can be made with presence of exudates, enlarged tonsils, and absence of nasal discharge. The diagnosis can be confirmed by throat swab culture. Now, a rapid diagnostic test based on latex agglutination is also available for diagnosis of streptococcal pharyngitis and can be carried out in office practice. A polymerase chain reaction-based test (multiplex PCR) on nasopharyngeal swab/aspirate can identify multiple pathogens including viruses and bacteria. However, its utility in clinical practice remains doubtful.[2]

Treatment

The major consideration in treatment of acute pharyngitis is to prevent acute rheumatic fever. If a clinical diagnosis of streptococcal pharyngitis is made, a throat swab should be taken, or rapid diagnostic test performed to demonstrate streptococci, and penicillin should be administered.

Penicillin can be given orally or by intramuscular route. The duration of oral penicillin is for 10–14 days. If compliance is a problem, a single injection of long-acting (benzathine) penicillin can be given. No significant difference has been found in the efficacy of different antibiotics.[3] The other alternative antibiotics are ampicillin, amoxicillin, or oral cephalosporins. If an individual is sensitive to penicillin, he/she may be treated with one of the macrolide antibiotics, such as erythromycin, roxithromycin, clarithromycin, or azithromycin.

ACUTE SUPPURATIVE OTITIS MEDIA

Acute suppurative otitis media (ASOM) is a common cause of morbidity in children specifically infants and young children. It is defined as inflammation of mucoperiosteal lining of the middle ear. If the duration of illness is more than 2 weeks, it is termed as *chronic suppurative otitis media (CSOM)*. Children are more prone for ASOM because the eustachian tubes communicating throat with ears are straight and short. Acute suppurative otitis media may be one of the complications of other respiratory infections.

Etiology

Acute suppurative otitis media in children is commonly caused by *Streptococcus pneumoniae, Haemophilus influenzae*, and *Moraxella catarrhalis*. Very rarely, it may be caused by *Staphylococcus* and gram-negative organisms. The latter is more common in immunocompromised hosts.

Clinical Features

Acute suppurative otitis media presents with fever, ear pain, ear discharge, and restlessness. In young children, this is a common cause of excessive crying. Once the tympanic membrane perforates, the child may get relief in pain but could develop pus discharge from ear. Acute suppurative otitis media may cause infection of mastoids in older children. The intracranial extension may lead to pyogenic brain abscess. Sometimes, ASOM may cause lower motor neuron facial palsy. Children may develop middle-ear effusion even after treatment with antibiotics; it is self-limiting and resolve in majority in a 12-week time. If it persists, these children should be sent to otolaryngologists for consideration of grommet insertion. Chronic middle-ear effusion may lead to hearing impairment.

Diagnosis

In a setting of URTI, if a child is crying excessively, his/her ears should be examined by otoscope. Eardrum may be inflamed and bulging with loss of normal anatomy with fluid in middle ear. Otoscopic examination should be part of routine examination in young children, presenting with fever without localization.

Treatment

Acute suppurative otitis media is a bacterial infection and should be treated with antibiotics. The antibacterial useful in ASOM includes ampicillin, amoxicillin, oral cephalosporins, or macrolide. Children below 2 years of age may be treated with antibiotics from the time of diagnosis. However, children above 2 years of age with mild disease may be treated with analgesics and for 2–3 days for improvement in clinical symptoms without antibiotics. In severe disease as indicated by presence of high fever (explosive onset, severe otalgia, and toxic appearance and high-grade fever more than 102°F) and children with mild disease in beginning but deterioration in 48–72 hours, one should consider starting antibiotics. The antibiotic of choice is amoxicillin. The antibiotics continued for 10 days to prevent recurrence and development of chronicity. If the child is not improving by 3–4 days, an alternative antibiotic, such as injectable third-generation cephalosporin or amoxicillin-clavulanic acid combination, may be started. In severe cases, injectable third-generation cephalosporin (cefotaxime or ceftriaxone) may be started.

For relief from pain, paracetamol or one of the nonsteroidal anti-inflammatory drugs, i.e., ibuprofen, may be given round the clock. Occasionally, tympanocentesis may be required to relieve pain. There is no role of local antibiotic drugs in ASOM.

For treatment of chronic otitis media, it is recommended to keep the ears dry by cotton wick. A course of oral antibiotics sometimes may be useful.

ACUTE SINUSITIS

In children, ethmoid and maxillary sinuses are present in infancy. Sphenoid sinuses are well developed by 3–5 years, and frontal sinus develops between 6 and 11 years of age. Infection of sinuses is common and associated with nasopharyngitis and pharyngitis.

Etiology

Commonly, the viruses causing pharyngitis and nasopharyngitis are responsible for sinusitis. Sometimes, they may be invaded by bacterial pathogens. The common bacterial pathogens include *S. pneumoniae, H. influenzae*, and *M. catarrhalis*. Gram-negative bacteria and fungi may invade paranasal sinuses in immunocompromised patients.

Clinical Features

Common presentation of sinusitis includes non-resolving rhinitis or common cold even after 7 days, thick purulent nasal discharge, fever, and tenderness over sinuses. In young infants, there may be swelling around the eyes. There may be headache—unilateral, bilateral, temporal, or occipital depending on sinus involvement.

Diagnosis

Usually, prolonged course of nasopharyngitis in the form of persistence of fever and nasal discharge could be due to sinusitis. If tenderness over sinuses can be demonstrated or periorbital puffiness is present in young children, a clinical diagnosis of sinusitis can be made. It can be confirmed by demonstrating opacity or mucosal thickening or fluid level in paranasal sinuses on X-ray films. Other imaging modalities, such as computed tomography or magnetic resonance imaging scan of sinuses, may be done in immunocompromised host or complicated cases.

Treatment

The clinical significance of sinusitis is due to bacterial invasion. A course of amoxicillin, ampicillin, or oral cephalosporin should be given to the child.[4] The supportive care includes normal saline in nostrils and paracetamol for fever and pain relief. There is no role of routine administration of antihistamines.

REFERENCES

1. Kumar P, Medigeshi GR, Mishra VS, Islam M, Randev S, Mukherjee A, et al. Etiology of Acute Respiratory Infections in Infants: A Prospective Birth Cohort Study. Pediatr Infect Dis J. 2017;36(1):25-30.
2. Bharaj P, Sullender WM, Kabra SK, Mani K, Cherian J, Tyagi V, et al. Respiratory viral infections detected by multiplex PCR among pediatric patients with lower respiratory tract infections seen at an urban hospital in Delhi from 2005 to 2007. Virol J. 2009;6:89.
3. Hedin K, Thorning S, van Driel ML. Different antibiotic treatments for group A streptococcal pharyngitis. Cochrane Database Syst Rev. 2023;11(11):CD004406.
4. Savage TJ, Kronman MP, Sreedhara SK, Lee SB, Oduol T, Huybrechts KF. Treatment Failure and Adverse Events After Amoxicillin-Clavulanate vs Amoxicillin for Pediatric Acute Sinusitis. JAMA. 2023;330(11):1064-73.

10.4 Croup

Deepak Ugra

INTRODUCTION

Croup is the most common infectious cause of upper respiratory obstruction amongst children, from 6 months to 6 years of age with the peak incidence at around 2 years of age. It is an acute and infectious process and is also termed as acute laryngotracheitis or laryngotracheobronchitis. It affects boys more often than girls. Traditionally, spasmodic croup and recurrent croup are considered as separate diagnoses, but many believe that they are a part of the spectrum of a single disease.

Croup occurs most commonly in winter but can occur throughout the year. Recurrences are frequent from 3 years to 6 years of age and decrease with age. Approximately 15% of patients have a strong family history of croup. Most children with croup have an uncomplicated course, managed with symptomatic treatment, and have complete recovery. <7% of children with croup require hospitalization and among those hospitalized only 1–2% require intensive care.[1] Mortality rate in croup is usually <0.5% even for intubated.

ETIOLOGY AND PATHOGENESIS

The parainfluenza viruses (types 1, 2, and 3) account for 75% of cases; other viruses associated with croup include influenza A and B, adenovirus, rhinovirus, respiratory syncytial virus, and measles.[1] Influenza A has been associated with severe laryngotracheobronchitis. Rarely, *Mycoplasma pneumoniae* has been isolated from children with croup.

Viral infection of the upper airway causes inflammation of pharynx, larynx, trachea, and bronchi. The subglottic inflammation compromises the airway in croup.

CLINICAL FEATURES

The diagnosis of croup is usually clinical. It presents with barking cough, hoarse voice and high-pitched inspiratory stridor, and respiratory distress. These symptoms usually follow a prodrome of mild fever, rhinorrhea, and sore throat for 2–3 days. The symptoms are characteristically worse at night. Occasionally, there may be wheezing. Immunity to viral infection is transient and repeat infections are common; however, in older children, symptoms are less severe.

The disease can be of varying severity from mild to severe. In most children, the illness is mild. The child appears happy, playful, and feeds well. The stridor appears on coughing and crying. There may be mild respiratory distress.

In moderate illness, the stridor is audible at rest and get worse on crying. Tachypnea, respiratory distress, and sometimes tachycardia are present. The child may be irritable but is alert and comforted by parents.

In severe cases, the child appears tired and exhausted due to labored breathing, has significant tachypnea and tachycardia, and is restless and agitated. Some of the children may have altered sensorium, hypotonia, cyanosis, and marked pallor due to severe airway obstruction and resultant hypoxia.

INVESTIGATIONS

Croup is a clinical diagnosis and does not require any investigation. Radiographs are used only if diagnosis is uncertain. The X-ray of the neck may show the typical subglottic narrowing or steeple sign on the posteroanterior view **(Fig. 10.4.1)**.[2] However, the steeple sign may be absent in patients with croup. Radiograph does not reflect the severity of airway obstruction. X-ray lateral view of neck may help in diagnosis of retropharyngeal abscess and epiglottitis. Throat swab culture and antigen test may help identifying bacterial organism responsible for upper respiratory infection other than croup.

DIFFERENTIAL DIAGNOSIS

The differential diagnosis includes conditions that cause obstruction in the region of larynx:[3]

- *Epiglottitis:* It is very rare in India.
- *Laryngeal foreign body:* Sudden onset of choking and coughing without prodromal signs of infection.

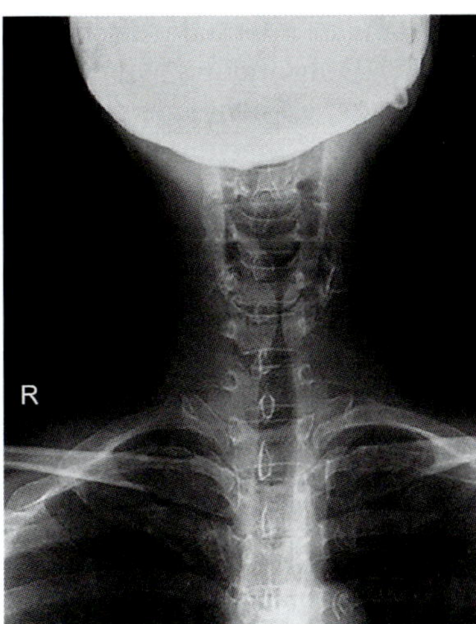

Fig. 10.4.1: Radiograph of an airway of a child with croup, showing typical subglottic narrowing (steeple sign).

- *Acute angioedema:* Usually, presents with swelling of the face and neck and other manifestations of allergic reactions.
- *Retropharyngeal and peritonsillar abscess:* A peritonsillar abscess is often a clinical diagnosis, whereas radiograph or computed tomography scan of upper airway helps in diagnosis of retropharyngeal abscess.
- *Bacterial tracheitis:* Although it is very rare, it is important differential diagnosis as it may have fulminant course and needs antibiotic.
- *Laryngeal diphtheria:* Early symptoms of diphtheria include malaise, sore throat, anorexia, and low-grade fever. Within 2–3 days, a typical gray-white membrane on tonsils and/or soft palate is seen on pharyngeal examination. The membrane is adherent to the tissue, and forcible attempts to remove it cause bleeding.
- *Measles croup:* It almost always has full manifestations of systemic disease and the course may be fulminant.
- *Bronchial asthma:* A croupy cough may be an early sign of asthma.
- *Subglottic stenosis:* It presents from early infancy and is not associated with prodromal symptoms.

TREATMENT

Children with mild croup do not need any specific treatment. They need minimal handling. They should be nursed with parents and should not be examined very often. They adopt the posture of maximum comfort; we should not change the posture forcibly. Intravenous access should be deferred.

Steam inhalation at home or saline nebulization in a clinic is often not effective in humidifying the airway and may not provide symptomatic relief.[4] Children with moderate-to-severe croup need definitive therapy **(Table 10.4.1)**. The components of definitive therapy are:

- Oxygen
- Corticosteroids
- Nebulized adrenaline
- Intubation.

Oxygen

Oxygen is the most important component of the definitive therapy of moderate-to-severe croup. Humidified oxygen is given to children with significant upper airway obstruction and SpO_2 <92%. Oxygen should be administered in a nonthreatening manner to maintain oxygen saturation (SpO_2) >95%.[5]

CORTICOSTEROIDS

Steroids are useful in moderate-to-severe croup. Nebulized budesonide 2 mg 12 hourly for up to 48 hours shows improvement in croup symptoms. The onset of action is seen

TABLE 10.4.1: Evaluation and management of children with croup.

	Croup severity (Westley score)		
	Mild (≤2)	***Moderate (3–7)***	***Severe (≥8)***
	Barking cough, hoarseness; no stridor, no or minimal chest wall retractions at rest	Stridor and chest wall retractions at rest, no agitation	Stridor, sternal contractions at rest, accompanied by agitation or fatigue
Therapy			
Decongestants, cough suppressants, antibiotics	Not recommended	Not recommended	Not recommended
Humidification	Not proven beneficial	Not effective	Not effective
Corticosteroids	Dexamethasone (0.6 mg/kg, one dose PO)	Dexamethasone (0.6 mg/kg, one dose PO or IM)	Dexamethasone (0.6 mg/kg, one dose PO or IM)
Nebulized epinephrine	Not recommended	Not recommended	Nebulized racemic epinephrine (2.25%), 0.5 mL in 2.5 mL of saline or L-epinephrine (1:1,000 dilution in normal saline with maximum volume 5 mL)
Disposition	Discharge to home	Discharge to home if no stridor, no retractions at rest. If no improvement in 4 hours, consider hospitalization	• Observe 2 hours • *Good response:* No recurrence, no stridor, and no retractions at rest. Discharge to home possible. • *Poor response:* Stridor, retractions at rest after two epinephrine doses • Hospitalize

(IM: intramuscular)

Source: Mandell GL: Douglas and Bennett's Principles and Practice of Infectious Disease, 5th edition. Philadelphia, PA: Churchill Livingstone; 2005.

within 30 minutes. Oral prednisolone (1–2 mg/kg) and oral or intramuscular dexamethasone (0.6 mg/kg—maximum 8 mg) are equally efficacious.[6] Steroids therapy causes significant decrease in the need for nebulized adrenaline, need and duration of intubation, and average stay in hospital.

Nebulized Adrenaline

It should be given immediately to children with severe croup. The doses are 0.5 mL/kg of body weight of 1:1,000 dilutions to a maximum of 5 mL. The onset of action is seen within 30 minutes and the effect lasts for about 2 hours. In case of persistent stridor, the dose can be repeated every 2–4 hours.

Intubation

Children with signs of impending respiratory failure should be intubated for a better control on airway. An endotracheal tube of 0.5 mm smaller than expected for the child's size is selected. Intubation is maintained till an air leak develops to a maximum of 5 days.

Discharge from the Hospital

The child who is given adrenaline nebulization can be discharged if he is stridor free at rest 4 hours after the dose, and the one who is given oral steroids is stridor free at rest posthalf an hour after the dose.

Reporting Back to the Hospital

Parents should be instructed to report back to the hospital in case stridor at rest reappears, irrespective of what treatment was given to the child.

OUTCOME

Croup is a common infectious condition amongst small children. Most children have mild symptoms and are treated at home and the illness resolves in 3–4 days. It is observed that if the child's symptoms are minimal at discharge, return within 24 hours is unlikely. Only about 5% of children discharged from the emergency department after corticosteroid therapy need to return because of worsening of symptoms. Intubation is rarely required.[7] In Canada, of all children with croup, about 4% have been estimated to require hospitalization, and intubation was required for only 1 of the 170 hospitalized children or 1 in 4,500 of all children with croup.[8]

REFERENCES

1. Sizar O, Carr B. Croup. In: StatPearls [Internet]. Treasure Island (Fl): StatPearls Publishing; 2024 Jan. 2023 Jul 24.
2. Marchessault V. Historical review of croup. Can J Infect Dis. 2001;12(6):337-9.
3. Rodrigues K, Roosevelt G. Acute inflammatory upper airway obstruction (croup, epiglottitis, laryngitis, and bacterial tracheitis). In: Kligeman R, St Geme III J (Eds). Nelson Textbook of Pediatrics, 21st edition. Philadelphia: Elsevier; 2020. pp. 2202-5.

4. Scarborough A, Scarborough O, Abdi H, Atkins J. Steam inhalation: More harm than good? Perspective from a UK burns centre. Burns. 2021;47(3):721-7.
5. Narayanan S, Funkhouser E. Inpatient hospitalizations for croup. Hosp Pediatr. 2014;4(2):88-92.
6. Shenoi RP, Timm N; Committee on Drugs; Committee om Pediatric Emergency Medicine. Drugs used to treat pediatric emergencies. Pediatrics. 2020;145(1):e20193450.
7. Rosychuk RJ, Klassen TP, Metes D, Voaklander DC, Senthilselvan A, Rowe BH. Croup presentations to emergency departments in Alberta, Canada: a large population-based study. Pediatr Pulmonol. 2010;45(1):83-91.
8. Wilmott RW, Deterding RR, Li A, Ratjen F, Sly P, Zar H, et al. Kendig's Disorders of the Respiratory Tract in Children, 9th edition. Amsterdam, Netherlands: Elsevier; 2019. pp. 406-12.

10.5 Pneumonia

Rohit C Agrawal

INTRODUCTION

Pneumonia probably is one of the oldest diseases, as old as antiquity known to humankind and has always remained a subject of challenge to medical science, despite extensive research. Pneumonia is number one cause of under-five childhood mortality across the globe, particularly in developing countries. Unfortunately, over the years the mortality remained almost the same, and hence, it has also been called as "forgotten killer" or "silent killer".

EPIDEMIOLOGY

Approximately 150 million episodes of childhood pneumonia are reported every year from the world, out of which 90% are from developing countries. A total of 15 countries account for nearly 75%, and 6 countries including India account for 50% cases. India alone bears the brunt of 20% pneumonia disease burden.

According to Million Death Study, out of the 6 million under-five childhood mortality world over (in 2019), pneumonia is 14%, i.e., 840,000 deaths are due to pneumonia (around 2,000 every day). This includes approximate 200,000 newborns. >90% of the deaths due to pneumonia among young children occur in 68 poor nations, mostly from Africa and Asia.[1,2]

In India, the disease burden is huge. 45 million episodes are estimated annually with 6.6 million hospitalizations, which contribute to around 20% national disease burden with 97,000–122,000 deaths annually.

DEFINITION

Pneumonia is defined as an inflammatory process involving lung parenchyma usually due to microorganisms. However, etiopathogenesis still remains ill-understood.

CLASSIFICATION

Pneumonia is a big basket containing varied varieties, broadly classified into three categories as mentioned below:

1. *Community-acquired:* Pneumonia acquired outside the hospital environment in a previously healthy immune-competent subject. The patient should not have been hospitalized within 14 days prior to the onset of symptoms or within 4 days of hospitalization for any cause.
2. *Nosocomial pneumonia:* Pneumonia acquired within hospital setting >48 hours after hospitalization (hospital-acquired pneumonia) or >48–72 hours after endotracheal intubation (ventilator-associated pneumonia).
3. *Necrotizing and complicated pneumonia:* Usually defined as fast progressing complicating pneumonia in an otherwise normal healthy immunocompetent subject. It is characterized by destruction of underlying lung parenchyma with multiple small thin-walled cavities within alveolar consolidations usually accompanied with parapneumonic effusions, empyema or bronchopleural fistula.

These categories can be further subclassified into:

- Bacteremic (invasive) pneumonia
- Mucosal (nonbacteremic) pneumonia
- Radiological pneumonia
- Nonradiological pneumonia

Pneumonia can be further classified on functional and behavioral patterns such as "recurrent pneumonia" which is defined as two episodes of documented pneumonia in a span of 1 year or 3 episodes in any timeframe with total clinicoradiological resolution in between the episodes. Another pattern is "nonresolving/persistent" pneumonia which is defined as failure in clinicoradiological resolution after 3–4 weeks of appropriate and optimum duration of antibiotic therapy. At times, pneumonia may be a manifesting presentation of a systemic disease, particularly in an immune-compromised subject or some genetic disorders such as cystic fibrosis and chronic granulomatous disease (CGD).

Pneumonia which are not caused due to microorganisms are called as pneumonitis. Classical examples of this condition are aspiration, inhalation, and chemical pneumonitis.

ETIOLOGY

It depends on various factors, such as age, immune status, underlying comorbidity, and various risk factors, as shown in **Figure 10.5.1**.[3]

The causative agents may be viral, bacterial, atypical pathogens, or fungal. They are usually age-specific as shown in **Table 10.5.1**.

Most common bacterial pathogens are *Streptococcus pneumoniae* and *Haemophilus influenzae*, which together are responsible for 60–70% of total pneumonia cases, followed by viruses, which account for remaining 30–35% cases.

Chlamydia in newborns and *Mycoplasma pneumoniae* in school-going children older than 5 years of age are most common causes of "atypical pneumonia" accounting for 11–24% cases. *Legionella* is infrequent but serious cause of atypical pneumonia. Significant proportion of pneumonia is due to mixed infection (8–40%), and in 20–60% of cases, pathogens are not identified. Mycoplasma usually involves interstitium and causes interstitial pneumonia. The symptoms usually are disproportionate and milder compared to the gravity of the disease. Child with substantial disease usually walks into the clinic with mildest symptoms and hence it is also known as walking pneumonia.

Staphylococcal pneumonias are rapidly progressive, more tissue destructive, toxin-producing usually with thin-walled cavities, and lung abscesses. If they are coinfected with viruses such as influenza or respiratory syncytial virus (RSV), they may lead to fast deterioration and may even be fatal.[4]

PATHOGENESIS

Pneumonia is usually preceded by a respiratory viral infection, which disturbs the defense mechanism of the lungs and disrupts the normal epithelial layer of respiratory tract and as a result there is dysfunction of ciliary brush border

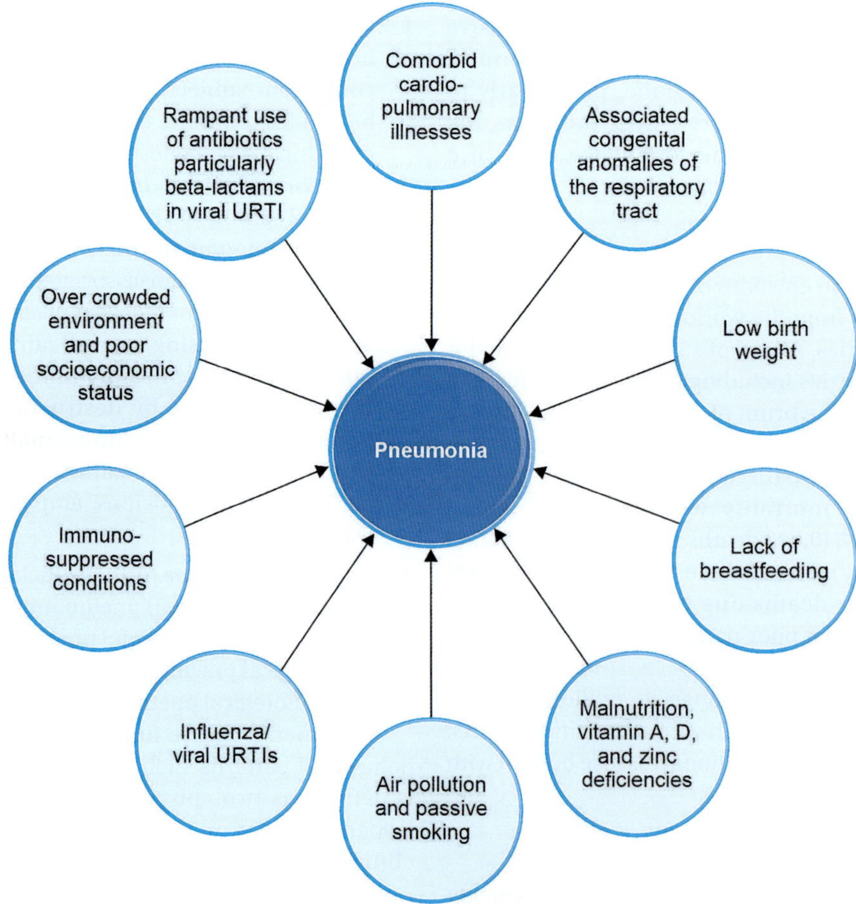

Fig. 10.5.1: Risks and predisposing factors. (URTIs: upper respiratory tract infections)
Source: Berman S. Epidemiology of acute respiratory infections in children of developing countries. Rev Infect Dis. 1991;13(6):S454-62.

TABLE 10.5.1: Etiology of pneumonia—relation to age.

Age group	*Etiology*
0–3 months	• Gram-negative *Enterobacteriaceae* • Enterococci • *Chlamydia trachomatis* • Group B streptococci • *Haemophilus influenzae* • *Streptococcus pneumoniae* • *Listeria monocytogenes*
3 months–5 years	• *Streptococcus pneumoniae* • Viruses • *Haemophilus influenzae* • *Staphylococcus* • *Mycoplasma pneumoniae*
>5 years	• *Streptococcus pneumoniae* • *Mycoplasma pneumoniae* • Viruses • *Staphylococcus* • *Streptococcus pyogenes*

TABLE 10.5.2: The World Health Organization (WHO) grading of pneumonia.

Pneumonia	Fever <38.5°C, cough and tachypnea, no feeding difficulties, no dehydration
Severe pneumonia	High-grade fever >39°C, difficulty in feeding, tachypnea, respiratory distress with ICR or SCR, dehydration, grunt, bronchial breath sounds on auscultation with or without crackles, SpO_2 ≥92 at room air, radiological opacity on chest X-ray +/–
Severe to very severe pneumonia	Inability to feed, altered sensorium, intermittent apneic spells, cyanosis, excessive diaphoresis, narrow pulse pressure, acidemia, and SpO_2 <92 at room air

Note: The recent WHO guidelines have removed the pneumonia category and retained only severe and severe to very severe pneumonia (ICR: intercostal retraction; SCR: subcostal retraction; SpO_2: peripheral capillary oxygen saturation)

clearing mechanism. There is inhibition of phagocytosis by alveolar macrophages. Thus, bacteria and other organisms invade the lung parenchyma and produce a pneumonic lesion with collection of secretions, forming microabscesses in the alveolar cavities, microthrombi and at times, microhemorrhages. The invasion could be either direct spread from nasopharyngeal tract through respiratory droplet infection or could be by invasion through hematogenous dissemination within the lung parenchyma. When the spread is hematogenous, it is called *invasive or bacteremic pneumonia* and when the spread is direct, it is called mucosal or *nonbacteremic pneumonia*. However, the pathogenesis is still ill understood.

CLINICAL FEATURES

Constellation of symptom triad of fever, cough, rapid breathing, and/or difficult breathing is classical clinical manifestation of pneumonia. Diagnosis of pneumonia is essentially clinical. Tachypnea is single most sensitive and specific sign to diagnose pneumonia, as sensitive as 66–88% of auscultation.

Clinical features may differ from neonate to older child. In an infant and young child, respiratory distress with intercostal retractions and at times, fine scattered crackles are the most common features. In an older child, localized bronchial breathing with/without increased vocal resonance is suggestive of lobar consolidation. In neonates, there could be absence of cough and fever, and common presenting features are excessive irritability or lethargy, difficulty in feeding, intermittent apneic spells, cyanosis ±, progressive air hunger, and rapid clinical deterioration with or without evidence of sepsis. In severely malnourished children, the breathing efforts will be poor. The World Health Organization (WHO) has graded pneumonia as given in **Table 10.5.2** based on symptoms. Assessment and grading of severity is most important for successful management.

DIAGNOSIS

Diagnosis of pneumonia is essentially clinical and seldom requires laboratory support. Absence of past history of recurrent cough and presence of fever with fast breathing is a hallmark presentation in clinical diagnosis of pneumonia. It should always be remembered that there are no definite differentiating markers between viral, bacterial, and atypical pneumonia. However, there are certain clinical clues, which can help to nail down on etiological diagnosis **(Table 10.5.3)**.[5]

Characteristics of Viral Pneumonia

- Acute—sudden onset
- Younger age
- Preceding upper respiratory catarrh
- Wheeze with crackles
- Clinical evidence of hyperinflation with scattered exudates on radiology due to segmental atelectasis.

For optimum antimicrobial management of pneumonia, it is prudent to differentiate between bacterial, viral, and atypical pneumonia clinically, as it is often very difficult to isolate the offending pathogen **(Table 10.5.4)**.

LABORATORY DIAGNOSIS

- *Acute phase reactants*, such as complete blood cell counts (CBC), C-reactive protein (CRP), erythrocyte sedimentation rate (ESR), have poor sensitivity and

TABLE 10.5.3: Clinical clues which help in diagnosis of etiological diagnosis of pneumonia.

Predisposing factors	*Organisms (apart from usual ones)*
Pyoderma, measles, pneumatoceles	*Staphylococcus*
Human immunodeficiency virus infection	*Pneumocystis carinii*
Neutropenia	Gram-negative, *Aspergillus*
Cystic fibrosis	*Pseudomonas, Staphylococcus*
Severe malnutrition	Gram-negative, *Staphylococcus*
Preceding coryza, wheeze	Viral
Young afebrile infant with neonatal conjunctivitis	*Chlamydia trachomatis*
Multisystem involvement (rash, anemia, hepatitis, encephalitis)	*Mycoplasma pneumoniae*
Marked leukocytosis	Bacteria
Acute otitis media	*Streptococcus pneumoniae/ Haemophilus influenzae*

TABLE 10.5.4: Differential diagnosis between typical and atypical pneumonia.

Features	*Typical pneumonia*	*Atypical pneumonia*
Age	More common in young infants, children, and in older children	School-going children, adolescents, and adults
Onset	Acute/sudden	Gradual/insidious
Facies	Toxic	Well
Rigors	Shaking chills	Chilliness
Wheeze	Rare or nil	Common
Cough	Productive	Nonproductive/ paroxysmal
Sputum	Purulent/bloody	Mucoid
Temperature	High 102–104°F	Mild-moderate <102°F
Pleurisy	Frequent	Rare
Consolidation	Frequent	Rare
Extrapulmonary manifestations	Uncommon	Common
Gram staining (sputum)	Neutrophils	Mononuclear cells
Sputum culture	Occasional growth of microbe	Rarely any growth
WBC count	>15,000/mm^3; shift to left	>15,000/mm^3; no shift
Chest radiography	Defined density	Nondefined infiltrates

(WBC: white blood cell)

specificity. They do not distinguish between viral and bacterial etiology, nor they help in making decision of antibiotic choice; however, they may be useful tools for monitoring the course of the disease.

- *Radiology* is not routinely required in nonsevere pneumonia to confirm the diagnosis. At times, it may not correlate with the clinical signs; there is also wide variation in the interpretation by radiologists. Moreover, reliability in predicting the etiology is poor. However, chest X-ray may be indicated in severe disease, ambiguous picture, no improvement/worsening even after 48–72 hours of therapy, suspected complications, and in a known immune-compromised child **(Figs. 10.5.2A to C)**.
- *Microbiology*—sputum culture or blood culture though more specific, but the yield is very poor (10–15%), as the most common organisms *S. pneumoniae* and *H. influenzae* are fastidious organisms to be grown easily. There is also a risk of growing normal nasopharyngeal flora.
- *Serology*—latex agglutination, urinary antigens for pneumococcus and *Haemophilus influenzae* b (Hib), rapid antigen detection test, and cold agglutinins for mycoplasma are not easily available, expensive with time lagging, and have poor sensitivity.
- *Invasive procedures,* such as bronchoscopy, bronchoalveolar lavage (BAL), and lung aspiration, have high sensitivity and specificity; however, lung aspiration is too invasive and unethical to be advised in office practice.
- *Pulse oximetry* is a mandatory tool for monitoring the course of the disease in all outpatient and hospitalized children.

DIFFERENTIAL DIAGNOSIS

Though symptom complex of fever, cough, and rapid/ difficult breathing is classical presentation of pneumonia; it should be differentiated from other masqueraders, which may mimic with same symptomatology. One should keep in mind to differentiate "pneumonia" from "noninfective pneumonitis" such as chemical, aspiration, and inhalation as the management would differ in such conditions. Some close differentials of community-acquired pneumonia (CAP) are interstitial pneumonia, hypersensitive pneumonitis, bronchiolitis, obliterans and persistent bacterial bronchitis. One should remember all cases of fever, cough, and breathlessness need not be pneumonia **(Fig. 10.5.3)**.

MANAGEMENT

The mainstays of management are antibiotics and supportive treatment. It is imperative to understand that all pneumonias deserve antibiotics for two reasons, one because pneumonia is number one cause of childhood mortality, particularly

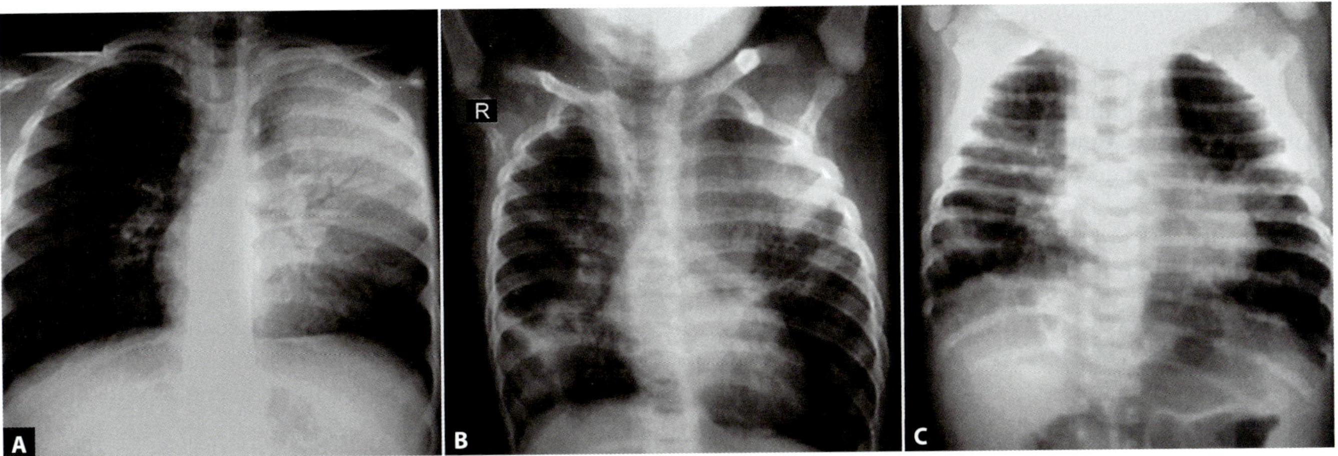

Figs. 10.5.2A to C: Radiologic findings in: (A) Bacterial lobar consolidation; (B) Bronchopneumonia; (C) Interstitial pneumonia.

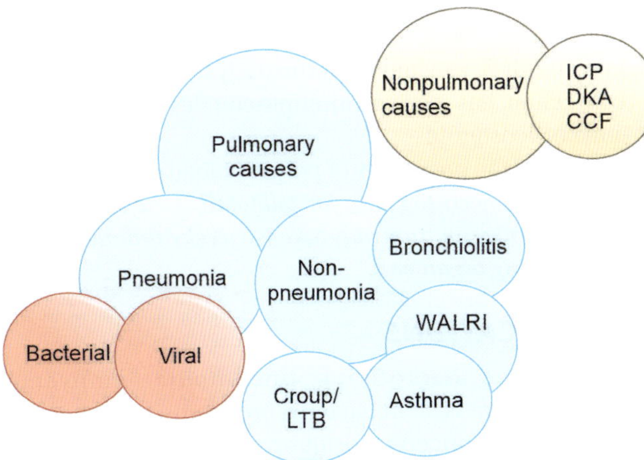

Fig. 10.5.3: Triad of fever + cough + tachypnea is symbolic of LRTI; but all LRTIs are not pneumonias. (CCF: congestive cardiac failure; DKA: diabetic ketoacidosis; ICP: intracranial pressure; LRTI: lower respiratory tract infection; LTB: laryngotracheobronchitis; WALRI: wheeze-associated lower respiratory infection)

in developing world where children die due to either nonavailability or delayed initiation of antibiotic therapy. Secondly, differentiation between viral and bacterial is difficult. Thus, empirical antibiotics are prudent and rational in pneumonia.

Nonsevere pneumonia above the age of 3 months can be managed at domiciliary level with oral antibiotics. However, any pneumonia below the age of 3 months should be hospitalized and treated with parenteral antibiotics. The choice of antibiotics though empirical should be determined by age, severity, predisposing conditions if any, local epidemiology, and drug resistance pattern.

Outpatient Management

All nonsevere pneumonias >3 months of age, when the child is not very sick, accepting oral feeds, not dehydrated, maintaining normal saturation, and fever <38.5°C can be managed at domiciliary level with oral antibiotics and supportive care, such as maintenance of hydration, nutrition, antipyretics, and adjuvants, if needed. The choice of first-line empirical oral antibiotic should always be amoxicillin because *S. pneumoniae* is the most common causative bug from 3 months onward till adolescence and adulthood. The optimum duration for first-line antibiotics should be 3–5 days and for second line should be 5–7 days. Since mycoplasma is an important organism for pneumonia in the age group of 5–15 years, macrolide should be considered alone or in combination with amoxicillin/coamoxiclav. The choice of antibiotics is as shown in **Table 10.5.5**.[6]

First-line oral antibiotics should be given minimum for 5 days and second line for 7 days. Child should be followed up after 48 hours, and if there is clinical improvement, the child should be continued with the same management. If the condition clinically deteriorates after 48 hours, one should revise the diagnosis, look for associated complications and comorbidities, changing the antibiotic to second line, and if be the need, the child should be hospitalized **(Box 10.5.1)**.[7]

Inpatient Management

Management comprises specific antimicrobial along with supportive care of nutrition, hydration, oxygen if needed, antipyretics (paracetamol), and nebulized bronchodilators along with chest physiotherapy if needed **(Table 10.5.6)**.

During the outbreak of influenza in the community and severe acute onset of pneumonia, viral infections like influenza should be covered with oseltamivir in the prescribed doses.

If the pneumonia is very severe, fast progressive, preceded by measles or pyoderma with cavitation or pneumatocele, *Staphylococcus aureus* is the causative organism. In case of *methicillin-sensitive Staphylococcus aureus* (MSSA), the antibiotic duration should be for 2 weeks, and in case of *methicillin-resistant Staphylococcus aureus* (MRSA), it should be 4–6 weeks.

The duration for intravenous antibiotics should be for 5–7 days in uncomplicated cases; however, switchover to oral antibiotics may be considered if accepted orally. The switchover therapy for injectable third-generation cephalosporins should be either cefpodoxime (10 mg/kg/day in two divided doses) or cefdinir (15 mg/kg/day in two divided doses) and should never be cefixime as it has no activity against *Pneumococcus* and poor activity against community pathogens responsible for pneumonia.[8] Vancomycin is not a preferred drug for pneumonia as it poorly penetrates into the lung tissues.

TABLE 10.5.5: Choice of antibiotics.

Age	First-line	Second-line
3 months–5 years	Amoxicillin*	Co-amoxiclav/Cefuroxime/+/– Macrolide
>5 years	Amoxicillin*	Macrolide†/Co-amoxiclav/ Cefuroxime

**Standard doses*: 40–45 mg/kg/day in two or three divided doses.
†*Erythromycin*: 30–40 mg/kg/day in three divided doses; *Clarithromycin*: 15 mg/kg/day in two divided doses; *Azithromycin*: 10 mg/kg/day in once a day dose.

BOX 10.5.1: Indications for hospitalization.

- Infants less than 3 months
- Severe malnutrition
- More than two risk factors
- Comorbidities
- Associated complications
- Respiratory rate more than 70 per minute in infants and more than 50 per minute in older children
- Respiratory distress—grunting, alae nasi flare, ICR, or SCR
- Cyanosis or SpO_2 less than 92% in room air
- Poor oral intake/dehydration
- Inappropriate observation or supervision at home

(ICR: intercostal retraction; SCR: subcostal retraction; SpO_2: oxygen saturation)

Despite rational choice of antibiotics in right dose and for optimal duration, if there is failure in clinical improvement (nonresolving pneumonia), one needs to:
- Check the diagnosis and rule out foreign body, aspiration pneumonia, and interstitial lung disease.
- Look for underlying comorbidity, such as lung abscess, empyema, bronchiectasis, left-to-right shunts, gastroesophageal reflux disease, asthma, cystic fibrosis, and ciliary dyskinesia.
- Evaluate immune suppression in the host, such as primary immunodeficiencies and hypogammaglobulinemia.
- Look for complement disorders and phagocytic dysfunctions like CGD.
- Look for drug resistance, particularly if child is from day-care center, has received multiple courses of beta-lactams and corticosteroids.
- Search for the possibility of polymicrobial etiology.
- *There is no need to chase for follow-up X-rays since total radiological resolution may take 4–8 weeks' time depending on offending organisms.*

COMPLICATIONS

These include necrotizing pneumonia, empyema, pneumothorax, persistent bacterial bronchitis, bronchogenic dissemination, septicemia, osteomyelitis, multiple systemic abscesses, septic arthritis, and meningitis.

PROGNOSIS

Prognosis is good provided there is appropriate recognition and proper referral by the healthcare provider and early

TABLE 10.5.6: Specific antimicrobial therapy in pneumonia.

Age	First-line	Second-line
<3 months	Cefotaxime‡/Ceftriaxone† ± Aminoglycosides‖	
3 months–5 years	Amoxicillin/Co-amoxiclav*	Ceftriaxone†/Cefotaxime‡
>5 years	• Ampicillin/Penicillin G • Co-amoxiclav/Cefuroxime/Macrolide (if mycoplasma suspected)	Ceftriaxone†/Cefotaxime‡ and Macrolides
Suspected staphylococcal infection	Co-amoxiclav or Cefuroxime§ (oral/IV) or 3rd generation Cephalosporins + Cloxacillin	Ceftriaxone†/Cefotaxime‡ and Vancomycin/Linezolid (In case of CA-MRSA, the drug of choice is Clindamycin as an add-on to the above antibiotics)

**Co-amoxiclav:* 30–40 mg/kg/day.
†*Ceftriaxone:* 50–100 mg/kg/day.
‡*Cefotaxime:* 100–200 mg/kg/day.
§*Cefuroxime:* 20–30 mg/kg/day.
‖*Aminoglycosides:* 15 mg/kg/day in single or two divided doses.

initiation of antibiotics. Unfortunately, only 15–20% cases of pneumonia receive proper and adequate antibiotics, particularly in rural areas of developing countries, which is the main reason for high infant mortality.

PREVENTION

A multifaceted approach is needed to prevent and control childhood pneumonia. These include:

- Exclusive breastfeeding for first 6 months of life
- Weaning to solid foods after 6 months of age, preferably with homemade foods
- Avoidance of risk factors, such as overcrowded environment, biofuels, exposure to pollution, and bottle-feeding
- Protection from malnutrition and supplementation of vitamin A and D
- Optimum immunization with diphtheria-pertussis-tetanus, measles, Hib, pneumococcal and influenza vaccines at appropriate ages.

CONCLUSION

Pneumonia is the number 1 cause of childhood mortality across the globe, particularly in developing countries. Hence, it has also been called the 'forgotten or silent killer'. *S. pneumoniae, H. influenzae* and viruses are the main causative agents. The symptoms triad of fever, cough, and rapid or difficult breathing is the classical clinical manifestation. Diagnosis of pneumonia is essentially clinical and laboratory investigations or imaging is seldom required. Empirical antibiotics are prudent in the management of pneumonia since it is very difficult to distinguish between viral and bacterial etiology. Amoxicillin is the drug of choice for the uncomplicated, domiciliary and indoor management of pneumonia, whereas ceftriaxone or co-amoxiclav is the second drug of choice. All the pneumonias, even if not severe, below the age of 3 months should be managed as indoor patients. Recurrent, nonresolving, necrotizing and complicated pneumonias require altogether different approaches. In a nutshell, early recognition, proper reference to an appropriate facility along with right choice of antibiotics with early initiation based on age, severity and epidemiological patterns, and prevention with appropriate vaccines can help in lowering mortality due to pneumonia.

REFERENCES

1. le Roux DM, Zar HJ. Community-acquired pneumonia in children-a changing spectrum of disease. Pediatr Radiol. 2017;47(11):1392-8.
2. McAllister DA, Liu L, Shi T, Chu Y, Reed C, Burrows J, et al. Global, regional, and national estimates of pneumonia morbidity and mortality in children younger than 5 years between 2000 and 2015: a systematic analysis. Lancet Glob Health. 2019;7(1):e47-e57.
3. Goyal JP, Kumar P, Mukherjee A, Das RR, Bhat JI, Ratageri V, et al. Risk Factors for the Development of Pneumonia and Severe Pneumonia in Children. Indian Pediatr. 2021;58(11):1036-9
4. Pneumonia Etiology Research for Child Health (PERCH) Study Group. Causes of severe pneumonia requiring hospital admission in children without HIV infection from Africa and Asia: the PERCH multi-country case-control study. Lancet. 2019;394(10200):757-79.
5. Das RR, Satapathy AK, Mukherjee a, Goyal JP, Bhat JI, Ratageri VH, et al. Role of Clinical Criteria and Oxygen Saturation Monitoring in Diagnosis of Childhood Pneumonia in Children Aged 2 to 59 Months. Indian Pediatr. 2021;58(11):1024-9.
6. Mathur S, Fuchs A, Bielicki J, Van Den Anker J, Sharland M. Antibiotic use for community-acquired pneumonia in neonates and children: WHO evidence review. Paediatr Int Child Health. 2018;38(Suppl):S66-S75.
7. Bhat JI, Charoo BA, Mukherjee A, Ahad R, Das RR, Goyal JP, et al. Risk of Hospitalization in Under-five Children with Community – A Multicentric Prospective Cohort Study. Indian Pediatr. 2021;58(11):1019-23.
8. Williams DJ, Creech CB, Walter EB, Martin JM, Gerber JS, Newland JG, et al; The DMID 14-0079 Study Team. Short- vs Standard-Course Outpatient Antibiotic Therapy for Community-Acquired Pneumonia in Children: The SCOUT-CAP Randomized Clinical Trial. JAMA Pediatr. 2022;176(3):253-61.

10.6 Bronchiolitis

A Balachandran

INTRODUCTION

Bronchiolitis is a common viral respiratory illness in children. It is an acute inflammatory condition of the bronchioles that is a result of virus-induced injury. It accounts for a substantial portion of the pediatric burden of illness all over the world; it is the most common and serious lower respiratory tract syndrome that results in hospital admission among infants and is associated with considerable morbidity. It is generally a self-limiting condition and is most commonly due to respiratory syncytial virus (RSV) infection. Babies with chronic lung disease are at risk for more severe RSV-associated illness. Bronchiolitis occurs most frequently among children younger than 12 months of age. Most cases occur between late autumn and early spring, with sporadic cases throughout the year.[1]

DEFINITION

Bronchiolitis is a clinical syndrome characterized by the acute onset of respiratory symptoms in a child younger than 2 years of age. Typically, the initial symptoms of upper respiratory tract viral infection, such as fever and coryza, progress within 4–6 days to include evidence of lower respiratory tract involvement with the onset of cough and wheezing.[1]

RISK FACTORS

In bronchiolitis, an increased risk for hospitalization is seen among infants attending daycare, those exposed to passive smoking and overcrowding in the household. Environmental and genetic factors may also contribute to the severity of disease. High-risk factors include age <3 months, premature delivery, low birth weight (LBW), congenital heart disease, chronic lung disease (e.g., cystic fibrosis), recurrent aspiration pneumonitis, bronchopulmonary dysplasia (BPD), congenital lung malformations, tracheoesophageal fistula, neurogenic disorders (interfering with pulmonary toilet), immunodeficiency, and malnutrition.

The high-risk groups are vulnerable for rapid deterioration and more severe disease. Children with a pulmonary patch (consolidation or atelectasis) on radiograph, hypoxia, repeat episodes of apnea, and extreme tachypnea at admission are at higher risk of admission to the pediatric intensive care unit (PICU) and may need mechanical ventilation.[1]

ETIOLOGY

Bronchiolitis is usually a result of a viral respiratory tract infection. RSV is the most common underlying infecting agent. Other viral pathogens, such as influenza, parainfluenza, adenovirus, coronavirus, and rhinovirus, can also cause bronchiolitis. *Mycoplasma* is also implicated in older children with lower respiratory tract infection and wheezing.[1,2]

PATHOLOGY

Respiratory syncytial virus infection results in the loss of epithelial cilia and sloughing of epithelial cells in the airways. This leads to the collection of desquamated airway epithelial cells, polymorphonuclear cells, and lymphocytes within the airway. There may also be cellular infiltration and airway mucosal edema with very little or no alveolar infiltration. In acute bronchiolitis, sloughed epithelial cells, neutrophils, and lymphocytes appear to be the major contributors to airway obstruction. The complete plugging of some airways and partial plugging of others may lead to localized atelectasis of some units of lung parenchyma and overdistention of other units. These results in ventilation-perfusion mismatch causing hypoxemia, which is generally relieved by the administration of oxygen (O_2).

CLINICAL FEATURES

Clinical features are quite variable. Initially, they present like any other viral upper respiratory tract infection with cough or cold with or without fever. Later, disturbing cough, tachypnea, respiratory distress, and poor feeding may develop depending on the severity of illness. Fever is present in almost 50% of the infants. In patients with adenovirus or influenza-associated bronchiolitis, fever is often higher than 39°C. On examination, infants typically may have tachypnea, respiratory distress, audible wheezing, rales or rhonchi, crackles, and poor air movement, and the expiratory phase is usually prolonged. Other concomitant findings, such as conjunctivitis, rhinitis, and otitis media, may be present. Once hypoxia sets in, it can lead on to cardiorespiratory compromise and there can be lethargy, seizure, hypoxia, apnea, shock, and death. Apnea may be the only presenting feature, particularly below 6 weeks of age.[1,2]

GRADING OF BRONCHIOLITIS

Based on the ability to feed, the respiratory effort, and O_2 saturation (SaO_2) observed at admission, each infant's condition can be clinically graded as mild, moderate, and severe bronchiolitis **(Table 10.6.1)**.

TABLE 10.6.1: Grading of bronchiolitis.

	Mild	*Moderate*	*Severe*
Ability to feed	Ability to feed normally	Appear short of breath during feeds	May be reluctant or unable to feed
Respiratory effort	Little or no respiratory distress	Moderate distress with some chest wall retractions and nasal flaring	Severe distress with marked chest wall retractions, nasal flaring, and grunting may have frequent or prolonged apneic episodes
Oxygen saturation	*Saturations*: SaO_2 >92%	Saturations <92%, correctable with oxygen	Saturations <92%, may or may not be correctable with oxygen

INVESTIGATIONS

Bronchiolitis is a clinical diagnosis. The specific and supportive investigations, which can be done in bronchiolitis, are discussed further.[3]

- *Nasopharyngeal aspirate* for RSV and viral culture
- *Complete blood counts* (CBCs)
- *Serum electrolytes,* to look for evidence of syndrome of inappropriate antidiuretic hormone secretion (SIADH), especially when intravenous (IV) fluids, are needed.
- *Blood culture* if temperature >38.5°C
- *Arterial blood gas* (ABG) analysis to look for carbon dioxide (CO_2) retention when there is evidence of respiratory failure.
- *The chest X-ray* need not be done routinely and is indicated only in children with severe respiratory distress or when there is diagnostic dilemma. The radiographic findings of bronchiolitis include hyperinflation, patchy infiltrates that are typically migratory and attributable to postobstructive atelectasis, and peribronchial cuffing. Because bronchiolitis is not a disease of the alveolar spaces, a secondary bacterial pneumonitis should be suspected if a true alveolar infiltrate is seen on chest radiograph.

DIFFERENTIAL DIAGNOSIS

Congenital anomalies, such as vascular ring, congenital heart disease, gastroesophageal reflux, aspiration pneumonia, bacterial pneumonia, and episodic viral wheeze or foreign body aspiration can mimic the symptoms of bronchiolitis.

MANAGEMENT

Supportive care is the mainstay of therapy for infants with bronchiolitis.[4] Children with mild bronchiolitis can be managed on outpatient basis. They need to be followed and reviewed earlier if there is clinical worsening. Infants in high-risk group are better hospitalized and managed even if they are graded as mild in view of their propensity to deteriorate rapidly, whereas moderate and severe cases have to be definitely admitted and monitored.[5] Considerable unexplained variation exists in the inpatient management of bronchiolitis.[1,3]

NONCONTROVERSIAL ISSUES [6]

Oxygen

The drug of choice in bronchiolitis is O_2. O_2 is used when the SaO_2 is <94% or in a combination of clinically significant respiratory distress, a respiratory rate above 60 breaths/min, and difficulty in feeding. The aim of humidified O_2 supplementation is to maintain SaO_2 above 95% using suitable device, preferably in a nonthreatening fashion. Noninvasive strategies that may be effective in reducing work of breathing, improving gas exchange, and avoiding the need for endotracheal intubation include heated humidified high-flow nasal cannula (HFNC) therapy and continuous positive airway pressure (CPAP) ventilation. During recovery, SaO_2 of 90–92% in room air is acceptable if baby is feeding well and not distressed except in children with chronic lung disease.[4]

Fluid Therapy

If the infant tolerates well, oral feeds are continued, as is the case with mild-to-moderate severity. Intravenous fluids are needed to maintain hydration in moderate-to-severe or severe respiratory distress (marked retractions and nasal flaring), marked tachypnea (>60 breaths/min), coughing and choking with feeds, vomiting, decreased intake, apneic episodes, and tiring during feeds. Normal general maintenance fluids with normal maintenance volumes are used with N/2 or N/4 dextrose saline.[4]

Nasogastric Feeding

Nasogastric (NG) feeding is avoided during acute phase and is reserved for recovery phase. During acute phase, the NG tube blocks one nostril and increases upper airway resistance, which in turn further increases the work of breathing.

Symptomatic Management

Symptomatic management, such as antipyretics, is needed to relieve fever.

CONTROVERSIAL ISSUES[6]

Bronchodilators

The role of bronchodilators (salbutamol and epinephrine) in acute bronchiolitis is controversial. Though there is no absolute contraindication, bronchodilators neither treats hypoxemia nor affects the duration or progress of bronchiolitis.

Inhaled beta-agonist therapy when used should be on a case-by-case basis, by critically evaluating its effectiveness in the individual patient. They might be of benefit in intermediate conditions, such as early wheezers or children with atopy.[7]

Beta-agonists: Optional single trial; may be continued if there is clinical response (a trial of bronchodilator therapy may be initiated, but should be discontinued if there is no objective improvement).

Since mucosal edema is an important component of airway obstruction in infants with bronchiolitis, a logical approach to therapy might be to use a combined (alpha-adrenergic and beta-adrenergic agonist), such as epinephrine (0.3 mL/kg of 1:1,000 solution). Till date there is no definitive evidence to support the use of nebulized epinephrine in all children with moderate or severe bronchiolitis. When the effect of epinephrine was compared with placebo, the improvement in respiratory symptoms across studies has been inconsistent and potentially short-lived. It may therefore be appropriate for clinicians to use nebulized epinephrine as a potential rescue medication which has inconsistent and short-lived improvement. This can be tried in patients who are to be admitted.[7,8]

There is no role for ipratropium bromide in the management of bronchiolitis.

Hypertonic Saline

Hypertonic saline has the potential to reduce airway edema and mucus plugging, the predominant feature of acute bronchiolitis. Several trials have indicated the potential benefit of hypertonic saline (3% NaCl) in acute bronchiolitis with conflicting results.[7]

Sedation

Sedation should be avoided in an irritable child as this may be a sign of hypoxia and sedation further compromises the respiratory drive of the child.[7]

Antibiotics

There is no role for routine or prophylactic antibiotics in bronchiolitis. Since secondary bacterial infections of the lower respiratory tract are unusual in children with bronchiolitis.[7]

Aerosolized Ribavirin

Respiratory syncytial virus is the most common cause of bronchiolitis but specific antiviral therapy for symptomatic infants has been of limited value. Aerosolized ribavirin, used to treat mild to moderately ill infants with laboratory confirmed RSV bronchiolitis neither prevents the need for mechanical ventilation nor reduces the length of hospital stay. It is not recommended at present for treatment of bronchiolitis.[7]

Noninvasive Ventilation

Humidified HFNC (HHFNC) or CPAP may potentially benefit infants with bronchiolitis, by tenting to open the smaller airways during all phases of respiration, preventing air trapping and obstructive disease, and by serving as a constant ipratropium stimulus in infants with a propensity to experience apnea.

Role of Steroids

There is no role of systemic (parenteral/oral) or inhaled steroids in the management of bronchiolitis.

Intensive Care Unit Management

It will be needed if there is:[5]

- Progression to severe respiratory distress, especially in high-risk group
- Any significant apneic episodes (>15 seconds or associated with desaturation) or frequent recurrent brief apneic episodes
- Persistent desaturation despite O_2; where ABG shows the evidence of respiratory failure, i.e., partial pressure of O_2 < 80 mm Hg; partial pressure of CO_2 > 50 mm Hg; pH < 7.25.

Other Nonstandard Therapies

Antirespiratory Syncytial Virus Preparation

The use of immunoglobulin with a neutralizing activity against RSV [RSV-immune globulin intravenous (IGIV)] or RSV-specific humanized monoclonal antibody (palivizumab) have failed to improve outcomes in infants with or without risk factors, hospitalized with RSV infection.[9]

Heliox

It is a mixture of helium and O_2 (80:20%). It can flow through airways with less turbulence and resistance than O_2. Only very small benefit is observed in a limited group of children who were administered heliox; hence, it is not recommended for routine use.

Management Summary

No role of:

- Chest physiotherapy
- Antibiotics
- Antivirals
- Montelukast
- Ipratropium bromide
- Systemic or inhaled steroids
- Steam inhalation
- RSV polyclonal immunoglobulin/palivizumab (no role in acute management but useful in prophylaxis)[9]

- Inhaled furosemide/inhaled interferon alpha-2a/inhaled recombinant human deoxyribonuclease (DNase)

Interventions which are possibly effective for most severe cases:

- HHFNC
- CPAP
- Surfactant
- Heliox
- Aerosolized ribavirin

DISCHARGE CRITERIA

The infant is considered fit for discharge if the child did not require supplemental O_2 for >10 hours, had minimal or no chest recession, and is feeding adequately, without the need for IV fluids.

COMPLICATIONS

Complication rates are higher in prematurely born infants with congenital heart disease and infants with other congenital abnormalities compared to infants without risk factors. Serious respiratory complications include respiratory failure, apnea, and pneumothorax. Others include secondary infection, cardiovascular involvement, and electrolyte imbalance.

Other Complications

- Acute respiratory distress syndrome (ARDS)
- Myocarditis
- Congestive heart failure
- Arrhythmias
- Bronchiolitis obliterans
- Secondary bacterial infection
- Predisposition to childhood asthma

PROGNOSIS

The need for supplemental O_2 (based on SaO_2 in room air) at admission is highly predictive of the length of the hospital stay. The case fatality rate for bronchiolitis is highest among infants <3-month age.

PREVENTION

Respiratory syncytial virus is highly contagious and spreads via inhalation of small particle aerosols or direct transfer via hand-to-hand contact. RSV cross infection is common but is largely preventable by:

- Simple hand washing by nursing, medical, other staff, and parents
- Isolation of RSV-infected cases will minimize this problem
- *Breastfeeding:* Threefold greater risk in nonbreastfed infant
- Avoiding passive smoking
- Palivizumab (RSV Ig) prophylaxis in BPD may be beneficial and has to be decided on case-by-case basis.[9]

In July 2023, the Food and Drug Administration approved *Nirsevimab,* a long-acting monoclonal antibody, for passive immunization in infants and children aged <24 months for prevention of RSV lower respiratory tract disease in infants.[10] This recombinant human immunoglobulin G1 kappa, a long-acting monoclonal antibody that binds to the RSV F protein. The risk of getting RSV again after an initial infection is about 70% lower within the first 6 months. Research suggests that your body starts to have an immune response to RSV within 5 to 10 days. That protection lasts anywhere from 3 to 12 months before it starts to decline. The recommended dosage for infants born during or entering their first RSV season and weighing <5 kg is 50 mg; for those weighing ≥5 kg; is 100 mg as intramuscular injection and can be administered with other routine vaccines.

REFERENCES

1. Balachandran A, Gowrishankar NC. Bronchiolitis. In: Subramanyam L, Shivabalan S, Gowrishankar NC, Vijayasekaran D, Balachandran A (Eds). Essentials of Pediatric Pulmonology, 3rd edition. New Delhi: Jaypee Brothers Medical Publishers (P) Ltd.; 2008. pp. 91-5.
2. Chatterjee P, Sehgal V, Shah S. (2022). Bronchiolitis. Indian Academy of Pediatrics (IAP) Standard Treatment Guidelines. [online] Available from https://www.iapindia.org/pdf/Ch-027-STG-Bronchiolitis.pdf [Last accessed December, 2024].
3. Christakis DA, Cowan CA, Garrison MM, Molteni R, Marcuse E, Zerr DM. Variation in inpatient diagnostic testing and management of bronchiolitis. Pediatrics. 2005;115(4):878-84.
4. Respiratory tract infection-group education module. IAP consensus protocol for the management of respiratory tract infection for children. IAP Action Plan; 2006.
5. Coffin SE. Bronchiolitis: inpatient focus. Pediatr Clin North Am. 2005;52(4):1047-57.
6. Dayan PS, Roskind CG, Levine D, Kuppermann N. Controversies in the management of children with bronchiolitis. Clin Pediatr Emerg Med. 2004;5(1):41-53.
7. King VJ, Viswanathan M, Bordley WC, Jackman AM, Sutton SF, Lohr KN, et al. Pharmacologic treatment of bronchiolitis in infants and children: a systematic review. Arch Pediatr Adolesc Med. 2004;158(2):127-37.
8. Wainwright C, Altamirano L, Cheney M, Cheney J, Barber S, Price D, et al. A multicenter randomized double-blind controlled trial of nebulized epinephrine in infants with acute bronchiolitis. N Engl J Med. 2003;349(1):27-35.
9. Grimaldi M, Gouyon B, Michaut F, Huet F, Gouyon JB; Burgundy Perinatal Network. Severe respiratory syncytial virus bronchiolitis: epidemiologic variations associated with the initiation of palivizumab in severely premature infants with bronchopulmonary dysplasia. Pediatr Infect Dis J. 2004;23(12):1081-5.
10. Jones JM, Fleming-Dutra KE, Prill MM, Roper LE, Brooks O, Sánchez PJ, et al. Use of Nirsevimab for the Prevention of Respiratory Syncytial Virus Disease Among Infants and Young Children: Recommendations of the Advisory Committee on Immunization Practices — United States, 2023. MMWR Morb Mortal Wkly Rep. 2023;72(34):920-5.

10.7 Empyema

Savneet Kaur, Varinder Singh

INTRODUCTION

Involvement of the pleural space with pulmonary infections has been recognized since the ancient times. Bacterial pneumonia with associated empyema is the most common cause of pleural effusion found in the pediatric population. They need to be understood differently from parapneumonic effusions (PPE), which are exudative thin effusion collection in pleural space in presence of underlying lung infection. Uncomplicated parapneumonic effusion (UPPE) is a sterile collection with low white cell count and free-flowing fluid without septations. Complicated parapneumonic effusion (CPPE) occurs due to invasion of bacteria into pleural space with high white cell count, fibrin deposition in pleural fluid, and septations seen. Empyema is the last stage of CPPE with pus in the pleural space, multiple loculations and often a thick pleural rind present. The stage of the effusion is best assessed using chest ultrasound. Importantly, a clinician must know that while most of the PPE resolve with an adequate and appropriate antimicrobial therapy, yet antibiotics alone are almost never sufficient to treat empyema and require drainage of the pus via an intercostal chest tube.

DISEASE BURDEN

The reported global incidence of PPE and empyema is 3.3 per 10,000 children, but this varies with different populace and economic level. Although the incidence is less in developed countries as compared to developing countries, some of the developed nations are showing an increased prevalence lately. It is more common in infants and young children under 5 years of age.[1]

ETIOPATHOGENESIS

Staphylococcus aureus, Streptococcus pneumoniae, and *Streptococcus pyogenes* are the most commonly implicated organisms in empyema thoracis. *S. pneumoniae* is the most common organism implicated in the most western and developed countries. In India, *S. aureus* continues to be the most common organism. The prevalence of *Haemophilus influenzae* pneumonia with empyema has decreased following *H. influenzae* type b vaccination. *S. pneumoniae, H. influenzae,* and gram-negative bacilli form rest of the burden. In recent years, infection by resistant bacteria, specifically methicillin-resistant *S. aureus* (MRSA) has increased. In immunocompromised patients, gram-negative organisms (*Pseudomonas aeruginosa, Klebsiella*) and fungi can be seen. Frank tuberculous empyema is very uncommon.[2-4]

TABLE 10.7.1: Stages of empyema development.

Stage 1	Exudative phase	First 1–3 days of PPE, usually a UPPE	• Clear free-flowing pleural fluid • Low white cell count • pH > 7.3 • Glucose >60 mg/dL • LDH < 1,000 IU/L • Bacteria-free
Stage 2	Fibrinopurulent phase	4–14 days	• High white cell count • Fibrin seen • Pleural fluid is purulent with pH < 7.2 • Glucose <40 mg/dL • LDH > 1,000 IU/L • Bacteria + on Gram stain or culture • Echogenic fluid, septations may be seen
Stage 3	Organizational phase	After 14 days	Fibroblasts grow and form exudates on visceral and pleural pleura to form an inelastic membrane "the peel", entrapping lung and preventing expansion

(LDH: lactate dehydrogenase enzyme; PPE: parapneumonic effusion; UPPE: uncomplicated parapneumonic effusion)

Various host factors like noninfectious inflammatory conditions, trauma, chronic infections, or malignancies may cause fluid accumulation in the pleural space, which later may get secondarily infected.

There are three stages of development of empyema as described in **Table 10.7.1**.

CLINICAL FEATURES

Clinical signs vary depending on the age of the patient, stage of the effusion, and type of prior antibiotic therapy. A high index of suspicion and appreciation of factors that predispose to development of empyema facilitates its recognition. Children usually present with a severe pneumonia, or a pneumonia that does not respond well to initial therapy. Lack of response to the antibiotics after 48 hours of treatment should raise the suspicion of an effusion. However, some may even present with a fever without clear focus, or with chest or abdominal pain.[3]

Usual features of pneumonia, such as high-grade fever, chest pain, breathing difficulty, loss of appetite, and refusal to feed may be present. Fever may not be present in the immunocompromised or debilitated patients. On physical examination, children may be sick and toxic-looking, tachypneic, often hypoxic, and in respiratory distress and/or respiratory failure. On systemic examination, decreased chest expansion on the affected side, dullness on percussion with decreased air entry or bronchial breath sound is seen. If the collection is large, there may also be tracheal and/or mediastinal shift to opposite side. Few may also have pleural friction rub, bronchophony or egophony above pleural effusion, bulge on the affected side of the chest, or a preference to lie on the affected side. Oxygen saturation ($SpaO_2$) levels below 92% in room air may indicate severe disease.

Some children may have other stigmata of staphylococcal infection, such as skin pustules or boils, infected scabies, pyomyositis, septic arthritis, pyopneumothorax, and pyopericardium.

DIAGNOSIS

Chest Skiagram: Frontal Views

Frontal views form the most important and first-line investigation for patients with pleural disease. There is no role for a routine lateral or decubitus views. The earliest sign to be seen is the obliteration of the costophrenic angle. White opacity of the lateral part or whole of hemithorax is usually seen. Skiagrams, however, cannot differentiate empyema from a PPE. Scoliosis may also be seen.[5,6]

Sonography of Chest

It is a very useful tool for the diagnosis, guidance for thoracocentesis, or intercostal chest tube placement. Sonography gives valuable information regarding size of the effusion, the presence of adhesions or loculations, and the echogenicity of the pleural fluid, suggesting presence of pus in the pleural cavity. It is especially helpful when the radiograph shows a white out and does not distinguish between pleural effusion and empyema, whereas sonography can. Furthermore, where chest skiagram can only detect pleural effusion minimum of 100–150 mL, ultrasonography can detect effusions as small as 5 mL, making it much more sensitive and effective investigation to detect small effusions/empyema.[7]

Sonographic appearance of pleural fluid varies according to the stage of effusion, ranging from an anechoic completely echo-free or sonolucent PPE to very echogenic fluid with septa as seen in frank empyema. Ultrasonography shows limiting membranes, suggesting the presence of loculated collections even when they are not so well seen on computed tomography (CT) scan. However, sonography cannot suggest the etiology of the effusion with certainty, for which a diagnostic thoracentesis is a must.[5]

Computed Tomography Scan

Empyema appears well-defined, smooth, round, or elliptical on CT scan. The parietal and visceral layers are separated by interposed empyema fluid, giving rise to the "split pleura sign" of empyema. The CT scan should not be performed routinely as it exposes the child to a very high radiation dose and other investigations provide better information for diagnosis and for guiding treatment decisions. It may have a limited role in the cases which do not respond to the initial medical management or before a surgery to delineate the anatomy and to rule out a lung abscess.[7]

Microbiological Diagnosis—Diagnostic Thoracentesis

The next most important investigation is the aspiration of the fluid and to confirm that it is pus. Fluid/pus aspirated should be sent for gram stain and culture to guide the therapy. In case of clear fluid is aspirated, it should also be subjected to cytological and biochemical examination to differentiate between the transudative and exudative effusions with cell count [white blood cells (WBCs)] is high, pH <7.2, lactate dehydrogenase (LDH) >1,000 IU/L, and glucose <40 mg/dL.[6]

MANAGEMENT

Supportive Management

All children with empyema should be hospitalized and started on supportive therapy, and antibiotic therapy.

Fluids and Hydration

If the child is toxic-looking with decreased oral intake, in severe respiratory distress or dehydrated, maintenance fluid should be provided.

Oxygen

Oxygen therapy is needed in cases with hypoxemia (peripheral $SpO_2 < 92\%$), or severe respiratory distress like in cases of massive empyema.

Antipyretics

Antipyretics should be judiciously used as fever is one of the parameters used to assess response.

Definitive Therapy

Management of empyema thoracis requires antibiotics, along with any of the following:[8]

- Insertion of intercostal chest tube for draining the pus
- Intercostal drainage with addition of fibrinolytics
- Open decortication
- Video-assisted thoracic surgery (VATS)
- Rib resection/thoracoplasty/lobectomy

And the decision is based on staging of the disease as shown in **Table 10.7.2**.

Antimicrobial Therapy

Antibiotics should be started on empirical basis initially and may need upgradation or change based on organism grown on the pus culture and its sensitivity pattern. The choice of empirical antibiotics is based on the likeliest causative organisms. Penicillin-group (cloxacillin 100–200 mg/kg/day) and third-generation cephalosporins (such as ceftriaxone 50–100 mg/kg/day) may be used as a first-line drugs. Co-amoxiclav is another good alternative drug. Upgradation to vancomycin/linezolid may be needed in patients not responding to the first-line therapy and in those MRSA is suspected/grown on culture or in hemodynamically unstable patients. Later, on the basis of organism grown and its sensitivity report, antibiotics can be upgraded. The preferred route of therapy is intravenous (IV) for initial 2 weeks or so, and it can then be replaced by oral therapy later once the patient is stable and accepting orally well. The total duration of therapy is 4–6 weeks. In case of complication like soft-tissue involvement, clindamycin may be required.[8,9]

Intercostal Chest Tube Drainage

Most of the symptomatic cases need drainage by an intercostal chest tube. Repeated thoracocentesis is not recommended except in a few with very thin pus. If the initial aspiration fails, the drainage may be done under the ultrasound guidance. Conscious sedation can be used for the chest tube insertion with all the personnel and equipment necessary for resuscitation. Small collections (<10 mm in a child below 2 years and <20 mm in a child above 2 years) with no significant symptoms or distress may respond to antibiotic therapy alone.[10]

TABLE 10.7.2: Management of empyema based on staging.

Stage	*Treatment*
Stage 1	Antibiotics, ± ICD if no clinical improvement and/or increasing fluid
Stage 2	Antibiotics + ICD ± fibrinolytics/VATS
Stage 3	VATS/thoracotomy

(ICD: intercostal chest drainage; VATS: video-assisted thoracoscopic surgery)

The chest tube is connected to an underwater seal bottle, which must always be kept below the level of the patient's chest. The drain should be clamped for 1 hour once 10 mL/kg of the initial fluid is removed. In older children and adolescents, not >1.5 L should be drained at once. Air column movement must be checked to ensure the correct positioning of the tube inside the pleural cavity. A chest radiograph is repeated after the chest drain insertion to check the placement of tube and lung expansion.[11]

The chest tube can be removed when the drain output decreases to <1–2 mL/kg/day (or <10–20 mL/day) for 2–3 consecutive days in presence of clinical and radiological improvement and there is no bubbling of air on coughing/crying/laughing. A nonfunctional drain (no air column movement) must be reassessed by a repeat imaging for need of repositioning or removal of tube. Loculation should be ruled out. The chest tube should be removed during expiration or a Valsalva maneuver. The chest X-ray is repeated after 24 hours to check for any recollection.

Role of Intrapleural Fibrinolytic Agents

The agents such as urokinase, streptokinase, and alteplase have been used to facilitate the drainage. Their use is recommended for CPPE (thick fluid with loculations) or empyema (frank pus), as it increases the drainage and obviates the need for surgical intervention. The treatment, however, is expensive and has side effects which can be serious.[8]

Response to Therapy

Children may continue to be febrile for initial 5–7 days of starting antibiotic therapy in case of *S. pneumoniae* and *H. influenzae* and a little longer in the case of *S. aureus* infection. The clinical response to therapy should be assessed with parameters, such as improvement in general condition, decreasing fever, improving air entry, normalization of laboratory parameters, such as white blood cell count, C-reactive protein, decrease in drain output and clearing on chest X-ray.[3,12]

A second-line treatment may be instituted in case of:

- Poor or no response after 96 hours of antibiotic therapy and drainage
- Persisting high spiking fever, and persistent drainage, a combination of vancomycin with piperacillin–tazobactam is suggested or else choice of antibiotics should be according to the culture report.

Parenteral therapy is continued till the child becomes afebrile or at least till the chest tube is removed and subsequently can be started on oral antibiotics to finish 4–6 weeks of therapy.

Failure of medical therapy, persisting sepsis, and large pleural collection beyond 10 days should prompt surgical referral. Cases of chronic empyema in a symptomatic child should be referred for open thoracostomy and decortication. Cases with persistent bronchopleural fistula is also an indication for surgical intervention. A symptom-free child with persistent radiological abnormality is not an indication for surgery.

COMPLICATIONS

Worsening sepsis can lead to septic shock. Due to intercostal tube malposition, complications like pneumothorax, bronchopleural fistulas, and pleural fibrosis may arise. Rarely, involvement of the subcutaneous tissue of chest wall may occur leading to empyema necessitans.[13]

KEY MESSAGES

- There is no "one size fits all" treatment for the PPE and empyema.
- *The pathology of empyema is a dynamic process:* It is not feasible to manage all stages of it with a single-therapeutic strategy.
- Management, therefore, needs to be tailor-made, using the broad principals described above on a case-by-case basis and requires clinical experience.
- Key steps in treatment are good antibiotic coverage with diagnostic thoracocentesis followed by insertion of drain.
- The outcome is usually good.
- The use of fibrinolysis in the early empyema stage may be guided by the user's experience, affordability, and cost versus benefit expected.
- Nonresolving cases may benefit from surgical intervention. However, efforts to achieve complete radiological clearance are largely nonproductive and inconsequential.
- In the long-term, most children will eventually show a complete expansion of the lung, if appropriately treated in the early phase.

CONCLUSION

Empyema refers to collection of pus in the pleural cavity. The common presentation is with high-grade fever, chest pain, breathing difficulty, and loss of appetite. On systemic examination, decreased chest expansion on the affected side and dullness on percussion with decreased air entry are often present. In a child with pneumonia, lack of response to the antibiotics within 48 hours of treatment should raise the suspicion of a complication like effusion. The earliest sign seen in X-ray chest is the obliteration of the costophrenic angle with white-out seen in later stages. Ultrasound chest is more sensitive in detecting smaller collections. CT scan of chest is indicated in those cases not responding to initial medical management or prior to surgery. Mainstay of the treatment is antibiotics. Drainage of pleural pus is required and ICD insertion to drain the pus from the pleural cavity is the mostcommon modality used. Timely management has good prognosis with complete resolution of the disease.

REFERENCES

1. Haggie S, Fitzgerald DA, Pandit C, Selvadurai H, Robinson P, Gunasekara H, et al. Increasing rates of pediatric empyema and disease severity with predominance of serotype 3 S. pneumonia: an Australian single-center, retrospective cohort 2011 to 2018. Pediatr Infect Dis J. 2019;38(12):e320-5.
2. Krenke K, Sadowy E, Podsiadły E, Hryniewicz W, Demkow U, Kulus M. Etiology of parapneumonic effusion and pleural empyema in children. The role of conventional and molecular microbiological tests. Respir Med. 2016;116:28-33.
3. Eastham KM, Freeman R, Kearns AM, Eltringham G, Clark J, Leeming J, et al. Clinical features, aetiology and outcome of empyema in children in the North East of England. Thorax. 2004;59(6):522-5.
4. Buckingham SC, King MD, Miller ML. Incidence and etiologies of complicated parapneumonic effusions in children, 1996 to 2001. Pediatr Infect Dis J. 2003;22(6):499-504.
5. Qureshi NR, Gleeson FV. Imaging of pleural disease. Clin Chest Med. 2006;27(2):193-213.
6. Na MJ. Diagnostic tools of pleural effusion. Tuberc Respir Dis (Seoul). 2014;76(5):199-210.
7. Colins JD, Burwell D, Furmanski S, Lorber P, Steckel RJ. Minimal detectable pleural effusions: a roentgen pathology model. Radiology. 1972;105(1):51-3.
8. Subhi R, Gelbart B, Ching N, Thompson J, Osowicki J, Rozen TH, et al. Characteristics, management and changing incidence of children with empyema in a paediatric intensive care unit. J Paediatr Child Health. 2022;58(6):1046-52.
9. Azoulay E. Pleural effusions in the intensive care unit. Curr Opin Pulm Med. 2003;9(4):291-7.
10. Shankar G, Sahadev R, Santhanakrishnan R. Pediatric empyema thoracis management: should the Consensus be different for the developing countries? J Pediatr Surg. 2020;55(3):513-7.
11. Menon P, Rao KL, Singh M, Venkatesh MA, Kanojia RP, Samujh R, et al. Surgical management and outcome analysis of stage III pediatric empyema thoracis. J Indian Assoc Pediatr Surg. 2010;15(1):9-14.
12. Proesmans M, Gijsens B, Van de Wijdeven P, De Caluwe H, Verhaegen J, Lagrou K, et al. Clinical outcome of parapneumonic empyema in children treated according to a standardized medical treatment. Eur J Pediatr. 2014;173(10):1339-45.
13. de Benedictis FM, Carloni I, Osimani P, Cobellis G, Martino A, Lanza C, et al. Prospective evaluation of Lung function in children with parapneumonic empyema. Pediatr Pulmonol. 2019;54(4):421-7.

10.8 Suppurative Lung Disease

L Subramanyam, NC Gowrishankar

INTRODUCTION

Suppurative disease of the lung includes bronchiectasis, lung abscess, and empyema. Bronchiectasis and lung abscess will be presented here. Empyema has been discussed separately in Chapter 10.7.

"Bronchiectasis" in children is one end of spectrum of chronic suppurative lung disease (CSLD). It is characterized by presence of persistent or recurrent cough, which is moist in nature associated with infection and/or inflammation of the airway along with evidence of abnormal dilatation of bronchi in computed tomography (CT) of chest.

"Chronic suppurative lung disease" is often used in the same context, with slightly different meaning. Bronchiectasis is a pathological diagnosis confirmed by a computed tomography (CT). CSLD is a clinical diagnosis secondary to endobronchial suppuration without CT evidence of bronchiectasis. Both bronchiectasis and CSLD are the end result of protracted bacterial bronchitis (PBB).

"Protracted bacterial bronchitis" progresses to bronchiectasis through stages of CSLD. PBB is characterized by isolated persistent wet cough lasting for >2 weeks that resolves with a course of oral antibiotics for 2–4 weeks. Bronchiectasis on the other hand is characterized by recurrent (>3) or persistent episodes of chronic productive cough (>4 weeks' duration) associated with coarse crackles and clubbing with or without hypoxemia. Two broad types of bronchiectasis are often described in clinical medicine—cystic fibrosis (CF)-related and non-CF related.

BRONCHIECTASIS

CAUSES

Etiological factors in bronchiectasis are traditionally classified as congenital and acquired. Congenital causes of bronchiectasis are usually associated with airway malformations, impaired mucociliary clearance, primary immunodeficiency, and genetic causes. Acquired bronchiectasis is due to postinfectious conditions, airway obstruction, autoimmune disorders, exposure to Inhaled toxins, and primary aspiration during swallowing causing progressive irreversible airway damage resulting in bronchiectasis. The conditions that predispose to bronchiectasis can be classified as in **Table 10.8.1**.[1]

TABLE 10.8.1: Causes of bronchiectasis.

Congenital	***Acquired***
Congenital anatomical defects: • Tracheobronchomalacia • Laryngeal cleft • Tracheoesophageal fistula (TEF-H type) • Bronchopulmonary sequestration • Congenital pulmonary airway malformation (CPAM)	*Infections*: • Persistent bacterial bronchitis (PBB) • Severe bacterial pneumonia (*Staphylococcus aureus, Streptococcus pneumoniae, Klebsiella, Pseudomonas*) • Tuberculosis • Human immunodeficiency virus (HIV) infection • Mycoplasma • Pertussis • Fungal infections • Measles • Varicella
Defective clearance of secretion: • Cystic fibrosis (CF) • Primary ciliary dyskinesia (PCD) • Alpha-1 antitrypsin deficiency	*Airway obstructions*: • Foreign body aspirations • Compression (lymph node, mass) • Vascular ring
Immunodeficiency state: • B-cell (IgG and IgA deficiency) • T-cell (Hyper-IgE and hyper-M syndromes) • Severe combined immune deficiency (SCID) • Ataxia telangiectasia (AT) • Chronic granulomatous disease (CGD)	*Allergy and autoimmune disease*: • Allergic bronchopulmonary aspergillosis (ABPA) • Rheumatoid arthritis, systemic lupus erythematosus
Genetic syndromes	*Recurrent aspirations*: • Neurological disorders (vocal card paralysis) • Swallowing dysfunction (direct/antegrade reflux) • Retrograde reflux—gastroesophageal reflux disease (GERD)
	Environmental: • Toxic inhalations • Smoke, irritant gases

The types of disorders that cause bronchiectasis vary among populations and age-groups. Infections and acquired causes of bronchiectasis predominate in developing nations, whereas CF, congenital anomalies of the airways, or immunodeficiency are more common in children of developed nations. The common syndromes associated with bronchiectasis are given below:[1]

- *Williams-Campbell syndrome:* Developmental defect of the tracheobronchial tree
- *Mounier-Kuhn syndrome:* Associated with tracheobronchomegaly
- *Kartagener syndrome:* A form of ciliary dyskinesia characterized by bronchiectasis, sinusitis and situs inversus
- *Middle lobe syndrome:* Compression of middle lobe bronchus by lymph node leading on to bronchiectasis
- *Yellow nail syndrome:* Characterized by yellow nail, bronchiectasis, pleural effusion, and lymphedema
- *Young syndrome:* Young syndrome describes patients with bronchiectasis, sinusitis, and obstructive azoospermia who have no evidence of CF and PCD.
- *Syndromes associated with immune deficiency:* Ataxia telangiectasia, DiGeorge syndrome.

PATHOGENESIS

The pathogenesis of bronchiectasis usually involves a combination of chronic or recurrent infection, airway inflammation, airway obstruction, and/or impaired mucociliary clearance, interacting in a vicious cycle that causes progressive damage to the lower airway structure. Chronic endobronchial suppurative disease represents a spectrum ranging from PBB to CSLD to bronchiectasis.[1]

While the relationship among these disorders has not been fully established, a pathobiologic model has been proposed which suggests that PBB, CSLD, and bronchiectasis represent a spectrum of disease with PBB at one end and irreversible bronchiectasis at the other. All three diseases have similar pathophysiology with airway inflammation **(Fig. 10.8.1)**.

Whatever be the disease, the common cause of bronchiectasis is repeated or persistent airway injury, mucus stasis, infections, and predominantly neutrophilic inflammation. There is infiltration of neutrophils and T lymphocytes in the airway as a result of infection. The inflammatory mediators released as a result of inflammation includes interleukin-8 (IL-8), neutrophil elastase, tumor necrosis factor (TNF), and prostanoids. The presence of large amount of these inflammatory mediators in the mucosa of the airway leads to a complex process of tissue destruction including the airway cartilage resulting in abnormal dilatation of bronchi. If this process is not stopped by proper anti-infective therapy and airway clearance, the continued inflammatory process leads to airway remodeling wherein the dilatation of airways become permanent.

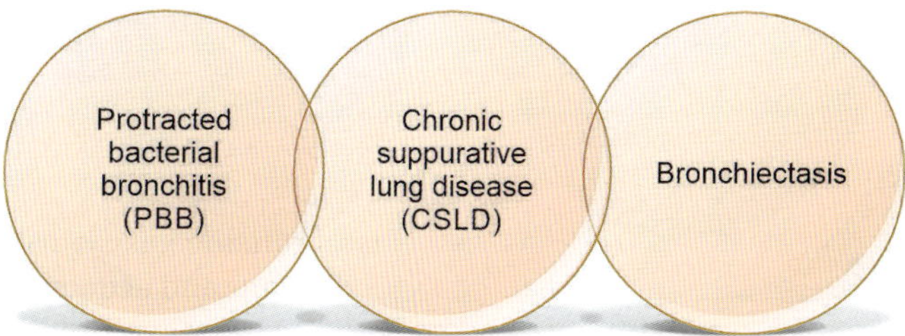

Fig. 10.8.1: Evolution of bronchiectasis.

The airways become collapsible, limiting airflow, especially with forced expiration. The lung parenchyma is often involved, developing areas of atelectasis, emphysema, and fibrosis. In addition, there is marked hypertrophy of the bronchial vasculature which is prone to rupture.

Morphologically bronchiectasis is classified as cylindrical, varicose, and saccular (cystic). Cylindrical is mildly enlarged bronchi that fails to taper distally; this is an early feature after an infection and can be reversed on appropriate management. Varicose type has a beaded appearance due to areas of constriction and dilation. Saccular is the most severe form, i.e., irreversible ballooning of airways.[1]

Bronchiectasis is sometimes classified by its anatomic distribution (generalized versus focal/segmental). Generalized bronchiectasis is typically seen in cases with an underlying systemic disease or condition, whereas focal bronchiectasis is usually the end result of a localized disease process such as bronchial obstruction.

CLINICAL MANIFESTATIONS

The most common symptom in children with bronchiectasis is *persistent cough*, and is typically "wet" or productive. The absence of sputum production does not exclude bronchiectasis, because children younger than 6 years old may not be able to expectorate sputum.[2]

Some patients present with episodic exacerbations of infection, characterized by increased cough and sputum production that may be associated with change in color of sputum, fever, and pleuritic chest pain and dyspnea. These exacerbations typically respond to antibiotic therapy. Dyspnea and exercise intolerance are uncommon at presentation but may develop as the disease progresses or may occur during an acute exacerbation of the disease due to intercurrent infection.

Hemoptysis is caused by erosion of inflamed airway tissue adjacent to pulmonary vessels. The amount of bleeding can range from mild with blood streaked sputum to profuse amounts of fresh bleeding if larger pulmonary vessels rupture.

Children with severe bronchiectatic lung disease may have clubbing, indicating severe hypoxemia due to mismatched pulmonary ventilation and perfusion. If the hypoxemia is prolonged and profound, it may lead to pulmonary hypertension and cor pulmonale.

The underlying disorder responsible for the bronchiectasis may also cause other symptoms at presentation and provide clues to the diagnosis. Failure to thrive is frequently seen in diseases such as CF and immunodeficiency disorders. Chronic sinusitis is common among children with CF, ciliary dysfunction disorders, and immunodeficiencies. The presence of congenital anomalies should alert the clinician to the possibility of associated anomalies that predispose to bronchiectasis (e.g., anomalies of the tracheobronchial tree).[2,3]

EVALUATION

The evaluation includes a complete medical history and physical examination, radiographic imaging, as well as laboratory testing and pulmonary function test.

A complete medical history including past medical, family, travel, and environmental history is a crucial part of the evaluation and can be helpful in identifying the underlying cause for bronchiectasis. Certain features of the history should raise concern for specific underlying disorders; for example, history of choking suggests foreign body aspiration and chronic aspiration should be considered in patients with recurrent pneumonia particularly those with neurologic dysfunction.

Pulmonary examination may reveal the following features: Crackles and rhonchi, which are often heard over the area of bronchiectasis, wheezing, which is less common; clubbing of the nailbed, a basic clinical sign of bronchiectasis and chest wall deformity, can be seen in obstructive lung diseases (e.g., CF), in which hyperinflation of the lungs results in increased anterior to posterior chest diameter.[3]

DIAGNOSIS

The suggestion for a possible diagnosis of bronchiectasis should occur if any child presents with moist cough persisting for 4 weeks or longer especially if there is inadequate response to treatment. Also if the child with moist cough has had hemoptysis and crackles which are persistent and have no obvious etiology for their presence, pneumonia which is recurring in nature, respiratory symptoms which are recurrent especially if there is accompanying esophagitis, the diagnosis of bronchiectasis become most probable.[3,4]

Chest imaging is the cornerstone of diagnosis of bronchiectasis and is the first investigation any child with moist cough is subjected to. Parenchymal infiltrates giving a clue to the diagnosis of pneumonia can be provided by X-ray chest. Unilateral hyperinflation or atelectasis in X-ray chest guides the clinician to proceed with further investigation to rule out possible intraluminal or extraluminal cause. If bronchiectasis is seen in chest X-ray, it indicates that the damage occurred is permanent and cannot be reversed. Findings in chest X-ray includes tram track which occurs due to thickened and dilated walls of the bronchi. Many a times ring-like structural changes may also be visible in those with long-standing bronchiectasis along with volume loss in the lungs **(Fig. 10.8.2)**.

Multidetector CT (MDCT) scan with high-resolution computed tomography (HRCT) reconstruction is the current imaging modality of choice. Contrast study may be required if tuberculosis (TB), mass lesion, or lymph nodes are suspected to be the underlying pathology. The pathognomonic finding in CT chest for a diagnosis of bronchiectasis is the increase in bronchoarterial ratio, which is the ratio of the internal diameter of the bronchi (airway) compared to the outer diameter of the accompanying artery. The normal ratio is below 0.8. If the ratio is above 0.8 in children, it indicates ectasia of bronchi and is diagnostic of bronchiectasis.

Other findings in CT suggesting bronchiectasis include signet rings wherein the airway which is dilated with the accompanying artery giving the characteristic appearance **(Fig. 10.8.3)**, failure of airways to taper toward the periphery,

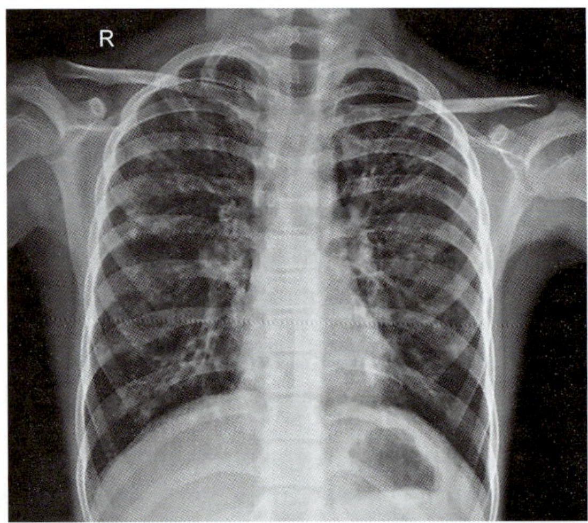

Fig. 10.8.2: Chest X-ray—bronchiectasis in right lower lobe.

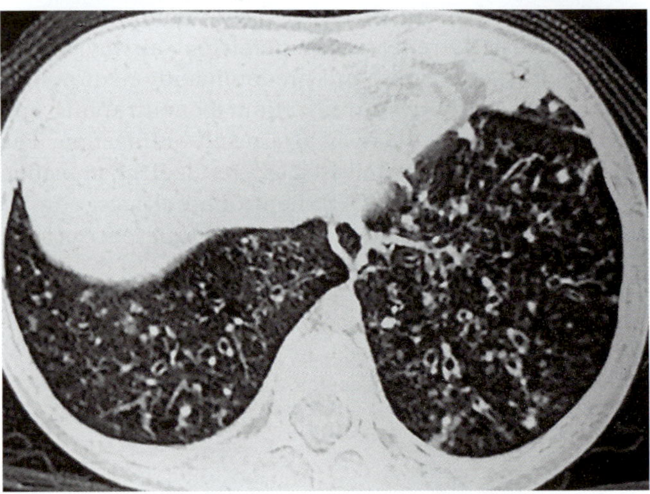

Fig. 10.8.3: Computed tomography (CT) chest—bronchiectasis—signet rings.

bronchial wall thickening, mucus impaction, air-fluid levels inside airway lumen and sometimes, frank cystic changes. Bronchography which was used previously to diagnose bronchiectasis is not used nowadays.

Once a diagnosis of bronchiectasis is made, further investigations are oriented to find out the etiology and should be prioritized based on the clinical picture. The panel of tests include sweat chloride estimation (to exclude CF), complete blood count (CBC), tests for immune function [immunoglobulin profile—IgG, IgA, IgM and IgE, flow cytometry for chronic granulomatous disease (CGD)] and tests to rule out TB and human immunodeficiency virus (HIV) infection.

Further, specialized tests like bronchoscopy and bronchoalveolar lavage (BAL) might be needed based on the yield from the initial tests. Structural alterations of airway can be easily identified by flexible bronchoscopy which can also help to get BAL samples. Primary ciliary dyskinesia (PCD) needs to be ruled out by demonstration of ciliary motility or structure (under electron microscope), nasal nitric oxide (NO) measurement, and genetic studies (clinical exome sequencing). As untreated allergic bronchopulmonary aspergillosis (ABPA) can lead to bronchiectasis, it needs to be ruled out while evaluating a child with bronchiectasis.

Bacterial culture of lower airway secretions is warranted at diagnosis, during exacerbations and sometimes, for routine surveillance. A spontaneously expectorated or induced sputum (following 3% saline nebulization) sample usually suffices. Otherwise, a BAL might help in organism isolation. Oropharyngeal and nasopharyngeal specimens are sometimes used as surrogate, but might lack specificity.

Monitoring a child with bronchiectasis is mainly by looking for control of symptoms and gain in weight along with assessment of respiratory function by spirometry every 3 to 6 months. This will help to find out if the interventions are able to modify the course of the disease. Culture of sputum can give insight about the microbial colonization in the diseased airway, which helps to choose the appropriate antimicrobials for any exacerbations if it is going to occur. Imaging may not be necessary during follow-up except in those whose response to treatment during exacerbations is inadequate.

MANAGEMENT

Mainstay of treatment in children with bronchiectasis is medical, with surgery being reserved for rare indications. Airway clearance technique to keep the airways free of secretions along with nutritional rehabilitation by advising intake of proteins with good net protein utilization will help to prevent frequent pulmonary exacerbation. Antimicrobial treatment is reserved for pulmonary exacerbations. All of the above form the framework of medical management.[3,5]

General Measures

These include adequate protein and calories intake, good hydration, vaccination against respiratory pathogens (pneumococcal, influenza, measles, *Haemophilus influenzae,* and pertussis) and avoidance of exposure to smoke (biofuel, tobacco) or environmental pollution.

Specific Therapy

It is possible in a handful of conditions like airway foreign body and active infections (e.g., TB). Children with aspiration syndromes may benefit from medical (treatment of reflux) or surgical treatment (in case no response to medical treatment). If bronchiectasis occurs in those with B-cell immunodeficiency, intravenous infusion of gamma globulin once in every 4 weeks can help to overcome frequent pulmonary infection.[3]

In case of evidence of reactive airway disease (e.g., presence of wheezing), inhaled steroids (ICS) and bronchodilators can be used. Treatment if started early in the course of disease, the airway changes can be reversed, especially in younger children.

Supportive Therapy

Airway Clearance Therapy

It is the mainstay of nonpharmacological treatment of bronchiectasis. Adequate intake of oral fluid can help to maintain the secretions of the airway in thin state. Physiotherapy for draining impacted secretions is an essential part of treatment and needs to be emphasized to the family early. A combination of cupped hand percussion, dependent drainage of the affected lobe of the lung along with coughing and chest wall vibration helps to clear the diseased airway of its increased secretions, which can be augmented by the use of oscillating positive expiratory pressure (OPEP). Improved ability to clear the increased secretions in the airway can be done the active participation of the affected child by techniques like active cycle of breathing which in association with high-frequency chest wall oscillation (HFCWO) by chest vest along with nebulized hypertonic saline during HFCWO helps in better airway clearance taking into consideration the age of the patient, compliance, and available resources. Hypertonic saline 3% nebulization 2–3 times as a mucoactive agent can be considered in selected patients.[3,5]

Pretreatment with a bronchodilator might be essential to avoid bronchospasm. Chest physiotherapy usually follows the mucoactive agent inhalation. Recombinant human DNase may worsen lung function and should be avoided.

Treatment of Infections

Both viral and bacterial infections may cause exacerbations and need to be treated aggressively. Efforts should be made for eradication after the first isolation of *Pseudomonas aeruginosa*. Inhaled antibiotics (tobramycin) may be added to systemic ones for this purpose. Intermittent exacerbations are also treated with systemic antibiotics for 14 days, guided by culture of sputum or BAL and sensitivity patterns. Severe exacerbations often require admission and intravenous antibiotics. Long-term macrolides are now a part of recommendation in patients with recurrent exacerbations.[3]

Surgical Treatment

The indications of surgery are limited. Surgical treatment may be needed if the disease is localized but medical management cannot bring it under control. Surgical treatment includes either removal of the affected lobe or lung. Surgery may be needed if there is uncontrolled localized bleed too. Lobectomy should be viewed only as a last resort and has few indications like poor control of symptoms and growth failure despite optimal medical management and uncontrolled hemoptysis despite bronchial artery embolization. Surgery is usually not a valid option in extensive or diffuse disease.[5]

PROGNOSIS

Overall the prognosis for patients with bronchiectasis has improved considerably in the past few decades. Early recognition of pneumonia, prompt treatment with appropriate antibiotics, prevention of predisposing conditions and improved surgical outcomes are the likely reasons. Poor prognostic factors include bilateral lung disease, saccular bronchiectasis, frequent exacerbations, and *Pseudomonas* colonization.

CONCLUSION

Bronchiectasis is a common chronic respiratory morbidity in children. The etiology depends on the geographic region and of underlying illness. Common causes of non-CF bronchiectasis in Indian children are postinfectious and airway obstructions. When any child presents with a wet cough lasting 4 weeks or longer, a diagnosis of bronchiectasis should be thought of. Depending on the underlying etiology, the presentation of bronchiectasis can vary. The investigation of choice for making a diagnosis of bronchiectasis is CT chest. Management is mainly medical with surgery reserved for localized disease, which is not responding to medical management. Long-term regular follow-up is usually essential for these patients with monitoring of growth, lung function, and airway microbiology.

LUNG ABSCESS

Lung abscess are cavities, one or more, in the lung due not only to destruction of tissues but also necrosis leading on to inflammatory cell accumulation in the cavities. A primary lung abscess occurs in a previously healthy patient with no underlying disorders. A secondary lung abscess occurs in a patient with underlying or predisposing condition. Lung abscess develops if there is inappropriate or late institution of antimicrobials while managing lobar pneumonia. Aspiration is the most important predisposing factor for lung abscess. The usual timeline for lung abscess to develop after an aspiration event is either 1 or 2 weeks. Important factors predisposing to development of lung abscess are obstruction in the airway or deviant development of lung.[6]

ETIOLOGY

Both anaerobic and aerobic organisms can cause lung abscesses. Common anaerobic bacteria that can cause a pulmonary abscess include Bacteroides spp., Fusobacterium spp., and Peptostreptococcus spp. Abscesses also can be caused by aerobic organisms such as Streptococcus spp., *Staphylococcus aureus, Escherichia coli, Klebsiella pneumoniae* and *P. aeruginosa*. Among these, *S. aureus* is the most common organism.[6]

CLINICAL FEATURES

There are no specific clinical manifestations peculiar to lung abscess. The symptoms of pneumonia including fever, fast breathing, and cough are the same symptoms with which a child with lung abscess presents with. In addition they can have chest pain, anorexia, hemoptysis, and foul-smelling breath. Physical examination typically reveals tachypnea, dyspnea, retractions with accessory muscle use, decreased breath sounds, and dullness on percussion in the affected area. Crackles may be heard on auscultation.

DIAGNOSIS

Chest X-ray can give a clue to the diagnosis of lung abscess, which can be confirmed by CT chest. Chest X-ray can show lung abscess like a thick-walled cavity **(Fig. 10.8.4A)**. The location, the size, and number of lung abscess cavities in the lungs are delineated by CT chest **(Fig. 10.8.4B)**. Persistence of clinical symptoms along with persisting radiological changes including consolidation, bulging fissure, etc., should make one think of the possibility of a lung abscess developing. Aspiration of the abscess under guidance of imaging can help to get fluid from abscess cavity for microbiological studies.

MANAGEMENT

Antibiotics covering the common organisms causing lung abscess need to started initially intravenously which can be modified to oral medication as the child improves. But the course of antibiotics need to be given for a longer duration.

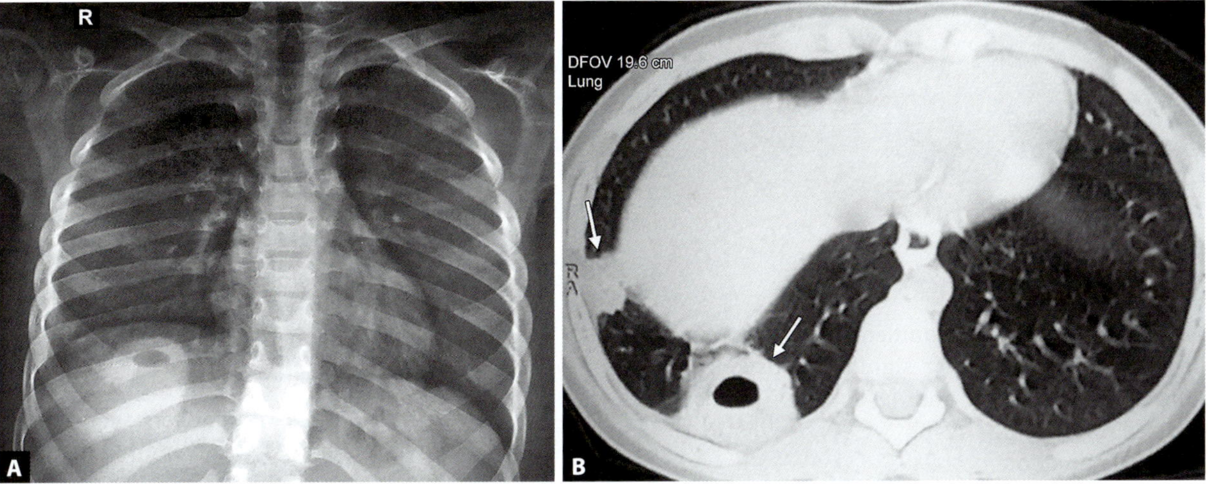

Figs. 10.8.4A and B: (A) Chest X-ray—lung abscess right lower lobe; and (B) CT chest—lung abscess right lower lobe.

Antibiotic choice should be guided by gram stain and culture but initially should include aerobic and anaerobic coverage. Treatment regimens should include agents active against a penicillinase-resistant *S. aureus* and anaerobes. If gram-negative bacteria are suspected or isolated, an aminoglycoside should be added. The duration is determined by the clinical response, but is usually a total of 4 or 2 weeks after the patient is afebrile. The average duration for fever to subside is 3–4 days. 80–90% of lung abscesses in children resolve with antibiotic therapy alone and spontaneous drainage through the tracheobronchial tree, provided that bronchial obstruction is cleared.[7]

In cases if it fails to improve or worsen after 72 hours of antibiotic therapy, needle aspiration or percutaneous catheter drainage may provide diagnostic information and therapeutic benefit without the increased risk of complications as occurs in children with necrotizing pneumonia. At least 3 weeks of IV/oral antibiotic therapy should be given before lobectomy is considered for treatment failure.

COMPLICATIONS

Hemorrhage occurring within the cavity of the lung abscess can present as hemoptysis and can also lead to spread of infection to other parts of the lungs. If not managed correctly, lung abscess can lead to empyema and bronchopleural fistula while septicemia and brain abscess are remote complications.

PROGNOSIS

Overall, prognosis for children with primary pulmonary abscesses is excellent. Most children become asymptomatic within 7–10 days. Radiologic abnormalities usually resolve in 1–3 months.

REFERENCES

1. Goyal V, Chang AB. Bronchiectasis in children: Pathophysiology and causes. In UpToDate. Chmiel JF, Hoppin AG (Eds). Topic 6358 Version 26.0 Accessed on 1st Nov 2023
2. Goyal V. Bronchiectasis in children: Clinical manifestations and evaluation In Uptodate Mallory GB, Hoppin GB (Eds). Topic 6360 Version 24.0 Accessed on 10th Nov 2023
3. Goyal V. Bronchiectasis in children without cystic fibrosis: Management. In UpToDate. Mallory GB, Hoppin AG (Eds). Topic 6355 Version 35.0 Accessed on 1st Nov 2024.
4. Das RR, Kumar K, Gulla KM. Bronchiectasis—Non-cystic fibrosis. Indian J Pract Pediatr. 2023;25(2):165-70.
5. Vijayasekaran D, Sivabalan S. Bronchiectasis. In: Subramanyam L, Sivabalan S, Gowrishankar NC, Vijayasekaran D, Balachandran A (Eds). Essentials of Pediatric Pulmonology. Chennai: Pediatric Pulmonology Foundation; 2008. pp. 196-200.
6. Patradoon-Ho P, Fitzgerald DA. Lung abscess in children. Paediatr Respir Rev. 2007;8(1):77-84.
7. Barson WJ. Pneumonia in children: Inpatient treatment. In: Edwards MS, Blake D (Eds). UpToDate. Topic 5986 Version 59.0. Accessed on 10th Nov 2023

10.9 Bronchial Asthma

H Paramesh

INTRODUCTION

Asthma is an early-onset environmental noncommunicable chronic lung disease, having significant psycho-socio-economic burden on family and the society. The disease is characterized by:

- Airway inflammation
- Airway obstruction mainly due to muscle spasm, associated with mucosal edema and accumulation of the mucus
- Airway hyperreactivity to aerobiologicals and irritants
- Airway remodeling in uncontrolled asthma

EPIDEMIOLOGY

The global prevalence of asthma varies from 1 to 29% of the population in different countries.[1] A hospital-based study in Bengaluru on children under 18 years of age from 1979, 1984, 1989 and 1999 showed a prevalence of 9%, 10.5%, 18.5%, 24.5% and 29.5% respectively. This was attributed to change in the demography of the city with increase in industries, density of population, and increased motor vehicles and air pollution.[2] However in the year 2004, the asthma prevalence decreased by 3% and further by 1% in 2009, which has been opined by experts due to saturation of the genetically predisposed population and one can expect small peaks in future but severity of the disease may be increased. True to the opinion the persistent asthma increased from 20 to 72% and persistent severe asthma by 4–11% between 1999 and 2009. The same trend been appreciated in Australia, Hong Kong, UK, Italy, and Mexico. Recent Indian Council for Medical Research (ICMR) data shows the asthma prevalence in India is 24% in 2014.[3]

The socio-economic burden of asthma from hospitalization, emergency room visits, clinic visits, and medication is 2% of healthcare budget, more than tuberculosis (TB) and human immunodeficiency virus (HIV) infections combined. The cost of management of asthma patient is $3,300 per patient per year; 69% of parents had taken time off from work; 13% of people lost their jobs and 70% of mild asthma patients account 20% of the cost.

The increased prevalence of asthma is noticed in the following situations:

- Urban children
- Rapid urbanization increasing prevalence in the semirural areas compared to rural
- Children attending schools in heavy traffic areas, especially from the lower socioeconomic population
- Children living in poorly ventilated homes and single room dwelling huts
- Children living in houses with smokers; there is a threefold increase in asthma if one person smokes tobacco in the house.
- Children living in houses where noncommercial cooking fuel like cow dung cakes, agricultural waste, and firewood are used as cooking fuel
- During *Diwali* and similar festivals, there is a 100% increase in emergency room visits for acute asthma episodes due to increase in sulfur dioxide (SO_2) in the air from bursting of the firecrackers.
- The prevalence in children <5 years is about 75%; above 5 years of age around 25%
- *Male predominance*: The male-to-female ratio is 2:1 owing to the relatively small airways with which boys are born and inherited as an autosomal dominant trait
- Positive family history of asthma either in parents, siblings, or grandparents
- Air pollution not only triggers asthma but also changes genetic pattern and change in nonatopic asthma to atopic asthma.[2]

ETIOPATHOGENESIS

The etiological factors can be classified as biologicals and irritants as shown in **Table 10.9.1**.

Aerobiologicals

Children develop sensitivity to indoor allergens, as they grow older in the atmosphere they are reared. The predominant indoor allergen is the house dust mite. It takes 100 dust mites/g of dust to get sensitized and 500 dust mites/g of dust to produce wheezing. About 50% of the perennial asthma is due to dust mites. The pollen and mold sensitivity is observed in 7.5% of asthmatics, whereas cockroach sensitivity is 25% and pets 5% of cases.

Viral Infection

The precipitating factor for an asthma attack in 40% of the children is viral upper respiratory tract infections (URTIs).

TABLE 10.9.1: Etiological factors in asthma.

Biologicals	*Irritants*
Dust mites (50%)	Tobacco smoke
Cockroaches (25%)	Cooking fuel smoke
Pollens (7.5%)	Mosquito coil smoke
Fungi (7.5%)	Sprays
Pets—saliva, urine (5.0%)	Perfumes
Viral infections (40%)	Formaldehyde and volatile organic compounds from compressed wood and panel board furniture, etc.

Most children develop rhinitis with or without fever, followed by cough. In these children, chest congestion persists over 10 days, often with wheeze. The incidence varies from 29% to 54% in both atopic and nonatopic individuals. Respiratory syncytial virus (RSV) and rhinoviruses are the predominant viruses triggering asthma.

Season

Seasonal variation of asthma attacks is experienced by 35% of the children. The incidence is higher during monsoon, followed by winter, and is less common in summer. An increase of asthma attacks in summer from 2% to 28.5% in 17-year period has been noted, which is attributed to an increase in automobile emission from slow traffic and the bright sun converting the oxides of nitrogen to ozone (O_3), which aggravates the asthma sensitivity; in addition, O_3 has the cumulative effect.[4]

Food

Diet plays a multifaceted role in shaping the observed worldwide trends of childhood allergies. Sensitivity can occur by ingestion, inhalation of cooking fumes, and from skin contact. Both early- and late-phase reactions are observed. Only 10% of the asthmatics react to food and drinks. Eight foods—groundnut, egg, crustaceans, milk, fish, tree nuts, wheat, and soybean—account for 90% of the food allergies globally. In our country, we can add lentils, black gram, and many legumes. The incidence of food allergy is 4–8% in children globally. A community survey done in Mysuru and Bengaluru showed an incidence of only 1.88%. However, many parents of asthmatic children have misconceptions and perceptions about food allergy, especially fruits, such as guava, banana, citrus fruits, grapes, and tomato.

Pets

Pets are not the major factor for the asthma in India. Cats are more allergic than dogs. The saliva, urine, and dander are the causes for allergy sensitization. Specific immunotherapy for cat's allergy is beneficial, but dogs are not established equally. Dogs are stress busters, and in some asthmatic children, pet therapy (dog) has been recommended.

Air Pollution

Air pollution is both outdoor and indoor. The important outdoor pollutants are black smoke, respirable suspended particulates, SO_2, nitric oxide (NO), carbon monoxide (CO), and O_3 produced by the combustion of fossil fuels, factories, mines, paper pulp mills, and automobile exhaust. Nitrogen oxide triggers asthma in 65% of the patients and also sensitizes to dust mites allergy. O_3 triggers asthma in 43% of the patients, and SO_2 sensitizes the asthmatics by tenfold.[2,4]

Recent observation shows outdoor air pollution increased by 115.3% while indoor air pollution decreased by 64.2% mainly by increased use of cooking gas and migration of people to urban areas.[2,5]

PATHOPHYSIOLOGY

Asthma is a complex condition where interaction of genetics and environment occurs involving many inflammatory cells, which release a wide range of mediators. These mediators act on the cells of the airway leading to smooth muscle contraction, mucus hypersecretion, plasma leakage, edema, activation of cholinergic reflexes, and activation of sensory nerves, which lead to amplification of the continuing inflammatory response. The chronic inflammation leads to the structural changes, including subepithelial fibrosis and smooth muscle hypertrophy and hyperplasia. This late process is less easily reversed than the acute changes and might end up with airway remodeling.

To mount an allergic response, one has to be sensitized to an allergen. When an allergen enters the epithelial cell, the dendritic cells below the epithelial cell act like a custom officer—catch the allergen by their long arms and break the allergen into small pieces called epitopes. These are handed over to the T-lymphocytes, the orchestrator of the immune system, which give the instruction to various cells for appropriate action. The B-lymphocytes are instructed to handle pollens, which produce interleukins (IL-4 and IL-13) to make immunoglobulin E (IgE) antibodies. The IgE arms the mast cell, the muscle man of immune system. The mast cell binds very large number of IgE molecules of various allergens. The activation of mast cell (mast cell degranulation) releases preformed histamine. The continued exposure to allergen brings eosinophils (dreaded cell for parasites) into action. The eosinophilic granules release toxic chemicals, such as eosinophil cationic protein, eosinophil-derived neurotoxin, and major basic protein, which damage the epithelium and sensory nerves causing hyperresponsiveness to nonallergic stimuli. The mast cells are responsible for the early-phase reaction and eosinophils for the late-phase reaction in general.

It is the imbalance in the reaction oxygen species (ROS) and antioxidants that produces the oxidative stress producing smooth muscle contraction increased permeability of vessels, impairment of beta-adrenergic receptors, mucus production altered release of inflammatory mediators, airway hyperresponsiveness, and epithelial damage.

CLINICAL FEATURES

All that wheezes is not asthma but most asthmatics do not wheeze. The common clinical features include the following:

- *Recurrent cough:* The majority of children present with recurrent cough 90% of the time. The cough is more at night or early morning; induced by physical or emotional stress (crying, laughing, and shouting).
- *Recurrent wheeze* is a prominent feature seen in 74% of asthmatic children. Many people mistake rattling in the chest as wheeze. Wheezing is not felt on palpation of the chest.
- *Retractions* are a common feature for airway obstruction, depending on the severity of asthma; they may be present over subcostal, intercostal, or suprasternal areas, with flaring of nostrils.
- *Post-tussive vomiting* (vomiting after a bout of coughing) occurs in 5% of the cases.
- Abdominal pain rarely occurs due to the overworking of expiratory abdominal muscles in 3% of the children.
- Chest pain is present rarely in 1% of the children.
- Other comorbid conditions, such as allergic rhinitis, sinusitis, serous otitis media, eczema, and conjunctivitis, may be present.

DIAGNOSIS

Diagnosis of asthma is mainly by the history and physical examination. The diagnosis of asthma in infants and preschoolers is often difficult due to poor cooperation for diagnostic procedures, hesitation by pediatricians, time-consuming and practicality, and ethical issues. However, an early diagnosis is essential for timely treatment to improve the quality of life, physical and psychological development; to prevent chronic pulmonary disease due to "airway remodeling"; to educate on the preventive measures; to cut the healthcare cost; and to prognosticate.

Preschool Children

The diagnosis of asthma is made based on clinical features only with following features:[6]

- *Variable respiratory symptoms of:*
    - Wheeze
    - Shortness of breath
    - Chest tightness
    - Cough persisting >2 weeks at night
- *Associated with other features:*
    - Having wheeze, cough with emotional stress, (crying laughing shouting) or physical stress (running, jumping playing) in the absence of any respiratory infections
    - Having eczema, allergic rhinitis, family history of atopy
    - Improvement with controller medicines during 2–3 months treatment and relapse after cessation
    - If lung function is normal, repeat reversibility testing when patient is symptomatic or [after withholding short-acting beta-2-agonists (SABA) for >4 hours, twice daily inhaled corticosteroids–long-acting beta-2-agonists (ICS–LABA) for >24 hours, and daily ICS–LABA for >36 hours]
- However, one has to document the variable expiratory airflow limitation at least once preferably before starting controllers.

In young infants who are wheezing, the healthcare personnel should observe for two clinical features of reversibility of airway obstruction following nebulization—whether the social smile of an infant to the mother returns and whether the infant starts feeding due to improvement in breathing with a decrease in wheezing. These may be documented as reversibility of airway obstruction.

The phenotype classification of asthma in children over 2 years of age helps the clinician to distinguish the types of asthma and provide appropriate management and prognostication as shown in **Flowchart 10.9.1**.

School-going Children[6]

- *Peak expiratory flow (PEF)* measurement before and after salbutamol nebulization with improvement (12–15%) is highly suggestive of reversible airway obstruction in asthma. This simple and less expensive procedure can be used to monitor the therapeutic response. Early asthma attack can be recognized by measuring diurnal variation in PEF. It measures the air coming out of larger- and medium-sized airways.
- *Spirometry* is the central tool for defining the obstructive airway disease. In asthma, there is decreased forced expiratory volume in 1 second (FEV_1), FEV_1/FVC ratio (forced volume in 1 second/forced vital capacity). It also measures small airway obstruction [forced expiratory flow (FEF 25–75)]. FEV_1/FVC ratio < 80% indicates airflow obstruction.
- *Eosinophil count:* The increased eosinophil count in the blood is suggestive of an allergic phenomenon.
- *Total IgE level:* It is beneficial only to recognize the atopic background of asthma. It helps to predict a response to steroids, the prognosis, and the possibility of development of persistent as well as strongly advocated environment control.

Flowchart 10.9.1: Identification of asthma phenotypes.

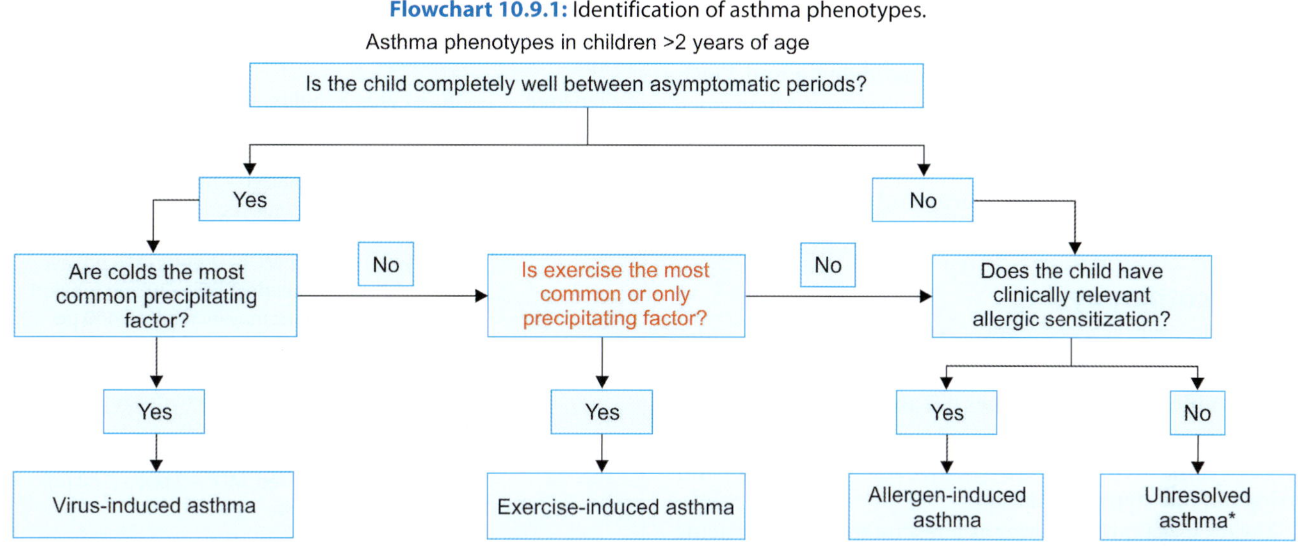

*Children may also be atopic. Different etiologies, including irritant exposure and as yet not evident allergies, may be involved here.
Source: Bacharier LB, Boner A, Carlsen KH, Eigenmann PA, Frischer T, Götz M, et al. Diagnosis and treatment of asthma in childhood: a PRACTALL consensus report. Allergy. 2008;63(1):5-34.

- *Specific IgE level:* It is needed for specific immunotherapy and before the use of anti-IgE antibody treatment.
- *Chest radiograph* is not routinely needed to diagnose asthma. It is needed only when the diagnosis is not clear, or any complications are suspected. Children below 5 years do not have lung collaterals, and as a result, one may see subsegmental, segmental, or lobar atelectasis quite often in radiographs, which might be misdiagnosed and treated as recurrent pneumonia.
- *Breath nitric oxide* is used in some pulmonary centers for monitoring the eosinophilic airway inflammation. It is not used much in children for various reasons.
- *Breath volatile organic compound (VOC) analysis* offers the possibility of a rapid straightforward and noninvasive method to measure the control of asthma in future.
- *Skin testing with allergens* is the gold standard to identify the specific allergens and used before immunotherapy for aeroallergens.
- *Bronchial challenge tests* and other physiological tests do not have a major role in the diagnosis of asthma in children.
- *Impulse oscillometry* is an attractive method to determine the respiratory resistance of the lungs with simple breathing giving details of the ventilation on the elastic properties of lung and homogeneity of the ventilation.

MANAGEMENT

The management of asthma includes efforts to minimize risk and control symptoms:[6]

- Education
- Environment control
- Pharmacotherapy
- Regular follow-up

Education

The pediatrician must spend time to clear the misconceptions about the disease, sexual bias, no communicability of the disease, fear of inhalers, steroids, etc. In India, doctors should always include the grandparents in counseling. Individual counseling is preferred in adolescents.[7,8]

Environment Control

Environmental control is the most important factor in the control of asthma. The aim should be to avoid allergens and irritants:

- *Dust mites:* Avoid carpets, upholstered furniture, use plastic covers to pillows and mattresses for easy washability, and expose them to sunlight once a week, wash soft toys periodically, and wet mop the floorings.
- *Cockroach:* Cover garbage and unused food containers.
- *Fungus:* Attend to damp walls, have good ventilation, and clean the shower curtains weekly.
- *Pets:* Ownership reduces asthma by having endotoxin with TH1 stimulation Our observation in Bangalore for the past 3 decades reveal that the prevalence of asthma is more in lower pet ownership and low in high pet ownership. Pets are stress buster and best companions in modern satellite families with working parents. We recommend pet therapy in children with persistent asthma. Global Initiative for Asthma (GINA) recommends two pets at home. Pets' saliva and urine need to be cleaned.[9]

- Avoid strong odors, smoke, mosquito coil burning, and especially tobacco smoke.
- Have indoor plants to absorb formaldehyde and VOCs from modern furniture, etc. and expose to sunlight once a week and remove the water from trays once a week. The recommended plants in our country are bamboo, *Anthurium*, money plant, fern, and chrysanthemum, snake plant, and *tulsi*.

Pharmacotherapy

The drugs used in the management of asthma include quick relievers, controllers, and long-term symptoms relievers as listed in **Table 10.9.2** and dosages in **Table 10.9.3**. The choice of the drugs depends on the age and severity of the wheezing episodes **(Fig. 10.9.1 and Table 10.9.3)**. It should be ideally carried out in a stepwise manner:[6]

- Always use a quick reliever as a rescue treatment in acute exacerbation of persistent asthmatics on preventers. Inhalation method is the best way to administer medication to avoid adverse reactions and for quick actions.
- Recent observation in the treatment from GINA-23 suggests following things:[9]
  - Patients with mild asthma can have severe exacerbations.
  - Low-dose ICS markedly reduces severe exacerbations, hospitalizations, death, and improves lung function.
- In patients who were on SABA alone or low-dose ICS or leukotriene receptor antagonists (LTRA) as needed low-dose ICS-formoterol reduces the risk of emergency room visits by about two-thirds compared to SABA alone and by over one-third compared to low-dose ICS plus as needed SABA.
- It is always preferable to use spacer for inhalation therapy by which one can expect quick results using 1/10th dose of oral medications with less adverse reaction.

TABLE 10.9.2: Classification of drugs used for the management of asthma.

Quick relievers	*Controller*	*Long-term symptoms relievers*
Used for acute attacks to relieve bronchospasm as and when needed	Used for long-term to control the inflammation and to prevent further attacks	Used to relieve bronchospasm for longer hours
• *Short-acting beta-2-agonists (SABA):* – Salbutamol – Terbutaline • Adrenaline • Aminophylline	• Leukotriene receptor antagonists (LTRA) • *Steroids:* – Oral – Inhaled corticosteroids (ICS) • Theophylline	• *Long-acting beta-2-agonists:* – Salmeterol – Formoterol – Bambuterol • Always use with ICS

TABLE 10.9.3: Dosage of drugs.

Drugs	*Dosage*
Salbutamol	• *<1 year:* Nebulizer—0.05–0.15 mg/kg/dose every 4–6 hours with subsequent doses titrated based on clinical response • *1–4 years:* Nebulizer—1.25–2.5 mg every 4–6 hours with subsequent doses titrated based on clinical response • *5 years or more:* MDI—2 puffs (216 µg) every 4–6 hours as needed; DPI—200 µg inhaled every 4–6 hours; may increase to 400 µg inhaled every 4–6 hours, if necessary • *5–11 years:* Nebulizer—2.5 mg every 4–6 hours with subsequent doses titrated based on clinical response • *12 years or more:* Nebulizer—2.5–5 mg every 6 hours as needed; MDI—2 puffs (180 µg) every 4–6 hours
Lev salbutamol	Half dose of salbutamol
Terbutaline	• *<12 years:* Nebulization—0.01–0.03 mg/kg/dose with the minimum dose of 0.1 mg; maximum dose is 2.5 mg diluted with 1–2 mL of normal saline every 4–6 hours • *>12 years:* Inhalation aerosol—2 inhalations separated by 60 second every 4–6 hours. Do not repeat more often 4–6 hours
Salmeterol	• 1 puff (50 µg) every 12 hours in >4 years • Combination with fluticasone propionate; 50 µg, 125 µg, 250 µg
Formoterol	12 µg (1 inhalation) every 12 hours (2 puffs—6 µg/puff) in children 5 years or more. Total daily dose should not exceed 24 µg. Combination available with budesonide or mometasone furoate as 100 µg, 200 µg, and 400 µg
Montelukast sodium	• *6 months to 5 years:* 4 mg OD • *6–14 years:* 5 mg OD • *15 years and above:* 10 mg OD
Theophylline	• *Age <1 year:* [0.2 × (age in weeks)] + 5 = mg/kg/day • *Age ≥1 year:* 16 mg/kg/day
Tiotropium bromide	Age 12 years and above 2.5 µg/day (2 inhalations orally of 1.25 µg OD)
Beclomethasone	100 µg
Budesonide	100 µg
Budesonide nebulized	250 µg
Fluticasone propionate	100 µg
Mometasone	100 µg
Ciclesonide	Low dose—100 µg, medium dose—double (200 µg), high dose—quadruple (400 µg)

(DPI: dry powder inhaler; MDI: metered dose inhaler)

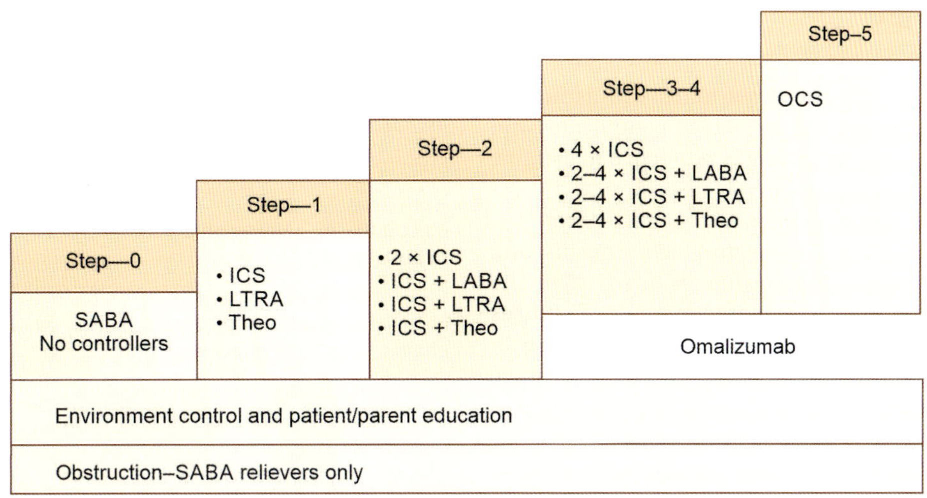

Fig. 10.9.1: Pharmacotherapy in bronchial asthma.

Note:
- The stepwise approach is meant to assist not to replace the clinical decision-making and required to meet individual patient needs.
- If alternative treatment is used and response is inadequate, discontinue it and use the preferred treatment before stepping up.
- *Quick-relief medication for all patients:*
  - Short-acting beta-2 agonist as needed for symptoms; intensity of treatment depends on the severity of symptoms: up to three treatments at 20-minute intervals as needed. Short course of oral systemic corticosteroids may be needed.
  - Use of SABA > 2 days a week for symptom relief [not prevention of exercise-induced bronchoconstriction (EIB)] generally indicates inadequate control and the need to step-up treatment.

(EIB: exercise-induced bronchoconstriction; ICON: International Consensus; ICS: inhaled corticosteroid; LABA: long-acting beta-2 agonist; LTRA: leukotriene receptor antagonist; OCS: oral corticosteroid; SABA: short-acting beta-2 agonist)

Source: Adapted from International Consensus On (ICON) Pediatric Asthma.

- In children, <5 years of age, static treated spacer and mask or a mouthpiece can be used whenever the child is capable of using the spacer; above 5 years, spacer with mouthpiece, dry powder inhaler (DPI), or breath-activated pressurized meter dose in inhaler are used.
- Nebulizer usage is a second choice; and 500 mL plastic bottle spacer is an effective spacer in all ages; and one should consider the child's ability to use the device, preference, and cost. Always rinse or gargle after the use of inhaled steroids in DPI.

Follow-up

Regular follow-up is needed to assess, adjust treatment, and review the response. The level of controlling of asthma by using the parameters as listed in **Table 10.9.4**. Always give hope, confidence, and encourage sports activities. The pneumonic for the follow-up would be:

- ILL—What makes you ill?
- HELL—When do you feel worst?
- PILL—Medication used dosage
- SKILL—Technique of inhalation and nasal spray

TABLE 10.9.4: Level of control of asthma.

Parameters	*Controlled*	*Partly controlled*	*Poorly controlled*
Daytime symptoms	<2 times/week	>2 times/week	Three or more features of partly controlled asthma in any week
Limitations of activities	None	Any	
Nocturnal symptoms of disturbed sleep	None	Any	
Need for relievers or rescue treatment	<2 times/week	>2 times/week	
Lung functions PEF or FEV_1	Normal	<80% of predicted or personal best	
Exacerbation	None	One or more per year	One in any week

(FEV_1: forced expiratory volume in 1 second; PEF: peak expiratory flow)

- WELL—Follow instruction of your physician, environment control, lifestyle, yoga exercise, and regular follow-up.

COMORBIDITIES

The most common comorbid conditions are as follows:

- *Allergic rhinitis:* Nearly the three-fourths of asthmatic children develop allergic rhinitis, which complicates and worsens asthma. Nasal breathing is protective to asthma. Always evaluate as a unified airway disease, and a successful treatment of allergic rhinitis can control asthma.[10]
- *Sinusitis:* Nearly 9% of the asthmatics have sinusitis, and the incidence in uncontrolled asthma is nearly 35%. The sinusitis is a result of blockage of ostomates of sinuses due to edematous nasal mucosa and compromise in the mucociliary function of sinus. Nearly 27% have conjunctivitis with rubbing of eyes with or without redness. We often brand as rhino-sino-conjunctivitis.[10]
- *Otitis media:* Nearly 25% of the children have serous otitis media due to the blockage of eustachian tube from edema of nasal mucosa.
- *Gastroesophageal reflux disease (GERD):* GERD is quite common in infants, which we need not be worried about, but GERD as a cause for worsening of asthma is seen only in the few cases of refractory asthma. It should be suspected in children with prominent asthma symptoms while eating or sleeping or who prop up in bed by themselves to relieve nocturnal symptoms. The gold standard for diagnosis is esophageal pH monitoring.
- *Acute severe asthma:* Asthma attacks can be very severe in untreated or improperly treated cases needing hospitalization for intensive treatment. This occurs when the early signs of severity are missed or ignored by the patients, parents, and physicians.

MANAGEMENT OF ACUTE SEVERE ASTHMA IN HOSPITALIZED PATIENT

To cover all aspects in acute severe attack of asthma and to prioritize the treatment, please remember six "M"s in aiming the therapy as shown in **Table 10.9.5**.

NUTRITIONAL MANAGEMENT OF ASTHMA CHILDREN

- Suggest smaller frequent meals for better diaphragmatic work and also to help to decrease the chances of gastroesophageal reflux.
- Always prefer homemade traditional food.
- Encourage fresh fruit, vegetables, butter, curd, pickles fish, and food with omega-3 fatty acids.
- Encourage traditional food habits.
- Avoid salty snacks, carbonated water.

ADVICE ON ASTHMA MANAGEMENT DURING THE COVID-19 PANDEMIC

- Overall people with asthma had lower risk of being infected and severity contrary to the prediction.

TABLE 10.9.5: Six "M"s in the management of acute severe asthma in children.

Principle of management	*Pathogenetic mechanism*	*Management*
Metabolic correction	Hypoxemia, metabolic acidosis	Warm humidified oxygen by mask, nasal prongs
Muscle spasm to be relieved	Airway obstruction	Beta-2-agonists + ipratropium bromide in O_2-driven nebulizers
Mucosal edema	Inflammation, airway obstruction	• Systemic or oral prednisolone or methylprednisolone • Intravenous (IV) or inhaled fluticasone 1,500 µg
Mucus secretions	Excess mucus secretion and airway obstruction	Appropriate hydration, staccato type of coughing
Monitor for infection	Pneumonia, otitis media, sinusitis	Antibiotics
Mechanical ventilation	Respiratory acidosis, apnea ventilation failure	Ventilatory care as last resort

- Patients are advised to take prescribed medicine, especially controller medicine inhaled steroids) regularly.
- Avoid spirometry in patients with suspected/confirmed coronavirus disease 2019 (COVID-19).
- Avoid nebulization in COVID-19-confirmed asthmatics to avoid the risk of transmitting infection to healthcare workers and other patients.
- Follow local infections control measures and encourage COVID-19 vaccine and influenza vaccine.

PROGNOSIS

Children with viral infection-triggered asthma tend to outgrow the disease by 5 years of age when the immune system attains adult levels. Some more outgrow the disease by 8 years when the airway caliber reaches adult levels, more so in boys. During adolescent period, the majority tends to outgrow the attacks. However, those with atopic asthma (high IgE level) and children with low lung capacities and girls have the tendency for asthma remaining for an indefinite period.

PREVENTION

The *primary prevention* is to prevent sensitization to allergens. Avoid unnecessary use of spectrum antibiotics.

Children born prematurely, small for date children and infants who gain weight more are prone for airflow limitation and a prelude for airway remodeling one has to guide them properly.

The *secondary prevention* is to prevent the occurrence of symptoms in sensitized child, which is to avoid environmental triggers predominantly the tobacco smoke and indoor pollutants, such as dust mites, cockroach, fungi, pollens, and other smokes.

The *tertiary prevention* is to control the symptoms by environment control and long-term use of anti-inflammatory drugs and quick relievers as rescue medicines in any exacerbations.

RECENT ADVANCES

- Recognition of unified airway disease and chronic inflammatory disease concept
- The asthma phenotypes based on inflammatory cells and mediators released by eosinophils, neutrophils, T-lymphocytes, and vascular endothelial cells
- The importance of environment control
- The use of breathing exercise or yoga to avoid chest and spinal deformity, which increases morbidity and mortality
- Use of anti-IgE antibody treatment in the difficult cases
- The use of immunotherapy preferably by sublingual route
- Obesity is recognized as a major risk factor for the development of asthma, especially in girls. A decrease in lung function is proportionately related to obesity.

PRACTICE GUIDELINES

Use quick reliever as and when necessary and use preventers in steps 2–5 as described in **Figure 10.9.1**. Depending on the response either step-up or step-down the dose of preventers, some studies recommend starting with high dose and then reducing the dose earlier.

PRACTICAL TIPS

- Aim at good control of asthma with good education and bonding with patient, parents, and grandparents for better compliance.
- Avoid prolonged use of systemic steroids or high dose of inhaled steroids.
- Always use spacer preferably clear, valved one for better delivery. For metered dose inhaler, slow inhalation, and for powder inhaler, faster inhalation is needed.
- Always assess the compliance and technique of inhalation during follow-up while infusing trust, hope, and confidence.
- Counsel the adolescent separately and stress on ill effect of tobacco smoke.
- Stress on good environment control and to have indoor plants, which need to be exposed to sunlight and to remove water from the tray once a week.
- Always use COVID-19 vaccine and influenza vaccine as recommended by local health authorities.

KEY MESSAGES

- Please keep it in mind that while dealing with a biological system based on expert opinion, there should be enough room for individualization.
- Always look for availability, accessibility, and affordability in managing our children with asthma.
- Do realize that different forms of asthma respond differently to drugs.
- Phenotype-based treatments are likely to be more effective and safer than standard uniform treatment that we currently offer to all asthma phenotypes.
- Be optimistic as newer research needs a link between clinicians, researchers, and pharmacological companies for better, cost-effective individual treatment of patients.

REFERENCES

1. Serebrisky D, Wiznia A. Pediatric Asthma: A Global Epidemic. Ann Glob Health. 2019;85(10):6.
2. India State-level Disease Burden Initiative Air Pollution Collaborators. Health and Economic impact of air pollution in the states of India: The Global burden of disease study 2019. Lancet Planet Health. 2021;5(1):e25-e38.
3. Central Bureau of Health Intelligence. (2018). National Health Profile 2018. Available from [online] https://cbhidghs.mohfw.gov.in/index1.php?lang=1&level=2&sublinkid=88&lid=1138 [Last accessed December 2024].
4. Paramesh H. Air pollution climate change on lung health. Curr Sci. 2022;122(5):499-500.
5. Paramesh H. Air pollution and allergic airway diseases: social determinants and sustainability in the control and prevention. Indian J Pediatr. 2018;85(4):284-94.
6. Papadopoulos NG, Arakawa H, Carlsen KH, Custovic A, Gern J, Lemanske R, et al. International consensus on (ICON) pediatric asthma. Allergy. 2012;67(8):976-97.
7. Paramesh H, Nagaraju K, Sukumaran TU, Agarkhedkar S, Bhakta S, Raj T, et al. Airway Diseases Education and Expertise (ADEX) in Pediatrics: Adaptation for Clinical Practice in India. Indian Pediatr. 2016;53(2):154-8.
8. Paramesh H, Mohanty NC, Kumar R, Kumar P, Sivabalan S, Vaidya PC, et al. Airway Disease Education & Expertise (ADEX) NEXT Working Group Recommendations-Persistent (Chronic) Cough In Pediatric Practice. J Pediatr Assoc India. 2017;6(4);230-43.
9. Global Initiative for Asthma (GINA). (2023). Global Strategy for Asthma Management and Prevention, 2023. [online] Available from https://ginasthma.org/wp-content/uploads/2023/07/GINA-2023-Full-report-23_07_06-WMS.pdf [Last accessed December 2024].
10. Paramesh H, Mahashur A, Talwar D, Bhagawa S, Lele J, Verma S, et al. Pollution-Induced Rhinitis and Nasal Health in India. J Indian Med Assoc. 2021;119(12):57-61.

10.10 Aerosol Therapy

Jagdish Prasad Goyal, Prawin Kumar

INTRODUCTION

Aerosol therapy is the delivery of aerosolized medication directly into the airways. It has been used as a part of the treatment for a variety of respiratory diseases in children. Current ongoing research has shown effectiveness of aerosol therapy in other systemic diseases. There are several types of aerosol devices with their advantages and disadvantages. Some of the devices can be used in ambulatory care while others are mainly suited for acute care settings including intubated children. The proper technique of device use varies from one device to another device. Therefore, it is critical to know the correct method of their use. These devices may easily get contaminated therefore it is mandatory to know proper cleaning methods.[1]

The drug used in aerosol forms include bronchodilators, steroids, and antibiotics. Aerosol therapy has revolutionized the care of asthma and other chronic respiratory diseases, viz., cystic fibrosis, primary ciliary dyskinesia, etc.[2]

BENEFITS OF AEROSOL THERAPY

The aerosol therapy delivers the drug directly into the lung and has several significant advantages over systemic drug delivery:[3,4]

- Smaller medication dose to achieve the desired therapeutic effect with lesser side effects as compared to oral or the parenteral route
- Faster onset action for the reversal of acute episodes of bronchospasm
- Easy and convenient to administer by patients, parents, and healthcare providers
- Aerosol therapy is painless as compared to the parenteral route of drug administration.

FACTORS AFFECTING AEROSOL THERAPY

Aerosol particle characteristics, including the size (diameter), density, electrical charge, hygroscopy, shape, and velocity of the aerosol, determine the efficacy of aerosol therapy.[3,4] Any particle size larger than 5 μm is likely to be filtered out in the upper airways and fail to reach to lower airways. Aerosol particles <5 μm in size readily reach the periphery of the lung.[5] The chemical and physical properties of the aerosolized drug also play an important role in drug delivery. Furthermore, the hygroscopic property of aerosolized drugs may have unfavorable effects on the drug delivery. The shape and velocity of particles eventually may affect drug deposition in airways. A high velocity of aerosolized drug particles may lead to drug deposition in the upper airway, while slow velocity enhances drug deposition in the lower airways.[3-5]

The host factors also play an important role in drug deposition in the lower airways. Patient's disease state and severity, breathing pattern, preference for device, and technique are important factors that affect drug delivery. It has also been observed that increased breath-holding time is associated with better drug deposition in the lungs.[2]

INDICATIONS OF AEROSOL THERAPY

Aerosol therapy is indicated in a variety of respiratory conditions. In children, the most common indication for use of aerosol therapy is in the long-term management of bronchial asthma in which both the inhaled corticosteroid (ICS) and long-acting β2-agonist (LABA) are used.[2] Short-acting β2-agonist (SABA) is used in the management of acute asthma. The use of inhaled tobramycin is now well established in cystic fibrosis. Other antibiotics (pentamidine, colistin, etc.) and antifungal agents (amphotericin B) have also been used as inhaled form. Hypertonic saline in aerosolized form is used in cystic fibrosis patients before chest physiotherapy and for inducing sputum in tuberculosis patients.[3,4] The drugs administered through the aerosol devices are summarized in **Table 10.10.1**.

AEROSOL DEVICES

In the last decade, there has been tremendous advance in aerosol devices with advent of new technology and newer therapeutic molecules. Aerosol devices can broadly be divided into four categories: Nebulizer, pressurized metered-dose inhaler (pMDI), dry powder inhaler (DPI), and soft mist inhaler (SMI). Each one of them has its own advantages and disadvantages **(Table 10.10.2)**.[5] These attributes should be taken into account during the selection of appropriate aerosol devices in children.[3,4]

NEBULIZERS

Nebulizers have been used widely to deliver aerosol therapy in children in a variety of respiratory conditions.[6] They are

TABLE 10.10.1: Different drugs used for aerosol therapy.

Type of drug	*Diseases*	*Aerosol device*
Beta-2 agonist	Asthma, bronchiectasis, CF, etc.	All types of devices
Anticholinergic	Asthma	All types of devices
Inhaled corticosteroids (ICS) (budesonide, fluticasone, etc.)	Asthma, bronchiectasis, CF, etc.	All types of devices
Inhaled antibiotics (tobramycin, colistin, etc.)	CF, bronchiectasis	Nebulizer
Inhaled antiviral (ribavirin)	RSV infection	Nebulizer
Mucolytics (hypertonic saline, dNAase, etc.)	CF, bronchiectasis, etc.	Nebulizer
Inhaled pulmonary vasodilator (treprostinil))	Pulmonary hypertension	Nebulizer
Drugs for nonrespiratory diseases (insulin, opiates, levodopa, etc.)	Systemic disease (diabetes mellitus, hypertension)	Nebulizer

(CF: cystic fibrosis; RSV: respiratory syncytial virus)

mostly available to use for the hospital setting but some of them can be used at home as well. The effective delivery of the drug depends on a number of factors, viz., dose, nebulization time, dead volume, flow of driving gas, density of gas, and breathing pattern of the child. The drugs through this device can be given intermittently or continuously in the emergency room and pediatric intensive care unit for severe diseases. The pediatrician must be aware of these devices. It will help them to select a specific nebulizer for a specific drug to be delivered to the child.

Indications

A nebulizer is indicated when a child is in respiratory distress and not able to take inhaled medication by other aerosol devices. It is also required for some medications, which are not available in a form suitable for other devices, including pentamidine, ribavirin, deoxyribonuclease, hypertonic saline, and tobramycin. The steps for the correct use of nebulizer are shown in **Box 10.10.1**.[3,4]

Types of Nebulizers

Three types of nebulizers are available:[6]

1. Jet nebulizers
2. Ultrasonic nebulizers
3. Mesh nebulizers

These three types of nebulizers work on different principles but have many common features **(Fig. 10.10.1)**.

TABLE 10.10.2: Advantages and disadvantages of different aerosol devices.

Type of device	*Advantages*	*Disadvantages*
Nebulizer	• No patient coordination is required • Can be used in all age-groups • Can be used for wide range of medications • Suited in emergency room specially for severe disease	• Large and cumbersome device • Treatment time is long • Costly device • Drug is required to add in chamber • Potential risk of drug delivery to the eye with a facemask • Cleaning is required after each use
pMDI	• Easy to use • Compact and portable • It takes short time • Multidose formulation, no need to fill each time	• Require hand breath coordination (use of spacer can overcome it) • Availability of limited drug/combination • Expensive as compared to DPI • It contains propellent which may be harmful for environment
DPI	• Compact and portable • Short treatment time • It does not contain propellent • Available in both single and multidose formulation	• High inspiratory flow is required • Large amount of drug gets deposited in oropharynx • Availability of limited drug/combination • Dose can be affected by humidity • Not suited for severe exacerbation
SMI	• Portable and easy to use • Short treatment time • Less drug deposition in oropharynx	• Expensive • Limited evidence to use in children • Availability of limited drug/combination

(pMDI: pressurized metered-dose inhaler; SMI: soft mist inhaler)

BOX 10.10.1: Steps for the correct use of nebulizer.

1. Hands should be washed prior to preparing each nebulizer treatment
2. Assemble tubing, nebulizer cup, and mouthpiece/mask
3. Place medicine into nebulizer cup (if using a multidose bottle of medicine, use correct amount of medication into the chamber along with saline solution)
4. Sit in upright position and hold the nebulizer vertically
5. Connect the nebulizer to power source
6. As the mist starts, encourage the child to take normal tidal breath with open mouth
7. Continue until the medicine is finished in the chamber. This may take 5–10 minutes

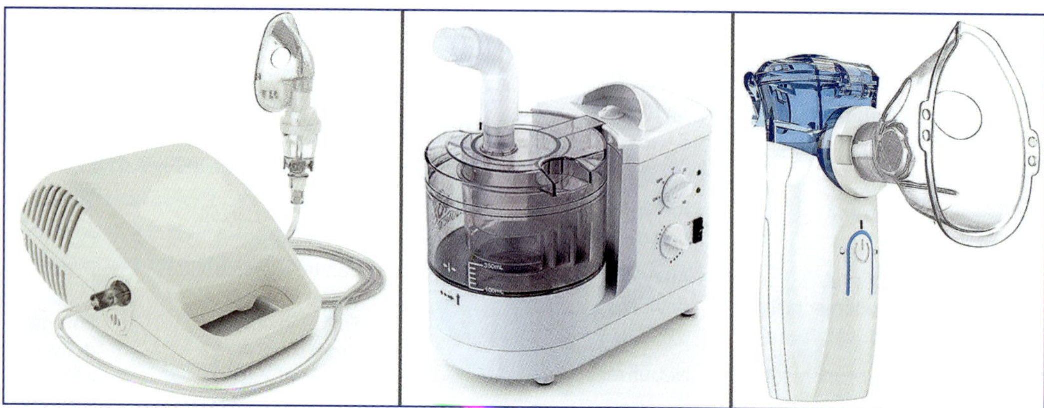

Fig. 10.10.1: Different types of nebulizers.

Jet Nebulizer

A jet nebulizer works on Bernoulli's principle and uses a compressed gas source (oxygen or air) to generate an aerosol that breaks up liquid into small droplets and suspends into the gas to be inhaled by the patient.[6] The smaller particles move through the outlet to the patient, whereas larger particles hold on to nebulizer chamber and get reaerosolized. The size of the nozzle and compressed gas flow determine the size of aerosol particles. The commonly used nebulizers deliver aerosol continuously, and only 10–20% of the aerosol drug reaches the airways. Jet nebulizers have been modified to overcome this problem in several ways including a one-way valve for inhalation and exhalation and a breath-actuated nebulizer where the aerosol is generated only during inspiration.[7] There is a possible risk of contamination due to a large amount of residual drug and open reservoir therefore it should be used after proper cleaning and drying.

Ultrasonic Nebulizer

An ultrasonic nebulizer produces aerosol by means of electricity-powered piezoelectric crystal to generate high-frequency vibration. The size of aerosol particles in ultrasonic nebulizers depends upon the frequency of vibration. It has been shown from studies that the size of the aerosol particles generated from ultrasonic nebulizers is larger than jet nebulizer. Therefore, drug deposition in the upper airway is more as compared to the jet nebulizer.[5] Recently, small handheld devices is available in the market, which may be helpful in ambulatory care.

Mesh Nebulizer

A mesh nebulizer is an aerosol device that uses a mesh with multiple, tiny openings to produce a liquid aerosol.[6] In this aerosol device, the liquid solution is passed through a fine mesh to produce aerosol. Mesh nebulizer generates aerosol with very small particle size. Research has shown that mesh nebulizer is superior to jet nebulizer in drug delivery due to small residual volume and particle size. Because of the effective drug delivery of mesh nebulizers, it is sometimes necessary to adjust the dose of inhaled medication in view of possible adverse effects due to high doses. It can be used in ambulatory care as well as in acute care settings. It has minimal residual volume and has faster drug delivery as compared to jet nebulizers. Both ultrasonic and mesh nebulizers are costlier than jet nebulizers.

Interface for Nebulizer

It is equipment applied in between the nebulizer and the patient to deliver aerosolized medications.[6] The proper selection of interface is very important for the proper delivery of aerosolized medications and the prevention of adverse events. It could be of different types, viz., blow-by, hood, face mask, and mouthpiece. The selection of interface will depend upon the age of the child, their ability to inhale, and disease severity.[1]

Disinfection and Cleaning

Jet nebulizers require periodic cleaning or disinfection to minimize the risk of contamination.[8] Jet nebulizers used in office practice should be discarded after each patient's use. The nebulizer parts should be cleaned with soap and water. It should also be disinfected as per the manufacturer's recommendations using boiled water, isopropyl alcohol, or hydrogen peroxide.

PRESSURIZED METERED-DOSE INHALER

The pMDI has become the most common aerosol device prescribed for pediatric patients with asthma after its development by George Maison in 1955. The basic components of pMDI include canister, propellant [chlorofluorocarbon (CFC)] or [hydrofluoroalkane (HFA)], drug formulation, metering valve, actuator, and dose counter.[9] In the past, CFC had been used as a propellant but due to the effect on the ozone layer, it has been replaced by HFA, which is considered safe. The device can be actuated by pressing the canister; the propellant gets exposed to atmospheric pressure, which leads to the aerosolization of the drug into fine particles. The commonly available pMDIs in India are shown in **Figure 10.10.2**. The drug delivery to the lung depends upon hand-breath coordination, and a significant amount of drug is deposited in the oropharynx without proper hand-breath coordination. To overcome the problem of hand-breath coordination, pMDI should always be used with a spacer, which decreases the particle velocity and minimizes oropharyngeal deposition.[5] The commonly available spacers in India are shown in **Figure 10.10.3**. The newer pMDI devices come with a dose counter, which helps patient to know when pMDI is becoming empty. Smart pMDI devices with patient tracking systems will revolutionize patient care in the future.

Indications

The pMDI with spacer is indicated for the long-term management of asthma in children.[9] It can also be used in

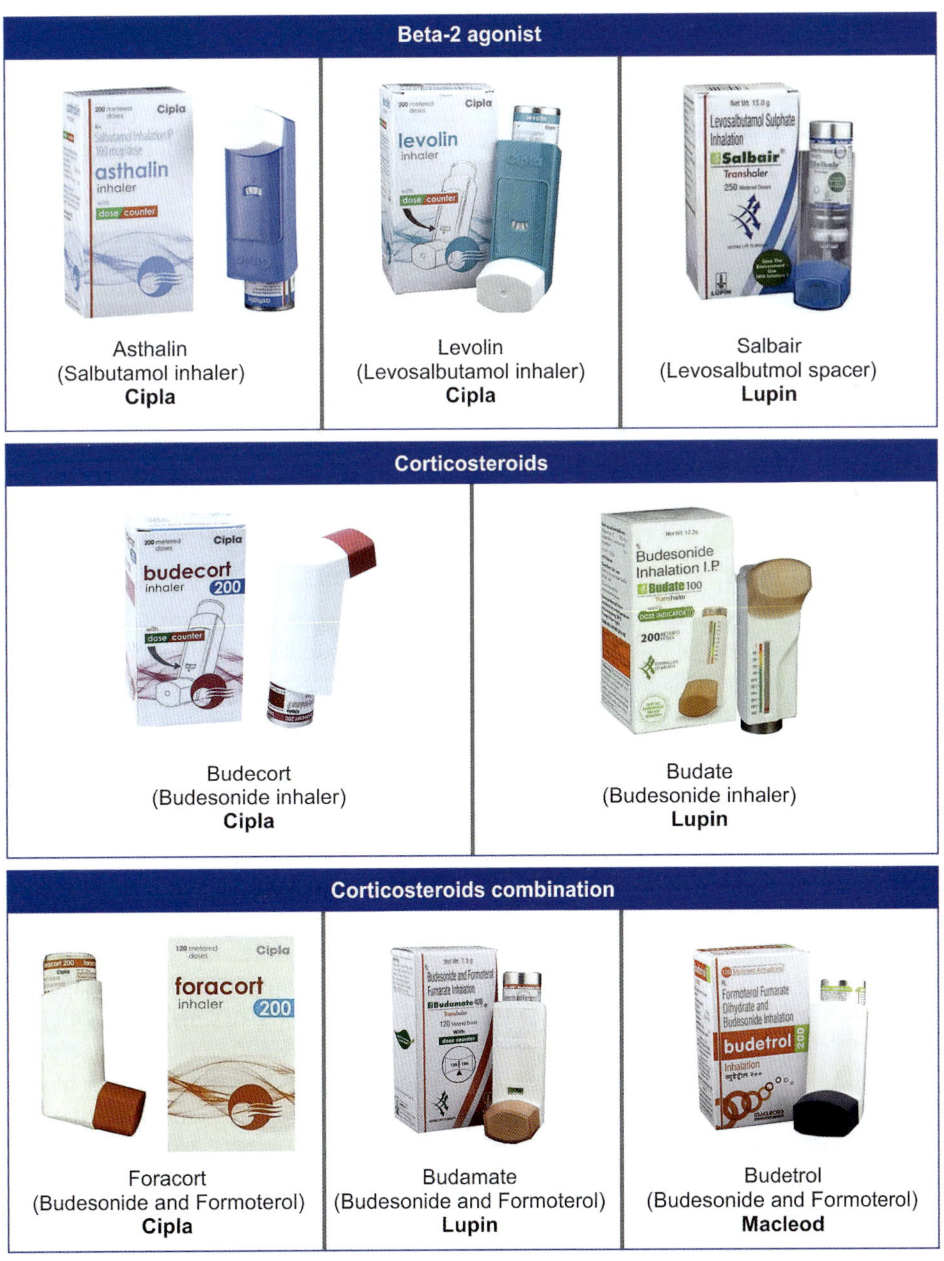

Fig. 10.10.2: Commonly available pressurized metered-dose inhalers (pMDIs).

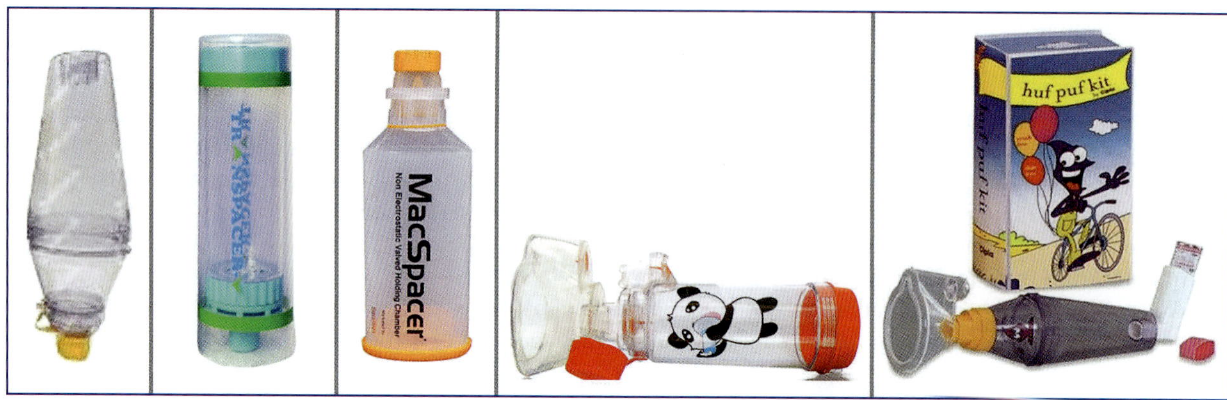

Fig. 10.10.3: Commonly available spacers.

BOX 10.10.2: Steps for the correct use of pMDI with spacer.

1. Assemble the spacer and pressurized metered-dose inhaler (pMDI)
2. Remove the cap of pMDI
3. Hold the pMDI in upright position and shake it well for four to five times
4. Stand or sit straight
5. Place the mouthpiece between teeth and close lips without leaving any gaps
6. Ask the patient to exhale into spacer
7. Actuate the pMDI in spacer
8. Take 5–10 tidal breaths
9. Wait for at least 60 seconds before the next puff and repeat steps 3–8
10. Gargle/rinse the mouth after taking steroid-containing pMDI

asthma exacerbation. The pMDI with a spacer is found to be equally effective as nebulizers in acute exacerbation. In children, pMDI with a spacer has also been used to document bronchodilator reversibility to diagnose asthma in spirometry. The steps for the correct use of pMDI are shown in **Box 10.10.2**.

Types of Pressurized Metered-dose Inhaler

There are two types of pMDIs: Conventional pMDIs and breath-actuated pMDI, which is also known as autohaler:[9]

1. *Conventional pMDI:* It is actuated by pressing the canister, which releases a drug propellant mixture. It requires hand-breath coordination if used without a spacer.
2. *Breath-actuated pMDI:* It is triggered by inhalation, and there is no need for hand-breath coordination.[7]

Disinfection and Cleaning

The plastic container of pMDI should be cleaned at least once a week or as needed. The spacer should be cleaned periodically as per manufacturer's recommendations.[8] It should be disassembled and soaked in warm water with liquid detergent, and both pieces should be gently shaken back and forth and air-dried. One should not rub the spacer with a dry cloth, as this will reduce drug delivery because of static charge.

DRY-POWDER INHALER

Dry-powder inhalers (DPIs) are portable, breath-actuated aerosolized devices that deliver the medication in the form of dry powder to the lungs **(Fig. 10.10.3)**.[10] It requires sufficient inspiratory flow to deliver the medication to lungs and may not be suitable for children with respiratory distress and <5 years of age. The fraction of drug delivery varies from 9% to 30% among different commercially available devices. The commonly available DPI in India are shown in **Figure 10.10.4**.

Indications

A DPI is also indicated for the long-term management of asthma, particularly in older children who can make enough inspiratory force.[10] The steps for the correct use of DPI are shown in **Box 10.10.3**.

Types of Dry-powder Inhaler

There are three types of DPIs available to use: Single dose, multiple single-dose, and multiple doses.[10]

1. *Single-dose DPI:* In this device a prefilled capsule is punctured that releases the medication. Patient needs to load the capsule each time into the device. One can see the empty capsule after the dosage has been delivered. A typical example of single-dose DPI is "Rotacap".
2. *Multiple single-dose DPI:* It has a wheel, which contains four to eight drug blisters. Each blister is punctured with one-time use. The example of this is "Diskhaler."
3. *Multiple-dose DPIs:* Multiple-dose DPIs deliver doses of medication from a reservoir of powder within the inhaler or from an individual premeasured blister strip. The preparation and use of medication is easy with multiple-dose DPIs. The dose counter is present in almost all

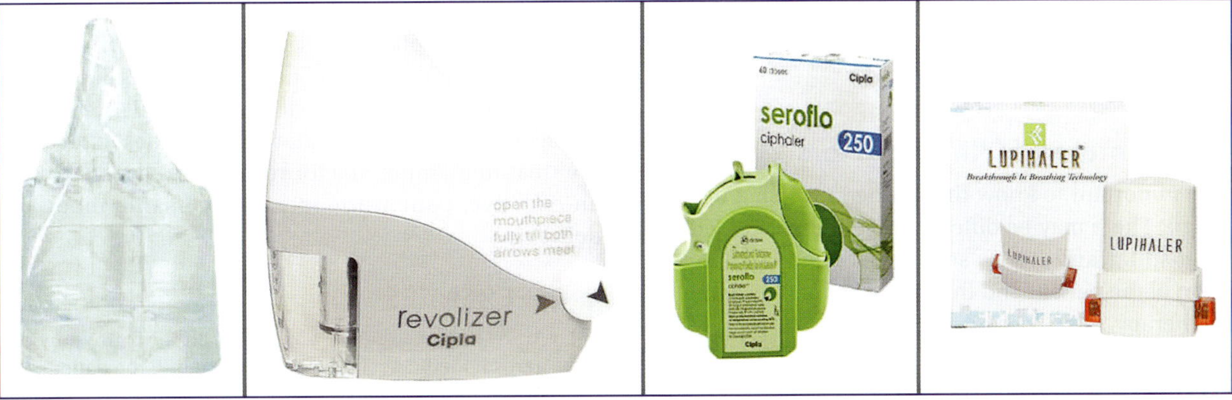

Fig. 10.10.4: Commonly available dry powder inhalers (DPIs).

BOX 10.10.3: Steps for the correct use of dry-powder inhaler (DPI).

1. Check the device and ensure that it is clean and mouthpiece is free from obstruction
2. Load a dose into the device as directed by the manufacturer
3. Breath out away from the mouthpiece
4. Put the mouthpiece of DPI between teeth without biting and close the lip to form a seal
5. Take a fast and deep breath through the mouth
6. Remove the device from the mouth
7. Hold breath for 5–10 seconds
8. Breath out gently
9. If an additional dose is required, follow steps 2–8
10. After inhaling steroid-containing DPI—gargle/rinse the mouth

TABLE 10.10.3: Age guidelines for preferred aerosol therapy in children.

Age of child	*Aerosol device*
Birth to 3 years	pMDI with spacer with mask or nebulizer with mask
4–5 years	pMDI with spacer, nebulizer with mask, DPI, breath-actuated pMDI (at the age of 5 years)
6–12 years	pMDI with spacer, nebulizer with mouthpiece, DPI, breath-actuated pMDI
>12 years	All devices

(DPI: dry powder inhaler; pMDI: pressurized metered-dose inhaler)

multiple-dose DPIs. Examples of multiple-dose DPIs are Diskus, Turbuhaler, Twisthaler, Flexhaler, etc.

Disinfection and Cleaning

Patients should be advised to wipe the mouthpiece of DPI with a dry and clean cloth after each use. Any kind of moisture may lead to a decrease in drug delivery, so a DPI should not be submerged in water.[10]

SOFT MIST INHALER (SMI)

This device works on a microelectronic dosimetric system. There is a mechanical spring that pressurizes the device; upon priming it draws up a measured amount of medication into the dosing system. When the spring is released, it generates soft mist aerosol 1 to 1.5 seconds. It has very fine particles and it delivers 2–3 times greater drug deposition into the lung compared to pMDI. It does not depend on inspiratory flow.[5]

Indication: SMI can be used in the management of asthma in children. Currently, bronchodilator and ICS can be given through this device.

Disinfection and cleaning: SMI is similar to a pMDI device.

CRITERIA FOR SELECTING APPROPRIATE DEVICE

It is important to select the correct device for the patient for their satisfaction and good compliance. The selection of appropriate devices will depend on patient, drug, device, as well as environmental and clinical factors.[11] The preferred device according to the patient's age has been shown in **Table 10.10.3**.

Patient-related Factors

The selection of the appropriate device depends upon the diagnosis. It should also be decided by the patient's age and physical and cognitive ability. Patient preference is also important in the selection of the correct device as patients tend to use the device more regularly which they prefer.

Drug-related Factors

Some medications, especially hypertonic saline and antibiotics, are available only in liquid form and can be delivered only through nebulizers.

Device-related Factors

Easy to use, portability and low maintenance cost are taken into account.

Environmental and Clinical Factors

It is very important to know the setting in which a device is to be used. There may be different requirements of a device in the hospital and home setting. Depending upon the condition of the patient and the frequency of requirement of aerosol therapy, the device may be selected.[11]

PATIENT EDUCATION FOR CORRECT USE OF THE DEVICE

It is important for healthcare providers to explain the advantages of aerosol therapy and dispel the myths and fears of patients and family. The healthcare provider should provide a demonstration for correct use and cleaning. Technique and compliance should be checked on every visit. The response to therapy and any adverse effects should be monitored.

CONCLUSION

Aerosol therapy has emerged as a cornerstone in the management of various respiratory and systemic diseases, particularly in children. The ability to deliver medications directly to the lungs offers numerous advantages, including targeted drug delivery, rapid onset of action, and minimized systemic side effects. Over the years, significant advancements in aerosol devices, such as nebulizers, pMDIs, DPIs and SMIs have enhanced their efficiency and broadened their applicability.

Understanding the nuances of aerosol particle dynamics, device-specific techniques, and proper cleaning protocols is essential for optimizing therapeutic outcomes and minimizing complications. Furthermore, the choice of device should be individualized, considering factors like patient age, disease severity, and personal preference.

In conclusion, aerosol therapy continues to revolutionize the treatment landscape for respiratory diseases, providing an effective, patient-friendly, and versatile mode of drug delivery.

REFERENCES

1. Ari A, Raghavan N, Diaz M, Rubin BK, Fink JB. Individualized aerosol medicine: Integrating device into the patient. Paediatr Respir Rev. 2024:49:14-23.
2. Berlinski A. Pediatric aerosol therapy. Respir Care. 2017;62(6):662-77.
3. Ari A, Fink JB. Aerosol therapy in children: challenges and solutions. Expert Rev Respir Med. 2013;7(6):665-72.
4. Ari A, Fink JB. Guidelines for aerosol devices in infants, children and adults: which to choose, why and how to achieve effective aerosol therapy. Expert Rev Respir Med. 2011;5(4):561-72.
5. Cheng YS. Mechanisms of pharmaceutical aerosol deposition in the respiratory tract. AAPS PharmSciTech. 2014;15(3):630-40.
6. Martin AR, Finlay WH. Nebulizers for drug delivery to the lungs. Expert Opin Drug Deliv. 2015;12(6):889-900.
7. Ibrahim M, Verma R, Garcia-Contreras L. Inhalation drug delivery devices: technology update. Med Devices (Auckl). 2015;8:131-9.
8. O'Malley CA. Device cleaning and infection control in aerosol therapy. Respir Care. 2015;60(6):917-27; discussion 928-30.
9. Myrdal PB, Sheth P, Stein SW. Advances in metered dose inhaler technology: formulation development. AAPS PharmSciTech. 2014;15(2):434-55.
10. Atkins PJ. Dry powder inhalers: an overview. Respir Care. 2015;50(10):1304-12; discussion 1312.
11. Rubin BK, Williams RW. Emerging aerosol drug delivery strategies: from bench to clinic. Adv Drug Deliv Rev. 2014;75:141-8.

SECTION

Disorders of Gastrointestinal System and Liver

Section Editor: **Riyaz Arakkal**

11.1 Recurrent Abdominal Pain

Riyaz Arakkal

INTRODUCTION

Recurrent abdominal pain (RAP) is one of the most common medical problems encountered in children. It is seen in almost 25% of children between 4 and 18 years, and accounts for almost 2–4% of all pediatric consultations.[1] It is characterized by poorly localized recurrent, or continuous abdominal pain. There may be waxing and waning of pain which may seriously affect the child's routine activities. In between, there may be asymptomatic periods also.

A large number of these children ultimately turn out to have functional pain, in which there is no evidence of any underlying anatomic, inflammatory, metabolic, or neoplastic disorders. Hence, this condition may also be called *functional abdominal pain* (FAP). It causes considerable anxiety in parents resulting in significant emotional disturbances as well as a huge financial burden due to the loss of work and the cost of expensive investigations. Therefore, the evaluation and management of a child with RAP can be a real challenge to patients, their parents and also pediatricians.

PATHOPHYSIOLOGY

John Apley, a British pediatrician, along with Nora Naish, published a ground-breaking paper in 1958, in which they studied children between 5 and 15 years with abdominal pain, and defined it as *"at least 3 episodes of abdominal pain, severe enough to affect routine activities over a period of more than 3 months."*[2] Since Apley's pioneer work, there has been extensive research all over the world on this intriguing problem. Various factors implicated in the pathophysiology of FAP include psychological stress, visceral hypersensitivity, disturbed gastrointestinal (GI) motility, altered gut biota, food intolerance, etc. Unfortunately, the exact pathophysiology of FAP continues to be elusive even 65 years after its original description.

The role of stress in the pathogenesis of RAP is emphasized by the famous statement, *"The more sophisticated the country is, the more bellyachers will it have, and little bellyachers develop into big bellyachers."*

The gut influences our brain, and therefore our behavior. The gut-brain axis **(Fig. 11.1.1)** is the constant bidirectional biochemical signaling that links the enteric nervous system (ENS) and the central nervous system (CNS) through millions of nerves, the most important being the vagus nerve. The ENS that regulates our GI tract is also known as the *"second brain."* The role of the ENS in FAP has been studied extensively recently, and the term "functional abdominal pain" has been renamed as *"gut-brain interaction disorders"* (GBIDs).

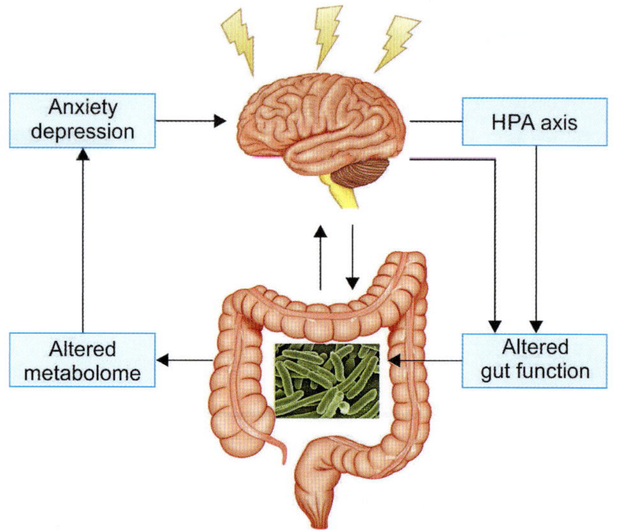

Fig. 11.1.1: Gut-brain axis.

In visceral hyperalgesia (decreased threshold of pain to changes in intraluminal pressure), the intensity of the signals from the GI tract to the brain by nerves, is exaggerated. Hence, even normal peristalsis may be perceived by the child as pain. This may occur secondary to inflammation of the gut due to infection, inflammatory bowel disorders (IBDs) or psychological stress such as failure in the examination, bullying, etc.[3] Gastric emptying and intestinal transit may be delayed by emotions such as anger, anxiety, fear, painful stimuli, and physical stress. They may stimulate colonic motor function resulting in decreased colonic transit time, increased contractile activity, and cause pain and diarrhea.[4]

The gut contains 10–100 trillion microbes, which is even 10 times more than the total number of cells in our body. The homeostasis of GI function is maintained by the microbiota-gut-brain axis. The gut microbiota which increases the synthesis of mucin and IgA, plays a crucial role in maintaining the intestinal barrier. FAP may be precipitated by events like GI infection that interrupt this axis.[5] Changes in the composition of intestinal microbiota may play a role in the pathophysiology of FAP.

Studies have shown that hyperactivity of the hypothalamic-pituitary-adrenal (HPA) axis increases cortisol secretion, which may alter both blood-brain barrier and intestinal mucosal permeability. This facilitates communication between the CNS and gut microbiota leading to pain.[6] Misuse of antibiotics for enteric or nonenteric infections that lead to dysbiosis may also disturb the microbiota contributing to pain.[7]

Ingestion of FODMAPs (**F**ermentable **O**ligo-, **D**i-, **M**ono-saccharides **A**nd **P**olyols) may also contribute to abdominal pain as the intestine cannot produce the enzymes needed to break down the sugars of FODMAPs, which are poorly absorbed resulting in osmotic diarrhea. The unabsorbed short-chain carbohydrates in them are fermented by colonic bacteria to short-chain fatty acids leading to increased synthesis of gas resulting in abdominal pain, bloating, and distension. These symptoms may be aggravated in patients with visceral hypersensitivity.

ROME IV CLASSIFICATION

As per the revised Rome IV criteria (2016), there are four different abdominal pain-related functional gastrointestinal disorders (FGIDs):[8]

1. Functional dyspepsia
2. Abdominal migraine
3. Irritable bowel syndrome (IBS)
4. Functional abdominal pain-not otherwise specified (FAP-NOS)

Functional Dyspepsia

The word dyspepsia means an "upset stomach." Here, the child has recurrent epigastric pain with a feeling of early satiety, i.e., feeling full earlier than expected when eating. The associated symptoms include belching, nausea, anorexia, and heartburn. Even though the pain is suggestive of peptic ulcer disease, endoscopy will be normal. Hence, it is called "nonulcer dyspepsia," and is caused by delayed gastric emptying. Almost 75% of these children have a functional problem while 25% may have an underlying organic cause such as gastroesophageal reflux disease (GERD), *Helicobacter pylori* gastritis, or appendicitis. Hence, children with dyspepsia require careful evaluation.

Abdominal Migraine

The term migraine refers to a type of headache, but abdominal migraine is a chronic recurrent abdominal pain. It differs from typical migraine as a headache may not be present. It is characterized by moderate to severe periumbilical pain, and photophobia and phonophobia as in classic migraine. The triggering factors include lack of sleep, tension, travel, missing meals, etc. Unfortunately, there are no tests to diagnose migraine. There may be a family history of migraine, and all organic causes should be excluded. These children should avoid the 5 C's of migraine—**C**affeine (coffee/tea), **C**hocolate, **C**itrus fruits, **C**hinese food, and **C**heese.

Abdominal Epilepsy

This is another uncommon cause of central neurogenic abdominal pain like abdominal migraine. In addition, they have CNS symptoms consistent with epilepsy like headache, confusion, syncope and transient blindness, and electroencephalogram (EEG) abnormalities.[9] The prognosis is usually good with a dramatic response to antiepileptic medication. Although epilepsy with GI symptoms is uncommon, an EEG should be considered in the diagnostic workup of all patients with unexplained paroxysmal GI complaints associated with CNS symptoms. **Table 11.1.1** lists the differences between abdominal migraine and abdominal epilepsy.

Irritable Bowel Syndrome

The IBS is characterized by abdominal pain which may be relieved by defecation, and may be associated with bloating/distension or passage of mucoid stools. Psychological or physical stress may aggravate symptoms. Parents or siblings may have symptoms of IBS. IBS may be mistaken for IBD, especially Crohn's disease and celiac disease.

TABLE 11.1.1: Abdominal migraine versus abdominal epilepsy.

Features	*Abdominal migraine*	*Abdominal epilepsy*
Family history	Vascular headache	Seizure disorder
Onset	Sudden	Sudden
Severity of pain	Very severe	Moderate
Periodicity	Present	Absent
Duration of pain	Minutes to hours	Transient
Site of pain	Periumbilical/upper abdominal	Periumbilical/upper abdominal
Associated symptoms	Headache, photophobia, phonophobia	Confusion, syncope, seizure, transient blindness
EEG	Normal	Temporal lobe abnormality
Treatment	Antimigraine	Antiepileptic

(EEG: electroencephalogram)

Functional Abdominal Pain–Not Otherwise Specified

There is always some degree of overlap between the four subtypes of FAP, especially between FAP-NOS and IBS. Children with FAP-NOS have features similar to IBS; hence, it may be difficult to differentiate them. Management includes dietary modifications, pharmacologic treatments, and psychotherapy. There may be a role for probiotics also.

Organic Causes

Organic causes of RAP are listed in **Box 11.1.1**. A detailed discussion of each cause is beyond the scope of this chapter.

DIAGNOSIS OF FUNCTIONAL ABDOMINAL PAIN

Pediatricians should always take a detailed history and make a meticulous physical examination which may take up to 45–60 minutes! This is because children and often parents are poor in giving a correct history, and the chronology of symptoms may be difficult to obtain. When evaluating adolescents, sufficient privacy should be ensured.

Apley's law states that *"the further the pain is away from the umbilicus, the more likely it is of organic pathology."*

BOX 11.1.1: Organic causes of recurrent abdominal pain.

Gastrointestinal causes

GERD:
- Eosinophilic esophagitis
- Hiatal hernia
- *Helicobacter pylori* infection
- Food intolerance
- Peptic ulcer disease
- Crohn's disease
- Celiac disease
- Anatomic malformations—Meckel diverticulum, malrotation
- Pancreatitis

Genitourinary causes:
- Recurrent urinary tract infection (UTI)
- Ovarian cyst
- Pelvic inflammatory disease
- Ureteropelvic junction obstruction

Metabolic causes:
- Diabetic ketoacidosis
- Porphyria
- Adrenal crisis

Neurologic disorders:
- Abdominal migraine
- Abdominal epilepsy
- Spinal cord tumor

Miscellaneous causes:
- Lead poisoning
- Sickle cell anemia
- Familial Mediterranean fever
- Polyarteritis nodosa

In other words, functional pain is usually periumbilical in location. However, it should be noted that organic conditions may also present as periumbilical pain.

The following clinical signs may be elicited in a child with FAP:[10]
- Umbilical sign
- Closed eye sign
- Stethoscope sign

- *Umbilical sign:* When asked to indicate the site of maximum pain, the child with FAP may draw a circle around the umbilicus **(Fig. 11.1.2)**.
- *Closed eye sign:* A child with FAP is aware that the examination will not hurt him/her. Hence, he/she may keep his/her eyes closed when being examined, while in organic pain, the patient is very anxious and will keep his/her eyes wide open to see if the examiner will hurt him/her **(Fig. 11.1.3)**.

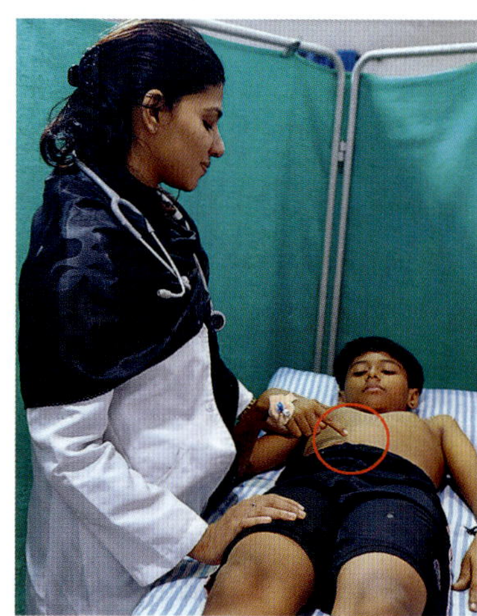

Fig. 11.1.2: Umbilical sign. When asked to show the site of maximum pain, the child with functional abdominal pain (FAP) may draw a circle around the umbilicus.

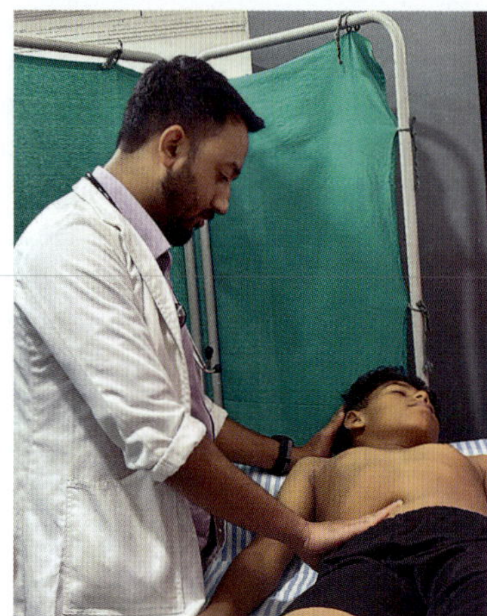

Fig. 11.1.3: Closed eye sign. The child with functional abdominal pain (FAP) may keep his eyes closed when examined.

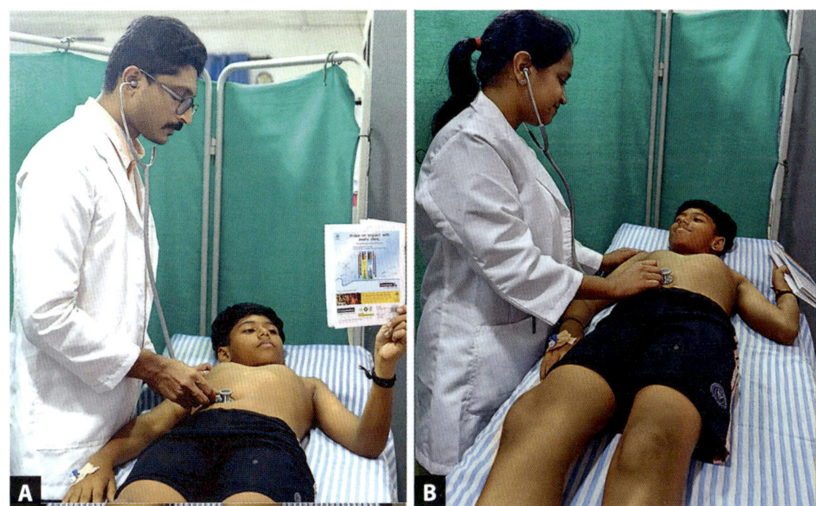

Figs. 11.1.4A and B: (A) Stethoscope sign. The child with functional abdominal pain (FAP) will allow even deep palpation with a stethoscope and continue reading his comic; (B) The adolescent boy with FAP may even smile when examined by a lady doctor.

- *Stethoscope sign:* The child should be reassured that you are only going to auscultate him/her. Begin from his/her chest and slowly come down to the abdomen, especially to the area where he/she has pain, and apply firm pressure with the diaphragm. In FAP, the child will allow even deep palpation and continue what he/she has been doing—reading his comic! **(Fig. 11.1.4A)**. The adolescent boy may even smile when examined by a lady doctor! **(Fig. 11.1.4B)**.

Almost 50% of children with RAP may have underlying chronic constipation and encopresis which may be picked up from history. There may be a palpable fecal mass, and rectal examination may reveal soiling, anal fissure, and a loaded rectum.

Surgical history is important as patients who have undergone abdominal wall surgeries earlier may have pain localized to the scar. FAP may be mistaken for *chronic abdominal wall pain (CAWP)* in which pain arises from the abdominal wall itself rather than from the underlying viscera. Pain may be aggravated by activities that tense the anterior abdominal wall such as sneezing or coughing. The most common cause of CAWP is *anterior cutaneous nerve entrapment syndrome* which can be diagnosed clinically by the *Carnett's test.* The area of maximum pain in the patient's abdomen is palpated and he is asked to tense the anterior abdominal wall muscle. If there is an abdominal wall pathology, pain is aggravated. These patients may respond dramatically to the injection of xylocaine with triamcinolone.[11]

Table 11.1.2 lists the red flag symptoms and signs in RAP.

INVESTIGATIONS

As there are no specific diagnostic tests, there is usually a tendency to do all possible investigations to exclude organic causes, which is very stressful to the child and expensive to parents, and hence should be avoided.

TABLE 11.1.2: Red flag symptoms and signs in recurrent abdominal pain (RAP).

Symptoms	*Signs*
Nocturnal pain; persistent fever	Recurrent oral ulcers
Pain localized away from the umbilicus	• Erythema nodosum in Crohn's disease, tuberculosis • Palpable purpura in Henoch–Schönlein vasculitis • Oral pigmentation in Peutz–Jeghers syndrome • Burton's line in plumbism
Radiation of pain	Pallor-plumbism, IBD, PUD
Significant vomiting	Jaundice-cholelithiasis, Crohn's disease
Unintentional weight loss	Arthritis, iridocyclitis–IBD
Chronic diarrhea/nocturnal diarrhea	Significant growth faltering
Hematochezia/hematemesis/melena	Hepatosplenomegaly
Delayed puberty/amenorrhea/short stature	Perianal lesions–fissure/fistula/tag

(IBD: inflammatory bowel disease; PUD: peptic ulcer disease)

Level I Investigations

These are sufficient if the pain has the characteristics of FAP, and no red flag signs or symptoms are present **(Table 11.1.2)**.

Complete Hemogram

The complete blood count (CBC) and erythrocyte sedimentation rate (ESR) should be normal in FAP. The following abnormalities indicate organic disease:

- *Hypochromic microcytic anemia:* IBD and peptic ulcer disease

- *Megaloblastic anemia (B_{12}/folate deficiency):* IBD, small bowel bacterial overgrowth
- *Basophilic stippling:* Lead poisoning
- *Neutrophilia:* Infections of GI tract or urinary tract
- *Eosinophilia:* Parasitic infections, eosinophilic esophagitis
- *High ESR:* Neoplasia, IBD, and abdominal tuberculosis (TB)

Urine Analysis

Urinary tract infection (UTI), hematuria for renal calculi.

Stool Examination

- Occult blood—peptic ulcer disease, IBD
- Ova, parasites—giardia, hookworms, etc.

Blood Biochemistry

Serum amylase/lipase/liver and renal function tests.

Mantoux Test

Tests for screening tuberculosis are helpful.

Ultrasonography

It is painless, noninvasive, and does not involve radiation. A normal ultrasonography (USG) reassures patients, parents, and physicians. USG also detects thickening of bowel (Crohn's disease); and pelvic/ovarian disease in adolescent girls; renal calculi, gallstones, pancreatic calculi, and hydronephrosis. *Disadvantage* is that incidental findings like small mesenteric lymph nodes may aggravate parental anxiety. They are significant only when their transverse diameter is >8.5 mm, or if there is matting/evidence of bowel thickening/ascites.

Level II Investigations

If the above investigations are normal, and the child has one or more red flag signs, additional investigations may be needed:

Contrast Studies of Upper and Lower Gastrointestinal Tract

These are mostly done to rule out the following:
- Malrotation with intermittent volvulus
- Congenital malformations of bowel
- Mucosal abnormalities of IBD
- Tuberculosis
- Immunoproliferative small intestinal disease (IPSID).

Endoscopy

Indications for endoscopy in RAP include the following:
- Associated dysphagia, chronic diarrhea, or growth retardation
- Dyspepsia not responding to proton pump inhibitors (PPI) or symptoms recurring on stoppage of PPI
- Celiac serology positive
- Raised inflammatory markers, stool occult blood positive

Several conditions can be diagnosed such as peptic ulcer, *Helicobacter pylori* infection, eosinophilic esophagitis, celiac disease, IBD, etc., by endoscopy. Only about 1% with RAP will require further tests.

Level III Investigations

- EEG to rule out abdominal epilepsy
- Serum lead level for lead poisoning
- Fecal calprotectin (Crohn's disease)
- "Watson-Schwartz test" test for porphyria
- Hydrogen breath test for lactose intolerance

MANAGEMENT

Management is hampered by the lack of effective treatment.[12] We should convince parents and older children that it is a benign condition and that he/she will gradually outgrow it. However, it should be emphasized that the child's pain is real and that he/she is not faking it, but he/she does not have a serious underlying disease. The known theories of FAP such as visceral hyperalgesia and brain-gut interaction may be explained to them in a simple language, with suitable illustrations.

Our aim should not be the complete eradication of pain. Children should be coaxed to normalize their daily activities—school, meals, play, etc. They should be encouraged to focus on studies, sports, and extracurricular activities rather than the pain. If parents are summoned to school, the child should not be brought back home as it may reinforce the symptoms. About 50–70% of patients will respond to this approach. Unfortunately, the remaining may continue to be symptomatic in their adolescence and adulthood.

Parents of some children with FAP are very eager to get the elusive "magic pill' which will cure their child. Medications that may worsen symptoms such as nonsteroidal anti-inflammatory drugs (NSAIDs) should be avoided in functional dyspepsia; instead simple analgesics such as paracetamol and antispasmodics may be tried. Proton pump inhibitors (PPI) and prokinetics may be beneficial in functional dyspepsia and GER. Some children with IBS improve with peppermint oil.[13] Dietary substances that precipitate pain (FODMAPS, caffeine, etc.) should be avoided.

Pain Diary

This is a record of the pain felt by the child. At the end of each day, the child or family member records information about the day's pain, including an indication of its severity (using a 1–10 or faces pain rating scale shown in **Fig. 11.1.5**). If the

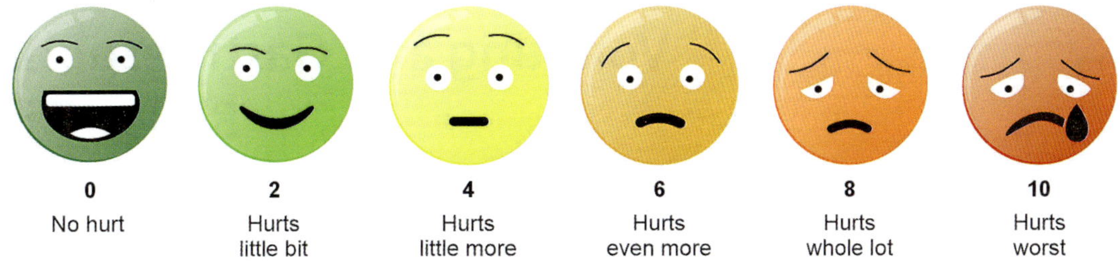

Fig. 11.1.5: Wong–Baker scale for pain.

child has associated depression or anxiety or when symptoms are disabling, preliminary investigations are normal, and he/she is not responding to first-line measures, he/she may be referred for psychological evaluation.

Psychological Interventions for Functional Abdominal Pain

- *Cognitive behavioral therapy (CBT):* Aims to modify thoughts, beliefs, and behavioral responses to symptoms and the effects of illness. This may require multiple sessions with a psychologist with or without some medications from a psychiatrist.
- *Relaxation technique:* Deep breathing exercises—10 minutes every day and also during the episode of pain.
- Hypnotherapy
- Distraction
- Biofeedback
- Meditation/Yoga

CONCLUSION

Recurrent abdominal pain is one of the most common medical problems in children. Most of these patients do not have any serious underlying organic disease. A detailed history and careful examination are vital. Investigations should be restricted to children with alarm symptoms or signs. Drug therapy is of limited use in FAP.

REFERENCES

1. Robin SG, Keller C, Zwiener R, Hyman PE, Nurko S, Saps M, et al. Prevalence of pediatric functional gastrointestinal disorders utilizing the Rome IV criteria. J Pediatr. 2018;195:134-9.
2. Apley J, Naish N. Recurrent abdominal pains: a field survey of 1,000 school children. Arch Dis Child. 1958;33(168):165-70.
3. Endo Y, Shoji T, Fukudo S, Machida T, Machida T, Noda S. The features of adolescent irritable bowel syndrome in Japan. J Gastroenterol Hepatol. 2011;26(Suppl 3):106-9.
4. Drossman DA. Functional gastrointestinal disorders: History, pathophysiology, clinical features, and Rome IV. Gastroenterology. 2016;150:1262-79.
5. Thapar N, Benninga MA, Crowell MD, Di Lorenzo C, Mack I, Nurko S, et al. Paediatric functional abdominal pain disorders. Nat Rev Dis Primers. 2020;6(1):89.
6. Huang TT, Lai JB, Du YL, Xu Y, Ruan LM, Hu SH. Current understanding of gut microbiota in mood disorders: an update of human studies. Front Genet. 2019;10:98.
7. Paula H, Grover M, Halder SL, Locke GR 3rd, Schleck CD, Zinsmeister AR, et al. Non-enteric infections, antibiotic use, and risk of development of functional gastrointestinal disorders. Neurogastroenterol Motil. 2015;27(11):1580-6.
8. Devanarayana NM, Rajindrajith S, Perera MS, Nishanthanie SW, Benninga MA. Gastric emptying and antral motility parameters in children with functional dyspepsia: association with symptom severity. J Gastroenterol Hepatol. 2013;28(7):1161-6.
9. Balagoni H, Mando R, Dhara Chaudhari D, Swenson JA, Young M. Abdominal Epilepsy: A rare cause of paroxysmal abdominal symptoms associated with epilepsy: 1699. Am J Gastroenterol. 2016;111(1):S809-10.
10. Riyaz A. Recurrent abdominal pain. In: Pediatric Gastroenterology and Hepatology, 4th edition. Hyderabad: Paras Publishers; 2019. pp. 117-30.
11. Schneiderman H, Lopetegui-Lia N, Nichols J. The enduring and practical power of physical examination: Carnett Sign. Am J Med. 2020;133(6):682-4.
12. Van den Houte K, Carbone F, Tack J. Postprandial distress syndrome: stratification and management. Expert Rev Gastroenterol Hepatol. 2019;13(1):37-46.
13. Rajindrajith S, Chiong-Meng Boey C, Devanarayana NM, Niriella MA, Thapar N, Benninga MA. Navigating through 65 years of insights: lessons learned on functional abdominal pain in children. Eur J Pediatr. 2024;183(9):3689-703.

11.2 Vomiting and Gastroesophageal Reflux Disease

Aathira Ravindranath

INTRODUCTION

Vomiting involves forceful expulsion of gastric contents through the mouth (may be associated with nausea and retching). *Nausea* is a subjective feeling of unpleasantness accompanied by pallor, hypersalivation, and anorexia. *Retching* encompasses spasmodic respiratory movements, contraction of abdominal muscles against a closed glottis without actually throwing out gastric contents.[1] *Regurgitation* is the passive effortless movement of gastric contents into the mouth without abdominal wall contractions. *Rumination* involves effortlessly bringing up recently ingested food through a voluntary increase in abdominal pressure, chewing, and sometimes reswallowing. Though definitions make our understanding easier, analyzing the symptoms in a child is a challenge in itself where a clear distinction between the above conditions cannot be made and parents often put everything in the basket of "vomiting." Thus, tweezing out the underlying cause requires thorough history from the child and the parents.

Vomiting can be acute or chronic. Though the ROME IV foundation defines the duration of chronic nausea and vomiting in children as 2 months, a more practical cutoff would be to take 4 weeks so that evaluation is not delayed. Chronic vomiting can further be classified as chronic continuous and chronic recurrent which helps in identifying the underlying cause.

ETIOLOGY

Acute Vomiting

Episodes of vomiting with onset <4 weeks with no significant past history can be classified as acute vomiting. The underlying causes are usually acute gastritis, infective gastroenteritis, foreign body ingestion, food bolus impaction, pancreatitis, urinary tract infection, diabetic ketoacidosis, and drug-induced.

Chronic Vomiting

The etiology of chronic vomiting in children is diverse, varies with age of the child, and includes extra-intestinal causes also. Differential diagnosis of chronic vomiting based on the age of the child is given in **Table 11.2.1**. The causes can be broadly divided as those arising due to gastrointestinal, metabolic, endocrine, neurological, and renal disorders.[2] Many of the

TABLE 11.2.1: Etiology of chronic vomiting based on age of the child.

Neonates	*Infants*	*Children*	*Adolescents*
Gastrointestinal			
Esophageal stenosis	GERD	GERD	Rumination syndrome
GERD	Cow's milk protein allergy	Cow's milk protein allergy	Gastritis
Cow's milk protein intolerance	Intestinal malrotation	Eosinophilic esophagitis	Peptic ulcer disease
Congenital microgastria	Duodenal web	Gastritis	Eosinophilic esophagitis
Hypertrophic pyloric stenosis	Esophageal stricture	Achalasia cardia	GERD
Duodenal web	Ileal jejunal stenosis	Esophageal, pyloric strictures	Esophageal, pyloric strictures
Intestinal malrotation	Intussusception	Foreign body ingestion	Achalasia cardia
Duplication cyst	Hirschsprung disease	Superior mesenteric artery syndrome	Crohn's disease
Annular pancreas	Annular pancreas	Crohn's disease	Intestinal tuberculosis
Ileal, jejunal stenosis	Very early onset inflammatory bowel disease	Intestinal tuberculosis	Gastrointestinal lymphoma
Hiatus hernia	Gastroparesis	Gastrointestinal lymphoma	Superior mesenteric artery syndrome

Contd...

Contd...

Neonates	***Infants***	***Children***	***Adolescents***
Hirschsprung disease	Duplication cyst	Rumination syndrome	Gastroparesis
Intestinal aganglionosis		Intestinal malrotation	Chronic pseudo-obstruction
		Intussusception	Distal intestinal obstruction syndrome
			Chronic pancreatitis
Metabolic			
Urea cycle defects	Hereditary fructose intolerance	Hereditary fructose intolerance	Urea cycle defects
Fatty acid oxidation defects	Urea cycle defects	Urea cycle defects	Fatty acid oxidation defects
Organic acidemias	Fatty acid oxidation defects	Fatty acid oxidation defects	Acute intermittent porphyria
Mitochondrial hepatopathies	Organic acidemias	Organic acidemias	
Gluconeogenic disorders	Mitochondrial hepatopathies	Mitochondrial hepatopathies	
Galactosemia			
Phenylketonuria			
Congenital lactic acidosis			
Endocrine			
Congenital adrenal hyperplasia	Hypercalcemia	Diabetic ketoacidosis	Diabetic ketoacidosis
Neonatal thyrotoxicosis	Addison disease	Hypercalcemia	Hypercalcemia
Hypercalcemia		Hyperthyroidism	Hyperthyroidism
		Addison disease	Addison disease
Neurological			
Congenital hydrocephalus	Intracranial tumors	Cyclical vomiting syndrome	Cyclical vomiting syndrome
Meningitis	Meningitis	Intracranial tumors	Intracranial tumors
Arnold–Chiari malformation	Pseudotumor cerebri	Meningitis	Meningitis
Intracranial hemorrhage		CNS tuberculosis	CNS tuberculosis
Pseudotumor cerebri		Neurocysticercosis	Neurocysticercosis
			Bulimia nervosa
			Functional vomiting
			Migraine
Others			
Hydronephrosis	UTI	Uremia	Uremia
UTI	Uremia	UTI	UTI
VUR	VUR	Hydronephrosis	Vestibular disorders
Neonatal abstinence syndrome	Renal tubular acidosis	Vestibular disorders	Cannabinoid hyperemesis syndrome
Munchausen syndrome by proxy	Munchausen syndrome by proxy		Glaucoma
			Drug-induced
			Testicular/ovarian torsion

(CNS: central nervous system; GERD: gastroesophageal reflux disease; UTI: urinary tract infection; VUR: vesicoureteric reflux)

obstructive causes have a dramatic presentation, however, noncritical narrowing can present as chronic vomiting, failure to thrive, and feed refusal. When one congenital anomaly of the gastrointestinal tract is diagnosed, other associated anomalies should be actively looked for, because they will cause persistent symptoms despite surgical correction of the obstruction.

Gastroesophageal reflux (GER) is a physiological phenomenon affecting 50% infants between 0 and 3 months, 67% in those between 4 and 6 months, and it decreases to 5% at 1 year. The majority are "happy spitters" and are otherwise normal. But 5–10% of them can have pathological *gastroesophageal reflux disease (GERD)* causing bothersome symptoms, failure to gain weight or complications. One of the manifestations of cow's milk protein allergy (CMPA) is recurrent vomiting and it can start in the first few days of birth after exposure to bovine milk protein. In all babies with GERD, CMPA ought to be considered as a possibility.[3] Eosinophilic esophagitis (EoE) is an emerging disease in children and 38% present with symptoms similar to GERD. In infants and older children, apart from the other anatomical causes of obstruction, intussusception can present with vomiting in 48% cases along with pain and incessant crying. Intestinal tuberculosis and Crohn's disease can have vomiting in 8–20% children.[4] In normal children and adolescents at least one episode of rumination is seen in up to 11% and recurrent rumination in 1.5%.

Though metabolic causes can present acutely, many of them can have recurrent vomiting as the initial manifestation. Diagnosing these disorders urgently is imperative to initiate treatment. Any cause of raised intracranial pressure can present with vomiting. In children with intracranial tumors, 30% have vomiting as the earliest symptom along with headache. Prevalence of cyclical vomiting syndrome (CVS) in normal children is only 0.3%, but it is important to recognize it as a specific cause of recurrent vomiting. Renal and endocrine diseases may also have vomiting as the sole symptom. Many of the extraintestinal causes have a recurrent pattern of vomiting as that seen in CVS, organic acidemia, hydronephrosis, urea cycle defects, diabetic ketoacidosis, and Addison disease. Intestinal malrotation with volvulus also may have a recurrent pattern. Most of the other causes have a chronic continuous pattern.

DIAGNOSTIC APPROACH TO VOMITING

Arriving at a clinical diagnosis and tailoring investigations in a child with vomiting are akin to solving a jigsaw puzzle. In most of the cases broad classification of etiology can be ascertained with clinical features and basic blood work which can be confirmed with specific investigations **(Flowchart 11.2.1)**.

Step 1: Gastrointestinal versus Extraintestinal Causes

Differentiating between gastrointestinal and extra-intestinal source is the foremost step. Children with raised intracranial pressure often present with early morning vomiting and headache. They may also have focal neurological deficits, seizures, macrocephaly, and behavioral problems. Recurrent episodes of vomiting along with encephalopathy triggered by minor infections, acidosis, hypoglycemia, and hyperammonemia indicate underlying inborn errors of metabolism. Vomiting may be induced by protein-rich diet in urea cycle defects and organic acidemias, and by sweets and juices in hereditary fructose intolerance. Acute intermittent porphyria can present with vomiting in association with hypertension and peripheral neuropathy. Hyponatremia, hyperkalemia, hypotension, and ambiguous genitalia suggest congenital adrenal hyperplasia. Fever, burning micturition, anemia, growth failure, normal anion gap acidosis, and elevated urea and creatinine suggest renal disorders. CVS occurs in stereotypical patterns with absolute normalcy in between episodes, and could be triggered by stressful events; there can associated family history of migraine, will be associated with intense nausea and severity of vomiting may be as high as 4 times in 1 hour.[5] Thus, basic metabolic workup will include arterial blood gas, lactate, electrolytes, blood glucose, arterial ammonia, liver enzymes, urea, creatinine, urine ketones, urine nonglucose reducing substances and urine porphyrins.

Step 2: Source in the Gastrointestinal Tract

Once the source is narrowed to the gastrointestinal tract, the next step is to ascertain the location of pathology. In an infant if the vomitus contains uncurdled milk, esophageal causes should be considered. If the vomitus is large quantity, contains curdled milk in infants or stale food in children etiology is localized to the stomach. Infantile hypertrophic pyloric stenosis (IHPS) presents with nonbilious projectile vomiting from 2 to 8 weeks of life, an olive may be palpable in the right upper quadrant in half of them, and dehydration and metabolic alkalosis is seen in 30%. CMPA can present with GERD, hematemesis and refusal to feed.

When anatomical obstruction is considered the site of block ought to be determined. Nonbilious vomiting suggests obstruction proximal to ampulla of Vater, while in bilious vomiting obstruction is distal to ampulla, and feculent suggests colonic stasis. Pain and visible bowel loops in the periumbilical area suggest small intestinal obstruction, while generalized distension and obstipation narrow down the cause to the colon. Children with intussusception may have a sausage shaped mass palpable in the right side of abdomen and "currant jelly" stools. Constitutional symptoms will accompany intestinal tuberculosis, Crohn's disease, and lymphoma. History of rapid weight loss preceding onset of vomiting is clue to superior mesenteric artery (SMA) syndrome. In rumination syndrome, regurgitation occurs immediately after eating, the act of vomiting can be controlled and reswallowing may also be present. In those with achalasia cardia, dysphagia is a predominant complaint along with regurgitation, and nocturnal cough. In children who have dysphagia, vomiting, skin pigmentation,

Flowchart 11.2.1: Approach to chronic vomiting.

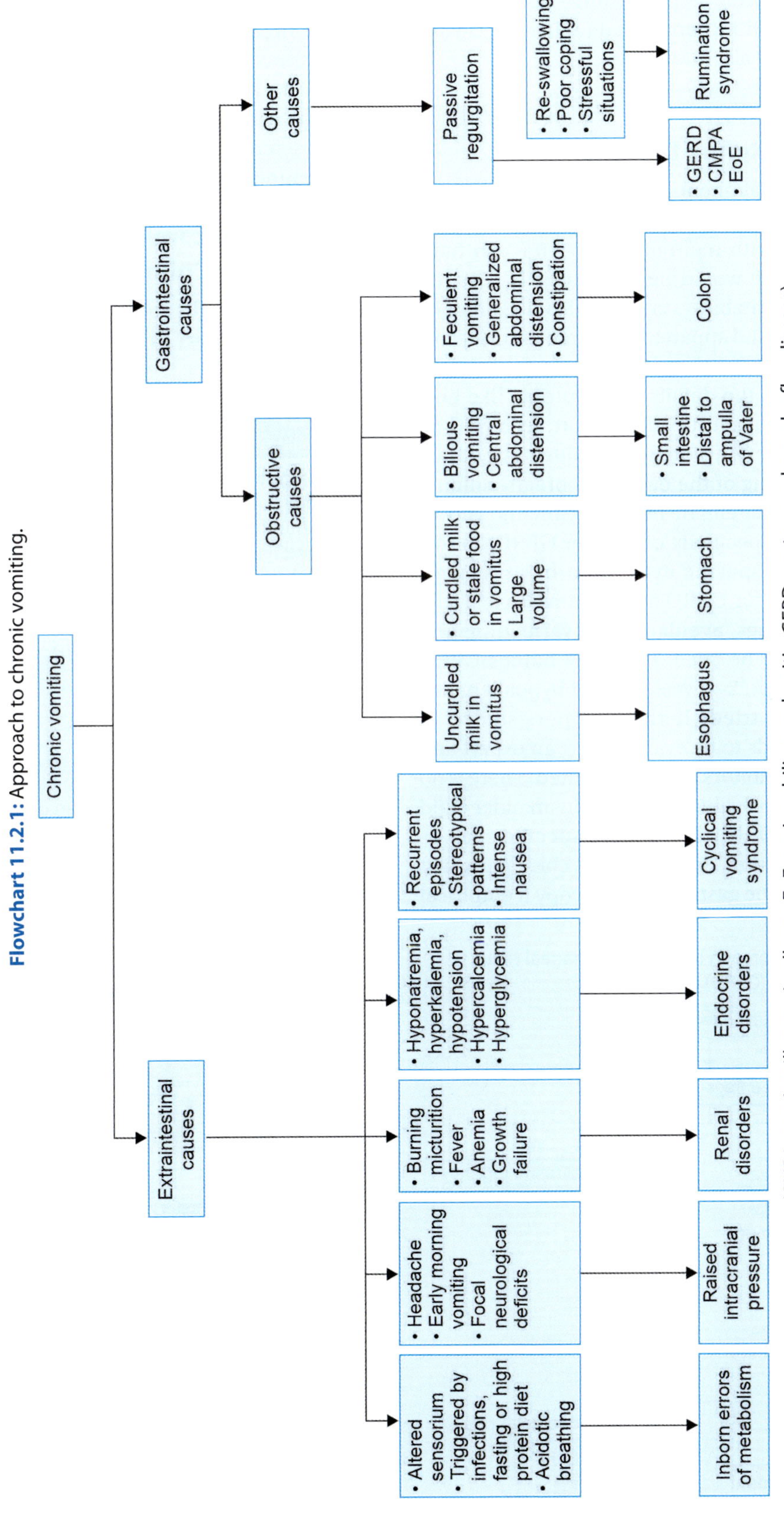

(CMPA: cow's milk protein allergy; EoE: eosinophilic esophagitis; GERD: gastroesophageal reflux disease)

hypotension, hyperkalemia, hypotension—possibility of Allgrove syndrome should be considered (achalasia cardia, adrenal insufficiency, and alacrimia).

Diagnostic Approach to Gastroesophageal Reflux Disease

The GER is a physiological phenomenon in infants peaking at 6 months of age and then gradually declines by one year of age. Among infants with regurgitation 5–10% can have pathological reflux which would be called GERD. The red flags are poor growth, irritability, crying episodes, anemia, choking, cough, wheeze, and apparent life-threatening events **(Flowchart 11.2.2)**. Orenstein's questionnaire (consists of questions with regard to the details of symptoms like how many spit-ups, quantity of spit-up, discomfort, feed refusal, failure to gain weight, crying or fussing during feeding, duration of crying, arching of the back, and breath holding spells) may be used to differentiate between GER and GERD. If the score is >7, it has specificity of 94% for GERD. In this case the child requires specific evaluation by an expert. Predisposing conditions for GERD are given in **Box 11.2.1**. In the absence of red flags, avoidance of overfeeding and thickening of feeds may be tried. In 1–10% babies GERD may be the result of CMPA, 2–4 weeks trial of hypoallergenic formula feeds may be tried. If there is persistence of symptoms, the child needs to be evaluated by an expert and empiric proton pump inhibitors are not indicated. There is no role for contrast studies in evaluating reflux. In an older child with symptoms of GERD which are more specific such as heartburn, sour regurgitation, dysphagia and chest pain, first step in evaluation would be gastroduodenoscopy if empirical acid suppression for 2–4 weeks has not yielded symptomatic relief or there is recurrence of symptoms on tapering. If there are no esophageal erosions, 24-hour pH metry can document acidic reflux. In the absence of acidic reflux with a positive symptom correlation, reflux hypersensitivity is to be considered, and in the absence of symptom correlation, it could be functional heartburn.[6]

Flowchart 11.2.2: Approach to gastroesophageal reflux disease (GERD) in an infant.

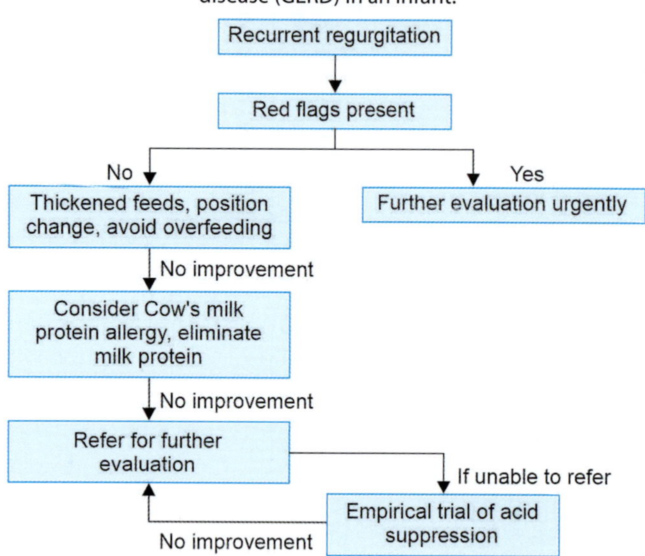

Step 3: Specific Investigations in a Vomiting Child

Investigations ought to be planned based on the clinical diagnosis **(Flowchart 11.2.3)**.

BOX 11.2.1: Predisposing factors for gastroesophageal reflux disease (GERD).

- Neurological impairment like cerebral palsy
- Obesity
- Neuromuscular disorders
- Repaired trachea-esophageal fistula, esophageal atresia
- Sliding hiatus hernia
- Caustic injury to esophagus
- Prematurity
- Chronic lung diseases
- Cystic fibrosis
- Scleroderma

Flowchart 11.2.3: Approach to gastroesophageal reflux disease (GERD) in an older child.

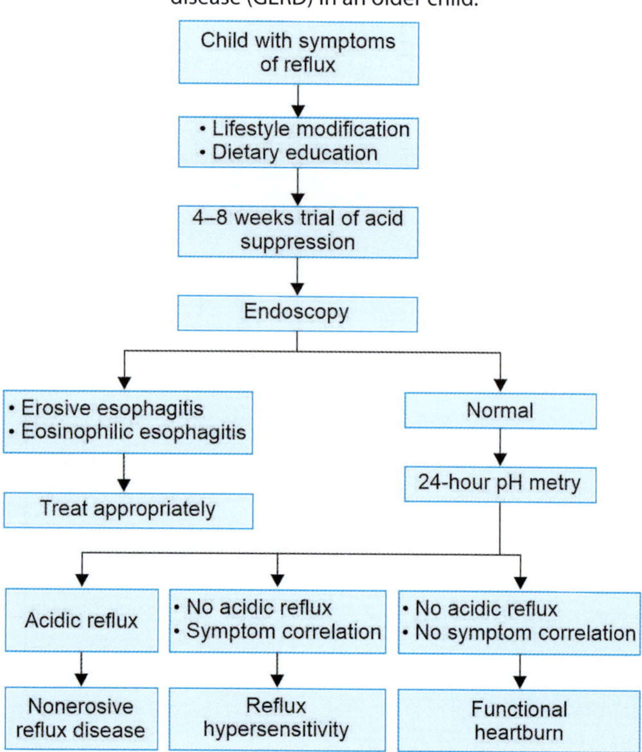

Radiological Investigations

Erect radiographs ought to be performed if obstructive causes are suspected. In the infant, single bubble and double bubble signs may be seen in pyloric and duodenal obstruction, respectively. Multiple air fluid levels may be seen in other causes of intestinal obstruction. Ultrasonogram is diagnostic in IHPS (pyloric muscle wall thickness >3 mm and pyloric canal length >12 mm), gut duplication (gut signature sign), intussusception (target sign, pseudo-kidney sign, and Doppler for vascularity), and malrotation with volvulus (relationship between superior mesenteric artery and vein). Upper gastrointestinal series best demonstrate malrotation and other causes of anatomical obstruction. Timed barium swallow studies would show hold-up of the contrast in achalasia cardia. Contrast-enhanced computed tomography will be needed in cases with intestinal tuberculosis, Crohn's disease, gastrointestinal lymphoma, and SMA syndrome.

Esophagogastroduodenoscopy

Of all children presenting to an endoscopy unit, 21% had persistent vomiting as the symptom. The overall yield of esophagogastroduodenoscopy (EGD) in children with vomiting is 67%.[7] Conditions that can be diagnosed on EGD are esophageal strictures, foreign body, erosive esophagitis, EoE, peptic ulcer disease, gastritis, and gastric outlet obstruction. In EoE, EGD will show linear furrows, trachealization of esophagus, whitish plaques, mucosal fragility, small luminal caliber and biopsy will demonstrate increase in eosinophils.

Manometry

High-resolution esophageal manometry can diagnose and classify achalasia cardia and other causes of esophageal dysmotility. However, in young children placement of catheter will require mild sedation. Swallows should be given after the effect of sedation is worn off. For antroduodenal manometry, placement of catheter usually requires deeper anesthesia which can affect digestive motility.[8] There are limited indications for antroduodenal manometry in children which include gastroparesis, pseudo-obstruction, and rumination syndrome.

Other Investigations

The CMPA is diagnosed by elimination of milk and milk products in the diet for 1–2 weeks, symptom resolution, and recurrence on rechallenge. 24-hour pH monitoring for acid reflux, nuclear studies for gastric emptying, breath tests for small bowel motility, and full thickness intestinal biopsy in pseudo-obstruction are specific tests that need to be done on a case-to-case basis. Bulimia nervosa, functional vomiting, rumination, migraine, and cyclical vomiting syndrome are diagnosed clinically but often additional tests have to be performed to rule out organic etiology.

MANAGEMENT

Primarily dehydration, electrolyte imbalances, hypoglycemia, and acid balance need to be corrected. Other management strategies depend on the underlying cause. Apart from medical and surgical management, endoscopic, dietary, and behavioral therapy are also a part of the therapeutic armamentarium in children with chronic vomiting. In case of obstructive causes child has to be kept nil per orally, gastric decompression with nasogastric tube, intravenous fluids, and antibiotics have to be started followed by surgical consultation.

In CMPA, therapeutic elimination of milk and milk products have to be done for a minimum of 6 months in IgE-mediated allergy and 12–18 months in non-IgE-mediated cases. In exclusively breastfed babies, mother ought to eliminate milk products from her diet, if the baby is formula fed extensively, hydrolyzed formula (eHF) feeds should be given. Amino acid-based formula may be considered in severe cases not responding to eHF.[9]

In babies with GERD, if there is no improvement after thickening feeds and elimination of milk, a 4–8 weeks trial of proton pump inhibitors (PPI) should be given **(Flowchart 11.2.2)**. In older children, if PPI trial is not successful or if weaning off PPI is difficult then EoE is a possibility **(Flowchart 11.2.3)**. Following the six-food elimination diet (cow's milk, soy, egg, fish, wheat, and nuts) can achieve remission in 74% cases of EoE in 6 weeks. Thereafter, sequential reintroduction will aid in identifying specific triggers. In the cohort that does not respond to PPI, viscous budesonide, or oral fluticasone has shown good efficacy. In SMA syndrome majority of the cases improve with conservative management by hyperalimentation, nasojejunal feeding, and only the resistant cases require duodenojejunostomy.

Pneumatic balloon dilatation has been the first line of treatment of achalasia followed by Heller's myotomy. But recently there are many reports of successful per oral endoscopic myotomy in children. Esophageal and pyloric strictures can be managed by endoscopic dilatations.

Diaphragmatic breathing is the cornerstone of therapy in rumination syndrome. Other behavioral modifications such as aversion techniques, general relaxation, and distraction may also be beneficial.[10] Making a positive diagnosis of CVS itself reduced the severity of vomiting in 78% children. During the acute episode abortive strategies include dextrose containing intravenous fluids, ondansetron, and sedation. Prophylactic measures comprise avoiding triggers, medications [*first line:* cyproheptadine, pizotifen (age <5 years), and amitriptyline (age >5 years), *second line:* propranolol] and supplements (carnitine and coenzyme Q).

For gastroparesis, management includes low fat, low fiber, small frequent feeds, prokinetics (erythromycin, azithromycin, domperidone, metoclopramide, and baclofen), gastric electric stimulation and in refractory cases botulinum toxin injection, pyloroplasty, or partial gastrectomy may be indicated.

CONCLUSION

Vomiting in children encompasses a whole gamut of causes. Reaching a clinical diagnosis guides further investigations for confirmation.

REFERENCES

1. Lacy BE, Parkman HP, Camilleri M. Chronic nausea and vomiting: evaluation and treatment. Am J Gastroenterol. 2018;113(5):647-59.
2. Ravindranath A. Chronic vomiting in children: Etiology, diagnosis, and management. Indian J Gastroenterol. 2020;39(2):117-22.
3. Rosen R, Vandenplas Y, Singendonk M, Cabana M, DiLorenzo C, Gottrand F, et al. Pediatric gastroesophageal reflux clinical practice guidelines: Joint recommendations of the North American Society for Pediatric Gastroenterology, Hepatology, and Nutrition and the European Society for Pediatric Gastroenterology, Hepatology, and Nutrition. J Pediatr Gastroeneterol Nutr. 2018;66(3):516-54.
4. Singh SK, Srivastava A, Kumari N, Poddar U, Yachha SK, Pandey CM. Differentiation between Crohn disease and intestinal tuberculosis in children. J Pediatr Gastroenterol Nutr. 2018;66(1):e6-e11.
5. Frazier R, Li BUK, Venkatesan T. Diagnosis and management of cyclic vomiting syndrome: A critical review. Am J Gastroenterol. 2023;118(7):1157-67.
6. Mohan N, Matthai J, Bolia R, Agarwal J, Shrivastava R, Borkar VV; For Pediatric Gastroenterology Chapter of Indian Academy of Pediatrics, Indian Society of Pediatric Gastroenterology, Hepatology and Nutrition (ISPGHAN). Diagnosis and Management of Gastroesophageal Reflux Disease in Children: Recommendations of Pediatric Gastroenterology Chapter of Indian Academy of Pediatrics, Indian Society of Pediatric Gastroenterology, Hepatology and Nutrition (ISPGHAN). Indian Pediatr. 2021;58(12):1163-70.
7. Mahoney LB, Walsh CM, Lightdale JR. Promoting research that supports high-quality gastrointestinal endoscopy in children. Curr Gastroenterol Rep. 2023;25(11):333-43.
8. Rosen R, Garza JM, Tipnis N, Nurko S. An ANMS-NASPGHAN consensus document on esophageal and antroduodenal manometry in children. Neurogastroenterol Motil. 2018;30(3):1-31.
9. Koletzko S, Niggemann B, Arato A, Diaz JA, Heuschkel R, Husby S, et al. Diagnostic approach and management of cow's-milk protein allergy in infants and children: ESPGHAN GI Committee practical guidelines. J Pediatr Gastroenterol Nutr. 2012;55(2):221-9.
10. Murray HB, Juarascio AS, Di Lorenzo C, Drossman DA, Thomas JJ. Diagnosis and treatment of rumination Syndrome: A critical review. Am J Gastroenterol. 2019;114(4):562-78.

11.3 *Helicobacter pylori* Infection in Childhood

Jagadeesh Menon VR

INTRODUCTION

Helicobacter pylori (*H. pylori*) is an important pathogen encountered in the pediatric age group.[1] The organism has not only been associated with disorders such as gastritis and peptic ulcer disease, but also with other extra gastrointestinal (GI) illnesses such as autoimmune thrombocytopenic purpura (AITP) and Henoch-Schönlein purpura (HSP).[2,3] The profile of *H. pylori* infection in children is considerably different from that of adults. This chapter focuses on the current aspects of *H. pylori* infection in children, including its management.

MICROBIAL ASPECTS

Helicobacter pylori was first described by Warren and Marshal in 1982, while they were studying gastric biopsies of patients suffering from gastritis, and this remarkable discovery procured them the Nobel prize for Medicine in 2005.[1] Later, an association of *H. pylori* with mucosa-associated lymphoid tissue lymphoma (MALToma) was described in 1991, and its association with peptic ulcer disease, gastric adenocarcinoma, and non-Hodgkin lymphoma was described in 1994.

Helicobacter pylori is the most common bacteria to infect human beings and is thought to be acquired around 60,000 years back during migration from Africa. It is a spiral-shaped microaerophilic gram-negative bacillus, which is predominantly found in the antrum of stomach. This organism is highly adapted to the gastric environment and has the ability to secrete the enzyme urease, which helps in neutralizing the acidic pH of the stomach. The urease also provides nitrogen for the protein synthesis of the bacterium. The lipopolysaccharide of *H. pylori* mimics blood group antigens, and this also gives survival benefit to the bacteria in the hostile gastric environment.

EPIDEMIOLOGY OF *HELICOBACTER PYLORI* IN CHILDREN

The prevalence of *H. pylori* in children is highly dependent on environmental factors and social striatization. Asymptomatic children from developing countries have a high prevalence of *H. pylori,* which shows that these children were exposed to this pathogen from early life. In one of the largest meta-analysis, including 632 data points and 152,650 children, it was seen that the global prevalence of *H. pylori* in children was 32.3%.[4] The more affected were older children and those from low and middle income countries. Lower income strata, no access to sewage, room sharing, more siblings, and at least one of the parents affected were the risk factors for acquiring *H. pylori* infection. Higher incidence of up to 85–90% has been reported from countries such as South Africa, Nigeria, Nicaragua, and Serbia. The prevalence is decreasing slowly with respect to the improving sanitation and social standards, with Japan having a steep decrease in its prevalence in the post-World war period.

Majority of the children acquire *H. pylori* usually by 3–4 years of age, and it remains lifelong in their gastric environment. Infants are rarely infected possibly due to the presence of maternal antibodies [immunoglobulin G (IgG)] against *H. pylori.*

Helicobacter pylori is transmitted between human beings, especially among family members. This human to human transmission can be either gastric-oral or feco-oral in which the former appears to be the most important route. This is supported by the fact that the only reservoir of this pathogen is human stomach, and *H. pylori* can be cultured in gastric juices of even young children.[2] Waterborne transmission has also been evaluated as one of the possible sources of transmission. The reinfection rate in children belonging to developing countries can be as high has 13% per year due to the predisposing social factors.

PATHOLOGY AND PATHOGENESIS

Helicobacter pylori is highly adapted to the extremely unfavorable acidic gastric environment. In the majority of individuals, the organism attaches to the gastric epithelium as a colonizer and remains asymptomatic. The ability of the organism to survive in gastric medium and also to invade the mucosa causing tissue injury is due to its various intrinsic factors **(Fig. 11.3.1)**.

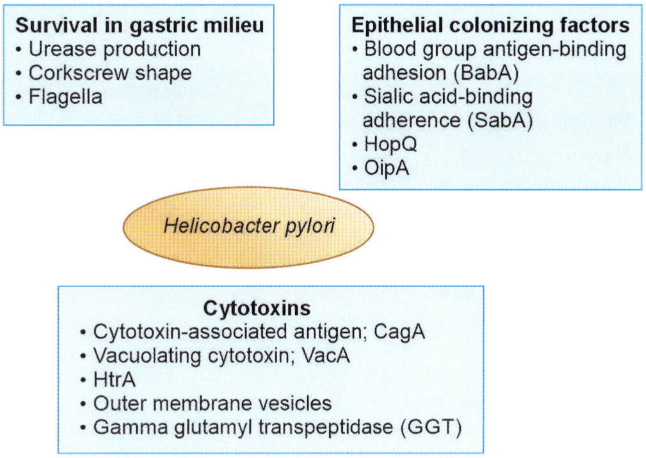

Factors to Survive the Gastric Acidic Environment

The bacterial urease splits urea to release ammonium ions, which neutralize the acidic media around the bacteria. This

Survival in gastric milieu
- Urease production
- Corkscrew shape
- Flagella

Epithelial colonizing factors
- Blood group antigen-binding adhesion (BabA)
- Sialic acid-binding adherence (SabA)
- HopQ
- OipA

Helicobacter pylori

Cytotoxins
- Cytotoxin-associated antigen; CagA
- Vacuolating cytotoxin; VacA
- HtrA
- Outer membrane vesicles
- Gamma glutamyl transpeptidase (GGT)

Fig. 11.3.1: Factors contributing to pathogenesis of *Helicobacter pylori* infection.

along with the inherent corkscrew shape of the organism and its flagella helps to breach the mucosal layer of the stomach, attach to the gastric epithelium and subsequently damage it. Urease has also been implicated in promoting tumorigenesis. Apart from this, *H. pylori* also produces epithelial cell colonizing factors [blood group antigen-binding adhesion (BabA), sialic acid-binding adherence (SabA) etc.], which help the pathogen to attach to gastric epithelium. *H. pylori* also produces cytotoxins, which induce tissue damage [e.g., cytotoxin-associated antigen (CagA) and vacuolating cytotoxin (VacA) causing cellular necrosis and apoptosis etc.].[1,2]

Once the bacteria transcend the host barrier or defense, it leads to significant gastric inflammation. Acute gastritis is usually associated with low acid secretion. Untreated acute gastritis progresses to a chronic active gastritis in the majority of patients. Three different patterns of gastritis have been described in association with *H. pylori.* The most common is the antral-predominant gastritis as this area has a slightly higher pH than other parts of the stomach. These patients usually have gastric hypersecretion, and they land up with duodenal ulcers. Another pattern is pangastritis, which can be atrophic (corpus-predominant) or nonatrophic. The atrophic pattern usually predisposes to developing gastric carcinomas and chronic gastric ulcers, whereas the nonatrophic pattern leads to MALTomas. These patterns of involvement are more clearly described in adults rather in pediatric population. Gastritis is the most common presentation of *H. pylori* in children, of which antral gastritis predominates. Children usually do not have atrophic gastritis or intestinal metaplasia.[5]

CLINICAL FEATURES (TABLE 11.3.1)

Gastritis

Helicobacter pylori is associated with acute and chronic gastritis in children.[6] However, the severity of inflammation is

TABLE 11.3.1: Disorders associated with *Helicobacter pylori* infection.

Strongly associated	Weak or no evidence	Potentially protective
• Gastritis • Peptic ulcer • MALToma • Gastric adenocarcinoma • Gastric lymphoma • Iron deficiency anemia • Autoimmune thrombocytopenia	• Gastroesophageal reflux disease • Recurrent abdominal pain • Henoch–Schönlein purpura • Short stature • Guillain–Barré syndrome • Diabetes mellitus/ metabolic syndrome	• Allergy/asthma • Inflammatory bowel disease

(MALToma: mucosa-associated lymphoid tissue lymphoma)

much lesser than adults with *H. pylori* gastritis. The pathogen leads to lymphonodular hyperplasia, which is predominantly seen in the antrum and along with neutrophilic infiltrates, which may represent the active gastritis component. Majority of these patients may remain asymptomatic and no studies conclusively prove that eradication of this bacteria would prevent the subsequent development of gastric cancers.

Peptic Ulcer

Helicobacter pylori can cause both gastric or duodenal ulcers, and the association is found to be very strong.[1] As mentioned previously, an antral-predominant gastritis leads to duodenal ulcer, whereas the corpus-predominant gastritis would lead to gastric ulcers. The dupA (duodenal ulcer-promoting) gene may confer the ulcer-forming potential for this bacterium.

Gastric Malignancies

The World Health Organization (WHO) has classified *H. pylori* as a class 1 carcinogen, and it is the first bacterium to be described an oncogen. *H. pylori* increases three times the risk of developing malignancies such as adenocarcinoma of stomach, non-Hodgkin lymphoma, and MALToma. All children with a MALToma should be investigated and treated for *H. pylori,* which may induce remission in up to 70%. Patients with MALToma who do not achieve remission with *H. pylori* eradication may have underlying chromosomal translocations, and may require chemotherapy.

Gastric carcinoma has a definite association with *H. pylori* infection, with an odds ratio varying from 2 to 9 when compared to those who are uninfected. Acquiring *H. pylori* infection at a very early age is associated with a higher gastric cancer risk, especially in the setting of a positive family history of gastric cancer.

Gastroesophageal Reflux Disease

The association of *H. pylori* to gastroesophageal reflux disease (GERD) is not convincing and may even have an inverse relationship. Analysis done in pediatric age group failed to show that eradication of *H. pylori* would improve symptoms of GERD.

Pain Abdomen

Recurrent abdominal pain (RAP) in children is often attributed to *H. pylori* infection in children, but a solid evidence in favor of this is lacking.[1,3] In a meta-analysis of 45 studies done in children, a definite association of RAP with *H. pylori* was not found. In a Polish multicentric study, it was seen that adults rather than children had higher incidence of *H. pylori* infection when they had symptoms of heartburn and pain abdomen. However, a few pediatric studies from India showed a possible association of pain abdomen with *H. pylori* and symptomatic response after eradication of the organism. However, due to the lack of a strong scientific evidence, the European Society of Pediatric Gastroenterology Hepatology and Nutrition (ESPGHAN) guidelines recommends to weigh the risk and benefits before testing for *H. pylori* in children in children with RAP. Children with recurrent pain abdomen may be recommended an endoscopy if the clinical features do not go in favor of a functional cause to diagnose specific pathologies such as duodenal ulcers and food allergies.

Iron Deficiency Anemia

Helicobacter pylori can cause iron deficiency anemia (IDA) by several mechanisms. The bacteria are known to possess genes, which can scavenge dietary iron, and hence extract it from the host. This becomes more profound in children, who are otherwise prone for iron deficiency due to various sociocultural factors and coexisting enteropathies. Other mechanisms by which *H. pylori* causes IDA include chronic blood loss from gastric erosions or peptic ulcer disease and longstanding gastritis leading to hypochlorhydria. *H. pylori* infection should be kept as a possible cause for IDA in a child, especially if its treatment is refractory, and ESPGHAN guidelines recommend a test and treat strategy in such scenarios.

Autoimmune Thrombocytopenia

There is a strong association of *H. pylori* infection with AITP in adults. However, there is no conclusive evidence for this in children.

Allergic Disorders

There is an inverse correlation between allergic disorders such as asthma, skin allergy, allergic rhinitis, and *H. pylori* infection in children. A protective role for *H. pylori* in inflammatory bowel disease has also been suggested.

Henoch–Schönlein Purpura

Henoch-Schönlein purpura may be triggered by *H. pylori*, and a study by Xiong et al. has shown that the risk may be doubled, and that its eradication may decrease the incidence of HSP. However, more evidence is needed to establish this.

Short Stature

Multiple analysis looking into *H. pylori* as a cause of short stature in children concluded by stating that confounding factors (such as socioeconomic status which can cause either of the aforementioned conditions) are likely responsible, rather the pathogen directly causing stunting in these children.

DIAGNOSIS (TABLE 11.3.2)

Tests for *H. pylori* can be classified as invasive or noninvasive.[7] The ESPGHAN guidelines recommend only testing of children with significant symptoms, not attributable to functional symptoms (e.g., abdominal pain).[3] Patients who have red flag symptoms, family history of gastric cancer, and those with refractory IDA are subjected to *H. pylori* testing including an upper gastrointestinal endoscopy (UGIE). However, those with AITP, growth faltering, food allergy, etc. are not tested for *H. pylori* infection.

It should be noted that the main aim of the investigation is to find the etiology of patient's symptom (given further), which could be related to *H. pylori* rather than looking for the bacteria and treating it (test and treat strategy).

Noninvasive Investigations

Urea Breath Test

Urea breath test (UBT) is considered to be the most accurate noninvasive investigation for *H. pylori* infection. This is performed by orally administering carbon isotope (either C13 or C14) tagged urea to the patient. C13 is a nonradioactive isotope and can be safely administered in children including infants. If the patient has *H. pylori* infection, the urease which is produced by this bacterium would release ammonia and carbon dioxide (CO_2). The tagged CO_2 rapidly diffuses into the blood and gets excreted in the breath, which can be detected using a mass spectrometer. The patients should be off proton pump inhibitors (PPI) as optimum results are obtained in a proper acidic gastric environment. With the current standards, the accuracy of this investigation is >95%. However, for practical reasons, this test cannot be used in children <6 years of age.[7]

TABLE 11.3.2: Investigations to diagnose *Helicobacter pylori* infection.

Noninvasive	*Invasive*
• Urea breath test (UBT) • Stool for *H. pylori* antigen • Serology for *H. pylori*: Blood, saliva, and urine	• Upper gastrointestinal endoscopy (UGIE) and biopsy • Histopathology • Rapid urease test (RUT) • *H. pylori* culture

Stool for Helicobacter pylori Antigen

Detection of the bacterial antigen in stool is another noninvasive investigation, which is widely used to diagnose *H. pylori* infection.[1,7] The most common and most widely used technique is ELISA based, which uses either monoclonal or polyclonal antibody. The former one has a higher specificity (97%) and sensitivity (94%). There are many advantages of stool antigen test when compared to UBT in children. The stool in children can easily be obtained, is cost-effective, and there are no operational difficulties with the equipment used for testing. Since this is not a quantitative test, the adult standard cut offs can be extrapolated to the pediatric age group. This investigation can also be used to demonstrate eradication of *H. pylori* post-eradication.

Helicobacter pylori Serology

This investigation tests for antibody against *H. pylori* (IgM, IgG, and IgA) in the serum, saliva, or urine of suspected patients. During the initial phase of infection, IgM becomes detectable in plasma, but the levels rapidly disappear; hence, these are not routinely monitored. Hence IgG (or sometimes IgA) is the antibody that is analyzed in these patients. The major drawback of this test is that it cannot be used for monitoring a therapeutic response or a recurrence of *H. pylori* infection, as the serological response (IgG) may last for months (serologic scar).[7] Serology is more of use in primary care settings as it is inexpensive, noninvasive, and provides results even in 30 minutes to 1 hour. The results of studies using saliva and urine samples have been largely disappointing.

Invasive investigations

Upper Gastrointestinal Endoscopy

Upper gastrointestinal endoscopy and biopsy are the gold standards to diagnose *H. pylori* infection. The major part of the stomach where the bacteria show characteristic pathological changes is in the antrum. Antral nodularity is the most specific finding in pediatric *H. pylori* infection. These nodules are usually <5 mm and resemble the color of surrounding mucosa (i.e., without hyperemia). Hence, biopsies from the gastric antrum (especially the prepyloric area) are a must in suspected patients. Patients on PPI usually have proximal migration of the bacteria, and hence findings are more commonly seen in the corpus of the stomach. It should also be noted that if an UGIE is performed for evaluation of refractory IDA, biopsies should also be obtained to rule out *H. pylori* infection.

Histopathology

The pathological findings (active inflammation with lymphocytes, plasma cells, and neutrophils) and the bacilli may be demonstrated with the routine hematoxylin and eosin staining, but specific stains such as Giemsa or silver stains like Genta, Warthin-Starry, or Steiner can also be used to detect the bacteria. The severity of histological findings usually correlates with the severity of antral nodularity seen on UGIE **(Fig. 11.3.2)**.

Bacterial Culture and Sensitivity

The endoscopic biopsy specimen taken from antrum and/or corpus of stomach should not come into contact with formalin, as this would kill the bacteria. It should be transported in a saline-filled container or in an appropriate culture medium and should be processed within 2–3 hours as the survival of the organism outside gastric environment is very short. If the cultures are negative, an alternate method such as fluorescence in situ hybridization (FISH) needs to be performed to look for antibiotic susceptibility, especially in those areas with a higher drug resistance to the commonly used anti *H. pylori* medications.

THERAPY OF *HELICOBACTER PYLORI* INFECTION (TABLE 11.3.3)

Indications

These include children with peptic ulcer disease associated with *H. pylori*:

- *H. pylori* colonization in patients with strong family history of gastric cancer
- *H. pylori* infection in the setting of refractory IDA

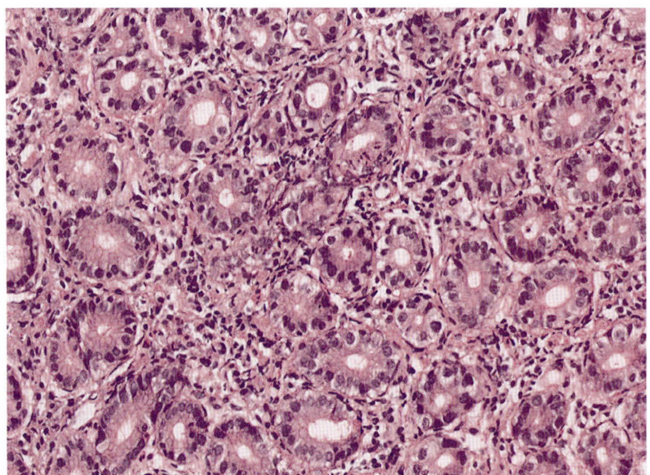

Fig. 11.3.2: Antral biopsy showing active inflammation with lymphomononuclear cells along with *Helicobacter pylori*.

- *H. pylori*-associated gastritis (after considering potential risk and benefits)

The standard recommendation from the EPSGHAN is a triple regimen, which includes two antibiotics, viz. clarithromycin and amoxicillin for 2 weeks, and a PPI for 6 weeks.[3,8,9] The rationale for PPI is that by decreasing acidity it helps faster eradication of *H. pylori*, and improves the efficacy of antibiotics. In the sequential regimen, the first antibiotic used is usually amoxicillin for the first 5 days, as this is known to reduce the resistance to clarithromycin, which is usually the second agent to be administered also for 5 days. Some studies have shown a higher eradication rate with the sequential regimen compared to the conventional 2-week

TABLE 11.3.3: Weight-based regimen for therapy of *Helicobacter pylori* in children and choice of regimen based on sensitivity pattern.

Drug	*Body weight*	*Morning dose*	*Evening dose*
Amoxicillin (AMO)	15–24 kg	500 mg	500 mg
	25–34 kg	750 mg	750 mg
	>35 kg	1,000 mg	1,000 mg
Clarithromycin (CLA)	15–24 kg	250 mg	250 mg
	25–34 kg	500 mg	250 mg
	>35 kg	500 mg	500 mg
Metronidazole (MET)	15–24 kg	250 mg	250 mg
	25–34 kg	500 mg	250 mg
	>35 kg	500 mg	500 mg
Bismuth subsalicylate	<10 years	262 mg QID	
	>10 years	524 mg QID	
Proton pump inhibitors (PPIs)	15–24 kg	20 mg	20 mg
	25–34 kg	30 mg	30 mg
	>35 kg	40 mg	40 mg
Antimicrobial susceptibility		*Regimen used*	
To CLA and MET		AMO-CLA-PPI 14 days, standard dose*	
Resistant to CLA, susceptible to MET		AMO-MET-PPI 14 days, or Bismuth**	
Resistant to MET, susceptible to CLA		AMO-CLA-PPI 14 days, or Bismuth**	
Resistant to both MET and CLA		AMO-MET-PPI 14 days; high dose for AMO# or Bismuth*,**	
Unknown		AMO-MET-PPT 14 days or Bismuth*,**	

*OR concomitant therapy (PPI-AMO-MET-CLA) for 14 days
***In the case of penicillin allergy:* If the strain is susceptible to CLA and MET, use standard dose triple therapy with MET in place of AMO; if the strain is resistant to CLA, then use bismuth-based therapy with tetracycline instead of AMO if over the age of 8 years old.
#*High dose for Amoxicillin:* 15–24 kg; 750 mg twice daily, 25–34 kg; 1,000 mg twice daily, >35 kg; 1,500 mg BD

antibiotic regimen. Drug resistance is least with amoxicillin.[10] Irrational use of antibiotics for trivial infections is known to increase the resistance and hence decrease the efficacy of *H. pylori* eradication. The usual cure rate of the conventional regimen is >80%. Alternate agents such as fluoroquinolones or bismuth salts are indicated in patients with antibiotic resistance, but palatability of bismuth can be an issue in the pediatric age group.

Eradication should be ensured 4–8 weeks post-therapy with a combination of stool antigen test and UBT. There is usually no role for endoscopy post therapy to demonstrate eradication of the bacilli.[3]

HELICOBACTER PYLORI VACCINE

Bacterial proteins such as VacA and CagA are known to be immunogenic in experimental models and ongoing trials using a mixture of multiple proteins are going on. As for now, there is no preventive vaccine available commercially against *H. pylori.*

CONCLUSION

H. pylori infection is an important cause of peptic ulcer disease in children and becomes a definite indication for antimicrobial therapy. However, more evidence is required in the pediatric age group to establish a link between *H. pylori* infection and recurrent abdominal pain. An effective vaccine against this pathogen can be a landmark discovery in medicine, as this could prevent a major fraction of gastric malignancies, which are otherwise directly associated with this microbial agent.

REFERENCES

1. Rajindrajith S, Devanarayana NM, de Silva HJ. Helicobacter pylori infection in children. Saudi J Gastroenterol. 2009;15(2):86-94.
2. Mehrabani S. Helicobacter pylori Infection in Children: a Comprehensive Review. Maedica (Bucur). 2019;14(3):292-7.
3. Jones NL, Koletzko S, Goodman K, Bontems P, Cadranel S, Casswall T, et al. Joint ESPGHAN/NASPGHAN Guidelines for the Management of Helicobacter pylori in Children and Adolescents (Update 2016). J Pediatr Gastroenterol Nutr. 2017;64(6):991-1003.
4. Balas RB, Meliț LE, Mărginean CO. Worldwide Prevalence and Risk Factors of *Helicobacter pylori* Infection in Children. Children (Basel). 2022;9(9):1359.
5. Sharndama HC, Mba IE. Helicobacter pylori: an up-to-date overview on the virulence and pathogenesis mechanisms. Braz J Microbiol. 2022;53(1):33-50.
6. Poddar U, Yachha SK. Helicobacter pylori in children: an Indian perspective. Indian Pediatr. 2007;44(10):761-70.
7. Ricci C, Holton J, Vaira D. Diagnosis of Helicobacter pylori: invasive and non-invasive tests. Best Pract Res Clin Gastroenterol. 2007;21(12):299-313.
8. Yang H, Hu B. Diagnosis of *Helicobacter pylori* Infection and Recent Advances. Diagnostics (Basel). 2021;11(8):1305.
9. Le Thi TG, Werkstetter K, Kotilea K, Bontems P, Cabral J, Cilleruelo Pascual ML, et al. Helicobacter pylori Special Interest Group of ESPGHAN. Management of Helicobacter pylori infection in paediatric patients in Europe: results from the EuroPedHp Registry. Infection. 2023;51(4):921-934.
10. Tshibangu-Kabamba E, Yamaoka Y. Helicobacter pylori infection and antibiotic resistance - from biology to clinical implications. Nat Rev Gastroenterol Hepatol. 2021;18(9):613-29.

11.4 Gastrointestinal Bleeding

Neelam Mohan

INTRODUCTION

Gastrointestinal (GI) bleeding could result from bleeding from esophagus to anus. It has been divided into upper, middle, and lower depending on the site of bleeding. GI bleeding may be overt or obscure. Overt bleeding may present as hematemesis, melenemesis, melena, or hematochezia. Obscure GI bleed is defined as bleeding from GIT that persists or recurs without any obvious etiology after a diagnostic endoscopy.[1] It accounts for around 5% of all GI bleeds. Occult bleeding may present as positive fecal occult blood test (e.g., guaiac testing), laboratory evidence of anemia and iron deficiency, or symptoms of anemia or blood loss (e.g., fatigue, light headedness, syncope, dyspnea, and angina).

DEFINITIONS

- *Upper GI bleeding* is defined as bleeding from a source in the esophagus, stomach, or duodenum proximal to the duodenojejunal junction (ligament of Treitz).
- *Mid-GI bleeding:* GI bleeding occurs between ampulla of Vater and terminal ileum.

- *Lower GI bleeding:* Refers to colonic GI bleeds.
- *Obscure GI bleeding* is overt GI bleeding from remote sites where both upper GI endoscopy and ileocolonoscopy do not reveal the cause for GI bleeding.[1]
- *Spurious hematemesis* can present as swallowed blood in a neonate or the source can be from oral cavity or as part of malingering/attention seeking ill health behavior.
- *Major GI bleeding is* alarming with overt clots of blood, tarry stools (melena) with over 100 mL of bleeding, and postural hypotension/shock.
- *Hematemesis:* Vomiting of fresh blood
- *Melenemesis:* Vomiting of altered blood
- *Melena:* Passage of black, tarry, sticky, offensive, and loose stools
- *Hematochezia:* Passage of fresh blood in stool. It is most commonly associated with a colonic source of bleeding. If hematochezia is from an upper GI site, it reflects major bleeding with rapid transit which present with hemodynamic instability and increased mortality.

EPIDEMIOLOGY

Upper GI bleed is an indication for upper GI endoscopy in 5% of children and 5% of total GI bleeding may present as obscure GI bleeding. Need for hospitalization in patients with Lower GI bleed is only one-third of upper GI bleeding patients. Etiological spectrum varies in neonates, infants, and older children **(Table 11.4.1)**. A meticulous history, physical examination, and step-by-step evaluation is necessary in a tertiary care center preferably by trained pediatric gastroenterologist along with team of imaging, nuclear medicine, intervention specialists, and sometimes surgeons.

TABLE 11.4.1: Causes of upper gastrointestinal bleed.

Newborn	Infant	Children
• Swallowed maternal blood • Hemorrhagic disease of newborn (HDN) • Stress gastritis • Cow's milk protein allergy (CMPA) • Acid-peptic disease (APD) • Vascular anomaly • Coagulopathy	• Stress ulcer/ gastritis • Acid-peptic disease (APD) • Mallory-Weiss tear • Vascular anomaly • Duplication cyst • Varices • Webs • Intestinal obstruction	• Mallory–Weiss tear • GERD/acid-peptic disease • Varices • Stress ulcer/ erosive gastritis • Caustic injury • Foreign body • Vasculitis–HSP • Crohn's disease • Intestinal obstruction • Dieulafoy lesion • Hemobilia • Pancreatic pseudoaneurysm

(GERD: gastroesophageal reflux disease; HSP: Henoch-Schönlein purpura)

ETIOLOGY

Tables 11.4.1 to 11.4.3 list the causes of GI bleeding from upper and lower GI tract in children.

Mallory–Weiss Tears

It occurs at the gastroesophageal (GE) junction primarily on the gastric side, resulting from retching or coughing followed by hematemesis. It is less frequently seen with children.

HEMORRHAGIC AND EROSIVE GASTROPATHY

It refers to subepithelial hemorrhage and erosions. These are restricted to the mucosa, where no large blood vessels are present and therefore do not cause major bleeding. Erosions are reported in around 2–10% of patients with upper GI bleeding. The most common causes are nonsteroidal anti-inflammatory drug (NSAID) use and stress. Prevalence in neonatal intensive care unit (NICU) is around 44% but only 5% are clinically significant.

PEPTIC ULCER

Incidence of bleeding due to NSAID-induced erosive gastritis is common but bleeding ulcers appears to be rare compared to

TABLE 11.4.2: Common causes of rectal bleeding in children.

Infant	Older child
• Anal fissure • Milk protein intolerance • Necrotizing enterocolitis • Swallowed maternal blood • Vitamin K deficiency	• Anal fissure • Intussusception • Infectious enterocolitis* • Amebiasis • Meckel diverticulum • Juvenile polyp

**Shigella*; *E. coli*; *Cl. difficile*; Salmonellosis.

TABLE 11.4.3: Less common causes of rectal bleeding in children.

Infant	Older child
• Vascular lesions • Bleeding diathesis • Hirschsprung enterocolitis • Meckel diverticulum • Malrotation with volvulus • Intestinal duplication • Intussusception	• Inflammatory bowel disease (IBD) • Ischemic/collagenous colitis • Vascular malformations • Intestinal duplication • Bleeding diathesis • Henoch-Schönlein purpura (HSP) • Hemolytic uremic syndrome (HUS) • Hemorrhoids, rectal varices • Perianal cellulitis • Rectal prolapse • Solitary rectal ulcer • Hereditary polyposis syndrome • Sexual abuse and anorectal trauma • Eosinophilic proctocolitis • Nodular lymphoid hyperplasia

adults. Approximately, one-third of patients found to have an ulcer with active bleeding or a nonbleeding visible vessel will have further bleeding requiring surgery if treated expectantly. These patients should receive endoscopic therapy and intravenous (IV) infusion of proton pump inhibitor (PPI). In <10 years of age, around 77% of the peptic ulcer disease (PUD) is in duodenum. Hematemesis and perforation are more in secondary PUD. Factors associated with PUD include:

- *Primary:* Related to *Helicobacter pylori*, bile reflux
- *Secondary:* Related to—
    - NSAID intake
    - *Stress:* Shock, ischemia
    - Drugs
    - Corrosives
    - Ménétrier disease
    - Zollinger-Ellison syndrome.

Variceal Bleeding

In India, portal hypertension in children is caused more often by extrahepatic portal vein obstruction [EHPVO (68–76%)], cirrhosis (24–28%); and infrequently due to congenital hepatic fibrosis (3%), noncirrhotic portal fibrosis (NCPF), and Budd-Chiari syndrome. In portal hypertension, there are several sites where natural portosystemic shunts appear **(Table 11.4.4)**, the most common sites are esophagus, stomach, and rectum. EHPVO is also the most common cause of GI bleeding in children (70%). Predictors of variceal bleed include large varices and presence of red color signs (red wale marking, diffuse redness, and hematocystic malformation).

Gastric varices are found most commonly with splenic vein thrombosis or after endoscopic sclerotherapy (EST) of esophageal varices.

Extrahepatic Portal Vein Obstruction and Portal Hypertension

The mean age of presentation is 5–6 years. In India, 83% of patients with EHPVO present with upper GI bleeding before the age of 20 years.[2] Hematemesis with or without melena is the most common presentation; only 8–10% patients may not bleed. Upper GI bleeding is massive and recurrent, but risk of rebleeding after major episode is less than in cirrhosis; though fairly uniform and occurs once in every 2 years. The average number of bleed is 2.5–5 episodes per patient.

Firm splenomegaly is almost universal in patient with EHPVO. It can be present as early as 1 month of age and is usually seen before 3 years of age. Splenomegaly is mild (<6 cm) in 42%, moderate (6–10 cm) in 40%, and massive (>10 cm) in 18%. Children with EHPVO do not grow as much as their healthy siblings.

Variceal bleeding in EHPVO is well tolerated with reference to the liver function, viz., following the GI variceal bleeding, they usually do not develop encephalopathy even with massive GI bleed and they have normal liver functions.[3] They may develop transient ascites following major bleeding episode. Persistent or massive ascites in children with EHPVO should make one doubt about the diagnosis or suggest the possibility of presence of coexistent cirrhosis. Recurrent GI bleeding in EHPVO decreases with age. Abdominal ultrasonography and Doppler study are diagnostic.

In portal hypertension occurring secondary to chronic liver disease (CLD), the presentation is usually dominated by manifestations of primary disease. The major causes in children are viral hepatitis, neonatal cholestasis, autoimmune liver disease, and metabolic liver disease such as Wilson disease and glycogen storage disease.

Children with EHPVO when compared to CLD have more chances of UGI bleed, more previous bleeding episodes, long duration of symptoms and absence of jaundice, preservation of liver function, and less Hb value.[2]

Esophageal varices can be classified as small (<5 mm), medium (5–10 mm), or large (>10 mm) according to size or graded by endoscopy according to Conn's classification **(Table 11.4.4)**.[3]

Gastric varices are found most commonly with splenic vein thrombosis or after EST of esophageal varices. It can be further classified **(Fig. 11.4.1)** endoscopically according to location (Sarin classification).

TABLE 11.4.4: Conn's classification of esophageal varices.

Grade 1	On inspiration only	Can be effaced	Straight	Red
Grade 2	Both on inspiration and expiration	Cannot be effaced	Straight	Red
Grade 3	Projecting into lumen <50%, wavy	Cannot be effaced	Straight	Blue
Grade 4	Projecting into lumen more than 50% and coiled	Tense	Tortuous	Blue

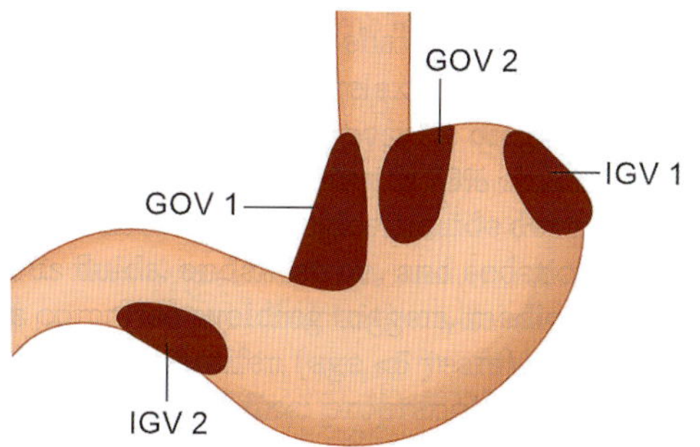

Fig. 11.4.1: Gastric varices (Sarin classification).
(GOV: gastroesophageal varices; IGV: isolated gastric varices)

- *Gastroesophageal varices (GOV):* Gastric varices continuing with esophageal varices—
  - *GOV1:* Extending toward lesser curvature
  - *GOV2:* Extending toward fundus
- *Isolated gastric varices (IGV):* Gastric varices discontinuous with esophageal varices or present in absence of esophageal varices—
  - *IGV1:* Fundal varices, tortuous, nodular
  - *IGV2:* Ectopic varices (body, antrum, and pylorus).

Ectopic varices account for 5% of all variceal bleed. Duodenum is a common site.

EVALUATION OF GASTROINTESTINAL BLEEDING

Vital signs include the pulse rate and the blood pressure (BP) in lying, sitting and if possible, in standing position for postural hypotension. It is essential to monitor urine output and fluid intake and respiratory rate throughout fluid resuscitation of patients in shock and altered sensorium/coma. Hyperventilation is an early sign of developing acidosis.

Physical examination to evaluate capillary perfusion, skin color for the presence of cyanosis, pulse, BP, respiratory pattern, and level of consciousness should continue on an ongoing basis during active bleeding. Nasogastric aspirations that are grossly blood confirm upper GI sources while a negative aspiration does not rule out.

Some clinical clues to etiology in a GI bleed patient are given in **Table 11.4.5**. Presence of melena followed by any bright-colored blood in stool indicates rebleed and these patients with melena should be monitored and managed in the pediatric intensive care unit (PICU). In patients with smaller amount of doubtful bleed, it is important to first confirm whether it is blood or something else by guaiac test **(Table 11.4.6)**.

Flowchart 11.4.1 provides a schematic approach to the diagnosis of etiology of upper gastrointestinal bleeding (UGIB).

MANAGEMENT

Management includes resuscitation, identification of the cause of bleed, control of bleed, and its prevention **(Box 11.4.1)**.

TABLE 11.4.5: Clinical clues to etiology in a gastrointestinal bleed patient.

Bleeding etiology	*Clinical clues*
Mallory-Weiss tear	Emesis before hematemesis, pain +
Esophageal ulcer	Odynophagia, GERD, H/O pill ingestion
Stress gastritis/PUD	Sick patient in ICU, respiratory failure/NSAID ingestion/pain
Angiodysplasia	Renal failure, hereditary hemorrhagic telangiectasia
Aortoenteric fistula	H/O aortic aneurysm or surgery
CLD	Variceal bleed significant, painless, splenomegaly, jaundice, stigmata of CLD, ascites

(CLD: chronic liver disease; GERD: gastroesophageal reflux disease; NSAID: nonsteroidal anti-inflammatory drug; PUD: peptic ulcer disease)

TABLE 11.4.6: Drugs used to stop variceal bleeding.

Drug	*Mechanism of action*	*Dose*	*Comments*
Vasopressin	• Potent nonselective vasoconstrictor • Lowers the portal pressure by causing splanchnic arterial vasoconstriction and reducing the splanchnic blood flow to the varices	Given in a bolus of 0.33 U/kg of body weight diluted with 2 mL/kg of 5% dextrose given over a period of 15–20 minutes	Nitroglycerine, a vasodilator, may reduce the cardiac side effects of vasopressin by increasing local concentration of NO and reducing cardiac output
Terlipressin	• Synthetic analog of vasopressin acts by immediate vasoconstriction • Its use in children requires further evaluation • It is more effective in controlling bleeding (up to 79%) than vasopressin without any adverse side effects	Given as IV injections (2 mg) every 4 hours till bleeding free interval of 24–48 hours is achieved	
Somatostatin	• Acts by inhibiting release of several vasodilatory hormones such as glucagon • It induces selective splanchnic vasoconstriction	Recommended dosage is 1–3 bolus injections (250 µg/bolus) during first hour of therapy followed by infusion of 250 µg/h of continuous infusion for 2–5 days	• There is lower failure rate and complications in comparison to vasopressin • Disadvantage is its short half-life
Octreotide	A synthetic analog of somatostatin with half-life of 90 minutes	1–2 µg/kg over 2–5 minutes, then 1–2 µg/kg/h for 5 days	Side-effects are uncommon

Flowchart 11.4.1: Approach to etiology for upper gastrointestinal bleed (UGI).

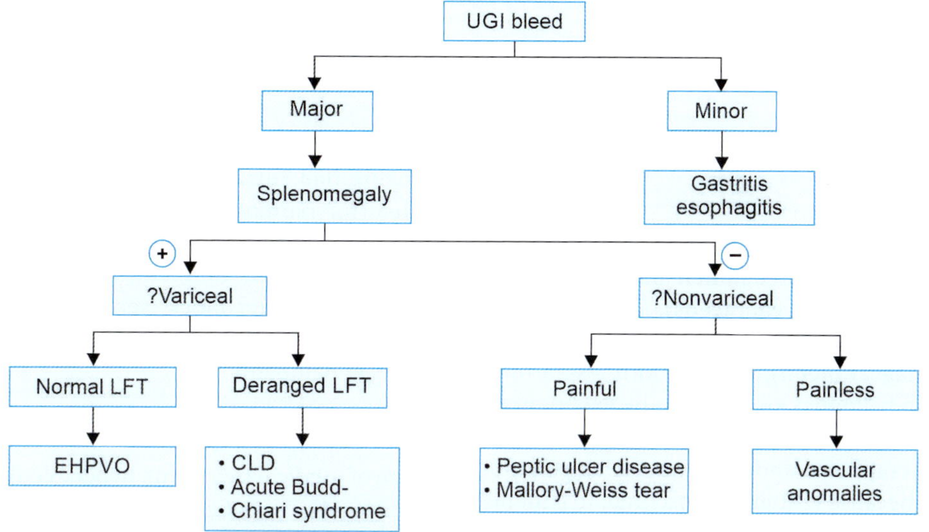

(CLD: chronic liver disease; EHPVO: extrahepatic portal vein obstruction; LFT: liver function test)

BOX 11.4.1: Treatment goals.

- Immediate assessment of severity and causes
- Establish and maintain the intravascular volume
- *Packed red blood cell transfusion:* Maintain Hb >8–10 g/dL
- FFP transfusion with INR >1.5–2, platelets transfusion if platelet <50,000/mm^3
- *Labs:* Hemogram, LFT, BUN, creatinine, PT, APTT, USG abdomen—Doppler, endoscopy
- Determine source and site of blood loss
- Stop gastrointestinal bleeding
- Prevention of further bleed

(APTT: activated partial thromboplastin time; BUN: blood urea nitrogen; FFP: fresh frozen plasma; INR: international normalized ratio; LFT: liver function test; PT: prothrombin time; USG: ultrasonography)

Resuscitation

This includes achieving hemodynamic stability and treatment of hypovolemic shock. Adequate IV access should be established and carefully monitor pulse, BP, and central venous pressure (CVP). Oxygen is given to counter hypoxia due to acute blood loss. An increase in the pulse rate of >20 beats per minute or a decrease in diastolic BP of >10 mm Hg or a decrease in systolic of >20 mm Hg within 3 minutes of standing, indicates a >20% loss of intravascular volume. As blood loss increases to 20–25%, the pulse rate increases >150 beats/min. When the intravascular volume deficit exceeds 25%, the capillary refill is prolonged as blood is shunted from the skin to the brain and kidneys. Urine output decreases with further compromise and metabolic acidosis result; in short, all features of hypovolemic shock develop. Urine output and fluid intake must be carefully monitored throughout fluid resuscitation in patients with shock. Urine output in children is normally 2–3 mL/kg/h, and urine output <1 mL/kg/h is indicative of renal hypoperfusion. As blood loss exceeds 40%, compensation fails, pulses are lost, cerebral perfusion decreases, and the patient passes from lethargy to coma. The respiratory rate should also be carefully monitored. Hyperventilation is an early sign of a developing acidosis induced by a decrease in central nervous systems pH.

Physical examination by an experienced observer to evaluate capillary perfusion, skin color for the presence of cyanosis, pulse, BP, respiratory pattern, and level of consciousness should continue on an ongoing basis throughout the hemorrhage to enable rapid recognition of shock. To enhance the ability to anticipate shock, it is helpful if the rate of bleeding is assessed periodically. In UGIB this is best accomplished through lavage of the stomach by means of a nasogastric tube placed in the stomach. Nasogastric aspiration that are grossly bleeding confirm upper GI sources but a negative aspiration does not rule out. Up to 15–18% of patients with UGIB have nonbloody nasogastric aspirate. The amount of blood lost in the stool should also be monitored, estimated, and recorded and any change in color from melena to bright red blood should be noted as a possible sign of increased blood loss and hypovolemic shock. It is prudent that all patients with significant GI bleeding be monitored in a PICU for changes in vital signs and urine output until they are stable and bleeding has ceased.

For calculating transfusion requirement, quantity of packed red blood cells [(70 mL/kg × weight in kg) (desired hemoglobin – present hemoglobin)]/23 g hemoglobin per 100 dL of packed red blood cells; rough guideline –5 mL of packed RBC/kg will raise the Hct. Three points and Hb 1 g/dL (5:3:1).

Control of Acute Variceal Bleeding

It can be by the following modalities:

Pharmacotherapy

The most widely used agents to stop variceal bleeds are given in **Table 11.4.6.**[4]

Balloon Tamponade

Sengstaken–Blakemore tube (three lumen and two balloons for esophageal and gastric variceal bleeds), Linton-Nachlas tube (three lumen and single balloon more effective for gastric variceal than esophageal bleed), and the Minnesota tube (four lumen and two balloons) are handled by experienced specialists as a lifesaver in active variceal bleeding if emergency sclerotherapy or banding is unavailable or not technically possible because visibility is obscured. In patients with active bleeding, an endotracheal tube should be inserted to protect the airway before attempting to place the esophageal balloon tube. Continued bleeding during balloon tamponade indicates an incorrectly positioned tube and bleeding from another source. After resuscitation, and within 12 hours, the tube is removed and endoscopic treatment repeated.

Endotherapy (Endoscopic Variceal Ligation or Sclerotherapy)

- *Endoscopic variceal ligation:* Using multiband ligator banding has less complications and is more effective than sclerotherapy. However, it is not possible in small children between 2 and 3 years of age **(Table 11.4.7)**.
- *Endoscopic sclerotherapy:* Injection of sclerosant into (intravariceal) or around (perivariceal) the varices. Various sclerosants used in esophageal varices are polidocanol, sodium tetradecyl sulfate, absolute alcohol, sodium morrhuate, and in bleeding gastric varices, injection of glue (N-butyl-2-cyanoacrylate) is done.

TABLE 11.4.7: Comparison of endoscopic variceal ligation (EVL) and endoscopic sclerotherapy (EST).

	EVL	*EST*
Indications	Large varices, difficult in small children	Any size
Complications	Less (4%)	More (25%)
Rebleeding rate	Low (4%)	More (25%)
Sessions needed	More (17%)	Less (10%)
Recurrence of varices	Increase	IGV and GOV
Gastric varices	Increase	Increase

(GOV: gastroesophageal varices; IGV: isolated gastric varices)

- *Complications of endotherapy:* Fever, chest pain, dysphagia, superficial mucosal ulcerations (6–70%), esophageal perforation, pulmonary complications, and esophageal stricture.

Transjugular Intrahepatic Portosystemic Shunt

Transjugular intrahepatic portosystemic shunt (TIPS) is ideal for patients whose bleeding is not controlled by endoscopy. It is effective only in portal hypertension of hepatic origin and contraindicated in portal vein thrombosis, biliary block, septicemia, and severe hepatic encephalopathy. Complications include thrombosis of stent and encephalopathy.

Indications for Surgery

Failure of medical treatment, hypersplenism, isolated splenic vein thrombosis, patients from remote and underprivileged places, and of rare blood group. Emergency devascularization and esophageal transection (modified Tanner) or elective Warren distal splenorenal shunt or rarely Rex shunt (superior mesenteric vein to left portal vein branch with venous graft) or liver transplantation is useful.

Prophylaxis

For secondary prophylaxis, beta-blockers (propranolol) may be used in a dose of 1 2 mg/kg lowers venous flow, and the portal pressure by decreasing the heart rate by 25% and the BP by 15 mm Hg and causing splanchnic vasoconstriction and decreasing portal venous flow.[3]

Control of Nonvariceal Bleeding

Treatment depends on the cause of the bleeding. Various treatment modalities are H_2 receptor antagonists/PPIs, vasoactive agents, endotherapy including electrothermal agents such as endoclips and argon plasma coagulation **(Table 11.4.8)**.

Identifying the other Sources of Gastrointestinal Hemorrhage

The other sources can be identified by esophagogastroduodenoscopy, colonoscopy, Meckel's scans (^{99m}Tc-pertechnetate scan) bleeding isotope scan, angiography, capsule endoscopy, double balloon enteroscopy, imaging, upper GI radiography, and barium enema, and preoperative endoscopy.

- *Endoscopy:* Esophagogastroduodenoscopy or colonoscopy is very useful to detect esophagitis, Mallory–Weiss tears, varices, gastritis, ulcer, vascular malformations, etc. Bleeding from an ulcer is controlled using injection with adrenaline and recently hemoclips

TABLE 11.4.8: Pharmacotherapy.

Drug	*Mechanism of action*	*Dose*	*Comments*
Ranitidine	H_2 receptor antagonist	20–40 mg/kg/day in 2–3 divided doses	
Famotidine	H_2 receptor antagonist	1–2 mg/kg/day in 2 divided doses	
Omeprazole	Proton pump inhibitor	1–3.3 mg/kg/day (<20 kg) 10 mg/day (>20 kg)	Approved for >2 years old
Esomeprazole	Proton pump inhibitor	0.2–1 mg/kg/day	Approved for >1 year old
Lansoprazole	Proton pump inhibitor	0.8–4 mg/kg/day (<30 kg) 15 mg/day (>30 kg)	Approved for >1 year old
Pantoprazole	Proton pump inhibitor	Adult dose—40 mg/day	
Sucralfate	Cytoprotective agent	40–80 mg/kg/day	

are also available for clipping at the site of vessel bleed at the base of the ulcer. Similarly, colonoscopy helps diagnosis and therapy of common causes such as polyps and the less common vascular malformations and diagnosis of colitis, inflammatory bowel disease (IBD), solitary rectal ulcer, vascular malformations, etc.

- *Angiography:* It is indicated in active GI bleeding and the rate of bleeding must be at least 0.5 mL/min. The diagnostic yield of emergency arteriography is low. Nowadays computed tomography (CT) angiography is preferred and conventional angiography is hardly used.
- *UGI radiology:* Radiographic studies are particularly useful in the diagnosis of esophageal strictures, malrotation of the bowel, or deep ulcerations.
- *Meckel's scan:* Because technetium (Tc) ^{99m}pertechnetate is actively accumulated by cells in gastric mucosa, it can be used to identify the presence of ectopic gastric mucosa in a Meckel's diverticulum or intestinal duplications. >90% of bleeding Meckel's diverticula do contain gastric mucosa. A Meckel's scan should be considered whenever significant lower GI has occurred.
- *Bleeding scan:* It is a noninvasive study with a low radiation exposure. Tc sulfur or Tc-pertechnetate-labeled red blood cell scan are used. Tc sulfur red cell scan can detect site of bleeding even when the rate of bleeding is as low as 0.1 mL/min. However, its half-life is only 2 minutes. Tc-pertechnetate-labeled red blood cell scan can visualize the site of bleeding when the bleeding rate is 0.5 mL/min or higher. However, the longer half-life of the labeled red blood cells enables the images of the GI system to continue for up to 24 hours. The Tc-pertechnetate-labeled blood cell scan should be considered when a small intestinal source of bleeding is suspected. In most institutions, the Tc-pertechnetate-labeled red blood cell scan is used to direct subsequent localized angiography. The nuclear scan can be readily repeated in patients with intermittent bleeding.
- *Barium enema:* Barium enema is useful in neonates and infants presenting with malrotation with secondary intestinal volvulus, intussusception which can be diagnosed and in many cases treated by barium enema. The barium enema is also effective in identifying the presence of polyps.

Specific Management of Common Conditions Presenting as Lower Gastrointestinal Bleeding

- *Anal fissure:* Treatment of constipation, laxatives, Sitz bath, topical 0.2% glyceryl nitrate twice daily
- *Solitary rectal ulcer syndrome:* Sucralfate enema, twice daily, for 3–6 weeks with training on "not to strain during defecation" and yttrium-aluminum garnet (YAG) laser treatment for severe bleeds
- *Hemorrhagic infective colitis:* Antimicrobials
- *Polyps:* Colonoscopic snare polypectomy
- *Inflammatory bowel disease and ulcerative colitis:* 5-amino-salicylic acid, steroids, cyclosporine, and total colectomy.
- *Crohn's disease:* Steroids, azathioprine, infliximab, metronidazole, and ciprofloxacin.
- *Vascular lesions:* Therapeutic endoscopy.
- *Portal colopathy and variceal bleed:* Octreotide, transjugular intrahepatic portosystemic stent shunt, and shunt surgery.

Indications for Surgery in Lower Gastrointestinal Bleeding

Intraoperative enteroscopy using pediatric colonoscope or enteroscope may be useful to identify small bowel lesions.

- Surgery of Meckel's diverticulum, duplication of small bowel, and Hirschsprung disease (HD)
- Portosystemic shunt, esophageal
- Liver transplantation may be necessary in the upper GI hemorrhage refractory to medical, endoscopic, and radiologic interventions.
- In lower GI hemorrhage, hemicolectomy or subtotal colectomy is occasionally required.
- Complications due to endotherapy such as perforation

Flowcharts 11.4.2 and 11.4.3 summarize the approach to a case of upper GI and lower GI bleed, respectively.

Flowchart 11.4.2: Approach to a case of upper gastrointestinal bleed.

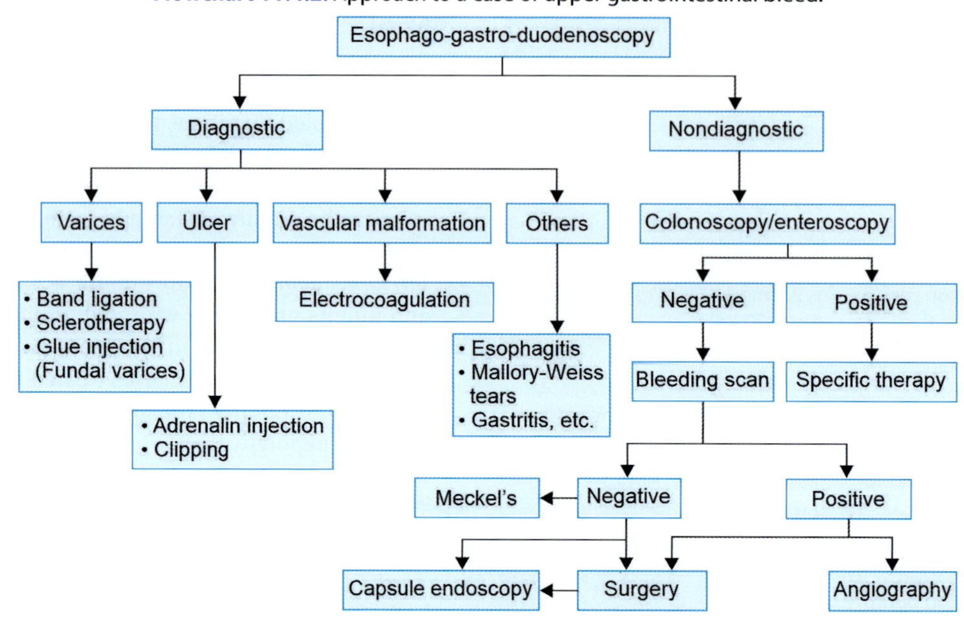

Flowchart 11.4.3: Approach to a case of lower gastrointestinal bleed.

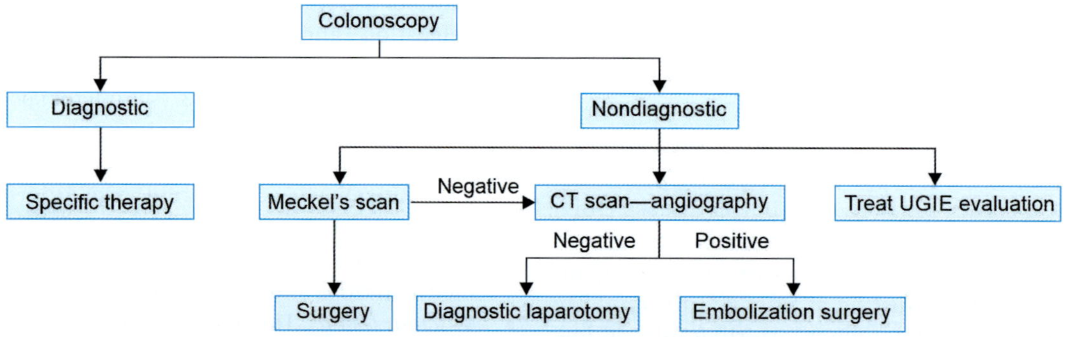

(CT: computed tomography; UGIE: upper gastrointestinal endoscopy)

Flowchart 11.4.4: Management of obscure bleeding transection, and TIPS.

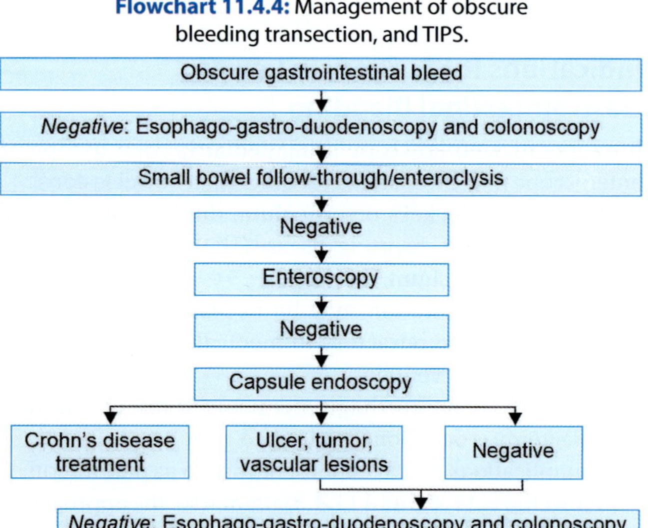

Obscure Gastrointestinal Bleed

It may occur as overt or occult bleed often in small bowel such as Crohn's disease, anastomotic, cytomegalovirus (CMV)/viral, or other infections such as vascular (angiodysplasia, Dieulafoy lesion, varices, or lymphangioma) or tumors (polyps, carcinoid, or lymphoma), and others such as Meckel's diverticulum and diverticulosis.[1]

Various diagnostic modalities include small bowel follow through, enteroclysis, push enteroscopy, and capsule endoscopy. Rarely, surgery with intraoperative endoscopy may be required **(Flowchart 11.4.4)**.

CONCLUSION

GI bleed could be UGI bleed proximal to duodenojejunal junction or lower GI bleed from colon. Mid-GI bleed includes the small bowel region. Focused history, examination and appropriate laboratory, endoscopic and radiological investigations are needed to identify the cause and severity of bleed. Most common cause of life-threatening upper GI bleed in children is variceal bleed. Endoscopy is the key to diagnosis in most cases therefore early referral to pediatric gastroenterologist is essential. In severe GI bleed stabilization of airways, breathing and circulation is essential before proceeding or referring for endoscopy. Vasoactive agents are used for variceal bleed till endotherapy is done.

REFERENCES

1. Raju GS, Gerson L, Das A, Lewis B; American Gastroenterological Association. American Gastroenterological Association (AGA) Institute medical position statement on obscure gastrointestinal bleeding. Gastroenterology. 2007;133(5):1694-6.
2. Poddar U, Borkar V. Management of extrahepatic portal venous obstruction (EHPO): Current strategies. Trop Gastroenterol. 2011;32(2):94-102.
3. Garcia-Tsao G, Sanyal AJ, Grace ND, Carey W; Practice Guidelines Committee of the American Association for the Study of Liver Diseases; Practice Parameters Committee of the American College of Gastroenterology. Prevention and management of gastroesophageal varices and variceal hemorrhage in cirrhosis. Hepatology. 2007;46(3):923-38.
4. D'Amico G, Pagliaro L, Bosch J. Pharmacological treatment of portal hypertension. An evidence based approach. Semin Liver Dis.1999;19(4):475-505.

11.5 Acute Diarrhea

Ashok K Patwari

INTRODUCTION

Diarrheal disease is the second leading cause of death in children under five years old and was responsible for the deaths of 370,000 children worldwide in 2019.[1] The most severe threat posed by diarrhea is dehydration. Standard case management with oral rehydration salts (ORS), oral zinc, and proper diet has drastically improved the outcome of acute diarrhea. Promotion of exclusive breastfeeding up to 6 months of age, improved complementary feeding practices, hand washing, and measles vaccination have significantly reduced the prevalence of acute diarrhea in young children. Diarrhea is also a major cause of malnutrition in low and middle-income countries, making children more susceptible to future bouts of diarrhea and other diseases.[2] It is essential to understand various types of diarrheas based on duration and etiology as the approach and management differ.

DEFINITION

Diarrhea is usually defined as the passage of three or more loose or watery stools in a 24-hour period, a loose stool being one that would take the shape of a container. However, for practical purposes, it is the recent change in consistency and character of stool and its water content rather than the number of stools that are important. Infants who are exclusively breastfed normally pass several soft or semiliquid stools each day; for them, it is practical to define diarrhea as an increase in stool frequency or liquidity that is considered abnormal by the mother/caregiver.

Acute Watery Diarrhea

It refers to diarrhea that begins acutely and lasts for <14 days, with the passage of frequent loose or watery stools without visible blood. Vomiting may occur and fever may be present. Loss of a large volume of water and electrolytes can result in dehydration and dyselectrolytemia.

Dysentery

It is the term used for diarrhea with visible blood and mucus. It is often associated with fever and tenesmus. Common clinical features of dysentery include anorexia, rapid weight loss, and complications, such as renal failure and encephalopathy.

Persistent Diarrhea

It represents diarrhea, presumed to be caused by infectious agents that begins acutely but is usually of a long duration (>14 days). The episode may begin either as acute watery diarrhea or as dysentery. Marked weight loss is common. Diarrheal stool volume may also be great, with a risk of dehydration. Persistent diarrhea should not be confused with "chronic diarrhea" which is recurrent or long-lasting diarrhea due to non-infectious causes such as sensitivity to gluten or an inherited metabolic disorder.

EPIDEMIOLOGY

Acute diarrhea constitutes a leading cause of morbidity and mortality among children below 5 years of age in low and middle-income countries including India where 13% of under-five children reportedly died as a result of diarrhea in 2010, based on the data from Child Health Reference Group (CHERG).[1] On average, 3.3 episodes of diarrhea are experienced per child per year, but in some areas, the average exceeds nine episodes per year. Recent data from some states in India reported as high as 6.2–13.7% of under-five children presenting with diarrhea two weeks preceding the survey.[3] More than 2 million deaths are estimated to result each year as a consequence of diarrheal disease in under-fives. Eighty percent of these deaths occur in the first 2 years of life, the main causes being dehydration, complications associated with dysentery, malnutrition, and serious infections, such as pneumonia.

Most of the diarrheal episodes occur during the first 2 years of life (highest incidence 6–11 months), in low socioeconomic status, in nonbreastfed infants, and in association with measles, severe malnutrition, and immunodeficiency.

ETIOLOGY

In low and middle-income countries, the organisms most frequently associated with acute watery diarrhea include enterotoxigenic *Escherichia coli* (ETEC), enteropathogenic *E. coli* (EPEC), *Shigella dysenteriae,* and *Campylobacter jejuni.* Rotavirus is a common cause of severe diarrhea, vomiting, and fever leading to rapid dehydration. *Vibrio cholerae* is an important organism in endemic areas and during epidemics. Nontyphoidal *Salmonella* is a common organism in areas where commercially processed foods are widely used and in hospital outbreaks. Most of these organisms produce watery diarrhea. The main causes of acute dysentery are *S. dysenteriae, C. jejuni,* and infrequently enteroinvasive *E. coli* (EIEC) or *Salmonella.* Epidemics of dysentery are usually caused by *S. dysenteriae* type 1. *Entamoeba histolytica* can cause dysentery in adults but is a less common cause in young children.

Diarrhea may also be caused by a number of antibacterial agents such as ampicillin, cotrimoxazole, chloramphenicol, amoxicillin, and clindamycin. Pseudomembranous colitis is the most severe form of antibiotic-associated diarrhea.

PATHOGENESIS AND CLINICAL FEATURES

Acute diarrhea in children usually results from inflammation of the intestines caused by offending agents (enteropathogens, toxins, or chemical agents). The other mechanism is noninflammatory in nature in which diarrhea results from disturbances of absorptive functions of the intestines due to a toxin (e.g., ETEC) or as a result of disturbances in the osmolality of the intestinal contents or normal absorptive functions of the intestines. Most enteropathogens cause diarrhea by more than one mechanism. The clinical presentation depends upon the underlying pathophysiological changes taking place in the gastrointestinal tract (GIT). Three clinical types of diarrheas have been defined, each reflecting a different pathogenesis and requiring a different approach to treatment.

Secretory Diarrhea

It is characterized by acute watery diarrhea with profound losses of water and electrolytes due to sodium pump failure as a result of the action of identified toxins. This group is at risk for rapid development of dehydration and electrolyte imbalance. Common causes are ETEC and *V. cholerae.*

Invasive Diarrhea (Dysentery)

Intestinal mucosal cells are actually invaded by microorganisms which set up an inflammatory reaction clinically presenting with blood and mucus in the stools. This group is prone to develop other complications like intestinal perforation, toxic megacolon, rectal prolapse, convulsions, septicemia, and hemolytic uremic syndrome (HUS).

Osmotic Diarrhea

Injury to enterocytes may result in brush border damage and epithelial destruction leading to decreased mucosal disaccharidase activity. Clinical presentation is characterized by the passage of large, frothy, explosive, and acidic stools. High osmolar solutions given orally [e.g., carbonated soft drinks and ORS with high sugar content] can also result in osmotic diarrhea. Another complication of osmotic diarrhea is hypernatremia.

Pathogenesis of Rotavirus Diarrhea

Rotavirus, the most common etiological organism resulting in severe diarrhea in young children, causes diarrhea by multiple mechanisms. Alteration of gastrointestinal motility and destruction of the intestinal epithelium with reduction of brush border enzymes is a common mechanism resulting in osmotic diarrhea. The nonstructural protein of rotavirus, rotavirus nonstructural protein 4 (NSP4) acts like an enterotoxin and causes secretory diarrhea by altering epithelial cell function and permeability. In addition, rotavirus may also increase fluid secretion by activating the enteric nervous system in the intestinal wall. There is also a possibility that the virus may escape the intestinal wall and result in antigenemia and viremia[4] **(Flowchart 11.5.1)**.

DIAGNOSIS

Diagnosis of acute diarrhea is based on the clinical history of passing frequent, loose, or watery stools, with or without vomiting, fever, pain in the abdomen, or blood in the stools. Many children may have symptoms and signs of other associated illnesses, such as cough, skin rashes/measles, and urinary symptoms. The clinical triad of rotaviral diarrhea is fever, vomiting, and profuse watery stools with a tendency for dehydration.

Dehydration is the most common and life-threatening consequence of diarrhea. Loss of water and electrolytes in the diarrheal stool results in depletion of the extracellular fluid (ECF) volume, electrolyte imbalance, and clinical manifestation of dehydration. The first symptom of dehydration appears after fluid loss of 5% of body weight. When fluid loss reaches 10%, shock often sets in, and the cascade of events that follow can culminate in death unless there is immediate intervention to rehydrate.

Routine stool examination is not recommended except in situations such as young infants (aged <2 months) with fever, suspected protozoan *Giardia* or *E. histolytica* as a cause, extragut infections or persistent colitis or disaccharide intolerance, and prolonged/persistent diarrhea with malnutrition. Stool culture is invariably noncontributory.

Flowchart 11.5.1: Pathogenesis of rotavirus infection.

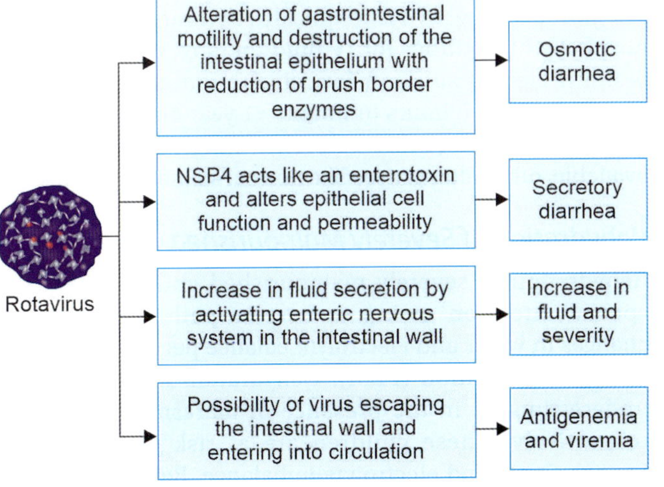

Diarrhea when prolonged or recurrent, is a major cause of malnutrition in children, owing to the use of bottle feeds, stoppage of breastfeeds, and lack of energy-dense feeds and hygiene such as hand washing, low food intake during the illness (poor appetite, vomiting, oral thrush, or stomatitis, diluting/withholding of food, etc.), reduced nutrient absorption in the intestines, and increased requirements as a result of infection. Repeated and prolonged episodes of diarrhea have even more deleterious effects and may eventually result in growth failure, intercurrent infections, and problems associated with severe malnutrition and even death.

MANAGEMENT[5,6]

Principles of Treatment

- General assessment of the child.
- *Assessment of hydration status:* A number of clinical signs and symptoms can help in detecting dehydration. However, a simple assessment chart based on a few reliable clinical signs can be referred for quick assessment of dehydration **(Table 11.5.1)** and administration of appropriate fluids for prevention and treatment of dehydration.
- Correction of electrolyte and acid-base imbalance.
- Proper feeding to provide normal nutritional requirements.
- Zinc supplementation.
- Treatment of associated problems, such as dysentery and persistent diarrhea.
- Nutritional rehabilitation.
- Health education for the prevention of diarrhea.

Oral Rehydration Therapy

The concept of oral rehydration therapy (ORT) has revolutionized the management of diarrhea with the discovery of coupled active transport of glucose and sodium in the small bowel, resulting in the passive absorption of

TABLE 11.5.1: Assessment of hydration status in a patient with diarrhea.*

Clinical signs			
General condition	Well, alert	Restless, irritable	Lethargic or unconscious
Eyes	Normal	Sunken	Sunken
Thirst*	Drinks normally, not thirsty	Drinks eagerly, thirsty	Drinks poorly, not able to drink
Skin pinch	Goes back quickly	Goes back "slowly"	Goes back "very slowly"**
Decide hydration status	The patient has "no signs of dehydration"	If the patient has two or more signs, there is "some dehydration"	If the patient has two or more signs, there is "severe dehydration"
Treatment plan	*Plan A*	*Plan B*	*Plan C*

*In a young infant <2 months of age, thirst is not assessed and a decision regarding "some" or "severe dehydration" is made if "two" of the three signs are present.

**Skin pinch takes longer than 2 seconds to go back.

water and other electrolytes even during copious diarrhea. Oral rehydration therapy includes:

- ORS solution of recommended composition
- Solution made from sugar and salt (if prepared correctly)
- Food-based solutions with appropriate concentrations of salt, such as lentil soup, rice, *kanji*, and buttermilk.
- Plain water was given along with continued feeding.

Low Osmolarity Oral Rehydration Salts Solution

The standard World Health Organization (WHO)-ORS, used for over three decades, has saved millions of lives but did not decrease diarrheal duration or stool output. More effective low osmolarity ORS **(Table 11.5.2)** is now recommended as the universal solution for the treatment and prevention of dehydration for all causes of diarrhea and at all ages.

Prevention and Treatment of Dehydration

Management of "No Dehydration"

The objective of the treatment is the prevention of dehydration and malnutrition (Plan A). The management can be successfully carried out at home, by the mother/caretaker who is advised to:

- Give more fluids than normal **(Table 11.5.3)**
- Continue feeding
- Bring the child back after 2 days, or earlier if he/she has any of the danger signs (thirsty, irritable/restless, fever, high purge rate, repeated vomiting, blood in the stool, eating or drinking poorly, and lethargic).

Management of "Some Dehydration"

The objective of treatment is to treat dehydration and electrolyte imbalance, and to continue feeding. These children should be rehydrated with ORS under supervision in a health facility (Plan B).

Correction of dehydration:

- For correction of fluid and electrolyte deficit on account of dehydration, 50–100 mL/kg body weight (75 mL/kg) of ORS must be administered, over a period of 4 hours. If the child wants more, more ORS should be given. Breastfeeding should be continued.
- Older children should have free access to plain water.
- Acceptance of ORS, purge rate, and vomiting should be closely monitored.

Reassess after 4 hours:

- If still dehydrated, deficit therapy should be repeated (Plan B), and milk/food should also be offered.
- If rehydrated, it is treated as "no dehydration" with maintenance therapy with ORS as in plan A.
- If ORT is not successful, it is treated as "severe dehydration" with intravenous (IV) fluids as in plan C.

Management of "Severe Dehydration"

The primary objective is to quickly rehydrate the child in a hospital with facilities for IV fluid therapy. Ringer's lactate is the preferred solution for rehydration and is given as 100 mL/kg over 6 hours in infants <1 year and over 3 hours in older children **(Table 11.5.4)**. If Ringer's lactate is not available, other alternatives like normal saline may be used.

Rehydration of Severely Malnourished Children

Rehydration of severely malnourished children deserves special attention owing to certain pathophysiological changes in water and electrolyte balance peculiar to protein energy malnutrition (PEM). Dehydration may be over or underestimated in the presence of marasmus or edema, respectively. These children are at risk of developing hypoglycemia and electrolyte imbalance. Rehydration with ORS solution should be preferred because IV fluids can easily cause overhydration and heart failure. Therefore, it is recommended that severely malnourished children are slowly rehydrated, carefully monitored and feeding is started early.

TABLE 11.5.2: Low osmolarity ORS formulation recommended by WHO/UNICEF.

Reduced osmolarity ORS	*g/L*	*Reduced osmolarity ORS*	*mmol/L*
Sodium chloride	2.6	Sodium	75
Glucose, anhydrous	13.5	Chloride	65
Potassium chloride	1.5	Glucose, anhydrous	75
Trisodium citrate, dihydrate	2.9	Potassium	20
		Citrate	10
		Total osmolarity	*245*

(ORS: oral rehydration salts; UNICEF: United Nations International Children's Emergency Fund; WHO: World Health Organization)

TABLE 11.5.3: Guidelines for replacement of fluid and electrolytes in children with "no dehydration" (Plan A).

Age	*After each loose stool, offer**
<6 months	Quarter glass or cup (50 mL)
7 months to 2 years	Quarter to half glass or cup (50–100 mL)
2–5 years	Half to one glass or cup (100–200 mL)
Older children	As much as the child can take

*Fluids that can be offered include ORS, lemon water, buttermilk, rice *kanji*, lentil soup, light tea, etc.

TABLE 11.5.4: Deficit fluid therapy for "severe dehydration" (Plan C).

	Infants (<1 year)	*Older child (>1 year)*
Volume of Ringer's lactate	30 mL/kg body weight within the first 1 hour, followed by 70 mL/kg body weight over the next 5 hours	30 mL/kg body weight within half an hour, followed by 70 mL/kg body weight over the next 2.5 hours
Monitoring	*Assess for improvement every 1–2 hours:* • If not improving, give IV infusion more rapidly • Encourage oral feeding by giving ORS 5 mL/kg/h, along with IV fluids, as soon as the child is able to drink • *Reassess hydration status:* After 6 hours (infants) and 3 hours (older children) assess hydration status and choose the appropriate plan for hydration (Plan A, B, or C)	

Children with severe acute malnutrition (SAM) need a separate rehydrating solution because of a higher risk of hypo- or hypernatremia and hypokalemia. WHO guidelines for the management of dehydration in children with SAM recommend oral rehydration with ReSoMal (REhydration SOlution for MALnutrition) which has lower sodium (45 mmol/L) and higher potassium (40 mmol/L) than the low osmolarity ORS recommended for oral rehydration of children. However, programmatically, the currently recommended low osmolarity ORS is considered safe and effective in these children.[6]

TABLE 11.5.5: Feeding during diarrhea.

Stage of hydration	*Recommended schedule of feeding*
During rehydration phase: • Breastfed infants	• Continue breastfeeding and resume normal feeding after rehydration is completed
• Nonbreastfed infants	• Should be preferably given only ORS till they are rehydrated • Animal milk/food should be offered if rehydration takes longer than 4 hours
• Severely malnourished children	• Offer some food as soon as possible
After the rehydration phase: • Breastfed infants	• Breastfeed more frequently
• Nonbreastfed infants	• Offer undiluted milk as before
• Infants 6–12 months	• Give easily digestible energy-rich complementary foods in addition to breast/animal milk
• For older children	• Give thick preparation of staple food with extra vegetable oil or animal fats, rich in potassium (legumes and banana), carotene (dark green leafy vegetables, red palm oil, carrot, and pumpkin) • Encourage them to eat at least six times a day

Feeding During Acute Diarrhea and Dysentery

Nutritional management of acute diarrhea and dysentery takes optimal advantage of intestinal absorption capacity, which is affected to some extent during diarrhea, by feeding small, frequent, energy-dense food taking into consideration the age, preillness feeding pattern, and state of hydration of the child **(Table 11.5.5)**. Feeding is continued in children with no dehydration and resumed as early as possible for some dehydration.

Zinc Supplementation for Treatment of Diarrhea

Zinc deficiency is common in children from low and middle-income countries because of the intake of predominant vegetarian diets and the high content of dietary phytates. Increased fecal losses during many episodes of diarrhea aggravate pre-existing zinc deficiency. WHO and the Indian Academy of Pediatrics (IAP) recommend zinc supplementation as an adjunct to ORS in the treatment of diarrhea. The National IAP Task Force recommends that all children older than 6 months suffering from diarrhea should receive a uniform dose of 20 mg of elemental zinc as soon as diarrhea starts and continues for a total period of 14 days. Children aged 2–6 months should be advised 10 mg/day of elemental zinc for a total period of 14 days.[5]

Use of Antimicrobial Agents

Antibiotic therapy should be reserved only for cases of dysentery and suspected cholera **(Table 11.5.6)**. Every case of diarrhea needs to be carefully evaluated for the presence of blood in the stools which indicates dysentery and to identify cases of suspected cholera (high purge rate with severe dehydration in a child above 2 years in an area where cholera is known to be present). No chemoprophylaxis is needed for contacts.

Associated nongastrointestinal infections such as pneumonia, meningitis, and urinary tract infections, should also be carefully looked for and appropriately treated. In severe malnutrition, the usual signs of infection such as fever are often absent, yet multiple infections are common in these children. Therefore, it is assumed that all severely malnourished children may have an underlying infection which should be treated with broad-spectrum parenteral antibiotics.

TABLE 11.5.6: Antimicrobials used to treat specific causes of diarrhea in children.

Cause	Drug of choice	Dose
Cholera	*First line:* Doxycycline *Second line:* Ciprofloxacin*	Single dose of 6 mg/kg PO Single dose 15 mg/kg
Dysentery	*First-line:* Ciprofloxacin** *Second line:* Pivmecillinam Ceftriaxone	15 mg/kg two times a day PO × 3 days 20 mg/kg four times a day PO × 5 days 50–100 mg/kg once a day IM × 2–5 days
Amebic dysentery	Metronidazole	30 mg/kg/day in three divided doses PO × 5–10 days
Acute giardiasis	Metronidazole or tinidazole	15 mg/kg/day in three divided doses PO × 5 days 15 mg/kg/day in three divided doses PO × 5 days

*Can be used if there is resistance to doxycycline or no clinical response.
**In view of widespread resistance to trimethoprim–sulfamethoxazole (TMP–SMX) and reported resistance to nalidixic acid, the Indian Academy of Pediatrics Task Force recommends ciprofloxacin as a first-line drug in areas where resistance rates to TMP–SMX exceed 30%.

Nutritional Rehabilitation

Nutritional support to a child following an episode of acute or persistent diarrhea is of immense importance in view of the known adverse impact of diarrheal diseases on the nutrition of a young child. The need for proper feeding after an episode of diarrhea has even greater importance particularly because the efforts made by the mother/caretaker to feed during convalescence are more rewarding when these children tend to have better appetites. Therefore, one extra meal, at least for 2 weeks after an episode of acute diarrhea and for at least 1 month after persistent diarrhea, stressing the need for "catch-up growth," is likely to help in the nutritional rehabilitation of these children.

COMPLICATIONS

Electrolyte Imbalance

With appropriate use of oral rehydration therapy, access to plain water, and continued feeding, the risk of electrolyte disturbances is minimized. However, following electrolyte disturbances may be encountered in some cases.

Hypernatremia

Some children with diarrhea, especially young infants, develop hypernatremic dehydration which usually follows the use of hypertonic drinks (canned fruit juices, carbonated cold drinks, and incorrectly prepared salt and sugar solutions, or ORS with high glucose content). Children with hypernatremic dehydration (serum sodium >150 mEq/L osmolality >295 mOsm/kg) are extremely thirsty, out of proportion to their other signs of dehydration, and sometimes have convulsions. These children can be successfully treated with low osmolarity ORS. However, if the child is unable to drink orally, Ringer's lactate can be initially given to treat shock and later switch over to ORT with low osmolarity ORS.

Hyponatremia

Patients who ingest only large amounts of water or watery drinks that contain very little salt may present with hyponatremia (serum sodium <130 mEq/L, osmolality <275 mOsm/kg), which may be clinically associated with lethargy and seizures. ORS is a safe and effective therapy for hyponatremia as well. For children who are unable to drink orally, IV infusion of Ringer's lactate can effectively treat hyponatremia.

Hypokalemia

Inadequate replacement of potassium losses during diarrhea can lead to potassium depletion and hypokalemia (serum potassium <3 mEq/L), which may result in muscle weakness, paralytic ileus, renal impairment, and cardiac arrhythmias. Severe potassium depletion particularly in malnourished children may lead to acute onset flaccid paralysis ranging from neck flop to quadriparesis and even respiratory paralysis. The potassium deficit can be corrected by using ORS solution for rehydration therapy and by feeding potassium-rich foods (e.g., banana or fresh fruit juices) during and after diarrhea. Oral potassium supplementation (2 mEq/kg/day) is indicated in malnourished children. In transient flaccid paralysis due to hypokalemia, potassium can be administered parenterally by using a 15% solution of potassium chloride (1 mL = 2 mEq of potassium) but not exceeding 40 mEq/L of IV fluids after ensuring adequate renal functions.

Hypoglycemia

Continued feeding during an episode of diarrhea minimizes the risk of getting hypoglycemia. However, some children, particularly those severely malnourished, are at risk of getting hypoglycemia. Early feeding can prevent hypoglycemia in these cases. Sick young infants (<2 months) who are not able to breastfeed or have low weight for their age and a child with symptoms of hypoglycemia should be given 20–50 mL (10 mL/kg) expressed breast milk or locally appropriate animal milk (with added sugar). If neither of these is available, give 20–50 mL (10 mL/kg) sugar water.

Metabolic Acidosis

During acute diarrhea, large amounts of bicarbonate may be lost in the stool. If the kidneys continue to function normally, most of the lost bicarbonate is replaced and a serious base deficit does not develop. Metabolic acidosis tends to correct spontaneously in most of the cases as the child is properly rehydrated. ORS solution contains adequate bicarbonate/citrate to counter acidosis in less severe cases. However, in severe dehydration, compromised renal function leads to rapid development of base deficit and metabolic acidosis. Hypovolemic shock occurs as a consequence of rapid loss of water and electrolytes in severe diarrhea. This results in excessive production of lactic acid, which may further contribute to metabolic acidosis. Rapid IV infusion of Ringer's lactate, containing 28 mEq/L of lactate (metabolized to bicarbonate), is recommended in severe dehydration. However, in the presence of circulatory failure, bicarbonate precursors (e.g., citrate and lactate) may not be readily metabolized in the body. If the patient presents with severe metabolic acidosis, (pH <7.20, serum HCO_3^- <8 mEq/L) sodium bicarbonate in a bolus dose of 2–3 mEq/kg can be given to correct acidosis. Attention should be paid to serum potassium concentration as correction of acidosis in a patient with low potassium can lead to life-threatening severe hypokalemia.

Acute Renal Failure

Severe dehydration and shock lead to a decrease in renal blood flow resulting in a prerenal type of acute renal failure. Immediate replacement of fluids is generally helpful to revive kidney functions unless renal failure is irreversible. In case of the fluid challenge, after rehydration fails to reverse the process, the child needs to be hospitalized and managed as per acute renal failure protocol.

Hemolytic Uremic Syndrome

Some children with invasive diarrhea due to *S. dysenteriae* or enteroinvasive *E. coli* may have HUS due to nephrotoxin liberated by these organisms. These children develop intravascular hemolysis with acute renal failure. This is a serious condition and needs to be managed in a hospital setting.

PROGNOSIS

Acute diarrhea is a self-limiting disorder. Early administration of ORS or home-available fluids prevents the onset of dehydration. Appropriate use of low osmolarity ORS in some dehydration and Ringer's lactate in severe dehydration can prevent all diarrheal deaths.

PREVENTION

Diarrheal diseases can be prevented to a great extent by improving infant feeding practices and personal and domestic hygiene. Some of the interventions which are feasible and cost-effective include:

- Promotion of exclusive breastfeeding up to 6 months of age
- Improved complementary feeding practices
- Use of clean drinking water and sufficient water for personal hygiene
- Hand washing
- Rotavirus vaccine
- Use of sanitary toilets
- Safe disposal of the stool of young children
- Measles vaccination

CONCLUSION

- Diarrhea is a self-limiting disorder and does not need any antibiotics for treatment.
- Oral rehydration with low osmolarity ORS continued feeding and zinc supplementation are the key to the treatment of diarrhea in children.
- Intravenous fluids are indicated in a few cases who have severe dehydration or are unable to drink orally. Ringer's lactate is the most suitable solution for IV therapy.
- A child with diarrhea should be thoroughly examined for associated illnesses.
- Exclusive breastfeeding up to 6 months of age and hand washing significantly reduce the incidence of diarrhea.
- The rotavirus vaccine is an effective way of preventing episodes of severe watery diarrhea and is included in the National Immunization Program.

REFERENCES

1. Kotloff KL, Nasrin D, Blackwelder WC, Wu Y, Farag T, Panchalingham S, et al. The incidence, aetiology, and adverse clinical consequences of less severe diarrhoeal episodes among infants and children residing in low-income and middle-income countries: a 12-month case-control study as a follow-on to the Global Enteric Multicenter Study (GEMS). Lancet Glob Health. 2019;7(5):e568-84.
2. World Health Organization. (2017). Diarrhoeal Diseases (Human). https://www.undrr.org/understanding-disaster-risk/terminology/hips/bi0028#:~:text=Diarrhoea%20is%20a%20leading%20cause,diarrhoea%20(WHO%2C%202017) [Last accessed December, 2024].
3. International Institute for Population Sciences (IIPS). National Family Health Survey (NFHS-5), 2019-20, March 2021. IIPS, Mumbai.
4. Blutt SE, Kirkwood CD, Parreno V, Warfield KL, Clarlet M, Estes MK, et al. Rotavirus antigenemia and viremia: a common event. Lancet. 2003;362(9394):1445-9.
5. Bhatnagar S, Bhandari N, Mouli UC, Bhan MK; IAP National Task Force. Consensus Statement of IAP National Task Force: Status Report on Management of Acute Diarrhea. Indian Pediatr. 2004;41(4):335-48.
6. Integrated Management of Neonatal and Childhood Illness. Physician Chart Booklet. Ministry of Health and Family Welfare, Govt. of India; 2021.

11.6 Chronic and Persistent Diarrhea

Sahana Shankar

INTRODUCTION

Diarrhea remains the second leading cause of mortality in children under 5 years of age killing nearly 5,00,000 children worldwide.[1] Although there is a significant decline in child mortality related to diarrheal diseases in India and worldwide, it remains an important cause for morbidity in low- and middle-income countries (LMICs) including India.

Acute diarrhea typically lasts 7–14 days and is often infectious in etiology.[2] Diarrhea with a presumed infectious etiology and lasting for longer than 14 days is defined as persistent diarrhea (PD).[2] Chronic diarrhea refers to diarrheal illness lasting for longer than 4 weeks.[2] Although these definitions are arbitrary, duration of diarrhea provides a clue to the underlying etiology of diarrhea and guides management. In this chapter, we discuss the etiology, pathophysiology, approach, and management of persistent and chronic diarrhea.

PERSISTENT DIARRHEA

Definition

According to World Health Organization (WHO), diarrhea is defined as passage of three or more liquid stools or more frequently than is normal for the individual.[1] Defining normal stooling pattern in children is challenging as stool frequency and consistency varies with age, type of feeding and geographical location.[3] A normal breastfed infant's bowel movements may vary from 12 stools in a day to one stool in a week whereas an older child rarely passes more than 3 stools per day **(Table 11.6.1)**.

Diarrhea is characterized by an increase in the volume and water content of stools. Hence, it is important to elicit consistency of stool in history. Bristol stool scale **(Table 11.6.2)** is a handy aid in office practice to establish stool consistency. Frequent passage of formed stools is not diarrhea. It is equally important to not confuse constipation-related overflow diarrhea with true diarrhea.

TABLE 11.6.1: Normal stool frequency in children.[3]

Age group	Average number of stools per day (Range)
Infants (0–14 weeks)	3.1 (0.6–5.0)
Breastfeeding	3.3 (1.3–5.4)
Formula feeding	2.0 (0.8–3.4)
Mixed feeding	3.0 (1.0–4.3)
Young children (14–4 years)	1.6 (0.8–2.4)

Pathophysiology and Etiology

Persistent diarrhea is a continuum of acute diarrhea. The pathogenesis of PD is multifactorial and includes (1) infection, (2) mucosal injury, (3) delayed regeneration of damaged intestinal mucosa, and (4) increased host susceptibility, all of which are driven by malnutrition. PD is a consequence of multiple simultaneous or sequential enteric infections which lead to mucosal injury resulting in malabsorption and nutrient deficiencies, thus perpetuating the vicious cycle of malnutrition, susceptibility to infections and further diarrhea **(Fig. 11.6.1)**. Nearly 90–95% of acute diarrheal episodes resolve within 7 days. Around 5–10% of diarrheal illnesses last longer than 5–7 days and constitute *"prolonged diarrhea"* (>7 days but <14 days) (ProD). It is important to recognize this entity and intervene early as it often progresses to PD resulting in significant morbidity. Children with ProD have a sixfold risk of progression to PD. They are stunted with poor neurodevelopmental outcomes.

Etiology of PD is often infectious and includes various bacteria, viruses, and protozoa **(Box 11.6.1)**. Enteropathogenic *Escherichia coli* (EPEC) and enteroaggregative *E. coli* (EAEC)

TABLE 11.6.2: Bristol stool scale.

Type 1	Separate hard lumps, like nuts	
Type 2	Sausage-shaped but lumpy	
Type 3	Like a sausage or snake but with cracks on its surface	
Type 4	Like a sausage or snake, smooth and soft	
Type 5	Soft blobs with clear-cut edges	
Type 6	Fluffy pieces with ragged edges, a mushy stool	
Type 7	Watery, no solid pieces	

are the commonly implicated bacterial pathogens while *Giardia, Cryptosporidium,* and *Entamoeba* are the common parasites causing PD among children in LMIC **(Box 11.6.2)**. In immunocompromised children, parasites followed by viruses are the most common cause of PD. However, demonstration of pathogens in stool may not indicate causality of PD, as the diarrhea is often a consequence of mucosal damage.

Epidemiology

PD accounts for 5–18% of diarrheal episodes, it contributes to nearly 50% of days with diarrhea and 35% of diarrhea-related mortality in children under 5 years of age.[5]

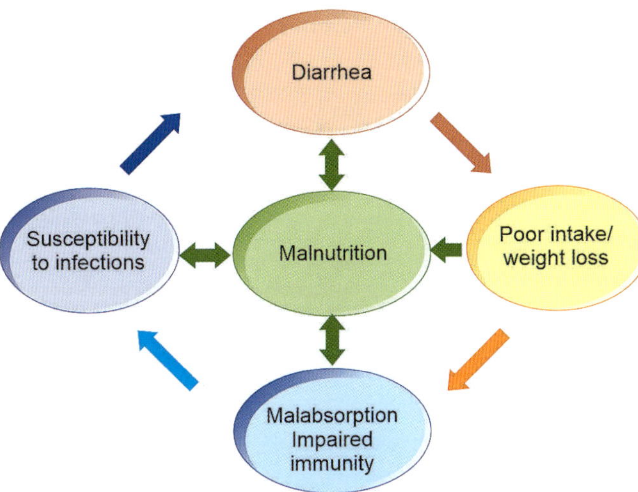

Fig. 11.6.1: The pathophysiology of persistent diarrhea.

BOX 11.6.1: Etiology of persistent diarrhea.

Infections:
- Bacteria—*Escherichia coli* (EPEC/EAEC), *Shigella, Salmonella, Campylobacter, Clostridium difficile,* and atypical mycobacteria*
- Parasites*—*Cryptosporidium, Giardia, Isospora,* Entamoeba, *Strongyloides,* and *Microsporidia*
- Viruses*—Norovirus, *Rotavirus, Sapovirus, Adenovirus,* and *Astrovirus*

Postinfectious irritable bowel syndrome (PI-IBS):
- Food allergy
- Secondary carbohydrate malabsorption
- Small intestinal bacterial overgrowth (SIBO)

*In immunocompromised patients

BOX 11.6.2: Risk factors for persistent diarrhea.[4]

- Prolonged diarrhea in first year of life
- Immunodeficiency—primary or acquired [human immunodeficiency virus (HIV)]
- Malnutrition—macro- and micronutrient deficiencies
- Early introduction of faulty complementary feeds
- Lack of exclusive breastfeeding up to 4 months of age
- Irrational antibiotic use during acute diarrheal episode
- Use of unsafe drinking water

About 60% of PD occurs before 6 months and 90% below 1 year of age.[6]

Management

Management of PD includes early recognition of children with ProD and PD, thorough physical examination to identify red flags of dehydration, severe malnutrition, and systemic infection and timely initiation of fluid and nutritional rehabilitation.

History and Physical Examination

A thorough history is mandatory with special attention to type of feeding (breastfeeding or formula feeding), type of formula (standard vs. lactose-free vs. soy-based/hydrolyzed), standard strength or dilute, mode of feeding (bottle or pallada or other), recent change in diet or introduction of new foods or milk, recent travel or sick contacts, recurrent antibiotic use, and growth of child prior to illness.

Physical examination of the child should be done to assess anthropometry (to assess growth failure—acute vs. chronic), hydration status, examination of oral cavity and perineum (for fungal infection), ear and chest (for otitis media or pneumonia), and abdomen (for organomegaly).

Investigations

Child needs hospitalization if there is severe malnutrition, moderate-to-severe dehydration or evidence of sepsis. Investigations in PD include the following:

- Complete blood counts (CBCs), C-reactive protein (CRP), total protein and albumin, blood glucose, electrolytes, blood and urine cultures, and chest radiograph.
- *Stool examination for opportunistic pathogens* is indicated in appropriate clinical setting such as suspected immunodeficiency states. Traditional laboratory methods of detection of stool pathogens include stool culture, but are limited by low yield, poor sensitivity, and long turnaround times. Culture-independent diagnostic tests (CIDT) such as multiplex PCR include testing for a panel of bacteria, viruses, and parasites in a single stool specimen. The advantages include quicker turnaround time, screening for multiple pathogens, and a higher sensitivity.[7] The limitation is the inability to perform antibiotic susceptibility assays. It is a useful tool to administer targeted antibiotic therapy in an immunocompromised or a critically ill child.

Treatment

The principles for optimal management of PD include the following:

Rehydration or fluid resuscitation: Management of dehydration in PD is similar to that of acute diarrhea based on the severity of dehydration. Correction of dyselectrolytemia and hypoglycemia is essential. In PD, low osmolarity glucose-based or rice-based oral rehydration salts (ORS) is preferred to standard ORS for oral rehydration therapy, as it is associated with significant reduction in total stool output and duration of diarrhea.

Dietary management: Diet is crucial and remains the cornerstone of management of PD **(Flowchart 11.6.1)**. Following stabilization with correction of dehydration and acidosis, children with PD should be commenced on low lactose or lactose-free rice-based home diets to meet an energy requirement of 75 kcal/kg/day, increasing with increments of 25 kcal/kg/day to a target of 150 kcal/kg/day by day 4–5 of illness to achieve weight gain of 10–20 g/kg/day. Based on tolerance, different diet plans have been formulated—diet A consists of low lactose-based regime of rice, milk, and sugar, whereas diets B and C consist of lactose-free diets containing rice, glucose, oil, and egg and chicken respectively as source of protein **(Table 11.6.3)**.[6]

Green banana diet, alone or mixed with rice, has been shown to be effective in reduction of stool volume and protection against recurrence in PD.[8] Mechanism of action of green banana is postulated to be mediated through conversion of starch in banana, which is amylase-resistant, to short chain fatty acids (SCFA) by colonic bacteria. Due to its resistant nature, nearly 84% of banana starch reaches terminal ileum intact and production of SCFA facilitates absorption of sodium and water in colon.

Micronutrient supplementation: Concomitant micronutrient deficiency is common in PD due to mucosal injury and malabsorption. Zinc supplementation is recommended in PD as it reduces duration of diarrheal episode and protects

Flowchart 11.6.1: Management algorithm of persistent diarrhea.

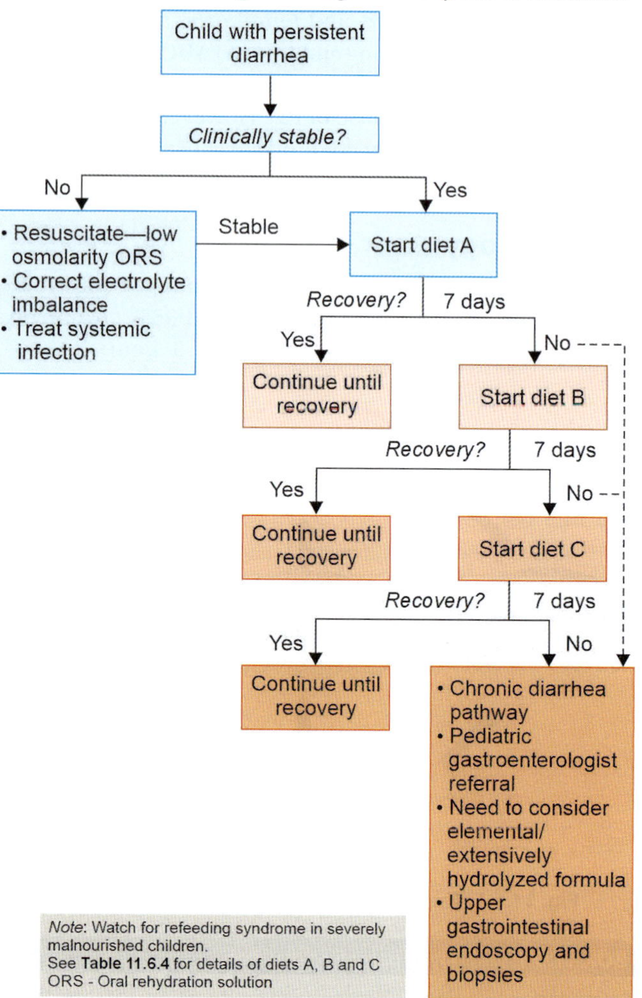

(ORS: oral rehydration salts)

TABLE 11.6.3: Diet plans in persistent diarrhea.

Type A diet (milk-based rice diet)		***Type B diet (milk-free, egg-based rice diet)***		***Type C (milk-free, chicken-based diet)***	
Ingredient	***Amount***	***Ingredient***	***Amount***	***Ingredient***	***Amount (/L)***
Puffed rice	12.5 g	Puffed rice	13.5 g	Chicken	100 g
Milk	40 mL	Egg white	11 g	Glucose	20–40 g
Sugar	2.25 g	Sugar/glucose	3.5 g	Oil	40–50 g
Oil	2 g	Oil	3.5 g	KCl (15%)	7.5 mL
Water	100 mL	Water	100 mL	$NaHCO_3$ (7.5%)	20–30 mL
Total calories	96 kcal/100 g	Total calories	92.2 kcal/100 g	Water	1,000 mL
Protein	10%	Protein	9.5%	This yields 720 kcal and 26 g/L of protein	
Fat	33%	Fat	33%		
Puffed rice is ground and mixed with sugar and oil. Boiled water is then added to make a thick gruel. This has a shelf life of 3 hours		Egg white is added to the mixture of weighed rice, sugar and oil. Boiled water is added to make a thick gruel weighing 100 g			

against recurrence. Combination of vitamin A and zinc supplementation was found to reduce the prevalence of PD. Although the evidence to suggest routine supplementation with folic acid, iron and vitamin D in PD is weak, it is prudent to start these supplements in children with PD at recommended dietary allowance (RDA) **(Table 11.6.4)**.

Antimicrobials: Routine empiric use of antibiotics is not indicated in PD. Indications for antibiotics include presence of gross blood in stools, children <3 months of age, immunocompromised states [primary or acquired immunodeficiency, corticosteroid or chemotherapy, solid organ transplant (SOT) or hematopoietic stem cell transplant (HSCT) recipients, chronic disease, and severe malnutrition], and presence of extraintestinal infection such as otitis media or pneumonia or urinary tract infection (UTI). Third-generation cephalosporin or quinolone is recommended as first line with addition of aminoglycoside or ampicillin in infants under 3 months of age. If there is evidence of fungal infection, fluconazole is added. Antibiotic therapy when indicated for PD has to be targeted based on identification of specific pathogens.

There is insufficient evidence to recommend probiotics and antisecretory agents such as racecadotril in management of PD.

CHRONIC DIARRHEA

Definition

Chronic diarrhea constitutes diarrhea without a demonstrable infectious etiology, lasting for >4 weeks, associated with malabsorption and growth failure. The cut-off of 4 weeks is debatable as some authors refer to diarrhea lasting longer than 2 weeks as chronic diarrhea. The 4-week threshold helps to exclude diarrhea of infectious etiology, as most enteric infections resolve within 1 month. The definition of chronic diarrhea was proposed based on studies done in industrialized countries where prevalence of enteric infections is low. In tropical countries such as India, it is prudent to remain vigilant about enteric infections as 10–20% of all infectious diarrhea can progress to chronic diarrhea.

TABLE 11.6.4: Nutritional supplementation in PD.[6]

Supplement	Dose	Duration
Elemental zinc	10 mg <6 months; 20 mg >6 months OD	2 weeks
Vitamin A	<6 months 50,000 IU; 6–12 months 100,000 IU; >12 months 200,000 IU	One stat dose
Multivitamins	2 × RDA	2–4 weeks
Iron	After cessation of diarrhea—3 mg/kg	3 months
Folic acid	1 mg/day	2 weeks
Vitamin D	200–400 IU/day	3 months
Potassium*	2–3 mEq/kg/day	2 weeks
Magnesium Sulfate*	0.2 mL/kg/day IM	2–3 days

*In severely malnourished children with dyselectrolytemia

Pathophysiology and Etiology

The etiologies of chronic diarrhea are several and require numerous diagnostic tests to narrow down the differentials. It helps to categorize chronic diarrhea based on pathophysiology into five large groups—(1) osmotic, (2) secretory, (3) inflammatory, (4) fatty, and (5) motility-related.[9]

Osmotic Diarrhea

Osmotic diarrhea results from unabsorbed osmotically active solutes or nutrients within the intestinal lumen which causes water retention in the lumen. It can be easily differentiated from non-osmotic causes by a trial of fasting. Osmotic diarrhea resolves with fasting or cessation of ingestion of the offending substance. Usually, stool is iso-osmolar to serum (290 mOsm) and is accounted for by major electrolytes (Na^+ and K^+) in stool. In osmotic diarrhea, the presence of osmotically active substance in stool results in an osmotic gap which can be confirmed by measurement of stool electrolytes and stool osmolality **(Box 11.6.3)**. Causes of osmotic diarrhea based on age of onset is listed in **Table 11.6.5**.

Secretory Diarrhea

Secretory diarrhea results from aberrant electrolyte transport. It is due to net secretion of anions (chloride or bicarbonate) or

BOX 11.6.3: List of investigations in chronic diarrhea.

Tests:
- Stool microscopy and culture
- Stool *Clostridium difficile* toxin (CD)
- Stool electrolytes
- Stool reducing substances and pH
- Stool pancreatic elastase
- 72-hour stool fat quantification
- Fecal calprotectin (FCP)
- Stool alpha-1-antitrypsin (α1-AT)
- Complete blood counts
- Renal function test (RFT)
- Inflammatory markers
- Liver function test (LFT)
- Celiac serology with IgA detection[10]
- Upper GI endoscopy and colonoscopy + light microscopy +/-Electron microscopy of duodenal biopsies
- CT abdomen
- Breath hydrogen test (glucose, lactose and fructose)
- Genetic testing (whole exome sequencing—WES and next-generation sequencing—NGS)

potassium across the intestinal epithelium or net inhibition of sodium absorption, thus resulting in large volume watery diarrhea. The mechanisms of secretory diarrhea are as follows:

- *Exogenous secretagogues:* Infections such as cholera, *E. coli,* and rotaviral gastroenteritis are the most common causes of acute secretory diarrhea. Enterotoxin produced by *Vibrio cholerae* is the prototype of secretagogue resulting in large volume secretory diarrhea. These infections rarely cause chronic diarrhea.
- *Endogenous secretagogues:* Neuroendocrine tumors such as VIPoma (vasointestinal peptide), carcinoid tumor, Zollinger–Ellison syndrome, etc., produce peptides or hormones which act as secretagogues.
- *Absence of ion transporter:* Absence/deficiency of electrolyte channels in the intestinal epithelial cells can result in congenital secretory diarrhea (e.g., congenital chloride diarrhea, congenital sodium diarrhea, etc.)
- *Loss of intestinal surface area:* Extensive intestinal resection results in diarrhea which has both secretory and osmotic components due to loss of surface area.

Inflammatory Diarrhea

GI infection is the most common cause of acute bloody diarrhea. It is important to have a high index of suspicion for *Clostridium difficile* infection (CDI) and test accordingly **(Box 11.6.3)**. Once infections are ruled out, etiology varies depending on the age of presentation **(Table 11.6.5)**.

Fatty Diarrhea or Steatorrhea

This is covered in Chapter 11.7: Maldigestion and Malabsorption Syndromes.

Protein-losing enteropathy is associated with hypoalbuminemia, lymphopenia, and hypogammaglobulinemia **(Table 11.6.5)**.

Motility-related Diarrhea

Normal gut motility allows optimal contact time between absorbable solutes and intestinal epithelium for net fluid reabsorption. Both rapid transit and slow transit cause diarrhea—by preventing reabsorption of normally secreted fluid in the small bowel and by resulting in bacterial overgrowth and bile acid deconjugation, respectively. Rapid transit is noted in functional diarrhea and inflammatory bowel disease (IBD) and slow transit contribute to diarrhea seen in chronic intestinal pseudo-obstruction (CIPO), postsurgical states, etc. **(Table 11.6.5)**.

Evaluation of a Child with Chronic Diarrhea

Age of Onset

Infection is the most common cause across all age groups. When onset of diarrhea is from birth or immediate postnatal period, prompt evaluation for congenital enteropathies, necrotizing enterocolitis (NEC) or anatomical abnormalities should be performed. Clues on history which indicate congenital enteropathies include consanguinity, polyhydramnios, and decreased fetal movements.

TABLE 11.6.5: Etiology of chronic diarrhea based on type of diarrhea and age of onset.

Osmotic	***Secretory***	***Inflammatory***
Neonate/infant: • Glucosegalactose malabsorption • Congenital sucrase-isomaltase deficiency • Primary lactase deficiency • Short gut syndrome	*Neonate/infant:* • Microvillous inclusion disease • Tufting enteropathy • Congenital chloride diarrhea • Congenital sodium diarrhea • Syndromic diarrhea of infancy • Primary bile acid diarrhea	*Neonate/infant:* • NEC • Cow's milk protein allergy • Very early onset IBD—autoimmune enteropathy/IPEX/primary immunodeficiency
Older child: • Postinfectious enteropathy/IBS • Secondary carbohydrate malabsorption—lactose/fructose • Small intestinal bacterial overgrowth • Celiac disease • Diet induced—apple, pears, carbonated drinks, dietetic foods containing sorbitol, mannitol or xylitol; antacids or laxatives containing lactulose or $Mg(OH)_2$; methylxanthines-containing drinks (cola, tea, and coffee); NSAIDs	*Older child:* • VIPoma (vasoactive intestinal polypeptide), carcinoid tumor, Zollinger–Ellison syndrome, and mastocytosis • Intestinal resection following trauma/vascular accident	*Older child:* • IBD • *Clostridium difficile* infection • Food protein allergy • Autoimmune enteropathy

(IBD: inflammatory bowel disease; IBS: irritable bowel syndrome; IPEX: immune dysregulation, polyendocrinopathy, enteropathy, X-linked; NEC: necrotizing enterocolitis; NSAIDs: nonsteroidal anti-inflammatory drugs)

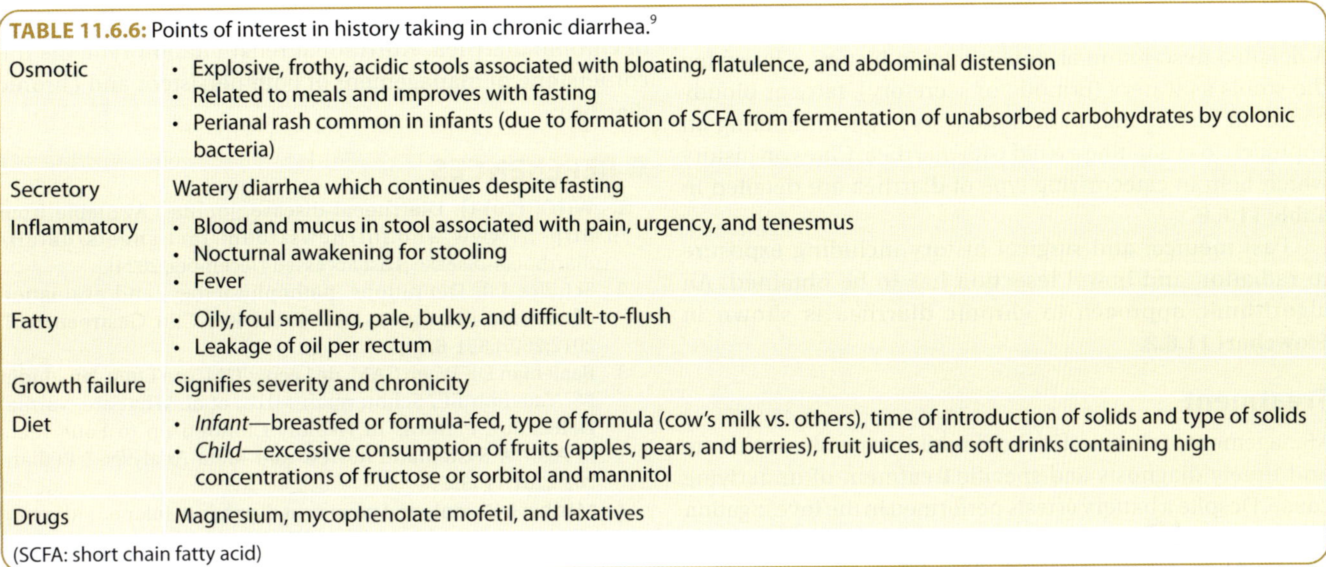

TABLE 11.6.6: Points of interest in history taking in chronic diarrhea.[9]

Osmotic	• Explosive, frothy, acidic stools associated with bloating, flatulence, and abdominal distension • Related to meals and improves with fasting • Perianal rash common in infants (due to formation of SCFA from fermentation of unabsorbed carbohydrates by colonic bacteria)
Secretory	Watery diarrhea which continues despite fasting
Inflammatory	• Blood and mucus in stool associated with pain, urgency, and tenesmus • Nocturnal awakening for stooling • Fever
Fatty	• Oily, foul smelling, pale, bulky, and difficult-to-flush • Leakage of oil per rectum
Growth failure	Signifies severity and chronicity
Diet	• *Infant*—breastfed or formula-fed, type of formula (cow's milk vs. others), time of introduction of solids and type of solids • *Child*—excessive consumption of fruits (apples, pears, and berries), fruit juices, and soft drinks containing high concentrations of fructose or sorbitol and mannitol
Drugs	Magnesium, mycophenolate mofetil, and laxatives

(SCFA: short chain fatty acid)

Flowchart 11.6.2: Approach to a child with chronic diarrhea.[9]

Diarrhea lasting >4 weeks

History and physical examination

Assess for red flags
• Age of onset-neonatal
• Presence of blood or mucus or fat, nocturnal diarrhea
• Unexplained fevers
• Persistent vomiting
• Growth failure and/or developmental delay/pubertal delay
• Arthritis, eye or skin involvement
• Hydration status
• Nutritional status—evidence of micronutrient deficiencies
• Presence of edema
• Abnormal perianal examination—rash, tags, fistulae, fissures
• Presence of abdominal distension and organomegaly

Unwell Dehydrated → Fluid resuscitation and stabilization as necessary

• Stool microscopy and culture/infectious workup, stool RS and pH
• *Clostridium difficile* toxin (>1 year of age)
• FCP (>4 years of age)—if available
• CBC, LFT, CRP, ESR, serum electrolytes, celiac serology, and TFT

→ • No red flags, normal stool and blood examination
• Likely functional diarrhea or irritable bowel syndrome

Positive infectious screen → Treat as appropriate

Positive celiac screen → Upper GI endoscopy

No WC or RC, fat globules ++ → 72 hours stool fat quantification or low fecal elastase → Fatty diarrhea

WC/RC ++ FCP >250 μg/g → Inflammatory/bloody diarrhea

Trial of fasting / Stool RS and pH OR Stool osmotic gap

Resolves with fasting OR Stool osmotic gap >100 mOsm Stool RS positive and acidic pH → Osmotic diarrhea

Minimal or no improvement OR Stool osmotic gap <50 mOsm Negative stool RS and normal pH → Secretory diarrhea

(CBC: complete blood count; CRP: C-reactive protein; ESR: erythrocyte sedimentation rate; FCP: fecal calprotectin; LFT: liver function test; RS: reducing substance; TFT: thyroid function test)

Stool Characteristics

A detailed description of stool is vital in history. Classifying the stools as watery (osmotic or secretory), fatty or bloody based on history and basic stool tests helps in defining an approach to evaluating a child with diarrhea. Clues on history which help in categorizing type of diarrhea are detailed in **Table 11.6.6**.

Past medical and surgical history including exposure to radiation and bowel resection has to be obtained. An algorithmic approach to chronic diarrhea is shown in **Flowchart 11.6.2**.

Treatment

Management of chronic diarrhea in children involves accurate and timely diagnosis and specific treatment of underlying cause. Despite a battery of tests performed in the investigation of a child with chronic diarrhea, specific etiology may be elusive. General principles include nutritional rehabilitation, dietary modification, drug therapy and parenteral nutrition, and intestinal transplantation in cases of intestinal failure. Treatment strategies for individual causes of chronic diarrhea are outside the scope of this chapter.

CONCLUSION

Persistent diarrhea is associated with significant morbidity and requires early recognition and timely nutritional intervention. Promotion of exclusive breastfeeding, proper weaning, and access to safe drinking water remains important preventative strategies. Chronic diarrhea is a challenging condition which requires exhaustive workup, not easily accessible to all centers. It requires early recognition and expeditious referral to a tertiary care center which has facilities for endoscopy, histology, and genetic testing. Advent of cost-effective PCR-based testing and next-generation sequencing has had a significant impact on management of chronic diarrhea. Nutritional rehabilitation remains the cornerstone of management of both persistent and chronic diarrhea.

REFERENCES

1. WHO. (2014). Diarrhoeal disease. [online] Available from https://www.who.int/news-room/fact-sheets/detail/diarrhoeal-disease [Last accessed December, 2024].
2. Schiller LR. Definitions, pathophysiology, and evaluation of chronic diarrhoea. Best Pract Res Clin Gastroenterol. 2012;26(5):551-62.
3. Baaleman DF, Wegh CAM, de Leeuw TJM, van Etten-Jamaludin FS, Vaughan EE, Schoterman MHC, et al. What are Normal Defecation Patterns in Healthy Children up to Four Years of Age? A Systematic Review and Meta-Analysis. J Pediatr. 2023;261:113559.
4. Matthai J. Chronic and persistent diarrhea in infants and young children: Status statement. Indian Pediatr. 2011;48(1):37-42.
5. Moore SR. Update on prolonged and persistent diarrhea in children. Curr Opin Gastroenterol. 2011;27(1):19-23.
6. Riyaz A, Gajera K, Biradar VD. Persistent Diarrhea. Standard Treatment Guidelines 2022. Indian Acad Pediat; 2022.
7. Ghoshal U, Tejan N, Sisodia J, Verma S, Prasad N, Ghoshal Uc. The utility of multiplex polymerase chain reaction for diagnosis of infectious diarrhoea in a tropical country. Indian J Med Microbiol. 2021;39(3):323-7.
8. Sarmin M, Hossain MI, Islam SB, Shikha SS, Alam NH, Sarker MSA, et al. Open-label, randomised controlled trial found that a green banana mixed rice suji diet was most effective for persistent diarrhoea in children in Bangladesh. Acta Paediatr. 2023;112(8):1755-63.
9. Shankar S, Rosenbaum J. Chronic diarrhoea in children: A practical algorithm-based approach. J Paediatr Child Health. 2020;56(7):1029-38.
10. Rubio-Tapia A, Hill ID, Semrad C, Kelly CP, Greer KB, Limketkai BN, et al. American College of Gastroenterology Guidelines Update: Diagnosis and Management of Celiac Disease. Am J Gastroenterol. 2023;118(1):59-76.

11.7 Maldigestion and Malabsorption Syndromes

Ujjal Poddar

INTRODUCTION

Malabsorption syndrome (MAS) is defined as the failure of absorption of one or more nutrients. Over the years, the spectrum of MAS in India has changed. Initial studies of the 1960s and 1970s were mainly on young (<5 years) malnourished children and the focus was on stool examination to isolate infections and infestations. Almost half of those cases were due to gastrointestinal (GI) infestations such as *giardiasis*. Nevertheless, with improvement in nutritional status, personal hygiene, and appropriate use of antimicrobials, the prevalence of GI infestations (especially *Giardia*) as a primary cause of MAS has decreased tremendously. Due to increasing awareness and easy availability of diagnostic tools such as serology and endoscopic biopsy, the focus has now shifted from infestation to celiac disease, especially in North India. Recent studies have shown that celiac disease is the most common cause of MAS in Western countries as well as in India (especially in North India) both in children as well as in adults.[1] With the improved survival of preterm babies due to improved neonatal care, short-bowel syndrome following surgical resection of small bowel due to necrotizing enterocolitis is no longer an uncommon entity. MAS is a common feature of short-bowel syndrome due to a lack of absorptive surface and failure of luminal digestion.[2] The severe form of small intestinal bacterial overgrowth (SIBO) can manifest as MAS and the entity is common with either surgical cause such as small bowel stricture, internal fistula, blind-loop syndrome, and diverticula or due to stasis caused by the reduced motility of the gut (pseudo-obstruction).[3] The severe form of cow's milk protein allergy (CMPA) can cause significant mucosal damage and can manifest as MAS in infants.[4]

PATHOGENESIS

Malabsorption syndrome is grossly divided into two categories:

1. Impaired breakdown of nutrients (*maldigestion*)
2. Defective mucosal uptake and transport of adequately digested nutrients (*true malabsorption*).

The latter may be specific malabsorption of a nutrient or a group of nutrients or generalized malabsorption or panmalabsorption (malabsorption of a broad range of nutrients).

Maldigestion

The luminal phase of digestion requires pancreatic enzymes and bile salts, and the absence of either of them gives rise to failure of digestion of carbohydrate (lack of pancreatic amylase), fat (pancreatic lipase and bile salts), and proteins (pancreatic trypsin and chymotrypsin). Similarly, SIBO can cause maldigestion by breaking down bile salts (deconjugation of conjugated bile salts) in the proximal small intestine by bacteria and thereby rendering them (conjugated bile salts) unavailable for mixed micelle formation for fat digestion. Even carbohydrate and protein malabsorption can happen in SIBO, primarily due to bacterial degradation of carbohydrates and mucosal injury by bacterial overgrowth, leading to brush-border enzyme deficiency. Another prominent feature of SIBO is vitamin B_{12} deficiency, as bacteria utilize vitamin B_{12}.

Malabsorption

Diseases that cause small intestinal mucosal damage such as celiac disease, tropical sprue, and food protein allergies such as CMPA give rise to panmalabsorption of carbohydrate, proteins, and fat due to deficiency of brush-border enzymes and lack of transport system located on the apical surface of enterocytes and in the cytosol of enterocytes. The important brush-border enzymes for carbohydrate digestion are lactase (lactose malabsorption), maltase (maltose: up to nine residue oligosaccharides), and sucrase (sucrose malabsorption). The end products of luminal digestion of proteins are amino acids (30%) and oligopeptides (2–6 amino acids). Brush border enzymes for proteins are oligopeptidases (cleave amino acids from 2 to 6 residue peptides), dipeptidases (on the brush border), and tripeptidases (in the cytosol of enterocytes). Fat (triglyceride) becomes monoglyceride and fatty acid in the luminal phase of digestion. There is no brush border enzyme for fat digestion but inside the enterocytes, fatty acids and monoglyceride reassemble to triglyceride and then bind to apolipoproteins and phospholipid to become chylomicron which is transported via lymphatics to the circulation. Hence, enterocyte damage or intestinal lymphatic obstruction causes fat malabsorption. In malabsorption, the unabsorbed carbohydrate (oligosaccharides, and disaccharides such as lactose and sucrose) and proteins (oligopeptides, dipeptides, and tripeptides) reach the colon, where colonic bacteria ferment carbohydrate and produce short-chain fatty acids (propionic acid, acetoacetic acid, and butyric acid), and gas (hydrogen, methane, and carbon dioxide). Short-chain fatty acids (2–4 carbon length) in the colon produce the osmotic effect and draw water into the lumen and the net result is diarrhea and bloating. Bacterial degradation of proteins (especially sulfur-containing amino acids) produces odor in flatus (hydrogen sulfide, mercaptan, etc.). Similarly, unabsorbed fat and bile salts produce a cathartic effect in the colon and cause diarrhea.

Congenital absence of selective brush-border enzymes such as congenital alactasia and sucrase-isomaltase deficiency give rise to selective malabsorption of lactose and sucrose, respectively.

The postmucosal phase of digestion is basically the transport of fat from mucosa through lymphatics. Lymphatic blockage (congenital: primary intestinal lymphangiectasia or acquired due to lymphoma, tuberculosis, retroperitoneal fibrosis, or surgery) gives rise to dilated lacteals in the intestinal mucosa which rupture due to overdistension leading to fat malabsorption (selective malabsorption).

ETIOLOGY

The etiology of malabsorption depends on the age and geographic location of the patient. In Western countries, celiac disease, cystic fibrosis, immune deficiency, and Crohn's disease are the main causes of MAS in children. In India, etiology is different in North from South and between younger (<2 years) and older children.[5] In North India, celiac disease is the most common cause but in South India, celiac disease is a rare entity. We do not have much information in the literature about the etiology of MAS from South India, it used to be the tropical sprue which is hardly seen at the present time. In a report from Delhi, it has been shown that most children (74%) with MAS were due to celiac disease, and GI infestations with pathogenic parasites (such as *Giardia*) are often associated with some underlying causes of MAS like celiac disease. However, a proportion of children (10%) with MAS were due to *giardiasis* and the other common infestation was *Cryptosporidium* (14%), which was seen, in malnourished young children of <2 years of age (71%).[6] CMPA is an important cause in <3 years of age, but tuberculosis is a rare cause of MAS even in developing countries like India. The recent data suggest that inflammatory bowel disease (IBD) and AIDS are becoming more common in India as well.[1] Short-bowel syndrome and SIBO are less common causes of MAS. The etiology of MAS in India is given in **Table 11.7.1**.

CLINICAL FEATURES

The most common presentation of MAS in children is chronic diarrhea. However, almost one-fifth to one-third of them present without diarrhea with nutritional deficiency signs and symptoms such as short stature, anemia, rickets, and even constipation. The diarrhea of MAS is usually of small bowel type, i.e., large volume stools with features of carbohydrate (explosive diarrhea, abdominal distension, and flatulence), proteins (offensive stools and edema), and fat (steatorrhea) malabsorption. The presence of chronic malnutrition with features of water-soluble vitamin deficiencies (anemia, glossitis, angular stomatitis, etc.) substantiates the clinical suspicion of MAS. In severe cases, features of fat-soluble vitamin deficiency such as night blindness, conjunctival xerosis, phrynoderma (vitamin A), rickets (vitamin D), skin bleeding (vitamin K), and rarely neurological manifestation (posterior column signs) of vitamin E deficiency. In selective malabsorption, like in lymphangiectasia, the predominant manifestations are fat malabsorption and loss of plasma proteins and lymphocytes due to rupture of intestinal lymphatic channels (diarrhea with disproportionate edema, lymphopenia, hypokalemia, and hypocalcemia).

Clinical Features of Celiac Disease

In Western countries, the age of onset of the disease in celiac disease is 6–12 months and the age of diagnosis is around 18 months. The latent period between the introduction of gluten and the onset of symptoms is variable (months to years). In India, it has been reported that the age of onset of symptoms is 2.4–3 years and the age of diagnosis is 6.3–8.3 years. This delay (3–6 years) in diagnosis is mainly due to lack of awareness among parents and pediatricians. The delay in the onset of symptoms may be due to prolonged breastfeeding and delayed weaning. Almost 60–90% of cases of celiac disease in India present with typical features (classical form) of chronic diarrhea (small bowel type with features of malabsorption), failure to thrive, and anemia **(Table 11.7.2)**. However, a proportion of celiac disease cases present with nutritional deficiency features without diarrhea (atypical or nonclassical celiac disease) and may attend various specialties **(Table 11.7.3)**. In the West, almost half of the cases of celiac disease do not present with diarrhea **(Table 11.7.2)**. With the increasing awareness and easy availability of diagnostic tests especially celiac serology, the ratio of classical to nonclassical form of celiac disease is fast

TABLE 11.7.1: Etiology of malabsorption syndrome in children in India.

Etiology	*Yachha, et al. (1993) PGI, Chandigarh*[5]		*Poddar, et al. (2010) SGPGI, Lucknow*[7]	*Behera, et al. (2008) AIIMS, New Delhi*[6]
	n = 62 (<2 years) %	*n = 75 (>2 years) %*	*n = 135 (<5 years) %*	*n = 50 (up to 12 years) %*
Protracted diarrhea	73	0	—	—
CMPA	13	0	29.6	—
Celiac disease	5	43	55.5	74
Parasites	3	15	4 (*Giardia*)	26 (*Giardia, Cryptosporidium, Isospora*)
IBD	—	—	6	—
AIDS			2	—
Tuberculosis	0	9	0.7	—
Miscellaneous*	6	9	1.5	—
Unknown	0	24	0	—

*Short bowel syndrome 2, acrodermatitis enteropathica 2, cystic fibrosis 2, tropical sprue 2, trichobezoar 1, nodular lymphoid hyperplasia 1, isolated lactase deficiency 1.

(AIDS: acquired immune deficiency syndrome; CMPA: cow's milk protein allergy; IBD: inflammatory bowel disease)

TABLE 11.7.2: Clinical presentation of celiac disease: East versus West.

Presentation	*George et al. (n = 185)*[8]	*Mohindra et al. (n = 42)*[9]	*Poddar et al. (n = 300)*[1]
Mean age at diagnosis (years)	3.1 ± 3	8.3 (3–14)	6.7 ± 3
Diarrhea	63%	88%	84%
Abdominal distension	55%	—	48%
Growth failure	50%	90%	91%
Undernutrition	60%	90%	92%
Short stature	5.4%	100%	80%
Anemia	5%	90%	84%

TABLE 11.7.3: Atypical presentations of malabsorption syndrome.

Presentation	*Primary specialty*
Short stature	Endocrinology
Refractory anemia	Hematology
Constipation with abdominal distension	Pediatric surgery
Rickets with fracture and deformity	Orthopedics
Neuropathy and ataxia	Neurology
Infertility, impotence, and amenorrhea	Gynecology

changing. In a study from Lucknow, we have shown that 44% of all celiac disease cases were atypical or nonclassical.

INVESTIGATIONS

The approach to MAS can be divided into three stages:

1. First, clinical suspicion of MAS is based on history and physical examination.
2. Second, confirmation of its presence by simple laboratory tests
3. Lastly, demonstrating its cause by structural tests such as endoscopy, mucosal biopsy, imaging, etc.

Clinical Suspicion of Malabsorption Syndrome

Clinical features of MAS have already been elucidated.

Confirmation of Malabsorption Syndrome

Simple laboratory tests help in finding out the presence or absence of malabsorption. The presence and type of anemia are assessed by complete blood counts (CBCs). Besides anemia, some specific features of MAS such as lymphocytopenia (in lymphangiectasia), thrombocytosis (in celiac disease and IBD), and acanthocytes in peripheral blood film (in abetalipoproteinemia) can be picked up in CBC. Stool pH (<5.5) and the presence of reducing substances confirm carbohydrate malabsorption. Similarly, fat malabsorption is diagnosed by fecal fat estimation (fat globules or fatty acid crystals on microscopy and quantitative fecal fat estimation). Though it is not easily available, fecal alpha-1-antitrypsin estimation is the test for intestinal protein loss. Other tests, that are commonly used in MAS, are the urinary D-xylose excretion test (mucosal malabsorption), lactose tolerance and lactose hydrogen breath test (lactose intolerance), glucose or lactulose hydrogen breath test (for SIBO), and Schilling test (for Vitamin B_{12} malabsorption).

Demonstrating the Cause of Malabsorption Syndrome

The third stage of the approach to MAS is to find out the cause. Tests to document structural changes in the intestine such as endoscopy with small intestinal biopsy, barium meal follow-through, and CT scan abdomen play an important role in finding out the causes of MAS. In addition to structural tests, some other specific tests, such as celiac serology, sweat chloride test, and molecular testing (clinical exome sequencing, whole exome sequencing, or next-generation sequencing) help in finding a specific cause. Upper gastrointestinal (UGI) endoscopy and duodenal biopsy are the mainstay of all investigations for MAS. The mere presence of villous atrophy does not give a diagnosis of MAS. Mucosal biopsy is diagnostic (means always positive) in abetalipoproteinemia (fat globule within enterocytes), Whipple's disease (finding a specific acid-fast organism), and agammaglobulinemia (absence of plasma cells in the lamina propria). There are conditions where biopsy changes are diagnostic but patchy (diagnostic if found) such as lymphangiectasia (dilated lacteals in lamina propria), *giardiasis*, strongyloidiasis, lymphoma, eosinophilic gastroenteritis, and Crohn's disease. However, in most cases of MAS, the mucosal biopsies are abnormal (show villous atrophy) but not diagnostic of a condition such as celiac disease, tropical sprue, CMPA, severe protein energy malnutrition (PEM), prolonged iron, and folate deficiencies. The approach to MAS is given in **Flowchart 11.7.1**. In a suspected case of CMPA, a simple proctoscopic rectal biopsy may help in reaching diagnosis (eosinophilic proctitis: >6 eosinophils per high power field).[7] However, the recent European Society of Pediatric Gastroenterology, Hepatology, and Nutrition (ESPGHAN 2023) guidelines suggested that all children with suspected CMPA should be subjected to diagnostic elimination of cow's milk for 2–4 weeks followed by oral milk challenge before embarking on a long-term (6 months or 12 months of age, whichever is earlier) therapeutic elimination diet.[4] Response to diagnostic elimination diet followed by a positive response to challenge is the cornerstone in the diagnosis of CMPA.

The duodenal biopsy is no longer essential in diagnosing celiac disease. As per ESPGHAN 2020 guidelines, in a suspected case of celiac disease, tissue transglutaminase

Flowchart 11.7.1: Approach to suspected malabsorption syndrome.

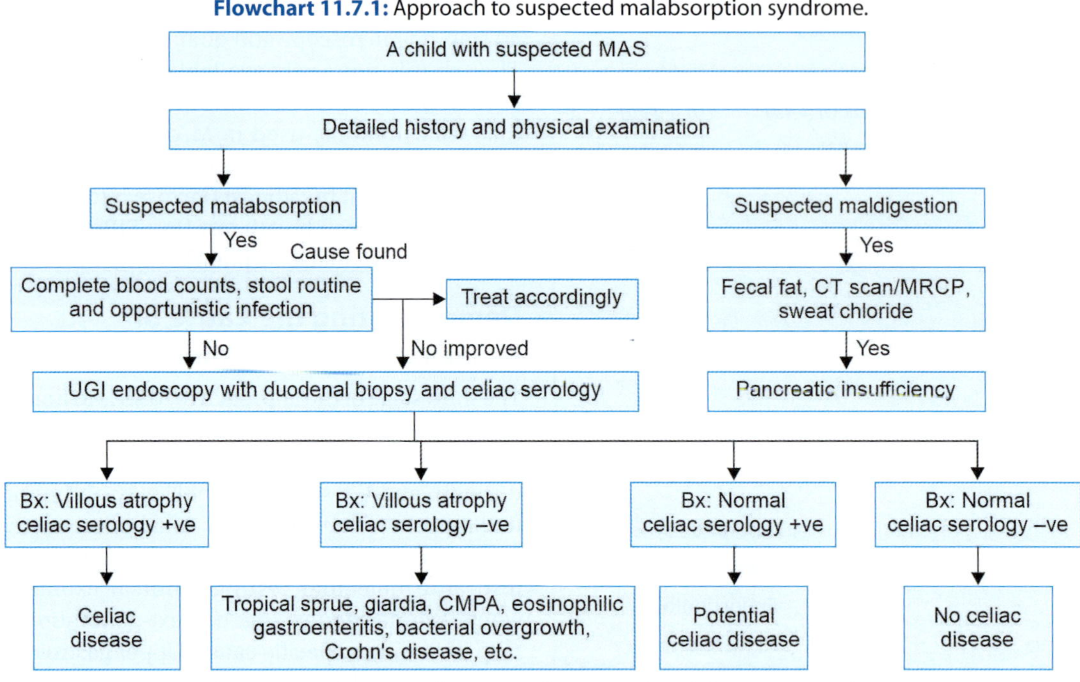

(Bx: biopsy; CMPA: cow's milk protein allergy; MAS: malabsorption syndrome; MRCP: magnetic resonance cholangiopancreatography; UGI: upper gastrointestinal tract)

(IgA-tTG) >10 times the upper limit of normal (ULN) and a positive anti-endomyseal antibody (IgA-EMA) in a separate sample is diagnostic of celiac disease.[10] In this era of sophisticated investigations, simple stool examination (consecutive 3 days) cannot be ignored especially in young malnourished children to document parasitic infestations.

Diagnosis of Celiac Disease

Celiac disease is diagnosed by modified European Society of Pediatric Gastroenterology and Nutrition (ESPGAN) criteria. According to these criteria, a small intestinal biopsy should be suggestive of celiac disease showing villous atrophy and the patient should show an unequivocal clinical response to a gluten-free diet (GFD) in weeks. However, there are many conditions other than celiac disease, which can give rise to villous atrophy, in developing countries like India. If these criteria are applied in our population, celiac disease will be over-diagnosed. To overcome this problem, additional criteria, over and above ESPGAN criteria are needed. The best option to confirm the diagnosis is gluten challenge but it is cumbersome and requires repeated endoscopic biopsies and needs cooperation of child and parents. On the contrary, celiac serology is simple and effective, and if positive at the time of diagnosis and becomes negative on follow-up on "GFD", it confirms the diagnosis.

There are several serological tests for celiac disease and the best antibody test is shown to be the anti-EMA with a sensitivity of >90% and specificity of 97%, but it is a technically demanding test (done by indirect immunofluorescent technique). On the other hand, anti-tTG is almost as good as EMA and it is done by enzyme-linked immunosorbent assay (ELISA) technique. The sensitivity and specificity of tTG are around 95%. In a prospective study of 180 children with celiac disease, it was shown that the tTG has 95% concordance with EMA and its sensitivity and specificity were 94% and 97%, respectively. Hence, in Indian setting tTG is the best antibody to diagnose celiac disease. Nevertheless, in first 2 years of life when IgA antibody titers against tTG and EMA may not be adequate to be detected by these tests, and in IgA deficiency state (which is 10 times more common in celiac disease than that in the general population), IgA plus IgG deamidated gliadin peptide (anti-DGP) antibody is shown to be superior to IgA-tTG and IgA-EMA tests.

Recently, ESPGHAN (2020)[10] has modified its criteria to diagnose celiac disease and as per these new criteria, a duodenal biopsy is not essential in all cases. In a suspected case of celiac disease, if IgA-tTG is 10 times or more than the ULN then IgA-EMA should be ordered in second blood sample. If both serological tests (IgA-tTG ≥10 times ULN and IgA-EMA) are positive then a patient can be labeled as celiac disease without a duodenal biopsy. However, this approach is not suitable in an Indian setting as IgA-EMA test is scarcely available and prohibitively expensive. Hence, we should stick to biopsy-based criteria.

Proposed criteria to diagnose celiac disease in India (all three need to be present):

1. *Positive celiac serology (tTG):* At least 10 times the ULN
2. Endoscopic duodenal biopsy showing villous atrophy

3. An unequivocal clinical response to a GFD in weeks along with the disappearance of celiac serology on follow-up (6–12 months)

MANAGEMENT

Besides managing the underlying cause of MAS, these patients need supplements with iron, folic acid, multivitamins, and calcium. Severely malnourished children should be supplemented with extracalories and proteins. Caution should be maintained to avoid being too aggressive in restarting feeding in severely malnourished MAS patients as they are at risk of developing "refeeding or nutritional recovery syndrome". In such a situation, the dictum is to "start low, go slow". All such patients should be supplemented with thiamine, calcium, phosphate, magnesium, and potassium, and feeding should be started with half of the daily requirements and to be increased gradually over a week.

Parasitic infestations are quite common in MAS patients but many of them are associated with another cause for MAS. Hence, just treatment of isolated parasites (like metronidazole for *Giardia*, nitazoxanide for *Cryptosporidium*) may not cure the condition. All such children should be followed up and if their symptoms persist despite antiparasitic treatment they should be investigated for underlying diseases such as celiac disease or CMPA.

In CMPA, besides stopping cow's milk attention should be paid to foods containing milk proteins such as biscuits, dairy products, butter, and ghee as even a minute quantity of milk proteins can cause persistence or flare of the disease. All such children should be supplemented with calcium as milk is the richest source of calcium. Fortunately, CMPA is a self-limiting condition and most children (>90%) grow out of this condition by 3–5 years of age.

On the contrary, celiac disease is a lifelong condition and the patient (and parents) should be given a clear understanding that gluten cannot be introduced at any stage of life.

KEY MESSAGES

- The etiology of MAS depends on age and geographic location.
- Protracted diarrhea due to CMPA and parasitic infestations are common causes in the first 2 years of life.
- Celiac disease is the most common cause of MAS in >2 years of age in North India.
- Consecutive 3-day stool examination needs to be done in all cases before embarking on sophisticated investigations.
- Endoscopy and duodenal biopsy play important role in the diagnosis of MAS.
- Nondiarrheal manifestations of celiac disease are not uncommon in India and a high index of suspicion is required to diagnose atypical/nonclassical celiac disease.
- Parasitic infestations are common in patients with MAS and many a time they are not the primary cause of malabsorption.
- Adequate supplements with minerals, and vitamins, and gradual introduction of feed are the key to prevent nutritional recovery syndrome in severely malnourished MAS patients.

CONCLUSION

The etiology of MAS has changed over the years from infection/infestations to celiac disease, short bowel syndrome and small intestinal bacterial overgrowth (SIBO). MAS is divided into two categories; maldigestion (impaired breakdown of nutrients) and malabsorption (defective mucosal uptake/transport). Though chronic diarrhea is the most common presentation, a quarter of them may present without diarrhea with short-stature, anemia, rickets, etc. The step-wise approach to MAS is—clinically suspect, laboratory confirmation of its presence and then etiological workup such as endoscopic mucosal biopsy, serology, imaging, etc. Besides managing the underlying cause, they need macro- and micronutrient supplementation.

REFERENCES

1. Poddar U, Thapa BR, Singh K. Clinical features of celiac disease in Indian children: Are they different from the West? J Pediatr Gastroenterol Nutr. 2006;43(3):313-7.
2. Caporilli C, Gianni G, Grassi F, Esposito S. An overview of short-bowel syndrome in pediatric patients: focus on clinical management and prevention of complications. Nutrients. 2023;15(10):2341.
3. Cho YK, Lee J, Paik CN. Prevalence, risk factors, and treatment of small intestinal bacterial overgrowth in children. Clin Exp Pediatrics. 2023;66(9):377-83.
4. Vandenplas Y, Broekaert I, Domellof M, Indrio F, Lapillonne A, Piennar C, et al. An ESPGHAN position paper on diagnosis, management and prevention of cow's milk allergy. J Pediatr Gastroenterol Nutr; 2023.
5. Yachha SK, Misra S, Malik AK, Nagi B, Mehta S. Spectrum of malabsorption syndrome in North Indian children. Indian J Gastroenterol. 1993;12(4):120-5.
6. Behera B, Mirdha BR, Makharia GK, Bhatnagar S, Dattagupta S, Samantaray JC. Parasites in patients with malabsorption syndrome: A clinical study in children and adults. Dig Dis Sci. 2008;53(3):672-9.
7. Poddar U, Yachha SK, Krishnani N, Srivastava A. Cow's milk protein allergy (CMPA): An entity for recognition in developing countries. J Gastroenterol Hepatol. 2010;25(1):178-82.
8. George EK, Mearin ML, Franken HC, Houwen RH, Hirasing RA, Vandenbroucke JP. Twenty years of childhood celiac disease in the Netherlands: a rapidly increasing incidence? Gut. 1997;40(1):61-6.
9. Mohindra S, Yachha SK, Srivastava A, Krishnani N, Aggarwal R, Ghoshal UC, et al. Celiac disease in Indian children: Assessment of clinical, nutritional, and pathologic characteristics. J Health Popul Nutr. 2001;19(3):204-8.
10. Husby S, Koletzko S, Korponay-Szabó IR, Kurppa K, Mearin ML, Ribes-Koninckx C, et al. European Society of Pediatric Gastroenterology, Hepatology and Nutrition guidelines for the diagnosis of celiac disease 2020. J Pediatr Gastroenterol Nutr. 2020;70(1):141-57.

11.8 Food Allergic Enteropathy

R Bhanu Vikraman Pillai

INTRODUCTION

Adverse reactions to food are common in children as well as adults. The adverse reactions include food allergies [immunoglobulin E (IgE)-mediated as well as non-IgE-mediated or mixed], intolerance to certain components causing symptoms (such as abdominal pain and diarrhea from lactose intolerance), or the adverse immune-mediated disorders in genetically susceptible individuals to certain food (e.g., celiac disease) or it can be the adverse reaction to certain food components (e.g., migraine precipitated by certain foods) or metabolic abnormality such as galactosemia. Detailed discussion regarding celiac disease and gluten sensitivity is dealt with in Chapter 11.7. This chapter will discuss the food allergic enteropathy only. As indicated in the previous text, the food allergic enteropathy includes the IgE-mediated food allergy, non-IgE-mediated as well as mixed reaction.

Allergy could happen to any food, but majority of significant allergic manifestations occur to a relatively smaller list of foods such as milk, soy, wheat, egg, peanuts and tree nuts, shellfish, and fish. There is difference in the prevalence depending on the geographical locations and is more common in the developed countries. The different components of the immune system, such as the epithelial barrier, innate immune cells, T cells, B cells, and effector cells (mast cells, eosinophils, and basophils), determine whether a person can either promote tolerance to food antigens or sensitization to them, which will then lead to allergic manifestations.[1] The types of food allergy are:

- IgE-mediated allergy;
- Non-IgE-mediated allergy;
- Mixed; and
- Oral allergy syndrome or food pollen syndrome.

IMMUNOGLOBULIN E-MEDIATED FOOD ALLERGY

This is caused by food-specific IgE and can be detected by tests and cause allergic reactions that are immediate and are reproducible. These food-specific IgE binds to basophils, mast cells, dendritic cells, and Langerhans cells in the gut, skin, or through the respiratory system. When exposed to the offending food, the specific food antigen is recognized by two or more specific IgE bound to the high affinity IgE receptor, FcεRI, resulting in activation of mast cells to release histamine and other mediators. These released chemical mediators will cause vasodilatation, hives, angioedema, hypotension, smooth muscle constriction, consequent bronchospasm, diarrhea, and vomiting.

Anaphylaxis to certain foods is IgE-mediated and occur in a previously sensitized person with food-specific IgE on mast cells and basophils; the food allergen when ingested and absorbed into the local tissue, cross-links with IgE resulting in immediate release of preformed mediators. This immune response is rapid; the onset of symptoms typically occurs within 5–60 minutes after exposure to the food. An anaphylactic reaction affects multiple organ systems and may rapidly develop severe symptoms (e.g., hypotension or respiratory collapse) and even death. They have varying symptoms, such as hives or pruritus, cough, wheezing, stridor, vomiting, diarrhea, and hypotension.[1]

NONIMMUNOGLOBULIN-MEDIATED FOOD ALLERGY

Allergic manifestations still can occur when there is no demonstrable food specific IgE in the serum or the skin. T-cell mechanism may be involved in this type. Several conditions such as eosinophilic esophagitis (EoE), food protein-induced enterocolitis (FPIES), and food protein-induced allergic proctocolitis (FPIAP) are considered to be through non-IgE-mediated mechanism.

MIXED IMMUNOGLOBULIN AND NONIMMUNOGLOBULIN-MEDIATED FOOD ALLERGY

Mixed and non-IgE-mediated food allergies, such as EoE, eosinophilic gastroenteritis (EGE), and atopic dermatitis (AD), have a more prolonged onset. This type of allergy manifests primarily in the gastrointestinal (GI) tract and skin. Atopic dermatitis is a common presentation. Milk, soy, egg, wheat, and peanut are the most common food antigens involved, and elimination of these antigens helps the resolution of the symptoms.

ORAL ALLERGY SYNDROME OR FOOD POLLEN SYNDROME

When the antigens in certain pollen share the epitopes in certain fruits and vegetables, the IgE produced against the pollen can cause allergic symptoms when the fruits and vegetables that share the epitopes in the pollen are eaten; symptoms then develop in addition to allergic rhinoconjunctivitis such as itching, redness, and edema of the lips, numbness in lips and tongue, itching, and swelling in the throat.

Food additives and coloring agents are well known to produce allergic or adverse reaction, for e.g., monosodium glutamate (MSG) or sulfites.

CLINICAL PRESENTATION

Immunoglobulin-mediated Food Allergy

The IgE-mediated food allergy present with urticaria, angioedema, allergic rhinitis, oral allergy syndrome, acute asthmatic attack, or in severe cases with anaphylaxis. Specific serum IgE is elevated in these children and skin prick test is positive to the specific food.

Nonimmunoglobulin-mediated Food Allergy

Non-IgE-mediated food allergy manifests with symptoms involving GI tract, skin, or respiratory tract. Atopic eczema/dermatitis, respiratory symptoms including cough, wheezing, and rhinitis are common in these children. GI presentation of non-IgE mediated food allergy may present with well described clinical picture such as FPIAP, FPIES, food protein-induced enteropathy (FPE), and eosinophilic gastrointestinal disorders (EGID). EGID include EoE, when involving only the esophagus, allergic eosinophilic gastroenteritis (EGE) when there is involvement of more than one area of the GI tract and eosinophilic colitis (EC) when affecting only the colon.[2] The symptoms include frequent vomiting/regurgitation, feeding refusal, dysphagia, failure to thrive, irritability, diarrhea, and blood in stools. These infants also could present with acute onset of severe vomiting, diarrhea, and shock-like appearance following the intake of the offending food item like in FPIES. Resolution of the symptoms occur after stopping the offending food protein, most often the cow's milk protein.

Food Protein-induced Allergic Proctocolitis Syndrome

The FPIAP usually present in the first few months, usually <2 months of life with diarrhea, rectal bleeding, and excessive mucus production. Similar symptoms can also occur in adolescence. Usually these infants otherwise look well, but can have irritability and also atopic eczema and reactive airways disease. Avoiding cow's milk protein in the diet either directly or in the mother if breastfed, resolves the problem. Improvement is seen within 3–5 days and visible blood disappears in 2–3 weeks. Stool occult blood may be positive for several weeks. If abstaining the cow's milk products does not cause improvement, one may have to avoid other allergens too including soy, wheat, or egg. Mother must take 1 g calcium tablets supplementation if avoiding the milk products.

Food Protein-induced Enterocolitis Syndrome

The FPIES presents usually acutely with a severe reaction with profuse vomiting and diarrhea and could present in a shock-like presentation with onset within 1–6 hours after ingestion of the offending food. Usual offending foods include milk, soy, rice, and oats. There could be multiple episodes before the actual offending agent is identified. Since non-IgE-mediated, skin prick testing is negative. Oral food challenge may be necessary for confirmation.

Food Protein-induced Enteropathy

The FPE presents with chronic diarrhea, failure to thrive (FTT) in infancy, with malabsorption often before 9 months of age, occurring after exposure to cow's milk. In addition, these infants usually have abdominal distension and poor appetite. They also can have iron deficiency anemia, with presence of occult blood in stools. Elimination of the offending agent, often milk, soy or egg, will heal the villous atrophy. Confirmation is by challenge and reappearance of the symptoms.

Eosinophilic Gastrointestinal Disorders

The EGID can be classified to EoE (when only the esophagus is involved), EC (when only the colon is involved), and EGE (when more than one area is involved—esophagus/stomach/small bowel/colon). Peripheral eosinophilia may be present.

Eosinophilic Esophagitis

Eosinophilic esophagitis is the most extensively studied. This occurs due to abnormal immunological response to specific antigens, most often food antigen and can be multiple food antigens. Infants and children with EoE present with frequent regurgitation and vomiting (often confused as gastroesophageal reflux disease or GERD), FTT, dysphagia, feeding refusal, irritability. EoE should be strongly suspected if the symptoms of GERD fail to respond to proton pump inhibitors (PPIs). Older children may come with dysphagia and food impaction as well as chest pain in addition to the above. Boys are more frequently affected with a ratio of 3:1. Often there is association with atopic eczema or allergic rhinitis. More than 50% children may have a family history of allergy.

Endoscopy with biopsy is necessary for diagnosis. Endoscopy may show linear furrowing, esophageal ring-like appearance, edema, whitish exudates as well as narrow caliber esophagus, but at times it could even appear normal. Multiple biopsies are necessary and show >15 eosinophils/high power field (HPF). Other conditions that cause EoE should be ruled out, including GERD and may require 24-hour esophageal pH metry.

Eosinophilic Gastroenteritis

Eosinophilic gastroenteritis (EGE) is much less common than EoE. Symptoms depend on the predominant site of involvement. These include nausea, vomiting, abdominal pain, diarrhea, weight loss, early satiety, anemia, GI bleeding, ascites, and hypoalbuminemia. Symptoms also depend on the extent of involvement, affecting different layers of the bowel wall. Gastric antrum is affected most commonly up to even 95% children. More than 50% children may have peripheral eosinophilia. Eczema and other allergic conditions may coexist. Clinically there can be three forms—mucosal, muscular, or serosal form depending on the depth of involvement and can affect anywhere from mouth to anus, just like Crohn's disease.[3]

Eosinophilic Colitis/Proctocolitis

Eosinophilic proctocolitis is one of the presentations of cow's milk protein allergy and presents with rectal bleeding, typically in young infant <2 months of age. The involvement is only in the rectum and colon, unlike the EGE. These infants present with diarrhea, rectal bleeding, and presence of mucus in the stools. The infants with EC otherwise look well and thriving well. Atopic symptoms can coexist. This usually happens to the baby who is exposed to milk-based formula. Cow's milk protein followed by soy protein is usually the offending agent and elimination of the offending agent results in resolution of the symptoms. The EC can also happen in the exclusively breastfed infant, typically due to passage of the offending antigen through the breast milk rather than to the breast milk protein itself. EC is a clinical diagnosis in the well appearing infant with diarrhea and blood in stools. However, if the infant looks toxic, one must rule out other clinical possibilities including necrotizing enterocolitis and infections.

Diagnosis

Flexible sigmoidoscopy and biopsy can be done to confirm EC if in doubt. Endoscopy could show erythema, friability, ulcerations, but at times may show lymphonodular hyperplasia or even normal. These findings may be patchy. The biopsy typically shows eosinophilic inflammation, focal aggregates, or eosinophilic micro abscess in the lamina propria.[4]

Treatment

Treatment is to avoid the offending protein and response can be prompt. Since there is significant cross reactivity with cow's milk protein and soy protein (up to 35–50%), it is not recommended to switch to soy formula. It will be appropriate to change to an extensively hydrolyzed formula resolution of the symptoms is expected in 95% of infants. In up to 3–5% of infants with EC, there could be continued symptoms and may require an elemental formula. In a breastfed infant, the mother should stop all the dairy products, and soy products as well as beef and continue to breastfeed the infant. If the mother is placed on the elimination diet, she should be advised to take 1 g of calcium tablets daily to safeguard her health. If the symptoms persist, one should consider other dietary antigens such as wheat or egg causing the symptoms in the infant. Resolution of rectal bleeding can occur within 3–5 days of eliminating the offending protein, but the stool occult blood may be positive for several weeks. Generally, EC has an excellent outcome with >70% outgrowing the condition by 1 year of age and up to 98% by 3 years of age.

INVESTIGATIONS IN FOOD ALLERGY

Several investigations can aid in the diagnosis in addition to appropriate history taking and physical examination.

Skin Prick Test

This is the most commonly used test and depends on the presence of food specific IgE and hence useful only for the IgE-mediated allergy. The standardized antigen solution is used for testing, a drop of which is applied on the forearm or the back and scratch is made. The excess solution is wiped off and the reaction or the wheal is measured. It must be compared with a positive control (histamine) and negative control (normal saline). If there is a reaction with negative control (dermographism) or negative reaction with the positive control (use of antihistamine), the test is discarded. Emergency equipment and drugs should be readily accessible in case of any systemic adverse reactions to the allergen solution. Skin prick test serve as a good guide for the family and the patients especially which foods to avoid and when to do the oral food challenge.[1]

Immunoglobulin–Radioallergosorbent Test

This measures the IgE against the food antigens and again is useful only for the allergies caused by IgE mediated mechanism, but the advantage is it can be easily performed in such cases, and can serve as a guide in the management of such cases and the timing of the oral food challenge.

Component-resolved Diagnostics

Component-resolved diagnostics (CRD) in food allergies is an approach utilized to characterize the molecular components of each allergen involved in a specific IgE (sIgE)-mediated response. This test is also IgE-dependent. CRD can improve diagnostic accuracy and assist the physician in many aspects of the allergy workup. CRD can be useful to stratify the clinical risk associated with a specific sensitization pattern, in addition to the oral food challenge (OFC).

Atopy Patch Testing

Atopy patch testing (APT) is another way of allergy testing and very useful in identifying delayed hypersensitivity reaction. Since the APT can identify T cell-mediated allergic response, it has found a value in non-IgE-mediated allergy.

Basophil Activation Test

The role of basophils is similar to mast cells in allergy. The degranulation of the basophils that occurs in the allergic response identifies allergy and not just sensitization. Lack of widespread availability limits its use at the present time.

Endoscopy

Upper endoscopy and colonoscopy have a great role in the workup of these children suspected to have EGID. Biopsy is necessary and available during the endoscopy to confirm the EGID, such as EoE, EGE as well as EC. Not only that, it helps to rule out or confirm other conditions that mimic these conditions including gastroesophageal reflux disease, inflammatory bowel diseases, and alike.

Oral Food Challenge

Double-blind placebo-controlled OFC is the standard gold test for diagnosing food allergies. It needs the oral administration of incremental doses of the suspected allergen, e.g., cow's milk. A physician, a nurse, resuscitation equipment, and rescue medications should be available. OFC is commonly performed in-office or clinic settings, especially for low-risk challenges. High-risk challenges, such as previous anaphylaxis and FPIES, should always be conducted in a hospital with full resuscitation facilities to treat anaphylaxis after informed consent. Before reintroduction of food that had caused allergic manifestations in the past, OFC can be extremely useful and gives the parents confidence in giving the suspected food after a negative OFC. In a child who had severe allergic reactions previously, the OFC is done after a negative skin prick test (SPT) and low levels of food specific serum IgE. OFC is done when the child is not having any concurrent illness. Any antihistamines, if the child had been taking should be stopped 48 hours before the OFC. The test is considered negative if no symptoms are observed following exposure to the problematic food, in an amount equivalent to a standard serving. If the child develops any untoward symptoms, such as hives, stridor, and breathing difficulty, the OFC should be aborted.

TREATMENT

Treatment remains primarily based on counseling the patients and their families to avoid offending food item. Parents and the family should be taught and counseled to read all the food labels to avoid the specific allergen, even if it is in small amounts.[4] During travel, they should keep a list of the allergic food items. In case of severe allergy, antihistamines and adrenaline autoinjector device should be handy all the time.

Oral Immunotherapy

Oral immunotherapy has been tried with partial success. This is based on the concept that the continuous introduction of small amounts of allergenic food would induce tolerance over weeks or months. This may take months or years.

Probiotics

Studies have shown that intestinal microbiota may have a role in supporting the early establishment of immune tolerance, and reducing the risk of developing food allergies in early life.

Most of the studies that looked at function of probiotics in food allergy have focused on their role in managing cow's milk protein allergy. *Lactobacillus rhamnosus* GG can help induce tolerance in infants with suspected cow's milk protein allergy.

Biologicals

Omalizumab is one of the biologicals investigated and shown encouraging results in desensitization. Dupilumab has shown benefit in treating EoE and atopic eczema.

Specific Situations

The EoE is treated with elimination diet, one food, two foods, four foods, and six food elimination diet. Also at times, especially in infants, it is treated with elemental formula feeding.

Proton pump inhibitor (PPI) including lansoprazole, omeprazole, esomeprazole, rabeprazole, and pantoprazole is also given to these children and has showed benefit in up to 50% of children with EoE, considered to be PPI-responsive esophageal eosinophilia (PPI-REE). Children with EoE are initially started on PPI and if there is response, continue close monitoring.

If there is inadequate response, one could try the elimination diet or *swallowed topical steroids* such as budesonide or fluticasone. If swallowed topical steroids are used, it is continued for 8 weeks in the twice a day dose and then decreased to once a day. Elimination diet or the swallowed topical steroids can be used depending on the patient's choice. Either pathway will require repeat endoscopy to assess the disease and then modify the treatment.

One food (milk) two foods (milk and soy) four foods (milk, egg, soy, and wheat) and six foods (milk, soy, egg, wheat, nuts/tree nuts, and fish/shellfish) elimination diets were studied and found to be useful. Dupilumab is recently approved for severe atopic eczema and EoE.

Endoscopy and dilatation may be required for stricture associated with EoE. Systemic steroids may be required in severe cases of EoE for short periods.

Eosinophilic gastroenteritis can be difficult to treat. In addition to elimination diet, if possible, systemic steroids are often required to control the disease and should be attempted to wean and stop. Azathioprine had been tried when steroids are difficult to wean and stop.

Most children with cow's milk and egg allergies grow out of their allergies, but tree nuts, peanut, fish, and shellfish allergies may persist. Peanut allergy can be stubborn and deadly.

REFERENCES

1. Elghoudi A, Narchi H. Food allergy in children-the current status and the way forward. World J Clin Pediatr. 2022;11(3):253-69.
2. Calvani M, Anania C, Cuomo B, D'Auria E, Decimo F, Indirli GC, et al. Non-IgE- or Mixed IgE/Non-IgE-mediated gastrointestinal food allergies in the first years of life: Old and new tools for diagnosis. Nutrients. 2021;13(1):226.
3. Chehade M, Furuta G, Klion A, Abonia JP, Aceves S, Bose P, et al. Enhancing diversity, equity, inclusion, and accessibility in eosinophilic gastrointestinal disease research: the consortium for eosinophilic gastrointestinal disease researchers' journey. Ther Adv Rare Dis. 2023;4:26330040231180895.
4. Markowitz JE, Venkatesh RD, Moye L, Liacouras CA. Allergic and eosinophilic gastrointestinal disease. In: Wyllie R, Hyams JS, Kay M (Eds). Pediatric Gastrointestinal and Liver Disease, 6th edition. Philadelphia, PA, USA: The Ohio State University; 2021. pp. 388-97.

11.9 Parasitic Bowel Disease

BD Gupta

INTRODUCTION

A parasite is an organism that grows, feeds, and is sheltered by or within a different organism while contributing nothing to survival of its host. The only possible exception is some protective role on inflammatory bowel disease (IBD) in human host by intestinal parasites. Unlike protozoa, most helminths do not multiply within the human body, except *Strongyloides stercoralis.*

EPIDEMIOLOGY

Intestinal parasitic infestation is more common in developing countries, though worldwide the vulnerable groups are children of both urban poor and rural population. Parasitic infestation was detected in asymptomatic as well as symptomatic children in a hospital-based study. In a study done in Ethiopia, the overall prevalence of intestinal parasitic infection was found to be 52.9%. *Entamoeba histolytica* (21.5%) was the leading cause of intestinal parasitosis followed by hookworm species (13.3%).[1]

Indian studies have recently reported higher incidence of protozoan parasitic infestation to be commoner than helminthic infestation. Among protozoans most commonly detected are *Giardia lamblia* (10–20%) and *E. histolytica* (3–6%); most commonly reported helminths are ascaris (1–52%) followed by hookworms (1.5–42%). Parasitic infections are commoner in schoolgoing children in rural areas than urban kids.[2,3]

Most often the larva or ova of intestinal parasites are passed intermittently in stools, and hence repeated examination of fresh stool is recommended for better yield rate, especially in immune-deficient children when we screen them for parasites causing diarrhea such as *G. lamblia, Cryptosporidium, S. stercoralis,* and so on.

CLASSIFICATION

Parasitic bowel diseases are a group of infectious diseases due to protozoa and helminths and are a major cause of morbidity in infants and children in many parts of the world. Parasitic bowel diseases may be classified according to their etiological agents as follows:

- *Protozoan diseases:* Due to *E. histolytica, G. lamblia, Balantidium coli, Cryptosporidium parvum, Blastocystis hominis, Isospora belli, Cyclospora cayetanensis,* and microsporidia
- *Helminthic diseases:*
    - *Due to Nematodes: Ascaris lumbricoides, Enterobius vermicularis,* hookworms, i.e., *Ancylostoma duodenale* and *Necator americanus, Trichinella spiralis,* and *Trichuris trichiura*
    - *Trematodes: Fasciolopsis buski. Nanophyetus salmincola,* and *Heterophyes heterophyes*
    - *Cestodes: Taenia solium, Taenia saginata, Diphyllobothrium latum, Hymenolepis nana,* and *Echinococcus granulosus*

ETIOPATHOGENESIS

Parasitic bowel diseases are endemic in areas of world with poor levels of sanitation and low socioeconomic standards. Two distinct modes of transmission are known, namely feco-oral route and cutaneous route.

1. Protozoa such as *E. histolytica, G. lamblia,* and *B. coli* infect humans by ingestion of cysts, while nematodes such as *A. lumbricoides, T. trichiura,* and *E. vermicularis,* and cestodes such as *T. saginata, T. solium,* and *D. latum* spread by ingestion of contaminated food and water with eggs of respective parasites.
2. Hookworms such as *A. duodenale* and *N. americanus* enter the human body through skin penetration by their larvae. These larvae undergo extraintestinal migration through the venous circulation and lungs before they are swallowed to reach intestines.

Various parasites localize themselves at various sites in small as well as large intestine as per their suitable environment, e.g., *E. histolytica* dwell in colon; *G. lamblia* colonize in the lumen of duodenum and proximal jejunum; *B. coli* infests the large intestine; *A. lumbricoides* in small intestine; *T. trichiura* in cecum and ascending colon, and *E. vermicularis* typically inhabits cecum, appendix, and adjacent areas of ileum and ascending colon.

Various parasites cause symptoms due to invasion (*E. histolytica*), obstruction (*A. lumbricoides*), reduced absorptive surface (*G. lamblia*), and blood loss (hookworms).

It has been observed that parasitic bowel diseases have a role in prevention of IBD such as Crohn's disease, which are most prevalent in highly industrialized countries with temperate climate and occur rarely in tropical third world countries with poor environmental sanitation.[4] Many helminths live within and migrate through human gut and interact with the mucosal immune system. The host mounts a mucosal response including Th2 cytokine production limiting helminthic colonization, as helminths and their eggs are probably most potent stimulus of mucosal Th2 response. This may modulate immune reaction to parasitic, bacterial, and viral infections. Perhaps, failure to acquire these parasites and experience mucosal Th2 conditioning predisposes to IBDs, i.e., Crohn's disease and ulcerative colitis, and celiac disease, which is an overtly active Th1 inflammation. In some countries, the patients intentionally infect themselves with worms such as *N. americanus,* and this is considered as a possible treatment for IBD and celiac disease. On the other hand, celiac disease may be aggravated by coexistent *G. lamblia* infestation and the disease may improve after treatment of giardiasis.

CLINICAL FEATURES

Parasitic bowel disease is associated with wide variety of clinical manifestations ranging from asymptomatic carrier stage to various intestinal and extraintestinal manifestations. The clinical features depend largely on the parasite, site of involvement, mechanical factors, and interference with host's nutrition.

General Symptoms

Most of the parasites present with pain abdomen and diarrhea, which can be acute, chronic, or recurrent; bloody or nonbloody; with or without tenesmus, abdominal cramps, bloating, and flatulence. Other symptoms include nausea, vomiting, anorexia, weight loss, fever, abdominal distension, malaise, myalgia, and headache. Various other clinical features caused by different parasites are summarized in **Table 11.9.1**.

LABORATORY DIAGNOSIS

Stool Microscopy

Parasitic bowel diseases can be diagnosed by examination of stool samples under direct microscopy. Repeated fresh samples (three times) may be required to reach the diagnosis of clinically suspected organisms. Stool examination along with endoscopically obtained smears and tissue biopsy helps a lot in the diagnosis of specific parasitic infestation. Ideally fresh stools should be examined within 30 minutes of passage for evidence of trophozoites/cysts in case of *E. histolytica* or *G. lamblia*. Stool samples preserved in polyvinyl alcohol helps in the diagnosis of these organisms. Stool examination and demonstration of oocysts help in the diagnosis of spore-forming intestinal protozoa such as *Cryptosporidium, Isospora,* and *Cyclospora.*

Demonstration of eggs of helminths in stool is the mainstay of diagnosis of most of parasites. For ascariasis, Kato's thick

TABLE 11.9.1: Clinical manifestations.

Clinical manifestation	***Parasitic bowel disease(s)***
Nutritional deficiency (Vitamin A deficiency)	Ascariasis, giardiasis, and infection by intestinal flukes
Anemia Iron deficiency	Hookworm disease
B_{12} or folic acid deficiency	Diphyllobothriasis and trichuriasis
Gastrointestinal involvement	
Malabsorption syndrome	Giardiasis, ascariasis, hookworm disease, infestation by intestinal flukes
Weight loss	Giardiasis, hookworm disease, diphyllobothriasis, and spore-forming protozoal infestations such as cryptosporidiosis, isosporiasis, and cyclosporiasis
Intestinal obstruction	Ascariasis and teniasis
Rectal prolapse	Giardiasis and trichuriasis
Perianal itching	Enterobiasis
Extraintestinal involvement	
Liver	Amebiasis and intestinal flukes infestation
Muscles	Trichinosis, flukes, spore-forming protozoa, e.g., microsporidia
Skin	Cutaneous larva migrans—hookworm and strongyloidiasis
Brain	Amebiasis, trichinosis, microsporidiosis, teniasis—neurocysticercosis
Lungs	Amebiasis, ascariasis, hookworm disease, and strongyloidiasis
Immunodeficiency states	*Associated parasites: Cryptosporidium parvum, Isospora belli, Cyclospora cayetanensis*, microsporidium (AIDS), giardiasis, and amebiasis

smear examination of stool is an easy and sensitive method. Fertilized eggs signify infection with both male and female worms, while unfertilized eggs show infection with female worm only. Enterobiasis can be diagnosed by examining cellophane tape imprint from perianal area.[3]

Hematology

The stool examination may be supported by peripheral blood film examination (for evidence of eosinophilia) and various serological tests (specifically designed for the organism under consideration). Serological tests such as indirect hemagglutination are available for *E. histolytica*. *Enterotest* on duodenal fluid for giardiasis is another alternative. Blood enzyme immunoassay (EIA) or direct fluorescent antibody test for *Giardia* antigen are now the tests of choice for giardiasis in most situations. For trichinosis, serologic tests such as bentonite flocculation test, muscle biopsy, and levels of muscle enzymes such as creatine kinase and lactic dehydrogenase (LDH) help in the diagnosis.

Other tests for detection of these parasites are indirect immunofluorescence and polymerase chain reaction (PCR). Species-specific PCR is helpful for detection of a single organism, while multiplex PCR testing for mixed parasitic infection with multiple pathogens may become a viable option for testing in future.[3]

Ultrasonography

Ultrasonography (USG) of abdomen may be helpful in the diagnosis of intestinal obstruction due to ascariasis.

MANAGEMENT

Treatment of various parasitic infestations is summarized in **Table 11.9.2**.[5,6]

PREVENTION AND CONTROL

Parasitic bowel diseases essentially are much more prevalent in areas of poor sanitation and environmental conditions. Hence, these diseases can be prevented by following certain

TABLE 11.9.2: Common parasitic infections and their treatment.

Etiological agent	***Major clinical features***	***Treatment***	***Alternative drug(s)***
Entamoeba histolytica	• Diarrhea • Dysentery • Liver abscess	• *Metronidazole* 35–50 mg/kg/day PO in three doses for 10 days • *Diloxanide furoate* 20 mg/kg/day PO in three doses for 10 days *Either is followed by:* • *Iodoquinol* 30–40 mg/kg/day PO in three doses for 20 days • *Paromomycin* 25–35 mg/kg/day PO in three doses for 7 days	• *Tinidazole* 50 mg/kg/day PO (maximum 2 g) OD for 3 days • *Ornidazole* 30–50 mg/kg/day PO in two doses for 5 days • *Nitazoxanide* 7.5 mg/kg twice daily for 3 days

Contd...

Contd...

Etiological agent	*Major clinical features*	*Treatment*	*Alternative drug(s)*
Giardia lamblia	• Diarrhea • Malabsorption	• *Metronidazole* 5–10 mg/kg tid PO for 5 days • *Nitazoxanide* 7.5 mg/kg twice daily for 3 days	• *Quinacrine* 2 mg/kg tid PO for 5 days • *Albendazole* 400 mg OD for 5 days • *Tinidazole* 50 mg/kg (maximum 2 g) once • *Furazolidone* 6 mg/kg/day q 6 hours for 10 days • *Paromomycin* 25–30 mg/kg/day PO in three doses for 7 days
Balantidium coli	• Diarrhea • Dysentery • Painful abdomen	*Metronidazole* 45 mg/kg/day q 8 hours PO for 5 days	• *Tetracycline* 40 mg/kg (maximum 2 g) q 6 hours for 10 days (>8 years) • *Iodoquinol* 40 mg/kg/day q 8 hours PO (20 days)
Cryptosporidium	Severe diarrhea with malabsorption in AIDS patients	*Nitazoxanide* 100 mg bid PO for 3 days (1–3 years); 200 mg bid for three days (4–11 years)	• *Paromomycin* 25–35 mg/kg/day in three doses for 7 days • *Azithromycin* 10–15 mg/kg/day PO for 4 weeks followed by *Paromomycin* 25–35 mg/kg/day in two doses PO for 8 weeks
Isospora belli	Severe diarrhea with malabsorption in AIDS patients	*Trimethoprim* 5 mg/kg/dose + *Sulfamethoxazole* 25 mg/kg/dose 8 hourly PO for 10 days; then bid for 3 weeks	*Ciprofloxacin* or *Pyrimethamine* ± *Folinic acid* in sulfa-intolerant patients
Cyclospora	Severe diarrhea with malabsorption in AIDS patients	*Trimethoprim* 5 mg/kg/dose + *Sulfamethoxazole* 25 mg/kg/dose bid PO for 7 days	*Ciprofloxacin* (adults)
Microsporidium	Severe diarrhea with malabsorption in AIDS patients	*Albendazole* 400 mg bid for 3 weeks	*Nitazoxanide* 7.5 mg/kg bid for 3 days *Atovaquone*
Ascaris lumbricoides	• Abdominal pain • Cough • Nausea	• *Albendazole* 400 mg PO once • *Mebendazole* 100 mg bid PO for 3 days or 500 mg once • *Pyrantel pamoate* 11 mg/kg once	• *Piperazine citrate* 75 mg/kg per day for 2 days, 65 mg/kg/dose 12 hourly for six doses • *Ivermectin* 200 µg/kg/day od PO for 1–2 days
Strongyloides stercoralis	• Loeffler-like syndrome • Abdominal pain • Diarrhea • Malabsorption	*Ivermectin* 200 µg/kg/day once PO for 1–2 days	• *Thiabendazole* 50 mg/kg bid PO for 2 days • *Albendazole* 400 mg bid for 7 days
Enterobius vermicularis	• Pruritus ani • Sleeplessness	• *Pyrantel pamoate* 11 mg/kg once (maximum 1 g) • *Mebendazole* 100 mg bid PO for 3 days • *Albendazole* 400 mg once (Therapy to be repeated after 2 weeks)	*Ivermectin* 200 µg/kg/day PO for 1–2 days
Trichuris trichiura	• Chronic dysentery • Rectal prolapse • Anemia	*Mebendazole* 100 mg bid PO for 3 days or 500 mg once	• *Albendazole* 400 mg once for 3 days • *Ivermectin* 200 µg per kg daily for 3 days
Hookworm infection (*Ancylostoma duodenale* and *Necator americanus*)	• Chronic dysentery • Rectal prolapse • Anemia	• *Albendazole* 400 mg/day PO once • *Mebendazole* 100 mg bid for 3 days	*Pyrantel pamoate* 11 mg/kg/day (maximum 1 g) once for 3 days
Hymenolepis nana	• Abdominal pain • Loss of appetite • Diarrhea • Anemia • Hypoalbuminemia	• *Praziquantel* 25 mg/kg PO once (if available) • *Nitazoxanide* 7.5 mg/kg bid PO for 3 days	*Albendazole* 400 mg/day for 3 days *Niclosamide* 11–34 kg–1 g PO on day 1 then 500 mg PO for 6 days >34 kg–1.5 g PO on day 1 and then 1 g/day PO for 6 days

Contd...

Contd...

Etiological agent	*Major clinical features*	*Treatment*	*Alternative drug(s)*
Trichinella spiralis	• Abdominal pain • Discomfort	• *Mebendazole* 200–400 mg tid PO for 3 days, then 400–500 mg tid for 10 days • *Steroids* to be given for severe symptoms	*Albendazole* 400 mg bid PO for 8–14 days
Diphyllobothrium latum	• Diarrhea • Fever • Periorbital edema • Myalgia • Megaloblastic anemia • Leukopenia • Thrombocytopenia	*Praziquantel* 5–10 mg/kg PO once	*Niclosamide* 50 mg/kg once

measures, viz. safe disposal of human excreta, safe water supply, proper food hygiene, personal and community hygiene, health education, and early diagnosis and treatment of symptomatic and asymptomatic cases.[7] Regular deworming of children between 1 and 19 years must be done every year (National Deworming Day, 10 February) even if they are asymptomatic.

REFERENCES

1. Evayu T, Kiros T, Workineh L, Sema M, Damtie S, Hailemichael W, et al. Prevalence of intestinal parasitic infections and associated factors among patients attending at Sanja Primary Hospital, Northwest Ethiopia: An institutional-based cross-sectional study. PloS One. 2021;16(2):e0247075.
2. Langbang D, Dhodapkar R, Parija SC, Premarajan KC, Rajkumari N. Prevalence of intestinal parasites among rural and urban population in Puducherry, South India - A community-based study. J Family Med Prim Care. 2019;8(5):1607-12.
3. Shivananda S, Chatterjee K, Srikrishna S. Common Worm Infestations. (2022). IAP Standard Treatment Guidelines. [online] Available from https://iapindia.org/pdf/Ch-125-Common-Worm-Infestations.pdf. [Last accessed December, 2024].
4. Mohammadi R, Hosseini-Safa A, Ardakani MJE, Rostami-Nejad M. The relationship between intestinal parasites and some immune-mediated intestinal conditions. Gastroenterol Hepatol Bed Bench. 2015;8(2):123-31.
5. Thielen BK, Schless MR. Antiparasitic Therapy. In: Kliegman RM, Geme III JW, Blum NJ, et al. (Eds). Nelson Textbook of Pediatrics, 21st edition. New Delhi: Elsevier; 2020. pp. 1812-28.
6. Tripathi KD. Antiamoebic and other antiprotozoal drugs and anthelmintic drugs. In: Tripathi KD (Ed). Essentials of Medical Pharmacology, 8th edition. New Delhi: Jaypee Brothers Medical Publishers (P) Ltd.; 2018. pp. 893-914.
7. Park K. Intestinal infections. In: Park K (Ed). Park's Textbook of Preventive and Social Medicine, 23rd edition. Jabalpur: Banarsidas Bhanot; 2015. pp. 202-45.

11.10 Inflammatory Bowel Disease

Moinak Sen Sarma

INTRODUCTION

Inflammatory bowel disease (IBD) is a chronic inflammatory disease of the gastrointestinal tract (GIT) and is of two main types: (1) Crohn's disease (CD) and (2) ulcerative colitis (UC). In about 10% cases, the findings are labeled as unclassified IBD. Nearly 25% of all IBD patients present in the pediatric age group. Worldwide the incidences of IBD, more so CD, are increasing in children. Large population-based studies have shown an incidence of 1.2–11.8 cases per 100,000 predominantly in the West. Higher latitude and northern hemisphere report higher incidences. There are population-based data available from India. The average age of presentation in children is 10–11 years. However, it is recently described in all the age groups including infancy.

PATHOPHYSIOLOGY

Being an immune-mediated disease, there is a complex interaction of innate and adaptive immunity, gut bacteria, genetic predisposition, and environmental factors **(Fig. 11.10.1)**. Genome-wide association studies have

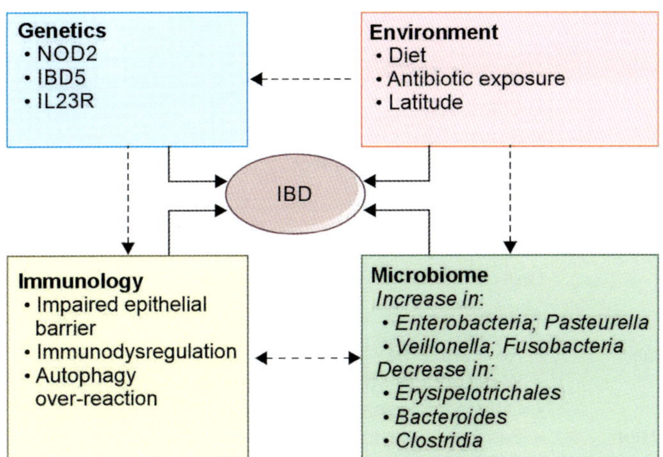

Fig. 11.10.1: Pathophysiology of inflammatory bowel disease (IBD): Complex interaction of diet, genetics, immunology, and gut microbiota.

revealed more than 200 genetic loci responsible for the pathogenesis of IBD. These genes that code for proteins modify the body's immunity. A dysregulation in the gut barrier integrity and immune homeostasis may lead to alterations in biodiversity (proliferation and suppression of various gut bacterial species) triggering a chronic inflammation in the gut. The microbiome change in CD is better documented than the other IBDs. The older concept of hygiene hypothesis (people raised in sanitary conditions have higher risk of immune-mediated diseases) is gradually receding as IBD is now being reported frequently in lower socioeconomic strata too.

Genetics is a very important risk factor for IBD and up to 19–41% children in the West may have an affected family member with IBD. Having a first-degree relative with IBD increases the risk to about 30-fold. Susceptibility has been linked to some human leukocyte antigen (HLA) subtypes, and linkage analysis has identified multiple other susceptibility loci on several chromosomes. Environmental factors (not yet identified) also seem to play a role, because there is often nonconcordance among monozygotic twins. It is possible that viral infections can initiate the inflammatory process. Dietary triggers are unproven. CD causes transmural (mucosa, submucosa, muscular layers, and serosa) inflammation of various part of GIT, whereas in UC the inflammation is limited to the colonic mucosa only. **Tables 11.10.1 and 11.10.2** summarize the disease distribution of UC and CD and classify the diseases based on their extent, respectively.[1-3]

TABLE 11.10.1: Disease distribution in inflammatory bowel disease (IBD).

Ulcerative colitis	*Crohn's disease*
Distal colitis (proctitis/ proctosigmoiditis): 5–20%	*Ileocolonic disease:* 50–70%
Left side colitis (up to splenic flexure): 10–40%	*Isolated colonic involvement:* 10–20%
Pancolitis: 50–90%	*Small bowel:* 10–15%
	Associated: • *Upper gastrointestinal involvement:* 30–40% • *Perianal disease:* 20–25%

TABLE 11.10.2: Paris classification for disease extent of inflammatory bowel disease (IBD).

Crohn's disease	*Ulcerative colitis*
Age at diagnosis: *A1a:* <10 years *A1b:* 10–17 years *A2:* 17–40 years *A3:* >40 years	*Extension*: *E1:* Proctitis *E2:* Left-sided colitis (distal to splenic flexure) *E3:* Extensive (up to hepatic flexure) *E4:* Pancolitis
Location: *L1:* Distal one-third ileum ± limited cecal disease *L2:* Colonic *L3:* Ileocolonic *L4:* Upper gastroenteritis (GI) or rest of small bowel involvement	*Severity:* *S0:* Never severe *S1:* Ever severe
Behavior: *B1:* Nonstricturing *B2:* Stricturing *B3:* Penetrating *B2B3:* Both stricturing and penetrating *P:* Perianal	
Growth: *G0:* No growth delay *G1:* Growth delay	

CLINICAL FEATURES

Children with CD present with abdominal pain, diarrhea (with or without blood), and constitutional symptoms (fever and anorexia).[4] The classical triad of diarrhea, abdominal pain, and weight loss is seen in only 25% of children. In contrast children with UC present with bloody diarrhea. In Asia, children with both UC as well as CD have growth failure or weight loss due to late referral. In the West, children with IBD present relatively early, and hence growth failure is more often encountered in CD than UC.[5] **Table 11.10.3** summarizes the clinical, histologic, and endoscopic differences between UC and CD.[1-3]

Extraintestinal manifestations **(Table 11.10.4)** are seen in 25–30% children with IBD. They can precede, follow, or occur concurrently with the intestinal disease and may be related or unrelated to activity of the intestinal disease. Of all the

TABLE 11.10.3: Differentiation between Crohn's disease and ulcerative colitis.

Parameters	***Crohn's disease***	***Ulcerative colitis***
Distribution	• Entire gastrointestinal (GI) tract • Transmural inflammation • Discontinuous lesions	• Colon only • Mucosal disease • Continuous involvement
Bloody diarrhea	Less common	Common
Abdominal pain	Common	Less common
Growth failure	Common	Less common
Perianal disease	Present [abscess, fistulae, tags **(Fig. 11.10.2A)**]	Absent
Histopathology	• Noncaseating ill-defined (<300 µm) granuloma (throughout GI tract) • No goblet cell dysplasia • Focal discontinuous crypt architectural distortion • Focal discontinuous chronic inflammation • Focally enhancing gastritis (biopsy of stomach) • Pyloric gland metaplasia (terminal ileum)	• No granuloma • Widespread crypt architectural distortion • Diffuse inflammatory infiltrate • Basal plasmacytosis • Goblet cell depletion • Crypt abscess • Paneth cell metaplasia
Endoscopy **(Figs. 11.10.2B to F)**	• Deep irregular serpiginous or aphthous ulcers • Normal intervening mucosa (skip lesion) • Ileal involvement, rectal sparing (60%) • Internal fistulae	• Diffuse superficial ulceration • Granularity, loss of vascular pattern, and friability • Rectal involvement (80–90%) ileal sparing (unless back-wash ileitis) and cecal patch in left-sided colitis

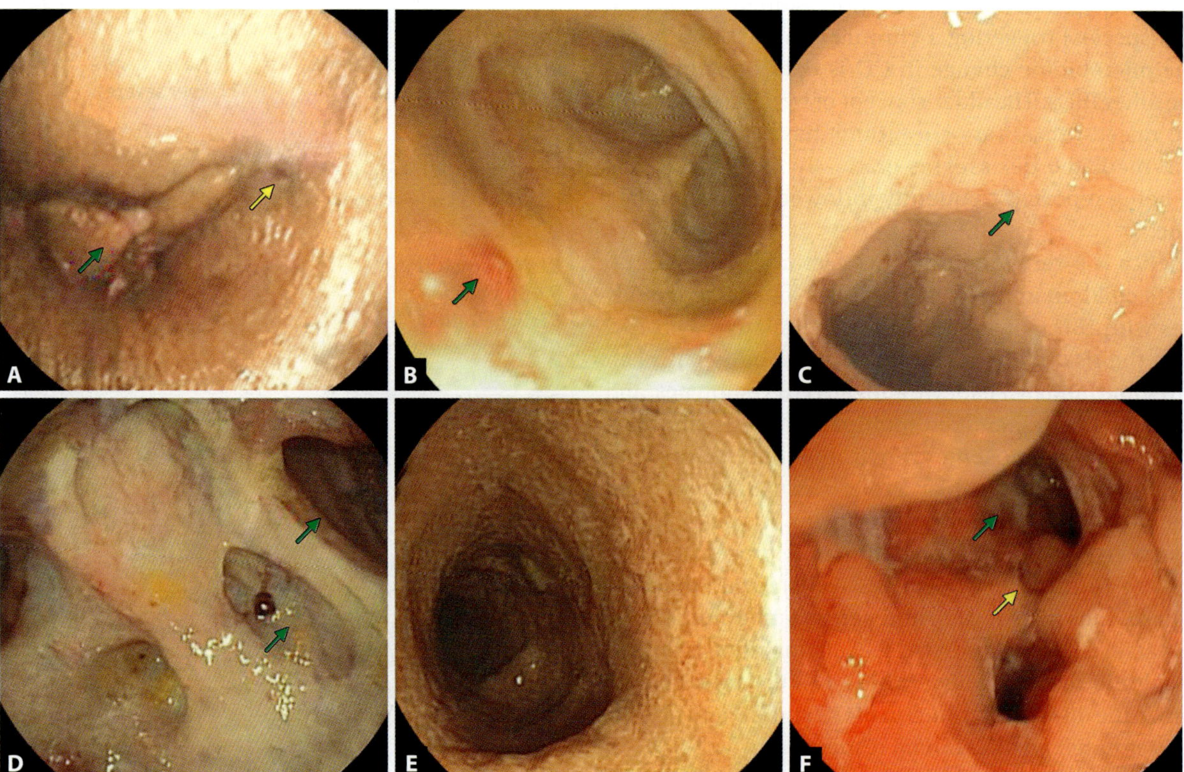

Figs. 11.10.2A to F: (A) Yellow arrow: Mucocutaneous fistula; green arrow: perianal tag in Crohn's disease (CD); (B) Green arrow: aphthous ulcers in CD; (C): Green arrow: linear serpiginous ulcer in CD; (D) Green arrows: internal fistulae of colon to small bowel; (E) Superficial continuous ulcers in ulcerative colitis (UC); and (F) Green arrow: ileal ulcer; yellow arrow: ileocecal valve destruction.

TABLE 11.10.4: Extraintestinal manifestations in IBD.

System	*Extraintestinal manifestation*
Joints	• Nondeforming arthritis (large joints > small joints) and arthralgia • Enthesitis • Sacroiliitis • Ankylosing spondylitis (HLA-B27 positive)
Skin/oral cavity	• Oral ulcers • Pyoderma gangrenosum • Erythema nodosum • Alopecia areata • "Metastatic" Crohn's disease (ulcers and granulomatosis of penis, vulva, and labia)
Eye	• Uveitis • Episcleritis
Liver/biliary tract	• Primary or autoimmune sclerosing cholangitis • Autoimmune hepatitis • Pancreatitis • Cholelithiasis • Fatty liver • Asymptomatic hypertransaminasemia • IgG4 cholangiopathy
Bones	Osteopenia and osteoporosis
Coagulation	Venous thrombosis (portal vein, hepatic vein, and mesenteric veins)
Kidneys	Renal stones (oxalate)

(HLA: human leukocyte antigen; IBD: inflammatory bowel disease; IgG: immunoglobulin G)

extraintestinal manifestations, arthralgia or arthritis are the most common manifestation (15%).

DIAGNOSIS

The initial evaluation of a child with suspected IBD includes a detailed clinical, family, and treatment history.[6] A complete examination includes growth charting, perianal, and rectal examination for fistulae, tags, and fissures. Laboratory tests may reveal anemia and thrombocytosis (67%), low albumin, high erythrocyte sedimentation rate (ESR), and C-reactive protein (CRP) in 40–60%, and these are reliable indicators of IBD.[7]

Fecal inflammatory markers such as fecal calprotectin are popular in the West for screening of IBD. However, it has many fallacies, especially in developing countries. Fecal calprotectin may not be sufficiently raised in early stage of disease, has poor specificity, and elevated in intercurrent GI infections (bacterial, parasitic, *H. pylori* infection, and small bowel bacterial overgrowth). *Antineutrophil cytoplasmic antibody (ANCA)* is found in about 66% of UC patients and in only a few CD cases. *Anti-Saccharomyces cerevisiae antibody (ASCA)* is present in about 50% of CD patients and is uncommon in UC. Because there is overlap between CD and UC, none of these tests can discriminate absolutely between

TABLE 11.10.5: Diagnostic modalities available for IBD.

Diagnostic modality	*Importance*
• Colonoscopy with ileal intubation • Multiple biopsies from disease sites • UGI endoscopy with biopsies	• Most important to differentiate UC vs. CD • To look for granulomas
• Small bowel imaging • Barium enteroclysis, CT, or MR enteroclysis	• For small bowel strictures fistula • Extramural complications may be seen in CT/MRI
MRI pelvis	Fistula, pelvic, and genitourinary abscess
Capsule endoscopy	• Ideal to evaluate small bowel involvement after excluding intestinal stricture that may result in retention of capsule • *Disadvantage:* Biopsies cannot be taken
Enteroscopy	Limitation of not able to pass bigger diameter enteroscope in younger children

(CD: Crohn's disease; CT: computed tomography; IBD: inflammatory bowel disease; MRI: magnetic resonance imaging; UC: ulcerative colitis; UGI: upper gastrointestinal)

the two conditions. The use of antibodies is complementary and ancillary in the diagnosis of IBD. In fact, they may have a role in prognostication of the disease. ASCA positive CD patients are likely to have ileal involvement and greater need for surgery in future. ANCA positive CD has left colonic disease, sparing of terminal ileum and lesser need for surgery.

Table 11.10.5 summarizes the diagnostic modalities available for IBD.[6] Upper gastrointestinal (UGI) endoscopy, colonoscopy, and small bowel imaging are mandatory for mapping of disease and confirmation of diagnosis. Biopsies from endoscopically involved and uninvolved sites at the onset are essential.

Basal plasmacytosis is the earliest diagnostic feature with the highest predictive value for the diagnosis of UC. Preserved crypt architecture does not rule out early UC. Therefore, repeat biopsies are recommended not sooner than 6 weeks after the initial assessment for the diagnosis of UC. At onset, CD in children is associated with more colitis and less ileitis. The frequency of granulomas is higher in the upper GIT and is of assistance in differentiating CD from UC.

MANAGEMENT

General Management

Classification of severity of disease is by pediatric ulcerative colitis activity index (PUCAI) and pediatric Crohn's disease activity index (PCDAI).[1-3] While PUCAI takes consideration of grading of clinical parameters (abdominal pain, rectal bleeding, stool number, consistency, nocturnal awakening, and daily activity), PCDAI is a much more elaborate grading that incorporates clinical as well as laboratory parameters (hematocrit, ESR, and albumin) and examination (height, weight, abdominal tenderness, perirectal disease, and extraintestinal manifestations). Both the indices are important for assessing response to therapy.[7,8]

The goals of treatment are to control inflammation, mucosal healing, improve growth, and ensure a good quality of life with the least toxic therapeutic regimen. Ensuring proper nutrition with caloric supplementation [120% of recommended daily allowance (RDA)] is a necessity for children with IBD. Calcium and vitamin D supplementation should be given as these children are at an increased risk of osteoporosis. As IBD is a chronic disease with remissions and exacerbations, proper counseling of both patient and family at diagnosis is essential. Exclusive enteral nutrition (EEN) with elemental, semielemental, or polymeric formulae are popular in the West to induce remission in mild-moderate CD compared to drug therapy. EEN may not be effective in severe pancolitis, fistulizing or perianal CD. Duration of EEN therapy should be 6–8 weeks. Drug therapy must be considered if there is no response by second week of EEN. EEN is not used as modality of therapy in UC.[7]

Drugs

The main drugs used for IBD are listed in **Tables 11.10.6 and 11.10.7**. There are two phases of therapy: (1) Induction and (2) maintenance.

Steroids have a central role, as they are the most commonly used induction agents in moderate to severe UC and all severities of CD and IBD-U. Prednisolone is started as 2 mg/kg (maximum 40 mg/day and 60 mg/day in case of unsatisfactory response in older children) for 2–4 weeks followed by gradual tapering over 6–8 weeks by which time clinical remission is seen in majority. Toxicity of steroids must be monitored from time to time (every 2–3 weeks) with mandatory examination of blood pressure, intraocular pressure, and cataract formation. Role of budesonide in place of prednisolone (for lesser steroid toxicity) in maintenance therapy in CD is not well established in children.

In cases of UC with steroid dependence, relapse or steroid refractory course, and invariably in all cases of CD, *azathioprine* (1–2 mg/kg) is added on for maintenance. A small dose of steroids may be additionally required in a minority along with azathioprine to maintain remission. Azathioprine is chosen as a steroid-sparing agent, which takes approximately 2–3 months for optimal action. On azathioprine, regular monitoring of blood counts for bone marrow suppression and liver enzymes for hepatotoxicity is required.

Second-line agents are used in select situations. Patients who are steroid-resistant and thiopurine-intolerant are invariably considered for *biologicals*. Infliximab and adalimumab have been used with response rates of 50–60% to achieve remission. Adalimumab has a better safety profile (infusion reactions) compared to infliximab and can be used if antibodies to infliximab have developed leading to infliximab nonresponse. Biologicals may be combined

TABLE 11.10.6: Drugs used in IBD (first-line therapy).

Drug	***Dosage and route***	***Indication***	***Main side effects***
Sulfasalazine *Or* 5-aminosalicylic acid or mesalamine *(active moiety of sulfasalazine)*	• 40–60 mg/kg/day oral • 50–100 mg/kg/day oral • Enema	• Anti-inflammatory (local action) in mild UC and maintenance • Enema in mild to moderate left sided colonic disease	• Folate deficiency • Pancreatitis • Stevens–Johnson syndrome • Hepatotoxicity • Oligospermia (with sulfasalazine)
Prednisolone	1–2 mg/kg oral	Induction therapy (first line) in all types of IBD	• Cushingoid facies • Hypertension • Glaucoma • Cataract • Fractures • Hyperglycemia • Growth impairment
Thiopurines: Azathioprine (AZA) 6-Mercaptopurine *(active moiety of AZA)*	• 2–3 mg/kg/day oral • 1–2 mg/kg/day oral	• Frequent relapses* • Steroid dependence# • Steroid resistance% • Maintenance in moderate to severe disease	• Myelosuppression • Hepatotoxicity • Pancreatitis

**Frequent relapses:* 2–3 relapses per year
#*Steroid dependency:* Initial remission but recurrence while tapering or inability to stop steroids in 14–16 weeks of initiation
%*Steroid resistance:* Nonresponse to optimal doses of oral steroids within 7–14 days of initiation and good compliance
(IBD: inflammatory bowel disease; UC: ulcerative colitis)

TABLE 11.10.7: Drugs used in IBD (second-line therapy).

Drug	Dosage and route	Indication	Main side effects
Methotrexate	15 mg/m^2 IM weekly	• Steroid sparing • Refractory disease and/or intolerant to thiopurines	• Hepatotoxicity • Myelosuppression • Folate deficiency
Cyclosporine Tacrolimus	• 2–4 mg/kg/d IV infusion followed by 5–8 mg/kg/d oral • 0.1 mg/kg oral	Rescue therapy for maximum 4 weeks in severe refractory UC	• Nephrotoxicity • Hypertrichosis • Gum hyperplasia • Hypertension • Paresthesia
Biological agents (infliximab and adalimumab)	• Infliximab 5 mg/kg IV at 0, 2, 6 weeks and thereafter 8–weekly • Adalimumab 2.4 mg/kg first dose followed by 1.2 mg/kg second dose followed by 0.6 mg/kg every 2 weekly	• Fistulating CD • Perianal disease • Severe disease not responding to immunomodulators	• Infusion reaction • Autoimmunity • Demyelination • Psychiatric problems • Flare infections • Hepatosplenic T-cell lymphoma
Thalidomide	1.5–2.5 mg/kg oral	Refractory CD and intolerant to biological agents (very selective group)	• Irreversible peripheral neuropathy • Agitation • Hallucination

(CD: Crohn's disease; IBD: inflammatory bowel disease; IM: intramuscular; IV: intravenous; UC: ulcerative colitis)

with immunomodulators in severe disease. In developing countries, biologicals can only be started if tuberculosis (TB) is ruled out. Biologicals are anti-tumor necrosis factor (TNF) alpha agents that will uncover a tubercular granuloma and allow the mycobacteria to disseminate. Biologicals are also contraindicated in the presence of active suppurative infections.

Additionally, for perianal fistulizing CD, antibiotics (ciprofloxacin 20 mg/kg, metronidazole 10–20 mg/kg, or rifaximin 10–30 mg/kg) for 4–6 weeks have shown good short-term response. In mild-moderate nonfistulizing, nonstricturing CD, EEN with polymeric, semielemental or elemental formulations may be used for 6–8 weeks for induction of remission, followed by a maintenance first-line immunomodulator. Oral 5-aminosalicylic acid (5-ASA) has a role in induction of remission in mild UC and maintenance phase of mild-moderate UC. Topical 5-ASA may be used in localized left-sided UC. 5-ASA has limited role in CD. Combining oral 5-ASA with topical 5-ASA is more effective than oral alone in UC. Rectal 5-ASA is superior and should be preferred over rectal steroid therapy in UC.

Surgery

In IBD, cumulative risk of surgery increases with duration of disease (CD: 18%, 27%, and 32% at 1, 5, and 10 years, respectively and UC: 8% and 20% at 1 and 5 years, respectively). Surgery is indicated in UC patients with severe acute colitis refractory to medical disease. Uncontrolled hemorrhage, perforation, toxic megacolon (TMC), abscesses, and obstruction are the other indications for surgery. Proctocolectomy is curative in UC but creating an ileal pouch for fecal continence is done with caution in a girl child due to reduced chances of fecundity later in adulthood. Since surgery is not curative in CD, its use must be limited, and the length of bowel resection must be minimized. Risk of adenocarcinoma colon is 8% after 20 years of disease in pediatric UC and should be suspected with new onset of symptoms after years of remission or features of large bowel obstruction and occult GI blood loss.

Acute Severe Ulcerative Colitis

Approximately 18–25% of UC may experience acute severe symptoms (PUCAI > 65) at any point of time during their disease course (>10 years) and will be transiently steroid refractory.[1,2] In this scenario, associated infections such as *Clostridium difficile* (stool toxin assay and passage of membranes per rectum), cytomegalovirus [(CMV) deep colonic ulcers, immunohistochemistry, and CMV inclusion bodies in colonic biopsies], concurrent fungal infections (stool for fungal hyphae), and infective colitis (stool culture for shigella, enterohemorrhagic *Escherichia coli*, etc.) must be considered and appropriately treated. TMC (see further) should be looked for.

Considering the case as a steroid refractory state, intravenous (IV) methylprednisolone 1–1.5 mg/kg/day should be started. If there is failure of response to methylprednisolone by day 5, then second-line rescue therapy with IV cyclosporine/oral tacrolimus or infliximab must be considered. Both cyclosporine and infliximab are equally efficacious with similar response (75–80%) for remission. Cyclosporine is given for 3–4 months but therapy with infliximab is indefinite and hence infliximab has lower future colectomy rates. Failure of second-line therapy by day 14 is an indication for colectomy. Colectomy is also indicated if during the course the patient develops perforation or hemorrhage. Response and failure in acute UC is monitored by PUCAI.

TOXIC MEGACOLON

Toxic megacolon is a complication seen in the setting of acute severe ulcerative colitis (ASUC).[2] It is to be diagnosed if transverse colon diameter in an erect X-ray abdomen is >40 mm (<10 years age) and >56 mm (>10 years age) with evidence of systemic toxicity (fever, tachycardia, dehydration, dyselectrolytemia, altered sensorium, hypotension, or shock). IV antibiotics (such as ampicillin, gentamycin, and metronidazole), correction of electrolyte imbalance, food restriction, and preparation for surgery compose the mainstay of initial therapy for TMC. Rectal decompression tube and positional changes have limited benefits. Failure of medical management is an indication for emergency colectomy.

VERY EARLY-ONSET INFLAMMATORY BOWEL DISEASE

Recently pediatric IBD has been reclassified as shown in **Figure 11.10.3**. Very early-onset inflammatory bowel disease (VEOIBD) is IBD occurring <6 years age.[9] In this bracket, infantile IBD (<2 years age) comprises <5% of all pediatric IBD. VEOIBD requires detailed immunological workup for immunodeficiencies of monogenic inheritance. Some of the notable genetic defects associated with the infantile-onset IBD are IL (interleukin)-10, IL-10 receptor A, IL-10 receptor B, ADAM-17, XIAP, TTC7A (apoptotic enterocolitis), IPEX syndrome, atypical severe combined immunodeficiency (Omenn syndrome), Wiskott–Aldrich syndrome, agammaglobulinemia, hyperimmunoglobulin M (IgM) syndrome, common variable immunodeficiency (CVID), and chronic granulomatous disease. The settings to suspect monogenic IBS are given in **Table 11.10.8**. The monogenic disorders and their disorder subtype is shown in **Table 11.10.9**. These diseases are primary immunodeficiencies, which

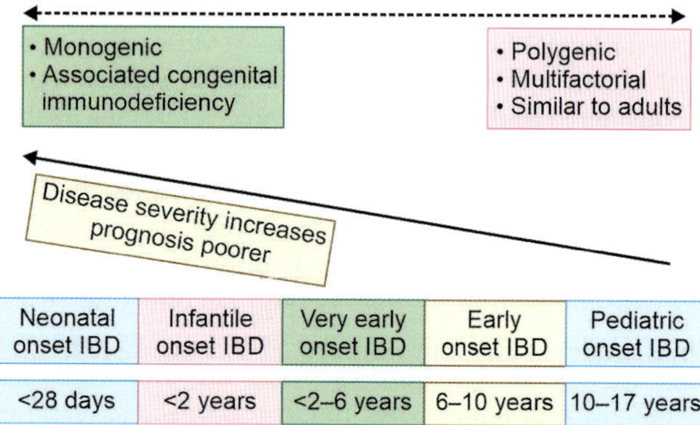

Fig. 11.10.3: New classification of pediatric inflammatory bowel disease (IBD).

TABLE 11.10.8: Settings to suspect monogenic inflammatory bowel disease (IBD) (one or more features).

Feature	*Comment*
Very early onset of symptoms	Most commonly <2 years age
Family history	Consanguinity, sib death, affected sib or multiple family members, known immunodeficiency state in family
Atypical endoscopy or histology	Apoptotic enterocolitis, unusual, and coalescent pattern of ulcers
Resistance to conventional therapies	Failure of response to steroids, immunomodulators, and biological therapy
Ectodermal defects	Skin lesions (epidermolysis bullosa, eczema), nail dystrophy, and hair abnormalities (wooly hair, trichorrhexis nodosa)
Early-onset perianal disease	Deep fistula (mucocutaneous and rectogenitourinary) and abscess
Reticuloendothelial abnormalities	Lymph node abscesses, splenomegaly, and cyclical neutropenia
Recurrent infections or unexplained fever	Deep-seated infections, atypical infections (intestinal or nonintestinal), and multisystemic life-threatening infections
Hemophagocytic lymphohistiocytosis	Induced by Epstein–Barr virus or cytomegalovirus
Associated autoimmunity	Arthritis, serositis, thyroiditis, and type 1 diabetes
Early-onset tumors	Non-Hodgkin lymphoma, hamartomas

TABLE 11.10.9: The monogenic disorders and their disorder subtype.

Disorder subtype	*Monogenic diseases*
Neutrophil production	Congenital, cyclic, and autoimmune neutropenia
Neutrophil migration	Leukocyte adhesion deficiency
Lysozyme trafficking	Hermansky–Pudlak syndrome
Respiratory burst	Chediak–Higashi syndrome Chronic granulomatous disease and deficit in components of the nicotinamide adenine dinucleotide phosphate (NADPH) oxidase complex
NOD2 pathways Adaptive immunity Regulatory immune response	Glycogen storage Ib XIAP defect Wiskott–Aldrich syndrome IPEX syndrome Interleukin 10 (IL-10) signaling defect

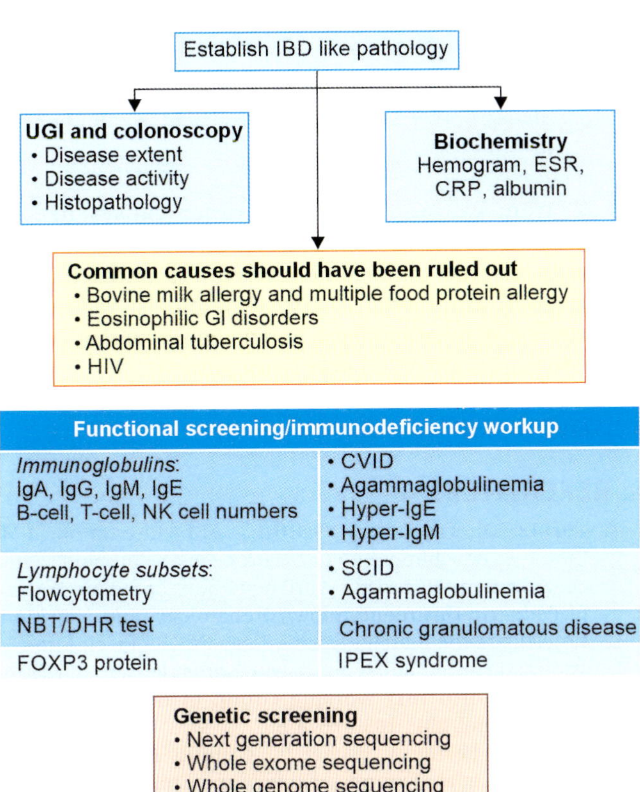

Fig. 11.10.4: Approach to VEOIBD in India. (CVID: common variable immunodeficiency; VEOIBD: very early-onset inflammatory bowel disease; CRP: C-reactive protein; UGI: upper gastrointestinal; DHR: dihydrohodamine; ESR: erythrocyte sedimentation rate; HIV: human immunodeficiency virus; Ig: immunoglobulin; NBT: nitroblue tetrazolium; NK: natural killer; SCID: severe combined immunodeficiency)

manifest as recurrent infections and IBD. An approach to workup of VEOIBD in India is shown in **Figure 11.10.4**. The very early-onset, infantile, and neonatal IBD have markedly poor prognosis. They have severe course, fistulizing disease, and resistance to biological therapy and often require colectomy or colonic diversion. Allogeneic hematopoietic stem cell transplants (HSCT) have shown to produce 80% remission in those who do not respond to standard therapy. In those with chronic granulomatous disorder, biologicals are contraindicated. Epithelial barrier defects such as NEMO will worsen after stem cell transplant.

Due to the significant risk associated with HSCT, including graft-versus-host disease and severe infections, it is important to determine the genetic basis for each patient's VEOIBD before selecting HSCT as a treatment approach.

BIOLOGICAL THERAPY IN INFLAMMATORY BOWEL DISEASE

The standard biologicals in IBD are infliximab and adalimumab, which are anti-TNF-α inhibitors. Ustekinumab

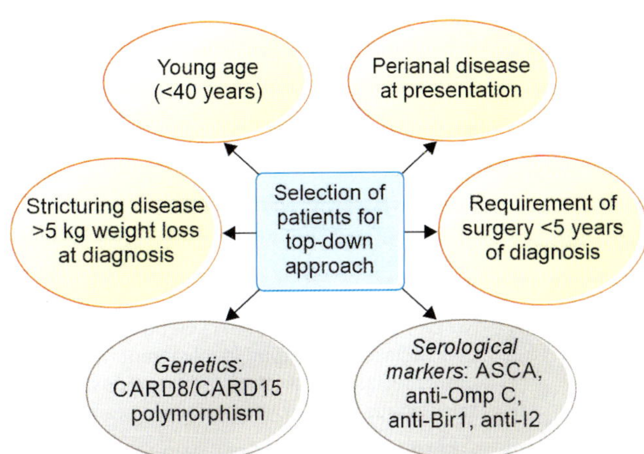

Fig. 11.10.5: Additional risk factors that require biologics. (ASCA: anti-Saccharomyces cerevisiae antibody)

and vedolizumab are newer biologicals acting by different pathways. Vedolizumab is a gut-selective drug. Indications for biologicals in CD include failure of standard immunosuppression, primary steroid failure, and perianal disease.[3] There are various risk factors that require use of biologicals shown in **Figure 11.10.5**. Top-down approach is a modality of therapy where biologicals are used as primary agents in the disease for aggressive control instead of immunomodulators. In UC, indications to use biologicals are uncontrolled disease and second-line therapy in acute severe disease.[1,2] Biologicals are monitored by trough levels and antibodies. Loss of response can be primary (at onset) or secondary (after a period of response). Drug monitoring can be proactive (periodic for drug titrations) or reactive (when there is loss of response). If there is loss of response, options are dose escalation, interval shortening, switching to alternative class, combination (dual) biologicals, or surgery.

DIFFERENTIAL DIAGNOSIS OF INFLAMMATORY BOWEL DISEASE

Abdominal Tuberculosis

In developing countries, tuberculous colitis is a very close differential diagnosis and possibly more common than IBD. Hence while working up for IBD, simultaneous evaluation for TB is mandatory. The discriminatory features are shown in **Table 11.10.10**. Basic workup required are chest X-ray, Mantoux test, and computed tomography (CT) enterography. In select scenarios and high index of suspicion, high-resolution CT (HRCT) of chest is required. Circular transverse ulcers are commonly seen in tubercular colitis. Tissue biopsies should also be processed for TB-polymerase chain reaction (TB-PCR), Ziehl–Neelsen (ZN) stain, TB culture, and GeneXpert/line probe assay. Interferon gamma release assay is not recommended due to poor sensitivity. Occasionally, it is very difficult to differentiate IBD vs. abdominal TB despite

TABLE 11.10.10: Discriminatory features favoring tuberculosis.

Clinical	Contact history, peripheral lymphadenopathy, disseminated disease [pulmonary and central nervous system (CNS)], and abdominal lymph nodal masses
Laboratory	Mantoux positivity and exudative ascites (lymphocyte predominant with high adenosine deaminase)
Imaging	Necrotic calcified or conglomerate abdominal lymph nodes, peritoneal thickening, pericardial effusion, lung involvement (military, bronchiectasis, mediastinal lymph nodes), and calcified space-occupying lesions in brain
Histopathology	Caseating large well-defined granulomas (>300 µm size)
Microbiology	Acid-fast bacilli in Ziehl–Neelsen (ZN) stain, culture positivity or positive GeneXpert/line probe assay

thorough workup and hence a trial and response to at least 8–12 weeks of antituberculosis therapy (ATT) is required. Paradoxically 20% of CD may report a transient clinical response to ATT, which leads to further confusion in a case scenario of diagnostic dilemma. In this scenario, objective findings (resolution of imaging and mucosal changes) is considered response to ATT and suggestive of TB (Logan's criteria of TB).

Bovine milk allergy, multiple food protein allergy, and eosinophilic colitis: This is to be considered in setting of infantile IBD. Temporal correlation with introduction of bovine milk or soy, colonic aphthous ulcers and eosinophilic infiltration of colonic biopsies are features.

Acquired Immunodeficiency Syndrome

Presentation may mimic IBD colitis. It is suspected in the presence of recurrent urinary, sinopulmonary or dermatological infections (extensive scabies and dermatophytoses), hepatosplenomegaly, generalized lymphadenopathy, thrombocytopenia, and hypergammaglobulinemia.

LONG-TERM ISSUES IN PEDIATRIC INFLAMMATORY BOWEL DISEASE

Bone density and linear growth (on steroids), nutrition (due to anorexia, recurrent pain abdomen, small bowel strictures, and malabsorption), immunizations (live vaccines contraindication due to immunosuppression), drug compliance (due to polytherapy, affordability of biologicals, and adolescence), psychosocial issues (due to cosmetic stigmata of surgery and recurrent infections), school absenteeism (recurrent hospital admissions), fertility potential (due to drug toxicity and colectomy), and cumulative cancer risks are some of the long-term issues prevailing in IBD.

CONCLUSION

- Pediatric IBD constitutes nearly 25% of all IBDs.
- Increase in incidence of pediatric IBD is seen over last 2–3 decades.
- It is crucial to make a timely diagnosis of IBD, differentiate UC from CD and also from other causes like GI tuberculosis, bovine milk intolerance, etc.
- Diagnosis and management need a multidisciplinary approach with pediatric gastroenterologist, radiologist, pathologist, microbiologist, and pediatric surgeon.
- Endoscopies are mandatory in the workup.
- Treatment should be done only in tertiary referral centers.
- Very early IBD is a challenging entity.

REFERENCES

1. Turner D, Travis SP, Griffiths AM, Ruemmele FM, Levine A, Benchimol EI, et al.; European Crohn's and Colitis Organization; Porto IBD Working Group, European Society of Pediatric Gastroenterology, Hepatology, and Nutrition. Consensus for managing acute severe UC in children: a systematic review and joint statement from ECCO, ESPGHAN, and the Porto IBD Working Group of ESPGHAN. Am J Gastroenterol. 2011;106(4):574-88.
2. Turner D, Levine A, Escher JC, Griffiths AM, Russell RK, Dignass A, et al.; European Crohn's and Colitis Organization; European Society for Paediatric Gastroenterology, Hepatology and Nutrition. Management of pediatric ulcerative colitis: joint ECCO and ESPGHAN evidence-based consensus guidelines. J Pediatr Gastroeneterol Nutr. 2012;55(3):340-61.
3. Vernier-Massouille G, Balde M, Salleron J, Turck D, Dupas JL, Mouterde O, et al. Natural history of pediatric Crohn's disease: a population-based cohort study. Gastroenterology. 2008;135(4):1106-13.
4. Gower-Rousseau C, Dauchet L, Vernier-Massouille G, Tilloy E, Brazier F, Merle V, et al. The natural history of pediatric ulcerative colitis: a population-based cohort study. Am J Gastroenterol. 2009;104(8):2080-8.
5. Sawczenko A, Sandhu BK. Presenting features of inflammatory bowel disease in Great Britain and Ireland. Arch Dis Child. 2003;88(11):995-1000.
6. Levine A, Koletzko S, Turner D, Escher JC, Cucchiara S, de Ridder L, et al.; European Society of Pediatric Gastroenterology, Hepatology and Nutrition. ESPGHAN revised porto criteria for the diagnosis of inflammatory bowel disease in children and adolescents. J Pediatr Gastroenterol Nutr. 2014;58(6):795-806.
7. Oliveira SB, Monteiro IM. Diagnosis and management of inflammatory bowel disease in children. BMJ. 2017;357:j2083.
8. Ruemmele FM, Veres G, Kolho KL, Griffiths A, Levine A, Escher JC, et al.; European Crohn's and Colitis Organization; European Society of Pediatric Gastroenterology, Hepatology and Nutrition. Consensus guidelines of ECCO/ESPGHAN on the medical management of pediatric Crohn's disease. J Crohns Colitis. 2014;8(10):1179-207.
9. Uhlig HH, Schwerd T, Koletzko S, Shah N, Kammermeier J, Elkadri A, et al.; COLORS in IBD Study Group and NEOPICS. The diagnostic approach to monogenic very early onset inflammatory bowel disease. Gastroenterology. 2014;147(5):990-1007.e3.

11.11 Functional Constipation and Incontinence

VR Ravikumar, VS Sankaranarayanan

INTRODUCTION

Constipation is a symptom of an underlying disorder seen in approximately 10–25% of all patients presenting in a pediatric gastroenterology clinic.[1] A normal bowel pattern is considered as a sign of good health. Constipation in children is common, often chronic (persisting for >2 weeks) associated with consequences such as chronic abdominal pain, fecal soiling, voiding dysfunction, psychosocial stress, and behavioral problems resulting in poor quality of life.[2]

DEFINITIONS

For practical clinical purposes, constipation is defined as infrequent defecation, painful defecation, or both. In most cases, stools are too large, too hard, not frequent enough, and/or painful to pass.[1] The North American Society for Pediatric Gastroenterology Hepatology and Nutrition (NASPGHAN) defines constipation as "a delay or difficulty in defecation, present for 2 weeks or more, and sufficient to cause significant distress to the patient".[3,4]

According to Rome III definition of chronic constipation, symptoms must include at least two of the following for the past 2 months:[3,5]

- Two or fewer defecations per week
- At least one episode of fecal incontinence per week in a toilet-trained child
- History of excessive stool retention or retentive posturing
- History of painful or hard bowel movements
- Presence of large fecal mass in the rectum
- History of large diameter stools that may obstruct the toilet.

CONSEQUENCES

Hard stools are difficult and painful to push leading to "pooping is pain" and stool withholding resulting in fecal retention. With rectal distension, excessive absorption of fluid and decreased sensory perception follow with hard stools. This leads to *fissure in ano*, painful defecation with partial evacuation. The vicious cycle results in "toilet-o-phobia", further impaction with fecaloma formation. This affects toilet training.[2,6]

Encopresis (Fecal Incontinence)

Defecation reflex is normal. Chronic fecal retention leads to megarectum and megacolon with involuntary overflow and fecal soiling or encopresis.

Obstipation

Obstipation is the absence of passage of both feces and flatus and indicates underlying organic obstruction or pseudo-obstruction.

Functional Constipation

Nearly 90% of children with constipation have functional constipation (c.f. for organic cause) at the school entry age.[2,6] The contributing factors include stool-withholding habits after experience of passing painful bowel movement, denying natural calls in the school or teachers not giving permission to defecate and retentive defecation posturing. Characteristically the "red flags" (vide infra) are absent.[7,8]

Currently, the diagnosis of functional constipation is based on the new Rome IV criteria, which are the updated version of the older Rome III criteria. Only minor changes have been made in the Rome IV diagnostic criteria compared to the previous Rome III criteria. In the group of neonate/toddlers, considering that the majority of toddlers aged <2.5 years are not toilet trained, a differentiation between toilet-trained and not toilet-trained children has been included. In the group of child/adolescent, the only modification is the decrease from 2 months to 1 month in the duration of symptoms needed to fulfill the criteria for the diagnosis.[8]

ETIOLOGY

The common causes of constipation are listed in **Table 11.11.1**. Neuronal intestinal dysplasia, visceral myopathy, Chagas disease, small left colon syndrome, and neurofibromatosis are some of the rare causes leading to pseudo-obstruction.[7]

CLINICAL FEATURES

Assessment of a Child with Constipation

A careful history and thorough physical examination including per rectal examination will suffice to diagnose functional constipation provided there are no "red flags".[2]

"Red flags" suggesting organic cause of constipation are failure to thrive, abdominal distension, lack of lumbosacral curve, sacral agenesis, flat buttocks, patulous or anteriorly placed anus, tight empty rectum, gush of air and liquid stool on withdrawal of finger per rectal examination and absent anal wink or cremasteric reflex, and lower limb weakness.

Timing of Constipation

At the time of initiating complementary feeds or toilet training (1–2 years); school entry or school age.

Hirschsprung Disease and Functional Constipation

Table 11.11.2 highlights the differences between Hirschsprung disease and functional constipation.[7]

INVESTIGATIONS

Good history and physical examination with rectal examination are essential.

- <5% organic—tests rarely needed
- *X-ray abdomen* may show loaded colon **(Fig. 11.11.1A)**.
- *Barium enema:* Dilatation from anal verge in habit constipation **(Fig. 11.11.1B)**; transition zone in Hirschsprung disease **(Fig. 11.11.1C)**; and rarely to look for strictures
- *Colonic manometry* may be helpful in refractory constipation.
- *Rectal mucosal biopsy* in Hirschsprung disease, intestinal neuronal dysplasia, and solitary rectal ulcer
- Do not forget to screen for hypothyroidism, diabetes mellitus, lead poisoning, celiac disease, and hypercalcemia.

MANAGEMENT

The main steps in the management of constipation are:

- Ensure there is no organic cause, treat if present
- Diet, fluids, exercise, and toilet training
- Pharmacotherapy
- Disimpaction
- Maintenance—prevention of reimpaction

TABLE 11.11.1: Common causes of constipation.

Newborn	***Infants and children***
Prematurity	*Diet:* Poor dietary habits, lack of fiber
Underfeeding, formula feeds	Weaning formulas
Hypothyroidism	Hypothyroidism
Hirschsprung disease	Hirschsprung disease
Low anorectal anomalies (e.g., anteriorly placed anus)	Functional or psychogenic
Spinal abnormalities	Irritable bowel syndrome (constipating type)
Meconium plug syndrome	*Central nervous system (CNS)*: Hypoxic ischemic encephalopathy, cerebral palsy, and mental retardation
Presacral/pelvic mass	*Drugs*: Antispasmodics, antimotility drugs, phenothiazines, codeine containing cough syrups, vincristine, and vinblastine

TABLE 11.11.2: Differences between Hirschsprung disease and functional constipation.

Functional constipation	***Hirschsprung disease***
More common	Less common
Meconium history—normal	Delayed passage
Onset beyond infancy	From birth
Fecal soiling	Spurious diarrhea
Abdominal distension—rare	Common
Loaded rectum	Empty rectum, grips finger, gush of air, and fluid on release
Failure to thrive or enterocolitis—rare	Common

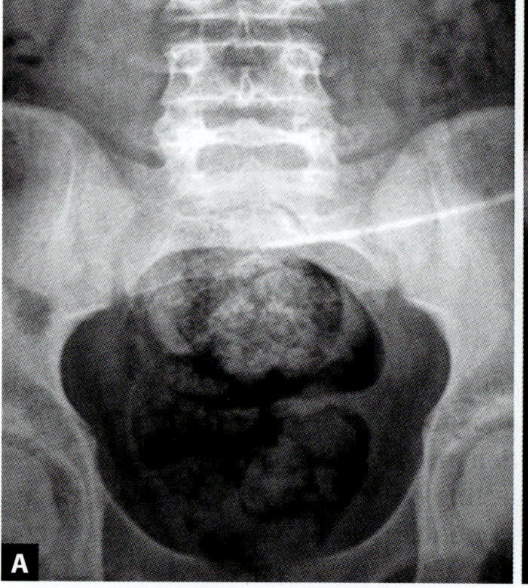

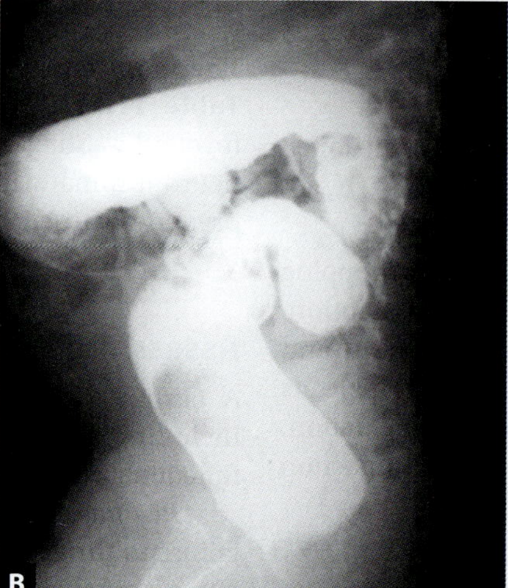

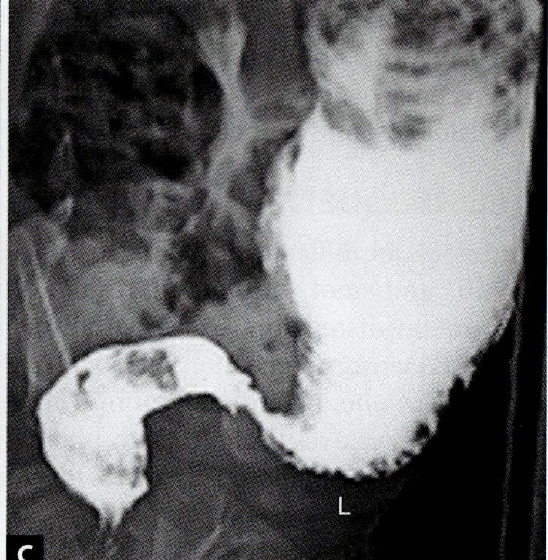

Figs. 11.11.1A to C: (A) Plain X-ray abdomen showing colon loaded with feces in a child with fecal impaction; (B) Habitual constipation with dilatation from anal verge; (C) Hirschsprung disease showing transition zone.

- Behavioral therapy
- Education and re-education (counseling).

Consultation with a pediatric gastroenterologist or pediatric surgeon is appropriate if the child's history or examination findings suggest an underlying organic cause (e.g., Hirschsprung disease). Also seek consultation when the child fails routine therapy or when management is otherwise complex.

Diet

Diet in constipation includes fiber-containing items such as sprouted whole grains, pulses, beans, and sorbitol-rich fruits (apple with peel, guava, pomegranate, pear, and prune juice), green leafy vegetables, and water. Fiber intake is recommended over 2 years of age and the dose is calculated as age in years plus 5 g/day. Involvement of dietician is beneficial.

Laxatives

Laxatives such as lubricants, osmotic, and stimulants for maintenance are required for a longer period over years to regulate the bowel habits. These should be explained to the parents at the onset. Guidelines for maintenance dose of commonly used drugs are given in **Table 11.11.3**.

Mechanism of Action of Fiber in Chronic Constipation

Fiber is a bulk laxative available as psyllium (Isphagol), methylcellulose, and polycarbophil.

TABLE 11.11.3: Laxatives dose and side effects.

Laxative	*Dose*	*Side effects*
Lubricant: Mineral oil	1–3 mL/kg/day once daily or in divided doses for a short period only	• Do not give to infants • Anal leakage, lipoid pneumonia
Osmotic: Lactulose, lactitol or sorbitol	1–3 mL/kg/day in two doses	Bloating, cramps, and diarrhea
Polyethylene glycol (PEG)	5–10 mL/kg/day	Nausea, vomiting, cramps, and diarrhea
Magnesium hydroxide	1–3 mL/kg/day in two doses	Hypermagnesemia, hypophosphatemia, and hypocalcemia
Stimulant: Bisacodyl	*>2 years*: 5–10 mg daily orally; 5 mg per rectally	Cramps, diarrhea, and anal irritation
Senna	• *>6 years:* 5–15 mL/day (8.8 mg/5 mL) • *2–6 years:* 2.5–7.5 mL/day	Melanosis coli and hepatitis

Dose: Age in years + g/day (1–1.5 g/kg). Bloating is the side effect. Commercial fiber preparations are recommended above 3 years of age only. Combinations of fiber with lactulose or lactitol/polyethylene glycol (PEG) preparations are available in the pharmacy. Fiber and excess dietary carbohydrates have the mechanical effect of water holding and increase the bulk of the stool and osmotic effect, respectively. The bulk of the stool is also increased by bacterial overgrowth, colonic bacterial fermentation, gas production, and production of short-chain fatty acids (SCFA). Both mechanisms will stimulate the faster transit of colonic fecal mass and also reduce the colonic absorption.

Disimpaction

- *Polyethylene glycol* is preferred as it is noninvasive. It is given orally in a dose of 20–25 mL/kg/h (up to 1,000 mL/h) until clear colonic content is evacuated.[9] It should be administered only under supervision in small children; Ryle's tube may be required for administration. Single dose of prokinetic and intravenous fluids may be needed in some children.
- *Mineral oil* is not recommended in infants.
- *Rectal suppositories* are useful in infants—glycerin suppository 1 g for pediatric size and 2–3 g for adolescents.
- *Rectal enema with* glycerin, sodium phosphate, saline, or dioctyl sodium sulfosuccinate is invasive; not preferred by most children—but may be required in some cases.
- *Rectal digital disimpaction* is quick but invasive; painful, increases defecation phobia though it is effective especially in stubborn children withholding stools. If necessary, it may be done under anesthesia (cases refractory to all measures).
- *Topical applications:* Twice daily anal applications of petroleum jelly, zinc oxide cream, diltiazem, nitroglycerine, or sucralfate with 2% xylocaine jelly using ear bud are effective for painful defecation due to anal cracks.

Maintenance Therapy

Maintenance therapy is aimed to avoid reimpaction and to ensure regular passage of stools with the help of diet modification, laxatives, and behavioral therapy. The caregivers are trained on a simplified use of stool diary and recording of daily stool and defecation details. These include:

- The parents are apprised about the need for long-term treatment and regular follow-up to make sure fecal impaction is not re-established
- Maintenance medication, diet, fluid intake, and exercise, toilet training to be continued for several weeks after regular bowel habits are established.
- *Medication:* PEG 3350 with electrolytes if no fecal impaction.[9]

- *Dose:* Half the dose used for disimpaction regimen (1 g/kg/day). Dose can be adjusted depending on symptoms and response.
- *Side effects:* Nausea, vomiting, and bloating (osmotic effects)
- Add stimulant laxative (lactulose or lactitol for hard stools), if PEG is not effective.
- No abrupt stoppage of treatment

- Initial weekly review for 2–3 weeks with parents and stool diary is helpful.

Fecal Impaction not Responding to PEG—What Next ?

- *Lactitol* should be preferred over lactulose in the management of chronic constipation because of its superior efficacy as adjudged by the physician, better palatability, lesser incidence of adverse events, better acceptance, and compliance reported by patients.
- A combined high dose of *PEG and sodium picosulphate (SPS)* on days 1 and 2 was effective in removing the fecaloma in half of the children.[9]
- Administering high doses for a longer period should be tested to provide outpatient disimpaction for severe fecalomas.
- *Prucalopride* (0.03 mg/kg/day) treatment for 8 weeks demonstrated an apparent favorable efficacy and tolerability profile in children with functional constipation.[10]
- *Lubiprostone* is another effective and well-tolerated agent in children and adolescents with functional constipation.[11]
- Bristol Stool Chart and Stool diary can be handed over to the parents for better follow-up of chronic functional constipation impaction.

Behavioral Therapy

Behavioral therapy includes proper toilet training after feeds, three times daily for 5–10 minutes. One word, one person, one year, one stool/day, one sitting posture policy is ideal. Schoolteachers should be informed about the child's problem and management.

Education and Counseling

- Explain physiological basis of constipation and soiling. The National Institute for Health and Care Excellence (NICE) guidelines recommend that the child should never be blamed for soiling.
- Need to adhere to long-term medication and a regular toilet pattern.[10]
- Avoid antispasmodics and antidiarrheal drugs for pain and fluid fecal soiling (pseudodiarrhea)
- If needed, meeting with teacher in school
- As optimum dose is unpredictable for any child, initial weekly meeting for 2–3 weeks is suggested to help family titrate the dose.

Follow-up Schedule

- *Monthly follow-up* till regular bowel movement is achieved. Check diary, physical, and rectal examination. Laxative dose is to be adjusted.
- *Follow-up of 3 months for next 2 years.* Continue same dose of laxative for at least 3 months (distended bowel to regain its function) and then slow tapering (early withdrawal of laxative is the most common cause of recurrence).
- *Yearly follow-up*

Refractory Constipation

Children with refractory constipation with recurrent impaction, not responding to routine use of laxatives, diet, and behavioral therapy need evaluation of organic diseases and timely referral for specific investigations such as rectal biopsy or to rule out anatomic defects by referral to pediatric surgeons or pediatric gastroenterologists for anorectal manometry, metabolic screen (hypothyroidism, cystic fibrosis, hypercalcemia, celiac disease, lead poisoning, mental retardation, etc.), colonic transit study, colonic manometry or ileo-colonoscopy, and magnetic resonance imaging (MRI) of lumbosacral spine for spinal dysraphism.

These patients, especially school-going children, may need to be diagnosed whether they are functional or organic, or have irritable bowel syndrome (IBS)-constipating type; or if functional whether they are of slow transit or normal transit type or pelvic floor dysfunction (rectoanal dyskinesia) which needs biofeedback training.[2,7]

KEY MESSAGES

- Constipation is a common problem in children and often presents as chronic periumbilical pain with difficulty and delay in passing dry stools.
- Nearly 95% are functional and often does not need any investigation; diagnosis is invariably clinical including rectal examination and long-term follow-up is essential.
- Management includes drugs, diet modification, toilet training, and regular follow-up and behavioral therapy.
- Refractory cases need referral to the pediatric gastroenterologist for further workup to know the cause and for management guidance.

REFERENCES

1. Medscape. (2017). Pediatric Constipation. [online] Available from: https://emedicine.medscape.com/article/928185-overview [Last accessed January, 2024].
2. Srivastava A. Management of functional constipation. Indian J Pediatr. 2008;(Suppl 75):519-25.

3. North American Society for Pediatric Gastroenterology, Hepatology and Nutrition. Evaluation and treatment of constipation in children: Summary of updated recommendations of the North American Society for Pediatric Gastroenterology, Hepatology and Nutrition. J Pediatr Gastroenterol Nutr. 2006;43(3):405-7.
4. Tabbers MM, DiLorenzo C, Berger MY, Faure C, Langendam MW, Nurko S, et al; European Society for Pediatric Gastroenterology, Hepatology and Nutrition; North American Society for Pediatric Gastroenterology. Evaluation and treatment of functional constipation in Infants and children: Evidence-based recommendations from ESPGHAN and NASPGHAN. J Pediatr Gastroenterol Nutr. 2014;58(2):258-74.
5. Aziz I, Whitehead WE, Palsson OS, Tornblom H, Simren M. An approach to the diagnosis and management of Rome IV functional disorders of chronic constipation. Expert Rev Gastroenterol Hepatol. 2020;14(1):39-46.
6. Schmulson MJ, Drossman DA. What is new in Rome IV. J Neurogastroenterol Motil. 2017;23(2):151-63.
7. Thapa BR. Constipation in children. In: Bavdekar A, Matthai J, Sathiyasekaran M (Eds). IAP Speciality Series on Pediatric Gastroenterology. New Delhi: Jaypee Brothers Medical Publishers (P) Ltd.; 2008. pp. 125-44.
8. Tran DL, Sintusek P. Functional constipation in children: What physicians should know. World J Gastroenterol. 2023;29(8):1261-88.
9. Lamanna A, Dughetti LD, Jordan-Ely JA, Dobson KM, Dynan M, Foo A, et al. Treatment of fecal impaction in children using combined polyethylene glycol and sodium picosulphate. JGH Open. 2018;2(4):144-51.
10. Winter HS, Di Lorenzo C, Benninga MA, Gilger MA, Kearns GL, Hyman PE, et al. Oral prucalopride in children with functional constipation. J Pediatr Gastroenterol Nutr. 2013;57(2):197-203.
11. Elkaragy ES, Shamseya MM, Metwally RH, Mansour ER, Lashen SA. Efficacy of lubiprostone for functional constipation treatment in adolescents and children: Randomized controlled trial. J Pediatr Gastroenterol Nutr. 2024;78(4):800-9.
12. National Institute for Health and Care Excellence. (2017). Constipation in children and young people: diagnosis and management. [online] Available from www.nice.org.uk/guidance/cg99 [Last accessed in December, 2024).

11.12 Hirschsprung Disease

Kanishka Das, Suravi Mohanty

INTRODUCTION

Hirschsprung disease (HD), named after Harald Hirschsprung (Danish pediatrician, 1886), is a disorder of bowel motility characterized by uncoordinated peristalsis and functional bowel obstruction. Important clinical observations (delayed neonatal passage of meconium, chronic infantile constipation, dependence on rectal stimulation to move bowels, episodic acute abdominal features suggesting enterocolitis) and operative/autopsy observations (dilated, thick walled sigmoid and transverse colon and a narrow rectum) have historically led to defining the disease. Interestingly, Sushruta's description of *'Baddha Gudodaram'* in 1200 BC resembles HD and was treated with a procedure akin to a colostomy. The first successful modern treatment of HD is credited to Orvar Swenson (1949) who also deduced that the narrow-collapsed segment, not the proximal dilated portion, was the diseased bowel. With a worldwide incidence of 1 in 5,000 livebirths and an overall 4:1 male preponderance, 80–90% of HD occurs sporadically in full-term births and the rest account for the rare genetic/familial/syndromic forms.

EMBRYOLOGY, ETIOPATHOGENESIS AND PATHOPHYSIOLOGY

The ganglion cells originate in the neural crest and migrate aborally along the bowel till the proximal anal canal; further they migrate centripetally into the myenteric plexus and then the submucous plexus. These parasympathetic ganglion cells of the intrinsic enteric nervous system employ nitric oxide as the neurotransmitter and modulate smooth muscle excitatory/inhibitory interactions in the bowel to effect a relaxation during rest and a coordinated antegrade peristalsis of a luminal bolus. HD results from a failure of such migration or destruction of the ganglion cells in a hostile local environment. Additionally, there is a deficiency of intestinal pacemaker cells—the interstitial cells of Cajal (ICC). The resultant loss of receptive relaxation of the distal aganglionic bowel in response to the antegrade propulsive peristalsis of the proximal ganglionic bowel leads to uncoordinated peristalsis and functional bowel obstruction. The extrinsic nerves supplying the bowel respond by proliferation and elaboration of both cholinergic (excitatory) and adrenergic (inhibitory and excitatory) neurotransmitters; the excitatory effects of both predominate to render the aganglionic colon and internal anal sphincter spastic.[1]

CLASSIFICATION

In the classic rectosigmoid form (85%) of HD, the aganglionosis commonly involves the anal canal and the rectum with a transition to normal ganglionic bowel at the sigmoid; rarely the aganglionosis extends proximally into the rest of the colon (long-segment, colonic), terminal ileum [total colonic aganglionosis (TCA)], or more proximally till the esophagus [total intestinal aganglionosis (TIA)]. Such 'long-segment disease' is characterized by relative female preponderance and association with familial, syndromic, and genetic forms. Ultrashort segment HD (USSHD) refers to a localized spasm/achalasia of the internal anal sphincter identifiable at manometry. Indeed, TCA and USSHD are now considered as entities biologically distinct from classical HD.[1]

CLINICAL FEATURES

A clinical presentation of large bowel obstruction presenting at any time from the postnatal period to adulthood, but dating back to infancy or early childhood is characteristic. Currently, nearly 90% is diagnosed in the neonatal period or early infancy. Failure to pass meconium within 48 hours of birth is a cardinal clinical feature seen in 80–90% infants with HD but also with 30–40% children without HD, and 30–35% healthy preterm babies. Symptoms of abdominal distension, poor feeding, nonbilious or bilious vomiting, and progressive constipation are characteristic. Infantile constipation often manifests at weaning, and the recurrent symptom complex of constipation-spurious diarrhea-abdominal distension culminates in failure to thrive during childhood.[1]

Hirschsprung enterocolitis is an immune-mediated toxic fulminant sepsis occurring at any age, even after definitive management is completed. It presents with fever, malaise, foul smelling, and often bloody diarrhea and abdominal distension; sometimes progressing to perforation of the cecum or appendix, particularly in the neonate.

Common associated anomalies include trisomy 21 (5–15%), bowel atresias, and anorectal malformations. HD may be associated with neoplastic or non-neoplastic manifestations of aberrant migration of neural crest cells into the skin, retina, thyroid, adrenal, etc., the "neurocristopathies" [e.g., multiple endocrine neoplasia (MEN) syndromes, neuroblastoma, and skin pigmentation].[2]

The physical findings vary with the presentation; typical features in nonacute states are anemia, malnutrition, gaseous abdominal distension, visible/palpable bowel loops, a spastic tight anus at per rectal examination, and a rectal blast of stool and gas at withdrawal of the finger after per rectal examination **(Figs. 11.12.1A to C)**.

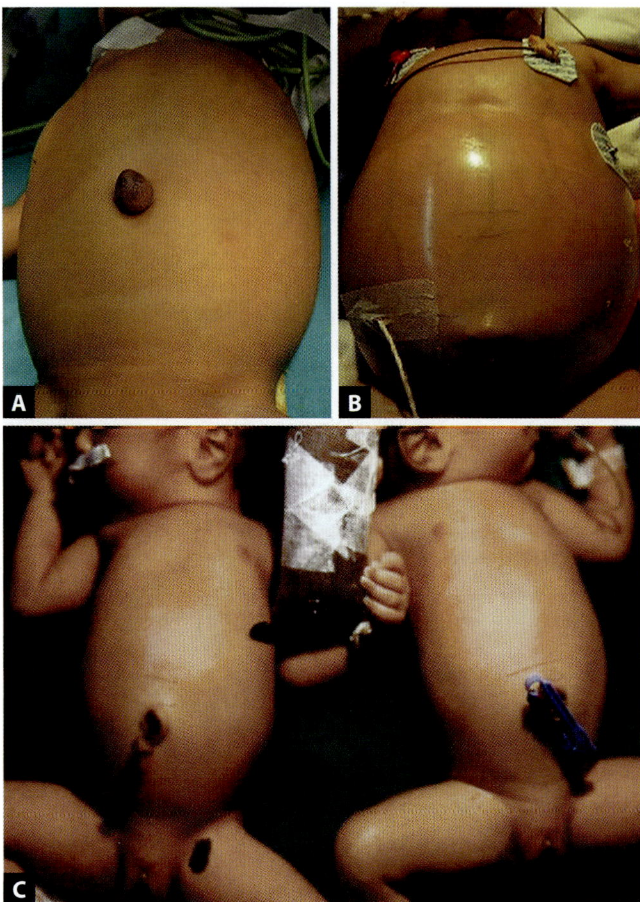

Figs. 11.12.1A to C: Clinical presentation in HD ranges from innocuous generalized abdominal distension in classical HD (A) to acute abdominal signs with enterocolitis; (B) Total colonic aganglionosis (TCA) in twin female neonates; (C) The pigmented skin lesions suggest a neurocristopathy.

DIFFERENTIAL DIAGNOSIS AND INVESTIGATIONS

Although HD is more common than several other conditions that may mimic it in the neonatal period, the differential diagnosis includes meconium plug syndrome, small left colon syndrome (diabetic mother), distal small bowel/ colonic atresia, meconium ileus-cystic fibrosis complex, and other medical conditions such as hypothyroidism and sepsis. Historical clues and clinical features direct the confirmatory investigations. Habitual constipation in the older child can be differentiated from HD by several factors that predominate in the former—a normal meconium history, secondary/ recent onset of constipation, lack of significant abdominal distension, fecal loading of rectum, perianal soiling, poor dietary fiber, evidence of associated voiding disturbances, and psychological overlay. The diagnosis of HD is based on an amalgamation of information from the following investigative modalities.[3]

Anorectal Manometry

The principle of anorectal manometry (ARM) is an absence of the normal rectoanal inhibitory reflex (RAIR)—inhibition of the resting rhythmic activity of the internal anal sphincter with rectal distension in HD (including USSHD). This is preserved in the normal and the habitually constipated child. Though it is minimally invasive and has 75–95% accuracy, it is not widely available and difficult in the young uncooperative child. It may be performed under sedation or anesthesia. Though the RAIR has been detected by 26 weeks of gestation, it is often poorly developed and inconsistent in the term neonate. Anyway, histopathological confirmation of the diagnosis is required prior to surgical intervention.

Radiography

Plain abdominopelvic X-ray and *contrast enema* remain the basic diagnostic investigations that are easily performed and interpreted. An erect plain X-ray showing generalized dilatation of bowel, especially the peripherally placed colonic loops, and an absence of the normal rectal gas shadow in the pelvis, suggest the common rectosigmoid form of HD.

The contrast enema is diagnostic in the majority of rectosigmoid disease **(Figs. 11.12.2A to C)**. A dilated sigmoid and a narrow rectum, a reversed rectosigmoid ratio, and a conical transition zone between the two are characteristic of rectosigmoid HD. The mixed barium-stool picture in the delayed contrast enema film at 24 hours is also reliable. In associated colitis, a saw tooth mucosal contour due to irregular uncoordinated contractions of the aganglionic segment is seen. In distal small bowel obstruction, it clarifies the wide differential diagnosis; the "question mark microcolon" of TCA is typical. Despite precautionary measures and guarded interpretation, a significant false positive/negative rate is recognized in diagnosis of long-segment colonic disease and TCA; further the site and extent of the transition zone is unpredictable on radiology. In conclusion, the contrast enema is a good screening investigation prior to histological confirmation of HD by rectal biopsy.

HISTOPATHOLOGY

Histopathological evaluation is the gold standard for diagnosis with a 93–98% sensitivity and specificity. A rectal biopsy is essential to confirm the diagnosis of all forms of HD and further colonic, appendicular, or ileal biopsies are examined to determine the proximal extent of aganglionosis (levelling). The rectal biopsy may be full or partial (mucosubmucosal) thickness and is taken at least 2 cm above the dentate line to avoid the physiological hypoganglionic anal zone. At laparotomy/laparoscopy, the gross transition zone, where evident, guides the siting of more proximal levelling biopsies. Various histopathological methods are in use (H&E, acetylcholinesterase histochemistry and calretinin immunohistochemistry) for accurate diagnosis and levelling.[4]

The characteristic features of HD on a rectal biopsy are depicted in **Figures 11.12.3A to C**. The histological features in the ganglionic segment (regularly distributed, normal

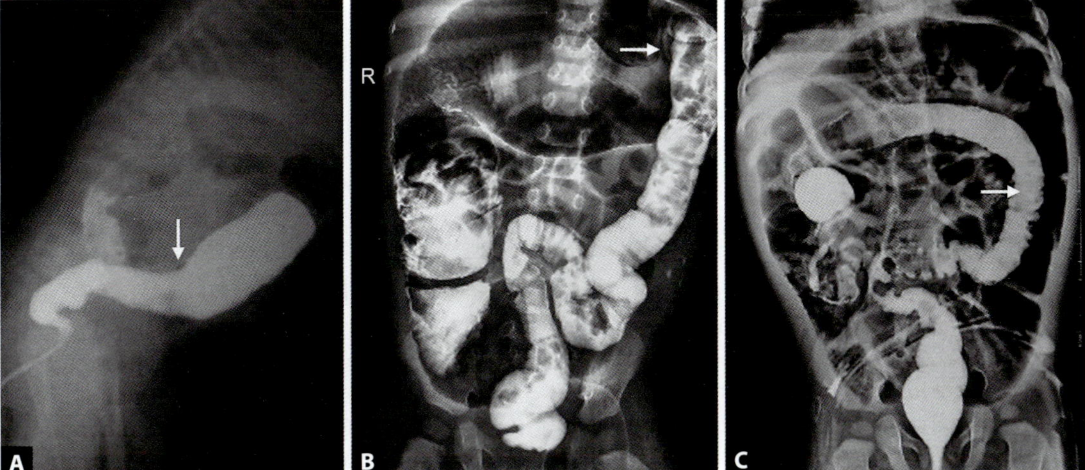

Figs. 11.12.2A to C: Contrast enema findings in varying extents of aganglionosis. Note the transition zone between the narrow rectum and dilated sigmoid in rectosigmoid HD (arrow, A). In this long segment colonic HD (B), the transition (arrow) is at the splenic flexure (arrow, B). The question mark microcolon (arrow, C) and the dilated small bowel in the background are typical of total colonic aganglionosis.

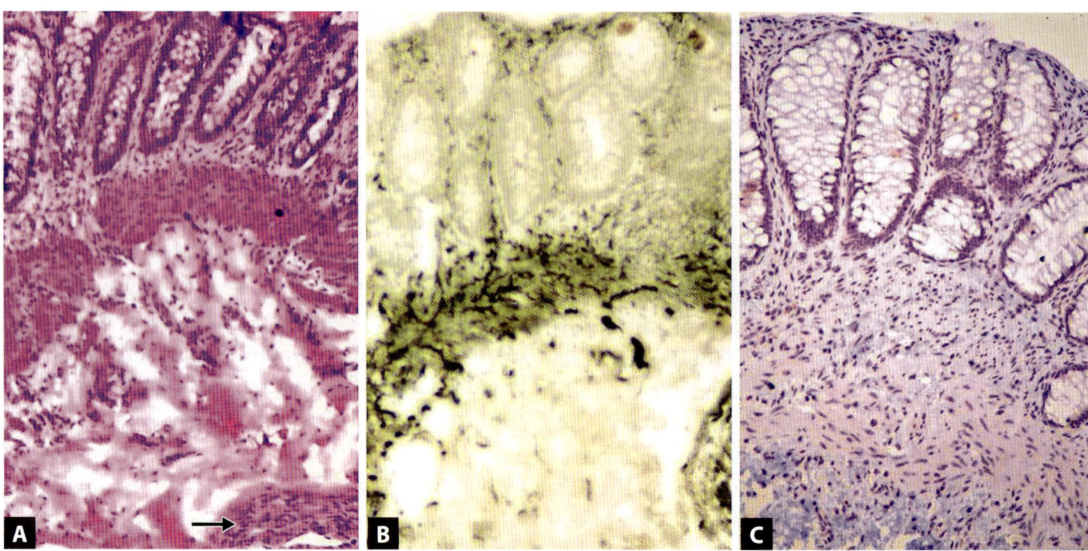

Figs. 11.12.3A to C: Histological confirmation of Hirschsprung disease on a biopsy of the aganglionic rectum. At frozen section evaluation, the H&E stain (A) shows rectal mucosa and submucosa with a hypertrophic nerve bundle in the submucosa (arrow) and absence of ganglion cells. Concurrent acetylcholinesterase stain (B) shows increased cholinergic activity in the mucosa in a typical pattern. Calretinin immunostaining (C) on formalin-fixed tissue shows lack of the normal intrinsic nerve fiber distribution in the muscularis mucosa and lamina propria.

morphology ganglion cells, and normal nerve fibers in the different plexus along the entire circumference), intervening transition segment (randomly present occasional ganglion cells, hypertrophic nerves), and the aganglionic segment (absence of ganglion cells, hypertrophic nerves) guide the levelling. The routine rectal biopsy is normal in USSHD.[3,4]

GENETICS

Hirschsprung disease is multifactorial state with a sex-modified heterogeneous inheritance involving dominant, recessive, and polygenic forms in multiple pathways and >10 genes. The two major gene loci for diagnostic purposes are the long arm of chromosome 10 and the 13q22-*EDNRB* gene. However, variable expressivity and incomplete sex-dependent penetrance have limited attempts at prenatal diagnosis, pedigree analysis, and genetic counseling.[5]

Management

The management of HD is based on the surgical principle of near total or total resection of the aganglionic bowel and apposition of the distal most ganglionic bowel within a centimeter of the dentate line, thus dividing the cranial half of the spastic internal anal sphincter. This may be achieved in a single stage pull through or a staged procedure with initial levelling stoma (ganglionated colostomy or ileostomy) and a subsequent pull through (Duhamel, Soave, Swenson/or their modifications) by an abdominal/transanal, combined, or laparoscopic-assisted procedure at any age depending on the modalities of diagnosis, levelling, and surgical expertise available at a center. Generally, an initial stoma is preferred in poor risk malnourished patients, massively dilated proximal bowel, emergency settings (enterocolitis, bowel perforation, and peritonitis), or nonavailability of intraoperative histological levelling. In TCA, conventional pull-through procedures are generally modified to patch a longitudinal strip of aganglionic colon along the ganglionic ileum to facilitate optimal fluid reabsorption and avert troublesome diarrhea. USSHD is usually amenable to botulinum injections or a transanal longitudinal myotomy/myectomy of the internal anal sphincter.[3]

In toxic acute states without bowel perforation, resuscitation with intravenous fluids, triple antibiotics (beta-lactam, aminoglycosides, and metronidazole), gentle rectal washes with warm saline, and other supportive critical care is vital prior to further surgical management.

PROGNOSIS AND OUTCOME

The majority of HD being sporadic rectosigmoid disease, early management with standard protocols outlined above yields an excellent outcome. Long-term complications or sequel-like frequency of bowel movement, incontinence—perianal soiling, anastomotic strictures, recurrent constipation, residual/secondary aganglionosis, and variable somatic retardation occur in <10%, especially in long-segment disease and TCA and those managed without accurate histological levelling. Associated anomalies and neurocristopathies also influence the outcome.

CONCLUSION

In conclusion, Hirschsprung disease is a common sporadic cause of functional large bowel obstruction in neonates and infants due to bowel aganglionosis. A typical history (delayed meconium passage, constipation, abdominal distension) and suggestive imaging (plain X-ray/contrast enema) is confirmed with histopathology (rectal biopsy) before surgical treatment (laparotomy/laparoscopy and levelling biopsies, single staged pull through or staged management—initial stoma and subsequent pull through) in classic rectosigmoid HD. The long-term outcome is excellent in the majority.

REFERENCES

1. Langer JC. Hirschsprung disease. Curr Opin Pediatr. 2013;25(3):368-74.
2. Teitelbaum DH. Hirschsprung disease and related conditions. Semin Pediatr Surg. 2012;21(4):281-3.
3. Das K, Mohanty S. Hirschsprung Disease—Current Diagnosis and Management. Indian J Pediatr. 2017;84(8):618-23.
4. Ambartsumyan L, Smith C, Kapur RP. Diagnosis of Hirschsprung Disease. Pediatr Dev Pathol. 2020;23(1):8-22.
5. Tang CS, Karim A, Zhong Y, Chung PH, Tam PK. Genetics of Hirschsprung's disease. Pediatr Surg Int. 2023;39(1):104.

SECTION

Disorders of Hepatobiliary System and Pancreas

Section Editor: **John Matthai**

12.1 Approach to Liver Disease

Bhaskar Raju, Sumathi Bavanandam

INTRODUCTION

Liver is the second largest organ in the body performing various functions such as metabolism of carbohydrates, proteins, fats, and drugs; storage of glycogen, fats, and vitamins; detoxification; synthesis of proteins and clotting factors; and excretion of bile. It is actually the metabolic engine of the body. It is no surprise that damage to the liver can cause not only liver-specific signs and symptoms but throw up evidence of dysfunction of other systems as well.

Many insults such as infection, inflammation, toxins, drugs, immune factors, genetic, ischemia, and blockage of venous drainage can affect the liver, manifesting clinically as hepatomegaly or hepatosplenomegaly (HSM) with various clinical symptoms and signs.

HEPATOMEGALY

The mere presence of a palpable liver does not mean pathological hepatomegaly. While in neonates the liver may be palpable 2–3 cm below the costal margin, this is usually <2 cm between 4 and 6 months of age and 1 cm in older children. In general, a liver edge >3.5 cm in newborns and >2 cm in children suggests enlargement.[1,2]

For palpation, wrist and forearm should be in the same horizontal plane. Examination should start from the right iliac fossa with warm fingers pointing toward upward and the sensing fingers (index and middle) lateral to rectus muscle parallel to rectus sheath. With stationary hands during inspiration, lower border of liver can be felt. The fingers should be moved progressively 1 cm at a time between each breath until the costal margin or liver edge is felt. If liver edge is felt it denotes either enlarged or displaced liver. A soft liver, however, may be normally palpable 3 cm in infants and 2 cm in older children, below the costal margin.

Liver Span

Liver span is a better way of defining hepatomegaly, since it helps differentiate between true hepatomegaly and pushed down liver. It is determined by measuring the distance between the upper edge, determined by percussion, and the lower edge, determined by palpation, in the mid-clavicular line. The liver span increases with body height and age **(Table 12.1.1)**. A perception of hepatomegaly can occur without enlargement of liver in inferior displacement by the following:

TABLE 12.1.1: Liver span at various ages.

Age	*Span (in cm)*
Birth	5.6–5.9
2 months	5
1 year	6
2 years	6.5
3 years	7
4 years	7.5
5 years	8
6–12 years	9
Adolescents	10–15

- Diaphragm
- Thoracic organs
- Fluid, pus, or air under diaphragm
- Chest wall deformities
- Riedel's lobe

Retroperitoneal masses, choledochal cysts, and perihepatic abscesses may be mistaken for hepatomegaly.[1,2]

Clinical Description of Hepatomegaly

Clinical description of hepatomegaly should include the following:

- *Size:* Mild/moderate/massive
- *Shape* (symmetric or asymmetric enlargement. Left lobe is enlarged in congenital hepatic fibrosis)
- *Consistency:* Soft/firm/hard
- *Surface:* Smooth/irregular/nodular
- *Edge:* Rounded or sharp
- Tenderness
- Pulsatile or not
- Hepatic rub
- Any bruit

SPLENOMEGALY

The normal spleen lies entirely within the rib cage and is usually not palpable. However, one-third of newborns, 5–15% of children and 3% of young adults, may physiologically have a palpable spleen. The tip of the normal, palpable spleen is soft, smooth, nontender and <1–2 cm below the left costal margin. Inspection may reveal fullness in the left upper quadrant that descends on inspiration indicating splenomegaly. *Bimanual palpation* is done to differentiate from kidney enlargement mimicking spleen. *Middleton maneuver* is done as follows—the examiner is positioned to the patient's left, facing the patient's feet. The fingers of both the examiner's hands are curled under the left costal margin, and the patient is asked to take a long, deep breath as the palpation of a descending spleen is sought. *Percussion* for splenic dullness is performed by one of the several methods (described by Nixon, Castell, and Barkun, or percussion of Traube's semilunar space). Studies have demonstrated sensitivity of 56–71% for palpation and 59–82% for percussion.[1,2]

Splenomegaly is usually secondary to one of the following mechanisms such as infections (malaria, enteric, leptospirosis, and scrub typhus), reticuloendothelial hyperplasia, congestion, or infiltration or space-occupying lesions such as hydatid, congenital cysts, abscesses, and very rarely tumors. However, a palpable spleen might also be the result of visceroptosis, pushed down in conditions in hyperreactive airway disease, pneumothorax, or secondary to malnutrition and rickets.

CLINICAL APPROACH TO HEPATOSPLENOMEGALY

Most cases of HSM are due to hepatobiliary, hematological, or systemic disease **(Table 12.1.2)**. A simple approach to differential diagnosis of HSM would be through the major presenting symptoms or the lack of any major presenting symptom and the age of the child **(Table 12.1.3)**.[1,2]

- *HSM with ascites* is common in cirrhosis, abdominal malignancies, and abdominal tuberculosis (TB).
- *HSM with arthritis* is seen in systemic lupus erythematosus (SLE), juvenile idiopathic arthritis (JIA), sickle cell disease (SCD), and leukemia.

Some children in clinical practice will present with predominantly one organ enlargement, like isolated hepatomegaly or isolated splenomegaly. The common causes of isolated hepatomegaly depending on consistency and tenderness are listed in **Table 12.1.4**.

The differential diagnosis of isolated splenomegaly without significant hepatomegaly is shown in **Table 12.1.5**.

TABLE 12.1.2: Common causes of hepatosplenomegaly.

Hepatobiliary disease	*Hematological disease*	*Systemic causes*
• High-colored urine and pale stools • Clinical evidence of portal hypertension • Cutaneous markers of liver disease • Signs of liver cell failure	• Absence of liver symptoms • Acholuric jaundice • Significant anemia	• Persistent fever • Absence of overt hepatic or hematological symptoms/signs • Generalized adenopathy • Central nervous system (CNS) symptoms

TABLE 12.1.3: Major presenting symptoms in hepatosplenomegaly.

Fever	*Gross pallor*	*Jaundice with high-colored urine*	*CNS symptoms*	*Lymphadenopathy*	*Silent HSM*
<3 years: • Immunodeficiency syndromes • Malignancies • IU infections • Sepsis	*<3 years:* • Beta-thalassemia • Osteopetrosis • Leukemias • Histiocytosis	*<3 years:* • NCS • IU infection • Galactosemia • ICC • Storage (Niemann–Pick disease) • Hepatoma	*<3 years:* • IU infections • Storage diseases • MPS • Mucolipidosis • Wolman disease	• Infectious mononucleosis • Leukemias • Lymphomas • Disseminated tuberculosis • Immune deficiency syndromes	*<3 years:* • Storage • IU infections • Histiocytosis • Rickets • Osteopetrosis
>3 years: • Malaria • Kala-azar • AI hepatitis • Collagen vascular disease/JIA • Tuberculosis	*>3 years:* • Thalassemia intermedia • Post-GI bleed • Lymphomas • AI hepatitis • Wilson disease	*>3 years:* • Wilson disease • Alpha-1-antitrypsin deficiency • Drug-induced CLD • Tyrosinosis • Other MLDs • Hepatitis B • AI hepatitis • Hemochromatosis	*>3 years:* • Wilson disease • Gangliosidosis • GM1/GM2/ Farber disease		*>3 years:* • Compensated cirrhosis any cause • Storage disorders • CAH • Chronic infections • Hepatitis B • Tuberculosis

(AI: autoimmune; CAH: chronic active hepatitis; CLD: chronic liver disease; GI: gastrointestinal; JIA: juvenile idiopathic arthritis; ICC: Indian childhood cirrhosis; IU: intrauterine; MPS: mucopolysaccharidosis; MLD: metabolic liver disease; NCS: neonatal cholestasis syndrome)

TABLE 12.1.4: Common etiologies of isolated hepatomegaly.

Isolated firm/hard hepatomegaly	***Isolated soft/tense/tender hepatomegaly***
• Glycogen storage disease (GSD) • Chronic active hepatitis (early stage) • *Infections:* Early tuberculosis (TB) • Budd–Chiari syndrome • Congenital hepatic fibrosis (left lobe enlargement) • Chronic congestive heart failure • *Space-occupying lesions*: – Hamartoma – Hepatoma – Other malignancies – AV malformations – Hydatid and other cysts	• *Infections:* – Viral hepatitis (A, B, C, D, and E) – Dengue illnesses – TORCH infections – *Bacterial:* Typhoid, leptospirosis, sepsis, abscess, etc. – *Parasites:* Ameba, acute malaria, toxoplasmosis, histoplasmosis, etc. • Ischemic or toxic hepatitis • Reye syndrome • Acute cardiac failure • *Fatty liver:* – Collagen vascular disorders

(AV: arteriovenous; TORCH: toxoplasmosis, rubella, cytomegalovirus, herpes, and other intrauterine infections)

TABLE 12.1.5: Differential diagnosis for isolated splenomegaly.

Isolated firm splenomegaly, without significant hepatomegaly	***Isolated soft splenomegaly, without significant hepatomegaly***
• Extrahepatic portal venous obstruction (EHPO) • Spherocytosis • Splenic vein thrombosis • *Cysts of the spleen*: – Hydatid cyst – Congenital lesions • Chronic malaria in endemic areas • Hemangioma/hamartoma • Hematological malignancies	• *Infections*: – Bacterial typhoid/ septicemia – Nonhepatotropic viral infections • May be normal

Clues in History to Arrive at a Diagnosis[1,2]

- Drug therapy, especially TB, malignancies, and antiepileptic drugs
- Consanguinity, sibling death due to liver disease [inborn errors of metabolism (IEM), e.g., Wilson disease]
- Risk factors for hepatitis B virus (HBV) and hepatitis C virus (HCV) infections
- History of frequent transfusions (e.g., thalassemia), bone marrow dysfunction syndromes, and postviral hepatitis
- History of developmental delay, seizures in glycogen storage disease (GSD), lipidosis, and mucopolysaccharidoses (MPS)
- History of meconium ileus, malabsorption, and recurrent lower respiratory tract infections (LRTI)—cystic fibrosis
- Major presenting symptom and age of onset (referred to above)
- Blindness or deafness [e.g., osteopetrosis, Hunter disease (deafness), and Hurler disease]
- Persistent ear discharge (e.g., Letterer-Siwe disease or histiocytosis)
- Maculopapular rash, infectious mononucleosis, cytomegalovirus (CMV), and hepatitis B (Gianotti–Crosti syndrome)
- Past history of jaundice, gastrointestinal (GI) bleed with or without decompensation in extra-/intrahepatic portal hypertension (PHT)

Clinical Examination (Signs) that Help in Arriving at a Diagnosis[1,2]

General Examination

Ideally children should be examined in a supine position in warm surroundings in a comfortable environment and in a good light. Abdomen should be exposed from xiphisternum to symphysis pubis. Inspection should start from oral cavity. Check the buccal mucosa, tongue and teeth, and oral hygiene. Abnormal odor due to fetor hepaticus is a manifestation of hepatic failure.

Eye Examination

- *Jaundice:* It is yellowish discoloration of mucus membranes and skin that can occur in hemolysis, hepatocellular disease, obstructive biliary disease, or due to inherited disorders of bilirubin metabolism (congenital jaundice). Look for scleral icterus by requesting the child to look up if possible and retract the lower eyelid in natural light.
- *Anemia* can be seen in chronic liver disease (CLD) either due to reduced iron absorption or reduced intake due to anorexia, or due to GI blood loss or hypersplenism.
- *Kayser-Fleischer (KF) ring* is hallmark of Wilson disease and can be identified with naked eye only in older patients, and a similar ring can also be seen in chronic cholestasis and is called as non-Wilsonian KF ring. Infants and toddlers will need slit lamp examination to identify KF ring **(Fig. 12.1.1A)**.
- *Cataract:* Sunflower cataract is typical of Wilson disease. Rarely, cataracts may be seen in intrauterine (IU) infections presenting as neonatal cholestasis.
- *Fundoscopic examination* can reveal bleed secondary to coagulopathy. In young infants and cherry-red spots may be seen in storage diseases such as Niemann-Pick disease, Tay-Sachs disease, and rarely in Gaucher disease **(Fig. 12.1.1B)**.

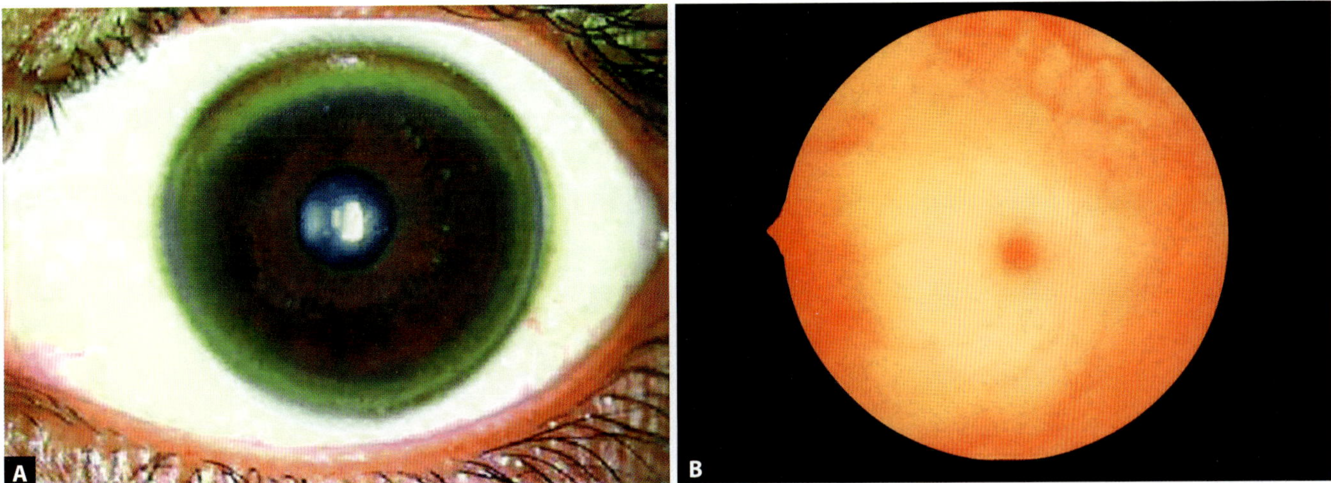

Figs. 12.1.1A and B: (A) Full Kayser–Fleischer (KF) ring, usually seen in untreated adults; (B) Cherryred spot in Tay–Sachs disease.

- *Signs of vitamin A deficiency* like conjunctival or corneal xerosis, Bitot spots, corneal scars, xerophthalmia, and fundal scars may be seen in chronic cholestasis with fat-soluble vitamin deficiencies.
- *Phlycten:* Sometimes phlycten can be seen in hepatobiliary TB.
- *Posterior embryotoxon* may be seen in Alagille syndrome. It often needs a slit lamb examination to visualize the embryotoxon.
- *Xanthelasma:* High-cholesterol levels in GSD and chronic cholestasis might produce xanthelasma visible on the eyelids.

Skin and Musculoskeletal System

- *Spider nevi* are abnormal collection of blood vessels on the skin with a red center and radiating vessels, such as a spider, formed when sphincteric muscles around a cutaneous arteriole fail and surrounding vessels drain the excess blood **(Fig. 12.1.2A)**. They are typically seen in CLD due to failure of liver to metabolize estrone.
- *Palmar erythema:* The same mechanism produces *palmar erythema* as well.
- *Blueberry muffins* may be seen in neonatal hepatitis due to IU infections, especially parvovirus. They indicate extramedullary dermal erythropoiesis **(Fig. 12.1.2B)**.
- *Leukonychia (white nails)* suggest hypoalbuminemia due to CLD **(Fig. 12.1.2C)**. Nails may also show blue lunules in Wilson disease.
- *Scratch marks* over the skin, shiny nails, and hyperpigmented and thick skin over fingers will be seen in chronic cholestatic liver disease caused by itching.
- *Bleeding:* Skin should be examined for *purpura* due to low platelet count, which is due to hypersplenism or functional defects of platelets in CLD. *Ecchymosis* may be seen due to coagulopathy.
- *Clubbing:* It refers to increase in the angle between the nail and nail bed, increased fluctuation in the nail bed, increased curvature of nail in later stages, and increased bulk of the soft tissues over the terminal phalanges. Clubbing is common in long-standing cirrhosis, cystic fibrosis, and in hepatopulmonary syndrome.

Other Common Features

Presence of thyromegaly and parotid enlargement may indicate autoimmune liver disease. Some important features seen on general examination in liver diseases and their probable etiology are listed in **Table 12.1.6**.

Abdominal Examination

Skin of the Abdomen

In tense ascites, skin will be stretched and shiny. Umbilicus will be slightly retracted and inverted in CLD, but may be bulgy in tense ascites. Presence of abnormally prominent veins over the abdomen indicates sinusoidal PHT or hepatic or vena caval obstruction. In PHT due to cirrhosis, recanalization of umbilical vein along the falciform ligament produces distended veins draining away from umbilicus called *caput medusae*. Umbilicus may appear bluish and distended due to umbilical varix **(Figs. 12.1.3A and B)**. Periumbilical erythema may be seen in spontaneous bacterial peritonitis. Scars if any should be noted.

Palpation and Percussion of Liver

If liver edge is felt, it denotes either enlarged or displaced liver. A soft liver, however, may be normally palpable 3 cm in

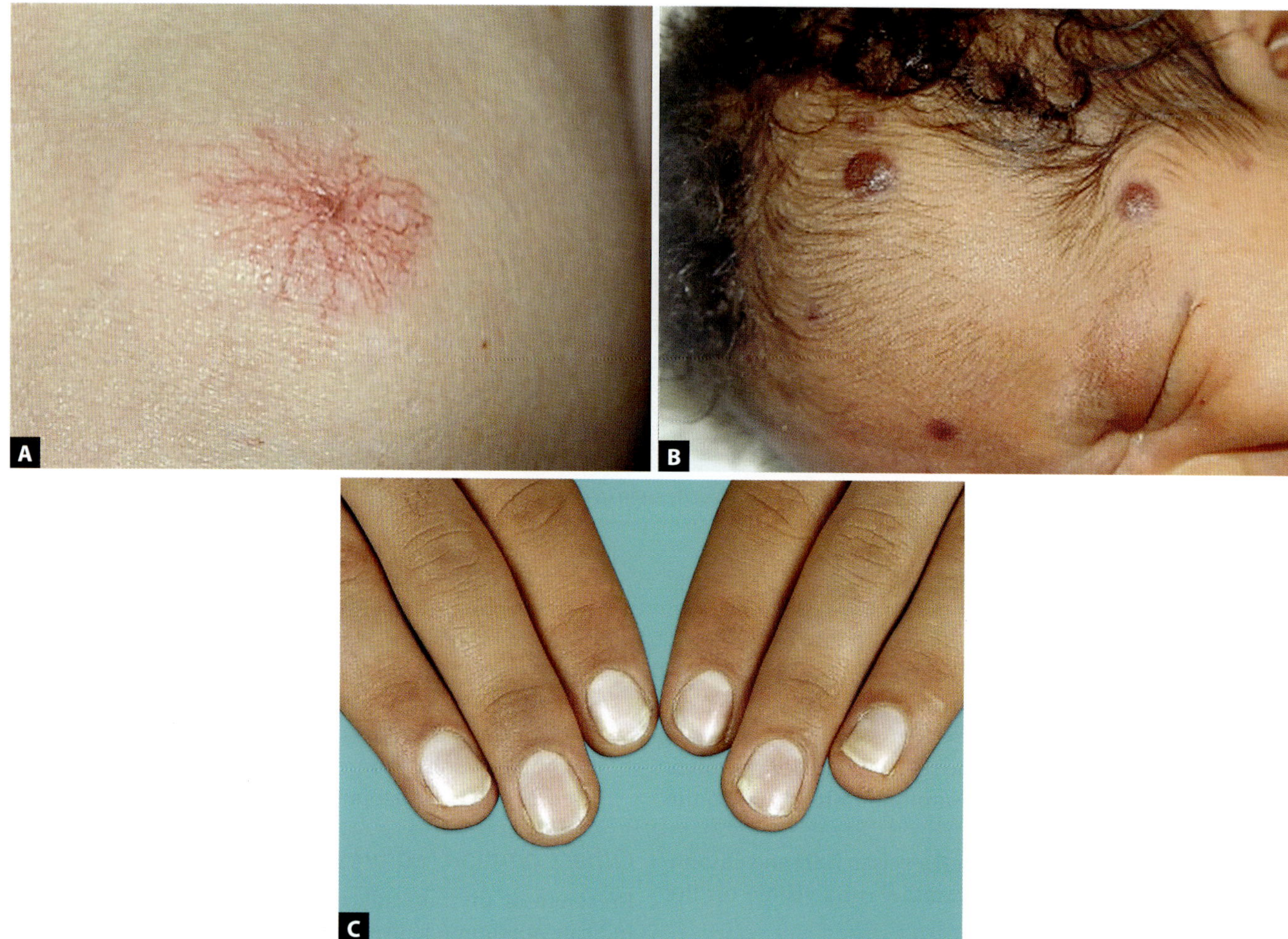

Figs. 12.1.2A to C: Skin manifestations of hepatic disease. (A) Spider naevi; (B) Blueberry muffin spots; (C) White nails or leukonychia.

TABLE 12.1.6: Some important general examination findings in liver disease.

Clinical finding	*Probable diagnosis*
Rickets: • Widening of wrist • Rachitic rosary • Bow legs	• Wilson disease • Tyrosinemia • Glycogen storage disorder (GSD) [glucose transporter, type 2 (GLUT-2) deficiency]
Flapping tremor	Hepatic encephalopathy
Wing beating tremor	Wilson disease
Parotid and/or thyroid swelling	Autoimmune hepatitis
Absent hepatojugular reflex	Budd–Chiari syndrome

infants and 2 cm in older children, below the costal margin. Liver span is a better indicator of pathological hepatomegaly.

Percussion will identify the upper border of the liver, which is usually at the fifth intercostal space at midclavicular line.

Once the liver edge is felt, consistency, size, surface, and tenderness if any should be looked for. *See* **Tables 12.1.4 to 12.1.6** for differential diagnosis.

Sudden inspiratory catch in right upper quadrant indicates acute cholecystitis (Murphy's sign).

Splenomegaly

The spleen has to increase three times the normal to be clinically palpable. Spleen enlarges from left costal margin down and medially toward umbilicus. Presence of splenic notch differentiates it from left kidney. Ischemic injury to spleen like in SCD might make a palpable spleen disappear over time.

Ascites

Fluid collection in abdominal cavity should always be looked for when suspecting liver disease. Shifting dullness and fluid thrill will confirm the presence of ascites. Positive

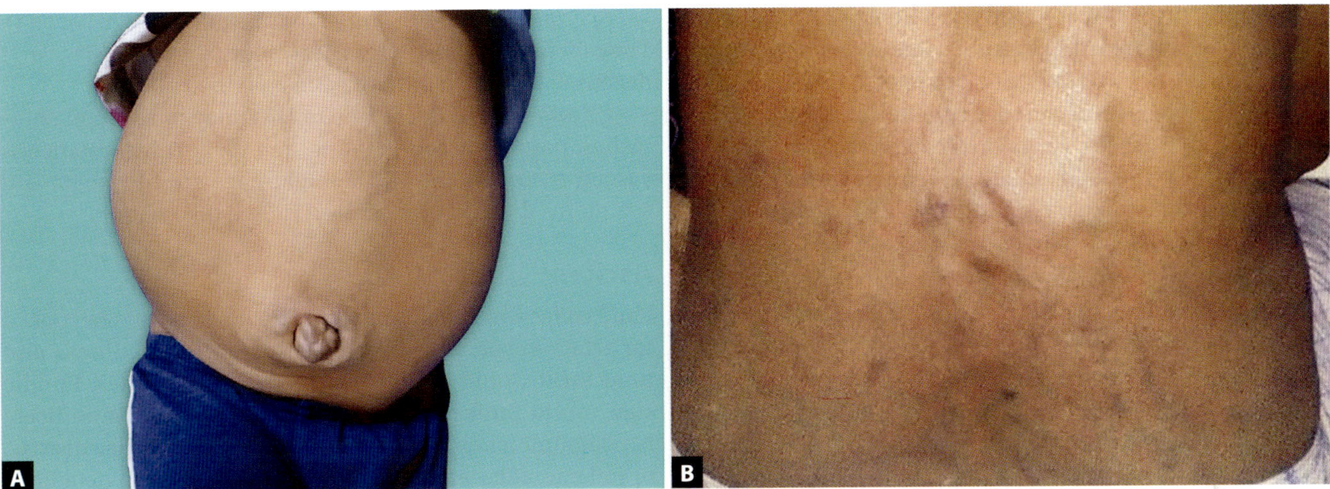

Figs. 12.1.3A and B: Examination of abdomen: (A) Abdominal veins; (B) Dilated veins at the back.

puddle sign indicates minimal ascites. Ascites indicates hypoalbuminemia, CLD with PHT, and associated renal disease, cardiac disease, or inflammatory pathology. They will be discussed in detail in a separate chapter.

Genitalia

Scrotal swelling can be seen with ascites and greenish scrotum would suggest spontaneous perforation of bile duct. Hernial orifices should be examined for any hernias. Complete the examination with a rectal examination for pale stools, fresh bleed, or melena.

Auscultation

With the child lying on the back, placing the diaphragm of the stethoscope to the right of the umbilicus, bowel sounds can be heard as gurgling noises from normal peristalsis. Normally, the bowel sound occurs every 5–10 seconds. Bowel sounds are said to be absent if not heard for 2 minutes. Auscultation of abdomen should include auscultation over liver area for any rub in liver abscess or hepatoma or bruit in vascular tumors and PHT.

SIGNS AND SYMPTOMS OF SPECIFIC LIVER DISORDERS[2]

Acute Hepatitis

Acute hepatitis is a common condition and in majority it is due to hepatotropic viruses and less commonly due to nonhepatotropic viruses. Acute hepatitis due to hepatitis A virus (HAV) can be mild, subclinical, or rarely severe. HCV is usually mild or asymptomatic in children. It may, however, slowly progress to CLD. Hepatitis E virus (HEV) is rare in early childhood, but can cause severe disease in adolescents. HBV runs the whole gamut of acute, subacute, chronic, and asymptomatic infection in pediatrics.

Symptoms of Acute Liver Disease

Acute liver disease particularly viral hepatitis presents with a classic progressive constellation of symptoms.[3]

Prodrome phase presents as fever nausea, vomiting, diarrhea, malaise, loss of appetite, lethargy, and myalgia and lasts 2–7 days. This is followed by the icteric phase, characterized by slow amelioration of prodromal symptoms along with deepening jaundice, high-colored urine, pale stools, and later pruritus if the disease progresses to a cholestatic phase. The icteric phase can last one or several weeks, especially in older children and adolescents. This is followed by recovery phase where the child feels well, eats well, but may be still icteric. The icterus too slowly resolves in 4–6 weeks in majority.

Extrahepatic manifestations can rarely occur in acute viral hepatitis; more commonly in HBV than HBA and more commonly in older children and adolescents. They include evanescent rash, arthritis, glomerulonephritis, leukocytoclastic vasculitis, and very rarely epidermal necrolysis, fatal myocarditis, renal failure, optic neuritis, transverse myelitis, polyneuritis, and cholecystitis.

Symptoms of Pediatric Acute Liver Failure

The causes of pediatric acute liver failure (PALF) include viral, rarely bacterial, ischemic hepatitis, metabolic liver diseases such as tyrosinemia, galactosemia, mitochondrial hepatopathy, urea cycle defects, Wilson disease, neonatal iron storage disease, hemophagocytic syndromes, drugs, and toxins. The signs and symptoms of PALF vary with age and etiology.[4]

A strong suspicion of progression of acute liver disease to acute liver failure (ALF) must be entertained if prodrome symptoms do not resolve with onset of icterus. PALF is recognized by deepening jaundice, rapidly shrinking liver size, development of ascites, coagulopathy, and neuropsychiatric manifestations. Unlike in adults, encephalopathy is not an invariable accompaniment of ALF, and ALF is better defined with alterations in post-vitamin K prothrombin time than presence of encephalopathy.[5]

Alterations in sensorium are used to grade hepatic encephalopathy, when present. Grading has strong connection to prognosis and need for liver transplantation.

- *Grade 1:* Alert restless irritable child with normal neurological reflexes
- *Grade 2:* Irritability increases with brisk reflexes including pupillary and hypertonia
- *Grade 3:* Child is stuporous with decreased tone and hyper-reflexia
- *Grade 4:* Unconscious child, often with evidence of cerebral edema (ALF is discussed in detail in another chapter.)

As hepatic failure progresses, symptoms and signs of coagulopathy, shock, acute renal injury, respiratory failure, and fluid retention, develop. Secondary infections are common and may manifest features of sepsis.

Symptoms of Chronic Liver Disease

Liver disease in children is considered chronic if symptoms referable to liver persist for 3 months or more, or disordered liver function lasts more than 3 months [e.g., increased alanine aminotransferase or aspartate aminotransferase (ALT/AST)]. Some symptoms and signs are specific to CLD and can be used for diagnosis even in the absence of history. Biopsy is the gold standard.[6]

Classic signs and symptoms of CLD include firm hepatomegaly with or without evidence of PHT. The liver, however, shrinks with progression of disease and development of ascites. Hematemesis and melena are common features of CLD. The GI bleed classically is massive, often has clots, always followed by melena and often precipitates encephalopathy, differentiating it from hematemesis due to other causes.

Other characteristics of CLD include firm splenomegaly, ascites (dealt in detail in a separate chapter) edema, anterior abdominal wall veins, periumbilical collaterals (look for veins at the back that enlarge in Budd-Chiari syndrome), growth failure, and muscle wasting. Rickets can occur and when it is obvious do screen for tyrosinosis and Wilson disease. Dupuytren's contracture of palmar facia is rare in pediatrics. Adolescents might show loss of pubic hair, testicular atrophy, and gynecomastia.

Specific skin manifestations may be the first signs of CLD. They include jaundice, xerosis, spider telangiectasias, stria distensae, leukonychia, and palmar erythema.

Chronic liver disease due to HBV may in addition show rashes, papular acrodermatitis, and necrotizing cutaneous vasculitis. Individual CLDs might have specific signs and symptoms that will be discussed later in this chapter.

Ascites

Fluid collection in abdominal cavity should always be looked for when suspecting liver disease. Shifting dullness and fluid thrill would confirm the presence of ascites. Puddle sign would indicate minimal ascites. Ascites can indicate hypoalbuminemia, CLD with PHT, renal and cardiac disease, or inflammatory pathology. They are discussed in detail in a separate chapter.

Extrahepatic Manifestations in Liver Disease

These are detailed in **Table 12.1.7**.

Wilson Disease

Even though Wilson disease usually presents as CLD, it should also be suspected when child presents like acute hepatitis but has palpable firm liver with or without splenomegaly. KF ring is diagnostic but might need slit lamp examination to identify in pediatric age group. KF ring is seen as a greenish yellow, sometimes brown ring 1–3 mm at the periphery of the cornea. It is usually partial in children, visible only in superior and inferior quadrants. Rarely sunflower cataract may be seen. Children with Wilson disease look very dark in complexion because of increased melanin synthesis. Blue lunulae due to copper deposition also may be seen on nails.

TABLE 12.1.7: Extrahepatic manifestations in liver disease.

Symptoms	*Suspect*
• Cataract • Cardiac dysfunction • Hypotonia • Developmental delay • Neuromuscular degeneration • Failure to thrive • Recurrent vomiting • Seizures • Renal involvement	Metabolic liver disease
• Severe abdominal pain • Neuropsychiatric manifestations • Hallucinations • Seizures	Porphyrias
• Failure to thrive • Recurrent vomiting • Irritability • Symptoms of hyperammonemia	Urea cycle disorders

Presence of anemia (hemolytic), arthritis, and bow legs help in the diagnosis of Wilson disease. Central nervous system (CNS) manifestations of Wilson disease such as dystonia and tremors are rare in childhood.

Hepatomegaly in other Diseases

Short stature, cushingoid features (doll-like facies), massive hepatomegaly **(Fig. 12.1.4)** without splenomegaly, early morning seizures, noncholestatic xanthomata, and easy bruising due to platelet dysfunction suggest GSD.

Chronic liver disease with recurrent wheeze suggests *alpha-1 antitrypsin deficiency* and *cystic fibrosis*. Cystic fibrosis often has history of meconium ileus.

Chronic liver disease with mild jaundice with disproportionate pruritus should raise suspicion of *Alagille syndrome*. Additional findings include cardiac lesions (pulmonary stenosis) and typical triangular facies (frontal bossing, deep eye sockets, hypertelorism, and small mandible with pointy chin). Posterior embryotoxon and high myopia may be present **(Fig. 12.1.5)**. While many typical bone changes are present in Alagille syndrome, they can be identified only by X-ray and not on clinical examination. Clinically, however, curved distal phalanges might be identifiable.

Neonatal Cholestasis

Cholestasis in neonates and infants are due to either hepatocellular damage, biochemical defects in bile secretion by hepatocytes (intrahepatic cholestasis), or physical obstruction (extrahepatic cholestasis) to bile flow. Clinical examination will need to focus on differentiating the three, since early diagnosis of biliary atresia is associated with better prognosis. Icterus with history of high-colored urine and pale stools with hepatomegaly or hepatosplenomegaly is sine quo non of cholestasis in neonatal period and infancy. **Table 12.1.8** details the differences between intrahepatic and extrahepatic cholestasis.

Presence of micro- or macrocephaly, cataract, growth retardation, petechia, purpura, HSM, and cardiac defects should raise suspicion of IU infections.

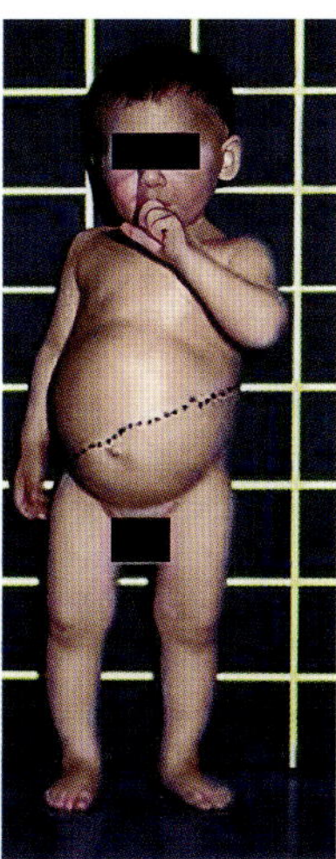

Fig. 12.1.4: Glycogen storage disease: Massive hepatomegaly with short stature.

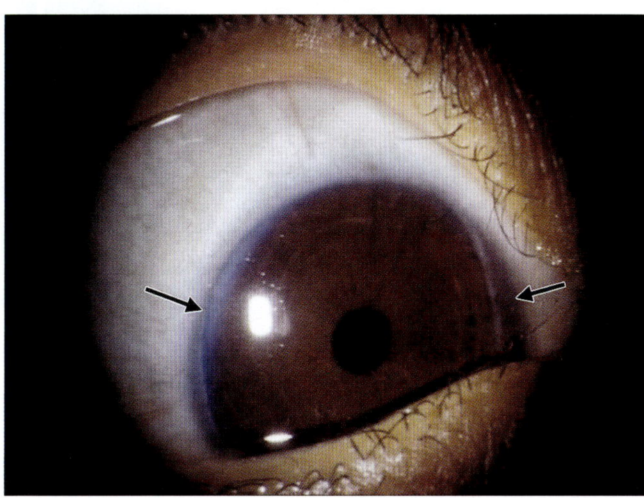

Fig. 12.1.5: Posterior embryotoxon with Schwalbe lines.

TABLE 12.1.8: Differences between intrahepatic and extrahepatic cholestasis.

Clinical features	*Intrahepatic cholestasis*	*Extrahepatic cholestasis*
Appearance	Usually sick-looking child, although in idiopathic giant cell hepatitis baby might appear normal	Well child except for icterus
Onset of jaundice	Early, soon after birth	Usually delayed by few weeks
Gestation	May be preterm or have intrauterine growth restriction (IUGR)	• Usually term • Normal birth weight
Skin	• Blueberry muffin spots may be seen in intrauterine infections • Rashes	Usually normal
Abdomen examination	Early splenomegaly	• Splenomegaly late • Asplenia possible
Other system involvement	May occur, especially in intrauterine infections	Other systems usually normal
Cataract	May occur	Not seen
Stools	Pale or light yellow	Clay colored
Growth retardation	Possible	Usually grow well first few months
Ecchymosis	Late	Early

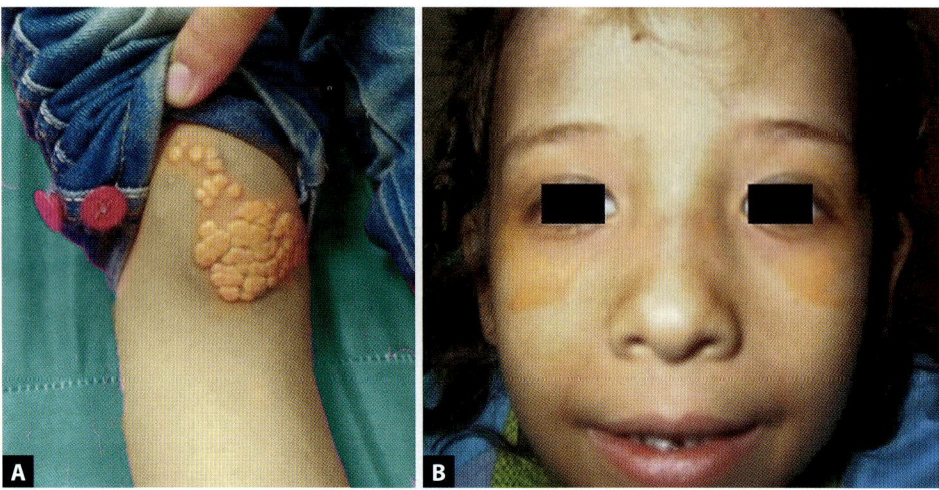

Figs. 12.1.6A and B: (A) Xanthomas; (B) Xanthelasma.

In older children presenting with jaundice of cholestatic type, look for Alagille syndrome (described earlier) and choledochal cyst (mass may be palpable).

Progressive Familial Intrahepatic Cholestasis

Progressive familial intrahepatic cholestases (PFICs) are important though rare causes of neonatal cholestasis.

- *PFIC 1 (mild):* Suspect when there is intermittent cholestasis with transient improvement in between.
- *PFIC 1 (severe):* Recurrent pancreatitis, recurrent diarrhea, failure to thrive, early rickets, and deafness are hallmarks.
- *PFIC 2:* Intense cholestasis like the PFIC 1 severe form, but no history of recurrent pancreatitis or diarrhea
- *PFIC 3:* Also presents with intense cholestasis and diagnosed by markedly raised gamma-glutamyl transpeptidase (GGTP), with normal cholesterol levels while the other two PFICs have normal GGTP.

Biopsy, blood investigations, and genetic studies help differentiate different PFICs.

Pruritus

Pruritus is hallmark of cholestatic liver disease, and its severity is unrelated to intensity of jaundice. Acute hepatitis in older children often goes into a cholestatic phase, which is benign. Chronic cholestasis presents with intense itching. Itching is rare in newborn period and soon after, but becomes obvious once baby develops hand control and starts scratching. In Alagille syndrome, intense pruritus is often the predominant symptom while icterus is minimal.

Xanthoma

Biliary obstruction blocks the only excretory pathway available for cholesterol excretion, and it is not surprising very high values are seen in chronic cholestasis. This leads to deposition of cholesterol in the dermis and subcutaneous tissue causing brownish nodules called xanthomas. They are seen early on the extensor surfaces of extremities, and later they may spread to rest of the body. Flat or slightly raised yellowish brown lesions may be seen on eyelids called xanthelasmas **(Figs. 12.1.6A and B)**.

CONCLUSION

A detailed history and a careful clinical examination are usually sufficient to arrive at a provisional diagnosis in hepatic disorders. First assess if it is liver disease, and if suggestive of liver disease, if it is acute or subacute (fluid retention within 8 weeks of liver-associated symptoms; rare in children) or chronic. Next step is defining if it is parenchymal disease or biliary disease. The third step would be to narrow down the etiology.

REFERENCES

1. Raju B, Bavanandam S. Examination. In: Mathai J, Sathiyasekaran M, Shanmugam N (Eds). Textbook of Pediatric Hepatology. Hyderabad: Paras Medical Publishers; 2023. pp. 24-7.
2. Raju B, Bavanandam S. Signs and symptoms of specific liver disorders. In: Mathai J, Sathiyasekaran M, Shanmugam N (Eds). Textbook of Pediatric Hepatology. Hyderabad: Paras Medical Publishers; 2023. pp. 28-32.
3. Devictor D, Tissieres P, Afanetti M, Debray D. Acute liver failure in children. Clin Res Hepatol Gastroenterol. 2011;35(6-7):430-7.
4. Alam S, Lal BB. Metabolic Liver Diseases Presenting as Acute Liver Failure in Children. Indian Pediatr. 2016;53(8):695-701.
5. Di Giorgio A, Bartolini E, Calvo PL, Cananzi M, Cirillo F, Della Corte C, et al. Diagnostic Approach to Acute Liver Failure in Children: A Position Paper by the SIGENP Liver Disease Working Group. Dig Liver Dis. 2021;53(5):545-57.
6. Mieli-Vergani G, Vergani D. Approach to a child with chronic liver disease. J Gastroenterol Hepatol. 2004;19(s7):S377-8.

12.2 Ascites

Lalit Bharadia

INTRODUCTION

Ascites is derived from Greek word "askites" and "askos" meaning bag, bladder, or belly and is defined as pathological accumulation of fluid in the peritoneal cavity.[1] Successful treatment of ascites depends upon an accurate diagnosis of its cause.

In the normal liver, blood flow from the hepatic artery and portal vein perfuses the hepatic sinusoids and then leaves the liver through the hepatic veins to the inferior vena cava. Hepatic lymph is formed by the filtration of sinusoidal plasma into the space of Disse (bordered by hepatocytes on one side and sinusoidal lining cells on the other). It drains from the liver via the transdiaphragmatic lymphatic vessels to the thoracic duct, which empties into the left subclavian vein. In the intestines, blood from the mesenteric capillaries drains via the mesenteric veins into the portal vein. Intestinal lymph drains from regional lymphatics and ultimately combines with hepatic lymph in the thoracic duct.

Ascites from portal hypertension occurs when high hydrostatic and osmotic pressures within hepatic and mesenteric capillaries produce a net transfer of fluid from blood vessels to lymphatic vessels at a rate that exceeds the drainage capacity of the lymphatics.

ETIOLOGY

The common causes of ascites in infants and children include liver, renal, and cardiac disorders. Other causes include hypoproteinemia, secondary to malabsorption or protein-losing enteropathy, serositis, abdominal tuberculosis, malignancy, and special types of ascites such as pancreatic, biliary, or chylous ascites. A list of causes of ascites in infants and children is given in **Table 12.2.1**.

Ascites can be broadly divided into portal hypertensive and nonportal hypertensive causes. Ascites due to portal hypertension may be due to either causes at the hepatic (sinusoidal) or posthepatic (postsinusoidal) levels. Extrahepatic or presinusoidal portal hypertension seldom causes ascites. While primary liver disease causing cirrhosis causes "sinusoidal" level portal hypertension, hepatic venous outflow tract obstruction state like Budd–Chiari syndrome and cardiac causes like constrictive pericarditis, causing congestive hepatomegaly may result in "postsinusoidal" portal hypertension.

TABLE 12.2.1: Causes of ascites in infants and children.

Hepatobiliary	***Gastrointestinal***	***Neoplasm***
Cirrhosis	Pancreatitis	Lymphoma
Congenital hepatic fibrosis	Peritonitis	Neuroblastoma
Budd–Chiari syndrome	Acute appendicitis	Wilms tumor
Bile duct perforation		Mesothelioma
Chylous ascites	***Genitourinary***	***Pseudoascites***
Intestinal lymphangiectasia	Nephrotic syndrome	Omental cyst
Lymphatic duct obstruction or trauma	Peritoneal dialysis	Ovarian cyst
Serositis	***Cardiac***	
Systemic lupus erythematosus (SLE)	Heart failure	
Henoch–Schönlein purpura (HSP)	Constrictive pericarditis	

Ascites is the most common complication of cirrhosis and indicates chronic liver disease (CLD). This usually marks the transition from compensated to decompensated stage of liver disease. Unless there is a treatable cause of liver disease such as Wilson disease, autoimmune hepatitis, hereditary fructose intolerance, or galactosemia, most children with decompensated liver disease will eventually need orthotopic liver transplantation.

The persistence of ascites in cirrhosis poses an increased risk for complication such as spontaneous bacterial peritonitis (SBP) and hepatorenal syndrome. SBP needs to be recognized even in the absence of fever and treated with antibiotics (usually third generation cephalosporin). In the initial stages, ascites in the compensated liver disease can be well managed or controlled with diuretic and/or albumin infusions. Large volume ascites causing respiratory distress may need therapeutic paracentesis. The ascites is called refractory when these measures fail to control the ascites. Children with refractory ascites often develop hepatorenal syndrome, and orthotopic liver transplantation remains the definitive curative procedure.

CLINICAL MANIFESTATIONS

The child is asymptomatic when ascites is mild. As ascites increases, abdominal fullness, distension, and difficulty in walking and breathing set in. Sometime ascites is associated with edema of feet, periorbital puffiness, or anasarca, depending upon the etiology of ascites. Abdomen is distended with everted umbilicus. Sometime there is presence of scrotal edema or development of abdominal hernias.

A grading system of ascites proposed by International Ascitic Club is as follows:[2]

- *Grade 1:* Mild ascites, detected only by ultrasound examination
- *Grade 2:* Moderate ascites, causing some abdominal distension and presence of flank dullness and shifting dullness
- *Grade 3:* Gross ascites causing significant abdominal distension and positive fluid thrill

An older system that grades ascites from 1+ to 4+ is also used. In this system 1+ is minimal and barely detectable, 2+ is moderate, 3+ is massive but not tense, and 4+ is massive and tense.

DIAGNOSIS

The diagnosis of ascites is established with a combination of physical examination and abdominal imaging (usually ultrasonography). Once the diagnosis of ascites is made, the next step is to look for the cause. An algorithmic approach for diagnosis of etiology of ascites is provided in **Flowchart 12.2.1**.

Paracentesis and Evaluation of Ascitic Fluid

Abdominal paracentesis and evaluation of ascitic fluid (AF) are the most useful tests to diagnose the cause of ascites. Paracentesis is indicated when ascites first appears, at the time of hospitalization or when there is clinical deterioration, unexplained fever, or abdominal pain. Bedside diagnostic paracentesis is a simple procedure that can be performed safely even in sick children with coagulopathy.

Two of the main issues that arise regarding ascites are:

1. Is the fluid infected?
2. Is portal hypertension present?

The routine tests to answer these questions are done on the first AF sample. Additional tests may be indicated based on the clinical setting and results of initial testing. Initial tests include:

- Appearance assessment (e.g., clear, bloody, cloudy, or milky)
- Serum-ascites albumin gradient (SAAG) determination
- Cell count and differential–absolute neutrophil count $\geq 250/mm^3$ is suggestive of SBP and needs starting of antibiotic therapy.
- Total protein concentration

The ascitic white blood cell and neutrophil counts need to be corrected in patients in whom the tap yielded a blood-stained sample. One white blood cell should be subtracted from the white blood cell count for every 750 red blood cells to yield the "corrected white blood cell count," and one neutrophil should be subtracted from the absolute neutrophil

Flowchart 12.2.1: Approach to etiological diagnosis of ascites based on ascitic fluid analysis.

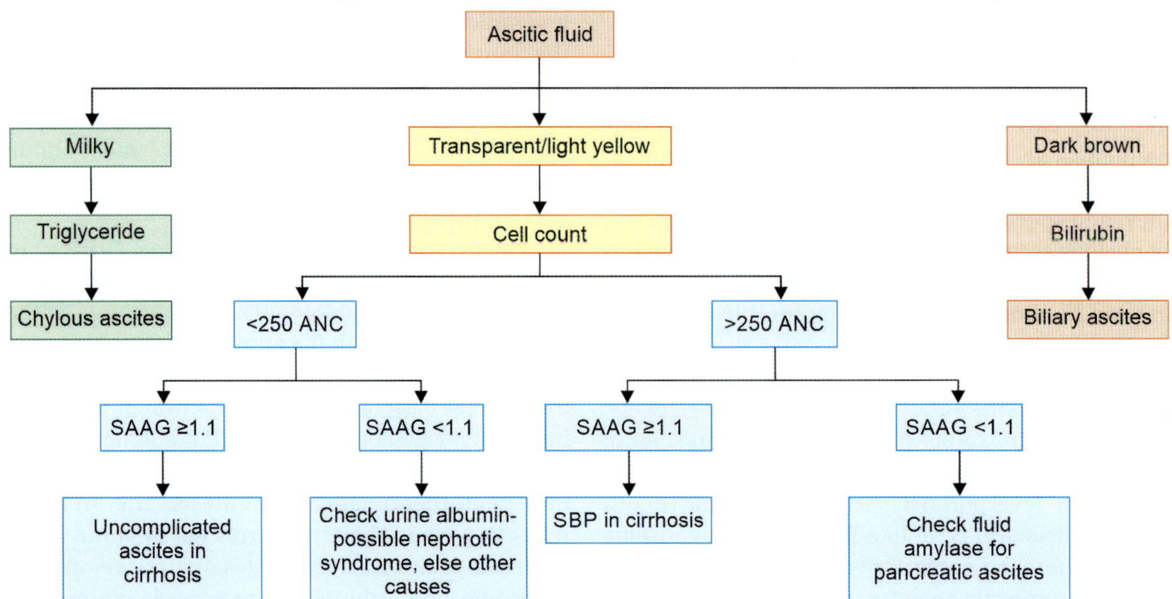

(ANC: absolute neutrophil count; SAAG: serum-ascites albumin gradient; SBP: spontaneous bacterial peritonitis)

count for every 250 red blood cells to yield the "corrected neutrophil count".

Patients with AF that has a corrected neutrophil count ≥250 cells/mm^3 and meets two out of the following three criteria are unlikely to have SBP and warrant immediate evaluation to determine if bowel perforation into ascites has occurred:

1. Total protein >1 g/dL
2. Glucose <50 mg/dL (2.8 mmol/L)
3. LDH greater than the upper limit of normal for serum

Additional tests that may be performed to aid in confirming a diagnosis include:

- Culture with bedside inoculation of aerobic and anaerobic blood culture bottles (infection, or bowel perforation)
- Glucose concentration (malignancy, infection, or bowel perforation)
- Lactate dehydrogenase (LDH) concentration (malignancy, infection, or bowel perforation)
- Gram stain (suspected bowel perforation)—approximately 10,000 bacteria/mL are required for detection by Gram stain.
- Amylase concentration (pancreatic ascites or bowel perforation)—in pancreatic ascites, the AF amylase concentration is approximately 2,000 IU/L, and the AF/serum ratio is approximately 6.0.[3]
- Tuberculosis smear, culture, and adenosine deaminase activity (tuberculous peritonitis)
- Cytology (malignancy)
- *Triglyceride concentration (chylous ascites):* Milky fluid usually has a triglyceride concentration that exceeds the serum concentration, is >200 mg/dL, and is often >1,000 mg/dL. Such specimens are referred to as "chylous ascites."[4]
- *Bilirubin concentration (bowel or biliary perforation):* AF bilirubin value greater than the serum suggests bowel or biliary perforation into ascites.

These additional tests may be performed with the initial paracentesis if there is clinical suspicion for a particular disorder, or they may be performed on a subsequent paracentesis based on the results of initial testing.

Serum-ascites Albumin Gradient

Serum-ascites albumin gradient is a very useful test for classification of ascites into portal hypertensive and nonportal hypertensive causes of ascites. **Table 12.2.2** shows common causes of these two groups. SAAG ≥1.1 suggests underlying portal hypertension with 97% accuracy, and SAAG <1.1 is nonportal hypertensive cause. The SAAG accurately identifies the presence of portal hypertension and is more useful than the protein-based exudate/transudate concept.[5] The SAAG is easily calculated by subtracting the AF albumin value from the serum albumin value, which should be obtained the same day.

TABLE 12.2.2: Causes of ascites based on serum-ascites albumin gradient (SAAG).

High SAAG ≥1.1	*Low SAAG <1.1*
Cirrhosis	Nephrotic syndrome
Budd–Chiari syndrome	Peritoneal tuberculosis
Congenital hepatic fibrosis	Pancreatitis
Portal vein thrombosis	Serositis
Noncirrhotic portal fibrosis	Tumors
Heart failure/constrictive pericarditis	

Imaging

Ultrasound is probably the most cost-effective modality.[6] Patients suspected of having ascites based on history and physical examination should undergo imaging to confirm the presence of ascites and to look for evidence of cirrhosis or portal hypertension. This includes assessment of the size and patency of portal vein, hepatic vein, and inferior vena cava.

DIFFERENTIAL DIAGNOSIS

The differential diagnosis of ascites includes abdominal obesity, giant ovarian or mesenteric cyst, and bowel obstruction (mechanical or functional). Obesity decreases the accuracy of the abdominal examination. These entities can typically be differentiated from ascites based on physical examination findings and abdominal imaging.

MANAGEMENT

Management of ascites involves symptomatic treatment and treatment of the underlying cause.

Cirrhotic Ascites

- *Salt restriction:* In infants and children, sodium is restricted to a maximum of 1–2 mEq/kg/day (1 g of table salt contains 17 mEq of sodium). Water restriction is necessary only if serum sodium is <125 mEq/L.
- *Diuretics:* Spironolactone in the dosage of 2–3 mg/kg/day is the first choice as a single dose in the morning. It counteracts hyperaldosteronism, which is responsible for renal sodium retention.
  Combination therapy of aldosterone antagonist and a loop diuretic may be beneficial in certain circumstances. Furosemide in the dosage of 1 mg/kg/day may be added to spironolocatone.
- *Albumin infusion* may be worthwhile if serum albumin is less to maintain it above 2.5 g/dL.
- *Large volume paracentesis* is reserved for diuretic-resistant severe ascites.
- *Refractory ascites*: Additional therapy in the form of transjugular intrahepatic portosystemic shunt (TIPSS) or liver transplantation is required.
- *Prevention of SBP:* Norfloxacin in a dosage of 5–7.5 mg/kg once daily is recommended long-term in cirrhotic patients.

The treatment of ascites due to nonliver disease depends on the underlying condition.

CHYLOUS ASCITES

The therapeutic options include a trial of conservative therapy with diet control with low-fat, medium-chain triglyceride (MCT) diet. If this is not helpful, one may need additional measures such as total parenteral nutrition, medical treatment with somatostatin analogs such as octreotide, and large volume paracentesis with the addition of sclerosing age.

CONCLUSION

Ascites in children occur due to a variety of causes within and outside the abdomen. Ascites can be broadly divided into portal hypertensive and nonportal hypertensive causes based on the serum ascites albumin gradient. The treatment depends upon the primary cause.

REFERENCES

1. Giefer MJ, Murray KF, Colletti RB. Pathophysiology, diagnosis, and management of pediatric ascites. J Pediatr Gastroenterol Nutr. 2011;52(5):503-13.
2. Moore KP, Wong F, Gines P, Bernardi M, Ochs A, Salerno F, et al. The management of ascites in cirrhosis: report on the consensus conference of the International Ascites Club. J Hepatol. 2003;38(1):258-66.
3. Runyon BA. Amylase levels in ascitic fluid. J Clin Gastroenterol. 1987;9(2):172-4.
4. Press OW, Press NO, Kaufman SD. Evaluation and management of chylous ascites. Ann Intern Med. 1982;96(3):358-64.
5. Runyon BA, Montano AA, Akriviadis EA, Antillon MR, Irving MA, McHutchison JG. The serum-ascites albumin gradient is superior to exudate-transudate concept in the differential diagnosis of ascites. Ann Intern Med. 1992;117(3):215-20.
6. Rudralingam V, Footit C, Layton B. Ascites matters. Ultrasound. 2017;25(2):69-79.

12.3 Portal Hypertension

Somashekara HR

INTRODUCTION

Portal hypertension (PHTN) occurs when there is increased portal resistance and/or increased portal blood flow. Normal portal venous pressure is 10 mm Hg (14 cmH_2O). Direct measurement of portal pressure is clinically impractical and cumbersome. The indirect way of estimating of portal pressure is by the measurement of the hepatic venous pressure gradient (HVPG), which is the difference between hepatic venous wedge pressure and free hepatic venous pressure. When the blood flow in the hepatic venous channels is obstructed by a catheter, the proximal static column of blood in the hepatic veins communicates with the hepatic sinusoids reflecting sinusoidal pressure. Normal HVPG is between 1 and 5 mm Hg. HVPG of 6 mm Hg or more suggests the presence of PHTN. Values ≥10 mm Hg suggests clinically significant PHTN, and those >12 mm Hg predisposes to rupture of esophageal varices.

Portal hypertension develops when resistance to portal blood flow increases. This resistance can be within the liver, as in cirrhosis. It can also be outside of the liver, such as prehepatic in portal vein thrombosis or posthepatic in the case of constrictive pericarditis or Budd-Chiari syndrome. Identification of the level of resistance to portal blood flow allows the determination of the cause of PHTN **(Fig. 12.3.1)**.

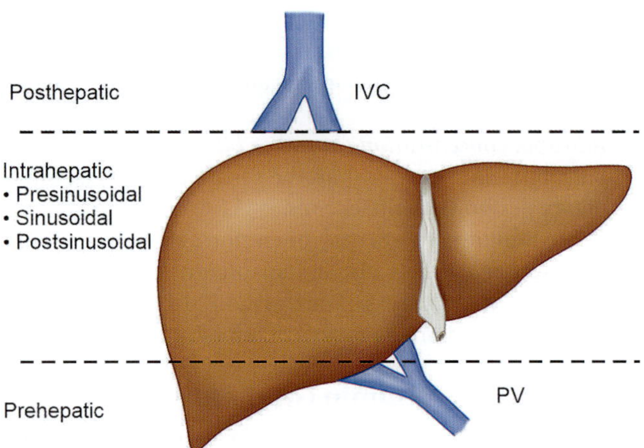

Fig. 12.3.1: Portal hypertension categories: (1) Prehepatic or (2) intrahepatic subcategorized into presinusoidal, sinusoidal, postsinusoidal, and (3) posthepatic. (IVC: inferior vena cava; PV: portal vein)

CAUSES OF PORTAL HYPERTENSION

There are numerous causes of PHTN. The etiology of PHTN can be classified as prehepatic, intrahepatic, or posthepatic causes **(Fig. 12.3.1 and Table 12.3.1)**.[1]

TABLE 12.3.1: Causes of portal hypertension in children.

Prehepatic		• Splenic vein thrombosis • Portal vein thrombosis • Congenital stenosis of the portal vein • Arteriovenous fistula • Tropical splenomegaly
Intrahepatic	Presinusoidal	• Noncirrhotic portal fibrosis (NCPF) • Congenital hepatic fibrosis • Early primary biliary cirrhosis • Schistosomiasis • Granulomatous disease
	Sinusoidal	• Autoimmune hepatitis • Hepatitis B and C • Alfa-1 antitrypsin deficiency • Wilson disease • Biliary atresia • Primary sclerosing cholangitis • Cystic fibrosis • Caroli disease • Familial cholestasis syndromes (Progressive familial intrahepatic cholestasis, PFIC)
	Postsinusoidal	• Veno-occlusive disease • Phlebosclerosis of hepatic veins • Primary vascular malignancies
Posthepatic		• Budd–Chiari syndrome • Congestive heart failure • Inferior vena cava obstruction • Constrictive pericarditis

- *Prehepatic PHTN:* This occurs due to increased blood flow or obstruction within the portal vein or splenic vein. Blockage of portal or splenic vein commonly occurs due to thrombosis known as extrahepatic portal vein obstruction (EHPVO) or it may be due to invasion or compression of these veins by tumors. Increased blood flow can be secondary to idiopathic tropical splenomegaly, arteriovenous malformations, or fistula.
- *Intrahepatic PHTN:* It is further subclassified into presinusoidal, sinusoidal, or postsinusoidal.
- *Posthepatic PHTN:* Posthepatic causes can be at the level of the heart, hepatic vein, as in Budd–Chiari syndrome, or inferior vena cava (IVC). Causes at the level of the heart are due to a rise in atrial pressure, as seen in constrictive pericarditis. Common reasons for IVC obstruction include stenosis, thrombosis, webs, or tumor invasion.

Irrespective of etiology, all forms of PHTN are characterized by the triad of (1) splenomegaly, (2) dilated, blocked, or transformed portal vein on ultrasonography, and (3) presence of varies on endoscopy.

CLINICAL FEATURES

The most common cause of PHTN in children in developing countries is EHPVO, wherein there are no signs and symptoms of liver disease. Patients may present with signs of liver disease, if the underlying cause of PHTN is the damage of liver parenchyma. Clinical features depend on two essential factors—the site of the obstruction and the presence or absence of cirrhosis.[1]

Gastrointestinal Bleeding

Gastrointestinal (GI) bleeding is a common presenting symptom in children, which can be potentially life-threatening. Bleeding from GI tract commonly presents as hematemesis or melena, usually from ruptured esophageal varix. GI hemorrhage can also be secondary to portal hypertensive gastropathy, gastric, duodenal, peristomal, or rectal varices. Variceal hemorrhage is the result of increased pressure within the varix, which leads to increased wall tension. When the tension exceeds the variceal wall strength, rupture of the varix occurs. The sentinel bleeding episode may occur across a wide range of ages, starting as early as 2 months of age. Variceal bleeding in children often follows an acute upper respiratory infection, fever, or drug ingestion. The combination of factors including increased abdominal pressure from coughing or sneezing, increased cardiac output from fever, and ulceration from medications such as nonsteroidal anti-inflammatory drugs or aspirin contribute to the rupture of varices. About 70% of the EHPVO patients present with upper GI bleeding. Since the liver parenchyma is not involved and well preserved in these patients, almost all children with EHPVO will have a normal liver function.

Portal Hypertensive Gastropathy

Portal hypertensive gastropathy refers to changes in the mucosa of the stomach in patients with PHTN. It ranges from erythema to diffuse gastritis. It is an occasional cause of upper GI bleeding. Most commonly it causes iron deficiency anemia due to chronic blood loss, which may also manifest as melena.

Splenomegaly

Splenomegaly is the second most common finding in children with PHTN. In many instances, an enlarged spleen is first discovered on routine physical examination. Many children may present with a vague fullness in the left upper quadrant for many years, prior to the diagnosis. Occasionally, manifestations of hypersplenism including thrombocytopenia, leukopenia, petechiae, or ecchymoses will prompt evaluation, leading to the discovery of PHTN.

Ascites

Ascites is more common in intrahepatic and posthepatic causes of PHTN and develops due to two important factors—decreased intravascular oncotic pressure secondary to impaired protein synthesis in the liver and increased portal hydrostatic pressure. It is the presenting sign of PHTN in 7–21% of children. Impaired lymphatic drainage also contributes to the development of ascites.

Abdominal Venous Patterning

Prominent venous markings on the abdomen are the features of significant PHTN. Dilated veins are a result of shunting of blood through portosystemic collaterals by subcutaneous vessels. PHTN decompression through the umbilical vein results in prominent periumbilical collaterals, referred to as *caput medusae*. An audible venous hum (Cruveilhier–Baumgarten murmur) may occasionally be heard over dilated abdominal veins. Caput medusae are not seen in children with portal vein thrombosis (EHPVO) as umbilical vein is usually obliterated in this condition. The direction of flow through these veins indicates the site of obstruction. In caput medusae, the blood flows in a cephalad and caudad direction (physiological direction with increased flow) from the umbilicus. In IVC syndrome, blood flows cephalad, whereas it flows caudad in superior vena cava syndrome. The abdominal veins are also more lateral compared to the more central abdominal veins seen in caput medusa.

Hepatic Encephalopathy

Hepatic encephalopathy is a known complication of cirrhosis and liver failure. However, it can also be seen in extrahepatic PH and is caused by port-systemic shunts. Early hepatic encephalopathy manifests as learning difficulty and behavior abnormalities.

Hepatorenal Syndrome

Portal hypertension can contribute to the development of hepatorenal syndrome, a condition which presents with kidney dysfunction in children with advanced liver disease.

Pulmonary Complications

Hepatopulmonary syndrome (HPS) and portopulmonary hypertension are rare but often underdiagnosed complications of PHTN in children.

DIAGNOSIS[2]

Investigations

- *Complete blood count (CBC):* It helps identify the presence of and type of anemia. It also guides assessment of the requirement of blood and blood product transfusion in the setting of acute variceal bleeding. The presence of thrombocytopenia and leukopenia usually indicates hypersplenism.
- *Liver function test (LFT):* LFT helps in evaluation of the underlying cause of PHTN and also the functional reserve of the liver. Low albumin level and prolonged coagulation profile indicate impaired synthetic function of the liver. Increased bilirubin level and hepatic enzymes indicate hepatocellular damage.
- *Renal function test (RFT):* RFT helps in the assessment of dehydration, especially in the setting of acute variceal bleeding. Impaired renal function is associated with liver diseases, such as congenital hepatic fibrosis, which is linked to polycystic kidney disease.
- *Radiology:* Abdominal ultrasound with Doppler is the choice of investigation in children with PHTN. It provides important and useful information, which includes the liver size, echogenicity, and presence of the nodules or cysts. It also delineates the status of the intra- and extrabiliary tree, the patency of the portal vein, the presence of the cavernoma, and presence of spontaneous portosystemic shunts.
- *Other investigations:* They are decided according to the clinical status of the patients. Blood glucose will be low in decompensated liver cirrhosis. Serum ammonia level is elevated in hepatic encephalopathy.
- *Upper GI endoscopy:* It is an essential tool in PHTN management. It confirms the presence of varices in the esophagus and the stomach and helps in differentiating variceal bleed from other causes such as hemorrhagic gastritis or Mallory–Weiss syndrome. In acute upper GI bleeding, unresponsive to medical management, endoscopy offers an important therapeutic option to control the variceal bleeding either via endoscopic variceal ligation (EVL), (preferred modality) or sclerotherapy.

MANAGEMENT

Therapy is primarily directed at the most dramatic manifestation, variceal hemorrhage. Management can be divided into primary prophylaxis, emergency therapy, and secondary prophylaxis. Also underlying cause of PHTN/liver disease should be treated.[1,3]

Primary Prophylaxis

Primary prophylaxis aims to prevent the first variceal bleeding and includes screening for varices by endoscopy and treatment with nonselective beta blockers.[2]

- *Endoscopy:* The efficiency of the primary prophylaxis is very well established in adults with chronic liver disease. However, there are no consensuses in children due to lack of substantial data on which patients need screening and what are the predictive factors for variceal presence. Endoscopy in children with liver disease and/or stigmata of PHTN is justified if the clinician anticipates high risk of bleeding. It is also advisable in patients who live in remote areas, far from emergency medical care.

- *Nonselective beta-blockers:* Nonselective beta-blockers act by decreasing the portal pressure (via unopposed action of alfa-receptor on the splanchnic arterioles) and decreasing the cardiac output, which in turn results in decreased portal pressure. Beta-blocker use in children results in decreased frequency of bleeding episodes and improved long-term survival. Propranolol is commonly used (see further).

Emergency Therapy of Variceal Bleeding

Variceal hemorrhage is a frequent complication and may be secondary to drugs or infection and may provoke encephalopathy. If hematemesis or melena occurs, the child requires urgent evaluation as the severity of bleeding may not be immediately obvious. It is also important to note that bleeding in patients with known PHTN may sometimes be due to a peptic ulcer.[2]

Evaluation

- Evaluate the child's clinical condition, and secure intravenous access immediately. Few children may require placement of a central line.
- Check hemoglobin levels and cross-match blood.
- Monitor cardiorespiratory rate, oxygen saturation, and central venous pressure (CVP). If child is encephalopathic, Glasgow Coma Scale (GCS) should be assessed to decide on ventilatory support.

Resuscitation

If there are signs of hypovolemia, resuscitate at once with blood. Normal saline or 4.5% human albumin solution may be used until blood becomes available.

Initial Management[4]

- Place a large-bore nasogastric tube and aspirate at frequent intervals to identify persistent/recurrent bleeding. This acts as early warning of bleeding and reduces the likelihood of vomiting. It also helps in removal of blood, a protein source that may precipitate encephalopathy. In addition, blood in the stomach increases splanchnic blood flow, aggravates PHTN, and promotes ongoing bleeding.
- Place urinary catheter and monitor urine output, which is a good indicator of intravascular volume status.

Pharmacotherapy

- *Octreotide:* Somatostatin and its synthetic homolog octreotide have shown to decrease splanchnic blood flow. Their beneficial effects on acute variceal hemorrhage appear to be similar to those of vasopressin, but with fewer side effects. Continuous infusion of 1–5 µg/kg/h of octreotide is effective in arresting variceal bleed.
- *H2-receptor blockers and proton pump inhibitors* are often used to decrease gastric acid secretion.

Endoscopy and Sclerotherapy

Approximately 15% of children will have persistent hemorrhage despite conservative management and octreotide therapy. They would need endoscopic sclerotherapy or EVL. Endoscopic therapy is very effective in controlling bleeding, although it may be technically challenging. It should be performed only after the child is hemodynamically stable.[4]

Sengstaken-Blakemore Tube

Sengstaken-Blakemore tube (SSBT) stops variceal hemorrhage by mechanically compressing esophageal and gastric varices. The device consists of a rubber tube with two balloons. It is passed into the stomach, where the first balloon is inflated and pulled up to snugly fit against the gastroesophageal junction. After the tube is secured in place, the second balloon in the esophagus is inflated to the pressure of 60–70 mm Hg that compresses the esophageal varices without necrosing the esophagus. A channel in the rubber tube allows gastric contents to be sampled for evidence of bleeding. SSBT is very effective in controlling acute bleeding. However, it is associated with significant number of complications and high incidence of rebleeding when the tube is removed. Most older patients find it uncomfortable, and children require sedation and/or endotracheal intubation. Rebleeding has been reported in 33–60% of patients. Given these problems, it is reserved for severe uncontrollable hemorrhage and generally acts as bridge therapy until a more definite procedure can be performed.

Emergency Surgical and Interventional Radiology Procedures

- *Surgery* is usually the last resort to control acute variceal hemorrhage. Surgical procedures and interventional shunts are associated with high mortality, increased incidence of encephalopathy, and greater difficulty for subsequent liver transplantation (if required). Surgical procedures available include transection, devascularization, and portosystemic shunting. Liver transplantation may be an effective means of treating uncontrolled esophageal variceal bleeding in intrahepatic causes of PHTN if an acceptable donor is readily available.
- *Variceal embolization* via a percutaneous transhepatic or trans-splenic approach is another method of controlling acute hemorrhage.
- *Transjugular intrahepatic portosystemic shunt (TIPS)* placement may be the optimal approach for intractable

bleeding, since it does not require surgery. Experience in young children is limited and expertise available only in select centers.

Secondary Prophylaxis

Secondary prophylaxis aims to prevent recurrence of bleeding after the first variceal bleeding. It is recommended in view of the high recurrence rate bleeding in children and includes:[5]

- *Surveillance endoscopy* at frequent specified intervals and EVL or sclerotherapy
- *Nonselective beta-blockers:* Propranolol is the most commonly used beta-blocker; started at the dose of 0.5 mg/kg/day (in 3–4 divided doses) and gradually increased every 5–7 days to maximum dose of 8 mg/kg/day to achieve a target decrease of 25% in heart rate from baseline.

Surgical Therapy

Endoscopy continues to be the first-line treatment in patients with GI bleeding.[4,6] A surgical shunt is considered pre-emptively if mesoportal bypass is feasible. Otherwise, main indication for surgical treatment remains recurrent/persistent bleeding following failure of medical management. The type of surgery depends on the level of obstruction (prehepatic, hepatic, and posthepatic). Different surgical procedures available for PHTN are outlined in **Box 12.3.1**. Shunts can be described as nonselective or selective.

Selective shunts: They preserve the majority of portal or mesenteric blood flow to the liver while shunting blood from regional gastroesophageal varices from a high-pressure system into the low-pressure systemic venous circulation. Selective shunts include:[5]

- *Distal splenorenal (Warren shunt):* Shunt between the portal end of the splenic vein and the side of the renal vein
- *Side-to-side splenorenal shunt (Mitra shunt):* The shunt is fashioned between the splenic vein and the left renal vein.

Nonselective shunts: They divert a large proportion of mesenteric blood flow away from the liver, so that the entire GI tract, including spleen and pancreas, is decompressed. Nonselective shunts include:[5]

- *End-to-side portacaval shunt:* Mesenteric end of the portal vein is anastomosed to the side of the IVC.
- *Proximal splenorenal shunt:* Proximal end of the splenic vein is anastomosed to left renal vein.
- *Side-to-side mesocaval shunt:* Side-to-side anastomosis of superior mesenteric vein and IVC
- *Portocaval shunt:* Anastomosis between portal vein and IVC

Mesorex shunt: It is indicated in children with EHPVO. Procedure involves the placement of an autologous venous graft from mesenteric vasculature to the left branch of intrahepatic portal vein. One of the major advantages of this approach is the restoration of normal portal blood flow, which eliminates the risk of hepatic encephalopathy and helps in preservation of hepatic function.

BOX 12.3.1: Surgical options for portal hypertension in children.

- *Shunt surgery:*
  - Nonphysiologic shunts (diverting blood away from liver):
    - Selective shunts
    - *Nonselective shunts:*
      - Partial shunting of portal blood
      - Complete shunting of portal blood
  - Physiologic shunts (restoring blood flow back to liver)—mesorex shunt (bypass)
- *Nonshunt surgery:*
  - Surgical ligation of varices
  - Sugiura procedure and others

REFERENCES

1. Sen Sarma M, Yachha SK. Portal Hypertension. In: Matthai J, Sathiyasekaran M, Shanmugam N (Eds). Textbook of Pediatric Hepatology. Hyderabad: Paras Medical Books; 2023. pp. 33-55.
2. Shneider BL, Bosch J, de Franchis R, Emre SH, Groszmann RJ, Ling SC, et al.; expert panel of the Children's Hospital of Pittsburgh of UPMC. Portal hypertension in children: expert pediatric opinion on the report of the Baveno v Consensus Workshop on Methodology of Diagnosis and Therapy in Portal Hypertension. Pediatr Transplant. 2012;16(5):426-37.
3. Gugig R, Rosenthal P. Management of portal hypertension in children. World J Gastroenterol. 2012;18(11):1176-84.
4. Grammatikopoulos T, McKiernan PJ, Dhawan A. Portal hypertension and its management in children. Arch Dis Child. 2018;103(2):186-91.
5. McKiernan P, Abdel-Hady M. Advances in the management of childhood portal hypertension. Expert Rev Gastroenterol Hepatol. 2015;9(5):575-83.
6. Scholz S, Sharif K. Surgery for portal hypertension in children. Curr Gastroenterol Rep. 2011;13(3):279-85.

12.4 Clinical Relevance of Liver Function Tests in Hepatobiliary Disorders

Geetha Mammayil

INTRODUCTION

Liver function tests (LFTs) are a set of basic investigations done in all suspected hepatobiliary diseases. However, it is actually a misnomer. In reality, the standard "liver function test" as done in the laboratory do not accurately reflect all the functions of the liver. In some cases, this test may be completely normal even in the presence of an underlying liver disease! Conversely, some of the values may be abnormal but there may be no underlying liver disease. Hence, these tests should be interpreted in the background of the clinical history and physical findings to yield meaningful conclusions.

WHAT ARE THE LIVER FUNCTION TESTS?

When you order for a "liver function test" or LFT as they are commonly called, most laboratories include:

- Serum bilirubin (total, direct, and indirect)
- Alanine aminotransferase—ALT [serum glutamic-pyruvic transaminase (SGPT)]
- Aspartate aminotransferase—AST [serum glutamic-oxaloacetic transaminase (SGOT)]
- Serum alkaline phosphatase (ALP)
- Serum proteins (total, albumin, and globulin).

The *prothrombin time (PT)* and International normalized ratio (INR) are very important tests of the liver function although they do not fall under the heading of "liver function tests." They have to be ordered separately.

In addition to these, there some tests which are not routinely done but actually reflect the liver functions in some part—for example, serum bile salts, serum ammonia, serum 5' nucleotidase, etc.

It is important to understand that these LFT give a picture of the liver function at a given point in time. However, to be able to reasonably predict involvement of the liver and the prognosis in various conditions, these tests must be repeated serially over time. The trend and pattern of the liver functions will give a clearer picture of the damage to the liver.

Let us first look at the different tests that are done under the heading of "Liver Function Tests" and then learn about the clinical interpretation.

SERUM BILIRUBIN

Bilirubin is formed by the degradation of the heme component of hemoglobin from red blood cells (RBCs) at the end of its life-cycle.[1] This bilirubin is transported to the liver in an insoluble or unconjugated form, where it gets converted into a soluble form by conjugation with glucuronic acid, facilitated by the enzyme uridine diphosphate glucuronosyl transferase.[2] This soluble form is then excreted into bile and removed from the body via the stool or urine. The conjugated and unconjugated bilirubin are also referred to as direct and indirect bilirubin based on its reaction with diazo dyes.[3]

Normal values of serum total bilirubin: 1–1.2 mg/dL; direct bilirubin <0.3 mg/dL.

This process of bilirubin metabolism—conjugation and excretion, is so efficient that the blood levels of bilirubin are normally maintained at <1 mg/dL. Of this <20% is conjugated or direct. When the normal process of metabolism is affected either due to genetic defects or illness, bilirubin levels can rise. A rise above 2.5–3 mg/dL results in yellow discoloration of sclera and jaundice.

Fractionation of bilirubin into direct or indirect helps categorize the type of jaundice as indirect, direct, or mixed hyperbilirubinemia.

Causes of Indirect Hyperbilirubinemia

- *Physiological jaundice of newborn:* In newborn babies a physiological rise in indirect bilirubin occurs due to the immaturity of the conjugation process. It peaks around day 3–5 of life and then spontaneously falls to normal by 10–14 days of life. However, in cases when indirect bilirubin rises above a critical level, it can cross the blood brain barrier and get deposited in the brain resulting in a permanent damage to the brain a condition called kernicterus.
- *Hemolytic anemia:* Examples include hereditary spherocytosis, sickle cell anemia, Glucose-6-phosphate dehydrogenase (G6PD) deficiency, etc. In these conditions, excessive hemolysis or breakage of RBCs results in excessive formation of unconjugated or indirect bilirubin. When this exceeds the capacity of the liver to conjugate it, there is a rise in indirect bilirubin and this is called hemolytic jaundice.
- *Gilbert syndrome* is a harmless genetic condition resulting in *decreased* activity of *uridine diphosphate glucuronosyl transferase* enzyme which is responsible for the conjugation of indirect bilirubin to direct. Hence, there is a mild build-up of indirect bilirubin in blood.

- *Crigler-Najjar syndrome types I and II:* This condition is a genetic defect causing *a decrease or absence* of the enzyme uridine diphosphate glucuronosyl transferase enzyme. This results in high levels of indirect bilirubin causing kernicterus. Type I is due to complete absence of the enzyme and is fatal in childhood while type II is due to partial deficiency.[4]

Causes of Direct Hyperbilirubinemia

- *Dubin-Johnson and Rotor syndromes.* These are genetically inherited mutations that affect the secretion of bilirubin into the canaliculi. They are usually mild and harmless and require no treatment.
- Obstruction of the common bile duct (CBD) due to stones or stricture, extrahepatic biliary atresia, etc.
- Cholestatic phase of viral hepatitis, drug-induced cholestasis, total parenteral nutrition associated cholestasis, etc.

Causes of Mixed Hyperbilirubinemia

- Systemic illness such as enteric fever, dengue fever, malaria, etc.
- Liver specific infections such as viral hepatitis A, B, E, cytomegalovirus (CMV), Epstein-Barr virus (EBV), etc.

TESTS OF LIVER INJURY: AMINOTRANSFERASES: ASPARTATE AMINOTRANSFERASE (SERUM GLUTAMIC OXALOACETIC TRANSAMINASE) AND ALANINE TRANSAMINASE (SERUM GLUTAMIC PYRUVIC TRANSAMINASE)

Aspartate transaminase earlier called serum glutamic oxaloacetic transaminase and alanine transaminase, earlier called serum glutamic pyruvic transaminase are referred to as *transaminases*. These enzymes are located in the mitochondria and/or cytoplasm of the hepatocytes and are released when there is cellular damage resulting in elevated serum levels. Hence, they reflect the degree of liver injury. The larger the number of cells that are damaged, the higher the value. However, this does not have any prognostic value. AST and ALT levels are found to be lower in renal disease.

Aspartate Transaminase (Serum Glutamic Oxaloacetic Transaminase)

Normal range: 8–33 IU/L.

As the name suggests, this enzyme catalyzes the transfer of an amino group from oxaloacetate to α-ketoglutarate to form pyruvate and glutarate. Besides liver it is also found in myocardium, skeletal muscle and smooth muscle, and RBC. Hence, conditions such as myocardial infarction, myositis, hemolysis, and renal damage can cause an isolated increase in AST.

In hepatitis, both AST and ALT are elevated. However in conditions such as alcoholic liver disease, Wilson disease, and nonalcoholic fatty liver disease (NAFLD), the AST levels are higher than ALT.

Alanine Transaminase (Serum Glutamic Pyruvic Transaminase)

Normal range: Males <30 IU/L, females <19 IU/L.[5]

This enzyme catalyzes the transfer of amino group from L-alanine to α-ketoglutarate. It is found mainly in the liver and in smaller quantities in intestine.

The degree of rise in ALT and AST is reflective of the severity of cellular damage. In cirrhosis, NAFLD, Wilson disease, and autoimmune hepatitis, etc., the rise is mild-to-moderate, i.e., 3–10 times the "upper limit of normal (ULN)." Conditions causing massive necrosis of hepatocytes such as acute liver failure, ischemic hepatitis, or toxic hepatitis, levels >100 times the ULN, i.e., >3,000 are characteristically seen. A gradual decrease in level with time carries a better prognosis when compared to sudden or rapid fall in enzyme levels.[6]

TESTS REFLECTING BILIARY PATHOLOGY OR CHOLESTASIS

This includes serum ALP, gamma glutamyl transferase (GGT), and 5' nucleotidase.

Alkaline Phosphatase

This consists of four isoenzymes which are named according to the tissue in which it is found—namely placental ALP, intestinal ALP, germ cell ALP, and tissue nonspecific ALP (TNSALP) found mainly in liver, kidney, and bone. Generally, laboratories estimate the blood levels of all the isoenzymes together. An electrophoresis can help isolate the isoenzymes individually.

The TNSALP is commonly found among the cholangiocytes lining the biliary tree, in the kidney and in bones. In preadolescent children, the ALP levels are characteristically high. This is mainly of bony origin and is most likely due to the mineralization of the growing bones. This can be confirmed by doing a GGT level which will be normal.

Normal range in adults: 20–140 IU/L; preadolescent children 150–450 IU/L.

Causes of Raised Alkaline Phosphatase

- Physiological
  - Children (bone mineralization)
  - Pregnant women (placental isoenzyme)

- Obstruction of the biliary tree—choledocholithiasis, primary sclerosing cholangitis (PSC), bile duct strictures, etc.
- Extrahepatic biliary atresia—infants
- Bony conditions—Paget's disease, bone metastasis.

Causes of Low Alkaline Phosphatase

- Hypophosphatasia
- Magnesium deficiency
- Anemia—aplastic, pernicious
- Wilson disease
- Estrogen therapy

Gamma Glutamyl Transferase

This enzyme is found in cholangiocytes of liver and are raised whenever there is an obstruction in the biliary tree, e.g., CBD stones or stricture. It is also present in kidneys, intestine, prostate, and pancreas but not in the bone. Hence, in conditions where ALP is raised, GGT can help differentiate if the source is from the liver or the bone. Since it is not present in the bone, raised ALP with normal GGT indicates a nonhepatic source and if both ALP and GGT are raised, it indicates a hepatic source.

In children, ALP is normally high due to the contribution from the growing bones. In children with cholestatic jaundice, measurement of GGT can help identify conditions like progressive familial intrahepatic cholestasis (PFIC). Types I and II PFIC are associated with normal or low GGT and type III is associated with high levels of GGT.

Normal range: <5–50 IU/L

Causes of Raised Gamma Glutamyl Transferase

- Cholestasis due to CBD stone/stricture
- Obesity
- Excess alcohol consumption
- Drug-induced—phenytoin or barbiturates
- PFIC type III

Causes of Decrease in Gamma Glutamyl Transferase

PFIC types I and II.

5′ Nucleotidase

This enzyme is located in canalicular and sinusoidal plasma membranes of the liver. It is also found in extrahepatic organs such as intestine, brain, heart, blood vessels, and pancreas. Serum levels are lowest in children and increases with age. Just like GGT, it also helps in identifying if the rise in serum ALP is hepatic or not.[7]

Normal range: 2–17 U/L

TESTS REFLECTING HEPATIC SYNTHETIC FUNCTIONS

The liver synthesizes proteins, especially albumin, and coagulation factors II, VII, IX, and X. When >75% of the hepatocytes are damaged, these synthetic functions are affected. This is reflected by a decrease in serum albumin and prolongation of prothrombin time (PT).

Serum Proteins/Albumin

Albumin plays a major role in maintaining the oncotic pressure of the serum. It also binds to bilirubin and several other drugs.

Normal range:

Total proteins: 6.7–8.6 g/dL
Serum albumin: 3.5–5.5 g/dL
Serum globulin: 2.0–3.5 g/dL
A:G ratio: 1.5–2.5: 1

Conditions Causing Decrease in Serum Albumin

- *Hepatic:*
  - Acute liver failure
  - Decompensated cirrhosis due to any cause
- *Extrahepatic:*
  - Sepsis—This is a catabolic state which causes fall in proteins and albumin
  - Malabsorption syndromes due to protein loss in stools—celiac disease
  - Nephrotic syndrome—loss of albumin in urine
  - Chronic malnutrition—due to poor nutrition

Hypoalbuminemia can occur due to hepatic or nonhepatic causes. Persistent low levels may indicate chronic liver disease especially if accompanied by prolonged PT or international normalized ratio (INR).

Prothrombin Time

This test measures the activity of pro-coagulation factors II, VII IX, and X (extrinsic coagulation pathway) which are produced by the liver and are also vitamin K-dependent. In the laboratory, it is measured as the time taken by a plasma sample to clot after the addition of a specific tissue factor. This tissue factor differs from one lab to another and hence affects the measurement of PT.

Normal value: Around 11–13 seconds

A prolongation of PT > 2 seconds of ULN which is not corrected by vitamin K injection is generally considered a poor prognostic factor in the background of a liver disease.

Causes of Prolonged Prothrombin Time

- Deficient of individual coagulation factors II, VII, IX, and X.

- Vitamin K deficiency
- Acute or chronic liver disease

Since the PT can vary from one laboratory to another, it needs to be standardized for proper interpretation. For this purpose, an INR was instituted. This is calculated as follows:

$$INR = \frac{PT\ (Patient)^{ISI}}{PT\ (Control)}$$

Normal INR value is 0.8–1.2.

The INR is taken as the standard for assessing the pediatric end-stage liver disease (PELD) or model for end-stage liver disease (MELD), which in turn is the criteria for listing a patient for liver transplant.[8]

RECOGNIZING PATTERNS

Since the LFT measure different aspects of liver activity, a combination of tests taken together helps identify a specific pattern which gives more information than the individual tests in isolation. These are discussed in the following text.

Hemolytic Pattern

In hemolytic anemia, lysis of the RBCs release hemoglobin which is then degraded to bilirubin and transported to the liver. The pattern seen is:

- Total bilirubin is raised and is predominantly *indirect.*
- Liver enzymes, ALP, albumin, and PT are *normal.*

A similar pattern is seen in Gilbert syndrome. However, a peripheral smear, serum lactate dehydrogenase (LDH), and reticulocyte count will be helpful in differentiating the two conditions. These will be normal in Gilbert syndrome while in hemolytic anemias, they show the typical features of hemolysis—polychromasia, target cells, and specific cells such as spherocytes (in hereditary spherocytosis), raised LDH, and reticulocyte count.

Cholestatic Pattern

This is seen in conditions causing obstruction of the biliary tree, e.g., CBD stones, strictures or growths, extrahepatic biliary atresia, or conditions affecting the canaliculi like certain drugs, sepsis, PFIC, etc. The pattern seen is as follows:

- Bilirubin (predominantly direct)—increased
- Transaminases (AST and ALT)—increased (3–10 times the upper limit of normal)
- ALP and GGT—markedly raised. An exception is PFIC type I and II where GGT is normal or low normal.
- PT—this may or may not be prolonged. In cases where it is prolonged, a single dose of injection vitamin K can typically normalize the values.

Hepatocellular Pattern

In conditions involving predominant damage to the hepatocytes—as in acute viral hepatitis, drug-induced hepatitis, etc., a hepatocellular pattern is seen. It is characterized by:

- Bilirubin—increased (both direct and indirect)
- Transaminases (AST and ALT)—moderate to massive rise in enzymes (10–100 times the upper limit of normal)
- PT—maybe prolonged in severe cases
- Albumin—reduced in severe cases.

These patterns are useful in clinical practice to help narrow down the differential diagnosis and to plan imaging studies to confirm the etiology.

CONCLUSION

- Always interpret LFTs in the clinical context.
- A series of tests over a period of time gives better information than a single one-point test.
- PT is the most important test for assessing liver function in acute or chronic liver disease and can predict prognosis.
- PT is included in the criteria for listing a patient for liver transplant.

REFERENCES

1. Gazzin S, Vitek L, Watchko J, Shapiro SM, Tiribelli C. A novel perspective on the biology of bilirubin in health and disease. Trends Mol Med. 2016;22:758-68.
2. Gartner LM, Arias IM. Formation, transport, metabolism and excretion of bilirubin. N Engl J Med. 1969;280(24):1339-45.
3. Vuppalanchi R, Chalasani N. Chapter 3. Laboratory Tests in Liver Disease. In: R Saxena (Ed) Practical Hepatic Pathology: A Diagnostic Approach, 2nd edition. Philadelphia: Elsevier; 2018. pp. 43-53.
4. Kliegman R, Toth H, Bordini BJ, Basel D. Nelson Pediatric Symptom-Based Diagnosis: Common Diseases and their Mimics, 2nd edition. Philadelphia: Elsevier; 2022. pp. 320-40.
5. Prati D, Taioli E, Zanella A, Torre ED, Butelli S, Vecchio ED, et al. Updated definitions of healthy ranges for serum alanine aminotransferase levels. Ann Intern Med. 2002;137:1-10.
6. Litin SC, O'Brien JF, Pruett S, Forsman RW, Burritt MF, Bartholomew LG, et al. Macroenzyme as a cause of unexplained elevation of aspartate aminotransferase. Mayo Clin Proc. 1987;62:681-7.
7. Pratt DS. Liver chemistry and function tests. In: Feldman M, Friedman LS, Brandt LJ (Eds). Sleisenger and Fordtran's Gastrointestinal and Liver Disease. Philadelphia: Saunders Elsevier; 2010. pp. 1227-37.
8. Taberner DA, Poller L, Thomson JM, Darby KV. Effect of international sensitivity index (ISI) of thromboplastins on precision of international normalised ratios (INR). J Clin Pathol. 1989;42:92-6.

12.5 Hepatic-Pancreato-Biliary Imaging

Komalavalli Subbiah

INTRODUCTION

Children are not miniature adults and their physiology and pathology are unique. It is very much true in the field of pediatric hepatobiliary diseases and knowledge of the disease, their embryo-pathophysiological origin and the morphology is important in deciding the appropriate imaging modality.

IMAGING MODALITIES

The common abdominal imaging modalities include ultrasonography (USG), X-ray radiography, computed tomography (CT), magnetic resonance imaging (MRI), and scintigraphy. USG and MRI are the preferred modalities for children in view of lack of ionizing radiation[1] **(Table 12.5.1)**.

USG is the primary screening modality in the antenatal as well as pediatric hepato-pancreatic-biliary (HPB) imaging in view of its ease of availability, repeatability, and portability. However, it is subject to interobserver variations and is less specific compared to CT or MRI for liver lesions.

Computer tomography (CT) is the most commonly performed axial imaging. Difference in the attenuation coefficient of X-ray for different tissues forms the basis of imaging in CT. Hepatobiliary CT imaging is based on differential perfusion of the liver lesion compared to the liver which helps in the diagnosis. Triple phase [arterial, portal, and equilibrium (hepatic venous) phases] CT is the commonly performed CT protocol for liver lesions **(Figs. 12.5.1A to D)**.

Magnetic resonance imaging is the second most commonly performed axial imaging for liver. It is a noninvasive, sophisticated imaging technology which is radiation-free. The two MRI sequences which are commonly performed are T1-weighted [fat tissue appears bright and cerebrospinal fluid (CSF) appears dark] and T2-weighted images (fat and water are bright and CSF appear bright) to characterize a lesion. In HPB imaging, apart from T2-weighted images which helps to differentiate cystic (bright) and solid liver lesions, magnetic resonance cholangiopancreatography (MRCP) which is a specialized heavy T2-weighted MRI sequence is also used routinely. It shows high signal in static or slow moving fluids such as bile within the gallbladder, biliary ducts, and pancreatic juice in pancreatic duct, with low signal of surrounding tissue. Rarely, extracellular and hepatobiliary specific contrast agents are used in specific conditions **(Figs. 12.5.2A to C)**.

The different terminologies used to describe a lesion differs between the various modalities such as *echogenicity* for ultrasound, *density* for CT, and *intensity* for MRI.

TABLE 12.5.1: Comparison of various HPB imaging modalities.

	USG	*CT*	*MRI/MRCP*	*Scintigraphy*
Indications	• Parenchymal and biliary evaluation • Doppler for vascular evaluation	• Characterization of liver lesion • Calcification, calculus, and bone lesions are better appreciated	• Bile duct and pancreatic duct evaluation • Quantification of fat, fibrosis, and iron deposition	Specific role in biliary atresia
Advantages	• Wide availability • Inexpensive • Easy to use • Faster to perform • No ionizing radiation	• Readily available • Objective • Easy to interpret • Less time consuming • Postprocessing techniques available	• Better soft tissue resolution • No ionizing radiation	Functional imaging
Disadvantages	• Interobserver variation • Lack of penetration through the bones and fat as in obese individuals and air filled bowel loops	• Ionizing radiation • Contrast reactions including its nephrotoxicity	• Not readily available • Difficult to interpret • More time consumption Claustrophobia • Increased cost	• Ionizing radiation • Handling of radioactive material

(CT: computed tomography; HPB: hepato-pancreatic-biliary; MRCP: magnetic resonance cholangiopancreatography; MRI: magnetic resonance imaging; USG: ultrasonography)

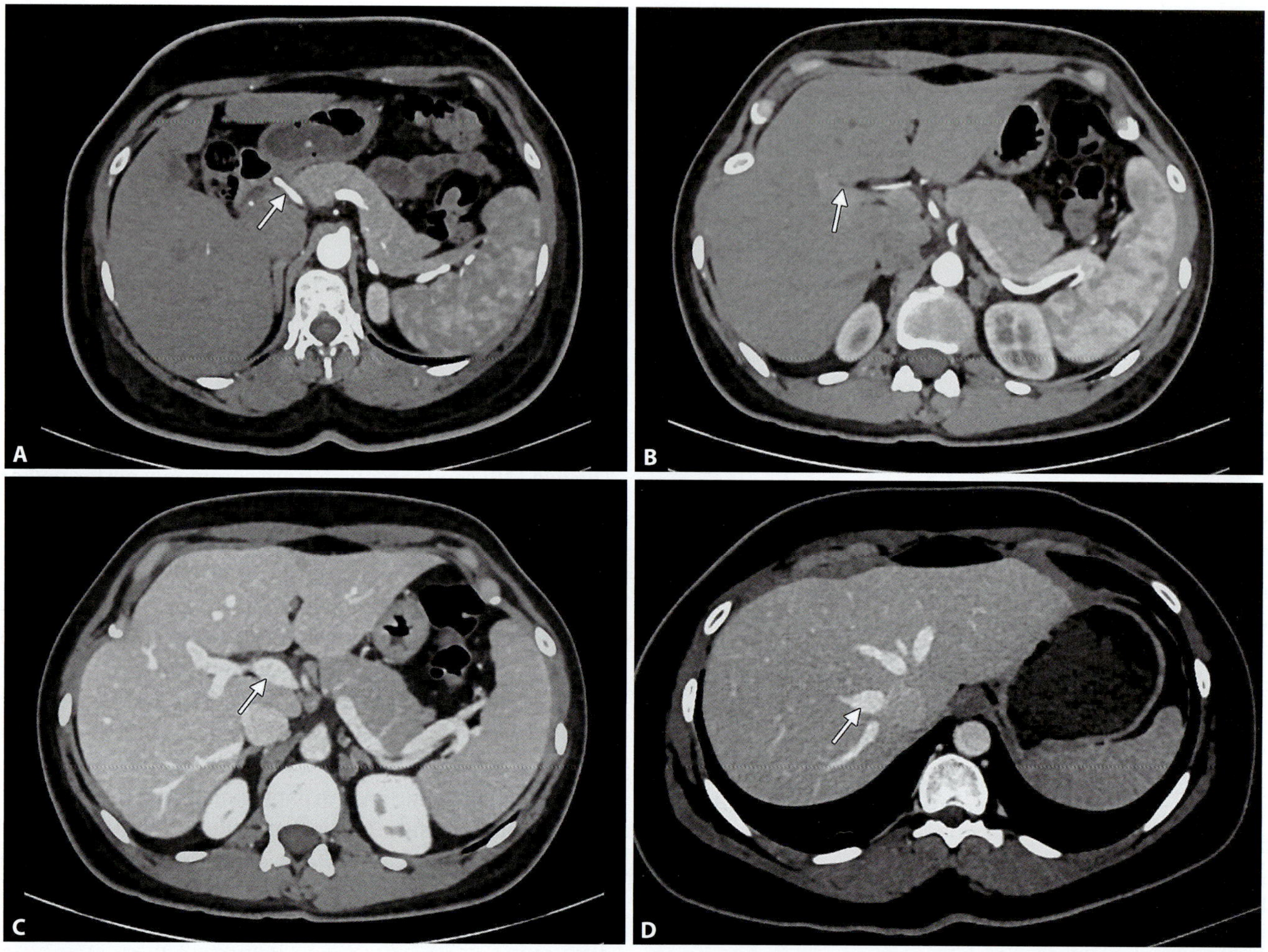

Figs. 12.5.1A to D: Triple phase contrast-enhanced computed tomography (CECT) abdomen showing: (A) Early arterial phase where hepatic artery (arrow) is opacified; (B) Late arterial phase (opacification of hepatic artery and portal vein); (C) Portal venous phase (portal vein is opacified); and (D) Hepatic venous phase (hepatic veins are opacified).

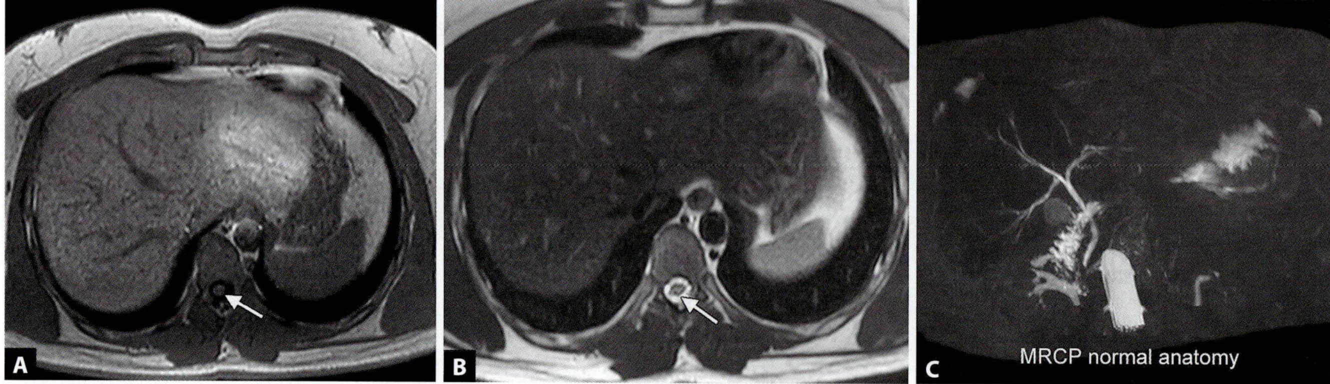

Figs. 12.5.2A to C: Magnetic resonance imaging (MRI) abdomen with: (A) T1-weighted [dark cerebrospinal fluid (CSF)]; (B) T2-weighted (bright CSF); and (C) Magnetic resonance cholangiopancreatography (MRCP) coronal image (demonstrating the bile ducts).

Scintigraphy uses radioisotope to expose its dynamic excretion in the HPB system in children suspicious of biliary atresia using derivatives of Tc-labeled iminodiacetic acid (IDA).

Imaging children under sedation/general anesthesia is the routine because it ensures patient conformity and provides a more controlled environment. Choice of the anesthesia depends on the duration of the imaging technique. Multislice CT being faster requires an oral or short intravenous (IV) sedation whereas for MRI, general anesthesia is preferred due to prolonged duration and noisy environment. Parental consent and adequate monitoring facilities are mandatory.

HEPATOBILIARY PATHOLOGIES

Normal Variants

Awareness about the normal variants is important to differentiate them from pathological process. Very often they are incidental findings. Agenesis or hypoplasia of the hepatic lobes or segments, sliver of the liver (hypertrophied left lateral segment), Riedel's lobe (tongue-like projection from the anterior aspect of the right hepatic lobe mimicking a mass or hepatomegaly), and enlarged papillary process of the caudate lobe which can mimic as nodal or pancreatic mass are few examples.

Diffuse Liver Diseases

Fatty Liver Disease (Steatosis)

Fatty acid (triacylglycerol) accumulation in the hepatocytes (called steatosis), in children is usually associated with viral hepatitis, inborn errors of metabolism (IEM), celiac disease, autoimmune hepatitis, hepatotoxic drug consumption, malnutrition, and parenteral nutrition, unlike obesity-related nonalcoholic fatty liver disease (NAFLD) which is common in adults. The most common imaging pattern is diffuse homogeneous fat deposition. Steatotic liver appears hypoechoic in USG and hypodense in CT. MR imaging is the best technique to accurately detect and quantify steatosis **(Figs. 12.5.3A and B)**.

Hepatitis

Hepatitis can be due to viral, fungal, and bacterial infections as well as exogenous toxic agents. In acute hepatitis, the imaging findings are nonspecific which includes hepatosplenomegaly, heterogeneous enhancement of the liver parenchyma, periportal edema, gallbladder wall edema, portal hilar nodes and mild ascites.

Cirrhosis

Cirrhosis is end stage fibrosis followed by nodular regeneration. They are usually parenchymal (e.g., Wilson disease, **Fig. 12.5.4**) or biliary (biliary atresia) in origin. Imaging is important to diagnose as well as assess the complications of cirrhosis such as portal hypertension (portosystemic collaterals and splenomegaly) and malignancies like hepatocellular carcinoma. Classical imaging findings are shrunken liver, nodular surface with volume redistribution in the form of hypertrophied caudate and left lateral segment with atrophied right lobe. USG and CT are the commonly used modalities.

Vascular Pathologies of the Liver

Portal Hypertension

Portal hypertension is defined as elevated portal venous pressure within the splanchnic venous system which is normally around 1–4 mm Hg. Based on the location of resistance, the pathologies are classified as either presinusoidal, sinusoidal, and postsinusoidal causes. The most common etiology causing portal hypertension in children is extrahepatic portal venous obstruction (EHPVO) which is characterized by portal cavernoma and portosystemic

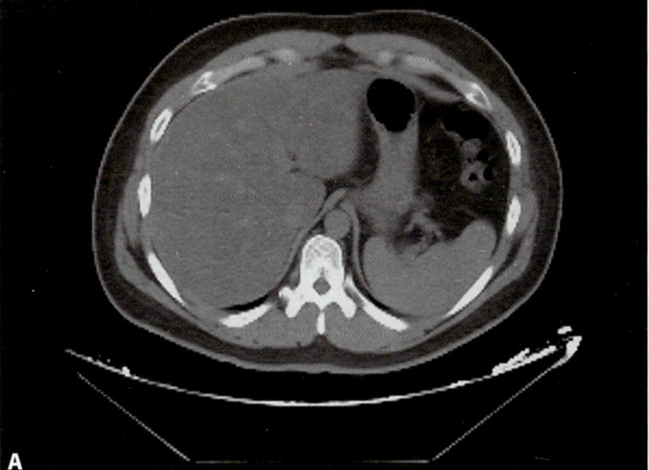

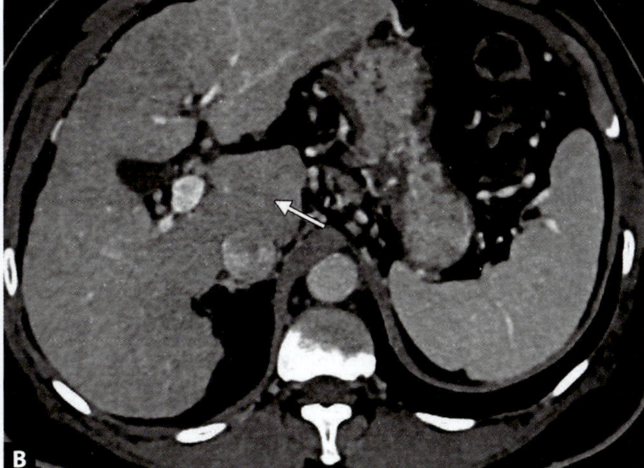

Figs. 12.5.3A and B: CECT showing: (A) Fatty liver has reduced density than spleen; and (B) Cirrhosis [Surface nodularity with caudate (arrow) and left lateral hypertrophy].

collaterals.[2] Imaging findings specific to various etiologies are discussed in **Table 12.5.2**.

Congenital Extrahepatic Portosystemic Shunts (Abernathy Malformation)

Although rare, due to the persistence of embryonic vessels, partial or total shunts can exist from birth between portal [portal vein (PV), splenic vein (SV), and superior mesenteric vein (SMV)] and the systemic circulation [inferior vena cava (IVC) and renal veins]. Usually they are at the level of liver hilum, where portal vein enters IVC partially or completely causing liver dysfunction and various lesions such as adenoma, hemangioma, and focal nodular hyperplasia due to altered liver perfusion. Doppler USG is the modality of choice to demonstrate the shunts and CT or MRI angiography for characterization.

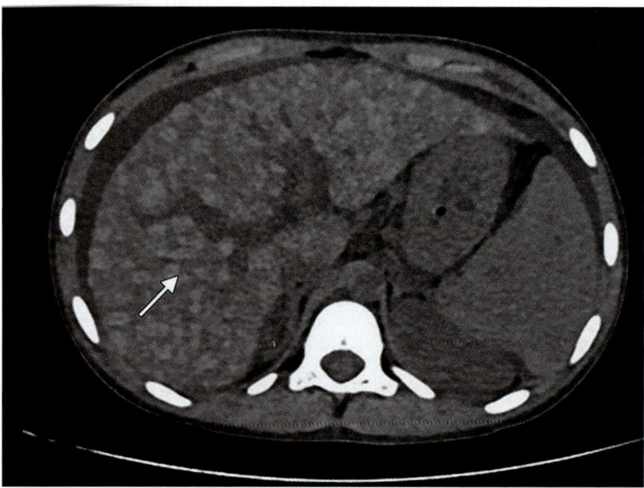

Fig. 12.5.4: Unenhanced CT in a 12-year-old male child shows cirrhosis (surface nodularity) due to Wilson disease (multiple hyperdense regenerative nodules).

Neonatal Biliopathies

Among infants with surgical causes of jaundice, about 80% have biliary atresia (BA), while the remaining have inspissated bile syndrome or choledochal malformation. Differential diagnoses in a jaundiced infant without biliary dilatation are biliary atresia, neonatal hepatitis, Alagille syndrome (paucity of bile ducts) and persistent familial intrahepatic cholestasis (PFIC). Differentiation between Alagille syndrome and BA is essential as the former needs medical management and Kasai procedure worsens its course. USG findings are similar to BA. The diagnosis of Alagille syndrome may sometimes be suspected clinically but is often based on liver biopsy and genetic testing.[3]

Biliary atresia is due to idiopathic, postinflammatory, and fibrotic obliteration of the extrahepatic or intrahepatic biliary tree. The overall incidence is approximately 1:15,000 births, but it is far more common in the Asian population and most common indication for liver transplantation in children. Kasai portoenterostomy performed within the 3 months of life halts the progression to cirrhosis and the need for liver transplantation. There may be atresia of the common bile duct (type I), common hepatic duct (type II), or intrahepatic ducts (type III). Specific findings in various imaging modalities aids in the diagnosis of biliary atresia **(Table 12.5.3 and Figs. 12.5.5A to E)**.

TABLE 12.5.2: Etiology specific imaging findings in portal hypertension.

Causes	*Disease*	*Clinical and imaging findings*
Extrahepatic (presinusoidal)	EHPVO (age 1–4 years)	• Normal liver with obliteration of main portal vein replaced with portal cavernoma (paracholedochal collaterals) • Porto-systemic collaterals especially coronary and splenorenal collaterals with moderate splenomegaly • They can have biliary dilatation due to cavernoma (portal biliopathy)
Intrahepatic (presinusoidal)	NCPF (age 15–25 years)	• Normal liver with grossly dilated main portal vein • Abrupt narrowing of the intrahepatic segmental portal veins (fibrosis of portal venules) • Massive splenomegaly is typical
Intrahepatic (sinusoidal)	Cirrhosis (age 2–5 years)	• Abnormal liver with classical imaging findings showing shrunken liver with volume redistribution • Porto-systemic collaterals/splenomegaly
Suprahepatic (postsinusoidal)	Budd–Chiari syndrome	• Mottled parenchymal enhancement • Nonvisualization of hepatic veins with abnormal intrahepatic and extrahepatic collaterals • Doppler is diagnostic
	Congestive hepatopathy (cardiac cause)	• Dilated right atrium with hugely distended hepatic veins and cava • Altered enhancement of the liver parenchyma is a classical finding

(EHPVO: extrahepatic portal venous obstruction; NCPF: noncirrhotic portal fibrosis)

TABLE 12.5.3: Diagnostic criteria for biliary atresia.

USG	• Gallbladder *ghost triad sign* [reduced gallbladder size (<15 mm), irregular wall, and absent smooth echogenic mucosa] • *Triangular cord sign* (liver hilum in the vicinity of the portal vein appears hyperechoic with thickness >4 mm) • Reduced gallbladder contractility, absence of common bile duct, hepatic artery diameter >1.5 mm, hypoplastic portal vein (<3 mm), and cysts in the portal hilum • Cirrhosis and portal hypertension features
CT	• To confirm the USG findings • Look for associated anomalies such as malrotation, polysplenia, annular pancreas, dorsal pancreatic agenesis, preduodenal portal vein, interrupted IVC, isomerism, situs inversus, etc. • Screening of HCC, though rare
HIDA scintigraphy	Nonvisualization of gallbladder, prolonged hepatic tracer retention and lack of intestinal excretion of tracer

(CT: computed tomography; HCC: hepatocellular carcinoma; HIDA: hepatobiliary iminodiacetic acid scan; IVC: inferior vena cava; USG: ultrasonography)

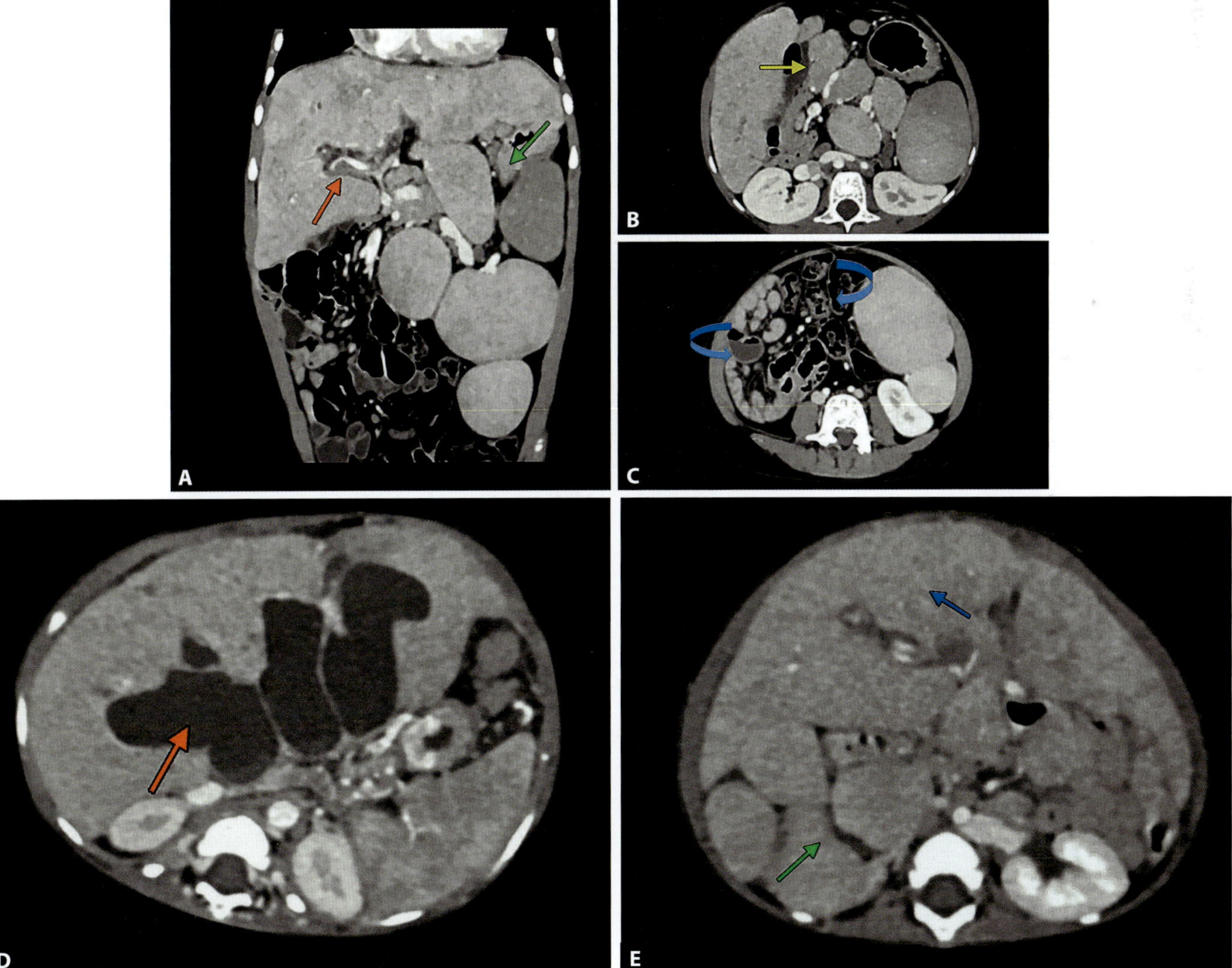

Figs. 12.5.5A to E: Biliary atresia (cystic form) and spectrum of associated anomalies: (A) Hypertrophied hepatic artery (red arrow) and polysplenia (green arrow); (B) Dorsal agenesis of pancreas; (C) Small bowel malrotation; (D) Cystic dilatation of peribiliary glands; (E) Situs inversus—midline liver (blue arrow) and right-sided spleen (green arrow).

Focal Hepatic Masses

Apart from USG which is the primary screening modality, contrast CT or MRI is the most common modality used for characterizing focal liver lesions based on perfusion. Congenital masses, infective lesions, and neoplasm are dealt in this subtopic.[4]

Congenital Hepatic Masses

Hepatic cysts: Simple cysts are common imaging findings which can be single or multiple with well-defined nonenhancing wall and clear internal content. Complex cyst may be of neoplastic, inflammatory, infectious or post-traumatic origin having thick enhancing wall with internal septa, mural nodularity with possible intracystic debris, proteinaceous or hemorrhagic contents.

Fibropolycystic liver disease: These are heterogeneous group of congenital fibrocystic liver diseases resulting from insult to the ductal plate at various stages of embryogenesis. They are classified depending on the involvement of extra/intrahepatic duct and small/large duct involvement **(Table 12.5.4)**.

- *Choledochal cyst (CDC) malformations:* Choledochal cysts are a congenital dilatation of the extrahepatic and/or intrahepatic bile ducts. MRI and MRCP are the diagnostic imaging modalities mapping the biliary dilatation (intra and extrahepatic) as well as detecting anomalous pancreaticobiliary junction, which are associated with this condition. Intraluminal portal vein sign on USG and central dot sign in CT (due to ectatic ducts surrounding portal vein radicles) are the hallmark of Caroli's disease (type V CDC). Associated imaging features are of cholangitis, cystolithiasis, pancreatitis, and rarely cirrhosis.
- *Polycystic liver disease:* This manifests as hepatomegaly with multiple liver cysts >10 in number along with multiple renal cysts. Complications are rare in children, but may include infection and rupture of cysts, bleeding, and mass effect.
- *Congenital hepatic fibrosis:* It is associated with autosomal recessive polycystic kidney disease (ARPKD). Hepatosplenomegaly with heterogeneous parenchymal echogenicity, hyperechoic portal triads, and regenerative nodules are the common findings.
- *Biliary hamartomas (Von Meyenburg complexes):* They are very common incidental insignificant imaging findings. Imaging shows uniform cystic lesions <15 mm in diameter with thin rim enhancement. MRCP is diagnostic by demonstrating that the cystic lesions have no biliary communications, thereby differentiating it from Caroli's disease.

TABLE 12.5.4: Classification of ductal plate malformation.

Extrahepatic bile duct	Choledochal cyst
Large intrahepatic ducts	Caroli's disease
Medium-sized intrahepatic ducts	Autosomal dominant polycystic liver disease
Small-sized intrahepatic ducts	Biliary hamartomas, congenital hepatic fibrosis

Infections

Pyogenic abscess are common with imaging showing a hypoechoic center with a rim in USG. The center of the lesion is usually necrotic filled with debris and/or air pockets. Contrast CT shows hypodense center with hyperdense wall enhancement. Air fluid level and intralesional air pockets are additional findings. Imaging features unique to various infections are summarized in **Table 12.5.5**.

Neoplasms of the Liver

Primary hepatic neoplasm constitutes 1–4% of solid tumors in children. Metastatic disease (from neuroblastoma, Wilms tumor, or lymphoma) is the most common neoplasm involving the liver in children. Important considerations when evaluating a child with a liver tumor are the age of the patient, laboratory findings, and specific imaging features.

Benign neoplasm: The most common benign lesion in pediatric population is infantile hepatic hemangioma **(Figs. 12.5.6A and B)**. Other lesions include mesenchymal hamartoma, focal nodular hyperplasia, and hepatic adenoma **(Table 12.5.6)**.[5]

Malignant neoplasm: The most common malignant tumors in decreasing order of frequency are hepatoblastoma (37%) **(Figs. 12.5.7A to D)**, hepatocellular carcinoma (HCC)

TABLE 12.5.5: Typical imaging findings of common hepatic infections.

Pyogenic	Cluster of grape appearance (coalescing lesions), double target sign
Amebic	85% solitary and 75% in the right lobe. Central hypoattenuation with peripheral enhancement
Fungal	Multiple small lesions with a wheel within wheel appearance and bull's eye appearance
Granulomatous (tuberculosis, sarcoid)	Hepatosplenomegaly with multiple tiny hypodense lesions and lymphadenopathy
Hydatid	Uni/multilocular complex cystic lesions with nonenhancing smooth wall, thin septa, daughter cysts, and peripheral calcifications

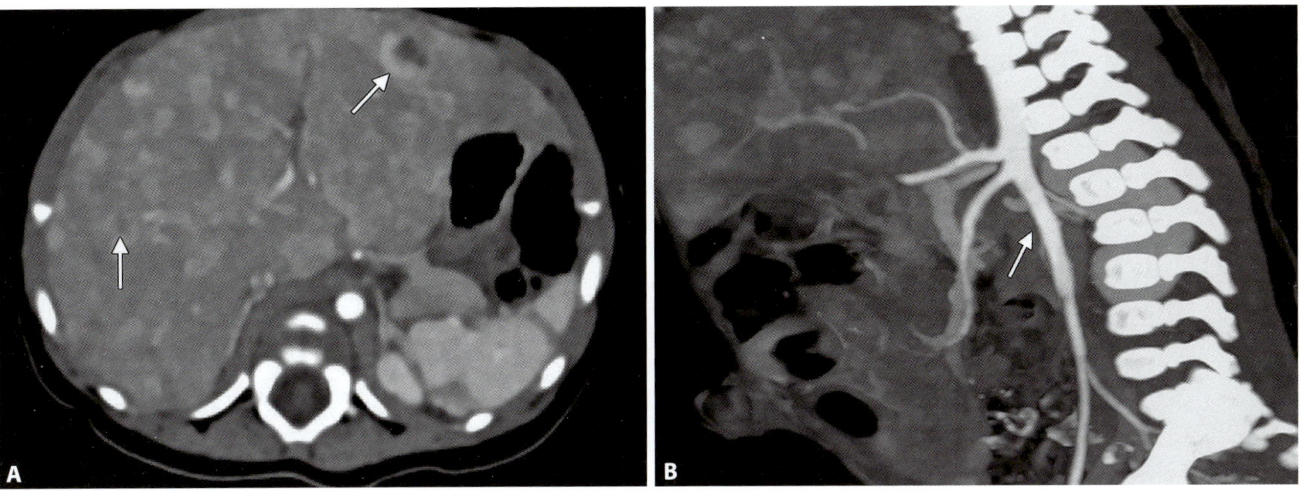

Figs. 12.5.6A and B: Triple phase computed tomography (CT) in a 2-year-old female child shows: (A) Multiple infantile hepatic hemangioma (peripherally enhancing lesions) with (B) Aorotogram sagittal images showing infraceliac aortic narrowing.

TABLE 12.5.6: Common hepatic benign neoplasms.

Lesion and its incidence	*Age*	*Clinical features*	*Imaging features*
Infantile hepatic hemangioma (15%)	• Congenital—at birth • Infantile—after 4–8 weeks, starts to regress after 1 year and resolves during puberty	Abdominal mass, cardiac failure, Kasabach–Merritt syndrome, and rarely hemoperitoneum	• *Contrast-enhanced computed tomography (CECT):* Large lesion with peripheral discontinuous nodular enhancement with progressive centripetal filling in • Infraceliac aortic narrowing due to shunting of blood to the liver • T2 light bulb sign in MRI
Mesenchymal hamartoma (7%)	<2 years	Abdominal distension and pain	• Well-circumscribed multilocular solid cystic lesion separated by thin enhancing septa • Calcification is rare
Focal nodular hyperplasia (5%)	All age groups, peak 7–8 years. Hyperplastic response to an increased arterial flow	Usually asymptomatic and found incidentally on imaging	• Lobulated lesion isodense to the liver in all the phases with a T2 hyperintense central scar showing delayed enhancement • Spoke wheel pattern in Doppler due to radiating vessels in the center
Hepatocellular adenoma (3%)	• Mean age is around 10–14 years • Associated with steroids usage, glycogen storage disease, tyrosinemia, portosystemic shunts, etc.	Abdominal mass, distension, pain due to hemorrhage	• Solitary mass in 70–80% • Arterial enhancing lesion with portal venous washout. Calcification/fat/hemorrhage/necrosis usually seen • Pseudocapsule in 25–30% • Malignant transformation is common

(21%) **(Figs. 12.5.8A to C)**, undifferentiated (embryonal) sarcoma (UES) (8%), and other rare tumors such as epithelioid hemangioendothelioma (EHE), angiosarcoma, and embryonal rhabdomyosarcoma constitutes around 4% **(Table 12.5.7)**.[6]

Hepatoblastoma is common during infancy up to 5 years of age. It presents as rapidly growing abdominal mass, hepatomegaly, pain, and weight loss. Serum α-fetoprotein (AFP) levels are grossly elevated in up to 90% of children. They are very chemo-responsive. On USG, it is seen as a well-defined, lobulated, heterogeneous mass with chunky calcifications (40%), hemorrhage, and necrosis within it. Contrast CT is the most useful modality for diagnosis, staging, and assessing response to treatment. It appears as a hypodense/heterodense lesion showing arterial enhancement, slightly less than the normal liver and delayed washout. Tumor invasion into the portal and hepatic vein is common. Pulmonary metastasis is seen in 10–20% at presentation **(Figs. 12.5.7A to D)**. Differential diagnosis include the following:

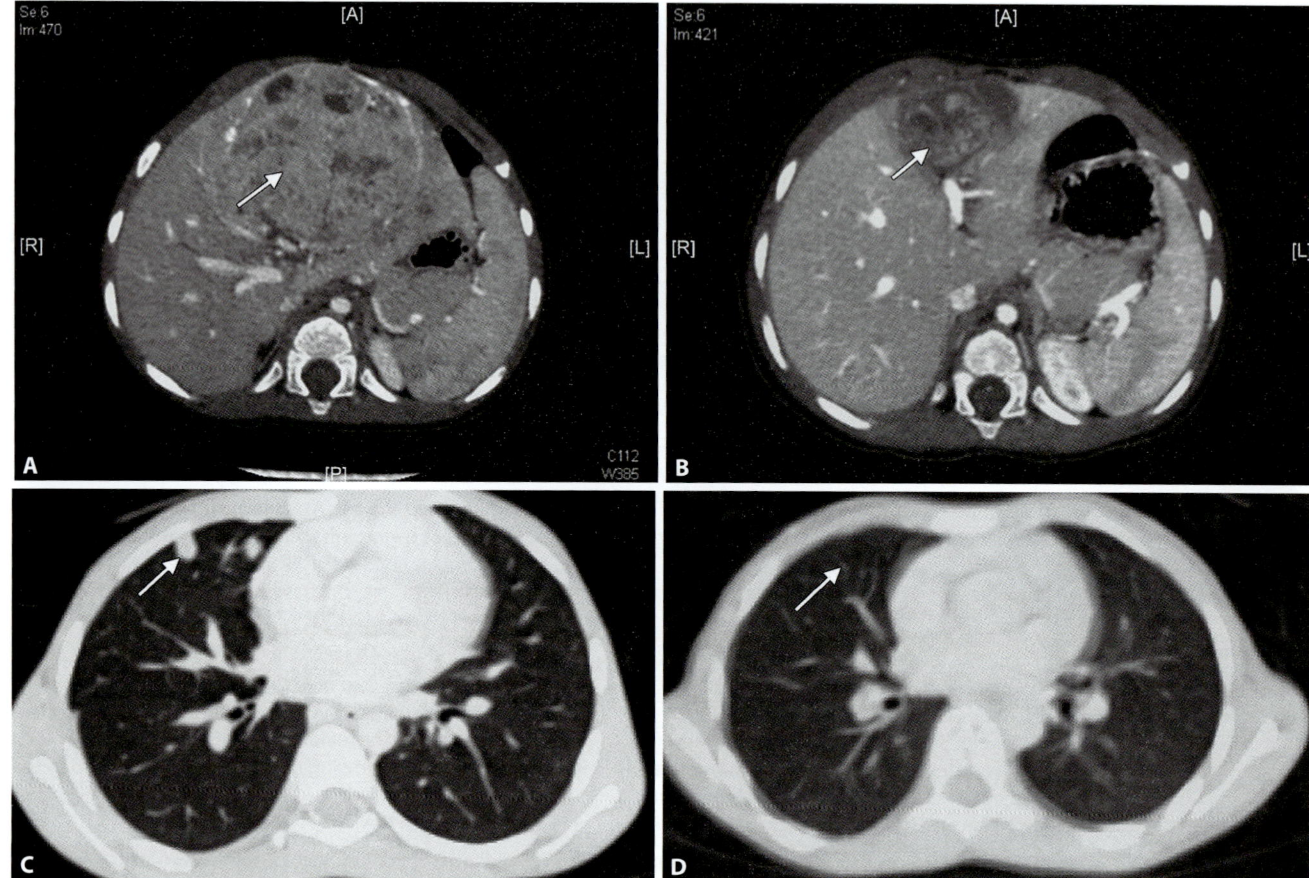

Figs. 12.5.7A to D: Contrast-enhanced computer tomography (CECT) abdomen in a 11-month-old child showing hepatoblastoma (arterial enhancing tumor in the left lobe of the liver)—prechemotherapy (A) and good response—postchemotherapy; (B) Right pulmonary metastasis (well-defined nodules in the lung)—prechemotherapy (C) and postchemotherapy, showing complete resolution (D).

- Infantile hepatic hemangioma which has fine granular calcifications, enhancement following the blood pool occurring exclusively <1 year.
- Mesenchymal hamartoma occurring at the same age group by their cystic nature and normal AFP.[7]

Liver Trauma

The liver is the most commonly injured organ (particularly the right lobe) in pediatric abdominal trauma due to the soft rib cage. Liver injuries range from a minor tear of the capsule to a full-blown laceration with injury of the vascular supply and/or bile ducts of the liver. USG is primarily used as the first screening modality however CT is used to grade the severity and to rule out other organ injuries.

IMAGING OF PANCREAS

Congenital Abnormalities

Congenital anomalies of the pancreas include pancreas divisum, annular pancreas, and agenesis of the dorsal pancreatic anlagen. MRI is the modality of choice to detect these pathologies.

Pancreatitis

Etiologies are different in children compared to adults. USG is the first choice imaging modality. Contrast CT/MRI is recommended in clinical deterioration to document pancreatic necrosis and other complications. The optimal timing of the scan is at least 72–96 hours after the presentation since early imaging may underestimate the extent of the disease and its complications.

Acute Pancreatitis

Modified CT severity score is used to grade the severity which takes into account pancreatic enlargement, peripancreatic inflammation, peripancreatic fluid, intrapancreatic necrosis, and extrapancreatic findings including vascular thrombosis, ascites, pleural fluid, gastrointestinal complications, etc.

The *Revised Atlanta classification of acute pancreatitis* from 2012 is an international multidisciplinary classification

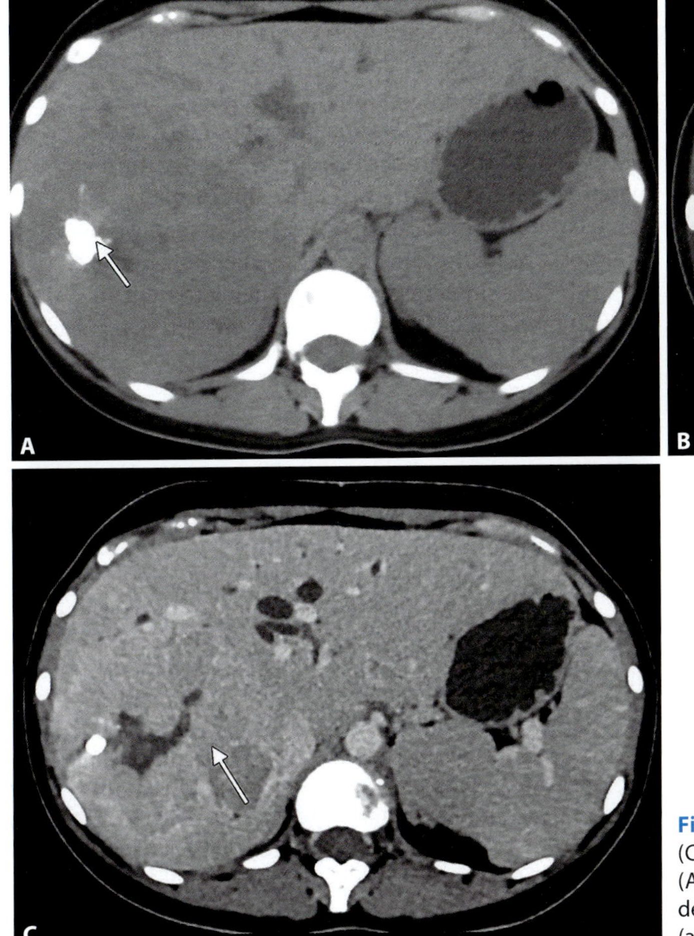
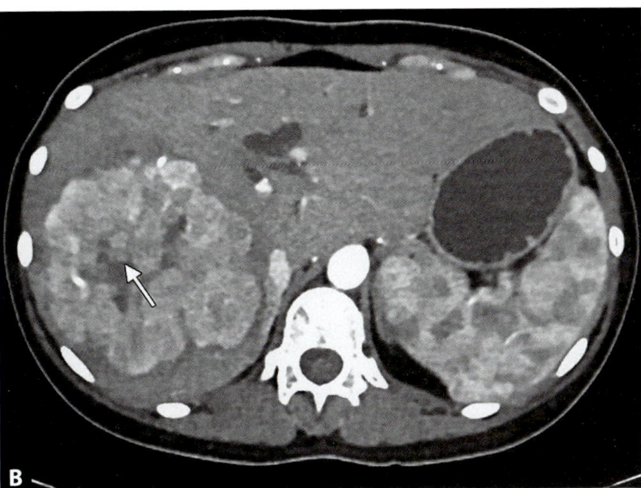

Figs. 12.5.8A to C: Contrast-enhanced computed tomography (CECT) of a 26-year-old female with fibrolamellar carcinoma. (A) Plain CT showing chunky calcification; (B) Arterial phase demonstrating enhancing lesion with a central nonenhancing scar (arrow); (C) Portal venous phase showing washout in the lesion.

TABLE 12.5.7: Common malignant hepatic neoplasms.

Pathology	*Age group*	*Clinical features*	*Biochemical parameters*	*Imaging findings*
Hepatocellular carcinoma (HCC): • Second most common primary pediatric malignancy • Preexisting liver disease is seen only in 30–50% • Predisposing factors are biliary atresia, cholestatic syndromes, hemochromatosis, hereditary tyrosinemia, glycogen storage disorders, Wilson disease, and hepatitis B infection	• Bimodal • First 2–5 years • Viral induced—adolescence	Abdominal mass, constitutional symptoms, and abdominal pain	Serum α-fetoprotein (AFP) levels are elevated in 55–65% of the cases	• Mosaic pattern due to fat, necrosis, and hemorrhage is the hallmark • Nonperipheral arterial enhancement with portal venous enhancement and a delayed enhancing pseudocapsule is the typical enhancement pattern • Metastasis to the nodes (50%), lungs, mediastinum, skeleton, and brain are observed
Fibrolamellar carcinoma: Fibrolamellar carcinoma is a rare variant of HCC without predisposing factors such as cirrhosis or viral hepatitis	Adolescents and young adults	Mass, pain	Serum AFP level is normal	• Well-defined lobulated lesion showing arterial enhancement with variable portal venous washout • Chunky calcification (35–68%) with a central nonenhancing T2 hypointense hyperechoic scar • Nodal metastases is common (65%).Other common sites are the lungs, peritoneum, and adrenal glands (20–30%) • Increased recurrence necessitates frequent follow-up imaging

TABLE 12.5.8: Revised Atlanta classification for acute pancreatitis 2012.

1. Interstitial edematous pancreatitis (IEP)		
Acute peripancreatic fluid collections (APFC)	<4 weeks	Nonencapsulated fluid peripancreatic collection
Pseudocysts	>4 weeks	Encapsulated fluid peripancreatic/remote fluid collection
2. Necrotizing pancreatitis (NP)		
Acute necrotic collection (ANC)	<4 weeks	Nonencapsulated nonfluid debris collection
Walled off necrosis (WON)	>4 weeks	Encapsulated nonfluid collection

of the severity of acute pancreatitis, with standardized terminology for pancreatitis and its complications **(Table 12.5.8)**.

Chronic Pancreatitis

Chronic pancreatitis is characterized by parenchymal atrophy, parenchymal, and ductal calcification, chain of lake appearance of main pancreatic duct (MPD) in MRCP due to irregularly dilated main duct along with branch duct dilatation (>1.5 mm at 1–6 years of age, >1.9 mm at 7–12 years, and >2.2 mm at 13–18 years).

Trauma

Children are more prone to pancreatic injury because of its fixed retroperitoneal position. Injury manifest as edema, laceration, transection, and/or acute pancreatitis. CT shows bulky hypoenhancing pancreas with adjacent fluid. MRCP is the best modality to evaluate ductal laceration. Pseudocysts develop in 50% of the patients.

CONCLUSION

Pediatric hepatobiliary imaging is important not only for evaluation of congenital or structural anomalies but also for diffuse/focal parenchymal and vascular lesions including neoplasms. The specific imaging characteristics of various pathologies are often distinctive. Recognition of these patterns, combined with correlative clinical data, is imperative for accurate diagnosis and proper patient management. USG is almost always the first imaging modality of choice, followed by MRI. CT is often reserved for imaging trauma and staging of malignancies although for the latter MRI is increasingly validated and used.

REFERENCES

1. Nievelstein RA, Robben SG, Blickman JG. Hepatobiliary and pancreatic imaging in children-techniques and an overview of non-neoplastic disease entities. Pediatr Radiol. 2011;41(1):55-75.
2. Arora A, Sarin SK. Multimodality imaging of primary extrahepatic portal vein obstruction (EHPVO): What every radiologist should know. Br J Radiol. 2015;88(1052):20150008.
3. Sureka B, Rastogi A, Bihari C, Bharathy KGS, Sood V, Alam S. Imaging in ductal plate malformations. Indian J Radiol Imaging. 2017;27(1):6-12.
4. Adeyiga AO, Lee EY, Eisenberg RL. Focal hepatic masses in pediatric patients. AJR Am J Roentgenol. 2012;199(4):W422-40.
5. Chiorean L, Cui XW, Tannapfel A, Franke D, Stenzel M, Kosiak W, et al. Benign liver tumors in pediatric patients—Review with emphasis on imaging features. World J Gastroenterol. 2015;21(28):8541-61.
6. Ng K, Mogul DB. Pediatric liver tumors. Clin Liver Dis. 2018;22(4):753-72.
7. Dhali A, Kumar H, Sengupta S, Biswas J, Kumar B, Dhali GK. Mesenchymal hamartoma versus hepatoblastoma: A diagnostic dilemma. Int J Surg Case Rep. 2023;112:108931.

12.6 Pediatric Liver Pathology

Pallavi Prasad, Mukul Vij

INTRODUCTION

An adequate needle liver biopsy must be at least 2.0 cm long, 0.2 mm wide, nonfragmented, and contain a minimum of ten portal tracts. An adequate surgical wedge biopsy should be deep enough to include six complete portal tracts independent of the liver capsule.

NORMAL HISTOLOGY

Lobule

The liver parenchyma is composed of lobules with a vein at its center and portal tracts at its periphery.[1] The lobules have thin-walled sinusoidal capillaries, lined by fenestrated endothelial cells, which drain the portal tract toward a central vein. The hepatocytes are arranged in cords surrounding individual sinusoidal capillaries.[1]

Portal Tracts

Portal tracts comprise of three structures—a portal vein, branch of the hepatic artery, and a bile duct, which define three different "zones"—zone 1, which is adjacent to the portal tract, zone 3 is nearest to the hepatic venule, and zone 2 lies in between **(Fig. 12.6.1)**. This arrangement of structures is known as an "acinus." The periportal, mid, and pericentral zones of the lobule are represented by the acinar zones 1, 2, and 3, respectively.[2] The connective tissue of portal tracts is formed mainly by type 1 collagen.

Hepatocytes

Hepatocytes are normally arranged in one-to-two cells thick cords, separated by sinusoids. Hepatocytes at the periphery of the portal tracts form a sheath-like layer called the "limiting plate." Hepatocytes are polygonal, measuring about 25–40 μm, having a central nucleus, and abundant eosinophilic cytoplasm, which is rich in endoplasmic reticulum and glycogen, the latter highlighted with a periodic acid-Schiff stain.[2]

Sinusoidal Lining Cells

They are lined by endothelial cells and Kupffer cells, resting on a layer of reticulin. Because of the fenestrated endothelial lining, blood, and hepatocyte exchange through the Disse space is facilitated. Kupffer cells have cytoplasmic extensions that enable phagocytosis, imparting them an uneven appearance.

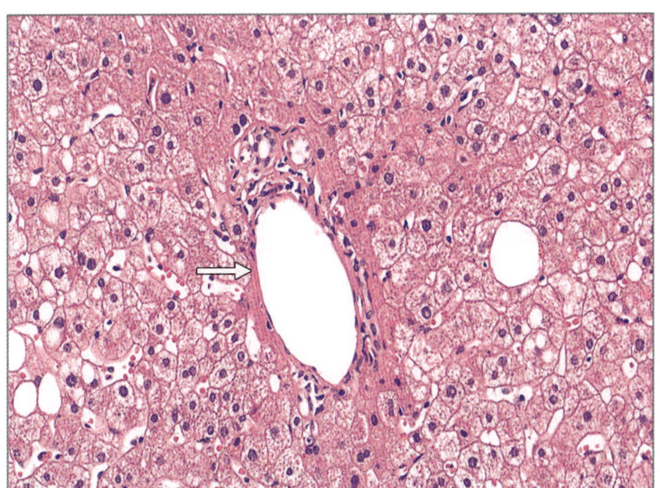

Fig. 12.6.1: Portal tract (arrow) with a bile duct, portal vein, and hepatic artery (H&E, ×16).

Space of Disse

Space of Disse lies between endothelial cells and hepatocytes. It contains plasma, connective tissue, and hepatic stellate cells (Ito cells).

Bile Ducts and Ductules

Bile ducts are lined by cuboidal to columnar epithelium, and are usually accompanied by an artery and a vein.[2] These anastomose to form larger ducts that leave at the hilum as right and left hepatic ducts. Bile ductules are present at the periphery of the tracts.[2]

Vasculature

The portal vein and bile duct are surrounded by terminal hepatic arterioles and plexuses, which mark the end of the hepatic arterial supply. Terminal portal venules mark the end of the portal vein. Both arterial and venous blood from portal tracts enters the terminal hepatic venule through the sinusoids after crossing the limiting plate in both arterial and venous forms. The inferior vena cava receives the larger hepatic veins formed by the combination of these venules.[2]

NEONATAL GIANT CELL HEPATITIS

Cholestasis in early infancy poses a diagnostic quandary. In around a quarter to half of infants presenting with conjugated hyperbilirubinemia within the first 3 months of life, no obvious cause is detected, and these are considered to have (idiopathic) neonatal giant cell hepatitis. It is believed to represent a form of neonatal hepatitis associated with an underlying condition (e.g., infection, inborn error of metabolism, etc.) which becomes apparent later after extensive evaluation. Histologically, it is characterized by the formation of syncytial hepatic giant cells, variable inflammation, and lobular cholestasis **(Fig. 12.6.2)**. Significant obstructive changes as seen in biliary atresia or paucity of intrahepatic bile ducts are not observed.[3] Liver biopsy is needed to differentiate between biliary atresia, paucity of intrahepatic bile ducts, and neonatal giant cell hepatitis (NGCH).

BILIARY ATRESIA

Biliary atresia (BA) is a progressive disease of extra- and intrahepatic bile ducts developing in the first weeks of life. It is the main cause of neonatal cholestasis and the most common indication of liver transplantation in children. The key histopathological findings include expansion of portal tracts and bile ductular proliferation, comprising of anastomosing ductules located at the periphery of the portal tracts **(Fig. 12.6.3)**.[4] Ductular cholestasis is an important diagnostic finding. Duct/ductal bile plugs and portal stromal edema are strong histologic predictors of BA. Neutrophils within

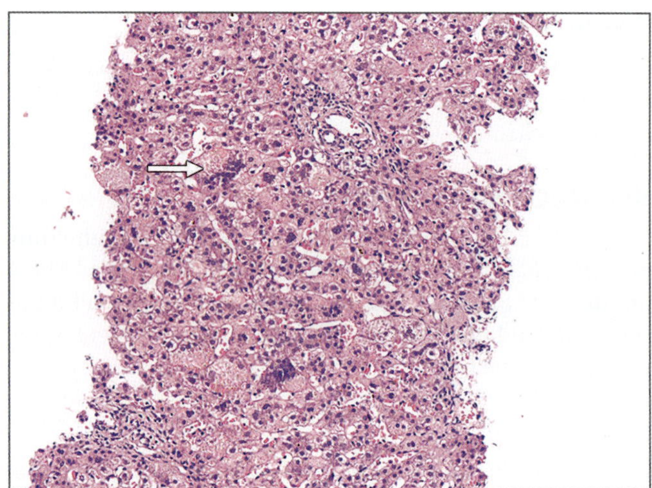

Fig. 12.6.2: Giant cell hepatitis with multinucleate giant cells (arrow) in an infant (H&E, ×12).

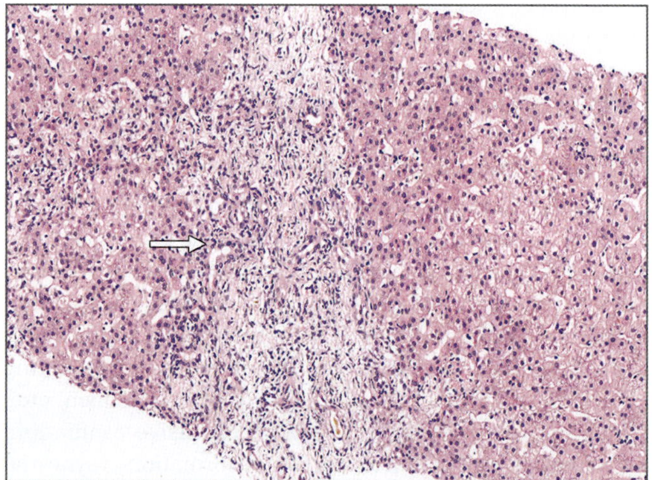

Fig. 12.6.3: Biliary atresia demonstrating expansion of portal tracts and bile ductular proliferation (arrow, H&E, ×12).

the lumen of the ducts suggest superimposed cholangitis.[4] The presence of ductal plate malformation (DPM) carries an unfavorable prognosis. DPM is characterized by circumferential biliary ductular structures within the connective tissue of the portal tract, which resembles primitive ductal elements. The incidence of DPM reported in most studies is 20–50%.[4] DPM results from improper remodeling of primitive fetal bile ducts during organogenesis. Lobular features include hepatocyte giant cell transformation, extramedullary hematopoiesis, ballooning degeneration, hepatic and canalicular bile plugs, rosetting, and patchy lobular inflammation with spotty necrosis.[4]

The BA is believed to be a multifactorial disease; factors include genetic predisposition with glypican 1, adducin 3, and ADP-ribosylation factor 6, genes vital in embryonic development and organogenesis, environmental factors (ex. biliary toxin biliatresone), infections, and immune dysregulation.

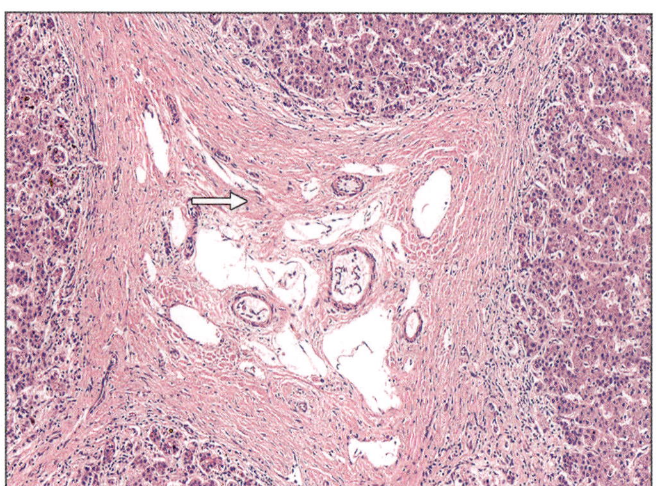

Fig. 12.6.4: An explant liver with paucity of bile ducts (arrow, H&E, ×13).

PAUCITY OF INTERLOBULAR BILE DUCTS

It constitutes a small proportion of neonatal obstructive cholangiopathy cases. Paucity of interlobular bile ducts (PILBD) can be nonsyndromic (idiopathic) or syndromic (Alagille's syndrome). Mutations in the *NOTCH2* or *JAG-1* genes result in Alagille syndrome or arteriohepatic dysplasia, which is a multisystem autosomal dominant disorder. The nonsyndromic form is less common and is poorly characterized.[5]

The differential diagnosis includes other metabolic and genetic disorders, infections, immune/inflammatory disorders, drugs, endocrinopathies, and idiopathic causes. A reduced number of interlobular bile ducts (BD) in the portal triad (PT) with a BD/PT of <0.9 in a liver biopsy with at least five portal tracts suggests a diagnosis of PILBD **(Fig. 12.6.4)**. A BD/PT <0.6 is highly likely and <0.5 is virtually diagnostic of PILBD.[5] Apart from hematoxylin and eosin (H&E) stain, Masson's trichrome stain, and cytokeratin-7 immunohistochemistry aid in better characterization of the bile ducts.

PROGRESSIVE FAMILIAL INTRAHEPATIC CHOLESTASIS

Progressive familial intrahepatic cholestasis (PFIC) is a heterogeneous group of autosomal-recessive disorders that impede bile formation and presents with hepatocellular cholestasis. PFIC3 may appear later in infancy, childhood, or young adulthood, while PFIC1 and PFIC2 typically manifest

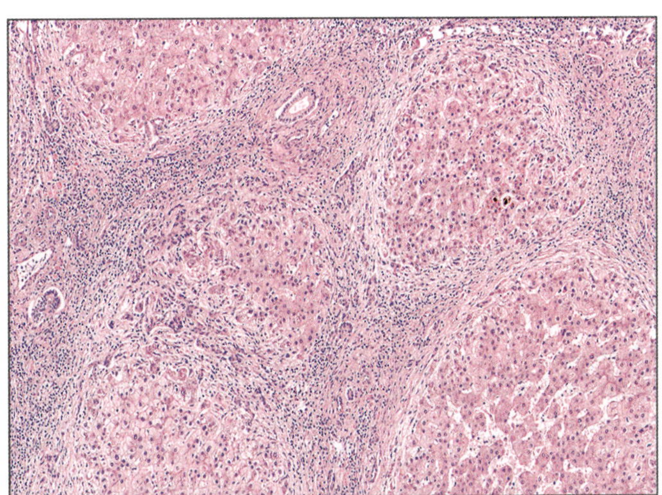

Fig. 12.6.5: An explant liver with multidrug-resistance protein 3 (MDR3) deficiency displaying cirrhosis (H&E, ×7).

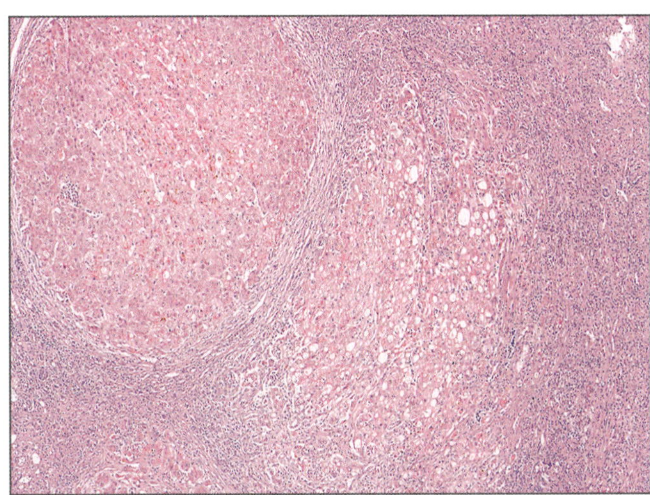

Fig. 12.6.6: Wilson disease with cirrhosis, cholestasis, and steatosis (H&E, ×5).

in the first few months of life. It begins initially as jaundice and itchy skin and then progresses from persistent cholestasis to cirrhosis and liver failure before late childhood. Based on the six mutated genes—*ATP8B1*, ATP-binding cassette subfamily B member 11 (*ABCB11*), ATP-binding cassette transporter A4 (*ABCB4*), *TJP2*, *NR1H4*, and *MYO5B*—six types of PFIC have been identified.

The PFIC is a diagnosis of exclusion. Patients with PFIC1 and PFIC2 usually have normal serum gamma-glutamyl transpeptidase (GGT), while patients with PFIC3 have elevated GGT. Multidrug-resistance protein 3 (MDR3) and bile salt export pump (BSEP) liver immunostaining help to select PFIC cases in whom molecular diagnosis can be proposed.

The liver histology of PFIC1 patients shows periportal biliary metaplasia of hepatocytes along with canalicular cholestasis and lack of true ductular proliferation.[6] In early PFIC2, histology displays features similar to neonatal hepatitis, including inflammation, giant cell transformation, and canalicular cholestasis. Fibrosis, ductular reaction, and canalicular cholestasis appear in later stages.[7]

Liver biopsy in PFIC3 reveals true ductular proliferation along with portal fibrosis. Lobular and canalicular cholestasis can occasionally be observed **(Fig. 12.6.5)**. Later stages are characterized by a typical picture of biliary cirrhosis and extensive portal fibrosis. Most portal tracts have interlobular bile ducts, but there is no evidence of periductal fibrosis or biliary epithelium damage.[8]

WILSON DISEASE

Wilson disease (WD) is a rare copper metabolism disorder. It is autosomal recessive. It was first identified by Kinnear Wilson in 1912 as "progressive lenticular degeneration," a familial neurological disorder that causes liver failure that eventually results in cirrhosis. Mutations in the *ATP7B* gene and resultant dysfunction in the *ATP7B* protein lead to defective biliary copper excretion, causing various hepatic, neurologic, and psychiatric disorders. These patients have hemolysis-related transient, unconjugated hyperbilirubinemia in addition to abnormal aminotransferase levels. A 24-hour urinary copper test is a useful diagnostic tool for WD and aids in measuring nonceruloplasmin-bound copper. For symptomatic patients, a urinary copper threshold of >100 μg/24 hour aids in the diagnosis of WD. Hepatic copper content in healthy individuals is <50 μg/g dry weight; in patients with WD, it is usually >250 μg/g dry weight. Although not to the same extent as in WD, cirrhosis and cholestatic disease also demonstrate increased hepatic copper content.

On histology, early cases show mild, nonspecific lobular changes. Scattered apoptotic hepatocytes, spotty necrosis, occasional ballooned hepatocytes, glycogenated hepatocyte nuclei, and mild macrovesicular steatosis may be present. In later stages, portal inflammation increases, interface activity develops, and hepatocyte ballooning increases. Bridging fibrosis and ultimately cirrhosis develop **(Fig. 12.6.6)**. Parenchymal apoptosis of hepatocytes is also a striking feature.[9] Rhodanine or rubeanic acid stains highlight increased hepatocytic copper accumulation. Mild copper accumulation may be seen in cholestatic diseases and is therefore not specific for WD.[9]

AUTOIMMUNE HEPATITIS

Autoimmune hepatitis (AIH) is a liver immune-mediated inflammatory disease. Clinical presentation is variable, ranging from liver enzyme alterations to fulminant hepatitis. Clinical symptoms include fatigue, nausea, anorexia, abdominal pain, weight loss, and arthralgia. Alanine aminotransferase (ALT), aspartate aminotransferase (AST), alkaline phosphatase (ALP), and GGT, serum immunoglobulin G (IgG) levels are elevated, the latter is usually 1.2–3 times the normal value. Serum antibodies such as antinuclear antibody (ANA), antismooth muscle antibody (SMA), and antiliver kidney microsomal antibody (LKM-1) are used for the diagnosis of AIH.[10]

Liver biopsy can be classified as:

- *Typical for AIH:* When all three features are present—typical interface hepatitis, with lymphocytic/lymphoplasmocytic infiltrate in portal tracts extending into the lobule, emperipolesis, and hepatic rosette formation.
- *Compatible with AIH:* Lack of all the features considered typical, i.e., chronic hepatitis pattern of injury with lymphocytic infiltration.
- *Atypical for AIH:* Signs suggestive of other diagnosis.

Differential Diagnosis

Since the pattern of injury and typical features of AIH are nonspecific, the histological differential diagnosis includes:

- *Viral hepatitis:* Serological testing, which is mandatory in all patients for whom an AIH diagnosis is being considered, helps in excluding viral infection.
- *Drug-induced liver injury (DILI):* DILI is the most difficult differential diagnosis to make because it can resemble the morphological, biochemical, clinical, and serological characteristics of AIH. Additionally, drugs have the potential to cause a de novo AIH or activate a latent one. The diagnosis of AIH is supported by severe portal plasma cell-rich inflammation, prominent intralobular plasma cells and eosinophils, rosette formation, absence of cholestasis, and presence of fibrosis; on the other hand, AIH-like DILI is more likely to be present in cases without cirrhosis or with advanced fibrosis. History of recent exposure to drugs should be elicited.[10]
- *Primary biliary cholangitis (PBC):* PBC is characterized by moderate-to-severe portal inflammatory inflammation with many plasma cells, interface hepatitis, and positive antimitochondrial antibodies (AMAs). Moreover, prominent bile duct loss and florid duct lesions may be observed (absent in AIH).
- *WD:* Serum ceruloplasmin levels and 24-hour urine copper levels are typically sufficient to rule out WD. Rhodanine stain may be useful in liver biopsies to detect copper.

DUCTAL PLATE MALFORMATIONS

Ductal plate malformations (DPM) was defined by Desmet as "the excessive presence of juvenile bile duct structures due to the absence of ductal plate remodeling that should differentiate into mature bile ducts during fetal life." The persistence of embryonic biliary structures after birth is a characteristic of DPM.[11] DPM is the cause of several congenital diseases such as congenital hepatic fibrosis and autosomal dominant polycystic liver disease. Low et al. first established the poor prognosis of BA in patients with DPM, thereafter, many other studies have shown similar findings.

GLYCOGEN STORAGE DISEASE

Glycogen storage disease (GSD) is caused by a genetically determined metabolic block involving enzymes that mediate glycogenesis or glycogenolysis, leading to impaired accumulation of abnormal metabolites of this branched polysaccharide. GSD is clinically characterized by hypoglycemia and hepatomegaly. Histopathological examination of the liver in patients with GSD-Ia characteristically reveals a mosaic pattern with pale-staining, distended glycogen-containing hepatocytes (periodic acid-Schiff (PAS)-positive and diastase-sensitive) **(Fig. 12.6.7)**. Steatosis and glycogenated nuclei may be noted. Fibrosis is not as prominent in GSD-I as in GSD types III, IV, and VI. Mutation analysis or an enzyme assay validate the final diagnosis. Electron microscopic evaluation can help differentiate GSD from other metabolic storage diseases or mitochondrial disorders.[12]

OTHER METABOLIC LIVER DISEASES

Alpha 1-antitrypsin deficiency is caused by mutations in the coding sequence of the serine protease inhibitor, alpha 1-antitrypsin, which prevents its export from the hepatocyte. Liver biopsy reveals periodic acid-Schiff-positive, diastase-resistant globules in hepatocytes.[13]

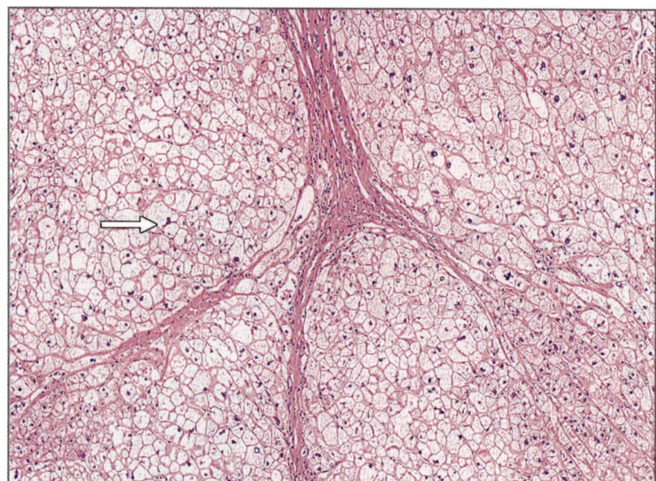

Fig. 12.6.7: Glycogen storage disease with enlarged pale hepatocytes and scarring (H&E, ×8).

Cystic fibrosis (CF) is caused by a mutation in the *CFTR* gene. Biliary obstruction and progressive periportal fibrosis lead initially to focal biliary cirrhosis, which may progress to multilobular biliary cirrhosis.[13] Steatosis is also a frequent finding.[13]

Hereditary fructosemia is caused by deficiency of aldolase B enzyme. Patients usually become symptomatic at the time of weaning with hypoglycemia, lactic acidosis, ketosis, and typical aversion to sweet foods. Biopsy findings include neonatal giant cell hepatitis, macrovesicular steatosis, portal or periportal fibrosis, cirrhosis, ductular proliferation, acinar transformation of hepatocytes, cholestasis, and collagenization of sinusoids.[14]

*Hereditary tyrosine*mia is an autosomal recessive inborn error of metabolism caused by the deficiency of fumarylacetoacetate hydrolase (FAH).

Hemochromatosis: The histology depends on the cells where iron accumulates and correlates with the disease etiology—parenchymal (in hepatocytes and bile duct epithelium) or Kupffer cells, portal macrophages, and endothelial cells (in secondary iron overload). The former is characteristic of hereditary hemochromatosis and should be supplemented with serum iron studies and *HFE* gene testing. Hemosiderin pigment appears as golden-brown refractile granules on hematoxylin and eosin stains and as bluish granules on Perls' Prussian blue stain.[15]

CIRRHOSIS

Cirrhosis is characterized by disruption of the lobular architecture as a result of fibrosis and nodular regeneration. Common causes in infants include biliary atresia and genetic-metabolic illnesses, whereas autoimmune hepatitis, WD, alpha-1-antitrypsin deficiency, and primary sclerosing cholangitis are the most common etiologies in older children. The "gold-standard" modality for diagnosing cirrhosis is liver biopsy, however, limited specimen size, sampling error, and fragmented biopsies constitute the important limitations.[16]

Several semiquantitative scoring systems have been established for grading fibrosis and cirrhosis—namely, Knodell, Batts-Ludwig, Scheuer, Ishak, and METAVIR systems. The basic grading concept is similar across all these systems, i.e., fibrosis begins in the portal tracts, and extends to adjacent portal tracts and terminal hepatic venules resulting in architectural distortion and finely cirrhosis.[17]

The histological patterns of liver fibrosis depend on the etiology.

- *Chronic hepatitis*—portal and periportal fibrosis, septal fibrosis, and cirrhosis.
- *Fatty liver disease*—pericentral fibrosis.
- *Biliary tract disease*—irregular-shaped nodules ("jigsaw" pattern).[17]

CONCLUSION

In conclusion, histologic study of liver tissue remains the cornerstone of diagnosing and treating liver disease in children. Meaningful interpretation of pediatric liver biopsies can only happen alongside a global assessment of the clinical scenario and other investigations.

REFERENCES

1. Juza RM, Pauli EM. Clinical and surgical anatomy of the liver: a review for clinicians. Clin Anat. 2014;27(5):764-9.
2. Krishna M. Microscopic anatomy of the liver. Clin Liver Dis (Hoboken). 2013;2(Suppl 1):S4-S7.
3. Torbenson M, Hart J, Westerhoff M, Azzam RK, Elgendi A, Mziray-Andrew HC, et al. Neonatal giant cell hepatitis: histological and etiological findings. Am J Surg Pathol. 2010;34(10):1498-503.
4. Vij M, Rela M. Biliary atresia: pathology, etiology and pathogenesis. Future Sci OA. 2020;6(5):FSO466.
5. Mohanty S, Das K, Anne Correa MM. Non Syndromic Paucity of Interlobular Bile Ducts in Children - A Clinicopathological Study. Fetal Pediatr Pathol. 2020;39(4):317-33.
6. Davit-Spraul A, Gonzales E, Baussan C, Jacquemin E. Progressive familial intrahepatic cholestasis. Orphanet J Rare Dis. 2009;4:1.
7. Evason K, Bove KE, Finegold MJ, Knisely AS, Rhee S, Rosenthal P, et al. Morphologic findings in progressive familial intrahepatic cholestasis 2 (PFIC2): correlation with genetic and immunohistochemical studies. Am J Surg Pathol. 2011;35(5):687-96.
8. Vij M, Safwan M, Shanmugam NP, Rela M. Liver pathology in severe multidrug resistant 3 protein deficiency: a series of 10 pediatric cases. Ann Diagn Pathol. 2015;19(5):277-82.
9. Schroeder SM, Matsukuma KE, Medici V. Wilson disease and the differential diagnosis of its hepatic manifestations: a narrative review of clinical, laboratory, and liver histological features. Ann Transl Med. 2021;9(17):1394.
10. Covelli C, Sacchi D, Sarcognato S, Cazzagon N, Grillo F, Baciorri F, et al. Pathology of autoimmune hepatitis. Pathologica. 2021;113(3):185.
11. Raynaud P, Tate J, Callens C, Cordi S, Vandersmissen P, Carpentier R, et al. A classification of ductal plate malformations based on distinct pathogenic mechanisms of biliary dysmorphogenesis. Hepatology. 2011;53(6):1959-66.
12. Roy A, Finegold MJ. Biopsy diagnosis of inherited liver disease. Surg Pathol Clin. 2010;3:743-68.
13. Ovchinsky N, Moreira RK, Lefkowitch JH, Lavine JE. Liver biopsy in modern clinical practice: a pediatric point-of-view. Adv Anat Pathol. 2012;19(4):250-62.
14. Menon J, Vij M, Sachan D, Rammohan A, Shanmugam N, Kaliamoorthy I, et al. Pediatric metabolic liver diseases: Evolving role of liver transplantation. World J Transplant. 2021;11(6):161-79.
15. Salomao MA. Pathology of hepatic iron overload. Clin Liver Dis. 2021;17(4):232.
16. Pinto RB, Schneider AC, da Silveira TR. Cirrhosis in children and adolescents: An overview. World J Hepatol. 2015;7(3):392-405.
17. Lo RC, Kim H. Histopathological evaluation of liver fibrosis and cirrhosis regression. Clin Mol Hepatol. 2017;23(4):302-7.

12.7 Viral Hepatitis

Malathi Sathiyasekaran

INTRODUCTION

Hepatitis or inflammation of the hepatocytes may be acute or chronic in its presentation. *Acute hepatitis* is a self-limiting liver disease characterized by an abrupt onset of symptoms with the hepatocellular inflammation usually resolving completely within 4 weeks. When there is a continuing inflammation beyond 6 months (3 months in children), it is labeled as *chronic hepatitis*. Viruses are the most important causative agents of hepatitis and the term viral hepatitis refers to the illness caused by the major hepatotropic viruses—hepatitis A, B, C, D, and E [(hepatitis A virus (HAV), hepatitis B virus (HBV), hepatitis C virus (HCV), hepatitis D virus (HDV), and hepatitis E virus (HEV)], though several other viruses such as Coxsackie virus, Epstein–Barr virus (EBV), *Herpes simplex*, cytomegalovirus (CMV), severe acute respiratory syndrome coronavirus 2 (SARS-CoV2), and adenovirus can also cause hepatitis. This chapter highlights the features of acute viral hepatitis (AVH) caused by the common hepatotropic viruses.

DEFINITION

Acute viral hepatitis is a systemic viral infection predominantly affecting the liver with a characteristic constellation of clinical (jaundice, nausea, vomiting, and right hypochondrial pain), biochemical (elevated serum bilirubin and/or transaminases more than twice upper limit of normal), and pathological (hepatocellular inflammation and necrosis) features, which resolves spontaneously or progresses to acute liver failure or chronic hepatitis.

EPIDEMIOLOGY

In India sporadic AVH is caused mainly by the two enterally transmitted viruses namely hepatitis A (60–70%) and hepatitis E (10–20%). The two parenterally transmitted viruses namely HBV (10–15%) and HCV (<1%) are less common causes of acute sporadic hepatitis. Improvement in socioeconomic status has resulted in a shift in epidemiology of HAV with older children being susceptible to the infection. The prevalence of HBV in India ranges from 2.4–16% to HCV 1–2.5%. HEV has been isolated in all the major epidemics in India and is more common in North India especially in regions around the river Ganges. Infections due to HAV and HEV are generally self-limiting and do not progress to chronicity. Chronic HEV (presence of HEV >3 months) though rare may occur in immunocompromised children or those with solid organ transplant. HBV and HCV infections may progress to chronic hepatitis, cirrhosis, and hepatocellular carcinoma.

ETIOPATHOGENESIS

- *Hepatitis A virus* is a 27 nm picornavirus spread by the orofecal route with an incubation period of 15–50 days. The necroinflammatory reaction is believed to be an immune response of the host to the HAV.[1] A child with HAV infection is usually infective from 2 weeks before the onset of symptoms to a few days after because of the high fecal viral shedding during this period **(Fig. 12.7.1)**.
- *Hepatitis E virus* is a 30 nm RNA virus of the *Genus Herpesvirus* with 8 genotypes (GT). HEV 1 and 2 are transmitted by the orofecal route with an incubation period of 15–40 days similar to HAV. The mechanism of hepatocyte injury is most likely due to an immune-mediated reaction.[2]
- *Hepatitis B virus* is a 42 nm virus of hepadnavirus family, which causes an immune-mediated injury. The severity of the illness depends on the degree of immune response produced by the host. HBV is a highly infective virus with an incubation period of 60–180 days and is transmitted by blood, blood products, and body fluids. The three antigens—hepatitis B surface antigen (HBsAg), envelope antigen (HBeAg), and core antigen (HBcAg)—and their corresponding antibodies and the viral HBV deoxyribonucleic acid (DNA) are useful biomarkers in diagnosis and monitoring therapy. HBsAg appears in the blood 6 weeks after infection and usually disappears within 6 months. Persistence of HBsAg beyond 6 months indicates chronicity. HBeAg appears soon after HBsAg and disappears within 6 weeks. Persistence of this antigen beyond 6 weeks indicates HBeAg positive chronic hepatitis. HBcAg is detected only in hepatocytes and not in the serum. The presence of anti-HBc immunoglobulin (Ig)M indicates recent infection, whereas presence of anti-HBc IgG indicates past infection. Anti-HBs is the protective antibody and may be present following immunization or natural infection. Quantification of HBV DNA is essential to determine the phase of chronic infection. The relaxed DNA of the HBV on entering the hepatocyte becomes a

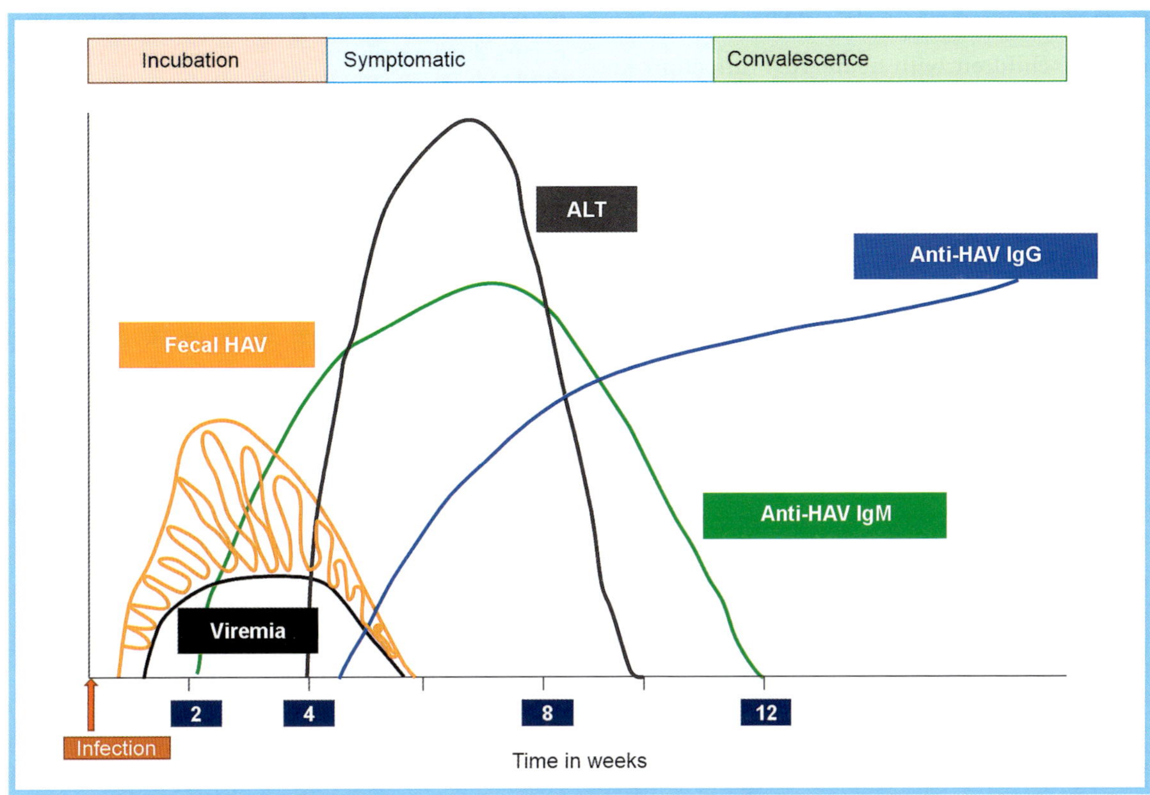

Fig. 12.7.1: Natural course of hepatitis A infection. (ALT: alanine transaminase; HAV: hepatitis A virus; IgG: immunoglobulin G; IgM: immunoglobulin M)

closed circular covalent DNA (cccDNA) and integrates with the host DNA.[3] Perinatal transmission of HBV is a unique problem seen in children and is more common in areas of high endemicity.

- *Hepatitis C virus* is a 30–80 nm RNA virus of Flaviviridae family and results in a complex immune response. HCV has an incubation period of 60–150 days and is less infective; but more sinister than HBV and is spread by blood and blood products. Perinatal transmission occurs when mothers have a high HCV viral load.
- *Hepatitis D virus* is a defective virus with a small ribonucleic acid (RNA) molecule and an envelope constituted by HBsAg. This virus infects only those who are HBsAg positive and presents either as superinfection or coinfection depending on whether HDV infects a child with preexisting chronic HBV infection or infects along with HBV.

CLINICAL FEATURES

In the majority of young children with AVH, the presentation may be subclinical or anicteric whereas in older children the three stages of AVH, viz., the prodrome, icteric stage, and convalescence may be more distinct. The clinical presentation is common to all the types of viral hepatitis with a prodrome, which usually lasts for 2–7 days characterized by nausea, vomiting, high-colored urine, fever, and right hypochondrial pain followed by jaundice, pale stools, and tender hepatomegaly. The icteric stage usually lasts for 7–14 days but may persist as long as 12 weeks in older children. The recovery is heralded by the disappearance of the constitutional symptoms, improvement in appetite, and decrease in the size of liver.

Hepatitis A Virus and Hepatitis E Virus

Older children with HAV infection may present with atypical manifestations[2] such as ascites, pleural effusion, firm hepatomegaly, relapsing hepatitis, and prolonged cholestasis.[4] Extrahepatic manifestations are uncommon and include evanescent skin rash, transient arthralgia, pancreatitis, vasculitis, thrombocytopenia, triggering of autoimmune hepatitis, red cell aplasia, myocarditis, nephritis, cryoglobulinemia, and Guillain-Barré syndrome. Acute liver failure occurs in <1% of children.

Infection due to HEV is similar to HAV. During HEV epidemics children usually have a milder or subclinical infection. HEV-related pancreatitis is seen in regions where HEV1 is endemic whereas neurological manifestations are seen with HEV genotype 3. Pregnant women present with acute liver failure associated with a high maternal mortality (1–20%) and stillbirths.[2]

Hepatitis B Virus and Hepatitis C Virus

The majority of children with acute HBV infection are anicteric. Those with icteric hepatitis may be symptomatic for 1–2 months. Immune-mediated extrahepatic manifestations such as maculopapular or urticarial rash, migratory arthritis, nephritis, and papular acrodermatitis of childhood (Gianotti–Crosti syndrome) may be present. Since the risk of chronicity is inversely proportional to the age of acquisition of the illness, a neonate has about 90% chance of acquiring the infection. This decreases to 30% if the age of acquisition is 1–5 years and 5–10% if acquired after the age of 5 years. The five stages in the natural history of HBV infection, viz., immune tolerant, immune-active HBeAg positive, immune-active HBeAg negative, inactive HBsAg carrier, and viral clearance are categorized according to the transaminase and HBV DNA levels. These terminologies have been changed to HBeAg positive chronic hepatitis B (CHB) infection or disease and HBeAg negative CHB infection or disease **(Table 12.7.1)**. At present treatment is recommended only for HBeAg positive or negative CHB hepatitis.[5]

Perinatal Transmission of Hepatitis B virus

In this condition the virus is transmitted from a HBsAg positive mother to her child. In India HBsAg positivity in pregnant women is 0.9 1.1% and vertical transmission (VT) has been reported to be as high as 45%. The risk of VT is as high as 58–90% if mother is HBsAg and HBeAg positive but is only 5–20%, if she is HBsAg positive and HBeAg negative. In perinatal transmission, the phase of immune tolerance characterized by high viral DNA, normal transaminases, and minimal hepatic inflammation lasts for many years. HBV infection due to VT is associated with a lower annual HBsAg, HBeAg, and HBV DNA clearance compared to horizontal transmission. The term "mother to child transmission (MTCT)" is preferred to perinatal transmission since VT is seen from 28 weeks gestational age to 28 days postnatal age. The transmission may be transplacental, during delivery (natal), or postnatal. However, most of the transmission occurs during delivery from cervical secretions or maternal blood. Hence, all babies born to HBsAg positive mothers should receive hepatitis B immunoglobulin within 6 hours of birth along with HBV vaccine. It is also recommended to give antiviral agent tenofovir antenatally for mothers who are HBsAg and HBeAg positive with high viral load to decrease the chance of VT.

Acute HCV hepatitis presents with a milder illness in children and acute liver failure occurs in <1%. The symptoms of malaise, fatigue, and jaundice are mild but the transaminases are elevated for a longer period. Approximately 40–50% may progress to chronicity and later to cirrhosis and hepatocellular carcinoma. Sporadic hepatitis in children due to HCV is rare and is reported in children receiving multiple blood transfusions. Chronic HCV infection is diagnosed if HCV RNA is present for >6 months.

DIAGNOSIS OF ACUTE VIRAL HEPATITIS

The basic investigations, such as urine for bile salts, bile pigments, total bilirubin with fractionation, alanine transaminase (ALT), and aspartate transaminase (AST) will suffice in most children with AVH. Prothrombin time (PT) and international normalized ratio (INR) are useful tests for assessing synthetic function of the liver and diagnosing acute liver failure. Complete blood counts, blood glucose, urea, creatinine, total protein, and albumin are checked when the child is hospitalized. Hepatitis is diagnosed only if the transaminases are more than twice the upper limit of normal. In viral hepatitis, ALT is markedly increased >20 times the upper limit of normal and is higher than AST indicating cytoplasmic rather than mitochondrial injury. Investigations for etiology are not necessary unless there are atypical manifestations or the child is hospitalized. All children should be screened for HBsAg. The presence of anti-HAV IgM or anti-HEV IgM confirms the diagnosis of acute HAV and HEV hepatitis, respectively. HBsAg positivity along with anti-HBc

TABLE 12.7.1: Interpretation of serologic markers in hepatitis B infection.

HBsAg	*HBeAg*	*Anti-HBe*	*Anti-HBc*	*Anti-HBs*	*HBV DNA*	*ALT*	*Significance*
+	+	–	IgM	–	>200,000 IU/L	>1,000 IU/L	Acute hepatitis
+	+	–	IgG	–	>200,000 IU/L	Normal	Immune tolerance (CHB HBeAg positive infection)
+	+	–	IgG	–	>20,000 IU/L	>2 UL/ N	Immune active HBeAg positive (CHB HBeAg positive hepatitis)
+	–	+	IgG	–	>2,000 IU/L	>2 UL/ N	Immune active HBeAg negative (CHB HBeAg negative hepatitis)
+	–	+	IgG	–	<2,000 IU/L	Normal	Inactive carrier (CHB HBeAg negative infection)
–	–	±	IgG	+	Not detected	Normal	Viral clearance
–	–	–	–	+	Not detected	Normal	Effective HBV vaccination

(ALT: alanine transaminase; CHB: chronic hepatitis B; Ig: immunoglobulin; HBsAg: hepatitis B surface antigen; HBeAg: hepatitis B envelope antigen; HBV: hepatitis B virus; ULN: Upper limit of normal range)

IgM indicates acute HBV hepatitis; whereas anti-HCV IgM and HCV RNA positivity indicates acute HCV hepatitis.

Infection due to nonhepatotropic viruses, such as measles, parvovirus B19, *Herpes simplex* 1 and 2, dengue virus, CMV, EBV, and human immunodeficiency virus (HIV) may present with jaundice and moderate elevation of transaminases. The associated clinical features of the underlying illness and specific serologic tests will help in diagnosis. Drug-induced liver injury presenting as acute hepatitis is a close mimic of AVH. Therefore, it is very essential to get a detailed history of medications including complementary alternative medicine (CAM). Other causes of noninfectious hepatitis such as leptospirosis, typhoid fever, Wilson disease (WD), and autoimmune hepatitis should be excluded if there are atypical manifestations.

Ultrasound examination is done when there is a possibility of acute on chronic liver disease or the child presents with persistent abdominal pain or fever to exclude liver abscess gallstones or pancreatitis. Liver biopsy is not recommended in children with AVH, but is essential in those with suspected acute on chronic liver disease or chronic hepatitis.

MANAGEMENT

The majority of children with AVH will recover spontaneously and require only supportive treatment. A nutritious diet should be provided and undue physical exertion, hepatotoxic drugs, and constipation should be avoided. Children with persistent vomiting, fever, fluid retention, altered sensorium, or gastrointestinal bleed require hospitalization.

Medications

Any child with deranged INR should be given injection vitamin K slowly and the test repeated. Severe cholestasis with itching can be managed with ursodeoxycholic acid (UDCA) in a dose of 20 mg/kg/day.

Antivirals

HAV and HEV hepatitis: There is no role for antiviral agents in acute HAV and HEV hepatitis. In patients with chronic HEV, the immunosuppression should be reduced. Oral ribavirin has been prescribed for 3–6 months in those in whom immunosuppression cannot be decreased or do not respond to the reduction.

HBV and HCV hepatitis: Antivirals are not recommended for acute HBV infection. Entecavir is recommended for CHB with acute liver failure awaiting liver transplant. Though interferon-based treatments may offer higher HBsAg and HBeAg seroconversion rates, the antivirals are preferred. Entecavir and tenofivir are the two antivirals which are approved in children. Functional cure may be attained (loss of HBeAg and undetectable HBV DNA off therapy) but complete cure (loss of HbsAg, undetectable HBV DNA, and the clearance of cccDNA off therapy) is rarely achieved.[6]

Children >3 years with acute HCV who have persistent viremia (i.e., HCV RNA positive for 12 weeks) following infection require treatment. Direct acting antivirals (DAAs) pan-genotypic are safe and may be given for 12 weeks. Similarly, children >3 years with chronic HCV infection (HCV RNA positive for >6 months) should also be treated with DAAs. Recommended drugs are combination of ledipasvir + sofosbuvir for GT 1, 4, 5, or 6 or sofosbuvir + velpatasvir or glecaprevir + pibrentasvir for any genotype for a duration of 12 weeks, and is very effective (>95%).[7]

Liver transplantation: This is the definitive therapy with excellent results for those who have progressed to acute liver failure.

COMPLICATIONS

The AVH is a self-limiting illness and most of the children recover without any sequel. Fever, hyperbilirubinemia, prolonged cholestasis, ascites, and coagulopathy may be a presentation in older children. The most important complication is acute liver failure. Chronic hepatitis, cirrhosis, and hepatocellular carcinoma are the complications seen in HBV and HCV infections.

PROGNOSIS

The majority of children with acute HAV and HEV hepatitis recover without any complications. Hepatotoxic drugs, indigenous medications, and underlying metabolic liver disease may precipitate acute liver failure. HBeAg negative and HBeAg positive chronic hepatitis need prolonged treatment with antivirals.

PREVENTION

General Measures

Infections due to HAV and HEV can be prevented by improving environmental sanitation and hygiene. Drinking clean water, washing hands, and hygienic preparation of food are essential in preventing the transmission of HAV and HEV. Since, HBV and HCV are spread parenterally, proper screening of blood and blood products is necessary prior to transfusion. Disposable needles should be used and unnecessary needle pricks including tattooing should be avoided.

Immunization

The HAV infection can be prevented by active immunization with two doses of inactivated hepatitis A vaccine given intramuscularly 6 months apart after the age of 12 months. A single dose of a live attenuated vaccine also can be administered with more or less the same efficacy.

Hepatitis B can be prevented by active immunization with three doses of HBV vaccine given at 0, 1, and 6 months. It is recommended with the first dose preferably given soon after birth.

At present no vaccines are available for HEV and HCV.

RECENT ADVANCES

Novel drugs for treating HBV infection are on the pipeline which will act on the cccDNA and achieve a complete cure. More potent vaccines, such as DNA vaccines and cell-based vaccines to increase the efficacy are undergoing trials. New biomarkers for monitoring end points for therapy such as HBV RNA, HBcrAg (considered surrogate for intrahepatic cccDNA), and qHBsAg (quantitative HBsAg) will soon be available.

Liver transplant is an excellent option in children with acute liver failure who fulfill the criteria for liver transplantation.

CONCLUSION

- HAV, HEV, and HBV are the most important causes of viral hepatitis. Specific serologic tests help in the etiological diagnosis.
- HAV and HEV hepatitis are self-limiting illnesses whereas HBV and HCV hepatitis may progress to chronic hepatitis, hepatocellular carcinoma, and cirrhosis.
- The incidence of acute liver failure in AVH is <1%.
- Perinatal transmission occurs in both HBV and HCV infections from mothers who are HBsAg and HBeAg positive or have high HCV RNA, respectively.
- Antivirals have no role to play in the management of acute HAV and HEV hepatitis. However, antivirals do play a definite role in chronic HBV hepatitis and HCV infection.
- Viral hepatitis though a communicable disease is preventable—HAV and HEV by improving water supply and environmental hygiene; and HAV and HBV by proper immunization. HBV and HCV transmission can be reduced by screening blood donors.

REFERENCES

1. Abutaleb A, Kottilil S. Hepatitis A: Epidemiology, natural history, unusual clinical manifestations, and prevention. Gastroenterol Clin North Am. 2020;49(2):191-9.
2. European Association for the Study of the Liver. EASL clinical practice guidelines on hepatitis E virus infection. J Hepatol. 2018;68(6):1256-71.
3. Indolfi G, Easterbrook P, Dusheiko G, Siberry G, Chang M-H, Thorne C, et al. Hepatitis B virus infection in children and adolescents. Lancet Gastroenterol Hepatol. 2019;4(6):466-76.
4. Singh SK, Borkar V, Srivastava A, Mathias A, Yachha SK, Poddar U. Need for recognizing atypical manifestations of childhood sporadic acute viral hepatitis warranting differences in management. Eur J Pediatr. 2019;178(1):61-7.
5. Huang DQ, Lim SD. Hepatitis B: Who to treat? A critical review of international guidelines. Liver Int. 2020;40(Suppl.1):5-14.
6. Reddy U, Poddar U. In: Mathai J, Sathiyasekaran M, Shanmugam N (Eds). Textbook of Hepatology, 1st edition. Hyderabad: Paras Medical Books Pvt Ltd; 2023. pp. 151-74.
7. Leung DH, Squires JE, Jhaveri R, Kerkar N, Lin CH, Mohan P, et al. Hepatitis C in 2020: A North American Society for Pediatric Gastroenterology, Hepatology, and Nutrition Position Paper. J Pediatr Gastroenterol Nutr. 2020;71(3):407-17.

12.8 Approach to Metabolic Liver Diseases

Moinak Sen Sarma

INTRODUCTION

Metabolic liver diseases (MLDs) are inborn errors of metabolism originating in the liver primarily or secondarily affecting the liver. They are characterized mainly by one or more of the following:

- Liver dysfunction and organomegaly
- Significant extrahepatic involvement
- Specific peculiarities of diet, odor, or examination
- Recurrent or unusual pattern of illness
- Familial or heritable tendencies

In this chapter, we understand the approach to MLD, how to identify a case of MLD and the general nuances in the management of the same. Details on specific diseases are beyond the scope of this chapter.

AGE OF PRESENTATION AND OUTCOME

The MLDs have a wide spectrum in the age of presentation. Most MLDs begin in infancy or early childhood. The lethal ones [(e.g., Wolman disease, Niemann-Pick disease (NPD) type C, and respiratory chain disorders] may succumb in this period. Others may persist through childhood and enter adulthood [e.g., glycogen storage disorders (GSDs), hereditary fructose intolerance (HFI), urea cycle defects, galactosemia, Wilson disease (WD), etc.]. Some disorders present for the first time in adulthood such as medium chain fatty acid oxidation defects (FAODs), urea cycle defects, citrullinemia type 2, etc. On careful history taking, there may be tell-tale subtle indications in the past or modifications in the diet that provide clues to the diagnosis. Through nature's own protective mechanisms, many of these disorders survive into adulthood with self-modifications in the diet, classically encountered in HFI where there is an aversion to sweet products (fructose and sucrose) since childhood. Others require specific therapy for survival, such as chelators in WD. Potentially lethal disorders, such as galactosemia, can be fatal on breastfeeds if unrecognized, but can survive for a lifetime if galactose is stopped. Hence, MLDs have mixed outcomes. Some are favorable for the liver but not for extrahepatic organs or vice versa. Others have an overall poor prognosis with or without therapy.

PATHOPHYSIOLOGY

Largely there are three groups of MLD:

1. *Synthesis or catabolism of complex molecules,* e.g., lysosomal storage disorders and peroxisomal disorders. Partly degraded molecules accumulate in the liver or other organs.
2. *Accumulation of toxic compounds or metals,* e.g., tyrosinemia and WD. Here, there is an excess of a by-product or end-product that accumulates in the liver or extrahepatic tissues.
3. *Disorders of intermediary metabolism,* e.g., FAODs and GSD. The disruption of a pathway is due to an enzyme defect, typically leading to energy depletion or excess of a physiological waste product.

Specifically, the energy depletion disorders typically cause glycopenia (hypoglycemia) (e.g., FAOD and galactosemia). Urea cycle disorders and FAOD cause intoxication due to accumulation of ammonia. Galactosemia causes neuroglycopenia resulting in seizures and also an osmotic damage from the toxic metabolites resulting in cataract, hemolysis, etc. Intermediary products in tyrosinemia lead to a neurological crisis mimicking porphyria.

PRESENTATION CATEGORIES

There are broadly four types of presentations based on the first organ of involvement:

1. *Hepatic first:* In this presentation, the first feature is liver dysfunction which may or may not be followed by extrahepatic symptoms, e.g., galactosemia, hepatic phenotype of WD, and tyrosinemia.
2. *Nonhepatic first:* The extrahepatic manifestation appears earlier; liver dysfunction may ensue later, e.g., neurological phenotype of WD. The condition may present exclusively as extrapyramidal features with subtle or overt liver manifestations over the years. In HFI, gastrointestinal symptoms may appear much earlier than liver dysfunction.
3. *Multisystemic:* The hepatic and extrahepatic features appear simultaneously, e.g., long-chain FAOD where the infant manifests with liver and neuromuscular symptoms together. In tyrosinemia, liver failure and rickets (renal tubular acidosis) may coexist together.
4. *Liver sparing:* In this situation the defect is primarily in the liver but liver dysfunction never occurs. The brunt of the defect is rather borne by a different organ. The classical example is primary hyperoxaluria where the liver enzyme alanine-glyoxylate aminotransferase (AGT), which converts glyoxylate to glycine, is absent. Hence, there are recurrent renal stones and end-stage renal disease but never liver disease.

HOW TO SUSPECT METABOLIC LIVER DISEASE?

Let us see the various settings to suspect MLD in a step-wise manner.

First Suspicion: Unusual Hepatic Manifestation

- Liver failure in neonates/infants
- Early cirrhosis in young children
- Neonatal cholestasis with decompensation
- Recurrent encephalopathy (Reye-like illness)
- Massive hepatomegaly
- Splenohepatomegaly (larger spleen as compared to liver)
- Steatosis in a young child

Liver Failure and Early Cirrhosis

Liver failure in children may arise due to multiple causes, the most common being hepatotropic viruses in developing countries. The MLDs that cause liver failure are shown in **Table 12.8.1**. MLD accounts for 2–13% of liver failures in older children, 15–30% in toddlers, and 20% in infants.[1] Infants have lower risk of liver failure from hepatotropic viruses due to protective factors from breast milk and relatively lesser frequency of feco-oral transmission of viruses. Hence, the younger the child with liver failure, the more is the suspicion for MLD. Mitochondrial hepatopathies (FAODs and respiratory chain defects) and galactosemia presenting as liver failure are most prominent in the early months of life. In infants, mitochondrial hepatopathies need to be differentiated from other conditions that have considerable overlap such as neonatal hemochromatosis, *herpes simplex* liver failure, and hemophagocytic lymphohistiocytosis. **Table 12.8.2** shows the clinical differentiation of these conditions.[2] Early cirrhosis suggests that either the liver damage has started in utero (e.g., neonatal hemochromatosis) or just after birth (e.g., galactosemia on exposure to milk). Ascites appearing in early infancy is highly suggestive of early-onset cirrhosis. Neonatal hemochromatosis may have nonpalpable or shrunken liver. Ultrasonography may show liver nodularity in cirrhosis. Recurrent acute liver failure (RALF) is a distinct and a rare entity where there are multiple episodes of liver failure with complete recovery of symptoms and biochemistry in between. RALF is caused by mitochondrial disorders such as FAOD, respiratory chain defects, citrullinemia and specific mutations (LARS, TRMU, NBAS, etc.).

TABLE 12.8.1: Causes of liver failure in children.

Neonates and infants	*Older children*
• Galactosemia • Tyrosinemia • Neonatal hemochromatosis (gestational alloimmune liver disease) • Hereditary fructose intolerance (HFI) • Urea cycle defects • Mitochondrial hepatopathies • Niemann–Pick disease (NPD) type C • Bile acid synthetic defects	• Wilson disease (WD) • Mitochondrial hepatopathies

Reye-like Illness

Classically described in earlier reports, Reye's syndrome was postulated to occur as a result of influenza infection and aspirin. This condition classically presents as:

- Age of onset <5 years
- Sudden onset, may be recurrent
- Anicteric encephalopathy
- Significant hepatomegaly
- Hyperammonemia
- Hypoglycemia
- High liver enzymes (3–10 times upper limit of normal)
- Elevated international normalized ratio (INR)
- With or without liver steatosis (on ultrasonography)
- Organic acids in urine and blood by mass spectrometry.

In the Indian subcontinent and developing countries, this condition should be differentiated from acute liver failure (ischemia or hepatotropic virus), septicemia, and other multisystemic illnesses. In toddlers and infants, Reye-like illness is one of the major manifestations of medium-chain FAOD and urea cycle defects. Urea cycle defects may present without jaundice, while FAOD may have mild jaundice.[3]

Cholestasis

Most causes of liver failure above may also present as cholestasis in the early period. In addition, progressive familial intrahepatic cholestasis (PFIC) types 1–8, bile acid synthetic, and conjugation defects are added to the list. NPD type C can also cause transient or progressive cholestasis and may culminate into decompensated liver disease. Citrin

TABLE 12.8.2: Differentiation of common causes of neonatal liver failure.

	Neonatal hemochromatosis	*HSV*	*HLH*	*Mitochondrial cytopathy*
Premature birth/IUGR	70–90%	Rare	Rare	Rare
Sib death	Common	No	May be	25%
Amniotic fluid	Oligohydramnios	Normal	Normal	Polyhydramnios
Ascites at birth	Common	Rare	Rare	Rare
Liver	Shrunken	Enlarged	Enlarged	Enlarged
Organ involvement	Renal tubular dysplasia, PDA	CNS; Skin	Bone marrow	Heart; CNS
Acidosis at presentation	–	–	–	++
Cholestasis	Not at birth	Minimal	Moderate	Moderate
Coagulopathy	Profound	+	+	+
ALT (U/L)	Low normal (<100)	High (>1,000)	High (>1,000)	Moderate (100–500)
Ferritin (ng/mL)	800–7,000	>20,000	>20,000	Variable
Alphafetoprotein (ng/mL)	80,000–300,000	<80,000	<80,000	Variable
Definitive test	Lip biopsy, MRI pancreas Complement C5b-9	HSV-PCR	Perforin levels Genetics	Genetics

(ALT: alanine transaminase; CNS: central nervous system; HLH: hemophagocytic lymphohistiocytosis; HSV: herpes simplex virus; IUGR: intrauterine growth retardation; MRI: magnetic resonance imaging; PCR: polymerase chain reaction; PDA: patent ductus arteriosus)

deficiency can also cause transient cholestasis in infancy, later returning as citrullinemia type 2 in adults.

Organomegaly

Most MLD have some degree of hepatomegaly and some alterations in the liver function tests (LFTs), most commonly raised liver enzymes. Massive hepatomegaly is seen in GSD (types 1, 3, 4, 6, 9, and 11), mucopolysaccharidoses and lysosomal acid lipase deficiency (LAL-D). **Figure 12.8.1** shows a typical case of glycogen storage disease (GSD). Larger splenomegaly than hepatomegaly (splenohepatomegaly) is seen with NPD and Gaucher disease, though the reverse is also well known. In NPD, it has been seen that the liver and spleen are 2 and 11 times the size of normal respectively.[4] Rest of the causes enlisted for liver failure and cholestasis also cause organomegaly. Renomegaly is specifically seen in GSD type 1 and tyrosinemia. Mucopolysaccharidoses cause hepatomegaly without any alteration in LFTs. Primary hyperoxaluria and a few urea cycle defects have no or minimal hepatomegaly without any appreciable LFTs. Similarly branched chain amino acid disorders (methylmalonic, propionic and isovaleric acidemias, and maple syrup urine disease (MSUD)] have mild hepatomegaly but do not cause liver dysfunction. Here, the liver is otherwise functionally normal but deficient in the enzyme. Hence, liver transplantation is curative.

Second Suspicion: Pattern of Involvement

Many of the MLD have a specific pattern of involvement. FAODs (especially medium chain) and urea cycle defects have an intoxicating illness precipitated by a febrile episode, stress, or surgery that results in rapid deterioration of sensorium. The encephalopathy is often mistaken as meningoencephalitis, uremic, hepatic, or vaguely referred to as a "sepsis-like illness." Metabolic changes predominate during this period. However, on initiation of dextrose-rich fluid and supplementation of electrolytes, there is quick recovery to baseline health, unlike the other differential diagnoses mentioned earlier. This pattern is recurrent, requiring multiple hospitalizations. A keen index of suspicion is required.[2,5,6]

Third Suspicion: Extrahepatic Involvement

One of the hallmarks of MLD is the extrahepatic involvement. A few examples are listed in **Table 12.8.3**.

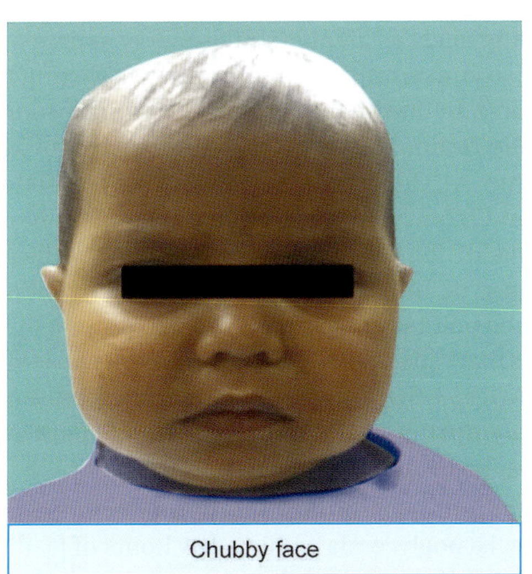

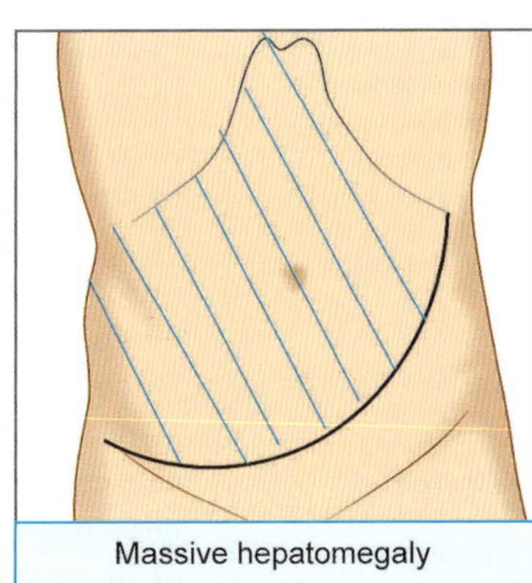

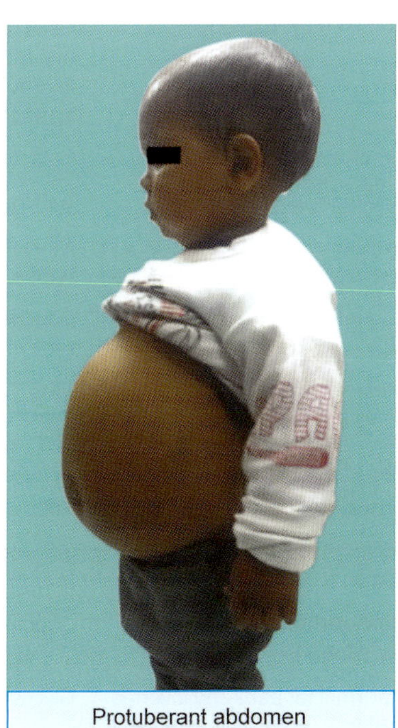

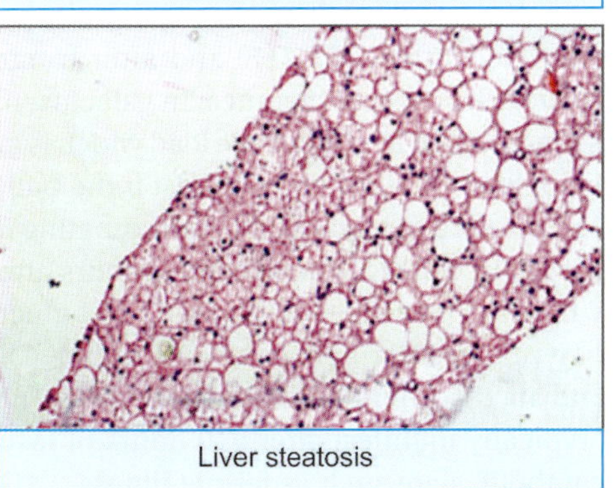

- Hypoglycemia
- Seizures
- Lactic acidosis
- Hypertriglyceridemia
- Hyperuricemia
- Diarrhea, neutropenia (type 1b)
- Myopathy (type III)

Fig. 12.8.1: Child with glycogen storage disease (GSD).
Courtesy: Dr Moinak Sen Sarma, Lucknow.

TABLE 12.8.3: Extrahepatic involvement of metabolic liver disease (MLD).

Feature/condition	***Disease***
Renal tubular acidosis Rickets **(Fig. 12.8.2)**	Tyrosinemia, HFI, WD, GSD type 11
Neurologic crisis	Tyrosinemia
Adrenal crisis	Wolman disease
Diarrhea	GSD type 1, HFI, PFIC types 1, 6
Steatorrhea	Bile acid synthetic defects, lysosomal acid lipase deficiency
Choreoathetosis	WD
Spasticity	NPD
Myopathies (skeletal/cardiac)	FAOD, GSD type 3
Developmental delay or regression	FAOD, NPD type A and C, MPS
Gaze palsy	• NPD type C (vertical palsy) • Gaucher disease type 3 (horizontal palsy)
Hypoglycemic seizures	Galactosemia, FAOD, GSD types 1, 3, 4, 6, 9, 11
Cataract **(Fig. 12.8.3)**	Galactosemia, peroxisomal disorders, cerebrotendinous xanthomatosis (bile acid synthetic defect)
Hemolysis	Galactosemia, WD
Bone marrow failure	Gaucher disease type 1
Lymphadenopathy	Gaucher disease type 1, NPD type A
Lung infiltration	Gaucher disease type 2, NPD type A
Coarse facies	MPS
Kayser–Fleischer ring **(Fig. 12.8.3)**	WD
Corneal clouding	MPS
Dysmorphism	Zellweger syndrome (peroxisomal disorder)
Cherry red spot (fundus) **(Fig. 12.8.3)**	Gaucher disease, NPD
Abnormal fat pads and inverted nipples	Glycosylation disorders
Chubby cheeks **(Fig. 12.8.1)**	GSD, citrin deficiency
Nephromegaly (palpable or sonological)	GSD type 1, tyrosinemia

(FAOD: fatty acid oxidation defects; GSD: glycogen storage disorder; HFI: hereditary fructose intolerance; MPS: mucopolysaccharidosis; NPD: Niemann-Pick disease; PFIC: progressive familial intrahepatic cholestasis; WD: Wilson disease)

Hypoglycemia

Hypoglycemia is a

- Hallmark manifestation of carbohydrate-related MLD (e.g.: GSD, galactosemia, and HFI);
- Energy depletion defect (e.g.: FAOD); or
- Occurs as a part of advanced liver disease and liver failure in any MLD.

Normally glucose that is not immediately used is stored as glycogen in the liver and muscle or converted to lipid. In normal individuals, there are compensatory mechanisms to compensate for the fall in blood glucose. These mechanisms are glycogenolysis, gluconeogenesis, and fatty acid oxidation (which is an alternative pathway to provide energy) as shown in **Figure 12.8.4**. Insulin secretion is suppressed, while glucagon is secreted, promoting glucose production from glycogen in the liver. The brain has limited glycogen stores and capacity for gluconeogenesis, and therefore requires a continuous glucose supply. In healthy children, after 12–16 hours of fasting, first the glycogen stores become depleted. Then glucose is produced by hepatic gluconeogenesis, primarily from amino acids and glycerol. Lipolysis increases the supply of fatty acids as an alternative energy source and reducing glucose consumption. After prolonged fasting (in excess of 24 hours), ketone bodies become the primary source of energy for the brain. Fatty acid oxidation also provides acetyl-coenzyme A (CoA) for ketogenesis. For practical purposes, beyond infancy, hypoglycemia is defined as blood glucose <59 mg/dL or 3.3 mmol/L. Maintenance blood glucose is >72 mg/dL or 4 mmol/L. There are many inborn errors of metabolism that cause hypoglycemia. Among these causes, the ones that cause liver dysfunction are galactosemia, tyrosinemia, FAODs, GSD, and HFI. There may be presence of hepatomegaly during acute attacks of hypoglycemia in fructose 1, 6, bisphosphatase deficiency.

The timing and precipitant of hypoglycemia are important clues. Hypoglycemia within a few hours of feeding suggests hyperinsulinism, though it is occasionally seen in mitochondrial defects (e.g., MPV17) and after fructose ingestion in hereditary fructose intolerance. In galactosemia, hypoglycemia is precipitated by a galactose load which is milk in a neonate. Hypoglycemia does not manifest if the baby is already on a galactose-free formula as the incriminating diet has been withdrawn. In GSD I, hypoglycemia occurs after a brief fast (1.5–4 hours), once exogenous sources of glucose are exhausted. Hypoglycemia occurs later in other GSDs (4–12 hours) and in disorders of gluconeogenesis (8–16 hours). FAODs typically manifest after >10 hours of fasting or earlier in a catabolic state such as febrile illness. FAODs typically present as hypoketotic hypoglycemia where as other causes are normo- or hyperketotic.[7]

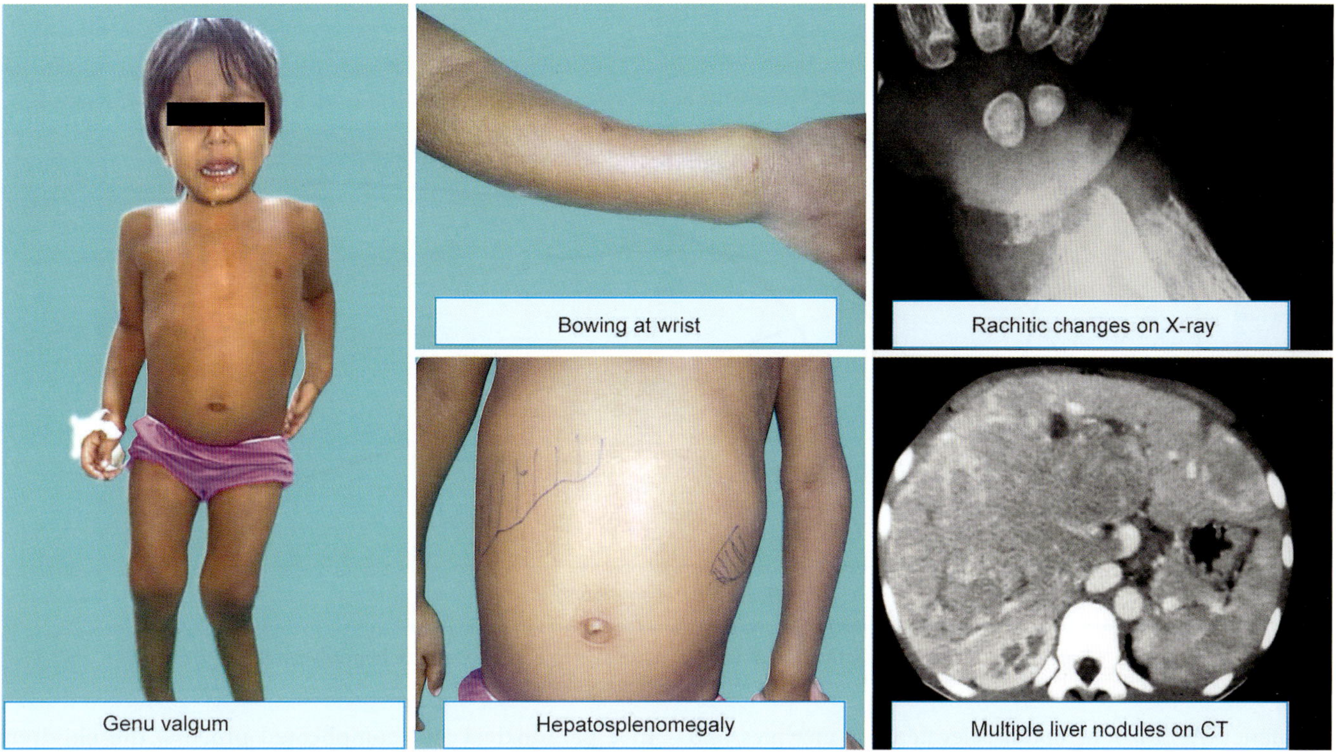

Fig. 12.8.2: Rickets and development of hepatocellular carcinoma in a child with tyrosinemia.
Courtesy: Dr Moinak Sen Sarma, Lucknow.

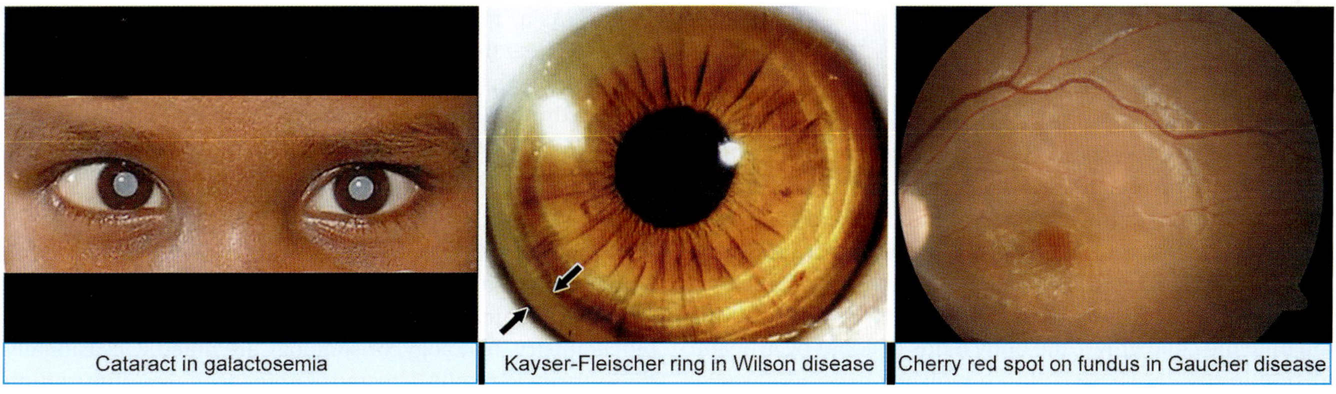

Fig. 12.8.3: Eye findings in metabolic liver diseases.
Courtesy: Dr Moinak Sen Sarma, Lucknow.

Fourth Suspicion: Family History

When an MLD is suspected, a 3-generation elaborate pedigree chart is recommended. Clues such as consanguinity, positive family history (neuropsychiatric illness, seizure disorder, myopathies, or cholestasis), and sibling deaths (sudden unexplained or similar phenotype of proband).

Fifth Suspicion: Maternal History

Prenatal or antenatal issues in the mother may indicate genetic problems in the neonate. Cholestasis during oral contraceptive pill intake (in mother or maternal female members), cholestasis during pregnancy and severe antenatal pruritus may suggest PFIC in the child. Oligohydramnios and mega placenta are seen in neonatal hemochromatosis. It is important for obstetricians to record the presence of mega placenta, send for histological analysis and alert the neonatologist. Some FAODs are associated with intrauterine growth restriction (IUGR), prematurity, and pregnancy complications in the heterozygous mother. These complications include severe preeclampsia, acute fatty liver of

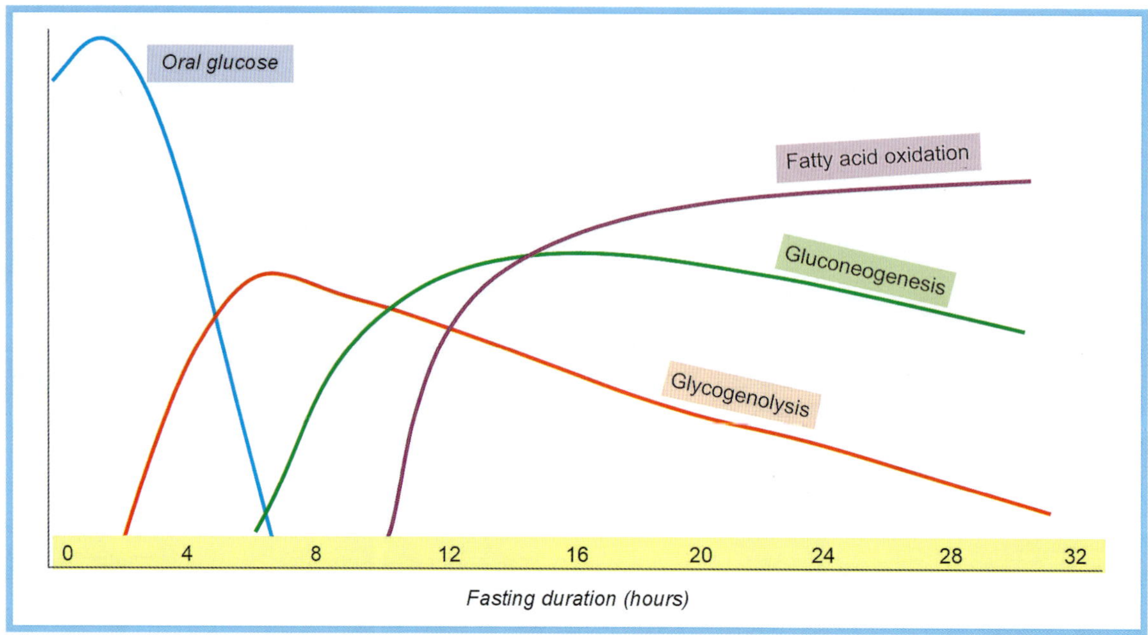

Fig. 12.8.4: Timeline of activation of various pathways to compensate for hypoglycemia.
Courtesy: Dr Moinak Sen Sarma, Lucknow.

pregnancy (AFLP), or hemolysis, elevated liver enzymes, and low platelets (HELLP syndrome). Pregnancy complications occur primarily in mothers carrying a fetus with FAOD like long chain L-3-hydroxyacyl CoA dehydrogenase deficiency or general trifunctional protein deficiencies.[2,5]

Sixth Suspicion: Diet History

Diet history is unique in MLD. Patients have symptom precipitation by ingestion of the incriminating agent. There may be symptom precipitation, craving, or aversion to various food products. It is important to remember that sucrose is fructose + glucose and lactose is galactose + glucose. Hence, symptoms of HFI (vomiting, diarrhea, and liver dysfunction) are precipitated by simple sugars, honey, juices, and fruits. By the time the child grows, the body tends to adapt by aversion to simple sugars. These children typically have an absence of caries.[8] Symptoms of galactosemia start from the neonatal period on breast milk and lactose-containing formula feeds. Therapy of galactosemia consists of soy-free formula in infancy and avoidance of lactose-containing products throughout life. Fruits containing small amounts of galactose are not enough to cause symptoms, hence they are allowed.[9] Proteins contain nitrogen and generate ammonia which is metabolized in the urea cycle. Hence, urea cycle defects have an aversion to proteins. High protein intake results in intoxication and encephalopathy.[6] Citrin deficiency is a problem of the glutamate-aspartate shuttle that participates in the urea genesis from ammonia and contributes further to the malate-aspartate shuttle which drives the electron transport system. In a paradoxical and complicated process, the children prefer protein-rich, fat-rich foods such as peanuts and beans but avoid carbohydrates like rice. High dose of glucose or dextrose infusion may precipitate hyperammonemia. Hence in East Asia, mothers typically complain that "the child chooses to eat the fish but leaves the rice in the bowl." Milk is well tolerated as the content of protein and fat is higher than carbohydrates. These children are often labelled as "picky-eaters." A child with dietary preferences must be examined for growth, hepatomegaly, and tested for liver functions.[10]

Seventh Suspicion: Workup During Basic Tests

Sometimes, history and general examination are inconclusive and the suspicion is fortified when specific changes in biochemistry, histology, or sonology are noted. Occasionally these are incidentally detected or noted while sending routine investigations for other differentials. These are briefly shown in **Table 12.8.4**. The next segment on workup will elaborate the same.

HOW TO WORKUP A CASE OF METABOLIC LIVER DISEASE?

Screening Tests

Other than routine tests such as hemogram and LFTs, there are some specific tests that have a role in the workup of MLD. Basic screening tests are blood glucose, pH (blood-gas analysis), blood or urine ketones, and serum lactate and serum ammonia. An arterial sample swiftly transported to the laboratory in an ice pack for analysis yields the best results. **Table 12.8.5** shows differentiation of some common conditions. Urine for nonglucose reducing substances is done by Benedict's solution and a glucose strip. A positive test indicates that a reducing substance, other than glucose is being excreted in urine. This is an important screening test in galactosemia (galactose in urine) and HFI (fructose in urine) while the patient is on the original diet. Once changed to an alternative diet, this test will no longer be positive. Hence, it is important to remember that galactosemia babies on soy milk will have a negative test. It is cautioned not to rechallenge with the original diet as it may be a provocative test and precipitate hypoglycemia and seizures. In galactosemia, three consecutive samples are tested; typically two or all three are positive. However, this urine test has a high false positivity (any cholestasis, preterm, sepsis, or cardiac issues).[9]

Urine Gas Chromatography-Mass Spectroscopy-Blood Tandem Mass Spectroscopy

Urine gas chromatography-mass spectroscopy (GCMS) and blood tandem mass spectroscopy (TMS) have mixed results. If sent during an acute crisis, it may lead to some specific diagnosis such as dicarboxylic aciduria in FAOD or various typical aciduria in organic acidemias. In settings of liver failure and severe liver dysfunction, the yield may be poor. Often the tyrosine pathway metabolites are elevated that lead to a false reporting of tyrosinemia. If the GCMS/TMS are sent in the resolving phase or baseline normal health, they may not reveal the abnormalities that are expected. In organic acidemias, baseline GCMS/TMS help in monitoring response to dialysis, and specific therapy at follow-up. Similarly, in FAOD, carnitine profiles can be checked on follow-up. The advantage of GCMS/TMS over genetics is the quick turnaround time and a guide for initiating therapy.

TABLE 12.8.4: Specific changes providing clues to diagnoses of metabolic liver disease (MLD).

Investigations	*Conditions*
Low gamma-glutamyl transpeptidase	Progressive familial intrahepatic cholestasis I, II, IV, V, XI Bile acid synthetic defects
High gamma-glutamyl transpeptidase	Progressive familial intrahepatic cholestasis III
Low alkaline phosphatase	Acute Wilson disease in liver failure
Neutropenia	GSD type 1b
Recurrent acidosis, high lactate	FAOD; respiratory chain defect
Hyperammonemia with normal liver function tests	Urea cycle defect
Hypo- or nonketotic hypoglycemia	FAOD
Fatty liver changes (sonology or histology)	Glycogen storage disorder, hereditary fructose intolerance, FAOD

(FAOD: fatty acid oxidation defect; GSD: glycogen storage disorder)

Enzyme Assays

Enzyme assays are particularly helpful in the diagnosis of lysosomal storage disorders such as Gaucher disease (glucocerebrosidase), NPD types A and B (acid sphingomyelinase), and lysosomal acid lipase deficiencies (cholesteryl ester storage disease and Wolman disease). It is to be remembered that NPD type C is NOT an enzyme deficiency state; it is a problem of intracellular transport of endocytosed cholesterol and sequestration of unesterified cholesterol in lysosomes. Chitotriosidase, which is an enzyme involved in the degradation of chitin, is expressed by activated macrophages. Hence, serum chitotriodisase may be used as a screening biomarker for lysosomal storage disorders.[4] Diagnosis of classical galactosemia is demonstrated by undetectable to deficient galactose-1-uridyl phosphatase enzyme (GAL-1-PUT) levels.[9]

Genetic Studies

Genetic studies are confirmatory but the turnaround time is approximately 4–6 weeks. Hence, empirical therapy must not be withheld until that time. Next generation sequencing (NGS) is recommended. It is preferred to perform a clinical exome or whole exome sequencing (WES) for MLD. Adequate clinical information needs to be provided to widen the search for the genes. For example, in a setting of neonatal cholestasis with pruritus, incriminating genes may vary from the ones that cause liver failure or storage disorders. Both sets of search may overlap with those who have a steatotic MLD. Variants of unknown significance (VUS) must be interpreted with caution

TABLE 12.8.5: Differentiation of common conditions.

<table>
<tr><th></th><th>Acidosis</th><th>Urine ketones</th><th>Blood glucose</th><th>Serum lactate</th><th>Serum ammonia</th></tr>
<tr><td>Fatty acid oxidation defect (FAOD)</td><td>++</td><td>Nil</td><td>Low (nonketotic hypoglycemia)</td><td>++</td><td>+</td></tr>
<tr><td>Respiratory chain defects</td><td>++</td><td>++</td><td>Normal</td><td>++++</td><td>±</td></tr>
<tr><td>Organic aciduria</td><td>+++ (persistent)</td><td>++/+++</td><td>Low/normal/high</td><td>Normal</td><td>++</td></tr>
<tr><td>Urea cycle defect</td><td colspan="4">Normal</td><td>++++</td></tr>
</table>

BOX 12.8.1: Clinical settings for genetic testing in neonatal cholestasis.

- Presentation as pruritus or steatorrhea (progressive familial intrahepatic cholestasis, bile acid synthetic defects)
- Low gamma-glutamyl transpeptidase (GGT) cholestasis (progressive familial intrahepatic cholestasis, bile acid synthetic defects)
- Suspected galactosemia where enzyme assay is fallacious (hemolysis, blood transfusion) or unavailable
- Suspected tyrosinemia where urinary succinylacetone is unavailable
- Neonatal liver failure where infectious causes have been ruled out (causes mentioned in text)
- Predominant extrahepatic manifestations (causes mentioned in text)
- Strong family or sibling history
- Significant clues on mass spectroscopy or gas chromatography

as it may be a pathogenic new mutant or a bystander in a larger disease. It is encouraged that all mutations should be reported by the clinician to update the phenotypic variability of rare disorders and augment the information into the global libraries. Though galactosemia is diagnosed by enzyme assay, there are few situations in which genetic confirmation is required. As the GAL-1-PUT assay is measured from red blood cells, this assay will be erroneous in the setting of hemolysis (known to occur in 25–30% of galactosemia) and blood transfusion. **Box 12.8.1** shows the settings of neonatal cholestasis in which genetic testing is indicated.

Tissue Biopsies

Due to invasiveness and newer modalities of diagnosis, such as enzyme assay and genetic studies, tissue biopsies by and large have been abandoned.

Steatosis in liver biopsy is seen in a number of conditions such as galactosemia, citrin deficiency, FAOD, respiratory chain defects, urea cycle defects hereditary fructose intolerance, GSD, and WD. Hence, steatosis is a nonspecific finding, presence of which indicates a possible MLD, absence of which does not rule out MLD. In WD, elevated hepatic copper and copper staining provides clues to diagnosis of the same.[11] In GSD, the liver shows hepatocytes filled with glycogen that is periodic acid-Schiff (PAS) positive and diastase sensitive. Earlier quantification of liver glycogen was performed. Specifically in GSD type 4, amylopectin inclusion bodies are pathognomonic.

In the past, bone marrow aspiration-biopsies or liver biopsies were routinely performed to diagnose lysosomal storage disorders. In NPD, histology shows lipid-laden macrophages in the marrow, also called foam-cells. Due to the accumulation of sphingomyelin and cholesterol and an ineffective transport system, the affected cells enlarge to approximately 90 μm in diameter. Numerous small vacuoles of relatively uniform size ensue within the cell cytoplasm giving a foamy appearance. Electron microscopy shows electron-opaque, concentrically laminated inclusions within the macrophage cytoplasm. In Gaucher disease, classic glycolipid-laden macrophages known as Gaucher cells in bone marrow samples. These cells have a characteristic wrinkled-paper appearance, resulting from intracytoplasmic substrate deposition, and stain positive with PAS. They may appear in liver biopsy (most evident in sinusoids) too but as such hepatocytes do not manifest overt glycolipid storage because of biliary excretion of glucocerebroside and ability of mononuclear phagocytes to handle exogenous glycolipid turnover. As hepatocytes are usually spared, liver failure is less in Gaucher than NPD. Overall yield of diagnosis in bone marrow and liver biopsies in lysosomal storage disorders is 40–80%. Splenic aspirates are no longer performed.[4]

In respiratory chain defects, the respiratory chain enzymes can be analyzed and quantified on tissue biopsy specimens. These disorders involve muscle, hence snap frozen skeletal muscle tissue (100–200 g of quadriceps) used to be a useful site for analysis. Due to its mutilating nature, concomitant coagulopathy and sickness of the infant, muscle biopsies have been abandoned. Cultured skin fibroblasts were an alternative option, but not all diseases are detected by the same.[5]

THERAPY

Nutrition

Nutritional intervention is an important therapy. Various disorders have various levels of intervention. Ingestion is targeted in galactosemia (galactose-free, lactose free), HFI (fructose-free), and tyrosinemia (phenylalanine- and tyrosine-free). The end product is targeted in glycogen storage therapy. Instead of simple sugars that are quickly metabolized and produce rebound hypoglycemia, slow sustained release of glucose is administered with corn starch therapy. Corn starch has a moderately high glycemic index (70–85) with abundant alpha 1, 4 and alpha 1, 6 bonds that release glucose with help of amylase and maltase. Corn starch is most suitable out of all other cereals. Tapioca, potato, and rice starch have glycemic index that causes quick increases in blood glucose levels. Corn starch is given as raw and uncooked in GSD. Since the final enzyme is affected in glycogenolysis, milk (lactose) is avoided in type 1 GSD. Corn starch can also be given in FAODs to sustain euglycemia.[12]

In type 3 GSD, additional protein is supplemented (3 mg/kg) to replenish the ongoing myopathy. Other supportive nutritional interventional measures include salt restriction in ascites, supplementation of branched chain amino acids in hepatic encephalopathy, supplementation of medium chain triglycerides in cholestasis, and restriction of dietary copper in the first year of therapy in WD (till chelation becomes effective).

Specific Drugs

The WD is treated with chelators such as D-penicillamine or trientine. Zinc is not effective in hepatic disease and reserved for presymptomatic siblings. Enzyme replacement therapy is available for lysosomal storage disorders (except NPD type C).[4] Nitisinone is the drug of choice in tyrosinemia along in synergy with the specific diet.[13] Cholic acid and/or chenodeoxycholic acid are used in bile acid synthetic defects.[14] Ammonia scavengers (sodium benzoate and phenylacetate) and supplements (L-arginine, L-citrulline, and N-carbamyl glutamate) are life-saving in urea cycle defects.[5] Similarly, carnitine is life-saving in primary carnitine transport defects. Oral mannose helps in congenital disorder of glycosylation type 1b.

Other Therapies

Hemodialysis helps in rapid clearance of elevated blood ammonia in urea cycle defects. Plasmapheresis is a bridge to liver transplantation in acute WD with liver failure and hemolysis. Partial biliary diversion (internal or external) is recommended for managing pruritus refractory to medical therapy in PFIC. Liver transplantation is curative in various MLD such as branched chain organic acidurias, urea cycle defects, and primary hyperoxaluria as the liver is the main area of the deficient enzyme.

In those with neurological setbacks and multisystemic issues (FAOD, respiratory chain defects and Wolman disease), liver transplantation is contraindicated or to be done with a guarded long-term prognosis. Combined liver-kidney transplantation is also required in primary hyperoxaluria with end-stage renal disease. In any end-stage liver disease or acute liver failure refractory to medical therapy (e.g.: WD, bile acid synthetic defects, and PFID), liver transplantation is the final solution.[15]

CONCLUSION

- Metabolic liver diseases should be suspected if there are peculiarities in the pattern of illness, positive family history, dietary preferences and specific clues on examination
- Workup requires a battery of tests such as tissue biopsy, enzyme assays and genetic profile
- Many of the metabolic liver diseases are treatable and merit a dedicated effort in procuring the specific drugs
- Metabolic liver diseases that are untreatable or refractory to medical therapy require liver transplantation if other systems are not involved.

REFERENCES

1. Squires RH Jr, Shneider BL, Bucuvalas J, Alonso E, Sokol RJ, Narkewicz MR, et al. Acute liver failure in children: the first 348 patients in the pediatric acute liver failure study group. J Pediatr. 2006;148(5):652-8.
2. Taylor SA, Whitington PF. Neonatal acute liver failure. Liver Transpl. 2016;22(5):677-85.
3. Ravindranath A, Sarma MS. Mitochondrial hepatopathy: Anticipated difficulties in management of fatty acid oxidation defects and urea cycle defects. World J Hepatol. 2022;14(1):180-94.
4. Sarma MS, Tripathi PR. Natural history and management of liver dysfunction in lysosomal storage disorders. World J Hepatol. 2022;14(10):1844-61.
5. Gopan A, Sarma MS. Mitochondrial hepatopathy: Respiratory chain disorders- 'breathing in and out of the liver'. World J Hepatol. 2021;13(11):1707-26.
6. Bigot A, Tchan MC, Thoreau B, Blasco H, Maillot F. Liver involvement in urea cycle disorders: a review of the literature. J Inherit Metab Dis. 2017;40(6):757-69.
7. Ghosh A, Banerjee I, Morris AAM. Recognition, assessment and management of hypoglycaemia in childhood. Arch Dis Child. 2016;101(6):575-80.
8. Singh SK, Sarma MS. Hereditary fructose intolerance: A comprehensive review. World J Clin Pediatr. 2022;11(4):321-9.
9. Sarma MS, Srivastava A, Yachha SK, Poddar U, Mathias A. Classical galactosemia among Indian Children: Presentation and outcome from a Pediatric Gastroenterology Center. Indian Pediatr. 2016;53:27-31.
10. Saheki T, Inoue K, Tushima A, Mutoh K, Kobayashi K. Citrin deficiency and current treatment concepts. Mol Genet Metab. 2010;100(Suppl 1):S59-64.
11. Ghosh U, Sarma MS, Samanta A. Challenges and dilemmas in pediatric hepatic Wilson's disease. World J Hepatol. 2023;15(10):1109-26.
12. Kishnani PS, Austin SL, Abdenur JE, Arn P, Bali DS, Boney A, et al; American College of Medical Genetics and Genomics. Diagnosis and management of glycogen storage disease type I: a practice guideline of the American College of Medical Genetics and Genomics. Genet Med. 2014;16(11):e1.
13. Kehar M, Sarma MS, Seetharaman J, Rivera CJ, Chakraborty P. Decoding hepatorenal tyrosinemia type 1: Unraveling the impact of early detection, NTBC, and the role of liver transplantation. Can Liver J. 2024;7(1):54-63.
14. Ravindranath A, Sarma MS, Yachha SK. Bile acid synthetic defects: Simplified approach in a nutshell. Hepatobiliary Pancreat Dis Int. 2020;19(1):80-4.
15. Squires RH. Ng V, Romero R, Ekong U, Hardikar W, Emre S, et al. Evaluation of the pediatric patient for liver transplantation: 2014 practice guideline by the American Association for the Study of Liver Diseases, American Society of Transplantation and the North American Society for Pediatric Gastroenterology, Hepatology and Nutrition. Hepatology. 2014;60(1):362-98.

12.9 Wilson Disease

Snehavardhan R Pandey, Ashish R Bavdekar

INTRODUCTION

Wilson disease (WD) is an inborn error of metabolism characterized by toxic accumulation of copper (Cu) in liver, brain, cornea, kidneys, and other tissues due to a mutation in the *ATP7B* gene (chromosome 13q). It occurs worldwide with an estimated prevalence of 1 in 30–50,000 and is one of the leading causes of chronic liver disease (7.6–19.7%) in children.[1]

PHYSIOLOGY OF COPPER METABOLISM

Copper is an essential trace element as it acts as a cofactor for many enzymes, viz., cytochrome c oxidase, superoxide dismutase, and lysyl oxidase. The human body contains about 110 mg of Cu of which 60–95% is bound to ceruloplasmin (Cp), which is a source of Cu for peripheral organs. Normal dietary intake of Cu is 1.5–5 mg/day. Of these, 50–60% is unabsorbed and excreted in feces while 25–40% is absorbed from the duodenum and stored in the enterocytes in a nontoxic form. From this intestinal pool, copper is bound to albumin and transported; 75% to the liver through the portal circulation (transcuprein) and 25% in the peripheral circulation. In the liver, 20% of Cu is reexcreted back into the gastrointestinal tract through bile (enterohepatic circulation) and 80% is transported to the periphery bound to Cp. Approximately 80% of the copper excreted in the bile is again reabsorbed by the intestinal mucosa. When copper is deficient in the diet, the affinity of the enterocytes to copper in increased thus increasing its absorption and vice versa. Compared to fecal excretion, urinary Cu excretion is low (10–100 µg/day).[1]

PATHOGENESIS OF WILSON DISEASE

Wilson disease is an autosomal recessive disorder that affects the *ATP7B* gene (chromosome 13q) expressed in hepatocytes, kidneys, and placenta which encodes for the copper transporting P-type ATPase or copper translocase *ATP7B*.[2]

Role of *ATP7B*

- When Cu levels are normal, *ATP7B* helps in transport of copper to the trans-Golgi network and its binding to Cp.
- When intracellular Cu is in excess, *ATP7B* facilitates biliary excretion of Cu.
- Binding of copper to *ATP7B* causes adenosine triphosphate (ATP) hydrolysis, which supplies energy for the transport of copper to the lysosome where it is incorporated into Cp, which is then released in the circulation.

Mutations in ATP7B result in increased cytosolic, mitochondrial and nuclear levels of copper by:

- Decreased synthesis of copper-bound Cp
- Impaired excretion of copper
- Although not yet fully understood, a postulated mechanism is that increased intracellular copper induces oxidative stress leading to the production of hydroxyl radicals and reduced superoxide dismutase and glutathione which leads to damage of cellular lipids, proteins, nucleic acids, and mitochondrial membrane.

CLINICAL FEATURES

The age of presentation can vary from 3 to 85 years. The manifestations are more likely to be hepatic in early childhood and neurological in adolescents; however, other forms of presentation are also seen. The spectrum of hepatic manifestations is very varied as asymptomatic hepatomegaly (3–40%), acute or chronic hepatitis (10–25%), portal hypertension with liver cirrhosis (35–60%), and sometimes in fulminant acute or acute on chronic hepatic failure (11–55%) with very high mortality.[1,3]

Neurological abnormalities can be equally varied and include clumsiness, speech or feeding difficulties, scholastic deterioration, behavior problems, choreoathetoid and dystonic movements, and rarely seizures. Psychobehavioral manifestations, viz., dementia, depression, psychosis, and anxiety are not uncommon and seen in 2.4–20% patients. Most of these patients have past or concurrent history or biochemical evidence of liver disease.

Other rare presentations are "osseomuscular" with resistant rickets, arthritis or arthralgias, unexplained anemia or hemolysis, ocular [sunflower cataract and Kayser–Fleischer (KF) rings], renal (renal tubular acidosis, renal calculi, or Fanconi syndrome), and endocrine (hypogonadism, pancreatic insufficiency, and hypoparathyroidism).

DIAGNOSIS

The key to diagnosis remains to be a high index of suspicion. A detailed family history for affected members and systematic evaluation is quintessential in the diagnosis of WD. No single test is diagnostic by itself. Serum Cp, 24-hour urinary copper and presence of KF ring are the three most common tests done for the diagnosis of WD. Presence of any two of these is highly suggestive of WD. In case of equivocal results, other investigations such as evidence of Coombs negative hemolysis, MRI brain, liver biopsy, and genetic mutation testing must be done and diagnosis could be reasonably made.[1,4,5]

The WD presenting as acute liver failure often presents a major diagnostic problem due to false positive or negative results in the primary tests.[6] In such cases, evidence of hemolysis, very high bilirubin compared to the liver enzymes, aspartate transaminase (AST) raised significantly more than alanine aminotransferase (ALT), low alkaline phosphatase (ALP), and low Cp in siblings might be very helpful.[7,8] **Table 12.9.1** shows the cutoffs for common diagnostic tests and difficulties in its interpretation. The consensus group of the Indian National Association for the study of Liver (INASL) in 2017 has modified the original Leipzig score to aid the diagnosis of WD, especially suitable to the Indian subcontinent.[9]

Serum Ceruloplasmin

It is reduced in most patients with WD. However, 5–40% of WD may have a normal Cp. Enzymatic methods which measure the copper dependent oxidase activity are preferred over immunological assays as the latter overestimates the Cp levels. Though a value of <20 mg/dL is significant, a value <10 mg/dL strongly favors WD.

24-hour Urinary Copper

In symptomatic patients with WD, the 24-hour urinary Cu excretion is >100 μg/day but a value >40 μg/day has also been found to be significant. It is absolutely prudent to ensure urinary collection in the recommended manner and to process the samples in reliable laboratories. Estimation of urinary Cu after a penicillamine challenge has been suggested as a test to differentiate WD from other causes of raised urinary Cu.

Kayser–Fleischer Ring

It appears as a golden brown or greenish-yellow discoloration in the limbus of the cornea **(Fig. 12.9.1)**. It is best seen on a slit lamp examination. Its presence indicates long-standing disease and severe Cu overload. It is positive in >90% patients with neurological WD and but only 50–60% in hepatic WD. The KF ring must be differentiated from the bilirubin ring seen in patients with high bilirubin with chronic cholestatic liver diseases.

Liver Biopsy and Hepatic Copper

There are no histopathological findings specific for WD. Presence of steatohepatitis, interface hepatitis, chronic hepatitis with Mallory's hyaline, bridging fibrosis, and cirrhosis are commonly found on liver biopsy. Histochemical staining for Cu is unreliable, due to the insensitivity of staining techniques to pick up cytosolic Cu, and the heterogeneity of Cu deposition within the liver. Hepatic copper is considered

TABLE 12.9.1: Diagnostic tests used in the evaluation of Wilson disease (WD).

Test	*Cutoff*	*False-positive test*	*False-negative test*
Serum ceruloplasmin (Cp)	<20 mg/dL	• Kwashiorkor • Nutritional copper deficiency • Protein losing states • Fulminant hepatitis/liver failure • Hereditary hypo-aceruloplasminemia or aceruloplasminemia • WD heterozygote • Menkes syndrome • Normal neonate	• Acute inflammation (hepatitis) • Malignancy • Pregnancy or estrogen therapy • Immunoassays of apoceruloplasmin
24-hour urinary copper	>100 μg/day >40 μg/day (children)	• Copper chelation therapy • Chronic cholestatic liver diseases • Hepatic failure • Nephrotic syndrome	Copper chelation therapy in WD
Kayser–Fleischer (KF) ring	Present	Chronic cholestatic liver diseases	Early WD
Hepatic copper estimation	>250 μg/g	• Chronic cholestatic liver diseases • Liver tumors • Newborn liver	Copper chelation therapy in WD
Genetic mutation testing	Pathogenic mutations of *ATP7B* gene	Laboratory error	Presence of unknown mutations

to be the gold standard for diagnosis of WD with values usually >250 μg/g dry weight.

MRI Brain

"Face of giant panda", tectal plate hyperintensity, central pontine myelinolysis-like abnormalities, and involvement of the basal ganglia, thalamus, and brainstem are pathognomonic findings of WD on MRI **(Figs. 12.9.2A to C)**.

Detection of Mutation in the *ATP7B* Gene

Mutational analysis and haplotype studies have been used for the diagnosis of symptomatic and pre-symptomatic patients. However, till date >600 mutations have identified in the large *ATP7B* gene making it more complex for analysis. Many patients are compound heterozygotes (carry two different mutations).

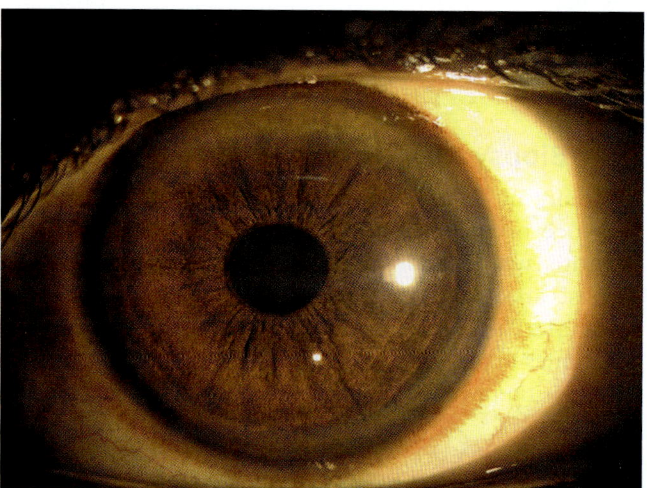

Fig. 12.9.1: Kayser–Fleischer (KF) ring.

Mutational testing has special importance in presymptomatic patients as well as in antenatal screening of high-risk families where the mutation of the proband is known.[2,7]

TREATMENT

Low Copper Diet

The WD cannot be prevented or controlled by a low Cu diet alone. However, it is advisable to avoid high Cu containing foods like organ meats (liver), chocolates, nuts dry fruits, mushrooms, and most importantly, Cu and brass vessels for water or cooking.[1,5,8]

Chelation Therapy

Continuous lifelong drug therapy is essential in the management of WD.[7]

- The *initial therapy* (4–6 months) aims to reduce the Cu to subtoxic threshold, i.e., urinary Cu < 500 μg/day and non-Cp bound Cu or serum free copper to <25 μg/dL.
- The *maintenance therapy* aims to maintain a slightly negative Cu balance so as to prevent Cu accumulation and toxicity.

D-penicillamine (DP), trientine, and zinc have been traditionally used as chelators of Cu in WD. There are no randomized controlled trials to prove the superiority of DP/trientine alone or zinc alone or its combination. The advantage of starting combination of DP/trientine with zinc is preferred. **Table 12.9.2** shows a tabulated description of the various chelating agents.

D-Penicillamine

It reduces protein bound Cu; binds and mobilizes Cu, and excretes it in the urine. It does so by inducing hepatic

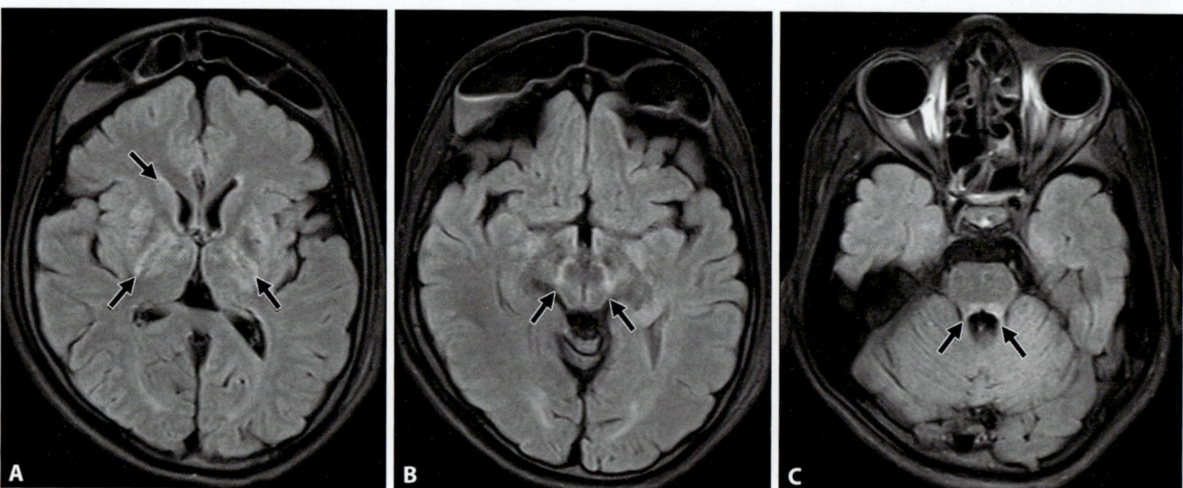

Figs. 12.9.2A to C: Axial fluid-attenuated inversion recovery (FLAIR) sequence showing hyperintensities at level of (A) Basal ganglia—bilateral lentiform nuclei; (B) Midbrain—bilateral tegmentum; (C) Posterior pons—near superior cerebellar peduncle.

TABLE 12.9.2: Drug therapy for Wilson disease (WD).

Name	Dosing and compounding	Side effects
D-penicillamine (DP)	• 5 mg/kg/day gradually escalated to 20 mg/kg/day (maximum dose 1,500 mg/day) in two to three divided doses • To ensure at least 2 hours fasting before and after each dose • Trientine to be stored at 2–8°C	Hypersensitivity reactions, proteinuria, cytopenias, skin toxicity, pyridoxine deficiency, and neurological worsening
Trientine		• Fewer than DP • In addition, sideroblastic anemia, iron and copper deficiency • Neurological worsening is less common DP
Zinc	In <50 kg: 75 mg/day >50 kg: 150 mg/day in two to three divided doses to be taken on empty stomach and not with DP/trientine	Gastritis and pancreatitis
Ammonium tetrathiomolybdate	20 mg six times a day (three doses to be taken premeals and three doses between meals)	Cytopenias and hepatoxicity

metallothionein, a cytosolic metal-binding protein that sequesters copper and renders it nontoxic. A large cupriuresis in the initial phase is followed by a decline in the maintenance phase. Although a powerful chelator, it has fallen into disrepute due to its many adverse effects, viz., hematological cytopenias, worsening of neurological features, allergic reactions, and renal side effects. Smaller initiating doses of DP to produce a cupriuresis of say 1–2 mg/day may prevent neurological deterioration.

Trientine

This is an alternative chelating agent, especially for children intolerant to DP. The mechanism of action of trientine is similar to that of DP. For some time now, trientine has been used as an alternative drug in children not tolerating DP. However, recently it is increasingly being used as a first line drug instead of DP, with good efficacy and fewer side effects.

Zinc

Zinc (Zn) acetate salts are preferred due to lesser incidence of gastric discomfort. Zn acts by inducing intestinal cell metallothionein, which binds Cu, Zn, and cadmium. The metallothionein bound Cu is held in the intestinal cells till it is sloughed out. Zinc also induces metallothionein in hepatocytes. Unlike DP and trientine, Zn acts by increasing the fecal excretion of Cu. However, Zn is slow acting and takes much longer to achieve a negative Cu balance, and hence is effectively used as maintenance therapy, especially because of its low cost and low toxicity.

Monitoring of Patients on Chelation Therapy

Patients on chelation therapy have to be monitored for new onset clinical features, allergic reactions, hematological cytopenias, and renal side effects after initiating therapy every 3–6 monthly. Adequacy of chelation is calculated with the help of 24-hour measurement urinary Cu, urinary Zn, and calculation of serum free copper (serum copper – 3 × serum Cp). After an initial phase of severe cupriuresis, good control is indicated with resolution of clinical and biochemical features with urinary Cu 200–500 µg/day and serum free Cu 10–15 µg/dL. Urinary copper (U Cu) < 200 µg/day can be seen in both noncompliance (or inadequate dosing) and overchelation.

Adjuvant Therapy

Pyridoxine and antioxidants like vitamin E act as adjunctive therapies in patients on chelation.

Role of Plasma Exchange in Wilson Disease

Extracorporeal therapies like high volume plasma exchange (PE) have shown considerable promise in patients with acute liver failure.[6] PE in WD is a category 1 indication as per the American Society for Apheresis (ASFA) (recommendation 1C), but this has not been substantiated with robust comparative data or randomized controlled trials. PE has proven to be an efficient bridge to liver transplant (LT), especially in those considered to be too sick for transplantation on admission.[10]

Management of Patients with Neurological Features

Patients with neurological features are best managed with the help of experienced neurologists and/or psychiatrists. Drugs such as trihexyphenidyl (for dystonia), baclofen (for muscle relaxants), propranolol and benzodiazepines (for tremors), levodopa (for parkinsonian features), selective serotonin reuptake inhibitors, and/or atypical antipsychotics (for behavioral abnormalities) are commonly used medications prescribed to these patients.

Liver Transplant

Liver transplant is the treatment of choice in children with acute onset liver failure or decompensated cirrhosis unresponsive to medical therapy.[6] LTs correct the metabolic defect and the transplanted children do not require any anti-Cu medications. In case of live related donors, it is imperative to screen for WD as many might be asymptomatic and may present later in life. Heterozygous relatives are suitable as donors without any risk of disease recurrence. The 5-year patient survival post LT was 96% in recently published study in a French cohort. The decision for LT in WD with neurological involvement is still challenging as LT may not completely reverse the neuropsychiatric manifestations.[11]

Management of Siblings of Wilson Disease

All siblings carry a 25% chance of having WD. Hence, they should undergo a detailed clinical examination, slit lamp examination for KF ring, liver function tests, serum Cp, and a 24-hour urinary Cu determination. If these are normal, the child is unlikely to have WD. This screening should be done initially at 3–5 years and repeated again at 15 years. As such, genetic linkage studies (haplotype analysis) are of great promise because the disease/normal/carrier status of sibs can be detected at birth or even earlier in antenatal period. The treatment of asymptomatic sibs is identical to that recommended for children receiving maintenance therapy viz., zinc, DP, or trientine.

PROGNOSIS OF WILSON DISEASE

Despite initiation and maintenance of adequate Cu chelation therapy, the outcome is unpredictable. The types of outcomes seen are:

- Rapid and complete improvement, especially of hepatic symptoms with reversal of parenchymal lesions including early cirrhosis
- Initial deterioration particularly of neurological symptoms with eventual improvement but with residual handicap (speech and handwriting)
- Relentless deterioration and death in spite of therapy as in fulminant hepatic failure. Patients with advanced cirrhosis and its complications may also succumb after prolonged survival.
- The best outcome is seen in asymptomatic siblings of index WD cases. If diagnosed early, these children have the best chance of normal health and longevity provided they take regular therapy.

REFERENCES

1. Pandit AN, Bavdekar AR, Bhave SA. Wilson's disease. Indian J Pediatr. 2002;69(9):785-91.
2. Wu F, Wang J, Pu C, Qiao L, Jiang C. Wilson's disease: a comprehensive review of the molecular mechanisms. Int J Mol Sci. 2015;16(3):6419-31.
3. Lin L, Wang D, Ding N, Zheng C. Hepatic manifestations in Wilson disease: report of 110 cases. Hepatogastroenterology. 2015;62(139):657-60.
4. Bavdekar AR. Wilson's disease–A diagnostic dilemma? Indian J Gastroenterol. 2003;22(1):2-3.
5. Roberts EA. Update on the Diagnosis and Management of Wilson Disease. Curr Gastroenterol Rep. 2018;20(12):56.
6. Alam S, Lal BB, Sood V, Rawat D. Pediatric Acute-on-Chronic Liver Failure in a Specialized Liver Unit: Prevalence, Profile, Outcome, and Predictive Factors. J Pediatr Gastroenterol Nutr. 2016;63(4):400-5.
7. Roberts EA, Schilsky ML. Current and Emerging Issues in Wilson's Disease. N Engl J Med. 2023;389(10):922-38.
8. European Association for Study of Liver. EASL Clinical Practice Guidelines: Wilson's disease. J Hepatol. 2012;56(3):671-85.
9. Nagral A, Sarma MS, Matthai J, Kukkle PL, Devarbhavi H, Sinha S, et al. Wilson's Disease: clinical practice guidelines of the Indian National Association for study of the liver, the Indian society of pediatric gastroenterology, hepatology and nutrition, and the movement disorders society of India. J Clin Exp Hepatol. 2019;9(1):74-98.
10. Tan EX, Wang MX, Pang J, Lee GH. Plasma exchange in patients with acute and acute-on-chronic liver failure: A systematic review. World J Gastroenterol. 2020;26(2):219-45.
11. Guillaud O, Dumortier J, Sobesky R, Debray D, Wolf P, Vanlemmens C, et al. Long term results of liver transplantation for Wilson's disease: experience in France. J Hepatol. 2014; 60(3):579-89.

12.10 Neonatal Cholestasis Syndromes

Riyaz Arakkal

INTRODUCTION

Cholestasis is defined as interference of bile flow anywhere from the basolateral membrane of hepatocytes to the entry of the common bile duct (CBD) into the duodenum. It is caused by diseases either in the hepatocytes, intrahepatic bile ducts, or extrahepatic biliary system. It can also be defined as follows:

- *Biochemically* as increased levels of conjugated bilirubin, bile acids or their intermediate metabolites, and other bile compounds
- *Clinically* as the accumulation in the blood and extrahepatic tissues of substances which are normally excreted in the bile (e.g., bilirubin, bile acids, and cholesterol).[1]

The term *neonatal cholestasis* (NC) refers to conjugated hyperbilirubinemia that is present at birth or develops within the first few months of life, rather than referring strictly to the neonatal period (the first 28 days of life). These disorders usually manifest within the first 2 months of life, which is the critical period for diagnosing and treating biliary atresia (BA). It is the duty of the pediatrician who sees the baby first to differentiate BA which requires surgery before 60 days, from the various nonsurgical causes which may require specific treatment urgently (congenital hypothyroidism, galactosemia, type 1 tyrosinemia and various infectious causes like herpes).

Neonatal cholestasis syndromes (NCS) present with prolonged conjugated hyperbilirubinemia beyond 2 weeks of life, and high colored urine with or without pale stools. The presence of high level of conjugated bilirubin (>20% of total bilirubin if serum bilirubin >5 mg/dL or >1 mg/dL if total serum bilirubin <5 mg/dL) is suggestive of NC.[2]

EPIDEMIOLOGY

About 60% of term babies and 80% of preterm babies develop physiologic jaundice which subsides by 2 weeks in at least 85%. Most infants in whom jaundice persists even after 2 weeks have some benign conditions such as breast milk jaundice, congenital hypothyroidism, or hemolytic jaundice. Only about 0.2–0.4% of them have conjugated hyperbilirubinemia due to BA or other life-threatening diseases that require prompt diagnosis and treatment to optimize outcomes. NC accounts for about 30% of all hepatobiliary disorders in children in India.

CLASSIFICATION

Based on the primary site of pathology, NC may be classified as intrahepatic (medical) or extrahepatic (surgical).

- *Intrahepatic cholestasis* is seen in toxoplasma gondii, other agents, rubella, cytomegalovirus (CMV), and herpes simplex virus (TORCH) infections, septicemia, during total parenteral nutrition (TPN), and various inborn errors of metabolism such as galactosemia, type 1 tyrosinemia, and various types of progressive familial intrahepatic cholestasis (PFIC).
- In the *extrahepatic group,* BA is the most important, followed by choledochal cyst.

The spectrum of diseases causing NCS in India and the West is quite different as shown in **Table 12.10.1**.

TABLE 12.10.1: The spectrum of neonatal cholestasis syndromes: West versus India.

Disease	*West*	*India (multicentric)*
Biliary atresia/choledochal cyst	25%	38%
Neonatal hepatitis (NH)	15%	37%
Metabolic diseases	20%	4%
PFIC/Alagille syndrome/bile acid synthesis disorders	25%	3%
Alpha-1 antitrypsin deficiency	10%	—
Viral infections	5%	10%
Others	—	2%
Unknown	—	6%

(PFIC: progressive familial intrahepatic cholestasis)

It is also useful to classify NC as babies who are sick and nonsick, as the sick babies require urgent workup for prompt therapy as shown in **Flowchart 12.10.1**.

Neonatal Cholestasis due to TORCH Infections

The TORCH infections are characterized by failure to thrive, purpura, microcephaly, chorioretinitis, and hepatosplenomegaly; and congenital heart disease in congenital rubella syndrome. In most children, CMV hepatitis is mild and resolves completely but a few may develop hepatic fibrosis, noncirrhotic portal hypertension, and cirrhosis. Neonatal hepatitis (NH) due to *herpes simplex* causes fulminant hepatitis and encephalitis. Intravenous (IV) acyclovir therapy may be lifesaving.

Galactosemia

Galactosemia is an autosomal recessive inborn error of galactose metabolism affecting one in 50,000 live births. Classic galactosemia is due to deficiency of galactose-1-phosphate uridyltransferase (GALT). The infant is normal at birth, but soon after breastfeeding he/she may develop severe hypoglycemia, convulsions, shock, disseminated intravascular coagulation (DIC), and even death, if not diagnosed and treated promptly. There is a striking association between galactosemia and neonatal *Escherichia coli* septicemia. This is because the bactericidal activity of leukocytes may be inhibited by galactose.

Diagnosis is usually established by a low red blood cell (RBC) GALT activity. Urine sugar may be negative if the baby has not been breastfed, or is only on IV fluids. All galactose-containing food items should be stopped and a galactose and lactose-free diet should be started immediately. If the diagnosis is delayed, the child may die of fulminant hepatic failure.

Progressive Familial Intrahepatic Cholestasis

These are a group of recently described rare autosomal recessive diseases due to mutations in specific canalicular

Flowchart 12.10.1: Classification of neonatal cholestasis syndromes.

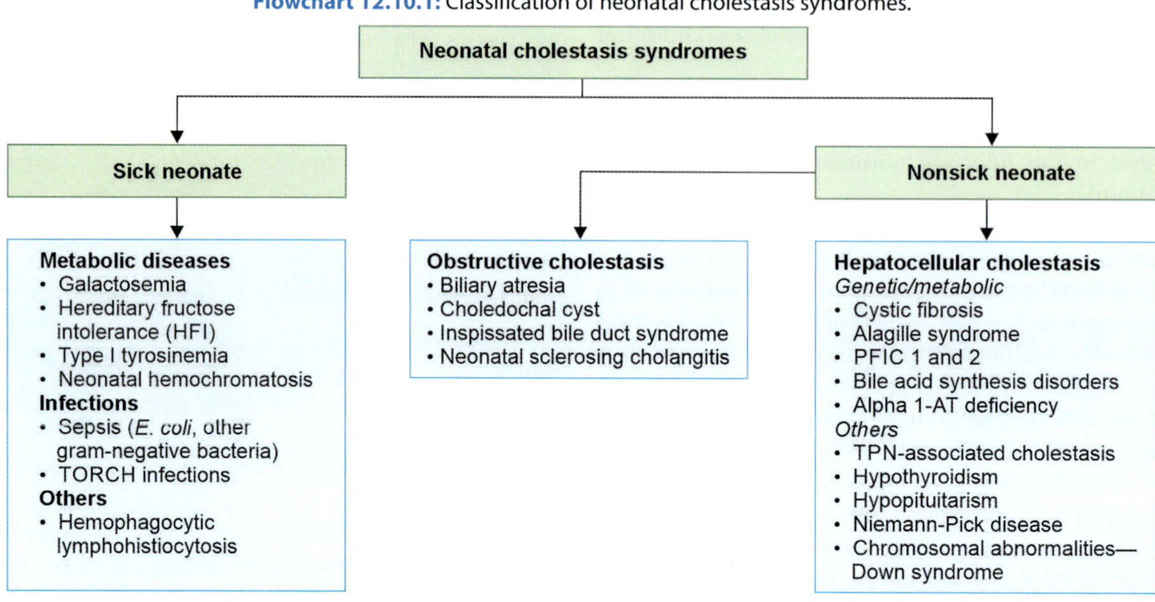

(AT: antitrypsin; PFIC: progressive familial intrahepatic cholestasis; TORCH: toxoplasma gondii, other agents, rubella, cytomegalovirus, and herpes simplex virus; TPN: total parenteral nutrition)

membrane transport proteins in which toxic bile acids accumulate in the hepatocytes resulting in liver injury. A total of seven types of PFIC have been described so far. They account for 10–15% of all NCS and 10–15% of all liver transplantation (LT) in children.

One of the hallmarks of these patients is the *intractable pruritus*, which is out of proportion to the intensity of icterus. These children should be managed symptomatically till they require LT. Biliary diversion procedures may help to relieve the intractable pruritus in some, but the ultimate answer is LT.

Alagille Syndrome (Figs. 12.10.1 and 12.10.2)

Alagille syndrome (AS) is an autosomal dominant disease, with mutations in the *JAGI* gene (90%) or *NOTCH2* gene (10%). It is associated with intractable pruritus, cirrhosis, congenital heart disease (peripheral pulmonary stenosis or tetralogy of Fallot), xanthomas, dysmorphism, and posterior embryotoxon. AS may be mistaken for BA with disastrous consequences, and hence it is very important to differentiate BA from AS **(Table 12.10.2)**.

Gestational Alloimmune Liver Disease or Neonatal Hemochromatosis

Gestational alloimmune liver disease (GALD) is the result of alloimmune liver injury due to transplacental passage of immunoglobulin G (IgG) antibodies from a mother sensitized to fetal-derived antigens which destroy fetal hepatocytes. The neonate presents with severe liver failure. Buccal mucosal biopsy which shows deposition of iron in minor salivary glands is a simple test for diagnosis.

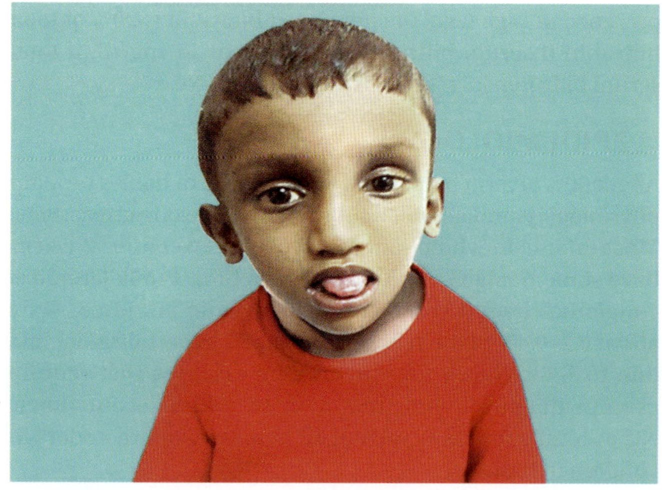

Fig. 12.10.1: Child with Alagille syndrome (AS) and tetralogy of Fallot.

Treating the mother with high-dose intravenous immunoglobulin (IVIG) can dramatically reduce the risk for recurrence of disease and also fetal loss. Neonates with GALD should be given the combination of exchange transfusion and IVIG. The only option for nonresponders to this regime is LT.

Biliary Atresia

Biliary atresia is the most common cause of NC, accounting for almost 30% of all cases. It is a fatal progressive fibroinflammatory cholangiopathy resulting in complete obliteration of the entire or portions of the extrahepatic and intrahepatic biliary tree within weeks of birth. Japan and Taiwan are the countries with the highest incidence of BA in the world.

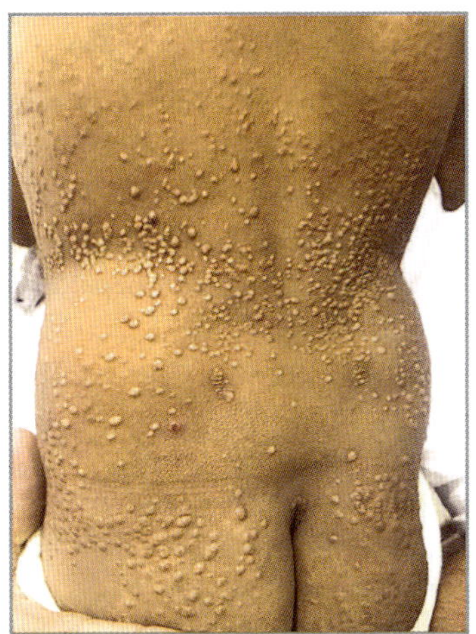

Fig. 12.10.2: Extensive xanthomas in Alagille syndrome (AS).

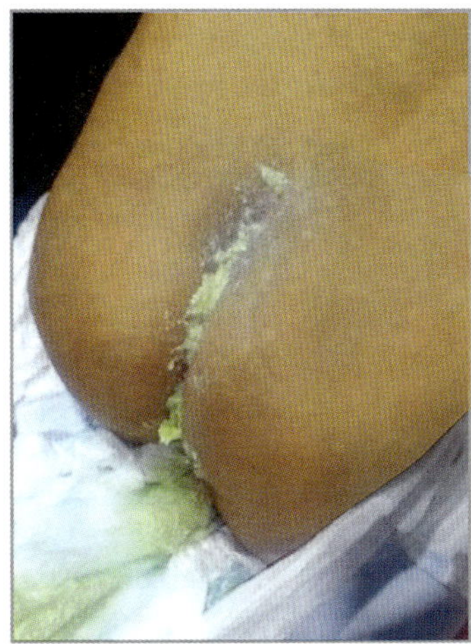

Fig. 12.10.3: Pale (acholic) stool of biliary atresia (BA).

TABLE 12.10.2: Biliary atresia (BA) versus Alagille syndrome.

Features	***Biliary atresia***	***Alagille syndrome***
Stools	Persistent acholic	Intermittent pale/ normal stools
Dysmorphism	Nil	Triangular face, pointed chin, deep-set eyes, etc.
Pruritus	Mild	Severe
Congenital heart disease	Rare, <10%	Common
Ophthalmology evaluation	Essentially normal	Posterior embryotoxon, Axenfeld anomaly
GGT	Very high	Very high
Dyslipidemia	Minimal	Severe
USG	GB absent/atretic; triangular cord sign; GB ghost triad; normal kidneys	GB may be atretic; increased renal echogenicity
Isotope (mebrofenin) scan	Usually, no excretion	Rarely, no excretion—hence mistaken for BA

(GB: gallbladder; GGT: gamma-glutamyl transpeptidase; USG: ultrasonography)

Biliary atresia is more common in term female babies with normal birth weight. The triad of BA includes jaundice, acholic stools **(Fig. 12.10.3)** and firm hepatomegaly. Splenomegaly is late and is a sign of hepatic fibrosis and portal hypertension. Bleeding may occur due to uncorrected vitamin K deficiency, especially in breastfed babies. BA should be ruled out in any neonate with conjugated jaundice persisting beyond 14 days of life.

Choledochal Cyst (Biliary Cyst)

Choledochal cysts are a rare but important treatable cause of NC. Like BA, this is also more common in females. Diagnosis is usually by ultrasonography (USG). Rarely, endoscopic retrograde cholangiopancreatography (ERCP) and percutaneous transhepatic cholangiography (PTC) may be necessary. Treatment is by complete surgical excision with drainage of the biliary tract into the jejunum.

EVALUATION OF NEONATAL CHOLESTASIS SYNDROME

Neonatal cholestasis is usually a sign of underlying serious hepatobiliary and/or metabolic disorders. If not diagnosed and treated promptly, these may be fatal. It is the duty of the primary pediatrician to pick up those cases which have a specific treatment. Many of these disorders cannot be diagnosed by liver biopsy or standard blood tests. The evaluation of NC is usually a tedious and laborious process in which a wide range of diseases that come in the differential diagnosis should be carefully excluded by a detailed history **(Table 12.10.3)**, meticulous physical examination **(Table 12.10.4)**, especially a detailed ophthalmologic evaluation **(Table 12.10.5)**, and relevant investigations **(Table 12.10.6)**.

There has been an exponential increase in our knowledge of NC in the last couple of decades due to the easy availability of genetic studies (targeted gene panels, whole-exome sequencing, and whole-genome sequencing) in our country at affordable costs. These help in the early diagnosis of potentially life-threatening conditions that need immediate intervention such as galactosemia, type 1 tyrosinemia, and mitochondrial hepatopathies. At the same time surgical conditions like BA should be ruled out. This approach will also help to decide on referral for LT.[3]

Neonatologists of Taiwan have introduced a novel screening program using an infant stool card with different stool colors, which can be compared with the baby's stool color. This helps in the early diagnosis of BA. This has been modified in India incorporating urine color also by

TABLE 12.10.3: Clues in history in NC.

Antenatal history	***Clues***
Consanguinity, similar illness in family	AR diseases such as galactosemia, type 1 tyrosinemia, and PFIC
Recurrent fetal loss or early demise	GALD
Intrahepatic cholestasis of pregnancy	PFIC, especially type 3
Acute fatty liver of pregnancy	Neonatal long-chain 3-hydroxyacyl CoA dehydrogenase deficiency
Antenatal USG	Choledochal cyst; cystic BA
Postnatal history	***Clues***
Female gender	BA, choledochal cyst
Delayed passage of meconium	Congenital hypothyroidism, cystic fibrosis
Appearance	*Well looking*—BA *Sick looking*—sepsis/metabolic liver disease
Intrauterine growth retardation	TORCH infections
Rh/ABO incompatibility	Inspissated bile duct syndrome
Escherichia coli sepsis	Galactosemia
History of prolonged stay in NICU	Rh/ABO incompatibility, inspissated BD syndrome, sepsis
Recurrent seizures, vomiting	Galactosemia, HFI, panhypopituitarism, intracranial hemorrhage
Precipitating factors	Milk feeds in galactosemia; fructose feeds in HFI
Persistent acholic stools	Biliary atresia
Intermittent pale stools	Medical causes of NC
Abnormal urine odor	Boiled cabbage/rancid butter odor in type 1 tyrosinemia
Older children with severe aversion for cereals and craving for protein and fat-rich food	Citrin deficiency
Chronic diarrhea, recurrent pancreatitis	PFIC1

(AR: autosomal recessive; BA: biliary atresia; BD: bile duct; GALD: gestational alloimmune liver disease; HFI: hereditary fructose intolerance; NC: neonatal cholestasis; NICU: neonatal intensive care unit; PFIC: progressive familial intrahepatic cholestasis)

Yachha et al. (integrated NC card), and is much superior compared to the Taiwan card.[4]

Metabolic Workup

- *Hypoglycemia:* Galactosemia, HFI, and hypopituitarism
- *High sweat chloride:* Cystic fibrosis

TABLE 12.10.4: Clues in clinical examination in NC.

Dysmorphism	Down syndrome, Zellweger syndrome, Alagille syndrome, citrin deficiency (chubby face)
Microcephaly	Congenital rubella, CMV, SLOS, Down syndrome
Sensory neural deafness	Congenital rubella syndrome, PFIC1, TJP2, PFIC7, mitochondrial hepatopathies
Relative bradycardia	Bile salts depress SA node Due to propranolol given for portal hypertension
Congenital heart disease	PDA and peripheral PS in congenital rubella syndrome; peripheral PS and Fallot in Alagille syndrome; PDA and ASD in SLOS
Genitalia and NC	Cryptorchidism in hypopituitarism and SLOS; biliscrotum in spontaneous perforation of bile duct
NC with spleno-megaly at birth	TORCH infections; Niemann–Pick C disease, Gaucher disease type 2
Hard liver and ascites	Ominous signs—cirrhosis has already set in
Lymphedema of extremities	Aagenaes syndrome
Vertical gaze palsy, gelastic cataplexy	Niemann–Pick C disease

(ASD: atrial septal defect; CMV: cytomegalovirus; NC: neonatal cholestasis; PDA: patent ductus arteriosus; PFIC: progressive familial intrahepatic cholestasis; PS: pulmonary stenosis; SLOS: Smith–Lemli–Opitz syndrome; TJP2: tight junction protein 2)

TABLE 12.10.5: Clues in ophthalmology in NC.

Epicanthic folds	Down syndrome, Zellweger syndrome
Brushfield spots	Down syndrome
Cataract	Galactosemia, HFI, congenital rubella syndrome, CMV hepatitis, SLOS, Zellweger syndrome
Chorioretinitis (salt and pepper appearance)	CMV, toxoplasmosis, rubella
Posterior embryotoxon, Axenfeld anomaly	Alagille syndrome
Microphthalmia	Congenital rubella, CMV
Cherry red spot	Niemann–Pick C disease
Retinitis pigmentosa, glaucoma	Zellweger syndrome

(CMV: cytomegalovirus; HFI: hereditary fructose intolerance; NC: neonatal cholestasis; SLOS: Smith–Lemli–Opitz syndrome)

- *Low RBC GALT:* Galactosemia
- *Serum alpha-fetoprotein* is normal in BA and high in NH; it is extremely high in type 1 tyrosinemia and GALD

TABLE 12.10.6: Clues from investigations in NC.

Finding	*Clue*
Urine examination "Owl-eye" bodies	• Pyuria and urine culture in urosepsis; positive Benedict's test in galactosemia • CMV hepatitis
CBC, differential	Low WBC count and low absolute neutrophil count in early neonatal sepsis
ESR, C-reactive protein (CRP)	High in sepsis
Fractionated bilirubin	Helps to confirm cholestasis
Serum bilirubin, ALT, AST	• Biliary pathology (BA)—SB relatively high • Hepatocellular cholestasis—ALT, AST higher
Low/normal GGT with high alkaline phosphatase (ALP)	• All PFIC except type 3 • BRIC • ARC syndrome; bile acid synthetic disorders
High GGT and ALP	BA, Alagille syndrome, PFIC3
Prothrombin time (PT)/ international normalized ratio (INR)	• Most important for prognosis • Prolonged PT/INR corrected by injection vitamin K is S/O malabsorption; if not corrected, hepatocellular failure
Alpha-fetoprotein (AFP)	• Very high in type 1 tyrosinemia and GALD >100,000 • High in citrin deficiency
High lactate >90 mEq/L	Mitochondrial hepatopathy
Low serum cholesterol	SLOS
Bone marrow	• Macrophages with "wrinkled tissue paper" appearance (type 2 Gaucher disease) • Foamy histiocytes (Niemann–Pick C disease, Farber disease)

(ARC: arthrogryposis-renal dysfunction-cholestasis; BRIC: benign recurrent intrahepatic cholestasis; CBC: complete blood count; CMV: cytomegalovirus; GALD: gestational alloimmune liver disease; GGT: gamma-glutamyl transpeptidase; NC: neonatal cholestasis; SLOS: Smith–Lemli–Opitz syndrome)

Radiological Workup

- *Diffuse cerebral calcification:* Congenital toxoplasmosis
- *Periventricular calcification:* Congenital CMV infection
- *Wimberger sign (erosion of the upper medial surface of tibia):* Congenital syphilis
- *Butterfly vertebrae, fused vertebrae, and spina bifida occulta:* AS

Ultrasonography

Among all noninvasive procedures, USG has the highest diagnostic accuracy in NC, and it helps to avoid unnecessary invasive procedures. It should be ensured that the baby is not fed for 4 hours before the scan.

- Nonimaged or small gallbladder (GB) in fasting state and invisible CBD are suggestive of BA, but not diagnostic.
- *If normal GB and CBD are visualized:* BA unlikely
- *Triangular cord sign:* A cone-shaped fibrotic mass of thickness >4 mm cranial to the bifurcation of the portal vein is highly suggestive of BA.
- *GB ghost triad of Kendrick in BA:*
    - Small GB (length <19 mm)
    - An irregular/lobulated contour
    - An indistinct and thin GB wall with a lack of a smooth mucosal lining.
- *Pseudo GB sign:*[5] Some infants with proven BA may have a GB-like structure, ≤15 mm in length. This is a small ovoid fluid-filled structure in the expected region of the GB—the pseudo GB sign. This may be mistaken for a normal GB by inexperienced radiologists, thus missing the diagnosis of BA.

Color Doppler Echo[6]

Hepatic artery is enlarged, and there is increased hepatic subcapsular flow—early and useful markers of BA.

Radionuclide Hepatobiliary Scintigraphy

Technetium-99m-labeled derivatives of iminodiacetic acid are used to assess the continuity of the biliary tract with the small intestine.

- In *medical cholestasis,* the uptake is decreased, but the excretion into the gut is normal.
- In BA, the uptake is normal but excretion into gut is decreased, so that there is no radioactivity in the gut, even after 24 hours.
- The presence of radioactivity in the gut is a strong point against the diagnosis of BA.

Liver Biopsy

Features of Biliary Atresia

- Marked bile ductular proliferation and fibrosis
- Minimal giant cell formation
- Presence of bile lakes

Features of Neonatal Hepatitis

- Very little bile ductular proliferation
- Striking giant cell formation
- Focal hepatocellular necrosis

Recent Advances in the Diagnosis of Biliary Atresia

Elevated serum levels of interleukin-33 and serum matrix metalloproteinase-7 (MMP-7) are suggestive of BA. MMP-7 has a sensitivity and specificity of 95–98%, and may help to avoid liver biopsy.[7]

MANAGEMENT OF NEONATAL CHOLESTASIS

An algorithm for management of NC is given in **Flowchart 12.10.2**.[8]

Nutrition

Cholestasis leads to maldigestion and malabsorption of fat, and fat-soluble vitamins due to diminished bile acid secretion. This leads to steatorrhea that aggravates malnutrition. The other causes of malnutrition are anorexia, recurrent infections, and early satiety secondary to compression of stomach by the enlarged liver and spleen, and ascites. Hence, all infants with cholestasis require nutritional support in the form of adequate calories to compensate for steatorrhea—125% of the recommended dietary allowance (RDA) based on ideal body weight; 5–10 times RDA of fat soluble vitamins; 2–3 g protein/kg/day; and sufficient water-soluble vitamins and minerals **(Table 12.10.7)**. Breastfeeding should be encouraged, except in galactosemia.

5 mg of vitamin K should be given intramuscularly (IM), subcutaneously (SC), or intravenously at diagnosis to all babies with NC to correct coagulopathy, and prevent fatal intracranial hemorrhage. IM route should be avoided if prothrombin time (PT)/international normalized ratio (INR) is prolonged.[9]

In NC, formula feeds that contain medium-chain triglycerides (MCTs) are well tolerated. This is because medium-chain fatty acids (MCFAs) in them are more water-soluble compared to long-chain fatty acids (LCFAs) and are absorbed from the gut by passive diffusion directly to the portal venous system, even in the absence of bile acids. In contrast, LCFAs are absorbed only into the lymphatics. MCFAs can reach mitochondria for beta oxidation even without the help of carnitine, unlike LCFAs. Hence, MCTs are very useful in NC.

Coconut oil is the richest natural source of MCTs, followed by palm oil **(Table 12.10.8)**. Pure MCT oil (100%) which is commercially available is a highly concentrated source of MCTs. 1–2 mL/kg of MCT oil may be given in two to four divided doses in expressed breast milk.

Treatment of Pruritus

Pruritus is believed to be due to the deposition of bile acids in the skin or due to increased endogenous opioids like met-enkephalins synthesized in the gut. Some of the treatment options are as follows:

- *Cholestyramine:* This nonabsorbable anion exchange resin in the dose of 250 mg/kg binds bile acids and cholesterol, and eliminates them in stool.
- Colestipol

Flowchart 12.10.2: Algorithm for management of neonatal cholestasis (NC).[8]

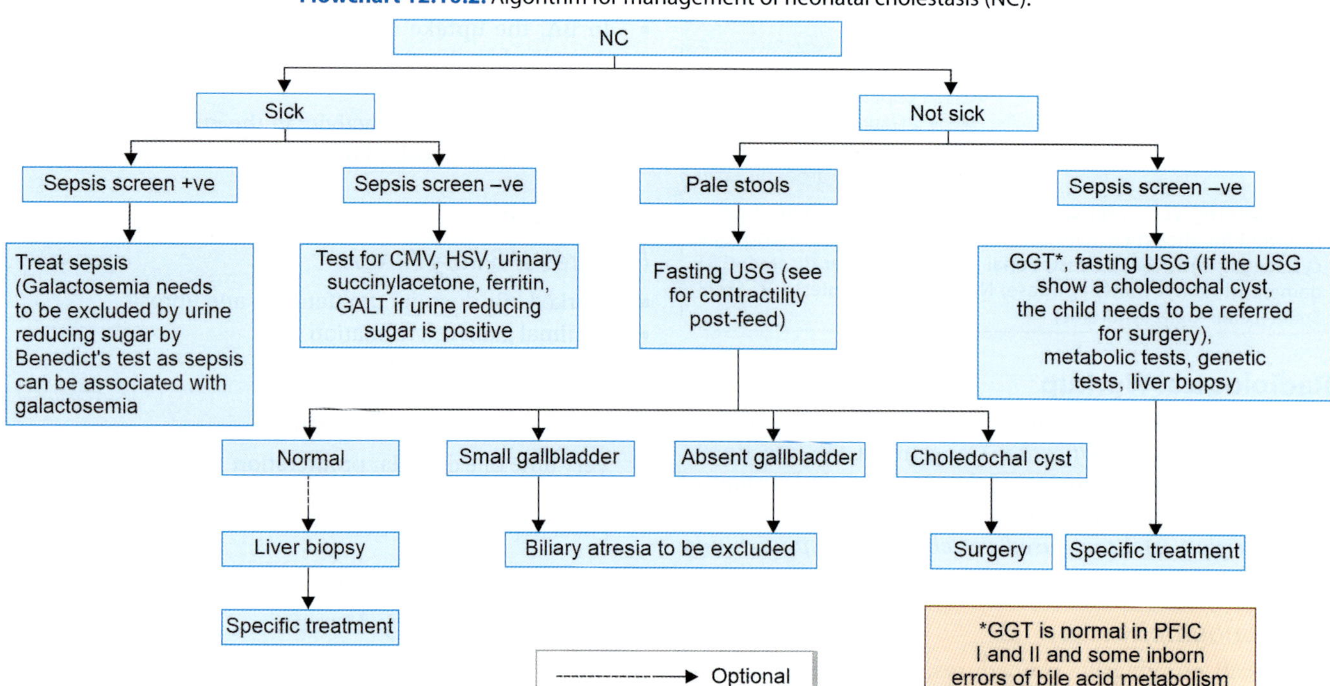

(CMV: cytomegalovirus; GALT: galactose-1-phosphate uridyltransferase; GGT: gamma-glutamyltransferase; HSV: herpes simplex virus; PFIC: progressive familial intrahepatic cholestasis; USG: ultrasonography)

- *Colesevelam hydrochloride:* This is a newer more powerful bile acid sequestrant.
- Phenobarbitone
- Ursodeoxycholic acid—a tertiary nontoxic hydrophilic bile acid is a powerful choleretic agent. Dose is 15–30 mg/kg/day.
- Opioid antagonists—IV naloxone or oral nalmefene
- Rifampicin, antihistamines, and carbamazepine
- Plasmapheresis and ultraviolet B light
- Bile diversion procedures

TABLE 12.10.7: Vitamin and mineral supplementation in NC.

Nutrients	*Dose*	*Route*
Vitamin A Serum retinol <20 μg/dL indicates deficiency	5,000–25,000 IU/day	Oral
Vitamin D	400–1,200 IU/day	Oral
1,25-dihydroxyvitamin D_3 If child has significant bone changes or severe cholestasis	0.05–0.2 μg/kg/day	Oral
Vitamin E	50–100 IU/day or 15–25 IU/kg/day of TPGS, if available	Oral
Vitamin K	2.5 mg twice weekly to 5 mg/day 2–5 mg Dose may be adjusted depending on PT/INR done monthly	Oral IM/SC/IV monthly
Water-soluble vitamins	1–2 times RDA	Oral
Elemental iron	5–6 mg/kg/day	Oral
Calcium	20–100 mg/kg/day	Oral
Phosphorus	25–50 mg/kg/day	Oral
Zinc	1 mg/kg/day	Oral
Magnesium	1–2 mEq/kg/day 0.3–0.5 mEq/kg over 3 hours of 50% solution	Oral IV

(INR: international normalized ratio; IV: intravenous; NC: neonatal cholestasis; PT: prothrombin time; RDA: recommended dietary allowance; TPGS: tocopherol polyethylene glycol succinate)

TABLE 12.10.8: Sources of medium-chain triglycerides (MCTs).

Type of oil	*Medium-chain fatty acid %*
Coconut oil	55
Palm oil	54
Whole milk	9
Butter	8
MCT oil	100

Recent Advances in Treatment of Pruritus

Bile acids are absorbed from the terminal ileum by apical sodium-dependent bile acid transporter (ASBT) which can be inhibited by new drugs such as maralixibat and odevixibat. They may relieve the intractable pruritus of AS and PFIC1 and 2. Sertraline, a selective serotonin reuptake inhibitor, may also relieve intractable pruritus in some cases.

Immunization

In general, all routine vaccines including hepatitis B virus (HBV) vaccine should be given to children with NCS. Hepatitis A vaccine should be given to children >1 year. Live vaccines are contraindicated in children who have undergone LT.

Surgery

In 1955, Morio Kasai, the famous Japanese surgeon **(Fig. 12.10.4)**, operated a 72-day-old infant with BA—Kasai portoenterostomy (KPE) **(Table 12.10.9)**. This surgery helps to slow down the rapid downhill course of unoperated BA by establishing bile flow by removing atretic bile ducts and creating a liver-intestine anastomosis.

The crucial factors that decide the success of KPE are:

- Age of infant at surgery (ideally <60 days)
- The presence of good bile flow at the porta hepatis during surgery
- Cholangitis following surgery
- Ductules within the biliary remnant are ≥150 μm
- The skill and experience of the surgical team

Kasai Portoenterostomy versus Primary Liver Transplantation for Biliary Atresia[10]

The morbidity following KPE is usually high, and most children will subsequently require LT. Hence, some

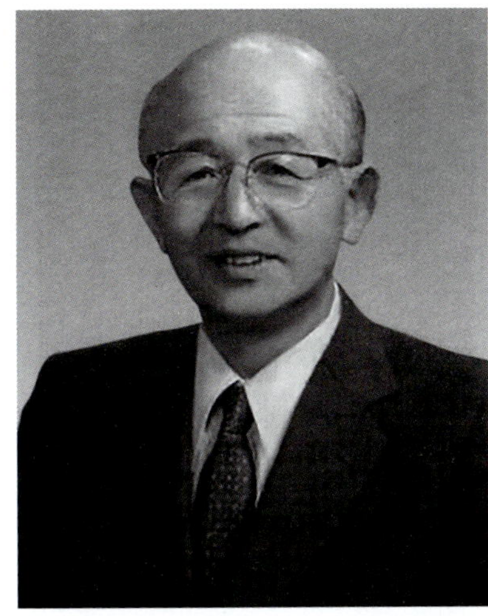

Fig. 12.10.4: Morio Kasai, Japanese surgeon (1922–2008).

TABLE 12.10.9: Outcome of Kasai portoenterostomy (KPE).[10]

Failed KPE (Fig. 12.10.5)	Successful KPE (Fig. 12.10.6)
• Infants who do not clear jaundice following surgery • Develop complications such as intractable ascites, portal hypertension, etc. • Require liver transplantation (LT) by 6–9 months of age	• In a small subset of children, the total serum bilirubin will be <2 mg/dL 3 months after surgery; the 10-year LT-free survival rate in them is 75–95% • These children grow well and can receive full immunization • Thus, it helps to delay LT to an older age when the surgery is relatively easier, and donor availability is better

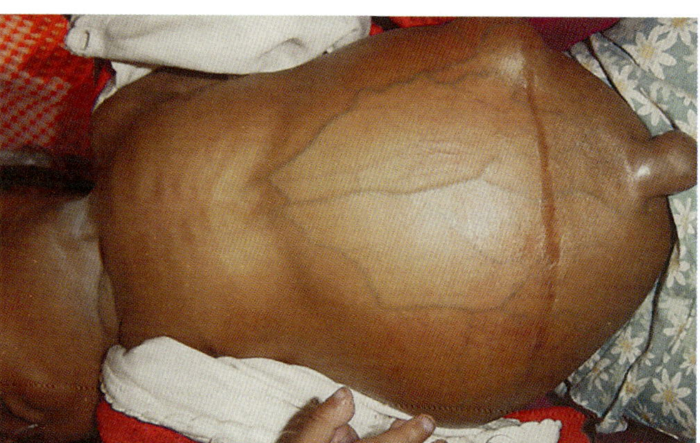

Fig. 12.10.5: Failed Kasai portoenterostomy (KPE)—massive ascites, dilated anterior abdominal wall veins.

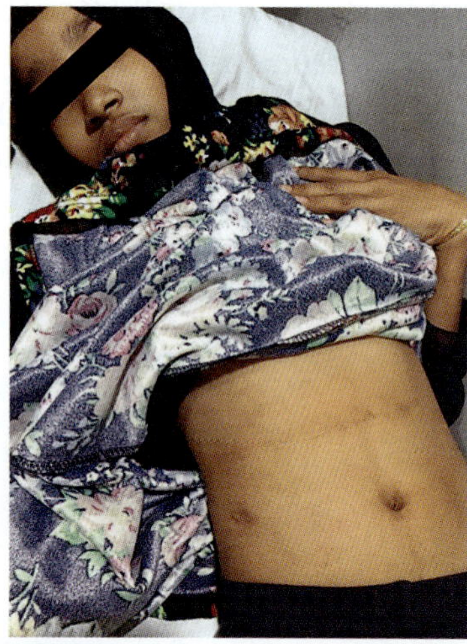

Fig. 12.10.6: A 14-year-old girl post-Kasai portoenterostomy; underwent liver transplantation (LT) at 16 years.

researchers believe that primary LT may be better compared to KPE, as surgery may be easier in the absence of adhesions due to a previous KPE. However, in developing countries, LT is technically more difficult in very young infants. Besides, availability of donors for very young infants is also of concern. Hence, a "sequential approach"—KPE followed by LT is better. Primary LT may be done in children with BA diagnosed after 120 days.

CONCLUSION

Conjugated jaundice is always abnormal in neonates. It may be due to surgical causes such as biliary atresia or various medical causes, some of which may require early treatment. It is vital to make a prompt diagnosis of BA as Kasai surgery, before 2 months of age, has a much better prognosis. The gold standard for the diagnosis of BA continues to be intraoperative cholangiography. The pediatrician must identify sick neonates with cholestasis, which may be due to sepsis, herpes, HLH, GALD, tyrosinemia, etc. Fractionation of bilirubin and GGT should be done in all infants; USG should be done only after 4 hours of fasting. Vitamin K should be given to all neonates with cholestasis to prevent intracranial hemorrhage.

REFERENCES

1. Riyaz A. Cholestatic liver disorders. In: Riyaz A (Ed). Paediatric Gastroenterology and Hepatology, 4th edition. Hyderabad: Paras Publishers; 2019. pp. 390-426.
2. Fernando M, Rajindrajith S. Neonatal and infantile cholestasis: An overlooked health burden with unmet needs. Indian J Gastroenterol. 2020;39(6):531-8.
3. Ibrahim SH, Kamath BM, Loomes KM, Karpen SJ. Cholestatic liver diseases of genetic etiology: Advances and controversies. Hepatology. 2022;75(6):1627-46.
4. Yachha, SK, Das MC, Kumar P, Sharma L, Singh SK, Sarma MS, et al. Development of integrated neonatal cholestasis card for early recognition and referral of neonatal cholestasis. Indian J Gastroenterol. 2020;39(6):584-90.
5. Aziz S, Wild Y, Rosenthal P, Goldstein RB. Pseudo gallbladder sign in biliary atresia—an imaging pitfall. Pediatr Radiol. 2011;41(5):620-6.
6. Kim SS, Kim MJ, Lee MJ, Yoon CS, Han SJ, Koh H. Ultrasonographic findings of type IIIa biliary atresia. Ultrasonography. 2014;33(4):267-74.
7. Nomden M, Beljaars L, Verkade HJ, Hulscher JBF, Peter Olinga P. Current concepts of biliary atresia and matrix metalloproteinase-7: A review of literature. Front Med. 2020;7:617261.
8. Bhatia V, Bavdekar A, Matthai J, Waikar Y, Sibal A. Management of neonatal cholestasis: Consensus statement of the pediatric gastroenterology chapter of Indian Academy of Pediatrics. Indian Pediatr. 2014;51(3):203-10.
9. Pediatric Gastroenterology Chapter of Indian Academy of Pediatrics; Bhatia V, Bavdekar A, Yachha SK. Management of acute liver failure in infants and children: Consensus statement of the Pediatric Gastroenterology Chapter, Indian Academy of Pediatrics. Indian Pediatr. 2013;50(5):477-82.
10. Sathiasekaran M, Matthai J. Biliary atresia. In: Matthai J, Sathiasekaran M, Shanmugam N (Eds). Textbook of Pediatric Hepatology, 1st edition. Hyderabad. Paras Medical books; 2023. pp. 318-28.

12.11 Immune-related Diseases of Liver

Rimjhim Shrivastava, Jaya Agarwal

INTRODUCTION

The liver is a distinct immunological organ with a unique anatomy which promotes the immune response to hepatotropic pathogens. Liver is constantly exposed to various food antigens, endotoxins, pathogens, etc., and it can develop immune tolerance to many or generate immune response to others. Immune-mediated injury of hepatocytes or bile ducts can be because of cellular immune attack on the hepatocytes, maternal-fetal alloimmune disorder or it can be a possible mechanism of injury in few other diseases leading to a progressive, inflammatory, and fibrotic disease **(Box 12.11.1)**. In recent years, the cross talk between the liver and the immune system is being increasingly recognized as liver involvement in primary immunodeficiencies (PID), human immunodeficiency virus (HIV) infection, and the alterations of the immune system following orthotopic liver transplantation (OLT).

This chapter covers autoimmune liver diseases, primary immune deficiency, and association of HIV with liver. Autoimmune diseases of liver were earlier considered relatively uncommon, but with the advent of better laboratory technologies the prevalence of autoimmune disorders is escalating.

AUTOIMMUNE HEPATITIS

Autoimmune hepatitis (AIH) is designated as immune-mediated chronic inflammatory condition of the liver of unknown etiology delineated by elevated serum transaminases and immunoglobulin G (IgG), detection of specific autoantibodies, and histologically by interface hepatitis with lymphoplasmacytic infiltration. On the basis of type of autoantibodies present, clinical features, and histology AIH is classified as types 1 and 2 **(Table 12.11.1)**. However, both the types may be associated with other autoimmune conditions, such as celiac disease, type 1 diabetes or thyroiditis, and can have a strong family history in up to 40% of children. A third type, type 3 AIH has also been proposed, which is characterized by presence of antisoluble

BOX 12.11.1: Classification of immune-related diseases of liver.

- *Autoimmune liver disease:*
  - Autoimmune hepatitis (AIH)
  - Primary sclerosing cholangitis (PSC)
  - Primary biliary cholangitis (PBC)
  - Immunoglobulin G4-associated cholangitis
  - Overlap syndrome
  - De novo AIH after liver transplantation
- *Alloimmune:* Gestational alloimmune liver disease (GALD)
- *Miscellaneous*
  - Human immunodeficiency virus (HIV) and liver
  - Primary immune deficiency
  - Nonalcoholic fatty liver disease (NAFLD)
  - Cirrhosis-associated immune dysfunction
  - Immune-mediated drug-induced liver injury
  - De novo AIH after liver transplantation

TABLE 12.11.1: Differences between type 1 and type 2 autoimmune hepatitis (AIH).

	Type 1 AIH	*Type 2 AIH*
Age group	All ages, two peaks: adolescence and around 40 years of age; commonly adolescents	Infants and younger children
Presentation	Mostly insidious	Acute liver failure
Prevalence	More common (two-thirds of pediatric cases)	Less common
Autoantibodies	ANA, SMA, and anti-SLA in all age groups	Anti-LKM1/anti-LC1 in pediatric population
Serum IgG	Higher levels present (normal in 15%)	High levels (normal in 25%)
Partial IgA deficiency	Less common	More common
Fulminant hepatic failure with encephalopathy	Less common (3%)	More common (25%)
Overlap with sclerosing cholangitis	Seen	Rare
Histology	Cirrhosis	
Duration of medication	Can be stopped after 3 years of remission	Generally, for indefinite period

(ANA: antinuclear antibody; LC1: liver cytosol type 1; LKM1: liver/kidney microsomal type 1; IgA: immunoglobulin A; IgG: immunoglobulinG; SLA: soluble liver antibody; SMA: smooth muscle antibody)

liver antigen/liver-pancreas antibodies. Prevalence of AIH in India among adult population has been reported as 1.3% and 8.74% in all liver disease patients and chronic liver disease (CLD), respectively. The data in pediatric population is scarce. AIH can have more aggressive course in the pediatric population as compared to adults therefore early diagnosis and treatment is key to better survival. Untreated cases may result in liver failure requiring liver transplantation.[1,2]

Clinical Features

The AIH is a disease of all ages and ethnic groups with a female predominance up to the tune of 60%. The incidence of pediatric AIH (3 per 100,000 persons) is lower as compared to the adults. The median age of diagnosis is 12.9 years and highest incidence is seen in the 10–30 years of age group. It is extremely rare below 2 years of age, however, it has been reported in infancy also. AIH is a complex genetic condition associated with major histocompatibility complex II and is related to human leukocyte antigen HLA-DR3 and HLA-DR4. Occurrence of AIH requires genetic predisposition and an interplay of epigenetic, immunological, and environmental triggers such as infections or xenobiotic exposures, which leads to loss of self- tolerance to autoantigens.

The AIH can be asymptomatic with raised transaminases in 2–35% of affected patients. They can develop symptoms (26–70%) within 2–12 months or improve spontaneously (12%). Few asymptomatic ones may have significant histological findings on liver biopsy. In 25–40% the onset can be insidious with nonspecific symptoms such as relapsing jaundice, fatigue, anorexia, headache, diarrhea, weight loss, etc., for 6 months or more. About 40–50% of children with AIH can present with nonspecific symptoms resembling viral hepatitis such as nausea, vomiting, malaise, anorexia, abdominal, or joint pain which may precede jaundice and pale stools. Nonresolution of symptoms after 4–6 weeks should raise suspicion of AIH. It can also present with acute liver failure followed by encephalopathy in 3–25% of children. Complications of cirrhosis and portal hypertension can be seen 10% of them.

The AIH being an immune-mediated disease, presence of other autoimmune conditions is commonly seen in 14–44% of cases. Autoimmune thyroiditis is the most common concurrent disease in type 1 AIH while type 1 diabetes, autoimmune thyroiditis, and autoimmune skin diseases are commonly seen along with type 2 AIH. Since AIH can have varied presentations, it should be suspected in all children with symptoms and signs of prolonged or severe liver disease. Even with acute presentation or recent onset the disease process is long standing with almost one-third of patients having cirrhosis at the time of diagnosis.[2,3]

Diagnosis

The diagnosis of AIH is based on clinical features, laboratory investigations, and histopathology. A modified scoring system is followed for the diagnosis of AIH.

Investigations

The AIH is characterized by three main findings:

1. High levels of transaminases and IgG, and presence of autoantibodies,
2. Presence of interface hepatitis on histology, and
3. Absence of a known etiology for hepatitis.

The simplified diagnostic criteria can be used for diagnosis **(Table 12.11.2)**, but it has got limitations.[4] It is not validated in pediatric population. It is not helpful in acute conditions as in acute presentation the IgG level is low. Also, children usually have low titers of antibodies which is reported as negative as per adult laboratory standardizations.

Following investigations would help in the diagnosis of AIH:[4-8]

- *Complete blood count:* It will help in identifying the anemia of chronic disease. AIH is strongly associated with other autoimmune disorders such as rare autoimmune hemolytic anemia and hepatitis-associated aplastic anemia. It can also identify pancytopenia due to hypersplenism as a result of portal hypertension and advanced cirrhosis.
- *Liver function tests (LFTs):*
  - Serum bilirubin levels are commonly 2–10 mg/dL.
  - Serum alkaline phosphatase (ALP) activity is normal or only slightly increased in AIH.

TABLE 12.11.2: Diagnostic criteria for autoimmune hepatitis (AIH).[4]

Features	*Levels*	*Score*
ANA or SMA	≥1:40	1
ANA or SMA	≥1:80	2
Anti-LKM1	≥1:40	2
Anti-SLA	Positive	
IgG	>ULN	1
	>1.1 times ULN	2
Liver biopsy (interface hepatitis)	Compatible with AIH	1
	Typical of AIH	2
Negative viral markers (IgM, anti-HAV, HbsAg, HBV DNA, HCV RNA)		2
Score: ≥6: Probable AIH; ≥7: Definite AIH		

(ANA: antinuclear antibody; LKM1: liver/kidney microsomal type 1; HAV: hepatitis A; HbsAg: hepatitis B surface antigen; HBV: hepatitis B virus; HCV: hepatitis C virus; SLA: soluble liver antigen; SMA: smooth muscle antibody; ULN: upper limit of normal)

- In AIH hepatocellular pattern of injury is seen where aminotransferases [alanine aminotransferase (ALT), aspartate aminotransferase (AST)] are elevated out of proportion to ALP, which is normal or mildly increased; and ALT is more than AST. Rise in aminotransferases is usually <1,000 IU/mL.
- In primary biliary cholangitis (PBC) and primary sclerosing cholangitis (PSC) cholestatic pattern of injury is seen where ALP, gamma-glutamyl transferase (GGT), and bilirubin are elevated out of proportion to AST and ALT.
- Elevated ALT and AST along with decrease in serum albumin indicates poor synthetic function and poor prognosis.
- Serum ALP and GGT are usually normal or mildly elevated.
- Serum albumin may be low.

▪ *Coagulogram:* International normalized ratio (INR) is an important marker for prognosis and further course of management. Acute liver failure is defined as an INR ≥2.0 without encephalopathy or INR ≥1.5 with encephalopathy. If INR is approaching ≥4.0, the child should be prioritized for liver transplantation.

▪ *Autoantibodies:*
- The detection of specific autoantibodies, viz., antinuclear antibodies (ANAs), antismooth muscle antibodies (anti-SMA), antiliver/kidney microsomal type 1 (anti-LKM1), antiliver cytosol type 1 (anti-LC1), and antisoluble liver antigen/liver-pancreas (anti-SLA/LP) is fundamental in the diagnosis of AIH.
- In children, lower titers of these antibodies are observed than the cutoff values set for adults. In adults, autoantibodies titers are significant if it is >1:40, while in children ANA and SMA in a dilution of >1:20 and anti-LKM1 titers >1:10 are considered clinically significant.
- ANA, SMA, and anti-SLA are often detected at the onset of the disease in all age groups while anti-LKM1 and anti-LC1 are mainly detected in pediatric patients.
- Presence of at least one of these antibodies is important for the diagnosis.
- In children positivity at dilution ≥1:20 for SMA and ANA or ≥1:10 for anti-LKM1 is considered clinically significant.
- Absence of these antibodies does not rule out the diagnosis of AIH, which may be seen in autoantibody-negative AIH or due to false negative results seen in case of high IgG or following immunosuppression.
- Anti-SLA/LP shows very high specificity among all autoantibodies. Presence of anti-SLA indicates severe clinical course and worse histology.
- Presence of ANA even in the absence of cholestatic features, suggest an overlapping AIH/primary biliary cirrhosis syndrome.

▪ *Serum immunoglobulin G:* IgG is a major antibody isotype in the blood that contribute to the immunopathogenesis of liver diseases. To some extent it is found raised in all the liver diseases but much higher levels are seen in AIH. Some studies have suggested that lower levels of IgG before treatment is associated with complete remission, and normalization after treatment may indicate transplant-free survival.

▪ *Viral markers:* Viral markers to detect hepatitis B and C should be done to rule out chronic viral hepatitis.

▪ *Markers for Wilson disease:* It is mandatory to rule out Wilson disease, which is the most common CLD in children, before arriving at the diagnosis of AIH. Serum ceruloplasmin and 24-hour urinary copper should be sent as screening tests.

▪ *Imaging:*
- *Ultrasonography:* Ultrasonography is not mandatory for the diagnosis of AIH. It should be done to know the echotexture and size of the liver, confirm ascites in ambiguous cases, portal cavernoma for portal hypertension, and it is a prerequisite for liver biopsy. Enlarged perihepatic lymph nodes are a typical ultrasound feature of PBC.
- *Elastography:* Ultrasound-guided elastography can be a useful noninvasive method detection and staging of liver fibrosis initially as well as during clinical follow-up.
- *Magnetic resonance cholangiopancreatography (MRCP):* It is recommended to detect PSC or concurrent overlap syndromes.

▪ *Liver biopsy:* Liver biopsy is advocated to establish the diagnosis of AIH and PBC, rule out other causes of CLD and overlap syndromes, and for prognostication of the disease. It is a gold standard for grading and staging AIH and can guide further management. Though there is no pathognomonic morphological feature of AIH on histology, in most of the patients features suggestive of chronic hepatitis is observed with portal and lobular inflammation with lymphoplasmacytic infiltrate, severe interface hepatitis, periportal hepatocyte rosette formation and presence of centrilobular and bridging necrosis.[9]

Treatment

Remission in AIH is defined as normalization of transaminases and IgG levels with low titers of autoantibodies and histological resolution. The standard treatment for AIH in children is immunosuppression using corticosteroids and azathioprine with a remission rate of about 80%. Corticosteroids should be initiated as soon as the diagnosis is established at a dose of 2 mg/kg/day (maximum 60 mg/day). It acts by reducing proinflammatory cytokine production and T-cell activation thus reducing transaminases by 80% in nearly 8 weeks. After 6–9 months of treatment 70–90% can achieve normal liver function. To avoid the side effects of steroids, azathioprine is usually added along with steroids or if side effects of steroids are evident, and steroids are gradually tapered over 4–8 weeks to a maintenance dose of 2.5–5 mg/day. Azathioprine is started at a dose of 0.5 mg/kg/day and gradually increased to 2–2.5 mg/kg/day. Frequent monitoring of LFTs should be done for timely detection of side effects of the drugs.

In type 1 AIH, medications can be stopped after 3 years of remission, with frequent monitoring for relapse, in which case high dose of immunosuppression should be started. In type 2, most of the patients need low dose of steroid for indefinite duration. Despite treatment almost 8.5% of children develop end stage liver disease which requires liver transplantation. One year patient survival after liver transplantation is excellent (95.4%).[3]

Prognosis

Normalization of LFT is achieved by almost 93% of children with sustained remission in 24%. The 30 years probability of survival with native liver is 61%. Progression to cirrhosis is more common in type 1 than in type 2 AIH. Persistent abnormal INR is associated with poor prognosis. Almost half of type 1 and type 2 children show presence of SLA which is associated with severe disease and high tendency for relapse.

PRIMARY SCLEROSING CHOLANGITIS

Primary sclerosing cholangitis is a cholestatic liver disease of unknown origin characterized by progressive multifocal strictures of the extra- and/or intrahepatic bile ducts. It has an insidious onset but the slow natural course leads to biliary cirrhosis and liver failure. The term "primary" is reserved for sclerosing cholangitis (SC) without any associated conditions. In most of the children SC is associated with biliary atresia, neonatal sclerosing cholangitis, defects in the *ABCB4 (MDR3)* gene, immunodeficiencies, Langerhans cell histiocytosis (LCH), psoriasis, cystic fibrosis, sickle cell anemia, and an overlap syndrome between AIH and sclerosing cholangitis. All these conditions should be ruled out before diagnosing PSC. Children present with intermittent jaundice, abdominal pain, and weight loss.

Laboratory investigations show a cholestatic profile of liver enzymes with elevation of ALP. The immune serology in PSC is generally nonspecific with antineutrophil cytoplasmic antibodies with perinuclear staining pattern (p-ANCA) being the most prevalent (93%), ANA (8–77%) and anti-SMA (0–83%). The diagnosis is established by MRCP where bile duct disease is evident. Liver biopsy may show biliary features and interface hepatitis but it is mandatory if there is suspicion of associated AIH. MRCP may be normal in small-duct PSC where chronic cholestasis and hepatic histology are compatible with SC.

Treatment predominantly aims at controlling the associated primary condition. No specific treatment is recommended in case of PSC. PSC is not responsive to standard immunosuppression. Ursodeoxycholic acid (UDCA) may be used in PSC, but its benefit is not established yet. Liver transplantation yields excellent result with 5-year survival about 90%.[10,11]

PRIMARY BILIARY CHOLANGITIS

Primary biliary cholangitis, formerly termed primary biliary cirrhosis, is another autoimmune liver disease of unknown origin, where chronic nonsuppurative granulomatous inflammation of the small intrahepatic bile ducts results in gradual destruction of intrahepatic bile ducts, periportal inflammation, and cholestasis. As a consequence of prolonged hepatic cholestasis, cirrhosis and portal hypertension may supervene. There is a strong female preponderance (>90%). It is postulated that in presence of strong genetic predisposition, some environmental triggers such as urinary tract infection, nail polish, xenobiotics, etc., can induce the autoimmune reaction.

Patients may remain asymptomatic and can be incidentally diagnosed with abnormal LFT or they may present with jaundice, pruritus (seen in 20–70%), which worsens when skin is dry, at night, or in hot and humid weather. Steatorrhea may be seen due to deficiency of fat-soluble vitamins. On examination they may have dry skin, hyperpigmentation, and dermatographism. Due to pruritus, scratch marks, and excoriations are commonly seen. Hepatomegaly can be seen in asymptomatic children as well. Splenomegaly is seen in later stage. PBC may be associated with other autoimmune conditions as celiac disease, rheumatoid arthritis, Hashimoto thyroiditis, etc.

PBC can be diagnosed on the basis two of the following three criteria and after excluding other CLDs:

1. Elevated ALP (at least 1.5 times upper limit of normal),
2. Presence of antimitochondrial antibody (AMA) (>1:40), and
3. Histological evidence.

Liver biopsy may show nonsuppurative destruction of interlobular bile ducts with a predominance of lymphocytic infiltration. Though liver biopsy is not required for the diagnosis in the presence of rest of the two criteria, but it helps in prognostication. In >90% of cases AMA is present but in AMA negative cases PBS-specific ANA should be tested as surrogate marker. In 10–20% of patients with PBC, features of AIH may be present. According to the Paris criteria, AIH can be diagnosed if two of three criteria are present:

1. Elevated f ALT >5 times upper limit the normal (ULN),
2. Elevated serum igG levels >2 times ULN or positive anti-SMA, and
3. Moderate-to-severe interface hepatitis on liver biopsy histology.

In suspected cases MRCP should be done to rule out extrahepatic biliary obstruction. They may also have deranged lipid profile.

The primary goal of management in PBC is to prevent the disease progression and manage cholestasis-induced pruritus and complications. UDCA is recommended at a dose of 13–15 mg/kg per day. Patients benefit most when UDCA is started at an earlier stage, which has been shown to delay the progression of the disease and the development of cirrhosis. UDCA can delay the progression of disease if started at an early age. Postliver transplant the outcome is very good with 5- and 10-year survival rates around 80% and 70%, respectively, but there is a high chance of recurrence of the disease after transplantation.[12,13]

OVERLAP SYNDROME

Overlap syndromes are clinical descriptions where features of AIH is associated with features of PBC or PSC. These are the children who do not respond to the conventional treatment of AIH. Overlap syndrome between AIH and SC, autoimmune sclerosing cholangitis (ASC) is more common seen in children than in adults. ASC has some peculiar features which can differentiate it from AIH or PSC. It is equally seen in males and females. Most common presentations are weight loss, abdominal pain, and intermittent jaundice. Almost 45% of children have associated inflammatory bowel disease. They have increased IgG levels, and p-ANCA is present in 75% of patients. They have autoimmune serology and histological characteristics similar to AIH-1 but MRCP may show evidence of bile duct disease. AIH-PBC overlap can be identified using Paris criteria where two out of the following three criteria are present: raised ALP or GGT, presence of AMA, and histological evidence of bile duct lesion.[3,10,11]

LIVER AND PRIMARY IMMUNE DEFICIENCIES

The PID is a rapidly growing group of >350 conditions, characterized by increased susceptibility to infections, autoimmunity, and even malignancy.[14] Most common are defects in T and B cells, innate immunity (including neutrophils and complement) or combinations of these. Some of the important PID associated with liver abnormalities are detailed in the following text.

Predominantly T-cell Abnormalities

Severe Combined Immune Deficiency

These include defects that severely compromise the generation and function of thymocytes and T cells. Serum levels of immunoglobulins are usually very low, and specific antibody responses are impaired. Severe and recurrent bacterial, viral, and fungal infections may occur from early infancy. Early recognition and prevention of complications followed by hematopoietic stem cell transplantation (HSCT) is the standard of care for affected children.

Hemophagocytic Lymphohistiocytosis

It is characterized by immune cell hyperproliferation due to either genetic defects in cytotoxicity (primary) or secondary to a precipitating infection like Epstein–Barr virus (EBV) [secondary hemophagocytic lymphohistiocytosis (HLH)]. Patients typically present as prolonged fever, cytopenia, hemophagocytosis in the bone marrow, hepatosplenomegaly, and raised inflammatory markers. Infrequently the damage to hepatocytes affected by HLH can lead to liver failure.[15]

Predominantly B-cell Abnormalities

Common Variable Immunodeficiency Disorders

Common variable immunodeficiency disorders (CVIDs) comprises of heterogeneous group of immune defects characterized by reduced immunoglobulin levels and impaired production of antibodies. Liver involvement in CVID is highly variable. Up to 50% of CVID patients present with elevation of liver transaminase associated with mild hepatomegaly. Nodular regenerative hyperplasia (NRH) is the most common liver histopathological change observed followed by infections of liver and biliary tract by opportunistic pathogens especially *Giardia lamblia*. Given the heterogeneity of liver disease and the possible impact on long term outcome, each CVID patient should be screened for a possible liver impairment through biochemical and radiological assessments at regular intervals.

CD40 Ligand Deficiency

Inherited defects in CD40 ligand cause an X-linked disease characterized by elevated (or preserved) levels of IgM with low IgG, IgA, and IgE, a condition known as hyper-IgM syndrome. The bile tract is the most frequent extra intestinal site to be infected. Patients suffer from increased susceptibility to infections and autoimmunity, including hepatitis, sclerosing cholangitis, often in association with *Cryptosporidium* infection.

Innate Immunity Defects

Chronic Granulomatous Disease

Chronic granulomatous disease (CGD) is attributed to impaired formation of reactive oxygen compounds by immune cells, such as neutrophils and macrophages. This is caused by X-linked or autosomal recessive mutations in genes important for the NADPH oxidase complex. Liver enzymes are elevated with persistent elevations of ALP. Liver abscesses are common in CGD. These may be recurrent and require prolonged therapy.

The prognosis of children with PID has improved significantly with use of intravenous immunoglobulins and antibiotic prophylaxis to prevent severe infections. It is important that HSCT is offered before significant liver disease has developed in children with PIDs. Severe liver disease prior to HSCT is likely to affect the success of even well matched HSCT and would require sequential liver and HSCT replacement.

ACQUIRED IMMUNODEFICIENCY SYNDROME

With the advent of efficacious antiretroviral therapy (ART), the prognosis of HIV infection has improved dramatically over the last few years resulting in prolonged survival of HIV-infected individuals.[16] This has led to decline in acquired immunodeficiency syndrome (AIDS)-associated morbidities and mortality, but emergence of HIV-related liver diseases as the most common cause of death in them. Among HIV-infected children, the prevalence rate of chronic hepatitis B may be as high as 49% in some regions, which is much higher than the 2–5% in HIV-negative. Most children with coinfection acquire them vertically from their mothers. Coinfections with HBV and HCV results in faster progression to liver cirrhosis and end-stage liver disease compared to patients with mono-infection, even though ART is also active against HBV. Apart from viral coinfections, liver disease in HIV-infected patients may result from hepatotoxic antiretroviral drugs manifesting as elevated liver enzymes, hepatomegaly, and liver steatosis, often labeled as drug-induced liver injury (DILI). As patients with HIV infection become older, early detection of liver disease is the key to improved clinical outcomes. Screening for metabolic complications and fatty liver in patients with HIV by noninvasive methods should be standard of care.

CONCLUSION

Interactions between the liver and the immune system manifests as a spectrum of liver diseases that lead to significant morbidity and mortality. Despite early detection and adequate treatment of complications, liver impairment may progress toward an end-stage disease in a few. A better understanding of these complex diseases in future will lead to personalized approaches to have a positive impact on their long-term outcome.

REFERENCES

1. Kerkar N, Chan A. Autoimmune hepatitis, sclerosing cholangitis, and autoimmune sclerosing cholangitis or overlap syndrome. Clin Liver Dis. 2018;22(4):689-702.
2. Gupta R, Agarwal SR, Jain M, Malhotra V, Sarin SK. Autoimmune hepatitis in the Indian subcontinent: 7 years experience. J Gastroenterol Hepatol. 2002;16(10):1144-8.
3. Mieli-Vergani G, Vergani D, Baumann U, Czubkowski P, Debray D, Dezsofi A, et al. Diagnosis and Management of Pediatric Autoimmune Liver Disease: ESPGHAN Hepatology Committee Position Statement. J Pediatr Gastroenterol Nutr. 2018;66(2):345-60.
4. Muratori P, Lenzi M, Cassani F, Lalanne C, Muratori L. Diagnostic approach to autoimmune hepatitis. Expert Rev Clin Immunol. 2017;13(8):769-79.
5. Muratori L, Deleonardi G, Lalanne C, Barbato E, Tovoli A, Libra A. Autoantibodies in Autoimmune Hepatitis. Dig Dis. 2015;33(Suppl 2):65-9.
6. Li Y, Yan L, Wang R, You Z, Li B, Zhang J, et al. Serum immunoglobulin g levels predict biochemical and histological remission of autoimmune hepatitis type 1: A single-center experience and literature review. Clin Rev Allergy Immunol. 2022;62(2):292-300.
7. Gerussi A, Halliday N, Saffioti F, Bernasconi DP, Roccarina D, Marshall A, et al. Normalization of serum immunoglobulin G levels is associated with improved transplant-free survival in patients with autoimmune hepatitis. Dig Liver Dis. 2020;52(7):761-7.
8. Hennes EM, Zeniya M, Czaja AJ, Parés A, Dalekos GN, Krawitt EL, et al. International Autoimmune Hepatitis Group. Simplified criteria for the diagnosis of autoimmune hepatitis. Hepatology. 2008;48(1):169-76.
9. Covelli C, Sacchi D, Sarcognato S, Cazzagon N, Grillo F, Baciorri F, et al. Pathology of autoimmune hepatitis. Pathologica. 2021;113(3):185-93.
10. Mieli-Vergani G, Vergani D. Sclerosing Cholangitis in Children and Adolescents. Clin Liver Dis. 2016;20(1):99-111.
11. Jossen J, Annunziato R, Kim HS, Chu J, Arnon R. Liver Transplantation for Children with Primary Sclerosing Cholangitis and Autoimmune Hepatitis: UNOS Database Analysis. J Pediatr Gastroenterol Nutr. 2017;64(4):e83-7.
12. Sebode M, Weiler-Normann C, Liwinski T, Schramm C. Autoantibodies in Autoimmune Liver Disease-Clinical and Diagnostic Relevance. Front Immunol. 2018;9:609.
13. Pandit S, Samant H. Primary Biliary Cholangitis. In: StatPearls [Internet]. Treasure Island (FL): StatPearls Publishing; 2024.
14. Sharma D, Ben Yakov G, Kapuria D, Rodriguez GV, Gewirtz M, Haddad J, et al. Tip of the iceberg: A comprehensive review of liver disease in Inborn errors of immunity. Hepatology. 2022;76(6):1845-61.
15. Canna SW, Marsh RA. Pediatric hemophagocytic lymphohistiocytosis. Blood. 2020;135(16):1332-43.
16. Berendam SJ, Nelson AN, Goswami R, Persaud D, Haigwood NNL, Chahroudi A, et al. Pediatric HIV: the Potential of Immune Therapeutics to Achieve Viral Remission and Functional Cure. Curr HIV/AIDS Rep. 2020;17(3):237-48.

12.12 Noninfectious Liver Diseases and Drug-induced Liver Injury

John Matthai, Prasanth KS

DRUG-INDUCED LIVER INJURY

INTRODUCTION

Drug-induced liver injury (DILI) is an important, often unrecognized adverse event caused by various medications and results in a spectrum of liver disease ranging from biochemical abnormalities to liver failure. DILI should be suspected whenever a child presents with unexplained liver disease, which has a temporal association to the ingestion of medications belonging to any system of medicine.

DEFINITION

Drug-induced liver injury is a predictable or unpredictable (idiosyncratic) adverse reaction to medications, herbal remedies, or other xenobiotics, presenting as acute or chronic liver disease (CLD), in the absence of other identifiable etiologies.[1]

EPIDEMIOLOGY

The incidence of idiosyncratic DILI in the adult population is around 13.9–19.1 per 100,000. In children it is not known, but constitutes 10% of all DILI reported. The lower incidence is probably because children metabolize drugs differently, medications are less often prescribed, and concomitant exposure to alcohol or cigarettes (two factors that alter drug metabolism) is either absent or less. In a retrospective study from India, DILI constituted 3.7% of all children with liver disease.

Data from the Pediatric Acute Liver Failure Study Group (PALFSG) showed that idiosyncratic DILI can trigger acute liver failure (ALF) at any age, and accounts for about 7% of ALF in children above 10 years of age. Acetaminophen (APAP) is one of the major causes of DILI-induced pediatric ALF. DILI may lead to ALF necessitating liver transplantation (LT) (5%) and chronic DILI (17%).[2]

In the US Drug-Induced Liver Injury Network (DILIN) study, antimicrobials (51%), antiepileptic agents (21%), and psychotropic agents were the most frequently implicated drugs in pediatric DILI. In India complementary and alternative medicines (CAMs) and drugs used in antitubercular treatment (ATT) were the cause in 75% of cases.[3] In a Chinese study (77 newborns and 261 children), the causes of DILI were medium- and long-chain fat emulsions (17%), sodium glycerophosphate (12%), and meropenem (9%) in newborns, while omeprazole (11%), methylprednisolone sodium succinate (10%), and meropenem (8%) were the causes in children.[4] **Table 12.12.1** lists the characteristic features of DILI.

TABLE 12.12.1: Characteristics of drug-induced liver injury (DILI).

Intrinsic DILI	*Idiosyncratic*
Dose-dependent	Metabolism-related and/or immune-mediated
Predictable	Unpredictable
Short latency period	Variable latency
Occurs in a large proportion of individuals, e.g., acetaminophen	Occurs in a small group of individuals, e.g., amoxycillin–clavulanate

The risk factors may be drug-related or host-related. The host factors are either genetic or nongenetic **(Table 12.12.2)**.

TABLE 12.12.2: Risk factors/predictors of susceptibility to drug-induced liver injury (DILI).

Drug-related factors	*Host-related factors*	
	Genetic factors	*Nongenetic*
• Daily dose • Lipophilicity • Reactive metabolites • Drug interactions • Hepatobiliary transport inhibition	• Human leukocyte antigen (HLA) polymorphisms • Metabolizing enzymes	• Age • Gender • Obesity • Comorbidities • Preexisting liver disease

PATHOGENESIS

Drug metabolism or biotransformation is one of the vital functions of the liver. Hepatic clearance depends upon the efficiency of the drug metabolizing enzymes, intrinsic blood flow, and plasma protein binding. This complex biochemical process can be divided into three phases—activation (phase I), detoxification (phase II), and excretion (phase III). The outcome of phase I biotransformation reactions is to make the substrate a more polar chemical for further modification via a phase II reaction. Phase II reactions complete the conversion of a hydrophobic chemical to a hydrophilic one, which can be excreted easily in urine or bile. The water-soluble product is transported into the canalicular space and secreted with bile. DILI most commonly occurs due to hepatocyte injury, due to its central role in drug metabolism. However biliary cells, Ito cells, and sinusoidal endothelium may also be sites of injury.

Adaptation

Adaptation is a transient moderate elevation of enzymes by a drug, which does not increase or may even decrease in spite of continuing medication. Adaptation serves as a barrier to hepatocyte dysfunction and injury from an inflammatory state. This develops in response to the constant exposure to ingested antigens. Several mechanisms including immune tolerance have been proposed for this protective phenomenon. In genetically susceptible individuals, overt liver injury may occur as a result of "defective adaptation".

Mechanisms of Drug-induced Liver Injury

A drug may cause DILI by itself or through an intermediate metabolite by:

- Impairment of cell structure
- Inhibition of enzyme activity
- Overwhelming glutathione cytoprotection
- Forming dysfunctional protein adducts (drug-binding to protein)
- Forming adducts that promote injurious immunological responses
- Impairment of bile transport leading to biliary injury
- Causing canalicular and hepatocyte injury
- Evoking a type IV systemic hypersensitivity reaction.

These mechanisms may occur in combination, and for many drugs the precise mechanism remains unknown. Apoptosis and necrosis are the two end results, which mediate hepatocyte death.

Toxic Metabolites

Most drugs implicated in DILI are lipophilic and metabolized by the liver. They undergo phase I reaction, which is usually mediated by the hepatic cytochrome p450 (CYP450) system. The generation of intermediate bioactive or reactive metabolites is an important step, leading to both intrinsic and idiosyncratic DILI. These toxic intermediate products are usually inactivated by phase II reactions, such as glutathione or sulfate conjugation. If conjugation pathways are overwhelmed by the excess production of the toxic reactive metabolites or caused by depletion of the conjugating factors, it results in covalent binding of the reactive metabolites to mitochondrial proteins. This leads to production of reactive oxygen species and adenosine triphosphate (ATP) depletion, causing cellular organelle dysfunction by the activation of stress kinase signaling pathways and disruption of membrane permeability pores resulting in hepatocyte dysfunction, necrosis, and/or apoptosis cell death. In dose-related APAP-related intrinsic liver injury, the conjugation pathways are saturated, thereby generating N-acetyl-p-benzoquinone-imine (NAPQI), a highly reactive toxic metabolite leading to hepatocellular necrosis.

Immune-mediated Injury

This is an important mechanism for idiosyncratic DILI. Two mechanisms have been hypothesized for idiosyncratic DILI—hapten hypothesis and pharmacologic interaction concept.

1. *Hapten hypothesis:* The reactive metabolites irreversibly bind with cellular proteins to form neoantigens (also referred to as haptens), which are presented to major histocompatibility complex (MHC) molecules on antigen-presenting cells, triggering an immune response against the hepatocyte by recruitment of cytotoxic T lymphocytes, natural killer cells, and B cells. The haptens can also induce development of autoantibodies against CYP450 enzymes, leading to cellular injury and death. In a prospective DILI study, 64% of the children had autoantibodies. Drugs associated with autoantibodies are minocycline, lamotrigine, azithromycin, and amoxicillin.
2. *The pharmacological interaction concept* proposes that a drug or its metabolite can bind directly to the human leukocyte antigen (HLA) molecule to trigger a T cell-mediated injury, especially in genetically susceptible individuals.

Drugs or Metabolites that Inhibit Bile Salt Export Pump Function

Drugs or metabolites that inhibit bile salt export pump (BSEP) function may cause DILI. BSEP dysfunction can cause excessive bile salt accumulation in hepatocytes inducing oxidative stress and hepatocyte death. Cyclosporine A, a potent BSEP inhibitor, is often implicated in the occurrence of cholestatic DILI. When a drug causes both mitochondrial injury and BSEP inhibition, there is a higher risk of inducing DILI. Dysregulation of mitochondrial function would reduce ATP production, which further exacerbates the inhibitory effects of BSEP. Liver transporter P-glycoproteins play an important role in mediating multidrug resistance to chemotherapeutic agents.

Coadministration of Drugs

Some drugs can increase hepatotoxicity when used in combination. Coadministered drugs can modulate the production of active metabolites via induction, inhibition, or substrate competition, particularly via CYP450 responses to certain drugs, thereby affecting an individual's risk of DILI. Rifampicin (RIF), a potent CYP450 enzyme inducer, has been shown to increase the risk of hepatotoxicity when combined with isoniazid (INH) for ATT. The combination of RIF and INH exerts a synergistic effect. Liver damage increases with the triple combination of INH, RIF, and pyrazinamide (PZA).[1]

CLINICAL FEATURES

Drug-induced liver injury has a wide spectrum of hepatic manifestations that mimics all forms of liver disease and may be acute or chronic. The term chronic DILI is used where there is persistent liver injury for >1 year after onset, or 6 months after withdrawal of offending drug.

The clinical presentation of DILI is not drug-specific and features may be primary hepatocyte dysfunction (hepatitis), cholestatic, or mixed **(Table 12.12.3)**. Many drugs cause more than one syndrome and some present with overlapping features. In most, the clinical symptoms resemble acute hepatitis with nonspecific symptoms like fatigue, nausea, malaise, pruritus, and jaundice. In those with immune-mediated DILI, rash and arthralgia are additional manifestations. Rarely abdominal pain resembling cholecystitis may be a presentation. Some drugs like phenytoin and phenobarbitone may cause isolated elevation of gamma-glutamyl transpeptidase (GGT).

- *Hepatitis:* Acute hepatitis is the most common type and occurs when drug metabolites damage hepatocytes. The symptoms of nausea, fever, vomiting, jaundice, and elevated transaminases are similar to acute viral hepatitis (AVH). Liver histology resembles AVH but the presence of eosinophils is characteristic of DILI. Presence of jaundice in hepatocellular DILI has much higher risk of ALF and mortality than other forms of DILI and this is called Hy's law. DILI constitutes nearly 10–20% of all ALF between the ages of 3 and 18 years in Western countries and is a result of acute hepatocellular necrosis. Hepatocellular injury is two to three times more likely to lead to LT unlike cholestatic DILI, which has a more protracted course.

TABLE 12.12.3: Clinical features of drug-induced liver injury (DILI).

Pattern of DILI	Hepatocellular	Cholestatic	Mixed
Symptoms	• Asymptomatic • Malaise • Nausea • Vomiting • Right upper quadrant (RUQ) pain • Low-grade fever • Rash • Coagulopathy • Encephalopathy	• Pruritus • Jaundice • Alcoholic stools • Dark urine	• Asymptomatic • Malaise • Nausea • Vomiting • RUQ pain • Low-grade fever • Coagulopathy • Encephalopathy • Pruritus • Jaundice • Acholic stools • Dark urine

- *Cholestatic:* When drug metabolites damage the cholangiocytes, a cholestatic pattern presenting with jaundice and pruritus is seen. It is usually self-limited and will resolve even if it takes a chronic course in some children. Recovery is faster if there is no associated hepatitis. Liver histology shows bland cholestasis and bile duct injury.
- *Mixed hepatitic-cholestatic:* When the drug affects multiple cell types within the liver, it results in a mixed hepatic-cholestatic clinical picture.

  In addition to the above patterns, specific systemic syndromes are also reported.
- *Systemic drug-induced hypersensitivity syndrome:* It presents with fever, inflammation of other organ systems (morbilliform rash or Stevens-Johnson syndrome/toxic epidermal necrolysis, renal dysfunction, and myocarditis), atypical lymphocytosis, and eosinophilia.
- *Autoimmune hepatitis (AIH)-like syndrome (mimicking AIH):* The presentation may be acute or chronic, associated with fatigue, anorexia, nonspecific autoantibodies, increased serum IgG with variable involvement of organ systems, lupoid rash, and arthralgia.

Less common clinicopathological features include granulomatous hepatitis (carbamazepine), chronic hepatitis (methyldopa, nitrofurantoin, and lamotrigine), sinusoidal obstruction syndrome (chemotherapy and immunomodulatory drugs), peliosis hepatis (anabolic steroids and cytotoxic chemotherapy), hepatic tumor (oral contraceptive steroids), microvesicular steatosis (aspirin and tetracycline), drug-associated fatty liver disease (DAFLD) resembling nonalcoholic fatty liver disease (NAFLD) (methotrexate or tamoxifen), macrovesicular steatosis (amiodarone), nodular regenerative hyperplasia [azathioprine, mercaptopurine, or thioguanine or by first-generation nucleoside antiretroviral agents (zidovudine, stavudine, or didanosine)], vanishing duct syndrome, and sinusoidal fibrosis (hypervitaminosis A and methotrexate).[1,5]

DIAGNOSIS

A high degree of suspicion is necessary for early diagnosis in view of the wide spectrum of presenting symptoms. There is no diagnostic test to confirm DILI and liver function tests at the onset of illness have no distinctive feature. The underlying disease for which medication is prescribed could itself have hepatic involvement.

Evaluation of Liver Dysfunction

Clinical Assessment

Clinical features are very nonspecific with subtle differences between the three patterns of liver injury **(Table 12.12.3)**.

Biochemical Assessment

The liver enzymes especially alanine transferase (ALT) and alkaline phosphatase (ALP) and calculation of the *R* ratio help in classifying the pattern of liver injury as hepatitis, cholestatic, and mixed. Three patterns of DILI are determined using the earliest identified elevation of liver enzymes levels and calculating the *R* value [serum ALT/ULN (upper limit of normal) divided by serum ALP/ULN].

1. *Hepatocellular pattern:* If ALT alone is elevated ≥5-fold above ULN or R ≥5
2. *Cholestatic pattern:* ALP alone is elevated ≥2-fold above ULN or R ≤2
3. *Mixed pattern:* ALT /ALP ratio >2 to <5

The use of GGT instead of ALP to calculate *R* value in children has been proposed, since ALP is higher in growing children. However, this has not been validated. The pattern of DILI for a certain drug may differ between adults and children, with the hepatocellular pattern being more common (82%).[6] In newborns, a mixed pattern is more common.

Estimating the total serum bilirubin and fractionation is better for assessing severity. Prothrombin time (PT) and international normalized ratio (INR) should be done to diagnose ALF. The severity of DILI is calculated based on the DILIN using the three parameters—bilirubin, ALT, and INR and classified as mild, moderate, moderate-to-severe, severe, or fatal. This is further divided as *S* (symptomatic) or *A* (asymptomatic).

Other Tests

Excluding other etiologies of liver disease is vital. A complete blood count (CBC) is done to check for anemia and thrombocytopenia to exclude hemophagocytic lymphohistiocytosis (HLH). The presence of autoantibodies such as antinuclear antibody (ANA), antimitochondrial antibody (AMA), and antismooth muscle antibody (SMA) helps to diagnose autoimmune hepatitis (AIH). Low serum ceruloplasmin indicates Wilson disease. Viral markers for hepatitis A, E, B, C (HAV, HEV, HBV, and HCV), cytomegalovirus (CMV), and Epstein–Barr virus (EBV) exclude common infective causes of liver disease.

Radiology

An ultrasound of the abdomen is done in all children with DILI to exclude other causes of liver disease. Coarse echotexture of liver indicates cirrhosis. Contrast-enhanced computerized tomography (CECT) with triple vessel arteriography is indicated when there are space-occupying lesions like vascular malformations or tumors. Magnetic resonance cholangiography (MRC) is indicated when there are features of sclerosing cholangitis.

Pathology

Liver biopsy is not indicated in all children suspected to have DILI. The procedure is invasive and there are no characteristic diagnostic features. Zonal necrosis, eosinophilia, and microvesicular steatosis are some features suggestive of DILI. However, liver biopsy is indicated when the diagnosis of DILI is not clear or other more serious diseases need to be ruled out. Liver biopsy is also indicated in children who do not respond to withdrawal of drug or show worsening of disease.[1,5]

Causality Assessment

Medication History

A detailed and careful history regarding all medications including combinations received in the preceding 12 months should be accurately noted. The precise date of start and stop of each medication should be enquired. Previous history of hepatotoxicity if present and the nature of the drug will help in diagnosis. Four important features should be recorded:

1. *Latency period:* The duration between the drug intake and onset of symptoms
2. *Pattern of liver injury,* since most drugs have a characteristic signature
3. *Dechallenge:* Time to recovery after discontinuation of drug
4. *Rechallenge:* When there has been past exposure to the drug being implicated for the present DILI.

Causality Assessing Methods

Several DILI specific causality methods are available. Roussel Uclaf Causality Assessment Method (RUCAM) is a structured, standardized, validated, and hepatoxicity-specific diagnostic approach that confers points for clinical, biochemical, and serological features.

Differential Diagnosis

The differential diagnosis depends on the pattern of liver injury and is shown in **Table 12.12.4**.

MANAGEMENT

Medical Management

The first step in the management of DILI is to withdraw the offending agent. The usual cutoffs for immediate withdrawal of the drug are:

- ALT or AST (aspartate aminotransferase) > 8 × ULN
- ALT or AST >5 × ULN for 2 weeks
- ALT or AST 3 × ULN with total bilirubin >2 ULN or INR >1.5
- ALT or AST 3 × ULN with progressive nonspecific symptoms

TABLE 12.12.4: Differential diagnosis of DILI according to pattern.

Hepatitic	*Cholestatic*	*Mixed*
• *Viral hepatitis:* Hepatotropic/nonhepatotropic • Wilson disease • Autoimmune hepatitis • NAFLD/MAFLD • Sepsis • Ischemic hepatitis	• *Biliary obstruction:* Cholelithiasis/ choledocholithiasis • Biliary tract malformation • Primary sclerosing cholangitis (PSC)	• Budd–Chiari syndrome • Total parenteral nutrition (TPN) • Congestive hepatopathy • Sickle cell hepatopathy

(DILI: drug-induced liver injury; MAFLD: metabolic dysfunction-associated fatty liver disease; NAFLD: nonalcoholic fatty liver disease)

Rechallenge is not advisable and should not be attempted unless there is no alternate therapy for the underlying disease. The only exceptions are oncology and ATT drugs.

Anti-tuberculous Treatment Drug Induced Liver Injury

When there is clinical evidence of acute hepatitis in a patient receiving ATT, it is essential to immediately stop all potentially hepatotoxic drugs such as INH, RIF, and PZA till complete clinical and biochemical resolution. This includes those with ALT elevation more than three times the ULN in the presence of hepatitis symptoms and/or jaundice, or five times the ULN in the absence of symptoms. In the interim period, at least three non-hepatotoxic drugs, viz., ethambutol, streptomycin, and quinolones can be used.

In most children, ATT can be safely restarted in a phased manner after complete resolution of hepatitis. After ALT returns to less than two times the ULN, RIF may be restarted with or without ethambutol. After 3–7 days, INH may be reintroduced, while monitoring ALT. If symptoms recur or ALT increases, the last added drug added should be stopped. For those with prolonged or severe hepatotoxicity, who tolerate reintroduction with RIF and INH, reintroduction of PZA may be hazardous. In this circumstance, PZA may be permanently discontinued, with treatment extended to 9 months.

N-acetyl Cysteine

In acetaminophen-induced DILI, N-acetyl cysteine is the mainstay of treatment and must be started within 12–24 hours for best results. It decreases mortality even in children with ALF and grade I–II encephalopathy.

Steroids

In drug-induced AIH and hypersensitivity reaction, steroids may be given for a shorter duration (6 months) compared to the classical AIH.

Ursodeoxycholic Acid

This has been used in cholestatic disease with variable results. It is also recommended as a pretreatment prophylaxis in myeloblastic hematopoietic stem cell transplantation (HSCT).

Cholestyramine

This is helpful to relieve pruritus in cholestatic injury. This bile acid binding resin has also been found beneficial in leflunomide and terbinafine toxicity because of its ability to bind the enterohepatically circulating metabolite.

Carnitine

This is indicated in valproate hepatotoxicity, because carnitine regulates mitochondrial CoA leading to beta-oxidation in the mitochondria.

Plasmapheresis

High-volume plasma exchange has been found to be effective in DILI-related ALF and may reduce the need for LT.

Liver Transplantation

Indications for LT is severe DILI with worsening ALF. Best results are reported in acetaminophen-related disease. LT is not generally recommended for valproate-induced ALF, in view of high possibility of underlying mitochondrial disease.[5]

PEDIATRIC FATTY LIVER DISEASE

INTRODUCTION

Liver steatosis (i.e., excessive triglyceride accumulation within the hepatocyte) has shown an alarmingly high prevalence, paralleling the ever-increasing rates of overweight and obesity among children in the last 2 decades. NAFLD is linked with the increased adiposity associated with obesity. NAFLD has become the most frequent cause of CLD in children worldwide.[6]

DEFINITION

Pediatric NAFLD has been traditionally used to denote a condition characterized by chronic hepatic steatosis in the absence of other causes of steatosis including genetic and metabolic disorders, infections, alcohol consumption, medications, and malnutrition. The histopathological spectrum of liver disease includes fat accumulation in >5% of hepatocytes, which progresses from simple steatosis to nonalcoholic steatohepatitis (NASH) and eventual fibrosis (steatofibrosis).

The main limitations lie in its negative definition (i.e., the diagnosis of NAFLD depends on the exclusion of other forms of liver disease and not on demonstrating its underlying causes), the possible stigma rising from the word "alcoholic", and its inability to reflect the strict relationship with insulin resistance and metabolic dysfunction. A panel of international experts have recently proposed a new definition of metabolic (dysfunction)-associated fatty liver disease (MAFLD) for both adult and pediatric patients to overcome these limitations. A new set of positive criteria has been proposed, in which the presence of liver steatosis has to be accompanied by at least one of the following features: Excess adiposity, (pre-) type 2 diabetes mellitus (T2DM), and metabolic dysregulation. MAFLD has started to supersede NAFLD as the preferred nomenclature due to aforementioned limitations.[7,8]

EPIDEMIOLOGY

Metabolic (dysfunction)-associated fatty liver disease is an increasing problem for children and adults worldwide. The prevalence of NAFLD varies widely depending on the definition used and the diagnostic methods employed like ALT, ultrasound, or histological confirmation by liver biopsy. Recent studies have demonstrated that the prevalence ranges from 5 to 10% in general pediatric population to 30% in obese children. Studies from India show that prevalence of NAFLD varies from 45 to 60% among obese children.

PATHOGENESIS

Pathophysiology of NAFLD is complex and is likely multifactorial. It includes interaction between environmental factors such as metabolic (obesity and insulin resistance) nutrient excess, gut microbiome, oxidative stress, and unfolded protein response in addition to genetic risk factors **(Table 12.12.5)**.

Interactions between the liver and two other organs, adipose tissue, and gut microbiome have been linked to the development of NAFLD. Adipocytokines like adiponectin, resistin, interleukin-1 beta (IL)-1β, IL-6, and tumor necrosis factor-alpha (TNF-α) play an important role in the pathogenesis of pediatric NAFLD.

TABLE 12.12.5: Risk factors implicated in the development of nonalcoholic fatty liver disease (NAFLD).[8]

Modifiable	***Nonmodifiable***
• *Diet and nutrition:* – High fructose foods – High glycemic index foods – Sugar-sweetened drinks – High omega-6 to omega-3 ratio diet – High total calorie consumption • *Exercise:* Sedentary lifestyle	• *Genetic predisposition:* – *PNPLA3* – *PARVB* – *MBOAT7* – *GCKR* – *TM6SF2* • Gut microbiome

There is also growing evidence on the role of the gut dysbiosis in the progression of NAFLD. Increased intestinal permeability allows bacteria or its products via portal circulation to interact with toll-like receptors on the hepatocytes, activating a chronic systemic inflammatory response and progression to NASH.[8]

NATURAL HISTORY

A retrospective study done from USA to assess the natural history of NAFLD revealed that children with NAFLD had 14 times increased risk of severe liver disease or death as compared to children without NAFLD. The TONIC trial showed that 20–30% of pediatric NAFLD progress to NASH, of which one-third develop fibrosis and 5–20% progress to cirrhosis. A recently published prospective 10-year follow-up study from Netherlands showed that one-third of the young adults who had childhood obesity developed steatosis. 6% of those with NAFLD developed advanced fibrosis at follow-up. These data underscore the importance of screening for NAFLD and monitoring for progression to advanced NAFLD in children with obesity.[6]

CLINICAL FEATURES

Children with NAFLD are nearly always asymptomatic at diagnosis. When symptoms are present, right upper quadrant pain has been thought to be a possible result of the hepatic capsule stretching from fat deposition, leading to hepatomegaly and/or elevated ALT. Acanthosis nigricans is a manifestation of insulin resistance. Children with NAFLD have higher rates of dyslipidemia, hypertriglyceridemia, hypertension, and diabetes. Children with obesity are at increased risk of poor quality of life, and patients with NAFLD specifically have lower physical and mental health.[7,8]

DIFFERENTIAL DIAGNOSIS

The latest guidelines from the North American Society of Pediatric Gastroenterology, Hepatology and Nutrition (NASPGHAN) suggest NAFLD is a diagnosis of exclusion that is defined as chronic hepatic steatosis in children (≤18 years) with exclusion of other causes, such as genetic or metabolic disorders, infections, use of steatogenic medications, ethanol consumption, or malnutrition.[6]

In children, the term NAFLD is a misnomer, since alcohol consumption is largely not a factor. Inherited metabolic disorders (IMDs) can sometimes present with fatty liver. Clues that point toward an underlying IMD include younger age (<5 years), lean body habitus, lack of risk factors for NAFLD,

BOX 12.12.1: Differential diagnosis in pediatric fatty liver.

- Viral hepatitis
- Autoimmune liver disease
- Celiac disease
- Hypothyroidism
- Drugs
- Inflammatory bowel disease
- Wilson disease
- Glycogen storage disorders
- Lysosomal acid lipase deficiency
- Niemann–Pick disease type C
- Cystic fibrosis
- Alpha 1-antitrypsin deficiency

consanguinity, and clinical phenotypes of ALF, neonatal/infantile conjugated jaundice, organomegaly, developmental delay, or psychomotor retardation.[7] **Box 12.12.1** lists the differential diagnosis of pediatric fatty liver.

DIAGNOSIS

Screening for NAFLD is recommended with ALT testing in overweight children [body mass index (BMI) > 95 centile] with other risk factors like central adiposity, prediabetes/diabetes, insulin resistance, obstructive sleep apnea, dyslipidemia, and family history of NAFLD. The ULN for ALT in male children is 26 U/L and in female children is 22 U/L.[6]

Detection of steatosis by imaging techniques is the hallmark of diagnosis of fatty liver, and the new definition of MAFLD invites the use of ultrasound scan given its wide availability. Ultrasound can detect >30% steatosis, which is around the level at which it is most clinically significant. However, it must be recognized that qualitative grades, labeled mild, moderate, and severe, may not be accurate and cannot differentiate steatosis from steatohepatitis or fibrosis, which are the main determinants of outcome. Therefore, ultrasound results must be interpreted with caution.

Increasingly, alternative, noninvasive modalities of assessment of hepatic steatosis are being used. In controlled attenuation parameter (CAP), which is based on ultrasound signals acquired by transient elastography (TE), detection of 10–30% steatosis is possible alongside fibrosis based on the principle of attenuation of ultrasound signal through fat. Normal values for children are yet to be firmly established, with one study looking at healthy children establishing a CAP ULN at 248 dB/m. Point quantification shear wave elastography (pSWE) is another ultrasound-based technology that involves acoustic radiation force impulse (ARFI).

Magnetic resonance (MR) imaging with or without elastography has shown high diagnostic accuracy for detection of steatosis. In the largest pediatric study, MR-estimated liver proton density fat fraction (PDFF) correlated well with histological steatosis grade. However, its use including MR spectroscopy, the imaging gold standard, is limited by availability.

Liver histology has traditionally been the gold standard for the assessment of steatosis. However, it is subject to sampling bias and inter- and intra-examiner variability let alone its invasive nature and possibility of complications. Grading is carried out according to the proportion of hepatocytes containing fat macrovesicles on hematoxylin and eosin staining (grade 0: <5%; grade 1: 5–33%; grade 2: 34–66%; and grade 3: >66%). In children, inflammation is often portal-based, steatosis may be periportal in distribution, located in acinar zone 3 or panacinar while ballooning is uncommon (type 2 NASH).[8]

NASPGHAN guidelines recommend performing a liver biopsy in patients who have increased risk of NASH and/or advanced fibrosis such as those with high ALT levels (>80 U/L), splenomegaly, or an AST to ALT ratio of >1. Histological sampling is prudent in cases where other clinical features (as mentioned above) are present in a child that may indicate an alternative or coexistent diagnosis.[6]

Numerous noninvasive fibrosis scores of fatty liver have been studied in adults, including AST to ALT ratio, AST to platelet ratio index (APRI), NAFLD fibrosis score, and Fib-4 Index. However, they remain unvalidated in children. The Pediatric NAFLD Fibrosis Index (PNFI) based on age, waist circumference, and triglycerides predicted advanced fibrosis. Several serum biomarkers of liver injury and extracellular matrix turnover, including cytokeratin-18 (CK-18), hyaluronic acid and enhanced liver fibrosis (ELF), have been studied in children. However, none of these biomarkers have been validated and are currently restricted to research purposes.[7]

MANAGEMENT

The goals of treatment are:

- Regression of NAFLD, defined as decrease in steatosis, inflammation, and/or fibrosis
- Resolution of NASH
- Decrease excess adiposity to improve dyslipidemia, insulin resistance, high blood pressure, and central adiposity

Sustained decline in ALT from baseline is commonly used as a surrogate marker of improvement in histology of NAFLD. Ultrasound is not able to reliably detect changes in steatosis and therefore does not have a role in assessing steatosis longitudinally.[6]

Lifestyle Interventions

Hypocaloric low-carbohydrate diet and low-fat diet, increasing physical activity, and gradual weight loss remain the mainstay of treatment in children with NAFLD. A weight loss of 7–10% is associated with improvement in hepatic steatosis, NASH remission, and even regression of fibrosis. Children with NAFLD should limit consumption of carbohydrates and foods with high glycemic index. Studies evaluating the role of physical activities including aerobic and resistance exercises demonstrated reduction in visceral adiposity, intrahepatic lipid accumulation, and insulin resistance. Increasing moderate- to high-intensity physical activity and limiting screen time activities to <2 hours/day is recommended for all children including those with NAFLD. Most relevant to the pediatric population, the treatment of NAFLD and obesity must include family-based sustained behavioral approaches, because parental habits are strongly embedded in cultural beliefs regarding health and weight.[6,8]

Pharmacotherapy

Due to limited pharmacologic options and evidence of improvement in liver histology, a trial of vitamin E (800 IU daily) in children with biopsy-proven NASH may be an acceptable option. Omega-3 fatty acids [docosahexaenoic acid (DHA) and eicosapentaenoic acid (EPA)] (250 and 500 mg/day) for 6 months in children with biopsy-proven NAFLD demonstrated significant reduction in hepatic steatosis. Omega-3 fatty acids is considered a safe and viable treatment option for NAFLD in children. Novel medications under investigation include obeticholic acid, elafibranor, selonsertib, cenicriviroc, aramchol, and liraglutide.

Bariatric Surgery

Bariatric surgery may be considered for selected adolescents with BMI > 35 kg/m^2, who have noncirrhotic NAFLD and other serious comorbidities (e.g., T2DM, severe sleep apnea, and idiopathic intracranial hypertension).

Long-term Care

Nonalcoholic fatty liver disease is associated with multiple extrahepatic complications, such as cardiovascular disease, T2DM, sleep disorders, and osteoporosis. Clinicians should be aware of these complications to ensure prompt screening and treatment. Children with NAFLD should be vaccinated against hepatitis A and B.[6]

INTESTINAL FAILURE-ASSOCIATED LIVER DISEASE

INTRODUCTION

Parenteral nutrition (PN) is a life-saving therapy for individuals with intestinal failure (IF), as it delivers vital nutrients directly into the bloodstream, thereby circumventing the digestive system when oral or enteral nutrition (EN) options are inadequate or restricted. Intestinal failure-associated liver disease (IFALD) is one of the most common and serious complications of IF and consequently of long-term PN. The term IFALD has replaced the old terminology "PN-associated liver disease/cholestasis (PNALD, PNAC)".[9]

DEFINITION

Intestinal failure-associated liver disease is defined as "hepatobiliary dysfunction as a consequence of medical and surgical management strategies for IF, which can variably progress to end-stage liver disease, or can be stabilized or reversed with promotion of intestinal adaptation".

EPIDEMIOLOGY

The true prevalence of IFALD is difficult to estimate due to the heterogeneity in its definition in different studies. IFALD occurs in 20–60% of pediatric patients receiving prolonged PN and manifests as cholestasis in 25–60% of cases. In neonatal population, the rates are increased, particularly in patients with necrotizing enterocolitis (NEC). When PN is required for >60 days, IFALD occurs in >75% of cases. Premature infants who develop NEC are at particular risk because, in addition to liver immaturity, they are exposed to multiple risk factors, which include a higher rate of sepsis from both the intestine and indwelling central venous catheter (CVC), intestinal obstruction and stasis and requirement for continuous rather than cyclical PN infusion.[9,10]

RISK FACTORS

The risk factors for IFALD relate to both patient characteristics and management of the IF **(Table 12.12.6)**.[10]

PATHOGENESIS

The pathogenic mechanisms for IFALD are multifactorial, which include an interplay of infections from indwelling CVC [downregulate Famesoid X receptor (FXR) activity

TABLE 12.12.6: Risk factors of intestinal failure-associated liver disease (IFALD).[10]

Treatment-related risk factors	*Patient-dependent risk factors*
• Composition of PN • Mode of administration (continuous/cyclical), • Duration of PN dependency • *Surgical interventions and their anatomical consequences:* Intestinal obstruction, disruption of enterohepatic circulation, resection of the terminal ileum or ileocecal valve • Use of antibiotics (liver/renal toxicity)	• Age (infants born <34 weeks of gestation) • Degree of liver maturation (prematurity) • Etiology of IF (NEC) • Site and frequency of infection [gastrointestinal tract, central venous catheter (CVC)], small bowel bacterial overgrowth (SIBO) • Enteral feed tolerance

(IF: intestinal failure; NEC: necrotizing enterocolitis; PN: parenteral nutrition)

via inflammatory cytokines], gut dysbiosis (leads to small intestinal bacterial overgrowth), disruption of the gut barrier (leads to bacterial translocation), and components of PN (lipid emulsions with soya bean oil contain high amount of proinflammatory phytosterols). Liver injury results from the release of proinflammatory cytokines like IL-β and TNF-α by activation of the innate immune system in the liver. Liver injury is also directly proportional to the dose of intravenous lipids used in PN though the optimum dose required to prevent liver injury is not known. Liver steatosis may also be caused by a deficiency in choline, carnitine, and essential fatty acids, which can be related to the amount and different types of lipid emulsions administered.[10]

CLINICAL FEATURES

Patients are often asymptomatic and the first sign of IFALD comes following a deranged blood test. Neonates often present with cholestatic jaundice. Usually, cholestasis is prominent in infants and young children whereas steatosis and steatohepatitis are more common in older children. These examination findings, in addition to laboratory abnormalities found in patients with IFALD, are summarized in **Table 12.12.7**. It is important to recognize that the presentation and severity of IFALD range from mild liver injury to end-stage liver disease.[10]

DIAGNOSIS

Mild conjugated hyperbilirubinemia may be the only initial sign. Patients with IF without IFALD can have an isolated mild-to-moderate increase of liver enzymes. Criteria for IFALD include a persistent elevation of transaminases and GGT >1.5 above the ULN and hyperbilirubinemia below 3 mg/dL for early IFALD. Histology of the liver reveals intracellular and canalicular cholestasis, bile duct proliferation, extramedullary hematopoiesis, periportal inflammation, portal tract bile duct plugging, and fibrosis. These findings are similar to other causes of neonatal cholestasis like biliary atresia.[9]

MANAGEMENT

Prevention

Prevention is based on early recognition and timely medical management of NEC, CVC care protocols, and early enteral feeding. As for parenteral nutrients, excessive energy intake, dextrose, and amino acids in high doses should be avoided because they are related to increased prevalence of IFALD.

Treatment

Nontransplant treatment of IFALD relies on two strategies, first one targeting enteral rehabilitation and second one to minimize further liver injury **(Table 12.12.8)**. It is vital to ensure that nutrition and growth are not compromised while implementing these measures.

Transplantation is indicated in children with severe IFALD. In cases where patients exhibit no or minimal signs of IFALD, isolated small bowel transplantation is a potential consideration. However, for severe IFALD cases characterized

TABLE 12.12.7: Clinical findings in intestinal failure-associated liver disease.[10]

Physical examination	*Laboratory findings*	*Imaging findings*
Physical examination findings may be normal, but can include the following: • Jaundice (most common physical examination finding) • Hepatomegaly • Splenomegaly	• Elevated total and direct bilirubin • Elevated AST and ALT • Elevated ALP • Elevated GGT • *Late findings*: Hypoalbuminemia, coagulopathy, thrombocytopenia	• Imaging is not necessarily indicated for evaluation if it is clear the diagnosis is PN-associated cholestasis, but it can be used to rule out other causes of cholestasis • *Abdominal ultrasonography* may show hepatomegaly, contracted gallbladder, biliary sludge, and/or splenomegaly

(ALP: alkaline phosphatase; ALT: alanine transferase; AST: aspartate aminotransferase; GGT: gamma-glutamyl transpeptidase; PN: parenteral nutrition)

TABLE 12.12.8: Treatment strategies for IFALD.

Enteral rehabilitation	*Minimize progressive liver injury*
• Early initiation of enteral feeding • Use breastmilk as far as possible • Greater initial EN volumes (20 mL/kg/day) and daily feeding advancement • Medications to help feed tolerance • Glucagon-like peptide analogs to enhance mucosal absorptive capacity (e.g., teduglutide) • Surgery to remove dysmotile bowel • Stoma closure to manage fluid shifts and promote enterohepatic circulation	• Cycling of PN (reduction in time on PN) • Reduction in amount of lipid emulsion • Use of fish oil containing lipid emulsions or mixture of different oils • Minimizing central line-associated blood stream infections (CLABSIs) • Reducing intestinal bacterial overgrowth • Promoting bile flow with use of ursodeoxycholic acid

(EN: enteral nutrition; IFALD: intestinal failure-associated liver disease; PN: parenteral nutrition)

by fibrosis or cirrhosis the most commonly performed procedure is a combined liver and intestine transplant.[9]

REFERENCES

1. Roberts EA. Drug-induced liver disease. In: Suchy F, Sokol R, Balistreri W (Eds). Liver Disease in Children, 4th edition. Cambridge: Cambridge University Press; 2021. pp. 348-82.
2. DiPaola F, Molleston JP, Gu J, Cirulli ET, Chalasani N, Barnhart H, et al; US Drug Induced Liver Injury Network. Antimicrobials and Antiepileptics Are the Leading Causes of Idiosyncratic Drug-induced Liver Injury in American Children. J Pediatr Gastroenterol Nutr. 2019;69(2):152-9.
3. Kumar A, Sood V, Khanna R, Verma SK, Mehra N, Rawat D, et al. Clinical Spectrum and Outcome of Pediatric Drug Induced Liver Injury. Indian J Pediatr. 2018;85(8):676-8.
4. Ye L, Feng Z, Huang L, Guo C, Wu X, He L, et al. Causality Evaluation of Drug-Induced Liver Injury in Newborns and Children in the Intensive Care Unit Using the Updated Roussel Uclaf Causality Assessment Method. Front Pharmacol. 2021;12:790108.
5. Monge-Urrea F, Montijo-Barrios E. Drug-induced Liver Injury in Pediatrics. J Pediatr Gastroenterol Nutr. 2022;75(4):391-5.
6. Vos MB, Abrams SH, Barlow SE, Caprio S, Daniels SR, Kohli R, et al. NASPGHAN Clinical Practice Guideline for the Diagnosis and Treatment of Nonalcoholic Fatty Liver Disease in Children: Recommendations from the Expert Committee on NAFLD (ECON) and the North American Society of Pediatric Gastroenterology, Hepatology and Nutrition (NASPGHAN). J Pediatr Gastroenterol Nutr. 2017;64(2):319-34.
7. Hegarty R, Kyrana E, Fitzpatrick E, Dhawan A. Fatty liver disease in children (MAFLD/PeFLD Type 2): unique classification considerations and challenges. Ther Adv Endocrinol Metab. 2023;14:20420188231160388.
8. Rupasinghe K, Hind J, Hegarty R. Updates in Metabolic Dysfunction-Associated Fatty Liver Disease (MAFLD) in Children. J Pediatr Gastroenterol Nutr. 2023;77(5):583-91.
9. Di Dato F, Iorio R, Spagnuolo MI. IFALD in children: What's new? A narrative review. Front Nutr. 2022;9:928371.
10. Fundora J, Aucott SW. Intestinal Failure-Associated Liver Disease in Neonates. Neoreviews. 2020;21(9):e591-e599.

12.13 Pediatric and Neonatal Acute Liver Failure

Seema Alam, Bikrant Bihari Lal, Vikrant Sood

INTRODUCTION

Pediatric acute liver failure (PALF) is characterized by an acute deterioration in liver function due to any cause resulting in altered mental status and coagulopathy in children without underlying chronic liver disease (CLD). It results from rapid and massive hepatocyte necrosis or injury, leaving behind liver parenchymal mass insufficient to sustain liver function, resulting in high rates of mortality.

DEFINITION

There is a lot of heterogeneity in definition of acute liver failure (ALF) in adults. Most definitions focus on the presence of coagulopathy [elevated prothrombin time (PT) or international normalized ratio (INR)], and the rapid onset of hepatic encephalopathy (HE). Identification of ALF in children is difficult and complex compared to adults, as identification of early signs of HE are challenging resulting in delayed diagnosis.[1] The Pediatric Acute Liver Failure Study Group (PALFSG) was formed in 1999 to develop a database of PALF cases all over the world for better characterization of the etiology, pathogenesis, treatment modalities, and outcome. The entry criteria for the PALF study are now universally used to define PALF.[1] These include:

- Children with no known evidence of CLD
- Biochemical evidence of acute liver injury, and
- Hepatic-based coagulopathy defined as a PT ≥15 seconds or INR ≥1.5 not corrected by vitamin K in the presence of clinical HE or a PT ≥20 seconds or INR ≥2.0 regardless of the presence or absence of clinical HE.

The standard adult West Haven Scale is used to stage HE in older children, while a modified scale was proposed by the PALF Study Group for identification and staging of HE in children up to 3 years of age **(Table 12.13.1)**.[1]

ETIOLOGICAL SPECTRUM

The acute insult or trigger for the development of PALF varies widely with age and geographical distribution. Gestational alloimmune liver disease (GALD), herpes simplex virus (HSV) infection, and metabolic liver diseases (MLDs) are the predominant causes of PALF in neonates.[2-5] MLD, certain nonhepatotropic virus infections, genetic intrahepatic cholestasis, and hemophagocytic lymphohistiocytosis (HLH) are the common causes of PALF in infancy beyond the neonatal period.[6-10]

Beyond infancy, the etiological spectrum varies considerably by geographical distribution. Drug-induced liver injury (DILI) predominantly caused by acetaminophen (APAP) is the leading cause of PALF in Western world followed by MLD, autoimmune hepatitis (AIH), and certain virus infections [adenovirus, Epstein–Barr virus (EBV), enterovirus, and HSV]. Compared to Europe and North America, antitubercular DILI is common in Asian population.[1,7] Hepatotropic viral infections (predominantly hepatitis A) are the leading cause of PALF in Indian subcontinent, Asia, and few South American nations.[7-10] Antitubercular drugs, antibiotics, antiepileptics, and complementary and alternative medicines (CAMs) are the common causes of DILI in India. Ischemic hepatitis caused by dengue hemorrhagic fever is common in northern parts of India. **Table 12.13.2** lists the common causes of PALF in various studies, sorted by geographical location and age.

TABLE 12.13.1: Modified hepatic encephalopathy assessment scale for children up to 3 years of age as recommended by the Pediatric Acute Liver Failure (PALF) Study Group.[1]

Grade	*Clinical*	*Asterixis/reflexes*	*Neurological signs*
Early (I and II)	Inconsolable crying, sleep reversal, and inattention to task	Unreliable/normal or hyper-reflexic	Untestable
Mid (III)	Somnolence, stupor, and combativeness	Unreliable/hyper-reflexic	Most likely untestable
Late (IV)	Comatose, arouses with painful stimuli (IVa), or no response (IVb)	Absent	Decerebrate or decorticate

TABLE 12.13.2: Age-wise etiologies of pediatric acute liver failure in various studies.

Study/Year	*Place*	*Age and number of subjects*	*Etiological profile*
		Neonates and infants	
Sundaram et al. (PALF study group) (2011)[2]	USA, Canada, and UK	<3 months (n = 148)	*Indeterminate:* 37.8% *Metabolic:* 18.9% *Viral (HSV and Enterovirus):* 16.2% *GALD:* 13.5%
Shanmugam et al. (2011)[3]	UK	Neonates (0–28 days) (n = 42)	*Metabolic:* 35.9% *Hypoxia-ischemia:* 19.2% *Infection:* 16.7% *GALD:* 9% *Indeterminate:* 6.4%
		Infants (1–12 months)	*Indeterminate:* 34.7% *DILI:* 26.1% *Viral:* 17.4% *Metabolic:* 13%
Antala et al. (2022)[4]	USA Database from 49 centers	Neonates (0–30 days) (n = 1,805)	*Indeterminate:* 32% *Cardiac and ischemia:* 36% *Viral (HSV and Enterovirus):* 10% *Metabolic:* 8.9% *GALD:* 2.7%
		31–120 days old infants (n = 889)	*Indeterminate:* 52% *Metabolic:* 13% *Viral:* 6.9%
		Infants (1–12 months)	*Indeterminate:* 34.7% *DILI:* 26.1%, *Viral:* 17.4% *Metabolic:* 13%
Bitar et al. (2017)[5]	UK	0–120 days (n = 78)	*Metabolic:* 35.9% *Hypoxia-ischemia:* 19.2% *Infection:* 16.7% *GALD:* 9% *Indeterminate:* 6.4%

Contd...

Contd...

Study/Year	Place	Age and number of subjects	Etiological profile
		Older children	
PALF Study Group (2006)[1]	21 sites in USA, 1 site in Canada, 2 sites in UK	<3 years (n = 127)	*Indeterminate:* 54% *Metabolic:* 18% *Viral:* 7% *Autoimmune:* 5%
		>3 years (n = 221)	*Indeterminate:* 46% *Acetaminophen:* 21% *Non-APAP DILI:* 7% *Autoimmune:* 7% *Metabolic:* 6%
Shanmugam et al. (2011)[3]	UK	1–18 years (n = 150)	*Indeterminate:* 38.7% *DILI:* 29.3% *Autoimmune:* 8.7% *Viral:* 6%, *Metabolic:* 4.7%
Ciocca et al. (2007)[6]	South America (Argentina and Brazil)	1–20 years (n = 88)	*HAV:* 43% *HBV:* 1%
Kayaalp et al. (2014)[7]	Turkey	0–18 years (n = 308)	*HAV:* 20.9% *Metabolic:* 14% *Indeterminate:* 18% *Mushroom poisoning:* 13%
Hegarty et al. (2015)[8]	UK	<5 years (n = 127)	*Indeterminate:* 32% *Metabolic:* 28% *Infections:* 12% *GALD:* 9% *HLH:* 6%
Alam S et al. (2015)[9]	India	<3 years (n = 30)	*Metabolic:* 33% *Viral:* 16.5% *HLH:* 16.5% *DILI:* 10% *Indeterminate:* 10%
Lal BB et al. (2020)[10]	India	0–18 years (n = 285)	*Viral:* 56% *HAV:* 45.9% *Indeterminate:* 20% *DILI:* 8% *Metabolic:* 7% *Autoimmune:* 5%

(APAP: acetaminophen; DILI: drug-induced liver injury; GALD: gestational alloimmune liver disease; HAV: hepatitis A virus; HBV: hepatitis B virus; HLH: hemophagocytic lymphohistiocytosis; HSV: herpes simplex virus; PALF: Pediatric Acute Liver Failure)

Indeterminate Liver Failure

Despite the advances in diagnostic modalities including genetic analysis, the etiology of PALF remains elusive in most patients (20–54%). A large majority of these children may represent missed diagnosis of viral infections, MLD, and genetic intrahepatic biliary transporters defects. Emerging evidence points toward the role of T cell-mediated immune injury to the liver in patients with indeterminate PALF. Mutations in neuroblastoma amplified sequence *(NBAS)* gene are known to result in recurrent PALF.

Severe Acute Hepatitis Outbreak (2021–2022)

Since early 2022, there has been a sudden surge in cases of acute hepatitis presenting as PALF. This includes cases with acute hepatitis without HE or coagulopathy. More than 1,000 cases have been reported from over 35 countries across the five World Health Organization (WHO) regions. Several viruses are implicated, the prominent among them being adenovirus type 41, adeno-associated virus-2, coronavirus disease-2019 (COVID-19), and coinfections. Adenovirus infection usually occurs in younger children who present with hyperacute liver failure (jaundice to HE interval <7 days) and predominance of gastrointestinal symptoms, with poor native liver survival (NLS).

PATHOGENESIS

Pediatric acute liver failure may develop due to direct [toxins, APAP, metabolic disorders (galactosemia and tyrosinemia), and viral] or indirect immune-mediated (autoimmune, DILI, and few viruses) injury. Innate immune-mediated injury occurs early and is usually followed by injury from adaptive immune responses. Pathogen-associated molecular patterns (PAMPs) are commonly implicated in injury caused by hepatotropic viruses, whereas damage-associated molecular patterns (DAMPs), endogenous signals derived from injured cells, are more important in toxic etiologies. Innate immune response is mediated by several cell types including monocytes, macrophages, dendritic cells, leukocytes, natural killer (NK) cells, and express receptors that can recognize both PAMPs and DAMPs. Monocytes, macrophages, and leukocytes also constitute the effector cells of innate immunity and regulate the inflammatory response by producing reactive oxygen radicals and pro- and anti-inflammatory cytokines. Dendritic cells present antigen and induce T cells through expression of costimulatory molecules and also produce cytokines, whereas NK cells provide interaction with virus-infected cells, T lymphocytes, and dendritic cells. Recognition of viral or other pathogens by a coordinated interaction of the cells of the innate immune system eventually leads to activation of adaptive immunity targeting viral- or drug-specific antigens. Of the various pattern recognition receptors, toll-like receptors (TLRs), ribonucleic acid (RNA) helicase receptors, and nucleotide-binding and oligomerization domain (NOD)-like receptors/inflammasomes sense endogenous and exogenous danger signals and induce proinflammatory cytokines and type I interferons. The specificity of ligands, pattern recognition receptors, intracellular adaptor molecules, and signal transduction pathways, and the relative concentration of each innate immune cell type determine the pattern of cytokines release locally within the liver, and eventually in the systemic circulation, defining the clinical characteristics and outcome.

CLINICAL PRESENTATION AND APPROACH

Approach to PALF in Older Children

A meticulous history and clinical examination would reveal several clues to the cause of PALF and the possible outcome. A typical prodrome characterized by a constellation of symptoms predominantly anorexia, vomiting, or low-grade fever preceding the onset of jaundice is strongly suggestive of viral hepatitis. Temporal clustering of cases in family or neighborhood also suggests a viral outbreak, commonly hepatitis A virus (HAV) among children. Predominance of gastrointestinal symptoms in a young child would point toward adenovirus infection. Personal or family history of autoimmune disorders would point toward immune dysregulation. History of prescription or nonprescription drugs (alternative medicines) should be sought very carefully. Clinician should be aware of possibility of accidental overdose of common drugs like paracetamol which are available over the counter in different concentrations. Usage of CAM should be specifically enquired. A meticulous central nervous system (CNS) examination is the key to identifying HE early and correctly staging it. Family history, intravascular hemolysis (cola-colored urine), and neuropsychiatric features suggest fulminant Wilson disease. **Flowchart 12.13.1** shows an algorithmic diagnostic approach in a case of PALF.

Investigative Workup of Acute Liver Failure

The etiologic profile of PALF includes drug and toxin exposures, metabolic and genetic disorders, infections, and immune-mediated disease. Prospective studies have found that a specific etiology is not identified in up to 49% of cases.[1] In a study from this center in India, the indeterminate etiology contributed about 14.6% of the total cohort.[10] The diagnostic work-up of the patient can be planned at admission of the patient and is depicted in the **Flowchart 12.13.1**. Rest of the investigative work-up for the monitoring of the patient will be dynamic, sometimes 2–6 hourly to identify the rapid changes in the severity of the disease.

OUTCOME AND PROGNOSTICATION IN PALF

Mortality rates were very high in the pretransplant era, with only about 25–30% children surviving. However, with advances in intensive care management of these children, and advent of liver transplantation (LT), both the NLS and overall survival of children with PALF has improved considerably.[1,7-10] Despite these advances, significant proportion of children with PALF die or require LT. **Table 12.13.3** describes the outcome of PALF in important literature worldwide.

Prognostic Models in PALF

An ideal prognostic model in PALF should be able to identify all those who are likely to die so that they could be offered a timely LT. At the same time, it should also identify all those likely to survive with their native liver so that an unwarranted LT is avoided in them. The ideal prognostic model should thus have 100% sensitivity, specificity and discriminatory value. Most of the adult ALF prognostic models such as King's College Hospital (KCH) criteria, Clichy criteria, and Liver Injury Unit (LIU) score have demonstrated poor discriminatory value in PALF. KCH criteria are the most widely used criteria to list children with PALF for LT. It was derived from a cohort of 588 patients with ALF, 310 of whom were APAP-induced ALF; it included only 29 children younger than 11 years and no infants.[13] KCH criteria has stood the test of time in APAP-induced ALF, but has been demonstrated to have very low sensitivity in identification of those who need transplant in non-APAP PALF. HAV is the most common

Flowchart 12.13.1: Approach to a case of pediatric acute liver failure (PALF).

Suspect PALF if: Presence of jaundice ± evidence of hepatic encephalopathy

Check LFT and PT-INR
Evaluate for HE

Confirm PALF as per definition

Historical evaluation
- Decreased appetite, malaise, and lethargy (viral prodrome)
- Interval between jaundice to ascites and jaundice to encephalopathy
- Skin or mucosal bleeds, abdominal distension, swelling over body, altered sensorium, and decreased urine output (underlying chronic liver disease)
- Past history of jaundice/BT/surgery/IV drug abuse/hospitalization/tattooing
- Family history of sibling death/liver disease/autoimmune disorder/neuropsychiatric illness/hemolytic disease

Examination
- General condition
- Vitals—evidence of raised intracranial pressure (ICP) (bradycardia and hypertension as per appropriate centiles)
- General examination—liver disease stigmata (palmar erythema, spider nevi, anasarca, icterus, gynecomastia), and lymphadenopathy, rash
- Systemic examination:
  - Abdomen—standard examination including liver span, abdominal veins especially over back, splenomegaly, hepatojugular reflex, and free fluid
  - Central nervous system—signs of raised ICP (pupillary changes, reflexes—deep and superficial, and tone), grade of encephalopathy, asterixis and cranial nerve function

Specific pointers

Autoimmune liver disease
- Rash, joint pains, and redness of eyes
- Increasing pallor, and cola-colored urine
- Family history of autoimmune diseases

Infectious etiology
- Environmental exposure/contact, viral prodrome (hepatotropic infections)
- Fever, rash, loose stools, vomits, redness of eyes, cough/coryza, and lymphadenopathy (viral)

Drug-induced injury
- Intake of drugs or alternative medications
- Prolonged paracetamol use in therapeutic doses with starvation or malnutrition

Mitochondrial hepatopathy
- Positive family history, and sibling deaths
- Developmental delay

Baseline

Liver function tests:
- Alanine aminotransferase (ALT)
- Aspartate aminotransferase (AST)
- Alkaline phosphatase (ALP)
- Total/direct/indirect bilirubin

Prothrombin time and INR
Hemogram
Serum electrolytes
Blood glucose
Blood urea, creatinine
Cultures
Blood group
Chest X-ray
Lactate
Lactate dehydrogenase
Retic count, direct Coombs test
Blood ammonia
Blood gas (arterial/venous)
Imaging: Bedside ultrasonography (Liver span, exclude chronicity of liver disease)

Specific

First line

Infectious
- IgM anti-hepatitis A
- IgM anti-hepatitis E virus
- Hepatitis B virus surface antigen, IgM anti-hepatitis B core antibody

*Wilson's disease**
- Serum ceruloplasmin
- 24-hour urinary copper estimation
- Kayser–Fleischer ring

Autoimmune#
- Immunoglobulin G levels
- Antinuclear antibody,
- Anti-liver kidney microsomal antibody,
- Anti-smooth muscle antibody
- Liver biopsy (percutaneous/transjugular route)

Metabolic screen (if younger age <5 years)
As in baseline testing + urine for reducing substance for galactose

Drug-induced liver injury (if history +)
Acetaminophen and valproate drug levels

Second Line Tests

Suspected Disorder	Tests
Adenovirus, CMV, EBV, dengue virus infection	Adenovirus PCR, IgM EBV, CMV PCR, IgM dengue
Parvovirus infection	IgM parvovirus (if bone marrow suppression +)
Hemophagocytosis	Serum triglyceride, fibrinogen, ferritin, bone marrow and/or lymph node biopsy (if fever + bicytopenia +)
Urea cycle defects	Plasma aminoacidogram and genetic testing
Fatty acid oxidation defects	Lactate/pyruvate levels, carnitine/acylcarnitine analysis, muscle biopsy, and genetic testing

*Clues: Alkaline phosphatase/bilirubin ratio <4.0, AST/ALT ratio > 2.2 ± Coombs negative hemolysis
#Clues: Coombs positive hemolysis, A:G reversal, family or personal history of autoimmune diseases (like thyroid, etc.)
(BT: blood transfusion; CMV: cytomegalovirus; EBV: Epstein–Barr virus; HE: hepatic encephalopathy; IgM: immunoglobulin M; IV: intravenous; LFT: liver function test; PCR: polymerase chain reaction; PT-INR: prothrombin time-international normalized ratio)

TABLE 12.13.3: Important studies describing the outcome of pediatric acute liver failure.

Study/Duration	*Country*	*Major etiology*	*Number of cases*	*Outcome*
Ciocca et al. 1982–2002[6]	Argentina	Hepatitis A Indeterminate	210	*Death:* 25.8% *LT:* 43%
Poddar et al. 1997–2000[11]	India	Hepatitis A Hepatitis E	67	*Death:* 24.4%
PALF Study Group 1999–2004[1]	USA, UK, and Canada	Indeterminate APAP	348	*Death:* 14.1% *LT:* 32.5%
Rajanayagam et al. 1991–2011[12]	Australia	Metabolic Infective	54	*Death:* 23% *LT:* 31%
Antala et al. (2004–2018)[4]	USA	Neonates Indeterminate	1,807	*Death:* 53% *LT:* 1.9%
		Infants Indeterminate	890	*Death:* 42% *LT:* 4.9%
Kayaalp et al. 2011[7]	Turkey	Hepatitis A Indeterminate Drugs	210	*Death:* 38.5% *LT:* 40%
Alam S, Lal BB et al. 2010–2020[9,10]	India	Hepatitis A Indeterminate	285	*Death:* 42.5% *LT:* 10%

(APAP: acetaminophen; LT: liver transplantation; PALF: pediatric acute liver failure)

cause of PALF in India, and Peds-HAV model, which is a HAV-specific model derived from a cohort of HAV-induced PALF, should be used to decide LT listing for HAV-related PALF.[9] **Table 12.13.4** summarizes the common prognostic models used in PALF.

GENERAL MANAGEMENT AND COMPLICATIONS

The PALFSG definition was meant to act as an indicator to refer the patient to the LT center since it can identify subjects with acute liver injury sufficiently severe to place the child at risk for progressive clinical deterioration that could result in LT or death.[1] PALF diagnosed in non-LT center should be referred to an experienced LT center as soon as possible as described in the **Figure 12.13.1**.

As PALF patients with coagulopathy usually do not bleed due to a balance between loss of both procoagulant and anticoagulant factors, there is no need to preemptively transfuse fresh frozen plasma (FFP) in these patients. Unwarranted FFP transfusion can cause fluid overload and worsen the intracranial pressure (ICP).

Proper management is dependent on intensive collaborative clinical and supportive care and for a small proportion of cases, specific therapy can be lifesaving. Collaborative efforts of the pediatric hepatologists, pediatric critical care experts, pediatric neurologist, pediatric nephrologist, infection control experts, and well-trained nursing staff are mandatory for the successful management of these patients. Moreover, detailed case information including the treatment received by the patient should accompany the patient's records. A telephonic sounding of the pediatric hepatologists at the LT center may help greatly in early as well as rapid assessment in the emergency room and early management for the patient.

Early and Rapid Assessment in the Emergency Room and Beyond

Check for Hemodynamic Instability

Manage shock if present, as early as possible, with inotropes but great caution should be exercised in transfusing fluids to avoid increased ICP. Prior information about the antibiotics received in the previous center can help decide the antibiotics keeping in view the antibiogram pattern of the area.

Check for the Presence of Raised ICP and Grade of HE

The risk factors associated with developing substantial cerebral edema are advanced HE, younger age, serum ammonia >150 μmol/L, presence of infections, and hyperacute presentation. Development of raised ICP should be suspected in presence of sudden-onset hypertension, bradycardia, changes in pupillary reactivity, irregular respiration, and worsening of HE. However, these signs and symptoms may be absent in many patients.

General Precautions to Avoid Raised Intracranial Pressure

The aim of these precautions is to prevent and treat cerebral edema as well as optimize neurological recovery. PALF

TABLE 12.13.4: Commonly employed prognostic models in pediatric acute liver failure.

Models	***Components***	***Strengths of the prognostic model***
KCH	*For APAP PALF:* LT listing if: • pH <7.3 (irrespective of grade of HE) Or • Prothrombin time >100 seconds and serum creatinine >300 µmol/L in patients with grade III or IV HE *For non-APAP PALF:* • Age <10 or >40 years • *Etiology:* Non-A, non-B, and drug-induced • Jaundice–HE interval >7 days • INR >3.5 • Bilirubin >17.5 mg/dL Presence of ≥3 out 5 criteria indicates need of listing for LT	• Most widely used • Excellent for prognostication in APAP-ALF • Acceptable specificity in non-APAP-ALF • Can be used dynamically to delist, relist a patient • Simple and bedside
PELD/MELD	PELD = 4.80 [Ln serum bilirubin (mg/dL)] + 18.57 [Ln INR] – 6.87 [Ln albumin (g/dL)] + 4.36 (<1 year old) + 6.67 (growth failure) MELD = 9.57 × loge (creatinine) + 3.78 × loge (total bilirubin) + 11.2 × loge (INR) + 6.43	• High sensitivity at lower cutoffs (PELD >27) • Can show interval change
Liver Injury Unit (LIU) Score	LIU = [3.584 × peak total bilirubin (mg/dL)] + [1.809 × peak prothrombin time (PT) (seconds)] + [0.307 × peak ammonia (µmol/L)]	• Good sensitivity and specificity • Externally and internally validated
Peds-HAV model	• INR >3.1 • Jaundice to HE interval >10 days • HE Grade III or IV Presence of ≥2 out of 3 criteria indicates need of listing for LT	• Etiology specific model for the most common etiology (hepatitis A) of PALF in Asia • Good sensitivity as well as specificity • Dynamic model • Simple and bedside

(ALF: acute liver failure; APAP: acetaminophen; HAV: hepatitis A virus; HE: hepatic encephalopathy; INR: international normalized ratio; IV: intravenous; LT: liver transplantation; KCH: King's College Hospital; MELD: Model for End-Stage Liver Disease; PALF: pediatric acute liver failure; PELD: pediatric end-stage liver disease)

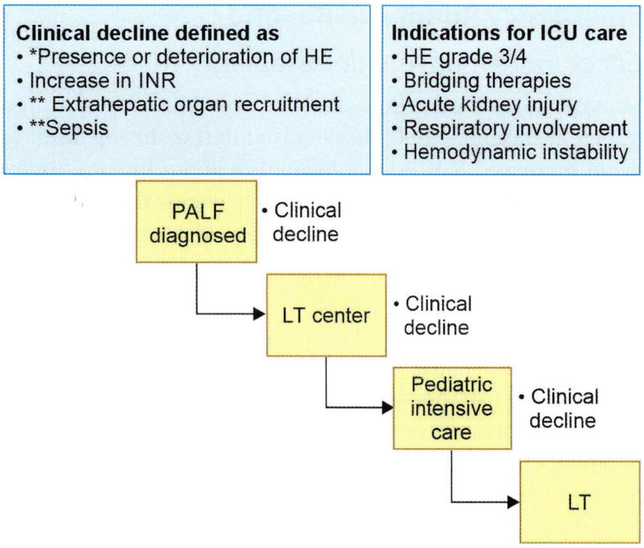

Fig. 12.13.1: Management approach to a case of pediatric acute liver failure.
*Presence of HE: Indicator to move the patient to a LT center
**Contraindication fo LT
(HE: hepatic encephalopathy; ICU: intensive care unit; INR: international normalized ratio; LT: liver transplantation; PALF: pediatric acute liver failure)

patients should have frequent examinations (at least every 2 hours) of pupil size and coma grade. All patients should be nursed in a quiet environment with 20–30° head up position to improve the venous drainage. Raising the head of the bed to 30° also decreases the risk of ventilator-associated pneumonia. However, some patients with markedly compromised cerebral perfusion may not tolerate elevation of the bed, and so it is always necessary to make individual assessments. Frequent suctioning, patient turning, and other tactile stimulation should be minimized. The patients should be kept well oxygenated. Avoid rectal enemas even in the presence of constipation and high ammonia. Ventilator settings should be adjusted to maintain normocarbia [partial pressure of arterial carbon dioxide ($PaCO_2$) 35–40 mm Hg] and higher positive end-expiratory pressure (PEEP) >8 mm Hg can raise ICP in these patients. Therapeutic hyperventilation must be reserved for patients with refractory raised ICP, and it should be used with caution because it induces cerebral vasoconstriction and may provoke ischemia. Body temperature must be closely monitored with a target temperature of 36°C. Fever and hyperthermia demands aggressive treatment because they can exacerbate ICP. Infections are common in patients with PALF and often trigger cerebral edema. Periodic surveillance cultures and chest X-rays are recommended in these patients, and broad-spectrum prophylactic antimicrobials (antibacterial and antifungal) should be considered if the patient develops fever or other signs of systemic inflammatory response syndrome. Severe hyperglycemia and even mild degrees of hypoglycemia should be promptly treated.

Hemodynamic Management

Patient should be kept euvolemic, and hypotension should be avoided to optimize cerebral perfusion pressure (CPP). Previously, the recommendations were to restrict the fluid to 70–80% of requirement, but later studies have identified the benefits of maintaining euvolemia on maintaining the CPP. Due to impaired cerebral autoregulation, systemic hypotension may reduce CPP and induce brain ischemia and hypertension may increase ICP. In adults, mean arterial pressure (MAP) should be sufficient to maintain a CPP above 60 mm Hg. In patients with persistent hypotension despite volume repletion, norepinephrine is usually the first choice inotrope, with or without vasopressin. In cases of circulatory collapse, the possibility of relative adrenal insufficiency has been documented in patients with PALF and a trial of hydrocortisone (300 mg/d) may be considered.

Management of Raised Intracranial Pressure

Refer to **Figure 12.13.2 and Flowchart 12.13.2** for mechanism of action of drugs and algorithmic approach in management of raised ICP. Clinical evidence of raised ICP should be quickly assessed and if present, decongestive therapy in the form of intravenous (IV) 20% mannitol (0.5–1 g/kg/dose) and IV 3% hypertonic saline (HTS) (dose 1.0–10 mL/kg bolus dose, maximum increase 10 mEq of serum sodium in 24 hours to maintain the range 149–155 mEq/L). While using mannitol, please ensure that the patient is not oliguric. The US Acute Liver Failure Study Group (ALFSG) guidelines recommend that mannitol therapy may be repeated so long as serum osmolality remains <320 mOsm/L. Repeated use of mannitol may be associated with serious adverse effects such as intravascular volume depletion, rebound ICP elevation, and renal failure from mannitol accumulation.

Hyponatremia should be avoided as it will worsen cerebral edema. Some guidelines advocate a target serum sodium at 145–155 mEq/L. In a randomized, placebo-controlled study, patients who were managed at serum sodium of 145–155 mEq/L after HTS boluses maintained lower ICP compared with patients managed at near-normal concentrations (137–142 mEq/L). Most studies using HTS report that sodium levels between 145 and 155 mEq/L to be safe and effective at reducing ICP in children with cerebral edema.

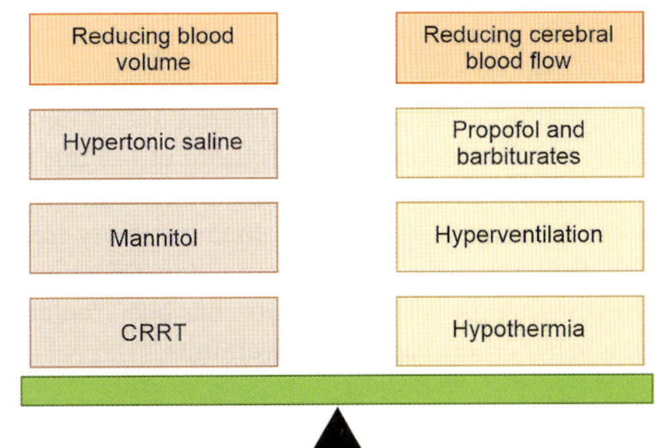

Fig. 12.13.2: Ways to reduce raised intracranial pressure. (CRRT: continuous renal replacement therapy)

Flowchart 12.13.2: Algorithmic approach to manage HE and ICP.

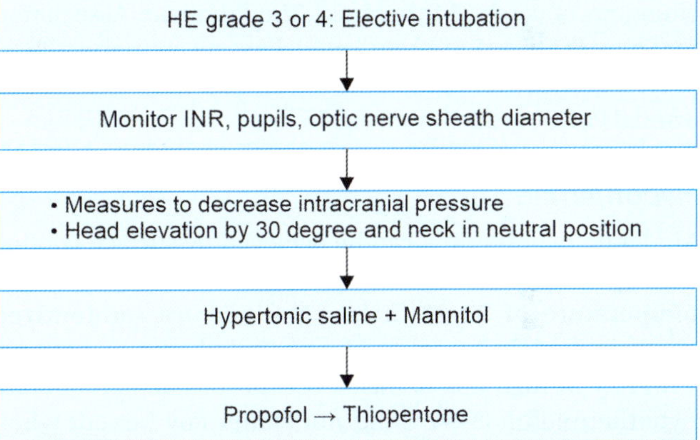

(HE: hepatic encephalopathy; ICP: intracranial pressure; INR: international normalized ratio)

Ventilatory Support and Pharmacologic Coma

In presence of HE grade 3 or 4, patient should be intubated which would help in controlling ICP with propofol and hyperventilation. Antiammonia measures such as lactulose and rifaximin can also be added. Lactulose may be associated with an increased risk of ileus and bowel dilation. In case of concern of seizure activity, electroencephalogram (EEG) monitoring should be undertaken and antiepileptic drugs administered; however, the prophylactic use of antiepileptic drugs is not warranted.

Propofol

Propofol is routinely chosen for sedation along with short-acting opioids such as fentanyl for adequate analgesia. Propofol (1–2 mg/kg IV, maximum of 5 mg/kg/day) is the induction agent of choice to facilitate intubation and ventilation. Propofol decreases the cerebral metabolic rate and cerebral oxygen demands and hence reduces cerebral blood flow and ICP. It also has anticonvulsant properties and permits a faster recovery, as its pharmacokinetics are not influenced by liver failure.

Barbiturates

In patients with refractory intracranial hypertension, barbiturate coma can be induced by thiopental (5–10 mg/kg IV bolus followed by a maintenance infusion of 1–3 mg/kg per hour). It reduces the cerebral metabolic rate and may be utilized to decrease ICP. Adverse effects are very frequent and include hypotension, cardiac depression, infections, and ileus. Rescue therapy with barbiturates has been replaced by therapeutic hypothermia in many liver units.

Hyperventilation

Forced hyperventilation induces hypocapnia and cerebral vasoconstriction and decreases cerebral blood flow and ICP. However, hyperventilation carries a serious risk of causing cerebral ischemia, and hence it should only be used in situations of cerebral hyperemia. The European Association for Study of Liver (EASL) 2017 guidelines recommend a short period of hyperventilation in resistant scenarios to reduce arterial $PaCO_2$ to 25–30 mm Hg.

Hypothermia

Moderate hypothermia can be achieved by surface cooling through the use of cooling blankets with targeted core temperature of 32–33°C. In a multicentre randomized controlled trial, Bernal et al. concluded that in patients with ALF at high risk of raised ICP, prophylactic moderate hypothermia of 33–34°C did not confer any benefit when compared to a temperature of 36°C to prevent raised ICP or in overall survival. The major adverse effect of moderate hypothermia includes worsening of coagulopathy, arrhythmia, increased chances of sepsis, and also chances of rebound increase in ICP during rewarming. Currently, moderate hypothermia remains a recommended treatment option, but only in those with refractory ICP elevation.[14]

Fluid and Electrolyte Management

Ensure arterial line and central venous catheter are in place. Maintaining CPPs is important, hence replete intravascular volume, but avoid large volume infusions of hypotonic fluids to prevent hyponatremia and cerebral edema. Correct any electrolyte abnormalities and acid base imbalance. Check serum osmolality and repeat mannitol provided it is below 320 mOsm/L. Monitor urine output along with serum creatinine levels. The FloTrac®/Vigileo device uses arterial pressure waveform analysis to calculate stroke volume and cardiac output; it does not require calibration against an independent measurement of cardiac output. If the stroke volume variation is >10%, then the patient might be fluid responsive **(Fig. 12.13.3 and Flowchart 12.13.3)**.

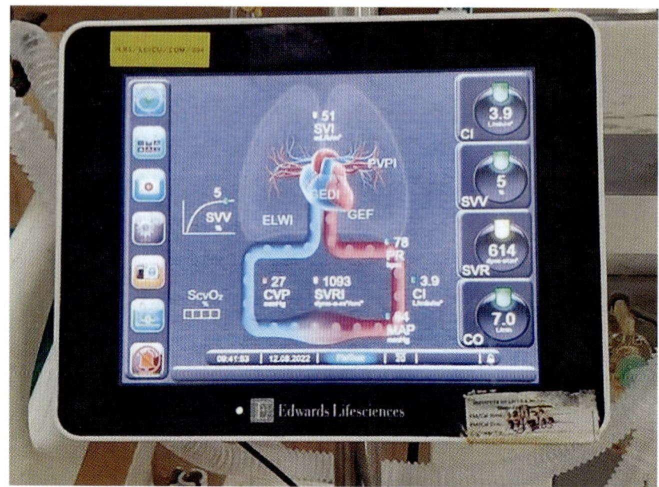

Fig. 12.13.3: Use of FloTrac to assess fluid responsiveness.

Enteral Nutrition

Adequate calories and protein (1–1.5 g/kg/day) can be safely given as tube feeds to the patients on ventilator support. To reduce fluid overload, avoid using IV 25 or 50% dextrose to maintain blood glucose, the same can be added in moderate amounts in the feeds. Keeping in view the inborn error of the metabolism suspected, the specific component can be removed from the diet till the disorder is confirmed, e.g., hereditary fructose intolerance, galactosemia, and fatty acid oxidation defect. Avoid hyponatremia and hypokalemia.

Extrahepatic Organ Involvement

Respiratory involvement in PALF can vary from ventilator-associated pneumonia to acute respiratory distress syndrome. Early institution of appropriate antibiotics guided by bronchoalveolar lavage culture keeping the local sensitivity pattern of emerging and extended drug resistance would improve outcomes. Early identification of acute kidney injury and appropriate management including antibiotics and continuous renal replacement therapy (CRRT) would help in avoiding renal failure and improve outcomes. Procalcitonin and galactomannan essay help in early identification of bacterial and fungal infections respectively.

Choice of Antimicrobials and Antifungals

Infections due to bacteria are more commonly seen compared to fungal or viral etiologies. Gram-negative enteric bacilli and gram-positive cocci are most frequently isolated. Among gram-positive bacteria, high frequency of infection with either methicillin-resistant *Staphylococcus aureus* and vancomycin-resistant *Enterococcus* are commonly encountered. Fungal infections occur in about one-third of patients requiring prolonged critical care support, largely with *Candida* species.

Flowchart 12.13.3: Suggested protocol for fluid management in PALF.

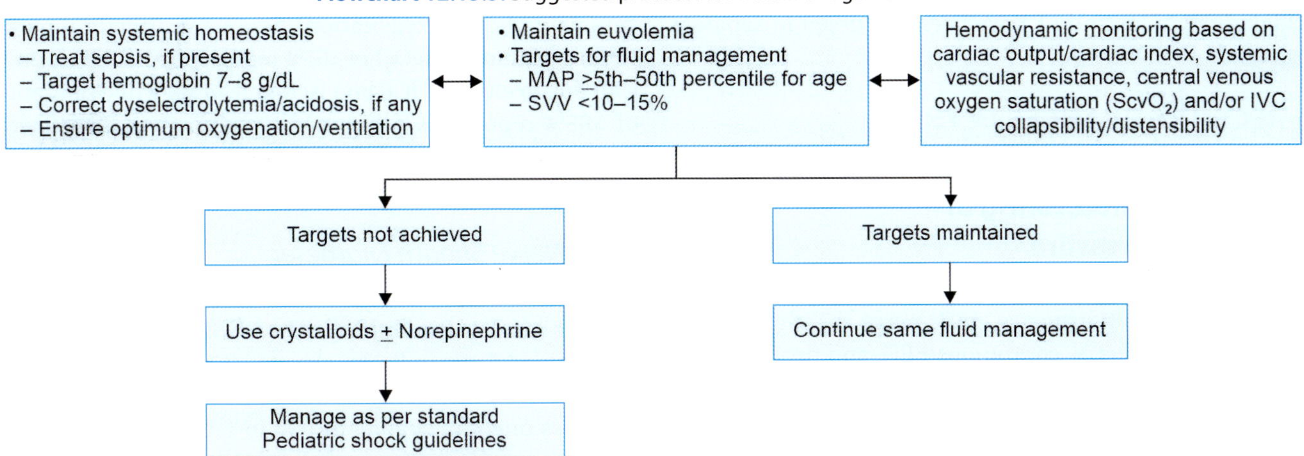

(IVC: inferior vena cava; PALF: pediatric acute liver failure; MAP: mean arterial pressure; SVV: stroke volume variation)

Source: Weiss SL, Peters MJ, Alhazzani W, Agus MSD, Flori HR, Inwald DP, et al. Surviving sepsis campaign international guidelines for the management of septic shock and sepsis-associated organ dysfunction in children. Intensive Care Med. 2020;46(Suppl 1):10-67.

The diagnosis of infection in PALF is a challenge as patients present with very nonspecific symptoms, culture positivity is low, blood cultures often turn out to be negative, and biomarkers such as C-reactive protein (CRP) and procalcitonin are not found to be very helpful. Frequent screening of blood, urine and appropriate samples for cultures should be performed as clinically indicated.

Broad-spectrum antibiotics against gram-negative and gram-positive bacteria should be used along with fluconazole. Choice of antibiotics should be decided based on whether the patient is coming from community or hospital setting, previous usage of antibiotics, present intensive care unit (ICU) sensitivity pattern as well as if there is any indwelling catheters which should prompt us to add anti-staphylococcal coverage. De-escalation or change of antibiotics is based on the antibiogram. Galactomannan essay should indicate upgradation or de-escalation of antifungal agents.

Specific Therapy

Specific therapy could be instituted in cases with PALF like N-acetyl cysteine (NAC) for APAP-related PALF. NAC should be started at the dose of 150 mg/kg/day as an infusion. In non-APAP PALF, NAC did not improve 1-year survival; while 1-year LT-free survival was significantly lower with NAC, particularly among those <2 years old. These results do not support broad use of NAC in non-APAP PALF.[15] Although NAC is antioxidant, anti-inflammatory, improves microcirculation, improves hemodynamics and improves regeneration, its benefits in PALF remain unproven in clinical trials.

Liver biopsy and immunosuppressives should be planned in cases of suspected AIH, if clinical condition permits. Wilson disease induced PALF should be treated with chelation therapy and plasmapheresis. If herpes simplex infection is suspected in a young infant, then IV acyclovir should be given (80 mg/kg/day in four divided doses). If an inborn error of metabolism is suspected, stop dietary ingredients for 48–72 hours till you have confirmed the diagnosis. Toxins and drugs, e.g., antitubercular drugs suspected to be the cause of PALF should be stopped immediately.

Bridging Therapies to Liver Transplantation

Continuous Renal Replacement Therapy and Plasmapheresis

The initiation of CRRT is primarily for fluid overload, hyperlactatemia, acute kidney injury, and hyperammonemia. CRRT can be used successfully in critically ill children with PALF to provide stability and bridge to transplantation. Inability to reduce ammonia by 48 hours confers poor prognosis. CRRT should be considered at an early stage to help prevent further deterioration and buy time for potential spontaneous recovery or bridge to LT. Therapeutic plasma exchange (TPE) in combination with CRRT can be used safely as a bridging therapy in children with PALF. Larsen et al. demonstrated the efficacy of TPE in improving the NLS in a large randomized controlled trial in adults.[16]

Liver Transplantation

Liver transplantation is the only proven treatment for PALF. Of late, spontaneous NLS is increasingly being reported, making one wonder if we are over-transplanting children with PALF. Only patients who have poor prognosis should undergo LT, and those who would spontaneously recover should avoid unnecessary LT. An effective prognostic model for PALF would help direct appropriate time for LT. Role of bridging therapies and LT have been discussed in separate chapters.

RECENT ADVANCES IN THE MANAGEMENT OF PALF

Noninvasive Monitoring of Intracranial Pressure

Several noninvasive techniques such as transcranial Doppler (TCD), jugular bulb oximetry, optic nerve sheath diameter (ONSD), pupillometry, continuous EEG, and near-infrared spectroscopy (NIRS) have recently come up as a good alternative to invasive ICP monitoring.

Transcranial Doppler Ultrasonography

Though still not universally validated in pediatric population, TCD is a useful noninvasive surrogate method of measuring ICP by assessing flow velocity characteristics in intracranial blood vessels (most commonly in the middle cerebral artery). Elevations in ICP can cause an increase in the extramural pressure, flow velocities and the pulsatility index (PI) [(Peak systolic velocity – end-diastolic velocity)/mean velocity]. The CPP, and thus the ICP, can be calculated based on the flow velocities and the arterial blood pressure **(Fig. 12.13.4)**.[17]

Near-infrared Spectroscopy

Near-infrared spectroscopy is a noninvasive, continuous monitoring technique that measures regional tissue oxygenation. NIRS that is placed over the internal jugular vein cutaneous area (NIRS-IJV) has the potential to show central venous catheter oxygenation ($ScvO_2$) indirectly. Jugular venous saturation (JvO_2) of <55% represents the reduction in CPP due to elevated ICP and ischemic brain while saturation of >85% represents a hyperemic brain. JvO_2 is a useful monitoring tool while using therapeutic hyperventilation and hypothermia **(Figs. 12.13.5A and B)**.

Optic Nerve Sheath Diameter

Optic nerve sheath diameter has also been used to monitor patients with PALF in children. The ONSD correlates with ICP and value >4.6 mm indicates elevated ICP.[18] ONSD is a simple, bedside, inexpensive, reproducible, and repeatable modality to assess ongoing change in ICP in PALF. ONSD >4.6 mm suggests raised ICP.[19] The goal should be to bring ONSD down to <4.6 mm within 24 hours by aggressive anti-ICP therapy to achieve favorable outcome. **Figure 12.13.6** shows ONSD measurement of a patient with cerebral edema in a case of hepatitis A-induced PALF.

Role of Histopathology

A key event in PALF is massive hepatic necrosis, a distinct pathophysiological process characterized by extremely rapid extensive and diffuse parenchymal necrosis spanning across multiple lobes of liver. Various previous studies conducted in predominantly adult subjects have established that a hepatocyte loss of >50–75% is usually associated with poor outcomes in ALF patients.[19,20] Incorporation of this information with the prognostic score may strengthen the prognostic ability of the score.

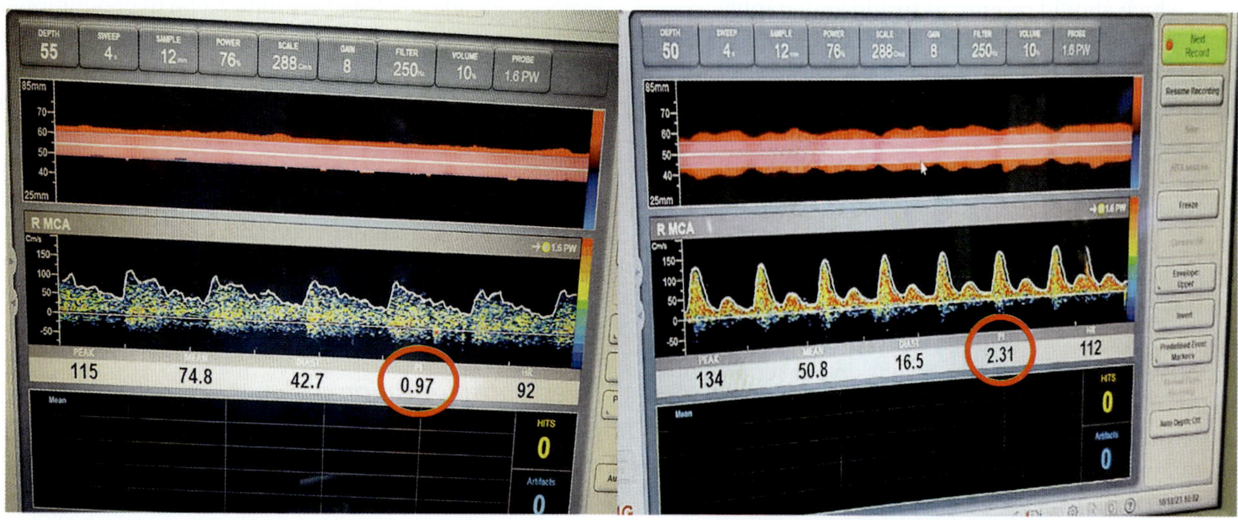

Fig. 12.13.4: Use of transcranial Doppler for measurement of intracranial pressure (ICP) using pulsatility index (PI) as a surrogate (though no standard pediatric cutoffs are defined, but usually PI <0.8–1.2 is normal; PI >1.2 is considered a surrogate for increased resistance to blood flow or raised ICP).

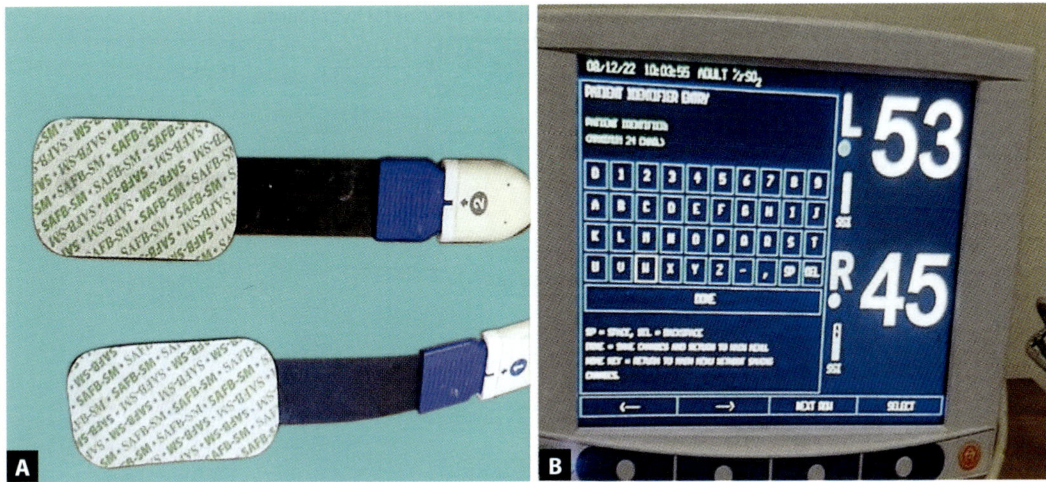

Figs. 12.13.5A and B: Near-infrared spectroscopy.

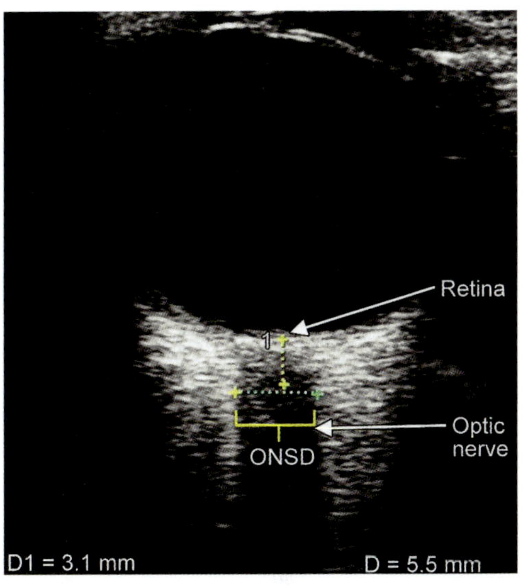

Fig. 12.13.6: Optic nerve sheath diameter (ONSD) being measured in a child with Pediatric acute liver failure (PALF). ONSD of 5.5 mm denotes that the child is having rise in intracranial pressure. The maximum diameter of optic nerve is measured 3 mm behind the retina of each eye.

Hepatocyte Transplantation

A potential alternative to LT is allogenic hepatocyte transplantation which has made the transition from bench to bedside. Standardized techniques have been established for isolation, culture, and cryopreservation of human hepatocytes. Clinical hepatocyte transplantation safety and short-term efficacy have been proven; however, some major hurdles—mainly concerning shortage of donor organs, low cell engraftment, and lack of a long-lasting effect—need to be overcome to widen its clinical applications. Current research is aimed at addressing these problems, with the ultimate goal of increasing hepatocyte transplantation efficacy in clinical applications.

Auxiliary Liver Transplantation

Auxiliary LT consists of implanting a healthy liver graft placed orthotopically while leaving all or part of the native liver. Favorable outcomes were reported in a European series using auxiliary partial orthotopic liver transplantation (APOLT). Complete regeneration of the native liver can be observed in >50% of patients, who can be withdrawn from immunosuppression which in turn will lead to atrophy of the graft liver and the regenerated native liver takes over the function.

NEONATAL LIVER FAILURE

Neonatal acute liver failure (NALF) is distinct from PALF seen in older children and adolescents. The diagnosis of HE is practically impossible in neonatal age group, hence uncorrectable coagulopathy defined as INR $\geq$2.0 after administration of parenteral vitamin K is used to define NALF. The mechanism of the disease, etiologic possibilities, and diagnostic approach of NALF are different from the PALF of older children and adolescents. The liver injury in NALF may have occurred in a fetal liver which may be functionally immature or in the neonatal liver. So the time of liver injury may influence the mechanism of the disease in NALF, e.g., gestational alloimmune liver disorder (GALD)-related immune injury causes failure of the fetal hepatocytes to develop into mature hepatocytes. This injury thus results in neonatal hemochromatosis (NH), which should be termed as GALD-NH and is responsible for 60% cases of NALF. **Flowchart 12.13.4** depicts the pathogenetic pathways of NALF and their associated etiologies. **Table 12.13.5** describes

Flowchart 12.13.4: Pathogenesis of neonatal liver failure.

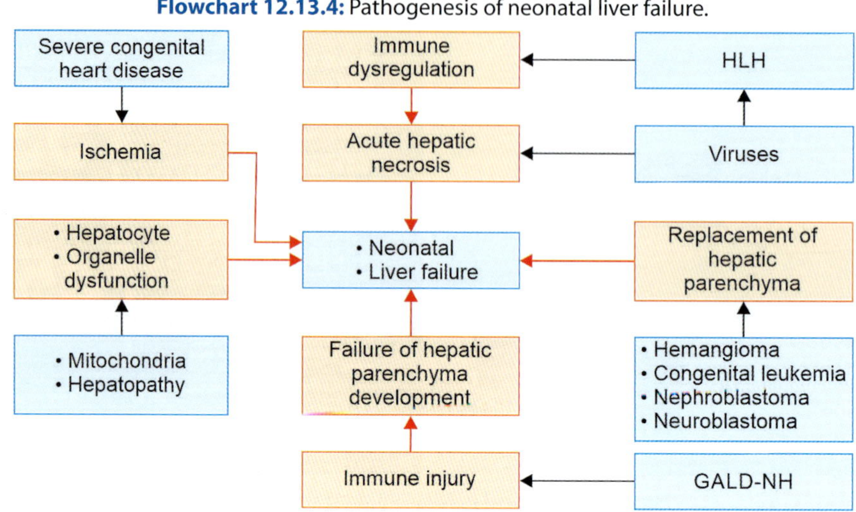

(GALD-NH: gestational alloimmune liver disease-neonatal hemochromatosis; HLH: hemophagocytic lymphohistiocytosis)

TABLE 12.13.5: Important causes of neonatal liver failure and their differentiating features on history and laboratory markers.

	GALD-NH	***Viral***	***HLH***	***Mitochondrial hepatopathy***
Age of onset	First 3 days	5–14 days	Variable	Variable
Sibling death	Yes	No	No	25% risk
IUGR	70–90%	No	No	20–30%
Ascites	40–60%	Uncommon	Uncommon	Uncommon
Hepatomegaly	10–20%	Common	Common	Common
Splenomegaly	10–20%	Common	Common	Uncommon
Coagulopathy	Profound	Moderate to profound	Moderate	Moderate to profound
Bilirubin	High	Mild	Moderate	Moderate
AST/ALT	Low	High	Moderately elevated	Moderately elevated
Ferritin	High	Very high	Very high	Variable
AFP	Very high	Normal	Normal	Variable
High lactate	Normal	Normal	Normal	High

(AFP: Alpha-fetoprotein; GALD-NH: gestational alloimmune liver disease-neonatal hemochromatosis; HLH: hemophagocytic lymphohistiocytosis; IUGR: intrauterine growth restriction; NALF: neonatal liver failure)

the various etiologies responsible for NALF and their clinical and biochemical differentiators.

Neonatal Hemochromatosis—Gestational Alloimmune Liver Disease

Gestational alloimmune liver disease is the most common cause of NALF. However, its incidence has decreased significantly since the use of intravenous immunoglobulin (IVIG) during pregnancy in mothers with previous affected offsprings, to prevent GALD. Hepatic injury results in decreased hepcidin production leading to uncontrolled iron transport across placenta from maternal to fetal side resulting in extrahepatic and hepatic siderosis. The typical histopathology of GALD-NH reflects this dynamic: absence of normal hepatocytes; normal portal areas; numerous tubules in parenchyma; extensive parenchymal fibrosis; and multinucleate giant cells as the only remaining hepatocyte forms. The retention of membrane attack complex (complement C5b-9 complex) in remaining hepatocyte forms is an evidence of alloimmune injury. Diagnosis of GALD is based on demonstration of extrahepatic siderosis in pancreas (on MRI abdomen) or in minor salivary glands (by buccal biopsy). A dose of IVIG should be given empirically if suspicion of GALD-NH is strong awaiting further tests. Once diagnosis is confirmed, double volume exchange transfusion should be done followed by another dose of IVIG. The affected babies are sick and small, making liver transplant a difficult proposition.

Viral Infections

Neonatal HSV infection is typically acquired during passage via the birth canal. History of herpes infection in mother may not be forthcoming. The disease has fulminant course and poor outcome. IV acyclovir should be started if there is suspicion of HSV-induced NALF. Serum transaminases are typically in thousands. Diagnosis can be made with polymerase chain reaction (PCR) from blood, skin, eye, cerebrospinal fluid (CSF), and mucous membranes. Early administration of acyclovir can change the outcome drastically.

Enteroviruses are another viral cause of NALF, present with more generalized symptoms including respiratory distress, diarrhea, poor feeding, rash, and fever. It should be suspected in neonates with necrotizing enterocolitis. Diagnosis can be made with PCR from blood, CSF, and stool. Treatment includes supportive care.

Mitochondrial Hepatopathy

Mitochondrial liver disease accounts for 2–12% of NALF. Mitochondrial diseases that may present as ALF include disorders of fatty oxidation (carnitine palmitoyl transferase II deficiency), mitochondrial deoxyribonucleic acid (DNA) depletion syndromes (DGUOK deficiency and *MPV17* mutation). DGUOK deficiency results in impaired energy production and organ dysfunction. It presents in the neonatal period or later infancy as a multisystem (hepatocerebral) disorder. There is variable phenotypic presentation even within siblings who have the same mutation. Patients can present with elevated tyrosine and phenylalanine on the newborn screen. Confirmation of DGUOK deficiency is through identification of the genetic mutation. Treatment of children with DGUOK deficiency is focused on supporting the hepatic and neurological manifestations.

MPV17 gene codes for mitochondrial DNA maintenance; thus, mutations lead to mitochondrial DNA depletion. Phenotypic presentation depends on the exact *MPV17* mutation and liver failure can precede neurological symptoms in some cases. Other respiratory chain defects, e.g., *BCS1L* mutation (GRACILE syndrome) can present with NALF.

Hemophagocytic Lymphohistiocytosis

Approximately 3% of NALF results from HLH which can be primary or secondary and results in altered NK cell and cytotoxic T cell function and decreased immune-mediated apoptosis. Treatment of HLH includes use of dexamethasone, IVIG, plasmapheresis, and etoposide as per established chemotherapy protocols. Children with primary HLH or those who do not respond to chemotherapy are candidates for hematopoietic stem cell transplant.

KEY POINTS

- High index of suspicion is needed in children as diagnosis of HE is difficult in them.
- The etiological spectrum varies by age at presentation and the geographical location.
- Outcome varies by age, etiology and management strategies. Several prognostic models are available. KCH criteria are most widely used to decide for LT listing.
- Early referral and close monitoring are the key points in the management of PALF.
- Very careful identification and monitoring of ICP using the recent advanced equipment can help greatly in the management of the PALF.
- Adequate coverage with appropriate antibiotics and antifungal drugs should be instituted.
- Bridging therapies should institute early, e.g., CRRT.
- Appropriate timing for the LT is very important.

TIPS FOR PEDIATRICIANS

- Always look for signs of HE and check INR. In case of coagulopathy or HE, refer the patient to a center equipped for LT.
- Pediatricians have a very important role to identify PALF and arrange early referral with appropriate information about the case.
- Refrain from FFP transfusion or any such treatment causing fluid overload and raised ICP.
- Parents' education regarding seriousness of the disease, potential need of LT and identification of a potential donor should be introduced by pediatricians.

REFERENCES

1. Squires RH Jr, Shneider BL, Bucuvalas J, Alonso E, Sokol RJ, Narkewicz MR, et al. Acute liver failure in children: the first 348 patients in the pediatric acute liver failure study group. J Pediatr. 2006;148(5):652-8.
2. Sundaram SS, Alonso EM, Narkewicz MR, Zhang S, Squires RH; Pediatric Acute Liver Failure Study Group. Characterization and outcomes of young infants with acute liver failure. J Pediatr. 2011;159(5):813-8.e1.
3. Shanmugam NP, Bansal S, Greenough A, Verma A, Dhawan A. Neonatal liver failure: aetiologies and management—state of the art. Eur J Pediatr. 2011;170(5):573-81.
4. Antala S, Whitehead B, Godown J, Hall M, Banc-Husu A, Alonso E, et al. Neonates with acute liver failure have higher overall mortality but similar posttransplant outcomes as older infants. Liver Transpl. 2022;29(1):5-14.

5. Bitar R, Thwaites R, Davison S, Rajwal S, McClean P. Liver Failure in Early Infancy: Aetiology, Presentation, and Outcome. J Pediatr Gastroenterol Nutr. 2017;64(1):70-5.
6. Ciocca M, Moreira-Silva SF, Alegría S, Galoppo C, Ruttiman R, Porta G, et al. Hepatitis A as an etiologic agent of acute liver failure in Latin America. Pediatr Infect Dis J. 2007;26(8):711-5.
7. Kayaalp C, Ersan V, Yılmaz S. Acute liver failure in Turkey: a systematic review. Turk J Gastroenterol. 2014;25(1):35-40.
8. Hegarty R, Hadzic N, Gissen P, Dhawan A. Inherited metabolic disorders presenting as acute liver failure in newborns and young children: King's College Hospital experience. Eur J Pediatr. 2015;174(10):1387-92.
9. Alam S, Khanna R, Sood V, Lal BB, Rawat D. Profile and outcome of first 109 cases of paediatric acute liver failure at a specialized paediatric liver unit in India. Liver Int. 2017;37(10):1508-14.
10. Lal BB, Sood V, Snehavardhan P, Khanna R, Pasupuleti SSR, Siloliya M, et al. A novel, bedside, etiology specific prognostic model (Peds-HAV) in hepatitis A induced pediatric acute liver failure. Hepatol Int. 2020;14(4):483-90.
11. Poddar U, Thapa BR, Prasad A, Singh K. Changing spectrum of sporadic acute viral hepatitis in Indian children. J Trop Pediatr. 2002;48(4):210-3.
12. Rajanayagam J, Coman D, Cartwright D, Lewindon PJ. Pediatric acute liver failure: etiology, outcomes, and the role of serial pediatric end-stage liver disease scores. Pediatr Transplant. 2013;17(4):362-8.
13. O'Grady JG, Alexander GJ, Hayllar KM, Williams R. Early indicators of prognosis in fulminant hepatic failure. Gastroenterology. 1989;97(2):439-45.
14. Bernal W, Murphy N, Brown S, Whitehouse T, Bjerring PN, Hauerberg J, et al. A multicentre randomized controlled trial of moderate hypothermia to prevent intracranial hypertension in acute liver failure. J Hepatol. 2016;65(2):273-9.
15. Squires RH, Dhawan A, Alonso E, Narkewicz MR, Shneider BL, Rodriguez-Baez N, et al.; Pediatric Acute Liver failure Study Group. Intravenous N-acetylcysteine in pediatric patients with nonacetaminophen acute liver failure: a placebo-controlled clinical trial. Hepatology. 2013;57(4):1542-9.
16. Larsen FS, Schmidt LE, Bernsmeier C, Rasmussen A, Isoniemi H, Patel VC, et al. High-volume plasma exchange in patients with acute liver failure: an open randomised controlled trial. J Hepatol. 2016;64(1):69-78.
17. Hunt A, Tasker RC, Deep A. Neurocritical care monitoring of encephalopathic children with acute liver failure: a systematic review. Pediatr Transplant. 2019;23(7):e13556.
18. Vijay P, Lal BB, Sood V, Khanna R, Patidar Y, Alam S. Dynamic Optic Nerve Sheath Diameter (ONSD) guided management of raised intracranial pressure in pediatric acute liver failure. Hepatol Int. 2021;15(2):502-9.
19. Donaldson BW, Gopinath R, Wanless IR, Philips MJ, Roberts EA, Grieg PD, et al. The role of transjugular liver biopsy in fulminant liver failure: relation to other prognostic indicators. Hepatology. 1993;18(6):1370-6.
20. Ndekwe P, Ghabril MS, Zang Y, Mann SA, Cummings OW, Lin J. Substantial hepatic necrosis is prognostic in fulminant liver failure. World J Gastroenterol. 2017;23(23):4303-10.

12.14 Chronic Liver Disease

Naresh Shanmugam

INTRODUCTION

Chronic liver disease (CLD) in children is an important cause of morbidity and mortality. The pathological spectrum ranges from simple steatosis to cirrhosis, which may progress to end-stage liver disease (ESLD) or hepatic malignancy. The liver is an organ that regenerates; but in the presence of persistent insult to the liver cells, formation of fibrous scars leads to cirrhosis. Cirrhosis completely distorts the liver architecture and also the increases the resistance to blood and bile flow through the liver. Cirrhosis interferes with hepatocyte regeneration and the hemodynamics of blood, flow resulting in complications such portal hypertension, ascites, and encephalopathy. This can lead on to a secondary cascade of events that affect the function of several end-organs such as brain, kidney, and lungs.

DEFINITION

Persistent liver disease of >6 *months* duration is considered as CLD.[1] ESLD is sometimes used interchangeably with the terminology CLD, suggesting decompensated liver disease. Cirrhosis is a term used to describe microscopic and/or macroscopic changes in liver characterized by aberrant nodule formation, vascular changes, and totally disturbed architecture associated with fibrosis.

ETIOLOGY

Chronic persistent insult to liver cells is associated with fibrosis, which can ultimately lead to cirrhosis. Some of the common diseases that cause chronic injury to liver in children leading to cirrhosis are outlined in **Box 12.14.1**. The common

BOX 12.14.1: Common etiologies of chronic liver disease (CLD).

- *Infections:* Hepatitis B virus (HBV) and hepatitis C virus (HCV) related
- *Metabolic:* Wilson disease, glycogen storage disorder, tyrosinemia, galactosemia, and nonalcoholic fatty liver disease (NAFLD)
- *Autoimmune hepatitis (AIH)* type I and II
- *Drug-induced liver injury (DILI)*
- *Cholestatic liver disease:* Biliary atresia and sclerosing cholangitis
- *Vascular:* Hepatic venous outflow tract obstruction (HVOTO), noncirrhotic portal fibrosis (NCPF), and extrahepatic portal venous obstruction (EHPVO)
- *Hematological:* Sickle cell disease
- *Miscellaneous:* Secondary to Langerhans's cell histiocytosis, juvenile rheumatoid arthritis, and Indian childhood cirrhosis (ICC)
- *Cryptogenic*
- *Structural:* Fibropolycystic disease of liver and Caroli disease

Note: The pattern of CLD may be either parenchymal or cholestatic. Infants usually have a cholestatic presentation and the most common cause is biliary atresia

conditions that lead on to progressive liver disease in children such as viral hepatitis (Chapter 12.7), Wilson disease (WD) (Chapter 12.9), neonatal cholestatic disorders (Chapter 12.10), and autoimmune liver disease (Chapter 12.11) are discussed in separate chapters and thus not discussed in detail in this chapter.

PATHOGENESIS OF CIRRHOSIS

Cell death or injury to hepatocytes is associated with release of several proinflammatory mediators [e.g., tumor necrosis factor (TNF)] that act on Kupffer cells, hepatocytes, cholangiocytes, etc., that release secondary mediators, which then activates hepatic stellate cells (HSCs) to produce extracellular matrix (ECM). Under normal conditions, HSCs are quiescent cells which reside in the space of Disse, that store lipids and vitamin A. When activated, HSC transdifferentiate to myofibroblast-like cells, acquiring fibrogenic and secretory properties. Mitogenic stimuli such as transforming growth factor-beta (TGF-beta), upregulate several precollagenous genes, and increase the secretion of collagen by myofibroblasts, particularly type 1 and 3.[2] There is gross imbalance between production and degradation of ECM. The fibrous tissue thus formed will interconnect the portal tracts, portal tracts, and central venules or a mixture of both patterns and progress to cirrhosis. As with any other multifactorial disease, both genetic and environmental factors play a role in the progression of cirrhosis. Contrary to the earlier belief, it has now been shown that liver fibrosis, even cirrhosis can regress to some extent on successful treatment of the underlying cause.[3]

CLINICAL PRESENTATION

- Initial presentation can be with jaundice but can also present with nonspecific symptoms such as failure to thrive, growth retardation, muscle weakness, or lethargy.
- Severe pruritus may be a feature of Alagille syndrome and progressive familial intrahepatic cholestasis (PFIC).
- As the disease progresses symptoms such as ascites, gastrointestinal (GI) bleed, abdominal pain, and altered sensorium appear, which are suggestive of decompensated liver disease or ESLD.
- Cyanosis and clubbing point toward development of hepatopulmonary syndrome (HPS) or portopulmonary hypertension.
- Nutritional manifestations such as malnutrition, malabsorption, steatorrhea, hypoalbuminemia, and fat-soluble vitamin deficiencies are common in CLD. Malnutrition is a common problem of CLD, especially when the onset of disease occurs in infancy. Vitamin A and D deficiencies commonly present as xerosis and rickets. Vitamin K deficiency presents as coagulopathy and is seen in CLD, more so in cholestatic liver disease.

CLINICAL EXAMINATION

A good clinical examination gives clues about disease severity and also the underlying etiology.

General Examination

- Dysmorphic facies can suggest some specific syndromes such as Alagille and Zellweger syndromes.
- Cataracts are a finding seen in galactosemia.
- Pigmented sclero-corneal ring or Kayser–Fleischer (KF) ring is seen in WD. Non-Wilsonian KF ring may also be seen in cholestatic liver disease.
- Cherry red spot may be seen in Gaucher disease and Niemann–Pick disease type C.
- Vertical gaze palsy is seen in Niemann–Pick disease.
- The examination of the eyes for vitamin A deficiency is important.
- Xanthoma suggesting hypercholesterolemia is seen in Alagille syndrome.

Abdominal Examination

- The liver may be firm with a sharp edge in chronic hepatitis whereas it is firmer and more nodular in cirrhosis.
- The liver size may not always be decreased in CLD and usually, the liver is enlarged in nonalcoholic liver fatty liver disease (NAFLD), glycogen storage disease (GSD), and biliary cirrhosis. The vertical span should be documented.

- Splenomegaly indicates portal hypertension.
- Ascites is a feature of decompensation.
- Prominent abdominal wall veins are seen in in sinusoidal and postsinusoidal portal hypertension.

Neurological Examination

- The neurological assessment is very crucial. Changes in sleep rhythm, tremors, flap, and reflexes indicate encephalopathy.
- Certain findings on neurologic examination could give clues to etiology such as vacuous smile, drooling of saliva, and choreoathetosis as in WD.

COMPLICATIONS OF CHRONIC LIVER DISEASE

Complications such as ascites (Chapter 12.2) and portal hypertension (Chapter 12.3) are dealt in separate chapters in this book and only other complications are dealt here.

Malnutrition

Due to prolonged course of illness, malnutrition is much more of a problem in CLD than in acute liver failure (ALF). Increased nutritional requirement due to increased resting energy expenditure (REE) and total energy expenditure (TEE) coupled with poor intake and poor absorption lead to malnutrition.[4] In children, CLD is mainly due to due to congenital malformations of liver or biliary system (e.g., biliary atresia and Caroli disease) and inherited metabolic disorders (e.g., PFIC, WD, and tyrosinemia). The nutritional requirement varies with disease type and severity. In a cohort of children awaiting orthotropic liver transplantation, it was found that their mean protein-energy intakes were 70% of recommended daily intake and all were deficient in essential fatty acids (EFAs), fat-soluble vitamins, and minerals such as zinc, selenium, and iron.[5] With the wide availability of liver transplantation for children with CLD, it is essential to optimize their nutritional status, since it is an important determinant of posttransplant mortality and morbidity.[6]

Hepatic Encephalopathy

The major neurological complication in CLD is hepatic encephalopathy (HE). It is defined as a metabolically induced, potentially reversible, and functional disturbance of the brain that may occur in acute or CLD.[7] Features of HE varies considerably between subtle behavioral alterations to overt coma. Sometimes patients with HE may have similar features of parkinsonism such as muscular rigidity, bradykinesia, hypokinesia, and monotony of speech and tremors.

Though ammonia is implicated in HE, the exact mechanism is still elusive. One such suggested mechanism is that increased intracellular glutamine due to raised ammonia in astrocytes raises the intracellular osmotic pressure, leading on to swelling of astrocytes, cerebral edema, and dysfunction.

TABLE 12.14.1: West haven criteria for grading of mental state.[9]

Grade	Features
Grade 0	Normal
Grade 1	• Euphoria or anxiety • Shortened attention span • Impaired performance of addition • Trivial lack of awareness • Inverted sleep pattern
Grade 2	• Subtle personality change • Minimal disorientation for time or place • Impaired performance of subtraction • Lethargy or slow response • Tremor and hypoactive reflexes
Grade 3	• Somnolence to semi-stupor, but responds to verbal stimuli • Confusion, gross disorientation • Inappropriate behavior • Brisk reflexes and Babinski sign • Muscle rigidity
Grade 4	Deep coma (unresponsive to verbal or noxious stimuli)

Diagnosis of encephalopathy is mainly based on clinical evaluation and so a good clinical history and thorough clinical examination must be performed.[8] Clinical grading using West Haven criteria **(Table 12.14.1)** should be carried out in all patients with HE and Glasgow Coma Scale (GCS) could be used to grade the conscious levels. Biochemical tests are of little value in making the diagnosis of HE as there is no specific biomarker. Arterial ammonia has poor correlation with the grade of encephalopathy.[9] Neuroimaging and electrophysiological studies of brain help in ruling out other causes of encephalopathy and give supportive evidence such as cerebral edema and specific electroencephalogram (EEG) changes rather than making the diagnosis of HE.

Hepatorenal Syndrome

Hepatorenal syndrome is a progressive, reversible functional renal impairment that occurs in patients with advanced liver cirrhosis or those with fulminant hepatic failure. Two forms of hepatorenal syndrome have been described. Type 1 hepatorenal syndrome is characterized by rapid progression of renal failure and has a precipitating factor in most cases. It is defined by a doubling of the initial serum creatinine to a level >2.5 mg/dL or 220 µmol/L in <2 weeks and carries a poor prognosis. Type 2 hepatorenal syndrome is characterized by a moderate renal failure (serum creatinine >1.5 mg/dL or 133 µmol/L) which follows a steady or slowly progressive course.

Hepatopulmonary Syndrome

Hepatopulmonary syndrome is characterized by triad of liver disease, arterial hypoxemia, and intrapulmonary vascular dilatation. The diagnostic criteria for HPS is the presence of CLD along with partial pressure of arterial oxygen (PaO_2) <70 mm Hg or alveolar-arterial oxygen gradient >15 mm Hg and intrapulmonary vascular dilatation.[10] Clinical manifestation of HPS is that of hypoxia such as dyspnea, clubbing, and cyanosis. Spider nevi are considered a sensitive marker of HPS. In HPS, dyspnea is more in upright position (orthodoxia), and is due to increased congestion because of gravity exaggerating the ventilation–perfusion mismatch. Children with saturation <94% should be screened with bubble echocardiography. Appearance of air bubbles on the left heart within five cardiac cycles is suggestive of intrapulmonary vascular dilatation. If the initial screening raises the possibility of HPS, technetium-99m macroaggregated albumin (Tc-99m MAA) lung perfusion scan should be considered, which is more sensitive and specific in diagnosis and quantification of shunt fraction.[10,11]

Hepatic Osteodystrophy

Hepatic osteodystrophy is a generalized term used to denote metabolic bone disease in CLD that occurs due to osteoporosis and osteomalacia in various proportions.[12] In children, hepatic osteodystrophy comprises of vitamin D deficiency rickets, low bone mass, spine abnormalities, and growth failure due to malnutrition and malabsorption.[13]

INVESTIGATIONS

Investigations are done to confirm diagnosis of CLD, identify etiology, and detect complications. Some of the common investigations are outlined in **Table 12.14.2**.

Histopathology

Liver biopsy helps in diagnosis of underlying etiology and also gives information about severity of fibrosis. Synthetic liver function or cholestasis has no correlation with the degree of fibrosis, as these parameters may be normal even in advanced fibrosis as in congenital hepatic fibrosis. Liver biopsy is considered to be the gold-standard method for the assessment of liver fibrosis as it provides necroinflammatory and the fibrosis grade. Scoring of degree of fibrosis is done using Metavir (stages I–IV) and Ishak score (stages I–V).

Transient Elastography

Due to invasive nature of the procedure, it is practically difficult to monitor fibrosis progression using liver biopsy. To overcome this problem, transient elastography (FibroScan®),

TABLE 12.14.2: Investigations in CLD.

To confirm diagnosis	1. Complete blood counts (CBC) 2. Urine routine 3. Liver function tests (LFTs) 4. Prothrombin time (PT) 5. Ultrasonography of abdomen (USG) and Doppler	1. *CBC:* a. *Anemia:* Iron deficiency, nutritional, and gastrointestinal (GI) bleed b. *Pancytopenia:* Hypersplenism c. *Thrombocytopenia:* Cirrhosis 2. *Urine:* Albumin ++: WD, AIH, and HBV 3. *SGPT (ALT)/SGOT (AST):* >5 UL: Acute hepatitis and cirrhosis 4. *PT:* Prolonged: Liver failure 5. *USG abdomen:* a. *Coarse echoes:* Cirrhosis b. *Dilated portal vein, portal hypertension (PHT), and free fluid:* Venous outflow obstruction such as Budd–Chiari syndrome
To identify the etiology	1. HBsAg, HBeAg, anti-HBe, HBV DNA 2. HCV, HCV RNA+ (>6 m) 3. Serum amino acid profile, 4. Tandem mass spectrometry 5. Exome sequencing 6. Diagnosis of Wilson disease and autoimmune liver disease discussed in other chapters	1. HBsAg +ve, HBeAg +ve, HBV DNA >20,000 IU/L. HBeAg +ve CHB (chronic hepatitis) 2. HBsAg +ve, HBeAg –ve, HBV DNA >2000 IU/L. HBeAg –ve: CHB 3. HCV RNA +ve—chronic hepatitis C 4. Specific increase in amino acids 5. Positive mutations
To identify complications	1. Blood glucose, electrolytes 2. Serum creatinine 3. Serum ammonia 4. Upper gastrointestinal GI endoscopy 5. Bubble echocardiography (ECHO)	1. *Persistently low blood glucose and low sodium:* Bad prognostic marker 2. *Elevated creatinine:* WD and acute kidney injury 3. *Elevated ammonia:* Hepatic encephalopathy 4. *Upper GI endoscopy:* Varices +: Portal hypertension (PHT) 5. *Bubble ECHO:* Hepatopulmonary syndrome

(AIH: autoimmune hepatitis; ALT: alanine aminotransferase; AST: aspartate aminotransferase; CLD: chronic liver disease; HBV: hepatitis B virus; WD: Wilson disease)

a noninvasive technique is used in serial monitoring of progress of fibrosis with good accuracy and has been validated even in children.[14]

MANAGEMENT OF CHRONIC LIVER DISEASE

General Management

All children with CLD should avoid prolonged periods of fasting, take small meals and snacks/day, and a late evening snack to reduce the duration of overnight fasting. Oral liquid supplements help in increasing calorie and protein consumption. Avoid unnecessary diet restrictions. Protein to be given is 2–2.5 g/kg but may be restricted to 0.5–1 g/kg/day during HE. The suggested form of vitamin D for both prophylaxis and treatment of hepatic osteodystrophy is either ergocalciferol (vitamin D_2) or cholecalciferol (vitamin D_3) targeting a 25-hydroxyvitamin D (25OHD) level of >50 nmol/L. Other fat-soluble vitamins also have to be supplemented.

All children with CLD should receive age-appropriate vaccines, especially hepatitis A and hepatitis B vaccines.

Management of Complications

Management of ascites, variceal bleed, and encephalopathy have been described in the respective sections.

Encephalopathy

Lactulose reaches the colon undigested where it is broken down by the by the intestinal flora to fructose and galactose which are further fermented to acids such as acetic and lactic acids that decrease the luminal pH to be around 5. In acidic environment, the ammonia produced in colon is converted to ammonium ion which is less diffusible back into circulation and thereby removed along with stools. Gut decontamination using various antibiotics is been used to eliminate ammoniagenic bacteria from the gut, to decrease the ammonia load in the intestine in HE. *L-Ornithine l-aspartate (LOLA)* can be beneficial and the protective effect on brain is probably due to overall decrease in ammonia level rather than direct effect on brain. Sodium benzoate (250 mg/kg/day) along with intravenous (IV) sodium phenylacetate (250 mg/kg/day) or oral sodium phenylbutyrate (250 mg/kg/day) can be used to eliminate ammonia by alternate pathways. Extracorporeal liver support such as continuous venovenous hemodialysis can help in removing ammonia, while liver transplantation remains the definitive treatment.

Hepatorenal Syndrome

The general principles include treating precipitating factors and avoiding agents and factors which can precipitate hepatorenal syndrome. Other causes of renal failure should be excluded. Dehydration, GI hemorrhage, and sepsis should be treated promptly. Two groups of medications namely renal vasodilators (dopamine and prostaglandins) and systemic vasoconstrictors (terlipressin and ornipressin) have been tried as treatment. Studies have shown that terlipressin when used alone or with albumin has higher efficacy in reversing the renal function in patients with hepatorenal syndrome.[15] Liver transplantation is the definitive treatment for patients with hepatorenal syndrome, as it corrects liver dysfunction and eliminates portal hypertension. For those who do not respond to vasoconstrictors or develop volume overload, intractable metabolic acidosis, or hyperkalemia, dialysis may be a reasonable option as a bridge to transplantation.

Hepatopulmonary Syndrome

Liver transplantation remains the only effective treatment that reverses HPS.

Definitive Treatment

Definitive disease-specific medical treatment for WD, autoimmune liver disease, and neonatal cholestatic disorders are outlined in respective chapters. There are certain prognostic models that have been developed to indicate when such patient with CLD would require a liver transplant. *Prognostic scores* that are generally used in children are Child–Turcott–Pugh (CTP) score and Pediatric End-Stage Liver Disease (PELD) score. These are used to prognosticate and register for liver transplantation **(Table 12.14.3)**.

Once the CLD progresses to ESLD where there are signs and symptoms of liver failure such as synthetic failure and detoxification failure, the only definitive treatment is liver transplantation. Indications for liver transplantation in CLD are outlined in **Box 12.14.2**.

TABLE 12.14.3: Prognostic scores for chronic liver disease (CLD) in children.

Score	*Parameters*	*Mortality risk or need for liver transplant*
PELD	• Bilirubin • Albumin • INR • Growth (weight and height) • Age <1 year	Score >12
CTP score	• Bilirubin • Albumin • INR • Hepatic encephalopathy • Ascites	Score >9

(CTP: Child–Turcott–Pugh; INR: international normalized ratio; PELD: Pediatric End-Stage Liver Disease)

BOX 12.14.2: Indications for liver transplantation in chronic liver disease.*

- *Life expectancy:* Anticipated length of life <18 months (because of liver disease)
- Unacceptable quality of life (because of liver disease)
- Growth failure or impairment due to liver disease
- Reversible neurodevelopmental impairment due to liver disease [hepatic encephalopathy (HE)]
- Likelihood of irreversible end organ damage (which may be renal, respiratory, or cardiovascular depending on underlying disorder)

*Operating Principles for Liver Transplant Centers in the UK and Republic of Ireland. Prepared by the NHSBT Liver Advisory Group.

KEY MESSAGES

- Unlike adults, in children, the causes of CLD are more varied and include several genetically inherited metabolic disorders.
- Some of the CLDs are preventable, while some are treatable with either diet modification, enzyme replacement, or specific medications.
- All children with CLD should be immunized with hepatitis A virus (HAV) and hepatitis B virus (HBV) vaccines.
- Liver transplantation should be offered whenever required at the appropriate time.

REFERENCES

1. Kuntz K. Clinical aspects of liver diseases. In: Kuntz K (Ed). Hepatology: Textbook and Atlas. Berlin: Springer-Verlag; 2008. pp. 397-417.
2. Ahmad A, Ahmad R. Understanding the mechanism of hepatic fibrosis and potential therapeutic approaches. Saudi J Gastroenterol. 2012:18(3):155-67.
3. Fallowfield J, Hayes P. Pathogenesis and treatment of hepatic fibrosis: is cirrhosis reversible? Clin Med (Lond). 2011;11(2):179-83.
4. Pierro A, Koletzko B, Carnielli V, Superina RA, Roberts EA, Filler RM, et al. Resting energy expenditure is increased in infants and children with extrahepatic biliary atresia. J Pediatr Surg. 1989;24(6):534-8.
5. Chin SE, Shepherd RW, Thomas BJ, Cleghorn GJ, Patrick MK, Wilcox JA, et al. The nature of malnutrition in children with end-stage liver disease awaiting orthotopic liver transplantation. Am J Clin Nutr. 1992;56(1):164-8.
6. Shepherd RW, Chin SE, Cleghorn GJ, Patrick M, Ong TH, Lynch SV, et al. Malnutrition in children with chronic liver disease accepted for liver transplantation: clinical profile and effect on outcome. J Paediatr Child Health. 1991;27(5):295-9.
7. Cash WJ, McConville P, McDermott E, McCormick PA, Callender ME, McDougall NI. Current concepts in the assessment and treatment of hepatic encephalopathy. QJM. 2010;103(1):9-16.
8. Quero Guillén JC, Herrerías Gutiérrez JM. Diagnostic methods in hepatic encephalopathy. Clin Chim Acta. 2006;365(1-2):1-8.
9. Ferenci P, Lockwood A, Mullen K, Tarter R, Weissenborn K, Blei AT. Hepatic encephalopathy–definition, nomenclature, diagnosis, and quantification: final report of the working party at the 11th World Congresses of Gastroenterology, Vienna, 1998. Hepatology. 2002;35(3):716-21.
10. Abrams GA, Nanda NC, Dubovsky EV, Krowka MJ, Fallon MB. Use of macroaggregated albumin lung perfusion scan to diagnose hepatopulmonary syndrome: a new approach. Gastroenterology. 1998;114(2):305-10.
11. El-Shabrawi MH, Omran S, Wageeh S, Isa M, Okasha S, Mohsen NA. (99m)Technetium-macroaggregated albumin perfusion lung scan versus contrast enhanced echocardiography in the diagnosis of the hepatopulmonary syndrome in children with chronic liver disease. Eur J Gastroenterol Hepatol. 2010;22(8):1006-12.
12. Goel V, Kar P. Hepatic osteodystrophy. Trop Gastroenterol. 2010;31(2):82-6.
13. Klein GL, Soriano H, Shulman RJ, Levy M, Jones G, Langman CB. Hepatic osteodystrophy in chronic cholestasis: evidence for a multifactorial etiology. Pediatr Transplant. 2002;6(2):136-40.
14. Goldschmidt I, Streckenbach C, Dingemann C, Pfister ED, di Nanni A, Zapf A, et al. Application and limitations of transient liver elastography in children. J Pediatr Gastroenterol Nutr. 2013;57(1):109-13.
15. Martín-Llahí M, Pépin MN, Guevara M, Díaz F, Torre A, Monescillo A, et al. Terlipressin and albumin vs albumin in patients with cirrhosis and hepatorenal syndrome: a randomized study. Gastroenterology. 2008;134(5):1352-9.

12.15 Pediatric Liver Transplantation

Neelam Mohan

INTRODUCTION

Liver transplantation (LT) or hepatic transplantation is the replacement of a diseased liver with a healthy liver allograft. The most commonly used technique is orthotopic transplantation, in which the native liver is removed and the donor organ is placed in the same anatomic location as the original liver. Dr Thomas Starzl performed the first pediatric liver transplant in 1963.[1] Since then, new advances and techniques in both surgical and medical management have increased the incidence and improved the outcomes of LT. While pediatric LT accounts for only a small proportion of all LTs, there are sufficient differences between pediatric and adult patients seeking LT. Pediatric LT constitutes approximately 10% of the transplants done in adults and children together. Etiology and the challenges following LT in children are much different from adults and require the specialized care by a team of pediatric transplantation physicians and pediatric hepatologists.

INDICATIONS FOR LIVER TRANSPLANTATION IN CHILDREN

Mostly, LT is indicated in children when the risk of mortality from the native liver disease is higher than the overall risk of transplantation. The indications for LT in children traditionally were end-stage liver disease (ESLD) with a predicted life expectancy <1 year, acute liver failure (ALF), nonresectable liver tumors in the absence of significant extrahepatic disease, and metabolic liver diseases (MLDs). With the improved survival of children undergoing LT for these conventional indications, LT is increasingly being done for nontraditional indications. These include growth failure, intractable pruritus or bone density loss from cholestatic liver disease, and intractable seizures due to MLD.

Generally, the indications for LT are divided into the following and the detailed causes are listed in **Box 12.15.1**:

- Cholestatic hepatic diseases
- MLD
- ALF
- Liver tumors
- Autoimmune or advanced chronic viral hepatitis
- Cryptogenic.

Cholestatic Liver Disease

Globally, biliary atresia (BA) is the most common indication for LT in children. Untreated BA is fatal. Early diagnosis of BA could result in Kasai portoenterostomy within 6–10 weeks of life which may give transplant-free survival in early childhood. Late diagnosis of BA would result in early biliary cirrhosis necessitating LT. Following hepatoportoenterostomy, these babies would fall in two groups:

1. *Recurrent cholangitis progressing to ESLD.* If serum total bilirubin is over 6 mg/dL 3 months after portoenterostomy, these children would need LT.
2. *Successful portoenterostomy leads to satisfactory biliary drainage* but most frequently these children end with cirrhosis and ESLD in adolescence or late childhood.

Recent concern among experts is to offer primary LT for delayed diagnosis of BA with advanced disease. Studies have shown that though there is no difference in survival in BA with/without prior Kasai surgery, morbidity is more in LT done before Kasai surgery.[2] Complications of post-hepatoportoenterostomy that require LT include failure of biliary drainage with progressive cholestasis, portal

BOX 12.15.1: Indications for pediatric liver transplantation.

Cholestatic disease
- Biliary atresia (BA)
- Progressive familial intrahepatic cholestasis (PFIC)
- Sclerosing cholangitis (primary/neonatal/Langerhans cell histiocytosis)
- Idiopathic neonatal hepatitis
- Alagille syndrome (bile duct paucity syndrome)

Metabolic liver disease (MLD)
- Wilson disease (WD)
- Tyrosinemia type I
- Glycogen storage disease (GSD) types I, III, and IV
- Crigler–Najjar syndrome type I
- Alpha1-antitrypsin deficiency
- Cystic fibrosis (CF)
- Urea cycle defects
- Primary hyperoxaluria
- Organic acidemia
- Familial hypercholesterolemia

Acute liver failure (ALF)
- *Neonates:*
  - *Infectious:* Herpes viruses, echovirus, adenovirus, and hepatitis B virus (HBV)
  - *Metabolic:* Galactosemia, tyrosinemia, neonatal hemochromatosis, mitochondrial disease, and fatty acid oxidation (FAO) defects
- *Older children:*
  - *Infectious:* Hepatitis A virus (HAV), hepatitis B virus (HBV), herpes viruses, sepsis, and other
  - *Drugs:* Acetaminophen, valproate, isoniazid, carbamazepine, halothane, and propylthiouracil
  - *Toxins: Amanita phalloides*, carbon tetrachloride, and phosphorus
  - *Metabolic:* WD, hereditary fructose intolerance, and tyrosinemia
  - Mitochondrial diseases
  - *Autoimmune:* Types 1 and 2

Hepatic tumors
- Nonresectable hepatoblastoma
- Nonresectable hepatocellular carcinoma
- Nonresectable large benign tumors (hemangioendothelioma)

Chronic hepatitis with decompensated liver diseases
- Autoimmune hepatitis
- Chronic viral hepatitis (B and C)
- Cryptogenic cirrhosis
- Nonalcoholic steatohepatitis (NASH) with cirrhosis

Others
- Budd–Chiari syndrome
- Polycystic liver disease
- Caroli disease
- Traumatic/postsurgical biliary tract diseases
- Factor VII deficiency
- Primary immunodeficiency with cirrhosis (combined liver and bone marrow transplantation)

hypertension, refractory ascites or gastrointestinal (GI) bleeding, recurrent cholangitis, or hepatopulmonary syndrome.

Other common cholestasis causes of liver transplant are:

- Alagille syndrome with either advanced liver disease or intractable pruritus
- Progressive familial intrahepatic cholestasis (PFIC)

Progressive Familial Intrahepatic Cholestasis and Liver Transplantation

The PFIC is a group of inherited cholestatic disorders in which bile salt, phospholipid, or cholesterol transport genes are affected resulting in abnormal or absent. The most common types include PFIC1 (deficiency of FIC1 protein), PFIC2 (bile salt export pump deficiency), and PFIC3. PFIC is a heterogeneous group of disorders characterized by defects in bile secretion and presentation with intrahepatic cholestasis in infancy or childhood. Newer variants of PFIC includes PFIC4 (loss of function of *TJP2*), PFIC5 *(NR1H4)*, PFIC6 *(MYO5B)* gene mutation, and PFIC7.[3]

The spectrum of clinical manifestations in PFIC varies from mild to severe leading to ESLD. Indications for LT in PFIC include decompensated chronic liver disease (CLD) (ESLD and advanced fibrosis), growth failure (not amenable to dietary modification), refractory pruritus despite biliary diversion surgery, and associated complications like hepatopulmonary syndrome. Recently, newer drugs are available in the West to control itching in PFIC. Around 15% of neonatal transplants are for PFIC. Outcomes of LT in PFIC1 patients have not been very favorable, as they may continue to present with diarrhea or have recurrence of disease with steatosis and cirrhosis, baseline high volume diarrhea, posttransplant steatosis, and eventual cirrhosis.

Metabolic Liver Disease

Metabolic liver disease is an important and often the second leading cause of LT in children. The disease may be limited to the liver, e.g., Crigler–Najjar syndrome or have multiple organ involvement, e.g., Wilson disease (WD) and tyrosinemia. These disorders result from mutations affecting amino acid, metal, lipid, or carbohydrate metabolism, or mitochondrial function. Broadly, LT in a setting of an inherited metabolic disorder is offered to children who can be cured or whose medical management can be significantly simplified with LT, LT is life-saving and achieves phenotypic and functional cure of MLD. LT to correct the metabolic defect should be considered before other organ systems are affected, or the consequences of the defect result in irreversible quality of life; or the complications become contraindications for transplantation. Thus, these patients should be referred to a transplant facility early so that timely intervention can be ensured before the occurrence of irreparable damage. The indications of performing LT in inborn errors of metabolism have been expanded now to improve the quality of life from being life-saving and to avoid long-term sequelae.

Pediatric Acute Liver Failure

Pediatric acute liver failure (PALF) is defined as per PALF Longitudinal Research Study criteria.[4] These include evidence of deranged liver function associated with liver-induced coagulopathy and international normalized ration (INR) >2 (nonresponsive to vitamin K) or an INR >1.5 along with evidence of encephalopathy in the absence of a known CLD.

Pediatric acute liver failure is a heterogeneous condition with many different etiologies. The etiology of PALF includes viral hepatitis, MLD, drugs or toxins, autoimmune liver disease, sepsis, hypoxia, or ischemia secondary to thrombosis of vasculature of liver. Rarely mitochondrial disorders and fatty acid oxidation defects could be the underlying cause in young children, and neonatal hemochromatosis in newborns. There could be few genetic diseases (e.g., *NBAS* gene) which may result in liver failure. Recently, immune disease has also been identified as an underlying etiology of PALF, which can respond to immunosuppressive therapy.[5] Often the underlying etiology of ALF may not be identified and these cases are labeled under cryptogenic category, which constitute as large as 20–30% of the cases globally. A significant proportion of children with ALF have spontaneous recovery of liver function depending on the age of the child and underlying etiology.

The decision to proceed with transplantation should be made at a point when there is no clinically significant evidence of liver regeneration or recovery of function. It is often difficult to identify the children who may not recover spontaneously and need LT. The King's College Hospital criteria **(Box 12.15.2)** have been extensively used and have been criticized for lack of sensitivity, though they have a high degree of specificity. More recent recommendation from the same group is to use an INR > 4 (though this is not appreciable in cases of viral hepatitis) or factor V concentration <20% as the best available criteria for listing for LT. In addition, several other criteria have been suggested based on bilirubin, INR, and ammonia or high lactate at presentation. The issues of identifying an appropriate criteria becomes difficult due to various factors including age, presentation, etiology, incorporation bias, blood product interventions, time points of studies (admission and peak), whether it is a multicentric study or single center enrolment, assessment and outcome as LT/death or death alone, calibration and discrimination cutoff used in the study and missing data due to retrospective validation on studies. Although these various criteria are helpful, careful observation for progression and clinical change is most rewarding. It is always important to refer PALF cases early to a center with facility for LT.

BOX 12.15.2: The King's College criteria transplantation in pediatric acute liver failure.

For acetaminophen poisoning:
- Arterial pH <7.3
- Or the following three factors:
  1. Prothrombin time (PT) >100 sec
  2. Creatinine >3.5 mg/dL
  3. Grade III or IV encephalopathy

For other causes:
- PT >100 sec
- Or any three of the following:
  1. PT >50 seconds
  2. Bilirubin >17.5 mg/dL
  3. Age <10 years
  4. Cryptogenic or drug-induced
  5. Jaundice for >7 days before onset of encephalopathy

Liver Tumors

The most common liver tumor in children is hepatoblastoma. In patients with nonresectable and chemoresistant tumors, with no extrahepatic metastasis, LT is a viable option. In children with hepatoblastoma and metastasis in lung, LT can be considered following chemotherapy if positron emission tomography-computed tomography PET–CT scan is clear of metastasis. Occasionally a pulmonary wedge resection may be performed and if the margins are free of tumor, one may proceed for LT.

Others Conditions

Autoimmune Hepatitis

Autoimmune hepatitis (AIH) is a progressive inflammatory liver disorder characterized by increase in serum levels of aminotransferases, immunoglobulin G (IgG), and the presence of autoantibodies such as anti-smooth muscle antibody (ASMA), antinuclear antibody (ANA), anti-liver-kidney microsomal antibody (LKM_1), and soluble liver antigen (SLA). LT is considered in patients with AIH who present with ALF or those who develop complications of ESLD. Post LT, these cases need to be monitored for recurrence of liver disease in graft. Hepatitis with autoimmune sclerosing cholangitis has a very high risk of recurrence.

Budd–Chiari Syndrome

Budd–Chiari syndrome (BCS) results from outflow tract obstruction of hepatic venous system at any level like intrahepatic hepatic vein or inferior vena cava (IVC) from any mechanism exclusive of cardiac disease. LT is a good option in selected case of BCS.

Inborn Errors of Metabolism

Inborn errors of metabolism can be divided into two types, those in which liver is the primary organ to be affected such as tyrosinemia, glycogen storage disease (GSD), or WD and in those where the primary organ affected is not the liver but the enzyme defect is in liver, necessitating the need of LT, e.g., primary hyperoxaluria, an autosomal recessive genetic disorder with lack of alanine-glyoxylate aminotransferase enzymes in liver leading to systemic oxalosis, renal calculi, and renal failure. Other organs such as heart and eyes may also be affected due to systemic oxalosis. Timely diagnosis of the condition may salvage these patients combined with heart and kidney transplant. In urea cycle defects and organic acidemias, neurological involvement is seen but hepatic enzyme deficiency exists. The purpose of LT in this group of diseases is to replace the missing hepatic enzyme to prevent or reverse extrahepatic disease. Other such conditions include Crigler–Najjar syndrome type 1, familial hypercholesterolemia and maple syrup urine disease.

In a large series of 200 pediatric LT reported by the author from India, the leading indications of LT were cholestatic liver disease (46%) followed by MLD (33%) and ALF/acute on chronic liver failure (28.5%).[6]

CONTRAINDICATIONS TO LIVER TRANSPLANTATION

Contraindications include extrahepatic malignance, advanced cardiopulmonary diseases, sepsis, and with ongoing multiorgan failure.

PRETRANSPLANT EVALUATION

Pretransplantation evaluation of the child is particularly important and should include the following:

- Assessment of the severity of the liver disease and the possibility for medical management
- Assessment of the technical feasibility of the operation
- Consideration of any contraindications
- Psychological preparation of the family and child

The assessment has been given in **Box 12.15.3**.

PREPARATIONS FOR LIVER TRANSPLANTATION

Immunization

Most units consider live vaccines to be contraindicated after LT because of the risk of dissemination, secondary to immunosuppression. It is therefore better to complete normal immunizations before transplant if feasible. All attempts should be made to immunize the child while waiting for LT; often an accelerated schedule may be needed. Ideally, LT should not be performed within 2–3 weeks following administration of a live vaccine.

Growth Monitoring

Growth failure is common in CLDs, due to malnutrition due to factors such as poor intake due to decreased appetite,

BOX 12.15.3: Pretransplant assessment.

- *Nutritional status:* Height, weight, triceps skinfold, midarm muscle area, midarm circumference
- *Identification of hepatic complications:* Ascites and varices
- *Cardiac assessment:* Electrocardiography (ECG), echocardiography (ECHO), chest radiography, and cardiac catheterization
- *Respiratory function:* Oxygen saturation, ventilation-perfusion scan, and lung function tests
- *Neurologic and developmental assessment:* EEG, Bayley developmental scales, and Stanford–Binet intelligence scales
- *Renal function:* Urea, creatinine, electrolytes, urinary protein-to-creatinine ratio, and chromium ethylene diamine-tetra-acetic acid (EDTA)
- *Serology:* Cytomegalovirus (CMV); Epstein–Barr virus (EBV); varicella zoster virus (VZV); herpes simplex virus (HSV); hepatitis A, B, and C; human immunodeficiency virus (HIV); and measles
- *Hematology:* Complete blood count (CBC), platelets, and blood groups
- *Radiology:* Ultrasonography (USG) of liver and spleen for vascular anatomy, wrist radiography for bone age, and rickets
- Dental assessment

abdominal distension, faulty feeding with vomiting, poor tolerance, and poor absorption. Children with CLD are at risk for malnutrition, as they need 20–80% more calories than normal children to achieve adequate growth. It has been demonstrated in several studies that nutritional status at LT is an important prognostic factor in survival. A high-calorie protein feed (150–200% of estimated average requirement) is required with high calorie supplements given orally or by nocturnal nasogastric enteral feeding or continuous enteral feeding. Fat-soluble vitamin deficiencies (A, D, E, and K) are common in CLD patients and they must be adequately supplemented besides water-soluble vitamins supplementation.

Management of Hepatic Complications

It is important to ensure that specific hepatic complications such as variceal bleeding, ascites, and spontaneous bacterial peritonitis are appropriately managed while the patient waits for LT.

Psychological Preparation

Liver transplant is a major undertaking for the child and family; thus, psychological counseling, information giving, and preparation of the child and family is an essential component of pretransplantation management.

LIVER TRANSPLANT SURGERY

The graft is either a cadaveric liver or a living related.

Cadaveric Liver Transplantation

Here, the liver of a brain-dead person is used for transplantation. Cadaveric transplants could be:

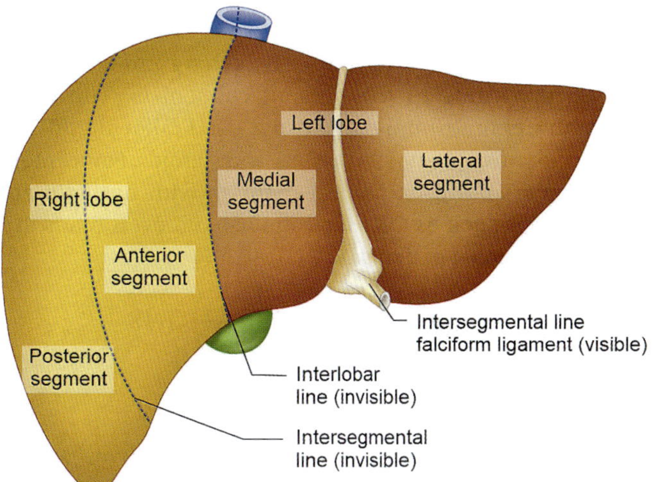

Fig. 12.15.1: Segments of liver.

- *Whole graft:* The entire graft is transplanted in the recipient.
- *Reduced graft:* When only a part of the cadaveric liver (i.e., right/left/left lateral part) is used for the recipient **(Fig. 12.15.1)**.
- *Split graft:* The shortage of suitable organs for young children led to development of split livers. The liver of the cadaveric donor is divided and used for two patients, usually the right lobe for adults and left lobe for children.

Living-related Liver Transplantation

This has been a further step to answer the shortage of organs for children. In living-related LT, a part of the liver from a living related donor is used in the child. This procedure is more popular in Eastern countries such as Japan, Korea, and India where cadaveric LT has not been possible until recently. To carry out living-related LT, two-transplant surgeons' teams are required as simultaneously surgery is being carried out on the donor and the recipient.

Mostly blood compatible transplants are done. However, in living-related LT scenarios, ABO incompatible transplants are also being done with preoperative use of plasmapheresis with rituximab in older children along with modified immunosuppression.

Auxiliary Liver Transplant

The term auxiliary liver transplant is referred when a part of the donor liver (usually segments 2 + 3) is implanted beside or in continuity with the native liver. The main purpose of this form of liver transplant is to ensure that the native liver is retained in the event of graft failure or for the future development of gene therapy. Auxiliary transplant is now accepted therapy for Crigler–Najjar syndrome type I and also for propionic acidemia and ornithine transcarbamylase deficiency while its role in the management of fulminant hepatic failure is more controversial.

Immunosuppression

Following LT, the patient requires lifelong immunosuppression according to the present consensus. The most common immunosuppressive drugs used following LT are tacrolimus, mycophenolate mofetil, and steroids. Few centers use steroid-sparing induction regimen with basiliximab. Newer drugs such as OKT3, sirolimus, and everolimus are used in occasional patients.

POSTOPERATIVE COMPLICATIONS

Early Postoperative Complications

Primary Graft Nonfunction

Primary nonfunctioning of the transplanted liver occurs within 48 hours. The cause is unknown and may be related to cadaveric donor factor; this is not seen in living-related transplant scenarios. The only appropriate management is retransplant.

Surgical Complications of Intra-abdominal Hemorrhage

- *Hepatic artery thrombosis (HAT):* HAT is a potentially life-threatening complication. Incidence of HAT ranges from 2 to 10% after LT in the pediatric population. Recent studies show decreased incidence. Improved outcomes are due to the progress made in surgical techniques. HAT may present as ALF with raised liver enzymes, sepsis, and biliary issues. HAT is typically diagnosed by absent hepatic artery flow in Doppler ultrasound, which can be further confirmed by a contrast-enhanced triphasic CT scan of abdomen. Treatment of HAT is by arterial thrombectomy performed by interventional radiology or surgical exploration. When revascularization fails, urgent retransplantation is mandatory. Monitoring for biliary complications/liver abscess is needed in HAT.
- *Portal vein complications:* Portal vein thrombosis (PVT) and portal vein stenosis (PVS) are common complications ranging between 4 and 12% of pediatric LT recipients. Younger recipient age, BA, variant graft, and prolonged warm ischemia are high risk factor. Early PVT occurs within 30 days of LT and late PVT beyond 30 days of LT. Treatment of PVT is usually radiological intervention or by surgical thrombectomy.[7]

Rejection

Acute cellular rejection may occur between 7 and 10 days postoperatively. The incidence of acute rejection varies. It is less common in infants (20%) but increases to 50–60% in older children and adults. In majority of the cases, it responds with increase in immunosuppression and high dose of steroids.

Biliary Complications

Biliary complications occur in approximately 10–30% of pediatric LT recipients and are risk factors for fungal infection. They include biliary strictures (BSs), bile leaks (BLs), bilomas, excluded ducts, stones, and cast formation. BLs occur more frequently in patients with bilioenteric anastomosis compared with that of duct-to-duct anastomosis. BL is treated often conservatively by maintaining the abdominal drain. Biliary complications are managed either by surgical, endoscopic, or radiological intervention.[8]

Enteric Complications

The incidence of the enteric complications after pediatric LT is reported in 6.4–20% of cases, especially in in post-Kasai children.[9]

Sepsis

Infection is still the most common complication following LT. Infections may be bacterial or fungal. Bacterial infections are most common immediately after LT and are related to the high doses of immunosuppressive drugs and central line infections. The mortality of patients with systemic infection is high.

Late Complications Post-transplant

These fall into two general categories:

1. *Complication related to allograft itself:* They include chronic rejection, cytomegalovirus (CMV) and Epstein–Barr virus (EBV) infection, late BS, hepatic artery or PVT, post-transplant lymphoproliferative disease, and de novo AIH.
2. *Those related to immunosuppressive drugs:* These include nephrotoxicity, hyperlipidemia, hypertension, hyperglycemia, food allergy, and hirsutism secondary mostly due to immunosuppressive drugs.

OUTCOME

Due to advances in liver surgery and immunosuppressant regimens, the survival rates have significantly increased than earlier with a 95% survival at 1 year post-LT and 85–90% at 10 years post-LT. In a large series of pediatric LTs from India, the overall 1-year survival rate was 94% and 5-year actuarial survival was 87% with no statistically significant difference between children with weight <10 kg versus those with >10 kg. Outcome in ALF did not differ significantly between those with ALF on CLF versus those with CLD.[10]

Quality-of-Life

It is now anticipated that children who survive LT will achieve a normal lifestyle despite the necessity for continuous monitoring of immunosuppressive treatment. An important aspect of long-term survival is the development of puberty. A long-term study from France has demonstrated that there are no differences between the genders in attaining puberty and developing secondary sexual characteristics.[11]

CONCLUSION

Liver transplantation in children is now a well-accepted treatment for end-stage liver disease. Surgical, medical and pharmacological advances contributed to significant improvement in the outcome of liver transplantation. Biliary atresia is the mostcommon cause of liver transplantation globally and in India. In India, pediatric liver transplant is being performed with excellent results in few centers in private sector. Liver transplantation in small babies is highly challenging and requires the expertise of a multidisciplinary team, including pediatric-trained anesthetists, intensivists, interventional radiologists besides transplant surgeons, and liver transplant hepatologist. In India, the liver transplantation program is predominantly living related and there is a huge need to promote cadaveric organ donation and eventually establish the program in public sector too.

REFERENCES

1. Schaefer F. Growth and development after organ transplantation. In: Kirk AD, Knechtie SJ, Larsen CP, Madsen JC, Pearson TC, Webber SA (Eds). Textbook of Organ Transplantation, 1st edition. Hoboken, New Jersey: Wiley-Blackwell; 2014. pp. 1435-42.
2. Lemoine CP, LeShock JP, Brandt KA, Superina R. Primary Liver Transplantation vs. Transplant after Kasai Portoenterostomy for Infants with Biliary Atresia. J Clin Med. 2022;11(11):3012.
3. Alam S, Lal BB. Recent updates on progressive familial intrahepatic cholestasis types 1, 2 and 3: Outcome and therapeutic strategies. World J Hepatol. 2022;14(1):98-118.
4. Shanmugam NP, Dhawan A. Selection criteria for liver transplantation in pediatric acute liver failure: The saga continues. Pediatr Transplant. 2011;134(15):5-6.
5. Chapin CA, Burn T, Meijome T, Loomes KM, Melin-Aldana H, Kreiger PA, et al. Indeterminate pediatric acute liver failure is uniquely characterized by a CD103+ CD8+ T cell infiltrate. Hepatology. 2018;68(3):1087-100.
6. Mohan N, Karkra S, Rastogi A, Dhaliwal MS, Raghunathan V, Goyal D, et al. Outcome of 200 Pediatric Living Donor Liver Transplantations in India. Indian Pediatr. 2017;54(11):913-8.
7. Alfares BA, Bokkers RPH, Verkade HJ, Dierckx RAJO, Gupte G, Franchi-Abella S, et al. Portal vein obstruction after pediatric liver transplantation: a systematic review of current treatment strategies. Transplant Rev. 2021;35(4):100630
8. Gheorghe G, Diaconu CC, Bungau S, Bacalbasa N, Motas N, Ionescu V-A. Biliary and Vascular Complications after Liver Transplantation–From Diagnosis to Treatment. Medicina (Kaunas). 2023;59(5):850.
9. Dehghani SM, Nikeghbalian S, Kazemi K, Dehghani M, Gholami S, Bahador A, et al. Outcome of bowel perforation after pediatric liver transplantation. Pediatr Transplant. 2008;12(2):146-9.
10. Gad EH, Sallam AN, Soliman H, Ibrahim T, Salem TAH, Ali MA, et al. Pediatric living donor liver transplantation (LDLT): Short- and long-term outcomes during sixteen years period at a single centre—A retrospective cohort study. Ann Med Surg (Lond). 2022;79:103938.
11. Hager A, Mager D, Robert C, Nicholas D, Gilmour S. Health-Related Quality of Life 10 Years after Liver Transplantation: A Longitudinal Retrospective Review. Diagnostics (Basel). 2021;11(1):111.

12.16 Diseases of the Gallbladder

Shrish Bhatnagar

DEVELOPMENT AND ANATOMY

The gallbladder diverticulum begins to form around 5 weeks of embryonic development, originating from a portion of the ventral foregut near the liver. This diverticulum branches into two parts: The "pars cystica", which develops into the cystic duct and gallbladder, and the "pars hepatica", which further divides to form the right and left lobes of the liver. Both structures interact with the proliferating mesenchymal components of the septum transversum to create the gallbladder, extrahepatic bile ducts, and liver.

Anatomically, the gallbladder consists of the fundus, body, infundibulum, and neck. Its blood supply comes from the cystic artery, while the vagus nerve provides parasympathetic innervation that regulates gallbladder motility. The primary function of the gallbladder is to store and concentrate bile, which can be concentrated by 5–20 times through an active sodium transport mechanism. Cholecystokinin, a hormone secreted by the duodenum, stimulates gallbladder contraction, facilitating the release of bile into the duodenum via the common bile duct (CBD). Any disruptions in these developmental processes can lead to various, though uncommon, congenital anomalies of the liver, gallbladder, and pancreas.[1] The type and severity of anomalies depend on the time at which disruption or alteration of the embryological mechanisms takes place.

CONGENITAL ANOMALIES

Congenital anomalies include double gallbladder, bilobed gallbladder, vestigial and absent gallbladder, and those related to extrahepatic biliary tree are namely biliary atresia (which is discussed in Chapter 12.10: Neonatal Cholestasis Syndromes) and choledochal cysts (congenital choledochal malformation).[2,3]

Choledochal Cysts

Choledochal cysts are a rare congenital anomaly of the bile ducts, characterized by cystic dilations of the extrahepatic and/or intrahepatic biliary systems. While the incidence in Western countries is about 1 in 150,000 live births, it is more common in Asia, particularly in Japan, with rates ranging from 1 in 1,000 to 1 in 1,750 live births. The condition has a male-to-female ratio of approximately 4:1, and although it is congenital, symptoms often do not manifest until childhood or adulthood.[4]

The classification of choledochal cysts follows the Todani system, which includes five main types. Type I is the most prevalent, characterized by cystic or fusiform dilation of the CBD, while the right and left hepatic ducts remain normal.

Patients typically fall into two age groups based on their presentation. Infants under 6 months often exhibit obstructive jaundice and hepatomegaly, with bile flow potentially ceasing due to angulation and obstruction of the dilated duct after 3–6 weeks. These infants may also experience fever due to cholangitis, making their condition difficult to distinguish from biliary atresia. In older children, usually after the age of two, symptoms such as abdominal pain and jaundice may arise, often due to cyst distension or cholangitis. Additionally, these patients may experience intermittent biliary obstruction or recurrent pancreatitis.

Laboratory tests may reveal conjugated hyperbilirubinemia and elevated amylase levels. Abdominal ultrasound is the preferred diagnostic tool, and some forms of choledochal cysts can be identified through antenatal ultrasound. MRI can be useful for detailing the anomaly and its relationship to surrounding structures. The recommended treatment involves complete excision of the cyst and the creation of a biliary-enteric anastomosis to restore normal bile flow.

GALLSTONE DISEASE

Gallstones (cholelithiasis) were once thought to be uncommon in infants and children, but their diagnosis has become more frequent, largely due to the increased use of ultrasonography (USG). The exact prevalence of gallstones in children remains unclear. A hospital-based study in India reported a prevalence of 0.3% among 13,675 children, with higher rates observed in obese children and adolescents.[5]

Etiology

Cholelithiasis in children can be categorized into three main groups: Hemolytic, other known causes, and idiopathic. Approximately 20–30% of pediatric gallstones are linked to hemolytic conditions, such as sickle cell disease, hereditary spherocytosis, and thalassemia. Around 40–50% of cases arise from other known factors, including total parenteral nutrition, prolonged fasting, ileal diseases or resections, the use of furosemide, congenital biliary disorders like choledochal cysts, chronic liver disease, and progressive familial intrahepatic cholestasis (PFIC). The remaining 30–40% of cases are classified as idiopathic, with adolescent girls often experiencing idiopathic gallstones similar to adults.[2]

Gallstones can be categorized as either cholesterol stones (pure or mixed) or pigment stones (black or brown). Cholesterol stones are formed when bile becomes supersaturated with cholesterol, often leading to stasis. Mixed cholesterol stones are the most common type found in adults and adolescent girls, while pigment stones are more prevalent in children. Black pigment stones result from the supersaturation of bile with calcium bilirubinate and are commonly associated with hemolytic disorders or total parenteral nutrition. Brown pigment stones, on the other hand, are linked to infections and biliary stasis and are more frequently found in the bile ducts rather than the gallbladder.

Biliary sludge, which consists of mucin, calcium bilirubinate, and cholesterol crystals, is typically seen in cases of prolonged fasting, total parenteral nutrition, pregnancy, sickle cell disease, and treatments involving ceftriaxone or octreotide. The natural progression of biliary sludge can vary; it may resolve on its own or progress to the formation of gallstones. Persistent sludge can lead to biliary complications such as obstruction or infection.

Clinical Presentations

- *Infants (<2 years):* 10%
  - *Symptomatic:* Cholestatic jaundice, transient acholic stools, abdominal pain, and sepsis
  - *Asymptomatic:* Incidental detected
- *Children (2–14 years):* 40%
  - *Typical biliary symptoms (40–50%):* Right upper quadrant or epigastric pain with or without nausea, vomiting, and fat intolerance
  - Nonspecific abdominal pain (20–30%)

- *Acute abdomen (5–10%):* Due to acute cholecystitis, pancreatitis, or cholangitis
- Asymptomatic (20%)

- Adolescents (14–18 years); 50%; present with same as in children but right upper quadrant pain and fatty food intolerance are more common in adolescents than in children and rest are asymptomatic with incidental detection.

Diagnosis

Ultrasonography is the most widely used and accurate method for detecting gallstones. Typically, gallstones are mobile and can be single or multiple, often producing an acoustic shadow. In contrast, biliary sludge appears echogenic on ultrasound but does not cast an acoustic shadow. Gallstones as small as 1.5 mm can be identified using this technique, which has a sensitivity and specificity exceeding 95% for gallbladder cholelithiasis. For diagnosing acute cholecystitis, cholescintigraphy using technetium-99m labeled diisopropyl iminodiacetic acid (DISIDA) is the most reliable method. Additionally, magnetic resonance cholangiopancreatography (MRCP) and endoscopic retrograde cholangiopancreatography (ERCP) are increasingly utilized for evaluating complicated gallstone disease.

Management

The management of gallstones in children depends on the presence of symptoms and the patient's age. The role of stone dissolution therapy in pediatric cases remains unclear. Symptomatic or complicated gallstones typically require cholecystectomy. However, there is no consensus on the management of asymptomatic gallstones; these children can often be monitored safely, particularly if their symptoms are nonspecific.

Laparoscopic cholecystectomy is the preferred treatment, offering benefits such as reduced invasiveness, lower morbidity and mortality rates, and shorter hospital stays.

Choledocholithiasis

Common bile duct stones are typically associated with gallbladder stones, though in cases of hemolytic disorders, they can occur as primary stones. While CBD stones are relatively rare in children, accounting for only about 10% of all gallstones, their incidence is higher in infants. The clinical symptoms of CBD stones include jaundice, cholangitis, and gallstone pancreatitis. A CBD stone should be considered in patients with gallstones who exhibit hyperbilirubinemia (total bilirubin levels exceeding 1.3 mg/dL) and/or a dilated CBD on ultrasound (measuring >6 mm). The recommended approach for managing CBD stones involves ERCP, followed by laparoscopic cholecystectomy with an intraoperative cholangiogram.[2]

Acute Hydrops

Acute hydrops is defined as a sudden, noncalculus, sterile, and noninflammatory distention of the gallbladder. This condition can be associated with systemic illnesses such as scarlet fever, Kawasaki syndrome, Epstein–Barr virus infection, and Henoch–Schönlein purpura. Symptoms typically include acute abdominal pain, nausea, vomiting, and sometimes fever and jaundice. On examination, there may be tenderness in the right upper quadrant, and the gallbladder may be palpable. Ultrasound imaging reveals a distended gallbladder without the presence of stones. Management is generally conservative, focusing on supportive care and treating the underlying illness. Cholecystostomy is warranted only if imaging suggests gangrenous changes in the gallbladder, such as significant distension, pericholecystic fluid collections, or gas within the gallbladder wall or lumen. The overall prognosis for acute hydrops is excellent, with the condition likely stemming from local lymph node enlargement and vasculitis leading to gallbladder ischemia.

Acalculous Cholecystitis

Acalculous cholecystitis is an acute inflammation of the gallbladder occurring without gallstones. While rare in children, it has been linked to infections such as typhoid fever and severe systemic inflammatory states.[6] Risk factors include infection, trauma, and systemic vasculitis. The condition's pathogenesis is multifactorial, with bile stasis contributing to local ischemia and inflammation. Symptoms often include right upper quadrant or epigastric pain, nausea, vomiting, and jaundice. Treatment typically involves conservative management with broad-spectrum intravenous antibiotics and fluids. A cholecystectomy is rarely required but may be considered if the patient's condition deteriorates. Distinguishing between acalculous cholecystitis and acute hydrops can be challenging, as acalculous cholecystitis usually occurs in critically ill patients, whereas acute hydrops is often seen in less severe cases.

Biliary Dyskinesia

Biliary dyskinesia is classified as a functional disorder of the gallbladder, characterized by decreased activity and contractility without obstruction. Patients typically experience chronic right upper quadrant or epigastric discomfort in the absence of gallstones.[7] This condition is thought to arise from increased pressure in the gallbladder lumen due to uncoordinated contractions. Diagnosis can be supported by a gallbladder emptying scan using a radioactive bile tracer to assess gallbladder evacuation. A gallbladder ejection fraction of <35% is indicative of biliary dyskinesia.[8] There has been an increasing trend toward performing cholecystectomy in children and adolescents diagnosed with this condition; however, this practice remains controversial, as many patients continue to experience symptoms even after surgery.

REFERENCES

1. Sontakke YA, Gladwin V, Chand P. Anatomic Variant of Liver, Gall Bladder and Inferior Vena Cava. J Clin Diagn Res. 2016;10(7):AD03-5.
2. Goldman DA. Gallbladder, Gallstones, and Diseases of the Gallbladder in Children. Pediatr Rev. 2020;41(12):623-9.
3. Keshav N, Verma N, Parisi MT, Matesan M, Elojeimy S. Pictorial Summary of Congenital Gallbladder and Biliary Duct Anomalies Presentation on HIDA Imaging. Curr Probl Diagn Radiol. 2022;51(2):282-7.
4. Ludwig K, Santoro L, Ingravallo G, Cazzato G, Giacometti C, Dall'Igna P. Congenital anomalies of the gastrointestinal tract: the liver, extrahepatic biliary tree and pancreas. Pathologica. 2022;114(1):55-63.
5. Poddar U. Gallstone disease in children. Indian Pediatr. 2010;47(11):945-53.
6. Poddighe D, Sazonov V. Acute acalculous cholecystitis in children. World J Gastroenterol. 2018;24(43):4870-9.
7. Lugo-Vicente HL. Gallbladder dyskinesia in children. JSLS. 1997;1(1):61-4.
8. Santucci NR, Hyman PE, Harmon CM, Schiavo JH, Hussain SZ. Biliary Dyskinesia in Children: A Systematic Review. J Pediatr Gastroenterol Nutr. 2017;64(2):186-93.

12.17 Pancreatitis

Nirmala Dheivamani

INTRODUCTION

Pancreatitis is an inflammation of the pancreas presenting as abdominal pain that is often severe, as well as nausea and vomiting. The disease can occur in three forms: Acute, acute recurrent (two or more acute episodes), and chronic. This chapter will predominantly cover acute pancreatitis.

Table 12.17.1 provides the definitions of pancreatitis in children.

TABLE 12.17.1: Definitions of pancreatitis in children.

Entity	*Clinical definition*
Pediatric onset	First episode of AP occurring before the patient's 19th birthday
Acute pancreatitis (AP)	Must meet at least two of the following: 1. Abdominal pain suggestive of or compatible with AP 2. Serum amylase and/or lipase activity at least 3 times greater than the upper limit of normal 3. Imaging findings characteristic of or compatible with AP
Acute recurrent pancreatitis (ARP)	Requires at least two distinct episodes of AP, along with: 1. Complete resolution of pain (≥1 month pain-free interval between diagnoses of AP) OR 2. Complete normalization of serum amylase and lipase levels between episodes

"Suggestive" imaging findings of chronic pancreatitis include ductal changes (irregular contour of the main PD or its radicles; intraductal filling defects; calculi, stricture, or dilation) and parenchymal changes [generalized or focal enlargement, irregular contour (accentuated lobular architecture), cavities, calcifications, and heterogeneous echotexture].

ACUTE PANCREATITIS

Acute pancreatitis is a disorder of varied etiologies with obscure pathogenesis presenting as both mild disease and multiorgan failure and is difficult to treat as there is no specific treatment and has an unpredictable outcome. It is relatively uncommon during childhood and there is a significant morbidity and mortality associated with it.

Acute pancreatitis is an acute inflammatory process of the pancreas resulting in edema, hemorrhagic, or fatty necrosis of pancreatic acinar cells and peripancreatic tissues and even remote organ involvement, which are often reversible. Mild acute pancreatitis is the term reserved for pancreatitis with minimal or no organ dysfunction, whereas severe pancreatitis should be considered if there is evidence of life-threatening complications such as organ failure (shock, pulmonary insufficiency, and renal failure) or local complications such as necrosis, abscess, or pseudocyst.

EPIDEMIOLOGY

The frequency and true incidence of pancreatitis in children are unknown due to limited case reporting and underdiagnosis, but recent studies have demonstrated that the incidence of acute pancreatitis has increased even in pediatrics. A review of pancreatitis in childhood over a 15-year period concluded that pancreatitis was not rare in childhood and had a significant overall mortality rate of 30% or greater as compared to 12% in adults. Pseudocysts complicate acute pancreatitis in approximately 10–23% of cases. The incidence of pancreatic pseudocysts is greater than 50% when associated with traumatic injury to the abdomen.

ETIOPATHOGENESIS

The causes of pancreatitis are as diverse or even more in children compared to adults as shown in **Table 12.17.2**.

Drugs and blunt trauma were the leading causes for acute pancreatitis in children followed by gallstone disease, tuberculosis, mumps, viral hepatitis, and hypertriglyceridemia, according to an Indian study, and the cause was not known in 35% of cases.[1]

Acute pancreatitis usually follows a complex cascade of events. The pancreas is protected from the harmful effects of its lytic enzymes by a series of highly compartmented systems. At each step of their formation and secretion, the enzymes are totally sequestrated in a membrane-bound space.

The various potent inhibitors of proteolytic enzymes present in many body fluids, and tissues constitute a second line of protection, defending the organism against inappropriate activation of the digestive proenzymes of the pancreas. These inhibitors bind strongly to the proteases and render them inactive.

Till now, the exact mechanisms of the development of acute pancreatitis are a matter of debate. The most common and widely accepted theory is that pancreatitis develops because of an injury to the pancreatic acini or disruption of the pancreatic duct, which permits the leakage of pancreatic enzymes (trypsin, chymotrypsin, and elastase) into pancreatic tissue. The leaked enzymes become activated in the tissue, initiating autodigestion and acute pancreatitis. The activated proteases (trypsin and elastase) and lipase break down tissue and cell membranes, causing edema, vascular damage, hemorrhage, ischemia, inflammation, and necrosis with

TABLE 12.17.2: Etiology of acute pancreatitis.

Physical injury: • Abdominal trauma (blunt or penetrating) • Abdominal surgery • Endoscopic retrograde cholangiopancreatography • Posterior penetrating duodenal ulcer	*Metabolic disorders:* • Hyperlipidemia (primary type I and IV) • Diabetes mellitus • Hypercalcemia • Hyperparathyroidism • Uremia	*Pancreatic-flow obstruction disorders:* • Cystic fibrosis • Pancreas divisum • Pancreatic/ductal anomalies • Annular pancreas
Multisystem diseases: • Crohn's disease • Hemolytic uremic syndrome • Reye syndrome • Sepsis • Sarcoidosis • Shock (hypoperfusion)	*Toxins*: • Alcohol • Boric acid • Carbamate • Organophosphorus • Yellow scorpion sting *Nutritional problems*: • Hyperalimentation • Malnutrition • Rapid refeeding after starvation	*Biliary tract obstruction*: • Biliary tract anomalies – Choledochal cyst • Gallstones • Parasites (Ascaris) *Vasculitis*: • Henoch–Schönlein purpura • Kawasaki disease • Systemic lupus erythematosus
Drugs: • L-asparaginase • Azathioprine • Corticosteroids • Didanosine • Estrogens • Ethacrynic acid • Furosemide • Procainamide • Sulfasalazine • Sulfonamides • Tetracyclines • Thiazides • Valproate • Zalcitabine	*Infections*: • *Campylobacter* • *Cryptosporidium* • *Leptospira* • *Mycoplasma* • *Salmonella typhi* • *Toxoplasma* • Viruses such as mumps, coxsackie, cytomegalovirus, herpes simplex virus, hepatitis B and varicella-zoster virus	*Miscellaneous*: • Graft-versus-host disease • Hereditary • Idiopathic • Renal transplantation

Flowchart 12.17.1: Pathogenesis of acute pancreatitis.

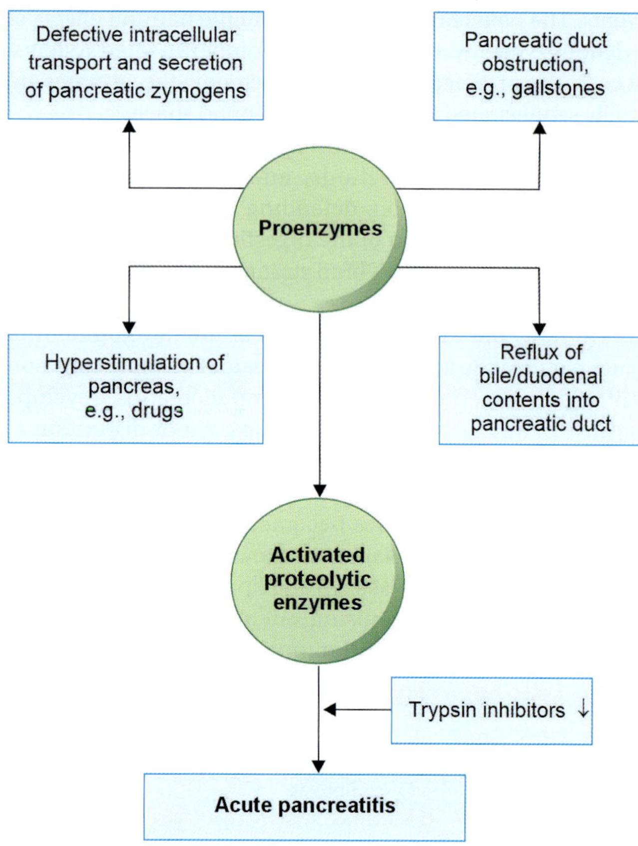

release of toxic factors in both pancreatic and peripancreatic tissues leading to systemic effects such as multiorgan failure. **Flowchart 12.17.1** illustrates the pathophysiology of acute pancreatitis.

CLINICAL FEATURES AND COMPLICATIONS

Abdominal pain with nausea and vomiting is the hallmark of pancreatitis in children as well as in adults. Abdominal pain is characteristically a sharp and steady epigastric pain of sudden onset, commonly aggravated by eating and improved by drawing the knees up to the chest. Radiation of pain to the back or pain in other sites of abdomen is rare in children unlike adults. The pain increases in intensity over 24–48 hours and the patient may require hospitalization.[2]

Infants and toddlers cannot verbalize abdominal pain, but vomiting, irritability, and lethargy are common. In severe acute pancreatitis, children may initially present with shock, followed by symptoms of multiorgan failure, including dyspnea, oliguria, hemorrhage, and mental status changes.

On physical examination, the child usually appears anxious and uncomfortable, particularly with any movement. Tachycardia and fever are common; diffuse abdominal tenderness, more marked in the upper abdomen, and quiet bowel sounds are the rule. However, the diagnosis is not always obvious, and the symptoms can easily be attributed to other acute abdominal emergencies.

Other possible findings include signs of pancreatic ascites, an epigastric mass suggestive of phlegmon or a pseudocyst formation, and bluish flanks (Grey Turner sign) or umbilicus (Cullen sign), indicating hemorrhagic pancreatitis. Evidence of pleural effusion, more commonly on the left side or dyspnea in the presence of acute respiratory distress syndrome (ARDS), may be found on examination of the chest.

Severe acute pancreatitis is rare in children. In this life-threatening condition, the patient may be acutely ill with severe abdominal pain and vomiting progressing to shock, high fever, jaundice, ascites, and pleural effusion. The mortality is highly related to systemic inflammatory response syndrome with multiple organ dysfunctions like shock, renal failure, ARDS, disseminated intravascular coagulation (DIC), and systemic infection.

Scoring Systems

There are several scoring indices that have been used as predictors of survival. Two such scoring systems are Ranson's criteria and Acute Physiology and Chronic Health Evaluation II (APACHE II) indices. Most but not all studies report that the APACHE score may be more accurate. These scoring systems are meant for adults and not well validated in children.

DeBanto Scoring

It is a prognostic scoring system to assess the severity of acute pancreatitis in children.[3] The factors identified in this study were age <7 years, weight <23 kg, admission white blood cell (WBC) >18,500, admission lactate dehydrogenase (LDH) >2,000 IU/L, ionized calcium <8.3 mg/dL at 48 hours, trough albumin <2.6 g/dL at 48 hours, 48 hours fluid sequestration >75 mL/kg/48 hours, and a 48-hour rise in blood urea nitrogen (BUN) >5 mg/dL. When the cutoff for predicting a severe outcome was set at 3 or more, the author's prediction rule was found to be more sensitive for predicting severe acute pancreatitis than Ranson scores (70 vs. 30%).

COMPLICATIONS

- *Local complications* include pancreatic pseudocyst, necrosis and phlegmon or abscess formation, splenic artery pseudoaneurysms, hemorrhage from erosions into splenic artery and vein, thrombosis of the splenic vein, superior mesenteric vein and portal veins (in descending order of frequency), duodenal obstruction, common bile duct obstruction, and progression to chronic pancreatitis.
- *Systemic complications* include ARDS, DIC, hypocalcemia (from fat saponification), hyperglycemia, multiple organ dysfunction syndrome, and insulin-dependent diabetes mellitus (DM; from pancreatic insulin-producing beta cell damage).

DIAGNOSIS

A high index of suspicion with a history of abdominal (even if trivial) trauma, drugs, or acute infections is stressed. Screening of family for hereditary or metabolic disorders associated with pancreatitis may be of help.

White blood cell counts may be increased with increased band counts, and these findings do not imply infection always. An increased hematocrit secondary to hemoconcentration, secondary to volume depletion, may be found. Also, 15% of children with pancreatitis develop hypocalcemia, and up to 25% have hyperglycemia during the acute attack. Blood urea nitrogen may be increased due to prerenal azotemia or acute renal injury, metabolic acidosis due to circulatory failure, and hypoxemia due to respiratory insufficiency.

The serum amylase concentration is elevated in at least 75% of cases of acute pancreatitis on the initial day of symptoms and remains elevated in most patients for 5–10 days. Protracted elevations of serum amylase are suggestive of pseudocyst or other complications of pancreatitis.

The serum lipase level is also usually elevated in acute pancreatitis, and serum lipase measurement is preferable to serum amylase because of its equal sensitivity and greater specificity because almost all lipase originates from the pancreas.[4] Urinary lipase levels may remain elevated for a few days longer than serum levels.

Additional tests, which have been used in the diagnosis of acute pancreatitis, include immunoreactive trypsinogen, elastase, ribonuclease, and phospholipase A, but these tests have no particular advantage. Levels of cationic trypsin are said to be a more sensitive and an early marker of pancreatic inflammation.

Radiography and Imaging

Plain X-ray Film of Abdomen

Though the abdominal plain film may be completely normal in patients with acute pancreatitis, the most commonly recognized radiologic signs associated with acute pancreatitis include the following:

- Air in the duodenal C-loop; the sentinel loop sign, which represents a focal dilated proximal jejunal loop in the left upper quadrant
- The colon cutoff sign, which represents distention of the colon up to the transverse colon with a paucity of gas distal to the splenic flexure
- One-fifth of children may show evidence of pleural effusion on chest films.

Ultrasonography

Ultrasonography (USG) is especially useful in the diagnosis of gallstones and follow-up observation of pseudocysts. An enlarged, edematous-appearing pancreas usually suggests pancreatitis on ultrasound, but the pancreas may appear completely normal in mild cases of acute pancreatitis.

Contrast-enhanced Computed Tomography

This is the standard imaging modality for the evaluation of acute pancreatitis and its complications. Using non-contrast-enhanced computed tomography (CT), clinicians can establish the diagnosis and demonstrate fluid collections but cannot evaluate for pancreatic necrosis or vascular complications.

Typical CT findings in acute pancreatitis include focal or diffuse enlargement of the pancreas, heterogeneous enhancement of the gland, irregular or shaggy contour of the pancreatic margins, blurring of peripancreatic fat planes with streaky soft tissue stranding densities, thickening of fascial planes, and the presence of intraperitoneal or retroperitoneal fluid collections. The fluid collections most commonly are found in the peripancreatic and anterior pararenal spaces but can extend from the mediastinum down to the pelvis.

Balthazar Scoring

Developed in the early 1990s by Balthazar et al., the CT Severity Index (CTSI) is a grading system used to determine the severity of acute pancreatitis.[5] The numerical CTSI has a maximum of 10 points and is the sum of the Balthazar grade points and pancreatic necrosis grade points.

CT Severity Index staging of acute pancreatitis severity has been shown by a number of studies to provide more accurate assessment than APACHE II, Ranson, and C-reactive protein level. However, a few studies indicate that CTSI is neither significantly associated with the prognosis of hospitalization in patients with pancreatic necrosis nor an accurate predictor of acute pancreatitis severity.

Magnetic Resonance Imaging

The diagnostic efficacy of MRI is comparable to that of CECT, although MRI examination is more time-consuming and costly. Magnetic resonance cholangiopancreatography (MRCP) should be performed before endoscopic retrograde cholangiopancreatography (ERCP) to detect any pancreatobiliary tract disease in children with the initial onset of acute pancreatitis of an unknown cause or if pancreatitis is recurrent.

Angiography

Angiography is primarily used to help diagnose the vascular complications of acute pancreatitis.

MANAGEMENT

The mainstay of treatment is supportive with fluid resuscitation, analgesia, and attention to nutritional needs

Flowchart 12.17.2: Management of acute pancreatitis.

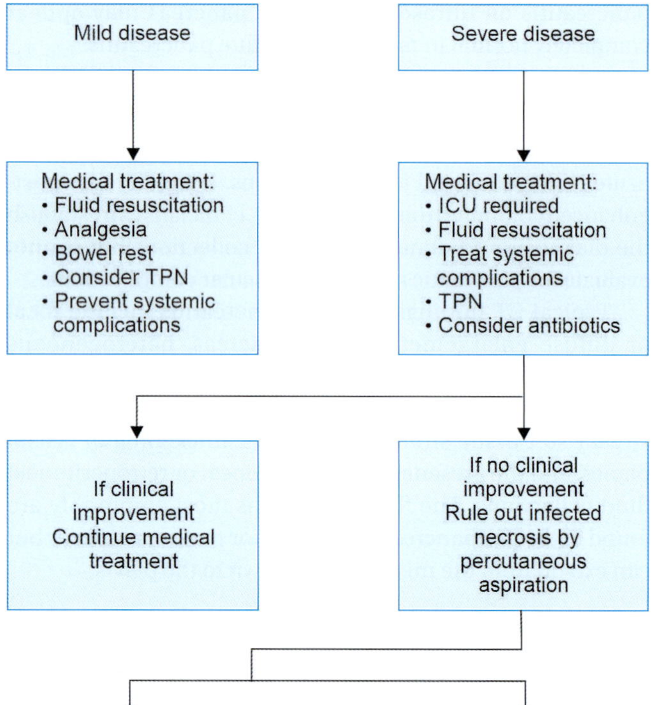

(ICU: intensive care unit; TPN: total parenteral nutrition)

and to limit systemic complications, prevention of pancreatic necrosis and infection once necrosis has occurred.[6] **Flowchart 12.17.2** depicts the protocol followed in the management of acute pancreatitis.

Fluid and Nutrition

In the management of acute pancreatitis, the treatment is to stop feeding the patient, giving him/her nothing by mouth, and giving IV fluids to prevent dehydration. Fluid administration must be sufficient to replace "third spacing" and to maintain good urine output. In prolonged cases, peripheral or central IV nutrition may be necessary because of the high metabolic rate that accompanies pancreatitis. Recently, there has been a shift in the management paradigm from total parenteral nutrition (TPN) to early enteral feeding. The advantage of enteral feeding is that it is more physiological, prevents gut mucosal atrophy, and is free from the side effects of TPN.

Pain Control

Pain in acute pancreatitis is very severe, and hence control of pain becomes necessary. The analgesics used include pentazocine, metamizole, and morphine.[7]

Treatment of Infection

The role of antibiotics is controversial. Antibiotics are generally unnecessary in mild cases even in the presence of elevated WBC counts and fever. In severe cases, antibiotics can reduce infectious pancreatitis complications and improve the prognosis.[8]

Management of Severe Pancreatitis

In severe pancreatitis, which forms a small percentage in children, the patient should be transferred to an intensive care unit for close monitoring. Fluid resuscitation helps to prevent hypotension and renal insufficiency; crystalloids may suffice but colloids may be necessary if there is hypoalbuminemia consequent to protein loss into the peritoneum. Cardiorespiratory monitoring is necessary to prevent hypoxemia, ARDS, and cardiac complications like heart failure, myocardial infarction, cardiac arrhythmia, and shock.

Surgical Treatment

Surgical management of acute pancreatitis is rarely required. Surgical intervention is only needed if the symptoms are severe and prolonged or complicated by necrosis or abscess formation that requires debridement. Peritoneal lavage has been used in adults in an effort to reduce the incidence of secondary infection; however, its efficacy has not been confirmed through clinical trials in children. If an underlying pancreatic or biliary disease is present, surgical intervention is required for cure. Surgery for pancreatic ductal disruption or compromise (i.e., acute traumatic pancreatitis with ductal injury) is indicated after medical failure.

Acute pancreatic pseudocysts, which are smaller than 5 cm in diameter, are managed with observation for 4–6 weeks. Most of them resolve spontaneously. Pancreatic pseudocysts larger than 5 cm in diameter may require surgical intervention.

Endoscopic sphincterotomy with stone extraction is the treatment of choice for pancreatitis secondary to obstruction of gallstone at the ampulla though it is found to be rare in children.

Cases of uncomplicated acute pancreatitis usually resolve within 2–4 days, but severe acute pancreatitis may require parenteral nutrition for long. Diagnosis of the specific cause of pancreatitis is important to elucidate as there is a 9% recurrence rate, most of which are diagnosed with idiopathic recurrent pancreatitis or structural anomalies.

ACUTE RECURRENT AND CHRONIC PANCREATITIS IN CHILDREN

Several studies indicate that 15–35% of children with acute pancreatitis will progress to ARP in contrary to the previous belief that most children who experienced one episode of acute pancreatitis did not go on to have additional episodes of acute pancreatitis. Acute recurrent pancreatitis (ARP) is defined as two distinct episodes of acute pancreatitis while chronic pancreatitis is caused by persistent inflammation of the pancreas **(Table 12.17.1)**.[9] Acute recurrent and pediatric (ARP) and chronic pancreatitis are relatively rare conditions and current knowledge on ARP and chronic pancreatitis are mainly derived from adult studies.

PATHOGENESIS AND RISK FACTORS

The differentiation between ARP and chronic pancreatitis is based on the morphology and/or histology of the pancreas, and ARP is considered an intermediary stage in the pathogenesis of chronic pancreatitis.[9] The basic pathogenesis of CP is persistent inflammation of the pancreas resulting in tissue injury. However, the risk factors for ARP and CP in children include:

- Genetic mutations
- Obstructive factors (e.g., pancreatic divisum and pancreaticobiliary maljunction)
- Additional risk factors (e.g., autoimmune pancreatitis and metabolic disease)

EVALUATION OF CAUSE OF ACUTE RECURRENT PANCREATITIS OR CHRONIC PANCREATITIS[9,10]

Imaging

Imaging has been used in pediatric patients and is useful in determining the cause of both ARP and CP [e.g., pancreatic divisum or pancreato-biliary malformation (PBM)], and in following its clinical course. ERCP is selectively performed in patients in whom there is a high index of suspicion of a pancreatic duct anomaly that was not detected via MRCP, as well as for therapeutic purposes. Imaging studies can confirm acute inflammatory or chronic irreversible changes, in the pancreas. Recent studies also have shown the effectiveness of endoscopic ultrasound (EUS) in the early diagnosis of CP in children with ARP, but its use remains limited.

Biochemical Tests

Abnormally low serum levels of trypsinogen, lipase, elastase-1, and pancreatic-amylase were observed during clinical remission of the disease. These lowered levels of serum pancreatic enzymes were highly specific (92–98%) but very insensitive (20–32%) in the diagnosis of chronic pancreatitis. Diabetes secondary to pancreatic disease is commonly referred to as pancreatogenic diabetes or type 3c DM. Regular annual checks of fasting blood glucose levels and hemoglobin A1c levels are used to determine disease progression.

Genetic Risk Evaluation

Recent data have demonstrated a high prevalence of genetic mutations among pediatric patients with ARP and CP. In the INSPPIRE cohort, genetic testing was encouraged only for *PRSS1* mutations.

Pancreatic Exocrine Function Tests

Flowchart 12.17.3 depicts the procedure for the evaluation of exocrine pancreatic function. In children with symptoms such as steatorrhea, diarrhea, poor weight gain and fat malabsorption, exocrine pancreatic insufficiency should be suspected. The fat digestion and absorption test, stool fat staining, 72-hour fecal fat assessment, oral fat loading test, and ^{13}C-mixed triglyceride breath test (^{13}C-MTBT) are all used to evaluate exocrine pancreatic function.

MANAGEMENT

Abdominal pain is a significant and debilitating symptom in pediatric ARP and chronic pancreatitis patients. To relieve pain, nonsteroidal anti-inflammatory drugs (NSAIDs) are commonly used as first-line treatment, progressing to opioids as necessary. An additional medical option for pain reduction is pancreatic enzyme replacement therapy (PERT). Meta-analysis of the data showed no significant benefit of PERT in pain reduction. PERT by nonenteric-coated enzymes would be considered an optional treatment for reduction of pain. PERT is also indicated in patients with exocrine pancreatic insufficiency and steatorrhea.

Endoscopic therapy of CP is an effective treatment in adults, and the evidence of its efficacy for pediatric populations has been growing. The indication for endoscopic therapy is for the management of CP complications such as pancreatic ductal stones and a narrowing pancreatic duct. Treatment involves ERCP with pancreatic sphincterotomy, pancreatic stent placement, and stone removal.

Surgery is the option when the pancreatic duct is markedly dilated due to pancreatic duct obstruction in patients with poorly controlled abdominal pain and/or

Flowchart 12.17.3: Evaluation of exocrine pancreatic function.

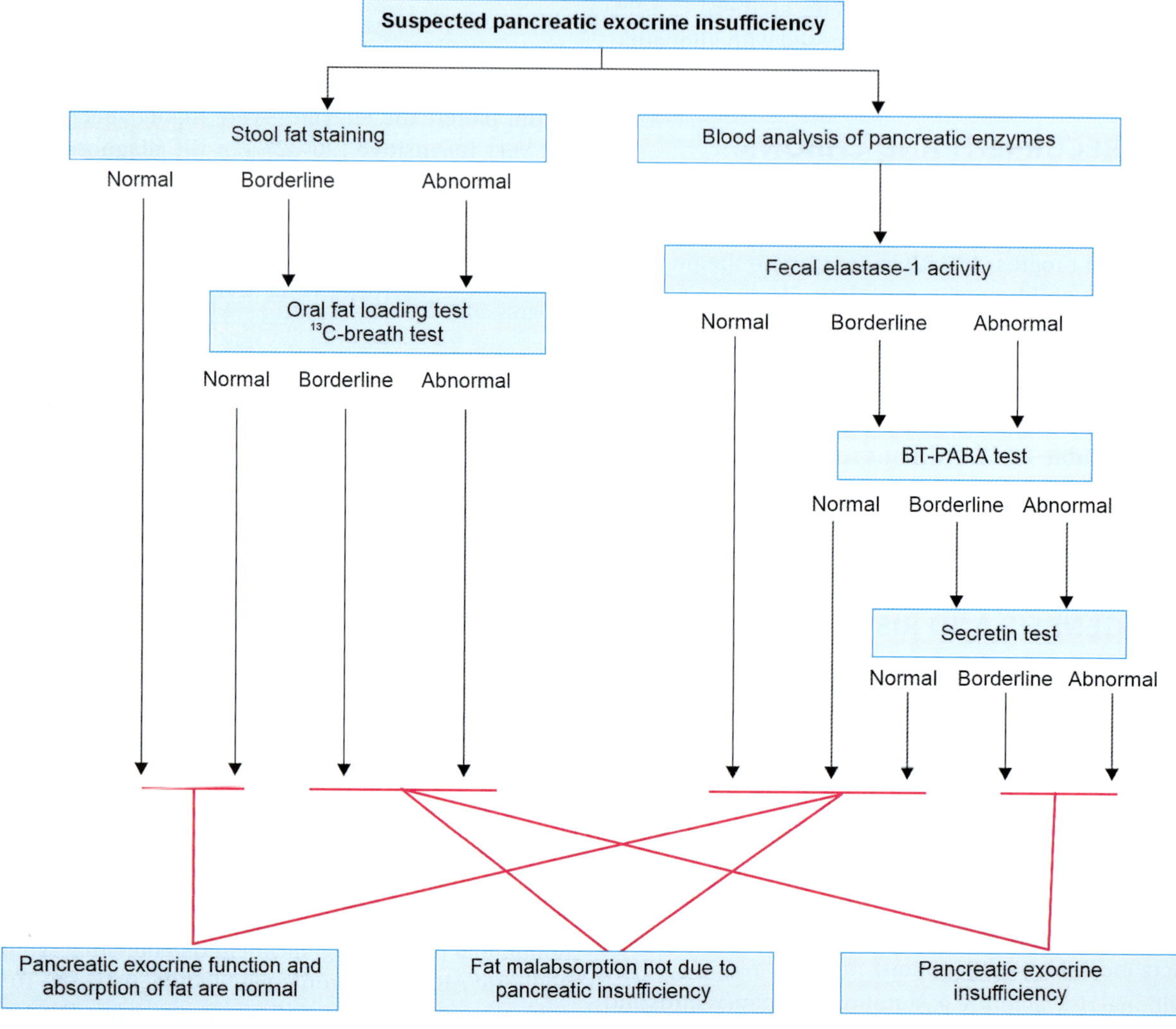

refractory main pancreatic duct strictures and longitudinal pancreaticojejunostomy (modified Puestow procedure) achieves maximum ductal drainage with minimal loss of pancreatic tissue,

CONCLUSION

- Acute pancreatitis, though rare in children, there is an increased incidence due to increased awareness among physicians.
- Causes are plenty but blunt trauma, systemic causes, and drugs are common etiologies.
- Pathogenesis still remains obscure in spite of many theories.
- Diagnosis is possible in the presence of clinical suspicion with elevated amylase and lipase, which is then confirmed by imaging.
- Management is essentially medical consisting of supportive care and prevention of complications and surgery is rarely needed.
- Mild acute pancreatitis carries good prognosis though severe pancreatitis carries high mortality.
- ARP and chronic pancreatitis in children are no more uncommon and clinicians should carefully follow up pediatric ARP and chronic pancreatitis patients, in particular patients with gene mutations indicating a potentially high risk of developing pancreatic exocrine insufficiency, DM, and pancreatic carcinoma (PC).

REFERENCES

1. Das S, Arora NK, Gupta DK, Gupta AK, Mathur P, Ahuja A. Pancreatic diseases in children in a North Indian referral hospital. Indian Pediatr. 2004;41(7):704-11.

2. Lautz TB, Chin AC, Radhakrishnan J. Acute pancreatitis in children: spectrum of disease and predictors of severity. J Pediatr Surg. 2011;46(6):1144-9.
3. DeBanto JR, Goday PS, Pedroso MR, Iftikar R, Fazel A, Nayyar S, et al. Acute pancreatitis in children. Am J Gastroenterol. 2002;97(7):1726-31.
4. Coffey MJ, Nightingale S, Ooi CY. Serum lipase as an early predictor of severity in pediatric acute pancreatitis. J Pediatr Gastroenterol Nutr. 2013;56(6):602-8.
5. Balthazar EJ. Acute pancreatitis: assessment of severity with clinical and CT evaluation. Radiology. 2002;223(3):603-13.
6. Koizumi M, Takada T, Kawarada Y, Hirata K, Mayumi T, Yoshida M, et al. JPN Guidelines for the management of acute pancreatitis: diagnostic criteria for acute pancreatitis. J Hepatobiliary Pancreat Surg. 2006;13(1):25-32.
7. Peiró AM, Martínez J, Martínez E, de madaria E, Llorens P, Pérez-Mateo M, et al. Efficacy and tolerance of metamizole versus morphine for acute pancreatitis pain. Pancreatology. 2008;8(1):25-9.
8. Manes G, Uomo I, Menchise A, Rabiti PG, Ferrara EC, Uoma G. Timing of antibiotic prophylaxis in acute pancreatitis: a controlled randomized study with meropenem. Am J Gastroenterol. 2006;101(60):1348-53.
9. Gariepy CE, Heyman MB, Lowe ME, Pohl JF, Werlin SL, Wilschanski M, et al. Causal Evaluation of Acute Recurrent and Chronic Pancreatitis in Children: Consensus From the INSPPIRE Group. J Pediatr Gastroenterol Nutr. 2017;64(1): 95-103.
10. Suzuki M, Minowa K, Isayama H, Shimizu T. Acute recurrent and chronic pancreatitis in children. Paediatrics Int. 2021;63(2): 137-49.

SECTION

Disorders of Kidney and Urinary Tract

Section Editor: Arvind Bagga

13.1 The Kidney: Structure and Function

Sudha Ekambaram, Sunil Reddy KG, BR Nammalwar

INTRODUCTION

The kidney presents in the highest degree the phenomenon of sensibility, the power of reacting to various stimuli in a direction which is appropriate for the survival of the organism; a power of adaptation which almost gives one the idea that is component parts must be endowed with intelligence. **E Starling 1909**. This chapter will focus on the anatomy, functions of the glomerulus and different part of the tubules.

ANATOMY

The kidneys are paired organs that lie on the posterior wall of the abdomen behind the peritoneum on either side of the vertebral column. They extend from T12 to L3, although the right kidney is often situated slightly lower due to the presence of liver. The kidneys grow rapidly in the first year of life, from 4.5 cm in length at birth to 6.5 cm in childhood and to 11 cm in adulthood. The weight of both kidneys at birth is about 23 g and increases to 150–200 g in adults. The renal artery and vein, nerves, and pelvis enter the kidney on the medial side, which is the hilum **(Fig. 13.1.1)**.

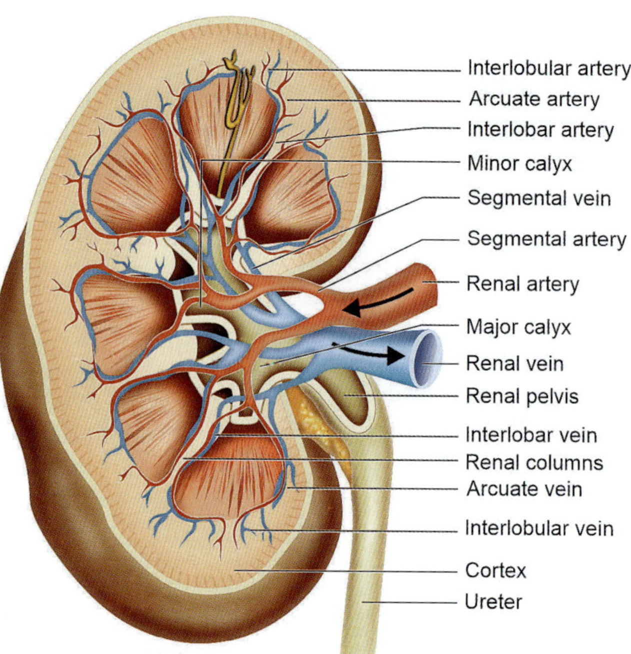

Fig. 13.1.1: Diagrammatic presentation of kidney anatomy and blood supply.

The renal tissue is divided into the outer cortex and the inner medulla, and both are composed of nephrons, blood vessels, lymphatics, and nerves. The medulla in the human kidney is divided into conical masses called renal pyramids with the intervening renal columns of Bertini, which is a medullary extension of the renal cortex in between the renal pyramids. It allows the cortex to be better anchored. The base of the pyramids originates at the corticomedullary border, and the apices are the papillae, which project into the minor calyces, wherein urine is collected from the papillae. The minor calyces are cup-like structures and join to form three or four major calyces. The major calyces in turn unite to form the pelvis, the upper expanded region of the ureter, which carries urine to the urinary bladder **(Fig. 13.1.1)**. The walls of the calyces, pelvis, and ureters contain smooth muscle that contracts to propel the urine toward the urinary bladder.

VASCULAR SYSTEM

Each renal artery branches off from the abdominal aorta just below the mesenteric artery and supplies the kidneys with blood. Renal blood flow (RBF) comprises roughly 20% of the total cardiac output. There may be one or more renal arteries supplying each kidney. The renal artery divides before entering the renal hilum into anterior and posterior divisions, which receive approximately 75% and 25% of the blood, respectively. The anterior division further divides into the upper, middle, lower, and apical segmental arteries, while the posterior division forms the posterior segmental artery. Segmental arteries subsequently divide into lobar, interlobar, arcuate, and interlobular arteries before forming the afferent arterioles, which feed into the glomerular capillaries of Bowman's capsule **(Fig. 13.1.1)**.[1]

The glomerular capillaries come together to form the efferent arterioles, which leads into a second capillary network, the peritubular capillaries, which supply blood to the nephron in the superficial cortical zone. Secondly, efferent arterioles of the nephrons that are located above the corticomedullary border (juxtamedullary nephrons) travel downward into the medulla. They further divide into straight arterioles and straight venules (vasa recta of the kidney), which surround the loop of Henle. The purpose of these vessels is to supply capillaries located in the medulla. This crucial difference plays a significant role in the medullary osmotic gradient and regulation of water excretion. Subsequently, the vessels of both venous systems run parallel to the arterial vessels and progressively form the interlobular, arcuate, interlobar, and renal veins. Blood then leaves the kidney and enters the renal vein. Sympathetic fibers originate in the lower splanchnic nerves and travel through the lumbar ganglion to the kidney. Stimulation of the sympathetic nervous system reduces RBF by causing intrarenal vasoconstriction. It also stimulates the local renin-angiotensin-aldosterone system (RAAS) and enhances Na^+ reabsorption. The kidney also receives input from the parasympathetic nervous system by way of the renal branches of the vagus nerve, which causes vasodilatation and increased blood flow of the afferent arterioles. Due to this mechanism, sympathetic nervous stimulation will decrease urine production, while parasympathetic nervous stimulation will increase urine production.[2-4]

FUNCTIONS OF THE KIDNEY[2-4]

- Regulates the volume and composition of the body fluids
- Maintains osmotic pressure (osmolality) of the body fluids by excreting osmotically dilute or concentrated urine
- Maintains volume of the extracellular fluid by controlling Na^+ and water excretion
- Maintains concentrations of numerous ions in blood plasma (sodium, potassium, chloride, bicarbonate, phosphate, sulphate, calcium, and magnesium)
- Maintains acid-base balance by excreting H^+ ions and synthesis of ammonia
- Regulates blood pressure by modulating the intraglomerular hemodynamics, adjusting Na^+ excretion, and producing various substances (e.g., renin) that can affect blood pressure
- Eliminates waste products of metabolism, such as urea, uric acid, the end product of purine metabolism, and creatinine and also certain drugs and toxic compounds
- Produces hormones like erythropoietin, calcitriol, renin, prostaglandins, endothelins, adrenomedullin, autocrine, and paracrine molecules
- Degrades several polypeptides and hormones such as insulin, glucagon, and parathyroid hormone
- Synthesizes substances that affect RBF and Na^+ excretion, viz. arachidonic acid derivatives, prostaglandins, thromboxane A2, and kallikrein
- Gluconeogenesis

MICROSTRUCTURE AND FUNCTION

Nephrogenesis begins at gestational age of 9 weeks and is completed by approximately 36 weeks. The nephron is the smallest functional unit, and each kidney at birth will have a million nephrons. The nephron is divided into a corpuscle (made up of glomerulus and Bowman space) and the tubule. The tubule comprises multiple functional units, namely proximal tubules, loop of Henle, distal tubule, juxtaglomerular apparatus (JGA), the collecting ducts, and the ductus of Bellini **(Fig. 13.1.2)**.

Glomerular Filtration[1]

The first step in the generation of urine is glomerular filtration.[1] Systemic hydrostatic pressure passively forces fluid and solute across glomerular filtration barrier (GFB), which is semipermeable in nature. The GFB consists of:

- Fenestrated endothelium of the glomerular capillaries, which allows blood components other than cells to pass through
- Basement membrane, a negatively charged physical barrier that prevents proteins from permeating
- Foot processes of the podocytes that produce more selective filtration **(Fig. 13.1.3)**.

The amount of water and solute passing through the filtration membrane is determined by the outward and inward forces within the capillaries. Hydrostatic pressure within the glomerular capillaries is the major filtration force. The hydrostatic pressure within the capsular space and the colloid osmotic pressure in glomerular capillaries negate the filtration force of the glomerular capillaries, resulting in a net filtration pressure of 10–20 mm Hg **(Fig. 13.1.4)**.

Renal Autoregulation

Blood flow through glomerular capillaries is regulated by increasing or decreasing its own blood flow resistance through myogenic and tubuloglomerular feedback mechanisms. When the vascular smooth muscle stretches as a result of elevated blood flow, the afferent arteriole feeding the glomerular capillaries is constricted by the myogenic mechanism, limiting the amount of blood passing through the glomerular capillaries. When the blood flow inside the afferent arteriole is low, it dilates the vascular smooth muscle, enabling more blood to pass through. Tubuloglomerular feedback mechanism senses the level of Na^+ inside the tubule in order to maintain the glomerular capillary blood flow. Na^+ is detected by macula densa cells of the JGA at the ascending limb of the nephron loop. An increase in Na^+ concentration at the macula densa constricts the glomerular afferent arteriole and thus decreases glomerular capillary blood flow. A decrease in Na^+ concentration increases glomerular capillary blood flow.

The renin-angiotensin-aldosterone axis is activated in three different steps:

1. If the perfusion decreases through the JGA, the granular cells in the macula densa release the enzyme renin
2. Renin cleaves angiotensinogen to form angiotensin I
3. Angiotensin I is converted to angiotensin II by angiotensin-converting enzyme (ACE) found mainly in endothelial cells of the capillaries throughout the body, within the lungs, and the epithelial cells of the kidneys. Angiotensin II

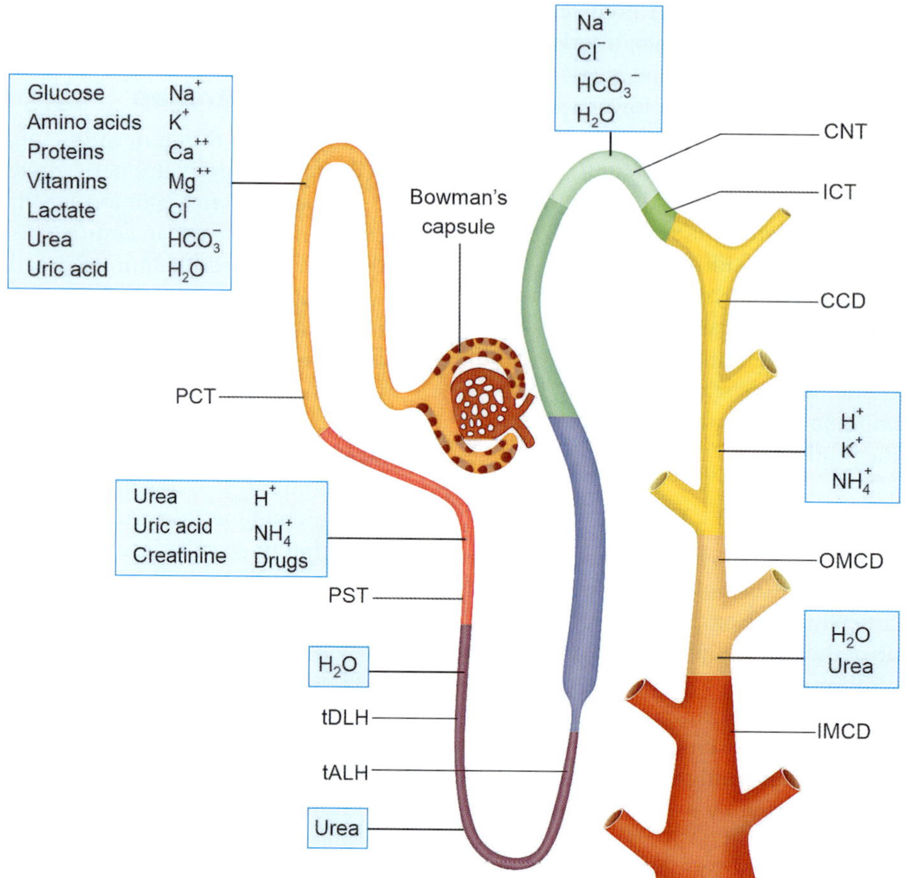

Fig. 13.1.2: Tubular segments with their reabsorption and secretion. (CCD: cortical collecting duct; CNT: connecting tubule; ICT: initial collecting tubule; IMCD: inner medullary collecting duct; OMCD: outer medullary collecting duct; PCT: proximal convoluted tubule; PST: proximal secretory tubule; tALH: thin ascending loop of Henle; tDLH: thin descending loop of Henle)

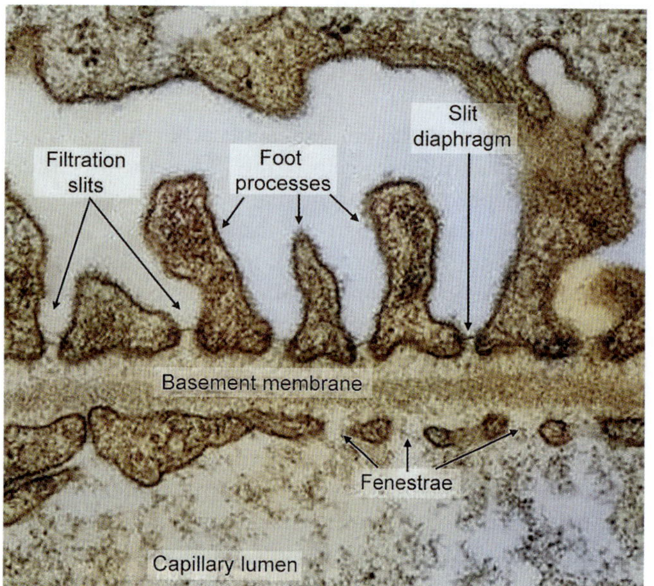

Fig. 13.1.3: Electron micrograph of the glomerular filtration barrier.

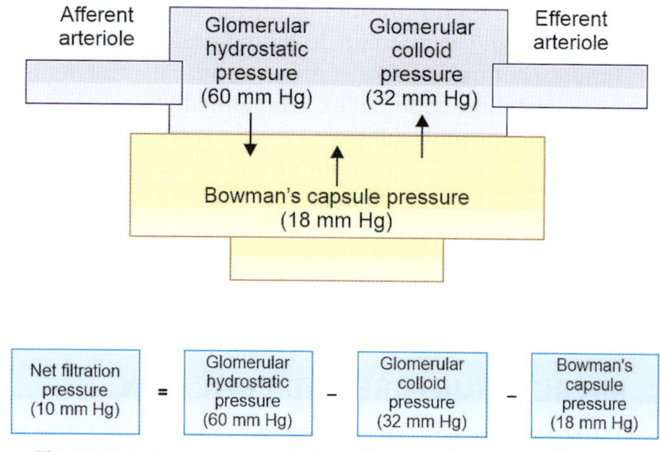

Fig. 13.1.4: Pressures regulating effective glomerular filtration.

acts on angiotensin receptors and releases aldosterone from the zona glomerulosa in the adrenal cortex, which constricts efferent arterioles and maintains glomerular filtration rate (GFR) **(Fig. 13.1.5)**.

Tubular Reabsorption[2-4]

Proximal Convoluted Tubule

The proximal convoluted tubule (PCT) is the first segment in the tubule with two distinctive regions, PCT1 and PCT2. PCT cells are characterized by the greatest capacity for absorption. The PCT reabsorbs almost all of the glucose, amino acids, 65% of Na^+, and most of the water. The basolateral Na^+/K^+-ATPase pumps 3 Na^+ out of the cell and 2 K^+ into the cell and activates the "secondary active" transport of a number of other solutes **(Fig. 13.1.6)**. Na^+ is reabsorbed through both a secondary active transport and a passive paracellular diffusion by an electrochemical gradient along with vitamins, amino acids, and glucose. Water is reabsorbed through osmosis. Additionally, passive diffusion is used to reabsorb lipid-soluble solutes. By means of passive paracellular diffusion, fueled by a chemical gradient, urea is also reabsorbed in the PCT.

Loop of Henle

This segment has a hairpin configuration with a thin descending limb and both a thin and a thick ascending limb (TAL). The thin descending limb is highly permeable to water, with reabsorption occurring passively via aquaporin 1 (AQP1) channels. Very low amounts of urea, Na^+, and other ions are reabsorbed into the tubule. This increases tubular fluid osmolarity to ~1,200 mOsm/L.

Water reabsorption is driven by the hyperosmotic environment due to active reabsorption of Na^+ in TAL. The TAL is impermeable to water but permeable to Na^+ and Cl^-. As the liquid returns through the thin ascending limb, the Na^+ and Cl^- diffuse paracellularly out of the tubule into the surrounding tissue. This is due to the difference in osmolarity between the tubule and the interstitium, where the Na^+ and Cl^- concentrations are lower. However, the primary site of Na^+ reabsorption in the limb of Henle is the TAL. Na^+/K^+/ATPase, located on the basolateral membrane, creates a negatively charged intracellular environment, thereby generating an electrochemical gradient. Na^+ ions then move into the cell (from the tubular lumen) down the electrical and chemical gradients through the Na/K/Cl cotransporter (NKCC) on the apical membrane **(Fig. 13.1.7)**. This transporter moves one Na^+ ion, one K^+ ion, and two Cl^- ions across the apical membrane. K^+ ions are transported back into the tubule by renal outer medullary potassium (ROMK) channels on the apical membrane. Cl^- ions are transported into the tissue fluid via chloride channel-Kb (ClC-Kb). The loop of Henle contributes to the absorption of approximately 25% of filtered Na^+. This leads to a drop in the osmolarity of fluid from 1,200 to 100 mOsm/L, and a hypotonic solution arrives at the distal tubule. In addition to the above concentrating mechanisms, there is significant paracellular reabsorption of Mg^{+2}, Ca^{+2}, Na^+, and K^+ and synthesis of uromodulin.

Juxtaglomerular Apparatus

The JGA **(Fig. 13.1.8)** is a specialized structure formed by the ascending limb of Henle, the glomerular afferent and efferent arterioles, and the extraglomerular mesangial cells. It is located near the vascular pole of the glomerulus, and its main function is to regulate blood pressure and the filtration rate of the glomerulus.

The macula densa is a collection of specialized epithelial cells in the distal convoluted tubule (DCT) that detect Na^+ concentration of the fluid in the tubule. In response to elevated

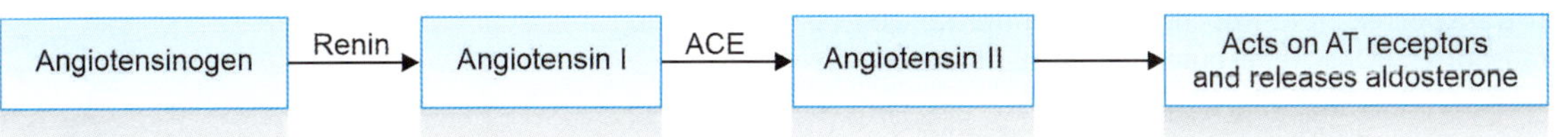

Fig. 13.1.5: Renin–angiotensin–aldosterone system. (ACE: angiotensin-converting enzyme; AT: angiotensin)

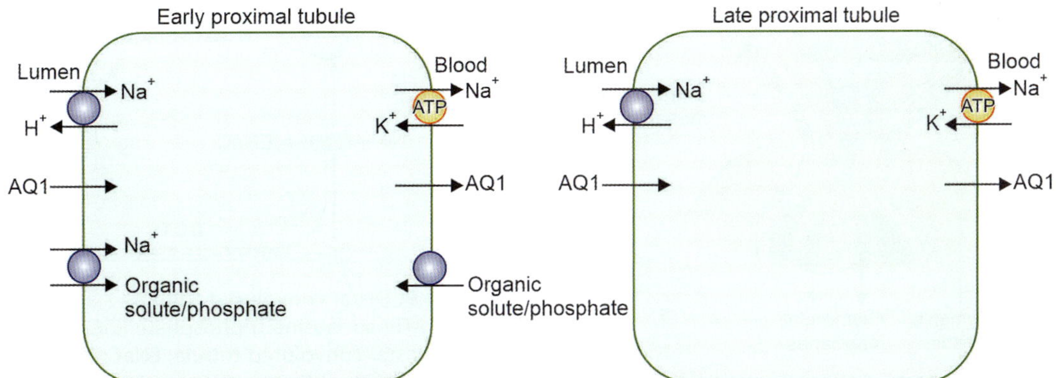

Fig. 13.1.6: Segments of the proximal tubule with their transcellular transporters. (AQ: aquaporin; ATP: adenosine triphosphate)

Na^+, the macula densa cells trigger the contraction of the afferent arteriole, reducing the flow of blood to the glomerulus and the GFR. The juxtaglomerular cells, derived from smooth muscle cells, of the afferent arteriole secrete renin when blood pressure in the arteriole falls. Renin increases blood pressure by RAAS. Lacis cells are flat and elongated and found outside the glomerulus near the macula densa.

Distal Tubules

The distal tubule starts shortly after the macula densa **(Fig. 13.1.9)** and comprises the DCT and the connecting tubule (CNT). The DCT is the shortest segment of the nephron, of about 5 mm in length, and consists of two distinct subsegments, DCT1 and DCT2. The role of the DCT is the absorption of Na^+, Cl^-, Mg^{+2}, and Ca^{+2} ions. The DCT1 and DCT2 together reabsorb roughly 5–10% of the filtered Na^+ load. Both are impermeable to water. The movement of these ions is dependent on the Na^+/K^+-ATPase transporter on the basolateral membrane of the cells. This excretes Na^+ ions into the extracellular fluid and brings K^+ ions into the cell. This process occurs via primary active transport, as ATP is directly needed to set up the gradient. The Na^+ concentration gradient generated allows Na^+ to enter the cell from the lumen of the DCT, along with Cl^- ions, which occurs through the sodium-chloride cotransporter (NCC). The Cl^- ions then exit the cell through a Cl^- ion uniporter on the basolateral membrane into the extracellular fluid, preventing accumulation within the cell. In addition to NCC, the DCT2 segment expresses the amiloride-sensitive epithelial Na^+ channel (ENaC) on the apical side.

Approximately 10% of filtered K^+ reaches the distal tubule and downstream. The luminal K^+ concentration progressively increases, indicating that a large amount of K^+ secretion occurs along the distal tubule. The K^+ secretion is mediated by the ROMK channel. In addition, the basolateral K^+ efflux into peritubular interstitium in the DCT is by K^+ transporters, ClC-Kb (voltage-gated Cl^- channel) and KCC4 (potassium chloride cotransporter).

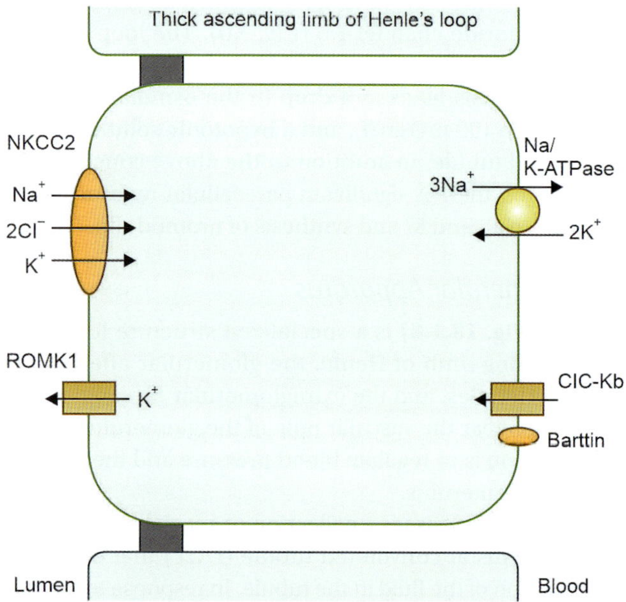

Fig. 13.1.7: Thick ascending limb of loop of Henle with their transcellular transporters. (ClC-Kb: chloride channel-Kb; NKCC2: Na/K/Cl cotransporter; ROMK: renal outer medullary potassium)

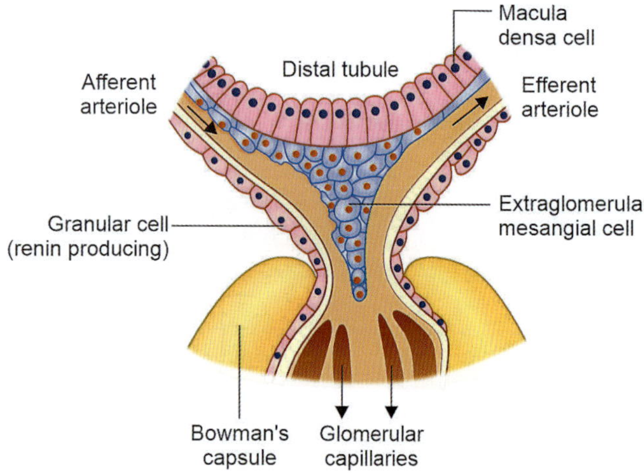

Fig. 13.1.8: Diagrammatic presentation of the juxtaglomerular apparatus.

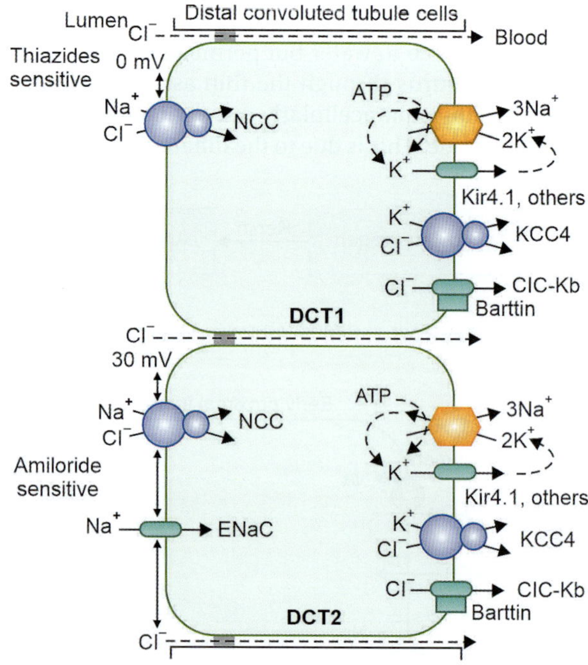

Fig. 13.1.9: Distal convoluted tubules 1 and 2 with their transporters. (ATP: adenosine triphosphate; ClC-Kb: chloride channel-Kb; DCT: distal convoluted tubule; ENaC: epithelial Na^+ channel; KCC4: potassium chloride cotransporter; NCC: sodium-chloride cotransporter)

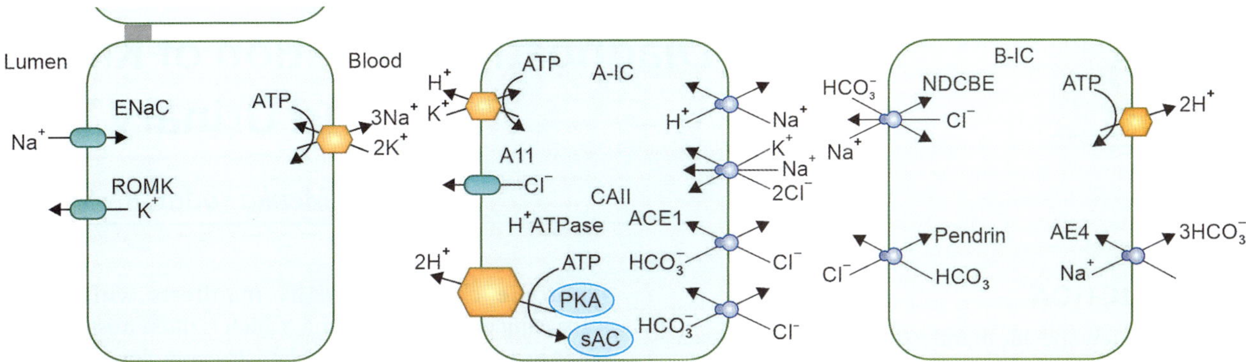

Fig. 13.1.10: Cortical collecting ducts and their transporters. (AE: anion exchanger; ATP: adenosine triphosphate; ENaC: epithelial Na^+ channel; IC: intercalated cells; NDCBE: sodium-driven Cl^-/HCO_3^- exchanger; PKA: protein kinase A; ROMK: renal outer medullary potassium; sAC: soluble adenylyl cyclase)

Connecting tubule (CNT) lies between the DCT and the initial portion of the collecting duct system (CDS) and functionally simulates both segments. The CNT (1) is impermeable to water even with antidiuretic hormone (ADH); (2) participates in active Ca^{2+} reabsorption, in response to PTH and calcitriol; (3) partially reabsorbs Na^+ by a thiazide-sensitive NaCl cotransporter (NCC); (4) reabsorbs Na^+ in exchange for K^+ secretion in principal cells; and (5) aldosterone stimulates uptake of Na^+ by the luminal ENaC and K^+ secretion by the luminal K^+ channels that are accumulated in the cell by the apical K^+ transporter Na^+ – K^+-ATPase.

Collecting Duct[4]

The CNT from different nephrons merge together to form the cortical collecting duct (CCD). The collecting duct system fine-tunes salt and water reabsorption and plays a major role in acid-base balance. The two main cell types of the CCD are principal cells and intercalated (IC) cells **(Fig. 13.1.10)**. The principal cells are responsible for Na^+ reabsorption via the amiloride-sensitive sodium channel ENaC. Principal cells also secrete K^+ via the ROMK potassium channel. The ability of the CCD to absorb water is controlled by antidiuretic hormone (ADH). In the presence of ADH, AQP2-containing vesicles fuse with the apical membrane, allowing water to enter the cell. Water exits from the basolateral aspect via AQP3 and AQP4 channels. The action of ADH on the CCD allows the production of concentrated urine and protects against dehydration.

In contrast to principal cells, IC cells express high levels of carbonic anhydrase (CA) and are involved in acid-base regulation. There are two types of IC cells, type A and B. Type A cells use cytoplasmic CA to produce H^+ and HCO_3^- ions. H^+ is secreted into the lumen by an apical H^+ ATPase pump and HCO_3^- is pumped out of the basolateral surface via an HCO_3^-/Cl^- exchanger. Type B intercalated cells have an inverse orientation of pumps and channels as compared to type A cells. In type B IC cells, the HCO_3^-/Cl^- exchanger (Pendrin) is located in the apical membrane and the H^+ ATPase pump is located in the basolateral membrane domain. Through the action of cytoplasmic CA, type B IC cells secrete HCO_3^- and reabsorb H^+. Experimentally induced metabolic acidosis results in conversion of type B IC cells to type A IC leading to H^+ secretion and returning pH to normal range.

The CCD continues into the outer medulla as the outer medullary collecting duct (OMCD). This tubular segment is lined by principal cells that are involved in Na^+ reabsorption and by type A IC cells. Type B IC cells are rarely found in the OMCD. Several OMCD contribute tributaries to the inner medullary collecting ducts (IMCD) that have correspondingly larger luminal diameters. The terminal portions of the IMCD (ducts of Bellini) are lined by taller columnar cells that open into the papillae. The IMCD epithelium expresses urea transporters that play an important role in maintaining the high medullary interstitial concentration of urea. It is this hypertonic interstitium that facilitates urine concentration by the countercurrent multiplication mechanism of the LOH and DT.

CONCLUSION

The kidney has two major functions (1) simple process of filtration, all the components of the blood except cells, and (2) tubules intelligently manipulates filtration, absorption, secretion, components of the blood to maintain internal milieu.

REFERENCES

1. Farquhar MG. The glomerular basement membrane: not gone, just forgotten. J Clin Invest. 2006;116(8):2090-9.
2. Eaton DC, Pooler JP. Vander's Renal Physiology, 7th edition. New York: McGraw Hill; 2009.
3. Koepen BM, Stanton BA. Renal Physiology, 4th edition. Philadelphia: Mosby; 2009.
4. Ekambaram S, Nammalwar BR. Structure and functions of the kidneys. In: Iyengar AA, Uthup S, Ekambaram S (Eds). BRN's Principles and Practice of Pediatric Nephrology, 3rd edition. New Delhi: Jaypee Brothers Medical Publishers; 2022. pp. 10-21.

13.2 Diagnostic Evaluation of Kidney and Urinary Tract

Menka Yadav, RN Srivastava

INTRODUCTION

There are only a few specific manifestations of kidney diseases in infants and children. Other clinical features are subtle or vague and may not lead to a suspicion of an underlying kidney disorder. Kidney diseases should be considered in children with failure to thrive, unexplained fever, obscure anemia, rickets, and dyselectrolytemia with acid-base abnormalities. A family history of kidney disease should always be obtained. A meticulous urinalysis is the crucial diagnostic investigation, and expert ultrasonography is required in most cases. Computed tomography (CT) and magnetic resonance imaging (MRI) and radionuclide studies must be used judiciously.

CLINICAL FEATURES

Common presenting features suggestive of an underlying kidney disease include gross hematuria, edema, hypertension, dysuria, flank pain, polyuria, urinary incontinence, and decrease in urine output.

Hematuria

Urine color may vary from frank red to shades of brown, described as cola- or tea-colored. A small amount of blood (1 mL in 1 L of urine) is sufficient to change the urine color. Concentrated urine looks like mustard oil and is often mistakenly reported as hematuria. Myoglobinuria, porphyria, or alkaptonuria may cause brown discoloration of urine, while administration of rifampicin and pyridium and ingestion of sugar beet or red dyes impart a reddish orange color. Hematuria should be confirmed by microscopy and differentiated from hemoglobinuria and methemoglobinuria. The dipstick test identifies heme and thus is not specific for red blood cells (RBCs). The supernatant in a centrifuged urine with hematuria is clear but is pink in hemoglobinuria and myoglobinuria. Urine microscopy is confirmatory, and the presence of dysmorphic red cells suggests the glomerular origin. Important causes of hematuria and the steps of evaluation are listed in the chapter "Asymptomatic Hematuria."

Edema

Facial edema is an important feature of kidney disease and is often ignored unless acute and associated with other abnormalities such as gross hematuria or oliguria. Nephrotic syndrome characteristically manifests with gradually increasing periorbital edema, which is often mistakenly attributed to an allergic or eye problem. In acute glomerulonephritis (GN), edema is turgid and persistent, whereas in nephrotic syndrome, the swelling is soft and pits on pressure. Nephrotic syndrome is easily differentiated from other causes of edema such as severe malnutrition, congestive cardiac failure, and cirrhosis of the liver.

Oliguria

A decrease in urine volume denotes kidney dysfunction. Oliguria is defined as a urine output <400 mL/day/1.73 m^2 or <0.5 mL/kg/h (<1 mL/kg/h in newborns). Anuria may result from severe dehydration and hypovolemia, complete obstruction of the urinary tract, or profound kidney parenchymal injury.

Polyuria

Urine volumes >2 L/m^2/day reflect impaired urinary concentration. Polydipsia is often associated. Conditions causing excessive solute excretion (osmotic diuresis, e.g., diabetes mellitus) or reduced proximal tubular reabsorption (Fanconi syndrome and isolated hypercalciuria) lead to mild polyuria. Impaired distal concentration due to vasopressin deficiency (central diabetes insipidus) or a lack of tubular response to vasopressin (nephrogenic diabetes insipidus) will lead to profound water losses. Distal tubular dysfunction may be inherited or result from obstructive uropathy, chronic hypokalemia, or interstitial nephritis. Polyuria and polydipsia are important features of nephronophthisis, a familial nephropathy that manifests during infancy.

Abdominal Pain

Flank pain is often present in acute pyelonephritis and nephrolithiasis. Young children may not be able to localize the pain. Ultrasonography is a useful tool for the evaluation of the anatomy of kidneys and urinary tract.

Abnormalities of Micturition

Constant bedwetting, weak urinary stream, dribbling, and crying during micturition are abnormal and require evaluation. Distal obstruction, most commonly from posterior urethral valve, should be excluded in male infants. Persistent dribbling suggests abnormal ureteric insertion distal to bladder neck. Spinal dysraphism should be excluded in patients with neurogenic bladder.

Enuresis and Daytime Symptoms

Involuntary voiding occurring only at night and being the only complaint (monosymptomatic nocturnal enuresis) is quite common in young children and does not require detailed investigation. Voiding problems during daytime, such as urgency, frequency, or holding maneuvers, suggest an underlying bladder dysfunction. Detailed history and examination, including neurological evaluation (anal tone, sensory loss over the perineum), are carried out. Constipation is frequently present (bladder bowel dysfunction) and should be treated appropriately. Recurrent urinary tract infections (UTIs) are commonly associated with voiding dysfunction and constipation. Voiding diary informs on type of bladder (overactive vs. underactive) and functional bladder capacity. Urine flowmetry and the study of bladder function may be required.

Abnormalities on Urinalysis

Microscopic hematuria [>3 RBC/high power field (HPF)] is occasionally detected in an asymptomatic child on routine urinalysis. It may be associated with mild-to-moderate proteinuria. The presence of these abnormalities should be confirmed on repeated, careful urine examination. Persistent microscopic hematuria or microscopic hematuria associated with proteinuria suggests an underlying glomerular, or occasionally tubulointerstitial abnormality.

Isolated microscopic hematuria is most commonly due to idiopathic hypercalciuria (defined as random urine calcium: creatinine ratio of >0.2 mg/mg in ≥2-year-olds or 24-hour urine calcium >4 mg/kg body weight).

Transient, mild proteinuria may be observed during fever, following exercise, and during infections. Persistent proteinuria is most commonly due to kidney disease and should always be investigated to find the cause. Orthostatic proteinuria, defined as elevated protein excretion in upright position but normal in recumbent position, is not uncommon (2–20%) and can be excluded using split 24 hours proteinuria assessment.

Other Features

The presence of dysuria, flank pain, and cloudy urine suggests UTIs. Tenderness in the Kidney angle and fever indicate pyelonephritis. Features suggestive of chronic kidney disease (CKD) include hypertension, growth retardation, normocytic normochromic anemia, and rachitic deformities. The presence of palpable kidney may suggest hydronephrosis, multicystic dysplastic kidney, polycystic kidney disease (kidneys being bilaterally enlarged), or Wilms' tumor.

LABORATORY EVALUATION

Urinalysis

A detailed examination of urine is crucial in the evaluation of kidney disease. The first morning specimen is more concentrated and preferred since formed elements lyse quickly in dilute urine. Urine is examined promptly or stored at 4°C. A clean catch midstream specimen can be obtained in older children, but in neonates and infants, transurethral catheterization or suprapubic bladder puncture is preferred, especially to confirm UTI.

Examination of urine specific gravity or osmolality aids the evaluation for polyuria, while the measurement of urine pH assists in determining tubular acidification abnormalities. Determination of urine electrolytes and fractional excretion is necessary for the diagnosis of various tubulopathies (e.g., Fanconi syndrome and Bartter syndrome). While dipstick can detect glucose, other reducing sugars require biochemical tests, e.g., Benedict's test for detection.

Proteinuria

Urine protein can be estimated with heat precipitation or sulfosalicylic acid as turbidity that is graded from trace, 1+ to 4+. Dipstick testing is more convenient and is graded similarly (trace: 15 mg/dL; 1+: 30 mg/dL; 2+: 100 mg/dL; 3+: 300 mg/dL; 4+: 2 g/dL). Prolonged immersion of the reagent strip and alkaline urine may cause a false-positive dipstick result. Composite sticks are available for examining pH, glucose, protein, RBCs, leukocyte esterase, and nitrite. The latter two tests help in the diagnosis of UTI. Normal children excrete <100 mg/m^2/day of protein in urine, which is chiefly tubular Tamm–Horsfall protein. Since collection of 24-hour urine specimens is often difficult, the ratio of protein to creatinine (mg/mg) in a random sample can be used. Normal values are <0.5 in infants and <0.2 in older children; values >2 suggest nephrotic range proteinuria. Urine protein-to-osmolality ratio, proposed as a useful alternative in children with poor muscle mass, is not commonly used in clinical practice.

Microscopic Examination

Fresh, centrifuged specimen should be examined. RBCs and leukocytes can be counted under microscope (count/HPF) in centrifuged sample and more accurately in a counting chamber (count/mm^3), which avoids the loss of red cells during centrifugation.[1] More than 5 neutrophils per HPF (leukocyturia) with bacteriuria suggest UTI. Microscopic hematuria is defined as the presence of >3 RBCs per HPF in a centrifuged specimen **(Figs. 13.2.1A to D)**. Phase contrast microscopy is helpful to examine red cell morphology, casts, and crystals. Dysmorphic RBCs showing fragmented, crenated appearance indicate glomerular source of red cells, whereas

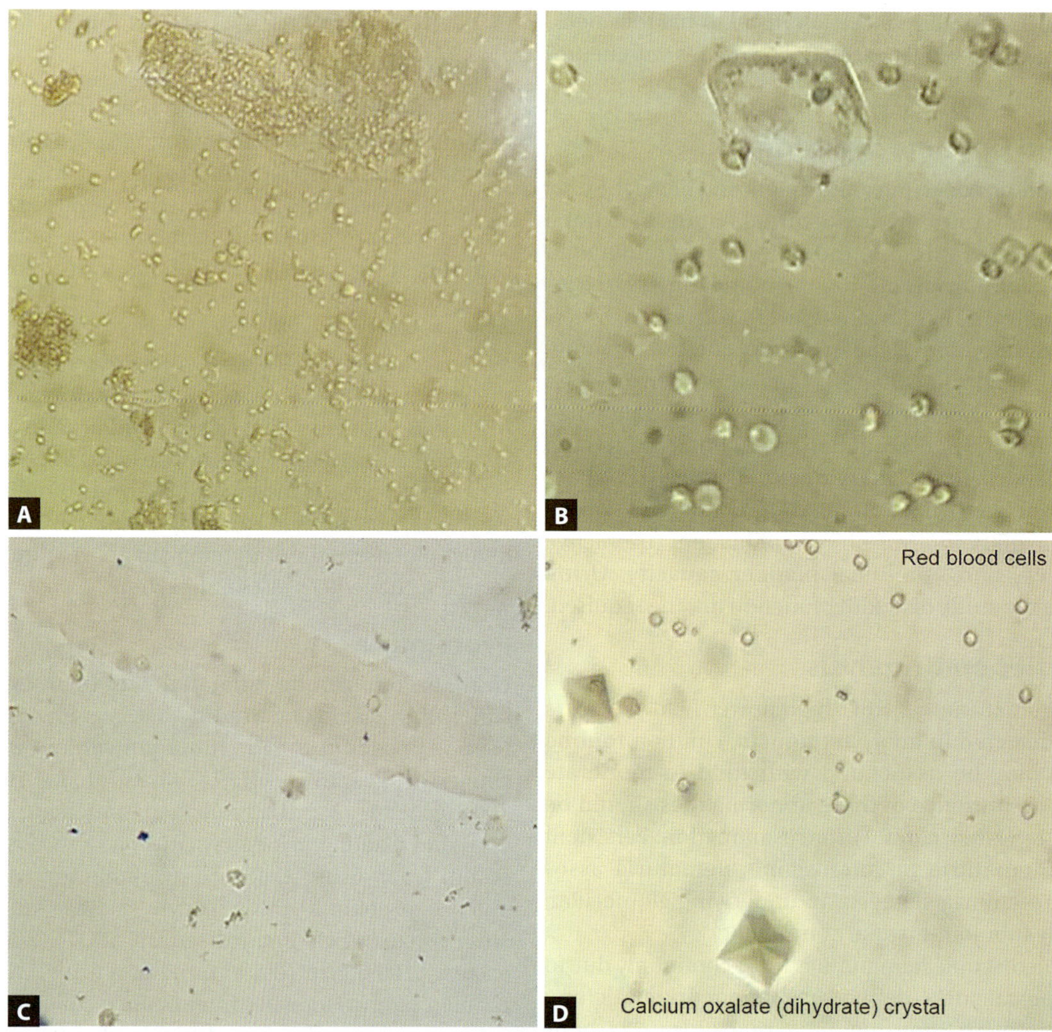

Figs. 13.2.1A to D: Urine microscopy shows the presence of (A) Dysmorphic red blood cells and a red blood cell cast in a patient with systemic lupus nephritis; (B) Epithelial cells and red blood cells in a patient with immunoglobulin A (IgA) nephropathy; (C) Waxy hyaline cast (normal finding); and (D) Calcium oxalate dihydrate crystal with red blood cells in a patient with hypercalciuria.

normal-looking cells are derived from pelvicalyceal or distal parts. Red cell casts indicate glomerular inflammation. White blood cell casts formed of clumped neutrophils suggest acute pyelonephritis. Hyaline casts (from Tamm–Horsfall protein in tubules) and epithelial cell casts can be identified. Fatty casts and oval fat bodies are commonly found in nephrotic syndrome. Crystals of various compositions (calcium oxalate, phosphate, uric acid, cystine, etc.) can be observed. While calcium oxalate, urate, and phosphate crystals can be seen in normal conditions, the presence of cystine and cholesterol crystals is pathological.

Timed Urine Collection

Because of difficulties in accurately collecting all specimens of urine, 12-hour or 24-hour collections are undertaken when definitely needed, e.g., for quantitative measurement of calcium, phosphate, creatinine, magnesium, or oxalate for the diagnosis of metabolic abnormalities underlying urolithiasis (refer to Chapter 13.13) or in evaluation of tubular dysfunction (refer to Chapter 13.11). Timed protein excretion is helpful in the assessment of response to therapy in secondary causes of nephrotic range proteinuria (>40 mg/m^2/h). The first morning void is discarded, followed by the collection of every voided sample till the first void of the subsequent day. The adequacy of collection can be confirmed using creatinine excretion of 10–15 mg/kg/day in girls and 15–20 mg/kg/day in boys.

Blood Tests

The normal level of blood urea ranges between 20 and 40 mg/dL. Factors that reduce kidney perfusion can cause a reversible increase in blood urea levels. The levels are also increased during excessive tissue breakdown, trauma, gastrointestinal bleeding, and the use of corticosteroids and tetracycline. Urea levels are low in the presence of hepatic failure and on a low protein diet. Normal blood urea level does not necessarily indicate normal kidney function since the glomerular filtration rate (GFR) must decline to about <75% of normal for the levels to increase.

The level of serum creatinine varies inversely with the GFR, of which it is a better indicator than blood urea. Serum creatinine is not readily affected by prekidney factors. However, these levels are related to the muscle mass and may overestimate GFR in the presence of malnutrition. Hyperbilirubinemia (bilirubin level >5 mg/dL) interferes with the measurement of creatinine. GFR may be estimated in children as follows:

$$\text{Glomerular filtration rate} = \frac{k \times \text{height (in cm)}}{\text{Serum creatinine (mg/dL)}}$$

where $k = 0.413$. Recently, serum cystatin C levels have been suggested to be a better marker of GFR. It is a protein secreted by all nucleated cells and is freely filtered, not secreted by tubules, and totally reabsorbed.[2]

Serum albumin is reduced in patients with nephrotic syndrome proteinuria, occasionally below 1.5 g/dL. In children with nephrotic syndrome, hypercholesterolemia is typically present.

The levels of complement factor 3 (C3) in blood are reduced in postinfectious GN, membranoproliferative glomerulonephritis (MPGN), and lupus nephritis. Estimation of C3 and C4 levels is helpful in GN and other complement-mediated disorders, e.g., atypical hemolytic uremic syndrome. In systemic lupus erythematosus (SLE), C3 levels reflect disease activity. The normal range varies as per laboratory reference.

Antinuclear antibodies (ANAs) are antibodies directed against chromatin-associated or ribonucleoprotein particles. They are not specific and may be increased in many autoimmune diseases such as SLE, juvenile rheumatoid arthritis, polyarteritis nodosa (PAN), and autoimmune hepatitis. ANA titers >1:100 form the entry criteria for SLE as per ACR-EULAR (American College of Rheumatology–European League Against Rheumatism) criteria. Antibodies to double-stranded DNA (anti-dsDNA) is specific to SLE, while increased titer of antineutrophil cytoplasmic antibody (ANCA) is seen in a group of small vessel vasculitis, including microscopic polyangiitis, granulomatosis with polyangiitis, and renal-limited vasculitis.

Tests of Tubular Function

Testing for specific tubular function is indicated by clinical features. For example, children with polyuria may require water deprivation test and vasopressin administration, and bicarbonate or ammonium chloride loading tests are performed in those with impaired urinary acidification. These tests are discussed in Chapter 13.11.

Estimation of Kidney Reserve

Once the decline in GFR is noted, significant decline in kidney function has already occurred. Similarly, after recovery from acute kidney injury, a certain level of kidney function is already lost despite an apparently normal serum creatinine. This lost kidney reserve is the ability of kidneys to increase basal GFR following stress, e.g., protein load. Kidney reserve can be measured using creatinine clearance following amino acid or protein load.

IMAGING STUDIES

Performance of diagnostic imaging in children requires expertise, experience, and patience. Appropriate sedation should be used whenever required. Care is taken to minimize exposure to both radiation and radiocontrast. The guiding principle of *A*s *L*ow *A*s *R*easonably *A*chievable (ALARA) must be followed. Common imaging techniques used are listed below.

Plain X-ray of the Abdomen

A plain radiograph has limited utility, chiefly in detecting small radiopaque kidney calculi and ureteric calculi without proximal ureteral dilatation. Radiographs also assist in the evaluation of the spine in children with neurogenic bladder, assessment for changes of kidney osteodystrophy, and screening for metastatic bone disease.

Intravenous Pyelography

The use of intravenous pyelography (IVP) or excretory urography has declined due to the advent of ultrasonography and radionuclide studies. It is currently indicated for detailed evaluation of structural anomalies, e.g., duplex kidneys and horseshoe kidneys, and for ureteric calculi. IVP requires bowel preparation and administration of an ionic contrast (urograffin, 3–4 mL/kg) with films taken at 1–5 minutes, 10–15 minutes, and a late pelvic film for the bladder. Hydration is necessary to avoid contrast nephropathy. The test is avoided in neonates since urinary concentration of the contrast is inadequate.

Micturating Cystourethrogram

Micturating cystourethrography (MCU), or voiding cystourethrography, is useful for the diagnosis and grading of vesicoureteric reflux (VUR) **(Figs. 13.2.2A to D)** and the detection of bladder and urethral abnormalities. Following urinary catheterization, radiocontrast agent is introduced

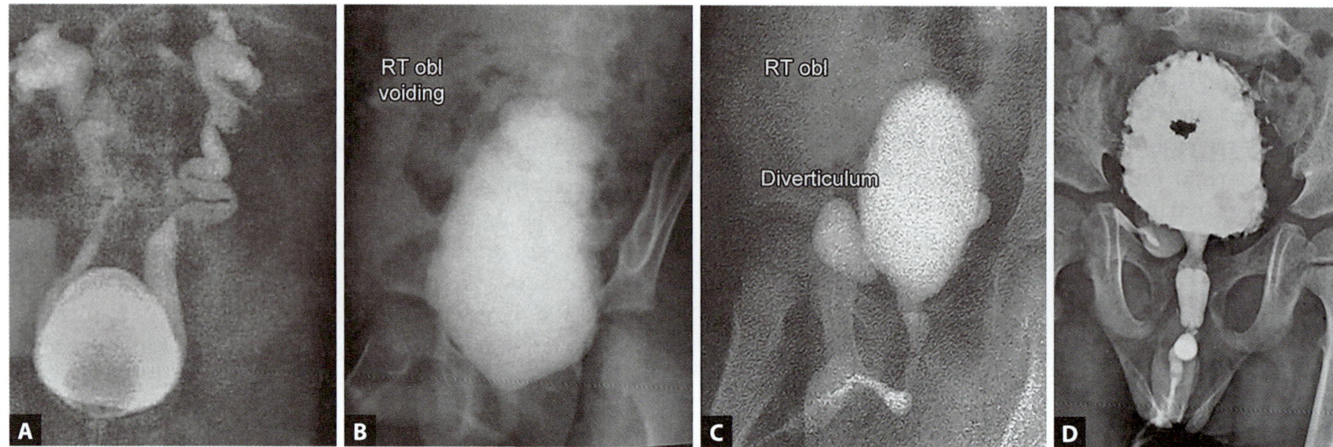

Figs. 13.2.2A to D: Micturating cystourethrogram showing (A) Bilateral grade 5 vesicoureteric reflux in a patient with primary vesicoureteric reflux; (B) Elongated bladder in a patient with neurogenic bladder; (C) Bladder diverticuli in a boy following ablation for posterior urethral valves (right oblique view); and (D) Dilated posterior urethra with trabeculated urinary bladder. (RT obl: right oblique view)

into the bladder; films are taken while the child is voiding. Voiding films provide information on the presence of dilated posterior urethra, bladder neck hypertrophy, and bladder trabeculations. Strict aseptic precautions are required. Oral amoxicillin or parenteral gentamicin (administered 30–60 minutes prior to the procedure and 6 hours afterward) may be administered prophylactically.

Ultrasonography

Ultrasound gives excellent information on anatomical aspects **(Fig. 13.2.3)**. It is especially suited for children.

Since it is painless, requires no sedation or radiocontrast administration, and can be repeated safely. Ultrasound is useful in guiding procedures such as kidney biopsy or fine needle aspiration. The major limitation of ultrasonography is that it is operator-dependent; interpretation in children requires considerable experience.

The kidney cortical echotexture is compared with the liver, spleen, and kidney medulla; nonspecific changes may occur with kidney parenchymal disease. Objective documentation of pelvicalyceal dilation using anteroposterior diameter helps in serial follow-up. Measurement of kidney size helps assess its growth. Doppler evaluation is useful for the assessment of blood flow. Large rectal diameter on ultrasound provides clue to underlying constipation in a child with voiding dysfunction.

Antenatal Ultrasonography

Evaluation in antenatal period allows detection of common abnormalities such as unilateral or bilateral hydronephrosis and multicystic dysplastic kidney. Particular attention is directed toward the amount of amniotic fluid, anteroposterior diameter of the kidney pelvis and pelviectasis, kidney echotexture, and the appearance of the ureters and urinary bladder. Distended bladder with bilateral hydronephrosis suggests distal obstruction as seen with posterior urethral valves, while unilateral hydronephrosis with normal ureters and bladder suggests pelviureteric junction obstruction.

Computed Tomography

Noncontrast helical CT scanning is useful in identifying very small calculi, which might not be detected on ultrasonography. CT provides excellent anatomical details, which is especially useful in evaluating abdominal masses (e.g., tumor or abscess). The disadvantages include radiation exposure, the need for sedation, and contrast administration.

Magnetic Resonance Imaging

Magnetic resonance imaging is used for the detection of spinal abnormalities such as tethered cord. MRI provides superior resolution and avoids radiation. Magnetic resonance urography is an alternative to IVP and provides clear information of kidney function and excretion. However, the procedure requires sedation.

Radionuclide Imaging

The term radionuclide refers to the radioactive substances that are the molecules containing radioactive atoms. When those atoms decay, they emit energy in the form of gamma rays or alpha or beta particles that are detected by the nuclear medicine camera. Radionuclide methods are increasingly replacing conventional radiocontrast studies such as IVP and angiography, since they are noninvasive, highly sensitive, and involve lower radiation exposures.[3] They are used to assess differential kidney function and kidney perfusion and to identify cortical scars, intrakidney masses, and upper tract dilatation. Radionuclide scans also provide valuable information on kidney allograft perfusion and function.

Renography

Renography, or kidney perfusion study, monitors the arrival, uptake, and elimination of a radiopharmaceutical by the kidney. Accordingly, it consists of a flow (perfusion) phase and a function (uptake and excretion) phase. Agents used include ^{99m}technetium (Tc)-labeled diethylenetriaminepentaacetic acid (DTPA), an agent excreted purely by glomerular filtration, and mercaptoacetylglycine (MAG-3) and LL-ethylene cysteine (LL-EC) dimer, excreted by glomerular filtration and tubular secretion.

Figures 13.2.4A and B show the three phases of a normal renogram. The peak of the curve depends on kidney blood flow, kidney function, tubular transit, and excretion. Therefore, the peak is delayed in kidney artery stenosis, kidney parenchymal disease, oliguria, and with obstruction. Dynamic scans are useful in identification of pelviureteric junction obstruction and renovascular stenosis, evaluation of differential and total kidney function, assessment of allograft function, and perfusion. Pitfalls such as distended bladder, severe hydronephrosis, poor kidney function, and patient positioning may limit the interpretation of observed renogram. A diuretic renogram helps differentiate obstructive dilatation of the upper urinary tract from nonobstructive hydronephrosis; in the latter, the radionuclide clears promptly following the injection of frusemide. Administration of captopril acutely reduces kidney blood flow and GFR, thus accentuating the abnormalities, which facilitates the diagnosis of kidney arterial stenosis.

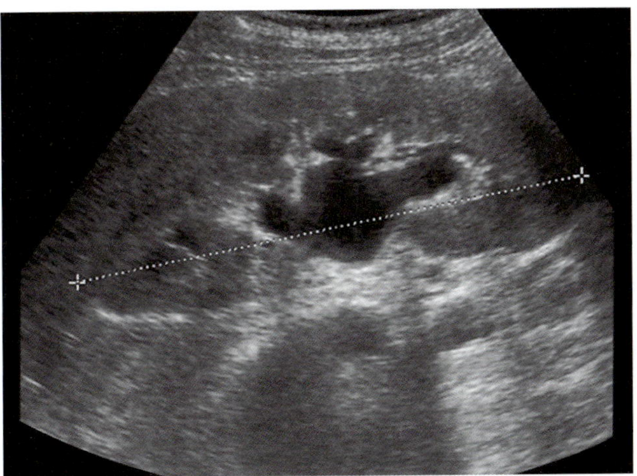

Fig. 13.2.3: Ultrasound study in a 6-year-old boy showing hydronephrosis; note enlarged kidney and dilated Kidney pelvis.

Kidney Static Imaging

Kidney static imaging provides a two-dimensional depiction of the concentration and distribution of radionuclide. ^{99m}Tc-labeled dimercaptosuccinic acid (DMSA) and glucoheptonate (GHA) are the cortical agents and provide excellent quality of images. ^{99m}Tc DTPA visualizes the pelvicalyceal collecting system and ureters well. Due to its concentration in the kidney cortex and a slow rate of urinary excretion, DMSA is particularly useful for the demonstration of kidney scarring **(Fig. 13.2.5)**, identification of ectopic and horseshoe kidneys, and in detecting damage from trauma. Imaging with GHA is useful when evaluating abnormalities in both the cortex and collecting system since it is filtered, partially reabsorbed, and retained in proximal tubular cells.

Clearance Studies

Agents such as ^{51}Cr-ethylene-diamine-tetra-acetic acid (EDTA) and ^{99m}Tc DTPA are used for the estimation of total

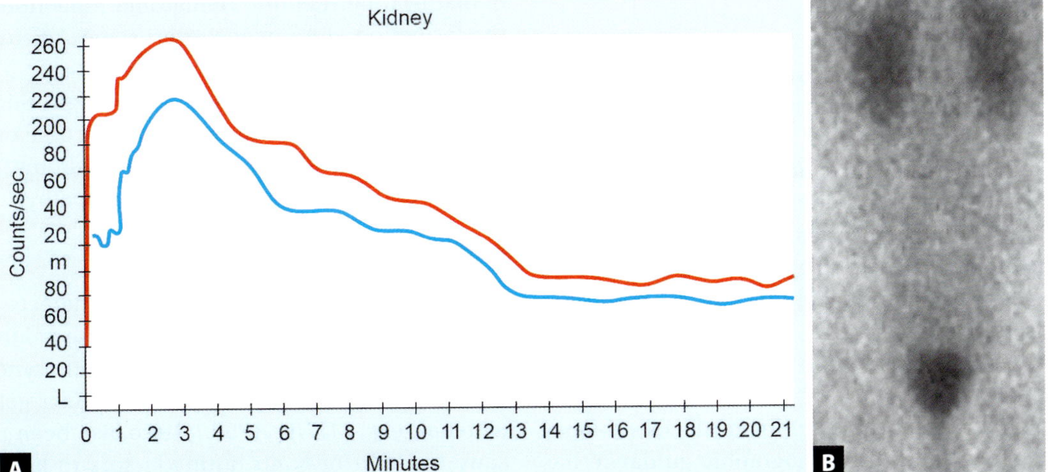

Figs. 13.2.4A and B: Diethylenetriaminepentaacetic acid renogram showing normal concentration and excretion of the radiolabeled agent through both kidneys. Note the three phases: (1) A rapid rise and fall due to first-pass perfusion, (2) a slow rise to a peak due to the arrival of the agent into the kidney, and (3) declining amplitude due to excretion. Delayed image shows clearing of the radionuclide from both kidneys and its presence in the urinary bladder.

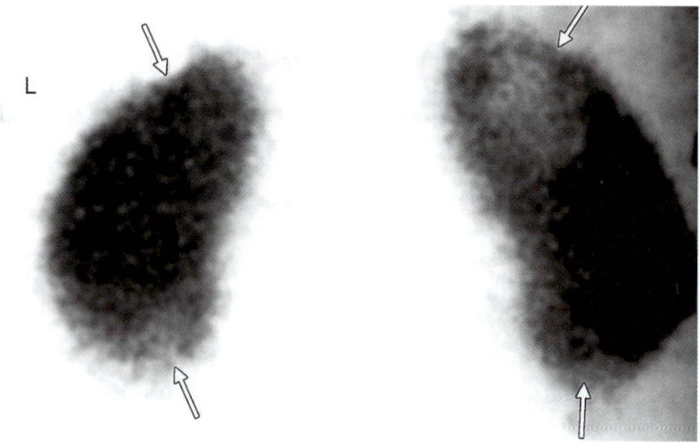

Fig. 13.2.5: Dimercaptosuccinic acid scan showing bilateral cortical scarring in a 7-year-old girl with recurrent urinary tract infections.

BOX 13.2.1: Indications of kidney biopsy.

Common or usually indicated:
- Steroid-resistant nephrotic syndrome
- Persistent acute kidney injury; unexplained acute kidney injury
- Rapidly progressive glomerulonephritis
- Systemic diseases [immunoglobulin A (IgA) vasculitis and systemic lupus erythematosus]
- Inherited nephropathies, e.g., Alport syndrome (less common with increasing availability of genetic tests)
- Kidney allograft dysfunction
- Detection of calcineurin inhibitors toxicity

Less common:
- Chronic kidney disease, to ascertain etiology
- Persistent non-nephrotic range proteinuria
- Persistent microscopic hematuria
- Steroid-sensitive nephrotic syndrome (prior to therapy with calcineurin inhibitors)

and differential glomerular filtration. ^{131}I orthoiodohippurate helps determine effective kidney plasma flow.

Direct Radionuclide Cystogram

Direct radionuclide cystography (DRCG) is a reliable and sensitive technique for the detection of VUR. It is performed by instilling radionuclide through a urethral catheter or by its injection into the bladder. Thereafter, rapid sequence images of the bladder are obtained while the patient voids. Indirect radionuclide cystourethrography may be used in cases of difficult catheterization. These provide a visual representation of the rate of bladder emptying, residual urine volume, and evidence of reflux. Compared to MCU, which provides superior anatomical information, DRCG involves lower radiation exposure, making it suitable for repeated follow-up examinations.

KIDNEY BIOPSY

Evaluation of kidney histology is an important tool for the diagnosis of various kidney parenchymal diseases involving glomeruli or tubule interstitium.[4] Indications for kidney biopsy are listed under specific conditions in **Box 13.2.1**. A kidney biopsy is not necessary in uncomplicated cases of poststreptococcal GN and corticosteroid-responsive nephrotic syndrome. The procedure should be performed early in case of rapidly progressive glomerulonephritis (RPGN), suspected SLE nephritis, kidney vasculitis, and kidney allograft dysfunction, where early institution of specific therapy may improve outcome.

The availability of disposable automatic devices (biopsy gun, 16 or 18 gauge) and ultrasonographic guidance has improved the yield of the procedure, with relatively less risks. Prior to biopsy, a normal coagulation profile and normal blood pressure must be ensured to reduce the risk of bleeding. Patients with marked azotemia should be dialyzed. Intranasal desmopressin may be administered 30–60 minutes prior to the procedure.

The procedure is performed on an empty stomach (4-hour fasting) under light sedation using intravenous midazolam and/or ketamine; atropine administration may be required to reduce the risk of secretions. The child lies in the prone position with a folded towel or bedsheet placed under his lower ribs and epigastrium to push the kidney posteriorly and stabilize its position. The biopsy site is the angle made by the lower edge of the 12th rib and the lateral border of sacrospinalis. The kidney is localized with a "probing" 23-gauge needle or visualized directly by ultrasound. The entry of the biopsy needle into the kidney when it pierces the kidney capsule is indicated by slight loss of resistance ("give way" feeling). Following biopsy, vital signs should be monitored closely for the next 6–8 hours. Complications include local pain, gross hematuria, perinephric hematoma, infection, and, rarely, the formation of traumatic arteriovenous fistula. Strenuous exercise should be avoided for a few days.

Kidney histology is examined by light microscopy and immunofluorescence. Electron microscopic examination is useful for precise diagnosis of Alport syndrome, dense deposit disease, and early transplant glomerulopathy.

GENETIC STUDIES

In the past few decades, single-gene defects (monogenic) have been well characterized as the cause of inherited kidney diseases, e.g., steroid-resistant nephrotic syndrome, cystic kidney disease, and Alport syndrome. Also, genetic variants in genes, e.g., *MYH9*, *APOL1*, have also been recognized as causative and/or contributing factors to kidney diseases.[5] With increasing availability and affordability of the genetic tests, e.g., next-generation (clinical/whole exome or whole genome) sequencing, inherited disorders may emerge as the chief contributor to the burden of CKD.

A careful and detailed pre- and post-test counseling is mandatory as the yield varies among various diseases. Nevertheless, genetic analysis has a role in confirmation of diagnosis and prenatal counseling, e.g., tubulopathies, and provides therapeutic (e.g., coenzyme Q-associated steroid-resistant nephrotic syndrome) and prognostic information (e.g., truncating vs. missense variant in Alport syndrome) to guide patient care. The significance of an observed variant may change with time, and thus careful correlation with phenotype and frequent reanalysis, as needed, is important.

CONCLUSION

A focused diagnostic evaluation enables timely identification and management of various kidney and urinary tract disorders. The approach begins with a careful clinical assessment, thorough laboratory testing of blood and urine samples, appropriate imaging studies, and in some cases, kidney biopsy. Advances in genetic testing have enhanced our ability to diagnose inherited disorders. The choice and sequence of diagnostic tests should be tailored to each patient's presentation and suspected underlying pathology.

REFERENCES

1. Cavanaugh C, Perazella MA. Urine sediment examination in the diagnosis and management of kidney disease: Core curriculum 2019. Am J Kidney Dis. 2019;73:258-72.
2. Schwartz GJ, Muñoz A, Schneider MF, Mak RH, Kaskel F, Warady BA, et al. New equations to estimate GFR in children with CKD. J Am Soc Nephrol. 2009;20:629-37.
3. Mendichovszky I, Solar BT, Smeulders N, Easty M, Biassoni L. Nuclear medicine in pediatric nephro-urology: An overview. Semin Nucl Med. 2017;47:204-28.
4. Najafian B, Lusco MA, Alpers CE, Fogo AB. Approach to kidney biopsy: Core curriculum 2022. Am J Kidney Dis. 2022;80:119-31.
5. Arora V, Anand K, Verma IC. Genetic testing in pediatric kidney disease. Indian J Pediatr. 2020;87:706-15.

13.3 Developmental Anomalies

Susan Uthup

INTRODUCTION

Congenital anomalies of the kidney and urinary tract (CAKUT) represent a broad range of disorders. Severe structural fetal anomalies occur in 1% of pregnancies, and defects of renal development might account for 30% of chronic kidney failure in children.[1] CAKUT is phenotypically variable and can affect the kidney(s) alone and/or the lower urinary tract. In young children, congenital anomalies are the leading cause of kidney failure and for kidney transplantation or dialysis. CAKUT can also lead to significant renal problems in adulthood, including hypertension and/or proteinuria.[2] Congenital renal anomalies can be sporadic or familial, syndromic or nonsyndromic. Anomalies of other organ systems may occur in association with renal anomalies.[3] Clues suggesting renal anomalies are given in **Box 13.3.1**.

BOX 13.3.1: Clues suggesting renal anomalies.

- Oligohydramnios
- Fetal compression syndrome (Potter sequence: Flat facies, low-set malformed ears, pulmonary hypoplasia, and limb anomalies)
- *Chromosomal disorders:* Trisomy 13, trisomy 18, and Turner syndrome
- Tuberous sclerosis
- Prune belly syndrome (absent/deficient abdominal muscles and cryptorchidism)
- Meningomyelocele
- Anorectal malformations
- Aniridia (Wilms' tumor)
- Family history of renal disease (Alport syndrome and polycystic kidney disease)

The development of kidneys begins at the fourth week of gestation from the intermediate mesoderm, which differentiates into pronephros, mesonephros, and metanephros. Pronephros and mesonephros degenerate. The metanephric kidney, definitive fetal kidneys, begins development during the fifth week of gestation. The ureteric bud, originating from the mesonephric (Wolffian) duct, penetrates the metanephric blastema, inducing its differentiation into the renal parenchyma.[4] In the absence of ureteric bud, metanephric kidneys will not form. The kidneys ascend from the sacral to the lumbar region, and nephrogenesis is complete by 36 weeks of gestation.[5]

Embryologically, the ureter begins development as a solid cord. As the collecting system lengthens and canalizes, anomalies can lead to transient or permanent, partial or complete obstruction to urine flow. This obstructive process, if significant and persistent, results in varying degrees of cystic dysplasia and renal dysfunction. The fetal kidneys start producing urine by the ninth week of gestation and contribute to the amniotic fluid. An adequate amniotic fluid volume is essential for normal lung development. Fetuses with oligohydramnios show pulmonary hypoplasia, deformities of the skeleton and soft tissues.[3]

Developmental anomalies of kidneys include malformation of renal parenchyma, abnormalities of migration, or in the development of collecting system. Derangements in cellular, molecular, and morphogenic mechanisms that direct normal renal system development are the major causes of CAKUT. Genetic, epigenetic, and environmental factors play a crucial role in the development of kidneys and urinary tract.[6,7]

RENAL AGENESIS

Renal agenesis is the complete absence of identifiable renal tissue due to failure of development of the ureteric bud or metanephros. It may be unilateral or bilateral. Bilateral renal agenesis is incompatible with life. The incidence is 1 in 3,000 births and is associated with pulmonary hypoplasia and facial appearance characterized by wide-set eyes, squashed flattened nose, receding chin, large low-set ears, small mandible, and deficiency of cartilage (Potter sequence). The absent renal echoes and urinary bladder can be detected at 12 weeks of gestation on ultrasound. Death occurs in the perinatal period due to respiratory insufficiency. Unilateral renal agenesis occurs in 1 in 500–1,000 births. Typically, the ureter and ipsilateral trigone of the urinary bladder are absent. In unilateral renal agenesis, the contralateral normal kidney hypertrophies.[5]

RENAL HYPOPLASIA

The hypoplastic kidney is small, but the shape and structure are normal. The functioning renal parenchyma is reduced as there is a reduction in the number of nephrons. Hypoplastic kidney may be unilateral or bilateral. Bilateral renal hypoplasia is an important cause of kidney failure in the first decade of life.[5,7]

RENAL DYSPLASIA

There is abnormal differentiation of renal parenchyma with the development of cysts, undifferentiated mesenchymal tissue, cartilage, primitive glomeruli, and primitive tubules. Dysplasia may be unilateral or bilateral and may be associated with other developmental abnormalities of the urinary tract. Intrauterine obstruction of the urinary tract may cause severe bilateral renal dysplasia. Severe bilateral dysplasia presents as Potter sequence and is incompatible with life.[3,5]

CYSTIC LESIONS

Multicystic Dysplastic Kidney

This is the most common renal cystic disease. The kidney is enlarged and presents as an abdominal mass in neonates. There is severe cystic renal dysplasia, with no functioning renal tissue. The cysts are randomly arranged. Multicystic dysplastic kidneys may be associated with developmental abnormalities of the urinary tract. Surgical removal is seldom necessary, as the dysplastic kidney usually involutes.[1,3]

Polycystic Kidney Disease

Inherited polycystic kidney disease is an important cause of end-stage renal disease. Two distinct patterns of inheritance have been described, autosomal dominant and recessive, each with different characteristics.

Autosomal Dominant Polycystic Kidney Disease

Autosomal dominant polycystic kidney disease is one of the common inherited disorders and the most frequent genetic cause of renal failure in adults. It often presents in adults but can occasionally be detected in children. Chief manifestations include palpable kidneys, hematuria, hypertension, urinary tract infections, and renal stones. The genetic loci are on chromosomes 16 and 4. The kidneys are enlarged with multiple cysts. Hepatic cysts, cysts in the pancreas, spleen, and cerebral aneurysms may also occur. End-stage kidney disease occurs in the fifth or sixth decade. Screening ultrasound examination of parents and siblings should be done.[1]

Autosomal Recessive Polycystic Kidney Disease

Autosomal recessive polycystic kidney disease, linked to chromosome 6, has a more severe clinical course. It may present as Potter sequence, with pulmonary hypoplasia, chronic kidney disease during childhood, or with liver disease in older survivors. The kidneys are enlarged with multiple cysts. The reniform shape is maintained.[1,3]

ABNORMALITIES IN POSITION

Renal Ectopia and Malrotation

During development, the kidneys ascend and rotate so that the renal pelvis faces medially. Renal ectopia occurs in 1 in 800 births. Pelviureteric junction obstruction and vesicoureteral reflux may occur in kidneys that fail to ascend.[1,8]

Horseshoe Kidney

In horseshoe kidneys, the lower poles of the kidneys commonly fuse in the midline. This anomaly occurs in 1 in 400 births. One-third of patients with Turner syndrome have horseshoe kidneys. Reflux, obstruction, infection, and stone formation are common; there is an increased risk of Wilms' tumor. Skeletal, cardiovascular, neural tube defects, and anorectal malformations are associated.[1]

Crossed Fused Ectopia

During the ascent, one kidney may cross the midline and fuse with the other. Patients with this condition often show anomalies of the collecting system, including reflux and obstruction.[1]

ANTENATAL HYDRONEPHROSIS

Antenatal ultrasonography can detect anomalies of kidneys as early as 16 weeks of gestation. Hydronephrosis is the most common renal anomaly detected on ultrasound in 3–5% of pregnancies. The dilatation may involve the calyces (caliectasis) or pelvis (pelviectasis) or both. Antenatally detected hydronephrosis may be the result of obstruction or nonobstructive causes **(Box 13.3.2)**. Obstructive lesions, particularly bilateral lesions, are harmful to the developing kidneys.[9]

The anteroposterior diameter of the fetal renal pelvis >4 mm below 20 weeks and >7 mm above 20 weeks of gestation is considered significant. In most cases (60%), antenatal hydronephrosis is physiological and resolves by the first year of life.[9,10]

Amniotic fluid volume is the chief determinant of fetal survival in these babies, oligohydramnios being associated with pulmonary hypoplasia. Oligohydramnios beyond the second trimester indicates urinary obstruction or renal failure in the fetus. The presence of bilateral upper tract dilatation and persistently distended bladder suggests the possibility of posterior urethral valves. Oligohydramnios and brightly echogenic kidneys, if detected on ultrasound prior to 24 weeks of gestation, predict fetal end-stage renal disease syndrome and poor postnatal survival.[9] In such cases, termination of pregnancy may be contemplated. Careful postnatal follow-up is needed in all children with CAKUT.[1,3]

BOX 13.3.2: Causes of antenatal hydronephrosis.

- Physiological
- *Obstructive lesions:*
  - Pelviureteric junction obstruction
  - Posterior urethral valve
- *Vesicoureteric reflux:*
  - Primary
  - Secondary to duplex collecting system, ectopic ureter, and prune belly syndrome
- Nonobstructive, nonrefluxing ureters
- Primary megaureter

CONCLUSION

Congenital kidney anomalies constitute the leading cause of CKD and kidney failure in the young. Early detection, evaluation, intervention and follow-up are required to prevent kidney failure. Antenatal ultrasound evaluation is extremely useful in assessing the status of the kidneys and urinary system. However, postnatal assessment of the newborn seldom receives as much importance as fetal assessment. Follow-up evaluation after initial assessment and intervention are also equally important. Genetics now play an important role in the diagnosis as well as prognosis of babies with cystic kidney diseases.

REFERENCES

1. Elder JE. Congenital anomalies and dysgenesis of the kidneys. In: Kliegman RM, St Geme JW, Blum NJ, Shah SS, Tasker RC, Wilson KM (Eds). Nelson Textbook of Pediatrics, 21st edition. Elsevier Saunders; 2021. pp. 2786-9.e1.
2. Toka HR, Toka O, Hariri A, Nguyen HT. Congenital anomalies of kidneys and urinary tract. Semin Nephrol. 2010;30(4): 374-86.
3. Goodyer P. Renal dysplasia/hypoplasia. In: Emma F, Goldstein SL, Bagga A, Bates CM, Shroff R. Pediatric Nephrology, 8th edition. Switzerland AG: Springer Nature; 2021. pp. 79-114.
4. Capone VP, Morello W, Taroni F, Montini G. Genetics of congenital anomalies of the kidney and urinary tract. Int J Mol Sci. 2017;18(4):796.
5. Shubha AM, Nandhini G, Prasad N. Congenital anomalies of kidneys and urinary tract. In: Iyenger AA, Uthup S, Ekambaram S (Eds). Nammalwar's Principles and Practice of Pediatric Nephrology, 3rd edition. New Delhi: Jaypee Brothers Medical Publishers; 2022. pp. 760-79.
6. Pohl M, Bhatnagar V, Mendoza SA, Nigam SK. Toward an etiological classification of developmental disorders of the kidney and upper urinary tract. Kidney Int. 2002;61(1):10-9.
7. Song R1, Yosypiv IV. Genetics of congenital anomalies of the kidney and urinary tract. Pediatr Nephrol. 2011;26(3):353-64.
8. Murugapoopathy V, Gupta IR. A primer on congenital anomalies of the kidneys and urinary tracts. Clin J Am Soc Nephrol. 2020;15(5):723-31.
9. Sinha A, Bagga A, Krishna A, Bajpai M, Srinivas M, Uppal R, et al. Revised guidelines on management of antenatal hydronephrosis. Indian J Nephrol. 2013;23(2):83-97.
10. Choi YH, Cheon JE, Kim WS, Kim IO. Ultrasonography of hydronephrosis in the newborn: a practical review. Ultrasonography. 2016;35(3):198-211.

13.4 Glomerulonephritis

Kamran Afzal

INTRODUCTION

Glomerulonephritis (GN) refers to disorders in which an immunologic insult triggers inflammation and proliferation of glomerular tissue, with damage to the glomerular basement membrane (GBM), mesangium, or capillary endothelium. GN may be *primary* (confined to the kidney) or *secondary* (part of a systemic disorder). Depending on the duration of disease onset and the rate of progression, GN could be acute, rapidly progressive, or chronic.

ACUTE GLOMERULONEPHRITIS

Acute GN, or the acute nephritic syndrome, is defined as the sudden onset of hematuria and proteinuria, accompanied by hypertension, edema, and impaired renal function.

Infection-related GN is the most common cause. Nearly 60–80% cases in developing countries follow streptococcal infections of the throat or skin, the so-called poststreptococcal glomerulonephritis (PSGN) **(Box 13.4.1)**.[1,2] Other organisms, chiefly *Staphylococcus aureus*, are increasingly recognized.

BOX 13.4.1: Etiology of acute glomerulonephritis.

Infection related:
- *Bacteria:* Streptococci (group A, beta-hemolytic), staphylococci, pneumococci, meningococci, *Treponema pallidum, Salmonella typhi,* and *Leptospira*
- *Viruses:* Hepatitis B and C, cytomegalovirus, parvovirus B19, Epstein–Barr virus, coxsackie virus, echovirus, varicella, rubella, rickettsiae, and mumps
- *Parasites: Plasmodium malariae, P. falciparum,* toxoplasmosis, filariasis, and *Schistosoma mansoni*
- *Others:* Infection of shunts and prosthesis and infective endocarditis

Noninfectious:
- *Primary renal diseases:*
  - Immunoglobulin A (IgA) nephropathy
  - Membranoproliferative immune complex glomerulonephritis and C3 glomerulopathy
- *Systemic diseases:*
  - *Vasculitis:* IgA vasculitis, microscopic polyangiitis, granulomatosis, and polyangiitis
  - *Collagen vascular disorder:* Systemic lupus erythematosus, Sjögren's syndrome, and mixed connective tissue disease

Pathogenesis

Most cases of GN are due to an immunologic response to a variety of etiologic agents. PSGN is associated with throat or skin infection with nephritogenic strains of group A streptococci. Their nephritogenicity is related to the M-protein serotype—types 2, 49, 56, and 60 are associated with pyoderma, while 1, 4, 12, and 25 are associated with throat infection. The process of renal injury begins with deposition of immune complexes formed either in the circulation or in situ by binding of antibodies to antigens trapped in the glomerulus or native glomerular components. The immune complexes and streptococcal antigens activate the complement pathways with recruitment of leukocytes and macrophages and release of growth factors and cytokines that together initiate and propagate glomerular inflammation and injury.

Pathology

Light microscopy shows diffuse proliferative and exudative changes, with polymorphonuclear infiltrate and variable mesangial matrix expansion. There is endothelial and mesangial cell proliferation, resulting in obliteration of the glomerular tuft. Severe injury results in the proliferation of parietal and visceral epithelial cells, resulting in crescents. Immunofluorescence reveals irregular immunoglobulin G (IgG) and C3 deposits along the capillary wall in early stages (starry sky appearance) and the mesangium later. Garland pattern of confluent deposits along capillaries correlates with heavy proteinuria.

Clinical Features

Poststreptococcal glomerulonephritis affects children in the age group of 5–12 years (rare below 2 years), with male preponderance. Asymptomatic disease is 4–5 times more common among sporadic PSGN, although less frequently during epidemics. Subclinical cases have microscopic hematuria and low complement with or without hypertension. Symptomatic cases have an abrupt onset with hematuria, proteinuria, and variable edema and hypertension. History of streptococcal infection may precede onset of clinical features by 1–2 weeks for throat infections and 3–4 weeks for skin infections. Anuria is rare, though transient oliguria may be noted.

The occurrence of symptoms within 3–4 days of a respiratory or gastrointestinal infection suggests IgA nephropathy and rarely other disorders, including Alport syndrome. The presence of rash, arthralgia, abdominal pain, and hemoptysis suggests diagnoses other than postinfectious GN **(Table 13.4.1)**. Family history of renal disease suggests hereditary nephropathies such as Alport syndrome. Systemic features are seen with vasculitis and systemic lupus erythematosus.

Complications

An occasional patient may present with nephrotic range proteinuria or hypertensive emergency. The latter is characterized by stage 2 hypertension, with clinical evidence of heart failure, pulmonary edema, or encephalopathy. Rarely, there is progressive worsening of renal functions with hypertension and oligoanuria.

Diagnosis

Normocytic, normochromic anemia correlates with expansion of the extracellular fluid. The presence of thrombocytopenia requires investigations for lupus or hemolytic uremic syndrome (HUS). On urinalysis, gross hematuria is present; dysmorphic red cells, red cell and hyaline casts, and occasional neutrophils are seen. While proteinuria is often mild, occasionally nephrotic range proteinuria may be observed.

Although most patients have mild-to-modest elevation in serum concentrations of creatinine and urea, these range from severe azotemia to even normal levels at presentation. Hyperkalemia, metabolic acidosis, and hyponatremia are present in patients with significant renal function impairment.

Antistreptolysin O (ASO) titers are elevated in up to 80% of cases, suggesting preceding streptococcal infection; antibiotic therapy may attenuate this response.

Total hemolytic complement and some components are low during acute PSGN, suggesting activation of the alternate pathway of the complement system. The concentration of C3 is reduced in >90% of patients and normalizes by 6–8 weeks. The level of C3 does not have prognostic significance; persistent low C3 suggests diagnoses such as lupus, membranoproliferative glomerulonephritis (MPGN), C3 glomerulopathy, or nephritis associated with bacterial endocarditis, visceral abscess, and shunt nephritis.

Kidney biopsy is not needed to confirm the diagnosis of PSGN. It is indicated in those with heavy proteinuria, suspected crescentic GN, or significant deviation from the natural course of the disease **(Box 13.4.2)**.

Treatment

Therapy is essentially symptomatic, with mild cases of PSGN requiring home-based treatment. Hospital admission is required for those with oligoanuria, moderate-to-severe edema, hypertension, and impaired kidney functions. Penicillin, administered for 5–7 days to those with residual pharyngitis or pyoderma, prevents the spread of streptococci to others but does not alter disease course in the index case.

TABLE 13.4.1: Clues to underlying etiology of GN.

Clinical presentation	***Investigations***	***Diagnosis***
Preceding sore throat or skin infection, abscess, endocarditis, infected shunt, prosthetic valves, and indwelling catheters	Hematuria, high blood creatinine, low serum C3, elevated ASO, anti-DNase B, and antihyaluronidase	Postinfectious GN
Palpable purpura, joint pain, abdominal pain, and hematuria	*Skin biopsy:* Leukocytoclastic vasculitis and IgA deposits *Renal biopsy:* Proliferative GN and mesangial IgA deposits	IgA vasculitis
Recurrent hematuria, proteinuria, following respiratory tract infection	Mesangial IgA deposits	IgA nephropathy
Hematuria following respiratory infections, sensorineural deafness, lenticonus, retinopathy, and family history	*Electron microscopy:* Irregular thickening, splitting, and lamination of GBM	Alport syndrome
Arthralgia, malar rash, and nephritis	Positive ANA, dsDNA, and low C3	Systemic lupus erythematosus
Sinusitis, pulmonary infiltrates, and nephritis	Positive cytoplasmic ANCA *Biopsy:* Pauci-immune necrotizing GN	Granulomatosis with polyangiitis
Nephritis, fever, rash, arthralgia, and pulmonary hemorrhage	Positive perinuclear ANCA *Biopsy:* Pauci-immune necrotizing GN	Microscopic polyangiitis
Hemoptysis, pulmonary hemorrhage, and nephritis	Anti-GBM antibody in serum Crescentic GN with linear IgG deposits on biopsy	Goodpasture syndrome

(ANA: antinuclear antibody; ANCA: antineutrophil cytoplasmic antibody; ASO: antistreptolysin O; dsDNA: double-stranded DNA; GBM: glomerular basement membrane; GN: glomerulonephritis; Ig: immunoglobulin)

BOX 13.4.2: Indications for kidney biopsy in acute glomerulonephritis.

During early phase of disease:
- Latent period between streptococcal infection and acute glomerulonephritis of <1 week, no serologic evidence of streptococcal infection, and normal serum complement C3
- *Extrarenal manifestations of systemic disease:* Rash, joint pain, fever, hepatosplenomegaly, lymphadenopathy, and hemoptysis
- Anuria and rapidly deteriorating kidney function

During recovery phase:
- Persistent hypertension or nephrotic range proteinuria beyond 2–3 weeks
- No improvement or continued decrease in the glomerular filtration rate beyond 2 weeks
- Persistent hypocomplementemia beyond 12 weeks
- Persistent gross hematuria >1 month and microscopic hematuria >6–12 months

Those with oliguria or anuria require control of fluid intake to insensible water losses along with replacement of urine output. The use of diuretics (frusemide 1–3 mg/kg) helps manage fluid overload and circulatory congestion. Salt and fluid intake should be limited in those with significant hypertension, edema, or kidney failure. Dialysis is required in patients with refractory or worsening acute kidney injury. Hypertension is treated with oral diuretics, calcium channel blockers, or β-adrenergic blockers. Severe hypertension requires oral or intravenous (IV) furosemide and oral or sublingual nifedipine. For those presenting with hypertensive emergencies, IV short-acting medications (sodium nitroprusside or labetalol) are used.

Patients with nephrotic range proteinuria or rapidly progressive glomerulonephritis (RPGN) require prompt therapy (see further). Patients with IgA nephropathy and microscopic or recurrent gross hematuria and minimal proteinuria (<0.3–0.4 g/m^2/day) do not require specific treatment.

Course

It is important to attempt to identify the etiology of infection-related GN. The course in patients with PSGN is almost always satisfactory. Edema usually resolves in 5–10 days, and the blood pressure returns to normal after 2–3 weeks, though persistence of hypertension for up to 6 weeks is compatible with complete resolution. Urinary abnormalities resolve at various times after onset: Gross hematuria and proteinuria resolve early, but microscopic hematuria might continue for 6–12 months. C3 concentration normalized in >95% of patients by 8–10 weeks. Clinical manifestations of the disease rarely recur, and second episodes of PSGN are rare. The clinical course in patients with nonstreptococcal GN is not always satisfactory, and a proportion might progress to chronic kidney disease.

RAPIDLY PROGRESSIVE GLOMERULONEPHRITIS

Rapidly progressive glomerulonephritis is characterized by the nephritic syndrome (hematuria, edema, and hypertension) and rapidly declining kidney functions with oligoanuria and azotemia, which typically happens over days to weeks. Extensive crescents, involving 50% or more of the glomeruli, are the histological hallmark.[3,4] Crescents are two or more layers of segmental to circumferential proliferation of parietal epithelial cells that completely or partially obliterate the Bowman space. Crescents can evolve from being chiefly cellular to fibrocellular and fibrous, especially with delayed treatment.

Crescentic GN is rare in children. Its causes are categorized based on findings on immunofluorescence: Immune, pauci-immune, and anti-GBM disease, reflecting different mechanisms of glomerular injury **(Table 13.4.2)**. Immune complex GN is common in children.

Diagnosis

Investigations include blood counts, urinalysis (hematuria, proteinuria, and red cell casts), and blood levels of urea, creatinine, and C3. Serology includes ASO for preceding streptococcal infection and antinuclear and anti-double-stranded DNA (anti-dsDNA) autoantibodies in lupus. Antineutrophil cytoplasmic antibody (ANCA) with specificity for proteinase-3 produce cytoplasmic staining on immunofluorescence (cANCA), as in granulomatosis with polyangiitis. Myeloperoxidase-specific ANCA produces perinuclear staining on immunofluorescence (pANCA) in renal-limited vasculitis and microscopic polyangiitis. A kidney biopsy is necessary to confirm the diagnosis of crescentic GN; occasionally, diffuse proliferative GN or thrombotic microangiopathy may have a similar clinical presentation.

Treatment

Early diagnosis and treatment are necessary, given the risk of poor outcome and progressive kidney failure. Initial therapy with IV methylprednisolone (15–20 mg/kg, maximum 1 g/day) for 3–6 days is followed by oral prednisolone (1.5 mg/kg daily) for 4 weeks, with tapering to 0.5 mg/kg daily by 3 months, and then on alternate days for 12 months. IV cyclophosphamide (500–750 mg/m^2) is administered monthly for six doses.

Plasma exchange for 7–14 days is recommended for patients with anti-GBM disease and dialysis-dependent pauci-immune crescentic GN. Maintenance immunosuppression with azathioprine (2 mg/kg) and alternate-day prednisolone is advised for 2–3 years in most patients; longer therapies may be necessary in ANCA-associated diseases. Therapy for immune complex disease depends on the underlying etiology.

TABLE 13.4.2: Common causes and histology of crescentic glomerulonephritis (GN).

Cause (prevalence)	***Histology***
Immune complex GN (50–70%) • Postinfectious (streptococci, staphylococci, infective endocarditis, shunt nephritis, visceral abscess, hepatitis B, hepatitis C, and HIV) • Systemic diseases [lupus, immunoglobulin A (IgA) vasculitis, and rheumatoid arthritis] • Primary renal disease (IgA nephropathy and C3 glomerulopathy)	• Cellular and fibrocellular crescents • *Immunofluorescence:* Granular deposits of complement and immune complexes along capillary wall and mesangium • *Electron microscopy:* Subepithelial electron-dense deposits
Pauci-immune (25–40%): Microscopic polyangiitis, granulomatosis with polyangiitis, and renal-limited vasculitis	• Focal necrotizing GN with crescents, vasculitis, fibrinoid necrosis in glomeruli, and blood vessels • *Immunofluorescence:* Minimal or no immune deposits
Antiglomerular basement membrane (GBM) disease (5–7%): Goodpasture syndrome (lung and kidney involvement), anti-GBM disease (kidney involvement), and post-transplant in Alport syndrome	• Severe histological disease and crescents in most glomeruli • *Immunofluorescence:* Linear deposits of IgG along GBM

Promising agents for induction and maintenance therapy include rituximab and mycophenolate mofetil, respectively.

Prognosis

Prognosis depends on:

- *Etiology:* PGN fares better than pauci-immune or anti-GBM nephritis.
- *Histology:* Fibrous crescents fare worse than cellular or fibrocellular crescents.
- *Severity* of renal failure and promptness of *initiating therapy*

CHRONIC GLOMERULONEPHRITIS

Chronic glomerulonephritis (CGN) is characterized by progressive glomerular and tubulointerstitial fibrosis, ultimately leading to a reduction in glomerular filtration rate and retention of uremic toxins. If disease progression is not halted, the net result is chronic kidney disease and kidney failure. Almost all the causes listed in **Box 13.4.1** can progress to CGN. Common causes include crescentic GN, immune complex MPGN and C3 glomerulopathy, IgA nephropathy, and lupus nephritis.

Clinical Features

Patients have variable combinations of proteinuria, hematuria, edema, and hypertension. Cause-specific symptoms can help determine the etiology. Once chronic kidney disease sets in, there is a progressive decline in glomerular filtration rate and azotemia with associated complications and fluid overload.

Diagnosis

Laboratory workup includes urinalysis (hematuria, proteinuria, and red blood cell casts) and the estimation of blood levels of creatinine, electrolytes, calcium, phosphorus, and alkaline phosphatase. Renal ultrasound is done to assess kidney size, followed by biopsy.

Treatment

Antiproteinuric treatment with angiotensin-converting enzyme (ACE) inhibitors or angiotensin receptor blocker (ARB) may be used to reduce heavy proteinuria and retard disease progression. Immunosuppressive therapy with mycophenolate mofetil and prednisolone has been advised for patients with immune complex MPGN and C3 glomerulopathy. Daily therapy with prednisolone is recommended for patients with IgA nephropathy and nephrotic range proteinuria. Immunosuppressive therapy is also recommended for patients with lupus nephritis and IgA vasculitis.

Prognosis

The outcome depends on the etiology, stage of disease, and renal histology. Those with significant obsolescent and sclerosed glomeruli with tubulointerstitial fibrosis fare worse with progression to end-stage renal disease (ESRD).

REFERENCES

1. Xu H, Somers MJG. Acute post-streptococcal glomerulonephritis. In: Emma F, Goldstein S, Bagga A, Bates CM, Shroff R (Eds). Pediatric Nephrology, 8th edition. Switzerland AG: Springer Nature; 2022. pp. 659-72.
2. Iyengar A, Kamath N, Radhakrishnan J, Estebanez BT. Infection-related glomerulonephritis. Semin Nephrol. 2023;43(5):151469.
3. Menon S, Bagga A. Rapidly progressive glomerulonephritis. In: Schafer F, Greenbaum LA (Eds). Pediatric Kidney Disease, 3rd edition. Philadelphia: Springer Link; 2023. pp. 575-90.
4. Roper T, Salama AD. ANCA-associated vasculitis: Practical issues in management. Indian J Nephrol. 2024;34(1):6-23.

13.5 Renal Vasculitis and Lupus Nephritis

Sushmita Banerjee

INTRODUCTION

Vasculitis is an inflammation of blood vessel walls that results in endothelial damage with ischemic injury to the end organ or tissue. Different vasculitides have predilection for involving specific organ systems, and the kidney is quite commonly affected. The majority of these conditions do not have a proven etiology. Evidence suggests a genetic predisposition with disease precipitated by an environmental trigger, resulting in an abnormal immune response.[1]

The vasculitic syndromes were classified according to the dimension of vessel affected during the International Chapel Hill Consensus Conference in 2012 **(Table 13.5.1 and Fig. 13.5.1)**.[2] Characteristics for specific diseases were further formulated by the EULAR/PRINTO/PReS-endorsed Ankara 2008 criteria.[3]

Clinical Features

Most vasculitides involve several organ systems resulting in variable patterns of clinical involvement. Anemia, fever, malaise, and weight loss may be present along with arthritis, skin rashes, purpura **(Fig. 13.5.2)**, abdominal pain, uveitis, and mucosal ulcers. Large vessel disease can cause absent or asymmetric arterial pulses and claudication. The respiratory and neurological systems may be involved. Hypertension is a common finding; patients with Takayasu arteritis often have abdominal bruit due to renal artery stenosis. Intrarenal involvement causes an acute nephritic or nephritic-nephrotic presentation with hematuria and edema.[1,4]

Investigations

Patients show evidence of raised acute phase reactants. Investigation of extrarenal manifestations is guided by clinical features, and may include chest X-ray, lung CT, brain imaging, and echocardiography. Biopsies of upper respiratory tract mucosa are performed for the diagnosis of granulomatosis with polyangiitis (GPA) where they show a granulomatous necrotizing vasculitis. Skin biopsies show leukocytoclastic vasculitis with immunoglobulin A (IgA) deposition in IgA vasculitis (IgAV) and necrotizing vasculitis in polyarteritis nodosa (PAN). Angiography shows changes such as thickening and narrowing of the aorta and its branches in Takayasu disease, or intrakidney aneurysms or vascular pruning in PAN **(Figs. 13.5.3 and 13.5.4)**.

Urinalysis might show an active sediment with hematuria, proteinuria, and casts. Urea and creatinine may be raised. antinuclear antibody (ANA), anti-double-stranded DNA (anti-dsDNA), antineutrophil cytoplasmic antibody (ANCA) serology, and complement levels are useful in ascertaining

TABLE 13.5.1: 2012 Revised International Chapel Hill Consensus Conference Nomenclature of Vasculitides.

Vessel size	*Disease*
Large	• Takayasu arteritis • Giant cell arteritis
Medium	• Polyarteritis nodosa • Kawasaki disease
Small	*Antineutrophil cytoplasmic antibody (ANCA)-associated vasculitis:* • Microscopic polyangiitis • Granulomatosis with polyangiitis (Wegener granulomatosis) • Eosinophilic granulomatosis with polyangiitis (Churg–Strauss) *Immune complex vasculitis:* • Antiglomerular basement membrane (anti-GBM) disease • Cryoglobulinemic vasculitis • Immunoglobulin A (IgA) vasculitis (Henoch–Schönlein syndrome) • Hypocomplementemic urticarial vasculitis (anti-C1q vasculitis)
Variable vessel vasculitis	• Behçet disease • Cogan syndrome
Single-organ vasculitis	• Cutaneous leukocytoclastic angiitis • Cutaneous arteritis • Primary central nervous system vasculitis • Isolated aortitis • Others
Vasculitis associated with systemic disease	• Lupus vasculitis • Rheumatoid vasculitis • Sarcoid vasculitis
Vasculitis associated with probable etiology	• Hepatitis C virus-associated cryoglobulinemic vasculitis • Hepatitis B virus-associated vasculitis • Syphilis-associated aortitis • Drug-associated immune complex vasculitis • Drug-associated ANCA-associated vasculitis • Cancer-associated vasculitis

Immune complex small vessel vasculitis
- Cryoglobulinemic vasculitis
- IgA vasculitis (Henoch-Schönlein)
- Hypocomplementemic urticarial vasculitis (Anti-C1q vasculitis)

Medium vessel vasculitis
- Polyarteritis nodosa
- Kawasaki disease

Anti-GBM disease

ANCA-associated small vessel vasculitis
- Microscopic polyangiitis
- Granulomatosis with polyangiitis (Wegener's)
- Eosinophilic granulomatosis with polyangiitis (Churg-Strauss)

Large vessel vasculitis
- Takayasu arteritis
- Giant cell arteritis

Fig. 13.5.1: The nomenclature of vasculitides by vessel size. (ANCA: antineutrophil cytoplasmic antibody; Anti-GBM: antiglomerular basement membrane)

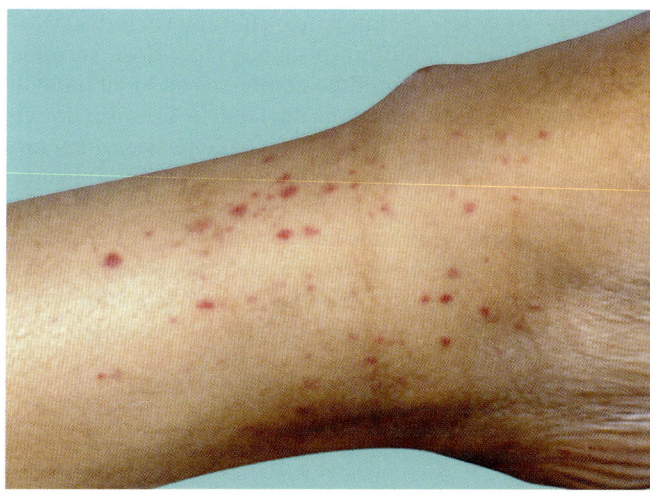

Fig. 13.5.2: Immunoglobulin A (IgA) vasculitis; note the palpable purpura.

the diagnosis. Kidney biopsy features are discussed in the sections on individual diseases below.[4,5]

Management

Supportive management with antipyretics, antibiotics, and antihypertensive agents are used as required. Kidney failure is managed with salt, potassium and fluid restriction, and dialysis when indicated. Management of extrarenal symptoms is done simultaneously. The specific management of the kidney disease in the majority of these conditions [PAN, Takayasu disease, systemic lupus erythematosus (SLE), and ANCA-related vasculitis] involves therapy with steroids and other immunosuppressive agents with regular monitoring to keep disease activity (clinical and serological) under control, and for adverse effects of therapy.[6] Kidney revascularization procedures (stenting, grafting, or autotransplantation) may be required in patients developing arterial stenosis or dilatation.

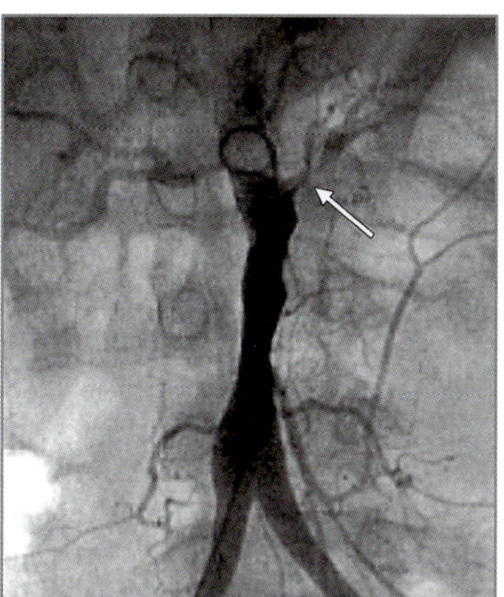

Fig. 13.5.3: Takayasu arteritis with left kidney artery stenosis.

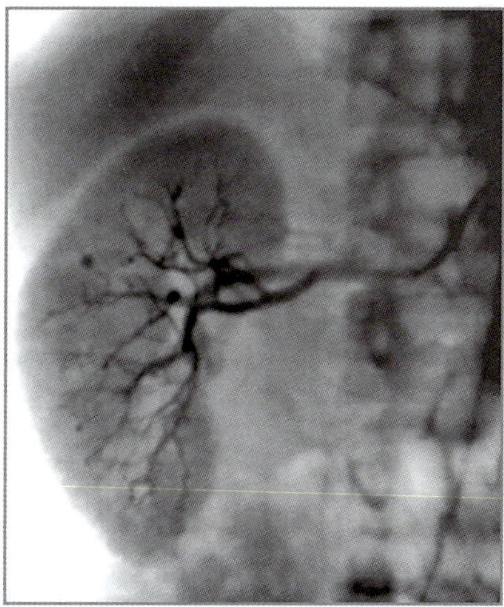

Fig. 13.5.4: Kidney aneurysms in polyarteritis nodosa.

IMMUNOGLOBULIN A VASCULITIS

Henoch-Schönlein purpura (HSP) or IgAV is the most common childhood vasculitis. Kidney involvement is reported to occur in 20–55% patients with risk of progression to end-stage kidney disease (ESKD) in 1–3%. Kidney manifestations in the majority occur within 4–6 weeks after onset of rash but may occur up to 6 months. Occasional late progression up to 2 years after onset has been documented in patients who have initially improved, making long-term follow-up essential.[1,7]

The most common renal finding is microscopic hematuria or minor proteinuria, which are generally self-limiting. The presence of kidney insufficiency, hypertension, or significant proteinuria indicates a poorer prognosis with increased likelihood of persistence and progression. Kidney biopsy findings are classified according to the International Study of Kidney Disease in Children (ISKDC) criteria and vary from mesangial and/or endocapillary proliferation to severe involvement with crescentic glomerulonephritis. Predominant IgA mesangial deposits on immunofluorescence, indistinguishable from IgA nephropathy, are characteristic. Studies examining the utility of MEST-C classification (used in primary IgA nephropathy) are ongoing. Recent European consensus-based recommendations (SHARE initiative 2019) has laid down criteria for defining disease severity and subsequent management.[7]

A short course of corticosteroids is recommended in patients with severe abdominal symptoms. The presence of microscopic hematuria alone does not warrant specific treatment. Prophylactic therapy with corticosteroids does not reduce the risk of HSP nephritis but may improve outcome in established cases. Patients with severe HSP nephritis, particularly rapidly progressive glomerulonephritis (RPGN), are treated with combinations of oral or intravenous (IV) corticosteroids, immunosuppressive agents [azathioprine, cyclophosphamide, and mycophenolate mofetil (MMF)], intravenous immunoglobulin (IVIG), and plasma exchange. IgAV may recur after kidney transplant.

NEPHRITIS ASSOCIATED WITH SYSTEMIC LUPUS ERYTHEMATOSUS

Systemic lupus erythematosus is a multisystem disease with kidney involvement occurring in 50–75% affected children, the majority within the first 2 years of presentation. Lupus nephritis is characterized by variable grades of hematuria, proteinuria, hypertension, and kidney functional impairment. Kidney tubular dysfunction occurs rarely. Clinical criteria suggesting kidney involvement [as per Systemic Lupus International Collaborating Clinics (SLICC), 2012] in SLE patients are 24-hour urine protein >500 mg (corresponding to spot urine protein creatinine ratio >0.5 mg/mg) or RBC casts.[1,8]

Multiple ANA are found in SLE, of which anti-dsDNA is the most specific. Activation of the classical pathway of complement results in low levels of C3 and C4 and the deposition of C3, C4, and C1q in kidney tissue. A kidney biopsy is indicated in all patients with kidney involvement, as there might be unsatisfactory correlation of clinical findings, serology, and pathology. The deposition of IgG, IgA and IgM immune-complexes, C3, C4, and C1q indicates a full house on immunofluorescence, characteristic of SLE nephritis. Histological grading influences management and prognosis **(Box 13.5.1)**. Class IV or diffuse proliferative glomerulonephritis is most common and may have a rapidly progressive course with devastating consequences if untreated.[1,8]

BOX 13.5.1: International Society of Nephrology/Kidney Pathology Society classification for lupus nephritis (2003, revised 2018).

- *Class I:* Minimal changes on light microscopy
- *Class II:* Mesangial hypercellularity
- *Class III:* Focal glomerulonephritis (<50% glomeruli involved)
- *Class IV:* Diffuse glomerulonephritis (>50% glomeruli involved)
- *Class V:* Membranous changes
- *Class VI:* Sclerosed lesions

Scores for activity and chronicity:
- Chronicity index (based on fibrous crescents/tubular atrophy/interstitial fibrosis)
- Activity index (based on endocapillary hypercellularity/glomerular neutrophils/karyorrhexis/fibrinoid necrosis/wire loop lesions/hyaline thrombi, cellular or fibrocellular crescent, and interstitial leukocytes)

Class I–II lupus nephritis is treated with corticosteroids with management aimed more at extrarenal disease. Patients with class III and IV nephritis and high activity indices are treated aggressively with combinations of high-dose steroids and cytotoxic agents. Commonly used protocols include induction agents such as IV or oral corticosteroids, cyclophosphamide, or MMF. Maintenance therapy includes MMF or azathioprine in addition to tapered low-dose steroids. Hydroxychloroquine should be administered in all patients with annual eye examination advised to monitor for its adverse effects. Treatment options in patients with refractory illness include calcineurin inhibitors, rituximab, plasmapheresis, and IVIG. Other biological agents are under trial and belimumab has recently been approved for use in active disease. Adjunct therapies such as aggressive control of hypertension and treatment of persistent proteinuria with renin-angiotensin system (RAS) inhibitors are recommended.[6,9]

ANTINEUTROPHIL CYTOPLASMIC ANTIBODY-ASSOCIATED NEPHRITIS

The common ANCA-associated kidney diseases are granulomatous polyangiitis (GPA, formerly known as Wegener granulomatosis) and microscopic polyangiitis (MPA), while Churg–Strauss syndrome is rare in children. The former are severe diseases that have a fulminant relapsing course with high risk of ESKD and mortality. Kidney disease presents with a nephritic-nephrotic syndrome, acute kidney failure, and RPGN.

Circulating ANCAs have a role in pathogenesis and correlate with disease activity. Immunofluorescence detects protoplasmic ANCA (p-ANCA or perinuclear pattern of staining) or cytoplasmic ANCA (c-ANCA with diffusely granular, cytoplasmic staining). Enzyme-linked immunosorbent assay (ELISA) may show antimyeloperoxidase (anti-MPO) specificity or antiprotease 3 (anti-PR3) specificity.[4]

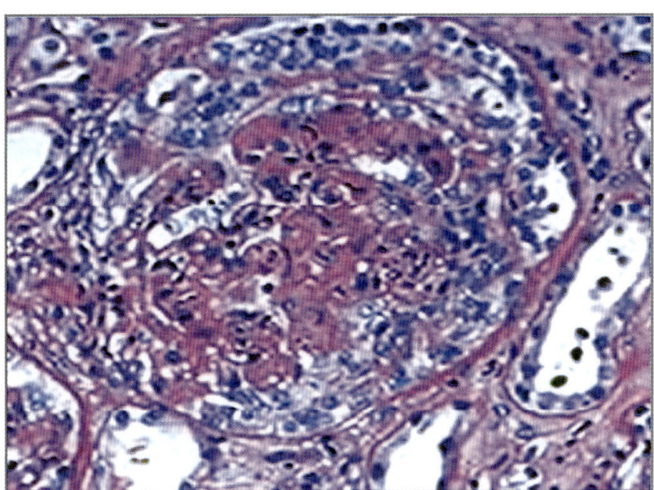

Fig. 13.5.5: Crescentic glomerulonephritis. Note the circumferential cellular crescent with collapse of the capillary tuft.

Kidney histopathology reveals a necrotizing, pauci-immune glomerulonephritis with crescents **(Fig. 13.5.5)**. Aggressive immunosuppression is required, the most common agents used for induction therapy are steroids and cyclophosphamide. Methotrexate, MMF, azathioprine have been used as maintenance therapies. Plasmapheresis, IVIG, rituximab, and other biological compounds are used in severe and resistant cases.[3,6]

CONCLUSION

The renal vasculitic diseases should be considered in the differential diagnosis of patients who present with nephritic or nephritic-nephrotic features, particularly when there are associated extrarenal manifestations. These potentially aggressive conditions need rapid workup so that an early diagnosis can be made and appropriate management initiated in order to limit kidney damage. Even after initial therapy of the specific disease, long-term follow-up is indicated for residual effects and for relapses.

REFERENCES

1. Schnabel A, Hedrich CM. Childhood vasculitis. Front Pediatr. 2019;6:421.
2. Jennette JC, Falk RJ, Bacon PA, Basu N, Cid MC, Ferrario F, et al. 2012 revised International Chapel Hill Consensus Conference Nomenclature of Vasculitides. Arthritis Rheum. 2013;65(1):1-11.
3. Ozen S, Pistorio A, Iusan SM, Bakkaloglu A, Herlin T, Brik R, et al. Pediatric Rheumatology International Trials Organisation (PRINTO) (2010). EULAR/PRINTO/PRES criteria for Henoch-Schönlein purpura, childhood polyarteritis nodosa, childhood Wegener granulomatosis, and childhood Takayasu arteritis: Final classification criteria. Ann Rheum Dis. 2010;69(5):798-806.
4. Ozen S, Orhan D, Marks SD. Renal vasculitis. In: Emma F, Goldstein SL, Bagga A, Bates C, Shroff R (Eds). Pediatric Nephrology, 8th edition. Switzerland: Springer Nature. 2021. pp. 490-507.
5. de Graeff N, Groot N, Brogan P, Ozen S, Avcin T, Bader-Meunier B, et al. European consensus-based recommendations for the diagnosis and treatment of rare pediatric vasculitides: SHARE initiative. Rheumatology. (Oxford) 2019;58(4):656-71. Erratum in: Rheumatology (Oxford). 2020;59(4):919.
6. Rovin BH, Adler SG, Barratt J, Barratt J, Bridoux F, Burdge KA, et al. Executive summary of the KDIGO 2021 guideline for the management of glomerular diseases. Kidney Int. 2021; 100(4):753-79.
7. Ozen S, Marks SD, Brogan P, Groot N, de Graeff N, Avcin T, et al. European consensus-based recommendations for diagnosis and treatment of immunoglobulin A vasculitis-the SHARE initiative. Rheumatology (Oxford). 2019;58(9):1607-16
8. Pennesi M, Benvenuto S. Lupus nephritis in children: Novel perspectives. Medicina (Kaunas). 2023;59(10):1841.
9. Scobell R, Pradhan M. Management of lupus nephritis in children. Indian Pediatr. 2020;57(5):401-6.

13.6 Acute Kidney Injury

Sumantra Kumar Raut, Arvind Bagga

INTRODUCTION

Acute kidney injury (AKI) is present when there is a rapid decline in kidney function. The "Kidney Disease: Improving Global Outcomes (KDIGO)" defines AKI as an absolute increase in serum creatinine of either ≥0.3 mg/dL within 48 hours or a percentage increase in serum creatinine of ≥50% over 7 days or less, and/or reduction in urine output to <0.5 mL/kg/h for >6 hours.[1]

If the diagnosis of AKI is based on the urine output criterion alone, urinary tract obstruction and other reversible causes of oliguria (dehydration) should be excluded. Patients meeting the definition of AKI are staged using KDIGO criteria **(Table 13.6.1)**.

TABLE 13.6.1: Staging of acute kidney injury.*

Stage	Serum creatinine criteria	Urine output criteria
1	Increase in serum creatinine by ≥0.3 mg/dL from baseline within 48 hours or to 150–200% (1.5 to 2-fold) of baseline within 7 days	<0.5 mL/kg/h for 6–12 hours
2	Increase in serum creatinine to >200–300% (>2 to 3-fold) from baseline	<0.5 mL/kg/h for >12 hours
3	• Increase in serum creatinine to >300% (>3-fold) of baseline or increase in serum creatinine by ≥4** mg/dL from baseline with acute increase of ≥0.5 mg/dL • Initiation of kidney support therapy or estimated glomerular filtration rate <35 mL/min/1.73 m^2	<0.3 mL/kg/h for 24 hours or anuria for 12 hours

*Only one criterion (creatinine or urine output) is required for staging.
**2.5 mg/dL in case of neonates

ETIOLOGY

Acute kidney injury occurs in a variety of settings with clinical features ranging from mild elevation in serum creatinine to anuric renal failure. The etiology of AKI is conventionally classified as prerenal, intrinsic renal, or postrenal **(Box 13.6.1)**. The index most useful in helping differentiate prerenal from renal azotemia is the fractional excretion of sodium. Patients with prerenal illness show a low fractional excretion of sodium (<1%); higher values are seen with acute tubular necrosis (ATN).

The chief causes of AKI include ATN secondary to hypovolemia, sepsis and nephrotoxic agents, acute glomerulonephritis (GN) and hemolytic uremic syndrome (HUS). ATN is quite common in sick hospitalized children and is associated with risk factors such as sepsis, hypotension, ventilation, and surgery. Almost one-third children admitted to the pediatric or neonatal intensive care units may show evidence of AKI; the risk is higher among patients undergoing cardiac or other complex surgeries.[2,3]

Perinatal asphyxia and respiratory distress syndrome are leading causes of AKI in neonates. In developing countries, AKI is chiefly community acquired and usually secondary to a single cause such as acute gastroenteritis or tropical infections such as malaria or dengue.

EVALUATION

A careful history provides clues to the underlying cause. A history of diarrhea, vomiting, fluid, or blood loss should be sought and an assessment of fluid intake in the previous 24 hours be made. Investigations in patients with AKI include the following:

- Complete blood counts (CBCs), urea, creatinine, sodium, potassium, calcium, phosphate, pH, and bicarbonate
- Urinalysis (for red cells, casts, and proteinuria); culture (if febrile); sodium, osmolality, and fractional excretion of sodium
- Peripheral smear examination, platelet and reticulocyte count, and lactate dehydrogenase

BOX 13.6.1: Important causes of acute kidney injury.

Prerenal failure:
- Hypovolemia (dehydration, blood loss, diabetic ketoacidosis, nasogastric drainage, and burns)
- Third space losses (septicemia and nephrotic syndrome)
- Congestive heart failure
- Hepatorenal syndrome
- Perinatal asphyxia
- *Drugs:* ACE inhibitors, diuretics, NSAID, and calcineurin inhibitors

Intrinsic renal failure:
- *Acute tubular necrosis:*
  - Prolonged prerenal insult (see earlier)
  - *Medications:* Aminoglycosides, radiocontrast agents, cisplatin, and amphotericin B
  - Disseminated intravascular coagulation
  - *Exogenous toxins:* Diethylene glycol, methanol, heavy metals, and snake venom
  - Intravascular hemolysis, hemoglobinuria, and tumor lysis syndrome
  - *Infections:* Malaria, leptospirosis, and dengue hemorrhagic fever; pyelonephritis
- *Rapidly progressive glomerulonephritis:*
  - *Immune complex:* Postinfectious glomerulonephritis; IgA nephropathy; C3 glomerulopathy; lupus nephritis and IgA vasculitis
  - ANCA-associated vasculitides
- *Thrombotic microangiopathy:*
  - Hemolytic uremic syndrome (Shiga toxin associated, secondary, and atypical forms)
  - Thrombotic thrombocytopenic purpura
- *Vascular causes:*
  - Renal artery stenosis
  - Renal artery or vein thrombosis
- *Interstitial nephritis:* Drug-induced and idiopathic

Postrenal failure:
- Posterior urethral valves and urethral stricture
- Ureteral obstruction (stenosis, stone, and ureterocele)
- Neurogenic bladder

(ACE: angiotensin-converting enzyme; ANCA antineutrophilic cytoplasmic antibodies; IgA: immunoglobulin A; NSAID: nonsteroidal anti-inflammatory drug)

- Screening for malaria, leptospirosis, or dengue (if suspected)
- *Chest X-ray:* For fluid overload and cardiomegaly
- Complement, C3 (HUS and GN); factor H antibodies (suspected HUS)
- Stool culture and screening for verotoxin (suspected Shiga toxin-associated HUS)
- Blood antistreptolysin O (ASO), antinuclear antibody (ANA), antineutrophil cytoplasmic antibody (ANCA): (suspected acute or rapidly progressive GN)
- *Abdominal ultrasonography:* Kidney size and structure; urinary tract dilatation; vena cava collapsibility
- *Doppler ultrasound:* Suspected arterial or venous thrombosis
- *Furosemide stress test (FST):* This can be done to differentiate prerenal from intrinsic renal AKI.[4] A normal saline bolus of 10 mL/kg over 20 minutes followed by intravenous (IV) furosemide 1 mg/kg. Patients with prerenal AKI usually show urine output of 2–3 mL/kg/hour over the next 2 hours.
- A *kidney biopsy* is not required in most patients with AKI. Indications for kidney biopsy are: Rapidly progressive or nonresolving GN; AKI associated with systemic lupus erythematosus or immunoglobulin A (IgA) vasculitis; suspected interstitial nephritis; or if the underlying cause of AKI is not apparent on clinical features and investigations.

MANAGEMENT

Specific management of the underlying disorder is possible in some cases **(Table 13.6.2)**. Fluid resuscitation in patients with septic shock or dehydration improves renal perfusion and improves urine output.[5] Patients with urinary tract obstruction need catheterization. It is important to manage life-threatening complications including hyperkalemia, pulmonary edema, hypertensive emergencies, and severe acidosis **(Table 13.6.3)**.

Hyperkalemia

Hyperkalemia is a serious emergency. Urgent treatment is instituted depending on blood potassium levels and electrocardiography (ECG) changes. Concomitant metabolic acidosis should be corrected. While salbutamol, insulin, glucose, and sodium bicarbonate reduce the extracellular concentration of potassium by moving the ion into the cells, calcium infusion decreases membrane irritability without altering serum potassium levels. The action of Kayexalate (sodium polystyrene sulfonate) or calcium resonium, which exchanges potassium for sodium or calcium ions, is slow and not useful in emergencies. Peritoneal or hemodialysis is the most effective method to remove excess potassium from the body.

Hypertension

Hypertension is commonly observed in patients with GN and HUS. The symptoms of hypertensive encephalopathy are related to rapidity of rise rather than absolute value of the blood pressure. These include headache, blurring of vision, convulsions, papilledema, cranial nerve palsies, vomiting, and altered sensorium. Blood pressure should be reduced slowly and carefully with sodium nitroprusside or labetalol infusion. In asymptomatic hypertension, oral nifedipine, amlodipine, prazosin, and labetalol may be used.

Hyponatremia

Hyponatremia (sodium <130 mEq/L) is usually the result of excessive fluid administration rather than salt loss. Patients with blood sodium concentration >125 mEq/L are rarely symptomatic. Hyponatremia is best managed by fluid restriction; patients with resistant hyponatremia can be satisfactorily managed by dialysis. Treatment with hypertonic saline (3%) is reserved for those with symptomatic hyponatremia (encephalopathy, lethargy, and seizures), but should be used cautiously because of complications of fluid overload and hypertension.

TABLE 13.6.2: Specific management of conditions causing acute kidney injury (AKI).

Prerenal AKI	Administer fluids and/or vasopressors to correct dehydration and maintain blood pressure; avoid NSAID, ACE inhibitors, and radiocontrast agents
Acute tubular necrosis	Supportive care; treat infections or underlying cause (e.g., circulatory failure)
Glomerulonephritis	Supportive care; plasma exchange; immunosuppression (IV corticosteroids and cyclophosphamide)
Hemolytic uremic syndrome	Supportive care; plasma exchanges/infusions or eculizumab for atypical HUS
Vasculitis	Immunosuppression (IV methylprednisolone, cyclophosphamide, and rituximab)
Interstitial nephritis	Discontinue offending drug; consider oral corticosteroids
Renal artery or vein occlusion	Anticoagulation; thrombolysis or surgery
Urinary tract obstruction	Bladder catheter, nephrostomy, and surgical treatment

(ACE: angiotensin-converting enzyme; HUS: hemolytic uremic syndrome; IV: intravenous; NSAID: nonsteroidal anti-inflammatory drug)

TABLE 13.6.3: Management of complications of AKI.

Complication	*Treatment*
Fluid overload	*Fluid restriction:* Insensible losses (400 mL/m^2/day, as 5% dextrose); add urine output and other losses (as half-normal saline); consider dialysis
Pulmonary edema	Oxygen; fluid restriction; furosemide 2–4 mg/kg IV; monitor CVP; consider dialysis
Hypertension	• *Symptomatic:* Sodium nitroprusside 0.5–8 µg/kg/min or labetalol 0.25–3 mg/kg/h as infusion; furosemide 1–4 mg/kg IV, if fluid overload; nifedipine 0.3–0.5 mg/kg oral/sublingual. Aim to reduce blood pressure by 25% of the desired reduction during first 8 hours, and remainder over next 12–24 hours • *Asymptomatic:* Amlodipine, prazosin, labetalol, and clonidine
Metabolic acidosis	Sodium bicarbonate (IV or oral) if bicarbonate <18 mEq/L; monitor for hypernatremia, hypocalcemia, and fluid overload; consider dialysis
Hyperkalemia	• *Calcium gluconate (10%):* 0.5–1 mL/kg over 5–10 minutes • *Salbutamol:* 5–10 mg nebulized over 10 minutes • *Dextrose (10%):* 0.5–1 g/kg and insulin 0.1–0.2 U/kg • *Sodium bicarbonate (7.5%):* 1–2 mL/kg over 5–15 minutes • *Calcium or sodium resonium (Kayexalate):* 1 g/kg orally or rectally every 4–6 hours
Hyponatremia	Fluid restriction; if sensorial alteration or seizures, give 3% saline 6–12 mL/kg over 30–90 minutes
Severe anemia	Packed red cells 3–5 mL/kg; monitor for hypertension, hyperkalemia, and fluid overload; consider exchange transfusion
High phosphate	Reduce dietary phosphate; consider phosphate binders (calcium carbonate; aluminum hydroxide)

(AKI: acute kidney injury; CVP: central venous pressure)

Fluid and Nutrition

Fluid and electrolyte intake in a patient with AKI should be regulated based on a clinical examination of extracellular fluid volume status, urine output, and daily weights. The daily fluid requirement amounts to insensible water losses (300–400 mL/m^2), urinary output, and extrarenal fluid losses. Insensible fluid losses are replaced with 5–10% dextrose or glucose solution. Urine output should be measured without resorting to catheterization. Urinary losses and those from extrarenal sources should have their composition analyzed and replaced accordingly. It is preferable to administer the required amounts of fluid by mouth, whenever feasible. If there is persistent vomiting, IV route may be necessary. Potassium containing fluids should not be given to patients with oliguria. Ongoing treatment is guided by intake output analysis, daily weight, physical examination, and serum sodium. If fluid in an appropriate volume and composition has been given, the patient should lose 0.5–1% of his weight every day. This weight loss is the result of caloric deprivation and not inadequate fluid therapy. Serum sodium concentrations should be maintained within the normal range.

Adequate nutritional support is preferred with maximization of caloric intake. A diet containing 1.2–2 g/kg of protein in infants and 0.8–1.2 g/kg in older children, and 60–80 Cal/kg should be given. Once dialysis is initiated, dietary protein, fluid, and electrolyte intake should be increased.

Diuretics and Drugs

Diuretics may be useful in instances where high urine flow is required to prevent intratubular precipitation as with intravascular hemolysis, hyperuricemia, and myoglobinuria.

Drugs that increase severity of renal damage, delay recovery of function, or reduce perfusion, e.g., aminoglycosides, radiocontrast media, nonsteroidal anti-inflammatory drugs, amphotericin B, angiotensin-converting enzyme inhibitors, and indomethacin, should be avoided. Standard charts are used for modifying the dose and dosing interval of antibiotics depending on the severity of renal injury.

There is no beneficial effect of dopamine infusion on the outcome of AKI. Its routine use for prevention or treatment of ATN is therefore not recommended. The role of other medications, including fenoldopam, atrial natriuretic peptide, calcium channel blockers, and other medications is investigational.

Kidney Support Therapy

Indications for initiating kidney support therapy (KST) include severe or persistent hyperkalemia (>7 mEq/L), fluid overload (pulmonary edema and severe hypertension), uremic encephalopathy, severe metabolic acidosis (bicarbonate <10–12 mEq/L), severe (<120 mEq/L) or symptomatic hyponatremia, or severe hypernatremia.[6]

The initial KST of choice in sick and unstable infants is often intermittent peritoneal dialysis (PD), since it is technically less challenging, can be performed in all settings and requires limited expertise. It is easy to initiate in children of all ages, including neonates. Peritoneal access can be obtained using a stiff catheter and trocar. While PD can be effectively performed with these catheters, these should be removed after 48–72 hours beyond which the risk of infection is very high. If the duration of AKI is prolonged, chronic PD may be performed, either manually (continuous ambulatory PD) or with the use of an automated device (continuous cycling PD).

Hemodialysis is more efficient for correction of fluid and electrolyte abnormalities. However, it is expensive to institute, requires expertise and skilled nursing and is not available at many centers. It is not suited for patients with hemodynamic instability, bleeding tendency, and in very young children where vascular access might be difficult. Continuous renal replacement therapy (CRRT) is useful when KST is necessary in sick and unstable patients. Special equipment and trained staff are necessary to provide CRRT in children. Hemodialysis is less expensive than CRRT and should be the first KST of choice in centers where it is available.

HEMOLYTIC UREMIC SYNDROME

Hemolytic uremic syndrome characterized by microangiopathic hemolytic anemia, thrombocytopenia, and renal impairment is one of the most common causes of AKI in children. The diarrhea-associated (classic) HUS occurs in childhood, usually caused by Shiga toxin (verotoxin) producing bacteria (*Escherichia coli* 0157:H7, *Shigella dysenteriae*) and is associated with a satisfactory prognosis. More than 90% of children recover normal renal function with supportive therapy.

Atypical HUS (aHUS) is a heterogeneous disorder with less favorable outcome. This condition is distinguished from Shiga toxin-associated HUS by absence of diarrheal prodrome, and often a chronic and relapsing course, with high mortality and risk of progressive kidney failure. Certain conditions (e.g., malignancy, pregnancy, systemic lupus erythematosus, and hematopoietic stem cell transplantation) and medications (cyclosporine, tacrolimus, and ticlopidine) are also associated with HUS, termed as secondary HUS.

Diagnosis

The diagnosis of HUS is made in presence of azotemia, thrombocytopenia (<100,000/mm^3), and microangiopathic hemolysis, occurring with or without history of preceding diarrhea or dysentery. The underlying histology is a thrombotic microangiopathy (TMA) involving capillaries and small arterioles in the kidney. While histological changes are most marked in the kidneys, evidence of TMA might be present in the brain, heart, lungs, gastrointestinal tract, and pancreas.

Atypical HUS is characterized by activation of the alternative complement pathway. Defects in the genes for multiple complement components have been identified. These include loss of function mutations of genes encoding factor H (*CFH*), membrane cofactor protein (*MCP*, CD46), factor I (*CFI*), *MMACHC*, and diacylglycerol kinase (*DGKE*), and gain of function mutations in *CFB* and *C3*. About 20–50% cases have been associated with autoantibodies against factor H (anti-FH antibodies), particularly in the background of homozygous deletion in *CFHR1/3*. Deficient activity of metalloproteinase with thrombospondin motifs 13 (ADAMTS13) is associated with thrombotic thrombocytopenic purpura, a distinct disorder but with features similar to HUS.

Enterohemorrhagic *E. coli* (EHEC) or *S. dysenteriae* is the likely cause of HUS in patients older than 6 months with history of bloody diarrhea in the preceding 2 weeks. Stool is examined for infection with EHEC and for presence of Shiga toxin. Serum levels of complement factors C3 and C4 are estimated. A low level of C3 in a patient with normal C4 indicates activation of the alternative pathway. In patients with suspected aHUS, blood samples are taken for estimation of anti-FH antibodies and flow cytometry for CD46. Patients with aHUS should undergo genetic screening for pathogenic variations in key complement genes.

Therapy

Therapy for HUS includes the management of AKI. Management of Shiga toxin-associated HUS includes maintaining appropriate hydration and use of appropriate antibiotics. Transfusion of packed red blood cells (RBCs) is needed in patients with severe anemia (hemoglobin <6 g/dL). Careful monitoring of blood pressure, urine output, and respiratory rate is necessary. Platelet transfusions are rarely necessary.

Guidelines on therapy for aHUS recommend the use of eculizumab, a monoclonal antibody against C5, that blocks the terminal complement cascade and enables recovery from the disease. However, this medication is not easily available in developing countries.[7] In absence of availability of complement blockers, double-volume plasma exchanges have increasingly been used for patients with aHUS. Plasma infusion is able to provide the deficient complement factor and help manage the acute disease. Patients with anti-FH antibodies benefit from the combination of plasma exchanges and therapy with immunosuppressive agents (corticosteroids, IV cyclophosphamide, and oral mycophenolate mofetil).

OUTCOME OF ACUTE KIDNEY INJURY

Long-term follow-up is necessary in children with severe AKI. Meta-analysis of pediatric studies shows ~10% mortality among hospitalized children with AKI.[8] Another 20–25% patients show progression to chronic kidney disease on long-term follow-up. Patients with HUS and GN may show persistent hypertension and variable degrees of proteinuria. Patients with AKI need to be followed up every 3–6 months with particular attention to urinalysis, blood pressure, and kidney function.

CONCLUSION

AKI is a rapid decline in kidney function and is diagnosed by elevation of serum creatinine and/or decreasing urine output.

AKI is staged as per its severity, and its etiology varies from prerenal causes, to primary kidney disease, and obstruction to urine flow. Various blood and urine investigations and imaging help to determine the cause of AKI, since treatment may vary with etiology; a kidney biopsy is rarely required. Treatment of AKI is chiefly conservative; RRT may be required in patients with severe AKI. The outcome of AKI is mostly favorable, but patients require long-term follow-up to diagnose progression to chronic kidney disease.

REFERENCES

1. Khwaja A. KDIGO clinical practice guidelines for acute kidney injury. Nephron Clin Pract. 2012;120(4):179-84.
2. Kaddourah A, Basu RK, Bagshaw SM, Goldstein SL; AWARE Investigators. Epidemiology of acute kidney injury in critically ill children and young adults. N Engl J Med. 2017;376(1):11-20.
3. Jetton JG, Boohaker LJ, Sethi SK, Wazir S, Rohatgi S, Soranno DE, et al. Neonatal Kidney Collaborative (NKC). Incidence and outcomes of neonatal acute kidney injury (AWAKEN): a multicentre, multinational, observational cohort study. Lancet Child Adolesc Health. 2017;1(3):184-94.
4. Chawla LS, Davison DL, Brasha-Mitchell E, Koyner JL, Arthur JM, Shaw AD, et al. Development and standardization of a furosemide stress test to predict the severity of acute kidney injury. Crit Care. 2013;17(5):R207.
5. Mehta R, Bagga A, Patibandla R, Chakravarthi R. Detection and management of AKI in the developing world: the 18th Acute Disease Quality Initiative (ADQI) International Consensus Conference. Kidney Int Rep. 2017;2(4):515-8.
6. Askenazi D, Basu RK. Kidney support therapy in the pediatric patient: unique considerations for a unique population. Semin Dial. 2021;34(6):530-6.
7. Khandelwal P, Bagga A. Guidelines on hemolytic uremic syndrome by Indian Society of Pediatric Nephrology: Key messages. Indian Pediatr. 2020;57(8):744-7.
8. Meena J, Mathew G, Kumar J, Chanchlani, R. Incidence of acute kidney injury in hospitalized children: A meta-analysis. Pediatrics. 2023;151(2).e2022058823.

13.7 Nephrotic Syndrome

Arvind Bagga, Aditi Sinha

INTRODUCTION

Nephrotic syndrome is characterized by heavy proteinuria (>1 g/m^2/day; early morning urine protein to creatinine ratio >2 mg/mg), hypoalbuminemia (albumin <3.0 g/dL), and edema. The incidence is 1–6 per 100,000 children, varying by ethnicity and region. The large majority is primary (idiopathic); a secondary cause [e.g., amyloidosis, lupus, and immunoglobulin A (IgA) vasculitis] is rare.[1]

The therapy and outcome of nephrotic syndrome is determined by corticosteroid responsiveness and frequency of relapses. Most (>80%) children with idiopathic nephrotic syndrome show remission following therapy with oral prednisolone (steroid-sensitive disease). The prognosis in these cases is favorable, compared to patients who do not respond to such therapy (steroid resistance). The disease course in patients with steroid-sensitive nephrotic syndrome is variable. While few children have no relapses or 1–2 relapses a year (~40%), about 40–50% patients show frequent relapses.[1] A small proportion shows resistance after initial steroid responsiveness (late steroid resistance). **Box 13.7.1** lists definitions that clarify the course of nephrotic syndrome.

BOX 13.7.1: Definitions for clarifying the course of nephrotic syndrome.

- *Remission:* Urine protein nil or trace by dipstick or first morning urine spot protein to creatinine ratio <0.2 mg/mg for 3 consecutive days; or 24-hour urine protein excretion <100 mg/m^2
- *Relapse:* In a child who is previously in remission, presence of either of the following: Urine protein 3+ or 4+ by dipstick or first morning urine spot protein to creatinine ratio >2 mg/mg, or 24-hour urine protein >1 g/m^2/day
- *Infrequent relapses:* Up to two relapses in any 12 months
- *Frequent relapses:* Two or more relapses within 6 months of discontinuing initial treatment; or three or more relapses in any 12 months
- *Steroid dependence:* Two consecutive relapses when on prednisolone on alternate days or within 14 days of its discontinuation
- *Steroid resistance:* Absence of remission despite therapy with daily prednisolone at a dose of 2 mg/kg or 60 mg/m^2 for 6 weeks, in the absence of significant infection

CLINICAL FEATURES AND EVALUATION

Patients usually present between 2 and 5 years of age with progressive edema that is initially periorbital and noticed in the morning. There may be an antecedent infection. Urine appears frothy and the output is reduced. Abdominal pain is usually attributed to mesenteric ischemia secondary to

BOX 13.7.2: Investigations at the first episode of nephrotic syndrome.

Essential:
- *Urinalysis*: Proteinuria, red cells, and casts
- Blood levels of urea, creatinine, albumin, and cholesterol
- Complete blood counts
- Tuberculin test

If required (indication):
- C3 and antistreptolysin O (gross or persistent microscopic hematuria)
- Chest X-ray (positive tuberculin test; history of contact with tuberculosis)
- Hepatitis B surface antigen (recent jaundice; raised levels of transaminases)
- Antinuclear antibodies (features of systemic lupus erythematosus)

hypovolemia but may also be due to gastritis or peritonitis. Evaluation of a patient with suspected nephrotic syndrome includes history and physical examination, with attention to etiology, prior therapies, edema, blood pressure, anthropometry, and evidence of infection(s).[1] Heavy (nephrotic range) proteinuria is presence of 3–4 + (300–1,000 mg/dL) protein by dipstick or spot urine protein to creatinine ratio >2 mg/mg on early morning urine, for 3 consecutive days; or 24-hour protein excretion >1 g/m^2. A precise quantitative assessment of proteinuria is not necessary. Relevant investigations are listed in **Box 13.7.2**.

Indications for Biopsy

Most children with nephrotic syndrome do not require a biopsy during the disease course. Indications for biopsy, either at onset or during the course of nephrotic syndrome, include:

- Gross or persistent microscopic hematuria, sustained stage 2 hypertension, or low C3
- Acute kidney injury, not attributed to hypovolemia
- Suspected secondary cause
- Initial or late steroid resistance, and
- Prolonged therapy with calcineurin inhibitors

MANAGEMENT OF INITIAL EPISODE

The adequacy of treatment of the initial episode, in terms of dose and duration of corticosteroids, is an important determinant of long-term course.[2,3]

Agents

Prednisolone and prednisone are of proven benefit in patients with nephrotic syndrome. Other agents such as deflazacort, methylprednisolone, dexamethasone, or triamcinolone should not be used. Prednisolone is given after meals to reduce gastrointestinal side effects; administration of antacids is usually not required.

Dose and Duration

Prednisolone is given at a dose of 2 mg/kg or 60 mg/m^2 daily (maximum 60 mg) in single or divided doses for 6 weeks, followed by 1.5 mg/kg or 40 mg/m^2 (maximum 40 mg) as single morning dose on alternate days for the next 6 weeks. Therapy with prednisolone is then stopped. Evidence from controlled studies suggests that 8–12 weeks of initial steroid therapy is associated with reduced risk for relapses than shorter regimens. Further prolongation of therapy has no effect on the disease course and carries risk of steroid adverse effects. Failure to achieve remission of proteinuria despite treatment with prednisolone in adequate doses for 6 weeks is labeled as steroid-resistant nephrotic syndrome.

THERAPY FOR RELAPSES

Relapses are often triggered by minor infections. Symptomatic therapy of infectious illness might result in remission of 1+/2+ proteinuria. However, persistence of 3+/4+ proteinuria denotes a disease relapse, which requires therapy. Prednisolone is given at a dose of 2 mg/kg/day until urine protein is trace or nil for 3 consecutive days (remission), and subsequently as a single morning dose of 1.5 mg/kg on alternate days for 4 weeks. Treatment for a relapse thus usually lasts for 5–6 weeks. The subsequent management of a patient with steroid-sensitive nephrotic syndrome depends on the course of the illness.[2,3]

Infrequent Relapses

Patients with infrequent relapses should receive treatment for each disease relapse as described above: Prednisolone at 2 mg/kg/day (single or divided doses) until remission, followed by the same agent given in a single morning dose at 1.5 mg/kg on alternate days for 4 weeks. Therapy is then discontinued.

Frequent Relapses and Steroid Dependence

These patients require prolonged treatment to maintain disease remission. The strategies are summarized here and in **Flowchart 13.7.1**. Patients are initially managed with low-dose prednisolone on alternate days; therapy with steroid-sparing agents is initiated when low-dose alternate-day steroid therapy fails or if adverse effects of steroids develop.

Long-term, Alternate-day Steroids

Following treatment of a relapse, prednisolone is tapered to a dose of 0.5–0.7 mg/kg on alternate days, which is given for 9–18 months. Relapses are often triggered by upper respiratory tract or other minor infections. Recent studies suggest that the risk of relapses is reduced if prednisolone is administered

Flowchart 13.7.1: Management of steroid-sensitive nephrotic syndrome. Prednisolone is the cornerstone of therapy for both the initial episode and relapses. While the initial episode is treated with prednisolone for 6 weeks each daily and on alternate days, therapy of relapse is briefer, typically about 6 weeks. Since frequent relapses carry risk of steroid toxicity as well as complications of relapse, these patients are managed differently. Low dose therapy with prednisolone on alternate days (AD; *with the same dose given daily during infections) is a satisfactory option in most cases. Patients who continue to relapse frequently or show features of steroid toxicity are considered for additional medications. The choice of medication depends on considerations of efficacy, adverse effects, cost, and feasibility as discussed in text. The management of steroid resistance is detailed in the text.

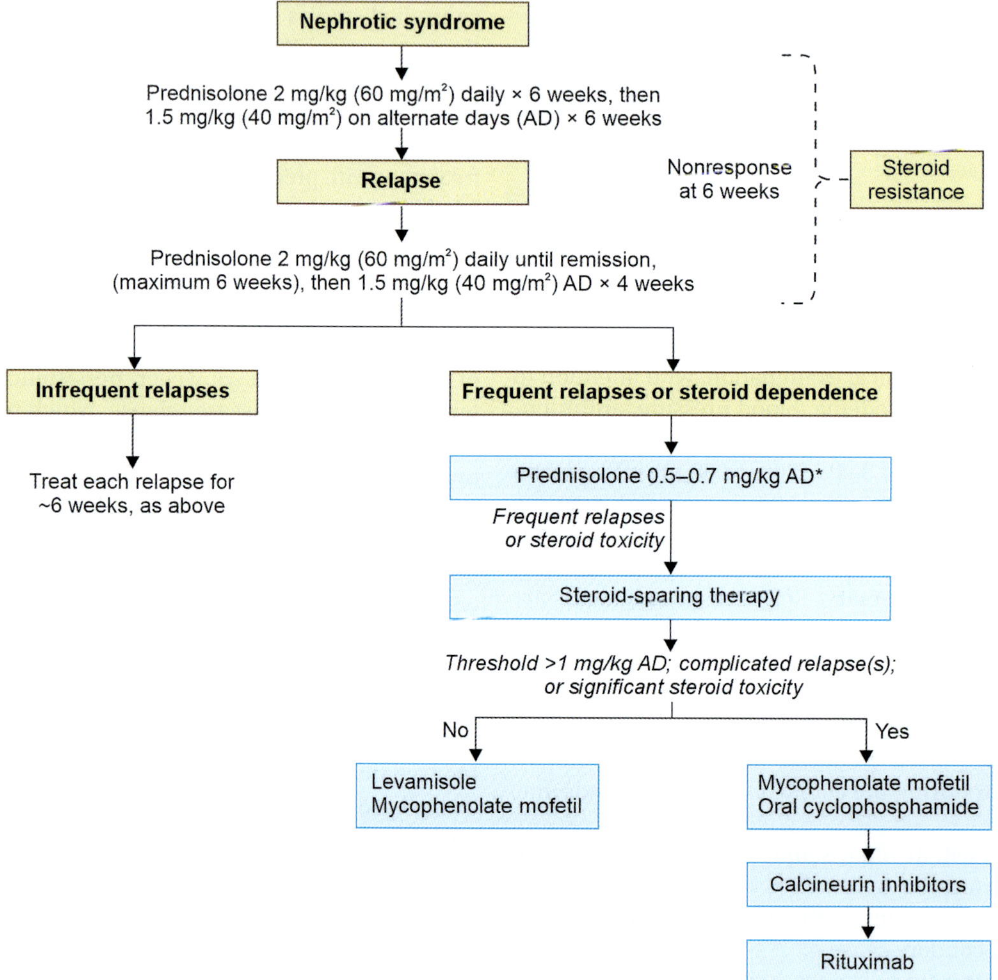

daily for 5–7 days at the onset of infection in patients receiving corticosteroids on alternate days.

Steroid-sparing Agents

Alternative agents are recommended, if prednisolone threshold to maintain remission is >0.5–0.7 mg/kg on alternate days, or if there are features of corticosteroid toxicity (growth failure, obesity, stage 2 hypertension, and cataract). The choice of medications depends on patient age, severity of illness, presence of adverse effects, and physician and patient preference.[2,3] Relapses during therapy are treated with daily steroids, followed by tapering doses of prednisolone on alternate days. The occurrence of frequent relapses is an indication for considering change of medication. The medications are summarized here.

Levamisole

- *Dose, duration:* 2–2.5 mg/kg on alternate days for 12–24 months
- *Adverse effects:* Flu-like symptoms, neutropenia, hepatotoxic, positive antineutrophil cytoplasmic antibody (ANCA) serology, and vasculitis
- *Monitoring:* Total and differential leukocyte count, q 3–4 months; ANCA q 6–12 months
- *Steroid therapy:* Prednisolone tapered to 0.25–0.5 mg/kg on alternate days; may be stopped.

Cyclophosphamide

- *Dose, duration:* 2–2.5 mg/kg/day for 8–12 weeks (cumulative dose should not exceed 168 mg/kg; repeat courses are avoided)
- *Adverse effects:* Leukopenia, alopecia, vomiting, hyperpigmentation, hemorrhagic cystitis, gonadal toxicity, and malignancies. Fluid intake should be increased; patients are encouraged to void frequently.
- *Monitoring:* Leukocyte counts are monitored every 2 weeks; cyclophosphamide is stopped, if the total count is <4,000/mm^3.
- *Steroid therapy:* Prednisolone is tapered and given on alternate days during cyclophosphamide therapy; subsequently prednisolone is tapered and discontinued over 2–3 months.

Mycophenolate mofetil

- *Dose, duration:* 800–1,200 mg/m^2/day or 20–30 mg/kg/day for 12–36 months
- *Adverse effects:* Abdominal pain, diarrhea, weight loss, exacerbation of warts, raised transaminases
- *Monitoring:* Leukocyte counts are monitored 1–2 months; treatment is withheld if count <4,000/mm^3.
- *Steroid therapy:* Prednisolone is tapered and discontinued over 3–6 months.

Calcineurin inhibitors (cyclosporine and tacrolimus)

- These agents are indicated in patients with steroid dependence that fails to benefit with levamisole, cyclophosphamide and/or mycophenolate mofetil.
- *Dose, duration:* Cyclosporine (CsA) 4–6 mg/kg/day; tacrolimus 0.1–0.2 mg/kg/day for 12–24 months
- *Adverse effects:* Nephrotoxicity, neurotoxicity (both); hirsutism, gum hyperplasia, hypertension and hypercholesterolemia (with CsA); hyperglycemia, headache and seizures, hypomagnesemia and diarrhea (with tacrolimus)
- *Monitoring:* Monitor kidney functions q 3–4 months, medication trough levels (CsA 80–120 ng/mL; tacrolimus 3–7 ng/mL), lipid profile and glucose. Repeat kidney biopsy after 2–3 years, particularly if prolonged therapy is planned.

Rituximab

- Rituximab, a monoclonal antibody that depletes B cells, is shown to have considerable steroid-sparing efficacy that is comparable to calcineurin inhibitors.
- *Dose, duration:* The medication is given IV at a dose of 375 mg/m^2 every week for 2–3 weeks, targeting CD19 depletion. The drug is effective in patients with steroid-dependent nephrotic syndrome, allows withdrawal of prednisolone, and enables sustained remission for many months. Some patients may require readministration of the medication after 9–12 months.
- *Adverse effects:* Infusion reactions that are minimized by appropriate premedication. More important complications include variable degree of hypogammaglobulinemia, acute lung injury, and anaphylaxis.

Flowchart 13.7.1 summarizes the protocol for managing patients with steroid-sensitive nephrotic syndrome.[2,3]

STEROID-RESISTANT NEPHROTIC SYNDROME

Initial resistance is defined by the lack of remission at the first episode of nephrotic syndrome, and late resistance is considered in patients who are steroid sensitive initially but show steroid resistance during a subsequent relapse **(Flowchart 13.7.1)**. All patients with steroid resistance (initial or late) should undergo kidney biopsy before instituting specific treatment. Histology shows minimal change disease (MCD) and focal segmental glomerulosclerosis (FSGS) in 30–40% and 40–45%, respectively.[4,5] A small proportion of patients shows variable mesangial proliferation. Patients with collapsing form of FSGS, tubular atrophy, and/or tubulointerstitial fibrosis show less satisfactory outcomes.

Genetic Studies

About one-third patients with initial steroid resistance show mutations in genes encoding podocyte proteins.[4,5] Although defects in over 80 genes are recognized, commonly implicated genes include those encoding podocin (*NPHS2*), nephrin (*NPHS1*), Wilms tumor 1 (*WT1*), collagen 4 (*COL4A3-5*), CD2-associated protein (*CD2AP*), transient receptor potential cation channel (*TRPC6*), and actinin 4 (*ACT4*). Patients with genetic mutations do not respond to immunosuppressive medications and progress rapidly to end-stage kidney disease. Unlike nongenetic FSGS, which recurs after transplant in 40–50%, patients with genetic mutations do not recur. Mutational analysis should be offered to patients with: (i) congenital nephrotic syndrome, (ii) infantile onset steroid resistance; (iii) family history of steroid resistance, (iv) initial resistance that does not show remission following therapy with calcineurin inhibitors, and (v) prior to kidney transplantation.

Management

Patients with steroid-resistance secondary to MCD or FSGS are treated similarly. The chief factor predicting outcome is the response of proteinuria to therapy rather than the precise renal histology.[4,5] These patients require prompt referral to a pediatric nephrologist. The aim of therapy is to induce and maintain remission of proteinuria, while avoiding adverse effects of medications. Most regimens use a combination of a calcineurin inhibitor (CsA or tacrolimus) with prednisolone and an angiotensin-converting enzyme inhibitor (ACEI) (or angiotensin receptor blocker).

TABLE 13.7.1: Agents used for management of steroid-resistant nephrotic syndrome.

Agent	Dose	Duration	Efficacy	Adverse effects
Cyclosporine (CsA)	4–5 mg/kg/day	12–36 months	60–70%	Acute, chronic nephrotoxicity (both agents); hirsutism and gum hyperplasia (CsA > Tac); hypertension; dyslipidemia (CsA > Tac); diarrhea, hyperglycemia, hypomagnesemia (Tac); neurotoxicity (Tac > CsA)
Tacrolimus	0.1–0.2 mg/kg/day			
Intravenous cyclophosphamide	500–750 mg/m^2	6 pulses once a month	30–35%	Leukopenia; alopecia; nausea and vomiting; gonadal toxicity; hemorrhagic cystitis
Rituximab	375 mg/m^2	2–4 doses once a week	25–30%	Infusion reactions; serum sickness like illness; leukopenia, neutropenia, acute lung injury, hypogammaglobulinemia

Therapy with CsA or tacrolimus results in complete or partial remission in almost 60–70% patients with steroid-resistance.[4,5] Adverse effects require close monitoring **(Table 13.7.1)**. Therapy with intravenous (IV) cyclophosphamide and tapering doses of prednisolone is less satisfactory, with remission in 30–35% patients. Most guidelines do not recommend the use of IV corticosteroids and oral cyclophosphamide. There is limited data on other forms of therapy, including rituximab, combination of calcineurin inhibitors and mycophenolate mofetil, and lipoprotein apheresis.

Prednisolone is a component of all regimens used in therapy of steroid-resistant nephrotic syndrome. The agent is given on alternate days at 1 mg/kg/day for 2 months, following which the dose is tapered, over the next 6–9 months.

Therapy with ACEIs (enalapril 0.3–0.6 mg/kg/day; ramipril 6 mg/m^2 q24h) is associated with decrease in proteinuria and control of hypertension. Adverse effects include dry cough, hyperkalemia and decline in renal function. Angiotensin receptor blockers (losartan, valsartan, and irbesartan) may be used in patients having persistent dry cough.[4]

Monitoring

Patients are monitored for proteinuria (dipstick, spot urine samples), blood levels of creatinine and albumin, and edema every 2–3 months. While the aim of treatment is complete remission, the occurrence of partial remission is satisfactory. Most patients who respond do so within the first 6 months of therapy. Therapy with calcineurin inhibitors is tapered and discontinued after 2–3 years if the response has been satisfactory.[5] It is advised that immunosuppressive therapy should be discontinued if nephrotic range proteinuria persists beyond 6 months. These patients are at risk of end-stage kidney failure and should be counseled appropriately.

Monitoring for drug levels is recommended when using CsA or tacrolimus, because variable bioavailability might result in either subtherapeutic or toxic levels. Trough level drawn 15–30 minutes prior to the due dose) is estimated 10–14 days after introducing therapy or suspecting toxicity or poor compliance. Trough levels of 80–120 ng/mL for CsA and 4–7 ng/mL for tacrolimus are acceptable.[5]

CONGENITAL NEPHROTIC SYNDROME

Congenital nephrotic syndrome presents with nephrotic syndrome within the first 3 months of life.[5] This condition has diverse etiologies. While inherited defects in genes encoding key podocyte, proteins underlie almost 85% cases, other causes include intrauterine infections. Sequencing of *NPHS1* enables precise genetic diagnosis in the majority. Mutations in *NPHS2, WT1, PLCE,* and *LAMB2* may also be detected. A correct diagnosis is important for prognosis, therapy, and prenatal genetic counseling. Immunosuppression has no role in managing infants with congenital nephrotic syndrome. ACEIs (enalapril 0.2–0.5 mg/kg/day) are effective in reducing proteinuria. Supportive care includes adequate nutrition, supplementation with vitamin D, thyroxine and multivitamins, judicious use of diuretics, and regular administration of IV albumin. Progression of end-stage kidney failure is usual during the first decade of life, and parents should be counseled about the need for kidney replacement therapy.

SUPPORTIVE CARE AND COMPLICATIONS

Edema

Daily administration of corticosteroids results in diuresis within 2–4 days. Therapy for edema is therefore not required in most patients with steroid-sensitive disease. Patients with significant edema (>7% weight gain) require treatment with diuretics. Anasarca results in discomfort and an increased risk of infections and should be avoided.[6]

Short-term therapy with furosemide (1–3 mg/kg/day, in 1–2 doses) is effective; therapy beyond 3–4 days is rarely necessary. Edema that does not respond to maximal doses of furosemide requires coadministration of thiazide. If furosemide is used for prolonged duration or at high doses, therapy with spironolactone (2–4 mg/kg/day) prevents the occurrence of hypokalemia. Patients with refractory edema are hospitalized and given IV furosemide either as bolus injections (1–3 mg/kg/dose, infused over 15–20 minutes) or as infusion (0.1–1 mg/kg/h) under close monitoring.

Infusions of albumin (20% albumin, 0.5–1 g/kg over 2–4 hours) with IV furosemide given at the end of the infusion are useful in patients with evidence of hypovolemia (see below) or severe hypoalbuminemia (albumin <1.5 g/dL). The effect is transient and repeat administration of albumin is often required. Albumin infusions should be given carefully in patients with respiratory distress, hypertension, and impaired kidney function.[6]

Hypovolemia

Hypovolemia may occur during a disease relapse or following administration of diuretics, particularly in children with poor oral intake, diarrhea, and vomiting. Patients complain of abdominal pain, lethargy, dizziness, and leg cramps. Signs include the presence of tachycardia, hypotension, delayed capillary refill, low volume pulses, and cold peripheries. An elevated ratio of blood urea to creatinine, rising hematocrit, urine sodium <20 mEq/L, or fractional excretion of sodium <0.2% suggest presence of hypovolemia. Patients require admission and rapid infusion of normal saline (10–20 mL/kg) over 20–30 minutes. Patients who do not respond to two saline boluses should receive infusion of 5% albumin (10–15 mL/kg) or 20% albumin (0.5–1 g/kg).[2,3]

Infections

Table 13.7.2 provides a summary of management of common bacterial infections in patients with nephrotic syndrome. During serious infections, steroids should be administered daily at stress doses **(Table 13.7.2)**.

Varicella may be a life-threatening illness in immunocompromised patients. All patients should receive oral acyclovir (80 mg/kg/day in four doses) for 7 days; severe illness requires admission and administration of IV acyclovir.[2,3] Administration of oral acyclovir (beginning 5–7 days after exposure), or varicella zoster immunoglobulin (single dose within 96 hours of exposure) might prevent or lessen the severity of the disease in susceptible individuals exposed to varicella. Children with nephrotic syndrome and positive tuberculin test in absence of evidence of tuberculosis should receive prophylaxis with isoniazid for 6 months.

Thrombosis

Children with nephrotic syndrome are predisposed to venous thrombosis during relapses, due to loss of antithrombin III, low-intravascular volume, immobilization, indwelling vascular catheters, puncture of deep vessels, and use of diuretics. Cerebral venous sinus thrombosis is the chief site; children present with headache that interferes with daily activities and/or sleep, during the first episode or an untreated relapse. Diagnosis requires confirmation with magnetic resonance imaging with venography. Therapy is with low molecular weight heparin initially, followed by oral warfarin. Patients with persistently low serum albumin levels (congenital nephrotic syndrome; refractory to calcineurin inhibitors) may benefit from prolonged therapy with aspirin or oral anticoagulants.

Hyperlipidemia

Patients with steroid resistance may show persistent dyslipidemia due to abnormal lipid metabolism, leading to hypercholesterolemia, hypertriglyceridemia, and lipoprotein abnormalities. Treatment is with atorvastatin (10–20 mg/day) with monitoring of liver function and creatinine kinase.

Vaccinations

Live vaccines (oral polio and varicella) are deferred until the child is off immunosuppressive medications for at least 4 weeks. Two doses of the varicella vaccine are given 4 weeks apart, while the child is in remission and off immunosuppressive medications. Injectable polio vaccine

TABLE 13.7.2: Management of systemic bacterial infections in nephrotic syndrome.

Infection	*Medication (dose)*	*Duration*
Peritonitis	Intravenous (IV) cefotaxime (100–150 mg/kg/day), or IV ceftriaxone (75–100 mg/kg/day)	7 days
Cellulitis	IV co-amoxiclav (100 mg/kg/day amoxicillin), or IV cloxacillin (100–200 mg/kg/day) and IV ceftriaxone (50–100 mg/kg/day) Shift to oral cloxacillin (100 mg/kg/day) or co-amoxiclav (30–40 mg/kg/day) once erythema and induration resolve	7 days
Pneumonia	Co-amoxiclav (30–40 mg/kg/day), or cefadroxil (30 mg/kg/day) *Atypical and nonsevere*: Azithromycin (10 mg/kg/day) *Severe*: IV cefotaxime (100–150 mg/kg/day) or IV ceftriaxone (75–100 mg/kg/day) *Severe infection with Staphylococcus aureus*: Teicoplanin (10 mg/kg/day) or vancomycin (40–60 mg/kg/day) with or without amikacin (15 mg/kg/day)	7–10 days 3–5 days 7–10 days 10–14 days

should be administered to children with nephrotic syndrome and their siblings.

The administration of pneumococcal vaccine is desirable. Children below 2 years of age should receive the pneumococcal conjugate vaccine. Above 2 years of age, two doses of the conjugate vaccine are followed 2 months later by the polysaccharide vaccine (PPSV23). Children who continue to have relapses of nephrotic syndrome may receive one repeat dose of PPSV23, 5 years after the first dose. Patients on prolonged immunosuppression should receive the killed influenza vaccine annually.[2-5]

Nutrition

During remission, children should eat a balanced and nutritious diet. Salt restriction is advised in patients with anasarca; undue restrictions that make food unpalatable are not required. Patients with persistent or recurrent proteinuria should increase their daily intake of proteins to 2–2.5 g/kg. Those receiving prolonged (>3 months) steroid therapy should receive supplements of calcium carbonate (250–500 mg) and vitamin D (125–250 IU).

Stress Doses of Steroids

Patients who have received steroids at high doses for >2 weeks in the past 1 year are at risk of suppression of the hypothalamic-pituitary-adrenal axis. These children require steroid supplements during surgery, anesthesia, or serious infections, which are given as parenteral hydrocortisone (2–4 mg/kg/day) followed by oral prednisolone (0.3–0.6 mg/kg/day). The medications are given for the duration of stress and tapered rapidly.

Parent Education and Counseling

Parents are explained the natural history of the disease, and the adverse effects of repeated courses of high-dose corticosteroids and other medications. The patient should return for follow-up at 2- and 4-week therapy of the initial episode, and during disease relapses. The need to examine urine protein at home (by either dipstick or boiling method) is emphasized. Parents should maintain a diary, recording urine protein excretion, intake of medications, and intercurrent illnesses. The record provides useful assessment of the disease status and course, including steroid threshold for relapses.

CONCLUSION

The management and outcomes of idiopathic nephrotic syndrome in children are determined by the response to corticosteroids. While patients with steroid-sensitive nephrotic syndrome have a favorable long-term outcome, almost half of them relapse frequently and are at risk of adverse effects of corticosteroids. Therapy with prednisolone in low doses on alternate days and various noncorticosteroid immunosuppressive agents are used to prolong disease remission, but require careful monitoring for potential adverse effects. The management of steroid-resistant nephrotic syndrome is challenging due to variable response to immunosuppression, therapy-related adverse effects and high rates of disease progression to end-stage kidney failure. The combination of calcineurin inhibitors, ACEI and alternate day prednisolone induces partial or complete remission in the majority of patients with steroid resistance, and is therefore the current choice of therapy. Patients with nephrotic syndrome require long-term monitoring, including home-based monitoring for proteinuria and follow-up to ensure appropriate growth and clinical and biochemical screening for complications of disease and therapies.

REFERENCES

1. Vivarelli M, Gibson K, Sinha A, Boyer O. Childhood nephrotic syndrome. Lancet. 2023;402(10404):809-24.
2. Sinha A, Bagga A, Banerjee S, Mishra K, Mehta A, Agarwal I, et al. Steroid sensitive nephrotic syndrome: Revised guidelines. Indian Pediatr. 2021;58(5):461-81.
3. Trautmann A, Boyer O, Hodson E, Bagga A, Gipson DS, Samuel S, et al. IPNA clinical practice recommendations for the diagnosis and management of children with steroid-sensitive nephrotic syndrome. Pediatr Nephrol. 2023;38(3):877-919.
4. Tullus K, Webb H, Bagga A. Management of steroid-resistant nephrotic syndrome in children and adolescents. Lancet Child Adolesc Health. 2018;2(12):880-90.
5. Vasudevan A, Thergaonkar R, Mantan M, Sharma J, Khandelwal P, Bagga A, et al. Consensus guidelines on management of steroid-resistant nephrotic syndrome. Indian Pediatr. 2021;58(7):650-66.
6. Meena J, Bagga A. Current perspectives in management of edema in nephrotic syndrome. Indian J Pediatr. 2020;87(8):633-40.

13.8 Urinary Tract Infection, Vesicoureteric Reflux, and Reflux Nephropathy

Jitendra Meena, Pankaj Hari

INTRODUCTION

Urinary tract infections (UTIs) are among the most common bacterial infections of childhood. About 2–8% of children develop UTI by the age of 7 years; the risk being approximately 1–3% in boys and 3–10% in girls. During infancy, the male-to-female ratio is 3–5:1. However, beyond 1–2 years, there is a female preponderance with male-to-female ratio of 1:10.[1] The diagnosis of UTI is challenging due to nonspecific symptoms especially in infancy and young age and hence is often missed. Prompt diagnosis and adequate management are mandatory to prevent kidney scarring, which can lead to progressive parenchymal damage and hypertension. Delayed or inadequate antibacterial therapy, recurrent infections, bladder-bowel dysfunction (BBD), and high grades of vesicoureteric reflux (VUR) are risk factors for development of kidney scarring in children.[2]

URINARY TRACT INFECTIONS

Clinical Features

Newborns with UTI present with septicemia, jaundice, vomiting, and shock. In infancy, symptoms are nonspecific, such as unexplained fever, diarrhea, vomiting, and failure to thrive. UTIs are an important cause of fever without focus in children younger than 2 years of age. Older children have dysuria, increased frequency, and suprapubic pain. Fever, flank pain, and toxic appearance suggest kidney parenchymal involvement. Any febrile UTI in a young child should be considered as acute pyelonephritis.

Examination should include evaluation for features suggesting underlying structural abnormalities, such as distended bladder, palpable enlarged kidney(s), tight phimosis in a boy, vulval synechiae in a girl, palpable fecal lump(s) in the abdomen, patulous anus, neurological deficit in lower limbs, urinary incontinence, and evidence of previous surgery of the urinary tract, anorectal malformation, or meningomyelocele.[3]

Etiology and Pathogenesis

Urinary tract infections are usually caused by ascending infection from the urethra to the bladder and/or kidneys while spread by hematogenous route is common in newborns. The most common cause of UTI in children is *Escherichia coli* (60–80%). Other organisms, such as *Proteus, Klebsiella, Staphylococcus saprophyticus, Streptococcus faecalis, Enterococcus,* and *Enterobacter*, are chiefly isolated in immunocompromized children, nosocomial setting, or following prolonged urinary catheterization. Preterm infants, immunocompromized children and those receiving prolonged antibiotics are at risk of *Candida* UTI.[4]

Diagnosis

Diagnosis of UTI is confirmed by significant bacterial growth in urine in presence of appropriate clinical setting. Urine specimens for analysis and culture should be collected by clean catch method in all stable children with suspected UTI but in case of failure of clean catch method, invasive methods (catheterization and suprapubic aspiration) can be used. In sick infants, invasive methods can be used initially to collect urine specimens to avoid delay in making diagnosis of UTI. Urine culture is not recommended on samples collected from the urinary bag.

The presence of *leukocytes at more than 5 white blood cells (WBCs) per high power field (HPF)* in centrifuged urine (spun at 2,000 rpm for 10 minutes), and bacteria on microscopic examination of a carefully collected fresh sample of urine are suggestive but not confirmatory for diagnosis of UTI. The presence of bacteriuria on uncentrifuged urine indicates $>10^4$ bacteria/mL. Enhanced urinalysis includes evaluation of uncentrifuged urine for leukocyturia (>10 WBC/mm^3 in Neubauer counting chamber) along with Gram staining (any bacteria per 10 oil immersion fields). Leukocyturia can be observed in diverse conditions such as interstitial nephritis and glomerulonephritis and hence cannot be used as a diagnostic test for UTI.[5] Presence of bacteriuria has excellent specificity (94%) and good sensitivity (86%); however, it may not always be feasible to perform in emergency departments.[3]

Rapid diagnostic tests based on urine dipstick which uses nitrite and leukocyte esterase are useful for presumptive diagnosis of UTI in children. The nitrite test based on the bacterial enzyme nitrate reductase that converts urinary nitrate to nitrite is 99% specific for UTI. However, it may be falsely negative in infants with urinary frequency resulting in insufficient time for incubation of bacteria in urine, or during infection with bacteria lacking nitrate reductase, e.g.,

Streptococcus. Staining for the neutrophil enzyme leukocyte esterase detects leukocyturia. However, a combination of these two rapid tests has high sensitivity (84%) and specificity (88%) for making a diagnosis of UTI.[3]

The gold standard for diagnosis of UTI is *urine culture.* The threshold of bacterial colony counts for making a diagnosis of UTI depends on the method of collection of urine. UTI is diagnosed in the presence of bacterial growth of $\geq 10^{4-5}$ colony-forming units (CFUs)/mL in a midstream clean-catch specimen. On samples collected by urethral catheterization, a colony count of $>10^4$ CFU/mL indicates UTI. A lower colony count usually indicates urinary contamination unless the child has received antimicrobial therapy. If a urine sample is obtained by suprapubic aspiration (e.g., infants), growth of any number of pathogens (corresponds to 10^3 CFU/mL) is diagnostic of UTI.[3-5]

Other investigations at evaluation of UTI may include complete blood counts, blood urea, serum creatinine, and electrolytes. Presence of leukocytosis, raised C-reactive protein, and procalcitonin suggest acute pyelonephritis; however, these are not necessary for diagnosis of UTI.

Definitions

The diagnosis of UTI requires demonstration of significant bacteriuria on urine culture in the presence of symptoms. Important definitions are listed here:

- *Significant bacteriuria:* Count of $>10^5$ CFU/mL of a single bacterial species in a midstream clean catch sample of urine.
- *Asymptomatic bacteriuria:* Significant bacteriuria without symptoms of UTI.
- *Recurrent UTI:* Occurrence of two or more episodes of UTI.
- *Complicated UTI or pyelonephritis:* Fever >39°C, systemic toxicity, persistent vomiting, dehydration, renal angle tenderness, or raised serum creatinine.
- *Simple UTI or cystitis:* Dysuria, frequency or urgency with or without fever, and none of the symptoms of complicated UTI.

Management

Prompt therapy of UTI is essential to reduce the morbidity of infection, minimize kidney damage, and prevent subsequent complications. Third-generation cephalosporins (as monotherapy) and co-amoxiclav are preferred empirical antibiotics for treatment of UTI. Therapy can be modified later according to antimicrobial sensitivity in patients with no clinical response. Oral administration of antibacterial therapy is preferred over intravenous in all children with UTI except in infants who are <2 months old or are unable to take oral medication and in severely ill patients. After 48–72 hours of parenteral therapy, once the patient improves, therapy is switched over to oral route. Hospitalization can be considered in young infants requiring intravenous antibiotics. With adequate therapy, fever resolves and symptoms reduce by 48–72 hours.

Failure to respond to therapy may be due to resistant pathogens, complicating factors, or noncompliance, and requires evaluation.

Most recent guidelines suggest that a total of 7–10 days therapy is adequate in most children with febrile UTI; therapy for even 3–7 days may suffice in lower tract infections (cystitis) in adolescents.

Supportive therapy includes maintenance of adequate hydration and control of fever. Parenteral fluids are indicated in febrile children within adequate oral intake or dehydration. A repeat urine culture is not necessary, unless there is persistence of fever and toxicity despite 72 hours of adequate antibiotic therapy.[3]

Imaging Following Diagnosis of Urinary Tract Infection

The aim of imaging following the diagnosis of UTI is to identify urinary tract abnormalities that predispose to UTI and to detect kidney scarring **(Flowchart 13.8.1)**. All children presenting for the first time with UTI should undergo an *ultrasonography,* which may demonstrate renal anomalies, and dilated pelvicalyceal system. However, ultrasound is insensitive for detecting VUR, acute pyelonephritis, and kidney scarring.

Flowchart 13.8.1: Evaluation following the first febrile urinary tract infection.

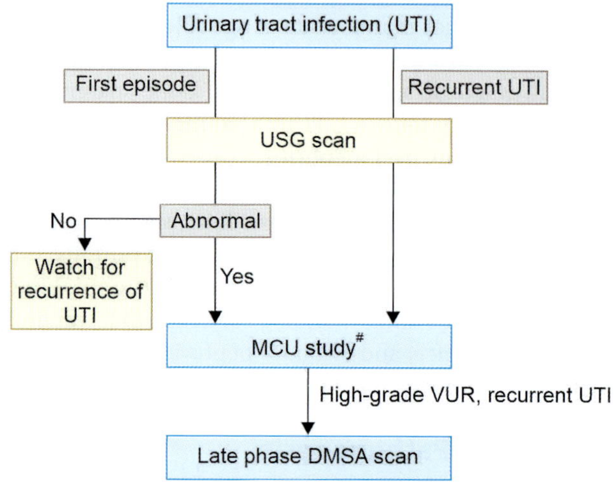

#Consider MCU study in children younger than 2 years with UTI caused by non-*Escherichia coli* uropathogens.

(DMSA: dimercaptosuccinic acid; MCU: micturating cystourethrogram; VUR: vesicoureteric reflux)

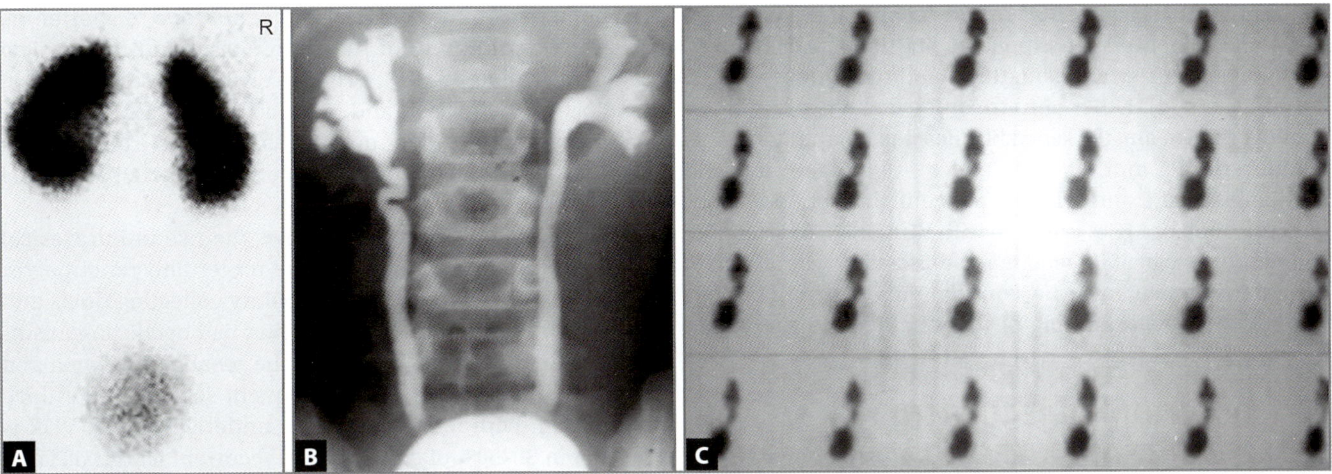

Figs. 13.8.1A to C: Imaging studies in an 18-month-old girl with recurrent urinary tract infections since 6 months of age. (A) Dimercaptosuccinic acid shows multiple scars and loss of volume in the right kidney while the left kidney is normal; (B) Micturating cystourethrography showed bilateral grade V vesicoureteric reflux; the ureters appear dilated and tortuous while the calyces show cupping; and (C) Direct radionuclide cystourethrography (DRCG) at 4 years of age shows persistence of severe reflux on the right side.

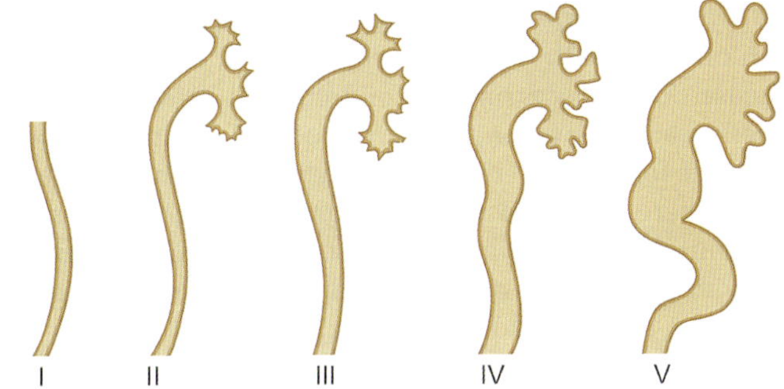

Fig. 13.8.2: Graphic representation of the grading of vesicoureteric reflux on micturating cystourethrogram.

Cystourethrography is an invasive procedure that requires catheterization, risking UTI, and exposes the child to radiation. Micturating cystourethrography (MCU) involves filling the bladder up with radiocontrast, followed by capturing of images during voiding. MCU is the gold standard for diagnosing and staging VUR **(Figs. 13.8.1B and 13.8.2)**. The anatomy of bladder and urethra are defined well during an MCU, helping to detect bladder abnormalities due to lower tract dysfunction caused by neurogenic bladder or obstruction by posterior urethral valves. Both MCU and ultrasound allow the assessment of residual urine. An MCU should be performed only after adequate control of infection.

Direct radionuclide cystourethrography (DRCG) detects VUR at a lower radiation exposure. It is a useful alternative to MCU for repeat evaluations for persistence of VUR during follow-up **(Fig. 13.8.1C)**. It is not recommended for initial screening as it does not provide detailed anatomy of bladder and urethra.

Demonstration of reduced cortical uptake by *^{99}Tc-dimercaptosuccinic acid (DMSA) scan* during the acute phase of UTI is sensitive and specific for detecting pyelonephritis; however, the diagnosis of acute pyelonephritis is clinical and DMSA scan is not necessary. More often, DMSA is used at 4–6 months of follow-up to identify permanent kidney scars **(Fig. 13.8.1A)**.

The approach to radiological evaluation following the UTI is based on the balance between risks with investigations and benefits of improving outcome by detecting abnormalities such as high-grade VUR **(Flowchart 13.8.1)**. Primary VUR and BBD are the two most important risk factors for recurrent UTI and kidney scarring. However, none of the existing interventions are effective in reducing the risk of kidney scarring and long-term outcomes in these patients. Hence, the overall approach to imaging following UTI has now become less aggressive and in mostly focused on detecting high-grade VUR. The recently updated Indian Society of Pediatric Nephrology guidelines suggest that all children with UTI should have an ultrasound scan of kidney, ureter, and bladder. Indications of MCU have been restricted to those with abnormal ultrasound scan, recurrent UTI, and in children <2 years with UTI caused by non-*E.coli* uropathogens. Similarly, indications to detect kidney scarring using late phase DMSA scan is restricted to those with recurrent UTI and high-grade VUR.[3]

RECURRENT URINARY TRACT INFECTION AND BLADDER–BOWEL DYSFUNCTION

About 20–30% children with UTI show recurrence of symptoms, usually within 6 months of the first UTI, and often by the same pathogen. All children with recurrent UTI should undergo thorough clinical examination and imaging studies to evaluate for risk factors such as VUR, BBD, obstruction of the urinary system, and neurogenic bladder.

Features that suggest BBD include constipation, impacted stools, and maneuvers to postpone voiding (holding maneuvers, e.g., Vincent curtsy and squatting) and infrequent voiding (<4 times a day). Other abnormalities include straining or poor urinary stream, thickened bladder wall (>3 mm for empty bladder and >5 mm for full bladder), significant postvoid residue (>20 mL), and spinning top configuration of bladder on ultrasound or MCU. Children with VUR, BBD, obstruction, and neurogenic bladder require multidisciplinary approach to their management, involving consultations with both urology and nephrology, retraining of toilet habits and therapy of constipation.[2]

PREVENTION OF RECURRENT URINARY TRACT INFECTION

Long-term daily administration of low-dose antibiotic prophylaxis has been the cornerstone of prevention of UTI in children at risk of recurrence. However, recently its efficacy and safety has been questioned due to increasing risk of antimicrobial resistance. Current evidence suggests that antibiotic prophylaxis is not effective in preventing UTI in children with normal urinary tract therefore recent guideline suggests limited indications where this intervention might be beneficial (i) high-grade VUR; and (ii) BBD, and (iii) infants with low-grade VUR.

Drugs used for prophylaxis include cotrimoxazole (1–2 mg/kg/day), cephalexin (10 mg/kg/day), cefadroxil (5 mg/kg/day), or nitrofurantoin (1–2 mg/kg/day) administered in a single dose at bedtime. Cephalexin is preferred in young infants (<3 months old) and in those with deficiency of glucose 6-phosphate dehydrogenase. Patients on antibiotic prophylaxis may have breakthrough UTI due to noncompliance or development of bacterial resistance. Antibiotic prophylaxis can be stopped in toilet-trained children if they are free of BBD and there is no recurrence of febrile UTI in the previous 1 year.[3]

ASYMPTOMATIC BACTERIURIA

Screening of normal school children may reveal significant bacteriuria in 0.05% boys and 1% girls. In most cases, the organism is *E. coli* of low virulence that colonizes the lower tract. Treating such colonization may lead to symptomatic infections with more virulent organisms. Hence, asymptomatic bacteriuria does not merit any treatment, even in the presence of VUR.

VESICOURETERIC REFLUX AND REFLUX NEPHROPATHY

Vesicoureteric reflux implies passage of urine into the ureter during micturition. Normally, the long submucosal and intravesical segment of the ureter at the ureterovesical junction closes when the bladder contracts, effectively preventing VUR. Incompetence of ureterovesical junction due to shortening and lack of obliquity of the submucosal and intravesical segments results in VUR. Primary VUR is an isolated defect that has a genetic basis and may occur in siblings. VUR may be secondary to bladder outflow obstruction (e.g., posterior urethral valves), neurogenic bladder, or a functional voiding disorder.

During micturition, VUR allows the rise in intravesical pressure to be transmitted to the ureter and renal pelvis, which enables urine to enter papillary collecting ducts and renal tubules (intrarenal reflux). Thus, pathogenic organisms present in the bladder can reach the renal parenchyma and initiate inflammation and subsequent scarring. One-third of children with febrile UTI have underlying VUR. VUR is present in 30–50% of children with recurrent febrile UTI and kidney scarring. Low grades (I-III) of VUR are likely to resolve over time. Moderate-to-severe VUR, particularly if bilateral, is an important risk factor for pyelonephritis and renal scarring, which leads to hypertension, proteinuria, and rarely progressive kidney disease.[6]

Reflux nephropathy refers to kidney damage associated with primary VUR. It accounts for 7–17% of end-stage renal disease. Kidney scarring in children with primary VUR is chiefly caused by congenital hypodysplasia rather than acquired, following a UTI. Many patients with renal dysplasia have severe VUR and no documented UTI. Patients with congenital hypodysplasia (congenital scarring) are more likely to progress to chronic kidney disease compared to those with acquired kidney scarring.[2,6]

Clinical Features

Children with VUR may present with recurrent febrile UTI with or without structural anomalies of the urinary tract.[7] VUR may be detected following evaluation of antenatally detected hydronephrosis or during screening of offsprings or siblings of patients with VUR (see below). Patients with reflux nephropathy may present with chronic acidosis, hypertension, and renal failure. A high proportion (~45–50%) of patients with VUR have BBD.[8] Symptoms to be enquired include urgency, holding maneuvers, nocturnal and diurnal incontinence, frequency, and constipation. Spinal dysraphism should be ruled out as a cause of secondary VUR.

Diagnosis

The severity of VUR is graded from I to V based on the appearance of the urinary tract on contrast MCU, using the International Reflux Study classification **(Fig. 13.8.2)**. Mild-to-moderate VUR (grades I–III) is characterized by reflux into nondilated or dilated ureter and upper collecting system. In severe VUR (grades IV–V), there is reflux into grossly dilated and distorted ureter(s), pelvis, and calyces. While DRCG entails significantly lower radiation than MCU, it cannot delineate anatomic abnormalities, and the grading is not reliable. Hence, the use of DRCG is limited to follow-up studies **(Figs. 13.8.1A to C)**. The DMSA scan is a sensitive technique to detect kidney scarring in reflux nephropathy; however, to ensure that it detects only permanent scars DMSA scan should be performed 4–6 months after the episode of febrile UTI. Patients with imaging evidence of scars on the background of VUR require evaluation for evidence of hypertension or proteinuria.[2,9]

Management of Vesicoureteric Reflux

Previously all children with VUR and otherwise normal urinary tract were managed with long-term prophylaxis with nitrofurantoin, cotrimoxazole, cephalexin, or cefadroxil while awaiting spontaneous resolution of VUR. However recently due to concern about efficacy and safety of this intervention, recent guidelines suggest a restrictive approach. Infants with VUR grades I and II detected following an episode of UTI or recurrent UTI may be given antibiotic prophylaxis up to 1 year of age. All children with high grades of VUR (III–V VUR), those with BBD, and any grade VUR should also receive antibiotic prophylaxis. Antibiotic prophylaxis can be discontinued in toilet-trained children if there is no bowel bladder dysfunction and no recurrence of febrile UTI in the preceding 1 year. Training the child for double or triple voiding reduces the residual urine and may be beneficial. Urine microscopy and culture are performed, whenever UTI is suspected.[3]

Surgery for primary VUR is indicated in patients with:

- Recurrent breakthrough febrile UTIs while on prophylaxis and optimal management of BBD
- By parental choice (remote residence and anxiety)

There are two surgical options for correction of VUR. Subureteric injection of dextranomer/hyaluronic acid polymer (Deflux) is a day-care technique, which is 70% effective in eliminating VUR in patients with grade III or IV VUR. A day-care minimal access extravesical ureteric reimplantation technique is also suitable for grades III or IV VUR. The cost of the implant and risk of failure, particularly in inexperienced hands or with BBD, limit its utility. The most effective method of reflux elimination is open surgical ureteric reimplantation.[3] Voiding dysfunction is an important reason for recurrences of UTI, particularly in children with VUR. Failure to manage this entity is a common cause of failure of antibiotic prophylaxis and/or surgery. Treating constipation and voiding dysfunction is an important component of the management of VUR in children.[6]

Patients with renal scarring should be monitored for hypertension, proteinuria, and for physical growth. Repeat cystography to assess for resolution of VUR is not required in all children as it does not alter the long-term management of these patients. However, if indicated can be performed 4–8 years after initial diagnosis in children with high-grade VUR. Late phase DMSA scan should be done to only in children with recurrence of febrile UTI during follow up. Most cases of grades I–III VUR resolve; higher grades of reflux may disappear in a small percentage of patients.[2,6]

Screening of Siblings and Offsprings

Vesicoureteric reflux is inherited in an autosomal dominant manner with incomplete penetrance. About 25% of siblings and 25–50% of offsprings of patients may have reflux. The majority of inherited VUR is of low grade and not associated with UTI. Ultrasonography is the modality of choice to screen these individuals. Further imaging is required, if ultrasonography is abnormal or on occurrence of febrile UTI.

Long-term Follow-up

Children with kidney scars (reflux nephropathy) are counseled regarding the need for early diagnosis and therapy of UTI, and regular follow-up. Physical growth and blood pressure should be monitored every 6–12 months through adolescence. Investigations include urinalysis for proteinuria and estimation of serum creatinine. Ultrasound scan can be performed once in 1–2 years to monitor renal growth. Patients with proteinuria and hypertension benefit from treatment with angiotensin-converting enzyme inhibitors (ACEIs) and angiotensin II receptor blockers.[10]

REFERENCES

1. Shaikh N, Morone NE, Bost JE, Farrell MH. Prevalence of urinary tract infection in childhood: a meta-analysis. Pediatr Infect Dis J. 2008;27(4):302-8.
2. Meena J, Hari P. Vesicoureteral reflux and recurrent urinary tract infections. Asian J Pediatr Nephrol. 2019;2(2):61-70.
3. Hari P, Meena J, Kumar M, Sinha A, Thergaonkar RW, Iyengar A, et al. Evidence-based clinical practice guideline for management of urinary tract infection and primary vesicoureteric reflux. Pediatr Nephrol. 2024;39(5):1639-68.
4. Tullus K, Shaikh N. Urinary tract infections in children. Lancet. 2020;395(10237):1659-68.
5. Kaufman J, Temple-Smith M, Sanci L. Urinary tract infections in children: an overview of diagnosis and management. BMJ Paediatrics Open. 2019;3:e000487.
6. Bortnick EM, Nelson CP. Vesicoureteral Reflux: Current Care Trends and Future Possibilities. Urol Clin North Am. 2023;50(3):391-402.
7. Garcia-Roig ML, Kirsch AJ. Urinary tract infection in the setting of vesicoureteral reflux. F1000Res. 2016;5:F1000.
8. Meena J, Mathew G, Hari P, Sinha A, Bagga A. Prevalence of Bladder and Bowel Dysfunction in Toilet-Trained Children With Urinary Tract Infection and/or Primary Vesicoureteral Reflux: A Systematic Review and Meta-Analysis. Front Pediatr. 2020;8:84.
9. Tullus K. Vesicoureteric reflux in children. Lancet. 2015; 385(9965):371-9.
10. Mattoo TK. Vesicoureteral Reflux and Reflux Nephropathy. Adv Chronic Kidney Dis. 2011;18(5):348-54.

13.9 Voiding Disorders and Disorders of Obstruction of the Urinary Tract

Jyoti Sharma, (Lt Gen) Madhuri Kanitkar

INTRODUCTION

This chapter deals with two topics, i.e., voiding disorders in children and conditions that cause obstruction of the urinary tract.

VOIDING DISORDERS

Voiding disorders (VDs) are functional, abnormal patterns of micturition that occur due to abnormalities in storage or voiding phase in *the absence of a neurological or anatomic lesion.*

Physiology of Voiding

The urinary bladder is a compliant organ that fills continuously with urine with a minimal rise in pressure. It functions as a coordinated unit with the urethra and sphincters for intermittent efficient voiding. In neonates and infants, the full bladder empties by contraction of the detrusor, mediated by the spinal reflex arc. Conscious control, achieved through central inhibition of this voiding reflex, ensures that voiding occurs at an appropriate place and time. By 2–3 years of age, this control is established, resulting in daytime dryness by this age and nighttime dryness by about 5 years. An aberration of this function results in either a *wet child* or a child unable to *void to completion.*

Classification

Voiding disorders are classified as *secondary* in the presence of an underlying neurological or structural abnormality of the urinary tract, *or as primary* or *functional* voiding disorder in their absence. The nomenclature for symptoms and the classification of VD has been standardized by the International Children's Continence Society (ICCS).[1]

Some of the VDs are associated with incontinence. Continuous incontinence is almost always due to an underlying anatomical or neurological anomaly. Intermittent incontinence is usually functional.

Enuresis

Enuresis refers to intermittent incontinence that occurs during periods of sleep. Though it causes no physical harm, the ICCS guidelines recommend that the condition should be treated once the child is 6 years old due to its considerable psychosocial impact on the child and caregiver distress.

Enuresis is termed *primary* when the child has never been dry and *secondary* when bedwetting starts after a minimum period of 6 months of dryness at night. A cause for the latter can usually be identified, and its management results in the resolution of enuresis. When associated with daytime symptoms, enuresis is referred to as *nonmonosymptomatic enuresis*, and as monosymptomatic enuresis in the absence of these symptoms **(Table 13.9.1)**. Differentiating the two conditions through detailed history taking is crucial as management is determined by this.

Factors implicated in the pathogenesis of enuresis include some combination of inadequate antidiuretic hormone secretion resulting in nocturnal polyuria (urine output exceeding 130% of expected bladder capacity for age), reduced nocturnal bladder capacity, and an increased arousal threshold from sleep.[2]

Comorbid conditions requiring concurrent or prior to management of enuresis include constipation, attention deficit hyperactivity disorder, and sleep disordered breathing. A familial association has also been noticed.

A meticulously obtained history and thorough examination can help rule out pathological conditions contributing to polyuria or incontinence manifesting as enuresis, such as myelomeningocele, diabetes mellitus, diabetes insipidus, tubular disorders, and chronic kidney disease of tubulointerstitial origin **(Fig. 13.9.1)**. Very few investigations are necessary for children with enuresis. A voiding diary, along with details of bowel movements, aids in identifying children

TABLE 13.9.1: Daytime symptoms that may be associated with enuresis.

Term	*Definition*
Storage symptoms	
Frequency	Increased if >8 times/day; decreased if <3 times/day
Urgency	Sudden, unexpected, and immediate need to void
Voiding symptoms	
Hesitancy	Difficult initiation of voiding
Straining	Child applies abdominal pressure to initiate and maintain voiding
Intermittency	Micturition in several discrete spurts

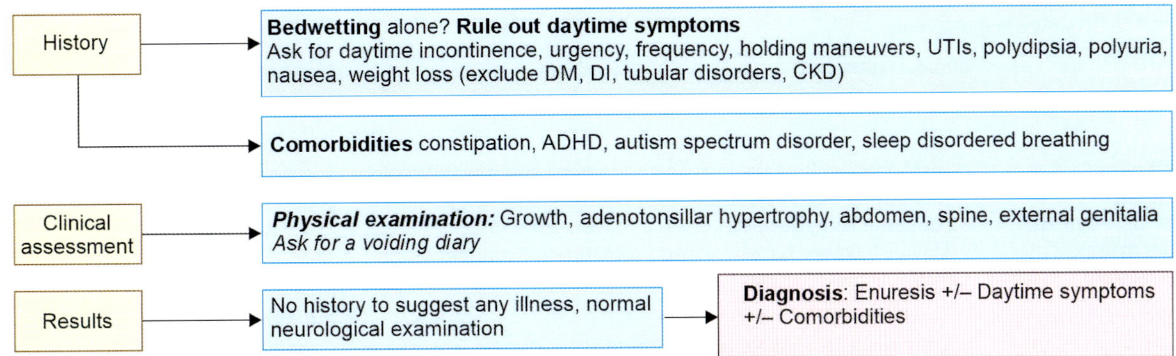

Fig. 13.9.1: Evaluation of a child with enuresis. (ADHD: attention deficit hyperactivity disorder; CKD: chronic kidney disease; DI: diabetes insipidus; DM: diabetes mellitus; UTIs: urinary tract infections)

Flowchart 13.9.1: Management of a child with enuresis.

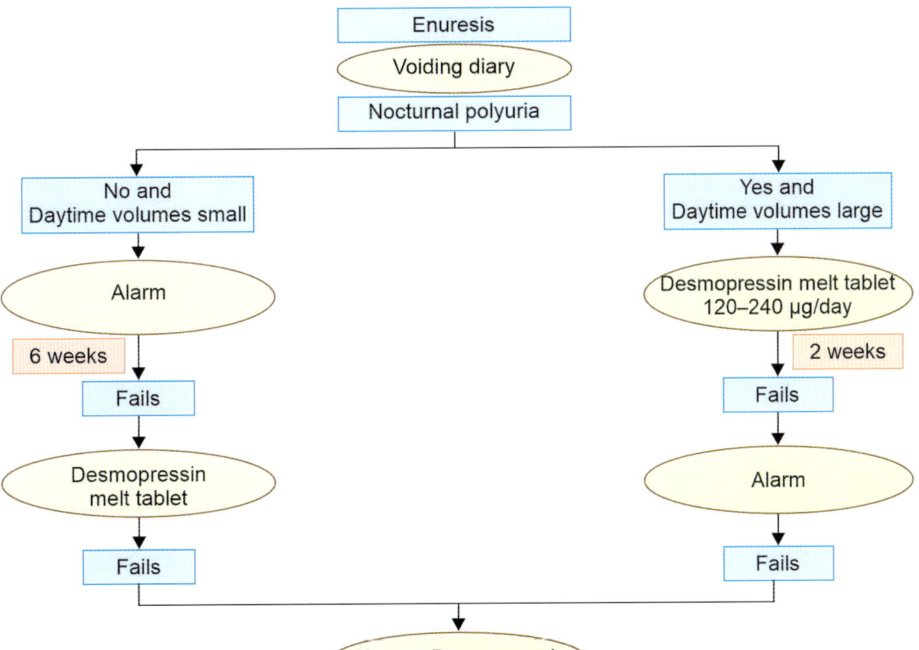

Anticholinergics (oxybutynin or tolterodine) can be considered as a second-line antineuritic therapy, in combination with desmopressin when bladder overactivity is suspected to contribute to enuresis

with nonmonosymptomatic enuresis and those experiencing constipation.[3]

Management of Enuresis

Management of enuresis entails management of comorbid conditions, urotherapy, and drug therapy.

Urotherapy involves discussions with parents and the child regarding pathophysiology of enuresis, emphasizing the importance of adequate fluid intake throughout the day, establishing good voiding practices (approximately six times a day), and promoting healthy bowel practices.[4] Initial management includes the use of an alarm or desmopressin with a possibility of adding anticholinergics to the latter **(Flowchart 13.9.1)**. The alarm device, positioned in the child's underclothes, triggers a conditioned response, initially awakening the child to moisture from urine and eventually to the sensation of a full bladder. The tricyclic antidepressant imipramine is considered a third-line drug.[5]

Other Voiding Disorders

Clinical features and management of other VDs are summarized in **Table 13.9.2**.

Constipation may be a concurrent comorbidity with these disorders, collectively termed as bladder bowel dysfunction.[1]

TABLE 13.9.2: Other voiding disorders.

Type	*Clinical features*	*Management*
1. Overactive bladder	Frequency, urgency, with or without incontinence	*Anticholinergics:* Oxybutynin, tolterodine, solifenacin, or β3-agonist mirabegron
2. Voiding postponement (a component of oppositional defiant disorder may exist in these children)	• History of habitual voiding postponement, often with holding maneuvers such as standing on tiptoe, crossing the legs, or squatting with the heel pressed into the perineum • May be followed by urgency and sometimes incontinence	*Specific urotherapy:* Psychotherapy and cognitive behavioral therapy
3. Extraordinary daytime only urinary frequency	• Seen in toilet-trained children • They need to void frequently during the day (at least once/hour), have small volume voids and no nocturia • Not associated with incontinence • Is self-limiting over a few days to weeks?	• Pathological conditions like diabetes mellitus, diabetes insipidus, psychogenic polydipsia and cystitis should be excluded by history and a urine dipstick evaluation • Reassurance of the child and parents
4. Vaginal reflux	Incontinence occurs soon after voiding. Usually seen in obese adolescent girls who void without adequate labial separation or in girls who have or develop labial adhesions	• Counseling about proper position while voiding; may be advised to face the wall when voiding to ensure labial separation • Surgical separation of labial adhesions and local application of an estrogen cream
5. Underactive bladder—a term used for children who strain to void; they need to raise intra-abdominal pressure to initiate, maintain, or complete voiding	• The voiding frequency may be <3 times a day or may be high due to incomplete voiding each time • *Diagnosis:* By invasive urodynamics	Clean intermittent catheterization if there is no response to urotherapy
6. Giggle incontinence—rare condition	There is sudden partial or complete evacuation of the bladder during an episode of laughter	• Cognitive behavioral therapy • Methylphenidate and oxybutynin have been tried
7. Dysfunctional voiding—a condition in which the external urethral sphincter contracts simultaneously with contraction of the detrusor	• Children present with suprapubic pain, voiding postponement, and/or recurrent urinary tract infections (UTIs) • Constipation is frequently present. Ultrasound may show a thickened bladder wall and significant postvoid residue • Micturating cystourethrogram (MCU) may demonstrate a dilated urethra and sometimes vesicoureteric reflux. Diagnosis is confirmed by uroflowmetry or urodynamic studies	• Management of constipation • Pelvic floor muscle relaxation by animated biofeedback • Antibiotic prophylaxis for UTI till the condition improves

Eliciting a history of constipation and/or encopresis is crucial; the parents and the child may be requested to maintain a 2-week bowel chart for validation. General urotherapy as a first step in management is applicable to all the conditions.

DISORDERS OF OBSTRUCTION OF THE URINARY TRACT

Obstruction of the urinary tract refers to a group of congenital or acquired disorders that cause anatomical or functional obstruction at different levels of the urinary tract. The clinical features depend on the site and severity of obstruction as well as the duration for which it has existed. For example, a child with postvoid residual urine in the bladder due to a bladder outlet obstruction is likely to present with recurrent urinary tract infections (UTIs). An undiagnosed pelviureteric junction obstruction (PUJO) may cause progressive thinning of the renal parenchyma and loss of function in the kidney. Common causes for obstruction of the urinary tract are enumerated in **Table 13.9.3**.

The most common acquired cause of obstruction is calculi which are likely to cause PUJO, midureteric obstruction, vesicoureteric junction obstruction (VUJO), and bladder outlet obstruction **(Figs. 13.9.2A to D)**. Children with calculi typically present with painful gross hematuria, passage of bright red blood in urine with clots and colicky pain.[6]

The aim of management of these conditions is often surgical, and aims to relieve obstruction, prevent UTIs

TABLE 13.9.3: Etiology and diagnosis of obstruction of the urinary tract.

Site/type of obstruction	*Suspect*	*Diagnosis*
Posterior urethral valves	Antenatal hydroureteronephrosis, oligohydramnios, poor stream, dribbling, recurrent UTI, palpable kidneys, and palpable urinary bladder	Characteristic findings on ultrasonography of kidneys ureter and bladder (USG KUB), micturating cystourethrogram (MCU), and cystoscopy
Urethral strictures/atresia	Straining, weak stream, history of urethral manipulations, and/or trauma	Cystoscopy and MCU
Urogenital sinus anomalies, bladder agenesis, and anorectal malformations	Continuous incontinence, abnormal external genitalia, and recurrent UTI	MCU, cystoscopy, and magnetic resonance urography (MRU)
Prune belly syndrome	Poorly developed abdominal muscles, nonrefluxing dilated ureters, hypoplastic kidneys, and urethral hypoplasia	USG and MCU
Congenital pelviureteric junction obstruction (PUJO)	Antenatal hydronephrosis, recurrent UTI, and abdominal mass	USG KUB and DTPA/EC scintigraphy
Congenital vesicoureteric junction obstruction (VUJO)	Antenatal hydroureteronephrosis	USG KUB and DTPA/EC scintigraphy
Calculi: Staghorn, or causing PUJO, VUJO, midureteric or bladder outlet obstruction	Ureteric colic, hematuria, and recurrent UTI	USG KUB and computed tomography (CT)
Neurogenic bladder (functional obstruction)	Urinary incontinence, UTI, fecal incontinence/constipation; sacral dimple; at the back, a midline tuft of hair or pad of fat, meningomyelocele, asymmetric gluteal folds, and neurological deficits in lower limbs	Magnetic resonance imaging (MRI) spine, USG KUB, MCU, and urodynamic studies

(DTPA: diethylenetriaminepentaacetic acid; EC: ethylene dicysteine; UTI: urinary tract infection)

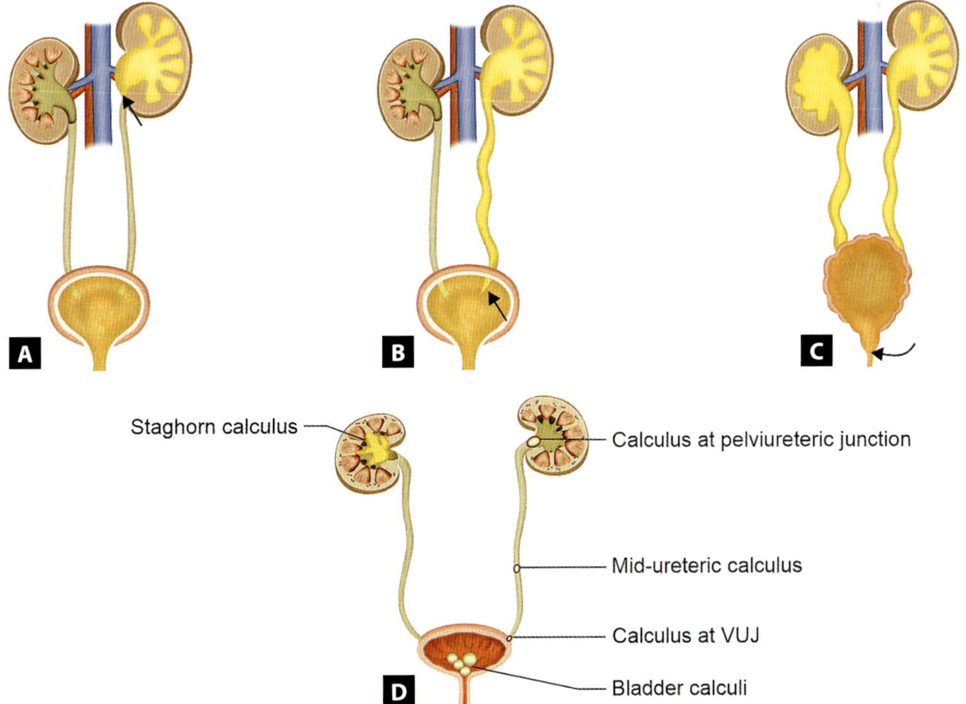

Figs. 13.9.2A to D: Common sites of obstruction of the urinary tract. Black arrows are at sites of obstruction. (A) Congenital pelviureteric junction obstruction (PUJO); (B) Congenital vesicoureteric junction obstruction (VUJO); (C) Posterior urethral valves (PUV); and (D) Sites of obstruction due to calculi.

or prevent adverse effects on kidney function due to back pressure changes. Some children like those with posterior urethral valves need long-term follow-up for growth, hypertension, bladder function, renal function, metabolic acidosis, and proteinuria.

ACKNOWLEDGMENT

We would like to acknowledge with gratitude the contribution of Dr Jyoti Singhal for creating the illustrations.

CONCLUSION

Voiding disorders manifest with various lower urinary tract symptoms (LUTS), e.g., incontinence, urgency, increased frequency of voiding or with recurrent UTIs. Enuresis is one of the most important and often overlooked VD. Constipation and behavioral disorders are associated comorbid factors. The mainstay of management is urotherapy; management of comorbid factors and specific treatments are recommended for each condition.

Obstruction of the urinary tract may be anatomical or functional; at different levels, affecting the urinary tract bilaterally or unilaterally. Anatomic obstructions present since birth are a part of a group of disorders referred to as congenital anomalies of the kidneys and urinary tract (CAKUT). Diagnosis is either on antenatal USG or postnatally with LUTS or UTI. Appropriate imaging is essential for an early diagnosis and surgery is required for relief of obstruction. Clinical clues of a neurogenic, functional obstruction must be borne in mind when examining a child with LUTS with or without bowel symptoms. These children need specialized management and long-term care.

REFERENCES

1. Austin PF, Bauer SB, Bower W, Chase J, Franco I, Hoebeke P, et al. The standardization of terminology of lower urinary tract function in children and adolescents: Update report from the standardization committee of the International Children's Continence Society. Neurourol Urodyn. 2016;35(4):471-81.
2. Nevéus T. Pathogenesis of enuresis: Towards a new understanding. Int J Urol. 2017;24(3):174-82.
3. Kanitkar M, Ramamurthy HR. Bed wetting - silent suffering: an approach to enuresis and voiding disorders in children. Indian J Pediatr. 2013;80(9):750-3.
4. Nieuwhof-Leppink AJ, Hussong J, Chase J, Larsson J, Renson C, Hoebeke P, et al. Definitions, indications and practice of urotherapy in children and adolescents: A standardization document of the International Children's Continence Society (ICCS). J Pediatr Urol. 2021;17(2):172-81.
5. Nevéus T, Fonseca E, Franco I, Kawauchi A, Kovacevic L, Nieuwhof-Leppink A, et al. Management, and treatment of nocturnal enuresis-an updated standardization document from the International Children's Continence Society. J Pediatr Urol. 2020;16(1):10-9.
6. Reddy PP, Minevich E. Renal calculus disease. In: Docimo SG, Canning DA, Khoury AE, Pippi Salle JL (Eds). The Kelalis King Belman Textbook of Clinical Pediatric Urology, 6th edition. Florida: Taylor and Francis Group; 2019. pp. 431-41.

13.10 Chronic Kidney Disease and Kidney Replacement Therapies

Soumya Reddy, Arpana Iyengar

INTRODUCTION

Chronic kidney disease (CKD), an important pediatric noncommunicable disease, is characterized by irreversible kidney damage over time and is associated with a high risk of morbidity, mortality, and poor quality of life. Children with CKD have a diverse spectrum of clinical manifestations, which are often subtle and nonspecific leading to a delay in diagnosis and management. CKD has replaced "chronic kidney failure" and "chronic kidney insufficiency" as the globally accepted terminology for persistent kidney dysfunction. Kidney failure (KF), previously referred to as end-stage kidney disease, is the most severe stage of CKD and children often present in this stage with significant life-threatening complications. The goals of therapy are to slow progression of early CKD to KF, identify and appropriately treat complications, and ensure timely initiation of dialysis or kidney transplantation.

This chapter deals with the basics of pediatric CKD, common etiologies, clinical features and complications, and management including kidney replacement therapies (KRTs) like dialysis and kidney transplant.

DEFINITION AND STAGING

Chronic kidney disease is defined as abnormalities of kidney structure or function, present for >3 months, with implications to health.[1] Criteria for diagnosing CKD include (any one of the following lasting for >3 months):

- *Markers of kidney damage:*
  - Abnormal urine analysis (albuminuria and hematuria)
  - Biochemical abnormalities (persistently elevated serum creatinine)
  - Structural malformations (solitary kidney and hydroureteronephrosis)
  - Histopathological diseases [focal segmental glomerulosclerosis and immunoglobulin A (IgA) nephropathy]
  - History of kidney transplantation
- Decline in glomerular filtration rate (GFR) to <60 mL/min/1.73 m^2

The classification of CKD proposed by the kidney disease Improving Global Outcomes (KDIGO): KDIGO has five stages based on estimated GFR and urinary albumin excretion **(Table 13.10.1)**. Estimated GFR is calculated using modified Schwartz formula (k × height (cm)/serum creatinine (mg/dL), where k is a constant = 0.413). Stage 1 CKD is difficult to identify as children rarely have symptoms and GFR is in the normal range, but the presence of an underlying structural malformation or persistent urinary abnormality can aid in making a diagnosis. The most severe stage of CKD is stage 5 (also known as KF), defined as GFR < 15 mL/min/1.73 m^2 or need for dialysis.

The KDIGO staging helps stratify the risk for progression of CKD and its complications based on GFR and is used to guide appropriate management and monitoring. However, this staging is not applicable in children aged ≤2 years (as normal physiological maturation of GFR occurs during this period and reaches adult values only by 2 years of age). Instead, in these children, GFR should be compared to age adjusted mean values and a level of more than one standard deviation above the mean indicates CKD. The normal values of GFR for age are given in **Table 13.10.2**.

EPIDEMIOLOGY

The term CKD defines kidney dysfunction as a *continuum*, rather than a discrete change in kidney function, making the epidemiology difficult to study. Since CKD in early stages is largely asymptomatic and challenging to detect clinically, the incidence and prevalence is commonly underestimated. In addition, there are limited national pediatric CKD registries. The estimated prevalence of CKD in children is around 30–100 per million age-related population (pmarp) per year based on international registries.[2]

ETIOLOGY

The most common causes of CKD in children are congenital anomalies of the kidney and urinary tract (CAKUT) such as hypodysplastic kidneys or posterior urethral valve accounting for approximately 50%, followed by hereditary nephropathies (congenital nephrotic syndrome, polycystic kidney disease, and primary hyperoxaluria) and glomerulonephritis (focal segmental glomerulosclerosis, IgA nephropathy, and hemolytic uremic syndrome).[3]

The etiology of CKD varies with age, as congenital malformations and metabolic/genetic disorders are common in younger children whereas in older children, glomerular and tubular diseases are more prevalent. **Table 13.10.3** highlights the common causes of CKD in children.

PATHOPHYSIOLOGY

Progressive loss of kidney function, irrespective of the etiology, leads to uremia and critical decline in homeostasis.

TABLE 13.10.1: Staging of chronic kidney disease (CKD) as per Kidney Disease: Improving Global Outcomes (KDIGO 2024).

Glomerular filtration rate (GFR) categories		
CKD stage	***Description***	***GFR category (mL/min/1.73 m^2)***
1	Kidney damage with normal or increased GFR	≥90
2	Kidney damage with mild decrease in GFR	60–89
3a	Mild-to-moderate decrease in GFR	45–59
3b	Moderate-to-severe decrease in GFR	30–44
4	Severe decrease in GFR	15–29
5	Kidney failure (KF)	<15 (or dialysis)

Albuminuria categories			
Albuminuria category	***Description***	***AER (mg/24 hour) or ACR (mg/g)***	***PER (mg/24 hour) or PCR (mg/g)***
A1	Normal to mildly increased	<30	<150
A2	Moderately increased	30–300	150–500
A3	Severely increased	>300	>500

(ACR: albumin creatinine ratio; AER: albumin excretion rate; PCR: protein creatinine ratio; PER: protein excretion rate)

TABLE 13.10.2: Normal glomerular filtration rate (GFR) in children.

Age	*Mean (± SD) GFR mL/min/1.73 m²*
1 week	41 ± 15
2–8 weeks	55 ± 25
2 months to 2 years	96 ± 22
2–12 years	133 ± 27
13–21 years:	
Males	140 ± 30
Females	126 ± 22

(SD: standard deviation)

TABLE 13.10.3: Common causes of chronic kidney disease in children.

<5 years of age	*>5 years of age*
Congenital malformations: • Hypoplastic/dysplastic kidneys • Reflux nephropathy • Obstructive uropathy (posterior urethral valves) *Metabolic/genetic disorders:* • Congenital nephrotic syndrome • Primary hyperoxaluria • Polycystic kidney disease • Wilms tumor	*Glomerular disease:* • Focal segmental glomerulosclerosis • *Chronic glomerulonephritis:* Immunoglobulin A (IgA) nephropathy and IgA vasculitis • Hemolytic uremic syndrome • Alport syndrome *Tubulointerstitial disease:* • Juvenile nephronophthisis • Polycystic kidney disease (autosomal recessive and dominant) • Cystinosis • Primary hyperoxaluria • Nephrotoxic medications

There are three phases involved in the deterioration of kidney function:

1. *First phase:* Initial injury [structural, metabolic, drugs, and systemic diseases (systemic lupus erythematosus)] and inflammation interferes with kidney function.
2. *Second phase:* Scarring occurs as a response to kidney injury.
3. *Third phase:* Maladaptive (disorganized) and incomplete repair leads to loss of nephrons resulting in fibrosis and thus, worsening kidney damage.

The factors responsible for CKD in children are distinctive and classified into nonmodifiable (primary kidney disease, preterm, low birth weight, and genetic predisposition) or modifiable (proteinuria, hypertension, anemia, obesity, dyslipidemia, recurrent urinary tract infections, and nephrotoxic medications). These factors contribute to progression to KF by causing direct damage to nephrons or by hyperfiltration injury (structural and functional hypertrophy of unaffected glomeruli causing damage to normal nephrons over time).[4]

Decline in glomerular filtration and tubular dysfunction results in symptoms and signs of CKD including uremia, polyuria, nocturia, and electrolyte or acid-base abnormalities. Metabolic complications typically become evident in stage 3 CKD. The most common complications seen in children with CKD include anemia, hypertension, growth failure, mineral bone disease (MBD), metabolic acidosis, electrolyte (potassium, sodium, calcium, and phosphate) imbalances, cardiovascular disease (left ventricular hypertrophy), dyslipidemia, delayed puberty, and neurocognitive impairment. The pathophysiological mechanisms of these complications are outlined in **Table 13.10.4**.

CLINICAL MANIFESTATIONS

The clinical features of CKD in children are related to both the underlying etiology and stage of CKD at the time of diagnosis. As children become symptomatic only when GFR declines to <30 mL/min/1.73 m², early stages of CKD have subtle nonspecific manifestations and are usually missed. Hence, it is crucial to have a high index of suspicion in children presenting with unexplained failure to thrive, anemia, bony deformities, history of antenatally detected hydronephrosis or polyhydramnios, as early diagnosis and prompt therapy may aid in retarding the progression of kidney damage. The spectrum of features suggestive of CKD is listed in **Box 13.10.1**.

Children with nonglomerular (tubule-interstitial) disease may often be identified by imaging techniques during routine antenatal screening or present with significant failure to thrive, polyuria, polydipsia, and recurrent urinary tract infections, while those with glomerular cause of CKD have more overt signs and symptoms such as edema, oliguria, frothy urine, hematuria, and hypertension.

EVALUATION OF CHRONIC KIDNEY DISEASE

Clinical

History regarding antenatal events, age of onset and duration of symptoms, significant past and family history and other additional information to identify CKD risk factors need to be enquired.

A comprehensive physical examination is essential to recognize features of CKD and screen for complications. Measurement of growth parameters and blood pressure (BP) and assessment for anemia, rickets, fluid retention cardiac dysfunction should be undertaken in all children with suspected CKD. Absence of oliguria does not rule out CKD as urine output may be preserved in children with nonglomerular cause of CKD till advanced stages. The relevant points in history and physical examination for evaluating CKD in children are depicted in **Figure 13.10.1**.

Biochemical

Measurement of serum creatinine is used for confirming diagnosis of CKD. However, serum creatinine is a late marker

TABLE 13.10.4: Pathophysiology of complications of chronic kidney disease.

Clinical manifestations	*Mechanisms*
Growth failure	• *Inadequate calorie intake:* Uremia and acidosis • Growth hormone resistance • Mineral bone disease • Anemia
Hypertension	• Volume overload • Vascular stiffness • Activation of renin-angiotensin-aldosterone axis
Anemia	• *Nutritional deficiency:* Iron, vitamin B_{12}, and folic acid • Decreased erythropoietin production • Decreased erythrocyte survival • Hemolysis • Gastrointestinal bleeding
Mineral bone disease (MBD)	• Hyperphosphatemia • Hypocalcemia/hypercalcemia • Impaired active D (1,25-hydroxyvitamin D) production • Secondary hyperparathyroidism • Metabolic acidosis
Metabolic acidosis	• Decreased ammonia synthesis, net acid excretion • Decreased bicarbonate reabsorption
Electrolyte abnormalities	• *Hyperkalemia:* Decreased GFR, metabolic acidosis, hyporeninemic hypoaldosteronism • *Hyponatremia:* Tubular dysfunction, solute diuresis
Predisposition to infections	• *Impaired immune response:* Decreased granulocyte function, reduced cellular response • Indwelling catheters • Anatomical issues with lower urinary tract
Cardiovascular disease	• Left ventricular hypertrophy due to hypertension • Volume overload • *Cardiomyopathy:* Hypertension and anemia • Pericarditis • Vascular calcifications
Endocrine disorders	*Delayed puberty:* Elevated luteinizing hormone (LH), follicle-stimulating hormone (FSH), loss of LH pulsatile pattern, reduced levels of testosterone, and dihydrotestosterone
Dyslipidemia	• Decreased plasma lipoprotein lipase activity • Abnormal high-density lipoprotein-C (HDL-C)
Neurocognitive impairment	• *Headache and seizures:* Hypertension, uremia, hypocalcemia, and other electrolyte imbalance • *Peripheral neuropathy:* Uremic toxins

(GFR: glomerular filtration rate)

BOX 13.10.1: Early clinical pointers to chronic kidney disease.

- Unexplained failure to thrive
- Short stature
- Unexplained anemia
- Hypertension
- Bony deformities or recurrent fractures
- Persistent proteinuria and abnormal urine analysis (hematuria)
- Recurrent urinary tract infection
- Recurrent kidney stones/nephrocalcinosis
- Abnormal urinary stream
- Family history of kidney disease
- Systemic disease with known kidney involvement
- Exposure to nephrotoxic drugs
- Previous acute kidney injury
- Abnormal kidney imaging

of kidney function as it rises only when GFR declines by 50%. There are no early biomarkers for CKD yet that can replace serum creatinine. For routine clinical practice, GFR is estimated with standardized serum creatinine levels [modified Jaffe or enzymatic methods with calibration traceable to isotope dilution mass spectrometry (IDMS)] using the modified Schwartz formula.

Blood levels of serum urea, electrolytes, acid-base, hemoglobin (Hb), calcium, phosphate, alkaline phosphatase (ALP), parathyroid hormone (PTH), vitamin D, and iron profile are commonly used to screen and monitor associated complications.

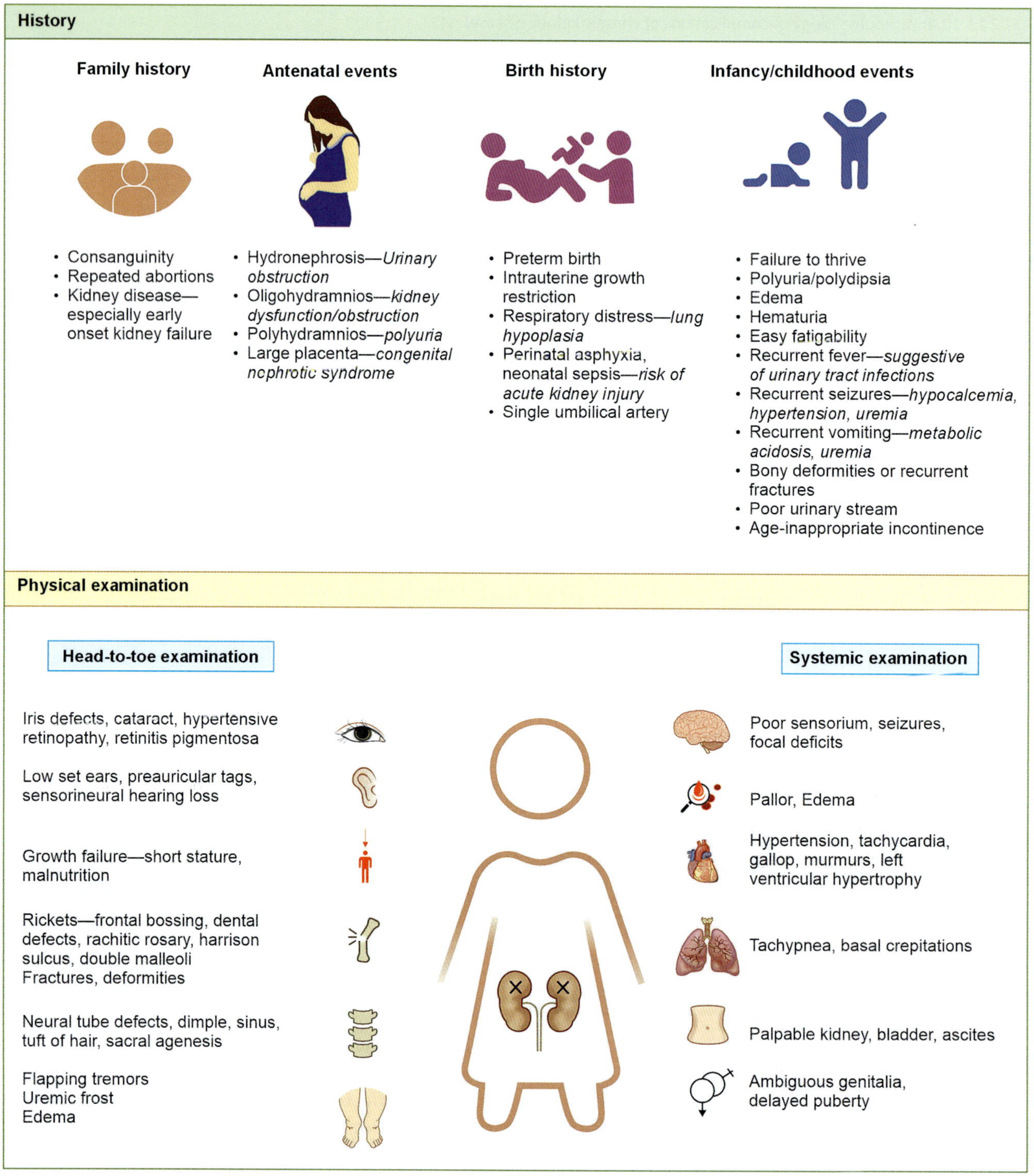

Fig. 13.10.1: Clinical evaluation of chronic kidney disease.

Urine Examination

Urinalysis may help in identifying the underlying cause of CKD and risk factors for progression. Isosthenuria (urine specific gravity of 1.010), a marker of loss of tubular concentration, favors the diagnosis of CKD.

Proteinuria is an important marker of progressive kidney damage. Urinary protein (or albumin) excretion is assessed either by estimating albumin or protein creatinine ratio (ACR or PCR) on the first morning urine sample or 24 hours urine protein quantification if feasible.

Screening for hematuria or urinary tract infection is undertaken in specific scenarios such as hereditary nephropathies (Alport syndrome) and obstructive uropathy, respectively.

Other urinary findings in CKD include presence of granular or waxy casts.

Imaging Studies

- *Ultrasonography* is the preferred imaging modality to assess kidney anatomy, kidney size, echotexture, corticomedullary differentiation, cystic changes, presence of stones, dilatation of pelvicalyceal system, and bladder wall thickness. In CKD, kidneys usually appear small (kidney length compared to normative age-appropriate values) with increased echotexture and loss of corticomedullary differentiation. Normal or large-sized kidneys are seen in nephronophthisis, polycystic kidney disease, and obstructive uropathy.
- *Micturating cystourethrogram (MCU)* is recommended for diagnosing posterior urethral valves, vesicoureteral reflux, and structural and functional bladder disorders.
- *Nuclear imaging studies* such as dimercaptosuccinic acid (DMSA) or diethylenetriamine pentaacetate (DTPA) scan are indicated for evaluation of kidney scars and differential kidney function.

Kidney Biopsy

Kidney biopsy is rarely done in advanced stages of CKD as histopathological examination is of limited use with nonspecific findings such as global glomerulosclerosis, extensive tubular atrophy, and interstitial fibrosis, and seldom yields information regarding the underlying etiology. Kidney biopsy in these children is also associated with high risk of significant postprocedural bleeding.

MANAGEMENT OF CHRONIC KIDNEY DISEASE

Management of a child with CKD requires a multidisciplinary team approach consisting of pediatric nephrologists, pediatric surgeons, trained nurses, dietician, and social worker to address the medical and social issues of the child and family. The key components of management include identification and treatment of primary kidney disease, adopting steps to retard progression, vigilant monitoring for complications, institution of appropriate therapy for metabolic derangements, and timely initiation of KRT.

Interventions to Slow Progression of Kidney Damage

The risk of progression to KF is related to the underlying cause and severity of CKD. At risk children must be identified and measures taken to avoid factors that might worsen kidney damage such as dehydration and nephrotoxic medications. In children with recurrent urinary tract infections, antibiotic prophylaxis may be indicated.

Hypertension, proteinuria, and dyslipidemia are some of the modifiable risk factors for CKD progression. Specific interventions proven to retard kidney damage include targeting BP to 50th centile for age, height, and gender and treatment of proteinuria with angiotensin-converting enzyme (ACE) inhibitors or angiotensin receptor blockers (ARBs).[5]

COMPLICATIONS OF CHRONIC KIDNEY DISEASE

Anemia

Anemia is a frequent complication in advanced stages of CKD (GFR < 45 mL/min/1.73 m^2).

Pathogenesis

The pathogenesis is multifactorial, though the root cause is decreased erythropoietin (EPO) production by the peritubular fibroblasts in the kidney cortex. An important contributing factor is iron deficiency secondary to decreased dietary intake, poor gastrointestinal absorption, and increased blood loss. Vitamin B_{12}, folate deficiency, reduced red blood cell survival, and bone marrow fibrosis due to hyperparathyroidism and chronic inflammation are other causes of anemia of CKD.

Clinical Features

Children present with weakness, fatigue, increased sleepiness, poor exercise tolerance, and anorexia.

Evaluation

The diagnosis of anemia is based on Hb level cut-offs according to age <5 years: Hb < 11 g/dL, 5–12 years: <11.5 g/dL, 12–15 years: <12 g/dL, >15 years (female): <12 g/dL, and >15 years (male): <13 g/dL. Evaluation includes complete hemogram, peripheral smear, iron studies, and stool for occult blood. Anemia of CKD is typically normocytic and normochromic with normal reticulocyte count. Iron deficiency, the most common contributing factor, is defined as transferrin saturation (TSAT) ≤20% and ferritin ≤100 ng/mL.

Treatment

Prior to starting recombinant EPO, iron supplementation should be initiated. The dose of oral iron therapy is 3–6 mg/kg/day. Intravenous iron therapy with iron sucrose or ferric carboxymaltose is indicated in children with poor response to oral iron or on dialysis. Supplementation with folic acid and vitamin B_{12} is also advised. Initiation of EPO stimulating agents are recommended when Hb is below 10 g/dL and after confirming iron-replete status. EPO is administered subcutaneously at 150–200 IU/kg/week and titrated to maintain Hb levels between 10 and 12 g/dL. Darbepoetin-α and CERA (methoxy polyethylene glycol-epoetin-β) are long-acting recombinant EPO formulations. In children with inadequate response to EPO, correction of micronutrient deficiencies, hyperparathyroidism, infections, hemolysis, and blood loss is advised. Blood transfusions are avoided to reduce risk of sensitization in children anticipating kidney transplant. If unavoidable due to critical situations, leukocyte filters should be used during transfusion.[6]

Mineral Bone Disease

Mineral bone disease, previously known as kidney osteodystrophy, is a systemic disorder of mineral and bone metabolism due to CKD characterized by abnormal metabolism of calcium, phosphorus, PTH or vitamin D, bone disorders, and soft tissue or vascular calcifications.

Pathogenesis

Elevated fibroblast growth factor (FGF23), hyperphosphatemia, reduced synthesis of 1,25-hydroxyvitamin D (calcitriol), hyperparathyroidism, and impaired bone mineralization are implicated in the pathogenesis of MBD.

Clinical Features

While biochemical alterations may present in early CKD stage 2, clinical manifestations of bone pains, recurrent fractures, deformities, abnormal gait, and rickets **(Figs. 13.10.2A and B)** become apparent when GFR is below 45 mL/min/1.73 m^2.

Evaluation

Monitoring for MDB should be commenced in stage 2 with serum calcium, phosphorus, ALP, PTH, and vitamin D levels.

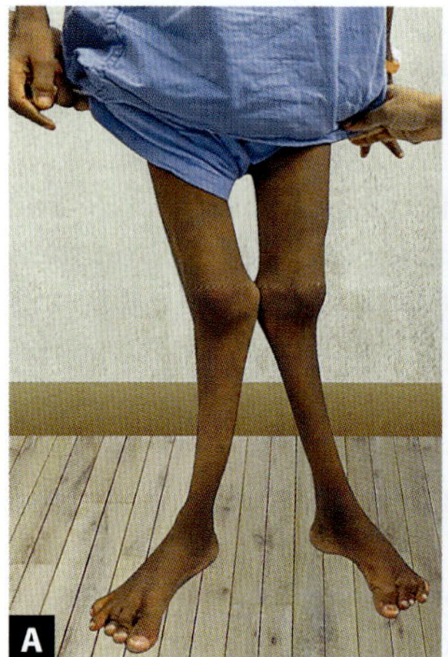

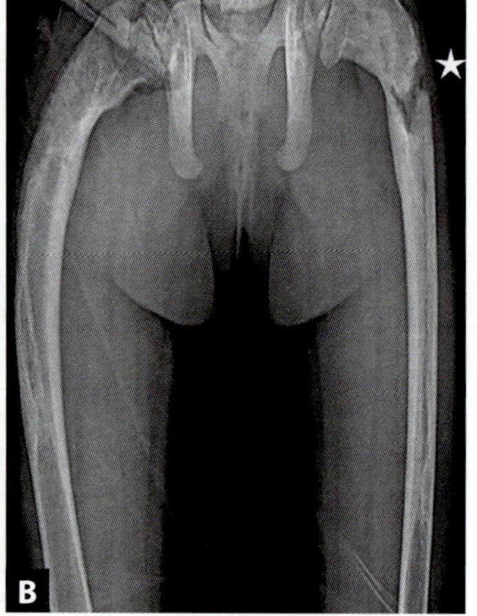

Figs. 13.10.2A and B: Severe rickets and X-ray of the femur showing fracture (asterisk) of neck of femur with severe osteopenia.

Hypocalcemia, hyperphosphatemia, elevated ALP, PTH, and low vitamin D are common. Radiographs of long bones reveal features of calcipenic rickets (subperiosteal bone resorption and metaphyseal widening, **Figures 13.10.2A and B**) and hyperparathyroidism.

Treatment

Maintaining normal serum calcium and phosphorus, appropriate PTH level (according to CKD stage), optimization of growth, limiting risk of deformities, and calcification are the main principles of treatment of CKD-MBD. Oral calcium supplements (50–100 mg/kg/day), dietary phosphate restriction, and oral phosphate binders (calcium carbonate, calcium acetate, and sevelamer) help in normalization of serum calcium and phosphorus. Oral vitamin D therapy with 25-hydroxyvitamin D (cholecalciferol) is instituted when levels are below 30 ng/mL. In children with hyperparathyroidism (PTH above the target range for CKD stage) or hypocalcemia despite adequate vitamin D levels, treatment with 1,25-hydroxyvitamin D (calcitriol) is recommended. In resistant hyperparathyroidism or side effects of calcitriol (hypercalcemia and hypercalciuria), calcimimetics such as cinacalcet should be considered. Parathyroidectomy is indicated for refractory hyperparathyroidism with PTH >800 ng/mL for 6 months despite maximal treatment. Corrective orthopedic surgeries may be indicated in children with progressive deformities after control of secondary hyperparathyroidism.[7]

Hypertension

Hypertension is a commonly encountered complication in pediatric CKD and is associated with cardiovascular morbidity and mortality. Volume overload, activation of renin-angiotensin-aldosterone, and vascular stiffness contribute to pathogenesis of hypertension. Measurement of BP is a critical component of routine examination in CKD. Hypertension is classified according to the American Academy of Pediatrics hypertension guidelines 2017 using appropriate age, height, and gender cut-offs. Ambulatory blood pressure monitoring (ABPM) is the gold standard for diagnosing and monitoring BP in these children.

Management of hypertension involves salt and fluid restriction, screening for left ventricular hypertrophy, and initiation of antihypertensive therapy (ACE inhibitors, ARBs, calcium channel blockers, α- and β-blockers) maintain mean arterial pressure (MAP) by ABPM to less than 50th percentile for age, sex, and height or target auscultatory systolic BP between 50 and 75th percentile when ABPM is not available.[8]

Growth and Nutrition

Short stature is one of the hallmarks of pediatric CKD. Relative growth hormone resistance, tubular dysfunction leading to electrolyte and fluid imbalance, MBD, poor dietary intake, and metabolic acidosis are a few factors responsible for growth failure. Younger children with nonglomerular cause of CKD are more severely affected. Early nutritional intervention and correction of metabolic derangements are key components in preservation of growth in these children. Recombinant growth hormone therapy is indicated in persistent growth failure in children with stage 3–5 CKD or on dialysis, with growth potential (open epiphysis), once other potentially treatable causes have been addressed. The recommended dose is 0.045–0.05 mg/kg/day subcutaneously with monitoring of growth parameters and side effects (intracranial hypertension and glucose intolerance).

Inadequate dietary intake, altered taste sensation, poor gastric emptying, tubular nutrient losses, anemia, and acidosis contribute to undernutrition in children with CKD. Dietary recall and regular assessment of anthropometric parameters once every 1–3 months in younger children and 3–6 monthly in older children is advised. To promote optimal growth, calorie, and protein intake of 100–120% of dietary reference intake (DRI) or upper limit of suggested dietary intake (SDI) is recommended.[9] Children with poor nutrition must be monitored closely under the supervision of a kidney dietician. Tube feeding with nasogastric or gastrostomy tube is necessary to meet nutritional needs in children with poor oral tolerance. In children with hyperkalemia, it is advised to avoid foods rich in potassium such as banana, coconut water, potato, drumstick, and gooseberries (amla). Phosphate-rich foods such as dairy products (milk, cheese, and ice cream), organ meats, processed or canned food, junk food, and aerated drinks should also be avoided in children with CKD and hyperphosphatemia.

Fluid, Electrolyte, and Acid–Base Disorders

Tubular dysfunction leads to lack of urinary concentrating ability resulting in polyuria, nocturia, and solute losses. These children require high volume of fluid and salt supplementation to prevent hypovolemia and complications of hyponatremia.

Children with primary glomerular disease or advanced CKD may develop fluid overload, requiring salt and fluid restriction.

Hyperkalemia is a life-threatening complication of CKD occurring due to worsening GFR, hyporeninemic-hypoaldosterone state, or increased intake. Electrocardiography (ECG) and cardiovascular monitoring are essential to identify arrhythmias. Emergency treatment with membrane stabilizers (intravenous calcium gluconate), β-agonists (salbutamol nebulization), correction of acidosis (bicarbonate infusion), and insulin-dextrose drip is instituted. Dietary restriction of potassium and oral potassium-binding resins (sodium polystyrene, patiromer, and sodium zirconium) are advised. In children with refractory hyperkalemia, KRT is recommended.

Children with CKD develop metabolic acidosis due to decreased net acid excretion and bicarbonate reabsorption and present with anorexia, recurrent vomiting, growth failure, bony deformities, and acidotic breathing. Treatment with oral sodium bicarbonate supplements or intravenous therapy in severe acidosis is warranted.

Urological Issues

Underlying urological disorders such as posterior urethral valve, hydronephrosis, vesicoureteric reflux, bowel-bladder dysfunction, and neurogenic bladder are noted in 50–60% of children with CKD. The common clinical features include abnormal urinary stream, recurrent urinary tract infections, age-inappropriate incontinence, dribbling of urine, bowel dysfunction, neural tube defects, and palpable kidney or bladder. Maintenance of bladder diary, urine analysis, ultrasound imaging, MCU, urodynamic studies, DMSA, and DTPA scan are some of the important tools to evaluate these children. Depending on the underlying disorder, interventions in the form of urotherapy (timed voiding and double voiding), clean intermittent catheterization (CIC), bladder relaxants (anticholinergics), and occasionally, surgical therapy are recommended.

SUPPORTIVE TREATMENT

Immunization

As children with CKD are at risking of contracting infections, standard immunization as per the national schedule and with special attention to influenza, pneumococcal, hepatitis B, and varicella vaccines is recommended. Frequent monitoring of hepatitis B titers in children on hemodialysis is advised. It is also important to ensure that potential kidney transplant recipients receive all live vaccines at least 4–6 weeks prior to transplantation.

Psychosocial Support

Children with CKD have poor health-related quality of life. Involvement of child psychiatrists, counselors, and social workers to address issues of low self-esteem, psychological stress, and compliance to treatment is crucial. Home-schooling to facilitate missed educational opportunities, vocational training services, and peer support groups may help tackle some of these problems. Families of children with CKD in developing countries experience severe caregiver burden and would benefit from financial and psychosocial support.

KIDNEY REPLACEMENT THERAPY

When a child with CKD progresses to KF (GFR <15 mL/min/1.73 m^2), only medical management will not suffice and initiation of KRT is essential for survival. KRT refers to treatments that replace the critical functioning of a child's own native kidney and includes kidney transplantation, peritoneal dialysis (PD) and hemodialysis (HD), of which kidney transplantation is the ideal choice offering better patient outcomes and quality of life.[10] Despite the benefits of preemptive transplantation, dialysis might have to be initiated in certain emergency situations as a temporary treatment while awaiting transplant or in those with contraindications to transplant. The decision regarding KRT is a shared exercise with the healthcare provider team and patient's family and counseling must begin when GFR declines to <30 mL/min/1.73 m^2.

Indications for Initiation of Dialysis

Clinical parameters are more important deciding factors for initiation of dialysis than a particular level of GFR. The indications for initiation of dialysis are listed in **Table 13.10.5**.

Peritoneal Dialysis

Chronic ambulatory PD or home dialysis is the most ideal modality of dialysis for children. In PD, the removal of fluid and solutes is achieved by infusing the peritoneal cavity with a dialysis solution and drainage after a certain "dwell" time as the peritoneum (semipermeable membrane) functions as the dialyzer. Chronic PD is performed with a surgically inserted Tenckhoff catheter **(Fig. 13.10.3A)**, and the parents are trained to perform exchanges at home. PD is usually a continuous form of therapy and consists of 3–5 exchanges lasting for a total duration of 12–24 hours. The main complications of PD include peritonitis and mechanical issues.

Advantages

- Home-based treatment
- Permits normal physical and scholastic activity
- Promotes better growth
- Lesser dietary and fluid restrictions

Limitations

- Requires the caregiver to be trained and committed to perform procedure at home daily
- Expensive therapy
- Contraindicated in intra-abdominal pathologies like omphalocele, gastroschisis, bladder exstrophy, and diaphragmatic hernia

Hemodialysis

Hemodialysis works on the principle of diffusion to clear solutes such as urea and potassium from the patient's blood compartment into the dialysis fluid compartment through

TABLE 13.10.5: Indications for initiation of dialysis.

Clinical	Fluid overload, anuria, severe hypertension, recurrent vomiting, tremors (uremia), encephalopathy, and refractory growth failure
Biochemical	Glomerular filtration rate <15 mL/min/1.73 m^2, refractory hyperkalemia, and refractory metabolic acidosis

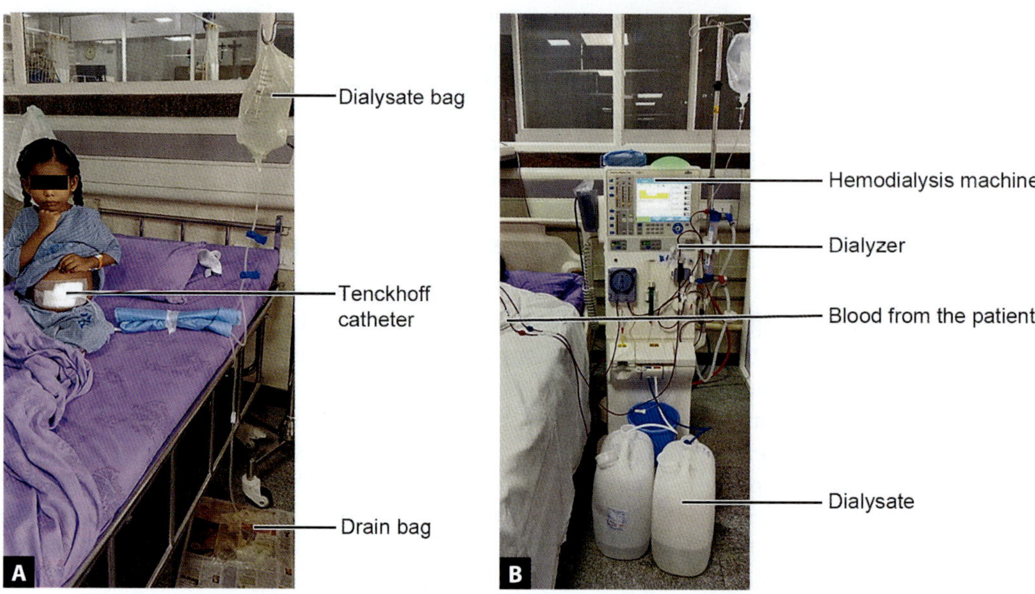

Figs. 13.10.3A and B: (A) Chronic ambulatory peritoneal dialysis and (B) Hemodialysis.

the dialyzer membrane. In addition, excess fluid is removed by ultrafiltration generated by a pressure difference between the compartments. After establishing a permanent vascular access (catheter in the internal jugular vein or arteriovenous fistula), dialysis is usually performed for 3–4 hours/session thrice a week. **Figure 13.10.3B** shows a dialysis machine with dialyzer.

Advantages

- Better dialytic therapy for acute on chronic problems such as fluid overload, hyperkalemia, and uremia
- Controlled fluid removal (ultrafiltration)

Limitations

- Frequent visits to dialysis center
- Challenges with securing a vascular access
- Technical difficulties in infants/young children
- Requirement of dialysis machine, trained technician, and continuous monitoring during the session
- Strict fluid and dietary restrictions

Kidney Transplant

Kidney transplantation is the optimal therapy for children with KF. Preemptive transplant (transplantation undertaken without going through dialysis therapy) has superior outcomes and should be considered in children with stage 4–5 CKD who might require dialysis within 1 year. Living related (parents, grandparents, and siblings) and deceased donor transplantation have been approved by the Government of India. A comprehensive pretransplant evaluation of the recipient and potential donor is essential. Technical expertise, vigilant perioperative monitoring, and use of induction immunosuppression (at the time of transplant) followed by lifelong maintenance immunosuppression with calcineurin inhibitors (tacrolimus/cyclosporine), antiproliferative agents (mycophenolate/azathioprine), and steroids have improved graft survival outcomes in pediatric transplants. Some of the complications that may be encountered after kidney transplant include graft rejection, thrombosis, recurrence of primary disease, hypertension, and steroid side effects.

BOX 13.10.2: Recent advances in chronic kidney disease and kidney replacement therapy.

Evaluation:
- *GFR estimation:* CKD-EPIcr-cys 2021 formula (based on creatinine and cystatin C), CKD-U25 formula (creatinine based)
- *Anemia:* Assessment of iron status—reticulocyte hemoglobin count, percentage of hypochromic red cells, soluble transferrin receptors, hepcidin
- *Hypertension:* Ambulatory blood pressure monitoring

Treatment:
- *Anemia:* Newer iron formulations (ferric maltol, sucrosomial iron), erythropoiesis stimulating agents [darbepoetin-α and CERA (methoxy polyethylene glycol-epoetin-β)], hypoxia-inducible factor-prolyl hydroxylase inhibitors (Roxadustat, Vadadustat, Daprodustat)
- *Phosphate binders:* Sucroferric oxyhydroxide, ferric citrate
- *Potassium binders:* Sodium zirconium cyclosilicate, patiromer
- *Prevention of progression to kidney failure/proteinuria:* SGLT2 inhibitors (dapagliflozin), glucagon-like peptide-1 receptor agonists (exenatide), mineralocorticoid receptor antagonist (finerenone)
- *Hemodialysis:* Hemodiafiltration, nocturnal hemodialysis

(GFR: glomerular filtration rate; SGLT2: sodium-glucose cotransporter 2)

CONCLUSION

Chronic kidney disease is a state of irreversible kidney damage with progressive loss of kidney function. Children with CKD are usually asymptomatic till they progress to advanced stages such as KF. Comprehensive evaluation through detailed history, focused examination, and thorough investigations helps in diagnosing CKD, identifying the underlying etiology, and associated complications such as anemia, MBD, hypertension, and growth failure. Early detection and timely therapy might slow the progression of kidney damage and reduce severity of complications. Evolving evidence continues to shape our understanding of CKD. The recent advances in evaluation and treatment are summarized in **Box 13.10.2**. Kidney transplant is the treatment of choice in children with KF, while dialysis is indicated in emergency situations or ideally as a temporary therapy while awaiting transplant.

REFERENCES

1. KDIGO 2024 Clinical Practice Guideline for the Evaluation and Management of Chronic Kidney Disease. Kidney Int Suppl. 2024;105(4):117-314.
2. Harambat J, Madden I. What is the true burden of chronic kidney disease in children worldwide. Pediatr Nephrol. 2023; 38(5):1389-93.
3. Kamath N, Iyengar AA. Chronic Kidney Disease (CKD): An Observational Study of Etiology, Severity and Burden of Comorbidities. Indian J Pediatr. 2017;84(11):822-5.
4. Becherucci F, Roperto RM, Materassi M, Romagnani P. Chronic kidney disease in children. Clin Kidney J. 2016;9(4):583-91.
5. Cirillo L, De Chiara L, Innocenti S, Errichiello C, Romagnani P, Becherucci F. Chronic kidney disease in children: an update. Clin Kidney J. 2023;16(10):1600-11.
6. Babitt JL, Eisenga MF, Haase VH, Kshirsagar AV, Levin A, Locatelli F, et al. Controversies in optimal anemia management: conclusions from a Kidney Disease: Improving Global Outcomes (KDIGO) Conference. Kidney Int. 2021;99(6):1280-95.
7. Kidney Disease: Improving Global Outcomes (KDIGO) CKD–MBD Update Work Group. KDIGO 2017 Clinical Practice Guideline Update for the Diagnosis, Evaluation, Prevention, and Treatment of Chronic Kidney Disease-Mineral and Bone Disorder (CKD-MBD). Kidney Int Suppl. 2017;7(1):1-59.
8. Mitsnefes MM. Cardiovascular disease in children with chronic kidney disease. J Am Soc Nephrol. 2012;23(4):578-85.
9. Shaw V, Polderman N, Renken-Terhaerdt J, Paglialonga F, Oosterveld M, Tuokkola J, et al. Energy and protein requirements for children with CKD stages 2-5 and on dialysis–clinical practice recommendations from the Pediatric Renal Nutrition Taskforce. Pediatr Nephrol. 2020;35(3):519-31.
10. VanSickle JS, Warady BA. Chronic Kidney Disease in Children. Pediatr Clin North Am. 2022;69(6):1239-54.

13.11 Renal Tubular Diseases

Arvind Bagga, Aditi Sinha

INTRODUCTION

In comparison to glomerular diseases, tubular disorders are less common. A high index of suspicion and correct diagnosis allow specific management in many patients. Tubulopathies should be suspected in children presenting with symptoms listed in **Box 13.11.1**. The diagnosis of a primary tubular disorder implies that there is no significant impairment of glomerular function or tubulointerstitial inflammation. The disorder may be congenital or acquired and involve a single tubular function (renal glucosuria, nephrogenic diabetes insipidus) or multiple functions (Fanconi syndrome). Most disorders can be diagnosed following careful interpretation of specific urine and plasma biochemical tests.[1]

RENAL TUBULAR ACIDOSIS

Renal tubular acidosis (RTA) includes conditions characterized by a defect of renal acidification resulting in impaired capacity for net acid excretion and hyperchloremic metabolic acidosis, in the presence of normal glomerular function.[1] Transport defects are usually secondary to reduced proximal tubular reabsorption of bicarbonate (HCO_3^-), as in proximal RTA, or the distal secretion of protons (hydrogen ion, H^+), as in distal RTA.[2] A third variety called type IV RTA is distinguished by the presence of hyperkalemia. These conditions may be primary, with or without known genetic defects, or secondary to other causes **(Table 13.11.1)**.[1]

Pathophysiology

In the proximal tubule, the reabsorption of filtered HCO_3^- is mediated by carbonic anhydrase in the tubular brush border. The primary defect in proximal (type II) RTA is reduced renal threshold for HCO_3^- reabsorption, leading to bicarbonaturia. Fanconi syndrome refers to a generalized proximal tubular dysfunction characterized by tubular proteinuria, aminoaciduria and variable bicarbonaturia, phosphaturia, and glucosuria.[1,3]

BOX 13.11.1: Presenting features of tubular disorders.[1]

- Growth retardation, poor weight, and height gain
- Delayed gross motor milestones
- Polyuria, excessive thirst
- Recurrent episodes of dehydration, vomiting, and/or fever
- Rickets, bone fractures
- Episodic muscle weakness or neck flop
- Constipation
- Craving for salt and savory foods
- Tetany, seizures, and/or muscle cramps
- Kidney stones or incidentally detected nephrocalcinosis

In the distal tubule, secreted H^+ ions combine with hydrogen phosphate (HPO_4^{2-}) and ammonia to form $H_2PO_4^-$ and NH_4^+, measured as titratable acidity and urinary ammonium ion, respectively. Additional factors that influence H^+ secretion and HCO_3^- reabsorption include extracellular fluid volume, potassium balance, and plasma aldosterone. Distal RTA is characterized by decreased distal tubular secretion of H^+, leading to low rates of excretion of NH_4^+ and titratable acidity. Hypokalemic distal (classic or type 1) RTA is usually a secretory defect, with decreased excretion of H^+ due to impaired function of one of the subunits of the anion channel H^+-adenosine triphosphatase (H^+-ATPase), or the Cl^-/HCO_3^- exchanger. Less often, it is a rate defect (lower rate of H^+ secretion), permeability defect (backleak of H^+) or an inability to generate the required voltage (voltage-dependent or hyperkalemic form). More recently, defects in *WDR72* and *FOXI1* are also described to cause distal RTA. In all forms, except mild rate defects, the urine pH cannot reach maximal acidity (i.e., remains >5.3) despite acidemia. Hypokalemia, a hallmark of distal RTA, is attributed to increased urinary losses of K^+, partially secondary to hyperaldosteronism in response to volume contraction and urinary losses of Na^+.[1,2]

Distal RTA with hyperkalemia may result from a voltage defect (hyperkalemic distal RTA), secondary to insufficient negative intraluminal potential in the cortical collecting duct, or a rate defect, due to aldosterone deficiency or resistance (type 4 RTA). Other than normokalemia or hyperkalemia, the findings in hyperkalemic distal RTA resemble classic distal RTA. Aldosterone resistance or deficiency decreases distal reabsorption of Na^+, which lowers the transtubular potential gradient for H^+ secretion. In addition, lack of aldosterone action decreases urinary excretion of K^+. Hyperkalemia in turn reduces ammoniagenesis. In type 4 RTA, maximally acidic urine (<5.3) can be formed, indicating intact ability to establish a maximal H^+ gradient.

Clinical Features

Features that suggest RTA are listed in **Box 13.11.1**. Children with proximal RTA present with failure to thrive, irritability,

TABLE 13.11.1: Inherited and acquired forms of renal tubular acidosis (RTA).[1]

Type of RTA	*Inherited: Gene affected (associated features or syndrome)*	*Acquired*
Type 1 (distal) RTA	• *SCL4A1* (hemolytic anemia) • *ATP6V1B1* (early onset hearing loss) • *ATP6V0A4* (no or delayed hearing loss) • *ATP6V1C2* • *FOXI1* (early onset hearing loss) • *WDR72* (amelogenesis imperfecta)	• Systemic lupus erythematosus, Sjögren syndrome • Obstructive uropathy, reflux nephropathy • Sickle cell anemia • Amphotericin B toxicity
Type 2 (proximal) RTA: Isolated Multiple tubular dysfunction (Fanconi syndrome)	• *SCL4A4* (band keratopathy, cataract or glaucoma; defective enamel; intellectual impairment; basal ganglia calcification) • *CTNS* (cystinosis) • *CLCN5* (Dent disease) • *Other syndromes:* Fanconi–Bickel syndrome; Fanconi renotubular syndromes 1–4; galactosemia; tyrosinemia; Wilson disease; hereditary fructose intolerance; Lowe syndrome; glycogen storage disease type I; mitochondrial disorders; arthrogryposis; cholestasis; microcephaly (ARC) syndromes	• Carbonic anhydrase inhibitors (acetazolamide) • Vitamin D-dependent rickets, vitamin D deficiency • Primary hyperparathyroidism • Focal segmental glomerulosclerosis • Acute tubulointerstitial nephritis with uveitis • *Drugs:* Ifosfamide, cisplatin, aminoglycosides • *Toxins:* Lead, cadmium, mercury, toluene
Type 3 (combined)	*CA2* (with osteopetrosis; blindness, deafness)	
Type 4 (hyperkalemic)	• *MR* (*NR3C2*), *SCNN1B* (Pseudohypoaldosteronism type 1) • *WNK4, WNK1, KLHL3, CUL3* (Pseudohypoaldosteronism type 2; Gordon syndrome) • *CYP11B2, CYP17A1* (congenital adrenal hyperplasia)	• *Aldosterone deficiency without renal disease* (Addison disease; adrenal tuberculosis; necrosis) • *Chronic renal insufficiency* (obstructive uropathy, interstitial nephritis) • *Aldosterone resistance* (amiloride, spironolactone) • Transient, following urinary tract infections in infancy

anorexia, listlessness, and uncommonly, with symptoms of hypokalemia (weakness, paralysis).[3-5] Patients with Fanconi syndrome may have features of the underlying disorder **(Table 13.11.1)**, as in patients with cystinosis (presentation in infancy, photophobia, hepatosplenomegaly, and blond hair)[3] or Lowe syndrome (presentation in infancy with severe rickets, cataract, buphthalmos, hypotonia, and developmental delay).[3-5] Boys with Dent disease may present with refractory rickets, nephrocalcinosis, and night blindness.[4] Features in distal RTA include impaired growth, polyuria, nephrocalcinosis **(Fig. 13.11.1)** or nephrolithiasis, symptoms of hypokalemia and/or hearing loss.[1,2,6] Children with type 4 RTA have milder acidosis without nephrocalcinosis, urolithiasis, or bone lesions. Underlying tubulointerstitial disease may be evident. The autosomal recessive form of pseudohypoaldosteronism (PHA) type 1, caused by inactivation of the epithelial sodium channel (*SCNN1A/B/G* variants) is an important differential diagnosis in infants presenting with salt loss, hypotension, hyperkalemia, and metabolic acidosis, and is a severe systemic disease, affecting sweat and salivary glands and colon. The autosomal dominant form of PHA type 1, involving the inactivation of the mineralocorticoid receptor (*NR3C2*), affects only the kidneys and is less severe than the recessive form.

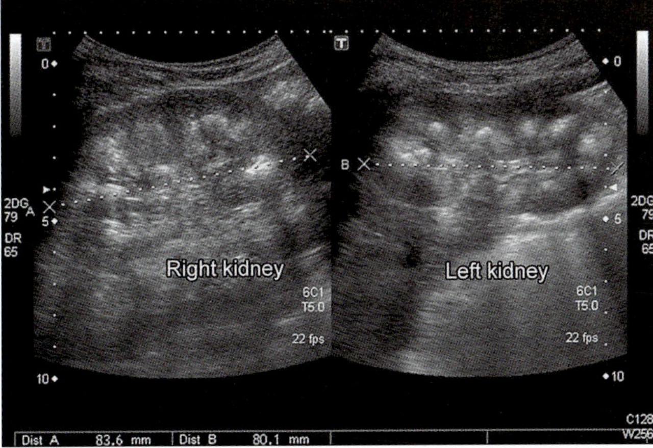

Fig. 13.11.1: Nephrocalcinosis in a 6-year-old girl with distal renal tubular acidosis, presenting with polyuria and failure to thrive.

Evaluation

Metabolic acidosis may result from either increased endogenous acid synthesis (e.g., ketoacidosis, lactic acidosis) or enhanced bicarbonate losses (diarrhea, intestinal tube drainage or fistula, ureterosigmoidostomy, cholestyramine). Since all types of RTA are associated with hyperchloremic metabolic acidosis, the initial step is the determination of the plasma anion gap, which is normal (8–12 mEq/L) in all types of RTA. **Table 13.11.2** lists important steps of evaluation.[1]

Elevated excretion of urinary NH_4^+ in patients with metabolic acidosis suggests extrarenal HCO_3^- losses (diarrhea), while low excretion points to RTA. Since the difference between urinary unmeasured anions (sulfates, phosphates, and organic anions) and cations (calcium, magnesium) is relatively constant (at ~80 mEq/L), the measurement of important ions as urine anion gap (UAG; urine net charge) effectively estimates NH_4^+ excretion.

Loading with sodium bicarbonate, performed orally (2–4 mEq/kg/day for 3 days) or intravenously (0.5 mEq/mL at 3 mL/min) to achieve urine pH >7.5 and normal serum HCO_3^- (>22 mEq/L), allows simultaneous measurement of fractional excretion of bicarbonate and urine to blood CO_2 gradient, which reflects proximal bicarbonate handling and distal tubular acidification, respectively.[1]

Table 13.11.3 summarizes the differences among various types of RTA.[1] Additional tests are required depending on the type suspected. In patients with proximal RTA, other proximal functions are evaluated, including for aminoaciduria, glucosuria, low molecular weight proteinuria, and calculation of fractional excretion of phosphate ($FEPO_4$) and tubular maximum for phosphate.[1] Patients are screened

TABLE 13.11.2: Evaluation in patients with suspected renal tubular acidosis (RTA).[1]

Test	*Comment*
Plasma anion gap	• Calculated as $[Na^+ - (Cl^- + HCO_3^-)]$ • Normal (8–12 mEq/L) in RTA and diarrhea • Elevated in patients with ketoacidosis, lactic acidosis, inborn errors of metabolism, poisoning, or uremia
Urine anion gap (UAG) or urine net charge	• UAG = Urinary $Na^+ + K^+ - Cl^-$ • Urinary NH_4^+ = 80 – UAG • Is positive in normal conditions; during systemic acidosis, negative UAG suggests extrarenal (diarrheal) HCO_3^- losses, while positive UAG reflects impaired urinary acidification (RTA)
Urine pH	• Is measured on fresh voided specimen with pH meter, not dipstick • Estimates <1% of urinary proton excretion • During systemic acidosis, pH >5.3 suggests distal RTA; value <5.3 suggests extrarenal cause or RTA type 2 or 4
Fractional excretion of bicarbonate ($FEHCO_3^-$)	$FEHCO_3^-(\%) = \frac{\text{Urine bicarbonate} \times \text{Plasma creatinine}}{\text{Plasma bicarbonate} \times \text{Urine creatinine}} \times 100$ After bicarbonate loading, value is >15% in proximal RTA; <5% in normal persons and distal RTA
Urine to blood pCO_2 gradient (U-B CO_2)	• Urine pCO_2 sensitively reflects distal H^+ secretion, rising to >70 mm Hg during alkalosis • U-B CO_2 = Urine pCO_2 – blood pCO_2 • After bicarbonate loading, value <10 mm Hg suggest classic distal RTA; value is >20 mm Hg in normal individuals, patients with permeability and voltage defects, and in types 2 and 4 RTA

TABLE 13.11.3: Investigations to differentiate types of renal tubular acidosis (RTA).*

		Distal RTA		
Investigation	***Proximal RTA***	***Classic***	***Hyperkalemic (voltage defect)***	***Type 4 RTA***
Plasma K^+	Normal/low	Low	High/normal	High
Serum bicarbonate, mEq/L	12–20	Usually <12	Usually >17	Usually >17
Urine pH	<5.3	>5.3	>5.3	<5.3
Urine anion gap	Positive	Positive	Positive	Positive
Urine NH_4^+	Low	Low	Low	Low
Fractional HCO_3^- excretion	>10–15%	<5%	<5%	>5–10%
U-B pCO_2, mm Hg	>20	<20	</>20	>20
Urine calcium	Normal	High	High/normal	Normal
Other tubular defects[1]	Often present	Absent	Absent	Absent
Nephrocalcinosis	Absent	Present	Present/absent	Absent
Bone disease	Common	Often present	Uncommon	Absent

[1]Includes phosphaturia, low molecular weight proteinuria, generalized aminoaciduria, and glucosuria
(U-B pCO_2: urine to blood pCO_2 gradient)

for cystinosis, Lowe syndrome, galactosemia, and Wilson disease.[1,7] Evaluation in patients with distal RTA includes ultrasonography (nephrocalcinosis, renal calculi) and measurement of urinary calcium and citrate excretion.[2,8] All patients should undergo hearing evaluation; older children are evaluated for secondary (e.g., autoimmune) causes.[2]

Workup in patients with type 4 RTA should include renal function tests and ultrasonography to identify structural or parenchymal disease. Measurements of plasma renin activity and aldosterone levels are required. Transtubular potassium gradient is a useful test in diagnosing type 4 RTA. When coupled to a mineralocorticoid challenge, this test allows distinction between aldosterone deficiency and resistance.

Treatment

Management of RTA involves correction of acidosis through administration of alkali supplements (Uriliser, Polycitra, and Shohl solution) and provision of adequate nutrition, fluids and deficient electrolytes. Patients with distal RTA require 2–3 mEq/kg/day of alkali. Urinary potassium losses decrease with correction of acidosis, but some patients require prolonged potassium supplementation. Similarly, rickets improves with management of acidosis. Urinary calcium excretion should be monitored; patients with persistent hypercalciuria require thiazides.[1,2]

The requirement of alkali supplements is higher (5–20 mEq/kg/day) in patients with proximal RTA.[1,3-5] This is given as a combination of sodium and potassium citrate, with restriction of dietary sodium. Supplements of phosphate (neutral phosphate, Joulie solution) are necessary in Fanconi syndrome. Small doses of vitamin D may enable healing of rickets. Specific treatment may be useful, such as therapy with cysteamine in patients with cystinosis, penicillamine in Wilson disease, nitisinone in tyrosinemia, and dietary interventions (galactosemia, hereditary fructose intolerance, and tyrosinemia).[1,3-5]

TUBULOPATHIES WITH URINARY CHLORIDE WASTING

Bartter and Gitelman syndromes are caused by defects in ion transporters resulting in increased urinary losses of chloride, accompanied by potassium and sodium wasting. **Table 13.11.4** lists salient features of tubulopathies presenting with hypokalemic metabolic alkalosis.[9-11]

Bartter Syndrome

Patients present with failure to thrive, polyuria, polydipsia, and recurrent episodes of dehydration. The neonatal form is particularly severe with maternal polyhydramnios, polyuria, dehydration, hypercalciuria, and nephrocalcinosis. Hypokalemia is marked and associated with hypochloremic metabolic alkalosis and increased levels of plasma renin and aldosterone.[9,11]

Bartter syndrome is differentiated from other conditions with persistent hypokalemic metabolic alkalosis by the presence of normal blood pressure, and high urinary excretion of chloride and calcium. Further characterization of the molecular defect is based on genetic testing. Differences in presentation may help characterize the defect **(Table 13.11.4)**.

Management of Bartter syndrome includes fluid replacement and supplementation of potassium chloride (1–3 mEq/kg/day). Administration of indomethacin (2–3 mg/kg/day) or ibuprofen (30 mg/kg/day) decreases elevated prostaglandins and ameliorates polyuria. Potassium-sparing diuretics and occasionally, angiotensin-converting enzyme (ACE) inhibitors, are used to aid potassium retention.[9,11]

TABLE 13.11.4: Tubular diseases presenting with hyperchloremic metabolic alkalosis with hypokalemia and normal or low blood pressure.[9,10]

Disorder: protein (gene)	***Presentation***
Antenatal Bartter syndrome: Types *1:* NKCC2 (*SLC12A1*) *2:* ROMK (*KCNJ1*) *4a:* Barttin, beta subunit of ClC-K (*BSND*) *4b:* ClC-Ka (*CLCNKA-CLCNKB*) *5:* Melanoma-associated antigen D2 (*MAGED2*)	• *Antenatal:* Polyhydramnios, prematurity • *Neonatal:* Failure to thrive, nephrocalcinosis; hypercalciuria • Sensorineural deafness in type 4 Bartter syndrome • Transient hyperkalemia in type 2 Bartter syndrome; transient Bartter syndrome in type 5
Classic Bartter syndrome or type 3: ClC-Kb (*CLCNKB*)	Growth retardation, hypercalciuria, no nephrocalcinosis, normal serum magnesium
Gitelman syndrome: NCCT (*SLC12A3*)	Episodic muscle weakness; mild polyuria; hypocalciuria, hypomagnesemia, chondrocalcinosis
EAST/SeSAME syndrome (*KCNJ10*)	Ataxia, seizures, sensorineural deafness, developmental delay; hypocalciuria, hypomagnesemia

Inherited in autosomal recessive manner, except type 5 Bartter syndrome, which is X-linked.
(ClC-Kb: chloride channel, kidney, B; EAST: epilepsy, ataxia, sensorineural deafness and salt-wasting tubulopathy; NCCT: sodium chloride cotransporter; NKCC2: sodium potassium chloride cotransporter-2; ROMK: renal outer medullary potassium channel; SeSAME: seizures, sensorineural deafness, ataxia, mental retardation, and electrolyte imbalance)

Gitelman Syndrome

Patients with Gitelman syndrome have abnormalities similar to Bartter syndrome, including hypokalemia, metabolic alkalosis, and hypomagnesemia.[10,11] However, symptoms, including polyuria and growth retardation, are milder and appear in older children. Episodes of weakness, vomiting, abdominal pain, and tetany may occur. The underlying mechanism is a defect in the thiazide sensitive, sodium chloride cotransporter in the distal tubule. Urinary calcium excretion is low but magnesium wasting is prominent. Treatment is with supplementation of potassium and magnesium (as oral magnesium oxide, chloride, gluconate, oxide, or hydroxide).[10,11]

POLYURIA

Polyuria is defined as urine output exceeding 6 mL/kg/h or 2 L/m^2 in children. Polyuria may accompany structural renal disorders including juvenile nephronophthisis, renal dysplasia (reflux nephropathy, obstructive uropathy) and chronic tubulointerstitial nephritis, or solute losses (RTA, Bartter-like syndromes, and diabetes mellitus).[12]

Nephrogenic diabetes insipidus (NDI), also termed arginine vasopressin (AVP) resistance, is a rare condition characterized by tubular unresponsiveness to the antidiuretic hormone (ADH, vasopressin). Most cases are inherited in an X-linked recessive pattern with mutations in the gene for the arginine vasopressin V2 receptor (*AVPR2*); 10% cases of NDI are inherited in an autosomal recessive manner through mutations in the gene for aquaporin 2 (*AQP2*). Infants present with irritability, failure to thrive, recurrent episodes of dehydration, and intermittent fever. NDI may also be acquired, as with obstructive uropathy, analgesic nephropathy, sickle cell disease, chronic pyelonephritis, sarcoidosis, in association with hypercalcemia or hypokalemia, or following use of lithium and tetracyclines.[12] Uncommonly, NDI may also be seen as a part of Bartter syndrome, distal RTA, Fanconi syndrome, or autosomal recessive polycystic kidney disease.

The diagnosis of diabetes insipidus requires confirmation of polyuria and exclusion of differential diagnoses. Useful investigations include measurement of urine osmolality, electrolytes, sugar and ketones; blood electrolytes, pH, bicarbonate, sugar, calcium and creatinine, and ultrasonography for the kidneys. Upon water deprivation, diabetes insipidus is suggested by plasma sodium of >145 mEq/L, plasma osmolality >295 mEq/kg, and urine osmolality <300 mEq/kg. A rise in urine osmolality to >150% of baseline following administration of desmopressin (DDAVP) suggests complete central diabetes insipidus (arginine vasopressin deficiency), while no change (<110% of baseline) suggests complete NDI. The plasma level of copeptin, which is secreted in an equimolar amount to AVP, satisfactorily discriminates between various forms of polyuria if measured at baseline and following water deprivation. However, the assay is not available routinely.[12]

Patients with diabetes insipidus require adequate intake of water. Restriction of dietary sodium to 1 mEq/kg/day and administration of hydrochlorothiazide (2–4 mg/kg/day), with or without amiloride (0.3 mg/kg/day) help reduce polyuria in patients with NDI. Indomethacin (2 mg/kg/day) is also useful.[12]

REFRACTORY RICKETS

Rickets results from a lack of adequate mineralization of growing bones. The diagnosis is based on clinical findings, radiological features **(Fig. 13.11.2)**, and blood biochemistry.[13] The term refractory rickets is used for patients who fail to show radiological healing and normalization of biochemical abnormalities despite therapy with two large doses of vitamin D; alternatively, it is diagnosed in presence of rickets despite normal serum 25-hydroxy vitamin D levels. The causes of refractory rickets are grouped into two categories according to the underlying defect, abnormal vitamin D metabolism or impaired renal tubular phosphate handling **(Box 13.11.2)**.[13,14] The former is characterized by low serum levels of calcium and phosphate, aminoaciduria, and high parathyroid hormone (PTH). The latter shows hypophosphatemia with normal serum calcium and PTH. Rickets in distal RTA is attributed to impaired renal hydroxylation of calcidiol and a negative calcium balance secondary to persistent metabolic acidosis.[13,14]

Clinical Presentations

Presentation varies by cause and severity. Patients with vitamin D-dependent rickets (VDDR) have onset in infancy with tetany, seizures, delayed dentition, and hypocalcemia.

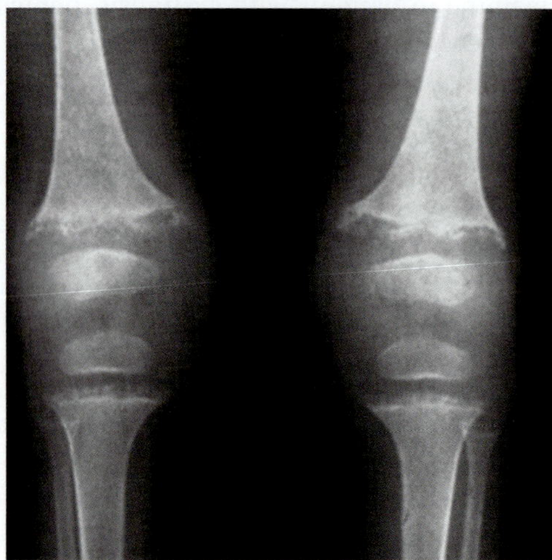

Fig. 13.11.2: Radiograph of both knees in a 4-year-old boy showing widening, flaring, and irregularity of the metaphyseal ends of long bones. Serum 25-hydroxyvitamin D levels were above normal limits due to past treatment and a diagnosis of refractory rickets was made.

BOX 13.11.2: Causes of refractory rickets.[13,14]

Calcipenic rickets
- *Vitamin D-dependent rickets, types 1A, 1B:* 1-alpha hydroxylase (*CYP27B1*), 25-hydroxylase (*CYP2R1*)
- *Vitamin D-dependent rickets, type 2:* Vitamin D receptor (*VDR*)

Hypophosphatemic rickets
- *X-linked familial:* Phosphate-regulating endopeptidase (*PHEX*)
- *Autosomal dominant:* Fibroblast growth factor 23 (*FGF23*)
- *Autosomal recessive:* Dentin matrix phosphoprotein 1 (*DMP1*), ectonucleotide pyrophosphatase/phosphodiesterase 1 (*ENPP*)
- *Hypophosphatemic rickets with hypercalciuria:* NaPi-2c (*SLC34A3*) defect
- McCune-Albright syndrome (*GNAS*)
- Fanconi syndrome; Dent disease **(Table 13.11.1)**

Distal renal tubular acidosis **(Table 13.11.1)**

Chronic kidney disease mineral bone disease

Note: Names after colon indicate the affected protein (gene)

Flowchart 13.11.1: Evaluation in patients with refractory rickets.

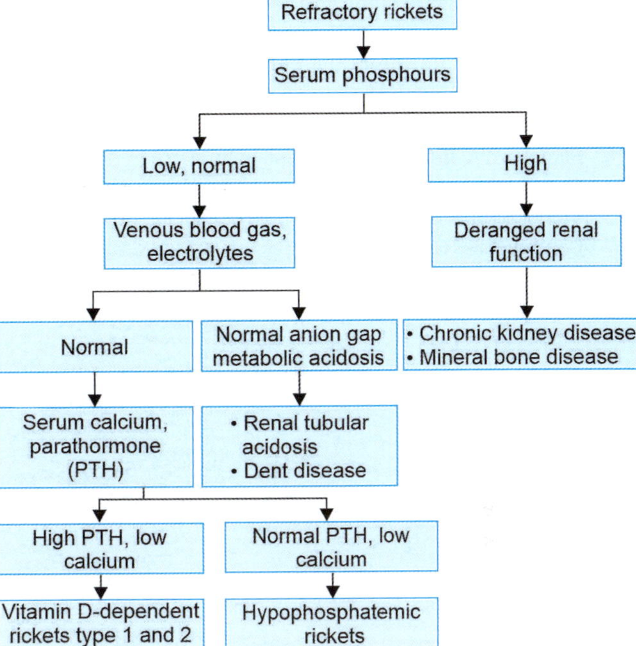

Patients with VDDR type 1 show enamel hypoplasia; those with VDDR type 2 may have alopecia and ectodermal defects (oligodontia, epidermal cysts). Presentation of hypophosphatemic rickets includes short stature, lower limb deformities, and dental abnormalities (pulp deformities, abscess).[15] Patients with hypercalciuric variant of hypophosphatemic rickets, distal RTA, or Dent disease may show nephrocalcinosis or nephrolithiasis. Presentation of RTA and Fanconi has been discussed.[13,14]

Evaluation

Evaluation should include estimation of blood levels of calcium, phosphorous, alkaline phosphatase, creatinine, pH, electrolytes, bicarbonate, 25-hydroxyvitamin D, and PTH; urinalysis; estimation of timed excretion of calcium, phosphate, protein, and creatinine; and ultrasonography of kidneys. While levels of fibroblast growth factor-23 (FGF-23) have satisfactory diagnostic utility, particularly for X-linked hypophosphatemic rickets, the assay is not available routinely. **Flowchart 13.11.1** provides a practical approach to diagnosis.[13,14]

Management

The therapy of rickets is tailored to the underlying cause. Patients with VDDR type 1 are treated with calcidiol or calcitriol (1–2 µg daily) and supplements of calcium and phosphate. Requirement of calcitriol is higher (0.05–0.2 µg/kg/day) in patients with VDDR type 2. These patients may benefit from administration of high-dose calcium infusions.[13]

Management of hypophosphatemic rickets involves supplementation of phosphate (30–50 mg/kg/day) as neutral phosphate or acid phosphate (Joulie solution).[14,15] Patients with X-linked hypophosphatemic rickets also require small doses of calcitriol (25–50 ng/kg/day; 0.25–0.5 µg daily). Burosumab, a recombinant human monoclonal antibody against FGF-23, has been approved for the therapy of X-linked hypophosphatemic rickets; however, therapy is not afforded by most patients.[14,15]

The rickets in RTA responds satisfactorily to correction of acidosis; patients with proximal RTA additionally require supplements of oral phosphate with or without vitamin D. Management of mineral bone disease associated with chronic kidney disease relies on control of hyperphosphatemia (dietary restriction, use of oral phosphate binders) and therapy with active vitamin D analogs.[13-15]

REFERENCES

1. Bagga A, Sinha A. Renal tubular acidosis. Indian J Pediatr. 2020; 87:733-44.
2. Trepiccione F, Walsh SB, Ariceta G, Boyer O, Emma F, Camilla R, et al. Distal renal tubular acidosis: ERKNet/ESPN clinical practice points. Nephrol Dial Transplant. 2021;36:1585-96.
3. Emma F, Nesterova G, Langman C, Labbé A, Cherqui S, Goodyer P, et al. Nephropathic cystinosis: An international consensus document. Nephrol Dial Transplant. 2014;29(Suppl 4):iv87-94
4. Jin YY, Huang LM, Quan XF, Mao JH. Dent disease: Classification, heterogeneity and diagnosis. World J Pediatr. 2021;17: 52-7.
5. Foreman JW. Fanconi syndrome. Pediatr Clin North Am. 2019; 66:159-67.
6. Alonso-Varela M, Gil-Peña H, Santos F. Incomplete distal renal tubular acidosis in children. Acta Paediatr. 2020;109:2243-50.
7. Kashoor I, Batlle D. Proximal renal tubular acidosis with and without Fanconi syndrome. Kidney Res Clin Pract. 2019;38: 267-81.
8. Giglio S, Montini G, Trepiccione F, Gambaro G, Emma F. Distal renal tubular acidosis: A systematic approach from diagnosis to treatment. J Nephrol. 2021;34:2073-83.

9. Konrad M, Nijenhuis T, Ariceta G, Bertholet-Thomas A, Calo LA, Capasso G, et al. Diagnosis and management of Bartter syndrome: Executive summary of the consensus and recommendations from the European Rare Kidney Disease Reference Network Working Group for Tubular Disorders. Kidney Int. 2021;99:324-35.
10. Blanchard A, Bockenhauer D, Bolignano D, Calò LA, Cosyns E, Devuyst O, et al. Gitelman syndrome: Consensus and guidance from a Kidney Disease: Improving Global Outcomes (KDIGO) Controversies Conference. Kidney Int. 2017;91:24-33.
11. Fulchiero R, Seo-Mayer P. Bartter syndrome and Gitelman syndrome. Pediatr Clin North Am. 2019;66:121-34.
12. Vaz de Castro PAS, Bitencourt L, de Oliveira Campos JL, Fischer BL, Soares de Brito SBC, Soares BS, et al. Nephrogenic diabetes insipidus: a comprehensive overview. J Pediatr Endocrinol Metab. 2022;35:421-34.
13. Michałus I, Rusińska A. Rare, genetically conditioned forms of rickets: Differential diagnosis and advances in diagnostics and treatment. Clin Genet. 2018;94:103-14.
14. Ackah SA, Imel EA. Approach to hypophosphatemic rickets. J Clin Endocrinol Metab. 2022;108:209-20.
15. Haffner D, Emma F, Eastwood DM, Duplan MB, Bacchetta J, Schnabel D, et al. Clinical practice recommendations for the diagnosis and management of X-linked hypophosphataemia. Nat Rev Nephrol. 2019;15:435-55.

13.12 Asymptomatic Hematuria

Indira Agarwal

INTRODUCTION

Hematuria is a sign of underlying renal disease; the cause of this may vary from benign to very serious disease. Urine color may vary from bright red to cola colored, depending on the underlying cause. When visible only under the microscope and not visible to the naked eye—it is called microscopic hematuria and is often incidentally detected on routine screening of urine for any reason. Gross hematuria, though uncommon, may be more serious, as it often originates from glomeruli or the urinary tract and needs immediate attention.

The persistent finding of five or more red cells per high power field (HPF) on a centrifuged urine specimen performed over 2–3 weeks warrants evaluation.[1] As little as 1 mL of blood is sufficient to make the urine color red. Dipsticks have good sensitivity and specificity in detecting 1–5 red blood cells (RBCs)/HPF but need confirmation by microscopy of the centrifuged specimen. The presence of dysmorphic RBC and granular casts with proteinuria >2+ suggest a glomerular cause.

A positive dipstick reaction in the absence of RBC and RBC casts in the urine suggests hemoglobinuria or myoglobinuria. This can be differentiated from hematuria by centrifugation where a clear pink supernatant with minimal or no deposits will suggest hemoglobinuria while cloudy red or dark brown supernatant will suggest hematuria. Phase-contrast microscopy helps to determine the site of origin of the bleeding as it distinguishes dysmorphic from normal RBCs. Presence of at least 100 RBCs which are dysmorphic or >5% are acanthocytes on phase contrast on original magnification of 3,400 or if there is >1 RBC cast on low power on at least 50 microscopic fields characterizes glomerular hematuria.[2] Automated flow cytometry and digitalized microscopy are two modern tools for counting urinary particles using very small volume of urine.[3]

EPIDEMIOLOGY

The estimated incidence of gross hematuria is 1.3/1,000 population,[4] and the prevalence is 0.15–2% with more than half being due to identifiable causes.[5,6] Asymptomatic microscopic hematuria is ten-fold as prevalent as gross hematuria; most often it is transient and on repeated evaluation the prevalence decreases to <0.5%.

The causes of hematuria may be varied. The approach involves differentiating true hematuria from causes which may discolor the urine and give a false appearance. Beets, dyes, medications (phenazopyridine), uric acid, and porphyrins can color urine red or pink. It also needs to be differentiated from myoglobinuria which also colors the urine red and gives a positive dipstick but under the microscope, only sparse RBCs are seen.

Onset of gross hematuria may be abrupt and suggest transient causes such as fever, severe infection, exercise, and trauma.[7] Symptoms resolve with symptomatic treatment. If there is persistence of gross or microscopic hematuria, further evaluation is warranted. Systemic causes for bleeding need to be considered in a sick patient where coagulopathy and platelet dysfunction and hematological disorders could be an underlying contributing factor. Once these are ruled out, evaluation for an underlying renal cause is required. A good clinical history and thorough physical examination will help in identifying the cause.

The first step is to identify the site of bleeding: glomerular or nonglomerular. If bleeding occurs in the upper tract the color of the urine is "cola-colored" or "tea-colored" and shows dysmorphic RBC (>30% by phase contrast microscopy). Urine from the lower tract is bright red, has clots and is eumorphic. Hematuria may be painless or painful and may or may not be associated with proteinuria.

Causes of glomerular hematuria include postinfectious glomerulonephritis (GN), immunoglobulin A (IgA) nephropathy, systemic lupus, Henoch–Schönlein purpura (HSP), hemolytic uremic syndrome (HUS), membranoproliferative glomerulonephritis (MPGN), and infections (malaria, leptospirosis, and endocarditis). Familial causes of hematuria include thin basement membrane disease (benign familial hematuria), Alport syndrome, cystic diseases of the kidney disease, and some types of renal stone disease. There may be recurrent episodes of gross hematuria precipitated by respiratory infections or may remain microscopic. The presence of significant proteinuria suggests more severe disease.

Nonglomerular causes include nephrolithiasis, hypercalciuria, viral hemorrhagic cystitis, urinary tract infection (UTI), and vascular abnormalities.

CLINICAL FEATURES

A good clinical history will help to identify the cause. A history of facial puffiness, oliguria, hypertension, and impaired renal function suggests a glomerular disease. Hematuria, hypertension, and edema mark the clinical triad of GN. Hematuria associated with infection or following a bacterial/viral infection is now termed as infection related glomerulonephritis (IRGN) and is commonly seen with postinfectious glomerulonephritis (PIGN).[8] Poststreptococcal GN is considered the prototype and is considered as the most common cause of hematuria in children. Seen in school going children, the onset is abrupt following a throat or skin infection. Low C3 which normalizes in 6–8 weeks is the norm. Presentation may vary from mild-to-severe but recovery in most cases is good and relapse very rarely occurs. IgA nephropathy can mimic postinfectious GN but can be differentiated by symptoms being "synpharyngitic", normal C3, and recurrent episodes with normal urine in between can occur. At times microscopic hematuria may persist.

The presence of fever, rash, and joint pains with or without abdominal pain suggests an underlying systemic disorder such as systemic lupus erythematosus and HSP. Patients with collagen vascular disorders may occasionally present with rapidly progressive glomerulonephritis (RPGN) and require urgent intervention. Pulmonary renal syndromes such as Goodpasture syndrome and microscopic polyangiitis present symptoms of epistaxis, hemoptysis, and exertional dyspnea. These may be missed if a careful history is not taken.

In the absence of systemic signs and symptoms, conditions such as benign familial hematuria or Alport syndrome should be considered. Family history of members with late onset hearing loss, renal failure, and dialysis should be enquired about. Urinalysis of family members, and eye (anterior lenticonus) and hearing assessments (high tone hearing deafness) are advised. Hematological conditions such as sickle cell disease and trait, coagulopathies, and thrombocytopenia may occasionally present with hematuria. Loin pain hematuria syndrome (LPHS) presents with recurrent episodes of loin pain (unilateral, bilateral) and hematuria (microscopic, gross) where investigations do not reveal any abnormality. Nutcracker syndrome due to entrapment of left renal vein between aorta and superior mesenteric artery presents similarly.

Patients with hematuria due to a disorder in the lower tract have symptoms of dysuria, burning, frequency, or hesitancy. Terminal hematuria suggests cystitis, while at initiation suggests urethritis. UTI presents with fever; and may be either localized to the bladder as in cystitis or may suggest pyelonephritis in a more toxic patient who also has loin pain. Adenovirus infection may result in hemorrhagic cystitis. Renal vein thrombosis may present with loin pain hematuria and palpable kidneys. It needs to be considered in all those with underlying hypercoagulable states. Cystic kidney disease may present with hematuria if there is hemorrhage and infection into the cysts. Children with nephrolithiasis present with renal colic, gross or asymptomatic microhematuria while those with hypercalciuria have hematuria without evident calculi. Prolonged immobilization or conditions such as hypervitaminosis D, hyperparathyroidism, and drugs may be associated with hypercalciuria or it may be idiopathic in origin. Interstitial nephritis may present with malaise, fatigue, and variable volumes of urine output.

Following confirmation of presence of hematuria and type of hematuria through urine analysis, further investigations are indicated to confirm the diagnosis as depicted in the given flowchart (**Flowcharts 13.12.1 and 13.12.2**, for gross hematuria and for microscopic hematuria, respectively).[8-10]

INVESTIGATIONS

Urine analysis is the key to analyzing the cause of hematuria and the first step in the clinic may be screening by urine dipsticks which have a sensitivity of 100% and specificity of 99.3%.[11] RBC morphology and presence of casts will help to elucidate the origin of hematuria. A centrifuged urine sample showing dysmorphic RBCs are the characteristic findings

Flowchart 13.12.1: Gross hematuria. Steps in urine analysis for evaluation of hematuria.

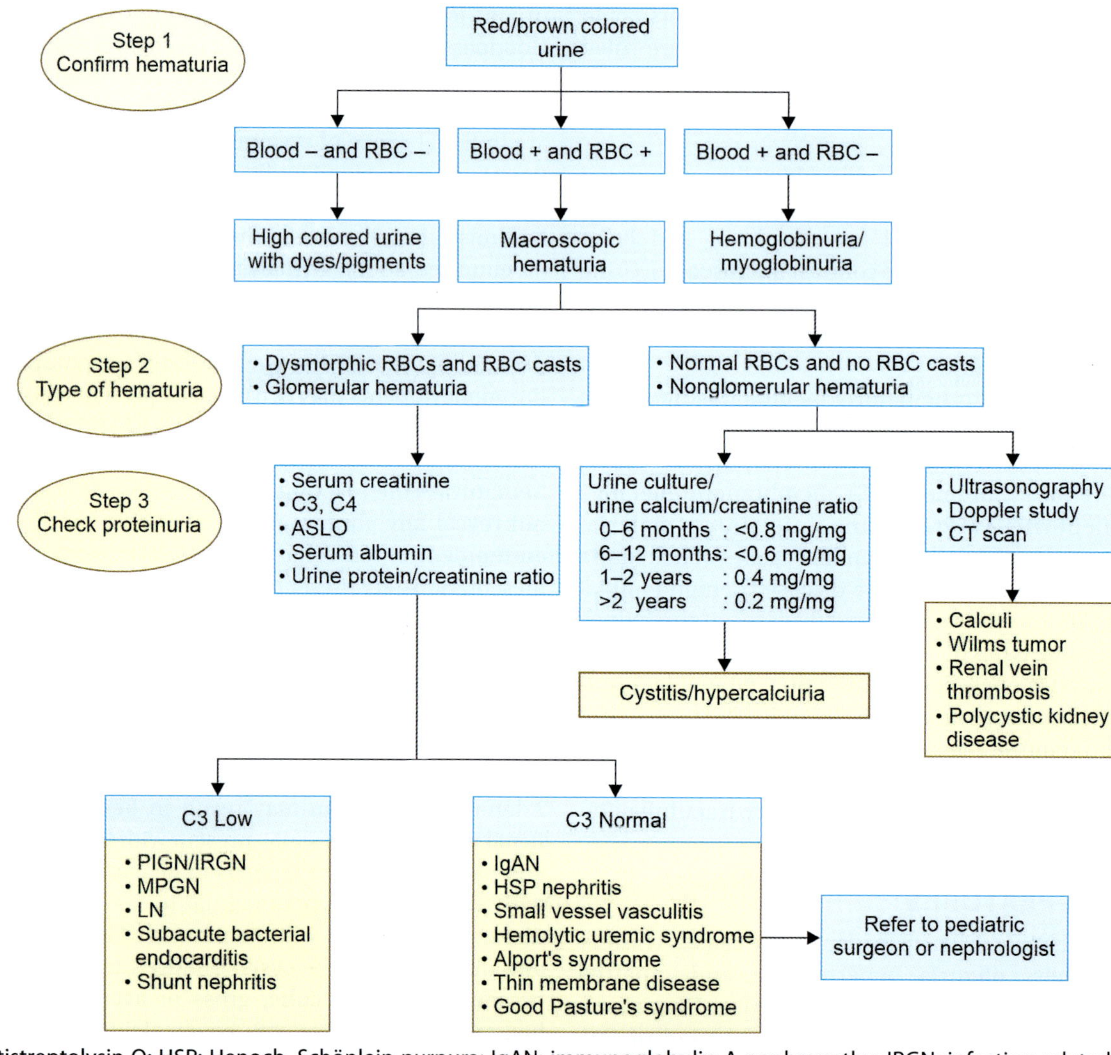

(ASLO: antistreptolysin O; HSP: Henoch–Schönlein purpura; IgAN: immunoglobulin A nephropathy; IRGN: infection-related glomerulonephritis; LN: lupus nephritis; MPGN: membranoproliferative glomerulonephritis; PIGN: postinfectious glomerulonephritis)
Source: Vedula R, Iyengar AA. Approach to diagnosis and management of hematuria. Indian J of Pediatr. 2020;87(8):618-24.

in glomerular hematuria. Mechanical damage of RBCs as they pass through the glomerular basement membrane and osmotic damage while traversing across the nephron results in changes in the RBC morphology. Typical dysmorphic RBCs and acanthocytes or G1 cells (vesicle-like protrusions) are the typical findings on phase contrast microscopy. Acanthocytes >5% is a specific indicator of glomerular disease.[12] **Table 13.12.1** lists out the differences between urinary findings of glomerular and nonglomerular hematuria.

The presence of an RBC cast is pathognomonic for glomerular hematuria. RBC cast appears cylindrical as they are usually formed within the tubule. They are comprised of RBCs that are bound to each other in a protein matrix. They are typically seen on the edge of the cover slip in an uncentrifuged urine.

Urinalysis and complete blood count (CBC) is the first step in evaluation, followed by electrolytes, creatinine, complement levels (C3, C4), and antistreptolysin O (ASO). Low C3 and evidence of streptococcal infection confirms the diagnosis of poststreptococcal GN. C3 levels are low in lupus nephritis, MPGN, and cryoglobulinemia and in some patients with hemolytic uremic syndrome. If there is no evidence of streptococcal infection, other infections, or alternative glomerular diseases need to be considered. If hematuria is persistent and accompanied by heavy proteinuria and reduced renal function, renal biopsy with immunofluorescence, and electron microscopy differentiates glomerular disease from inherited nephropathy. Indications for renal biopsy are shown in **Box 13.12.1**. Genetic studies may also be considered as it may help in characterizing the

Flowchart 13.12.2: Microscopic hematuria.

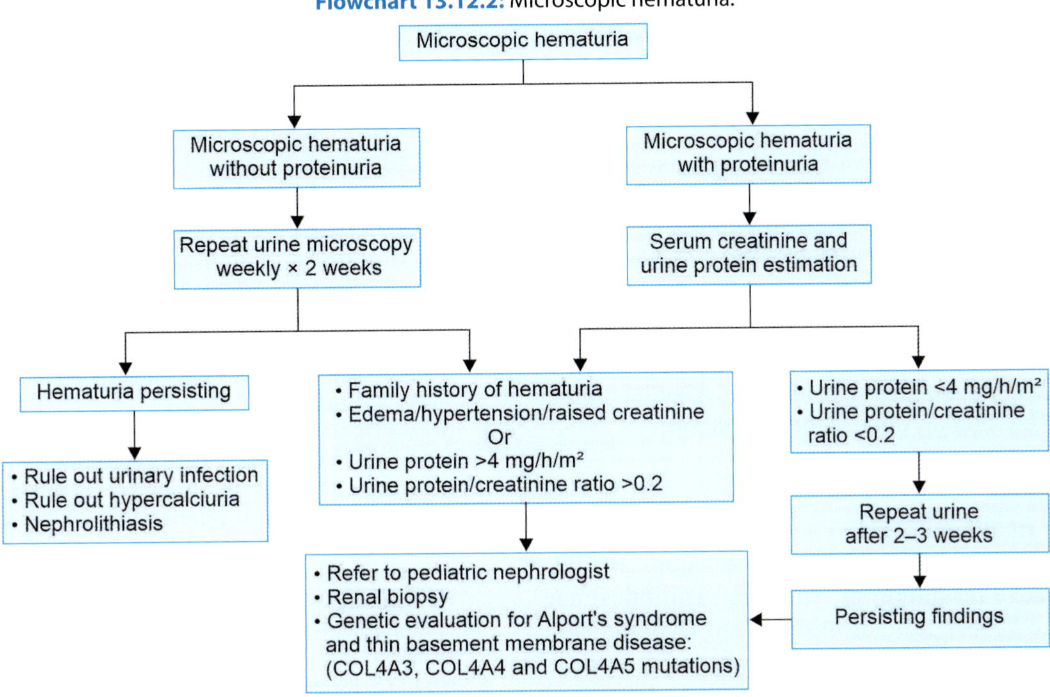

Source: Vedula R, Iyengar AA. Approach to diagnosis and management of hematuria. Indian J of Pediatr. 2020;87(8):618-24.

TABLE 13.12.1: Differences between glomerular and nonglomerular hematuria.[14,15]

Urinary findings	*Glomerular hematuria*	*Nonglomerular hematuria*
Color	Brown, cola colored	Bright red
Proteinuria	+++	–
Red blood cell (RBC) morphology	Dysmorphic	Normal
Centrifugation	Pink supernatant	Dark brown supernatant
Cast	RBC casts +	Nil
Crystals	Nil	±

BOX 13.12.1: Indications of renal biopsy.

- Persistent gross hematuria >3 weeks or recurrent episodes
- Microscopic hematuria >2 years
- Nephrotic proteinuria >3 weeks, subnephrotic proteinuria >6 months
- Severe or progressive renal failure
- Presence of systemic symptoms such as skin rash, joint pains, hemoptysis, or heart disease
- Normal serum complement or failure of complement to normalize after a suspected AGN
- Family history of renal disease, renal failure, dialysis, or transplant
- Persistent hypertension >3 weeks

(AGN: acute glomerulonephritis)

disease, assess its severity, outcome, and risk of recurrence in subsequent pregnancies.

Minor trauma can precipitate hematuria in children with renal cysts and hydronephrosis. Arteriovenous malformations and hemangiomas, which cause episodic gross hematuria, may be difficult to diagnose even by cystoscopy or angiography. Further evaluation by computed tomography (CT) or magnetic resonance (MR) may be required if initial imaging and tests are inconclusive.

Eumorphic RBC suggest nonglomerular hematuria. If white cells are present, a clean-catch urine culture is indicated. If genitourinary tuberculosis is suspected, then urine is cultured for acid-fast bacilli. Urine calcium/creatinine ratio is estimated for hypercalciuria and if high may be considered to be idiopathic if all other causes are ruled out. Idiopathic hypercalciuria may be familial and increase predisposition to nephrolithiasis and osteoporosis.[13] If calculi are not visualized by ultrasound abdomen, a spiral CT scan should be done. Stone analysis is useful, but a metabolic workup is necessary to determine the underlying cause. Genetic testing may also be helpful; with its increased availability and affordable cost, may be considered as an early option in evaluation.

The discovery of asymptomatic hematuria with proteinuria though a rare finding in school going children could suggest a significant underlying renal disease. The first step in this category is to quantitate the urine protein at the initial or follow-up visit. If the child has significant proteinuria (i.e., >4 mg/m^2 per hour or urine protein/Cr >0.2), they should be referred to the nephrologist for further evaluation. In some instances, proteinuria may be transient and hence warrants reevaluation in 2–3 weeks' time.

Referral to a pediatric surgeon/urologist may be considered if an underlying structural abnormality such as hydronephrosis, renal mass, or obstruction is suspected. Cystoscopic evaluation rarely reveals a cause for hematuria but should be considered. If bladder pathology is suspected, it is best done when there is active bleeding. In young girls with recurrent gross hematuria, child abuse, or insertion of vaginal foreign body should not be forgotten. Genital examination should be carefully done in these situations.

TREATMENT

Symptomatic treatment is given and may depend on the underlying cause. Glomerular diseases may require steroids which may cause resolution of symptoms. Diuretics may be required to relieve tubular obstruction. Hypertension management with calcium channel blockers and β-blockers is indicated. Hyperhydration and modification of diet may be required in those with hypercalciuria and nephrolithiasis. Those with inherited disorders will require close follow for risk of progression to renal failure. Angiotensin-converting-enzyme inhibitors (ACEi) and angiotensin II receptor blockers (ARBs) may have a renoprotective effect and help to delay progression.

Early referral to a pediatric nephrologist is advisable when symptoms persist, are severe, have systemic involvement, associated hypertension and proteinuria, progressive renal impairment, or are of familial nature.

CONCLUSION

Hematuria is a sign of underlying renal disease; the cause of this may vary from benign to very serious disease. Asymptomatic microscopic hematuria is more prevalent than gross hematuria; most often, it is transient, and on repeated evaluation, the prevalence may decrease. Differentiation of glomerular from nonglomerular causes is important and familial causes need to be identified early. A good clinical history and a detailed evaluation are imperative. Referral to a pediatric nephrologist or urologist may be required if symptoms are persistent or severe, as a kidney biopsy and further treatment may be required. If a structural cause is suspected, surgical intervention may be required. Treatment and final outcome will depend on the underlying cause.

REFERENCES

1. Fitzwater DS, Wyatt RJ. Hematuria. Pediatr Rev.1994;15(3):101-8.
2. Fogazzi GB, Edefonti A, Garigali G, Giani M, Zolin A, Raimondi S, et al. Urine erythrocyte morphology in patients with microscopic hematuria caused by glomerulopathy. Pediatr Nephrol. 2008;23(7):1093-100.
3. Becker GJ, Garigali G, Fogazzi GB. Advances in urine microscopy. Am J Kidney Dis. 2016;67(6):954-64.
4. Ingelfinger JR, Davis AE, Grupe WE. Frequency and etiology of gross hematuria in general pediatric setting. Pediatrics. 1977;59(4):557-61.
5. Vehaskari VM, Rapola J, Koskimies O, Savilahti E, Vilska J, Hallman N. Microscopic hematuria in school children: epidemiology and clinicopathologic evaluation. J Pediatr. 1979;95:676-84.
6. Hisano S, Kwano M, Hatae K, Kaku Y, Yamane I, Ueda K, et al. Asymptomatic isolated microhematuria. Natural history of 136 children. Pediatr Nephrol. 1991;5(5):578-81.
7. Chung H-M, Liao Y-M, Tsai Y-C, Liu M-C. Microscopic hematuria in children. Urol Sci. 2011;22:93-6.
8. Vedula R, Iyengar AA. Approach to diagnosis and management of hematuria. Indian J of Pediatr. 2020;87(8):618-24.
9. Phadke KD, Goodyer P, Bitzan M. Glomerular diseases. In: Phadke KD, Goodyer P, Bitzan M (Eds). Manual of Pediatric Nephrology, 1st edition. New York: Springer; 2014.
10. Diven SC, Travis LB. A practical primary care approach to hematuria in children. Pediatr Nephrol. 2000;14(1):65-72.
11. Moore GP, Robinson M. Do urine dipsticks reliably predict microhematuria? The bloody truth! Ann Emerg Med. 1988; 17(3):257-60.
12. Kohler H, Wandel E, Brunck B. Acanthocyturia - a characteristic marker for glomerular bleeding. Kidney Int. 1991;40(1):115-20.
13. Brown DD, Reidy KJ. Approach to child with hematuria. Pediatr Clin N Am. 2019;66(1):15-30.
14. Phadke KD, Vijayakumar M, Sharma J, Iyengar A; Indian Pediatric Nephrology Group. Consensus statement on evaluation of hematuria. Indian Pediatr. 2006;43(11):965-73.
15. Meyers KE. Evaluation of hematuria in children. Urol Clin North Am. 2004;31(3):559-73.

13.13 Nephrolithiasis

Sriram Krishnamurthy

INTRODUCTION

The term nephrolithiasis (or urolithiasis) refers to kidney stone formation in the pelvicalyceal system. This term should be distinguished from a related entity known as *nephrocalcinosis,* in which deposits of calcium salts form in the renal parenchyma, principally the tubulointerstitial compartment. The causes of both the entities overlap to a significant extent.

Since pediatric nephrolithiasis often has genetic or metabolic causes, a thorough metabolic and genetic workup of these cases is necessary as it helps in the commencement of specific therapeutic strategies, retards progression to end-stage kidney disease (ESKD), and facilitates prenatal counseling.

EPIDEMIOLOGY

Childhood nephrolithiasis is reported to have a 5-fold rise in the incidence of hospitalization in the last decade.[1] The most commonly discussed environmental causes for the increase in the reported incidence of pediatric nephrolithiasis are obesity, increased intake of fructose-containing energy drinks, increased sodium content in junk foods, decrease in oral calcium intake and water; and increasing usage of antibiotics. Monogenic and metabolic causes of nephrolithiasis are being recognized increasingly. Overall, the proportion of various types of stones in children is as follows:

- Calcium oxalate (45–65% of all pediatric stones)
- Calcium phosphate (14–30%)
- Uric acid, struvite, and cystine (5–10%).

ETIOLOGY

The causes of stones are as given in the following text.

Monogenic and Metabolic Causes

These causes account for >40% of pediatric kidney stones.[1] The causes of urolithiasis and nephrocalcinosis overlap to a significant extent. While the principal causes of nephrocalcinosis include distal renal tubular acidosis (dRTA), primary hyperoxaluria (PH), Bartter syndrome, Dent disease, and hypercalcemic states; the causes of urolithiasis include hyperoxaluria (including primary hyperoxaluria, dietary hyperoxaluria, and enteric hyperoxaluria), hypercalciuria (including monogenic and idiopathic types), hyperuricosuria (including Lesch–Nyhan syndrome, tumor lysis syndrome, urate transporter defects, etc.), adenine phosphoribosyl transferase (APRT) deficiency (leading to 2, 8 dihydroxyadenine stones), cystinuria, xanthinuria, etc.[2-4]

Entities causing both nephrocalcinosis and urolithiasis include PH, Dent disease, familial hypomagnesemia with hypercalciuria and nephrocalcinosis (FHHNC), and hypercalcemic states.

Neonates and Premature/Very Low Birth Weight Infants

Neonates and especially premature/very low birth weight (VLBW) infants are vulnerable to nephrolithiasis, owing to renal tubule immaturity. The resultant hypercalciuria and hyperoxaluria act as promoting factors for stone formation. Similarly, hypocitraturia is known in sick preterm and low birth weight infants; this results from more citrate reabsorption by the proximal tubules to compensate for the often observed metabolic acidosis in sick neonates. Urinary citrate acts as an inhibiting factor for kidney stone formation, thereby resulting in predisposition to nephrolithiasis.[1] Additionally, usage of furosemide, dexamethasone, methylxanthines, and total parenteral nutrition also contribute to nephrolithiasis.

Environmental Causes

These include low intake of water, environmental heat/ episodes of dehydration, immobilization (leading to hypercalcemia), and increased intake of sodium and fructose energy drinks (promoting hypercalciuria). High salt intake in the diet causes hypercalciuria. Decrease in the intake of calcium leads to enteric hyperoxaluria, since calcium binds to dietary oxalate preventing its intestinal absorption. Increasing use of antibiotics prevents *Oxalobacter formigenes* colonization, thereby promoting greater intestinal oxalate absorption, since this bacteria degrades intestinal oxalate. Low fruit/citrus fruit intake (causing hypocitraturia) and low phosphate intake (leading to hypercalciuria) are other predisposing factors. Single cereal intake or consumption of acidogenic rice leads to high serum acid load, leading to endemic vesical calculi formation, comprising of ammonium urate.

Drugs

Drugs such as topiramate, zonisamide, ceftriaxone, furosemide, vitamin D, steroids, indinavir, sulfonamides, allopurinol, triamterene, acetazolamide, guaiphenesin, and pseudoephedrine (present in cough syrups), efavirenz, amoxicillin, and ampicillin are known to be associated with hypercalciuria; while the usage of mannitol, losartan, radiocontrast agents, high dose salicylates, and probenecid leads to hyperuricosuria.[1]

Urinary Tract Infections and Struvite Stones

Congenital anomalies of the kidney and urinary tract (CAKUT) are associated with interruption of the normal urinary flow from the kidney to the bladder and constitute important risk factors for kidney stone formation and urinary tract infection. These urinary tract infections may be associated with urease-splitting organisms such as, e.g., *Proteus* or *Pseudomonas,* leading to the formation of struvite stones or staghorn calculi comprising of calcium-magnesium-ammonium phosphate (triple phosphate) in an alkaline urinary milieu. These stones have decreased in prevalence due to widespread antenatal screening for CAKUT, as well as increased antibiotic usage for urinary tract infections.

BOX 13.13.1: Monogenic causes of renal stones accompanied by hypercalciuria.

- Distal renal tubular acidosis (dRTA)
- Dent disease types 1 and 2
- Hypophosphatemic rickets with hypercalciuria
- Familial hypomagnesemia with hypercalciuria and nephrocalcinosis (FHHNC)
- Primary hyperoxalurias 1, 2, 3
- Infantile idiopathic hypercalcemia types 1 and 2
- Hypophosphatemic nephrolithiasis/osteoporosis 1
- Wilson disease
- Lowe syndrome
- Tyrosinemia type 1
- Glycogen storage disease (GSD) type 1a
- Bartter syndrome
- Familial isolated hypoparathyroidism
- Liddle syndrome
- Pseudohypoaldosteronism type 2
- Autosomal dominant hypocalcemia (calcium sensing receptor mutations)
- Syndrome of apparent mineralocorticoid excess

BOX 13.13.2: Monogenic causes of renal stones due to purine/pyrimidine metabolism abnormalities.

With hyperuricosuria
- Lesch–Nyhan syndrome (complete HPRT deficiency)
- X-linked hyperuricemia (Kelley–Seegmiller syndrome) (partial HPRT deficiency)
- Renal hypouricemia types 1 and 2
- PRPP synthase overactivity

Without hyperuricosuria
- Hereditary xanthinuria
- APRT deficiency
- Orotic aciduria

(APRT: adenine phosphoribosyl transferase; HPRT: hypoxanthine phosphoribosyl transferase; PRPP: phosphoribosyl pyrophosphate)

MONOGENIC CAUSES OF KIDNEY STONE DISEASE

Box 13.13.1 summarizes the monogenic causes of renal stones accompanied by hypercalciuria, while **Box 13.13.2** summarizes monogenic causes of renal stones due to purine/pyrimidine metabolism abnormalities. A few monogenic disorders are described in the following text.

Primary Hyperoxaluria

Primary hyperoxaluria are rare autosomal recessive diseases of glyoxylate metabolism, causing increased urinary oxalate excretion leading to nephrolithiasis, nephrocalcinosis, and chronic kidney disease (CKD).[2] Three subtypes of PH are known: PH1, PH2, and PH3.

- PH1 comprises 80% of cases, and often has poor clinical outcomes. PH1 is a rare, autosomal recessive disorder of glyoxylate metabolism caused by deficiency of the peroxisomal liver-specific enzyme alanine-glyoxylate aminotransferase, which is under the control of the *AGXT* gene. Systemic oxalosis affecting many vital organs such as the skeleton, eyes, and heart may develop gradually once kidney dysfunction sets in. The age at onset is variable: 15% of children are symptomatic during infancy and 50% before 5 years of age.[2] The infantile form is severe and associated with failure to thrive, nephrocalcinosis, kidney, bladder or urethral stones, and might present with dysuria, hematuria, urinary tract infection, and colic. End-stage renal failure finally occurs. The childhood and adolescent forms of PH1 are characterized by recurrent nephrolithiasis and progressive kidney dysfunction. An early diagnosis is essential to prevent or slow down the ESKD. PH1 is confirmed by recognition of pathogenic/likely pathogenic biallelic variants in *AGXT* gene.
- PH2, the second most common subtype of PH, results from *GRHPR* gene mutations, causing glyoxylate reductase/hydroxy-pyruvate reductase enzyme deficiency and a subsequent rise in the urine L-glycerate and oxalate excretion. PH3 is caused by hydroxy-oxo-glutarate aldolase 1 (HOGA 1) gene mutations. PH2 and PH3 are generally milder as compared to PH1.
- The diagnosis of PH is suspected with an elevated urinary oxalate excretion (45 mg/1.73 m^2/day), after excluding enteric hyperoxaluria (due to inflammatory bowel disease,

cystic fibrosis, pancreatitis, short bowel syndrome, etc.) and confirmed by genetic testing.[2]

Hereditary Xanthinurias

Xanthine stones due to hereditary xanthinurias (HX) are rare in infants and children, and could be due to HX type I and HX type II.[3] The affected infants and children in HX type I and type II may present with renal colic, inconsolable cry, urinary tract infections, hematuria; and exhibit low serum uric acid (hypouricemia) and hypouricosuria (low urinary uric acid excretion) due to failure of conversion of xanthine to uric acid.

HX type I occurs due *XDH* gene mutations that encode the enzyme xanthine dehydrogenase (responsible for conversion of xanthine to uric acid). HX type II occurs due to molybdenum cofactor sulfurase (*MOCOS*) gene mutations that lead secondarily to xanthine dehydrogenase and aldehyde oxidase deficiency.[4]

Molybdenum-cofactor-deficiency (sometimes known as HX type III) can also cause xanthine renal stones, and is much rarer compared with the other two types. It is an autosomal recessive defect of the molybdenum containing cofactor (under control of *MOCS1*, *MOCS2*, *MOCS3*, and *GEPH* genes) that is necessary for the function of xanthine dehydrogenase, aldehyde oxidase, and sulfite oxidase. Spasticity and microcephaly are known in molybdenum-cofactor deficiency.

Cystinuria

Cystinuria is an autosomal recessive disorder due to mutation in *SLC3A1* and *SLC7A9* genes, leading to poor proximal tubular reabsorption of dibasic amino acids such as cystine, lysine, ornithine, and arginine.[5] Cystine is insoluble in urine, and forms kidney stones. As per the current classification, cystinuria is classified as: Type A (*SLC3A1* mutations), Type B (*SLC7A9* mutations), and a possible third type AB (compound heterozygous mutations in these 2 genes). Both cystinuria types A and B have comparable outcomes. Hexagonal crystals of cystine may be seen in the urine of children with cystinuria.

Lesch–Nyhan Syndrome

Lesch–Nyhan syndrome [complete hypoxanthine-guanine phosphoribosyltransferase (HPRT) deficiency, an X-linked disorder of purine metabolism] leads to uric acid urolithiasis of early onset, intellectual disability, and self-mutilating behavior. Laboratory investigations show hyperuricemia and hyperuricosuria. Enzyme analysis in erythrocyte lysates or skin fibroblasts, and genetic analysis using next-generation sequencing can confirm the diagnosis.

Renal Hypouricemia

Idiopathic renal hypouricemia is an autosomal-recessive disease wherein there is decreased reabsorption of renal tubular uric acid leading to hyperuricosuria.[6] Many affected patients are asymptomatic, but a higher risk of kidney stones, obstructive uropathy, hematuria, and acute kidney injury have been reported. Two types of idiopathic renal hypouricemia have been reported: Type 1 due to mutations in the *SLC22A12* gene, encoding the urate transporter 1 protein, and type 2 caused by *SLC2A9* gene mutations. The diagnosis of renal hypouricemia is considered in the presence of hypouricemia (<2.0 mg/dL) and increased fractional excretion of uric acid (>10%), followed by molecular genetic analysis targeting the causative genes.

Familial Hypomagnesemia with Hypercalciuria and Nephrocalcinosis

The FHHNC is caused by mutations in the CLDN16 (FHHNC type 1) and *CLDN19* genes (FHHNC type 2). The gene products are claudin-16 and claudin-19, found in thick ascending limb of the loop of Henle where they are responsible for the paracellular reabsorption of calcium and magnesium. The clinical phenotype is characterized by cramps, tetany, nephrolithiasis, and nephrocalcinosis. Ophthalmological findings in FHHNC type 2 include high myopia, pigmentary retinitis, coloboma involving the macula, tapetoretinal degeneration, strabismus, nystagmus, and astigmatism.[6]

PATHOGENESIS: MECHANISMS OF KIDNEY STONE FORMATION

There are three pathways of stone formation:[1,6]

1. The first pathway is Randall's plaques which are interstitial apatite or calcium phosphate plaques on renal papillae that have their origins in the thin loops of Henle's basement membranes where they originate and then spread to the suburothelial space from the interstitium.
2. The second pathway is through Randall's plugs which are formed when salts precipitate in and ultimately obstruct the collecting ducts, and protrude into the pelvis of the kidney creating sites for kidney stone growth. They are associated with kidney tubular injury and focal inflammation.
3. The final pathway of stone formation is precipitation and crystallization of poorly-soluble stone-forming salts, e.g., cystine, dihydroxyadenine, or xanthine.

It is notable that cystine and uric acid get supersaturated in acidic pH (pH <7.5 and pH <6, respectively); while calcium phosphate gets precipitated in alkaline urine (pH >6). Urine citrate, pyrophosphate, and magnesium are important low molecular weight crystal inhibitors.

Clinical Risk Factors for Kidney Stone Formation

The known urinary risk factors for calcium kidney stone formation (after exclusion of systemic disorders) include familial (idiopathic) hypercalciuria, hypocitraturia, hyperoxaluria, low urinary volume, and hyperuricosuria.[1,6]

Hypercalciuria

Idiopathic hypercalciuria is the most common underlying risk factor for nephrolithiasis, found in 75–80% of pediatric renal stone patients.[1,6] It has an autosomal dominant inheritance. Idiopathic hypercalciuria can be divided into the following varieties:

- *Absorptive*—due to (1) *Type 1 absorptive hypercalciuria:* Direct absorption of excessive calcium from the gut (2) *Type 2 absorptive hypercalciuria:* 1, 25-dihydroxyvitamin D3-mediated excessive reabsorption of calcium from the gut (3) *Type 3 absorptive hypercalciuria:* Due to increased urinary phosphorus loss resulting in calcitriol upregulation and increased absorption of calcium from the gut.
- *Renal hypercalciuria*—due to increased calcium loss into the urine.
- *Resorptive hypercalciuria*—due to increase calcium reabsorption from the bones.

Hypercalciuria can be secondary to loop diuretics, immobilization, hypercalcemia, vitamin D excess, sarcoidosis, milk alkali syndrome, phosphate depletion, increased sodium or calcium in diet, ketogenic diet, hyperthyroidism, hypothyroidism, primary hyperparathyroidism, or monogenic disorders.

Hyperoxaluria

Hyperoxaluria is reported in 4–40 % of childhood nephrolithiasis.[1,6] It can occur due to:

- *Dietary hyperoxaluria* (excessive intake of oxalate rich foods such as tomatoes, spinach, broccoli, chocolate, cocoa, coffee, tea, etc., in presence of low water intake or hypocitraturia).
- *Enteric hyperoxaluria* (due to inflammatory bowel disease, short bowel syndrome, pancreatitis, celiac disease, cystic fibrosis, biliary tract disease, gastric bypass surgery, bariatric surgery, etc., since malabsorbed fatty acids bind to intestinal calcium leading to greater absorption of oxalate from the gut).
- Renal tubular immaturity in children <2 years of age.
- *Accidental ingestion of ethylene-glycol* leading to transient oxaluria.
- *Primary hyperoxaluria* types 1, 2, and 3.

Hypocitraturia

Hypocitraturia has been found in 13–70 % of pediatric nephrolithiasis.[1,6] Urine citrate lowers the urinary calcium supersaturation by binding or complexing with urine free calcium. Hence, hypocitraturia promotes hypercalciuria.

Hyperuricosuria

It is seen in 4–27% of pediatric stone formers.[1,6] Risk factors include family history of hyperuricosuria, high dose pancreatic enzyme therapy, diabetes, tumor lysis syndrome, and monogenic disorders like HPRT deficiency.

CLINICAL FEATURES

Abdominal pain or loin pain, colicky in nature, is the most common presenting feature of nephrolithiasis in older children, described in about 50–80% of cases; whereas nonspecific pain in abdomen and irritability are usually noticed in infants and younger children. Children may be referred for evaluation of hydronephrosis with pain in the loin.

Gross hematuria is the prominent presenting feature in 30–50% of patients, with microscopic hematuria being seen in most patients. Other important clinical features are urinary tract infection or frequency, dysuria, and voiding dysfunction, or even severe acute kidney injury due to obstruction by the stones (urinary retention) if stone formation occurs in the distal ureter, urethra, or urinary bladder. CKD or ESKD may be a presenting feature of monogenic or inherited metabolic disorders. At the other end of the spectrum, some children might be referred for asymptomatic incidental detection of stones during an ultrasound done for some other reason. Thus, renal stones may have protean clinical manifestations.[1,6]

DIAGNOSTIC EVALUATION

History Taking and Examination

A thorough history taking and a meticulous physical examination, a robust laboratory evaluation, and imaging using ultrasound are indispensable for diagnostic evaluation of children with nephrolithiasis **(Box 13.13.3)**.

Laboratory Evaluation

Urinalysis (hematuria, proteinuria, or pyuria), urine microscopic examination for crystals, renal ultrasonography, and stone analysis by Fourier transform infrared spectroscopy (FTIR), and serum and urinary metabolite estimation are required to ascertain the etiology. Stone analysis by FTIR helps makes a definite diagnosis of cystinuria, xanthinuria, or APRT deficiency (2, 8, dihydroxyadenine stones).[3-6]

The normal values of urinary solute excretion are described in **Table 13.13.1**. The laboratory evaluation of children with renal stones (including serum and urinary biochemical parameters) is presented in **Box 13.13.4**. Analysis of urinary biochemical parameters such as oxalate, calcium, citrate, uric acid, etc., should preferably be done in 24-hour samples. However, these may be replaced with

BOX 13.13.3: Clinical evaluation in nephrolithiasis.

Medical history
- History of consanguinity
- Positive family history for renal tubular dysfunction or kidney stone disease or CKD
- Review of nutritional intake (high salt, fructose containing high energy drinks)
- Medical conditions associated with stone disease or nephrocalcinosis (e.g., prematurity, subcutaneous fat necrosis)
- Drug history (glucocorticoids, furosemide, topiramate, zonisamide, etc.)
- Ketogenic diet
- History of cystic fibrosis, short bowel syndrome, cystic fibrosis for hyperoxaluria

Physical examination
- Weight, height, blood pressure
- For features suggestive of an underlying genetic disorder such as Williams–Beuren syndrome
- Rickets, dehydration, failure to thrive, short stature, hypokalemic features
- Abnormal neurological examination (spasticity, microcephaly, intellectual disability, self- and mutilating behavior): Lesch–Nyhan syndrome, molybdenum cofactor deficiency
- Tetany (e.g., in familial hypomagnesemia with hypercalciuria or nephrocalcinosis)

TABLE 13.13.1: Normal values of 24-hour and spot urine solutes.

24-hour urine solute excretion	
Calcium	<4 mg/kg/day
Oxalate	<40 mg/1.73 m²/day
Uric acid	<815 mg/1.73 m²/day
Cystine	<75 mg/1.73 m²/day
Creatinine	10–15 mg/kg/day
Citrate	>400 mg/g creatinine
Spot urine values	
Calcium: Creatinine ratio	<0.2 (<0.6–0.8 for infants)
Oxalate: Creatinine ratio >4 years	<0.1
Oxalate: Creatinine ratio <6 months	<0.3
Oxalate: Creatinine ratio 6 months–4 years	<0.15
Citrate: Creatinine ratio	>0.51

random urine samples (such as spot calcium: creatinine ratios, etc.) in children not yet toilet trained. Several collections are required to confirm a normal or abnormal value since there is variation in urinary solute excretion in individuals.[1,6]

Finally, it is important to consider inherited metabolic disorders and monogenic disorders in the differential diagnosis of nephrolithiasis and/or CKD in children. Sodium nitroprusside test can be performed to screen for cystinuria as an initial test. Dent disease can be considered in boys with

BOX 13.13.4: Laboratory evaluation in nephrolithiasis.

Serum investigations: Serum creatinine, sodium, potassium, bicarbonate, chloride, uric acid, calcium, phosphorus, and magnesium

Urine investigations:
- 24-hour urine calcium, oxalate, creatinine, uric acid, bicarbonate, phosphorus, citrate, and protein as indicated
- Urine calcium: Creatinine ratio; urine oxalate: Creatinine ratio
- Fractional excretion of magnesium (FEMg) if hypomagnesemia (<1.5 mg/dL)
- Urine pH, urinalysis for hematuria, pyuria, and crystals
- Urine sodium nitroprusside test (for cystinuria screening)
- Urine culture if indicated

Imaging:
- Renal ultrasound
- Plain X-ray abdomen

Stone analysis by Fourier transform infrared spectroscopy
Next-generation sequencing if monogenic disorder suspected on metabolic evaluation

Note:
1. Defer metabolic evaluation till renal colic and urinary tract infection are cured
2. 24-hour urine oxalate is not reliable when eGFR is low. Plasma oxalate may be indicated if hyperoxaluria is suspected in this situation
3. Oxalate crystals are dumb-bell shaped or enveloped-shaped crystals, uric acid crystals are rhomboid or needle shaped, cystine crystals are hexagonal, while 2–8 dihydroxyadenine crystals are round and brown on light microscopy and Maltese-cross shaped on polarized light

hypophosphatemic rickets, hypercalciuria, nephrocalcinosis, urolithiasis, and low-molecular-weight (LMW) proteinuria. FHHNC should be considered if there is hypomagnesemia and hypercalciuria with kidney stones or nephrocalcinosis. Serum 25-hydroxyvitamin D and serum parathormone may be required for evaluation of hypocalcemia or hypercalcemia with kidney stones. Next-generation sequencing helps establish a definitive diagnosis in monogenic causes of stones.

Imaging

In adults, computed tomography (CT) imaging of the kidneys is considered important for the evaluation of nephrolithiasis. However, the radiation delivered by the CT scans is a major concern for growing children. Renal ultrasounds are the preferred first-line imaging for nephrolithiasis in children; even plain X-rays or intravenous urography (IVU) are not routinely required.[6]

MANAGEMENT OF KIDNEY STONE DISEASE

Acute Management

For acute management of renal stones presenting as renal colic, intravenous ketorolac (0.75–1.5 mg/kg) or intravenous morphine (0.1 mg/kg) can be used for pain relief, with ketorolac being proven to be superior in the form of lesser incidence of postoperative vomiting. Ondansetron (in inpatient setting) or promethazine (in an outpatient setting) can be used for management of vomiting associated with renal colic.[6] Paracetamol too can be used for pain relief. Urinary tract infections should be treated with appropriate antibiotics. It is important to maintain hydration.

Surgical Management

Stones of size 5–10 mm can be treated with extracorporeal shock wave lithotripsy (ESWL) or ureteroscopic lithotripsy. ESWL is advised for upper urinary tract stones up to even 15 mm in largest diameter; nevertheless, a significant proportion of such cases may need repeated treatments. Large stones such as staghorn calculi are treated with percutaneous nephrolithotomy. Urgent decompression in the form of percutaneous nephrostomy or stent insertion is required if obstructive uropathy or acute kidney injury or single renal system is present.[6]

Medical Expulsive Therapy

Treatment with α- or calcium channel blockers to cause ureteral stone passage (for distal ureteral stones) constitutes "medical expulsive therapy." The mechanism is that α-blockers and calcium channel blockers dilate the ureter due to abundant α-receptors and calcium channel receptors in the smooth muscle of the distal one-third of the ureter and the vesicoureteric junction. Tamsulosin and doxazosin are popular agents for medical expulsive therapy. Medical expulsive therapy is acceptable when:[6]

- Stones <4–5 mm in diameter
- When infection is not suspected
- When there is no acute kidney injury
- When pain control is acceptable
- There is no single renal system

General Measures to Prevent Stone Formation

Adequate fluid intake is the universal advice for children with nephrolithiasis, and the fluid intake that is advised in children with kidney stone disease is a minimum of 1.5–2 L/m^2/day. Fructose and glucose "energy drinks" should be curtailed. Children with calcium stone disease may benefit from intake of citrate juices such lemonade and orange juices.[1,6]

Since high sodium diet can worsen urinary calcium excretion, reducing dietary sodium intake to 2–3 mEq/kg/day is advised. In children, the recommended calcium intake in nephrolithiasis should be 100% of the recommended daily allowance (RDA), and both calcium restriction and excessive intake should be discouraged. Similarly, a protein intake in diet of 100% of RDA is recommended, and excessive protein consumption is to be avoided since excessive protein intake parallels purine intake.[1,6] A diet rich in fruits and vegetables may be useful for children with hypocitraturia.

Pharmacotherapy to Prevent Stone Formation

The goal of pharmacotherapy is to decrease the urinary concentration and supersaturation of lithogenic ions and their salts. Hypocitraturia is common in nephrolithiasis and alkalinization with oral potassium citrate (2–4 mEq/kg/day) is beneficial for prevention of recurrent stones. Care should be taken to prevent a urine pH > 6.5, as calcium phosphate can precipitate in alkaline pH. In idiopathic hypercalciuria, oral hydrochlorthiazide (0.5–2 mg/kg/day) is administered which reduces urinary calcium excretion.[6] Care must be taken to monitor serum potassium, magnesium, and sodium during thiazide therapy as hypokalemia, hypomagnesemia, and hyponatremia can ensue.

Alkalinization is to be avoided in situations such as struvite calculi (wherein the urease-splitting organisms thrive in an alkaline milieu) and Bartter syndrome (which has metabolic alkalosis).[6]

Specific Measures to Prevent Stone Recurrence in Monogenic Nephrolithiasis

Primary Hyperoxaluria

In PH1, at least 3 L/m^2/day of fluid intake is recommended.[2,6] Vitamin B_6 (pyridoxine—which is a cofactor for *AGXT*) is prescribed in confirmed PH1; at a dose of 5 mg/kg/day and might require escalation of doses up to 20 mg/kg/day, with the objective of reducing the urinary oxalate concentration by 30%. Alkalinization with oral potassium citrate (0.3–0.5 mmoL/kg) is advised until the estimated glomerular filtration rate (eGFR) is normal. This may be substituted by sodium bicarbonate once the patient progresses to CKD stage 4. Some experts recommend avoiding oxalate-rich diet (e.g., spinach, tomato, chocolate, and beetroot) based on principles of precautionary measures, although this may not be of much use. In addition, a low-salt diet, avoiding too much of vitamin C and D, and not reducing dietary calcium; are useful strategies.

In PH type 2 and type 3, potassium citrate therapy and intake of fluids is beneficial, but pyridoxine therapy has no role.

Hereditary Xanthinurias

There is no specific treatment that is effective enough for xanthinuria management, and therefore the strategies for management are mostly conservative. Increase in fluid intake (1.5–2 times daily maintenance and increasing water intake in the evening to prevent dehydration) and restriction of purine in diet are advised. A diet that is low in purine (e.g., eggs, grains, cheese, fruits, vegetables, and nuts) may be advised.[3,4,6] Alkalinization of urine is usually ineffective as xanthine is insoluble even in alkaline pH. Purified cyclic pyranopterin-monophosphate therapy in patients with molybdenum cofactor-A deficiency has been found to be useful.

Cystinuria

Cystinuria is managed with urinary alkalinization using potassium citrate, restriction of salt in diet, increased intake of fluids, and avoiding high purine diet. Tiopronin and D-penicillamine are specific drugs used for cystinuria management.[5] These drugs undergo a thiol-disulfide exchange with cystine which leads to formation of a water-soluble mixed disulfide complex.

Hyperuricosuric States

Hyperuricosuric states include Lesch–Nyhan syndrome, Phosphoribosyl pyrophosphate (PRPP) synthase overactivity, tumor lysis syndrome, renal hypouricemia, and glycogen storage disease type 1, etc. In these situations, restricting purine in the diet (e.g., avoiding red meat) is advised. In addition to increasing oral fluid intake and potassium citrate therapy, allopurinol therapy is advised which decreases the conversion of xanthine to uric acid.

Allopurinol therapy is also advised in 2, 8-dihydroxyadenine stones (a rare form of nephrolithiasis due to APRT deficiency in which urine examination may show "Maltese crosses").[6]

Familial Hypomagnesemia with Hypercalciuria and Nephrocalcinosis

Treatment is with magnesium supplements and alkalinization with potassium citrate, and increase the intake of fluids.

OUTCOME AND FOLLOW-UP OF CHILDREN WITH KIDNEY STONES

The recurrence rate for kidney stones is 16–67% in different studies.[7] The risk of CKD or ESKD dependent on etiology; e.g., primary hyperoxaluria type 1 is associated with high risk of progression to ESKD. ESKD is possible in neglected struvite stones too. Alkalinization and increased fluid intake is associated with reduced risk of progression to ESKD.[7] Regular follow-up required in children with nephrolithiasis to check serum and urine laboratory parameters, growth, compliance with medications, and urine pH.

CONCLUSION

Monogenic and metabolic etiologies account for more than 40% of cases of nephrolithiasis in children. The evaluation of pediatric nephrolithiasis includes a detailed history taking, examination, basic imaging using renal ultrasound, metabolic and genetic testing. The recurrence risk for kidney stone occurrence in children is high, placing them at risk for severe morbidities including renal colic, urinary tract infections, acute kidney injury and chronic kidney disease. The management of pediatric nephrolithiasis necessitates a multidisciplinary approach involving pediatricians, pediatric nephrologists and urologists. Effective medical and surgical treatments are available for children with kidney stones.

REFERENCES

1. Copelovitch L. Urolithiasis in children: medical approach. Pediatr Clin N Am. 2012;59:881-96.
2. Cochat P, Hulton SA, Acquaviva C, Danpure CJ, Daudon M, De Marchi M, et al. Primary hyperoxaluria type 1: Indications for screening and guidance for diagnosis and treatment. Nephrol Dial Transplant. 2012;27:1729-36.
3. Arikyants N, Sarkissian A, Hesse A, Eggermann T, Leumann E, Steinmann B. Xanthinuria type I: a rare cause of urolithiasis. Pediatr Nephrol. 2007;22:310-4.
4. Ichida K, Matsumura T, Sakuma R, Hosoya T, Nishino T. Mutation of human molybdenum cofactor sulfurase gene is responsible for classical xanthinuria type II. Biochem Biophys Res Commun. 2001;282:1194-200.
5. Font-Llitjós M, Jiménez-Vidal M, Bisceglia L, Di Perna M, de Sanctis L, Rousaud F, et al. New insights into cystinuria: 40 new mutations, genotype-phenotype correlation, and digenic inheritance causing partial phenotype. J Med Genet. 2005; 42:58-68.
6. Edvardsson V. Urolithiasis in children: In: Avner ED, Harmon WE, Niaudet P, Yoshikawa N, Emma F, Goldstein SL (Eds). Pediatric Nephrology, 7th edition. Hiedelberg, Germany: Springer; 2017. pp. 1831-58.
7. Pietrow PK, Pope JC 4th, Adams MC, Shyr Y, Brock JW 3rd. Clinical outcome of pediatric stone disease. J Urol. 2002; 167(2 Pt 1):670-3.

13.14 Hypertension

Jitendra Meena

INTRODUCTION

The prevalence of hypertension is increasing in children. Approximately 3–4% of children and adolescents have hypertension while elevated blood pressure is reported in 10%. Essential hypertension is less common in younger children, but it is being increasingly recognized in adolescents. Children with persistent severe hypertension are at increased risk of adverse outcomes, such as hypertensive encephalopathy, retinopathy, congestive heart failure, and chronic kidney disease.[1,2]

DEFINITIONS AND STAGING OF HYPERTENSION

Unlike adults, hypertension in children is defined based on age, sex, and height specific percentile for blood pressure.[2] Hypertension is defined as blood pressure >95th percentile for age, height, and sex. Normative reference data for blood pressure is reported clinical practice guidelines (CPGs) for screening and management of high blood pressure in children and adolescents by American Academy of Pediatrics (AAP) 2017.[2-4] Reference data have been developed from previous normative data of fourth report, after excluding data of overweight and obese children, as adiposity is strongly associated with higher blood pressure.[3,4] The tables in latest guidelines provide blood pressure values, based on sex, age, and height percentiles, at 50th, 90th, 95th, and 95th + 12 mm Hg, and should be used to define and stage the high blood pressure **(Table 13.14.1)**. Based on new normative blood pressure data, **Figures 13.14.1 and 13.14.2** provide charts for screening and staging of hypertension in boys and girls, respectively. **Table 13.14.2** provides screening blood pressure cutoffs for identification of the children who require further evaluation, and it is based on 90th centile blood pressure for age and gender at 5th centile of the stature. White coat hypertension refers to high office blood pressure in a child who has normal blood pressures in a familiar setting. Masked hypertension defined as normal clinic blood pressures, but the child actually having hypertension. Ambulatory blood pressure monitoring (ABPM) is a useful tool to confirm diagnosis of masked and white coat hypertension.[5]

TABLE 13.14.1: Definition and staging of hypertension in children.

Elevated blood pressure	≥90th–<95th percentile or 120/80 mm Hg to <95th percentile (whichever is lower)*
Hypertension	SBP or DBP ≥ 95th percentile or >130/80 mm Hg*
Stage 1 hypertension	SBP or DBP between ≥95th percentile and <95th percentile +12 mm Hg, or 130/80–139/89 mm Hg (whichever is lower)*
Stage 2 hypertension	SBP or DBP ≥95th percentile +12 mm Hg, or ≥140/90 mm Hg (whichever is lower)*

*For adolescent aged ≥13 years.
(DBP: diastolic blood pressure; SBP: systolic blood pressure)
Source: Adapted from 2017 clinical practice guideline by American Academy of Pediatrics.

DIAGNOSIS OF HYPERTENSION

To diagnose hypertension blood pressure either systolic or diastolic >95th percentile should be documented on at least three separate occasions unless patient is symptomatic.[1,2] Blood pressure should be measured annually in all children and adolescents ≥3 years of age, and at every healthcare visit in children, if they have specific conditions associated with increased risk of hypertension. These conditions include prematurity, obesity, kidney disorders, heart disease, diabetes, systemic illnesses associated with hypertension (neurofibromatosis, tuberous sclerosis, sickle cell disease), history of solid organ transplant, and taking drugs that are known to raise blood pressure such steroids, tacrolimus, etc.[1]

MEASUREMENT OF BLOOD PRESSURE

Table 13.14.3 shows a comparison of various techniques for measurement of blood pressure. Blood pressure measurement by auscultation should be the preferred method for confirmation of abnormal blood pressure as normative data is based on auscultated measurements. Blood pressure measurement in children should be performed after adequate rest of 3–5 minutes while sitting in an upright position with the back supported, feet uncrossed on the floor, and the cubital fossa at the level of the heart. The right arm is preferred to avoid falsely low readings in patients with coarctation of the aorta and for consistency. At least three measurements are taken on a visit, for confirming reproducibility of the result and for decreasing the effect of white coat hypertension. An appropriate cuff size with an inflatable bladder width that is at least

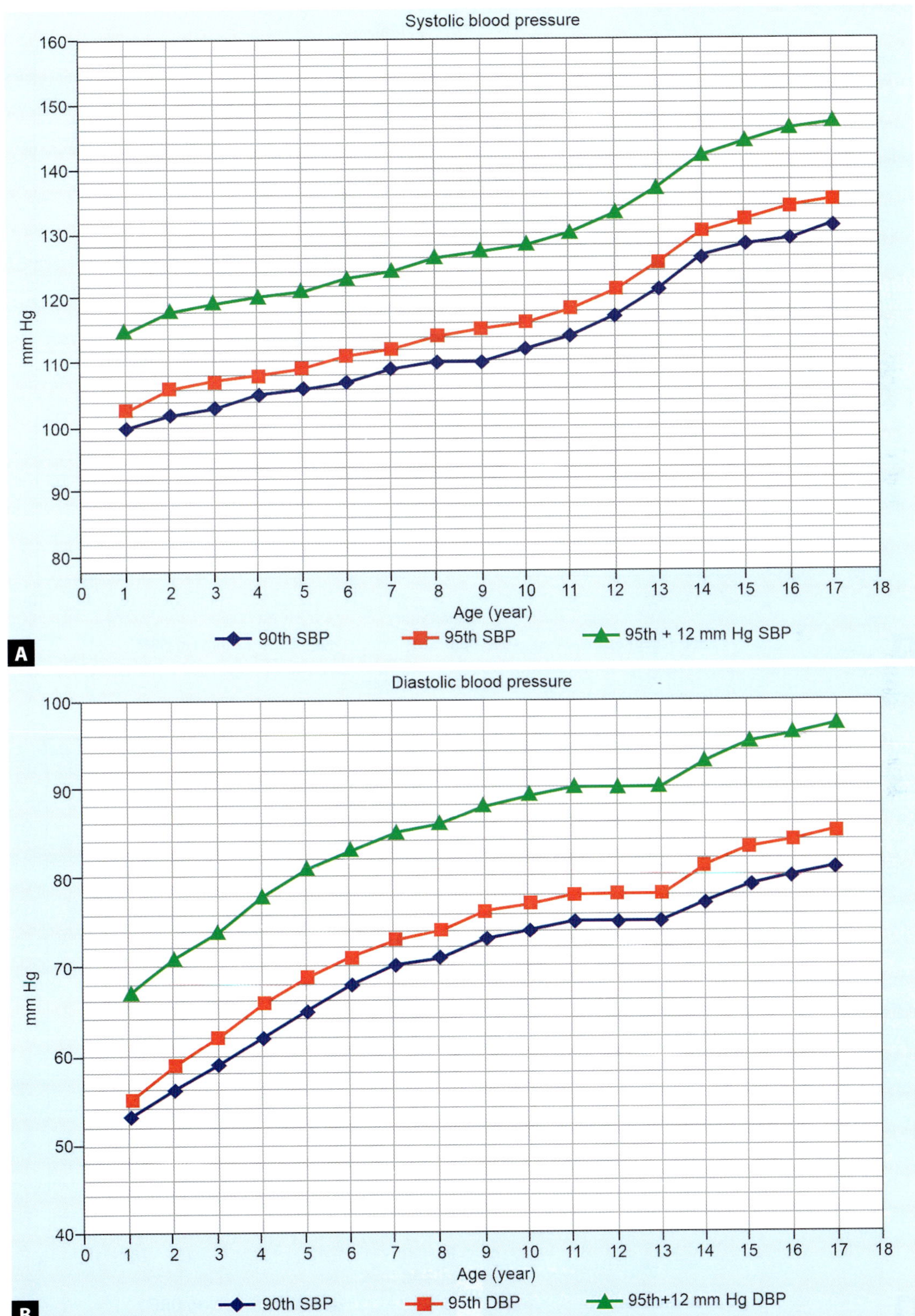

Figs. 13.14.1A and B: Blood pressure levels for boys at 50th percentile for height. Chart depicting 90th (closed diamonds), 95th (open squares) and 95th +12 mm Hg (closed triangles) percentile values for (A) Systolic and (B) Diastolic blood pressures, representing cutoff values for the diagnosis of elevated blood pressure, stage 1 and stage 2 hypertension respectively in boys (based on AAP clinical practice guideline for screening and management of high blood pressure in children and adolescents 2017).

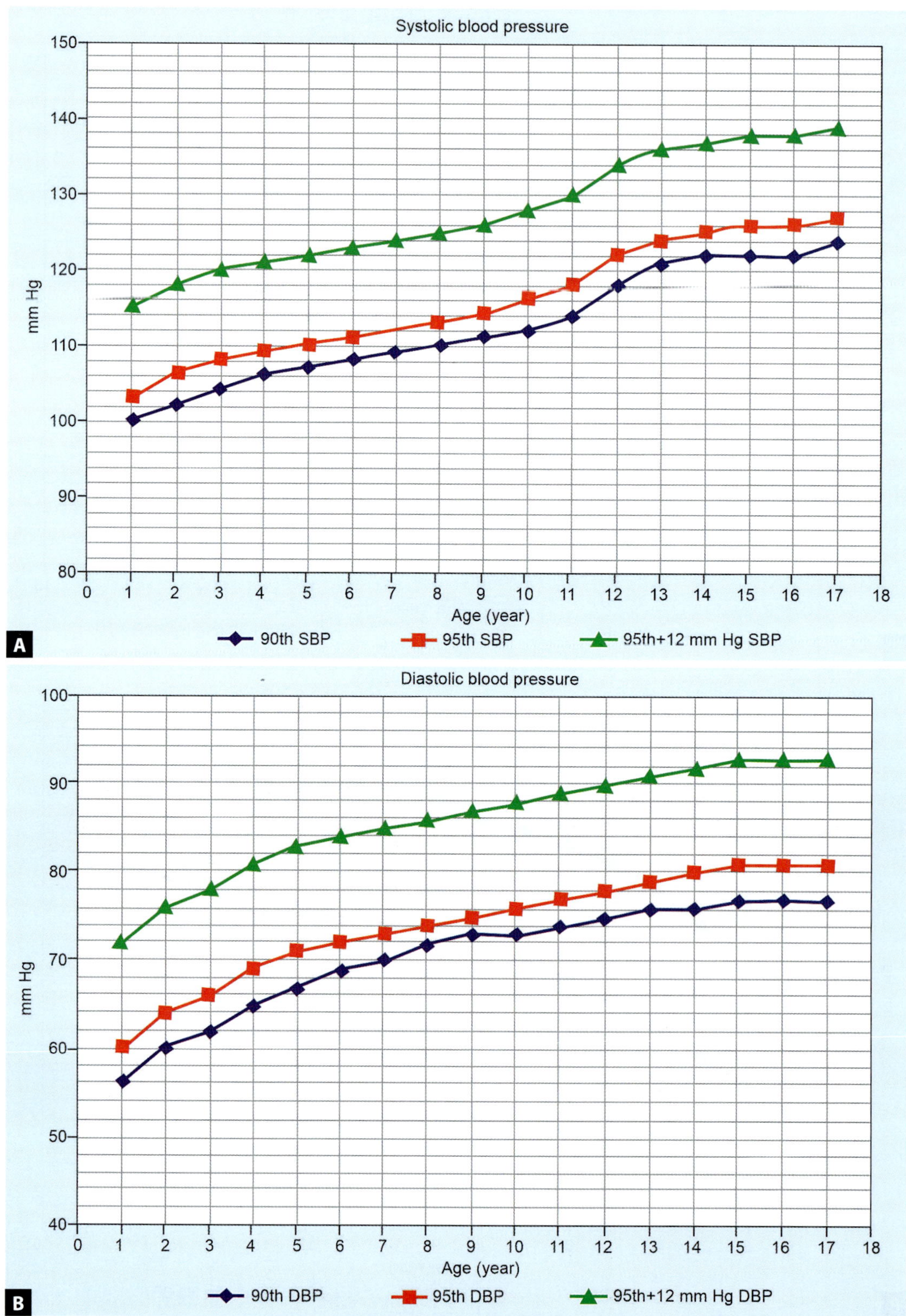

Figs. 13.14.2A and B: Blood pressure levels for girls at 50th percentile for height. Chart depicting 90th (closed diamonds), 95th (open squares) and 95th + 12 mm Hg (closed triangles) percentile values for (A) Systolic and (B) Diastolic blood pressures, representing cutoff values for the diagnosis of elevated blood pressure, stage 1 and stage 2 hypertension respectively in girls (based on AAP clinical practice guideline for screening and management of high blood pressure in children and adolescents 2017).

TABLE 13.14.2: Screening blood pressure for children.

Age (year)		1	2	3	4	5	6	7	8	9	10	11	12	≥13
Girls	SBP (mm Hg)	98	101	102	103	104	105	106	107	108	109	111	114	120
	DBP (mm Hg)	54	58	60	62	64	67	68	69	71	72	74	75	80
Boys	SBP (mm Hg)	98	100	101	102	103	105	106	107	107	108	110	113	120
	DBP (mm Hg)	52	55	58	60	63	66	68	69	70	72	74	75	80

(DBP: diastolic blood pressure; SBP: systolic blood pressure)

TABLE 13.14.3: Blood pressure monitoring techniques.

Technique	Advantages	Drawbacks
Auscultatory (Mercury sphygmomanometer)	• Most evidence based • Noninvasive • Quick to perform • Easily available	• White coat effect • Observer bias • Terminal digit preference • *Safety hazard:* Mercury spill
Aneroid manometer	• Easily portable • Mercury free	Needs frequent calibration
Oscillometric devices	• Easy to use • Useful in infants, where auscultation is difficult • No observer bias	• Limited reference data • Values of diastolic pressure derived from mean pressure; may be inaccurate • Requires repeated validation • Cost and availability
Ambulatory blood pressure monitoring (ABPM)	For white coat, masked hypertension, data on diurnal variability	• Considerable cost • Needs patient cooperation and training

40% of the arm circumference, and bladder length sufficient to cover 80–100% of the arm circumference should be used.[1]

Ambulatory blood pressure monitoring refers to the continuous recordings of blood pressure over 24 hours; it is believed to reflect true blood pressures accurately, is more reproducible and correlates with target organ damage.[5] Data is interpreted in terms of mean ambulatory blood systolic or diastolic pressure. Blood pressure load (percentage of readings above the ambulatory 95th percentile) is no longer used for classification as this does not correlate with long-term adverse outcomes. Hence a child with both mean ambulatory blood pressure and clinical blood pressure ≥95th percentile classified as ambulatory hypertension, while a child with clinical blood pressure <95th centile but ≥95th percentile mean ambulatory blood pressure is classified as masked hypertension. The reverse of masked hypertension is white coat hypertension. ABPM is indicated for diagnosis of masked hypertension, white coat hypertension, and nocturnal hypertension and to assess the effectiveness of antihypertensive therapy for control of hypertension.

ETIOLOGY

Sustained hypertension in children is often secondary to an underlying etiology **(Box 13.14.1)**; in approximately 90% of patient's secondary hypertension is due to kidney parenchymal or renovascular abnormalities.[1,3] In recent years, essential hypertension has become an important health concern. Patients with essential hypertension are usually postpubertal and overweight and typically show stage 1 hypertension.

CLINICAL FEATURES

Patients with elevated blood pressure and stage 1 hypertension are usually asymptomatic. Symptoms are more common in patients with secondary hypertension. Symptoms such as headache, dizziness, vomiting, irritability, epistaxis, flush, visual disturbances, and vertigo usually occur with significant elevation of blood pressure.[2,3]

Hypertensive Crisis

Patients with stage 2 hypertension may manifest with hypertensive crises, which are classified as emergency or urgency.[6] Hypertensive emergency is associated with acute target organ damage such as encephalopathy, intracranial hemorrhage, acute left ventricular failure with pulmonary edema, dissecting aortic aneurysm, papilledema, and acute kidney injury. Hypertensive urgency is severe hypertension without end organ damage. The occurrence of these complications is related to the rate of rise and duration of hypertension, rather than absolute blood pressure values.

BOX 13.14.1: Causes of hypertension.

Transient hypertension
- Acute renal failure; acute glomerulonephritis
- Increased intracranial pressure
- Acute intermittent porphyria
- Guillain–Barré syndrome
- Hyperthyroidism

Persistent hypertension

Renal parenchymal disease:
- Glomerulonephritis
- Hemolytic uremic syndrome
- Reflux nephropathy; obstructive uropathy
- Polycystic kidney disease, renal dysplasia
- Postkidney transplantation

Renovascular:
- Renal vein thrombosis
- Renal artery stenosis
- Fibromuscular dysplasia
- Takayasu arteritis
- Tumors compressing on renal vessels
- Syndromes (William, Turner, and neurofibromatosis type 1)

Cardiovascular: Coarctation of aorta

Primary (essential) hypertension:
- Isolated
- With metabolic syndrome

Endocrine:
- Cushing syndrome
- Congenital adrenal hyperplasia
- Primary hyperaldosteronism
- Hyperthyroidism, hypothyroidism
- Liddle syndrome
- Syndrome of apparent mineralocorticoid excess
- Glucocorticoid remediable aldosteronism

Tumors
- *Renal:*
  - Wilms' tumor
  - Reninoma
  - Hemangiopericytoma
  - Hamartoma
- *Extrarenal:*
  - Pheochromocytoma
  - Neuroblastoma
  - Paraganglioma

Medications/iatrogenic:
- Corticosteroids
- Substance abuse
- Nasal decongestants (phenylephrine, pseudoephedrine, and oxymetazoline)
- Nonsteroidal anti-inflammatory drugs
- *Others:* Erythropoietin, calcineurin inhibitors, theophylline, caffeine, antidepressants

Complications of sustained hypertension includes hypertensive retinopathy, albuminuria, left ventricular hypertrophy, diastolic dysfunction, and premature atherosclerosis as evidenced by increased carotid intima media thickness.

EVALUATION

Careful history and physical examination may provide important clues to the underlying etiology **(Table 13.14.4)**. Family history is taken for hypertension, diabetes, dyslipidemia, obesity, premature cardiovascular or cerebrovascular disease, and renal disorders. Assessment of body mass index and measurement of blood pressure in all four limbs are necessary.[2,3]

INVESTIGATIONS

Since most patients with hypertension have underlying renal or renovascular etiology, screening tests (urinalysis, blood urea and creatinine, electrolytes, lipid profile, and renal ultrasound) are designed to evaluate for these conditions **(Box 13.14.1)**.[1] Patients with hypertension should also be screened for target organ damage. Based on clinical features and initial evaluation, a cause for hypertension is suggested in most instances. Confirmation of the diagnosis of underlying etiology requires specific investigations tailored to specific needs **(Tables 13.14.4 and 13.14.5)**. However, recent AAP guideline recommends that children >6 years of age, who are obese or overweight and if they have family history of hypertension, do not require comprehensive investigation in the absence of physical finding suggestive of a cause for secondary hypertension.[4,5]

MANAGEMENT

Management of high blood pressure should begin with therapeutic lifestyle modification, especially in children who have modifiable risk factors. The indications for pharmacological therapy are listed in **Box 13.14.2**.[2,4,5]

Target Blood Pressure

American Academy of Pediatrics (2017) CPGs recommend lowering systolic and diastolic blood pressure to below 90th percentile in all children and <130/80 mm Hg in adolescent >13 years old. However, guidelines recommend that in hypertensive children with chronic kidney disease target blood pressure should be between 50th and 75th percentile of mean 24-hour ambulatory blood pressure to reduce the rate of decline in kidney function.

Elevated Blood Pressure

These patients are managed by lifestyle modifications (see later) and reevaluated 3–6 months later. Medications are not required unless the patient has comorbid conditions.

Essential Hypertension

Patients with essential hypertension are initially managed with lifestyle modifications and pharmacological therapy is

TABLE 13.14.4: Clinical features and investigations for secondary hypertension.

Condition	*Clinical features*	*Investigations*
Glomerulonephritis	Facial puffiness, edema, hematuria and oligoanuria	Urinalysis, 24-hour urine protein, C3, antinuclear antibody, antineutrophil cytoplasmic antibody, renal biopsy
Reflux nephropathy	Dysuria, frequency, history of urinary tract infections	Renal ultrasound, micturating cystourethrography, renal scintigraphy
Renovascular disease	Asymmetric pulses, abdominal/neck bruit, weak femoral artery pulses	Doppler ultrasound, captopril renography, computed tomography (CT), magnetic resonance imaging angiography or digital subtraction angiography (DSA)
Coarctation of aorta	Weak femoral artery pulses	Echocardiography, DSA
Metabolic syndrome	Adolescent age, obesity	Blood sugars, HbA1c, lipid profile, aspartate transaminase and alanine transaminase
Endocrine	Muscle weakness, cramps, episodic fever, flushing, tachycardia, polyuria, polydipsia, failure to thrive, ambiguous genitalia	Plasma renin, aldosterone, plasma and urinary cortisol, plasma and urine metanephrines, metaiodobenzyl guanidine (MIBG) scan, CT/magnetic resonance imaging (MRI) scan

TABLE 13.14.5: Diagnostic workup.

Evaluation for etiology	*Screen for target organ damage*
Hemogram	Retina fundus examination
Blood urea, creatinine, electrolytes	Urinalysis, urine spot protein to creatinine ratio
Lipid profile, uric acid, HbA1c (if patient is obese)	Chest X-ray
Urinalysis, culture 24-hour protein	Electrocardiogram (ECG)
Renal ultrasonography and Doppler	Echocardiography

initiated later. Thiazide diuretics and β-blockers, especially in combination, should be avoided due to their significant diabetogenic potential. Therapy may be initiated with calcium-channel blockers (CCB) or angiotensin-converting enzyme inhibitor (ACEI). Screening for dyslipidemia, fatty liver, and impaired glucose tolerance should be done.

Secondary Hypertension

Patients with sustained secondary hypertension require therapy with antihypertensive agents. The treatment plan should incorporate nonpharmacological measures in all patients.

NONPHARMACOLOGICAL THERAPY

Major lifestyle modification recommended for management of hypertension is weight reduction, improving physical activity, stress reduction, and dietary approach to stop hypertension (DASH).[2,4,5] Weight reduction in overweight and obese patients with hypertension results in significant reduction in blood pressure as well as also reduces other cardiovascular risk factors, i.e., hyperlipidemia and insulin resistance. Recent CPGs recommend 30–60 minutes per session of moderate-to-vigorous aerobic physical activity 3–5 days per week with limitation of sedentary activity to 2 hours per day. Children with hypertension may benefit from DASH, which includes increasing the intake of fresh fruit, fiber, low fat dairy products, and whole grains with reduction in sugar and salt consumption.

BOX 13.14.2: Indications for drug therapy.

- Stage 2 hypertension without modifiable risk factors
- Symptomatic hypertension
- Secondary hypertension
- Hypertension in patient with diabetes and chronic kidney disease
- Persistent hypertension despite nonpharmacological measures
- Hypertension with additional risk factors (i.e., obesity, hyperlipidemia)

Pharmacological Therapy

Study of antihypertensive drugs regarding safety and their impact on cardiovascular outcomes is limited in children. Pharmacological therapy should be initiated with single medication at low end of dosing range while continuing lifestyle modification. Dosing recommendations are shown in **Table 13.14.6**. Drugs with a longer duration of action are preferred for better compliance. When required, dose should be increased every 2–4 weeks until blood pressure is controlled, or adverse effects occur. Patients should have a clinic visit every 4–6 weeks until blood pressure is normalized. A second medication with a complementary mechanism of action should be added if blood pressure control is still not achieved and dose increased to maximum, if necessary. If blood pressure is not controlled, a third antihypertensive drug of a different class may be added. Therapy in children is often started with a CCB or ACEI. The choice of initial medication often depends on the cause of hypertension and associated comorbidities and complications. In hypertensive

TABLE 13.14.6: Commonly used drugs for treatment of hypertension in children.

Agents	Dose	Side effects/comments
Angiotensin-converting enzyme inhibitors (ACEIs) • Captopril • Enalapril • Lisinopril • Ramipril	 0.05–6 mg/kg/day 0.08–0.6 mg/kg/day 0.06–0.6 mg/kg/day 1.6–6 mg/m^2	• Use cautiously if glomerular filtration rate (GFR) <30 mL/min/1.73 m^2 • Avoid in renal artery stenosis • Use smaller doses in neonates • Monitor serum potassium, creatinine, contraindicated in pregnancy
Angiotensin receptor blockers (ARBs) • Losartan • Olmesartan • Valsartan • Candesartan	 0.75–1.4 mg/kg/day 10–40 mg/day 1.3–2.7 mg/kg/day 0.02–0.4 mg/kg/day	Similar to ACEI; cough, angioedema not seen
Calcium-channel blockers • Amlodipine • Nifedipine • Isradipine	 0.05–0.6 mg/kg/day 0.25–3 mg/kg/day 0.15–0.6 mg/kg/day	• Headache, flushing, tachycardia, edema, dizziness • May increase proteinuria
β-blockers • Atenolol • Labetalol • Metoprolol	 0.5–2.0 mg/kg/day 1–40 mg/kg/day 1–6 mg/kg/day	• Avoid in asthma, heart failure • Reduce dose of atenolol in renal dysfunction
Central α-agonist Clonidine	 5–25 µg/kg/day	Rebound hypertension when withdrawn
Peripheral alpha-antagonists Prazosin	 0.05–0.5 mg/kg/day	Syncope
Diuretics • Hydrochlorothiazide • Furosemide • Amiloride • Spironolactone	 1–2 mg/kg/day 0.5–6 mg/kg/day 0.4–0.6 mg/kg/day 1–3 mg/kg/day	• *Thiazide:* Hyperuricemia, hyperlipidemia, hyperglycemia, hypokalemia, ineffective at GFR <30 mL/min/1.73 m^2 • *Loop diuretics:* Alkalosis, hypokalemia • *Potassium-sparing diuretics:* Hyperkalemia especially with ACEI, ARB
Vasodilators • Hydralazine • Minoxidil	 1–8 mg/kg/day 0.1–1.0 mg/kg/day	• Headache, palpitation • Hypertrichosis, fluid retention, pericardial effusion

children with chronic kidney disease, proteinuria and diabetes ACEI are the preferred drugs unless there is an absolute contraindication.

Follow-up and Monitoring

After initiation of drug therapy, follow-up visits should be frequent (every 4–6 weeks) until blood pressure is controlled. Once blood pressure is optimized patient can be followed up once in every 3–4 months. At every follow-up visit adherence to medication, home blood pressure monitoring and assessment for side effects should be done. ABPM can be used to assess the control of blood pressure especially in a patient with chronic kidney disease and/or target end organ damage. After successful blood pressure control, "step down" of therapy may be attempted. Monitoring for target organ damage should be done at regular intervals.

MANAGEMENT OF HYPERTENSIVE CRISES

Hypertensive emergency requires immediate reduction in blood pressure in order to prevent or limit target organ damage. These patients require constant monitoring and supportive care, necessitating hospitalization.[6] Patients with hypertensive emergency are treated with a potent intravenous antihypertensive medications titrated to produce a controlled reduction in blood pressure, with the aim of reducing the mean arterial blood pressure up to ~95th percentile. Up to 25% of the planned reduction should be done over the first 8 hours of presentation and then the remainder reduction gradually over next 12–24 hours. Rapid reduction of blood pressure may compromise blood flow to important organs causing ischemic damage, especially since autoregulation may be impaired or altered. Therapy with oral antihypertensive drugs should be commenced as soon as patient can take

TABLE 13.14.7: Commonly used drugs for hypertensive emergency.

Drug	*Onset*	*Route*	*Dose*	*Side effects*
Labetalol	5–10 minutes	Intravenous (IV) infusion	0.25–3 mg/kg/h	• Orthostatic hypotension, bradycardia, pallor, abdominal pain, diarrhea • Asthma and overt heart failure are relative contraindication
		IV bolus	0.2–1 mg/kg/dose q 5–10 minutes (maximum 40 mg)	
Sodium nitroprusside	30 seconds	IV infusion	0.5–10 µg/kg/min (in 5% dextrose)	Nausea, vomiting, headache, tachycardia, cyanide toxicity (dizziness, confusion, seizures, jaw stiffness, and lactic acidosis)
Nicardipine	1–10 minutes	IV infusion	0.5–4 µg/kg/min (maximum 5 mg/h)	Flushing, reflex tachycardia, phlebitis, edema, headache, nausea, vomiting
		IV bolus	30 µg/kg (max 2 mg/dose) q 15 min	
Esmolol	60 seconds	IV infusion	Loading with 100–500 µg/kg over 1–2 minutes; then maintain at 25–100 µg/kg/minutes	Bradycardia, orthostatic hypotension, pallor
Hydralazine		IV bolus or intramuscular Oral	• 0.1–0.2 mg/kg/dose, maximum 0.4 mg/kg Bolus dose every 4 hour • 0.25 mg/kg/dose every 6–8 hours	Tachycardia
Sodium nitroglycerin	2–5 minutes	IV infusion	1–3 µg/kg/min	Methemoglobinemia, headache, tachycardia
Nifedipine	10–30 minutes	Oral	0.2–0.5 mg/kg (maximum 10 mg) q 4–6 hour	Excessive hypotension, peripheral edema
Minoxidil		Oral	0.1–0.2 mg/kg/dose up to 10 mg per dose; every 8–12 hours	

orally, in order to permit withdrawal of intravenous therapy. The drug therapy of hypertensive emergency is summarized in **Table 13.14.7**. Intravenous nitroprusside and labetalol are the preferred antihypertensive drugs for management of the hypertensive emergency. Alternatively intravenous nicardipine or esmolol may be used. Hypertensive urgency can be treated with oral medications over 24–48 hours.

REFERENCES

1. Robinson CH, Chanchlani R. High Blood Pressure in Children and Adolescents: Current Perspectives and Strategies to Improve Future Kidney and Cardiovascular Health. Kidney Int Rep. 2022;7(5):954-70.
2. Thomas J, Stonebrook E, Kallash M. Pediatric hypertension: Review of the definition, diagnosis, and initial management. Int J Pediatr Adolesc Med. 2022;9(1):1-6.
3. Falkner B, Gidding SS, Baker-Smith CM, Brady TM, Flynn JT, Malle LM, et al. Pediatric Primary Hypertension: An Under recognized Condition: A Scientific Statement from the American Heart Association. Hypertension. 2023;80(6):e101-11.
4. Flynn JT, Kaelber DC, Baker-Smith CM, et al. Subcommittee on screening and management of high blood pressure in children. Clinical practice guidelines for screening and management of high blood pressure in children and adolescents. Pediatrics. 2017;140(3):e20171904.
5. Flynn JT, Urbina EM, Brady TM, Baker-Smith C, Daniels SR, Hayman LL, et al. Ambulatory Blood Pressure Monitoring in Children and Adolescents: 2022 Update: A Scientific Statement from the American Heart Association. Hypertension. 2022; 79(7):e114-24.
6. Bertazza Partigiani N, Spagnol R, Di Michele L, Santini M, Grotto B, Sartori A, et al. Management of hypertensive crises in children: A review of recent literature. Front Pediatr. 2022;10:880678.

SECTION

Disorders of Hemopoietic System

Section Editor: Ved Prakash Choudhry

14.1 ABC of Complete Blood Counts

(Col) Jyoti Kotwal, Surbhi Dahiya

INTRODUCTION

Modern automated hematology analyzers are routinely used to count blood cells and study blood cell histograms. This state-of-the-art technology which has been continuously evolving with the dawn of latest technologies provides a plethora of information on many hematological conditions that help to slender down the differential diagnosis even before ancillary testing is performed. They usually work on the Coulter's principle along with others like flowcytometry, optical light scattering, optical absorbance, radiofrequency and VCS (*V*olume, *C*onductivity, and *S*catter) technology. In general, the analyzers can be three-part (measures granulocytes, monocytes + eosinophils + basophils and lymphocytes), five-part (granulocytes, lymphocytes, monocytes, eosinophils, and basophils separately), or seven-part (in addition to above, also measures immature cells, abnormal lymphocytes, and large immature cells like blasts).[1]

An automated hematology analyzer has three detector blocks: RBCs and platelets are counted in the same block whereas WBCs are counted in a separate block. The third chamber is used for the hemoglobin estimation. Cells are counted by passing a dilute solution of the blood through an aperture across which an electrical current is flowing. The sizing and counting of blood cells is based on this measurable change in the electrical impedance (Coulter principle) **(Figs. 14.1.1A and B)**.

Typically, the histogram provides RBC, WBC, and platelet distribution curves which are derived by plotting the size of each cell on X-axis and their relative number on Y-axis. Each graph has a lower discriminator (LD) and an upper discriminator (UD) and always start and end at the baseline.[2] Over the last few years several new parameters have been introduced. Some abnormal cells that were previously only identified by the generation of an abnormal cell flag are now quantified. These include nucleated red blood cells (NRBCs), immature granulocytes (IG), activated/abnormal lymphocytes, and fragmented red cells (FRC), reticulocyte hemoglobin equivalent (RET-He)/CHr, immature platelet fraction (IPF) **(Table 14.1.1)**.[3]

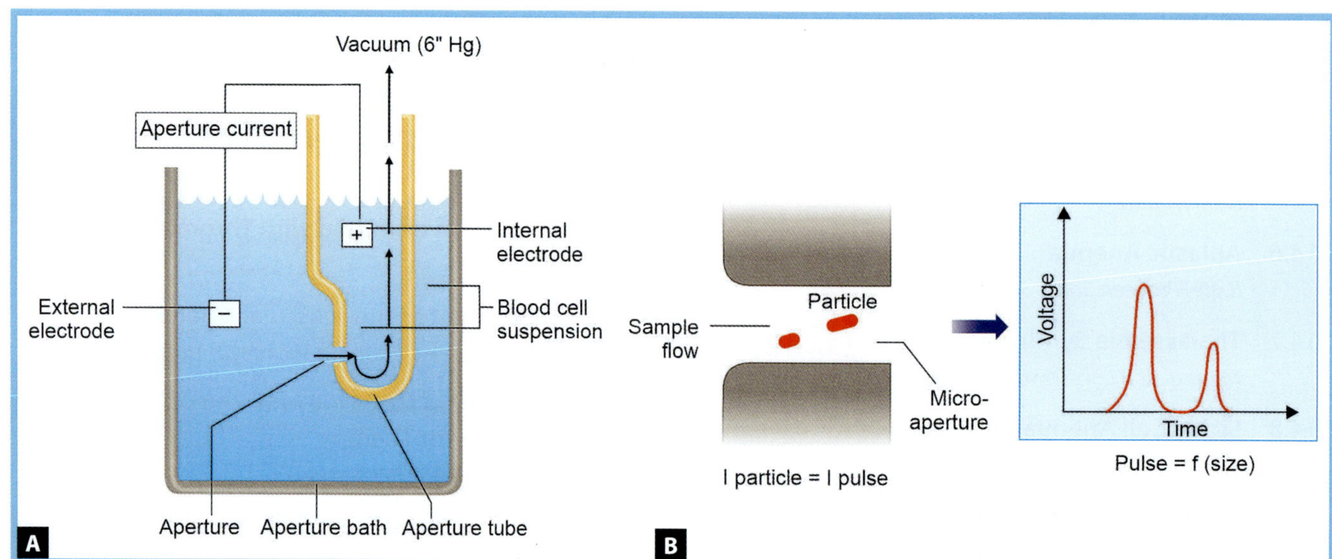

Figs. 14.1.1A and B: Coulter principle: The particle, liquid, and electric current are pumped through an orifice of an exact diameter. The particles when pass through the orifice, produce a change in electric current which is monitored to count and size the particles by plotting curves.
Source: https://www.beckman.com

TABLE 14.1.1: Newer parameters that are now routinely reported in the complete blood counts (CBCs).

Red cell	*WBC*	*Platelet*
Nucleated red blood cells (NRBCs)	Immature granulocytes	Immature platelet fraction
Immature reticulocyte fraction (IRF)		
Fragmented red cells (FRC)		
Reticulocyte hemoglobin equivalent (RET-He)		

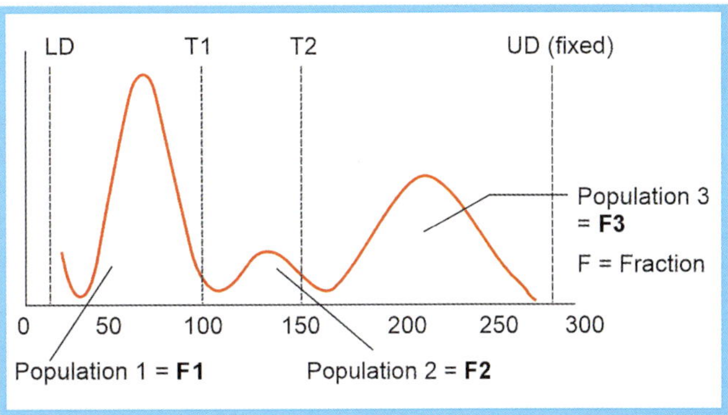

Fig. 14.1.2: WBC histogram. The leukocytes are separated in three parts: Lymphocytes (F1), mixed cells—monocytes, eosinophils, basophils (F2), and granulocytes (F3) by two discriminators: T1 and T2. (LD: lower discriminator; UD: upper discriminator)

WHITE BLOOD CELLS HISTOGRAM

In a normal WBC histogram **(Fig. 14.1.2)**, the lymphocytes are distributed between 50 and 100 fL, mixed cell population (monocytes, basophils, and eosinophils) between 100 and 150 fL, and neutrophils between 150 and 300 fL.[2]

Any deviation from the normal will reflect as a flag **(Table 14.1.2)**.

- *Neutrophilia* can suggest a bacterial infection, sepsis, steroid intake, inflammation, or malignancy such as chronic myeloid leukemia or a leukemoid reaction in the background of appropriate clinical details.
- In cases of *lymphocytosis,* one must investigate for any chronic infection or viral infections (one may find reactive lymphocytes in the smear). In case of persistent lymphocytosis without any evidence of infection, further testing to rule out chronic lymphoproliferative neoplasm is warranted.
- *Monocytosis* is usually seen in some chronic infections, viral infections such as infectious mononucleosis, during recovery from chemotherapy and also in some hematological disorders like chronic myelomonocytic leukemia (CMML) and juvenile myelomonocytic leukemia (JMML). Examination of the peripheral smear and its correlation with clinical profile and molecular testing is needed for confirmation of the diagnosis.
- *Eosinophilia* is seen in allergic conditions, parasitic infections, secondary to drugs. If persistent without any cause mentioned above, primary eosinophilia with molecular testing for FIP1L1-PDGFR mutation should be considered.

Similarly, the flag is generated in leukopenia.

- *Neutropenia* can be seen due to drugs, severe infections, and even in bone marrow failure (if associated with thrombocytopenia and anemia). It can also be seen in some rare inherited disorders like Kotsman syndrome where the cyclical trend of neutropenia is watched by follow-up complete blood counts (CBCs).
- *Promyelocytes, myelocytes, and metamyelocytes* are all included in the automated immature granulocytes (IG) count. It can be seen in various conditions such as infection, trauma, cancer, steroid intake, and myeloproliferative neoplasms.[3]
- Another flag appears as "atypical lymphocytes" whenever there are reactive lymphocytes or lympho-monocytoid cells as seen in viral infections such as dengue and Epstein–Barr virus (EBV).

RED BLOOD CELLS HISTOGRAM

RBCs and platelets are counted in the same chamber and plotted in a same graph. An arbitrary line is drawn through the trough of the curve usually in the 25–30 fL region which separates the platelets from RBCs. The RBC histogram has two discriminators: Upper discriminator (UL) between 200 and 250 fL and lower discriminator (RL) between 25 and 75 fL. Normal RBC curve is a symmetrical bell-shaped (Gaussian curve) **(Figs. 14.1.3A and B)**. Hemoglobin, hematocrit, total RBC count, and mean cell volume (MCV) are directly derived parameters, whereas mean cell hemoglobin (MCH) (Hb/RBC) and mean cell hemoglobin concentration (MCHC) (Hb/Hct) are the calculated parameters generated by the analyzers.[4] Low MCV indicates microcytic RBC whereas high MCV indicates macrocytes or polychromatophils. The MCH is high in dense RBCs and can be seen in macrocytes and spherocytes. Spuriously high levels of MCV, MCH, and MCHC which tend to disobey the "rule of 3" (Hct = 3 × Hb and Hb = RBC count × 3) indicates RBC agglutination and appears as a flag of agglutination in the analyzers. As this is usually secondary to the cold agglutinins, the sample is incubated for about 1–2 hours at 37°C to dissolve these agglutinates and repeat run shows corrected red cell indices following the "rule of 3". Refer to **Table 14.1.3** for the pediatric reference ranges.

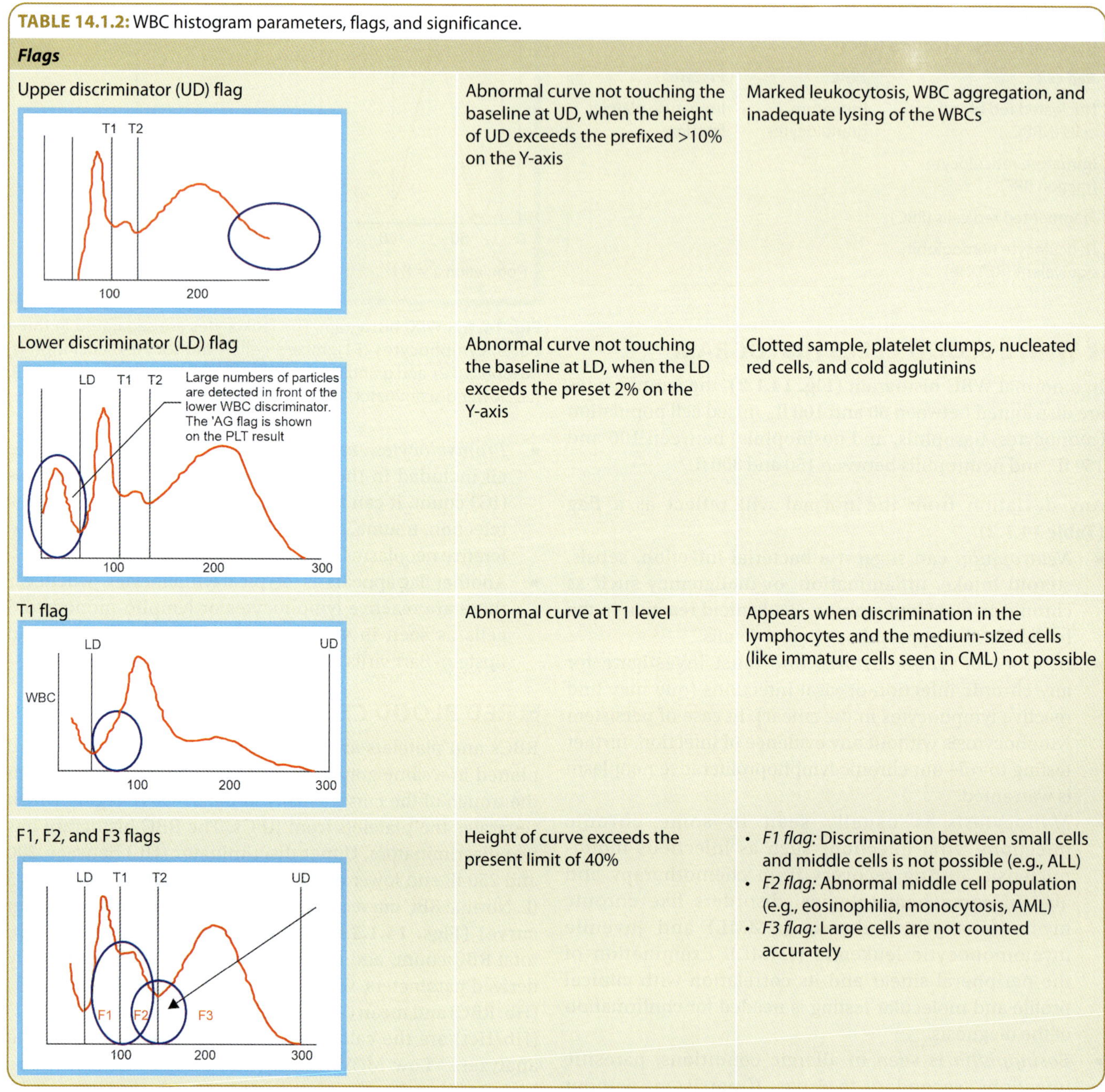

TABLE 14.1.2: WBC histogram parameters, flags, and significance.

Flags		
Upper discriminator (UD) flag	Abnormal curve not touching the baseline at UD, when the height of UD exceeds the prefixed >10% on the Y-axis	Marked leukocytosis, WBC aggregation, and inadequate lysing of the WBCs
Lower discriminator (LD) flag	Abnormal curve not touching the baseline at LD, when the LD exceeds the preset 2% on the Y-axis	Clotted sample, platelet clumps, nucleated red cells, and cold agglutinins
T1 flag	Abnormal curve at T1 level	Appears when discrimination in the lymphocytes and the medium-sized cells (like immature cells seen in CML) not possible
F1, F2, and F3 flags	Height of curve exceeds the present limit of 40%	• *F1 flag:* Discrimination between small cells and middle cells is not possible (e.g., ALL) • *F2 flag:* Abnormal middle cell population (e.g., eosinophilia, monocytosis, AML) • *F3 flag:* Large cells are not counted accurately

Red cell distribution width (RDW) is measurement of the width of the bases of the RBC histogram and depicts the RBC size distribution. It is of two types: (1) RDW-CV and (2) RDW-SD. RDW-SD is the arithmetic width of the distribution curve measured at the 20% frequency curve (normal range is 39–47 fL). RDW-CV is the coefficient of variation percentage (normal range is 11.5–14.5%) **(Figs. 14.1.3A and B)**.

Table 14.1.4 details the various flags produced by the RBC histogram and their interpretation.

PLATELET HISTOGRAM

Platelet-derived histograms are obtained from volume sizes of 2 to 30 fL (lower and upper discriminator, respectively) using electrical impedance and optical system reflecting the cell size. The actual size is derived from the log normal curve and generally falls between 2 and 20 fL. The platelet histogram is normally left skewed and lies between the lower discriminator (LD) and upper discriminator (UD), starting and ending at

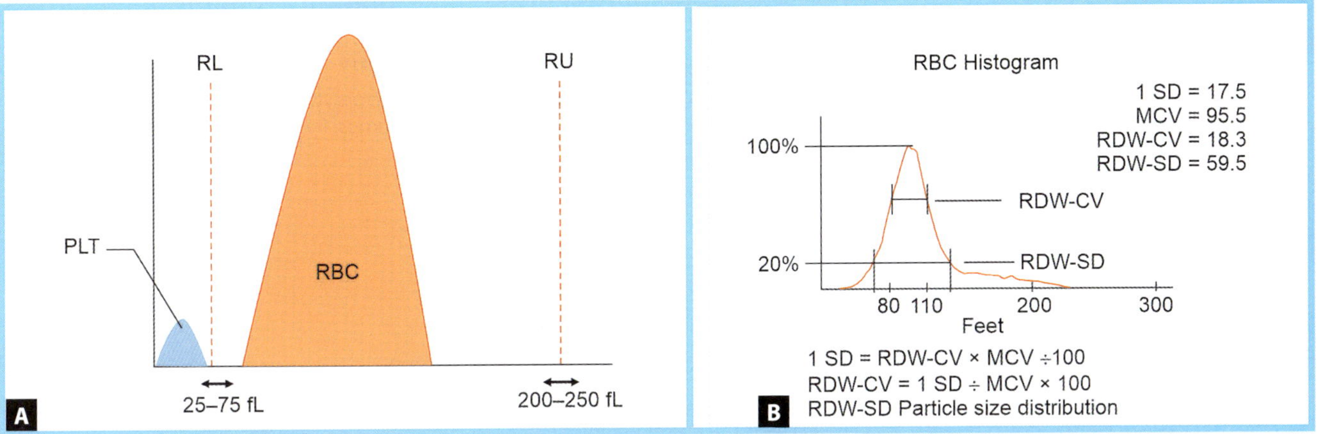

Figs. 14.1.3A and B: RBC and platelet histogram. RBC detected between 25 fL and 250 fL and is separated by flexible discriminators RL and RU. RBC histogram describing the calculation of red cells distribution width (RDW).

TABLE 14.1.3: Hematological values for normal infants (amalgamation of data derived from various sources; expressed as mean ± 2 SD of 95% range.[5]

	Birth	*Day 3*	*Day 7*	*Day 14*	*1 month*	*2 months*	*3–6 months*
Red blood cell count (RBC) ($\times 10^{12}$/L)	6.0 ± 1.0	5.3 ± 1.3	5.1 ± 1.2	4.9 ± 1.3	4.2 ± 1.2	3.7 ± 0.6	4.7 ± 0.6
Hemoglobin concentration (Hct) (L/L)	180 ± 40	180 ± 30	175 ± 40	165 ± 40	140 ± 25	112 ± 18	126 ± 15
Mean cell volume (MCV) (fL)	110 ± 10	105 ± 13	107 ± 19	105 ± 19	104 ± 12	95 ± 8	76 ± 8
Mean cell hemoglobin (MCH) (pg)	34 ± 3	34 ± 3	34 ± 3	34 ± 3	33 ± 3	30 ± 3	27 ± 3
Mean cell hemoglobin concentration (MCHC) (g/L)	330 ± 30	330 ± 40	330 ± 50	330 ± 50	330 ± 40	320 ± 35	330 ± 30
Reticulocyte count ($\times 10^9$/L)	120–400	50–350	50–100	50–100	20–60	30–50	40–100
White blood cell (WBC) count ($\times 10^9$/L)	18 ± 8	15 ± 8	14 ± 8	14 ± 8	12 ± 7	10 ± 5	12 ± 6
Neutrophils ($\times 10^9$/L)	4–14	3–5	3–6	3–7	3–9	1–5	1–6
Lymphocytes ($\times 10^9$/L)	3–8	2–8	3–9	3–9	3–16	4–10	4–12
Monocytes ($\times 10^9$/L)	0.5–2.0	0.5–1.0	0.1–1.7	0.1–1.7	0.3–1.0	0.4–1.2	0.2–1.2
Eosinophils ($\times 10^9$/L)	0.1–1.0	0.1–2.0	0.1–0.8	0.1–0.9	0.2–1.0	0.1–1.0	0.1–1.0
Platelets ($\times 10^9$/L)	100–450	210–500	160–500	170–500	200–500	210–650	200–550

the baseline **(Fig. 14.1.4)**. Small particles can overlap with the lower discriminator of the curve, e.g., bubbles and dust, whereas microcytic erythrocytes can interfere with the upper end. The analyzers commonly use impedance method for platelet counts which differentiate the platelets from red cells based upon their size and may give false low platelet counts in the presence of large or giant platelets which are falsely counted as red cells. To overcome this, new technologies like optical counts (platelet-O mode) and fluorescent platelet counts (platelet-F mode) are now being evaluated and have been found to be more precise **(Table 14.1.5)**.[6]

The Derived Platelet Parameters

Mean Platelet Volume

Mean platelet volume (MPV) is a mathematically derived parameter that determines the average size of the platelets. Normal range of MPV is 7.4–10.4 fL. MPV is a marker of platelet function.

An increase in MPV has been observed in patients at risk of myocardial infarction and cerebral infarction, inherited congenital macrothrombocytopenias such as Bernard–Soulier syndrome and familial platelet disorders with myosin

TABLE 14.1.4: Various flags produced by the RBC histogram and their interpretation.

Flags	*Description*	*Causes*
Lower discriminator (RL) flag 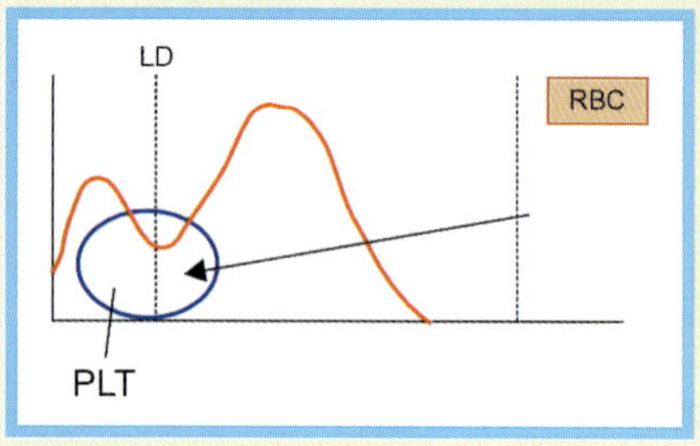	Abnormal height at lower discriminator, exceeds the preset height by >10%	Microerythrocytes, giant platelets, platelet clumps, fragmented red cells, and in CLL
Upper discriminator (RU) flag 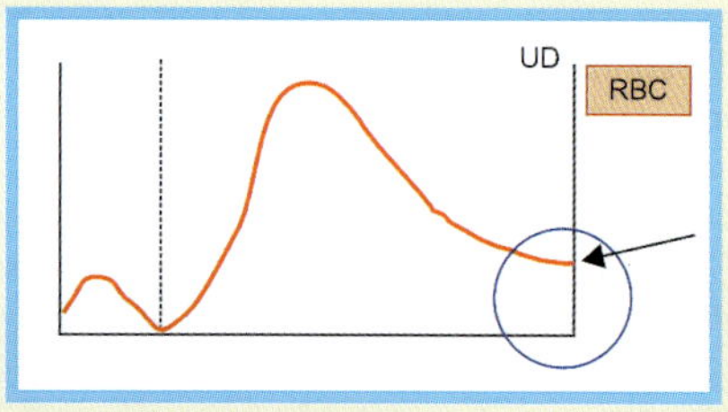	Abnormal height at upper discriminator, exceeds the preset height by >5%	Cold agglutinins and Rouleaux formation
Multiple peak (MP) flag 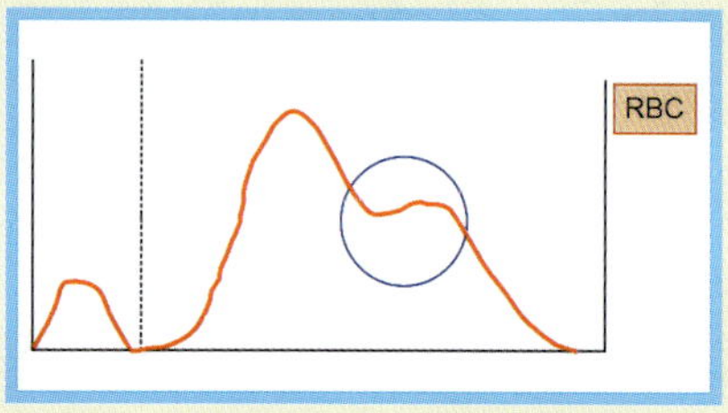	Multiple peaks in the curve	Due to significant anisocytosis possibly due to post transfusion or under the effect of hematinics therapy and dimorphic anemia
Abnormal distribution width (DW) flag	RBC curve not touching the baseline and ends above the 20% mark, RDW is not calculated	All causes as above

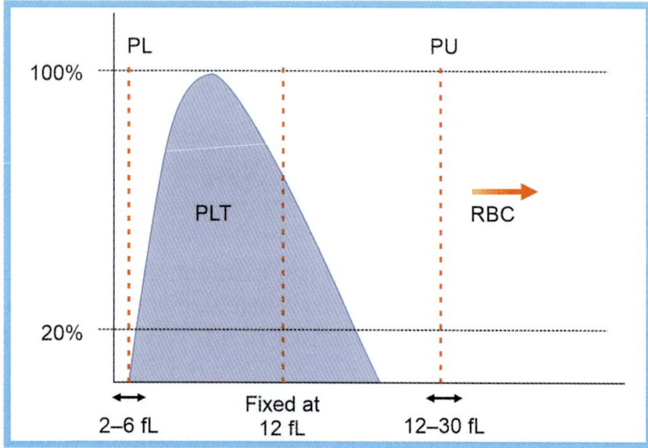

Fig. 14.1.4: The platelet histogram. Platelets are measured between 2 and 30 fL with a fixed discriminator at 12 fL.

heavy chain 9 (MYH9). It is also commonly seen in the Eastern part of India, particularly Assam and West Bengal, known as Harris syndrome, where the platelet count is spuriously low in the automated analyzers due to the large sized functionally normal platelets. Other causes include splenectomy, immune thrombocytopenic purpura, chronic myeloproliferative neoplasm. A low MPV has been reported in thrombocytopenic patients with marrow disease, hypersplenism, megaloblastic anemia, and Wiscott-Aldrich syndrome.

Platelet Distribution Width

It is the width of the curve of distribution of platelets and depicts their anisocytosis. It is calculated at 20% peak height of the distribution curve with a normal reference range of 9–14%. The role of MPV and platelet distribution width (PDW) has also been established in the risk stratification to

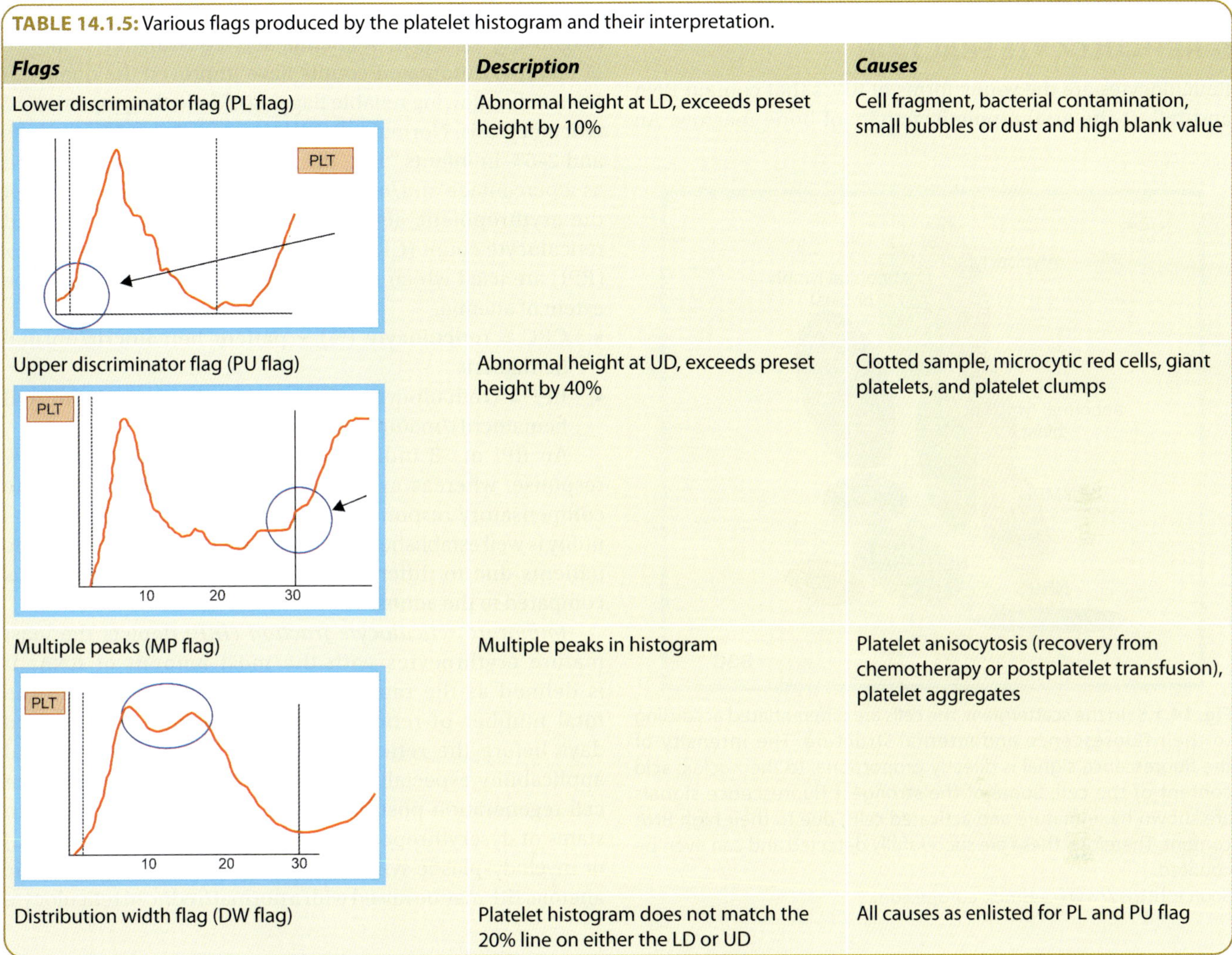

TABLE 14.1.5: Various flags produced by the platelet histogram and their interpretation.

Flags	*Description*	*Causes*
Lower discriminator flag (PL flag)	Abnormal height at LD, exceeds preset height by 10%	Cell fragment, bacterial contamination, small bubbles or dust and high blank value
Upper discriminator flag (PU flag)	Abnormal height at UD, exceeds preset height by 40%	Clotted sample, microcytic red cells, giant platelets, and platelet clumps
Multiple peaks (MP flag)	Multiple peaks in histogram	Platelet anisocytosis (recovery from chemotherapy or postplatelet transfusion), platelet aggregates
Distribution width flag (DW flag)	Platelet histogram does not match the 20% line on either the LD or UD	All causes as enlisted for PL and PU flag

predict acute coronary events and response to therapy in such patients.[7]

NEWER PARAMETERS

Above were the histograms of a three-part analyzer, but in the recent times with the growing technology, many centers are now using 5- or 7-part hematology analyzers that provide several parameters which give a more detailed insight. The various technologies used are volume conductivity scatter (VCS), peroxidase staining (Advia), multi-angle polarized scatter separation (MAPPS—Abott) and fluorescence flowcytometry (Sysmex).

The 5-part analyzers have different types of channels that measure various parameters **(Fig. 14.1.5)** and generate flags. The WNR channel measures WBC, NRBC, and basophils. The WDF channel measures granulocytes, lymphocytes, eosinophils, monocytes, and immature granulocytes (IG). RET channel measures reticulocyte and RET-He. Platelet-F channel provides platelet count and measures the IPF **(Figs. 14.1.6A to C)**.

NUCLEATED RED CELLS

Nucleated red blood cells/erythroblasts are normally only found in bone marrow except, during the immediate neonatal period. Their presence in peripheral blood is abnormal which could reflect either a significant increase in erythropoietic activity (hemolytic anemia, thalassemia major, sepsis, massive acute hemorrhage, hypoxia, etc.) or could be secondary to bone marrow damage (e.g., malignancies, fibrosis, necrosis, etc.).[3] In ICU patients, presence of NRBCs indicates increased mortality risk. In areas with high prevalence of sickle cell anemia, CBC with presence of NRBCs despite normal red cell indices, may be an indicator of sickle cell disease and calls in for a sickling test or Hb-HPLC.

RETICULOCYTE COUNT AND IMMATURE RETICULOCYTE FRACTION

Reticulocytes are the young forms of RBCs that contain RNA and reflect the erythropoietic activity of bone marrow. An assessment of reticulocyte maturation is thus important for diagnosing the cause of anemia and assessing the response of therapy. Automated counts have improved the quality of the results allowing reliable flagging of reticulocytopenia and reticulocytosis. Normal reference range is 0.5–2.5% in adults and 2–6% in infants.[8] But, the reticulocyte count (expressed as a percentage and/or a count) does not accurately depict the erythropoietic activity of marrow and thus corrected reticulocyte count (CRC) and reticulocyte production index (RPI) are used which relate the reticulocyte count with the extent of anemia.

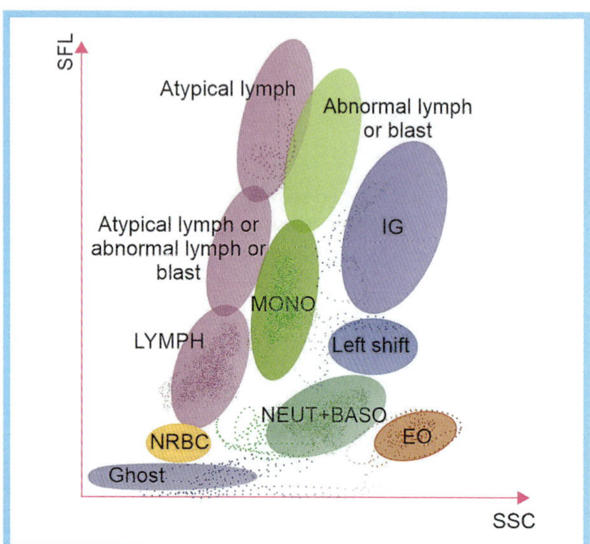

Fig. 14.1.5: In the scattergram, the cells are differentiated according to their fluorescence and internal structure. The intensity of the fluorescence signal is directly proportional to the nucleic acid content of the cell. Some of the strongest fluorescence signals are shown by immature and activated cells, due to their high RNA content. Therefore, these are successfully detected and can even be counted.
Source: https://www.sysmex-europe.com.

- CRC = reticulocyte (%) × patient hematocrit/normal hematocrit
- RPI = (reticulocyte (%) × patient hematocrit/normal hematocrit)/maturation time

An RPI of >3 indicates an appropriate bone marrow response, whereas an RPI of <2 indicates an inadequate compensatory response to correct the anemia. Though its utility is well established, it is not an adequate tool in pediatric patients due to differences in the hematologic values as compared to the adults.[9]

Immature reticulocyte fraction (IRF) depicts the least mature erythrocytes with the most amount of RNA. It is defined as the ratio of immature reticulocytes to the total number of reticulocytes. As IRF increases several days before the reticulocyte count, it has great clinical applicability especially in monitoring the marrow or stem cell regeneration posttransplantation or chemotherapy. In states of dyserythropoiesis [acute myeloid leukemia (AML) or myelodysplastic syndromes (MDS)] and in megaloblastic anemia, IRF may be raised with a normal/reduced reticulocyte

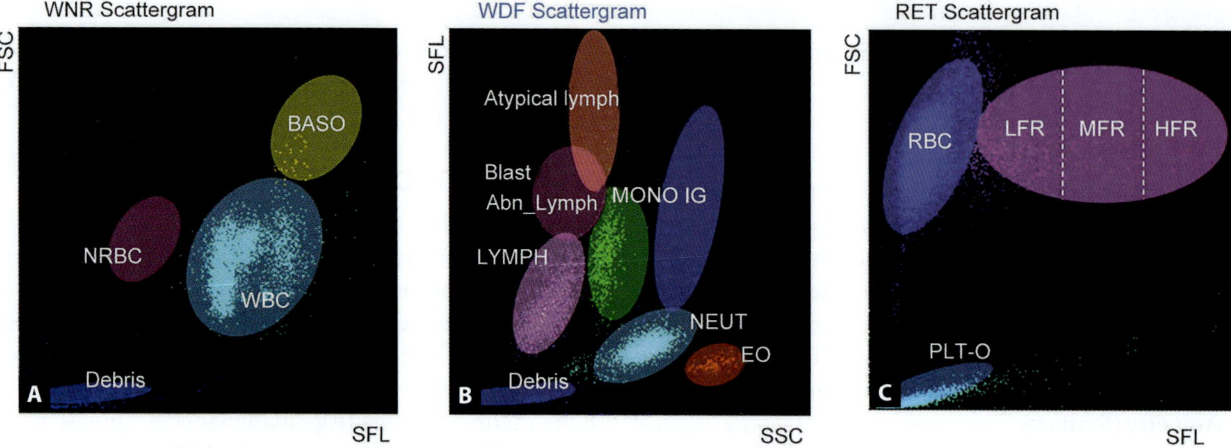

Figs. 14.1.6A to C: The different channels and parameters measured in a Sysmex 5-part hematology analyzer. Ret scattergram measures reticulocytes on the basis of their RNA content into high fluorescent reticulocytes (HFR: the most immature reticulocytes with the most amount of RNA), Medium fluorescent reticulocytes (MFR) and the low fluorescent reticulocytes (LFR—the most mature reticulocytes with the least amount of RNA). HFR + MFR = IRF (immature reticulocyte fraction).
Source: https://www.sysmex-europe.com.

count. In iron deficiency or anemia of chronic disease, the reticulocyte count is reduced but the IRF is normal.[3]

FUNCTIONAL IRON DEFICIENCY AND THE RETICULOCYTE HEMOGLOBIN EQUIVALENT OR MEAN RETICULOCYTE HEMOGLOBIN CONTENT

Functional iron deficiency (FID) occurs when reticuloendothelial iron stores are normal, or high, but the iron is not delivered to the bone marrow and is unavailable for erythropoiesis. This is often seen in patients with chronic inflammation, cancer, those undergoing long-term renal dialysis. RET-He reflects the actual iron supply for hemoglobin synthesis in the bone marrow over the previous 3–4 days and thus aids in quick screening of erythropoietic status. With the development of flow cell hematology analyzers, it is now possible to measure the volume and hemoglobin content of reticulocytes. It is available on the Siemens (CHr: mean reticulocyte hemoglobin content) and Sysmex analyzers (RET-He: the reticulocyte hemoglobin equivalent). The reference values in health for both parameters are the same, for adult it is 28–35 pg or >29 pg and for pediatric population it is >27.5 pg. It is often used together with ferritin: High or normal ferritin together with a low RET-He is suggestive of functional iron deficiency whereas low ferritin together with low RET-He is suggestive of classic iron deficiency.[10] It is reliably used as a marker to distinguish iron-deficiency anemia (IDA) from FID and is also utilized in the monitoring of erythropoietin (EPO)/iron therapy in chronic kidney diseases.

A new research parameter, δ-He gives information about the Hb content of mature RBCs. δ-He = [(RET-He) - (RBCs-He)]. The normal range is 0.268–0.451 f/mol (4.31–7.26 pg). δ-He above normal range suggests improvement in erythropoiesis whereas if below normal range for longer periods predicts onset of anemia.[11]

Red blood cells extended parameters and include the percentages of microcytic (%micro R) and hypochromic red cells (%hypo-He) that are now gaining importance. Percentage of micro R indicates the percentage of microcytic red cells with a volume <60 fL. % hypo-He indicates the percentage of microcytic hypochromic red cells with a Hb content of <17 pg (Sysmex) and <28 g/dL (Siemens). They are sensitive indicators for quantification of hemoglobinization of red cells and %hypo-He value >10% is highly suggestive of iron-deficiency anemia.[12] Together with RDW-CV, %micro R and %hypo-He are utilized in Urrechaga index, a sensitive index used to differentiate between iron deficiency anemia and thalassemia trait. It is calculated as: %microR - %hypo-He - RDW-CV. A value higher than –7.6 is highly suspicious of β-thalassemia trait, and the HbA_2 level must be quantified to confirm the same.[13]

FRAGMENTED RED CELLS

Fragmented red cells are normally not seen in the peripheral blood. In adults/neonates >1% and in premature babies >5% fragmented cells become clinically significant and should always be considered for the possibility of thrombotic microangiopathy (TMA).[14] They are found in microangiopathies (HUS and TTP), disseminated carcinoma, transplant-associated thrombotic microangiopathy (TMA), cytotoxic chemotherapy, disseminated intravascular coagulation (DIC), and immune disorders and infection. Their manual microscopic counting is subjective and imprecise. FRC count has significant impact in both for screening in neonatal coagulopathies and infections and for monitoring, thus potentially reducing serial phlebotomies.[15] The use of the IPF and the FRC count together may be helpful for the early differential diagnosis of immune thrombocytopenia (ITP) and microangiopathies.

IMMATURE PLATELET FRACTION

Newly released platelets have more RNA content compared to the mature platelets and are larger and more reactive.[3] The content of RNA is directly proportional to the marrow megakaryocytic activity and thus offers the ability to determine whether thrombocytopenia is due to marrow failure or due to increased peripheral platelet destruction/loss, thus avoiding the need for bone marrow examination. The normal range has been reported as 1.1–6.1%. The IPF is raised in patients with peripheral consumption/destruction of platelets (e.g., ITP and TTP) and is normal or low in patients with marrow failure. The IPF rises 1–2 days prior to the platelet count following peripheral blood stem cell transplantation and 4–4.5 days prior to the platelet count following allogenic bone marrow transplantation, thus, helps to reduce prophylactic platelet transfusions in patients undergoing transplants. The use of the IPF and the FRC count together may be helpful for the early differential diagnosis of ITP and microangiopathies.

Case 1

A 4-year-old female child presented with petechiae over face and lower limb for 1 month. On investigation, she was found to have thrombocytopenia. She received IVIG for the same. Hemogram received 3 days after with bone marrow studies. Urrechaga Index (MicroR-Hypo-He-RDW-CV) = 7.5 - 3.0 - 17.1 = -12.6. Ret-He was 24.3 pg. Platelet count: 36,000/uL with IPF: 13% **(Figs. 14.1.7A to D)**. Marrow iron stores: Nil.

Impression: ITP with iron-deficiency anemia.

Case 2

A 9-year-old female child had complaints of weakness and pallor. CBC with peripheral smear revealed the following:

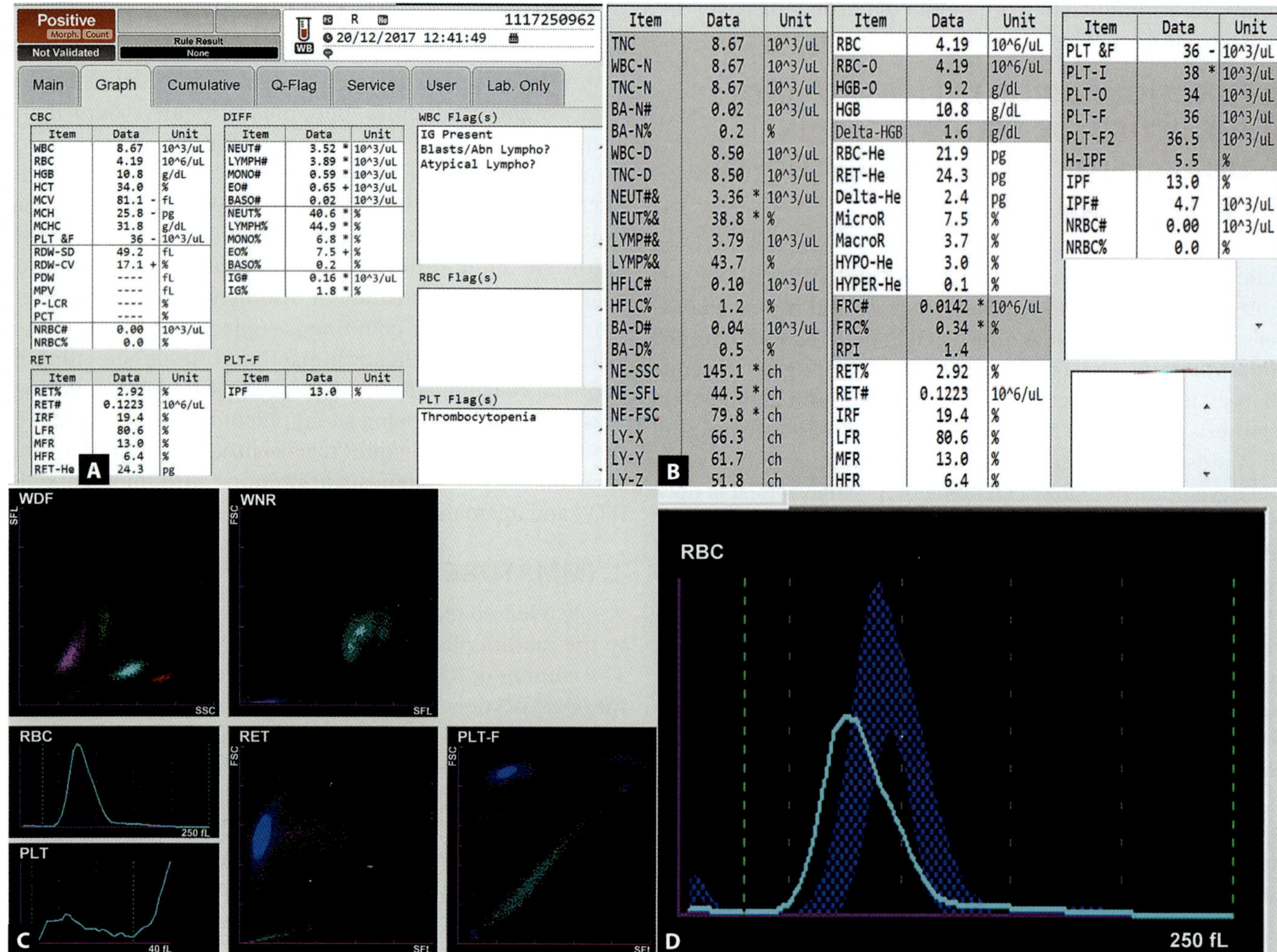

Figs. 14.1.7A to D: Data shows low Hb (10.8 g/dL), reduced MCV, MCH, MCHC, raised RDW-CV, reduced RET-He, raised MicroR%, reduced platelet counts with raised IPF%. (MCH: mean cell hemoglobin; MCHC: mean cell hemoglobin concentration; MCV: mean cell volume; RDW: red cell distribution width; RET-He: reticulocyte hemoglobin equivalent)

RBC—mild-to-moderate anisocytosis, normocytic normochromic to macrocytic normochromic red cells noted. Polychromasia +. Schistocytes seen. Schistocyte index 7%. WBC—mild neutrophilic leukocytosis with increased granulations. Platelets—Decreased and large platelets seen. MPV = 12.3 fL. Suggesting peripheral destruction **(Figs. 14.1.8A to C)**.

Impression: PBF suggestive of microangiopathic hemolysis. In view of age of child, it was suggested to rule out HUS if acute case. If chronic case, rule out TMA-associated kidney disease.

Case 3

A 15-year-old girl presented to the OPD with complaints of generalized weakness and lethargy. Her CBC revealed; Hb: 6.1 g/dL, RBC count: 0.20 × 10^6/uL, MCV: 115 fL, MCH: 305 pg, MCHC: 265.2 g/dL. Platelet count: 158,000/uL and a flag for abnormal RBC distribution. The smear revealed RBC agglutination leading to the erroneous red cell indices **(Figs. 14.1.9A to C)**. The sample in such cases is to be incubated for 2 hours at 37°C to remove the effect of cold agglutinins. The post-incubated sample showed correction of red cell indices (MCV: 88.1 fL, MCH: 28.9 pg, MCHC: 32.9 g/dL) and improvement in the red cell agglutination. DAT was positive (4+) with reticulocytosis, raised serum LDH levels, and unconjugated hyperbilirubinemia.

Impression: Autoimmune hemolytic anemia (DAT-IgM positive)

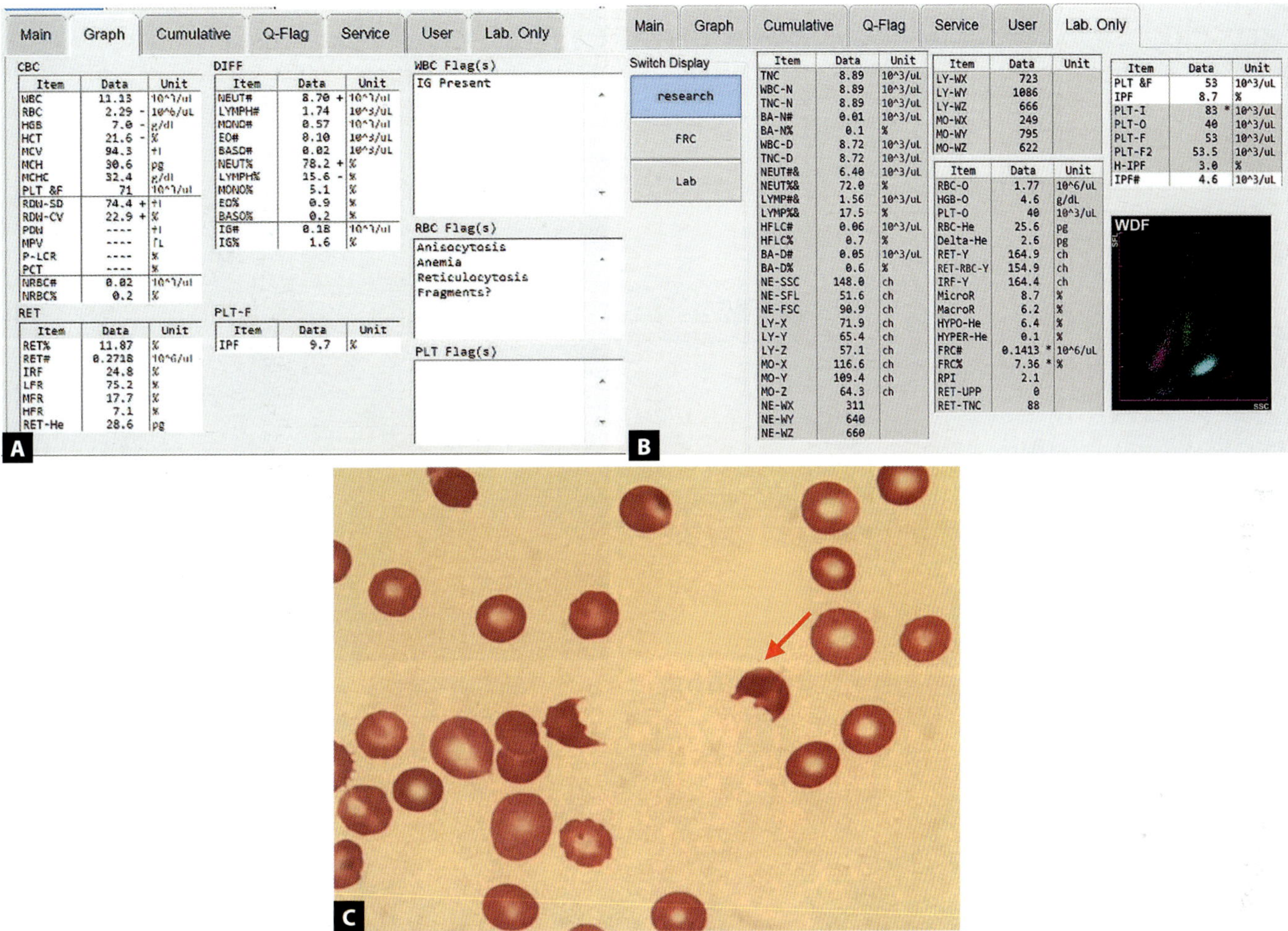

A

CBC

Item	Data	Unit
WBC	11.13	10^3/ul
RBC	2.29 -	10^6/uL
HGB	7.0 -	g/dl
HCT	21.6 -	%
MCV	94.3	fl
MCH	30.6	pg
MCHC	32.4	g/dl
PLT &F	71	10^3/ul
RDW-SD	74.4 +	fl
RDW-CV	22.9 +	%
PDW	----	fl
MPV	----	fL
P-LCR	----	%
PCT	----	%
NRBC#	0.02	10^3/ul
NRBC%	0.2	%

DIFF

Item	Data	Unit
NEUT#	8.70 +	10^3/ul
LYMPH#	1.74	10^3/uL
MONO#	0.57	10^3/ul
EO#	0.10	10^3/uL
BASO#	0.02	10^3/uL
NEUT%	78.2 +	%
LYMPH%	15.6 -	%
MONO%	5.1	%
EO%	0.9	%
BASO%	0.2	%
IG#	0.18	10^3/ul
IG%	1.6	%

WBC Flag(s)
IG Present

RBC Flag(s)
Anisocytosis
Anemia
Reticulocytosis
Fragments?

PLT Flag(s)

RET

Item	Data	Unit
RET%	11.87	%
RET#	0.2718	10^6/ul
IRF	24.8	%
LFR	75.2	%
MFR	17.7	%
HFR	7.1	%
RET-He	28.6	pg

PLT-F

Item	Data	Unit
IPF	9.7	%

B

Item	Data	Unit
TNC	8.89	10^3/uL
WBC-N	8.89	10^3/uL
TNC-N	8.89	10^3/uL
BA-N#	0.01	10^3/uL
BA-N%	0.1	%
WBC-D	8.72	10^3/uL
TNC-D	8.72	10^3/uL
NEUT#&	6.40	10^3/uL
NEUT%&	72.0	%
LYMP#&	1.56	10^3/uL
LYMP%&	17.5	%
HFLC#	0.06	10^3/uL
HFLC%	0.7	%
BA-D#	0.05	10^3/uL
BA-D%	0.6	%
NE-SSC	148.0	ch
NE-SFL	51.6	ch
NE-FSC	90.9	ch
LY-X	71.9	ch
LY-Y	65.4	ch
LY-Z	57.1	ch
MO-X	116.6	ch
MO-Y	109.4	ch
MO-Z	64.3	ch
NE-WX	311	
NE-WY	640	
NE-WZ	660	

Item	Data	Unit
LY-WX	723	
LY-WY	1086	
LY-WZ	666	
MO-WX	249	
MO-WY	795	
MO-WZ	622	

Item	Data	Unit
RBC-O	1.77	10^6/uL
HGB-O	4.6	g/dL
PLT-O	40	10^3/uL
RBC-He	25.6	pg
Delta-He	2.6	pg
RET-Y	164.9	ch
RET-RBC-Y	154.9	ch
IRF-Y	164.4	ch
MicroR	8.7	%
MacroR	6.2	%
HYPO-He	6.4	%
HYPER-He	0.1	%
FRC#	0.1413 *	10^6/uL
FRC%	7.36 *	%
RPI	2.1	
RET-UPP	0	
RET-TNC	88	

Item	Data	Unit
PLT &F	53	10^3/uL
IPF	8.7	%
PLT-I	83 *	10^3/uL
PLT-O	40	10^3/uL
PLT-F	53	10^3/uL
PLT-F2	53.5	10^3/uL
H-IPF	3.0	%
IPF#	4.6	10^3/uL

Figs. 14.1.8A to C: The data shows low Hb (7 g/dL), increased RET% (11.87), low platelet count (71,000/uL), raised IPF% (9.7) and raised FRC% (7.36). The smear shows presence of schistocytes (red arrow).

CONCLUSION

So, whenever a CBC or peripheral smear is interpreted, besides seeing the conventional values of Hb, WBC count, and the platelet counts, look for the red cell indices if they are following the rule of 3, if violated then incubate the sample at 37°C for 2 hours and see for the correction of indices which may be correlated in the slide by disappearance/reduction of red cell agglutinates. Look at the RBC histogram for any shift (microcytic cells or macrocytes), multiple peaks or hump in the curve. If there is microcytic hypochromic anemia with erythrocytosis, one must calculate the Mentzer's index/Urrechaga index for the possibility of thalassemia syndromes and order Hb-HPLC. In smear look for spherocytes, schistocytes, polychromatophils, NRBC, sickle cells, etc., all of which carry their own significances. For a patient with low platelet counts, look at the IPF, if it is more (normal reference range: 1.1–6.1%), then thrombocytopenia is more likely secondary to the peripheral destruction (e.g., ITP, sepsis, hypersplenism, dengue, etc.).

The awareness of the possibilities and scope of the modern analyzers is imperative both to the laboratory physicians and the clinicians as it allows us time to evaluate abnormal blood films, consider diagnostic clues, and correlate clinical findings to histograms and other hematologic parameters with greater confidence and efficiency, all of which produce high returns in terms of patient's healthcare by reducing the cost to the diagnosis and avoiding other unnecessary tests together helping in timely management of the disease states.

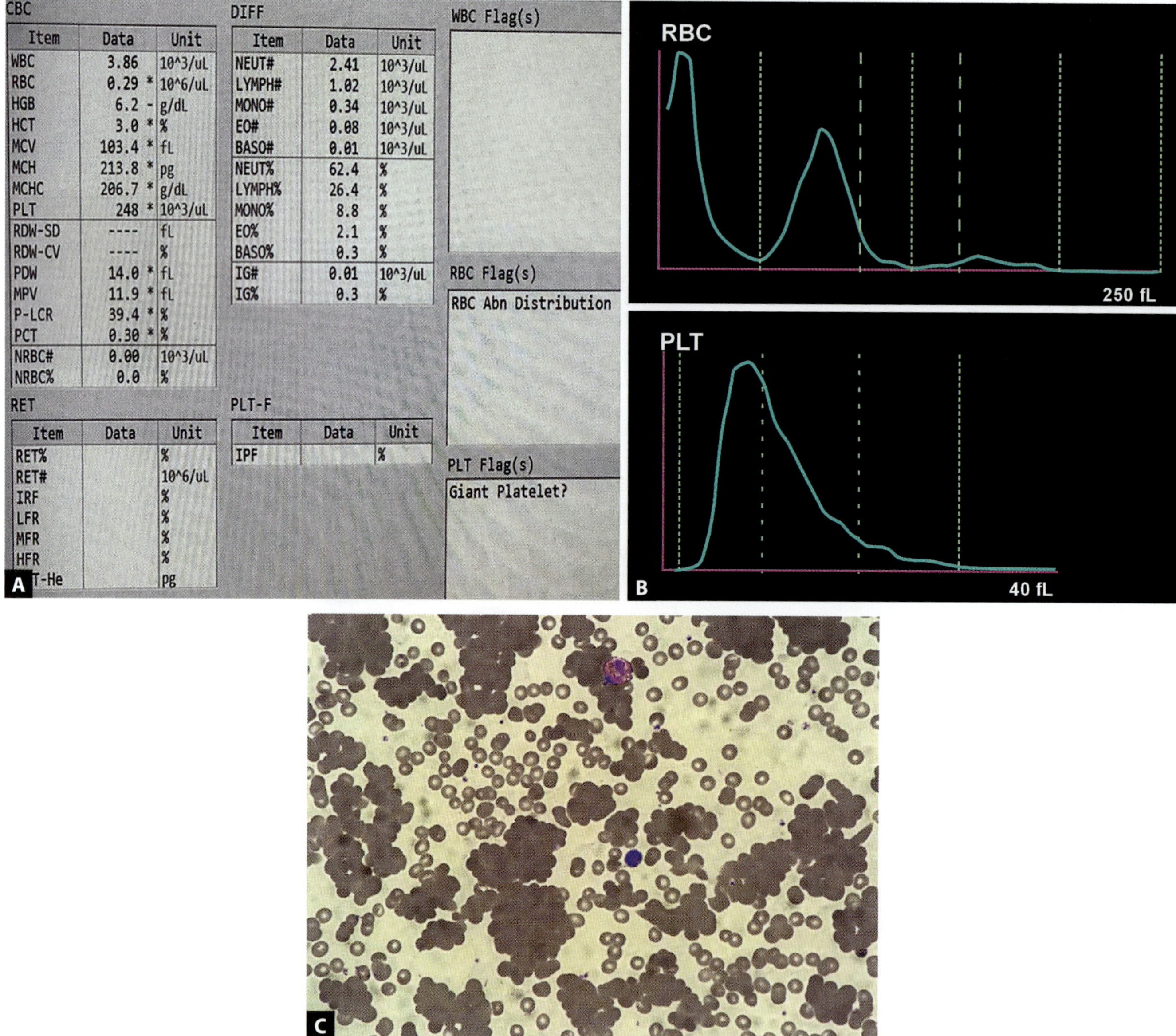

Figs. 14.1.9A to C: The data shows deranged red cell indices with violation of "rule of 3". The RBC histogram shows two peaks with abnormal lower discriminator. Smear (40x) shows red cell agglutination.

REFERENCES

1. Green R, Wachsmann-Hogiu S. Development, history, and future of automated cell counters. Clin Lab Med. 2015;35(1):1-10.
2. Thomas ETA, Bhagya S, Majeed A. Clinical Utility of Blood Cell Histogram Interpretation. J Clin Diagn Res. 2017;11(9):OE01-OE04.
3. Briggs C. Quality counts: new parameters in blood cell counting. Int J Lab Hematol. 2009;31(3):277-97.
4. Chhabra G. Automated hematology analyzers: recent trends and applications. J Lab Physicians. 2018;10(1):15-6.
5. Bates I. Reference ranges and normal values. In: Bain BJ, Bates I, Michael A Laffan MA (Eds). Dacie and Lewis Practical Haematology, 12th edition. Netherlands: Elsevier; 2017. pp. 8-17.
6. Schoori R, Schoori M, Oomes J, Van Pelt J. New fluorescent method (PLT-F) on Sysmex XN2000 hematology analyzer achieved higher accuracy in low platelet counting. Am J Clin Pathol. 2013;140(4):495-9.
7. Rigvardhan, Kumar N, Girish R, Taur N, Kotwal J. Correlation of platelet volume indices (PVI) with spectrum of coronary artery disease: a prospective study in Indian scenario. J Evolution Med Dent Sci. 2016;5(35):1969-72.

8. Briggs C, Bain BJ. Basic haematological techniques. In: Bain BJ, Bates I, Laffan MA (Eds). Dacie and Lewis Practical Haematology, 12th edition, Vol. 3. Netherlands: Elsevier; 2017. pp. 18-49.
9. Bracho FJ, Osorio IA. Evaluation of the Reticulocyte Production Index in the Pediatric Population. Am J Clin Pathol. 2020;154(1):70-7.
10. Weimann A, Cremer M, Hernáiz-Driever P, Zimmermann M. Delta-He, Ret-He and a New Diagnostic Plot for Differential Diagnosis and Therapy Monitoring of Patients Suffering from Various Disease-Specific Types of Anemia. Clin Lab. 2016;62(4):667-77.
11. Urrechaga E, Borque L, Escanero JF. Biomarkers of hypochromia: The contemporary assessment of iron status and erythropoiesis. Biomed Res Int. 2013;2013:603786.
12. Urrechaga E, Borque L, Escanero JF. The role of automated measurement of red cell subpopulations on the Sysmex XE 5000 analyzer in the differential diagnosis of microcytic anemia. Int J Lab Hematol. 2011;33(1):30-6.
13. Urrechaga E, Borque L, Escanero JF. The Role of Automated Measurement of RBC Subpopulations in Differential Diagnosis of Microcytic Anemia and β-Thalassemia Screening. Am J Clin Path. 2011;135(3):374-9.
14. Zini G, d'Onofrio G, Briggs C, Erber W, Jou JM, Lee SH, et al. International Council for Standardization in Haematology (ICSH). ICSH recommendations for identification, diagnostic value, and quantitation of schistocytes. Int J Lab Hematol. 2012;34(2):107-16.
15. Judkins AJ, MacQueen BC, Christensen RD, Henry E, Snow GL, Bennett ST. Automated Quantification of Fragmented Red Blood Cells: Neonatal Reference Intervals and Clinical Disorders of Neonatal Intensive Care Unit Patients with High Values. Neonatology. 2019;115(1):5-12.

14.2 Approach to Anemia in a Newborn

Vivek Kumar, Ramesh Agarwal

INTRODUCTION

Anemia is a common problem in the neonatal period as almost all neonates experience a physiologic fall in hemoglobin (Hb) immediately after delivery. It is commonly defined as Hb or hematocrit <5th percentile for a particular gestational and postnatal age. It is important to recognize that anemia cut-offs in neonates are not static, but change with gestation and postnatal age. For example, a neonate at 28 weeks with a venous hematocrit of 38% at birth will be within normal range while a 38-week neonate with same hematocrit would be in anemic range. Similarly, a term neonate at birth will have a higher hematocrit cut-off for defining anemia than at the postnatal age of 60 days. Further, severe anemia is defined as Hb/hematocrit less than the 1st percentile of the reference population.[1] This use of "reference intervals" for neonatal anemia in place of the commonly used "normal ranges" for adults highlights the need to keep developmental physiology into consideration.

EPIDEMIOLOGY

Although the exact incidence of neonatal anemia is not known, studies have reported a prevalence between 20 and 25% in term neonates. Preterm neonates have a much higher prevalence with up to 50% very low birthweight (<1,500 g) neonates and up to 90% extremely low birthweight (<1,000 g) neonates requiring blood transfusions.[2]

The etiology of neonatal anemia is often multifactorial and includes prenatal factors such as maternal malnutrition, infections, and iron-deficiency anemia as well as neonatal factors such as poor iron stores, low erythropoietin (EPO) levels, decreased red blood cell (RBC) lifespan, and frequent blood sampling.[3] Thus, a combination of physiologic and various nonphysiologic factors determine the onset and severity of neonatal anemia.

HEMATOLOGIC PHYSIOLOGY IN NEWBORN

Before proceeding ahead, let us recapitulate a few points worth remembering regarding developmental hematological physiology while evaluating neonatal anemia:

- *The intrauterine transition of hematopoiesis:* While initial erythropoiesis starts in the yolk sac, the liver becomes the predominant site for erythropoiesis from 6 to 8 weeks till 28–30 weeks when bone marrow takes over as the major site. Also, in utero liver is the major site for EPO production. This has important implications for anemia among preterm neonates as we will see later.

- *Transfer of iron during the third trimester:* Transfer of iron from mother to fetus occurs efficiently due to abundant transferrin receptors present in the placenta. However, the majority of iron is transferred during the third trimester. Thus, sudden abruption in this transfer due to preterm delivery contributes significantly to causing anemia.
- *Postnatal fall in hemoglobin:* The mean hematocrit in the fetus rises steadily from around ~33 at 18 weeks to a hematocrit of ~52 at 40 weeks' gestation. Thereafter, postnatally, all infants experience a physiological fall of Hb/hematocrit due to:
    - Initial physiological hemolysis
    - Decreased RBC production and shortened neonatal RBC survival compared to adults (~60 days versus ~120 days), and
    - Lower plasma concentrations of EPO to degree of anemia compared to adults.

  Thus, Hb is at its peak in term neonates at the time of birth, decreasing on either side of it.
- *Progressive right shift of oxygen dissociation curve:* After birth, there is a progressive switch from high oxygen-affinity fetal hemoglobin (HbF) to low oxygen-affinity adult hemoglobin (HbA) and there is an increase in 2,3-diphosphoglycerate (DPG) within RBCs. Both these factors result in a right shift of the oxygen dissociation curve, allowing greater ease in releasing oxygen from Hb.
- Timing of umbilical cord clamping: The amount of blood transferred to the neonate at delivery is dependent on the time of clamping of the umbilical cord. It is estimated that delayed cord clamping of 60–90 seconds transfers ~10–15 mL/kg of blood to the newborn, while if the cord is not cut until pulsations cease, ~20–30 mL/kg blood is transferred to the neonate. This is equivalent to almost 30–35 mg of additional iron. To put this in context, this amount of iron is equivalent to the amount found in 100 L of human breast milk!
- *Capillary versus venous Hb/hematocrit*: The Hb/hematocrit of capillary blood can be 5–10% higher than from venous blood, especially hours immediately after birth or during skin cooling. This difference typically disappears by about 3 months of age. This fact needs to be kept in mind while interpreting serial Hb/hematocrit observations.

PHYSIOLOGICAL ANEMIA IN NEONATE

Physiologic Anemia of Infancy

- Due to the reasons discussed above, almost all neonates experience a progressive fall in Hb levels starting immediately after birth.
- However, due to the right shift of the Hb oxygen dissociation curve, this physiological anemia is not accompanied by a functional anemia as oxygen delivery to the tissues is adequate.
- By 8–12 weeks, the Hb reaches its nadir of 10–11 g/dL.
- This decreases the oxygen delivery to tissues thus stimulating EPO production and RBC production. Rapid erythropoiesis uses up the iron stores.
- As term neonates have sufficient stores for 15–20 weeks, this anemia is tolerated well and usually requires no treatment. However, beyond this period they may need iron supplementation.
- Laboratory investigations reveal a hypogenerative marrow with decreased hematocrit, decreased reticulocyte count, and low EPO.

Anemia of Prematurity

- Seen exclusively in preterm neonates, anemia of prematurity (AoP) is an exaggeration of physiologic anemia.
- The Hb nadir in AoP is lower (7–8 g/dL) than the term infants (10–11 g/dL). Also, the nadir is reached earlier (at 6–8 weeks of age) than in the term infants because of the following:[4]
    - Decreased RBC mass and iron stores due to deprivation of third-trimester iron transport to the fetus
    - Shorter half-life of RBC than term neonates
    - More rapid body growth which requires iron, and
    - Lower EPO compared to term neonates

  Nonphysiological factors such as infections, inadequate nutrition, and phlebotomy losses further exaggerate the condition.
- While low EPO in physiologic anemia of infancy is proportionate to the degree of anemia, in AoP the EPO levels are disproportionately low compared to the degree of anemia. Think why?

  Recall that the liver is not only the predominant site of erythropoiesis till the second trimester, but also a major source of EPO. EPO production switches from the liver to the kidney near term gestation and the "hypoxia sensor" of the liver is much less sensitive than the kidney. Thus, while a term neonate's kidney responds to tissue hypoxia due to anemia by increasing EPO production, the preterm liver is less responsive leading to disproportionately lower levels of EPO to the hematocrit seen in AoP.
- *Laboratory investigations* are similar to physiologic anemia of infancy, however unlike term infants, the more rapid and profound fall in Hb may be accompanied by clinical signs of anemia.
- *Management:* It is important to note that AoP is not due to nutrient deficiency and thus not responsive to iron or folate supplementation. Thus, iron supplementation in

early infancy (2–3 months age) does not prevent a fall in Hb. EPO is also not routinely used.[4] Preventive strategies such as delayed cord clamping, and reducing phlebotomy losses are helpful. In severe cases causing symptoms, packed red blood transfusion(s) may be required.

ETIOLOGY OF ANEMIA IN NEONATE

The nonphysiologic causes of anemia in neonates can be broadly remembered by "triple H"—*H*emorrhage, *H*emolysis, and *H*yporegeneration.

Hemorrhage (Anemia Due to Blood Loss)

These are characterized by negative direct Coombs' test (DCT) with normal peripheral smear. Bilirubin levels are generally normal unless hemorrhage is retained. Acute cases have normal hematocrit and reticulocyte count though infants may have features of shock. In chronic cases, hematocrit is low with increased reticulocyte count.

- *Obstetric causes:* Abruptio placenta, malformations of cord and placenta, rupture of cord (more common in short or dysmature cords), inadvertent incision of placenta at the time of cesarean section
- *Occult blood loss:*
  - *Fetomaternal bleeding:* This can be acute or chronic. Chronic fetal to maternal transfusion has a reticulocyte count >10%. Placental malformations, obstetric procedures, or spontaneous fetomaternal bleeding may cause this type of bleeding.
  - *Fetoplacental bleeding:* This may be associated with occult cord prolapse, cesarean section with infant held above placenta, and chorioangioma.
  - Twin-to-twin transfusion (TTTS) and twin anemia polycythemia sequence (TAPS)
- *Bleeding in the neonatal period:*
  - *Intracranial bleed:* This may be associated with prematurity, traumatic delivery especially vacuum extraction, and coagulation disorders.
  - *Bleeding from different sites:* Cephalohematoma, subgaleal hemorrhage, gastrointestinal bleeding (rule out swallowed maternal blood by Apt test), bleeding from umbilical catheters, or cord clamp.
  - *Iatrogenic:* It is one of the most common causes of anemia in neonatal intensive care units (NICU).

Hemolysis (Hemolytic Anemia)

These are characterized by decreased hematocrit, increased reticulocyte count, and increased (indirect) bilirubin level. DCT is positive in immune-mediated cases.

- *Immune hemolysis:*
  - Rh or ABO incompatibility
  - Minor blood group incompatibility (e.g., C, E, Kell, and Duffy)
  - Maternal autoimmune disease such as lupus, autoimmune hemolytic disease
- *Hereditary RBC disorders:*
  - *RBC membrane defects:* Hereditary spherocytosis and elliptocytosis
  - *Metabolic defects:* Glucose-6-phosphate dehydrogenase (G6PD) and pyruvate kinase deficiency
  - *Hemoglobinopathies:* α- and γ-thalassemia.
- *Infections:* Sepsis and disseminated intravascular coagulation.

Hyporegeneration (Decreased RBC Production)

These are characterized by decreased hematocrit and reticulocyte count with negative DCT. Bilirubin levels are normal. This includes:

- Physiologic anemia of infancy
- Anemia of prematurity
- Infections such as rubella and parvovirus
- Diamond–Blackfan syndrome
- Bone marrow infiltrative disorders.

DIAGNOSTIC APPROACH TO ANEMIA IN NEWBORN

While anemia is common in newborns especially preterm neonates, ascertaining the etiology of anemia in these vulnerable groups can be challenging. A good history and examination is always the initial guide toward diagnostic evaluation and determining possible etiology. The family history should enquire about anemia, jaundice, gallstones, and splenectomy, while the obstetric history should look for evidence of abruption or intrapartum blood loss.

Clinical features of anemia in newborns depend upon the chronicity and severity of anemia. Acute anemia such as due to blood loss or hemolysis presents as tachycardia, tachypnea, metabolic acidosis, poor perfusion, and signs of shock, while chronic cases may manifest as poor weight gain, increase in apnea or bradycardia, increased oxygen, or respiratory support requirement, unexplained tachycardia, and metabolic acidosis. These features of chronic anemia are more pronounced in preterm neonates.

It is important to note that not every newborn with anemia requires a diagnostic evaluation to determine the cause. If the newborn is appearing well and the Hb/hematocrit is not significantly below the 5th centile or there is a clear history of blood loss, no further workup is usually required.

Laboratory investigations are required to ascertain the cause of anemia when hematocrit is significantly below the 5th centile and the cause is not clear from history and examination. A stepwise approach to testing minimizes unnecessary pricks and blood loss **(Table 14.2.1)**.

Level 1 investigations are the first line of investigations done in cases of significant neonatal anemia. A simple peripheral smear often can reveal very important clues to diagnosis. Note that the mean corpuscular volume (MCV) values tend to be higher in neonates, thus microcytic anemia with iron deficiency seen in children is not that common in neonates. Level 2 investigations, guided by history and clinical examination, are often required while looking for

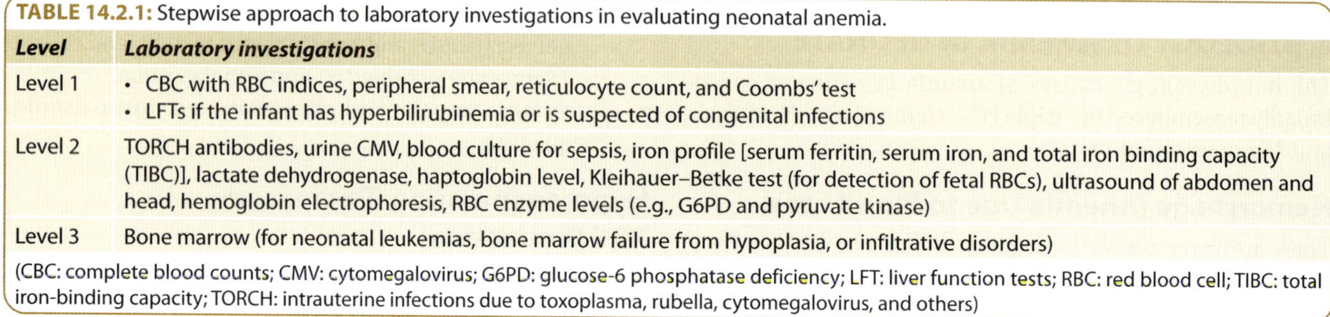

TABLE 14.2.1: Stepwise approach to laboratory investigations in evaluating neonatal anemia.

Level	*Laboratory investigations*
Level 1	• CBC with RBC indices, peripheral smear, reticulocyte count, and Coombs' test • LFTs if the infant has hyperbilirubinemia or is suspected of congenital infections
Level 2	TORCH antibodies, urine CMV, blood culture for sepsis, iron profile [serum ferritin, serum iron, and total iron binding capacity (TIBC)], lactate dehydrogenase, haptoglobin level, Kleihauer–Betke test (for detection of fetal RBCs), ultrasound of abdomen and head, hemoglobin electrophoresis, RBC enzyme levels (e.g., G6PD and pyruvate kinase)
Level 3	Bone marrow (for neonatal leukemias, bone marrow failure from hypoplasia, or infiltrative disorders)

(CBC: complete blood counts; CMV: cytomegalovirus; G6PD: glucose-6 phosphatase deficiency; LFT: liver function tests; RBC: red blood cell; TIBC: total iron-binding capacity; TORCH: intrauterine infections due to toxoplasma, rubella, cytomegalovirus, and others)

Flowchart 14.2.1: A simplified diagnostic approach to anemia in newborns.

Complete blood count (CBC) (confirm anemia: Hemotocrit <5th centile for age)

'Significant' anemia and cause unknown

No → Monitor closely, repeat CBC in few days/weeks

Yes → **Reticulocyte count**

Decreased →
Physiologic anemia of infancy
Anemia of prematurity
Congenital hypoplastic anemia
Other cases of decreased production
Infections (rubella, parvovirus)

Increased → **Direct Coombs' Test (DCT)**

DCT positive → Immune hemolysis (Rh or ABO incompatibility or maternal autoantibody)

DCT negative → **Mean corpuscular volume (MCV)**

Low MCV → Chronic intrauterine blood loss (Twin-to-twin transfusion, Fetomaternal hemorrhage, Abruptio placenta)
α or γ-thalassemia

Normal/High MCV → **Peripheral smear**

Normal and no hemolysis → Blood loss due to:
- Obstetric causes
- Neonatal period (massive cephalohematoma, subgaleal, intracranial bleed, GI, or other site bleed, etc.)
- Iatrogenic

Normal and hemolysis present →
- Infections (Bacterial, viral, fungal, and toxoplasma)
- Galactosemia
- Hypothyroidism
- Some cases of congenital
- RBC enzyme defects

Abnormal →
- *Spherocytes:* Hereditary spherocytosis
- *Elliptocytes:* Hereditary elliptocytosis
- *Spiculated RBCs*: PK deficiency
- *Schistocytes and RBCs fragments:* DIC and other microangiopathic processes
- *Bite cells:* G6PD deficiency

focused etiology, while level 3 investigation (bone marrow) being more invasive is used sparingly.

A simplified diagnostic approach to anemia in newborns is provided in **Flowchart 14.2.1**.

THERAPY

While packed red blood cell (PRBC) transfusion remains the mainstay of treatment, there is a lack of consensus about the threshold and timing of PRBC transfusions, due to its associated complications.[2] Apart from different reference intervals for different gestation and postnatal age, another problem encountered is that unstable and sick neonates may have hematocrit values within the reference interval, yet those values may not be optimal for patient's care. As an example, a neonate on room air born at 26 weeks' gestation with a hematocrit of 25% on day 28 has hematocrit which is within the reference interval. However, if same neonate was hypoxemic and on ventilator, the hematocrit of 25% might be too low for optimal care. As a result, just because hematocrit falls within the reference interval does not mean it is appropriate for the clinical situation.

Therefore, determining whether a hematocrit value indicates need for PRBC transfusions often requires cognizance of the gestational age, the postnatal age at sample collection, the anatomical site of the blood sampling (venous, arterial, or capillary) as well as illnesses involved and the level of intensive care support. The latest Indian guidelines for the use of blood components in neonates have been published by the National Neonatology Forum of India in 2020.[5]

CONCLUSION

Neonatal anemia is a multifactorial condition influenced by physiological, developmental, and pathological factors. Understanding the variations in hematologic physiology across gestational ages is key to accurate diagnosis and management. While physiologic anemia is often well-tolerated, conditions like anemia of prematurity require targeted interventions. Preventive strategies such as delayed cord clamping and minimizing blood loss, combined with a systematic diagnostic approach, ensure effective identification and care for affected neonates.

REFERENCES

1. Christensen RD, Bahr TM, Tweddell SM, Ohls RK, Henry E. Diagnosing Anemia in Neonates: An Evidence-Based Approach. NeoReviews. 2023;24(6):e343-55.
2. Bell EF. Red cell transfusion thresholds for preterm infants: finally some answers. Arch Dis Child Fetal Neonatal Ed. 2022;107(2):126-30.
3. Kalteren WS, Verhagen EA, Mintzer JP, Bos AF, Kooi EMW. Anemia and Red Blood Cell Transfusions, Cerebral Oxygenation, Brain Injury and Development, and Neurodevelopmental Outcome in Preterm Infants: A Systematic Review. Front Pediatr. 2021;9:644462.
4. Aher SM, Ohlsson A. Early versus late erythropoietin for preventing red blood cell transfusion in preterm and/ or low birth weight infants. Cochrane Database Syst Rev. 2020;2020(2):CD004865.
5. Pandita A, Kumar A, Gupta (Chairperson) G, Taligasalam V, Tewari VV. Use of Blood Components in Newborns. J Neonatol. 2020;34(4):199-217.

14.3 Approach to Diagnosis of Anemia in Children

Ved Prakash Choudhry

INTRODUCTION

A person is considered anemic when the amount of hemoglobin (Hb), the oxygen-carrying pigment of the red blood cells (RBCs), is reduced from the normal value for that age and gender. Anemia is characterized by abnormally low levels of healthy RBCs, reduced Hb, or red cell blood volume (hematocrit). The reduction of any or all the three blood parameters affects the oxygen-carrying capability of blood adversely. **Table 14.3.1** provides the mean Hb concentration levels along with two standard deviations (SD) below the mean for normal population for gender and age, defined as normal blood levels by the World Health Organization (WHO), the United Nations Children's Fund, and the United Nations University.

The levels of Hb below which child is considered to have anemia as per the WHO criteria are given in **Table 14.3.2.**[1]

EPIDEMIOLOGY

Anemia is widely prevalent and is a major cause of morbidity. Globally, anemia affects 1.62 billion people which correspond to 24.8% of the population.[2] The highest prevalence is seen in preschool-age children (47.4%), and the lowest prevalence is

TABLE 14.3.1: Normal hemoglobin, hematocrit, or packed cell volume at different ages.

Age	Hb (g/dL)		PCV (%)		RCC (10^{12}/L)	
	Mean	±2 SD	Mean	±2 SD	Mean	±2 SD
Birth (cord blood)	16.5	13.5	51	42	4.7	3.9
1–3 days	18.5	14.5	56	45	5.3	4.0
7 days	17.5	13.5	54	42	5.1	3.9
14 days	16.5	12.5	51	39	4.9	3.6
1 month	14.0	10.0	43	31	4.2	3.0
2 months	11.5	9.0	35	28	3.8	2.7
6 months	11.5	9.5	35	29	3.8	3.1
1 year	12.0	10.5	36	33	4.5	3.7
2–6 years	12.5	11.5	37	34	4.6	3.9
6–12 years	13.5	11.5	40	35	4.6	4.0
12–18 years:						
Girls	14.0	12.0	41	36	4.6	4.1
Boys	14.5	13.0	43	37	4.9	4.5

(Hb: hemoglobin; PCV: packed cell volume; RCC: red cell count; SD: standard deviation)

TABLE 14.3.2: World Health Organization criteria for hemoglobin below which person is anemic.

Age/gender groups	Hb (g/dL)
Children 6 months to 5 years	<11
Children 6–14 years	<12
Adult males	<13
Females (nonpregnant)	<12
Females (pregnant)	<11

(Hb: hemoglobin)

seen in men (12.7%). Various surveys, including the National Family Health Survey (NFHS), have revealed that anemia is highest in children below 6-59 months of age.[3] The data given in **Table 14.3.3** indicates that the prevalence of anemia in India has increased over the last decade. It is more common in rural areas as compared to urban population.[4]

ETIOLOGY

The etiology of anemia is variable. It may occur because of:

- Decreased erythropoiesis either due to the deficiency of nutrition or the defect in erythropoiesis
- Increased blood loss
- Diminished red cell survival as result of immune disorders and chronic infections.

  The etiology of anemia is given in **Box 14.3.1**.[1]

TABLE 14.3.3: Prevalence of anemia in different groups as per surveys in India.

Group	Reference	Prevalence (%)
Early childhood	NFHS 1, 1998–99	74
Preschool children (6–35 months)	NFHS 3, 2006–7	79
Children (6–59 months who are anemic (<11.0 g/dL)	NFHS 4, 2015–16, Total	58.6
	NFHS 5, 2019–21, Urban	64.2
	NFHS 5, 201–21, Rural	68.3
	NFHS 5, 2019–21, Total	67.1
Adolescent girls	Seshadri, 1999, Rural Gujarat	62
	Seshadri, 1999, Urban affluent	22
	ICMR, 2001, Rural India	90

(ICMR: Indian Council of Medical Research; NFHS: National Family Health Survey)

CLASSIFICATION

It is preferable to classify anemia based on the pathophysiologic effects for its better understanding **(Table 14.3.4)**. The classification based on red cell morphology (red cell size and Hb content) is useful in determining the etiology and is helpful in investigating the cause of anemia with minimal investigations **(Flowcharts 14.3.1 to 14.3.4)**.

BOX 14.3.1: Etiology of anemia.

- Inadequate dietary intake of iron and other nutrients (vitamin B_{12} and folic acid)
- *Inadequate supply of iron at birth:* Prenatal or maternal nutrition deficiency, prematurity, low birthweight, multiple births, and prenatal blood loss
- *Inadequate absorption of iron:* Gluten-induced enteropathy, atrophic gastritis, and postgastrectomy, presence of phytates and calcium in the diet, and presence of recurrent or chronic diarrhea
- Excessive physiological demands of iron associated with rapid growth periods—prematurity, preschool period, and adolescence
- *Hemolytic anemias:*
  - *Extracorpuscular:* Autoimmune hemolytic anemia, microangiopathic hemolytic anemia, toxic effects due to infection, due to splenomegaly, paroxysmal nocturnal hemoglobinuria, hematopoietic disorders (e.g., leukemia, aplastic anemia, and myelodysplastic anemia), blood loss (acute or chronic), chronic illnesses, such as juvenile rheumatoid arthritis, renal disease, heart diseases, poisoning (lead, arsenic, and other heavy metals)
  - *Intracorpuscular:* Red cell membrane disorders (hereditary spherocytosis, hereditary elliptocytosis, and hereditary stomatocytosis), red cell enzyme deficiencies (G6PD deficiency, PK deficiency), thalassemia, and hemoglobinopathies
- Hematopoietic disorders (leukemia, aplastic anemia, and myelodysplastic anemia)
- Blood loss (acute or chronic), secondary to parasitic infections such as hookworm, giardiasis, gastritis, peptic ulcer, polyps, etc.
- Chronic illnesses such as juvenile rheumatoid arthritis, renal disease, heart diseases, etc.
- *Poisoning:* Lead, arsenic, and other heavy metals

(G6PD: glucose-6-phosphate dehydrogenase; PK: pyruvate kinase)

CLINICAL FEATURES

Presence of anemia is associated with significant morbidity and mortality. The symptoms depend on the severity of anemia and whether it develops over a short or long period of time. Children may remain asymptomatic for long duration if the onset of anemia is insidious. When the onset of anemia is acute, children develop significant pallor, exertional dyspnea, and restlessness. Severe anemia also leads to cardiac enlargement, flow murmurs, and even chronic heart failure.[1]

The tongue papillae are atrophied. The structural changes in the intestine may result in malabsorption and even protein enteropathy. Nails may become brittle and flat with longitudinal ridges (koilonychia). The work capacity or the

TABLE 14.3.4: Pathophysiologic classification of anemia.

Anemia due to increase blood loss	• Acute posthemorrhagic anemia • Chronic blood loss due to some chronic disease, e.g., hookworm infestation, ulcerative colitis, polyps, etc.
Anemia due to impaired red cell production	*Deficient heme synthesis:* • Iron-deficiency anemia • Vitamin B_{12} or folic-acid deficiency (megaloblastic anemia) *Deficient globin synthesis:* • Thalassemia • Aplastic anemia (acquired or hereditary) • Pure red cell aplasia • Anemia of chronic disorders (chronic renal failure and cardiac disorders)
Anemia due to increased red cell destruction (hemolytic anemia)	• Sickle cell anemia, thalassemia, and hemoglobinopathies • Autoimmune hemolytic anemia • Hereditary spherocytosis • Paroxysmal nocturnal hemoglobinuria

Flowchart 14.3.1: Clinical approach to a child with anemia.

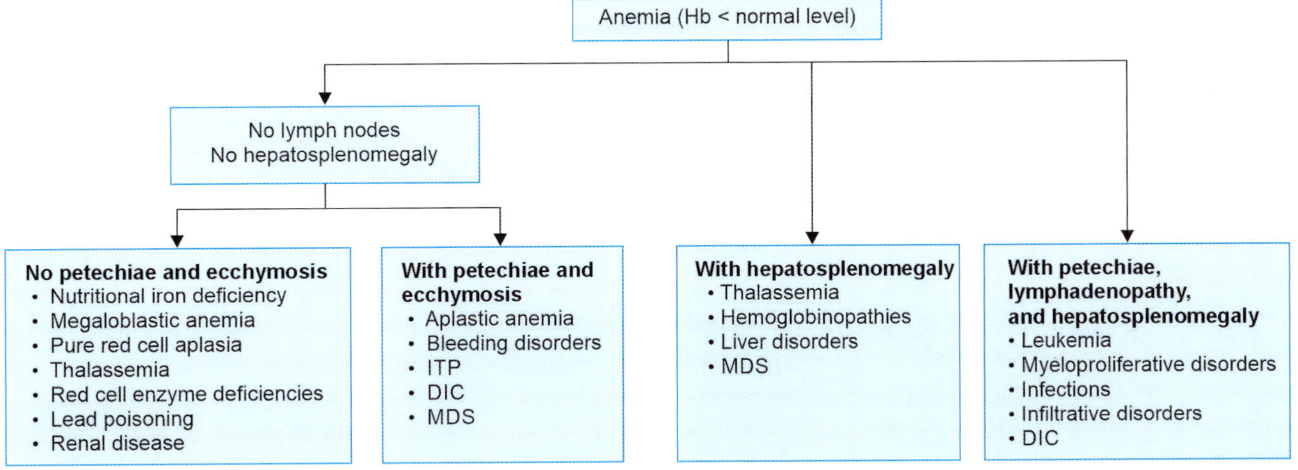

(DIC: disseminated intravascular coagulopathy; Hb: hemoglobin; ITP: immune thrombocytopenic purpura; MDS: myelodysplastic syndrome)

Flowchart 14.3.2: Algorithm for microcytic and hypochromic picture on peripheral blood.

- Microcytic and hypochromic anemia (MCV <80 fL)
  - Serum iron
    - Serum iron normal/high
      - Hemoglobin electrophoresis (High-pressure liquid chromatography)
        - Normal
          - Congenital dyserythropoietic anemia
          - Sideroblastic anemia
        - Abnormal
          - Thalassemia
          - Hemoglobinopathies (HbE, HbS, HbD, etc.)
    - Serum iron low
      - Serum ferritin levels
        - Low ferritin
          - Iron-deficiency anemia
        - Normal/high ferritin
          - Anemia of chronic disorders
          - Rheumatoid arthritis
          - Chronic renal failure
          - Anemia of chronic infection

(HbD: hemoglobin D; HbE: hemoglobin E; HbS: Sickle cell hemoglobin; MCV: mean corpuscular volume)

Flowchart 14.3.3: Algorithm for macrocytic picture on peripheral blood.

- Macrocytic picture (MCV >100 fL)
  - Reticulocyte count
    - Reticulocytes high
      - History of blood loss
        - Present
          - Acute blood loss
          - Chronic blood loss
        - Absent
          - AIHA
          - Hemoglobinopathies
          - Thalassemia
          - Hereditary spherocytosis
          - CDA
    - Reticulocytes normal/low
      - Bone marrow
        - Nonmegaloblastic
          - Normoblastic
            - Liver disease, e.g., cirrhosis
            - Hypothyroidism
          - Dyserythropoietic
            - CDA
            - Myelodysplastic anemia
        - Megaloblastic
          - Folate and B_{12} level
            - Folate low
              - Folate deficiency
            - Vitamin B_{12} low
              - Vitamin B_{12} deficiency

(AIHA: autoimmune hemolytic anemia; CDA: congenital dyserythropoietic anemia)

Flowchart 14.3.4: Algorithm for normocytic and normochromic picture on peripheral blood.

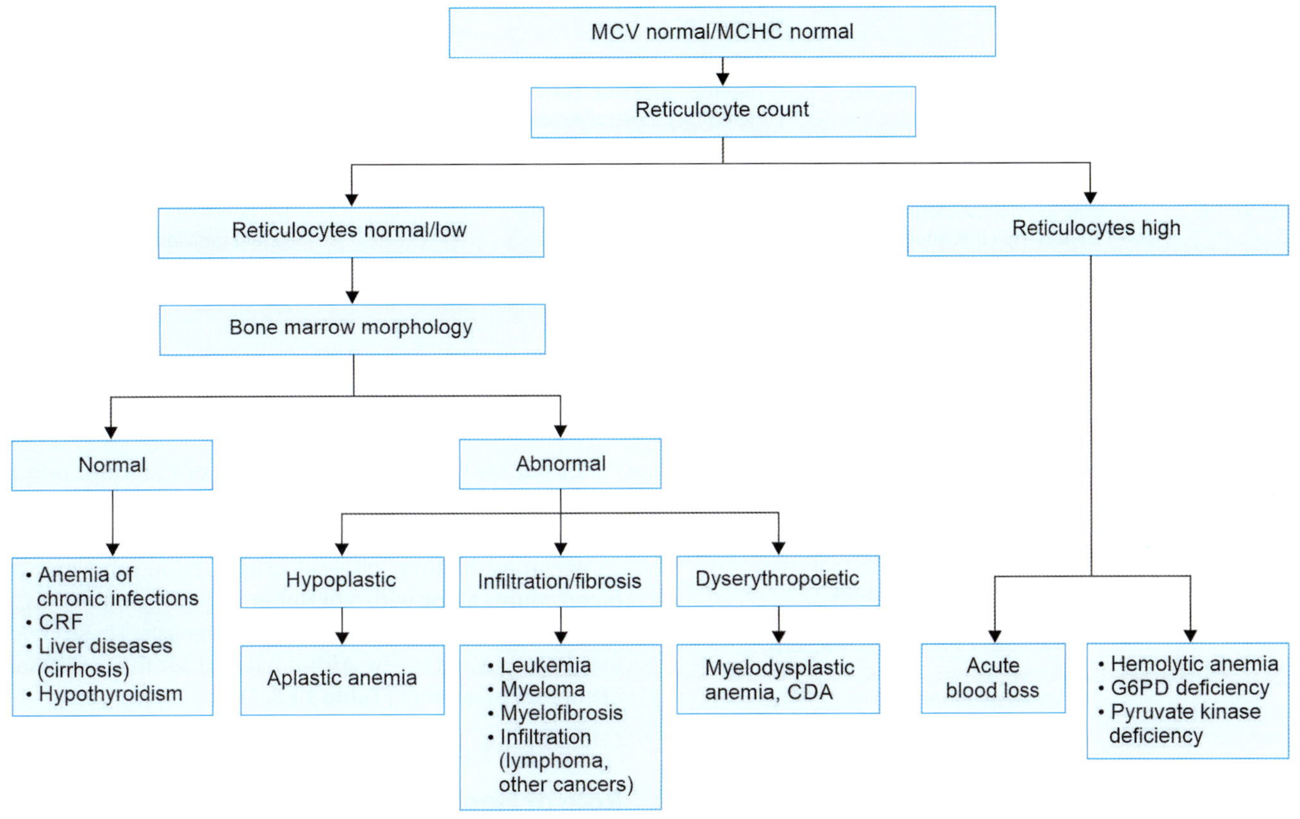

(CDA: congenital dyserythropoietic anemia; CRF: chronic renal failure; G6PD: glucose-6-phosphate dehydrogenase; MCHC: mean corpuscular hemoglobin concentration)

activity of the child gets impaired. Persistence of anemia leads to neurophysiological and developmental deficits.[5] Children may have reduced motor development, muscle power, and coordination with behavioral effects. The intelligence quotient of children may be reduced by 5–7 points.

Persistence of anemia has adverse impact on the bactericidal activity of neutrophils and impairs cell immunity leading to recurrent infections. In addition, children may develop lymph node enlargement, petechiae, ecchymosis, or bleeding symptoms. Presence of liver and spleen enlargement should be observed during the examination of child.

Clinical Approach to Anemia

The causes of anemia are variable; hence, family history of anemia, jaundice, race, and area of origin should be recorded. Detailed clinical history should be taken, including dietary habits and chronic diarrhea. Evaluation of growth retardation and organomegaly is of utmost importance. A simple algorithm for clinical diagnosis is given in **Flowchart 14.3.1**.[6]

Laboratory Approach to Anemia

The objectives of laboratory tests are to determine the type, severity, and the etiology of anemia. The severity of anemia is determined by the Hb level. The examination of peripheral blood film identifies the morphological type of anemia. Based on the red cell morphology and red cell indices, such as mean corpuscular volume (MCV), the anemia has been classified as microcytic hypochromic, macrocytic, and normocytic normochromic. Simple algorithms toward the diagnosis of various etiological conditions are given in **Flowcharts 14.3.2 to 14.3.4**.

Reticulocyte count indicates the erythropoietic activity and serves as a useful indicator for diagnosis. Recently red cell distribution width (RDW) is provided by most cell counters. RDW along with MCV helps in differentiating various etiological conditions **(Table 14.3.5)**.

Detailed peripheral smear examination is of utmost importance. This not only helps in the classification of anemia but the presence of red cell abnormalities gives clue to the underlying diagnosis.

TABLE 14.3.5: Diagnosis of anemia on mean corpuscular volume and red cell distribution width.

RDW	*Low MCV*	*Normal MCV*	*High MCV*
RDW <15	• Thalassemia trait • Heterozygous HbE, HbC, etc. • ACD	• ACD • Heterozygous HbE, HbS, HbC, etc. • Hereditary spherocytosis • Acute hemorrhage	• Aplastic anemia • MDS • Myeloma • Liver disease • Hyperthyroidism
RDW >15	• Iron-deficiency anemia • Thalassemia intermedia • Sideroblastic anemia • ACD • RBC fragmentation	• Early nutritional deficiency • Myelodysplasia • Myelophthisic anemia • Sickle cell disease	• B_{12} deficiency • Folate deficiency • AIHA • *Drugs:* Hydroxyurea

(ACD: anemia of chronic disease; AIHA: autoimmune hemolytic anemia; MCV: mean corpuscular volume; MDS: myelodysplastic syndromes; RBC: red blood cell; RDW: red cell distribution width)

TABLE 14.3.6: Abnormal cells on peripheral smear and underlying disorders.

Characteristics	*Underlying disorders*
Spherocytes	• Hereditary spherocytosis • Autoimmune hemolytic anemia • Hemolytic transfusion reactions • Severe burns • Hypersplenism • *Clostridium welchii* septicemia
Target cells	• Hemoglobinopathies S, C, D, and E • Thalassemia • Postsplenectomy
Elliptocytes	• Hereditary elliptocytosis • Thalassemias • Myelofibrosis • Myelophthisic anemia
Schistocytes and fragmental red cells	• Disseminated intravascular coagulopathy • Hemolytic uremic syndrome • Prosthetic heart valve • Malignant hypertension
Basophilic stippling	• Thalassemia • Poisoning (arsenic or lead) • Sideroblastic anemia • Unstable hemoglobins • Hemolytic anemias

- Presence of spherocytes in high number (15–20/100 RBC) is suggestive of hereditary spherocytosis or immune hemolytic anemia, while the presence of a few spherocytes is suggestive of other states **(Table 14.3.6)**.
- Presence of schistocytes suggests life-threatening conditions, such as disseminated intravascular coagulopathy or hemolytic uremic syndrome.
- Presence of basophilic stippling is suggestive of various types of hemolytic anemia, lead or arsenic poisoning, and sideroblastic anemia **(Table 14.3.6)**.

Based on the peripheral blood examination, one may proceed to undertake specific tests to confirm the etiology of the disease process.

Detailed history, clinical examination, and complete blood counts along with a peripheral blood examination, and various algorithms aid in reaching a diagnosis. These children may be subjected to few additional tests for the confirmation of etiology of anemia **(Table 14.3.7)**.[7]

RECENT ADVANCES

Role of Hepcidin in Iron Metabolism

Several studies have demonstrated that hepcidin controls the release of iron from variety of cells, such as macrophages, hepatocytes, and enterocytes into plasma.[8] However, the recycling of iron from RBC lysis and release of iron from tissue iron stores are carried by the interaction of hepcidin with ferroportin which is a cellular iron exporter in vertebrates.

It has been shown that the release of ferroportin is primarily expressed by enterocytes and macrophages, which is also controlled by hepcidin.

Iron homeostasis in the body is controlled by very complex mechanism, and the main components include:

- Erythropoietic activity
- Hypoxia
- Iron stores
- Inflammation

All these components act through common pathways of hepcidin. Enhanced erythropoiesis and the presence of tissue hypoxia decrease the hepcidin production by the liver, resulting in enhanced iron absorption. In contrast, increased iron stores and the presence of infection reduce the hepcidin production by the liver, which causes internalization and degradation of ferroportin by the target cells, leading to decrease or total inhibition of iron absorption by the enterocytes and release of iron by the macrophages and other cells. Thus, hepcidin primarily controls the iron absorption.

TABLE 14.3.7: Diagnostic tests to confirm the etiology of anemia.

Bone marrow aspiration	Type of erythropoiesis (normocytic or megaloblastic), leukemia, hemolytic anemia, etc., and marrow iron stores
Bone biopsy	Aplastic anemia, infiltrative disorders (lymphoma or secondaries), and myelofibrosis
Iron-deficiency anemia	• Serum iron and total iron-binding capacity • Percent saturation of transferrin • Serum ferritin • Serum transferrin receptor assays • Red cell protoporphyrin levels
Megaloblastic anemia	• Serum folate levels • Serum vitamin B_{12} levels • Schilling test of vitamin B_{12} absorption
Pernicious anemia	• Estimation of intrinsic factor in gastric juice • Intrinsic factor antibodies levels • Parietal cell antibodies • Plasma (or serum) vitamin B_{12}-binding capacity
Hemolytic anemia	• Estimation of serum haptoglobin levels • Demonstration of hemosiderin in urine • Serum bilirubin, total and indirect, serum urobilinogen • Serum lactic dehydrogenase levels
Hereditary hemolytic anemia	• Detection of enzyme deficiency, such as G6PD assay and pyruvate kinase assay • Glutathione stability test for G6PD-deficient patients • Coomb's test (direct and indirect) • Hemoglobin electrophoresis (high-pressure liquid chromatography) • Hemoglobin fetal and hemoglobin A2 estimation
Acquired hemolytic anemia	• Warm and cold autoantibodies detection • Detection of incomplete antibodies by the Coomb's test • Ham test for paroxysmal nocturnal hemoglobinuria • Flow cytometry evaluation of G-PI-linked proteins on neutrophils • CD-55 and CD-59 markers

(CD: clusters of differentiation; G6PD: glucose 6-phosphate dehydrogenase; G-PI: glycophosphatidylinositol)

Infections and Anemia

Children, particularly infants, living in the developing countries are highly vulnerable to infectious diseases. Iron deficiency is associated with the impairment of innate (natural) immunity and cell-mediated immunity, thereby contributing to increased risk of infections.[9] The iron acquisition by the microbes and their virulence is determined by various host and microbial mechanisms which are given here:

- Reduced neutrophil function with decreased enzymatic activity
- Impaired natural killer cell activity and impaired bactericidal activity
- Depression of T-lymphocyte numbers/defective T-lymphocyte response, impaired interleukin-2 production
- Reduced production of macrophage migration inhibition factor
- Impaired or delayed cutaneous hypersensitivity tuberculin reactivity

Developmental and Neurophysiological Deficits in Iron Deficiency

Recently, iron deficiency has been shown to have effect on brain metabolism, neurotransmitter function, and myelination.[5] These changes lead to neurophysiological and developmental deficits in infants and children, which may have adverse effect even during adulthood. Motor development and coordination are reduced. In addition, there is impaired language development, scholastic achievement, psychological and behavioral effects, such as insecurity, fatigue, poor attention, etc. These children have decreased physical activity. Changes in brain iron content caused by early iron deficiency are not reversible on iron therapy in animals in spite of correction of anemia and other tissue iron deficits. These observations provide explanation why some effects of iron deficiency are irreversible even after complete correction of iron deficiency. Thus, the timing of iron deficiency during infancy and its severity have critical impact even in adult life.

KEY MESSAGES

- Anemia is widely prevalent in the world. It is more common in the developing countries.
- Children and women are worst affected.
- Iron-deficiency anemia (IDA) is the most common cause of anemia.
- Persistence of severe IDA has adverse effects in adult life.
- Detailed history, examination, and use of simple tests are essential for early diagnosis.
- Simple algorithms are helpful for early diagnosis of anemia.

REFERENCES

1. Galllagher PG. Anemia in the pediatric patient. Blood. 2022;140:571-93.
2. Choudhry VP. Hematological disorders. In: Ghai OP, Gupta P, Paul VK (Eds). Essential Pediatrics, 6th edition. New Delhi: CBS Publishers and Distributors; 2004. pp. 298-307.
3. National Family Health Survey-5 (NFHS-5) 2019–2021. Key Indicators. India and 14 States/UTs (Phase II). New Delhi: Ministry of Health & Family Welfare, Government of India; 2021.

4. Yadav S, Chandra J. Iron deficiency: beyond anemia. Indian J Pediatr. 2011;78(1):65-72.
5. Madan N, Rusia U, Sikka M, Sharma S, Shankar N. Developmental and neurophysiologic deficits in iron deficiency in children. Indian J Pediatr. 2011;78(1):58-64.
6. Oski FA, Brugnara C, Nathan DG. A diagnostic approach to the anemic patient. In: Nathan DG, Orkin SH (Eds). Hematology of Infancy and Childhood, 5th edition. Philadelphia, PA: WB Saunders; 1997. pp. 375-84.
7. Chandra J, Dewan P, Kumar P, Mahajan A, Singh P, Dhingra B, et al. Diagnosis, treatment and prevention of nutritional anemia in children: Recommendations of the Joint Committee of Pediatric Hematology-Oncology Chapter and Pediatric and Adolescent Nutrition Society of Indian Academy of Pediatrics. Indian Pediatr. 2022;59:782-801
8. Choudhry VP. Hepcidin and its role in iron metabolism. Indian J Pediatr. 2010;77(7):787-8.
9. Kumar V, Choudhry VP. Iron deficiency and infection. Indian J Pediatr. 2010;77(7):789-93.

14.4 Nutritional Anemias in Infancy and Childhood

Niranjan G Shendurnikar, Tushar P Shah

INTRODUCTION

Nutritional anemias are conditions in which hemoglobin (Hb) concentration of a given individual is below the normal level for the age, due to the deficiency of one or more bioavailable nutrients needed for hematopoiesis, i.e., nutrients required for Hb synthesis and/or maintenance are insufficient and the Hb can be increased by the supplementation of the deficient nutrient(s).[1] The most common cause of nutritional anemia is due to the deficiency of iron, vitamin B_{12} (cobalamin, Cbl) and/or folic acid. In addition, the role of other nutrients such as vitamin D, vitamin A, vitamin C, pyridoxine, and proteins in erythropoiesis is being recognized.[2]

EPIDEMIOLOGY

As per the National Family Health Survey-5 (NFHS-5; 2019–21) data, a rising prevalence of anemia across all ages with the highest spike in children (6–59 months) with a rise to 67.1% (NFHS-5) from 58.6% (NFHS-4, 2015–16) followed by in adolescent girls aged 15–19 years is observed. Whereas as per Comprehensive National Nutrition Survey (CNNS) conducted in 2016–18, it revealed that 41% of preschoolers (1–4 years), 24% school age children (5–9 years) and 28% of adolescents (10–19 years) in India have anemia. It was observed that nutritional anemia was responsible as cause in 68.9, 50.9, and 65.1% in children aged 1–4 years, 5–9 years, and 10–19 years, respectively. Iron deficiency was common in children under 5 years of age, while folate and vitamin B_{12} deficiency was higher among schoolgoing and adolescent age groups. 10–18% of children and adolescents with anemia had combined iron and folate or vitamin B_{12} deficiencies.[3,4]

CONSEQUENCES OF ANEMIA ON HEALTH

Anemia is an indicator of both poor nutrition and poor health. Nutritional anemias lead to impaired cognitive function and diminished attention span in children, which affect learning, physical strength, lowered immunity as well as decreased productivity and an increased economic burden to the country. These changes may be irreversible in younger children thus emphasizing the need for timely prevention, diagnosis, and treatment.

The World Health Organization (WHO) suggests the use of Hb cut-off levels below two standard deviations (SD) from the population mean (in a representative healthy population) to define anemia and its severity as shown in **Table 14.4.1**.[5]

For Indian children, cutoffs of Hb in healthy children are lower, by 1–2 g/dL based on the large scale, nationally representative survey of children and adolescents aged 0–19 years conducted (Comprehensive National Nutrition Survey) in 2019.[6,7]

CLASSIFICATION

Nutritional anemia can be classified based on the morphological features of red blood cells (RBCs). Cases with iron deficiency have microcytic anemia and are characterized by smaller sized RBCs with low mean corpuscular volume (MCV). The lower limit of MCV (fL) in children below 2 years is 70 fL **(Table 14.4.2)**.[8] For children between 2 and 10 years, a lower limit of MCV is 70+ age in years. In older children and adolescents (≥10 years), the MCV cutoff value is <80 fL.[8]

TABLE 14.4.1: Hemoglobin thresholds (g/dL) to define severity of anemia as per the world health organization.[5,8]

	Nonanemic[#]	*Mild*	*Moderate*	*Severe*
Children 6–59 months	>11	10–10.9	7–9.9	<7
Children 5–11 years	>11.5	11–11.4	8–10.9	<8
Children 12–14 years	>12	11–11.9	8–10.9	<8
Men aged ≥15 years	>13	11–12.9	8–10.9	<8
Women aged >15 years	>12	11–11.9	8–10.9	<8
Pregnant women	>11	10–10.9	7–9.9	<7

[#]Nutritional anemias: tools for effective prevention and control. Geneva: World Health Organization; 2017.

TABLE 14.4.2: Cutoffs for laboratory estimates for the diagnosis of nutritional anemia.[7,8]

Parameter	*Cut-off*
Microcytosis, MCV (fL)	
Up to 2 years	<70
2–10 years	<70 plus age (years)
>10 years	<80
Macrocytosis, MCV (fL)	
2–10 years	>84 plus 0.6 × Age (years)
>10 years	>90
Serum ferritin (μg/L)	
<5 years	<12 (IDA)
>5 years	<15 (IDA)
With infection	<30 (IDA)
Serum transferrin saturation	<16% (IDA)
Reticulocyte Hb content (CHr) (pg)	<29 (IDA)
% hypochromic cells	>5% (IDA)
Free erythrocyte protoporphyrin level (FEP) (μg/dL)	
<5 years	>70 (IDA)
>5 years	>80 (IDA)
Serum folate (ng/mL)	<4 (Folate deficiency)
RBC folate (ng/mL)	<100 (Folate deficiency)
Vitamin B_{12} (pg/mL)	<200 (Vitamin B_{12} deficiency)
Homocysteine (mol/L)	>15 (Folate deficiency)
Methyl malonic acid (nmol/L)	>750 (Vitamin B_{12} deficiency)

IRON-DEFICIENCY ANEMIA

Iron deficiency is the most common cause (nutritional or otherwise) of anemia and is estimated to contribute to approximately 50% of all cases of anemia among nonpregnant and pregnant women, and 42% of cases in children under 5 years of age worldwide. About one-third of world population suffers from iron-deficiency anemia (IDA) of which 90% lives in the third-world countries. Infants, preschool children, adolescents, and women of child-bearing age are at the greatest risk. The WHO estimates that roughly 50% of anemia prevalence can be attributed to iron deficiency.[5]

IRON REQUIREMENTS DURING CHILDHOOD

Understanding the requirements, intake and bioavailability of iron is essential to explain the vulnerability of some individuals to develop IDA. The iron released from senescent red cells during the first 8–12 weeks of life (a period of quiescent erythropoiesis) is stored in the body and helps to maintain erythropoiesis up to 4–6 months in a normal term baby and up to 2 months in a low-birth-weight baby.

- Normal infants have about 75 mg of iron per kg bodyweight, two-thirds of which is present in RBCs.
- Infants and young children should continue to absorb 0.8–1.0 mg of iron daily to reach the adult level of stores of 4–5 g.
- The majority of body iron is in the form of Hb with about 10% in iron-containing proteins in nonheme tissues (myoglobin and cytochromes).
- Further 10–15% is stored intracellularly as ferritin or its degradation product, hemosiderin.
- Iron requirements are highest in infancy during the period of rapid growth, and these are also increased during adolescence, menstruation, pregnancy, and lactation.
- The iron requirement is crucial for the physiologic and metabolic processes which are involved with oxygen transport, oxidative metabolism, and the cellular growth. Though anemia is the end result of continued iron deficiency, it must be remembered that iron deficiency that suboptimal iron levels affect all the tissues.

Normal body loss of iron is about 20 μg/kg/day, but this may increase manifold during the episodes of diarrhea, dysentery, and parasitic infestations. Factors, such as preferential delivery of iron to fetus during the third trimester, delayed cord clamping, and exclusive breastfeeding in the first 6 months of life, protect infants from becoming iron deficient. Malnutrition, chronic infections, and worm infestations also contribute to a high prevalence of anemia.

ETIOLOGY

The causes of IDA are listed in **Box 14.4.1**. These are dependent on three main principle factors of pathogenesis such as inadequate intake and/or assimilation of iron or increased physiologic requirements or chronic ongoing blood loss.[9]

Source of Iron

Iron in the diet is contained in two forms: Heme iron (in animal products such as meat, poultry, and fish) and nonheme (mainly from plants products). Iron is also contained in tissues as ferritin in liver, spleen, and bone marrow and myoglobin in muscles. Heme iron is better absorbed than nonheme iron and is not influenced by dietary factors. Breastmilk in spite of low levels of iron (0.5 mg/L) has a better absorption and bioavailability as compared to cow's milk. Good sources of iron in the diet include pulses, dals, green leafy vegetables, bajra, dates, nuts, jaggery, meat, and fish. The administration of 50 mg of vitamin C daily increases iron absorption by twofold.

CLINICAL MANIFESTATIONS

Iron deficiency is a systemic disorder involving multiple systems rather than being an isolated hematological condition associated with anemia. The peak incidence of iron deficiency in children occurs between 6 months and 3 years, followed by adolescents 11–17 years. Children between 6 months and 24 months are a particularly high-risk group for the development of iron deficiency due to the low content of bioavailable iron in the weaning foods in the developing countries. It is important to take dietary history of excessive milk intake (>500 mL/day).

BOX 14.4.1: Causes of iron deficiency.

Decreased iron stores
- Preterm
- Small-for-date babies
- Twins

Decreased intake/assimilation
- Delayed introduction of complementary feeds
- Malnutrition/iron-poor diet/malabsorption syndromes
- Chronic infection/chronic diarrhea
- Gastrointestinal surgery

Increased losses
- Gastrointestinal bleeding (e.g., esophageal varices, Meckel's diverticulum, peptic ulcer, and intestinal polyps)
- Malaria
- Worm infestations (Hookworm and whipworm)
- Bleeding diathesis
- Fetomaternal hemorrhage
- Repeated venous sampling

Increased demands
- Prematurity
- Low birthweight (LBW)
- Recovery from severe malnutrition
- Adolescents (due to pubertal growth spurt and excessive menstrual blood loss)

The appearance of symptoms depends upon the rate of fall of Hb and hemostatic adjustment of various organs systems. As the fall of Hb is often gradual, the onset of symptoms is insidious. Given the gradual development of IDA, pediatric patients rarely exhibit significant physiological consequences of decompensation.

Initial manifestations include irritability, anorexia, and pallor. Later hyperdynamic circulation leads to palpitation, shortness of breath, easy fatigability, reduced exercise tolerance, and heart failure. Gradual onset of pallor may escape notice of the caregivers even when the Hb falls to 4 g/dL. Platonychia, koilonychias, glossitis, stomatitis, and angular cheilitis may be observed, especially with long-standing anemia **(Fig. 14.4.1)**. Pica is a well-documented feature of anemia in children and manifested as craving for inedible things, such as dirt, clay (geophagia), ice (pagophagia), laundry starch (amylophagia), salt, cardboard. Pica is seen in almost 70–80% of patients and is usually cured by prompt iron therapy.

Growth retardation and altered host immune responses are other associated features of IDA in children. Blue sclera is also occasionally observed in iron deficiency in children and adolescents.

Iron-deficiency anemia is associated with impaired performance on a range of mental and physical functions, including physical coordination and capacity, mental development, cognitive abilities, social and emotional development. Iron deficiency leads to impaired growth,

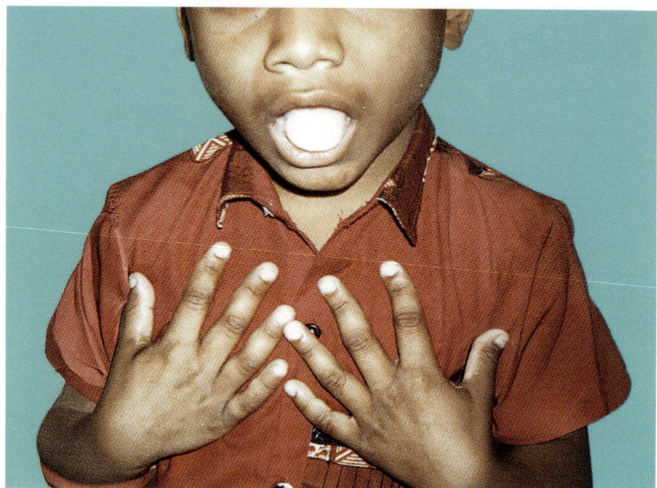

Fig. 14.4.1: Pallor in iron-deficiency anemia.
Courtesy: Dr MR Lokeshwar, Mumbai, India.

BOX 14.4.2: Nonhematologic features of iron deficiency in children.

- Koilonychia, glossitis, and esophageal web
- Pica
- Reduced work capacity
- Reduced exercise performance
- Decrease attention span/cognition

compromises cognitive development, and contributes to shortened attention span and scholastic failure **(Box 14.4.2)**.

Other health consequences include reduced immunity, increased morbidity, and increased susceptibility to heavy metal (including lead) poisoning. These changes may be related to functional changes in iron-containing enzymes at cellular level. IDA at the time of crucial brain growth and development may produce permanent and irreversible abnormalities in these functions.[3,8,10]

The triad of dysphagia due to esophageal webs, koilonychia, and splenomegaly with IDA is known as Plummer-Vinson or Paterson-Kelly syndrome and is not common in children. Mild hepatosplenomegaly is not uncommon in IDA, but significant hepatosplenomegaly is not a clinical feature of IDA. Atrophy of tongue papillae giving an appearance of a smooth tongue, malnutrition and other vitamin deficiencies may be coexistent.

INVESTIGATIONS IN IRON DEFICIENCY ANEMIA

- Iron-deficiency anemia develops sequentially from the depletion of iron stores, iron-deficient erythropoiesis to the resultant anemia **(Box 14.4.3)**. Laboratory evaluation in IDA is required to diagnose, assess the severity of anemia and iron status, and to establish its cause.[8]
- Hb, RBC count, and hematocrit are decreased in IDA along with low mean corpuscular volume (MCV), mean corpuscular hemoglobin (MCH), and MCHC concentration.
- Blood smear shows hypochromia, microcytosis, poikilocytosis, and target cells **(Fig. 14.4.2)**.
- Reticulocyte count is usually normal unless the child has an acute or recent blood loss or has received hematinics. However, in mild iron deficiency, RBC morphology and indices are not altered.
- Thrombocytosis is a common associated feature of IDA in children.
- Low serum iron, increased total iron-binding capacity (>470 μg/dL), and low transferrin saturation.
- Serum ferritin levels may be normal, if there is an associated illness (e.g., infectious and inflammatory diseases) as ferritin is an acute phase reactant.
- A low MCV with an elevated red cell distribution width (RDW) is strongly suggestive of IDA. RDW is highly sensitive (>90%) but low in specificity (50–70%) in detecting IDA.
- Bone marrow studies for the depletion of stainable iron are not recommended as other noninvasive investigations are available for the diagnosis.
- Soluble transferrin receptor measures the severity of IDA, and values >9 mg/L are considered abnormal.
- Newer red cell indices such as reticulocyte Hb have the advantage of estimation of availability of iron to form Hb.[8]

BOX 14.4.3: Summary of laboratory tests in iron-deficiency anemia.

- Depletion of stainable iron from BM
- Reduction of serum ferritin levels (<15 ng/mL)
- Increased RDW (>14.5%)
- Low serum iron (<75 mg/dL)
- Increased TIBC (>470 μg/dL)
- Low transferrin saturation (<12 and 14% for infants and children)
- Increased red cell protoporphyrin concentration

(BM: bone marrow; RDW: red cell distribution width; TIBC: total iron-binding capacity)

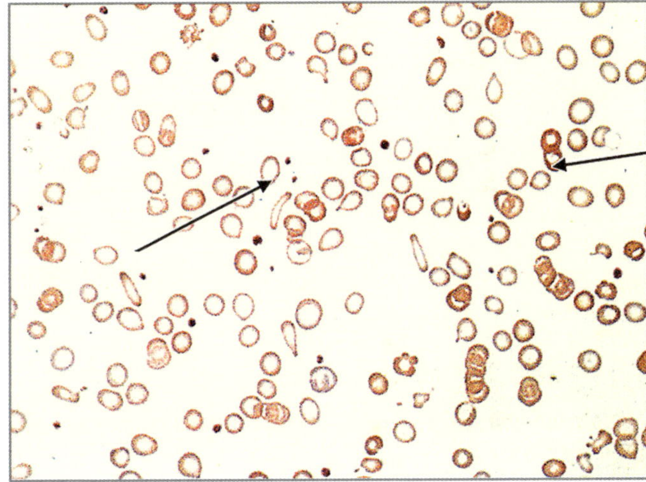

Fig. 14.4.2: Hypochromia and microcytosis in iron-deficiency anemia.
Courtesy: Dr MR Lokeshwar, Mumbai, India.

DIAGNOSIS AND DIFFERENTIAL DIAGNOSIS

A presumptive diagnosis of IDA can be made based on dietary history, clinical features, and the peripheral blood picture suggestive of microcytic hypochromic anemia with anisopoikilocytosis. The classical triad of low MCV, MCH, and MCHC for age is diagnostic and is often confirmed in a clinical setting by assessing response to empirical iron therapy. The diagnosis is confirmed if a trial of oral iron

Flowchart 14.4.1: A diagnostic approach for a child with microcytic hypochromic anemia.

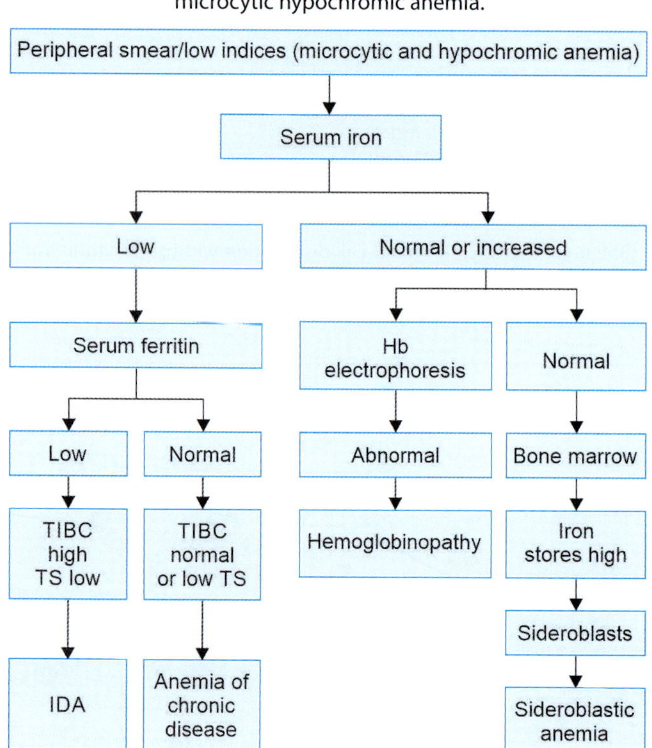

(IDA: iron-deficiency anemia; TIBC: total iron-binding capacity)

(3 mg/kg elemental iron per day) results in an Hb rise of >1 g/dL within 4 weeks for children with mild anemia or within 2 weeks for those with severe anemia.[11]

Though IDA is the most common cause of childhood microcytic hypochromic anemia, other important differentials of microcytic anemia include thalassemia syndromes, lead poisoning, sideroblastic anemia, and anemia of chronic disease. A diagnostic approach or a child with microcytic hypochromic anemia is shown in **Flowchart 14.4.1**.

MANAGEMENT

The basic principle of management of IDA is the correction of anemia and the eradication of underlying cause.[5,8,11]

Oral Iron Therapy

Bivalent iron salts, such as ferrous sulfate, fumarate, gluconate, succinate, and lactate, are preferred over ferric preparations as these are 4–10 times better absorbed than ferric compounds. In general, the solubility and the bioavailability of iron from ferric salts is 3–4 times less than that of ferrous sulfate. Iron salts of carbonate, citrate, choline citrate, and pyrophosphates are not efficiently absorbed. Hb-containing preparations do not offer additional advantage over simple ferrous salts and thus ferrous sulfate is a commonly used cost effective iron preparation over other alternatives. While prescribing oral iron, the amount of elemental iron in the preparation should be noted, and the dose should be calculated accordingly.[5,8,11] Newer iron preparations, such as ferrous ascorbate and ferrous bisglycinate, have a high bioavailability and are less affected by the dietary factors and have fewer gastrointestinal side effects.

TABLE 14.4.3: Response to iron therapy in iron-deficiency anemia.

12–24 hours	Replacement of iron enzymes, subjective improvement, decreased irritability, and increased appetite
36–48 hours	Initial bone marrow response and erythroid hyperplasia
48–72 hours	Reticulocytosis, peaking at 5–7 days
2–3 months	Repletion of stores

The recommended dosage of elemental iron is 3 mg/kg/day. Higher doses may increase side effects and reduce patient compliance. Iron preparations should not be given on a full stomach but are rather best given on empty stomach or in between the meals.[9,12] The side effects of oral iron therapy may include altered taste, staining of teeth, gastrointestinal upsets, and dark-colored stools.

Iron therapy needs to be continued for 3 months after the blood values have returned to normal to replenish the iron stores. Suboptimal response to iron therapy may be due to poor compliance, inadequate dosage, associated infections, occult blood loss, or other causes of microcytic hypochromic anemia and conditions such as coexisting folate or vitamin B12 deficiency. Celiac disease should be a consideration for underlying cause of iron deficiency if the anemia is not responding to appropriate dosing and is refractory to therapy. Information regarding the elemental iron content of the preparation is very important to ensure the adequate intake of therapeutic dose of iron and get an optimal response.

The assessment of response to treatment is made by reticulocyte count which rises in 2–3 days of therapy which indicates a bone marrow response and it becomes maximal at 5–7 days. **Table 14.4.3** shows the response to iron therapy in IDA.

A single daily dosing is considered as an equally effective option as compared to divided doses or alternate day options as they are reported to ensure a long-term compliance. An alternate day regimen may be given in gastrointestinal intolerance though it may result in a slower response. Along with the therapy of iron deficiency, a timely introduction of complementary feeds, diet with a rich source of iron for the child and the family, avoidance of excess of milk and phytates should be advised, and any underlying cause of the nutritional anemia must be addressed and treated simultaneously.[8]

TABLE 14.4.4: Supplementation of iron + folic acid: The intensified National Iron Plus Initiative.[11]

Age	Frequency of administration of iron + folic acid	Preparation	Albendazole (tablet: 400 mg), twice a year
6 months to 5 years	Twice a week (fixed days)	1 mL IFA = 20 mg elemental iron + 100 µg folic acid	• 1–2 years:1/2 tablet • >/2 years: 1 tablet
5–10 years	Once a week	45 mg elemental iron + 400 µg folic acid	
10–19 years		100 mg elemental iron + 500 µg folic acid	

(IFA: iron and folic acid)

Iron supplement should be started in a term and breastfed baby at 6 months of age as recommended by Intensified-National Iron Plus Initiative of Ministry of Health and Family Welfare (I-NIPI of MoHFW). In preterm babies, iron supplementation should be started at 2 weeks of age in dose of 2–4 mg/kg/day (maximum 15 mg) of elemental iron due to their inadequate body iron stores.[11]

Parenteral Iron Therapy

Parenteral iron is rarely administered in children. The response is not more rapid than oral iron. The indications include inflammatory bowel disease with blood loss, bowel resection, epidermolysis bullosa, heart failure, iron refractory IDA, and rarely poor tolerability to oral iron. The US Food and Drug Administration has approved use of iron sucrose, ferric gluconate, and iron dextran in children. Ferric carboxymaltose is approved in the USA for children ≥1 year.

Iron dextran is a complex of ferric hydrochloride and high molecular weight dextran. This needs to be given by IV route either by infusion or bolus (single total) dose. The dosage is calculated as: Iron (mg) = Weight in kg × Hb deficit (g/dL) × 4.

Life-threatening anaphylactic reactions may occur; and hence, parenteral iron should be given in hospital setting only. Other side effects may include fever, abdominal cramps, pain, skin rash, arthralgia, and serum sickness like illness. The use of iron dextran has decreased because of the risk of anaphylaxis. Ferric carboxymaltose injection has a better safety and tolerability profile than existing products and has little toxicity. High doses can be administered with good local tolerance.[8]

Prevention of Iron Deficiency

Appropriate nutritional strategies are important factors in the prevention of IDA. These include:

- Protection and promotion of breastfeeding with timely introduction of complementary feeding at 6 months of age.
- Early supplementation of preterm babies and low-birthweight infants from 4 to 6 weeks of age.
- Processes, such as germination (sprouting of green grams) and intake of green leafy vegetables, are also helpful in prevention of IDA.
- Periodic (once every 6 months) deworming should be considered in endemic area.

NATIONAL ANEMIA CONTROL PROGRAM

The National Anemia Control Program has now been adopted as Iron Supplementation: Anemia Mukt Bharat: The Intensified National Iron Plus Initiative (I-NIPI). The I-NIPI of the Ministry of Health and Family Welfare (MoHFW), Government of India, recommendations include iron and folic acid supplementation throughout childhood as stated in **Table 14.4.4.**[11] The program is to encourage and implement the recommendations of I-NIPI in everyday practice to reduce the burden of IDA in the community.

It is to be emphasized that iron supplementation has to follow a lifecycle approach as it starts in infancy and continues into the end of adolescence for boys and into adulthood for girls. Notably, all children, 6 months to 19 years, should receive regular iron supplementation. Bi-annual deworming with oral albendazole is done for all children between the age of 1 and 19 years. The iron supplementation is continued till 45 years in women. The practice of delayed cord clamping is encouraged and recommended.[8]

REFRACTORY IRON DEFICIENCY ANEMIA: IRON DEFICIENCY ANEMIA NOT RESPONDING TO ORAL IRON THERAPY

- Ensuring compliance to therapy with adequate dosages should be an integral part of follow-up evaluation and a prerequisite before labeling nonresponse to oral iron therapy.
- Conditions interfering with iron absorption such as celiac disease, *Helicobacter pylori* infection, autoimmune gastritis, or anemia of chronic disease may be underlying cause of IDA and must be considered after thorough evaluation.
- All such nonresponsive patients should be evaluated for ongoing/occult gastrointestinal blood loss such as cow's milk protein intolerance, Meckel diverticulum, and inflammatory bowel disease. Three consecutive stool samples should be evaluated for occult blood.

- Other causes of microcytic anemia such as anemia of chronic infection, thalassemia minor, lead poisoning, and sideroblastic anemia must be excluded.
- Iron-refractory and iron-deficiency anemia (IRIDA) is a rare inherited disorder in which absorption of oral iron is markedly impaired. IRIDA is caused by loss of function of the *TMPRSS6*/matriptase-2 gene, which causes iron deficiency due to inappropriately high hepcidin levels with markedly reduced iron absorption and increased sequestration of iron in macrophages. Such patients present with a mild hypochromic, microcytic anemia with very low serum iron levels, and low transferrin saturation. Serum ferritin levels are mostly within the normal range or even slightly elevated following treatment with intravenous iron. The diagnosis of IRIDA is confirmed by demonstrating biallelic mutation in the *TMPRSS6* gene. These patients can be treated with a trial of intravenous iron therapy.[8]

MEGALOBLASTIC ANEMIA

INTRODUCTION

Megaloblastic anemia is a macrocytic anemia caused by ineffective erythropoiesis due to vitamin B_{12} (cobalamin) or folate deficiency or both. Though both of these micronutrients are a common cause of megaloblastic anemia of childhood, vitamin B_{12} deficiency is more common than folate deficiency and infants born to B_{12}-deficient mothers and adolescents are more vulnerable to develop anemia due to B_{12} deficiency.[8] Other causes include drugs (e.g., methotrexate, phenytoin, and hydroxyurea) and liver diseases. Rarely, it can be caused by defective transport mechanism of vitamin B_{12} or folate gene mutation. Certain inborn errors of metabolism of vitamin B_{12} and folate lead to disorder of DNA synthesis contributing to megaloblastic anemia.

The anemia is thus named due to the classical presence of megaloblasts in bone marrow and macrocytes (large, structurally abnormal, and immature red blood cells) in the blood. These are formed as a result of asynchronous maturation between the nucleus and cytoplasm due to defective deoxyribonucleic acid (DNA) synthesis.[9] These deficiencies are enumerated in **Table 14.4.5**.

CLINICAL FEATURES

These children appear sicker than the degree of anemia warrants. Anorexia, mental apathy, and fatigability are early symptoms, while glossitis and diarrhea can also occur. Hyperpigmentation of dorsum of hands and knuckles are important findings **(Fig. 14.4.3)**. Tremors, hypotonia, failure to thrive, and developmental regression are also observed. Petechiae and other hemorrhagic manifestations may be seen due to associated thrombocytopenia. A mild degree of hepatosplenomegaly may also be clinically observed thus mimicking acute leukemia.[8,13]

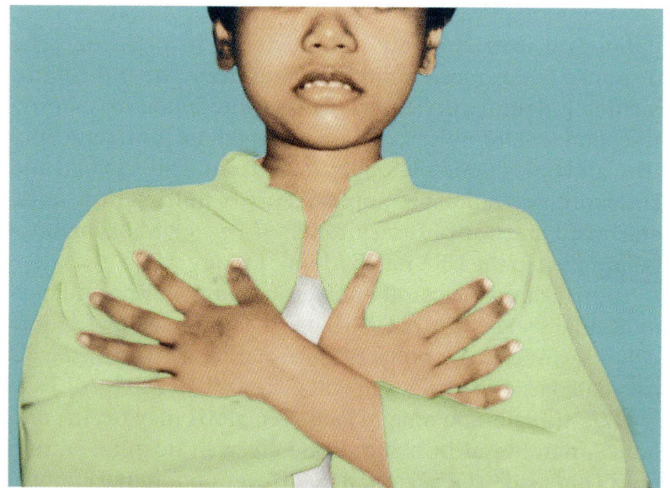

Fig. 14.4.3: Hyperpigmentation of dorsum of hands and knuckles. *Courtesy: Dr MR Lokeshwar, Mumbai, India.*

TABLE 14.4.5: Causes of vitamin B_{12} and folate deficiencies.[12]

Causes of deficiency	*Vitamin B_{12}*	*Folate*
Inadequate intake	• Dietary (<2 mg/day) • Vegetarian diets • Maternal deficiency	• Maternal deficiency with prolonged breastfeeding • Goat's milk feeding • Prematurity • Increased requirements—chronic hemolysis
Defective absorption	• Congenital intrinsic factor deficiency • Pernicious anemia • Imerslund–Grasbeck syndrome • Malabsorption due to various intestinal pathologies	• Congenital • Acquired—postintestinal surgeries, antibiotics and other drugs
Defective transport	• Transcobalamin deficiency	• *FOLR1* gene mutation
Disorders of metabolism	• Methylcobalamine deficiency • Liver disease • Protein energy malnutrition	• Congenital—methylenetetrahydrofolate reductase deficiency • Acquired—vitamin B_{12} deficiency and liver disease

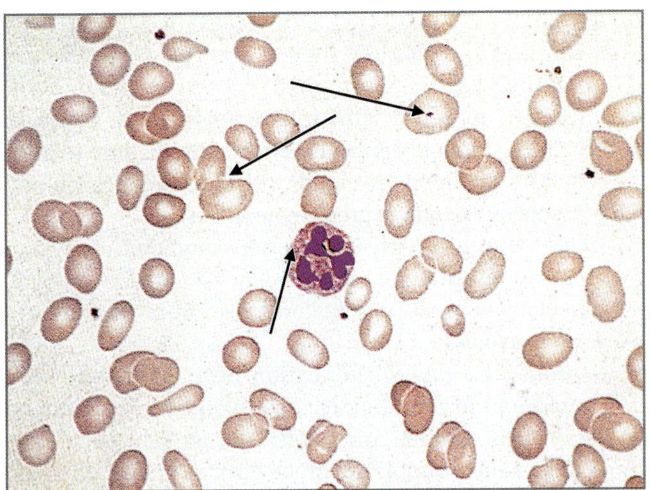

Fig. 14.4.4: Peripheral smear showing macro-ovalocytes and hypersegmented neutrophils.
Courtesy: Dr MR Lokeshwar, Mumbai, India.

LABORATORY DIAGNOSIS

Peripheral blood smear is one of the best indicators of megaloblastic anemia with the presence of macro-ovalocytes, hypersegmented neutrophils (at least 5% with more than five lobes or single cell with six or more lobes) are a cardinal feature, and a raised MCV >110 **(Fig. 14.4.4)**. There may be evidence of leukopenia and thrombocytopenia in severely deficient cases. Macrocytosis precedes anemia, and the MCV may be in the range of 110–130 fL. However, it may be masked by the concomitant presence of IDA. Red blood cells folate level and low B_{12} levels more accurately reflect the folate and vitamin B_{12} balance, respectively. Elevated lactate dehydrogenase (LDH) is a marker of ineffective erythropoiesis and often seen in megaloblastic anemia. Holotranscobalamin (HoloTC) is the "active" fraction of serum cobalamin and is more specific than serum cobalamin levels. It may be used as a routine diagnostic test in the future. Estimation of serum vitamin B_{12} and folate levels alone have limitations and need to be clinically interpreted. In general, vitamin B_{12} levels <200 pg/mL are considered deficient **(Flowchart 14.4.2)**.[8,9]

MANAGEMENT

Vitamin B_{12} and folic acid can be given either orally or parenterally. Parenteral administration is necessary in patients with malabsorption due to various causes, or intrinsic factor deficiency. Intravenous route should be used in patients with thrombocytopenia. In cases of confirmed deficiency, cobalamin deficiency should be corrected first for a few days before starting folate, as folate alone may precipitate or aggravate neurologic symptoms, if present.

Flowchart 14.4.2: Basic laboratory investigations in megaloblastic anemia.[12]

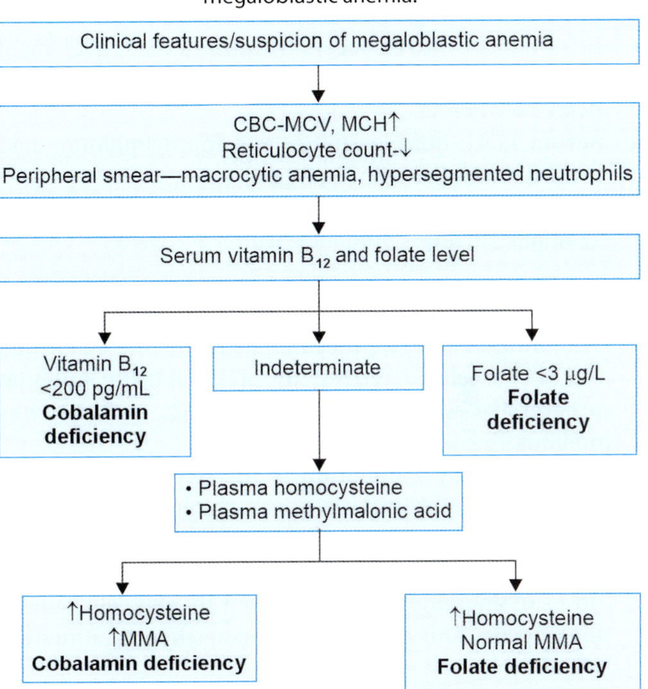

(CBC: complete blood count; MCH: mean corpuscular hemoglobin; MCV: mean corpuscular volume; MMA: methylmalonic acid)

Cobalamin

The dosages, schedules, and formulations used (cyanocobalamin, methylcobalamin, and hydroxycobalamin) widely vary in individual practice and their treatment regimens in children have not been studied well with variable recommendations for the dosage and routes of administration of vitamin B_{12}.[14] In a child with neurological symptoms due to B_{12} deficiency who needs a quick therapeutic response, initial parenteral route may be preferred. The recommended dose of vitamin B_{12} is 500–1,000 µg/day orally daily to be given in a fasting state as food interferes with the absorption of vitamin B_{12}, for 4–6 weeks, then once a week (or) 1,000 µg/day intramuscular/intravenous for 2 weeks or thrice weekly for 2 weeks followed by weekly for another six doses till hematocrit returns to normal.[8]

Folic Acid

Dose in children above 1 year of age and adults is oral folic acid 1–5 mg daily; in infants, 50 µg/day may suffice. Recently, dose of 0.2 mg/day over at least 6 months has shown optimal results. The British Society for Hematology Guidelines recommends dose of 5 mg of for 4 months in adults. In children with malabsorption, higher daily doses of 5 mg are preferred. The treatment duration should be 3–4 months to replenish the depleted stores.[7]

Response to Treatment

- Symptomatic response is usually seen within 48–72 hours.
- Brisk reticulocytosis occurs within 2–3 days, peaking at 5–8 days—degree of response is inversely proportional to degree of anemia.
- Serum LDH, homocysteine, and methylmalonic acid (MMA) normalize within a week.
- Bone marrow ineffective erythropoiesis is reversed within 72 hours; Hb levels normalize within 4–8 weeks.

Thiamine-responsive Megaloblastic Anemia

- Thiamine-responsive megaloblastic anemia syndrome (TRMA) is characterized by megaloblastic anemia, progressive sensorineural hearing loss, and diabetes mellitus.
- It is caused by a mutation in the *SLC19A2* gene and inherited in autosomal recessive fashion.
- Onset of megaloblastic anemia occurs between infancy and adolescence. The anemia is corrected with high doses of thiamine (vitamin B_1), but the red cells remain macrocytic, and anemia can recur when treatment is withdrawn.
- Lifelong supplementation of thiamine (50–100 mg/day) is required.[13]

BLOOD TRANSFUSIONS IN NUTRITIONAL ANEMIAS

- Severe anemia with no cardiac decompensation may be managed successfully with supplementation therapy, provided compliance is ensured.
- As recommended by the WHO, the indications for blood transfusion for children are with Hb ≤ 4 g/dL or Hb between 4 and 6 g/dL associated with cardiac decompensation.
- Packed red cells may be transfused at a volume of 5–10 mL/kg over 4 hours under close cardiac monitoring with the administration of furosemide, if required.[8,11,13]

PREVENTION OF NUTRITIONAL ANEMIA

- *Diet:* Iron rich diet and iron food fortification is important.
- *Infectious diseases*—Malaria control: chemoprophylaxis/ intermittent preventative treatment, insecticide-treated nets, and vector elimination.
- *Deworming:* Periodic treatment with anthelminthic (deworming) medicines should be given once a year when the prevalence of soil-transmitted helminth infections in the community is over 20%, and twice a year when the prevalence exceeds 50%.
- *Hygiene:* WASH strategy, safe water, sanitation, and hygiene have been successful in reducing the prevalence of anemia in children.
- *Neonatal care:* Delayed cord clamping (by at least 3 minutes, not earlier than 1 minute, or until cord pulsations cease after birth) is recommended for improved maternal and infant health and nutrition outcomes, including increased iron stores in term infants, reducing the need for blood transfusions for low blood pressure or anemia in preterm neonates.
- *High-risk groups*: Early interventions targeting adolescent girls for prevention of iron deficiency anemia are critical, especially in areas with high adolescent birth rates and early marriages.
- *Reproductive health:* Education must encompass the component of reproductive health and family planning services for women and adolescent girls, to encourage dialogue and promote adequate birth spacing. Education will help to promote gender equality and female empowerment.

CONCLUSION

Iron deficiency is a systemic disorder involving multiple systems rather than being an isolated hematological disorder associate with anemia. A long-standing iron deficiency in children can cause alterations in physiological contributing to impaired cognitive function and learning and lowered immunity and these changes may be permanent in young children. Such changes may be permanent in younger children thus emphasizing the importance of timely prevention, diagnosis and treatment. (I-NIPI) aims to reduce the burden of iron deficiency in the community.

REFERENCES

1. Ministry of Health and Family Welfare. (2013). Guidelines for Control of Iron Deficiency Anaemia: National Iron + Initiative. [online] Available from https://www.nhm.gov.in/images/pdf/programmes/child-health/guidelines/Controlof-Iron-Deficiency-Anaemia.pdf [Last accessed Dec., 2024].
2. Onyeneho NG, Ozumba BC, Subramanian SV. Determinants of childhood anemia in India. Sci Rep. 2019;9:16540.
3. Ministry of Health and Family Welfare. (2019–2020). National Family Health Survey (NFHS-5). Compendium of Fact Sheets: Key indicators India and 14 states/UTs (phase II). [online] Available from https://main.mohfw.gov.in/sites/default/files/NFHS-5_Phase-II_0.pdfphase1 [Last accessed Dec., 2024].
4. Comprehensive National Nutrition Survey (2016–18) reports: National Health Mission [Internet]. [online] Available from https://nhm.gov.in/index1.php?lang=1&level=2&sublinkid=1332&lid=713 [Last accessed Dec., 2024].
5. World Health Organization. (2017). Nutritional Anemias: Tools for Effective Prevention and Control. Geneva: World Health Organization; 2017. [online] Available from http://apps.who.int/iris/bitstream/handle/10665/259425/9789241513067-eng.pdf?sequence =1 [Last accessed Dec., 2024].
6. Sachdev HS, Porwal A, Acharya R, Ashraf S, Ramesh S, Khan N, et al. Haemoglobin thresholds to define anaemia in a

national sample of healthy children and adolescents aged 1-19 years in India: a population-based study. Lancet Glob Health. 2021;9:e822-e31.

7. Ministry of Health and Family Welfare. (2018). Anemia Mukt Bharat: Intensified National Iron Plus Initiative; 2018. [online] Available from https://anemiamuktbharat.info/dashemoglobinoard/#/ [Last accessed Dec., 2024].
8. Chandra J, Dewan P, Kumar P, Mahajan A, Singh P, Dhingra B, et al. Diagnosis, Treatment and Prevention of Nutritional Anemia in Children: Recommendations of the Joint Committee of Pediatric Hematology-Oncology Chapter and Pediatric and Adolescent Nutrition Society of the Indian Academy of Pediatrics. Indian Pediatr. 2022;59(10):782-801.
9. Dewan P, Trivedi M. Iron Deficiency Anemia. In: Gupta P (Ed). UG Textbook of Pediatrics, 1st edition. New Delhi: Jaypee Brothers Medical Publishers (P) Ltd.; 2023. pp. 526-30.
10. Powers JM. (2021). Iron deficiency in infants and children <12 years: Screening, prevention, clinical manifestations, and diagnosis. [online] Available from https://www.uptodate.com/contents/irondeficiency-in-infants-and-children-less-than12-years-screening-prevention-clinical-manifestationsand-diagnosis. [Last accessed December, 2024].
11. Bansal D, Radhakrishnan N, Prakash A. Iron Deficiency Anemia. Chandigarh: IAP Standard Treatment Guidelines Committee; 2022.
12. Powers J, Buchanan GR, Adix L, Zhang S, Gao A, McCavit TL. Effect of low-dose ferrous sulfate vs iron polysaccharide complex on Hb concentration in young children with nutritional iron-deficiency anemia: a randomized clinical trial. JAMA. 2017;317:2297-304.
13. Dheenadayalan, Abhilasha S, Gupta A. Megaloblastic Anemia. Chandigarh: IAP Standard Treatment Guidelines Committee; 2022.
14. Lee CKK. Drug Doses. In: Hughes HK, Kahl LK, The Johns Hopkins Hospital (Eds). The Harriet Lane Handbook, 21st Edition. Netherlands: Elsevier; 2018. pp. 842-3.

14.5 Bone Marrow Failure Syndrome

Nitin K Shah

INTRODUCTION

Aplastic anemia (AA) is an uncommon but potentially serious hematological disorder caused due to pancytopenia with a hypocellular bone marrow (BM) without infiltration or fibrosis with annual incidence of about 2–6/million population. It affects all the age-groups, and a small peak occurs at the age of 5–6 years due to inherited causes of AA. It results in decreased production of one or more hematopoietic lineages—mature red cells, granulocytes, and platelets leading to pancytopenia, i.e., AA or mono- or bicytopenia (e.g., agranulocytosis and red cell aplasia)—and is characterized by hypocellular (or fatty) marrow.

Aplastic anemia is defined as the presence of any two peripheral blood criteria [absolute neutrophil count (ANC) <1,500/mm^3, platelet count <150,000/mm^3, and reticulocyte count <40,000/mm^3] in the presence of BM hypocellularity on BM biopsy. Severe AA is characterized by the presence of any two of the peripheral blood criteria (ANC <500/mm^3, platelet count <20,000/mm^3, corrected reticulocyte count <1%) along with the presence of either of the marrow criteria—severe hypocellularity (<25%), moderate cellularity with <30% of hematopoietic cells. All nonsevere AA cases are defined as moderate AA. If left untreated, 80–90% of patients with severe AA will die within a year.

ETIOLOGY

Aplastic anemia is classified as acquired or inherited. Inherited cases may or may not be present at birth (congenital).[1] The etiological classification of AA is shown in **Box 14.5.1**. There is also a genetic predisposition for the development of marrow aplasia seen in patients with human leukocyte antigens (HLA) class II antigens DR2 and DPW3 **(Box 14.5.1)**. With the availability of genetic studies like whole exome sequencing, more and more cases of genetic defects leading to AA are being recognized. Some of these mutations are important to recognize as they have direct bearing on the choice of management. For example, if the patient with AA has homozygous mutation in *THPO* gene, all he needs is thrombopoietin mimetic agents like "Romiplostim" and "Eltrombopag" and stem cell transplantation, which is the treatment modality for severe AA will miserably fail in this case.

ACQUIRED APLASTIC ANEMIA

Pathophysiology

Seed Theory

Hematopoietic stem cell has tremendous proliferative capacity and has potential, not only to differentiate into various cell lineages, but also has property of self-renewal.[2,3]

It has been observed that primitive progenitor cell number is significantly reduced in all patients with severe AA. Seed theory contemplates that AA is caused due to the lack of pluripotent stem cells/progenitor cells or a qualitative defect of common stem cell population.

Soil Therapy

Survival and proliferation of hematopoietic cells are dependent on stroma cells.[2] Lack of surrounding microenvironment or stromal support (a soil or microenvironment deficiency) leads to AA. Success of BM transplantation favors seed theory, whereas success of immunotherapy proves that in some patients it is the soil which is at fault. Probably, there are different mechanisms of damage in different patients.

BOX 14.5.1: Etiology of aplastic anemia.

Acquired:
- Idiopathic
- Secondary
  - *Drugs:* Sulfa, anticancer drugs, antiepileptic agents, chloramphenicol, gold, carbamazepine, indomethacin, and phenylbutazone
  - *Chemicals:* Benzene, sniffing glue, insecticides, and dyes
  - Radiation
  - *Viruses:* Hepatitis, Epstein–Barr virus, and parvovirus
  - Pregnancy
  - Paroxysmal nocturnal hemoglobinuria (PNH)
  - *Miscellaneous*: Hypogammaglobulinemia, thymoma, eosinophilic fasciitis, preleukemic syndromes

Inherited:
- Fanconi anemia
- Dyskeratosis congenita
- Reticular dysgenesis
- Shwachman syndrome
- Diamond–Blackfan syndrome

Miscellaneous:
- Familial aplastic anemia
- Monosomy 7
- Down syndrome
- Amegakaryocytic thrombocytopenia

Clinical Presentation

Symptoms and signs depend on cell line involved. The onset is usually insidious.[3]

- Thrombocytopenia will lead to bleeding manifestations, such as skin bleeds, mucosal bleeds, gastrointestinal (GI) tract bleeding, hematuria, menorrhagia, and rarely intracranial hemorrhage **(Figs. 14.5.1A and B)**.
- Neutropenia will lead to infection and fever with or without localization of infection.
- Anemia appears last and, if severe, will lead to fatigue, breathlessness, puffiness, edema of feet, and congestive cardiac failure. One should look for evidence of etiological factors, such as viral hepatitis, past history of drugs use, etc. **(Fig. 14.5.2)**.
- Presence of hepatomegaly, splenomegaly, lymphadenopathy, bone pains, etc. usually rules out AA and suggests more sinister disease, such as leukemia. A child with AA is usually a sick looking child compared to a well looking child with immune thrombocytopenic purpura (ITP).

The differential diagnosis of pancytopenia is shown in **Box 14.5.2**.

Diagnosis

Diagnosis of AA is one of exclusions, and proper examination of BM is essential.[3]

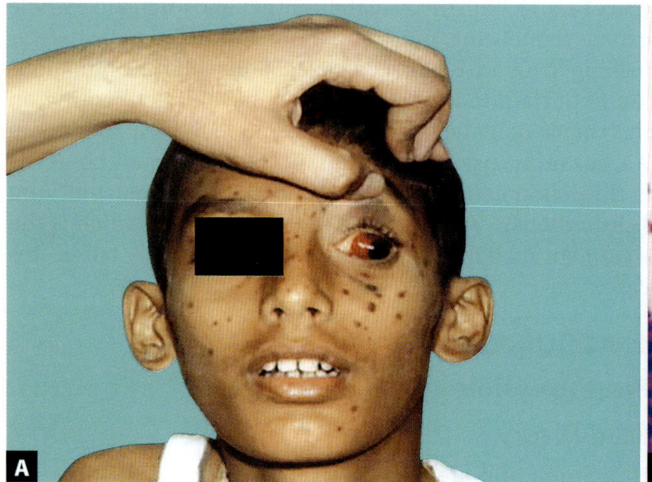

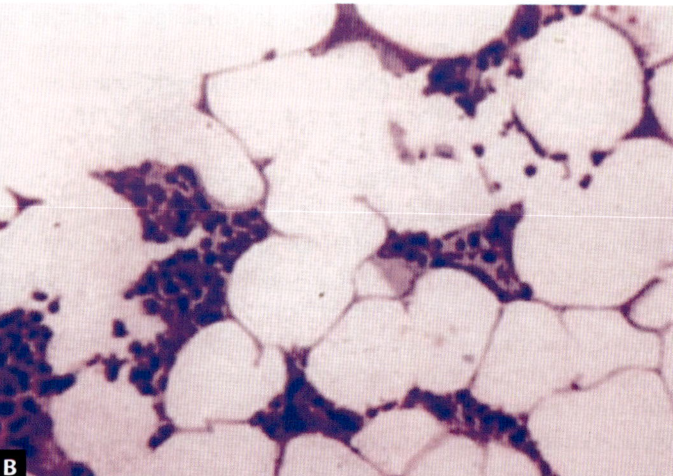

Figs. 14.5.1A and B: (A) A well child with ITP with purpura; and (B) Trephine biopsy in aplastic anemia.
Courtesy: Dr MR Lokeshwar and Dr Nitin Shah, Mumbai.

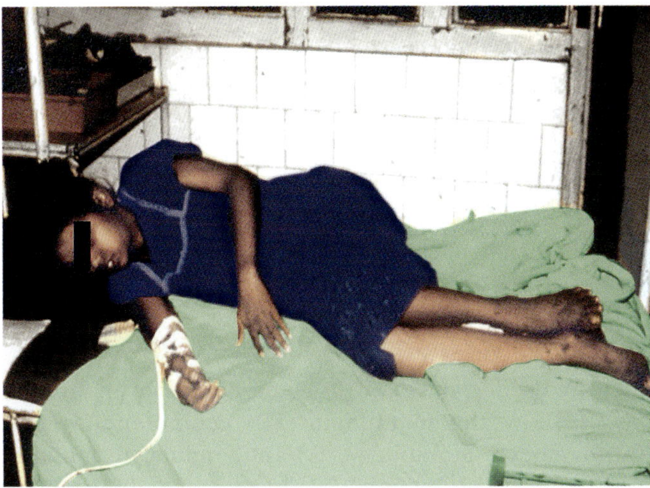

Fig. 14.5.2: Aplastic anemia. Sick-looking child, anemia, ecchymosis, petechiae, purpura, bleeding tendency, no hepatosplenomegaly, or bony tenderness.
Courtesy: Dr MR Lokeshwar and Dr Nitin Shah, Mumbai.

BOX 14.5.2: Differential diagnosis of pancytopenia in children.

- *Artifact*: Clot in sample
- *Genuine*: Central (bone marrow involved)
- *Replacement*: As in leukemia and other malignancies
- *Infections*: Kala-azar and severe malaria
- Myelosclerosis, osteopetrosis, myelofibrosis, HLH, and severe megaloblastic anemia
- *Peripheral*: Sequestration and hypersplenism (portal hypertension)
- *Destruction of mature elements*: Infection (most commonly viral), immune (SLE), complement-mediated (PNH)
- *Mechanism obscure*: Organic acidemias

(HLH: hemophagocytic lymphohistiocytosis; PNH: paroxysmal nocturnal hemoglobinuria; SLE: systemic lupus erythematosus)

Peripheral Blood

- Anemia with normal red cell distribution width, normocytic normochromic red blood cells (RBCs), occasional macrocytosis with low-corrected reticulocyte count.
- Leukopenia with decreased ANC.
- *Thrombocytopenia:* Decreased platelet count with normal mean platelet volume.
- *Stress erythropoiesis:* Raised fetal hemoglobin (HbF) and I antigen in some patients, especially in Fanconi's anemia which are phenotypically normal and may be confused with acquired AA.
- Coagulation parameters are generally normal.
- Pancytopenia with low reticulocyte count and without blasts in the blood is most likely due to marrow aplasia, but diagnosis requires aspirate and trephine biopsy of BM.
- Iron study may show iron overload.

The first sign of recovery after successful therapy is a rise in reticulocyte count, followed by increase in hemoglobin (Hb) levels, then neutrophils, while platelets are the slowest to recover if at all.

Bone Marrow and Trephine Biopsy

It is mandatory to do BM trephine biopsy as well as an aspiration to diagnose AA. It will show hypocellular marrow with empty spicules, increased fats spaces, hypoplasia may be patchy, especially early in the disease. Marrow consists of little more than fat, stromal cells, lymphocytes, and plasma cells; mast cells may be prominent. Because of diminution in the erythron, storage iron and sideroblasts may be increased; ring sideroblasts are not seen, except in rare specific syndromes **(Fig. 14.5.1B)**.

- *Stress cytogenetics:* It should always be done to rule out Fanconi anemia (FA) which will show increased spontaneous and clastogen-induced chromosomal breaks [like with mitomycin (MMC) or diepoxybutane (DEB)].
- *Others*: This includes tests to find out etiological factors, such as liver function test (LFT). It is prudent to do viral polymerase chain reactions (PCRs) for cytomegalovirus (CMV), Epstein–Barr virus (EBV), and parvovirus as these are treatable causes of AA. Bone marrow should also be subjected to cytogenetics studies as myelodysplastic (MDS) can present as AA earlier. Genetic studies like whole exome sequencing should be done especially in a child with early onset and born to consanguineous marriage to rule out genetic basis for AA. When I doubt about diagnosis, especially in those treated with steroids before BM studies, one should repeat BM after few weeks to rule out evolving leukemia.

Treatment

Curative Therapy

Curative therapy for AA involves the use of stem cell transplantation (SCT), immunomodulating therapy, and rarely other modalities of treatment.[2,3] With the availability of thrombopoietin mimetic agents such as "Romiplostim" and "Eltrombopag" many children can be tried on these agents along with cyclosporine with good results obviating the need for stem cell transplantation.[4-6]

Supportive Therapy

Supportive care provides the backbone of any therapy. It includes the use of appropriate antimicrobial therapy and occasional use of colony-stimulating factors for the control of infections, use of blood components to tackle anemia and thrombocytopenia, and management of iron overload.

- *Anemia*: Leukodepleted packed cell transfusion should be given to maintain Hb above 7–8 g/dL avoiding the use of relative donor for the fear of HLA sensitization and graft-versus-host disease (GVHD). Iron chelation is started when serum ferritin level is >500–1,000 ng/mL.
- *Bleeding*: Platelet transfusion is given when the patient has acute mucosal bleeds or severe internal bleeding. Isolated skin bleeds do not merit use of platelets, howsoever, grotesque and frequent they may be.

Prophylactic platelets may be used when the platelet count falls below <5,000/mm^3. However, misuse of platelets for minor or skin bleeds may lead to refractoriness. General measures, such as local pressure, use of epsilon-aminocaproic acid or tranexamic acid, dental care, avoiding use of nonsteroidal anti-inflammatory drugs, also help to prevent or minimize bleeding.

Infections

Standard protocols of febrile neutropenia should be followed in patients with AA who develop fever.

One can use 5–10 days of granulocyte-colony-stimulating factor (G-CSF) in 5 µg/kg/day subcutaneous to tide over crisis in a sick severely neutropenic child with fever.

Asepsis precautions, such as sterile diet, chlorhexidine mouthwashes, betadine bath, clean drinking water, and hand sanitization, go a long way in preventing infections in neutropenic patients.

Stem Cell Transplantation

Stem cell transplantation has become treatment of choice for patients with severe AA who are young and have HLA-matched sibling donor.[7] However, problem of SCT includes nonavailability of HLA-matched donor with small family size, nonaffordability of procedure, higher complications, especially in older than 40-year-old patients and poor response in previously heavily transfused patients and high mortality in patients who are sick with uncontrollable infection at the time of transplant. Use of matched unrelated donor [(MUD) through BM registries] or use of one of the parents as a haplo-identical matched donor has helped many patients with AA who do not have a matched sibling donor.

Cure rates in young patients with HLA-matched donors are over 80%. Complications of procedure include acute and chronic GVHD, interstitial pneumonia, other infections, veno-occlusive disease.

Other long-term problems secondary to SCT are those due to chemotherapy and radiation. These include poor pulmonary function, endocrine dysfunction, including infertility, cognitive disorders, leukoencephalopathy, and occurrence of second malignancy.

Immunomodulatory Therapy

It involves use of drugs, such as cyclosporine A (CsA), antithymocyte globulin, antilymphocyte globulin, and steroids used in combination.[6] One can use these agents alone if the patient cannot afford all the drugs; however, the response is not as well as when used in combination.

Antithymocyte Globulin/Antilymphocyte Globulin

They are used in doses of 10–40 mg/kg/day given for 5–10 days (follow the manufacturer's recommendations).[8] Antithymocyte globulin (ATG)/antilymphocyte globulin (ALG) can lead to anaphylaxis but fortunately it is rare. One should run the infusion slowly initially to look for hypersensitivity. Premedication with antihistamines will help to reduce other minor sensitivity reactions, such as fever, chills, and urticaria. Serum sickness after about 10 days of therapy is also common. 1 mg/kg of prednisolone is started on day 5 till 15 days and tapered over the next 7 days to counter these side effects.

Cyclosporin A

It is usually started on day 21 after steroids are stopped to avoid overlapping toxicities, such as hypertension. It is used in the doses of 5–10 mg/kg/day to keep a trough level of 100–150 ng/mL and continued for up to 6 months. Nephrotoxicity can be dose limiting. All patients on CsA must receive *Pneumocystis carinii* prophylaxis. Side effects, such as electrolyte disturbance, renal toxicity, liver toxicity, hirsutism, gingival hypertrophy, can occur.

Response to Immunosuppressive Therapy (Antithymocyte Globulin Plus Cyclosporine A)

It should be assessed after 3–4 months of treatment. Response is divided as follows:[6,9]

- *Complete response*: Defined as response to therapy where patient is free from transfusion support, Hb is maintained at normal level for age and gender, ANC is maintained >1.5 × 10^9/L, and platelets >150 × 10^9/L on repeated counts 4 weeks apart.
- *Partial response*: Defined as response to therapy where the patient is transfusion independent for RBC and/or platelets but does not have complete recovery of counts and does not anymore meet the criteria for severe AA.
- *No response*: The patient continues to fulfill criteria for severe AA. Overall long-term survival after immunomodulatory therapy is comparable to SCT in Western world for moderate AA. However, late clonal

hematological diseases, such as paroxysmal nocturnal hemoglobinuria, MDS syndromes, can occur after apparent recovery from aplasia. The success rate is 60–70%.

Androgenic Steroids

They stimulate erythropoiesis.[10] Nandrolone enanthate is used in a dose of 2–5 mg/kg/day as injectable form once in 10 days and continued till response is evident. Some response is seen in 20–30% of patients of moderate AA. Side effects are many, especially masculinization, stunted growth, hepatotoxicity, liver carcinoma, etc. Androgens have a mixed reputation. Probably dose makes the difference. One can use nandrolone decanoate at 5 mg/kg/week intramuscularly for at least 3 months. The advantage of this preparation is freedom from hepatotoxicity.

Corticosteroids

Steroids stimulate erythropoiesis. It also stabilizes capillary membrane and decreases bleeding. They are useful to counteract side effects of androgenic steroids on growing epiphysis and the serum sickness of immunotherapy.

Oral prednisolone is used in the dose of 0.5–1 mg/kg/day and tapered to a minimum effective dose.

Pulsed intravenous methylprednisolone in doses of 30 mg/kg has been used by some with limited success.

Side effects include hypertension, fluid electrolyte imbalance, infections, suppression of neuroendocrine axis, psychosis, avascular necrosis of femur, etc.

Colony-stimulating Factors

Hematopoietic growth factors, such as G-CSF and granulocyte-macrophage CSF, have been used to counter neutropenia in patients with severe AA, especially neutropenia following SCT. It helps to control infections when added to antibiotics and is helpful in the management of infected neutropenic patients. They may also be useful as a part of immunosuppressive regimen as they promote hematopoietic regeneration.

Thrombopoietin Mimetic Agents Like Eltrombopag and Romiplostim

Recently, two drugs are available which are thrombopoietin (TPO) agonists. They induce thrombopoiesis by stimulating the megakaryocytes by attaching to the TPO receptor. They also induce stem cells to improve erythropoiesis and granulopoiesis. Hence, these agents overall help to improve all three cell lines. They have been used extensively in ITP patients. We have used eltrombopag orally along with cyclosporine in AA patients and have found good results in 2 years follow-up without the need for stem cell transplantation.[6] They are, of course, the only treatment that a child with AA due to *THPO* mutation.

SECONDARY APLASTIC ANEMIA

Paroxysmal Nocturnal Hemoglobinuria

It is rare cause of acquired AA in childhood. A variety of cells are abnormally sensitive to lysis by complement, due to a defect in the glycosylphosphatidylinositol anchor, which binds proteins to the cell membrane (including those which protect against complement). We do PNH workup in many AA children but do not find PNH as a cause in majority.

Diagnosis might be considered for hemolysis of obscure origin. Chronic hemolysis is more common than sleep-induced hemoglobinuria, and hemosiderinuria is constant. Diagnosis is achieved by molecular testing for CD56.

Inherited Bone Marrow Failure Syndrome

This includes various inherited causes of mono-/bi-/tricytopenia, such as Fanconi anemia (FA), dyskeratosis congenita, congenital amegakaryocytic thrombocytopenia, Shwachman–Diamond syndrome and Diamond–Blackfan syndrome.

INHERITED APLASTIC ANEMIA

Fanconi Anemia

Fanconi anemia is inherited autosomal recessively, which is the most common cause of constitutional AA caused by defect in deoxyribonucleic acid that repairs leading to spontaneous or induced breaks in chromosomes.[11] Mean age at diagnosis is 7–8 years with 4% cases <1-year-old and 10% cases >16-year-old in age. Male-to-female (M:E) ratio is 1.06:1.0.

Clinical Features

Characteristic physical anomalies seen include generalized or perioral hyperpigmentation; Café-au-lait spots; short stature; microcephaly; mental retardation; skeletal anomalies, such as absent or hypoplastic thumb, bifid or triphalangeal thumb, absent radius, hypogonadism; spinal anomalies; renal anomalies, such as ectopic kidney; eye anomalies; deafness; ear malformations; and GI anomalies and cardiopulmonary anomalies. Around 15–30% of patients with FA are physically normal or have only short stature and/or skin changes **(Figs. 14.5.3A to C)**.

Thrombocytopenia is usually the first sign and may be misdiagnosed as immune-mediated thrombocytopenia if the association with somatic anomalies is not recognized; granulocytopenia and then anemia follows, evolving over months to years.

Macrocytosis and increased HbF levels are common, even before the onset of anemia. There is a risk (about 20%)

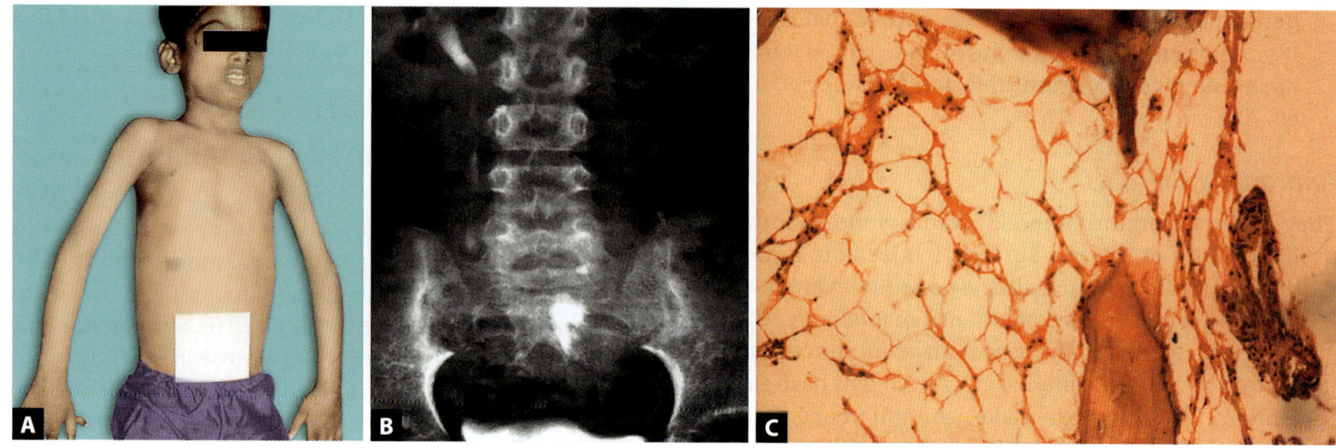

Figs. 14.5.3A to C: (A) Fanconi anemia; (B) Ectopic kidney; and (C) Trephine biopsy-hypocellular marrow.
Courtesy: Dr MR Lokeshwar and Dr Nitin Shah, Mumbai.

of malignancy, especially acute myelomonocytic leukemia (AML)-M4 and squamous cell carcinoma.

Diagnosis

It is achieved by stress cytogenetic study on peripheral blood induced by clastogen like mitomycine (MMC) or diepoxybutane (DEB), which will show increased chromosomal breaks. Homozygotes will show 8–9 breaks per cell compared to 0.06 in non-FA persons.

Prognosis

Without therapy, 80% FA patients die at mean age of 16 years or 2 years following the onset of aplasia and most by 4 years following aplasia. About 25% survive beyond the third decade.

Therapy

Androgens are helpful in FA patients with the mean age of survival being 17 or 7 years following the onset of aplasia, which is little better than no therapy. Around 50–75% of FA patients respond to androgens, and it may take 6–12 months for peak response to occur.

Stem Cell Transplantation

However, mainstay therapy is SCT which gives the only hope of long-term survival. Due to inherent chromosomal instability, these patients are sensitive to radiation and chemotherapy used for conditioning. Accordingly, low doses of cyclophosphamide should be used for better outcome.[7] The success of BM transplantation is 78% with modified conditioning regimen. One must screen the sibling donor to rule out occult FA.

Complications

Fanconi anemia patients are prone to develop malignancies, 20% chances of leukemia are mainly due to AML and liver cancers mainly due to androgens. Rare cancers include preleukemia, gynecological tumors, Wilms' tumor, medulloblastoma, etc.

DYSKERATOSIS CONGENITA

It is characterized by ectodermal dysplasia with changes in skin, nails, teeth, and hair. Leukoplakia of squamous surfaces may produce stricture of hollow viscera (e.g., esophagus), and there is a risk of about 10% for malignancy. Growth retardation is common. Most cases are X-linked recessive, but some are autosomal recessive or dominant **(Fig. 14.5.4)**.

CONGENITAL AMEGAKARYOCYTIC THROMBOCYTOPENIA

A rare disorder with severe diminution in megakaryocytes in marrow, attributed to stem cell defect, occurs without associated physical defects or abnormal chromosome fragility. About 80% evolve, at a median age of about 3 years, into aplastic anemia.

SHWACHMAN SYNDROME

It is characterized by pancreatic insufficiency (fatty replacement), neutropenia, metaphyseal dyschondroplasia, and growth retardation.

Neutropenia

It is intermittent rather than constant, but it may be cyclic, though not with the same predictability as true cyclic neutropenia. The neutrophil count may rise with infection

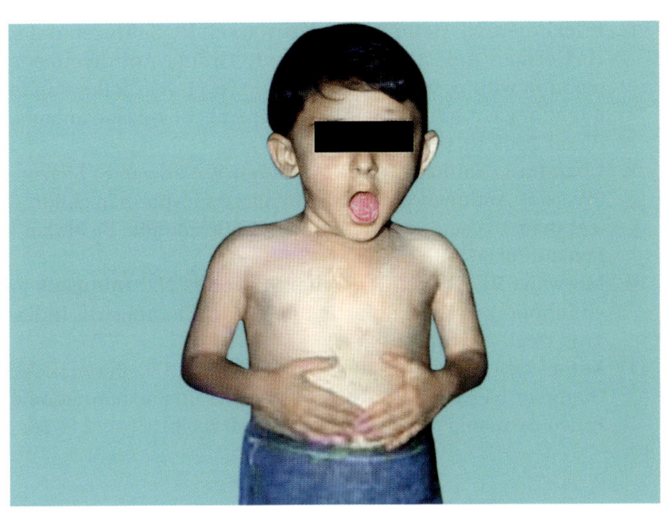

Fig. 14.5.4: Dyskeratosis congenita.
Courtesy: Dr MR Lokeshwar and Dr Nitin Shah, Mumbai.

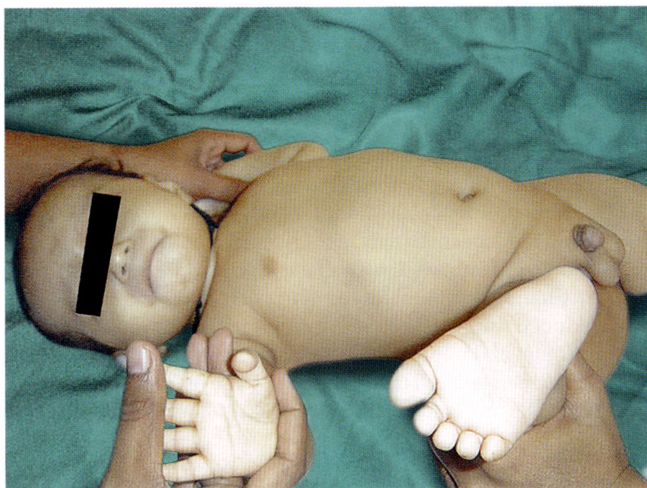

Fig. 14.5.5: Diamond–Blackfan syndrome.
Courtesy: Dr MR Lokeshwar and Dr Nitin Shah, Mumbai.

and is responsive to administration of G-CSF. About 50% of patients have anemia, 70% have thrombocytopenia, and 10% have pancytopenia. Inheritance is thought to be autosomal recessive. There is a risk of about 5% for development of leukemia.

DIAMOND–BLACKFAN SYNDROME

Diamond–Blackfan syndrome or constitutional chronic pure red cell aplasia is characterized by isolated erythroid hypoplasia occurring in early childhood, inherited as autosomal dominant or recessive condition. A variety of congenital abnormalities may be associated, such as strabismus, webbed neck, deformed thumb, bony abnormalities of finger and ribs, double ureter with hydronephrosis. Investigations suggest normochromic, macrocytic anemia with marked reticulocytopenia **(Figs. 14.5.5 and 14.5.6)**. Marrow aspiration characteristically discloses cellular marrow with profound erythroid hypoplasia with markedly increased M:E ratio. HbF is elevated in most cases as also I antigen on the red cell surface. Mainstay of treatment is transfusion therapy and corticosteroid. In some cases, cyclosporine may help.[6]

Hemosiderosis is unavoidable complication and may also eventually lead to portal hypertension and hypersplenism; and hence, chelation therapy and splenectomy may be required. Dose of steroid is 1–2 mg/kg of prednisolone for 4–6 weeks, and if unsuccessful, then may be discontinued. Steroid therapy may have to be maintained to the minimal required dose for years. Successful SCT has been reported in patients' refractory to above therapy and having HLA identical sibling. Intravenous gammaglobulin has been found to be useful. In most of the patients, carefully adjusted steroid therapy has been found successful.

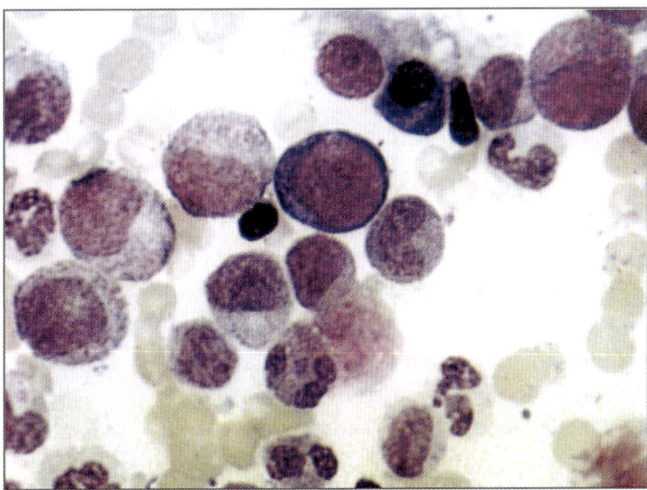

Fig. 14.5.6: Diamond–Blackfan syndrome cellular marrow with profound erythroid hypoplasia.
Courtesy: Dr MR Lokeshwar and Dr Nitin Shah, Mumbai.

REFERENCES

1. Bhatnagar SK, Chandra J, Narayan S, Sharma S, Singh V, Dutta AK. Pancytopenia in children: etiological profile. J Trop Pediatr. 2005;51(4):236-9.
2. Young NS, Calado RT, Scheinberg P. Current concepts in the pathophysiology and treatment of aplastic anemia. Blood. 2006;108(8):2509-19.
3. Marsh JC, Ball SE, Darbyshire P, Gordon-Smith EC, Keidan AJ, Martin A, et al; British Committee for Standards in Haematology. Guidelines for the diagnosis and management of acquired aplastic anaemia. Br J Haematol. 2003;123(5):782-801.
4. Davies JK, Guinan EC. An update on the management of severe aplastic anaemia in children. Br J Haematol. 2007;136(4):549-64.

5. De Latour RP, Kulsekararaj A, Lacobelli S, Terwel SR, Cook R, Griffin M, et al; Severe Aplastic Anemia Working Party of the European Society for Blood and Marrow Transplantation. Eltrombopag Added to Immunosuppression in Severe Aplastic Anemia. N Engl J Med. 2022;386(1):11-23.
6. Chen M, Liu Q, Gao Y, Suo X, Ding X, Wang L, et al. Cyclosporine plus eltrombopag in the treatment of aplastic anemia with or without antithymocyte immunoglobulin: A multicenter real-world retrospective study. Eur J Haematol. 2023;111(3):407-13.
7. George B, Mathews V, Viswabandya A, Kavitha ML, Srivastava A, Chandy M. Fludarabine and cyclophosphamide based reduced intensity conditioning (RIC) regimens reduce rejection and improve outcome in Indian patients undergoing allogeneic stem cell transplantation for severe aplastic anemia. Bone Marrow Transplant. 2007;40(1):13-8.
8. Frickhofen N, Heimpel H, Kaltwasser JP, Schrezenmeier H; German Aplastic Anemia Study Group. Antithymocyte globulin with or without cyclosporin A: 11-year follow-up of a randomized trial comparing treatments of aplastic anemia. Blood. 2003;101(4):1236-42.
9. Chandra J, Naithani R, Ravi R, Singh V, Narayan S, Sharma SW, et al. Antithymocyte globulin plus cyclosporin in children less than 12 years with acquired aplastic anemia. Br Indian J Pediatr. 2008;75(3):229-33.
10. Marwaha RK, Bansal D, Trehan A, Verma N. Androgens in childhood acquired aplastic anemia in Chandigarh, India. Trop Doct. 2004;34(3):149-52.
11. Kutler DI, Singh B, Satagopan J, Batish SD, Berwick M, Giampietro PF, et al. A 20-year perspective on the International Fanconi Anemia Registry (IFAR). Blood. 2003;101(4):1249-56.

14.6 Aplastic Anemia

(Late) Praveen Sobti, Shruti Kakkar

INTRODUCTION

Aplastic anemia (AA) is characterized by peripheral blood pancytopenia in the presence of a hypocellular bone marrow and the absence of any abnormal infiltrate or increased reticulin. Pancytopenia is defined as the presence of ≥2 of the following on a peripheral blood evaluation:

- Hemoglobin (Hb) <10 g/dL;
- Platelet count ≤100,000/mm^3; and
- Absolute neutrophil count (ANC) ≤1,500/mm^3

The AA was first described in a young pregnant woman by Ehrlich in 1988 by demonstrating an empty bone marrow. AA can be inherited or acquired.[1,2] Inherited bone marrow failure syndromes have already been discussed in the previous chapter; hence, this section refers to acquired AA only.

EPIDEMIOLOGY

Acquired AA is a rare disorder affecting 1–2 cases per million per year in developed countries. The incidence is 2–3 times higher in South-East Asia, however, data from developing countries is lacking. AA has a biphasic age distribution with one peak seen in adolescents and young adults and the other in the elderly population. There is no sex predilection.[3,4]

ETIOPATHOGENESIS

The disease could result from abnormalities in either the hematopoietic stem cells or the bone marrow (BM) stroma (seed and soil theory). Immune-mediated alteration in the bone marrow microenvironment by cytotoxic T cells and cytokines can suppress BM lymphocytes. The etiology of AA is described in **Table 14.6.1**.

Genetic susceptibility plays an important role in the development of AA. An increased risk of AA has been associated with human leukocyte antigen alleles (HLA-A) and HLA-DRB1 polymorphism. The etiology of AA in children is different from that in adults. Inherited AA accounts for 25–30% of AA in children.[2,5]

CLINICAL FEATURES

The signs and symptoms of AA arise from cytopenias. Anemia is usually well tolerated by children but can present with pallor, fatigue, and exercise intolerance as the severity increases. Children with severe anemia may present with features suggestive of congestive heart failure. Easy bruisability, petechiae, and ecchymosis occur due to thrombocytopenia. Menorrhagia can be a presenting symptom in adolescent girls. Children with AA are at risk of life-threatening hemorrhage such as intracranial bleeding.[1,4]

Patients may present with frequent infections due to neutropenia. Fever is usually an uncommon symptom at initial presentation and should raise a suspicion of alternate diagnosis such as leukemia, hemophagocytosis, etc. History of jaundice 2–3 months before onset of symptoms may be present in hepatitis-associated AA. History of onset of symptoms, exposure to medications, recreational drugs, chemicals, and any preceding infections must be enquired about. It is not uncommon to find the child has received multiple transfusions before presentation. A history of diarrhea, steatorrhea, or a family history of chronic lung disease, premature graying, or cancers may point toward inherited marrow failure syndrome (IBMFS). A history of joint pains, rash, or photosensitivity may point toward an immunological disorder.[3,6,7]

Hepatosplenomegaly and lymphadenopathy are typically absent in patients with AA and their presence points at alternative diagnosis. The presence of limb abnormalities, and skin, mucosal, or nail abnormalities suggest an inherited marrow failure, but the absence of these external stigmata does not rule out the possibility of an IBMFS. An algorithm with an approach to pancytopenia is shown in **Flowchart 14.6.1**.

TABLE 14.6.1: Etiology of aplastic anemia in children.

Infections	• Hepatitis A, B, C, non-A, non-B • Dengue • EBV • CMV, HHV6 • Parvovirus B_{19} • HIV • Measles, mumps, rubella, varicella • Influenza A, adenovirus
Nutritional	Copper deficiency
Drugs	• Nonsteroidal anti-inflammatory drugs • Chloramphenicol • Anticonvulsants • Sulfonamides • Gold • Chemotherapeutic drugs
Toxins	Benzene, insecticides, solvents
Radiation	
Others	Pregnancy, autoimmune disorders, GVHD
Idiopathic	Unknown etiology

(CMV: cytomegalovirus; EBV: Epstein–Barr virus; GVHD: graft versus host disease; HHV6: human herpesvirus type 6; HIV: human immunodeficiency virus)

DIFFERENTIAL DIAGNOSIS

The differential diagnosis in a child presenting with pancytopenia in the absence of lymphadenopathy or hepatosplenomegaly apart from AA may include:

- *Transient bone marrow suppression* due to viral infections.
- *Nutritional anemia (B_{12} or folate deficiency):* A history of a strict vegan diet or an eating disorder may give a clue to an underlying nutrition deficiency.
- *Infiltrative disorders:* Children with malignancies, acute lymphoblastic leukemia, or acute myeloid leukemia (AML) and pediatric solid tumors infiltrating the marrow present with pancytopenia; however, bone marrow examination reveals a hypercellular marrow with abnormal cells.

Flowchart 14.6.1: Approach to a child with pancytopenia.

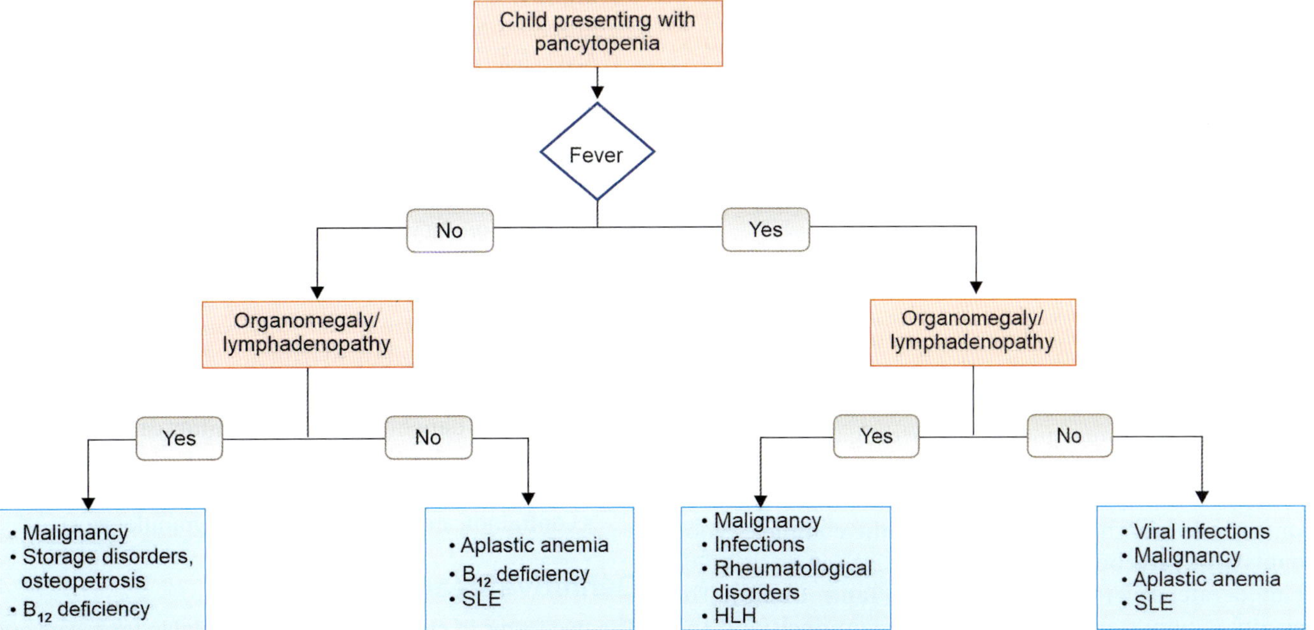

(HLH: hemophagocytic lymphocytosis; SLE: systemic lupus erythematosus)

Flowchart 14.6.2: Etiological classification of pancytopenia based on bone marrow examination.

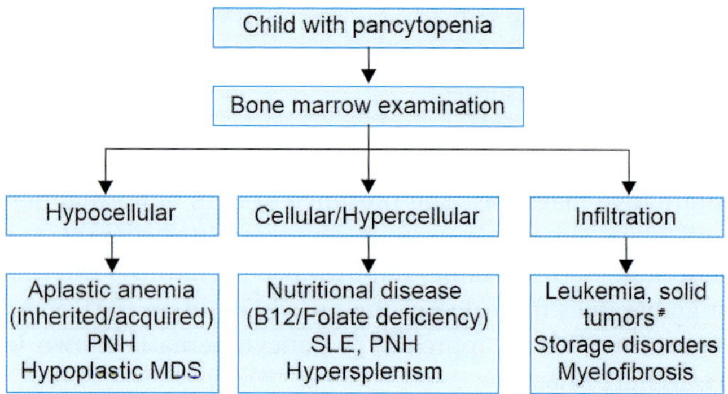

#Neuroblastoma, retinoblastoma, Ewing's sarcoma, rhabdomyosarcoma

(HLH: hemophagocytic lymphocytosis; MDS: myelodysplastic syndrome; PNH: paroxysmal nocturnal hemoglobinuria; SLE: systemic lupus erythematosus)

- *Immunological disorders:* Systemic diseases like systemic lupus erythematosus (SLE) can present with pancytopenia due to bone marrow suppression or due to macrophage activation syndrome.
- *Myelodysplastic syndrome (MDS), especially refractory cytopenia of childhood (RCC),* may mimic AA clinically. Bone marrow may be hypocellular or hypercellular. Bone marrow aspirate may show dyserythropoiesis along with the presence of small mononuclear or aberrant megakaryocytes.

Bone marrow can be hypo- or hypercellular in a child presenting with pancytopenia and is the most important investigation to diagnose AA **(Flowchart 14.6.2)**. A trephine bone marrow biopsy is mandatory for diagnosis. It is important to differentiate between inherited and acquired AA as it has important implications for management. Patients with IBMFS may not respond to immunosuppressive therapy (IST), are at a higher risk of toxicity with a conditioning regimen, for hematopoietic stem cell transplant (HSCT) and need an appropriate long-term follow-up.[3,4,6,7]

DIAGNOSIS

A thorough history and clinical examination followed by appropriate investigations are required to establish the diagnosis, assess severity, elaborate etiology, and make an appropriate treatment plan. The investigations required have been mentioned in **Table 14.6.2**. A bone marrow biopsy is essential for the diagnosis of AA as the involvement of bone marrow can be patchy. Based on the complete blood counts (CBC) and bone marrow findings, AA can be classified as moderate, severe, and very severe **(Table 14.6.3)**. The severity is important for making treatment decisions and prognostication. **Figures 14.6.1A to D** demonstrates the peripheral smear and bone marrow smears from a normal 10-year-old as well as a child with severe AA.

MANAGEMENT

Early diagnosis and prompt intervention are crucial for optimal outcomes in children with AA. The interval between diagnosis and treatment negatively correlates with response to treatment.

The treatment in AA can be classified as supportive and definitive treatment. It is improvement in supportive care over the years that has led to better outcomes in acquired AA.

Supportive Treatment (Fig. 14.6.2)

- *Packed cell transfusion:* A restrictive transfusion policy is followed in patients with AA, i.e., transfuse if hemoglobin (Hb) <6 g/dL or the patient has symptomatic anemia. Packed cells should be leukoreduced and irradiated to prevent HLA sensitization and transfusion-associated graft versus host disease (TA-GVHD). Directed donations from family members should be avoided to prevent HLA sensitization and graft rejection.
- *Platelet transfusion:* Transfuse if platelets are below 10,000/mm^3 or in the presence of bleeding. A higher transfusion cutoff (<20,000/mm^3) can be kept in febrile and sick patients.
- *Neutropenic precautions:* Prevention of infections by simple measures such as hand washing, wearing masks in crowded places, and avoiding unpasteurized milk and uncooked food may help prevent infections till ANC improves. Prophylactic antifungal and *Pneumocystis jirovecii* prophylaxis is recommended for patients with ANC <500/mm^3.
- *Management of febrile neutropenia:* Prompt initiation of broad-spectrum antibiotics is necessary in a febrile child. Granulocyte transfusions help supplement neutrophils in children with sepsis.
- *Use of granulocyte-colony stimulating factor (G-CSF):* G-CSF may be used in a febrile patient. There is a concern regarding an increased risk of clonal hematopoiesis and malignant transformation to MDS or AML with the use of G-CSF in this subgroup of patients.
- *Iron chelation therapy* may be required if a child is transfusion-dependent. Iron chelation can be initiated once serum ferritin >1,000 ng/mL. Deferasirox or desferrioxamine are the preferred drugs and deferiprone is contraindicated due to the risk of agranulocytosis.[3,4,6,7]

Definitive Treatment

The two forms of curative treatment available for severe and very severe AA are IST and HSCT **(Flowchart 14.6.3)**.

TABLE 14.6.2: Recommended investigations in a child with pancytopenia.

Investigation	*Relevance*	*Findings*
Complete blood count (CBC) and peripheral blood film (PBF)	Establish diagnosis and determine the severity	• Macrocytic anemia • Thrombocytopenia • Leukopenia with relative lymphocytosis
Bone marrow aspiration and biopsy	Establish diagnosis	• Hypocellular with prominent fat spaces • Reduced hematopoietic elements
Reticulocyte count	Determine severity	Reticulocytopenia
Viral serology	To establish etiology	Hepatitis A, B, C, parvovirus, Ebstein–Barr virus (EBV), Cytomegalovirus (CMV)
Flow cytometry for CD55/59	Establish etiology (to rule out PNH)	
Autoimmune disease evaluation	To establish etiology	
Bone marrow (BM) cytogenetics	To rule out MDS	12% of patients have cytogenetic anomalies (trisomy 8, trisomy 6,5q)
Chromosomal breakage studies	To distinguish IBMFS	Increased chromosomal breaks in Fanconi's anemia under the effect of mitomycin c and diepoxy butane
Telomere length analysis by FISH	To distinguish IBMFS	
Next generation sequencing	To distinguish IBMFS	
HLA typing	To aid in the treatment	
Liver and kidney function tests	To aid in the treatment	

(FISH: fluorescent in situ hybridization; HLA: human leukocyte antigen; IBMFS: inherited bone marrow failure syndromes; MDS: myelodysplastic syndromes; PNH: paroxysmal nocturnal hemoglobinuria)

TABLE 14.6.3: Severity of aplastic anemia (Modified Camitta's criteria).

Severity	*Criteria*
Severe (SAA)	Bone marrow cellularity <25% (or 25–50% with <30% hematopoietic stem cells) along with at least 2 of the following • Absolute neutrophil count <500/mm^3 • Platelet count <20,000/mm^3 • Absolute reticulocyte count <20,000/mm^3
Very severe (VSAA)	Criteria for SAA with absolute neutrophil count <200/mm^3
Non-severe	Decreased bone marrow cellularity and peripheral blood cytopenia, not fulfilling the criteria for SAA

Severe and Very Severe Aplastic Anemia

Hematopoietic stem cell transplant is the preferred treatment for children with AA if a matched sibling donor is available. The recommended conditioning regimen is a combination of fludarabine-cyclophosphamide and antithymocyte globulin (ATG). The stem cells can be collected from bone marrow as well as peripheral blood apheresis. Post-transplant immunosuppression includes cyclosporine and methotrexate. Major challenges with a HSCT include chemotherapy-related side effects, GVHD, graft failure, and secondary malignancies. In the absence of a matched sibling donor, alternative

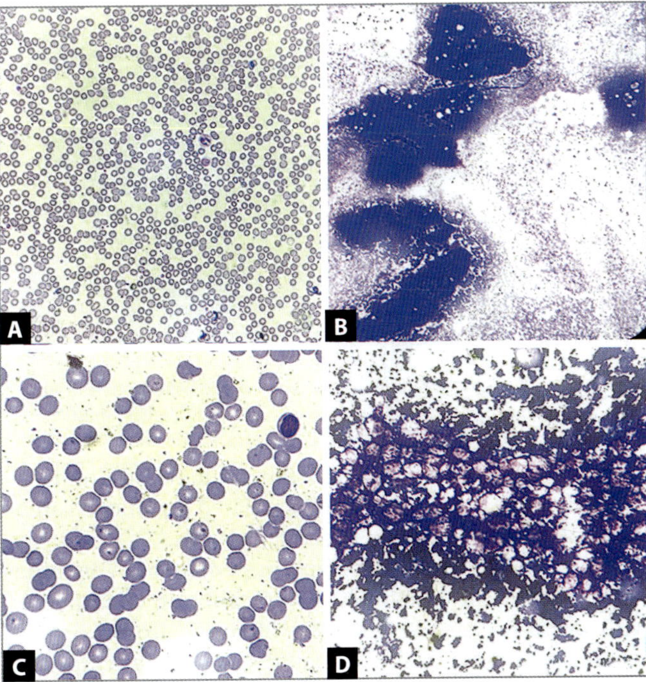

Figs. 14.6.1A to D: (A) Peripheral smear normal 10-year-old child; (B) Bone marrow aspirate smear exhibiting normal for age; (C) Peripheral smear of a 10-year-old child exhibiting pancytopenia and neutropenia; and (D) Bone marrow aspirate smears showing hypocellular marrow (cellularity 10%).

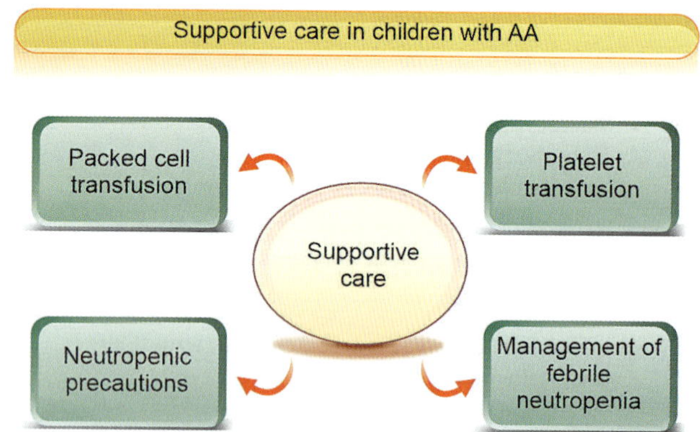

Fig. 14.6.2: Supportive care in children with aplastic anemia (AA).

Flowchart 14.6.3: Algorithm for definitive care in children with aplastic anemia.

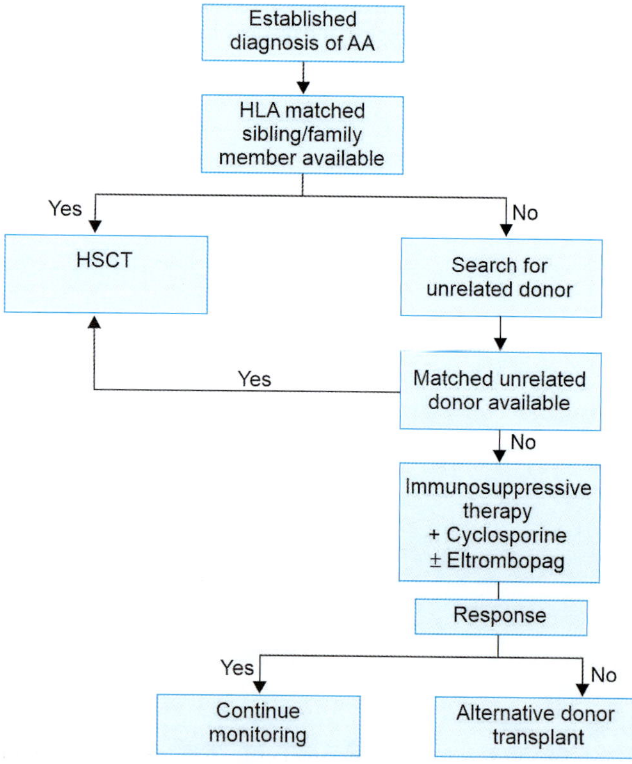

donors can be used such as matched unrelated donors or haploidentical donors. Matched unrelated donations can be processed through various stem cell registries.[3,4,6,8]

Immunosuppressive therapy in pediatric AA includes antithymocyte or antilymphocyte globulin in combination with cyclosporine. ATG can be obtained from horse or rabbit. Equine ATG results in better responses as compared to rabbit ATG, hence is preferred for the upfront treatment. The criteria for response evaluation are mentioned in **Table 14.6.4**. In case of no response or relapse, a second course can be administered using rabbit ATG. The response rate to IST is 60–75%. The major concerns with IST include

TABLE 14.6.4: Response evaluation in aplastic anemia.

Complete response	• Red cell and platelet transfusion independent • Absolute neutrophil count (ANC) >1,500/mm^3 • Platelet count >150,000/mm^3
Partial response	• ANC >500/mm^3 • Platelet count >20,000/mm^3 • May or may not be red cell and platelet transfusion-independent
No response	Transfusion dependent and meets severe aplastic anemia (SAA) criteria

anaphylactic reactions, serum sickness, lack of response, relapse, and clonal evolution. A short course of steroids is given with ATG as prophylaxis for serum sickness.[2,8,9]

Eltrombopag, a thrombopoietin analog, has been shown to improve response to IST in combination with ATG and cyclosporine in adult patients with AA.[3,4]

Androgens can be used alone or in combination with cyclosporine in patients where HSCT or IST is not feasible.[3,6]

Moderate Aplastic Anemia

The treatment is less defined for patients with moderate AA. Patients with moderate AA may improve spontaneously or progress to severe AA. Patients who are transfusion-independent can be observed closely. Cyclosporine, androgens, and eltrombopag have been used as single agents. If the patient is transfusion-dependent or progresses to severe AA, IST, or HSCT can be offered.[3,4,6]

PROGNOSIS

The outcome of AA in developed countries has reached >90% due to the wide availability of bone marrow transplants (BMTs) and improved supportive care. The survival in India is nearly 50%. The poor outcomes are related to late diagnosis and referrals. Early IST within 4 weeks of diagnosis and early BMT at 12 weeks is associated with improved survival. Infection and bleeding are the two main causes of morbidity and mortality in patients with severe AA.[1,3,8,10]

FOLLOW-UP

Patients with AA need long-term follow-up to monitor for relapse and later clonal disorders, such as MDS, leukemia, paroxysmal nocturnal hemoglobinuria (PNH), and solid tumors. Long-term survival is higher in patients undergoing a BMT as compared to IST. The development of clonal hematopoiesis is observed in 10–20%, autoimmune disorders in 10%, and solid tumors in 10% of patients.[3,6]

Social Support

Coal India Limited under its corporate social responsibility (CSR) initiative grants financial support for HSCT for a child with AA. The eligibility criteria include age <18 years, family income <8 lakhs per annum, and availability of a matched family donor.[11]

CONCLUSION

Acquired aplastic anemia is a rare condition marked by pancytopenia and decreased bone marrow cellularity. Diagnosis is confirmed through a trephine bone marrow biopsy. Children with this disorder require urgent referral and management. The two curative options are hematopoietic stem-cell transplantation (HSCT) and immunosuppressive therapy (IST). Supportive care is essential while awaiting these treatments.

REFERENCES

1. Hartung HD, Olson TS, Bessler M. Acquired aplastic anemia in children. Pediatr Clin North Am. 2013;60(6):1311-36.
2. Young NS, Calado RT, Scheinberg P. Current concepts in the pathophysiology and treatment of aplastic anemia. Blood. 2006;108(8):2509.
3. Iftikhar R, Ahmad P, de Latour R, Dufour C, Risitano A, Chaudhri N, et al. Special issues related to the diagnosis and management of acquired aplastic anemia in countries with restricted resources, a report on behalf of the Eastern Mediterranean blood and marrow transplantation (EMBMT) group and severe aplastic anemia working party of the European Society for blood and marrow transplantation (SAAWP of EBMT). Bone Marrow Transplant. 2021;56(10):2518-32.
4. Peslak SA, Olson T, Babushok DV. Diagnosis and treatment of aplastic anemia opinion statement. Curr Treat Options Oncol. 2017;18(12):70.
5. Schoettler ML, Nathan DG. The pathophysiology of acquired aplastic anemia: Current concepts revisited. Hematol Oncol Clin North Am. 2018;32(4):581-94.
6. Danewa A, Kalra M, Sachdeva A, Sachdeva P, Bansal D, Bhat S, et al. Diagnosis and management of acquired aplastic anemia: Consensus statement of Indian Academy of Pediatrics. Indian Pediatr. 2022;59:467-75.
7. Shimano KA, Narla A, Rose MJ, Gloude NJ, Allen SW, Bergstrom K, et al. Diagnostic work-up for severe aplastic anemia in children: Consensus of the North American Pediatric Aplastic Anemia Consortium. Am J Hematol. 2021;96(11):1491-504.
8. Yoshida N. Recent advances in the diagnosis and treatment of pediatric acquired aplastic anemia. Int J Hematol. 2024;119(3):240-7.
9. Jain R, Trehan A, Bansal D, Varma N. Aplastic anemia in children: How good is immunosuppressive therapy? Pediatr Hematol Oncol. 2019;36(4):211-21.
10. Schoettler ML, Nathan DG. The Pathophysiology of acquired aplastic anemia: Current concepts revisited. Hematol Oncol Clin North Am. 2018;32(4):581-94.
11. CIL. Thalassemia Bal Sewa Yojana. [online] Available from https://www.coalindia.in/tbsy/about-us/ [Last accessed December, 2024].

14.7 Thalassemia Syndromes

Madhukar R Lokeshwar, Swati R Kanakia

INTRODUCTION

Thalassemia syndromes constitute a heterogeneous group of hematologic disorders characterized by defects in the synthesis of one or more of the globin chains that form the hemoglobin tetramer. This results in reduced or complete absence of production of one or more of the globin polypeptide chains of the hemoglobin molecule leading to an imbalance in alpha (α) and non-α-chains of hemoglobin. Depending upon the chains affected, the disorder is named as α- or β-thalassemia. They are single gene disorders inherited in an autosomal recessive manner and represent a major health burden worldwide.[1]

The disease was first described by Thomas B Cooley and Pearl Lee in 1925 and it was initially known as Cooley's anemia. Whipple and Bradford first used the term "Thalassemia" in 1932; *"Thalassa"* in Greek meaning sea and *"-emia"*, meaning anemia around the sea. It was also known as "Mediterranean anemia". It was soon realized that it occurs not only around Mediterranean regions but also in Southeast Asia, Indian subcontinent, and Middle East. The first case of thalassemia from India was reported by M Mukherjee. PK Sukumaran from Mumbai did pioneering works in the field of diagnosis of thalassemia syndromes in India.

EPIDEMIOLOGY

All over the world, there are >250 million (1.5% of world population) carriers of β-thalassemia gene and in Southeast Asia, there are 40 million carriers of this gene.[2] Approximately,

5% of the world's population are carriers of α-thalassemia and around 1,000,000 patients are affected by various forms of α-thalassemia syndromes worldwide. They are most prevalent in Southeast Asia, Southern China, the Middle East, the Mediterranean region, and Africa. Thalassemia belt stretches across African continent, Mediterranean regions, Middle East, Indian subcontinent, Southeast Asia, Southern China, Europe, and Melanesia. However, population migration has not restricted the gene frequency to above tropical areas and hence seen all over the world **(Fig. 14.7.1)**.

In India, prevalence of the β-gene (trait) varies from 1 to 17%. Incidence varies in various communities, religions, and ethnic groups in India. A higher frequency is noted in Sindhis, Punjabis, migrants from Pakistan such as Khatris and Khukrejas in north, Bhanushalis, Lohanas, Kutchis, and baniyas from Gujarat, neo-Buddhists, Mahars, Chamars, Buddhists, Kolis, Agris, and Kunbis from Maharashtra, Reddys, Gowdas, Lingayats, and Kurgs from Andhra Pradesh and Karnataka and Gowd Saraswats from Goa. With a birth rate of 22.8 per 1,000 in India, it is estimated that there are about 9,000–10,000 cases being added every year, and there are around 65,000–67,000 β-thalassemia patients in our country at given time.

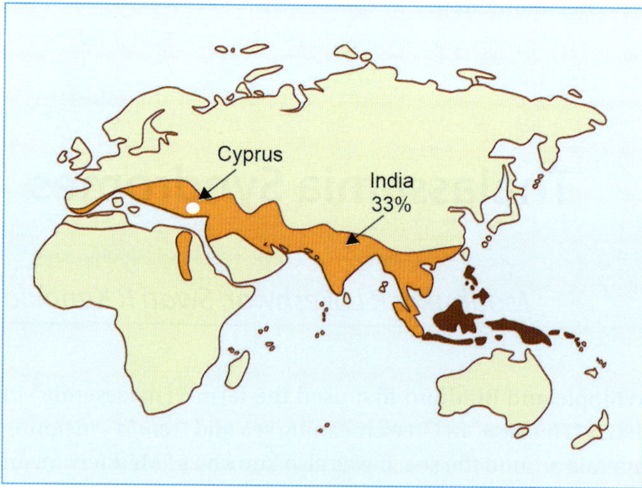

Fig. 14.7.1: Thalassemia incidence: World scenario of the thalassemia belt.

ETIOPATHOGENESIS

Thalassemia is an inherited disorder of hemoglobin. The hemoglobin consists of two pairs of amino acid chains.[1-3] Adult hemoglobin (HbA) consists of two pairs of α-chains and β-chains. Hemoglobin A2 (HbA_2), a variant of HbA, consists of two pairs of α-chains and δ-chains. Fetal hemoglobin (HbF) is constituted by two pairs of α-chains and γ-chains. In α-thalassemia, α-chain synthesis is affected. They are classified into four different categories depending on the number of genes affected **(Table 14.7.1)**. In β-thalassemia, there is reduced or absent production of β-chains, leading to excess α-chains with reduced or absent β-(non-α) chains **(Table 14.7.2)**.

Excess α-chains that have no complementary non-α-chains with which to pair, form insoluble inclusions that precipitate on red cell membrane and damages it, leading to premature destruction of red blood cells (RBCs) in bone marrow (ineffective erythropoiesis) and in peripheral circulation, particularly in reticuloendothelial system of spleen (extravascular hemolysis) resulting in persistent progressive anemia **(Flowchart 14.7.1)**.[4] Extramedullary erythropoiesis results in expansion of bone marrow spaces. Due to reduced production of HbA in postnatal life, the normal switch mechanism leading to reduction in β-chain synthesis does not occur. This leads to higher HbF in postnatal life. The precise mechanism controlling the switch from fetal to HbA is not fully understood.

However, the degree of ineffective erythropoiesis appears to be less in α-thalassemia compared to β-thalassemia.

CLINICAL MANIFESTATIONS

Based on the clinical severity and transfusion requirement, thalassemia syndromes are classified phenotypically into two main groups:

1. Transfusion-dependent thalassemia (TDT)
2. Nontransfusion-dependent thalassemia (NTDT)

Main clinical features are characteristic hemolytic facies—frontal, parietal, and occipital bossing, malar prominence, and malocclusion of teeth—along with distortion and osteoporosis of ribs and vertebrae, pathological fracture/s of long bones; splenomegaly with its complications such as hypersplenism, hepatomegaly, gallstones, and chronic leg ulcers.

TABLE 14.7.1: Classification of α-thalassemia syndromes.

Syndrome	*Clinical features*	*Hemoglobin pattern*	*α-globin genes affected*
Silent carrier	No anemia, normal red cells	1–2% Hb Bart's (γ_4) at birth	1
α-thalassemia trait	Mild anemia, hypochromic microcytic red cells	5–10% Hb Bart's (γ_4) at birth	2
Hemoglobin H (HbH) disease	Moderate hypochromic, microcytic anemia	5–30% HbH (β_4) red cells	3
Hydrops fetalis	Death in utero caused by severe anemia	Mainly Hb Bart's, small amount of HbH	4

TABLE 14.7.2: Classification of β-thalassemia.

Syndrome	*Clinical features*	*Hemoglobin pattern*	*β-globin genes affected*
Silent carrier	Asymptomatic No anemia	Normal, diagnosed by chain synthesis or identification of mutation	Heterozygous state
Thalassemia trait	Mild anemia, hypochromic microcytic red cells	Elevated HbA_2 > 3.4%	Heterozygous state
Thalassemia intermedia	• Moderate, not dependent on blood transfusion for their survival • May require transfusion occasionally	HbF or HbA_2 elevated	Homozygous/double heterozygous state
Thalassemia major	Dependent on regular blood transfusion for survival	HbF markedly elevated	Homozygous state

(HbA_2: hemoglobin A_2; HbF: fetal hemoglobin)

Flowchart 14.7.1: Pathophysiology of β-thalassemia.

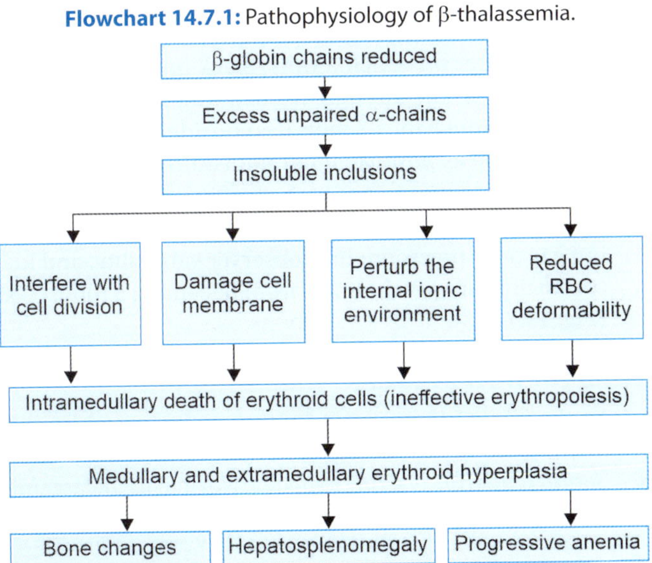

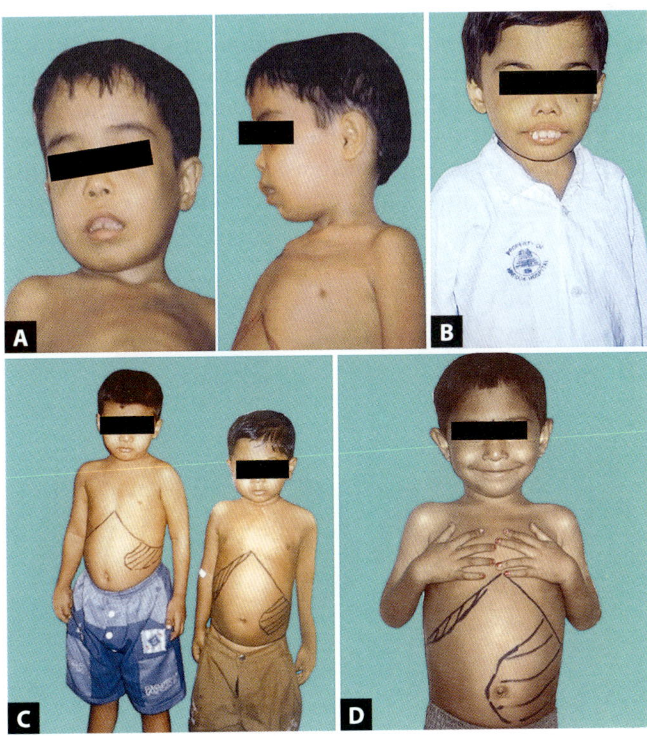

Figs. 14.7.2A to D: Transfusion-dependent thalassemia.

Transfusion-dependent Thalassemia

Children with TDT are generally diagnosed between 6 months and 2 years of life. In India, many children born with thalassemia major die undiagnosed or due to lack of ideal treatment. The spectrum of clinical manifestations of β-thalassemia varies widely. The serious homozygous form (*thalassemia major*) presents in early infancy (6–18 months) with progressive pallor, hepatosplenomegaly, and bony changes and if untreated, is invariably fatal during first few years of life, whereas at the other end of the spectrum is a heterozygous form (*thalassemia minor*) in which the patient can lead a practically normal life except for a mild persistent anemia **(Figs. 14.7.2A to D)**. In between these two extremes are forms with varying degrees of clinical manifestations of anemia, splenohepatomegaly, and bony changes who maintain their life fairly comfortably and are not dependent on blood transfusions for their survival and are called *thalassemia intermedia*.

Nontransfusion-dependent Thalassemia

The major pathophysiological processes underlying these thalassemias are ineffective erythropoiesis and peripheral hemolysis. This in turn gives rise to various pathologies such as anemia, extramedullary hematopoiesis, hypercoagulability, iron overload, and decreased bone densities. This group, however, does not have a uniform presentation but encompasses highly variable clinical phenotypes. This can be asymptomatic with no/or occasional requirement of blood transfusion, no/minimal iron overload, no growth retardation, or general debility **(Figs. 14.7.3A and B)**.

DIAGNOSIS

It is important to correlate clinical profile and ethnicity of the individuals, with the blood counts and blood film evaluation and do further investigations to confirm the diagnosis.

Blood Counts and Film Evaluation

- *Complete blood counts (CBCs)* reveals generally severe anemia, a high leukocyte count (due to immature myeloid cells as well as nucleated red cells—also known as "leukoerythroblastic reaction").
- *White blood cell (WBC) and platelets* may decrease if there is accompanying hypersplenism.
- *Reticulocyte count* ranges from 2 to 4%. It is generally low to normal in thalassemia major, whereas in thalassemia intermedia, it increases from 3 to 6% **(Fig. 14.7.4A)**.
- *Peripheral blood film examination* is diagnostic and has a characteristic bizarre picture with microcytic, hypochromic RBCs with striking number of normoblasts. In addition, there may be target cells, macrocytosis, poikilocytosis, polychromasia, moderate basophilic stippling, Cabot rings, and fragmented erythrocytes **(Fig. 14.7.4B)**.

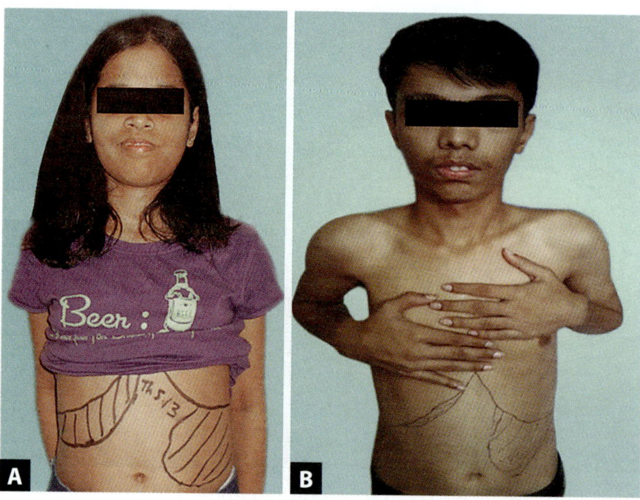

Figs. 14.7.3A and B: Nontransfusion-dependent thalassemia.

- *Mean corpuscular volume (MCV)* is reduced in thalassemia minor.
- *RBC count* reveals a severe hypochromia with microcytosis. In thalassemia minor, a high RBC count relative to Hb concentration and hematocrit (Hct) is seen.
- *Red cell distribution width (RDW):* RDW in thalassemia major is significantly high (ranging from 30 to 40% for a normal value of 11.5 to 14.5%), suggesting a very high degree of anisocytosis. RDW is normal in thalassemia trait as well as in anemia of chronic infection.
- *Osmotic fragility* is reduced.
- *Naked-eye single tube red cell osmotic fragility test (NESTROFT) for thalassemia minor:* A drop of blood is added to two tubes containing 2 mL of buffered saline (BS 0.36%) and distilled water and kept for an hour at room temperature. Then the tubes are shaken and held against a white paper on which a thick black line is drawn. The line will be visible through distilled water tube. It the line is visible through the BS tube, it is considered *negative* and if not visible as *positive*. If left undisturbed, in a positive case a clear supernatant with a sediment at the bottom is seen at 3 hours. The test has a high sensitivity of 95%, but gas poor precision, interobserver variability, and low specificity have precluding it from becoming a robust test **(Fig. 14.7.5)**.

Tests for Iron Status

- *Serum iron and transferrin saturation:* Increased/normal in thalassemia depending on iron overload
- *Serum total iron-binding capacity:* Normal in thalassemia and anemia of chronic infection.

Methods of Measurement of Hemoglobin A_2

The methods available for qualitative and quantitative hemoglobin analysis include isoelectric focusing, microcolumn chromatography, cellular acetate electrophoresis **(Fig. 14.7.6)**, paper electrophoresis **(Fig. 14.7.7)**, and automated high-performance liquid chromatography (HPLC).

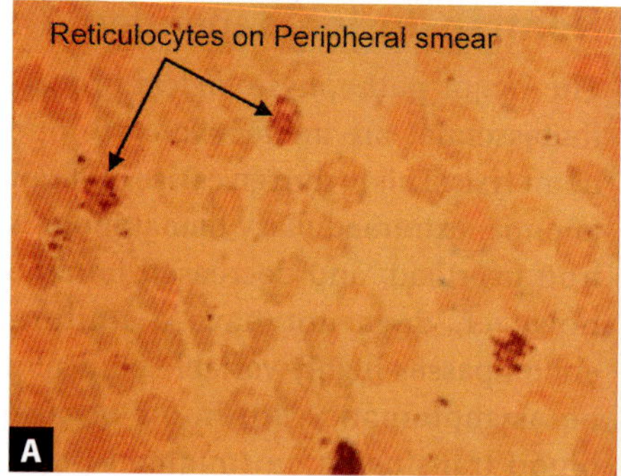

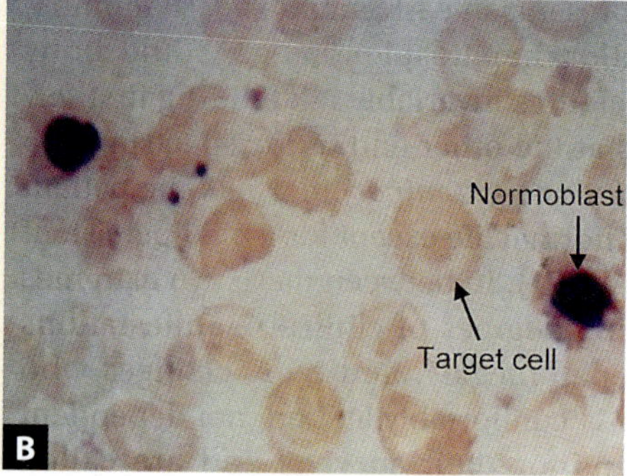

Figs. 14.7.4A and B: (A) Reticulocytes in peripheral smear (arrows); (B) Normoblast and target cell.

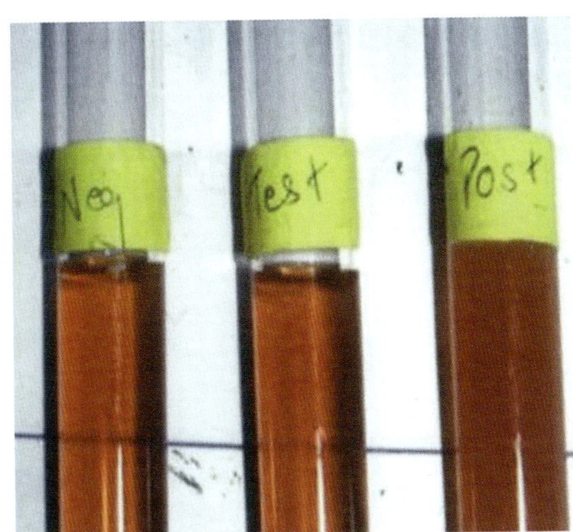

Fig. 14.7.5: NESTROFT test. The tube on the left is negative and on the right is positive.

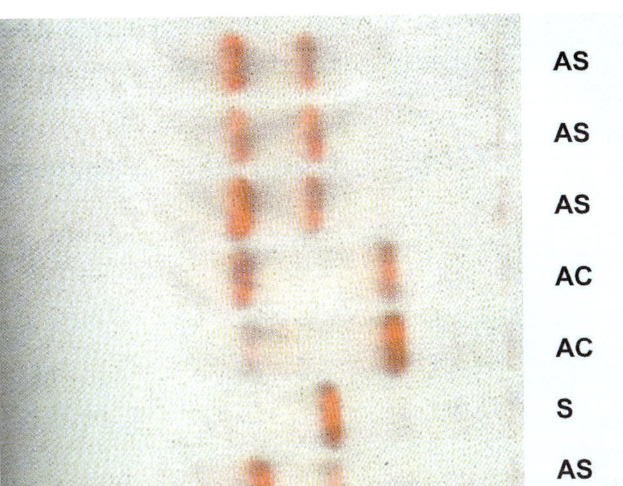

Fig. 14.7.6: Cellulose acetate electrophoresis.

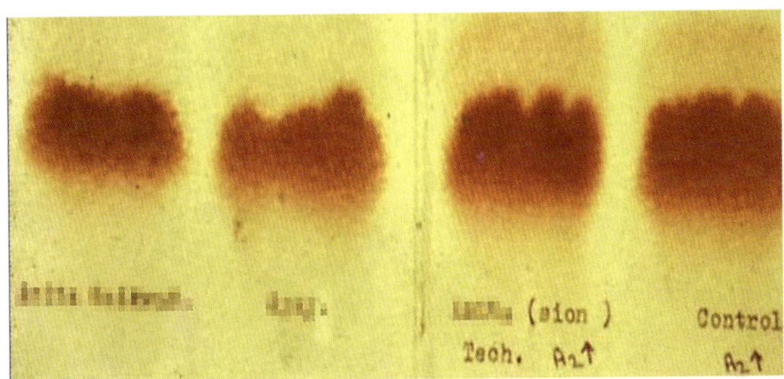

Fig. 14.7.7: Paper electrophoresis.

Microcolumn chromatography and HPLC by automated (BIORAD) machines are the most popular methods for measurement of HbA_2. It has thus become the gold standard for diagnosis of thalassemia syndromes. It generates graphs depicting various abnormal and normal hemoglobins with quantification **(Fig. 14.7.8)**.

- *In TDT,* hemoglobin pattern reveals HbA_2 of 5% or more, HbF up to 95%, with no HbA.
- *In NTDT,* there is HbA_2 of 4% or more, HbF up to 50%.
- *Thalassemia minor* is characterized by elevated HbA_2 of 4% or more, HbF up to 5%.
- HbA_2 value of >9% indicates the presence of a coeluting abnormal hemoglobin such as HbE, HbD Iran, and Hb Lepore.
- *In hydrops fetalis* with Hb Barts, HPLC reveals Hb Barts (γ globin tetramers); Hb Portland, no HbF, HbA_2, or HbA.
- *In HbH disease,* there is elevated HbH up to 30%, HbA_2 up to 4%.

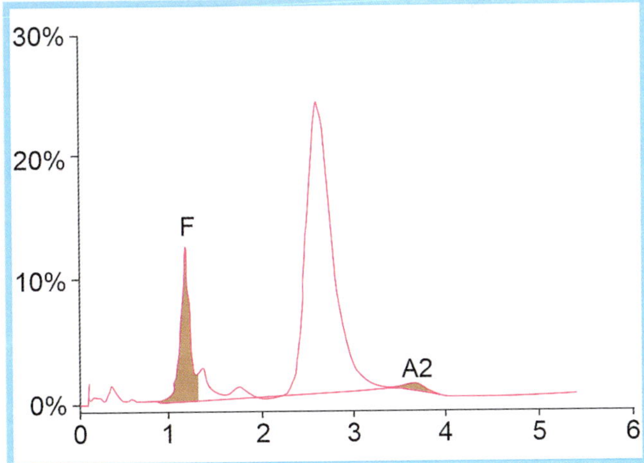

Fig. 14.7.8: Graphic pattern of hemoglobin in thalassemia minor/trait.

Radiological Findings

These include widening of medulla due to bone marrow hyperplasia, thinning of the cortex and trabeculations and fracture in long bones, metacarpals, and metatarsals **(Figs. 14.7.9A to C)**.

Tests Used for Estimating Iron Overload

- *Serum ferritin*: It is high in children with thalassemia major and normal to increased or decreased when there is concomitant iron deficiency associated with thalassemia minor. The values of ferritin are proportionate to the iron overload due to multiple transfusions. It is the commonly used test for diagnosing iron overload. It should be assessed every 3–6 months in order to avoid overchelation in patients with ferritin levels <1,000 ng/mL.
- *Liver iron concentration (LIC):* LIC provides a reliable estimate of total body iron stores. Any level above 7 mg/g of dry liver tissue is indicative of significant iron overload. Levels above 15 mg/g are associated with cardiac iron overload.

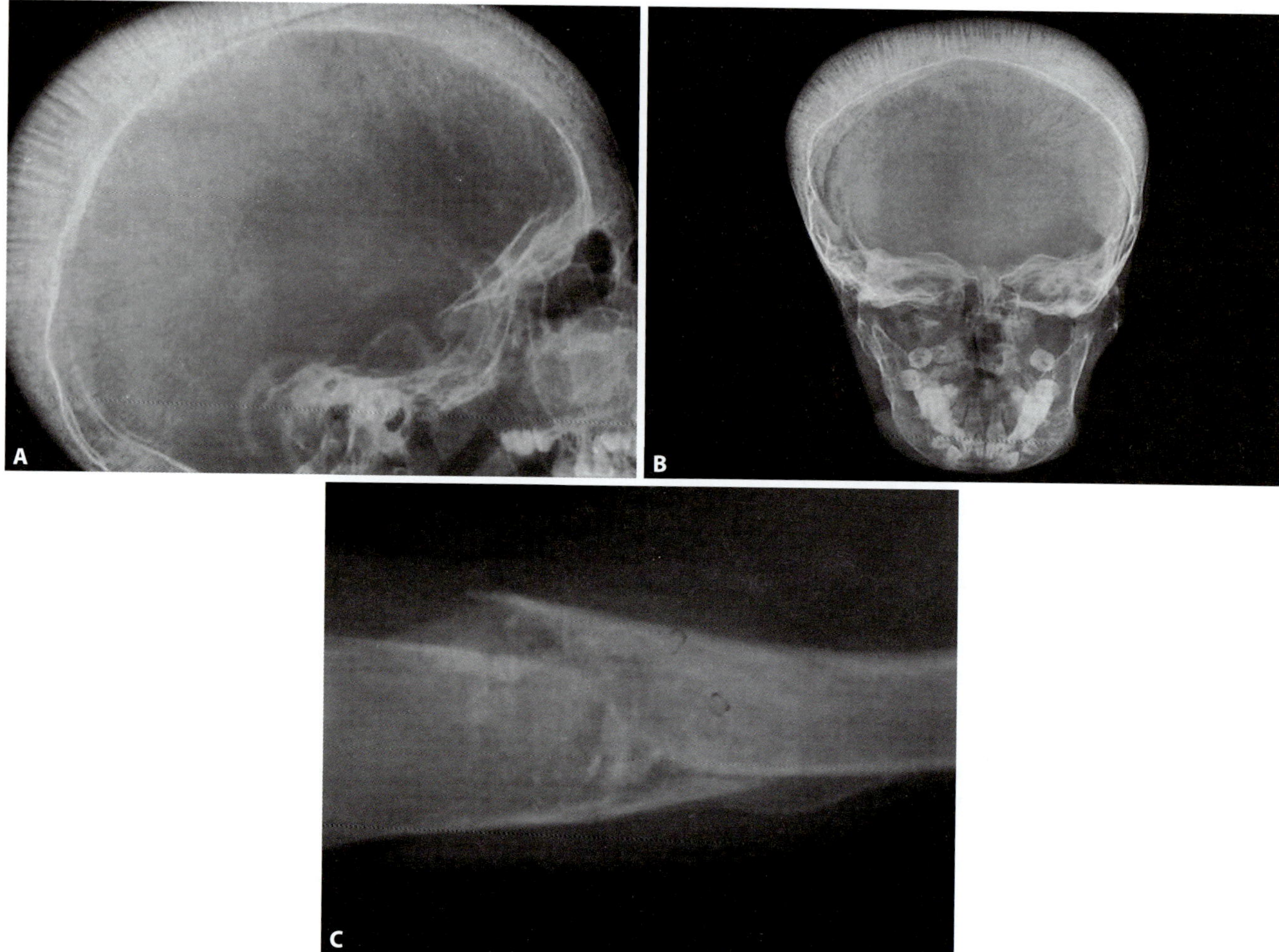

Figs. 14.7.9A to C: X-ray of skull AP (A) and lateral views (B) show "hair on end" appearance. Widening of medulla, thinning of the cortex and trabeculations, and fracture in the long bones (C).

- *Magnetic resonance imaging (MRI):* It has generally replaced the more invasive liver biopsy. Liver and cardiac iron imaging by MRI are the standard of care. Cardiac iron is typically measured with T2 images and this technique is widely available and highly reproducible. Mild cardiac iron overload is defined as T2 of 10–20 ms and severe cardiac overload is <10 ms. Cardiac MRI should be performed annually in all patients; every 6 months in high-risk patients and every 2 years in well-chelated low-risk patients.
- *Superconducting quantum interference device (SQUID):* It is a noninvasive method of estimating liver iron. SQUID remains reserved for experimental purpose and only few machines are available worldwide.
- *Bone marrow examination:* It is not indicated for the diagnosis of thalassemia major. It shows normoblastic erythroid hyperplasia with excessive iron on iron staining with Prussian blue.

Molecular Tests

Recently, next-generation sequencing (NES) and long-read sequencing (LRS) are emerging as new techniques in genetic testing for thalassemia.

Artificial Intelligence in Diagnosis of Thalassemia

The importance of artificial intelligence (AI) in diagnosing thalassemia is increasing and different indices and web-based prediction tools are being developed to aid in the diagnosis of thalassemia.[5]

Periodic Tests for Organ Dysfunction

While diagnosis of thalassemia major can be achieved by the tests, it is also mandatory to do baseline screening of various parameters listed in **Table 14.7.3**.

TABLE 14.7.3: Periodic tests for organ dysfunction. Bone densitometry by DEXA scan.

Test	*Frequency of monitoring*
Alpha- and beta-globin genotyping	Once at diagnosis
High-resolution HLA typing	Once at diagnosis
Growth parameters: Height, weight, and head circumference	Every 3–6 months
Complete blood count (CBC)	Every 6 months if no transfusion/ every 3–5 weeks if on transfusion
Comprehensive biochemistry panel	Every 6 months
Iron panel	Every 6 months
Serum ferritin	Every 3 months (monthly if on aggressive chelation)
Echocardiogram	Annually starting at 10–14 years
Tanner staging and menstrual assessment	Every 6 months starting at 8–10 years
TSH and free T4 (FT4)	Annually starting at 6 years
Hormonal profile	Annually starting at 10 years
Vitamin D, serum calcium, PTH	Annually starting at age of 10 years
Bone densitometry by dual-energy X-ray absorptiometry (DXA) scan	Annually starting at 10 years
Fasting blood glucose	Annually starting at 10 years

(PTH: parathyroid hormone; TSH: thyroid-stimulating hormone)

BOX 14.7.1: Multidisciplinary of thalassemia.

- Transfusion therapy—packed red cell transfusion
- Iron overload—removal of iron with iron chelating agents
- Transfusion transmitted infections—hepatitis B and C, HIV, *Yersinia* species, malaria, and CMV
- Hypersplenism—role of splenectomy
- Cardiac complications
- Leg ulcers
- Gallstones and hepatic dysfunction
- Endocrine evaluation and assessment of growth and development
- Curative treatment—bone marrow transplantation
- Future treatment—pharmacologic manipulation of HbF/gene therapy
- Prevention of the disease by antenatal diagnosis and genetic counseling

(CMV: Cytomegalovirus; HIV: human immunodeficiency virus)

TABLE 14.7.4: Transfusion therapy.

Test	*Frequency of monitoring*
Red blood cell genotype	Once at start of transfusion
Pretransfusion CBC	Every 3–5 weeks
Transfusion history including volume transfused, presence of red cell antibody	Every 3–5 weeks
Triple H (HIV/HBsAg/HCV)	Annually

(CBC: complete blood count; HBsAg: hepatitis B surface antigen; HCV: hepatitis C virus; HIV: human immunodeficiency virus)

MANAGEMENT OF THALASSEMIA

It involves a multidisciplinary therapeutic team approach and should be preferably done at a comprehensive thalassemia children care center with outdoor transfusion facilities **(Box 14.7.1)**.

Transfusion Therapy

The decision to initiate lifelong regular transfusion in patients with β-thalassemia should be based on the molecular defect, severity of symptoms, and clinical criteria, such as failure of growth and development, bone changes, and endocrine involvement. The diagnosis of thalassemia intermedia can be ascertained by observing the rate of fall of Hb without transfusions. If the Hb drops to below 7 g/dL without transfusion, in the absence of any concurrent illness, it is imperative to put the child on a regular transfusion program **(Table 14.7.4)**.

It is ideal to use optimally screened (ideally leukodepleted) packed red cells, cross matched, and negative for cytomegalovirus (CMV), human immunodeficiency virus (HIV), malarial parasite (MP), hepatitis C virus (HCV), and hepatitis B surface antigen (HBsAg). These red cells are transfused, 10–15 mL/kg, at the rate of 3–5 mL/kg/h every 2–4 weeks to maintain the hemoglobin. A goal of pretransfusion Hb of 9.5–10.5 g/dL is advocated. Patients with cardiac decompensation should be given red cells at the rate of not >1–2 mL/kg/h. Higher pretransfusion Hb levels may be needed for patients with heart complications. Packed red cells should be extended phenotype-matched (for ABO and Rh, C, C, D, E, E, and Kell where feasible) to limit the chances of alloimmunization. The alternative to this is Coombs crossmatch for each transfusion.

The next best is to use leukodepleting filters at bedside, but they are also costly. Another alternative is to use triple saline washed red cells in cold centrifuge. The red cells should be fresh, not older than 2 weeks with Hct > 60%. Various other methods of leukodepletion are available, including use of frozen red cells.

The transfusions are given on an outdoor basis in a daycare transfusion center.

Iron Overload and Chelation Therapy

Two factors contribute to iron overload in a thalassemic child:

1. Enhanced gastrointestinal absorption of iron
2. Transfusional siderosis

Chelation Therapy

Iron chelation should be initiated after age of 2 years when there is evidence of significant iron overload (10–20 transfusions, serum ferritin >1,000 ng/mL and LIC >5–7 mg/g dry weight). The standard available chelators used are listed in **Table 14.7.5**.

- *Deferasirox (Asunra, Desirox, and Defrijet)*: Deferasirox is the current drug of choice. The drug is available as a dispersible tablet (to be dissolved in water/orange juice or apple juice) or as film-coated tablet given orally once preferably in the morning on empty stomach. It has better bioavailability. The recommended dose ranges from 20 to 40 mg/kg/day once daily.
- *Deferoxamine (DFO, Desferal)*. Though, DFO is the gold standard, it has not become popular particularly in the developing countries and is preferred by only 10–15% of thalassemia patients in our country. This is mainly due to its high cost and the need for continuous subcutaneous (SC) injection over 6–8 hours with the Desferal pump. Dose is 30–40 mg/kg/day for 5–7 days/week SC over 8–10 hours. In recent times, methods of administration have improved with better, more convenient smaller, and lighter infusion pumps with LCD display. Balloon pumps, prefilled syringes of Desferal, are available though they are prohibitively costly. Intravenous (IV) Desferal can be given particularly in those with very high iron overload through port-a-caths (central line).
- *Deferiprone (L1) or 1,2-dimethyl-3-hydroxypyridin-4-one (DFP, Kelfer):* It has a better protective effect on myocardial tissue. The recommended dose is 75–100 mg/kg/day in three divided doses orally.

Role of Vitamin C

Ascorbic acid (vitamin C) helps in conversion of hemosiderin into ferritin from which iron can be chelated. Addition of vitamin C 100 mg daily prior to DFO therapy increases iron excretion.

Combination Therapy

If the iron overload is not adequately controlled in spite of using optimal doses and good compliance, two chelators can be combined, but need close monitoring. Most strong data is available for deferasirox and DFO, but the two oral chelators can also be combined. The dose of DFO is 50 mg/kg/day as overnight SC infusion through pump for 2 days a week and DFP at 50 mg/kg/day orally in three divided doses for rest of the 5 days a week. In case of cardiac failure, DFO can be given at a dose of 80 mg/kg/day along with DFP.

Nontransfusion-dependent Thalassemia

In NTDT, deferasirox therapy should be started at a dose of 10 mg/kg/day. Consider dose escalation to 20 mg/kg/day in patients with serum ferritin level >1,500–2,000 ng/mL. Chelation should be discontinued at serum ferritin <300 ng/mL. The Thalassemia International Federation guidelines do not recommend the use of other chelators such as DFO and DFP for management of iron overload in NTDT.

Newer Iron Chelators being Studied in Animals as well as in Humans

These include hydroxybenzyl-ethylenediamine-diacetic acid, pyridoxal-isonicotinoyl-hydrazone (PIH), desferrithiocin (DFT), GT56-252, and 40SD02 (CHF1540).

Transfusion-transmitted Infections

Hepatitis B Virus

All thalassemias who are negative for the HBsAg and antibody should receive hepatitis B virus (HBV) vaccine, four doses at day 0, at 1 month, 2nd month, and 12th month intramuscularly (IM). Medications approved by Food and Drug Administration (FDA) for the treatment of children with HBV include interferon (IFN)-alpha, lamivudine, and adefovir.

TABLE 14.7.5: Chelation therapy and complications.

Chelator	Deferasirox	Deferoxamine (DFO)	Deferiprone (DFP)
Molecule	Tridentate	Hexadentate	Bidentate
Route	Oral—dispersible tablet (DT) or film-coated tablet (FCT)	SC/IV if intensive chelation required	Oral
Dose	DT: 20–40 mg/kg/day FCT: 14–28 mg/kg/day	30–40 mg/kg/d, 5–7 days/week	75–100 mg/kg/day
Frequency	Daily once	12-hour infusions	Three divided doses
Side effects	Gastrointestinal (GI) disturbances, microalbuminuria transaminitis, and azotemia	Local reactions, ototoxicity, retinopathy, and sensory neural hearing loss	GI symptoms, agranulocytosis, and arthralgias
Monitoring	LFT/serum creatinine, urine monthly to begin with then 3 monthly	Annual ophthalmic slit lamp examination and audiometry	CBC every 2 weeks

(CBC: complete blood count; IV: intravenous; LFT: liver function test; SC: continuous subcutaneous)

Human Immunodeficiency Virus in Thalassemia

Patients with thalassemia identified with HIV infection should be managed in collaboration with an infectious diseases unit with expertise in HIV. Advances in drug treatment have revolutionized the care of patients.

Hepatitis C Virus Infection in Thalassemia

Patients treated with peg-IFN-α (PegIFN) and ribavirin (RBV) combination therapy demonstrate overall 50–55% sustained viral response (SVR) with rates as high as 80% in patients with genotypes 2 and 3.

Cytomegalovirus

Transfusion-associated CMV has a wide clinical spectrum. As CMV is WBC-associated virus, the widespread use of leukocyte filtration, in recent years recommended for all patients with thalassemia, no matter what their condition, constitutes an effective preventative measure. The increasing use of bone marrow transplantation (BMT) as a treatment for thalassemia demands special attention to the serological status of CMV.

Bacterial Infections

Yersinia species are common cause of infection in severe iron overloaded patients or in those undergoing iron chelation with desferrioxamine. Main treatment is to stop injection DFO, immediately, IV cotrimoxazole, gentamycin, ceftriaxone, doxycycline, and ciprofloxacin are the common antibiotics used.

Hypersplenism and Splenectomy

Hypersplenism may occur due to inadequate transfusions, alloimmunization, and rarely autoimmune hemolysis complicating thalassemia major and chronic liver disease. With the advent of hyper- and supertransfusion therapy, splenomegaly and hypersplenism have become a rarity and hence splenectomy is usually not needed in these patients. If the child has already developed splenomegaly and signs of hypersplenism and is above 5 years of age, splenectomy is indicated. Splenectomy should be considered when:

- Annual blood requirement exceeds 1.5 times the basal requirement for a patient maintaining pretransfusion Hb about 10 g/dL (transfusion requirement increases to more than 200–220 mL/kg/year of packed red cells).
- Massive spleen enlargement posing a risk of splenic rupture or when splenic enlargement is associated with left upper quadrant pain or early satiety.
- Presence of leukopenia or thrombocytopenia

Prophylaxis

All patients undergoing splenectomy should receive immunization to protect against capsulated organisms. These include pneumococcal, *Haemophilus influenzae* type B (Hib), meningococcal vaccines, and *Salmonella typhi,* which should be given at least 4 weeks before surgery. Lifelong postsplenectomy penicillin prophylaxis 125 mg twice a day for children up to 2 years and 250 mg twice a day for children 2 years and above is recommended.

Chemoprophylaxis is recommended for at least 2 years while some advocate this for whole life. In the presence of early signs of infection, treatment should be started immediately with broad-spectrum antibiotics without waiting for the result of laboratory tests. Postsplenectomy, there may be transient or persistent thrombocytosis. Aspirin therapy should be considered in splenectomized NTDT patients with elevated platelet counts ($\geq 500 \times 10^9$) in a dose of 50–100 mg/day is recommended. In endemic areas, prophylactic antimalarial treatment may be given to prevent malaria.

Osteopenia and Osteoporosis

This can be diagnosed by dual-energy X-ray absorptiometry (DEXA) scan for bone density and biochemical studies of serum calcium, inorganic phosphate, alkaline phosphatase, urinary calcium/creatinine ratio (>0.2), and urinary phosphorus/creatinine ratio (>0.6) **(Figs. 14.7.10A and B)**. DEXA scan is recommended beginning by the age of 10 years. Bone density T score >1.5 SD below the mean is diagnostic of osteopenia whereas T score >2.5 SD below the mean is termed osteoporosis.

Treatment

- Diet, rich in calcium and vitamin D as well as calcium supplementation (500–1,000 mg/day and vitamin D 800–1,000 units/day)
- Calcitonin-inhibitor of osteoclasts
- IV pamidronate (15 mg/kg, every 3 months for 1 year)
- Bisphosphonates like Osteofos 75 mg once a week
- Moderate and high impact activities—walking, ballet dancing, aerobics jogging, etc.

Cardiac Complications

Cardiac decompensation secondary to myopathy, iron overload, and congestive cardiac failure resulting from anemia should be treated promptly. Adequate chelation and symptomatic therapy can reverse the cardiac damage caused by iron overload.

Leg Ulcers

Leg ulcers are more common in thalassemia intermedia and thalassemia minor **(Fig. 14.7.11)**. Bed rest, regular transfusions, and wound care are adequate. Local infiltration of growth factors such as granulocyte-colony stimulating factor (G-CSF) has been found to be useful.

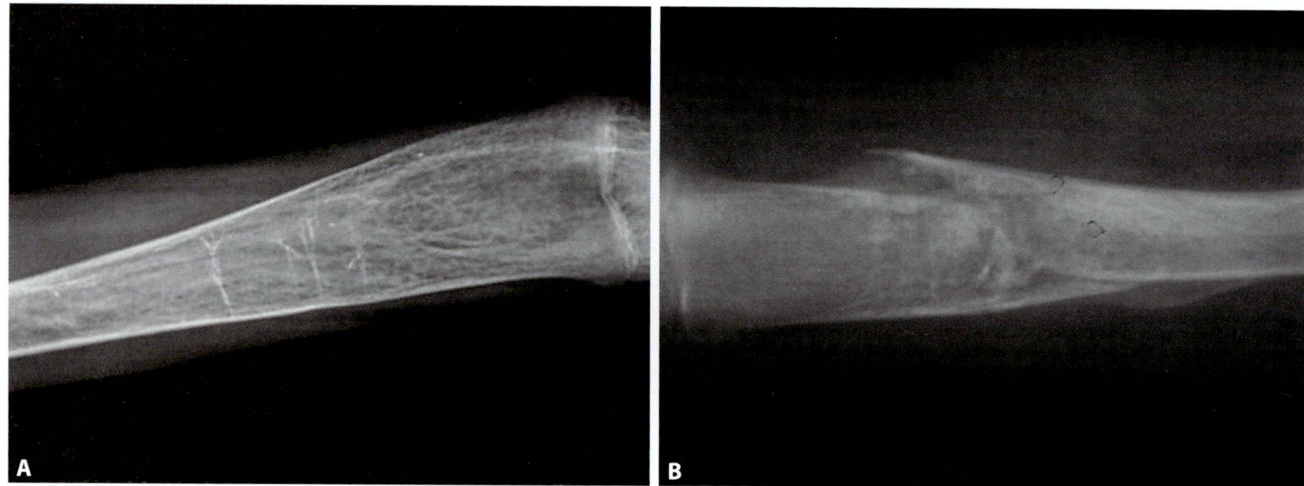

Figs. 14.7.10A and B: Osteopenia and osteoporosis of the long bone.
Courtesy: Dr MR Lokeshwar and Dr Mamta Manglani.

Gallstones and Hepatic Dysfunction

Gallstones are more commonly seen in children receiving irregular treatment as well as in thalassemia minor. In asymptomatic cases, no active treatment is required. However, they may be removed along with splenectomy (if splenectomy is indicated).

Liver dysfunction is secondary to plasma-borne infections and iron overload. It is thus necessary to do the liver function tests and hepatitis markers particularly HBsAg and HCV antibodies every 6 months.

Endocrine Evaluation and Assessment of Growth and Development

Growth retardation, hypogonadotropic hypogonadism, diabetes mellitus, hypothyroidism, hypoparathyroidism, osteopenia, and osteoporosis are the common endocrine abnormalities of thalassemia. Iron deposition in the pituitary, pancreas, and other endocrine organs leads to significant morbidity in transfusion-dependent thalassemic patients.

Curative Options—Bone Marrow Transplant or Stem Cell Transplant

Bone marrow transplantation is effective and offers the potential permanent cure if an HLA-matched sibling donor is available. The credit of first BMT in thalassemia major goes to E Donald Thomas who performed this procedure in an 18-month-old thalassemic child in 1982 using HLA matched elder sister as donor. This child was cured of thalassemia. The first BMT in thalassemia in India was successfully done by Dr M Chandy at Christian Medical College, Vellore. All over the world, transplantations have been done with a 70–80% cure rate.

The BMT is most successful in patients who are young, properly transfused and well-chelated, and in good clinical shape without hepatomegaly. Ideal age of transplantation is between 2 and 5 years. Younger the child lesser the iron overload and other complications, hence better the results. Transplant outcomes are better with a fully HLA-matched related donor; cord blood from a matched related donor can also potentially provide good outcomes. The cost of BMT in India is around INR 10–1,500,000 and is being done at Vellore, Mumbai, Chennai, Ahmadabad, Bangaluru, etc.

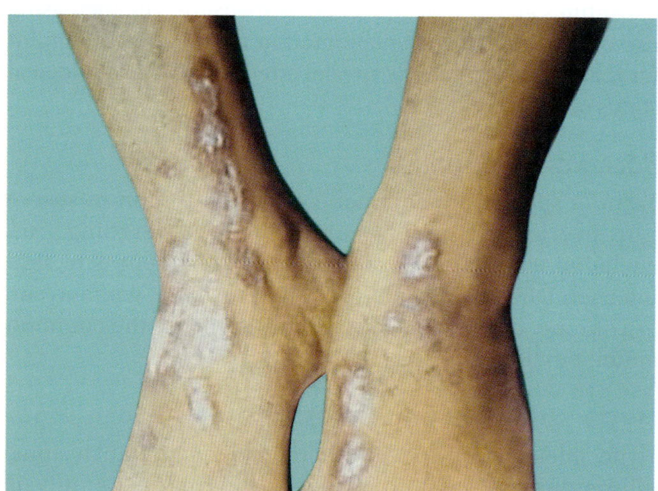

Fig. 14.7.11: Leg ulcers.

Allogeneic hematopoietic stem cell transplantation (HSCT) is the only curative option currently available for long-term survivors of hemoglobin Barts hydrops fetalis.

Pharmacological Methods to Increase Gamma Chain Production and Gene Manipulation

Drugs such as hydroxyurea, butyrate, 5-azacytidine, and erythropoietin have been tried to induce HbF production with varying success.

Hydroxyurea is a short-acting cytotoxic drug and is the only FDA-approved drug for the treatment of thalassemia. It is more useful in thalassemia intermedia. Dose is 5–10 mg/kg per day and slowly escalated as tolerated to 20 mg/kg/day. HbF induction with hydroxyurea may increase HbF and thus reduce transfusion requirements, decrease extramedullary erythropoietic masses, and decrease leg ulcers.

Thalidomide is a drug known for its immunomodulating and antiangiogenic properties. There are not enough clinical data to prove the efficacy. The combination of hydroxyurea with thalidomide reduced the need for transfusions among pediatric patients with β-thalassemia, according to the results of a single-arm study. The maximum response was achieved at the dose of 2–3 mg/kg of thalidomide.[6]

Erythropoietin has shown no benefit when used alone but in combination with hydroxyurea an additive effect has been found.

Metformin: In a phase I study conducted in children >12 years with NTDT and sickle cell disease, metformin-induced expression of HbF in primary erythroid cell cultures and is additive with hydroxyurea.

Amlodipine: In a small phase III trial, amlodipine at a dose of 5 mg per day >30 kg or 2.5 mg/day <30 kg improved the myocardial iron overload without increasing the adverse effects when given in combination with standard iron chelation therapy.

Wheatgrass acts as an antioxidant and detoxifier. Oral intake of aqueous extract of *Triticum aestivum* has shown to reduce transfusion requirement in TDT in children with thalassemia receiving chronic blood transfusions.

Fetal globin reactivation: BCL11A is being currently studied as a therapeutic target in β-thalassemia.

Gene Therapy

Among the novel gene therapies, lentiviral vector gene therapy has shown to provide adequate clinical efficacy and safety. The European Commission granted conditional approval, in June 2019, for the Bluebird bio gene therapy product (autologous CD34+ cells encoding the β A-T87Q-globin gene) under the commercial name Zynteglo, to treat transfusion-dependent β-thalassemia in patients 12 years and older, for whom HSCT is appropriate but an HLA-matched, related donor is not available.

Gene Addition and Gene Editing

In the last decade, new curative strategies have been developed—gene addition and gene editing, the former acting by adding a copy of a gene into the genome of the cells in the target organ or tissue, the latter by altering the DNA sequence of a gene and thus modifying its expression.[7,8] These techniques target specific mutation sites and replace them with the normal sequence.

UK Medicines and Healthcare Products Regulatory Agency (MHRA) has granted conditional marketing authorization for CASGEVY™ (Exa-cel, a CRISPR/Cas9 gene-edited therapy, for the treatment of TDT (patients >12 years of age) for whom a HLA-matched donor not available.

EMERGING THERAPIES[7]

Activin Receptor–II Ligand Traps

Sotatercept (ACE-011) showed improvement in hemoglobin level and decreased transfusion burden in NTDT and TDT in phase II study with a dose of ≥0.3 mg/kg and ≥0.5 mg/kg, respectively. Doses were administered by SC injection every 3 weeks. However, the trials were terminated due to binding of sotatercept to activin A.

Luspatercept (ACE-536, Reblozyl) has been permitted official authorization by European Medicines Agency (EMA) and FDA. Luspatercept seems to be promising, with significant improvement in hemoglobin levels and reduction in transfusion requirements. The recommended starting dose of luspatercept is 1 mg/kg once every 3 weeks by SC injection. The dose is increased to 1.25 mg if reduction in red cell transfusion burden is not achieved by 6 weeks. Luspatercept is not currently indicated in the pediatric population because no data are available yet. Clinical trials are underway to evaluate the efficacy and safety in this population (NCT04143724).[9]

Pyruvate Kinase Activators

Mitapivat (AG-348) is an oral, small-molecule activator of wild-type, and mutant forms of PKR. In studies of adult patients with pyruvate kinase (PK) deficiency, twice daily dosing with mitapivat reduced hemolysis and improved anemia.

Etavopivat (FT-4202) is another oral private kinase activator currently under evaluation.

Janus Kinase Inhibitor (Ruxolitinib)

A recent study looked at the efficacy and safety of ruxolitinib in IE suppression as a pretransplantation treatment in 10 pediatric patients with TDT. The outcomes of HSCT post-ruxolitinib treatment were favorable in seven of eight cases.[10]

Glycine Transporter-1 Inhibitors

Bitopertin (RO-4917838): The phase 2 trial was prematurely terminated as there was no improvement in the hematological and chemical biomarkers.

Role of Macrophage Manipulation Therapy

It is still under experimental stage.

Hepcidin Targeting Drugs

There are ongoing trials for hepcidin mimetics (LJPC-401,PTG-300), agonists of hepcidin regulator TMPRSS6

(Ionis-TMPRSS6-LRx), and ferroportin inhibitors (VIT-2763). Other approaches targeting iron dysregulation as minihepcidins, exogenous transferrin, erythroferrone inhibitors, and AG-348 (an oral, small molecule, allosteric activator of the red cell-specific form of PK) are in preclinical studies. Different agents are studied in α-thalassemia, with the most promising being luspatercept and mitapivat.

PREVENTION OF THALASSEMIA

Prenatal Diagnosis

It is conventionally based on molecular or cytogenetic analysis of fetal cells from chorionic villi, amniotic fluid, or fetal blood obtained from invasive obstetric procedures. The discovery of fetus-originated cell-free fetal DNA (cff-DNA) in maternal plasma of pregnant females has opened a new approach for noninvasive prenatal testing (NIPT).

Preimplantation Genetic Testing For Monogenic Disease

Preimplantation genetic diagnosis has been used not only to avoid the risk of having an affected child, but it also offers, using HLA matching, preselection of potential HLA-genoidentical healthy donor progeny for an affected sibling who requires BMT.[11]

BMT in Utero

Research is underway on BMT in utero, at 14 weeks of gestation. Intrauterine HSCT is another promising approach.

In Utero Stem Cell Transplantation

It may enable treatment of life-threatening disorders before birth, ameliorate in utero damage, and potentially provide curative treatment.[12] Two clinical trials of in utero stem cell transplantation (IU-SCT) are in progress (NCT02986698 and NCT03706482).

GOVERNMENT INITIATIVE

Thalassemia Bal Sewa Yojana

The Coal India CSR-funded HSCT program is a unique initiative aimed to help underprivileged thalassemia patients who have a matched sibling donor but do not have the financial resources to cover the cost of the procedure.

CONCLUSION

Until the last few decades, thalassemia was regarded as uniformly fatal disease and death was expected during the second decade of life before adulthood. However, progress in the understanding and management of the disease has brought brighter prospects of survival extending into the third and fourth decades of life, provided, they receive the latest treatment with good compliance. This has opened a new chapter in the management of thalassemia beyond blood transfusion and chelation therapy.

The availability of hematopoietic stem cell transplant (HSCT) and advances in this field with gene therapy in the last two decades has immensely changed the outlook of families with children afflicted with thalassemia and given them hope regarding a permanent cure for the disease.

REFERENCES

1. Lokeshwar MR, Kanakia S. Thalassemia Syndromes. Parthasarathy A, Menon PSN (Eds). IAP Recent Advances in Pediatrics, 1st edition. New Delhi: Jaypee Brothers Medical Publishers Pvt Ltd.; 2020. pp. 340-70.
2. Lokeshwar MR. Thalassemia Syndromes. Parthasarathy A, Menon PSN, Nair MKC (Eds). IAP Textbook of Pediatrics, 7th edition. New Delhi: Jaypee Brothers Medical Publishers Pvt Ltd.; 2019; pp. 881-98.
3. Lokeshwar MR, Sharma R, Pandrowala A, Manglani MV. Thalassemia Syndromes. In: Lokeshwar MR, Shah NK, Sachdeva A, Agarwal BR, Manglani MV (Eds). Textbook of Pediatric Hematology and Hemato-Oncology. New Delhi: Jaypee Brothers Medical Publishers Pvt Ltd.; 2016;17:163-89.
4. Sanchez-Villalobos M, Blanquer M, Moraleda JM, Salido EJ, Perez-Oliva AB. New Insights Into Pathophysiology of β-Thalassemia. Front Med (Lausanne). 2022;9:880752.
5. Ferih K, Elsayed B, Elshoeibi AM, Elsabagh AA, Elhadary M, Soliman A, et al. Applications of Artificial Intelligence in Thalassemia: A Comprehensive Review. Diagnostics. 2023;13(9):1551.
6. Ansari SH, Ansari I, Wasim M, Sattar A, Khawaja S, Zohaib M, et al. Evaluation of the combination therapy of hydroxyurea and thalidomide in β-thalassemia. Blood Adv. 2022;6(24):6162-8.
7. Bou-Fakhredin R, Kuo KHM, Taher AT. Emerging Therapies in β-Thalassemia. Hematol Oncol Clin North Am. 2023;37(2):449-62.
8. Christakopoulos GE, Telange R, Yen J, Weiss MJ. Gene therapy and Gene Editing for β-Thalassemia. Hematol Oncol Clin North Am. 2023;37(2):433-47.
9. Viprakasit V, Coates TD, Musallam KM, Buerki JV, Patturajan M, Holot N, et al A Phase 2a Study Evaluating the Safety and Pharmacokinetics (PK) of Luspatercept in Pediatric Patients with Transfusion-Dependent β-Thalassemia (TDT). Blood. 2021;138(Suppl 1):4161.
10. Ovsyannikova G, Balashov D, Demina I, Shelikhova L, Pshonkin A, Maschan M, et al. Efficacy and safety of ruxolitinib in ineffective erythropoiesis suppression as a pretransplantation treatment for pediatric patients with beta-thalassemia major. Pediatr Blood Cancer. 2021;68(11):e29338.
11. Parikh FR, Athalye AS, Kulkarni DK, Sanap RR, Dhu, Warang DJ, et al. Evolution and Utility of Preimplantation Genetic Testing for Monogenic Disorders in Assisted Reproduction—A Narrative Review. J Hum Reprod Sci. 2021;14(4):329-39.
12. Sagar RL, Walther-Jallow L, Götherström C, Westgren M, David AL. Maternal and fetal safety outcomes after in utero stem cell injection: a systematic review. Prenat Diagn. 2023;43(13):1622-37.

14.8 Sickle Cell Anemia

Vibhawari S Dani, Dipty L Jain

INTRODUCTION

Sickle cell disease (SCD) is the most common inherited hemoglobinopathy. In 1910, Dr. James Herrick described the characteristic sickle-shaped red blood cells (RBC) on the blood smear of a 20-year-old dental student from Grenada.[1] In 1952, Lehmann and Cutbush described the presence of sickle hemoglobin (Hb) in the tribal population of Nilgiri hills in South India. It is characterized by a point mutation in β-globin gene located on short arm of chromosome 11, where the base adenine is replaced by thymine in the coding sequence of DNA that results in the substitution of glutamic acid with valine on the sixth amino acid of β-globin chain.

EPIDEMIOLOGY OF SCD IN INDIA

India is the second-largest hub for SCD after Africa. About 15% of the total newborns with SCD in the world belong to India with an overall prevalence of 4.3%. Majority of these patients reside in tribal population in states of Gujarat, Maharashtra, Madhya Pradesh, Chhattisgarh, Odisha, and Telangana **(Fig. 14.8.1)**.[2]

INHERITANCE

Sickle cell anemia is called an autosomal recessive condition because you must have two copies of the sickle hemoglobin gene to have the disorder. Sickle hemoglobin is often shortened to S or sickle hemoglobin (HbS). If you have only one copy of the HbS along with one copy of the more usual hemoglobin (A or HbA), you are said to have sickle cell trait or sickle cell carrier state. If both parents have sickle cell trait (HbAS), there is a one-in-four (25%) chance that any given child could be born with sickle cell anemia (HbSS). There is also a one-in-four chance that any given child could be completely unaffected. There is a one-in-two (50%) chance that any given child will get the sickle cell trait **(Fig. 14.8.2)**.[3]

PHENOTYPE HETEROGENEITY IN INDIAN CONTEXT

First reported among tribal people in southern India, there was an early misconception that the *SS* gene was linked to the tribal origin, but later it was found to be widespread among nontribals too. The polymorphisms in DNA surrounding the β-globin locus are different from those observed in African peoples, most readily explained as an independent occurrence of the HbS gene, known as the Asian haplotype. This haplotype occurs in 91–100% of Indian patients with SS disease and is typical of the disease in the eastern province of Saudi Arabia.[4]

PATHOPHYSIOLOGY

Sickle cell disease causes polymerization of the hemoglobin molecule that alters the erythrocyte shape. This in turn leads to the inability of RBC to deform. Hence, there is increased adhesion of erythrocytes which causes small vessel occlusion resulting in hypoxia. This process triggers a vicious cycle of increased HbS formation, the release of inflammatory mediators, and free radicals that contribute to reperfusion injury. Erythrocytes are more likely to sickle and become rigid in the presence of dehydration. Other associated pathological events include increased neutrophil adhesiveness, nitric oxide binding, increased platelet activation, and hypercoagulability, all of which leads to increased sickling. The damage caused to the microcirculation in turn leads to vaso-occlusive crisis, endothelial dysfunction, or hemolysis **(Fig. 14.8.3)**.[3]

LABORATORY TESTS FOR SICKLE CELL DISEASE

Sickling Test

Sickling test is a part of the diagnostic workup in patients suspected of having a sickle cell syndrome. Sodium metabisulfite reduces the oxygen tension inducing the typical sickle shape of red blood cells. It is important to let the preparation stand for 24 hours before declaring the test negative. However, it does not distinguish homozygous from heterozygous sickle cell cases **(Fig. 14.8.4)**.

Solubility Test

It is an easy and inexpensive method for rapid detection of HbS. HbS is quite insoluble in a high phosphate buffer solution in the reduced state. It forms water crystals (tactoids) which refract and deflect light rays and produce a turbid solution. False-negative results are seen when the HbS is <10% of the total hemoglobin, and also in patients with coinheritance of β-thalassemia trait and severe anemia. In contrast, false

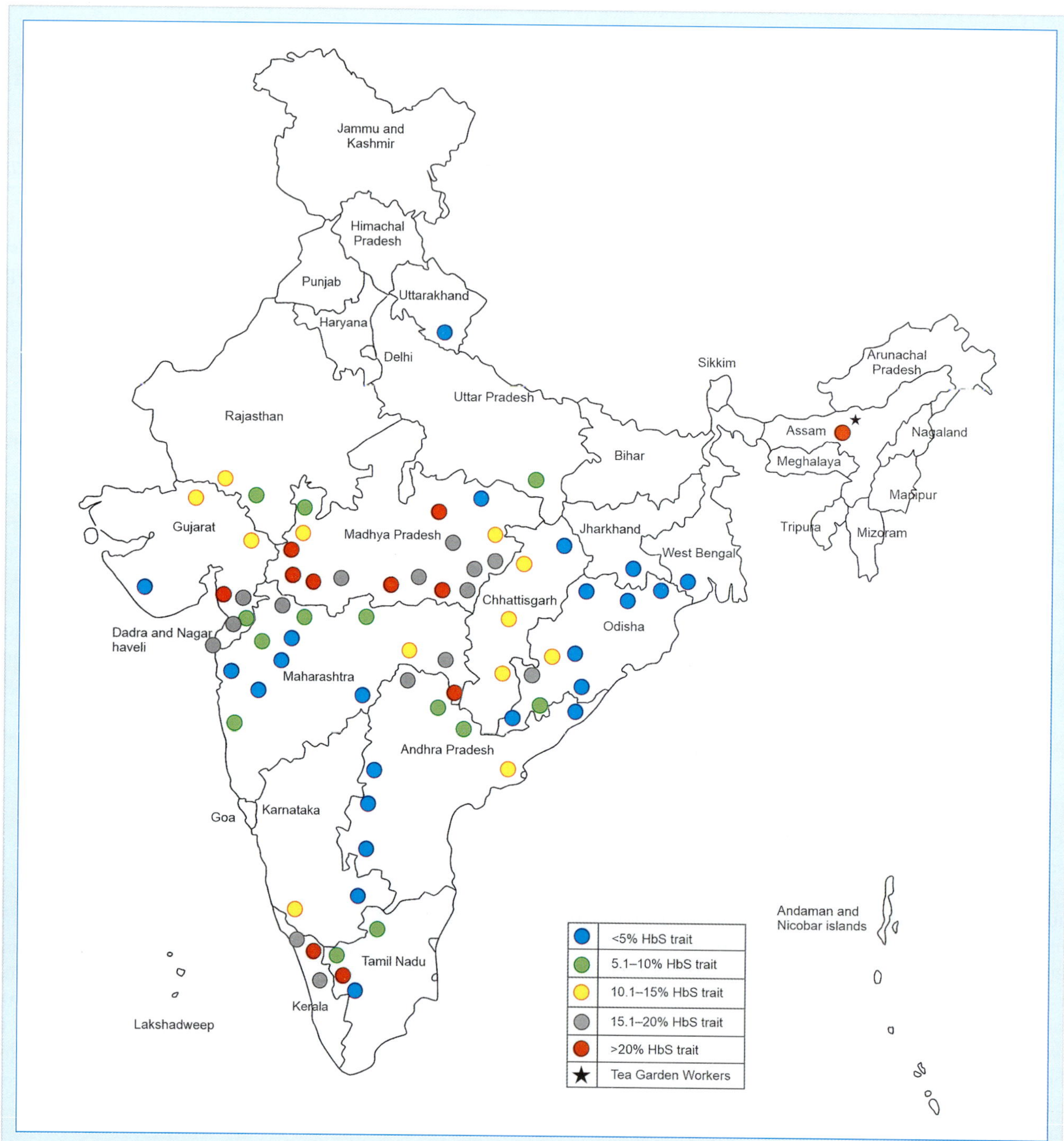

Fig. 14.8.1: District-wise distribution of sickle cell trait among the tribal communities in different states of India.

positives are observed in patients with high serum viscosity, erythrocytosis, and highly marked leukocytosis and in some cases of anemia **(Fig. 14.8.5)**.

Sickling and solubility tests should not be done in infancy due to higher fetal hemoglobin (HbF).

Hemoglobin Electrophoresis

Hemoglobin electrophoresis uses the principles of gel electrophoresis to separate the various types of hemoglobin (A, F, A2, S, and others). Sample is treated to release the hemoglobin from the red cells, introduced into a porous

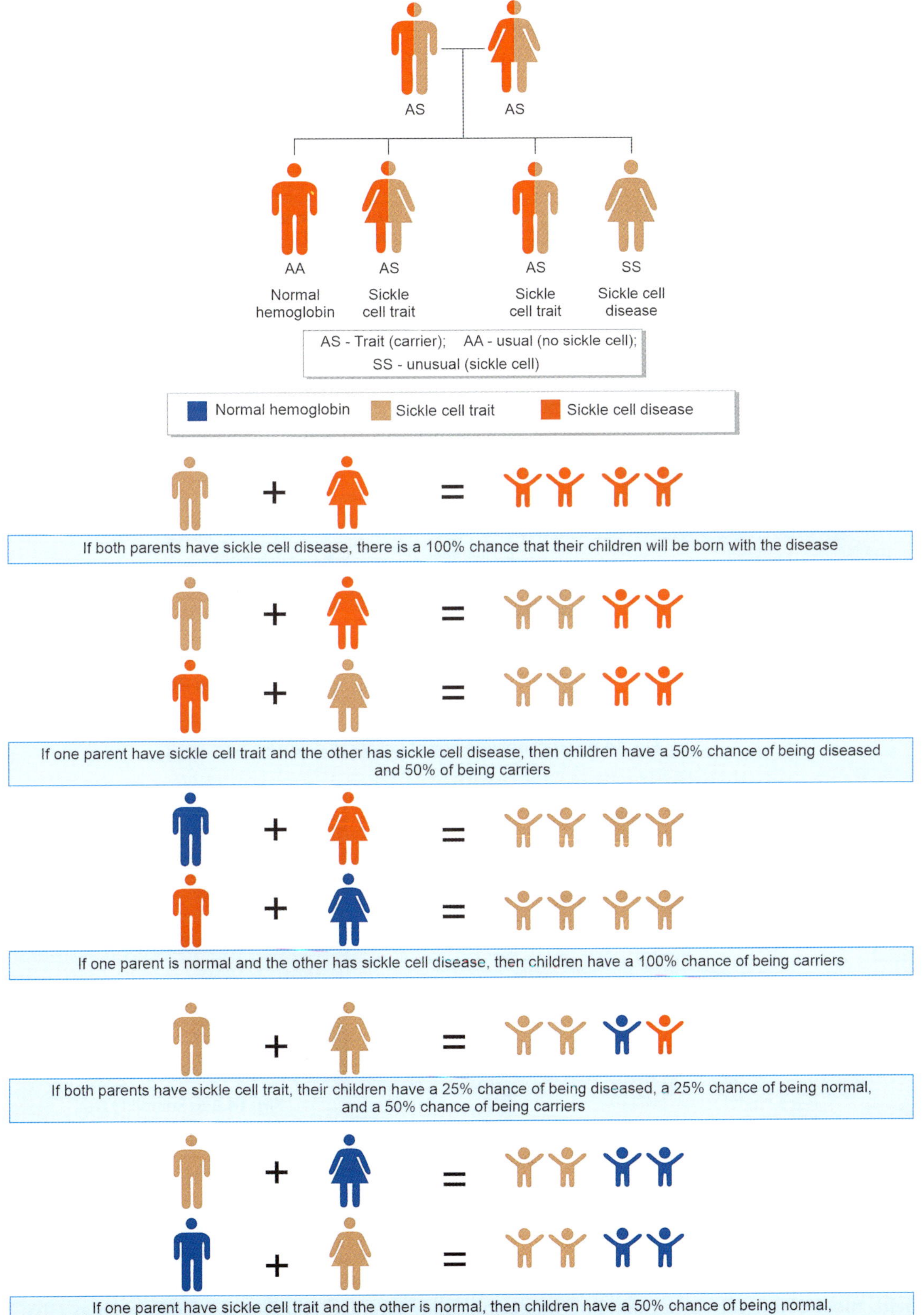

Fig. 14.8.2: Autosomal recessive pattern of inheritance of sickle cell disease.

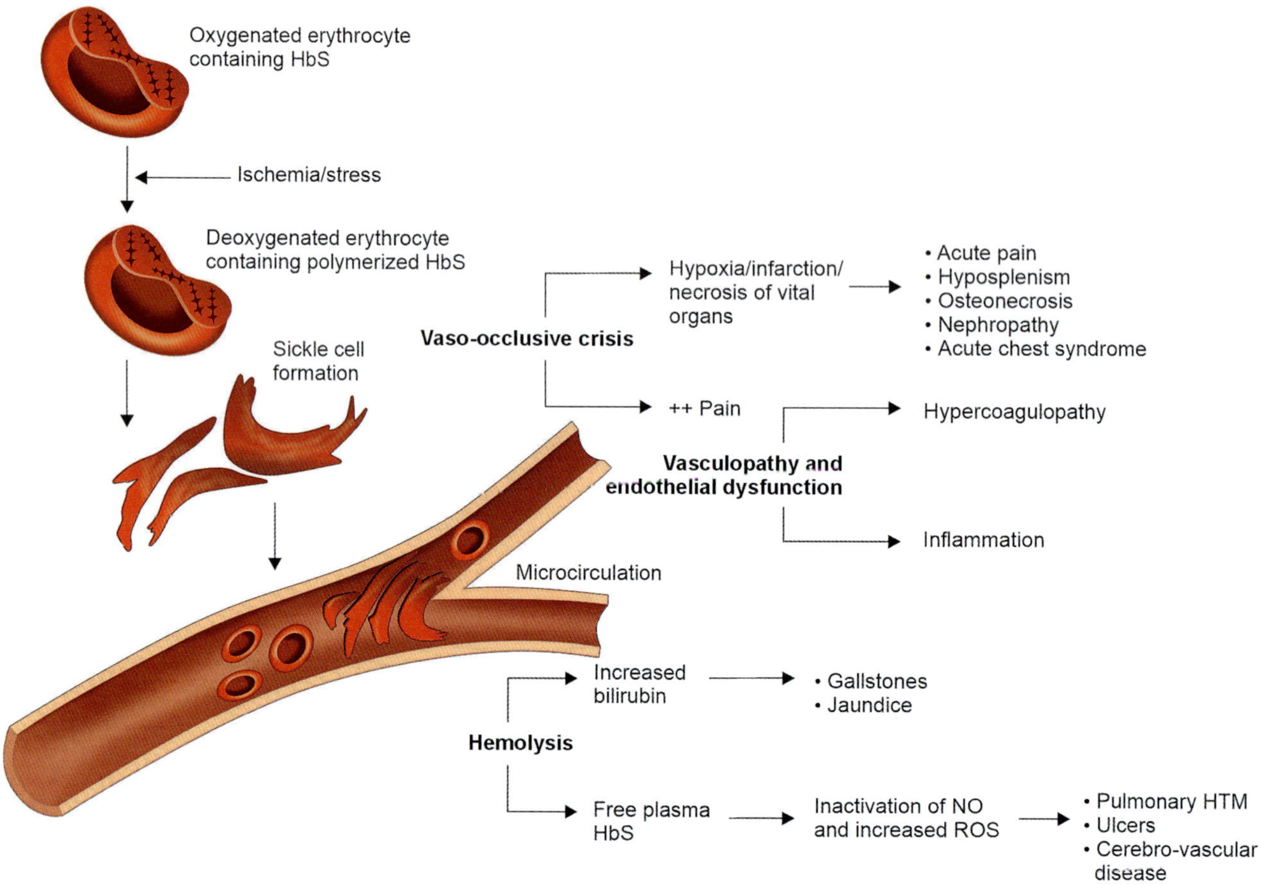

Oxygenated erythrocyte containing HbS

Ischemia/stress

Deoxygenated erythrocyte containing polymerized HbS

Sickle cell formation

Microcirculation

Vaso-occlusive crisis

Hypoxia/infarction/ necrosis of vital organs

- Acute pain
- Hyposplenism
- Osteonecrosis
- Nephropathy
- Acute chest syndrome

++ Pain

Vasculopathy and endothelial dysfunction

Hypercoagulopathy

Inflammation

Hemolysis

Increased bilirubin

- Gallstones
- Jaundice

Free plasma HbS

Inactivation of NO and increased ROS

- Pulmonary HTM
- Ulcers
- Cerebro-vascular disease

Fig. 14.8.3: Pathophysiology of sickle cell disease.

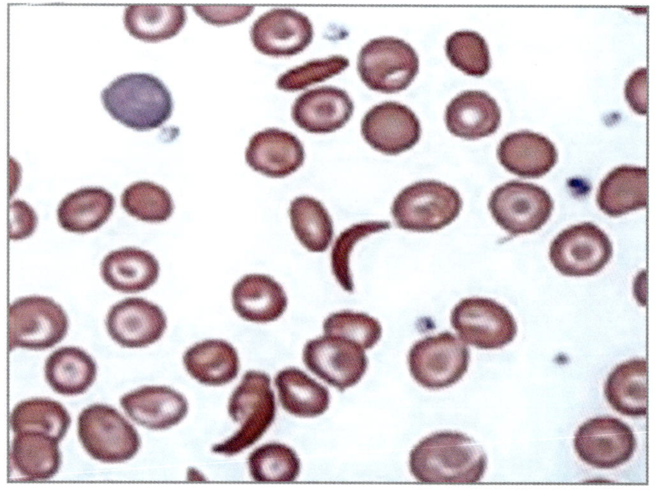

Fig. 14.8.4: Sickling test showing typical sickle shaped red blood cells (RBCs).

gel (usually made of cellulose acetate) and subjected to an electrical field, most commonly in an alkaline medium. HbS, HbD-Punjab, and HbD-Iran comigrate at alkaline pH. This method cannot quantify the Hb variant and thus

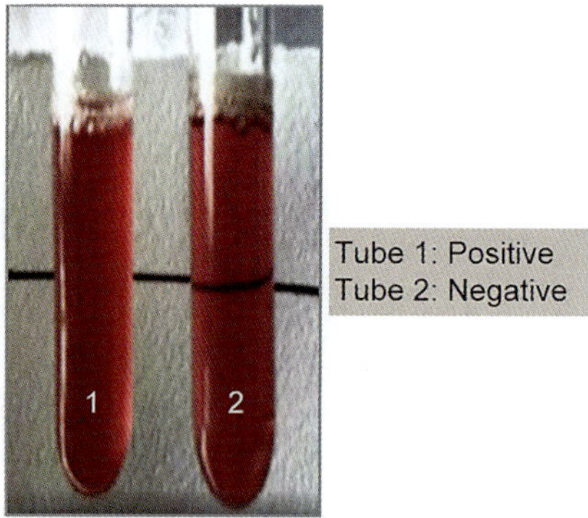

Fig. 14.8.5: Solubility test.

distinguishing carrier state from disease is not possible **(Fig. 14.8.6)**.[3]

High Performance Liquid Chromatography

This is the method of choice for quantitation of HbA2, HbF, and for detection and quantitation of the Hb variants, which may interact with β-thalassemia such as HbS, HbE, HbD-Punjab, and Hb-Lepore. This is based on the principle that positively-charged hemoglobin molecules adsorb onto a

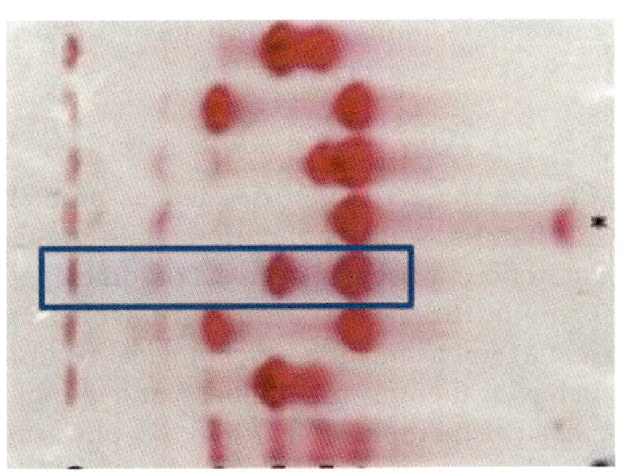

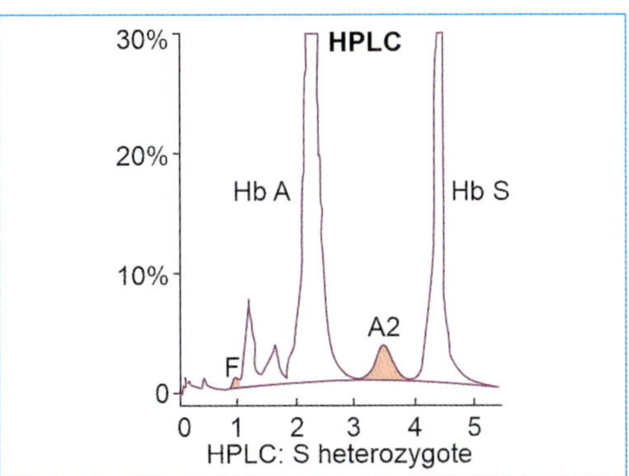

Fig. 14.8.6: Laboratory diagnosis of sickle cell disease showing Hb electrophoresis and high performance liquid chromatography (HPLC).

negatively-charged stationary phase in a microbore precision column till they are eluted out into a high-precision gradient-generating liquid buffer (mobile phase). A chromatogram of absorbance versus duration of adsorption "retention time" is displayed. Windows are set for common hemoglobin variants based on their retention times **(Fig. 14.8.6)**.[3]

No test for diagnosis of sickle cell disease should be performed till 3 months after the transfusion.

Capillary Electrophoresis

Capillary electrophoresis combines two principles of separation of hemoglobins, the electrophoretic mobility in alkaline buffer and the electro-osmotic flow. It is performed in a capillary that is filled with an electrolyte solution. Detected hemoglobin fractions can be relatively quantified and produce an electropherogram. In the presence of different Hb variants, capillary zone electrophoresis (CZE) is better than high performance liquid chromatography (HPLC) for quantifying HbA2 except in the presence of HbC.

Point of Care

Point of care devices have been tested and validated in the field in setting where they are required to be used. Devices which have been field tested and used for new born screening include Sickle SCAN, HemoTypeSC, Gazelle (Hemex Dx), etc.

SickleSCAN (BioMedomics™) is based on lateral flow chromatographic qualitative immunoassay. It utilizes Hb variant-specific polyclonal antibodies. The test is completed within 10–15 minutes and is easily interpretable and minimal training is required for conduct and interpretation of results. Presence of a line indicates the presence of Hb type. It can differentiate AS with SS. Newborn screening is possible with this test.

HemoTypeSC assay based on monoclonal antibody-based distinction of adult hemoglobin versus hemoglobin S and C by a competitive enzyme-linked lateral-flow immunoassay. Fetal hemoglobin does not affect results. Phenotype HbS/β0-thalassemia produces the same result as HbSS while other hemoglobin variants (HbD and HbE) produce the same result as HbA by HemoTypeSC assay.

Gazelle (Hemex Dx) is battery operated HemeChip cellulose acetate paper-based microchip electrophoresis system which yields results in ~8 minutes. However, it cannot be included in point of care test. Quantitative analysis of HbA, HbF, and HbS% is possible. It is a good confirmatory test for school screening and institution screening.

Molecular Diagnosis

It is the confirmatory method for diagnosis in neonatal screening program for SCD and mostly indicated in couples requiring prenatal diagnosis, patients in whom the diagnosis is uncertain (usually due to ambiguous results on screening tests or after a recent transfusion or if parental studies not possible) and genotype/phenotype discorrelation. Commonly used methods are PCR-RFLP (by DdeI, MstII, Bsu 361) (presence of HbS, zygosity), ARMS-PCR for b-mutations (co-inheritance of β-thalassemia), PCR-RFLP (by EcoRI) (co-inheritance of HbD Punjab), and Sanger sequencing. Less commonly used tests include ARMS-PCR for βS allele or ASO-PCR or reverse dot-blot hybridization (RDB) assay.[3]

CLINICAL MANIFESTATIONS

Vaso-occlusive Crisis

Vaso-occlusive crisis (VOC) is acute painful episode most commonly occurring in bones, lungs, liver, spleen, brain, and penis, due to intravascular sickling and tissue infarction. It is mainly localized to hand and foot in patients aged 2–5 years, large joints after 5 years of age and ribs and vertebrae in adolescents.

Hand and Foot Syndrome

This painful hand-foot syndrome is typically the first clinical manifestation of SCD. It occurs in about 50% of children by the age of 2 years. Small bones of hands and feet are often affected in children younger than 5 years of age. Involvement varies from individual bone to multiple small bones of hands

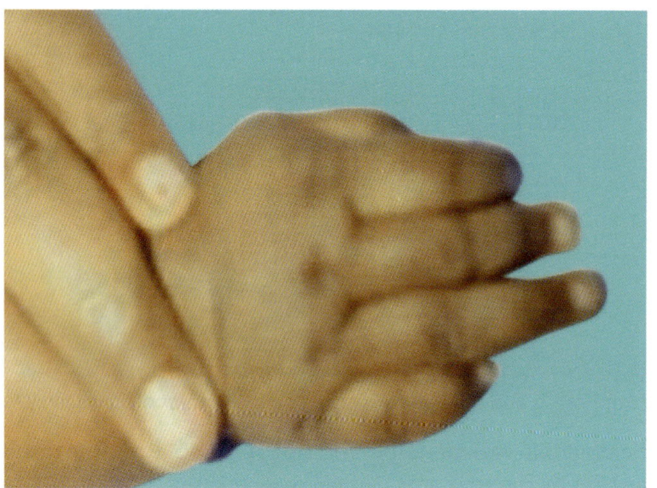

Fig. 14.8.7: Dactylitis.

and feet **(Fig. 14.8.7)**. They become mildly to extremely painful and may also become swollen or tender, or both. The age at which a child experiences the hand-foot syndrome is a strong predictor of overall severity by 10 years of age.

Unilateral dactylitis should be differentiated from osteomyelitis as the treatment differs significantly. Dactylitis requires pain medications such as acetaminophen with codeine, whereas osteomyelitis requires at least 6 weeks of antibiotics. Hand-foot syndrome disappears when bone marrow from small bones of hands and feet stop erythropoietic activity. These episodes resolve completely but attacks tend to recur.

Pain

Pain in SCD can be classified into three types and should be treated as a disease.[5-7]

Acute Pain

It is evoked by VOC in which sickle RBCs adhere to the activated endothelium leading to vaso-occlusion of blood vessels and bone marrow ischemia.[6-7] The pain is rapid-onset, continuous, and deep throbbing in nature.[5] Pain should be assessed using Wong-Baker Faces Pain Rating Scale to see severity. The scale shows a series of faces ranging from a "happy face" at 0, or "no hurt", to a crying face at 10, which represents "hurts like the worst pain imaginable." Acute pain in sickle can be precipitated by physical stress, infection, dehydration, hypoxia, local or systemic acidosis, exposure to cold, and swimming for prolonged period.

Specific therapy for pain varies greatly and includes the use of acetaminophen or nonsteroidal anti-inflammatory drug (NSAID) early in the course followed by escalation to opioids if the pain does not get relieved. Intravenous (IV) hydration does not relieve or prevent pain and is appropriate only in conditions when the patient is dehydrated or unable to drink because of severe pain.[6]

Chronic Pain

Chronic pain is often defined as pain that persists for ≥3 months. Sources of chronic pain in SCD include bone infarction, avascular necrosis of joints, leg ulcers, chronic osteomyelitis, etc.[5,7] Nonpharmacological strategies of management include psychological techniques (cognitive behavior therapy, mindfulness, and coping skills training), physical therapies (e.g., exercise, physical activities, and yoga), integrative medicine approaches (e.g., massage and acupuncture) and initiation of chronic opioid therapy if pain is refractory to multiple other treatment modalities.[6]

Neuropathic Pain

Neuropathic pain is described as numb, tingling, shooting, or paroxysmal in nature associated with a sensation of pins and needles, hyperalgesia, and allodynia.[5] Its severity is also enhanced by exposure to either cold or heat. This pain could be secondary to nerve injury or nerve dysfunction whether peripheral or central. Anecdotally, neuropathic pain in SCD may be the result of tissue damage after vaso-occlusion of blood vessels of nerves (vasa vasorum). It is usually treated with gabapentin (GABA analog).[6,7]

Acute Chest Syndrome

Acute chest syndrome (ACS) is an episode of acute lung injury that occurs with alveolar-capillary leak and neutrophilic inflammation, which may be radiographically and clinically indistinguishable from multi-lobar pneumonia.[8] It is the most common cause of death and the second most common cause of hospital admission.

The clinical diagnosis of ACS is defined as an acute illness with a new pulmonary infiltrate [chest X-ray and computed tomography (CT])] consistent with consolidation, but not atelectasis, along with one of the following symptoms: chest pain, fever (>38.5°C), cough, tachypnea, wheezing, rales, appearance of an increased work of breathing, and hypoxemia relative to baseline (>2% decrease in SpO_2 from steady state on room air, and PaO_2 <60 mmHg).[8]

Fat embolism has also been considered as a cause of ACS and should be considered in any patient presenting with rapid onset of respiratory distress and altered mental state changes. The treatment is multimodal and blood transfusion (either simple or exchange) is the only method to abort a rapidly progressing ACS episode.

Acute Episodes: Priapism

Priapism is a painful, prolonged erection of the penis. It may occur starting in early childhood, and the estimated prevalence in males with HbSS is 30–40% by 18 years of age. Episodes occur in two patterns: prolonged, lasting >4 hours, and shorter "stuttering" episodes. Stuttering priapism may occur in cluster and sometimes daily. A prolonged episode of priapism requires rapid intervention to prevent ischemic damage to the penis and erectile dysfunction. Management includes hydration, pain control, and oral adrenergic medications such as pseudoephedrine. If an episode lasts longer than 4 hours, aspiration of the corpora cavernosa and irrigation with a dilute solution of phenylephrine or epinephrine is indicated. Chronic transfusion may prevent recurrent events, but the use of simple transfusion for an acute event is unproven.

Neurological Complication

The incidence of stroke is 300 times higher in HbSS than HbAA children. The most common underlying lesion is internal carotid stenosis or obstruction but proximal medial carotid artery and anterior carotid artery can also be involved. Hemiplegia, speech defect, seizures, and gait dysfunction may occur. Cognitive impairment may occur due to silent cerebral infarct.

The Stroke Prevention Trial in Sickle Cell Anemia (STOP) study, was the first primary prevention trial for stroke in HbSS and the first randomized controlled trial of chronic transfusion for any indication in HbSS.

Primary Prevention of Stroke

Transcranial Doppler (TCD) screening of children with SCD-SS is recommended to start at 2 years of age and continue annually till 18 years to identify those with a high risk of developing stroke. If TCD velocity is 170–99 cm/s (conditional), then repeat in 3 months. If time averaged mean maximum velocity (TAMMV) ≥200 cm/s (abnormal) is detected in the anterior or middle cerebral artery on two occasions 6 weeks apart, this is an indication for a transfusion program to prevent primary stroke.

Another indication for primary stroke prevention is occurrence of transient ischemic attacks (TIAs). In those identified with the high risk, stroke should be prevented with hydroxyurea or transfusion. If blood transfusion is used, to be effective, the circulating HbS should be reduced to <30%.

Magnetic resonance imaging (MRI) with magnetic resonance venography/or angiography (MRV/MRA). Diffusion-weighted MRI (DW MRI is highly sensitive in detecting early ischemic changes in first 4–6 hours. Administer oxygen to maintain SpO_2 above 96%. Initially, simple (top-up) blood transfusion within 1 hour of presentation, with goal of increasing Hb to maximum of 11 g/dL is effective. If baseline Hb is >11 g/dL, then standard approach is exchange transfusion to reduce HbS by at least <50%, if not 30%. The aim of the maintenance blood transfusion program, preferably exchange transfusion, is to keep the proportion of HbS below 30% in the patient's blood indefinitely, to prevent secondary stroke.

Acute Splenic Sequestration Crisis

This event is defined as decrease of hemoglobin or packed cell volume (PCV) of at least 20% from the baseline along with increase in the palpable spleen size of >2 cm from baseline due to trapping of large amount of red cell mass in spleen or less commonly in liver **(Fig. 14.8.8)**. On presentation, patients appear weak and dyspneic with sudden, rapidly enlarging spleen, anemia, and shock. This is associated with increase in nucleated RBCs, reticulocytosis to 20–30% and moderate-to-severe thrombocytopenia. Sequestration may recur within 4 months of initial episode. In emergency, blood transfusion should be given only at 5 mL per kg and/or a post-transfusion Hb target of 8 g/dL, keeping in mind that the goal of transfusion is to prevent hypovolemia. Blood transfusion that results in Hb >10 g/dL may put the patient at a risk of hyperviscosity syndrome because blood may be released from the spleen post-transfusion. Elective splenectomy after second episode is recommended to eliminate recurrence. Pneumococcal vaccine and prophylactic penicillin for 3 years is recommended following splenectomy.

Infection and Bacteremia

Fever alone is considered a potential emergency situation and fever associated with pain should not be considered a VOC until infection is ruled out. Predisposing factors include functional asplenia (hyposplenism), impaired complement activity, zinc deficiency, iron overload, hypoventilation, and the presence of necrotic tissue. High grade fever (>39°C or 102.4°F) is potentially serious in children with homozygous

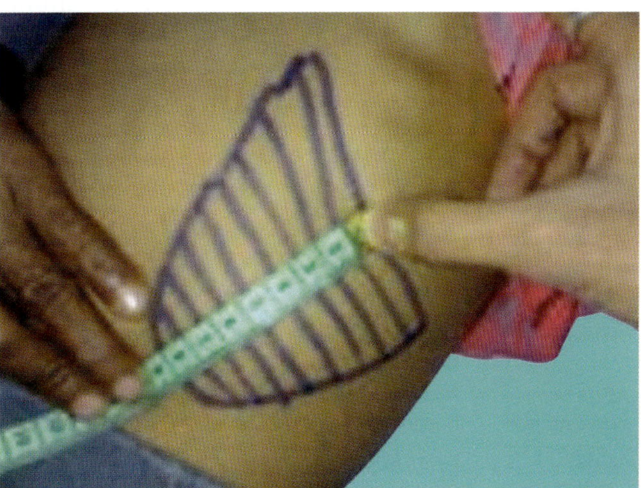

Fig. 14.8.8: Splenic sequestration.

"SS" disease and possible septicemia must be investigated. Organisms most commonly involved are *Streptococcus pneumoniae, Haemophilus influenzae,* and gram-negative enteric organisms. Osteomyelitis and septic arthritis can occur, and patients with pain should be investigated for avascular necrosis or bone infarcts. Osteomyelitis is most often caused by *Salmonella*. These children should be managed with IV third-generation cephalosporins. Prophylaxis with oral penicillin, erythromycin up to 5 years of age and pneumococcal vaccination is advised.

Aplastic Crisis

Human parvovirus B19 infection poses a unique threat for patients with SCD because this results in temporary red cell aplasia. Any child with SCD, fever and reticulocytopenia should be presumed to have parvovirus B19 infection until proven otherwise. In addition, acute infection with parvovirus B19 is associated with pain, splenic sequestration, ACS, glomerulonephritis, arthropathy, and stroke. Many of these patient`s aplastic crisis is contagious and infection precaution should be taken to avoid nosocomial spread of infection.

Renal Disease

The SCD nephropathies include gross hematuria, papillary necrosis, nephrotic syndrome, renal infarction, hyposthenuria, pyelonephritis, and renal medullary carcinoma. The clinical presentation includes hematuria, proteinuria, renal insufficiency, concentrating defects, and hypertension. Nocturnal enuresis has also been encountered in about 33% of children with SCD which is usually troublesome for the child as well as the parent.

Sickle Hepatopathy

Sickle hepatopathy is a broad term for a range of hepatic complications from mild liver dysfunction to chronic liver failure and cirrhosis **(Table 14.8.1)**.[9] Management is supportive with hydration, pain control, or transfusion as needed for symptomatic anemia.

Hyperhemolytic Crisis

Hyperhemolytic crisis refers to the sudden exacerbation of hemolysis with worsening anemia despite ongoing reticulocyte production. Serial hemoglobin levels, reticulocyte counts, and hemoglobin electrophoresis may be helpful in making a diagnosis of hyperhemolysis in the post-transfusion setting. Delayed hemolytic transfusion reaction (DHTR) is often associated with a positive antiglobulin test (DAT). Corticosteroids (methylprednisolone 500 mg/day for 2 days) and intravenous immunoglobulin (IVIG; 0.4 g/kg daily for 5 days) are the mainstays of treatment. In some cases, rituximab may be required after specialist consultation.

Leg Ulcers

Leg ulcers are a chronic painful problem. They result from minor injury to the area around the malleoli. Because of relativity poor circulation, compounded by sickling and microinfarcts, healing is delayed, and infection becomes established.

Orthopedic Complications

Orthopedic complications are one of the most common sources of long-term morbidity in patients with SCD, typically chronic osteomyelitis and avascular necrosis of the head of the femur **(Table 14.8.2)**. The presentation is characterized by pain in the hips, limping, and progressive deformity of the hip joints. Management includes prolonged analgesics, which only provide temporal relief of pain. The standard treatment for these patients should include physical therapy and surgical intervention.

Table 14.8.3 lists the chronic clinical complications of SCD affecting kidneys, hearts, lungs, brain, and other organs.

MANAGEMENT OF SICKLE CELL DISEASE

Routine Healthcare and Monitoring

All the newly diagnosed patients and newborns should be enrolled and registered in SCD registry. Document the

TABLE 14.8.1: Acute hepatobiliary manifestations of sickle cell disease.

Acute manifestations of SCD	*Clinical presentation*	*Biochemical changes*			*Management*
		Transaminase (AST, ALT) levels	*Bilirubin*	*Alkaline phosphatase*	
Acute sickle cell hepatic crisis	Fever, acute onset RUQ pain, jaundice, and tender hepatomegaly	Normal to 3 × upper normal	Up to 15 mg/dL, mainly conjugated	Normal to slight elevation	Supportive with treatment of SCD crisis
Acute hepatic sequestration	Acute onset RUQ pain, hepatomegaly and anemia	Normal	Up to 24 mg/dL, mainly conjugated	Can go up to 650 IU/L	Supportive with blood or exchange transfusion
Acute intrahepatic cholestasis	Fever, RUQ pain rapidly progressing to acute liver failure	Elevated usually >1,000	Elevated in 100s, mostly conjugated	Normal or elevated >1,000 IU/L	Supportive exchange transfusion, correction of coagulopathy? Liver transplant

(AST: aspartate transaminase; ALT: alanine transaminase; RUQ: right upper quadrant; SCD: sickle cell disease)

TABLE 14.8.2: Acute clinical orthopedic complications of sickle cell disease.

	Manifestations	*Pathophysiology*	*Treatment*
Painful event	Dactylitis, pain in the sternum/ribs, pain in the long bones, priapism	Vaso-occlusion, hypoxia, ischemia-reperfusion	Hydration, analgesia
Infection	Bacteremia/sepsis, meningitis, osteomyelitis, pneumonia, malaria	Splenic dysfunction, defective alternate pathway for complement-mediated lysis due to deficient levels of serum opsonin, inflammation, necrotic bone	Antibiotics, surgery
Anemia	Splenic sequestration, transient aplastic crisis	Erythrocyte sickling, infection, sequestration	Transfusion
Hyperhemolytic crisis	Sudden worsening anemia post-transfusion	Delayed hemolytic transfusion reaction (DHTR)	Corticosteroids, intravenous immunoglobulin (IVIG)
Organ damage	Stroke, acute chest syndrome, splenic infarction, renal papillary necrosis, priapism	Ischemia, infarction, hemorrhage	Hydration, transfusion

TABLE 14.8.3: Chronic clinical complications of sickle cell disease.

	Manifestations	*Treatment*
Kidneys	Hyposthenuria, glomerular hyperfiltration, glomerulosclerosis, albuminuria, end-stage renal disease	ACE inhibitors, hydroxycarbamide, dialysis, renal transplant
Heart/ lungs	Restrictive lung disease, elevated tricuspid jet velocity, pulmonary hypertension, restrictive cardiomyopathy	Bronchodilators, hydroxycarbamide, transfusion
Brain	Ischemic stroke, hemorrhagic stroke, silent infarction, neurological decline	Transfusion, hydroxycarbamide
Liver	Jaundice, pigmented gall stone	Cholecystectomy
Spleen	Infarction, hypersplenism	Splenectomy
Bones/ skin	Avascular necrosis, leg ulcers	Physical therapy, cord decompression, wound care, surgery
Eyes	Retinopathy	Laser therapy
Penis	Impotence, infertility	Surgery (if needed)

HPLC pattern, HbF level, patient's baseline clinical disease status, baseline laboratory parameters, vaccine records and past history of complications, and their ongoing treatment **(Table 14.8.4)**.

Penicillin Prophylaxis (Penicillin V Potassium)

It is given since screening to children <5 years. The dose is 65 mg BD for children <12 months, 125 mg BD till 2 years, then 250 mg BD after 2 years till the age of 5 years. Erythromycin is recommended for patients who are allergic to penicillin. Discontinue penicillin prophylaxis in children with HbSS at age 5 years, unless they have had splenectomy; then it should be continued lifelong.

Folic Acid Supplementation

In children <1 year of age 2.5 mg daily; in those >1 year of age 5 mg daily.

Treatment of Acute Crises and Complications

Fluid Management in Vaso-occlusive Crisis

Give 100–120 mL/kg/day fluids orally (if there is no vomiting or if patient can drink that volume). Can use normal saline 0.9%. Avoid overhydration as it can cause pulmonary edema.

Pain Management

Early pain management should be done with oral analgesics at start point to cutoff the pain cycle. For mild pain, paracetamol 15 mg/kg 4–6-hourly or ibuprofen 10 mg/kg 8-hourly, or diclofenac 1 mg/kg 8-hourly orally. For severe pain it is advised to give diclofenac or paracetamol suppositories; Injection paracetamol, injection tramadol, or opioids are useful. Vasodilators such as pentoxifylline, nifedipine, and buflomedil increase microvascular circulation.[6]

Simple Blood Transfusion

Transfusion is an important therapy for SCD, but not needed in all patients. It is indicated in severe anemia (i.e., Hb <5 g/dL), preoperative transfusion to reduce complications postsurgery, patients who have Hb <10 g/dL with symptoms of anemia without any acute complications. Contraindications to simple transfusion are patients with SCD complications whose hemoglobin level is near their baseline (Hb 7–9 g/dL) and avoid use of simple blood transfusion therapy in individuals who have a Hb >10 g/dL and an HbS percentage >50% of total Hb due to the risk of hyperviscosity.

Exchange Transfusion

Management of acute emergency for rapid reduction in HbS concentration to <30% in multiorgan failure, suspected stroke,

TABLE 14.8.4: Ideal health maintenance for children with sickle cell disease.

Physical examination	*Age*	*Frequency*
All systemic examination	0–24 months	Every month till 3 months if possible
	>24 months	Every 3 months
Laboratory tests		
Complete blood count (CBC)/platelet/reticulocyte	3–24 months	Every 3 months
	>24 months	Every 3 months (monthly if on hydroxyurea)
Renal function tests	12 months	Annually (every 3 months if on hydroxyurea OR if microalbuminuria present)
Liver function tests	12 months	Annually (every 3 months if on hydroxyurea)
Urine analysis for microalbuminuria	>6 years	Annually; if abnormal repeat every 3 months
Serum ferritin	Iron deficiency and iron overload are both seen, if iron overload regular monitoring needed	Every 6 months for those on regular blood transfusions
Screening test		
Physical examination	*Age*	*Frequency*
Transcranial Doppler	2–18 years	Annually, if borderline repeat every 4 months, if abnormal repeat after 2–4 weeks. Do magnetic resonance imaging (MRI) if abnormal
Pulmonary function tests	>6 years	Annually based on clinical course
Echocardiogram	>12 years	Annually or depending on symptoms

ACS, and regularly scheduled exchange transfusions used in the prevention of stroke, ACS, and recurrent painful episodes.

Selection of blood component [packed red blood cell (PRBC)] requires the following:

- Matching for patient ABO and minor antigens (at minimum RH D, C, c, E, e and K)
- Matched for any alloantibodies
- Cross matched using antihuman globulin (AHG) technique
- Leukoreduced
- Preferably within 7–10 days of collection
- Negative for sickle cell trait

TABLE 14.8.5: Blood Transfusion for acute and chronic complications in sickle cell disease (SCD).

Complication	*How to transfuse*
Acute chest syndrome: Symptomatic, with decreased Hb of 1 g/dL below baseline	Simple
Anemia, symptomatic	Simple
Aplastic crisis	Simple
Splenic sequestration + severe anemia	Simple
Acute chest syndrome: Symptomatic, severe (oxygen saturation <90% despite supplement oxygen)	Exchange
Hepatic sequestration	Exchange or simple
Intrahepatic cholestasis	Exchange or simple
Multisystem organ failure	Exchange or simple
Stroke, acute	Simple or exchange
Chronic: Stroke risk	• Chronic program • Exchange or simple

- Irradiation not necessary unless planned for hemopoietic stem cell transplant (HSCT)

Table 14.8.5 lists how blood transfusion is performed for acute and chronic complications in SCD.

Vaccination for Sickle Cell Disease in India

Table 14.8.6 provides the current recommendations for immunization in addition to routine immunization for children with SCD.

Hydroxyurea

It is a ribonucleotide reductase inhibitor, increases γ-globin gene expression, which causes a shift in gene expression away from the β-globin gene. It also causes arrest of the cell cycle in S phase of replicating cells, which results in myelosuppression, which also contributes to stress erythropoiesis causing a further increment in HbF production.

In USA, SCD patients are offered hydroxyurea starting from 9 months. In India, hydroxyurea is started before 2 years except for patients with severe presentation (stroke, acute chest syndrome).

Infants and children: 10–15 mg/kg/day. Dose escalation by 5 mg/kg every 4–6 weeks only if a definite indication is present.

Adults: 15 mg/kg/day (round up to the nearest 500 mg)

In patients with chronic kidney disease: 5–10 mg/kg/day. Complete blood count (CBC) and reticulocyte count should be monitored at least every 4 weeks once. Avoid having absolute neutrophil count (ANC) <2 × 109/L and platelet count <80,000/µL. If neutropenia or thrombocytopenia is encountered, hold hydroxyurea and monitor CBC weekly.

TABLE 14.8.6: Immunization schedule in addition to routine immunization for children with sickle cell disease.

Vaccine	*Age/frequency route intramuscular (IM)*
Pneumococcal vaccine (conjugated) (PCV13/10) and pneumococcal vaccine (polysaccharide) (PPSV23)	Starting at 6 weeks, 10 weeks, 14 weeks and booster 15 months (4 doses of PCV13/10); then administer PPSV23 at 2 years
Pneumococcal vaccine (conjugated) (PCV13/10) and pneumococcal vaccine (polysaccharide) (PPSV23)	*(Sickle cell disease)* (In IAP this schedule for 1–2 years of normal children only) *If child 1 year old till 5 years:* Give at least 2 doses of PCV13/PCV10 at intervals of 4 weeks, followed by booster PPSV23 after at least 2 months gap (CDC recommendation)
	• *(Sickle cell disease)* (In IAP this schedule for all normal children >2 years old) • *6 years till 18 years:* Then only one dose PCV13/PCV10 is required, followed by booster with PPSV23 after 2 months of the PCV13/10 • After 5 years of last PPSV23 should receive booster of PPSV23 (CDC recommendation)
H-influenza vaccine	• <1 year, 3 doses at an interval of 1 month; <2 years, 2 doses at an interval of 1 year • >2 years, 1 dose
Typhoid vaccine (conjugate) (TCV)	First dose from 6 months of age till any age
Typhoid polysaccharide vaccine	Given >2 years and booster dose every 3 every year
Influenza vaccine	Annually
COVID 19 vaccine	As per government guidelines

When the counts recover, restart the treatment at 5 mg/kg/day lower than the previous dose on which patient had cytopenia.

Hydroxyurea dose escalation: Dose escalation should be slow. Every 2 months increase the dose by 5 mg/kg/d up to maximum of 35 mg/kg/d if symptomatic or complications. During dose escalation the CBC should be monitored at least every 4 weeks and checked to keep ANC >2.0 × 109/L.

Self-management and Care for Sickle Cell Disease

The guardians of the children suffering from SCD should be sensitized about requirement of routine follow-up. They should be taught method of self-palpation of spleen which should be done daily or more often if the child is sick. Attention to fever and grade of fever, regular vaccination schedules, recognition of pain, and home remedies should be well emphasized. Promote a healthy lifestyle and to drink plenty of oral fluids at home to avoid dehydration and further sickling.

Pregnancy and Sickle Cell Disease

Women with SCD are at high risk of preeclampsia, maternal mortality, intrauterine growth restriction (IUGR), preterm labor, and spontaneous abortion. All women with SCD in reproductive age group should be informed regarding the need of special precautions during pregnancy, and end organ damage workup should be done. Hydroxyurea should be stopped 3 months prior to conception. These patients need to be monitored for SCD symptoms, blood pressure, and urine examination. Aspirin 75 mg per day should be started to all women with SCD from 12 weeks of gestation onward. Postpartum anticoagulation and contraception should be planned accordingly.

NATIONAL SICKLE CELL DISEASE ELIMINATION MISSION

Government of India has launched a mission to eliminate sickle cell anemia by 2047 led by Ministry of Health and Family Welfare (MoHFW) through National Health Mission (NHM) and Ministry of Tribal Affairs (MoTA). The five pillars of the mission are awareness and counseling, screening, management of patients in health facilities along with creation of center of competence, data management, and research.[10] This involves screening of 70 million people in the age group of 0–40 years in affected tribal areas of 17 states through collaborative efforts of central ministries and state governments.

COMPREHENSIVE CARE MODEL FOR SICKLE CELL DISEASE: PUBLIC HEALTH AND SICKLE CELL DISEASE

The overall aim is to enable access to affordable and quality healthcare for all SCD patients, and to lower the prevalence through awareness, change of practices, and screening interventions. At individual level, accredited social health activists (ASHAs), community health volunteers, local nongovernmental organizations (NGOs), etc., shall be engaged in raising awareness toward SCDs through home visits. At community level, awareness modalities such as street plays, wall writings and paintings, quizzes, etc., shall be undertaken to raise community awareness. At school level, disease prevention information in the form of interesting activities will be provided and teachers shall be educated to identify early symptoms of crisis in SCD children so that they can provide paracetamol and hydration in emergency cases. Counselors at the primary healthcare centers shall be using sickle cell cards. The card will show the status of the individual, viz., normal, carrier, or diseased. The cards are color coded separately for male (blue) and female (pink). Based on the card's status, the individual will receive treatment and counseling services.[10]

NEWBORN SCREENING FOR SICKLE CELL DISEASE

The objective is to detect newborns from high-risk population for SCD. This is intended to improve outcomes through early treatment and care. The dried blood spot card is used for sickle screening. Blood is obtained from umbilical cord or heel prick on filter paper (Guthrie cards) and sent to central laboratory for HPLC analysis. If screening shows "F" and "S" hemoglobin with baseline hemoglobin range between 6 and 12 g/dL, the diagnosis is likely to be homozygous SCD or sickle β-thalassemia while hemoglobin analysis of "F", "A", or "S" hemoglobin the diagnosis is likely to be heterozygous SCD or sickle cell trait. Reconfirmation of diagnosis is advisable at 6 months by HPLC preferably along with molecular studies.[3]

Newborn screening should not be done with solubility or sickling tests.

Antenatal Screening for Sickle Cell Disease

Screening for SCD is of immense importance because it is a monogenic disorder with high carrier frequency. Sickle cell carriers can be diagnosed by simple tests and even antenatal diagnosis is available. Thus, prevention and significant reduction of birth of affected child is possible **(Table 14.8.7)**. Cost of population screening is profitable than treatment and prevents psychosocial and economic burden.

TABLE 14.8.7: Screening test for SCD.

Target group to be screened	*Tests/remarks*
Antenatal mothers or prepregnancy planning	• Complete blood count (CBC) all women in first trimester • *In endemic pockets/high risk population:* solubility test/point-of-care (POC) tests for sickle cell • Or HPLC and electrophoresis, if available – If mother is a sickle cell carrier/disease – Then testing of father is mandatory – Ideally by HPLC, if not available refer to higher center – If father tests positive, counseling and prenatal testing should be performed (at centers with necessary facilities) to prevent risk of birth of affected newborn
Newborn	• POC tests to initiate penicillin prophylaxis in baby and enrolling vaccination program • High performance liquid chromatography (HPLC) and electrophoresis, if available or at later date
Population screening/patient of any age	*In endemic pockets/high risk population:* Solubility test/POC tests for sickle cell

Prenatal Diagnosis

Table 14.8.8 describes the various procedures used for prenatal diagnosis in SCD.

Genetic Counseling in Sickle Cell Disease

Genetic counseling aims at providing information and support to individuals and families about genetic risks of passing on the gene/disorder to the children.[10] SCD is a recessive gene disorder. A baby inherits two copies of the gene (one from each parent) to have the disorder or one copy to have a trait/be a carrier. Parents can face the following scenarios, depending on their own hemoglobin status:

- Both parents have normal hemoglobin (AA), there is nothing to worry since the children will be fine.
- If only one parent is AS/has a sickle cell trait, then there is a 25% chance that a child might also be a carrier.
- If both parents are AS/has a sickle cell trait, then there is a 25% risk that a child might have SS, 25% chance that it will be AA, and a 50 % that it might have a trait (AS).
- If one parent is SS and the other is AS, a child will have a 50% risk of inheriting a trait (AS) and 50% risk of having SS.
- If both parents have SCD then all children have the same, 100% risk of having the SS **(Fig. 14.8.2)**.

Since the disease is transmitted to the children only from their parents, genetic counseling becomes extremely important in the management of SCD.[10] Genetic counseling should be "nondirective", where the counselor presents the information regarding patterns of inheritance and allows the individual or the couple to make their own decisions on marriage and procreation.

RECENT ADVANCES IN SICKLE CELL DISEASE MANAGEMENT–SCOPE AND CHALLENGES

Novel Therapies

Newer therapies include novel medications such as L-glutamine that are currently FDA approved, hematopoietic stem cell transplantation, gene editing, and the latest been gene therapy.[11,12]

L-glutamine

It was approved by US FDA in children 5 years and older with SCD in 2017.[11] It increases the proportion of the reduced form of nicotinamide adenine dinucleotides in sickle cell erythrocytes which probably decreases the oxidative stress and contributes to reduction of pain. A placebo-controlled phase III study with 230 subjects, evaluated the impact of

TABLE 14.8.8: The procedures used for prenatal diagnosis in Sickle cell disease.

Chorionic villus sampling (CVS)	*Amniocentesis*	*Fetal blood sampling (Cordocentesis)*
10–12 weeks' gestation CVS for DNA analysis or for mutation study	16–20 weeks' gestation for DNA analysis or for mutation study	At approximately 20 weeks' gestation by fetoscopy

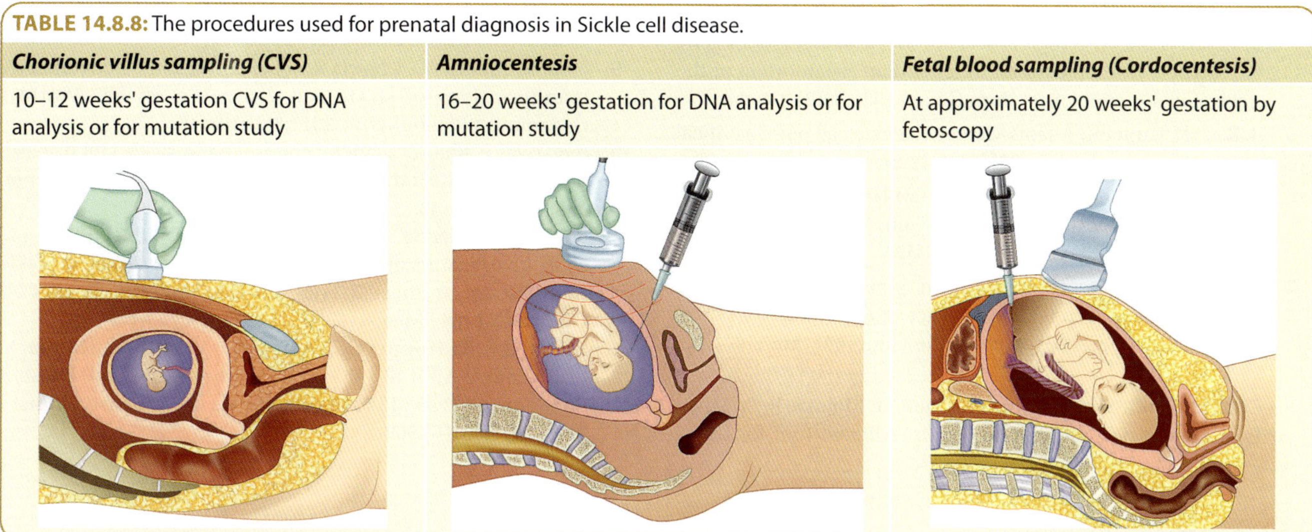

l-glutamine administered twice daily on reducing VOCs in subjects ≥5 years of age with SCD who experienced at least two crises during the previous year.[12]

Hematopoietic Stem Cell Transplant

Allogeneic stem cell transplant remains the only widely available curative option for patients with SCD. HSCT performed at a younger age between 2 and 5 years of age, had best results as compared to older children or adults. The best donor while planning HSCT is a matched sibling donor (MSD) followed by matched unrelated donor (MUD) and then haploidentical donor. Careful assessment of relative risks and benefits should be emphasized before taking up the patient for MUD or haplotransplants. Bone marrow and cord blood (related) are the preferred options as stem cell source.

Indications of HSCT in SCD include:

- Stroke or central nervous system (CNS) event lasting >24 hours
- ACS with recurrent hospitalizations or previous exchange transfusions
- Recurrent VOC (≥2/year) for several years or recurrent priapism
- Impaired neuropsychological function or abnormal brain MRI
- Stage I or II sickle lung disease
- Sickle nephropathy [moderate to severe proteinuria or glomerular filtration rate (GFR) 30–50% of predicted]
- Bilateral proliferative retinopathy and major visual impairment in at least one eye
- Red cell alloimmunization (≥2 alloantibodies) during long-term transfusion therapy.

Gene Therapy

Gene therapy is an alternative potentially curative therapy for SCD. It uses the stem cells of the recipients, corrects the genetic defect with the help of a viral vector, and is reinfused into the patient after a conditioning regimen. There is no risk of graft versus host disease. The types of gene therapy currently being evaluated for SCD can be broadly categorized into four main groups:

1. *Gene addition therapy:* This is the most widely studied and is already available in clinical trials. In this technique, HbS gene is added into hematopoietic stem cells in vitro with the help usually of a lentiviral vector. The native HbS gene is not altered.
2. *Gene editing therapy:* In this method, usually an unrelated gene that regulates phenotype by altering; for example the HbF levels is targeted. Current available therapies target the *BCL11A* gene, a negative regulator of HbF and by the gene editing technology is used to turn off the regulation of HbF to increase HbF production and ameliorate the phenotype.
3. *Gene silencing therapy:* Like gene editing the *BCL11A* gene, the respective gene the gene product is silenced by introducing a gene to produce an antisense strand to messenger ribonucleic acid (RNA) of interest to silence the gene product.
4. *Gene correction therapy*: The mutated native HbS gene is corrected by various techniques.

REFERENCES

1. Herrick JB. Peculiar elongated and sickle-shaped red blood corpuscles in a case of severe anemia. 1910. Yale J Biol Med. 2001;74(3):179-84.
2. Jain D, Warthe V, Dayama P, Sarate D, Colah R, Mehta P, et al. Sickle cell disease in central India: a potentially severe syndrome. Indian J Pediatr. 2016;83(10):1071-6.
3. Kato GJ, Piel FB, Reid CD, Gaston MH, Ohene-Frempong K, Krishnamurti L, et al. Sickle cell disease. Nat Rev Dis Primers. 2018;4:18010.

4. Kulozik AE, Wainscoat JS, Serjeant GR, Kar BC, Al-Awamy B, Essan GJ, et al. Geographical survey of beta S-globin gene haplotypes: Evidence for an independent Asian origin of the sickle-cell mutation. Am J Hum Genet. 1986;39(2):239-44.
5. Ballas SK, Gupta K, Adams-Graves P. Sickle cell pain: a critical reappraisal. Blood. 2012;120(18):3647-56.
6. Ballas SK, Eckman JR. Biology of pain and treatment of the sickle cell pain. Disorders of Hemoglobin: Genetics, Pathophysiology and Clinical Management. 2009:497-524.
7. Benjamin LJ, Payne R. Pain in sickle cell disease: a multidimensional construct. In: Pace, B (Ed). Renaissance of Sickle Cell Disease Research in the Genomic Era; 2007. pp. 99-118.
8. Colla JS, Kotini-Shah P, Soppet S, Chen YF, Molokie R, Prajapati P, et al. Bedside ultrasound as a predictive tool for acute chest syndrome in sickle cell patients. Am J Emerg Med. 2018;36(10):1855-61.
9. Shah R, Taborda C, Chawla S. Acute and chronic hepatobiliary manifestations of sickle cell disease: a review. World J Gastrointest Pathophysiol. 2017;8(3):108-16.
10. Aggarwal P, Bhat D. Genetic counseling in sickle cell disease: Insights from the Indian tribal population. J Community Genet. 2023;14(4):345-53.
11. Niihara Y, Miller ST, Kanter J, Lanzkron S, Smith WR, Hsu LL, et al.; Investigators of the Phase 3 Trial of l-Glutamine in Sickle Cell Disease. A Phase 3 Trial of l-Glutamine in Sickle Cell Disease. N Engl J Med. 2018;379(3):226-35.
12. Vichinsky E, Hoppe CC, Ataga KI, Ware RE, Nduba V, El-Beshlawy A, et al.; HOPE Trial Investigators. A Phase 3 Randomized Trial of Voxelotor In Sickle Cell Disease. N Engl J Med. 2019;381(6):509-19.

14.9 Red Cell Membrane Disorders

Rashmi Dalvi

INTRODUCTION

The erythrocyte membrane structure comprises an outer lipid bilayer of phospholipids and glycolipids, with integral proteins which penetrate or span this bilayer. These include glycoproteins and glycophorins for MNS blood group and others interacting with the inner cytoskeleton. Important among these are the band three proteins, which are vital for anion transport in cellular respiration and contain ABO blood group antigens on their outer surface. Inner to the lipid bilayer is a separate network of proteins forming a membrane cytoskeleton, viz., spectrin, ankyrin, actin, protein 4.1, protein 4.2, actin, and many others. A normal intact membrane structure is critical to red cell deformability, stability, and membrane permeability. A hereditary or acquired defect in any of these structural components destabilizes the cytoskeleton, alters red cell morphology, and shortens the red cell lifespan resulting in variable degrees of anemia.[1]

HEREDITARY SPHEROCYTOSIS

This is the most common of red cell membranopathies, characterized by the following:[2]

- Hemolysis, intermittent jaundice, splenomegaly with the spherocytes in the peripheral smear being its morphologic hallmark.
- It is inherited as an autosomal dominant trait in most patients, although de novo sporadic mutations are also seen and rarely may be recessively inherited.
- Hereditary spherocytosis (HS) results from a deficiency or defect in spectrin or its anchoring proteins, ankyrin, band 3 protein, or protein 4.2. Molecular defects causing these deficiencies are now known **(Fig. 14.9.1)**.[3]
- However, most mutations though common within a family almost always vary between families.
- Deficient cytoskeleton results in the loss of membrane lipids and converts red cells into rigid, osmotically fragile spherocytes which get sequestered in the spleen. In the process, they undergo various metabolic changes, nutrient loss, and lose other membrane components. These deformed red blood cells (RBCs) are susceptible to destruction by splenic macrophages.

CLINICAL FEATURES

There is marked heterogeneity of clinical presentation from the asymptomatic to a transfusion-dependent hemolytic anemia:[1,2]

- Most patients present during infancy or childhood with anemia, although presentation in the fourth or fifth decade is also known.
- Typically, there is a history of mild jaundice, mild or absent anemia, or intermittent anemia and jaundice.
- However, mild-to-moderate splenomegaly is always present **(Fig. 14.9.2)**.
- More severe forms may present in the newborn period with anemia and severe hyperbilirubinemia necessitating exchange transfusion.

- As in other hemolytic anemias, they are prone to aplastic crisis following parvovirus infection, or megaloblastic crisis due to folate deficiency.
- Some patients may develop or rarely even present with symptomatic gallstones.
- Rarely leg ulcers and growth retardation can also complicate the course.

LABORATORY FEATURES

- The hemoglobin (Hb) is usually mildly decreased or normal, with normal mean corpuscular volume (MCV) and typically high mean corpuscular Hb (MCH) content.
- Most patients however exhibit marked reticulocytosis indicating compensatory erythroid hyperplasia.
- Red cell morphology is distinctive with 15–20% being hyperchromatic spherocytes lacking central pallor **(Fig. 14.9.3)**. There is variable polychromatophilia and even spherocytosis in peripheral smear. Poikilocytosis in severe HS is due to combined spectrin-ankyrin deficiency or in recessive variants.

The most common diagnostic screening test used is osmotic fragility test.[2] Red cells in HS show increased osmotic fragility when incubated with hypotonic NaCl solutions in vitro, yielding a diagnostic osmotic fragility curve **(Fig. 14.9.4)**.

- In most cases, a definitive diagnosis of HS can be made based on family history, red cell indices and morphology, and a positive screening test.
- However, quantitation of membrane proteins, especially spectrin content, is possible by flow cytometric or gel electrophoretic analysis, and characterization of molecular lesions is done in the research setting.
- Patients can be classified into clinical severity phenotypes based on Hb, reticulocyte count, serum bilirubin, and spectrin content **(Box 14.9.1)**.

Clinically HS should be differentiated from other inherited disorders presenting with episodic anemia, jaundice, and splenomegaly, such as other red cell membranopathies, enzymopathies, unstable Hb, and autoimmune hemolytic anemia.

MANAGEMENT

Basic supportive care is advised to all patients in the form of:[2]

- Lifelong folate supplementation
- Prevention of iron deficiency
- Prompt treatment of infections
- Blood transfusion may be required on a regular basis in severe phenotypes, in individuals in a steady state during the episodes of acute hemolysis, or during aplastic crisis.
- Regular follow-up is recommended to monitor growth, spleen size, Hb trend, and occurrence of gallstones.
- Splenectomy prolongs RBC survival to almost 80% of normal and prevents other complications, however, is recommended only in clinically severe phenotype.[4]
- Because of the higher risk of postsplenectomy sepsis, it should be postponed to at least 5 years of age.[4]

Acquired Spherocytosis

Certain acquired conditions may also cause reduction in membrane surface area with resultant spherocyte formation, such as:[1]

- Immune adherence and thermal injury
- Mechanical injury (microangiopathic anemia)
- Clostridial sepsis
- Certain snake, bee, and spider venoms

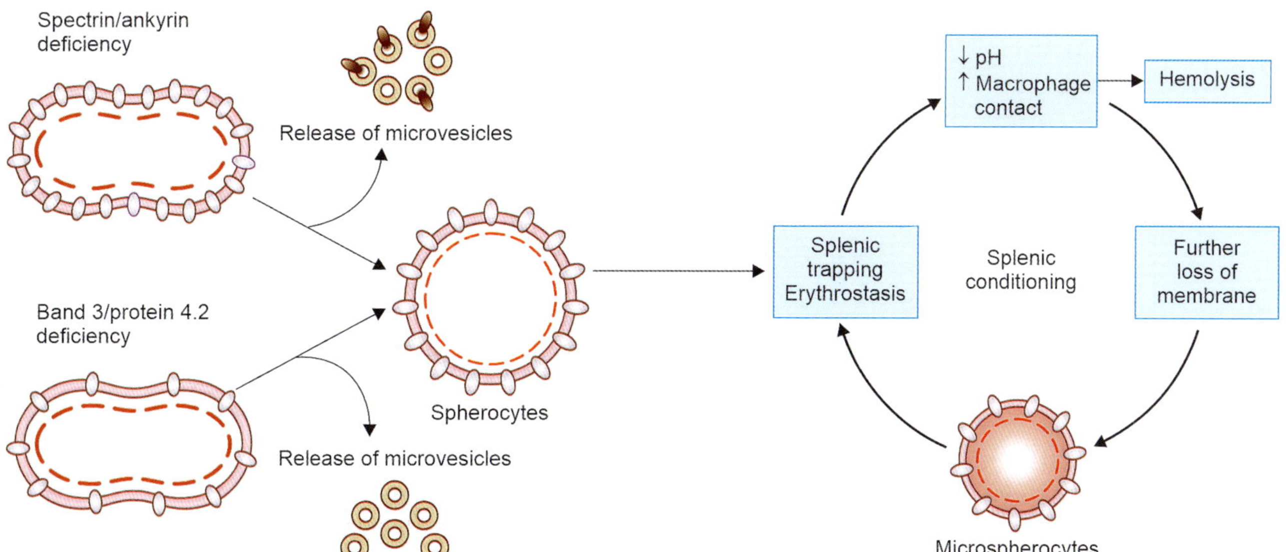

Fig. 14.9.1: Molecular defects and pathogenesis in hereditary spherocytosis.

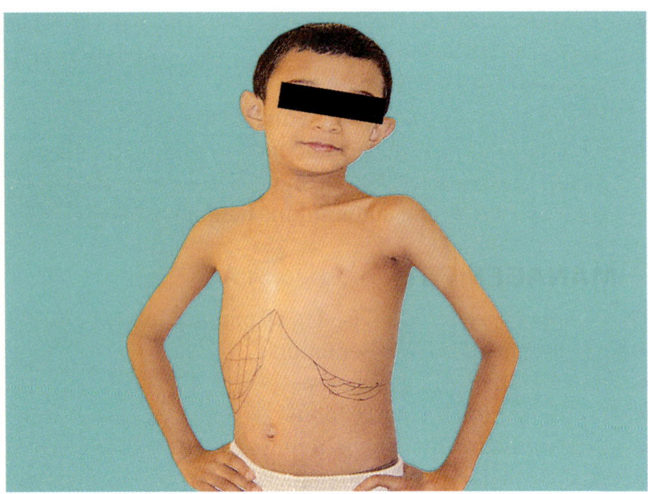

Fig. 14.9.2: Anemia with hepatosplenomegaly, jaundice (indirect type), and hereditary spherocytosis.

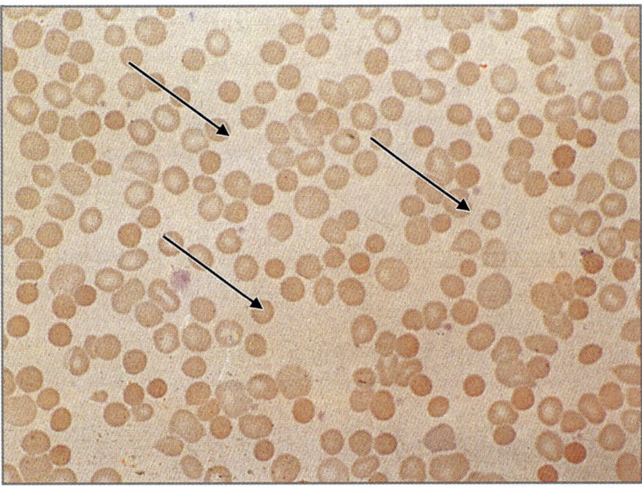

Fig. 14.9.3: Peripheral smear showing microspherocytes.

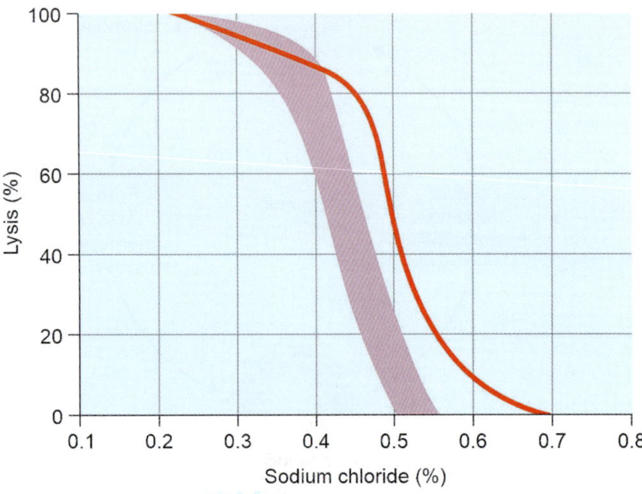

Fig. 14.9.4: Osmotic fragility curve.

BOX 14.9.1: Differential diagnosis of spherocytes.

Spherocytes are also seen in other states, such as:
- ABO incompatibility
- Immune-mediated hemolytic anemia
- Burns
- *Clostridium perfringens* sepsis

HEREDITARY ELLIPTOCYTOSIS SYNDROMES[1]

- Hereditary elliptocytosis (HE) designates a group of inherited disorders that have in common the presence of elliptical RBCs.
- Characterized by defects in spectrin binding with other membrane proteins.
- In most patients, it is inherited as an autosomal dominant trait with a striking molecular heterogeneity, having a variable clinical spectrum ranging from the asymptomatic trait to a life-threatening hemolysis.
- Members of the same family may exhibit different clinical courses, and an individual's frequency and severity may change with time.
- Although mutations of α-spectrin are responsible for most cases of dominantly inherited common HE, it is also seen due to deficiencies in protein 4.1 or glycophorin C or with defects in band 3 protein/β-spectrin impairing ankyrin binding.[3,5,6]
- These defects in the cytoskeleton make the red cells less tolerant to shear stress during circulation. Red blood cell precursors here are round initially but become more elliptical as they age.
- In children and adults, common HE is usually asymptomatic often discovered accidentally on a peripheral smear showing 15–20% elliptocytes.
- Others many have a mild hemolytic anemia and splenomegaly, sometimes with gallstones.
- Common HE is asymptomatic in the neonatal period with elliptocytes appearing only by 4–6 months of age.

HEREDITARY PYROPOIKILOCYTOSIS

Hereditary pyropoikilocytosis (HPP) is a recessively inherited form of hemolytic anemia biochemically related to common HE, having a severe clinical phenotype. They typically present in the newborn period with severe anemia and neonatal jaundice, with red cell fragmentation, poikilocytosis, elliptocytosis, and microspherocytosis.[1]

South East Asian ovalocytosis is another variant of HE seen in malaria-endemic regions of South East Asia and is characterized by red cells with a broad oval shape and the presence of stomatocytes. It is clinically a benign disorder **(Fig. 14.9.5)**.

Laboratory Diagnosis

Hemoglobin may be normal or decreased, and the reticulocyte count will reflect the severity of hemolysis. Other

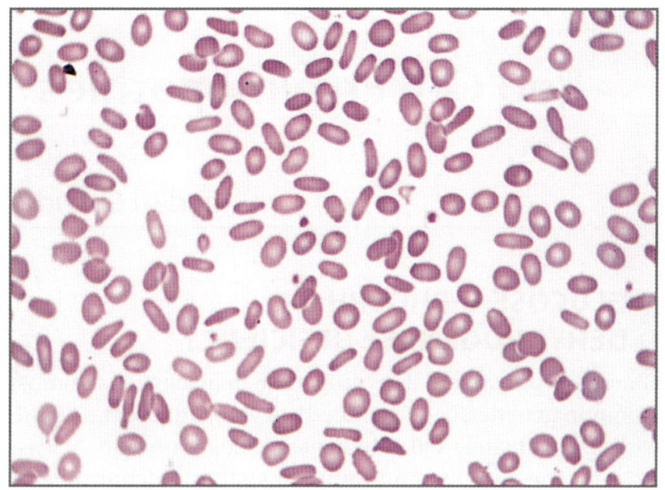

Fig. 14.9.5: Ovalocytes in peripheral smear.

evidence of hemolysis may be present, such as reduced serum haptoglobin, elevated serum lactate dehydrogenase, serum bilirubin, and urinary urobilinogen levels.

Osmotic fragility testing is not required although it is increased in severe HE/HPP. Red cells in HPP also show increased thermal instability as red cells undergo lysis at lower temperatures.

Management

- Treatment is rarely indicated for mild HE or its variants.
- Daily folate supplementation is recommended in patients with significant hemolysis.
- Acute hemolysis during viral infections or other febrile illnesses may need attention.
- Vigilance for gallstones is required.
- Splenectomy may be indicated in severe HE/HPP wherein it results in increase in Hb, decrease in reticulocyte counts, and improved symptoms.[4]

RED CELL PERMEABILITY DISORDERS

Hereditary Stomatocytosis

It is a rare heterogeneous group of autosomal dominant hemolytic anemia characterized by marked increase in RBC membrane permeability to sodium and an increase in red cell water content.[1]

This results in cup-shaped red cells that have a mouth, such as slit in place of the normal central pallor on stained blood films.

Most patients have a very mild hemolytic anemia and jaundice with variable reticulocyte increase, high MCV, 10–50% red cells as stomatocytes, and an increased osmotic fragility.

Splenectomy is contraindicated as these stomatocytic red cells are abnormally adherent, thereby increasing the risk of thrombosis in conjunction with postsplenectomy thrombocytosis.[4]

Hereditary Xerocytosis

It is a rare autosomal dominantly inherited hemolytic anemia characterized by increased red cell permeability to potassium ions and thereby leakage of potassium and water out of the cell. This results in cellular dehydration and is also known as dehydrated stomatocytosis. Laboratory features are characterized by elevated MCH content and mildly elevated MCV.

DISORDERS OF RED CELL MEMBRANE LIPID BILAYER

Red blood cell membrane lipid disorders are characterized by the presence of acanthocytes, echinocytes, and target cells.[1]

Acanthocytic Disorders

Acquired acanthocytes are seen in hypothyroidism, anorexia nervosa, postsplenectomy, severe hepatocellular disease, vitamin E deficiency (especially in neonates/preterms), and inherited neurological disorders, such as abetalipoproteinemia and McLeod syndrome.

Echinocytes are seen in hemolytic anemia associated with hypophosphatemia, pyruvate kinase deficiency, uremia, and long-distance runners.

Target cells are formed due to increased ratio of cell surface compared to volume and are seen in thalassemia, HbC disease, familial lecithin-cholesterol acyltransferase deficiency, and obstructive liver disease.

REFERENCES

1. Golan DE. Hemolytic anemias: Red cell membrane and metabolic disorders. In: Goldman L, Ausiello D (Eds). Cecil Medicine, 23rd edition. Philadelphia, PA: Saunders Elsevier; 2007.
2. Perrotta S, Gallagher PG, Mohandas N. Hereditary spherocytosis. Lancet. 2008;372(9647):1411-26.
3. Hassoun H, Palek J. Hereditary spherocytosis: a review of the clinical and molecular aspects of the disease. Blood Rev. 1996;10(3):129-47.
4. Abdullah F, Zhang Y, Camp M, Rossberg MI, Bathurst MA, Colombani PM, et al. Splenectomy in hereditary spherocytosis: review of 1,657 patients and application of the pediatric quality indicators. Pediatr Blood Cancer. 2009;52(7):834-7.
5. Maciag M, Płochocka D, Adamowicz-Salach A, Burzynska B. Novel beta-spectrin mutations in hereditary spherocytosis associated with decreased levels of mRNA. Br J Haematol. 2009;146(3):326-32.
6. Perrotta S, Della Ragione F, Rossi F, Avvisatti RA, Di Pinto D, De Mieri G, et al. Beta-spectrinBari - a truncated beta-chain responsible for dominant hereditary spherocytosis. Haematologica. 2009;94(12):1753-7.

14.10 Red Cell Enzymopathies

Jagdish Chandra

INTRODUCTION

Defects in various enzymes associated with the red blood cell (RBC) glycolytic pathway, hexose monophosphate (HMP) shunt, or pentose phosphate pathway (PPP), leading to the development of hemolytic anemias of varying severity, are defined as red cell enzymopathies or erythroid enzymopathies (EEPs). These anemias are mostly congenital nonspherocytic hemolytic anemias. The enzymopathies are linked to the prevention of oxidative damage or the generation of energy in the RBCs.

INHERITANCE

Glucose-6-phosphate dehydrogenase (G6PD) deficiency and phosphoglycerate kinase deficiency are chromosome X-linked recessive, and the other EEPs are usually inherited in an autosomal recessive manner.

PENTOSE PHOSPHATE PATHWAY (HEXOSE MONOPHOSPHATE SHUNT)

Glucose-6-phosphate dehydrogenase is the first enzyme involved in the PPP and controls the flux through this pathway. **Figure 14.10.1** depicts the PPP, and **Figure 14.10.2** shows the glutathione cycle and synthetic pathways along with the various enzymes involved in different reactions.

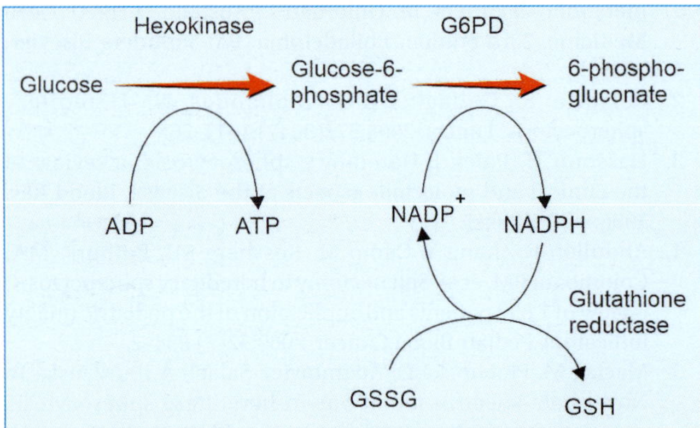

Fig. 14.10.1: Pentose phosphate pathway. (ADP: adenosine diphosphate; ATP: adenosine triphosphate; $NADP^+$: reduction of nicotinamide adenine dinucleotide phosphate; NADPH: nicotinamide adenine dinucleotide phosphate-oxidase; G6PD: glucose-6-phosphate dehydrogenase)

GLUCOSE-6-PHOSPHATE DEHYDROGENASE DEFICIENCY

Glucose-6-phosphate dehydrogenase deficiency is the most common genetically determined enzymopathy in the world, with approximately 440 million people being affected. At least 127 enzyme variants and numerous other polymorphisms that do not affect enzyme activity have been described. The gene for G6PD is located on the X-chromosome at Xq28 and comprises 13 exons and 12 introns. It helps in the conversion of glucose-6-phosphate to 6-phosphogluconate through the reduction of nicotinamide adenine dinucleotide phosphate ($NADP^+$) to nicotinamide adenine dinucleotide phosphate-oxidase (NADPH).

The 6-phosphogluconate is also a substrate for the glycolytic pathway. Under normal conditions, only 10% glucose is metabolized by the PPP, and its activity is governed by the availability of nicotinamide adenine dinucleotide (NAD^+) and its feedback inhibition by adenosine triphosphate (ATP).

Nicotinamide adenine dinucleotide phosphate availability is dependent on the activity of the glutathione pathway, which is linked to the PPP through the enzyme glutathione reductase **(Fig. 14.10.2)**. The availability of $NADP^+$ is the major rate-limiting step for PPP. Nicotinamide adenine dinucleotide phosphate oxidase is required to keep glutathione in reduced form, which prevents red cells from oxidative damage. The clinical consequences of G6PD deficiency are virtually limited to the RBCs, with occasional malfunction of the leukocytes, in some variants, as RBCs cannot generate NADPH in any other way. The majority of the mutations affect the stability of the transcribed enzyme, so that the activity declines rapidly in the mature enucleate RBCs.

Being an X-linked disorder, males are commonly affected, and females are heterozygous carriers. These heterozygous females are often susceptible to oxidative stress because of the effects of X-inactivation and marked lyonization in leaving a significant population of deficient red cells.

Epidemiology

Glucose-6-phosphate dehydrogenase deficiency is widely disseminated throughout Africa, the Mediterranean basin,

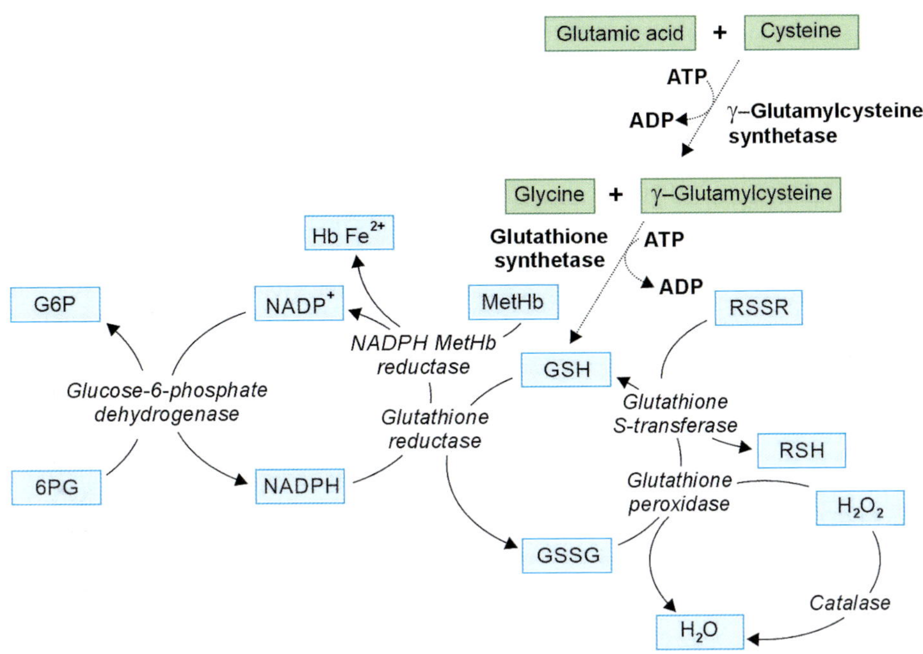

Fig. 14.10.2: The glutathione cycle and synthetic pathways. (ADP: adenosine diphosphate; ATP: adenosine triphosphate; NADP$^+$: reduction of nicotinamide adenine dinucleotide phosphate; NADPH: nicotinamide adenine dinucleotide phosphate-oxidase)

the Middle East, Southeast Asia, and among the indigenous populations of the Indian subcontinent.[1] In Southeast Asia the prevalence varies widely in different ethnic groups—10–20% in certain Cambodian groups to 1–3% in Vietnamese population groups. G6PD deficiency was reported about 40 years ago from India, and varying prevalence rates of 0–27% have been reported from diverse ethnic, caste, linguistic, and tribal groups. The most common variants are:

- Mediterranean variant among the caste groups
- Odisha variant among the Indian tribals[1]
- Kerala-Kalyan is the third most common variant seen in India.

A higher incidence of G6PD deficiency has been observed in north and west India (15% in Parsees to 27% in Angami Nagas), compared to the south (1–2%), except in the tribal belt of Tamil Nadu and Andhra Pradesh (5–13%).[2]

Glucose-6-phosphate Dehydrogenase and Malaria

It has been hypothesized that the distribution of G6PD deficiency equates with areas where *Plasmodium falciparum* malaria is common, and this is thought to be the evolutionary drive that produced such widespread polymorphisms.[3] It has subsequently been confirmed that G6PD deficiency does indeed protect against lethal falciparum malaria, particularly in childhood. This hypothesis has been called G6PD/malaria or "malaria hypothesis". Malarial parasite grows less well in red cells deficient in G6PD. Decreased parasitemia has been documented in these individuals in various studies.

Variants of Glucose-6-phosphate Dehydrogenase

Based upon biochemical and other characterizations, 442 different variants of G6PD have been identified. Of them, 299 have been characterized with the methods recommended by the World Health Organization (WHO). About 100 biochemical variants are thought to be polymorphic in human populations. A total of 13 biochemically characterized variants have been reported from India.[1] The 1986 classification has recently given way to newer classification proposed by WHO 2022 technical consultation based on enzymatic activity and clinical presentation **(Table 14.10.1)**.[4] The expert group emphasized that this system is meant for classifying genetic variants of G6PD and not classifying individual patients with G6PD deficiency.

- *Polymorphic variants:* These variants have achieved a high frequency in some populations and represent balanced polymorphisms, e.g., G6PD Mediterranean, G6PD African, and oriental variants.
- *Sporadic variants:* These are characterized by chronic nonspherocytic hemolytic anemia (CNSHA) and get exacerbated by oxidant stress. These are not limited to a particular population alone. A total of 13 such variants have been reported from the Indian subcontinent, though

TABLE 14.10.1: The WHO classification of variants of G6PD deficiency.

Class	Median G6PD Enzyme activity	Clinical presentation
A	<20%	CNSHA, acute exacerbations
B	<45%	Acute, triggered
C	60–150%	No hemolysis
U	Any	Uncertain significance

(CNSHA: congenital nonspherocytic hemolytic anemia; G6PD: glucose-6-phosphate dehydrogenase; WHO: World Health Organization)

all of these have not been characterized at the molecular level.[1]

- *G6PD mutations in India:* Mutations in the Indian subcontinent in the G6PD are seen in exon 6 and 7, which is near G6PD-binding site.[1] G6PD Mediterranean (563 C-T) is the most common polymorphism in India, and it is a severely deficient variant associated with drug-induced hemolytic anemia, favism, and neonatal jaundice (NNJ); G6PD Kerala-Kalyan (949 G-A) and G6PD Odisha (131 C-G) are the other common variants in India. G6PD Chatham (1003 G-A) with undetectable enzyme activity and G6PD Insuli (989 G-A) with normal enzyme activity are very rare in Indian population.[2]

Clinical Presentation

There are four main syndromes associated with G6PD deficiency. In G6PD-deficient individuals, hemolysis is aggravated by exposure to oxidative stress through infection or ingestion of oxidative foods or drugs. The four syndromes are:

1. NNJ syndrome
2. Favism
3. Chronic nonspherocytic hemolytic anemia
4. Drug-induced hemolytic anemia

The NNJ syndrome has been described in class I, II, and III variants; favism in mainly, although not exclusively, class II; CNSHA in class I; and the drug-induced hemolysis in mainly class III.

Neonatal Jaundice and Glucose-6-phosphate Dehydrogenase Deficiency

Neonatal jaundice is a severe manifestation of G6PD deficiency, and resultant kernicterus is the main cause of morbidity and mortality.[5] Most common variants have been associated with NNJ, including the A- and Mediterranean variants. The jaundice probably starts in utero in the perinatal period, but the clinical problem becomes apparent only about the second day or third day after birth.[6] Between 10 and 50% of the deficient infants are affected. Phototherapy or exchange transfusion (ET) may be required to prevent neurological sequelae. Anemia is usually absent, and it is thought that this is a manifestation of liver enzyme deficiency, along with the physiological underdevelopment of neonatal liver function or the coinheritance of uridine diphosphate glucuronyl transferase-1 deficiency of Gilbert syndrome though the Gilbert syndrome association has not been consistently observed to increase the severity.[7] Acute hemolytic crises may occur in G6PD-deficient infants, usually through exposure to oxidative stress, including nitrites or nitrates in water or the ingestion of fava beans by the mother, which may result in severe intrauterine hemolysis and hydrops fetalis. In some cases, idiopathic severe and sometimes fatal hemolysis has been reported. In an Indian series, in 12 out of 100 neonates with jaundice, G6PD deficiency was the cause, of them 10 being G6PD Mediterranean type.[2]

Acute Intravascular Hemolysis

Glucose-6-phosphate dehydrogenase deficiency was first described during investigation for “primaquine sensitivity”. Since then many drugs have been incriminated to result in intravascular hemolysis in individuals with G6PD deficiency. Children with certain variants of G6PD deficiency are clinically in a steady state till they develop anemia of sudden onset under the effect of some oxidative stress. Within 24–48 hours of exposure to such stress, the child suddenly becomes pale and has cola-colored or dark-colored urine. Depending upon the severity of hemolysis and the resultant anemia, the child may present with incipient or frank congestive cardiac failure. Depending upon the degree of extravascular hemolysis, splenic enlargement may be noticed. Hemolysis occurs after the exposure to stressor but does not continue with continued exposure. This is thought to be because of older RBCs being damaged first as they have most severe deficiency of enzyme. Once the population of deficient RBC is hemolyzed, the juvenile RBCs and reticulocytes withstand, the stress as they have typically higher levels of enzyme activity. Hemoglobinemia and hemoglobinuria may result in azotemia and/or acute renal failure.

Laboratory findings during intravascular hemolysis include moderate-to-severe anemia, which is usually normocytic-normochromic. RBC morphology shows anisocytosis due to increased number of juvenile red cells and contracted cells. Poikilocytosis with the presence of “bite cells” may be seen. Intense reticulocytosis is present. Plasma hemoglobin (Hb) level is increased and so is unconjugated bilirubin level. Haptoglobin and other Hb-binding proteins are decreased.

Box 14.10.1 lists the drugs that need to be avoided in G6PD-deficient individuals and the risk of hemolysis

BOX 14.10.1: Drugs to be avoided in patients with glucose-6-phosphate dehydrogenase deficiency.

- Acetanilide
- Acetylphenylhydrazine (2-phenyl-acetohydrazide)
- Aldesulfone sodium (sulfoxone)
- Aminophenazone (aminopyrine)
- Antazoline (antistine)
- Arsine
- Ascorbic acid
- Beta-naphthol (2-naphthol)
- Chloramphenicol
- Chloroquine
- Ciprofloxacin
- Colchicine
- Dapsone (diaminodiphenyl sulfone)
- Dimercaprol
- Diphenhydramine
- Dopamine (L-dopa)
- Doxorubicin
- Furazolidone
- Glibenclamide
- Glucosulfone sodium
- Isobutyl nitrite
- Isoniazid
- Menadiol sodium sulfate
- Menadione (menaphtone)
- Menadione sodium bisulfite (vitamin K_3 sodium bisulfite)
- Mepacrine (quinacrine)
- Mesalazine 5-aminosalicylic acid (paraminosalicylic acid)
- Methylthioninium chloride (methylene blue)
- Nalidixic acid
- Naphthalene, pure (naphthalene)
- Niridazole
- Nitrofural (nitrofurazone)
- Nitrofurantoin
- Norfloxacin
- *O*-acetylsalicylic acid (acetylsalicylic acid)
- Oxidase, urate (urate oxidase)
- Phenazopyridine
- Phenylbutazone
- Phenytoin
- Pamaquine
- *Para*-aminobenzoic acid (4-aminobenzoic acid)
- Paracetamol (acetaminophen)
- Pentaquine
- Phenacetin (acetophenetidin)
- Phenylhydrazine
- Phytomenadione (vitamin K_1)
- Primaquine
- Probenecid
- Procainamide
- Proguanil (chlorguanidine)
- Pyrimethamine
- Quinidine
- Quinine
- Stibophen
- Streptomycin
- Sulfacetamide

Contd...

Contd...

- Sulfacytine
- Sulfadiazine
- Sulfadimidine
- Sulfafurazole (sulfafurazole, sulfisoxazole)
- Sulfaguanidine
- Sulfamerazine
- Sulfamethoxazole
- Sulfamethoxypyridazine
- Sulfanilamide (sulfanilamide)
- Sulfapyridine
- Sulfasalazine
- Salazosulfapyridine (salazopyrin)
- Thiazosulfone (thiazolesulfone)
- Tiaprofenic acid
- Tolonium chloride, tolonium chloride (toluidine blue)
- Trihexyphenidyl (benzhexol)
- Trimethoprim
- Trinitrotoluene (2,4,6-trinitrotoluene)
- Tripelennamine

associated with these drugs. In an Indian series, bacterial sepsis, malaria, and hepatitis were identifiable triggers other than drugs. Alpha-hydroxy acids following ingestion of soft drinks containing ascorbate have also been reported from India.

Chronic Nonspherocytic Hemolytic Anemia

Chronic anemia with normal/near normal red cell morphology is the most severe form of G6PD deficiency and is usually seen in infancy or childhood. CNSHA develops in a minority of cases with G6PD deficiency (class I variants). Most of the mutations causing CNSHA are seen on exon 10 and affects the formation of dimers and tetramers. Clinical presentation is variable. CNSHA affects only male patients, and these patients usually have history of NNJ necessitating therapeutic intervention. The patient presents later with anemia and jaundice. Splenomegaly is variable. Anemia is normocytic, normochromic, and slight macrocytosis may be observed due to reticulocytosis. Unconjugated hyperbilirubinemia, increased levels of lactate dehydrogenase (LDH), and decreased levels of haptoglobin are present. Hemolysis is usually extravascular, although additional oxidant stress may precipitate intravascular hemolysis. Continuous hemolysis in these patients results from red cell membrane damage due to oxidation of sulfhydryl group of Hb, resulting in its precipitation.

Association with Other Hemolytic States

In the cases with sickle cell disease (SCD), the presence of G6PD deficiency has been found to be an independent risk factor for abnormally high cerebral velocities as assessed by transcranial Doppler assessment.[8] In another study, association of G6PD deficiency did not influence the severity and frequency of painful crisis, anemic episodes, or infections in patients with SCD.[9]

Role of Glucose-6-phosphate Dehydrogenase Deficiency in Other Diseases

Interactions of G6PD deficiency in other diseases are increasingly being reported. Viral infections are long been recognized to result in intravascular hemolysis. G6PD deficiency leading to increased susceptibility to viral infections such as hepatitis B virus (HBV), dengue virus, enteroviruses, and coronavirus is being recognized. Presence of G6PD deficiency in individuals with diabetes mellitus may result in enhanced β-cell dysfunction predisposing to diabetic complications.[10]

Laboratory Diagnosis

Acute *intravascular hemolysis* raises the suspicion of G6PD deficiency. The peripheral blood smear shows red cells with contracted Hb in "ghost" membrane. *Hemoglobinuria* may be gross, producing almost black urine without red cells in the centrifuge deposit. Several screening tests have been devised to identify G6PD deficiency in RBCs. The most widely used tests are the brilliant cresyl blue decolorization test, the methemoglobin reduction test, and an ultraviolet spot test. These are good qualitative tests that can differentiate between the deficient and nondeficient cases but do not provide quantitative data.

If a screening test indicates deficiency or is doubtful, the ideal follow-up test for definitive diagnosis is quantification of G6PD activity by spectrophotometric assay. The quantification is essential in the case of hemolytic attack, wherein the oldest red cells (with the least G6PD activity) are destroyed selectively, and the surviving red cells have a relatively higher (but still deficient) G6PD activity. This increases further as the reticulocyte response evolves. During this time, a screening test might yield a false-normal result and, rarely, even a quantitative test might do so. In such cases, it is best to repeat the test a couple of weeks later. The oldest remaining cells can be isolated by differential centrifugation, and they can be shown to have a low G6PD activity.

Quantitative estimation is also important for the diagnosis of heterozygous females; the probability of clinically significant hemolysis in a heterozygote roughly correlates with the proportion of G6PD-deficient red cells in her blood. Thus, the demonstration of a normal level of G6PD activity in a heterozygote makes it unlikely that the affected individual will be at risk of G6PD-related hemolysis. In regions where G6PD has a high prevalence and the main variants are known, DNA analysis is the most effective way of identifying heterozygotes.

Enzyme-linked immunosorbent assay-based methods have been developed for field use. A recent study reported a good sensitivity and specificity of this test and recommended for use in resource-limited settings. Another test for field studies is NADPH fluorescence test on paper (NFP test). This test was compared with polymerase chain reaction (PCR)-based G6PD genotyping also using blood samples on filter papers. There was good agreement between the NFP test results and the PCR findings. The estimate of the sensitivity of the NFP test was 98.2% (95.8–99.6%), and the specificity was 97.1% (94.2–99.2%). In cases with indeterminate results, molecular diagnosis using next-generation sequencing (NGS) can be resorted to (this will also map for other red cell enzymes, which may result in hemolysis).

Preventive and Therapeutic Strategies

Preventing the development of hemolysis is of key importance in managing patients with G6PD deficiency, along with appropriate treatment of acute and chronic anemia and NNJ. The WHO recommends screening all newborns for G6PD deficiency population groups with prevalence rates of 3–5% or more in males. Identifying the affected newborns early makes it easier to take due precautions for preventing the development of NNJ. Avoidance of the known oxidative stresses and drugs in G6PD-deficient individuals can help prevent the development of hemolytic anemia.

Management of NNJ should be as per the standard protocols, including phototherapy and ET.[12] Phototherapy in these neonates may be started at a lower level than otherwise recommended.

Treatment of acute episode of intravascular hemolysis includes transfusion support to correct anemia and supportive care. Adequate fluid therapy during hemolytic episodes is crucial for prevention and treatment of acute renal failure.

Patients with CNSHA require meticulous monitoring. In most cases, occasional exacerbation may require blood transfusion. During steady state, administration of folic acid is recommended to meet the increased demands due to increased red cell turnover. Occasional patient may need to be started on chronic transfusion therapy. Splenectomy may be required due to large size, development of hypersplenism, or to decrease the transfusion requirement. Splenectomy has been described to result in clinical improvement in most of the transfusion dependent patients.

There has been a growing interest in research for increasing G6PD levels with the use of drugs. Antioxidants (ascorbate, vitamin E, α-lipoic acid, and β-carotenoids) have been tried in subjects with G6PD deficiency for improving total antioxidant capacity of RBC but have not resulting in meaningful improvement. N-acetyl-cysteine (NAC), a prodrug of L-cysteine, has been used and has been found to be useful in cases with AHA. G6PD enzyme upregulation using Histone deacetylase inhibitors (HDACis) and other drugs is being explored.

OTHER ENZYMOPATHIES OF THE GLUTATHIONE PATHWAY

- *Gamma-glutamyl cysteine synthetase deficiency:* It is the rate-limiting enzyme in glutathione biosynthesis. Patients may present with CNSHA, oxidative hemolytic anemia, basophilic stippling, and spinocerebellar degeneration in adulthood. The genetic locus is identified on chromosome 6p12.
- *Glutathione peroxidase deficiency:* This enzyme is responsible for the elimination of hydrogen peroxide from the erythrocytes, and its production depends on adequate selenium supply. Moderate deficiency may result in nonspherocytic hemolytic anemia in infants or self-limited NNJ, and Heinz bodies. Oxidizing drugs need to be avoided. The genetic locus is localized to chromosome 3p21.3.
- *Glutathione synthetase deficiency:* Mutations in the glutathione synthetase gene lead to low levels of this enzyme in the RBCs, leading to 5-oxoprolinemia and oxoprolinuria. The classical triad of presentation is hemolysis, metabolic acidosis, and mental deterioration. The affected gene is located at chromosome 20q11. Treatment is to supplement vitamin C, vitamin E, bicarbonate, and avoidance of oxidative drugs.
- *Glutathione reductase deficiency:* This enzyme is responsible for the reduction of oxidized glutathione in the presence of flavin adenine dinucleotide, and its deficiency leads to increased susceptibility to drug-induced hemolysis and favism. Its activity increases with dietary riboflavin supplementation in a few patients. In patients with a 2,246 base pair gene deletion in the glutathione reductase gene, riboflavin supplementation does not lead to its increased activity.

ENZYMOPATHIES OF THE GLYCOLYTIC PATHWAY

Pyruvate kinase (PK) deficiency is the well-recognized enzymopathy of glycolytic pathway, and along with G6PD deficiency **(Fig. 14.10.3)**.[13] It is the most common cause of CNSHA. In contrast to G6PD deficiency, patients with deficiency of enzymes of glycolytic pathway usually have CNSHA with the onset in neonatal period. Drug-induced hemolytic anemia is not a common problem in these patients. **Table 14.10.2** lists the important features of important enzymopathies of the glycolytic pathway.

With the easy availability of genetic testing by NGS, cases with hemolytic anemia due to other rare enzymopathies are increasingly being reported.

PYRUVATE KINASE DEFICIENCY

Pyruvate kinase enzyme catalyzes the final step of the glycolytic pathway, leading to overall net gain of ATP from

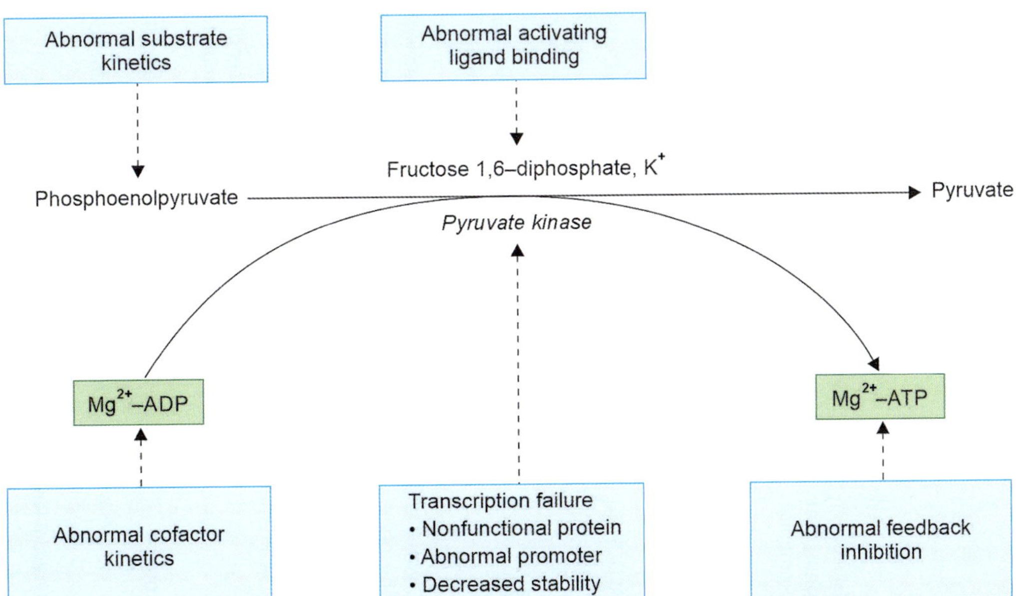

Fig. 14.10.3: The reactions of pyruvate kinase and the sites affected by various mutations in pyruvate kinase deficiency. (ADP: adenosine diphosphate; ATP: adenosine triphosphate)

TABLE 14.10.2: Enzymopathies of the glycolytic pathway.

S. no.	Enzyme	Genetics (chromosome/ inheritance)	Clinical features	Other systems affected	Hematological/ other laboratory findings	Treatment	Comments
1.	Hexokinase	10q11.2/AR	• NNJ • Anemia • Splenomegaly • CNSHA • Gallstones • Hyperhemolytic episodes • High O_2 affinity	None directly	Red cell morphology unremarkable	• Packed RBC transfusions • Folic acid • Splenectomy	• Very rare • Occasional AD
2.	Glucose phosphate isomerase	19 cen-q12/AR	• NNJ • Hydrops • CNSHA • Hyperhemolytic episodes	None directly	• Erythrocytosis • Very high • Reticulocyte count • High MCV	• Packed RBC transfusions • Folic acid • Splenectomy	Most common after PK deficiency
3.	Phosphofructokinase	1(M) and 21(L)/ complex	• Erythrocytosis (Type VII glycogen storage disease) • Mild hemolytic anemia	Dominant myopathy	• No lactate production in "ischemic arm test" • Muscle biopsy	Unsatisfactory	Tarui's disease, subunit genes
4.	ALDOA	16q22-q24/AR	Severe CNSHA	• Myopathy • Dysmorphism • Intellectual retardation	Normal red cell morphology	Undefined	Very few cases
5.	TPI	12p13/AR	• Moderate-to-severe CNSHA • Neonatal anemia	• Neuromuscular • Cardiac	Very high reticulocyte count	• Transfusions • Folic acid • Splenectomy	Sudden death
6.	Glyceraldehyde-3 phosphate dehydrogenase	12p13/AD	None/associated with other defects, such as hereditary spherocytosis	None	Nonspecific	Nonspecific	Gene syntenic with TPI, membrane protein band 6
7.	Phosphoglycerate kinase	Xq13/X-linked	CNSHA NNJ	• CNS, myopathy • Rhabdomyo-lysis	Reticulocytosis	Splenectomy	Rare, variable systems involved
8.	2,3-DPG mutase	7q23-q34/AR	• Polycythemia • Neonatal onset of progressive anemia described with 50% activity	None	Erythrocytosis	Phlebotomy for symptomatic polycythemia	Very rare
9.	Enolase		• Shortened red cell survival not necessary • Nitrofurantoin-induced • hemolysis	None	Spherocytosis	Undefined	
10.	Pyruvate kinase	1q21-q22 (PKLR)/ AR rarely AD	See text				Most common CNSHA
11.	Lactate dehydrogenase		Decreased levels not associated with anemia				

(AD: autosomal dominant; ALDOA: fructose diphosphate aldolase; AR: autosomal recessive; CNS: central nervous system; CNSHA: chronic nonspherocytic hemolytic anemia; DPG: diphosphoglycerate; MCV: mean corpuscular volume; NNJ: neonatal jaundice; PK: pyruvate kinase; PKLR: pyruvate kinase, liver, and RBC; RBC: red blood cell; TPI: triose phosphate isomerase)

this pathway. This enzyme is a tetramer with four tissue-specific subunits: R (RBC), L (liver), M1-muscle, and M2 for platelets and leukocytes.[13] Genetic control is separate for R-L subunit and M1-M2 subunits. Deficient PK activity leads to the accumulation of substrates upstream, including 2,3-diphosphoglycerate (DPG), which shifts the oxygen dissociation curve to the right, indicating low oxygen affinity. PK activity decreases during RBC aging, as the enzyme is gradually denatured, and after the activity falls below a critical level, glycolytic failure and ATP depletion result. Over 300 genetic mutations (mostly missense mutations) are associated with PK deficiency. Most patients are compound heterozygotes for the two most common mutant forms of the enzyme. This deficiency is common in people of northern European lineage. Prevalence of PK deficiency has varied from 0.14 to 6%. PK deficiency provides some protection against malaria. **Figure 14.10.3** depicts the biochemical role of PK.

Clinical Features

Chronic nonspherocytic hemolytic anemia with extravascular hemolysis is the hallmark of clinical presentation in PK deficiency. Around one-third of patients present with jaundice in the newborn period, and one-third of these cases are severe enough to warrant packed RBC transfusions and/or ET.[7] Severe anemia and hydrops are the usual cause of death during this period. Milder variants usually present in late childhood with nonsevere anemia, unconjugated hyperbilirubinemia, and splenomegaly, which may be massive at times. Chronic leg ulcers are a complication in some individuals. Aplastic crisis due to parvovirus infection can occur. Gallstones are increasingly seen after the first decade. The prognosis is confounded by the lack of good correlation between PK activity level and the severity of clinical hemolysis. Association of Gilbert syndrome with PK deficiency has been described leading to significant hyperbilirubinemia and increased risk of gall stones.[7]

Laboratory Features

Red cell morphology is normocytic-normochromic. Active regeneration of RBCs leading to macrocytosis and acanthocytosis may be observed. Reticulocyte count is increased but not proportionate to the extent of hemolysis, due to selective sequestration of young RBCs and reticulocytes in the spleen. A paradoxical rise in reticulocytes after splenectomy therefore is commonly seen. Hepatic PK deficiency leads to elevated liver enzymes. Iron overload disproportionate to transfusions is sometimes observed and has been explained based on associated hemochromatosis mutations.

Usually, the diagnosis is suspected after more common and easily investigated causes of hereditary hemolytic anemia including G6PD deficiency have been excluded. Enzymes estimation is the laboratory test ordered, which is becoming more widely available. However, the test is dependent on availability of transfusion-free window and may be spuriously normal following an acute episode of hemolysis. NGS is the test for making the molecular diagnosis. NGS is not dependent on transfusion status and requires smaller volume of blood.[13]

Treatment

Treatment of PK deficiency includes transfusion support, folate supplementation, splenectomy, and cholecystectomy for gallstones. Anemia is better tolerated in patients with PK deficiency compared to other conditions associated with chronic hemolysis such as thalassemia syndromes. Transfusion requirement also varies with age as infections precipitating hemolysis and aplastic crisis decrease with age. The use of salicylates may lead to hyperhemolytic crisis in patients with PK deficiency. The role of splenectomy as a therapeutic measure is not well established, and variable response rates are reported.

Over the last 10–15 years, attempts have been made to boost the enzyme activity. Mitapivat (AG-348) is an allosteric activator of red cell PK. It is administered orally and has a favorable safety profile. Studies have shown good hematological response in about 40% of the patients.[14]

ENZYMOPATHIES OF THE NUCLEOTIDE METABOLISM

Pyrimidine 5′ Nucleotidase (Uridine 5′ Monophosphate Hydrolase) Deficiency

It is probably the third most common EEP, probably equal to glucose phosphate isomerase deficiency. Pyrimidine 5′ nucleotidase deficiency is inherited in an autosomal recessive manner, and the gene is located on chromosome 7p15-14. The accumulation of pyrimidine nucleotides in high concentration leads to marked basophilic stippling in the RBCs. Diagnosis is confirmed by a decrease in the nucleotide OD260:OD280 ratio and decreased enzymatic activity. Patients present with hemolysis of varying severity and its sequelae. Splenectomy is usually of little value, though some cases have reported benefit.

Adenosine Deaminase Excess

Adenosine deaminase (ADA) is a purine catabolic enzyme that leads to the conversion of adenosine to inosine. Its deficiency leads to severe combined immunodeficiency, while its excess due to increased amplification of the ADA, messenger ribonucleic acid, produces hemolytic anemia.

OTHER ENZYMOPATHIES ASSOCIATED WITH HEMOLYSIS

Heme-oxygenase-1 Deficiency

Heme-oxygenase-1 converts heme to bilirubin and is protective against oxidative stresses. Clinical presentation is in early childhood with hemolytic anemia, abnormal coagulation/fibrinolytic system, asplenia, and marked growth retardation. It can present as intravascular hemolysis with RBC fragmentation in the absence of hyperbilirubinemia and decreased haptoglobin.

Lecithin Cholesterol Acyltransferase Deficiency

This enzyme is involved in lipoprotein metabolism, and its deficiency leads to erythroid membrane defects due to excess of unesterified cholesterol. These patients may have renal disease with proteinuria and corneal opacifications, and the lipid profile shows decreased high-density lipoprotein levels.

Clinical Approach

The diagnosis of enzymopathy should be suspected in all cases with chronic hemolysis and unexplained unconjugated hyperbilirubinemia, particularly if red cell morphology is unremarkable.[15] Intense reticulocytosis supports the diagnosis of various enzymopathies. In the cases presenting with acute intravascular hemolysis, history of exposure to trigger drugs helps in the diagnosis. Family history of jaundice, anemia, splenectomy, and cholelithiasis may also point toward such a disease. In the absence of such history, the diagnosis may be difficult. The diagnosis can be confirmed by appropriate enzyme assays or by the demonstration, accumulation of proximal, or depletion of distal intermediary compounds of the glycolytic pathway. The diagnostic tests need to be made available more widely, and a high index of suspicion is needed to suspect these conditions.

REFERENCES

1. Mohanty D, Mukherjee MB, Colah RB. Glucose-6-phosphate dehydrogenase deficiency in India. Indian J Pediatr. 2004;71(6): 525-9.
2. Sukumar S, Mukherjee MB, Colah RB, Mohanty D. Molecular basis of G6PD deficiency in India. Blood Cells Mols Dis. 2004;33(2):141-5.
3. Mohanty D, Sukumar S, Mukherjee MB, Colah RB. G6PD deficiency and malaria in India. Am J Hematol. 2003;72(2): 150-1.
4. World Health Organization. (2022). Malaria policy advisory group meeting. Meeting report of the technical consultation to review the classification of glucose-6-phosphate dehydrogenase (G6PD). [online] Available from https://www.who.int/publications/m/item/WHO-UCN-GMP-MPAG-2022.01 [Last accessed December, 2024].
5. Ip S, Chung M, Kulig J, O'Brien R, Sege R, Glicken S, et al. An evidence-based review of important issues concerning neonatal hyperbilirubinemia. Pediatrics. 2004;114(1):e130-53.
6. Steiner LA, Gallagher PG. Erythrocyte disorders in perinatal period. Semin Perinatol. 2007;31(4):254-61.
7. Sampietro M, Tavazzi D, Fermo E, Bianchi P, Zanella A. Hyperbilirubinemia in pyruvate kinase deficiency: the role of Gilbert's Syndrome. Blood 2003;102:258a (abstract).
8. Bernaudin F, Verlhac F, Chevret S, Torres M, Coic L, Arnaud C, et al. G6PD deficiency, absence of alpha thalassemia and hemolytic rate at baseline are significant independent risk factors for abnormally high cerebral velocities in patients with sickle cell anemia. Blood. 2008;112(10):4314-7.
9. Memon MJ, Gahine R, Hussain N, Gupta Y. Influence of glucose-6-phosphate-dehydroginase (G-6-PD) deficiency upon clinic-haematological and biochemical expression of patients with sickle cell disease. Int J Adv Med. 2017;4(2):573-80.
10. Cappai G, Songini M, Doria A, Cavallerano JD, Lorenzi M. Increased prevalence of proliferative retinopathy in patients with type 1 diabetes who are deficient in glucose-6-phosphate dehydrogenase. Diabetologia. 2011;54(6):1539-42.
11. Roper D, Layton M, Rees D, Lambert C, Vulliamy T, De la Salle B, et al. Laboratory diagnosis of G6PD deficiency. A British Society for Haematology Guideline. Br J Haematol. 2020;189(1):24-38.
12. Frank JE. Diagnosis and management of G6PD deficiency. Am Fam Physician. 2005;72(7):1277-82.
13. Zanella A, Fermo E, Bianchi P, Valentini G. Red cell pyruvate kinase deficiency: molecular and clinical aspects. Br J Haematol. 2005;130(1):11-25.
14. Fattizzo B, Cavallaro F, Luisa Mercello APM, Vercellati C, Barcellini W. Pyruvate Kinase Deficiency: Current challenges and Future Perspectives. J Blood Med. 2022;13: 461-71.
15. Sivasankaran M, Reddy VK, Kumar V, Munirathnam G. Hereditary Non-Spherocytic Hemolytic Anemia (HNSHA): Four children with rare hereditary red cell enzymopathies. Indian Pediatr. 2021;58(10):993-4.

14.11 Autoimmune Hemolytic Anemia

Bharat R Agarwal

INTRODUCTION

Hemolytic anemia can be due to defects within the red blood cells (RBCs) or due to damage from external forces. In children, hemolytic anemia is usually due to intrinsic RBC defects, leading to hemolysis and anemia as seen typically in RBC membranopathy or RBC enzymopathy; most of these are inherited in nature. Occasionally hemolytic anemia can result due to factors extrinsic to RBC; most of these causes are acquired in nature. Autoimmune hemolytic anemia (AIHA) is one such cause resulting from interaction of RBC with the immune system. It is characterized by shortened RBC life, hemolysis, and anemia. It is caused by autoantibodies to RBC antigens.

Keen clinical observations led to the concept of AIHA as a disease different from the congenital causes, such as hereditary spherocytosis (HS). Invention of Coomb's reagent and testing led to detection of the "incomplete" autoantibodies as seen in AIHA. The detection of complement components on RBC membrane in AIHA further expanded the understanding of the pathophysiology. Improved understanding of the spleen and its functions helped to understand the mechanism of RBC clearance in AIHA. Focus for current research is on the role of immunity (T-cell and B-cell) in AIHA, reasons for failure of self-tolerance and uncontrolled production of autoantibodies, and possible therapeutic options based on molecular pathophysiology.[1]

CLASSIFICATION

Autoimmune hemolytic anemia can be classified in various ways, depending on the type of autoantibody, site of hemolysis, or the precipitating illness. However, the most practical classification of AIHA is whether it is primary or secondary as shown in **Box 14.11.1**.[2]

BOX 14.11.1: Classification of AIHA.

Primary AIHA:
- Warm-reactive antibody (mainly IgG)
- Cold agglutinin disease (mainly IgM and complements)
- Paroxysmal cold hemoglobinuria (mainly IgG and complements)

Secondary AIHA:
- Underlying autoimmune disorders, e.g., systemic lupus erythematosus and Evan's syndrome
- Drug-induced, e.g., penicillin
- Immunodeficiency, e.g., HIV and primary immunodeficiency
- Specific infections, e.g., mycoplasma infection
- Malignancies, e.g., lymphomas and leukemia

(AIHA: autoimmune hemolytic anemia; HIV: human immunodeficiency virus; IgG: immunoglobulin G; IgM: immunoglobulin M)

Primary Autoimmune Hemolytic Anemia

Primary AIHA is not uncommon in children and is next to immune thrombocytopenic purpura in its occurrence as an immune hematological disorder.

- Primary AIHA occurs without any baseline immune disorder or obvious precipitating factors, though many of the primary AIHA cases occur following nonspecific viral infections, and cold agglutinin disease in children usually follows specifically mycoplasma infection.
- In the West, it is more common than hypoplastic anemia, but in our country, hypoplastic anemia is more common due to rampant misuse of drugs and highly prevalent viral infections.

Secondary Autoimmune Hemolytic Anemia

- Secondary AIHA occurs as a part of some systemic illness or a wider baseline immune disease.
- It occurs more commonly in adolescents and young adults and is more common in females, as are other immune disorders.
- Cold agglutinin disease has abrupt onset of symptoms, short history, need aggressive short-term treatment, and ultimately recovery.
- Paroxysmal cold hemoglobinuria (PCH) is caused by autoantibody of immunoglobulin G (IgG) class that binds to RBC antigen at below 37°C, efficiently fixes complements, and leads to intravascular hemolysis.

CLINICAL FORMS OF AUTOIMMUNE HEMOLYTIC ANEMIA

Warm-reactive Autoantibody

- It is caused by autoantibody of IgG class that binds the RBC antigens at 37°C, sometimes fixes complements, and leads to extravascular hemolysis.[2]

- Autoantibody IgG molecule binds firmly to RBC antigens, which may or may not fix complements. The reticuloendothelial (RE) system recognizes the fragment crystallizable (Fc) segment of the bound IgG through its interaction with the Fc receptor present on the surface of the RE cells. The sensitized RBC if engulfed completely is removed from circulation leading to extravascular hemolysis. However, if only a part of the RBC membrane is bitten off, it will form a spherocyte which will return to circulation.[3]
- Warm-reactive IgG antibody-sensitized RBCs are preferentially removed in spleen. If IgG antibody also fixes and activates complements, it will be recognized by the macrophages with receptor to C3b, mainly in the liver.

Cold-reactive Autoimmune Hemolytic Anemia

- It is caused by autoantibody of IgM class that binds RBC antigen at below 37°C; efficiently fixes complements and leads to intravascular hemolysis.[2]
- It reacts with the RBC antigen at 4°C and fixes complements; however, at body temperature, the antibody dissociates, and there is hardly any antibody attached to RBCs. However, the complement activation continues. If the complement activation is complete, the RBC will lyse and lead to intravascular hemolysis. If the complement activation stops at C3b, it will be recognized by the receptor to C3b present on the surface of the macrophages of the RE system, preferentially in liver.
- Often have chronic illnesses with intermittent relapses and remissions, need long-term therapy, and develop treatment-associated complications. However, overall mortality in children with AIHA is usually <10%. Children between 2 and 12 years seem to have best prognosis.

CLINICAL EVALUATION

- Patients with AIHA usually have typical history and physical findings. The patient will present with anemia, acholuric jaundice, and organomegaly. There may be presence of fever in some patients.
- History suggestive of nonspecific viral infection in recent past. Being an acquired disorder, the family history is usually not contributory.
- Anemia will present with fatigue, lassitude, and giddiness.
- Acholuric jaundice due to indirect hyperbilirubinemia following hemolysis (icterus in eyes without dark urine). The presence of dark urine is usually due to intravascular hemolysis; cola-colored urine with the presence of hemoglobin (Hb) without the presence of RBCs on urinalysis.
- Organomegaly in the form of enlarged liver and spleen, which occur due to hyperplasia of RE system, the site of extravascular hemolysis. Marked hepatosplenomegaly should arouse suspicion of some other disease like leukemia. Always look for secondary cause such as systemic lupus erythematosus (SLE), malignancy, human immunodeficiency virus (HIV), or recent ingestion of certain drugs.

LABORATORY WORKUP

Investigations are targeted to look for:

- Presence of hemolysis
- Presence of autoantibody
- Presence of secondary cause, if any

Complete Blood Count

- *Hemoglobin* may fall as low as 3–5 g/dL without many symptoms or cardiac failure as there is adequate cardiovascular compensation.
- *White blood cell (WBC) count and platelet count* should be normal as low platelet count may suggest microangiopathic anemia, and the presence of low WBC counts and platelet counts will suggest other causes like aplastic anemia; though in rare cases of Evans' syndrome, the platelet count as well as Hb may be low due to autoimmune pancytopenia.
- *The RBC indices*: The RBC indices, such as mean corpuscular volume (MCV) and mean corpuscular Hb concentration (MCHC), will be normal as the large reticulocytes are balanced by the presence of microspherocytes; however, the RBC distribution width (RDW) will be high due to the presence of marked anisocytosis. High MCHC should arouse suspicion of HS.
- *Reticulocyte count:*
    - Reticulocyte count will be high indicating the presence of hemolysis with normal marrow response. It will be seen as polychromasia on peripheral smear (PS) stained with Wright's stain. Very high reticulocyte count with the presence of nucleated RBCs on smear may suggest more severe disease with propensity to chronicity.
    - Reticulocyte count may be low due to autoantibody also affecting the RBC precursors in bone marrow (BM) or due to associated parvovirus B19 infection.

Peripheral Smear

Peripheral smear will show the presence of macrocytosis, polychromasia, anisocytosis, nucleated RBCs, and microspherocytes. In extreme cases, autoagglutination may be present. Features of microangiopathy, such as schistocytes and helmet cells, will be absent differentiating it from other causes of hemolytic anemia (microangiopathic hemolytic anemia). The presence of significant target cells would suggest hemoglobinopathy.

Other Tests

- There will be other markers of hemolysis, such as high *serum lactate dehydrogenase* (LDH) levels and increased *serum bilirubin* with high indirect component.
- *Intravascular hemolysis* will lead to hemoglobinuria with the presence of Hb in urine without RBCs, hemoglobinemia, low hemalbumin and low hemopexin levels, and in the long run hemosiderinuria.
- Bone marrow is not indicated in the clinical setup of suspected hemolytic anemia. However, if BM study is done, it will show erythroid hyperplasia.
- *Presence of autoantibody*: The direct evidence of AIHA is to detect the presence of autoantibody and/or complement component C3 on RBC. This is done by direct antiglobulin test (DAT) also known as Coombs' test **(Fig. 14.11.1)**.[4]
- While IgM antibody-coating RBC membrane can be detected by saline agglutination tests, IgG antibody is an incomplete antibody not detectable easily. In DAT, polyspecific sera-containing antihuman IgG and anticomplement rabbit globulin are added. This helps "bridge" the autoantibodies present on the RBC and leads to agglutination. Once DAT is positive, one can characterize the presence of autoantibody or complement C3, or both by using monospecific test. This will also help characterize cold agglutinin disease where IgM may not be attached to RBC at 37°C or the presence of Donath-Landsteiner antibody.
- Direct antiglobulin test is usually reported on a scale of 1–4 depending on the strength of reaction. One can estimate titers of the autoantibody involved. DAT may be false negative, if the steps of the tests are not followed properly.[4]
- In 10% of patients of AIHA, DAT may be truly negative either due to scanty number of autoantibodies or due to the presence of IgA antibody.[4]
- Direct antiglobulin test may also be false positive in some otherwise normal patients who never progress to develop AIHA. It can also be positive following recent blood transfusion. However, in both these cases, it is weakly positive.[4]

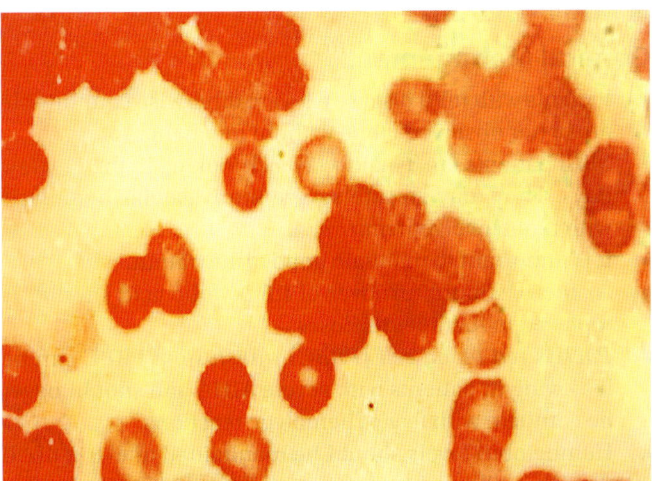

Fig. 14.11.1: Positive direct antiglobulin test.

DIFFERENTIAL DIAGNOSIS

- The presence of anemia, acholuric jaundice, splenohepatomegaly, and reticulocytosis in PS showing changes of hemolysis with positive DAT clinches the diagnosis of AIHA.
- *Hereditary spherocytosis:* The presence of microspherocytes may lead to confusion with HS. Clinical settings are totally different in these conditions. Microspherocytes are not the prominent feature in AIHA, and DAT is negative in HS. In addition, MCHC will be high in HS. Microspherocytes may also be seen in other conditions.
- Microangiopathy may be confused with AIHA; however, platelets will be low and DAT negative in microangiopathic hemolytic anemia.
- Secondary cause of AIHA should be looked for, such as SLE, malignancies, immunodeficiency syndromes, especially HIV, and incriminating drugs. AIHA with low reticulocyte count should be investigated for parvovirus B19 infection.

PATHOPHYSIOLOGY

Both primary and secondary AIHA are caused by the presence of autoantibodies that bind the RBC antigens. This leads to intravascular hemolysis (as in cold agglutinin disease or PCH) or extravascular clearance of the sensitized RBCs in spleen or liver (as in warm-reactive antibody). Hence, it is important to understand the role of the autoantibody and the RE system in AIHA.

- *Autoantibody:* It is important to understand the characteristics of the autoantibody, including its isotype, thermal range, capacity to fix complements, binding affinity, and antigenic specificity.
- *Antibody isotype:* In most cases of AIHA, the antibody is of IgG class. Most of the IgG autoantibodies are warm-reactive, though some may be cold-reactive as seen in PCH or rarely cold agglutinin disease. In others the autoantibody is of IgM type as seen classically in cold agglutinin diseases following mycoplasma infections

TABLE 14.11.1: Essential characteristics of different autoantibody isotypes seen in autoimmune hemolytic anemia.

Characteristic	*Warm-reactive*	*PCH*	*Cold agglutinin*
Isotype	IgG	IgG	IgM
Temperature	37°C	4°C	4°C
Complement fixation	Variable	Yes	Yes
Antigen specificity	Rh	P	I/i
Site of destruction of RBC	Extravascular	Intravascular	Intravascular/liver
DAT			
• *At 37°C*	IgG ± C3	C3	C3
• *At 4°C*	No need	IgG ± C3	C3
Titers of antibody	Low	Moderate	High
Treatment	• Steroids/intravenous immunoglobulin splenectomy • Plasmapheresis	Avoid cold Steroids	Avoid cold
Outcome	Chronic	Short term	Short term

(DAT: direct antiglobulin test; IgG: immunoglobulin G; IgM: immunoglobulin M; PCH: paroxysmal cold hemoglobinuria; RBC: red blood cell; Rh: Rhesus)

in children. Rarely the autoantibody is of IgA class, which is not detectable by standard DAT. The essential characteristics of these different autoantibody isotypes seen in the three clinical forms of primary AIHA are shown in **Table 14.11.1**.

In 70% of the cases with IgG autoantibody, IgG1 is the only subtype, in 20%, it is IgG1 plus some other subtype. In rest, subtypes other than IgG1 are involved. IgG1 and IgG2 are better capable to bind complement than IgG3 or IgG4.

Thermal Amplitude

Warm-reactive IgG autoantibody has thermal reactivity at 37°C, which means that it shows activity at body temperature.

Cold-reactive IgG autoantibodies of PCH show thermal reactivity at 4°C. They bind the RBC antigen at 4°C and bind complements. At body temperature the IgG antibody dissociates and cannot be detected by DAT at 37°C, but the complement cascade gets amplified leading to hemolysis. Hence, this antibody is demonstrated by a special biphasic test. IgM autoantibody seen in cold agglutinin disease has thermal activity <37°C and is best at 4°C. The clinical disease also depends on the antigenic specificity and the complement-binding capacity.

Complement-binding capacity, RBC antigen specificity, and antibody-binding affinity: Bound immunoglobulin binds complement C1q via its Fc portion. This leads to further cascade effect up to the formation of C3b. At this juncture, either the RBC is cleared by the RE system that recognizes the C3b via specific surface receptor leading to extravascular hemolysis, or the complement cascade activation continues till the RBC is destroyed leading to intravascular hemolysis. As IgG autoantibody has specificity to Rhesus (Rh) system, which has sparse distribution on RBC surface, and as two molecules of IgG antibodies are needed nearby to bind C1q, the complement capacity binding of IgG autoantibody is inefficient leading to extravascular hemolysis, whereas IgM autoantibody being a pentamer binds complement efficiently leading to intravascular hemolysis. IgM antibody has antigen specificity against I/i antigen. Similarly, as the cold-reactive IgG autoantibody has specificity against P antigen, which is densely present on the RBC membrane; it binds the complements efficiently leading to intravascular hemolysis. IgG antibody binds the RBC antigen with high affinity compared to IgM antibody.

MANAGEMENT

General Management[5]

- Patients with mild disease who are otherwise comfortable are better observed alone without much therapy.
- Most patients are usually very sick looking in the first few days. They may go into severe intravascular hemolysis with renal involvement.
- It is important to maintain good urine output.
- As there is rapid turnover of RBCs, folic acid should be replaced in therapeutic doses.
- *Packed red blood cell (PRBC) transfusion*: PRBC can be lifesaving in patients with severe AIHA and should never be withheld with fear of hemolytic reactions.[6]
- Hemoglobin levels should be maintained at 6–8 g/dL. If the Hb is allowed to drop lower than that, it can lead to cardiovascular decompensation.

Two problems may occur with transfusion in patients with AIHA:

1. There is usually a problem with cross-matching the unit.
2. There are chances of hemolysis following transfusion.

As most of the warm-reactive antibodies are against Rh system, they are pan-reactive and will react with all the units of PRBC. One can use the pack that is found to be "least incompatible" on cross-matching and start the transfusion at very slow rate initially to see for hemolytic reaction.

Always watch for hemolysis, which will be evident with fever, restlessness, loin pain, hemoglobinuria (dark urine), and check for hemoglobinemia in plasma and hemoglobinuria in urine tests.

Steroids

Corticosteroids are the first line and the mainstay in the definitive therapy of AIHA. It is indicated for moderate-to-severe disease. They are effective in 80% of warm-reactive antibodies and occasionally even in cold agglutinin disease. For initial few days, one can use intravenous (IV) methylprednisolone in the dose of 1–2 mg/kg 6–8 hourly. Once the patient is stable, one can switch over to high-dose oral prednisolone in the dose of 2 mg/kg/day for 2–4 weeks, followed by gradual tapering over 3 months based on the symptoms, Hb levels, evidence of hemolysis, serum LDH levels, reticulocyte count, and DAT grade.

While tapering, one may switch over to daily or alternate single dose of steroids. Steroids work by blocking the Fc receptor as well as suppressing the antibody production. Hence, the effect is usually seen in few days of therapy. One should regularly monitor with blood pressure, blood glucose, and weight recordings for common side effects **(Fig. 14.11.2)**.

Intravenous Immunoglobulin

Intravenous immunoglobulin (IVIg) in high doses of 2–5 g/kg has only limited response and is exorbitantly expensive and has potential side effects. It has shown benefit only in 30–50% of AIHA treated with IVIg. It is not the standard of care as the first-line therapy in AIHA.[7]

Other Modes

- *Exchange transfusion:* It is beneficial as it removes the antibody, complements, and the sensitized RBCs. However, it is labor-intensive and hazardous.[8]
- *Plasma exchange:* It is found to be very successful in IgM antibody-induced AIHA. IgM being a large molecule stays in the circulation and does not leak into the tissues. As IgM does not bind to RBCs at body temperature, it is likely to be free in plasma available for exchange, especially in warm atmosphere.

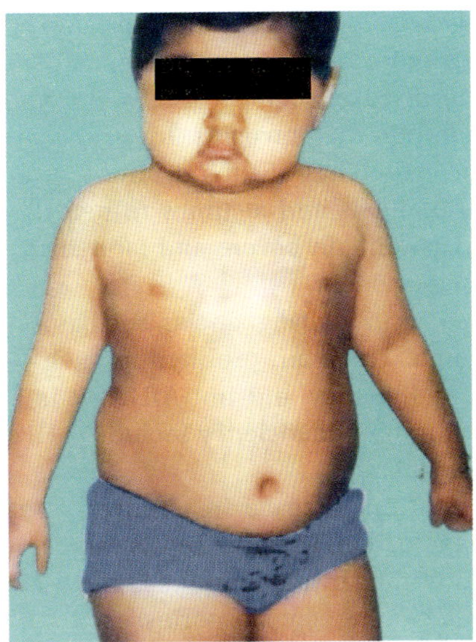

Fig. 14.11.2: Autoimmune hemolytic anemia on steroid therapy. *Courtesy:* Dr MR Lokeshwar and Dr Bharat Agarwal, Mumbai, Maharashtra, India.

Splenectomy

Warm-reactive AIHA is likely to be chronic despite steroids and IVIg use. Many such patients who are perpetually sick and need repeated admissions and packed RBC transfusions with its own therapy-related complications, and splenectomy is the ultimate therapy of choice and works better in patients with IgG-induced AIHA than IgM-induced AIHA. Nearly 60% respond very well, and another 20% have satisfactory response. All the precautions, such as immunization against capsulated organisms before splenectomy and penicillin prophylaxis for life after splenectomy, must be followed. Splenectomy is avoided as far as possible till the age of 5 years.

Other Modalities

- High-dose dexamethasone
- Cytotoxic drugs, such as vincristine, cyclophosphamide, and azathioprine
- Immunomodulators, such as danazol and cyclosporine
- Rituximab, the monoclonal anti-CD20 antibody, has been used as off-label in many autoimmune disorders, including AIHA with anecdotal reports of success. There is limited experience to use these drugs in children with AIHA. They also have limited success and are toxic in children.

SECONDARY AUTOIMMUNE HEMOLYTIC ANEMIA

Autoimmune hemolytic anemia can occur as a part of underlying autoimmune disease or because of a specific precipitating cause, which must be looked for in every case. Secondary AIHA can occur in patients with underlying autoimmune disease, such as SLE, scleroderma, Sjögren syndrome, and dermatomyositis. It can occur as a part of autoimmune cytopenias—Evans' syndrome where one sees antibody to platelets and at times to neutrophils. Evans' syndrome is potentially severe and fatal and hence needs aggressive management.

It can also occur in malignancies, such as acute leukemia and lymphoma. The main problem in such patients is of course the malignancy and not AIHA. It is also seen in patients with immunodeficiency including HIV because of immune dysregulation.

Cold agglutinin disease in children usually follows mycoplasma infection. Bacterial sepsis can lead to exposure of the cryptic T antigen and immune hemolysis. Drugs, such as penicillin including cephalosporins, can induce AIHA.

Secondary AIHA needs twofold therapy, treatment of AIHA and treatment of the baseline disease. Attention should be paid to remove the offending drugs. Steroids are equally useful in secondary AIHA as in primary AIHA and can be used without fear even in the cases of immunodeficiency.

REFERENCES

1. Ware RE. Autoimmune hemolytic anemia. In: Nathan DG, Ginsburg D, Orkin SH, Look AT (Eds). Hematology of Infancy and Childhood. Philadelphia, PA: Saunders; 2019. pp. 521-59.
2. Engelfriet CP, Overbeeke MAM, von dem Borne AE. Autoimmune hemolytic anemia. Semin Hematol. 1992;29(1):3-12.
3. Salama A, Mueller-Eckhardt C. Autoimmune haemolytic anemia in childhood associated with non-compliment binding IgM autoantibodies. Br J Haematol. 1987;65(1):67-71.
4. Kowal-Vern A, Jacobson P, Okuno T, Blank J. Negative direct antiglobulin test in autoimmune hemolytic anemia. Am J Pediatr Hematol Oncol. 1986;8(4):349-51.
5. Collins PW, Newland AC. Treatment modalities of autoimmune blood disorders. Semin Hematol. 1992;29(1):64-74.
6. Salama A, Berghofer H, Mueller-Eckhardt C. Red blood cell transfusion in warm-type autoimmune haemolytic anaemia. Lancet. 1992;340(8834-8835):1515-7.
7. Hilgartner MW, Bussel J. Use of intravenous gamma globulin for the treatment of autoimmune neutropenia of childhood and autoimmune hemolytic anemia. Am J Med. 1987;83(4A):25-9.
8. Heidemann SM, Sarnaik SA, Sarnaik AP. Exchange transfusion for severe autoimmune hemolytic anemia. Am J Pediatr Hematol Oncol. 1987;9(4):302-4.

14.12 Approach to a Child with Coagulation Disorders and Hemophilia

Pravas Mishra

INTRODUCTION

Congenital coagulation defects present variably from simple bruising or epistaxis to more severe bleeds into joints or organs. The bleeding history includes the duration, age of presentation, sites of bleed, exposure to trauma and surgery, family history, and need for transfusions. There are validated questionnaires from international societies as well. The investigation screen includes the hemogram, peripheral smear, prothrombin time (PT), and activated partial thromboplastin time (aPTT). Platelet disorders and the laboratory approach are discussed separately. Acquired causes are rare in children, and this section will discuss the congenital coagulation defects and their management.

Our country faces challenges in uniformity of diagnosis and care. At the time of drafting this article, availability of factor prophylaxis for hemophilia is not universal. Even blood product supply could be unreliable. This poses challenges to the hemophiliac, for whom home care is the norm in developed economies. The recent approval for gene therapies in the USA and Europe has made the contrast in available treatment options even more stark. However, there has been a concerted push in our country toward making treatment available for all and therefore knowledge of the following disorders and their management is extremely important.

HEMOPHILIA

Hemophilia A and B are congenital X-linked coagulation disorders of factors VIII and IX, respectively. These are produced in the liver sinusoidal endothelial cells and hepatocytes, respectively.

Epidemiology

The incidence is about 1:5,000 males for hemophilia A and 1:30,000 males for hemophilia B. Epidemiological data from India is lacking, Indian Council for Medical Research (ICMR) estimates that there could be 80,000–100,000 severe hemophilia cases in India.

Genetics

The long arm of the X chromosome Xq28 and Xq27 carries the gene loci for factors VIII and factor IX, respectively. It is transmitted to 50% of children of a career mother; 50% of daughters will be hemophilia carriers, and 50% of sons will be hemophiliac. A hemophiliac male does not transmit to male offspring, who has normal maternal X chromosome. However, 30% of the new mutations result in a male hemophiliac or a female carrier with no family history of bleeding. A female hemophiliac is possible in the event of skewed lyonization of the normal X chromosome, and in cases of Turner syndrome and homozygous transmission (affected father and carrier mother).

Pathophysiology

Factors VIII and IX are components of the *intrinsic system* of coagulation cascade. Exposed tissue factor (TF) and activated factor VII activate factors X and V. The Xa-Va complex generates thrombin which in turn activates factors VIII and IX, which together activate factor X. Thus, these factors are part of a positive feedback loop system. Patients with mild (levels >5% of normal) or moderate hemophilia (between 1 and 5%) bleed only after trauma. Severe hemophiliacs (<1%) are also prone to spontaneous bleeds. Repeated joint bleeds lead to synovial thickening and restricted movements. The local joint inflammation and breakdown of blood products release cytokines stimulating further synovial thickening, loss of the cartilage, subchondral cysts, and bone damage leading to fixed flexion deformities. Joint damage sets in after 3–6 consecutive bleeds.

Clinical Presentation

The child has mucocutaneous bleeds by the age of 1 month. Joints generally bleed after 1 year of age. Bleeds into soft tissues present as pseudotumor, psoas bleeds, and intracranial bleeds. Gastrointestinal (GI) bleeds (10%) and genitourinary bleeds (5%) are uncommon. Signs of joint bleeds include crepitus and a reduction in the range of movement.

Investigations

A prolonged aPTT triggers search for deficiencies of factor VIII, factor IX, factor XI, and factor XII. A deficient von Willebrand factor (VWF) (typically type 2N or type 3) could prolong the aPTT owing to rapid degradation of factor VIII in the absence of VWF.

Treatment

General Care of a Hemophiliac Child

Hemophilia care is undertaken as a comprehensive care by a team comprising hematologists, physiotherapists, orthopedician, blood bank experts, among others. Physiotherapy to strengthen muscles around joints is crucial. Vaccines are traditionally given subcutaneously using a fine needle, 23-guage or smaller, with local pressure for 5–10 minutes after the injection. Intramuscular (IM) injections are given within 24 hours of prophylactic factor dose, with local icepacks applied for 5 minutes postinjection. The child must avoid contact sports and activities with significant risk of trauma such as football and cricket. Protective gear such as helmets, knee, and elbow pads are essential. Nonsteroidal anti-inflammatory agents are best avoided.

First Aid

In case of a joint or limb bleed, the patient is advised RICE (*R*est, *I*ce, *I*mmobilization, *C*ompression, and *E*levation) therapy **(Table 14.12.1)**. RICE therapy must be accompanied by factor replacement for successful bleed management.[1]

Factor Replacement Therapy: Basic Considerations

Table 14.12.2 describes recommended factor support for acute bleeds and surgical procedures. This is adapted from the World Federation of Hemophilia guidelines.[2] Commercial viral-inactivated factor concentrates, plasma-derived or recombinant, including the extended half-life products are preferred. In their absence, one uses fresh frozen plasma (FFP) (all factors) or cryoprecipitate (factor VIII, fibrinogen, VWF, and factor XIII). *Examples:* A 100% correction in a 30-kg

TABLE 14.12.1: RICE (Rest, Ice, Immobilization, Compression, Elevation) therapy.

Rest	The joint should be rested till it heals. If knee or ankle is involved, then walking must not be allowed
Ice	Use crushed ice wrapped in a damp towel for 10–15 minutes at a time. Ice baths are useful for ankle, wrist, or hand involvement
Immobilization	A half cast or splint is used to limit movement
Compress	Wrap the foot or muscle starting well below the affected area and ending well above the affected area, using crisscross pattern
Elevation	Elevate the affected limb above the level of the heart using cushions

TABLE 14.12.2: Suggested correction of factor deficiency in hemophilia.

	Hemophilia A		*Hemophilia B*	
Type of bleed	***Desired level (%)***	***Duration (days): Adjusted as per response***	***Desired level (%)***	***Duration (days): Adjusted as per response***
Joint	10–20	1–2 days	10–20	1–2 days
Major bleeds				
Initial	50–80	1–3	50–80	1–3
Maintenance	30–50	4–7	30–50	4–7
	20–40	8–14	20–40	8–14
Major surgery	*Central nervous system (CNS), intra-abdominal, orthopedic, and intrathoracic*			
	60–80	Preoperative	50–70	Preoperative
	30 40	1–3	30–40	1–3
	20–30	4–6	20–30	4–6
	10–20	7–14	10–20	7–14
Minor surgery, minor bleeds	*Including tooth extraction*			
	40–80	Preoperative	40–80	Preoperative
	20–50	1–5	20–50	1–5

Source: Adapted from World Federation of Hemophilia guidelines.[2]

child with severe hemophilia requires 3,000 units of factor (30 × 100).

- *Hemophilia A*: In case of hemophilia A, each unit of factor VIII raises the factor levels to 0.02 U/mL. Therefore, the required dose would be 1,500 units. However, as the median half-life of factor VIII is 12 hours, another dose of 750 units is required after 12 hours to maintain 100% factor levels.
- *Hemophilia B*: Each unit of factor IX raises the levels to 0.01 U/mL and the median half-life of factor IX is 24 hours. A single dose of 3,000 units is required in this case, administered once every 24 hours, to maintain 100% factor levels.

If factor concentrates are required on subsequent days as for a major bleed or surgery, one would need to make allowance for residual factor activity from the previous day's administration. It is necessary to monitor factor levels daily for the first 3–4 days followed by a reduced frequency of testing. This would ensure that target levels are maintained and both overdose and wastage of factor are avoided. Overdosage runs the risk of thrombosis postoperatively.

Prophylaxis—Prevention of Bleeds

Prophylaxis avoids fatal bleeds and chronic arthropathy in patients with severe hemophilia by raising the factor level >1%. Primary prophylaxis is recommended before 3 years old and any clinical or radiological evidence of joint damage. This standard of care enables hemophiliacs to lead a near normal life. Prophylaxis with plasma-derived and recombinant products are given thrice (hemophilia A) or twice (hemophilia B) a week at doses of 20–30 IU/kg/dose. Improved factor half-life achieved via pegylation or binding to albumin or Fc receptors enables less frequent dosing. *Efanesoctocog-alfa,* a recombinant B domain deleted factor VIII Fc protein bound to D′D3 domain of *VWF*, is given once weekly for hemophilia A prophylaxis.

Novel Agents

Emicizumab is a humanized bispecific monoclonal antibody that binds factor IXa with X bypassing factor VIII.[3] It achieves factor VIII activity levels of 15%, and additional support is still required for breakthrough bleeds and surgery. It interferes with the aPTT and other assays. It is approved for subcutaneous (SC) use, 3 mg/kg, in patients with hemophilia A once a week for the first 4 weeks followed by either of the following: 1.5 mg/kg per week or 3 mg/kg every 2 weeks or 6 mg/kg every 4 weeks.

Fitusiran inhibits production of antithrombin (reduces antithrombotic action to compensate for loss of procoagulant) in the liver via inhibition of ant-thrombin mRNA and can be used in both hemophilia A and B. It is administered once a month.[4] Both fitusiran and emicizumab are effective in the presence of inhibitors. Recent data has shown benefit for more intensive doses in patients with acquired inhibitors as well. Fitusiran and monoclonal antibodies against antitissue factor pathway inhibitors (TFPIs) such as concizumab and marstacimab are under clinical trials for both hemophilia A and B.[3]

Pharmacological Agents

Desmopressin (DDAVP) is an alternative to plasma or factor concentrate administration in case of minor bleeds or minor surgical procedures in mild/moderate hemophiliacs and patients with type 1 von Willebrand disease (VWD). Vasopressin acts on vascular endothelial cells to release high-molecular-weight multimers of VWF to 2–5 times normal levels.[5] This also increases factor VIII, which is bound to VWF. The VWF so released increases platelet adhesion and function at sites of tissue injury. DDAVP is administered intravenously (IV) at a dose of 0.3 µg/kg. It is contraindicated in children <2 years of age due to risk of seizures. The DDAVP nasal spray for hemophilia supplies 150 µg/metered dose/per nostril. One must note that the DDAVP metered dose for diabetes insipidus has lower doses.

Other useful adjuncts in minor bleeds are epsilon aminocaproic acid (EACA) administered orally or IV every 4–6 hours to total dose not exceeding 24 g/day or tranexamic acid (25 mg/kg orally every 6–8 hours).[5] They could predispose to thrombosis if used in conjunction with factor concentrates and are contraindicated for use in hematuria as blood clots could cause ureteric obstruction.

Inhibitors

Twenty percent of severe hemophilia A and 3% of severe hemophilia B develop alloantibodies to exogenous factor and no longer respond appropriately.[2] Patients with large deletions such intron 22 inversion are more likely to develop inhibitors. These patients have very little factor and thus would develop antibodies more readily on exposure to exogenous products. Treatment options for bleeds include bypassing agents [recombinant factor VII, factor VIII bypassing agents, and prothrombin complex concentrates (PCC)] and the novel agents described earlier. Prolonged exposure to high doses of factor is required to reduce the inhibitors. Acquired inhibitors are rare in children and need in addition, immunosuppressant therapy with steroids, rituximab, and cyclophosphamide.

Gene Therapy for Hemophilia

Valoctocogene roxaparvovec (hemophilia A) and *Etranacogene dezaparvovec* (hemophilia B) are adenovirus-associated virus 5 (AAV5) packaged gene products that have been approved for use in 2022.[6] Valoctocogene roxaparvovec has a gene for B domain deleted human factor VIII. B domain deletion results in smaller gene size and more efficient packaging. Both products are given as a single IV dose, resulting in elevated levels of factor, which comes down over time. However, the levels remain in the moderate range (>5%) in two-thirds cases.[7] Even those patients with <5% maintain a less severe phenotype compared to baseline. These products are not given to patients with inhibitors.

All recipients develop antibodies to AAV5, and hence repeat doses are not possible in case of failure. Transaminitis is the most common side effect. Gene therapy is currently not approved for pediatric use where the liver is still developing. It is not administered in those with baseline antibodies to AAV5 and also in those with inhibitors. Though not described in clinical trials, there is a theoretical risk of oncogenesis.

VON WILLEBRAND FACTOR DEFICIENCY

von Willebrand factor is a multimeric protein encoded by *178 kb* gene on the short arm of chromosome 12. It is secreted from the vascular endothelium. VWF multimers bind to circulating factor VIII and increase its half-life from 2 hours to 12–20 hours.[8]

Pathophysiology

Following vascular damage, VWF binds to exposed collagen fibers. The high shear stress of flowing blood initiates a confirmational change that exposes the platelet glycoprotein GP1bα-binding site within the multimer. This binds circulating platelets to the damaged endothelium, activating them in the process. The GPIIb-IIIa and phosphatidyl serine on the surface of activated platelets attach VWF/fibrinogen and factor VIII, respectively.

Inheritance and Classification of von Willebrand Disease

Types 1 and 3 are qualitative defects with partial and complete deficiency of VWF, respectively. Type 2 defects are qualitative, resulting in reduced activity. VWF activity is measured by the VWF:ristocetin cofactor assay (VWF:RCo), which tests the ability of VWF to agglutinate platelets exposed to ristocetin. Type 1 and most of the type 2, except type 2N, are autosomal dominant, whereas type 2N and type 3 are autosomal recessive.[8]

Type 1 VWD is the most common VWD variant (75% cases). Genetic defects, mostly missense mutations, reduce the protein production/secretion from endoplasmic reticulum, Golgi bodies, and Wiebel Palade bodies. Laboratory testing shows proportionately reduced VWF antigen and VWF activity.

Type 2 VWD, on the other hand, is a qualitative defect, and the activity is suppressed in excess to the reduced antigen levels (VWF:RCo to VWF antigen levels <0.7). The type 2 defect is further subdivided into:

- Type 2A—reduced multimers
- Type 2M—normal multimer pattern
- Type 2N—reduced binding to factor VIII, presents with reduced factor VIII:C but normal multimer pattern; and
- Type 2B—increased affinity to GP1bα bypassing the need for collagen. It differs from 2A in demonstrating increased

sensitivity to ristocetin. This results in aggregates of VWF multimers, which are cleared from the circulation along with the platelets causing thrombocytopenia as well.

- Type 3 is associated with complete absence of VWF and thereby reduced levels of its binding protein, factor VIII.

Clinical Presentation

von Willebrand disease typically presents with mucocutaneous bleeds, excessive bruising, epistaxis, bleeds from wounds, dental procedures, and postsurgery in both males and females. Affected women, 75–100% of whom present with menorrhagia, are also at risk of peripartum bleeding. Women and girl children remain at risk of underdiagnosis. The long-term effects of bleeding resulting in iron deficiency anemia including poor obstetric outcome is cause for concern and VWD must be thought of. Hemophilia-like joint and soft tissue bleeds are seen in type 2N and type 3 defects.

Management

Mild bleeding and planning for minor surgeries with low bleeding risk.[5]

- *Desmopressin (DDAVP):* It is useful in type 1 defects and does not work in type 3 where there is no VWF to be released from endothelial cells and in most types of type 2 as well. It could cause thrombocytopenia in type 2B and hence not recommended in these patients.
- *Antifibrinolytics* in minor mucocutaneous bleeds (avoid in urinary bleeds) and hormonal therapies in women are other measures, which could help in addressing bleeds without recourse to factor support.

Major bleeds, planning for surgery, and cases where pharmacological methods are inappropriate:

- *Cryoprecipitate and FFP* have VWF and are commonly used in resource-poor settings. They have the risk of volume overload and risk of infection.
- *Factor concentrates:* One needs to choose factor concentrates with both VWF and factor VIII as some of the newer highly purified options would not contain VWF. The initial dose is 40–60 units/kg to target VWF and factor VIII levels between 80 and 100 IU/dL followed by 20–40 units/kg every 12–24 hours to keep both VWF and factor VIII levels 50–100 IU/dL for 5–10 days. Minor surgeries need a preoperative level of 30–50 IU/dL (both VWF and factor VIII) with postoperative levels of >30 IU/dL for 3–5 days. Enthusiastic overdosing must be avoided as case reports of thrombosis have been reported. Regular monitoring of VWF:RCo and VIII:C levels is required to ensure appropriate hemostatic levels.

RARE INHERITED BLEEDING DISORDERS

Epidemiology and Inheritance

Rare inherited coagulation disorders (RICDs) comprise deficiencies of factors I (fibrinogen), II, V, VII, X, XI, XIII, combined deficiencies of vitamin K-dependent factors, and combinations of factor with VIII. These constitute 5–8% of coagulation defects. Factor XII deficiency, although prolonging aPTT, is not associated with clinical bleeding. Defects in factor I, II, and factor V Leiden mutation are also associated with thrombotic tendency. These disorders are autosomal recessive.[9]

Clinical Presentation

These disorders, having a variable phenotype, present at any age.

- *Hypofibrinogenemia* presents at birth with umbilical cord bleed.
- *Factor X deficiency* is associated with hematomas, GI, and other soft tissue bleeds. Factor X deficiency has been associated with other congenital defects such as absent radius, valvular defects, and hypertrophic cardiomyopathy.[9]
- *The vitamin K-dependent deficiencies,* documented in about 50 families, manifest in infancy and early childhood, and are associated with skeletal defects. Young females after menarche and women of childbearing age have menorrhagia.
- *Deficiencies of factors I, X, and XIII* are also associated with early pregnancy losses owing to their role in placental implantation.

Management

Unlike hemophilia A and B, factor activity levels do not always correlate with bleeding tendency. **Table 14.12.3** summarizes the key features of RICD including half-life and hemostatic levels. There are commercial factor concentrates for all factors, except factors II and V. Commercial prothrombin complex concentrates (PCC—obtained from pooled normal plasma, has FII, FIX, FX, and FVII) are indicated for factor II and factor X. In case of the combined factor V and VIII deficiency, recombinant factor VIII along with FFP are used to provide the respective deficient factors.

Fresh frozen plasma (all factors) and cryoprecipitate (VWF, factor VIII, and factor XIII factor I) can be used for management of acute bleeds, surgical management, and prophylaxis wherever specific factor concentrates are unavailable. These carry the risk of transfusion-transmitted infections and transfusion-associated lung injury. The transfusion of FFP/cryoprecipitate needs ABO matching

TABLE 14.12.3: Rare inherited coagulation disorders (RICDs).

Factor	*Prevalence (%age of all RICD)*	*Half-life of factor*	*Target level for hemostasis*	*Prophylaxis dose*
I (Fibrinogen): • Afibrinogenemia—absent • Severe hypofibrinogenemia—<0.5 g/L • Hypofibrinogenemia—0.5–1.5 g/L • Dysfibrinogenemia—antigen activity ratio <0.7	7–10	2–4 days	Minor bleed 1g/L Major bleed 1.5 g/L Maintain >1g/L throughout pregnancy	15–30 mL/kg cryoprecipitate or FFP every 7–10 days
II (Prothrombin): • Severe: Undetectable • Moderate: <10% • Mild: >10%	2	3–4 days	Minor bleed >10% Major bleed >20%	Prothrombin complex concentrate: 20–40 IU/kg once a week or 15–30 mL/kg FFP
V: • Severe: Undetectable • Moderate: <10% • Mild: >10% • Poor clinical correlation with factor levels	7–10	36 hours	Minor bleed >10% Major bleed >15–20% >15% levels at onset of labor	FFP: 20–30 mL/kg twice a week only in those with severe bleeding
VII: • Severe: <10% • Moderate: 10–20% • Mild: >20% • Weak correlate with bleed	28–36	4–6 hours	>20%	Recombinant factor VII: 20–40 µg/kg 2–3 times a week for those with severe bleeds
X: • Severe: <10% • Moderate: 10–40% • Mild: >40%	7–10	40–60 hours	Minor bleed >20% Major bleed >40% Prophylaxis in pregnancy for those with past bleeding history	FFP: 20–30 mL/kg twice a week (if plasma-derived factor unavailable)
XI: Severity: Weak laboratory correlation	23–32	40–70 hours	15–20%	No data
XIII: • Abnormal clot solubility • Severe: Undetectable • Moderate: 30% • Mild: >30%	6	11–14 days	30%	Cryoprecipitate 2–3 units 3 times a week. Prophylaxis throughout pregnancy
V + VIII: • Severe: <20% • Moderate: 10–40% • Mild: >40%	2–3	36 hours (factor V) 10–12 hours (factor VIII)	Major bleeding: • FVIII > 40% • FV > 15–20% Desmopressin to increase VIII levels prior to minor procedures	Vitamin K 5–20 mg once a week orally
VKCFD: Severity: No laboratory correlation	50 families worldwide	As per each factor	No data	Vitamin K 5–20 mg once a week orally

(FFP: fresh frozen plasma; VKCFD: combined vitamin K-dependent clotting factors deficiency)

and avoiding volume overload. These also need to be thawed prior to infusion. They must be transfused at once after thawing and not stored in the refrigerator or left unattended for prolonged periods in the ward. In general, most infusions raise the factor level by approximately 2 IU/dL per IU/kg of infused factor, except for factor V (1 IU/dL rise) and factor VII (0.44 IU/kg rise). Each unit of FFP/cryoprecipitate has 1 U/dL of each factor per mL.

In case of minor mucosal bleeds, antifibrinolytics such as EACA or tranexamic acid can also be used. These are avoided in urinary bleeds. These can be used in females to reduce the menstrual bleed, thereby avoiding need for factor infusions with an option to add on hormonal therapies.

PREVENTIVE ASPECTS

Congenital coagulation disorders are potentially fatal in their severe forms without appropriate life long and expensive factor support. In cases with a positive family history, it is possible to do a prenatal diagnosis on chorionic villus samples at 10–12 weeks or amniocentesis at 15–18 weeks. The fetal DNA, if 46, XY, is further analyzed for disease causing mutations or informative markers by linkage analysis. Thereafter, the decision to continue pregnancy rests with the mother.[10]

HEMOPHILIA IN INDIA: CURRENT STATUS ON CARE AND AWARENESS

From humble beginnings in 1983 when Hemophilia Federation of India (HFI) was established in Delhi with 12 families, patient advocacy in hemophilia has come a long way in working for the cause of persons with hemophilia and other bleeding disorders. It has engaged with international bodies for training and support. It has worked with corporate and governmental agencies at state and national level for funding of treatment. It is aptly described as a low volume, high-cost problem.[11] The high cost pushes this down in priority when government funds are allocated. It does not help that almost all newer therapies are beyond reach of most patients. Prevention of hemophilia births is the key to reduce the prevalence and awareness is being spread through the HFI and its chapters that have tried to garner funding for prenatal diagnosis and carrier detection.

CONCLUSION

Congenital coagulation disorders result in impaired blood clotting, leading to prolonged bleeding or spontaneous bleeding episodes. Severe deficiencies of factors VIII, IX, X, and V mainly present with joint and organ bleeds. VWD could present as both primary and/or secondary hemostasis defect depending on the type. Diagnosis involves bleeding history, laboratory, and genetic testing. Treatment typically involves factor replacement therapy, or novel nonfactor agents for hemophilia A and B. Gene therapy for hemophilia A and B is now approved.

REFERENCES

1. Sachdeva A, Gunasekaran V, Ramya HN, Dass J, Kotwal J, Seth T, et al.; 'Consensus in Diagnosis and Management of Hemophilia' Committee*, Indian Academy of Pediatrics. Consensus Statement of the Indian Academy of Pediatrics in Diagnosis and Management of Hemophilia. Indian Pediatr. 2018;55(7):582-90.
2. Srivastava A, Santagostino E, Dougall A, Kitchen S, Sutherland, Pipe SW, et al. WFH Guidelines for the Management of Hemophilia, 3rd edition. Haemophilia. 2020;26(Suppl 6):1-158.
3. Ozelo MC, Yamaguti-Hayakawa GG. Impact of novel hemophilia therapies around the world. Res Pract Thromb Haemost. 2022;6(3):e12695.
4. Srivastava A, Rangarajan S, Kavakli K, Klamroth R, Kenet G, Khoo L, et al. Fitusiran prophylaxis in people with severe haemophilia A or haemophilia B without inhibitors (ATLAS-A/B): a multicentre, open-label, randomised, phase 3 trial. Lancet Haematol. 2023;10(5):e322-e332.
5. Connell NT, Flood VH, Brignardello-Petersen R, Abdul-Kadir R, Arapshian A, Couper S, et al. ASH ISTH NHF WFH 2021 guidelines on the management of von Willebrand disease. Blood Adv. 2021;5(1):301-25.
6. VandenDriessche T, Tatsumi K, Shima M. Should patients with haemophilia receive gene therapy? Lancet Haematol. 2022;9(10):e722-e723.
7. Mahlangu J, Kaczmarek R, von Drygalski A, Shapiro S, Chou S-C, Ozelo MC, et al.; GENEr8-1 Trial Group. Two-Year Outcomes of Valoctocogene Roxaparvovec Therapy for Hemophilia A. N Engl J Med. 2023;388(8):694-705.
8. Weyand AC, Flood VH. Von Willebrand Disease: Current Status of Diagnosis and Management. Hematol Oncol Clin North Am. 2021;35(6):1085-101.
9. Menegatti M, Biguzzi E, Peyvandi F. Management of rare acquired bleeding disorders. Hematology Am Soc Hematol Educ Program. 2019;2019(1):80-7.
10. Lavery, S. Preimplantation genetic diagnosis of haemophilia. Br J Haematol. 2009;144(3):303-7.
11. Ghosh K. Evolution of Hemophilia Care in India. Indian J Hematol Blood Transfus. 2019;35(4):716-21.

14.13 Laboratory Approach to Coagulation Disorders and Its Role in Management

Udayakumar DS, Renu Saxena

INTRODUCTION

Evaluating a patient with a suspected bleeding disorder is one of the more challenging endeavors. After a thorough bleeding history, family history, and physical examination, the extent of diagnostic testing is individualized as per a patient's clinical presentation.[1]

To recap the fundamentals of coagulation, *primary hemostasis* involves the formation of the platelet plug. The essential components of this process include platelets, the blood vessel wall and von Willebrand factor (VWF). Hence, disorders of primary hemostasis include quantitative and/or qualitative platelet defects and von Willebrand disease (VWD).[2]

Secondary hemostasis involves the formation of fibrin through the coagulation cascade. Disorders of secondary hemostasis include coagulation factor deficiencies or connective tissue diseases (CTDs).

Bleeding manifestations provide an essential clue regarding primary and secondary hemostatic disorders and direct the clinician to order appropriate tests. Disorders of primary hemostasis typically present as epistaxis, petechiae, menorrhagia, melena, and intraoperative or immediate postoperative bleeding. In contrast, disorders of secondary hemostasis manifest as spontaneous hemarthrosis, intramuscular bleeds, and delayed postoperative bleeding.

Certain tests are mandatory for hemostasis screening and are widely available in most centers. Hemostasis screening tests include a complete blood count (CBC) for platelet count and morphology of red blood cells (RBCs) and white blood cells (WBCs), prothrombin time (PT), activated partial thromboplastin time (aPTT), and fibrinogen. Some centers routinely include thrombin time and/or clot solubility testing using 5M urea in their initial screening panel.[1]

Differential diagnoses can be generated based on the results of these screening tests to assist in evaluating patients with bleeding disorders **(Table 14.13.1)**. Further workups involving specialized testing must be performed on a patient-by-patient basis.[1]

Based on the screening assay results, common scenarios that depict a methodical approach to diagnosing the bleeding disorder are presented below.

SCENARIO 1: BLEEDING HISTORY WITH ISOLATED aPTT PROLONGATION

Prolonged apt indicates inherited or acquired deficiencies of the factors in the intrinsic pathway—the type of bleeding, age of presentation, and most importantly, the sex of the patient—and guides further workup.[3] Hemophilia and VAD are the most common differential diagnoses in children; however, in patients receiving immune checkpoint inhibitors (ICIs), acquired inhibitors against factors should also be considered.[4] Specific factor levels (factor VIII, IX, and XI) by factor assays are commonly done either by clot-based assays or rarely by chromogenic assays. The factor levels determine the severity of the disease.

von Willebrand disease is the most common inherited bleeding disorder and is often underdiagnosed. Only a fraction of these individuals come to medical attention since the bleeding severity is variable. A rare acquired von Willebrand syndrome (AVOWS) may occur in malignancies, autoimmune diseases, cardiovascular disorders, especially valvular disorders such as aortic stenosis and may be induced by drugs such as valproate.[5]

The aPTT may be prolonged in severe cases of VWD or AVWS and may be normal in mild cases (especially if the factor VIII activity is above 40–50%).

Testing for VWF function typically includes ristocetin-induced platelet agglutination (RIPA) using light transmission aggregometry (LTA) using standard and low-dose ristocetin, plasma VWF antigen (VWF:Ag) levels, and plasma VWF activity [ristocetin cofactor activity (VWF:RCo) and collagen-binding activity (VWF:CB)]. Using the above tests might help to identify the type of VWD. Analysis of multimers should be done if there is low VWF antigen or activity or if the ratio of VWF:RCo to VWF:Ag is <0.7, suggesting the presence of a dysfunctional VWF (type 2 VWD). Type 2b VWD shows hyperagglutination with low-dose ristocetin.

Repeat testing may be required in cases with a strong family history as VWF levels fluctuate with stress, pregnancy, exercise, and inflammatory processes and show some differences based on gender and blood group type.

SCENARIO 2: BLEEDING HISTORY WITH ISOLATED PROTHROMBIN TIME PROLONGATION

An abnormal PT, with or without an abnormal aPTT, indicates an abnormal reduction in the vitamin K-dependent clotting factors (II, VII, IX, and X) or factor V. PT prolongation should always prompt a search for liver function tests and a history of anticoagulation.

Role of Mixing Studies/Inhibitor Screening Test in PT/aPTT Prolongation

Abnormal PT or aPTT results are due to factor deficiency or an inhibitor (antibody against a specific factor or heparin).

The mixing study helps to distinguish between factor deficiency and inhibitors. The test is performed by mixing patient plasma with normal plasma in a 1:1 ratio, followed by performing PT or aPTT immediately after mixing (0 hours) and repeating the test after incubation at 37°C for 120 minutes (2 hours). Sample mixes that correct to normal at both intervals suggest a factor deficiency, while sample mixes that fail to correct to normal at one or both intervals suggest the presence of an inhibitor **(Table 14.13.2)**.

Most prolonged PT samples result from factor deficiency. Hence, the mixing test is most helpful in evaluating prolonged aPTT. Factor VIII inhibitors are time-dependent compared to factor IX (FIX) inhibitors, which act immediately and require an incubation step.[6]

SCENARIO 3

When the thrombin time (TT) is abnormal, disseminated intravascular coagulation (DIC), the presence of plasma

TABLE 14.13.1: Interpretation of screening assays in patients with bleeding history.

Platelet count	PT	aPTT	Fibrinogen	TT	Differential diagnoses		Further testing
Normal	Normal	Normal	Normal or increased	Normal	• Vasculitis or connective tissue disorders (CTDs) • Platelet function defects (inherited or acquired)		• Platelet aggregation studies [using agonists such as ADP, arachidonic acid (AA), epinephrine, collagen, and ristocetin] • ANCA and work-up for CTD • Genetic testing
Decreased	Normal	Normal	Normal	Normal	Acquired or congenital causes of thrombocytopenia		• Bone marrow examination • Viral/autoimmune workup • Genetic testing
Normal	Normal	Pro-longed[##]	Normal	Normal	*Inherited*: • Factor deficiencies (VIII, IX, and XI) • VWD (variable)	*Acquired*: • Anticoagulants (heparin, dabigatran, and argatroban) • Acquired inhibitor of factor VIII, IX, XI, or XII • Acquired von Willebrand syndrome (AVWS) • Lupus anticoagulant	• Family and drug history • Mixing study • Factor assays • VWD workup • DRVVT • Autoimmune workup
Normal[**]	Normal	Normal or prolonged	Normal	Normal	von Willebrand disease (VWD)		VWD workup
Normal	Prolonged	Normal	Normal	Normal	*Inherited*: Factor VII deficiency	*Acquired*: • Mild vitamin K deficiency • Liver disease • Warfarin • Acute DIC[@]	• Family and drug history • Liver function tests • Factor assay • Vitamin K trial
Decreased	Prolonged	Prolonged	Decreased	Prolonged	*Inherited*: • Deficiency of prothrombin, fibrinogen, factor V, or factor X • Combined factor deficiencies [familial multiple coagulation factor deficiency (FMCFD), combined factor V and VIII deficiency]	*Acquired*: • Liver disease • Acute DIC[@] • Severe vitamin K deficiency • Anticoagulants[$$] (warfarin, DTIs, and others) • Acquired inhibitor of prothrombin, fibrinogen, factor V, or factor X	• Family and drug history • Liver function tests • Mixing test • Factor assays

[##]Isolated aPTT prolongation: 1. aPTT might be normal in VWD. 2. Factor XII, prekallikrein, or HMW kininogen deficiencies are not associated with a bleeding diathesis. 3. Lupus anticoagulant (associated with thrombosis).

[**]In VWD Type 2b: Platelet count is reduced.

[@]In chronic DIC (also called compensated DIC), both the PT and aPTT may be normal.

[$$]Warfarin typically prolongs the PT. Heparin typically prolongs the aPTT alone. Most PT reagents contain heparin-binding agents that block the heparin effect. However, high levels of heparin can prolong both PT and aPTT. Anticoagulants can prolong both the PT and the aPTT if present at high levels. Direct thrombin inhibitors (DTIs) such as argatroban and dabigatran, typically prolong both tests. Direct factor Xa inhibitors (apixaban and rivaroxaban) can variably prolong the PT and aPTT.

(ADP: adenosine diphosphate; ANCA: anti-neutrophil cytoplasmic antibody; aPTT: activated partial thromboplastin time; DIC: disseminated intravascular coagulation; DRVVT: Dilute Russell's Viper Venom Time; HMW: high molecular weight; PT: prothrombin time; TT: thrombin time; VWD: von Willebrand disease)

TABLE 14.13.2: Interpretation of aPTT mixing study (inhibitor screen).

aPTT test plasma	*1:1 Mix (0 hour)*	*1:1 Mix (2 hours) at 37°C*	*Interpretation*	*Further testing*
Normal	No need to perform mixing test		Normal	None
Prolonged	Normal	Normal	Factor deficiency	Factor assays (VIII, IX, XI) and VWF antigen levels
Prolonged	Prolonged	Prolonged	Immediate acting inhibitors (antibodies, heparin, and lupus anticoagulant)	Bethesda assay and DRVVT
Prolonged	Normal	Prolonged	Time-dependent inhibitor	Bethesda assay

(aPTT: activated partial thromboplastin time; DRVVT: Dilute Russell's Viper Venom Time; VWF: von Willebrand factor)

heparin or hepatopathy should be suspected. Most often, the PT and aPTT will also be deranged.

SCENARIO 4: BLEEDING HISTORY WITH NORMAL INITIAL SCREENING TESTS

Uncommonly, a positive bleeding history can be seen in individuals with normal initial screening tests with or without a high score on a bleeding assessment tool (BAT) such as the International Society on Thrombosis and Hemostasis (ISTH) BAT.[2] These individuals should be evaluated for other bleeding disorders, such as inherited platelet function disorders (IPFDs), VWD, and vascular and connective tissue disorders (CTDs).

Platelet aggregation studies by LTA measure platelet-platelet cohesion induced by platelet agonists.[2] These specialized tests are usually available at tertiary care centers. Standard agonists such as adenosine diphosphate (ADP), arachidonic acid (AA), collagen, epinephrine, and ristocetin in standard concentrations are used to induce aggregation of platelets in platelet-rich plasma (PRP) of a patient with suspected IPFD. The addition of agonists to PRP increases light transmission in a spectrophotometer-based assay. Furthermore, if necessary, testing is also performed in higher or lower concentrations of agonists. Since ristocetin causes agglutination and not aggregation of platelets, it is described as RIPA.

Light transmission aggregometry is considered thè gold standard for platelet function testing. Excellent guidelines are in place from the British Society of Haematology (BSH) and the ISTH for LTA and its use in diagnosing IPFD.[2]

Out of the many inherited platelet function defects, the two common diseases that are routinely and confidently diagnosed by LTA are Glanzmann thrombasthenia (GT) and Bernard–Soulier syndrome (BSS).[2] In GT, a platelet GPIIb-IIIa complex defect results in absent platelet aggregation to ADP, AA, epinephrine, and collagen but will show agglutination in response to ristocetin **(Fig. 14.13.1)**. In BSS, a defect in the platelet GPIb-IX complex results in normal platelet aggregation in response to ADP, AA, collagen, and epinephrine but not to ristocetin (RIPA). In some granule disorders, platelets may show abnormal aggregation tracing, especially loss of the second wave of aggregation in response to weaker platelet agonists.[3]

Flowcytometric immunophenotyping for platelet glycoproteins can further confirm these diseases with or without additional genetic testing.[2]

A workup for factor XIII deficiency and α2-antiplasmin deficiency are warranted in patients with a history of bleeding and normal screening tests. 5M urea clot solubility test for factor XIII deficiency and a chromogenic assay for α2-antiplasmin deficiency can be performed in such individuals.

Lastly, vascular wall abnormalities due to hereditary hemorrhagic telangiectasia (HHT) and Ehlers–Danlos syndrome (EDS), Henoch–Schönlein purpura, scurvy, Cushing's syndrome, and osteogenesis imperfecta (OI) should be considered, and necessary workup carried out for the same.

MANAGEMENT OF BLEEDING DISORDERS

As discussed earlier, screening assays are primarily used in an individual with a positive bleeding history. These tests are also routinely done as a part of preoperative assessment. Factor assays, VWF:Ag testing, are also frequently done to assess response to the treatment of patients with hemophilia and VWD.

The mainstay treatment of hemophilia is factor replacement using recombinant-derived factor VIII and IX concentrates, either prophylactically or need-based. The therapy monitoring is done by measuring the factor levels as and when required using specific factor assays.[7]

Inhibitory alloantibodies against factors VIII or IX can develop during treatment with factor concentrates and may cause increased bleeding and prolongation of aPTT that does not improve with factor replacement.[8] In such cases, the mixing studies/inhibitor screen is performed as described above, and inhibitor quantitation is done using the Nijmegen–Bethesda assay (NBA).[8]

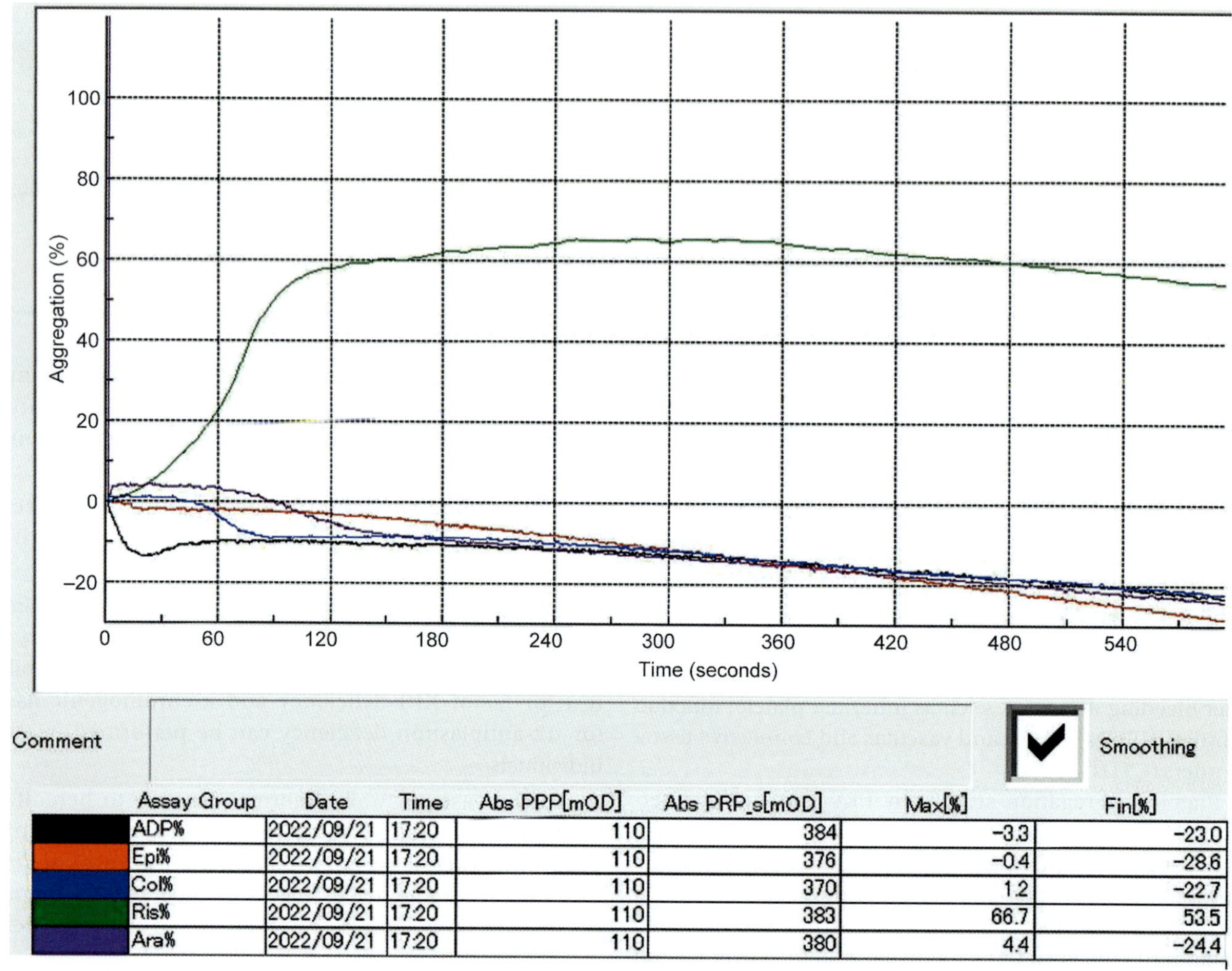

Assay Group	Date	Time	Abs PPP[mOD]	Abs PRP_s[mOD]	Max[%]	Fin[%]
ADP%	2022/09/21	17:20	110	384	−3.3	−23.0
Epi%	2022/09/21	17:20	110	376	−0.4	−28.6
Col%	2022/09/21	17:20	110	370	1.2	−22.7
Ris%	2022/09/21	17:20	110	383	66.7	53.5
Ara%	2022/09/21	17:20	110	380	4.4	−24.4

Fig. 14.13.1: LTA tracing of a 6-month-old male child with Glanzmann thrombasthenia (GT) showing absent aggregation with standard concentrations of ADP, AA, epinephrine and collagen and a normal RIPA (test performed in Sysmex CS-2400). (AA: arachidonic acid; ADP: adenosine diphosphate; LTA: light transmission aggregometry; RIPA: ristocetin-induced platelet agglutination)

The inhibitor titer is the reciprocal of the dilution of patient plasma that results in 50% factor activity. Inhibitor titer is expressed as Bethesda units (BUs) or Nijmegen-Bethesda units (NBUs). Inhibitor titer is important since a patient with a high responding inhibitor (>5 BU) has a greater likelihood of increase upon reexposure to the factor than a low responding inhibitor (<5 BU).[6,8]

Nijmegen–Bethesda assay is used to assess response to immune tolerance induction (ITI). Guidelines are in place for the timing of screening for inhibitors in hemophilia by the United Kingdom Haemophilia Centre Doctors' Organisation (UKHCDO) and United States guidelines from the International Immune Tolerance Induction Study Investigators.[6]

Other than alloantibodies in hemophilia patients, several reports of autoantibodies against factor VIII or IX have been reported in patients treated with ICIs for various malignancies.[4] A mixing study/inhibitor screen and NBA are used for diagnosis and follow-up of such patients developing acquired hemophilia. In hemophilia A patients with inhibitors receiving emicizumab, factor VIII levels should be monitored by chromogenic assays.

Viscoelastic tests (VETs) such as thromboelastogram (TEG) or rotation thromboelastometry (ROTEM) are point-of-care tests that strongly correlate with results from standard laboratory tests and, most importantly, enable clinicians to make timely decisions in the management of a bleeding patient.[7,9] VETs are included in transfusion algorithms in several centers since they provide a more individualized and goal-oriented approach to patient blood management.

Flowchart 14.13.1: Simplified algorithmic approach using PT, aPTT, and platelet count.

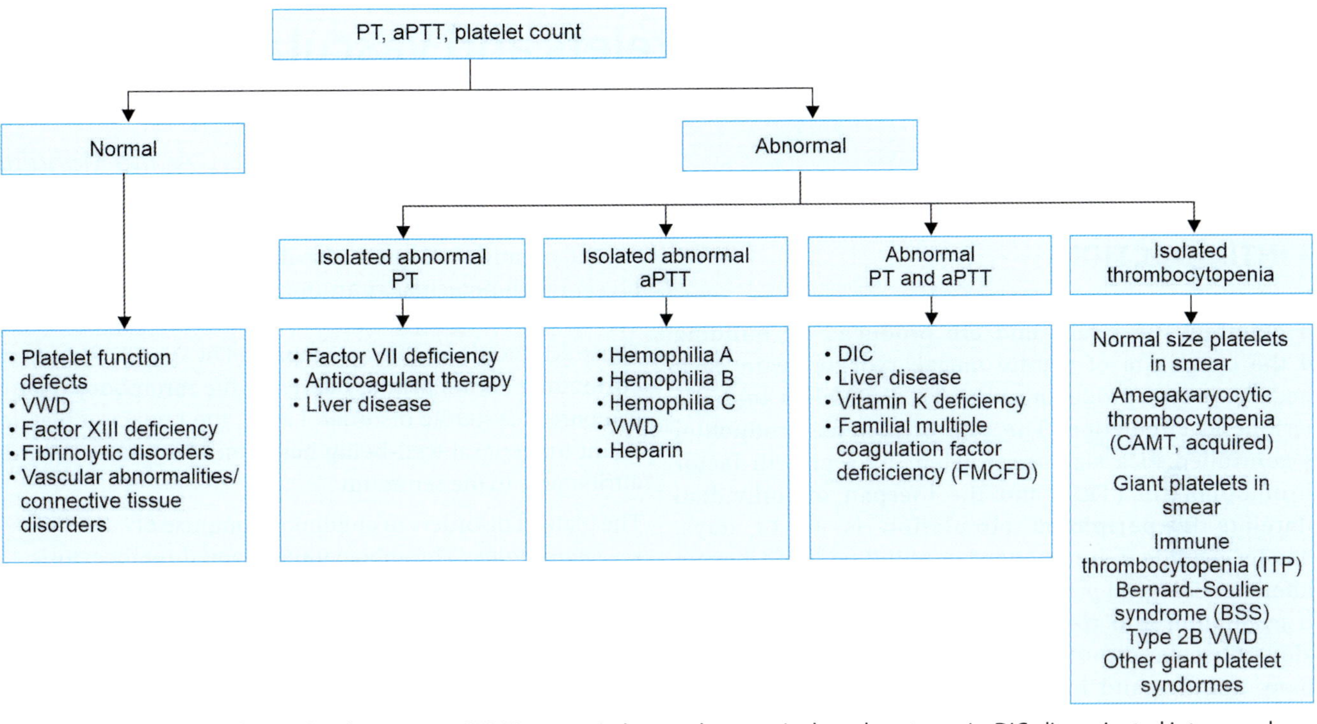

(aPTT: activated partial thromboplastin time; CAMT: congenital amegakaryocytic thrombocytopenia; DIC: disseminated intravascular coagulation; PT: prothrombin time; VWD: von Willebrand disease)

CONCLUSION

- Evaluation of an individual with a bleeding disorder begins with a detailed history, including family history and a thorough clinical examination.
- The use of a BAT is recommended.
- Testing should begin with screening assays (PT, aPTT, and CBC) with or without fibrinogen, TT, and 5M urea clot solubility test.
- Further, specialized testing, such as mixing studies, VWF workup, LTA, and factor assays, should be tailored on a patient-by-patient basis.
- A systematic, algorithmic approach helps evaluate a bleeding disorder patient **(Flowchart 14.13.1)**.
- Laboratory tests are also used to monitor responses to treatment in coagulation disorders and diagnose and follow-up on patients with inhibitors.
- More recently, VETs have been incorporated into transfusion algorithms for a more individualized management of a bleeding patient.

REFERENCES

1. Hayward CPM. How I investigate for bleeding disorders. Int J Lab Hematol. 2018;40 Suppl 1:6-14.
2. Gresele P; Subcommittee on Platelet Physiology of the International Society on Thrombosis and Hemostasis. Diagnosis of inherited platelet function disorders: guidance from the SSC of the ISTH. J Thromb Haemost. 2015;13(2):314-22.
3. Gomez K, Anderson J, Baker P, Biss T, Jennings I, Lowe G, et al. Clinical and laboratory diagnosis of heritable platelet disorders in adults and children: a British Society for Haematology Guideline. Br J Haematol. 2021;195(1):46-72.
4. Archibald WJ, Kouides PA, Refaai MA, Lachant NA. Acquired bleeding disorders secondary to immune checkpoint inhibitors: a case report and systematic literature review. Blood Coagul Fibrinolysis. 2023;34(7):427-31.
5. Franchini M, Mannucci PM. Acquired von Willebrand syndrome: focused for hematologists. Haematologica. 2020;105(8):2032-7.
6. Collins PW, Chalmers E, Hart DP, Liesner R, Rangarajan S, Talks K, et al. Diagnosis and treatment of factor VIII and IX inhibitors in congenital haemophilia: (4th edition). UK Haemophilia Centre Doctors Organization. Br J Haematol. 2013;160(2):153-70.
7. Matkovic E, Lindholm PF. Role of Viscoelastic and Conventional Coagulation Tests for Management of Blood Product Replacement in the Bleeding Patient. Semin Thromb Hemost. 2022;48(7):785-95.
8. Garagiola I, Palla R, Peyvandi F. Risk factors for inhibitor development in severe hemophilia a. Thromb Res. 2018;168:20-7.
9. Whiting D, DiNardo JA. TEG and ROTEM: technology and clinical applications. Am J Hematol. 2014;89(2):228-32.

14.14 Platelets and Vascular Disorders

Amita Mahajan

INTRODUCTION

Platelets play a vital role in achieving primary hemostasis in children and adults and are produced by budding of the cytoplasm of mature megakaryocytes with each megakaryocyte producing numerous platelets into the peripheral circulation. The rate of platelet production is controlled to a significant extent by a growth factor thrombopoietin (TPO) and the lifespan of individual platelets in peripheral circulation is 10–14 days. Platelet disorders are frequent in childhood and have a different etiological profile and consequently the approach to evaluation and treatment is different from those in adults. Vascular disorders, while less frequent, may mimic many findings and indeed in some conditions may be associated with platelet disorders.

HEMOSTATIC FUNCTION OF PLATELETS

The hemostatic effect of platelets is attributable to a number of factors such as surface proteins von Willebrand factor (VWF), fibrinogen, thrombin, collagen, and adenosine diphosphate (ADP). Following any injury to the blood vessel wall or endothelial injury, the extracellular matrix releases these adhesive proteins promoting platelet adhesion and activation generating thromboxane A2. Activated platelets release ADP, adenosine triphosphate (ATP), calcium, serotonin, and coagulation factors. This is followed by binding of fibrinogen to the surface receptors on the activated platelets resulting in aggregation and a hemostatic plug. The serotonin and histamine released in this process lead to vasoconstriction and the platelet surface provides the platform on which the coagulation factors assemble and following a cascade of steps lead to thrombin generation completing the secondary hemostasis. Finally, the contractile proteins of the platelets facilitate clot retraction.[1] **Figure 14.14.1** depicts this complex interaction that is requisite for the hemostatic function of the platelets.

Thrombopoietin controls platelet production and is raised to varying levels in thrombocytopenic states. It is highest in patients with bone marrow (BM) failure or other disorders of reduced production and is raised variably in the setting of platelet destruction.

Quantitative and qualitative disorders of platelets usually present with petechiae, purpura, ecchymosis, and mucosal bleeds such as gum bleeds, epistaxis, and menorrhagia. These symptoms may be accompanied by specific symptoms attributable to the primary illness if the thrombocytopenia is a part of systemic disorder. Lately, the impact of platelet count on general well-being has been identified primarily attributable to the serotonin.

The platelet disorders in childhood comprise of:

- *Quantitative:* Thrombocytopenia and thrombocytosis
- *Qualitative:* Disorders of platelet function

QUANTITATIVE DISORDERS OF PLATELETS/ THROMBOCYTOPENIA

Thrombocytopenia is defined as a platelet count <100,000/μL. The etiology may be congenital sequestration. **Box 14.14.1** lists the most common causes with acquired immune thrombocytopenia being the most common entity in childhood. Many of these conditions are covered in separate sections in this textbook and only specific conditions will be covered in this chapter.

It is important to remember the phenomenon of "pseudothrombocytopenia". This refers to thrombocytopenia as assessed in the ethylenediaminetetraacetic acid (EDTA) specimen and is due to agglutination of platelets in vitro mediated by the EDTA. The patient is clinically asymptomatic. A peripheral smear can clarify this and should be the first investigation if thrombocytopenia is reported in an asymptomatic patient.

The causes of thrombocytopenia in neonates may have a different etiological profile and may sometimes be indicative of a transfer of maternal antibodies. **Box 14.14.2** lists the etiological conditions associated with thrombocytopenia specific to the neonatal period.

IMMUNE THROMBOCYTOPENIC PURPURA

This is, by far, the most common cause of thrombocytopenia in childhood and the peak age is 1–5 years. The condition is characterized by isolated thrombocytopenia in a well child. It is autoimmune in origin with the development of antibodies mostly directed to the GP IIb/IIIa complex. There may be history of a viral infection or immunization in

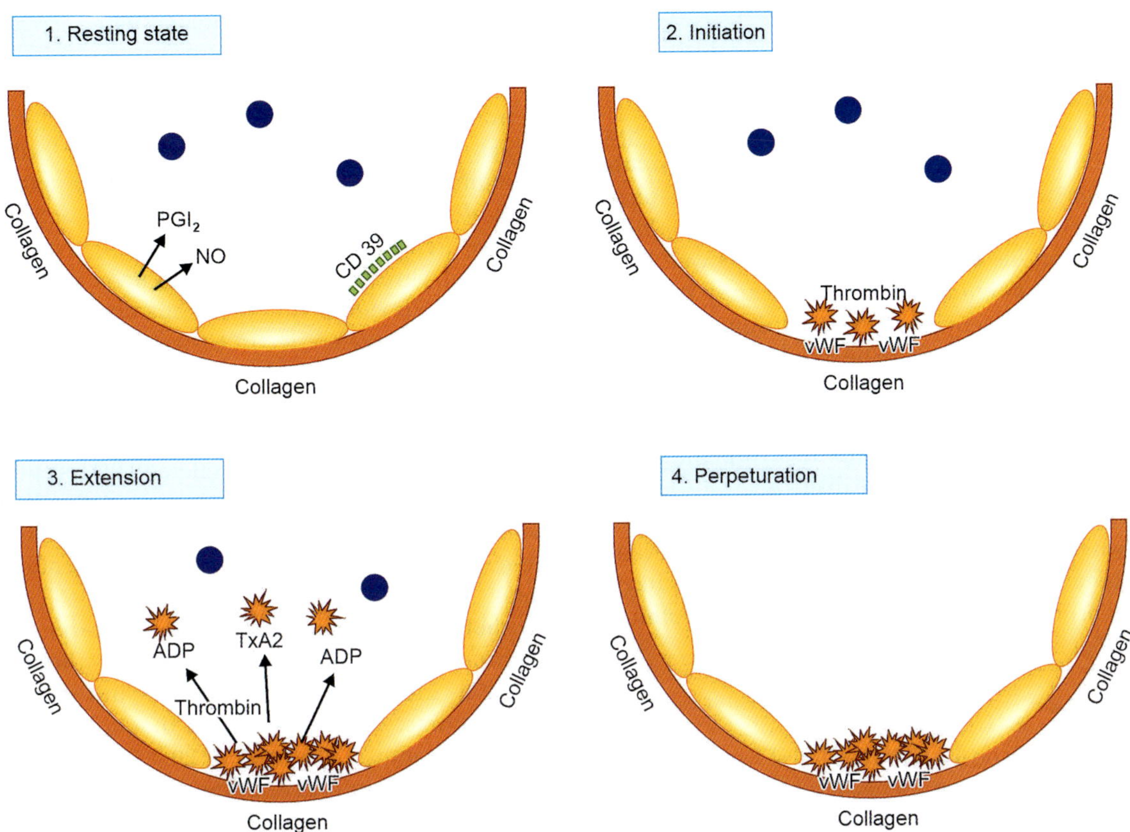

Fig. 14.14.1: Steps in platelet plug formation. (1) Resting state; (2) Development of platelet plug initiated by exposure of collagen following endothelial injury and generation of thrombin leading to platelet adhesion in the presence of collagen and von Willebrand factor (vWF) establishing a monolayer; (3) Additional platelets in response to thromboxane A2, adenosine diphosphate (ADP), and other platelet agonists; (4) Growing hemostatic plug and fibrin meshwork perpetuate and stabilize the platelet aggregate.

BOX 14.14.1: Etiology of thrombocytopenia in childhood.

Decreased production:
- Megaloblastic anemia
- Congenital bone marrow (BM) failure syndromes/amegakaryocytic thrombocytopenia/Wiskott–Aldrich syndrome
- Acquired aplastic anemia
- Lympho-/myeloproliferative disorders
- Storage disorders
- *Infections:* Viral (CMV, hepatitis C, and HIV), bacterial (typhoid/paratyphoid fever), and parasitic (malaria)
- *Secondary to drugs:* Chemotherapy, targocid, and anticonvulsants

Increased peripheral destruction:
- Immune thrombocytopenic purpura
- Autoimmune disorders like SLE
- Mechanical valves
- *Microangiopathic states:* Hemolytic uremic syndrome/thrombotic thrombocytopenic purpura/disseminated intravascular coagulation
- Hemophagocytic lymphohistiocytosis

Sequestration:
- Hypersplenism, e.g., in hemoglobinopathies/portal hypertension
- Kasabach–Merritt syndrome

(CMV: cytomegalovirus HIV: human immunodeficiency virus; SLE: systemic lupus erythematosus)

BOX 14.14.2: Etiology of thrombocytopenia in the neonatal period.

- Maternal ITP/SLE
- Neonatal alloimmune thrombocytopenia
- Congenital infections (CMV, toxoplasmosis, rubella, and HIV)
- Placental insufficiency/perinatal asphyxia
- Bacterial and fungal sepsis
- Bone marrow failure syndromes/congenital leukemia
- Metabolic diseases, e.g., propionic and methylmalonic acidemia
- Kasabach–Merritt syndrome
- Thrombotic thrombocytopenic purpura

(CMV: cytomegalovirus HIV: human immunodeficiency virus; ITP: immune thrombocytopenic purpura; SLE: systemic lupus erythematosus)

the days and weeks preceding the onset of thrombocytopenia. The presence/absence of antibodies does not equate with active disease or remission suggesting that alternate pathways may be at play. Indeed, patients with chronic immune thrombocytopenic purpura (ITP) have been demonstrated to have increased numbers of terminally differentiated effector memory $CD8^+$ T cells.

Clinical Features

The child usually presents with sudden onset of ecchymosis and petechiae and may have mucocutaneous bleeds. Clinically, there are usually no other findings apart from bruising. Complete hemogram reveals *isolated thrombocytopenia* with the other cell lines and peripheral smear being normal. In addition, the *mean platelet volume* (MPV) on the complete hemogram as well as the *immature platelet fraction* (IPF) is significantly increased which helps to differentiate this condition from other causes of thrombocytopenia. The presence of systemic symptoms, adenopathy, organomegaly, bleeding at other than mucocutaneous sites or any abnormality on complete hemogram apart from isolated thrombocytopenia should prompt the search for an alternative diagnosis.

Immune thrombocytopenic purpura is referred to as being "newly diagnosed" if the diagnosis has been made in the preceding 3 months. Patients are labeled as having "persistent" or "chronic" ITP if the duration of symptoms is 3–12 months or over 12 months, respectively.

Management

The diagnosis is made on the basis of clinical symptomatology and a complete hemogram inclusive of peripheral smear. BM examination is indicated if there are any systemic symptoms and signs as organomegaly or adenopathy or if there are any doubts about the diagnosis.[2] If done, the BM usually shows increased megakaryopoiesis confirming peripheral destruction as the etiology of thrombocytopenia. However, in a proportion of patients, the antibodies can also lead to the destruction of developing megakaryocytes in the BM and the classical picture of increased megakaryocytes in the BM may not be evident. Children who go on to develop persistent or chronic ITP warrant evaluation for infections such as hepatitis B and C and human immunodeficiency virus (HIV), and for broader autoimmune disorders such as systemic lupus erythematosus (SLE). It may also be prudent to assess the immunoglobulin levels especially if contemplating treatment with intravenous immunoglobulin (IVIG).

Childhood ITP is a self-limiting condition, and most children may not warrant active intervention apart from clinical surveillance. In general, the risk of visceral or intracranial bleed in this condition is very low despite very low counts.[3] Active treatment may achieve a platelet count >100,000/μL faster but does not alter the clinical course of this condition or the proportion of patients who go on to develop chronic ITP.

Indications to intervene with medical treatment include:

- Bleeding other than bruising
- Mucosal bleeds as this correlates with increased risk of intracranial bleed
- Lack of access to immediate medical attention or distance from a medical center

Patients with no or mild bleeding (skin bleeds only) do not require admission. Hospitalization may be offered if there is any doubt about the diagnosis, there is active bleeding or there are any social concerns. Where active treatment is warranted, current guidelines recommend a short course of corticosteroids with prednisolone at a dose of 2–4 mg/kg for 5–7 days as the preferred corticosteroid with an 80% chance of response. Patients who have any contraindication or poor response to steroids, may be offered single dose of IVIG at a dose of 1 g/kg. Patients warranting treatment and poor response to steroids or IVIG are offered TPO receptor agonists (TPO-RAs) discussed below. Response is defined as a platelet count of 30,000/μL or doubling of the baseline counts. Prolonged courses of steroids are actively discouraged as are platelet transfusions.

About 15–20% patients will go on to develop persistent or chronic ITP. While it is difficult to predict the clinical course in individual patients, those with subacute onset of symptoms, age >10 years at diagnosis, and platelet count at diagnosis in excess of 20,000/μL are more likely to develop chronic ITP.[4] Again management for these patients depends on the presence on the symptomatology rather than the platelet count alone. It is increasingly being highlighted that a proportion of patients with ITP report fatigue correlating with the severity of thrombocytopenia and is thought to be due to low serotonin levels.[5] If this is impacting the health-related quality of life, it may also be an indication to consider treatment.

If treatment is warranted due to symptoms, the treatment of choice currently is TPO-RA such as eltrombopag or romiplostim. While the etiology is largely peripheral destruction, there is also an element of inadequate thrombopoietic response despite severe thrombocytopenia. The TPO while elevated may not be elevated commensurate with the degree of thrombocytopenia which forms the basis of employing TPO agonists in this setting. Eltrombopag is given via the oral route daily in the fasting state and romiplostim is given subcutaneously (SC) weekly. Current evidence confirms the safety and efficacy of these agents in children. However, it must be borne in mind that these agents, while effective in achieving remission are not curative in nature.

Patients with suboptimal response and persistent symptoms may be offered rituximab, a CD20 antibody, weekly for four doses. A significant proportion of children with chronic ITP are expected to go into a remission after 2–5 years. Splenectomy is hardly ever indicated in the current era.

NEONATAL ALLOIMMUNE THROMBOCYTOPENIA

This is a serious condition encountered in the early neonatal period and is because of transplacental transfer of maternal antibodies against antigens present on fetal platelets shared with the father and recognized as foreign by the immune system of the mother. In some ways, it is similar to the phenomenon of rhesus isoimmunization. The incidence of clinically significant neonatal alloimmune thrombocytopenia (NAIT) is approximately 1 in 1,500 live births. The clinical presentation is that of an otherwise well newborn with generalized petechiae with moderate-severe thrombocytopenia in the early neonatal period. Up to 20–30% may develop intracranial hemorrhage (ICH) and the risk of ICH is much higher than seen in infants born to mothers with ITP or SLE. Unlike rhesus isoimmunization, the presentation may be severe even in the first pregnancy itself, but the severity is enhanced in subsequent pregnancies.[6] The diagnosis is established by evaluation the mother for alloantibodies directed against the father's platelet antigens, the most common being human platelet antigen 1a (HPA-1a).

Management comprises platelet transfusion, ideally washed maternal platelets. Random donor platelets may be given if this is not feasible. For subsequent pregnancies, the mother should receive IVIG prenatally from the second trimester till delivery.

CONGENITAL THROMBOCYTOPENIC SYNDROMES

Congenital thrombocytopenic syndromes are rare but the presence of other physical anomalies, abnormal platelet morphology, poor response to frontline therapy, and a positive family history should prompt consideration of these rare conditions. Some of the more significant conditions are listed below:

- *Congenital amegakaryocytic thrombocytopenia:* Skin and mucosal bleeds may proceed to aplasia. Treatment is hematopoietic stem cell transplantation (HSCT).
- *Thrombocytopenia-absent radius (TAR) syndrome:* Bilateral radius abnormalities but preservation of thumbs. The thrombocytopenia can remit spontaneously.
- *Wiskott–Aldrich syndrome:* X-linked microthrombocytopenia, eczema, thrombocytopenia, and severe immunodeficiency. Treatment is HSCT.
- *DiGeorge syndrome:* Right-sided cardiac lesions, cleft lip, severe immunodeficiency, and thrombocytopenia. The thrombocytopenia is usually mild and immune in nature.
- *Familial thrombocytopenia syndrome:* A number of thrombocytopenic syndromes of varying severity have been identified, the most common being MYH9-related thrombocytopenia. The platelets are large (macrothrombocytopenia); thrombocytopenia is usually mild and may be discovered incidentally. Individual conditions may be associated with involvement of other organs such as kidneys and ears and eyes.[7]
- *von Willebrand disease (VWD) 2B:* This is an autosomal dominant (AD) disorder wherein an abnormal VWF molecule promotes clumping. The platelet counts may fluctuate especially in relation to hormonal changes, e.g., menstrual cycle and pregnancy. The other variants of VWD affect platelet function but do not have thrombocytopenia. Patients do respond to desmopressin.

DRUG-INDUCED THROMBOCYTOPENIA

Thrombocytopenia secondary to drugs may be due to myelosuppression (e.g., chemotherapy) or immune-mediated injury following sodium valproate, carbamazepine, vancomycin, and sulfonamides. It usually resolves after withdrawal of the offending drug.

Heparin-induced thrombocytopenia (HIT) is rare in childhood. It develops as a consequence of the development of an antibody directed against the heparin-platelet factor 4 complex. The incidence is lower in patients on low molecular weight heparin rather than standard heparin. Management of HIT includes removal of all possible sources of heparin including heparin flushes of lines and direct thrombin inhibitors such as danaparoid and argatroban.[8]

THROMBOTIC THROMBOCYTOPENIC PURPURA

This is a rare condition in childhood and may be congenital or acquired. It refers to a thrombotic microangiopathy characterized by a constellation of fever, microangiopathic hemolysis, thrombocytopenia, renal abnormalities akin to those seen in hemolytic uremic syndrome (HUS), and neurological symptoms. Neurological symptoms may include visual deficits, aphasia, and seizures. Congenital thrombotic thrombocytopenic purpura (TTP) is a rare disorder secondary to deficiency of ADAMTS13 protein. Acquired TTP is seen in patients on immunosuppression wherein there is an antibody-mediated destruction of ADAMTS13.[9]

Early recognition is important. Laboratory findings include macroangiopathic anemia with schistocytes on peripheral smear, helmet cells, thrombocytopenia, and derangement of renal function tests. Prothrombin time/activated partial thromboplastin time (PT/aPTT) may be mildly elevated due to consumptive coagulopathy.

Patients with congenital TTP respond to infusions of fresh frozen plasma repeated every 4 weeks. Treatment comprises plasmapheresis with corticosteroids, rituximab, and sometimes splenectomy employed in patients with refractory disease. A monoclonal antibody directed against anti-VWF can yield rapid resolution of TTP but access to this agent is limited.

Hemolytic Uremic Syndrome

The pathophysiology is very similar to TTP in terms of microangiopathic hemolysis but the lesions are largely confined to the kidney. In young children, it usually presents after a brief diarrheal illness usually due to *Escherichia coli* O157: H7 strain, but may be seen without this preceding illness. The treatment is largely supportive. Eculizumab, a monoclonal antibody, is licensed for both children and adults with atypical HUS, but access is limited.

SEQUESTRATION

The most common etiology of sequestration is massive splenomegaly in the context of hemoglobinopathies or portal hypertension. Under normal circumstances, about 30% of platelets are located in the spleen. In massive splenomegaly, this could be as high as 80–90%. Treatment is usually directed at reducing the splenic size wherever feasible by medical measures and if unsuccessful, splenectomy. It must be borne in mind that splenectomy is associated with a lifetime increased risk of fulminant infection that is only partially attenuated by vaccination prior to procedure. In addition, patients have an increased risk of thromboembolic phenomenon and pulmonary hypertension. Efforts should therefore be aimed at preventing the development of massive splenomegaly in these settings thereby averting the need for splenectomy.

Another condition encountered in children is presence of large congenital arteriovenous malformations that can lead to sequestration and consumption of platelets. Treatment options include propranolol, corticosteroids, laser photocoagulation, surgery, intralesional sclerosing agents, local radiation, and interferon-α.

QUALITATIVE DISORDERS OF PLATELETS

There are a number of platelet function disorders where the platelet numbers may be adequate or mildly reduced or in fact even higher. The symptoms are usually those similar to thrombocytopenia with bruising and mucosal bleeds but chronic in nature and often associated with a family history of similar symptoms in the absence of severe thrombocytopenia. In some cases, there may be a dramatic presentation with severe menorrhagia at menarche prompting workup and diagnosis.

Screening Tests[10]

Platelet morphology: On peripheral smear, the platelets may have unusual size (significantly increased in Bernard-Soulier syndrome) or shape.

Bleeding time (BT): It measures the interaction of the blood vessels with platelets and is deranged in both qualitative and quantitative disorders of platelets. A significantly prolonged BT in the absence of thrombocytopenia is therefore likely to indicate a platelet function disorder. The test is highly operator-dependent. It is ideally performed by measuring the time required for bleeding to stop after a superficial cut 1 mm deep and 1 cm long (IVY's template) made on the flexor surface of the forearm. It is prolonged if the platelet count is <75,000/µL and in the absence of thrombocytopenia is indicative of a functional disorder. The sensitivity and specificity are low especially in very young children and may be at best be used as a screening tool.

Platelet function analyzer (PFA-100): This measures platelet adhesion and aggregation when the blood is exposed to collagen-epinephrine or collagen-ADP. Like the BT, it is relatively nonspecific and when considering a significant platelet function disorder, platelet aggregometry should be used.

Platelet aggregometry: Agents such as ristocetin, ADP, collagen, epinephrine, and arachidonic acid are added to platelet-rich plasma and an automated machine measures the clumping of platelets over time. Specific patterns point to the underlying diagnosis **(Fig. 14.14.2)**.

Finally, a mutational analysis, molecular testing, and flowcytometry can offer a definitive diagnosis.

Table 14.14.1 enumerates the common platelet function disorders. von Willebrand disorder is the most common disorder of platelet function wherein either a reduced VWF or functionally defective VWF (type IIA) leads to impaired aggregation of platelets.

Management of platelet function disorders depends on the severity of bleeds and the underlying diagnosis. Antifibrinolytic agents such as tranexamic acid can be used both as a preventive modality as well for treating mild bleeds. For mild bleeds and defects, desmopressin 0.3 µg/kg given intravenously (IV) is usually effective.

For severe bleeds as seen in Glanzmann thrombasthenia platelet transfusions can lead to cessation of bleeding but repeated use can lead to development of platelet refractoriness. Recombinant factor VIIa can be used in these settings. HSCT can be curative for these patients but only a small number have been transplanted to date.

ACQUIRED DISORDERS OF PLATELET FUNCTION

Many systemic illnesses may be associated with platelet function defect, most significantly chronic renal and liver disease. Desmopressin may at least partially correct this. Rarely, platelet or cryoprecipitate infusions may be needed.

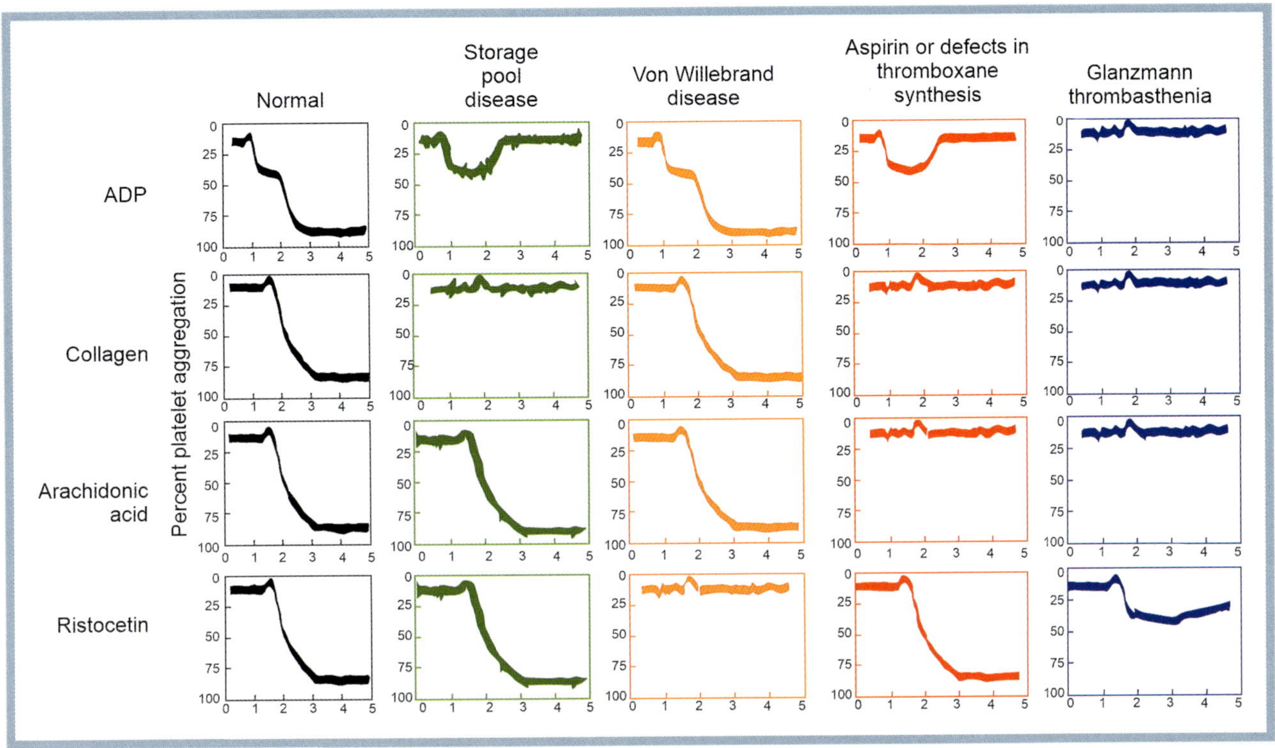

Fig. 14.14.2: Patterns of specific platelet function disorders on platelet aggregometry. (ADP: adenosine diphosphate)

TABLE 14.14.1: Lists of the common disorders of platelet function with the characteristic abnormalities.

Condition	*Inheritance*	*Platelet size*	*Platelet number*	*Clinical picture*	*Diagnosis*
Von Willebrand disease	AD	Normal	Normal/reduced	Mild symptoms	Impaired ristocetin-induced aggregation
Bernard–Soulier	AR	Large	Reduced	Mucocutaneous/GI bleeds	Absent ristocetin-induced aggregation but normal to other agents
Glanzmann thrombasthenia	AR	Normal	normal	Bruising/epistaxis/menorrhagia	Absent aggregation with all disorders
Chediak-Higashi syndrome	AR	Normal with granules	Normal	Oculocutaneous albinism, immunodeficiency, mucocutaneous bleeds, CNS symptoms	Impaired aggregation to adrenaline

(AD: autosomal dominant; AR: autosomal recessive; CNS: central nervous system; GI: gastrointestinal)

A number of drugs such as aspirin, clopidogrel, nonsteroidal anti-inflammatory drugs, penicillin, and valproic acid may impact platelet function. Aspirin and clopidogrel are used prophylactically to prevent thrombosis either by irreversibly acetylating cyclooxygenase critical in the formation of thromboxane A2 as in aspirin or block the platelet ADP receptor, αIIb-β3 receptor, as in clopidogrel. Drug-induced platelet dysfunction is usually mild in nature but may be enhanced in the presence of other abnormalities of the coagulation pathway.

THROMBOCYTOSIS

In the vast majority of patients, this is reactive in nature, the most common cause being iron-deficiency state with/without anemia. It may also be seen with ongoing losses, infections, chronic inflammation and following splenectomy. Very rarely, it may be a manifestation of a chronic lymphoproliferative disorder. In most cases, the thrombocytosis is mild-moderate <700,000/μL but may exceed >1,000,000/μL. Reactive thrombocytosis resolves following correcting the cause and hardly ever requires prophylaxis for thrombosis.

VASCULAR DISORDERS

Certain disorders of the vascular system can mimic the clinical picture of a bleeding disorder although platelet number, function, and the coagulation system are essentially normal. The purpura associated with these conditions is essentially consequent to vasculitis.

HENOCH–SCHÖNLEIN PURPURA

This is a unique entity wherein medium vessel vasculitis can lead to the development of "palpable purpura" almost exclusively on the extensor surfaces of the lower extremities and buttocks though other parts of the body may be involved as well. This is often accompanied by joint swelling in the knees and ankle, nephritis, gastrointestinal, and sometimes central nervous system (CNS) symptoms secondary to the vasculitic process. The diagnosis is generally based on the clinical features but may sometimes require confirmation with a skin biopsy. This is a self-limiting condition and most cases require supportive treatment only. Patients with severe symptoms of gastrointestinal tract (GI) tract or CNS may warrant a short course of steroids.

A number of autoimmune disorders may also occasionally have a similar rash which is vasculitic in nature but may have an appearance similar to purpura.

EHLERS–DANLOS SYNDROME

Ehlers–Danlos syndrome (EDS) is a group of hereditary connective tissue disorders that manifests clinically with skin hyperelasticity, hypermobility of joints, atrophic scarring, and fragility of blood vessels.

The pathophysiology of most subtypes of EDS involves heritable mutations in collagen synthesis and/or processing. The inheritance pattern of these mutations is variable, including AD and recessive patterns. However, it is worth noting that there are reports of spontaneous mutations causing identical genotypes and phenotypes. The collagen affected by these mutations is integral to everybody system, from the skin to the integrity of the vasculature, and as such, the symptoms of the disease can be variable and widespread. Vascular and organ rupture are the two most feared and mortal complications of EDS.

SCURVY

This is consequent to insufficient dietary vitamin C and is fortunately encountered rarely now. Suboptimal collagen production in the body results in fragile skin and blood vessels, gingival hemorrhages, and petechiae. Symptoms such as fatigue, malaise, lethargy, and anorexia of scurvy can emerge after 4–12 weeks of insufficient intake of vitamin C. Eventually patients with scurvy experience bleeding gums, easy bruising, skin rashes, delayed wound healing, and bone and joint aches. The bone pains are due to perifollicular hemorrhages and are usually limited to the lower extremities. Apart from mucocutaneous bleeds, patients may have hemarthroses, and subperiosteal hematomas due to impaired collagen formation. Treatment with oral vitamin C can lead to rapid resolution of symptoms.

KEY MESSAGES

- Quantitative and qualitative disorders of thrombocytopenic disorders are common in childhood.
- Thrombocytopenia may be secondary to decreased production, enhanced destruction, or sequestration.
- Immune thrombocytopenic purpura is the most common disorder seen in childhood and usually has a benign self-limited clinical course.
- Platelet function disorders are increasingly being identified.
- Thrombocytosis is usually reactive and resolves spontaneously.

REFERENCES

1. Periayah MH, Halim AS, Mat Saad AZ. Mechanism Action of Platelets and Crucial Blood Coagulation Pathways in Hemostasis. Int J Hematol Oncol Stem Cell Res. 2017;11(4):319-27.
2. Neunert C, Terrell DR, Arnold DM, Buchanan G, Cines DB, Cooper N, et al. American Society of Hematology 2019 Guidelines for immune thrombocytopenia. Blood Adv. 2019;3(23):3829-66.
3. Neunert C, Buchanan GR, Imbach P, Bolton-Maggs PHB, Bennett C, Neufield E, et al. Bleeding manifestations and management of children with persistent and chronic immune thrombocytopenia: data from the intercontinental cooperative ITP Study Group (ICIS). Blood. 2013;121(22):4457-62.
4. Heitnik-Polle KM, Njisten J, Boonacker CW, Hass MJ, Bruin MCA. Clinical and laboratory predictors of chronic immune thrombocytopenia in children: a systematic review and meta-analysis. Blood. 2015;124(22):3295-307.
5. Grace RF, Klaassen RJ, Shimano KA, Lambert MP, Grimes A, Bussel JB, et al. Fatigue in children and adolescents with immune thrombocytopenia. Br J Haematol. 2020;191(1):98-106.
6. Curtis BR. Recent progress in understanding the pathogenesis of fetal and neonatal alloimmune thrombocytopenia. Br J Haematol. 2015;171(5):671-82.
7. Balduini CL, Savoia A. Genetics of familial forms of thrombocytopenia. Hum Genet. 2012;131(12):1821-32.
8. Greinacher A. Heparin-induced thrombocytopenia. N Engl J Med. 2015;373(13):252-60.
9. Kapler S, Ronan-Bentle S, Graham A. Thrombotic microangiopathies (TTP, HUS, HELPP). Hematol Oncol Clin North Am. 2017;31(6):1081-103.
10. Lasila R. Platelet function tests in bleeding disorders. Semin Thromb Hemost. 2016;42(3):185-90.

14.15 Evaluation of a Child with Thrombosis

Tulika Seth

INTRODUCTION

Thrombosis can cause significant morbidity and mortality in newborns and children. Excessive coagulation or abnormal hemostasis leading to the formation of a thrombus can potentially obstruct blood flow. Thrombosis may be venous or arterial. This is a relatively uncommon emergency in pediatrics. However, it is important to ensure early diagnosis and a proper management to reduce permanent sequelae.

EPIDEMIOLOGY

- Critically ill children may develop thrombosis due to inflammation, infection, disseminated intravascular coagulation (DIC), and impaired liver function and from central venous or arterial catheters.
- Sick newborns are at higher risk as children till 6 months of age have lower levels of the vitamin K-dependent coagulation factors II, IX, and X, compared to adults.
- Thrombin inhibitors, such as antithrombin and heparin cofactor II, and proteins C and S are low at birth. Protein S levels reach adult levels by 1 year of age, but protein C levels remain low throughout childhood.
- Plasminogen levels are low in newborns and infants.
- Thrombin generation is decreased (due to low prothrombin levels) and delayed in newborns compared with adults.
- The incidence of thrombosis peaks in infants younger than 1 year and again during adolescence.

ETIOPATHOGENESIS

The process of hemostasis is divided into a *cellular* and *fluid* phase. The former involves platelets and the vascular wall, while the latter involves plasma proteins. The *fluid phase* is divided into three processes:[1]

1. The multiple-step zymogen pathway that leads to thrombin generation
2. Thrombin-induced formation of fibrin clot
3. Complex fibrinolytic mechanisms which limit clot propagation.

Current evidence suggests that there is an overlap between the previously described intrinsic and extrinsic pathways and an important interaction between cells directly involved in hemostasis [i.e., tissue factor (TF)-bearing cells and platelets] and the coagulation factors. Tissue factor-VIIa complex activates factors in both extrinsic and intrinsic systems. The cell-based model of coagulation identifies the membranes of TF-bearing cells and platelets as the site of activation of specific coagulation factors. It has three phases:[1]

1. Initiation
2. Amplification
3. Thrombin production and action

The *initiation* occurs after a vascular injury, with the binding of cells that bear tissue, which activates factor VII. This produces a small amount of thrombin, which activates platelets and cofactors in the *amplification* phase. The prothrombinase complex (factor Xa + cofactors bound to activated platelets) is responsible for the burst of *thrombin production*, which leads to the third phase of *clot formation*.

The coagulation cascade is triggered after injury to a blood vessel allowing exposure to TF-bearing cells. The factor Xa and activated factor V (Va) as a cofactor propagate coagulation by converting prothrombin (factor II) to thrombin (factor IIa). Factor Xa is central to the amplification of this process. This process may be set off by inherited prothrombotic factors **(Box 14.15.1)** but are more commonly due to inflammation, vasculitis, infection, malignancy, etc.[1]

CLINICAL FEATURES

- Symptoms of thrombosis vary with the site and type—whether venous or arterial **(Figs. 14.15.1A and B)**.[2]
- In deep vein thrombosis (DVT), there may be pain and swelling of the limb. Pulmonary embolism (PE) may present with anxiety, breathlessness, pleuritic chest pain, fever, and cough; and a high index of suspicion is required to identify this early.
- Symptoms of central nervous system (CNS) thrombosis include vomiting, lethargy, seizures, or weakness in an extremity.
- Stroke may occur in utero, in newborns may present with seizures and lethargy. In older children, the presentation is with headaches and acute onset of weakness in an extremity/hemiplegia, with a preceding episode of infection, dehydration, or trauma.
- Patients with renal vein thrombosis may present with flank pain and hematuria.

BOX 14.15.1: Risk factors for thrombosis in children.

- *Time-limited risk factors:*
  - Indwelling catheters
  - Infections
  - Surgery
  - Disseminated intravascular coagulation
  - Postinfectious transient antiphospholipid antibodies
  - Surgically correctable congenital heart disease (risk decreases once corrected)
    - Ongoing risk factors
    - Inherited thrombophilias
  - Factor V Leiden
  - Deficient antithrombin, protein C, and protein S
  - Elevated homocysteine level
  - Elevations in lipoprotein (a)
  - Other less common genetic disorders of coagulation regulation or fibrinolysis
- *Acquired thrombophilias and prothrombotic states:*
  - Primary antiphospholipid antibody
  - Acquired decrease in coagulation regulatory proteins (nephrotic syndrome, protein-losing enteropathy)
  - Indwelling catheters
  - Leukemia, solid tumors, and chemotherapy (e.g., L-asparaginase)
  - Inflammatory diseases (e.g., Systemic lupus erythematosus and inflammatory bowel disease)
  - Prosthetic cardiac valves
  - Sickle-cell anemia
  - Thalassemia intermedia
  - Diabetes mellitus

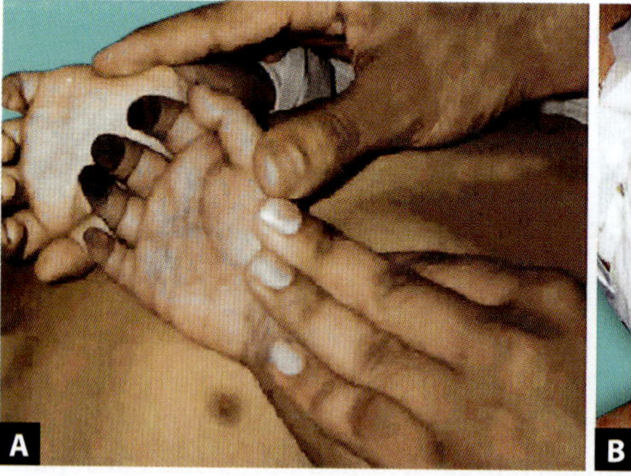

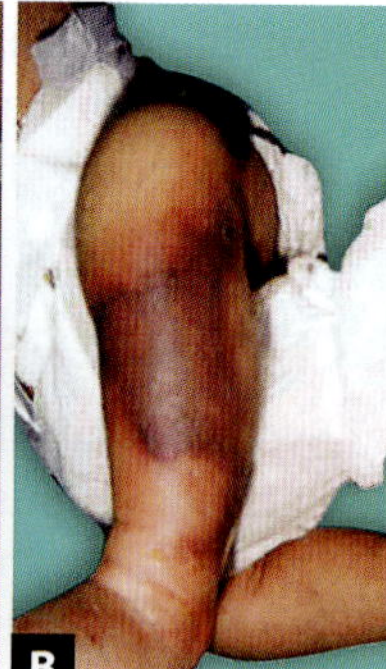

Figs. 14.15.1A and B: Children with thrombosis. (A) Gangrene following microvascular thrombosis; (B) Purpura fulminans.
Courtesy: Dr MR Lokeshwar, Mumbai, Maharashtra and Dr A Sachdeva, New Delhi, India.

- Signs, such as limb edema, erythema, and tenderness on dorsiflexion of the foot (positive Homan's sign), are present in DVT but are difficult to elicit in young children.
- Thrombosis of the inferior vena cava (IVC) and/or renal vein can cause flank tenderness.
- Signs of PE are nonspecific and include diaphoresis, tachycardia, and tachypnea.
- Signs of arterial thrombosis include diminished or absent peripheral pulses and a coolness of extremity skin, with ischemic changes if not diagnosed early.

Some important sites and their clinical features and risk factors are described below.

Cerebral Sinovenous Thrombosis

The cerebral sinovenous system comprises superficial cortical veins, superior sagittal sinus, lateral sinuses and deep, straight sinus, vein of Galen, internal cerebral, and jugular veins. The important risk factors for thrombosis are infection and trauma of the head and neck. Other factors include perinatal complications in newborn infants (e.g., hypoxia and placental abruption), bacterial sepsis, connective tissue disorders, hematologic disorders (e.g., sickle-cell disease, leukemia, pediatric myelodysplasia, and paroxysmal nocturnal hemoglobinuria), solid tumors, cardiac disease, indwelling vascular catheter, prothrombotic states (antiphospholipid antibodies or lupus anticoagulant; factor V Leiden or prothrombin *G20210A*; acquired deficiency of protein S, protein C, or antithrombin III), procoagulant drugs (e.g., L-asparaginase). A small percentage of patients (2%) will not have any identifiable risk factor.[2]

Renal Vein Thrombosis

Neonates may develop thrombosis of a renal vein. Risk factors are polycythemia, dehydration, gestational diabetes (as it is associated with polycythemia and respiratory distress), asphyxia, sepsis, and hypercoagulable states (protein C deficiency and antithrombin III deficiency).[3] The newborn presents with flank mass, hematuria, hypertension, thrombocytopenia, and oliguria. Diagnosis requires a high clinical suspicion with appropriate diagnostic tests, e.g., ultrasonography. The infant should be evaluated for a hypercoagulable state if no other causative factor is identified.

Protein C Deficiency

This usually presents in early infancy or childhood. There may be a history of consanguinity in the family. The parents are heterozygous for the protein C defect. A marked deficiency of protein C (<1% of normal) is usually associated with a homozygous or double heterozygous deficiency. Recurrent episodes of purpura fulminans and/or DVT will occur unless anticoagulation therapy is given. It may be difficult to differentiate this from DIC in a newborn.[2]

Activated Protein C Resistance Ratio

Activated protein C (APC) normally has an anticoagulant effect. Some patients with recurrent venous thrombosis do not show the expected anticoagulant effect when APC is added to clotting tests, and these persons are termed "resistant" to the anticoagulant effect of APC. This is usually due to an autosomal dominant inherited mutation in factor V (factor V Leiden), which resists proteolysis by APC when activated to factor Va.[3]

Antiphospholipid Syndrome

Antiphospholipid syndrome (APS) is a disorder that manifests clinically as recurrent venous or arterial thrombosis and/or fetal loss. If either lupus anticoagulants or increased anticardiolipin antibodies levels are present, APS should be suspected. The diagnosis should not be made on a single abnormal test. It is important to demonstrate that the antibody is persistent in a patient with appropriate clinical findings, with at least two positive values at least 6 weeks apart.[4]

The diagnosis of the APS (according to the Sydney criteria or Sapporo classification) requires at least one of the clinical criteria and one of the four laboratory criteria listed below.

Clinical Criteria[4]

- One or more vascular thrombosis in any artery, vein, or small vessel in the absence of vasculitis
- Three or more unexplained consecutive abortions before the 10th week of gestation with normal maternal and paternal cytogenetics and normal maternal anatomy
- One or more unexplained fetal death after the 10th week of gestation with normal fetal morphology
- One or more premature birth before the 34th week of gestation because of eclampsia or severe preeclampsia
- One or more premature birth before the 34th week of gestation with placental insufficiency

Laboratory Criteria

- Lupus anticoagulant on two or more occasions 12 or more weeks apart
- Immunoglobulin G (IgG) and/or IgM anticardiolipin antibody at moderate-to-high titers (>40 G phospholipids or M phospholipids units) on two or more occasions 12 or more weeks apart
- Immunoglobulin G and/or IgM anti-β-2-glycoprotein antibody on two or more occasions 12 or more weeks apart
- Mixed (more than one of the above)

Portal Vein Thrombosis

In children, portal vein thrombosis is rare, it may occur if certain risk factors are present. These may involve the liver, the portal vein, or the intra-abdominal structures drained by the portal vein. Known risk factors are intra-abdominal infection or inflammation; decreased blood flow due to cirrhosis with portal hypertension or fibrosis; mass lesion interfering with blood flow including congenital anomalies; hypercoagulable states—protein S or protein C deficiency, antithrombin III deficiency, or factor V Leiden; vascular injury from blunt abdominal trauma, catheterization, and infusion of drugs or hyperosmolar glucose into the umbilical vein and exchange transfusion via umbilical vein.[3]

MODALITIES OF DIAGNOSIS[2]

- If venous thrombosis is present, look for fever, recent surgery, trauma, central venous catheter use, nephrotic syndrome, varicella, and other infections.
- Elicit a history of any previous thrombosis. Obtain a thorough family history to suggest inherited thrombophilia states **(Box 14.15.2)**.
- Inquire for a history or symptoms suggestive of congenital heart disease and/or recent cardiac catheterization, which are the most common causes of arterial thrombosis in children.

Laboratory Studies

- Many clotting factors are consumed in the clot formation, and some tests are hindered by the concomitant use of heparin or warfarin, and the reported low protein C and

BOX 14.15.2: Initial workup for thrombosis to evaluate for hypercoagulable state.

- Complete hemogram (Hb/TLC/platelet count, DLC, peripheral blood film)
- PT/aPTT
- Radiology as indicated by symptoms
- Activated protein C resistance and/or factor V Leiden mutation
- Antithrombin
- Lupus anticoagulant (which may be screened by using the dilute Russell viper venom test)
- Anticardiolipin antibodies
- Lipoprotein (a) level
- Plasma homocysteine values
- Prothrombin gene *20210A* mutation (infrequent in India)

Some tests are difficult in the acute period after thrombosis:

- Protein C (usually decreased in acute thrombosis)
- Free and total protein S (usually decreased in acute thrombosis)

Anticoagulation therapy can interfere with the validity of tests:

- Warfarin therapy affects protein C, protein S, and antithrombin assay
- Heparin therapy (both unfractionated and low molecular weight) affects antithrombin, protein C, protein S, and APC resistance assays *However, neither drug treatment nor an acute thrombosis affects the results of anticardiolipin antibodies, factor V Leiden, prothrombin mutation, lipoprotein (a), nor homocysteine levels. Hence, these tests can be done at any time.*

(APC: activated protein C; aPTT: activated partial prothrombin time; DLC: differential leukocyte count; Hb; hemoglobin; PT: prothrombin time; TLC: total leukocyte count)

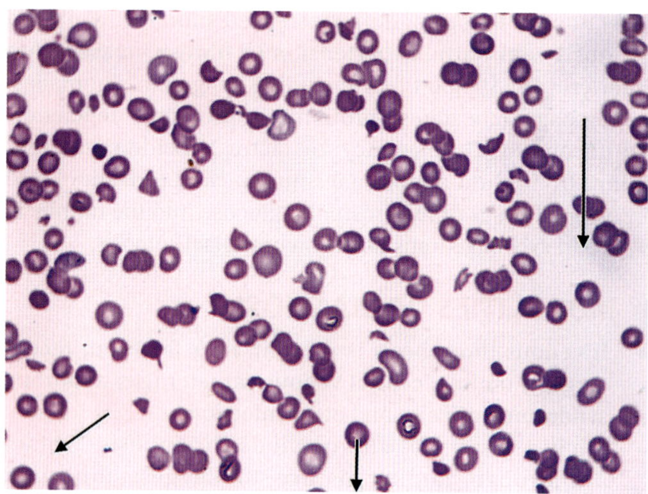

Fig. 14.15.2: Picture of DIC. This picture shows decreased platelets, spherocytes, and fragmented red cells. (DIC: disseminated intravascular coagulation)

protein S level may be the result of the existing thrombosis. Hence, tests need to take account of the current status and type of antithrombotic medications being given.

- The child should be evaluated to rule out DIC, complete blood counts with peripheral blood smear, prothrombin time (PT), activated partial thromboplastin time (aPTT), and fibrinogen level **(Box 14.15.2 and Fig. 14.15.2)**.[5]

Imaging Studies

Imaging studies are difficult as the child requires sedation, and the small size of blood vessels makes the imaging even more complex.

- *Color Doppler imaging* is performed in vessels with thrombosis. The Doppler signals are absent, and the lumen cannot be compressed with direct pressure in a thrombosed vessel. However, this may not be sufficiently sensitive to detect thrombosis in certain vessels, such as subclavian veins, superior vena cava, or brachiocephalic veins.
- *Echocardiography* is of great utility in detecting vena caval and proximal subclavian vein thrombosis.
- *Central nervous system imaging:* A contrast-enhanced head computed tomography (CT) is useful for detecting venous sinus thrombosis. However, both magnetic resonance imaging (MRI) and magnetic resonance angiography are better at detecting early arterial ischemic strokes and suspected CNS thrombosis.
- *Chest radiography* can show the classic findings of PE, including small pleural effusions with a wedge-shaped pleural-based opacity of pulmonary infarction, but frequently the X-ray of chest may be normal.
- *Pulmonary imaging:* Multirow detector CT pulmonary angiography and pulmonary CT angiography studies are successful in visualizing arteries to the level of segmental pulmonary arteries, but the evaluation of subsegmental pulmonary arteries is limited to 80% visualization.
- *Ventilation-perfusion (V/Q) scanning* is the procedure of choice in children with suspected PE. As an alternative, if D-dimer levels are elevated and if the V/Q scan indicates intermediate probability, spiral CT may be useful.

MANAGEMENT

Once a diagnosis of thrombosis is made, the child needs urgent management to prevent mortality and late sequelae.[6] If sick, stabilization is required, and if respiratory distress or neurological problems exist, management in an intensive care unit is required. Screening tests for hypercoagulable state should be sent prior to initiating anticoagulation therapy if possible. Initial therapy requires heparin [unfractionated heparin (UFH) or low-molecular-weight heparin (LMWH)], followed by oral warfarin therapy **(Table 14.15.1)**.[7]

Close monitoring is required to prevent overdosage and the risk of bleeding. Underdosing will hamper resolution of the thrombus; most early recurrent thrombosis is due to inadequate therapy. The decision for long-term thrombosis depends on the risk of recurrence; this can be assessed by testing for thrombophilia status after 3 months of event and after stopping anticoagulants. The *international normalized ratio (INR)*, which is the ratio of PT of patient to standard, is the most useful test for monitoring oral anticoagulation. The INR therapeutic range is 2–3. Because the effects of LMWH on thrombin are minimal, the aPTT prolongation by LMWH is also correspondingly small. Hence, aPTT can be used for the monitoring of UFH only, and for LMWHs, the antifactor Xa assay may be needed in the presence of renal compromise or extreme obesity, and in newborns.

Newer guidelines recommend that UFH should also be monitored by anti-Xa activity; however, this is available in only few hospitals in India. Thrombolytic agents can be administered systemically or locally. The most relevant monitoring during thrombolytic therapy is clot lysis as determined by objective imaging. Clots should be imaged prior to and at the end of thrombolytic therapy.

Some children may need special care in the selection of anticoagulant medication or may need alternative therapy due to contraindications to anticoagulation; these children may benefit from the placement of a temporary IVC filter **(Box 14.15.3)**. Any IVC filter should be removed as soon as possible, as prolonged placement may make removable impossible and require lifelong anticoagulation due to the IVC filter.

TABLE 14.15.1: Dosage for antithrombotic therapy in children.

Oral vitamin K antagonists (warfarin/acitrom)		
Age	***Dose***	***Monitoring***
Infants younger than 1 year	Up to 0.5 mg/kg/day	• The *INR* is first measured after 3–5 days of therapy. • Warfarin should be overlapped with heparin. Heparin should not be discontinued until the INR is in therapeutic range for two consecutive readings. • INR between 2 and 3 is therapeutic range
Older children	0.1–0.15 mg/kg/day	
LMWH (enoxaparin) q12h subcutaneous route		
Age	***Dose***	***Monitoring (necessary in neonates or if obesity. Avoid using, if renal failure)***
Newborns <1-month old	1.625 mg/kg	Antifactor Xa activity 0.5–1.0 U/mL
Infants between 1 month and 1 year of age	1.5 mg/kg	
Children of 1–5 years of age	1.375 mg/kg	
Children of 6–18 years of age	1.25 mg/kg	
UFH by continuous intravenously (Loading dose, U/kg initial maintenance dose) (Used less due to risk of heparin-induced thrombocytopenia and safety and experience with LMWH)		
Age	***Loading (maintenance dose)***	***Monitoring***
Neonates 28–37 weeks of gestation	100 U/kg (28 U/kg/hour)	• Baseline aPTT is prolonged in neonates and infants, may be difficult to monitor. • Therapeutic range aPTT is 2× of normal
Infants at least 37 weeks of gestation	75 U/kg (20 U/kg/hour)	
Infants and children older than 1 month	50 U/kg (15 U/kg/hour)	
Dabigatron	• Recommended 3 months and above • See package insert for weight-based dosing	
Rivaroxaban dosing	• Recommended 6 months onward • Twice a day for children <30 kg, modification for creatinine clearance • See package insert for weight-based dosing	Monitoring is recommended in children, however, unavailable
Apixaban	Studies in adolescents available	

(aPTT: activated partial thromboplastin time; INR: international normalized ratio; LMWH: low-molecular-weight heparin; UFH: unfractionated heparin)

BOX 14.15.3: Contraindications to antithrombotic treatment in infants and children.

For unfractionated heparin:
- Known allergy to heparin
- History of heparin-induced thrombocytopenia

For low-molecular-weight heparin:
- Known allergy to low-molecular-weight preparation
- History of heparin-induced thrombocytopenia
- Plan to perform an invasive procedure within 24 hours
- Thrombolysis by interventional radiology
- Limitations due to small size of involved vessels
- Known allergy
- Systemic tissue plasminogen activator
- Active bleeding
- Central nervous system ischemia/hemorrhage/surgery (includes birth asphyxia) in last 7–10 days
- Seizures within the last 48 hours
- Had an invasive procedure within the last 3 days

History of heparin-induced thrombocytopenia:
- Argatroban (not available in India) or fondaparinux may be used—this product is available in India.

Antithrombin activity is necessary to mediate the anticoagulant effect of heparin. This is decreased physiologically in well-term infants, more so in sick preterm infants, and low in children with extensive thromboses, nephrotic syndrome, or on L-asparaginase chemotherapy. A baseline aPTT within the normal range for age can be used to monitor UFH with a target aiming for a prolongation to 2–3 times the baseline value. If LMWH is used in newborns, it is essential to monitor with the specific assays, else it is best to use the UFH in these cases.

COMPLICATIONS

The sequelae can be devastating and permanent; they will depend on the site, extent, and duration of thrombosis.

- *In utero*, CNS thrombosis or placental thrombosis may lead to severe, irreversible neurologic damage.
- Superior sagittal vein thrombosis, if managed early, may have only slight residual weakness which may resolve.
- Arterial thrombosis may lead to vascular compromise and even loss of limb.

- Postthrombotic syndrome is characterized by persistent swelling, skin discoloration, and pain. It is very common if delayed treatment of DVT and is difficult to treat. This may cause significant stress and impairment in the quality of life.

PROGNOSIS

Predictors of a poor outcome in a child with thrombosis can be evaluated by factor VIII and D-dimer levels. The factors found to correlate with a poor thrombotic outcome are:[8]

- The presence of residual thrombosis at 3 months or 6 months after onset
- Recurrent thromboembolism within 2 years in a previously unaffected venous system
- Development of postthrombotic syndrome

Children with elevated factor VIII and/or D-dimer at presentation with thrombosis or persisting after 3–6 months after standard duration of anticoagulant therapy need close follow-up and longer therapy.

RECENT ADVANCES

- Factor Xa activates clotting over a wider concentration range than thrombin. New *direct factor Xa inhibitors or direct-acting oral anticoagulants* (DOAC) possess many properties of an ideal anticoagulant, including oral administration, rapid onset of action, and predictable pharmacokinetics and pharmacodynamics, with reduced need for monitoring. These include rivaroxaban, apixaban, and edoxaban. Rivaroxaban, apixaban, etc. have been approved in Europe for the management and prevention of venous thromboembolism in adult patients.[9,10]
- Parenteral direct *thrombin inhibitors* are currently available for clinical use—lepirudin, bivalirudin, dabigatran, and argatroban. However, even though they have been available for some time, pediatric use is limited due to safety issues and lack of approval for children. Bleeding episodes can be as severe as with other agents and are difficult to control; Dabigatran has a specific antidote—idarucizumab (a monoclonal antibody); others will need prothrombin complexes to control bleeding.
- Thrombin has a central role in the coagulation cascade. Produced in small amounts in the initiation phase and large amounts in the propagation phase, thrombin is essential for the amplification of coagulation and fibrin formation. Parenteral direct *thrombin inhibitors* currently available are argatroban or fondaparinux and can be used for anticoagulation in patients with heparin-induced thrombocytopenia.
- However, DOACs/novel oral anticoagulants are still not routinely used in children; they are not well studied in children with cancer. Risk of bleeding is present, and they are difficult to reverse; this makes these agents less useful for sick children.[9,10]
- An anticoagulant protein isolated from mosquito saliva inhibits thrombosis by blocking platelet adhesion. *Anopheline antiplatelet protein* interferes with the link between collagen and the platelet glycoprotein VI receptor.
- Adenosine diphosphate (ADP) is the ligand for both P2Y1 and P2Y12 receptors. Stimulation of P2Y1 receptors initiates platelet activation and aggregation. Activation of P2Y12 amplifies the process. *The P2Y12 receptor* is the target for the thienopyridines group of drugs—clopidogrel and ticlopidine. Prasugrel, a new thienopyridine, binds P2Y12 more avidly than clopidogrel.
- A different approach to platelet inhibition involves the hydrolysis of ADP into inactive adenosine monophosphate, thereby removing this potent stimulant from the platelet's microenvironment. Cluster of differentiation (CD)-39, found on epithelial surfaces, has a hydrolytic function that confers both anti-inflammatory and antithrombotic properties. Recombinant human CD39 has been shown to inhibit platelet aggregation in vivo.

CASE SCENARIO

A 15-month-old boy presented with lethargy and seizures after 3–4 days low-grade fever, vomiting, and diarrhea. Initial examination showed responsiveness only to painful stimuli, extensor posturing, and hyperreflexia of the lower extremities (left greater than right) with bilateral clonus. Hemoglobin was 12.9 g/dL, total leukocytes count 5,000/mm^3, and platelet count was 325,000/L. Cerebrospinal fluid showed normal white and red cell counts and glucose and a protein level of 262 g/dL. An MRI showed thrombosis of the straight sinus and internal cerebral veins, hemorrhage in the posterior limb of the left internal capsule. The patient was started on continuous UFH infusion. Increased intracranial pressure was treated with dexamethasone and mannitol.

A partial workup for hypercoagulable disease was performed. Factor V Leiden, anticardiolipin antibodies, β-2 glycoprotein, and serum homocysteine were within normal limits. The patient was discharged on warfarin with regular monitoring of INR from the outpatient department. On follow-up, after 6 months of oral anticoagulation, his complete thrombophilia workup was performed. Protein C, protein S, and antithrombin were found to be normal. Repeat MRI showed resolution, and anticoagulation was stopped. On follow-up at 4 years of age, the child had a normal neurologic examination, except for a slight terminal tremor in the right upper extremities.

PRACTICE GUIDELINES

- Early initiation of treatment is required for good outcome.
- Standard dosing and monitoring are essential.
- Lifelong anticoagulation is not needed in all children.
- Consultation with a hematologist for severe thrombosis and to get the appropriate thrombophilia tests performed, as this may be a life-threatening condition.
- The baseline aPTT is prolonged in neonates and infants.
- Unfractionated heparin does not result in a linear prolongation of the aPTT, and regular monitoring is essential.

PRACTICE POINTS/TIPS

- Inadequate dosing results in recurrent thrombosis and frequent boluses may put the child at risk for hemorrhage.
- Unfractionated heparin and LMWH have similar results; the clinical scenario will dictate which will be used.
- The need for monitoring depends on the underlying disease and risk for bleeding in the individual case.
- Due to fear of bleeding complications associated with anticoagulants, clinicians are reluctant to treat neonates and children with thrombosis aggressively, despite a high prevalence of short- and long-term sequelae in this age-group.

KEY MESSAGES

- Thrombosis needs treatment.
- Investigate to find the underlying cause.
- Treat other comorbid factors.
- Initial thrombophilia workup prior to anticoagulation (if possible).
- Repeat thrombophilia workup after 3–6 months.

CONCLUSION

By a good history and examination and simple tests the diagnosis and management of thrombosis in children can be done effectively. Knowing the limitations of the tests is important to prevent falsely labeling the child with a deficiency or defect. Understanding the underlying condition and identifying any comorbid states helps in selection of appropriate anticoagulation. Selecting the right dose and duration of anticoagulation is important and hematology consultation beneficial, when in doubt.

REFERENCES

1. Hoffman M, Monroe DM. Coagulation 2006: a modern view of hemostasis. Hematol Oncol Clin North Am. 2007;21(1):1-11.
2. Tormene D, Gavasso S, Rossetto V, Simioni P. Thrombosis and thrombophilia in children: a systematic review. Semin Thromb Hemost. 2006;32(7):724-8.
3. Seth T. Thrombosis in neonates and children. East J Med. 2009;14:36-45.
4. Miyakis S, Lockshin MD, Atsumi T, Branch DW, Brey RL, Cervera R, et al. International consensus statement on an update of the classification criteria for definite antiphospholipid syndrome (APS). J Thromb Haemost. 2006;4(6):295-306.
5. Sharma SK, Kumar S, Seth T, Mishra P, Mahapatra M. Eosinophilia: rare cause of arterial thrombosis and cardioembolic stroke in childhood. World J Cardiol. 2012;4(4):128-9.
6. Manco-Johnson MJ. How I treat venous thrombosis in children. Blood. 2006;107(1):21-9.
7. Kearon C, Akl EA, Ornelas J, Blaivas A, Jimenez D, Bounameaux H, et al. Antithrombotic therapy for VTE disease: CHEST guideline and expert panel report. Chest. 2016;149(2): 315-52.
8. Goldenberg NA, Knapp-Clevenger R, Manco-Johnson MJ; Mountain States Regional Thrombophilia Group. Elevated plasma factor VIII and D-dimer levels as predictors of poor outcome of thrombosis in children. N Engl J Med. 2004;351(11):1081-8.
9. Al-Ghafry M, Sharathkumar A. Direct oral anticoagulants in pediatric venous thromboembolism: Review of approved products rivaroxaban and dabigatran. Front Pediatr. 2022;10:1005098.
10. Whitworth H, Raffini L. Practical Considerations for Use of Direct Oral Anticoagulants in Children. Front Pediatr. 2022;10:860369.

14.16 Disseminated Intravascular Coagulation

Divij Sachdeva, Anupam Sachdeva, Manas Kalra

INTRODUCTION

Disseminated intravascular coagulation (DIC) is a systemic disorder that is usually not a single entity in itself but a result of widespread endothelial damage due to underlying uncontrolled systemic illnesses. This can be due to varied disorders such as sepsis, trauma, malignancy, and connective tissue disorders. The endothelial activation in turn activates the coagulation cascade and platelets, which leads to deposition of fibrin. Thus, a vicious loop of endothelial activation and clotting ensues which causes consumption of clotting factors and platelets leading to the classical clinical picture of a child with bleeding and thrombosis at the same time. This can have a fulminant course affecting multiple organs of the body with multiorgan dysfunction and death if not attended to.

EPIDEMIOLOGY

Disseminated intravascular coagulation can occur across hospitalized patients with a variable frequency of around 1–3%.[1,2] Out of all the etiologies, sepsis is the most common cause especially in lower and medium income countries. The rates of DIC are highest for patients with gram-negative septicemia, with around 30–50% developing it.[1] There is no sex predisposition and DIC occurs across all age groups.

ETIOLOGY

As summarized above, DIC is not a disease in itself but a culmination of a severe systemic illness. Hence, it always has a preexisting pathology. Many systemic illnesses can contribute to endothelial injury and systemic activation of coagulation and cytokines by exposure to procoagulant proteins. The causes can vary according to the age group of the individual with neonates developing it secondary to hyaline membrane disease, hypoxic ischemic encephalopathy, meconium aspiration syndrome, and early and late onset sepsis. In patients that are older, it is usually secondary to septicemia **(Box 14.16.1)**.[1,3]

PATHOPHYSIOLOGY[4]

Disseminated intravascular coagulation is the result of several simultaneously occurring mechanisms **(Flowchart 14.16.1)**. The systemic formation of fibrin is a result of tissue factor-mediated thrombin generation and the simultaneous suppression of physiologic anticoagulation mechanisms such as the antithrombin system and the protein C system. The activation of the intravascular coagulation system initiates the following processes:

- *Endothelial damage:* Tissue damage from the primary systemic disorder causes endothelial injury which exposes the subendothelial matrix uncovering von Willebrand factor (vWF) and activating platelets.

BOX 14.16.1: Systemic conditions associated with DIC.[3]

Infectious triggers:
- *Bacteria: Neisseria meningitis*, scrub typhus, and gram-negative and gram-positive sepsis
- *Viruses:* Human immunodeficiency virus (HIV), dengue virus, and cytomegalovirus (CMV)
- *Fungal infections:* Candidiasis and aspergillosis
- *Parasites:* Malaria and leishmaniasis

Neonates:
- Hypoxic ischemic encephalopathy (HIE)
- Necrotizing enterocolitis (NEC)
- Hyaline membrane disease (HMD)
- Meconium aspiration syndrome (MAS)
- Intrauterine infections (TORCH group)

Trauma:
- Severe crush injury
- Burns
- Fat embolism

Organ dysfunction:
- Severe pancreatitis
- Severe hepatic failure

Malignancy:
- Solid tumors
- Lymphoproliferative malignancies

Immunologic:
- Hemolytic transfusion reaction
- Bone marrow and solid organ transplant rejection

Vascular abnormalities:
- Kasabach–Merritt syndrome
- Large vascular aneurysm

Severe toxic reactions:
- Snake bite
- Drugs

Hemorrhagic skin necrosis:
- Purpura fulminans

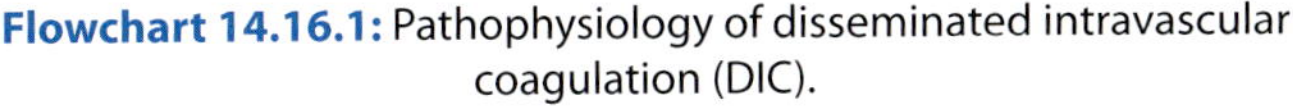

Flowchart 14.16.1: Pathophysiology of disseminated intravascular coagulation (DIC).

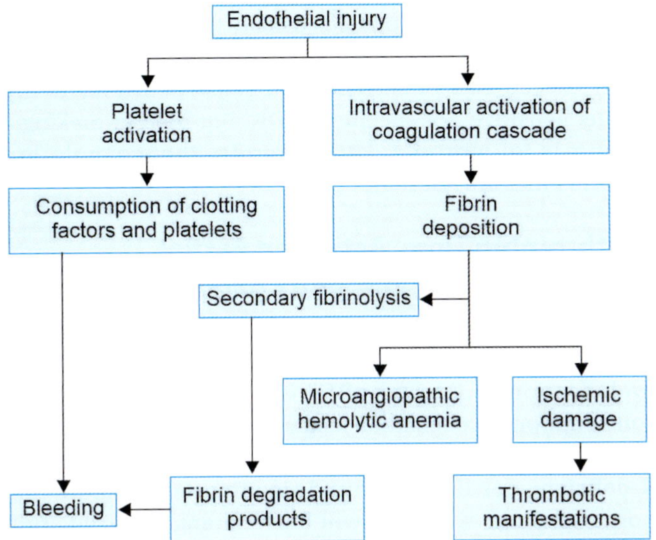

- *Procoagulant state:* Tissue damage further releases procoagulants in the bloodstream.
- *Fibrin plug formation:* Coagulation cascade is activated by exposure of the subendothelial matrix and platelets. The cascade is initiated by the interaction of tissue factor and factor VII; a thrombin plug is generated which propagates conversion of fibrinogen to fibrin which gets deposited in the microvasculature. The loop is amplified by activated factor VIII, V, XI, and XIII.
- *Fibrinolysis:* Once fibrin starts depositing, fibrinolytic pathways are triggered simultaneously to limit the thrombi formation. The main stimulus for this is plasmin, which cleaves both fibrinogen and fibrin. Excessive fibrin degradation products (FDP) are then released which interfere with polymerization of fibrin and inhibit platelet aggregation.
- *Depletion of clotting factors and platelets:* Excessive activation of platelets and clotting factors causes secondary depletion leading to increased risk of bleeding.
- *End-organ damage:* The fibrin clots get deposited into the microvasculature of the end organs leading to ischemia and necrosis.
- *Hemolysis:* The deposition of fibrin also causes the flow inside the blood vessels to become turbulent. Hence, it increases the mechanical shearing forces on the red blood cells resulting in microangiopathic hemolytic anemia.

SEPSIS AND DISSEMINATED INTRAVASCULAR COAGULATION[2]

As mentioned above, the most common cause of DIC in the developing countries is sepsis. Gram-negative sepsis is associated with higher rates of DIC with around 30–50% patients having clinical signs and symptoms of it. The primary trigger for DIC in patients with sepsis is the massive release of proinflammatory cytokines which initiate the loop by enhancing tissue injury and activation of coagulation pathways.[3] Interleukin-6 has been shown to be one of the principal mediators of this.

TYPES OF DISSEMINATED INTRAVASCULAR COAGULATION

Disseminated intravascular coagulation is commonly seen in two clinical forms—uncompensated or acute DIC and compensated or chronic DIC.[3-5] The compensation in the term is reflective of the body's mechanisms to control the cascade.

- *Uncompensated DIC:* Sudden and massive exposure of blood to procoagulants which generates intravascular coagulation and resultant consumptive hemorrhagic manifestations. End-organ damage can rapidly ensue if not dealt adequately and emergently.
- *Chronic disseminated DIC:* When the exposure to the trigger is slow, a chronic state of slow thrombi generation and compensated bleeding is ensued. The liver and bone marrow are able to cope with this enhanced production. Clinical signs and symptoms are usually subtle. This clinical scenario is seen in patients with malignancies, connective tissue disorders, and vasculitis.[3]

CLINICAL MANIFESTATIONS

The clinical presentation and prognosis of DIC all depend on the initiating event and its rapidity. All share in common the same pathophysiology—a deranged hemostatic system which is unable to cope and compensate with the ongoing thrombosis and bleeding.

Background symptoms are usually specific to the underlying etiology. Patients mostly have bleeding manifestations, especially in fragile areas such as oral cavity and the alimentary tract. Hematuria is also common. Acute manifestations can range from petechiae on the oral cavity and body and massive sites of subcutaneous hemorrhage at vascular access sites or catheters. Blood might ooze from surroundings of the intravenous (IV) cannulations, catheters, or surgical sites.[5] Serious bleeding might also ensue in serous cavities. Patients with bleeding from at least three sites that are unrelated to each other should be evaluated for DIC.

Multiple organs can get affected; lung involvement is heralded by complaints of cough, difficulty in breathing, and hemoptysis. Patients with accelerated hemolysis can present with signs of jaundice which can rapidly get complicated once secondary liver dysfunction settles in. If the cascade is not halted, patients can rapidly deteriorate and develop neurological signs and symptoms such as delirium, altered sensorium, and coma. Thrombi formation can occur both in smaller vessels and larger vessels; the common manifestations include deep vein thrombi and renal failure due to involvement of the kidney microvasculature. Renal failure can complicate DIC is as much as 25% of patients.[2] Venous thromboembolism is a common manifestation in patients with chronic DIC as the consumption of platelets and clotting factors is not rampant enough to cause bleeding.

Bleeding might not be an alarming clinical manifestation early on in the course of DIC. Hence, clinicians should be aware that patients might still develop extensive thrombi which may embolize to different organs and cause ischemic damage resulting in multiorgan dysfunction. This can evolve rapidly as seen in patients with *N. meningitidis* infections and associated Waterhouse-Friedrichsen syndrome.

On the other end of the spectrum are patients with malignancies such as acute promyelocytic leukemia, where hyperfibrinolysis dominates the pathophysiology of DIC. These patients are more likely to present with symptoms of bleeding which requires extensive supportive therapy.

APPROACH TO DIAGNOSIS

Diagnosis of a patient with DIC is usually clinical along with laboratory findings that corroborate the presence of both thrombosis and bleeding. There is no laboratory test or assay that is pathognomonic to the diagnosis of DIC. Laboratory test values may change rapidly due to the dynamic nature of the disease; hence, supportive investigations need to be repeated and intensively monitored to watch out for signs of deterioration. In patients with DIC, the common laboratory derangements that are seen include a low platelet count or a rapid fall in it, prolonged prothrombin time (PT) or activated partial thromboplastin time (aPTT), elevation of the levels of FDP and the resultant lowering of antithrombin III, protein C and S due to consumption.[3]

In the appropriate clinical scenario, a patient having DIC will have prolonged PT, aPTT, low fibrinogen levels, and thrombocytopenia; these point to extreme activation of the coagulation pathway and excessive thrombin generation. Testing for increased fibrinogen turnover—FDP or D-dimer is an adjunct to the diagnosis.

INVESTIGATIONS[6]

Platelet Count

A declining platelet count is a sensitive indicator of DIC, through lacking specificity. Thrombin generation is reliably depicted by the platelet count and its fall. It is important to monitor serial fall in the platelets even when it is in normal range to pick up deteriorating patients early.

Peripheral Blood Smear

There can be a myriad of abnormalities that can occur in patients with DIC; cytopenia is usually apparent. Abnormal cells like schistocytes may also be present; however, they rarely exceed 10% of all red blood cells.[6] Schistocytes are neither sensitive nor specific for DIC but help in making a diagnosis of chronic DIC wherein the coagulation abnormalities are not stark.

Prothrombin Time, Activated Partial Thromboplastin Time, and Coagulation Factors

Coagulation abnormalities are common in patients with DIC, with around 50–75% patients developing it.[3] The prolongation of PT and aPTT is a sensitive measure of consumption of coagulation factors, and in addition, patients might have impaired synthesis of them due to vitamin K deficiency or liver disease. It is important to note that not all patients with DIC will have deranged coagulation profiles, as circulating activated clotting factors normalize these assays. Individual factor levels will show decreased activity of V, VII, and VIII. Serial measurement of clotting factors is more helpful than a single test done in helping the diagnosis of DIC.

Fibrin Degradation Products and D-dimer

The excessive generation of fibrin is a key component of DIC. Elevated levels of soluble fibrin can be seen in 90–100% of patients with DIC but is limited by its low specificity. Another caveat in this is the standardization of the test and its availability.[3,7]

Excessive fibrin generation is then followed by enhanced fibrinolysis which can be measured by the help of elevated FDP and D-dimer. These tests are again limited by their applicability as they lack specificity. D-dimer can be elevated in patients with thromboembolism, trauma, surgery, and inflammatory conditions. In addition, renal and hepatic insults can also influence their levels.

Fibrinogen

Hypofibrinogenemia is a common manifestation in patients with DIC, with up to 30–40% children having it. This is due to excessive consumption. As it is an acute phase reactant, levels may be erroneously high or normal in patients having inflammatory conditions. Sequential monitoring helps in detecting consumptive coagulopathy in patients with DIC.

Anticoagulants

As a compensatory mechanism to the excessive intravascular thrombosis, proteins C and S, and antithrombin-III are upregulated; however, these rapidly get consumed and levels in patients are usually low especially late in the disease.

As mentioned above, DIC is a dynamic condition and the tests depict the patient's condition at that time. Another caveat of the tests is the limited sensitivity and specificity as they can be altered in a variety of conditions. Hence, serial monitoring of the tests is important rather than a single measurement to pick up deteriorating patients early. PT, aPTT, CBC with peripheral smear, platelet count, FDP, and D-dimer are commonly available tests at most hospitals and are useful adjuncts to a clinical diagnosis of DIC.

SCORING SYSTEM

There are multiple scoring methods that are available to score the severity of DIC. The most routinely used score is the International Society on Thrombosis and Hemostasis (ISTH) scoring for DIC.[8] This score uses the commonly available coagulation tests like platelet count, PT, fibrinogen, and FDP (**Table 14.16.1**).[9] These tests are graded based on the degree of abnormality. The test is known to be highly sensitive and specific for patients with DIC. The major drawback of all such tests is that they convey the status of the patient in that particular time point when the test was taken, hence, in a dynamic condition like DIC there is a need to revisit the score again if the patient deteriorates.

The other scores that are used for DIC are similar to the ISTH in that they all use similar parameters to quantify the severity. The other common scoring system that is used in clinical practice is the Japanese Association for Acute Medicine (JAAM) for DIC. The major deviation that the JAAM score has to the ISTH score is that it takes into consideration the trend of platelet counts rather than a single measurement, hence, it might be a better test to prognosticate patients with DIC. The score is still to be validated in pediatric patients.

TABLE 14.16.1: International Society on Thrombosis and Hemostasis (ISTH) scoring system for disseminated intravascular coagulation (DIC).[9]

1. *Risk assessment:* Does the patient have an underlying disorder known to be associated with overt DIC?* – If yes, proceed. – If no, do not use this scoring system.	
2. *Obtain the following laboratory tests:* – Platelet count – Fibrin related markers [e.g., fibrin degradation products (FDP), soluble fibrin monomers, D-dimer] – Prothrombin time (PT) – Fibrinogen	
3. *Assign score for each laboratory parameter*	*Score*
Platelet count:	
– >100,000/μL	0
– 50,000–100,000/μL	1
– <50,000/μL	2
Fibrin-related markers (e.g., FDP, D-dimer):*	
– No increase	0
– Moderate increase	2
– Strong increase	3
Prothrombin time (PT):	
– Prolonged <3 seconds	0
– Prolonged 3–6 seconds	1
– Prolonged >6 seconds	2
Fibrinogen level:	
– >100 mg/dL (>1.0 g/L)	0
– <100 mg/dL (>100 g/L)	1
4. *Calculate total score: Add individual scores for each laboratory parameter.*	
5. *Score interpretation:* – ≥5: Compatible with overt DIC. Repeat scoring daily. – <5: Suggestive (not affirmative) for nonovert DIC. Repeat in 1–2 days	

*Although D-dimer is not explicitly included in this scoring system, elevated D-dimer is a strong indicator of fibrinolysis and is more specific than FDPs.

Source: Reproduced from Taylor FB, Toh CH, Hoots WK, et al. Towards definition, Clinical and Laboratory Criteria, and a Scoring System for Disseminated Intravascular Coagulation. Thromb Hemost. 2001;86:1327. Copyright © 2001 Schattauer GmbH.[9]

DIFFERENTIAL DIAGNOSIS

There are a multitude of clinical conditions that share clinical manifestations and laboratory abnormalities in patients with DIC. The common conditions include acute liver failure, hemolytic uremic syndrome, and thrombotic thrombocytopenic purpura.

In patients with *acute liver failure,* the coagulation abnormalities are due to altered synthesis of clotting factors. The major differentiating factor in patients with DIC is low levels of factor VIII which can be confirmed by doing a factor assay. In contrast, patients with liver disease will have a normal level. Furthermore, D-dimer assays are abnormal in DIC but normal in liver disease.

Hemolytic uremic syndrome, another clinical and laboratory mimic which commonly presents with anemia and renal dysfunction does not have accompanied coagulopathy.

TREATMENT OF DISSEMINATED INTRAVASCULAR COAGULATION[8,10]

Patients with DIC usually settle on giving treatment for the enticing cause of the DIC—in case of infections triggering DIC, rapid treatment with antibiotics, and chemotherapy or surgery in patients with malignant causes. Patients with DIC

TABLE 14.16.2: Replacement products to be used in disseminated intravascular coagulation (DIC).

Replacement product	*Indication*	*Dose*
Platelets	Active bleed/high risk with platelet count <50 × 10^9/L	10 mL/kg IV over 30 minutes *or* 1 unit for every 10 kg of body weight (adult dose)
Fresh frozen plasma (FFP)	Prolonged PT, aPTT, and in need of invasive procedure	15 mL/kg IV at <1 mL/kg/min using an infusion set with a filter can be repeated in 24 hours
Cryoprecipitate	Severe hypofibrinogenemia (<1 g/L)	10 mL/kg per infusion (1 unit for every 10 kg) can be repeated every 6 hours. It is generally provided in donor pools (each containing 5 units)
Fibrinogen concentrate	Severe hypofibrinogenemia (<1 g/L)	20–50 mg/kg (total dose of 2–3 g)
Unfractionated heparin	Thrombotic event associated with DIC	5–10 IU/kg/hour as continuous infusion

(aPTT: activated partial thromboplastin time; PT: prothrombin time)

will require intensive support of blood products including packed cell transfusions, platelets, fresh frozen plasma (FFP) and cryoprecipitate transfusions **(Table 14.16.2)**.

Blood Component Therapy

Patients with DIC are at high risk of bleeding, the need of replacement therapy is based on the bleeding phenotype of the patient. Prophylactic blood product transfusion is discouraged unless the patient is at very high risk of bleeding. Our goals are usually to keep a platelet count of above 50,000/cumm and fibrinogen >1 g/dL. Patients who are on chemotherapy require platelets at a cut of 10,000–20,000/cumm as they are not expected to rise on their platelet count due to effect of the medication.

Prophylactic FFP transfusion are not to normalize the coagulation profile but to minimize the risk of bleeding; this can be attained by keeping the aPTT and PT at around 1.5 times the normal value. A patient who is bleeding and has low fibrinogen levels requires cryoprecipitate transfusion. As these patients are sick and may require repetitive use of blood products, careful assessment of fluid balance is required. Administration of factor VIIa for bleeding which is refractory to multiple blood product transfusions has been described but has to be tested in a randomized clinical trial setting.

Packed cell transfusion is required for patients who are bleeding and have low hemoglobin levels.

It is important to take cognizance of the fact that the response to blood component therapy should be gauged on the basis of the bleeding phenotype of the patient rather than just the laboratory parameters.

Anticoagulants

Considering that there is extreme activation of the coagulation system in patients with DIC, the administration of anticoagulants in patients appears to be a rational approach, however, the use of heparin and its analogs is not recommended universally for all DIC patients due to risk of bleeding.

Therapeutic doses of heparin should be considered in patients with DIC in whom thrombosis is the primary feature. A low dose of 10 IU/kg/hour can be ensued for patients with DIC who have arterial or venous thrombotic events. Some randomized control trials (RCT) have shown the superiority of giving low molecular heparin versus unfractionated heparin in patients with DIC. If patients are being given heparin, they should be monitored to keep the aPTT around 60–90 seconds (1.5–2.5 times normal). As patients with DIC have abnormal coagulation profiles, monitoring of APTT might be complicated and clinical signs of bleeding should be watched out for.

Conceptually, the use of anticoagulant agents effective against tissue factor activity seems to be most logical. Although, phase II trials of recombinant tissue factor pathway inhibitor (TFPI) in patients with sepsis showed encouraging results, a phase III trial did not show an overall survival benefit. Recent trials of recombinant human thrombomodulin suggest that this compound may reduce mortality and may reduce the severity of organ failure significantly.

Concentrate of Coagulation Inhibitors

The use of anticoagulant factors such as antithrombin and activated protein C to restore the dysfunctional anticoagulant pathway in DIC is not recommended in pediatric patients. Antithrombin concentrate has been available since 1980s and most trials with this compound show some benefit in terms of improvement of laboratory parameters but no clinical trial has been able to demonstrate improved mortality. Based on the logic that there is depression of the protein C pathway in DIC, it has been suggested that supplementation of activated protein C might potentially be of benefit. Some studies have shown the ability of activated protein C to normalize coagulation activation during severe sepsis, but it has also been reported to increase the risk of major bleeding. Unlike in adults, use of activated protein C is not recommended in children with DIC. In fact, because of an increased risk of bleeding and lack of efficacy, a randomized clinical trial of activated protein C in children with severe sepsis was terminated early.

Antifibrinolytic Agents

The use of antifibrinolytic agents such as tranexamic acid in patients with DIC is generally not recommended because DIC has hypofibrinolysis and antifibrinolytic agent might worsen the condition by prothrombotic effect. The only exception may be made in patients with primary or secondary hyperfibrinolysis (e.g., coagulopathy associated with promyelocytic leukemia or in some cases of DIC secondary to other malignancies), where antifibrinolytic treatment has been shown to control coagulopathy. The use of procoagulant factor concentrate like prothrombin complex or recombinant factor VIIa is not recommended for the treatment of DIC patients with coagulopathy as they may worsen the condition.

PROGNOSIS

In general, presence of DIC worsens prognosis in all disorders. Development of complications such as shock, hemorrhage, thrombosis, and renal failure are associated with increased mortality. DIC is an independent predictor of mortality in patients with sepsis and trauma. It is difficult to state the mortality and morbidity of DIC as both DIC and its underlying conditions contribute to these. Overall mortality of severe acute DIC ranges from 50 to 70%. However, if the underlying condition is self-limiting or can be controlled, DIC will disappear and the coagulation status will be normalized. With the early recognition of systemic abnormalities and the introduction of new therapies, the prognosis for many patients with DIC has improved over the last several years.

CONCLUSION

- Disseminated intravascular coagulation never occurs alone, it usually is a secondary disorder with a preexisting trigger.
- Patients with DIC usually have signs and symptoms both of thrombosis and bleeding at the same time.
- Infections and sepsis are the most common trigger in patient with DIC. Prompt identification and rapid administration of antibiotics is of utmost importance.
- Excessive coagulation activation, secondary consumption of physiological anticoagulants and clotting factors and resulting bleeding are the key features in the pathophysiology of DIC.
- There is no single test or assay that can diagnose DIC. The diagnosis is usually established by the help of clinical findings of bleeding and microthrombi along with a low platelet count and abnormal coagulation profile.
- A combination of prolonged PT, aPTT, low platelet count, elevated D-dimers along with a clinical profile corroborating the above is sufficient to make diagnosis of DIC.
- Disseminated intravascular coagulation should be identified early and treatment of the triggering cause is paramount to stop the cascade.
- Clinical condition of the patient (e.g., bleeding) should guide replacement therapy rather than laboratory values.
- Presence of DIC worsens prognosis in all disorders.

REFERENCES

1. Chichra A, Mahajan A. Disseminated intravascular coagulation. In: Sachdeva A, Dutta AK (Eds). Advances in Pediatrics, 2nd edition. New Delhi: Jaypee Brothers Medical Publishers (P) Ltd; 2012. pp. 720-4.
2. Dalainas I. Pathogenesis, diagnosis and management of disseminated intravascular coagulation: a literature review. Eur Rev Med Pharmacol Sci. 2008;12(1):19-31.
3. Bick RL. Disseminated intravascular coagulation current concepts of etiology, pathophysiology, diagnosis, and treatment. Hematol Oncol Clin North Am. 2003;17(1): 149-76.
4. Franchini M, Lippi G, Manzato F. Recent acquisitions in the pathophysiology, diagnosis and treatment of disseminated intravascular coagulation. Thrombosis J. 2006;4:4.
5. Baglin T. Disseminated intravascular coagulation: diagnosis and treatment. Br Med J. 1996;312(7032):683-7.
6. Levi M, Toh CH, Thachil J, Watson HG. Guidelines for the diagnosis and management of disseminated intravascular coagulation. Br J Haematol. 2009;145(1):24-33.
7. Levi M, Schmaier AH. (2014). Disseminated intravascular coagulation. [online] Available from http://emedicine.medscape.com/article/199627-overview. [Last accessed Dec., 2014].
8. Wada H, Matsumoto T, Yamashita Y. Diagnosis and treatment of disseminated intravascular coagulation (DIC) according to four DIC guidelines. J Intens Care. 2014;2(1):15.
9. Taylor FB Jr, Toh CH, Hoots WK, Wada H, Levi M; Scientific Subcommittee on Disseminated Intravascular Coagulation (DIC) of the International Society on Thrombosis and Haemostasis (ISTH). Towards definition, clinical and laboratory criteria, and a scoring system for disseminated intravascular coagulation. Thromb Haemost. 2001;86(5):1327-30.
10. Levi M, Scully M. How I treat disseminated intravascular coagulation. Blood. 2018;131(8):845-54.

14.17 Transfusion Medicine and Component Therapy

Deepak Bansal, Rekha Hans

INTRODUCTION

Blood is categorized as a drug as per the "Drugs and Cosmetic Act 1940" by the Government of India and rules therein because of its use in treating diseases. The demand for this life-sustaining drug invariably exceeds the amount collected. Despite this, one-fourth of the country's annual collection is wasted as a single unit of whole blood transfusions **(Table 14.17.1)**. Advances in transfusion therapy have improved blood preservation techniques and enabled the separation of whole blood into its components. Component therapy has enabled the optimal use of every donation as specific components can be transfused selectively to different patients, depending on the actual needs of an individual patient.[1,2]

BLOOD COMPONENTS AND SEPARATION TECHNIQUES

Whole blood is made up of cellular elements [red blood cells (RBCs), leukocytes, and platelets] and plasma. Whole blood can be separated into components depending on their specific gravity by centrifugation techniques, as illustrated in **Flowchart 14.17.1**.[1]

Apheresis is a specialized procedure wherein whole blood is removed from the donor and is then separated into its components by centrifugation in a cell separator **(Fig. 14.17.1)**. The desired components (e.g., platelets/granulocytes/mononuclear cells/RBCs/plasma) are collected, and the remainder returned to the donor. The procedure allows selective collection of platelets, RBCs, granulocytes, or plasma in sufficient amounts from a single matched, ABO-compatible donor. The term "plateletpheresis" is used for the collection of platelets by apheresis; "granulocytapheresis" is used for the collection of granulocytes; "erythrocytapheresis" is collection of RBCs and "plasmapheresis" is used for collection of plasma by apheresis. Volume, storage temperature, and shelf life of different blood components are tabulated in **Table 14.17.2**.[1,3]

TABLE 14.17.1: Blood component use in various countries.

Country	% Used as whole blood	% Used as components
India	22	78
Myanmar	38	62
Sri Lanka	–	100
Nepal	30	70
Thailand	20	80

Flowchart 14.17.1: Separation of components from blood.

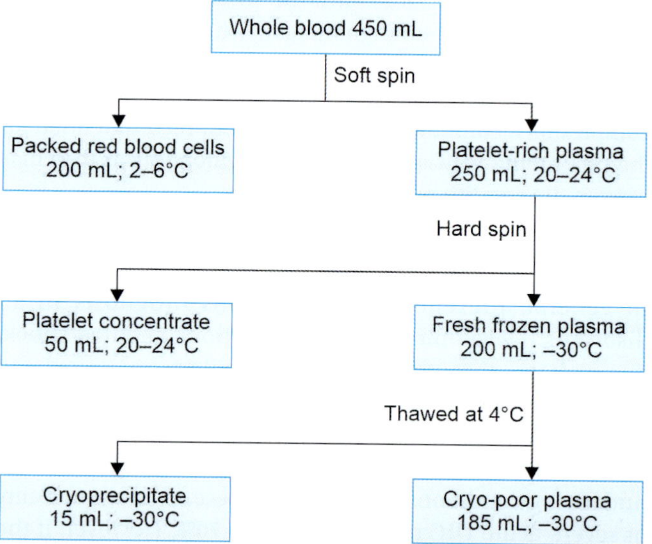

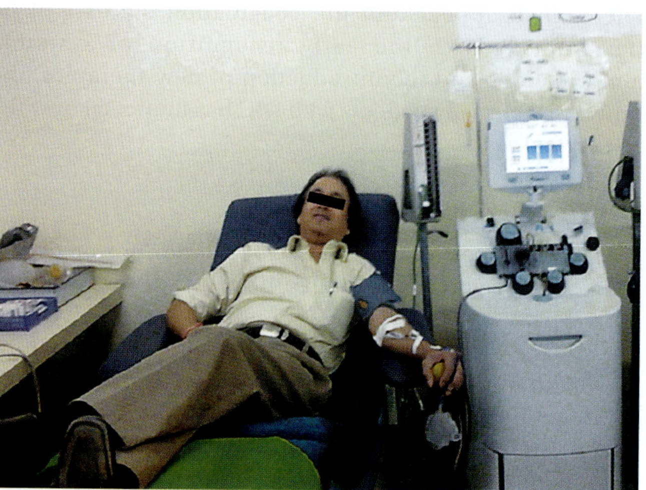

Fig. 14.17.1: Cell separator for the collection of specific components from whole blood (Apheresis procedure).

TABLE 14.17.2: Volume, storage temperature, and shelf life of blood and components.

	Volume (mL)	Storage temperature (°C)	Shelf life
Whole blood	400–500	2–6	35 days
Packed RBC (CPDA-1)	200–300		
Packed RBC—SAGM (nutrient solution)	250–350	2–6	42 days
Platelet concentrates	50–90 (RDP) 200–250 (SDAP)	20–24	5 days
Fresh frozen plasma	150–220	<–30	1 year
Cryoprecipitate	15–20	<–30	1 year

(CPDA: citrate phosphate dextrose adenine; RBC: red blood cell; RDP: random donor platelets; SAGM: saline, adenine, glucose, and mannitol; SDAP: single donor apheresis platelets)

Whole Blood

There are very few indications for the use of whole blood, including cardiac surgery, extracorporeal membrane oxygenator (ECMO), or massive hemorrhage, as in trauma. The usage of whole blood has re-emerged as an option for trauma patients. It may be the only choice for life-threatening hemorrhage when RBC component therapy is not available. Whole blood or reconstituted whole blood may be used for exchange transfusion in neonates and for therapeutic whole blood exchange.[1,4]

BOX 14.17.1: Indications for packed red blood cell transfusion for neonates.

- Transfusion need is based on presence or absence of cardiac, respiratory, or hemodynamic instability, prematurity, gestational age, hypotension, and inotropic or vasopressor support Tabulated guidelines are available for reference
- A Hb threshold of <7 g/dL (Hct <21%) is appropriate for most neonates ≥ 35 weeks' gestation who are >7 days old provided they are not small for gestational age
- A Hb <7 g/dL threshold applies to hemodynamically stabile critically ill neonates

Fresh Whole Blood

It is a myth that whole blood collected within 24 hours is the best. It is often requisitioned in bleeding disorders in the erroneous belief that it provides platelets and clotting factors. Almost 90% of platelets and 40% of factor VIII activity are lost within 24 hours of storage at 4°C. In addition, time is required for mandatory screening for infections. This age-old practice, therefore, has no role in modern times. Specific blood component therapy should be requested depending on the etiology of bleeding. For neonatal exchange transfusion, blood up to 7–10 days old is good enough to prevent hyperkalemia.[1,4]

Packed Red Blood Cells

The usual dose for packed RBCs (PRBCs) is 10–15 mL/kg but varies according to clinical indications **(Boxes 14.17.1 and 14.17.2)**.[5,6]

- In severe chronic anemia [hemoglobin (Hb) <5 g/dL], the child should receive 2–3 aliquots of 3–5 mL/kg over 2–3 hours, separated by a few hours.
- A partial exchange transfusion may be considered in those presenting with overt features of congestive heart failure (CHF). It corrects the anemia rapidly and isovolumetrically. Each unit of transfused PRBC is expected to increase the Hb level by 1 g/dL and hematocrit level by 3% in a 70-kg adult. A dose of 10–15 mL/kg in a pediatric patient will increase the Hb by about 2–3 g/dL or hematocrit by 6–9%.[1,3]

Saline Washed Red Blood Cells

Patients who have severe allergic reactions to RBC transfusion may benefit from washed RBCs, as washing removes plasma, the cause of allergy. RBCs are washed using 1–2 L of 0.9% normal saline by centrifugation at 4°C. It removes electrolytes and 99% of plasma proteins. Washed RBCs should be used within 6–24 hours.[5]

Platelet Transfusion and Plateletpheresis

The process of obtaining platelet-rich plasma and platelet concentrate is outlined in **Flowchart 14.17.1**.[1]

Random Donor Platelets

Platelets derived from whole blood are known as random donor platelets (RDPs). Random donor platelets must contain at least 5.5×10^{10} platelets. RDPs can be prepared by two methods: the platelet-rich plasma (PRP) method and the buffy coat (BC) method. In the PRP method, a soft spin is followed by a hard spin, whereas it is the opposite in the BC method. RDPs prepared by the BC method are preferred.

BOX 14.17.2: Indications for PRBC transfusion for children older than or equal to 4 months.

- *In deficiency anemia,* with features of overt CHF. Often, children with iron deficiency anemia are treated with oral iron alone, even with Hb <5 g/dL
- *Thalassemia major*: Attempt should be made to maintain a pretransfusion Hb >9–10 g/dL
- *Aplastic anemia*: Children often do well with Hb >6 g/dL Leukocyte filters **(Fig. 14.17.2)** should be utilized to prevent alloimmunization and graft rejection if a BMT is planned
- *Malignancies*: Hb <8 g/dL. Factors influencing decision include the intensity of chemotherapy and timing (counts expected to rise or fall)
- *Significant preoperative anemia*: An individual approach is necessary; most children who do not have cardiorespiratory disease do not require Hb >8 g/dL
- *Postoperative Hb <8 g/dL with symptoms/signs of anemia.* Most children can quickly restore Hb with oral iron. There should be a compelling reason to administer a postoperative red cell transfusion
- *Pediatric ICU*: Restrictive strategy is favored in the PICU. It has been demonstrated that in stable and critically ill children, the Hb of 7 g/dL is as good as 9.5 g/dL (children with severe hypoxia, hemodynamic instability, and cyanotic heart disease were excluded from the study). Blood is immunosuppressive. Cytokines released following the transfusion may contribute to enhanced inflammatory response and increased morbidity[6]

(BMT: bone marrow transplantation; CHF: congestive heart failure; Hb: hemoglobin; ICU: intensive care unit; PICU: pediatric intensive care unit; PRBC: packed red blood cell)

Caution: PRBC transfusion should be started within 30 minutes of removal of the unit from the refrigerator, and transfusion should be complete within 4 hours of commencement.

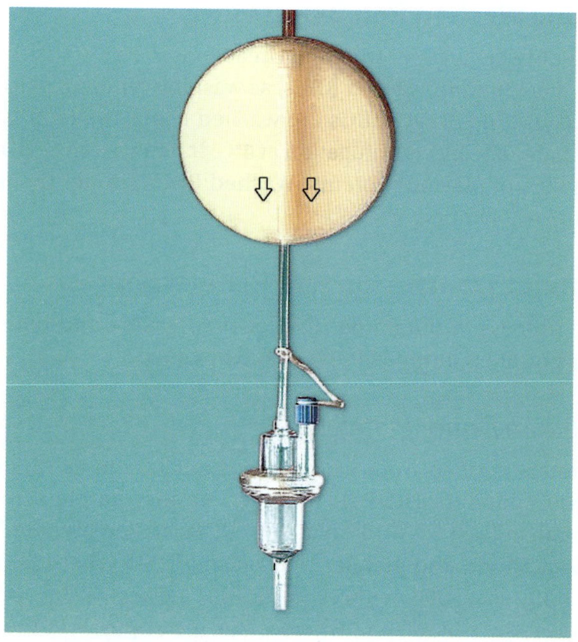

Fig. 14.17.2: A bedside leukocyte filter.

BOX 14.17.3: Indications of platelet transfusion in neonates.

- *<100 × 10^9/L:*
  - Prior to major surgery
- *<50 × 10^9/L:*
  - *Preterm infant (<33 weeks):* First week of life
  - *Clinically unstable term infants:* First week of life
  - Invasive procedure (e.g., ventricular tap)
  - *Preterm neonate:*
    - To be started on ibuprofen or indomethacin
    - Recent onset grade 3 or 4 intraventricular hemorrhage
- *<20 × 10^9/L:*
  - Stable infants beyond the first week of life without active bleeding

Pooled Platelet Concentrates

Pooled platelet concentrates may be prepared by pooling six units of ABO and Rh (D) blood group-matched random donor platelets prepared either by buffy coat method or by platelet-rich plasma method in a closed system.

Single Donor Apheresis Platelets

The alternative approach involves the collection of single-donor platelets by apheresis using a cell separator **(Fig. 14.17.1)**. A single unit obtained from apheresis has 3×10^{11} platelets, which equals 5–6 RDPs. The yield is higher with single-donor platelets; in addition, the donor exposure is reduced. Platelets are stored at 20–24°C, under constant agitation for 5 days. Beyond this duration, the risk of bacterial contamination increases excessively. The dose of RDP is 1 U/10 kg of body weight or 5–10 mL/kg for newborns. Indications include disseminated intravascular coagulation (DIC) with bleed (50 × 10^9/L), major surgery (50–100 × 10^9/L), leukemia, aplastic anemia (10 × 10^9/L; each unit may have its policy; lower threshold if concomitant fever or sepsis), and platelet function defects with severe bleeding. Indications in neonates are listed in **Box 14.17.3**.

Fresh Frozen Plasma

Indications

- Coagulopathy with bleeding (e.g., hemorrhagic disease of newborn and liver disease)
- Hemophilia A/B (if factors unavailable or cannot be afforded)
- Deficiency of antithrombin III and protein C/S
- Warfarin overdose
- Factor XI deficiency
- Vitamin K deficiency (for severe bleeding, in addition to injection vitamin K)

- Massive transfusion
- Replacement fluid for plasma exchange in the cases of thrombotic thrombocytopenic purpura and hemolytic uremic syndrome, liver failure.

The use of fresh frozen plasma (FFP) is not justified for hypovolemia (use crystalloids), prolonged international normalized ratio in the absence of bleeding, and hypoalbuminemia (use albumin). The dose is 10–20 mL/kg for infants/children and 5–10 mL/kg for newborns. FFP must generally be ABO compatible to avoid the risk of hemolysis in the recipient and should be transfused within 6 hours of thawing.[1,3]

Cryoprecipitate

The contents include fibrinogen, von Willebrand factor (VVF), and factors VIII and XIII. The corresponding indications are fibrinogen <1.0 g/L (e.g., DIC with bleeding), hemophilia A (only if factor concentrates are unavailable), von Willebrand disease (VWD), and factor XIII deficiency. It does not contain factor IX and, thus, is not indicated in hemophilia B. The average dose is 1 U for 5–10 kg bodyweight.

Cryoprecipitate can be transfused across the ABO barrier (as it contains a scant amount of RBCs) and should be transfused immediately after thawing.[1,3]

Granulocytes

Granulocyte transfusion is used for septic, neutropenic patients not responding to antibiotics or antifungals. The efficacy is not clearly established. Granulocytes can be prepared either by pooling multiple units of buffy coat or by apheresis technology.[2] Granulocytes must be irradiated and can be stored at 20–24°C without agitation and used within a maximum period of 24 hours. It is prepared on request for a specific patient.[7]

Irradiated Blood Products

Under normal circumstances, T-lymphocytes in donor blood are destroyed by the recipient. They can survive and proliferate if they are not recognized as foreign (e.g., related donor) or if the recipient is immunocompromised. The proliferating T-cells cause graft-versus-host disease (GVHD).[8] It is a rare, however, a frequently fatal complication that occurs 3–30 days following blood transfusion. As there is no effective treatment, the aim is to recognize high-risk patients and to administer blood products with T-cells that have been rendered ineffective **(Boxes 14.17.4 and 14.17.5)**. It is done by exposing the blood bag to ionizing radiation. Facilities for irradiating blood are gradually increasing at centers in India. Irradiation does not reduce the risk of transmission of cytomegalovirus (CMV).[7]

BOX 14.17.4: When to ask for irradiated blood products?[7]

- Donations from relatives (directed donation)
- *Intrauterine transfusion:* Neonatal exchange transfusion
- *Immunocompromised patients:* BMT, SCID, and Hodgkin lymphoma
- Granulocyte transfusion

(BMT: bone marrow transplantation; SCID: severe combined immunodeficiency)

BOX 14.17.5: Conditions where irradiated blood is not required.[7]

- Newborns for top-up transfusion
- HIV and AIDS[10]
- Solid organ transplantation
- Autoimmune diseases

(AIDS: acquired immunodeficiency syndrome; HIV: human immunodeficiency virus)

Leukoreduction

It refers to the removal of white cells from a blood product.[3] Deleterious effects caused by leukocytes include:

- Febrile nonhemolytic reactions
- Human leukocyte antigen (HLA) alloimmunization
- Platelet refractoriness
- Transmission of CMV, Epstein–Barr virus (EBV), human immunodeficiency virus (HIV), and human T-cell lymphotropic virus (HTLV)[9]
- Possibly immunosuppression, organ dysfunction, and increased mortality

A unit of whole blood contains approximately 2×10^9 leukocytes. These can be removed soon after collecting blood (prestorage) or at the bedside. Prestorage leukoreduction is superior, as inflammatory cytokine accumulation following release from white blood cells (WBCs) during storage is avoided. Though leukoreduction significantly reduces the number of leukocytes, the few remaining leukocytes can replicate and cause transfusion-associated graft-versus host disease (GVHD) in susceptible individuals.[8] Therefore, leukoreduction alone is inadequate to prevent GVHD. The patients at risk for GVHD should be transfused leukoreduced and irradiated RBC units.[7] Prestorage leukoreduction is often unavailable in India; therefore, bedside leukocyte filters **(Fig. 14.17.2)** should be considered for patients receiving multiple transfusions, e.g., thalassemia major. Nowadays, blood bags with inline leukofilters are also available but are expensive.

Autologous Blood

It is the collection and reinfusion of the patient's own blood. It is possible for some children who have to undergo elective surgery for which transfusion is anticipated. The advantage is a reduction in the risk of transfusion-transmitted viral diseases. Blood, proportionate to the child's size, is collected 4–5 weeks before surgery. All risks are not avoided: the stored unit could still be contaminated with bacteria, or the wrong unit could be inadvertently transfused. It is rarely used in the modern era as the safety of blood products has improved.

HAZARDS OF BLOOD TRANSFUSION

Adverse reactions to blood transfusion can be subdivided according to whether they are immediate or delayed and whether they are immunologically mediated **(Table 14.17.3)**. Acute hemolytic reaction is the dreaded complication of blood transfusion, one of the common causes being clerical errors of mislabeling or misidentification, resulting in the infusion of a wrong patient's blood. Signs and symptoms include fever, chills, back or chest pain, flushing, nausea, and hemoglobinuria. These can progress to shock with acute renal failure. Management is outlined in **Box 14.17.6**. Two common but less known adverse effects are detailed here. All the transfusion reactions should be recorded and reported to the blood transfusion services.

TABLE 14.17.3: Adverse effects of transfusion.

Adverse effect	*Usual cause*
Immunological	
Hemolysis	Red cell incompatibility
Anaphylaxis	Antibody to IgA in donor plasma
Febrile, nonhemolytic	Antibody to donor leukocyte antigen
Urticaria	Antibody to donor plasma proteins
Transfusion-related acute lung injury	Donor antibody to leukocyte of patient
Graft-versus-host disease	Functional lymphocytes in the blood
Post-transfusion purpura (PTP)	Antibody in the patient-directed against the human platelet antigen (HPA) system
Nonimmunological	
Transfusion-associated circulatory overload (TACO)	Volume overload
Fever with shock	Bacterial contamination
Hypothermia	Rapid infusion of cold blood
Air embolus	Air infusion in line
Hyperkalemia	Rapid infusion of multiple units of stored blood
Hypocalcemia	Massive transfusion of citrated blood
Disease transmission	HIV, hepatitis B and C, CMV, malaria, and syphilis[9]
Iron overload	Multiple transfusions in chronically anemic patients without blood loss

(CMV: cytomegalovirus; HIV: human immunodeficiency virus; IgA: immunoglobulin A)

Bacterial Contamination of Blood Products

It is a relatively common, however, poorly recognized complication. The source of contamination could be the donor (skin commensals or unrecognized bacteremia), environment, or improper product handling. The clinical profile often resembles an acute hemolytic reaction. Platelets are most commonly implicated as they are stored at room temperature. Broad-spectrum antibiotics should be initiated at the earliest suspicion.

Transfusion-related Acute Lung Injury

It is characterized by acute onset hypoxemia in the absence of circulatory overload and is one of the leading causes of transfusion-related mortality. It results from plasma-containing transfusions (RBCs, platelets, or FFP) and typically occurs during or within 6 hours of completion of a transfusion. Chest X-ray shows bilateral lung infiltration. It usually resolves in 24–72 hours. Management is supportive. Mechanical ventilation may be required. There is no role for steroids. Mortality is 5–10%. Antibodies (HLA or WBC) from donors are implicated in causing pulmonary capillary leak. Avoiding plasma components from multiparous female donors has reduced the incidence of transfusion-related acute lung injury (TRALI).

Transfusion-associated Circulatory Overload

It refers to circulatory volume overload resulting from the transfusion of any blood component and is a leading cause of transfusion-related mortality. It is defined as new onset dyspnea within 12 hours of transfusion. Risk factors include preexisting cardiac/renal dysfunction, a large number of units transfused, and a faster rate of infusion. Diuretics can be used for prevention as well as treatment.

BOX 14.17.6: Management of acute hemolytic transfusion reaction.

- Discontinue blood transfusion; however, maintain IV access
- Alert blood bank and return unit of blood along with BT set
- Draw clotted and anticoagulated blood specimens from a vein other than the one being used for transfusion. Send an anticoagulated sample with a compatibility form to the blood bank, mentioning transfusion reaction details. Request the following tests: DCT, plasma Hb, blood counts, urea, creatinine, and bilirubin
- Collect urine sample for urinary Hb
- Investigate for DIC; blood culture if fever is a prominent feature
- Monitor urine output
- *Treatment is mainly supportive*: Infusion of normal saline to maintain adequate urine output, furosemide to enhance renal cortical perfusion. Dialysis may be required if acute tubular necrosis develops

(BT: blood transfusion; DCT: direct Coombs' test; DIC: disseminated intravascular coagulation; Hb: hemoglobin; IV: intravenous)

CASE SCENARIOS AND FREQUENTLY ASKED QUESTIONS

1. A 1.5 kg preterm neonate, 5 days old, Hb: 9 g/dL, on a ventilator, is to be given packed red cells of 25 mL. What should be done with the remaining bag?

Ans. The best option is to request the blood bank to issue blood in a pediatric bag. One RBC unit can be divided into several pediatric bags for a single neonate/infant over an extended period **(Figs. 14.17.3A and B)**. It reduces donor exposure and prevents wastage. The remaining unit should never be stored in a refrigerator **(Fig. 14.17.4)**.

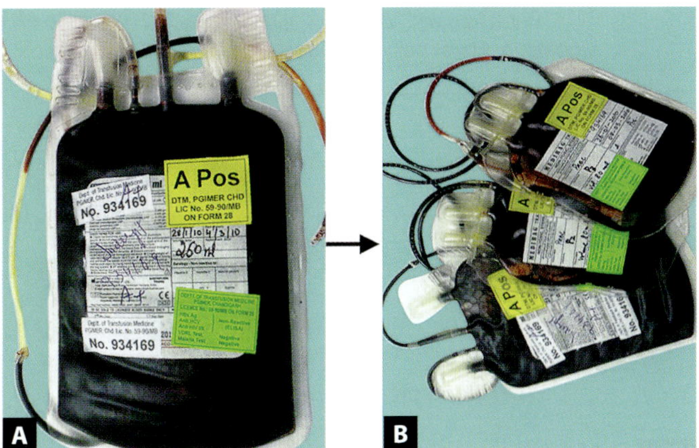

Figs. 14.17.3A and B: The use of blood can be optimized in neonates and infants by the use of pediatric bags.

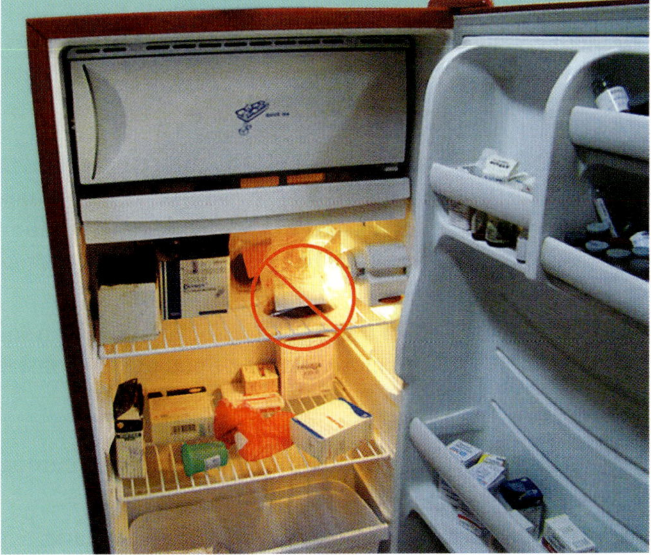

Fig. 14.17.4: Blood is never to be stored in the fridge.

2. I requested blood for an anticipated use; however, the unit was not administered. Can the blood be returned to the blood bank?

Ans. Inform the blood bank staff. Every blood bank should have a policy for unused products. The ideal policy is that the blood components outside a temperature-controlled environment for >30 minutes must be discarded.[10]

3. Red cell transfusion is on flow for a child. He deveops a fever of 39°C after 30 minutes. What should be done?

Ans. The algorithm is illustrated in **Flowchart 14.17.2**.

Flowchart 14.17.2: Algorithm for management of fever while a blood transfusion is running.

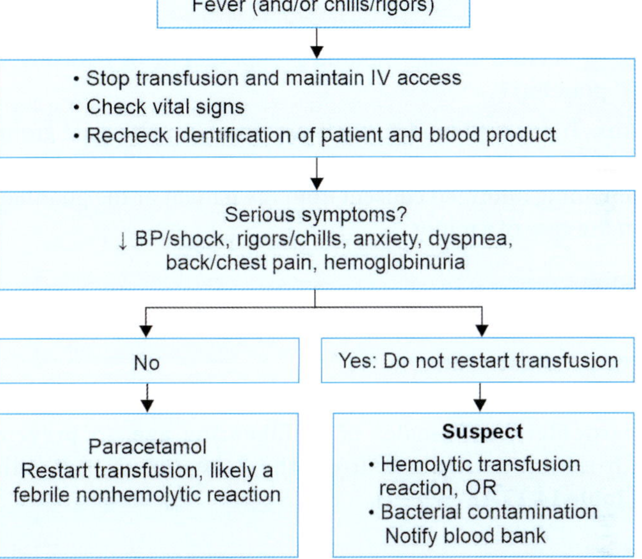

4. How long can one wait to start a blood transfusion after obtaining the bag from the blood bank?

Ans. If transfusion is not initiated within 30 minutes of removal from a blood bank or an approved temperature-controlled blood product refrigerator, the unit should be returned immediately to the blood bank to prevent wastage.[10]

5. There is an 11-year-old boy with thalassemia major. He receives 3–4 weekly blood transfusions. Hb is 8 g/dL on a visit for transfusion to the hospital. How slowly should one transfuse a unit of packed red cells?

Ans. It is appropriate to transfuse over 2–3 hours. No diuretic is required unless the Hb has been low for a prolonged duration. No transfusion should take >4 hours because of the risk of bacterial proliferation at room temperature.

6. Platelets were transfused to a patient; however, the posttransfusion count did not increase significantly. What are the common causes and remedial measures?

Ans. Sepsis, fever, idiopathic thrombocytopenic purpura (ITP), DIC, splenomegaly, amphotericin, and alloimmunization.

Remedial measures include ordering ABO-compatible product, single-donor apheresis platelets, increasing the number of units transfused, and requesting HLA or cross-matched platelets.[2]

7. I ordered platelets at 9 PM but decided to transfuse them the following day. In which compartment of the fridge should I store them until the next day?

Ans. Platelets are stored under continuous agitation in a platelet shaker at 20–24°C (room temperature) to prevent clumping. Do not store it in the refrigerator.[10]

8. A child has an A⁺ blood group. Can he be transfused B⁺ platelets?

Ans. The same blood group is preferred. An alternate group can be transfused if the plasma volume is limited after obtaining informed consent from the patient or the guardian in the case of a minor.[10]

9. B⁺ platelets are transfused to a B⁻ patient inadvertently. The patient is asymptomatic. Does anything need to be done?

Ans. Rhesus (Rh) immunoglobulin should be administered, particularly to females of childbearing age, to prevent Rh-alloimmunization from the transfused red cells **(Table 14.17.4)**.[10]

TABLE 14.17.4: Requirement of ABO and Rh (rhesus) compatibility for transfusing blood components.

	ABO compatibility	Rh compatibility
Red cells	Must	Must
Platelets	Preferred	Preferred
Plasma	Must	No
Cryoprecipitate	Preferred, but not required	

10. How should fresh frozen plasma (FFP) be thawed?

Ans. Ideally, it would be by a plasma thawer (nonaqueous). It may not be available in most units; the bag may be thawed by placing it over a clean surface. If using water, ensure that the ports are above the water level. Blankets, body surfaces (e.g., armpits), or heaters should not be used.[10]

11. I diagnosed a 7-month-old infant with thalassemia major. Is there anything that should be requested from the blood bank before the first transfusion?

Ans. Extended red cell phenotyping (Rh, Kell, Kidd, and Duffy) should be performed. Attempts should be made to match minor blood group antigens in patients who receive multiple transfusions to prevent alloimmunization later.

12. A child develops urticarial lesions while blood is running. Should I hold or discontinue the transfusion?

Ans. The algorithm is illustrated in **Flowchart 14.17.3.**

Flowchart 14.17.3: Algorithm for management of allergic reactions while blood is being transfused.

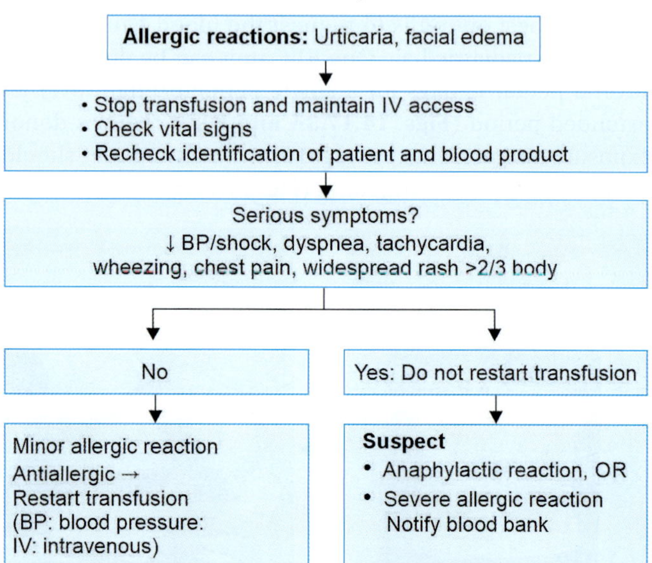

(BP: blood pressure: IV: intravenous)

13. A child with thalassemia major has frequent "reactions" to blood. What can be done?

Ans. Prophylactic antihistaminic and paracetamol can be given. A leukocyte filter should be used if finances are not a limitation. Request blood matched for C, E, and Kell antigens. Washed red cells may be required (saline washing removes plasma proteins).

14. A child needs a blood transfusion. His father is an engineer. Fearing the risk of transmission of human immunodeficiency virus (HIV), the concerned father offers to donate blood for his baby. Should such a directed donation be encouraged?

Ans. No, there is a risk of transfusion-associated GVHD from products obtained from close relatives. Such transfusions, if given, must be irradiated.[7,9]

15. What are the tests mandatory for infection screening of blood in India?

Ans. HIV 1 and 2, hepatitis B and C, syphilis, and malaria.[9]

16. What are the additional tests performed in the developed world?

Ans. Nucleic acid testing for HIV-1 and -2, hepatitis B, hepatitis C virus, HTLV, CMV, West Nile virus, etc.

17. A child develops dyspnea during transfusion. What are the possible causes?

Ans. Transfusion-related acute lung injury, circulatory overload, and anaphylaxis.

18. A 3-year-old child is diagnosed with idiopathic thrombocytopenic purpura (ITP). He has widespread skin bleeds and epistaxis. The platelet count is 2×10^9/L. A decision is taken to administer intravenous immune globulin. Should platelets be transfused?

Ans. No, it is a common error to transfuse platelets for ITP. Transfused platelets are rapidly destroyed due to circulating antibodies. Platelet transfusion is rarely indicated for life-threatening situations (e.g., intracranial bleed) along with steroids/intravenous immune globulin.

19. What are the prerequisites for a plateletpheresis procedure? How long does it take?

Ans. Request the patient's attendants to arrange 2–3 donors (excluding first-degree relatives) of the same blood group as the patient. Counsel the attendants about the cost of the disposable kit for the procedure (~₹ 8,000 in a government hospital). The donors are asked to contact the blood bank along with a requisition for plateletpheresis. The procedure takes ~2–3 hours.[2]

20. How can I improve transfusion practice in my unit?

Ans. Cordial and regular communication with the blood bank personnel is the key. Avoid the blame game. Accept limitations and frame guidelines after mutual discussion.

21. Why is it necessary to report adverse transfusion reactions to blood banks?

Ans. Under the "Hemovigilance program of India", blood banks must report adverse transfusion reaction data to a central reporting authority.[11]

22. I need to transfuse a patient. What is the prerequisite documentation needed?

Ans. Document the indication(s) and type of blood component(s) to be transfused in the patient's file. Before sending the blood requisition to the blood bank, obtain written consent from the patient or the guardian (in the case of a minor) after explaining the indication and the associated risks.

CONCLUSION

Blood and blood products should be transfused only when there are clear and specific therapeutic indications. The risk of transfusion reactions and transfusion-related infections deserves careful consideration. Specific blood component therapy suited to the requirements of an individual patient must be recommended whenever possible.

REFERENCES

1. Kennedy MS. Transfusion therapy. In: Harmening DM (Ed). Modern Blood Banking and Transfusion Practices, 6th edition. New Delhi: Jaypee Brothers Medical Publishers (P) Ltd.; 2013. pp. 352-66.
2. Sharma RR, Hans R, Lamba DS. Apheresis. In: Gupta S, Marwaha N, Chaudhary R, Rajan S, Gupta D, Kaur R (Eds). Transfusion Medicine Technical Manual, 3rd edition. New Delhi: Directorate General of Health Sciences Ministry of Health and Family Welfare, Government of India; 2022. pp. 180-94.
3. Sloan SR. Transfusion Medicine. In: Orkin SH, Fisher DE, Ginsburg AT, Lux SE, Nathan DG (Eds). Nathan and Oski's Hematology and Oncology of Infancy and Childhood, 8th edition. Philadelphia, PA: Elsevier Saunders; 2015. pp. 1127-64.
4. Marwaha N. Whole blood and component use in resource poor settings. Biologicals. 2010;38(1):68-71.
5. Carless PA, Henry DA, Carson JL, Hebert PP, McClelland B, Ker K. Transfusion thresholds and other strategies for guiding allogeneic red blood cell transfusion. Cochrane Database Syst Rev. 2010;(10):CD002042.
6. Lacroix J, Hébert PC, Hutchison JS, Hume HA, Tucci M, Ducruet T, et al; TRIPICU Investigators; Canadian Critical Care Trias Group; Pediatric Acute Lung Injury and Sepsis Investigation Network. Transfusion strategies for patients in pediatric intensive care units. N Engl J Med. 2007;356(16):1609-19.
7. Treleaven J, Gennery A, Marsh J, Norfolk D, Page L, Parker A, et al. Guidelines on the use of irradiated blood components prepared by the British Committee for Standards in Haematology Blood Transfusion Task Force. Br J Haematol. 2011;152(1):35-51.
8. Gupta A, Bansal D, Dass R, Das A. Transfusion associated graft versus host disease. Indian Pediatr. 2004;41(12):1260-4.
9. National AIDS Control Organisation, Ministry of Health and Family Welfare, Government of India. Annual report 2016–2017. [online] Available from http://naco.gov.in/NACO/Quick_Links/Publication/Annual_Report/NACO_Annual_Report/Annual_Report_NACO_2016-17_English/ [Last accessed December, 2024].
10. Funk MK, Grossman BJ, Westhoff CM (Eds). Technical Manual, 18th edition. Bethesda MD. AABB Press; 2014.
11. Jain A, Kaur R. Hemovigilance and blood safety. Asian J Transfus Sci. 2012;6(2):137-8.

14.18 Hematopoietic Stem Cell Transplant

Rahul Naithani

INTRODUCTION

Hematopoietic stem cells (HSCs) are multipotent cells found in bone marrow (BM), and cord blood (CB) that can develop into all types of blood cells like red blood cells (RBCs), platelets, white blood cells (WBCs), etc. HSCs proliferate by self-renewal and differentiation. Any defect in differentiation or further downstream till the final blood cell (say RBC) leads to the evolution of hematological disease. For example, globin gene defect leads to hemoglobinopathies. Other examples are diseases of WBCs such as leukemia, aplastic anemia, and other bone marrow failure syndromes. The word "transplant" means to lift and reset in another soil or situation as is common in plantation. Replacing fresh HSCs from a normal donor is likely to take care of defects downstream and lead to the resolution of disease. Similarly, immunodeficiency disorders due to deficiency of T and/or B lymphocytes are amenable to cure by hematopoietic stem cell transplantation (HSCT). In some metabolic disorders like Hurler disease (mucopolysaccharidosis type 1), a deficiency of enzyme α-L-iduronidase deficiency leads to lysosomal storage disease. An allogeneic transplantation by generating donor-derived cells will be able to produce normal enzymes and cure this before permanent damage happens.

Preparation for HSCT involves the administration of high doses of therapy. Patients become immunocompromised. Infections along with other complications, namely graft rejection, graft versus host disease (GVHD), and relapse of the primary disease have been major obstacles to the success of HSCT. However, recent advances in understanding the biology and immunology of underlying transplantation, improvements in supportive care and clinical management of complications have made HSCT an increasingly effective modality for many diseases.[1] The commonly used terminology about HSCT is described in **Table 14.18.1**.

TABLE 14.18.1: Terminology often used with hematopoietic stem cell transplantation.

Term	*Meaning*	*Remark*
HSC	Hematopoietic stem cells	
HSCT	Hematopoietic stem cell transplantation	Interchangeably used with BMT, PBSCT, or CBT depending on source
BMT	Bone marrow transplantation	When source of HSC is bone marrow
PBSCT	Peripheral blood stem cell transplantation	HSC collected by apheresis
CBT	Cord blood transplantation	When source of HSC is cord blood
Allogeneic	When the HSCs come from a donor	
MSD	Matched sibling donor	
MRD	Matched related donor	Matched family member
MUD	Matched unrelated donor	
Haploidentical	Donor having HLA half-match or <9/10 matched with recipient	E.g., parent donor to child recipient
Autologous	Patient's own HSCs are used for transplantation	Not useful in benign or genetic diseases
Engraftment	Recovery of blood counts post-HSC infusion	
Graft rejection	Graft failure	Recipient immune cells act against the donor HSCs failing the transplantation and potential death of the recipient
GVHD	Graft versus host disease	Immune reaction of donor T cells against organs of recipient
GVL	Graft versus leukemia effect	Favorable immune reaction of donor T/NK cells against hematological malignancy
HLA	Human leukocyte antigen	• Immune protein cluster associated with histocompatibility • Mismatches in HLA between donor and recipient cause GVL or GVHD

INDIAN SCENARIO

From 2012 to 2021, 5,734 pediatric allogeneic HSCTs have been performed by 110 centers across India as per the Indian Society for Blood and Marrow Transplant Registry (ISBMTR). Thalassemia (35%), aplastic anemia and other bone marrow failure syndromes (20%), acute lymphoblastic leukemia (ALL) (14%) and acute myeloid leukemia (AML) (11%) account for 80% of these transplants. The number of haploidentical HSCTs has rapidly risen over the last 10 years to 33% of total allogeneic BMTs while matched unrelated donor (MUD) transplants stand at 11%. During the same 10-year period 902 autologous HSCTs were performed. Neuroblastoma (37%), Hodgkin lymphoma (28%), and other solid tumors (18%) accounted for 83% of indications. Stratified survival outcomes were not available (Data from ISBMTR-Personal Communication).

INDICATIONS FOR HEMATOPOIETIC STEM-CELL TRANSPLANTATION

Indications for HSCT can be broadly divided into two groups: (1) benign and (2) malignant diseases. **Table 14.18.2** lists the indications for allogeneic and autologous HSCT. Allogeneic BMT is the only curative treatment for thalassemia, sickle-cell anemia, aplastic anemia, and immune-deficiency diseases. High-risk ALL, such as BCR-ABL-positive ALL, induction failure, minimal residual disease-positive leukemia, or complex karyotype leukemia may benefit from allogeneic HSCT. Similarly, allogeneic HSCT is indicated in high-risk AML such as complex karyotype, MDS-related or therapy-related AML or induction failure. All children with relapsed AML need bone marrow transplant (BMT).

Some patients relapsing after autologous HSCT can be salvaged by allogeneic HSCT.[2] Success rates depend on several patient and disease-related factors such as remission status, number of previous therapies, number of previous transfusions, active infection at the time of HSCT, and degree of mismatch between donor and recipient. Early transplants usually result in better outcomes than late HSCT.

TABLE 14.18.2: Indications of hematopoietic stem cell transplant in children.

Allogeneic hematopoietic stem cell transplantation	
Severe aplastic anemia	All patients
Thalassemia major	All patients
Sickle-cell anemia	Specific indications
Congenital immuno-deficiency syndromes	Severe combined immunodeficiency, hemophagocytic lymphohistiocytosis
Inborn errors of metabolism	Hurler syndrome and Krabbe disease
Acute myeloid leukemia	• High-risk acute myeloid leukemia • Relapsed acute myeloid leukemia
Acute lymphoblastic leukemia	• High-risk acute lymphoblastic leukemia • Relapsed acute lymphoblastic leukemia
Chronic myeloid leukemia	• Blast crisis • Refractory to tyrosine kinase inhibitors
Myelodysplastic syndrome	All patients
Juvenile myelomonocytic leukemia	All patients
Myeloproliferative neoplasm	High-risk
Autologous hematopoietic stem cell transplantation	
Hodgkin lymphoma	Relapsed Hodgkin lymphoma
Non-Hodgkin lymphoma	• High-risk non-Hodgkin lymphoma • Relapsed non-Hodgkin lymphoma
Solid tumors	• Neuroblastoma • Germ cell tumor • Brain tumor • Wilms tumor • Ewing sarcoma

HEMATOPOIETIC STEM CELL SOURCES

There are three main sources of HSCs: (1) bone marrow, (2) peripheral blood stem cells (PBSc), and (3) cord blood.

Bone Marrow

Bone marrow harvest requires an operating room where two operators perform repeated aspiration from the iliac crest under general anesthesia **(Fig. 14.18.1A)**. The bone marrow is then filtered through a fine metal mesh to remove bone and tissue pieces. A bone marrow volume of 20 mL/kg of donor body weight can be collected safely. This becomes a challenge in situations where the donor is smaller than the recipient. A surrogate marker for stem cells is CD34. There are approximately 1–3 × 10^6 $CD34^+$ cells per 10^8 bone marrow cells. Donor bone marrow is usually collected on the day of transplantation, but can also be cryopreserved if necessary.

Peripheral Blood Stem Cells

Administration of granulocyte colony-stimulating factor and plerixafor increases the exit of HSCs from the bone marrow niche, increasing their numbers in the peripheral blood. These cells are then collected by high-volume apheresis **(Fig. 14.18.1B)**. This process is similar to single-donor platelet apheresis. This procedure requires good venous access and takes 3–4 hours. This procedure saves the donor or patient (in autologous HSCT) the risk of anesthesia and pain caused by the aspiration of bone marrow. PBSCs induce faster hematopoietic recovery compared to bone marrow. However, it is associated with an increased incidence of chronic graft versus host disease (GVHD).

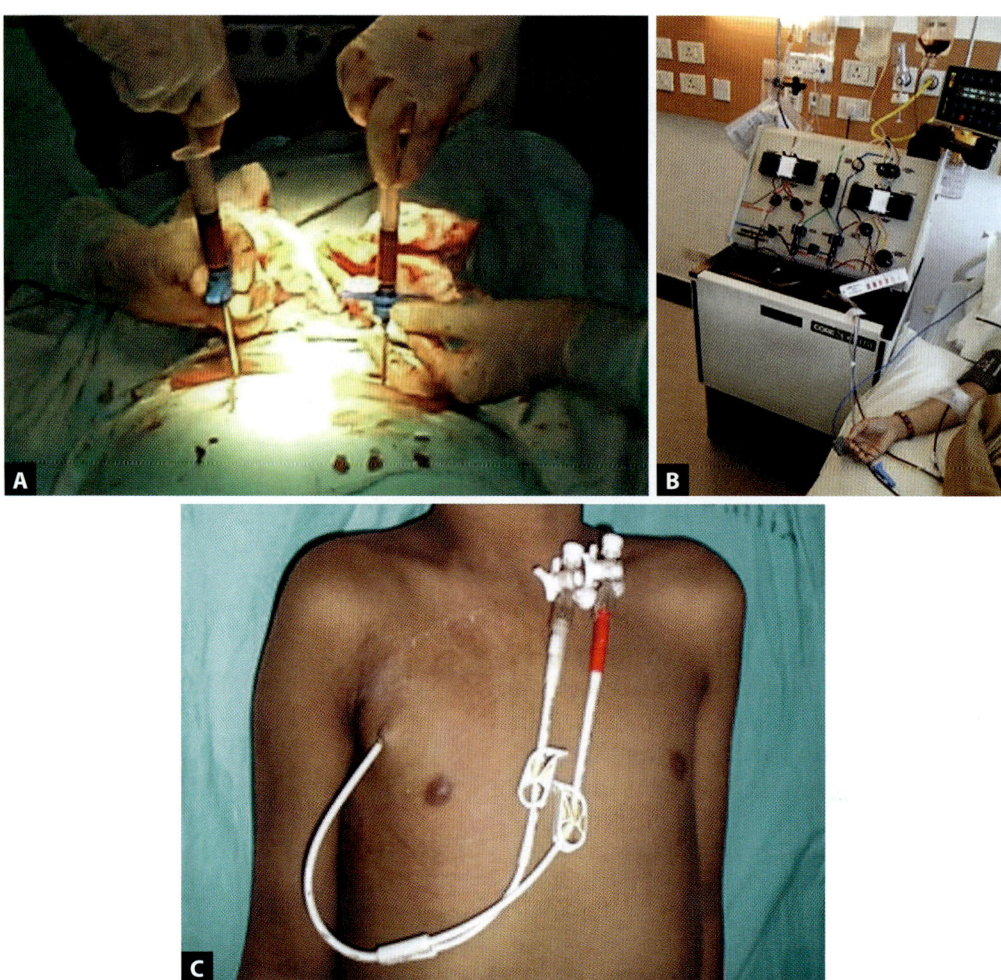

Figs. 14.18.1A to C: (A) Bone marrow harvest under general anesthesia in operation theater (OT); (B) Peripheral blood stem cell (apheresis) harvest in room; (C) Subcutaneously tunneled catheter.

Cord Blood

Cord blood collected shortly after birth contains large numbers of potent hematopoietic stem cells. Cord blood is cryopreserved and used when a close or unrelated donor is not available. Cord blood contains fewer HSCs compared to bone marrow or PBSC products. Therefore, the risk of risk of nonengraftment is higher. UCB cells have reduced alloreactivity, so the incidence of GVHD is lower.[3]

TYPES OF HEMATOPOIETIC STEM CELL TRANSPLANTATION

Hematopoietic stem cell transplantation is broadly divided into two types: (1) allogeneic HSCT (here a donor is required) and (2) autologous HSCT (self-stem cells are used).

Autologous Stem Cell Transplantation

The technical name for autologous HSCT is high-dose therapy with stem cell rescue. This is useful for diseases sensitive to chemotherapy such as neuroblastoma and lymphoma. The main hypothesis is that administering very high doses of chemotherapy will improve cure rates even further. Such intensive therapy is usually fatal for patients due to bone marrow aplasia. This toxicity can be mitigated by infusion of preharvested autologous HSCs. The HSC dose of 2×10^6/kg is considered an adequate dose for bone marrow recovery within 2–3 weeks.

Peripheral blood stem cell transplantation has replaced bone marrow in autologous stem cell transplantation. Hematopoietic recovery occurs faster when PBSCs are used compared to bone marrow HSCs. This results in shorter hospital days, shorter duration of neutropenia, antibiotic use, and the need for appropriate support services. Autologous transplantation has no risk of GVHD and graft rejection is unlikely. Thus, autologous stem cell transplantation is associated with fewer complications than allogeneic transplantation. It is important to note that autologous HSCT will not work in benign or genetic diseases. Some autoimmune diseases are offered autologous HSCT. Here, the concept is rebooting the immune system which may resolve autoimmune manifestations on immune reconstitution.[3]

Allogeneic Stem Cell Transplantation

For allogeneic HSCT, the purpose of HSCs is to shorten the duration of neutropenia, act as a carrier of replacing defective genes as in β-thalassemia, provide sufficient blood-forming stem cells as in aplastic anemia and immune reconstitution in cases of immune deficiency diseases or to produce competent T cells that can keep leukemia in check.[3]

Increasing genetic disparity between recipient and donor, known as histocompatibility or human leukocyte antigen (HLA) mismatch, is an important factor leading to an increased incidence of graft rejection and GVHD and is a critical factor in donor selection. HSCT does not require ABO/Rh blood group matching. After a successful allogeneic HSCT, the recipient's blood group also changes to that of the donor.

An HLA-identical sibling is an ideal donor for allogeneic HSCT and must be identical at the HLA-A, B, and DR loci. Even HLA-identical siblings have differences at minor histocompatibility sites that lead to complications. Due to improvements in immunosuppression and prevention and treatment of GVHD, unrelated donors, umbilical cord blood, and partially mismatched and haploidentical donors are now increasingly used.

Matched Unrelated Donor Bone Marrow Transplantation

Most international bone marrow donor registries are now linked. High-resolution HLA typing for HLA-A, B, C, DQ, and DR is required to begin the search for a matched unrelated donor (MUD). One can find out within 2–4 days if a suitable matched donor is available or not. It usually takes about 2–3 months to get the HSCs.

Haploidentical (Half-matched) Bone Marrow Transplantation

Only 30% of children have a fully HLA-identical sibling. Even MUD may not be available to everyone in a timely manner, especially in high-risk situations where HSCT is urgent. A haploidentical transplantation is universally available in parents or children and those can be mobilized fairly quickly. A major challenge of HLA-haploidentical HCT is strong bilateral alloreactivity, leading to high graft rejection and GVHD.[4]

CONDITIONING REGIMENS AND COMPLICATIONS

Conditioning regimen refers to chemotherapy, immunosuppression, and/or total body irradiation (TBI) administered prior to HSCT. The purpose of conditioning is to eradicate any malignant cells or clones of abnormal cells; second, to prevent allograft rejection by suppressing the recipient's immune system and to create a physical space by inducing sufficient bone marrow aplasia to allow adequate growth of donor stem cells. The full-intensity therapy that completely wipes out bone marrow is called myeloablative conditioning (MAC). In addition to myelotoxicity, the conventional regimen before HSC infusion also causes organ toxicity resulting in a mortality rate of 10–20%.[3]

Hepatic venoocclusive disease (VOD), also known as sinusoidal obstruction syndrome (SOS), is characterized by hepatomegaly, right upper quadrant pain, jaundice, and ascites or unexplained weight gain. VOD is a consequence of chemotherapy or radiation-mediated endothelial and hepatocyte damage. It occurs within the first 30 days of stem cell infusion and causes significant morbidity and mortality. Hemorrhagic cystitis is characterized by hematuria, dysuria, and urinary frequency in a patient with sterile urine. High-dose cyclophosphamide used during treatment and infection with adenovirus and BK virus are common causes of this complication. Neurotoxicity is a known complication of high doses of busulfan, and seizures occur in approximately 7.5% of children without anticonvulsant prophylaxis. Mucositis, hair loss, and nail changes are common after BMT conditioning. Most patients who undergo HSCT become sterile. So, sperm or egg banking options should be offered to these patients.

An important development in the last 20 years has been the introduction of reduced-intensity conditioning (RIC) regimens. The concept of RIC in patients with malignancy is to use donor immune cells for tumor eradication based on the allogeneic graft versus tumor effect. The safety and effectiveness of RIC must be balanced against an increased risk of acute leukemia relapses and an increased risk of chronic GVHD. **Box 14.18.1** shows how a typical HSC is performed.

DONOR SAFETY

Bone marrow or hematopoietic stem cell donation is remarkably safe for donors. For bone marrow donors, routine preanesthesia check-ups are required. A BM donor is left with a small puncture mark at bone marrow harvest sites as commonly happens during routine bone marrow testing. For PBSc apheresis, donors are administered 4 days of subcutaneous granulocyte colony-stimulating factors (G-CSF) injections on an outpatient basis. Low back pain

BOX 14.18.1: A typical hematopoietic stem cell transplantation procedure.

Allogeneic hematopoietic stem-cell transplantation
- Admission to the BMT unit
- Central venous catheter insertion like dialysis or angiography catheter
- Transplant conditioning therapy is started which lasts 4–10 days depending on the protocol
- Stem cells (collected from a donor) are administered for over 30 minutes intravenously like a blood transfusion once conditioning therapy is completed
- Supportive medicines including antimicrobial prophylaxis continue
- Mucositis (oral ulcers) develops 3–4 days after stem cells are infused which usually lasts for 1 week. One may also get diarrhea during that time
- Higher-grade mucositis can cause pain requiring analgesics and many times enteral/parenteral nutrition
- Generally, 90–95% of patients get a fever during this week. IV antibiotics and antifungals as per febrile neutropenia protocol are started
- Blood and platelet transfusions are required during this phase. On average 2–3 units of blood and 2–3 units of single donor platelets are required
- Recovery starts after this. Once adequate neutrophils are attained (generally 2–3 weeks after BMT) then patient is discharged

Autologous hematopoietic stem-cell transplantation
- 4 days of subcutaneous Injection G-CSF. Some patients receive plerixafor subcutaneous 12 hours before stem cell collection
- Admission to BMT unit on 4th day
- Central catheter insertion like dialysis or angiography catheter
- Collection of hematopoietic stem cells from the patient on the 5th day and cryopreserved as appropriate
- If the stem cell dose is adequate, then BMT conditioning therapy is started
- Subsequent steps are similar to steps 5–10 as above

(BMT: bone marrow transplantation; G-CSF: granulocyte colony-stimulating factors)

and/or low-grade fever up to 100°F may occur with these injections which respond to paracetamol. HSCs are collected on the 5th day. In both situations, donors are discharged the same day and are usually fit to resume school, college, office, or homework the next day. Sometimes in cases of large-volume bone marrow harvest (where the donor weighed less than the recipient), a packed red blood cell transfusion may be required.

SUPPORTIVE CARE

Hematopoietic stem cell transplantation is usually performed in isolation rooms with high-efficiency particulate air filters and laminar airflow. A subcutaneously tunneled long-term, flexible, double-lumen catheter is usually required for chemotherapy, HSC infusion, supportive care, regular blood sampling, transfusion of blood products, intravenous antibiotics, and parenteral nutrition **(Fig. 14.18.1C)**. The incidence of infection varies in different stages with bacterial infections especially gram-negative infections being the most common in the early stages. Fungal infections mainly aspergillosis and candida and viral infections occur in the early and late transplantation stage. The practice of screening for carbapenem-resistant *Enterobacteriaceae* in stool is largely abandoned. Uses of prophylactic antibacterial usually fluoroquinolone, antifungals (fluconazole and posaconazole), and antivirals (acyclovir and ganciclovir) have significantly reduced the incidence of bacterial, fungal and viral infections, respectively during and after HSCT.[5] Early institution of broad-spectrum empirical antibiotics to cover gram-negative bacteria as per institutional antibiograms, with the addition of antifungal drugs if fever persists, is the usual practice. After engraftment, viral infections with cytomegalovirus (CMV), *Herpes simplex, Varicella zoster*, and *Pneumocystis jerovicii* are common and prophylaxis as appropriate is part of the BMT protocols. Patients require multiple transfusions of red blood cells and platelets.[5] All blood products must be leukodepleted to prevent transmission of CMV. Blood products must be γ-irradiated to prevent transfusion-associated GVHD which is mediated by live lymphocytes in the blood product that recognize HLA differences in the host. G-CSF is often administered to patients after HSC infusion to shorten the duration of neutropenia. In the allogeneic setting, G-CSF is usually started on day +10 of HSCT. In autologous HSCT, some centers start G-CSF on day +1 and some start on day +6 of HSCT. Nutritional status is compromised by direct effects of the regimen (mucositis) and complications of HSCT. Enteral nutrition is effective and safe, with fewer complications. Parenteral nutrition is for patients who cannot tolerate enteral feeding.[6] Initial admission for HSCT is typically 3–4 weeks. Unlike solid organ transplantations, most patients are off therapy by 6–12 months post-BMT.

GRAFT FAILURE/REJECTION

Primary graft rejection (or failure of BMT) is defined as failure of (recovery of blood counts) to restore the hematopoietic function of the stem cell graft before day 30. The risk is increased in patients who undergo unrelated donor HSCT, are HLA-incompatible, receive an inadequate stem cell dose, have multiple prior transfusions, or have storage diseases like osteopetrosis.[7]

GRAFT VERSUS HOST DISEASE

The greater the genetic differences between the donor and recipient, the greater the risk and severity of GVHD. The donor T cells recognize these antigens as foreign and then mount an immune response against the recipient cells. The incidence of GVHD in allogeneic HSCT patients ranges from 20 to 60%. Severe GVHD is a major cause of morbidity and mortality in HSCT patients. Patients with hematological malignancies who develop mild to moderate GVHD have a lower risk of disease relapse due to the graft versus leukemia effect. Acute GVHD (aGVHD) develops within 100 days after allogeneic HSCT. Classically, it involves the skin (rashes especially on palms and soles), liver (hyperbilirubinemia) and lower gastrointestinal tract (large volume diarrhea), although the degree of involvement of each organ varies. Severity can be classified according to the extent of skin damage, degree of hyperbilirubinemia, and severity of diarrhea. Chronic GVHD (cGVHD) develops approximately 100 days after transplantation. It can follow a progressive expansion of aGVHD or develop de novo. cGVHD resembles autoimmune systemic collagen vascular diseases, and the manifestations can affect almost any organ, including the skin, eyes, oral cavity, gastrointestinal tract, urinary tract, liver, and lungs. Morbidity and mortality are highest in patients with progressive cGVHD. Steroids are usually the first line of treatment for both acute and chronic GVHD. Other immunosuppressive agents used include cyclosporine, azathioprine, methotrexate, and mycophenolate, etc. in various combinations. Newer oral medications like ruxolitinib are highly effective in the management of GVHD.[8]

LATE EFFECTS

Many long-term side effects have been observed after HSCT. There are hormonal dysfunction, cardiac, pulmonary issues, marital and fertility problems, psychosocial issues, and risk of second malignancies. Data are suggesting a small decrease in IQ in transplanted children, especially when cranial irradiation was used. Poor housing and difficulty finding work are other negative consequences.[6]

PRIVATE CORD BLOOD BANKING

At present cord blood transplantation is approved only for treating hematological diseases, immune deficiencies, and genetic diseases. Misunderstanding and misrepresenting the usage, a lot of private cord blood banks have come up and offer storage of child's cord blood as a biological insurance for possible future use. The chance of using umbilical cord blood for autologous use of hematopoietic stem cells is effectively between 1:75,000 and 1:100,000. The Indian Council of Medical Research (ICMR) has raised ethical concerns about promotional advertisements by private cord blood banks for future self-use. There is no scientific basis for preservation of cord blood for future self-use and this practice is not recommended. There are also concerns regarding the quality and viability of private cord blood.

Rarely, there may be a family where a child is already suffering from a disease requiring HSCT like leukemia or thalassemia and next child may not be fully HLA identical. These are rare special situations where private cord blood banking may be recommended.[9]

ROLE OF PEDIATRICIANS

Identify and Refer Early

Pediatricians are the first point of contact for children with hematological diseases. Pediatricians must be aware of diseases that can be cured by transplantation. Factors associated with high-graft rejection rates include long intervals between diagnosis and transplantation, increased number of pretransplantation blood transfusions (>20), infections, and multiple treatments including immunosuppressive therapy before transplantation. Multiple transfusions can lead to alloimmunization to leukocytes present in red cell and platelet transfusion. This includes both HLA and non-HLA antibodies. Preformed HLA antibodies can lead to primary transplantation rejection. This can be prevented by treating pediatricians by using leukocyte-depleted blood products (at the time of collection, or issue or by using blood filters during transfusion). We should avoid family-directed blood transfusion for the same reason. In case there is an emergency then family-directed blood product needs to be irradiated. An early referral to a BMT center helps to streamline a lot of issues.

During Bone Marrow Transplantation

Various pediatric subspecialty support is required for good outcomes for children. These include but are not limited to pediatric critical care, pulmonology, gastroenterology, neurology and transfusion medicine.

Post-transplantation Infections

Once a child is successfully transplanted the early immune recovery takes a few weeks, the bulk of immunity is back by 6 months and complete T cell repertoire recovery may take up to 1–2 years. When these children present with a fever early in the course (first month of autologous BMT and first 100 days in allogeneic BMT) then the majority will require hospitalization and parenteral antimicrobials even if the child is not neutropenic.

Post-transplantation Immunization

During the conditioning regimen the preexisting immunity to polio, hepatitis B, etc. is wiped out. These children need to be re-immunized. For allogeneic BMT, this usually starts 1 year after BMT and for autologous BMT the gap is 6 months. These children are given vaccination schedules by BMT centers which can be easily followed by the primary pediatrician.

Late Effects

Many survivors will be living in a community after a successful HSCT. These children are to be regularly followed by the primary pediatrician for the emergence of late effects as described above.

CONCLUSION

- Hematopoietic stem cell transplantation is curative in many benign and malignant hematological diseases due either to the replacement of the diseased HSCs in the recipient or to the antitumor activity of specific immune cells in the donor graft against the recipient's malignancy.
- Toxicities including immune reactions (rejection, engraftment syndrome, and GVHD) and organ toxicities of the transplantation regimen (sinusoidal obstruction syndrome and late effects) limit the full benefits of HSCT in curing pediatric patients.
- Hematopoietic stem cell transplantation outcomes are improving with improvements in diagnostics, supportive care, and therapeutic agents.
- Hematopoietic stem cell or bone marrow donation is safe for donors.
- Private cord blood banking is not recommended.
- Pediatricians play an integral role in management of children with BMT—both in pre- and post-transplantation stage.

REFERENCES

1. Indian Council of Medical Research. (2024). National guidelines for hematopoietic stem cell transplant. [online] Available from https://main.icmr.nic.in/sites/default/files/upload_documents/Nat_Guide_HCT.pdf. [Last accessed Dec., 2024].
2. Snowden JA, Sánchez-Ortega I, Corbacioglu S, Basak GW, Chabannon C, de la Camara R, et al; European Society for Blood and Marrow Transplantation (EBMT). Indications for haematopoietic cell transplantation for haematological diseases, solid tumours and immune disorders: current practice in Europe, 2022. Bone Marrow Transplant. 2022;57(8):1217-39.
3. Naithani R, Ortiz D, Webster-Carrion AM, Joshi S, Pillai AB. Hematopoietic Stem Cell Transplantation and Immunotherapy for Pediatric Hematologic Malignancies. In: Reis RL (Ed). Encyclopedia of Tissue Engineering and Regenerative Medicine, 1st edition. Cambridge, Massachusetts: Academic Press; 2019. pp. 65-79.
4. Shyr D, Davis KL, Bertaina A. Stem cell transplantation for ALL: you've always got a donor, why not always use it? Hematology Am Soc Hematol Educ Program. 2023;2023(1):84-90.
5. Borah P, Jeyaraman P, Pathak S, Dayal D, Tarai B, Naithani R. Quinolone Prophylaxis Prevents the Development of Carbapenem-Resistant Infection in Patients Undergoing Hematopoietic Stem Cell Transplant. Authorea. 2022.
6. Saglio F, Pagliara D, Zecca M, Balduzzi A, Cattoni A, Prete A, et al; AIEOP BMT Group. Long-Term Complications after Allogeneic Hematopoietic Stem Cell Transplantation with Treosulfan- or Busulfan-Based Conditioning in Pediatric Patients with Acute Leukemia or Myelodysplastic Syndrome: Results of an Associazione Italiana Ematologia Oncologia Pediatrica Retrospective Study. Transplant Cell Ther. 2024:S2666-6367(23)02410-7.
7. Müskens KF, Lindemans CA, Dandis R, Nierkens S, Belderbos ME. Definitions, incidence and outcome of poor graft function after hematopoietic cell transplantation: A systematic review and meta-analysis. Blood Rev. 2023;60:101076.
8. Watkins B, Qayed M. Novel approaches to acute graft-versus-host disease prevention. Hematology Am Soc Hematol Educ Program. 2023;2023(1):155-63.
9. Devi S, Bongale AM, Tefera MA, Dixit P, Bhanap P. Fresh Umbilical Cord Blood-A Source of Multipotent Stem Cells, Collection, Banking, Cryopreservation, and Ethical Concerns. Life (Basel). 2023;13(9):1794.

SECTION

15 Pediatric Malignancies

Section Editor: Purna A Kurkure

15.1 Malignancies in Children: An Introduction

Purna A Kurkure

INTRODUCTION

The recent understanding and advances in the total management of pediatric cancers form one of the most exciting chapters in the entire field of oncology. With increasing control of infectious diseases, eradication of malnutrition, and the rapid strides of the pediatric surgeons in correcting benign surgical problems, more children are now living to be diagnosed with cancer.

In the United States of America, cancer is second to accidents as a cause of mortality in children beyond the first year of life. There is a paucity of accurate statistics in our country. Children constitute approximately one-third of India's population, which is more than 1.2 billion. The annual incidence rates of cancer are about 75 and 80 per 100 men and women, respectively, or around 8,00,000 new cancers per year. Approximately 5% of these are in the pediatric age group as estimated by population-based cancer registries. Thus, approximately 40,000 new pediatric cancers are estimated to be diagnosed annually. Leukemias and lymphomas comprise nearly half of the pediatric cancers followed by tumors of the central nervous system (CNS), sympathetic nervous system, soft tissues, kidney, bone, eye, liver, and germ cells. "Child is not a miniature adult." The types of childhood cancers and response to therapy totally differ from those in adults.

The hallmark of success in pediatric oncology is the multidisciplinary approach executed through a carefully orchestrated multimodality team comprising a pediatric oncologist, a pediatric surgeon/pediatric oncosurgeon, a radiation oncologist, various diagnostic specialists (pathologist, hematopathologist, molecular pathologist, and radiologist), and supportive care services (registered dietician, physical therapist, occupational therapist, and psychologist). Burchenal succinctly characterized the basic tenet of multidisciplinary approach by stating "the pride of discipline must be put aside."[1,2] All the experts should work together, keeping the well-being of the child as the focus.

The first chance is the best chance, and giving optimum treatment at the outset is the most important factor in deciding the outcome. Any advances in health care are only as valuable as its availability and accessibility to those who need it. It has been well documented that organized and coordinated treatment programs carried out by experienced pediatric oncologists in well-staffed and well-equipped pediatric cancer units are the most effective. But the community pediatrician's role is crucial for a prompt diagnosis, early referral, and to ensure efficient follow-up.

The National Training Project in Practical Pediatric Oncology (NTPPPO) has been initiated under the auspices of Pediatric Hematology Oncology (PHO) chapter of the Indian Academy of Pediatrics (IAP) in collaboration with the International Society of Paediatric Oncology (SIOP) since 1998 with the aim to train, educate, and encourage pediatricians to participate in shared care of childhood cancer patients.[3]

Advances in the treatment of childhood cancers have dramatically increased survival rates to more than 70% in the developed countries. It has been estimated that by the year 2020, approximately 1 in 750 young adults in the society will be a survivor of childhood cancer in the United States of America. In India, children treated at comprehensive pediatric cancer units also stand an equal chance of being survivors. Childhood cancer survivors are unique and precious. Their contributions to the future are priceless. For each child who survives cancer, on average, 71 years of life will be saved.

Although this constitutes a remarkable medical achievement, the late morbidity in this growing survivor population has become an area of concern. The need to predict the future impact of current therapeutic strategies is a major challenge for the pediatric oncologist. A balance of reassurance to the survivor and vigilance in monitoring for late relapse, second malignancies, and other sequel is required. The recent concept of a truly "cured child" in pediatric oncology envisages not only a biological cure of the disease but also a child on par with peers in growth and development physically and in achievements and aspirations, both mentally and emotionally.

REFERENCES

1. Burchenal JH. The historical development of cancer chemotherapy. Semin Oncol. 1977;4(2):135-46.
2. Mendelsohn J. Blockade of receptors for growth factors: an anticancer therapy--the fourth annual Joseph H Burchenal American Association of Cancer Research Clinical Research Award Lecture. Clin Cancer Res. 2000;6(3):747-53.
3. NTP-PPO. (2024). Indian National Training Project in Practical Pediatric Oncology. Available from https://www.phoindia.org/cms/ntp-pponcology. [Last accessed December, 2024].

15.2 Epidemiology of Pediatric Malignancies in India

Payal Malhotra, Ramandeep Singh Arora

BURDEN AND INCIDENCE OF CHILDHOOD AND ADOLESCENT CANCER

According to the recent Global Cancer Observatory (GLOBOCAN) estimates, there were 19.3 million incident cancer cases worldwide for the year 2020. India ranked third after China and the United States of America (USA) and it is predicted that cancer cases in India would increase to 2.08 million, accounting for a rise of 57.5% in 2040 from 2020. Globally, more than 400,000 children and adolescents of 0–19 years old develop cancer per year, as per the World Health Organization (WHO) estimates.[1] Of note, >80% of all childhood cancer cases occur in low- and middle-income countries (LMICs). The estimated number of children (0–14 years) and, children and adolescents (0–19 years) that may develop cancer every year in India is 52,366 and 76,805 persons respectively.[2]

The incidence of childhood cancer in most populations in the world ranges from 7/100,000 to 16/100,000 person years (PYs). In childhood populations of Europe, North America and other developed regions of the world, cancer incidence rates are around 14/100,000 PYs and cancer in children and adolescents <19 years of age constitutes 1–2% of the overall cancer burden.[3] Cancer incidence in the developing countries is less well known, because there have been fewer population-based cancer registries (PBCRs) with adequate completeness. In India, the systematic collection of data on cancer through the PBCRs and hospital-based cancer registries (HBCRs) is in existence since 1981 under the National Cancer Registry Programme (NCRP) of the Indian Council of Medical Research-National Centre for Disease Informatics and Research (ICMR-NCDIR), Bengaluru. The age-adjusted incidence rate varies across the country and New Delhi recorded the highest among boys [20.3 per 100,000 PYs] and girls [12.5 per 100,000 PYs]. Recently published data from 96 HBCRs suggested that 3.2% and 4.6% of all cancer cases in India were among children in the 0–14 year and 0–19 year age groups respectively.[4]

DISTRIBUTION OF COMMON CHILDHOOD AND ADOLESCENT CANCERS

Unlike adult cancers which are mainly carcinomas, childhood cancers have a diverse histology and are hence grouped into 12 main cancer groups [International Classification of Childhood Cancer (ICCC)] based on morphology. Overall, leukemias, central nervous system (CNS) tumors and lymphomas predominate during childhood **(Figs. 15.2.1A and B)**. A recent study from India, published from 96 HBCRs revealed that the most common major groups of cancer among the 0–19 year age group were leukemias (36%), lymphomas (12%), bone tumors (11%), and CNS tumors (10%) **(Figs. 15.2.1A and B)**.[4]

Leukemia accounts for largest (35–50%) proportion of childhood cancer burden in India with acute lymphoblastic leukemia (ALL) being the most common type.[3,4] The overall incidence of childhood lymphoma in India is similar to that of the West. On the other hand, relative proportion of Hodgkin lymphoma (HL) is higher. In 0India, HL is characterized by younger age of presentation and predominance of mixed cellularity histopathology which may be due to subclinical Epstein–Barr virus infection in childhood. Among the no-Hodgkin lymphomas (NHLs), Burkitt's lymphoma (BL) (40–60%) and lymphoblastic lymphoma (30–40%) remain the predominant subtypes followed by anaplastic large cell lymphoma (ALCL) and diffuse large B-cell lymphoma (DLBCL) which is similar to the West.[3,4]

The CNS tumors account for 8–12% of total childhood cancer cases. Astrocytoma and medulloblastoma remain the two most common pediatric brain malignancies followed by primitive neuroectodermal tumor, craniopharyngioma, and ependymal tumors.[3,4] The lower incidence of CNS tumors in India may be due to poor recognition and missed diagnosis as the common presenting symptoms are headache, vomiting, and seizures, which can often be nonspecific in younger children. Hence, in the absence of readily available neuroimaging and neurosurgical facilities which is limited to predominantly tertiary care institutions, a large proportion of cases may be misdiagnosed and treated as meningoencephalitis.

There is a reported excess of retinoblastoma in India (also seen in Pakistan and sub-Saharan Africa). It is likely that some of this excess is, because of better diagnosis and recognition of retinoblastoma, which, once at an advanced stage, is easy to identify.[3,4]

VARIATION IN DISTRIBUTION BY GENDER AND AGE

The sex predilection among the boys and girls has been skewed toward the former in most part of the world, which

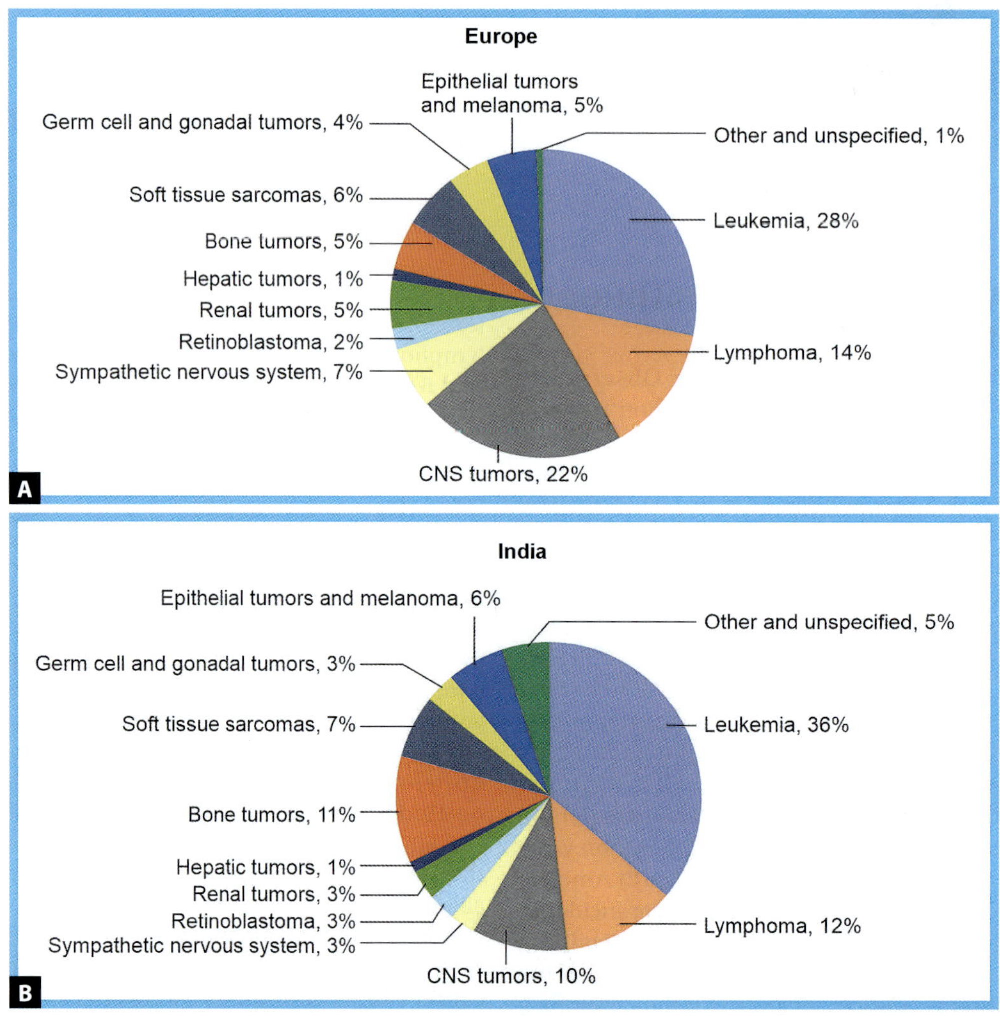

Figs. 15.2.1A and B: Distribution of childhood and adolescent cancer based on International Childhood Cancer Classification in Europe and India.

could possibly be due to biology, ethnicity or other factors which are still unknown. Data from the US Surveillance, Epidemiology, and End Results (SEER) 18 registries (2000–2015) showed that the incidence rate ratios for male to female childhood cancer overall was 1.19 [95% confidence interval (CI), 1.18–1.20].[5] This study also witnessed some correlation between diagnosis and its association with gender. Increased incidence was observed among males for ALL, HL, NHL and medulloblastoma. Male sex displayed a consistent inverse association (female preponderance) with nephroblastoma and thyroid carcinoma over the ages studied.

A recent descriptive cross-sectional analysis which was based on eight-year data (2012–2019) on childhood cancers from 96 HBCRs showed that the male-to-female ratio (MFR) was 1.72 in the 0–14 and 1.73 in the 0–19 age groups.[4] The proportion of boys seeking treatment was higher in northern India than southern India ($p < 0.0001$).[6] This data clearly signifies a skewed distribution, highlighting an increased prevalence among male, which may be due to bias in parents seeking treatment or gender preference in addition to the biological possibilities.

The distribution of childhood and adolescent cancers also varies by age **(Fig. 15.2.2)**. Children 0–4 years old frequently present with embryonal tumors including sympathetic nervous system tumors, nephroblastoma, retinoblastoma, and hepatoblastoma; adolescents 15–19-year-old children have more epithelial, germ cell, and gonadal tumors.

ETIOLOGY OF CHILDHOOD CANCER

The causes of childhood cancer have been systematically studied for several decades, and have been divided as genetic and nongenetic or external and inherent factors. Childhood malignancies are rarely related to known environmental exposures. Apart from rare cancers that are

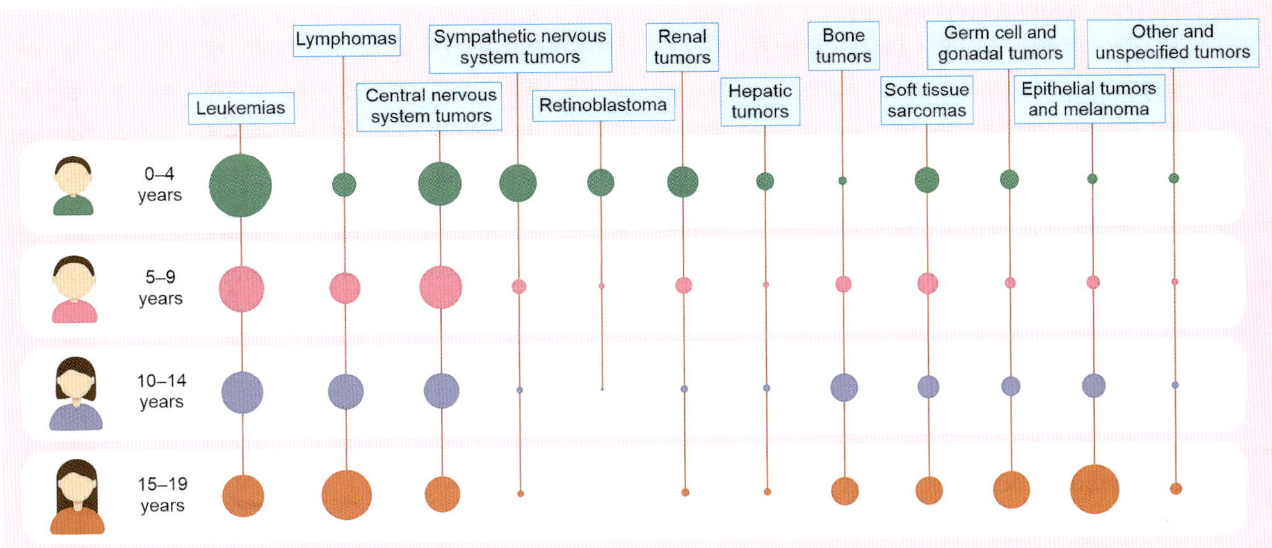

Fig. 15.2.2: Distribution of childhood and adolescent cancers by age.
Source: World Health Organization. (2024). International Childhood Cancer Day 2024. [online] Available from https://www.iarc.who.int/infographics/international-childhood-cancer-day-2024/. [Last accessed December, 2024].

TABLE 15.2.1: Common cancer predisposing syndromes and their associations.

Cancer predisposing syndrome	*Cancers with increased risk*
Down syndrome	Leukemia, lymphomas, and myelodysplastic syndrome
Ataxia telangiectasia	Leukemia, lymphoma, and breast cancer
Bloom syndrome	Leukemia, lymphoma, osteosarcoma, colon, breast, skin, lung, auditory canal, gastrointestinal tract, and uterine cancer
Fanconi anemia	Leukemia, testicular tumors, urogenital cancers, and liver tumor
Hereditary polyposis syndrome	Colorectal, endometrial, ovarian, gastrointestinal tract (stomach and small intestine, pancreas, and biliary tract), urinary tract, brain (glioblastomas), and skin (keratoacanthomas and sebaceous adenomas)
Li–Fraumeni syndrome (gene *TP53*)	Sarcomas, breast cancers, brain tumors, and adrenocortical carcinomas
Nijmegen breakage syndrome	Lymphoid cancers
Werner syndrome	Soft tissue sarcoma, colorectal, skin, thyroid, and pancreas cancers
Xeroderma pigmentosum	Skin cancer (melanoma and nonmelanoma)

caused by radiation, oncological, or immunosuppressive therapy, no major environmental causes are proven to be involved in pediatric malignancies. A number of other environmental risk factors have been studied including nonionizing radiation, maternal smoking, alcohol consumption and diet, paternal occupation, and exposure to various chemicals such as benzene, nitrosamines, pesticides, hair dyes, and some medications. Till date, their role in the causation of various childhood cancers has not been established.

It has become increasingly evident that inherited genetic factors play a substantial causal role. Large-scale sequencing studies have shown that approximately 10% of children with cancer have an underlying cancer predisposition syndrome. The number of recognized cancer predisposition syndromes and cancer predisposition genes are constantly growing.[7] Inherited syndromes, caused by high-penetrance germline deoxyribonucleic acid (DNA) mutations, chromosomal aneuploidy, or epigenetic disorders, are known to cause a minority of childhood cancers (<5%) including those having syndromic association. However for rare cancers, such as pediatric adrenocortical carcinoma, the proportion can be much higher. Highly-penetrant syndromes (Rothmund–Thomson, Neijamen breakage, and Blooms syndromes) have long been known to cause a small proportion of cancers but recently the contribution of common genetic variation to etiology has come gained its significance through genome wide association studies **(Table 15.2.1)**.[8]

CHILDHOOD AND ADOLESCENT CANCER OUTCOMES (MORTALITY AND SURVIVAL)

Cancer is an important contributor to death in children but its relative contribution varies. In the United Kingdom (UK), cancer is the most common cause of disease-related death (20%) in children and after injuries (21%) and the most common cause of death in children overall. Although cancer is the most common cause of disease-related death in children in the developed world, with improving survival rates, the mortality rate has declined to approximately 2/100,000 children/year **(Fig. 15.2.3)**.

In contrast to the developed world, cancer accounts for <1% of childhood deaths in developing countries, where deaths from infectious diseases are much more prominent. The global age-standardized rates (ASRs) of mortality for childhood cancer were 4.1 for both sexes. Notably, Eastern Africa (ASR = 5.6), Central America (ASR = 4.8), and South-Eastern Asia (ASR = 4.5) reported the highest mortality of childhood cancer.[9] In India, the mortality rate (adjusted to world standard population) is estimated to be 3.9 per 100,000 children PYs.

Since the 1960s, when most children who were diagnosed with cancer died, in the 21st century, nearly 80% of children are cured when timely and optimal treatment is available, accessible, and completed. Thus, improvement of survival reported from developed countries has resulted from use of intensive chemotherapy combined with other modalities of treatment, improved generalized supportive management, application of results of clinical trials and centralization of care permitting each patient to benefit from the best of multidisciplinary expertise and technology available for these rare conditions. The prognosis differs by tumor type. Currently, in high-income countries (HICs), childhood cancers with 5-year survival >80% include ALL < HL, NHL, retinoblastoma, nephroblastoma, hepatoblastoma, and germ cell tumors. Childhood cancers with 5-year survival >50 to <80% include acute myeloid leukemia, CNS tumors, nephroblastoma, bone tumors, and soft tissue sarcomas. Childhood cancers with 5-year survival 0 to ≤50% include high grade gliomas, infant ALL < metastatic soft tissue sarcomas.

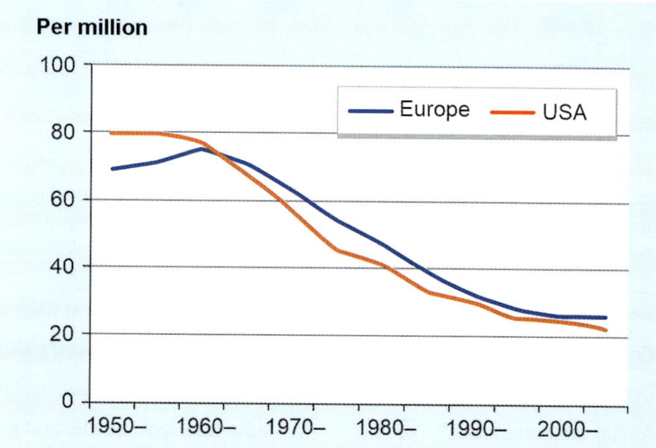

Fig. 15.2.3: Cancer mortality in children (aged 0–14 years) in three European countries (Ireland, the Netherlands, and the United Kingdom combined) for 1950–2009 and in the USA for 1950–2007. *Source*: Stewart BW. World Cancer Report 2014. Geneva: World Health Organization; 2014.

TABLE 15.2.2: Comparison of published data in India on 5-year overall survival of all main and selected extended categories of International Childhood Cancer Classification.

Data source	*Bengaluru PBCR*	*Chennai PBCR*	*New Delhi HBCR*
Time period	1982–1989	1990–2001	2013–2021
Cohort size	532	1274	705
Age group	0–14 years	0–14 years	0–17 years
All cancers combined	37%	40%	66%
Leukemia, myeloproliferative, and myelodysplastic diseases		36.3%	63.3%
Lymphoid leukemia	35%	38.7%	66.1%
Acute myeloid leukemia	10%	30.3%	41.2%
Chronic myeloproliferative diseases	26%	25.7%	100%
Lymphoma and reticuloendothelial neoplasms		55.3%	83.3%
Hodgkin lymphoma	72%	65%	100%
Non-Hodgkin lymphoma (except Burkitt's lymphoma)	33%	46.6%	46.1%

Contd...

Contd…

Data source	Bengaluru PBCR	Chennai PBCR	New Delhi HBCR
Burkitt's lymphoma	33%	46.6%	72.2%
CNS and miscellaneous intracranial and intraspinal neoplasms		26.8%	67%
Astrocytoma	40%	38.7%	79.5%
Intracranial and intraspinal embryonal tumor	43%		63.2%
Neuroblastoma and other peripheral nervous cell tumors		25.7%	64.5%
Neuroblastoma and ganglioneuroblastoma	28%	36.9%	62.9%
Retinoblastoma	71%	48.1%	50%
Renal tumors		58%	73.2%
Nephroblastoma and other nonepithelial renal tumors	27%	64.2%	84.4%
Hepatic tumors		10.5%	80%
Malignant bone tumors		30.6%	47.6%
Osteosarcoma	44%	43.6%	49.3%
Ewing tumor and related sarcomas of bone		23.4%	47.3%
Soft tissue and other extraosseous sarcomas		36.3%	52%
Rhabdomyosarcoma	13%	36.4%	47.1%
Germ cell tumor, trophoblastic tumor, and neoplasms of gonads	36%	38%	92.6%
Other malignant epithelial neoplasms and malignant melanomas	61%	35.1%	87.5%
Other and unspecified malignant neoplasms	17%		0%

(HBCR: hospital-based cancer registry; PBCR: population-based cancer registry)

These great leaps in childhood cancer survival seen in HICs have not been replicated to the same extent in LMICs like India where the improvement in survival is much more modest. The low survival rate is mainly attributed to weak health systems in LMICs. Childhood treatment services are primarily available at tertiary care facilities and display an urban skewing regarding availability and ease of accessibility, infrastructure, and manpower. Access to childhood cancer care is characterized by weak infrastructure, lack of supportive care, and poorly defined care pathways. Many children have advanced disease at the time of presentation.

Registry based data from India on childhood cancer survival from is scant. As shown in **Table 15.2.2**, the overall 5-year survival has improved from 37% to 66%, this is still not representative of the entire country.[3,10] The recent initiative by the Indian Pediatric Hematology Oncology Group to start HBCRs across the country would give us better estimates of childhood cancer survival in India.

REFERENCES

1. Jonston WT, Erdmann F, Newton R, Stellarova-Foucher E, Schüz J, Roman E. Childhood cancer: Estimating regional and global incidence. Cancer Epidemiol. 2021;71(Pt B):101662.
2. Arora RS, Bagai P, Bhakta N. Estimated National and State Level Incidence of Childhood and Adolescent Cancer in India. Indian Pediatr. 2021;58(5):417-23.
3. Arora RS, Eden TO, Kapoor G. Epidemiology of childhood cancer in India. Indian J Cancer. 2009;46(4):264-73.
4. Kapoor G, Arora RS, Radhakrishnan V, Natha A, Malhotra P, Cyriac SL, et al. Profile of Childhood Cancers From Hospital-Based Cancer Registries in India, 2017-19. Indian Pediatr. 2024;61(1):39-44.
5. Williams LZ, Richardson M, Marcotte EL, Poynter JN, Spector LG. Sex ratio among childhood cancers by single year of age. Pediatr Blood Cancer. 2019;66(6):e27520.
6. Bhatia KP, Ganguly S, Sasi A, Kumar V, Deo S, Agarwala S, et al. Sex disparity in childhood cancer in India: a multi-centre, individual patient data analysis. Lancet Oncol. 2013;24(1):54-63.
7. Kratz CP, Longmans MC, Cavé H, Wimmer K, Behjati S, Guerrini-Russseau L, et al. Predisposition to cancer in children and adolescents. Lancet Child Adolesc Health. 2021;5(2):142-54.
8. Garutti M, Foffano L, Mazzeo R, Michelotti A, Da Ros L, Viel A, et al. Hereditary Cancer Syndrom4es: A Comprehensive Review with a Visual Tool. Genes (Basel). 2023;14(5):1025.
9. Huang J, Chan SC, Ngai CH, Lok V, Zhang L, Lucero-Prisno 3rd DE, et al; NCD Global Health Research Group, Association of Pacific Rim Universities (APRU). Global incidence, mortality and temporal trends of cancer in children: A joinpoint regression analysis. Cancer Med. 2023;12(2):1903-11.
10. Arora RS, Kumari R, Adhana A, Tripathi R, Sachdev M, Jain P. Overall and Event Free Survival of Childhood Cancer—Report From a Hospital-based Cancer Registry in Northern India, 2013-12. Indian Pediatr. 2023;60(7):531-6.

15.3 Impact of Risk Stratification on Outcomes of Pediatric Malignancies

Nidhi Dhariwal, Badira C Parambil

INTRODUCTION

Pediatric cancers encompass a diverse array of hematolymphoid malignancies and solid tumors, each of which presents with unique challenges in diagnosis, treatment, and prognosis. Treatment of pediatric malignancies is multimodal and can include chemotherapy, radiation therapy, surgery, immunotherapy, and hematopoietic stem cell transplantation (HSCT). The outcomes of these malignancies have dramatically improved in the last five decades with 5-year survival reaching 90% for some. This leap in survival is the result of prospective trials conducted by pediatric oncology co-operative groups, advancing therapies, establishing standard of care, development of innovative and multimodal treatments, improvements in supportive care and better diagnostics. More than 80% of children with cancer who have access to contemporary therapies are expected to survive to adulthood.

These improved outcomes of childhood cancer have led to an increase in number of long-term survivors who are at a risk of late-effects of chemotherapy, radiotherapy and surgery. These late-effects are a cause of potential morbidity and mortality in childhood cancer survivors (CCSs). About 60–90% of the CCSs develop one or more chronic health conditions with >20% developing life-threatening complications in adulthood.[1] For instance, according to reports, one in 10 CCSs who had received an anthracycline will develop symptomatic cardiac event over time.[2] By identifying good risk cohort in certain malignancies, as described later, the risk of these sinister late-effects can be mitigated. Various clinical and biological factors could be used to stratify patients into risk groups for tailoring treatment strategies to maximize efficacy while minimizing potential toxicities.

RISK STRATIFICATION IN HEMATOLYMPHOID MALIGNANCIES

Acute Lymphoblastic Leukemia

Childhood acute lymphoblastic leukemia (ALL) has 5-year survival rates exceeding 90%. Risk stratification of pediatric ALL has also evolved over the last few decades to tailor treatment strategies and indications for HSCT **(Table 15.3.1)**. Factors incorporated include clinical and laboratory factors such as age at presentation, baseline white blood cell (WBC) count, testicular, and central nervous system (CNS) involvement and immunophenotype; leukemia genetics comprising of translocations and ploidy status; and early response to chemotherapy measured by flow cytometry as minimal residual disease (MRD).[3] Childhood ALL has been risk stratified into standard, intermediate and high-risk groups. While standard-risk ALL has excellent outcomes with less intensive chemotherapy thereby minimizing toxicities, intermediate, and high-risk groups require intensified chemotherapy protocols for achieving optimal survival rates. Standard-risk ALL has less anthracycline exposure when compared to other risks, thereby minimizing acute toxicities such as myelosuppression and risk of neutropenic sepsis, especially in induction phase; and long-term cardiotoxicity in this subset. Treatment of high-risk ALL is also associated with increased risk of mucositis and renal toxicities in the interim maintenance phase of treatment while receiving high-dose methotrexate chemotherapy.

Again, such encouraging outcomes of de novo ALL have led to an increase in number of long-term survivors and thereby relapse. Relapsed ALL is now the fourth most common malignancy seen in children. Risk stratification of relapsed ALL is essential to identify patients who can be treated with curative intent with available treatment options, those who require use of additional modalities for cure and those who continue to have dismal outcomes despite use of stem cell transplantation and hence are candidates for palliation. This pragmatic approach to triage patients is especially important in low-middle income countries (LMICs). Time to relapse, site of relapse, immunophenotype, and response to chemotherapy are used to classify relapsed ALL into standard-risk, intermediate-risk, and high-risk groups.[4] Most standard- and intermediate-risk relapses are usually managed with chemotherapy alone unlike high-risk relapses which would require immunotherapy and HSCT to achieve optimal outcomes.

Acute Myeloid Leukemia

Outcome of pediatric acute myeloid leukemia (AML) have dramatically improved in the last 40 years, with current outcomes reaching 70–80% in developed countries

TABLE 15.3.1: Risk stratification and risk group directed treatment of pediatric malignancies.

Disease	*Factors affecting risk stratification*	*Risk groups*	*Risk group directed treatment*	*Risk group-wise outcomes*	*Long-term morbidities*
ALL[3]	• Age • Baseline • WBC count • Immunophenotype • Testicular involvement • CNS status • Prednisolone response • Cytogenetics • Ploidy • MRD	Standard-risk	3-drug induction→ consolidation→ IM →DI	85%	• Anthracycline-related cardiotoxicity • Steroid-induced osteonecrosis • Neurocognitive impairment • Second malignant neoplasm
		Intermediate-risk	4-drug induction→ BFM consolidation→ Capizzi IM→ DI	75–80%	
		High-risk	4-drug induction→ augmented BFM consolidation→ high dose methotrexate based IM→DI	65–70%	
Relapsed ALL[4]	• Time to relapse • Site of relapse • Immunophenotype • Response to chemotherapy	Standard-risk	Chemotherapy only	70–80%	• Anthracycline-induced cardiotoxicity • Steroid-induced metabolic syndrome • Post-transplant acute/chronic GVHD
		Intermediate-risk	Chemotherapy only, HSCT if postinduction MRD positive	50–60%	
		High-risk	Chemotherapy + HSCT ± immunotherapy	20–30%	
AML[5]	• Cytogenetic abnormalities • Molecular markers	*Good-risk abnormalities:* • CBF-AML • Mutated NPM1 • Biallelic CEBPA	4 cycles of chemotherapy	80%	• Cardiotoxicity • Transplant-related complications/ chronic GVHD
		Intermediate-risk abnormalities: • t(9,11) • t(11,19) • Non-good/poor risk abnormalities	4–5 cycles of chemotherapy	50%	
		Poor-risk abnormalities: • Inv 3 • Monosomy 5/ del(5q) • Monosomy 7 • t(6,9) • t(4,11) • t(6,11) • t(10,11) • t(5,11) • t(7,12) • CBFA2T3::GLIS2 • FLT3-ITD • 12p abnormalities • MRD positive post-2 cycles of chemotherapy	4–5 cycles of chemotherapy and HSCT	30–40%	
APL[6]	Baseline WBC count	Low-risk	ATRA + ATO	95%	Anthracycline-induced cardiotoxicity
		High-risk	ATRA + ATO + anthracyclines	85%	

Contd...

Contd…

Disease	Factors affecting risk stratification	Risk groups	Risk group directed treatment	Risk group-wise outcomes	Long-term morbidities
Hodgkin lymphoma[7]	• Ann-Arbor stage • B-symptoms • Presence of bulky disease • Extranodal disease	Low-risk Intermediate-risk High-risk	2–4 cycles of chemotherapy 4 cycles of chemotherapy ± RT 6 cycles of chemotherapy ± RT *RT to bulky sites and sites of inadequate response depending on the protocol used	95% 90% 90%	• Cardiotoxicity due to anthracyclines and mediastinal RT • Bleomycin-induced pulmonary toxicity • Hypothyroidism due to RT to cervical nodes • Second malignant neoplasm
NHL[8]	St Jude staging degree of resection	Group A/R1 Group B/R2 Group C/R3/R4	2 cycles of chemotherapy 4 cycles of chemotherapy 6–8 cycles of chemotherapy	95% 90% 80%	• Anthracycline-induced cardiotoxicity • Infertility
Neuroblastoma[9]	• Age • INRG stage • Tumor histology • MYCN status • Ploidy • Segmental chromosomal aberrations	Low-risk Intermediate-risk High-risk	Surgery only Surgery + chemotherapy ± RT Chemotherapy + Surgery + HDCT/ASCT + RT+ immunotherapy	>90% 90% 50–60%	Anthracycline-induced cardiotoxicity
Wilms tumor[10]	• Age • Tumor stage • High-risk histological subtype • Response to chemotherapy	Low-risk Intermediate-risk High-risk	2-drug chemotherapy 2- or 3-drug chemotherapy + RT in stage 3/4 5-drug chemotherapy + RT in selected stages based on histology	90% 80% 60–70%	• Anthracycline-induced cardiotoxicity • End-stage renal disease
Rhabdomyosarcoma[11]	• Pretreatment • TNM staging • Clinical group • FOXO1 fusion status • Age	Low-risk Intermediate-risk High-risk	8 cycles of chemotherapy with lower CED 12 cycles of 3-drug chemotherapy 12 cycles of 3-drug chemotherapy or more intensive protocols depending on institutional practice	90% 70% <20%	Infertility (due to cumulative dose of alkylators)
Hepatoblastoma[12]	• PRETEXT staging • Vascular invasion • Extrahepatic extension • Metastatic disease • AFP < 100 ng/mL	Standard-risk High-risk	6 cycles of single drug Cisplatin 10 cycles of 3-drug chemotherapy (cisplatin alternating with doxorubicin/carboplatin)	90% 50–70%	• Cisplatin-induced ototoxicity • Cardiotoxicity

Contd…

Contd...

Disease	Factors affecting risk stratification	Risk groups	Risk group directed treatment	Risk group-wise outcomes	Long-term morbidities
Germ cell tumor[13]	• Staging • Site of primary	Low-risk	No chemotherapy	90%	• Cisplatin-induced ototoxicity • Bleomycin-related pulmonary toxicity • Second malignant neoplasm
		Intermediate-risk	4 cycles of 3-drug chemotherapy (cisplatin–etoposide–bleomycin)	80%	
		High-risk	4–6 cycles of 3-drug chemotherapy (cisplatin–etoposide–bleomycin)	70%	
Medulloblastoma[14]	• Presence of metastasis • Postoperative residual tumor volume • Histology	Average-risk	Surgery → 23.4 Gy CSI + 30.6 Gy TBB → 6 cycles of chemotherapy	85%	• Neurocognitive dysfunction • Abnormalities in growth and development • Endocrine dysfunction • Hearing defects • Visual disturbances • Cardiac toxicity • Gonadal dysfunction • Radiation-induced second malignancies
		High-risk	Surgery → 36 Gy CSI + 19.8 Gy TBB → 6 cycles of chemotherapy	70%	

(AFP: alpha-fetoprotein; ATO: arsenic trioxide; ATRA: all-trans retinoic acid; BFM: Berlin–Frankfurt–Munster; CSI: craniospinal irradiation; DI: delayed intensification; GVHD: graft-versus-host disease; HDCT/ASCT: high dose chemotherapy and autologous stem cell rescue; IM: interim maintenance; INRG: International Neuroblastoma Risk grouping; MRD: minimal residual disease; PRETEXT: pretreatment extent of tumor; RT: radiotherapy; TBB: tumor bed boost; TNM: tumor-node-metastasis)

and 50–60% in developing countries. Though upfront chemotherapy regimen remains same for all subtypes of AML, risk stratification is necessary to identify patients who require treatment intensification. Overall impact of patient associated factors such as age and ethnicity is not as large as disease related factors in children with AML. These disease-related factors include leukemia-specific cytogenetics, molecular genetics, and treatment response including MRD.[5] Children who fall in high-risk category need consolidation with HSCT once they achieve remission with chemotherapy.

Acute Promyelocytic Leukemia

Acute promyelocytic leukemia (APL) is a rare disease accounting for 5–10% of pediatric AML characterized by t(15;17) with resultant *PML-RARA* gene fusion driving the leukemia. Over the years, with combined use of differentiating agents such as all-trans retinoic acid (ATRA) and arsenic trioxide (ATO), outcomes of APL have improved drastically with survival rates of 95%. Baseline WBC count is used to risk stratify APL into low-risk and high-risk groups. Anthracyclines were the mainstay of treatment of APL previously but with current ATRA-ATO based protocols, high cure rates are achieved with reduced anthracycline exposure in high-risk APL and anthracycline-free regimens in low risk APL.[6]

HODGKIN LYMPHOMA

Hodgkin lymphoma (HL) is one of the most curable pediatric malignancies. With the expectation on long-term survival comes the responsibility to use treatment modalities that reduce risk of side effects such as cardiovascular disease, infertility, pulmonary complications, and second malignant neoplasms. Current use of risk adapted and response-based protocols have minimized late-effects while preserving high cure rates. The risk stratification of HL depends on Ann Arbor stage, B-symptoms, presence of bulky disease, and extranodal extension.[7] The duration of chemotherapy as well as need for consolidative radiotherapy depend on the risk group.

Non-Hodgkin Lymphoma

Outcomes of pediatric B-cell non-Hodgkin lymphoma (B-NHL) have dramatically improvements over the last 30 years with limited stage NHL (stage I to II) having approximately 5-year event-free survival of 95–100%.

Outcomes of advanced stage NHL have also improved from 40% 30 years back to 80% currently. Risk stratification of pediatric B-NHL is on the basis of stage and degree of resection, limiting the cumulative anthracycline, cyclophosphamide, and methotrexate exposure and total duration of treatment across these risk groups.[8]

RISK STRATIFICATION OF SOLID TUMORS

Neuroblastoma

The International Neuroblastoma Risk Grouping (INRG) uses an array of prognostic factors such as age, stage, tumor histology, MYCN status, tumor cell ploidy, and segmental chromosomal aberrations, to risk stratify neuroblastoma into low-risk, intermediate-risk, and high-risk groups.[9] While children with low-risk disease can treated with surgery only or can be observed alone, those with intermediate-risk require chemotherapy along with surgical resection. Both these risk groups have survival rates of >90% with current treatment. High-risk neuroblastoma, on the other hand, requires intense multimodality treatment that includes chemotherapy, surgery, high-dose chemotherapy with autologous stem cell rescue, radiotherapy, and immunotherapy in the form of anti-GD2 antibody, with event-free survival of 30–40%. These varied outcomes make it imperative to identify the risk group in which the child falls before starting treatment.

Wilms Tumor

With survival rates of >90%, the risk stratification of Wilms tumor (WT) has helped in concomitantly reducing therapy in most patients thereby leading to more healthier survivors by decreasing exposure to anthracyclines and abdominal radiotherapy. Tumor stage, presence of anaplasia, age and molecular markers such as loss of heterozygosity (LOH) 1p and 16q are used for risk stratification of WT.[10] Low-risk group has favorable outcomes without the use of anthracyclines and/or radiotherapy while high-risk groups require augmentation of therapy.

Rhabdomyosarcoma

Rhabdomyosarcoma (RMS) is the most common soft tissue sarcoma in children and adolescents with outcomes ranging from 20% (high-risk) to 90% (low-risk) with multimodality treatment that includes chemotherapy, surgery, and/or radiation therapy. With these varying outcomes, it is pertinent to identify patients with low-risk of relapse to minimize exposure to cyclophosphamide equivalent dose (CED) and radiation therapy. More nuanced risk stratification can also identify patients who may benefit from therapy intensification and/or use of novel agents. Risk stratification is based on pretreatment site, size, lymph nodal status, distant metastasis, extent of surgical resection, FOXO1 fusion status, and age.[11]

Titrating treatment according to risk groups in RMS helps in prevention of late-effects like infertility in survivors. A CED of >7.5 g/m^2 is associated with irreversible gonadal toxicity and sterility in males. Low-risk group receive a CED of 4.8 g/m^2, thereby decreasing risk of infertility without compromising outcomes.

Hepatoblastoma

Hepatoblastoma is the most common liver malignancy and children with surgical resection and chemotherapy being the mainstay of treatment and survival as good as 90% in low risk disease. Factors impacting risk stratification includes PRETEXT (preoperative evaluation of the tumor extent) staging, metastasis, and histology.[12] At present the SIOPEL group stratifies patients with hepatoblastoma into two categories: Standard-risk and high-risk. Standard-risk group has excellent outcomes with single agent cisplatin while chemotherapy for high-risk group includes a combination of cisplatin, carboplatin, and doxorubicin thereby subjecting survivors to potential risk of cardiotoxicity.

GERM CELL TUMOR

Risk groups for pediatric germ cell tumors (GCTs) have been developed based on factors known to influence outcomes such as age, site of primary, and staging.[13] Low-risk GCT do not require any adjuvant chemotherapy with excellent outcomes with surgery only. With a reported 40–60% incidence of cisplatin-induced ototoxicity in CCSs, omission of chemotherapy in this subset prevents survivors from this sinister late-effect.

Medulloblastoma

Childhood medulloblastoma (MB) (age >3 years), over the last 20 years, has been risk stratified on the basis of clinical, not biologic, criteria with 5-year survival rates for average-risk MB being over 80% and for high-risk, approximately 60%.[14] High-risk group requires higher dose of craniospinal irradiation in comparison to the average-risk group and thereby predisposes to higher risk of late effects such as decline in neurocognitive function, abnormalities in growth and development, endocrine dysfunction, hearing defects, visual disturbances, gonadal dysfunction, and radiation-induced second malignancies. With the advent of molecular classification of MB in 2010, the risk stratification was further refined in the context of subgroups and the following risk groups were identified based on current survival rates: Low-risk (>90% survival), average-(standard) risk (75–90% survival), high-risk (50–75% survival), and very high-risk (<50% survival). While low-risk tumors qualify for reduction in therapy, very high-risk tumors mandate identification of novel therapies.

CONCLUSION

With dramatic improvement in outcomes of most of the pediatric malignancies over last few decades, risk stratification of these cancers to identify patients eligible for escalation and de-escalation of therapy is of utmost importance to further improve outcomes, and decrease acute toxicities and late-effects, respectively.

REFERENCES

1. Hudson MM, Ness KK, Gurney JG, Mulroney DA, Chemaitilly W, Krull KR, et al. Clinical ascertainment of health outcomes among adults treated for childhood cancer. JAMA. 2013;309(22):2371-81.
2. Bertorello N, Luksch R, Bisogno G, Haupt R, Spallarossa P, Cenna R, et al. Cardiotoxicity in children with cancer treated with anthracyclines: A position statement on dexrazoxane. Pediatr Blood Cancer. 2023:e30515.
3. Das N, Banavali S, Bakhshi S, Trehan A, Radhakrishnan V, Seth R, et al. Protocol for ICiCLe-ALL-14 (InPOG-ALL-15-01): a prospective, risk stratified, randomised, multicentre, open label, controlled therapeutic trial for newly diagnosed childhood acute lymphoblastic leukaemia in India. Trials. 2022;23(1):102.
4. Hunger SP, Raetz EA. How I treat relapsed acute lymphoblastic leukemia in the pediatric population. Blood. 2020;136(16):1803-12.
5. Tomizawa D, Tsujimoto SI. Risk-Stratified Therapy for Pediatric Acute Myeloid Leukemia. Cancers (Basel). 2023;15(16):4171.
6. Kutny MA, Alonzo TA, Abla O, Rajpurkar M, Gerbing RB, Wang YC, et al. Assessment of Arsenic Trioxide and All-trans Retinoic Acid for the Treatment of Pediatric Acute Promyelocytic Leukemia: A Report From the Children's Oncology Group AAML1331 Trial. JAMA Oncol. 2022;8(1):79-87.
7. Mauz-Körholz C, Landman-Parker J, Balwierz W, Ammann RA, Anderson RA, Attarbaschi A, et al. Response-adapted omission of radiotherapy and comparison of consolidation chemotherapy in children and adolescents with intermediate-stage and advanced-stage classical Hodgkin lymphoma (EuroNet-PHL-C1): a titration study with an open-label, embedded, multinational, non-inferiority, randomised controlled trial. Lancet Oncol. 2022;23(1):125-37.
8. Thacker N, Bakhshi S, Chinnaswamy G, Vora T, Prasad M, Bansal D, et al. Management of Non-Hodgkin Lymphoma: ICMR Consensus Document. Indian J Pediatr. 2017;84(5):382-92.
9. Cohn SL, Pearson AD, London WB, Monclair T, Ambros PF, Brodeur GM, et al.; INRG Task Force. The International Neuroblastoma Risk Group (INRG) classification system: an INRG Task Force report. J Clin Oncol. 2009;27(2):289-97.
10. Dome JS, Perlman EJ, Graf N. Risk stratification for Wilms tumor: current approach and future directions. Am Soc Clin Oncol Educ Book; 2014. pp. 215-23.
11. Borinstein SC, Steppan D, Hayashi M, Loeb DM, Isakoff MS, Binitie O, et al. Consensus and controversies regarding the treatment of rhabdomyosarcoma. Pediatr Blood Cancer. 2018;65(2).
12. Meyers RL, Maibach R, Hiyama E, Häberle B, Krailo M, Rangaswami A, et al. Risk-stratified staging in paediatric hepatoblastoma: a unified analysis from the Children's Hepatic Tumors International Collaboration. Lancet Oncol. 2017;18(1):122-31.
13. Frazier AL, Hale JP, Rodriguez-Galindo C, Dang H, Olson T, Murray MJ, et al. Revised risk classification for pediatric extracranial germ cell tumors based on 25 years of clinical trial data from the United Kingdom and United States. J Clin Oncol. 2015;33(2):195-201.
14. Gajjar AJ, Robinson GW. Medulloblastoma-translating discoveries from the bench to the bedside. Nat Rev Clin Oncol. 2014;11(12):714-22.

15.4 Leukemia

Anupama S Borker

INTRODUCTION

Leukemias are malignant neoplasms arising from the uncontrolled proliferation and loss of differentiation of hematopoietic stem cells. Depending on the lineage of the progenitor stem cell involved, they are classified as lymphoid or myeloid. Depending on the natural history of the leukemia, they are classified as acute or chronic.

Acute leukemia accounts for about 40% of childhood cancers. Acute lymphoblastic leukemia (ALL) comprises about 70–80% and acute myeloid leukemia (AML) comprises about 10–15% of childhood leukemia. The remaining subset consists of the uncommon childhood leukemia.

ETIOPATHOGENESIS

The exact etiology of acute leukemia is unknown. Several genetic conditions are known to predispose to leukemia. These include Down syndrome (trisomy 21), Fanconi syndrome, Bloom syndrome, Shwachman syndrome, Klinefelter syndrome, Turner syndrome (45,XO), neurofibromatosis, ataxia telangiectasia, severe combined immunodeficiency, and Li-Fraumeni syndrome (p53 deletion). Exposure to ionizing radiation, benzene, and certain drugs such as alkylating agents, nitrosourea, and epipodophyllotoxins has been clearly associated with the development of leukemia. Certain environmental factors, viral infections, and immunodeficiency disorders may also predispose to leukemia.

Leukemia arises following certain carcinogenic stimuli that lead to the malignant transformation of hematopoietic cells rendering them capable of unregulated proliferation (self-renewal) coupled with loss of differentiation and loss of apoptosis (programmed cell death). The uncontrolled proliferation of these malignant cells leads to the expansion of marrow cavity with resultant suppression of normal cell lines.

CLASSIFICATION OF LEUKEMIA

Acute leukemia in children is classified according to their lineage as ALL and AML. The further subclassification of ALL and AML depends on the characteristics of leukemia cells at the cytogenetic and molecular level. A simplified classification on the basis of the surface markers as those derived from "B" or "T" cell precursors is shown in **Table 15.4.1**.

Common chromosomal aberrations that are known to influence outcomes in ALL are shown in **Table 15.4.2**. The World Health Organization (WHO) classification of lymphoid and myeloid neoplasms classifies leukemias according to the number of chromosomes or the recurrent molecular rearrangement.[1,2]

CLINICAL FEATURES

The common age group for acute leukemia is 2–5 years, and boys are often slightly more affected than girls. *Fever* is the most common presenting feature of acute leukemia. The other features usually reflect the suppression of one or more hematopoietic cell lines. Anemia may present with progressive pallor, weakness, fatigue, lethargy, refusal to feed, or shortness of breath. Thrombocytopenia leading to petechiae, ecchymosis, or gum bleeds is common. Neutropenia with resultant infections may present with fever, pneumonia, otitis; or with skin, soft tissue, or perianal infections. Mucositis with oral ulcers and thrush is a common finding in neutropenic patients. Hepatosplenomegaly and lymphadenopathy, secondary to leukemic infiltration, are common. The lymphadenopathy can be generalized and sometimes massive. Mediastinal lymphadenopathy mostly occurs in T-cell ALL. The resultant obstruction of the superior vena cava and the airway can present as medical emergencies. Children and adolescents with the superior vena cava syndrome present with edema and suffusion of the face and upper extremities, headache, and dilated neck veins. The superior mediastinal syndrome resulting from compression of the trachea leads to cough, breathlessness, and air hunger; and if untreated may progress to hypoxia with cyanosis, altered sensorium, and seizures.

Children with large tumor burden may sometimes develop spontaneous tumor lysis syndrome leading to acute renal failure, secondary to uric acid nephropathy.

Less common presenting features include bone and joint pains with tenderness, and rash or eruption, which may be due to cutaneous involvement. About 5–10% of patients have central nervous system (CNS) involvement at diagnosis

TABLE 15.4.1: Classification of acute lymphoblastic leukemia.

ALL subtype	Surface markers	Significance
Pre-B-cell	$CD10^+$, $CD19^+$, $CD20^+$, $CD21^+$, HLA^-DR^+	The most common subtype with good prognosis
B-cell	$CD19^+$, $CD20^+$, $CD21^+$, sIg^+	Burkitt leukemia (L3), good prognosis with short duration intensive chemotherapy
T-cell	$CD3^+$, $CD5^+$, $CD7^+$	Common in older boys, associated with high WBC counts, mediastinal mass, and CNS involvement

(ALL: acute lymphoblastic leukemia; CD: cluster of differentiation; CNS: central nervous system; HLA: human leukocyte antigen; WBC: white blood cell)

TABLE 15.4.2: Common chromosomal abnormalities in acute lymphoblastic leukemia.

Chromosomal abnormality	Fusion protein	Clinical significance
t(9;22)	BCR/ABL	Considered very high risk. Therapy with imatinib along with chemotherapy has improved survival
t(4;11)	MLL	Common in infantile leukemia, associated with high tumor burden, intrinsically drug resistant. Connotes poor prognosis
t(1;19)	PBX1/E2A	Associated with higher rates of CNS relapse
t(12;21)	TEL/AML-1	Good prognosis, needs minimal therapy
t(8;14)	MYC/IgL	Burkitt leukemia, needs short duration intensive chemotherapy

(AML-1: acute myeloid leukemia-1; BCR: B-cell receptor; CNS: central nervous system; IgL: immunoglobulin L; MLL: mixed lineage leukemia; PBX1: pre-B-cell leukemia transcription factor 1)

and may present with cranial nerve palsies or seizures. Signs of raised intracranial pressure such as headache and papilledema may be present. Painless testicular enlargement suggestive of testicular involvement is extremely rare at diagnosis.

Gum hypertrophy is rather a common presentation of AML, especially M4 subtype. Extramedullary myeloid cell tumors or chloromas can occur at a variety of locations and may sometimes precede the development of marrow involvement in AML. Disseminated intravascular coagulation is more common in AML, especially in M3 subtype or acute promyelocytic leukemia (APML).

DIFFERENTIAL DIAGNOSIS

The differential diagnosis of ALL includes several benign and malignant conditions.

- Viral infection-induced cytopenias in infectious mononucleosis, cytomegalovirus infection, and other viral infections
- Immune thrombocytopenia
- Drug-induced cytopenias
- Bone marrow failure syndromes, myelodysplastic syndromes, and hypoplastic/aplastic anemia
- Collagen vascular disorders such as juvenile idiopathic arthritis and systemic lupus erythematosus
- Langerhans cell histiocytosis
- Metastases from solid tumors such as neuroblastoma and rhabdomyosarcoma and marrow involvement in non-Hodgkin lymphoma (NHL).

LABORATORY FEATURES AND DIAGNOSIS

The complete blood count may reveal anemia and/or thrombocytopenia. The white blood cell (WBC) count may be increased or decreased; in either case, it is characterized by neutropenia. Hyperleukocytosis (WBC count >100,000/mm^3) is seen more commonly in ALL than AML. The peripheral blood smear may or may not reveal blasts. Often, they may be reported as atypical lymphocytes or immature cells. Coagulopathy may be present with elevated prothrombin time (PT), partial thromboplastin time (PTT), and fibrinogen degradation products (FDPs).

The diagnosis of leukemia is established by bone marrow aspiration. The presence of 20% blasts confirms the diagnosis of acute leukemia. In case of dry tap, a bone marrow biopsy is needed.

In patients with high WBC, there may be elevation of uric acid and lactate dehydrogenase (LDH). Tumor lysis syndrome is characterized by elevated potassium, phosphorus, uric acid, and depressed calcium.[3] Elevated transaminases and hyperbilirubinemia may, occasionally, be present in cases of extensive liver involvement.

BOX 15.4.1: Investigations recommended for the diagnosis of acute leukemia.

- Complete blood counts with peripheral smear
- *Bone marrow aspiration*: Morphology, immunophenotyping, cytogenetic analysis, FISH, or PCR for specific translocations
- Bone marrow biopsy, if dry tap
- *Cerebrospinal fluid examination*: To look for the presence of blasts
- *Serum electrolytes*: Serum sodium, potassium, chloride, calcium, phosphorus, and magnesium
- Renal function tests
- Liver function tests
- Serum lactate dehydrogenase (LDH)
- Serum uric acid
- *Coagulation profile*: Prothrombin time (PT), activated partial thromboplastin time (APTT), fibrinogen, and D-dimer
- Serology for HIV, HBsAg, anti-HBsAb, and anti-HCV
- Blood grouping
- Quantitative serum immunoglobulin
- Chest X-ray
- Ultrasound of abdomen

(FISH: fluorescence in situ hybridization; HBsAb: hepatitis B surface antibody; HBsAg: hepatitis B surface antigen; HCV: hepatitis C virus; HIV: human immunodeficiency virus; PCR: polymerase chain reaction)

Chest X-ray may reveal a mediastinal mass, more often, in T-cell ALL. Hepatosplenomegaly and, occasionally, nephromegaly may be documented by sonography.

Box 15.4.1 shows the investigations needed for the diagnosis of acute leukemia.

MANAGEMENT

The treatment of acute leukemia involves specific antileukemic therapy and supportive care. Specific antileukemic therapy depends on the subtype of leukemia. At diagnosis, the leukemic tumor burden is approximately 10^{12} cells. Chemotherapy given in phases reduces the leukemia cells exponentially with each cycle.[4,5]

Acute Lymphoblastic Leukemia

In ALL, antileukemic therapy is given in phases with specific aims.

- *Induction chemotherapy* refers to the first 4–6 weeks of chemotherapy designed to induce a remission in the marrow. It typically uses three to four drugs including a steroid (prednisone or dexamethasone), vincristine, and daunorubicin or L-asparaginase along with weekly doses of intrathecal methotrexate. About 90–95% patients achieve a remission at the end of induction chemotherapy.
- *Consolidation chemotherapy* has 16–20 weeks of intensive chemotherapy administered to further decrease the leukemic cell burden in the body. It uses combinations of drugs including cyclophosphamide, cytosine arabinoside, methotrexate, vincristine, and daunorubicin.

- *CNS-directed therapy* is aimed at eliminating the leukemic cells from within the CNS, which are usually shielded by the blood–brain barrier. The components of CNS-directed therapy include cranial irradiation, intrathecal chemotherapy, and high-dose systemic chemotherapy. Cranial irradiation is associated with serious long-term toxicity including neurocognitive dysfunction and secondary malignancies. Newer protocols have documented equivalent results with prolonged intrathecal chemotherapy and high-dose systemic chemotherapy, thus eliminating the use of radiotherapy (RT).
- *Maintenance chemotherapy* is low-dose oral chemotherapy administered for 24–30 months after completion of intensive chemotherapy to clear the marrow of residual leukemic cells. Methotrexate and 6-mercaptopurine are used for maintenance therapy.

Acute Myeloid Leukemia

In AML, induction chemotherapy uses two to three drugs, viz., daunorubicin, cytosine arabinoside, and etoposide. The remission rate is approximately 70%. This is followed by two to four cycles of consolidation chemotherapy usually with cytosine arabinoside. Intrathecal chemotherapy with methotrexate or cytosine arabinoside is used for CNS therapy. There is no established role of the maintenance chemotherapy in AML.

Acute Lymphoblastic Leukemia with t(9;22)

Acute lymphoblastic leukemia with t(9;22), also known as Philadelphia chromosome positive ALL is an aggressive leukemia. Imatinib mesylate is a tyrosine kinase inhibitor (TKI) that binds the adenosine triphosphate (ATP)-binding site of the tyrosine kinase molecule and disrupts its downstream enzymatic activity, thereby inhibiting cell division. Given in combination with chemotherapy, imatinib induces lasting remissions in patients.[6]

Acute Promyelocytic Leukemia

Acute promyelocytic leukemia is a type of AML with a distinct cytogenetic abnormality t(15;17) with the promyelocytic leukemia (PML)/retinoic acid receptor-alpha (RAR-α) fusion. It is characterized by the proliferation of promyelocytes rich in granules that result in disseminated intravascular coagulation. Treatment with all-trans-retinoic acid (ATRA) results in the differentiation of promyelocytes into mature neutrophils leading to the resolution of coagulopathy and to remission.[7]

Minimal Residual Disease

Minimal residual disease (MRD) is the presence of residual leukemic cells below the threshold that can be detected by light microscopy. These low levels of leukemic blasts can be detected by flow cytometry technique or by reverse transcription polymerase chain reaction (RT-PCR). The presence of MRD at the end of induction calls for augmentation of therapy to get rid of these persistent leukemic cells. Risk stratification of the patients on the basis of MRD status is now considered a standard of care in treatment of ALL.[8]

Hematopoietic Stem Cell Transplantation

Most children with leukemia can be cured with chemotherapy. The indications for hematopoietic stem cell transplantation (HSCT) in childhood leukemia are as follows:

- *Very high risk ALL*: Those with poor cytogenetic features or those who fail induction therapy
- Early relapse of ALL
- Late relapse of ALL who fail to respond to chemotherapy
- Second or subsequent relapses of ALL
- AML with poor cytogenetic features or failure of induction therapy

An HLA-matched sibling is the best possible donor for an allogeneic transplant. In the absence of a matched sibling donor, matched unrelated donor from donor registries can be used. Haploidentical bone marrow transplant (BMT) using either of the parents has widened the scope of transplant, especially when matched sibling is not available. The success rate of BMT for relapsed leukemia is about 50%.[9]

Recent Advances

Targeted Therapy

Targeted therapy recognizes and attacks certain targets on the surface of tumor cells such as certain receptors or chromosomal alterations. As a result, the action is very specific, and it spares normal cells.

- *Imatinib,* which targets the *BCR/ABL1* gene rearrangement in the Philadelphia chromosome, has been used successfully along with chemotherapy in the treatment of Ph+ ALL. The development of second-generation TKIs (dasatinib and nilotinib) has helped to overcome imatinib resistance.
- *Nelarabine* has been found effective in the treatment of relapsed T-cell ALL but has a high risk of neurotoxicity.
- *Venetoclax,* a BCL2 inhibitor, is effective in children with relapsed refractory AML. It is being used in clinical trials for children with newly diagnosed AML.

Other new agents with potential role in ALL therapy include FLT3 (FMS-like tyrosine kinase receptor-3) inhibitors, farnesyltransferase inhibitors, proteasome inhibitors (bortezomib), demethylating agents (decitabine), and histone deacetylase inhibitors (vorinostat).

Monoclonal antibody therapy with promising results includes rituximab (anti-CD20 antibody) and epratuzumab (anti-CD22).

Antibody-drug conjugate inotuzumab ozogamicin (anti-CD22 antibody conjugate) has been approved for the treatment of relapsed refractory ALL, and gemtuzumab ozogamicin (anti-CD33 antibody conjugate) has been approved for the treatment of relapse refractory AML in children.

Immunotherapy

Our body's immune surveillance mechanism is responsible for suppressing thousands of potentially carcinogenic events every day. Since cancer is caused by the failure of immune surveillance to thwart these events, immunotherapy aims to activate the immune system and eliminate the cancer cells from the body.

Chimeric Antigen Receptor T-cell Therapy

In chimeric antigen receptor (CAR) T-cell therapy, patients' T-cells are collected by apheresis and modified in vitro to alter their antigen receptor. When reintroduced in the patient's body, these modified cells recognize the leukemic cells and mount an immune response to eliminate them.[10]

Tisagenlecleucel is an anti-CD19 CAR T-cell drug that is effective and is approved for the treatment of relapse refractory B-cell ALL in children.

Blinatumomab, a bispecific anti-CD19/CD3 chimeric antibody (BiTE), helps to bring malignant cells and T-cells in close proximity, resulting in cell lysis. It has shown encouraging results in relapsed/refractory disease and those with persistent MRD.

SUPPORTIVE CARE

Supportive care involves the management of emergencies that the patient may present with at diagnosis and the management of complications during therapy.

Emergencies

Emergencies at diagnosis include obstructive conditions such as the *superior vena cava syndrome* and the *superior mediastinal syndrome*, metabolic conditions such as *tumor lysis syndrome* and hematological conditions such as *severe anemia and bleeding*.

Children with superior vena cava and superior mediastinal syndrome need prompt care in the intensive care unit (ICU) with close monitoring. Patients should be kept in the propped-up position to prevent the mediastinal mass from further compressing the airway and the great vessels.

Intravenous (IV) hydration should be started using a leg vein to avoid aggravating the congestive symptoms in the upper body. Once a diagnostic specimen has been obtained, the patient can be started on steroids, which give rapid relief by shrinking the mass.

Patients with hyperleukocytosis (WBC count >100,000/mm^3) may present with symptoms of thrombosis or with tumor lysis syndrome with hyperkalemia, hyperuricemia, hyperphosphatemia, and hypocalcemia.

Tumor lysis syndrome occurs within 7 days of starting cytotoxic therapy or due to spontaneous cell lysis even before starting the treatment.

Allopurinol, a xanthine oxidase inhibitor, helps to prevent the formation of uric acid. Rasburicase, a urate oxidase helps in degrading uric acid converting it into the water-soluble allantoin, which is easily excreted by the kidneys.

Supportive care during therapy includes blood component therapy and aggressive management of infectious complications.

Packed red blood cell (RBC) transfusions are indicated to maintain hemoglobin over 8 g/dL. Platelet transfusions are indicated if platelet count is <10,000/mm^3 or in the case of overt bleeding, especially in patients with fever and infection.

Every episode of febrile neutropenia should be treated aggressively with broad-spectrum antibiotics.

All patients should receive prophylaxis for *Pneumocystis carinii* pneumonia with cotrimoxazole and for oral candidiasis with clotrimazole lozenges.

Maintenance of oral and perianal hygiene reduces the risk of infections to a significant extent. The use of hematopoietic growth factors [granulocyte colony-stimulating factor (GCSF) reduces the period of neutropenia.

PROGNOSIS AND OUTCOME

Treatment outcomes in ALL depend on several factors:

- *Patient-related factors*—age, sex, ethnicity, and underlying immunodeficiency
- *Disease-related factors*—presenting WBC count, CNS involvement, lineage, subtypc, chromosomal abnormality, and ploidy
- *Treatment-related factors*—chemotherapy regimens and their intensity

The early response to treatment as judged by the clearance of blasts from the peripheral blood by day 7 of therapy is a good indicator of prognosis.

The presence of MRD at the end of induction is now considered the best predictor of outcome. Risk stratification based on the earlier-mentioned features helps tailor therapy to ensure the best results with the least toxicity.

Table 15.4.3 shows the risk stratification of ALL.

Presently, the cure rates in ALL in developed countries are as high as 79–86%. Studies from India have reported cure rates of 40–60%. Cure rates for AML are about 60–80% in developed countries and around 30–40% in developing countries.

TABLE 15.4.3: Risk stratification of acute lymphoblastic leukemia.

Risk stratification	Features
Low risk	Age 1–9 years, WBC count <50,000/mm^3, pre-B ALL, trisomy 4 and 10, hyperdiploidy, t(12;21)
Standard risk	Age 1–9 years, WBC count <50,000/mm^3, pre-B ALL, normal cytogenetics
High risk	Age <1 year and >9 years, WBC count >50,000/mm^3, T-cell ALL, CNS involvement, hypodiploidy, positive MRD after induction
Very high risk	t(9;22), t(4;11), induction failure

(ALL: acute lymphoblastic leukemia; CNS: central nervous system; MRD: minimal residual disease; WBC: white blood cell)

PRACTICE GUIDELINES

- Always establish a complete and accurate diagnosis before committing a patient to therapy.
- Treat the patient according to published protocols without undue deviations to ensure the best outcomes.
- Promptly initiate broad-spectrum antibiotics during febrile neutropenia treating it as a medical emergency.
- Lifelong follow-up of leukemia survivors is important to monitor for late effects and secondary malignancies.

KEY MESSAGES

- The incidence of leukemia is high enough for all pediatricians to maintain a high index of suspicion in children with unusual symptoms.
- Refer a suspected case of leukemia early to a tertiary center, as early diagnosis can make a significant difference in the outcome of this curable disease.
- Be wary of administering steroids to a patient suspected of having leukemia. It can precipitate tumor lysis syndrome, and sometimes, mask the diagnosis.
- If a patient is severely anemic, packed RBC transfusion can be given before transfer to a tertiary center as it can be lifesaving.

REFERENCES

1. Alaggio R, Amador C, Anagnostopoulos I, Attygalle AD, de Oliveira Araujo IB, Berti E, et al. The 5th edition of the World Health Organization Classification of Haematolymphoid Tumours: Lymphoid Neoplasms. Leukemia. 2022;36(7):1720-48.
2. Khoury JD, Solary E, Abla O, Akkari Y, Alaggio R, Apperley JF, et al. The 5th edition of the World Health Organization Classification of Haematolymphoid Tumours: Myeloid and Histiocytic/Dendritic Neoplasms. Leukemia. 2022;36(7):1703-19.
3. Howard SC, Jones, DP, Pui C-H. The Tumor Lysis Syndrome. N Eng J Med. 2011;364(19):1844-54.
4. Cooper SL, Brown PA. Treatment of pediatric acute lymphoblastic leukemia. Pediatr Clin North Am. 2015;62(1):61-73.
5. Kim H. Treatments for children and adolescents with AML. Blood Res. 2020;55(S1):S5-S13.
6. Ganguly S, Sasi A, Pushpam D, Bakhshi S. Philadelphia Chromosome Positive and Philadelphia-Like Acute Lymphoblastic Leukemia in Children and Adolescents: Current Management, Controversies and Emerging Concepts. Indian J Pediatr. 2024;91(1):37-46.
7. Gurnari C, Voso MT, Girardi K, Mastronuzzi A, Strocchio L. Acute Promyelocytic Leukemia in Children: A Model of Precision Medicine and Chemotherapy-Free Therapy. Int J Mol Sci. 2021;22(2):642.
8. Campana D, Pui CH. Minimal residual disease-guided therapy in childhood acute lymphoblastic leukemia. Blood. 2017;129(14):1913-8.
9. Truong TH, Jinca C, Mann G, Arghirescu S, Buechner J, Merli P, et al. Allogeneic Hematopoietic Stem Cell Transplantation for Children with Acute Lymphoblastic Leukemia: Shifting Indications in the Era of Immunotherapy. Front Pediatr. 2021;9:782785.
10. Boettcher M, Joechner A, Li Z, Yang SF, Schlegel P. Development of CAR T Cell Therapy in Children-A Comprehensive Overview. J Clin Med. 2022;11(8):2158.

15.5 Hodgkin Lymphoma

Amita Mahajan

INTRODUCTION

Hodgkin lymphoma (HL) was one of first cancers for which cure could be achieved both in adults and children. It continues to be the malignancy with overall cure rates exceeding 80% even in resource-limited settings. This condition, because of such high survival rates and availability of long-term follow-up of previously treated cohorts has also given us valuable lessons on the late effects of cancer treatment and the importance of survivorship clinics. A significant proportion of children and adults treated a few decades ago were detected to have serious side effects many years after completion of therapy attributable both to radiotherapy (RT) and chemotherapy. This has led to significant modifications and evolution of therapeutic strategies to ensure limiting the late-effects as much as possible. In the current era HL is the best example on how the focus is as much on curing the disease as much as limiting the late side effects secondary to treatment. This has meant that the treatment approach in children and adolescents is now considerably different than that employed in adults with HL.

The successful management of HL also highlights the importance of multicentric collaborative research that allows us to answer specific questions in relatively a short span of time for rare conditions like childhood cancer. Whilst research from the developed world often guides management in our setting, it is important to evaluate the management strategies in our patients as there may be biological differences and limitations in access to treatments used in the developed countries.

Prospective collaborative research has also come of age in India with the development of the Indian Pediatric Hematology Oncology Group (INPHOG) and HL is one of the first conditions for which such work has yielded important information regarding epidemiology and outcomes in our setting.[1]

EPIDEMIOLOGY

The HL comprises of 6% of all childhood cancer with approximately 4,500 new cases in India each year in the 0–18 years age group. In the developed countries, the median age at diagnosis is 15 years with M:F ratio of 1.2:1. Epidemiological data from India and other low-middle income countries consistently shows that the median age at diagnosis is much lower with a significantly higher male predominance. This is attributed to the underlying etiology. The vast proportion of patients in low/middle-income countries (LMICs) have Epstein–Barr virus (EBV) driven disease with its predilection for the younger male child.[2]

ETIOLOGY

The vast majority of patients from India have EBV-driven disease. In addition, patients with immunodeficiency have a higher incidence of HL. Specifically patients with human immunodeficiency virus (HIV), and posttransplant immunosuppression have a higher incidence of HL than the general population.

CLINICAL PRESENTATION

Patients usually present with painless lymphadenopathy, most often involving the cervical and supraclavicular lymph nodes, but may involve any lymph node region sometimes reaching very large dimensions or bulky disease. The patients may otherwise be entirely asymptomatic. Mediastinal adenopathy is seen more often in adolescents and is unusual in younger children. Involvement of the spleen can be seen at all ages. HL may also involve extralymphatic sites such as the liver, spleen, lungs, bones, bone-marrow, pleural, and pericardium.

Patients may have systemic symptoms, i.e., fever, weight loss, anorexia, fatigue, pruritus, and night sweats due to the cytokines released from the Reed–Sternberg (RS) cells, the hallmark cells of HL on histopathological examination.

DIAGNOSIS

The diagnosis is based on excision biopsy of a peripheral node. Excision biopsy is preferred over fine needle aspiration cytology, as the disease originates from the germinal centers and a fine-needle aspiration cytology (FNAC) may be falsely negative and miss the diagnosis **(Fig. 15.5.1)**. However, clinical situations wherein this is not feasible or may require a major surgical procedure, for e.g., when disease is confined to the mediastinum or retroperitoneal region, an image-guided core biopsy may be performed. In LMIC, it continues to be common practice to commence patients on empirical

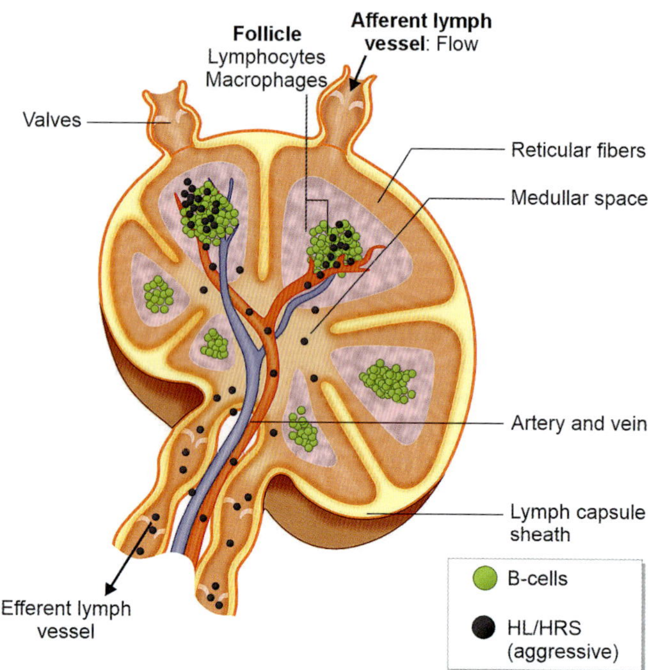

Fig. 15.5.1: Structure of a lymph node with HL. The black dots represent the Hodgkin Reed–Sternberg cells. The diagram depicts their origin and exemplifies why a fine-needle aspiration cytology (FNAC) can miss the diagnosis. (HL: Hodgkin lymphoma; HRS: Hodgkin and Reed–Sternberg)

antitubercular treatment based on clinical picture alone despite clear guidelines to the contrary and should be actively discouraged.[3]

The biopsy procedure may warrant general anesthesia for excision biopsy or sedation for a core biopsy. It is important to remember that in patients with large mediastinal masses, the airway may be compromised and sedation may be hazardous precipitating a respiratory arrest. In such patients, search for an alternative site to biopsy or doing the procedure without any sedation should be explored as this site is involved in relatively older children.

Histology

The classical RS cell is the hallmark of HL. HL is characterized by multinucleated giant Hodgkin and Reed–Sternberg (HRS) cells **(Fig. 15.5.2)** surrounded by inflammatory cells comprising of lymphocytes, histiocytes, eosinophils, and plasma cells. The HRS cell is binucleate or multinucleate cell with a characteristic bilobed nucleus.

In HL tissue, the RS cells are just a small minority and the vast majority are inflammatory cells. Patients are classified as having as "classical HL" or a more indolent subtype known as "nodular lymphocytic predominant HL" (NLPHL). Patients with classical HL are further classified as having lymphocyte

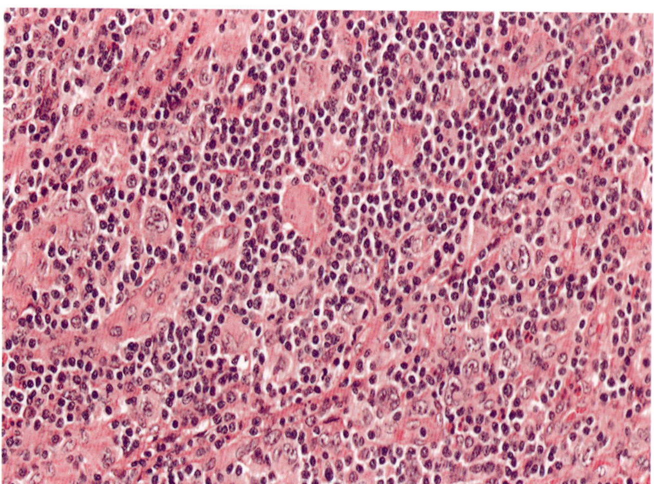

Fig. 15.5.2: Reed–Sternberg cells surrounded by inflammatory cells.

predominant, mixed cellularity, nodular sclerosis, and lymphocyte depleted variants. On immunohistochemistry, the HL cells are always positive for CD30 and about 70% are positive for CD15. The NLPHL variants are, positive for CD20 but negative for CD30.

There are again geographical variations with mixed-cellularity being the most common histology in LMIC due to high prevalence of EBV-driven disease in contrast to the developed countries wherein, nodular sclerosis is the most common histology in children. The histology within the classical HL cohort does not impact treatment or prognosis in contemporary protocols.

Staging

The ideal modality for staging and indeed assessment of response in patients with HL is 18F-fluorodeoxyglucose positron emission tomography (18F-FDG PET) which integrates functional and anatomical characteristics of the tumor. It identifies areas with anaerobic glycolysis and increased metabolic activity. In addition, children with disease that is staged IIB and above warrant bone marrow (BM) aspiration and biopsy to identify BM involvement. PET-computed tomographies (CTs) are sensitive in identifying marrow involvement but there are studies underway whether this procedure can be omitted if a PET-CT is available. The Lugano classification for staging has replaced the Ann Arbor classification which was more widely used previously.[4]

Patients are classified as having B symptoms if they have unexplained fever, unexplained weight loss >10% in the preceding 6 months and drenching night sweats. In the pre-FDG era, bulky disease was a significant risk factor and patients with bulky disease received radiation in addition to

TABLE 15.5.1: Staging in patients with Hodgkin lymphoma.

Stage I	Involvement of a single nodal or extralymphatic side
Stage II	Involvement of two/more nodal or extralymphatic sites on the same side of the diaphragm
Stage III	Involvement of nodal/extralymphatic sites on both sides of the diaphragm
Stage IV	Involvement of liver, lungs, bones, bone marrow
E	Involvement of an extralymphatic site
S	Splenic involvement

chemotherapy. Bulk is defined as peripheral adenopathy in excess of 6 cm or mediastinal adenopathy greater than one-third of the maximal diameter on a posteroanterior upright radiograph or volume of a contiguous lymph node mass in excess of 200 mL at any site.

Patients with Stage I or II without B symptoms (weight loss, fever, and night sweats) are classified as having early stage disease, Stage IIB and IIIA as intermediate stage, and Stage III with B symptoms or Stage IV as advanced disease. Some groups incorporate erythrocyte sedimentation rate (ESR), and bulk in the risk stratification **(Table 15.5.1)**.

MANAGEMENT

Current management employs a *risk-stratified* and *response-adapted* approach. Whilst different groups have minor differences in their approach to risk-stratification, factors that impact risk are stage, presence or absence of B symptoms, and bulky disease, involvement of extranodal sites, and raised ESR. All patients receive similar therapy initially but the number of cycles of chemotherapy is based on the initial risk-stratification and response to the initial cycles of chemotherapy.

Patients are reassessed after the first phase of chemotherapeutic treatment, usually after two cycles and further treatment is adapted to the early-interim response assessment (ERA). It is increasingly recognized that ERA is the most significant prognostic indicator and guides clinical management in individual patients. 18F-FDG-PET is now the standard of care for response evaluation.[5,6] A semiquantitative scoring system Deauville score (DS) is used to quantify response. Patients with DS 1 to 3 at ERA are deemed to have adequate response and those with DS 4 or 5 as having a suboptimal response. When done at the end of treatment, patients with DS 1 and 2 are qualified as having complete response. Whilst access to this modality is improving rapidly, sites where this modality is not available can employ contrast-enhanced computed tomography (CECT) for staging and reassessment. Patients with suboptimal response at ERA receive additional therapy usually in the form of radiation therapy after the completion of chemotherapy.

The HL is the perfect example of a risk-stratified, response-adapted therapeutic strategy aimed at achieving high cure rates but limiting the intensity of treatment for those with favorable disease to minimize the late-effects seen previously.[7] At the same time, this strategy allows the option of intensifying treatment for patients with unfavorable disease and optimize the outcome.

Chemotherapy

This forms the backbone of current treatment protocols. All patients except a minority with NLPHL receive chemotherapy. All groups employ a combination of noncross-resistant drugs. Also the doses of anthracyclines are much lower than those used in the past in an attempt to eliminate the risk of late cardiotoxicity. The most commonly used drugs are adriamycin, bleomycin, vinca alkaloids, dacarbazine, corticosteroids, cyclophosphamide, and etoposide. Increasingly, the focus is on limiting exposure to alkylating drugs and bleomycin which are believed to contribute significantly to the late morbidity seen in the past. The duration and intensity of therapy is titrated based on the stage at diagnosis and response at ERA with patients with advanced stage at diagnosis receiving higher number of chemotherapy cycles. Some collaborative groups incorporate gender and age in decision-making as male gonads are far more susceptible to the gonadotoxic effects of chemotherapy, and adolescent females at a much risk of carcinoma breast following radiation.

Contemporary protocols are largely chemotherapy based with radiation reserved for patients with suboptimal ERA.

Radiation

The HL is a very radiosensitive disease and in the past cure has been achieved by using radiation alone in selected cases. The recognition that much of the late morbidity noted in survivors of HL such as hypothyroidism, cardiopulmonary toxicity, and second malignant neoplasms is, at least in a significant measure, secondary to the radiation exposure has led to the restricted use of this modality in HL.[8] In children with HL as in many other diseases, efforts are made to omit or limit radiation to the proportion of children for whom it meets the risk-benefit ratio. A number of studies have been undertaken to identify the cohort of patients in whom it can be safely omitted without compromising the cure rates. Currently, in most protocols, RT is limited to patients with suboptimal response at ERA. Some groups use it for patients with bulky disease at the sites of bulky disease.

Where radiation is deemed necessary for cure, the doses as well as the fields are much lower (15–25 Gy) than the significantly higher doses (35–40 Gy) employed in the past. Where needed, the doses and the radiation fields are limited to the involved site (ISRT) or involved nodal region (INRT).

Treatment of Patients with Nodular Lymphocytic Predominant Hodgkin Lymphoma

This entity is rare in children and patients tend to have localized disease without systemic symptoms. In a small minority of patients with NLPHL, excision of the involved itself may be curative. Other patients where this is not feasible can be cured with short duration chemotherapy with or without immunotherapy or involved node RT.

PROGNOSIS

Overall, patients with HL have excellent outcome and over 80–90% can hope to achieve long-term cure with contemporary management strategies. Factors that impact prognosis at diagnosis adversely are incorporated in the risk-stratification and can be overcome with risk-directed therapy. Pleural and pericardial effusion are unusual but associated with inferior prognosis as are lower hemoglobin and albumin. Response to initial treatment (ERA) has emerged as the most important prognostic indicator and allows the opportunity to titrate subsequent therapy.

MANAGEMENT OF RELAPSED DISEASE

Most patients with relapsed disease can be salvaged using intensive salvage chemotherapy, radiation, and hematopoietic stem cell transplant (HSCT). The treatment strategy in individual patients depends on the timing of relapse since completion of therapy (less than vs. more than 12 months), site of relapse, systemic symptoms, and treatment given initially. Myeloablative chemotherapy with autologous HSCT is recommended for patients with refractory disease, early relapse or relapse in patients who have received adjuvant RT in the frontline setting. Those who relapse following HSCT can increasingly be salvaged employing novel therapeutic strategies now available to us and sometimes allogeneic HSCT. Whilst access to these modalities is currently limited owing to their high costs, this is expected to improve in the future.

NOVEL TREATMENTS

Monoclonal Antibody

Brentuximab vedotin is a monoclonal antibody against CD30 surface receptor which is positive in all patients with HL. There is now adequate evidence regarding the safety and efficacy of this agent in combination with chemotherapy. To begin with, this agent was employed in the setting of relapsed and refractory disease defined as inability to achieve remission with frontline therapy. There is now clinical experience with this agent in front-line setting as well which allows omission of certain chemotherapy drugs thereby limiting chemotherapy associated toxicity in these young patients. It may also help improve outcomes in patients with advanced disease.

Immunotherapy

This is a novel approach currently being used or evaluated for a number of cancers with the most robust evidence in HL. Agents that block the interaction between programmed death-1 (PD-1) and its ligands have shown high levels of activity in adults and children with HL. The two agents with the most evidence are nivolumab and pembrolizumab. They are currently approved for use in relapsed/refractory setting but in view of their safety and efficacy ongoing studies are evaluating their role in front-line therapy.

Chimeric antigen receptor (CAR) T-cell therapy using patient's autologous T-cells and genetically modifying them to attach to specific receptors on the cancer cells to kill them, has shown impressive results in relapsed or refractory B-lineage acute lymphoblastic leukemia. CAR T-cells targeting CD30 are currently being evaluated.

SURVIVORSHIP

Longitudinal cohort studies of patients with HL treated in the past highlights the significance of survivorship clinics and life-long follow-up of these patients.[9] Surveillance for recurrent disease can be carried out with clinical examination and conventional imaging. Depending on treatment received, they also need to be screened for late complications of treatment related both to specific chemotherapeutic exposures and radiation.[10] The late effects include cardiomyopathy (secondary to anthracyclines), restrictive lung disease, hypothyroidism, gonadotoxicity, and most devastatingly second malignant neoplasms.

CONCLUSION

- HL is a highly curable disease even in resource-limited settings.
- The clinical presentation is usually of painless adenopathy with or without systemic symptoms and an excision biopsy is warranted.
- The treatment paradigm is risk-stratified and response adapted.
- Early response to treatment is the best prognostic indicator.
- Contemporary protocols are focused on limiting long-term treatment-related toxicity without compromising the excellent outcomes.

REFERENCES

1. Arora RS, Raj R, Mahajan A, Radhakrishnan N, Chinnaswamy G, Banavali S. Collaborative cancer research: progress report from the Indian Pediatric Oncology Group. Lancet Child Adolesc Health. 2021;5(4):239-40.

2. Rani P, Jain M, Verma N, Kumar A, Jain A, Tripathi AK, et al. Epstein-Barr Virus Expression in Classic Hodgkin Lymphoma in an Indian Cohort and its Association with Clinical and Histomorphological Parameters. Indian J Hematol Blood Transfus. 2021;37(3):372-8.
3. Mahajan A, Bakhshi S, Singh M, Seth R, Verma N, Jain S, et al. Empirical Antitubercular Treatment for Lymphadenopathy: Are We Missing Lymphoma? Indian J Pediatr. 2023;90(8): 761-5.
4. Cheson BD, Fisher RI, Barrington SF, Cavalli F, Schwartz LH, Zucca E, et al. Recommendations for initial evaluation, staging, and response assessment of Hodgkin and non-Hodgkin lymphoma: the Lugano classification. J Clin Oncol. 2014;32(27):3059-68.
5. Hutchings M, Loft A, Hansen M, Pedersen LM, Buhi T, Jurlander J, et al. FDG-PET after two cycles of chemotherapy predicts treatment failure and progression-free survival in Hodgkin lymphoma. Blood. 2006;107(1):52-9.
6. Younes A, Hilden P, Coiffier B, Hagenbeek A, Salles G, Wilson W, et al.. International Working Group consensus response evaluation criteria in lymphoma (RECIL 2017). Ann Oncol. 2017;28(7):1436-47.
7. Kelly KM. Hodgkin lymphoma in children and adolescents: improving the therapeutic index. Hematology Am Soc Hematol Educ Program. 2015;2015:514-21.
8. Giulino-Roth L, Pei Q, Buxton A, Bush R, Wu Y, Wolden SL, et al. Subsequent malignant neoplasms among children with Hodgkin lymphoma: a report from the Children's Oncology Group. Blood. 2021;137(11):1449-56.
9. Castellino SM, Geiger AM, Mertens AC, Leisenring WM, Tooze JA, Goodman P, et al. Morbidity and mortality in long-term survivors of Hodgkin lymphoma: a report from the Childhood Cancer Survivor Study. Blood. 2011;117(6):1806-16.
10. Ng AK. Current survivorship recommendations for patients with Hodgkin lymphoma: focus on late effects. Blood. 2014;124(23):3373-9.

15.6 Non-Hodgkin Lymphoma

Ruchira Misra

INTRODUCTION

Non-Hodgkin lymphomas (NHLs) were first described by Denis Parson Burkitt, an Irish surgeon working in Africa in the 1950s.[1] Since then, many advances have occurred in the classification and treatment of NHL. It is the third most common disease in children and adolescents.[2] The incidence of NHL in Western countries is approximately 5–6 per million children younger than 15 years, and 10–17 per million between the ages of 15 and 19 years.[2] Approximately 2,500 cases of childhood NHL are estimated to occur annually in India. Age-related changes in the incidence, biology, distribution, and treatment affect the survival of these children. It occurs most commonly in the second decade of life and less frequently in children younger than 3 years. Immunodeficiency, both congenital (e.g., ataxia-telangiectasia and Wiskott–Aldrich syndrome) and acquired [human immunodeficiency virus (HIV) infection or post-transplant], increases the risk of NHL. Indeed, NHL is the most frequent malignancy in children with acquired immunodeficiency syndrome (AIDS). With current treatment modalities, about 80% of children and adolescents with NHL will survive at least 5 years.

CLASSIFICATION

Rappaport, in 1966, gave the first classification of NHL, dividing them into nodular and diffuse. Since then, the classification has changed, with the most recent classification being provided by World Health Organization (WHO). **Table 15.6.1** summarizes the commonly used classification systems.[3]

CHROMOSOMAL TRANSLOCATIONS IN NON-HODGKIN LYMPHOMAS

The theory in the development of pediatric cancers postulates that several "hits" occur in a normal cell, which alters the functions such as cell cycle control, proliferation, apoptosis, and cell death. These hits could happen in the oncogenes, tumor suppressor genes, or passenger genes. Different genomic aberrations, such as chromosomal translocations, single nucleotide variants, or copy number changes, lead to oncogene activation and tumor-suppressor gene inactivation. In pediatric B-cell NHL, some of these translocations have been identified **(Table 15.6.2)**.[3]

CLINICAL PRESENTATION

The NHL is a heterogeneous disease and may have a varied presentation. In children, the clinical presentation may differ from that in adults as the disease has a more aggressive course and usually an extranodal presentation. Presentations may also vary on the type of NHL. The disease is seen more in males than females.

TABLE 15.6.1: Different classifications of non-Hodgkin lymphoma over time.

Rappaport, 1956 (1966)	***Working formulation (1982)***
Well-differentiated lymphocytic lymphoma	Large cell immunoblastic
Poorly differentiated lymphocytic lymphoma	Lymphoblastic
Histiocytic/mixed lymphoma	Small noncleaved cell (Burkitt and non-Burkitt type)
Burkitt lymphoma	Diffuse large cell
Lukes and Collins classification, 1974	
B-cell	*T-cell*
Large noncleaved follicular center cell (FCC)	Convoluted lymphocytic
Small noncleaved FCC	Undefined
Burkitt type	Unclassifiable
Immunoblastic	Immunoblastic
REAL classification, International Lymphoma Study Group (1994)	
B-cell	*T-cell*
Precursor B-cell neoplasm	*Precursor T-cell neoplasm:* T-cell and natural killer cell neoplasm
Precursor B-lymphoblastic leukemia/lymphoma	Precursor T-lymphoblastic lymphoma/leukemia
Mature (peripheral) B-cell lymphoma/leukemia	Mature (peripheral) T-cell lymphoma/leukemia
Diffuse large B-cell lymphoma	Anaplastic large cell lymphoma (ALCL), T-/null cell, primary cutaneous type
Mediastinal large B-cell lymphoma	ALCL, T-/null cell, primary systemic type
Burkitt lymphoma/Burkitt cell leukemia	Peripheral T-cell lymphoma, not otherwise characterized
World Health Organization (WHO) 2008; Revised 2016	
B-cell	*T-cell*
Precursor B-cell neoplasm	Precursor T-cell neoplasm
Precursor B-lymphoblastic leukemia/lymphoma	Precursor T-lymphoblastic leukemia/lymphoma
Precursor B-cell acute lymphoblastic leukemia	Precursor T-cell acute lymphoblastic leukemia
Mature (peripheral) B-cell neoplasm	Mature (peripheral) T-cell neoplasm
Diffuse large B-cell lymphoma	Peripheral T-cell lymphoma, not otherwise characterized
Mediastinal large B-cell lymphoma	Anaplastic large cell lymphoma, T-/null cell, primary cutaneous type
Burkitt lymphoma/Burkitt cell leukemia	Anaplastic large cell lymphoma, T-/null cell, primary systemic type
Pediatric follicular lymphoma (2016)	EBV + T-cell lymphoma of childhood (2016)

(EBV: Epstein–Barr virus)
Source: Abla O, Attarbaschi A. Non-Hodgkin's Lymphoma in Childhood and Adolescence, 1st edition. Cham, Switzerland; Springer Nature; 2019.

Aggressive NHLs typically present as a rapidly growing mass with systemic symptoms such as fever, night sweats, and weight loss (B symptoms). Indolent lymphomas often present only with slow-growing lymphadenopathy, hepatomegaly, splenomegaly, or cytopenia. The less common presentations include skin rash, pruritus, hypersensitivity to insect stings and bites, generalized fatigue, malaise, fever of unknown origin, ascites, and effusions. Those with involvement of the gastrointestinal (GI) system may present with anorexia, weight loss, abdominal distention, nausea, vomiting, respiratory compromise due to mass effect, and even GI bleeding or perforation. Those with central nervous system (CNS) lymphoma may have headaches, lethargy, facial neurologic symptoms, seizures, paralysis, spinal cord compression, and features of meningitis. Anaplastic large cell lymphoma (ALCL) and lymphoblastic lymphoma have a propensity for skin involvement or present as a mediastinal mass. These patients tend to present with oncological emergencies such as superior vena cava (SVC) syndrome or with tumor lysis syndrome (which may be spontaneous also).

TABLE 15.6.2: Translocations associated with non-Hodgkin lymphoma.

Disease	*Translocation*	*Partner gene*
Large B-cell lymphoma (LBCL) with IRF4 rearrangement	p12; q25	*IRF4*
Large B-cell lymphoma (LBCL) with IRF4 rearrangement	t (6;22) (p25; q11)	*IRF4*
Large B-cell lymphoma (LBCL) with IRF4 rearrangement	t (6;14) (p25; q32)	*IRF4*
Burkitt lymphoma	t (2;8) (p12; q24)	*MYC*
Burkitt lymphoma Diffuse large B-cell lymphoma	t (8;14) (q24; q32)	*MYC*
Burkitt lymphoma Aggressive B-cell lymphoma	t (14;16) (q32; q24)	*CBFA2T3*
Diffuse large B-cell lymphoma	t (9;14) (p13; q32)	*PAX5*
Diffuse large B-cell lymphoma Follicular lymphoma	q32; q21	*BCL2*
Diffuse large B-cell lymphoma Follicular lymphoma	t (3;14) (q27; q32)	*BCL6*

Source: Abla O, Attarbaschi A. Non-Hodgkin's Lymphoma in Childhood and Adolescence, 1st edition. Cham, Switzerland; Springer Nature; 2019.

EVALUATION

Pediatric NHLs are aggressive tumors; hence, a rapid diagnosis is imperative. The evaluation should include the tests mentioned in **Box 15.6.1**. If the patient is sick and decompensating, do the least invasive tests needed to establish the diagnosis. For those who present with mediastinal masses and SVC syndrome, sedation for procedures may be risky, as intubation and ventilation may be difficult because of tumor compression of the big and small bronchi and bronchioles, and hence, it should be avoided if possible.[4]

BOX 15.6.1: Evaluation of a child suspected to have non-Hodgkin lymphoma.

- *Good history and impeccable physical examination* (including the testes and the fundus)
- *Complete blood counts (CBCs) with a peripheral smear*
- *Biochemistry:* Blood urea, uric acid, lactic dehydrogenase (LDH), calcium, phosphorus, sodium, and potassium
- *Radiology:* X-ray chest, ultrasound, contrast-enhanced computed tomography (CT) scan or magnetic resonance imaging (MRI) of the primary site, positron emission tomography (PET) scan
- *Biopsy:* Adequate tissue must be collected for morphology, immunohistochemistry, and for cytogenetics/molecular studies
- *Cerebrospinal fluid (CSF) for malignant cytology*

Source: Arora B. Lymphoma. In: Parthasarathy A, Menon PSN, Nair MKC (Eds). IAP Textbook of Pediatrics, 7th edition; 2019. pp. 957-64.

Burkitt Lymphoma

Burkitt lymphoma accounts for about 50% of childhood NHL and exhibits consistent, aggressive clinical behavior. The malignant cells show a mature B-cell phenotype, and the tumor has a "starry sky" appearance. Burkitt lymphoma expresses a characteristic chromosomal translocation, usually t(8;14) and rarely t(8;22) or t(2;8). Each of these translocations juxtaposes the *c-myc* gene, the gene involved in cellular proliferation, to immunoglobulin locus regulatory elements, resulting in the inappropriate expression of *c-myc*. The two most common primary disease sites are the head and neck region and the abdomen.

In India, these patients usually present with abdominal pain, vomiting, abdominal distension, palpable mass, intussusception, ascites, obstructive jaundice, or hepatosplenomegaly (sporadic presentation). Endemic Burkitt lymphoma is common in Africa, presents as jaw mass in most cases, and is usually associated with Epstein-Barr virus (EBV) infection. Burkitt lymphoma is also common with immunodeficiencies like the HIV. Other sites of involvement include testes, bone, peripheral lymph nodes, skin, bone marrow, and central nervous system (CNS). Burkitt lymphoma is famous for its aggressive presentation and rapid tumor lysis. These tumors are very responsive to chemotherapy and have good cure rates.

Diffuse Large B-cell Lymphoma

Diffuse large B-cell lymphoma (DLBCL) is a mature B-cell neoplasm representing 10–20% of pediatric NHL. DLBCL occurs more frequently during the second decade of life than the first. Pediatric DLBCL may present clinically similar to Burkitt lymphoma, though it is more often localized and less usually involves the bone marrow or CNS. Outcomes for children with DLBCL are more favorable than those observed in adults, with overall 5-year event-free survival (EFS) rates of approximately 90% at 5 years. About 20% of pediatric DLBCL present as a primary mediastinal disease [primary mediastinal B-cell lymphoma (PMBCL)]. This presentation is more common in older children and adolescents and is associated with an inferior outcome compared with other types of pediatric DLBCL.

Lymphoblastic Lymphoma

Lymphoblastic lymphoma (LL) makes up approximately 20% of childhood NHL. More than 75% of LL have a T-cell immunophenotype; the remainder have a precursor B-cell phenotype. Nearly 75% of patients with LL present with an anterior mediastinal mass and symptoms of dyspnea, wheezing, stridor, dysphagia, or swelling of the head and neck suggestive of SVC syndrome. Pleural effusion may be present, and the involvement of lymph nodes, usually above the diaphragm, maybe a prominent feature. There may also be involvement of bone, skin, bone marrow, CNS, abdominal organs (but rarely bowel), and occasionally, other sites such as lymphoid tissue of Waldeyer's ring and testes. Patients with >25% marrow blasts are considered to have leukemia, and those with fewer than 25% marrow blasts are deemed to have lymphoma.

Anaplastic Large Cell Lymphoma

Anaplastic large cell lymphoma (ALCL) accounts for approximately 10% of childhood NHL. While the predominant immunophenotype of ALCL is mature T-cell, null-cell disease [i.e., no T-cell, B-cell, or natural killer (NK)-cell surface antigen expression] does occur. More than 90% of ALCL cases have the translocation t(2;5)(p23;q35) leading to the expression of the fusion protein nucleophosmin (NPM)/anaplastic lymphoma kinase (ALK). Clinically, ALCL has a broad range of presentations, including involvement of lymph nodes and various extranodal sites, particularly skin, bone, gastrointestinal tract, lung, pleura, and muscle. Involvement of the CNS and bone marrow is uncommon. ALCL is often associated with systemic symptoms (e.g., fever and weight loss) and a prolonged waxing and waning course, making diagnosis difficult and usually delayed.

STAGING AND PROGNOSTICATION

It is essential to stage these neoplasms, as this defines their prognosis and the treatment we can offer. The St. Jude classification for staging NHL was developed over 35 years ago. It is primarily based on clinicopathologic features of childhood Burkitt lymphoma and LL. Staging is determined by the number and anatomic pattern of disease sites, their resectability, and the involvement of marrow and the CNS. Since then, the pathologic classification of NHL has changed significantly. New subtypes of pediatric NHL have been identified, some of which display unique patterns of organ involvement, including mucosal sites, skin, bone, ovary, and kidney.

Murphy's Classification or St Jude Classification

This is detailed in **Table 15.6.3**.[5]

Therapy Stratification by Group

Group A: Completely resected stage I or completely resected abdominal stage II lesions.

Group B: All cases not eligible for Group A or Group C (Murphy Stage III and non-CNS Stage IV).

Group C: Any CNS and/or bone marrow involvement ≥25% blasts. For CNS involvement, one or more of the following applies:

- Any L3 blasts in cerebrospinal fluid
- Cranial nerve palsy (if not explained by extracranial tumor)

TABLE 15.6.3: Murphy's staging system for non-Hodgkin's lymphoma.

Stage	*Criteria for the extent of disease*
I	A single tumor (extranodal) or single anatomic area (nodal) with the exclusion of the mediastinum and abdomen
II	• A single tumor (extranodal) with regional node involvement • Two or more nodal areas on the same side of the diaphragm • Two single (extranodal) tumors with or without regional node involvement on the same side of the diaphragm. • A primary gastrointestinal tumor, usually in the ileocecal area, with or without involvement of associated mesenteric lymph nodes only, grossly completely resected
III	• Two single tumors (extranodal) on opposite sides of the diaphragm • Two or more nodal areas above and below the diaphragm • All the primary intrathoracic tumors (mediastinal, pleural, and thymic) • All extensive primary intra-abdominal disease, unresectable • All paraspinal or epidural tumors, regardless of other tumor site(s)
IV	Any of the above with initial central nervous system (CNS) and/or bone marrow involvement

Source: Rosolen A, Perkins SL, Pinkerton CR, Guillerman RP, Sandlund JT, Patte C, et al. Revised international pediatric non-Hodgkin lymphoma staging system. J Clin Oncol. 2015;33(18):2112-8.

- Clinical spinal cord compression
- Isolated intracerebral mass
- *Parameningeal extension:* Cranial and/or spinal

Recently, the International Pediatric NHL Staging System (IPNHLSS) was published **(Table 15.6.4)**. The intention is to have one standard staging system and incorporate the newer disease subtypes.[5] Stages I and II or group A are considered good-risk diseases with high survival rates. Stages III and IV are considered disseminated diseases, but they still have a fair chance of survival.

TABLE 15.6.4: The revised international pediatric non-Hodgkin lymphoma (NHL) staging system [International Pediatric Non-Hodgkin Lymphoma Staging System (IPNHLSS)].

Stage	*Criteria for the extent of disease*
I	Single tumor with the exclusion of mediastinum and abdomen (N; EN; B or S: EN-B, EN-S)
II	• Single EN tumor with regional node involvement • More than or two N areas on the same side of diaphragm • Primary GI tract tumor (usually in the ileocecal area), involvement of associated mesenteric nodes, that is completely resectable (if malignant ascites or extension of tumor to adjacent organs, it should be regarded as stage III)
III	• More than or two EN tumors (including EN-B or EN-S) above and/or below the diaphragm • More than or two N areas above and below the diaphragm • Any intrathoracic tumor (mediastinal, hilar, pulmonary, pleural, or thymic) • Intra-abdominal and retroperitoneal disease, including liver, spleen, kidney, and/or ovary localizations, regardless of degree of resection [except primary GI tract tumor (usually in ileocecal region) involvement of associated mesenteric nodes that is completely resectable] • Any paraspinal or epidural tumor, regardless of whether other sites are involved • Single B lesion with concomitant involvement of EN and/or nonregional N sites
IV	Any of the above findings with initial involvement of *CNS (stage IV CNS), BM (stage IV BM), or both (stage IV combined)* based on conventional methods. BM involvement is defined by the morphologic evidence of ≥5% blasts or lymphoma cells by BM aspiration *CNS is considered involved in case of:* • Any CNS tumor mass [identified by imaging techniques (i.e., CT, MRI)] • Cranial nerve palsy that cannot be explained by extradural lesions • Blasts morphologically identified in CSF *Condition that defines CNS positivity should be specified:* CNS positive/ass, CNS positive/palsy, CNS positive/blasts *CSF status: CSF positivity is based on morphologic evidence of lymphoma cells* • CSF should be considered positive when any number of blasts is detected • CSF unknown (not performed, technical difficulties) *Note:* The type of examination and degree of *BM and CNS involvement* should be specified for each stage using the following abbreviations: • *BMm:* BM positivity by morphology (specify percentage of lymphoma cells) • *BMi:* BM positivity by immunophenotypic methods (immunohistochemical or flow-cytometric analysis; specify percentage of lymphoma cells) • *BMc:* BM positivity by cytogenetic or FISH analysis (specify percentage of lymphoma cells) • *BMmol:* BM positivity by molecular techniques (PCR-based; specify level of involvement) *Same approach should be used for PB involvement* (i.e., PBm, PBi, PBc, PBmol) bilateral BM aspirates and BM biopsy need to be performed *Similarly to BM, type of CSF involvement should be described whenever possible:* • *CSFm:* CSF positivity by morphology (specify number of blasts/μL) • *CSFi:* CSF positivity by immunophenotype methods (immunohistochemical or flow cytometric analysis; specify percentage of lymphoma cells) • *CSFc:* CSF positive by cytogenetic or FISH analysis (specify percentage of lymphoma cells) • *CSFmol:* CSF positivity by molecular techniques (PCR based; specify level of involvement)

(B: bone; BM: bone marrow; CNS: central nervous system; CSF: cerebrospinal fluid; CT: computed tomography; EN: extranodal; FISH: fluorescent in situ hybridization; GI: gastrointestinal; MRI: magnetic resonance imaging; N: nodal; PB: positivity by cytogenetic or FISH analysis; PCR: polymerase chain reaction; S: skin)

Source: Rosolen A, Perkins SL, Pinkerton CR, Guillerman RP, Sandlund JT, Patte C, et al. Revised international pediatric non-Hodgkin lymphoma staging system. J Clin Oncol. 2015;33(18):2112-8.

TREATMENT

The conventional treatment for NHL is chemotherapy. These tumors respond well to chemotherapy and radiation, and surgery is usually not the standard of care. The FAB/LMB protocol was the standard of care for Burkitt lymphoma and DLBCL. However, recent reports have suggested that adding rituximab improved the survival of patients in groups B and C.[6]

Primary mediastinal large B-cell lymphomas are usually treated with the DA-EPOCH (dose-adjusted etoposide, prednisone, vincristine, cyclophosphamide, doxorubicin) regimen.[7] While radiation therapy is used in adults, this modality is not commonly used in pediatric and adolescent patients. Lactic dehydrogenase (LDH) has been shown to have a prognostic impact, with levels >2 upper limit of normal having poorer survival rates. Studies have shown that adding rituximab may not have any survival advantage.[8]

The APO (adriamycin, prednisone, oncovin) regimen is considered the standard of care for ALCL. Recent studies have tried to prove that adding vinblastine to the treatment of ALCL did not improve survival and that vincristine was as effective as vinblastine.[9]

Lymphoblastic leukemias are best treated with the leukemia treatment protocols, which include an initial intense phase followed by maintenance chemotherapy. **Table 15.6.5** gives a synopsis of the treatment regimens of each subtype.[10]

Relapsed Refractory Non-Hodgkin Lymphomas

While front-line therapies offer good survival benefits for NHL, the treatment outcomes of relapsed refractory disease are only 30–40%. R-CYVE and R-ICE are the usual first salvage chemotherapy regimens, but these need to be consolidated with a hematopoietic stem cell transplant (HSCT). Both autologous and allogeneic HSCT are treatment options for those with relapsed refractory disease and have similar outcomes except for relapsed lymphoblastic lymphomas, which do better with allogeneic transplants. Some recent studies say that R/R ALCL may also benefit from allogeneic HSCT.

Newer Agents

Rituximab

Though we still describe it as a newer agent, rituximab, an anti-CD20 molecule, has long been shown to offer better cure rates for pediatric patients. A COG pilot study (AANHL01P1) showed that rituximab is safe when combined with standard chemotherapy and resulted in 3-year EFS rates of 95% for patients with intermediate-risk FAB group B (stage III/IV) disease and 90% for those with high-risk FAB group C disease.[6] The FDA has approved using rituximab for CD20-positive NHL based on the Inter B NHL-ritux 2010 trial.[11]

Nelaribine

Nelaribine is a purine analog that has been effective in managing T-cell leukemias. Though very effective in adult NHL, it has not shown similar impressive results in pediatric lymphoma patients as found in the AALL0434 study, where it was used with standard chemotherapy and did not significantly impact.[12]

Crizotinib

Crizotinib is a tyrosine kinase inhibitor that targets the ALK-NPM protein in patients with ALCL tumor cells. In a COG study, crizotinib showed efficacy even as monotherapy, suggesting that it may be used in children as a bridge to immunotherapy. The FDA has approved the use of crizotinib for relapsed refractory disease.

Blinatumumab

Blinatumumab is an anti-CD19 antibody that engages the T-cells and is currently used to treat relapsed leukemias. It can have severe toxicity, especially cytokine release syndrome and neurotoxicity. Though it is still not approved for use in relapsed/refractory NHL, it does show promise. Further clinical trials are warranted, especially in pediatrics.

Brentuximab Vedotin

Brentuximab vedotin is an anti-CD30 monoclonal antibody that induces apoptosis in lymphoma cells. It has been shown to improve survival without increasing the regimen's toxicity for both Hodgkin lymphoma and ALCL. Brentuximab can also be used as an adjunct therapy to induce remission and sustain it while the patient awaits an HSCT.

Other Agents

Inotuzumab ozogamicin is another monoclonal antibody that targets CD22-positive lymphoma/leukemia cells. Trials are currently underway to showcase its effectiveness in leukemia. Clinical studies are needed for the pediatric population.

Glofitamab and Mosunetuzumab have also emerged as bispecific antibodies against CD3 and CD20 surface antigens on lymphoma cells, showing promise in treating R/R NHL. They have been reported to have a lesser incidence of CRS than Blinatumumab. Pediatric trials with these two drugs are still awaited.

Ruxolitinib is a JAK 2 inhibitor with excellent efficacy in posttransplant graft versus host disease (GVHD). It is helpful in PMLBCL in children but not adults, underscoring the need for more extensive studies.

TABLE 15.6.5: The molecular biology, genetics, and most common treatment regimens for common non-Hodgkin lymphoma (NHLs) in the pediatric and adolescent population.

NHL subtype	*Molecular markers/genetic abnormalities*	*Treatment regimens*
Burkitt lymphoma	• CD19 • CD20 • Immunoglobulin kappa or • Gamma light chains, IgM • CD10/CALLA • MYC translocations • TP53 mutation • t(8:14)(q24: q32), t(8;22)(q24;q11)	• *FAB/LMB regimen:* Intravenous (IV) formulations of cyclophosphamide (CPM), vincristine, prednisone/prednisolone, doxorubicin along with intrathecal (IT) methotrexate (MTX); IV Ifosfamide, etoposide, MTX in higher risk group only (Group C) • *Inter-B-NHL Ritux 2010:* Addition of rituximab to the FAB/LMB backbone • *BFM regimen:* Involve IV formulations of doxorubicin and CPM with doses lower than FAB/LMB; addition of ifosfamide, etoposide, and IV MTX, including in lower and intermediate risk groups
Diffuse large B-cell lymphoma	• *Germinal center B-cell type:* CD10 and BCL6 • Activated B-cell type: MUM1 • MYC locus translocations involving chromosome 8q24 • Primary mediastinal large B-cell lymphoma • CD19, CD20, CD30, CD79 • JAK2, STAT, PDL1/2 mutations	Regimens like that used in Burkitt lymphoma
Primary mediastinal large B-cell lymphoma	• CD19, CD20, CD30, CD79 • JAK2, STAT, PDL1/2 mutations	• *DA-EPOCH-R:* Etoposide, doxorubicin, CPM vincristine, rituximab • Dismal response to FAB/LMB in comparison to responses seen in DLBCL (EFS of 66%) • No protocolized regimen
Anaplastic large cell lymphoma	CD30, t(2;5) translocations encoding NPM-ALK	• *NHL-BFM studies:* PO dexamethasone, IV MTX, IV etoposide, IV doxorubicin, IV vincristine, IV vindesine and IT triple chemotherapy with MTX, cytarabine, and prednisone • *APO regimen:* IV doxorubicin, PO prednisone, IV vincristine, PO 6-mercaptopurine and IT/IV MTX
Lymphoblastic lyphoma	• *B-cell type:* CD19, cytoplasmic CD79a, cytoplasmic CD22 CD10, CD24, PAX5, CD20 and CD34 expression is variable • *T-cell type:* CD3, CD1a, CD2, CD4, CD5, CD7, CD8, CD10, CD44	• Leukemia protocols like *COG AALL0434 (T-LL regimen): Augmented BFM regimen* – IV vincristine, IV doxorubicin, IV daunorubicin, IT MTX, IT cytarabine, PO prednisone, IM peg-asparaginase, PO dexamethasone, IV/IM cytarabine, Capizzi-style IV MTX (C-MTX), PO 6-mercaptopurine, PO thioguanine • *C-MTX:* Escalating doses of IV MTX with initial dose of 100 mg/m^2/day; no leucovorin rescue • *NHL-BFM-95 (including B-type LL), BFM IC 2002 , ICICLE COG-A5971 (including B type LL):* Similar to COG AALL0434, except does not include C-MTX; use high dose MTX
Pediatric follicular lymphoma	• Few cases with IRF4/MUM1 expression. • No widespread genetic abnormalities have been identified	• *NHL-BFM studies*: 2–4 cycles of IV doxorubicin, CPM, ifosfamide • Surgery in localized cases • *R-CHOP*

Source: Sheikh IN, Elgehiny A, Ragoonanan D, Mahadeo KM, Nieto Y, Khazal S. Management of Aggressive Non-Hodgkin Lymphomas in the Pediatric, Adolescent, and Young Adult Population: An Adult vs. Pediatric Perspective. Cancers (Basel). 2022;14(12):2912.

CAR T-cell Therapy

Chimeric antigen receptor (CAR) T-cell therapy uses the patient's autologous T-cells and genetically modifies them to attach to specific receptors on the cancer cells and then kill them. CAR T-cell therapy research is growing in leaps and bounds, with very promising results in pediatric and adult leukemia and adult lymphomas. CAR T targeting the CD19 or even CD22 receptors has been effective in adult settings. Four CD19 targeting CAR-T cells are approved for use in the adult ALL; only one is approved for use in adult NHL **(Table 15.6.6)**.

TABLE 15.6.6: CAR-T cells licensed for use in leukemia and lymphoma.

Drug	*Other terms*	*Construction*
Axicabtagene ciloleucel	Axi-cel, Yescarta, KTE-CD19	CD19-CD28-CD3ζ
Tisagenlecleucel	Tisa-cel, Kymriah, CTL019	CD19-4-1BB-CD3ζ
Brexucabtagene autoleucel	Tecartus, KTE-X19	CD19-CD28-CD3ζ
Lisocabtagene maraleucel	Liso-cel, Breyanzi, JCAR017	CD19-4-1BB-CD3ζ

While CAR T therapy is much talked about in pediatric leukemias, trials are still awaited in the pediatric population. The BIANCA study, which completed its recruitment in 2023, used Kymriah in eight pediatric patients. The results of this study are still awaited. Studies are also underway using cytotoxic T lymphocytes targeting the latent membrane proteins on EBV-associated NHL or NK Cells with anti-CD19 CAR cells, but the numbers are still small.

Immune Checkpoint Inhibitors

Nivolumab is a PD-1 inhibitor that has shown efficacy in pediatric Hodgkin lymphoma; however, its role in NHL is still unclear.

Pembrolizumab is a small-molecule inhibitor targeting programmed cell death protein-1 (PD-1) in lymphocytes. This prevents tumor-secreted programmed cell death protein ligand-1 (PD-L1) from attaching, leading to lymphocyte deactivation and tumor evasion of the immune system. Trials are underway with rituximab and other drugs/CAR T-cells to improve the outcomes of relapsed/refractory PMLBCL. However, most of these are in adults and not pediatrics.

Atelzolizumab, a PD-L1 inhibitor, was also well tolerated in a significant phase 1/2 study in pediatric patients with solid tumors, classical Hodgkin lymphoma, and NHL, but its responses were also suboptimal, as only 5% of patients had a partial response at 6 months.

CONCLUSION

Non-Hodgkin lymphomas are among the most common malignancies in pediatrics. The classification system has recently changed; however, four common variants are seen. These aggressive tumors need to be diagnosed quickly and safely. Also, treatment by the right person (pediatric oncologist) at the right time (early detection and initiation of therapy) and at the right place (in centers that are equipped to look after pediatric malignancies) will go a long way to improve further survival and decrease toxicities associated with the regimens. Newer therapies, especially CAR T-cell therapy, hold much promise.

REFERENCES

1. Burkitt D. A sarcoma involving the jaws of African children. Br J Surg. 1958;46(197):218-23.
2. Reedijk AMJ, Beishuizen A, Coebergh JWW, Hoeben BAW, Kremer LCM, Hebeda KM, et al. Progress against non-Hodgkin's lymphoma in children and young adolescents in the Netherlands since 1990: Stable incidence, improved survival, and lower mortality. Eur J Cancer. 2022;163:140-51.
3. Abla O, Attarbaschi A. Non-Hodgkin's Lymphoma in Childhood and Adolescence, 1st edition. Cham, Switzerland; Springer Nature; 2019.
4. Arora B. Lymphoma. In: Parthasarathy A, Menon PSN, Nair MKC (Eds). IAP Textbook of Pediatrics, 7th edition. New Delhi: Jaypee Brothers Medical Publishers; 2019. pp. 957-64.
5. Rosolen A, Perkins SL, Pinkerton CR, Guillerman RP, Sandlund JT, Patte C, et al. Revised international pediatric non-Hodgkin lymphoma staging system. J Clin Oncol. 2015;33(18):2112-8.
6. Goldman S, Smith L, Anderson JR, Perkins S, Harrison L, Geyer MB, et al. Rituximab and FAB/LMB 96 chemotherapy in children with Stage III/IV B-cell non-Hodgkin lymphoma: A Children's Oncology Group report. Leukemia. 2013;27:1174-7.
7. Giulino-Roth L. How I treat primary mediastinal B-cell lymphoma. Blood. 2018;132(8):782-90.
8. Burke GAA, Minard-Colin V, Aupérin A, Aupérin A, Alexander S, Pillon M, et al. Dose-Adjusted Etoposide, Doxorubicin, and Cyclophosphamide With Vincristine and Prednisone Plus Rituximab Therapy in Children and Adolescents With Primary Mediastinal B-Cell Lymphoma: A Multicenter Phase II Trial. J Clin Oncol. 2021;39(33):3716-24.
9. Advanced stage anaplastic large cell lymphoma in children and adolescents: Results of ANHL0131, a randomized phase III trial of APO versus a modified regimen with vinblastine: A children's oncology group report. Pediatr Blood Cancer. 2014;61(12):2236-42.
10. Sheikh IN, Elgehiny A, Ragoonanan D, Mahadeo KM, Nieto Y, Khazal S. Management of Aggressive Non-Hodgkin Lymphomas in the Pediatric, Adolescent, and Young Adult Population: An Adult vs. Pediatric Perspective. Cancers (Basel). 2022;14(12):2912.
11. Minard-Colin V, Aupérin A, Pillon M, Burke GAA, Barkauskas DA, Wheatley K, et al. Rituximab for High-Risk, Mature B-Cell Non-Hodgkin's Lymphoma in Children. New Eng J Med. 2020;382(23):2207-19.
12. Berg SL, Blaney SM, Devidas M, Lampkin TA, Murgo A, Bernstein M, et al. Phase II study of nelarabine (compound 506U78) in children and young adults with refractory T-cell malignancies: A report from the children's oncology group. J Clin Oncol. 2005;23(15):3376-82.

15.7 Wilms Tumor

Sachit Anand, Sandeep Agarwala

INTRODUCTION

Wilms tumor (WT), one of the common solid tumors of childhood, accounts for up to 6% of the pediatric malignancies. It is primarily a disease of the kidney, but few rare extrarenal locations have been reported, such as retroperitoneum, sacrococcygeal region, testis, uterus, inguinal canal, and mediastinum. The first detailed description of WT was provided by Max Wilms, a German surgeon and pathologist in 1899. The first nephrectomy for WT was performed by Jessop in 1877. Till 1950s, the overall survival of WT was only 22%. Most children who survived the surgery quickly succumbed to recurrent and metastatic disease. Radiotherapy (RT) was the only adjuvant therapy at that time. It was only after the introduction of chemotherapeutic agents (actinomycin-D and vincristine) in the 1960s, that an improvement in the overall survival of children with WT was observed.[1]

With the current multidisciplinary approach and the efforts of various cooperative study groups, it has been possible to achieve >90% 5-year overall survival rates. Better understanding of the disease process, discovery of effective chemotherapeutic agents and improved surgical techniques have all contributed to this excellent survival of children with WT. Globally, the current focus has now shifted toward the reduction of short-term and long-term morbidity in these patients, particularly those with low-risk disease. Most pediatricians are focused on reducing the chronic health conditions secondary to the treatment, e.g., renal failure, infertility, cardiac toxicity, restrictive pulmonary disease, and the development of subsequent malignancies.

EPIDEMIOLOGY

The WT is the most common renal tumor of childhood. It is known to affect 1 in 10,000 children under the age of 15 years. No reliable Indian statistics are available in terms of the incidence of WT. At our center, the proportion of WT is around 15% of all pediatric malignancies (including leukemia and lymphoma, brain tumor, etc.). The median age of presentation is 3.5 years. About 50% of the patients present before the age of 3 years and 90% before the age of 6 years. Worldwide, no gender or side predilection has been noted for WT. However, compared to the Asians, it is slightly more common in the black population.[2]

ETIOPATHOGENESIS

The WT appears to result from changes in one or more of several genes. Most cases of WT are sporadic and occur due to mutations in the tumor tissue which cannot be transmitted to the progeny. Less than 10% of the tumors appear to be a result of germ-line mutations. The *WT1* gene, the first WT suppressor gene, is located in the chromosomal band 11p13. Mutations in one of the two alleles of this gene may contribute to abnormal cell growth and genitourinary abnormalities. This gene has also been implicated in the etiopathogenesis of syndromic cases of WT, i.e., Denys–Drash syndrome and WAGR (Wilms tumor, aniridia, growth retardation, genitourinary anomalies, and mental retardation) complex. Loss of heterozygosity (LOH) at 11p15, the site of the second WT suppressor gene (*WT2*), leads to Beckwith–Weideman syndrome (BWS). Loss of heterozygosity at 1p (LOH 1p) is present in 11% of cases and that at 16q (LOH 16q) in 20% cases of WT. Apart from the genetic abnormalities, several environmental factors have also been implicated in the complex etiopathogenesis of WT. The role of air pollutants such as benzopyrene, a polycyclic aromatic hydrocarbon, carbon monoxide, and chromium (more VI compounds than III compounds) which can cross the placenta has also been questioned.[3]

CLINICAL FEATURES

The most common and classic presentation of WT is palpable flank mass in an otherwise healthy toddler. The mass is often incidentally noticed by mother while giving bath to the child or subsequent to a trivial abdominal trauma. Abdominal pain or hematuria is found in another quarter of the patients. Urinary tract infection and varicocele are less common and are confined to cases of left side tumor. Hypertension, seen in 25% of cases, is attributed to either increased renin activity or renal vascular compression by the mass.

Associated findings in syndromic WT may be aniridia, hemihypertrophy, hypospadias, facial dysmorphism, cryptorchidism, or differences in sex development (DSD). Occasionally, various syndromes are associated with the tumor and they can be broadly divided into two subgroups:

1. *Group I:* Syndromes that are associated with overgrowth such as hemihypertrophy, BWS, Perlman syndrome, and Simpson–Golabi–Behmel syndrome.

2. *Group II:* Syndromes not associated with overgrowth such as Denys-Drash syndrome, WAGR syndrome, neurofibromatosis, Sotos' syndrome, and Klippel-Trenaunay-Weber syndrome.

DIFFERENTIAL DIAGNOSIS

The differential diagnosis of WT includes neoplastic lesions such as mesoblastic nephroma (the most common renal tumor of neonatal period), clear cell sarcoma of kidney, rhabdoid tumor of the kidney, renal cell carcinoma, neuroblastoma, and retroperitoneal teratoma. In addition, nonmalignant renal lesions such as hydronephrosis, solitary renal cyst, multicystic (or polycystic kidney disease), and renal dysplasia may also be confused with WT.

DIAGNOSIS

Laboratory Investigations

Basic evaluation includes a complete blood count, liver and renal function tests, serum calcium levels (elevated in rhabdoid tumor and congenital mesoblastic nephroma), and coagulation profile (acquired von Willebrand disease may coexist in 8% at the time of diagnosis).

Radiological Imaging

Ultrasonography and Doppler Studies

Ultrasonography (USG) including a Doppler study of the renal veins, and inferior vena cava (IVC) is usually the screening investigation of choice in any suspected solid renal mass. It provides valuable information about the organ of origin of the mass, differentiation between solid versus cystic mass, tumor dimensions and relationship with the adjacent organs (including invasion), details of the contralateral kidney, involvement of the liver, tumor thrombus extending into IVC, renal vein or renal pelvis, the presence of hemoperitoneum, or tumor rupture, etc.

Contrast-enhanced Computed Tomography

Contrast-enhanced computed tomography (CECT) scans of the abdomen and chest are always performed in these cases for confirming the USG findings. The relationship of the mass to the adjacent structures and pulmonary metastasis are better delineated on CECT than in USG or chest radiograph, respectively. Due to this, a CECT chest is ordered in all cases of WT prior to starting therapy as only a chest radiograph is not optimal to rule out pulmonary metastases.

Magnetic Resonance Imaging

Magnetic resonance imaging (MRI) of the abdomen is an alternative to CECT scan and it is particularly useful in assessing nephrogenic rests. MRI has the advantage of multiplanar imaging, appropriate delineation of vascular thrombus and avoidance of contrast and radiation. However, it is much more expensive, less easily available, requires general anesthesia in children, and is not appropriate for pulmonary evaluation (for which a CECT chest is anyway required). Therefore, as of now, MRI is not the preferred radiological investigation.

Functional Imaging

Although WT is known to concentrate fluorodeoxyglucose (FDG), a definite role of functional imaging with FDG-positron emission tomography (PET) has not been established till date. The situation is further complicated in view of the routine excretion of FDG by the kidneys. Therefore, PET or PET-CT is not included as a routine workup of WT.

Cytogenetic Studies

Loss of heterozygosity (LOH) at 1p and 16q needs to be done to risk stratify the patients into appropriate treatment groups. Patients with LOH at both 1p and 16q have a high rate of recurrence and death; hence, they require more aggressive chemotherapy.

MANAGEMENT

Staging

Accurate staging of the tumor is necessary to provide optimal management. Different tumor groups use different staging systems. The staging system used by the North American Children's Oncology Group (COG) is based on surgical findings while that of the Société Internationale D'Oncologie Pédiatrique (SIOP) group is based on information gathered from neoadjuvant chemotherapy and nephrectomy specimens **(Table 15.7.1)**.[4] Any one of the staging systems should be followed consistently to avoid confusion. It has been a general observation that the patients of WT in India present at relatively advanced stages and an upfront surgery may not be feasible in a significant majority.[5,6]

Treatment Modalities

The current management of WT includes a multimodality treatment including neoadjuvant chemotherapy, surgery, and adjuvant therapy (chemotherapy and RT). At present, different protocols of management are utilized by different centers across the globe.[7] These are largely based on the contrasting treatment philosophies of cooperative tumor groups.[5] While COG believes in upfront surgery for all patients, SIOP offers neoadjuvant chemotherapy to all.[4]

TABLE 15.7.1: Staging of Wilms tumor.

Stage	NWTS staging system*	SIOP staging system
I	The tumor is limited to the kidney and excised completely. The renal capsule has an intact outer surface. The tumor was not ruptured or biopsied prior to removal (fine-needle aspiration biopsies are excluded from this restriction). The vessels of the renal sinus are also free. There is no evidence of tumor at or beyond the margins of surgical resection	The tumor is limited to the kidney and is completely excised
II	The tumor extends beyond the kidney but excised completely. However, there may be regional extension of tumor in the form of renal capsule penetration or extensive renal sinus invasion. The blood vessels outside the renal parenchyma, including those of the renal sinus may also contain tumor. The tumor was biopsied (except for fine-needle aspiration). There must be no evidence of tumor at or beyond the margins of resection	• The tumor is extending beyond the kidney and is completely excised • Invasion beyond the capsule, perirenal/perihilar involvement • Invasion of the regional lymph nodes (hilar nodes and/or periaortic nodes at the origin of the renal artery) is included in stage II • Invasion of the extrarenal vessels • Invasion of the ureter
III	Residual no-hematogenous tumor confined to the abdomen in any one of the following forms: 1. Lymph nodes within the abdomen or pelvis are found to be involved by tumor (renal hilar, para-aortic, or beyond). (Lymph node involvement in the thorax, or other extra-abdominal sites would be a criterion for stage IV) 2. Breach of the peritoneal surface 3. Tumor implants are found on the peritoneal surface 4. Positive margins of the specimen on histopathological examination 5. Unresectable tumor 6. Tumor spill occurred either before or during surgery	• Invasion beyond the capsule with incomplete excision • Preoperative or perioperative biopsy • Preoperative/perioperative rupture • Peritoneal metastases • Invasion of para-aortic lymph nodes (below the renal artery) • Incomplete excision
IV	Hematogenous metastases (lung, liver, bone, brain, etc.), or lymph node metastases outside the abdominopelvic region are present	Distant metastases
V	Bilateral renal involvement is present at the time of diagnosis. An attempt should be made to stage each side according to the above criteria on the basis of the extent of disease prior to biopsy or treatment	Bilateral renal tumors

*NWTS merged in 2000 and known as the Children's Oncology Group (COG).
(NWTS: National Wilms Tumor Study; SIOP: Société Internationale D'Oncologie Pédiatrique)

Surgery

According to the COG protocol, upfront surgery is the initial treatment of choice in most of the children with unilateral WT. Nephroureterectomy with adequate lymph node sampling is recommended.[8] Gentle handling of the tumor throughout the surgery is necessary to prevent tumor rupture and spillage which would upstage the tumor.[9] The renal vein and the inferior vena cava should be palpated to rule out the presence of any intravascular tumor thrombus prior to the ligation of the hilar vessels. It is important to assess the liver and regional periaortic lymph nodal involvement.[9,10]

Chemotherapy

The past six decades have witnessed dramatic changes as far as the chemotherapy for WT is concerned. This has been made possible by the efforts of various study groups and their clinical study trials. In general, two chemotherapy regimens by COG, i.e., EE4A, DD4A, are sufficient for an optimal management in majority of the cases. The former is a two-drug regimen including actinomycin D and vincristine and is used for adjuvant treatment in cases where the tumor is upfront resectable. The latter is a three-drug combination and is ideal for children requiring neoadjuvant chemotherapy. The chemotherapy regimens for special scenarios such as progressive disease, bilateral or metastatic disease with no response to initial neoadjuvant chemotherapy, anaplastic histology, and recurrent WT are complicated and beyond the scope of this chapter.[7,11]

Radiotherapy

Flank RT is given to all cases with a local stage III disease. The standard flank RT field is based on the original CECT scan and always goes across the midline to include the entire vertebral body (to decrease the incidence of scoliosis). Whole abdominal irradiation is indicated in scenarios of diffuse tumor spillage, intraperitoneal tumor rupture, and peritoneal tumor seeding/hemorrhagic or cytology positive ascites. Lung irradiation is given to patients with stage IV disease whose lung lesions do not show a complete response to neoadjuvant chemotherapy.

OUTCOMES

With the current multimodal management, the outcomes of children with WT have improved significantly. It has been possible to achieve >90% 5-year overall survival rates in cases with unilateral disease. However, the outcomes remain poor for children with anaplastic histology, bilateral tumors, syndromic presentation, and metastatic disease not responding to chemotherapy or showing a rapid progression.

LATE COMPLICATIONS

Improved survival rates have led to a dramatic increase in the number of long-term survivors and hence an increase in the incidence of long-term complications of WT. Common long-term complications are discussed in the following text:[12]

Renal Insufficiency

The overall incidence of renal insufficiency is only 0.25%. Notably, patients who developed renal failure are mostly those who underwent bilateral surgery for synchronous or metachronous WT, or those with associated syndrome, e.g., Denys–Drash syndrome, WAGR syndrome, and other genitourinary anomalies.[13]

Second Malignancy

The patients with WT have a 1.6% risk of developing a second malignancy after 15 years of diagnosis. Increased radiation dosage, use of drugs such as etoposide and cyclophosphamide are an important risk factor of secondary malignancy. About three-fourths of all secondary tumors occur in the field of radiation.

Infertility and Hypogonadism

Dose-dependent temporary azoospermia and hypogonadism occur in males exposed to irradiation therapy. About 80% of boys treated for WT develop oligospermia and azoospermia despite lead shielding of gonads during RT. Use of additional drugs such as etoposide and cyclophosphamide are also an important contributor to infertility.

Cardiotoxicity

Anthracyclines (doxorubicin) are particularly notorious of causing cardiac dysfunction. The combination of doxorubicin and radiation therapy is more harmful than either modality alone. Cardiac failure due to cardiotoxicity can be acute, subacute, or late. Therefore, repeated evaluations are mandated for at-risk survivors.

CONCLUSION

Wilms tumor is one of the most common solid tumors of childhood. Contrast-enhanced CT scan of thorax, abdomen and pelvis is the imaging modality of choice. Although surgery is the cornerstone of treatment, WT is an extremely chemosensitive and radiosensitive tumor. Therefore, the current multimodality treatment approach offers an excellent survival benefit for children with WT.

Pulmonary Toxicity

Pulmonary function can be seriously affected by radiation as well as chemotherapeutic agents. Radiation pneumonitis was common and was reported in 12% of patients with metastatic pulmonary disease in the past. However, this complication is now infrequently seen due to improvements in the RT techniques and reduction in the doses of radiation and chemotherapeutic agents.

REFERENCES

1. Aldrink JH, Heaton TE, Dasgupta R, Lautz TB, Malek MM, Abdessalam SF, et al.; American Pediatric Surgery Association Cancer Committee. Update on Wilms tumor. J Pediatr Surg. 2019;54(3):390-7.
2. Israels T, Bailey S, Verschoor R, Kaspers GJ, Kennedy N, Molyneux EM. Management of children with Wilms tumor in Africa and Europe; thoughts about costs, priorities and collaboration. Pediatr Hematol Oncol. 2014;31(5):395-9.
3. Cone EB, Dalton SS, Van Noord M, Tracy ET, Rice HE, Routh JC. Biomarkers for Wilms Tumor: A Systematic Review. J Urol. 2016;196(5):1530-5.
4. Godzinski J. The current status of treatment of Wilms' tumor as per the SIOP trials. J Indian Assoc Pediatr Surg. 2015;20(1):16-20.
5. Prasad M, Vora T, Agarwala S, Laskar S, Arora B, Bansal D, et al. Management of Wilms Tumor: ICMR Consensus Document. Indian J Pediatr. 2017;84(6):437-45.
6. Sarin YK, Bhatnagar SN. Wilms' tumor- roadmaps of management. Indian J Pediatr. 2012;79(60):776-86.
7. PDQ Pediatric Treatment Editorial Board. Wilms Tumor and Other Childhood Kidney Tumors Treatment (PDQ®): Health Professional Version. Bethesda: National Cancer Institute; 2002.
8. Murphy AJ, Davidoff AM. Bilateral Wilms Tumor: A Surgical Perspective. Children (Basel). 2018;5(10):134.
9. Kieran K, Ehrlich PF. Current surgical standards of care in Wilms tumor. Urol Oncol. 2016;34(1):13-23.
10. Vanden Berg RN, Bierman EN, Noord MV, Rice HE, Routh JC. Nephron-sparing surgery for Wilms tumor: A systematic review. Urol Oncol. 2016;34(1):24-32.
11. Dome JS, Graf N, Geller JI, Fernandez CV, Mullen EA, Spreafico F, et al. Advances in Wilms Tumor Treatment and Biology: Progress Through International Collaboration. J Clin Oncol. 2015;33(27):2999-3007.
12. Irtan S, Ehrlich PF, Pritchard-Jones K. Wilms tumor: "State-of-the-art" update, 2016. Semin Pediatr Surg. 2016;25(5):250-6.
13. Romao RL, Lorenzo AJ. Renal function in patients with Wilms tumor. Urol Oncol. 2016;34(1):33-41.

15.8 Neuroblastoma

Vignesh Subramani, Maya Prasad

INTRODUCTION

Neuroblastoma (NBL) is the most common intra-abdominal and extracranial solid tumor of childhood. It is an embryonal tumor derived from the sympathetic nervous system. It originates from the primordial neural crest cells that give rise to the adrenal medulla and sympathetic ganglia and may arise from several widely separated anatomical sites along the craniospinal axis.

Neuroblastoma accounts for 8–10% of all pediatric cancers. NBL is predominantly a disease of early childhood, with up to 90% of patients presenting before 5 years of age and 50% within the first 2 years of life, and it is also the most common cancer diagnosed during infancy. NBL is one of the few cancers that may undergo spontaneous regression or may mature into a benign ganglioneuroma, whereas high-risk NBLs tend to be aggressive and progress relentlessly. Advances in the treatment of children with these tumors have improved outcomes, although many with high-risk diseases still succumb despite intensive therapy.

EPIDEMIOLOGY

Neuroblastoma accounts for 8–10% of all childhood cancers in the developed world. The age-adjusted incidence of NBL is 10.6 cases per one million children aged 0–14 years. The prevalence is about 1 case per 7,000 live births. In India, the relative proportion of NBL (and ganglioneuroblastoma) in childhood (0–14 years) varied from 2.4% to 7.5% of all cancers.[1] NBL accounts for >15% of the mortality from cancer in children. The peak age of incidence is 22 months. The male-to-female ratio ranges from 1.2:1 to 1.3:1.

ETIOPATHOGENESIS

The etiology of NBL is unknown. A family history of NBL is identified in only 1–2% and exhibits an autosomal dominant inheritance, the majority being associated with a mutation in the anaplastic lymphoma kinase (*ALK*) gene. NBL may also be seen in children with Hirschsprung disease and congenital central hypoventilation syndrome; these are associated with loss of function mutations in the homeobox gene *PHOX2B*.

Neuroblastoma originates from the primordial neural crest cells; therefore, NBL can arise anywhere along the sympathetic nervous system. There are two clinically relevant aspects regarding the pathophysiology of NBL.

- Because of their adrenergic derivation, NBLs typically express essential enzymes involved in catecholamine synthesis. Because monoamine oxidase and catechol-O-methyltransferase enzymes are typically expressed, the metabolites homovanillic acid (HVA) and vanillylmandelic acid (VMA) have the highest sensitivity and specificity for tumor detection. Approximately 90% of NBL tumors secrete these byproducts. The quantitative levels of urinary catecholamines—mainly urinary VMA and HVA—are a supportive and noninvasive method for diagnosing and monitoring the disease.
- Because NBL arises from the developing sympathetic nervous system, the majority of tumors express norepinephrine receptors on their cell surface. Metaiodobenzylguanidine (MIBG) is a norepinephrine analog; radiolabeled MIBG has been used to localize tumors that express norepinephrine receptors and also for targeted treatment in patients with MIBG-avid tumors. Around 90% of NBLs are MIBG-avid.

BIOLOGY

Some of the important biomarkers implicated in the pathogenesis of NBL include:

- *Amplification of MYCN locus at 2p24 (more than fourfold MYCN copies when compared with control 2p probe)*: This occurs in approximately 20% of NBL (40–50% in high-risk cases) and is associated with advanced disease at diagnosis, aggressive and rapid tumor progression, and is an independent predictor of poor outcome. Amplification of the *MYCN* gene strongly predicts a poorer prognosis.[2]
- *The presence of segmental chromosomal aberrations (SCA)—unbalanced gain of 17q, deletion of 1p, and allelic loss of 11q*—has been associated with advanced age at diagnosis, advanced stage, and higher risk of relapse.
- *Trk expression*: Expression of neurotrophin receptor kinases and their ligands varies between high-risk and low-risk tumors. High levels of TrkA expression are highly correlated with favorable outcomes, whereas expression of TrkB is strongly associated with aggressive tumor behavior and poor outcomes.

- *Tumor ploidy:* Tumors that have a hyperdiploid DNA content (DI > 1) are more likely to have lower stages of disease and respond well to therapy, and diploid DNA content of tumor cells is associated with poor outcomes.

PATHOLOGY

Biopsy from a tumor suspected to be NBL is important not only for diagnosis but also for staging and for the study of biological markers, which can be used for risk stratification. Histopathological characteristics of NBL are generally defined on tumor tissue prior to the administration of chemotherapy; tumors undergo differentiation after treatment, and this may confound pathological examination.

The three classic histopathologic patterns of NBL, ganglioneuroblastoma, and ganglioneuroma reflect a spectrum of neuronal differentiation. NBL is the most primitive entity—composed of small, uniformly sized cells containing dense, hyperchromatic nuclei and scant cytoplasm. The presence of neuropil and Homer-Wright pseudorosette (ring of neuroblasts surrounding a central core of eosinophilic neuropil) is a characteristic feature. The fully differentiated counterpart is ganglioneuroma, composed of mature ganglion cells, neuropil, and Schwannian stroma. Between these two extremes is the transitional form known as ganglioneuroblastoma. The three classic histopathologic patterns reflect a spectrum of maturation and differentiation **(Fig. 15.8.1)**.

There are two commonly used histopathological classification systems:

1. *Shimada histology classification* utilizes patient's age and the presence or absence of Schwannian stroma, the degree of differentiation, and the mitosis-karyorrhexis index (MKI) to assign tumors to a favorable or unfavorable category.
2. More recent studies have used *the International Neuroblastoma Pathology Classification (INPC)*, which is a modification of the Shimada system and places pretreatment tumors into two broad categories of *favorable* and *unfavorable* histology based on the amount of Schwannian stromal component, degree of differentiation, MKI, and patient's age.

Neuroblastoma is one of several small blue round cell tumors (SBRCTs) of childhood, and it may be difficult to differentiate from non-Hodgkin's lymphoma (NHL), Ewing sarcoma, and rhabdomyosarcoma by light microscopy alone **(Fig. 15.8.1)**. The definitive diagnosis is commonly made by immunohistochemistry (IHC) as well as supporting clinical features and ancillary investigations. On immunohistochemical staining, NBLs are positive for neurofilament proteins, CD56, chromogranin, synaptophysin, and neuron-specific enolase (NSE) **(Table 15.8.1)**.

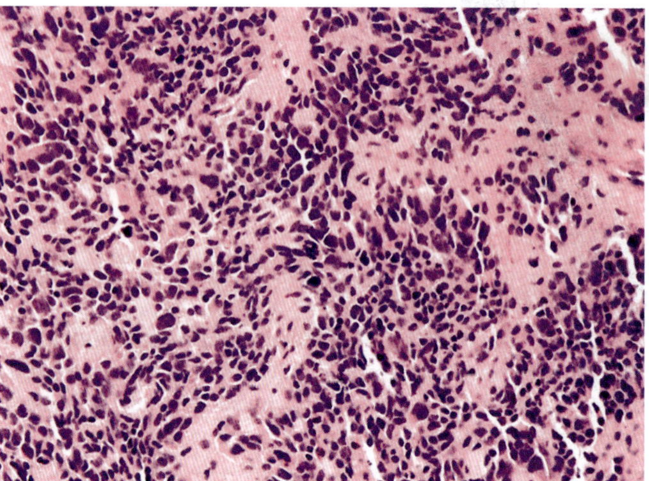

Fig. 15.8.1: Microscopy [hematoxylin and eosin (H&E) staining] of neuroblastoma, seen as a small round blue cell tumor.

TABLE 15.8.1: Immunohistochemical features of pediatric small round cell tumors that can present as abdominal mass.

Tumor	*Immunohistochemical markers*
Neuroblastoma	Neuron-specific enolase, chromogranin, synaptophysin, TrkA, ganglioside (GD2)
Rhabdomyosarcoma	Myogenin, desmin, muscle-specific actin, vimentin, and MyoD1
Ewing sarcoma/ primitive neuroectodermal tumors (PNETs)	CD99, β2 microglobulin, and vimentin
Lymphoma	CD45 (LCA), CD3, CD5, CD7, CD19, and CD20
Synovial sarcoma	Epithelial membrane antigen (EMA), cytokeratin, Bcl-2, TLE-1
Desmoplastic small round cell tumors (DSRCTs)	Desmin, cytokeratin, WT-1, EMA, and CD57

CLINICAL FEATURES

Neuroblastoma may develop at any site of the sympathetic nervous system. Approximately half the cases of NBL arise in the adrenal glands, and the remainder originate in the paraspinal sympathetic ganglia. Thoracic and cervical primary tumors are more common in infants. Physical examination of a child with NBL should include a detailed evaluation of the primary mass as well as draining lymph node structures. The general examination could reveal subcutaneous nodules, proptosis, or Horner syndrome. Detailed neurologic examination of a patient with a spinal lesion may detect impending neurological compromise. The manifestations of NBL are varied and can be broadly divided as those due to primary tumor or metastasis.

Clinical Features due to Primary Tumor

Neuroblastoma can originate from anywhere along the sympathetic chain, presenting as a cervical, cervicothoracic, thoracic, thoracoabdominal, abdominal, or pelvic mass. The most frequent anatomical sites of primary tumors are the adrenal gland (32%), paravertebral retroperitoneum (28%), posterior mediastinum (15%), pelvis (5%), and cervical area. Nearly two-thirds of primary tumors occur within the abdomen. Abdominal tumors may present as a mass that is usually firm and irregular and often crosses the midline **(Fig. 15.8.2)**. The mass may cause compression of neighboring abdominal structures and lead to complications such as hydronephrosis and bowel obstruction. Hypertension is common. Tumors with intraspinal extension or spinal cord compression lead to neurological symptoms such as flaccid paralysis of the legs and/or bladder or bowel dysfunction. Cervical masses from primary or metastatic NBL may cause Horner syndrome.

Clinical Manifestations due to Metastasis

Metastatic spread, which is more common in children >1 year old at diagnosis, occurs through local invasion or distant hematogenous or lymphatic routes. Lung and brain metastases are rare, occurring in <3% of cases. Characteristic descriptions of metastatic NBL include *raccoon eyes* due to periorbital edema and ecchymosis **(Fig. 15.8.3)**, *pepper syndrome (hepatomegaly)* due to liver involvement, and subcutaneous nodules (*blueberry muffin nodules*). Persistent anemia and thrombocytopenia due to bone marrow infiltration may also be a presentation. The paraneoplastic syndromes associated with NBL are listed in **Table 15.8.2**.

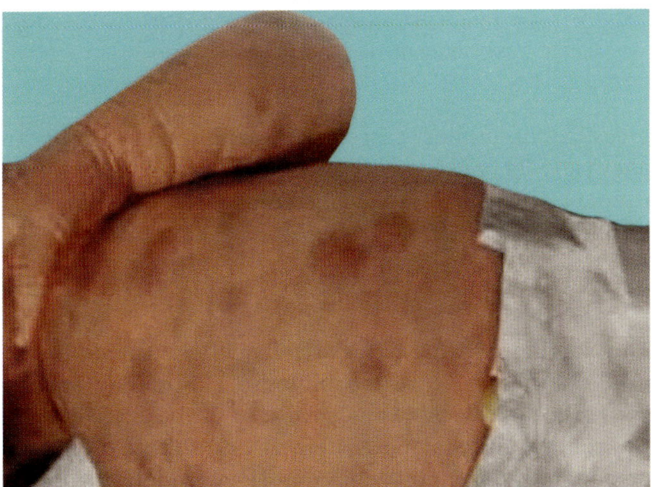

Fig. 15.8.2: Infant with neuroblastoma presenting with gross abdominal distension and blueberry muffin skin nodules.

DIFFERENTIAL DIAGNOSES

Several conditions may mimic the presentation of NBL. In a young child with a large abdominal mass, the differentials include other neoplasms such as Wilms' tumor and hepatoblastoma. Children with disseminated bone disease may mimic acute leukemia or other infectious/inflammatory diseases. Other metastatic sites like cranial bones/paraspinal soft tissue may mimic primary tumors arising from those areas. Histologically, NBL needs to be distinguished by IHC from other SBRCTs. The distinguishing features on IHC are detailed in **Table 15.8.1**.

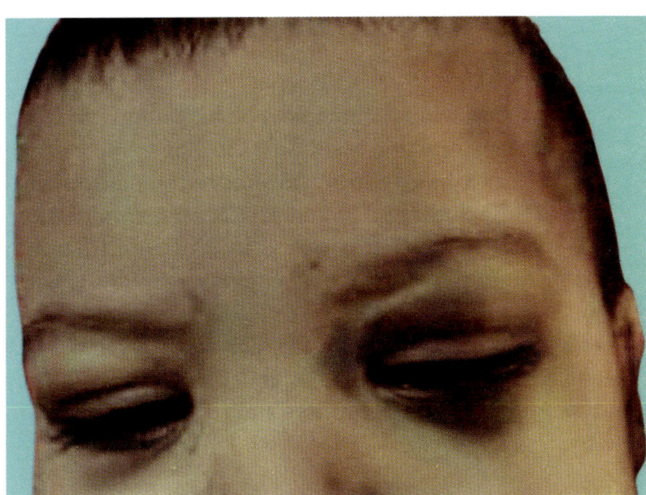

Fig. 15.8.3: Child with metastatic neuroblastoma presenting with *raccoon eyes*.

TABLE 15.8.2: Paraneoplastic syndromes associated with neuroblastoma.

Pepper syndrome	Massive involvement of the liver with metastatic disease, with or without respiratory distress
Horner syndrome	Unilateral ptosis, myosis, and anhidrosis associated with a cervical primary neuroblastoma
Opsoclonus–myoclonus syndrome (OMS)	Myoclonic jerking and random conjugate eye movements with cerebellar ataxia
Kerner–Morrison syndrome	Intractable secretory diarrhea caused by secretion of vasoactive intestinal peptide (VIP)

APPROACH TO DIAGNOSIS

A detailed physical examination, including neurologic examination, is essential in the evaluation of a child suspected to have NBL.

Diagnostic Criteria

The international criteria for the diagnosis of NBL state that diagnosis must be based on one of the following:

- An unequivocal pathologic diagnosis made from tumor tissue by light microscopy, with or without IHC, or increased levels of serum catecholamines or urinary catecholamine metabolites (VMA or HVA)
- The combination of bone marrow aspirate or trephine biopsy containing unequivocal tumor cells (e.g., syncytia or immunocytologically positive clumps of cells) and increased levels of serum catecholamines or urinary catecholamine metabolites

Initial Evaluation

Initial evaluation includes complete blood count (CBC) and liver and kidney function tests. Specific diagnostic workup of NBL includes biopsy from the tumor for pathological examination (including IHC) and *MYCN* gene amplification studies [usually by fluorescence in situ hybridization (FISH) or quantitative polymerase chain reaction (PCR)]. Lactate dehydrogenase (LDH) and ferritin are surrogate markers for identifying high-risk patients.[3] Levels of urinary catecholamine metabolites, HVA and VMA, are commonly measured for diagnostic purposes and to follow response to therapy.

Staging Workup

Ideally, imaging of the primary tumor should be done by either a computed tomography (CT) scan or magnetic resonance imaging (MRI) of the local region, depending upon the site. In practice, a CT scan of the thorax and/or abdomen and pelvis will be useful in most cases of NBL **(Figs. 15.8.4 and 15.8.5)**. MRI is preferred for paraspinal tumors to assess spinal cord compression. Essential staging/metastatic workup consists of bilateral bone marrow biopsies and imaging studies, preferably an MIBG scan, which applies to all sites of disease (primary as well as metastatic sites). MIBG scan using either ^{123}I-MIBG or ^{131}I-MIBG radionucleotide is the most sensitive metastatic investigation for skeletal and soft tissue and is now considered an essential part of staging workup as well as response evaluation in NBL (90% NBLs are MIBG-avid). Positron emission tomography (PET)-CT is gaining acceptance in the staging workup of NBL. The use of a PET-CT with contrast may suffice as a one-stop radiological investigation in most cases. ^{99}Technetium bone scan is an alternative for bony lesions if an MIBG scan is unavailable (but cannot be used for re-evaluation). The workup is summarized in **Table 15.8.3**.

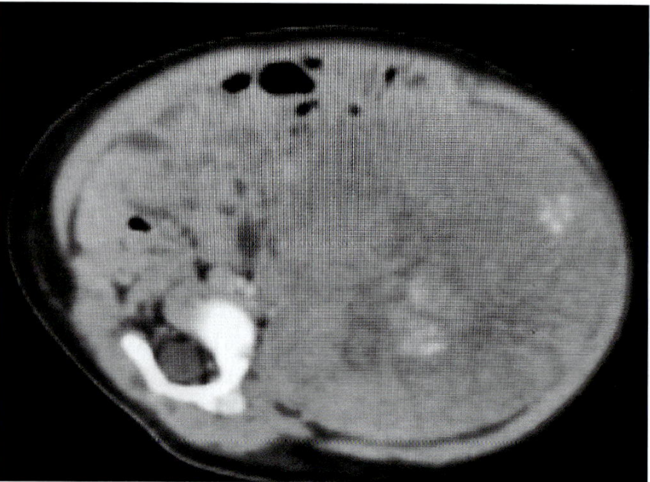

Fig. 15.8.4: Computed tomography (CT) scan of large left-sided abdominal neuroblastoma with calcifications.

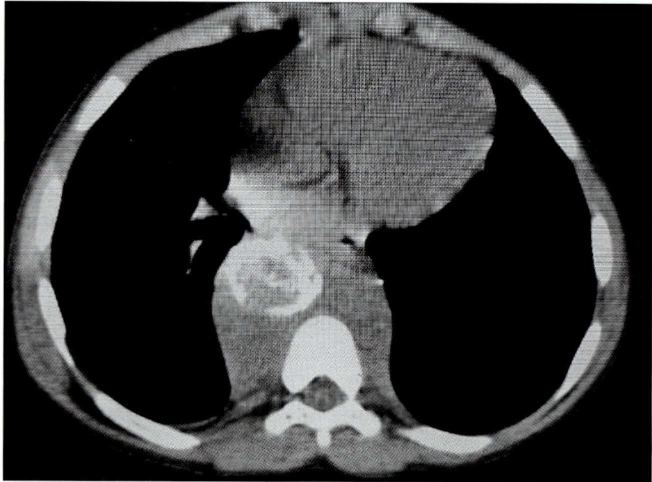

Fig. 15.8.5: Computed tomography (CT) scan of thorax showing posterior mediastinal neuroblastoma.

STAGING OF NEUROBLASTOMA

The staging of NBL has evolved with advances in the understanding of disease biology. The classic staging system proposed by Evans gave way to the International Neuroblastoma Staging System (INSS) **(Table 15.8.4)**, a postoperative staging system that is commonly used now. The International Neuroblastoma Risk Group Staging System (INRGSS) is outlined in **Table 15.8.5**.

TABLE 15.8.3: Evaluation of a child with suspected neuroblastoma.

Essential investigations	*Desirable investigations*
CBC	Urinary VMA and HVA
Serum electrolytes and renal and liver function tests	Segmental chromosomal aberrations
PT, aPTT, and INR (prior to invasive procedure/biopsy)	
Contrast-enhanced CT of primary tumor	
Tumor biopsy with IHC markers	
MIBG/FDG–PET	
Bilateral bone marrow aspiration and biopsy	
MYCN gene amplification (FISH/ MLPA)	

(aPTT: activated partial thromboplastin time; CBC: complete blood count; CT: computed tomography; FDG–PET: ^{18}fluorodeoxyglucose–positron emission tomography; FISH: fluorescence in situ hybridization; HVA: homovanillic acid; IHC: immunohistochemistry; INR: international normalized ratio; MIBG: metaiodobenzylguanidine; MLPA: multiplex ligation-dependent probe amplification; PT: prothrombin time; VMA: vanillylmandelic acid)

TABLE 15.8.4: International Neuroblastoma Staging System (INSS).

Stage 1	Localized tumor with complete gross excision, with or without microscopic residual disease; representative ipsilateral lymph nodes negative for tumor microscopically (nodes attached to and removed with the primary tumor may be positive)
Stage 2A	Localized tumor with incomplete gross excision; representative ipsilateral nonadherent lymph nodes negative for tumor microscopically
Stage 2B	• Localized tumor with or without complete gross excision, with ipsilateral nonadherent lymph nodes positive for tumor • Enlarged contralateral lymph nodes must be negative microscopically
Stage 3	Unresectable unilateral tumor infiltrating across the midline, with or without regional lymph node involvement; localized unilateral tumor with contralateral regional lymph node involvement; or midline tumor with bilateral extension by infiltration (unresectable) or by lymph node involvement
Stage 4	Any primary tumor with dissemination to distant lymph nodes, bone, bone marrow, liver, skin, and/or other organs (except as defined for stage 4S)
Stage 4S	Localized primary tumor (as defined for stage 1, 2A, or 2B), with dissemination limited to skin, liver, and/or bone marrow (limited to infants <1 year of age)

TABLE 15.8.5: International Neuroblastoma Risk Group Staging System (INRGSS).

L1	Localized tumors not involving vital structures as defined by IDRF and confined to one body compartment
L2	Locoregional tumor with the presence of one or more IDRF
M	Distant metastatic disease except for stage MS
MS	Metastatic disease in children younger than 18 months, with metastases confined to the skin, liver, and/or bone marrow

(IDRF: image-defined risk factors)

RISK STRATIFICATION

Risk stratification in NBL is based on variables such as age, clinical stage, histopathology, and biology.

The INRGSS is a preoperative staging system, where the extent of disease is determined by the presence or absence of image-defined risk factors (IDRFs) and/or metastatic tumor at the time of diagnosis before any treatment **(Table 15.8.5)**.

The International Neuroblastoma Risk Group (INRG) consensus pretreatment classification takes into account the molecular biology of the disease (DNA ploidy, *MYCN* amplification status, and 11q aberration), apart from the conventional factors such as age, INRG stage, and grade of tumor differentiation. Tumors are classified into 16 statistically distinct groups, under four broad categories: (1) very low, (2) low, (3) intermediate, and (4) high risk.

PROGNOSTIC FACTORS

Several prognostic factors have been identified in NBL—the most consistent being age at diagnosis, stage at presentation, and *N-myc* amplification.[4]

- *Stage of disease*: The stage of disease by the INSS is correlated with patient outcome (higher stages have poorer outcomes) and is used to stratify therapy.
- *Age at diagnosis*: Age <18 months confers a superior prognosis when there is no *MYCN* amplification.
- *Biological features*: *N-myc* amplification is a powerful, independent adverse prognostic marker. SCAs, found most frequently in 1p, 1q, 3p, 11q, 14q, and 17p, are being increasingly recognized as adverse prognostic factors and are being incorporated into risk stratification schema.
- *Tumor pathology*: The INPC involves the evaluation of tumor specimens obtained before therapy into favorable and unfavorable based on analysis of stromal components, degree of differentiation, MKI, and patient age.

TREATMENT OF NEUROBLASTOMA

Various modalities including surgery, radiation therapy, and chemotherapy are all used in the treatment of NBL. Treatment of NBL is tailored to the risk category and varies from cautious observation alone to aggressive multimodal treatment.[5]

Surgery

Surgery plays a pivotal role in the management of NBL, both for diagnosis and for treatment. Apart from helping to establish the diagnosis, the postoperative specimen also provides tissue for genetic studies. Although the excision of a tumor is essential, a maximal safe resection (rather than a radical surgery) is often considered adequate. Delayed surgery after chemotherapy is performed with a low rate of complications, achieving good local control of the disease.

Chemotherapy

Chemotherapy is the predominant modality of management in NBL, which is an exquisitely chemosensitive disease. The drugs commonly used include a combination of cyclophosphamide, cisplatin, doxorubicin, and etoposide. Other drugs such as ifosfamide, carboplatin, topotecan/irinotecan, and temozolomide are also used as second-line or salvage agents. Late effects of chemotherapy include sensorineural hearing loss (platinum analogs), cardiotoxicity (anthracyclines), and sterility.

Radiotherapy

Radiation therapy is an essential part of the management of high-risk NBL for local control of primary tumors as well as for control of metastatic sites. In the current treatment paradigm, radiation therapy for patients with low- or intermediate-risk NBL is reserved for symptomatic life-threatening tumors not responding to chemotherapy. Radiation is also a means of symptom control (palliation) of painful end-stage disease and may be combined with MIBG as a targeted therapy.

Risk-stratified Treatment of Neuroblastoma

Low-risk Disease

In patients with low-risk disease, surgery alone is adequate. In certain situations, a combination of surgery and chemotherapy is used (e.g., spinal cord compression and respiratory compromise secondary to hepatic infiltration). Some groups have reported observation alone without surgery for localized, suspected adrenal NBL in infants.

Treatment of Stage 4S Neuroblastoma

Most patients in this subgroup are classified as low-risk and can be managed by observation alone, as these tumors tend to regress spontaneously. Asymptomatic infants with 4S disease have been reported to have 100% survival with supportive care only. Symptomatic patients (huge hepatomegaly, respiratory, or impending neurological compromise) require short courses of low-dose chemotherapy.

Intermediate-risk Neuroblastoma

This group consists of infants with metastatic disease and patients of all ages with unresectable tumors at diagnosis. 4–8 cycles of chemotherapy followed by maximal safe resection is the recommended approach.

High-risk Neuroblastoma

The treatment of high-risk NBL remains a challenge worldwide, with outcomes of 30–50% even at the best centers. The intensive multimodality approach consists of:

Induction chemotherapy, followed by:

- Consolidation with surgery, myeloablative chemotherapy, followed by stem cell transplant, and radiation therapy
- Treatment of minimal residual disease using differentiating agents (cis-retinoic acid) and/or immunotherapy

Local Control of High-risk Neuroblastoma

Maximum safe resection with as much preservation of organ/neurologic function as possible is attempted postinduction chemotherapy. Vascular encasement, a common finding in NBL, is not a contraindication for surgery. All patients with high-risk NBL need to undergo radiation to the primary tumor site and metastatic sites.

Myeloablative chemotherapy, as well as control of minimal residual disease using differentiation agents such as 13-cis-retinoic acid, has also been shown to improve survival significantly. Immunotherapy using antigangliosidase (GD2) antibodies is also being incorporated into standard treatment protocols and is increasingly being used in India as well. Despite this aggressive approach, outcomes in high-risk NBL remain dismal. This has led to continued efforts to improve outcomes using other experimental therapies such as aurora kinase inhibitors, antiangiogenic agents, and MIBG therapy.

OUTCOMES

Various studies show a uniformly excellent prognosis (>90%) for low-risk NBL; some studies show >95% survival. Patients with intermediate-risk NBL also do well, with 80–90% cure rates. However, even at the best centers, patients with high-risk NBL do poorly with approximately 40–50% survival rates. Asymptomatic patients with stage 4S disease have nearly 100% survival.

Late diagnosis, malnutrition, improper local treatment, limited availability of autologous stem cell transplant (ASCT) and immunotherapy, and treatment abandonment contribute to further dismal outcomes in India. Hopefully, improvement in diagnostic and treatment facilities as well as financial and social support (to prevent treatment refusal and abandonment) will see an improvement in outcomes across the country.

FUTURE CONSIDERATIONS

Neuroblastoma remains the most fascinating pediatric tumor. Outcomes in low- and intermediate-risk NBL are good with existing treatment protocols. However, the treatment of high-risk NBL remains a challenge, and the long-term goal is to develop more effective and less toxic therapy. Several newer therapeutic options are being studied. It is hoped that further understanding of the molecular biology of the disease will lead to improved prognostication and subsequently more effective and less toxic therapy.

CONCLUSION

- Neuroblastoma is the most common intra-abdominal solid tumor in childhood, accounting for 8–10% of all pediatric cancers in the West (2.4–7.5% in India).
- Around 90% of patients present before 5 years of age.
- Neuroblastoma is one of the few cancers that may undergo spontaneous regression or may mature into a benign ganglioneuroma, whereas certain high-risk NBLs tend to be aggressive and progress relentlessly.
- Amplified *MYCN*—with an overall prevalence of 20% of NBL—is associated with advanced disease at diagnosis and poor outcome.
- Outcome in low- and most intermediate-risk NBL is excellent; however, the treatment of high-risk NBL remains quite challenging.
- Advances in research will lead to an improved understanding of the biology of this disease and hence to refined risk stratification and improved therapeutic approaches.

REFERENCES

1. Bansal D, Totadri S, Chinnaswamy G, Agarwala S, Vora T, Arora B, et al. Management of Neuroblastoma: ICMR Consensus Document. Indian J Pediatr. 2017;84(6):446-55.
2. Park JR, Hogarty MD, Bagatell R, Shleiermacher G, Mosse YP, Maris JM. Neuroblastoma. In: Pizzo PA, Poplack DG (Eds). Principles and Practice of Pediatric Oncology, 8th edition. Lippincott Williams & Wilkins; 2020.
3. Parikh NS, Howard SC, Chantada G, Israela T, Khattab M, Alcasabas P, et al.; International Society of Pediatric Oncology. SIOP-PODC adapted risk stratification and treatment guidelines: recommendations for neuroblastoma in low- and middle-income settings. Pediatr Blood Cancer. 2015;62(8):1305-16.
4. PDQ Pediatric Treatment Editorial Board. Neuroblastoma Treatment (PDQ®): Health Professional Version. 2024. In: PDQ Cancer Information Summaries [Internet]. Bethesda (MD): National Cancer Institute (US); 2002.
5. Matthay KK, Maris JM, Schleiermacher G, Nakagawara A, Mackall CL, Diller L, et al. Neuroblastoma. Nat Rev Dis Primers. 2016;2:16078.

15.9 Retinoblastoma

Amita Trehan, Richa Jain

INTRODUCTION

Retinoblastoma (RB) is the most common primary intraocular malignancy of childhood, affecting around 8,000 children annually and accounting for 1% of tumors in infancy. When the disease is diagnosed in its early intraocular stages, as is usual in developed countries, the probability of disease-free survival is around 90%. In developing countries, the diagnosis of RB is frequently made at later stages of the disease when extraocular dissemination has occurred, resulting in poor survival rates, estimated to be 60% and 30% in low-middle and low-income countries, respectively.[1,2]

EPIDEMIOLOGY

The incidence of sporadic RB is 1 in 15,000–20,000 live births, with no gender or racial predilection. It typically presents in the first 2–3 years of life, the median age being 12 months in heritable cases and around 24 months in sporadic cases. Presentation after 6 years of age is rare.[2]

GENETICS AND INHERITANCE PATTERN

The tumor arises from primitive cells of the developing retina with the loss of function of the RB tumor suppressor gene (*RB1*), which is located within the q14 band of chromosome 13 (Ch13q14). There are two copies (alleles) of the *RB* gene in every cell in the body. At least one functioning allele is required to prevent the development of RB in a retinal cell. Loss of both the alleles results in RB tumors. Identification of the genetic mutation is important to enable screening of family members for the mutation. In addition to *RB* gene mutation, p53 pathway is also affected in approximately 66% patients. In a small subset of patients, *MYCN* gene amplification may be noted.[2,3]

Retinoblastoma may be inherited or occur sporadically and may occur unilaterally or bilaterally. Approximately 60% cases are nonhereditary and unilateral, 15% are hereditary and unilateral, and 25% are hereditary and bilateral. The inheritance is autosomal dominant with incomplete penetrance and is identified by the presence of a germline mutation of the *RB1* gene. The significance of germline mutations lies in the possibility of transmission to the next generation and the need for genetic testing of the affected family members. Over 90% of children carrying the *RB* gene defect will develop RB. Inherited form of RB is seen at a younger age, and these children are also at the risk of developing new tumors over time.

Mutation analysis in the index case can be performed in the blood or the tumor tissue; it should ideally be done in all patients of RB regardless of the pattern of presentation. This is essential for genetic counseling and testing in future pregnancies. Patients who have germline *RB* gene mutation are at a later risk of sarcomas, including osteosarcoma, soft tissue sarcomas, melanoma, and other malignancies. This may be further potentiated by the use of radiotherapy (RT). Patients with nonheritable RB, on the other hand, do not have an increased risk of secondary malignancies.[1-3]

ANATOMY

The tumor arises from the retina and grows toward the vitreous. This is known as endophytic growth and is associated with vitreous seeding. Occasionally, there is growth in the subretinal space, and this is called exophytic growth. Progression of the tumor results in the involvement of ocular coats and the optic nerve, which may subsequently lead to scleral, orbital, and central nervous system (CNS) involvement. It progresses through the choroid and can invade the bloodstream with resultant distant metastasis.[2]

PATHOLOGY

Retinoblastoma is a small blue round cell tumor. It shows abundant mitosis and necrosis due to its rapidly proliferating nature. Flexner–Wintersteiner rosettes and Homer–Wright rosettes may both be present in the tumor. The dual presence of both types of rosettes is pathognomonic for RB. The degree of anaplasia in the tumor is associated with prognosis, with a worse prognosis in a highly anaplastic tumor.[3]

CLINICAL FEATURES

The most frequent presenting symptoms are leukocoria, a white reflex in the pupil, followed by squint, noted by family members or the child's pediatrician. In the era of smartphones, an important symptom is the presence of a white reflex in the eye instead of the usual red reflex on taking a picture of the child. This has at times been noted by the parents and brought to the attention of doctors. Several smartphone apps use this feature and are now freely available to help medical personnel in the field determine the presence of a white reflex in the eye of a child. This may help determine the need for an early referral to a specialized center where further assessment can be performed for the confirmation of diagnosis.[3,4]

Other clinical features include redness and pain, secondary to tumor deposits and increased intraocular pressure. Bilateral cases often present with poor vision and nystagmus or searching eye movements as a result of tumor involving the central part of the retina (macula) in both the eyes.

Massive proptosis or a fungating mass with lymphadenopathy is frequently seen at presentation in developing countries (including India) because of late presentation **(Fig. 15.9.1)**. Metastases occur by spreading of the tumor along the optic nerve to involve the CNS or through the choroid, resulting in hematogenous spread to bones, bone marrow, lungs, and liver. Associated CNS tumor may be present in the pineal gland, suprasellar, or intrasellar region. This is called trilateral RB. This is essentially an inheritable form of the disease and frequently has CNS dissemination.[3] Rarely quadrilateral RB (both pineal and suprasellar region involvement) may occur. Both trilateral and quadrilateral RB have worse prognosis than localized RB.

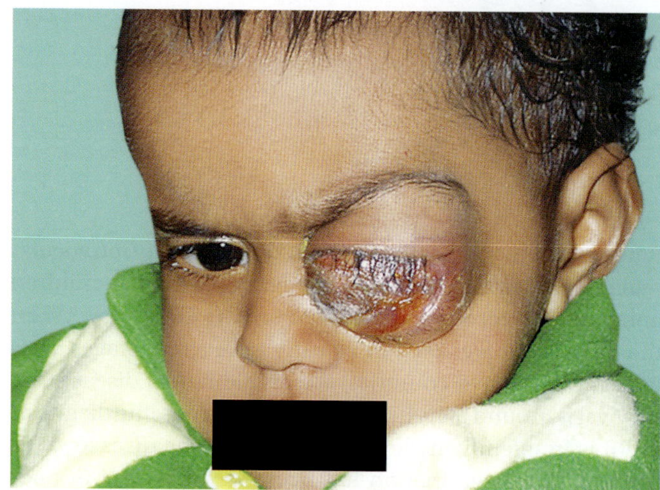

Fig. 15.9.1: Large mass is the presenting feature in developing countries.

CATEGORIZATION[1,2]

Retinoblastoma is categorized as intraocular or extraocular:

- *Intraocular*: Tumor is localized to the eye and may be confined to the retina. It may involve the choroid, ciliary body, anterior chamber, and optic nerve head, which are considered to be high-risk features. However, there should not be any evidence of disease at the optic nerve resection margin or beyond the sclera.
- *Extraocular*: Tumor has extended beyond the eye. It may be localized to the tissues around the eye (orbital RB); it may have spread to the CNS or systemically (metastatic RB).

DIFFERENTIAL DIAGNOSIS[2,3]

The important differential diagnoses of intraocular RB include:

- Coats' disease (a telangiectatic neovascular disease of the retina of unknown etiology)
- Persistent fetal vasculature
- Toxocariasis
- Cellulitis
- Metastasis
- Cataract
- Coloboma
- Retinopathy of prematurity
- Retinal detachment

In extraocular disease with proptosis, differential diagnoses include:

- Langerhans cell histiocytosis
- Rhabdomyosarcoma
- Acute myeloid leukemia or granulocytic sarcoma
- Burkitt lymphoma
- Arteriovenous malformations (AVM) or lymphangiomatosis of the eye
- Staphyloma

INVESTIGATIONS

The diagnosis is essentially clinical, with the support from imaging. Intraocular RB typically does not require tissue diagnosis. Tissue diagnosis may cause seeding or extraocular spread of the tumor.[2-5]

- *Indirect ophthalmoscopy:* This is generally performed under anesthesia. This includes the assessment of intraocular pressure. A manual examination is aided by real-time retinal imaging systems such as RetCam, which can provide digital recording.
- *Optical coherence tomography (OCT)* is a diagnostic tool using differential near-infrared light reflection. It has a higher resolution than ultrasonography (USG) or magnetic resonance imaging (MRI) and is used to image the disc and the macula in small intraocular tumors.
- *B-scan USG:* This confirms the presence of masses and calcification in the posterior segment of the eye. Calcification is characteristic of this tumor. USG is also helpful in monitoring the response to treatment, which will be seen as a reduction in the size of the tumor.
- *Computed tomography (CT) or MRI scan:* Imaging is done for visualization of the globe, orbit, CNS, and the pineal region (to look for pinealoblastoma, trilateral RB). MRI is preferred, as there is limited radiation exposure and improved visualization of the periorbital structures and orbital portion of the optic nerve.
- *Cerebrospinal fluid (CSF) examination for malignant cytology:* This is indicated in microscopic or overt extraocular disease or the presence of optic nerve thickening on neuroimaging. It is not required in intraocular RB.
- *Bone marrow:* This is performed in patients with extraocular disease (stage II and above) and/or those with altered complete blood counts (CBCs). Typically, a bilateral trephine along with bone marrow aspirate is done.
- *Abdominal USG*: This is performed when there is suspicion of metastasis to the liver.
- *Biopsy or fine-needle aspiration cytology (FNAC)*: This is a contraindication; occasionally, FNAC or vitreous tap may be performed when there is doubt in the primary diagnosis.

In children with overt extraocular disease, a fundus examination may not be possible due to the mass distorting the eye architecture. In such cases, a detailed history and a good clinical examination supported by imaging are sufficient to establish a diagnosis. Tissue diagnosis is required rarely.

STAGING

There are separate staging systems for intraocular and extraocular RB. The current staging system for intraocular RB is known as the International Classification of Intraocular Retinoblastoma **(Table 15.9.1)**.[6] It is based on the extent of

TABLE 15.9.1: International Classification of Intraocular Retinoblastoma.

Group A	No tumor >3 mm in dimension; away from fovea and optic nerve
Group B	Any eye not in Group A with no vitreous seeding, and subretinal fluid is <5 mm from the base of the tumor
Group C	Tumors with focal fine vitreous seeding or subretinal fluid (less than one quadrant)
Group D	Massive or diffuse vitreous seeding and extensive subretinal masses
Group E	Unsalvageable eyes, neovascular glaucoma, tumor touching the lens, anterior segment tumor, phthisis, and diffuse-infiltrating retinoblastoma

TABLE 15.9.2: Staging: International Retinoblastoma Staging System (IRSS).

Stage 0	Patients treated conservatively
Stage I	Eye enucleated, completely resected histologically
Stage II	Eye enucleated, microscopic residual tumor
Stage III	• Regional extension • Overt orbital disease • Preauricular or cervical node extension
Stage IV	Metastatic disease: *Stage IVa*: Central nervous system extension (with or without any other site of regional or metastatic disease): • Prechiasmatic lesion • Central nervous system mass • Leptomeningeal and cerebrospinal fluid (CSF) disease *Stage IVb*: Hematogenous metastasis (without central nervous system involvement): • Single lesion • Multiple lesions

tumor seeding in the vitreous and subretinal space and helps in predicting success of therapy. The older Reese–Ellsworth classification is no longer practiced. Another staging system exists for patients undergoing enucleation. This system is known as the International Retinoblastoma Staging System (IRSS); it also helps in defining and prognosticating extraocular RB **(Table 15.9.2)**.[7] A TNM (tumor, node, and metastasis) staging system has also been described recently by the American Joint Committee on Cancer (AJCC), making RB the only CNS tumor to have a TNM staging. The TNM staging system also incorporates the heritable nature of tumor. The International Classification of Retinoblastoma (ICRB) and IRSS are currently the more commonly used staging systems world over.[8]

TREATMENT

The therapy aims at:

- Eradication of disease
- Preservation of vision
- Preservation of life

Limited stage intraocular disease may be treatable only by focal therapy (detailed further). In the case of advanced-stage (Group D or E) intraocular disease, enucleation may be required. Alternative therapies include the combination of chemotherapy and focal therapies, intra-arterial chemotherapy, and newer modalities in a bid to preserve the eye.[2,9]

Treatment of extraocular RB, which has locoregional extension, includes initial neoadjuvant chemotherapy followed by enucleation, further chemotherapy, and radiation therapy (RT). Metastatic disease has poor outcome, and patients with CNS metastasis fare the worst, with dismal survival despite multimodality therapy and autologous stem cell transplantation.[3,10]

Types of Focal Therapy

- *Photocoagulation* is the primary treatment in smaller tumors. It may also be used after chemoreduction. The argon laser is used for photocoagulation. Laser treatment is not effective for vitreous seeds.
- *Cryotherapy*: A special probe is applied through the sclera to produce temperatures as low as –60°C to –80°C resulting in cryonecrosis of the tumors. This is suitable for tumors smaller than 4-disc diameters close to the retina.
- *Thermotherapy*: Diode laser is used for thermotherapy at temperatures just below the photocoagulation range.

Intra-arterial Chemotherapy

Intra-arterial chemotherapy is a modality used for advanced-stage intraocular disease. This involves direct delivery of chemotherapy into the eye via cannulation of the ophthalmic artery. Typically, one to six courses of such therapy may be required. Melphalan is the most commonly used chemotherapeutic agent. Intra-arterial chemotherapy helps in preserving the eye by preventing enucleation, even though vision may not always be salvaged. Other agents, such as topotecan and carboplatin, are also being tested and administered as single agents or in combination. This has shown high success in intraocular unilateral tumors.[9,10]

Chemotherapy

The main role of chemotherapy is in the treatment of extraocular disease; it is also used for intraocular advanced-stage disease. It helps to shrink the tumors to a size where local treatment can be effective. The most commonly used drugs include carboplatin, etoposide, vincristine, anthracyclines, and cyclophosphamide. In intraocular disease, only high-risk cases are candidates for chemotherapy. High risk includes the presence of anterior chamber involvement with or without buphthalmos, choroidal involvement, postlaminar optic nerve, or scleral involvement. Extraocular disease is treated with a multimodality approach consisting of combination chemotherapy, delayed surgery, and RT. In addition, metastatic RB also requires adjuvant high-dose chemotherapy with hematopoietic stem cell transplantation (HSCT).[3,9,10]

Surgery

Enucleation is the common surgical modality. It is the treatment of choice for advanced uniocular disease, with no hope for vision or the worse eye of bilateral cases. The eye is removed with a long segment of optic nerve. Chemotherapy may be required in cases with high-risk features. Orbital exenteration is almost never used in the current scenario.[3]

Radiotherapy

Retinoblastoma is a radiosensitive tumor. In combination with chemotherapy, RT is used for the treatment of extraocular disease. This is in the form of external beam RT. Brachytherapy can be used to treat small intraocular tumors, which have not responded well to chemotherapy or other forms of focal therapy. Proton beam therapy, though not available widely, has a role in the treatment of bilateral disease, as there is less chance of secondary malignant neoplasm.[10]

Newer Modalities

- *Subtenon (subconjunctival) chemotherapy*: Periocular injections of carboplatin/other agents to increase levels of the drug and enhance efficacy, particularly in high-tumor burden
- *Intravitreal chemotherapy*: Direct injection of drugs into the vitreous cavity has been attempted. Studies suggest that direct intravitreal injection of melphalan, topotecan, or a combination of both may be effective in controlling active vitreous seeds. The injections can be given at 1–4 weekly intervals for up to six injections.
- *Gene therapy*: "Suicide gene therapy" has been tried in early clinical trials in children with advanced intraocular disease **(Fig. 15.9.2)**.

Treatment schema for children with unilateral RB is demonstrated in **Flowchart 15.9.1**.[10]

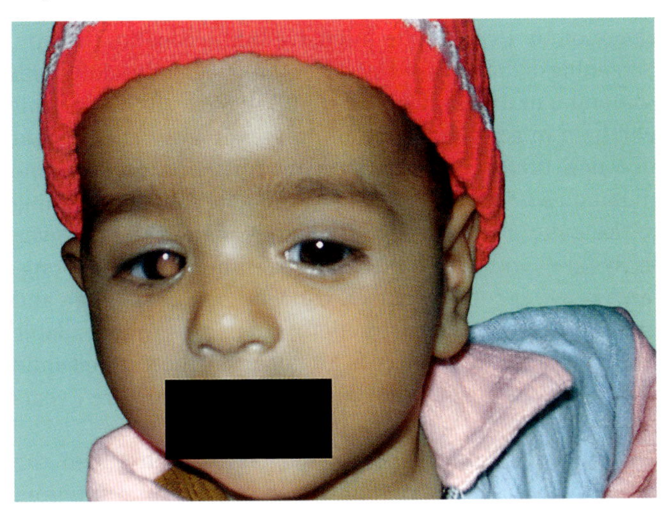

Fig. 15.9.2: White eye reflex along with squint in a case of intraocular retinoblastoma.

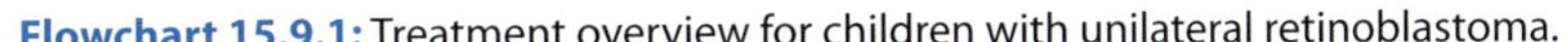

Flowchart 15.9.1: Treatment overview for children with unilateral retinoblastoma.

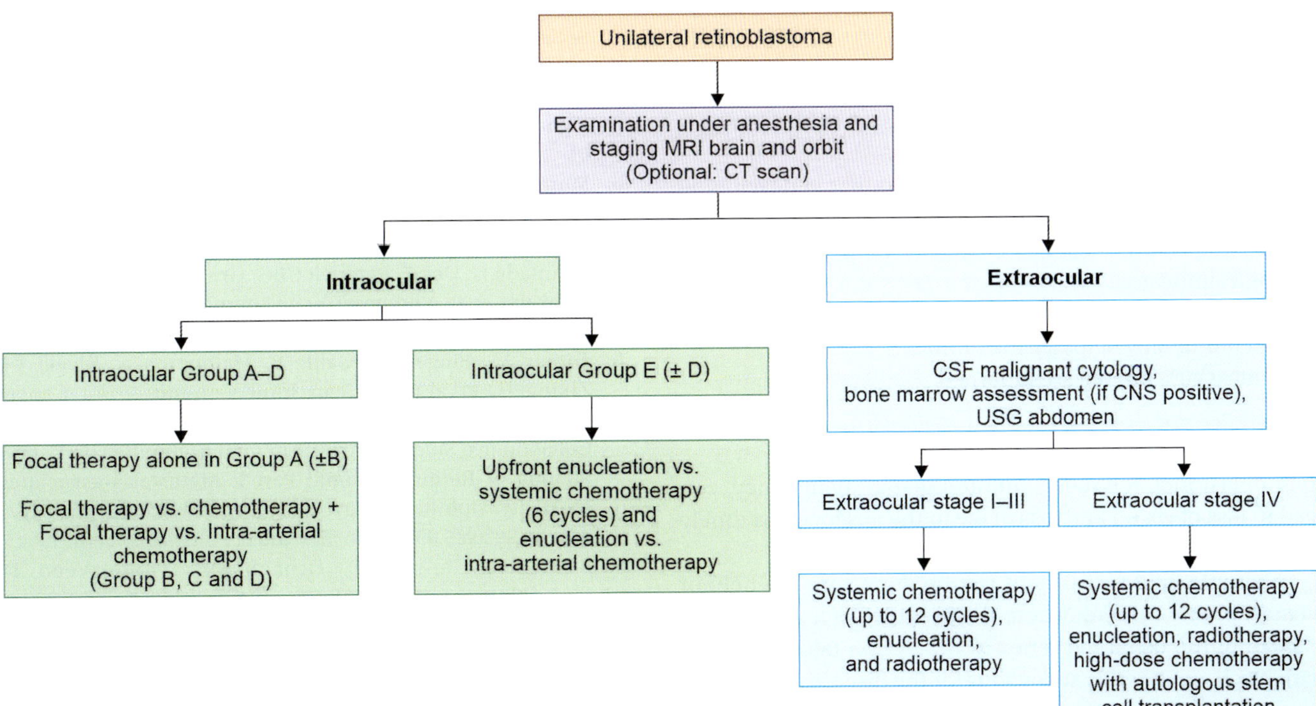

(CNS: central nervous system; CSF: cerebrospinal fluid; CT: computed tomography; MRI: magnetic resonance imaging; USG: ultrasonography)

OUTCOME

While the outcome of intraocular and nonmetastatic RB ranges from 40 to 80%, the presence of metastatic or trilateral disease is associated with exceedingly poor prognosis. Prognosis is worse for CNS disease than it is for systemic disease, as chemotherapy does not effectively cross the blood–brain barrier. These patients have outcomes in the range of 10–15% despite intensive multimodality therapy. Screening of the salvaged eye is required regularly, along with screening of the uninvolved eye till the age of 7 years. This will help in early detection of progression or development of a new tumor. Genetic screening for heritable *RB1* gene mutation is advisable, as it helps formulate plan for screening of the index case as well as the family members. Moreover, individuals with inherited *RB1* gene mutation require long-term screening for secondary cancers such as sarcoma and epithelial cancers. In case genetic screening is not available or prohibitive due to the cost, all siblings of the affected child should be screened for the presence of RB till they are 7 years of age.[3,10]

The important problems associated with RB in the developing countries are advanced stage of presentation, poor socioeconomic status of the majority of patients, and, most importantly, treatment abandonment due to fear of enucleation. Early detection of RB and emphasis on regular screening of the other eye of the patient as well as siblings of patients with RB are modalities that would help improve outcomes.

KEY MESSAGES

- Retinoblastoma has a good prognosis when the tumor is intraocular at diagnosis.
- Advanced stage of presentation is frequent in developing countries.
- Essentially, it is a clinical diagnosis; biopsy or FNAC are contraindicated.
- Small intraocular tumors may be cured by focal therapy.
- Chemotherapy helps shrink tumors.
- Almost 40% tumors are inherited.

CONCLUSION

Retinoblastoma, the most common ocular malignancy, can lead to loss of vision and loss of life in the absence of a timely diagnosis and appropriate treatment.

A simple field assessment can be done with the help of a smart phone camera; where the presence of a white reflex instead of the usual red reflex in the eye on taking a photo with 'flash' on is highly suspicious for the disease.

Diagnosis is made by examining the eye under anesthesia, without a biopsy. Imaging of brain and orbit (CT or MRI) is required to stage the disease.

Intraocular retinoblastoma in early stages may be treatable with focal laser treatment, cryotherapy or thermal therapy. Vision may be salvaged.

Extraocular retinoblastoma requires a combination of systemic chemotherapy, enucleation, and radiotherapy for successful treatment; though the vision is not salvageable.

It is heritable in approximately 40% cases. Screening of uninvolved eye as well as screening of siblings' eyes is required from an early age till approximately 7 years.

Genetic testing for germline RB gene mutation is advisable. It helps in planning family screening as well as screening for secondary malignancies in the index case.

REFERENCES

1. Chevz-Barrios P, Gimbos DS. Clinical features, diagnosis, pathology. In: Rodriguez-Galindo C, Wilson MW (Eds). Retinoblastoma, 1st edition. New York: Springer; 2010. pp. 25-40.
2. Leahey AM, Gombos DS, Chevez-Barrios P. Retinoblastoma. In: Blaney SM, Adamson PC, Helman LJ (Eds). Principles and Practice of Pediatric Oncology, 8th edition. Philadelphia: Lippincott Williams and Wilkins; 2021. pp. 868-88.
3. Dimaras H, Corson TW. Retinoblastoma, the visible CNS tumor: A review. J Neurosci Res. 2019;97(1):29-44.
4. Singh L, Chinnaswamy G, Meel R, Radhakrishnan V, Madan R, Kulkarni S, et al. Epidemiology, Diagnosis and Genetics of Retinoblastoma: ICMR Consensus Guidelines. Indian J Pediatr. 2024;91(11):1147-56.
5. Chantada GL, Dunkel IJ, Abramson DH. Management of high-risk retinoblastoma. Expert Rev Ophthalmol. 2012;7(1): 61-72.
6. Murphree AL. Intraocular retinoblastoma: the case for a new group classification. Ophthalmol Clin North Am. 2005;18(1):41-53, viii.
7. Chantada G, Doz F, Antoneli CBG, Grundy R, Stannard FFC, Dunkel IJ, et al. A proposal for an international retinoblastoma staging system. Pediatr Blood Cancer. 2006;47(6):801-5.
8. Tomar AS, Finger PT, Gallie B, Mallipatna A, Kivelä TT, Zhang C, et al. American Joint Committee on Cancer Ophthalmic Oncology Task Force. A Multicenter, International Collaborative Study for American Joint Committee on Cancer Staging of Retinoblastoma: Part I: Metastasis-associated Mortality. Ophthalmology. 2020;127:1719-32. doi: 10.1016/j.ophtha.2020.05.050. Epub 2020 Jun 6. PMID: 32512116.
9. Rodriguez-Galindo C, Orbach DB, VanderVeen D. Retinoblastoma. Pediatr Clin North Am. 2015;62(1):201-23.
10. Wilson MW. Treatment of intraocular retinoblastoma. In: Rodriguez-Galindo C, Wilson MW (Eds). Retinoblastoma, 1st edition. New York: Springer; 2010. pp. 91-101.

15.10 Soft-tissue Sarcoma

Gauri Kapoor

INTRODUCTION

Pediatric soft-tissue sarcomas (STS) are a group of malignant tumors that originate from primitive mesenchymal tissues and account for 7% of all childhood tumors. Rhabdomyosarcomas (RMS) are the most common of these and constitute about half of all cases of all STS in children. The remaining nonrhabdomyosarcomatous soft-tissue sarcomas (NRSTS) account for approximately 3% of all childhood tumors. The latter constitute a heterogeneous group of tumors and are rare in children. They include fibrosarcoma, neurofibrosarcoma, leiomyosarcoma, liposarcoma, synovial sarcoma, hemangiopericytoma, alveolar soft part sarcoma, and malignant fibrous histiocytoma, of which the synovial sarcoma, fibrosarcoma, and malignant peripheral nerve sheath tumor predominate in pediatric patients.

EPIDEMIOLOGY

- About 3% of all childhood cancers are RMS.[1]
- About 400–500 new cases of RMS occur each year in the United States of America. The number of new cases has not changed much over the past few decades.[1]
- Most RMS cases are diagnosed in children and teenagers. About 6 out of 10 of these tumors are diagnosed in children under the age of 10 years.
- These tumors are usually embryonal RMS and occur in the head and neck area (25%), in the genital and urinary tracts (31%), or in extremity (13%).[2]
- Adolescents and adults are more likely than younger children to have alveolar RMS, found more often in the arms, legs, or trunk.
- This disease is slightly more common in boys than in girls.
- There is no particular geographic location or ethnic group that has an unusually high rate of RMS.
- Children 1–9 years of age usually have a better outcome than infants and older children (≥10 years) and adolescents.

ETIOPATHOGENESIS

No known environmental factors are known to cause RMS in children. Some genetic and environmental factors have been associated with the development of NRSTS: Li–Fraumeni syndrome and neurofibromatosis type 1 (NF1). Members of the Li–Fraumeni families have an increased risk of developing soft-tissue tumors, bone sarcomas, breast cancers, brain tumors, and acute leukemias and have heritable mutations in the p53 tumor suppressor gene. Approximately 4% of patients with NF1 develop malignant peripheral nerve sheath tumors. Patients with familial adenomatous polyposis are at an increased risk of developing desmoid tumors. The malignant fibrous histiocytoma can develop within a previously irradiated site; others (e.g., leiomyosarcoma) have been linked to Epstein–Barr virus (EBV) infection in patients with acquired immune deficiency syndrome (AIDS).[2-4]

CLINICAL FEATURES

The most common sign of childhood STS is a painless lump or swelling, which may occur anywhere in the body. There may be no other symptoms at first; however, as the sarcoma grows, it may manifest with pressure symptoms on adjacent organs, nerves, muscles, or blood vessels, leading to pain or weakness, etc. Systemic symptoms (e.g., fever, weight loss, and night sweats) are rare. Hypoglycemia and hypophosphatemic rickets have been reported in cases of hemangiopericytoma, whereas hyperglycemia has been noted in patients with fibrosarcoma of the lung.

Rhabdomyosarcomas may originate in different sites of the body depending upon the age of the child. Most head and neck tumors occur in children under the age of 8 years, while those of the extremity are most commonly found in adolescents. Less common primary sites for this cancer are the genitourinary tract, including the bladder and prostate in the male and the vagina in the female.[4]

Nonrhabdomyosarcomatous soft-tissue sarcomas arise most commonly in the trunk and extremities. These neoplasms can present initially as an asymptomatic solid mass or may be symptomatic because of local invasion of the adjacent anatomical structures. Synovial sarcomas, the most common NRSTS, reported in children, most commonly occur in the lower extremity followed by upper extremity, trunk, abdomen, and head and neck. Approximately 30% of patients with synovial sarcoma are younger than 20 years. The most common site of metastasis is the lung.[5]

DIAGNOSIS

In STS as in all cancers, the first step in management is to establish a confirmed histological diagnosis. A thorough clinical examination helps the clinician plan the imaging investigations. Often the initial imaging is a plain X-ray (extremity) or ultrasound (for visceral masses) which gives an idea about the organ of origin of the tumor. This is followed by a computed tomography (CT) scan or magnetic resonance image (MRI) of the tumor prior to planning a biopsy. Obtaining adequate tissue is essential for diagnosis which may be image-guided biopsy (tru-cut needle biopsy), incisional biopsy, or excisional biopsy.

Rhabdomyosarcomas is a malignant round cell tumor and can appear very similar to other childhood cancers at the microscopic level, and immunohistochemistry (IHC) and molecular genetic tests are required to establish a firm diagnosis. Hence, obtaining sufficient tissue for histology, IHC, and molecular studies (if required) is very important to accurately characterize the STS as RMS or NRSTS.

Biopsy

The technique of biopsy is critically important in the diagnosis and management of STS. As discussed in the preceding text, adequate tissue may be obtained by core-needle biopsy, incisional biopsy, or excisional biopsy. It is recommended that planning and execution of biopsy be done by the surgeon who will perform the definitive resection as poorly planned biopsies may violate tissue planes, thereby compromising the performance of resection of the primary tumor.

Classification of STS according to histological type with corresponding chromosomal aberration is given in **Table 15.10.1**.

STAGING

Approximately 15–25% of patients present with metastatic disease at the time of diagnosis, which determines the stage of the tumor. The most common site of spread is lung, followed by bone, bone marrow, and lymph nodes. Hence, once a histological diagnosis is confirmed, further tests are done to determine the stage of the disease. Clinical staging has an important role in predicting the clinical outcome and determining the most effective therapy for pediatric STS. In RMS, CT chest, bone marrow aspiration and biopsy and bone scan are done to look for metastatic disease at these sites while for NRSTS, only CT chest is required. Whole-body positron-emission tomography (PET) scan may also be done as a single imaging to look for metastatic disease. The staging systems used are the Intergroup Rhabdomyosarcoma Study Group (IRSG), tumor, node, metastases (TNM) for RMS, and the Children's Oncology Group (COG) staging system for children with NRSTS **(Tables 15.10.2 and 15.10.3)**.

PROGNOSIS

The treatment outcome for pediatric RMS depends on anatomic site, patient age, stage, and histology, on the basis of which they are risk stratified. The various unfavorable prognostic factors include older age (>10 years), metastatic disease, large tumor (>5 cm), alveolar histology, and primary tumor at unresectable sites like trunk or pelvis. Based on the above factors, the patients are risk stratified as low risk, intermediate risk, and high risk and have a 3-year failure-free survival rate of 88%, 55–75%, and <30%, respectively **(Table 15.10.4)**.

MANAGEMENT

The treatment for childhood STS requires a multidisciplinary oncology team comprising pediatric oncologists, surgeons, and radiotherapists. All children require systemic chemotherapy in addition to either surgery or radiotherapy or both.

TABLE 15.10.1: Classification of soft tissue sarcomas (STS) according to histological type with corresponding chromosomal aberration.

Group	*Histological type*	*Chromosomal aberration*
Rhabdomyosarcomas (RMS)	• Embryonal RMS • Alveolar RMS • Spindle cell sclerosing RMS • Pleomorphic RMS	*Embryonal:* LOH of 11q15 *Alveolar*: t(2;13)(q35;q14), t(1;13)(p36;q14)
Nonrhabdomyosarcomatous soft-tissue sarcomas (NRSTS)	• Fibrosarcoma • Neurofibrosarcoma • Infantile fibrosarcoma • Malignant fibrous histiocytoma • Dermatofibrosarcoma protuberans • Kaposi sarcoma • Hemangioendothelioma • Leiomyosarcoma • Liposarcoma myxoid • Angiosarcoma • Synovial sarcoma • Alveolar soft part sarcoma • Epithelioid sarcoma	Deletion 17q11.26.2 t(12,15)(p13:q25) (qp+, ring chromosome) t(17;22)(q22;q13) t(12;14) (LM): t(12;22) or t(12;16) (Ss): t(x;18)(p11.2;q11.2) (Alv): t(x;17)(p11.2;q25)

TABLE 15.10.2: Children's Oncology Group-Soft Tissue Sarcoma (COG-STS) pretreatment staging system for rhabdomyosarcoma (RMS).

Stage	Sites of primary tumor	T stage	Tumor size	Regional lymph nodes	Distant metastasis
I	Favorable sites Orbit Head and neck Genitourinary	T1 or T2 T1 or T2 T1 or T2 T1 or T2	Any size	N0 or N1 or Nx	M0
II	Unfavorable sites Bladder/prostate Extremity Cranial Parameningeal	T1 or T2 T1 or T2 T1 or T2 T1 or T2 T1 or T2	≤5 cm	N0 or Nx	M0
III	Other unfavorable sites Bladder/prostate Extremity Cranial Parameningeal	T1 or T2 T1 or T2 T1 or T2 T1 or T2 T1 or T2	a. ≤5 cm b. ≥5 cm	N1 N0 or N1 or Nx	M0
IV	*Other* Any site All	T1 or T2 T1 or T2	Any size	N0 or N1 or Nx	M1

(M0: absence of metastatic spread; M1: presence of metastatic spread beyond the primary site; N0: absence of nodal spread; N1: presence of nodal spread beyond the primary site; Nx: unknown N status; T1: confined to anatomic site of origin, T2: extension and/or fixative to surrounding tissue)

TABLE 15.10.3: Children's Oncology Group-Soft Tissue Sarcomas (COG-STS) surgicopathologic group system for rhabdomyosarcoma (RMS).

Group		Definition
I	Approximately 13% of all patients are in this group	A localized tumor that is completely removed with pathologically clear margins and no regional lymph node involvement
II	Approximately 20% of all patients are in this group	A localized tumor that is grossly removed with: a. Microscopic disease at the margin b. Involve, grossly removed regional lymph nodes – Both (a) and (b)
III	Approximately 48% of all patients are in this group	A localized tumor with gross residual disease after incomplete removal or biopsy only
IV	Approximately 18% of all patients are in this group	Distant metastases are present at diagnosis

TABLE 15.10.4: Children's Oncology Group-Soft Tissue Sarcomas (COG-STS) rhabdomyosarcoma risk group classification.

Risk group prognosis (event-free survival)	Histology	Stage	Group
Low-risk Excellent (70 to ≥85%)	Embryonal	1	I, II, III
	Embryonal	2, 3	I, II
Intermediate-risk Good (50–70%)	Embryonal	2, 3	III
	Alveolar	1, 2, 3	I, II, III
High-risk Poor (≤30%)	Embryonal or alveolar	4	IV

Rhabdomyosarcoma

Chemotherapy

Rhabdomyosarcoma is a chemosensitive disease, and micrometastatic disease is believed to be present from its onset. Hence, all children with RMS receive chemotherapy, which forms the backbone of treatment, and the dose and duration depend on various risk factors. The most effective drugs include cyclophosphamide, vincristine, dactinomycin, doxorubicin, ifosfamide, and etoposide. The total duration of treatment ranges from 6 to 12 months based on the risk group.

Surgery

All children diagnosed with RMS also require surgery, either to remove all or part of the primary tumor or to perform an incisional or needle biopsy to reach a definitive diagnosis. Only about 10% of newly diagnosed children have tumors that can be completely removed. Every attempt should be made to resect the primary tumor with negative margins before or after chemotherapy (second-look surgery) and while causing minimum cosmetic and functional impairment.

Radiation Therapy

Radiation therapy is an important local control measure for all children with RMS except those with completely resected stage I and II disease. The total radiation dose ranges from 4,000 to 5,500 cGy over a period of 4–6 weeks. It is usually planned approximately 9 weeks after chemotherapy has begun and earlier for those with parameningeal disease. With the use of both surgery and radiation therapy, local control of the primary tumor can be achieved in more than 80% of patients.

Outcome

Childhood RMS is a curable disease. With appropriate treatment, the 5-year survival of low-, intermediate-, and high-risk RMS is 90%, 70%, and 30%, respectively.

Nonrhabdomyosarcomatous Soft-tissue Sarcomas

Surgery

For NRSTS, surgery is the cornerstone of the treatment. Ideally, an attempt is made to completely remove the mass with wide margins (portions of the surrounding tissue) to ensure that no microscopic disease remains. The most important prognostic factor is the ability to completely remove the primary tumor.

Radiation Therapy

Radiation therapy is indicated for patients with inadequate surgical margins and for larger, high-grade tumors. This is particularly important in high-grade tumors with tumor margins <1 cm. Brachytherapy and intraoperative radiation may be applicable in select situations.

Chemotherapy

Chemotherapy is sometimes used to shrink large tumors to make them operable. The two most active agents are ifosfamide and adriamycin. The role of adjuvant (postoperative) chemotherapy remains controversial for NRSTS.

Targeted Therapy

The role of antiangiogenesis agents and mammalian target of rapamycin (mTOR) inhibitors has been explored in adults but not in children.

Outcome

Long-term survival is dependent on the presence of metastatic disease and completeness of the surgical excision.

LATE EFFECTS

Improved outcomes with multimodality therapy in children with STS have caused increasing concern about the potential long-term side effects of therapy, especially when considering the expected longer life span of children. Late effects including consequences on growth and development, cardiac function, second malignancy, fertility, musculoskeletal hypoplasia, etc., all need to be considered when planning the treatment.

CONCLUSION

- STS comprise the fifth most common type of childhood solid tumor, of which RMS is the most common.
- It can arise at any site and in any tissue in the body except bone; hence, it may present as a mass or lump.
- Confirmation of histology and staging workup are essential prior to starting the therapy.
- The treatment for childhood STS is a coordinated multidisciplinary team effort comprising pediatric oncologists, surgeons, and radiotherapists.
- Chemotherapy is an essential component of therapy for RMS along with surgery and/or RT for local control. Survival depends on the risk group.
- For NRSTS, surgery is the mainstay of treatment with or without RT.

REFERENCES

1. American Cancer Society. (2020). Rhabdomyosarcoma. [online] Available from https://www.cancer.org/cancer/types/rhabdomyosarcoma.html [Last accessed December, 2024].
2. National Cancer Institute. Childhood Rhabdomyosarcoma Treatment (PDQ®)–Health Professional Version. [online] Available from https://www.cancer.gov/types/soft-tissue-sarcoma/hp/rhabdomyosarcoma-treatment-pdq [Last accessed December, 2024].
3. National Cancer Institute. Soft tissue sarcoma—Patient version. [online] Available from www.cancer.gov/cancertopics/types/soft- tissue-sarcoma [Last accessed December, 2024].
4. Linardic CM, Wexler LH. Rhabdomyosarcoma. In: Pizzo PA, Poplack DG (Eds). Principles and Practice of Pediatric Oncology, 8th edition. Philadelphia, PA: Lippincott Williams and Wilkins; 2021. pp. 2142-260.
5. Hawkins DS, O'Black J, Orbach D, et al. The nonrhabdomyosarcoma soft tissue sarcoma. In: Pizzo PA, Poplack DG (Eds). Principles and Practice of Pediatric Oncology, 8th edition. Philadelphia, PA: Lippincott Williams and Wilkins; 2021. pp. 2261-98.

15.11 Late Effects of Treatments in Survivors of Childhood Cancers

Purna A Kurkure, Vandana Dhamankar

INTRODUCTION

Surviving childhood cancer marks a profound victory over illness, yet it often heralds the beginning of a new journey filled with challenges after treatment ends. While advances in treatment have dramatically improved survival rates, studies show that survivors frequently face enduring complications that significantly impact their quality of life. As highlighted by the Children's Oncology Group (COG), late effects—such as cardiovascular, endocrine, neurological, and psychosocial issues—are common, necessitating lifelong surveillance and individualized care.[1] Findings from the "After Completion of Treatment (ACT) Clinic" in India echo these observations, documenting a 30-year experience in prevalence of such late effects.[2] These physical, psychological, and social challenges often emerge months or years after therapy concludes, underscoring the need for comprehensive, ongoing care to ensure that survivors not only achieve prolonged lifespans but also engage in healthier, more fulfilling lives. Continuous research and integrative care frameworks are essential to optimizing long-term outcomes and supporting survivors on their unique journey of healing and growth.[3] Curing more children and, even more importantly, without recurrence, has become the goal to be achieved. The concept of a truly "cured child" in pediatric oncology envisages not only eradication of the cancer but a surviving child at par with peers in growth and development, physically, mentally, and emotionally. Survivorship also includes new methods to estimate the burden of late effects and genetic susceptibility toward late effects. The development of surveillance guidelines for childhood cancer survivors and early toxicity signals from novel agents are now being tested and used increasingly to treat pediatric and adult cancers.[4]

SURVIVORS, LONG-TERM EFFECTS, AND LATE EFFECTS

It is often difficult for the cancer patients and his or her family to make the transition from active patient to survivorship, the fear of relapse being always intense despite counseling. While some risk of relapse is always present, it is safe to say that for most childhood cancers "cure" means disease-free survival of 2 years from cessation of therapy or 5 years after the diagnosis. A review of 5-year survivors of childhood cancers revealed that 92% of patients who were relapse-free at 5 years were alive at 15 years after diagnosis. Any side effect that does not resolve after completion of treatment is a "long-term effect of therapy". "Late effects" refer specifically to those unrecognized toxicities that are absent or subclinical at the end of therapy but manifest later with the unmasking of unseen injury because of multiple factors such as developmental processes, failure of compensatory mechanisms with time, and organ senescence. The type, dose, and target site of treatments such as chemotherapy and radiation play a crucial role, with younger children especially susceptible to radiation due to their developing bodies. According to the COG guidelines, certain agents, like anthracyclines and alkylating agents, carry a heightened risk of complications across multiple organ systems, including cardiovascular, endocrine, and psychosocial issues.[2] Patient-related factors—such as gender, health history, family cancer history, and socioeconomic status—further influence these outcomes. Addressing these complex needs requires a dedicated, multidisciplinary approach involving oncologists, psychologists, nutritionists, and social workers, with consensus in India favoring separate survivorship clinics that specifically focus on long-term health and well-being distinct from initial cancer care.[5]

CURRENT KNOWLEDGE OF LATE EFFECTS

Late effects in childhood cancer survivors can be broadly categorized as medical or psychosocial. Medical effects impact various organ systems, often including the musculoskeletal, cardiopulmonary, central nervous, endocrine, renal, gastrointestinal, and immune systems. Psychosocial effects may manifest as mental health issues (e.g., anxiety and depression), challenges with social integration, employment barriers, and family dynamics. The COG guidelines categorize these effects based on systems at risk, with particular emphasis on cardiovascular, endocrine, neurocognitive, and musculoskeletal issues. Studies at All India Institute of Medical Sciences (AIIMS), New Delhi, show high rates of organ-specific late effects like hypothyroidism and cardiac dysfunction, especially in those treated with cardiotoxic drugs such as anthracyclines.[6] Similarly, findings from the ACT Clinic of Tata Memorial Hospital, India, 30-year

TABLE 15.11.1: Summary of commonly encountered late effects.

Organ system	Late effects of chemotherapy	Late effects of radiotherapy
Bone and soft tissues	Avascular necrosis (steroids)	Short stature, limb length discrepancy, scoliosis, osteonecrosis, soft-tissue atrophy, second cancers
Cardiovascular system (CVS)	Cardiomyopathy (anthracyclines)	Pericardial effusion, early-onset coronary artery disease
Pulmonary system	Pulmonary fibrosis (bleomycin)	Decreased lung volumes, fibrosis
Central nervous system (CNS)	Neuropsychiatric issues, peripheral neuropathy	Neurocognitive deficits, structural brain changes
Renal/genitourinary system	Renal dysfunction	Bladder fibrosis, hypertension
Endocrine system	Metabolic syndrome, diabetes mellitus	Hypothyroidism, pituitary failure, pubertal development issues
Gonads	*Male:* Sterility *Female*: Premature ovarian failure	Infertility, early menopause
Ophthalmology	Cataracts (steroids)	Cataracts, retinopathy

data highlight that while 62.4% of survivors experience no or mild late effects, metabolic syndromes and neurocognitive challenges are significant concerns for others, underscoring the need for regular, targeted surveillance across affected systems to manage these complex health risks effectively **(Table 15.11.1)**.[2]

MUSCULOSKELETAL LATE EFFECTS

Growth disturbances, osteoporosis, and bone deformities are common in childhood cancer survivors, particularly among those treated with radiation or steroid-based chemotherapy. Radiation exposure to bones can result in asymmetric growth, scoliosis, and decreased bone density, while steroids further compromise bone health.[3] The COG guidelines highlight these risks, noting that survivors are especially susceptible to osteoporosis, growth hormone (GH) deficiency, and scoliosis.[1] Findings from recent research corroborate this, showing that radiation targeting bone structures can stunt growth and reduce bone density, especially in younger patients. This underscores the importance of routine physical assessments and interventions like exercise and calcium supplementation to help optimize long-term musculoskeletal health.

CARDIOPULMONARY LATE EFFECTS

Anthracyclines and thoracic radiation are linked to significant cardiopulmonary toxicity in childhood cancer survivors. A history of anthracycline use increases the risk of heart failure, while thoracic radiation can lead to pulmonary issues such as fibrosis, limiting lung function.[7] The COG guidelines recommend regular echocardiograms to detect and manage cardiomyopathy proactively, along with pulmonary function tests to monitor lung health.[1] Recent data aligns with these guidelines, showing a high prevalence of myocardial dysfunction in survivors treated with cardiotoxic chemotherapy, underscoring the importance of ongoing cardiac and pulmonary care to mitigate these long-term risks.[5]

NEUROCOGNITIVE LATE EFFECTS

Cognitive impairment is a significant concern for childhood cancer survivors, particularly those with CNS tumors or leukemia. Factors like age at treatment, tumor characteristics, cranial radiation dose, and chemotherapy agents such as methotrexate can negatively affect cognitive function, often impacting memory, learning, and attention. This emphasizes the importance of structured interventions to help manage educational and social difficulties that may arise from these impairments.

PSYCHOSOCIAL AND BEHAVIORAL LATE EFFECTS

Psychosocial issues among childhood cancer survivors extend beyond medical concerns, encompassing challenges like uncertainty, fear, and an altered life trajectory. Conditions such as post-traumatic stress disorder (PTSD) have been observed not only in survivors but also in their families, and long-term health-related challenges often hinder social and vocational integration. Experience from the ACT Clinic, Mumbai, shows that more than half of survivors experience anxiety, depression, and difficulties with social integration, underscoring the need for comprehensive support. The COG guidelines also stress the importance of addressing psychosocial concerns within survivorship care, recommending counseling and social support programs to help survivors manage these complex adjustments and improve their overall quality of life.[1]

ENDOCRINE AND FERTILITY LATE EFFECTS

Endocrine disruptions, including GH deficiency, thyroid dysfunction, and reproductive challenges, are common. Treatment with cranial irradiation poses risks for precocious puberty or growth inhibition, requiring endocrine monitoring. Gonadal dysfunction is another concern, often impacting fertility in survivors of childhood cancer.

SECOND MALIGNANCIES

Secondary cancers are a major long-term risk, with cumulative incidences of 3–10% within 20 years post-treatment. Radiation and alkylating agents are strongly linked to secondary malignancies, including thyroid and breast cancers. Survivors require lifelong vigilance and education on early detection strategies to mitigate these risks.

SURVEILLANCE OF LATE EFFECTS

Surveillance of late effects is a critical component of long-term survivorship care, as many cancer treatments, including chemotherapy, radiation, and surgery, can lead to delayed health complications that affect vital organs, cognitive and physical functions, and mental health. These risks necessitate careful, systematic monitoring over time through follow-up consultations, diagnostic screenings, and evaluations tailored to each survivor's treatment history and individual risk factors.[7]

Routine Evaluation

Routine evaluation of the survivors includes the following:

Clinical Evaluation

- Measurement of height, weight, and maintaining growth charts
- Assessment of pubertal development
- Monitoring for relapse/second malignancy
- Assessment of neuropsychological, social status, and rehabilitation needs

Investigations

- Investigations for confirmation of disease-free status to designate survivor status
- Screening for transfusion transmitted diseases, namely hepatitis B virus (HBV), hepatitis C virus (HCV), and human immunodeficiency virus (HIV)
- Baseline complete blood count
- Baseline biochemical profile
- X-ray chest
- Late-effect screening based on previous therapeutic exposure and organs/organ systems at risk of developing these late effects

Screening tests as depicted in **Table 15.11.2** may help to detect subclinical late effects that could become clinically

TABLE 15.11.2: Organ/organ system-specific late-effects screening.

Organ/organ system at risk	*Screening tests*	*Previous therapeutic exposure*
Musculoskeletal	• Physical examination annually to include height, weight, and growth velocity • X-ray as and when needed (p.r.n.)	Local radiotherapy (RT) + Surgery
Cardiac	2D-echo baseline for all; at 1 year, then q2–5 yearly (p.r.n.)	Anthracyclines + Cardiotoxic Chemotherapy ± Mediastinal RT
Pulmonary	PFT baseline, then q3–5 years (p.r.n.)	Bleomycin ± Mediastinal RT
CNS	• Neurocognitive testing at baseline, then q3–5 years (p.r.n.) • MRI brain (p.r.n.)	Cranial RT
Neuroendocrine	• Growth curve q1 year, bone age (age 9), free T3, T4, and TSH at baseline q2–5 years (p.r.n.) • LH, FSH, testosterone/estradiol, prolactin (baseline; p.r.n.) • GH stimulation test, morning cortisol (p.r.n.)	Hypothalamic–pituitary RT RT to thyroid (neck, craniospinal)
Renal	• Creatinine clearance baseline and q3–5 years (p.r.n.) • Urea, creatinine, serum electrolytes, Ca^{2+}, $MgPO_4$ 1–2 years, urinalysis 1–2 years	Cisplatin, carboplatin, ifosfamide RT
Ovary	Menstrual history annually, LH, FSH, estradiol baseline, AMH (age >12 years) and (p.r.n.)	Alkylating agents, RT
Testes	• LH, FSH, testosterone baseline (age >12 years) and (p.r.n.) • Sperm analysis (p.r.n.)	Alkylating agents, RT
Breast	• Breast examination • Mammography beginning age 25–30 years	Mediastinal RT

[AMH: anti-Müllerian hormone; CNS: central nervous system; FSH: follicle-stimulating hormone; LH: luteinizing hormone; PFT: pulmonary function test; p.r.n.: "when necessary" (from the Latin "prorenata," for an occasion that has arisen, as circumstances require, as needed)]

relevant in the future. A balance of reassurance to the survivor and his/her family and vigilance in monitoring recurrence such as SMN and late relapse are of utmost importance.

AFTER COMPLETION OF TREATMENT

Drawing inspiration from the model of care established at St. Jude Children Research Hospital (SJCRH), USA, a follow-up clinic for long-term survivors of childhood cancer was initiated at Tata Memorial Hospital (TMH) in February, 1991. This clinic was appropriately named *After Completion of Treatment (ACT)* clinic to emphasize that ACTs are needed beyond therapy treatment to achieve "cure" in its full dimensions. The aim of this clinic is to monitor growth, development, sexual maturation, and late effects of therapy and to apply corrective measures whenever feasible. Other objectives are to rehabilitate survivors for useful, productive adult life and collect data for future protocol modifications so as to obviate/minimize late effects. A team approach is adapted with pediatric oncologist, clinical psychologist, and medical social worker as a core group interacting with an array of specialists from medical and rehabilitation fields to deal with issues effectively.[8]

The training and resources for survivorship care are lacking. No national- or state-level policy addresses ongoing medical care, employment, or health insurance barriers for survivors of childhood cancer. Several initiatives aim to improve this scenario: Indian Cancer Society's Project PICASSO (Partnership in Cancer Survivorship Optimization) promotes and facilitates hospital-based ACT clinics at high-volume centers. *Ugam*, an advocacy and support group for survivors of childhood cancers created under the umbrella of the Indian Cancer Society, currently engages and works with survivors for their rehabilitation and advocacy; many more support groups are formed inspired by Ugam.[9,10] The Indian Pediatric Hematology Oncology Group of the Indian Academy of Pediatrics has formed a late-effects study group to promote survivorship research.[5]

CONCLUSION

Pediatric oncologists, in developing countries, are currently preoccupied with refining delivery of care to attain survival rates, which are comparable to the developed countries. However, they have an obligation to remember the lessons learned from the developed countries and actively build long-term follow-up and survivorship programs as an integral part of pediatric oncology initiative.

Cancer survivors will be increasing in number as the time passes. In spite of their overall wellness, they are at risk of complications and need close supervision. It will be the responsibility of health professionals, at both primary care and tertiary levels, to assess and care for these long-term issues and aid these survivors in realizing their optimum potential. To know more about childhood cancer survivorship refer to the website below:

https://www.cancer.gov/types/childhood-cancers/late-effects-hp-pdq

REFERENCES

1. Children's Oncology Group. Long-term follow-up guidelines for survivors of childhood, adolescent, and young adult cancers (Version 6.0) 2023. [online] Available from http://www.survivorshipguidelines.org/pdf/2023/COG_LTFU_Guidelines_Only_v6.pdf [Last accessed December, 2024].
2. Prasad M, Goswami S, Chinnaswamy G, Banavali SD, Kurkure PA. Long-term Outcomes in Survivors of Childhood Cancer: A 30-Year Experience From India. JCO Glob Oncol. 2022;8.8:e2200044.
3. Arora RS, Arora PR, Seth R, Sharma S, Kumar C, Dhamankar V, et al. Childhood cancer survivorship and late effects: The landscape in India in 2020. Pediatr Blood Cancer. 2020;67(9):e28556.
4. Chow EJ, Ness KK, Armstrong GT, Bhakta N, Yeh JM, Bhatia S, et al. Current and coming challenges in the management of the survivorship population. Semin Oncol. 2020;47(1):23-39.
5. Seth R, Prasad M, Kapoor G, Das G, Prasanth S, Dhamankar V, et al. Establishing childhood cancer survivorship clinics in India: A consensus statement. Pediatr Hematol Oncol J. 2024;9(3):138-42.
6. Seth R, Singh A, Seth S, Sapra S. Late effects of treatment in survivors of childhood cancers: A single-centre experience. Indian J Med Res. 2017;146(2):216-23.
7. Maeda M. Late effects of childhood cancer: life-threatening issues. J Nippon Med Sch. 2008;75(6):320-4.
8. Kurkure PA, Achrekar S, Uparkar U, Dalvi N, Doswami S. Surviving childhood cancer: what next? Issues under consideration at the After Completion of Therapy (ACT) clinic in India. Med Pediatr Oncol. 2003;41(6):588-9.
9. Tonorezos ES, Barnea D, Cohn RJ, Cypriano MS, Fresneau BC, Haupt R, et al. Models of care for survivors of childhood cancer from across the globe: advancing survivorship care in the next decade. J Clin Oncol. 2018;36(21):2223-30.
10. Singh A, Mudliar S, Sharma S, Chandrakala S, Kapoor G, Mandol J, et al. Partnership in cancer survivorship optimization (PICASSO) project: Roadmap for survivorship program in India. Pediatr Hematol Oncol J. 2020;5(4):S14-5.

SECTION

Disorders of Endocrine System and Diabetes Mellitus

Section Editors: Vijayalakshmi Bhatia, PSN Menon

16.1 Disorders of the Anterior Pituitary

Reetha Gopinath

INTRODUCTION

The pituitary gland, also known as the master gland of the endocrine system, is situated in the sella turcica at the base of the skull. It has two anatomically and functionally distinct parts—the adenohypophysis or anterior pituitary and neurohypophysis or posterior pituitary. Both these parts secrete several hormones. The anterior pituitary secretes six hormones **(Table 16.1.1)**.

Secretion of hormones from the anterior pituitary is controlled by the hypothalamus through another set of hormones, which includes growth hormone-releasing hormone (GHRH), thyrotropin-releasing hormone (TRH), gonadotropin-releasing hormone (GnRH), corticotropin-releasing hormone (CRH), prolactin-inhibiting hormone, and somatostatin.

GROWTH HORMONE

Physiology

Human growth hormone (HGH) is a 191 amino acid polypeptide secreted by the somatotropic cells of the anterior pituitary. The development of the pituitary gland and the somatotropes is mediated by several transcription factors. These include factors such as POU1F1, PROP-1, LHX3, LHX4, and SOX3. Mutations in these transcription factors affect the development of the pituitary gland and cause some genetic forms of pituitary hormone deficiencies.

Growth hormone is secreted in a pulsatile manner—about 10 pulses per day, the number of pulses increases after the onset of deep sleep and during puberty. Its secretion is regulated by multiple feedback signals, the most important being two hypothalamic factors—GHRH, which is stimulatory, and somatostatin, which is inhibitory. Ghrelin produced from the gastrointestinal tract in response to hunger is also an important regulator of GH secretion. The majority of the secreted GH circulates bound to growth hormone-binding protein (GHBP). GH exerts its action on the liver, muscle, and bone where it mediates the production of insulin-like growth factor-1 (IGF-1) **(Fig. 16.1.1)**. Hepatic IGF-1 circulates in the blood bound to binding proteins, the most important being insulin-like growth factor-binding protein 3 (IGFBP-3). The growth effect of GH is mainly mediated by IGF-1. The GH–IGF-1 axis plays a main role in the linear growth of children. In addition to its effect on growth, GH has an important role in the metabolism of carbohydrates, lipids, and proteins.[1]

TABLE 16.1.1: The hormones of the anterior pituitary.

Anterior pituitary hormones	*Target organ*
Growth hormone or somatotropin (GH)	Most of the tissues in the body
Prolactin (PRL)	Mammary gland
Thyroid-stimulating hormone (TSH)	Thyroid follicular cell
Adrenocorticotropic hormone (ACTH)	Cortex of the adrenal gland
Follicle-stimulating hormone (FSH)	Gonads (ovaries and testes)
Luteinizing hormone (LH)	Gonads (ovaries and testes)

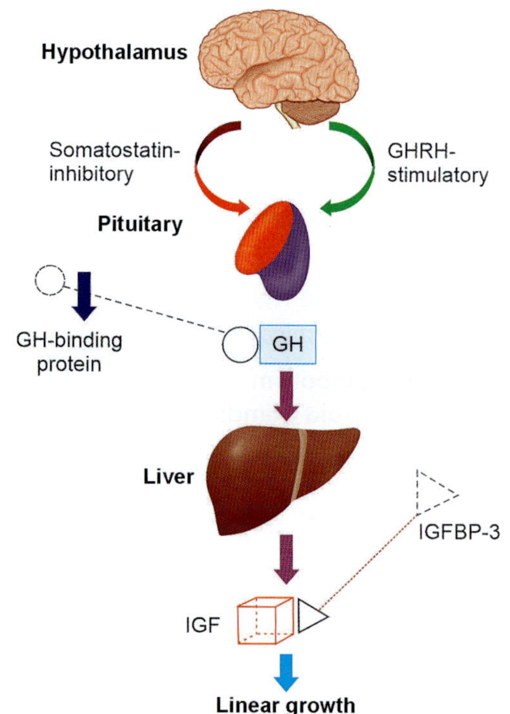

Fig. 16.1.1: The hypothalamic-pituitary-growth hormone axis. (GH: growth hormone; GHRH: growth hormone-releasing hormone; IGF: insulin-like growth factor; IGFBP-3: insulin-like growth factor-binding protein 3)

Courtesy: Dr Jijesh A, Department of Pediatrics, Government Medical College, Kannur

GROWTH HORMONE DEFICIENCY

Causes of Growth Hormone Deficiency

Growth hormone deficiency (GHD) can be congenital or acquired, or isolated or associated with multiple pituitary hormone deficiencies (MPHD) **(Box 16.1.1)**.

BOX 16.1.1: Causes of growth hormone deficiency (GHD).

Congenital GHD

- *Genetic forms:*
  - *Isolated GHD:* Mainly due to mutations in *GH1, GHRHR, SOX3,* and *HESX1* genes—can be autosomal recessive, autosomal dominant or X-linked
  - *Multiple pituitary hormone deficiencies*: Autosomal recessive (mutations in *PIT-1, PROP-1, LHX3, LHX4,* and *HESX1* genes)
- *Developmental defects of the hypothalamus or pituitary:*
  - Holoprosencephaly
  - Septo-optic dysplasia (*HESX1, OTX2,* and *SOX2* genes)
  - Aplasia or hypoplasia of the anterior pituitary
  - Interruption of stalk (*HESX1* and *LHX4* genes)
  - Empty sella syndrome
- *Associated with syndromes:*
  - Pallister–Hall syndrome (*GLI3* gene)
  - Prader–Willi syndrome (15q11 deletion/imprinting)

Acquired GHD

- *Tumors:* Craniopharyngioma, pituitary adenoma, germinoma, meningioma, glioma
- *Cystic lesions:* Rathke's cleft cyst, arachnoid cyst
- *Infiltration:* Langerhans cell histiocytosis, hemochromatosis
- *Trauma:* Road traffic accident, neurosurgery, child abuse
- *Cranial irradiation:* Hematological malignancies, CNS tumors
- *CNS infections:* Tuberculosis, meningitis

(CNS: central nervous system)

Clinical Features

Short stature is the hallmark clinical feature of GHD. However, this is a rare condition, the estimated prevalence being 1:4,000 to 1:10,000. Therefore, before embarking on detailed investigations for GHD in a short child, it is important to rule out more common causes, based on history and physical examination. Birth weight and length are usually normal in these children. Severe GHD may manifest in the neonatal period as hypoglycemia, prolonged jaundice, micropenis, and cryptorchidism. In toddler age, growth velocity is reduced and children usually present with proportionate short stature. They are usually plump with pot belly, immature facies, broad forehead, depressed nasal bridge, infantile voice, and may have associated midline craniofacial defects such as single central incisor, cleft palate, micropenis, meningocele **(Figs. 16.1.2A and B)**.

Short stature is diagnosed when the height is below–2 standard deviations (SD) for age- and sex-appropriate population norms. Based on the consensus guidelines by the Growth Hormone Research Society, GHD should be suspected if any one of the following criteria is present:[2]

1. Height below –3 SD for age-and sex-appropriate population norms
2. Height below –1.5 SD of the midparental height
3. Height below –2 SD and height velocity below –1 SD for age and sex, or a decrease in height SD of >0.5 over 1 year in children aged >2 years
4. Children who are not short, but have height velocity below –2 SD over 1 year, or below –1.5 SD sustained over 2 years (can occur in organic acquired GHD)
5. Features of multiple pituitary hormone deficiencies

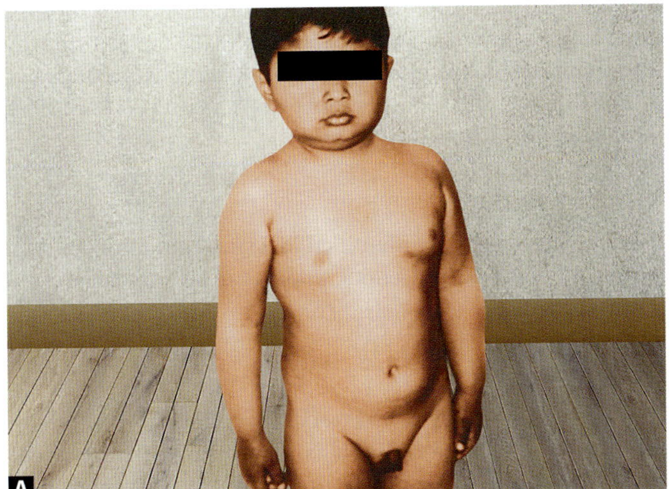

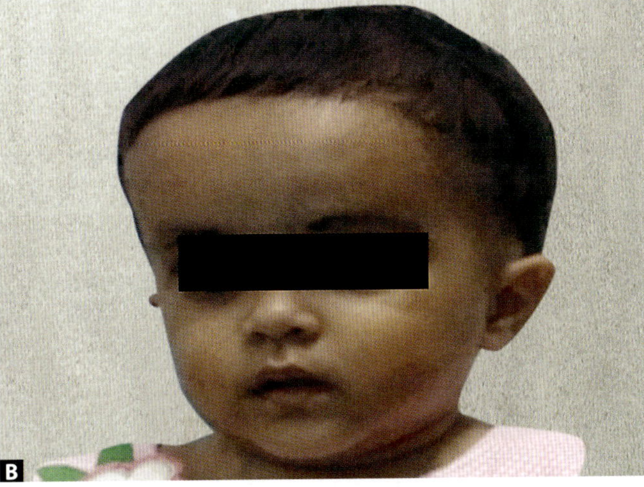

Figs. 16.1.2A and B: (A) A 9-year-old boy with growth hormone deficiency. Note immature facies, hypoplastic scrotum, and micropenis; (B) A 2-year-old girl with GHD. Note the prominent forehead, depressed nasal bridge, and frontal bossing.

6. Neonatal symptoms such as hypoglycemia, prolonged jaundice, micropenis, and craniofacial midline abnormalities
7. Signs of an intracranial lesion

Diagnosis of Growth Hormone Deficiency[2,3]

Growth hormone testing can be planned in a suspected case after general investigations to rule out other common causes of short stature. Bone age is significantly delayed in GHD, compared to conditions such as Turner syndrome, intrauterine growth restriction (IUGR)-related short stature, Cushing syndrome, and systemic diseases. Measurements of IGF-1 and its binding protein (IGFBP3) can be used as a convenient screening test for the functional assessment of GH. These molecules show little circadian variation and therefore, measurement can be done from a single sample taken at any time of the day. One major limitation of IGF-1 is that it is dependent on the nutritional status of the child and other factors such as age, pubertal status, thyroid status, and liver function. The values have to be compared with specific normative reference data and there are no single cut-offs.

Growth Hormone Stimulation Test

Since GH secretion occurs in pulses, a single random test report has no value in diagnosing GHD. Provocative testing is recommended **(Table 16.1.2)**. The test is done in the morning after a period of overnight fasting. Euthyroid status of the patient should be ensured before the procedure. In the peripubertal age, priming with sex steroids should be done. Boys who are still prepubertal at >11 years can be primed with depot testosterone given intramuscularly (IM) 50–100 mg 1 week before the test, and girls >10 years with estradiol valerate 1–2 mg on two evenings before the test. Priming is necessary as this will reduce the chances of misdiagnosing constitutional delay of growth and puberty as GHD.

There are various stimuli used for provocative testing, clonidine being most commonly used. Insulin should be used with caution for testing due to the likelihood of hypoglycemia. The tests are not foolproof and there can be overlap between normal short children and children with GHD. Hence, it is recommended that at least two different tests be done and GHD should be diagnosed only if both the tests are showing low peak GH values.

Interpretation: A peak GH value of >7 ng/mL is considered as normal.

There are certain situations where provocative testing is not needed for diagnosing GHD.[4] In neonates with high suspicion of GHD, a random GH <7 ng/mL in the first week of life supports the diagnosis. In infants with a combination of hypoglycemia, hyperbilirubinemia, poor growth, midline defects, micropenis, low IGF-1 and IGFBP3, multiple pituitary hormone deficiencies, or abnormal cranial neuroimaging, provocative testing is not needed.

Children with GHD may have other pituitary hormone deficiencies as well. So a complete evaluation of the anterior pituitary hormones should be done in every child diagnosed with GHD.

TABLE 16.1.2: Commonly used growth hormone stimulation tests.

Stimulus	*Dose and route*	*Time of sampling*	*Side effects*
Insulin	0.05–0.1 Units/kg IV	0, 30, 60, 90, 120 minutes	Hypoglycemia
Clonidine	0.15 mg/m² PO	0, 30, 60, 90 minutes	Hypotension, drowsiness
Glucagon	0.03 mg/kg SC or IM	0, 1, 2, 2.5, 3 hours	Hypoglycemia
Levodopa	125 mg for children with weight <13.5 kg 250 mg for weight 13.5–31.5 kg 500 mg for weight >31.5 kg	0, 30, 60, 90, 120 minutes	Headache, vomiting
Arginine	0.5 mg/kg in IV infusion		Not available in India

(IV: intravenous, PO: per oral, SC: subcutaneous, IM: intramuscular)

Neuroimaging

In patients with confirmed GHD or multiple pituitary hormone deficiencies, neuroimaging with computed tomography (CT) or magnetic resonance imaging (MRI) should be done. It helps in identifying intracranial tumors, and developmental malformations. MRI helps identify developmental abnormalities including pituitary hypoplasia, empty sella, and ectopic posterior pituitary and stalk abnormalities **(Figs. 16.1.3A and B)**.

Genetic Studies

Genetic mutations are identified in a small group of children with congenital GHD. Genetic studies can be done in relevant cases if feasible.

Treatment[4]

Recombinant HGH is the recommended treatment for confirmed cases of GHD. It is given daily, in the evening, subcutaneously, and the dose recommended is 25–50 μg/kg/day. Treatment can be restarted at a lower dose and gradually titrated to the optimal levels. Lower doses, i.e.,

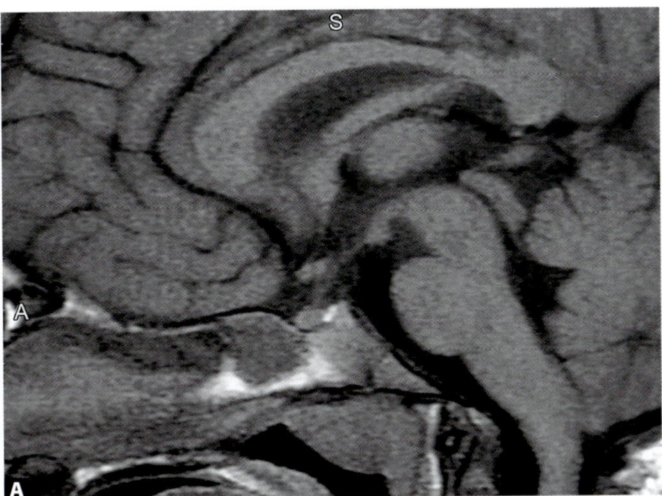

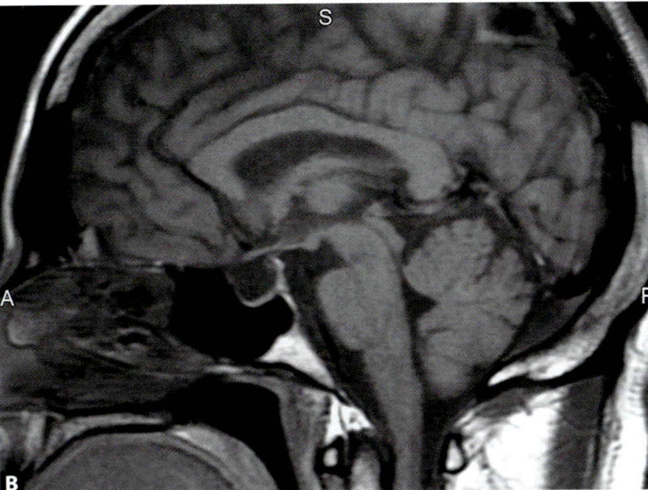

Figs. 16.1.3A and B: (A) T1-weighted MR image showing normal pituitary gland; (B) T1-weighted MR image showing empty sella.
Courtesy: Dr Mahesh P, Department of Radiodiagnosis, Government Medial College, Kannur

17–35 μg/kg/day, initially give good response in children with severe forms of GHD. Children who have very low GH levels on stimulation tests and younger age show better height increments. So, it is important to make a diagnosis early.

It is a relatively safe drug. The adverse effects include impaired glucose tolerance, fluid retention, and pseudotumor cerebri, slipped capital femoral epiphysis, worsening of scoliosis, prepubertal gynecomastia, and edema. There is no evidence to support the earlier concerns regarding the risk of leukemia, and brain tumor recurrence following long-term GH therapy. Side effects are dose related. So, reduction of the dose or temporary cessation of treatment will help to manage these issues.

Monitoring During Therapy

Children should be followed up once every 3–6 months. Maximum height increase is noted during the first 2 years of treatment. Average height gain during first year is 10–14 cm and during the next 2–3 years 6–8 cm/year. Thereafter, height gain follows the normal growth pattern. Measurement of IGF-1 levels can be used during treatment to guide GH dosing. IGF1-levels should be in the normal range to ensure drug safety. Regular monitoring of thyroid functions during therapy is needed. The pituitary axis should be checked annually.

Cessation of therapy should be considered if any one of the following criteria is met: Height gain <1 cm/year, attainment of acceptable height close to target height, and bone age over 16 years in boys and 14 years in girls. Children diagnosed with GHD in childhood may have sufficient GH levels during adulthood. So, retesting for GHD is recommended 1-3 months after stopping treatment.

Long-acting Growth Hormone[5]

A recent development in the treatment of GHD is long-acting, once-weekly preparations. The current evidence shows similar or even better height increments compared to daily recombinant GH injections. Compliance to therapy is better with LAGH. Studies are underway regarding the long-term safety profile of LAGH.

Multiple Pituitary Hormone Deficiencies

Adrenocorticotropic hormone (ACTH) deficiency should be treated with hydrocortisone at a dose of 10 mg/m^2/day. Hypothyroidism due to TSH deficiency is managed by levothyroxine. Sex steroids should be started for pubertal induction.

INDICATIONS FOR GH IN NON-GH-DEFICIENT CHILDREN[6,7]

Currently, GH has been approved for use in some other conditions causing short stature in which GH tests show normal values. These include:

- *Small for gestational age children who fail to catch up:* If they fail to catch up, i.e., height <–2 SD at 2 years or <–2.5 SD at 3–4 years should be evaluated. Treatment with GH is recommended at a dose of 35–70 μg/kg/day. Improvement in final height of 7–12 cm was noted.
- *Chronic renal failure:* Children with chronic renal failure with poor height velocity can be given GH at a dose of 40–50 μg/kg/day before undergoing transplantation.

TABLE 16.1.3: Causes of acquired hypopituitarism.

Tumors	Craniopharyngioma, adenoma, germinoma, glioma
Infections	Meningitis, encephalitis, tuberculosis,
Infiltration	Lymphocytic hypophysitis, Langerhans cell histiocytosis (LCH), hemochromatosis
Trauma	Head injury
Vascular	Pituitary apoplexy, Sheehan syndrome
Psychologic	Anorexia nervosa
Iatrogenic	Postradiotherapy, chemotherapy

- *Idiopathic short stature (ISS)*: ISS is a condition where the height of a child is below 2 SD and investigations show no identifiable cause. GH therapy has been recommended at a dose of 35–50 µg/kg/day to improve final height.
- *Prader-Willi syndrome:* Growth hormone therapy improves phenotypic appearance, body composition, and physical strength. The dose is 20–35 µg/kg/day.
- *Turner syndrome:* Growth impairment in Turner syndrome is partly due to *SHOX* gene haploinsufficiency and partly due to the involvement of the GH–IGF1 axis. GH therapy at a dose of 45–50 µg/kg/day is recommended for improving final height in Turner girls by about 5–8 cm.
- *Noonan syndrome:* GH therapy can improve final height by 5–13 cm. The dose recommended is 45–50 µg/kg/day.

ACQUIRED HYPOPITUITARISM

Table 16.1.3 highlights the important causes of acquired hypopituitarism in children. Some of these are discussed in specific chapters in the sections on Hematology, Malignancies or Infectious Diseases.

Craniopharyngioma

Craniopharyngioma is an embryonic malformation of the sellar and parasellar areas. It is a rare pediatric intracranial tumor with a peak incidence between 5 and 14 years. The symptoms of craniopharyngioma arise due to pressure effects involving the visual pathways, ventricular system, brain parenchyma, hypothalamus, and HP axis. They may present with growth failure, obesity, delayed puberty, signs of raised intracranial pressure, visual field defects, cranial nerve palsies, or rarely as precocious puberty. MRI is the imaging modality for diagnosis. Treatment of choice is surgery. After surgery, the child would require hormonal supplementation.

GROWTH HORMONE INSENSITIVITY AND IGF-1 DEFICIENCY[8]

Growth hormone insensitivity (GHI) is a group of rare genetic conditions that presents as proportionate short stature and typical clinical features of GHD. It is also known as Laron syndrome since it was first reported by Laron and colleagues in 1966. The genetic mutation could be in the GH receptor or the pathway after the GH binds to its receptor, impairing the release of IGF-1. Bone age will be delayed. Investigations show high basal as well as stimulated GH values along with low levels of IGF-1 and IGFBP3. The diagnosis can be confirmed by doing IGF generation test. For the test, recombinant GH is given at a dose of 33 µg/kg daily for 4–7 days and IGF-1 is checked. Low levels are diagnostic.

Recombinant GH is not effective in this condition. Treatment with biosynthetic IGF-1 has shown promising results. One major drawback is the high cost and limited availability of IGF-1.

GIGANTISM AND ACROMEGALY

Excess GH production causes gigantism in childhood and acromegaly in adults. This is a very rare condition.

Etiology

Causes of GH excess include tumors such as pituitary macro- or microadenomas, genetic abnormalities such as McCune-Albright syndrome, and Carney complex.

Clinical Features

The common symptom is excess growth. Children with pituitary tumors can have visual symptoms, headache, vomiting, amenorrhea, precocious puberty, and hypogonadism. Acromegalic features occur in adolescents and adults. This includes overgrowth of the mandible causing prognathism, soft-tissue growth of hands and feet, deepening of voice, excessive sweating, arthropathy, and impaired glucose tolerance.

Diagnosis

Diagnosis is made by clinical features, growth monitoring, and biochemical tests. Levels of IGF1 are raised. A GH suppression test with oral glucose load at a dose of 1.75 g/kg will show non-suppressed GH levels (<1 ng/mL). After biochemical confirmation, imaging should be done with magnetic resonance imaging.

Management

Management of pituitary tumors causing gigantism includes three modalities: medical, surgical, and radiotherapy.

- *Medical management:* The choice of drugs includes dopamine agonists (cabergoline, and bromocriptine), somatostatin analogs (octreotide, pasireotide, and lanreotide), and GH receptor antagonists (pegvisomant).

- *Surgical management:* Transsphenoidal surgery is the primary surgical option. In cases where total resection is not possible, surgical debulking can be done followed by medical therapy.
- *Radiotherapy:* If medical therapy is not feasible, then radiotherapy can be tried.

ADRENOCORTICOTROPIC HORMONE, CORTISOL, AND CUSHING DISEASE[9]

Cushing disease is caused by excess production of ACTH from the pituitary gland. It is a rare disorder in children, the incidence being 2–3 cases/million/year.

Causes

More than 70% of cases are due to pituitary microadenoma. Rare causes are pituitary corticotroph hyperplasia, and as part of multiple endocrine neoplasia.

Clinical Features

Growth retardation is the most common symptom. Weight gain with central obesity, facial changes, hirsutism, acne, dermatological manifestations such as skin thinning, broad purple striae, easy bruising, proximal myopathy, osteoporosis, frequent infections, hypertension, high blood glucose, and dyslipidemia are seen in children.

Investigations

The first step in case of suspected Cushing is to confirm excess cortisol production after ruling out exogenous source of cortisol from history. Any one of the following screening tests can be done.

- *24-hour urinary free cortisol excretion (At least 2 measurements):* Diagnostic cutoff is >70 μg/m^2/day.
- *Late night salivary cortisol or midnight serum cortisol:* A value >1.45 ng/mL is taken as positive.
- *Overnight dexamethasone suppression test (ONDST):* Dexamethasone 0.3 mg/m^2 (maximum 1 mg is given at 11 PM) and serum cortisol is measured at 8 AM the next day. A value >1.8 μg/dL is considered as abnormal.
- *Standard 2-day dexamethasone suppression test (LDDST):* Dexamethasone 0.5 mg is given every 6 hours for 2 days for children weighing >40 kg (30 μg/kg/day for children <40 kg) and serum cortisol is estimated 6 hours after the last dose. A value <1.8 μg/kg excludes endogenous Cushing syndrome.

Any two among these tests should be positive for confirmation of Cushing syndrome. A high-dose dexamethasone suppression test can be used for localization of the disease to pituitary or adrenal. Other tests include plasma ACTH, MRI of the pituitary gland and bilateral inferior petrosal sinus sampling to identify the source of excess cortisol.

Treatment

Transsphenoidal surgery for pituitary adenoma is the preferred treatment. Radiotherapy is also considered effective though it is associated with side effects. Medical therapy includes a combination of dopamine receptor agonist cabergoline, somatostatin analog octreotide or pasireotide, and/or ketoconazole.

REFERENCES

1. Tidblad A. The history, physiology and treatment safety of growth hormone. Acta Paediatr. 2022;111(2):215-24.
2. Collett-Solberg PF, Ambler G, Backeljauw PF, Bidlingmaier M, Biller BMK, Boguszewski MCS, et al. Diagnosis, genetics, and therapy of short stature in children: A Growth Hormone Research Society International perspective. Horm Res Paediatr. 2019;92(1):1-14.
3. Blum WF, Alherbish A, Alsagheir A, El Awwa A, Kaplan W, Koledova E, et al. The growth hormone-insulin-like growth factor-I axis in the diagnosis and treatment of growth disorders. Endocr Connect. 2018;7(6):R212-22.
4. Ranke MB. Short and long-term effects of growth hormone in children and adolescents with GH deficiency. Front Endocrinol. 2021;12:720419.
5. Grillo MS, Frank J, Saenger P. Long acting growth hormone (LAGH), an update. Front Pediatr. 2023;11:1254231.
6. Consensus guideline on small for gestational age: Etiology and management from infancy to early adulthood. Endocr Rev. 2023;44(3):539-65.
7. Angulo M, Abuzzahab MJ, Pietropoli A, Ostrow V, Kelepouris N, Tauber M. Outcomes in children treated with growth hormone for Prader-Willi syndrome: data from the ANSWER Program® and NordiNet® International Outcome Study. Int J Pediatr Endocrinol. 2020;20:2020(1):20.
8. Mastromauro C, Giannini C, Chiarelli F. Short stature related to growth hormone insensitivity (GHI) in childhood. Front Endocrinol. 2023;14:1141039.
9. Lodish MB, Keil MF, Stratakis CA. Cushing syndrome in children. Endocrinol Metab Clin North Am. 2018;47(2):451-62.

16.2 Disorders of the Posterior Pituitary and Diabetes Insipidus

Rajni Sharma

INTRODUCTION

The posterior pituitary gland (neurohypophysis) secretes two major hormones—(1) arginine vasopressin (AVP) (also known as antidiuretic hormone or ADH) and (2) oxytocin. ADH has a major role in regulating total body water and plasma osmolality.

The posterior pituitary is formed by a downgrowth of the diencephalon and mainly consists of axonal projections of neurosecretory cells originating in the hypothalamus. Unlike the anterior pituitary where the hormones are synthesized within the gland under control of hypothalamic stimuli, the posterior pituitary hormones are synthesized in the hypothalamus and transported via axons through the pituitary stalk or infundibulum and stored in the posterior pituitary.

DIABETES INSIPIDUS

A lack of ADH or its action results in a condition called "diabetes insipidus (DI)." ADH is a small peptide consisting of nine amino acids. As mentioned above, it is synthesized in the supraoptic and paraventricular nuclei of the hypothalamus and transported to and stored in the posterior pituitary. The preprohormone protein of ADH contains AVP, copeptin, and neurophysin that are cleaved during their course in the pituitary stalk and concurrently released into the bloodstream in equimolar amounts.

The main stimulus for ADH release is a rise in plasma osmolality and dehydration. ADH acts on vasopressin receptors (V2) located in the collecting ducts of the kidney and V1a receptors on the vascular smooth muscles. Binding of ADH to the V2 receptor leads to formation of cyclic AMP and of the surface protein aquaporin-2, which facilitates transport of water in the kidney.

Diabetes insipidus is a rare disorder and can result either from vasopressin deficiency (central DI) or vasopressin resistance at the level of kidney (nephrogenic DI). It manifests clinically as polyuria with increased serum osmolality and low urine osmolality.

Etiology of Diabetes Insipidus

Both central and nephrogenic diabetes can be partial, complete, or transient. The etiology may be congenital or acquired **(Table 16.2.1)**.[1]

Central Diabetes Insipidus

Congenital deficiency of ADH can arise from developmental malformations of the brain or inherited deficiency of vasopressin (familial forms due to autosomal dominant mutation of vasopressin gene on chromosome 20). Wolfram syndrome also known as DI with diabetes mellitus, optic atrophy, and deafness (DIDMOAD syndrome) is a rare inherited neurodegenerative disorder associated with DI.

Acquired deficiency of ADH can result from injury or lesions in the hypothalamus, pituitary stalk, or neurohypophysis. These include trauma, surgery, suprasellar tumors (craniopharyngioma, optic glioma, and germinoma), infiltrative conditions such as Langerhans cell histiocytosis, sarcoidosis, encephalitis, tuberculosis, and granulomas. DI can occur in the newborn following asphyxia, intracranial bleeding, and meningitis.

TABLE 16.2.1: Etiology of diabetes insipidus (DI).

Central DI	***Nephrogenic DI***
Genetic: • Genetic mutation in vasopressin gene • Wolfram syndrome	*Genetic:* • *X-linked:* Mutation of V2 receptors (*AVPR2* gene) • *Autosomal dominant or recessive:* Mutation in aquaporin-2 gene
Congenital malformation: • Holoprosencephaly • Septo-optic dysplasia • Empty sella syndrome • Agenesis of corpus callosum	*Congenital malformations of kidney:* • Polycystic kidney disease • Medullary cystic kidney disease
Trauma: • Accidental • Surgery	*Drugs:* Lithium, clozapine, demeclocycline, amphotericin B, methicillin, and rifampicin
Intracranial pathology: • *Brain tumor:* Craniopharyngioma, optic glioma, and germinoma • *Infiltrative disorder:* Langerhans cell histiocytosis and sarcoidosis • *CNS infections:* Tuberculosis, meningitis, and encephalitis	*Electrolyte abnormalities:* • Hypercalcemia • Hypokalemia
Idiopathic: • Autoimmune • Unknown cause	

(CNS: central nervous system)

Nephrogenic Diabetes Insipidus

Congenital nephrogenic DI can result from developmental (polycystic) disorders of the kidney or inherited ADH resistance. Hereditary nephrogenic DI is mostly X-linked due to vasopressin V2 receptor gene mutations (*AVPR2* gene located on the X chromosome). Secondly, mutations in the *aquaporin-2* gene that encodes the ADH-sensitive water channels in the collecting tubule cells can result in autosomal dominant or recessive forms of DI.

Lithium ingestion and toxicity can result in degradation of aquaporin-2 protein in the renal collecting tubules resulting in an acquired and reversible form of nephrogenic DI.

Clinical Features

Polyuria is a classical feature of DI. Children with DI pass large quantities of urine throughout the day and are chronically thirsty. Parents of infants may report unusually heavy diapers. Often, the symptoms go unnoticed by the parents and infants present with dehydration, intermittent fever, irritability, weight loss, and vascular collapse. Older children may develop secondary enuresis as the initial feature. Hypothalamic lesions may result in growth retardation, obesity, visual disturbances, precocious puberty, and change in appetite and sleep. Patients with histiocytosis may have additional features such as scalp seborrhea, chronic ear discharge, and lytic bony lesions.

Diagnosis

The diagnosis of DI is confirmed by laboratory tests. Presence of hypernatremia (serum sodium >150 mEq/L) and increased plasma osmolality (>300 mOsm/L) with a low urine osmolality (<200–300 mOsm/L) confirms the diagnosis of DI. Urine is very dilute with a specific gravity between 1.001 and 1.005. Often, a patient drinks excess water due to thirst which prevents dehydration and hypernatremia, and maintains the plasma osmolality in the normal range. The only presenting feature could be polyuria and polydipsia and further workup is required to ascertain the diagnosis.

APPROACH TO A CHILD WITH POLYURIA

Polyuria is defined as urine output >2 L/m^2/24 hours (>6 mL/kg/24 hours at birth, >4 mL/kg/24 hours up to 2 years, >2.5 mL/kg/24 hours older children).[2] Urine output should be confirmed by a 24-hour intake and output chart. Routine tests such as renal function tests and blood glucose should be documented. Osmotic diuresis due to hyperglycemia or mannitol should be ruled out. Polyuria may arise from compulsive water drinking or psychogenic forms of polydipsia which can be diagnosed by a water deprivation test.

Laboratory investigations and diagnostic criteria for DI are mentioned in **Box 16.2.1 and Table 16.2.2**, respectively.

Water Deprivation Test

This test is performed in patients with polyuria where DI is suspected **(Box 16.2.2)**. It helps to diagnose DI as well as to distinguish between central and nephrogenic forms.

BOX 16.2.1: Laboratory investigations in a case of polyuria.

- Serum electrolytes, urea, creatinine, calcium, and blood gas
- Blood glucose and glycosylated hemoglobin A1C (HbA1C)
- Paired urine and serum osmolality
- Urine specific gravity
- Magnetic resonance imaging (MRI) brain in case of central diabetes insipidus (DI)
- Renal imaging (Ultrasound)

TABLE 16.2.2: Diagnosis of diabetes insipidus.

Laboratory measurement	***Diagnosis***
• Plasma osmolality >300 mOsm/kg, *or* • Serum sodium >147 mEq/L, *with* • Urine osmolality <300 mOsm/kg, *or* • Urine specific gravity <1.005	Diabetes insipidus
Urine osmolality >750 mOsm/kg	Excludes diabetes insipidus
Urine osmolality <300 mOsm/kg *with* normal plasma osmolality	Go for water deprivation test and vasopressin challenge test

BOX 16.2.2: Procedure of water deprivation test.

- Child should avoid tea and coffee for 24–36 hours prior to procedure
- Test should be started early in the morning by 8–9 AM
- Patient should be asked to void at the start of procedure
- Stop all fluid intake once the procedure is started and insert an IV cannula
- Take blood sample for urea, creatinine, serum sodium, and osmolality and urine sample for osmolality and specific gravity
- Check bodyweight, vitals, blood pressure, and urine output hourly
- Watch for signs of dehydration
- Monitor urine and serum osmolality and serum sodium hourly
- Stop the test if there is loss of >5% bodyweight, or serum osmolality is >300 mOsm/kg, or serum sodium is ≥150 mEq/L or urine osmolality is >750 mOsm/kg (s/o psychogenic polydipsia)
- If goals of DI are achieved—proceed to vasopressin challenge test
- Give aqueous vasopressin (1 U/m^2 SC), take samples for urine osmolality after 30 minutes. A rise in urine osmolality >50% from baseline suggests central DI.

Note: Conversion of urine osmolality to urine specific gravity: 300 mOsm/kg ≥1.005; 750 mOsm/kg ≥1.010.
(DI: diabetes insipidus; IV: intravenous; SC: subcutaneous)

Prerequisites include documenting normal renal function tests, venous blood gas, and blood glucose. A renal ultrasound should also be done prior to the test to rule out scarred kidneys. The patient is admitted for a trial of water withdrawal. If the patient is called in the morning, do not ask the patient to withhold water intake overnight as it could lead to severe dehydration in a child with DI. Baseline electrolytes with paired plasma and urine osmolality are checked. In case the patient fulfills the criteria for DI at baseline, vasopressin is administered to distinguish between nephrogenic and central forms. Otherwise, water is withdrawn for a few hours while maintaining strict supervision and frequent monitoring of the patient's vitals, blood pressure, hydration status, and weight and urine output. Serum sodium, plasma, and urine osmolality are measured hourly. Children with DI fail to concentrate their urine and may continue to pass large amounts of dilute urine whereas those with primary polydipsia are able to pass concentrated urine. In case the patient fulfills the criteria for DI, vasopressin is administered. Failure to concentrate urine after vasopressin indicates ADH resistance and nephrogenic form of DI.

Copeptin Measurement

The water deprivation test can be cumbersome and investigators have tried to look for alternative tests to diagnose DI. Serum AVP levels have not been found useful as it has a very short half-life and is technically difficult to measure in commercially available immunoassays. Copeptin is the C-terminal segment of the AVP precursor peptide and is cosecreted from the posterior pituitary in equimolar concentrations with vasopressin.[3] Being a more stable peptide, copeptin can be more easily measured with available immunoassays. In a patient with polyuria, nephrogenic DI can be diagnosed by using a single baseline copeptin level with a value >21.4 pmol/L being highly accurate for the diagnosis.

However, there is great overlap in baseline copeptin levels in patients with central DI and primary polydipsia. Saline loading to raise the serum sodium ≥150 mmol/L can help to distinguish between the two. Osmotically stimulated copeptin levels of >4.9 pmol/L is seen in patients with primary polydipsia whereas lower level indicates central DI. Hypertonic saline stimulated copeptin level is a promising tool to diagnose central DI with high diagnostic accuracy and may supplant the water deprivation test in future.

Workup for Etiological Diagnosis of Central Diabetes Insipidus

MRI of brain helps to diagnose intracranial pathology including tumors and pituitary stalk thickening (seen in germinoma or Langerhans cell histiocytosis).[2,3] Vasopressin stored in the posterior pituitary results in the classical bright spot visible on MRI T1 images in normal individuals **(Fig. 16.2.1A)**. DI is characterized by an absent or ectopic posterior pituitary bright spot on MRI with or without other pituitary abnormalities such as hypoplastic anterior pituitary/empty sella or transection of pituitary stalk **(Fig. 16.2.1B)**. However, absence of posterior pituitary bright spot is nonspecific finding and can be seen in

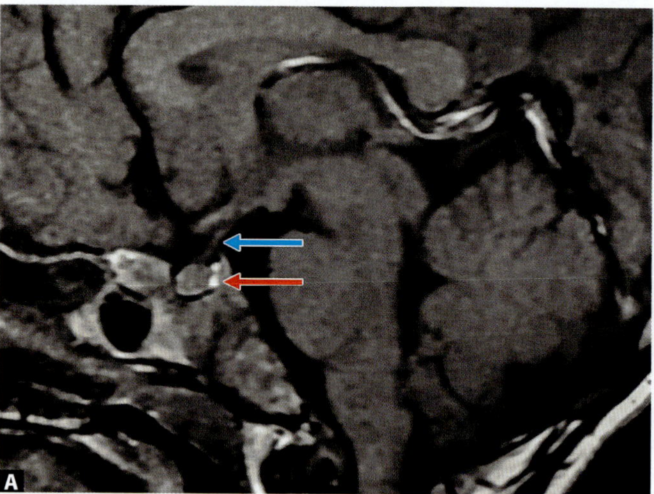

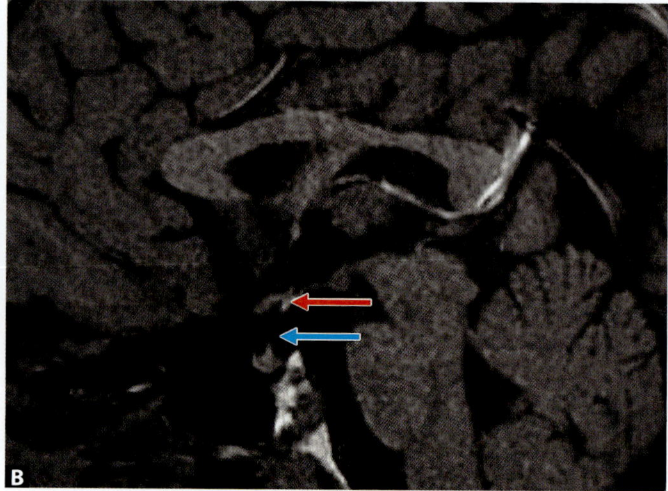

Figs. 16.2.1A and B: (A) MRI brain T1-weighted image showing normal anterior pituitary and pituitary stalk (blue arrow) with a normally positioned posterior pituitary bright spot (red arrow). The bright spot indicates the presence of stored vasopressin in the posterior pituitary; (B) Brain T1-weighted image showing pituitary stalk transection (blue arrow) with ectopic pituitary bright spot (red arrow) in a patient with central diabetes insipidus.

nephrogenic DI as well due to excessive secretion of vasopressin (secondary to nephrogenic resistance) and lack of posterior pituitary stores. Serum and cerebrospinal fluid (CSF)-α-fetoprotein and β-hCG levels can be measured in patients with central DI for central nervous system (CNS) germinoma.

Management

For central DI, treatment includes use of desmopressin which is a long-acting vasopressin analog.[4] It is available as intranasal spray (10 µg/0.1 mL) and sublingual (30–60 µg) or oral tablets (25–100 µg every 8–12 hourly). Urine output should be monitored and diuresis ensured prior to intake of the next dose to avoid fluid overload. Infants are generally not treated with DDAVP due to the risk of hyponatremia and better managed with increased provision of free water, restriction of salt intake and oral chlorothiazide.

Treatment of nephrogenic DI includes eliminating the cause such as drugs or electrolyte imbalance, maintenance of adequate hydration, and calories to promote growth, thiazide diuretics (hydrochlorothiazide), indomethacin, and salt restriction.

CONCLUSION

DI is characterized by passage of large amounts of dilute urine due to the inability of the kidneys to concentrate urine. The etiology of DI could be central (lack of ADH) or nephrogenic (ADH resistance) in etiology. A systemic approach should be followed in a patient presenting with polyuria to rule out all other causes such as diabetes mellitus and renal failure. Water deprivation test can help diagnose and distinguish between central and nephrogenic DI but must be performed with utmost care and good monitoring. Copeptin test is a promising test to diagnose DI.

REFERENCES

1. Weiner A, Vuguin P. Diabetes insipidus. Pediatr Rev. 2020;41(2):96-9.
2. Patti G, Napoli F, Fava D, Casalini E, Di Iorgi N, Maghnie M. Approach to the pediatric patient: central diabetes insipidus. J Clin Endocrinol Metab. 2022;107(5):1407-16.
3. Christ-Crain M, Winzeler B, Refardt J. Diagnosis and management of diabetes insipidus for the internist: an update. J Intern Med. 2021;290(1):73-87.
4. Di Iorgi N, Napoli F, Allegri AE, Olivieri I, Bertelli E, Gallizia A, et al. Diabetes insipidus–diagnosis and management. Horm Res Paediatr. 2012;77(2):69-84.

16.3 Disorders of Puberty

Prisca Colaco

INTRODUCTION

Puberty is the period of life which marks the transition of a child into an adult. It is accompanied by dramatic physiological and psychological changes. Its onset is marked by the appearance of secondary sexual characters. This is associated with an increase in the frequency and amplitude of gonadotropin-releasing hormone (GnRH) pulses, which precedes the rise in luteinizing hormone (LH) and follicle-stimulating hormone (FSH). GnRH neurosecretion appears to be under the control of many excitatory and inhibitory neurotransmitters and neuropeptides.

Puberty starts on an average between the ages of 8 and 13 years in girls and 9 and 14 years in boys and is typically complete in 2–5 years. Chapter 3.2 deals with the details of normal puberty. The onset is controlled by both genetic and environmental factors and has been shown to vary with race, ethnicity, geographical location, and environmental and nutritional conditions. This explains the 4–5-year physiological variation in the age at onset of puberty observed among normal individuals.

PRECOCIOUS PUBERTY

DEFINITION

Puberty is considered precocious if its onset is before the lower limits of normal [2 standard deviations (SD) below the mean age of pubertal onset in normal children].[1] Traditionally, this is considered to be 8 years in girls and 9 years in boys. A secular trend has been reported in the onset of puberty in girls and it was recommended that puberty be considered precocious if the onset is before the age of 7 years in white girls and 6 years in black girls. However, as a significant incidence of underlying pathology was found in the 6–8-year age group, many still use the traditional threshold of 8 years to define precocious pubertal development in girls. For boys, the onset of puberty before the age of 9 years is considered precocious.

Precocity may be isosexual (the secondary sexual characters are true to the gender of that child), or heterosexual (virilization in a girl or feminization in a boy). **Box 16.3.1** depicts the classification and causes of precocious puberty.

CENTRAL PRECOCIOUS PUBERTY

Central precocious puberty (CPP) is the most common form of precocious puberty and is about five times more common in girls than in boys.[2] CPP in girls is most often idiopathic (about 75%) **(Fig. 16.3.1)**. In contrast, about two thirds of boys with CPP have some underlying central nervous system (CNS) pathology. The younger the child, the greater the risk of underlying pathology. Hypothalamic hamartoma is the most common abnormality causing precocious puberty. In India, CNS infections are important causes of CPP. Some familial forms and association with *KISS1* and *MKRN3* genes and their receptors have been reported. It is more common in children who were internationally adopted. Childhood obesity is associated with the development of CPP in girls.

In idiopathic CPP, the appearance of secondary sexual characters is merely a normal event occurring early and puberty progresses normally.

BOX 16.3.1: Causes of precocious puberty.

- *Gonadotropin-dependent or central precocious puberty (due to premature activation of the HPG axis and therefore isosexual)*
  - *Idiopathic*
  - *Neurogenic:*
    - Congenital
      - *Cerebral malformations:* Hydrocephalus, arachnoid cyst
      - *Neurocutaneous syndromes:* Neurofibromatosis type 1, Sturge–Weber syndrome, tuberous sclerosis
    - Acquired
      - *Tumors:* Hypothalamic hamartoma, glioma, astrocytoma, ependymoma, germ cell tumor, pinealoma
      - Infections
      - Perinatal insults, trauma
      - Cranial irradiation
  - *Genetic:*
    - Loss of function mutation in the *MKRN3* (makorin ring finger 3) gene
    - Gain of function mutation encoding the kisspeptin (*KISS1*) and its receptor (*KISSR*) genes
  - *International adoption*
  - *Secondary to peripheral precocity*
- *Gonadotropin-independent or peripheral precocious puberty (Results from gonadal hormone production independent of the HPG axis, and may be isosexual or heterosexual)*
  - *Autonomous gonadal activation*
    - Ovarian cysts
    - McCune–Albright syndrome
    - Familial male-limited precocious puberty (testotoxicosis)
    - *Tumors of the ovary or testis:* Granulosa cell tumor, androgen-secreting ovarian tumors, testicular Leydig cell tumors, hCG-secreting tumors
  - *Adrenal disorders*
    - Congenital adrenal hyperplasia
    - Adrenal tumors
  - *Exogenous hormones*
  - *Severe untreated primary hypothyroidism*
- *Pubertal variants*
  - *Premature thelarche*
  - *Premature pubarche*
  - *Premature menarche*

(hCG: human chorionic gonadotropin; HPG: hypothalamic-pituitary-gonadal)

PERIPHERAL PRECOCIOUS PUBERTY

Peripheral precocious puberty (PPP) is only one-fifth as common as CPP. While CPP is always isosexual, PPP may be isosexual or heterosexual. It may be due to adrenal or gonadal causes.

Peripheral precocious puberty is much more common in boys than in girls as adrenal causes, most commonly congenital adrenal hyperplasia (CAH), cause PPP in boys **(Fig. 16.3.2)**. The prepubertal size of the testes suggests the diagnosis of PPP. Some forms of PPP predominate in boys, such as human chorionic gonadotropin (hCG)-secreting tumors and familial gonadotropin-independent precocious puberty or testotoxicosis, which is caused by an activating mutations of the LH receptor.

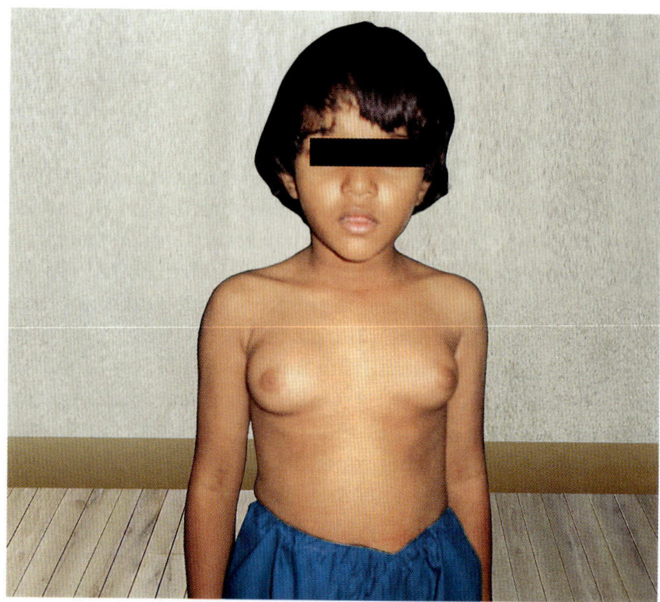

Fig. 16.3.1: A 4-year-old girl with idiopathic central precocious puberty.

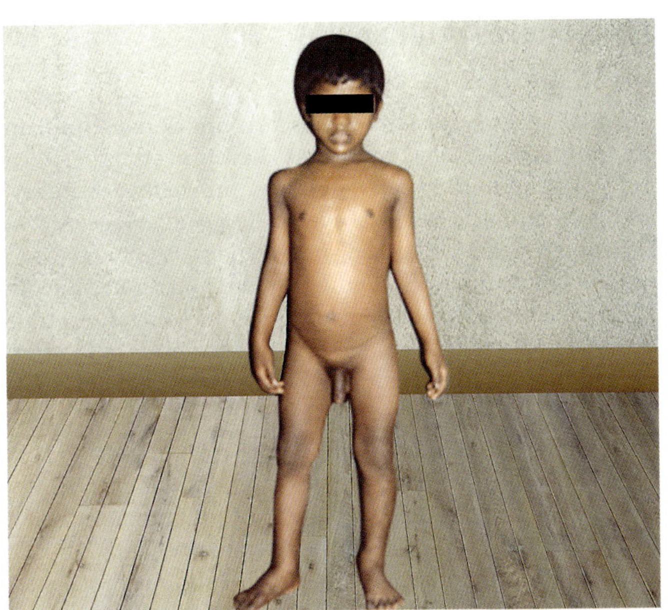

Fig. 16.3.2: A 3-year-old boy with peripheral precocious puberty due to congenital adrenal hyperplasia. Sexual maturity rating stage 4. Testicular volume: 2 mL. Note the generalized hyperpigmentation.

Ovarian rather than adrenal disorders are much more common in girls with isosexual PPP. Autonomous secreting follicular cysts of the ovary are the most common cause of PPP in girls even without any evidence of McCune-Albright syndrome (MAS), characterized by fibrous dysplasia, skin pigmentation, and precocious puberty. These cysts are often >2 cm in diameter in contrast to the smaller cysts, which are normally present in the prepubertal ovary or in CPP. Pubertal signs often develop rapidly. Subsequent atresia of the cysts results in withdrawal bleeding. MAS predominantly affects girls.[3]

Adrenal causes such as CAH and tumors result in heterosexual puberty in girls. Hypothyroidism, untreated or inadequately treated, is sometimes associated with precocious puberty. It is thought to be due to the effect of markedly elevated TSH levels on the FSH receptor.

PUBERTAL VARIANTS

The incomplete forms of sexual precocity can be differentiated from precocious puberty by the absence of other signs of puberty and a normal growth rate.

Premature Thelarche

Premature thelarche refers to the early appearance of breast development in girls with no other estrogen effects such as increase in uterine size, changes in external genitalia, growth acceleration, or bone age advancement. Breast development persists beyond 6 months of age or occurs anew usually before 3 years of age and rarely after 4 years. The cause is unknown. Postulations include increase in breast sensitivity to estrogen, transient estrogen secretion from follicular cysts of the ovary, increased estrogen from adrenal precursors, and transient partial activation of the hypothalamic-pituitary-gonadal (HPG) axis. Early breast development has also been linked to exogenous estrogen in food or in the environment and exposure to endocrine disruptors. Premature thelarche usually undergoes spontaneous regression during the first 2–3 years of life. However, in some cases, when its onset occurs after 2–3 years of age, a certain percentage develops CPP.

Premature Pubarche and Adrenarche

Premature pubarche refers to the appearance of pubic hair without other signs of puberty or virilization before the age of 8 years in girls and 9 years in boys. The precise etiology of premature pubarche is not known. It is generally attributed to early maturation of the zona reticularis of the adrenal cortex as adrenal androgen levels [dehydroepiandrosterone (DHEA), its sulfate (DHEAS), androstenedione and testosterone] increase to early pubertal levels (adrenarche). Alternatively, hypersensitivity of the hair follicle to steroid hormones is sometimes postulated, as androgen levels are normal in some patients.

It is much more commonly seen in girls in the 3–8-year age group. Pubarche is not progressive. These children may develop slight acne, axillary hair, and adult-type body odor but no other secondary sex characters. Linear growth and skeletal maturation may be slightly increased but the onset and progression of puberty and final height are not affected. Signs of severe androgen excess should prompt a search for a virilizing adrenal tumor or CAH.

Premature Menarche

Premature menarche is the onset of a single or few cycles of vaginal bleeding in girls unaccompanied by other signs of puberty. This is a rare condition and local lesions such as vaginal infections, foreign body, or sexual abuse must be ruled out. There is normal progression to puberty with no effect on final height. It is due to transient ovarian activity resulting in an isolated follicular cyst. Functioning ovarian cysts associated with MAS also may present with isolated menses.

EVALUATION

A detailed history and clinical examination are helpful in arriving at a diagnosis and directing investigations.

History

The age at onset is earlier with an underlying organic cause of precocious puberty. Idiopathic CPP usually presents between 6 and 7 years of age. Hypothalamic hamartoma and familial testotoxicosis present very early, in the first 3–4 years of life. The rate of pubertal progression may provide a clue. In idiopathic CPP, the rate of progression may sometimes be very slow, with menarche occurring up to 5 years after breast development. Very rapid progression of puberty is seen in androgen-producing tumors, ovarian cysts, and some CNS tumors such as hypothalamic hamartoma.

Accelerated growth is a feature of both CPP and PPP, but is not seen in the pubertal variants. Irregular vaginal bleeding is more common in ovarian tumors and hypothalamic hamartoma. History of a past CNS infection, headaches, visual disturbances, personality changes, developmental delay, and seizures should be sought, as a clue toward CPP. Drug exposure should be enquired into. Symptoms suggestive of hypothyroidism are important, especially in the case of precocious puberty without tall stature. A family history of precocious puberty would suggest constitutional precocious puberty, or familial testotoxicosis or a genetic variety of CPP. A history of precocious puberty in boys and genital ambiguity in girls of the same family would suggest CAH.

Clinical Examination

Staging of breast development as per Tanner staging, and changes in vaginal mucosa color from red to moist pink when estrogenized, should be recorded. The presence of acne, hirsutism, increased muscle mass, and clitoromegaly suggest androgen action. In boys, testicular volume of 4 mL or greater marks true puberty, and increasing volume provides the staging of puberty. Penis length and girth, and glans development, should be recorded as pubic hair stage. Testicular tumors may be palpated. Inspection of the skin is helpful in MAS, neurofibromatosis, and tuberous sclerosis. Neurologic examination should include fundus examination and perimetry. Signs of hypothyroidism should be looked for.

INVESTIGATIONS

It is recommended that all boys with precocious pubertal development should be investigated for etiology. For girls, those with the following features should be evaluated for the mechanism and potential for progression of puberty: puberty stage 3 or higher; stage 2 with additional criteria such as increased growth velocity; evidence of CNS dysfunction; or PPP.

Hormonal Evaluation

Sex Steroids

In girls, serum estradiol levels are not very helpful in determining the stage of puberty. Levels overlap between normal prepuberty, early puberty, precocious puberty, and premature thelarche. Levels >20 pg/mL suggests that puberty has started. Markedly elevated levels (>100 pg/mL) are seen in estrogen-secreting tumors and sometimes in follicular cysts. In contrast, in boys, rising serum testosterone can be tallied with the stage of puberty. Levels <10 ng/dL (depending on the sensitivity of the assay) are generally prepubertal.

Serum Gonadotropins

Gonadotropin levels are elevated in CPP and suppressed in PPP. An LH level <0.1 IU/L is prepubertal and 0.3 IU/L or more is compatible with puberty. Random FSH levels are not helpful in discriminating between prepubertal and pubertal children. GnRH stimulation test is more helpful in distinguishing CPP from PPP. In CPP, an LH predominant response is seen. Stimulated FSH levels do not distinguish CPP and PT. In PPP, gonadotropin levels do not rise in response to GnRH stimulation.

Serum DHEAS

Levels >50 µg/dL are consistent with the stage of pubic hair in premature adrenarche and can be very high (five-fold or more than the upper limit of normal) in virilizing adrenal conditions such as androgen-secreting adrenal tumors and CAH.

Serum 17-hydroxyprogesterone

Serum 17-hydroxyprogesterone (17OHP) and its response to ACTH or serum 11-deoxycortisol (DOC) may be required to rule out CAH due to 21-hydroxylase deficiency or 11-hydroxylase deficiency, respectively.

Serum Human Chorionic Gonadotropin

This is useful if an hCG-secreting tumor is suspected in boys.

Thyroid Hormone

In suspected hypothyroidism, TSH and T4 are useful.

Radiology

Bone Age

Bone age assessment is helpful in diagnosing precocious puberty and predicting adult height. Skeletal maturation is advanced in all cases of precocious puberty, except if associated with hypothyroidism, but remains normal in the incomplete forms.

Computed Tomography or Magnetic Resonance Imaging of the Brain

Both CT and MRI help to determine the etiology of CPP.

Pelvic and Abdominal Sonography

This helps to evaluate the size and morphology of the uterus, ovaries, and adrenals. This is essential in PPP to find the cause. In CPP, the size of the uterus is increased (>2 mL in volume or >3.4 cm in length) and an endometrial shadow is seen. The ovaries will also be bilaterally enlarged and may show multiple small follicular cysts.

Testicular Sonography

It is performed if a tumor is suspected.

Radionuclide Bone Scan or Skeletal Survey

It is done in suspected cases of MAS.

MANAGEMENT

Surgery

Any underlying cause should be identified and treated, e.g., intracranial, gonadal, or adrenal tumors. Surgery of hypothalamic hamartoma is hazardous and not recommended because they do not grow or become malignant. Surgery may not affect pubertal development. Ovarian cysts usually regress spontaneously and tend to be recurrent. Surgery should be avoided, or, when required as in cases of ovarian torsion, it should be conservative.

Medical Treatment

Not all cases of precocious puberty need to be treated. The goals of therapy should be clear. The only long-term complication of CPP which may improve with treatment is compromised adult height. Treatment of progressive CPP is indicated if:[4]

- There is evidence that adult height may be significantly compromised.
- Pubertal development is psychologically distressing to the child.
- Pubertal development is progressing rapidly over an observation period of about 6 months.

Gonadotropin-releasing Hormone Analog Therapy

This therapy aims at reversing the development of sexual characteristics and decreasing the acceleration of growth and bone age by using GnRH analogs.[2] GnRH analogs act by suppressing pulsatile GnRH secretion. Mean gains over predicted adult height in several studies range from 3 to 10 cm. Factors which affect height gain include baseline bone age and duration of treatment. Discontinuation of therapy at 11 years is associated with optimum height outcomes. Pubertal manifestations reappear within months of stopping treatment with a mean time to menarche of 16 months.

Antigonadotropic and Antiandrogen Drugs

Drugs such as medroxyprogesterone and cyproterone acetate cause regression of pubertal signs but have no effect on growth acceleration and bone age progression.

Treatment of Peripheral Precocious Puberty

This includes treatment of the cause as in hypothyroidism or CAH. Drugs used in gonadotropin-independent precocious puberty include androgen and estrogen receptor blockers and aromatase inhibitors.

Psychological Support

Psychological support for the child and parents is part of the general management scheme. The child's psychological development corresponds with the chronologic age. No major psychopathology is associated with precocious puberty. Future fertility is maintained,

DELAYED PUBERTY

DEFINITION

Delayed puberty is defined as the lack of specific pubertal signs, which is defined by breast budding in girls, and a testicular volume of 4 mL or more in boys; at an age that is 2–2.5 standard deviations later than the population mean, typically by the age of 13 years in girls and 14 years in boys.[5] The absence of menarche by the age of 16 years or within 5 years of pubertal onset is also included in the diagnosis. In males, a pubertal delay is evident by a lack of testicular enlargement by 14 years or >5 years between testicular enlargement and completion of puberty.

Puberty is usually completed within a period of 5 years and is considered "stalled" if there is no progression over a period of 2 years.

CLASSIFICATION

Delayed puberty results from inadequate gonadal steroid secretion caused by hypothalamic, pituitary, and gonadal disorders and is classified according to the circulating levels of the gonadotropins; FSH and LH as shown in **Box 16.3.2**.

EVALUATION

History

A good history should focus on a review of symptoms, which may indicate a chronic systemic disease, prolonged drug

BOX 16.3.2: Causes of delayed puberty.

- *Hypergonadotropic (primary gonadal failure)*
  - *Congenital*
    - Sex chromosome anomalies, e.g., Turner, X/XY, Klinefelter syndromes
    - Anomalies of testosterone synthesis or action
    - Pure gonadal dysgenesis
    - Associated with other syndromes, e.g., Noonan, Alström, Smith–Lemli–Opitz syndromes
  - *Acquired*
    - Surgical or traumatic castration
    - Orchitis/oophoritis
    - Chemotherapy, radiotherapy
    - Idiopathic
- *Hypogonadotropic (secondary hypogonadism)*
  - *Temporary causes (Functional)*
    - CDGP—sporadic or familial
    - Nutritional disorders
    - Chronic systemic disease
    - Hormonal disturbances, e.g., hypothyroidism, isolated GHD, excess glucocorticoids
    - Psychosocial problems
    - Intense exercise
  - *Permanent causes*
    - Congenital
      - » Isolated gonadotropin deficiency
      - » LH deficiency
      - » Associated with syndromes, e.g., Kallmann, Prader–Willi syndromes
      - » Panhypopituitarism
    - *Acquired:*
      - » Tumors, surgery
      - » Irradiation
      - » Trauma
      - » Hemochromatosis
      - » Hyperprolactinemia

(CDGP: constitutional delay in growth and puberty; GHD: growth hormone deficiency; LH: luteinizing hormone)

therapy, poor nutrition, head trauma, and anosmia. A history of any malignancy and cranial irradiation, cryptorchidism or orchidopexy should be noted. A family history of delayed puberty or hypogonadism and a history of parental consanguinity should be enquired into. Constitutional delay in growth and puberty (CDGP) is the most common cause of delayed puberty and is much more common in boys than girls. A family history of delayed puberty is seen in half of the CDGP cases and strongly suggests CDGP.[6]

Clinical Examination

Growth Assessment

This is an important part of the evaluation. The height of those with primary gonadal failure is usually normal unless associated with specific syndromes **(Fig. 16.3.3)**. Children with functional delay are commonly short. CDGP is a delay

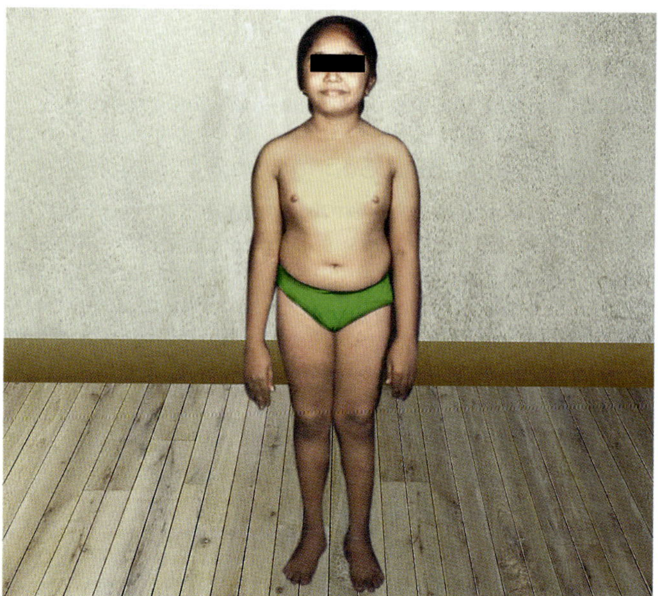

Fig. 16.3.3: A 14-year-old girl with hypergonadotropic hypogonadism—Turner syndrome.

of growth in otherwise healthy adolescents with stature reduced for chronologic age but appropriate for bone age and stage of pubertal development, both of which are usually delayed. The growth velocity is appropriate for bone age rather than chronologic age. In isolated gonadotropin deficiency, childhood growth is normal but the pubertal growth spurt does not occur. Growth is subnormal if there is associated growth hormone deficiency (GHD) or secondary hypothyroidism.

Body Proportions

Children with isolated gonadotropin deficiency and Klinefelter syndrome have eunuchoid proportions due to delayed epiphyseal closure.

Weight related to Height

It is decreased in malnutrition and chronic disease and increased in most hormonal disorders. Obesity is a feature of many syndromes associated with hypogonadism.

Pubertal Assessment

Puberty should be staged according to Tanner staging. The spontaneous start of puberty by 18 years of age is the gold standard to distinguish CDGP from gonadotropin deficiency. In gonadotropin deficiency, pubertal development is absent or incomplete. Slow progression suggests a partial gonadotropin deficiency. In CDGP, the rate of pubertal progression is normal.

Search for the Presence of Chronic Disease, Malnutrition, Anosmia, Midline Defects, Endocrine Disorders, and Dysmorphic Syndromes

Male babies born with congenital gonadotropin deficiency have normal sexual differentiation but micropenis.

Neurological Assessment

It includes fundus examination and evaluation of visual fields.

Investigations[6,7]

The child's predicted target height based on the parents' adult heights should be plotted.

Hormonal Evaluation

Serum gonadotropin levels: FSH and LH distinguish between hypogonadotropic and hypergonadotropic hypogonadism.

Serum gonadotropin response to stimulation with GnRH: It may show a pubertal response in CDGP but is not usually helpful in distinguishing it from isolated gonadotropin deficiency.

Serum testosterone and estradiol: As mentioned above under precocious puberty, serum testosterone measurement is useful to document start and progress in stages of puberty in boys; however, measurement of serum estradiol is less useful in girls.

Serum DHEAS levels: They are usually normal for chronologic age in hypogonadotropic hypogonadism but are low for age and correspond with the bone age in CDGP, where the tempo of maturation is delayed.

Inhibin B levels are low in congenital gonadotropin deficiency and may be helpful in distinguishing it from CGDP.

Serum thyroxine (T4), thyroid-stimulating hormone (TSH), prolactin, insulin-like growth factor-1 (IGF-1), and GH stimulation tests are performed, if indicated.

Radiographic Investigations

Bone age: In CDGP, the bone age corresponds with the height age and stage of puberty. Signs of sexual maturation should be evident by a bone age of 13 years. In isolated gonadotropin deficiency, bone age is usually slightly delayed. But with multiple pituitary hormone deficiency, the bone age is markedly delayed.

Pelvic sonography: It provides information about the development of the uterus and ovaries.

Computed tomography and magnetic resonance imaging are performed, if indicated.

MANAGEMENT

Treatment of the cause whenever possible will result in subsequent pubertal development.[8] Patients with CDGP require reassurance that there is nothing wrong and that puberty though delayed will progress normally. In a few cases of profound delay, short-term low-dose hormonal treatment with testosterone or estrogens for 3–6 months may occasionally be required, if the patient is psychologically stressed. In males, testosterone treatment to induce puberty is recommended only if the bone age is >12 years to avoid the risk of inappropriate bone age advancement and thus, compromised adult height. In girls, therapy is recommended only after careful consideration of the effect of even small amounts of estrogen on skeletal maturation and epiphyseal fusion. The anabolic steroid, oxandrolone in appropriate doses, might also be used to stimulate growth without compromising adult height.

Permanent hypogonadism (primary or secondary) requires long-term replacement therapy with gradually increasing doses of sex steroids over 2–3 years. In males, intramuscular testosterone is the treatment of choice starting with a low dose and gradually increasing over time till adult levels are achieved. In females, estrogen is started in low doses orally or through transdermal patches, and increased incrementally over time until breakthrough vaginal bleeding occurs, or 12–24 months of treatment have passed. Patients are then started on combination estrogen–progesterone therapy for normal monthly withdrawal bleeding.

REFERENCES

1. Carel JC. Leger J. Clinical practice. Precocious puberty. N Engl J Med. 2008;358(22):2366-77.
2. Eugster EA. Treatment of central precocious puberty. J Endocr Soc. 2019;3(5):965-72.
3. Corica D, Aversa T, Pepe G, De Luca F, Wasniewska M. Peculiarities of precocious puberty in in boys and girls with McCune-Albright syndrome. Front Endocrinol (Lausanne). 2018;9:337.
4. Chen Y, Liu J. Do most 7- to 8-year-old girls with early puberty require extensive investigation and treatment? J Pediatr Adolesc Gynecol. 2021;34(2):124-9.
5. Howard SR, Dunkel L. Delayed puberty–phenotypic diversity, molecular genetic mechanisms, and recent discoveries. Endocr Rev. 2019;40(5):1285-317.
6. Persiani L, Bonomi M, Cools M, Dattani M, Dunkel L, Gravholt CH, et al. ENDO-ERN expert opinion on the differential diagnosis of pubertal delay. Endocrine. 2021;71(3):681-8.
7. Harrington J, Palmert MR. Clinical review: Distinguishing constitutional delay of growth and puberty from isolated hypogonadotropic hypogonadism: Critical appraisal of available diagnostic tests. J Clin Endocrinol Metab. 2012;97(9):3056-67.
8. Gaudino R, De Filippo G, Bozzola E, Gasparri M, Bozzola M, Villani A, et al. Current clinical management of constitutional delay of growth and puberty. Ital J Pediatr. 2011;48(1):45.

16.4 Disorders of the Thyroid Gland

Sukanya Priyadarshini, Vandana Jain

INTRODUCTION

Disorders of the thyroid gland in children include congenital and acquired hypothyroidism, hyperthyroidism, and thyroid nodules. This chapter presents the key aspects of normal thyroid physiology, newborn screening for congenital hypothyroidism, and the diagnostic approach and management guidelines for important disorders.

DEVELOPMENT AND PHYSIOLOGY

The thyroid gland originates from an outpouching of the foregut at the base of the tongue (foramen caecum) in the 3rd week of gestation, and descends to its final position in front of the trachea by the end of 7th week. Thyroxine synthesis and secretion can be observed as early as 12 weeks of gestation. During its migration, the thyroid gland is connected to the floor of the pharynx via the *thyroglossal duct,* which later gets obliterated. Remnants of thyroglossal duct can give rise to thyroglossal cysts.[1]

Thyroid hormone is synthesized and stored in the colloid of thyroid follicles, and released when required. The process of thyroid hormone synthesis is illustrated in **Figure 16.4.1**. The key steps include trapping of iodine by the thyroid follicular epithelial cells, its incorporation into tyrosine residues of the thyroglobulin protein in the lumen of the thyroid follicles, coupling of tyrosine residues to form tri-iodotyrosine (T3) and tetra-iodotyrosine (T4); and finally, release of T3 and T4 from thyroglobulin.[1] The approximate concentrations of T4 and T3 in the plasma are 10 µg/dL and 100 ng/dL respectively, with a T4:T3 ratio of 100:1 in the circulation.

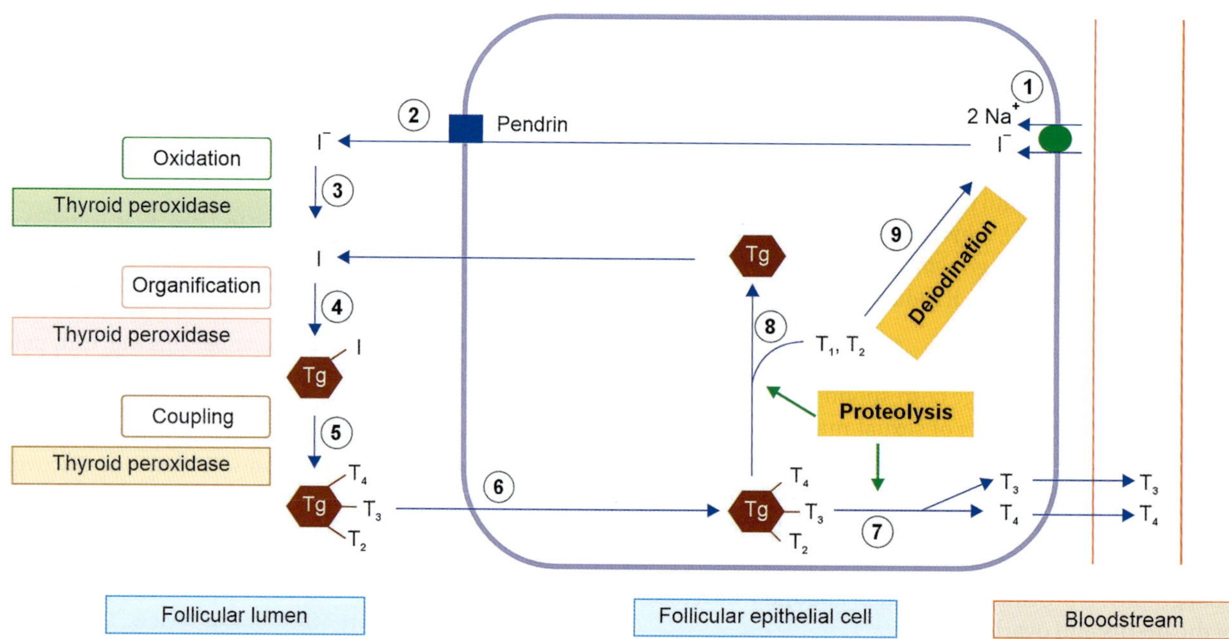

Fig. 16.4.1: The pathway of thyroid hormone synthesis involves the following steps. (1) Iodide uptake into thyroid follicular cell using sodium-iodide symporter; (2) Transport of iodide across the apical membrane into the lumen using pendrin; (3) Oxidation of iodide to iodine using thyroid peroxidase (TPO); (4) Incorporation of iodine into tyrosine residues (organification, also catalyzed by TPO) of thyroglobulin protein (synthesized by follicular cells and transported into the lumen), leading to synthesis of monoiodotyrosine (MIT) and diiodotyrosine (DIT); (5) Coupling of iodinated tyrosine residues leading to the formation of tri-iodotyrosine (T3) and tetraiodotyrosine (T4) residues, also catalyzed by TPO; (6) Uptake of iodinated thyroglobulin into follicular cells; (7 and 8) Proteolysis of iodinated thyroglobulin leading to the release of T3, T4, MIT (T1), and DIT (T2); and (9) MIT (T1) and DIT (T2) are deiodinated to release iodine which can be reused for thyroid hormone synthesis.

More than 99% of circulating T4 and T3 are bound to plasma proteins: albumin, thyroxine-binding globulin (TBG), and transthyretin; with albumin having the maximum capacity and TBG, the maximum affinity for binding to T4. T3 is the more physiologically active thyroid hormone. Several factors, including illness, drugs and conditions affecting serum protein levels such as nephrotic syndrome can affect the concentration of TBG, and hence the levels of total T4. Thus, it is important to interpret levels of total T4 in the appropriate context, and assess levels of free T4 when required.

Intracellular T4 is converted to T3 by types 1 and 2 deiodinase (D1 and D2). T3 then binds to the nuclear thyroid hormone receptor, and brings about gene transcription and protein synthesis.

The thyroid gland is regulated by thyroid stimulating hormone (TSH), a glycoprotein hormone produced by the anterior pituitary gland, which, in turn, is regulated by the hypothalamic peptide thyrotropin-releasing hormone (TRH). These are under negative feedback regulation of thyroid hormones; such that in primary hypothyroidism, TSH is high, while in central hypothyroidism, TSH is decreased.

HYPOTHYROIDISM

Hypothyroidism results when there is decreased production of thyroid hormones. Primary hypothyroidism occurs due to a defect in the thyroid gland itself, whereas central hypothyroidism occurs due to defects at the level of the pituitary gland (secondary hypothyroidism) or the hypothalamus (tertiary hypothyroidism). Both primary and central hypothyroidism may be congenital or acquired **(Table 16.4.1)**.

Etiology and Epidemiology

With a prevalence of 3–8 per 1,000 school-age children, acquired hypothyroidism due to autoimmune thyroiditis is the most common etiology of hypothyroidism in children.

TABLE 16.4.1: Etiologies of hypothyroidism in children.

Congenital hypothyroidism	
Primary	***Central***
Permanent: • Thyroid dysgenesis (responsible for about 70% of CH, mostly sporadic) • Ectopia, hypoplasia, and agenesis • Thyroid dyshormonogenesis	*Permanent:* • Isolated TSH deficiency • Multiple pituitary hormone deficiencies (e.g., due to defects in *PROP1*, *POU1F1*, *HESX1*, etc.)
Transient: • Iodine deficiency • Iodine exposure (maternal or neonatal) • Maternal blocking antibodies • Maternal antithyroid drugs • *DUOX2* and *DUOXA2* variants (dyshormonogenesis)	*Transient:* • Maternal thyrotoxicosis • Transient hypothyroxinemia of prematurity • *Drugs:* Dopamine, steroids, and somatostatin analogs • Sick euthyroid syndrome
Acquired hypothyroidism	
Primary	***Central***
Autoimmune: • Hashimoto thyroiditis *Drug-induced:* • *Iodine-containing drugs:* Amiodarone and expectorants • *Antiseizure medications:* Oxcarbazepine, phenytoin, phenobarbitone, and valproate • *Miscellaneous:* Lithium, dopamine, and tyrosine-kinase inhibitors *Systemic diseases:* • Nephropathic cystinosis • Multisystem Langerhans cell histiocytosis • Hemangiomas (especially those of the liver) *Treatment related:* • Antithyroid drugs • Postthyroidectomy • Posthead and neck irradiation • Postradioactive iodine ablation using ^{131}I	*Sellar-suprasellar injury* • Central nervous system tumors (e.g., craniopharyngioma) • Surgery/radiation • Trauma *Infiltration:* • Langerhans cell histiocytosis (LCH) • Lymphocytic hypophysitis • Tuberculosis

Note: Full forms of genes associated with thyroid dyshormonogenesis are provided in **Table 16.4.2**.
(*HESX1:* HESX homeobox 1; *POU1F1:* pituitary-specific positive transcription factor 1; *PROP1:* PROP paired-like homeobox 1; *TSHB*: TSH-β subunit).

TABLE 16.4.2: Genetic etiologies of congenital hypothyroidism due to dyshormonogenesis.

Gene	Protein	Inheritance	Key features
SLC5A5	Sodium iodide symporter	AR	Absent radioactive I or ^{99m}Tc uptake
SLC26A4	Pendrin	AR	Sensorineural hearing loss with enlarged vestibular aqueduct, mild CH
DUOX2, DUOXA2	Dual oxidase, dual oxidase associated protein	AR or AD, AR	May cause transient or permanent CH
TPO	Thyroid peroxidase	AR	The most common cause of CH due to dyshormonogenesis, CH may be severe
TG	Thyroglobulin	AR	CH may be severe
IYD	Iodotyrosine deiodinase (dehalogenase)	AR or AD with incomplete penetrance	Usually associated with mild CH

(AD: autosomal dominant; AR: autosomal recessive; CH: congenital hypothyroidism)

Congenital hypothyroidism (CH) is estimated to be present in approximately 1:2,500 newborns with thyroid dysgenesis being the most common cause. The types of thyroid dysgenesis include ectopic thyroid (e.g., lingual thyroid), agenesis, and hypoplasia. Dysgenesis is usually sporadic and has a 2:1 female to male ratio. Thyroid dyshormonogenesis (defect in thyroid hormone biosynthesis) is the next common cause and is characterized by enlarged (goitrous) thyroid gland. The genetic defects that can lead to dyshormonogenesis are summarized in **Table 16.4.2**. Dysgenesis and dyshormonogenesis lead to permanent primary CH, while conditions such as primary myxedema or atrophic thyroiditis associated with TSH receptor blocking immunoglobulins, maternal exposure to antithyroid medications, maternal iodine deficiency/excess, and neonatal iodine deficiency/excess cause transient CH. These conditions may be detected through newborn screening but often resolve on their own within the first few weeks to months of life. Maternal and/or neonatal exposure to excess iodine results in transient suppression of thyroid hormone synthesis (Wolff-Chaikoff effect).

Central hypothyroidism is usually associated with deficiency of other pituitary hormones as well. Congenital central hypothyroidism may be isolated TSH deficiency or associated with multiple pituitary hormone deficits due to defects in genes involved in development of the pituitary gland. Acquired central hypothyroidism may be due to a hypothalamic-pituitary tumor (e.g., craniopharyngioma), resection of such a tumor, cranial irradiation, head trauma, meningitis, or diseases affecting the pituitary gland such as tuberculosis or Langerhans cell histiocytosis.

Congenital Hypothyroidism

Clinical Features

Congenital hypothyroidism is asymptomatic at birth. This is due in part to passage of maternal thyroid hormones across the placenta, and the fact that several forms of CH

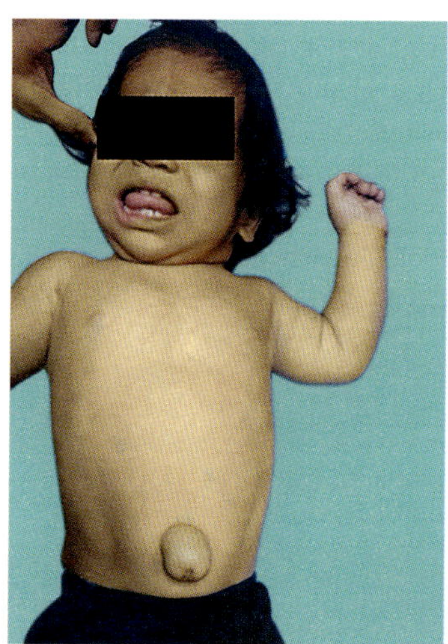

Fig. 16.4.2: A 2-and-a-half-year-old child with congenital hypothyroidism. Note the coarse faces, the large protruding tongue, and the umbilical hernia.

(such as ectopic thyroid, hypoplasia, or milder forms of dyshormonogenesis) have some residual thyroid function. Chief symptoms that become manifest over the first few months of life include prolonged jaundice due to immaturity of bilirubin uridine diphosphate (UDP) glucuronosyl transferase enzyme, poor feeding, lethargy, little cry with excessive sleeping, noisy breathing (macroglossia and nasal obstruction), and constipation.

Signs include hypothermia, bradycardia, cold and mottled skin, slightly increased head size with wide open anterior and posterior fontanels, protuberant abdomen with umbilical hernia, and hypotonia with delayed reflexes. When hypothyroidism is untreated; growth is stunted with short extremities; fontanels fail to close; the skin becomes pale and sallow; dentition and development are delayed; and in some instances, generalized muscular pseudohypertrophy develops. Thyroid dyshormonogenesis also usually presents with goiter.[1] **Figure 16.4.2** shows the picture of a child with untreated CH.

Laboratory Findings

Patients with primary hypothyroidism have elevated TSH with low total and free T4, whereas those with central hypothyroidism have low total and free T4 with inappropriately normal or low or even mildly elevated (possibly bioinactive) TSH.

A delay in skeletal maturation may be obvious wherein plain radiographs at birth show absent distal femoral and proximal tibial epiphyses. The underlying etiology of CH can be arrived at with the help of imaging modalities such as scintigraphy and ultrasonography. Scintigraphy using ^{123}I-sodium iodide or ^{99m}Tc-sodium pertechnetate is the imaging modality of choice in CH, but has the drawback that it needs to be done before starting treatment with levothyroxine. The radionuclide is transported by the sodium-iodide symporter **(Fig. 16.4.1)** into the thyroid gland. It can diagnose agenesis, ectopia, and dyshormonogenetic forms of CH. Apparent athyreosis (i.e., presence of gland on ultrasonography but no uptake on scintigraphy) can be seen in CH due to defective sodium-iodide symporter or TSH receptor, presence of maternal anti-TSH receptor antibodies, or if the scan has been done >5–6 days after starting treatment with levothyroxine. Therefore, all cases of "agenesis" on scintigraphy should be evaluated by ultrasonography. In no case should treatment of CH be delayed for waiting to arrange for scintigraphy. Ultrasonography is a more readily available investigation that can be done at any time irrespective of treatment. Absence of thyroid gland in its usual location or the presence of a hypoplastic thyroid gland on ultrasonogram suggests the diagnosis of thyroid dysgenesis. However, being operator-dependent, it has low specificity for diagnosing dysgenesis. Ectopic thyroid gland also is typically not identified on ultrasonogram.

Newborn Screening

If treatment for severe CH is not started by the age of 2 weeks, the infant will develop irreversible neurodevelopmental retardation. Relying on clinical features of CH, which are not evident till well beyond this time, to make a diagnosis and start therapy, will result in poor outcome in an otherwise easily treatable disorder. Newborn screening (NBS) programs address this gap. NBS is performed for conditions associated with high mortality or morbidity that are not clinically evident early on. These conditions must have reliable diagnostic modalities, effective therapies and be common enough to make screening cost-effective for every newborn in a given state or country. Thus, CH is the foremost among a growing list of disorders taken up in NBS programs worldwide.[2]

There are two main screening strategies for CH: primary T4 testing, and primary TSH testing. **Table 16.4.3** highlights the advantages and disadvantages of both screening strategies. In India, primary TSH screening strategy is recommended for NBS, but unfortunately is as yet not universal.

TABLE 16.4.3: Advantages and disadvantages of the primary TSH and primary T4 testing strategies.

Screening strategy	*Advantages*	*Disadvantages*
Primary TSH testing	High sensitivity for detection of both uncompensated (low T4 and high TSH) as well as compensated (normal T4 and high TSH) primary hypothyroidism	• May miss preterm/sick neonates with immaturity of the hypothalamic-pituitary-thyroid axis (A second screening should therefore be repeated in all such newborns at 2–4 weeks of age) • May miss central hypothyroidism
Primary T4 testing	Identifies neonates with both primary and central hypothyroidism	• High rate of false positivity in preterm and sick newborns, and newborns with TBG deficiency • High rate of false negativity due to infants with compensated hypothyroidism (normal T4 at the expense of high TSH)

(TSH: thyroid-stimulating hormone)

Following delivery, there is a massive surge in neonatal TSH concentration at 30–60 minutes, with gradual decline over 48–72 hours. This is due to sudden interruption in the supply of maternal thyroid hormones, and exposure of the neonate to the relatively hypothermic ex-utero environment. Following the rise in TSH, T4 and T3 also peak at around 24 hours of life and fall back to normal infant ranges at 5–7 days. Therefore, the appropriate time for NBS is after 72 hours of life, or at the time of birth. The latter is achieved by drawing whole blood from the placental end of the umbilical cord, which is largely spared of the neonatal surge.[3-5] **Flowchart 16.4.1** shows an algorithm based on the recommendations by the Indian Society for Pediatric and Adolescent Endocrinology and the American Academy of Pediatrics for screening and confirmation of CH.

Treatment and Follow-up

Treatment with oral levothyroxine (T4) should preferably be started within the first 2 weeks of life with a dose of 10–15 μg/kg orally once daily. Levothyroxine tablet is crushed, mixed with a small amount of expressed breastmilk and given, taking care to not give iron or calcium supplement at the same time.

T4/free T4 and TSH should be assessed after 2 and 4 weeks of starting treatment, with the goal of having achieved normalization of T4/free T4 by 2 weeks, and TSH

Flowchart 16.4.1: Screening algorithm for congenital hypothyroidism in neonates. Low T4 is <8 µg/dL and low fT4 is <1.1 ng/dL.

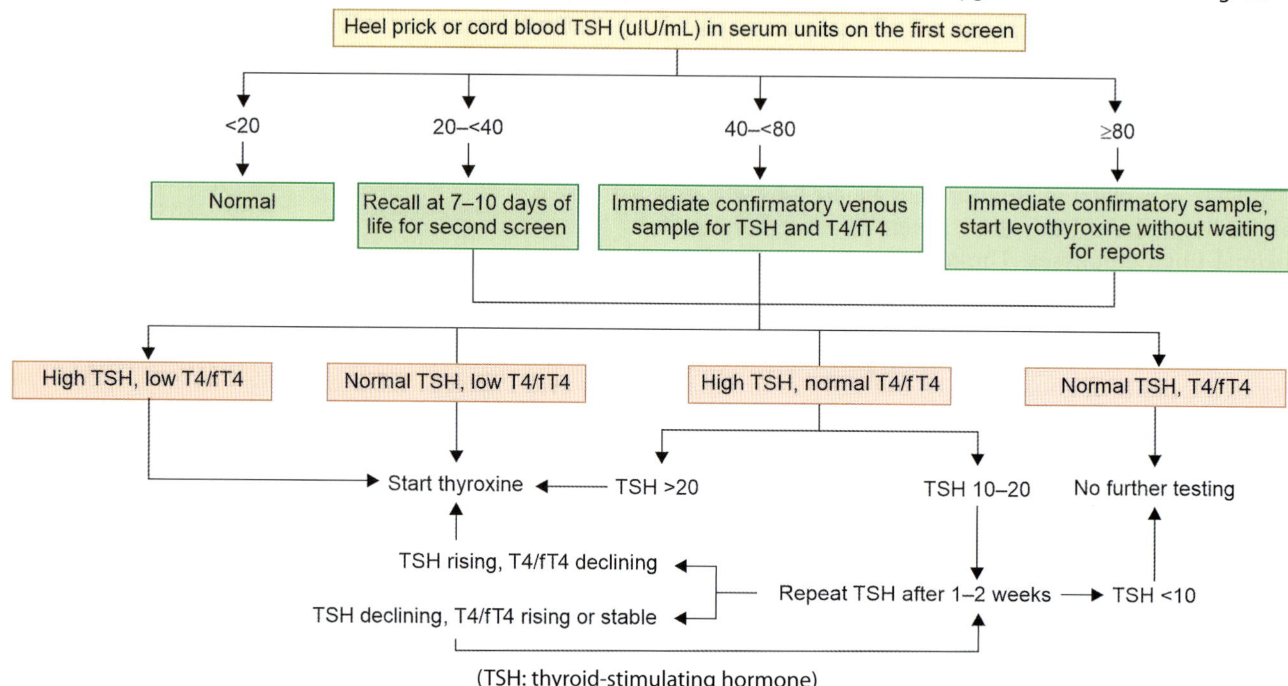

(TSH: thyroid-stimulating hormone)

by 1 month. Subsequent testing should be done 2-monthly till 6 months of age, and 3-monthly thereafter till 3 years of age, after which the testing frequency can be 3–6 monthly. Serum T4/free T4 should be maintained in the upper half of the normal age-based reference ranges.

During each visit, anthropometry and development of the child should be recorded, with prompt action in case of any deviation from normal. This may be in the form of ensuring compliance, adjusting the dose, and providing early stimulation. The per kg dose of levothyroxine reduces as the child becomes older, with the average dose being 4–6 µg/kg in children aged 1–4 years, 3–5 µg/kg in children aged 5–12 years, 2–3 µg/kg in children aged 12–18 years, and 1–2 µg/kg in adulthood.[4,5]

Trial Off Treatment

Repeat thyroid function test (TFT) at 3 years of age after stopping thyroid supplement for 4 weeks is recommended in cases where treatment was initiated in the neonatal period without imaging evaluation, or in preterm or sick neonates, or when the thyroid gland is present in its normal location, and the child has low thyroxine requirement (<2 µg/kg).[4,5]

Acquired Hypothyroidism

The most common etiology of acquired hypothyroidism in children is autoimmune thyroiditis (Hashimoto thyroiditis) with a female preponderance of 4:1. Most cases have a positive family history for autoimmune thyroid disease. Iodine deficiency, once thought to be the most common cause of acquired hypothyroidism, now contributes little to the burden of acquired hypothyroidism, chiefly because of widespread implementation of universal salt iodization. Children with Down, Turner, and Klinefelter syndromes, type 1 diabetes mellitus, celiac disease, and other autoimmune disorders are at an increased risk of autoimmune thyroid disease. Often, a child with CH due to an ectopic gland or dyshormonogenesis presents for the first time in mid-childhood, with "juvenile" hypothyroidism. The well-preserved IQ despite lack of therapy may prevent one from suspecting CH. The gland has produced enough thyroid hormone during the age of rapid brain development, thereafter, the production is insufficient to maintain physical growth but the child is spared from neurodevelopmental insufficiency. **Table 16.4.1** provides a list of causes of acquired hypothyroidism in children.

Clinical Features

The most common symptoms of acquired hypothyroidism in children are faltering of linear growth, lethargy, constipation, and cold intolerance. Children may present with mild weight gain due to fluid retention but hypothyroidism per se is not a cause of significant obesity. While delay in pubertal development is more common in children with hypothyroidism, some girls may present with gonadotropin-independent precocious puberty due to a specificity spill-over of TSH with follicle-stimulating hormone (FSH). TSH in excess binds to FSH receptors on the granulosa cells in the ovaries leading to development of estradiol producing cysts in the ovaries, thelarche, and vaginal bleeding. Contrary to popular belief, school performance is usually not affected in children with acquired hypothyroidism.[1]

Examination findings include bradycardia, hypertension, paradoxical pulse, short stature, coarse skin and facies, loss of lateral eyebrows, alopecia, carotenemia, signs of precocious/delayed puberty, pseudohypertrophy of calves and other muscles, and delayed relaxation of deep tendon reflexes. Goiter (usually soft in dyshormonogenesis, and firm in Hashimoto thyroiditis associated hypothyroidism) may be present in several children.

Laboratory Findings

Children with primary hypothyroidism have low T4 and high TSH. Detection of antithyroid peroxidase (anti-TPO) or antithyroglobulin (Tg) antibodies is diagnostic of Hashimoto thyroiditis. Ultrasonogram reveals diffuse enlargement of the thyroid gland with heterogeneous echotexture. Other laboratory abnormalities in hypothyroidism include macrocytic anemia, hyponatremia, hypercholesterolemia, and acquired von Willebrand disease.

Subclinical Hypothyroidism

An elevated TSH in the setting of normal T4 indicates subclinical hypothyroidism, which typically does not warrant treatment in children, unless TSH is >10 uIU/mL, or between 5 and 10 uIU/mL with presence of goiter. Children with subclinical hypothyroidism with positive anti-TPO antibodies, history of Hashimoto thyroiditis in first-degree relatives, or syndromes that are associated with hypothyroidism (such as Down syndrome), who do not currently fulfill the criteria for treatment should be kept under follow-up with serial testing every 6–12 months.

Treatment and Follow-up

Levothyroxine tablets should be administered once daily 30 minutes prior to meals. TSH and T4 (or free T4) should be checked 6–8 weeks after initiating or adjusting therapy. Once a therapeutic dose has been established, the thyroid function test should be checked every 4–6 months. The goals of treatment are to maintain normal growth, normal development, and clinical and biochemical euthyroidism.

HYPERTHYROIDISM

Hyperthyroidism is characterized by excessive production of thyroid hormones T4 and T3. Thyrotoxicosis, on the other hand, refers to a state of thyroid hormone excess regardless of the underlying function of the thyroid gland, as occurs in thyroid hormone overdosage, and subacute thyroiditis (where the prepared hormone in the thyroid gland gets leaked out into the blood, during an inflammatory state of the thyroid gland). The most common cause of pediatric hyperthyroidism is Graves' disease.[1]

Graves' Disease

Graves' disease is an autoimmune disorder characterized by presence of TSH receptor antibody (TRAb), which is a stimulatory antibody to TSH receptor, and results in thyroid hypertrophy and an overactive thyroid gland. Other causes of pediatric thyrotoxicosis and hyperthyroidism are listed in **Table 16.4.4**.

Clinical Features

The symptoms of thyrotoxicosis include anxiety, disturbed sleep, poor concentration, tremors, heat intolerance, emotional lability, palpitations, diarrhea, and weight loss despite increased appetite. Many children are often evaluated and treated for attention-deficit hyperactivity disorder (ADHD) for months before being diagnosed with thyrotoxicosis. Growth may be accelerated with advancement in skeletal age. Examination reveals tachycardia, systolic hypertension, widened pulse pressure, eyelid retraction with a staring look, warm and moist skin, fine hand tremors, and proximal muscle weakness.[1]

Children with thyrotoxicosis due to Graves' disease often have a large symmetric diffuse goiter with audible bruit on auscultation. Ocular examination reveals cardinal signs of inflammation involving the eyelids, conjunctiva, cornea, optic nerve, retro-orbital fat, and extraocular muscles. The presence of TSH receptor on retro-orbital fibroblasts and extraocular muscles explains the frequency of eye signs in patients with Graves' disease. Stimulated fibroblasts synthesize glycosaminoglycans and cytokines, leading to proptosis and inflammation, respectively.[1]

TABLE 16.4.4: Etiologies of pediatric thyrotoxicosis.

Thyrotoxicosis with hyperthyroidism	*Thyrotoxicosis without hyperthyroidism*
• Graves' disease • Toxic adenoma • Toxic multinodular goiter • McCune–Albright syndrome • hCG-secreting tumors • TSH-secreting pituitary adenomas	• Hashitoxicosis • Acute thyroiditis • Subacute thyroiditis • Drug-induced thyroiditis (amiodarone and lithium) • Radiation thyroiditis • Exogenous intake of thyroid hormone • Extrathyroidal source of thyroid hormone production (struma ovarii and metastases of thyroid cancer)

(hCG: human chorionic gonadotropin; TSH: thyroid stimulating hormone)

Laboratory Findings

T4 and T3 are elevated and TSH is suppressed in thyrotoxicosis. The additional finding of positive TRAb is diagnostic of Graves' disease. Negative TRAb with a positive anti-TPO or anti-Tg is suggestive of Hashitoxicosis. Nuclear studies with ^{123}I or ^{99m}Tc show diffusely increased uptake in Graves' disease, and focal increased uptake in case of solitary toxic nodule. In other causes of thyrotoxicosis, there is reduced uptake of the radionuclide. Sonographic characteristics of Graves' disease include a normal-sized or symmetrically enlarged hypoechoic thyroid gland, with increased vascularity on Doppler imaging.

Treatment and Follow-up

Once a diagnosis of Graves' disease is established, treatment with antithyroid drugs (ATDs) such as carbimazole or methimazole should be initiated. These are thionamides which inhibit the enzyme thyroid peroxidase, thereby limiting the production of thyroid hormones. Propylthiouracil has a similar mechanism of action with the additional function of preventing T4 to T3 conversion in the peripheral tissues. However, its use is not recommended due to the risk of hepatic failure. The goal of treatment is to establish clinical and biochemical euthyroidism. β-blockers, such as propranolol, are also used for the initial 2–4 weeks of treatment for symptomatic relief. Selective β-1 blocker such as atenolol may be preferred in children with asthma or cardiac disease.

Adverse effects of thionamides include agranulocytosis and hepatotoxicity. In case a child on a thionamide presents with fever, an absolute neutrophil count should be obtained to rule out febrile neutropenia.

Most children attain remission within a few weeks of starting treatment with ATDs, after which they need to be continued on a very low dose of the drug for 1–2 years to maintain remission. Children who do not attain remission but do well on ATDs may continue the same for years. The ones who relapse on or after discontinuing ATDs, or have adverse events on ATDs are candidates for definitive therapies such as radioactive iodine ablation (RAI) with ^{131}I or total thyroidectomy. ATDs should be discontinued 3–7 days prior to RAI to enable ^{131}I to be taken up by the thyroid gland, incorporated into thyroglobulin, and cause destruction of thyroid gland from within. Active Graves' orbitopathy is an absolute contraindication, whereas inactive Graves' orbitopathy is a relative contraindication to RAIU. This is because RAI-associated spill of thyroid antigens into the circulation exacerbates TSH-receptor antibody production, and worsening of immunological injury and inflammation in the setting of Graves' orbitopathy.[6]

GOITER AND THYROID NODULES

A goiter is defined as a diffuse enlargement of the thyroid gland. The most common etiologies are autoimmune thyroiditis and iodine deficiency. In children presenting with goiter, the focus is on assessing thyroid function, determining the etiology, evaluating for compressive symptoms and instituting appropriate management. When there is a localized discrete swelling of the thyroid, it may be a cyst or an abscess or a neoplasm. Although thyroid malignancies are rare in the pediatric age group, there is a higher rate of malignancy among solitary thyroid nodules identified in childhood as compared to those identified in adulthood.[7] Previous radiation exposure, family history of neoplasia, and certain syndromes confer a higher risk of thyroid malignancy. **Box 16.4.1** shows a list of etiologies causing thyromegaly in children.[8]

The most common pediatric thyroid malignancy is *papillary carcinoma,* constituting 80–90% of all cases, followed by follicular carcinoma. Sonographic findings that suggest malignancy include a solitary solid hypoechoic nodule, irregular margins, presence of calcifications, nodule being taller than wider, presence of abnormal lymph nodes in the vicinity, and progressive enlargement of the nodules with time. Whenever there is suspicion of a malignancy, a fine-needle aspiration cytology should be performed. The definitive treatment of thyroid malignancies is total thyroidectomy with or without cervical lymph node dissection. Following surgery, radioactive iodine (^{131}I) ablation is used to target locoregional invasion not amenable to surgical resection and distant metastases. Multiple endocrine neoplasia (MEN)-2A and -2B are syndromes associated with increased risk of medullary thyroid carcinoma, and warrant prophylactic thyroidectomy.

BOX 16.4.1: Etiologies of thyromegaly in childhood.

Diffuse:
- Autoimmune (Hashimoto) thyroiditis
- Iodine deficiency
- Dyshormonogenesis
- Graves' disease
- McCune–Albright syndrome

Nodular:
- Multinodular goiter
- Solitary nodule
- Toxic nodule
- Cyst and abscess
- Follicular adenoma
- Papillary carcinoma
- Follicular carcinoma
- Medullary carcinoma

CONCLUSION

To summarize, pediatric thyroid disease constitutes a broad spectrum of entities. CH has excellent prognosis when identified and treated in time. While newborn screening is recommended, it is not universally followed in our country. Therefore, a high index of suspicion should be kept for CH in infants and young children presenting with suggestive clinical features. Hashimoto thyroiditis is the most common cause of hypothyroidism in older children, and can have myriad presentations, the most common being growth deceleration, goiter, and myxedema. It is equally important to be aware of the symptoms and signs of the uncommon, yet sight-threatening Graves' disease, for which prompt identification and referral to a pediatric endocrinologist will be warranted. While thyroid nodules per se are not very common in childhood, the risk of malignancy is higher than in adults. An algorithmic approach should be adopted for their evaluation, so as not to miss the devastating yet curable differentiated carcinomas of the thyroid gland.

REFERENCES

1. Hanley P, Lord K, Bauer AJ. Thyroid Disorders in Children and Adolescents: a review. JAMA Pediatr. 2016;170(10):1008-19.
2. van Trotsenburg P, Stoupa A, Léger J, Rohrer T, Peters C, Fugazzola L, et al. Congenital Hypothyroidism: A 2020-2021 Consensus Guidelines Update-An ENDO-European Reference Network Initiative Endorsed by the European Society for Pediatric Endocrinology and the European Society for Endocrinology. Thyroid. 2021;31(3):387-419.
3. Desai MP, Sharma R, Riaz I, Sudhanshu S, Parikh R, Bhatia V. Newborn Screening Guidelines for Congenital Hypothyroidism in India: Recommendations of the Indian Society for Pediatric and Adolescent Endocrinology (ISPAE)—Part I: Screening and Confirmation of Diagnosis. Indian J Pediatr. 2018;85(6): 440-7.
4. Rose SR, Wassner AJ, Wintergerst KA, Yayah-Jones NH, Hopkin RJ, Chuang J, et al. Section on Endocrinology Executive Committee; Council on Genetics Executive Committee. Congenital Hypothyroidism: Screening and Management. Pediatrics. 2023;151(1):e2022060420.
5. Paul PG, Jain V. Congenital hypothyroidism. In: Agarwal R, Deorari AK, Paul VK, Sankar J, Sachdeva A (Eds). AIIMS Protocols in Neonatology, 3rd Edition. New Delhi: Noble Publishers; 2024.
6. Mooij CF, Cheetham TD, Verburg FA, Eckstein A, Pearce SH, Léger J, et al. 2022 European Thyroid Association Guideline for the management of pediatric Graves' disease. Eur Thyroid J. 2022;11(1):e210073.
7. Lebbink CA, Links TP, Czarniecka A, Dias RP, Elisei R, Izatt L, et al. 2022 European Thyroid Association Guidelines for the management of pediatric thyroid nodules and differentiated thyroid carcinoma. Eur Thyroid J. 2022;11(6):e220146.
8. Jain V. Goiter, Thyroid Nodules and Thyroid Neoplasia. In: Desai MP, Menon PSN, Bhatia V, Seth A (Eds). Pediatric Endocrine Disorders, 4th edition. Hyderabad: Universities Press; 2022.

16.5 Mineral Metabolism and Disorders of the Parathyroid Glands

Anju Seth, Preeti Singh

INTRODUCTION

Mineral metabolism is a finely regulated process essential for maintaining physiological homeostasis, involving the dynamic balance of calcium, phosphorus, and magnesium. These minerals play critical roles in skeletal development, neuromuscular function, enzymatic activity, and cellular signaling. The parathyroid glands are central to this regulation, primarily through parathyroid hormone (PTH) secretion, which modulates calcium and phosphate balance by acting on the bones, kidneys, and intestines. Disorders of the parathyroid glands can significantly disrupt mineral homeostasis, leading to a wide spectrum of clinical manifestations ranging from asymptomatic biochemical abnormalities to life-threatening complications like severe hypocalcemia or hypercalcemia. This chapter describes the mechanisms of mineral metabolism, and disorders related to these.

CALCIUM

Calcium (Ca) is among the most abundant mineral ions in the body. Over 98% of the total Ca is present as mineral salts in the bone while serum Ca accounts for 1% of total body Ca. The serum Ca exists in equilibrium with Ca present in extracellular and intracellular spaces and that in the recently accumulated surface of bone. It is the main regulator of bone formation and turnover and modulates vital body functions including neural transmission, blood clotting, intracellular signal transduction, as well as maintenance of cardiac rhythm and muscle contractility.[1] About 40–60% of serum Ca is the metabolically active ionized form (iCa), which is tightly regulated. The chief mechanisms regulating serum Ca involve the Ca-sensing receptor (CaSR) located on the chief cells of the parathyroid glands and renal tubules; parathyroid hormone (PTH) and its receptor; and the vitamin D hormone system.

Regulation of Calcium Homeostasis

With a drop in iCa concentration, the CaSR on the parathyroid glands gets inhibited and PTH is released.[1] PTH induces bone mineral release, thereby increasing circulating Ca and phosphate (P). In the kidney, PTH increases renal tubular Ca reabsorption and increases P excretion. The net effect of PTH on bone and kidney is to increase plasma Ca and decrease plasma P. In addition, PTH stimulates the conversion of 25-hydroxyvitamin D (25OHD) to its active form, 1,25 dihydroxyvitamin D [1,25$(OH)_2$D or calcitriol], which increases intestinal Ca and P absorption. A fall in iCa concentration also directly enhances renal Ca reabsorption by inhibition of CaSR located in renal tubules.

HYPOCALCEMIA

Definition

Total serum Ca (tCa) level is age-dependent. Normal tCa for 1–5 years is 9.4–10.8 mg/dL, 6–12 years 9.4–10.2 mg/dL and >20 years 8.8–10.2 mg/dL. Since Ca exists in serum both in free and albumin bound forms, for every 1 g/dL fall in serum albumin, serum tCa falls by 0.8 mg/dL. However, Ca binding to albumin is also altered by many factors like alkalosis, increase in free fatty acids (FFA) in serum, lipid infusion etc.; therefore, it is desirable to measure iCa while diagnosing hypocalcemia in the setting of acute illness or hypoalbuminemia. Normal serum iCa level ranges between 4.4 and 5.2 mg/dL (1.1–1.3 nmol/L).[2]

Hypocalcemia is defined as serum Ca <8.8 mg/dL (2.2 mmol/L) in the postneonatal period. For neonates, cut-off values <8 mg/dL (2 mmol/L) in the term and <7 mg/dL (1.75 mmol/L) for the preterm are accepted. The corresponding values for iCa are <4.7 mg/dL (1.17 mmol/L) in the postneonatal period and <4.4 mg/dL (1.1 mmol/L) in the neonatal period.

Requirement for Calcium

As per the recent Indian Council for Medical Research (ICMR) guidelines, the estimated average requirement (EAR) of Ca for children varies by age group: infants (AI-adequate intake)—300 mg/day, 1–3 years: 400 mg/day, 4–6 years: 450 mg/day, 7–9 years: 500 mg/day, 10–12 years: 650 mg/day, 13–18 years: 800 mg/day. Milk and milk products are the major sources of dietary Ca. When consumption of milk is low, cereals become the major dietary source of Ca. Ragi, *rajkeera* (amaranth), gingelly seeds, sea food, fish, mutton, and green leafy vegetables are good sources of Ca.[3] Cow milk contains approximately 120 mg Ca and buffalo milk approximately 210 mg/100 mL. Presence of P in milk and oxalates and phytates in grains decrease Ca absorption. The calcium and phosphorus concentration in breastmilk is 252 mg/L and 143 mg/L, respectively. This ratio of 2:1 in breastmilk is optimal for Ca absorption.

Causes of Hypocalcemia

Hypocalcemia is most commonly observed in the neonatal period and early infancy. In the neonate, there is a physiological dip in serum Ca levels 1–3 days after birth. Various situations commonly encountered in the neonatal period exaggerate this dip, leading to *transient hypocalcemia*. Depending on the time of occurrence, neonatal hypocalcemia is classified as early (within 72 hours of birth) or late (>72 hours of birth) **(Table 16.5.1)**.

Early Neonatal Hypocalcemia

Early neonatal hypocalcemia (ENH) is usually secondary to maternal illness or certain perinatal conditions (perinatal asphyxia, infant of a diabetic mother, small for gestational age, and prematurity) which exaggerate the physiological postnatal dip in serum Ca. This results from a suboptimal release of PTH or unresponsiveness of renal tubule cells to PTH. Neonatal hypocalcemia may be the first manifestation of maternal hyperparathyroidism. Intrauterine hypercalcemia inhibits the PTH release from the fetal parathyroid gland, resulting in parathyroid unresponsiveness to hypocalcemia after birth.

Late Neonatal Hypocalcemia

Late neonatal hypocalcemia (LNH) is often due to a high dietary P load as might occur in infants on cow milk, vitamin D deficiency, hypomagnesemia, and transient hypoparathyroidism.[4] Though classically described as occurring toward the end of 1st week, the nadir in serum Ca often occurs several weeks after birth. Vitamin D deficiency in infancy is usually associated with subclinical maternal deficiency common among Indian women due to skin pigment, modest clothing, and thus poor sun exposure.

Hypocalcemia in Older Children and Adolescents

The etiology of hypocalcemia in older children and adolescents can be broadly classified into three groups based on the key regulators of plasma Ca, i.e., PTH, CaSR, vitamin D, and the miscellaneous causes **(Table 16.5.1)**. Chronic

TABLE 16.5.1: Etiology of hypocalcemia in infants and children.

Infants <72 hours	*Infants >72 hours*	*Older children and adolescents*
Neonatal illness: • Prematurity • Birth asphyxia • Intrauterine growth retardation • Sepsis • Respiratory distress • Citrated blood/alkali • Phototherapy *Maternal illness:* • Diabetes mellitus • Toxemia of pregnancy • Hyperparathyroidism	• High dietary phosphate load • *Hypomagnesemia:* Transient/metabolic disorder • *Hypoparathyroidism:* Transient/permanent • Chronic renal insufficiency • Pseudohypoparathyroidism • Maternal vitamin D deficiency	*Vitamin D related:* • Vitamin D and/or calcium deficiency—nutritional, malabsorption, chronic liver disease, etc. • Drugs—antiepileptic drugs and antitubercular • Defects in vitamin D action—VDDR-I and VDDR-II *Parathyroid related:* • Hypoparathyroidism—congenital/acquired defects • Target organ resistance to PTH—hypomagnesemia or pseudohypoparathyroidism *Hypomagnesemia:* • Malabsorption states • Bartter syndrome • Renal tubular acidosis • Diuretics *Mutations in CaSR:* Autosomal dominant hypocalcemia *Hyperphosphatemia:* • Renal failure • Tumor lysis • Phosphate administration

(CaSR: calcium-sensing receptor; VDDR: vitamin D-dependent rickets)

hypocalcemia is most often due to deficiency of PTH or 1,25$(OH)_2$D or to resistance to their biological effects.[4] In our population vitamin D deficiency is the most common cause of symptomatic hypocalcemia, especially during infancy and adolescence.

Clinical Manifestations

ENH is often asymptomatic. When present, the symptoms are neither specific for hypocalcemia nor related to its severity. These include jitteriness, irritability, and focal, or generalized seizures. Hypocalcemia may thus be mistaken for other conditions like hypoglycemia, meningitis, and intracranial bleeding. On the other hand, LNH is often symptomatic, commonly with convulsions, less commonly with stridor due to laryngospasm, apnea, cyanosis, dilated cardiomyopathy, and arrhythmias.

In older children and adolescents, hypocalcemia manifestations range from an asymptomatic state to numbness and tingling in the circumoral region, fingers or toes, or severe neuromuscular symptoms such as seizures, tetany, and laryngospasm. In cases where hypocalcemia is secondary to vitamin D deficiency, classical signs of rickets may be present, especially in toddlers and young children. On the other hand, young infants and adolescents with vitamin D deficiency may present with hypocalcemic convulsions as a sole manifestation. Latent tetany can be demonstrated by Chvostek sign (twitching at the ipsilateral corner of the mouth with a light tap over the facial nerve just below the maxilla) and Trousseau sign (carpal spasm produced by inflating a blood pressure cuff around the arm to 10 mm Hg above systolic for 3 minutes) (**Fig. 16.5.1**). Chronic hypocalcemia may lead to dental enamel hypoplasia, basal ganglia calcification, and cataract, if associated with hyperphosphatemia (as in hypoparathyroidism or PTH resistance).

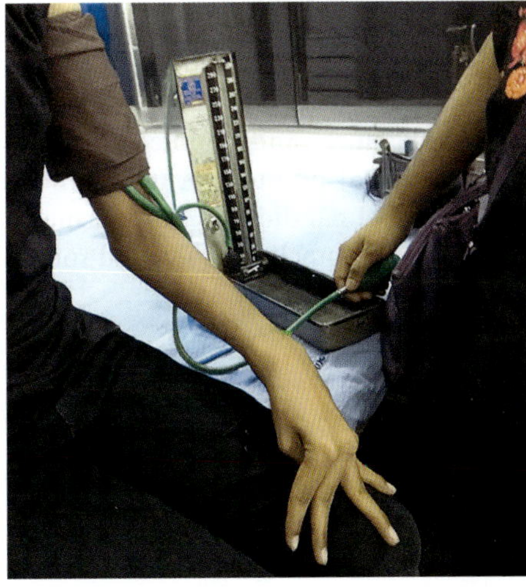

Fig. 16.5.1: Demonstration of trousseau sign in hypocalcemia.

Diagnostic Approach to a Case with Hypocalcemia

A thorough history and clinical examination are of utmost importance in the evaluation of a child with hypocalcemia, and provide the basis for planning the investigations.

Important Clues in History

Neonate: Age at onset of symptoms (ENH/LNH), gestational age (prematurity), perinatal events (birth asphyxia, jaundice, or respiratory distress), type of feeding (high P load), maternal illness (diabetes, hyperparathyroidism, or toxemia) and drug intake, and family history of hypocalcemic seizures (hypoparathyroidism).

Older child: Age, clinical symptoms, history suggestive of a chronic disease such as renal failure, malabsorption, thalassemia, other endocrine disorders (autoimmune polyglandular syndrome), medication history (antiepileptics), surgery, irradiation (parathyroid gland destruction), repeated infections with cardiac disease (DiGeorge syndrome), family history of seizures or hypocalcemia (hypoparathyroidism, autoimmune polyglandular syndrome, or pseudohypoparathyroidism).

Examination

Newborn: Gestation, systemic sickness, facial dysmorphism, and other malformations especially cardiac in DiGeorge syndrome, must be documented.

Older child: Features of rickets, and those suggestive of an underlying chronic systemic disease: anemia, hypertension, short stature (renal failure), and jaundice (liver disease) must be sought. The clinical pointers of metabolic conditions include alopecia, oral candidiasis/ectodermal dystrophy, heart disease, cataract, brachydactyly, and round face with obesity **(Table 16.5.2)**.

TABLE 16.5.2: Clinical pointers toward the etiology of hypocalcemia in children and adolescents.

Clinical evaluation	*Possible etiology*
Wrist widening, frontal bossing, rachitic rosary, double malleoli, Harrison sulcus, and genu valgum/varus	Rickets
Alopecia, epidermal cysts along with bony deformities of rickets	VDDR II
Recurrent infections, typical facies (mandibular hypoplasia, hypertelorism, short philtrum, and low set ears), and heart murmur	DiGeorge syndrome
History of neck surgery/irradiation, cataract, and deafness	Hypoparathyroidism and PHP
Mucocutaneous candidiasis, alopecia, and vitiligo	Polyglandular syndrome-I
Family history, short stature, brachydactyly, round facies, and obesity	Albrights hereditary osteodystrophy

(PHP: pseudohypoparathyroidism; VDDR: vitamin D dependent rickets type II)

Investigations

Level I

Serum Ca (total and ionized), P (fasting), alkaline phosphatase (ALP), magnesium, total protein, albumin, and serum creatinine should be done in all cases and values compared with age-specific norms in a case of suspected hypocalcemia. Further evaluation would depend upon the results obtained on these tests. Hypomagnesemia should be looked for in all cases of refractory hypocalcemia as it leads to both impaired PTH release and resistance to PTH action. ALP is a sensitive marker of bone turnover, being increased in disorders related to vitamin D and within normal range when hypocalcemia is secondary to hypoparathyroidism. Liver function tests, venous blood gas analysis, X-ray chest (thymic shadow and cardiac disease), and X-ray wrist (to look for signs of rickets) may be needed on a case-to-case basis.

Level II

Serum PTH is the key investigation in determining the etiology of hypocalcemia. A high PTH in the setting of hypocalcemia indicates secondary hyperparathyroidism (usually due to vitamin D deficiency), or PTH resistance (pseudohypoparathyroidism). A low PTH suggests hypoparathyroidism or hypomagnesemia. An inappropriately normal PTH in the setting of hypocalcemia indicates likelihood of an activating mutation involving the CaSR (autosomal dominant hypocalcemia) wherein PTH secretion gets inhibited at a relatively lower level of serum Ca. Assessment of serum 25OHD and 1,25$(OH)_2$D is essential for diagnosing disorders related to vitamin D metabolism. An assay of the mother's serum for Ca, P, ALP, and 25OHD may be required when suspecting maternal vitamin D deficiency or hyperparathyroidism. A stepwise approach to a child with hypocalcemia is shown in **Flowchart 16.5.1.**

Treatment of a Child with Hypocalcemia

Acute Management

Symptomatic children should be managed with intravenous (IV) Ca infusion of 0.2–0.5 mL/kg of 10% Ca gluconate (up to 2 mL/kg in neonates; maximum 10 mL) given over 10–20 min under cardiac monitoring. This is followed by a continuous IV infusion of 10% Ca gluconate 5 mL or 50 mg elemental Ca/kg/day for neonates and 2–3 mL or 20–30 mg elemental Ca/kg/day for older infants and children. A secure IV line is mandatory to avoid subcutaneous necrosis from extravasation. Ca infusions should not be mixed with solutions containing phosphates, to avoid precipitation. Once stabilized, the infusion is tapered over 24–48 hours, with the simultaneous introduction of oral Ca 50–75 mg/kg/day (up to 100 mg/kg/day in neonates). In case of refractory hypocalcemia with documented hypomagnesemia,

Flowchart 16.5.1: Algorithmic approach to hypocalcemia.

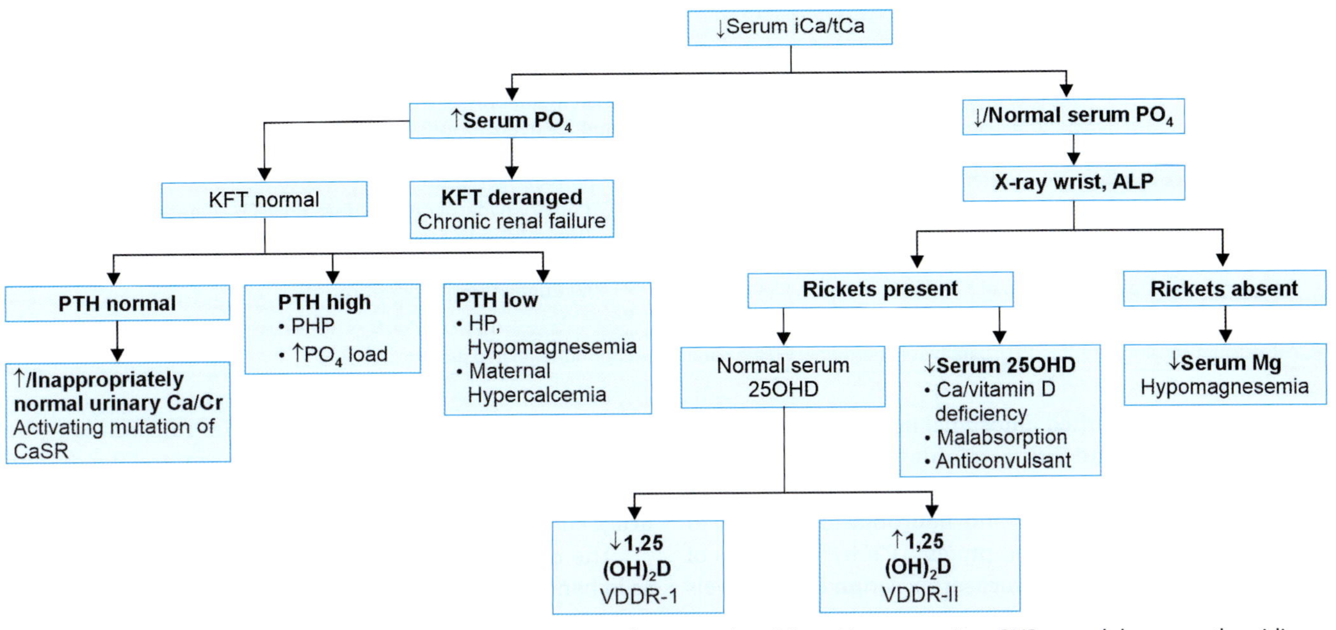

(ALP: alkaline phosphatase; CaSR: calcium-sensing receptor; HP: hypoparathyroidism; Mg: magnesium; PHP: pseudohypoparathyroidism; PTH: parathyroid hormone; VDDR-I and II: vitamin D-dependent rickets types I and II)

magnesium sulfate ($MgSO_4$) 50% is given IM in a dose of 0.2 mL/kg 12 hourly for 24 hours. Asymptomatic hypocalcemia is treated with oral Ca supplements at a rate of 50–75 mg/kg/day divided every 6 hours; duration depends on the underlying etiology.

Management of Underlying Cause

Children and adolescents with nutritional vitamin D deficiency are managed with age-appropriate oral cholecalciferol (2,000 IU/day for infants, 3,000–6,000 IU/day for ages 1–12 years, 6,000 IU/day for age >12 years), and Ca supplements (at a rate of 50–75 mg/kg/day) for 3 months.[5] Once normal serum 25OHD levels are achieved a preventive dose of vitamin D 400 IU/day and 600 IU/day for infants and older children respectively should be given to prevent recurrence of deficiency.

Mothers of young infants with vitamin D deficiency should also be investigated and treated with Ca and vitamin D. Chronic hypocalcemia resulting from hypoparathyroidism and pseudohypoparathyroidism [due to chronic kidney disease (CKD), and vitamin D dependent rickets (VDDR) types] is managed with active vitamin D analogs calcitriol (15–25 ng/kg/day) or alfacalcidol (25–40 ng/kg/day) with (if the child's diet is poor in dairy products) or without Ca supplements.[6]

HYPERCALCEMIA

Serum Ca levels are higher in children compared to adults and age-appropriate cut-offs should be taken to diagnose hypercalcemia. In neonates and infants, serum Ca >10.8–11.3 mg/dL and in older children and adolescents, values >10.3 mg/dL are considered as hypercalcemia.[7]

Causes of Hypercalcemia

Hypercalcemia is much less often encountered in children than hypocalcemia. Hypercalcemia can be classified as being PTH-independent (low or suppressed PTH) or PTH-dependent (PTH levels high), the former being more common during childhood.[8] The most common cause of hypercalcemia in pediatric practice is hypervitaminosis D (serum 25OHD level >100 ng/mL), due to the administration of excessive vitamin D, often to a child with nonnutritional or misdiagnosed rickets. Subcutaneous fat necrosis is associated with hypercalcemia in newborns with predisposing factors like birth asphyxia, meconium aspiration, and hypothermia. Prolonged immobilization results in disuse atrophy and decreased bone deposition with increased resorption resulting in hypercalcemia. The causes of hypercalcemia are given in **Table 16.5.3**.

A heterozygous loss-of-function mutation in the *CaSR* gene causes familial hypocalciuric hypercalcemia (FHH), an autosomal dominant disorder characterized by mild and asymptomatic hypercalcemia. A homozygous loss-of-function mutation in the same gene leads to neonatal severe hyperparathyroidism (NSHPT), a life-threatening condition with severe hypercalcemia in newborns. Primary hyperparathyroidism (PHPT) in children is mostly sporadic and often results from a parathyroid adenoma, but it can

TABLE 16.5.3: Etiology of hypercalcemia in children.

PTH-independent (low or suppressed PTH level)	*PTH-dependent (normal to high PTH level)*
• Hypervitaminosis D • *Dietary:* High-calcium load, low-phosphate diet (breastmilk/standard formula in preterm babies, total parenteral nutrition) • Subcutaneous fat necrosis (birth trauma and birth asphyxia) • Hypercalcemia in inflammatory/granulomatous states • *Drugs:* Thiazides and chronic ingestion of vitamin A • Williams syndrome and Jansen metaphyseal dysplasia (activating PTH receptor mutation) • Malignancy (ectopic production of PTHrP) • Immobilization	• Neonatal severe hyperparathyroidism (homozygous inactivating *CaSR* mutation) • Familial hypocalciuric hypercalcemia (heterozygous inactivating *CaSR* mutation)—normal to mildly elevated PTH level • Hyperparathyroidism: – Primary hyperparathyroidism (PHPT)—parathyroid adenoma (sporadic), and carcinoma – Multiple endocrine neoplasia types I and II – McCune–Albright syndrome

(CaSR: calcium-sensing receptor; PTH: parathyroid hormone; PTHrP: parathyroid hormone-related protein)

also be linked to inherited autosomal dominant syndromes such as multiple endocrine neoplasia (MEN). Rarely, hypercalcemia in children can be caused by malignancies (e.g., leukemia, lymphoma, and neuroblastoma) due to the production of PTH-related protein (PTHrP). In cases of unexplained hypercalcemia, measuring serum PTHrP levels can help to detect occult tumors.

Clinical Features of Hypercalcemia

Clinical features are generally seen when serum Ca exceeds 12 mg/dL with an insidious onset over a few weeks. Children present with nonspecific symptoms such as vomiting, irritability, hypotonia, constipation, polyuria, and dehydration. Children with chronic hypercalcemia have failure to thrive, abdominal pain, bone pains, and nephrocalcinosis. In severe cases, renal failure, pancreatitis, and reduced consciousness may occur. A serum Ca and P product exceeding 56 can cause soft-tissue and vascular calcification (manifesting with hypertension).

Diagnostic Approach

The history includes review of symptoms of hypercalcemia, intake of vitamin D and Ca, signs and symptoms of malignancy, family history of renal stones, MEN, and parathyroid surgery. The child should be examined for bony deformities (Jansen metaphyseal dysplasia and rickets in hypophosphatasia), dysmorphism (William syndrome), and hard mobile subcutaneous lumps (subcutaneous fat necrosis).

Laboratory tests should include Ca, phosphorus, 25OHD, $1,25(OH)_2D$, PTH, and urinary Ca levels. Family members should be screened for hypercalcemia and hypocalciuria. A technetium-99 (Tc-99) sestamibi scan is useful for localizing parathyroid adenomas before surgery.

Treatment

Treatment of hypercalcemia is aimed at both lowering the serum Ca concentration and correcting the underlying disease. General measures include minimizing the Ca concentration in enteral and parenteral feeds and discontinuing oral Ca and or vitamin D supplements and drugs known to cause hypercalcemia.

The management of mild asymptomatic hypercalcemia as in benign FHH does not require any specific management apart from periodic monitoring. Symptomatic patients with serum Ca >12 mg/dL and all patients with levels >14 mg/dL need urgent treatment regardless of underlying cause. Hypercalcemia in the acute phase is managed by parenteral rehydration with normal saline and loop diuretics, which increases urinary Ca excretion. For severe hypercalcemia, bisphosphonates, and calcitonin can be used. Hemodialysis is needed in acute severe life-threatening hypercalcemia unresponsive to medical management. Glucocorticoids have been used to treat hypercalcemia in granulomatous conditions such as tuberculosis and subcutaneous fat necrosis. Surgical removal is indicated in parathyroid adenoma. Parathyroidectomy may be required in cases with primary hyperparathyroidism or NSHPT. Cinacalcet is a calcimimetic agent that activates CaSR and suppresses PTH secretion.[9] It can be used for acute stabilization of NSHPT cases while awaiting surgery.

OSTEOPENIA OF PREMATURITY OR METABOLIC BONE DISEASE OF PREMATURITY

Metabolic bone disease (MBD) of prematurity is characterized by decreased bone mineral content or osteopenia relative to the gestational or postnatal age that is observed during the early postnatal weeks. This condition develops as the postnatal bone mineralization lags behind the high rates of intrauterine bone mineral accrual enabled by active transport across the placenta. This rich amount of mineral accrual during the 3rd trimester is not available to the prematurely born infant.[10] This low mineral state predisposes preterm infants, particularly those who receive breastmilk without any fortifier, inappropriate preterm formulae, or prolonged parenteral nutrition, to osteopenia. Other factors that compound the problem are critical illness, mechanical ventilation, immobilization, and the use of steroids or ionotropic support, furosemide, aminoglycosides, and methyl xanthine.

The primary pathophysiologic mechanism may be P depletion, though mixed P and Ca deficiency is more common.

Clinical Features

The clinical features can range from being asymptomatic to respiratory insufficiency or failure to wean from a ventilator (poor chest wall compliance). Other associated features include decreased linear growth with sustained head growth, hypotonia, and pain on handling due to pathologic fractures. Signs of rickets (metaphyseal dysplasia and skeletal deformities such as frontal bossing; enlarged anterior fontanel and widened cranial sutures; and craniotabes) usually become evident after 6 weeks postnatal age or by term-corrected gestational age.

Diagnosis

Serum Ca cannot be solely utilized for identifying the newborn at risk of MBD as serum Ca levels can be low to normal or high. A combination of low serum P (<5.6 mg/dL) and elevated ALP (>900 IU/L where the laboratory normal for adults is <25–125 IU/L) is a fairly sensitive and specific tool to identify infants at risk of osteopenia. Other biochemical features include a low or normal serum PTH, normal 25OHD, and elevated 1,25$(OH)_2$D. The characteristic radiological changes are not visible before 30–40% loss in bone mineralization occurs. Radiographic signs include widening of epiphyseal growth plates; cupping, fraying, and rarefaction of the metaphyses; subperiosteal new bone formation; osteopenia, particularly of the skull, spine, scapula, and ribs; and sometimes pathological fractures.

Management

The goal of management is to achieve normal blood mineral homeostasis and simulate the intrauterine bone mineral accretion rates. It is essentially achieved by the use of mineral-fortified human milk or "premature" formulae with an appropriate proportion of Ca and P to mineralize the growing bones. P supplementation promotes bone mineralization, but serum Ca may fall to subnormal levels ("hungry bones" syndrome) unless supplemental Ca is also provided. Therefore, both Ca and P intake of 150–220 mg/kg/day and 75–140 mg/kg/day respectively is recommended to optimize the Ca-to-P ratio of 1.5–2. Periodic monitoring of linear growth and serum phosphorus, ALP, and urinary Ca/creatinine is necessary to assess the therapeutic response and screen for complications.

PHOSPHATE

A normal serum level of P is essential for cellular functions such as intracellular signaling, energy metabolism as well skeletal mineralization. Dietary P is absorbed from the duodenum and jejunum through the action of 1,25$(OH)_2$D. PTH, by causing inhibition of its reabsorption in the proximal renal tubules is the key physiological regulator of P. Fibroblast growth factor (FGF-23), a protein produced by osteocytes, also regulates serum P levels by inhibiting P reabsorption in the proximal renal tubule. It also suppresses the renal production of 1,25$(OH)_2$D by inhibiting the enzyme 1α-hydroxylase and thus reducing intestinal P absorption.

Serum P concentration varies according to the time of day and dietary intake, and samples should be drawn in the morning in a fasting state. Phosphorus levels are higher in infants, ranging 4.8–7.4 mg/dL up to the age of 3 months, 4.5–5.8 mg/dL from 1 to 2 years, 3.5–5.5 mg/dL in mid-childhood, and reaching the adult range of 2.5–4.5 mg/dL by late adolescence. Changes in serum P levels are seldom symptomatic per se and are usually detected during evaluation of disorders in which they constitute part of metabolic abnormalities.

HYPOPHOSPHATEMIA

Transient hypophosphatemia is common in critically ill children and those with severe malnutrition. This is due to a combination of factors that lead to shift of P from extracellular to intracellular space. These include glucose infusion, insulin infusion, refeeding syndrome, mechanical ventilation, and respiratory alkalosis. The clinical features attributable to hypophosphatemia in this situation are nonspecific and usually difficult to differentiate from those of the primary illness.

Chronic hypophosphatemia, on the other hand, is usually due to increased renal P wasting secondary to either an FGF23-induced mechanism, primary/secondary hyperparathyroidism, or a primary renal tubular defect.[11] Important conditions with hypophosphatemia include caused by disorders of vitamin D metabolism such as vitamin D dependent rickets (VDDR) types 1 and 2, X-linked hypophosphatemic (XLR), and other inherited forms of hypophosphatemic rickets, renal tubular transport defects like proximal RTA (Fanconi syndrome) (*see* Chapter 16.6).

Management

Treatment essentially requires P supplementation as per the etiology. Oral P supplements along with 1,25$(OH)_2$D (calcitriol) or 1α(OH)D (alfacalcidol) are used for the management of hereditary hypophosphatemic rickets associated with raised serum FGF-23 levels. Burosumab, an FGF23-neutralizing antibody (administered fortnightly by subcutaneous injection), is approved by the Food and Drug Administration (FDA) for the management of XLR in children older than 1 year of age.[12]

HYPERPHOSPHATEMIA

The most frequent cause of hyperphosphatemia is impaired renal excretory functions due to an underlying renal disease or a critical illness. Other causes include acute cell lysis (tumor lysis, rhabdomyolysis, and hemolysis) magnesium deficiency (impairs PTH release), and hypoparathyroidism. A newborn receiving cow milk-based diet on the background of immature parathyroid function can also develop hyperphosphatemia due to a high-dietary load. Acute hyperphosphatemia has no specific features. However, high-serum P can interfere with absorption of other minerals especially Ca due to suppression of PTH and lead to hypocalcemia which can be symptomatic, especially in young infants. Chronic hyperphosphatemia may result in ectopic soft-tissue calcifications. They can present with symptomatic or asymptomatic late onset of hypocalcemia.

Management

Management essentially involves treatment of underlying disorders. Hyperphosphatemia can be managed with dietary P restriction, use of P binders, and in case of renal disease, dialysis. Oral Ca carbonate can be used as a P-binding agent. In children with chronic kidney disease, $1,25(OH)_2D$ or its analog is supplemented to maximize intestinal Ca absorption and prevent renal osteodystrophy.

CONCLUSION

A comprehensive understanding of mineral metabolism and function is vital for accurately diagnosing and effectively managing related disorders. Early recognition and prompt treatment are key to preventing severe complications. Continuous research into molecular mechanisms and novel treatments holds the potential to enhance patient care and optimize long-term outcomes.

REFERENCES

1. Root AW, Levine MA. Disorders of mineral metabolism. Abnormalities of mineral homeostasis in the newborn, infant, child and adolescent. In: Sperling MA, Majzoub JA, Menon RK, Stratakis CA (Eds). Sperling Pediatric Endocrinology, 5th edition. Philadelphia: Elsevier; 2020. pp. 705-813.
2. Shaw NJ. A Practical Approach to Hypocalcaemia in Children. In: Allgrove J, Shaw NJ (Eds). Calcium and Bone Disorders in Children and Adolescents, 2nd edition. Basel: Karger Publishers; 2015. pp. 123-34.
3. ICMR-NIN Expert Committee. (2024). Dietary Guidelines for Indians-2024. [online] Available from https://main.icmr.nic.in/sites/default/files/upload_documents/DGI_07th_May_2024_fin.pdf. [Last accessed Dec., 2024].
4. Chinoy A, Mughal Z, Padidela R. Hypocalcemia, hypercalcemia and disorders of parathyroid gland. In: Desai M, Menon PSN, Bhatia V, Seth A (Eds). Pediatric Endocrine Disorders, 4th edition. Telangana, India: University Press; 2022. pp. 473-85.
5. Munns CF, Shaw N, Kiely M, Specker BL, Thatcher TD, Ozono K, et al. Global consensus recommendations on prevention and management of nutritional rickets. J Clin Endocrinol Metab. 2016;101(2):394-415.
6. Khan AA, Bilezikian JP, Brandi ML, Clarke BL, Gittoes NJ, Pasieka JL, et al. Evaluation and management of hypoparathyroidism: Summary Statement and Guidelines from the Second International Workshop. J Bone Miner Res. 2022;37(12):2568-85.
7. Davies JH. Approach to the child with hypercalcaemia. Endocr Dev. 2015;28:101-18.
8. Stokes VJ, Nielsen MF, Hannan FM, Thakker RV. Hypercalcemic disorders in children. J Bone Miner Res. 2017;32(11):2157-70.
9. Gulcan-Kersin S, Kirkgoz T, Eltan M, Rzayev T, Ata P, Bilgen H, et al. Cinacalcet as a first-line treatment in neonatal severe hyperparathyroidism secondary to calcium sensing receptor (CaSR) mutation. Horm Res Paediatr. 2020;93(5):313-21.
10. Chinoy A, Mughal MZ, Padidela R. Metabolic bone disease of prematurity: causes, recognition, prevention, treatment and long-term consequences. Arch Dis Child Fetal Neonatal Ed. 2019;104(5):F560-6.
11. Haffner D, Emma F, Eastwood DM, Duplan MB, Bacchetta J, Schnabel D, et al. Clinical practice recommendations for the diagnosis and management of X-linked hypophosphataemia. Nat Rev Nephrol. 2019;15(7):435-55.
12. Mughal MZ, Baroncelli GI, de Lucas-Collantes C, Linglart A, Magnolato A, Raimann A, et al. Burosumab for X-linked hypophosphatemia in children and adolescents: Opinion based on early experience in seven European countries. Front Endocrinol (Lausanne). 2023;13:1034580.

16.6 Metabolic Rickets and Disorders of Bone Fragility

Siddhnath Sudhanshu

INTRODUCTION

The role of the skeletal system as an important metabolic organ for bone and mineral metabolism, vital for maintaining serum calcium within a narrow range, is highlighted in Chapter 16.5. The traditional role of the skeleton in maintaining mechanical stability of the body and aiding locomotion is more easily appreciable.

Bone consists of an organic matrix (osteoid) made up of a ground substance (mostly chondroitin sulfate and osteocalcin) and collagen fibrils, and an inorganic mineral compound the deposition of which results in further hardening of the skeleton. The mineral is calcium hydroxyapatite, a salt of calcium, phosphorus, and hydroxyl ions. Osteoblast cells are responsible for bone formation; osteocytes are the mature bone cells and osteoclasts bring about bone resorption to restore serum calcium as well as to enable bone remodeling. Laying down of mineral is brought about via the action of the hormone calcitriol (the active form of vitamin D) [1,25-dihydroxycholecalciferol (1,25(OH)$_2$D) which is synthesized by the action of 1α-hydroxylase on 25-hydroxycholecalciferol (25(OH)D)], and resorption is brought about via parathyroid hormone (PTH).

Defect in mineralization results in soft bones which have poor strength and are prone to bend on weight bearing. This state of soft bones with deformity due to bending is known as rickets. Such bones with inadequate mineralization and poor strength are fragile and are prone to fracture as well. Defect in organic matrix formation and development, as in osteogenesis imperfecta, leads to severe primary bone fragility. Further, demineralization and osteoporosis secondary to glucocorticoids, systemic inflammatory disorders, and/or hyperparathyroidism also make the bones fragile and prone to fractures. Disorders of bone mineralization and bone strength are discussed in this chapter.

RICKETS

EPIDEMIOLOGY

Nutritional rickets is the most common cause of rickets in India and worldwide. Vitamin D deficiency (25(OH)D <30 nmol/L or <12 ng/mL) is highly prevalent (63–90%) in India and is thought to be the most common cause of nutritional rickets. The largest study from India reported the prevalence of rickets as 7.6%. The cause of low incidence of rickets in developed countries is primarily the food (milk) fortification with vitamin D. The current prevalence rate in the USA and Europe is reported to be 2.9–27 per 100,000 individuals.[1,2]

ETIOPATHOGENESIS

Inadequate mineralization of the metaphyseal cartilage and osteoid matrix is central to the pathophysiology of rickets. Poor mineralization results in soft bones and the resultant soft bones bend and produce the hallmark deformities such as genu varum (bow legs) and genu valgum (knock knees). Areas of excess osteoid formation manifest as swollen and widened wrist, double malleoli at the ankle joints, and prominent costochondral junctions (rachitic rosary). Harrison's sulcus identified as retraction of the chest wall at the sites of insertion of the diaphragm occurs due to the constant pull of the strong muscle insertions on soft bones. The biochemical hallmarks of rickets are elevated serum alkaline phosphatase (ALP), low serum phosphorus, and in severe cases (especially in infancy and adolescence), low serum calcium. The causes of poor bone mineralization and rickets have been broadly categorized as nutritional and non-nutritional.

NUTRITIONAL RICKETS

Nutritional deficiency of calcium and vitamin D is the most common etiology for poor bone mineralization. Additionally, rise in PTH due to calcium and vitamin D deficiencies causes demineralization which results in further weakening and softening of bones and make them more fragile and prone to fracture as well. Nutritional deficiency of phosphorus leading to rickets is found only in special circumstances, such as prematurity or parenteral nutrition. In India, vitamin D deficiency is particularly encountered in the neonate or infant, due to poor maternal stores. Thereafter, it is prominent during adolescence, especially in girls, who cannot take advantage of the sunshine due to modest clothing and poor outdoor activity. Of note is the fact that dietary sources of vitamin D are fatty fish and organ meats, items not commonly consumed in vast regions of India. In toddlers and mid-childhood (and also in older age groups), dietary calcium deficiency plays a predominant role, along with vitamin D deficiency.[3] Nutritional rickets is discussed in detail in the chapter on fat soluble vitamins.

NON-NUTRITIONAL RICKETS

Among non-nutritional causes, vitamin D metabolism/action disorders known as vitamin D-dependent rickets (VDDR; VDDR-1A and B due to reduced 1-α or 25-hydroxylase enzyme resulting in inadequate active vitamin D/calcitriol, VDDR-2A and B due to reduced/absent vitamin D receptors causing the end-organ resistance to calcitriol, and VDDR-3 due to enhanced clearance of vitamin D and active vitamin D from the body); hypophosphatemic rickets (X-linked and autosomal inherited disorders causing increased loss of phosphorus from the kidneys) and renal tubular acidosis (RTA) are common causes of poor bone mineralization and development of rickets.[4-6] When vitamin D and calcium supplementations have been given in adequate doses for 12 weeks without onset of radiological healing or improvement in serum ALP, non-nutritional or resistant rickets should be suspected. Non-nutritional rickets may be categorized into calcium deficiency or phosphorus deficiency rickets for ease of differential diagnosis and diagnostic workup **(Table 16.6.1)**.

CLINICAL FEATURES

The deformities due to soft and weak bones like widened wrist, genu varum and valgum, rachitic rosary, Harrison's sulcus, and infants with soft skull in infants are common to all forms of rickets. However, there are clinical features which may provide clues toward a specific non-nutritional rickets and suggest early and specific diagnostic workup. Such clues include alopecia (in vitamin D-dependent rickets type 2), features of malabsorption such as anemia, abdominal pain, diarrhea (celiac disease), hypokalemia, nephrocalcinosis, polyuria (in distal RTA), dense bones (hypophosphatemic rickets), or glycosuria and proteinuria (in proximal RTA), among others **(Figs. 16.6.1A to E)**.

TABLE 16.6.1: Causes of non-nutritional rickets.

Calcipenic rickets	*Phosphopenic rickets*
Vitamin D/calcium deficiency	Prematurity (calcium plus phosphorus deficiency)
Distal renal tubular acidosis	Fanconi syndrome (proximal renal tubular acidosis)
1-α-hydroxylase defect: VDDR-1A 25-hydroxylase defect: VDDR-1B	Hypophosphatemic rickets (X-linked/AD/AR) (mutations in *PHEX*, *FGF-23*, *DMP1*, or *ENPP1* genes)
Calcitriol receptor defect: VDDR-2	Hypophosphatemic rickets with hypercalciuria (*SLC34A3* gene mutation)
Activating mutation in vitamin D degrading enzyme *(CYP3A4)*: VDDR-3	McCune–Albright syndrome-associated hypophosphatemic rickets
Chronic renal failure	Tumor-induced (mesenchymal tumor and epidermal nevus)
Malabsorption disorders	
Anticonvulsant-induced vitamin D deficiency and rickets	

(AD: autosomal dominant; AR: autosomal recessive)

DIFFERENTIAL DIAGNOSIS

Clinical history taking usually reveals the underlying nutritional deficit as the cause of nutritional rickets. The cases of rickets initially suspected to have nutritional rickets but having not responded to 12 weeks of vitamin D and calcium treatment are suspected to have non-nutritional cause of rickets. Broadly the clinical phenotypes of non-nutritional rickets have been categorized as calcipenic or phosphopenic rickets. The common differential diagnosis of these two clinical phenotypes of rickets has been shown in **Table 16.6.1**. The two distinct entities have many overlapping clinical features but there are many differentiating clinical features as well. Typical clinical differentiating features of calcipenic versus phosphopenic rickets are highlighted in **Table 16.6.2**.

DIAGNOSIS

A case of nutritional rickets is characterized by raised ALP (the upper normal limit of ALP in pediatric age group is three times of that in adults), raised PTH (secondary hyperparathyroidism) and low phosphorus due to high PTH. In severe cases sometimes, low calcium can also be found. Routine serum 25(OH)D estimation is not needed if clinical history is suggestive of poor vitamin D status. A plain radiograph will show typical features of rickets like metaphyseal growth plate widening with metaphyseal cupping and fraying. In addition, radiological features of secondary hyperparathyroidism are also seen like lucent bones with thin cortex due to osteopenia, Looser's zones as well as osteitis fibrosa cystica in severe cases. When a suspected case of nutritional rickets does not show improvement after vitamin D and calcium treatment for 12 weeks in terms of radiological healing (a dense calcification band in the provisional zone of calcification at the metaphyseal end known as "white line of Frankel") and lowering of ALP, one must suspect and start investigation for non-nutritional/resistant rickets. Serum PTH should guide further workup. Both primary and secondary hyperparathyroidism result in increased phosphorus leak from the proximal tubule. Thus, a child with any cause of calcipenic rickets, such as malabsorption or distal RTA, due to concomitant secondary hyperparathyroidism, may appear to

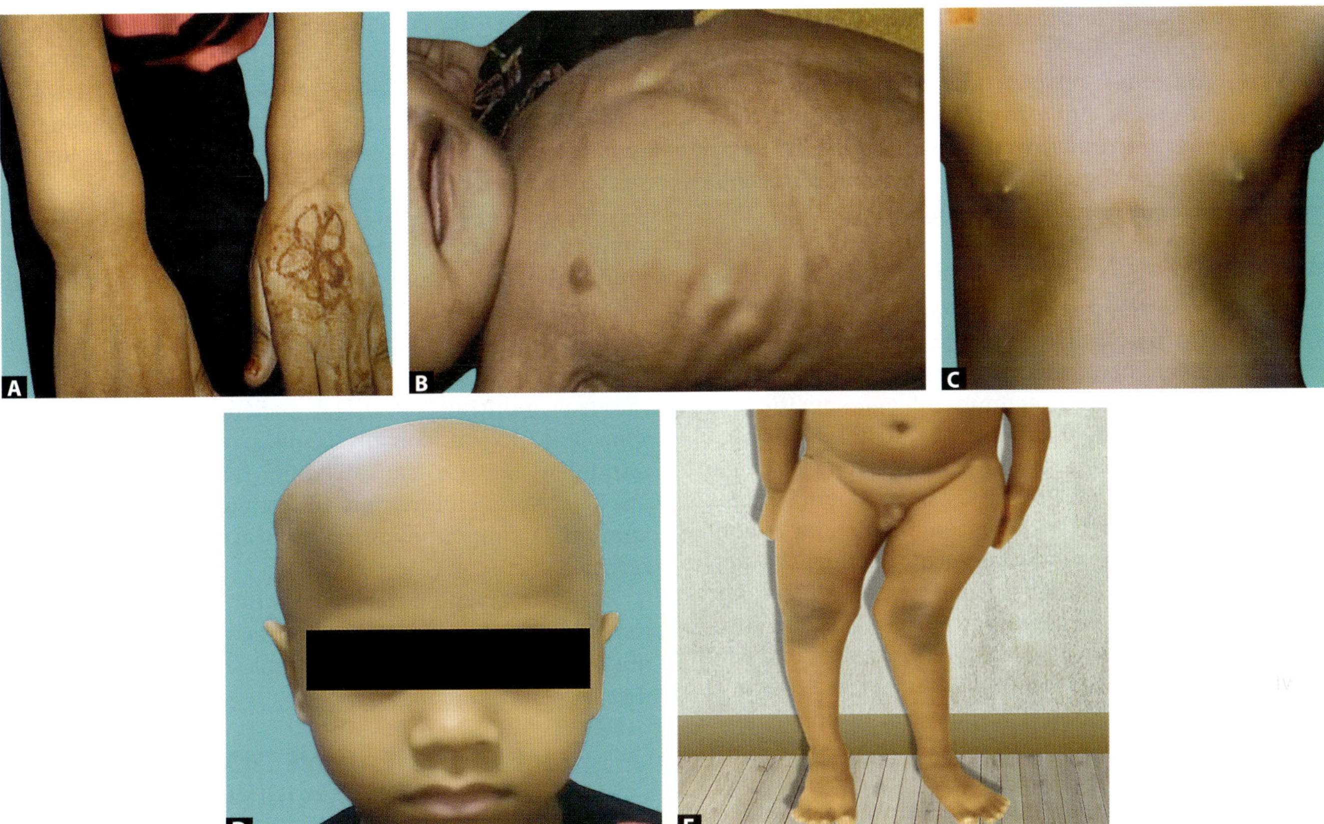

Figs. 16.6.1A to E: (A) Widened or swollen wrists; (B) Rachitic rosary (swollen costochondral junctions; (C) Harrison's sulcus (indrawing of the soft lateral chest wall); (D) Alopecia in VDDR-2; (E) Windswept deformity (genu varum in one limb and genu valgum in the other limb). *Courtesy:* Prof Vijayakumar M, Government Medical College, Kozhikode, for picture E.

TABLE 16.6.2: Features of calcipenic versus phosphopenic rickets.

Features	*Calcipenic rickets*	*Phosphopenic rickets*
Hypotonia	Present	Absent
Bone pain	Present	Absent
Tetany/seizure	Present	Absent
Dental enamel hypoplasia	Present	Absent
Dental caries	Absent	Present
Serum calcium	Low	Normal
Serum phosphorus	Low	Low
Serum alkaline phosphatase	Markedly raised	Moderately raised
Parathyroid hormone	Raised	Normal/minimally raised
Plain radiology	Lucent bone, Looser's zone, and osteitis fibrosa cystica	Dense bone

have hypophosphatemic rickets or proximal RTA. Serum PTH is a useful investigation at this juncture, being only marginally elevated in hypophosphatemic rickets and significantly raised in calcipenic rickets.

Cases with high PTH should be investigated for the etiologies mentioned in **Table 16.6.1**. Tests for malabsorption include erythrocyte sedimentation rate, anti-endomyseal or tissue transglutaminase antibodies, D-xylose test, and endoscopic duodenal biopsy. Distal RTA is characterized by hypokalemia, polyuria, nephrocalcinosis, and normal anion gap hyperchloremic metabolic acidosis, with concurrent urinary pH >5.5. A case of proximal RTA would show acidic urine pH and bicarbonaturia, along with, in Fanconi syndrome, glycosuria, aminoaciduria, uric aciduria, and phosphaturia with hypophosphatemia. Proximal RTA is confirmed by bicarbonate loading test.

If these are negative, serum 25(OH)D and $1,25(OH)_2D$ (calcitriol) can throw light on 1α-hydroxylase defect (VDDR-1) and calcitriol receptor defect (VDDR-2). Here, it is important to note that the estimation of calcitriol is most reliable if it is measured by liquid chromatography mass spectrometry (LCMS) method.

Normal to low PTH type resistant rickets should be worked up for phosphate clearance (phosphate clearance/creatinine clearance) and tubular maximum reabsorption of phosphate/glomerular filtration rate measurement. A renal phosphate leak with low/normal PTH level is confirmative of hypophosphatemic rickets.

Plain radiology reveals coarse trabecular pattern in RTA, and dense bone in hypophosphatemic rickets. In other non-nutritional rickets with high PTH (except RTA), the plain radiograph will show features of secondary hyperparathyroidism similar to nutritional rickets.

MANAGEMENT

Nutritional rickets is treated with vitamin D (cholecalciferol) and calcium. The Indian Academy of Pediatrics revised (2021) guidelines on prevention and treatment of vitamin D deficiency and rickets recommend age-specific doses of cholecalciferol for treatment of nutritional rickets as shown in **Table 16.6.3**. Along with vitamin D, calcium supplementation of 50–75 mg/kg/day elemental calcium (not exceeding 500 mg/day) is recommended for 3 months and thereafter daily requirement of calcium should be provided through diet rich in calcium such as dairy products, green leafy vegetables, ragi, and pulses. The response to treatment is documented by radiological healing in the form of white line of calcification (to be assessed at 4 weeks and 12 weeks) and biochemical response in normalization of ALP (at 12 weeks). Inadequate or no response by 12 weeks suggests the possibility of non-nutritional rickets.[3]

The treatment of non-nutritional rickets is planned as per the specific etiology. Renal tubular acidosis is treated with alkali in daily divided doses, the distal variety requires 2–8 mEq/kg/day and proximal RTA requires a higher dose of 6–18 mEq/kg/day of sodium bicarbonate or alkali. In general, the alkali dose requirement (per kg body weight) is higher at younger age and less in older children and young people. Citrate as the source of alkali is useful in distal RTA, as it counterbalances hypocitraturia in distal RTA and reduces the risk of nephrocalcinosis and nephrolithiasis. Potassium replenishment is required in the doses of 1–4 mEq/kg/day. Proximal RTA, when it is a part of Fanconi syndrome, is also associated with phosphaturia and hypophosphatemia. Phosphate replacement in such cases is needed in divided doses and slowly built-up doses of 30–50 mg/kg/day. Maintenance cholecalciferol supplementation should be continued in all non-nutritional cases of rickets. Investigation and treatment of the primary disease, if any, causing RTA, must be performed.[4]

Vitamin D-dependent rickets type 1 is treated with calcitriol in physiological or minimally higher doses of 20–70 ng/kg/day and VDRR-2 with a higher dose of calcitriol (2–5 times higher than physiological doses) and/or with intravenous calcium. Prevention of hypocalcemic tetany and seizures is a priority in VDDR-2.[5]

Hypophosphatemic rickets requires phosphorus supplementation in divided doses of 30–50 mg/kg/day to produce healing of bone and calcitriol supplementation with routine monitoring for PTH and hypercalciuria.[6]

Enzyme-inducing anticonvulsants (phenobarbitone, phenytoin, etc.) are known to cause vitamin D deficit and rickets by inducing 25(OH)D degradation, but some nonenzyme-inducing anticonvulsants like sodium valproate have also been shown to cause vitamin D deficiency and rickets. Therefore, children on anticonvulsants should be on vitamin D supplementation to prevent development of rickets.[7]

Deformities often normalize with years of growth and remodeling, in all etiologies of rickets. Therefore, one need not rush for corrective osteotomy unless deformities come in the way of locomotion.

METABOLIC BONE DISEASE OF PREMATURITY

The preterm baby is deprived of the large supply of calcium normally accrued during the 3rd trimester of pregnancy via active transport across the placenta. Breastmilk is not adequate to supply similar amounts of calcium and phosphorus. The resulting bone disease presents with fractures upon minimal handling and X-ray picture showing lucent bones.

It can be prevented by using commercially available human milk fortifiers providing the required 200 mg/kg/day of calcium and 100 mg/kg/day of phosphorus along with maintenance vitamin D.

DISORDERS OF INCREASED BONE FRAGILITY

Fractures are common in children, but minimal trauma fractures (such as those from standing height) must alert the pediatrician to an abnormality. "Clinically significant fracture" includes the presence of any vertebral

TABLE 16.6.3: Cholecalciferol doses (IU) for management of nutritional rickets in children.

Age	*Daily dose for 12 weeks*	*Alternative intermittent dose regimen (if compliance is not good)*	*Maintenance dose (daily)*
<6 months	2,000	Not recommended	400
6–12 months	2,000	Equivalent of 2,000 IU/day may be given on a monthly or weekly basis	400
>12 months	3,000	60,000 IU fortnightly (after every 2 weeks) × 5 doses	600

(IU: international units)

crush fracture, or at least two long bone fractures by the age of 10 years or three long bone fractures by the age of 19 years.

The prototype of primary disorder of bone fragility in children is osteogenesis imperfecta (OI), the clinical syndrome, which is known to occur from mutations of 20 distinct genes identified as of now.[8] However, >85% of the cases occur due to mutations in *COL1A1* and *COL1A2* genes and are classified as OI type I to IV. Mutation in these genes may cause quantitative as well as qualitative defect in collagen, leading to weak and fragile bone development. Type II OI is the most severe form and is lethal in perinatal age whereas, in alive children, type III is the most severe form with progressive course. Type I has mild clinical course with blue sclera and hearing loss and type II has mild to moderate clinical course with normal sclera. Other classified variants of OI have varied clinical associations and course. Some of them may have specific clinical and radiological clues toward a specific type of OI, but genetic testing is often needed for a final diagnosis. Low BMD (Z-score less than –2 SDS) is a characteristic feature of OI.[9] A multidisciplinary approach is required for the management of OI, which includes regular bisphosphonate (antiresorptive) therapy till puberty before weaning off the dose and frequency of bisphosphonate administration; regular physiotherapy and occupational therapy; and deformity correction and prevention by skilled pediatric orthopedician.

However, conditions of secondary bone fragility disorders are much more common than primary bone fragility disorders. A common condition in this category encountered by pediatricians is glucocorticoid-induced osteoporosis (GIO). Since pharmacological doses of glucocorticoids are used in children for diverse pediatric disorders, pediatricians must be aware of the side effects of systemic glucocorticoid therapy and especially on the bone health and thus, they must take the precautions needed to prevent or minimize GIO. These precautions include adequate calcium, protein, and vitamin D supplementation; institution of gonadal steroids in a timely manner in adolescents to induce and maintain puberty, in whom pubertal delay has occurred due to the underlying systemic disease; avoiding immobilization and encouraging regular and appropriate weight-bearing exercise. Needless to say, the minimum effective dose of glucocorticoid should be used for the minimum required duration to minimize bone fragility as well as other side effects of systemic glucocorticoid therapy.[10] Other conditions of secondary bone fragility include inflammatory bowel disease, other autoimmune disorders, immobilization, and cerebral palsy, among others.

A more detailed discussion on OI and other primary bone fragility disorders (fibrous dysplasia and osteopetrosis), as well as all the conditions causing secondary bone fragility disorders, is beyond the scope of this book.

CONCLUSION

Nutritional rickets is the most common cause of rickets worldwide and can be successfully prevented and managed with timely preventive and therapeutic measures. Suspecting and identifying the non-nutritional rickets is equally vital for timely commencement of specific and appropriate therapeutic interventions. Bone fragility disorders, most commonly OI as primary and GIO as secondary causes of bone fragility, need to be identified and intervened early to prevent life-long morbidity.

REFERENCES

1. Gentile C, Chiarelli F. Rickets in Children: An Update. Biomedicines. 2021;9(7):738.
2. Khadilkar A, Kajale N, Oza C, Oke R, Gondhalekar K, Patwardhan V, et al. Vitamin D status and determinants in Indian children and adolescents: a multicentre study. Sci Rep. 2022;12(1):16790.
3. Gupta P, Dabas A, Seth A, Bhatia VL, Khadgawat R, Kumar P, et al. Indian Academy of Pediatrics Revised (2021) Guidelines on Prevention and Treatment of Vitamin D Deficiency and Rickets. Indian Pediatr. 2022;59(2):142-58.
4. Wagner CA, Unwin R, Lopez-Garcia SC, Kleta R, Bockenhauer D, Walsh S. The pathophysiology of distal renal tubular acidosis. Nat Rev Nephrol. 2023;19(6):384-400.
5. Miller WL. Genetic disorders of vitamin D biosynthesis and degradation. J Steroid Biochem Mol Biol. 2017;165(Pt A):101-8.
6. Ackah SA, Imel EA. Approach to Hypophosphatemic Rickets. J Clin Endocrinol Metab. 2022;108(1):209-20.
7. Holick MF, Binkley NC, Bischoff-Ferrari HA, Gordon CM, Hanley DA, Heaney RP, et al.; Endocrine Society. Evaluation, treatment, and prevention of vitamin D deficiency: an Endocrine Society clinical practice guideline. J Clin Endocrinol Metab. 2011;96(7):1911-30.
8. Panzaru MC, Florea A, Caba L, Gorduza EV. Classification of osteogenesis imperfecta: Importance of prophylaxis and genetic counseling. World J Clin Cases. 2023;11(12):2604-20.
9. Khadilkar AV, Sanwalka NJ, Chiplonkar SA, Khadilkar V, Mughal MZ. Normative data and percentile curves for Dual Energy X-ray Absorptiometry in healthy Indian girls and boys aged 5-17 years. Bone. 2011;48(4):810-9.
10. Bell JM, Shields MD, Watters J, Hamilton A, Beringer T, Elliott M, et al. Interventions to prevent and treat corticosteroid-induced osteoporosis and prevent osteoporotic fractures in Duchenne muscular dystrophy. Cochrane Database Syst Rev. 2017;1(1):CD010899.

16.7 Disorders of Adrenal Glands

Preeti Dabadghao, Sapna Nayak

INTRODUCTION

The adrenal or suprarenal glands are small, triangular-shaped glands located on the superomedial aspect of both kidneys. Each adrenal gland is made up of two distinct parts—(1) the cortex and the (2) medulla, having different embryonic origins. The adrenal cortex is mesenchymal in origin, developing from the adrenogenital primordium, while the medulla is neuroectodermal in origin. The cortex in turn is comprised of three distinct anatomical areas:

- Outer *zona glomerulosa* secretes mineralocorticoids
- Middle *zona fasciculata* produces glucocorticoids
- Inner *zona reticularis* secretes androgens

The adrenocortical hormones are lipophilic steroid hormones and are crucial for maintenance of fluid and electrolyte balance (mineralocorticoids), intermediary metabolism (glucocorticoids), and sexual development (androgens).

Steroidogenesis (synthesis of steroid hormones) involves conversion of cholesterol to steroid hormones through a series of intermediate metabolites catalyzed by the sequential action of six enzymes, a group of P450 enzymes. The hypothalamic-pituitary-adrenal (HPA) axis is responsible for the maintenance of normal cortisol levels. This involves close interaction of three hormones:

1. *Corticotropin-releasing hormone (CRH)* produced by the hypothalamus
2. *Adrenocorticotropic hormone (ACTH)* produced by the anterior pituitary
3. *Cortisol* secreted by the adrenals

The CRH stimulates the release of ACTH, which in turn drives the synthesis and secretion of cortisol from the adrenal gland. The cortisol thus released has a negative feedback effect on the secretion of CRH and the ACTH. The secretion of aldosterone is independent of the HPA axis and is regulated by the renin-angiotensin-aldosterone system (RAAS), which is activated by low blood volume or blood pressure or high potassium levels.

Adrenal androgen secretion occurs with the onset of adrenarche and excess androgen secretion can be driven by ACTH in pathological states.

The adrenal medulla secretes the catecholamines—epinephrine, norepinephrine, and dopamine.

ADRENAL INSUFFICIENCY

Adrenal insufficiency (AI) is a condition caused by the lack of adrenal cortical steroids, glucocorticoids with or without mineralocorticoid deficiency. It can be classified as *primary adrenal insufficiency (PAI),* due to abnormal development or destruction of adrenal gland or defects in steroid synthesis pathway and *central adrenal insufficiency,* due to impaired production or release of ACTH from the pituitary gland *(secondary AI)* or CRH from the hypothalamus *(tertiary AI).*

Primary adrenal insufficiency can be congenital related to specific gene abnormality or acquired due to infection, infiltration, or hemorrhage in the adrenal glands. In these cases, there is an increase in ACTH and CRH due to loss of negative feedback of cortisol on the pituitary and hypothalamus, respectively. Compared to primary, secondary form of AI is much more common. Central AI such as PAI can be congenital due to hypothalamic and pituitary defects (holoprosencephaly and septo-optic dysplasia) or secondary to acquired organic lesions (tumor, surgery, irradiation, infections, etc.) or more commonly due to HPA axis suppression following prolonged exogenous steroid intake. The common causes of adrenal cortical insufficiency are given in **Box 16.7.1**. In a large pediatric series, congenital adrenal hyperplasia (CAH) accounted for over 70% of cases of PAI, autoimmune being the second most common cause.[1]

BOX 16.7.1: Etiology of adrenal insufficiency.

Primary

Congenital

Congenital adrenal hyperplasia (CAH):
- 21α-hydroxylase deficiency
- 11β-hydroxylase deficiency
- 3β-hydroxysteroid dehydrogenase deficiency
- *Other rare CAH forms due to mutations in:*
  - *CYP17A1*
  - *CYP11B1*
  - *POR* (P450 oxidoreductase)
  - *CYP11A1*/steroidogenic acute regulatory protein
- Smith–Lemli–Opitz syndrome

Congenital adrenal hypoplasia: NR0B1 mutations

Triple-A or Allgrove syndrome

ACTH resistance/familial isolated glucocorticoid deficiency

Contd...

Contd...

Glucocorticoid resistance

Metabolic diseases:
- Adrenoleukodystrophy
- Zellweger syndrome
- Wolman disease

Mitochondrial diseases: Kearns–Sayre syndrome

Acquired

Autoimmune adrenalitis:
- Isolated
- *Polyglandular syndromes:* Types I, II, and IV

Hemorrhage and infarction:
- Trauma
- Waterhouse–Friderichsen syndrome

Drugs:
- Aminoglutethimide
- Mitotane
- Ketoconazole
- Metyrapone

Infections:
- *Viral:* HIV and cytomegalovirus
- *Fungal:* Coccidioidomycosis and histoplasmosis
- *Mycobacterial:* Tuberculosis

Infiltration:
- Histiocytosis
- Amyloidosis
- Sarcoidosis
- Neoplasm

Secondary

Hypothalamus

Congenital:
- Septo-optic dysplasia (*HESX1*)
- CRH deficiency
- Pallister–Hall syndrome

Acquired:
- Steroid withdrawal after prolonged administration
- Inflammatory disorders
- Trauma
- Radiation therapy
- Surgery
- Tumors

Infiltrative disease: Sarcoidosis and histiocytosis X

Pituitary

Congenital:
- Aplasia/hypoplasia
- Multiple anterior pituitary hormone deficiencies
- Isolated ACTH deficiency

Acquired:
- Steroid withdrawal after prolonged administration
- Trauma
- *Tumors:* Craniopharyngioma
- Radiation therapy
- Lymphocytic hypophysitis
- Hemochromatosis

(ACTH: adrenocorticotropic hormone; CRH: corticotropin-releasing hormone; HIV: human immunodeficiency virus)

Clinical Features

Clinical features of AI depend on the severity, the onset (acute or chronic), and the etiology (primary or secondary) of the disease. Early onset (in neonatal or infantile) period may point toward a congenital etiology, while acquired causes have variable age of onset.

The symptoms of chronic AI are nonspecific and include fatigue, muscle weakness, dizziness, nausea, vomiting, loss of appetite, loss of weight or poor weight gain, and recurrent abdominal pain. As a result, the diagnosis may be delayed; a median delay of 2.3–3 years has been reported between the onset of symptoms and diagnosis. If unrecognized, AI may present with acute life-threatening cardiovascular collapse (acute adrenal crisis). Acute AI may be triggered by infection, trauma, or abrupt cessation of steroid replacement in children on long-term replacement therapy. Children with acute AI generally present with acute dehydration, hypotension, hypoglycemia, or altered mental status.

Additionally, PAI may have hyperpigmentation, generalized or localized to knuckles, palmar creases, axillae, joints, nipples, umbilicus, genitalia, recent scars, or mucosal surfaces such as lips and tongue **(Figs. 16.7.1A and B)**. Enhanced ACTH synthesis due to loss of feedback inhibition on the pituitary is accompanied with the elevation of its byproducts, proopiomelanocortin (POMC) and melanocyte-stimulating hormone (MSH), causing the hyperpigmentation. Patients with aldosterone deficiency may exhibit salt craving.

On the other hand, central AI may have associated symptoms of raised intracranial pressure like headache, seizures, projectile vomiting, and visual disturbances. Presence of these features or previous history of cranial surgeries or irradiation point toward a central cause. These children may, in addition, exhibit signs of other pituitary hormone deficiencies, such as growth failure, delayed puberty, diabetes insipidus (polyuria and polydipsia), and secondary hypothyroidism. However, they do not have hyperpigmentation. A history of recent pharmacologic glucocorticoid therapy for a prolonged duration (usually >2 weeks) is indicative of secondary AI due to HPA axis suppression. These patients may have features of hypercortisolism such as excess weight or poor height gain.

Common Causes of Primary Adrenal Insufficiency

Congenital Adrenal Hyperplasia

It is the most common group of disorders associated with PAI. CAH is a group of inherited disorders of adrenal steroid synthesis leading to cortisol deficiency due to enzymatic defects in the steroidogenesis pathways. It is discussed in Chapter 16.8.

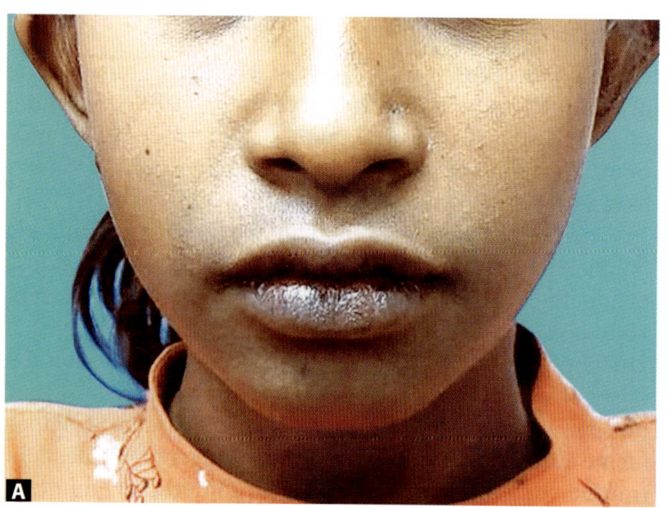

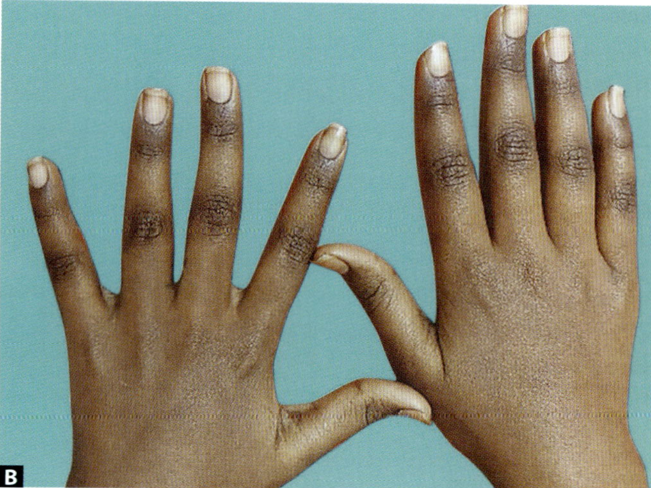

Figs. 16.7.1A and B: Hyperpigmentation of lips (A) and knuckles (B) in a 12-year-old girl with newly diagnosed primary adrenal insufficiency.

Congenital Adrenal Hypoplasia (Adrenal Hypoplasia Congenita)

This refers to abnormal development of the adrenal gland due to mutations in the genes involved in adrenal development. X-linked adrenal hypoplasia congenita (AHC) is the most common form and results from hemizygous mutations in the *NR0B1* (nuclear receptor subfamily 0, group B, member 1) gene encoding the nuclear receptor protein DAX-1 (dosage-sensitive sex reversal, adrenal hypoplasia critical region, on X chromosome, gene 1). This condition typically affects boys with early infantile or childhood onset PAI, and hypogonadotropic hypogonadism presenting at or after pubertal age. Heterozygous or less commonly homozygous mutations in *SF1* (steroidogenic factor-1) gene may cause PAI and may be associated with testicular dysgenesis in 46,XY individuals.[2]

Other rare syndromic forms of primary adrenal hypoplasia are seen in *IMAGe syndrome* (intrauterine growth retardation, metaphyseal dysplasia, adrenal hypoplasia, and genitourinary anomalies) due to mutations in *CDKN1C* (cyclin-dependent kinase inhibitor 1C) gene and *MIRAGE syndrome* (myelodysplasia, infections, restricted growth, adrenal insufficiency, genital anomalies, and enteropathy).

Disorders of Adrenocorticotropic Hormone Resistance

Allgrove syndrome (AS) or triple A syndrome: This condition is a triad of ACTH-resistant adrenal glucocorticoid insufficiency, alacrima, and achalasia cardia. Mineralocorticoid deficiency has been reported in about 15% of cases. About 60% may have progressive neurological impairment including cranial and peripheral neuropathy, sensorineural hearing loss, and autonomic dysfunction. It is caused due to autosomal recessive inheritance of mutations in *AAAS* (achalasia-addisonianism-alacrima syndrome) gene that codes for a nuclear envelope protein named ALADIN (alacrima-achalasia-adrenal insufficiency neurologic). Alacrima is present since early infancy while AI and achalasia generally develop during first two decades of life with neurological features appearing toward adolescence. Glucocorticoid with or without mineralocorticoid replacement is required in patients with AI.[3]

Familial glucocorticoid deficiency: This results in isolated glucocorticoid deficiency due to inherited unresponsiveness to ACTH. It results from mutations in the ACTH receptor, *MC2R (melanocortin receptor) gene,* its accessory protein *MRAP*, *NNT* (nicotinamide nucleotide transhydrogenase), and other newer genes. Mineralocorticoid axis is not affected.

Metabolic Disorders

X-linked adrenoleukodystrophy (ALD): ALD is the most common metabolic cause of PAI. It is inherited in an X-linked recessive manner and the defect lies in the *ABCD1* (ATP-binding cassette subfamily D member 1) gene that codes for a peroxisomal membrane protein called ALDP (adrenoleukodystrophy protein).[4] It is characterized by impaired peroxisomal β-oxidation of very long-chain fatty acids (VLCFAs), resulting in their accumulation in the plasma and various tissues including the white matter of cortex, spinal cord, and the adrenal gland. It typically affects males, who present with progressive neurological manifestations varying from cognitive decline, behavioral disturbances, seizures or peripheral neuropathy, or features of PAI or both. Different forms based on the neurological involvement and the age of onset include the *cerebral ALD* (childhood, adolescent, and adult onset), *adrenomyeloneuropathy (AMN),* and *the Addison-only type*. PAI generally occurs after onset of neurological symptoms but may occur earlier too. Depending on the primary presentation, screening for involvement of the other system should be done, even if asymptomatic. Diagnosis is established by estimation of VLCFA levels and genetic analysis for mutations in *ABCD1* gene. Magnetic resonance imaging (MRI) of the brain should be done to diagnose the neurological involvement. This condition is amenable to hematopoietic stem cell transplant (HSCT) before neurological deterioration. Females act as carriers but may manifest with AMN-like symptoms occurring in late adulthood. Cerebral form and PAI are rare in carrier females.

Other metabolic disorders causing PAI are rare and include Zellweger syndrome, Wolman disease, Niemann–Pick disease type B, and mitochondrial disorders such as Kearns–Sayre syndrome.

Infiltrative Disorders

Infections: Adrenal tuberculosis (TB), human immunodeficiency virus (HIV), and fungal infections such as histoplasmosis are important acquired causes of PAI in developing countries like India. Adrenal involvement should be considered in patients with disseminated TB. Imaging findings show enlarged adrenals with calcification.

Autoimmune Adrenalitis or Addison Disease

Autoimmune adrenalitis or Addison disease (AAD) is the most prevalent cause of PAI in developed countries. The autoantibodies are directed against the adrenal cortex and 21-hydroxylase enzyme. The condition may manifest as chronic AI or with acute adrenal crisis. AD can be isolated or a part of the APS (autoimmune polyglandular syndrome, APS-1, or APS-2). Diagnosis is by biochemical evaluation as detailed further, but ascertainment of autoimmune etiology may be difficult in isolated AAD, as there are no diagnostic criteria and commercial autoantibody assays are not easily available. Diagnosis is by exclusion of other acquired and inherited causes of PAI.

Type 1 Autoimmune Polyendocrine Syndrome

Autoimmune polyendocrinopathy-candidiasis-ectodermal dysplasia (APECED syndrome) or type 1 autoimmune polyendocrine syndrome (APS1) is a rare inherited autoimmune condition due to mutations in *AIRE* (autoimmune regulator) gene. Clinical diagnosis is established when at least two of three features that include chronic mucocutaneous candidiasis, autoimmune PAI, and hypoparathyroidism are present. PAI may develop during childhood or adolescence while candidiasis and hypoparathyroidism generally manifest earlier. Other autoimmune disorders include insulin-dependent diabetes mellitus (DM), hypothyroidism, hypergonadotropic hypogonadism, vitiligo, hepatitis, pernicious anemia, and others.[5]

Type 2 Autoimmune Polyendocrine Syndrome (APS2)/Schmidt Syndrome

Unlike APS1, type 2 autoimmune polyendocrine syndrome (APS2) occurs more frequently in adults but may occur during childhood. It is the association of autoimmune adrenalitis with thyroiditis and/or type 1 DM. Other manifestations such as pernicious anemia, vitiligo, alopecia, etc., may occur.

Other than these disorders, destruction of adrenal gland may result from adrenal hemorrhage associated with abdominal trauma, acute meningococcemia (Waterhouse–Friderichsen syndrome), or unilateral or bilateral adrenalectomy for tumors. Certain drugs such as ketoconazole and mitotane inhibit adrenal steroid synthesis and should be used with caution.

Diagnosis

Hyponatremia and hyperkalemia are characteristically seen in PAI when there is associated aldosterone deficiency. There may be associated metabolic acidosis. Hypoglycemia is common in both primary and secondary adrenal insufficiency. Hyponatremia may occur in secondary AI too.

Diagnosis of primary AI is based on an elevated plasma ACTH level (more than twofold increase above the upper limit of normal range) along with a low serum cortisol level (generally <5 μg/dL). A basal cortisol value of >18–20 μg/dL rules out AI. The cut-offs vary depending on the laboratory assay used to measure cortisol. In equivocal cases, the diagnosis is confirmed by ACTH (cosyntropin) stimulation test. Blood samples are obtained at 0 minute and 60 minutes after ACTH administration [250 μg or 15 μg/kg for infants <2 years, intravenous (IV)]. In AI, the peak cortisol level is <18 μg/dL. Mineralocorticoid deficiency is confirmed by relatively low aldosterone levels, compared to age-related cut-offs with high renin concentration or plasma renin activity (PRA), with or without hyponatremia and/or hyperkalemia.

Secondary AI is associated with low serum cortisol and low plasma ACTH levels. Confirmation of HPA axis insufficiency is done by insulin-induced hypoglycemia or CRH test. However, since insulin-induced hypoglycemia has a potential risk of hypoglycemic seizure, and CRH is not easily available, these tests are not routinely performed.

Adrenal imaging by ultrasonography or computed tomography (CT) and autoantibody testing or genetic analysis is indicated in AI to establish etiology.

In the cases of secondary AI, evaluation for other pituitary hormone deficiencies and MRI brain is recommended to look for any developmental defects or space-occupying lesion.

Management

Management of acute adrenal crisis should be immediate to restore intravascular volume with IV rapid bolus of 20 mL/kg of 0.9% saline. Dextrose bolus is given in the presence of hypoglycemia. After resolution of shock, infusion of dextrose containing isotonic saline is used at 1.2–1.5 times maintenance requirement for the next 24–48 hours.

Glucocorticoid in stress doses should be given simultaneously. Hydrocortisone is the treatment of choice because it has mineralocorticoid activity also. The recommended stress dose of hydrocortisone is 50–75 mg/m^2 IV initially, followed by 50–75 mg/m^2/day IV divided in four doses or as a continuous infusion. Once acute manifestations are controlled, oral steroid therapy with hydrocortisone 8–10 mg/m^2 in 2–3 divided doses is started. Long-acting steroids such as prednisolone or dexamethasone are not preferred in children as they have major inhibitory effect on the growth plate.

The 9-α-fluorocortisol acetate or fludrocortisone is the only available mineralocorticoid. It is given in a dose of 0.05–0.2 mg/day in children with aldosterone deficiency. Extra salt is required in early infancy for effective action of fludrocortisone (1–2 g/day). Fludrocortisone is not required in cases of secondary AI as the aldosterone pathway is independent of the HPA axis and hence unaffected. Children with established causes of permanent AI require lifelong steroid replacement and clinical and biochemical monitoring in 3–6 monthly intervals during childhood and less frequently after adolescence.[6]

Stress Doses of Glucocorticoids

Dose of steroids should be increased to 2–3 times the physiological dose in stress situations like febrile or diarrheal illness, trauma or minor surgery and is given only for the short period until that stress lasts. In major surgeries or persistent vomiting, a higher dose (50–75 mg/m^2) through parenteral route will be required. Educating the family regarding stress dosing is crucial in prevention of acute adrenal crisis that may result in death.

CESSATION OF GLUCOCORTICOID THERAPY

Exogenous steroid usage in pharmacological doses (doses above 8–10 mg/m^2/day of hydrocortisone equivalent) for prolonged duration (over 2 weeks) for various disorders suppresses CRH and ACTH secretion leading to decreased production of adrenocortical hormones and in the long-term cortical atrophy. The degree of suppression depends on the drug used, dosage, and duration of therapy. After stopping steroid therapy, recovery usually occurs in half of the patients by 6 weeks and in almost all by 6 months. ACTH stimulation test should be performed to check recovery of the adrenal glands prior to cessation of steroids. Sometimes the baseline cortisol value may be normal with low-stimulated value; in these cases, stress dose of glucocorticoids should be advised.

HYPERFUNCTION OF THE ADRENAL CORTEX

Hyperfunction of the adrenal cortex may be associated with excess production of glucocorticoids, mineralocorticoids, androgens, or estrogens. These disorders are rare in childhood. A high index of suspicion is essential for diagnosis as most of them present with nonspecific features.

GLUCOCORTICOID EXCESS STATES: CUSHING SYNDROME

Cushing syndrome (CS) is the most common disorder of adrenocortical hyperfunction. It is a generic term used to describe clinical findings caused by prolonged glucocorticoid excess.

Etiology

Increased blood cortisol levels or hypercortisolism in CS may be due to increased endogenous production or exogenous administration of glucocorticoids, which could be prescribed in various chronic illnesses such as nephrotic syndrome, acute lymphoblastic leukemia or as over-the-counter medication including creams and ointments for dermatological conditions. Exogenous CS is the most common cause of CS in all age-groups. Increased adrenal glucocorticoid production, i.e., endogenous CS, might occur in response to increased ACTH levels or represent autonomous adrenal hyperfunction **(Box 16.7.2)**.

The etiology of endogenous CS varies according to age; adrenal pathology is more likely in young children, while pituitary causes are more common after puberty. About 75–90% of cases of CS are due to pituitary cause.[7] Adrenal adenomas are pure secretors, secreting cortisol, aldosterone, or androgen while carcinomas are plurihormonal, i.e., they secrete more than one hormone.

Cushing syndrome may be secondary to an ACTH-secreting tumor of the pituitary, termed as Cushing disease (CD), often a basophilic pituitary adenoma. It leads to bilateral adrenal hyperplasia. CS due to ectopic ACTH production is extremely rare in children.

Autonomous secretion of cortisol from adrenal glands accounts for nearly 15% cases of CS. Adrenocortical carcinoma (ACC) has bimodal distribution with peak incidence at 3 years of age and the other peak in the fourth to fifth decade. In children, ACC may be associated with Li–Fraumeni or Beckwith–Wiedemann syndromes. Primary pigmented nodular adrenal hyperplasia is due to usually mutations in the *PRKAR1A* gene, regulatory α-subunit of protein kinase A. It is associated with Carney's complex, multiple endocrine neoplasia, myxomas, and lentigenes. McCune–Albright syndrome due to a somatic mutation of G-protein α-subunit may present with ACTH-independent CS due to constitutional activation of ACTH receptor. It is associated with fibrous dysplasia, *café au lait* spots, and other endocrinopathies, including precocious puberty and hyperthyroidism.

BOX 16.7.2: Etiology of Cushing syndrome in children.

ACTH-dependent:
- *Hypothalamic:* Increased CRH production by tumor
- *Pituitary:* Increased ACTH production—microadenoma and macroadenoma
- *Ectopic:* Carcinoids, neuroblastoma, Wilms tumor, and islet cell tumor

ACTH-independent:
- *Adrenal tumors:* Carcinoma and adenoma
- Primary pigmented nodular adrenal hyperplasia
- Macronodular adrenal hyperplasia
- McCune–Albright syndrome

Exogenous:
- *Glucocorticoid:* High dose or prolonged oral, parenteral, topical, inhaled
- ACTH

(ACTH: adrenocorticotropic hormone; CRH: corticotropin-releasing hormone)

Clinical Features

The classical features, such as central obesity, striae, moon facies, and buffalo hump, are uncommon in children. Growth failure coupled with weight gain is the most common feature. However, it is an extremely rare cause of childhood obesity. The fat distribution is often centripetal with accumulation on the face, neck, and abdomen. The extremities appear wasted with muscle weakness **(Figs. 16.7.2A and B)**.

Other clinical features include proximal myopathy, hypertension, delayed puberty, lethargy, bone pain, and obsessive-compulsive behavioral disorders. There may be thinning of skin with violaceous striae (frequently seen on the abdomen, buttocks, thighs, and axillae) and easy bruising. ACTH-dependent CS is characterized by hyperpigmentation. Androgen excess leads to hirsutism, acne, deepening of voice, and rarely clitoral hypertrophy.

Children with ectopic ACTH production usually present with hypertension and hypokalemic alkalosis.

Diagnosis

The diagnostic algorithm consists of biochemical evaluation followed by imaging studies as shown in **Flowchart 16.7.1**.

The first step in the diagnosis of CS is to rule out exogenous CS. A thorough history and review of prescriptions to identify prolonged intake of steroids is essential. Estimation of 8.00 AM basal serum cortisol will identify HPA axis suppression after prolonged steroid intake. Serum cortisol is typically undetectable with an unstimulated response on ACTH stimulation. These patients would require replacement of steroids in physiological doses until the recovery of HPA axis is documented. Once exogenous CS is ruled out, the further steps are directed toward documentation of autonomous

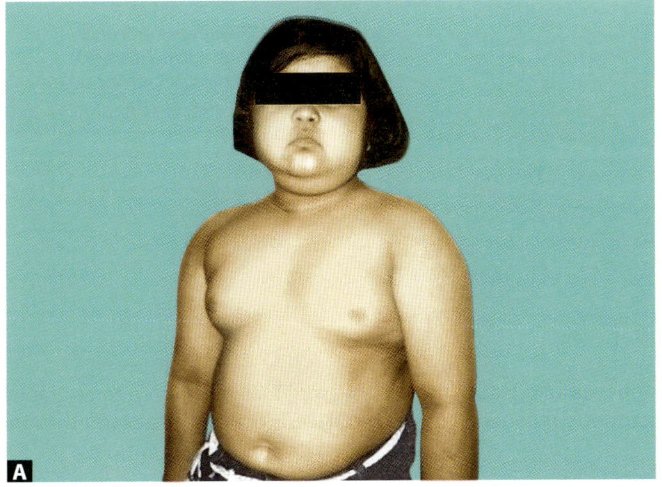

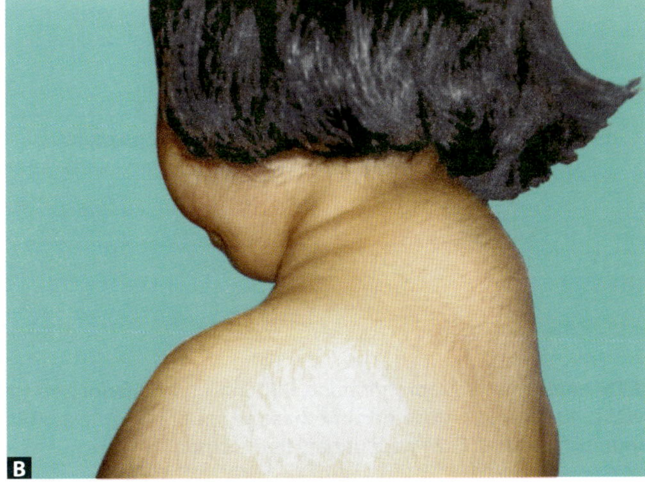

Figs. 16.7.2A and B: An 8-year-old girl with Cushing syndrome (CS) due to pituitary microadenoma. Note central obesity and moon facies (A) and buffalo hump and hypertrichosis (B).

Flowchart 16.7.1: Approach to a child with Cushing syndrome.

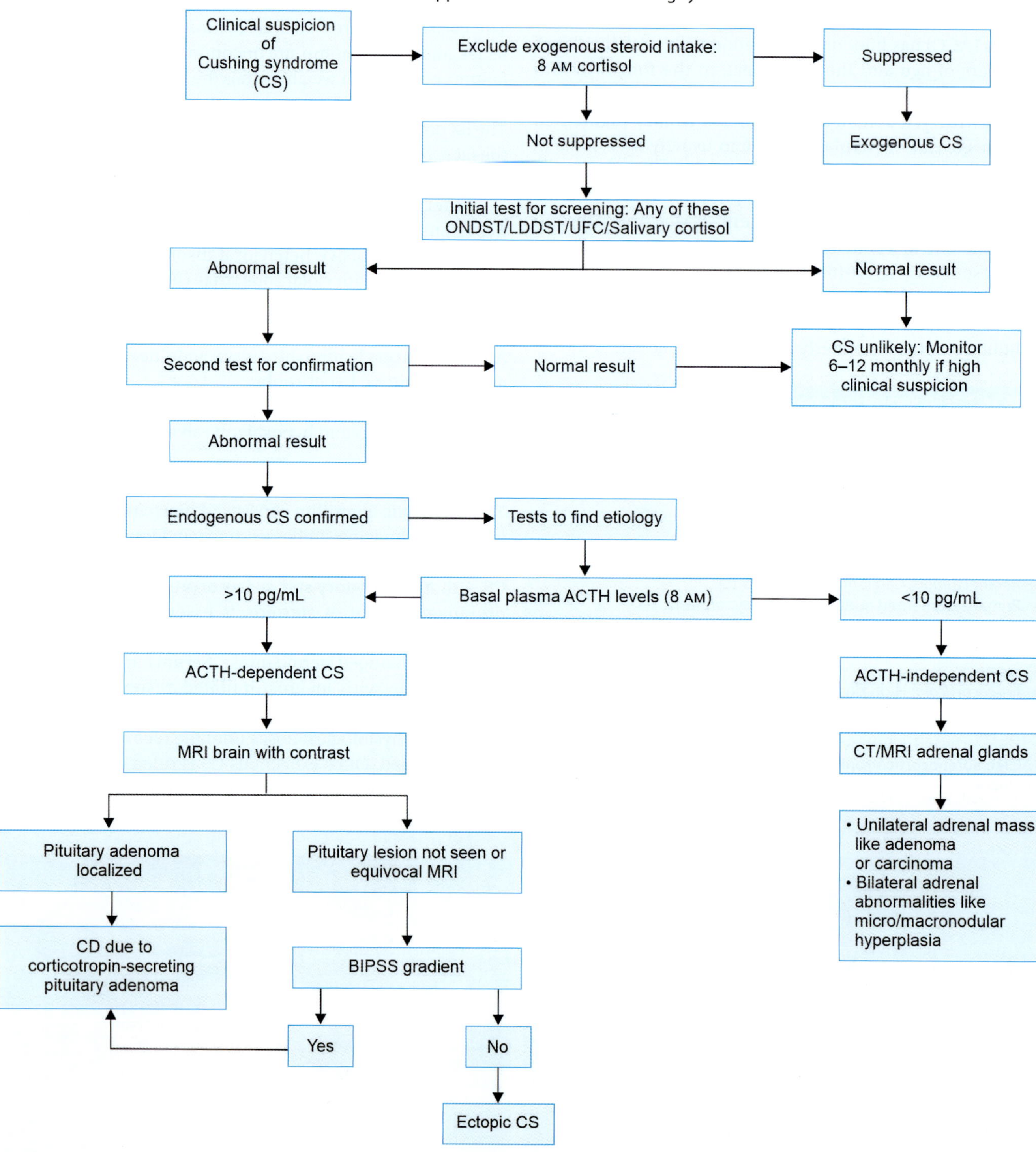

(ACTH: adrenocorticotropic hormone; BIPSS: bilateral inferior petrosal sinus sampling; CD: Cushing disease; CT: computerized tomography; LDDST: 48-hour low-dose dexamethasone suppression test; MRI: magnetic resonance imaging; ONDST: overnight dexamethasone suppression test; UFC: 24-hour urinary free cortisol)

BOX 16.7.3: Tests used in the establishment of hypercortisolism.

- *Loss of diurnal rhythm of cortisol* is the earliest biochemical marker of hypercortisolism. Usually, cortisol is highest around 8–9 AM and lowest at midnight. The normal plasma cortisol levels range between 5 µg/dL and 25 µg/dL (140–690 nmol/L) in the early morning, which is reduced to less than half by 11 PM. Morning cortisol levels are not elevated in many patients with CS, whereas late-night cortisol is usually increased
- *Overnight dexamethasone suppression test (ONDST):* Following administration of dexamethasone (10 µg/kg, maximum of 1 mg) at 11 PM to 12 midnight, plasma cortisol is estimated in the morning sample. Cortisol levels above 1.8 µg/dL (50 nmol/L) are suggestive of CS. This is a screening test and has lower specificity (80%)
- *Low-dose dexamethasone suppression test (LDDST):* This test involves the measurement of serum cortisol before and after oral dexamethasone (5 µg/kg/dose, every 6 hours for 2 days or 1.25 mg/m^2/day divided into four doses given over 2 days). Serum cortisol levels >1.8 µg/dL is diagnostic of CS
- The above suppression tests are based on the principle that dexamethasone will suppress ACTH, and hence cortisol release in normal subjects, whereas patients with autonomous cortisol production will not suppress below the specified cut-off
- *Estimation of excretion of urinary free cortisol (UFC)* is a good screening test for CS. Normal levels vary between 25 µg/m^2/day and 75 µg/m^2/day, and UFC levels >75 µg/m^2/day are suggestive of CS
- *Late-night salivary cortisol* is a better alternative and cortisol level >1.45 ng/mL (4 nmol/L) is suggestive of CS. Cut-offs may vary based on the assay methods used

cortisol production followed by identification of the source of production (adrenal or pituitary).

Two out of the following tests, namely overnight dexamethasone suppression test (ONDST), low-dose dexamethasone suppression test (LDDST), 24-hour urinary free cortisol (UFC), late-night salivary cortisol, should be abnormal for a diagnosis of CS. Loss of diurnal rhythm of cortisol secretion is an early biomarker of CS **(Box 16.7.3)**.

Once hypercortisolism is established, the next step is to differentiate whether CS is ACTH-dependent or independent by the estimation of plasma ACTH. If circulating early morning or 8 AM, ACTH is suppressed to <10 pg/mL, it suggests autonomous secretion of cortisol from the adrenals, i.e., ACTH-independent CS. Plasma ACTH value >10 pg/mL suggests ACTH-dependent CS due to ACTH release from a pituitary lesion or an ectopic source. There is a wide overlap in ACTH values in pituitary and ectopic ACTH production.

Further steps include localization of the anatomical site of the lesion by radiological imaging. If biochemical evaluation suggests ACTH-independent CS, adrenal CT or MRI is performed to detect the type of adrenal lesion: unilateral or bilateral, or benign adenoma or carcinoma. In cases of ACTH-dependent CS, pituitary MRI is recommended. The use of dynamic MRI (with IV gadolinium) with spoiled gradient sequences may increase the sensitivity. Bilateral inferior petrosal sinus sampling (BIPSS) is the test available for identifying the source of ACTH production and is performed in children with ACTH-dependent CS with normal neuroimaging.[8] This is a complex radiologically guided procedure available only at few specialized centers. However, the experience with children is limited. CT or MRI of chest and abdomen or rarely neck or functional imaging such as labeled octreotide scanning or gallium-68 labeled positron emission tomography CT imaging is used to determine the source of ectopic ACTH production **(Flowchart 16.7.1)**.

Management

Resection of adrenal lesion—unilateral adrenalectomy for adenoma or carcinoma and bilateral adrenalectomy for bilateral lesion is recommended. Prolonged cortisol excess causes suppression of the normal contralateral adrenal. Hence, close monitoring for adrenal insufficiency in the perioperative period is necessary. Physiological steroid replacement until the HPA axis recovery may also be required. Recovery of HPA axis may be delayed up to 6 months after surgery.

Adrenal carcinoma is highly malignant with a high rate of recurrence. Combination of chemotherapy with surgery is needed.

Medical management of childhood CS with inhibitors of steroidogenesis (ketoconazole, cyproheptadine, and mitotane) has been tried but is largely disappointing.

Transsphenoidal resection of pituitary adenoma is recommended for children with CD. The success rate varies from 66 to 80%. Pituitary irradiation or bilateral adrenalectomy is recommended in children with failed pituitary surgery or recurrent disease.[9] *Nelson syndrome* characterized by the enlargement of the pituitary and sella with autonomous ACTH secretion and hyperpigmentation is a dreaded complication after bilateral adrenalectomy in these patients.

HYPERALDOSTERONISM

Primary hyperaldosteronism due to increased adrenal aldosterone production is extremely rare in children. The causes include aldosterone-producing adrenal adenoma, familial primary hyperaldosteronism, and very rarely adrenal carcinoma. Secondary hyperaldosteronism results from factors that activate renin-angiotensin system. The most common clinical features of primary hyperaldosteronism are due to hypertension and hypokalemic alkalosis manifesting as fatigue, muscle cramps and weakness, polyuria, nocturia, and poor growth. This condition needs to be differentiated from Bartter syndrome, in which PRA is elevated with normal blood pressure.

Hyperaldosteronism should be managed with salt restriction and antialdosterone agent, spironolactone. Surgery is indicated only if an aldosterone-producing adenoma has been conclusively proven.

ANDROGEN AND ESTROGEN-SECRETING ADRENAL TUMORS

Although rare, sex hormone secreting tumors may arise from the zona reticularis of the adrenal cortex. Androgen-secreting tumors may present with isosexual peripheral precocious puberty in boys and virilization in girls while estrogen-secreting tumors result in isosexual peripheral precocity in girls and gynecomastia in boys.

PHEOCHROMOCYTOMA

Pheochromocytoma is a catecholamine-secreting tumor, which arises from the chromaffin cells of adrenal medulla. Tumors can also arise from abdominal sympathetic chain, periadrenal area, urinary bladder, thoracic cavity, or cervical region and extra-adrenal tumors are called paragangliomas. It is rare in children and accounts for only 0.5–2% of cases of secondary hypertension in children. It usually coexists with other familial syndromes, such as neurofibromatosis (von Recklinghausen disease) and von Hippel–Lindau disease, and multiple endocrine neoplasia type II. Genetic screening for mutation detection in the genes associated with these familial syndromes is recommended in childhood pheochromocytoma.

Clinical Features

Clinical features are due to hypersecretion of catecholamines. These include hypertension, sustained more often than paroxysmal. There may be associated headache, palpitation, pallor, flushing, sweating, nausea, vomiting, visual disturbances, polyuria, and polydipsia. Convulsions due to hypertensive encephalopathy may occur and may be the initial mode of presentation. Unexplained fever and weight loss due to hypercatabolism are seen more commonly in children than adults.

Diagnosis

Demonstration of increased plasma or urinary catecholamine levels or their metabolites, metanephrines, and normetanephrines confirm the diagnosis. Abdominal imaging with ultrasound, CT scan, or MRI is done to localize the lesion. Radionuclide imaging with iodine-123-metaiodobenzylguanidine (MIBG) or 18F-fluorodeoxyglucose (FDG) or 18F-fluoro-dihydroxyphenylalanine (F-DOPA) is also used for localization of the tumor. Often the tumors are multiple. Family screening is required, if stigmata of syndromes are present.

Management

Surgical removal of the tumor is the treatment of choice after adequate α-blockade with phenoxybenzamine or prazosin. Multiple antihypertensives may be required for control of blood pressure. β-blockers are added only after α-blockade is achieved.[10]

REFERENCES

1. Bowden SA. Current Screening Strategies for the Diagnosis of Adrenal Insufficiency in Children. Pediatric Health Med Ther. 2023;14:117-30.
2. Suntharalingham JP, Buonocore F, Duncan AJ, Achermann JC. DAX-1 (NR0B1) and steroidogenic factor-1 (SF-1, NR5A1) in human disease. Best Pract Res Clin Endocrinol Metab. 2015;29(4):607-19.
3. Flokas ME, Tomani M, Agdere L, Brown B. Triple A syndrome (Allgrove syndrome): improving outcomes with a multidisciplinary approach. Pediatric Health Med Ther. 2019;29;10:99-106.
4. Engelen M, Kemp S, de Visser M, van Geel BM, Wanders RJ, Aubourg P, et al. X-linked adrenoleukodystrophy (X-ALD): clinical presentation and guidelines for diagnosis, follow-up and management. Orphanet J Rare Dis. 2012;13;7:51.
5. Ferré EMN, Schmitt MM, Lionakis MS. Autoimmune polyendocrinopathy-candidiasis-ectodermal dystrophy. Front Pediatr. 2021;9:723532.
6. Bornstein SR, Allolio B, Arlt W, Barthel A, Don-Wauchope A, Hammer GD, et al. Diagnosis and Treatment of Primary Adrenal Insufficiency: An Endocrine Society Clinical Practice Guideline. J Clin Endocrinol Metab. 2016;101(2):364-89.
7. Lodish MB, Keil MF, Stratakis CA. Cushing's Syndrome in Pediatrics: An Update. Endocrinol Metab Clin North Am. 2018;47(2):451-62.
8. Nayak S, Dabadghao P, Dixit P, Dwivedi V, Srivastava AK, Behari S. Cushing's Disease in Children: A Review. Neurol India. 2020;68(Supplement):S52-S65.
9. Nieman LK, Biller BM, Findling JW, Murad MH, Newell-Price J, Savage MO, et al. Treatment of Cushing's Syndrome: An Endocrine Society Clinical Practice Guideline. J Clin Endocrinol Metab. 2015;100(8):2807-31.
10. Bholah R, Bunchman TE. Review of Pediatric Pheochromocytoma and Paraganglioma. Front Pediatr. 2017;5:155.

16.8 Congenital Adrenal Hyperplasia

Raghupathy Palany

INTRODUCTION

Congenital adrenal hyperplasia (CAH) includes a group of rare genetic disorders that affect the adrenal cortex causing a wide spectrum of clinical manifestations. The most common among these is due to 21-hydroxylase deficiency (21-OHD), an autosomal recessive disorder of adrenal steroidogenesis. Impaired cortisol synthesis is the end result, but this occurs due to the involvement at different segments of adrenal steroid biosynthetic pathway.

STEROIDOGENESIS

The adrenal cortex produces several steroid hormones, such as cortisol, aldosterone, and androgens. The conversion of cholesterol into steroidal hormones (steroid biosynthesis) takes place in the adrenal cortex but also in the gonads of both genders, and the placenta. An enzymatic defect of steroidogenesis may not affect the adrenal cortex and gonads equally. Hence, disorders of sex development (DSD) may result from the biosynthetic pathway defects in the adrenal cortex or the gonads, or both.

The adrenal cortex functions as two separate units because of the enzymatic differences between the zona glomerulosa and the inner two zones—(1) zona fasciculata and (2) zona reticularis. These two inner zones produce cortisol, androgens, and small quantities of estrogens and are directly controlled by adrenocorticotropic hormone (ACTH). They lack 18-hydroxylase and so cannot synthesize aldosterone.

The various enzymes involved in the biosynthetic pathway of cortisol are given in **Flowchart 16.8.1**. Corticotropin-releasing hormone (CRH) produced by the hypothalamus regulates pituitary ACTH. ACTH in turn induces synthesis and secretion of steroids within minutes. The conversion of cholesterol to pregnenolone is the major site of ACTH action on the adrenal cortex and is the rate-limiting step.

The zona glomerulosa lacks 17α–hydroxylase activity and, therefore, cannot synthesize 17α–hydroxypregnenolone and 17α–hydroxyprogesterone (17-OHP), the precursors of cortisol and androgens. The synthesis of aldosterone by this zone is regulated by the renin-angiotensin system and by potassium, in addition to that by ACTH.

CONGENITAL ADRENAL HYPERPLASIA

In CAH, cortisol synthesis from cholesterol is affected due to deficiency of one of the several enzymes in the adrenal cortex (**Flowchart 16.8.1**). Reduced cortisol level through the negative feedback mechanism leads to increase in hypothalamic CRH and pituitary ACTH, which induces adrenal cortex hyperplasia. Overproduction of the hormonal precursors proximal to the block and deficiency of the hormones distal to the blocked enzymatic step are responsible for the various clinical features encountered. The enzymatic defects are inherited by an autosomal recessive mode and produce characteristic clinical and biochemical pictures. The genes and enzymes involved in adrenal steroidogenesis are listed in **Table 16.8.1**.[1-3]

21-HYDROXYLASE DEFICIENCY

The 21-OHD is the most common enzyme deficiency seen in >90% of individuals with CAH. In Caucasians of European descent, prevalence of 21-OHD reported to be 1 in 15,000 to 1 in 20,000. In India, it is reported to be higher especially in regions high in consanguineous unions. The absence of 21-hydroxylase causes decreased synthesis of glucocorticoid and mineralocorticoid with elevated precursors. The precursor, 17-OHP accumulates in serum because it is not converted to 11-deoxycortisol. Similarly, progesterone accumulates following lack of conversion to 11-deoxycorticosterone (DOC) (**Flowchart 16.8.1**). The ultimate effects are:

- Cortisol deficiency and ACTH elevation giving rise to adrenocortical hyperplasia
- Mineralocorticoid deficiency causing salt loss, dehydration, and shock

As the formation of mineralocorticoids and glucocorticoids from cholesterol is blocked, the conversion of cholesterol flows largely into the androgen pathway without hindrance because adrenal androgen synthesis is not blocked. This causes virilization of the external genitalia of a female infant seen at birth.

Clinical Features

The classic clinical varieties of this deficiency are as follows:

- *Salt-wasting type* in nearly 75% of 21-OHD. This is the classic disorder. It presents usually between 1 week and

Flowchart 16.8.1: Scheme of adrenal steroidogenesis. Chemical names of enzymes are shown next to the arrows; enclosed numbers indicate traditional names of the enzymes: (1) 20,22-desmolase; (2) 3β-hydroxysteroid dehydrogenase/isomerase; (3) 17α-hydroxylase; (4) 17,20-lyase; (5) 21-hydroxylase; (6) 11β-hydroxylase; (7) 18-hydroxylase; (8) 18-oxidase; (9) 17β-hydroxysteroid dehydrogenase; (10) aromatase.

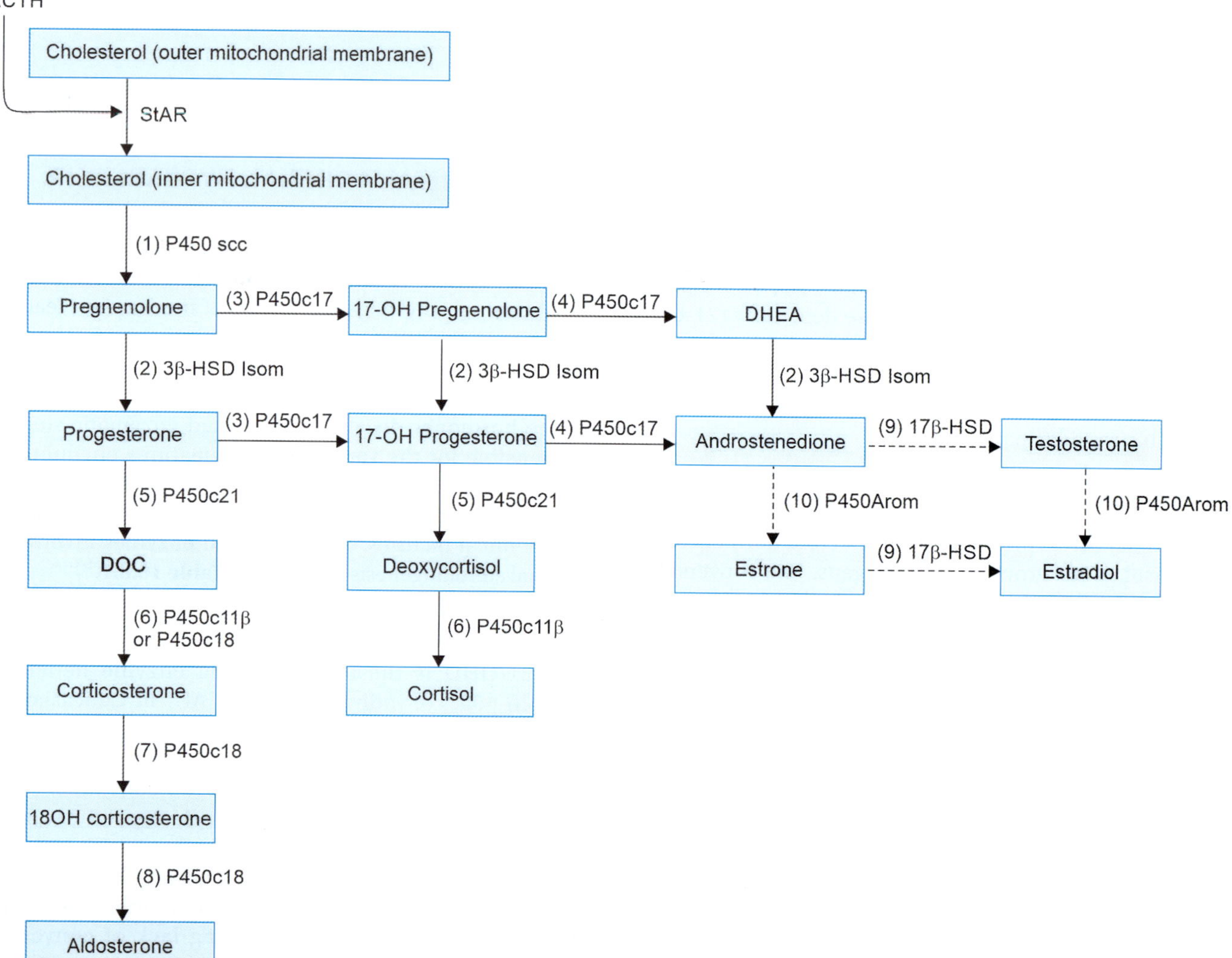

(ACTH: adrenocorticotropic hormone; DHEA: dehydroepiandrosterone; DOC: 11-deoxycorticosterone; StAR: steroidogenic acute regulatory protein)

TABLE 16.8.1: Genes and enzymes involved in adrenal steroidogenesis.

Gene	*Chromosomal location*	*Enzyme*	*Enzymatic activity*	*Cellular location*
CYP11A1	15q23-q24	P450scc (*CYP11A1*)	Cholesterol desmolase (side chain cleavage)	Mitochondrion
HSD3B2	1p13.1	3βHSD (*3βHSDII*)	3β-hydroxysteroid dehydrogenase	Endoplasmic reticulum
CYP17	10q24.3	P450c17 (*CYP17*)	17α-hydroxylase/17,20-lyase	Endoplasmic reticulum
CYP21A2	6p21.3	P450c21 (*CYP21A2*)	21-hydroxylase	Endoplasmic reticulum
CYP11B1	8q21-22	P450c11 (*CYP11B1*)	11β-hydroxylase	Mitochondrion
CYP11B2	8q21-22	P450c18 (*CYP11B2*)	Aldosterone synthase (corticosterone 18-methylcorticosterone oxidase/lyase)	Mitochondrion

1 month of age but may also occur beyond the neonatal period during infection-induced stress situations. Salt wasting and hypovolemia arise from aldosterone deficiency and the natriuretic effect of accumulated precursors, such as 17-OHP. Elevated ACTH results in pigmentation.

- *Simple virilizing type* without salt loss. Nonsalt losers with virilization account for nearly 25% of cases. The absence of salt loss can be explained by a partial defect in 21-OHD, since only a minimal 21-hydroxylase activity is needed for mineralocorticoid production. Virilization is seen at birth in girls.
- *Nonclassic (late onset) type,* wherein 50% of enzyme activity is retained. Salt wasting is absent, and cortisol deficiency is rare. The presentation is characterized by hyperandrogenism such as mild-to-moderate hirsutism, virilism, acne, menstrual irregularities premature adrenarche, early growth spurt, or accelerated skeletal maturation. The manifestations can also occur for the first time during adulthood as hirsutism in women or reduced fertility in both sexes.

The diagnosis of 21-OHD is easily identified in girls because of genital ambiguity. The degree of genital ambiguity does not correlate with the form of 21-OHD. Virilization in the female may present as mild clitoral hypertrophy, varying degrees of ambiguity, or complete masculinization with normal-looking male genitalia but with an empty scrotum. Thus, the absence of testes would be helpful in diagnosis.

In boys with simple virilizing form and absence of salt loss, however, the condition can go unnoticed until androgen excess causes increased height velocity, increase in the size of the external genitalia, appearance of pubic hair, and other signs of male secondary sexual characteristics are observed. Hyperpigmentation involving external genitalia, nipples, and umbilicus may be a very important clue for early diagnosis in these children.

Apart from the external virilizing and biochemical features, there are no abnormalities in genetic sex, gonadal differentiation, or development of the internal genitalia. The female infant will have normal ovaries, fallopian tubes, uterus, and proximal vagina. Postnatally, in untreated cases, there will be continued virilization effects with clitoromegaly or penile enlargement, accelerated growth, advanced skeletal maturation far in excess of the height age, and early appearance of secondary sexual characteristics. Untreated males will have advanced penile enlargement with disproportionately small testes. Because of the absence of testicular enlargement as observed in puberty, this is often referred to as precocious pseudopuberty. Untreated females have clitoromegaly, hirsutism, male-type baldness, menstrual irregularities, and impaired fertility. Short adult height resulting from premature epiphyseal fusion is a regular feature in all untreated cases. Even with regular therapy and good control, predicted adult height is not always achieved in CAH, and bone age may be advanced.

Laboratory Features

Hyponatremia, hyperkalemia, acidosis, and uremia are the biochemical features in salt-wasting type. Hypoglycemia may also be present. Elevated serum 17-OHP, elevated plasma renin (PR), serum dehydroepiandrosterone sulfate (DHEAS), and testosterone are diagnostics. On short Synacthen (synthetic ACTH) stimulation test, serum 17-OHP and DHEAS rise more than two- to-threefold.

Nonclassic 21-OHD is a very mild form of 21-OHD. This may be picked up only as an increased response of 17-OHP to ACTH stimulation or during genetic family studies.

Treatment

The essential principles of treatment are to replace the deficient hormones and to suppress the overproduction of precursor hormones.[4] Hydrocortisone is required in the dose of 8–15 mg/m^2/day in two or three divided doses. Constant monitoring is required to arrive at the right dose to facilitate normal growth and also the lowest possible dose in order to prevent central obesity, growth retardation, and decreased bone mineral density. Salt wasters require, in addition, 9α-fluorohydrocortisone 0.1–0.3 mg (50–200 μg)/day and need to be monitored for hypertension, edema, and suppressed PR. Sodium chloride supplementation up to 1–2 g daily is needed along with feeds. This is generally not required beyond infancy but may be encouraged in hot weather conditions and in situations with excessive sweating.

In the newborn period at presentation, a large dose of hydrocortisone and fluorohydrocortisone may be required. Dosages are modified by monitoring serum sodium and potassium daily and ideally, by frequent serum 17-OHP and PR estimations. Dose of hydrocortisone is gradually reduced and changed over to 5 mg twice a day orally.

The hormonal profile reverts to the normal range with appropriate treatment, which is monitored 3–6 monthly by estimating 17-OHP and PR values and when appropriate dosage adjustment is carried out.

Early epiphyseal fusion in both sexes will eventually cause short stature, if treatment is irregular and incomplete, with the disease being poorly controlled.

In stress situations, e.g., febrile infections, gastrointestinal illness, major trauma, surgery, or shock, large amounts of glucocorticoids are required to combat the stress. The daily dose of hydrocortisone may be doubled or tripled and given orally or intramuscularly, if oral administration is not tolerated. Fludrocortisone dose remains unchanged.

Glucocorticoid treatment may be required for nonclassic CAH for inducing ovulation. Hirsutism seen in this form requires antiandrogen and other measures as in polycystic ovarian syndrome.

Appropriate Sex Assignment

Assigning the appropriate sex is of paramount importance. The affected female with CAH has the potential for a normal fertile female role. Surgical correction of the genital abnormality (feminizing genitoplasty) is carried out in girls at around 1 year of age by doing reduction clitoroplasty. Definitive vaginoplasty with routine dilatation will also be required in late adolescence.

Parent Education

It is essential that the parents are given adequate health education regarding this condition. They will need to understand the nature of the disease, chronicity of the treatment required lifelong, the complications arising from poor compliance, and how increased dose of steroids play an essential role in stress situations, such as surgery, infection, or shock, which can be life-threatening, if inappropriately managed.

Newborn Screening for Congenital Adrenal Hyperplasia

Screening of all newborns with filter paper 17-OHP is carried out in many countries and some parts of India. This newborn screening is helpful:

- To identify infants with the classic form 21-OHD who carry the risk of developing life-threatening salt-wasting crisis
- To make a rapid diagnosis in cases of female infants with ambiguous genitalia

11β-HYDROXYLASE DEFICIENCY

In this disorder, which accounts for nearly 5% of cases of CAH, cortisol and corticosterone are deficient with low aldosterone and overproduction of 11-deoxycortisol and DOC. The precursor hormones are shunted into the androgen pathway causing prenatal and postnatal virilization. The accumulation of DOC results in sodium and water retention, increased plasma volume, and hence causes hypertension. Serum level of 11-deoxycortisol elevation is diagnostic. PR is suppressed, serum aldosterone is lowered, and hypokalemia may be present. Glucocorticoid therapy is effective in reversing all the abnormalities causing remission.

17-HYDROXYLASE/17,20-LYASE DEFICIENCY

This is a rare disorder occurring with cortisol deficiency, ACTH excess, overproduction of DOC causing hypertension and hypokalemia. Affected males are incompletely virilized (undervirilized male) owing to diminished androgen production and may be phenotypically female or ambiguous. In addition, ACTH excess driven by cortisol deficiency causes mineralocorticoid excess (as 17-hydroxylation is not needed in the mineralocorticoid pathway), with sodium retention, hypokalemia, and hypertension. Both sexes present with female external genitalia at birth and usually manifest at puberty with absence of secondary sexual characteristics. The serum levels of PR and aldosterone are low. Glucocorticoid therapy suppresses overproduction of the hormones and ameliorates the hypertension.

3β-HYDROXYSTEROID DEHYDROGENASE/4, 5 ISOMERASE DEFICIENCY

Classic and nonclassic forms are seen in this disorder. Salt wasting, deficiency of cortisol, and aldosterone are the usual manifestations of this condition. In the nonclassic form, there is no aldosterone deficiency. Males with this condition may show undervirilization with ambiguity of external genitalia owing to underproduction of testosterone in utero. Pseudovaginal hypospadias may be present in the males due to absence of potent androgens. But the excessive collection of the weak androgen, DHEAS, may cause clitoral enlargement in the female. Most of them have aldosterone deficiency with elevation of PR. Serum ACTH level is high and hyperpigmentation is seen. Treatment is with glucocorticoids.

P450 OXIDOREDUCTASE DEFICIENCY

Several enzymes including 17-hydroxylase, 21-hydroxylase, and aromatase depend on P450 oxidoreductase (POR) for their catalytic activity. The action of POR at multiple sites of steroidogenesis **(Flowchart 16.8.1)** explains multiple hormonal deficiencies. The action of POR at nonadrenal sites further explain the occurrence of skeletal dysplasia, which is seen as an associated finding in some patients (the Antley–Bixler syndrome). 17-hydroxylase deficiency may cause hypertension.

LIPOID ADRENAL HYPERPLASIA

This rare disease involves the steroidogenic acute regulatory (StAR) protein. Deficiency of StAR protein affects the adrenal cortex and gonads, and there is a global deficiency of all adrenal hormones—glucocorticoids, mineralocorticoids, and sex hormones. Presentation is very early in life with salt-wasting crisis. Later presentation up to 1 year of age has also been described. Females have no abnormality of internal or external genitalia. Males are phenotypically female but may have inguinal gonads. Sex hormone replacement will be necessary in those with undervirilization or in those with delayed puberty with the objective of achieving normal pubertal development, normal sexual function, and fertility.

CONCLUSION

Knowledge regarding CAH is widening constantly. The chromosomal locations and nature of the genes encoding the various enzymes needed for adrenocortical biosynthesis, the cellular locations, functions and abnormalities of these enzymes, the pathophysiology of adrenocortical disorders, the clinical features, and laboratory parameters have been documented further. Prenatal diagnosis and newborn screening are practiced widely. New therapeutic development, including ways of administering cortisol in a more physiological way is being tried. Control of excess androgens to enable optimal glucocorticoid doses are also being tried.[5]

REFERENCES

1. Ahmed SF, Rodie M. Investigation and initial management of ambiguous genitalia. Best Pract Res Clin Endocrinol Metab. 2010;24(2):197-218.
2. El-Maouche D, Arlt W, Merke DP. Congenital adrenal hyperplasia. Lancet. 2017;390(10108):2194-210.
3. White PC. Alterations of cortisol metabolism in human disorders. Horm Res Paediatr. 2018;89(5):320-30.
4. Speiser PW, Arlt W, Auchus RJ, Baskin LS, Conway GS, Merke DP, et al. Congenital adrenal hyperplasia due to steroid 21-hydroxylase deficiency: An Endocrine Society Clinical Practice Guideline. J Clin Endocrinol Metab. 2018;103(11):1-46.
5. White PC. Update on diagnosis and management of congenital adrenal hyperplasia due to 21-hydroxylase deficiency. Curr Opin Endocrinol Diabetes Obes. 2018;25(3):178-84.

16.9 Differences (Disorders) of Sex Development

Abraham Paulose, Raghupathy Palany

INTRODUCTION

"Differences or disorders of sex development" (DSD) are congenital anomalies in which there is a discordance between chromosomal, genetic, gonadal, and/or internal/external genital sex. The etiologies and related pathogeneses of DSDs can be comprehended once the developmental physiology of fetal sex differentiation is understood, as described in the following text.

NORMAL SEX DETERMINATION AND DIFFERENTIATION

The process of sexual differentiation in fetal life can be divided into three stages:

1. The formation of the undifferentiated gonads and the anlagen of the genitalia, internal (Müllerian and Wolffian ducts, urogenital sinus) and external (genital tubercle, urethral folds, labioscrotal folds)
2. Gonadal differentiation and
3. Male or female differentiation of the internal and external genitalia **(Flowchart 16.9.1)**.

It is a tightly controlled and highly complex process and any deviation from the intricate sequence of sexual differentiation may give rise to differences of sex development.[1]

The undifferentiated human embryos of the two genders differ only by their karyotypes. The gender of the individual is normally determined by factors that direct the gonads as early as the third gestational week in the male to differentiate along male line, and the process is continued in turn, by gonadal hormones which determine the development of the phenotypic sex. The *SRY* (sex-determining region on the Y-chromosome) gene residing in the Y-chromosome has now been documented as the mammalian sex-determining gene, which actively induces the formation of the testis and the male phenotype during embryonic life. The gonads, internal genitalia (genital ducts), and the external genitalia, which are all bipotential, are influenced by several genes and other factors necessary for sex differentiation.

Gonads

The gonads in the embryo remain undifferentiated until the 6th week of gestation. Subsequent development into either a testis or ovary is directed by the genetic sex (XY or XX).

Flowchart 16.9.1: Overview of normal sex determination and differentiation during fetal life.

1. *Formation of undifferentiated gonads:* Bipotential gonads are developed by 5 weeks of life, as well as two pairs of genital ducts (Müllerian and Wolffian ducts), common external genitalia comprise the genital tubercle, the urethral fold, the urogenital groove, and the labioscrotal folds. This stage ends by the 6th week.
2. *Gonadal differentiation* starts between 6th and 7th week when somatic cells and gonocytes in the bipotential gonad begin to differentiate into testicular or ovarian cells, depending on the presence and activation or repression of signaling pathways.
3. *Sex differentiation:* Internal and external genitalia differentiation depends on the presence or absence of testicular hormones—anti-Müllerian hormone (AMH), testosterone, and dihydrotestosterone (DHT).

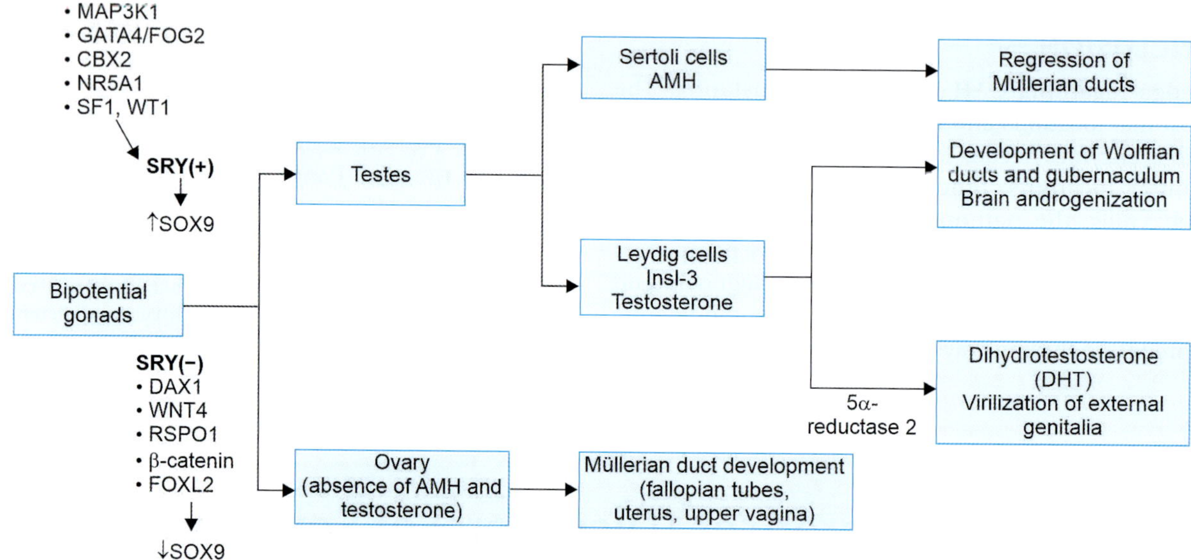

(SRY: Sex-determining region on the Y-chromosome; *SOX9*: SRY-box transcription factor 9; MAP3K1: Mitogen-activated protein kinase 1; GATA4: GATA binding protein 4; FOG2: Family member 2; CBX2: Chromobox 2; NR5A1: Nuclear receptor subfamily 5 group A membrane 1; SF1: Splicing factor 1; WT1: Wilms tumor 1 transcription factor; DAX1: Dosage-sensitive sex reversal, adrenal hypoplasia critical region, on chromosome X, gene 1; WNT4: Wnt Family member 4; RSPO1: Human R-spondin 1; FOXL2: Forkhead box protein L2; Insl-3: Insulin-like peptide 3)

The testis develops more rapidly than the ovary. Fetal testicular differentiation begins in the 7th week of gestation, whereas ovarian development begins not earlier than the 16th week of gestation. Female sex differentiation is not dependent on ovarian hormones, but there is evidence that *Wnt* signaling molecules play a role in Müllerian duct development and suppression of Leydig cell differentiation in ovary.[1]

Testicular Differentiation

The *SRY* gene (with 204 amino acids) located on the short arm of Y-chromosome (Yp11.3) is the trigger for testicular differentiation, by inducing the development of Sertoli cells, and subsequently, seminiferous tubules and Leydig cell formation in that order. *SRY* activates *SOX9* (SRY-homeobOX-like gene), an autosomal gene (chromosome17q24), and *SF1* (steroidogenic factor 1) to induce differentiation of the bipotential gonad into a testis. *SRY* suppresses dosage-sensitive sex reversal, adrenal hypoplasia critical region, on chromosome X, gene 1 (*DAX1*), which normally inhibits *SOX9*. The testis induces male sex differentiation including testicular descent through a hormone-mediated process.[1]

Ovarian Differentiation

DAX1, *SOX3*, and *Wnt4* are the three candidate genes currently known to suppress testicular differentiation. *DAX1* and *SOX3* inhibit *SF1* and *SOX9*, preventing Sertoli cell differentiation, favoring granulosa cell development. *Wnt4* arrests the Leydig cell precursors and induces development of Müllerian ducts into fallopian tubes, uterus, cervix, and upper third of vagina. Though the effects of these genes have been considered to result in ovarian differentiation, it should be remembered that active testicular differentiation occurs much earlier when compared to the ovarian.

Internal Genitalia

Testosterone initially under the control of human chorionic gonadotropin (hCG) is produced locally (paracrine) by Leydig cells of the fetal testis on either side. It helps in ipsilateral differentiation of the Wolffian ducts into epididymis, vas deferens, seminal vesicles, and ejaculatory ducts.

Anti-Müllerian hormone (AMH), secreted by the Sertoli cells, causes ipsilateral involution of the Müllerian structures.

In female fetuses, Wolffian structures regress in the absence of testosterone, and Müllerian ducts persist in the absence of AMH. However, *Wnt4* gene appears to play an important role in Müllerian duct differentiation and fetal ovarian function.[1]

External Genitalia

From the initial undifferentiated stage of the external genitalia, masculinizing features develop in the male under the influence of dihydrotestosterone formed peripherally from testosterone by the action of 5α-reductase. This process is dependent on an adequate number of functioning androgen receptors in the pubic skin. Formation of the female external genitalia does not require any active process and will persist with normal ovaries, in androgen insensitivity or even in the absence of gonads, sex chromosome abnormalities, streak gonads, or nonfunctioning testes.[1]

TABLE 16.9.1: Revised nomenclature.

Previous	*Revised*
Intersex	Differences or disorders of sex development (DSD)
Male pseudohermaphrodite: Undervirilization of an XY male, undermasculinization of a XY male	46,XY DSD
Female pseudohermaphrodite: Virilization of an XX female, masculinization of a XX female	46,XX DSD
True hermaphrodite	Ovotesticular DSD
XX male or XX sex reversal	46,XX testicular DSD
XY sex reversal	46,XY complete gonadal dysgenesis

Terms, such as intersex, hermaphroditism, pseudohermaphroditism, sex reversal, and gender-based diagnostic conditions, are currently recommended to be avoided. These terms may be deemed derogatory and confusing to parents and practitioners as well. Hence, changes in terminology have been proposed **(Table 16.9.1)**.

It is advisable to use terminology that is precise, descriptive, clear in expressing the genetic, etiologic, or diagnostic condition, and at the same time, sensitive to the concerns of parents. The consensus statement addressing the approach and care of DSD suggests the following broad classification for DSD:

- Sex chromosome DSD,
- 46,XY DSD, and
- 46,XX DSD.[2,3]

The revised classification of DSD is presented in **Table 16.9.2**.

When *SRY* gene undergoes mutation in its high-mobility group box protein, testicular failure, or genital ambiguity will result. *SOX9* mutation in 46,XY males leads to a female phenotype and streak ovarian-like gonads. Chromosomal abnormalities may lead to disorders of male gonadal differentiation or give rise to ovotesticular differentiation.[1]

Wolffian development and Müllerian regression on each side are dependent on the ipsilateral production of testosterone and AMH, respectively. Hence, abnormalities of the internal genitalia will be encountered, based on the presence of gonadal elements on that side. A streak gonad, which produces neither testosterone nor AMH, will give rise to poorly formed Müllerian structures,

TABLE 16.9.2: Revised classification of disorders of sex development (DSD).

Sex chromosome DSD	*XY DSD*	*XX DSD*
• 45,X (Turner syndrome and variants) • 47,XXY (Klinefelter syndrome and variants) • 45,X/46,XY (Mixed gonadal dysgenesis, ovotesticular dysgenesis) • 46,XX/46,XY (Chimeric, ovotesticular dysgenesis)	*Disorders of gonadal (testicular) development:* • Complete gonadal dysgenesis • Partial gonadal dysgenesis • Gonadal regression • Ovotesticular DSD *Disorders in androgen synthesis or action:* • Androgen biosynthesis defect (e.g., 17β-hydroxysteroid dehydrogenase deficiency, 5α-reductase deficiency, *StAR* mutations) • Defects of androgen action (e.g., CAIS, PAIS) • LH receptor defects (e.g., Leydig cell hypoplasia/aplasia) • Disorders of AMH and AMH receptor (persistent Müllerian duct syndrome) *Others:* (e.g., Severe hypospadias, cloacal exstrophy)	*Disorders of gonadal (ovarian) development:* • Ovotesticular DSD • Testicular DSD (e.g., SRY, dupSOX9) • Gonadal dysgenesis *Androgen excess:* • Fetal (e.g., 21-hydroxylase deficiency, 11β-hydroxylase deficiency) • Fetoplacental (aromatase deficiency, POR) • Maternal (luteoma, exogenous, etc.) *Others:* (e.g., cloacal exstrophy, vaginal atresia, MURCS, other syndromes)

(AMH: Anti-Müllerian hormone; CAIS: complete androgen insensitivity syndrome; DSD: disorders of sex development; LH: luteinizing hormone; MURCS: Müllerian, renal, cervicothoracic somite dysplasia; PAIS: partial androgen insensitivity syndrome; POR: P450 oxidoreductase; SOX: SRY-homeobOX-like gene: SRY: sex-determining region on the Y-chromosome; StAR: steroidogenic acute regulatory protein)

such as a hypoplastic or hemiuterus on the side of the defective gonad.[1]

Variable degrees of virilization of the female external genitalia leading to gender ambiguity will result when exposed to androgens, either from the mother (intake or excessive production of androgens in her body) or from the fetus [congenital adrenal hyperplasia (CAH), aromatase deficiency, ovotesticular DSD, or mixed gonadal dysgenesis]. Partial virilization producing ambiguity of the external genitalia or complete virilization with normal-looking male external genitalia (penis and a fully formed but empty scrotum) may occur in a genetic female with CAH due to 21-hydroxylase deficiency. A normal-looking female external genitalia (with testes in the labioscrotal folds) may be a case of complete androgen insensitivity syndrome. A genetic male may have undervirilization and present with underdeveloped and ambiguous genitalia as in 17α-hydroxylase deficiency or 3β-hydroxysteroid dehydrogenase deficiency. The appearance of the external genitalia does not always give any diagnostic clinical clues, e.g., an infant with ovotesticular DSD and a virilized female with genital ambiguity may look similar.[2,3]

Atypical Genitalia

Atypical or ambiguous genitalia may be defined as discordance between the external genitalia and the gonads. If the genotype is XX **(Fig. 16.9.1)**, and the impalpable gonads are ovaries, but the external genitalia are virilized partially or fully, this is likely to be due to the exposure of a female fetus to excessive androgens during the period of sex differentiation in early gestation, e.g., CAH due to 21-hydroxylase deficiency **(Flowchart 16.9.2)**, 11β-hydroxylase deficiency **(Fig. 16.9.2)**, 3β-hydroxysteroid dehydrogenase deficiency, or maternal androgen excess due to a tumor or therapy.

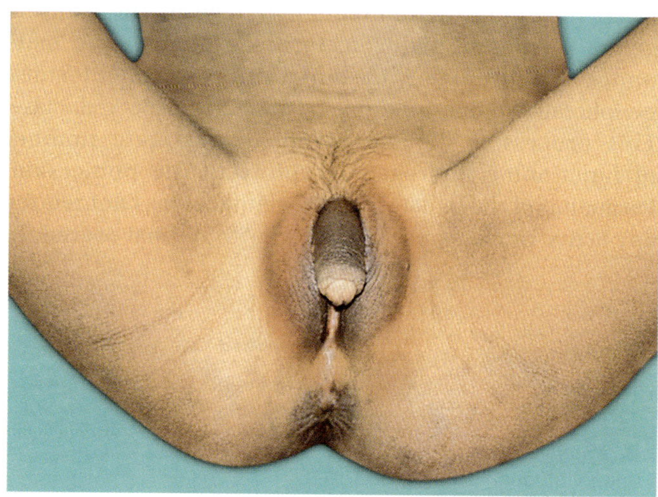

Fig. 16.9.1: A 3-year-old-girl with marked clitoromegaly due to untreated congenital adrenal hyperplasia—21-hydroxylase deficiency (nonsalt-loser).

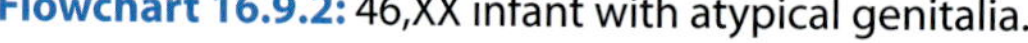

Flowchart 16.9.2: 46,XX infant with atypical genitalia.

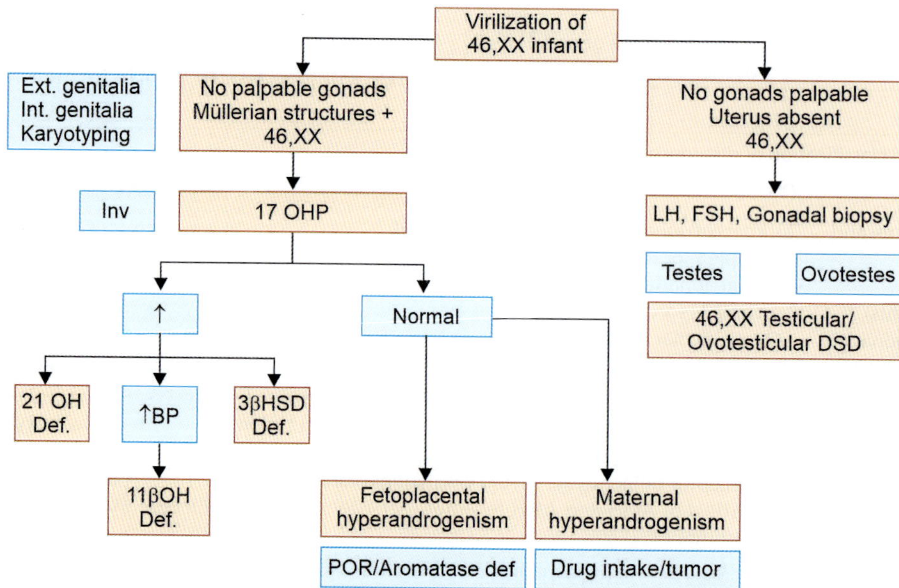

[Ext: External; Int: Internal; Inv: Investigations; 17 OHP: 17-hydroxyprogesterone; 21OHD: 21-hydroxylase (CYP21A2) deficiency; 11βOHD: 11β-hydroxylase (CYP11B1) deficiency; 3βHSD: 3β-hydroxysteroid dehydrogenase (HSD3B2) deficiency; POR: P450-oxidoreductase (POR) deficiency; LH: Luteinizing hormone; FSH: Follicle stimulating hormone]

If the genotype is XY **(Flowchart 16.9.3)**, the gonads which are palpable are testes, and the external genitalia is incompletely virilized or ambiguous; this may be due to a testosterone biosynthetic defect, or if the external genitalia is completely female, this may be a case of complete androgen insensitivity syndrome. If both ovarian and testicular tissues are present either in the same gonad (ovotestis) or opposite gonads—one gonad may be palpable or both gonads impalpable—this may be a case of ovotesticular DSD.[2,3]

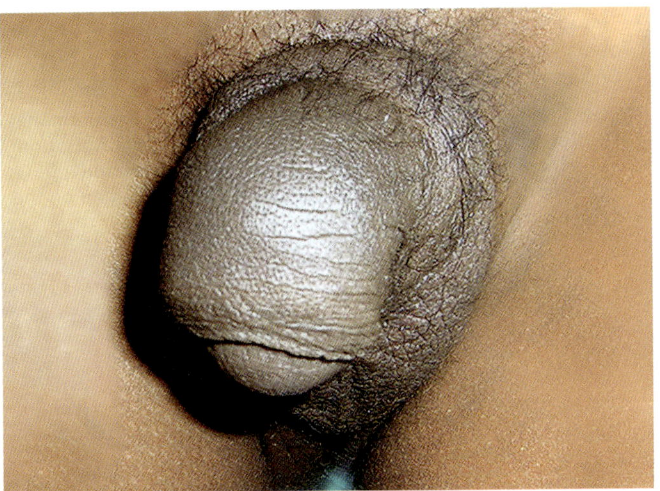

Fig. 16.9.2: Marked virilization external genitalia in a 4-year-old girl with 11β-hydroxylase deficiency.

CLINICAL APPROACH TO AN INFANT WITH DIFFERENCES OR DISORDERS OF SEX DEVELOPMENT

Clinical evaluation of the infant with a suspected DSD **(Box 16.9.1)** should be done to decide assignment of sex and to plan the long-term management of the infant's condition.[2,3] However, it is highly essential to rule out associated life-threatening metabolic conditions, like adrenal insufficiency.

History taking should include details regarding parental consanguinity, maternal drug intake, maternal condition wherein there is excessive production of androgens (uncontrolled CAH, androgen producing tumor), history of previous sibling deaths due to salt loss in the neonatal period, affected siblings or family members with DSD, history of low birth weight or intrauterine growth restriction (IUGR), and X-linked mode of inheritance and infertility (in the cases of androgen insensitivity).[2,3]

Physical assessment should include examination for dysmorphic features, midline defects in the cases of microphallus due to pituitary defects **(Figs. 16.9.3 and 16.9.4)**; hypo- or hypertension, dehydration, virilization in the case of girls; undervirilization in the case of boys; presence or absence of gonads, and hyperpigmentation of the skin.

Severe hyponatremia, hyperkalemia, dehydration, hypotension, and shock usually in the second week after birth, with increased pigmentation of the skin in a virilized female infant or an infant with normal male genitalia

Flowchart 16.9.3: 46,XY infant with atypical genitalia.

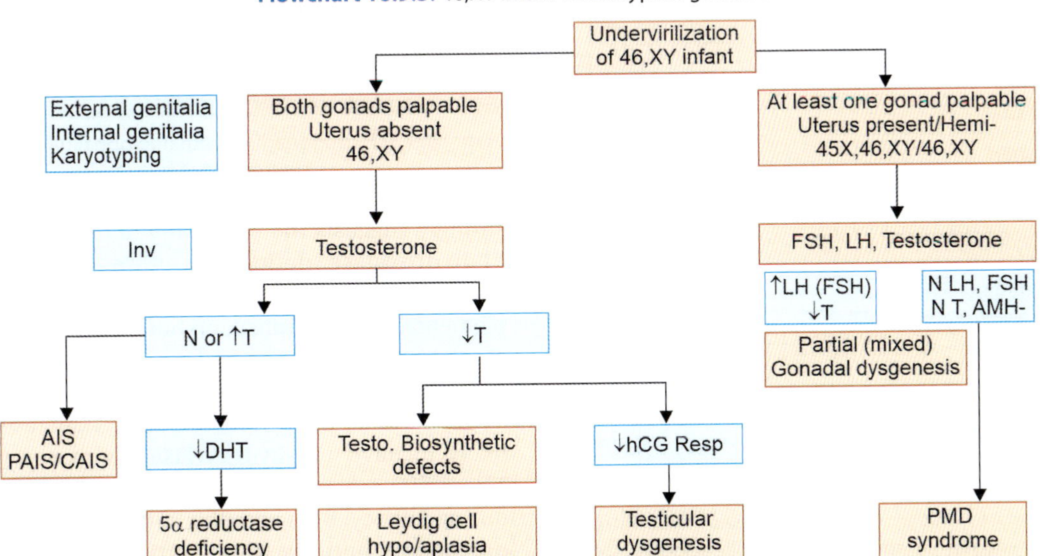

(T: Testosterone; AMH: Anti-Müllerian hormone; DHT: Dihydrotestosterone; AIS: Androgen insensitivity syndrome, PAIS: Partial AIS; CAIS: Complete AIS; LH: Luteinizing hormone; FSH: Follicle stimulating hormone; hCG: Human chorionic gonadotropin; PMDS: Persistent Müllerian duct syndrome)

BOX 16.9.1: Evaluation of an infant with a suspected disorders of sex development (DSD).

When to suspect?
- *Male appearance of the external genitalia and any of the following:* Bilaterally nonpalpable gonads; severe hypospadias; microphallus or perineal hypospadias with bifid scrotum
- *Apparent female appearance of the external genitalia and any of the following:* Clitoromegaly; posterior labial fusion; gonads palpable in the labioscrotal folds or inguinal region; and genital appearance discordant with sex chromosomes
- Overt atypical genitalia (ex. cloacal exstrophy)

History
- *Symptoms of adrenal crisis:* Circulatory collapse, hyperpigmentation, failure to thrive, persistent vomiting, and recurrent hospitalizations
- Maternal history of exposure to drugs (androgens), symptoms suggestive of androgen excess (acne, hirsutism, deepening of voice, and increased muscle mass)
- Family history of consanguinity, infertility or amenorrhea, gonadal/urogenital malformations, abortion/early infant death
- Virilization at puberty

Physical examination
- General condition
- Hyperpigmentation
- Dysmorphic features; skeletal/anatomic malformations
- Prader score/external masculinization score/external genitalia score
- Blood pressure
- Midline defects, neurocutaneous markers (*café-au-lait* macules, neurofibromas)
- Abdominal bimanual examination
- Height and weight measurements plotted on age-specific growth charts
- Hearing and eyes
- Cardiac and renal systems
- Limbs, digits, and spine

Gonads
- Palpable or not?
- Location and size?

Genital examination
- Size of phallus/glans well-formed?
- Location of the urethral meatus
- Degree of fusion of labioscrotal folds
- Scrotum well or poorly developed and rugosity/symmetry/hyperpigmentation
- Position of anus/anal abnormality
- Anogenital distance

Baseline tests
- Karyotype (or SRY FISH)
- Pelvic and abdominal ultrasound scan to assess for gonads/Müllerian structures
- Monitor blood glucose (hypoglycemia); serial monitoring of serum electrolytes and arterial blood gases (hyponatremia, hyperkalemia, and normal anion gap metabolic acidosis)
- *Adrenal steroids:* Serum 17-hydroxyprogesterone (17OHP)
- *Gonadal function:* Serum testosterone/LH/FSH, DHT, AMH

Contd...

Contd...

Hormonal evaluation
- Cortisol, ACTH, plasma renin activity (PRA)
- ACTH (cosyntropin) stimulation test
- hCG stimulation test in 46,XY DSDs for evaluation of testicular function (T:DHT <10:1 normal when expressed in same units)
- Serum dehydroepiandrosterone sulfate (DHEAS)
- 11-deoxycortisol, deoxycorticosterone (DOC)

Further testing
- Magnetic resonance imaging (MRI sensitive for gonadal tissue identification)
- Laparoscopic gonadal biopsy
- Retrograde genitogram (to determine genital anatomy, useful in operative planning)
- Genetic studies (target gene sequencing, whole genome sequencing)

(ACTH: Adrenocorticotropic hormone; AMH: Anti-Müllerian hormone; DHT: Dihydrotestosterone; FISH: Fluorescent in situ hybridization; LH: Luteinizing hormone; FSH: Follicle stimulating hormone; hCG: Human chorionic gonadotropin; SRY: sex-determining region on the Y-chromosome)

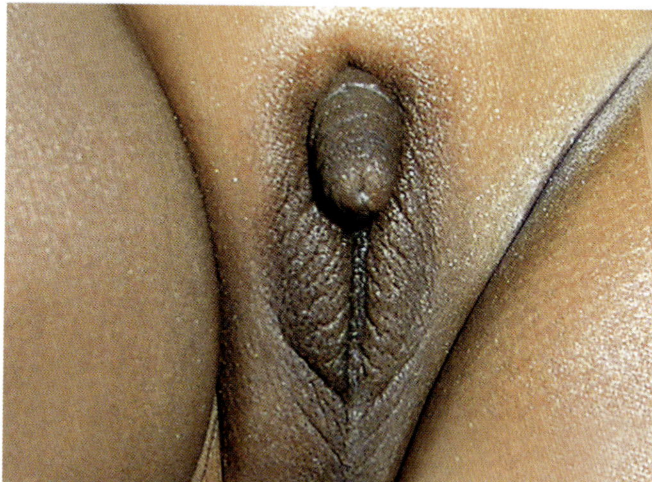

Fig. 16.9.3: Hypogonadism with microphallus in a 2-year-old boy with panhypopituitarism.

strongly suggests the possibility of CAH due to salt-losing 21-hydroxylase deficiency.[4] Non-salt-losers with this condition will present with the combination of increased pigmentation and virilization but without the dramatic signs of salt loss.[4]

Female infants presenting with increased pigmentation, hypokalemia, hypertension, and virilization are most likely to have 11β-hydroxylase deficiency **(Fig. 16.9.2)**. These signs may not be present universally, especially during infancy. Boys with this condition will have peripheral precocious puberty. Low cortisol and renin values are encountered.

If physical examination reveals the presence of a gonad, it is most often a testis, and the infant is a case of 46,XY DSD.

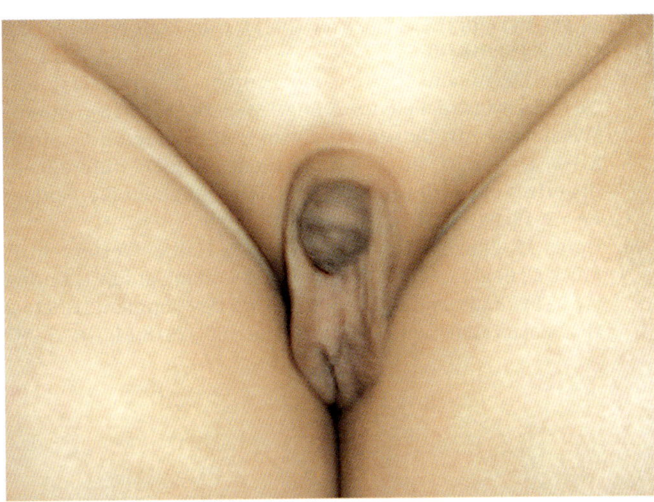

Fig. 16.9.4: A 1-year-old boy with severe hypogonadism due to panhypopituitarism.

If there is no gonad palpable, the genetic sex cannot be identified clinically, and further workup is essential.[2,3]

The phallus is measured for its length and width of erectile tissue and examined for chordee. Presence of separate openings of vagina and urethra should be looked for as also pigmentation and rugosity of labioscrotal folds.

It is often the responsibility of the pediatric endocrinologist or primary care physician to inform the parents of an infant born with uncertain gender and to discuss with them in detail about the nature of the defect observed, the need for the investigations to establish the diagnosis, the gender of rearing best suited for the infant. It is important to allay the anxiety and guilt of the parents and other family members in repeated sessions and to explain the available modalities and plan of treatment. To deal with the DSD optimally, a full team is ideal, viz., pediatric endocrinologist, neonatologist, family pediatrician, pediatric surgeon or urologist. Gynecologist, radiologist, ultrasonologist, biochemist, cytogeneticist, pediatric psychologist/psychiatrist as well as nursing colleague, and social worker.[5,6] Support group of parents with similarly affected children will also be helpful. Most importantly, the parents should be included in all discussions concerning the evaluation and management of the infant with DSD. It is always important to collect together all possible evidences for arriving at a diagnosis and then have discussions with the parents. Although urgency is still necessary, most parents will be willing to wait for a few days longer before making their decision about their child's gender and future. Until the decision is made, it is better to refer to the infant as "baby", and not as "he" or "she".[5,6]

INVESTIGATIONS

The workup of a child with a DSD is complex, and requires a specialist's inputs. However, all efforts should be made to diagnose CAH (the common variety 21-hydroxylase deficiency is responsible for 95% of CAH cases) so as to start life-saving hydrocortisone. Serum 17-hydroxyprogesterone (17OHP), electrolytes, blood gas, blood glucose, and serum cortisol, can be done immediately. The reader is referred to **Box 16.9.1** for baseline tests, hormonal evaluation, and further investigations.

MANAGEMENT

The management should focus on initial stabilization, accurate diagnosis, and decisions on the gender of rearing and planning of surgical interventions and/or hormonal treatment.[5,6]

The most common cause of atypical genitalia is 21-hydroxylase deficiency in genetic females. Nearly 75% present with salt loss typically during the second week of life. Hyperpigmentation of the skin, especially the nipples, umbilicus, and external genitalia should alert one to the diagnosis even before salt-losing manifestations appear. This clinical sign is particularly useful in males with CAH as they do not present with any abnormality of the external genitalia but have a high risk of shock due to salt loss. In the presence of the history of a previous sibling or family member involved, biochemical investigations may be performed earlier to hasten the diagnosis.[4]

Virilized females with CAH having a uterus and ovaries are assigned the female gender. Clitoral reduction and genitoplasty are usually undertaken around 1 year of age. Recommendations for assignment of gender in an individual with fully virilized male external genitalia and presence of female internal sex structures are still controversial.[5,6] Reconstructive surgery for hypospadias is needed in those with conditions like 5α-reductase deficiency. Assignment of a female gender to an individual with microphallus and fused scrotum, which was common practice in the past in Western societies, is being reconsidered and not always accepted today by many. This is often because gender identity in many individuals with a DSD may evolve at puberty to be discordant from gender of rearing. Thus, current guidelines go against irrevocable surgery of reproductive organs until past puberty and at the age of legal consent.[5,6] Testosterone therapy is recommended for microphallus and fused scrotum. In summary, there are no easy answers always for the assignment of gender in DSD.

CONCLUSION

Understanding normal sex determination and differentiation is essential for clinical approach of a child with disordered sex development in order to plan the line of investigation and to arrive at the right diagnosis for ideal management and optimal outcome.

REFERENCES

1. Grinspon RP, Bergadá I, Rey RA. Male hypogonadism and disorders of sex development. Front Endocrinol (Lausanne). 2020;11:211.
2. Grinspon RP, Castro S, Rey RA. Up-to-Date clinical and biochemical workup of the child and the adolescent with a suspected disorder of sex development. Horm Res Paediatr. 2023;96(2):116-27.
3. Ahmed SF, Achermann J, Alderson J, Crouch NS, Elford S, Hughes IA, et al. Society for Endocrinology UK Guidance on the initial evaluation of a suspected difference or disorder of sex development (Revised 2021). Clin Endocrinol (Oxf). 2021;95(6):818-40.
4. Merke DP, Auchus RJ. Congenital adrenal hyperplasia due to 21-hydroxylase deficiency. N Engl J Med. 2020;383(13):1248-61.
5. Wisniewski AB, Batista RL, Costa EMF, Finlayson C, Sircili MHP, Dénes FT, et al. Management of 46,XY differences/disorders of sex development (DSD) throughout life. Endocr Rev. 2019;40(6):1547-72.
6. Cools M, Nordenström A, Robeva R, Hall J, Westerveld P, Flück C, et al.; COST Action BM1303 working group 1. Caring for individuals with a difference of sex development (DSD): a Consensus Statement. Nat Rev Endocrinol. 2018;14(7):415-29.

16.10 Diabetes Mellitus

Medha Mittal, Vijayalakshmi Bhatia

INTRODUCTION

Diabetes mellitus is a group of metabolic disorders that manifest as hyperglycemia and result from defects in insulin secretion, action, or both. Apart from its short-term and long-term complications, it has significant impact on the growth and puberty of the child, besides having far reaching implications for the quality of life of the entire family. The classification of diabetes is as mentioned in the **Box 16.10.1**. Diabetes in childhood is mainly type 1 and will be the main focus of this chapter.

TYPE 1 DIABETES MELLITUS

EPIDEMIOLOGY

The prevalence of type 1 diabetes mellitus (T1D) is quite varied, maximum in Finland and least in China and Japan.[1,2] In USA, the prevalence in the age group below 20 years is 3.5 per 1,000. As per estimates of the International Diabetes Federation, there are about 16,000 new cases of T1D of age group 0–14 years in India every year, and we already have the second largest number of children with diabetes

BOX 16.10.1: Classification of diabetes.

Type 1 diabetes (T1D)

IA: Immune mediated

IB: Idiopathic

Type 2 diabetes (T2D)

Others

- *Monogenic diabetes:*
  - Maturity-onset diabetes of the young (MODY)—HNF4A, HNF1A, GCK, HNF1B
  - Neonatal diabetes—KCNJ11, ABCC8, GATA6, 6Q24, EIF2AK3
- *Defects in insulin action—INSR*, congenital generalized lipodystrophy, familial partial lipodystrophy, PIK3R1
- *Diseases of pancreas (exocrine part)*—Pancreatitis, pancreatectomy, neoplasia, cystic fibrosis, and hemochromatosis (thalassemia)
- *Endocrinopathies*—Acromegaly, Cushing syndrome, hyperthyroidism, pheochromocytoma, and glucagonoma
- Drug/chemical induced insulin deficiency and/or resistance—Glucocorticoids, statins, protease inhibitors (first generation), L-asparaginase, diazoxide, phenytoin, pentamidine, cyclosporine, tacrolimus, and atypical antipsychotics
- *Infections*—Rubella, enterovirus
- *Polyendocrinopathies*—Autoimmune polyendocrine deficiency syndromes (APS1 and 2)
- *Genetic syndromes associated with diabetes*—Down, Turner, Prader–Willi, Wolfram, Lawrence–Moon–Biedl, and Klinefelter syndromes
- *Immune-mediated diabetes*—Immune dysregulation, polyendocrinopathy, enteropathy and X-linked (IPEX) syndrome, and autoimmune polyendocrinopathy candidiasis ectodermal dysplasia (APECED) syndromes

living in a single country, in this age group. The peak age of onset of diabetes is between 5–8 years and 10–14 years. The presentation is often with diabetic ketoacidosis (DKA), especially in developing countries.

ETIOPATHOGENESIS

The T1D is a chronic disease, causing gradual destruction of pancreatic β cells, resulting in partial or complete deficiency of insulin. The underlying etiology is autoimmunity or in some cases, idiopathic. Certain factors influence the pathogenetic process including environmental factors, genetic background, age, and ethnicity. T lymphocytes, that mediate the damage, recognize a β cell antigen when it is presented bound with a human leukocyte antigen (HLA) molecule. The presence of the HLA molecules and their type will hence influence the susceptibility to develop T1D with HLA class II molecules (DR and DQ) having the strongest association. Among Caucasians, the association is strongest with DR3/DQ2 and DR4/DQ8 while among Indians, strong association has been found with DR3/DQ2. The other genetic predispositions have been attributed to insulin gene, the *PTPN22* gene and about 60 other minor alleles. How the environmental factors act is not quite clear. The "hygiene hypothesis" suggests that exposure to environmental factors such as viruses improves innate immunity and their absence might trigger autoimmunity. On the other hand, certain viruses may directly destroy pancreatic β cells, the most notable being congenital rubella infection. A shorter duration of breastfeeding and exposure to cow milk might also be a trigger.

With a trigger, there is initiation of β cell death that releases β cell autoantigens. These reach the draining lymph nodes where there are T cells that get activated and proliferate and initiate damage. B cells also get activated and produce autoantibodies, which are markers of autoimmunity but not the mediators of destruction. Cytokines produced during destruction of beta cells further increase the damage.

T1D has a long latent period before the manifest stage of hyperglycemia. An individual who is genetically predisposed and exposed to environmental factors develops autoantibodies to β cells, initially one and thereafter more. There are typically four stages in the build-up to overt diabetes:[3]

1. *Stage 1:* ≥2 islet autoantibodies, normal blood glucose (BG) (fasting plasma glucose <100 mg/dL)
2. *Stage 2:* ≥2 islet autoantibodies, abnormal glucose tolerance (fasting plasma glucose 100–125 mg/dL)
3. *Stage 3:* Stage of hyperglycemia, BG above American Diabetes Association (ADA) diagnostic thresholds, initially asymptomatic, symptomatic later (fasting plasma glucose ≥126 mg/dL)
4. *Stage 4:* Established T1D

In stage 1, there is a 44% 5-year risk of progression to stage 3 while in stage 2 the risk is 75%.

PATHOPHYSIOLOGY

Insulin being an anabolic hormone promotes glucose utilization by muscle and adipose tissue and keeps a check on activity of counter-regulatory hormones. Lack of insulin results in a catabolic state and unopposed action of glucagon, catecholamines, and cortisol. The reduced glucose uptake coupled with increased production by glycogenolysis and gluconeogenesis results in hyperglycemia. The hormonal imbalance also causes increased proteolysis and lipolysis that lead to muscle wasting, loss of subcutaneous fat, and increased output of free fatty acids from adipose tissue. These fatty acids accumulate in liver as triglycerides causing fatty liver and get oxidized to ketone bodies. The buffer systems of the body attempt to neutralize the ketoacids with a resultant decrease in serum bicarbonate along with hyperventilation causing fall in CO_2.

The classical symptoms of diabetes and its dreaded complication of DKA result from the high osmolar load causing diuresis (polyuria) leading to dehydration, and loss of electrolytes and minerals. This prompts the urge to have more water (polydipsia) and the loss of glucose prompts the urge to have more food (polyphagia).

CLINICAL FEATURES

The classical features of diabetes are polyuria, polyphagia, and polydipsia. Despite the polyphagia there is weight loss. Frequent urination or nocturnal enuresis in a previously dry child, ants noticed around urine, or a genital infection may bring the child to medical attention. The presentation may be with respiratory distress (hyperventilation) or with abdominal pain or vomiting. It may be mistaken for bronchial asthma, gastroenteritis, or meningoencephalitis. Hence, it is important to do a BG in every such condition. Often the initial presentation is with deep sighing respiration (Kussmaul respiration) with a fruity odor of ketones, vomiting, dehydration, and altered sensorium, suggestive of DKA.

DIAGNOSIS

With a child having classical symptoms, the diagnosis may be straightforward with the demonstration of hyperglycemia (random plasma glucose >200 mg/dL) **(Box 16.10.2)**. Routine testing for autoantibodies and C-peptide is not needed unless there is suspicion of type 2 diabetes (T2D) or maturity-onset diabetes of the young (MODY). Screening for other autoimmune conditions, such as thyroiditis, celiac disease should be planned. Glycosylated hemoglobin, HbA1c, indicates the glucose tolerance

BOX 16.10.2: Criteria for diagnosis of diabetes mellitus.

Any of the following criteria would classify the child as diabetes:
- Classic symptoms of diabetes or hyperglycemic crisis with plasma glucose ≥200 mg/dL
- Fasting plasma glucose ≥126 mg/dL
- HbA1c >6.5% along with presence of symptoms
- Oral glucose tolerance test (OGTT) result demonstrating 2-hour postload glucose ≥200 mg/dL. This is usually not indicated for diagnosing T1D though may be useful in diagnosing other forms such as type 2 diabetes (T2D) or cystic fibrosis-related diabetes

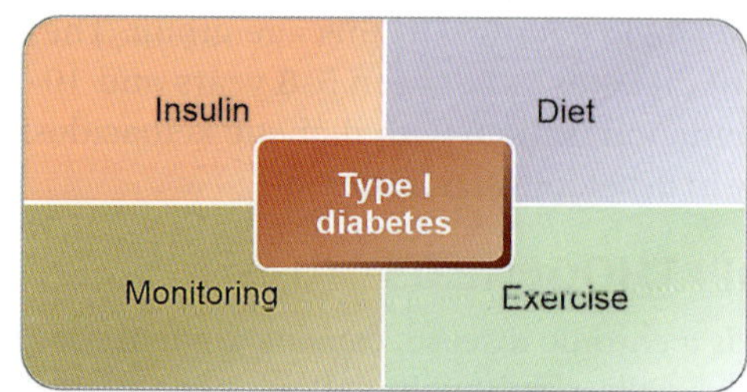

Fig. 16.10.1: Four important aspects of diabetes management.

over past 3 months and is useful for both diagnosis and monitoring the control.

If the child is brought with a report of glycosuria, other features should be carefully assessed and renal conditions ruled out. Sometimes, a sick child may have temporary stress-induced hyperglycemia but it settles gradually.

A child brought with altered sensorium, and hyperventilation (acidotic breathing), should be assessed for presence of blood or urine ketones by bedside ketone meter or dipsticks, respectively and for presence of acidosis (by venous blood gas) so as not to miss DKA.

MANAGEMENT

The management of the child has to be planned as per the presentation. If the child is stable and not in DKA, insulin therapy can be advised on an outpatient basis with education and counseling though it is often better to admit for a few days so that the nuances of diabetes management can be learnt well by the family. If the child has presented acutely with DKA, emergency measures have to be taken for stabilization—securing the airway, supporting the breathing with oxygen or assisted ventilation, and the circulation with intravenous fluids—before initiating insulin therapy.

The four pillars of diabetes management are insulin therapy, medical nutrition therapy (MNT), exercise, and monitoring **(Fig. 16.10.1)**.[4,5] A team of an experienced pediatrician/pediatric endocrinologist, diabetes educator, motivated family, a dietician, social worker, and a psychologist, would be best to enable optimum management with help from patient support groups if available. The goal of management is to gradually achieve a good glycemic control through the day and an optimum growth and development, keeping in mind the child's and family's customs and choices so as to have a good quality of life and minimize complications.

Insulin Therapy[4,5]

Insulin, discovered by Banting and Best about 100 years ago, is the cornerstone of management. The aim of insulin therapy is to match as closely as possible the physiologic insulin secretion from the pancreas which has a steady continuous secretion all through the day and peaks in response to glycemic surge after ingestion of food. Rapid-acting or short-acting insulin injections are given subcutaneously (SC) at mealtimes (bolus) and long-acting insulin is given once or twice a day to achieve a steady continuous insulin level (basal). The initial requirements may be high at 1.0–1.2 units/kg/day thereafter stabilizing at 0.5–1.0 units/kg/day. If the child is not in DKA, 0.5–0.7 units/kg/day may be started.

Types of Insulin

The various insulin types available to us are tabulated in **Table 16.10.1.** The older insulins or conventional insulin are regular (short-acting, natural insulin of the human islet) insulin and neutral protamine Hagedorn (NPH, intermediate-acting). They can be used in different combinations but premixed insulin combinations are not appropriate for use in children as one cannot modify the dose of one of the insulin types individually. Various insulin analogs are now available that allow greater flexibility of use with meals. Rapid-acting insulin analogs include lispro, aspart, glulisine, and recently developed fast-acting insulin aspart (Fiasp). These can be injected 10–15 minutes before meals, (or sometimes part of dose could be injected postmeal, when not sure of intake in toddlers). However, due to short duration of action, additional doses may be required for snacks. The long-acting insulin analogs have a relatively peakless action profile that avoids the hypoglycemia seen with NPH based regimes. Regular and NPH are available as 40 IU/mL or as 100 IU/mL preparations (and should be administered with the appropriate U40 or U100 syringe if in vials or may be available as cartridges to be used with injector pens) while the analogs are available as 100 IU/mL preparations, mostly as cartridges, to be used with their injection pens **(Fig. 16.10.2)**. NPH needs additional care that it has to be shaken well before each use as it tends to precipitate.

Insulin Regimens

- *Split mix regimen:* This was the earlier used regimen and has fallen out of favor due to the marked glycemic

TABLE 16.10.1: Action profile of different types of insulin preparations.

Insulin type	*Onset of action (hours)*	*Peak effect (hours)*	*Duration of action (hours)*
Bolus insulin			
Ultra-rapid acting aspart	0.1–0.2	1–3	3–5
Lispro/aspart/glulisine	0.2–0.3	1–3	3–5
Regular	0.5–1.0	2–4	6–8
Basal insulin			
NPH	2–3	4–6	12–14
Glargine/Detemir	2–4	8–10	22–24
Glargine U300	2–4	Peakless	30–36
Degludec	0.5–1.5	Peakless	>42

(NPH: neutral protamine Hagedorn)

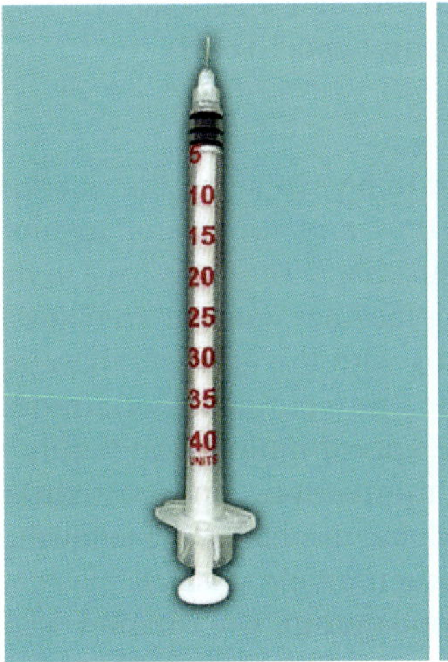

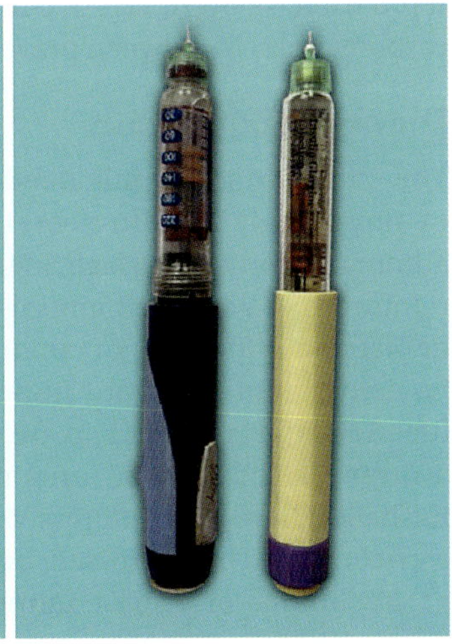

Fig. 16.10.2: Different insulin administration devices—syringe and injector pens (loaded with cartridge). The syringe shown here is for 40 IU/mL insulin. 100 IU syringes also available.

variability seen with it. Regular insulin was administered twice a day along with NPH which was mixed in the same syringe. The regular insulin covered glycemic excursions at breakfast and dinner and NPH provided the basal insulin with its daytime peak expected to cover lunch. However, the NPH peaks often caused hypoglycemia in the evening and at midnight. Further, since syringes are reused a few times for cost saving, a little NPH is always inadvertently introduced into the vial of regular insulin, rendering it partially intermediate-acting. Thus, a few modifications are necessary to use these cost effective insulins:

- Use of different syringes may be considered for regular and NPH insulins
- A dose of regular insulin at lunch will give better glucose control, and will allow the morning NPH dose to be smaller;
- Delaying the night NPH dose to bedtime rather than with regular insulin before dinner may decrease midnight hypoglycemia, and
- Bedtime snack is given to counter midnight NPH related hypoglycemia.

- *Basal bolus regimen:* Bolus dose of regular insulin or rapid-acting analog is given thrice a day to cover for each major meal and the basal requirement is met with a long-acting analog. This regimen provides a better glycemic control through the day. Basal insulin is started at 40–60% of the total dose (less in toddlers) while the rest is given as bolus doses with subsequent modifications as required.
- *Continuous subcutaneous insulin infusion (insulin pumps):* This battery-operated device uses continuous infusion of rapid-acting insulin at a low basal rate to provide the basal needs as well as bolus doses premeal. They provide a better glycemic control with fewer episodes of hypoglycemia. At the time of writing, pumps with an integrated continuous glucose monitoring systems (CGMS), which will automatically modulate basal insulin injection rate based on the ambient BG, (artificial pancreas), are already in use in India.[6] Only the prandial doses have to be enabled by the patient. However, at present, their cost may be prohibitive for use by most patients.

Precautions with Use of Insulin

- *Storage:* Unopened insulin vials should be stored at 2–8°C but never frozen. The ones in use can be kept at 15–30°C. If there is no refrigerator it can be kept in an earthenware clay vessel kept inside a larger pot.
- *Rotation of injection site:* The suitable injection sites include the lateral sides of abdomen avoiding the area just below the umbilicus, front and outer aspects of thighs, and the buttocks. Arm is not a preferred site due to the paucity of subcutaneous tissue. Care has to be taken to rotate the injection site for each prick to avoid lipohypertrophy that might otherwise result **(Figs. 16.10.3A and B)**.
- *Disposal of needles:* All used needles must be collected in a puncture proof plastic container and safely disposed in a medical facility and not in general garbage.

Medical Nutrition Therapy for Type 1 Diabetes Mellitus

The total recommended caloric intake is similar to any other child. The meal plan for the day is divided into three major

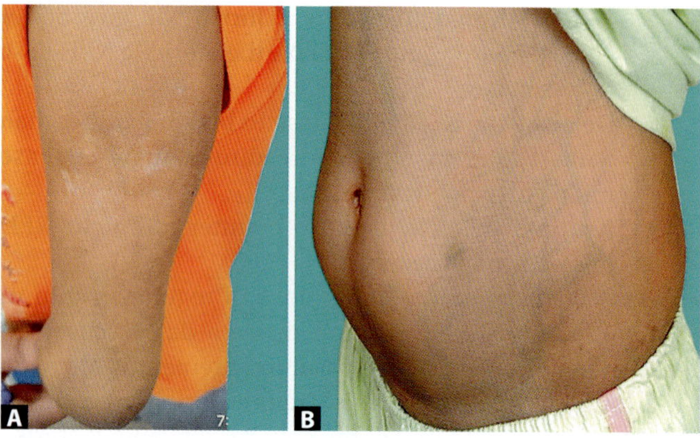

Figs. 16.10.3A and B: Complications of repeated insulin injections. (A) Fibrosis and scarring on left arm; (B) Lipohypertrophy on lower abdominal wall.

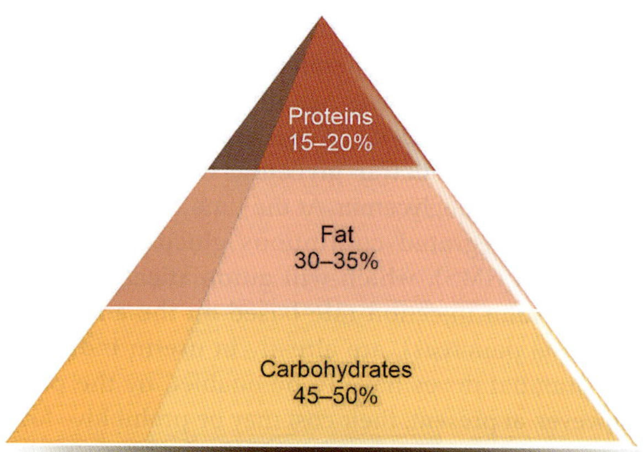

Fig. 16.10.4: Recommended macronutrient distribution for medical nutrition therapy for type 1 diabetes.

meals with 2-3 snacks. A balanced diet providing 45-50% caloric intake as carbohydrates, 30-35% as fats, and 15-20% as proteins should be planned.[4,5] **(Fig. 16.10.4)**. Carbohydrates have the greatest impact on immediate BG excursion. Fiber rich and complex carbohydrates with low glycemic load (the rise in BG with the food intake) and glycemic index (the rapidity of rise of BG) should be emphasized. Saturated fats must be limited to 10% of caloric intake and trans fats avoided. Carbohydrate counting and food groups and exchanges/ portion size recognition can be taught to parents and for occasions where extra carbohydrates may be taken, increased insulin dose can be given. This allows flexibility in the child's daily schedule and improves quality of life and compliance to the management plan.

Monitoring[4,5]

- *Anthropometry*
- *Glycemic control*, glycosylated hemoglobin gives an estimate of average BG over the preceding 8-12 weeks. The aim is to keep the HbA1c at <7%. In addition, BG 6-7 times daily (before meal and 2 hours after and often at 2-3 AM) or as often as feasible, by finger prick and glucometer, aids good BG control without too much hypoglycemia. The glycemic targets are to keep the BG between 80 and 160 or 180 mg/dL after meals and between 70 and 140 mg/dL before meals. During illnesses, more frequent testing is necessary.
- *Continuous glucose monitoring systems,* a boon for patients with T1D, enable frequent BG checks without finger-prick, the tissue glucose reading via a subcutaneous sensor filament being a fairly accurate surrogate for BG.[7]
- *Ketones* can also be checked during times of illness either by urine ketostrips or blood ketone meters (more reliable).

Exercise

Physical activity should be encouraged as it improves insulin sensitivity and lipid profile. Moderate physical activity of 60 minutes is recommended as for any other child. A pre-exercise BG of 150-200 mg/dL or a small snack (5-15 g carbohydrate) in between prevents hypoglycemia.

Diabetes Education

The child and the family need to be explained the science of physiologic insulin secretion and the art of insulin administration and dosage adjustment. The skills have to be reinforced at each visit aiming for finer control. The initial denial and difficulties of coping with the diagnosis have to be gently guided toward hope and confidence of a fuller life. The approach has to be appropriate to the family's awareness, education, and motivation. Any particular misbeliefs have to be addressed and dispelled. The following aspects should be addressed, over multiple sessions:

- Technique of insulin administration, site rotation, and storage
- Dosage adjustment when there is hyperglycemia, for exercise
- Hypoglycemia prevention and treatment
- Dietary counseling including carbohydrate counting and exchange
- Sick day management
- Importance of regular exercise

In brief, the family and child are entrusted and empowered to handle the entire management with guidance from the diabetes management team. The school teacher should also be informed and guided regarding the management in general and hypoglycemia in particular.

ACUTE COMPLICATIONS

Diabetic Ketoacidosis

This is a life-threatening emergency and the most common reason for admission to hospital. It is characterized by

BG >200 mg/dL, acidosis (venous pH <7.3 or bicarbonate <18 mmol/L), and ketonuria (moderate to large) or ketonemia (serum ketones >3 mmol/L). The common symptoms include nausea, vomiting, abdominal pain, rapid and deep breathing (Kussmaul breathing) that has a fruity odor and altered sensorium. Often the initial presentation of diabetes, it may be misinterpreted as respiratory distress, acute abdomen, gastroenteritis, or encephalitis. Signs of dehydration are relatively less due to hyperosmolality. A history of good urine output in a child with dehydration may point to the diagnosis of DKA.

DKA may be classified as:

- *Mild:* pH <7.3 or serum bicarbonate <18 mmol/L
- *Moderate:* pH <7.2 or serum bicarbonate <10 mmol/L
- *Severe:* pH <7.1 or serum bicarbonate <5 mmol/L.

Treatment of Diabetic Ketoacidosis[8]

- *ABC:* Airway, breathing, and a stable intravenous (IV) access are secured.
- *Fluid bolus:* 10–20 mL/kg over 20–30 minutes followed by IV fluids for maintenance and deficit correction at 6–10% over 36–48 hours. Usual fluids are normal saline for initial 6 hours followed by either N/2 or NS (with dextrose added as per BG levels).
- *Insulin:* Insulin is always started after an hour of fluid therapy. Regular insulin given IV at 0.1 unit/kg/h, constituted as infusion in normal saline. Lower dose infusion (0.05 unit/kg/h) is started in milder acidosis where pH is >7.15. An IV bolus may rapidly decrease intravascular osmotic pressure and precipitate shock and hence never given. Infusion is continued at same rate until resolution of acidosis (pH >7.3 and serum bicarbonate >15 mEq/mL) and thereafter stopped, overlapping it with subcutaneous insulin.
- *Hyperglycemia* settles earlier than acidosis and hence insulin infusion needs to be continued. When BG falls <250 mg/dL, 5% dextrose (or sometimes 10%) is added to IV fluids to prevent hypoglycemia.
- *Potassium* is added to IV fluids at 40 mEq/L (higher than usual concentration of 20 mEq/L) as insulin causes extracellular potassium to move intracellular.
- *Monitoring* sensorium, heart rate, BG hourly, serum electrolytes and blood ketones 4–6 hourly.
- With resolution of acidosis and improvement in general condition, the child would be able to take orally and is shifted from insulin infusion to subcutaneous (SC) injections.

Hypoglycemia

The BG levels below 70 mg/dL indicate hypoglycemia. The symptoms may be headache, nausea, irritability, autonomic symptoms such as sweating, trembling, palpitations and pallor, or neuroglycopenic symptoms (at BG <54 mg/dL) such as poor concentration, blurred vision, weakness, dizziness, loss of sensorium, or even seizures. These may occur due to excessive insulin doses, exercise uncompensated with food, or missed meals.

Treatment

The child should be administered oral glucose (10–15 g) followed by any carbohydrate snack if he/she can take orally. If not able to swallow or unconscious, injectable glucagon can be administered subcutaneously (SC) and can be taught to the caregivers. Dextrose containing fluids are administered in hospital settings.

Prevention

- Use of inappropriate syringe (use of 40 IU syringe for 100 IU/mL insulin) can result in inadvertently high insulin dose and should always be checked for.
- Using regular insulin and intermediate-acting insulin before dinner may cause nocturnal hypoglycemia as the latter has a peak effect in the middle of the night. For this, the intermediate-acting insulin is given as a separate injection at bedtime (to stagger its effect from that of the regular insulin) or replaced by a long-acting analog.
- A carbohydrate snack should be taken before moderate exercise.
- Regular BG monitoring
- A few months after the initiation of insulin in a new onset diabetes, the β-cell inflammation reduces and the insulin requirement significantly declines. Reduction of insulin doses is required for a few months till this "honeymoon phase" lasts (and then the requirement goes up again).

Precautions

Children with T1D should always carry a small snack and a sachet or tablet of glucose along with a diabetes identification card. Parents and caregivers must be trained to administer glucagon.

LONG-TERM COMPLICATIONS

Longstanding diabetes especially with poor glycemic control leads to various microvascular and macrovascular complications and these should be screened for as mentioned in **Table 16.10.2.** Along with these other autoimmune conditions should be screened for. Growth parameters should be assessed at every visit.

The mechanism underlying the microvascular complications are still not completely understood. Advanced glycation end products, sorbitol, and oxidant tissue injury

TABLE 16.10.2: Screen for complications.

Parameter	*Evaluate*	*Frequency*
Growth and development	Weight, height, body mass index (BMI), pubertal development	At every visit
Autoimmunity	Screen for thyroid function, celiac disease	At diagnosis and every 2 years
	Adrenal function, autoimmune hepatitis	As clinically indicated
Microvascular complications	*Kidney disease:* Urine albumin: creatinine ratio	Start from age 11 years or puberty whichever is earlier, after 2–5 years of diabetes duration, then annually for kidney disease and neuropathy; every 2 years for retinopathy >10 years age—annually
	Retinopathy: Retinal examination	
	Neuropathy: Examine clinically; nerve studies if indicated	
Cardiovascular risk	Serum lipid profile	Begin after 11 years age and every 3 years if results are normal
	Blood pressure	Every visit

have been variously implicated. There are organ-specific changes such as mesangial hypertrophy in the kidney, basement membrane thickening, hyperfiltration, hyperperfusion, and glomerular hypertrophy that precede the development of albuminuria. Overt proteinuria or kidney failure are rare in children and adolescents with T1D.

Neuropathy manifests as tingling and numbness with involvement of distal unmyelinated nerve fibers in a classic glove and stocking distribution. Involvement of motor nerves is rare. Involvement of retinal neurovasculature could result in retinopathy with potential threat to vision. Increased duration of diabetes, poor glycemic control, hypertension, and albuminuria are known risk factors.

All adolescents with T1D should be screened for early signs of microvascular complications and identification of modifiable risk factors. Atherosclerosis starts in childhood with increased intima media thickness detected in carotids and aorta. Poor glycemic control is associated with dyslipidemia and further increases the cardiovascular risk. Overweight/obesity and hypertension are also common in youth and together with other factors contribute to risk of cardiovascular disease related mortality.

OTHER COMMON TYPES OF DIABETES MELLITUS IN CHILDREN

TYPE 2 DIABETES

While a few decades back all diabetes in children was considered T1D, it is no longer so. Type 2 diabetes (T2D) is being increasingly reported with onset in early teens and constitutes about 8% of pediatric diabetes. The demographic pattern is quite different between the West and Asia with as many as 15–50% of the patients in the latter being of normal weight.

BOX 16.10.3: Criteria for screening for type 2 diabetes (T2D) in children after the onset of puberty or after age 10 years, whichever is earlier.[9]

- Overweight or obese
- One or more of the following:
  - T2D in a first or second degree relative
  - High risk racial and/or ethnic status
  - Signs of insulin resistance or conditions associated with insulin resistance: Acanthosis nigricans, dyslipidemia, hypertension, polycystic ovarian syndrome or small for gestational age at birth or high birth weight
  - Maternal T2D or gestational diabetes
  - Current use of weight promoting atypical antipsychotic agents

While in T1D the main pathology lies in reduced insulin secretion from the β-cells of pancreas, in T2D there is end-organ resistance (hepatic, adipose, and peripheral tissue) to insulin prompting further insulin secretion and thus hyperinsulinemia. There may be additional β-cell dysfunction causing insulin deficiency and α-cell dysfunction causing hyperglucagonemia. The importance of making a correct diagnosis lies in the risk of complications which are much more in T2D. Indians are ethnically a high-risk group for T2D and overweight children above the age of 10 years need to be screened **(Box 16.10.3)**.[9] Youth-onset T2D is more frequent in females and familial clustering of cases is known. In utero exposure to maternal overnutrition and diabetes lead to fetal overnutrition and are risk factors for T2D in the offspring. On the other hand, maternal undernutrition, intrauterine growth restriction, and rapid catch-up growth in the infant are also known risk factors. Breastfeeding may reduce the risk.

Diagnosis and Complications

The lab criteria for diagnosis of T2D are similar to that of T1 along with absence of islet cell antibodies. The target glycemic ranges are also similar. Complications include hypertension, dyslipidemia, nephropathy, nonalcoholic fatty liver disease, polycystic ovarian syndrome, retinopathy, and neuropathy and have to be screened for at diagnosis and regularly thereafter.

Management

Diet and lifestyle modifications constitute the main focus of management with at least 1 hour of moderate to vigorous physical activity and <2 hours of television/screen time. The diet should be rich in fiber with reduced carbohydrate and fat intake targeted at reducing weight.

Pharmacologic therapy is used in those not controlled. Biguanides (metformin) act by reducing hepatic gluconeogenesis and stimulating peripheral glucose uptake and are the main line of therapy. Insulin may need to be started initially in those who present in ketoacidosis and basal insulin is continued for a few months along with oral metformin and later metformin is increased and insulin withdrawn. Others include glucagon-like-peptide 1 (GLP-1) receptor agonists that act by increasing insulin secretion in response to BG rise, suppress glucagon, and prolong gastric emptying promoting satiety and weight loss. Liraglutide, administered as daily SC injections, has been approved for use in 12–17 year olds.

MONOGENIC DIABETES

Diabetes resulting due to mutations in genes causing beta cell loss or dysfunction is known as monogenic diabetes. It may present before 6 months of age (neonatal diabetes) or as autosomal dominant familial diabetes of the young known as maturity onset diabetes of the young (MODY).[10]

Neonatal Diabetes

Diabetes presenting before the age of 6 months is known as neonatal diabetes and these infants should have immediate molecular genetic testing. Those presenting between 6 and 12 months of age and are negative for islet cell antibody should also be tested. The genetic testing would allow prediction of the clinical course as some may be transient neonatal diabetes that would resolve eventually whereas others may be permanent neonatal diabetes. Of the permanent ones some may be amenable to treatment by oral drugs (such as sulfonylureas) and can be taken off insulin. Most of these mutations arise de novo but do have a 50% risk of recurrence in the offspring.

Maturity-onset Diabetes of the Young

This presents as mild hyperglycemia in the adolescent or young adult with a family history of diabetes and transmitted as an autosomal dominant trait. They rarely go into ketosis because of residual insulin secretion that persists for many years. There are different subtypes with slightly differing features and risk of complications. Most of these may also respond to sulfonylureas. In peripubertal children diagnosed as T1D or T2D without obesity, one should keep a possibility of MODY and undertake appropriate genetic testing.

CONCLUSION

Each physician needs to be aware of the varied manifestations of diabetes in children. Insulin remains the cornerstone of management. With the increasing prevalence of overweight and obesity, prevalence of T2D is rising at an alarming rate and has a more aggressive course and earlier onset of complications. With availability of molecular genetics, advancements have been possible to recognize the genetic forms and undertake appropriate management.

REFERENCES

1. Karvonen M, Viik-Kajander M, Moltchanova E, Libman I, LaPorte R, Tuomilehto J. Incidence of childhood type 1 diabetes worldwide. Diabetes Mondiales (DiaMond) Project Group. Diabetes Care. 2000;23(10):1516-26.
2. Knip M. Type 1 diabetes in Finland: past, present, and future. Lancet Diab Endocrinol. 2021;9(5):259-60.
3. Besser REJ, Bell KJ, Couper JJ, Ziegler AG, Wherrett DK, Knip M, et al. ISPAD Clinical Practice Consensus Guidelines 2022: Stages of type 1 diabetes in children and adolescents. Pediatr Diabetes. 2022;23(8):1175-87.
4. Limbert C, Tinti D, Malik F, Kosteria I, Messer L, Jalaludin MY, et al. ISPAD Clinical Practice Consensus Guidelines 2022: The delivery of ambulatory diabetes care to children and adolescents with diabetes. Pediatr Diabetes. 2022;23(8): 1243-69.
5. Virmani A. Ambulatory Management of Type 1 Diabetes Mellitus. In: Desai MP, Menon PSN, Bhatia V, Seth A (Eds.). Pediatric Endocrine Disorders, 4th edition. Hyderabad: Universities Press India Pvt Ltd; 2022. pp. 394-410.
6. Bionic Pancreas Research Group; Russell SJ, Beck RW, Damiano ER, El-Khatib FH, Ruedy KJ, et al. Multicenter, Randomized Trial of a Bionic Pancreas in Type 1 Diabetes. N Engl J Med. 2022;387(13):1161-72.
7. Fonseca VA, Grunberger G, Anhalt H, Bailey TS, Blevins T, Garg SK, et al. Continuous glucose monitoring: A Consensus Conference of the American Association of Clinical Endocrinologists and American College of Endocrinology. Endocr Pract. 2016 A;22(8):1008-21.
8. Glaser N, Fritsch M, Priyambada L, Rewers A, Cherubini V, Estrada S, et al. ISPAD Clinical Practice Consensus Guidelines 2022: Diabetic ketoacidosis and hyperglycemic hyperosmolar state. Pediatr Diabetes. 2022;23(7):835-56.
9. American Diabetes Association Professional Practice Committee. Classification and Diagnosis of Diabetes: Standards of Medical Care in Diabetes. Diabetes Care. 2022;45 (Suppl 1):S17-S38.
10. Nair VV, Chapla A, Arulappan N, Thomas N. Molecular diagnosis of maturity onset diabetes of the young in India. Indian J Endocrinol Metab. 2013;17(3):430-41.

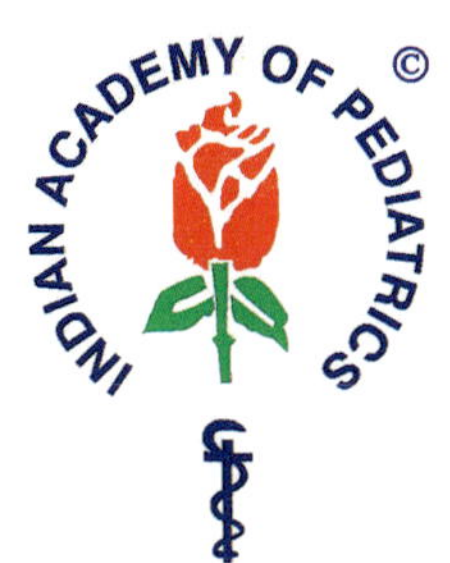

Partha's

IAP Textbook of PEDIATRICS

Eighth Edition

Volume 3

Founder Editors

(Late) A Parthasarathy, PSN Menon, MKC Nair

Editor-in-Chief

PSN Menon MD MNAMS
Former Professor
Department of Pediatrics
Sub-Dean, Consultant-In-Charge
Pediatric Endocrinology and Genetics
All India Institute of Medical Sciences
New Delhi, India

Academic Editors

MKC Nair MD PhD DSc FIACAM FAMS
Director, NIMS-Spectrum
Child Development Research Centre (CDRC)
Thiruvananthapuram, Kerala, India
Formerly Vice Chancellor, KUHS
Formerly Director, CDC Kerala (Adolescent Health)

Piyush Gupta MD FRCPCH FAMS
Former Principal, Professor and Head
Department of Pediatrics
University College of Medical Sciences
and Guru Teg Bahadur Hospital
New Delhi, India

Ramachandran Padmanabhan MD DNB
Professor of Eminence, Department of Pediatrics
Head, Division of Clinical Research and Head, Bioethics Unit
Sri Ramachandra Institute of Higher Education and Research
Chennai, Tamil Nadu, India

Ritabrata Kundu MD
Professor
Department of Pediatric Medicine
Institute of Child Health
Kolkata, West Bengal, India

Executive Editor

Alok Gupta MD
Pediatrician, Counselor and Environmentalist
Pediatric Specialities Clinic, Jaipur
Former Assistant Professor of Pediatrics
MGM University
Jaipur, Rajasthan, India

Ex-Officio Editorial Advisers

GV Basavaraja MD DNB
Professor Department of Pediatrics
Indira Gandhi Institute of Child Health
Bengaluru, Karnataka, India
IAP National President 2024

Vasant M Khalatkar MD PGDID FICMCH
Consultant Pediatrician and Neonatologist
Khalatkar Hospital
Nagpur, Maharashtra, India
IAP National President, 2025

Yogesh N Parikh MD
Associate Professor
Department of Pediatrics
Government Medical College
Surat, Gujarat, India
Secretary General, IAP (2024–2025)

Atanu Bhadra DCH
Medical Superintendent
ESI Hospital
Asansol, West Bengal, India
National Treasurer, IAP (2024–2025)

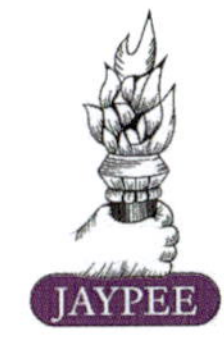

JAYPEE BROTHERS MEDICAL PUBLISHERS
The Health Sciences Publisher
New Delhi | London

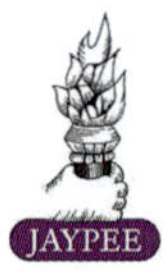

Jaypee Brothers Medical Publishers (P) Ltd

Headquarters
Jaypee Brothers Medical Publishers (P) Ltd
EMCA House, 23/23-B
Ansari Road, Daryaganj
New Delhi 110 002, India
Landline: +91-11-23272143, +91-11-23272703
+91-11-23282021, +91-11-23245672
Email: jaypee@jaypeebrothers.com

Corporate Office
Jaypee Brothers Medical Publishers (P) Ltd
4838/24, Ansari Road, Daryaganj
New Delhi 110 002, India
Phone: +91-11-43574357
Fax: +91-11-43574314
Email: jaypee@jaypeebrothers.com

Overseas Office
JP Medical Ltd
83 Victoria Street, London
SW1H 0HW (UK)
Phone: +44 20 3170 8910
Fax: +44 (0)20 3008 6180
Email: info@jpmedpub.com

Website: www.jaypeebrothers.com
Website: www.jaypeedigital.com

Inquiries for bulk sales may be solicited at: jaypee@jaypeebrothers.com

Partha's IAP Textbook of Pediatrics (3 Vols)

First Edition: 1999, 2000; Second Edition: 2002, 2003; Third Edition: 2006; Revised Reprint: 2007;
Fourth Edition: 2009; Fifth Edition: 2013; Sixth Edition: 2016; Seventh Edition: 2019

Eighth Edition: **2025**

ISBN: 978-93-5696-806-6

Printed at: Samrat Offset Pvt. Ltd.

Contents

Volume 1

SECTION 1: Basic Concepts of Child Care

Section Editor: Piyush Gupta

SECTION 2: Care of the Newborn

Section Editor: Rhishikesh P Thakre

SECTION 3: Growth

Section Editor: Anju Seth

SECTION 4: Development and Developmental Disorders

Section Editor: Samir Hasan Dalwai

SECTION 5: Nutrition and Nutritional Disorders

Section Editor: Praveen Kumar

SECTION 6: Immunity and Immunization

Section Editor: Srinivas G Kasi

SECTION 7: Infectious Diseases

Section Editor: Ritabrata Kundu

SECTION 8: Diseases of Central Nervous System

Section Editor: Sheffali Gulati

Volume 2

SECTION 9: Diseases of Cardiovascular System

Section Editor: S Srinivasan

SECTION 10: Disorders of Respiratory System

Section Editor: Sushil K Kabra

SECTION 11: Disorders of Gastrointestinal System and Liver

Section Editor: Riyaz Arakkal

SECTION 12: Disorders of Hepatobiliary System and Pancreas

Section Editor: John Matthai

SECTION 13: Disorders of Kidney and Urinary Tract

Section Editor: Arvind Bagga

SECTION 14: Disorders of Hemopoietic System

Section Editor: Ved Prakash Choudhry

SECTION 15: Pediatric Malignancies

Section Editor: **Purna A Kurkure**

SECTION 16: Disorders of Endocrine System and Diabetes Mellitus

Section Editors: **Vijayalakshmi Bhatia, PSN Menon**

Volume 3

SECTION 17: Genetics and Genetic Disorders

Section Editor: **Madhulika Kabra**

SECTION 18: Rheumatological Disorders and Allergy

Section Editor: Sathish Kumar

SECTION 19: Adolescent Health

Section Editor: MKC Nair

SECTION 20: Intensive Care and Emergencies

Section Editor: Jayashree Muralidharan

SECTION 21: Pediatric Subspecialties

Section Editor: Ramachandran Padmanabhan

SECTION 22: Community Pediatrics

Section Editor: Alok Gupta

SECTION 23: Pediatric Procedures

Section Editor: Baldev S Prajapati

SECTION 24: Pediatric Therapeutics

Section Editor: **Jeeson C Unni**

SECTION

Genetics and Genetic Disorders

Section Editor: Madhulika Kabra

17.1 Basic Genetics

Sankar VH

INTRODUCTION

Genetics is the science of human biologic variation. Medical genetics is the application of this knowledge for understanding health and disease, while clinical genetics is the application for diagnosis, prevention, and management of patients with genetic disorders.[1]

Deoxyribonucleic acid (DNA) is the hereditary material, which is present in the nucleus of the cell. The DNA is packaged into 23 pairs of chromosomes in each cell. Nucleic acid is composed of a long polymer of individual molecules called nucleotides. Each nucleotide is composed of a nitrogenous base, a sugar molecule, and a phosphate molecule. The nitrogenous base falls into two types:

1. Purines (adenine and guanine)
2. Pyrimidines (cytosine, thymine, and uracil)

Gene, which is the fundamental unit of heredity, is a segment of DNA molecule, which codes for a polypeptide. Each human is estimated to have approximately 24,000 genes. Alterations in these genes alone or in combinations of them can produce genetic disorders. These disorders are classified into the following major groups:

- *Chromosomal disorders:* Entire chromosome or segments of them are missing, duplicated, or altered. *Examples:* Down syndrome (DS), Turner syndrome
- *Single-gene disorders (also known as monogenic disorders):* Disorders in which single genes are altered—often called "Mendelian" conditions since they follow Mendelian mode of inheritance. *Examples:* Thalassemia, spinal muscular atrophy (SMA), hemophilia
- *Mitochondrial disorders:* A relatively small number of diseases are caused by alterations in the small cytoplasmic mitochondrial DNA and are inherited in a non-Mendelian fashion.[2]
- *Multifactorial disorders:* Results from a combination of multiple genetic and environmental causes. Examples: Birth defects like cleft palate/cleft lip, neural tube defect, and common diseases like diabetes, psychiatric illnesses, and hypertension.
- *Somatic cell genetic disorders:* Cancers are caused by additive effects of mutations in several genes in a somatic cell. Other disorders included in this group are autoimmune disorders and aging process.

IMPACT OF GENETIC DISEASES

The incidence of genetic disorders and their impact on health can be gauged from the following observations:[3]

- A chromosomal abnormality is present in 40–50% of all recognized first-trimester pregnancy losses.
- In neonates, 2–3% have at least one major congenital malformation.
- The incidence of chromosomal abnormalities and that of single-gene disorders in neonates are approximately 0.5% and 1%, respectively.
- Genetic disorders account for 50% of all cases of intellectual retardation and 50% cases of childhood deafness.
- Approximately 5–10% of common cancers such as breast, colon, and ovary have a strong genetic component.
- All common disorders like hypertension, psychiatric illnesses, diabetes, and coronary artery disease have a strong genetic susceptibility factor.

CHROMOSOMES AND CELL DIVISION

At conception, a human cell zygote consists of a single cell. This undergoes rapid division leading ultimately to the mature human adult, consisting of approximately 30 trillion cells. This process of cell division is called mitosis. During mitosis, each chromosome divides into two daughter chromosomes and one will segregate to each cell. Mitosis is a continuous process lasting for 1–2 hours. However, for convenience of description, it is divided into five distinct stages:[1]

1. Prophase
2. Prometaphase
3. Metaphase
4. Anaphase
5. Telophase **(Fig. 17.1.1)**

Meiosis is a specialized cell division process in which a diploid cell gives rise to haploid gametes. This occurs only in the final division of gametogenesis. In contrast to mitosis, meiosis occurs as two rounds of cell division (meiosis I and meiosis II) **(Fig. 17.1.2)**.

The word "chromosome" is derived from the Greek words for "colored body". Human cells contain 46 chromosomes comprising 22 pairs of autosomes numbered from 1 to 22 and

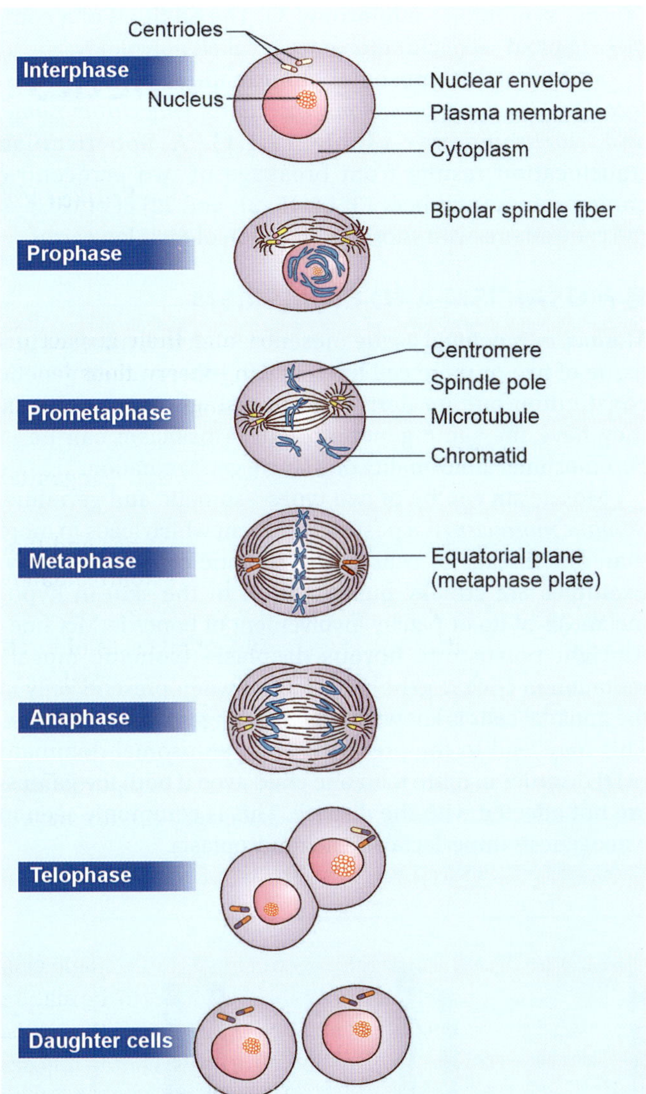

Fig. 17.1.1: Stages of mitosis resulting in two identical diploid cells formed from one original diploid cell.

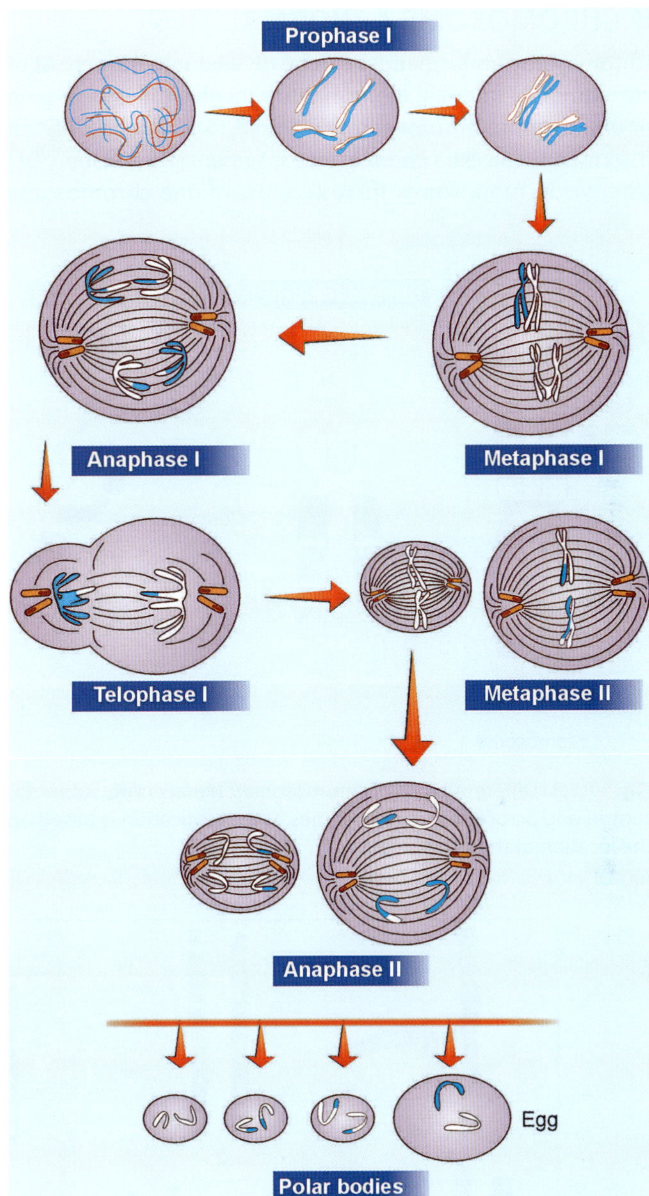

Fig. 17.1.2: Stages of meiosis during which haploid gametes are formed from a diploid cell.

a pair of sex chromosomes (two X chromosomes in females and one X and one Y in males). The numbers are assigned in a descending order of lengths of chromosomes and are classified into groups depending on the sizes of chromosomes and position of centromere in each chromosome. Each chromosome is made up of a short "p" arm and the longer "q" arm joined at the centromere. Various types of chromosomes are shown in **Figure 17.1.3**. The study of chromosomes is referred to as cytogenetics.

Karyotype refers to the orderly arrangement of chromosomes of one cell starting from the largest chromosome 1 to chromosome 22 followed by sex chromosomes. Chromosomes can be analyzed from any actively dividing cells. **Figure 17.1.4** shows a G-banded normal karyotype. The word "karyotype" is also used to describe the chromosome complement of an individual. For example, 46,XY means that the individual has normal 46 chromosomes with one X and one Y chromosome. Newly developed molecular cytogenetic techniques such as fluorescent in situ hybridization (FISH) and microarray-based cytogenetic analysis do not need live dividing cells and can detect chromosomal abnormalities of a very small size, which are not detectable by traditional karyotyping.

CHROMOSOME ABNORMALITIES

Chromosome abnormalities can be divided into numerical or structural.[4] Numerical abnormalities involve the loss or gain of one or more chromosome, referred to as *aneuploidy*. In trisomy, a single extra chromosome is present (DS—trisomy 21) whereas in monosomy, there is a loss of one chromosome (Turner syndrome—monosomy X). The addition of a complete haploid set of chromosomes is called polyploidy.[1]

Structural chromosomal abnormalities include *translocation, deletions, inversions, insertions, ring chromosome,* and *isochromosome* **(Table 17.1.1)**. A Robertsonian translocation results from breakage of two acrocentric chromosomes (numbers 13, 14, 15, 21, and 22) at or close to the centromere, with subsequent fusion of their long arms.

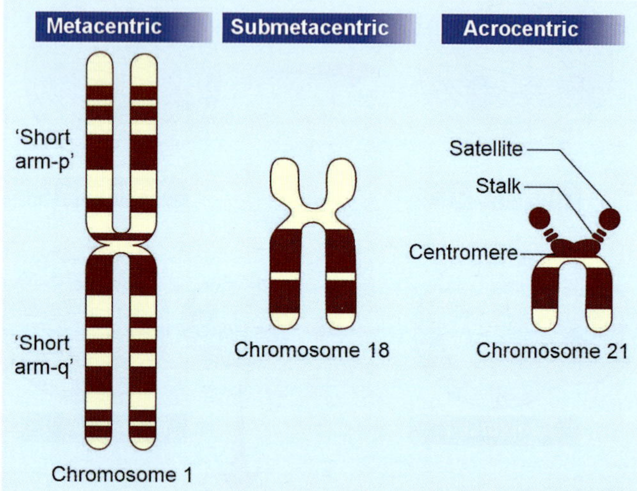

Fig. 17.1.3: Different types of chromosomes: Metacentric, submetacentric, and acrocentric chromosomes. The classification is based on the location of the centromere.

MOSAICISM AND CHIMERISM

Mosaicism is defined as the presence in an individual or in a tissue of two or more cell lines, which differ in their genetic constitution but are derived from a single zygote; that is, they have the same genetic origin. Mosaicism can be of chromosomal abnormality or a single gene mutation.[3]

Mosaicism can be of two types—somatic and germline. *Somatic mosaicism* is a postzygotic event which leads to more than one lineage of cells in the somatic cells of the body. Examples are streaky pigmentation in the skin in hypomelanosis of Ito or patchy involvement of bones in McCune-Albright polyostotic fibrous dysplasia (somatic mosaic mutation in *GNAS1* gene). Mosaicism when presents only in the gonadal cells is known as *gonadal or germline mosaicism*. This may lead to the presence of an autosomal dominant (AD) disorder in more than one child even if both the parents are not affected with the disease. This is commonly seen in osteogenesis imperfecta and achondroplasia.[5]

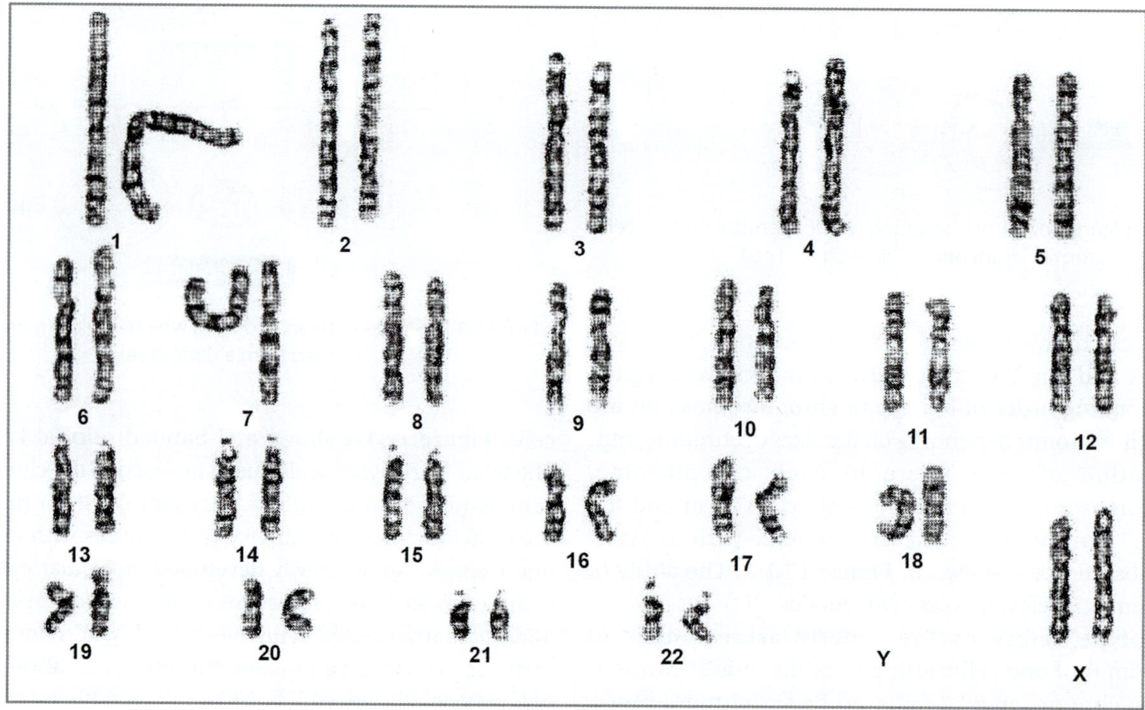

Fig. 17.1.4: G-banded karyotype of a normal female.

TABLE 17.1.1: Structural chromosomal abnormalities.

Type	*Description*	*Examples*
Deletions	A deletion involves loss of part of a chromosome resulting in monosomy for that segment of the chromosome	• Wolf–Hirschhorn syndrome (partial monosomy involving short arm of chromosome 4) • Cri-du-chat syndrome (partial monosomy involving short arm of chromosome 5)
Robertsonian translocation	This results from breakage of two acrocentric chromosomes (13, 14, 15, 21, and 22) at or close to the centromere with subsequent fusion of their long arms	Down syndrome due to translocation between chromosomes 14 and 21
Reciprocal translocation	This involves breakage of at least two chromosomes with exchange of the fragments	*Philadelphia (Ph) chromosome:* Involving chromosomes 9 and 22
Insertion	An insertion occurs when segment of one chromosome becomes inserted into another chromosome	
Inversion	An inversion is a two-break rearrangement involving a single chromosome in which a segment is reversed in position, i.e., inverted	Inversion can be pericentric inversion (involving centromere) or paracentric inversion (only one arm of the chromosome)

Chimeras can be defined as the presence in an individual of two or more genetically distinct cell lines derived from more than one zygote; that is, they have different genetic origins. Dispermic chimeras result from double fertilization of two different ova by two different sperms, and the resulting zygotes will fuse to form one embryo. Blood chimers are due to in utero exchange of red blood cells through placental circulation in nonidentical twins.

SINGLE-GENE DISORDERS

Disorders caused by alterations in single genes are often called "Mendelian" conditions since they follow the Mendelian mode of inheritance. Examples are thalassemia, SMA, and hemophilia. Gregor Johann Mendel, who is considered to be the "father" of genetics, designed experiments on garden peas and formulated a series of fundamental principles of heredity. Two important principles include:[6]

1. *Principle of segregation*, which states that sexually reproducing organisms possess genes that occur in pairs and that only one member of this pair is transmitted to the offspring (i.e., alleles on homologous chromosomes segregate)
2. *Principle of independent assortment*, which states that genes at different loci are transmitted independently

BASIC CONCEPTS

Pedigree

A diagrammatic representation of family history is known as a pedigree. The symbols are used to depict males, females, their relationships, and disease status **(Fig. 17.1.5)**. The affected individual who brings the family to notice is called "*proband*" and the one who comes for genetic counseling is the "*consultand*".[5,6]

Genotype and Phenotype

The term "*genotype*" has been defined as an individual's genetic constitution at a locus. The "*phenotype*", which is physically observable, results from the interaction of genotype and environment.

Locus and Allele

The site of a gene on a chromosome is *locus* and *allele* is the alternative form of a gene found at the same locus on homologous chromosomes.

Dominance

Dominance is not a property intrinsic to a particular allele but describes the relationship between it and the corresponding allele on the homologous chromosomes.[5]

Heterozygote and Homozygote

An individual who possesses two different alleles (different versions of a gene) at one particular locus on a pair of homologous chromosomes is called *heterozygote*, whereas an individual who possesses two identical alleles at a particular locus on a pair of homologous chromosomes is called *homozygote*.[6]

Sequence Variation: Mutations and Polymorphism

Sequence variation can be a single base substitution, insertion, or deletion of one or more base pairs. A permanent change in the nucleotide sequence or the DNA arrangement is called *mutation*. Some of the mutations cause diseases, whereas some may cause a predisposition to various diseases.

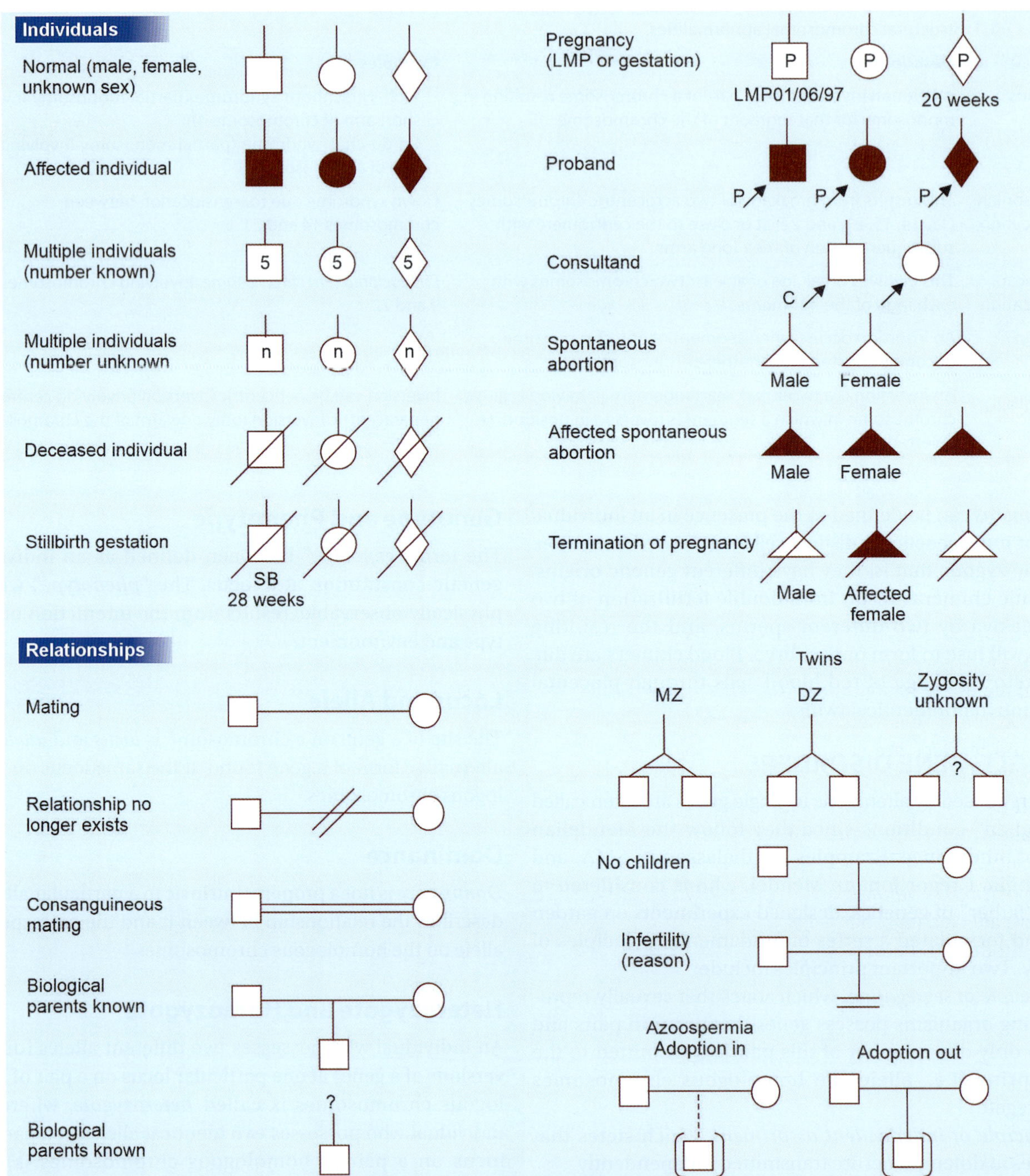

Fig. 17.1.5: Symbols for pedigree drawing.

Sequence variation with no obvious disease-causing effect is known as *polymorphism*. Common *single nucleotide polymorphisms (SNP)* are found in >1% of the population.

PEDIGREE ANALYSIS

The pedigree of at least three generations is to be constructed using a standard set of pedigree symbols **(Fig. 17.1.5)**. It illustrates the relationship among family members and their disease status. The individual affected with a genetic disease who brings the family to notice is described as the "proband" for the family and indicated by an arrow. Roman numerals are used for labeling generations, whereas Arabic numerals are used to indicate each individual within the generation.[5]

MENDELIAN INHERITANCE

A trait or disorder which is determined by a gene on an autosome is said to be followed an autosomal inheritance, whereas a trait or disorder determined by a gene on one of the sex chromosomes is said to be a sex-linked disorder.[6]

Autosomal dominant disorders are those in which both heterozygous and homozygous individuals show the abnormal phenotype, and the disease is transmitted from one generation to the other **(Fig. 17.1.6)**. One copy of the mutant gene is sufficient for expression of the abnormal phenotype.

An *autosomal recessive disorder* manifests only when both the copies of a gene are mutated in an individual and manifestations are seen in both male and female progeny of unaffected individuals. The autosomal recessive disorders usually manifest in the siblings, and there is no clinically affected individual in generations above and below **(Fig. 17.1.7)**. However, clinically normally both the parents of an individual with an autosomal recessive disorder are always heterozygous carriers.

X-linked recessive inheritance is due to a gene present on the X chromosome and manifest only in males **(Fig. 17.1.8)**. Affected males are related through carrier females.

The X-linked disorders which manifest in heterozygous males and females are called *X-linked dominant disorders* **(Fig. 17.1.9)**. In this mode of inheritance, males and females are both affected, but the severity of disorder is usually less in females than males. The number of affected females is more than that of affected males.

The *Y-linked (holandric inheritance)* implies that only males are affected (e.g., hairy ears). The characteristic pattern of each mode of inheritance is explained in **Table 17.1.2**.

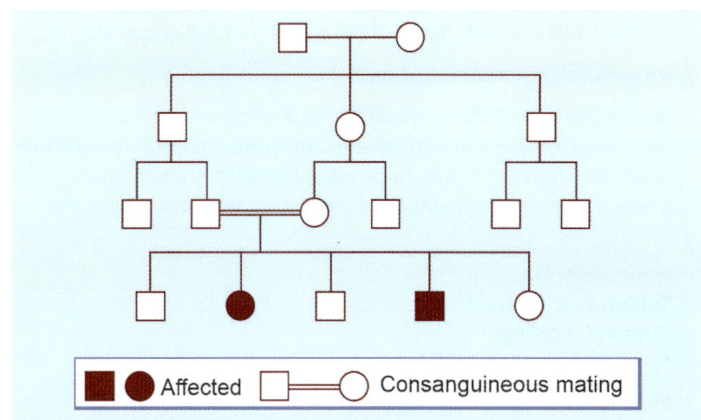

Fig. 17.1.7: A pedigree showing the inheritance of an autosomal recessive inheritance. Solid symbols represent affected individuals and double line indicates consanguinity. Note the horizontal transmission.

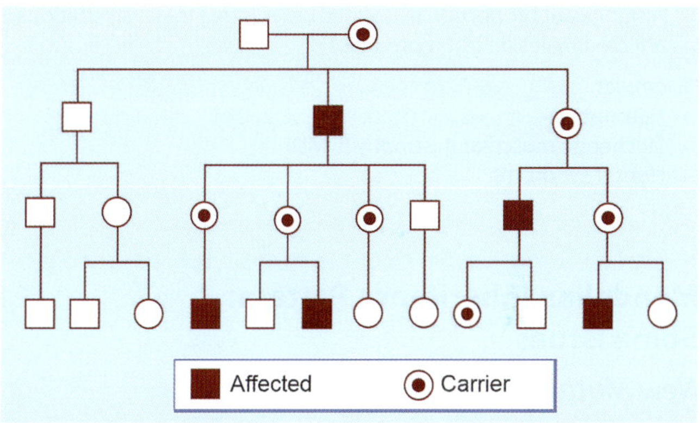

Fig. 17.1.8: A pedigree showing the inheritance of an X-linked recessive inheritance. Solid symbols represent affected individuals and dotted symbols represent heterozygous carriers. Note the oblique transmission.

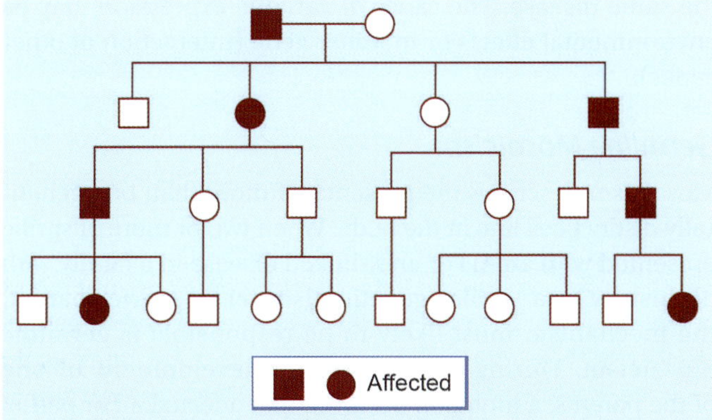

Fig. 17.1.6: A pedigree showing the inheritance of an AD inheritance. Solid symbols represent affected individuals.

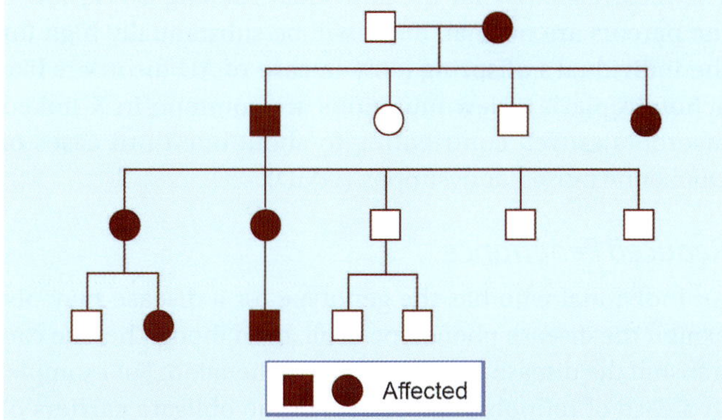

Fig. 17.1.9: A pedigree showing the inheritance of an X-linked dominant inheritance. Solid symbols represent affected individuals. It is almost similar to AD but has no male-to-male transmission.

TABLE 17.1.2: Characteristics of different inheritance patterns with examples.

Autosomal dominant inheritance	*Autosomal recessive inheritance*
• Successive or multiple generations in a family are affected • Males and females are both affected in approximately equal proportions • Males and females can both be responsible for transmission • There is at least one instance of male-to-male transmission *Examples:* • Neurofibromatosis (NF) • Tuberous sclerosis (TS) • Marfan syndrome • Familial hypercholesterolemia	• The disorder normally occurs in only one generation, usually within a single sibship • Both males and females are affected • The parents may be consanguineous *Examples:* • Thalassemia • Spinal muscular atrophy • Mucopolysaccharidosis
X-linked recessive inheritance	***X-linked dominant inheritance***
• Males are affected and females are carriers • No male-to-male transmission • 50% of the sons of the carrier females are affected; 50% of the daughters are carriers • All daughters of affected male are carriers • Affected individuals are related through transmitting (carrier) females • Pedigree is described as oblique transmission • A significant proportion of isolated cases is due to new mutations (some affected males do not reproduce) *Examples:* • Hemophilia • Duchenne muscular dystrophy (DMD) • Hunter syndrome	• Looks like autosomal dominant (AD) • Daughters of affected male always inherit the disorder • More females are affected, but have milder phenotype • No male-to-male transmission • Affected males with normal mates have no affected sons and no normal daughters • Some disorders may be lethal in males *Examples:* • Familial hypophosphatasia • Rett syndrome • Aicardi syndrome

Mendelian Inheritance Pattern: Some Issues

New Mutations

A child may be born with an AD disorder without any similar diseases in parents or other family members (a sporadic case). This is usually due to new mutation in the affected child. A large proportion of observed AD disorders are due to a new mutation. For example, it is estimated that seven out of eight cases of achondroplasia are caused by a new mutation. The recurrence risk for the individual's sibling is very low if the parents are normal, but it will be substantially high for the individual's offspring (50% in case of AD disorders like achondroplasia). New mutations are common in X-linked disorders as well contributing to about one-third cases of Duchenne muscular dystrophy (DMD).

Reduced Penetrance

An individual who has the genotype for a disease may not exhibit the disease phenotype at all, even though he/she can transmit the disease gene to the next generation. For example, in a case of retinoblastoma, 10% of the obligate carriers of mutation in the retinoblastoma susceptibility gene do not get the disease and the penetrance of the gene is then said to be 90%. In some genetic conditions like Huntington chorea, a delay in the age of onset of the disease may occur which is described as age-dependent penetrance.

Variable Expression

Here, penetrance may be complete, but the severity of the disease among affected family members may vary. The classic example is of tuberous sclerosis where a parent with milder manifestations like adenoma sebaceum may not be aware of the disease till his or her offspring develops seizures or rhabdomyosarcoma, which are severe manifestations of the same disease. The cause of variable expression may be environmental effects or modifier gene (interaction of other genes).

Germline Mosaicism

Mosaicism describes the presence of more than one genetically distinct cell line in the body. When two or more offspring presented with an AD or an X-linked disease in a family with no history of a similar genetic disorder or carrier parent, the mechanism most likely to be responsible is germline mosaicism. During the embryonic development of one of the parents, a mutation occurred that affected all or part of the germline but few or none of the somatic cell of the body. This mechanism is extensively studied in osteogenesis imperfecta type II and also described in DMD and hemophilia A.

Locus Heterogeneity

The causation of the same disease phenotype by mutations at distinct loci is termed locus heterogeneity. Genetic conditions with significant locus heterogeneity are sensorineural deafness, retinitis pigmentosa, and Charcot–Marie–Tooth disease.

Pleiotropy

Genes that have more than one discernible effect on the body are said to be pleiotropic. A classic example of pleiotropic effects is Marfan syndrome. Gene mutation affects eye, skeletal system, and cardiovascular system.

Consanguinity

Because relatives share disease-causing genes inherited from a common ancestor, consanguinity is likely to be more frequent among the parents of an individual with an autosomal recessive disorder, especially so if the disorder in concern is rare. For genetic counseling, it is considered that the prevalence of genetic diseases is roughly one to two times in the offspring of first-cousin marriages as compared to non-consanguineous population. Quantification of sharing of genes between two relatives can be done by estimating the coefficient of relationship. This shows that siblings share half of their genes (first-degree relatives), uncle/aunt shares a quarter (¼) of their genes (second-degree relatives), first cousins share 1/8th of their genes (third-degree relatives), and so on.

Manifesting Female Carriers of X-linked Recessive Disorders

Although female carriers of X-linked recessive disorders are usually asymptomatic, they can manifest the disease in the following situations:

- *Homozygous for X-linked recessive disorders:* Female offspring of an affected father and a carrier mother
- *Numerical X chromosome abnormalities:* Female carrier with only one X chromosome (Turner syndrome)
- *Female carrier with nonrandom or skewed X-inactivation:* In this situation, there is a departure from the normal random process of X-inactivation, with a greater proportion of normal X chromosome getting inactivated than the other one with a mutation of an X-linked disease.
- *X-autosome translocation when the breakpoint of the translocation disrupts a gene on the X chromosome*

X-inactivation (Lyon Hypothesis)

This states that one X chromosome in each cell is randomly inactivated early in the embryonic development of females. This would result in dosage compensation, an equalization of X-linked gene products in males and females.

NONMENDELIAN INHERITANCE

Genomic Imprinting

One of Mendel's laws states that the phenotype is the same, whether a given allele is inherited from the father or the mother. Now, it has been recognized that different clinical features can result depending on whether the gene is inherited from the father or the mother. This "parent of origin" effect is referred to as genomic imprinting. Evidence of genomic imprinting has been classically observed in two dysmorphic syndromes associated with learning difficulties known as the Prader–Willi syndrome and Angelman syndrome. Prader–Willi syndrome is caused by the absence of a small part of chromosome 15 of paternal origin, whereas the deletion of the same region on chromosome 15 from maternal origin gives rise to Angelman syndrome.

Uniparental Disomy

An individual normally inherits one of the pair of homologous chromosomes from each parent. On the contrary, if an individual inherits two copies of the same homologue from one parent, through an error in meiosis, this is called uniparental disomy (UPD). This mechanism has been identified as molecular pathology from a situation where a child with cystic fibrosis had only one parent who was the carrier of cystic fibrosis mutation and the other parent was not a carrier of cystic fibrosis. This mechanism is a cause in disorders of growth disturbances like Beckwith–Wiedemann syndrome (UPD of chromosome 11) and Silver–Russell syndrome (UPD chromosome 7).

Mitochondrial Inheritance

Each human cell contains several hundreds of mitochondria in the cytoplasm. Mitochondria produce adenosine triphosphate (ATP), the energy source essential for cellular metabolism. They have their own DNA molecule (mtDNA). Some important principles in mitochondrial inheritance are as follows:[2]

- Since mtDNA is present in the cytoplasm, it is exclusively derived from the maternal side. The pattern of inheritance shown in the pedigree **(Fig. 17.1.10)** suggests that only females can transmit the disease to their offspring.
- The mutation rate in mitochondrial DNA is 10 times higher than that of nuclear DNA. The reason for this is a high replication rate, lack of DNA repair, and damage by oxygen-free radicals in mtDNA.[2]
- Heteroplasmy indicates a cell with heterogeneous population of mitochondria with or without mutations.

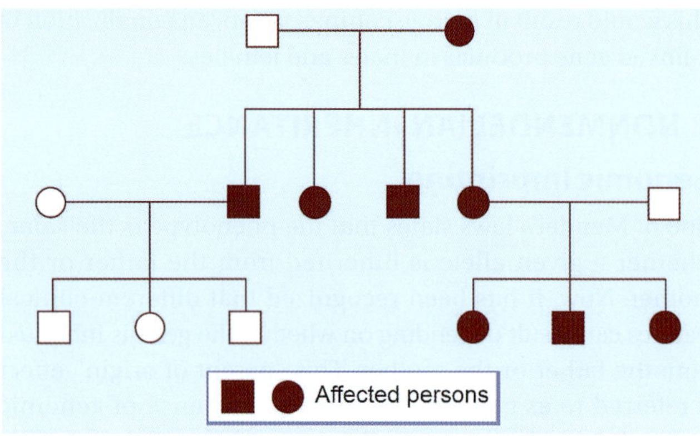

Fig. 17.1.10: A pedigree showing the inheritance of a disease caused by mitochondrial DNA mutation.

TABLE 17.1.3: Triplet repeat disorders.

Genetic disorder	*Gene*	*Repeat*
Fragile X syndrome (FXS)	*FMR 1*	CGG
Myotonic dystrophy	*DMPK*	CTG
Huntington disease	*HD*	CAG
Friedreich ataxia	*X5*	GAA
Spinocerebellar ataxia 1	*FRATAXIN*	CAG

It often results in incomplete penetrance of mitochondrial inheritance.

- At the cellular level, the proportion of mutated mtDNA (mutation load) determines phenotypic expression called threshold of expression. Central nervous system (CNS) and heart that need high energy are commonly involved in mitochondrial disorders.

Triplet Repeat Disorders

One assumption of Mendelian genetics is that a mutant allele which is transmitted from parent to offspring remains unchanged. Recently, an increasing number of disorders were identified in which the underlying mutation is an expansion of a triplet nucleotide repeat sequence that is unstable and can change in size on transmission from parent to offspring. The disorders with triplet repeat disorder are summarized in **Table 17.1.3**.

MULTIFACTORIAL DISORDERS

Multifactorial disorders are the result of a combination of small variations in genes, which predispose to a serious defect, often in combination with environmental factors. This group includes common diseases like diabetes mellitus, hypertension, obesity, schizophrenia. Another important group of multifactorial disorders include congenital malformations like neural tube defects and congenital heart disease (CHD). For counseling of multifactorial disorders, the empiric recurrence risk derived from observational studies in families with the given disorder is used.

Major characteristics of multifactorial disorders are as follows:[7]

- Affected individuals tend to cluster in families.
- The disease is more common among the close relatives of the proband and becomes less common as the relationship becomes distant.
- Heritability is defined as the function of the total phenotypic variance of a quantitative trait that is caused by genes. For a condition like bronchial asthma it is 0.80 whereas for CHD it is 0.35.

GENOMIC ALTERATIONS IN DISEASES

Genetic disorders are a spectrum of disorders and a result of genomic alterations. While Down syndrome occurs due to an extra copy of the chromosome 21, Turner syndrome is due to loss of one sex chromosome. DiGeorge syndrome and William syndrome are microdeletion syndromes due to large deletions involving multiple genes, which cannot be detected by conventional karyotype.

Variations in a particular gene result in single-gene disorders. Beta-thalassemia is due to point mutations in the beta globin gene, whereas deletion or duplications of single or multiple exons is the most common genetic abnormality (70%) in DMD. In some conditions like sickle cell anemia and achondroplasia, one or two missense mutations will be present in all cases. In conditions like thalassemia and cystic fibrosis, different mutations are present in different individuals. There are more than 300 different mutations, which cause beta-thalassemia.

A genetic disease can be caused by different mutations in the same gene—allelic heterogeneity (e.g., thalassemia)—or by mutations in several genes—locus heterogeneity (e.g., retinitis pigmentosa, deafness). On the other hand, different diseases or phenotypes can be caused by mutations in a single gene as well. Hence, it is vital to confirm the genetic disorder by genetic testing before genetic counseling.[7]

GENETIC TESTING IN PRACTICE

Analysis of human genome is an important investigation during evaluation of a genetic disorder. The selection of genetic tests depends on the probable genomic alterations in that condition.

The chromosomal abnormalities (numerical and structural) can be identified by karyotype. Microdeletions, which cannot be detected by conventional karyotype, can be demonstrated by locus-specific FISH or multiplex ligation-dependent probe amplification (MLPA).[8]

TABLE 17.1.4: Common clinical scenarios in clinical practice and rational genetic tests in the situation.

Clinical scenario	***Rational genetic tests***
Characteristic chromosomal abnormalities like Down syndrome, Turner syndrome, Klinefelter syndrome	Conventional karyotype
Parents of a child with chromosomal abnormalities, couple with recurrent pregnancy loss, infertility	Conventional karyotype
Microdeletion syndrome (DiGeorge syndrome, William syndrome), rapid aneuploidy testing in prenatal sample	Fluorescent in situ hybridization (FISH)
Multiple malformation, intellectual disability, autism spectrum disorders	Microarray
Single-gene disorders with specific point mutation like sickle cell disease, achondroplasia	Restriction fragment length polymorphism (RFLP)-based polymerase chain reaction (PCR) technique for specific mutation
Single-gene disorders with deletion/duplication of exons like spinal muscular atrophy and Duchenne muscular dystrophy	Multiplex ligation-dependent probe amplification (MLPA)
Single-gene disorders with different types of mutation in a single gene like thalassemia and cystic fibrosis	Sanger sequencing of the entire gene
Single-gene disorder due to trinucleotide repeat mutations like Huntington's chorea and fragile X syndrome	Triplet prime PCR (TP-PCR)
Hemophilia A to detect inversion mutation	Inverse PCR
Viral infections like COVID-19 and hepatitis B	RT-PCR (for RNA virus) and real-time PCR for viral load determination
Rapid prenatal diagnosis for aneuploidy detection	Quantitative florescent PCR (QF-PCR)
Single-gene disorders with different mutations in different patients (private mutation) like neurofibromatosis; same phenotype with mutation in multiple genes like deafness and muscular dystrophy	Next-generation sequencing (NGS)-based panel testing with multiple genes or clinical exome sequencing
Specific phenotype probable genetic disorder not fitting into known genetic disorder and other common genetic testing does not shown any abnormality	Whole exome sequencing (WES) and whole genome sequencing (WGS)

Microarray technology can detect copy number variations (CNV) in genome. A CNV may vary in size from 1 kb to several megabases and can occur anywhere in the genome. This can cause a spectrum of abnormalities like intellectual disability and multiple malformations.

Deletion/duplication in a single gene can be demonstrated by MLPA, whereas point mutations can be detected by sequencing of the specific gene. This can be a mutation-specific test in sickle cell anemia or achondroplasia or sequencing of the entire gene as in thalassemia where different mutations can lead to the phenotype.

In conditions like deafness where mutations in multiple genes cause the phenotype, panel testing for all involved genes is more cost-effective. This can be done with next-generation sequencing (NGS) technology where massively parallel sequencing of multiple genes can be done which will reduce the cost and turnaround time of sequencing. Whole exome sequencing (WES) targets the subsets of human genome that is protein coding (3% of the human genome). While whole genome sequencing (WGS) holds great promise for clinical practice, cost and availability set a limit for its widespread use.

Mutations of triple repeat disorders like fragile X syndrome and disorders of genomic imprinting (Prader–Willi syndrome) can be detected by specific polymerase chain reaction (PCR)-based tests like triple primed PCR and methylation-sensitive PCR, respectively.[7]

Common clinical scenarios in clinical practice and the rational genetic tests in each situation are depicted in **Table 17.1.4**.

GENETIC COUNSELING

The American Society of Human Genetics in 1975 has defined genetic counseling as a communicative process, which deals with human problems associated with the occurrence and/or recurrence of a genetic disorder in a family. This process involves an attempt by one or more appropriately trained persons to help the individual or family to:

- Comprehend the medical facts, including diagnosis, probable course of disorder, and available management.
- Appreciate the way heredity contributes to the disorder and the risk of recurrence in relatives.
- Understand the alternatives for dealing with the risk of recurrence.

BOX 17.1.1: Clinical situations where genetic counseling is important.

- Congenital malformations
- Unexplained stillbirth with or without malformations
- Developmental delay/intellectual retardation
- Neurodegenerative diseases
- Myopathy, neuropathy, seizures, focal neurological abnormality, abnormalities of tone and power
- Ambiguous genitalia
- Hypogonadism
- Recurrent reproductive losses, infertility
- *Short stature:* Proportionate or disproportionate
- *Acutely sick infant, neonate:* Inborn error of metabolism (IEM)
- *Known genetic disease:* Wilson disease, Down syndrome (DS), mucopolysaccharidosis, etc.
- Relatives of a person with chromosomal translocation
- Childhood deafness
- Familial cancer or cancer prone disease
- Any familial disease
- Any unusual disease of skin, bones and eyes
- Advanced maternal age
- Positive screening test for a genetic disorder, e.g., triple test, increased alpha-fetoprotein (AFP) in mother
- Prenatal diagnosis of malformation
- Exposure to known or suspected teratogen in pregnancy

- Choose the course of action, which seems appropriate to them in view of this risk, their family goals, and their ethical and religious standards and act in accordance with that decision.
- Make the best possible adjustments to the disorder in an affected family member and/or to the risk of recurrence of that disorder.[7]

Accurate and definitive diagnosis is the prerequisite for the prediction of prognosis and recurrence risk. Like any other clinical specialty, history taking including three-generation pedigree and clinical examination is important. Various hematological, biochemical, and imaging investigations are needed. Specialized tests like chromosomal analysis, enzyme analysis, metabolic studies, and DNA analysis are important for definitive diagnosis. Clinical situations where genetic counseling is important are listed in **Box 17.1.1**.[8]

THERAPY IN GENETIC DISORDERS

With improvements in understanding the pathogenesis of genetic disorders, a remarkable stride has been made in their treatment. Enzyme replacement therapy (ERT) for lysosomal storage disorders is one of the success stories of the last decade. ERT is available for Gaucher disease, Pompe disease, Fabry disease, and mucopolysaccharidosis. Regular administration of bisphosphonates (alendronate, pamidronate, and zoledronate) is the standard of care in osteogenesis imperfecta to prevent recurrent fractures. Stem cell therapy is a definitive treatment for conditions such as thalassemia and osteopetrosis. Metabolic and pharmacological therapy is available for some of the metabolic disorders.[7]

The ultimate treatment in genetic disorders is gene therapy. This may involve replacing the defective gene or suppressing the expression of gene that contributes to the phenotype. Gene therapy has proved successful in some conditions such as DMD, SMA, hemophilia B, primary immunodeficiency, etc. However, more refinements are required for regular use of this therapy in clinical practice.[8]

KEY MESSAGES

- Taking detailed three-generation family history and drawing in the form of pedigree is the first step in the evaluation of a case with a probable genetic disorder.
- Chromosomal disorders are an important cause of malformations and intellectual retardation and chromosomal study needs to be ordered in these situations.
- Single-gene disorders follow Mendelian inheritances: AD, autosomal recessive, X-linked recessive, and X-linked dominant.
- Factors complicating Mendelian inheritance such as new mutations, reduced penetrance, variable expression, and locus heterogeneity need to be considered while providing genetic counseling.
- Genomic imprinting, UPD, mitochondrial inheritance, and triple repeat disorders are non-Mendelian forms of inheritances.
- Multifactorial disorders are the result of a combination of small variations in genes that predispose to a serious defect, often in combination with environmental factors.
- Genetic counseling should be an integral part of management of any disorder with genetic or probable genetic etiology.

REFERENCES

1. Jorde LB, Carey JC, Bamshad MJ. Medical Genetics, 6th edition. Philadelphia: Elsevier; 2019.
2. Koene S, Smeitink J. Mitochondrial medicine. J Inherit Metab Dis. 2011;34(2):247-8.
3. Keagle MB, Gersen SL. Principles of Clinical Cytogenetics, 2nd edition. New Jersey: Humana Press; 2005.
4. Gardner RJM, Amor DJ. Chromosome Abnormalities and Genetic Counseling, 5th edition. Oxford: Oxford University Press; 2018.
5. Phadke SR. Genetics for Clinicians, 1st edition. Bangalore: Prism Books; 2007.
6. Nussbuam RL, McInnes RR, Willard HF. Thompson & Thompson Genetics in Medicine, 7th edition. Philadelphia: Saunders Elsevier; 2007.
7. Strachan T, Read AP. Human Molecular Genetics, 5th edition. Oxford: Garland Publishing; 2018.
8. Turnpenny PD, Ellard S. Cleaver R Emery's Elements of Medical Genetics, 16th edition. Philadelphia: Elsevier; 2020.

17.2 Clinical Dysmorphology

Muralidhar L Kulkarni

It does not matter what you see in the genome if you can't see the patient.

—Anna C E Hurst, Nathaniel H Robin

INTRODUCTION

Dysmorphology is a word coined by Dr David W Smith in 1966 and is derived from the Greek words *"dys"* (disordered, abnormal) and *"morph"* (shape, form). Simply, it is the study of human congenital defects—abnormalities of body structure that originate before birth.[1]

Individual birth defects are rare, but together they account for a large proportion of childhood mortality and morbidity. More than 7,000 dysmorphic, multiple congenital anomalies and intellectual retardation syndromes have been reported with more being added with time. About 1–3% of children are born with multiple or serious congenital defects. Knowledge and expertise are needed for identification not only of these serious defects but also of other minor anomalies, which may give clues to a more serious underlying pathology. Prompt recognition of the condition helps in prognostication, investigation, and treatment and also helps the family by way of genetic counseling about recurrence risk and prevention.

CLASSIFICATION OF DYSMORPHIC DEFECTS[1]

It is probably impossible to know all the congenital defects and the associated conditions by heart; hence, it is necessary to categorize them into manageable subdivisions. A *dysmorphic feature or anomaly* is an abnormality of shape, size, or structure. These features are traditionally classified as *major* or *minor* anomalies. A *major anomaly* is one that has severe medical or cosmetic consequences if untreated, such as a congenital heart defect or a cleft lip. A *minor anomaly* represents a medically insignificant departure from normal development, such as wide-set eyes or a single palmar crease. Three or more minor malformations are associated with multiple major anomalies in 90% of the patients and hence warrant a thorough evaluation. Before ascribing an anomaly to be significant, an astute clinician should first take into consideration the ethnical background and the familial occurrence.

Based on the pathogenesis, birth defects can be classified as follows:[2,3]

- *Malformation:* Early embryological developmental error (e.g., cleft palate)
- *Deformation:* Internal or external mechanical forces alter normally forming structure (e.g., clubfoot)
- *Disruption:* Breakdown of a previously normal tissue (e.g., amniotic band sequence) **(Fig. 17.2.1)**
- *Dysplasia:* Abnormal cellular organization within a tissue resulting in structural changes of organs containing the tissue involved (e.g., achondroplasia)

When multiple birth defects are encountered, it is useful to classify them first in order to arrive at an appropriate diagnosis. The most commonly used system for classification is as follows:

- *Syndrome ("running together" in Greek):* A pattern of features, often with a unifying underlying cause that arises from several different errors in morphogenesis (e.g., Down syndrome). Most dysmorphic syndromes are a constellation of major and minor anomalies. The presence of only one feature is never diagnostic, but the unique combination gives the diagnosis of a syndrome.
- *Sequence:* A pattern of multiple anomalies derived from a single prior anomaly or mechanical factor

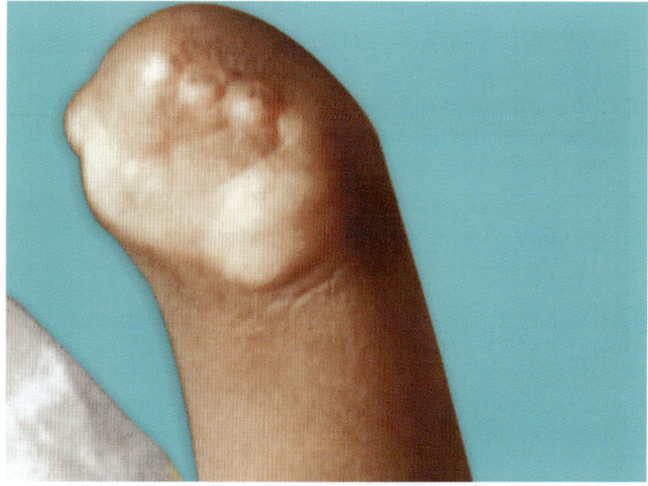

Fig. 17.2.1: Amnion rupture sequence. Note the amputation and disruption of the finger morphogenesis.

Example: In case of the Pierre–Robin sequence (micrognathia, glossoptosis, and U-shaped cleft palate), the primary anomaly is the early mandibular hypoplasia, which results in a posteriorly located tongue (secondary anomaly), thereby impairing the closure of palatal shelves resulting in a cleft palate (tertiary anomaly) **(Figs. 17.2.2A and B)**. Roughly 17% of Pierre–Robin sequence cases are isolated and nonsyndromic; in the remaining cases, it is a part of syndromes such as Stickler syndrome, velocardiofacial syndrome, and Beckwith–Wiedemann syndrome.

- *Association:* Nonrandom tendency of some malformations to occur together more commonly than would be expected by chance, without being part of a syndrome.
  Examples: VATERR association (*V*ertebral defects, *A*nal atresia, cardiovascular anomalies, *T*racheoesophageal fistula, *E*sophageal atresia, *R*adial dysplasia, *R*enal dysplasia) and MURCS association (*Mü*llerian duct aplasia, *R*enal aplasia, *C*ervicothoracic *S*omite dysplasia)
- Many cases of CHARGE association (*C*oloboma of the eye, *H*eart defects, *A*tresia of the nasal choanae, *R*etardation of growth and/or development, *G*enitourinary abnormalities, and *E*ar abnormalities and deafness) have recently been found to be caused by *CHD7* gene and hence, CHARGE is now grouped as a syndrome and not an association.

APPROACH TO A CHILD WITH MULTIPLE ANOMALIES[4-6]

Suspicion

The first step in the evaluation of a dysmorphic child is "suspicion of genetic etiology", which should be suspected in any child who presents with:

- *Congenital anomalies*: Major anomaly or more than two minor anomalies
- *Growth deficit:* Short stature or failure to thrive
- *Developmental delay, intellectual subnormality, or developmental regression*
- *Failure to develop secondary sexual characteristics*
- *Ambiguous genitalia*
- Or simply the child "does not look right"

History

Any mystery can be solved with a proper history. Some of the important historical points to be elicited are mentioned in **Tables 17.2.1 and 17.2.2**.

Physical Examination

In addition to routine examination, certain additional examination should be performed in a child with dysmorphic features. **Table 17.2.3** lists some of the salient features that point to an underlying dysmorphic syndrome.

The importance of major anomalies is well known in syndrome delineation. When it comes to minor anomalies, the presence of two or more features warrants further evaluation for syndrome association.

RECOGNITION OF GENETIC SYNDROMES[1,4-6]

Some syndromes are so striking to the eye of the pediatrician that a diagnosis is made instantaneously based on the general gist of the patient. This, termed "gestalt diagnosis", is exemplified in the diagnosis of a patient with Rubinstein–Taybi syndrome **(Figs. 17.2.3A to E)**, wherein multiple minor anomalies make a combination so unique that a diagnosis is rarely missed. In order to have expertise in this mode of "gestalt diagnosis", one has to have a vast experience in

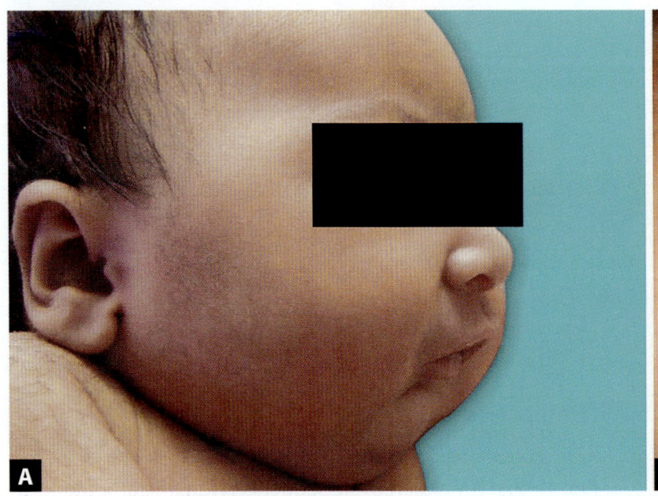

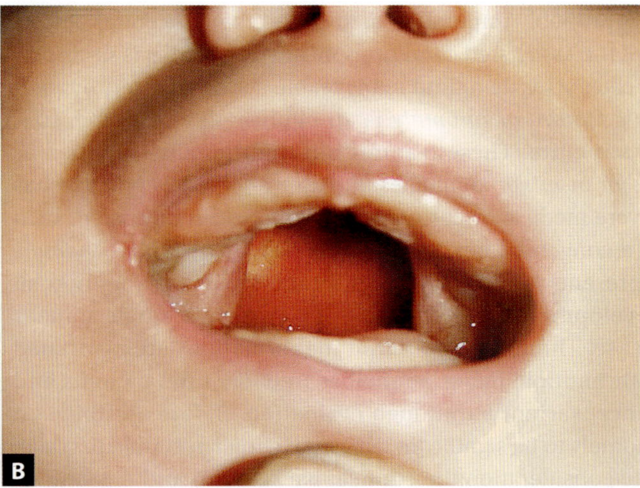

Figs. 17.2.2A and B: Pierre–Robin sequence. Note the micrognathia and unusual round-shaped palatal cleft unique to this sequence.

TABLE 17.2.1: Personal/family history.

History	*Significance*
Three-generation pedigree chart using standard symbols	Indicates pattern of inheritance
Elderly mother (>35 years)	Chromosomal aneuploidy *Example:* Down syndrome
Elderly father (>45 years)	New AD mutation *Examples:* Achondroplasia and Marfan syndrome
Maternal disease *Example*: Diabetes mellitus	• Known associated fetal abnormalities • Diabetic embryopathy (caudal regression, congenital heart defects, ear anomalies)
Poor social history	Possible alcohol/drug ingestion
Racial origin of parents	Known genes of high frequency in certain racial groups *Example*: Ellis–van Creveld syndrome in the Amish population
Parental consanguinity	Autosomal recessive disorders
Possible maternal uterine abnormalities	Deformations
Other affected family members or multiple single gene or chromosomal disorder	For diagnostic purpose and to know the pattern of inheritance

TABLE 17.2.2: Pregnancy history.

History	*Significance*
Antenatal ultrasound	Aids prenatal diagnosis, holds clues to the diagnosis and to assess fetal growth
Maternal drug or alcohol ingestion *Examples*: Warfarin, anticonvulsants, cocaine	Teratogenic effects *Examples*: • Warfarin—hypoplasia of nasal cartilage, CNS abnormality • Valproate—spina bifida, craniofacial dysmorphism • Cocaine—vascular disruptions
Exposure to radiation (especially therapeutic)	Possible mutagenic or teratogenic effects
Early rupture of membranes	Possible fetal compression leading to deformation
Oligohydramnios	Renal agenesis or outflow obstruction with Potter sequence
Polyhydramnios	Esophageal atresia, neuromuscular disorders
Poor fetal movements	Fetal compression, neuromuscular disorders
Breech presentation	Neuromuscular disorders

TABLE 17.2.3: Findings that suggest underlying genetic etiology.

General	• Short stature or tall stature • Failure to thrive or obesity • *Unusual head circumference*: Microcephaly or macrocephaly • *Unusual head shape*: Brachycephaly, scaphocephaly, trigonocephaly • *Altered body proportion*: Short spine, short limbs, long limbs
Facial features	• Synophrys (fused eyebrows) • Hypotelorism or hypertelorism* • Palpebral fissures that are up-slanting or down-slanting* • Short palpebral fissures (normally the length of palpebral fissure is equal to the distance between two eyes) • Short or long nose (the nose is usually 2/3rd to 3/4th the length of the distance between the nasal bridge and the upper lip) • Ears that are low set or posteriorly rotated* • Ears that are simple or abnormally shaped • Lips that are thin/full, tented, downturned or cleft • Philtrum that is long or smooth • Palate that is high arched or cleft • Uvula that is bifid or absent • Prognathia or micrognathia*
Hands and feet	• Brachydactyly (short fingers) • Arachnodactyly (long fingers) • Clinodactyly (incurved fingers, usually the fifth)* • Syndactyly (fusion of digits) • Polydactyly (extra digits) • Dysplastic nails • Abnormal creases*

Contd...

Contd...

Skin and hair	• Abnormal skin pigmentation, e.g., hemangioma, café au lait spots, streaks, or whorls • Abnormal amounts of hair, e.g., alopecia, hirsutism, or hypertrichosis • Abnormal hair line, e.g., low hairline (posteriorly or anteriorly) or receding hairline • Altered hair color, e.g., white forelock
Musculoskeletal	• Short neck • Abnormal chest shape or size, e.g., pectus carinatum, pectus excavatum, short sternum • Abnormalities of nipples, e.g., widely spaced, supernumerary* • Inverted nipples • Abnormalities of the spine, e.g., anencephaly, encephalocele • Myelomeningocele or stigmata of spina bifida occulta (hair, lipoma, deep dimple)* • Unusual joint shape, e.g., flaring • Abnormal joint mobility, e.g., hypermobility or reduced range of motion
Abdomen	• Abdominal wall defects, e.g., omphalocele, gastroschisis • Hepatosplenomegaly • Nephromegaly • Ambiguous genitalia

*Indicate minor anomalies.

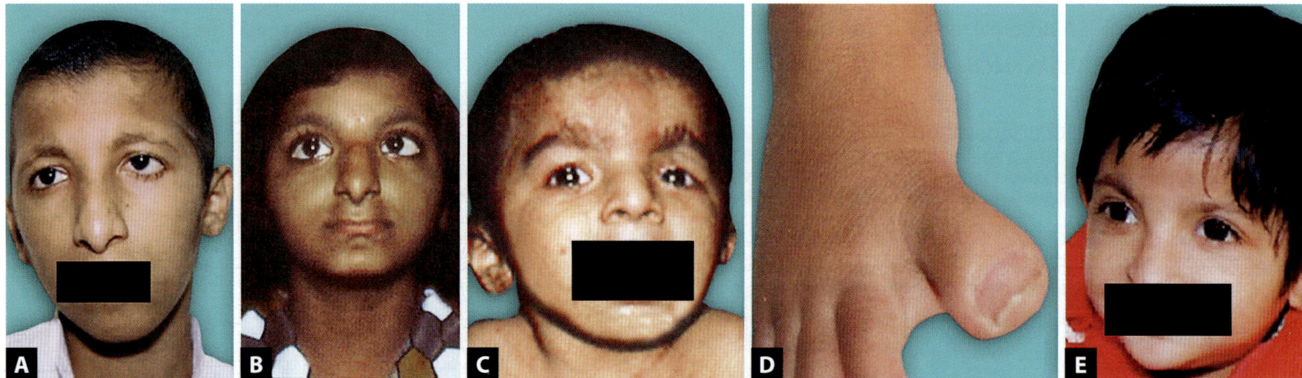

Figs. 17.2.3A to E: Unrelated children with Rubinstein–Taybi syndrome. Note the facial characteristics—downslanting palpebral fissures and overhanging columella of nose. Great toe is broad and medially rotated.

seeing similar patients previously in order to create a mental snapshot of the condition. Given the rarity of individual syndromes, such an experience is seldom gained but by a few; hence, repeated visual scanning of pictures of various syndromes from authoritative resources will have to suffice.

- Whenever an anomaly is noted, it should be described by keeping in mind the following directives:
  - Appropriate terminology
  - Minor or major anomaly
  - *Etiology:* Malformation/disruption/deformation
  - Time of onset
- Examination should not be restricted to the patient but should be extended to include all the available family members.
- Whenever feasible objective criteria should be used in diagnosing anomalies. The reader can refer to various Indian and foreign data useful in anthropometry.
- Cross-consultation should be taken from specialists of other fields in medicine when dealing with a child with multiple anomalies (e.g., ophthalmology consults in Rieger syndrome).
- Consultation with a specialist in the field of dysmorphology is of utmost importance for prompt diagnosis and further evaluation.
- The camera plays the role of a stethoscope in the field of dysmorphology. Pictures are not only useful for record purposes and second opinions, but also help in the appraisal of the morphological evolution of a syndrome.
- Radiography goes hand in hand with physical examination when it comes to anomalies, since they are diagnostic in several conditions such as the group of skeletal dysplasia.

When immediate recognition is not possible, it is necessary to identify one or more features (handles), which might lead to syndrome diagnosis. The best handle or

TABLE 17.2.4: Some clinical features which suggest specific diagnosis.

Clinical sign	*Specific diagnosis*
Pursed lips	Whistling face syndrome
Broad thumbs and great toes	Rubinstein–Taybi syndrome
Absent clavicle	Cleidocranial dysostosis
Heterochromia iridis	Waardenburg syndrome
Mitten hands	Apert syndrome
Inverted nipples	Congenital disorder of glycosylation
Webbing of neck	Turner and Noonan syndromes
Eversion of the lateral third of lower eyelid	Kabuki make-up syndrome

anomaly to be taken to consideration is one which is least likely to be a normal variant. Features such as intellectual retardation, microcephaly, simian crease, and clinodactyly are nonspecific and act as poor handles for syndrome delineation. The anomalies that are less common but more specific are more useful for the search of diagnosis. Examples are microphthalmia, preaxial polydactyly, midline cleft lip, etc. Once a suitable handle is identified, reference should be made to a standard monograph on syndromology or computer databases.

Sometimes, some clinical features suggest specific diagnosis, which could be called "pearls of dysmorphology", and few examples are mentioned here **(Table 17.2.4)**.

The "Smith's approach" to a child with multiple malformations is a way of classifying syndromes based on the combination of major handles. The author considers this particular approach to be extremely effective and time tested. A major list of classification that is used in the "Smith's approach" is as follows **(Table 17.2.5)**:

- Very small and proportionate stature, not skeletal dysplasia (e.g., Seckel syndrome) **(Fig. 17.2.4)**
- Moderate short stature, facial ± genital (e.g., Aarskog syndrome, Williams syndrome) **(Figs. 17.2.5 and 17.2.6)**
- Senile-like appearance (e.g., Cockayne syndrome, Werner syndrome) **(Figs. 17.2.7A and B)**
- Unusual brain and/or neuromuscular findings, with associated defects (e.g., acrocallosal syndrome) **(Figs. 17.2.8A and B)**
- Early overgrowth with associated defects (e.g., Sotos syndrome) **(Fig. 17.2.9)**
- Facial defects as major feature (e.g., frontonasal dysplasia syndrome) **(Fig. 17.2.10)**
- Facial–limb defects as a major feature (e.g., Hay–Wells syndrome of ectodermal dysplasia) **(Fig. 17.2.11)**
- Limb defects as a major feature (e.g., femoral hypoplasia) **(Fig. 17.2.12)**

TABLE 17.2.5: Important textbooks and online databases of genetic syndromes.

*Reference texts**	*Online and computerized databases*
Smith's recognizable pattern of human malformations *(Editor: Jones KL)*[1]	Online Mendelian inheritance in man (www.ncbi.nlm.nih.gov/Omim)
Atlas of skeletal dysplasias *(Editors: Wynne-Davies, Hall and Apley)*[2]	GeneClinics and GeneTests (www.geneticsclinic.com)
Syndromes of the head and neck *(Editors: Gorlin, Cohen, and Hennekam)*[4]	London dysmorphology database (www.lmdatabases.com)
Management of genetic syndromes (*Authors:* Cassidy and Allanson)[6]	POSSUM (Pictures of Standard Syndromes and Undiagnosed Malformations) (www.possum.net)
	TERIS (The teratogen information system) (depts.washington.edu/terisweb/teris)

**See* References for details.

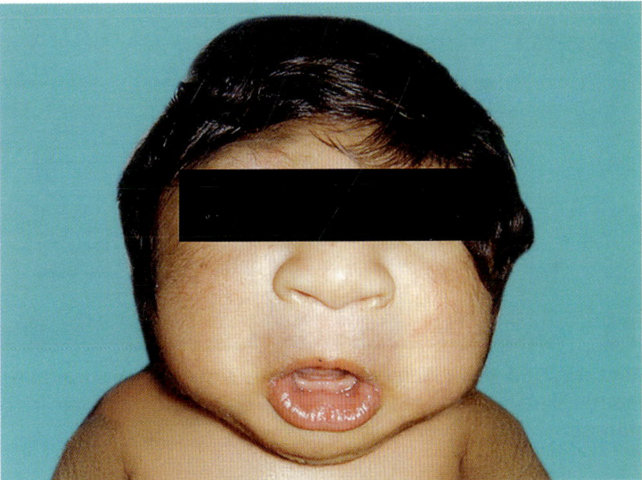

Fig. 17.2.4: Seckel syndrome. Note the severe microcephaly with prominent nose.

- Craniosynostosis syndromes (e.g., Apert syndrome) **(Figs. 17.2.13A and B)**.

A special mention is warranted in the case of skeletal dysplasia, since the huge list and the varied presentations of this group of enigmatic condition is a challenge even to the astute clinician. The following approach based on that suggested by Bryan D Hall is considered to be extremely effective in reaching a diagnosis:

- Diagnosing short stature
- Diagnosing disproportionate short stature

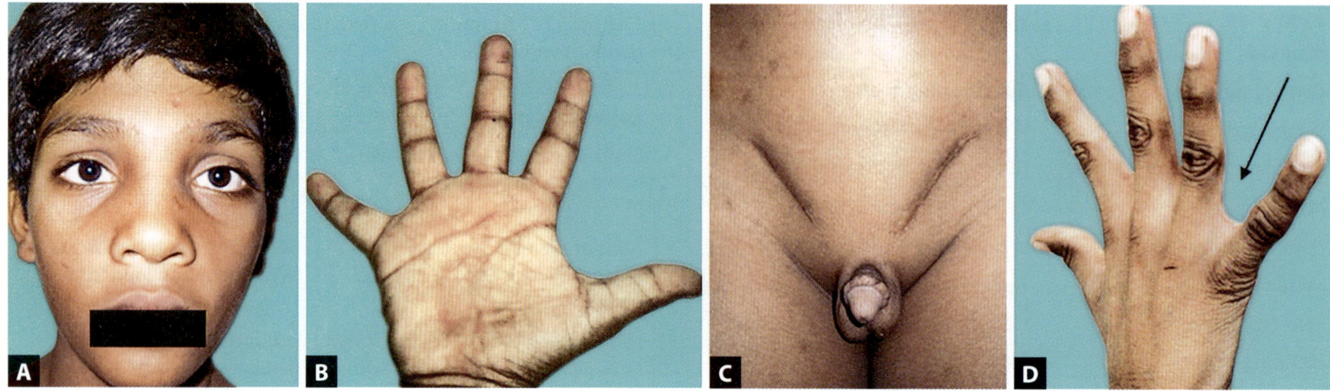

Figs. 17.2.5A to D: Aarskog syndrome. Note the hypertelorism and broad philtrum, hand showing brachydactyly with mild interdigital webbing (arrow), swan neck deformities of fingers, and characteristic shawl scrotum. Scars due to operation for bilateral inguinal hernia are also seen. The patient was of moderate short stature.

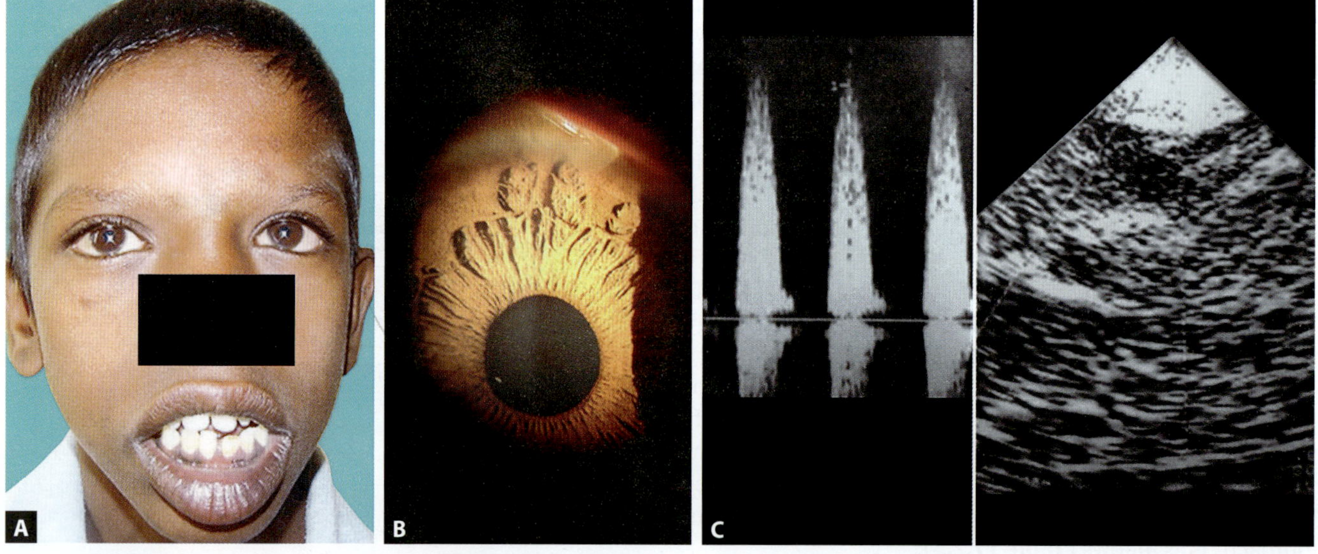

Figs. 17.2.6A to C: Williams syndrome. Note the periorbital fullness with medial eyebrow flare and prominent lips with an open mouth. Slit-lamp examination revealed a characteristic stellate iris pattern. Echocardiogram confirmed the diagnosis of supravalvular aortic stenosis.

- Diagnosing what causes this disproportion, is it short trunk (e.g., spondyloepiphyseal dysplasias) or short limbs (e.g., achondroplasia)
- If short-limbed, which part of the limbs are affected:
  - *Rhizomelia:* Proximal shortening, i.e., humerus and femur (e.g., chondrodysplasia punctata)
  - *Mesomelia:* Shortening of the middle segment, i.e., radius, ulna, tibia, and fibula (e.g., mesomelic dysplasia)
  - *Acromelia:* Distal shortening, i.e., hand and foot (e.g., acromesomelic dysplasia)
  - *Combination:* Ellis-van Creveld syndrome, achondroplasia
- Diagnosing deformations caused by the osseous abnormalities (e.g., craniosynostosis in thanatophoric dysplasia)
- Diagnosing associated malformations, which herald a clue to the actual condition (e.g., heart defects in Ellis-van Creveld syndrome)
  - *Categorizing based on the areas involved radiologically:* Epiphyseal dysplasias, diaphyseal dysplasias, metaphyseal dysplasias, spine involvement, cranial involvement, hand involvement
  - *Categorizing based on clinical and radiological grounds:* Pure skeletal dysplasia (e.g., achondroplasia)

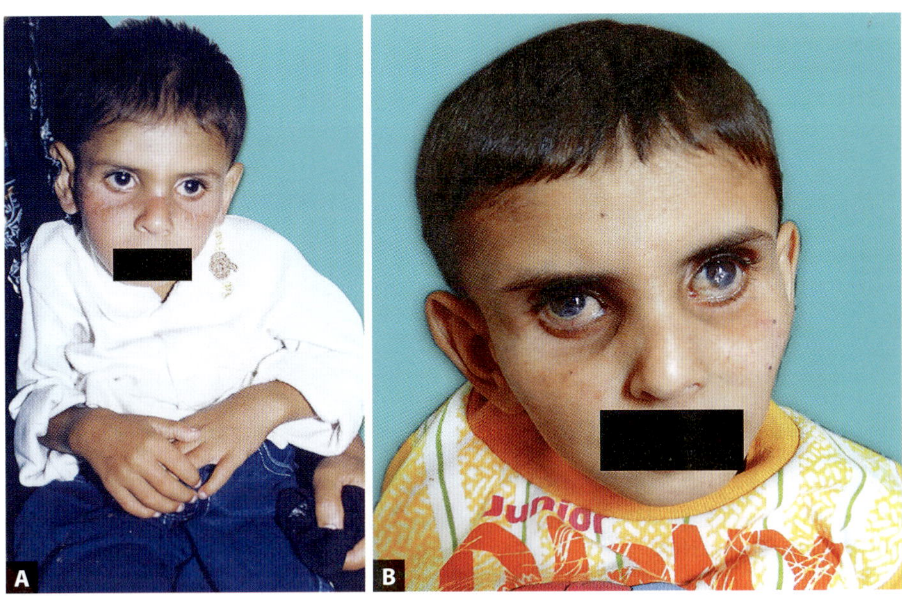

Figs. 17.2.7A and B: Cockayne syndrome: Deep set eyes, rash on cheeks, and changes of premature aging. The same child at (A) 5 years and (B) 12 years of age.

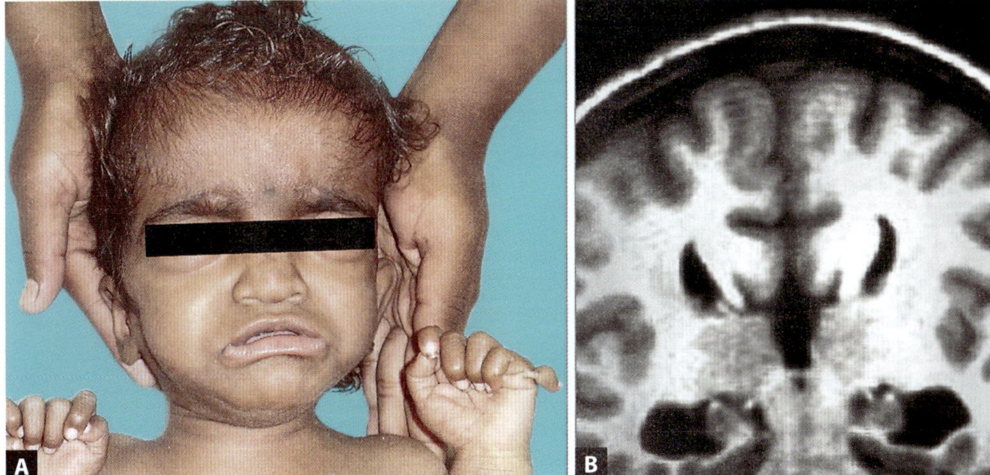

Figs. 17.2.8A and B: Acrocallosal syndrome: The hypertelorism, downslanting palpebral fissures, broad nasal bridge and short philtrum. (A) Postaxial polydactyly is seen in both the upper limbs; (B) Magnetic resonance imaging revealed absent corpus callosum.

- Malformations associated (e.g., Stickler syndrome)
- Malformation/mental retardation associated (e.g., campomelic dysplasia)

Attributes of a Dysmorphologist

- He/she should be a meticulous and keen observer and must record any deviation from the norms.
- He/she must see a number of cases and if not possible, must visually scan photographs and pictures.
- Always use objective criteria and appropriate terminology.
- As in any field a person interested in dysmorphology should be a learner forever.
- One has to be honest in his/her approach, hungry for knowledge, and humble in acquiring it.

Intuition (the Unteachable and the Undefinable)

Irrespective of their experience, training, extent of reading, clinical ability and observational skills, there exists a small group of individuals whose instinctive ability gives them

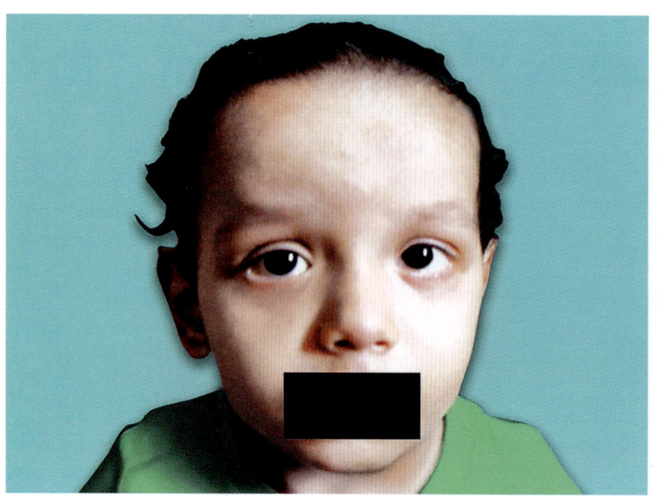

Fig. 17.2.9: Sotos syndrome: Macrocephaly, mild hypertelorism, prominent forehead and chin.

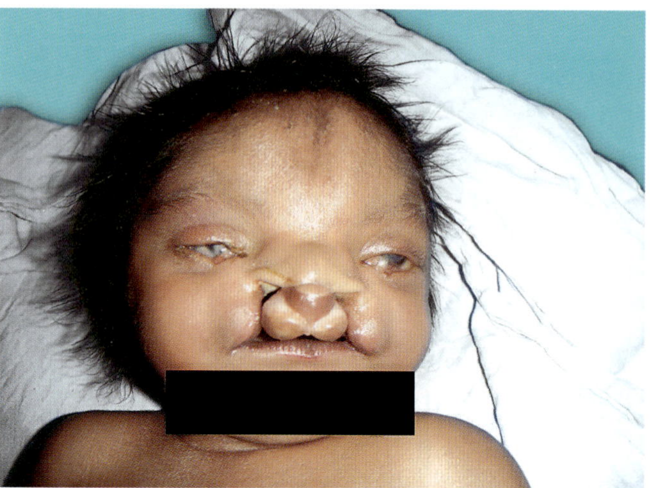

Fig. 17.2.11: Hay–Wells syndrome of ectodermal dysplasia: The obvious ankyloblepharon, broad nasal bridge with bilateral cleft lip and palate. Child had associated dystrophic nails and supernumerary nipples.

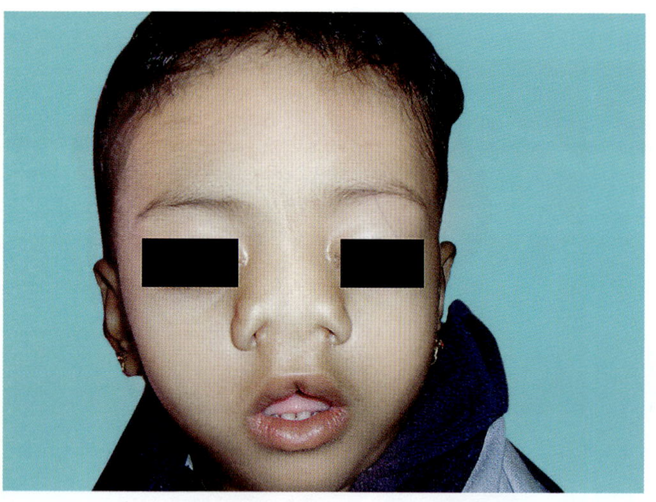

Fig. 17.2.10: Frontonasal dysplasia sequence: The completely divided nostrils with hypoplasia of the prolabium with a median cleft lip.

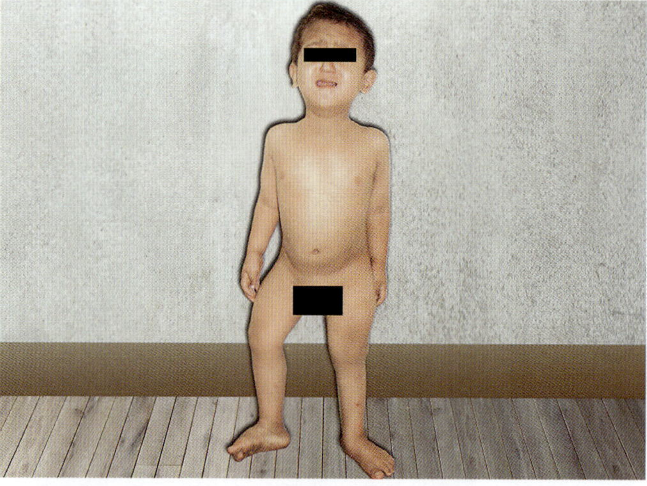

Fig. 17.2.12: Femoral hypoplasia—unusual facies syndrome: The short lower limbs; upslanting palpebral fissures with a short nose, hypoplastic alae nasi, and low-set ears.

better diagnostic expertise than their counterparts. Such individuals stand out in the field of dysmorphology.

LABORATORY EVALUATION

Deformations seldom require any laboratory-based diagnostic evaluation, whereas in this postgenomic era genetic testing plays a key role in the evaluation of malformations and associated syndromes. In addition to investigations to identify the etiology, investigations play an important role in detecting internal malformations of heart, brain, kidneys, etc. Diagnosis of malformation is not only useful in providing clue to the etiology but also important as the malformation may be surgically treatable.

Karyotyping

Unless a nonchromosomal etiology is apparent in a child with multiple malformations, it is a useful diagnostic approach to start with a karyotype (chromosome analysis). It is the definitive diagnostic test for aneuploidy syndromes such as Down syndrome, Turner syndrome, and other structural abnormalities of chromosomes.

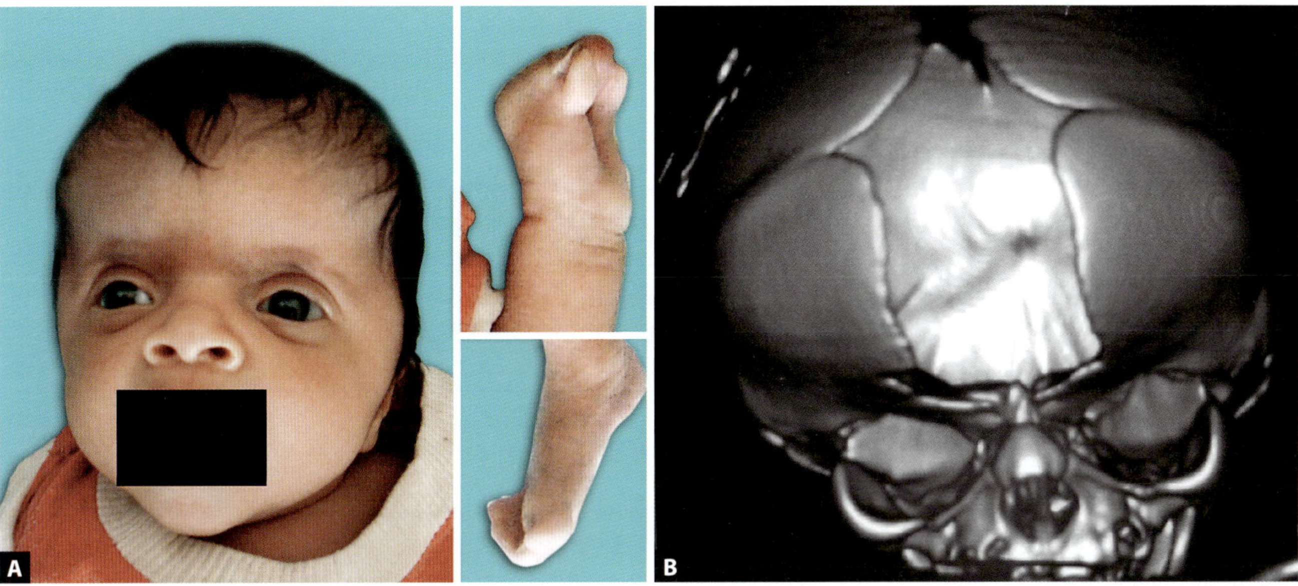

Figs. 17.2.13A and B: Apert syndrome: (A) High full forehead, hypertelorism, and downslanting palpebral fissures. Limbs show varying degrees of syndactyly (mitten hand); (B) Computed tomography (CT) head reconstruction showing bilateral coronal suture synostosis.

Fluorescent in situ Hybridization

The fluorescent in situ hybridization (FISH) technique has revolutionized the field of cytogenetics having tremendous implications in the diagnosis of malformation syndromes. FISH probes by their ability to attach to specific locus on a chromosome bring to light microdeletions that are not visible in the standard karyotype **(Fig. 17.2.14)**. **Table 17.2.6** lists the more commonly used and available FISH probes for syndrome delineation. As FISH can look at only a specific area of a chromosome, it is important to clinically suspect the condition before ordering the FISH test.

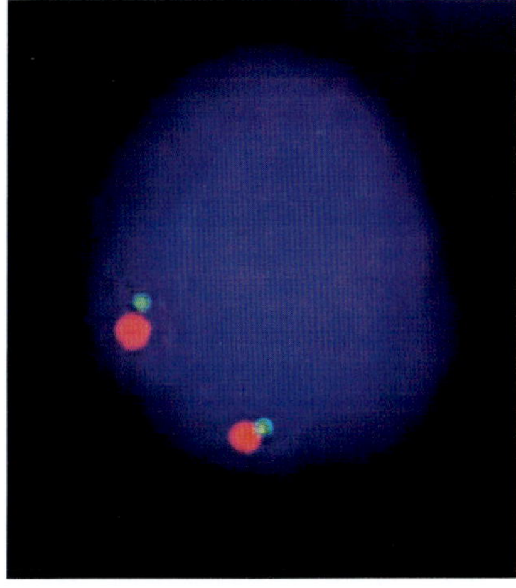

Fig. 17.2.14: Normal result of FISH technique. Two red (target region) and green (control probe) signals indicate the presence of two copies of a particular region of interest in the interphase nucleus and absence of microdeletion.

New Genetic Tests

Comparative Genomic Hybridization

Comparative genomic hybridization (CGH) combined with the microarray technique is a newer addition to the armamentarium of the dysmorphologists. It can detect very small deletions/duplications anywhere in the genome in one test. The microarray-based cytogenetic analysis has been advocated as a first line of test for cases with intellectual retardation/malformation without an obvious cause, and the diagnostic yield of the test is 7–10%.

Biochemical Testing

Many biochemical genetic defects are associated with dysmorphic features such as mucopolysaccharidosis, Zellweger syndrome, and Smith-Lemli-Opitz syndrome. Testing for a specific enzyme defect may be diagnostic in these conditions and can be supplemented by finding the underlying genetic defect.

Mutation Detection

Genes for many malformation syndromes such as Cornelia de Lange syndrome, Apert syndrome, and Treacher-Collins syndrome are known and many others are getting identified. However, due to a large size of genes and large number of mutations observed in each syndrome, the use of mutation detection by DNA-based techniques in clinical practice is

TABLE 17.2.6: Microdeletion syndromes commonly diagnosed using the FISH technique.

Syndrome	*Chromosomal region*	*Clinical features*
Angelman syndrome	15q11–q13	Magnetic resonance imaging (MRI), spastic gait, happy temperament
Prader–Willi syndrome	15q11–q13	MRI, hypotonia, hypogonadism, obesity, almond-shaped eyes
Williams syndrome	7q11.2	Aortic stenosis, facial dysmorphism, friendly behavior
Cri-du-chat syndrome	5p15.2	MRI, cat-like cry in infancy, microcephaly
Miller–Dieker syndrome	17p13.3	MRI, microcephaly, lissencephaly, furrowing of forehead while crying
Rubenstein–Taybi syndrome	16p13.3	MRI, beaked nose, broad thumbs and toes
Velocardiofacial syndrome	22q11.2	Conotruncal heart defects, cleft palate, prominent nose

(FISH: fluorescent in situ hybridization)

TABLE 17.2.7: Summary of approach to a dysmorphic child.

Suspicion	*Analysis*	*Previous laboratory and X-ray studies*	*Physical examination*
• Congenital abnormalities • Growth problems • Mental deficit	• History • Pedigree • Family • Pregnancy and birth • Health • Growth and development		• Anatomic regions • Organ systems • Measurements • Photographs
Other	***Synthesis***	***Confirmation***	***Intervention***
• Family investigation • Watchful waiting	• "Pivotal" findings • Pattern recognition • Comparison with known cases: – Personal experience – Literature	• Laboratory • Clinical course • Birth of affected relatives	• Treatment • Counseling
Follow-up	• Lack of diagnosis • Counseling other family members • New diagnostic technique • Natural history		

not easy. For some disorders such as Apert syndrome and achondroplasia, only one common mutation is identified in most of the cases. That is why mutation detection for such disorders is easy and available in India.

Now the sequencing of whole genome (WGS) has become possible and if there are 2–3 patients of a disorder in a family, the causative gene can be identified using DNA samples of such a few cases.

Table 17.2.7 provides a summary of the approach to diagnosis and management of common genetic disorders in children.

PRENATAL DIAGNOSIS

In essence, it is determination of the status (genetic or otherwise) of the fetus by a variety of techniques [ultrasonography (USG), chromosomal, biochemical, DNA, etc.], using a variety of procedures. These include chorionic villus sampling (CVS) (8–11 weeks), amniocentesis (11–16 weeks), and blood analysis by cordocentesis. Radiological investigations such as antenatal ultrasound, fetal magnetic resonance imaging (MRI), and fetal echocardiogram (ECHO) play an important role in the prenatal diagnosis of malformations.

GENETIC COUNSELING[7-9]

Genetic counseling is the process of helping people understand and adapt to the medical, psychological, and familial implications of genetic contributions to the disease. The counselor offers investigations, options, and support whereas the "consultand" (the person who seeks the advice) makes his/her own decision, which is known as nondirective counseling. The essential steps include accurate diagnosis of the affected member in the family, risk assessment, proper communication, discussion of options, and long-term contact and support. Assistance in enrolment of the patient in support groups may be paramount in this era of global communication.

DIFFICULTIES IN DYSMORPHOLOGY

Neonatal Period

It is a common occurrence in India to be faced with a neonate with no antenatal ultrasound presenting with gross dysmorphic features. This is exemplified in cases such as thanatophoric dysplasia **(Figs. 17.2.15A and B)**, where early neonatal death is the rule. The attending pediatrician should be able to quickly assess such a condition so as to stop futile resuscitation measures. Neonatal presentation of certain conditions such as Pierre-Robin sequence may be with feeding difficulties or failure to thrive with metabolic encephalopathy in cases such as Smith-Lemli- Opitz syndrome or Zellweger syndrome. Adequate expertise is needed for anticipation of difficulties in these conditions.

Evolution of Morphology

Some phenotypes evolve with time, such as *Proteus* syndrome; it is the rule in many of the metabolic conditions such as the group of mucopolysaccharidosis and hence a diagnosis is rarely made in the neonatal period, whereas in certain conditions such as the Beckwith-Wiedemann syndrome the phenotype tends to dissolve as the age progress. These caveats reinforce the need for proper documentation and photography to study the evolving nature of the condition.

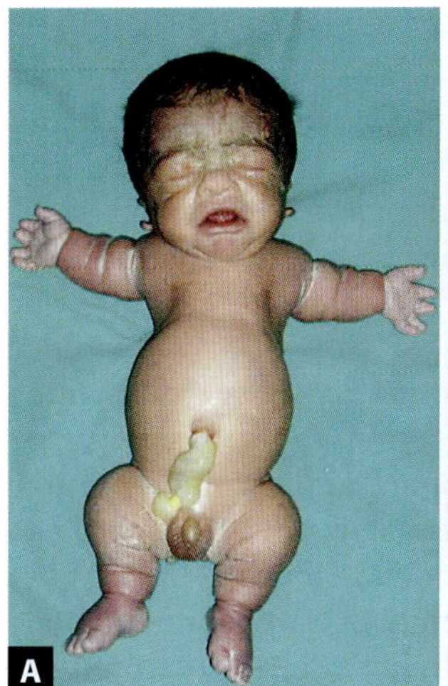

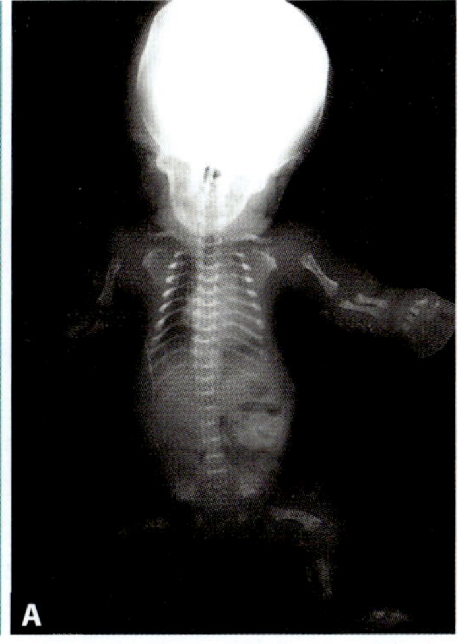

Figs. 17.2.15A and B: (A) Thanatophoric dysplasia, severe shortening of the limbs, i.e., acromesorhizomelic, loose folds of skin, macrocephaly with low nasal bridge, and narrow thorax; (B) Curved femora and flat vertebrae are seen in the radiograph.

RECENT ADVANCES

Facial Recognition Software in Clinical Dysmorphology[10,11]

Facial recognition software can help identify rare genetic diagnosis using two-dimensional photography of affected patients. Machine-learning algorithms allow for improvement in a tool's accuracy over time. Facial recognition software identify rare syndromic diagnosis in patients with dysmorphic findings at times comparable to or better than standard clinical examinations. Algorithms using two-dimensional images are more accessible than three-dimensional which currently require specialized equipment. Facial recognition software are useful to clinicians, researchers, laboratories, and pharmaceutical companies.

Behavioral Phenotypes

A well-known phenomenon is the unique behavior associated with specific syndrome. This is exemplified in the friendly social nature of patients with Williams syndrome, tendency to overeat in case of Prader-Willi syndrome, self-mutilating and destructive behavior of Lesch-Nyhan syndrome, autistic behavior in Fragile-X syndrome and Rett syndrome, happy nature of Angelman syndrome, and the lovable, friendly and music-loving nature of Down syndrome. This old phenomenon, termed as the "behavioral phenotype", is gaining more interest, not only as an aid to diagnosis but also in the comprehensive treatment of the patient.

Dysmorphology in the Era of Genomic Diagnosis[12,13]

Dramatic changes in sequencing technologies and in the introduction of artificial intelligence have changed the field of dysmorphology in the last two decades.

When a patient with a suspected genetic disorder arrives, the first thing they do is *genotype analysis* using a newer technique of *next-generation sequencing (NGS)* like *exome* (part of gene synthesizing proteins) *sequencing and whole genome* (all the DNA in a cell, both nuclear and mitochondrial) *sequencing. Clinical sequencing* involves workup of certain clinical syndromes such as deafness workup, hypotonia workup, skeletal dysplasia multigene panel, and familial aortopathy panel. These technologies sequence hundreds to thousands of genes. If the pathogenic gene is detected, the same gene is searched in parents and other family members. Once the genotype is fixed, a detailed examination of the patient and families is done to fix the phenotype. This is *genotype to phenotype approach* which is the reverse of the earlier approach of phenotype to genotype.

However, one should remember that clinical evaluation and genetic evaluation are complementary to each other.

Therefore, there will still be a need for dysmorphologists to bridge the gap between pure genetic testing results and predicted clinical consequences. The main difference may be that the dysmorphology examination occurs after genetic testing instead of prior to it.

REFERENCES

1. Jones KL. Smith's Recognizable Pattern of Human Malformation, 6th edition. Philadelphia: Elsevier Saunders; 2006.
2. Wynne-Davies R, Hall CM, Apley AG (Eds.). Atlas of Skeletal Dysplasia. Churchill Livingston, Edinburgh, London, Melbourne, New York; 1985.
3. Allanson JE, Biesecker LG, Carey JC, Hennekam RC. Elements of morphology: introduction. Am J Med Genet A. 2009;149A(1):2-5.
4. Falk MJ, Robin NH. The primary care physician's approach to congenital anomalies. Prim Care. 2004;31(3):605-19.
5. Gorlin RJ, Cohen MM, Hennekam RCM. Syndromes of the Head and Neck, 4th edition. New York: Oxford University Press; 2001.
6. Hall J, Allanson J, Gripp K, Slavotinek A. Handbook of Physical Measurements, 2nd edition. New York: Oxford University Press; 2006.
7. Cassidy SB, Allanson JE. Management of Genetic Syndromes, 3rd edition. New York: Willey Blackwell; 2010.
8. Toriello HV. Role of the dysmorphic evaluation in the child with developmental delay. Pediatr Clin North Am. 2008;55(5):1085-98.
9. Kulkarni ML. An Atlas of Neonatology. New Delhi: Jaypee Brothers Medical Publishers (P) Ltd; 2005.
10. Peter Hammond. The use of 3D face shape modelling in dysmorphology. Arch Dis Child. 2007;92(12):1120-6.
11. Hurst ACE. Facial recognition software in clinical dysmorphology. Curr Opin Pediatr. 2018;30:701-6.
12. Robin NH. Teaching dysmorphology in the era of genomes: New technologies, new learners. Curr Opin Pediatr. 2018;30(6):699-700.
13. Soloman BD, Ada MP, Fong CT, Girisha KM, Hall JG, Hurst ACE, et al. Perspectives on the future of dysmorphology. Am J Med Genet Part A. 2022;191(3):659671.

17.3 Common Genetic Disorders

Mounika Endrakanti, Madhulika Kabra

INTRODUCTION

With the increasing recognition that most disorders have a probable genetic basis; no clinician can escape learning about the diagnosis and management of common genetic disorders. The fact that some of these disorders are now amenable to therapy and most of the severe/lethal disorders can be prevented; it is all the more important that pediatricians, who are usually the first contact of children with likely genetic disorders, expand their knowledge and interest in this field.

Genetic disorders can be classified as follows:

- Chromosomal disorders
- Single-gene disorders
- Polygenic or multifactorial disorders
- Mitochondrial disorders
- Somatic cell (genetic) disorders (resulting in cancer)

In this chapter, we have discussed the clinical features, diagnosis, management, and counseling issues of common genetic disorders encountered in clinical practice.

CHROMOSOMAL DISORDERS

Chromosomal disorders account for approximately 6% of all recognized congenital abnormalities. They can be broadly categorized as numerical and structural abnormalities. Chromosomal mosaicism constitutes the third category, consisting of different chromosomal constitutions in two or more cell lines. Although chromosomal abnormalities are common at conception, their incidence declines with advancing gestation, as most imbalances that are not compatible with survival result in spontaneous pregnancy loss.

- *Numerical chromosomal abnormalities* (aneuploidies) are characterized by the presence of an extra chromosome, referred to as *trisomy* or, the presence of only one chromosome of the pair, referred to as *monosomy*. Autosomal trisomies commonly observed among liveborn infants include trisomy 21 (Down syndrome), trisomy 18 (Edward syndrome), and trisomy 13 (Patau syndrome). They differ in phenotype, disease course and severity. Other trisomies are less common in live-born infants because they are lethal in early embryonic life and are not compatible with life at birth. The presence of an additional sex chromosome (X or Y) has only mild phenotypic effects. Monosomy for an autosome is almost always incompatible with survival to term. Monosomy X (karyotype 45,X or Turner syndrome) is a frequent chromosomal aberration diagnosed in the postnatal period.

- *Structural chromosome rearrangements* result from chromosomal breakage with subsequent reunion in a different configuration or orientation. These are broadly categorized as balanced and unbalanced rearrangements, based on the absence or presence of net loss or gain of chromosomal material respectively and include translocations, inversions, deletions, duplications, insertions, etc.

CHROMOSOMAL ANEUPLOIDIES

Down Syndrome

Down syndrome (DS) is the most common autosomal trisomy with an incidence of about 1 per 800–1,200 live births. It is characterized by the presence of an extra copy of chromosome 21, arising most commonly as a result of nondisjunction in maternal meiosis I. About 95% of cases of DS result from trisomy 21, and the remaining 5% of cases comprise either mosaicism or Robertsonian translocation involving acrocentric chromosomes. There is a strong association between the incidence of DS and advancing maternal age.

Clinical Features

The phenotype of DS is well characterized and easily identifiable clinically. Though the diagnosis may be difficult in a neonate, especially a preterm, identification of characteristic dysmorphism, and constellation of associated clinical features often aid clinical diagnosis. Characteristic facial features of a child with DS include upslanted palpebral fissures, small ears, and protruding tongue. **Table 17.3.1** provides a short checklist of clinical features in these children. **Figures 17.3.1A to C** show a child with DS with characteristic facies.

TABLE 17.3.1: Checklist for clinical diagnosis of Down syndrome.

System/organ affected	***Abnormality detected***
Head	Brachycephaly with flat occiput, wide open fontanel
Face	Flat facial profile,* flat nasal bridge
Mouth	Habitually open furrowed/protruding tongue
Ears	Dysplastic,* small, and low set
Eyes	Upward slant of palpebral fissures,* epicanthic folds, squint, and speckled iris
Neck	Short and broad and abundant neck skin*
Hands	Short and broad, small fingers especially 5th finger, hypoplastic middle phalanx of 5th finger (clinodactyly),* and simian crease*
Feet	Increased space between 1st and 2nd toes,* furrow on the sole extending from the space between 1st and 2nd toes
Joints	Hypotonia*
Muscles	Hyperextensibility/hyperflexibility*
Heart	Murmur, cyanotic, or acyanotic congenital heart defect
Reflexes	Lack of Moro reflex*

*Useful for making a diagnosis in the newborn.

Associated problems:

- *Intellectual disability:*
  - Down syndrome is the most common genetic cause of moderate intellectual disability (IQ range 25–75).
  - Developmental delay in these patients is universal with variable cognitive impairment. They often have preserved social skills with a happy demeanor.
- *Congenital heart disease (CHD):*
  - About 40–50% of children with DS have CHD, with endocardial cushion defects accounting for about 40–60% of CHD.
  - Congenital heart disease constitutes the most common cause of morbidity and mortality in infants with DS. The presence of CHD is the most significant factor in determining survival.
  - Atrioventricular septal defect (AVSD), ventricular septal defect (VSD), and patent ductus arteriosus (PDA) are the most common CHD in patients with DS.
  - All children with DS should have a cardiac evaluation during the neonatal period or as early as possible and it should ideally include an echocardiogram.
- *Gastrointestinal (GI) malformations:*
  - Structural GI disorders including duodenal and small bowel atresia, annular pancreas, imperforate anus, and Hirschsprung disease occur more commonly in patients with DS as compared to the general population.
  - They are also prone to develop gastroesophageal reflux, intermittent diarrhea, chronic constipation, and celiac disease.
  - Celiac disease is strongly associated with DS, affecting up to 5% of the patients. Hence, it is recommended to screen them for celiac disease at 2 years of age or with symptoms using serum IgA levels and tissue transglutaminase antibodies.
- *Eye problems:*
  - Increased risk of refractory errors (50%), cataracts (15%), nystagmus, and strabismus
  - Routine ophthalmologic evaluation is recommended at birth or by 6 months of age, and annually thereafter.

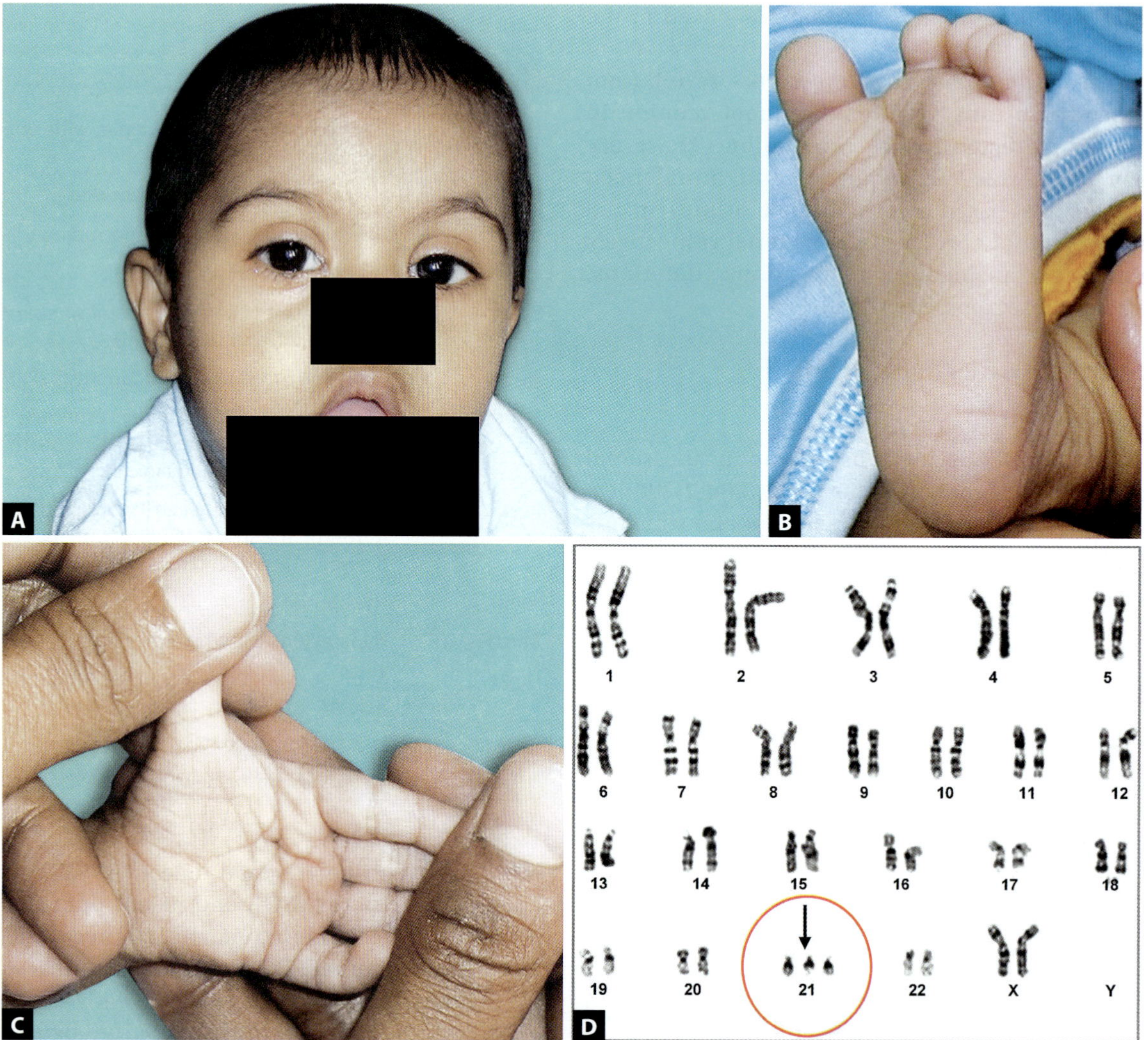

Figs. 17.3.1A to D: (A) Facial phenotype of Down syndrome (DS); (B) Increased gap in between first and second toes; (C) Single palmar crease; and (D) Karyotype of DS showing trisomy 21.

- *Hearing impairment or loss:*
  - About 40–60% of patients have conductive hearing loss and are also prone to serous otitis media (50–70% during 1st year).
  - Routine evaluation is indicated in the 1st year and then every year, including examination for otitis media at each visit.
  - Audiologic evaluation at least once between 5 years and 13 years and then every year is recommended.
- *Thyroid dysfunction:*
  - About 15–30% of children with DS have hypothyroidism, which can be either congenital or acquired.
  - Thyroid function tests [thyroxine (T4) and thyroid-stimulating hormone (TSH)] are recommended once in the neonatal period/at first contact, twice a year in the 1st year and then once every year.
- *Atlanto-occipital subluxation:*
  - A serious but infrequent complication of DS with variable incidence—reported in 10–30%.
  - Evaluation by CT scan is recommended before surgery, for participation in special games or in the presence of signs and symptoms suggestive of cord compression.
- *Physical growth:*
  - Regular follow-up for height and weight is recommended.
  - Linear growth is less as compared to normal children and these children tend to become obese with age.
  - Special growth charts for children with DS should ideally be used. As special growth charts for Indian children with DS are not available; growth charts published in Western literature may be used.

- *Malignancy:*
  - Hematological malignancies are more common in DS than in the general population.
  - In newborns and infants with DS, transient myeloproliferative disorder, a self-limiting condition can be seen.
  - They also have an increased incidence of acute leukemia during the first decade of life.
- *Immunity and infections:*
  - Pneumonia and other infections are more common in DS.
  - Respiratory tract infections are more frequent due to associated CHD and hypotonia.
  - Defects in the immunological system, involving both B-cells and T-cells contribute to infections.
- *Sexual development:*
  - Both males and females with DS display fairly normal sexual development.
  - The girls attain menarche and can be fertile, but males are always infertile.

Laboratory Diagnosis

Diagnosis is confirmed by karyotype testing, i.e., chromosomal analysis. In about 94% of cases, the cause of DS is trisomy 21 **(Fig. 17.3.1D)**, about 1% of cases are mosaics and the rest 4% are due to translocations, most commonly involving chromosomes 21 and 14. Karyotyping of the parents is only required if baby has DS due to translocation.

Management

Apart from the investigations and monitoring as described above, early stimulation and counseling are important components of management.[1]

Early stimulation: Early stimulation is recommended for all children with DS and should be started as early as possible with the active involvement of the parents. Ideally, it should be done by a child psychologist, but any pediatrician can guide the parents for the same. The basic objectives of early stimulation are as follows:

- To involve parents in effectively teaching the relevant skills in different areas of development.
- To individualize the training program.
- To impart basic knowledge and change unfavorable attitudes of parents toward children with DS.

Counseling

Counseling of parents having a child with DS varies with the age at presentation for consultation and their preparedness. It is important that the counsellor be passionate and truthful in discussing the attributes of patients with DS and not just the problems. The diagnosis should be disclosed as early as one is sure, preferably after karyotyping particularly in a neonate. It is preferred to discuss with both parents together using simple language and giving sufficient time. It is usually not necessary to discuss rare complications such as malignancies. One should give hope and emphasize the need for early stimulation and its benefits. Counseling regarding the risk of recurrence is important but may be postponed for a future date if the baby is very young. Parents should be encouraged to join a local parent group if existing. A regular follow-up needs to be ensured.

Risk of Recurrence

The risk of recurrence of DS predominantly varies according to the mother's age (at the time of delivery), chromosomal constitution of the previous affected child with DS (trisomy vs. translocation) and the balanced chromosomal translocation carrier status of parents.

- Women aged 35 years or less who have a previously affected child with trisomy 21 have about 1% risk of having another affected child, which is significantly greater than the general population.
- The risk increases a little, if any, over the usual maternal age-dependent frequency if the mother at risk is aged 35 years or older.
- The risks are higher in familial translocation cases where either the mother or the father is a balanced translocation carrier involving chromosome 21 and other acrocentric chromosomes. The risk of recurrence of DS in the next pregnancy is about 10% if the mother is a balanced chromosomal translocation carrier, and about 4–5% if the father is a balanced chromosomal translocation carrier respectively.
- The risk is 100% if either of the parents is a carrier of Robertsonian translocation involving two chromosomes 21.

Prenatal Screening and Prenatal Diagnosis

Prenatal screening for DS aims to assess the risk of having a baby with DS during pregnancy. It involves testing for various biochemical parameters and ultrasonogram (USG) during 1st and 2nd trimesters. Mothers having a child with DS and those conceiving after the age of 35 years can opt for definite prenatal diagnosis by invasive techniques. In other women with lesser a priori risk, or who do not wish to go for invasive testing, biochemical screening for chromosomal abnormalities can be carried out.

First-trimester screening: This includes maternal serum screening for human chorionic gonadotropin (hCG) and pregnancy-associated plasma protein-A (PAPP-A) (dual marker), and nuchal translucency (NT) or nasal bone (NB) assessment on USG (at 11–13^{+6} weeks of pregnancy). An increased NT (defined as NT greater than 99th percentile for gestational age) and an absent or hypoplastic nasal bone on 1st-trimester USG may indicate a high risk for DS in addition to other aneuploidies or single gene disorder, and needs confirmatory testing. Combined 1st-trimester screening analysis includes a combined assessment of the NT value and dual markers to assess the likelihood of the fetus of having risk for chromosomal aneuploidies involving chromosome 21, 18, and 13. It has a detection rate of up to 95%. A risk of 1 in 250 or higher is considered to be at high risk of having a baby with DS.

Second-trimester screening: This includes Quadruple marker screening [maternal serum α-fetoprotein (MSAFP), hCG, inhibin A, and unconjugated estriol (uE3) assays] and level II USG between 16–20 weeks of gestation. In DS pregnancies, the levels of MSAFP and uE3 are low, whereas hCG is high. Second-trimester serum screening (between 16 and 20 weeks of gestation) gives a detection rate of about 80%. Level II USG (around 18–21 weeks of gestation) is useful to assess fetal structural abnormalities and soft markers including nuchal fold thickness, short femur, duodenal atresia, renal pyelectasis, ventriculomegaly, etc. that may indicate an increased likelihood of fetal chromosomal abnormalities. Couples in whom the risk cut-off is high are offered prenatal diagnosis by invasive testing.

Noninvasive prenatal screening (NIPS): A recent noninvasive test referred to as NIPS is presently being used extensively in high-risk cases with a very high negative predictive value (close to 98%). This technique utilizes next generation sequencing (NGS) technologies on cell-free fetal DNA isolated from maternal blood for detecting common aneuploidies involving chromosomes 21, 18, 13, and sex chromosomes. Presently, the cost is prohibitive for the test to be used as a screening test universally.

Invasive testing: Invasive prenatal testing may be indicated in women at high risk of fetal aneuploidy (aged >35 years, abnormal serum screening/combined screening, previous pregnancy with chromosomal aneuploidy, or abnormal ultrasonogram).

Prenatal karyotyping can be done by various invasive procedures. Chorionic villus sampling (CVS) can be carried out between 10 weeks and 12 weeks of pregnancy (transcervical or transabdominal). This allows diagnosis in the first trimester. The options for the couples coming late or opting for the initial screening with serum markers and USG are karyotyping by amniocentesis (16–18 weeks), transabdominal placental biopsy, or cordocentesis (after 18 weeks). The karyotype results are available within a week with cord blood samples and direct CVS preparations. Amniotic fluid cultures take about 2–3 weeks for the results. The risk of fetal loss after CVS and amniocentesis is about 0.5–1% and with cordocentesis, it is about 3%. Rapid prenatal diagnosis of trisomy 21 can be done by FISH or quantitative fluorescent polymerase chain reaction (QF-PCR) on amniotic fluid sample, as these test results are available in 2 days.

Edward Syndrome or Trisomy 18

Edward syndrome is the second most common autosomal trisomy, with an incidence of about 1 in 3,000 newborn babies. These babies have high mortality early in life. Half of them may die within the 1st week and many of the remaining die in the next 1 year. Only 5–10% survive beyond the 1st year with profound physical and intellectual disability. Most of the surviving individuals have partial trisomies.

Cytogenetics

Most cases have full trisomy 18 with advanced maternal age being a risk factor. Mosaicism or partial trisomy or translocation cases are rare. The extra chromosome in trisomy 18 is usually of maternal origin, resulting from maternal meiosis II nondisjunction.

Clinical Features

This disorder is characterized by developmental retardation, hypertonia, characteristic craniofacial features including occipital prominence, dolichocephaly, high forehead, triangular face with low set and malformed ears and micrognathia, shield-shaped chest and short sternum, hypoplastic nails, joint abnormalities including flexion deformity of fingers resulting in overlapping fingers, limited hip abduction, prominent heels, rocker bottom feet, and short dorsiflexed hallux. Congenital heart diseases are also common, most commonly including VSD and PDA.

Recurrence Risk

The recurrence risk is lower than the 1% unless one of the parents is a carrier of balanced chromosomal rearrangement involving chromosome 18. Most trisomy 18 fetuses are spontaneously aborted.

Prenatal Diagnosis

Biochemical screening in the 1st and 2nd trimester is useful for detecting mothers at high risk for trisomy 18. Classically, all three maternal serum markers (hCG, AFP, and uE3) are low. Definitive prenatal diagnosis can be offered using the same (including NIPT) modalities as for DS.

Patau Syndrome or Trisomy 13

Patau syndrome has an incidence of about 1 in 5,000 births. Most babies would die in the first few days of life. Only 5% survive the first 6 months and have severe developmental delays, seizures, and failure to thrive.

Cytogenetics

Most cases have full trisomy 13. Mosaicism or partial trisomy or translocation cases are rare. About 20% of cases have Robertsonian translocation involving chromosome 13 or rarely other acrocentric chromosomes. Advanced maternal age is an important risk factor.

Clinical Features

It is characterized by severe developmental delays, postnatal growth retardation, microcephaly, and hypertonia. Holoprosencephaly with varying degrees of incomplete development of forebrain and olfactory and optic nerves is noted in about 66% of cases. Ocular manifestations including anophthalmia or microphthalmia, coloboma of iris, retinal dysplasia; ear malformations, cleft lip with or without cleft palate are common and many children are deaf. Capillary hemangiomas and scalp defects in the region of the posterior fontanel are characteristic. There are frequent abnormalities of fingers and toes such as postaxial polydactyly of hands and feet, flexion deformities, and long and hyperconvex nails. Congenital heart defects are present in almost 80% of cases, commonly including VSD, PDA, and ASD. It is important to suspect trisomy 13 in an infant with holoprosencephaly, cleft lip, and/or palate and other associated anomalies.

Recurrence Risk

Risk of recurrence in subsequent pregnancies is <1%.

Prenatal Diagnosis

Prenatal screening by biochemical screening and NIPT are helpful to detect mothers at high risk for fetal trisomy 13. Confirmatory testing is possible by doing a karyotype on CVS or amniotic fluid sample.

Turner Syndrome

Turner syndrome (TS) is characterized by complete or partial monosomy of chromosome X. It has an incidence of about 1 in 5,000 female live births but is much more common at conception and in spontaneous abortions. About 50% of patients with TS have monosomy X (45,X), most commonly the lost X chromosome being of paternal origin, with mosaicism being observed in the remaining. Maternal age is not a predisposing factor for TS.

Clinical Features

The clinical picture is highly variable. At birth, these girls may be phenotypically normal or may show nonpitting edema of hands and feet, neck webbing, deep-set nails, etc. **Box 17.3.1** mentions the list of suggestive clinical features. Common features in older children include short stature with variable

BOX 17.3.1: Clinical features of Turner syndrome.

- *Retarded growth and reduced final height:*
- *Gonadal dysgenesis:*
  - No pubertal development/lack of secondary sexual characters
  - Infertility
  - Gonadoblastoma (presence of Y chromosome material associated with increased risk)
- *Endocrine disturbances:*
  - Glucose intolerance (adults)
  - Type 2 diabetes mellitus
  - Type 1 diabetes mellitus
  - Autoimmune hypothyroidism (adults)
  - Thyroid autoantibodies (15–30%)
- *Physical abnormalities:*
  - *Mouth:*
    - Triangular facies
    - Micrognathia (small mandibular bone)
    - High-arched palate
    - Abnormal dental development
  - *Eyes:*
    - Epicanthic folds
    - Nearsightedness
    - Strabismus
    - Ptosis
  - *Ears:*
    - Prominent anomalous ears
    - Hearing impairment
    - Infection of middle ear
  - *Neck:*
    - Low posterior hair line
    - Short broad appearing neck
    - Pterygium colli (webbed neck)
    - Excess loose skin in the back of the newborn
  - *Thorax:*
    - Broad chest (shield chest) with widely spaced nipples
    - Inverted nipples
    - *Skin, nail, and hair:*
      - Lymphedema of hands and feet at birth or later
      - Multiple pigmented nevi
      - Nail hypoplasia and deep set nails
      - Vitiligo
      - Alopecia
    - *Skeleton:*
      - Delayed bone age
      - Decreased bone mineral content
      - Cubitus valgus
      - Short fourth metacarpal
      - Genu valgum
      - Congenital hip subluxation
      - Scoliosis
      - Madelung deformity

Contd...

Contd...

- *Heart:*
    - Bicuspid aortic valve
    - Coarctation aorta
    - Hypoplastic left heart syndrome and other left-sided cardiac abnormalities
- *Kidneys:*
    - Horseshoe kidney
    - Abnormal positioning or duplication of renal pelvis, ureter, or vessels
    - Renal aplasia or hypoplasia
- *Psychological problems*
- *Others:*
    - Failure to thrive during 1st year of life
    - Developmental delay (10%)
    - Learning disability (nonverbal motor and visuospatial skills, 70%)
    - Celiac disease
    - Inflammatory bowel disease
    - Sensorineural hearing loss

dysmorphic features, low posterior hairline, webbing of neck, shield chest, cubitus valgus, gonadal dysgenesis (streak ovaries) with primary amenorrhea, lack of secondary sexual characters, CHD, renal anomalies, and behavioral problems. All prepubertal girls with short stature and girls with primary amenorrhea should be investigated for TS.

A girl with TS with a characteristic phenotype is shown in **Figures 17.3.2A to C**.

Diagnosis

Karyotype from peripheral blood is diagnostic and commonly shows 45,X. Other karyotype abnormalities in these patients include 46,X,i(Xq); 45,X/46,XX; 45,X/46XY; 45,X/46,X,i(Xq). Mosaicism involving Y chromosome is observed in 5%. Search for Y-cell line is warranted, especially in the presence of masculinization or karyotyping findings of mosaicism, an unidentified marker or ring chromosome X. Routine scoring of 20 metaphases is recommended but if karyotype is normal and there is high index of suspicion score 100 metaphases.

Once the diagnosis is established, screening to look for associated abnormalities is important. Plasma gonadotropin levels show a high follicle-stimulating hormone (FSH) and luteinizing hormone (LH) suggestive of hypergonadotropic hypogonadism. USG of pelvis commonly shows hypoplastic uterus and streak ovaries. Structural abnormalities of the urinary tract are frequently noted. It is also important to evaluate for thyroid function, antithyroid peroxidase antibodies and celiac disease.

Management[2]

- *Height monitoring* to check height velocity.
- *Cardiac evaluation* includes measurement of the blood pressure and echocardiography—baseline and annual evaluation.
- *Growth hormone (GH) therapy* is beneficial and has been recommended by the Food and Drug Administration (FDA). The decision to treat should be left to the parents as the cost of treatment is high and height gain may be up to 10 cm.
- Counsel regarding *behavioral problems* due to short stature, amenorrhea, and infertility (usually) and provision of psychosocial support.
- *Evaluation for thyroid dysfunction:* Infancy and early childhood especially after 10 years of age. Hypothyroidism is often autoimmune and needs periodic evaluation. Replacement therapy should be given accordingly.
- *Ovarian hormone replacement:*
    - Start at 14 years (12 years, if the patient has received and completed GH therapy).
    - Start with conjugated estrogen at 0.3 mg/day or ethinyl estradiol 5–10 µg/day for 36 months; then increase to 0.625 mg or 1.25 mg (conjugated estrogen) or 20–50 µg/day (ethinyl estradiol)
    - After *6 months to 1 year:* Cyclical therapy with adding progesterone.
- *Regular audiometry* in adults or earlier, if indicated.
- *Evaluation for renal malformation* by USG, and, if abnormal, manage accordingly.
- *Prophylactic gonadectomy* in Turner syndrome patients with Y chromosome.

Prenatal Diagnosis

The risk of recurrence in subsequent pregnancies is low (<1%). Diagnosis of TS can be suspected prenatally on 1st trimester USG with increased nuchal translucency or in 2nd trimester USG showing cystic hygroma, generalized hydrops, or swelling localized to the neck (increased nuchal fold thickness). Confirmation can be done by karyotype of fetal sample collected by CVS, amniocentesis, or cordocentesis.

Klinefelter Syndrome

It is one of the most common sex chromosomal aneuploidies in males affecting about 1.32 per 1,000 among newborns. It is the most common cause of hypogonadism and infertility in males, characterized by failure of development of secondary sex characteristics and increased gonadotropin levels. The diagnosis is rarely before puberty. The affected individuals tend to have tall and slim stature with low upper and lower segment ratio, testis, and penis being smaller in size for their age. Pubertal development is delayed. The growth of pubic and facial hair is often late, with a generally feminine distribution of pubic hair. Infertility is present with hyalinization and fibrosis of seminiferous tubules. Virilization is partial and inadequate with gynecomastia occurring in one-third of adolescents.

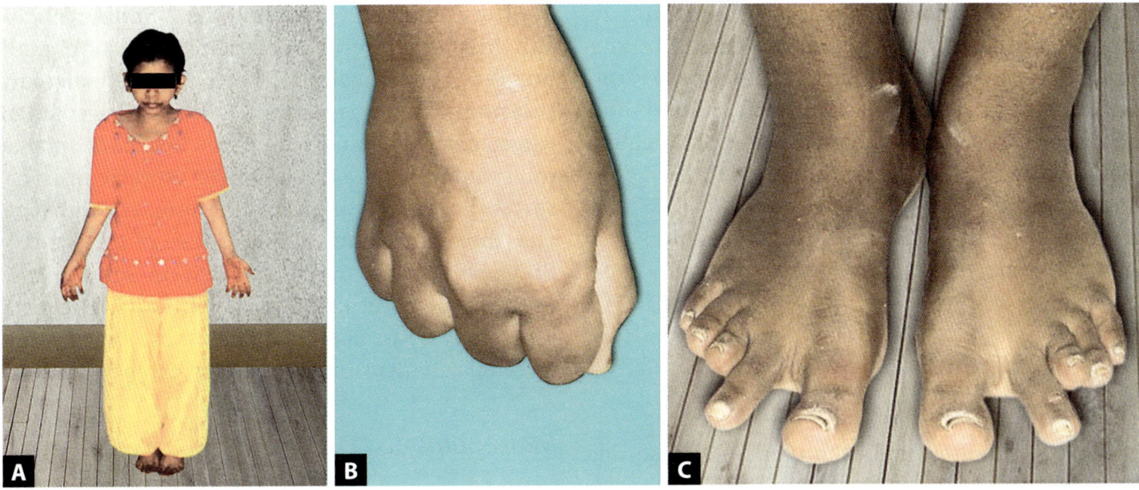

Figs. 17.3.2A to C: Girl with Turner syndrome: (A) Short stature, neck webbing and increased carrying angle; (B) Short 4th and 5th metacarpals; (C) Short 4th and 5th metatarsals.

Chromosomal Analysis

Chromosomal analysis reveals 47,XXY karyotype. Errors in paternal meiosis I account for about one-half of 47,XXY males while the remainder are due to maternal meiosis II errors, and a very small number of cases to a postzygotic mitotic error. Individuals with XXY/XY mosaicism have a better potential prognosis.

Structural Abnormalities

Structural chromosome rearrangements result from chromosomal breakage with subsequent reunion in a different configuration or orientation. These are broadly categorized as balanced and unbalanced rearrangements, based on the absence or presence of net loss or gain of extra chromosomal material respectively and include translocations, inversions, deletions, duplications, insertions, etc. These patients usually present with multiple major or minor malformations and developmental delays or mental retardation. Karyotyping is useful to detect large chromosomal rearrangements (usually >5 Mb) and balanced rearrangements. Chromosomal microdeletions and microduplications (smaller than 5 Mb) need higher resolution testing by chromosomal microarray for diagnosis.

SINGLE GENE DISORDERS

To date over 5,000 single gene traits and disorders have been identified. Each of these single gene disorders, often called Mendelian traits or diseases, is relatively uncommon. Most Mendelian diseases are rare, affecting about 1/10,000 to 1/100,000 live births as an order of magnitude estimate. In total, they will add to about 1% of live births. Since only a single gene is involved in each case, these diseases generally have simple inheritance patterns in family pedigrees. This means they can be traced through families and their occurrence in later generations can be predicted. The defective version of the gene responsible for the disease is known as a mutant allele or disease allele. Details of Mendelian inheritance are discussed elsewhere. At a minimum, a three-generation pedigree includes details about first-degree relatives (parents and siblings), second-degree relatives (aunts and uncles), and third-degree relatives (cousins and grandparents). The mode of inheritance is often recognizable from the pedigree. The various modes of inheritance are as follows:

- *Autosomal dominant traits* manifest in the heterozygous state, i.e., in a person possessing both an abnormal or mutant allele and the normal allele. Examples of autosomal dominant disorders include neurofibromatosis (NF), achondroplasia, Marfan syndrome, etc.
- *Autosomal recessive disorders* manifest when both the alleles of a gene carry a mutation in either homozygous or compound heterozygous state. Examples of autosomal recessive disorders are thalassemia, spinal muscular atrophy, sickle-cell anemia, and almost all inborn errors of metabolism.
- Sex-linked inheritance refers to the pattern of inheritance shown by genes, which are located on either of the sex chromosomes. *X-linked dominant inheritance* although is uncommon; is observed in disorders that manifest in the heterozygous female as well as in the male who has the mutant allele on his single X chromosome. Examples include hypophosphatemic type of vitamin D-resistant rickets, orofaciodigital syndrome, etc.
- *X-linked recessive diseases* usually manifest only in males. A male with a mutant allele on his single X chromosome is said to be hemizygous for that allele. Examples include hemophilia A and B, Duchenne muscular dystrophy, etc.

- *Mitochondrial inheritance* is due to mutations in mitochondrial genes. Typically, they are passed from a mother to all her children; her sons will not pass it on, but daughters will pass it on to all of their children and so on. Examples include mitochondrial encephalopathy, lactic acidosis, and stroke like syndrome (MELAS), Leber hereditary optic neuropathy (LHON), etc.

In this chapter, we have discussed clinical features and management of some of the most common single gene disorders.

AUTOSOMAL DOMINANT DISORDERS

Achondroplasia

Achondroplasia is an autosomal dominant (AD) disorder caused by a common point mutation c.1138 G > A (*p.Gly380Arg*) in fibroblast growth factor receptor 3 *(FGFR3)* gene. More than half of the cases are due to de novo mutations. Other mutations in the same gene cause allelic disorders with variable severity—a lethal skeletal dysplasia called thanatophoric dysplasia and a relatively mild skeletal dysplasia known as hypochondroplasia.

Clinical Manifestations

The clinical manifestations include disproportionate short stature with predominant short limbs. There is rhizomelic shortening, large head, frontal bossing, depressed nasal bridge, short and broad trident-shaped hands, lumbar lordosis, hypotonia, and delayed motor development. Cognitive development is usually normal.

Complications include hydrocephalus, otitis media, and hearing loss in adulthood, craniocervical junction compression, lumbar cord, and nerve root compression syndromes. **Figures 17.3.3A to C** show the typical phenotype of achondroplasia.

The characteristic radiological findings include small cuboid-shaped vertebral bodies with short pedicles and progressive narrowing of lumbar interpedicular distance (normally there is caudal widening), rectangular iliac wings, narrow greater sciatic notches, horizontal acetabular roofs, anterior breaking of lower thoracic or upper lumbar vertebrae, small foramen magnum, metaphyseal flaring, and short and wide tubular bones of the hands and feet. **Figures 17.3.4A to D** show characteristic radiological findings of achondroplasia. Although the diagnosis is essentially clinical-radiological, molecular testing through targeted variant testing is easily available and is confirmatory.

Management

Periodic evaluation is important to monitor height, weight, and head circumference. Assessment of the craniocervical junction should be performed soon after diagnosis through detailed neurologic history and examination, and neuroimaging of the craniocervical junction (CT or MRI). A baseline neuroimaging of the brain is also indicated soon after diagnosis to assess the ventricular size. They should also be monitored for features suggestive of complications including obstructive sleep apnea, middle ear dysfunction, obesity, and spinal stenosis.

Vosoritide, a C-type natriuretic peptide, administered as a subcutaneous daily injection has been recently approved for children with achondroplasia aged 5 years or more, to be continued till the closure of the growth plate. Additionally, prompt recognition and appropriate treatment of complications including obstructive sleep apnea, middle ear dysfunction, and spinal stenosis, management of psychological problems due to unusual appearance and prevention of obesity is important. GH therapy though may add a few inches to the final height, is not recommended.

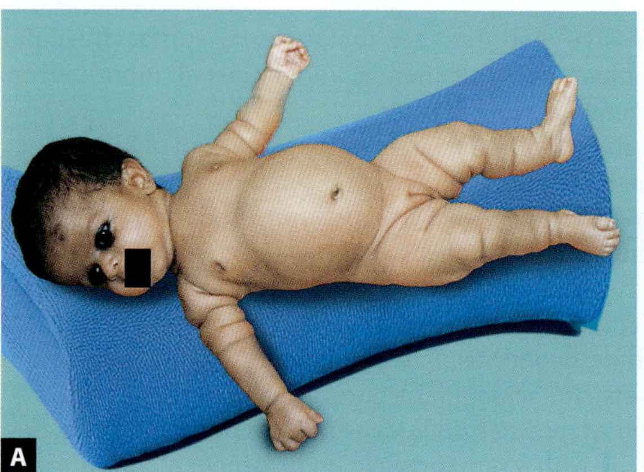

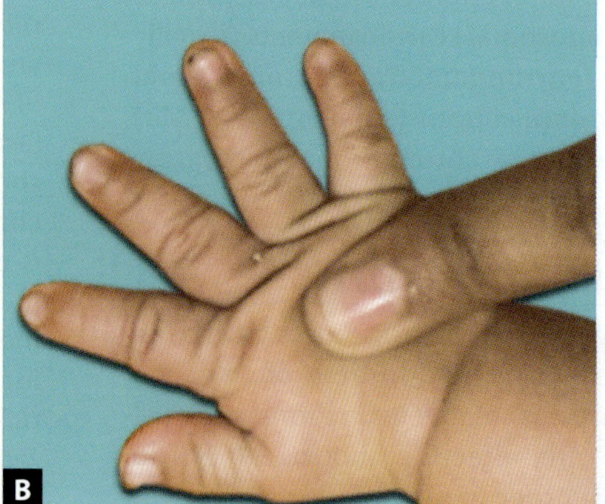

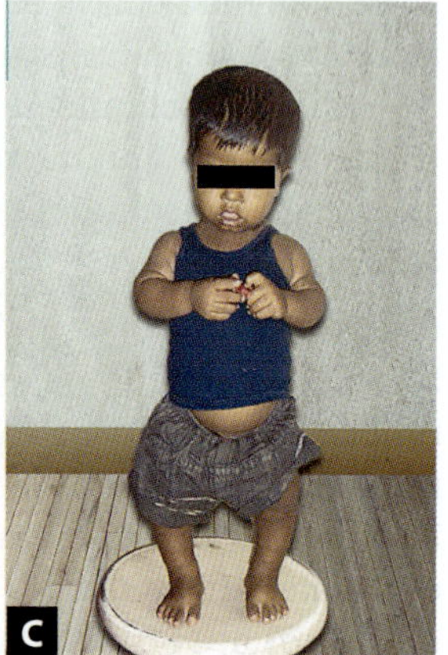

Figs. 17.3.3A to C: Achondroplasia: Short-limbed short stature, large head with frontal bossing, depressed nasal bridge, and trident hand. (A) Skin folds on the thighs and arms; (B) Trident hand; and (C) Genu varum.

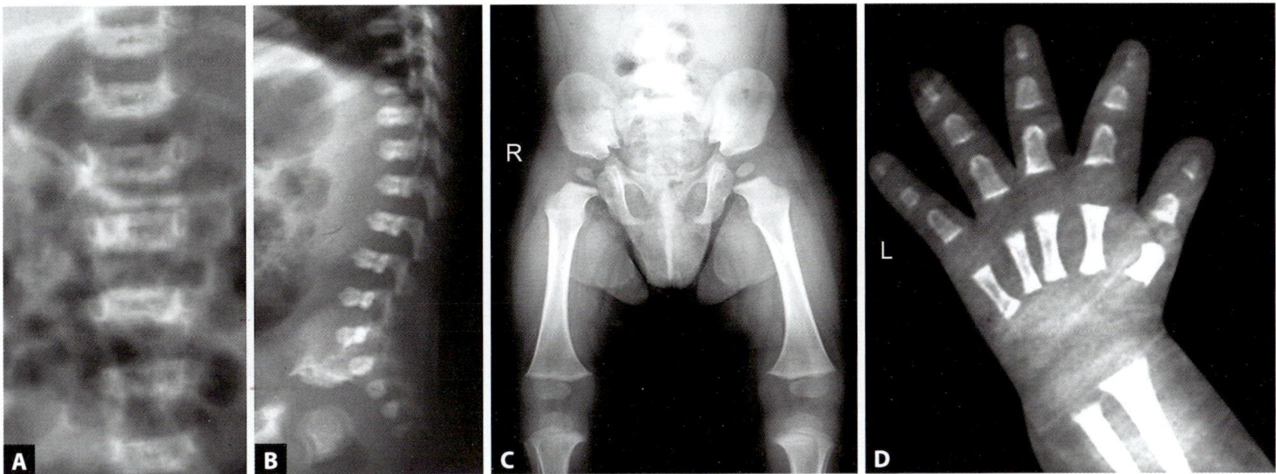

Figs. 17.3.4A to D: Radiological features of achondroplasia: (A) Small cuboid-shaped vertebral bodies with short pedicles and progressive narrowing of lumbar interpedicular distance (normally there is caudal widening); (B) Scalloping of posterior borders of vertebrae and anterior breaking of lower thoracic or upper lumbar vertebrae; (C) Rectangular iliac wings, narrow greater sciatic notches, horizontal acetabular roofs, metaphyseal flaring; and (D) Short and wide tubular bones of the hands with trident appearance.

Limb lengthening procedure, though very cumbersome, has been tried to improve height.[3]

Risk of Recurrence

The risk of recurrence is 50% if either of the parents is affected, but is very low if the disorder is caused by a de novo mutation.

Marfan Syndrome

Marfan syndrome is a systemic connective tissue disorder inherited in an AD manner. It is caused by mutations in the fibrillin gene (*FBN1*) located on chromosome 15q21.1. It has a high penetrance, but expression may be variable.

Clinical Manifestations

The disorder primarily involves the skeletal, ocular, and cardiovascular system. The common skeletal manifestations include tall stature, disproportionately long limbs with increased arm span (dolichostenomelia), arachnodactyly, joint laxity, scoliosis, kyphosis, decreased subcutaneous fat, pectus deformities (excavatum/carinatum), and flat feet (pes planus). The characteristic eye abnormality is superotemporal lens subluxation (noted in 60% of patients). Myopia, increased axial length of the globe, glaucoma, and retinal detachment may also be present. Cardiovascular involvement is responsible for major morbidity and mortality in these individuals and includes dilatation and aneurysm of the aorta (commonly ascending) predisposing to rupture of the aorta, aortic and mitral regurgitation, mitral valve prolapse, etc. **Figures 17.3.5A to C** show a patient with Marfan syndrome.

Diagnosis

The diagnosis of Marfan syndrome is suspected based on clinical evaluation. The clinical diagnostic criteria (Revised Ghent Nosology) also aid in the diagnosis of Marfan syndrome where a systemic score cut-off of ≥7 is taken as diagnostic. Molecular confirmation may be performed using exome sequencing as single gene testing may be cumbersome considering the large size of the gene.

Management

Following an initial diagnosis, these patients need to be evaluated for baseline skeletal manifestations including scoliosis and dural ectasia (MRI spine if symptomatic), cardiovascular (echocardiogram to assess aortic root Z-score), and ophthalmologic involvement. They need regular follow-up for early detection and prevention of complications, primarily cardiac. β-blockers are used to reduce cardiac complications. Recently, losartan, an angiotensin II type 1 receptor antagonist has been found useful to prevent cardiac complications of Marfan syndrome. Surgical repair of the aorta is indicated in children and adults with aortic root dilation of >5 cm, a rate of aortic root dilation of >1 cm/year, and progressive and severe aortic regurgitation.

Risk of Recurrence

The risk of recurrence in subsequent pregnancies is 50% if either of the parents is affected.

Tuberous Sclerosis

Tuberous sclerosis (TS) is an AD neurocutaneous syndrome with multisystem involvement resulting from mutations in

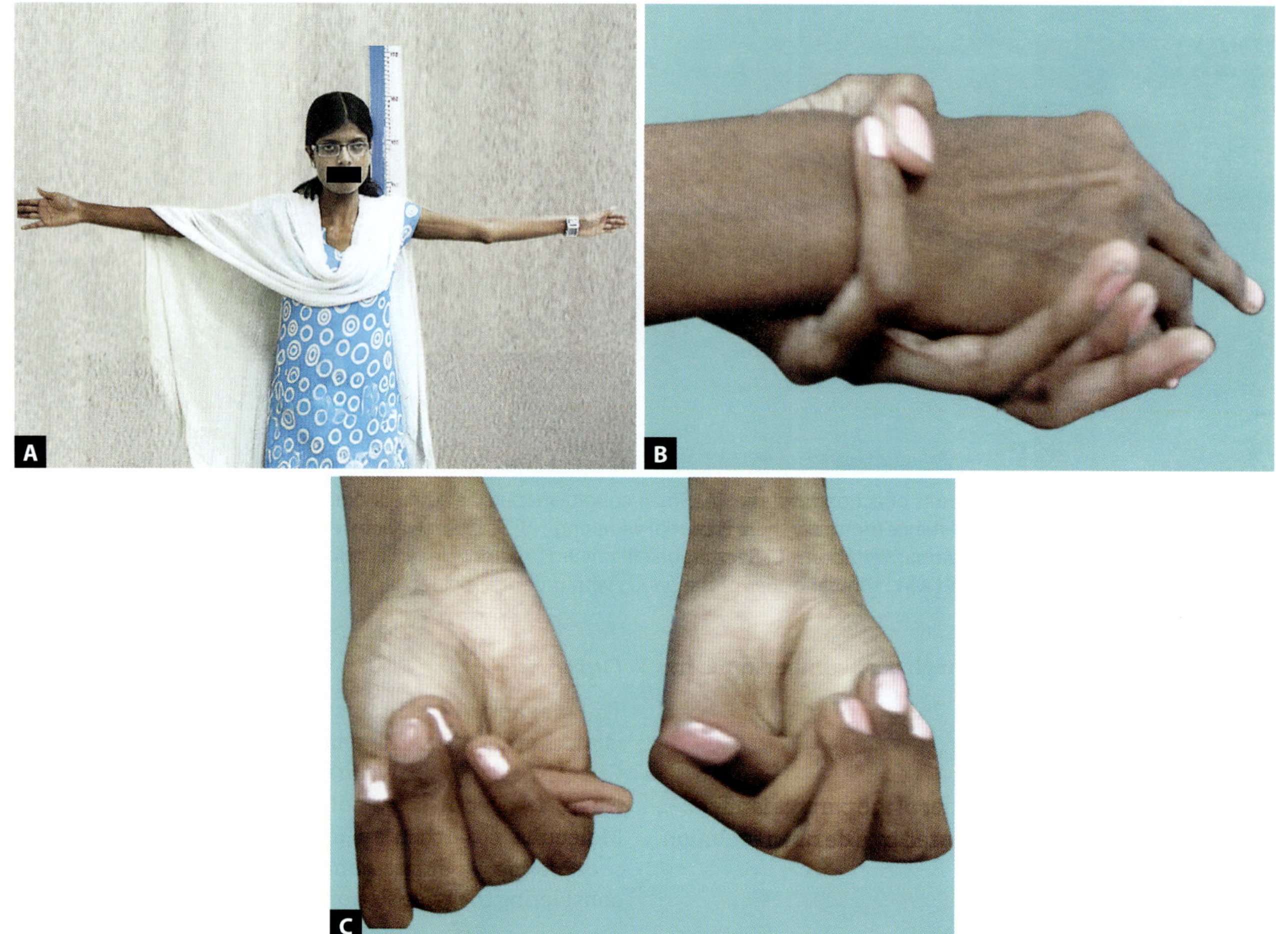

Figs. 17.3.5A to C: Marfan syndrome: (A) Increased arm span; (B) Wrist sign; and (C) Thumb sign.

tuberous sclerosis type 1 *(TSC1)* and tuberous sclerosis type 2 *(TSC2)* genes.

Clinical Features

Tuberous sclerosis is characterized by the involvement of the brain, skin, kidney, lungs, eyes, and cardiovascular system. The clinical features are categorized as major and minor criteria and aid in the diagnosis. The major criteria include facial angiofibromas (≥3) or forehead plaque, subungal fibromas (≥2), hypomelanotic macules (≥3) typically described as "ash leaf", shagreen patch (flesh-colored elevated orange peel-like lesions), retinal hamartomas, cortical tubers and/or radial migration lines (on neuroimaging), subependymal nodules (≥2), subependymal giant cell astrocytomas (SEGA), cardiac rhabdomyoma, renal angiomyolipoma (≥2), and pulmonary lymphangioleiomyomatosis. The minor criteria include sclerotic bone lesions, dental enamel pits, confetti skin lesions, multiple renal cysts, intraoral fibromas, nonrenal hamartomas, and retinal achromatic patch. Half of the patients have developmental delay. Seizures are difficult to control, behavioral problems, and autistic features are common. **Figures 17.3.6A and B** show skin manifestations in a patient with TS.

The unique skin lesions and neuroimaging findings are most helpful for confirming diagnosis. A clinical diagnosis of TS is established in the presence of two major or one major with two or more minor features. Confirmation of the diagnosis can be made by mutation testing for the two genes, *TSC1* and *TSC2*, through exome sequencing. For detailed discussion, please refer to Chapter 8.5.

Management

Following an initial diagnosis, it is important to evaluate and ensure timely surveillance for systemic involvement including the brain (MRI for tubers, SEGA, etc.), kidneys (renal function and angiomyolipoma), eye, heart (echocardiogram in children <3 years of age) and pulmonary involvement. Treatment of TS is largely symptomatic. Seizures may be refractory to treat. Some patients show a good response to vigabatrin therapy. Surgical interventions may be required for some patients.[4]

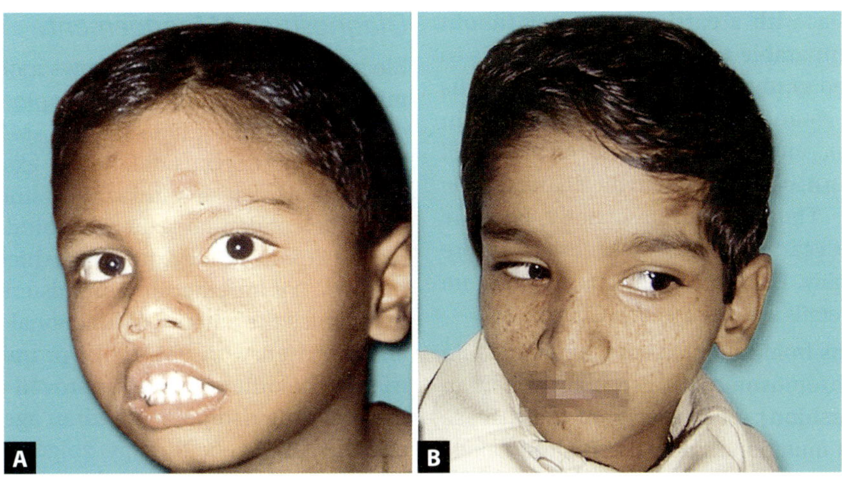

Figs. 17.3.6A and B: Skin lesions in a patient with TS: (A) Hyperpigmented thickened (Shagreen) patch on forehead; and (B) Adenoma sebaceum on cheeks in butterfly distribution.

Risk of Recurrence

The risk of recurrence is 50% if one of the parents is affected. Parents should be examined carefully and investigated for stigmata of tuberous sclerosis as some of them may have very few features.

Neurofibromatosis

Neurofibromatosis (NF) is a common AD neurocutaneous syndrome with variable expression. It is classified into two types: (1) neurofibromatosis type 1 (NF1) and (2) neurofibromatosis type 2 (NF2).

Clinical Features

Clinical features of NF1 include *café-au-lait* spots (six or more, 1.5 cm or larger in postpubertal patients, 0.5 cm or larger in prepubertal patients), two or more neurofibromas, or one plexiform neurofibroma, freckling of axillary or inguinal regions, optic glioma, iris hamartomas (Lisch nodules), pseudoarthrosis of tibia, and family history of an affected first-degree relative. For labeling as NF, two or more of these features should be present. **Figure 17.3.7** shows a patient with NF1. They are at an increased risk of developing benign/malignant tumors including optic nerve gliomas, malignant peripheral nerve sheath tumors, etc.

The most characteristic feature of NF2 is the development in early adult life of tumors involving eighth cranial nerve commonly called "acoustic neuromas", which may require surgical intervention. Skin manifestations are less common in NF2.

For detailed discussion, please refer to Chapter 8.5.

Diagnosis

Diagnosis is invariably clinical but can be confirmed by molecular studies.

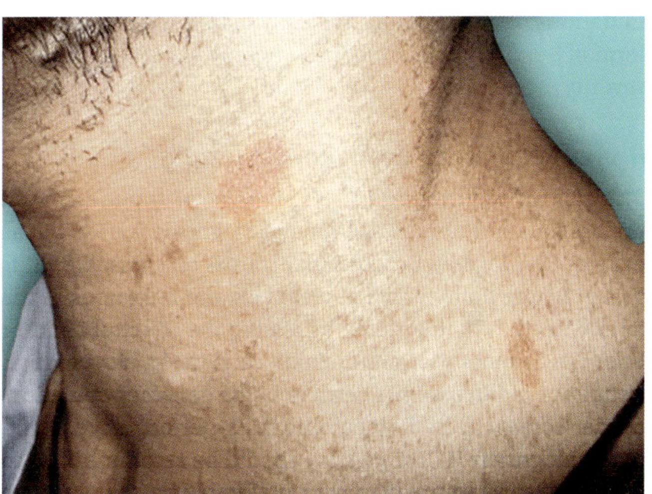

Fig. 17.3.7: Skin lesions in neurofibromatosis type 1 (NF1) (Café-au-lait spots).

Management

The management in NF1 is mainly supportive and consists of regular follow-up and evaluation for complications such as focal neurological dysfunction, optic gliomas, skeletal abnormalities, cognitive/learning problems, hypertension, and provision of symptomatic therapy. Recently, selumetinib, an MEK inhibitor has been approved by the FDA for treatment of NF1-related inoperable plexiform neurofibroma.[5]

AUTOSOMAL RECESSIVE DISORDERS

β-thalassemia

β-thalassemia is an inherited autosomal recessive hematological disorder characterized by reduced rate of synthesis of β-globin chains that make up adult hemoglobin (HbA). It is probably the most common autosomal recessive disorder in North India, with a carrier frequency (about 3%) approximately comparable to that of cystic fibrosis in Caucasians. The reduced synthesis of β-globin chains results in imbalance between α- and β-globin chains, resulting in ineffective erythropoiesis, increased peripheral red blood cell destruction which, in turn, causes anemia, the characteristic presenting symptom. These children usually become symptomatic in the 1st year of life and present with severe anemia and splenomegaly. Repeated blood transfusions are required for survival. Details are discussed in Chapter 14.7.

β-thalassemia results from mutations in the hemoglobin beta *(HBB)* gene on chromosome 11 (also inherited in an autosomal-recessive fashion). The severity of the disease depends on the type of mutation. If only *one* β-globin allele bears a mutation, the individual is clinically asymptomatic and is called β-*thalassemia minor* (or sometimes called β-*thalassemia carrier/trait*). If both the *HBB* alleles have mutations, the individuals typically manifest disease in the form of β-*thalassemia major* or *intermedia* depending on the severity of anemia.

Risk of Recurrence and Prenatal Testing

The risk of recurrence in the siblings of a patient with thalassemia major is 25%. Prenatal diagnosis is possible as early as 10–11 weeks by molecular studies on chorionic villus tissue. Before doing prenatal diagnosis, the mutations in the family need to be identified by testing the affected child or both the parents who are obligate carriers. In view of high frequency of thalassemia carriers in the general population, carrier screening by hemoglobin high-performance liquid chromatography (HPLC) testing should be recommended to all, either early in pregnancy or preferably before planning pregnancy.

Spinal Muscular Atrophy

Spinal muscular atrophy is an autosomal recessive disorder caused by mutations in survival motor neuron 1 (*SMN1*) gene. Disorders of varying severity manifesting with muscle weakness and atrophy due to loss of the motor neurons of the spinal cord and brainstem are grouped under SMA. The severe fetal form (SMA type 0) is characterized by severe neonatal hypotonia and is usually fatal in the perinatal period. Children with severe infantile SMA (type 1) present in first few weeks/months of life (usually <6 months) with motor delay and floppiness and die in early infancy. Characteristic tongue fasciculations are seen in most cases. Spinal muscular atrophy types II (late infantile and more slowly progressive form) and III (chronic juvenile form) are milder forms presenting beyond infancy (>18 months and in later childhood/adulthood respectively).

Diagnosis and Management

Electromyography (EMG) shows a neurogenic pattern, and muscle biopsy shows group atrophy. In most cases (>95%) diagnosis can be made by the *SMN* gene testing, which shows a homozygous deletion of exon 7 of the *SMN1* gene. Recently, the drug spinraza (nusinersen) is an antisense oligonucleotide that selectively binds and targets RNA and regulates *SMN2* gene expression which has been approved by the FDA. It is intrathecally administered and has the potential to enhance the amount of functional SMN protein in infants and children with SMA with promising results in recent trials.[6] The other recently approved drugs for SMA include the oral drug risdiplam (children aged 2 months and older) and the *AAV9* gene therapy, zolgensma administered as an intravenous infusion (for children aged <2 years). The cost of therapy is currently prohibitive.

Risk of Recurrence

The risk of recurrence is 25% in subsequent pregnancies and prenatal diagnosis is possible using chorionic villus tissue. Details of SMA are discussed in Chapter 8.19.

X-LINKED DISORDERS

Duchenne/Becker Muscular Dystrophy

Muscular dystrophies form a group of genetically determined progressive disorders primarily involving the muscles. The various forms of muscular dystrophies are distinguished by a combination of clinical, pathological features, and genetic investigations. The common muscular dystrophies following an X-linked pattern of inheritance are Duchenne muscular dystrophy (DMD) and Becker muscular dystrophy (BMD).

DMD is a severe muscle wasting disorder, and BMD is a milder form of the disease with later onset and slow progression. In DMD, the children usually present around 3–4 years of age with calf hypertrophy and proximal muscle weakness. Gower's sign is characteristically seen. DMD is also discussed in Chapter 8.19.

The dystrophin gene (*DMD*) responsible for DMD/BMD maps to the short arm of the X chromosome at band Xp21. DMD, being a severe form, has little or no functional dystrophin protein. In BMD, the milder form, dystrophin may be reduced in amount or altered in size. Approximately 60% of the affected males have a deletion of one or more exons of the *DMD* gene, while the remaining patients have duplications and point mutations. Recently, antisense oligonucleotide therapies based on exon skipping have been approved by the FDA for exon 51 (eteplirsen or exondys 51), exon 45 (casimersen or amondys 45) and exon 53 (golodirsen or vyondys 53, viltolarsen). Vamorolone, a novel dissociative oral steroid with reduced steroid toxicity and givonostat, an oral histone deacetylase inhibitor, have also been approved for DMD. Other therapies under investigation include ataleuren that acts through stop codon read-through mechanism.[7]

Risk of Recurrence

The risk of recurrence in subsequent pregnancies is 50% for a male offspring, if the mother is a carrier. There is 50% chance of the daughters being a carrier. Prenatal diagnosis is possible on chorionic villus tissue using molecular techniques.

Fragile X Syndrome

Fragile X syndrome (FXS) is an X-linked semidominantly inherited disorder with reduced penetrance and does not follow the classical Mendelian pattern of inheritance. Initially, it was thought to be a chromosomal disorder because of the presence of a fragile site at Xq27.3. FXS is the most common heritable form of moderate intellectual retardation and is second only to DS among all causes of moderate intellectual retardation in males. It occurs due to CGG repeat expansion in the 5′ untranslated region of the first exon of the fragile X mental retardation 1 *(FMR1)* gene on the X chromosome.

The inheritance of this X-linked disorder is unusual, where it is passed on by an unaffected transmitting male but only can be expressed after being passed through a female. The normal CGG repeat size is <50. In permutation carriers of FXS, the number of repeated CGG sequences is >50 but <200. In the full mutation, the number of repeats is >200. In general, the expression of phenotypic manifestations is less severe in females, as seen in an X-linked dominant inheritance.

Clinical Features

The clinical features are nonspecific and include overgrowth, large dolichocephalic head, large ears, joint hyperextensibility, hyperactivity, autistic features, and behavioral problems. Large testes become evident around puberty. Various scoring systems for the clinical phenotype have been used but it should be suspected and tested in all males with idiopathic intellectual disability with a normal or increased head size. **Figure 17.3.8** shows the typical facial features of FXS. Individuals with *FMR1* premutation are characterized by late onset cerebellar ataxia, tremors, and cognitive impairment, termed as "Fragile X-associated tremor/ataxia syndrome (FXTAS)." Also, female premutation carriers are at a risk of premature ovarian insufficiency.

Diagnosis and Management

Diagnosis is confirmed by DNA testing which has now replaced the cytogenetic analysis. The gold standard for testing is Southern blotting, which can differentiate normal genotype, premutation, and the full mutation. Polymerase chain reaction-based screening tests are available and are very reliable.

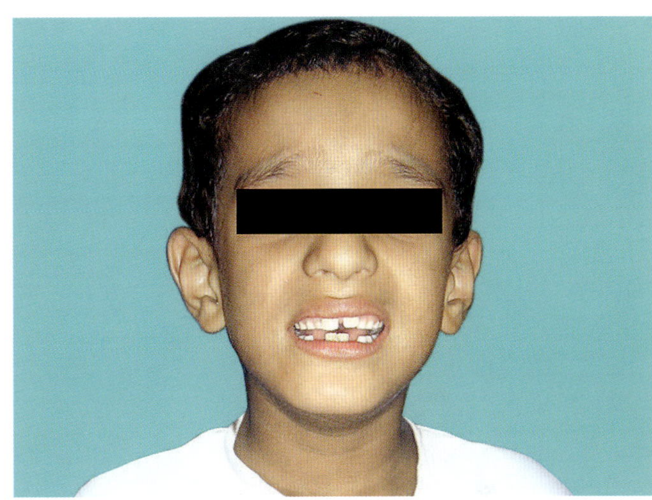

Fig. 17.3.8: A child with Fragile X syndrome (FXS) showing long face, large head, and large ears.

Treatment includes supportive measures and symptomatic therapy for psychological and behavioral disorders.

Rett Syndrome

Rett syndrome is an X-linked dominant pervasive neurodevelopmental disorder. The majority of Rett syndrome cases are caused by sporadic mutations in the gene methyl-CpG-binding domain protein 2 *(MECP2)* located on the long arm of X-chromosome at Xq28. It almost exclusively affects girls—male fetuses with the disorder rarely survive to term. Recently, *MECP2* mutations have also been identified in some males with intellectual disability. An atypical form of Rett syndrome, characterized by infantile spasms or early onset epilepsy, can also be caused by a mutation to the gene encoding cyclin-dependent kinase-like 5 (*CDKL5*).

Clinical Features

The revised clinical criteria for Rett syndrome are as follows:

- *Main criteria:*
  - Partial or complete loss of acquired purposeful hand skills.
  - Partial or complete loss of acquired spoken language.
  - *Gait abnormalities*: Impaired (dyspraxic) or absence of ability.
  - Stereotypic hand movements such as hand wringing/squeezing, clapping/tapping, mouthing, and washing/rubbing automatisms.
- *Exclusion criteria:*
  - Brain injury secondary to trauma (perinatally or postnatally), neurometabolic disease, or severe infection that causes neurological problems.
  - Grossly abnormal psychomotor development in first 6 months of life.

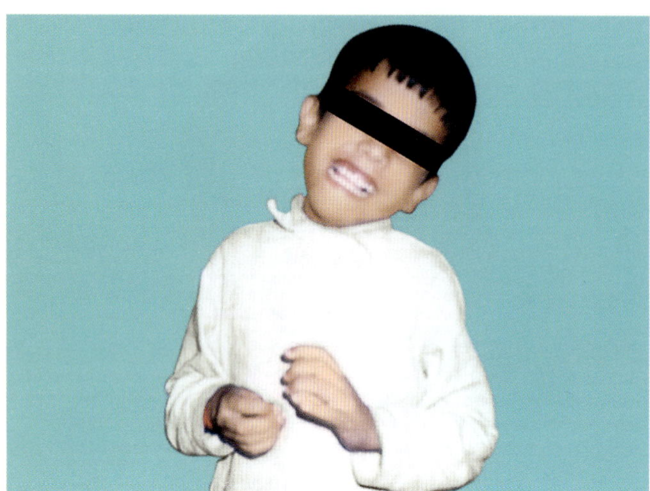

Fig. 17.3.9: A girl with Rett syndrome: characteristic hand stereotype.

- *Supportive criteria:*
    - Breathing disturbances when awake
    - Bruxism when awake
    - Impaired sleep pattern
    - Abnormal muscle tone
    - Peripheral vasomotor disturbances
    - Scoliosis/kyphosis

Diagnosis and Management

Important criteria for diagnosis include a period of regression followed by recovery or stabilization, all main criteria and all exclusion criteria but supportive criteria are not required. **Figure 17.3.9** shows a girl with Rett syndrome.

The treatment is essentially symptomatic and supportive. The risk of recurrence in subsequent pregnancies is low as most mutations are de novo.[8]

POLYGENIC DISORDERS

The expression of a phenotype determined by multiple genes at different loci, each exerting a small additive effect is called polygenic or quantitative inheritance. *Additive effect* implies that the effects of the genes are cumulative, i.e., no one gene is dominant or recessive to another. A trait is called *multifactorial* if multiple genes are assumed to interact with environmental factors. Since neither the environmental factors nor the genetic factors can be identified individually, the differentiation of polygenic and multifactorial is somewhat arbitrary. Few common examples include single malformations such as neural tube defects, CHD, cleft lip/palate, diabetes mellitus, ischemic heart disease, etc. Congenital malformations are seen in about 3% of newborns. Neural tube defects are the most common major malformation reported in India. **Table 17.3.2** lists common malformations and their risk of recurrence.

TABLE 17.3.2: Empiric risk of recurrence of isolated malformation.

Malformation	*Frequency per 1,000 births*	*Recurrence for normal parents of one affected child (%)*
Anencephaly/Spina bifida	4–5	5
Cardiac malformation	6–8	3–4
Cleft lip and cleft palate	2	4–5
Cleft palate alone	0.5	2–6
Pyloric stenosis	2–3	3
Talipes equinovarus	3–4	2–8
Dislocation of hip	3–4	3–4
Hirschsprung disease	0.1	6

Management in these situations involves surgical correction and symptomatic therapy. Many of these defects can be detected antenatally by USG. Antenatal screening with maternal serum AFP is very useful for open neural tube defects. More than 90% of anencephaly and about 80% of open neural tube defects can be detected by high AFP levels between 16 and 18 weeks of pregnancy.

Folic acid supplementation (4 mg/day) started 2 months before to 3 months after conception (periconceptional) prevents recurrence in about 72% of cases of neural tube defects. Primary prevention (about 50%) by use of 0.4 mg of folic acid periconceptionally has also been recommended.

CONCLUSION

- Pediatricians need to be vigilant for the red-flags that might suggest an underlying genetic disorder.
- Timely recognition and diagnosis can significantly improve prognosis and quality of life through early intervention and management strategies in children with common genetic disorders.
- Genetic counseling helps in educating and guiding parents regarding implications of the condition in the affected child, and also about the recurrence risk and options of prenatal diagnosis thereby aiding informed decision making.
- Multidisciplinary collaboration is essential to ensure holistic care in these children.

REFERENCES

1. American Academy of Pediatrics. Committee on Genetics. American Academy of Pediatrics: Health supervision for children with Down syndrome. Pediatrics. 2001;107(2):442-9.
2. Frías JL, Davenport ML. Committee on Genetics and Section on Endocrinology. Health supervision for children with Turner syndrome. Pediatrics. 2003;111(3):692-702.

3. Trotter TL, Hall JG. American Academy of Pediatrics Committee on Genetics. Health supervision for children with achondroplasia. Pediatrics. 2005;116(3):771-83.
4. Kandt RS. Tuberous sclerosis complex and NF type 1: the two most common neurocutaneous diseases. Neurol Clin. 2003;21(4):983-1004.
5. Hersh JH. American Academy of Pediatrics Committee on Genetics. Health supervision for children with neurofibromatosis. Pediatrics. 2008;121(3):633-42.
6. Wurster CD, Ludolph AC. Nusinersen for spinal muscular atrophy. Ther Adv Neurol Disord. 2018;11:1756285618754459.
7. Aartsma-Rus A, Straub V, Hemmings R, Haas M, Schlosser-Weber G, Stoyanova-Beninska V, et al. Development of exon skipping therapies for Duchenne muscular dystrophy: a critical review and a perspective on the outstanding issues. Nucleic Acid Ther. 2017;27(5):251-9.
8. Neul JL, Kaufmann WE, Glaze DG, Christodoulou J, Clarke AJ, Bahi-Buisson N, et al. Rett syndrome: revised diagnostic criteria and nomenclature. Ann Neurol. 2010;68(6):944-50.

17.4 Genetic Metabolic Disorders

Shubha R Phadke

INTRODUCTION

The body of a living organism is a biochemical factory with complex metabolic pathways working simultaneously and maintaining life processes in an efficient manner. The metabolism proceeds in steps—each step being governed by an enzyme. Usually, there is *one gene for one enzyme*. If a gene gets mutated, the enzyme will not be synthesized or will lose its function and the disease will manifest. These diseases are collectively known as *"inborn errors of metabolism (IEM)"*. The enzymes are required in a very small quantity and hence most of the genetic metabolic disorders manifest only when both copies of a gene for an enzyme are mutated or abnormal. Thus, most genetic metabolic disorders are inherited in *autosomal recessive mode* indicating that both the parents of an affected individual are clinically normal but carry one mutated copy of the gene in concern; that is, they are carriers of the disease. Some types of porphyria due to abnormalities in heme metabolism are inherited in an *autosomal dominant* fashion.

Genes for few enzymes are located on X chromosome. Examples of IEMs transmitted in an *X-linked manner* include mucopolysaccharidosis type II (Hunter syndrome), Fabry disease, ornithine transcarbamylase deficiency, and Lesch–Nyhan syndrome. The X-linked IEMs usually manifest only in males, and females usually are asymptomatic carriers who can transmit the disorder to the sons. The clinical presentations of these disorders can involve any organ of the body and signs and symptoms overlap with nongenetic disorders and hence, all clinicians need to be aware of these rare disorders.[1]

The first IEM was described by Sir Archibald Garrod in 1902. The disorder was alkaptonuria, in which nappies of children suffering from the disease turned black on exposure to air. This was due to excretion of homogentisic acid in urine due to a block in the metabolism of tyrosine **(Flowchart 17.4.1)**. Later, inborn errors of various pathways

Flowchart 17.4.1: Metabolism of phenylalanine and tyrosine. On the left is an enzyme catalyzing the step and on the right is the disease *(italics)* caused by deficiency of the enzyme.

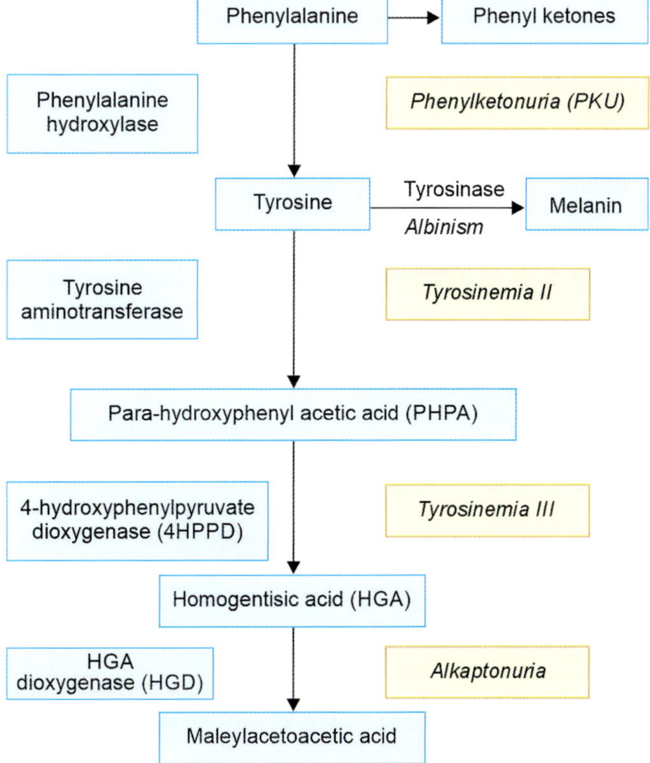

involving metabolism of amino acids, carbohydrates, fatty acids, lipids, trace minerals, and various complex molecules such as lipoproteins, mucopolysaccharides, and oligosaccharides were identified. Thus, the clinical manifestations are due to deficiency of the downstream product of the enzymatic reaction (as in albinism or hemophilia) or may be due to accumulation of metabolic products of the substrate [as in phenylketonuria (PKU)]. Tyrosine is required for the synthesis of skin pigment and deficiency of enzyme; tyrosinase leads to block in the synthesis of melanine pigment in skin and eyes **(Fig. 17.4.1)**.

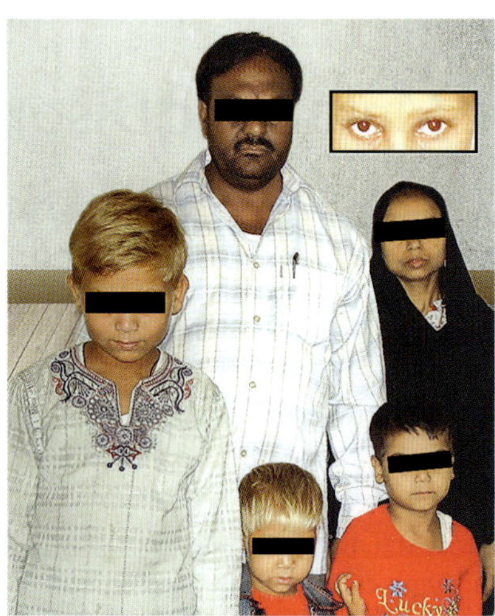

Fig. 17.4.1: A family with two children with oculocutaneous albinism. The parents and one child are normal. Note the light color of skin, hair, and eyes (inset). They have vision problems.

In lysosomal storage disorders, the intracellular accumulation of complex molecules due to lack of their degradation leads to signs and symptoms of the disease.

CLASSIFICATION

In addition to enzyme deficiencies, biochemical abnormalities of various proteins such as transport proteins, hormones, immunoglobulins, and coagulation factors also give rise to diseases. The metabolic disorders are classified into categories as given in **Table 17.4.1**.[2]

WHEN TO SUSPECT INBORN ERRORS OF METABOLISM?

The clinical features of category I group of genetic metabolic disorders depend on the function of the organ or system involved **(Table 17.4.1)**. The category II disorders affect multiple organ systems in the body because the enzyme or metabolites of the enzyme pathway affect many organs of the body. These are traditionally described as IEM and this chapter discusses this group of disorders. The clinical features of IEMs are varied and usually involve many systems. Involvement of the nervous system is common. Many of these disorders manifest in the neonatal period, infancy, or early childhood. However, many disorders, e.g., hyperlipidemias, Fabry disease, and some mitochondrial disorders, may present at a later part of life. Manifestations can be intermittent as well as dependent on exposure to an offending agent as in porphyria and some cases of urea cycle

TABLE 17.4.1: Classification of genetic metabolic disorders.

Category	*Group*	*Clinical manifestations*	*Examples*
I. Disorders that involve only one functional system or one organ		Symptoms characteristic for the system/organ involved	Immunodeficiency disorder, hemophilia, renal tubular acidosis
II. Diseases due to defects in the basic metabolic pathway common to a large number of cells or organs, or the pathway is restricted to one organ but has systemic effects	Defects affecting the synthesis or catabolism of complex molecules; defects of intracellular trafficking and processing	Progressive manifestations not affected by diet or environmental factors	Lysosomal storage disorders such as Gaucher disease, Hunter syndrome, peroxisomal disorders, alpha-l-antitrypsin deficiency
	Defects of intermediary metabolism that leads to acute or progressive intoxication due to accumulation of toxic compounds proximal to the block	Acute or intermittent manifestations. Onset may be late. Central nervous system involvement is frequent	Amino acidurias, urea cycle defects
	Disorder due to deficiency in energy production or utilization	Hypoglycemia, lactic acidosis, involvement of heart muscles, brain, liver and multiple organs	Mitochondrial disorders, disorders associated with lactic acidosis, defects of neoglucogenesis

Source: Saudubray JM, Garcia-Cazorla À. Inborn Errors of Metabolism Overview: Pathophysiology, Manifestations, Evaluation, and Management. Pediatr Clin North Am. 2018;65(2):179-208.

disorders. Acute illness with neurological deterioration in a neonate or an infant is a presentation of many IEMs such as aminoacidopathies, organic acidemias, galactosemia, disorders with lactic acidosis, glycogen storage disorders, and fatty acid oxidation defects. As neonates have limited manifestations and respond to any type of insult in the same way, the clinical picture of IEM, septicemia, birth asphyxia, and intracranial hemorrhage may superficially look similar. If a clinician is aware of various presentations of IEM, he or she can suspect the possibility of IEM in appropriate clinical situations. A high level of suspicion is the first step toward the diagnosis of IEMs which individually are rare. Other indicators to point toward IEM are the presence of consanguinity in parents and family history of similar illness.

In addition to acute presentation, some of the clinical manifestations suggestive of IEM are given in **Table 17.4.2**. Some disorders have intermittent acute presentation due to exposure to precipitating causes such as high protein diet or fasting. Many storage disorders have a chronic progressive course.

DIAGNOSIS

Inborn errors of metabolism are many and rare, and the manifestations are overlapping. These make diagnosis difficult. Clinical diagnosis is not possible and diagnostic tests are often not easily available. History and clinical examination are hence extremely important to search for diagnostic clues **(Fig. 17.4.2)**. **Table 17.4.3** lists some characteristic features of common IEMs.

Routine investigations showing liver involvement or high value of creatinine phosphokinase may give clues to the diagnosis.[3] MRI brain is useful, especially if white matter disease of brain is suspected **(Figs. 17.4.3A and B)**. Bone marrow examination may help in the diagnosis of Gaucher and Niemann–Pick diseases. However, confirmation of diagnosis is needed using specialized tests like enzyme assays, metabolite profile of plasma and urine using tandem mass spectrometry (TMS), and gas chromatography mass spectrometry (GCMS). Specific enzyme assays on white blood cells or cultured fibroblasts are necessary for confirmation of the diagnosis of lysosomal storage disorders.

TABLE 17.4.2: Common clinical presentations of inborn errors of metabolism.

Presentations	*Representative Diseases*
Development delay, seizures, regression of milestones, tone abnormalities	• Biotinidase deficiency • Tay–Sachs disease • Metachromatic leukodystrophy
Coarse facies, hepatosplenomegaly, joint contractures, corneal clouding	Mucopolysaccharidosis
Hepatosplenomegaly, neonatal cholestasis	• Galactosemia • Tyrosinemia • Niemann–Pick disease
Hepatosplenomegaly	• Glycogen storage diseases • Gaucher disease • Niemann–Pick disease
Cardiomyopathy	• Pompe disease • Mitochondrial diseases
Extrapyramidal manifestation and neuroregression	Wilson disease
Hepatic failure, hypoglycemia	Fatty acid oxidation defects
Vomiting, diarrhea, failure to thrive	• Wolman disease • Abetalipoproteinemia • Lactase deficiency

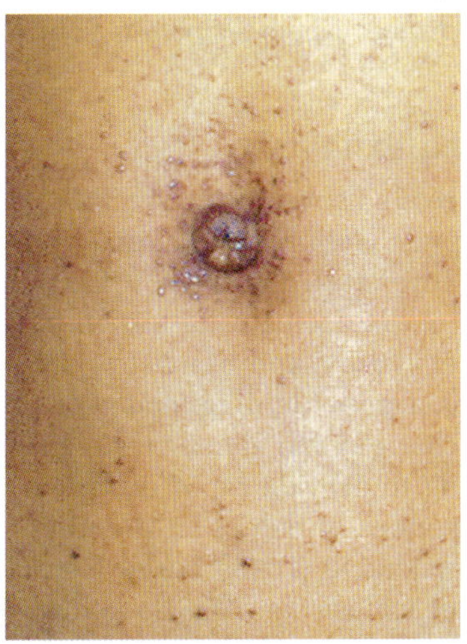

Fig. 17.4.2: Angiokeratomas characteristic of Fabry disease (also seen in fucosidosis).

TABLE 17.4.3: Characteristic manifestations of some inborn errors of metabolism.

Clinical manifestation	*Disease*
Cherry-red spot in fundus of eye	• Tay–Sachs disease • Niemann–Pick disease
Cataract	Galactosemia
Corneal opacities	• Cystinosis • Mucopolysaccharidosis
Alopecia, skin rash	Biotinidase deficiency
Macrocephaly (large head)	• Tay–Sachs disease • Canavan disease • van der Knapp disease
Rickets	• Tyrosinemia type I • Renal tubular acidosis
Macrocytic anemia	B1 responsive macrocytic anemia

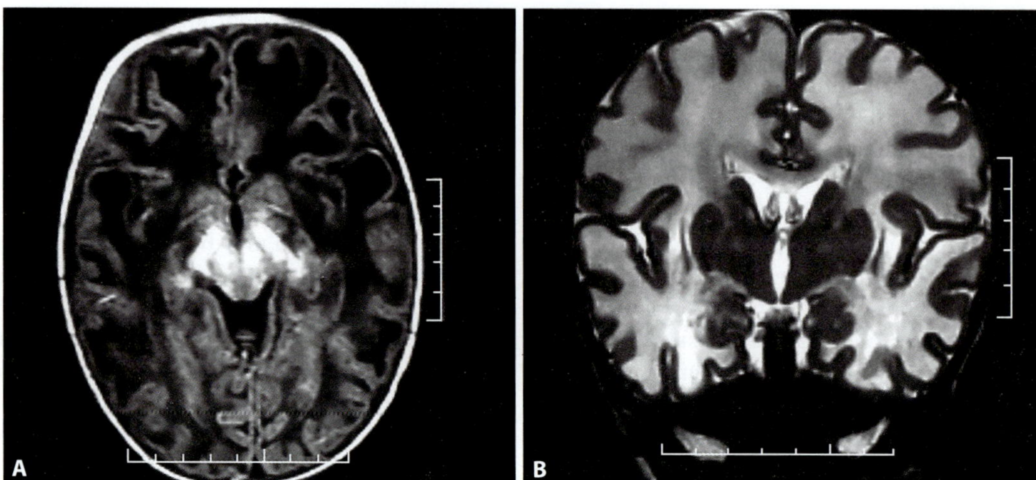

Figs. 17.4.3A and B: MRI brain showing cystic changes and leukodystrophy characteristic of van der Knaap disease. (A) Axial T1 FLAIR image showing cystic changes in both temporal regions; (B) Coronal T2 images showing extensive involvement and hyperintensity of central and peripheral white matter.

Genetic Diagnosis

Causative genes are known for most the IEMs and mutation detection helps in confirmation of diagnosis. It also helps in providing prenatal diagnosis. The genetic test for identification of disease-causing mutation was previously done only after clinical and biochemical testing provided a diagnosis or a possible diagnosis was made. Now the situation has changed and genetic testing can be used as a first-tier testing to provide rapid diagnosis and can help in the management of babies in the neonatal care unit. Deoxyribonucleic acid (DNA) based testing is done by a *next-generation sequencing (NGS)-based testing* which can sequence all genes or the whole genome in one go. This can also provide a diagnosis when the biochemical profile is not characteristic due to sample collection at an inappropriate time or the secondary metabolic changes complicating the scenario. Being multitargeted, NGS can make diagnosis even when the clinical suspicion is not possible. NGS is a powerful technology, but the results should be carefully evaluated and correlated with clinical and biochemical phenotypes.

MANAGEMENT

Successful treatments with various strategies have been available for some disorders for decades **(Table 17.4.4)**. Over the last few decades, the number of disorders for which partial improvement is possible is increasing. However, there is no curative treatment for many IEMs. Successful *enzyme replacement therapy (ERT)* as in Gaucher disease[4] **(Figs. 17.4.4A to D)**, mucopolysaccharidosis I SH (Scheie - Hurler), mucopolysaccharidosis II, glycogen storage disease type II (Pompe disease), and Fabry disease has brought hope that similar success stories may be repeated for other 40 lysosomal storage disorders. ERT cannot prevent neurological involvement yet as the modified enzymes cannot cross the blood–brain barrier.

TABLE 17.4.4: Treatment of inborn errors of metabolism.

Disorder	*Treatment*
Phenylketonuria	Phenylalanine restricted diet, tetrahydrobiopterin
Galactosemia	Lactose free diet
Biotinidase deficiency	Biotin
Tyrosinemia I	NTBC
Mucopolysaccharidosis	BMT, ERT
Wilson disease	Penicillamine, zinc
Pompe disease	ERT
Gaucher disease	BMT, ERT
Fatty acid oxidation defects	Prevent fasting, carnitine
Cobalamin metabolism disorder	Vitamin B_{12}
Homocystinuria	Pyridoxine
Porphyria	Load of glucose and acid hematin
Glycogen storage disorder type I	Corn starch

[BMT: bone marrow transplantation; ERT: enzyme replacement therapy; NTBC: 2-(2-nitro-4-trifluoromethyl benzoyl)-1,3-cyclohexanedione]

Bone marrow transplantation (BMT) is successful in preventing central nervous system involvement if done in early stages of mucopolysaccharidosis. Similarly, *liver transplantation* to replace the damaged liver or as a source of enzyme is successful in some disorders. Successful *gene therapy* for immunodeficiency disorders, beta thalassemia, sickle cell disease, and hemophilia has shown the hope that the gene therapy may be an option for many disorders soon.

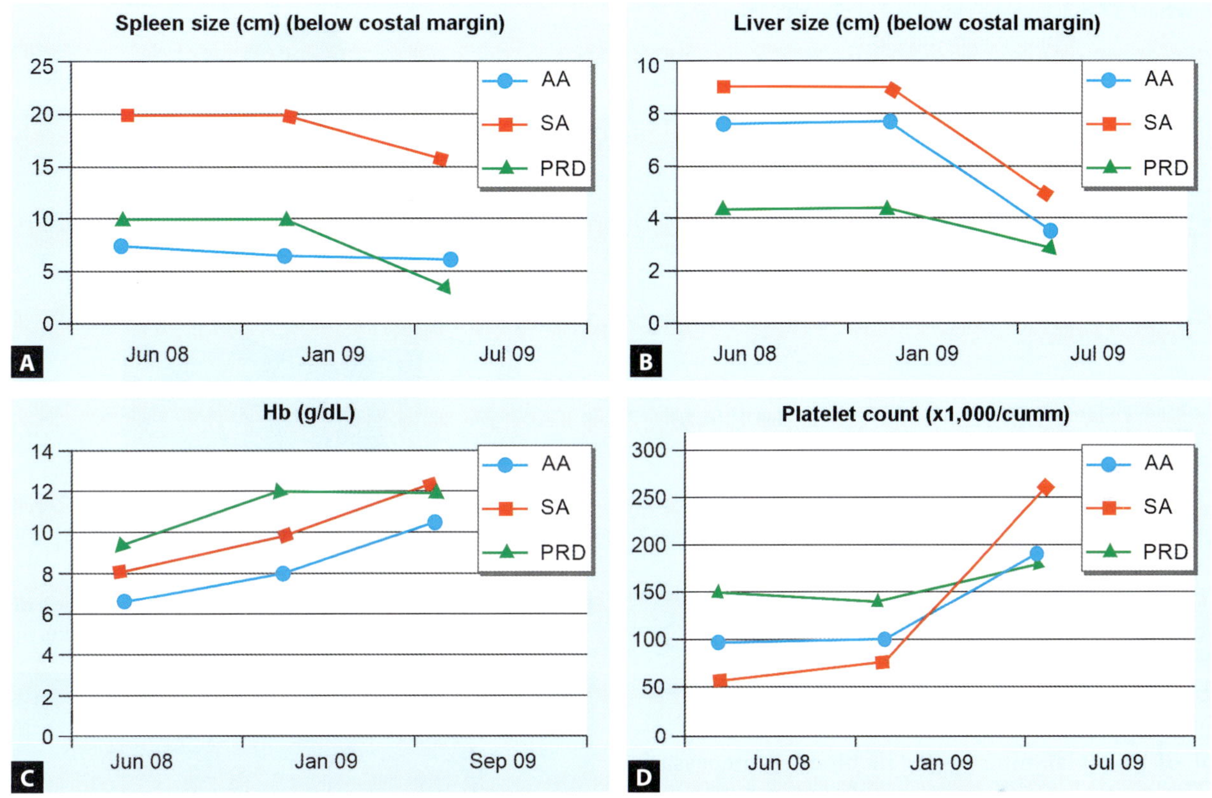

Figs. 17.4.4A to D: Response to enzyme replacement therapy (ERT) in three patients with Gaucher disease type I (different colors are used for different patients).

Lack of curative treatment; difficult, lifelong, costly treatment; and poor outcomes in many IEMs make *genetic counseling and prenatal diagnosis* important components of management. Accurate diagnosis of the affected patient in the family is the prerequisite for prenatal diagnosis. Hence, even if the child appears to be too serious to survive, all attempts should be made to confirm the diagnosis. Urine, plasma, and blood for DNA should be stored for future analysis even if the affected child dies before diagnosis. In the era of NGS, if the affected child is not alive but thought to be likely a case of a recessive genetic disorder, the parents can be investigated for a carrier status of genetic disorder and the surrogate diagnosis of the child can be done. This can help the family for genetic counseling and prenatal diagnosis. The limitations of such testing need to be explained to the family.

Deoxyribonucleic acid test for mutation in the chorionic villi or amniotic fluid cells is the best option for prenatal diagnosis.

SOME REPRESENTATIVE INBORN ERRORS OF METABOLISM

Phenylketonuria

Phenylketonuria (PKU) is one of the best studied IEMs. Still, there is limited understanding of pathology about how phenylalanine metabolites lead to neurological abnormalities. The history of PKU starting from diagnosis, diet therapy, newborn screening, and fetal effects of maternal PKU reflects the developments in IEM. PKU is an autosomal recessive disorder caused by the deficiency of phenylalanine hydroxylase (PAH), an enzyme which converts phenylalanine to tyrosine **(Flowchart 17.4.2)**.

In the absence of PAH, the phenylalanine accumulates in the body and some of it gets metabolized by alternate pathways to produce an increased amount of phenylpyruvic acid (a keto acid) which gets excreted in urine. That is why the name "phenylketonuria". The disease was described by Folling in 1934. In 1950, Horst Bickel performed successful intervention with dietary phenylalanine restriction in a patient with PKU. The phenylalanine levels in blood reduced and there was clinical improvement. However, soon it became obvious that the treatment unless started during the neonatal period could not prevent neurocognitive disability. This led to the beginning of newborn screening in the early 1960s. The prevalence of PKU varies from 1 in 10,000 to 100,000. Identification of PKU neonates through newborn screening and institution of diet therapy successfully prevented intellectual disability. However, if diet therapy is relaxed after childhood, hyperphenylalaninemia leads to dysfunction of adult brain and lifelong continued

Flowchart 17.4.2: Enzymes involved in phenylalanine and biopterin metabolism.

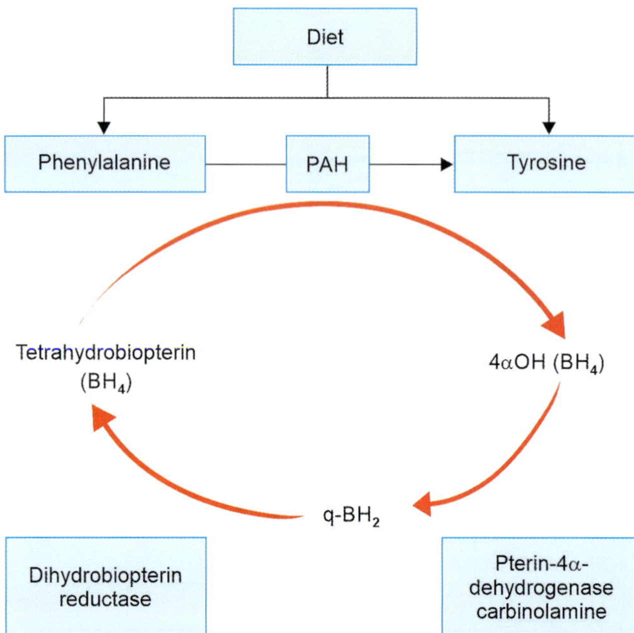

(PAH: phenylalanine hydroxylase)

control of phenylalanine levels in blood is necessary. Strict diet control is also necessary during pregnancy as hyperphenylalaninemia invariably leads to microcephaly, intellectual disability, and cardiac malformation in the baby. The diet management is a challenging issue, and other treatments like tetrahydrobiopterin and phenylalanine ammonia lyase enzyme can decrease the need of strict diet control in some cases.

Glycogen Storage Disease IA (von Gierke Disease)

Glycogen storage disease IA (GSD-IA) is an autosomal recessive disorder caused by the deficiency of glucose-6-phosphatase. Affected children present with hepatomegaly and episodes of seizures, sweating, and tachycardia due to hypoglycemia **(Fig. 17.4.5)**. Treatment is simple with frequent daytime feeds and a diet rich in uncooked corn starch (to release glucose slowly) at night to prevent hypoglycemia.

Glycogen Storage Disease Type II (Pompe Disease)

Pompe disease is an autosomal recessive disease caused by deficiency of the enzyme alpha-glucosidase. It primarily involves muscles. The manifestations start in the first 6 months of life. There is developmental delay, hypotonia, macroglossia, cardiomegaly, and congestive cardiac failure. The diagnosis is confirmed by enzyme assay on lymphocytes or fibroblasts or mutation detection. Late-onset variants presenting with limb girdle muscles predominantly are also described. Treatment

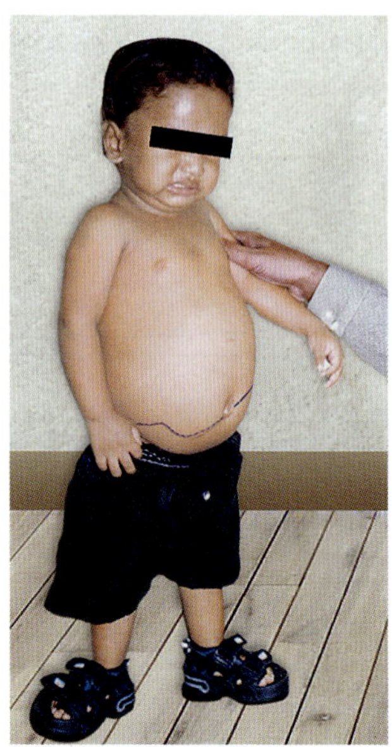

Fig. 17.4.5: An 18-month-old child with glycogen storage disease I (GSD I). A doll-like face is a characteristic feature.

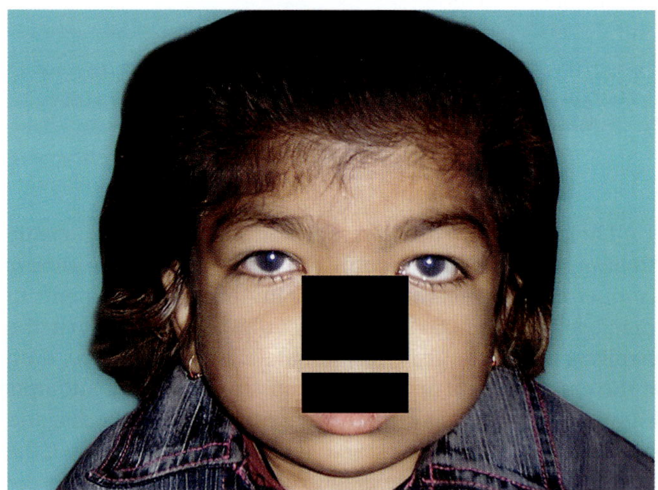

Fig. 17.4.6: A child with characteristic features of mucopolysaccharidosis I. She is I SH type with normal IQ.

with ERT has shown good results, especially when started early in the course of disease. For this reason, some countries have included Pompe disease in newborn screening program and shown absolutely normal outcomes in patients who were started on ERT during the neonatal period.[5]

Mucopolysaccharidosis

Hurler syndrome (HS) is type I mucopolysaccharidosis (MPS I). It is a prototype of lysosomal storage disorders. Clinical features include coarse facies, joint contractures, thickened skin, short stature, corneal clouding, and intellectual disability **(Fig. 17.4.6)**. There is cardiac involvement in the form of thickening of valves. The age of

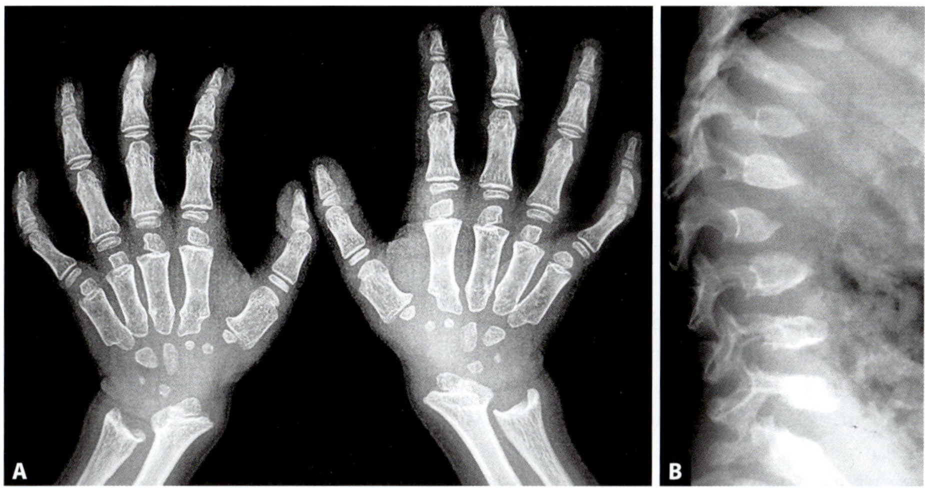

Figs. 17.4.7A and B: Dysostosis multiplex: (A) Radiograph of hands showing modeling deformities of metacarpals; (B) Lateral radiograph of spine showing oval-shaped vertebrae and anterior tongue-like process.

onset is usually 1–2 years. Mild forms of MPS I-Scheie type (MPS I S) and MPS I SH are known and may be difficult to diagnose. Characteristic radiological changes **(Figs. 17.4.7A and B),** known as dysostosis multiplex, can help in diagnosis. ERT with recombinant iduronidase (enzyme which is deficient in patients with MPS I) has become available at the beginning of the 21st century. It has shown remarkable results in the form of improvement in joint contractures and decrease in the sizes of liver and spleen. However, it is not useful if the patient has a classic Hurler variety because the recombinant enzyme cannot cross the blood–brain barrier.

Respiratory Chain Disorders

Oxidative phosphorylation, i.e., ATP synthesis through the respiratory chain in mitochondria, is a ubiquitous pathway that supplies energy to all organs and tissues. A defect of the respiratory chain can affect any organ system at any age. The oxidative reaction takes place in mitochondria giving the name "mitochondrial disorders". Mitochondria have their own DNA. Some of the genes of the respiratory chain pathway are coded by mitochondrial DNA, while many of the genes of this pathway are coded by nuclear gene. Hence, both mitochondrial (also known as maternal) and autosomal modes of inheritance are observed. The manifestation can be varied and can involve heart, brain, muscles, and any system of the body and can present at any age. Symptoms involving multiple systems strongly suggest the possibility of a mitochondrial disorder.

CASE SCENARIOS

Case I

A nonconsanguineous couple was referred for genetic counseling and prenatal diagnosis. The wife was 8 weeks pregnant. They had a 17-month-old daughter with spasticity and scissoring of both lower limbs **(Fig. 17.4.8)**. The child was normal till 1 year of age and had started standing and walking with support. She stopped that and the tone increased in lower limbs. The MRI brain showed demyelination of white matter consistent with leukodystrophy. The clinical features, history of regression of milestones after normal development up to 1 year, and MRI picture were consistent with metachromatic leukodystrophy (MLD). MLD is a progressive disease with no curative treatment currently. The risk of recurrence in the siblings of the affected child is 1 in 4 or 25%. For counseling and prenatal diagnosis, confirmation

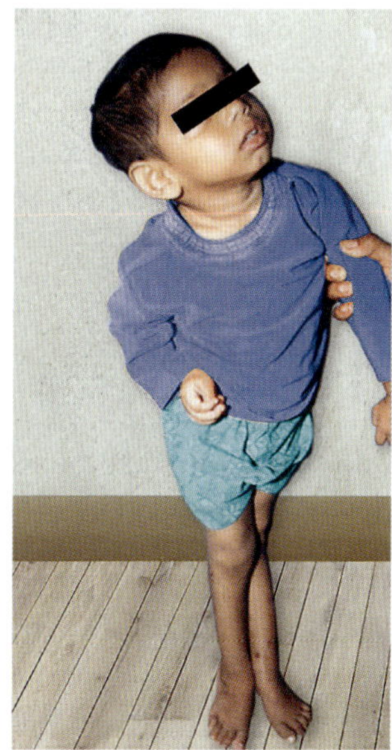

Fig. 17.4.8: A child with metachromatic leukodystrophy, superficially looking like cerebral palsy.

of the diagnosis by assay of arylsulfatase A enzyme on the white blood cells of the proband (affected child in the family) was done, which was very low confirming the diagnosis of MLD. After identification of DNA defect in the gene, prenatal diagnosis can be done at 13 weeks. If the fetus in the womb is found to be affected with the disease, the family may consider discontinuation of the pregnancy.

Case II

An 18-year-old medical student was admitted in the intensive care unit with coma and acute renal failure. She was fine a week ago and then developed diarrhea and was given intravenous (IV) fluids. During childhood, she was frequently hospitalized with documented attacks of hypoglycemia. Her brother also had attacks of hypoglycemia and died at 3 years of age. After early childhood, she stopped getting hypoglycemia. After 24 hours of IV fluids, she was discharged and then was readmitted in a serious condition. With this past history and family history, the most likely diagnosis is a fatty acid oxidation defect. There are many types of fatty acid oxidation defects and the treatment is to prevent fasting and give carnitine supplementation during attacks. She recovered with supportive treatment and was advised tandem mass spectrometry of plasma to study acylcarnitine profile. These groups of disorders are included in newborn screening programs of developed countries.

Case III

A couple came with the history that their two sons died of septicemia during the first month of life. The mothers of the husband and wife were sisters. There were no investigation reports of the babies. No blood or any other sample of the babies were available. Presence of consanguinity and recurrence in two children suggested the possibility of autosomal recessive IEM or immune function in the children and septicemia as the sole cause may be less likely. Hence, the option of sequencing all coding regions of known disease-related genes (clinical exome sequencing) by NGS was discussed with the family. Both of them were detected to harbor a known disease causing mutation (pathogenic sequence variation) in *BCKDHB* gene known to cause maple syrup urine disease, type Ib. They were informed that the possibility that the next baby is not affected with the same disease is 75% and the possibility that the baby will have the same disease will be 25%. The family decided that during the next pregnancy they will get prenatal testing done and if the baby is found to be affected (homozygous for the same mutation) they will avoid the birth of the child by opting termination of the pregnancy.

It should be noted that for sick babies in the intensive care unit, NGS-based testing can provide diagnosis in up to 30–50% cases and may open an option of treatment.[6] A small amount of blood sample in the EDTA tube should be stored and it may turn out to be very useful later for reaching the correct etiological diagnosis even after the demise of the child and help to prevent recurrence in the family.

KEY MESSAGES

- Though individually rare, IEMs contribute significantly to childhood mortality and morbidity.
- High level of suspicion of IEMs is necessary, especially in acutely sick neonates and children.
- As new therapies have become available for IEMs, timely diagnosis is important.
- In addition to biochemical techniques such as GCMS, TMS, and enzyme assays, NGS-based testing should be used as a complementary and adjunct technique.
- Genetic counseling should be a part of management of any child with IEM.

REFERENCES

1. Agana M, Frueh J, Kamboj M, Patel DR, Kanungo S. Common metabolic disorder (inborn errors of metabolism) concerns in primary care practice. Ann Transl Med. 2018;6(24):469.
2. Saudubray JM, Garcia-Cazorla À. Inborn Errors of Metabolism Overview: Pathophysiology, Manifestations, Evaluation, and Management. Pediatr Clin North Am. 2018;65(2):179-208.
3. Balakrishnan U. Inborn Errors of Metabolism: Approach to Diagnosis and Management in Neonates. Indian J Pediatr. 2021;88(7):679-89.
4. Muranjan M, Patil S. Outcome of Gaucher Disease in India: Lessons from Prevalent Diagnostic and Therapeutic Practices. Indian Pediatr. 2016;53(8):685-8.
5. Gragnaniello V, Pijnappel PWWM, Burlina AP, in 't Groen SLM, Gueraldi D, Cazzorla C, et al. Newborn screening for Pompe disease in Italy: Long-term results and future challenges. Mol Genet Metab Rep. 2022;33:100929.
6. Borghesi A, Mencarelli MA, Memo L, Ferrero GB, Bartuli A, Genuardi M; their respective Scientific Societies. Intersociety policy statement on the use of whole-exome sequencing in the critically ill newborn infant. Ital J Pediatr. 2017;43(1):100.

SECTION

18

Rheumatological Disorders and Allergy

Section Editor: Sathish Kumar

18.1 Approach to Child with Musculoskeletal Pain

Anju Gupta

INTRODUCTION

Musculoskeletal (MSK) pain is a common childhood complaint.[1] Etiologies can be diverse ranging from benign causes such as growing pains to serious causes such as malignancies. Basic clinical skills of history taking and physical examination are useful to differentiate benign etiologies from malignant causes in most cases. All physicians should master and apply p-GALS (pediatric gait, arms, legs, and spine), which is a quick, structured, and evidence-based screening method for assessing the spine, limbs, and joints in children.[2] Any abnormality noticed in p-GALS should be followed by a focused examination.

Musculoskeletal pain can arise from multiple origins such as muscles, joints, ligaments, tendons, bursae, etc. For a physician, it is essential to answer following three questions after history taking and physical examination:

1. Whether the pain is articular?
2. If the pain is articular, is there evidence of arthritis?
3. If there is evidence of arthritis, then define:
   a. Acute versus chronic
   b. Pattern of joint involvement
      i. Number of joints involved
      ii. Symmetrical versus asymmetrical involvement
      iii. Large joint versus small joint versus both
      iv. Migratory versus additive versus fixed involvement
      v. Peripheral versus axial involvement
      vi. *Periarticular involvement:* Enthesitis and muscular atrophy
   c. Systemic features

We shall discuss all these features separately in order to reach a differential diagnosis for MSK pain.

QUESTION 1: WHETHER PAIN IS ARTICULAR?

Musculoskeletal pain can broadly be divided into nonarticular, periarticular, and articular **(Flowchart 18.1.1)**.

Differentiating features are depicted in **Table 18.1.1.** We shall discuss etiologies of nonarticular and periarticular pain in brief here:

Growing Pains

Growing pains, also known as benign nocturnal limb pains of childhood, are a common cause of MSK pain.[3] Typically seen

Flowchart 18.1.1: Causes of musculoskeletal (MSK) pain in children.

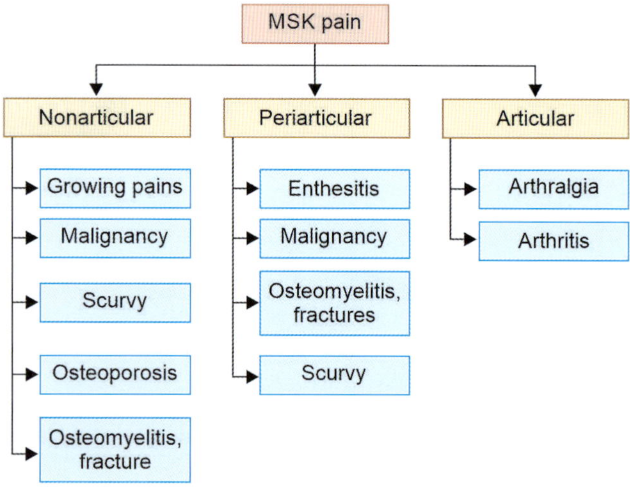

between the ages of 3 and 12 years, presenting features include intermittent, mild-to-moderate discomfort or aching in the legs (thighs, calves, and sometimes, behind the knees) during evening or night. Pain may last for several minutes to a few hours. Typically, children are well during day and indulge in physical activities. No investigations are required. Treatment is supportive and includes gentle massages, warm baths, and analgesics like acetaminophen or ibuprofen. Parental reassurance, that the pain is temporary and harmless, is essential and helps reduce anxiety.

Malignancy

Musculoskeletal pain is an important presenting feature of childhood malignancies like leukemia and neuroblastoma.[4] Pain is usually diffuse and nonspecific. Children often point to shafts of long bone when asked to pinpoint the site of pain. This occurs due to diffuse infiltration and expansion of bone marrow. This pain is typically of few weeks' duration, severe in intensity affecting daily activities, and associated with peculiar nocturnal worsening. Often the pain is severe enough to affect weight bearing and child requires intravenous analgesics with only partial relief. Presence of hematological manifestations such as anemia, thrombocytopenia, leukopenia, or leukocytosis with lymphocyte predominance aid in diagnosis. However, absence of hematological

TABLE 18.1.1: Differentiating features of various types of musculoskeletal (MSK) pain.

	Nonarticular pain	*Periarticular pain*	*Articular pain*
Characteristics of pain	Anywhere in the limb	• Pinpoint around the joint • Focal pain • Worsens with active movements in few planes only	• Across joint line (line across which joint movement occurs) • Diffuse and deep pain • Worsens with active and passive movements in all planes *Exceptions* • Referred pain of hip (can be referred to anterior thigh and ipsilateral knee) • Referred pain of sacroiliac joint (lower back, gluteal region, and posterior thigh)
Common causes	• Growing pain • Malignancy • Osteomyelitis • Scurvy • Osteoporosis	• Osteomyelitis • Fractures • Enthesitis • Bursitis • Scurvy • Osteoporosis	• Arthralgia • Arthritis

BOX 18.1.1: Red-flag signs in musculoskeletal (MSK) pain.

Red-flag signs in MSK pain
- Pain causing significant impairment in daily activities
- Pain with nocturnal exacerbation (especially after the child has slept)
- Bone pain
- Hepatosplenomegaly
- Lymphadenopathy
- Hematological involvement (anemia, thrombocytopenia, and leukopenia or leukocytosis with lymphocyte predominance)

manifestations should not lead the physician away from this diagnosis in the presence of the red-flag signs depicted in **Box 18.1.1**.

Occasionally focal infiltrative bone lesions are also seen in childhood malignancies and these may cause localized bone pain, swelling, and pathological fractures. This can also be seen in primary bone malignancies. Rarely, patients with leukemia can present with joint swelling and pain due to infiltration of synovial membrane.

In nutshell, malignancies can present with MSK pain, which may be nonarticular, periarticular, or articular. Physician should be aware of red-flag signs that could alert to this possibility.

Osteomyelitis

Infection of bone occurs commonly due to bacteria. In children, metaphysis of long bones such as femur and tibia are predisposed to develop osteomyelitis.[5] Rich blood supply, slower blood flow, and presence of trabecular bone are responsible for this predisposition. Hematogenous spread is most common mode of bacterial colonization in bone in children and occurs commonly due to *Staphylococcus aureus* (**Flowchart 18.1.2**). Bacterial multiplication and inflammatory response both contribute to osteomyelitis. If not treated appropriately in time, this can lead to chronic osteomyelitis with localized abscess formation in bone, which can exude pus intermittently through sinus tract. Chronic osteomyelitis can also occur due to mycobacterial infection.

Flowchart 18.1.2: Pathophysiology of osteomyelitis.

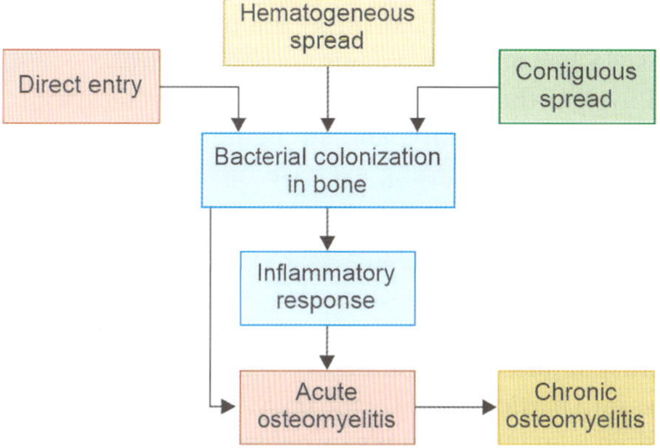

Children with acute osteomyelitis present with high-grade fever, toxic look, localized severe bone pain and swelling, and inability to bear weight on the limb for a short duration over a few hours to days. Polymorphonuclear leukocytosis and raised inflammatory parameters [erythrocyte sedimentation rate (ESR) and C-reactive protein (CRP)] are seen in all children with acute osteomyelitis. Blood cultures should be sent at presentation. X-ray of the involved bone may not show specific radiologic changes early and this should not delay treatment with appropriate antibiotics. Magnetic resonance imaging (MRI) is more sensitive but may not be available easily.

Treatment of acute osteomyelitis is a medical emergency. Appropriate intravenous antibiotics should be started at clinical suspicion. Surgical intervention to drain abscesses and remove necrotic tissue may be required. Treatment of chronic osteomyelitis is more complex with requirements of both medical and surgical interventions.

Enthesitis

Enthesitis refers to inflammation of entheses, which are the sites where tendons, ligaments, and joint capsules attach to bone.[6] Children typically present with pain and tenderness at affected sites. Pain is usually worse on waking up in the morning like any inflammatory pain. Swelling and warmth are uncommon. Common sites of pain include heels (Achilles tendon or plantar fascia), knees (patellar tendon), hips (iliac crest), and the bottom of the feet. Enthesitis is commonly seen in enthesitis-related arthritis, which we shall discuss later under juvenile idiopathic arthritis.

Treatment includes use of nonsteroidal anti-inflammatory drugs (NSAIDs) in acute phase. Disease-modifying antirheumatic drugs (DMARDs) and biologic therapies may be used when other treatments are not effective.

Physical therapy can be used to alleviate symptoms, improve joint mobility, and strengthen muscles. Lifestyle modifications, including exercise, maintaining a healthy weight, and using proper footwear to reduce strain on affected entheses are useful in long-term.

Overuse Injuries

Overuse injuries in children occur as a result of repetitive stress on a particular part of the body. These occur typically in children who indulge in organized sports.[7] They can involve various parts of the body (around the kneecap, calcaneum, just below the kneecap, insertion of Achilles tendon, etc.). Pain is pinpointed at a specific site and can be mild to severe. It is further worsened by a particular movement. Treatment involves rehabilitation and gradual return to play and modification of the activity to prevent further injury. Prevention includes proper training, rest, and monitoring for early signs of injury.

Bursitis

Bursitis refers to inflammation of a bursa, which is a small fluid-filled sac that serves as a cushion between a bone and a tendon or muscle. It is less common in children as compared to adults. It involves the bursae located near joints that are subjected to repetitive stress or trauma. In children, commonly, bursae around the knee, elbow, and hip are affected. Symptoms include pain, swelling, and tenderness around the joint. Pain is often worse with movement or pressure on the area. Imaging with ultrasound or MRI is useful to assess the extent of inflammation and rule out other potential causes of joint pain. Treatment is similar to treatment of overuse injuries with rest, application of ice, and use of analgesics in acute phase. This is followed by gradual physical therapy and modification of activities once acute stage is over.

Scurvy

Scurvy occurs due to lack of vitamin C, which is an essential vitamin for humans. Vitamin C plays an important role in collagen synthesis, which is an essential component of connective tissue. Lack of this vitamin in diet for 8–12 weeks can result in clinical manifestations.[8] Children with neurological conditions with very restricted diets are particularly predisposed. Clinical manifestations include swollen bleeding gums, skin, and mucosal bleeds; joint and bone pains resulting in difficulty in movements; increased risk of fractures; and swollen and tender ends of ribs (scorbutic rosary). All clinical features may not be present in every patient. Supplementation of vitamin C results in a quick recovery.

Osteoporosis

Osteoporosis is an important emerging cause of nonspecific MSK pain. >95% of skeleton is formed before the age of 19 years. Nearly 80% bone in adult human is cortical bone. However, trabecular bone which is only 20% bone by mass, occupies greater surface area and has more dynamic turnover (resorption followed by new bone formation). Due to this reason, fractures due to osteoporosis are seen most frequently in bones with more trabecular bone content such as vertebrae and hip.[9]

As depicted in **Flowchart 18.1.3**, bone structure and quality are affected by many factors such as genetic factors, chronic systemic illnesses, medications, and immobilization.

Flowchart 18.1.3: Pathophysiology of osteoporosis in children.

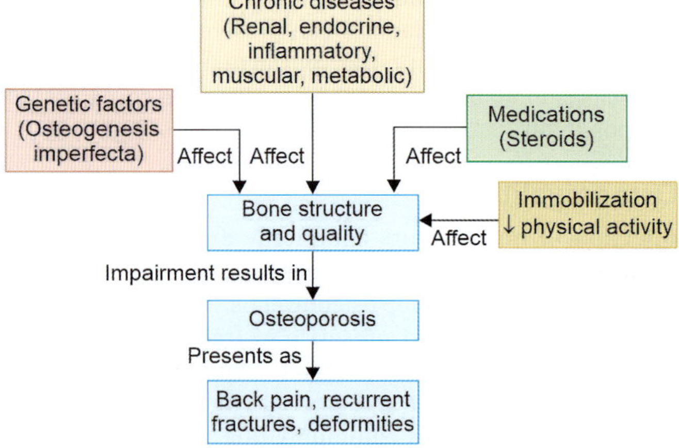

All these factors predispose to osteoporosis, which can present with back pain, recurrent fractures without significant trauma, or local disease and deformities.

QUESTION 2: IF PAIN IS ARTICULAR, IS THERE EVIDENCE OF ARTHRITIS?

Articular pain can occur both due to arthralgia and arthritis. Arthritis means inflammation of joint. It manifests clinically as swollen joint or presence of at least two of the following features: limited range of motion, redness, and warmth over the joint. Joint swelling is not obvious in deep joints like hip, shoulder, spine, and sacroiliac joint. Redness over the joint is also rare and can be occasionally seen in septic arthritis and reactive arthritis.

Early morning stiffness is another clinical feature of inflammatory joint pain. It refers to pain and difficulty in moving the joints in the morning on waking up and it usually lasts for half an hour or more.

Differentiating features between inflammatory and noninflammatory joint pain are depicted in **Table 18.1.2**.

Noninflammatory articular pain is typical of hypermobility and certain orthopedic conditions such as Perthes disease (idiopathic avascular necrosis of the femoral head). Features of inflammation are absent. Children with hereditary coagulopathy may show features of inflammation like warmth, swelling, and limitation of movements in a joint with acute hemarthrosis.

TABLE 18.1.2: Differentiating features between inflammatory and noninflammatory joint pain.

Clinical feature	*Inflammatory articular pain*	*Noninflammatory articular pain*
Pain	More in morning and after rest	More in evening and after movement
Swelling	Common and nonbony	Uncommon and bony
Redness	Occasional	Absent
Warmth	Sometimes	Absent
Limitation of joint movements	Frequent	Absent
Early morning stiffness	Prominent	Absent
Systemic features	Sometime	Absent
Inflammatory markers	May be elevated	Not elevated
Causes	Arthritis	• Hypermobility • Avascular necrosis of femoral head (Perthes disease) • Infective endocarditis

Perthes Disease

Perthes disease, also known as Legg-Calvé-Perthes disease, is a noninflammatory disorder of hip. Main pathophysiology implicated is avascular necrosis of femoral head.[10] Exact cause of this disease is not fully understood. Disease typically progresses through initial "necrosis" stage (disruption of blood supply), followed by a "fragmentation" stage (breakdown of the bone), and finally a "reossification" stage (healing and reformation of bone).

It is seen typically in children between the ages of 4 and 10 years. Children present with pain in the hip or groin and limp. Pain worsens typically after prolonged walking or running. Internal rotation of hip elicits pain. X-rays and MRI can help assess the condition of the hip joint and femoral head; however, X-rays may be normal early on in the disease.

The goal of treatment is to maintain the shape of the femoral head and prevent long-term joint problems. Treatment includes rest, activity modification to minimize stress on the hip, and physical therapy to maintain joint mobility and strength. Some children may need bracing or casting to maintain the position of the femoral head in the hip socket. Surgery may be considered in severe cases or when conservative treatments are not effective.

Most children with Perthes disease improve over time and return to normal activities. The condition typically resolves in 2–3 years. Long-term outcomes may vary and some individuals may experience early-onset osteoarthritis due to a significant residual hip deformity.

Hypermobility

Children with hypermobility may experience a range of MSK complaints due to increased joint flexibility.[11] Generalized or localized joint pains are common and can occur in different joints, including the knees, hips, elbows, and shoulders. Pain is usually episodic and gets aggravated by physical activity. These children are also prone to recurrent joint subluxations, overuse injuries, and growing pains. Treatment includes physical therapy (to strengthen muscles and improve joint stability), custom orthotic devices (e.g., shoe inserts for flat feet), management of pain, and adjustment of physical activities.

Hemarthrosis

Acute hemarthrosis (bleeding into the joint) is commonly seen in children with hereditary coagulopathies such as deficiency of clotting factors VIII or IX. These children present with severe pain, swelling, and limitation of joint movement of acute onset, usually after trauma. Usual joints affected are large joints that are prone to injury such as knees and elbows. Preceding history of bleeds and/or family history of bleeding disorder should point to this possibility.

The clinical presentation closely mimics septic arthritis except for absence of fever and toxic look.

If this is first presentation of a child with suspected hereditary coagulopathy, abnormal coagulogram with deranged activated partial thromboplastin time (aPTT) followed by correction studies help in diagnosis. Treatment including rest, application of ice, compression, and elevation of joint helps in reducing pain and swelling of joint. Replacement of deficient clotting factors helps in controlling further bleeding into the joint.

QUESTION 3: IF THERE IS EVIDENCE OF ARTHRITIS, THEN DEFINE THE FOLLOWING

- *Acute versus chronic*
- *Pattern of joint involvement*
- *Systemic features*

As we have seen before, arthritis is characterized by joint swelling, redness and warmth over the joints, limitation of joint movements, and early morning stiffness. It is important to remember that all these clinical features may not be present. Once diagnosis of arthritis is made, the physician needs to look at duration of illness, pattern of joint involvement, and presence of systemic features.

Acute Versus Chronic

Chronic arthritis is described as persistent arthritis lasting for >6 weeks. Juvenile idiopathic arthritis (JIA) is the most common cause of chronic arthritis in children and shall be discussed further in Chapter 18.2. Presence of systemic features in a child with chronic arthritis should take the physician away from a diagnosis of JIA.

Other causes include chronic infections [such as tuberculosis and human immunodeficiency virus (HIV)], autoimmune diseases [systemic lupus erythematosus (SLE) and chronic vasculitis], and autoinflammatory conditions.

Any arthritis of <6 weeks duration is defined as acute arthritis. Acute arthritis in children can result from various causes:

- Infectious causes (Infectious agent in the joint)
  - Septic arthritis
  - Viral infections such as parvovirus B19, rubella, mumps, and chikungunya
- Noninfectious causes
  - Rheumatic fever
  - Reactive arthritis
  - Autoimmune conditions such as SLE, Henoch-Schönlein purpura (IgA vasculitis)
  - Autoinflammatory syndromes
  - *Drug reactions:* Penicillin, sulphonamides, antiepileptic drugs, isoniazid, D-penicillamine, etc.

Pattern of Joint Involvement

Pattern of joint involvement is a very useful tool for differential diagnosis of arthritis.

- Number of joints involved
  - *Oligoarthritis:* Involvement of <5 joints
  - *Polyarthritis:* Involvement of ≥5 joints
- Symmetrical versus asymmetrical involvement
  - Symmetrical small joint arthritis of hands is typical of rheumatoid-factor positive polyarthritis in children.
  - Asymmetrical large-joint arthritis is typically seen in oligoarthritis, enthesitis-related arthritis (ERA), and juvenile psoriatic arthritis.
- Large joint versus small joint versus both
  - Large joints include shoulders, elbows, hips, knees, and ankles. Large-joint arthritis is typically seen in rheumatic fever, ERA, juvenile psoriatic arthritis, and oligoarthritis.
  - Small joints include wrists and all joints of hands and feet. Small-joint arthritis is typically seen in viral arthritis, rheumatoid-factor positive polyarthritis, rheumatoid-factor negative polyarthritis, and juvenile psoriatic arthritis.
- Migratory versus additive versus fixed involvement
  - Migratory arthritis is typically described in rheumatic fever, though can also be seen in viral infections and reactive arthritis. Inflammation moves from one joint to other and first joint becomes normal as the next joint gets affected.
  - Additive involvement is described as joint involvement wherein more joints get involved with time.
  - Fixed involvement is described as joint involvement wherein no further joints are involved after initial involvement.
- Peripheral versus axial involvement
  - Axial skeleton includes skull, ribs, spine, and sacroiliac joints. Its involvement is seen in ERA, reactive arthritis, juvenile psoriatic arthritis, and arthritis associated with inflammatory bowel disease.
  - Peripheral skeleton includes all the joints of appendages.
- Periarticular involvement
  - *Enthesitis:* Enthesitis is seen in ERA and reactive arthritis in children.
  - *Muscular atrophy:* Periarticular muscle atrophy is common in children with chronic arthritis and is an important determinant of long-term prognosis.

Presence of Systemic Features

Systemic features play an important role in differential diagnosis of arthritis. It is essential that a physician should do a thorough physical examination for every child with arthritis.

Systemic involvement in a child with chronic arthritis should alert the physician to a diagnosis other than JIA. Systemic manifestations are common in other autoimmune conditions such as SLE and vasculitis. We shall discuss these manifestations further in the following section.

SOME IMPORTANT CAUSES OF ARTHRITIS

Viral Infections

Viral infections are the most common causes of acute, self-limiting arthritis in children. Both small and large joints may be involved. History of fever and other systemic features help in diagnosis. Arthritis usually improves spontaneously within a few days to weeks; however, some children may continue to have arthritis for months.

Septic Arthritis

Septic arthritis, like acute osteomyelitis, is a medical emergency in childhood. Bacterial infection of the joint space leads to rapid joint destruction and systemic illness. *Staphylococcus aureus* is the most frequent bacterial pathogen. Though it can occur at any age, is more common in infants and young children. These children present with high grade fever with a toxic look and joint pain with refusal to move the affected joint. Commonly, a single large joint becomes swollen, red, and warm to the touch. Most children do not allow any movement of the joint.

Hemogram shows neutrophilic leukocytosis with raised inflammatory parameters. Blood culture should be sent at presentation. Joint fluid aspiration helps to identify the organism and reduce pain by relieving the pressure inside the joint. Ultrasound may help confirm joint effusion but is not essential.

Treatment should be initiated without delay to prevent joint destruction and systemic complications. Broad-spectrum intravenous antibiotics (with antistaphylococcal cover) should be initiated immediately, pending culture and sensitivity results. The affected joint is immobilized to reduce further damage and pain. Surgical intervention may be necessary in select patients.

Rheumatic Fever

Rheumatic fever is a postinfective inflammatory condition seen 2–4 weeks after untreated or inadequately treated streptococcal infection. It is commonly seen after the age of 5 years. Typically, children present with low-to-moderate fever and arthritis of large joints. Joint involvement is migratory, i.e., joint pain often migrates from one joint to another. Inflammation is severe and children often do not tolerate even a cloth over the inflamed joint.

Other clinical features include carditis (chest pain, heart murmurs, palpitations, fatigue, and congestive heart failure), erythema marginatum (painless, pink, and raised skin rash with clear centers and irregular borders over the trunk), painful subcutaneous nodules over bony areas, and chorea. A history of recent streptococcal infection may be present. While most clinical features are self-limiting, cardiac involvement can cause long-term complications.

Treatment of acute episodes includes antibiotics (penicillin) and anti-inflammatory medications to manage symptoms. Prevention of recurrences is achieved by long-term antibiotics to prevent recurrent streptococcal infections.

Reactive Arthritis

Reactive arthritis typically develops as a reaction to a bacterial infection in the gastrointestinal or genitourinary tract. Clinical features include arthritis of both large and small joints. Some children with reactive arthritis may develop uveitis. Enthesitis is a common feature of reactive arthritis and can lead to localized pain and tenderness at tendon insertion sites. Fever is usually not very impressive. Inflammatory parameters such as ESR and CRP are usually raised. HLA-B27 positivity is seen in a subset of children. Treatment is primarily supportive. It is self-limiting in many children. However, some individuals may experience recurrent episodes or persistent symptoms.

CONCLUSION

Musculoskeletal pain in children can occur due to multiple reasons, which could be as benign as growing pains and as life-threatening as malignancies. A physician should be able to answer three important questions **(Flowchart 18.1.4)** after

Flowchart 18.1.4: Algorithm for diagnosis of musculoskeletal (MSK) pain

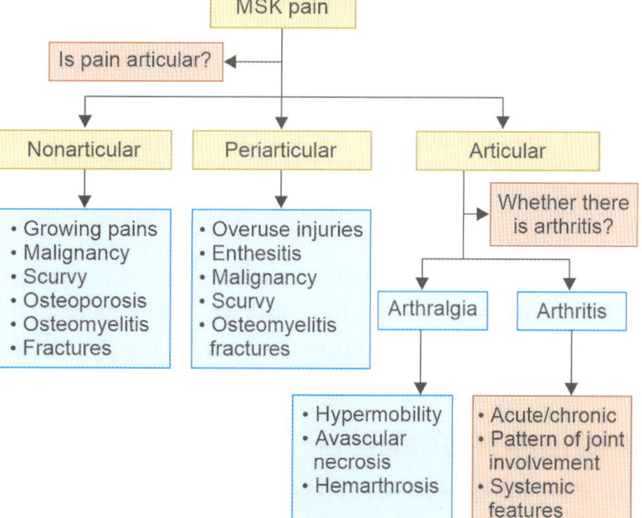

a meticulous history and a thorough physical examination. These three answers would help physicians in a judicious use of laboratory investigations and appropriate management.

REFERENCES

1. Kamper SJ, Williams CM. Musculoskeletal pain in children and adolescents: a way forward. J Orthop Sports Phys Ther. 2017;47(10):702-4.
2. Foster HE, Jandial S. pGALS-paediatric gait arms legs and spine: a simple examination of the musculoskeletal system. Pediatr Rheumatol Online J. 2013;11(1):44.
3. O'Keeffe M, Kamper SJ, Montgomery L, Williams A, Martiniuk A, Lucas B, et al. Defining growing pains: a scoping review. Pediatrics. 2022;150(2):e2021052578.
4. Barzilai-Birenboim S, Yacobovich J, Zalcberg Y, Arad-Cohen N, Avrahami G, Gilad G, et al. Bone pain at leukemia diagnosis and other risk factors for symptomatic osteonecrosis in children with acute lymphoblastic leukemia. Pediatr Blood Cancer. 2021;68(8):e29033.
5. Gornitzky AL, Kim AE, O'Donnell JM, Swarup I. Diagnosis and management of osteomyelitis in children: a critical analysis review. JBJS Rev. 2020;8(6):e1900202.
6. Schett G, Lories RJ, D'Agostino MA, Elewaut D, Kirkham B, Soriano ER, et al. Enthesitis: from pathophysiology to treatment. Nat Rev Rheumatol. 2017;13(12):731-41
7. Rodenberg RE, Bowman E, Ravindran R. Overuse injuries. Prim Care. 2013;40(2):453-73.
8. Trapani S, Rubino C, Indolfi G, Lionetti P. A narrative review on pediatric scurvy: The last twenty years. Nutrients. 2022;14(3):684.
9. Ciancia S, Högler W, Sakkers RJB, Appelman-Dijkstra NM, Boot AM, Sas TCJ, et al. Osteoporosis in children and adolescents: How to treat and monitor? Eur J Pediatr. 2023;182(2):501-11.
10. Rodríguez-Olivas AO, Hernández-Zamora E, Reyes-Maldonado E. Legg–Calvé–Perthes disease overview. Orphanet J Rare Dis. 2022;17(1):125.
11. Tinkle BT. Symptomatic joint hypermobility. Best Pract Res Clin Rheumatol. 2020;34(3):101508.

18.2 Juvenile Idiopathic Arthritis

Chandrika S Bhat

INTRODUCTION

Juvenile idiopathic arthritis (JIA) encompasses a heterogeneous group of conditions characterized by chronic arthritis of unknown origin, lasting for more than 6 weeks, with onset occurring before the age of 16 years. Arthritis is defined as the presence of joint swelling or effusion, increased warmth, and/or painful restricted movement, with or without joint line tenderness. According to the classification by the International League Against Rheumatism (ILAR), there are 7 distinct and mutually exclusive categories of JIA determined by the disease manifestations during the first 6 months.[1]

EPIDEMIOLOGY

The global prevalence of JIA has been estimated to range from 0.07 to 4.01 per 1,000 children, with an incidence of 1.6 to 23/100,000. The estimated prevalence of JIA was 48/100,000 in Indian children.[2]

ETIOPATHOGENESIS

The etiopathogenesis of JIA involves a complex interplay of genetic factors, environmental triggers, and a dysregulated immune response. Despite ongoing research, the precise pathogenesis remains elusive. It is hypothesized that environmental exposure in a genetically susceptible child leads to an altered immune response. Dysregulation in the adaptive immune system involving regulatory T-cells, Th1 [interferon-gamma (IFN-γ)-secreting T-cells], and Th17 [interleukin-17 (IL-17)-secreting T cells] is a shared characteristic across various subtypes of JIA. In oligoarticular, polyarticular, and psoriatic arthritis, IL-17 triggers the production of proinflammatory cytokines and matrix metalloproteinases, causing joint damage. In enthesitis-related arthritis, the pivotal cytokine is IL-23, which induces inflammation through IL-17 and tumor necrosis factor (TNF), as well as promotes new bone formation through IL-22. Persistent activation of innate immunity, including monocytes, macrophages, and neutrophils with elevation of cytokines such as IL-1β, IL-6, and IL-18, is the hallmark of systemic arthritis. The ensuing inflammation consisting of T and B lymphocytes, plasma cells, macrophages, and dendritic cells concentrates in the synovium and leads to synovial hypertrophy along with increased vascularization (hyperemia).

CLINICAL FEATURES

The manifestations can vary between the various subtypes of JIA (**Table 18.2.1**). Extraarticular involvement can occur in all types of JIA, but the frequency and severity may be different.[1,3]

- *Joint pain and swelling:* Persistent pain and swelling in one or more affected joints are hallmark symptoms of JIA. The skin overlying the affected joint may be warm to the touch.

TABLE 18.2.1: 2001 ILAR JIA definitions and exclusion criteria.[1,4]

JIA categories	*Definition*	*ILAR exclusion criteria*
Oligoarticular JIA: Persistent and extended	Arthritis affecting 4 or fewer joints during the first 6 months of disease • *Persistent oligoarthritis:* Arthritis in four or fewer joints for the entire disease course • *Extended oligoarthritis:* Arthritis in 5 or more joints after the initial 6 months of disease	• Psoriasis in the patient or a history of psoriasis in a first-degree relative or • Arthritis in an HLA-B27 male beginning after his sixth birthday or • 2 positive tests for RF obtained at least 3 months apart OR • HLA-associated disease* in a first-degree relative or • Systemic arthritis
RF-negative polyarticular JIA	Arthritis affecting 5 or more joints during the first 6 months of disease, with an RF negative test	• Psoriasis in the patient or a history of psoriasis in a first-degree relative or • Arthritis in an HLA-B27 male beginning after his sixth birthday or • 2 positive tests for RF obtained at least 3 months apart or • HLA-associated disease* in a first-degree relative or • Systemic arthritis
RF-positive polyarticular JIA	Arthritis affecting 5 or more joints during the first 6 months of disease, with 2 or more positive tests for RF at least 3 months apart during the first 6 months of disease	• Psoriasis in the patient or a history of psoriasis in a first-degree relative or • Arthritis in an HLA-B27 male beginning after his sixth birthday or • HLA-associated disease* in a first-degree relative or • Systemic arthritis
Systemic arthritis	Arthritis in 1 or more joints with or preceded by fever of at least 2 weeks duration that is documented to be daily for at least 3 days and accompanied by 1 or more of the following: • Evanescent erythematous rash • Generalized lymph-node enlargement • Hepatomegaly and/or splenomegaly • Serositis	• Psoriasis in the patient or a history of psoriasis in a first-degree relative or • Arthritis in an HLA-B27 male beginning after his sixth birthday or • Two positive tests for RF obtained at least three months apart; or • HLA-Associated disease* in a first-degree relative
Psoriatic arthritis	Arthritis and psoriasis, or arthritis and at least two of the following: • Dactylitis • Nail pitting or onycholysis • Psoriasis in a first-degree relative	• Arthritis in an HLA-B27 male beginning after his sixth birthday or • Two positive tests for RF obtained at least 3 months apart or • HLA-associated disease* in a first-degree relative or • Systemic arthritis.
Enthesitis-related arthritis	Arthritis and enthesitis or arthritis or enthesitis with at least 2 of the following: • Presence or a history of sacroiliac joint tenderness and/or inflammatory lumbosacral pain • The presence of HLA-B27 antigen • Onset of arthritis in a male over 6 years of age • Acute anterior uveitis • History of ankylosing spondylitis, ERA, sacroiliitis with inflammatory bowel disease, Reiter's syndrome, or acute anterior uveitis in a first-degree relative	• Psoriasis in the patient or a history of psoriasis in a first-degree relative or • Arthritis in an HLA-B27 male beginning after his sixth birthday; or • Two positive tests for RF obtained at least three months apart; or • Arthritis that fits 2 or more categories
Undifferentiated arthritis	Arthritis that fulfills criteria in no category or 2 or more of the above categories	

*HLA-associated disease includes ankylosing spondylitis, ERA, sacroiliitis with inflammatory bowel disease, reactive arthritis, or acute anterior uveitis. (ERA: enthesitis-related arthritis; HLA: human leukocyte antigen; ILAR: International League of Associations for Rheumatology; JIA: juvenile idiopathic arthritis; RF: rheumatoid factor;)

TABLE 18.2.2: Differential diagnosis of juvenile idiopathic arthritis (JIA).

Infections	• Septic arthritis • Reactive arthritis • Osteomyelitis • Viral arthritis
Connective tissue diseases	• Systemic lupus erythematosus (SLE) • Dermatomyositis • Scleroderma
Autoinflammatory syndromes	• Familial Mediterranean fever (FMF) • Tumor necrosis factor receptor-associated periodic syndrome (TRAPS)
Hematologic disorders	• Hemophilia • Leukemia
Gastrointestinal disorders	Inflammatory bowel disease (Crohn's disease and ulcerative colitis)
Structural disorders	• Skeletal dysplasia • Hypermobility syndromes

- *Morning stiffness:* Children with JIA may experience morning stiffness, where the affected joints are stiff and difficult to move after waking up or after prolonged inactivity.
- *Limited range of motion:* Joint stiffness and inflammation can lead to a limited range of motion in affected joints.
- *Limping:* Children with JIA may develop a limp or start favoring one limb due to pain or discomfort in the affected joint.
- *Fatigue:* Chronic inflammation in children with JIA can lead to fatigue, more pronounced in children with systemic onset JIA.
- *Fever:* Systemic JIA, one subtype of JIA, may be associated with systemic symptoms, including fever, rash, and general malaise.

Table 18.2.2 lists common conditions that should be considered in the differential diagnosis of children with chronic arthritis.

DIAGNOSIS OF JUVENILE IDIOPATHIC ARTHRITIS

The diagnosis of JIA is based on clinical criteria and investigations are done to exclude conditions that can mimic JIA. A detailed history and clinical examination are therefore of paramount importance in making the diagnosis. Initial evaluation may include:[4,5]

- Full blood count and peripheral smear to exclude infections or malignancy.
- C-reactive protein to exclude infection or to assess the degree of inflammation.
- Prothrombin time (PT)/activated partial thromboplastin time (aPTT) may be considered, especially in boys with monoarthritis, to exclude hemophilia.
- Immunological tests such as antinuclear antibody (ANA), rheumatoid factor, and human leukocyte antigen (HLA-B27) may be required based on the subtype of JIA.
- Liver and renal function tests are done prior to commencing treatment.
- Urine analysis for proteinuria.
- Synovial fluid analysis may be done to exclude septic arthritis.
- *Imaging*
  - Ultrasonography may be performed to ascertain inflammation of the synovium or to determine the degree of effusion.
  - *Magnetic resonance imaging (MRI):* Although not routinely performed, MRI is usually done when the diagnosis is unclear.
- *Other tests:* Eye screening for uveitis at baseline, and further frequency would depend on the age, gender of the child, and subtype of JIA.

MANAGEMENT

The management of JIA usually requires a combination of medications, physiotherapy, occupational therapy, and psychological support. Therefore, a multi-disciplinary team is of utmost importance in ensuring good outcomes. Parents and caregivers should be reminded of the need for regular follow-ups to assess whether joint inflammation is in remission and to promptly identify any potential flares.[4,5]

- *Medications* ***(Table 18.2.3)****:*
  - *Nonsteroidal anti-inflammatory drugs (NSAIDs):* These drugs help reduce pain and inflammation. Naproxen (5–15 mg/kg/day) is the preferred NSAID.
  - *Disease-modifying antirheumatic drugs (DMARDs):* Drugs like methotrexate, sulfasalazine, leflunomide, and others are used to control inflammation and prevent joint damage.
  - *Biologics:* Targeted cytokine blockade with drugs such as etanercept, adalimumab, and infliximab that block TNF-alpha or rituximab, which is an anti-CD20 monoclonal antibody, are often used in more severe cases.
- *Physical therapy:* Physiotherapy is crucial to maintain joint function, improve flexibility, and strengthen muscles.
- *Joint injections*: Intra-articular corticosteroid injections with triamcinolone hexacetonide or triamcinolone acetonide can also be used to reduce inflammation in the joint.
- *Patient education:* Educating both the patient and their family about the condition, treatment options, and self-management strategies is essential.
- *Nutrition:* Chronic inflammation can predispose children to undernutrition. A healthy balanced diet that meets

TABLE 18.2.3: Various agents used in the treatment of JIA in India.

Nonsteroidal anti-inflammatory drugs (NSAIDs)					
Medication	***Preparation***	***Dose range***	***Interval***	***Major side effects***	***Laboratory monitoring***
Ibuprofen	• *Liquid:*100 mg/5 mL • *Tablets:* 200 mg, 400 mg, 600 mg, and 800 mg	30–40 mg/kg/day	Three times a day	Gastrointestinal (GI), renal, and hepatic	Every 4–6 months
Naproxen	• *Liquid:*125 mg/5 mL • *Tablets:* 250, 500 mg	10–15 mg/kg/day	Twice daily	GI, renal, hepatic, and pseudoporphyria	Every 4–6 months
Indomethacin	*Capsule:* 25 mg, 75 mg (sustained release)	1–3 mg/kg/day	Three times a day	Renal toxicity and GI irritation	Every 4–6 months
Salicylates, e.g., aspirin	*Tablets:* 75 mg, 150 mg, and 325 mg	70–100 mg/kg/day	Four times a day	GI, renal, hepatic, tinnitus, caries, and association with Reye syndrome	Every 4–6 months
Conventional disease-modifying antirheumatic drugs (DMARDs)					
Methotrexate	• *Tablets:* 2.5 mg, 5 mg, and 10 mg • *Parenteral:* 15 mg/mL or 25 mg/mL (IV, IM, and SC)	10–15 mg/m^2/week	Weekly	• GI, hepatic, bone marrow suppression, acute pulmonary insufficiency, immunosuppression, teratogenicity, and alopecia • Incidence of most of above is very low in children at doses used, thereby making it a rather safe drug • The most common adverse effects in children are gastrointestinal and mouth ulcers	• *At onset:* As given above *plus* renal function if history of kidney disease (excreted by kidneys) • *Follow-up:* CBC and LFT 8–12 weekly
Sulfasalazine	*Tablets:* 500 mg and 1,000 mg	Start at 5–10 mg/kg/day for 1 week and gradually increase up to 20 mg/kg/day	Twice weekly	GI, hepatic, rash, allergic reactions, Stevens–Johnson syndrome, bone marrow suppression, associated with Reye syndrome. Contraindicated in G6PD deficiency	CBC and LFT 8–12 weekly
Leflunomide	*Tablets:* 10 mg, 20 mg	• *<20 kg:* 10 mg alternate day • *20–40 kg:* 10 mg daily • *>40 kg:* 20 mg daily	Once daily	Hepatotoxicity (more when combined with methotrexate), nausea, diarrhea, alopecia, and mild weight loss	CBC and LFT 8–12 weekly
Thalidomide	*Capsule:* 50 mg and 100 mg	2.5–4 mg/kg/day	Once daily, preferably at bedtime	Drowsiness, tingling numbness, peripheral neuropathy (irreversible), hypothyroidism, hypoglycemia, stimulation of ACTH, prolactin	Enquire about tingling numbness and check deep tendon reflexes
Biologic DMARDs					
Intravenous immunoglobulin (IVIG)	5 g or 10 g/100 mL intravenously	1–2 g/kg	Monthly	Allergic reactions, headache, and risk of blood-borne disease	

Contd...

Contd...

Etanercept (anti-TNF)	25 mg or 50 mg vial or prefilled syringe SC	0.4 mg/kg Maximum 50 mg/week	Twice weekly	Irritation at injection site and increased frequency of infection	Screen for tuberculosis prior to initiation, CBC and LFT 8–12 weekly
Infliximab (monoclonal antibody to TNF)	100 mg vial IV	3–10 mg/kg IV infusion	Every 4–8 weeks	Headache, dizziness, nasal and throat irritation. Irritation at injection site	Screen for tuberculosis prior to initiation, CBC and LFT 8–12 weekly
Anakinra (anti-IL1)	100 mg prefilled syringe or vial IV or SC	100 mg	Daily	Fever, flu-like reactions, and MAS	Screen for tuberculosis prior to initiation, CBC and LFT 8–12 weekly
Tocilizumab (anti-IL6)	80 mg vial, IV 162 mg prefilled syringe, SC	8–12 mg/kg	Fortnightly	Infusion reactions, rashes	Screen for tuberculosis prior to initiation, CBC and LFT 8–12 weekly
Targeted DMARDs					
Tofacitinib	*Tablet:* 5 mg and 11 mg	10–20 kg 3.2 mg/dose; 20–40 kg 4 mg/dose; >40 mg 5 mg/dose	Twice daily	Infections, hepatitis, and venous thromboembolism	Screen for tuberculosis prior to initiation, CBC and LFT 8–12 weekly

(ACTH: adrenocorticotropic hormone; CBC: complete blood count; IL: interleukin; JIA: juvenile idiopathic arthritis; LFT: liver function test; MAS: Macrophage activation syndrome; TNF: tumor necrosis factor)

the daily calorie and protein requirements should be provided to children with JIA.

- *Immunization:* Live vaccines are not administered to children on systemic immunomodulation.

COMPLICATIONS[4,5]

- *Growth problems:* Some children with JIA may experience growth problems, potentially due to the effects of chronic inflammation of the affected joint.
- *Macrophage activation syndrome (MAS)* is a severe and potentially life-threatening complication associated with systemic onset JIA (sJIA). Uncontrolled systemic inflammation or infections can act as triggers for MAS, which may manifest either at the initial presentation or subsequently in children with sJIA. A shift from a quotidian to a continuous fever pattern, evanescent to fixed rash, hepatosplenomegaly, lymphadenopathy, and a characteristic laboratory profile showing cytopenias, elevated liver enzymes, and hyperferritinemia typically indicate the onset of MAS. Prompt recognition and immunomodulation with drugs such as corticosteroids can be life-saving.
- *Uveitis:* Eye inflammation is a potential complication of JIA, especially in young girls with ANA-positive oligoarticular JIA. The inflammation is painless and the sole symptom that young children may exhibit is the presence of floaters in their vision, which might go unnoticed or unreported. Regular eye examinations are, therefore, extremely important for early detection and management.
- *Infections:* Medications used to treat JIA, particularly immunosuppressive drugs, may increase the risk of infections.

REFERENCES

1. Ravelli A, Martini A. Juvenile idiopathic arthritis. Lancet. 2007;369(9563):767-78.
2. Abujam B, Mishra R, Aggarwal A. Prevalence of musculoskeletal complaints and juvenile idiopathic arthritis in children from a developing country: a school-based study. Int J Rheum Dis. 2014;17(3):256-60.
3. Martini A, Ravelli A, Avcin T, Beresford MW, Burgos-Vargas R, Cuttica R, et al.; Pediatric Rheumatology International Trials Organization (PRINTO). Toward new classification criteria for juvenile idiopathic arthritis: First steps, Pediatric Rheumatology International Trials Organization International Consensus. J Rheumatol. 2019;46(2):190-7.
4. Martini A, Lovell DJ, Albani S, Brunner HI, Hyrich KL, Thompson SD, et al. Juvenile idiopathic arthritis. Nat Rev Dis Primers. 2022;8(1):5.
5. Zaripova LN, Midgley A, Christmas SE, Beresford MW, Baildam EM, Oldershaw RA. Juvenile idiopathic arthritis: From aetiopathogenesis to therapeutic approaches. Pediatr Rheumatol Online J. 2021;19(1):135.

18.3 Systemic Lupus Erythematosus

Amita Aggarwal

INTRODUCTION

Systemic lupus erythematosus (SLE) is an autoimmune disease characterized by multisystem involvement associated with presence of multiple autoantibodies. The disease affects girls more often than boys and presents usually after the age of 5 years though monogenic lupus can present earlier.

EPIDEMIOLOGY

The prevalence of SLE varies between 1 and 3/10,000 population and the incidence in children is between 0.28 and 0.48/100,000 children. The disease is more prevalent as well as more severe in Afro-Americans and Asians.[1] About 15–20% of SLE starts in childhood. The gender bias increases toward females as the age of the child increases. It varies from 3:1 in 5 to 7-year-olds to about 7–8:1 in adolescents.

PATHOGENESIS

Systemic lupus erythematosus is characterized by the presence of a plethora of autoantibodies directed against different components of cell, the most important of which is antibodies to double-stranded DNA (dsDNA). In SLE, due to decreased disposal of DNA (generated during normal cell death), an excess of DNA and modified DNA accumulates leading to the production of anti-dsDNA antibodies. When these antibodies bind to extracellular DNA, they form immune complexes. These immune complexes get deposited in small blood vessels such as glomerular tuft, pulmonary capillaries, and skin, leading to immune complex-mediated complement activation and release of proinflammatory mediators. This also results in consumption of complement, which is hallmark of active SLE. Further DNA–anti-DNA antibody complexes or RNA–anti-RNA associated protein complexes enter the cells via Fc receptors and reach the endosome where they activate Toll-like receptor-7 (TLR7), 8, and 9, which finally results in production of type I interferon, another hallmark of SLE pathogenesis. In addition to this, patients with SLE have abnormalities in T cells and B cells, which reduce their threshold of activation resulting in activation of autoreactive T and B cells **(Fig. 18.3.1)**.[2]

In children, defects in any of these pathways can result in monogenic lupus **(Table 18.3.1)**.

CLINICAL FEATURES

Systemic lupus erythematosus is a multisystem disease, thus a typical patient usually has fever, joint pains, skin rash, anemia, and leukopenia. If the patient has classical butterfly rash on the malar area sparing the nasolabial folds, the diagnosis is easy **(Fig. 18.3.2A)**. However a significant proportion of patients present with single organ involvement like nephritis, neuropsychiatric manifestations, or immune cytopenias.

Systemic Features

Fever is one of the common symptoms and is seen in around 80% of children. Usually, it is low grade but rarely it can be of moderate-to-high intensity. Other systemic features include weight loss, anorexia, myalgias, and lymphadenopathy.

Mucocutaneous Manifestations

The mucocutaneous manifestations occur in about three-fourths of patients. Though malar rash is the most typical, other lesions include discoid lupus (plaques with scaling and atrophy on healing), oral ulcers (painless, superficial, and located on hard palate), subacute lupus (annular, psoriasiform lesions located in sun-exposed area usually above the waist), and alopecia (usually nonscarring but discoid lesions on the scalp can result in scarring) **(Figs. 18.3.2A to C)**. Rarely digital gangrene, palpable purpura, skin infarcts, erythema nodosum, chilblains, and panniculitis can also be seen.

Musculoskeletal Manifestations

Polyarthralgia is the usual symptom in SLE; however, a significant proportion of patients have joint swelling due to synovitis and it can simulate polyarticular juvenile idiopathic arthritis. A few patients can have oligoarthritis or tenosynovitis. Though correctable deformities can occur in SLE, destructive arthritis is rare. Myalgias are common but significant muscle weakness due to inflammatory myopathy is seen only in 5–7% of patients. Occasionally, SLE patients can develop avascular necrosis of bones like hip or bone infarcts due to vascular occlusion.

Renal Manifestations

Renal disease can vary from asymptomatic urinary abnormalities to rapidly progressive renal failure. Children

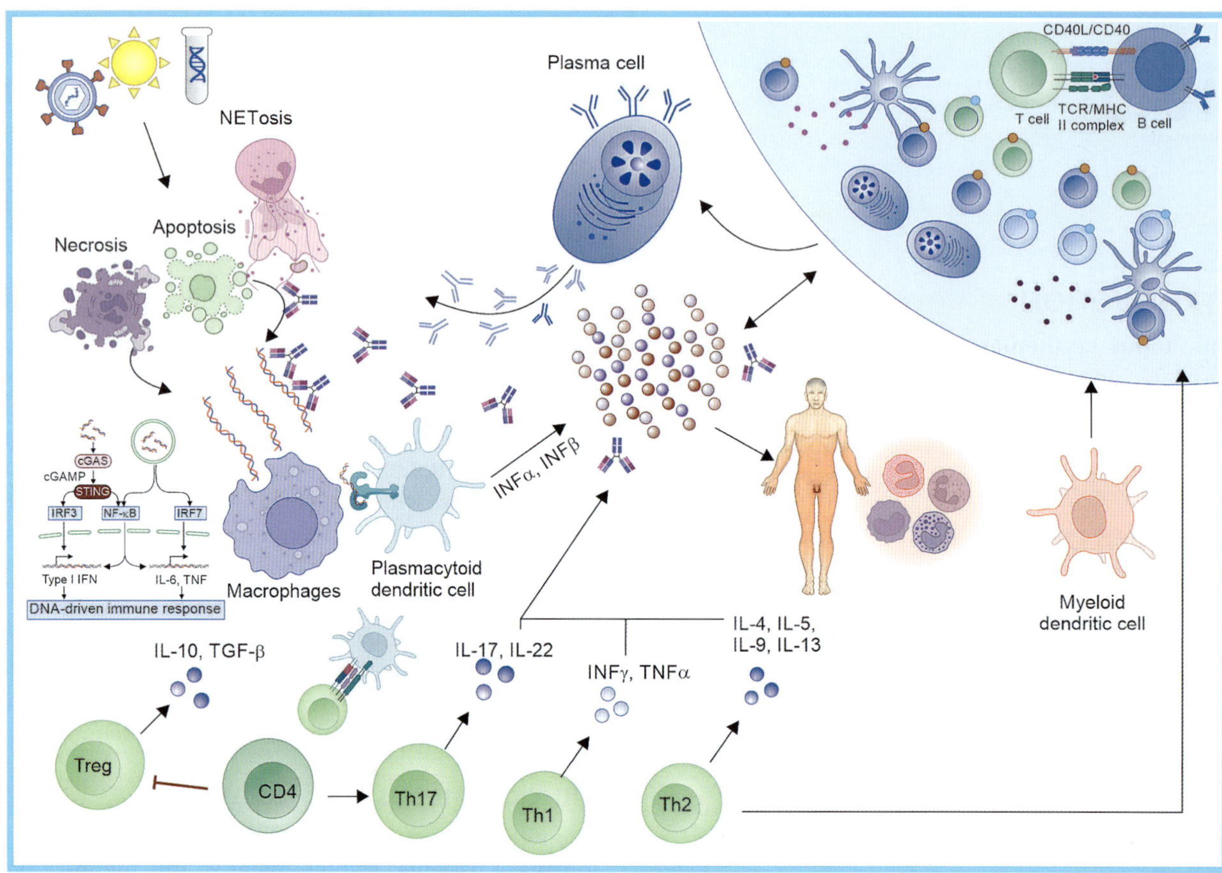

Fig. 18.3.1: Pathogenesis of systemic lupus erythematosus.
Source: Chandwar K, Aggarwal A Systemic lupus erythematosus. Indian J Pediatr. 2024;91(10):1032-40.
(cGAMP 2′3′: cyclic GMP–AMP; cGAS: cyclic GMP–AMP synthase; IRF3: interferon regulatory factor 3; IRF7: interferon regulatory factor 7; INF: interferon; IL: interleukin; MHC: major histocompatibility complex; NETosis: neutrophil extracellular trap, NF: nuclear factor-κB; STING: stimulator of interferon genes; TCR: T-cell receptors; TGF: tumor growth factor; Th1: T helper 1 cells; Th2: T helper2 cells; Th17: T helper 17 cells; TNFa: tumor necrosis factor a; Treg: T-regulatory cells)

usually present with pedal edema, hypertension, or nephrotic syndrome. Rarely, they can present with rapidly rising serum creatinine with nephritic picture. Renal disease has a major impact on the outcome of SLE in an individual.

Cardiopulmonary Manifestations

Pericardial involvement in SLE presents with acute pericarditis, pericardial effusion, or pericardial tamponade. Myocarditis can present with biventricular failure, arrhythmia, etc. Endocardial involvement due to antiphospholipid antibodies can give rise to nonbacterial thrombotic endocarditis. About 3–5% patients can have pulmonary artery hypertension due to pulmonary vasculitis.

Pleural effusions, usually bilateral, exudative with low complements are seen in about 15–20% of patients with SLE. Other rare pulmonary manifestations are acute pneumonitis, diffuse alveolar hemorrhage due to pulmonary capillaritis, and interstitial lung disease. Airway disease is uncommon in SLE.

Gastrointestinal Manifestations

Liver involvement is not uncommon with hepatomegaly seen in about 15–20% of patients. Peritonitis as part of serositis is an uncommon manifestation. Ascites usually occurs due to hypoproteinemia (due to poor intake, loss through the kidney in patients with nephrotic syndrome, or rarely, due to Budd-Chiari syndrome). Gastrointestinal (GI) tract involvement can rarely present as an emergency in lupus like pancreatitis, gangrene of the bowel, intestinal obstruction due to bowel-wall ischemia, acalculous cholecystitis, etc.

Hematological Manifestations

Blood abnormalities are invariably present in patients with SLE. Anemia due to chronic inflammation, autoimmune

TABLE 18.3.1: Monogenic causes of systemic lupus erythematosus (SLE).

Mutation	*Mechanism*	*Clinical manifestations*
Complement deficiencies (C1q, C1r, C1s, C2, and C4)	Impaired clearance of apoptotic cells and immune complexes	• Recurrent infections • Early onset • Prominent cutaneous manifestations • *Absence of anti-dsDNA antibodies* • Anti-Ro and La antibodies (>70%)
PKCδ deficiency	Excessive B-cell proliferation	• *Hepatosplenomegaly* • *Lymphadenopathy* • EBV or CMV infection
Prolidase deficiency	Alteration in C1q	• Recurrent infections • Elevated IgE • *Leg ulcers* • Cutaneous manifestations (telangiectasias) • Facial dysmorphia
Interferonopathy (TREX1, IFIH1, and ADAR)	Increase in IFNα	• Lupus pernio • *Basal ganglion calcification*
RASopathy (RAS/MAPK pathway)	• Leukocyte prolifera-tion • Defective apoptosis	• Increased rate of pericarditis • *Little skin involvement* • Splenomegaly • Lymphadenopathy • Risk of malignant transformation
Mutation in *DNASE1L3*	Alteration in DNA removal	• Urticaria • *Cutaneous vasculitis* • Recurrent abdominal pain • Uveitis and episcleritis • Glomerulonephritis with anti-C1q antibodies
Mutation in *ACP5* (SPENDI)	• Defect in TRAP • Increase in IFNα	• *Spondyloenchondrodysplasia* • Immune dysregulation • *Basal ganglion calcification*

(CMV: cytomegalovirus; DNA: deoxyribonucleic acid; EBV: Epstein–Barr virus; IFN: interferon; TRAP: tartrate-resistant acid phosphatase)

hemolysis, renal disease or nutritional deficiency or drugs is the most common. Leukopenia, lymphopenia and thrombocytopenia are seen in about one-third of patients. Other manifestations include presence of thrombosis in arterial and venous systems due to presence of anti-phospholipid antibodies or thrombotic thrombocytopenic purpura due to antibodies to ADAMTS13.

Neuropsychiatric Manifestations

Neuropsychiatric manifestations vary in severity from headache to a cerebrovascular accident. Mild abnormalities like anxiety, mood disorders, headache, and cognition abnormalities are common but are difficult to attribute to the disease. Central nervous system (CNS) disease can present as seizures, psychosis, stroke, movement disorders, and longitudinal myelitis while peripheral nervous system disease usually presents with mononeuropathy, mononeuritis multiplex, or demyelinating disorders.

Neonatal Lupus

Neonatal lupus can present in utero or at birth. In utero, it can present with heart block starting in second trimester of pregnancy at around 20 weeks. It can either stay static or progress to third-degree block. If the rate is slow, baby can have hydrops fetalis and intrauterine growth restriction (IUGR).

At birth, the child may have congenital heart block or may have a skin rash like subacute cutaneous lupus, thrombocytopenia, leukopenia, and rarely transaminitis. This is due to transplacental transfer of maternal antibodies and usually resolves spontaneously over a few weeks.

DIFFERENTIAL DIAGNOSIS

As lupus is a multisystem disease, therefore, many systemic diseases like chronic infections (tuberculosis, fungal or bacterial), hematological malignancies, other rheumatological diseases, metabolic diseases, etc. need to be considered in differential diagnosis. Infections can have rash, fever, cytopenias, and organomegaly but presence of significant renal disease makes infection less likely. Similarly, if a child has hypertension, then leukemia is less likely.

Juvenile dermatomyositis (JDM) can have malar rash, fever, arthritis with antinuclear antibodies (ANAs) and difficulty to move around, and thus can simulate SLE; however, a detailed muscle examination and typical rashes of JDM can easily clinch the diagnosis. In addition, renal and neuropsychiatric diseases are not seen in JDM.

LABORATORY INVESTIGATIONS

In any child suspected to have SLE, *ANA* should be ordered, as it has a sensitivity of 97–98%. A negative ANA should alert you to an alternative diagnosis. If the diagnosis of SLE is clinically certain like presence of multisystem disease with malar rash, one should repeat ANA in dilution. ANA should preferably be done by indirect immunofluorescence assay rather than by enzyme-linked immunosorbent assay (ELISA). ANA is not specific for SLE, and it can be present in SLE mimics like dermatomyositis, autoimmune hepatitis, chronic infections, etc.

In addition, laboratory tests need to be done to see the extent of involvement like *complete blood count* to look for immune cytopenias, *serum creatinine, and urine examination* for renal involvement, *chest X-ray and an electrocardiograph (ECG)* to look for cardiopulmonary disease, *liver function tests* for presence of hepatitis, *transaminitis* due to myositis, and also prior to starting immunosuppressive treatment. If patient has significant renal disease, then a *24-hour or timed*

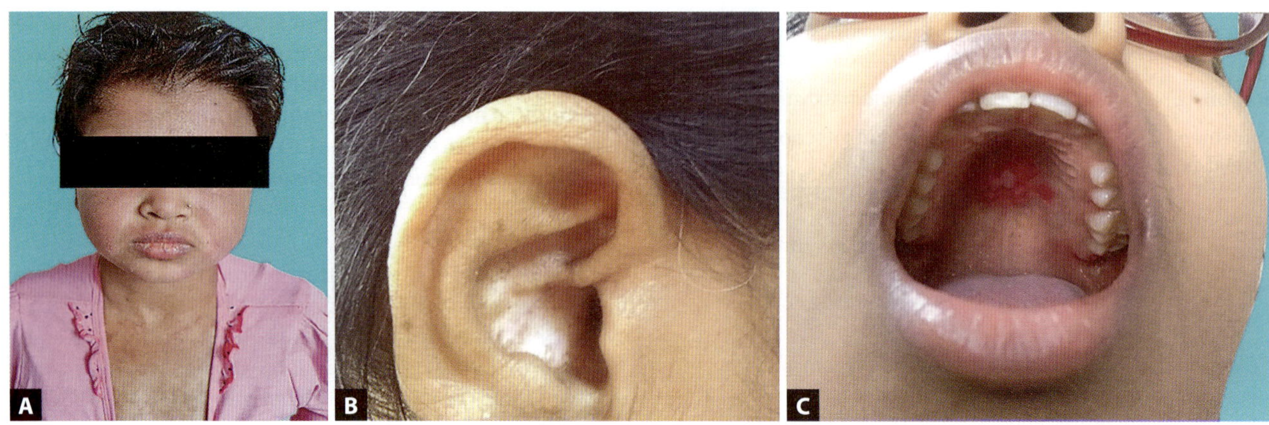

Figs. 18.3.2A to C: (A) Malar rash on the face sparing nasolabial fold; (B) Discoid lupus leading to hypopigmentation in the ear; and (C) Hard palate ulcer in a child with systemic lupus erythematosus (SLE).

collection of urine for protein and creatinine should be done to assess the degree of proteinuria. *Renal biopsy* is indicated in all children with significant proteinuria (>500 mg/24 hour) and/or urine sediment abnormalities or unexplained rise in creatinine. It helps to know the class as well as activity and chronicity of nephritis. Kidney biopsy also helps in guiding the therapy.

Other tests are done based on organ involved, when indicated: Such as echocardiography, cerebrospinal fluid (CSF) examination, magnetic resonance imaging (MRI) brain, ultrasound abdomen, and contrast-enhanced computed tomography (CECT).

To assess disease activity, levels of *anti-dsDNA* and *serum complement* should be done **(Table 18.3.2)**. Further, ANA specificity can be done to look for antibodies to Smith antigen (Sm), ribonucleoprotein (nRNP), and Ro and La. *Anti-phospholipid antibodies* are also present in about 30-40% of children with SLE. *Coomb's test* must be done in a child suspected to be having immune hemolysis.

MANAGEMENT

Children with SLE need a multidisciplinary approach starting with education of the family regarding the course of disease, need for adherence to drugs, sun protection as well as need for regular follow-up.[3] The current approach is to treat to target (T2T) and try to achieve remission, as remission has been shown to reduce damage over time **(Flowchart 18.3.1)**.[4]

Corticosteroids

Though corticosteroids have significant side effects, still they are the cornerstone of SLE management. The dose of prednisolone varies with organ involvement. In minor organ involvement, 0.25 mg/kg dose can be started while with major organ disease, 0.5–1 mg/kg dose may be required. In life and organ-threatening disease, intravenous (IV)

TABLE 18.3.2: Autoantibodies in systemic lupus erythematosus.

Autoantibody	*Antigenic target*	*Clinical association*
Antinuclear antibody (ANA)	Multiple antigens in the nucleus	Screening test, positive in nearly 98% patients
Antibodies to double-stranded DNA (dsDNA)	dsDNA	Seen in 55–60% patients, association with nephritis, and disease activity
Antibodies to Sm antigen	RNA-associated proteins	Specific for SLE, present in 20–30% patients, higher prevalence in India
Antibodies to RNP	U1RNA-associated proteins	Seen in 40–45% of SLE patients. Also seen in many connective tissue diseases
Antibodies to Ro	52, 60 kilodaltons RNA-associated protein	Seen in 30–40% patients; Associated with subacute cutaneous lupus, sicca symptoms, congenital heart block, and neonatal lupus
Antibodies to La	RNA-associated protein	Seen in 15–18% patients, association same as anti-Ro antibodies
Antibodies to ribosomal P	Ribosomal P protein	Seen in 10–12% patients, debatable association between hepatitis and psychosis
Antiphospholipid antibodies	Multiple phospholipids including beta 2 glycoprotein 1, cardiolipin, and annexin	Seen in 25–30%; association with thrombosis, cytopenias and fetal loss

(DNA: Deoxyribonucleic acid; RNA: ribonucleic acid; RNP: ribonucleoprotein)

Flowchart 18.3.1: Management of a child with systemic lupus erythematosus (SLE).

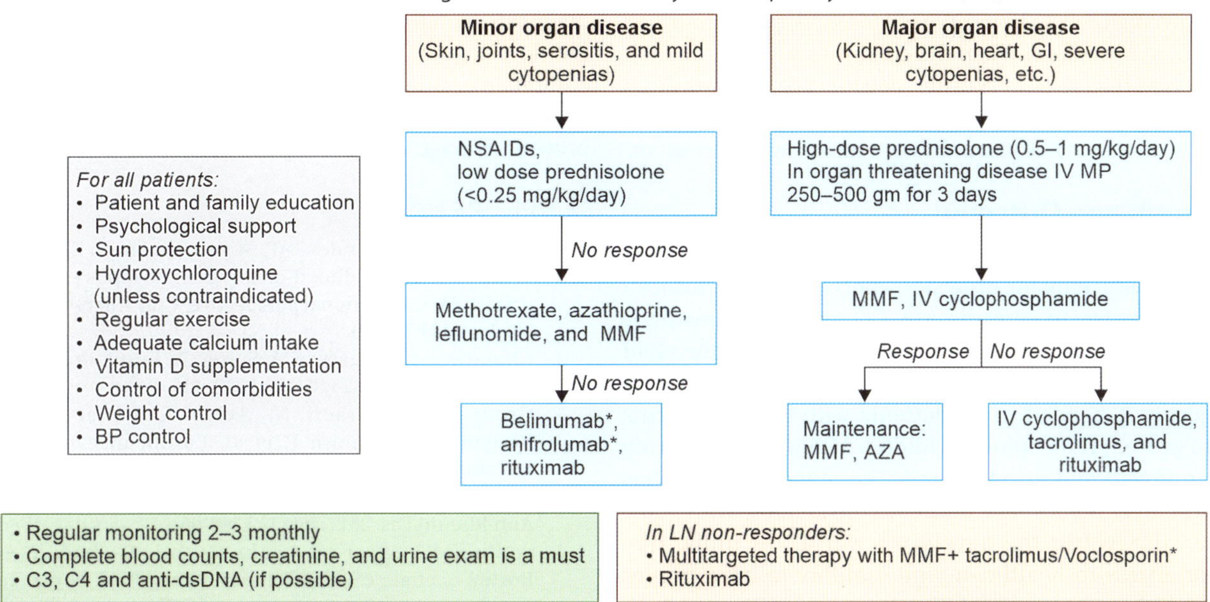

(AZA: azathioprine; GI: gastrointestinal; LN: lupus nephritis; MP: methylprednisolone pulses; MMF: mycophenolate mofetil; NSAIDs: nonsteroidal anti-inflammatory drugs)
*Not available in India.

methylprednisolone 15 mg/kg is generally used for 3 days. In the last decade, the attempt has been made to reduce the maintenance dose of prednisolone with the use of immunosuppressive agents. This helps to reduce long term side-effects of corticosteroids.

HYDROXYCHLOROQUINE

Hydroxychloroquine (HCQ) has multiple effects like reduced antigen presentation, improved endothelial function, antiplatelet effect, good effect on lipids, as well as anti-inflammatory effects. It is the most important background drug for SLE and should be given to all children unless contraindicated. The dose is 5 mg/kg/day preferably given at night. HCQ can lead to skin hyperpigmentation and can cause retinal toxicity on chronic use.[3] It is recommended to have a baseline eye examination and then repeat yearly after 5 years of therapy.

IMMUNOSUPPRESSIVE AGENTS

The list of immunosuppressive (IS) drugs that are currently being used in lupus includes mycophenolate mofetil (MMF), cyclophosphamide, azathioprine, methotrexate, leflunomide, and calcineurin inhibitors (cyclosporin, tacrolimus, and voclosporin). The choice of agent depends on organ involved, severity of disease, and choice of the patient and availability.

In case of skin, joint or constitutional symptoms, methotrexate is the preferred drug. While in renal disease, MMF is the drug of choice due to its good efficacy with minimal toxicity; calcineurin inhibitors are used in combination with MMF if there is an inadequate response. IV cyclophosphamide (500 mg every 15 days × 6 doses) is preferred in children with renal disease due to its safety profile. In patients with life-threatening complications like lupus enteritis, diffuse alveolar hemorrhage, etc., cyclophosphamide in a dose of 0.5–1 g/m^2 can be used monthly.

Azathioprine in a dose of 2–4 mg/kg is used for maintenance of remission for a period of 3–5 years. In refractory cases, leflunomide can also be tried for nephritis or arthritis.

Biologicals

Though multiple biologicals like belimumab (anti-B lymphocyte stimulator) and anifrolumab (antibodies to interferon alpha receptor) have been licensed for use in adults with SLE, their use in pediatrics is limited. Rituximab, anti-CD20 antibody, failed in clinical trials but has been used in children as a rescue therapy and has shown good benefit. The dose is 750 mg/m^2 IV and at induction, 2 doses are given 2 weeks apart. Maintenance therapy can be given at 6 months with a single dose. Rituximab is very useful in refractory cytopenias, renal disease, demyelinating disease, and severe vasculitis, etc.[5]

Adjunctive Therapy

All children should be given balanced diet, adequate calcium, and vitamin D supplements if the diet is deficient. Regular physical activity helps in keeping the morale up as well as improves muscle strength. All children with proteinuria should get angiotensin blockers as these reduce proteinuria as well as blood pressure. When the child is receiving induction therapy with high dose of IS drugs, cotrimoxazole prophylaxis can be used. Children should receive their scheduled vaccines *except* the live vaccines when they are receiving IS treatment.

Follow-up and Outcome

All patients with SLE need regular follow-ups to assess disease activity, look for drug side effects, and psychosocial impact of disease. In early disease, 1–2 monthly follow-up is recommended and as the disease activity reduces, the child can be followed every 3 months. Regular blood pressure monitoring is needed in all patients with lupus nephritis (LN) to prevent renal injury.[6] Children also need monitoring of their growth and development. The outcome of SLE has improved over the last five decades considerably with >90% 10-year survival in the developed world.[6] In India, due to poor access to healthcare and inability to have proper follow-up, the outcome is inferior. In a recent meta-analysis, patients with class IV LN in middle-income countries showed 5-and 10-year risk of end-stage renal disease of 14 and 30%, respectively, while in developed countries it was much lower (8 and 17%, respectively).[7]

CONCLUSION

Though SLE is a rare disease, early recognition and effective treatment has improved long-term outcome. SLE should be considered in differential diagnosis of a child with multisystem inflammatory disease. Presence of cytopenias, urinary abnormalities along with autoantibodies help in making a diagnosis. Treatment includes IS drugs along with adjunctive therapy. Regular follow up is needed for monitoring of drug compliance, side effects of drugs as well as early recognition of flares. The aim is to have long-term disease control to prevent damage with good quality of life.

REFERENCES

1. Aggarwal A, Fernandes TAP, Migowa A, Smith EMD, Hanif M, Webb K, et al. Childhood-onset systemic lupus erythematosus (cSLE): An international perspective. Curr Allergy Asthma Rep. 2024;24(10):559-69.
2. Chandwar K, Aggarwal A Systemic lupus erythematosus. Indian J Pediatr. 2024;91(10):1032-40.
3. Groot N, de Graeff N, Avcin T, Bader-Meunier B, Brogan P, Dolezalova P, et al. European evidence-based recommendations for diagnosis and treatment of childhood-onset systemic lupus erythematosus: The SHARE initiative. Ann Rheum Dis. 2017;76(11):1788-96.
4. Smith EMD, Aggarwal A, Ainsworth J, Al-Abadi E, Avcin T, Bortey L, et al.; cSLE T2T International Task Force. Towards development of treat to target (T2T) in childhood-onset systemic lupus erythematosus: PReS-endorsed overarching principles and points-to-consider from an international task force. Ann Rheum Dis. 2023;82(6):788-98.
5. Sawhney S, Agarwal M. Rituximab use in pediatric systemic lupus erythematosus: Indications, efficacy, and safety in an Indian cohort. Lupus. 2021;30(11):1829-36.
6. Silva CA, Aikawa NE, Bonfa E. Updates in the care and management of children and adolescents with systemic lupus erythematosus. Curr Opin Rheumatol. 2024;36(5):315-21.
7. Khandelwal P, Govindarajan S, Bagga A. Management and outcomes in children with lupus nephritis in the developing countries. Pediatr Nephrol. 2023;38(4):987-1000.

18.4 Approach to a Child with Vasculitis

Suma Balan

INTRODUCTION

Vasculitis refers to a group of disorders characterized by inflammation of blood vessels, leading to a spectrum of clinical manifestations ranging from mild skin lesions to life-threatening systemic involvement. The inflammation of blood vessels potentially leads to reduction in the size of lumen with stagnation or obstruction of blood flow which may lead to many significant manifestations. While vasculitis may affect individuals of any age, its presentation and management in childhood pose unique challenges. Vasculitis disorders may arise as primary diseases or as secondary diseases—secondary to infections (due to *Mycoplasma pneumoniae*, hepatitis B, etc.), connective tissue diseases [systemic lupus erythematosus (SLE), juvenile dermatomyositis, etc.], drugs (amphetamines, cocaine, etc.), and malignancies (lymphoma, lymphoreticular malignancies, etc.). This chapter aims to provide an overview of childhood primary systemic vasculitides, including their epidemiology, etiology, pathogenesis, clinical features, diagnosis, and management.

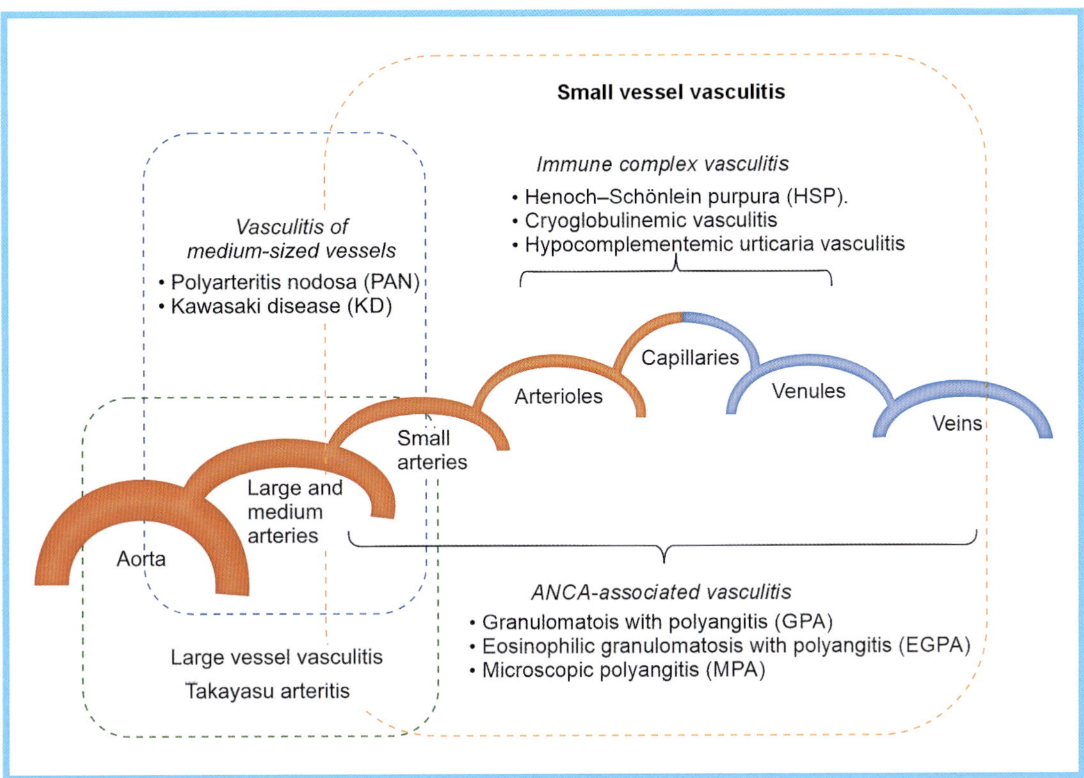

Fig. 18.4.1: Classification of primary childhood vasculitis based on revised Chapel Hill criteria (2012) and the EULAR/PRES classification.[2-4] (EULAR: European Alliance of Associations for Rheumatology PRES: Pediatric Rheumatology European Society)

CLASSIFICATION

Primary systemic vasculitis disorders are often classified according to the size of the vessel they involve **(Fig. 18.4.1)**:[1-4]

- *Large vessels*—aorta, its major branches and analogous veins
- *Medium vessels*—main visceral arteries, their veins, and their initial branches
- *Small vessels*—intraparenchymal arteries, arterioles, and venules

EPIDEMIOLOGY

The spectrum of childhood vasculitis in children is different compared to adults. In adults, large vessel vasculitis can occur due to giant cell arteritis or Takayasu arteritis (TA) but in children, only TA has been described. The exact prevalence and incidence of childhood vasculitis depend on the specific subtype and geographic region. Kawasaki disease (KD), the most common form of childhood vasculitis, has the highest incidence in East Asian populations, particularly in Japan. Other forms, such as Henoch-Schönlein purpura (HSP) and polyarteritis nodosa (PAN), also exhibit variability in prevalence among different ethnic groups. Similarly, monogenic forms of vasculitis such as deficiency of adenosine deaminase 2 (DADA2) or sting associated vasculopathy of infancy (SAVI) often present in childhood and have to be considered in the differential diagnosis of a vasculitic presentation.

The HSP [or immunoglobulin A (IgA) vasculitis] is the most common childhood vasculitis worldwide, however in countries like Japan, KD is the most common with an incidence of 239/100,000.[5] Antineutrophilic cytoplasmic antibody (ANCA)-associated vasculitis in children has an incidence of 1/1,000,000.[5] TA has an incidence of 0.8/million in UK compared to 2 per million in Asia with 10–20% childhood origin of disease.[5]

ETIOLOGY AND PATHOGENESIS

The etiology of childhood vasculitis is multifactorial and incompletely understood. In general, vasculitic disorders are thought to result from an abnormal immune response triggered by an infectious agent in genetically susceptible individuals. In many cases, the exact trigger remains elusive, although infectious agents, environmental factors, and genetic predisposition are believed to play roles in disease pathogenesis. Both KD and HSP often present in crops with seasonal incidence giving further evidence for that hypothesis.

CLINICAL FEATURES

Childhood vasculitis may manifest with a wide array of clinical features depending on the specific subtype and organs involved. Common presenting symptoms may include fever, rash, arthralgia, myalgia and abdominal pain, and constitutional symptoms such as fatigue and malaise.

Vasculitis must be suspected in the following clinical situations:

- Pyrexia of unknown origin (PUO)
- PUO with rash
- PUO with multisystem manifestations
- A child with hypertension
- Persistently raised inflammatory markers with nonspecific symptoms of unwellness.

Specific features can depend on the type of vessel involved as given in the following text:

- *Large vessel involvement:* Absent pulses, Bruits over aorta and vessels, Congestive heart failure and cardiomyopathy, Discrepant four limb blood pressure, and Elevated blood pressure (BP).
- *Medium vessel involvement:* Abdominal pain (celiac axes), Blindness, Claudication (subclavian, femoral, or iliac vessels), Chest pain (coronaries), Deep skin changes, Elevated BP (renal vessels), Focal deficits, Gangrene, Orchitis (testicular), and neuropathy.
- *Small vessel involvement:* Petechiae, purpura, superficial ulcers, mucosal ulcers, pulmonary and/or renal syndrome, ear-nose throat disease, and asthma.

The clinical course can be acute, subacute, or chronic, with some forms of vasculitis exhibiting relapsing-remitting patterns. It is essential for clinicians to recognize the diverse clinical presentations of childhood vasculitis to facilitate timely diagnosis and appropriate management.

DIAGNOSIS

Diagnosing childhood vasculitis requires a comprehensive approach that integrates clinical evaluation, laboratory investigations, imaging studies, and histopathological findings when available. *Pattern recognition*—the skill of identifying clinical patterns—helps rheumatologists to recognize the various vasculitic syndromes and venture to perform the appropriately confirmatory tests. There are classification criteria for the various primary systemic vasculitis that are shared in the following text which may help to make diagnoses.

Laboratory tests may reveal nonspecific markers of inflammation, such as elevated acute-phase reactants [e.g., erythrocyte sedimentation rate (ESR) and C-reactive protein (CRP)] and leukocytosis. Specific serological tests, such as ANCA in specific settings of ANCA-associated vasculitis, skin or organ biopsies (e.g., renal) may be required to make a diagnosis of IgA vasculitis (HSP), deep skin biopsies in PAN (systemic or cutaneous), and sometimes, muscle or nerve biopsies. In large vessel vasculitis as well as in PAN, imaging [computed tomography (CT) aortogram] may make the diagnosis. Echocardiography is an essential investigation in KD to monitor coronary aneurysms.

Imaging modalities, including ultrasound, CT, MRI, and angiography, play crucial roles in assessing the extent of vascular involvement and guiding targeted organ biopsies when indicated. Histopathological examination of affected tissues remains the gold standard for confirming the diagnosis of vasculitis and distinguishing between different subtypes.

VASCULITIS CLASSIFICATION CRITERIA

A brief account of the major primary systemic vasculitic syndromes in children is given in the following text.

Large Vessel Vasculitis

Takayasu Arteritis

About 10–20% of TA begins in childhood. While some children may present with an inflammatory PUO and weight loss (these children can be diagnosed in the prepulseless phase), most children present due to symptoms resulting from various stenotic lesions—hypertension, headaches, dyspnea, and claudication. The presence of elevated inflammatory markers indicate active disease, however they can be deceptively normal as well. There are clinical disease activity and damage scores which help to monitor treatment and prognosis **(Box 18.4.1)**. The treatment involves the use of systemic corticosteroids and steroid-sparing agents (methotrexate, mycophenolate mofetil, azathioprine, or biological medications) as well as medications to control hypertension, cardiac failure, etc. Revascularization procedures (interventional or surgical) may be required for severe and troublesome features not amenable to medical therapy alone like renal artery balloon dilatation for severe hypertension, but are recommended to be performed when disease activity is controlled by immunosuppressive therapy. The steroid-sparing medications are required for several

BOX 18.4.1: Classification criteria for childhood primary systemic vasculitis due to Takayasu arteritis.

Angiographic abnormalities of the aorta or its major branches and pulmonary arteries showing aneurysm/dilatation (mandatory) plus one of five:

1. Pulse deficit or claudication
2. Four limbs blood pressure discrepancy
3. Bruits
4. Hypertension
5. Elevated acute phase reactants

BOX 18.4.2: Criteria description of Polyarteritis nodosa.

Histopathology or angiographic abnormalities (mandatory) plus one of the following five:

1. Skin involvement
2. Myalgia or muscle tenderness
3. Hypertension
4. Peripheral neuropathy
5. Renal involvement

years to maintain disease remission. Delayed diagnosis and severe complications are sadly common and lead to a 5-year mortality rate of up to 27%.[2]

Medium Vessel Vasculitis

Polyarteritis Nodosa

Cutaneous PAN is more common in children than adults and present with painful subcutaneous nodules or panniculitic lesions along with some systemic symptoms and elevated inflammatory markers. A deep skin biopsy of the lesion is often confirmatory. Rarely peripheral vasculitic neuropathy of the affected region can also be seen. These patients respond well to treatment. Some children are easily managed on nonsteroidal anti-inflammatory agents (NSAIDs) such as naproxen and colchicine, whereas many children require systemic corticosteroids with steroid-sparing immunosuppressive agents such as methotrexate and mycophenolate or intravenous immunoglobulin.

Systemic PAN is commoner in adults than children and present as a PUO with a poorly thriving child or symptoms dependent on the affected medium vessels as elaborated in the **Box 18.4.2** with classification criteria.

A biopsy of skin lesion or nerve or involved muscle may give the diagnosis as also CT aortography or a digital subtraction angiogram showing the classic medium vessel involvement. This must be differentiated from congenital noninflammatory fibromuscular dysplasia or monogenetic vasculitis like DADA2 deficiency.

Kawasaki Disease

This is a medium vessel vasculitis presenting mostly in children under 5 years of age. It presents as a high-grade fever with significant clinical features as present in the diagnostic criteria as defined by the American Heart Association given below in **Box 18.4.3**.

This disease might present especially in young infants in an incomplete form which also needs to be recognized. The deadly complication of this disease is the occurrence of coronary artery aneurysms in about 25% of children if not diagnosed in time and treated adequately. The younger child and the male sex are at higher risk for aneurysms. Systemic inflammation on blood tests including a neutrophilic

BOX 18.4.3: Criteria description for Kawasaki disease.

Fever duration of 5 days or more plus four out of the following five:

1. *Conjunctivitis:* Bilateral, bulbar, nonsuppurative
2. *Lymphadenopathy:* Cervical, often >1.5 cm
3. *Rash:* Polymorphous, no vesicles or crusts
4. *Changes of lips or oral mucosa:* Red cracked lips; "strawberry" tongue; or diffuse erythema of oropharynx
5. *Changes of extremities:* Initial stage of erythema and edema of palms and soles, and convalescent stage: Peeling of skin from fingertip

leukocytosis, anemia, and thrombocytosis with extremely high erythrocyte sedimentation rate (ESR) and C-reactive protein (CRP) are observed and there is no response to anti-infection measures. Echocardiography should be performed by a cardiologist with good experience in imaging young children for recognition of subtle and overt coronary artery inflammation and aneurysms. Coronary artery aneurysms, especially giant aneurysms are associated with a high risk of sudden death or rupture which necessitate early diagnosis and appropriate management.

Treatment with intravenous immunoglobulin (IVIG) 2 g/kg given continuously intravenously has been shown to be effective in reducing the risk of coronary aneurysms significantly but today there is increased awareness of the possibility of early detection of IVIG resistance and therefore intensifying the immediate management with corticosteroids or antitumor necrosis factor (anti-TNF) blockade like infliximab along with IVIG. The acute vasculitic phase needs skilled management by a pediatrician or pediatric rheumatologist and the long-term cardiac monitoring phase is done by a pediatric cardiologist under ideal circumstances.

Immunoglobulin a Vasculitis or Henoch–Schönlein Purpura

This is the most common primary childhood vasculitis in most parts of the world, and nearly 90% of cases occur in children with the vast majority presenting between 6–10 years of age. Crops of purpura appear, usually on the lower limbs quickly progressing to buttocks and elsewhere along with musculoskeletal symptoms such as cutaneous vasculitic peripheral edema and peripheral arthritis which is very painful **(Box 18.4.4)**. Small vessel vasculitis in the bowel wall can present as acute abdominal pain leading to intussusception or bowel gangrene and needs close attention with appropriate imaging and treatment. Other acute presentations with orchitis mimicking torsion, lung hemorrhage, and central nervous system (CNS) vasculitis may occur. The renal involvement on the milder end of spectrum with a transient microscopic proteinuria or hematuria may present silently with progressive proteinuria with a slow and inexorable

BOX 18.4.4: Criteria description of immunoglobulin A (IgA) vasculitis/Henoch–Schönlein purpura (HSP).

Purpura or petechia (mandatory) with lower limb predominance plus one of the following four:
1. Abdominal pain
2. Histopathology (IgA deposit in a biopsy)
3. Arthritis or arthralgia
4. Renal involvement

progression to chronic kidney disease (CKD) and end-stage renal disease if not detected early. The diagnosis is based on clinical features, baseline blood tests which are often normal, a skin biopsy (indicated if skin lesions are atypical) or a renal biopsy in a nephritic syndrome or in persistent proteinuria or hematuria. While around 70% completely resolve in a period of 6 weeks, for 30% of children this is a recurrent disease. Recurrences are often seen as skin rash and perhaps milder versions of musculoskeletal or abdominal features.

Treatment depends on the symptom with no active systemic management required for skin lesion, easy response to NSAIDs for musculoskeletal features and the requirement of systemic corticosteroids (total course of up to 2–4 weeks) for documented bowel vasculitis not responding to pain relief. The treatment of renal disease or other severe systemic involvement will require aggressive management with systemic corticosteroids and steroid-sparing drugs along with supportive management for hypertension and proteinuria. It is recommended that all children who develop IgA vasculitis are encouraged to have at least 6 months of follow-up with regular urinalysis and blood pressure (BP) estimation to pick up silently progressing kidney disease.

Antineutrophilic Cytoplasmic Antibody-associated Vasculitis

These are rare diseases in childhood and only childhood granulomatosis with polyangiitis (CGPA) has its own classification criteria. The other two, eosinophilic granulomatosis with polyangiitis (EGPA) and microscopic polyangiitis (MPA) are even more rare, hence adult criteria are used **(Box 18.4.5)**. The patients usually present with characteristic clinical features as elaborated in the classification criteria, systemic inflammation, and multisystem involvement. Though rare, they can cause much morbidity and mortality and hence must not be missed. Children present with general systemic symptoms of fever, loss of weight, and fatigue as well as symptoms suggestive of the organ involved in the form of chronic nasal ulceration with saddle nose deformity, chronic rhinitis/sinusitis/mastoiditis, and stridor due to upper airway involvement as detailed in the following text. Serological tests for cytoplasmic-ANCA (cANCA) and perinuclear-ANCA (pANCA) as well as their direct antigenic targets, anti-proteinase-3 (anti-PR3) and anti-myeloperoxidase (anti-MPO) are significantly positive in this group of patients and biopsies of the affected sites can also yield the presence of a necrotizing granulomatous vasculitis that is pauci-immune on immunofluorescence.

BOX 18.4.5: Criteria description of granulomatous polyangiitis and childhood Wegener's granulomatosis (GPA/cWG).

At least three of the following six criteria:
1. Histopathology (granulomatous inflammation)
2. Upper airway involvement
3. Laryngo-tracheo-bronchial stenosis
4. Pulmonary involvement
5. ANCA positivity
6. Renal involvement

BOX 18.4.6: Criteria description of Behçet disease.

- *Recurrent oral aphthous:* At least three attacks/year
- *Genital ulceration or aphthous:* Typically with scar
- *Skin involvement:* Necrotic folliculitis, acneiform lesions, and erythema nodosum
- *Ocular involvement:* Anterior uveitis, posterior uveitis, retinal vasculitis
- *Neurological signs:* With the exception of isolated headaches
- *Vascular signs:* Venous thrombosis, arterial thrombosis, and arterial aneurysm.

Three or more items are needed for diagnosis.

Behçet Disease[1,5]

This is a vasculitis that affects all vessels (arteries, veins, venules, arterioles, capillaries) causing inflammation leading to endothelial proliferation, thrombosis and aneurysms. Chronic and recurrent oral and/or genital ulcers with typical involvement of cutaneous, ocular, gastrointestinal, neurological and other systems is seen. Pediatric Behçet classification criteria were created in 2015 and are listed in **Box 18.4.6**.

Rare Vasculitic Disorders

- Cogan's syndrome with multisystem inflammation of eye, inner ears which can occasionally cause a large vessel vasculitis.[5]
- Monogenic vasculitis and vasculitic illnesses that can present due to single gene mutations.[5-7] For example, recurrent deep brain infarcts should prompt investigation for DADA2. Such conditions have targeted therapies which can transform the long-term outlook for the patient.

MANAGEMENT

The management of childhood vasculitis aims to achieve two primary goals, controlling inflammation to prevent end-organ damage and minimizing treatment-related complications.

Treatment strategies vary depending on the specific subtype, disease severity, and organ involvement. In general, pharmacotherapy often involves the use of corticosteroids as first-line agents to induce remission, followed by adjunctive immunosuppressive agents such as methotrexate, azathioprine, mycophenolate mofetil, or biologic agents (e.g., rituximab) for refractory or severe cases.

In addition to pharmacological interventions, supportive care and multidisciplinary management are essential components of the treatment approach. This may include pain management, nutritional support, physical therapy, and psychosocial support to address the holistic needs of pediatric patients with vasculitis.

CONCLUSION

Childhood vasculitis encompasses a heterogeneous group of disorders characterized by inflammation of blood vessels, with diverse clinical presentations and outcomes. Early recognition and prompt initiation of appropriate treatment are crucial for optimizing outcomes and reducing morbidity and mortality associated with childhood vasculitis. It is important that physicians and primary pediatricians are aware of these disorders, consider the possibility when a child presents with suitable findings and appropriate referral to a pediatric rheumatologist. Continued research efforts are needed to better understand the underlying pathogenic mechanisms, refine diagnostic approaches, and develop targeted therapies to improve the management of these complex conditions in pediatric patients.

REFERENCES

1. Sag E, Batu ED, Ozen S. Childhood systemic vasculitis. Best Pract Res Clin Rheumatol. 2017;31(4):558-75.
2. Jennette JC. Overview of the 2012 revised International Chapel Hill Consensus Conference nomenclature of vasculitides. Clin Exp Nephrol. 2013;17(5):603-6.
3. Ozen S, Pistorio A, Iusan SM, Bakkaloglu A, Herlin T, Brik R, et al. EULAR/PRINTO/PRES criteria for Henoch-Schönlein purpura, childhood polyarteritis nodosa, childhood Wegener granulomatosis and childhood Takayasu arteritis: Ankara 2008. Part II: final classification criteria. Ann Rheum Dis. 2010;69(5):798-806.
4. Ozen S, Ruperto N, Dillon MJ, Bagga A, Barron K, Davin JC, et al. EULAR/PReS endorsed consensus criteria for the classification of childhood vasculitides. Ann Rheum Dis. 2006;65(7):936-41.
5. Schnabel A, Hedrich CM. Childhood Vasculitis. Front Pediatr. 2019;6:421.
6. Weiss PF. Pediatric vasculitis. Pediatr Clin North Am. 2012;59(2):407-23.
7. Petty RE, Laxer RM, Lindsley CB, Wedderburn L, Fuhlbrigge RC, Mellins ED. (Eds). Childhood Systemic Vasculitis. In: Textbook of Pediatric Rheumatology, 8th Edition; Elsevier, 2021.

18.5 Other Rheumatic Disorders

Tanya Singla, Narendra Kumar Bagri

INTRODUCTION

The list of immune-mediated rheumatic disorders is widely increasing. This chapter focuses on the rheumatic disorders which have not been covered elsewhere in this section.

JUVENILE DERMATOMYOSITIS

Juvenile dermatomyositis (JDM) is the most common inflammatory myositis in children. The mean age of diagnosis is 7.6 years. It is characterized by proximal muscle weakness and characteristic skin rash. The underlying pathogenesis is systemic vasculopathy which results in inflammation in muscles, skin, and other tissues. In the current era, the Bohan and Peter's diagnostic criteria proposed in 1975 which incorporates electromyography and muscle biopsy for demonstration of myositis is less relevant. The 2017 European Alliance of Associations for Rheumatology EULAR/American College of Rheumatology (ACR) classification criteria is based on web based scoring system (http://www.imm.ki.se/biostatistics/calculators/iim/) accounting for proximal muscle weakness, characteristic skin rash, laboratory evidence of myositis (elevated muscle enzymes), and muscle biopsy features.[1]

In clinical practice JDM is diagnosed in presence of proximal muscle weakness, characteristic skin rash along with elevated muscle enzymes [serum levels of creatine kinase (CK) or lactate dehydrogenase (LDH) or aspartate aminotransferase (AST) or alanine aminotransferase (ALT)]. The characteristic skin rash include:

- *Heliotrope rash:* Violaceous edematous erythema around the eyelids **(Fig. 18.5.1A)**
- *Gottron's papule:* Erythematous or violaceous papules over dorsal aspect of metacarpophalangeal or interphalangeal joints **(Fig. 18.5.1B)**.

In few children (around 5%) these cutaneous features may be present in isolation without muscle weakness which is classified as amyopathic (with normal muscle enzymes) or hypomyopathic (with elevated muscle enzymes) JDM.

In the current era, muscle magnetic resonance imaging (MRI) has replaced muscle biopsy or electromyography (EMG) to demonstrate muscle inflammation. T-2 weighted (T2W) MRI sequence can detect muscle inflammation, while T1W sequence can show muscle atrophy or fatty infiltration.

Nail fold capillaroscopy is an important adjunct for diagnosis and may also help in assessment of disease activity in follow-up. The characteristic finding include structural derangement, enlarged capillaries, tortuosity, and arborization of capillaries **(Fig. 18.5.1C)**.

The use of muscle specific autoantibodies (MSA) such as anti-melanoma differentiation-associated protein 5 (MDA-5), anti-nuclear matrix protein 2 (NXP2), transcriptional intermediary factor 1 (TIF-1), etc., may predict clinical phenotype and prognosis, for e.g., anti-MDA5 positive JDM is associated with interstitial lung disease and poor prognosis.

Treatment: The initial treatment include intravenous methylprednisolone (10–30 mg/kg/day) for 3–5 days followed by oral steroids (1–2 mg/kg/day) which are gradually tapered. The concomitant disease modifying antirheumatic drug (DMARD) of choice is methotrexate (15–25 mg/m^2/week) administered either subcutaneously (preferred route during initial phase of treatment) or orally. For severe/life-threatening or refractory disease, intravenous cyclophosphamide, mycophenolate mofetil (MMF), intravenous immunoglobulin (IVIG), or rituximab may be considered. The usual duration of treatment is 18–24 months.[2]

Complications involve skin ulceration, calcinosis **(Fig. 18.5.1D)**, lipodystrophy, progressive lung disease, gastrointestinal vasculopathy, etc. The overall prognosis is favorable with timely institution of therapy, the mortality in JDM has reduced to around 1%.

JUVENILE SYSTEMIC SCLEROSIS

Juvenile systemic sclerosis (JSScl) is a chronic, multisystem, and connective tissue disease characterized by symmetrical fibrous thickening and hardening of skin with widespread visceral involvement such as lung, heart, and gastrointestinal tract. The mean age of disease onset is 8–11 years. Girls are affected more than boys (3:1). The pathogenic mechanism includes immune activation leading to endothelial vascular damage and excessive extracellular matrix with collagen deposition leading to fibrosis. JSScl is classified as:

- Diffuse cutaneous
- Limited cutaneous disease; fibrosis is restricted proximal to knees and elbows.

Diffuse cutaneous disease is characterized by involvement proximal to elbow and wrists, Raynaud phenomenon, sclerodactyly **(Fig. 18.5.1E)**, skin ulceration **(Fig. 18.5.1F)**, characteristic mask like facies, and pinched nose **(Fig. 18.5.1G)**. The other cutaneous findings include telangiectasia. The nail fold capillary changes consistent with scleroderma include reduced density and giant capillaries. Other systemic features include interstitial lung disease, pulmonary arterial hypertension, dysphagia, bloating, arthritis, and myositis. The 2013 ACR/EULAR classification criteria includes major criteria of skin thickening and at least 2 of 20 minor criteria for diagnosis of SScl.[3] The characteristic autoantibodies include antinuclear antibody (ANA) in high titers and antibody to Scl70 or centromere.

Treatment: The treatment depends on the extent of organ involvement. Methotrexate is used for skin limited disease whereas cyclophosphamide, MMF, or rituximab are used for end organ involvement such as interstitial lung disease (ILD).[4] Nonpharmacological measures; cold protection, gloves and pharmacological management with calcium channel blockers, and phosphodiesterase-5 inhibitors are used for management of Raynaud phenomenon.

JSScl has a variable prognosis and depends on visceral organ involvement. The most common cause of morbidity and mortality in JSScl is cardiopulmonary involvement. Interstitial lung disease is the leading cause and accounts for nearly 30–50% of cases. The 10 year prognosis is better than adult systemic sclerosis. Most common cause of mortality is cardiopulmonary involvement.

LOCALIZED SCLERODERMA

Localized scleroderma (also known as *morphea*) is usually confined to cutaneous manifestation and characterized by skin hardening. It can be subdivided into various subtypes depending on the extent of involvement; circumscribed, linear, generalized, pansclerotic, and mixed morphea. **Fig. 18.5.1H** shows linear morphea involving lower limb and **Fig. 18.5.1I** shows Parry-Romberg syndrome which is a localized scleroderma resulting in localized morphea which causes hemifacial atrophy and may involve nervous system. The localized scleroderma is insidious in onset and leads to disfigurement and disability. Treatment of localized scleroderma includes corticosteroids and methotrexate.

OVERLAP/MIXED CONNECTIVE TISSUE DISEASE

Mixed connective tissue disease (MCTD) is a systemic rheumatic disease characterized by presence of anti-U1 ribonucleoprotein (RNP) antibodies in combination with clinical features of two or more diseases such as systemic lupus erythematosus (SLE), systemic sclerosis (SScl), juvenile idiopathic arthritis or dermatomyositis. Overlap syndrome is presence of features of two rheumatic conditions [SLE, SScl, juvenile idiopathic arthritis (JIA), or JDM] in absence of anti-U1 ribonucleoprotein (RNP). Treatment is individualized and directed at the specific disease manifestation.

SARCOIDOSIS

It is a multisystem granulomatous disease with variable clinical features. Noncaseating epithelioid granulomas in the affected organ are the cardinal feature of sarcoidosis. Fever, weight loss, and general malaise are nonspecific symptoms in children. Older children may present with isolated hilar lymphadenopathy and pulmonary infiltrates. Blau syndrome is an autosomal dominant form of sarcoidosis caused by mutation in *NOD2* gene, presenting during early childhood. The classic triad of Blau syndrome include uveitis, arthritis, and rash **(Figs. 18.5.1J and 18.5.1K)**.

Treatment is based on severity and extent of disease. Corticosteroids are the mainstay of treatment. DMARDs and biological agents in wide spread disease or if the disease is not controlled on steroids alone.[5] Prognosis depends on organ involvement. Disease may be self-limited with complete recovery and may have less favorable outcome in the setting of multiorgan involvement. Anti-tumor necrosis factor (TNF) agents are preferred agents for management of Blau Syndrome.

AUTOINFLAMMATORY SYNDROMES

Autoinflammatory syndrome comprises a wide spectrum of diseases characterized by spontaneous episodes of systemic inflammation involving multiple organ systems and results from an exaggerated innate immune system. These episodes are accompanied by elevated inflammatory markers, viz., erythrocyte sedimentation rate (ESR), C-reactive protein (CRP), and serum amyloid.[6] These disorders result from defects in innate immune system,

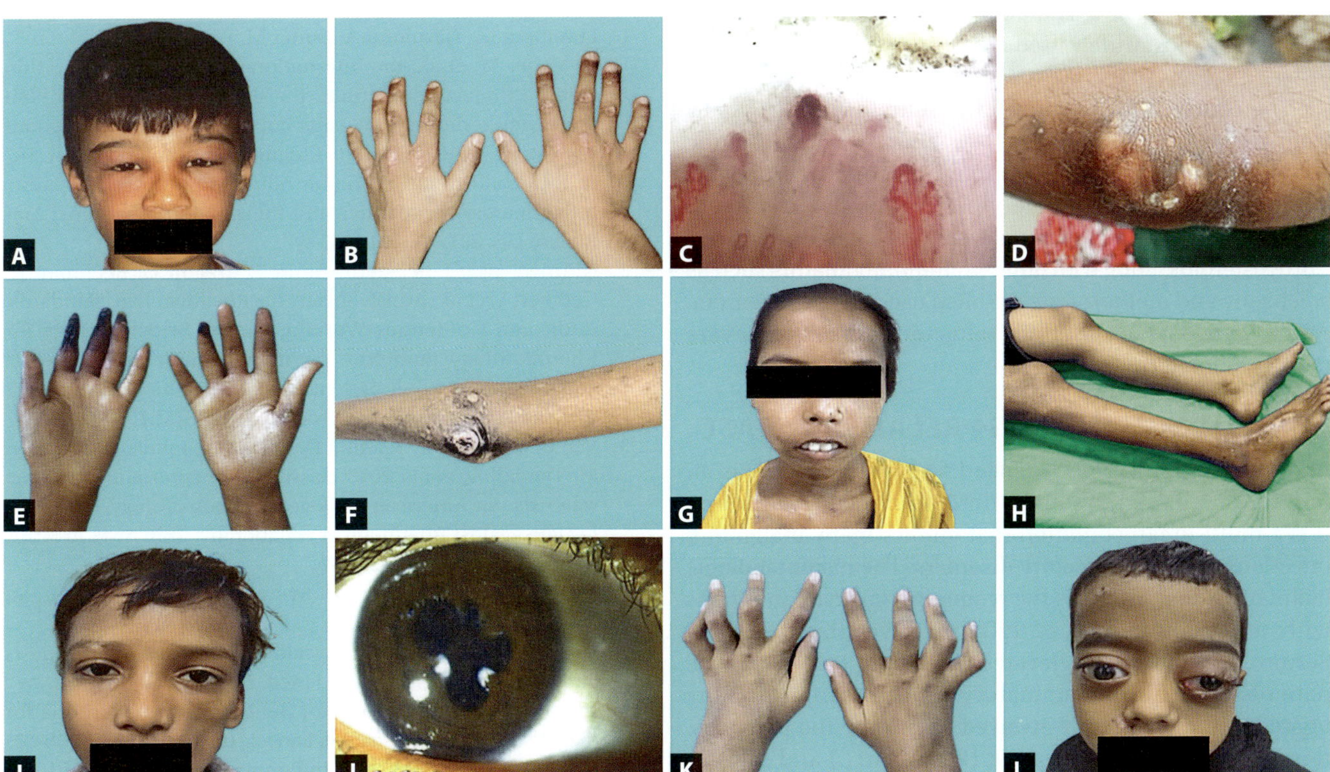

Figs. 18.5.1A to L: Clinical features of various rheumatic disorders. (A) Heliotrope rash; (B) Gottron's papules; (C) Arborization of nail fold capillaries; (D) Calcinosis cutis; (E-G) Sclerodactyly with gangrene, cutaneous ulcerations, and mask like facies in systemic sclerosis; (H) Linear scleroderma involving right leg; (I) Parry–Romberg syndrome; (J-K) Festooned pupil ophthalmic complication due to uveitis and arthritis along with boggy synovial swelling in Blau syndrome; (L) Proptosis due to orbital immunoglobulin G4-related disease (IgG4RLD).

unlike autoimmune disorders which have an underlying aberration in adaptive immune system and accordingly, there are no associated autoantibodies in autoinflammatory syndromes. The common features include episodes of fever, rash, arthritis, myositis, serositis, and uveitis. The monogenic autoinflammatory syndromes result from single gene defect and include disorders such as familial Mediterranean fever (FMF), TNF receptor-1 associated periodic fever syndrome (TRAPS), hyperimmunoglobulin D syndrome (HIDS), or mevalonate kinase deficiency, cryopyrin-associated periodic fever syndrome (CAPS), and deficiency of adenosine deaminase type 2 (DADA2). While the multifactorial disorders include systemic onset juvenile idiopathic arthritis, periodic fever-aphthous stomatitis-pharyngitis and adenitis (PFAPA) syndrome, and Behçet's disease. The treatment of these disorders includes anti-inflammatory drugs, DMARDs such as colchicine and wide spectrum of biological DMARD targeting specific pathway.

BEHÇET'S DISEASE

Behçet's disease is a type of variable vessel vasculitis and is also recognized as an autoinflammatory syndrome. The exact etiopathogenetic is not known, however there is some evidence of HLA-B51 as a genetic risk factor. **Box 18.5.1** outlines the most widely used diagnostic criteria for Behçet's disease.

The course is characterized by multiple relapses. Apart from mucocutaneous lesions, systemic features include ocular lesions, arthritis, gastrointestinal, and neurological manifestations and variable vessel vasculitis. Treatment is tailored according to the severity of clinical features. Corticosteroids along with other immunomodulators such as colchicine and methotrexate are often used for management. Anti-TNF agents are used for refractory disease or severe manifestations.

IMMUNOGLOBULIN G4-RELATED DISEASE

Immunoglobulin G (IgG)4-related disease (IgG4RLD) is an immune-mediated systemic fibroinflammatory disease. It is a multi-organ condition that mimics many malignant, infectious, and inflammatory disorders. The histopathologic hallmark of the disease is the lymphoplasmacytic infiltrates with a predominance of IgG4-positive plasma cells.[8] Serum IgG4 levels are elevated in around 60–70% of the patients. The fibroinflammatory process can affect any organ but the commonly involved organs are the pancreas, retroperitoneum, kidneys, orbit **(Fig. 18.5.1L)** and salivary glands. Treatment includes corticosteroids and other conventional (methotrexate, azathioprine etc.) and biological (rituximab) DMARDs depending on the extent of the disease.

BOX 18.5.1: International Study Group (ISG) criteria for Behçet's disease.[7]

Recurrent oral ulcers (at least 3 times per year) *Plus*
Two out of following major features:
- Genital ulcers
- Positive pathergy test
- Uveitis
- Characteristic skin lesions (necrotic folliculitis, acneiform lesions, and erythema nodosum)

CONCLUSION

This chapter gives a brief overview of various other immune-mediated rheumatic disorders that have distinct clinical presentations, diagnostic challenges, and treatment approaches. The diagnosis of these conditions require a high index of suspicion. Although these disorders can have potentially serious complications, opportune treatment with a combination of corticosteroids and disease-modifying antirheumatic drugs (conventional and biologics), can significantly improve outcomes.

REFERENCES

1. Lundberg IE, Tjärnlund A, Bottai M, Werth VP, Pilkington C, de Visser M, et al.; the International Myositis Classification Criteria Project consortium, the Euromyositis register, and the Juvenile dermatomyositis cohort biomarker study and repository (JDRG) (United Kingdom and Ireland). EULAR/ACR Classification Criteria for Adult and Juvenile Idiopathic Inflammatory Myopathies and their Major Subgroups. Ann Rheum Dis. 2017;76(12):1955-64.
2. Oldroyd AGS, Lilleker JB, Amin T, Aragon O, Bechman K, Cuthbert V, et al.; British Society for Rheumatology Standards, Audit and Guidelines Working Group. British Society for Rheumatology guideline on management of paediatric, adolescent and adult patients with idiopathic inflammatory myopathy. Rheumatology (Oxford). 2022;61(5):1760-8.
3. Van den Hoogen F, Khanna D, Fransen J, Johnson SR, Baron M, Tyndall A, et al.; 2013 classification criteria for systemic sclerosis: an American College of Rheumatology/European League against Rheumatism collaborative initiative. Arthritis Rheum. 2013;65(11):2737-47.
4. Denton CP, Khanna D. Systemic sclerosis. Lancet. 2017;390(10103):1685-99.
5. Drent M, Crouser ED, Grunewald J. Challenges of Sarcoidosis and Its Management. N Engl J Med. 2021;385(11):1018-32.
6. International Study Group for Behçet's Disease. Criteria for diagnosis of Behçet's disease. Lancet. 1990;335(8697):1078-80.
7. Schutt C, Siegel DM. Autoinflammatory Diseases/Periodic Fevers. Pediatr Rev. 2023;44(9):481-90.
8. Kamisawa T, Zen Y, Pillai S, Stone JH. IgG4-related disease. Lancet. 2015;385(9976):1460-71.

18.6 Allergic Disorders

Anu Kiruba Devi Gunasekaran, Dharshini Sathishkumar

INTRODUCTION

The term "allergy" refers to an aberrant state of immune reactivity against certain environmental triggers called *allergens*. These allergens are protein molecules derived from various sources such as plants, insects, mites, animals, food, etc. The allergic symptoms have manifestations of varying severity affecting different organ systems.

The term *"atopy"* refers to an inherent genetic tendency to develop allergy on exposure to allergens. The various allergic disorders include atopic dermatitis, urticaria, angioedema, anaphylaxis, food allergy, allergic rhinitis (AR), allergic conjunctivitis, bronchial asthma, drug allergy, and contact dermatitis. Allergic reactions can be triggered by ingestion, inhalation, contact with the allergen, drug intake, bites, and stings.[1]

Atopic march **(Fig. 18.6.1)** is characterized by age-wise sequential progression of allergic disorders with atopic dermatitis and food allergy in infancy and childhood to allergic asthma and rhinitis in childhood and early adolescence. Atopic dermatitis usually goes into remission in >50% of individuals by adolescence.[2] Most children outgrow food allergies to cow's milk and egg with age; however, nut and seafood allergies persist lifelong.[3]

The global prevalence of allergic disorders ranges from 8 to 10% with varying disease severity. The prevalence of allergic disorders is increasing worldwide, especially in developing countries like India due to industrialization and urbanization.[1]

Detailed evaluation regarding clinical features, family history, and environmental exposures with relevant examination and laboratory investigations help to clinch the diagnosis. Most of these disorders are chronic with remitting and relapsing course, significantly impacting the quality of life, requiring adequate counseling and education regarding preventive and protective measures.

ETIOPATHOGENESIS

Allergic disorders have a complex pathogenesis with multifactorial involvement. The primary mechanism is considered to be sensitization to various environmental allergens. Immunoglobulin E (IgE) antibody plays a critical role in the immunological mechanism of allergy. On initial exposure to the allergen, an immune sensitization occurs through resident dendritic cells, which, on repeat exposure, trigger immediate or delayed immunological hypersensitivity reaction through memory T cells affecting different organ systems.[1]

The host risk factors involved are genetic predisposition, variation in filaggrin gene (*FLG*), age, sex, stress, cutaneous and gut microbiome as well as bacterial and viral infections. The environmental risk factors include climate, smoking, pollution, indoor and outdoor dust or pollen exposure, pets, and irritant exposure.[4]

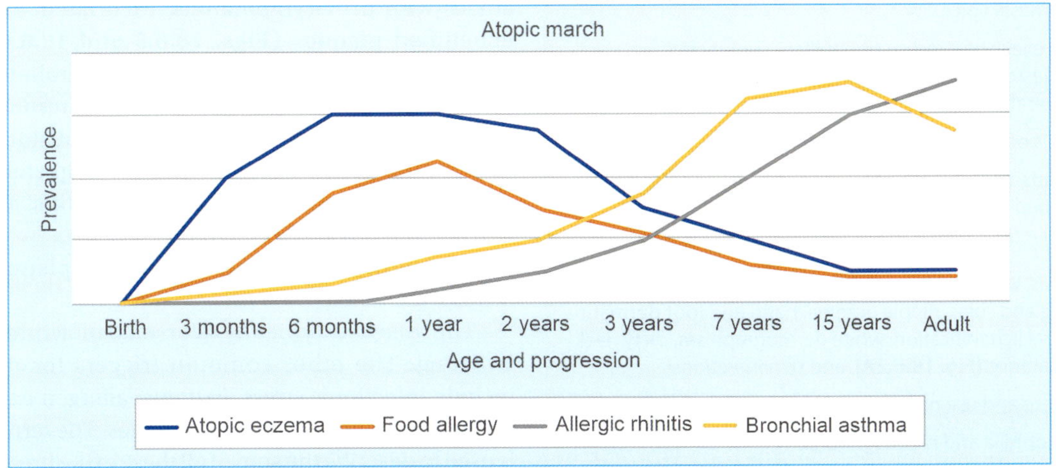

Fig. 18.6.1: Progression of atopic march.

MARKERS OF ATOPY

The various clinical symptoms and signs of atopy are listed in **Table 18.6.1** and depicted in **Figures 18.6.2 and 18.6.3**.

ATOPIC DERMATITIS

Atopic dermatitis (AD) is a chronic eczematous dermatitis with a remitting and relapsing course predominantly affecting children and is characterized by an itchy rash.

Epidemiology

Atopic dermatitis is the initial starting point of atopic march with a global prevalence of 17–24% among children and a peak prevalence at 2 years of age.[2] Indian studies have reported a prevalence between 3.1 and 7.21% among children.[5]

Etiopathogenesis

Atopic dermatitis has a complex pathogenesis with the interaction of skin barrier defect, genetic predisposition, altered cutaneous microbiome, and immune dysfunction involving both adaptive and innate immunity (Th2 cell-skewed immune dysregulation) leading to inflammation. The loss-of-function mutation in *FLG* coding for the protein filaggrin appears to be the key factor responsible for barrier dysfunction. Variations in *FLG* are associated with other atopic stigmata such as ichthyosis vulgaris, palmar hyperlinearity and keratosis pilaris **(Figs. 18.6.3A to C)**. Whether AD is primarily driven by immune abnormalities (inside-out theory) or epidermal barrier dysfunction (outside-in theory) is highly controversial. Skin microbiome alteration with reduced microbial diversity, increased staphylococcal peptides and their superantigens are implicated in driving the inflammation. The combination of all the above leads to varied AD phenotypes and endotypes.

TABLE 18.6.1: Atopic stigmata.

Face	Dennie–Morgan infraorbital folds **(Fig. 18.6.2B)**, allergic shiners **(Fig. 18.6.2A)**, allergic salute, allergic mannerisms, long face, facial erythema, perioral pallor, pityriasis alba **(Fig. 18.6.2C)**, Hertoghe sign (lateral madarosis) **(Fig. 18.6.2A)**
Nose	Pale mucosa, hypertrophied inferior turbinates, and hypernasal voice
Eyes	Long eyelashes, recurrent papillary conjunctivitis, cobblestone conjunctiva, anterior subcapsular cataract, and keratoconus
Ears	Serous otitis media (glue ear)
Mouth	Cheilitis, cobblestone pharynx, allergic cluck, and dry-chapped lips
Neck	Lymphadenopathy and anterior neck folds
Skin	Xerosis, keratosis pilaris, ichthyosis vulgaris, hyperlinear palms and soles, nipple eczema, hand and foot dermatitis, flexural lichenification, white dermographism, dirty neck appearance **(Fig. 18.6.2A)**, and skin infections
Chest	Wheeze and use of accessory muscle of respiration
Blood	Eosinophilia and raised IgE levels

(IgE: immunoglobulin E)

Clinical Features

The disease has three distinct stages of presentation—acute, subacute, and chronic with distinct morphology depending on the age of presentation: Infantile, childhood, and adolescence/adult onset **(Flowchart 18.6.1)**.[6]

- Acute AD—crusted, oozy, edematous, and erythematous papules and plaques
- Subacute AD—erythematous and scaly papules and plaques with or without crusting
- Chronic AD—lichenified and excoriated papules and plaques

The disease often presents in infancy in 60% of cases.[4] There is a slight female to male preponderance.

Infantile AD starts around 3–6 months of age with eczema affecting cheeks, scalp, trunk, and extensor aspect of elbows and knees **(Figs. 18.6.4A and B)**. It is often associated with xerosis, palmar hyperlinearity, ichthyosis vulgaris, and other atopic markers. In nearly 40% of cases, the disease goes into remission by 3 years of age while others may have intermittent disease with seasonal variation and progression to childhood and adolescent disease. Those with early onset of AD, family history of atopy and severe AD have a poorer prognosis.[6] Infantile seborrheic dermatitis can overlap with infantile AD presenting with cradle cap and intertriginous maceration. Scalp scaling is also a common feature in Indian population.

Childhood AD affects the face and flexures of the body such as neck, antecubital fossa, wrists, popliteal fossa, and ankles with dry erythematous, excoriated, and scaly and lichenified plaques **(Figs. 18.6.5 and 18.6.6)**. However, involvement of flexures like axillae and groin is uncommon in AD, hence we should prompt an alternate diagnosis. Pruritus is a striking feature with sleep disturbances.[6] The other morphological phenotypes of AD in children include eyelid dermatitis, head and neck dermatitis, and hand and foot eczema **(Figs. 18.6.7A to C)**.

In adulthood, chronic lichenified plaques involving flexures are noted.[6]

The disease typically worsens in winters and with sweating. The other common triggers for disease flares include infections, stress, irritants, allergen exposure (dust, pollen, etc.), and certain food allergies. The term "exposome" is used to describe the sum of all these exposures an individual is subjected to in his/her lifetime.[6]

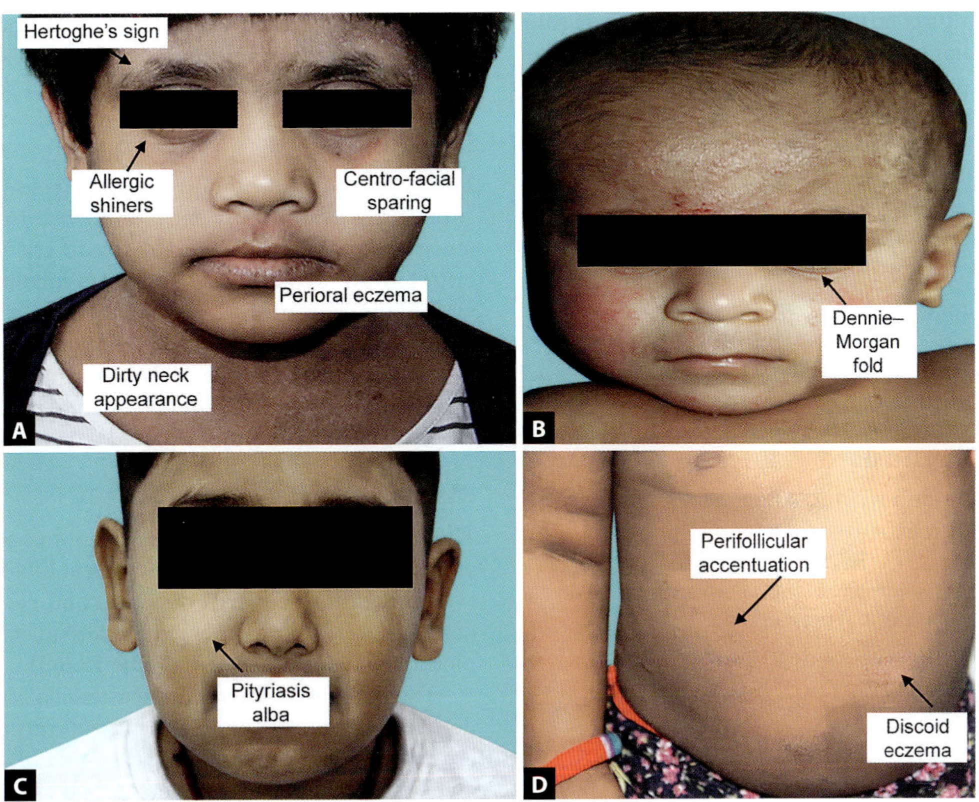

Figs. 18.6.2A to D: Markers of atopy. (A) Allergic shiners—periorbital hyperpigmentation, atopic dirty neck appearance, Hertoghe sign—lateral madarosis, cheilitis with perioral eczema; (B) Dennie–Morgan infraorbital folds; (C) Pityriasis alba—ill-defined hypopigmented macules involving bilateral cheeks; and (D) Follicular prominences in the trunk with discoid eczema.

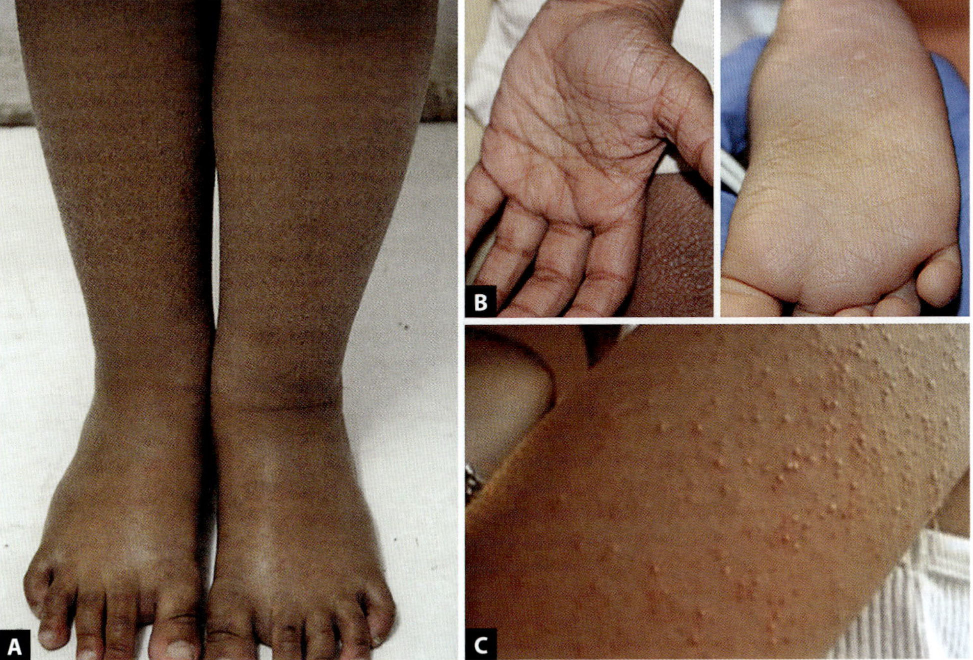

Figs. 18.6.3A to C: Markers of variants in Filaggrin gene associated with atopy. (A) Ichthyosis vulgaris (dry fish-like scaling of skin) involving bilateral extensor aspect of legs; (B) Hyperlinear palms and soles; and (C) Keratosis pilaris (rough spiny follicular papules) involving arms.

Atopic dermatitis is further classified into intrinsic (non-IgE-mediated inflammation) and extrinsic (IgE-mediated inflammation) types. Those with extrinsic AD have a higher propensity to develop asthma and AR.[6]

Complications

- Growth failure and malnutrition
- Recurrent skin infections (*Staphylococcus aureus* and *Herpes simplex* virus)
- Sleep disturbances
- Depression, anxiety, attention-deficit hyperactive disorder, and learning disability
- Other allergic disorders

Differential Diagnosis

- *Infantile AD*—seborrheic dermatitis, insect bite hypersensitivity reaction, scabies, and impetigo

Flowchart 18.6.1: Classification of atopic dermatitis based on age of onset and presentation.

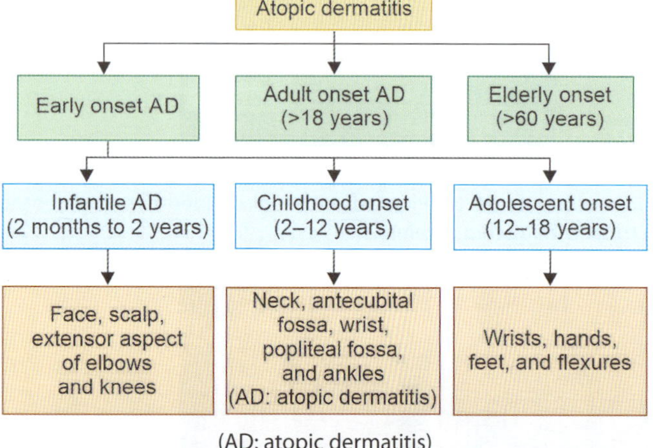

(AD: atopic dermatitis)

- *Childhood AD*—allergic contact dermatitis (ACD), psoriasis, seborrheic dermatitis, nutritional dermatitis, and metabolic disorders.

Diagnosis

The diagnosis is solely made based on clinical features with supporting evidence of peripheral eosinophilia, raised IgE levels, and raised inflammatory markers. Many diagnostic criteria have evolved over the years for diagnosis of AD of which the commonly employed ones are described in **Table 18.6.2**. In children with severe, persistent and recalcitrant AD with failure to thrive and recurrent infections, primary immunodeficiency disorders (e.g. hyper IgE syndrome and Wiskott-Aldrich syndrome) should be ruled out.

Management[6-8]

The treatment aims to restore the epithelial barrier, prevent exposure to irritants or allergens, treat infection, and reduce inflammation. It consists of parent and patient's education, disease severity assessment, general skin care measures, and pharmacological measures **(Table 18.6.3)**.

The quantity of topical corticosteroids (TCS) to be applied depends upon the age of the patient and the body surface area involved. In general, the "finger-tip unit (FTU)" is used to guide the safe use of topical steroids and 1 FTU is defined as the quantity of TCS delivered from a tube with a 5-mm nozzle from the distal crease to the tip on the pulp side of an adult's forefinger and is approximately equivalent to 0.5 g. This can cover two palm areas of an adult (equal to 2% of body surface area).

URTICARIA, ANGIOEDEMA, AND ANAPHYLAXIS

Urticaria is characterized by the development of wheals (hives), angioedema, or both.[9] Anaphylaxis is a serious

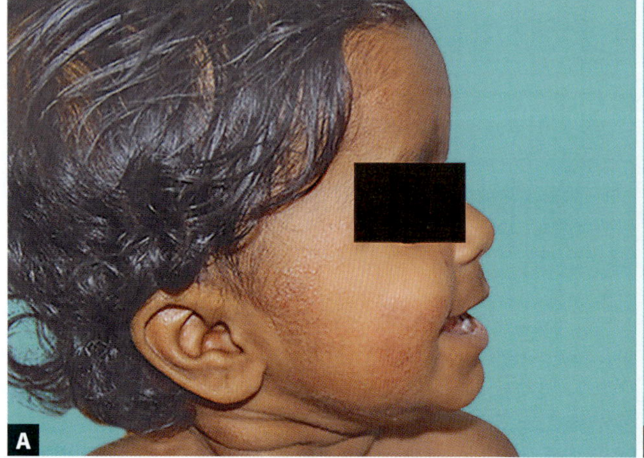
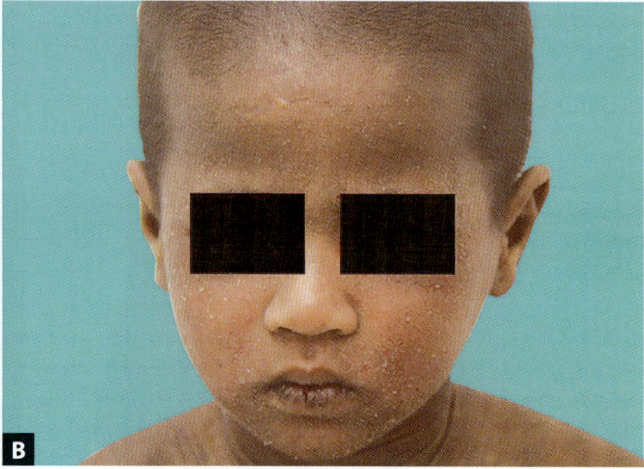

Figs. 18.6.4A and B: (A) Infantile atopic dermatitis with eczematous papules involving cheek; (B) Diffuse facial involvement with erythema and scaling, cheilitis, and sparing of the tip of nose in infantile atopic dermatitis.

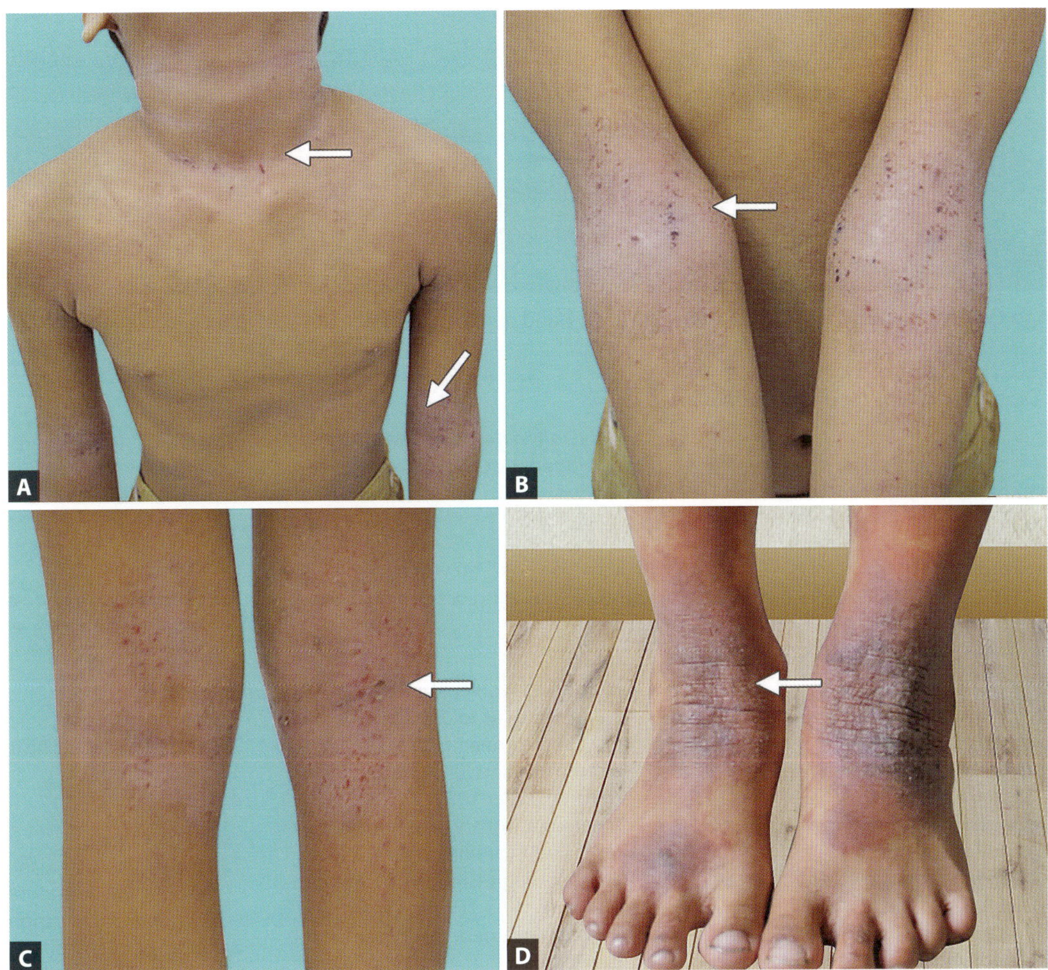

Figs. 18.6.5A to D: Childhood atopic dermatitis with flexural involvement. (A to C) Excoriated and scaly erythematous plaques involving neck, bilateral antecubital fossa, and popliteal fossa; and (D) Lichenified eczematous plaques involving both ankles.

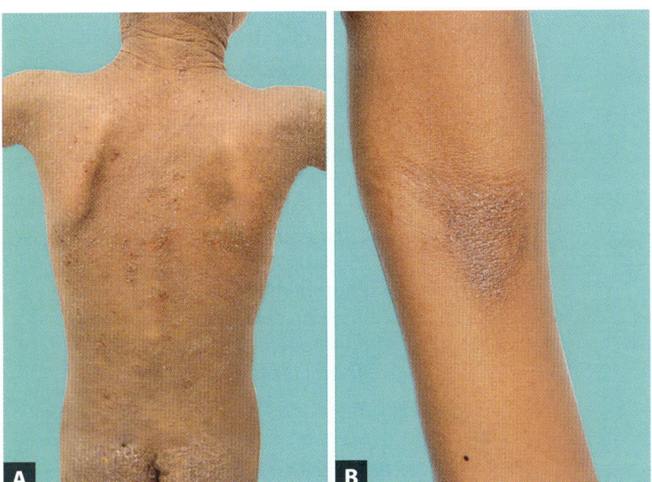

Figs. 18.6.6A and B: (A) Severe childhood atopic dermatitis with diffuse dermatitis involving trunk and flexures; (B) Lichenification of antecubital fossa in chronic stage of atopic eczema.

life-threatening hypersensitivity reaction affecting skin, respiratory, gastrointestinal, and cardiovascular system occurring within minutes to few hours following exposure to potentials triggers.[10]

Epidemiology

Acute urticaria affects 10–20% of pediatric population and chronic urticaria affects 0.1–0.3% of children.[11] Incidence of anaphylaxis in children based on various studies ranges from 1 and 761 per 100,000 person years.[10]

Etiopathogenesis

It is characterized by type 1 hypersensitivity reaction and the clinical features occur due to chemical mediators released following mast cell degranulation. Acute urticaria in children is commonly triggered by infections (respiratory tract, urinary tract, or gastrointestinal infections). The other triggers include food, drugs, bites, and stings. Food triggers

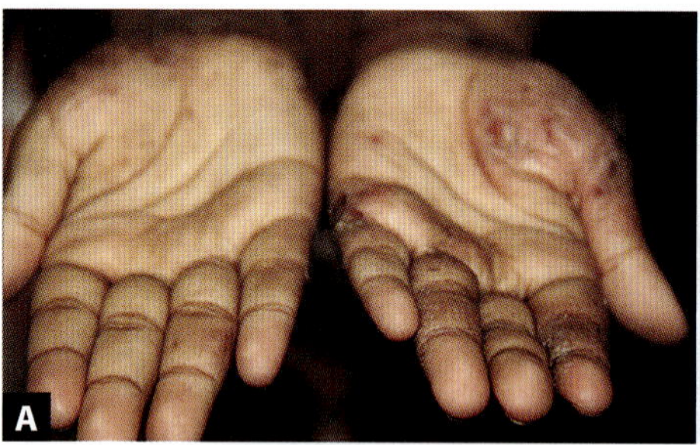

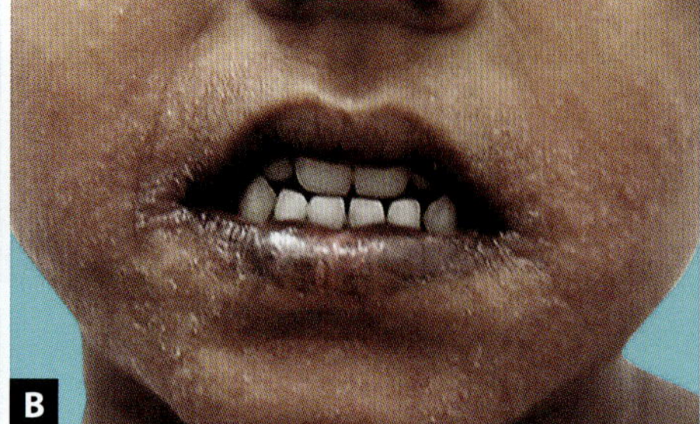

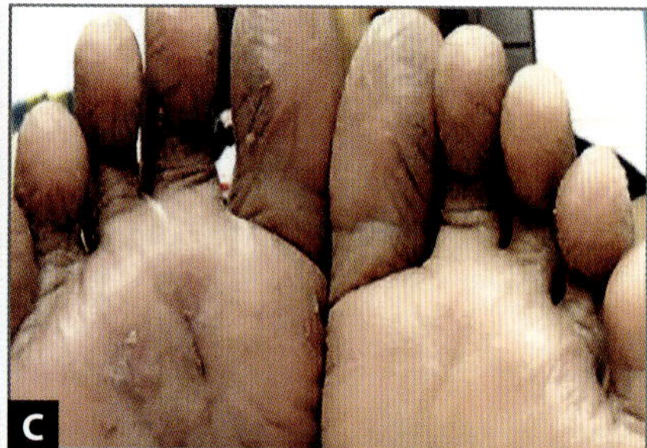

Figs. 18.6.7A to C: Other phenotypes of atopic dermatitis. (A) Hand dermatitis; (B) Cheilitis with perioral eczema; and (C) Foot eczema.

TABLE 18.6.2: Diagnostic criteria for Atopic dermatitis

Name	***Hanifin and Rajka criteria***	***The UK (United Kingdom) Working Party Diagnostic Criteria for Atopic dermatitis***	***AAD (American Academy of Dermatology) consensus criteria for Atopic dermatitis***
Year	*1980*	*1994*	*2003*
Major/ essential features	1. Pruritus 2. Typical morphology and distribution 3. Chronic relapsing dermatitis 4. Personal or family history of atopy	An itchy skin condition (or parental report of scratching or rubbing in a child)	1. Pruritus 2. Eczema—chronic or relapsing, typical morphology and age-specific patterns
Minor/ supporting features	1. Xerosis 2. Ichthyosis/palmar hyperlinearity/ keratosis pilaris 3. Immediate (type 1) skin test reactivity 4. Raised serum IgE 5. Early age of onset 6. Tendency toward cutaneous infections (*S. aureus* and Herpes simplex virus)/impaired, cell-mediated immunity 7. Hand or foot dermatitis 8. Nipple eczema 9. Cheilitis 10. Recurrent conjunctivitis 11. Dennie-Morgan fold 12. Keratoconus 13. Anterior subcapsular cataract 14. Orbital darkening 15. Facial pallor/facial erythema 16. Pityriasis alba 17. Anterior neck fold 18. Itch provoked by sweat 19. Intolerance to wool and lipid solvents 20. Perifollicular accentuation 21. Food intolerance 22. Course influence by environmental/ emotional factors 23. White dermographism/delayed blanch response	1. History of involvement of the skin creases such as folds of elbows, behind the knees, fronts of ankles or around the neck (including cheeks in children under 10). 2. A personal history of asthma or hay fever (or history of atopic disease in a first- degree relative in children under 4). 3. A history of a general dry skin in the last year. 4. Visible flexural eczema (or eczema involving the cheeks/forehead and outer limbs in children under 4). 5. Onset under the age of 2 (not used if child is under 4).	*Important features:* 1. Early age of onset 2. Personal or family history of atopy 3. Ig E reactivity 4. Xerosis *Associated features:* 1. Atypical vascular response (facial pallor/white dermographism/ delayed blanch response) 2. Keratosis pilaris/pityriasis alba/ hyperlinear palms/ichthyosis 3. Ocular/periorbital changes 4. Others: Perioral changes/ periauricular lesions 5. Perifollicular accentuation/ lichenification/prurigo lesions *Conditions to exclude:* • Scabies • Seborrhoeic dermatitis • Contact dermatitis (irritant and allergic) • Ichthyosis • Cutaneous T-cell lymphoma • Psoriasis • Photodermatoses • Immune deficiency syndromes • Erythroderma caused by skin disorders other than AD
Diagnostic points	3 major criteria + ≥3 minor criteria	Essential feature + ≥3 minor criteria	Both the essential features must be present + important features which may support the diagnosis

(IgE - immunoglobulin E; AD – atopic dermatitis)

TABLE 18.6.3: Management of atopic dermatitis.

Investigations:
- Complete blood count
- Absolute eosinophil count
- Serum immunoglobulin E—elevated levels seen in 80% of cases of AD
- Skin biopsy (if indicated to rule out non-eczematous disorders)
- Skin prick test/specific IgE testing—not routinely indicated. Considered in severe/refractory disease with reliable history of worsening with certain food or aeroallergens exposure
- Patch test (if allergic contact dermatitis is suspected)
- Skin swabs from involved areas for pus culture to treat accordingly
- Nasal swab to look for Staphylococcus aureus colonization if there is history of recurrent infections

Disease severity assessment tools:
- SCORing Atopic Dermatitis (SCORAD) index
- Eczema Area Severity Index (EASI)
- Physician global assessment (PGA)
- Children's Dermatology Life Quality Index (CDLQI)
- Visual Analog Scale (VAS) for pruritus and for sleep disturbance

General measures:
- Patient and parent education
- Avoidance of disease-provoking factors and exposure to dust, detergents, fragrances
- Take short showers in lukewarm water using fragrance-free hypoallergenic soap
- Frequent, liberal and regular application of emollients or fragrance-free moisturizers to hydrate the skin, irrespective of disease severity. It is to be applied at least two times per day and preferably immediately after bathing.
- Avoid exposure to extremes of temperature (hot or cold)
- Prefer loose cotton clothing. Avoid woolen, fur and synthetic clothes
- Antiseptic compresses/baths for oozy skin lesions
- Antihistamines, for pruritus (preferably sedative antihistamines)
- Infection if any, to be treated with antibiotics

Pharmacological measures

Mild disease	***Moderate disease***	***Severe disease***
• *Acute treatment:* – Low-to-moderate potency topical corticosteroids for affected areas once or twice daily till 3–5 days after clearance or upto a maximum of 2 weeks* – Topical calcineurin inhibitors (Pimecrolimus or Tacrolimus)$ – Topical Crisaborole 2% ointment (Phosphodiesterase 4 inhibitor, approved for age ≥3 months) • *Maintenance treatment:* – Emollients or moisturizers – Proactive therapy**	• *Acute treatment:* – Medium-to-high potency topical corticosteroids twice daily for up to 1–2 weeks • *Maintenance treatment:* – Emollients or moisturizers – Topical calcineurin inhibitors (Pimecrolimus or Tacrolimus)$ or – Topical Crisaborole – Proactive therapy** – Diluted bleach baths twice weekly#	• *Acute treatment:* – Medium-to-high potency topical corticosteroids twice daily for up to 1–2 weeks • *Maintenance treatment:* – Emollients or moisturizers – Topical calcineurin inhibitors (Pimecrolimus or Tacrolimus) or – Topical Crisaborole – Proactive therapy** – Diluted bleach baths twice weekly – Phototherapy – Consider wet wrap therapy – Systemic immunomodulators (azathioprine, methotrexate, cyclosporine – not to be combined with phototherapy) – Dupilumab injection (Anti-IL-4 antibody approved for children aged ≥6 months)

Contd...

Contd...

- *Other newer agents recently approved for AD:*
  - Topical Roflumilast 0.15%—phosphodiesterase 4 inhibitor for children aged ≥6 years with mild-to-moderate AD
  - Topical Ruxolitinib 1.5%—JAK inhibitor for children aged ≥12 years with mild-to-moderate AD
  - Topical Tapinarof—aryl hydrocarbon receptor agonist for children aged ≥2 years
  - *Oral JAK inhibitors for moderate-to-severe AD:*
    - Abrocitinib (JAK1 inhibitor)—for children aged ≥12 years
    - Upadacitinib (JAK1 inhibitor)—for children aged ≥12 years
  - *Other biologics for moderate-to-severe AD:* Tralokinumab (anti-IL-13 antibody for children aged ≥12 years) and Lebrikizumab (anti-IL-13 antibody for children aged ≥12 years)

*The potency of topical corticosteroid should be decided based on patient's age, site involved, and degree of inflammation. For face, genitalia and flexures, low-potent topical corticosteroids have to be used (*Example:* Desonide 0.05%, Hydrocortisone 2.5%). Prolonged use of topical corticosteroids and unsupervised use of high-to-very high potent corticosteroids in children should be avoided due to the risk of cutaneous and systemic adverse effects. Ointment formulations tend to be more potent than creams and lotions.

$Topical calcineurin inhibitors are used as alternatives to topical corticosteroid for mild-to-moderate AD involving face and flexures—Tacrolimus 0.03% ointment and Pimecrolimus 1% cream are approved for children aged ≥2 years and have to be applied twice daily over affected areas. Tacrolimus 0.1% ointment is approved for use in individual aged 16 years and above.

#Bleach baths are recommended in children with moderate-to-severe atopic dermatitis with recurrent skin infections. It exerts benefits by reducing the burden of *S. aureus* colonizing the skin. It is prepared by adding 120 mL of 6% household bleach in 150 L of water. The affected areas from the neck below is soaked for 10–15 minutes in the prepared solution and rinsed off with water.

**Proactive therapy is the use of long-term, intermittent use (such as weekend treatment) of low-dose, anti-inflammatory therapy (e.g., topical steroids/topical calcineurin inhibitors) in previously affected areas prone for frequent relapses, after obtaining remission with intense use of the anti-inflammatory agents.

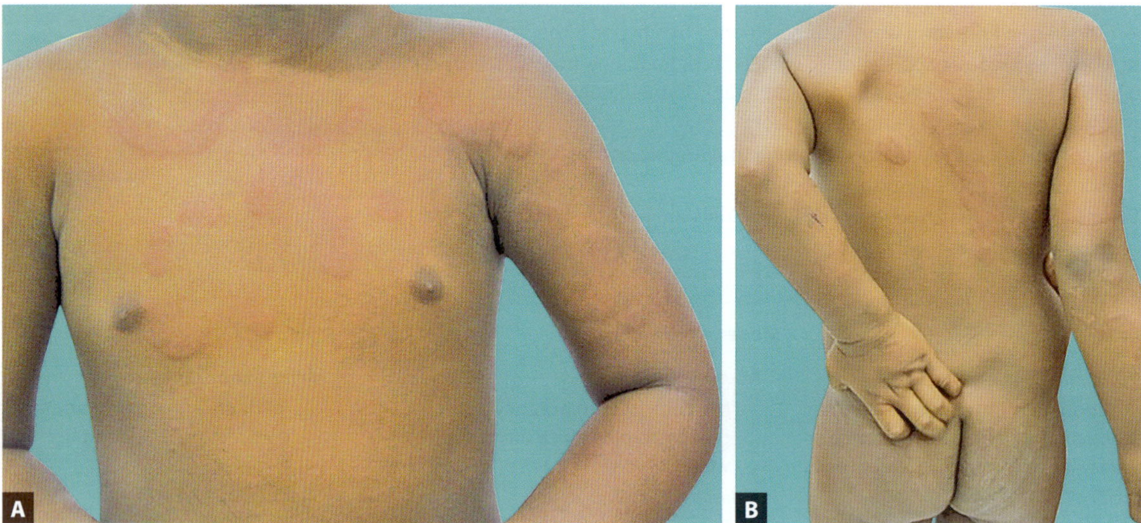

Figs. 18.6.8A and B: Multiple wheals involving the trunk in a child with acute urticaria.

commonly implicated are nuts, egg, and seafood. Drugs commonly associated with acute urticaria are nonsteroidal anti-inflammatory drugs (NSAIDs) and β-lactam antibiotics. Chronic urticaria can have associated autoimmune thyroid and rheumatological disorders.[9]

Worldwide, the most common cause of anaphylaxis in children is food (nuts, milk, and hen's egg) followed by insect venom and drugs.[10]

Clinical Features

Urticaria can be classified into:

- *Acute urticaria:* Occurrence of wheals, angioedema, or both for <6 weeks
- *Chronic urticaria:* Occurrence of wheals, angioedema, or both for >6 weeks. It is further subdivided into *chronic spontaneous urticaria* and *chronic inducible urticaria* (e.g., dermographism, cold urticaria, delayed pressure urticaria, etc.).

Wheal is characterized by transient, itchy, blanchable, erythematous, edematous, papules, and plaques which occur due to dermal edema **(Figs. 18.6.8A and B)**. Angioedema involves edema of deep dermis and subcutaneous tissue and affects lips, eyelids, hands, feet, and mucosal surfaces. In children with recurrent angioedema without wheals, hereditary angioneurotic edema should be ruled out.[9]

Anaphylaxis is characterized by stridor, bronchospasm, hypotension, abdominal pain, wheals, flushing, and angioedema.[10]

Differential Diagnosis

Urticaria mimics: Urticarial vasculitis, autoinflammatory syndromes, serum sickness, such as reactions, cutaneous mastocytosis, connective tissue disorders like SLE.

Angioedema mimics: Granulomatous cheilitis, and ACD.

Diagnosis

The diagnosis is made solely based on clinical presentation. For those with atypical features (joint pain, abdominal pain, nonitchy wheals, Raynaud's phenomenon, family history of similar illness, etc.) urticaria and angioedema mimics should be considered and relevant investigations to be carried out.

Management

For nonanaphylactic episodes, second-generation antihistamines form the cornerstone of management. For severe acute urticaria, short-course systemic steroids can be given for 3–5 days after ruling out infections. However, the use of long-term systemic steroids is strongly discouraged due to varied side effects including stunting of growth. Infections, if any, should be identified and treated.

Chronic urticaria requires long-term administration of antihistamines. For those with suboptimal control, cyclosporine is a second-line drug. Omalizumab is approved for the treatment of chronic urticaria as a second line agent in children aged 12 years and above.[9]

Children with anaphylaxis need intensive care with stabilization of vitals and airway management. They need to be administered the injection adrenaline immediately, (0.01 mg/kg of 1:1000, subcutaneous or intramuscular injection) along with antihistamines and short-acting systemic steroids.[10]

The dose of common antihistamines used in children is enlisted in **Table 18.6.4**.

TABLE 18.6.4: Antihistamines used in children.

Drug	*Dose and frequency*
Hydroxyzine	• *≤40 kg:* Oral 2 mg/kg/day divided every 6–8 hours, maximum 25 mg/dose • *>40 kg:* Oral 25–50 mg once daily at bedtime or twice daily
Chlorpheniramine maleate	• *2 to <6 years:* 1 mg every 4–6 hourly, maximum of 6 mg/day • *6 to <12 years:* 2 mg every 4–6 hourly, maximum of 12 mg/day • *≥12 years:* 4 mg every 4–6 hourly, maximum of 24 mg/day
Diphenhydramine	1–2 mg/kg/dose every 6 hours, maximum of 50 mg/dose and 300 mg/day
Cetirizine	• *2–5 years:* 2.5 mg once daily, can be increased to up to a maximum of 2.5 mg twice daily or 5 mg once daily • *≥6 years and adolescents:* 5–10 mg daily
Levocetirizine	• *Infants ≥6 months and children ≤5 years:* 1.25 mg once daily • *6–11 years:* 2.5 mg once daily • *≥12 years:* 5 mg once daily
Loratadine	• *2–11 years:* up to 31 kg 5 mg daily; >31 kg 10 mg daily • *12–17 years:* 10 mg daily
Desloratadine	• *1–5 years:* 1.25 mg daily • *6–11 years:* 2.5 mg daily • *12–17 years:* 5 mg daily
Fexofenadine	• *Infants ≥6 months and children <2 years:* Oral suspension 15 mg twice daily • *≥2 to <12 years:* Oral suspension 30 mg twice daily • *≥12 years:* Oral suspension 60 mg twice daily or once daily formulation 120–180 mg once daily
Bilastine	• *6 to <12 years:* 10 mg once daily • *≥12 years:* 20 mg once daily

FOOD ALLERGY

Food allergy is a hypersensitivity reaction that occurs following exposure to specific sensitized food items. It has an estimated global prevalence of 6–8%, but the data on prevalence in Indian children is lacking.[3] Food allergy is six times more prevalent among children with atopic dermatitis, especially those with moderate-to-severe disease and recalcitrant dermatitis.

Etiopathogenesis

Epicutaneous sensitization through impaired skin barrier has been proposed to be the underlying mechanism for food allergy in the recent past rather than gut sensitization.[2] The reactions can be IgE-mediated, non-IgE mediated, or a combination of both. "Major allergens" most commonly responsible for significant reactions include milk, egg, peanut, tree nuts, fish, wheat, and soya. In India, chickpea is a common allergen as it is consumed in various forms.[3]

Early introduction of potentially allergenic food (cow's milk, egg, and peanuts) in infancy between 6 months and 1 year may prevent the development of food allergies later according to recent studies and is being explored further.[3]

Clinical Features

Table 18.6.5 lists the common clinical manifestations of food allergy based on IgE-mediated or not.

TABLE 18.6.5: Clinical manifestations of food allergy.

IgE-mediated food allergy	*Mixed (IgE/non-IgE mediated)*	*Non-IgE-mediated*
• Acute urticaria/ angioedema • Pruritus • Anaphylaxis • Food-induced asthma • Pollen-food allergy syndrome	• Pruritus • Atopic dermatitis • Allergic eosinophilic esophagitis/ gastroenteritis	• Celiac disease • Protein-induced enterocolitis syndrome

Diagnosis

Diagnosis of food allergy is complex. It requires a detailed and focused history to identify the possible allergens. Although there can be flare of atopic dermatitis with certain food items and children with AD have specific IgE to many common food allergens, the evidence is inconclusive because most children tend to tolerate the food on oral challenge without any reaction.

The European Association of Allergy and Immunology (EAACI) Task Force recommends that allergy evaluation should be considered only in children ≤6 years of age with moderate-to-severe or persistent AD despite optimal treatment or if there is a reliable history of an immediate skin rash after ingestion of specific food or both.[12]

The double-blind placebo-controlled food challenge remains the gold standard to confirm food allergy, but it is not frequently performed due to its inherent risks, inconvenience, and cost. Skin prick testing, allergen-specific IgE testing, and component resolved diagnostics are the common methods employed to detect IgE-mediated food allergies. However, only 30–40% of children with positive IgE to specific food develop a reaction on oral challenge. Hence, blanket avoidance of food items showing positive IgE should not be done before clinical relevance is established.[13]

For those children with negative skin prick tests and allergen-specific IgE tests, elimination of suspected food from diet for 2 weeks is advised to look for clinical improvement. Atopic patch test is used to identify non-IgE-mediated food allergies. Other evaluations including upper and lower GI endoscopy are warranted for children with gastrointestinal symptoms.[3]

Management

Nearly 50% of children tend to outgrow food allergy to cow's milk, egg, wheat, and soya. However, nut and seafood allergy tend to persist lifelong.

There is no cure for food allergy. Elimination diet is recommended for clinically proven food allergy by oral challenge and for those with a history of severe reactions. Education of the family members regarding food avoidance, careful food labeling, emergency medications, and early identification of reactions is essential.

Desensitization using oral immunotherapy of allergenic food is not recommended.[3]

DRUG ALLERGY

Adverse drug reaction (ADR) is defined by the World Health Organization as "a response to a drug which is noxious, and unintended, which occurs at doses normally used in man for prophylaxis, diagnosis or therapy of disease, or for the modification of physiological function."[14] Drug hypersensitivity reactions (DHR) are uncommon in children. Labeling a child to have drug allergy without proper evaluation can lead to higher medical costs, limited treatment options, and higher incidence of antibiotic resistance. Hence, detailed history regarding all the drugs taken, previous history of similar reaction, severity of clinical symptoms, timeline of various drugs introduced, and temporal correlation along with relevant laboratory testing is mandatory.

Classification

Adverse drug reaction can be classified depending on predictability, pathogenesis, and morphological presentation as depicted in **Flowcharts 18.6.2 and 18.6.3.**[15]

The common drugs causing DHRs in children are antibiotics, NSAIDs, antiepileptic drugs, and vaccines.[14] It has to be remembered that any drug (allopathic/alternative medicines), food additives, and preservatives can cause a drug reaction, and the clinical suspicion of a drug reaction has to be considered in appropriate clinical scenarios. A good drug history, a well-drawn drug timeline and early withdrawal of all suspected drugs is of utmost importance. Cutaneous hypersensitivity with maculopapular rash is the most common presentation in children followed by urticaria, angioedema, and fixed drug eruption (FDE).[14] Severe cutaneous adverse reactions (SCARs) such as DRESS (Drug related eosinophilia with systemic symptoms), SJS/TEN (Steven-Johnson syndrome,/toxic epidermal necrolysis), AGEP (Acute generalized exanthematous pustulosis), and anaphylaxis though rare need to be identified at the earliest. The second most common system involved is the gastrointestinal system presenting as nausea, vomiting, diarrhea, or constipation.

For children with suspected drug allergy, allergy workup can be performed 4–6 weeks after resolution of clinical symptoms.[14] The recommended investigations for IgE-mediated immediate hypersensitivity reactions include skin prick test (SPT), intradermal test (IDT), and basophil activation test (in vitro). SPT and IDT are in vivo tests and carry risk of histamine release during the procedure. They have to

Flowchart 18.6.2: Classification of adverse drug reaction.[14,15]

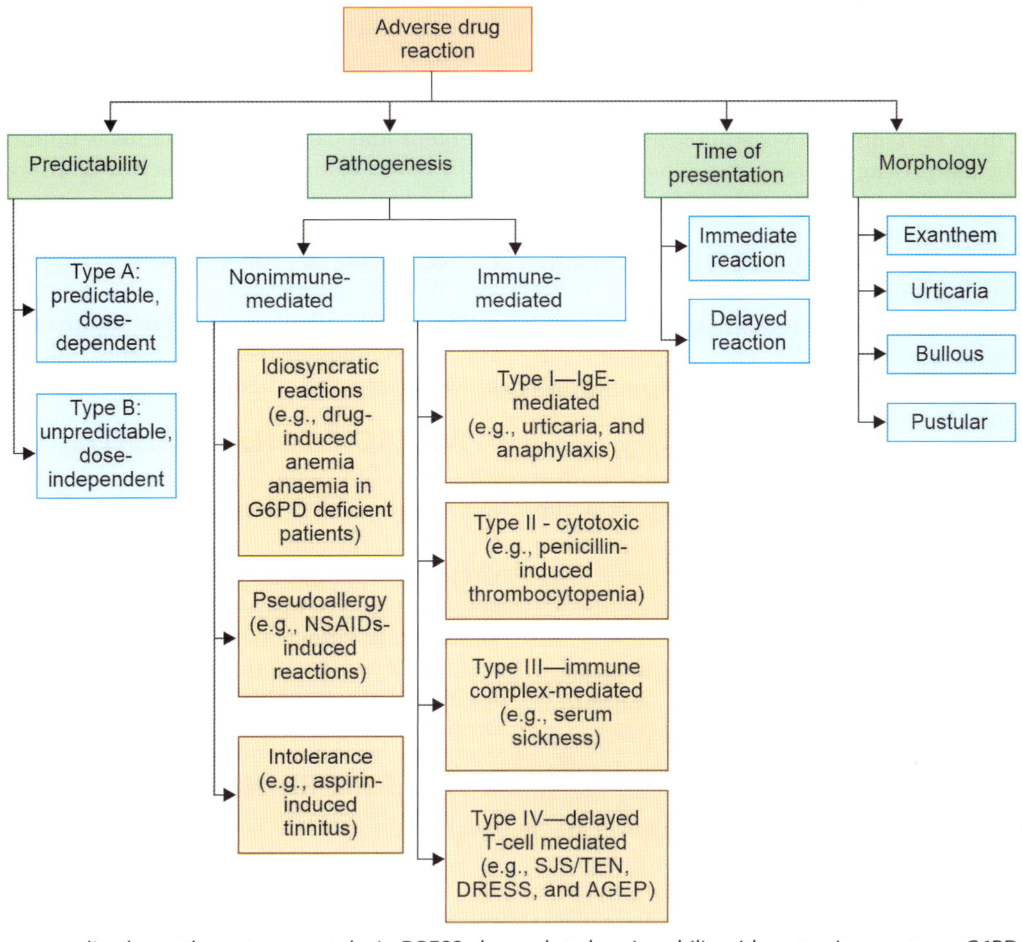

(AGEP: acute generalized exanthematous pustulosis; DRESS: drug-related eosinophilia with systemic symptoms; G6PD: glucose-6-phosphate dehydrogenase; IgE: immunoglobulin E; SJS: Steven–Johnson syndrome; TEN: toxic epidermal necrolysis)

Flowchart 18.6.3: Classification of adverse drug reaction based on rash morphology.[15]

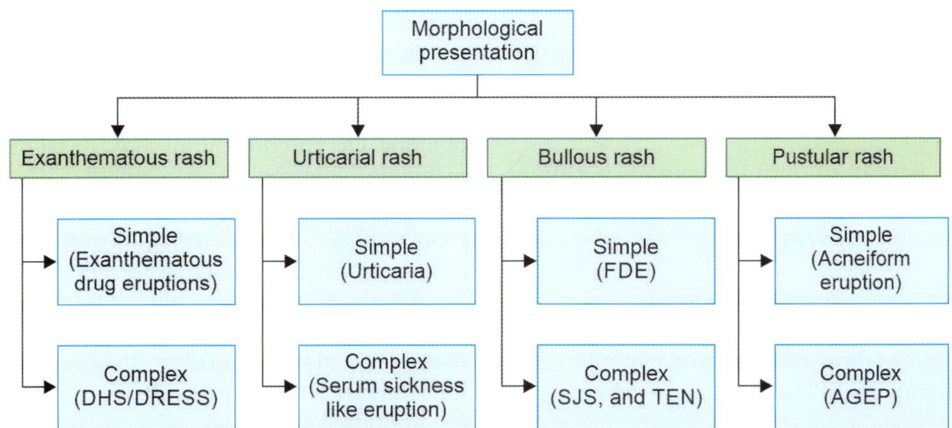

(AGEP: acute generalized exanthematous pustulosis; DHS: drug hypersensitivity syndrome; DRESS: drug-related eosinophilia with systemic symptoms; FDE: fixed drug eruption; SJS: Steven–Johnson syndrome; TEN: toxic epidermal necrolysis)

be carried out under strict monitoring with precautions. In patients with anaphylaxis, these tests should be avoided. The results also can be modified by concurrent antihistamines, requiring prior stoppage of these drugs.

Drug patch test is done to confirm the etiology in FDE. For maculopapular drug rash, drug provocation tests and drug patch tests can be done. Drug provocation testing should be avoided in severe drug reactions like SJS, TEN, etc. In vitro tests like lymphocyte transformation assay, drug induced cytokine assay - ELISPOT can be carried out in SCARs, although they have a low sensitivity.

Treatment relies on avoiding the offending drug and the use of drug from an alternate class with similar efficacy. Drug desensitization can be performed for certain drugs when the indication is absolute. Maculopapular rash can be managed with oral antihistamines, topical soothing agents like calamine lotion, emollients with or without topical corticosteroids. Severe reactions like SJS/TEN, DRESS, AGEP, etc., require treatment with systemic steroids, cyclosporine or Intravenous immunoglobulins.

ALLERGIC CONTACT DERMATITIS

Allergic contact dermatitis accounts for nearly 20% of pediatric dermatitis. It occurs following contact sensitization during initial exposure which on subsequent exposure to the specific allergen molecules (haptens) triggers an immune response with inflammatory skin rash. It is characterized by a type IV hypersensitivity reaction. Clinically, dermatitis involves areas that come in contact with the allergen. There are different morphological variants: Airborne contact dermatitis, photoallergic contact dermatitis, mixed pattern contact dermatitis, hand eczema, eyelid dermatitis, discoid eczema, lichenoid contact dermatitis, etc. The rash is characterized by pruritic erythematous to hyperpigmented, lichenified, oozy, scaly papules, and plaques depending on the stage of eczema. Thorough knowledge of commonly implicated allergens is essential as the first line of management is allergen exposure prevention.[16,17]

The most common contact allergens implicated in children are:[16,18]

- *Metals:* Nickel (jewelry, toys, coins, belts, zipper, etc.), cobalt, and gold
- Fragrance mix, Balsam of Peru (cosmetics, perfumes, lotions, shampoos, detergents, etc.)
- Thiomersal (vaccines and local antiseptics)
- Rubber
- Lanolin (used in topical creams and balms)
- Methylisothiazolinone (glue/slime, wet wipes and baby products, cosmetics, fabric softeners, and paints)
- Paraphenylenediamine (PPD)—used in dyes, henna, and tattoos
- Potassium dichromate (cement and leather)
- *Medications:* Neomycin, benzocaine, and corticosteroids
- Propylene glycol (moisturizers, cleaning products, etc.)
- Formaldehyde (preservative in baby wipes, cosmetics, adhesives, paints, etc.)
- Paraben (preservative)

Hence, a targeted history of exposure to particular allergens and pattern of dermatitis is important to suspect ACD. Patch testing with the series of allergen is the gold standard for diagnosis.

For treatment, patient and parent's education regarding the possible sources of allergen and exposure prevention is the key. Topical steroids and calcineurin inhibitors are used for mild-to-moderate dermatitis. For severe cases, short course systemic steroids are used. Emollients and antihistamines are provided for symptomatic treatment.[16,17]

ALLERGIC CONJUNCTIVITIS

Allergic conjunctivitis is common in children, especially males with seasonal variations.[19] Clinical manifestations include ocular itching and discomfort, periorbital edema, conjunctival congestion, watering of eyes, and foreign body sensation. Severe disease can lead to complications such as keratoconus, corneal ulcers, corneal ectasia, and diminished vision. Treatment modalities include trigger avoidance, avoidance of eye rubbing, cold compresses, olopatadine eye drops, mast cell stabilizers, and topical steroids.

ALLERGIC RHINITIS

Allergic rhinitis is a common disorder affecting between 10 and 30% of children and adolescents.[20] AR and asthma develop in 50–75% of children with atopic dermatitis, especially in those with severe AD.[2]

The clinical features include:[20]

- Rhinorrhea
- Recurrent sneezing
- Nasal itching
- Nasal congestion
- *Other associated symptoms:* Itching and watering of eyes, headache, and postnasal drip (if there is an associated allergic sinusitis).

Most patients have a positive family history of atopy, seasonal variation of symptoms, raised IgE levels, and markers of atopy. On anterior rhinoscopy, nasal mucosal pallor with turbinate hypertrophy can be noted.

It can be classified as intermittent and persistent rhinitis. Intermittent AR is defined as having symptoms present for <4 consecutive weeks per year and for <4 days per week. Persistent AR occurs when symptoms are present for >4 consecutive weeks per year and >4 days per week. The disease is said to be moderate-to-severe if one or more of the following features are present:

1. Abnormal sleep
2. Impairment of daily activities, leisure, or sports involvement

3. Troublesome symptoms
4. Impairment of school/work performance.[20]

The common triggers include dust mites, pollen, animal dander, fungal molds. To identify potential allergens, skin prick test and allergen specific IgE testing are carried out. X-ray paranasal sinuses and nasal endoscopy are other investigations required.

Treatment is mainly aimed at avoidance of offending allergens and symptomatic management.[20] Allergen avoidance measures include the following:[20]

- Avoidance of pet
- Regularly cleaning, washing, and sun-drying of bedding and mattresses, and humidity control
- Remove carpets
- Use of air conditioners/air filters
- Staying indoors in high-pollen days
- Wearing face masks

Pharmacological Treatment[20]

- *Main drugs:* Nasal saline, second-generation antihistamines, intranasal steroids (fluticasone propionate, fluticasone furoate, mometasone furoate, budesonide, and triamcinolone)
- *Others:* Mast cell stabilizers, montelukast, and nasal adrenergic decongestants
- *Allergen-specific immunotherapy (subcutaneous or sublingual)*—it has shown good efficacy for pollen, animal dander, dust mites, fungal molds, and cockroaches.
- *Newer agents:* Omalizumab (expensive and not routinely recommended)

BRONCHIAL ASTHMA

Allergic asthma is another common disorder affecting the respiratory system in children. It is discussed separately in Chapter 10.10.

CONCLUSION

Allergic disorders are common in children and have a wide spectrum of presentation, and varying severity. Atopic dermatitis is a common manifestation of allergy in young children. Some allergic disorders, grow out with age, while some may persist into adulthood; some disorders have a chronic remitting and relapsing course and few disorders may coexist. A systematic approach would aid in early diagnosis and initiate appropriate preventive and therapeutic measures to avoid complications and improve the quality of life.

REFERENCES

1. Aldakheel FM. Allergic Diseases: A Comprehensive Review on Risk Factors, Immunological Mechanisms, Link with COVID-19, Potential Treatments, and Role of Allergen Bioinformatics. Int J Environ Res Public Health. 2021;18(22):12105.
2. Tsuge M, Ikeda M, Matsumoto N, Yorifuji T, Tsukahara H. Current Insights into Atopic March. Children (Basel). 2021; 8(11):1067.
3. Devdas JM, Mckie C, Fox AT, Ratageri VH. Food Allergy in Children: An Overview. Indian J Pediatr. 2018;85(5):369-74.
4. Chad Z. Allergies in Children. Paediatr Child Health. 2001;6(8):555-66.
5. De A, Karekar S, Adhav C. Current Burden of Atopic Dermatitis in India: A Systematic Literature Review. Indian J Dermatol. 2023;68(4):487.
6. Kulthanan K, Tuchinda P, Nitiyarom R, Chunharas A, Chantaphakul H, Aunhachoke K, et al. Clinical practice guidelines for the diagnosis and management of atopic dermatitis. Asian Pac J Allergy Immunol. 2021;39(3):145-55.
7. Eichenfield LF, Stripling S, Fung S, Cha A, O'Brien A, Schachner LA. Recent developments and advances in atopic dermatitis: a focus on epidemiology, pathophysiology, and treatment in the pediatric setting. Paediatr Drugs. 2022;24(4):293-305.
8. Sathishkumar D, Gupta A, Saini K. Atopic dermatitis in children: an update for pediatricians. Curr Med Issues. 2020;18(4):317-25.
9. Zuberbier T, Abdul Latiff AH, Abuzakouk M, Aquilina S, Asero R, Baker D, et al. The international EAACI/GA²LEN/EuroGuiDerm/APAAACI guideline for the definition, classification, diagnosis, and management of urticaria. Allergy. 2022;77(3):734-66.
10. Tarczoń I, Cichocka-Jarosz E, Knapp A, Kwinta P. The 2020 update on anaphylaxis in paediatric population. Postepy Dermatol Alergol. 2022;39(1):13-9.
11. Pier J, Bingemann TA. Urticaria, Angioedema, and Anaphylaxis. Pediatr Rev. 2020;41(6):283-92.
12. Ramirez-Marin HA, Singh AM, Ong PY, Silverberg JI. Food allergy testing in atopic dermatitis. JAAD Int 2022;9:50-6.
13. Campbell DE. Role of food allergy in childhood atopic dermatitis. J Paediatr Child Health. 2012;48:1058-64.
14. Park JS, Suh DI. Drug Allergy in Children: What Should We Know? Clin Exp Pediatr. 2020;63(6):203-10.
15. Del Pozzo-Magaña BR, Liy-Wong C. Drugs and the skin: A concise review of cutaneous adverse drug reactions. Br J Clin Pharmacol. 2024;90(8):1838-55.
16. Bhat YJ, Akhtar S, Hassan I. Contact dermatitis in pediatric age group: Indian scenario. Indian J Paediatr Dermatol. 2019;20(3):205-11.
17. Belloni Fortina A, Caroppo F, Tadiotto Cicogna G. Allergic contact dermatitis in children. Expert Rev Clin Immunol. 2020;16(6):579-89.
18. Neale H, Garza-Mayers AC, Tam I, Yu J. Pediatric allergic contact dermatitis. Part I: Clinical features and common contact allergens in children. J Am Acad Dermatol. 2021;84(2):235-44.
19. Vazirani J, Shukla S, Chhawchharia R, Sahu S, Gokhale N, Basu S. Allergic conjunctivitis in children: current understanding and future perspectives. Curr Opin Allergy Clin Immunol. 2020;20(5):507-15.
20. Schuler Iv CF, Montejo JM. Allergic Rhinitis in Children and Adolescents. Pediatr Clin North Am. 2019;66(5):981-93.

SECTION

19

Adolescent Health

Section Editor: MKC Nair

19.1 Why Adolescent Care Counseling?

MKC Nair

INTRODUCTION

Adolescence is that period in our life where nothing seems to go smoothly and yet our best memories are about those wonderful days. The present-day adolescent is considered to be more knowledgeable about world affairs, thanks to the onslaught of the media. On the other hand, some feel disillusioned about the way things are going, and hence, point out the futility of any intervention program at this level. Adolescence is also that period in our lives where contradictions are the rule and not the exception. A period when they demand independence, yet are mostly dependent; period when maximum hostility is shown to the parents, yet want to be loved and cared for; a period with maximum rebellion shown, yet want to be the pet baby of their mothers; a period when they reject advice outright, yet love to be guided through difficulties. Surely any conventional approach is likely to fail with this group. Special problems of vulnerable and marginalized groups and problems of adolescent boys have to be addressed separately. Apart from these, we need to have a strategy for adolescents as a group in India, which should focus on:

- Malnutrition, anemia, iodine, deficiency, etc.
- Obesity, diabetes, hypertension, and all foundation for future heart problems
- Adolescent reproductive sexual health service delivery
- Scholastic backwardness issues and improving study habits
- Adolescent counseling services in the community
- Life skills and career guidance (employability training)
- National capacity building for delivery services

ADOLESCENT CARE COUNSELING

Child, adolescent, and youth mental health is probably a continuum from a child development perspective—normal and abnormal, evolution of problems, causative and risk factors, and ultimately the outcome. It is said that many of the adult psychiatric disorders have their onset in adolescence. Mental health issues of adolescents have to be addressed in the primary care setup itself, because there are far too many adolescents with behavioral and emotional problems in the community and only limited number of psychiatrists, clinical psychologists, and trained counselor being available. An adolescent's pediatrician can screen the adolescents for mental health problems using teen screen questionnaire for mental health (TSQ-M), a simple screening tool and making both parents and adolescents comfortable in nonstigmatizing way.[1] TSQ-M short has an overall diagnostic accuracy better than the original TSQ-M. Although the original version includes symptoms for more mental health disorders, providing a wider screen, the short version would prove useful in big community studies.

All of us have fond memories of our adolescences. Traditionally, the societal norms were such that we mostly tried to limit our activities within the acceptable norms of the society. Our parents and teachers tried to instill in us the correct moral values as thought appropriate for the day. Time has changed. Very little societal control is perceived now, and whatever is still left is not appreciated. With the present-day fast-changing norms of society, they are not sure about how to guide the youngster. Teachers, our traditional source of wisdom, are often confused about their role in society at least vis-à-vis the problems of adolescents. Yet, they have the best opportunity to guide the destiny of millions of youngsters, only if we could empower them their legitimate role in the society as guidance teachers and counselors.

The commonly used words related to counseling situations are;

- *Advice:* An opinion that someone offers you about what you should do or how you should act in a particular situation—something not often acceptable to adolescents.
- *Guidance:* An expert/experienced person helps and advices about how to do something or about how to deal with problems connected with your work, education, or personal relationships, e.g., career guidance.
- *Negotiation:* The process of discussing something with someone in order to reach an agreement with them, or the discussions themselves—marriage counseling.
- *Psychotherapy:* A variety of treatments that aim to help a person to identify and change troubling emotions, thoughts, and behaviors—by trained professionals.
- *Counseling:* The provision of professional assistance and guidance in resolving personal or psychological problems—leading on to improved personal growth.

COUNSELING

Counseling is not advising, do not solve all life's problems, aimed at helping people make choices and act on them, a learning process, and enables personality development.[2] Core conditions for counseling include:

- *Empathy*—a sense of caring and understanding
- *Unconditional positive regard*—focusing on value and worth
- *Congruence*—feeling, thinking, and actions match
- *Respect*—making positive statements
- *Immediacy*—direct, mutual communication
- *Confrontation*—pointing out discrepancies
- *Concreteness*—discuss in specific terms, and self-disclosure—making self-known to others.

Counseling Process—Practical Steps[2]

- *Positive relationship building*—differ with each individual adolescent
- *Ventilation*—meaning, an adolescent's full and free expression of feelings or emotions, especially in session or catharsis—meaning a powerful emotional release that, when successful, is accompanied by cognitive insight and positive change.
- *Prioritize problems*—from so many reduce to 3 and then to 1 or 2.
- *Adolescent's role in the problem*—we always blame the other person, forgetting our own role in creating the problem—self-evaluation.
- *Context of the problem*—the gravity of the problem and the probable solutions would depend on the circumstances or the context in which the adolescent is placed.
- *Prioritize solutions*—the adolescent himself/herself have to come out with possible solutions keeping in mind the feasibility in their own context.
- *Help implement solutions*—supporting the adolescent to go through all the six steps in a smooth manner is the responsibility of the counselor.
- *Termination of counseling*—at some point or other counseling sessions have to be terminated.

Effective Counselors

Effective counselors are those; personally integrated and having self-awareness; value the client as a unique person; understand how and what client is experiencing; identify "Hidden shame," unacknowledged, repressed, or defended against; client revelations must be protected from therapists "personal reactions," especially rejection; and have empathy towards the client.

Empathy involves:

- Empathic rapport meaning accurately sensing and being able to see the client's world the way they do.
- Communicative attunement meaning verbally sharing your understanding with the adolescent.
- Therapist senses accurately and communicates back to the client the feelings and meaning of experiences.
- Cultural empathy includes context and society in which both the counselor and client live.

Therapeutic Relationship

Therapeutic relationship is one which is perceived by adolescents to encompass caring, and supportive nonjudgmental behavior, embedded in a safe environment during an often-stressful period. Personhood of therapist is a key factor for the quality of the relationship, successful outcome; effectiveness that is related to mutual respect, caring, and trust creating safety for clients to share their deepest concerns. Adolescent's willingness to act and achieve a positive outcome is based on his/her view that the environment/relationship is safe.

Self-counseling

Self-counseling refers to the practice of examining one's own behavior, using psychoanalytical methods of free-thinking and free association that can help the adolescent take more effective control of everyday situations, and enable him/her to make continued progress. A successful self-counseling practice needs finding strength in not just oneself but also the support system which may include the family and/or friends.[3]

CONCLUSION

Adolescent counseling is crucial for addressing the various emotional, mental, and social challenges faced during this critical developmental stage. It emphasizes on building a supportive, empathetic, and nonjudgmental therapeutic relationship while empowering adolescents to find solutions within their own context. Effective counseling with professional guidance and strategies like self-counseling plays a vital role in shaping adolescents into confident and responsible individuals.

REFERENCES

1. Nair MKC, Rajaraman V, Chacko D, Russell S, George B, Samara L, et al. Comparison of the diagnostic accuracy and validity of a short version of teen screen questionnaire-mental health (TSQ-M-short) for use in community. Indian J Psychol Med. 2015;37(2):201-4.
2. Nair MKC. Adolescent Counselling, 1st edition. New Delhi: Jaypee Brothers Medical Publishers; 2016.
3. Nair MKC, Kumar S, Lukose R, Girish CS, Binod D, Sreejith S. Self-counselling. Pediatr Companion. 2022;1:16-20.

19.2 Family Life Education

MKC Nair, Gurmeet Kaur

INTRODUCTION

Family life education (FLE) is a more preferred term as compared to sex education that may provoke anxiety in the parents' mind as to what is being taught to the adolescents. The need to impart FLE is very pertinent as adolescents need authentic knowledge that help them to understand the process of growing up from childhood to adulthood. FLE is the platform where adolescent can learn accurate information about physiological processes in one's body, right from human conception and birth. It also creates awareness about the consequence of adolescent pregnancy and parenting. Risky sexual behavior and lack of knowledge on sexuality-related topics are among the leading problems associated with mortality and morbidity. Knowledge about sexuality is an important tool for primary prevention and possibly counter many related problems.

Family life education helps in:

- Decreasing the anxieties and confusion among adolescents about various aspects of growing up.
- Developing positive attitude sex and inculcate responsible behavior.
- Developing ability to deal with family relationship and responsibility of family.
- Establishing and maintaining satisfying relationship with members of family, with friends and with others whom they come into contact within the context of family life.
- Learning about coping with changes in one' own life and changes in the society.
- Raising awareness about the concept of family, its roles and functions, to recognize the various tasks that need to be observed for the well-being and maintenance of the family.
- Meeting the ultimate aim of FLE, is to create responsible and productive young citizens.

The Adolescence Education Program guided by National Curriculum Framework, launched by Government of India (GOI) in 2005, is a large scale school-based life skills education intervention for the holistic development of adolescents. It is an informal education which consists of experiences and actually living in the family or community. Globally, FLE program studies show the increased knowledge and use of contraceptives by adolescents and the increased understanding and positive attitude toward sexual behavior and sexuality. In India, although traditional norms oppose premarital sex, some studies indicate a growing trend toward premarital sexual activities and every day newspaper show growing incidences of sexual crimes, which have become a matter of great concern. Through FLE, adolescents can be taught how to channelize their minds into creative things as well as safeguard themselves against such inhuman incidents.[1]

In 2014, GOI launched the *Rashtriya Kishor Swasthya Karyakram (RKSK)* for adolescent health and development, focusing on sexual and reproductive health (SRH), nutrition, mental health, injuries and violence, substance abuse, and noncommunicable diseases.[2,3] The family is the center of personal affection that enables and enriches human life. India has 243 million adolescents constituting 21% of the total population and FLE has been implemented within middle schools over decades, but its impact on health and well-being has not been studied.[4]

Adolescents have unique SRH needs and risks. The emerging issues in child sexuality are child pornography, prostitution, child sexual abuse, poor parenting, adolescent dating violence or intimate partner violence, boy image disorders, rape and abortions, female feticide and psychosexual disorders, homosexuality, masturbation, and substance abuse.

COMPONENTS OF FAMILY LIFE EDUCATION

Adolescent Nutrition

Nutritional monitoring of preadolescents and adolescents should form part and parcel of any adolescent program. Adolescent nutrition should focus on both malnutrition (more important in the case of females) and obesity, in view of associated polycystic ovary syndrome. Obesity is now seen with increasing frequency and may be due to urbanization, less physical activity at school and home, and changing food habits. Childhood-onset adult diseases such as hypertension, diabetes mellitus, and heart disease should be prevented by reducing intrauterine growth restriction. The most significant community factors that predict low birthweight are prepregnant weight of mother <40 kg and height <140 cm and hence the need for nutritional intervention in the prepubertal stage of growth spurt.

Personal Hygiene

Many schoolgirls do not drink water adequately, nor pass urine frequently at school because of the poor hygiene of school toilets and this contributes toward silent urinary tract infection. Hence immediate attention is needed to overcome this problem. In many residential institutions for girls, proper menstrual hygiene is not taught to the girls. They also need to be made aware that some amount of vaginal discharge and dysmenorrhea is within normal limits.

Understanding One's Emotions

An adolescent with a wholesome personality is one, who has strong mental, physical, and cognitive skills, which enable her/him to behave, relate to and act effectively in the family and in the society at large. FLE is an acceptable mode of introducing what is essential for adolescents to understand and appreciate.

Life Skills Development

Life skills development emphasizes the links between knowledge, attitude, values, and positive health behavior. Life skill education can be acquired and learnt by practicing various scenarios. It is a continuous process and is based on social learning theory. Actual practice of skills is done in small groups or in pairs by various techniques such as brainstorming, role plays, games, and debates.

Saying "NO" to Alcohol, Smoking, and Substance Abuse

The capacity to say "NO" to unwanted influences from peers and even from persons of authority is one of the many life skills that an adolescent should learn and practice, especially to avoid the menace of substance abuse.

Awareness of One's Own Sexuality, HIV/AIDS, and Substance Abuse

For young adolescents' sexual matters should be presented in a way that is acceptable to the local community, emphasizing the advantages of practicing abstinence and dangers of irresponsible behavior. For older adolescents, the program should lay emphasis on understanding and appreciating one's sexuality and fostering the attitude that sexual relationship is like any other relationship where the feelings and needs of both partners are equally important.

Interpersonal Problems

Adolescents share their thoughts and feelings with their peers. They give great importance to friendship, but get easily hurt due to peer conflicts. Some students complain that their academic performance is disrupted because the teachers unduly favor some students. There is a need to develop strategies that would help adolescents handle interpersonal difficulties.

Love Affairs

Many adults dismiss teen love as love that is not real. While feelings aroused in some adolescents are of infatuation and are immature, those in others may signal a mature love. People of all ages can have either of the above, and teens especially need to know the difference.

Body Image

During adolescence, there is increased concern about one's body image. This may be due of personality factors, over consciousness about one's looks, or because of a desire to appeal to the opposite sex.

Developing Self-counseling Skill

Self-counseling is the process of examining one's own behavior, using psychoanalytical methods of free-thinking and free association. Self-counseling can help one take more effective control of everyday situations and enable to make continued progress or personal growth. The principles of self-counseling would be:

- Do not bluff to yourself, may have to bluff to others.
- *Not God—likely to make mistakes*: Take precaution
- *Don't think others have to like you always*: Self-love
- *Caring and not love*: More appropriate
- Kill enemy by caring them when they need.
- *Refuse to take insult*: Feeling 30 seconds then cognitive pathway
- Don't think others are lesser than you.
- *Think of other person's point of view*: Be a third party.
- Do not hurt someone if possible, do not hurt yourself ever.
- I am the custodian of my mind, body and spirit, I will protect, persevere, and enhance it.

A study on understanding the lives of adolescents and young adults (UDAYA), to evaluate the health and development of adolescents, was conducted in 2015–16 with a representative sample of 9,353 adolescents from 10–19 years old in Bihar.[5] The finding were that only 21.7% unmarried females, 10.98% married females, and 4.7% of males participated in an FLE program conducted by the school, community, and local organization. Adolescent males and females who attended the school, were more likely to receive FLE participation ($p < 0.0001$). The quality of FLE programs and other barriers have to be understood for better participation in these programs by adolescents. Another study on 160,551 unmarried young women aged 15–24 years from the District Level Reproductive and Child Health Survey (DLHS

2007–2008), evaluated the demographic and socioeconomic differentials in the access to family life/sex education among youth in India. They reported that 48% of unmarried young women received some form of FLE, and also found that a significantly higher proportion young women who had received FLE, had positive attitude toward reproductive processes, knowledge on transmission of reproductive tract infections and sexually transmitted infections (RTI/STI) including human immunodeficiency virus (HIV).[6]

IMPLEMENTING FLE IN SCHOOLS

A study done in Thiruvananthapuram to understand the problems of school going adolescents in selected schools in the first phase and to provide class-based FLE in the second phase had the following steps:

- Identification of the study sample
- Each adolescent was individually administered Teenage Screening Questionnaire-Trivandrum (TSQ-T) by trained project staff.
- FLE sessions were held for the whole class together.
- Queries were collected on a slip of paper without writing their names.
- Those needing medical attention was seen by a medical doctor and psychologist.
- Preparation of a guidebook named "101 questions", and
- Upscaling the project as a service component to government schools

Screening of adolescents using TSQ-T was found to be useful in identifying adolescents with nutrition and lifestyle issues, scholastic problems, mental health problems, and reproductive health problems, so that remedial measures could be taken, the very purpose of FLE.[7]

CONCLUSION

Family life education (FLE) is a comprehensive approach that emphasizes critical topics such as personal hygiene, nutrition, emotional well-being, sexual and reproductive health, fostering responsible attitudes and behaviors. By promoting awareness and self-counseling, FLE empowers adolescents and contributes positively to their development and societal well-being.

REFERENCES

1. Nair MKC, Leena ML, Menon P, George B, Indira MS, Russell PS. ARSH 8: Family life education and counseling: a school based model. Indian J Pediatr. 2013;80 Suppl 2:S234-9.
2. World Health Organization. Government of India launches new health programme for adolescents. Delhi, India: Partnership for Maternal, Newborn & Child Health; 2014.
3. Government of India. Rashtriya Kishor Swasthya Karyakram (RKSK). National Health Mission Ministry of Health & Family Welfare, Government of India 2014; Website:http://nhm.gov,in/rashtriya-kishor-swasthya-karyakram.html [Last accessed December, 2024].
4. Khubchandani J, Clark J, Kumar R. Beyond controversies: Sexuality education for adolescents in India. J Family Med Prim Care. 2014;3(3):175-9.
5. Wyss N, Bhadra K, Rao N, Bhan N, Raj A. (2019). Adolescent participation in Family Life Education Programs in Bihar, India. Center on Gender Equity and Health. University of San Diego School of Medicine. [online] Accessed From https://gehdev.ucsd.edu/wp-content/uploads/2019/05/final_fle-brief_up_template_5.9.2019_.pdf [Last accessed December, 2024].
6. Tripathi N. Does family life education influence attitude towards sexual and reproductive health matters among unmarried young women in India? PLoS One. 2021;16(1):e245883.
7. Nair MKC. (2024). Family Life & Life Skills Education for Adolescents: Trivandrum Experience. [online] Available from https://core.ac.uk/reader/86381 Accessed on 06/01/2024 [Last accessed December, 2024].

19.3 Adolescent Nutrition

Jugesh Chhatwal

INTRODUCTION

Growth is a hallmark of adolescent period. For adequate and appropriate growth, nutrition is vital. There are major growth tasks to be completed during adolescence as given below.[1]

- *Increase in height:* Nearly one-fifth (20%) of the adult height is gained during adolescence.
- *Weight gain:* About 25–50% of the final adult, ideal weight is gained during adolescence.
- *Muscles mass:* A little less than half (45%) of skeletal muscle mass is added.
- *Bone mass:* Almost 50% of bone mass is accumulated by the end of the second decade of life, 90% of total bone mass is gained.

For children entering the adolescent phase with a growth deficit carried over from childhood malnutrition, the adolescent period provides another opportunity to correct the deficiencies, catch up, improve growth, and attain their full potential. Adolescent nutrition can have significant consequences on the life course. This phase also sets the foundation for future nutritional health and adult eating patterns and behaviors. The aftermath of inadequate or inappropriate dietary intake during adolescence will be visible later in adult life. Adolescent nutrition impacts not only the physical growth measures as above but also has strong influence on puberty, neurodevelopment, immunity, and cardiorespiratory fitness.[2] Associated micronutrient deficiencies can cause anemia, stunting, and poor bone health. All these will eventually affect their adult life and lead to poor health outcomes, diminished work capacity, skills, and cognitive functioning. In addition, among malnourished females, there can be increased obstetrical risk with poor pregnancy outcome and higher maternal morbidity and mortality and intergenerational effects on future offspring.

ADOLESCENT NUTRITION: CURRENT STATUS

Various surveys have shown that the dietary intakes of Indian adolescents are significantly inadequate. Earlier, National Nutrition Monitoring Bureau Survey (2002) had shown that 30–40% of girls and 33–66% of boys consume <70% of the recommended daily allowance (RDA) for calories. Protein intake is also significantly less in more than half of the adolescent girls and boys. The intake of micronutrients is much more seriously reduced with the majority taking <50% of RDA for iron and >80% taking grossly inadequate amounts of vitamin A.[3] The recent Comprehensive National Nutrition Survey (CNNS 2016–18) from Birth to Adolescence has reported the dietary intakes of adolescents 10–19 years of age.[4] The consumption of the various food items at least once per week was, viz., milk 60.5%, pulses 85%, green leafy vegetables 88.2%, fruits 41.4%, eggs 34.9%, and flesh foods 36.2%. Adolescent girls' consumption of most food items was lower than boys.[4]

The nutritional status of the adolescent was also assessed in the CNNS using WHO child growth standards median (WHO, 2007). The prevalence of "thin for age [body mass index (BMI) <–2SD]" was 24% and 6.5% were at <–3SD. Stunting (height for age Z score < –2SD) was present in 30% by age of 18 years. Parallel to the problems of inadequate food intake obesity and overweight are also seen in substantial proportion of the population, especially among urban youth. Prevalence of adolescent overweight and obesity has shown a wide range from different parts of the country. The CNNS reported overweight (BMI for age > +1SD) 5%, obesity (BMI for age > +2SD) at 1%, and abdominal obesity as 2% (waist circumference for age > +1 SD).

In addition to the deviations of weight and height, micronutrient deficiencies are also a considerable problem. CNNS reported micronutrient deficiencies among adolescents aged 10–19 years. Anemia was found to be a moderate-to-severe problem in 20 states of the country with 28% anemic adolescents. 40% percent of the adolescent girls were anemic.[4] NFHS-5 also reported prevalence of anemia for 15–19 years old girls at 59.1% and boys at 31.1%.[5] The other micronutrients deficiencies observed were vitamin A 16%, vitamin D 24%, zinc 32%, B_{12} 31%, and folate 37%.[4]

ADOLESCENT NUTRITIONAL NEEDS

Early adolescence is marked by rapid growth phase and pubertal changes during which time the nutrient requirement is different as compared to late adolescence when growth has stabilized and the micronutrients have an important role. The current weight, gender, growth phase, and the level of physical activity have a major influence on energy needs of the teenager. Daily requirements for adolescent age-group as per the revised Indian Council of Medical Research Guidelines (2020) are given in **Tables 19.3.1 and 19.3.2**.[6]

Micronutrient Requirements

The most important micronutrients during adolescent period are iron, calcium, and zinc. At the onset of puberty, the preadolescent child may already have a preexisting iron deficiency, and most Indian diets, even if adequate otherwise, are not a good source of iron. Iron is essential for both girls and boys. Postmenarche girls will have additional requirements. Boys require iron as they are adding muscle bulk (myoglobin)

TABLE 19.3.1: Recommended daily allowance (per day) for adolescents (Indian Council of Medical Research, 2020).

Gender	*Age (years)*	*Proteins (g)*	*Calories*	*Fat (g)*	*Calcium (mg)*	*Iron (mg)*	*Zinc (mg)*	*Magnesium (mg)*
Boys	10–12	31.8	2,190	35	850	16	8.5	270
Girls	10–12	32.8	2,010	35	850	28	8.5	255
Boys	13–15	44.9	2,750	45	1,000	22	14.3	355
Girls	13–15	43.2	2,330	40	1,000	30	12.8	325
Boys	16–18	55.4	3,020	50	1,050	26	17.6	405
Girls	16–18	46.2	2,440	35	1,050	32	14.2	335

TABLE 19.3.2: Recommended daily allowance (per day) for adolescents (Indian Council of Medical Research, 2020).

Gender	*Age (years)*	*Thiamin (mg)*	*Riboflavin (mg)*	*Niacin (mg)*	*Pyridoxine (mg)*	*Vit B_{12} (µg)*	*Vit A (µg)*	*Vit C (mg)*	*Vit D (IU)*	*Folate (µg)*
Boys	10–12	1.5	2.1	15	2.0	2.5	770	54	600	220
Girls	10–12	1.4	1.9	14	1.9		790	52		225
Boys	13–15	1.9	2.7	19	2.6		930	72		285
Girls	13–15	1.6	2.2	16	2.2		890	66		245
Boys	16–18	2.2	3.1	22	3.0		1,000	82		340
Girls	16–18	1.7	2.3	17	2.3		860	68		270

and also increase in red cell mass increases the demand for iron (hemoglobin). Calcium is essential for the bone mineral accretion, which reaches peak in mid-adolescence. Accelerated muscular and skeletal development increases the demand for dietary calcium at this age. Inadequate calcium intake during this period can decrease the bone mineral mass with sometimes lifelong consequences in the form of increased risk of osteoporosis. Zinc is required for physical growth as well as sexual development, and deficiency can impair these processes.[6]

NUTRITIONAL DISORDERS

Adolescent period has its own behavioral complexities, which are closely linked with dietary intake. The growing teenager is breaking free from parental control, and this is reflected in the decision-making for food intake and accepting the norms and dietary guidelines. Dissatisfaction with body image, peer conformity, search for self-identity, and a busy schedule add to the nutritional problems. The onslaught of media along with the nutritional transition in the country has had a major impact on how the adolescents eat. Some of the common characteristics of food habits of adolescents are as follows:

- Missing meals, especially breakfast
- Frequent out of home meals
- Snacking, especially on calorie-dense fast foods
- Consumption of ultraprocessed foods and sugar sweetened beverages
- Fad diets

The important nutritional disorders seen in adolescents are as below:

- Undernutrition
- Iron deficiency anemia
- Obesity
- Eating disorders

Undernutrition

Undernutrition is a significant problem among adolescents in India (*See* Chapter 5.4). A number of studies have observed that the mean intake of energy, protein, iron, and other micronutrients is less than RDA for adolescents.[7] The prevalence of undernutrition manifesting as stunting and thinness was assessed in CNNS 2016–18. The findings showed that at national level 27.2% of the adolescents were stunted and 24.1% were thin. Correlating with gender, it was noted that thinness was significantly higher among girls especially 15–19 years old. Prevalence of stunting amongst adolescent boys and girls did not show any significant difference (25.4% vs. 28.9%).[8] The thin-stunted girls are at risk for poor growth into adulthood and also contribute to the intergenerational malnutrition cycle. The causation of undernutrition is multifactorial and includes economic and social disparities, dietary intake and patterns, water, and sanitation. Disadvantaged and vulnerable social groups, adolescent girls are at greater risk. Diet diversity, hygiene, maternal education, and adolescents in school were associated with lower prevalence.[8] Improving adolescents' nutrition is in national interest as these are the future adult wealth of a nation.

Iron Deficiency Anemia

Anemia among adolescents is a common nutritional problem (*See* Chapter 14.4). As per CNNS, 28.5% of the adolescents studied were anemic with 39.6% girls affected. The onset of menarche will further add to the burden of anemia among adolescent girls. Iron deficiency was evaluated separately and found to be 22% among total and 31% among girls and also noted to be more among urban adolescents.[4] Iron deficiency and anemia both can lead to poor growth and intellectual functioning in addition to making the girls more vulnerable to reproductive and maternal complications as they enter adulthood.

Obesity

Adolescent obesity has been a cause for concern in the developed nations and also emerging as an important problem in the developing countries. It frequently tracks into adulthood and can lead to related lifestyle disorders. Adolescence provides an opportunity to prevent adult obesity and future noncommunicable diseases. Different criteria have been used to define obesity (*See* Chapter 3.6). BMI cutoffs are most frequently used in clinical setting, although addition of skinfold thickness is reported to make the assessment better. Prevalence of obesity among Indian adolescents has a wide range related to the definitions and the populations studied. CNNS observed overweight at 5% and obesity 1%.[4] Obese adolescent needs a detailed dietary and clinical assessment, and usually, this is sufficient to rule out any significant pathological causes of obesity. Moderate-to-severe obesity can lead to a number of systemic and psychological disorders. Managing an obese teenager requires empathy as they usually have significant psychological problems. The first step is to motivate, as without motivation all modalities of treatment are likely to give poor results. Decreasing calorie intake along with increasing physical activity is the basis for management. Dietary and activity management are essential for other modalities of treatment, such as pharmacological interventions or bariatric surgery also.

Eating Disorders

Eating disorders are a group of complex conditions defined by abnormal eating behaviors which can lead to significant health and medical problems. Some of the better-known eating disorders are anorexia nervosa, bulimia nervosa, binge-eating disorder, and eating disorders not otherwise specified. These are more common in the developed countries but with the onset of nutritional transition and media influences, they are being reported from low- or middle-income countries (LMIC) also. Adolescents are at risk for these due the developmental process and changes in their food environment. A combination of biological, psychological, and environmental factors plays a role in causation. Young girls are at particular risk. Multiple organ systems can get affected and there is a risk of mortality. Screening and early diagnosis of eating disorders are important to prevent long-term effects on the adolescents' health. The treatment involves behavioral therapy along with nutritional rehabilitation and pharmacotherapy and may require hospitalization in unstable critical patients.[9]

Some practical tips for optimum adolescent nutrition are as follows:

- Ensure balanced and diverse diet
- Follow traffic light diet:
  - Green—part of all meals, and includes fruits and vegetables, lean meats and fish, eggs, nuts, seeds, wholegrain products, and water
  - Orange—eat sometime not daily and includes reduced fat products, breads, and processed meats
  - Red—meat less frequently, once a week and includes deep fried foods, bakery products, chocolates, confectionary, and sugary drinks
- Morning breakfast is very vital and all children must have a habit of eating before going to school.
- Avoid empty-calorie foods, such as carbonated drinks/ sugar sweetened beverages.
- Iron-rich foods must be included in the diet.
- An adolescent boy should eat as much as father eats (2,400 calories).
- An adolescent girl should eat a little more than what the mother eats (2,100 calories).
- Take enough calcium-rich foods for optimal bone growth and density.
- Avoid junk foods as they are poor source of nutrition, unsafe, unhygienic and high in salt, sugar, preservatives, and carcinogens
- Ensuring maternal and adolescent education and providing safe water and hygienic practices are important measures to reduce adolescent malnutrition.
- Practice mindful eating.

NATIONAL PROGRAMS ON ADOLESCENT HEALTH

The important national programs on adolescent health especially adolescent nutrition include:

- *Poshan Abhiyaan:* Anemia Mukt Bharat
- Kishori Shakti Yojana (KSY)
- Rajiv Gandhi Scheme for Empowerment of Adolescent Girls—SABLA
- Weekly iron and folic acid Supplementation (WIFS)
- Rashtriya Kishor Swasthya Karyakram (RKSK)
- School Health Programme

These programs are discussed in detail in Section 22 Community Pediatrics.

REFERENCES

1. Norris SA, Frongillo EA, Black MM, Dong Y, Fall C, Lampl M, et al. Nutrition in adolescent growth and development. Lancet. 2022;399:172-84.
2. Patton GC, Neufeld LM, Dogra S, Frongillo EA, Hargreaves D, He S, et al. Nourishing our future: the Lancet Series on adolescent nutrition. Lancet. 2022;399:123-5.
3. National Institute of Nutrition. National Nutrition Monitoring Bureau: Diet and nutritional status of rural population. Hyderabad: Indian Council of Medical Research; 2002.
4. Ministry of Health and Family Welfare (MoHFW), Government of India, UNICEF and Population Council. Comprehensive National Nutrition Survey (CNNS) National Report. New Delhi: Ministry of Health and Family Welfare; 2019.
5. National Family Health Survey (NFHS-5) 2019-2021, Fact Sheet India. India: Ministry of Health & Family Welfare, Government of India; 2021.
6. ICMR-National Institute of Nutrition, Indian Council of Medical Research, Department of Health Research Ministry of Health

and Family Welfare, Government of India. Recommended Dietary Allowances and Estimated Average Requirement: Nutrient Requirements for Indians. New Delhi: ICMR; 2020.
7. Locks LM, Shah M, Bhaise S, Hibberd PL, Patel A. Assessing the Diets of Young Children and Adolescents in India: Challenges and Opportunities. Front Pediatr. 2022;10:725812.
8. Kumar M, Mohanty PC. Undernutrition and anaemia among Indian adolescents: role of dietary diversity and hygiene practices. J Nutr Sci. 2023;12:e33.
9. Hornberger LL, Lane MA; AAP The Committee on Adolescence. Identification and management of eating disorders in children and adolescents. Pediatrics. 2021;147(1):e2020040279

19.4 Adolescent Counseling

Sushila Russell, MKC Nair

INTRODUCTION

Adolescents are diverse in their age and developmental stage, social and geographical environments, economic circumstances, subculture, ethnicity, gender, sex, sexual orientation, disabilities, and marital status. Despite all these variations, adolescence is a period of exaggerated physical, emotional, social, intellectual, and spiritual growth with their complexities often resulting in a need for counseling. Adolescents might require preventive and therapeutic counseling to address their mental health needs.[1]

Counseling, with its elements of science and art, is one of the major interventions in helping adolescents with mental health needs and includes as many as 400 different types of therapies.[2,3] Regardless of the different types, counseling is an interactive process involving a trained professional counselor and an adolescent with the aim of enhancing the adolescent's level of functioning. Although counseling is a part of any clinician-patient interaction, counseling using formal principles in an organized manner is seldom a part of the primary care pediatrician's therapeutic armamentarium. Globally, 20% of children and adolescents suffer from a major mental illness and 75% of them present to the primary care pediatrician. However, only about 17% of these children are identified by their primary care physicians, and even if recognized, only a small fraction receives appropriate mental health treatment, including counseling. In this section, the different types of counseling, their indication as well as the evidence to support their effectiveness, are presented.[4] It is important to remember that counseling should be a dialogue and is different from advice which is a monologue.

COGNITIVE DEVELOPMENT AND COUNSELING

The choice and modality of providing the counseling depend on the developmental age of the adolescent.

- *Children in early adolescence* (10–13 years of age) typically are concrete thinkers and are unable to clearly understand the cause and effect between their behaviors and their health. Therefore counseling for in early adolescence should be clear and direct. These children may also be relatively attached to their primary caregivers who can help reinforce counseling at home settings and should therefore be ideally empowered as cotherapists. In view of their developing cognitive abilities, play and behavioral therapies are used to modify behaviors in older childhood and early adolescence.
- *Children in mid-adolescence* (14–17 years of age) are able to think more abstractly; typically, they are capable of complex, logical thinking, and sometimes, are allowed to make their own healthcare decisions.
- *Children in late adolescence* (18–19 years of age) have a longitudinal understanding of how their behaviors can affect their health than do children in early or mid-adolescence. Counseling during late adolescence should continue to focus on risky behaviors (e.g., substance abuse, violence, and sexual behaviors) and coping skills.

It should be noted that the confidentiality requirements may change when working with mid-adolescence and late adolescence (15 years and above) or emancipated minors (17-year-old living on his/her own, away from parents) and most of the sessions with older adolescents are confidential unless there is a threat of suicide or homicide. Cognitive behavioral techniques are used in early and mid-adolescence and cognitive techniques with late adolescence. While being invited into the counseling room for a therapy session, adolescents are invited first before their caregiver to overcome their autonomy-related issues and enhance their cooperation.

TYPES OF COUNSELING

Based on the process and function of the therapy being used, the counseling techniques could be generically classified as supportive counseling that provide support, guidance, advice, and reassurance (e.g., guidance, milieu therapy); re-educational counseling that attempts to teach individuals new patterns of behavior and social functioning (e.g., cognitive therapy and behavior therapy) as well as reconstructive counseling that aims to dismantle and rebuild a new personality (e.g., psychoanalysis and psychodynamic therapy). More details about these forms of counseling are summarized in **Table 19.4.1**. Counselors in the primary care settings, more frequently and effectively, use supportive psychotherapy than re-educational or reconstructive therapies as they need extensive training.

Preventive Counseling

Commonly, preventive counseling is provided for health-related concerns associated with lifestyle issues (e.g., obesity, nutrition, and reproductive health) and substance abuse in primary care pediatric settings. Unfortunately, even when adolescents visit physicians, valuable opportunities for prevention are missed in >50% of routine visits. It is partly, because the recommendations for screening and prevention are clear for adults and children, but are less clear for adolescents. The broad categories for which preventive counseling can be given from a mental health perspective are for adolescents who go through normative crises and who have significant life events or accumulation of daily hassles.[4]

Normative Crises

Normative crises happen as a part of the adolescent constructing oneself. Resolving this identity crisis successfully during the separation-individuation process gives the adolescent a coherent, purposeful sense of self. However, during this process of psychosocial growth while attempting autonomy and separation from his or her family of origin, the individual problems of identity confusion, lack of self-esteem, problems with group and peer identity, troubles with gender identity, difficulties in organizing daily tasks, and strained and disconnected family relationships can happen among other problems. The core issues in counseling normative crises of adolescence, using supportive principles, are summarized in **Table 19.4.2**.

Life Events

Life events, such as domiciliary violence, parental death or separation, teenage pregnancy, serious illness requiring hospitalization, and relationship problems, have been reported among adolescents in India and often had been associated with suicidal behaviors.[5] They often unsettle the homeostatic mechanisms in the adolescent and his family. These adolescents need supportive counseling addressing the adjustment difficulty because of the changed life situation in addition to appropriately using crises intervention to resolve the crises. The basic techniques of crisis intervention are summarized in **Table 19.4.2**.

Therapeutic Counseling

Indications for Psychotherapy in Primary Care

Knowledge of the indications of therapeutic counseling, in treating the emotional problems and psychiatric illness, is essential for offering adolescents with counseling options.[6] The basic indications include those circumstances where the only intervention available is nonpharmacological (e.g., dissociative and somatoform disorders and attachment disorders). When an adolescent presents with stress-related physical symptoms or worsening of physical illness (e.g.,

TABLE 19.4.1: Classification of counseling—based on its therapeutic process.

Types	*Function*	*Examples*	*Indications*
Reconstructive therapies	Gives insights by focusing on psychological mechanisms, unlearning and relearning healthy relationships, behavior, and handling of emotions	• Psychoanalysis • Psychodynamic counseling	Personality disorders
Re-educative therapies	Emphasize on teaching alternative techniques that are often problem specific	• Behavioral therapy • Cognitive therapy • Interpersonal • Family therapy • Play therapy	• Anxiety disorders • Depressive disorder • Conduct disorder
Supportive therapies	Relief from the immediate crisis and removal of symptoms to premorbid levels using adolescents' own emotional, intellectual, and social skills	• Crisis intervention • Grief support	• Suicidal attempt • Grief

TABLE 19.4.2: Preventive counseling for normative crises and life events.[5]

Indication	Focus of counseling	General principles in crisis management
Normative crises	• Accepting one's body as it is and using the body effectively • Help form new and more mature relationship with age- mates of both sexes • Achieve gender appropriate social role • Achieve emotional independence from parents and other adults • Prepare oneself to have economic independence through an enjoyable and productive career, prepare for marriage and family life • Help to desire for and achieve socially responsible behavior • Assist to acquire a set of values and ethical system and develop an ideology as a guide to one's behavior	• Be nonjudgmental • Treat the adolescent's problems seriously and take all threats seriously • Do not try to talk the person out of it • Ask direct questions, such as "Have you been thinking of killing yourself?" • Communicate your concern and support, offer yourself as a caring listener until professional help can be arranged (e.g. in the case of imminent suicide) • Try to evaluate the seriousness of the risk in order to make the appropriate referral to a mental healthcare professional • Do not swear to secrecy, especially when there is a threat of suicide or homicide • Do not leave the person alone, if you feel the threat is immediate
Life events	• Help adolescent to realize the maladaptive response to the crisis (e.g. suicidal behavior for failing in board exam) • Assist one in crisis to identify the steps that lead to the crisis, identify the alternate steps that will not end in a crisis (e.g. failure in board exam) • Special attention on identifying the first step in the pathway that leads to the crisis and changes to the adaptive pathway, termination of counseling	

worsening of asthma or diabetes with stress), counseling is required. When psychotropic medications are expected to interact with prescribed medication(s), and therefore, they have to be avoided, if intolerance for psychotropic adverse effects is noted or when potentiating of the psychotropic is required with combined interventions (e.g., psychotherapy for refractory symptoms in depression or for obsessive compulsive disorder), counseling has a significant role in minimizing or eliminating the symptoms among adolescents.

Counseling for adolescents is prescribed when there is a high risk of deliberate self-harm (e.g., potential to overdose on psychotropic medication as with tricyclic antidepressants), medication abuse (e.g., prescription medications, such as psychostimulants being misused), and to improve treatment compliance or the illness has been controlled but the impairment of the illness persists in the patient (e.g., depression is treated with antidepressant but the child has school refusal as an impairment of the mood disorder). Therapeutic counseling for priority mental health disorders of adolescents recommended by the World Health Organization is presented in **Table 19.4.3**.[4]

RELATIONSHIP COUNSELING

Counseling as a collaborative effort between the counselor and client, aims at identifying goals and potential solution to problems which causes emotional conflicts in a human relationship. What bothers parents most often, rightly or wrongly is premature boy-girl relationship that had always been there, but parents take it too seriously.[7] A boy-girl relationship follows certain laws—"laws of attraction", "laws of difference", and "laws of self-image" that cannot be wished away. Relationship counseling not only aims at identifying the problems but also provides insight into the type of relationship between boys and girls some beneficial in the academic context, yet some harmful.[7] Based on this knowledge and years of experience, a counselor can seek to improve in their client, communication, and coping skills, strengthen self-esteem, and promote behavioral changes that in turn help develop strong interpersonal relationships that are mutually beneficial. The boys and girls coming in contact with the counsellor in the school or college need to be empowered on the following points:

- Boy-girl relationship can be of multiple types, and these have their own set of relationship issues.
- *Boy-girl relationship follows certain laws*: "Laws of attraction, difference, and self-image".
- Healthy boy-girl relationship is formed on the grounds of honesty, compassion, finding right balance, talking openly, and having mutual respect.
- Human relationship counseling model follows Roger's client-centered approach, where the client forms the core part of therapy process.

TABLE 19.4.3: Therapeutic counseling for priority mental health disorders of adolescents as recommended by the World Health Organization (WHO)*.[4]

Disorders	Treatment modality as recommended by WHO					
	Family therapy	School intervention	Counseling	Specialized interventions	Others	CBT
LD	–	–	Yes	Yes	–	Yes
ADHD	Yes	–	Yes	–	–	–
Tics	Yes	Yes	–	–	–	–
Depression	Yes	Yes	–	–	–	–
Psychoses	–	Yes	Yes	–	Yes	–
Schizophrenia	–	Yes	–	–	–	–

Note: *Because of the propensity of the illnesses of childhood to progress into adolescence, nonpharmacological intervention strategies for childhood disorders have also been included.
(ADHD: attention-deficit hyperactivity disorder; CBT: cognitive behavioral techniques; LD: learning disability)

- Physical relationship before marriage can affect postmarriage relationship.

CONCLUSION

Psychotherapy has a principled tradition and a theoretical basis for their use. A number of techniques of proven effectiveness are available for helping adolescents with their normative crises, life event provoked difficulties, or mental illnesses. Primary care pediatricians should be able to include simple counseling strategies in their therapeutic options for adolescents with mental health needs.

Existing literature readily supports to the evidence that various forms of counseling strategies are effective among adolescents with mental health needs. However, it should be noted that many of the current effectiveness evidence are a generalization of findings from the adult or childhood studies. It also seems that these therapies are acceptable and feasible in the primary care settings in different cultural contexts.

REFERENCES

1. Neinstein LS. Adolescent Health Care: A Practical Guide, 4th edition. Philadelphia, PA: Lippincott Williams and Wilkins; 2002. pp. 11-7.
2. Russell PS, Nair MK. Strengthening the Pediatricians Project 1: The need, content and process of a workshop to address the priority mental health disorders of adolescence in countries with low human resource for health. Asia Pac Fam Med. 2010;9(1):4.
3. Russell PS, Nair MK. Strengthening the Pediatricians Project 2: The effectiveness of a workshop to address the priority mental health disorders of adolescence in low-health related human resource countries. Asia Pac Fam Med. 2010;9(1):3.
4. Russell S, Russell PS, Kaur MS, Nair MK, Darlin D. Priority mental health disorders of children and adolescents in primary-care pediatric settings in India 3: psychotherapy and other non- pharmacological interventions. Indian J Pediatr. 2012;79(Suppl 1):S33-8.
5. Russell S, Subramanian B, Russell PS, Nair MK. Psychopathology, traumatic life events, and coping skills among patients attending a primary-care adolescent clinic. Indian J Pediatr. 2012;79(Suppl 1):S52-9.
6. Russell S, Subramanian B, Russell PS. Psychopathology and functional impairment among patients attending an adolescent health clinic: Implications for healthcare model reform. Osteopath Med Prim Care. 2008;2:3.
7. Nair MKC, Kumar S, Lukose R. Relationship Counselling. Indian J Practical Pediatr. 2021;23(2):200-3.

19.5 Adolescent Mental Health

Paul SS Russell, MKC Nair

INTRODUCTION

At present, we have the largest adolescent generation ever in the human history. Noncommunicable diseases among adolescents and mental health illnesses, in particular, have been documented to result in high levels of medical, social, and economic burden. Most of the adult mental health disorders have their onset during their childhood or adolescence. In the low- and middle-income countries, including India, with paucity as well as skewed distribution of resources for health, adolescents with mental health needs become doubly disadvantaged and often remain or perilously drift outside the safety of any healthcare system.[1] An effective way to address the resource paucity is by enhancing the primary care pediatrician (PCP) in the recognition, treatment, and when needed, referral of the adolescents to mental health specialists. This section will, therefore, brief the reader on the clinical skills of diagnosis, medical management, and referral protocols for the priority mental health disorders (PMHD) in PCP settings.

PRIORITY MENTAL HEALTH DISORDERS

Mental and behavioral disorders are common among adolescents in the community and in primary healthcare settings. Among the plethora of mental health illnesses, the adolescents present with, the World Health Organization (WHO) has suggested the gatekeeping physicians to apply their resources, on a group of illnesses identified as the PMHD.[2,3] PMHDs have been targeted for identification and intervention based on their higher prevalence, propensity to progress into adulthood, enduring impairment and therapeutic potentials in the primary care settings. Although during adolescence, WHO suggests to address depression and attempted suicide, as psychiatric disorders of childhood onset having a continuous course and will often continue into adolescence, other disorders, such as autism and attention-deficit hyperactivity disorder, will also have to be addressed but in decreasing priority.[3] The epidemiology and their intervention strategies are mentioned in **Table 19.5.1**.[4,5]

DIAGNOSTIC PRACTICE

Missed diagnosis and misdiagnosis often result in failure to involve adolescents in treatment and poor follow-up care. These diagnostic difficulties by PCP can be minimized in several ways.[6,7] Firstly, it is important to maintain a high index of suspicion for PMHD, which are widely prevalent in primary care settings. Secondly, the PCP should be enabled to clinically recognize the common overt, and if possible, the covert symptom presentations of PMHD. Thirdly, training the pediatrician in using a two-tier diagnostic approach might lessen the diagnostic errors. As an initial approach, the PCP should administer a general psychiatric screening questionnaires (self, parent, or clinician rated) routinely, or certainly, when a mental health need is suspected. The use of screening instruments has been documented to improve the case identification among those who are suffering from mental disorders, and clinicians support the use of screening instruments, as they are usually brief and easy-to-use in busy primary care practice. As using only brief screening measures can result in both under- or over-recognition of the PMHD, it is a good practice to confirm the potential mental illness with diagnostic clinical criteria.[8]

TABLE 19.5.1: The epidemiology and management of priority mental health disorders.[3-5]

Stage	*PMHD*	*Prevalence*	*Medication*	*Nonpharmacological*
Adolescence	Depression	0.1	Yes	Yes
	Psychoses*	–	Yes	Yes
	Mania*	–	Yes	Yes
	Conduct disorder	1.1	Yes	Yes
	OB syndromes*	–	Yes	Yes
Childhood	Tic	0.2	Yes	Yes
	Enuresis	6.2	Yes	Yes
	Anxiety disorder	4.1	Yes	Yes
Toddler	ID	2.3	No†	Yes
	Autism		No†	Yes
	ADHD	1.7	Yes	Yes

*No recent epidemiological data from India is available.
†Medication is prescribed only for targeted symptoms.
(ADHD: attention-deficit hyperactivity disorder; ID: intellectual disability; OB: organic brain; PMHD: priority mental health disorders)

Among the screening measures available, the most favored instruments for use in primary care settings are pediatric symptom checklist, the child and adolescent psychiatric screen, and child behavior checklist. It should, however, be noted that none of the above or other measures (scales, inventories, and questionnaires) in the mental health field is diagnostic in nature, and only the clinical diagnostic criteria [e.g. International Classification of Diseases and Diagnostic and Statistical Manual of Mental Disorders (DSM) systems] supported with extensive field trials have the diagnostic accuracy, reliability, and validity characteristics to act as diagnostic tools.

For the confirmatory assessment, using the DSM fifth edition (DSM 5) is recommended. The difficulty in using these clinical criteria is that it needs an extensive degree of training to achieve high interrater reliability in diagnosing adolescent psychiatric disorders, and hence, in primary care settings, untrained PCP may attain only low interrater reliability. But if DSM 5 can be used effectively, with training for PCP during their pediatric training or with follow-up workshops, then the advantages are the ability to confirm the primary diagnosis, identify comorbidities (as presence of comorbidity is a rule than an exception in child and adolescent psychiatry), quantify the impairments (in the areas of education, peers, and home), and recognize the unhealthy psychosocial situations (such as unstable family background) to help formulate a multiaxial treatment approach, the norm in treating adolescent mental health issues. The various characteristics of these screening and confirmatory measures are summarized in **Table 19.5.2**.

MEDICATION USE

All PMHDs, except the developmental disabilities (such as intellectual disability and autism), need pharmacological treatment and can be effectively treated in the primary care setting. However, even adolescents with developmental disabilities will require medications if medication-responsive symptom (such as self-injurious behaviors or stereotypic movements) is documented or a superimposed mental illness is diagnosed. The PCP can effectively treat all PMHDs with a thorough knowledge in using five psychotropic medications at the appropriate dose and dosing schedules **(Table 19.5.3)**. Best psychopharmacologic treatment in this population requires an appreciation that adolescents have an increased disposition to comorbidities, awareness of pharmacokinetic and pharmacodynamic aspects of specific medications and medication classes, in particular the elimination half-life, developmental considerations, drug interactions, and adverse effects. In this context, it should also be noted that many of the psychotropic drugs prescribed for adolescents have not been tested for their use in well-controlled trials. Instead, from the evidences available with adults, a weight-based dosing is used to estimate the necessary dosage in this population.

REFERRAL PATTERN

Majority of the mental health problems are managed in primary care, and only a handful of adolescents are referred to expert mental healthcare providers. However, not all cases of PMHD are suited for treatment in a primary care setting, and the PCP should be aware of the indications to refer an adolescent to a specialist adolescent psychiatric care.

If there is poor response to pharmacotherapy or failure to attain remission status (such as in refractory depression), or a rapidly deteriorating clinical picture, then the adolescents need to be referred to a specialist setting. Adolescents with comorbidities that significantly complicate treatment with the need for a complex regimen (such as depression with substance abuse) or multiple medications (such as depression with catatonic symptoms), disorders that require high doses of psychotropic medication (such as acute psychosis), and

TABLE 19.5.2: Screening and confirmatory instruments for priority mental health disorders.

Screening measures	***Number of PMHD addressed***	***Brevity***	***Age***	***Availability***	***Psychometric properties***
PSC	Not specific	35 items; 5–10 min	6–16 years	Available free of cost in public domain	Strong
CAPS	10/11 disorders except attachment disorders	85 items; 15–20 min	3–21 years	Available free of cost in public domain	Published data could not be located
CBCL	5/11 disorders	96 items; 15–20 min	5–14 years	Has to be purchased	Strong
Confirmatory measure	Number of PMHD addressed	Brevity	Age	Availability	Psychometric properties
ICD-10	All PMHD	Reference criteria	All ages	Has to be purchased	Strong
DSM-PC	All PMHD	Reference criteria	All ages	Has to be purchased	Strong

(CAPS: child and adolescent psychiatric screen; CBCL: child behavior checklist; DSM-PC: diagnostic and statistical manual for primary care; ICD-10: International Classification of Diseases-10; PMHD: priority mental health disorders; PSC: pediatric symptom checklist)

TABLE 19.5.3: Pharmacological treatment for the priority mental health disorders in primary-care pediatric setting.

Stages	*Disorders*	*Medications*	*Doses/day*	*Dosing/day*
Adolescence	Depression	Fluoxetine	10–20 mg	OD (breakfast)
	Psychoses	Risperidone	2–4 mg	OD–TID
	Mania	Risperidone ± sodium valproate	2–4 mg 20 mg/kg	OD–TID OD (dinner)
	Conduct disorder	Sodium valproate	20 mg/kg	OD (dinner)
	OB syndromes	Risperidone	0.25–1 mg	OD–TID
Childhood	Tic	Risperidone	0.25–2 mg	OD (dinner)
	Enuresis*	Imipramine/Vasopressin	According to the drug and route	OD (dinner)
	Anxiety disorder	Fluoxetine	10–40 mg	OD (breakfast)
Toddler	Autism	Risperidone	0.25–1 mg	OD–BD
	ADHD	Atomoxetine	1.2–1.8 mg/kg	OD–BD (breakfast, lunch)

*Enuresis is not a PMHD, but it is added in this schedule because of its high prevalence in primary-care settings.
(ADHD: attention-deficit hyperactivity disorder; BW: body weight; OB: organic brain; OD: one day; OD–BD: one day–twice a day; OD–TID: one day–three times a day)

treatment that can result in significant side effects (such as monoamine oxidase inhibitors) should be referred. When the patient requires specialized psychotherapy as the only modality of treatment (such as conflict resolution in dissociative disorder) and when the adolescent needs a strong component of adjuvant psychotherapy (such as exposure and response prevention in obsessive compulsive disorder) or formal family support (such as empowering parents for conduct disorder), an appropriate referral is needed. Psychiatric disorders with significant impairment (such as school or occupational impairment), atypical presentation (such as atypical depression), cases with diagnostic uncertainties (such as the overactivity disorder with stereotypic movements), multiple axis I or multiaxial comorbidities, primary care treatment failure in the past, those who had been in contact with specialist mental health care, need of mental health referral of parent, patients with homicidal or suicidal risk, adolescents with serious abuse, inability to maintain self-care or survival skill, and polysubstance abuse need referral to specialist adolescent psychiatric care.

In addition, it is known that despite the appropriate referral, many families are not effectively engaged in mental health services. To minimize this therapy attrition along the referral pathway, prior to the referral, the PCP has to, first, establish a good working relationship with a psychiatrist knowledgeable in current psychiatric diagnosis and pediatric psychopharmacology, and second, prepare the adolescent and his family to visit the mental health expert in a collaborative manner.

SELF-COUNSELING

With the increase in mental health conditions in the post-COVID era and with the limited availability of trained physicians to deal with it, self-counseling has been thought off as an effective method to help candidates with mild issues. Self-counseling helps to analyze oneself, allowing one to take control of oneself; self-evaluate and rediscover oneself. The theoretical basis for self-counseling essentially involves the basic processes of counseling. However, the prerequisite for an effective self-counseling includes self-awareness, self-motivation, and self-screening. A successful self-counseling session needs finding strength in not just oneself but also the support system which may include the family and/or friends.

Self-counseling is the process of examining one's own behavior, using psychoanalytical methods of free-thinking and free association.[9] Self-counseling can help one take more effective control of everyday situations and enable to make continued progress or personal growth. Self-counseling takes you on a journey of self-discovery. You work at your own pace and in the directions, you most feel comfortable with. Self-counseling may be considered as an alternative to a counseling relationship with a counsellor. The only difference is that in self-counseling, relationship is with one's inner self. Thus, the concept behind self-counseling is to bring out the better of oneself, every time you assess yourself, meaning you should be better than your "past-self." Overall, self-counseling is an effective method of exploring how one's mind works and how it behaves in varied situations. However, some problems may be too deep-seated for self-counseling, and these may require additional forms of therapy.

TEN PRINCIPLES OF SELF-COUNSELING

1. Do not bluff to yourself, though you may have to bluff to others sometimes for survival.
2. You are not God and likely to make mistakes; hence, take precaution always.

3. Do not think that others have to like you always, instead learn "self-love."
4. *Caring and not love*: Love can fade, but not caring with affection.
5. *Refuse to take insult*: Feeling pathway for only 30 seconds; shift to cognitive pathway—see reason.
6. Do not keep grudge; it only eats you up emotionally.
7. Disarm your perceived enemy by caring when they really need.
8. Don't think others are lesser than you, as you are also lesser than someone else.
9. *Think of other person's point of view*: Be a third party when analyzing yourself.
10. Take the pledge "I am the custodian of my mind, body and spirit—I will protect, preserve and enhance it."

CONCLUSION

Priority mental health disorders affect a substantial number of adolescents. Making an accurate diagnosis, using appropriate psychotropic medications and proper referral when required, is an important part of the clinical practice of PCPs, well supported by ten principles of self-counseling.

REFERENCES

1. Nair MKC, Russell PS. Adolescent health care in India: progressive, regressive or at the cross-roads? Indian J Pediatr. 2012;79(Suppl 1):S1-5.
2. Patel V, Flisher AJ, Hetrick S, McGorry P. Mental health of young people: a global public-health challenge. Lancet. 2007;369:1302-13.
3. World Health Organization. Caring for children and adolescents with mental disorders. Geneva: World Health Organization; 2003.
4. Russell S, Russell PS, Kaur MS, Nair MK, Darilin D. Priority mental health disorders of children and adolescents in primary-care pediatric settings in India 3: psychotherapy and other non- pharmacological interventions. Indian J Pediatr. 2012;79:S33-8.
5. Srinath S, Girimaji SC, Gururaj G, Seshadri S, Subbakrishna DK, Bhola P, et al. Epidemiological study of child and adolescent psychiatric disorders in urban and rural areas of Bangalore, India. Indian J Med Res. 2005;122(1):67-79.
6. Russell PS, Mammen P, Nair MKC, Minju KA. Priority mental health disorders of children and adolescents in primary-care pediatric setting in India 1: developing a child and adolescent mental health policy, program, and service model. Indian J Pediatr. 2012;79(Suppl 1):S19-26.
7. Russell PS, Nair MKC, Mammen P, Shankar SR. Priority mental health disorders of children and adolescents in primary-care pediatric settings in India 2: diagnosis, pharmacological treatment and referral. Indian J Pediatr. 2012;79(Suppl 1):S27-32.
8. Russell PS, Tsheringla S, Nair MKC, Minju KA. Priority mental health disorders of children and adolescents in primary-care pediatric settings in India 4: training and capacity building. Indian J Pediatr. 2012;79:S39-44.
9. Nair MKC, Kumar S, Lukose R, Girish CS, Binod D, Sreejith S. Self-counselling. Pediatr Companion 2022;1:16-20.

19.6 Adolescent Sexuality

MKC Nair

INTRODUCTION

As per the global and Indian scenario; children between 0 and 14 years constitute 25%, adolescents and young adults between 10 and 24 years constitute 24%, and those between 10 and 19 years constitute 16% of the world population, as of 2022.[1] Our children and young adults have specific sexual reproductive health (SRH) needs. A few studies that have examined the sexual knowledge and attitude of the Indian youth found that sexual knowledge is limited and that most hold a conservative attitude toward sexuality.[2] This poor knowledge and attitude reflect among youth as high-risk sexual behaviors and practices.

SEX VERSUS GENDER

Sex is physiological differences among male, female, and intersex bodies. Biological sex is conceptualized primarily as binary—male and female, though nowadays the third sex has become equally important. Sex is determined at birth by chromosomes, gonads, hormones, external genitalia, and secondary sex characteristics. On the other hand, gender is behavioral, social or cultural distinctions associated with being male, female, or indeterminate gender. Most civil societies try to bring their children to binary gender similar to sex through even corrective methods.[3] Gender is a social construct having links to emotional frame of the individual and exists within cultural and societal norms. Gender identity is a person's sense of self with some peculiarities and commonalities in perception, thoughts, expression, and enjoyments in day-to-day living.

HUMAN SEXUALITY

Sexuality encompasses the whole range of thoughts, feelings, fantasies, emotions, desires, and language along with action, as special behavior is only a part of it.[4] Thus, sexuality is an integrated part of every individual's personality and includes men, women as well as children. There is an energy that drives us to seek out love, contact and warmth, closeness that is expressed in our way to feel and to awake feelings as well as contact with each other. Our sexuality is expressed in the way we dress, the way we walk, and relate to people. It makes us feel alive and good about ourselves. Hence, sexual behavior is only a part of the whole sexuality of an individual.

The concepts pertaining to the development of human sexuality may need to address many theoretical foundations including:

- Theoretical underpinnings, based on Darwin's theory of sexual selection and transitions from a potential chimpanzee-like ancestor to the long-term bonded sociosexual partnerships,
- New findings in biology and genetics, e.g., comparative methods to identify signs of selection in phenotypes related to sexuality and investigations of human neuroendocrine reactions to sexual stimuli,
- Reviewing a few of the most comprehensive, large-scale, and contemporary research on human sexuality, e.g., perceptions regarding sexual conduct on the internet and in other country samples, and
- Taking a life course perspective—people are sexual beings from conception to death, despite the fact that this manifests itself differently at each stage of life.

CONCEPTS IN SEXUALITY

Sexual behavior of people finds many expressions, and it seems extremely difficult to classify behavior as normal or abnormal. However, it can be said that sexual behavior is inappropriate when it is uncomfortable for the other person and has the intention of doing harm either physically or psychologically on self or others. Socialization and related processes may be quite influenced by the norms surrounding sexuality in the society. Those who were fortunate to have a healthy childhood environment do not consider sex as sin, do not approach it with guilt, or go through it as a traumatic experience but will only have positive concepts about sexuality. Sexual right is the freedom to be enjoyed by an individual to decide without any compulsion, when, where, how, and with whom sexual acts are to be performed or not.

DIMENSIONS OF SEXUALITY

We often tend to forget that sexuality has eight other dimensions apart from physical, yet we often focus only on the physical dimension. Dimensions of sexuality that could be related to Maslow's hierarchy of needs theory as follows:

- *Physical:* The biological need to be satisfied as per age.
- *Legal:* Need for safety and security in both private and public space.
- *Romantic:* Need for love and belonging to give as well as to take.
- *Social/cultural:* Need for acceptance by others in a positive way.
- *Aesthetic:* Need for development of self-esteem at home/at work
- *Emotional:* Need for caring and affection and not "superficial love"
- *Existential:* Need for self-awareness, self-understanding, and self-counseling
- *Psychological:* Need for self-actualization to realize fully one's potential
- *Spiritual:* Need for transcendence—motivated by values going beyond personal self

DEVELOPMENT OF SEXUALITY

Sexuality Concepts in Boys versus Girls

Boys and girls develop gender-based differences in their sexual selves. Men are often bombarded with sexual information from childhood. Society's view that men are sexual by nature is in contrast with a women's sense of herself, in which her sexuality is usually kept private even from her partner, many a times.

Puberty

Puberty is the stage of physical maturation in which an individual becomes physiologically capable of sexual reproduction. The biological changes that occur during puberty are mainly indicated by the development of the sexual characteristics. Secondary sexual development in girls involves the enlargement of the ovaries, uterus, vagina, labia, breasts, and growth of pubic hair. Secondary sexual development in boys involves the enlargements of the testes, penis, and growth of pubic hair. Reassurance that the sexual development is normal; enhances body image, self-esteem, and self-confidence.

Concept of Virginity

The concept of virginity is an emotional issue with a lot of gender bias and an obsession for an intact female hymen. Hence, one's viewpoint may not be acceptable to all. A person who has never undergone sexual intercourse is considered a virgin, male or female. The customs and traditions of our society consider marriage as a religious ceremony conducted invoking blessings of God. To be or not to be a virgin is a personal choice, but the concept of keeping oneself for the one and only one person in your life can be a pleasant decision. However much the younger generation may want to disagree, it is a fact that we tend to get more emotionally attached to the first person with whom we have physical or sexual relationship, but it is your personal choice.

Female virginity is counted unnecessarily as the presence of a thin-skin membrane in the outer vagina, the hymen. But, there are situations in which this skin can be destroyed by heavy works, athletes, cyclists, dancers, vigorous exercises, swimming, bicycling, horse riding, use of tampons, menstrual cup, or introduction of objects into the vagina for self-stimulation.

Functions of Sexual Relation

- *Procreative:* Rewarding for those who want to have children.
- *Recreative:* Sexual pleasure, orgasm (physical), ecstasy (mental), and fulfillment (spiritual).
- *Relational:* Ensures a rewarding life-long partner relationship based on mutual respect.

Sex is not just a means of procreation, sex, after all is the art of enhancing love. Human sexual arousal is a primitive physiological response that cannot be consciously willed. Every partner may have different preferences from time-to-time. Good sex involves finding out what the partner wants to happen before, during, and after love making.

Genital Response

The biological function of the genital response in the male and female is to enable entry of the penis into vagina, with the consequent deposition of semen in the vagina.

- *Genital response in boys:* In the male, the principal response is erection of the penis, due to filling of the erectile tissue with blood. In addition to penile erection, the testes become somewhat enlarged, and the walls of the scrotum becomes thicker and tighter.
- *Genital response in girl:* In the female, the principal response is vaginal. The lining of the vagina is normally moist. This results in part from fluid from the uterus and mucus secretion from the cervix as well as from the vaginal wall. The cervical fluid varies in amount and consistency through the ovarian cycle, i.e., close to ovulation; there is marked increase in volume and has water consistency. This facilitates entry of the sperm from the vagina to uterus. Without sexual stimulation, the vagina is not sufficiently lubricated for comfortable entry of an erect penis. It is generally assumed that the sole function of the clitoris is to provide sexual pleasure for the woman as it contains large number of nerve endings.

SEXUALITY EDUCATION

Sexuality education, better termed "family life education", is important at all ages. It is more important if it is imparted during childhood and adolescence, but in a graded fashion and appropriate to the age. Many parents feel that knowing too much may lead to sexual misbehavior on the part of the youngsters. But, this is not true. Studies have shown that by offering sex education and correct scientific information, premature involvement in sex has been delayed as discussing the subject satiates curiosity and removes the compulsive motive to experiment. On the other hand, ignorant children are more prone to sexual abuse and sex-related crimes and teenage pregnancy risk.[5] Sex education should be targeted at individuals in the highest risk group, i.e., pubertal, prepubertal, and young adults. But before attempting to do so, we need to understand adolescent sexuality.

Sexuality education programs are typically aimed to the age and developmental stage of the adolescents. Younger children receive age-appropriate information about body parts and personal boundaries, while older adolescents also should receive more in-depth detailed age-appropriate information about sexual health, boundaries in relationships, and contraception, sexually transmitted infections (STIs), etc. Comprehensive sexuality education package can include a wide range of topics, such as basic structural and developmental anatomy of reproductive organs, reproductive health and hygiene, puberty and sexual development, setting relationships boundaries, significance of communication and consent, development of value system, safe and consensual sexual behaviors, secondary sexual characteristics, pregnancy and childbirth, complications of early/teenage pregnancy and delivery, contraception and STIs, sexual orientation and gender identity, sexual harassment and violence, and legal and ethical considerations related to sexuality [Protection of Children from Sexual Offences (POCSO)].[5]

Components of Adolescent Sexuality Education

- *Providing parental support and guidance:* Some programs encourage open communication between parents or caregivers and their children regarding sexuality education. They provide resources and guidance for parents to discuss these topics with their children. The parental concerns and consent are also important. Parents need to take effort to make them understand what constitutes a healthy and respectful relationship.
- *Abstinence and safer sex:* Education about abstinence (not engaging in sexual activity) is often included, along with information about safer sex practices for those who do choose to engage in sexual activity and its consequences.
- *Awareness on resources:* It should provide information about where to access healthcare services, contraception,

and counseling concerns, if needed. They must know this as where, who, when, how, why, should I contact, and importance and pattern of health checkup.

- *Cultural, legal, and ethical considerations:* Sexuality education should be sensitive to cultural and religious beliefs and practices, while still providing accurate information. The legal aspects of adolescent sexual activity, including age of consent and laws regarding sexual harassment etc. need to be discussed with them.
- *Media influence in behavior and attitude of teenagers:* Concerns around how young people are exposed to sexual content on television and in other electronic media, and how this may affect their attitudes, beliefs, and behaviors around sexuality, are becoming more and more prevalent. Teenagers may be exposed to sexual content in the media at a time when their sexual views, behaviors, and gender roles are still evolving.[6]
- *Neosexual revolution:* While the old sexuality was based primarily upon sexual instinct, orgasm, and the heterosexual couple, neosexualities revolve predominantly around gender difference, thrills, self-gratification, and prosthetic substitution. "Lean sexuality" and "self-sex" are two terms used to characterize the results of the neosexual revolution.
- *Priority on consent:* A key focus of sexuality education is teaching the importance of consent in sexual relationships and how to recognize and establish boundaries.
- *Respect for diverse gender identities:* A good sexuality education program respects and affirms the diversity of sexual orientations, gender identities, and cultural backgrounds.[7] It promotes acceptance and understanding of "LGBTIQA+", an evolving acronym that stands for;
    - *Lesbian:* A woman who is romantically, sexually, or emotionally attracted to other women.
    - *Gay:* Men who are romantically, sexually, or emotionally attracted to other men.
    - *Bisexual:* Are attracted to people of more than one gender both their own gender and other genders.
    - *Transgender:* A transgender person's gender identity differs from the sex assigned to them at birth.
    - *Intersex:* Intersex is a group of conditions in which there is a discrepancy between the external genitals and the internal organs, the testes, and ovaries. The older term hermaphroditism has now been replaced by disorders of sex development (DSDs).[8]
    - *Asexuality:* Is the lack of sexual/emotional attraction to others. Respect for each individual's self-identified gender and sexual orientation is a fundamental aspect of creating an inclusive and accepting society.
- *Premarital sex education:* Sex education focuses, largely though not exclusively, on self-awareness, personal relationships, human sexual development, reproduction, and sexual behavior.[3] Human sexuality is a function of the total personality, which includes reproductive system and processes, attitudes toward being a man or woman, and relationships among members of the same sex and the opposite sex. It embraces the biological, psychological, sociocultural, and ethical aspects of human sexual behavior.[7] It helps people to understand their sexuality learn to respect others as sexual beings, and to make responsible decisions about their behavior. Sex is considered to have an inseparable role in married life, and it makes the bond between the couple stronger and healthier. Sexual relationship involves respect, trust, and caring of partner perceiving the needs of the partner and feeling free to communicate desires and feelings.

CONCLUSION

Adolescent sexuality education is vital in fostering understanding of physical, emotional, and ethical aspects of relationships. It emphasizes critical topics such as abstinence, safer sex practices, consent, and respect for diverse gender identities and orientations. Providing comprehensive education on sexuality helps adolescents develop positive attitudes, make informed decisions, and understand cultural, legal, and ethical considerations better. Sex education can ensure a well-informed approach to sexual health and relationships, empowering young individuals for future challenges.

The Oath: I am the custodian of my mind, body, and spirit; I will protect, preserve, and enhance it—*MKC Nair*.

REFERENCES

1. United Nations Population Fund. (2024). World Population Dashboard. [online] Available from https://www.unfpa.org/data/world-population-dashboard. [Last accessed December, 2024].
2. Pal A, Shankar R, Ahmed SM, Malhotra N, Taneja N, Janardhanan R. A study on sexual behaviour and sexual knowledge among students of a private University of Delhi, NCR. Int J Sci Res. 2020;9(10):10-4.
3. Harikumar SK, Nair MKC. Sexuality in marriage counselling. In: Nair MKC, Leena ML, Russell PS (Eds). Premarital Health, 1st edition. Delhi: Noble Medical publishers; 2023. pp. 63.
4. Gray PB. Evolution and human sexuality. Am J Phys Anthropol. 2013;152 (Suppl 57):94-118.
5. Moni SA, Nair MKC, Devi RS. Pregnancy among unmarried adolescents and young adults. J Obstet Gynaecol India. 2013;63(1):49-54.
6. Gruber E, Grube JW. Adolescent sexuality and the media: a review of current knowledge and implications. West J Med. 2000;172(3):210-4.
7. Sigusch V. On cultural transformations of sexuality and gender in recent decades. Ger Med Sci. 200;2:Doc07.
8. MedlinePlus. (2024). Differences of sex development. [online] Available from https://medlineplus.gov/ency/article/001669.htm. [Last accessed December, 2024].

19.7 Common Health Problems in Adolescents

Sukanta Chatterjee

INTRODUCTION

Adolescence is the period of least physical health diseases in human life span. Mental health and social health issues become important. The significant amount of growth and developmental maturation in this period makes the adolescents vulnerable to growth and nutritional disorders. The development of sexual instinct with yet to complete self-protective mental maturation leads to unwanted pregnancy and sexually transmitted infections. Tendency to explore and adaptation of risk-taking behavior increase the incidence of accidents or unintentional injuries. Problem of social adaptation leads to intentional injuries, such as suicide attempts and homicide. Abuse of substance, such as smoking and consumption of alcohol, also starts at this age. Many controllable chronic diseases of adult life might be detected at this age, such as juvenile diabetes mellitus, bronchial asthma, epilepsy, and obesity. Acute infections of any system, although not specific for adolescents, commonly affect this population as well. This section deals with those health problems prevalent in adolescents excluding issues described in other sections, such as nutrition, sexuality, gynecology, mental health, and counseling.

Table 19.7.1 shows common adolescent problems presenting in a Teaching Medical College in Kolkata, India.

ACNE

Acne is a nodular cutaneous lesion consisting of multilobular sebaceous gland that drains its products into the follicular canal. More than 80% of adolescents and young adults are affected.[1]

Etiopathogenesis

Abnormal keratinization at the lower infundibulum of the hair follicle causes plugging of the follicular duct. This leads to impaction and distention of the duct giving rise to open or closed comedones. At puberty, sebum secretion is increased by androgenic stimulation. *Propionibacterium acnes* hydrolyze sebum and secrete proinflammatory and

TABLE 19.7.1: Patient profile of adolescent health clinic, Medical College Kolkata, 2023 (n = 1,247).

	Male			*Female (m/um = married/unmarried)*		
Name of the disease/problems	***10–14 years***	***15–19 years***	***Total***	***10–14 years***	***15–19 years***	***Total***
Menstrual problem *n* = 348/1,247 (27.9%)				198 um	116 um, 34 m	348
RTI/STI (10%)	24	5	29	46	48 um, 3 m	97
Skin problem (10.3%)	55	24	79	38	12	50
Anemia (8.1%)			35			67
Learning issues (11.1%)	62	17	79	41	19	60
Anxiety and depression (7.9%)			57			42
Behavior disorders (5.8%)			47			26
Growth problem (6.6%)			35			48
Seizure disorder (4%)			26			24
Asthma (3.8%)			27			21
Goiter (2%)			6			19
Vision problem (1.7%)			9			12
Autism (1%)			9			3
ADHD (0.7%)			6			3

(ADHD: attention-deficit hyperactivity disorder; RTI: reproductive tract infection; STI: sexually transmitted infection)

chemotactic factors to attract neutrophils, which release lysosomal enzymes leading to rupture of the follicles causing inflammatory papules, and pustules.

Clinical Features

Basic lesion of acne is comedone, which may be blackhead (open type) or whitehead (closed type). Subsequently, it may turn into papules, pustules, or cysts. Acne is distributed in areas having largest number of sebaceous glands, such as face, chest, back, and shoulder. It may be secondarily infected by scratching due to itch. Resolution after infection occurs with dyspigmentation and indented or hypertrophic scar.

Treatment

Topical treatment alone may be indicated for mild to moderate comedonal lesions, superficial inflammatory lesions either papular or pustular, and usually nonscarring lesions. Systemic treatment may be indicated in addition to local one for severe lesions with or without scarring or that in patients with persistent hyperpigmentation. Systemic treatment alone is needed in patients who are intolerant of topical treatment or in whom such treatment has failed. When antibiotics are used for the treatment of moderate-to-severe acne, it is recommended that topical therapy be used at the same time. Once a course of antibiotics is complete, patients should continue using topical treatments to manage their condition. Topical medications, such as retinoids and benzoyl peroxide may be combined with one another to create an effective treatment regimen. In addition, some female patients may see their acne improve with the use of oral contraceptives, which can be combined with other treatments.

The most commonly used treatment options are mentioned here.

Topical Therapy

- *Benzoyl peroxide:*
  - Benzoyl peroxide gel alone
  - Combination of benzoyl peroxide gel with erythromycin
  - Benzoyl peroxide gel along with sulfur
- *Antibiotics (topical):* Tetracycline, clindamycin, erythromycin, and meclocycline in the form of lotion, gel, or cream
- All-trans retinoic acid and salicylic acid are other options
- Sulfur and resorcinol are also used
- *Miscellaneous:* Astringents, soaps, and cleansers

Systemic Therapy

Most used are as follows:

- Oral antibiotics such as tetracycline, erythromycin, minocycline, and trimethoprim-sulfamethoxazole
- Isotretinoin—only prescribed when conventional anti-acne treatment with topical measures and systemic antibiotics fails. Because this medication carries a high risk of birth defects, females must take careful steps to prevent pregnancy while on isotretinoin.
  Hormonal treatments may include the oral contraceptives that exert their therapeutic effect by decreasing sebum production. Glucocorticoids will have anti-inflammatory action in addition to adrenal suppression of androgen production.
  Other tried options: Diet modification, controlled ultraviolet light exposure, superficial exfoliation, and carbon dioxide-acetone slush.

Surgical Therapy

It depends on the indications. Closed comedones may require content extraction; pustules and cysts may need drainage or excision of sinus tracts and cysts. Instillation of corticosteroids within the lesion may prevent scars. Cryotherapy and surgical repairs of scars are tried in selected cases.

During follow-up drug compliance, response to treatment and any adverse effect of therapy should decide the frequency of visit.

Approach to Treatment

General approach: An example of an initial approach to acne based upon the principles mentioned earlier is outlined here. Additional therapeutic options are reviewed in a table derived from the 2016 acne treatment guidelines from the American Academy of Dermatology.[2]

- *Comedonal (noninflammatory) acne:*
  - Topical retinoid (alternatives include azelaic acid and salicylic acid)
- *Mild papulopustular and mixed (comedonal and papulopustular) acne:*
  - Topical antimicrobial (e.g., benzoyl peroxide alone or benzoyl peroxide ± topical antibiotic) and topical retinoid

    or
  - Benzoyl peroxide and topical antibiotic (for patients who cannot tolerate a retinoid *or* who require a simplified treatment regimen)
- *Moderate papulopustular and mixed acne:*
  - Topical retinoid and oral antibiotic and topical benzoyl peroxide
- *Severe acne (e.g., nodular acne):*
  - Topical retinoid and oral antibiotic and topical benzoyl peroxide

    or
  - Oral isotretinoin monotherapy

The oral hormonal therapy is an alternative to oral antibiotic therapy in postmenarche females with moderate-to-severe acne. Consistent adherence to acne therapy is critical for achieving clinical improvement. When recommending topical therapy, the clinician should design a regimen that is feasible for the patient. This should involve a discussion with the patient to ensure that each component of the treatment regimen is acceptable to the patient. We typically design regimens that require the patient to treat no more than once or twice daily.

A sample regimen for a patient with mild inflammatory facial acne who is using a topical retinoid, topical benzoyl peroxide, and topical clindamycin is as follows:

- *Morning:* Wash face with a gentle facial cleanser. Apply a thin layer of a fixed-dose combination of benzoyl peroxide/clindamycin gel to the entire face (an alternative regimen could require the patient to wash the face with a benzoyl peroxide cleanser, followed by application of a thin layer of topical clindamycin to the entire face).
- *Night:* Wash face with a gentle facial cleanser. Apply a thin layer of the topical retinoid to the entire face. Some patients may prefer the use of fixed-dose combination of products to simplify treatment. However, the cost of such treatments may be higher than single-active ingredient agents.

The selection of the delivery system for topical acne medications also may help to improve the likelihood of adherence to treatment. The choice depends upon the patient's skin type (dry vs. oily) and preference. Some gels have a drying effect; patients with oily skin may prefer them. Creams and lotions tend to be moisturizing. Solutions are drying but they cover large areas more easily than other preparations, and foams are easy to apply to hair-bearing areas. Pledgets are single-use absorbent pads impregnated with medication. They are convenient to use and facilitate the spreading of medication over large areas.

Mild Acne

They are small papular lesions without cutaneous inflammatory erythema and tenderness. It is treated with topical agents, such as: (1) Topical antibiotics, e.g., clindamycin (1% solution, lotion, gel, foam; once or twice daily application), erythromycin (2% gel or liquid once daily), or sodium sulfacetamide; (2) benzoyl peroxide agents comedolytic and bactericidal (2.5%, 5%, 10% gel or wash once or twice daily), side effects are irritation and pigmentary changes. Combinations of topical antibiotic and benzoyl peroxide are available; (3) topical retinoids prevent follicular hyperkeratosis. It is the mainstay for the treatment of comedonal acne. Gels are better on oily skin but may cause irritation due to alcohol base. Lowest strength preparations should be used initially, increasing concentration, if comedones persist. Application on dry skin may avoid irritation and erythema. Small amount (pea size) is sufficient to cover the entire face and apply only once at night. Preparations available are: (i) Topical tretinoin, e.g., 0.025%, 0.05%, 0.1% cream, gel, or liquid and (ii) adapalene (0.1% gel or cream). Combinations of benzoyl peroxide + topical antibiotic and tretinoin are beneficial by synergistic action but they should be applied separately at different time of the day since benzoyl peroxide may deactivate tretinoin; and (4) other topical agents are salicylic acid: Comedolytic, found in many over the counter creams, washes, solutions or azelaic acid: Comedolytic, anti-inflammatory, and used twice daily for postinflammatory hyperpigmentation as 20% cream.

Moderate Acne

They are also known as inflammatory or nodular acne. It is treated with oral antibiotics to decrease inflammation and suppress *P. acnes* organisms. Oral dose of a tetracycline (250–500 mg twice daily), erythromycin (250–500 mg twice daily), doxycycline (100 mg once or twice daily), and minocycline (50–100 mg twice daily). All of them carry a risk of photosensitivity except erythromycin. Antibiotics should be used for a minimum of 5–8 weeks before progress is evaluated. All antibiotics carry a risk of vulvovaginal candidiasis and risk of decreased efficacy of birth control pill. Oral contraceptives, e.g., *Ortho-Tri-Cyclen*, may also be used.

Severe Nodulocystic Acne

This may be treated with isotretinoin (1 mg/kg/day orally, given as a 4–5-month course). Most important side effect involves teratogenicity.

Prevention

Diet and climate has little evidence to influence acne. Cleansing of skin is recommended. Greasy cosmetics and hair preparations should be avoided. Manipulation and squeezing of facial lesions leads to rupture of intact lesions and provokes a localized inflammatory reaction.

BREAST ENLARGEMENT

Breast enlargement as a small mass is often a presenting problem in preadolescents and also in boys during adolescence.[3] Girls and boys have the potential of full breast development by appropriate stimulation. Circulating estradiol along with that produced in the breast tissue by aromatase enzyme activity stimulates proliferation and differentiation of parenchymal epithelium. Fibrocystic changes and fibroadenoma are the most common masses. In girls, it might start as a unilateral swelling at the onset of puberty (thelarche) around 7 years of age. In boys,' benign breast enlargement or puberty gynecomastia is common and may last for 6 months to 2 years, but when it persists after achieving Tanner stage V, surgical opinion is recommended. Gynecomastia is palpable breast enlargement in boys beyond 2 cm around areola margin. Lipomastia is fatty tissue which is nonpalpable with flat surface of the hand. The breast mass should be palpated by gentle squeezing between thumb and forefinger. Clinical history must include onset and duration of gynecomastia, sexual development, substance abuse, and systemic disease. Detailed local examination is essential for any eccentric, heterogeneous mass, genitalia and testicular palpation, and systemic examination. Laboratory evaluations include ultrasonography (USG) testes, hormonal assay for testosterone, estradiol E_2, sex hormone-binding globulin, luteinizing hormone, follicle-stimulating hormone, thyroid-stimulating hormone, prolactin, human chorionic gonadotropin, alpha-fetoprotein, and liver and renal function tests.[4] Obesity and hereditary factor may be responsible for the gynecomastia due to increased aromatase activity. Differential diagnosis includes normal variant, recreational drug abuse, testicular malignancy, chronic renal failure, and Klinefelter's syndrome.

Treatment

Normal variant does not require any treatment except reassurance and follow-up. Breast mass should not be squeezed. Specific etiology as mentioned earlier needs to be managed appropriately.

NOCTURNAL ENURESIS

Definition

Involuntary voiding of urine at night after 4–6 years is called nocturnal enuresis. Incidence: It is seen in 5% of 10 years old. Male-to-female ratio is 3:2 with a spontaneous resolution of 15% per year.[5]

Etiology

It may be genetic, 15% in nonenuretic families, 44% and 77% when one or both parents, respectively, are enuretic. Stress, fear, insecurity, and psychological factors are common factors associated with it. Constipation, urinary tract infection (UTI) and worms, neurogenic bladder, and diabetes may contribute. Urinary tract anatomical anomaly is unlikely in the absence of daytime incontinence.

Diagnosis

Family history, primary or secondary enuresis, and presence of other medical conditions are noted, such as distended bladder or colon. Urinalysis and culture sensitivity are helpful investigations with renal USG and voiding cystourethrogram in the case of obstructive manifestations or previous UTI.

Treatment

Combined approach with supportive education, behavior modifications, and pharmacotherapy are important components of its treatment.

Supportive Education

- No punishment since bedwetting is not under conscious control.
- It is common and adolescents often get better of their own.
- Involve the adolescent in working toward a cure, praise for success, encouragement for lack of control and attach responsibility, such as change of bed clothes.
- Record keeping by calendar or star chart for success and lapse with agreed-on rewards for success.
- Bed-wetting alarm is good with 65–100% cure after 4–6 months.

Drugs

- Desmopressin (nasal spray or 0.2 mg tablet)—one spray in each nostril or one tablet at bedtime initially and may be increased to two sprays each nostril or three tablets. If successful, continue for 3–6 months and then taper. Success rate is 75% with high relapse.
- Imipramine (25–75 mg at bedtime) has high success rate but with possibility of relapse on discontinuation. Side effects are anxiety, dry mouth, and sleep disturbance.

CONCLUSION

Common physical health problems are discussed here although mental health issues outnumber physical health issues at this age group.

REFERENCES

1. Joseph G, Morelli JG. Acne. In: Kliegman RM, Behrman RE, Jenson HB, Stanton BF (Eds). Nelson Textbook of Pediatrics, 18th edition. Philadelphia, PA: Saunders, Elsevier; 2008. pp. 2759-64.
2. Zaenglein AL, Pathy AL, Schlosser BJ, Schlosser BJ, Alikhan A, Baldwin HE, et al. Guidelines of care for the management of acne vulgaris. J Am Acad Dermatol. 2016;74(5):945-73.
3. Limaye A. Gynecomastia. In: Desai MP, Menon PSN, Bhatia V (Eds). Pediatric Endocrine Disorders, 4th edition. Chennai: Orient Longman; 2022. pp. 170-5.
4. Xia Z, Ding N, Kang Y, Guan A, Wen J, Xuda Ma, et al. Is Breast Magnetic Resonance Imaging Superior to Sonography in Gynecomastia Evaluation and Surgery Planning. Aesthetic Plast Surg. 2023;47(5):1759-70.
5. Carlsen AR. Enuresis. In: Alario AJ, Brinkrant JD (Eds). Practical Guide to the Care of the Pediatric Patients, 2nd edition. Philadelphia, PA: Mosby, Elsevier; 2008. pp. 668-71.

19.8 Adolescent Gynecology

Suneeta Mittal

INTRODUCTION

The transition from childhood to adolescence in girls is marked by various changes in physiology. As the physiology changes and girls mature, various disorders may manifest which are unique for this age. It is imperative that one should have a clear idea of the common gynecological diseases that adolescent girls may encounter in the process of reaching adulthood.

EPIDEMIOLOGY

Girls and adolescents between 0 and 19 years make up almost 30% of worlds female population.[1] India has the largest population of adolescents aged 10–19 years in the world. Adolescents constitute about 22.8% of India's population and almost half of these are girls.

Adolescent gynecology is an emerging specialty, involving pediatrics, endocrinology, gynecology, pediatric surgery, dermatology, psychiatry, public health medicine, and genetics. The relatively common complaints in adolescents are dysmenorrhea, pelvic mass or pain, genital irritation, menstrual irregularities, and amenorrhea. There may be some uncommon etiologies, such as Müllerian anomalies, ovarian tumors, foreign bodies, labial hypertrophy, dermatopathies, genital ulcers, and imperforate hymen manifesting during adolescence. Common problems observed in an adolescent gynecology clinic, adolescent contraception, vaccination, and pregnancy are discussed here.

POLYCYSTIC OVARY SYNDROME

Definition

The Rotterdam criteria define polycystic ovary syndrome (PCOS) when two of the three primary features are present: Unexplained clinical or biochemical signs of hyperandrogenism, oligo-anovulation, and/or a polycystic ovaries on sonography.[2]

Prevalence

Prevalence of PCOS in Indian adolescents is 9.13%.[3] The pathogenesis is unknown; however, both genetic and environmental factors play a role, resulting in disordered gonadotropin release, dysregulated steroidogenesis, ovarian and adrenal hyperandrogenism, and hyperinsulinism. It is important to appreciate that PCOS is a syndrome, not a disease, reflecting multiple potential etiologies and variable clinical presentations. Adolescent girls with PCOS may present with hirsutism, menstrual irregularities, obesity, acne, and/or signs of insulin resistance (IR), such as acanthosis nigricans. There may be no evidence of clinical and biochemical hyperandrogenism; ovarian volume and morphology may be of limited use. Hyperandrogenism and IR are more severe in obese adolescents with PCOS. Adolescents who have irregular menstrual cycles have higher serum androgens than those who have regular menstrual cycles.

Treatment

Treatment of PCOS is symptomatic plus targets on correction of abnormal hormones. Early intervention, counseling, lifestyle changes, and weight management may be preferable as first line in adolescents, because it targets both menstrual dysfunction and long-term associated morbidity. The use of combined oral contraceptives (COCs) is recommended as first-line treatment for adolescents who suffer from the menstrual and cutaneous symptoms of PCOS.[4] Other therapeutic options for menstrual irregularities include progestin alone and the low-dose oral contraceptives containing estrogen and progesterone. The COCs containing drospirenone have a better outcome than with desogestrel containing pills. Adding spironolactone or cyproterone is sometimes required, if the hirsutism is severe. Metformin or myoinositol can be used in obese adolescents with PCOS as an adjunct to weight-control measures and to treat coexistent insulin-resistant metabolic abnormalities.

MENSTRUAL DISORDERS

Dysmenorrhea

Dysmenorrhea (33–67.2%) is common, and premenstrual syndrome (PMS) affects daily routine in 50–60% girls. If dysmenorrhea occurs early with menarche, Müllerian anomalies must be suspected. For primary dysmenorrhea, analgesics with fixed-dose combination of aceclofenac and drotaverine are a suitable, effective, and well-tolerated treatment option.

Menstrual Irregularity

Cycles are often irregular in the first few months after menarche. Most cases of abnormal uterine bleeding (AUB) in adolescents are caused by anovulatory cycles during the first 12–18 months after menarche, which is related to immaturity of the hypothalamic-pituitary-ovarian axis. Other common causes include pregnancy, infection, the irregular use of hormonal contraceptives, stress (psychogenic or exercise induced), bleeding disorders, and endocrine disorders (e.g., hypothyroidism and PCOS). Once pregnancy has been excluded, it is helpful to determine whether the bleeding is cyclic (regular) or acyclic (irregular) in nature. The differential diagnosis varies accordingly. Blood dyscrasias and structural anomalies (e.g., polyps and fibroids) are common with cyclic bleeding. Bleeding disorders should be considered in all adolescents with AUB, who present with extremely heavy first menses, bleeding requiring blood transfusion and patients with refractory menorrhagia and concomitant anemia. Sexually transmitted infections (STIs) and pelvic inflammatory disease (PID) should be considered in all sexually active (or sexually abused) adolescents who complain of irregular, breakthrough, or postcoital bleeding.

Investigations should be done to establish the cause. If there is no obvious cause, the diagnosis is dysfunctional uterine bleeding (DUB) and is due to anovulation.

Mild DUB can usually be managed with iron supplementation and observation. Hormonal therapy is sometimes necessary for controlling moderate or severe DUB. Combined oral contraceptive pills (OCPs) or progesterone alone can be given. Red blood cell transfusion may be necessary for patients who are hemodynamically unstable, have extremely low hemoglobin concentrations, or have symptomatic anemia. Peripheral blood should be obtained from the patient for the evaluation of bleeding disorders, including von Willebrand disease, before the blood is transfused. Puberty menorrhagia can be severe, sometimes requiring blood transfusion. Anovulation or DUB is the most common cause but bleeding disorders, other medical and organic conditions must be ruled out. The treatment includes hematinics, tranexamic acid, and hormones. Tranexamic acid in 2 g/day dosage is an effective and safe option to control bleeding, while waiting for complete evaluation. Hormones are the mainstay of treatment in DUB.

Such children need thorough gynecological examination and evaluation to arrive at a correct diagnosis. Understanding the proper technique of gynecological examination including making the patient comfortable and relaxed is important in this age group. Surgical intervention is required very infrequently.

PRECOCIOUS PUBERTY

Pubertal growth below the age of 8 years is labeled as precocious puberty. Early maturation can occur in girls with central nervous system abnormalities, family history of the disorder, certain rare genetic syndromes, and girls with tumors of the ovary, pituitary gland, or brain. Investigations are tailored based on symptoms and treatment is done as per diagnosis.

In *central precocious puberty* sometimes, the cause may not be identified and treatment is given to delay it by suppressing gonadotropin-releasing hormone (GnRH), In *peripheral precocious puberty,* usually estrogen or testosterone is high and GnRH is normal. The cause may be ovarian or adrenal tumor or exogenous use of hormones. Children with peripheral precocious puberty need more testing to find the cause of their condition. This might include more blood tests to check hormone levels or, in girls, an ultrasound to check for an ovarian cyst or tumor. Early judicious treatment is essential to prevent shortening of height.

DELAYED PUBERTY AND PRIMARY AMENORRHEA

If girls have not started to develop breasts by 14 years of age, or they have developed breasts but their periods have not started by 16 years, it is considered delayed puberty. This delay may be due to individual genetic variations, known as constitutional delay, undernutrition or chronic illness or variety of hypothalamic, pituitary, and gonadal disorders.

For primary amenorrhea (no periods till 18 years) common causes are hypothalamic amenorrhea, PCOS, hyperprolactinemia, Müllerian agenesis, and ovarian failure. A careful medical history and clinical examination, distinction between primary and secondary amenorrhea, together with the presence or absence of secondary sexual characteristics are essential. The presence or absence of uterus and ovaries is evaluated with transabdominal sonography. Other investigations include measurement of follicle-stimulating hormone (FSH), prolactin, and androgen levels if acne or hirsutism is present. If Turner syndrome or androgen insensitivity is suspected, a karyotype is done.

The analysis of 48 patients of primary amenorrhea in a tertiary hospital over 3 years showed 54.2% Müllerian anomalies, 22.9% hypogonadotropic hypogonadism, 16.6% hypergonadotropic hypogonadism, and 6.3% genital tuberculosis.[5]

Obstructive vaginal anomalies such as imperforate hymen, transverse vaginal septum, and vaginal or cervical atresia may manifest as absence of menstruation.[6] Here functional uterus is there and reconstructive surgery is required, Surgical vaginoplasty is done for complete or partial

Müllerian agenesis and is carried out after marriage is fixed. Patients with Müllerian agenesis are counseled regarding opportunities for adoption or surrogacy.

SECONDARY AMENORRHEA

Cessation of menstrual periods for >6 months may occur with genital tuberculosis or PCOS. Identifying the cause and appropriate treatment is important. This may also be due to primary or early premature ovarian failure. The administration of hormone treatment is remarkably beneficial for young women with primary or very premature ovarian failure resulting in restoration of menstrual cycles and the prevention of short-term and long-term hormonal imbalance consequences.

SEXUALLY TRANSMITTED INFECTIONS

In India, 26% girls are married before 15 years and 54% before 18 years. Multiple partners, new partners, and inconsistent use of condoms are well-known risk factors for acquiring STI among adolescents. Sexually transmitted diseases increase the rate of transmission of human immunodeficiency virus (HIV), and 50% of all HIV-positive new infections are in the age group of 10–25 years.

The evaluation and treatment of STI in adolescents raises a number of unique issues, including consent for diagnosis and treatment, confidentiality, parental notification, and mandatory reporting of sexual abuse in unmarried girls. Sexual history should be taken, with appropriate counseling regarding risk-taking behaviors. Sexually active adolescents should be screened for gonorrhea and chlamydia. Symptomatic genital herpes and primary syphilis are important diagnostic considerations. PID is a common sequel of genital gonorrhea and chlamydia infections. Microscopic examination of vaginal fluid mixed with saline and with potassium hydroxide, and Gram stain is useful for the diagnosis of trichomoniasis, bacterial vaginosis, and candidiasis. Culture is used widely for the diagnosis of gonorrhea, chlamydia, and genital herpes.

For treatment of STI, syndromic approach with single dose, observed therapy is preferable. Three bacterial STIs (chlamydia, gonorrhea, and syphilis) and one parasitic STI (trichomoniasis) are generally curable with existing, effective single-dose regimens of antibiotics. Syndromic management is simple, assures rapid, same-day treatment, and avoids expensive or unavailable diagnostic tests.

ADNEXAL AND PELVIC MASSES

A variety of ovarian and paraovarian lesions may occur in adolescents presenting as pelvic mass and/or pain. There may functional, benign, or malignant ovarian tumors or the girl may present with acute torsion of ovarian cyst.[7] Adnexal masses may be due to inflammatory pathology like salpingitis or tubercular tubo-ovarian mass, endometriosis, and rarely an ectopic pregnancy. Ultrasound imaging and or magnetic resonance imaging can help in clinching the diagnosis which helps in carrying out appropriate management.

VULVOVAGINITIS AND UROLOGIC ISSUES

Vulvovaginitis is mainly nonspecific but is a common gynecological problem in adolescents. Perineal pain, interlabial masses, urinary tract infections, and daytime incontinence are commonly seen. Improving hygiene, avoiding irritants, and keeping vulva dry are the basic principles of treatment.

ADOLESCENT ENDOMETRIOSIS

Endometriosis is a progressive disease that can cause chronic pelvic pain and infertility. The most immediate issue in adolescents is to relieve pain. Ultrasound will usually diagnose the condition when there are chocolate cysts. Usually, medical management is preferred in an adolescent but laparoscopy may be required in the case of large chocolate cysts or intractable pain.

ADOLESCENT VACCINATION

It is important to vaccinate all girls during adolescence against *rubella* if the same has not been done earlier. This is essential to prevent fetal damage in subsequent pregnancy due to rubella infection.

Human papilloma virus (HPV) vaccination is another important requirement of preventive health services during this period. In 2007, adolescents were designated as a special population for prevention of HPV related cervical cancer. Vaccination before the initiation of sexual activity is important. Cervical cancer, one of the leading causes of cancer-related mortality among women worldwide, is mainly caused by persistent HPV infection. The World Health Organization (WHO) has prequalified and widely licensed the bivalent (HPV 16/18), quadrivalent (HPV 6/11/16/18), and nonavalent (HPV 6/11/16/18/31/33/45/52/58) vaccines. According to the WHO recommendations, girls aged 9–14 years prior to sexual activity are the primary target population for HPV vaccination and the recommendation is one- or two-dose schedule for girls aged 9–14 years, one or two-dose schedule for girls and women aged 15–20 years and two doses with a 6-month interval for women aged >21 years. Immunocompromised patients should receive at least two doses and three doses.[8]

India's first indigenously developed quadrivalent HPV vaccination against cervical cancer is approved by the Drug Controller General of India and the Union Health Ministry has rolled out the HPV vaccine against cervical cancer for girls aged 9 to 14 years in the National Immunization Programme in February 2024.

ADOLESCENT CONTRACEPTION

There is an unmet need of contraception and misinformation requiring urgent intervention. Both married and unmarried adolescents may be in need for contraception, and depending on requirement, may be counseled regarding the use of COC pill and condoms. Dual protection against pregnancy and STI is important. Given the transience of many adolescent relationships and the high probability of multiple, sequential sexual partners prior to marriage, condom is the single best protective option for many adolescents. But it may be best to combine with an OCP, if possible. Emergency contraception as an emergency backup should also be available to young women.

TEENAGE PREGNANCY

Adolescent girls face considerable health risks during pregnancy and childbirth, accounting for 15% of the global burden of disease for maternal conditions and 13% of all maternal deaths.[9] The risk of medical complications, such as high blood pressure, iron-deficiency anemia, and eclampsia, is greater among adolescent mothers. An underdeveloped pelvis can lead to obstructed labor and grave complications, such as vesicovaginal fistula, infant mortality, or maternal death. Teenage mothers also have a high risk of genital tract infection, preterm labor, and intrauterine growth restricted babies. Early booking, adequate prenatal care, and delivery by trained obstetrician can improve the obstetric and perinatal outcome in teenage pregnancies.

Pregnancy may be unwanted resulting in unsafe abortion. Girls from troubled family backgrounds are at 11 times higher risk of unmarried teenage pregnancy than those from happy family circumstances, according to a new study in Kerala. As much as 64.5% of the unmarried pregnant girls or young women covered by the study came from "problem families". The problems included divorced or separated parents, polygamous families, parents with marital disharmony, mentally challenged parents, old and debilitated parents, and single parent with little other support.[10]

PRACTICE GUIDELINES

- Normal sexual development depends on normal karyotype, presence or absence of genes for testicular determination, and appropriate endocrinal milieu.
- Management of menorrhagia aims to find cause and institute appropriate treatment. Some adolescents require medical intervention for PMS.
- Hirsutism is a common disorder causing considerable psychological embarrassment. It may signify benign conditions, such as idiopathic hirsutism or PCOS and malignant neoplasms of ovaries or adrenals.
- PCOS may first manifest as persistent menstrual disorder, obesity, and/or hirsutism.
- Suspect endometriosis, if progressively severe dysmenorrhea is occurring for increasing number of days.
- Breast problems are common in young girls. About 1–5% have developmental defects and 5–10% present with benign breast disorders.
- Amenorrhea demands evaluation if there is no menstruation up to 15 years of age with normal puberty; up to 13 years in the case of delayed pubertal development and cessation of menstruation for three cycle lengths or 6 months. In the cases of normal uterus but delayed puberty, bone age assessment rules out constitutional delay.
- Tuberculosis in India is very common, and the aim is to diagnose and treat early to avoid long-term sequelae.
- In the absence of functioning uterus, the usual age for vaginal reconstruction is 16–20 years or 6 months before the marriage date. First operation has the best chance of success.

PRACTICE POINTS OR TIPS

- Preventive health services are important in this age group.
- Clinical examination and counseling should be done in a friendly environment with confidentiality.
- Malnutrition is a major health problem, and 50% of adolescent girls are anemic in India.
- Besides caring for diseases, attention to nutrition, exercise, and lifestyle is important. Correction and prevention of anemia and obesity will go a long way.
- A high degree of suspicion of sexual abuse to be kept in mind in all cases of genital tract trauma in young girls.
- Imaging is an important adjunct in the diagnosis of adolescent gynecologic disorders.

REFERENCES

1. Sanfilippo JS, Lara-Torre E. Adolescent Gynecology. Obstet Gynecol. 2009;113(4):935-47.
2. Rotterdam ESHRE/ASRM-Sponsored PCOS Consensus Workshop Group. Revised 2003 consensus on diagnostic criteria and long-term health risks related to polycystic ovary syndrome. Fertil Steril. 2004;81(1):19-25.
3. Nidhi R, Padmalatha V, Nagarathna R, Amritanshu R. Prevalence of polycystic ovarian syndrome in Indian adolescents. J Pediatr Adolesc Gynecol. 2011;24(4):223-7.
4. Formuso C, Stracquadanio M, Ciotta L. Myo-inositol vs. D-chiro inositol in PCOS treatment. Minerva Gynecol. 2015;67(4):321-5.

5. Kumar A, Verma A, Mittal A. Gynaecological disorders in girls less than 20 years of age. J Obstet Gynae India. 1998;48(1):60-3.
6. Mentessidou A, Mirilas P. Surgical disorders in Pediatric and adolescent gynecology: vaginal and uterine anomalies. Int J Gynaecol Obstet. 2023;160(3):762-70.
7. Mentessidou A, Mirilas P. Surgical disorders in pediatric and adolescent gynecology: Adnexal abnormalities. Int J Gynecol Obstet. 2023;161(3):702-10.
8. World Health Organization. (2022). WHO updates recommendations on HPV vaccination schedule. [online] Available from https://www.who.int/news/item/20-12-2022-WHO-updates-recommendations-on-HPV-vaccination-schedule. [Last accessed December, 2024].
9. Moni SA, Nair MKC, Devi RS. Pregnancy among unmarried adolescents and young adults. J Obstet Gynaecol India. 2013;63(1):49-54.
10. Sagili H, Pramya N, Prabhu K, Mascarenhas M, Rani PR. Are teenage pregnancies at high risk? A comparison study in a developing country. Arch Gynecol Obstet. 2012;285(3):573-7.

19.9 Adolescent-friendly School Initiatives

Abraham K Paul

INTRODUCTION

Children and adolescents are the wealth of nation and future citizens of our country; hence, it is imperative that they be brought up in a healthy, stimulating, and safe environment. Adolescents complete their physical, emotional, and psychological journey to adulthood in a fast changing world. Such an environment will positively contribute to their physical, mental, cognitive, emotional, spiritual, and social development. Since children and adolescents spend a considerable period of time in schools and colleges, these places should definitely provide such a positive environment. There are certain issues that particularly pertain to adolescents as compared to their younger counterparts, which include emotional problems, high-risk behavior, sexual matters, unwanted peer influence, and mental health issues. A school that addresses all these issues may be considered an adolescent-friendly school.

Addressing the needs of adolescents is a challenge that goes well beyond the role of adolescent-friendly school alone. The legal frame work, social policy, the safety of communities and opportunities for education, and recreation are just some of the factors key to adolescent development. The following may be adopted by the schools to make it an adolescent-friendly school.[1]

HEALTH CHECKUP AND MONITORING, LIFESTYLE DISEASE PREVENTION, MENTAL HEALTH, AND RISK BEHAVIORS

A good health depends on a proper diet, a positive attitude, and exercise. The major killer disease, the coronary artery disease, and its risk factors, such as hypertension, diabetes, dyslipidemia, and obesity, have their origin in childhood. All children before admission to school or college should have weight, height, blood pressure (BP) check, and a general medical examination once in a year. Nutritional advice should be given to all children and adolescents by a professional on a regular basis. Discourage eating excess snacks, confectionaries, fast food, soft drinks, and fun drinks. Routine dental checkup and eye checkup should be compulsory. Lapsed immunization, if any, should be completed, and adolescent immunization schedule should be followed. Psychological, emotional, and social problems, if any, should be evaluated and necessary referrals made.

Mental health problems frequently start to make themselves felt in this age group. Depression is common, especially for young who have low self-esteem and can lead to suicide. School authorities and parents have to be vigilant about this. Risk behaviors should be identified and dealt with appropriately.

Health services should be made available to treat conditions that give rise to ill health, to prevent health problems and to make links with other services, such as counseling services which can support adolescents.

SAFE TRANSPORT TO AND FROM SCHOOL

Considering the risk-taking behavior peculiar to this age group, strict monitoring of those using two-wheelers should be supervised for over-speeding and careless and rash driving. Use of helmet should be made compulsory. Safety measures for other modes of transport should also been forced.[2]

COUNSELING SERVICES

Teenagers experience stress on various situations related to education, psychological or emotional, physical, and environmental or social problems. As part of a normal developmental process also adolescents experience adjustment problems with peers, parents, and sometimes teachers. Scholastic expectations from parents, examination stress, learning disabilities, and attention-deficit disorders, all may require professional assessment, remedial measures, and counseling, and these services should be made available in the schools or colleges.

SAFE AND HEALTHY ENVIRONMENT

Schools or colleges and their neighborhood should be safe and healthy, free from environmental and sound pollution. Silent zone should be maintained near schools as per government rules. Since children and adolescents are particularly vulnerable to initiate use of tobacco, alcohol, and drugs at this age, their nonavailability near schools should be strictly ensured. Children with signs of depression, emotional problems, and low self-esteem should be closely monitored since they are at high risk for taking up tobacco and drug use.

GAMES PERIOD AND EXERCISE

Adolescence is a period, particularly prone to obesity. The hormonal changes, erratic dietary habits, lack of exercise, and sedentary habits make an adolescent highly susceptible to obesity. Decreasing caloric intake and increasing physical activity are the basis for prevention and management. Four games period per week must be made compulsory in schools and colleges. There should be adequate playground area (10 acres land for high schools). Provision of health club with equipment, such as treadmill, will motivate adolescents to a healthy lifestyle.

CLEAN AND HEALTHY EATING PLACE

Academic institutions with canteen should have clean kitchen and a clean place wherein children can bring in home-made food and eat. Outside vendors should not be allowed in the campus. Fast food, fried items, oily food, and aerated drinks should be discouraged in the canteen. Advertisements of aerated drinks should be prohibited in the canteen and neighborhood. Ensure that child labor is prohibited in the canteen and other workplaces.

FACILITIES FOR PERSONAL HYGIENE

Since children and adolescents spend about 5–6 hours in the schools, there should be adequate facilities for personal hygiene. Provision for adequate hygienic drinking water is a must to prevent waterborne diseases and to prevent urinary tract infection. Water requirement per person is more because of the excess physical activity peculiar to this age-group.

There should be minimum one urinal for 60 students and one latrine for every 100 students. Schools and colleges with a greater number of girls should have a proportionately higher number. There should be adequate supply of water in the toilets for maintaining genital hygiene and for washing hands. Sanitary napkins may be made available through school store or office. One may also consider napkin-vending machines, and facility for disposing sanitary napkins should be made available. Toilets should be kept neat and clean so that children will not hesitate to make use of the facility.

CAREER GUIDANCE

Many adolescents require help and guidance to select a career of their interest and choice. A career guidance program will go a long way in building a secure future for him or her and the family.

MEDIA LITERACY

Apart from all the benefits of the television (TV), the ill effects of media cannot be overlooked. Many studies have shown constant watching of violent scenes on TV, and fantasy violence make children more aggressive in their behavior to others. Media is certainly the one factor contributing to early sexual behavior. Since teenagers tend to follow the behavior they observe in the media without seeing the known consequences, they may end up pregnant with human immunodeficiency virus (HIV) or with other sexually transmitted diseases. Considering all these, counseling on the appropriate use of TV and other media should be a part of the school or college program.

FAMILY LIFE EDUCATION

Regular classes on family life education consisting of classes on adolescent nutrition, personal hygiene, menstrual hygiene for girls, emotional support, awareness on one's own sexuality, HIV or acquired immunodeficiency syndrome, and substance abuse should be conducted in schools or colleges. Classes may be conducted once a month by a specialist.[3]

ADOLESCENT HEALTH CARD AND IMMUNIZATION

Adolescent health card developed at Child Development Center, Thiruvananthapuram, may be issued to all children and adolescents on admission to school or college and relevant data, such as weight, height, BP, immunization status, body mass index, to be recorded **(Fig. 19.9.1)**. Health checkup as prescribed could be conducted by the school.[4,5]

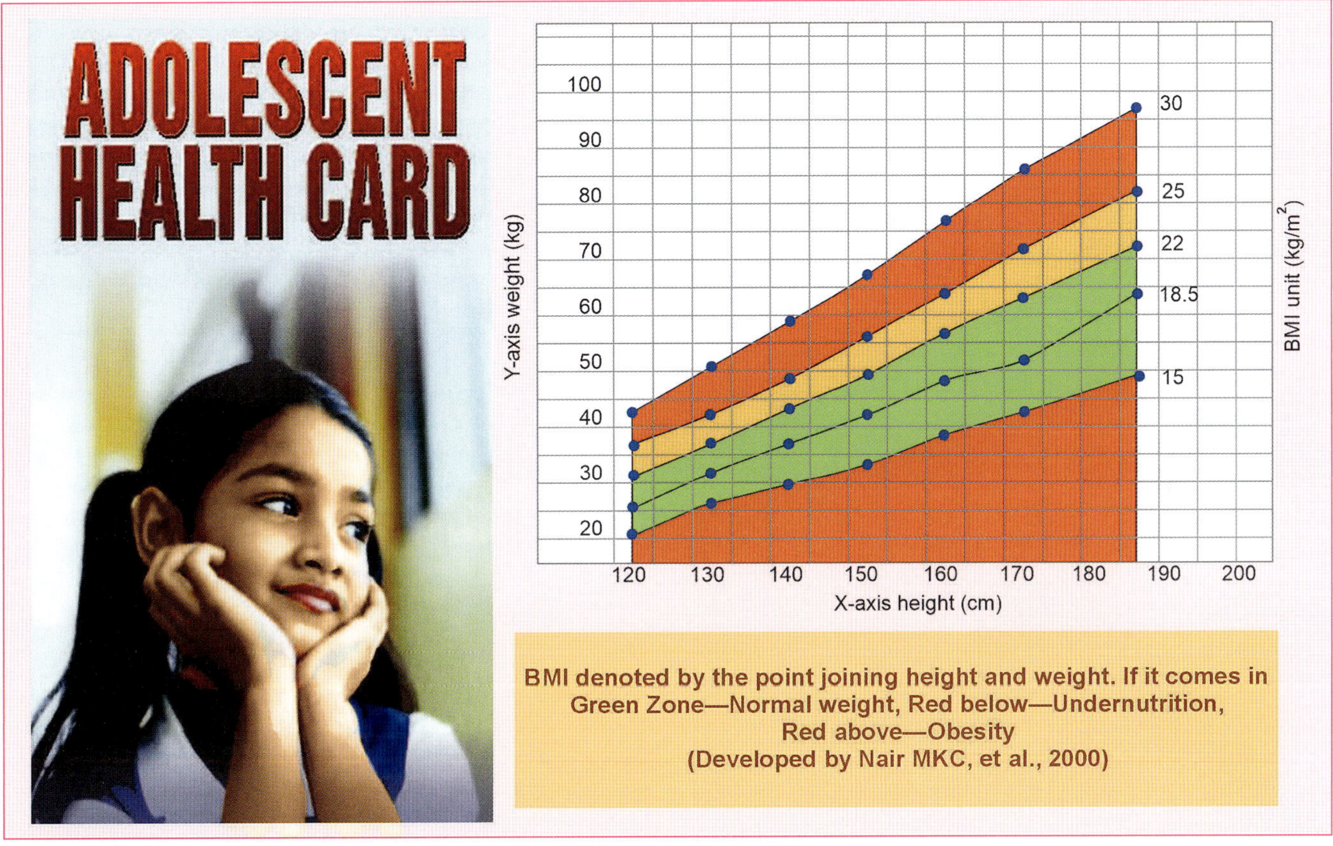

Fig. 19.9.1: Adolescent health card. (BMI: body mass index)

LIFE SKILL TRAINING: TEENAGE CLUBS

Life skill training should be conducted in school or college on a yearly basis or more often to prevent substance abuse, smoking, alcoholism, sexual contact, and adolescent pregnancy. It should also enable children and adolescents to deal actively with various demands of life.

LEARNING PROBLEMS

Learning problems are being increasingly recognized among school children. Early identification of scholastic backwardness is absolutely vital as early remediation and intervention has the best chance of favorable outcome.

Learning problems unidentified in early childhood may continue to manifest in later childhood and adolescence and should be recognized and interventional strategies instituted.

CONCLUSION

A school that addresses the issues, which particularly pertain to adolescents as compared to their younger counterparts, may be considered an adolescent-friendly school. The issues mainly include emotional problems, high-risk behavior, sexual matters, unwanted peer influence, and mental health issues. Regular health checkup and immunization also should be an integral part.

REFERENCES

1. World Health Organization. Adolescent Friendly Health Services: An agenda for change. Geneva: World Health Organization; 2002.
2. Agarwal RK. Promoting adolescent friendly reproductive and sexual health services. Indian Pediatr. 2008;45(1):881-2.
3. Bansal CP. Adolescent friendly school initiative program under IAP Vision—2007 module.
4. Nair MKC, George B, Sharma PS. Nutrition, Health and Psychological Status of Teenage Girls. Thiruvananthapuram, Kerala: UNICEF and Child Development Centre; 2003. pp. 8-9, 22-3.
5. Verma M, Chhatwal J. Common health problems in adolescents. In: Parthasarathy A (Ed). IAP Textbook of Pediatrics, 3rd edition. New Delhi: Jaypee Brothers Medical Publishers (P) Ltd.; 2006. pp. 943-50.

SECTION

20 Intensive Care and Emergencies

Section Editor: Jayashree Muralidharan

20.1 Setting Up a Triage and Pediatric Intensive Care Unit in Tertiary Care Hospitals

Lalit Takia, Rakesh Lodha

SETTING UP A TRIAGE

INTRODUCTION

Triage, derived from the French word "*trier*" denoting sorting and organization, is a critical process in healthcare for categorizing patients based on the severity of their illness or injuries. This classification drives the prioritization and order of care and monitoring, for multiple patients. The historical roots of emergency triage trace back to its inception in military settings, particularly for field doctors.[1] Documented practices from the 18th century reveal early triage forms employed by field surgeons assessing wounded soldiers. Baron Dominique Jean Larrey, a notable French military surgeon, pioneered a systematic triage system during Napoleon Bonaparte's era.[2] The formal integration of triage into civilian emergency departments (EDs) occurred in 1964 through Weinerman et al.'s systematic interpretation. Today, triage remains an integral component of healthcare protocols. Establishing an effective triage system in pediatric emergency settings is paramount to providing timely and tailored care for children in critical situations.

In contrast to adult triage, pediatric triage demands a more tailored approach that delicately balances the unique physiological needs of children. The fundamental principles and considerations in establishing a pediatric screening system emphasize the importance of age-appropriate assessments and continuous monitoring of pediatric patients in emergencies.

DEFINITION OF TRIAGE

Triage entails the systematic prioritization of individuals needing medical care, particularly in the setting of influx of many patients in emergency or mass casualty. This process is contingent upon factors such as the nature and severity of illness or injury, the anticipated prognosis, and the availability of resources.[3]

PRINCIPLES AND PURPOSE OF PEDIATRIC TRIAGE SYSTEM

Age-appropriate assessment: Pediatric triage systems are designed to consider children's specific physiological and developmental aspects. The assessment takes into account age-specific vital signs, symptoms, and responses to better understand the severity of their conditions.

Identification of critical cases: The primary purpose of pediatric triage is to quickly identify and prioritize critically ill or injured children so that immediate interventions are directed toward those requiring urgent attention.

Effective resource utilization: By categorizing children according to the urgency of their clinical conditions, the triage system helps optimize resource utilization and prevent delays in providing essential care.

Minimizing overcrowding in pediatric EDs: Efficient triage prevents pediatric emergency overcrowding by streamlining patient in-flow. This improves the overall effectiveness of emergency care delivery.

Reducing anxiety for children and families: Triage in pediatric emergencies acknowledges children's and their families' emotional and psychological needs. A prompt and organized triage process can help alleviate anxiety and uncertainty during critical situations.

Continuous monitoring and reassessment: Pediatric triage is an ongoing process that allows for continuous monitoring and reassessment of children's conditions. As their status changes, adjustments can be made to the level of care they receive.

TRIAGE CATEGORIES AND PRIORITIZATION

The triage process in a pediatric emergency should be designed to rapidly assess and categorize sick children upon arrival at the emergency room.[4]

Pediatric Triage Assessment/Categories

The triage evaluation process is conducted in a methodical and structured manner by utilizing general assessment tools, specifically the *pediatric assessment triangle* (PAT) and the primary assessment approach known as *ABCDE* (Airway, Breathing, Circulation, Disability, and Exposure). These details are fully outlined in the triage form provided.

It is crucial to note that the triage assessment differs significantly from the diagnostic evaluation. The primary objective of triage assessment is to promptly identify

Flowchart 20.1.1: Pediatric assessment triangle (PAT) to guide initial emergency treatment.

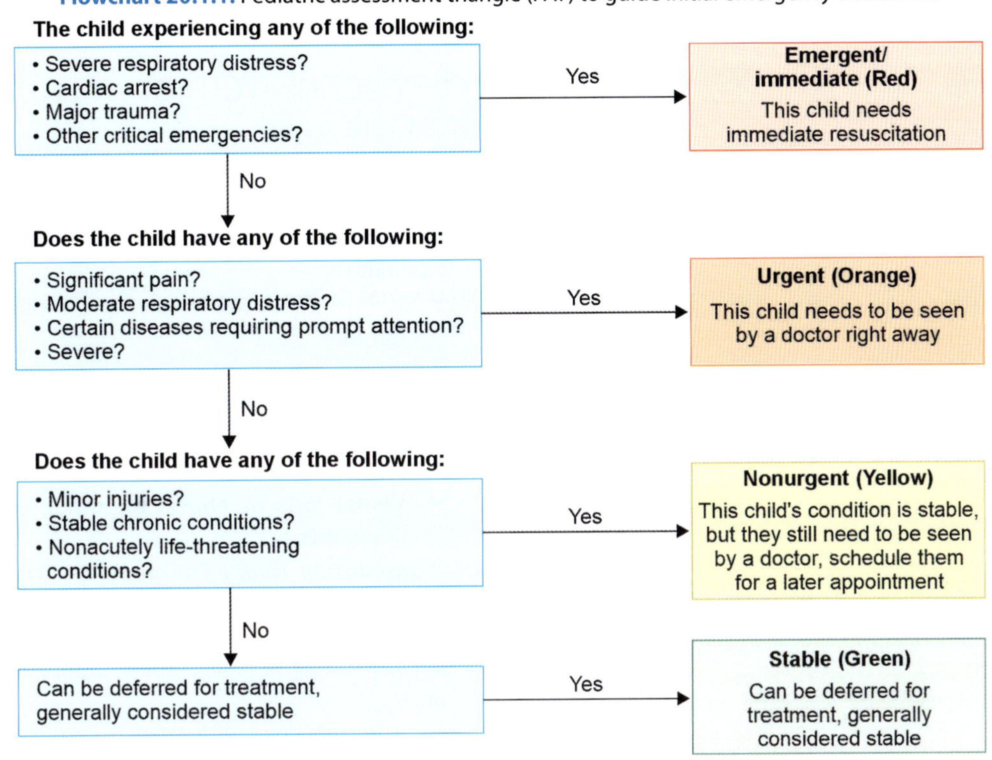

anatomical or functional abnormalities, assess their severity, and formulate a plan to *guide initial emergency treatment*, as succinctly depicted in **Flowchart 20.1.1**.

In the emergency room, triage assessment and management should optimally be assigned to resident doctors and nursing staff with Pediatric Advanced Life Support (PALS) training for proficient handling of pediatric emergencies. Additionally, this process is systematically supported and supervised by the on-duty senior resident or faculty who is also trained in PALS.

General Assessment

The PAT **(Flowchart 20.1.1)** involves immediate visual and auditory evaluation upon arrival of the patient, focusing on the appearance, breathing, and circulation triad. This rapid assessment within 30–40 seconds aids in identifying patients who need to make urgent life-saving decisions.

Pediatric assessment triangle concludes by categorizing the patient's illness as *stable* or *unstable*. Unstable conditions are further classified into *life-threatening* and *non-life-threatening*. Patients in the former category, such as cardiac arrest, cardiorespiratory failure, decompensated shock, deep coma, and severe stridor, require immediate treatment/resuscitation before proceeding to primary assessment.

GENERAL ASSESSMENT CATEGORIZING THE PATIENT ILLNESS

Primary Assessment

Primary assessment encompasses the assessment pentagon, which is conducted once a child is *en route* to stabilization. It includes a detailed examination of:

- A—Airway
- B—Breathing
- C—Circulation
- D—Disability and neurologic abnormalities
- E—Head-to-toe examination (Exposure)

Completion within 1-3 minutes is crucial. This process also involves additional recording of parameters such as peripheral oxygen saturation (SpO_2), electrocardiogram (ECG), and blood glucose for a comprehensive evaluation.

Primary Assessment (ABCDE): Assessment Pentagon

This is detailed in **Box 20.1.1 and Flowchart 20.1.2**.

TEAM COMPOSITION OF PEDIATRIC TRIAGE

The team composition for pediatric triage involves a collaborative effort among healthcare professionals with

BOX 20.1.1: Primary assessment—ABCDE.

1. *Airway:*
   Open and stable: Yes/no
   If No: ....
2. *Breathing*:
   RR...... breaths/min
   Efforts: Normal/poor/increased
   Auscultation:
   Air entry: Normal/decreased/differential
   Added sounds: None/stridor/wheeze/crackles
   SpO_2 on room air......
3. *Circulation:*
   HR............. beats/min
   CFT......... secs
   BP....../...... mm Hg
   Peripheral pulses: Poor/good
   Central pulses: Poor/good
   Skin temperature: Warm/cool
   Others:
4. *Disability*:
   GCS............
   Pupil size......... mm
   Pupillary reactions...........
   Motor activity: Normal and symmetrical/asymmetrical/posturing/seizure
   Blood glucose.......... mg/dL
5. *Exposure*:
   Temperature:.......
   Color: Normal/pallor/cyanosis/mottled
   Any other skin lesion...................

(BP: blood pressure; CFT: capillary refill time; GCS: Glasgow Coma Scale; HR: heart rate; RR: respiratory rate; SpO_2: peripheral oxygen saturation)

specialized training in pediatric care. All team members, including nurses and doctors, should have specialized training in PALS to ensure proficiency in handling pediatric emergencies. This team typically includes:

- *Pediatric emergency physician:* A pediatric emergency physician oversees the triage process, provides guidance, and makes critical patient prioritization and treatment decisions.
- *Resident doctors:* Junior and senior resident doctors play a crucial role in conducting initial assessments, managing patient care, and collaborating with the rest of the team under the guidance of the pediatric emergency physician.
- *Pediatric triage nurse:* An experienced nurse trained in pediatric triage is responsible for the initial assessment of patients, gathering vital information, and determining the urgency of care.
- *Ancillary support staff:* Depending on the healthcare facility, other healthcare professionals such as technicians and healthcare assistants may provide support as needed.
- *Administrative staff:* Personnel responsible for maintaining records, managing patient flow, and ensuring efficient communication within the team

However, the composition may be modified based on the available resources.

PHYSICAL LAYOUT OF A PEDIATRIC TRIAGE AREA

- *Reception/check-in area:*
  - Marked entrance for easy access
  - Reception desk to check in patients with trained staff
  - Waiting area with seating for patients and their families
- *Triage assessment zone:*
  - Designated space for initial patient assessments
  - Individual assessment stations equipped with necessary tools
  - Visual aids or charts for quick reference during assessments
- *Resuscitation room*: The pediatric triage resuscitation room is a vital frontline in emergencies, requiring meticulous design and organized tools for high-quality patient care. The resuscitation room should be made up of:
  - *Adjustable bed with safety rails and overhead lighting*: Beds should have the ability to maneuver the head end and foot end.
  - *Oxygen and suction outlets:* Easily accessible at various points around the bed
  - *Defibrillator:* Mounted on the wall with readily available electrodes and pads in different sizes
  - *Crash cart:* Mobile cart stocked with additional emergency medications, airway management devices, and resuscitation aids
  - *Monitoring equipment:* Vital signs monitor with display screen, pulse oximeter, and potentially EKG machine
  - *Storage cabinets:* Accessible and stocked with emergency medications, resuscitation equipment, and supplies
  - *Waste disposal:* Sharps container and biohazard bin placed safely
  - *Sink and countertop:* For handwashing, sterile procedures, and medication preparation
- *Privacy considerations:*
  - Curtained areas or partitions to ensure patient privacy during assessments
  - Separate areas for different acuity levels (e.g., critical, urgent, nonurgent)
- *Medical equipment and supplies:*
  - Easily accessible storage for medical supplies and equipment

Flowchart 20.1.2: Scheme for initial assessment and resuscitation in emergency room (ER).

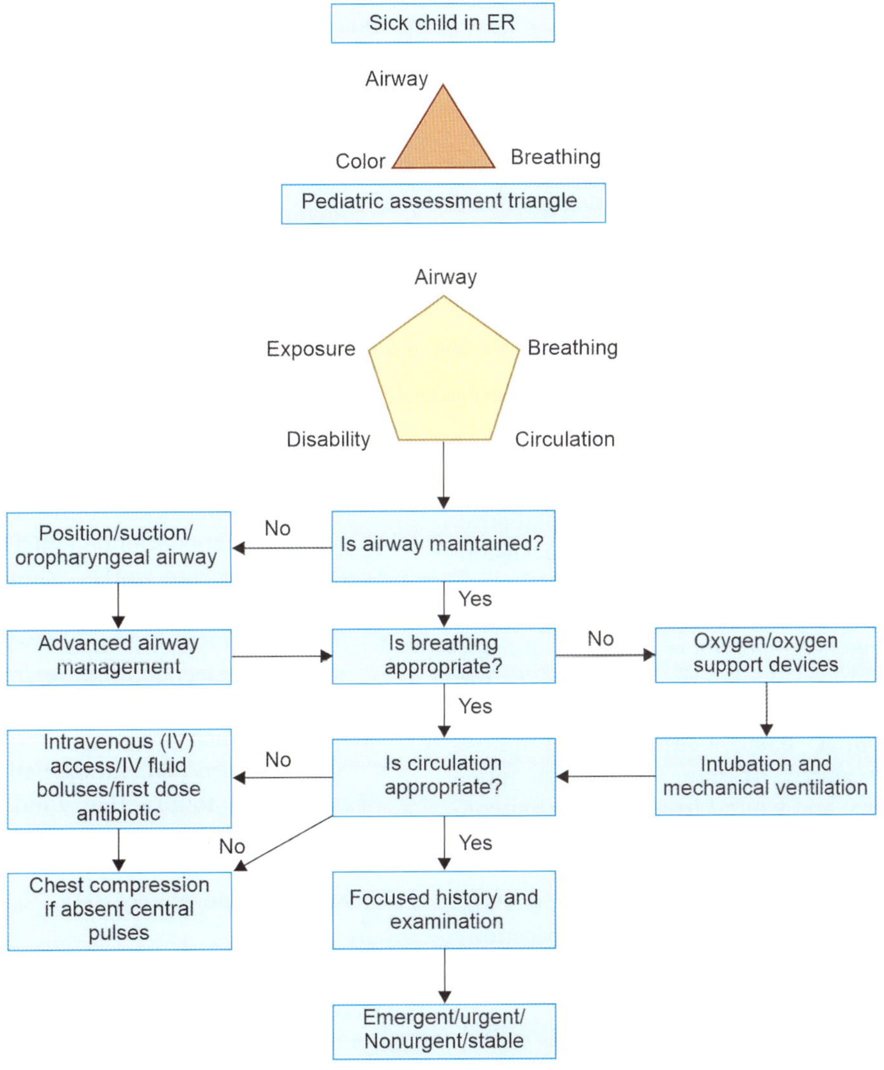

- Integration of pediatric-specific equipment, such as smaller-sized blood pressure cuffs and thermometers
- A communication station is used for staff to coordinate and communicate effectively.
- Access to phone, intercom, or other communication devices

▪ *Documentation area:*
  - Designated space for the maintenance of patient records and documentation
  - Computers or tablets for electronic record-keeping, if applicable

▪ *Isolation area:*
  - Designated area for potentially contagious cases
  - Adequate infection control measures

▪ *Emergency equipment:* Access to emergency equipment such as crash carts

▪ Clearly marked exits for rapid transport to other areas of the facility

▪ *Child-friendly environment:*
  - Use colorful and child-friendly decor to create a less intimidating atmosphere.
  - Age-appropriate distractions or entertainment to comfort pediatric patients

▪ *Staff workstations:*
  - Workstations for healthcare professionals involved in triage assessments
  - Adequate space for collaboration and communication among team members

NECESSARY EQUIPMENT AND SUPPLIES

In a pediatric triage setting, ensuring the availability of essential equipment and supplies is crucial for effectively assessing and managing pediatric patients. The following list outlines the necessary equipment and supplies:

- *Vital signs monitoring equipment:* Multipara monitors, especially for pediatric patients
- *Resuscitation equipment:* A well-equipped resuscitation area tailored for pediatric patients, such as appropriately sized medical equipment for managing pediatric emergencies, including basic and advanced airway management devices, oxygen delivery systems, suction devices, chest compression equipment, and defibrillator.
- *Emergency medications:* This may include managing respiratory distress, allergic reactions, seizures, cardiac emergencies, and pain relief. Medications should be age-appropriate, and dosages should be readily available for quick administration.
- *Intravenous (IV) access supplies:* Access to IV fluids and equipment for establishing IV access is essential for administering medications and fluids to pediatric patients. This includes IV catheters, IV fluids, extension sets, and infusion pumps.
- *Diagnostic equipment:* Basic diagnostic equipment such as thermometers, glucometers for blood glucose monitoring, and pulse oximeters are necessary for assessing the patient's condition quickly and accurately.
- *Wound care supplies:* Basic wound care supplies, including sterile gauze, dressings, adhesive tape, antiseptic solutions, and wound irrigation equipment, should be readily available for managing minor injuries and wounds.
- *Personal protective equipment (PPE):* Adequate PPE, including gloves, masks, gowns, and eye protection, should be available to ensure the safety of healthcare providers and prevent the spread of infections.
- *Communication devices:* Access to communication devices such as phones is essential for coordinating care among triage team members and other healthcare providers.
- *Documentation tools:* Supplies for documentation, such as paper charts, pens, and electronic devices for recording patient information, are essential for maintaining accurate records of patient assessments and interventions.

By ensuring the availability of these essential equipment and supplies, pediatric triage teams can effectively assess, stabilize, and manage pediatric patients presenting to the triage area, optimizing patient outcomes, and ensuring efficient healthcare delivery.

The triage area in any healthcare setting, especially one dealing with pediatrics, is the first point of contact for potentially infectious patients. Implementing infection control measures in this crucial space is vital to protect patients and healthcare workers. Some key measures to consider are given in the following text.

Infection Control Measures

- *Environmental measures:*
  - *Hand hygiene:* Alcohol-based hand-rub dispensers at the entrance, exit, and near each triage station. Encourage frequent hand hygiene for both staff and patients/guardians.
  - *Cleaning and disinfection:* Regularly clean and disinfect frequently touched surfaces in the triage area.
  - *Ventilation and air quality:* Maintain proper ventilation in the triage area to dilute and remove airborne contaminants. Consider using air purifiers with HEPA (high-efficiency particulate air) filters.
  - *Waste management:* Provide designated bins for regular waste and sharps disposal.
- *Patient management:*
  - *Screening and risk assessment:* Implement a system for screening patients for potential infectious diseases.
  - *PPE:* Healthcare workers should wear appropriate PPE based on the risk assessment of each patient.
  - *Patient cohorts:* If possible, segregate patients with suspected infectious diseases from others in the triage area. Utilize dedicated waiting areas or examination rooms for such patients.
  - *Source control:* Encourage patients with respiratory symptoms to practice good cough and sneeze etiquette, such as covering their mouth and nose with tissues or their elbow. Provide disposable tissues and masks whenever necessary.

CONCLUSION

The triage is a vital gateway to the healthcare system, facilitating streamlined patient flow, effective resource utilization, and improved outcomes for pediatric patients. Moreover, by adhering to established guidelines, incorporating infection control measures, and promoting multidisciplinary collaboration, pediatric triage units can enhance patient safety, minimize wait times, and optimize care delivery to pediatric populations within the hospital setting.

SETTING UP A PEDIATRIC INTENSIVE CARE UNIT

INTRODUCTION

Pediatric intensive care unit (PICU) is an essential requirement in any tertiary care hospital. These units care for pediatric patients who require intensive monitoring, advanced interventions, and multidisciplinary care within the PICU setting. PICU beds should approximately be 10–20% of the overall pediatric bed strength.[5,6]

ASSESSMENT AND ADMISSION CRITERIA IN THE PEDIATRIC INTENSIVE CARE UNIT

The usual admission criteria for PICU are outlined below:[7,8]

- *Requirement for mechanical ventilation:* Patients requiring mechanical ventilation due to respiratory failure or impending respiratory compromise are admitted to the level 3 care PICU. This includes those with upper or lower airway obstruction, alveolar disease, unstable airways, and impending respiratory failure.
- *Postresuscitation patients:* Pediatric patients requiring intensive monitoring and support following successful resuscitation efforts are admitted to the PICU. This includes patients with comatose states resulting from conditions such as meningitis, encephalitis, hepatic encephalopathy, cerebral malaria, head injury, poisonings, or status epilepticus.
- *Shock/hemodynamic instability:* Patients presenting with various types of shock or hemodynamic instability, including septic shock, hypovolemic shock, bleeding emergencies, cardiogenic shock, neurogenic shock, or multiple trauma, require immediate intensive care management in the PICU.
- *Cardiac arrhythmias and hypertensive emergencies:* Pediatric patients with cardiac arrhythmias or hypertensive emergencies necessitating urgent intervention and close monitoring are admitted to the level 3 care PICU.
- *Metabolic and renal disorders:* Severe acid–base disorders, electrolyte abnormalities, and acute renal failure requiring acute renal replacement therapies, such as hemodialysis, hemofiltration, or peritoneal dialysis, mandate admission to the PICU for specialized management.
- *Postoperative patients:* Pediatric patients requiring intensive monitoring and support following various surgical procedures, particularly those with potential for respiratory or hemodynamic instability, including open heart surgery, neurosurgery, thoracic surgery, or major general surgery, are admitted to the PICU.
- *Specialized therapies:* Patients requiring advanced therapies such as extracorporeal membrane oxygenation (ECMO), nitric oxide therapy, or management of conditions like malignant hyperpyrexia or acute hepatic failure necessitate admission to the level 3 care PICU.
- *Post-transplant patients:* Pediatric patients who have undergone organ transplantation and require intensive postoperative monitoring and management are admitted to the PICU, if applicable.

These admission criteria reflect the complexity and acuity of medical conditions requiring specialized care within the PICU setting, to optimize the patient outcomes with proper resource utilization.

PEDIATRIC INTENSIVE CARE UNIT DESIGN

Location

The selection of an appropriate location of PICU is a critical aspect of its establishment. Several factors need to be considered in this process:[9]

- *Proximity to ED:* The PICU should ideally be located in close proximity to the ED to ensure easy access and transfer of critically ill pediatric patients requiring intensive care.
- *Proximity to radiodiagnosis facilities* ensures prompt access to imaging modalities such as ultrasounds, computed tomography (CT) scans, and magnetic resonance imaging (MRI) scans. This enables rapid diagnostic radio-interventional procedures in critically ill pediatric patients, facilitating timely decision-making and treatment initiation.
- *Accessibility:* The location should be easily accessible for ambulance transport facilitating rapid response in emergency situations.
- *Adjacency to operating rooms:* Placing the PICU near the operating rooms allows for seamless coordination in cases requiring immediate surgical intervention.

DESIGN

Rooms

Regarding the rooms within the PICU, a conference or duty room is deemed mandatory to facilitate team meetings, discussions, and administrative tasks. Additionally, clean and dirty utility rooms are essential for maintaining cleanliness and infection control standards. The inclusion of a library is considered desirable, providing healthcare professionals with access to educational resources and research materials. Moreover, toilets for patients are mandatory to meet basic hygiene needs.[9,10]

Spacing

Initially, PICUs were typically designed with large, ward-type layouts. However, contemporary recommendations advocate for individual rooms that prioritize infection control, staff visibility of patients and monitors, and privacy for patients and families. Recognizing the significance of family involvement in pediatric patient care within the PICU, modern room designs often incorporate additional space to accommodate sleeping arrangements and private areas for parents or caregivers. Furthermore, the design must allow for flexibility to cater to varying patient ages, sizes, and medical conditions. The minimum recommended area per bed is specified at about 150 square feet per bed for cubicle-style beds and about 250 square feet for pediatric patient rooms; each room must be spacious enough to comfortably accommodate the patient's bed along with the increasing array of medical equipment.

Monitoring

Monitoring equipment is essential for patient assessment and management, with requirements including ECG, respiratory rate (RR), peripheral oxygen saturation (SpO_2), and noninvasive blood pressure (NIBP) monitoring for all beds. Additionally, invasive blood pressure monitoring should be available for at least 50% of beds to facilitate closer hemodynamic monitoring.

Ventilator

Availability of mechanical ventilators is mandatory, with invasive ventilators, noninvasive ventilation (NIV), and high-flow nasal cannula (HFNC) listed as mandatory equipment. High-frequency oscillatory ventilation (HFOV) is considered desirable for its potential benefits in certain cases.

Equipment

The PICU must be equipped with essential medical equipment, including infusion pumps, warmers, neonatal open care systems, electroencephalogram (EEG) facilities, and defibrillators, to support critical care interventions. Additionally, a fully stocked crash cart is mandatory to ensure immediate access to emergency medications and equipment.

Crash Cart

The crash cart must be appropriately stocked and readily accessible at all times within the PICU to ensure prompt and effective response to emergencies. Standardized guidelines dictate the contents of the crash cart, which typically include medications such as epinephrine, atropine, naloxone, and benzodiazepines, as well as airway management devices, defibrillation equipment, IV access supplies, and cardiac monitoring tools.

Laboratory Facility

On-site/near-site laboratory facilities with 24-hour availability for essential tests such as complete blood count (CBC), renal function tests (RFTs), liver function tests (LFTs), coagulation studies, arterial blood gas (ABG) analysis, and lactate measurement are mandated. Other investigations may be outsourced as needed.

Support Services

Support services, including access to the blood bank, pharmacy, neurosurgery, pediatric surgery, and ear, nose, and throat (ENT) surgical facilities, must be available 24 hours a day to facilitate prompt and comprehensive patient care.

Infection Control

Concerning infection control, evidence suggests that certain design measures can significantly improve outcomes. Among these measures:

- *Effective air quality control* emerges as a paramount consideration, especially during construction or renovation projects, to mitigate the risk of airborne infections.
- *Alcohol-based hand-rub dispensers* in easily accessible areas, particularly at the bedside, to promote regular hand hygiene among healthcare providers and visitors.
- *Coverings for floors, millwork, and furniture* that are easy to clean facilitate efficient infection control practices.
- *Ensuring the installation of an appropriate water system* is also imperative, encompassing proper temperature, pressure, and drainage mechanisms. Regular maintenance of the water system, including routine cleaning of point-of-use fixtures, helps prevent the proliferation of waterborne pathogens.
- *Single rooms instead of shared spaces* can significantly reduce the risk of patient-to-patient transmission of infections. Single rooms not only minimize the likelihood of airborne infection transmission but also facilitate more effective and thorough cleaning practices, thereby enhancing overall infection control efforts.

Storage

Storage for essential supplies should be conveniently located within or near the PICU. A refrigerator is necessary for storing certain pharmaceutical products. Additionally, provision must be made for storing large patient care equipment items when not in use, as well as for stretchers and wheelchairs.

Clean and Dirty Utility Room

Clean and dirty utility rooms must be separate to maintain infection control standards. The clean utility room is designated for storing clean linen, while the dirty utility room should contain a separate sink. Covered bins are essential for storing soiled linen and waste materials. An area for emptying and cleaning bedpans and urine bottles is also necessary. Both the dirty utility area and toilets should have independent exhaust systems with visible indicators.

Waste Disposal

Disposal of contaminated waste, including segregation of garbage and medical waste, must adhere to standard pollution control guidelines. Proper disposal of needles and sharp objects is paramount for safety.

Conference Room and Library

A dedicated conference room for intensivist and staff education, discussion of complex cases, and quality improvement meetings is desirable. This room should include a small library with access to scientific literature and a computer with reliable internet connectivity for accessing online resources and point-of-care management tools.

Counseling Room

A designated room for intensivist-parent counseling sessions regarding the patient's condition and treatment plan is essential. Audio-video recording facilities for counseling sessions, with consent from the family, are recommended.

Equipment

Equipment selection should be based on factors including cost-benefit analysis, accuracy and suitability for pediatric patients, ease of use, troubleshooting requirements, maintenance needs, and availability of biomedical support.

Noise

Pediatric intensive care units, are often noisy environments due to the presence of equipment, alarms, and staff required for patient care and safety. Excessive noise levels can have adverse effects on patients, such as decreased oxygen saturation, disrupted sleep, and increased blood pressure and heart rate. The World Health Organization (WHO) recommends that ambient noise levels should not exceed 35 dB, yet levels in hospitals often range from 45 to 70 dB. To mitigate noise, high-performance sound-absorbing materials should be used for floor coverings and ceilings, balancing noise reduction with ease of cleaning and infection control.

Lighting

Lighting also significantly impacts patient outcomes. Studies on adult patients have shown that exposure to natural sunlight correlates with shorter lengths of stay and improved mental status. Guidelines suggest a minimum of one window per patient bed area in ICU settings. Additionally, recommended lighting levels for patient rooms are typically below 30 foot candles (fc), with the ability to dim to as low as 6.5 fc at night. Adequate lighting is essential for charting, emergencies, and procedures, necessitating lighting systems with multiple types of lights to meet various needs throughout the day and night.

Bedside Facilities

In PICU, bedside facilities play a crucial role in providing comprehensive care to critically ill children. These facilities include a range of equipment, supplies, and amenities designed to support patient monitoring, treatment, and comfort.

- Each child bed should be equipped with essential features such as adjustable height and side rails for safety.
- Multipara monitoring to continuously monitor the child's condition
- Mechanical ventilators are readily available for needy patients.
- IV infusion pumps to facilitate accurate medication and fluid administration.
- Bedside procedures, including central line insertion and chest tube placement, can be promptly conducted when needed.
- Effective communication tools like nurse call systems and patient communication boards enable seamless interaction between patients, families, and healthcare providers.
- Adequate storage space ensures efficient organization of medical supplies and equipment, while infection control measures such as hand hygiene stations and easy-to-clean surfaces mitigate the risk of healthcare-associated infections.

PEDIATRIC INTENSIVE CARE UNIT STAFF

Pediatric Intensivist

In the PICU, the pediatric intensivist assumes a pivotal role in the comprehensive care of critically ill children. With specialized training and expertise, the pediatric intensivist serves as the primary overseer of the child, encompassing not only specific organ failures but also the intricate interactions of whole-body systems.

Pediatric intensivists are uniquely qualified to address the complex needs of critically ill children, possessing in-depth knowledge of pediatric physiology, pathophysiology, and pharmacotherapy. They are adept at managing various organ failures, such as respiratory, cardiovascular, neurological, and renal dysfunction, utilizing evidence-based interventions tailored to each patient's condition.

Nurses

Pediatric intensive care unit nurses play a vital role in delivering specialized care to medically unstable infants and children. Their duties encompass continuous, vigilant, and compassionate care tailored to the unique needs of each patient and their family. This involves ongoing physiological assessments, implementation and evaluation of treatment plans, and devising strategies to address the family's needs. Effective communication with the healthcare team is paramount, enabling prompt responses to changes in the child's condition. PICU nurses possess essential skills to ensure optimal patient outcomes and family support through comprehensive care and effective teamwork.

In Indian tertiary care hospital PICU, nurse-to-patient ratios are crucial determinants of the quality of care provided to critically ill children. These ratios are primarily influenced by patient census and acuity levels, with typical ratios ranging from 1:3 to 2:1, as observed globally. However, several additional factors specific to the Indian context must be taken into consideration when determining staffing needs; these include the level of experience and expertise of the nursing staff, and the availability and utilization of advanced medical technology within the PICU. Units equipped with state-of-the-art technology may require fewer nurses per patient due to the efficiency and support provided by these advancements. Conversely, units with limited access to advanced technology may necessitate higher nurse-to-patient ratios to ensure adequate monitoring and intervention.

Respiratory Therapist

They are indispensable members of the interdisciplinary team in the pediatric intensive care setting, providing essential respiratory care services tailored to the unique needs of critically ill children. Their diverse responsibilities encompass the entire spectrum of respiratory management, from airway interventions to ventilation support, transport assistance, and continuous monitoring, thus contributing significantly to the holistic care of pediatric intensive care patients. One respiratory therapist should be present round the clock in PICU.

Physiotherapists

The role of physiotherapists in the PICU setting encompasses a range of interventions aimed at optimizing mobility and functional outcomes. These interventions may include passive range of motion exercises, active-assisted exercises, bed mobility training, sitting balance exercises, and ambulation assistance.

Perfusionist

In units providing ECMO or extracorporeal life support (ELS) services in the PICU, the expertise of a perfusionist is essential.

Other Ancillary Staff

Numerous other healthcare professionals are essential for providing comprehensive care to patients in the PICU. Pharmacists play a vital role in medication management, with a satellite pharmacy ideally located near the PICU for immediate medication dispensing. Nutritionists, occupational therapists, speech therapists, and social workers are integral members of the PICU team, each contributing specialized skills to patient care. It is crucial for these professionals to have training in pediatric environments to effectively address the unique needs of pediatric patients.

QUALITY IMPROVEMENT

Quality improvement measures are integral to ensuring the delivery of high-quality care in the PICU. Regular audits of key quality indicators, such as catheter-associated urinary tract infections (CAUTIs), central line-associated bloodstream infections (CLABSIs), ventilator-associated pneumonia (VAP) rates, medication errors, readmission rates, and reintubation rates, are mandated. Additionally, the use of severity of illness scoring systems such as Pediatric Risk of Mortality (PRISM) or Pediatric Index of Mortality (PIM) is required to assess patient acuity and guide clinical decision-making.

POLICIES AND PROTOCOLS

In PICU policies and protocol (international/national/institutional) are essential for ensuring standardized practices, promoting patient safety, and optimizing clinical outcomes.[8]

CONCLUSION

Establishing a PICU within a tertiary care center in India is essential for addressing the specialized needs of critically ill children. By adhering to international standards and guidelines, while also considering the unique challenges, PICU setups can effectively enhance the quality of pediatric critical care services. Robust infrastructure, including state-of-the-art equipment, adequate staffing, and well-designed facilities, is paramount to ensure optimal patient outcomes.

REFERENCES

1. Robertson-Steel I. Evolution of triage systems. Emerg Med J. 2006;23(2):154-5.
2. Crumplin MK. The Myles Gibson military lecture: surgery in the Napoleonic Wars. J R Coll Surg Edinb. 2002;47(3):566-78.
3. Iserson KV, Moskop JC. Triage in medicine, part I: Concept, history, and types. Ann Emerg Med. 2007;49(3):275-81.
4. Jayashree M, Singhi SC. Initial assessment and triage in ER. Indian J Pediatr. 2011;78(9):1100-8.
5. Khilnani P, Ramachandran B, Shaikh F, Sharma R, Sachdev A, Deopujari S, et al; Indian Academy of Pediatrics College Council of Pediatric Intensive Care Chapter. Consensus Guidelines for Pediatric Intensive Care Units in India, 2020. Indian Pediatr. 2020;57(11):1049-54.
6. Rungta N, Zirpe KG, Dixit SB, Mehta Y, Chaudhry D, Govil D, et al. Indian Society of Critical Care Medicine Experts Committee Consensus Statement on ICU Planning and Designing, 2020. Indian J Crit Care Med. 2020;24(Suppl 1):S43-S60.
7. Moss M, Simone S. Pediatric intensive care unit organization and physical design. In: Shaffner DH, McCloskey JJ, Hunt EA, Tasker RC (Eds). Rogers' Textbook of Pediatric Intensive Care, 6th edition. Philadelphia: Wolters Kluwer; 2023. pp. 48-62.
8. Frankel LR, Hsu BS, Yeh TS, Simone S, Agus MSD, Arca MJ, et al. Criteria for Critical Care Infants and Children: PICU Admission, Discharge, and Triage Practice Statement and Levels of Care Guidance. Pediatr Crit Care Med. 2019;20(9):847-87.
9. Tiwari L, Jayashree M, Jindal A, Khera D, Banerjee A, Bhatt G, et al. Practical guideline for setting up a comprehensive pediatric care unit for critical care delivery at district hospitals and medical colleges under ECRP-II. J Pediatr Crit Care. 2023;10(2):63.
10. Rosenberg DI, Moss MM. American Academy of Pediatrics Section on Critical Care; American Academy of Pediatrics Committee on Hospital Care. Guidelines and Levels of Care for Pediatric Intensive Care Units. Pediatrics. 2004;114:1114-25.

20.2 Poisoning and Envenomation

Mahesh A Mohite, Sheikh Minhaj Ahmed

INTRODUCTION

Poisoning and envenomation are the common emergencies for pediatricians and intensive care practitioners. Due to improper storage, easy availability, and curious behavior, accidental poisonings are relatively common in children. Majority of them are accidental in nature but can have cases of suicidal poisoning in adolescent age-group or homicidal cases in any age-group.

Poisoning in children should be suspected in an acute setting with sudden-onset symptoms in a previously healthy child presenting with unexplained altered mental status, hypertension, cardiorespiratory insufficiency, new-onset seizures, or nonspecific symptoms not fitting in any known natural course of disease. Many poisons do not have specific treatment and stabilizing the child on principles of emergency care, supporting the tissue function till recovery is the basic principle of their management.

EPIDEMIOLOGY

Incidence of poisoning in children is variable in different units and different geographical areas. It is influenced by socioeconomic and cultural practices in a given region. The incidence of childhood poisoning in various studies ranges from 0.33 to 7.6%. Poisoning is most commonly observed in children at 1–5 years of age and constitutes 80% of all poisoning cases. The mortality rate due to poisoning is 3–5%.[1] Most of the times, circumstantial evidence guides you to the possible offending agent. In infants, toddlers, and children usually it is a household substance that is accidentally consumed. Type of poison is also influenced by geographical factors as urban cases and rural cases have different poisoning agents.

CLINICAL PRESENTATIONS

Clinical presentations are varied depending upon the agent causing the poisoning. **Table 20.2.1** lists some common toxic substances and their clinical manifestations. A particular offending agent disturbs the physiology, expressing as a group of symptoms and signs. This toxin-induced syndrome complex is called as *toxidrome*. There are different toxidromes such as cholinergic, anticholinergic, opioids, and autonomic storms **(Table 20.2.2)**. A practitioner must learn to recognize these toxidromes so as to diagnose the cause of poisoning in

TABLE 20.2.1: Common toxic substances and their clinical manifestations.

Physical sign	***Poison***
Odors	
Bitter almonds	Cyanide
Acetone	Isopropyl alcohol, methanol, paraldehyde, salicylates
Alcohol	Ethanol
Oil of wintergreen	Methyl salicylate
Garlic	Organophosphates, arsenic, thallium
Eyes	
Miosis	Narcotics, OPC, mushrooms (muscarine), clonidine phenothiazines, barbiturates (late)
Mydriasis	Atropine, alcohol, cocaine, amphetamines, antihistamines, cyclic antidepressants, cyanide, carbon monoxide
Nystagmus	Phenytoin, barbiturates, ethanol, carbon monoxide
Lacrimation	OPC irritant gas/vapors
Skin	
Dry, hot skin	Anticholinergics, botulism
Diaphoresis	OPC mushrooms (muscarinic), aspirin, cocaine
Erythema	Anticholinergics, boric acid, mercury
Oral cavity	
Salivation	OPC, corrosives, salicylates
Dry mouth	Anticholinergics, antihistamines, amphetamines
Burns	Corrosives, oxalate-containing plants
Gastrointestinal	
Cramps	OPC arsenic
Diarrhea	Antibiotics, iron, boric add
Constipation	Narcotics, botulism, codeine, lead
Hematemesis	Corrosives, iron, salicylates and aminophylline
Cardiovascular	
Tachycardia	Atropine, aspirin, amphetamines, cocaine, cyclic antidepressants, theophylline
Bradycardia	Digitalis, narcotics, mushrooms, clonidine, OPC beta blockers, calcium channel blockers

Contd...

Contd...

Physical sign	*Poison*
Hypertension	Sympathomimetics, anticholinergics, MAO inhibitors
Hypotension	Phenothiazines, barbiturates, cyclic anti-depressants, iron, beta blockers, calcium channel blockers
Respiratory	
Hypopnea/ apnea	Alcohol, narcotics, barbiturates
Tachypnea	Amphetamines, aspirin, ethylene glycol, CO, cyanide
Pulmonary edema	Hydrocarbons, heroin, OPC
Neuromuscular	
Coma	Sedatives, narcotics, barbiturates, OPC, salicylates, cyanide, CO, lead, cyclic antidepressants
Hyperpyrexia	Anticholinergics, quinine, salicylates, phenothiazines, amphetamines, cocaine
Ataxia	Alcohol, antidepressants, barbiturates, anticholinergics, phenytoin, narcotics
Muscle fasciculation	OPC, theophylline
Paralysis	OPC, mercury, arsenic
Altered behavior	Anticholinergics, alcohol, camphor, amphetamines

(CO: carbon monoxide; MAO: monoamine oxidase; OPC: organo-phosphate compound)

TABLE 20.2.2: Common toxidromes.

Toxins	*Toxidrome*
Cholinergic (organophosphates, carbamates)	(Dumbbells) diarrhea, diaphoresis, urination, miosis, bradycardia, bronchial secretions, emesis, lacrimation, lethargic, salivation
Anticholinergics (antihistamines, cyclic antidepressants, atropine, phenothiazines, scopolamine)	Hyperthermia (hot as a hare), flushed (red as a beet), dry skin (dry as a bone), dilated pupils (blind as a bat), delirium, hallucinations (mad as a hatter), tachycardia, urinary urgency and retention
Sympathomimetics (cocaine, ephedrine, pseudoephedrine)	Mydriasis, tachycardia, hypertension, hyperthermia, seizures
Opioids (heroin, morphine, codeine, methadone, fentanyl, hydrocodone)	Miosis, bradycardia, hypotension, hypoventilation, coma
Opioid withdrawal	Diarrhea, mydriasis, goose flesh, tachycardia, lacrimation, hypertension, yawning, cramps, hallucinations, seizures

index case. This will help decide specific treatment early in the course of management, improving the overall outcome.

In a suspected case of poisoning or envenomation, detail history regarding child's daily activity, his/her visits to various parts of house and outside, neighbor's visits, relatives' visits, school schedule, visit to farm or ponds are needed to be asked. Any storage of household poisons for various reasons are required to be enquired, e.g., storage of paints by painter and battery by mechanics may expose child to lead and chemical caustics leading to accidental ingestion. Household medications that can be consumed accidentally or intentionally by children include sedatives, antipsychotics, antihypertensives, etc. Accidental consumption of kerosene stored in fancy storage bottles is a common occurrence.

For early appropriate management, recognition of poisoning agent is desirable and this can be achieved by good history-taking and clinical examination to recognize the toxidrome. We will discuss further the toxidromes in specific poisoning.

DIAGNOSIS

Diagnosis of poisoning and envenomation may not be straightforward and needs high index of suspicion and good clinical acumen. Circumstances, symptoms, clinical examination, and laboratory tests are the keys to diagnosis. Many a time, caretakers know the agent. When it is not known, the clinical features may give clues about possible poison. Laboratory tests seldom help in the specific management. Gastric lavage sample needs to be preserved for forensic analysis and medicolegal purposes. Usually, these reports are available late which do not help in active management. For monitoring the clinical condition, routine emergency laboratory tests including serum electrolytes, blood glucose, arterial blood gases (ABG), liver function tests (LFTs), kidney function tests (KFTs), and bleeding profiles need to be performed. Few toxicology panels are available in advance laboratories; levels of benzodiazepines in urine sample, methemoglobin levels on spectrophotometry and co-oximetry, and red blood cell (RBC) acetylcholinesterase (AChE) levels in organophosphate poisoning can help in specific diagnosis and appropriate treatment.

GENERAL APPROACH TO A POISONED CHILD (FLOWCHART 20.2.1)

First Aid

Only 20–30% of known poisons have specific antidote. Majority need support of airway, breathing, hemodynamics, and neurological system till the effect of the poison wanes off from the body by natural process or facilitated by other techniques as described in the following text.

Emesis

Emesis is making the patient to vomit the toxin. This method is found to be unsafe and at times dangerous due to risk of aspiration and stomach and esophageal injury. Guidelines no longer recommend emesis in cases of poisoning.

Gastric Lavage

If a patient is brought to emergency room (ER) early, gastric lavage can help removing the toxin to the extent of 20–70%. It can be done if patient presents within 2 hours of consumption of the toxin. It is associated with risk of aspiration, more so in a patient with altered sensorium. In such cases, intubation with a cuffed endotracheal tube is preferable prior to gastric lavage. Lavage should be done with 0.9% saline with a quantity appropriate to stomach capacity. Gastric lavage is contraindicated in hydrocarbon ingestion as risk of aspiration and aggravation of chemical pneumonitis is very high in these cases.

Flowchart 20.2.1: General approach to a poisoned child.

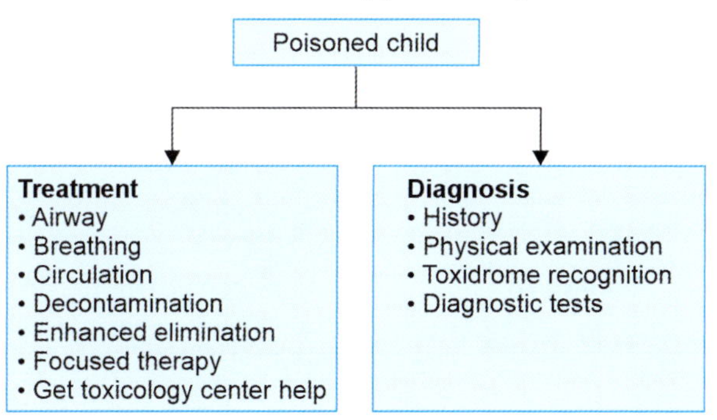

Activated Charcoal

Activated charcoal powder subjected to high temperature makes it porous increasing its surface area to adsorb the toxin in gastrointestinal (GI) system. It is to be given as 250 mg/kg immediately after lavage and repeated after 6 hours. It can be used for few toxins injected parenterally, e.g., digoxin and aminophylline. These toxins are secreted in stomach and can be adsorbed on activated charcoal. Activated charcoal is, however, ineffective in case of cyanide, hydrocarbon, ethanol, methanol, and iron and heavy metal poisoning.

Whole Bowel Lavage

This method irrigates the bowel to wash out the remanent toxin. It is done with polyethylene glycol solution given as 30 mL/kg at the maximum rate of 500 mL/h and continued till the effluent is clear (this is akin to preoperative preparation of bowel). This is contraindicated if serious GI injury is suspected.

Specific Management

When a child is brought to the outpatient clinic, ER, or pediatric intensive care unit (PICU), if poison is known and definite antidote is available, then antidote becomes priority while basic airway, breathing, and hemodynamic support is being provided to the child **(Table 20.2.3)**.

SUPPORTIVE CARE

If patient has respiratory insufficiency, then he/she may need oxygen, noninvasive or invasive ventilatory support as per clinical need. If patient is in shock, then volume resuscitation and appropriate vasoactive drugs become the priority. Shock and respiratory compromise need to be managed as for other

TABLE 20.2.3: Antidotes.

Toxin	*Antidote*	*Dose and route*
Paracetamol	N-acetyl cysteine	140 mg/kg stat orally followed by 70 mg/kg Q 4 h for 17 doses (in chronic poisoning only 12 doses); IV administration within 8–10 hours of ingestion, loading dose of 150 mg/kg infused over 15–60 minutes, followed by an initial maintenance dose of 50 mg/kg over 4 hours, followed by 100 mg/kg over 16 hours
Anticholinergics (atropine)	Physostigmine	0.02 mg/kg IV
Benzodiazepines	Flumazenil	0.01 mg/kg IV (maximum 3 mg)
Beta blockers	Glucagon	0.15 mg/kg IV stat followed by 0.1 mg/kg/h
Calcium channel blockers	Calcium chloride 10%	0.1–0.2 mL/kg IV
	Glucagon	0.15 mg/kg IV stat followed by 0.1 mg/kg/h
Carbamates	Atropine	0.1 mg/kg/dose (repeated till atropinization)

Contd...

Contd...

Toxin	*Antidote*	*Dose and route*
Organophosphates	Atropine	0.05 mg/kg/dose (repeated till atropinization)
	Pralidoxime	50 mg/kg IV stat followed by 25 mg/kg Q 4 h
Cyanide	Amyl nitrite inhalation	
	3% sodium nitrite	0.15–0.3 mL/kg IV infusion (maximum 300 mg)
	Sodium thiosulfate	400 mg/kg (maximum 12.5 g)
Digoxin	Digibind (digoxin immune antibody fragment)	1 mL binds 0.6 mg digoxin
Methanol	10% ethanol	10 mL/kg IV stat followed by 1–2 mL/kg/h
Ethylene glycol	10% ethanol	10 mL/kg IV stat followed by 1–2 mL/kg/h
	Fomepizole	15 mg/kg/dose IV
Iron	Desferrioxamine	5–15 mg/kg/h IV infusion
Isoniazid	Pyridoxine	1 g per g ingested
Methemoglobinemia	Methylene blue	1–2 mg/kg/dose IV
Opioids	Naloxone	0.5–2 mg IV titrated to effect
Salicylates	Sodium bicarbonate	150 mEq + 40 mEq KCl in 1 L of 5% dextrose infused to maintain a urine output of 1–2 mL/kg/h and a urine pH of 7.5
Tricyclic antidepressants	Sodium bicarbonate	1–2 mEq/kg
Warfarin/super warfarin	Vitamin K_1	0.5 mg/kg IV/SC/PO
	FFP	15 mL/kg/dose till PT normalizes
Botulism	Botulinum antitoxin	
Heparin	Protamine	
Type 1 antiarrhythmics	Sodium bicarbonate	1–2 mEq/kg

(FFP: fresh frozen plasma; PT: prothrombin time)

indications. Few patients may need renal replacement therapy (RRT) or liver support. RRT will help in removing the toxin as well as supporting the renal, cardiac, neurological functions till the natural system starts functioning adequately.

COMMON POISONING AND ENVENOMATION

ORGANOPHOSPHORUS POISONING

Organophosphates (OPs) are the compounds of phosphoric acid with alkyl or alkylamino side chains, and used as insecticides worldwide. An estimated 3,000,000 people are exposed to OP or carbamate agents each year worldwide, with up to 300,000 fatalities.[2] It is a popular suicidal poison in the world, with children and women being the common victim. Children are particularly prone for poisoning and higher exposure due to greater dose to body mass ratio, shorter height, and higher minute ventilation.

Pathophysiology

Table 20.2.4 lists common OP substances. OP compounds bind to AChE, making this enzyme nonfunctional, thus increasing the synaptic levels of acetylcholine (ACh). Increased ACh levels have following effects:

- *Muscarinic effects:* Postganglionic parasympathetic stimulation leads to increased exocrine secretion. The smooth muscles of sweat gland, salivary gland bronchial tree, gastrointestinal tract (GIT), urinary bladder, and ureter contract. The net effect is "SLUDGE", i.e., salivation, lacrimation, urination, diarrhea, GI upset, and emesis. Large-dose intoxication may lead to tachycardia, hypertension, and arrythmia.
- *Nicotinic effects:* Increased stimulation of neuromuscular junctions at skeletal muscles causes fasciculations and cramps followed by paralysis and weakness.
- *Central effect:* Direct effect on the brain leads to ataxia, disorientation, drowsiness, seizures, and coma.

TABLE 20.2.4: Common organophosphorus substances.

Natural	*Organophosphorus*	*Organochlorine*	*Carbamates*	*Repellents*	*Synthetic pyrethroids*
Pyrethrum	Chlorthion	DDT	Carbaryl	Benzyl benzoate	Resmethrin
Nicotine	Fenthion	BHC	Dimetilan	Indalone	Bioresmethrin
Mineral oils	Malathion	Chlordane	Pyrolan	Diethyl-meta-toluamide	Pothrin
Rotenone	Parathion	Aldrin	Propoxur	Dimethyl phthalate	
Derris	• Methyl parathion • Fenitrothion • Dioxathion • Diazinon • Dicapthon • Chlorpyrifos • Dichlorvos • Trichlorfon • Abate • Dimethoate • Gardena	• Dieldrin • Methoxychlor • Heptachlor • Toxaphene • Kepone • Mirex		Ethyl hexanediol	

Flowchart 20.2.2: Clinical features of organophosphorus poisoning.

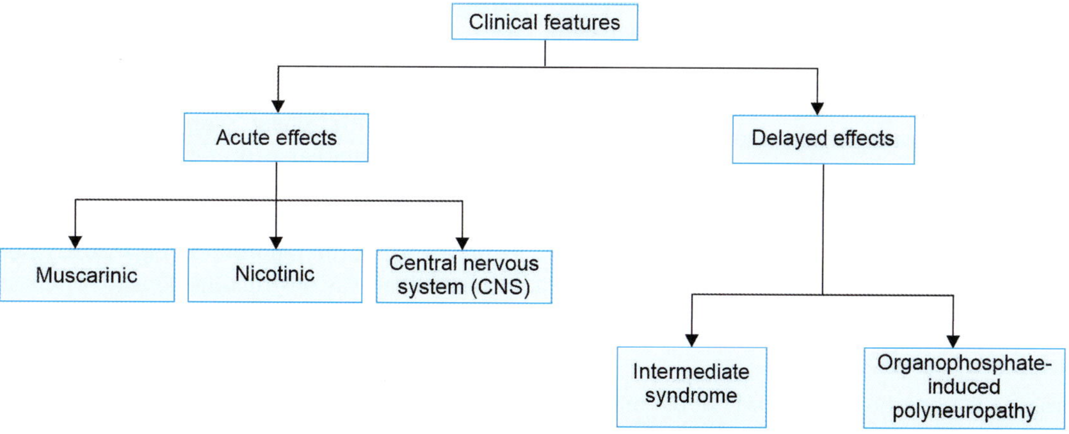

Clinical Features

Organophosphate poisoning should be suspected in a child with the cholinergic toxidrome that may comprise of muscarinic and/or nicotinic signs and symptoms. Clinical features include (**Flowchart 20.2.2**):

- *GIT:* Nausea, vomiting, abdominal cramps, and excessive salivation
- *Central nervous system (CNS):* Headache, giddiness, weakness, vertigo, confusion, disorientation, and drowsiness
- *Respiratory system:* Chest tightness, difficulty in breathing, excessive bronchial secretion, and pulmonary edema
- *Heart:* Bradycardia and heart blocks
- *Eye:* Miosis, blurred vision, and lacrimation

Diagnosis

The diagnosis of OP poisoning is made on the basis of history and clinical presentation. A history of a known or suspected exposure is helpful, but often may not be available. The diagnosis is largely clinical, ascertained by serum or RBC cholinesterase level when the OP poisoning is not evident or when toxicity is mild. Get the electrocardiogram (ECG) for conduction disturbances and cardiac arrhythmias, which may occur in OP poisoning.

Management

Patient is evacuated from the exposure source, clothing removed, and body washed thoroughly with mild soap and water. Airway, breathing, and circulation (ABC) assessed and stabilized as per the clinical status. OP poisoning results in significant GI fluid losses. Optimize circulation with volume resuscitation and vasopressors as per need. Frequent suctioning, respiratory support, and ventilation with escalating care as may be required. For ingestion, gastric lavage followed by activated charcoal (0.5–1 g/kg) is indicated, may be repeated after 24 hours.

Antidote

Rapid administration of atropine is indicated in the acutely symptomatic patient. Atropine may be administered in a dose of 0.05 mg/kg intravenously and repeated every 5–15 minutes until all secretions are dry.

Pralidoxime (PAM): PAM is nucleophilic oxime that regenerates AChE at the muscarinic and nicotinic synapses by reversing phosphorylation of the active site of the enzyme.[2] PAM therapy is effective in early course of disease. The dose of PAM is 25–50 mg/kg (maximum 1 g) in 100–150 mL NS/D5W (normal saline/dextrose 5% in water) intravenous infusion over 30 minutes, may be repeated every 6–8 hourly as may be required.

Prognosis

Organophosphate-induced delayed peripheral neuropathy occurs 1–3 weeks after exposure, begins as sensory symptoms, progresses to motor involvement, and may recover after 12 months of exposure. Severe OP poisoning may need prolonged respiratory support. Aggressive respiratory management, timely antidote, and intensive appropriate supportive care may lead to improved outcome.

KEROSENE POISONING

The word kerosene is from the Greek word "*keros*", meaning "wax". It is an aliphatic hydrocarbon consisting of straight-chain compound. Accidental kerosene poisoning is relatively common in children below 5 years of age due to easy availability of kerosene in rural households and the exploratory nature of young children. The inflammatory reaction in the lungs depends on the degree of exposure, volatility, surface tension, and viscosity. The low viscosity of kerosene makes penetration to more distal airways easy causing necrotizing pneumonia and liquefaction of the lipid surfactant layer.

Clinical Features (Table 20.2.5)[3]

- Asymptomatic
- GI irritation
- Immediate symptoms of aspiration—coughing, choking, tachypnea, grunting respiration
- Later symptoms of aspiration—2–6 hours

TABLE 20.2.5: Scoring for grading of severity.[3]

Parameter	*Absent*	*Present*
Fever	0	1
Malnutrition	0	1
Respiratory distress	0	2
Neurological symptoms	0	2
Cyanosis	0	4
Convulsion	0	4

Note: Score >4 = Observe; >7 = Poor prognosis

- Progressive lung disease with manifestations of hypoxia, cardiorespiratory failure
- Cardiac arrythmias
- Convulsions, drowsiness, and coma
- Fever in first 48 hours
- Fever beyond 48 hours suggestive of bacterial super infection

Diagnosis

Radiological Abnormalities

A chest X-ray must be taken in all victims of kerosene poisoning. Initial chest X-ray may be normal; however, findings may appear within 2–12 hours in majority of the victims. The radiological findings may include multiple small opacities, atelectasis progressing to pneumatoceles, emphysema, or pneumothorax **(Figs. 20.2.1A and B)**. Long-term small airway obstruction signs may persist for decades in severe injury.

Arterial Blood Gas Analysis

It may reveal hypoxemia or hypocarbia, which may progress to hypercarbia due to abnormalities in gas exchange. Increased anion gap metabolic acidosis may denote presence of coingestants, such as methanol or ethylene glycol.

Management

Assess ABC and stabilize the child with supportive care as may be required. Management is guided by the clinical condition at variable intervals as 2 hours, 6 hours, 24 hours, 48 hours and associated X-ray picture **(Flowchart 20.2.3)**. Most critical period is the first 24–48 hours. If the child is stable in first 6 hours, then he/she usually does not deteriorate later. There is no role of activated charcoal, gastric lavage, cathartics and steroids in the treatment of kerosene poisoning. In the initial asymptomatic child, 24-hour observation period is suggested as the child may develop full blown clinical symptoms over period of time.

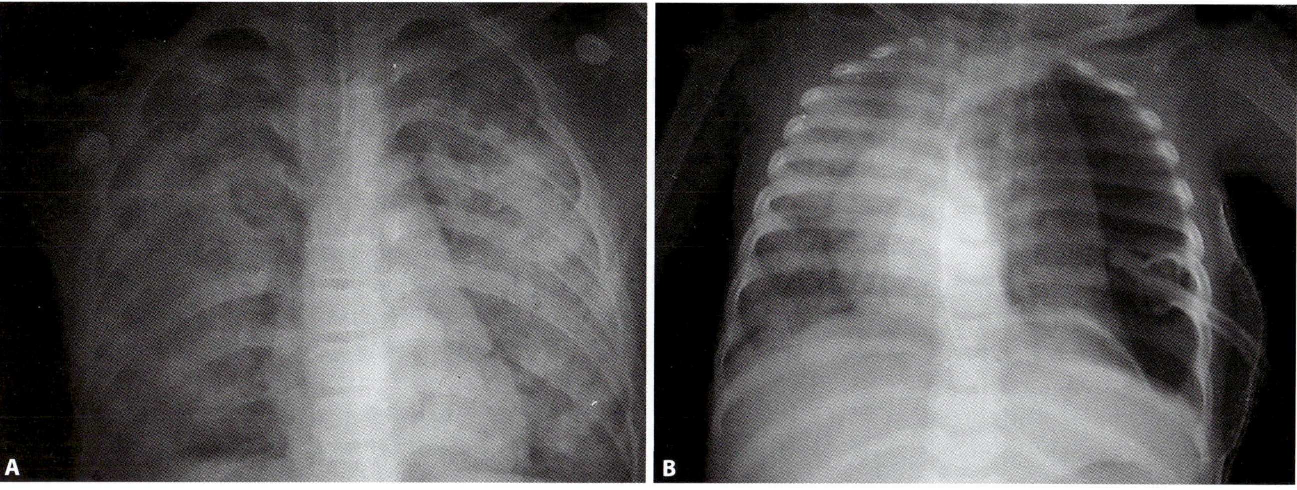

Figs. 20.2.1A and B: X-ray changes in kerosene poisoning.

Flowchart 20.2.3: Management of kerosene poisoning.

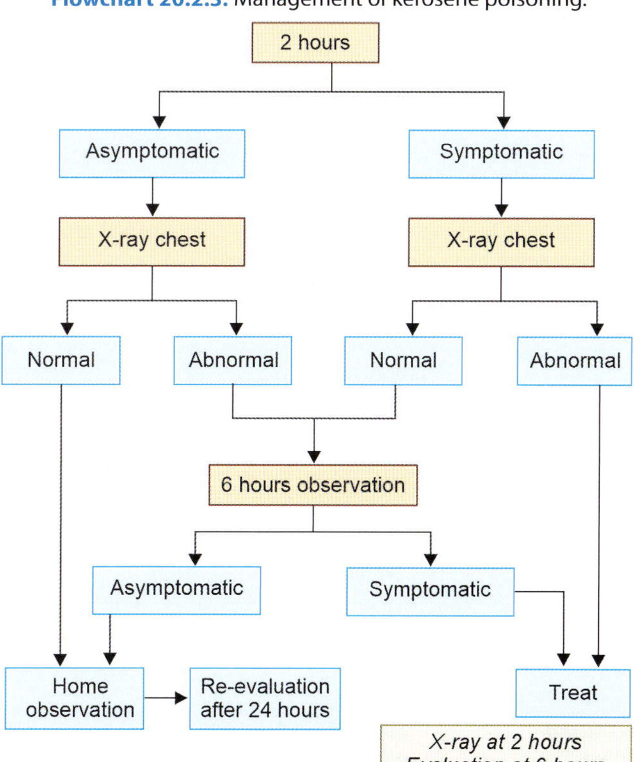

PARACETAMOL POISONING

Paracetamol (PCM) is a commonly used analgesic and antipyretic agent and in recommended therapeutic doses, its safety and efficacy is well established. Many formulations with variable dosage forms are easily available for over-the-counter sale. PCM poisoning may be unintentional due to exploratory nature of young children or inappropriate dosing by the caregiver; or it can be intentional among older children and adolescents. PCM toxicity is the leading cause of acute liver failure (ALF) in North America, Europe, and Australia.

Pathophysiology

Following oral ingestion, PCM is absorbed with peak concentration at 45 minutes. In slow released formulations, time to peak concentration may be delayed 8 hours or more. After absorption PCM is mainly metabolized inside the liver into two nontoxic metabolites, sulfate (30%) and glucuronide (55%) conjugates, which are excreted in the urine.[4] N-acetyl-p-benzoquinone imine (NAPQI), a highly reactive toxic metabolite formed by cytochromes P-450 2E1 and 3A4, is detoxified by glutathione (GSH)-dependent reactions to two nontoxic metabolites, mercapturic acid and cysteine conjugates. GSH combines with NAPQI resulting in nontoxic compound eliminated in urine. Depleted GSH with excess of NAPQI level is responsible for the liver cell injury that occurs with PCM toxicity.

Toxic Dose

In children younger than 12 years, the recommended maximum therapeutic dose is 90 mg/kg/day (15 mg/kg/dose, q 4 hourly). The therapeutic dose for children 12 years and older and adults is 325–1,000 mg per dose every 4–6 hours (maximum daily dose 4 g). Therapeutic serum concentrations range from 10 to 20 µg/mL (66–132 µmol/L). An acute ingestion is defined as any number of ingestions that occur within a period of up to 8 hours. Acute toxic dose of PCM is 200 mg/kg in children. Among infants of 6–9 weeks, even lower doses (of 60–100 mg/kg/day) may cause liver cell injury. Repeated supratherapeutic ingestion involves multiple ingestions over a period of >24 hours that results in a total dosage of >4 g/day.

Clinical Course

Table 20.2.6 shows the stages with clincal features of of acute acetaminophen intoxication.

Management

The management of PCM poisoning requires following risk assessment:

- Dose and time of ingestion
- Type of ingestion, that is acute (deliberate) versus repeated supratherapeutic ingestion
- Preparation ingested, i.e., immediate release versus slow release
- Laboratory results that guide antidote use, i.e., initial PCM and alanine transaminase (ALT)/aspartate transaminase (AST) levels
- Clinical and laboratory features to monitor for acute liver injury (ALI) or ALF (late) or hepatic encephalopathy—ALT/AST, blood glucose, arterial/venous blood gases, coagulation profile, renal function, and phosphate

Patients who present early within 1–2 hours of ingestion should receive activated charcoal, which may reduce the gut absorption of PCM. Patients at risk of hepatotoxicity should receive intravenous n-acetylcysteine (NAC) **(Table 20.2.7)**.[5] The PCM nomogram is used to assess the need for treatment in acute PCM ingestions where the time of ingestion is known **(Fig. 20.2.2)**. Value above the line indicates need for NAC infusion, which is most effective when started within

TABLE 20.2.6: Stages of acute acetaminophen intoxication.

Stage	*Hours after ingestion*	*Clinical features*
I	0.5–24 hours	• Nausea, vomiting, pallor, lethargy, malaise • Some patients remain asymptomatic • Laboratory studies are typically normal
II	24–72 hours	• Stage I symptoms resolve • Hepatotoxicity and nephrotoxicity become evident • Right upper quadrant pain, liver enlargement and tenderness • Elevation of aminotransferases occurs within 36 hours of ingestion in patients with hepatic injury • Elevation of prothrombin time (PT) and international normalized ratio (INR) of PT • Oliguria, abnormalities of renal function • Elevation of serum amylase with or without clinical pancreatitis
III	72–96 hours	• Liver enzyme and function abnormalities peak • Recurrence of stage I symptoms • Jaundice, hepatic encephalopathy, hyperammonemia, bleeding diathesis, hypoglycemia, lactic acidosis • Renal failure • Death, from multiorgan failure, occurs most commonly in this stage
IV	04–14 days	• Recovery phase • Symptoms and laboratory values may not normalize for several weeks • Histologic recovery lags behind clinical recovery

TABLE 20.2.7: N-acetylcysteine dose and dilution as per body weight.

Body weight	*Bag 1 (loading dose) 150 mg/kg in 3 mL/kg of diluent* infused over 1 hour*		*Bag 2 (second dose) 50 mg/kg in 7 mL/kg of diluent* infused over 4 hours*		*Bag 3 (third dose) 100 mg/kg diluted in 14 mL/kg of diluent* infused over 16 hours*	
	Loading dose	*Diluent volume*	*Second dose*	*Diluent volume*	*Third dose*	*Diluent volume*
5 kg[†]	750 mg	15 mL	250 mg	35 mL	500 mg	70 mL
10 kg	1,500 mg	30 mL	500 mg	70 mL	1,000 mg	140 mL
15 kg	2,250 mg	45 mL	750 mg	105 mL	1,500 mg	210 mL
20 kg	3,000 mg	60 mL	1,000 mg	140 mL	2,000 mg	280 mL

Contd...

Contd...

Body weight	Bag 1 (loading dose) 150 mg/kg in 100 mL of diluent* infused over 1 hour	Bag 2 (second dose) 50 mg/kg in 250 mL of diluent* infused over 4 hours	Bag 3 (third dose) 100 mg/kg in 500 mL of diluent* infused over 16 hours
21 kg	3,150 mg	1,050 mg	2,100 mg
30 kg	4,500 mg	1,500 mg	3,000 mg
40 kg	6,000 mg	2,000 mg	4,000 mg

*Dilute acetylcysteine in one of the following three solutions: Sterile water for injection, 0.45% sodium chloride injection, or 5% dextrose in water.
†Recommended dosing for those <5 kg has not been studied.

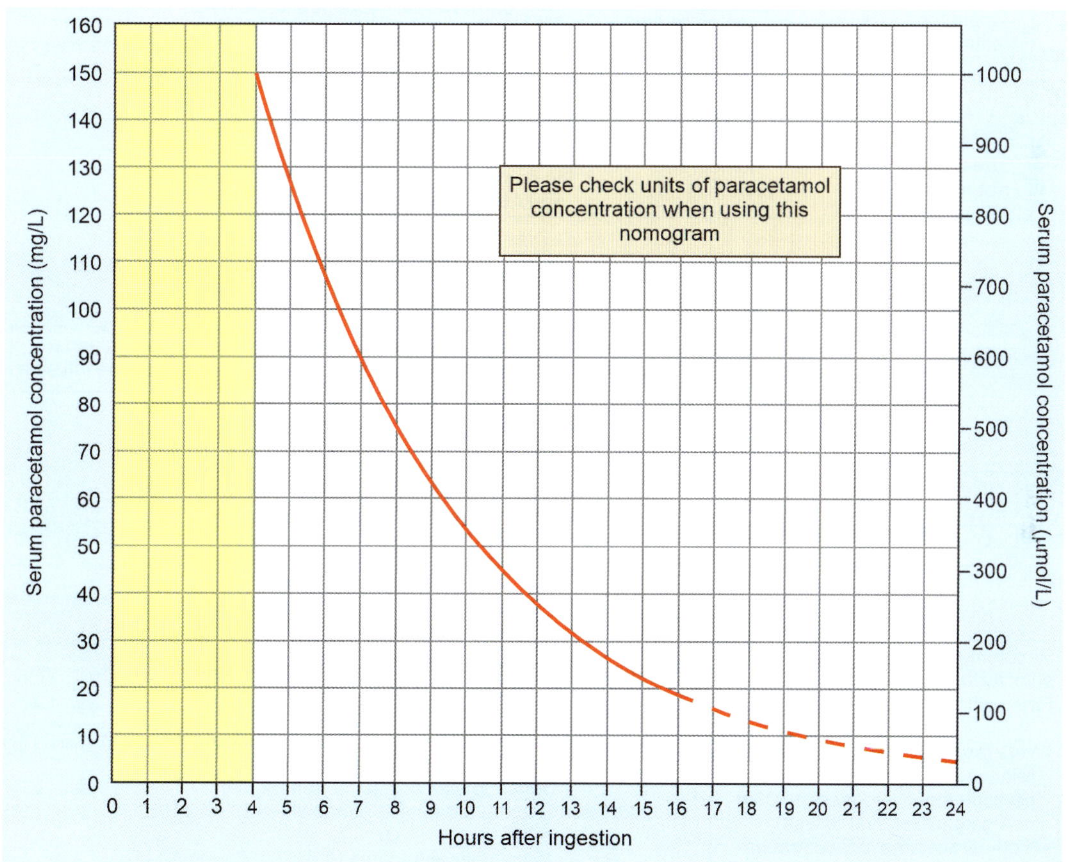

Fig. 20.2.2: Paracetamol treatment nomogram (Rumack–Matthew nomogram).

8 hours of ingestion. In children who require NAC beyond 20 hours, NAC can be stopped if ALT or AST are decreasing, international normalized ratio (INR) <2.0, PCM level returned to <10 mg/L, and child is clinically better (**Flowchart 20.2.4**).[6]

Prognosis

Many children with an acute overdose can be safely and effectively managed with NAC to prevent ALF. If treated early within 8 hours of ingestion, outcome is generally favorable. Hepatotoxicity occurs with increased frequency (20–30%) when administration of NAC is delayed >10 hours from ingestion. The poor prognostic factors in PCM-induced hepatic failure are pH below 7.3, serum creatinine above 300 mmol/L, and prothrombin time (PT) above 100 seconds in grade III to IV encephalopathy. Factor VIII to factor V ratio above 30 is the best poor prognostic indicator.

SNAKE BITE

As per World Health Organization (WHO) estimates, globally each year 5.4 million people are bitten by snakes with 1.8–2.7 million cases of envenomation, causing around 81,410–1,38,000 snake bite deaths annually.[7] India contributes to

Flowchart 20.2.4: Management algorithm for acute immediate release paracetamol ingestion.[6]

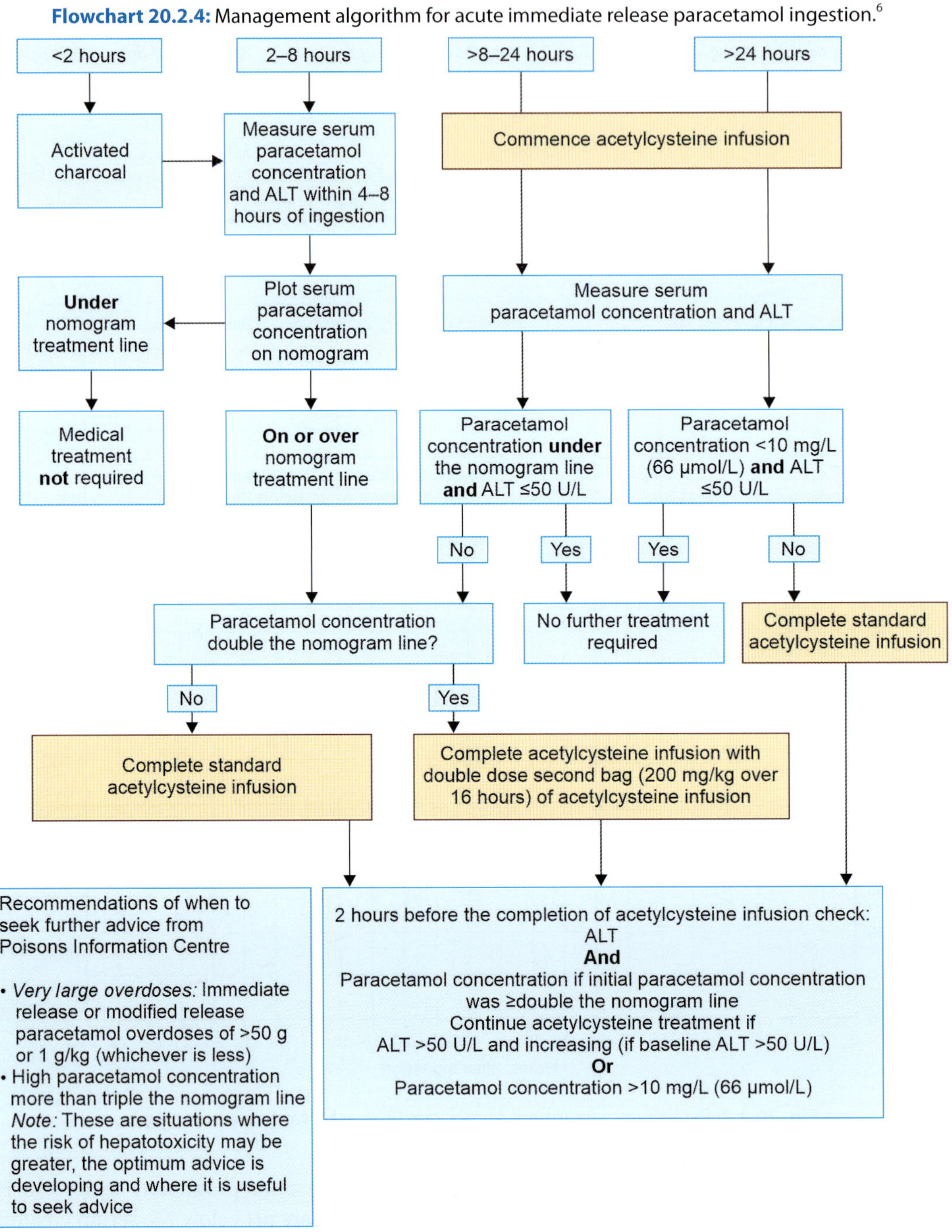

about half of global snake bite deaths amounting to around 46,000 annual snake bite deaths in 2005.[8]

There are 3,500 known snakes species of which around 300 species of snakes are poisonous; among which the common krait (*Bungarus caeruleus*), Indian cobra (*Naja naja*), saw-scaled viper (*Echis carinatus*), and Russell's viper (*Daboia russelii*) are the common snakes responsible for 95% of snake bite deaths (**Fig. 20.2.3**).

Venomous snake bites can cause neuroparalysis, respiratory failure, bleeding disorders that can lead to a fatal hemorrhage, irreversible kidney failure and tissue damage causing permanent disability and limb amputation. Children and agricultural workers are the most vulnerable population for snake bites. Children suffer more severe effects than adults, due to their smaller body mass.

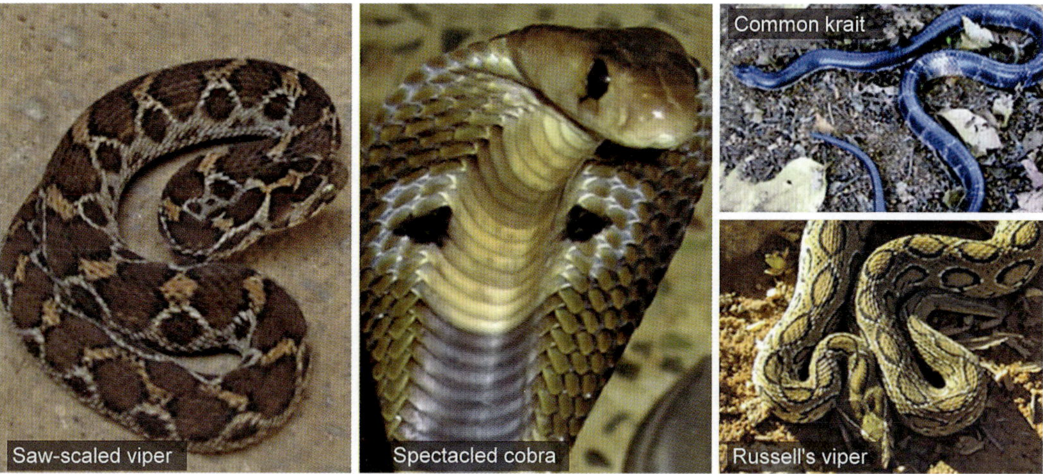

Fig. 20.2.3: Common snake species in India.

Snake Venom

Snake venom is a complex mixture of various enzymes, nonenzymatic proteins, and polypeptides. The clinical features are based on the predominance of a particular component of the snake venom compound.

Enzymes: Snake venom contains hydrolases, hyaluronidase, and proteases. These cause local injury at the site of bite and augment the damage caused by other components of venom.

Nonenzyme proteins:

- *Nerve growth factor:* Seen in elapid and viperid venom
- *Hemorrhagins*: Seen in viper venom
- *Neurotoxin and cardioaxins*: Seen in elapids and hydropids

Nonenzyme polypeptides:

- *Neurotoxins*: Lethal neurotoxins are seen in venom of cobra (cobra toxin), krait (alpha, beta and gamma bungarotoxin), and sea snakes (erabutoxins)
- *Vasculotoxin*: It causes endothelial (vipers) and basement membrane injury leading to capillary leak, edema, and shock.
- *Hemorrhagins*: Mainly exhibited by vipers; they work at various levels of coagulation cascade producing disseminated intravascular coagulation (DIC)-like picture. Snake venom-related coagulopathy differs from classical DIC in that platelets are not overconsumed; thrombin and D-dimer levels remain normal.
- *Cardiotoxin*: Venom molecule has direct effect on cardiac cell membranes, smooth muscles, and skeletal muscles, depolarizing the membrane and causing arrest in systole.

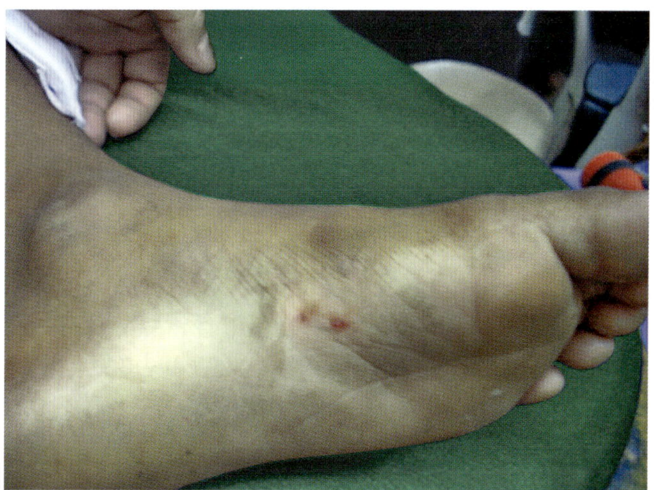

Fig. 20.2.4: Local fang marks.

Clinical Features

Local Features

Symptoms appear within 10–30 minutes of bite. Cobra bites have rapid onset of local swelling, pain, and bleeding. Krait bites have only local mark and no other signs (**Fig. 20.2.4**). Local findings are severe in case of vipers such as edema, pain, bleeding, gangrenous patch, compartment syndrome, bullae, etc. Nonpoisonous bites also cause local symptoms but usually they are not progressive.

Systemic Manifestation

It usually starts within 15 minutes to 1 hour, but may appear as late as 12 hours in cobra bite and up to 48 hours in viper bite. Hence, cobra bite should be observed for at least 24 hours and viper bite for at least 72 hours owing to their delayed manifestations.

Cobra bite: Abdominal pain may start within 1 hour due to submucosal intestinal bleed. Neuromuscular blockade may gradually cause ptosis, difficulty in swallowing, broken neck, weakness of limbs, respiratory failure, and death if not treated on time.

Krait bite: It has typical history wherein an asymptomatic child who is asleep at night, gets up at midnight due to abdominal pain and is found in respiratory failure early morning. This is because krait is a nocturnal species that chases rodents and mice in the house at night.

Vipers: They exhibit vasculotoxicity, hemolysis, and coagulopathy. Bleeding from local sites, progressive swelling with hemorrhagic bullae can be seen. Bleeding time (BT), clotting time (CT), PT, and partial thromboplastin time (PTT) are prolonged. Progressive bleeding may lead to shock and multiorgan dysfunction and death.

Diagnosis

- *20-minute whole blood clotting test (20WBCT)*: Simple bedside test where 3–5 mL blood is collected in a test tube, left undisturbed for 20 minutes at ambient temperature; after 20 minutes the test tube is turned upside down. If blood is not clotted, coagulopathy is confirmed necessitating antisnake venom (ASV) therapy **(Fig. 20.2.5)**.
- *Tests for bleeding and clotting assessment*: PT, activated partial thromboplastin time (aPTT), INR, platelet count, fibrin degradation products (FDP), D-dimer, complete blood count (CBC), peripheral smear, and reticulocyte count are done based on availability as appropriate.
- *Tests for organ involvement*: These include renal function test for kidney injury, ECG for arrythmias, and tests for rhabdomyolysis as urine for blood and myoglobin, RBCs, and serum creatinine kinase.

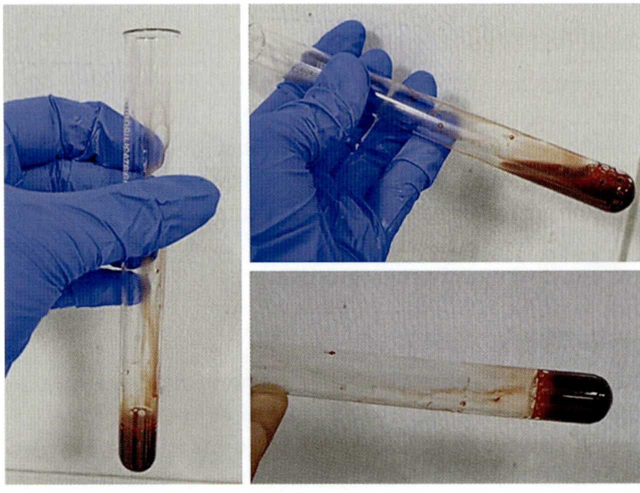

Fig. 20.2.5: 20-minute whole blood clotting test (20WBCT).

Management

Prehospital First Aid (Do It RIGHT)[9]

R—Reassure the patient.
I—Immobilize in the same way as a fractured limb. Use bandages or cloth to hold the splints, not to block the blood supply or apply pressure.
GH—Get to hospital immediately. Traditional remedies have *no proven* benefit in treating snake bite.
T—Tell the doctor of any systemic symptoms such as ptosis that may manifest on the way to hospital.

Limb Immobilization

The affected (bite) area should be immobilized and splinted if required **(Fig. 20.2.6)**. Any movement is going to rapidly aggravate spread of the venom proximally. Also, the paralytic effect of elapid venom is aggravated by repeated movements and depolarization of presynaptic plate.

Pressure Immobilization Method

Pressure immobilization method (PIM) is advised to prevent venom flow into the system. It involves crepe bandage tied around the limb, loose enough to allow two fingers slipping underneath **(Fig. 20.2.7)**. It should not be kept in place for a long period and should be removed only after ASV injection has been administered.

Acute Care

- *Airway stabilization*: Ensure the airway is clean and maintainable. There may be oral secretions due to palatal weakness, weak cough reflex, and inability to clear secretions.
- *Breathing*: Watch for efforts of breathing and provide respiratory support based on degree of breathing compromise.
- *Circulation*: It needs to be optimized with volume resuscitation, blood products, and vasoactive agents as may be required.

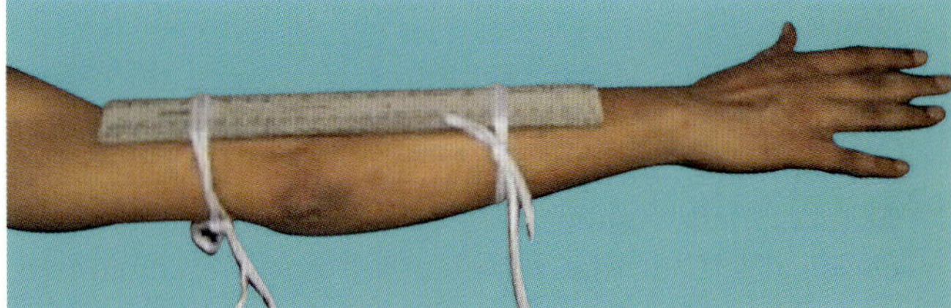

Fig. 20.2.6: Limb immobilization.
Source: Ministry of Health and Family Welfare. (2016). Standard Treatment Guidelines—Management of Snake Bite. [online] Available from https://nhm.gov.in/images/pdf/guidelines/nrhm-guidelines/stg/Snakebite_Full.pdf [Last accessed December, 2024].

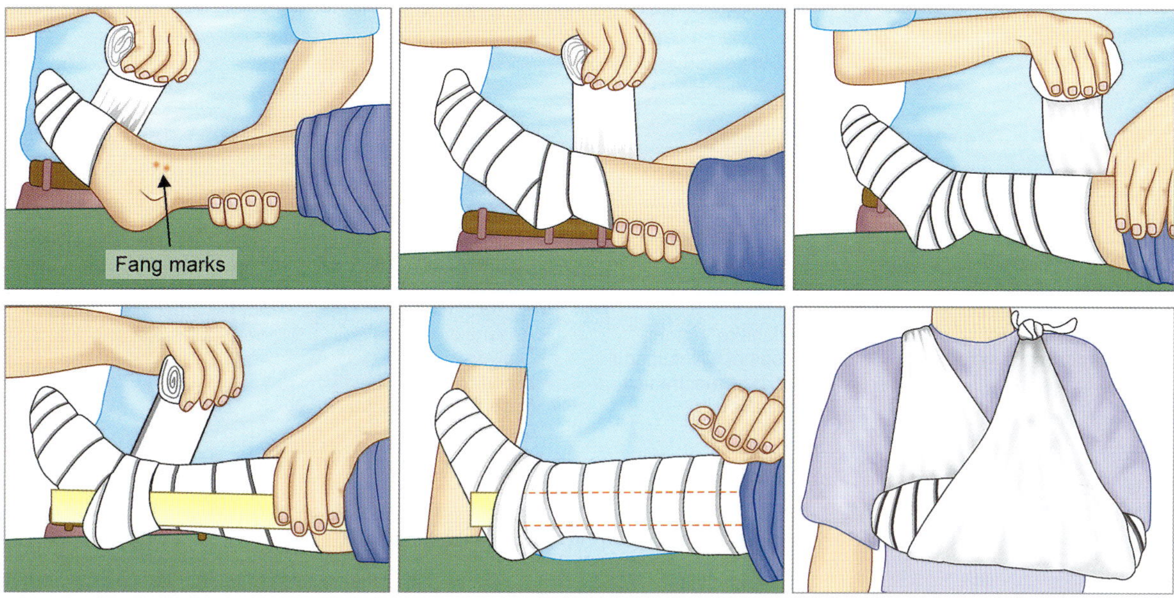

Fig. 20.2.7: Pressure immobilization methods.

Antisnake Venom

Two types of ASVs are available—the monovalent and polyvalent. ASV available in India is polyvalent and available as 10-mL vials in liquid and lyophilized forms and is useful toward the big four common snakes. The liquid form has a shelf life of around 2 years and requires good cold chain system whereas lyophilized form has a longer shelf life of around 5 years and can be stored at cool dark place to avoid exposure to heat. Each mL of polyvalent ASV neutralizes 0.60 mg of cobra, 0.45 mg of common krait, 0.6 mg of Russell's viper, and 0.45 mg of saw-scaled viper venom.

Antisnake Venom Indications

Local indications include rapid extension of local swelling and enlargement of draining lymph nodes of the bitten part. Systemic indications are neurotoxicity, hematological manifestations, cardiovascular abnormality, acute kidney injury (AKI), and hemoglobinuria or myoglobinuria.

Antisnake Venom Dose

Antivenin therapy should be started as soon as possible, latest by 4 hours after bite. Initial dose depends upon the approximate estimate of volume of envenomation as under **(Table 20.2.8)**. In children and small adults (body weight <40 kg) up to 50% greater doses of ASV should be administered. Each ASV vial is dissolved in 10 mL saline. Total dose is then diluted in 5–10 mL/kg 0.9% saline or 5% dextrose and given as an infusion over 30 minutes to 1 hour with close bedside monitoring, keeping injection adrenaline 0.01 mg/kg of 1:1,000 ready. Local-site infiltration of ASV is not advisable. Test doses have been shown to have no predictive value in detecting anaphylactoid or late serum reactions, hence it may not be administered. The clinical response to ASV is observed in the form cessation of bleeding, improvement of clotting, neurological recovery with decrease in local swelling, and recovery of other affected organ functions **(Flowcharts 20.2.5 and 20.2.6)**.[10]

TABLE 20.2.8: Envenomation.

Envenomation	*Dose*
Minimal (progressive local sweelling, no systemic symptoms)	5 vials (50 mL) are usually sufficient
Moderate (swelling beyond the site of the bite, mild systemic symptoms and/or neurological, hematological abnormalities)	5–10 vials (50–100 mL)
Severe (rapidly progressive and extensive local effects, systemic symptoms and neurological, hematological abnormalities)	10–20 vials (100–200 mL) or more

Prognosis

Not all the snake bites are venomous. The outcome of snake bite depends on the snake species, body part bitten, and the injected venom volume. The mortality and morbidity associated with snake bites can be minimized with timely administration of safe and effective ASV. Prevention and treatment interventions may substantially reduce snake bite mortality in India.

CONCLUSION

Poisoning and envenomation are the important clinical conditions encountered by pediatricians. Young children are susceptible to poisoning and envenomation due to their curious exploratory behavior. Early recognition and

Flowchart 20.2.5: Treatment algorithm for snake bite.[10]

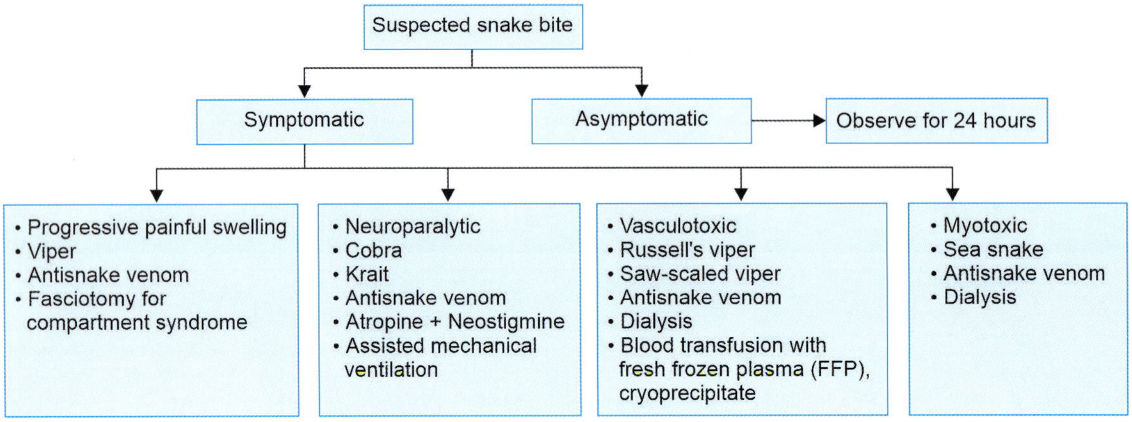

Suspected snake bite
- Symptomatic
- Asymptomatic → Observe for 24 hours

Symptomatic:

- • Progressive painful swelling • Viper • Antisnake venom • Fasciotomy for compartment syndrome
- • Neuroparalytic • Cobra • Krait • Antisnake venom • Atropine + Neostigmine • Assisted mechanical ventilation
- • Vasculotoxic • Russell's viper • Saw-scaled viper • Antisnake venom • Dialysis • Blood transfusion with fresh frozen plasma (FFP), cryoprecipitate
- • Myotoxic • Sea snake • Antisnake venom • Dialysis

Flowchart 20.2.6: Approach to snake bite.[10]

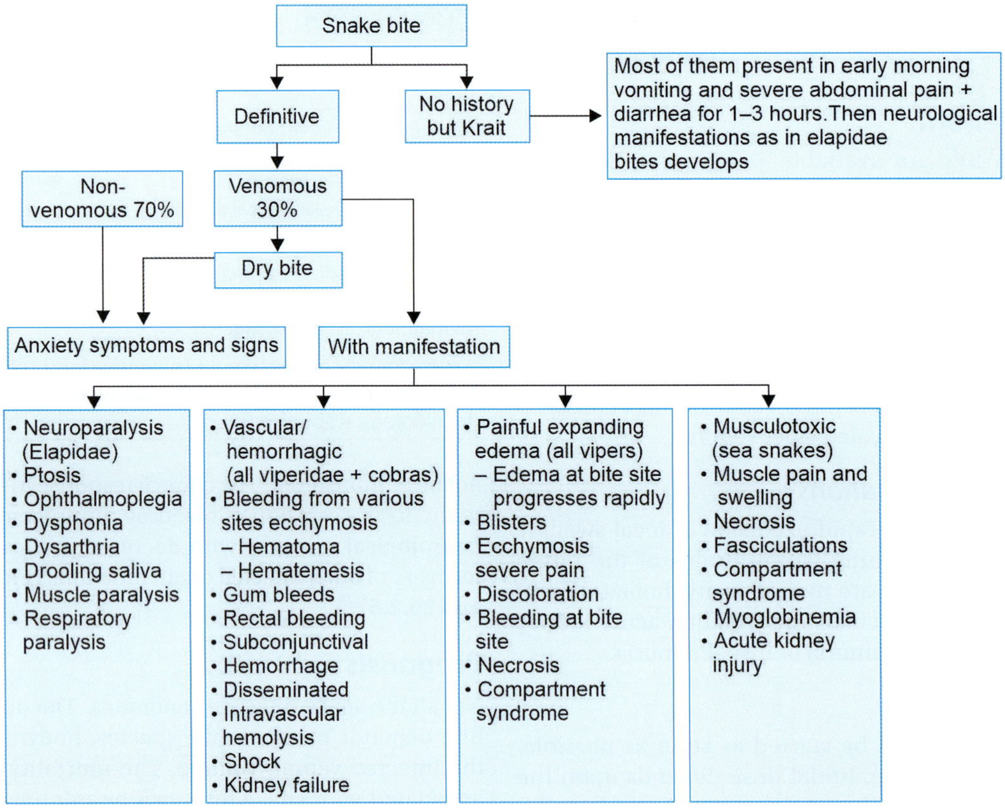

Snake bite
- Definitive → Venomous 30%
- No history but Krait → Most of them present in early morning vomiting and severe abdominal pain + diarrhea for 1–3 hours. Then neurological manifestations as in elapidae bites develops

Non-venomous 70% → Anxiety symptoms and signs

Venomous 30% → Dry bite → Anxiety symptoms and signs

Venomous 30% → With manifestation

With manifestation:

- • Neuroparalysis (Elapidae) • Ptosis • Ophthalmoplegia • Dysphonia • Dysarthria • Drooling saliva • Muscle paralysis • Respiratory paralysis
- • Vascular/hemorrhagic (all viperidae + cobras) • Bleeding from various sites ecchymosis – Hematoma – Hematemesis • Gum bleeds • Rectal bleeding • Subconjunctival • Hemorrhage • Disseminated • Intravascular hemolysis • Shock • Kidney failure
- • Painful expanding edema (all vipers) – Edema at bite site progresses rapidly • Blisters • Ecchymosis severe pain • Discoloration • Bleeding at bite site • Necrosis • Compartment syndrome
- • Musculotoxic (sea snakes) • Muscle pain and swelling • Necrosis • Fasciculations • Compartment syndrome • Myoglobinemia • Acute kidney injury

timely treatment is crucial for the favorable outcome. Pending the specific identification of the type of poison and or envenomation and treatment thereupon; stabilizing the child, supporting the organ functions remain the basic essence of management. Parental education is desirable for age appropriate preventive measures for poisoning and envenomation in children.

ACKNOWLEDGMENT

Tables 20.2.1 to 20.2.4 and **Flowcharts 20.2.1 and 20.2.2** have been reproduced from IAP Text Book of Pediatrics, Edition 7, Chapter 17.2, page no. 1169–77; authored by S Balasubramanian and Jaydeep Choudhury. We sincerely acknowledge their contribution for the same.

REFERENCES

1. Reddy KS, Kishor M, Manjunath VG. Poisoning in Children – A Study from Tertiary Care General Hospital. J Med Sci Health. 2020;6(3):14-8.
2. Eyer P. The role of oximes in the management of OP pesticide poisoning. Toxicol Rev. 2003;22(3):165-90.
3. Gupta P, Singh RP, Murali MV, Sharma PP. Prognostic score for kerosene oil poisoning. Indian Pediatr. 1992;29(9):1109-12.
4. Prescott LF. Kinetics and metabolism of paracetamol and phenacetin. Br J Clin Pharmacol. 1980;10(Suppl 2):291S-8S.
5. Cumberland Pharmaceuticals Inc. Acetadote—Acetylcysteine Injection. [online] Available from https://dailymed.nlm.nih.gov/dailymed/getFile.cfm?setid=472f158a-5ab9-4308-8e49-1116e6ea3d39&type=pdf [Last accessed December, 2024].
6. Chiew AL, Reith D, Pomerleau A, Wong A, Isoardi KZ, Soderstrom J, et al. Updated guidelines for the management of paracetamol poisoning in Australia and New Zealand. Med J Aust. 2020;212(4):175-83.
7. World Health Organization.. (2023). Snakebite envenoming. [online] Available from https://www.who.int/news-room/fact-sheets/detail/snakebite-envenoming [Last accessed December, 2024].
8. Mohapatra B, Warrell DA, Suraweera W, Bhatia P, Dhingra N, Jotkar RM, et al; Million Death Study Collaborators. Million Death Study Collaborators Snakebite Mortality in India: a nationally representative mortality survey. PLOS Negl Trop Dis. 2011;5:e1018.
9. Simpson ID. The pediatric management of snakebite: The national protocol. Indian Pediatr. 2007;44:173-6.
10. Rathinasamy M, Mithuna M, Ramasamy S, Antony J, Jaishree V, Alexander M. Identification and management of snake bite in Asia: A narrative review. J Sci Soc. 2023;50(2):147-54.

20.3 Pediatric Trauma and Foreign Bodies

Arun Kumar L, Ebor Jacob G James

PEDIATRIC TRAUMA

INTRODUCTION

Trauma is one of the leading causes of morbidity and mortality in the pediatric age group around the world. Unintentional injuries form a heavy economic, social and healthcare burden especially in low- and middle-income countries. India accounts for 11.1% of mortality and 17.6% of disability-adjusted life years (DALYs) in the world for injuries in children <14 years.[1] Hence, prompt and effective management is crucial to optimize outcomes and minimize long-term sequelae. This chapter aims to provide a comprehensive overview of the early management of pediatric trauma, including initial assessment, resuscitation, diagnostic evaluation, and specific considerations for different types of injuries.

UNIQUE PEDIATRIC CONSIDERATIONS

Children have specific anatomical and physiological differences when compared to adults that significantly impacts the early assessment and management in trauma.[2]

Anatomical Considerations

- *Airway:* Children have smaller airway, larger tongue, larger occiput, and floppy epiglottis making them more susceptible to obstruction. Larynx is more cephalad and anterior.
- *Head and brain:* Head is disproportionately larger than rest of the body and have weak neck musculature. The open fontanels result in more tolerance to rising intracranial pressure (ICP) resulting in diagnostic delays.
- *Spinal cord:* Spinal cord injury without radiographic abnormality (SCIWORA) is more common in children younger than 8 years of age.
- *Chest:* Ribs are positioned more horizontally and are pliable. Risk of pulmonary contusions without rib fracture or pneumothorax is higher.
- *Abdomen:* The solid organs such as liver, spleen, and pancreas are more exposed especially in infants and toddlers. They are more prone to direct injury and hemorrhage after blunt trauma.
- *Musculoskeletal system:* Immature growth plates with more pliable skeletal structure results in more physeal injuries, greenstick, and buckle fractures.
- *Vascular system:* Intraosseous access is required due to difficulty in securing peripheral venous access in emergency resuscitation.

Physiological Considerations

- *Vital signs:* The normal heart rates (HR), respiratory rates (RR), and blood pressure (BP) vary with age and appropriate scales or formulas to be used when performing assessment.

- *Breathing:* Hypoventilation or hypoxia is the most common cause of cardiorespiratory arrest. Children are diaphragmatic breathers and have fewer type 1 respiratory muscles and fatigue faster than adults. Decreased functional residual capacity and increased oxygen utilization means hypoxia occurs quickly when ventilation is inadequate.
- *Metabolism:* Larger body surface area to weight ratio can cause insensible fluid loss and more chances of hypothermia. Basal metabolic rate (BMR) is also higher.
- *Shock:* Higher physiological reserve results in uncompensated shock manifesting only after >30–45% loss of total blood volume. Tachycardia and poor skin perfusion are early signs which should be recognized and managed with fluid resuscitation.

PREHOSPITAL CARE

Initial care at the site of trauma consists of oxygen administration, airway adjuncts, bleeding control, spine stabilization, and temperature maintenance. *Broselow tape* is used to estimate medication doses, size of equipment, and other critical values. The child should be immediately shifted to a center equipped to provide care for critically ill children.

PRIMARY SURVEY

The initial assessment of a pediatric trauma patient follows the principles of the *advanced trauma life support (ATLS)* protocol. The primary survey, focusing on the ABCDEs (Airway, Breathing, Circulation, Disability, and Exposure), should be conducted rapidly but cautiously to avoid exacerbating injuries.[3]

Airway with Cervical Spine Stabilization

- *Relieve obstruction:* The airway should be examined for presence of foreign bodies in mouth or pharynx to establish patency. Presence of facial, mandibular, or tracheal fractures can lead to a potentially unstable airway.
- *Cervical spine stabilization:* Cervical spine injury should be assumed till ruled out in any multiple trauma patient. Rigid cervical collars are used to achieve cervical spine motion restriction. The child should be kept in a "sniffing position" with paddings under the shoulder and back. This places the cervical spine in a neutral position and opens the airway maximally.
- *If the airway is inadequate or unstable*, the following maneuvers have to be done in sequence—chin lift or jaw thrust, suctioning of secretions with oropharyngeal or nasopharyngeal airways as adjuncts to bag-valve-mask ventilation.
- *Endotracheal intubation* needs to be done early, if needed to avoid or manage hypoxemia and hypercarbia. Common indications include airway compromise, hypoxemia, major maxillofacial trauma, flail chest, hemorrhagic shock, and severe head injury.[4]

Breathing with Oxygen Support

Breathing assessment includes inspection of neck and thorax to look for any tracheal deviation, abnormal chest wall movement, use of accessory muscles, and external contusions or lacerations. The RR is measured and breath sounds auscultated. Tension pneumothorax presents with tracheal deviation, hyper-resonant chest and unilateral decreased, or absent breath sounds with obstructive shock. Massive hemothorax also has unilateral decreased breath sound but is dull on percussion. Asymmetric chest movements are suggestive of flail chest.

All children with multiple trauma should be started on oxygen by appropriate delivery systems. Any suspicion of tension pneumothorax, needle thoracostomy at second intercostal space in the anterior chest wall should be done followed by formal intercostal drainage tube.[5]

Circulation and Bleeding Control

Pediatric total blood volume averages between 80 and 90 mL/kg. Therefore, what appears to be a relatively small external blood loss is still very significant.[6] Tachycardia and poor skin perfusion are the first signs of hypovolemia in children. Any child who is cold and has tachycardia should be considered to be in shock until proven otherwise. Cardiac tamponade is rare in children but should be kept in mind and checked for in suspected cases. The assessment should also focus on any large external bleeding, significant chest trauma, abdominal signs suggestive of internal hemorrhage, pelvic fractures, and long bone fractures.[4]

Any site of external hemorrhage needs to be controlled with manual compression at the site or by applying a temporary tourniquet proximal to it. Reduction and splinting of long bone fractures may also provide hemostasis. Vascular access is established with two large bore intravenous (IV) cannulas in the upper extremities within 90 seconds of presenting. Intraosseous cannulas are a valid option in situations where rapid peripheral access could not be achieved.

Once access is secured, fluid bolus of 20 mL/kg with warmed normal saline or Ringer lactate (RL) is administered over 10–15 minutes. In children, three boluses or 60 mL/kg of normal saline or RL (maximum dose: 3 L total volume) would balance a blood loss of 20 mL/kg (approximately one-third of blood volume), assuming that bleeding is controlled. A transfusion of 10 mL/kg of packed red blood cells (PRBC) should be considered if there is inadequate clinical improvement after IV boluses of 40–60 mL/kg of normal saline.

Massive transfusion protocol is triggered when red blood transfusion is 50% of total blood volume in 3 hours, 100% in 24 hours.[7]

Disability Assessment

Pediatric Glasgow Coma Scale (GCS) is used to the determine the level of consciousness. Rapid resuscitative efforts are required if GCS is ≤8. Additional neurologic findings to elicit during the primary survey include pupillary responsiveness and brainstem reflexes. Secondary brain injury from hypoxia, ischemia, and cerebral edema should be prevented. Supplemental oxygen should be provided to keep saturation over 95%.[8]

Exposure and Environment

Complete exposure of the child should be done to avoid missing out any injuries. Log roll while maintaining cervical spine immobilization is done to assess the back and spine. Rectal examination is indicated in cases of pelvic fractures and bleeding per rectum. Hypothermia should be avoided with the use of increased ambient room temperature, radiant warmers, warmed IV fluids/blood, warm and humidified inspired oxygen, and covering the patient with warm blankets after full assessment.

Adjuncts to Primary Survey

Urinary catheterization is done to monitor urine output if there are no contraindications like suspected urethral injuries. A suprapubic cystostomy under guidance can be an option if there is indication of urethral transection. A orogastric or nasogastric tube is also inserted considering the risk of gastroparesis and aspiration in major trauma. However in children with oromaxillary trauma and suspected cribriform plate fracture, the insertion of nasogastric tube should be withheld till imaging is done.

Blood investigations include hematocrits, blood glucose, creatinine, liver enzymes, and cross matching for RBC. Arterial or venous blood gas in combination with pulse oximetry helps in identifying hypoxemia.

Screening radiographs along with primary survey including cross-table lateral cervical spine (C-spine), anteroposterior (AP) chest, and, in selected patients, AP pelvis help identify immediately life-threatening injuries.[4]

Extended focused assessment with sonography for trauma (e-FAST) is a rapid ultrasound examination of four abdominal locations—right upper quadrant, left upper quadrant, subxiphoid region, and pelvis; lungs; and heart. It aids in detecting and also in ruling out significant intra-abdominal or thoracic injuries.[9]

RESUSCITATION

Resuscitation happens in conjunction with primary survey. High-flow oxygen devices such as high-flow nasal cannula therapy, nonrebreather mask is sufficient in a child with respiratory distress after ensuring the airway is open and breathing is spontaneous. Endotracheal intubation with rapid-sequence induction techniques is necessary in respiratory failure. The first step in management of the circulation is control of bleeding. Direct pressure using sterile dressings is applied to all actively bleeding external wounds. Blind clamping is avoided, owing to the potential risk of injury to neurovascular bundles.

Volume resuscitation is then performed as explained above. Initial fluid resuscitation include 20–40 mL/kg bolus. Hypotensive shock (defined clinically by a systolic BP <70 mm Hg plus twice the age in years) requires higher volumes along with blood products if needed. The evidence for use of tranexamic acid (TXA) is limited in pediatric trauma. The loading dose is 15 mg/kg up to a maximum 1 g diluted in 0.9% sodium chloride and is given over 10 minutes within 3 hours of injury.[10] The adequacy of perfusion is monitored by urine output of 1–2 mL/kg/h. If a child initially is in shock, has no signs of intrathoracic, intra-abdominal, or intrapelvic bleeding, but fails to improve despite seemingly adequate volume resuscitation, other forms of shock (obstructive, cardiogenic, or neurogenic) should be considered. Most children in hypotensive shock are victims of unrecognized hemorrhage that can be reversed by means of rapid blood transfusion and immediate intervention, particularly if major intrathoracic or intra-abdominal vessels are injured.

SECONDARY SURVEY

Once resuscitation is underway and child is being stabilized, secondary survey is initiated. The components of secondary survey include Symptoms, Allergies, Medications, Past illnesses, Last meal, Events and Environment (SAMPLE).[5] This is combined with an extensive head-to-toe physical examination. The purpose of this repeat examination is to identify injuries that may have been overlooked by primary survey. The following components deserve special focus:

- *Head and neck:* Any drainage from ears or nose can be a marker for basilar skull fracture. Eyes should be checked for pupillary size, conjunctival hemorrhage, and periorbital ecchymoses. Crepitus in the neck is indicative of subcutaneous emphysema from esophageal or laryngeal injury.
- *Chest:* Repeat inspection and auscultation of chest should be done looking for any tenderness, crepitus, or step offs.
- *Abdomen:* Evaluate for any distension, ecchymoses, tenderness, rebound, or guarding. *Seat belt sign* (linear contusion across abdomen) has increased risk of bowel

injuries. Hollow viscus injuries and pancreatic injuries require high degree of clinical suspicion based on the mechanism of injuries. Inspection of the perineum is important for the identification of contusions, hematomas, lacerations, or urethral bleeding (in the male).

- *Musculoskeletal:* Bony point tenderness, hematoma, skin discoloration, and spasm of muscles can reveal an underlying fracture. Ecchymosis over the iliac wings, pubis, labia, or scrotum is suspicious for pelvic fractures.
- *Neurologic:* Sensory and motor deficits should be assessed. Due to higher risk of SCIWORA in children, trauma patients with brief or sustained sensory or motor deficits and decreased level of consciousness must be assumed to have a cervical spine injury, and cervical spine protection and motion restriction must be maintained.

Radiological Evaluation

Radiological evaluation forms an important part of secondary survey. Initial radiographs of cervical spine, chest, and pelvis are done now if not performed as an adjunct to primary survey.

The utility of *e-FAST* for the detection of intra-abdominal injury (IAI) in hemodynamically stable children with blunt abdominal trauma and no other injury is less clear. Studies have shown that e-FAST is insensitive for detecting important IAI. So e-FAST in combination with physical examination findings guides the clinical decisions and further imaging.

The use of CT scans should be judicious, balancing the short-term benefit of accurate diagnosis with long-term risk of late malignancy. When necessary, CT should be performed using radiation doses "as low as reasonably achievable" (ALARA), consistent with the "image gently" protocols advocated by The Alliance for Radiation Safety in Pediatric Imaging.[4]

The CT of the head is done whenever there is loss of consciousness and GCS is <15. CT can be avoided if mental status is normal, injury mechanism is nonsevere, and there are no obvious external injuries. CT of cervical spine is considered when there is focal neurologic findings, neck pain, torticollis, and high velocity motor vehicle accidents. CT of thorax adds little to chest radiographs with detection of incidental pulmonary contusions not significantly affecting long-term morbidity or mortality. CT of the abdomen is done for all intubated patients, any suspicion of internal bleeding (abdominal tenderness, distention, bruising, or gross hematuria), hypotensive shock, and significant mechanism of injury. Extremity radiographs is done for evaluation of suspected fractures.[4]

Tetanus immunization and pain control should also be addressed as a part of secondary survey. Open wounds should have appropriate wound care, and IV antibiotics should be given if necessary.

DEFINITIVE CARE

A flowchart showing the initial trauma management in children is shown in **Flowchart 20.3.1**. Further management depends on the type of injury and the anatomical location.

HEAD TRAUMA

Blunt injury to head requires neuroimaging to be done at the earliest. It can be avoided in children with minor or low-risk injury. The criteria for low-risk injury include normal mental status, no loss of consciousness, no vomiting, no scalp hematoma, no evidence of basilar skull fracture, and the mechanism of injury are not severe. The children are observed in the emergency department and do not require any further intervention as per PECARN criteria.[11] However, prompt neurosurgical consultation should be obtained in patients with clinically important traumatic brain injuries. These include any parenchymal injuries, intracranial hemorrhage, depressed or widely diastatic skull fractures. Any child with deteriorating GCS score or conscious level should also be seen by a neurosurgeon, irrespective of the neuroimaging results. Penetrating trauma with entry into cranial vault is a neurosurgical emergency and any protruding object should be left in place till definitive surgical management can be done. Puncture wounds and lacerations with an intact calvarium can be repaired primarily.[11]

NECK TRAUMA

Cervical collars are placed for any child presenting with a high-risk mechanism of injury. Clinical evidence of cervical spine injury includes neck pain, difficulty with neck motion, and presence of neurological deficits. Presence of posterior midline neck tenderness or step off sign on palpation can also be indicative of underlying cervical spine injury. Collar is kept in place till imaging of the cervical spine is done and any underlying injury is ruled out clinically.

Children with injuries penetrating the platysma may require emergency surgical consultation. Penetrating neck injury may cause life-threatening hemorrhage, injury to larynx or trachea, and the spine. These children require surgical neck exploration. Injuries superficial to the platysma can be repaired in the emergency department.

THORACIC TRAUMA

Children with low-velocity injuries, normal vital signs, breathing, and no chest wall injuries, require no further radiological imaging. However, abrasions or lacerations over the chest wall, significant bony tenderness, abnormal breath, or cardiac sounds can be suggestive of an intrathoracic injury. Clinical manifestations of intrathoracic injuries include tachypnea, hypoxemia, crepitus in the chest wall, and

Flowchart 20.3.1: Flowchart on timelines of initial trauma management in children with polytrauma.

Child with polytrauma

- Immobilize cervical spine
- Assess vital signs

Actions	Time
Airway: Open airway, suction secretions, administer oxygen *Breathing*: Assess need for ventilation/intubation. Needle thoracostomy/chest tube if needed *Circulation*: Secure IV/IO access, fluid resuscitation, and control obvious hemorrhage *Disability*: Identify GCS, pupillary response, signs of impending herniation, and signs of spinal cord injury *Exposure*: Remove clothing, examine, and initiate warming	0–5 mintues
• Repeat vital signs every 5 minutes • Reassess response to interventions • Nasogastric tube placement if not contraindicated • Urinary catheter placement • FAST examination • Blood sampling	5–15 minutes
• Reassess response to interventions • Reassess levels of consciousness • Continue care of airway, breathing, circulation and disability • Logroll patient • Screening radiographs	15–30 minutes
• Reassess response to interventions • Reassess levels of consciousness • Perform complete physical examination—secondary survey • Provide analgesia/tetanus immunization/splint fractures • Computed tomography scans of the head, neck, chest, abdomen, or pelvis as indicated by clinical signs	30–60 minutes
• Transfer to center with facilities for pediatric trauma care • Initiate definitive care for injuries identified	

paradoxical chest wall movements. Tension pneumothorax, when present, leads to marked hypotension, distended neck veins due to blockage of extrathoracic venous return, and may cause tracheal deviation away from the affected lung. Chest radiograph and bedside ultrasound can be done in unstable patients to avoid delay in placement of chest tubes. CT of the thorax has to be done in stable patients to rule of pneumothorax, hemothorax, rib fractures, pulmonary, and cardiac contusions. Penetrating injuries of the thorax can lead to exsanguinating hemorrhage and require emergency surgical exploration **(Fig. 20.3.1)**.

ABDOMINAL TRAUMA

Blunt injury to the abdomen can be suspected based on the mechanism of injury. However, in children, serious injuries such as splenic laceration or hematoma can happen following trivial injuries to the left upper quadrant also. Hence, a thorough physical examination is mandatory even in accidents with minimal force. The following clinical symptoms and signs have been identified to predict the risk of IAI—abdominal wall trauma or seat belt sign, abdominal tenderness, abdominal pain, vomiting, concomitant thoracic injury, and decreased breath sounds.[12]

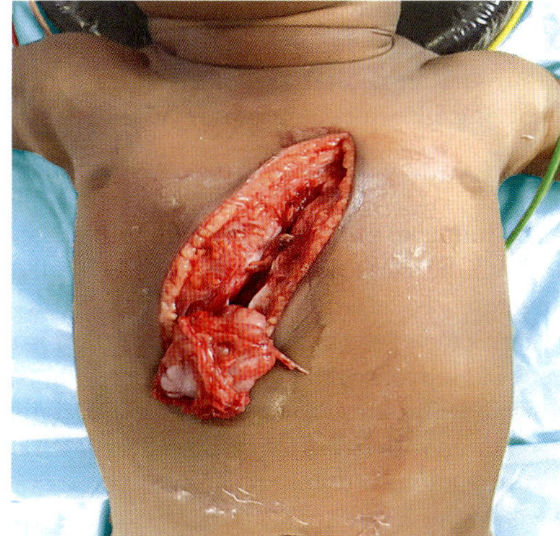

Fig. 20.3.1: Open chest wall injury secondary to accidental fall of an ax on a 2-year-old boy.

Use of FAST in children has a relatively lower sensitivity for IAI compared to adults and a contrast enhanced CT is warranted if FAST is positive or clinical suspicion is high. CT is sensitive and specific in diagnosing liver, spleen, and

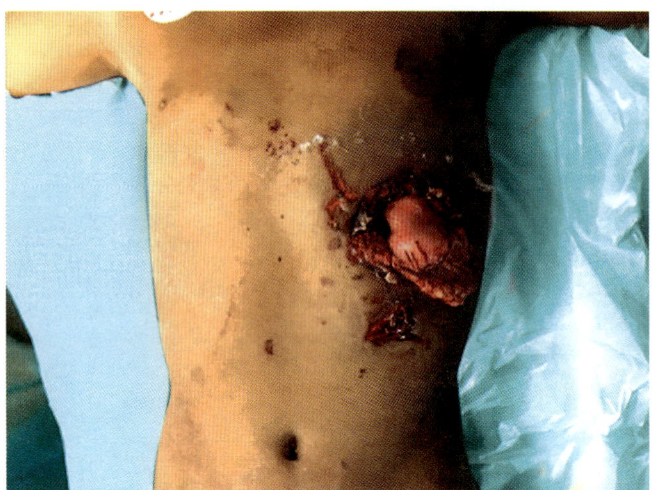

Fig. 20.3.2: Penetrating injury (Bull gore injury) of the abdominal wall in a 8-year-old boy requiring emergency laparotomy and exploration.

TABLE 20.3.1: A summary of broadly used scoring systems.

Physiological systems (Triage scoring systems)	• Glasgow Coma Scale (GCS) • Trauma score (TS) • Revised trauma score (RTS) • Pediatric trauma score (PTS) • Age-specific pediatric trauma score (ASPTS)
Anatomic systems (Severity assessment and risk prediction)	• Abbreviated injury scale (AIS) • Injury severity score (ISS) • Anatomic profile (AP)
Combined systems	• Trauma injury severity score - TRISS - (RTS + ISS) • Pediatric age-adjusted trauma injury severity score - PAAT - (ASPTS + ISS) • A severity characterization of trauma (ASCOT) • Pediatric risk of mortality (PRISM III) • Pediatric index of mortality 3 (PIM3) • Pediatric trauma BIG score • Shock index pediatric adjusted (SIPA)

retroperitoneal injuries. Injuries of the pancreas, intestinal tract, bladder, and lumbar spine may be missed however. Based upon a systematic review of observational studies that reported outcomes on over 9,000 children, asymptomatic children with a negative abdominal CT are very unlikely to have intra-abdominal injuries.[13] Nonoperative management is the gold standard for solid organ injuries with stable hemodynamic status in children irrespective of the grade of injury.

Penetrating injuries to the abdomen can be superficial or deep. Wounds where the peritoneum is not breached can be repaired in emergency department. Any peritoneal breach requires surgical consultation followed by a diagnostic laparoscopy or exploratory laparotomy **(Fig. 20.3.2)**.

EXTREMITY TRAUMA

Low-energy trauma to the extremities with children should be evaluated with radiological examination to look for possible physeal fractures. Focal tenderness at the physis can indicate a Salter–Harris type I fracture even if radiograph is normal. The chance of neurovascular compromise and compartment syndrome following fracture or dislocation is significantly higher in children with risk of loss of limb function. Clinically, apparent dislocations and fractures should be reduced and immobilized at the earliest.

Clinical features of *acute compartment syndrome* (ACS) include:

- Persistent pain, burning pain, or pain out of proportion to injury
- Paresthesia
- Indurated or wood-like feeling
- Pallor with prolonged with capillary filling time of fingers or toes
- Muscle weakness and paralysis—late finding

If ACS is suspected, urgent surgical intervention with fasciotomy is needed.[4]

Open fractures and penetrating injuries in the extremity will require detailed peripheral nerve and vascular assessment, control of hemorrhage, and surgical correction.

CLASSIFICATION SYSTEMS

Trauma classification systems were created for two primary objectives:

1. Triage decision support
2. Severity of illness, morbidity, and mortality prediction

These scoring systems can be based on physiology or anatomy or combination of both and take into consideration the body regions involved, the mechanism of injury and the severity. A summary of the broadly used scoring systems is given in **Table 20.3.1**.

Scores designed for pediatric use were found to have similar value as general trauma scores. Physiologic scores were better suited for morbidity and mortality prediction compared to anatomic scores.

FOREIGN BODIES

FOREIGN BODY IN AIRWAY

Foreign body aspiration is one of the common problems seen in pediatric emergency department. It is an important cause of accidental mortality in children <5 years. The incidence is maximum between 1 and 5 years of age. Inadequate chewing and uncoordinated swallowing mechanisms in younger children also increase the chance of aspiration. Boys are affected twice as often as girls.[14]

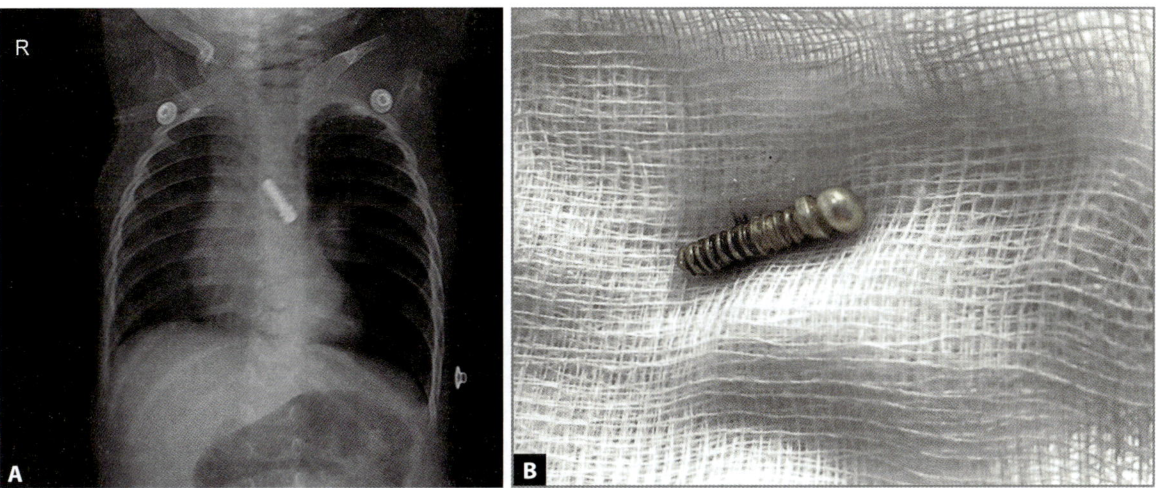

Figs. 20.3.3A and B: (A) Chest X-ray of 1-year-old boy showing foreign body in the trachea; (B) Rigid bronchoscopy and removal done.

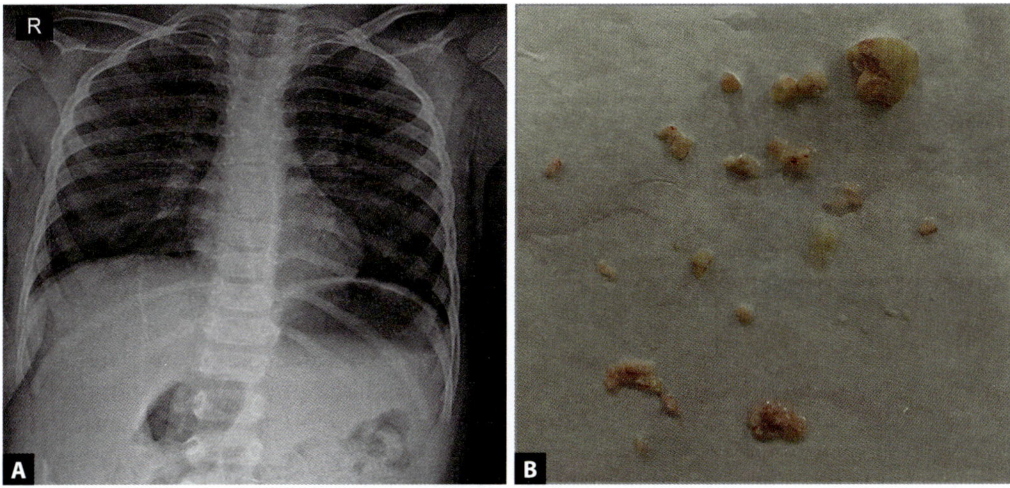

Figs. 20.3.4A and B: Chest X-ray of 6-year-old girl presenting with acute-onset respiratory distress showing bilateral hyperinflated lungs; (B) Pieces of almond removed from the trachea by rigid bronchoscopy.

Organic foreign bodies such as peanuts, seeds, and food particles are the usual culprits. They can absorb water and obstruction symptoms develop over time. They induce granulomatous reactions and rarely can also precipitate anaphylactic reactions. Aspiration of inorganic foreign bodies such as parts of toys, whistles, springs, magnets, and button batteries is increasing in recent times. While these are inert and do not cause inflammation, they are more difficult to extract **(Figs. 20.3.3A and B)**.

Clinically, children with foreign body aspiration present with sudden onset breathlessness. The onset is usually preceded by an episode of choking or vomiting. Majority of times the choking episode is witnessed by a caregiver or guardian. However, it is possible that the child aspirated while no one was around. In such scenarios, there can be difficulty in differentiating from other causes of acute respiratory distress such as asthma. The predictors include *new-onset distress* in an otherwise well child, no history of fever, no recent history of cough or cold, and no past history of reactive airway disease. Examination can show reduced air entry on one side with new-onset wheeze or crepitations. Dysphonia, subtle change in voice or cry may be the only signs in some children. The findings are usually unilateral. Right side bronchus is the most common site. The diameter of the right bronchus is larger than the left and it has smaller angle of divergence than the left. Chest radiograph both AP and lateral can help in diagnosis if the foreign body is radiopaque or if there is unilateral atelectasis or hyperinflation **(Figs. 20.3.4A and B)**. Large foreign bodies obstructing the glottis or the trachea cause sudden hypoxemia and respiratory arrest if not intervened immediately. Laryngeal pathology usually will manifest as inspiratory stridor while tracheal foreign bodies cause expiratory stridor.

Chronic foreign bodies often masquerade as respiratory illnesses with persistent cough and atelectasis, recurrent pneumonia, or hoarseness. Other late findings include the development of granulation tissue, strictures, perforation, and bronchiectasis. Contrast-enhanced high-resolution CT can be done in such situations to make the diagnosis.

The foreign body can cause airway obstruction in one of the following ways:

- *Bypass valve:* Air moves freely around the foreign body causing partial obstruction and radiograph appears normal.
- *Check valve:* There is obstruction in the exhalation phase leading to hyperinflation on the side of the foreign body.
- *Ball valve:* Air escapes out during expiration but there is obstruction during inspiration resulting in atelectasis.
- *Stop valve:* There is complete obstruction leading to atelectasis. Any of the above conditions can progress eventually to stop valve status.

In any child with suspicion of foreign body aspiration, an emergency bronchoscopy is warranted. If the history or findings are definitive, rigid bronchoscopy and removal of foreign body are done. If the history is chronic and suspicion is low, an initial flexible bronchoscopy can be done and if foreign body is seen it can be removed using rigid bronchoscope.[14]

FOREIGN BODY INGESTION

Foreign body ingestions are common between 6 months and 3 years of age due to the oral phase of the psychological development wherein they explore their surroundings orally. Majority of the children are asymptomatic and brought to hospital by caregiver or guardian following a witnessed or reported ingestion. The exact incidence is not really known due to high number of missed events and the very low morbidity with most ingested objects. Ingestion of multiple foreign objects or repeated occurrences can point to an underlying developmental delay or behavioral problems. Most of the ingested foreign bodies pass spontaneously with <20% requiring endoscopic removal. The need for surgical extraction is seen in less than one percent of the cases.

The clinical manifestation and management guidelines are different for esophageal impaction and objects passed into the stomach and small bowel.[15]

Esophageal Foreign Bodies

The risk factors for impaction in esophagus include younger age, congenital malformation, prior esophageal surgery, or neuromuscular disorders. The areas of physiological narrowing where impaction occurs include the upper esophageal sphincter, the level of aortic arch, and the lower esophageal sphincter. Symptomatic children can present with refusal to eat, drooling, dysphagia, and in older children a feeling of something stuck in neck or chest. Sharp objects and batteries can cause perforation and develop neck swelling, crepitus, and pneumomediastinum. Rarely, there can be erosion into trachea causing a fistula. Erosion into aorta is associated with life-threatening bleeding.

Stomach and Intestines

Foreign bodies in stomach do not usually cause any symptoms and those that crossed the stomach nearly always pass spontaneously. Endoscopic removal is warranted only for certain objects such as sharp objects, magnets, and batteries. Rarely some foreign body may be retained in the distal gastrointestinal tract causing delayed complications

Imaging

A conventional radiograph, both anteroposterior and lateral, of the neck, chest and abdomen should be done. Radiopaque foreign bodies are seen in 60–70% of children. If radiopaque object is seen in the neck or upper chest the location has to be differentiated between esophagus and trachea. Flat objects (e.g., coins or disk batteries) in the esophagus usually orient in the coronal plane and appear as a circular object on an anteroposterior radiograph, whereas objects lodged in the trachea tend to orient in the sagittal plane and are best seen in lateral radiographs. It is also important to differentiate between a coin and button battery (double ring or halo sign) on the radiography, since any battery impacted in the esophagus requires immediate removal.

Management

Based on the type of foreign body and the location, either expectant management or urgent removal is done. The indications for urgent endoscopic or surgical removal include:

- Airway compromise secondary to upper esophageal impacted foreign body
- Large foreign body completely obstructing the esophagus causing drooling of saliva
- Button batteries in the esophagus and stomach
- Long (>5 cm) and sharp objects in the esophagus and stomach
- Multiple magnets anywhere in the gastrointestinal tract. Single magnets if crossed stomach, can be managed expectantly.
- Any signs of gastrointestinal tract obstruction or perforation.

If any of the above indications are present, the patient should immediately be transferred to a center with facilities for upper gastrointestinal endoscopy. Children with known battery ingestion, which is impacted in the esophagus, if endoscopic facilities are not available, can be given honey orally to reduce the incidence of mucosal injury and perforation.

Removal can be done using Magill forceps and bougienage, if impaction is in upper esophagus and with flexible or rigid endoscopy if its beyond mid esophagus or in the stomach. Foley balloon extraction under fluoroscopy can be done for coins stuck in the upper esophageal sphincter. The Foley balloon extraction technique should be limited to round, smooth objects that have been impacted for <1 week in appropriately selected children without any evidence of complications.

Long-term follow-up is essential in these children even after successful extraction due to the high chance of strictures.

Children with none of the above indications can be managed expectantly. The majority of foreign bodies that pass into the stomach will usually pass through the remainder of the gastrointestinal tract uneventfully. These children can be managed on outpatient basis. There are no role for use of laxatives or prokinetic agents. The parents are asked to notice for passing of the object in the stools. However, this is successful only in 50% of the cases. If the child remains asymptomatic and the object has not been identified in stools, a repeat abdominal radiograph can be performed at 2–3 weeks intervals. Intervention is done if there any symptoms or if the object is retained beyond 4–6 weeks.[15]

REFERENCES

1. Amato S, Culbreath K, Dunne E, Sarathy A, Siroonian O, Sartorelli K, et al. Pediatric trauma mortality in India and the United States: A comparison and risk-adjusted analysis. J Pediatr Surg. 2023;58(1):99-105.
2. McFadyen Jg, Ramaiah R, Bhananker S. Initial assessment and management of pediatric trauma patients. Int J Crit Illn Inj Sci. 2012;2(3):121-7.
3. Hannon MM, Middelberg LK, Lee LK. The initial approach to the multisystem pediatric trauma patient. Pediatr Emerg Care. 2022;38(8):290.
4. American College of Surgeons Committee on Trauma. Advanced Trauma Life Support (ATLS) Student Course Manual, 10th edition. Chicago: American College of Surgeons; 2018.
5. Lavoie M, Nance ML. Approach to the injured child. In: Shaw KN, Bachur RG (Eds). Fleisher and Ludwig's Textbook of Pediatric Emergency Medicine, 7th edition. Philadelphia: Lippincott Williams and Wilkins; 2016. p. 9.
6. Gonzalez K, Desai A, Dalton B, Juang D. Hemorrhagic shock. J Pediatr Intensive Care. 2015;4(01):4-9.
7. Principi T, Schonfeld D, Weingarten L, Schneeweiss S, Rosenfield D, Ernst G, et al. Update in Pediatric Emergency Medicine: Pediatric Resuscitation, Pediatric Sepsis, Interfacility Transport of the Pediatric Patient, Pain and sedation in the Emergency Department, Pediatric Trauma. Update Pediatr; 2018. pp. 223-49.
8. Kochanek PM, Carney N, Adelson PD, Ashwal S, Bell MJ, Bratton S, et al. Guidelines for the Acute Medical Management of Severe Traumatic Brain Injury in Infants, Children, and Adolescents-Second Edition. Pediatr Crit Care Med. 2012;13 (Suppl 1):S1-82.
9. Kornblith AE, Addo N, Plasencia M, Shaahinfar A, Lin-Marttore M, Sabbineni N, Gold D, et al. Development of a Consensus-Based Definition of Focused Assessment With Sonography for Trauma in Children. JAMA Netw Open. 2022;5(3):e222922.
10. Beno S, Ackery AD, Callum J, Rizoli S. Tranexamic acid in pediatric trauma: why not? Crit Care. 2014;18(4):313.
11. Kuppermann N, Holmes JF, Dayan PS, Hoyle JD, Atabaki SM, Holubkov R, et al. Identification of children at very low risk of clinically-important brain injuries after head trauma: a prospective cohort study. Lancet. 2009;374(9696):1160-70.
12. Drucker NA, McDuffie L, Groh E, Hackworth J, Bell TM, Maarker TA. Physical Examination is the Best Predictor of the Need for Abdominal Surgery in Children Following Motor Vehicle Collision. J Emerg Med. 2018;54(1):1-7.
13. Braungart S, Beattie T, Midgley P, Powis M. Implications of a negative abdominal CT in the management of pediatric blunt abdominal trauma. J Pediatr Surg. 2017;52(2):293-8.
14. Rovin JD, Rodgers BM. Pediatric foreign body aspiration. Pediatr Rev. 2000;21(3):86-90.
15. Kramer RE, Lerner DG, Lin T, Manfredi M, Shah M, Stephen TC, et al; North American Society for Pediatric Gastroenterology, Hepatology, and Nutrition Endoscopy Committee. Management of Ingested Foreign Bodies in Children: A Clinical Report of the NASPGHAN Endoscopy Committee. J Pediatr Gastroenterol Nutr. 2015;60(4):562-74.

20.4 Drowning and Submersion Injury, and Burns

Mihir Sarkar

DROWNING AND SUBMERSION INJURY

INTRODUCTION

Drowning is one of the major global public health problems, and according to the World Health Organization (WHO) 2019 report, drowning accounts for estimated 236,000 deaths. Over 90% of drowning deaths are from low- and middle-resource countries.[1]

DEFINITION

Drowning is the process of experiencing respiratory impairment from submersion or immersion in liquid. Terminologies such as wet drowning, dry drowning, near drowning, and drowning injury are no longer used.[2]

PATHOPHYSIOLOGY

Drowning can lead to hypoxemia and subsequent apnea, and, if not rapidly addressed, culminates in cardiac arrest. The aspiration of fluid into the lungs induces pulmonary injury and can precipitate the onset of acute respiratory distress syndrome. Additionally, cerebral hypoxic-ischemic injury significantly contributes to both morbidity and mortality in such incidents.[3]

RISK FACTORS

Risk factors vary according to the age, geographical location, and underlying medical conditions. In our country, the most common sites for drowning are unprotected water bodies around the household (ponds, lakes, rivers, pools, underground sumps, open manholes, and septic tanks). **Table 20.4.1** summarizes the risk factors for drowning in children and adolescents.

TABLE 20.4.1: Risk factors of drowning.

Age	Infants	• Bathtub, large household buckets—*fall head first* • *Exclude child abuse in case of infant drowning*
	1–4 years	• Drowning rate is highest in this age group • Curious nature, rapid escalation of physical activity • Incidence happens in a water body near to the house—pools, ditches, ponds, and river • May be due to child neglect or abuse
	Adolescents	• Second major peak of drowning incidence and death • Male gender accounts for 80% fatal drowning • High-risk behavior, alcohol use, substance abuse, diminished awareness of risks, and lack of adult supervision
Underlying medical conditions	• Seizures • Hypoglycemia • Arrhythmias and long QT syndrome • Intoxication • Trauma while swimming	

EVALUATION AND MANAGEMENT[3]

History

Most cases of drowning do not result in respiratory impairment in children and do not require hospital admission beyond a period of observation. The following details in history should be obtained as soon as possible to evaluate and initiate treatment in a child with drowning or submersion injury.

Timeline

- Time and duration of immersion—outcome is generally good with submersion duration <5 minutes.
- The time to and type of basic life support (BLS)—delivered by the bystanders or emergency medical team before arrival to the healthcare facility
- Time to first respiratory effort following attempts to resuscitation
- Details of treatment received at the spot and during transport of the child

Circumstances Leading to the Drowning

Consider the following details during evaluation:

- Inconsistencies in history by the relatives or bystanders who have brought the child
- Whether the history is compatible with the developmental age of the child or not

Examination

Children who are alert and asymptomatic do not need investigation, except observation for a short period. The following points are important in evaluating a child with submersion injury:

- Evidence of hypoxic brain injury if any
- Evidence of respiratory compromise if any
- Signs of trauma particularly head and cervical spine trauma. Cervical spine injury is uncommon but should be considered if there is history of trauma or diving.

Management

The key to successful resuscitation of a drowning patient is following advanced life support (ALS) guidelines, correction of hypoxemia, providing organ support, and effective rewarming.[3] *The management should start at prehospital settings and continue at emergency room (ER) and subsequently in pediatric intensive care unit (PICU).* Clinical outcome largely depends on the duration of submersion, speed of recovery, and effective resuscitation at the scene of accident. **Flowchart 20.4.1** describes the important elements of management at the site of drowning.

Key Points[4]

- Management must begin at the prehospital setting in a coordinated manner pursuant to the ABCs (airway, breathing, and circulation) of resuscitation.
- Rescue breathing and chest compressions sequence should be followed rather than chest compressions alone in a state of cardiac arrest.
- Restoration of respiration and circulation are the primary goals at the scene.
- Rapid transportation to a hospital with ongoing resuscitation is essential for those who remain "lifeless" for definitive care (cerebral resuscitation).
- Support of lungs and cardiovascular system contributes to the potential for brain resuscitation.

Hospital Management at Emergency Department

For Unstable Patient[4]

- Initiate ALS for patient presenting in arrest state, unconscious, severe respiratory distress, and circulatory failure.
- Intubation and mechanical ventilation—if unable to protect airway
- Invasive or noninvasive ventilation/bi-level ventilation—if impaired gas exchange
- Fluid resuscitation, vasopressors, and inotropes—to maintain adequate circulation
- Temperature control:
  - Monitor core temperature—rectal or esophageal
  - Avoid aggressive rewarming in *cold water immersion*
  - Active rewarming (if core temperature <30°C)—warm intravenous (IV) fluids (39°C) and warm saline (42°C) gastric or bladder lavage
- *Changes in ALS guidelines in hypothermia, if the core temperature is <30°C:* Defibrillation is less effective in hypothermic myocardium. Limit the number of defibrillation shocks to less than three shocks. Do not use inotropes or antiarrhythmic agents, as they may precipitate arrhythmias. If the core temperature is 30–35°C, double the dose interval of inotropic or antiarrhythmic drugs (e.g., epinephrine or norepinephrine).

Flowchart 20.4.1: Important elements of management at the site of drowning.

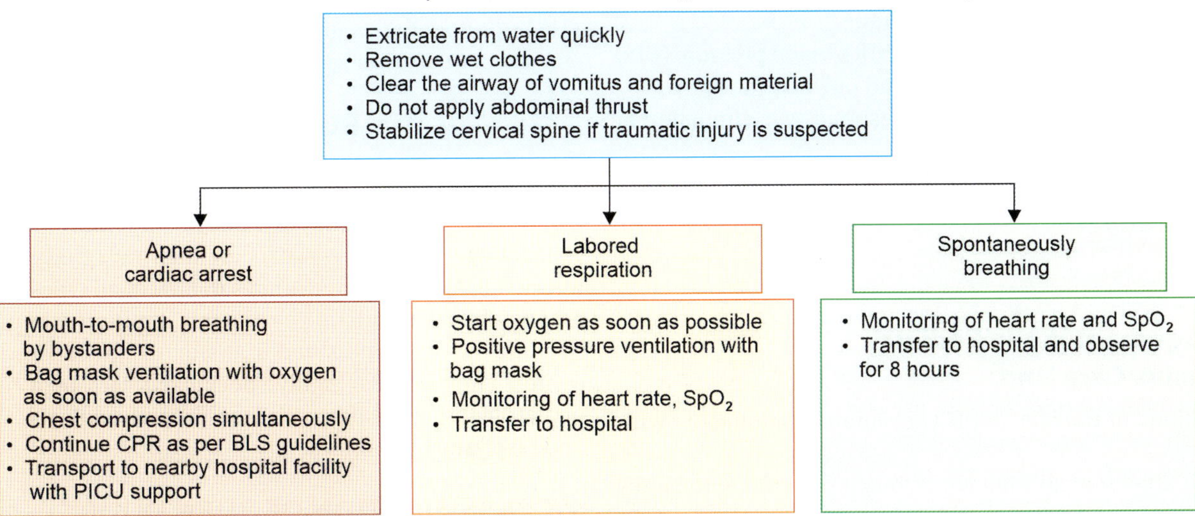

(BLS: basic life support; CPR: cardiopulmonary resuscitation)

TABLE 20.4.2: Key issues of management in pediatric intensive care unit (PICU).

Cerebral protection	• Seizures and fever should be aggressively and appropriately treated • Electroencephalography (EEG) is useful to detect nonconvulsive status and to titrate antiepileptic therapy • *Brain cooling has shown better neurological outcome in adult patients with cardiac arrest* • Maintain mild hypothermia (core temperature (32–34°C) for 12–72 hours in comatose children • Neuromuscular blocking agents
Respiratory support	• For ARDS—lung protective strategy according to second Pediatric Acute Lung Injury Consensus Conference (PALICC-2) guidelines • Low tidal volume (TV)—6–8 mL/kg • Optimum PEEP • Plateau pressure (Pplat) <28 cmH_2O • *Permissive hypercapnia*: • *Alter ventilator management if significant brain injury is detected* – Avoid permissive hypercapnia—risk of intra-cranial pressure surge • Avoid high PEEP—high PEEP diminishes cerebral venous return • Do not administer exogenous surfactant routinely
Cardio-vascular support	• Fluid resuscitation—avoid overzealous fluid bolus • Infusion of vasoactive agent—start early to treat hypoxic myocardial dysfunction • Normalize blood pressure, organ perfusion, and gas exchange
Metabolic	• Maintain euglycemia—both hypo- and hyperglycemia are detrimental • Correct dyselectrolytemia

(ARDS: acute respiratory distress syndrome; PEEP: positive end-expiratory pressure)

For Stable Patient[4]

- Observe at least 8 hours even for stable patients. Risk of pulmonary edema up to first 8 hours
- Serial monitoring of heart rate (HR), blood pressure (BP), respiratory rate, temperature, and pulse oximetry
- Neurological assessment and respiratory examination at frequent intervals
- Provide oxygen and other respiratory support (high-flow nasal oxygen and noninvasive ventilation at emergency as per the severity)
- Obtain chest X-ray

Management in the Pediatric Intensive Care Unit[5]

Indications to transfer to PICU or appropriate facility with PICU:

- Not able to regain full consciousness in the emergency department
- Concerns for severe injuries and life-threatening complications

Table 20.4.2 summarizes the key issues of management in a PICU.[4]

Poor Indicators of Prognosis[5]

- Submersion for >10 minutes is related to poor outcome.
- Duration >25 minutes is invariably fatal.
- A delay in the start of cardiopulmonary resuscitation (CPR) or no return of spontaneous circulation within 30 minutes of CPR
- Glassgow Coma scale (GCS) <5
- Rectal temperature <30°C
- Arterial blood pH <7.1 on arrival

Prevention of Drowning in Children

- *Supervision:* Provide constant supervision for children in or near water environments, ensuring that they are never left unattended, even momentarily.
- *Fencing:* Erect a 4-sided barrier around pools and hot tubs, with a minimum height of 4 feet.
- *Swim lessons:* Enrol children in swim lessons when they are developmentally prepared.
- *Life jackets:* Mandate the wearing of life jackets for boating or other water sports activities.
- *CPR knowledge:* BLS mass awareness training to start bystander CPR
- *Water safety rules:* Develop and strictly enforce water safety protocols.

CONCLUSION

Drowning among children constitutes an international issue, with risk factors differing based on age and preexisting health conditions. Immediate and appropriate resuscitation at the drowning location, along with consistent continuity of care during transportation to the hospital, is crucial for survival. The implementation of preventive strategies and rigorous enforcement of water safety regulations are essential.

BURN INJURY

INTRODUCTION

One-fourth of all burn injuries occur in children under 16 years of age. Children <5 years are high-risk group for burn injuries. Scald injury contributes to 65% of all types of burns among children under 5 years.[6] Only a minority of patients become critical and need transfer to specialized burn center. They require highly specialized care by a team of pediatricians, intensivists, surgeons, anesthesiologist, nurses, and respiratory therapists.

CLASSIFICATION OF BURN INJURY

Burn injury is classified according to the depth and extend of the injury. The classification of burns by depth is summarized

TABLE 20.4.3: Classification of burn by depth.

Depth	*Surface appearance*	*Pain*	*Healing time*
First degree, only epidermis	• No or minimal edema • Erythematous, dry • No blister	Very painful	2–5 days, no scarring
Second degree—entire epidermis and variable thickness of dermis	• Formation of blisters, moist blebs • Bleeding present	Very painful	• *Superficial:* 5–21 days • *Deep:* 21–35 days with no infection
• Third degree, full-thickness—entire epidermis and dermis destroyed • May include subcutaneous tissue, fascia, muscle, and bones	• Dry, leathery eschar • Mixed white, waxy • No bleeding or blanching	Insensate	• Never heals • Require grafting • Small area may heal from the edges

TABLE 20.4.4: Modified Lund–Browder chart for assessing percentage of total body surface area burn in children.*

Areas	*Birth to 1 year*	*1–4 years*	*5–9 years*	*10–14 years*
Head	9.5	8.5	6.5	5.5
Neck	1	1	1	1
Trunk	13	13	13	13
Upper arm	2	2	2	2
Forearm	1.5	1.5	1.5	1.5
Hands	1.25	1.25	1.25	1.25
Thigh	2.75	3.25	4	4.25
Leg	2.5	2.5	2.5	3
Foot	1.75	1.75	1.75	1.75
Buttock	2.5	2.5	2.5	2.5
Genitalia	1	1	1	1

*Values listed are for one surface area and each individual extremity. Anterior and posterior surface area values are equivalent in estimating total body surface area (TBSA). For circumferential burns, multiply surface area burned by two.
Source: Adapted from Lund CC et al.[7]

in **Table 20.4.3**, and the modified Lund-Browder chart for assessing burns according to percentage of total body surface area (BSA) burn in children is given in **Table 20.4.4.**[7] **Figure 20.4.1** describes the distribution of burn surface area according to age and surface area of the part of the body and age.

Following burns, inflammatory and vasoactive mediators including histamines, cytokines, and prostaglandins are released leading to sever systemic capillary leak, intravascular fluid loss, and large volume fluid shift within the first 24 hours, with peak in the first 6–8 hours. Decreased cardiac output ensues along with increased vascular resistance with resultant hypovolemia and hypoperfusion. This is known as "burn shock", which needs appropriate management with early rapid fluid replacement with monitoring.

PRINCIPLES OF ACUTE TREATMENT OF BURNS

Quite a few cases of small burns in children can be managed as an outpatient; however, very young children with >10% total BSA burned, especially with involvement of face, eyes, ears, joints, and genitalia, are better managed in a hospital setting. The initial resuscitation includes the following steps:[8,9]

1. Provide first aid at the site of occurrence.
2. Take an appropriate and quick history and assess ABCD, look for inhalation injury followed by appropriate examination and intervention for resuscitation.
3. Estimate the area of burn and decide whether the child requires aggressive fluid resuscitation.
4. Wash the wound and eliminate devitalized tissue.
5. Protection of airway, place nasogastric tube if necessary
6. Fluid resuscitation, especially in those with >20% total BSA burns. Be careful about overhydrating the child.
7. Cardiac and pulse oximetry as required
8. Adequate calorie and protein supplementation
9. Adequate analgesia
10. Prevention of infection and regulation of bacterial flora in wounds
11. Use of synthetic or biological dressing

Outpatient Management of Minor Burns[8,9]

- First- or second-degree burn with <10% BSA is managed in outpatient clinic.
- Adequate family support should be ensured, especially in very young children.
- Tetanus immunization is not required if the child is fully immunized as per the immunization schedule.
- The blisters should be as left intact as far as possible.
- Dress the burn areas with silver sulfadiazine cream, and the area should be washed with lukewarm water daily.

First Aid Treatment

The stepwise management to provide first aid at the site of burns is listed here:[8]

1. Roll the patient on the ground; cover with a blanket to extinguish flame.
2. Eliminate garments that are smoldering or saturated with hot liquid.
3. Jewellery should be removed.
4. Chemical burn—brush off any remaining chemical followed by irrigation or wash with water.

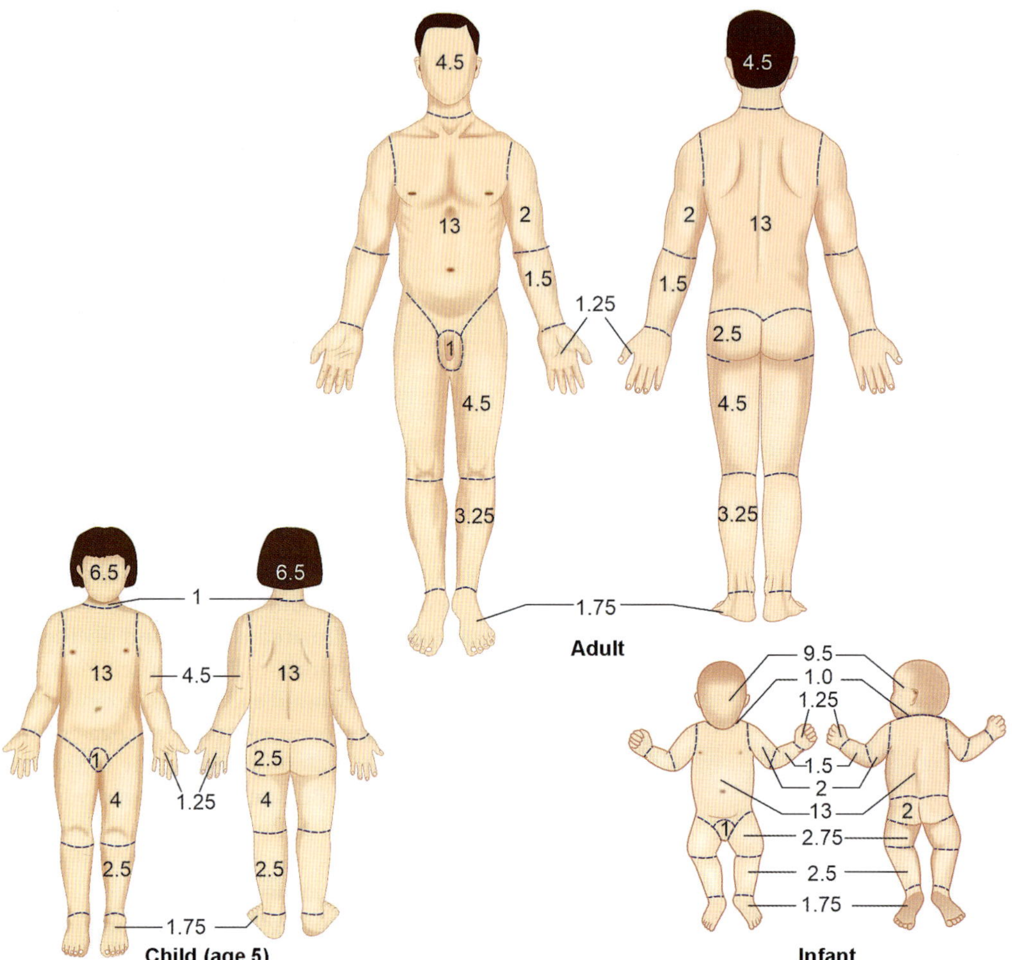

Fig. 20.4.1: Distribution of percentage of burn body surface area according to age and the part of the body.
Source: Modified Lund–Browder chart (Adapted from Lund CC et al.[7])

5. Call the local poison control center.
6. Cover with clean, dry sheeting.
7. Apply cold (not iced) wet compresses to small injuries.
8. Large burn injury (>15–20% of BSA) contraindicates the use of cold compresses.
9. If a burn results from hot tar exposure, utilize mineral oil to effectively remove the tar.
10. Dispense analgesic.

Indications for Hospitalization for Burns

A child with burns will require hospitalization if the child has the following:[8,9]

- Burns affecting >10% of BSA
- Third-degree burns
- Electrical burns due to high-tension wires or lightening
- Chemical burns
- Inhalation injury
- Suboptimal home or social environment
- Suspected child abuse or neglect
- Burns over the face, hands, feet, major joints, perineum, or genitals
- Burns in patients with pre-existing medical conditions that may complicate the acute recovery.

Emergency Care

The various steps in the management of burns in children are detailed in **Table 20.4.5**.[8,9]

Complications[9]

- Anemia may result from full-thickness burns of >10% total BSA.
- Compartment syndrome or rhabdomyolysis is common in electrical burns.
- Venous thrombosis may occur in 6–25% of patients with extensive burns.
- A hypermetabolic state is known to persist for years after a major burn in children; it may decrease bone density and muscle mass on follow-up.

TABLE 20.4.5: Steps in management of burns.

Airway	Compromised or at risk (facial burn, laryngeal edema, and inhalation of carbon monoxide)	Intubate and oxygenate
Breathing	Smoke inhalation—pulmonary edema, acute respiratory distress syndrome (ARDS)	• Oxygen and nebulization • Noninvasive or invasive ventilation
	Carboxyhemoglobin (>60% severe)	Ventilation with 100% O_2
	Mechanical obstruction	Escharotomy
Circulation	Lines	• Obtain IV/IO access—two wide-bore cannula • Central venous access to administer high volume fluid in burns >30%
	Fluid resuscitation—assess BSA of burn correctly	• Bolus of Ringer's lactate 10–20 mL/kg for shock • Parkland formula—4 mL/kg body weight/% • BSA—Ringer's lactate (RL) • Add dextrose in children <5 years • Target urine output—0.5–1 mL/kg/h
	Fluid in second 24 hours	• Adjust fluid according to urine output • May need restriction as patient begins to reabsorb fluid
	Colloids—5% albumin over 24 hours	• 30–50% of BSA—0.3 mL/kg/% BSA • 50–70% of BSA—0.4 mL/kg/% BSA • 70–100% of BSA—0.5 mL/kg/% BSA
Nutrition	Burn is a hypercatabolic state	Calorie—1.5 times of basal metabolic rate, Protein—3–4 g/kg
		Early enteral feeding from 12 hours
Wound management	FACED—first aid, analgesia, clean, assess, dress, and elevate	• Clean with saline • Blisters >5 mm and crossing joints should be deroofed • Topical application of silver sulphadiazine or mafenide acetate or 0.5% silver nitrate
	Surgical management	• Debridement and dressing • Circumferential burn—escharotomy • Autograft or biological graft to cover excised areas
Pain management	Provide adequate analgesia, anxiolytics, and psychological support	• Oral/IV/per rectal paracetamol • Oral/IV—morphine • IV ketamine/propofol—wound dressing
Infection control	Risk of infection—large open wound, suppressed immunity and malnutrition	• Routine use of antibiotics is not recommended • Barrier nursing, prevent cross infection • Early excision of burn tissue before bacterial colonization • Topical antiseptic cream with tissue penetrating capacity—0.5% silver nitrate lotion, mafenide acetate, and silver sulfadiazine cream

(BSA: body surface area; IV: intravenous)

- Keloids formation is common, and it may be associated with pain and disfiguration due to scarring.
- Psychological trauma and post-traumatic stress disorder are common, following extensive burns and long-term management.
- Burns result in significant scarring, leading to social isolation with resultant poverty, and child abandonment in low-income group countries.
- Make every effort to return the child to school and mix with peer group.

CONCLUSION

Children under the age of five represent a demographic with an elevated risk of experiencing burn injuries. The assessment of burn severity, determined by the degree and extent of body surface area affected, aids in the prioritization of patient treatment. The effective management of severe burn cases necessitates the collaboration of a multidisciplinary team.

REFERENCES

1. World Health Organization. (2024). Drowning. [online] Available from https://www.who.int/news-room/fact-sheets/detail/drowning [Last accessed December, 2024].
2. Van Beeck EF, Branche CM, Szpilman D, Modell JH, Bierens JJ. A new definition of drowning: Towards documentation and prevention of a global public health problem. Bull World Health Organ. 2005;83:853-6.
3. Kaglar D, Quan L. Drowning and submersion injury. In: Kliegman RM, Stanton BF, Geme III JWS, Schor NF, Behrman RE (Eds). Nelson Textbook of Pediatrics, 21st edition. Philadelphia: Elsevier; 2020. pp. 561-8.
4. Slonieewsky DE, Biagas KV. Drowning. In: Shaffner DH, McCloskey JJ, Huny EA, Tasker RC (Eds). Rogers' Textbook of Pediatric Intensive Care, 6th edition. Philadelphia: Wolters Kluwer; 2024. pp. 477-83.

5. Pellegrino F, Raffaldi I, Rossi R, De Vito B, Pagano M, Garelli D, et al. Epidemiology, clinical aspects, and management of pediatric drowning. Ital J Pediatr. 2023;49(1):74.
6. Krishnamoorthy V, Ramaiah R, Bhananker SM. Pediatric burn injuries. Int J Crit Illn Inj Sci. 2012;2(3):128-34.
7. Lund CC, Browder NC. The estimation of areas of burns. Surg Gynecol Obstet. 1944;79:352-8.
8. Antoon AY, Donovan MK. Burn injuries. In: Kliegman RM, Stanton BF, Geme III JWS, Schor NF, Behrman RE (Eds). Nelson Textbook of Pediatrics, 21st edition. Philadelphia: Elsevier; 2020. pp. 568-76.
9. Schaefer TJ, Nunez Lopez O. (2023). Burn resuscitation and management. Treasure Island (FL): StatPearls Publishing. [online] Available from https://www.ncbi.nlm.nih.gov/books/NBK430795. [Last accessed December, 2024].

20.5 Cardiopulmonary Resuscitation

Mounika Reddy, Suresh Kumar Angurana

INTRODUCTION

Cardiopulmonary resuscitation (CPR) is a crucial life-saving technique in those with cardiac arrest. Cardiac or cardiopulmonary arrest is the cessation of clinically detectable cardiac mechanical activity, leading to the stoppage of blood circulation (oxygen and nutrients) to various organs, including the brain. Clinically, cardiac arrest is characterized by unresponsiveness, apnea, and the absence of palpable central pulses. CPR is the only effective method to maintain circulation to the brain and heart in such situations. The primary goal of CPR is to quickly restore oxygenation and perfusion to vital organs by supporting the airway, breathing, and circulation. Time is critical in cardiac arrest situations; the brain starts to suffer damage within 3–5 minutes after cardiac arrest, and each minute of delay in initiating CPR reduces the chances of intact survival and increases the risk of long-term neurological damage.

EPIDEMIOLOGY

The incidence of pediatric out-of-hospital cardiac arrest (OHCA) in developed countries is 8.04 per 100,000 person-years. Among these cases, 12.1% survive to hospital discharge, and 4% survive with intact neurological function. Outcomes improve with witnessed arrests and bystander CPR.[1] In contrast, the incidence of in-hospital cardiac arrest (IHCA) in developed countries ranges from 2.8 to 12.6 events per 1,000 children, with survival rates at discharge between 25 and 50%.[2] In India, the actual incidence and outcomes of pediatric OHCA and IHCA are not well-documented due to the lack of CPR registries and central reporting systems. However, single-center studies in India report IHCA event rates between 67 and 83.7 per 1,000 infants and children admitted to hospitals, with survival rates at discharge ranging from 1.8 to 14%.[3]

ETIOPATHOGENESIS

In adults, cardiac arrest is often due to primary cardiac problems, and defibrillation is crucial for good outcomes. However, most pediatric arrests result from the progression of respiratory failure or shock, leading to hypoxemia and bradycardia. Tissue hypoperfusion and hypoxemia favor anaerobic metabolism, and along with the resultant lactic acidosis, contribute to myocardial depression and cardiac arrest. Common causes include respiratory failure due to upper or lower airway obstruction, lung parenchymal disease, or disordered control of breathing, and circulatory failure due to hypovolemic, distributive, cardiogenic, or obstructive shock. Primary cardiac arrhythmias as a cause of cardiac arrest are uncommon in children, with shockable rhythms like ventricular fibrillation (VF) accounting for only 10–15% of cardiac arrests **(Flowchart 20.5.1)**. Therefore, ventilation

Flowchart 20.5.1: Pathways to pediatric cardiac arrest.[4]

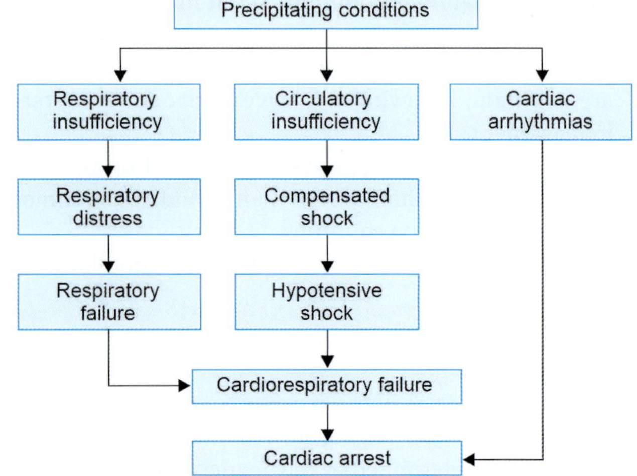

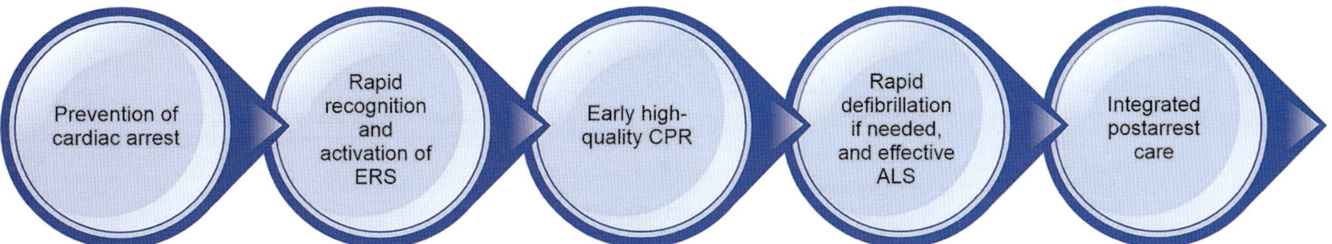

Fig. 20.5.1: Chain of survival for pediatric cardiac arrest.[5] (ALS: advanced life support; CPR: cardiopulmonary resuscitation; ERS: emergency response systems)

is of greater importance during the resuscitation of pediatric arrests. In a seriously ill or injured child, early recognition and aggressive treatment of respiratory failure and shock are crucial to prevent progression to cardiac arrest. Common upstream precipitating etiologies for pediatric cardiac arrest include pneumonia, diarrhea, sepsis, trauma, poisoning, and cardiac diseases, most of which are preventable.[4]

CHAIN OF SURVIVAL

The chain of survival refers to a sequence of events that must occur in rapid succession to maximize the chances of intact survival from cardiac arrest **(Fig. 20.5.1)**. Each element in this chain is crucial, interlinked, and interdependent. CPR is just one link in the chain, and any weakness in one of the linkages decreases the chances of intact survival. Prevention is a particularly important component of the pediatric chain of survival.[5]

TIERS OF CARDIOPULMONARY RESUSCITATION

There are three tiers of CPR, which vary based on the site of the cardiac arrest (IHCA vs. OHCA), the number and proficiency of rescuers, local protocols, and the availability of equipment.[5]

- *Tier 1 or hands-only CPR* is applicable for an OHCA where the rescuer is a layperson with limited basic life support (BLS) skills. The emphasis is on chest compressions only until further help arrives or the victim is taken to a healthcare facility. Most arrests occur at home and are witnessed, so the person next to the victim has the best chance to provide CPR. Early bystander CPR significantly increases the chances of survival in OHCA.
- *Tier 2 or compression and breathing CPR* is performed by skilled BLS rescuers who provide coordinated chest compressions and rescue breaths.
- *Tier 3 or multirescuer coordinated CPR* involves a team approach where multiple life-saving actions such as compressions, ventilation, and defibrillation are performed simultaneously by multiple skilled rescuers using effective team dynamics with a high chance of successful resuscitation, typically in an IHCA situation.

BASIC LIFE SUPPORT

Basic life support comprises the knowledge and skills necessary for providing life-sustaining support to an unresponsive victim in emergencies, either within or outside the hospital setting. The International Liaison Committee on Resuscitation (ILCOR) regularly reviews the science behind CPR and updates guidelines based on the latest research.[6-8] Early administration of high-quality CPR, along with early defibrillation if indicated, improves outcomes in cardiac arrest. The two major goals of CPR are the return of spontaneous circulation (ROSC) and survival with favorable neurological outcomes. The steps in BLS are depicted in **Flowchart 20.5.2** and are detailed below. For BLS purposes, anyone less than 1-year-old, excluding neonates, is considered an infant. A child is considered to be from 1 year of age until the onset of external signs of puberty. Anyone older than this is considered an adult.[5]

Scene Safety and Assessment

In any potential cardiac arrest situation, first ensure that the scene is safe. Look for circumstantial evidence of drug abuse or poisoning. Then assess the victim for unresponsiveness by tapping the shoulders or soles of the feet and asking loudly, "Are you alright?" Assess breathing and the central pulse simultaneously, taking no >10 seconds. In adults and children, palpate the carotid pulse using 2–3 fingers in the groove between the muscles at the side of the neck. In infants, palpate the brachial pulse above the cubital fossa. This assessment should be quick to minimize delays in starting CPR. Unresponsiveness, abnormal (gasping) or absent breathing, and no detectable pulse within 10 seconds indicates a cardiac arrest situation.

Activate the Emergency Response System

Upon identifying a cardiac arrest situation, shout for help and send someone to get an automated external defibrillator (AED) or activate the emergency response system (ERS) using a mobile phone (e.g., dial 108) or social media where appropriate without leaving the victim's side. In single-rescuer CPR for a child or infant, call for help after performing

Flowchart 20.5.2: Basic life support algorithm.

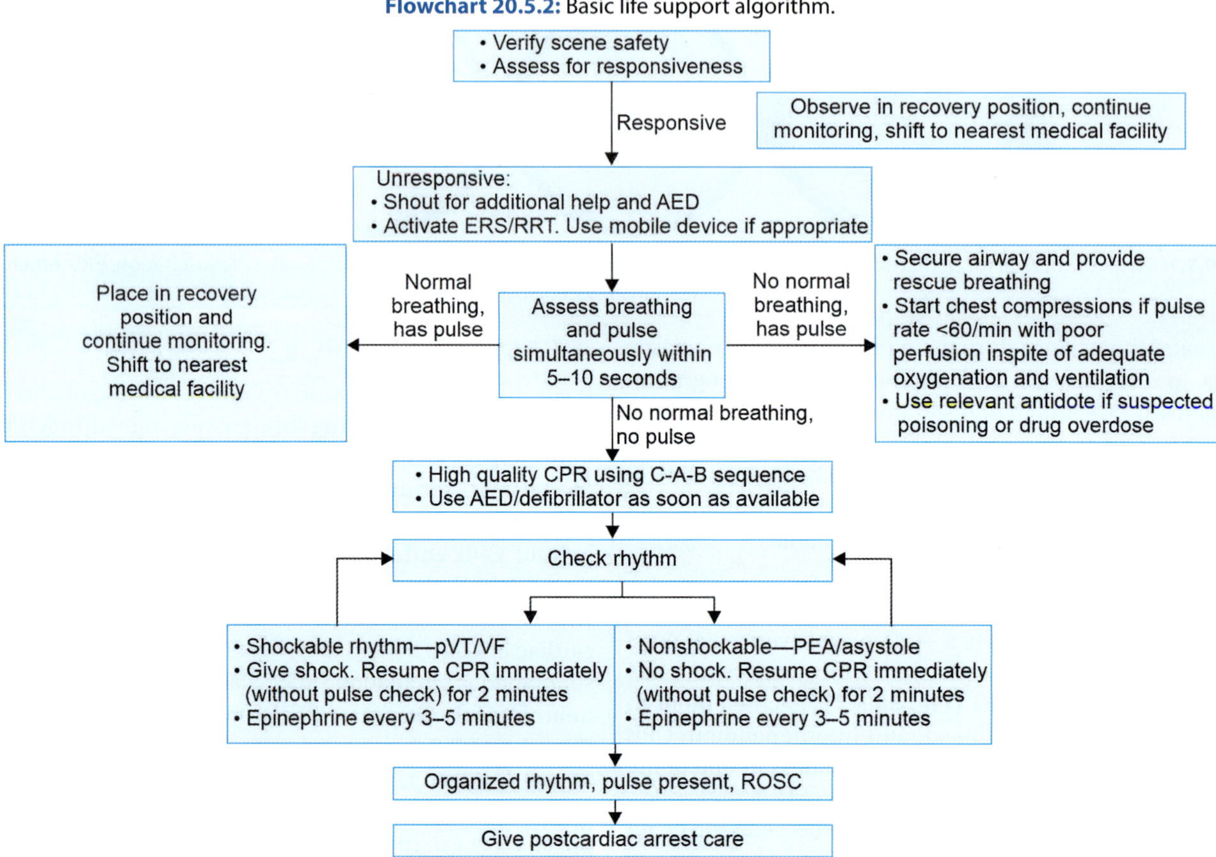

(AED: automated external defibrillator, CPR: cardiopulmonary resuscitation; C-A-B: compression-airway-breathing; ERS: emergency response system; PEA: pulseless electrical activity; ROSC: return of spontaneous circulation; RRT: rapid response team; VF: ventricular fibrillation; VT: ventricular tachycardia)

2 minutes of CPR. When at least two rescuers are available, one rescuer should initiate CPR while the second rescuer activates the ERS and brings the AED.

Chest Compressions

Place the victim in a supine position on a flat surface. Position yourself beside the victim and remove clothing to ensure the bare chest is visible. Start high-quality CPR **(Box 20.5.1)** following the C-A-B (compression-airway-breathing) sequence. For chest compressions, place the heel of one hand over the lower half of the breastbone, just below the nipple line, with the other hand on top of it. Keeping the hands locked, and hands, elbows, and shoulders aligned in a straight line above the chest, deliver smooth, and regular compressions **(Fig. 20.5.2A)**. The one-hand technique may be used for small children **(Fig. 20.5.2B)**. For infants, use the two-finger technique for single rescuer CPR: place the index and middle fingers of one hand on the chest, and use the other hand to slightly tilt the head back to keep the airway open **(Fig. 20.5.2C)**. For two or more rescuers, use the two-thumb encircling hands technique **(Fig. 20.5.2D)**. Ensure that the time for chest compression and recoil is approximately equal. Minimize interruptions in chest compressions to <10 seconds for procedures such as rhythm checks, shock delivery, or placing an advanced airway. Avoid pressing directly over the xiphisternum, as it can cause serious injury. A hard backboard under the patient and a step stool can facilitate good chest compressions if the patient is on a bed.

BOX. 20.5.1: The five components of high-quality cardiopulmonary resuscitation.

- *Push fast:* Ensure chest compressions at an adequate rate of 100–120 per minute
- *Push hard:* Ensure chest compressions of adequate depth of at least one-third of the anteroposterior diameter of the chest
- *Allow complete chest recoil* between compressions for adequate cardiac refilling
- *Minimize interruptions* in chest compressions to <10 seconds
- *Avoid hyperventilation*

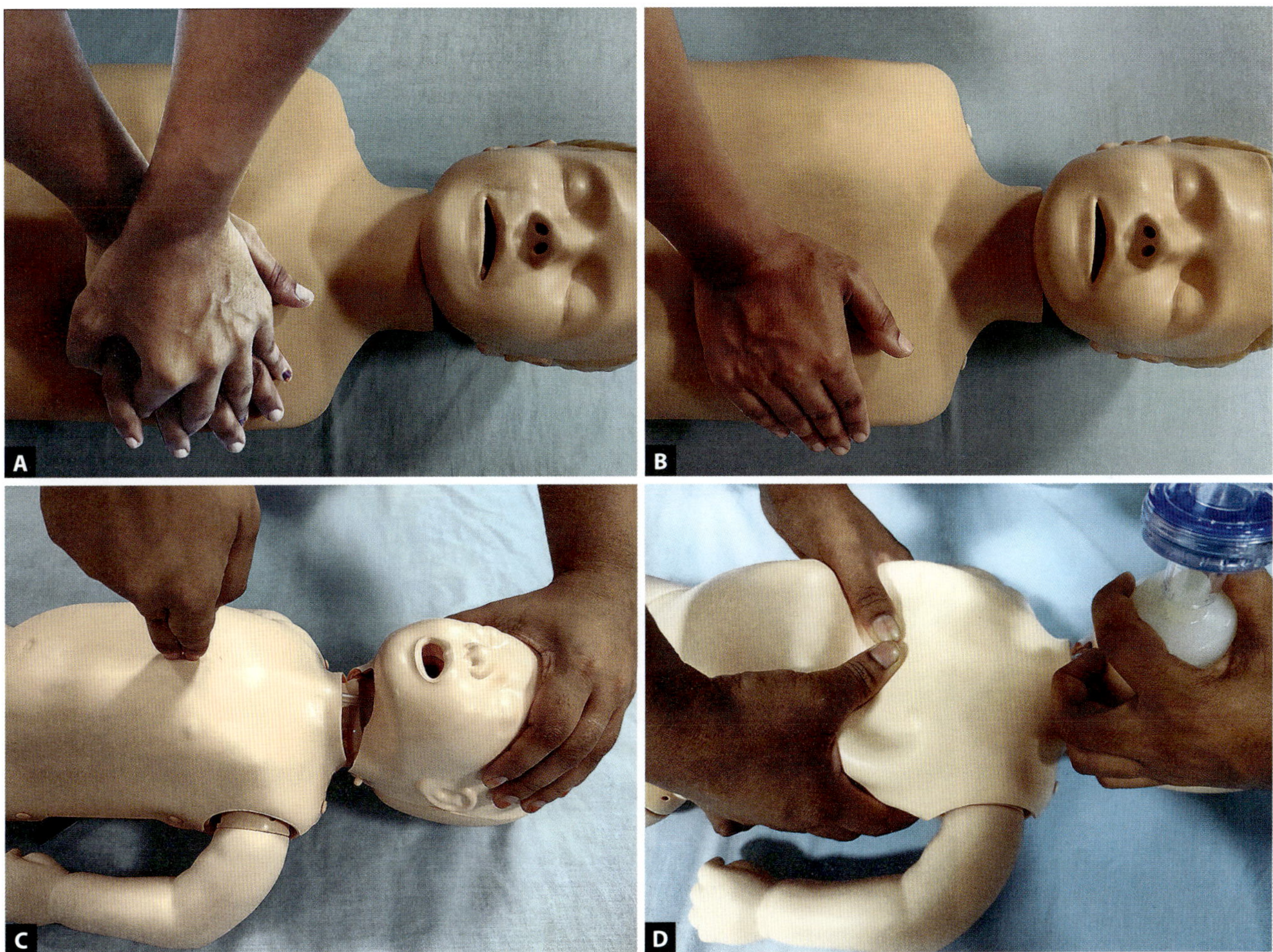

Figs. 20.5.2A to D: Hand placement and technique for chest compressions. (A) In an older child or adult; (B) In a small child; (C) In an infant with a single rescuer; (D) In an infant with two or more rescuers.

Effective chest compressions improve survival by providing blood flow to vital organs during CPR. Good-quality chest compressions provide nearly 20% of cardiac output. Adequate coronary artery perfusion pressure is essential for myocardial preservation and the ROSC.

Ventilation (Rescue Breaths)

Open the airway using the head-tilt-chin-lift maneuver **(Fig. 20.5.3A)** or the jaw thrust maneuver in cases of suspected cervical spine injury **(Fig. 20.5.3B)** to keep the tongue away and allow effective delivery of breaths. Check the oropharynx for any visible foreign objects. Pinch the victim's nose with your thumb and forefinger, take a normal breath, cover the victim's mouth with yours, and deliver two breaths, blowing for one second each, with just enough volume to create a visible chest rise. In infants, cover both the mouth and nose of the infant with your mouth to deliver breaths. The risk of contracting a communicable disease from the victim during mouth-to-mouth breathing is extremely small and should not deter from providing help when needed. Barrier devices like a pocket mask and bag-mask ventilation (BMV) **(Fig. 20.5.3C)** should be used where available. If chest expansion is inadequate, reassess the patient's position, and the adequacy of the seal. Compressions should be paused while giving ventilation. Adequate ventilation is a critical component of pediatric CPR, as most pediatric cardiac arrests are secondary to hypoxia. However, caution must be taken to avoid hyperventilation, as it increases intrathoracic pressure, impedes venous return to the heart, and reduces cardiac output and coronary perfusion pressure. Respiratory alkalosis due to hyperventilation also reduces cerebral perfusion. The chest compression-to-ventilation ratio for infants and children is 15:2, while for adults it is 30:2. This applies to both single-rescuer and two-rescuer CPR. If the rescuer or

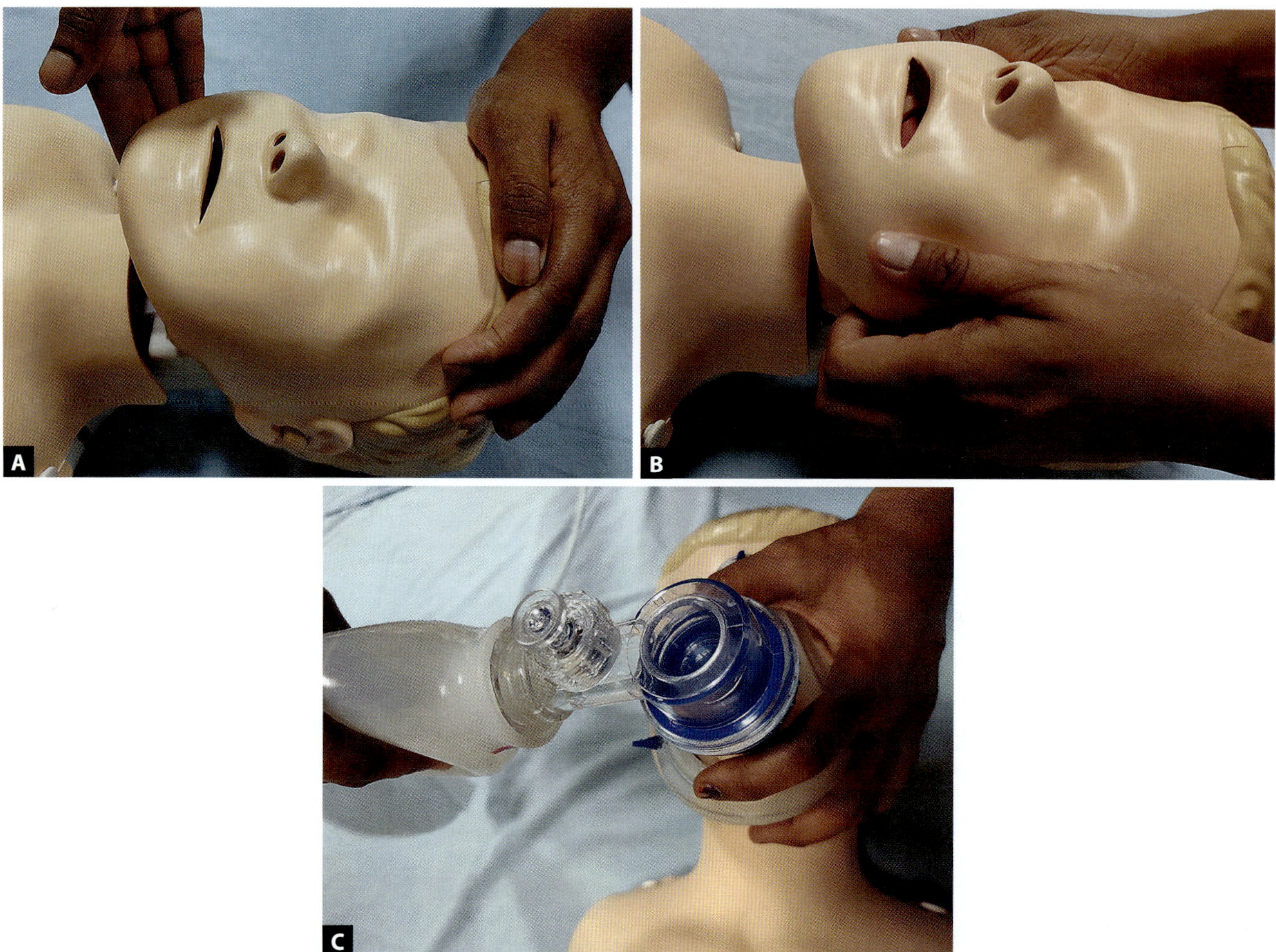

Figs. 20.5.3A to C: Maneuvers to open the airway and deliver rescue breaths. (A) Head-tilt-chin-lift maneuver: Place one hand over the forehead to gently tilt or extend the head, and use fingers of the other hand to lift the jaw forward, without pressing over soft tissues of the neck; (B) Jaw thrust maneuver: Stabilize the head in the neutral position, place fingers of both hands behind the jaw angles, and lift upward to open the airway without tilting the head; (C) Bag-and-mask ventilation with E-C clamp.

bystander is unwilling or unable to deliver rescue breaths, chest compressions alone can be provided. In a child with no or inadequate breathing but with a central pulse, deliver only rescue breaths (one breath every 2–3 seconds with respiratory rate of 20–30 breaths per minute) without chest compressions to support oxygenation and ventilation until spontaneous breathing resumes. In infants and children with an advanced airway (e.g., endotracheal tube), give one breath every 2–3 seconds (20–30 breaths/min) without interrupting chest compressions.

Defibrillation

Defibrillation is the delivery of an unsynchronized shock to terminate an abnormal electrical rhythm and allow the sinus node to resume normal pacemaker activity. Shockable cardiac arrest rhythms include pulseless ventricular tachycardia (VT) and VF, while asystole and pulseless electrical activity (PEA) are nonshockable rhythms. Use an AED or a manual defibrillator as soon as available to analyze the rhythm and determine if a shock is needed. Apply the pads to the victim's bare chest: one on the right side below the collarbone and lateral to the sternum, and the other lateral to the left nipple in the anterior axillary line **(Fig. 20.5.4)**. Adult pads may be used for children 8 years and above. For infants, a manual defibrillator is preferred. If unavailable, use an AED with a pediatric dose attenuator. If neither is available, standard AED pads may be applied in the anteroposterior direction. Do not stop compressions while attaching the pads. Turn on the defibrillator, analyze the rhythm, and deliver a shock if needed. An AED will automatically analyze the rhythm and deliver a shock, if indicated, within 5–15 seconds. If a manual defibrillator is used, the pediatric dose for defibrillation is

2 J/kg for the initial shock and 4 J/kg for subsequent shocks. Resume CPR immediately after defibrillation and continue for at least 2 minutes before the next rhythm check. This continuous CPR maintains oxygen and substrate supply to the heart muscle, enhancing its responsiveness to defibrillation.

Ongoing Cardiopulmonary Resuscitation

Complete five cycles of 30:2 or ten cycles of 15:2 compressions-to-ventilations within 2 minutes of CPR. After every 2 minutes of CPR, perform a pulse and rhythm check lasting 5–10 seconds. Rescuers should switch roles every 2 minutes to reduce fatigue, typically when the AED is analyzing the rhythm. The switch should be done in <10 seconds to minimize interruptions. Effective communication and coordination between rescuers are crucial for seamless transitions and maintaining CPR quality. Continue the cycles of compressions and ventilations until the victim becomes responsive (e.g., moving, coughing, or vocalizing), a pulse or breathing returns, or the child is transferred to a medical facility for advanced life support (ALS). The ROSC is indicated by the presence of a central pulse. The differences in CPR across age groups are outlined in **Table 20.5.1**.

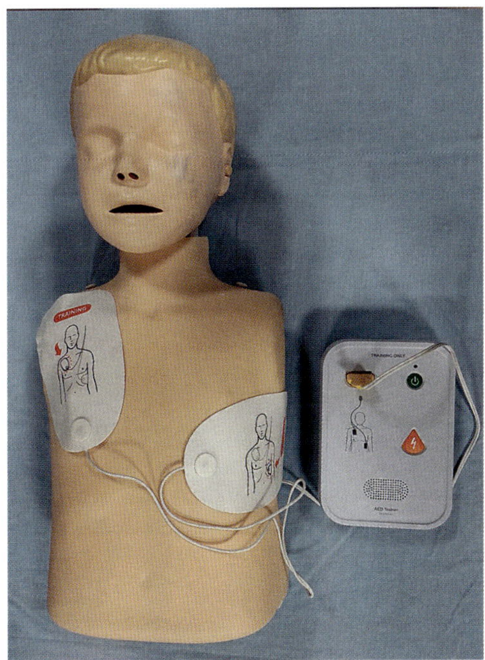

Fig. 20.5.4: Automated external defibrillator and pads placement for defibrillation.

Relief of Choking

Choking occurs when food or another object gets stuck in the airway, causing obstruction. Severe choking can be fatal. The universal sign of choking is holding the neck with one or both hands. The signs and actions for relief of choking are given in **Table 20.5.2**. For Heimlich maneuver, stand behind the victim and wrap your hands around them. Place the fist of one hand between the belly button and breastbone, and grasp with the other hand. Give quick, forceful upward thrusts until the object is forced out or the patient becomes unresponsive **(Fig. 20.5.5A)**. For obese or pregnant persons, use chest thrusts. In infants, perform back slaps and chest thrusts. Kneel or sit with the infant in your lap. Hold the infant facedown with the head slightly lower than the chest, resting on your forearm. Support the head and jaw with your hand. Deliver five back slaps between the infant's shoulder blades with the heel of your hand. Turn the infant and provide five quick downward chest thrusts. Repeat the sequence of five back slaps and five chest thrusts until the object is removed or the infant becomes unresponsive **(Figs. 20.5.5B and C)**. If the victim becomes unresponsive, activate ERS and start CPR. Each time you give a breath, open the mouth, and if a foreign body is visualized, remove it. Do not perform a blind sweep.

PEDIATRIC ADVANCED LIFE SUPPORT

In pediatric cardiac arrest situations, BLS transitions to ALS once trained providers are available in a hospital setting. One must always look for and treat the reversible causes of cardiac arrest **(Table 20.5.3)**.[7,8]

Advanced Airway

Endotracheal intubation is needed if BMV is inadequate or in prolonged CPR. It should be done as soon as possible to maximize oxygenation and ventilation and minimize the risk

TABLE 20.5.1: Differences in cardiopulmonary resuscitation across ages.

Steps in cardiopulmonary resuscitation	***Adults***	***Children (age 1 year to puberty)***	***Infants (less than 1 year of age excluding neonates)***
Hand placement for chest compressions	2 hands on the lower half of the sternum	2 hands or 1 hand (for small children) on the lower half of the sternum	• *1 rescuer:* 2 fingers of a hand in the center of the chest just below the nipple line • *2 rescuers:* 2 thumbs with encircling hands
Compression depth	2–2.4 inch or 5–6 cm	2-inch or 5cm	1.5-inch or 4 cm
Compression-ventilation ratio	30:2 (1 or 2 rescuer)	15:2 (1 or 2 rescuer)	

TABLE 20.5.2: Signs and actions for relief of choking.

Signs	*Airway obstruction*	*Rescuer action*
Can cough/make sound, good air exchange	Mild/partial	Encourage spontaneous breathing and coughing to expel the foreign body. Do not interfere with the victim's attempts
Cannot breathe, talk, cough, or make sound; ineffective cry or sound; possible cyanosis; universal choking sign	Severe	• *Responsive child or adult:* Heimlich maneuver • *Responsive infant:* Five back slaps and five chest thrusts • *Unresponsive victim:* Activate emergency response systems (ERS) and start cardiopulmonary resuscitation (CPR)

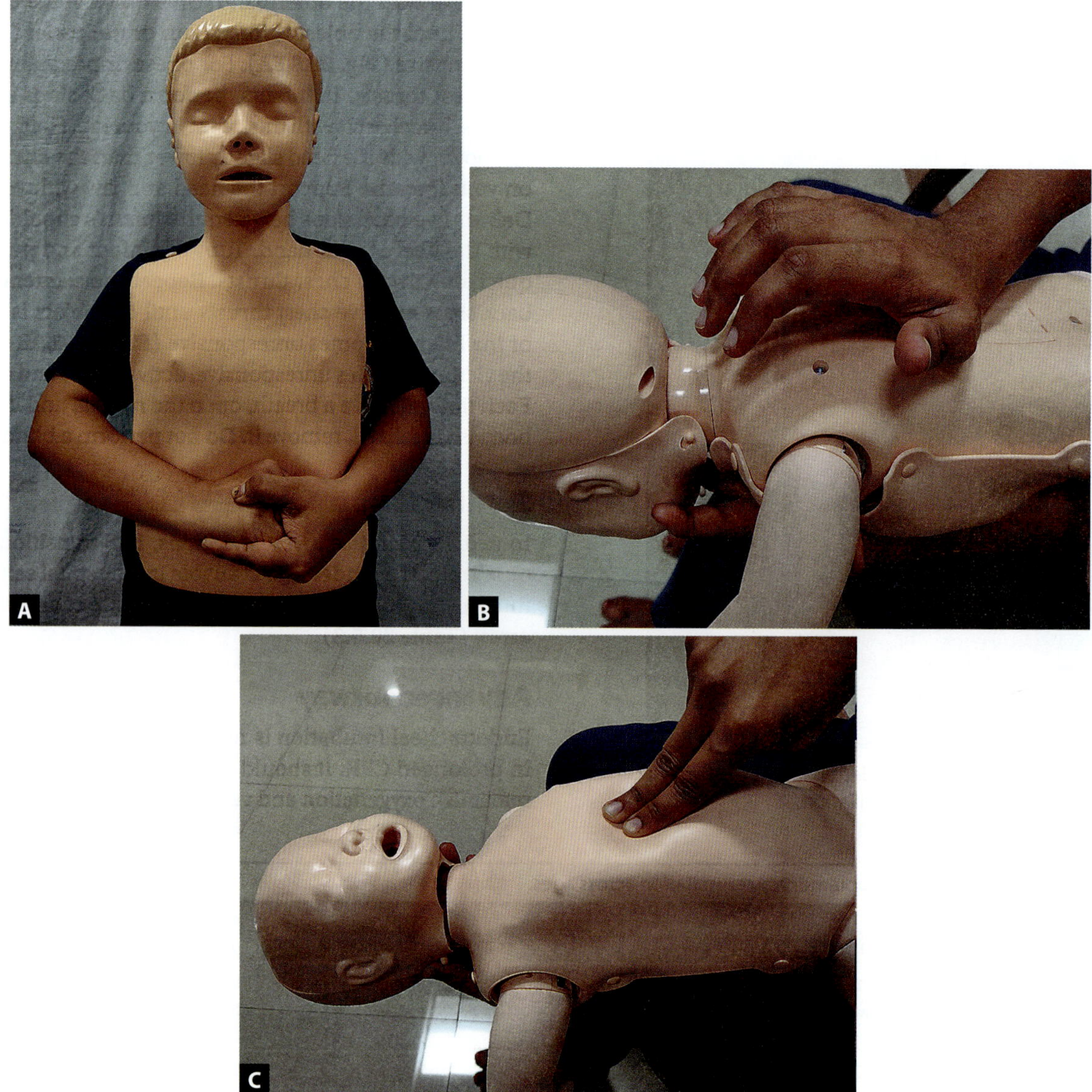

Figs. 20.5.5A to C: Maneuvers for relief of choking. (A) Heimlich's maneuver; (B and C) Back slaps and chest thrusts in an infant.

of aspiration. Insertion of an endotracheal tube during CPR may cause some interruption in chest compressions, hence, the risks and benefits should be weighed. Gastric distension leading to compromised ventilation and aspiration can be prevented by the insertion of an orogastric or nasogastric tube.

Vascular Access and Medications During CPR

Vascular access is needed during CPR for the administration of drugs and fluids **(Table 20.5.4)**. Intraosseous (IO) access is the preferred route, as obtaining peripheral intravenous (IV) access is difficult in a cardiac arrest situation. All resuscitation drugs and fluids can be delivered rapidly and safely via the IO route. If vascular access is unavailable, lipophilic drugs such as lidocaine, epinephrine, atropine, and naloxone (mnemonic LEAN) can be administered through the endotracheal tube at higher doses. Drug delivery should not interrupt CPR. Epinephrine is recommended to be administered soon after starting CPR in all cases, ideally within 5 minutes as it improves coronary and cerebral perfusion during CPR.

TABLE 20.5.3: Reversible causes of cardiac arrest (H's and T's).

Hs	*Ts*
• Hypoxia • Hypoglycemia • Hypovolemia • Hydrogen ions (Acidosis) • Hypocalcemia • Hypo/hyperkalemia • Hypomagnesemia • Hypo/hyperthermia	• Toxins (drug/poison) • Trauma • Tamponade (cardiac) • Tension pneumothorax • Thrombosis (pulmonary or coronary arteries)

CRASH CART

A crash cart or a code cart is a wheeled cart with medical equipment, medications, and supplies necessary for responding to medical emergencies, particularly cardiac arrest. The contents of a typical crash cart are given in **Box 20.5.2**.

POSTRESUSCITATION CARE

Aggressive multidisciplinary postresuscitation care after the ROSC is essential for improving survival rates and neurological outcomes. It focuses on stabilizing the child, identifying and treating the underlying cause of the arrest, preventing secondary injury, and supporting recovery and rehabilitation. In the postarrest phase, secondary neuronal and multiorgan injury due to ischemia-reperfusion influences the severity of encephalopathy and overall outcomes, compounded by ongoing pathophysiological

TABLE 20.5.4: Drugs commonly used during cardiopulmonary resuscitation.

Drug	*Indication*	*Dosage*
Adenosine	Supraventricular tachycardia	0.1 mg/kg (max 6 mg) given as a rapid bolus using a 2-syringe technique. 0.2 mg/kg (max 12 mg) may be used for a repeat dose
Amiodarone	VF or pulseless VT refractory to defibrillation	5 mg/kg over 20 minutes followed by 5 mL saline flush. May be repeated up to two more times (total dose 15 mg/kg)
Atropine	Bradycardia caused by increased vagal tone (e.g., infants and near drowning)	0.02 mg/kg/dose. No recommended minimum dose
Calcium gluconate	Hypocalcemia, calcium channel blocker overdose, hypermagnesemia, and hyperkalemia	1 mL/kg (maximum 10 mL) of 10% calcium gluconate diluted in an equal volume of distilled water given slowly
Dextrose	Hypoglycemia	2 mL/kg 25% dextrose or 5 mL/kg 10% dextrose or 10 mL/kg 5% dextrose
Epinephrine	In all cardiac arrests	0.1 mL/kg/dose (0.01 mg/kg) of 1:10,000 strength via IV/IO route, with a maximum single dose of 1 mg, repeated every 3–5 minutes 0.1 mg/kg/dose (0.1 mL/kg) of 1:1,000 strength if administered via endotracheal route
Lidocaine	VF or pulseless VT refractory to defibrillation	1 mg/kg/dose given undiluted over 2–3 minutes
Magnesium sulphate	Torsades de pointes	25–50 mg/kg (max 2 g) given slowly
Naloxone	Suspected opioid poisoning	0.04–0.1 mg/kg (max 2 mg)
Sodium bicarbonate	Hyperkalemia, tricyclic antidepressant overdose	1 mEq/kg/dose diluted in an equal volume of distilled water, given slowly Use only if ventilation is established

(IO: intraosseous; IV: intravenous; VF: ventricular fibrillation; VT: ventricular tachycardia)

BOX. 20.5.2: Composition of a crash cart.

- Personal protective equipment for providers including goggles, face shield, N95 mask, splash gown/apron, gloves, and footwear
- AED or manual defibrillator with pads

Airway and breathing:

- Self-inflating resuscitation bags with reservoir and face masks of all sizes
- Laryngoscopes with straight and curved blades of all sizes (video laryngoscope if available)
- Stylet or bougie
- Laryngeal mask airway (all sizes)
- Cuffed and uncuffed endotracheal tubes (all sizes)
- Oro/nasopharyngeal airway (all sizes)
- Oro/nasogastric tubes (all sizes)
- Oxygen tubings and oxygen source (cylinder)
- Portable suction
- Surgical airway kit

Circulation:

- Intraosseous needles and insertion set
- Cannula and syringes (all sizes)
- *Medications*: Epinephrine, atropine, amiodarone, adenosine, sodium bicarbonate, calcium gluconate, magnesium sulphate, lidocaine, naloxone, midazolam, fentanyl, vecuronium, ketamine, normal saline, and 10% dextrose
- ECG electrodes
- Broslow's (length-based weight) tape
- Miscellaneous
- Stethoscope, pulse oximeter, and blood pressure apparatus ($EtCO_2$ monitor if available)
- Adhesive tape
- Batteries
- CPR board
- Step stool

TABLE 20.5.5: Postcardiac arrest management bundle.

Evaluate	***Identify and intervene***
A and B: Oxygenation and ventilation	• Ensure airway patency, secure advanced airway, and mechanical ventilation as needed • Maintain normoxia and normocarbia. Avoid hyperoxia and hypercarbia
C: Circulation	• Monitor and maintain hemodynamic stability • Fluid resuscitation and vasoactive medications may be required to maintain systolic blood pressure more than 5th percentile for age • Anticipate and manage postarrest myocardial dysfunction. Epinephrine is the preferred agent • Monitor for and manage metabolic abnormalities
D: Neuroprotection	• Reduce metabolic demand and secondary brain injury • Maintain normoglycemia • Monitor for and treat seizures aggressively • Use appropriate sedoanalgesia to ensure comfort • *Targeted temperature management (TTM):* Target normothermia and strictly control fever. For those who remain comatose after cardiac arrest, consider either 2 days of initial continuous therapeutic hypothermia (32–34°C) followed by 3 days of continuous normothermia (36–37.5°C) or 5 days of continuous normothermia (36-37.5°C)[9] • Measures to prevent or treat raised intracranial pressure
E: Others	• Adequate nutrition is crucial for recovery • Strict adherence to infection control protocols

disturbances from the initial trigger. Progressively, worsening hypoxic-ischemic encephalopathy and postarrest myocardial dysfunction are the major causes of death after initial recovery from cardiac arrest. Management should take place in a pediatric intensive care unit **(Table 20.5.5)** with continuous monitoring of vital parameters, neurological status, and organ functions, with early detection and treatment of complications and multiple organ dysfunction syndrome (MODS).

TEAM DYNAMICS AND COMMUNICATION

A successful resuscitation attempt requires simultaneous concerted efforts of multiple healthcare providers with different levels of skills and expertise. Effective team dynamics are essential to ensure the delivery of high-quality CPR. The multirescuer CPR team composition with specific roles is represented in **Figure 20.5.6**. In situations where enough team members are not there, the existing members double up for certain tasks. The team leader is usually the most experienced person on the team who understands the strengths and weaknesses of all team members and allocates roles and responsibilities accordingly. He guides and monitors the quality of CPR. The elements of effective team dynamics are presented in **Box 20.5.3**. At the end of CPR, debriefing should be done to discuss the actions and remedial measures to enhance future team performance.

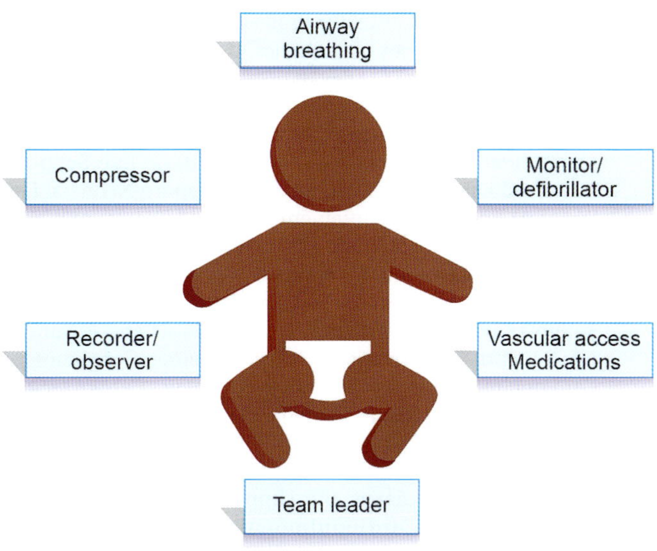

Fig. 20.5.6: Ideal team composition and positions of team members.

BOX. 20.5.3: Elements of effective team dynamics.

- Clear roles and responsibilities
- Clear messages (simple, specific, and loud)
- Closed loop communication
- Knowing your limitations
- Knowledge sharing
- Constructive intervention
- Mutual respect
- Summarizing and reevaluating

Effective communication with family members during ongoing CPR is crucial. They should be briefed at frequent intervals, and their concerns addressed appropriately. The presence of a nurse or a social worker is helpful. Following unsuccessful resuscitation efforts, death disclosure should be done by a senior team member in a compassionate and empathic manner. Spending adequate time, communicating in a private, quiet location, using active listening techniques, and clear understandable language are essential. Family presence during CPR is being increasingly recommended by several guidelines. However, it requires balancing their need for information and proximity with the medical team's operational needs.

Prognostication

There is no single parameter that can reliably predict prognosis after cardiac arrest. Multiple clinical and laboratory parameters are considered for prognostication. Neuroimaging, biomarkers, and electroencephalogram (EEG) can aid in prognostication. Shorter duration of cardiac arrest, early CPR, shockable rhythm, hypothermia as cause of arrest, IHCA, pupillary reaction at 12–24 hours after cardiac arrest, and lower lactate after 12 hours of cardiac arrest may be associated with better prognosis. There are no consistent guidelines as to when to stop resuscitation. There are reports of prolonged arrest with minimal sequelae, especially when good CPR is performed.

Ethical and Legal Considerations

Cardiopulmonary resuscitation involves several ethical and legal considerations, including do not resuscitate (DNR) orders, goals of care, end-of-life decision-making, and organ donation. These decisions are often influenced by religious and cultural norms and beliefs about death and dying. Termination of CPR or withdrawal of life-sustaining treatments requires ethical deliberation and shared decision-making with families, considering the likely prognosis.

TRAINING AND CERTIFICATION

The success of CPR is dependent on the immediate actions of the first responders. Enhancing community awareness and engagement and early CPR by bystanders significantly improves survival rates. Thus, there's a growing emphasis on community CPR training and public access defibrillation programs. Regular retraining and skill refreshments for healthcare providers are essential to maintain high standards of care and adherence to the latest evidence-based protocols. Simulation-based training can be particularly effective in preparing healthcare providers for real-life emergencies. Collecting and analyzing data on cardiac arrest and postresuscitation care can help identify areas for improvement.

RECENT ADVANCES

Ongoing research aims to make high-quality CPR accessible and effective worldwide. Real-time monitoring of CPR quality with feedback on compression depth, rate, and recoil, technological innovations such as automated CPR devices have the potential to improve outcomes. The use of high-fidelity simulation in training has been a gamechanger, providing realistic scenarios and allowing practitioners to hone their skills in a risk-free environment. The increasing use of point-of-care ultrasound (POCUS) allows for quicker diagnosis and management of conditions such as cardiac tamponade, pneumothorax, and internal bleeding. The integration of new technologies, such as advanced monitoring and telemedicine is an evolving frontier.

CONCLUSION

Cardiopulmonary resuscitation is a critical skill that requires specific knowledge and techniques. The key to successful pediatric resuscitation and optimal outcomes lies in early recognition, prompt initiation of CPR, and effective teamwork. As guidelines evolve, ongoing education and practice are vital in ensuring that healthcare providers and the public are prepared to respond effectively in these life-threatening situations. Adapting these practices to the local context, especially in diverse and resource-variable settings like India, is essential to improve outcomes in pediatric emergencies.

REFERENCES

1. Atkins DL, Everson-Stewart S, Sears GK, Daya M, Osmond MH, Warden CR, et al; Resuscitation Outcomes Consortium Investigators. Epidemiology and outcomes from out-of-hospital cardiac arrest in children: the Resuscitation Outcomes Consortium Epistry–Cardiac Arrest. Circulation. 2009;119(11):1484-91.
2. Nadkarni VM, Larkin GL, Peberdy MA, Carey SM, Kaye W, Mancini ME, et al. First documented rhythm and clinical outcome from in-hospital cardiac arrest among children and adults. JAMA. 2006;295(1):50-7.
3. Rathore V, Bansal A, Singhi SC, Singhi P, Muralidharan J. Survival and neurological outcome following in-hospital paediatric cardiopulmonary resuscitation in North India. Paediatr Int Child Health. 2016;36(2):141-7.
4. Jayashree M, Kulgod V, Sharma AK. IAP ALS Handbook, 2nd edition. New Delhi: Indian Academy of Pediatrics ALS BLS Group; 2020.
5. Taneja LN, Tiwari L. BLS for Professionals, 3rd edition. New Delhi: Indian Academy of Pediatrics ALS BLS Group; 2018.
6. Berg KM, Bray JE, Ng KC, Liley HG, Greif R, Carlson JN, et al. 2023 International consensus on cardiopulmonary resuscitation and emergency cardiovascular care science with treatment recommendations: summary from the Basic Life Support; Advanced Life Support; Pediatric Life Support; Neonatal Life Support; Education, Implementation, and Teams; and First Aid Task Forces. Circulation. 2023;148:e187-e280.
7. Topjian AA, Raymond TT, Atkins D, Chan M, Duff JP, Joyner BL Jr, et al; on behalf of the Pediatric Basic and Advanced Life Support Collaborators. Part 4: Pediatric Basic and Advanced Life Support: 2020 American Heart Association Guidelines for Cardiopulmonary Resuscitation and Emergency Cardiovascular Care. Circulation. 2020;142(Suppl 2):S469-S523.
8. Maconochie IK, Aickin R, Hazinski MF, Atkins DL, Bingham R, Couto TB, et al; on behalf of the Pediatric Life Support Collaborators. Pediatric life support: 2020 International Consensus on Cardiopulmonary Resuscitation and Emergency Cardiovascular Care Science with Treatment Recommendations. Circulation. 2020;142(Suppl 1):S140-84.
9. Scholefield BR, Silverstein FS, Telford R, Holubkov R, Slomine BS, Meert KL, et al. Therapeutic hypothermia after paediatric cardiac arrest: Pooled randomized controlled trials. Resuscitation. 2018;133:101-7.

20.6 Shock

Rajalakshmi Iyer, Jayashree Muralidharan

DEFINITION

Shock is a state of impaired tissue perfusion resulting in an imbalance between oxygen demand and supply. The widespread reduction in effective tissue perfusion causes inadequate delivery and distribution of oxygen and nutrients, the end result of which is altered cellular and subcellular function leading to anaerobic metabolism, accumulation of lactic acid, and consequently, cellular damage, and multiple organ dysfunction. Clinically, shock is characterized by tachycardia, bounding or feeble pulses, flash or prolonged capillary refill, with or without hypotension, and evidence of organ hypoperfusion (altered sensorium, reduced urine output, impaired gut motility, etc.).[1]

CLASSIFICATION OF SHOCK

A patient with shock can have abnormalities of:

- Circulating blood volume
- Pumping function of heart or
- Blood flow distribution

Accordingly, shock can be classified into the following groups:[1]

- Hypovolemic (decreased circulating blood volume)
- Cardiogenic (impaired myocardial function)
- Distributive (inappropriate distribution of blood flow); and
- Obstructive [mechanical obstruction to cardiac output (CO)]

Several etiologies, which fall into these broad groups, are outlined in **Box 20.6.1**.

PATHOPHYSIOLOGY OF SHOCK

The primary pathophysiological event in shock, regardless of its inciting etiology is tissue hypoperfusion, leading to tissue hypoxia, acidosis, and end-organ dysfunction.

The pathway to cardiovascular failure results from either impairment of CO or systemic vascular resistance (SVR) or both. CO is the product of heart rate and stroke volume

BOX 20.6.1: Etiology of shock.

Hypovolemic
- *Fluid and electrolyte loss:*
  - Diarrhea and vomiting
  - Excessive sweating
  - Pathologic renal loss
- *Blood loss:*
  - External—laceration, open fractures
  - Internal—ruptured viscera, gastrointestinal (GI) bleed
  - Intracranial bleed (neonates and infants)
- *Plasma loss:*
  - Burns
  - Leaky capillaries—sepsis, inflammation
  - Nephrotic syndrome
  - Third space loss—intestinal obstruction, peritonitis
- *Endocrine:*
  - Diabetes mellitus
  - Diabetes insipidus
  - Adrenal insufficiency

Cardiogenic
- *Myocardial insufficiency:**
  - Congestive heart failure (congenital or acquired heart disease)
  - Cardiomyopathies—myocarditis
  - Arrhythmias
  - Hypothermia
  - Drugs, toxins

Obstructive
- *Outflow obstruction:*
  - Cardiac tamponade
  - Pneumopericardium
  - Tension pneumothorax
  - Pulmonary embolism

Distributive
- Septic shock
- Anaphylaxis
- Drugs/toxin
- Tissue injury
- Prolonged hypoxia of ischemia

Note: *Myocardial depressant effect of hypoglycemia, acidosis, and hypoxia.

while stroke volume is determined by left ventricular filling pressure and myocardial contractility. SVR, on the other hand, represents the impedance to left ventricular ejection (afterload) as well as the tone of the peripheral vasculature. When the CO is unable to meet the demands of the tissues, compensatory sympathetic activity produces selective vasoconstriction of the skin and splanchnic vessels to divert the blood flow to vital organs, namely brain, heart, and kidney. Patients in hyperdynamic or warm shock are peripherally vasodilated with high CO (e.g., septic shock) whilst patients in hypodynamic or cold shock are peripherally vasoconstricted with low CO (e.g., cardiogenic shock).

Three pathophysiological concepts that need understanding especially in septic shock are detailed here.

Myocardial Dysfunction

It develops in nearly all patients with septic shock. This dysfunction peaks soon after the onset of sepsis and resolves within 7–10 days in survivors. Sepsis stimulates the release of inflammatory mediators that can compromise cardiac function. Reduced myocardial contractility and decreased ventricular compliance may be seen. Both systolic and diastolic dysfunctions are well described in septic shock. Diminished responsiveness of the myocardium to alpha-1 agonists is secondary to down-regulation of alpha-1 receptors, uncoupling of receptors from adenylate cyclase or depressed generation of cyclic adenosine monophosphate (cAMP). The myocardium is dysfunctional despite an increase in CO during the hyperdynamic phase of sepsis.

Mean Arterial Pressure

It is important to recognize that oxygen distribution is nonuniform in the body. When the CO falls, the body's primary compensatory mechanisms modulate SVR in such a way that blood is preferentially shunted from skin and gut to vital organs such as the heart and brain. The increase in SVR also maintains a normal blood pressure (BP) in the face of impaired peripheral perfusion. Maintenance of an adequate mean arterial pressure (MAP) is fundamental for organ perfusion. When MAP falls below the autoregulatory range of an organ, blood flow decreases, resulting in tissue ischemia and organ failure. As the kidneys receive the second highest blood flow of any organ in the body, measurement of urine output (with the exception of patients with hyperosmolar states, or diabetic ketoacidosis with osmotic diuresis) is a good surrogate for adjudging adequacy of perfusion.

Oxygen Delivery versus Consumption

Oxygen delivery is primarily dependent on CO. Enhancing CO by increasing preload and contractility or by decreasing afterload will increase oxygen delivery. Contrary to adults, oxygen delivery, not oxygen extraction, is the major determinant of oxygen consumption in children. Attainment of the therapeutic oxygen consumption goal of >200 mL/min/m^2 has been found to be associated with improved outcome. In normal circumstances, there is a coherence between macrocirculation and microcirculation. However, in patients with septic shock, this coherence is disturbed due to changes at microcirculatory level. As a result, there is pathological oxygen utilization, i.e., dependence of oxygen consumption on oxygen delivery even at supernormal oxygen delivery. The goal therefore is to increase oxygen delivery to avoid flow-dependent tissue hypoxia without overdoing it to supranormal levels.

Hypovolemic Shock

Hypovolemic shock is the most common form of shock in children worldwide. It is usually caused by hemorrhage or dehydration. Relative hypovolemia may occur secondary to "third spacing" of fluids (extravascular fluid shifts) as it is seen in children with burns, sepsis, or dengue shock syndrome. Depending on the severity and rate of development of hypovolemia, the shock may appear abruptly or evolve gradually over several stages. Regardless of etiology, the final common pathway to circulatory insufficiency is diminished intravascular volume. This volume reduction results in decreased systemic venous return and ventricular filling pressure (preload), thereby decreasing the stroke volume. Children with hypovolemia due to fluid and electrolyte losses have both intravascular and interstitial depletion.

Clinical findings include sunken eyes, depressed anterior fontanel, dry mucous membrane, poor skin turgor, delayed capillary refill, and cool extremities. On the other hand, patients with hypovolemia due to increased capillary permeability such as in burns or sepsis, may have intravascular hypovolemia in the setting of interstitial euvolemia or hypervolemia. This clinically manifests as signs of decreased end-organ perfusion that include altered mentation, decreased urine output, and cool, but often turgid extremities. The classical signs of dehydration based on interstitial fluid depletion are absent in relative hypovolemia states. Once again, hypotension is a late finding and may not occur until intravascular volume has decreased by about 25% of the total. Once this occurs, the compensatory mechanisms fail, and profound reduction of CO and fall of BP occur.

Cardiogenic Shock

Cardiogenic shock is commonly described as "pump failure". The common causes include myocarditis, dysrhythmias and drugs with a myocardial depressant action, acidosis, congenital heart lesions, and sepsis. It can also result from obstruction to the outflow tract, e.g., coarctation of aorta or aortic stenosis or in states of increased afterload like hypertension. Cardiogenic shock will have low CO, hypotension, and clinical signs of inadequate tissue perfusion. Typically, intravascular volume is adequate or even increased, but cardiac dysfunction limits CO.

Distributive Shock

The most common prototype of distributive shock is sepsis. Sepsis is a systemic disease caused by microorganisms or their products in the blood. Gram-negative bacilli predominate as a cause for sepsis and septic shock, other pathogens being gram-positive, rickettsial, fungal, and viral. The common pathophysiology is leakage of intravascular fluid through capillary bed into interstitial space known as "third spacing" of fluids. This occurs due to sepsis-induced disruption of the glycocalyx layer of endothelium resulting in increased transcapillary flow that leads to global increased permeability syndrome (GIPS).[2]

CLINICAL FEATURES AND STAGES OF SHOCK

Shock refers to a dynamic state ranging from early, compensated to refractory or irreversible state. This progression can occur over a span of few minutes to hours, e.g., hemorrhagic shock. The progression can be arbitrarily divided into three stages:

1. Compensated shock
2. Hypotensive shock
3. Irreversible or refractory shock

Compensated Shock

Compensated shock refers to preserved vital organ functions secondary to effective compensatory mechanisms. BP is maintained although signs of inadequate tissue and organ perfusion are observed. The early physical signs are that of an exaggerated sympathetic response to stress. Tachycardia and signs of decreased peripheral perfusion namely cold, clammy skin, capillary refill time (CRT) >2 seconds and difference between core and surface temperature ≥2°C are the most important clinical pointers to early shock. A CRT of 3 seconds or more denotes impaired skin perfusion. It is a valuable sign during assessment and monitoring. Tachypnea may be seen without evidence of an underlying pulmonary disease.

Hypotensive Shock

In this stage, the BP and CO fall, as they cannot be sustained by the intense peripheral vasoconstriction. The patient presents with poor pulses, peripheral cyanosis, cold extremities, hypotension, and acidosis. Vital organ perfusion gets progressively compromised. A cascade of anaerobic tissue metabolism and multiorgan dysfunction sets in. Oliguria or anuria results from diminished renal perfusion. Diminished cerebral perfusion manifests as lethargy, confusion, and disorientation. Rapid aggressive intervention is required to halt the progression to irreversible stage. **Table 20.6.1** summarizes the clinical features of different stages of shock.

Stages of Septic Shock

Septic shock is known to progress through stages; "early septic shock" also known as "warm shock" or hyperdynamic phase is characterized by warm extremities, low SVR, bounding pulses, high or normal cardiac CO, normal BP, and increased pulse pressure. Despite high CO, blood flow is inappropriately distributed to tissues due to sepsis-related microcirculatory

TABLE 20.6.1: Clinical stages of shock and physical signs.

Clinical parameters	*Stage I (compensated)*	*Stage II (hypotensive)*	*Stage III (irreversible)*
Heart rate	Tachycardia	Marked tachycardia	Severe tachycardia and bradycardia
Respiration rate	Normal	Tachypnea	Tachypnea/apnea
Blood pressure	Normal	Hypotension	Severe hypotension
Pulse pressure	Normal	Low	Markedly low
Skin	Cool	Mottled	Cold and cyanotic
Mental status	Anxious	Obtunded	Coma
Urine	Normal	Oliguria	Anuria

changes resulting in derangement of downstream markers such as lactate and mixed venous oxygen saturation ($ScVO_2$). Adequate and early treatment at this stage is crucial to prevent progression to "cold" shock that is characterized by cold extremities, high SVR, low CO, narrow pulse pressure, and hypotension.

Refractory Shock

This is an irreversible stage of shock in which there is progressive reduction in CO, fall in BP and worsening metabolic acidosis, and multiorgan failure.

Difference between Pediatric and Adult Shock

The compensatory cardiovascular responses of a child with decreased preload, impaired myocardial contractility, and alterations in vascular tone differ from those of an adult. In children, the CO is predominantly heart rate-dependent owing to the lack of adequate ventricular muscle mass. Therefore, a child in shock maintains an adequate CO by mounting a tachycardic response. Children maximize SVR mediated by the sympathetic response to maintain a normal BP, when there is significant decrease in the CO. This tends to preserve relatively normal BP till very late stages of shock. BP hence remains a poor surrogate of impaired cardiovascular homeostasis in children especially in early shock. The evaluation of other hemodynamic variables such as heart rate and end-organ perfusion, including CRT, the quality of the peripheral pulses, mentation, urine output, and acid–base status, is more reliable than BP in determining the adequacy of hemodynamic status in a child. Presence of hypotension is not a must for diagnosis of shock in children.

COMPLICATIONS OF SHOCK

Myocardial depression, acute respiratory distress syndrome (ARDS), acute renal failure, and disseminated intravascular coagulation (DIC) are the most dreaded and life-threatening complications of shock.[1]

TABLE 20.6.2: Laboratory investigations in shock.

Cardiovascular system: • ECG • Chest X-ray • Point of care USG/ echocardiogram	*Gastrointestinal and hepatobiliary:* • Stool occult blood • Gastric pH • Liver function test • Pancreatic functions
Respiratory system: Blood gases (arterial and mixed) venous	*Metabolic:* • Serum Na^+, K^+, Ca^{++}, Mg^{++}, and phosphorus • Blood glucose
Renal system: • Serum urea/creatinine • Urine Na^+/specific gravity/ sediments • Urine protein/sugar	*Infection screen:* • Cultures: Blood, CSF, urine, stool, and pus • Rapid diagnostic tests for tropical infections such as dengue, malaria, scrub typhus, and leptospirosis • Biomarkers like CRP/ procalcitonin • USG to screen for deep seated foci of infection
Hematologic system: • Hematocrit, TLC, DLC • Coagulation parameters • Platelet counts	Toxicology screen

(CRP: C-reactive protein; CSF: cerebrospinal fluid; DLC: differential leukocyte count; ECG: electrocardiogram; TLC: total leukocyte count)

DIAGNOSIS

Shock is a clinical diagnosis. Laboratory investigations are required to ascertain the etiology and monitor the progression and severity of organ dysfunction. The investigations that should be obtained in a patient with shock are shown in **Table 20.6.2**.

MANAGEMENT OF SHOCK

The goals of management in shock include:

- Rapid assessment, identification, and intervention (resuscitation)

- Achievement of cardiopulmonary stability (with fluids and vasoactives)
- Monitor the therapeutic response to interventions
- Initiate specific targeted therapy (antibiotics, source control, surgery, etc.)

Irrespective of the etiology, the initial resuscitation and stabilization should always focus on *A*irway, *B*reathing, and *C*irculation in all forms of shock. Stabilization of airway, provision of oxygen, and establishment of vascular access are immediate goals followed by fluid resuscitation and cardiovascular support.

Oxygen Administration

Supplemental oxygen should be administered to all patients in shock to improve oxygen content and delivery to the tissues. Intubation and mechanical ventilations are indicated in children with altered sensorium (for airway stabilization), and those with increased work of breathing or respiratory failure (to give rest to respiratory muscles).

Vascular Access

Immediate intravenous (IV) access needs to be established. Obtaining rapid vascular access with at least two wide bore peripheral lines is extremely crucial. Vascular access may be 20.6 extremely difficult in children with shock, as they have collapsed veins. Since time is extremely crucial, pediatric advanced life support (PALS) guidelines recommend placement of an intraosseous (IO) access in infants and children for volume resuscitation, if *peripheral access is not readily obtained (within 3 attempts or 90 seconds, whichever is earlier)*. Central venous access should be considered in fluid refractory shock for infusion of vasoactive drugs and monitoring of $ScVO_2$.[3]

Fluid Resuscitation

Type of Fluid

Optimization of circulating volume with fluids is the most important step in shock management. Correction of intravascular hypovolemia always requires crystalloids. However, the choice of crystalloids has been a subject of ongoing debate.[4-6] Traditionally, normal saline (0.9%) has always been used as resuscitation fluid owing to its easy availability, low cost, and compatibility with most medications. However, there is increasing evidence to suggest that normal saline is linked to a greater risk of hyperchloremic metabolic acidosis and acute kidney injury (AKI).

Balanced crystalloids (Ringer's lactate and plasmalyte) on the other hand, by virtue of their restrictive chloride content have been demonstrated to mitigate these effects. Colloids and blood products may be required in select situations; packed red blood cells (PRBCs) as volume expander in traumatic hemorrhagic shock or bleeding secondary to coagulopathies. Even in these situations, crystalloids are the first choice for volume expansion, while we await a PRBC bag.

In septic shock, colloids can be more harmful than crystalloids due to the GIPS. Hydroxyethyl starches are not to be used in septic shock, kidney injury, oliguria unresponsive to fluids, or burns. Current recommendations do not favor the use of colloids except in dengue shock syndrome not responsive to crystalloids, where albumin may be considered.

Dextrose-containing fluids should be avoided during shock resuscitation unless there is documented hypoglycemia. This is because dextrose-containing fluids cause hyperglycemia and osmotic diuresis, which can further aggravate shock.

Volume of Fluids

The earlier practice of rapid large volume fluids boluses, has given way to a more conservative approach following the results of the Fluid Expansion as Supportive Therapy (FEAST) trial that randomized children with febrile illness and poor perfusion to a bolus or no-bolus fluid strategy. This trial, conducted in a resource-limited setting in sub-Saharan Africa, compared 20 mL/kg of 0.9% saline or 5% albumin with no bolus and found an increased 48-hour mortality in the bolus arm (RR 1.45; 95% CI, 1.13–1.86; $p = 0.003$). Based on the findings of FEAST trial, the Surviving Sepsis Campaign Guidelines (SSC 2020) recommended a cautious approach based on the availability of intensive care services as given below:[7]

- *In healthcare facilities with a pediatric intensive care unit (PICU) back up,* up to 40–60 mL/kg of fluid bolus may be administered in aliquots of 10–20 mL/kg, carefully monitoring for fluid overload signs that include hepatomegaly, worsening respiratory distress, and basal crepitations. Fluid responsiveness may be aided by point-of-care ultrasound (POCUS) assessment of inferior vena cava (IVC) diameter, which is elaborated later in this chapter.
- *In healthcare facilities without a PICU back-up* fluid boluses are to be avoided in nonhypotensive children. Instead, maintenance fluids may be commenced. In hypotensive patients, fluid bolus may be administered up to 40 mL/kg, in aliquots of 10–20 mL/kg, while assessing for signs of fluid overload as mentioned above.

In a nutshell, these recommendations emphasize the need for a conservative fluid strategy in children with underlying comorbidities such as anemia, malnutrition, those without hypotension, and in facilities where intensive care unit (ICU) back-up is not available. Further pediatric trials are, however, needed to determine the optimal volume of boluses for children in septic shock and other critical states.

TABLE 20.6.3: Vasoactive drugs.

Class of drug	*Drug*	*Mechanism*	*Receptors*	*Dose*
Catecholamines	Adrenaline/epinephrine	Vasopressor Inotrope	α, β	*High dose:* >0.3 μg/kg/min *Low dose:* 0.05–0.3 μg/kg/min
	Noradrenaline/norepinephrine	Vasopressor	α	0.05–0.3 μg/kg/min
	Dopamine	Vasopressor	α, β, D	5–20 μg/kg/min
	Dobutamine	Inotrope	β_1, β_2	5–20 μg/kg/min
Noncatecholamine	Milrinone	Inodilator	PDE-3 inhibitor	0.25–0.75 μg/kg/min
	Levosimendan	Inodilator	Ca channel sensitizer	0.1–0.4 μg/kg/min
	Vasopressin	Vasopressor	V1 receptor	0.0005–0.002 U/kg/min

(PDE-3: phosphodiesterase-3; Ca: calcium; α, β: adrenergic receptors; D: dopamine receptors)

In cardiogenic shock or in a child with known cardiac disease, fluid boluses should be initiated cautiously, giving smaller aliquots of 5 mL/kg, and instituting inotropic therapy earlier.[3]

Therapeutic Endpoints of Shock

Fluid therapy should also be titrated to achieve therapeutic endpoints of shock as listed below:[1,8]

- CRT of ≤2 seconds
- Normal pulses with no difference between central and peripheral pulses
- Warm extremities
- Normal range of systolic BP and pulse pressure
- Urine output >1 mL/kg/h
- Normal mental status
- Decreased lactate
- Mixed SVO_2 >70%.

If endpoints of shock are not achieved with fluids, shock is labeled as fluid refractory and vasoactive therapy should be commenced immediately.

Cardiovascular Support

Following adequate intravascular volume repletion, continued presence of hypotension and/or poor perfusion warrants the initiation of vasoactive therapy, which should be goal directed. Vasoactive drugs augment CO, oxygen delivery, and/or organ perfusion. *Optimal preload is essential for all patients in shock before vasoactive therapy is contemplated.*

Vasoactive drugs can broadly be classified as vasopressors, inotropes, vasodilators, and inodilators, and chemically as catecholamine and noncatecholamine drugs.

Vasopressors increase SVR, thereby increasing MAP. Clinically, this translates into higher BP, but may lead to cold extremities. Inotropes increase cardiac contractility, allowing the heart to pump better, increasing stroke volume, and therefore, CO. Both, vasopressors and inotropes usually have the adverse effect of tachycardia, with the exception of noradrenaline. Vasodilators reduce systemic and pulmonary vascular resistance, reducing myocardial oxygen demand thereby improving CO. This effect may, however, be achieved at the cost of falling BP. Some drugs have actions on multiple receptors, acting as inotropes and vasodilators, increasing CO and peripheral vasodilation—these are commonly referred to as inodilators. **Table 20.6.3** summarizes the action, receptors and doses of commonly used vasoactive drugs in pediatrics.

How to Choose the Appropriate Drug?

The first-line vasoactive drug currently recommended in fluid refractory septic shock is epinephrine. Earlier, the drug of choice was dopamine, but studies in pediatrics have shown that epinephrine is better than dopamine as first-line agent owing to its inotropic and vasopressor effect.

Once the child is commenced on epinephrine, frequent reassessments are required to check for attainment of endpoints of shock, increasing dose if necessary. However, a second or third drug may be needed, especially in septic shock. The choice of the second drug will depend on the clinical picture and has to be guided by advanced monitoring.

Adequate CO is more important than BP alone, as adequate tissue oxygen delivery is the underlying goal. However, increasing CO above physiologic levels is not recommended. Two recent prospective clinical trials in critically ill patients with sepsis have failed to demonstrate benefit from increasing oxygen level to supernormal levels. The goal of resuscitation should be to achieve adequate levels of oxygen delivery to avoid flow-dependent tissue hypoxia.[1,8]

When should We Consider Inotropes?

Inotropes are needed upfront in children with known cardiac disease such as cardiomyopathy or suspected myocarditis, with or after a cautious fluid bolus.

In a child with septic shock, low-dose epinephrine started as a first-line agent provides inotropy. If BP is maintained, and cardiac contractility still requires some augmentation, an inodilator such as milrinone (or dobutamine, if milrinone is not available) can be added based on clinical monitoring, POCUS and surrogates like $ScVO_2$, and lactate. This will give added advantage of lowering the peripheral vascular resistance, thus reducing myocardial oxygen demand. Milrinone is also a lusitropic agent, helping the heart relax during diastole.[1,8]

When should We Consider Vasopressors?

Vasopressors are required for increasing MAP to a level that allows appropriate distribution of CO for adequate organ perfusion and oxygen delivery. Children with septic shock having warm peripheries and bounding pulses (suggestive of high CO, and low SVR), and fluid refractory hypotension, may benefit with vasopressors such as norepinephrine. The caveat that most children with septic shock have cardiac dysfunction needs to be kept in mind, and therefore, epinephrine may be needed as a second addition. Combining a vasopressor with an inotrope will also work to this effect. Vasopressin is a second-line agent to be considered in such scenarios if response to norepinephrine is not good. Titration of vasoactives should be again carefully guided by clinical, POCUS, and laboratory findings.[1,8]

When should We Consider Vasodilators?

Vasodilators are drug of choice in increased afterload situations such as hypertensive cardiac failure. The prerequisite for using vasodilators is adequate BP or perfusion pressure. Inodilators such as milrinone having dual action of inotropy and afterload reduction may be a good choice in myocarditis and dilated cardiomyopathy. Prostaglandin E1, a potent vasodilator is indicated in newborns with ductus-dependent lesion presenting in cardiogenic shock due to ductus closure.

Correction of Metabolic Derangements

Metabolic Acidosis

Poor tissue perfusion and resultant anaerobic metabolism lead to significant metabolic acidosis. Uncorrected acidosis can lead to further cellular damage and myocardial depression. Sodium bicarbonate as a rescue therapy for acidosis is indicated only in desperate situations where imminent myocardial failure secondary to severe and persistent acidosis (pH is below 6.9–7) is suspected. In all other situations, bicarbonate must be avoided and all attempts must be taken to correct the underlying shock. Overcorrection with sodium bicarbonate can be hazardous leading to CNS acidosis, coma, and death.

Calcium

Acute hemodynamic deterioration in various types of shock can decrease the ionized Ca^{++} level. This hypocalcemia leads to tachycardia, hypotension, alteration in sensorium, and motor nerve excitability. An IV infusion of 1–2 mL/kg of 10% calcium gluconate should be given when ionized Ca^{++} level falls below 0.8 mEq/L. Target calcium should be between 0.8 and 1.2 mEq/L.

Acute Kidney Injury

Acute kidney injury can be multifactorial in origin. The management of AKI in children with shock has been revolutionized with the use of continuous renal replacement therapy (CRRT), which allows fluid replacement and removal at a gentle rate, akin to the function of the normal kidney. In addition to solute removal (nitrogenous waste like urea, electrolytes like potassium, etc.), CRRT also contributes to removal of inflammatory cytokines and lactate. The indications for CRRT are hyperkalemia, refractory acidosis, and fluid overload. In resource-limited settings, peritoneal dialysis may be used instead. Conventional hemodialysis is much more difficult to use in children with shock, as massive volume shifts precipitate hypotension, with potentially disastrous consequences—therefore, it is used very sparingly in children in shock.

Hematologic Support

Hematocrit needs to be maintained between 35 and 45% with the help of transfusions during resuscitation of shock. However, in hemodynamically stable patients, the current recommendations favor a restrictive transfusion trigger at 7 g/dL to prevent transfusion-related complications such as transfusion-related acute lung injury (TRALI), transfusion-associated circulatory overload (TACO), and other transfusion-related cytokine-mediated multiorgan dysfunction. Bleeding, which complicates shock may need management with fresh frozen plasma (FFP), vitamin K, and platelet concentrates. However, it is important to remember that platelet transfusions are indicated only when counts are <5,000/mm^3 regardless of apparent bleeding. Platelet counts >50,000/mm^3 are required when some surgical or invasive procedure is contemplated in a child. Similarly, FFP is only indicated in select patients like those with active bleeding, before invasive procedures and to reverse warfarin effect.

Gastrointestinal Support

Prophylactic use of proton pump inhibitors or an H_2-receptor antagonist is commonly used in critically ill children to prevent stress ulcers. Although it is a practice followed widely, recent studies question this practice as they have demonstrated some increase in hospital-acquired infections.

Nutritional Support

Shock leads to excessive catabolism; hence nutritional support is one of the important pillars in the management. Nasogastric feeding should start as soon as patient can accept enteral feeds.

Respiratory Support

Mechanical ventilation is indicated for acute respiratory failure, to improve oxygenation and to decrease work of breathing.

Antibiotic Therapy and Source Control

Appropriate empiric antibiotics should be started in suspected septic shock. It should provide broad-spectrum coverage depending upon site of infection, local epidemiologic data, and sensitivity pattern. An aminoglycoside (gentamicin or amikacin) and a third-generation cephalosporin (cefotaxime or ceftriaxone) should be used for suspected gram-negative sepsis. Combination of cloxacillin and an aminoglycoside should be used if staphylococcal sepsis is suspected. Source control or source reduction such as abscess drainage, debridement, is very important.

Adjunctive Therapies

Corticosteroids

Corticosteroids have always been a controversial therapy in pediatric shock. Steroids as an adjunctive therapy for shock refractory to fluids and vasoactive support have not been conclusively proven. The current recommendations are against use of hydrocortisone in children with septic shock if endpoints of shock are attained using fluids and vasopressors. If they are not achieved, IV hydrocortisone may be used.[7]

Immunoglobulin

Intravenous immunoglobulin may be considered in children with suspected staphylococcal or streptococcal toxic shock syndrome.

Extracorporeal Membrane Oxygenation

After adequate treatment and correction of all possible reasons for refractory shock [such as source control, drainage of pleural or pericardial effusions/pneumothorax, adrenal or thyroid hormone replacement (if indicated), and ongoing blood loss], if endpoints of shock are not attained, one must consider extracorporeal membrane oxygenation (ECMO) in healthcare facilities where it is available. Although survival in pediatric septic shock on ECMO is around 50%, it has been shown to decrease vasoactive-inotropic requirement and hasten recovery of shock.

MONITORING OF SHOCK

The objectives of monitoring a patient with shock are:

- To assess the efficacy of the therapeutic interventions (e.g., response to fluid bolus or vasoactive therapy)
- To recognize complications and correct them; and
- To assess the degree of associated organ dysfunctions that will help in prognostication.

Monitoring involves careful and repeated examination of the child's physiological status that includes vital parameters such as heart rate, pulse volume, respiratory rate, BP, MAP, temperature (skin and core) and capillary refill, continuous ECG monitoring, and a strict intake or output record.[1,2,7,8] An important bedside adjunct to clinical assessment is the POCUS that can give valuable information regarding fluid responsiveness (IVC collapsibility or distensibility, aortic flow velocity, variability or left ventricular outflow tract velocity time integral (VTI)], cardiac contractility and fluid overload status of the lung.

Mixed venous oxygen saturation monitoring gives an idea about adequacy of CO. The normal value is >70% in critically ill patients. The $ScVO_2$ will fall in low CO states. Persistent low $ScVO_2$ while other endpoints of shock resuscitation have corrected, indicates more oxygen extraction and inadequate resuscitation. Central SVO_2 is being increasingly used as an alternative to $ScVO_2$ as it correlates well with mixed venous saturation and can be obtained from a central venous catheter.

Another surrogate used to assess resolution of shock is serum lactate and its clearance. Although there are no established cut-offs, a serum lactate level of >4 mmol/L is associated with higher mortality (studies have shown values ranging from 3.3 to 5.5 mmol/L). A more clinically relevant approach is the reduction of lactate by >10% in the first 6 hours of resuscitation of shock, which has been shown to be associated with better outcome. However, these levels are not yet established as guidelines or targets in the treatment of pediatric septic shock.

Invasive Hemodynamic Monitoring

The central venous pressure (CVP) is no longer used as a measure of right ventricular function and preload as studies have shown a poor correlation with blood volume; being a static parameter it is a poor predictor of volume status, especially in children with pulmonary hypertension, noncompliant right ventricle, poor right ventricular function, tricuspid regurgitation, pericardial tamponade, and high positive end-expiratory pressure (PEEP).

Multilumen pulmonary artery catheters (Swan-Ganz catheter) use for pulmonary artery occlusion pressure (PAOP), pulmonary artery pressure, mixed venous saturation, CO, vascular resistance, oxygen delivery, and consumption similarly has been abandoned in most units due to studies showing poor correlation of PAOP with volume status.

Noninvasive Hemodynamic Monitoring

Noninvasive tools for assessing fluid responsiveness, myocardial function, lung dynamics, and diaphragmatic function are being increasingly used as point of care assessment in ICU setting and have replaced the invasive monitoring tools for determination of volume status in critically ill children.[9] Important dynamic indices are pulse pressure variation (PPV) derived from analysis of arterial waveforms and stroke volume variation (SVV) derived from pulse contour analysis. IVC diameter (IVC collapsibility index) is another measure used to determine fluid responsiveness; a collapsed IVC indicative of volume depletion while a distended IVC suggests high right atrial pressure.

PROGNOSIS

Better outcome depends on early recognition and aggressive intervention in the stage of compensated shock. The mortality also depends on the etiology of shock; septic shock has mortality up to 50%. Hypothermia, decreased CO, decreased O_2, and development of multiple organ dysfunctions are poor prognostic indicators in shock.

KEY MESSAGES

- Shock is a state of impaired tissue perfusion resulting in an imbalance between oxygen demand and supply.
- Causes include hypovolemia, septic (distributive), cardiogenic, and obstructive.
- The diagnosis is clinical, based on a constellation of altered hemodynamic parameters such as tachycardia, poor peripheral perfusion, and evidence of organ hypoperfusion.
- Blood pressure is relatively well-preserved till late stages of shock. Presence of hypotension is therefore not a must for clinical diagnosis of shock.
- The management goals include early recognition, resuscitation, monitoring therapeutic response, and treating the underlying etiology.
- Crystalloids are fluids of choice for volume expansion. Balanced crystalloids are coming up as preferred agent for volume expansion due to their lower chloride content and lesser complication rates.
- The rate and volume of fluid bolus depend on presence or absence of comorbidities, hypotension, and ICU facilities.
- Epinephrine is first-line vasoactive agent for pediatric septic shock.
- Further requirement of fluids and titration of vasoactive medications depend on therapeutic response, fluid responsiveness, and myocardial function as judged by POCUS and laboratory parameters.
- Look for etiology and treat underlying cause, e.g., broad-spectrum antibiotics and source control for suspected septic shock, urgent pericardiocentesis for obstructive shock due to pericardial tamponade.

REFERENCES

1. Davis AL, Carcillo JA, Aneja RK, Deymann AJ, Lin JC, Nguyen TC, et al. American College of Critical Care Medicine Clinical Practice Parameters for Hemodynamic Support of Pediatric and Neonatal Septic Shock. Crit Care Med. 2017;45(6):1061-93.
2. Woodcock TE, Woodcock TM. Revised Starling equation and the glycocalyx model of transvascular fluid exchange: an improved paradigm for prescribing intravenous fluid therapy. Br J Anaesth. 2012;108(3):384-94.
3. de Caen AR, Berg MD, Chameides L, Gooden CK, Hickey RW, Scott HF, et al. Part 12: Pediatric advanced life support: 2015 American Heart Association Guidelines Update for Cardiopulmonary Resuscitation and Emergency Cardiovascular Care. Circulation. 2015;132(18 Suppl 2):S526-42.
4. Yunos NM, Bellomo R, Hegarty C, Story D, Ho L, Bailey M. Association between a chloride-liberal vs chloride-restrictive intravenous fluid administration strategy and kidney injury in critically ill adults. JAMA. 2012t;308(15):1566-72.
5. Sankar J, Muralidharan J, Lalitha AV, Rameshkumar R, Pathak M, Das RR, et al. Multiple Electrolytes Solution Versus Saline as Bolus Fluid for Resuscitation in Pediatric Septic Shock: A Multicenter Randomized Clinical Trial. Crit Care Med. 2023;51(11):1449-60.
6. Chowdhury AH, Cox EF, Francis ST, Lobo DN. A randomized, controlled, double-blind crossover study on the effects of 2-L infusions of 0.9% saline and plasma-lyte® 148 on renal blood flow velocity and renal cortical tissue perfusion in healthy volunteers. Ann Surg. 2012;256(1):18-24.
7. Weiss SL, Peters MJ, Alhazzani W, Agus MSD, Flori HR, Inwald DP, et al. Surviving Sepsis Campaign International Guidelines for the Management of Septic Shock and Sepsis-Associated Organ Dysfunction in Children. Pediatr Crit Care Med. 2020;21(2):e52-e106.
8. Lodha R, Oleti TP, Kabra SK. Management of septic shock. Indian J Pediatr. 2011;78(6):726-33.
9. Marik PE. Techniques for assessment of intravascular volume in critically ill patients. J Intensive Care Med. 2009;24(5):329-37.

20.7 Respiratory Failure: Clinical Recognition and Management

Madhusudan Samprathi, Karthi Nallasamy

INTRODUCTION

Case Vignettes

- *Case 1:* A 10-month-old boy is brought to the emergency room (ER) with fever, cough, and cold for 3 days and fast breathing from the previous night. He has irritability, tachypnea with respiratory rate of 70 breaths per minute, intercostal and subcostal retractions, and bilateral crackles and wheeze; oxygen saturation (SpO_2) on room air is 88%.
- *Case 2:* A 5-year-old girl is brought to the ER with fever, seizures, and altered sensorium for 2 days. She has a respiratory rate of 18 breaths per minute, Glasgow Coma Scale (GCS) score of 10, and neck rigidity is present; chest auscultation reveals no added sounds, and SpO_2 on room air is 90%.
- *Case 3:* A 12-year-old boy is brought with progressive, symmetrical, ascending weakness involving both lower limbs. He is alert, anxious, and obeys commands; power in lower limbs is 1/5, and in upper limbs 3/5, and deep tendon reflexes are absent. He has pooling of oral secretions, with respiratory rate of 12 breaths per minute, shallow breathing, and SpO_2 on room air is 88%.

What is common to these three patients? As you can see, they have presented with an acute illness, with different symptoms and signs. The similarity is that they are hypoxic, i.e., SpO_2 on room air is below the lower limit of the normal range, i.e., 94%, and hence respiratory failure. Subsequently, arterial blood gas (ABG) analysis revealed the results given in **Table 20.7.1**.

As can be noted from **Table 20.7.1**, though the values of partial pressure of oxygen (PaO_2) and partial pressure of carbon dioxide ($PaCO_2$) were variable, all three children were clinically in respiratory failure.

Respiratory distress or failure is one of the most common problems encountered in the pediatric ER. Acute lower respiratory infections are the most common causes of under-five mortality across the world.[1] Pediatricians and physicians managing children must therefore be well-versed in the clinical recognition and management of respiratory distress and failure.

TABLE 20.7.1: Arterial blood gas analysis results of the three patients.

	Case 1	*Case 2*	*Case 3*
pH	7.40	7.29	7.35
pO_2	108	88	99
pCO_2	29	49	42
Bicarbonate	22	22	23
SaO_2	98	90	98

DEFINITIONS

Respiratory Distress

Respiratory distress is increase in the respiratory rate and/or increase in respiratory effort or work of breathing (WOB). Respiratory rate has age-based cutoffs. Tachypnea is defined as respiratory rate >60 breaths/min for children <2 months, >50 breaths/min for children 2–12 months, >40 breaths/min for children 1–5 years, and >30 breaths/min for children >5 years. Increased respiratory effort manifests with increased depth of breathing or visible use of accessory muscles of inspiration or expiration.

Respiratory Failure

Respiratory failure refers to the failure of the above compensatory mechanisms leading to a decompensated stage where impaired oxygenation or ventilation leads to vital organ dysfunction. However, there is no single accepted cutoff in oxygenation or ventilation to define respiratory failure.

Oxygenation Failure

Oxygenation failure (type 1 respiratory failure) is defined as PaO_2 below 60 mm Hg. Usually, advanced life support guidelines define hypoxemia as pulse oximetry SpO_2 below 94% in a child breathing room air. However, this cutoff is not applicable to children with underlying chronic respiratory (chronic lung disease) or cardiac diseases (cyanotic heart disease) that tend to have a low baseline SpO_2.

Ventilation Failure

Ventilation failure or pump failure (type 2 respiratory failure) is generally defined as $PaCO_2$ above 50 mm Hg. However, acceptable $PaCO_2$ levels are variable and often depend on the nature and duration of the disease. Acute ventilation failure develops quickly over minutes to hours leading to hypercapnia and acidosis (pH below 7.35), while chronic respiratory failure can evolve gradually over several days to weeks.

ETIOLOGY

The etiological spectrum of respiratory distress or failure is wide and extends to several organ systems other than the respiratory system itself (**Box 20.7.1**). Children with cardiac disease or cardiac failure often present with respiratory distress or failure and do not have many of the classical cardiac symptoms seen in adults, i.e., chest pain, edema, palpitations, or syncope. Hence, they may commonly mimic a respiratory emergency like pneumonia. Neurological disorders may also present with respiratory failure. While disorders of the central nervous system (CNS) cause disordered control of breathing leading to bradypnea, or abnormal breathing patterns, disorders of the peripheral nervous system or motor unit lead to respiratory muscle paralysis, leading to inadequate respiratory effort and respiratory failure.

While respiratory distress of other causes can progress to failure when the underlying cause is untreated, neurological problems, when severe, can directly present with respiratory failure, as the compensatory mechanisms of increase in rate or effort are disabled. Metabolic acidosis, commonly due to diabetic ketoacidosis (DKA) or acute metabolic crisis, presents with Kussmaul breathing, i.e., increased rate and depth of breathing without increased use of accessory muscles.

BOX 20.7.1: Etiology of respiratory distress or failure.

Respiratory system
- *Upper airway obstruction:* Viral croup, epiglottitis, diphtheria, bacterial tracheitis, and retropharyngeal abscess
- *Lower airway obstruction:* Bronchiolitis, viral wheeze, asthma, and foreign body airway
- *Lung parenchymal disease:* Pneumonia, ARDS, collapse, and noncardiogenic pulmonary edema
- *Pleural disease:* Pneumothorax, pleural effusion, empyema, and hemothorax

Cardiovascular system: Congestive cardiac failure of any etiology—congenital or acquired heart disease

Neurological cause
- *Central causes:* CNS infections, drug poisoning, and traumatic brain injury
- *Peripheral causes:* Guillain–Barré syndrome, neurotoxic snake envenomation, congenital and acquired neuropathies, and myopathies

Metabolic causes: Acidotic breathing of any cause—diabetic ketoacidosis, poisoning, and inborn errors of metabolism

(ARDS: acute respiratory distress syndrome; CNS: central nervous system)

Within the respiratory system, based on localization of the underlying cause, respiratory distress or failure can be due to upper airway obstruction, lower airway obstruction, lung parenchymal disease, or pleural diseases. Localizing the problem and classifying the severity of the problem are basic prerequisites to instituting the correct line of management and ensuring a good outcome. This requires a good history and a meticulous examination. Recognition of respiratory distress or failure and stabilization in the ER are completely clinical processes with no need for any investigations. Blood gas, chest X-ray, and other investigations are required to confirm the severity of the problem and for definitive diagnosis of the underlying etiology.

CLINICAL APPROACH AND EVALUATION

As in any critically ill child, the pediatric advanced life support (PALS) guidelines and format for assessment must be followed. Accordingly, children are triaged in the ER, and the sickest ones are seen and evaluated first. The initial assessment comprising a few seconds of obtaining visual and auditory cues can identify respiratory distress and failure even before the hands-on primary assessment. The primary assessment (ABCDE) starts with the airway assessment, an integral prerequisite before assessing breathing.

Airway

Abnormal airway is suggested by increased inspiratory effort with retractions, or abnormal inspiratory sounds (stridor), or no breath sounds despite respiratory effort. Airway status is classified as clear, maintainable (by position, suction, and oral airway), or not maintainable (needs endotracheal intubation, tracheostomy, or cricothyroidotomy).

Breathing

Breathing is assessed by five parameters—respiratory rate (increased, decreased, irregular, or "quiet"), work of breathing (normal, high, or low), air entry (tidal volume, adequacy of ventilation, and chest rise), airway/lung sounds (crackles, wheeze, stridor, or grunting) and oxygen saturation (by pulse oximetry).

Respiratory Rate

Counting the respiratory rate for 1 full minute when the child is calm or asleep without crying is essential to document respiratory distress and for further monitoring and assessment of response to therapy. Tachypnea is the first compensatory mechanism, especially in infants, to maintain gas exchange. It can indicate pathology in any part of the respiratory system (airway obstruction, parenchymal, or pleural inflammation) or extrapulmonary causes including fever, anxiety, metabolic acidosis, or heart disease. Bradypnea and apnea in children are late signs suggesting advanced respiratory failure or arrest due to respiratory muscle fatigue.

As mentioned above, children with neurological and neuromuscular disorders may not mount this compensatory response and instead present with bradypnea. In such children, close monitoring for respiratory rates lower than normal and reduced efforts is essential.

Respiratory distress or failure has to be distinguished from "effortless tachypnea" where the respiratory rate alone is increased, with normal work of breathing (WOB), no noisy breathing, no respiratory findings on auscultation, and normal SpO_2 in room air. It occurs due to nonrespiratory causes (DKA, renal failure, poisoning with salicylates or isoniazid, etc.).

Work of Breathing

Increased work of breathing or distress is identified by the use of accessory muscles during respiration. Children use accessory muscles to generate greater negative pleural pressures and increase airflow into lungs. Mild respiratory distress manifests with tachypnea or difficult breathing. This can progress to moderate distress with nasal flaring and intercostal and subcostal recessions. Supraclavicular tugging and head bobbing are signs of severe distress. Occasionally, in severe respiratory distress, the sternum and chest wall may move inward during inspiration instead of the usual outward, which is referred to as paradoxical breathing. Paradoxical breathing is also a feature of neuromuscular weakness, especially of the intercostal muscles, where inspiration is being handled by the diaphragm alone.

Sometimes, posture can give a clue to the severity of distress. Children often assume a position of comfort while having increased work of breathing. The tripod position where children sit in a leaning forward position with arms placed over thighs to support upper body indicates use of the thoracoabdominal muscles to ease work of breathing. This is a sign of severe distress preceding the onset of respiratory failure.

Air Entry

Shape and symmetry of the chest and chest expansion should be assessed by inspection and auscultation. Children with severe bronchiolitis may have a hyperinflated chest. Unilateral involvement (consolidation, pleural effusion, and collapse) may lead to reduced expansion on that side, along with reduced air entry on auscultation. Though a detailed examination of the respiratory system is not warranted in the ER, a quick correlation of findings of inspection, percussion, and auscultation may be diagnostic and aid the emergency management. For example, reduced chest movements and air entry on one side that is hyperinflated, along with tympanic note on percussion indicate a pneumothorax, but reduced chest movements and air entry with dull note may suggest a collapse or effusion.

Airway/Lung Sounds

Audible sounds include:

- *Nonspecific sounds of the nasal secretions*
- *Snoring:* Low-pitched, inspiratory sounds originating in the pharynx
- *Stridor:* Inspiratory, low, or high-pitched sounds suggesting upper airway obstruction
- *Wheeze:* Expiratory, high-pitched, musical sounds along with prolonged expiration suggesting lower airway obstruction
- *Grunt:* End-expiratory sighing sound suggesting alveolar disease, where the child breathes out against a partially closed glottis to increase the positive end-expiratory pressure and maintain the functional residual capacity, in an attempt to preserve oxygenation.

Auscultation may detect crackles, wheeze, or other sounds like pleural rub, bronchial breathing, etc., which will be helpful when corroborated with other clinical signs.

Oxygen Saturation

Assessing and documenting a reliable, baseline oxygen saturation with a potable pulse oximeter or a monitor is important to define respiratory failure, as well as to assess progression and response to treatment. Awareness of the caveats that can lead to false readings is essential.

Circulation, Disability, and Exposure

Tachycardia commonly accompanies tachypnea in a child with respiratory distress due to increased sympathetic tone. It may also be associated with fever, pain, or dehydration. Bradycardia in children with respiratory distress is an ominous and a late sign that suggests impending cardiorespiratory arrest.

Proper hemodynamic assessment is a must in any critically ill child, as circulatory compromise can coexist and mandate immediate intervention.

Assessing sensorium with the GCS or AVPU (Alert, Voice, Pain, Unresponsive) scale is important. Altered sensorium can be a result of the hypoxemia or hypercarbia, manifesting with irritability or drowsiness.

It is important to recognize cyanosis (peripheral/central), clubbing, and presence and severity of pallor as these signs may impact diagnosis and management decisions. Drooling can occur due to pooled secretions in the oral cavity. This may be a sign of severe upper airway obstruction.

BOX 20.7.2: Categorization of type and severity of respiratory failure.

Type:
- Upper airway obstruction
- Lower airway obstruction
- Lung tissue (parenchymal disease)
- Disordered control of breathing
- Effortless tachypnea (Acidosis)

Severity:
- Respiratory distress
- Respiratory failure

By the end of the primary assessment (ABCDE), the type and severity of the physiological abnormality identified must be clear **(Box 20.7.2)**.

MANAGEMENT

In any critically ill child, evaluation and management go hand-in-hand. Clinical recognition of the physiological abnormalities and stabilization are the foremost priority. Detailed history and examination and planning investigations to uncover the correct diagnosis are secondary.

Airway abnormality must be corrected before proceeding to assess breathing. Simple measures to maintain airway include positioning (head-tilt and chin-lift or jaw lift/jaw thrust in suspected cervical spine injury), suctioning, and in comatose children, insertion of oropharyngeal/nasopharyngeal airway. Advanced measures include endotracheal intubation, tracheostomy, cricothyrotomy, and use of laryngeal mask airway.

Breathing is supported depending on spontaneous efforts and desired FiO_2. Increasing the alveolar oxygen will increase the alveolar-arterial oxygen gradient ($PA\text{-}aO_2$) gradient and improve oxygenation. When spontaneous efforts are present, oxygen has to be delivered in a nonthreatening manner. When spontaneous efforts are inadequate, mere supplementation of oxygen is deleterious and assisted ventilation has to be started immediately.

Low-flow Devices

Oxygen can be provided effectively to most children with respiratory distress with nasal cannula, nasal prongs, or face mask. The flow rate generally used is 0.5–1 L/min for infants and 1–2 L/min for older children. Flow rates beyond 2 L/min may not be well tolerated and may lead to drying and discomfort of the nasal mucosa and other mucosal complications. Nasal cannula and prongs are widely available and can be easily used; for older children, a face mask is better.

High-flow Devices

High-flow nasal cannula (HFNC), a noninvasive form of respiratory support, delivers heated and humidified oxygen through a nasal cannula interface. This prevents drying and discomfort of the nasal mucosa. Flow can be adjusted independent of FiO_2, unlike a nasal cannula. Weight-based dosing, such as 1–2 L/kg/min is generally followed. HFNC delivers positive airway pressure to some extent based on flow rate but the pressure is variable and unpredictable.

Selecting the right size of the nasal prong is crucial as it determines the success of HFNC. Nasal prongs should ideally occupy less than two-thirds of the area of the nasal cavity opening. Larger prongs covering most of the nostril may cause inadvertent high airway pressures, decrease the expiratory gas washout, and increase the risk of gastric distention and air leaks. Smaller prongs may cause failure in achieving higher flows.[2]

High-flow nasal cannula has been commonly studied as an alternative to continuous positive airway pressure (CPAP). The primary and most widespread use of HFNC is in infants and young children with bronchiolitis, pneumonia, or wheezing. Use of HFNC and other forms of noninvasive positive pressure ventilation has reduced the need for intubation and mechanical ventilation.[3]

Noninvasive Ventilation

Continuous Positive Airway Pressure

Continuous positive airway pressure is an alternative form of respiratory support for children presenting with moderate or severe respiratory distress. Through continuous end-expiratory pressure, it stents open the alveoli so that a larger surface area is recruited for ventilation and oxygenation. CPAP can be delivered through nasal prongs with a gas flow of 3–15 L/min from wall-mounted oxygen/medical air ports, using a bubble chamber with an adjustable water column in the expiratory limb. Indigenous bubble CPAP systems can be developed from commonly available items in hospitals and are effective in resource-limited settings. A bubble chamber may be insufficient for older children and piston/turbine-based CPAP systems with expiratory valves may be needed.

Several interfaces are available, including nasal plug, nasal mask that covers the nares, face mask that covers both the nares and the mouth, or a complete face mask that covers the entire face. When CPAP is used, it is recommended to start with lower pressures of about 5 cmH_2O and gradually increase in increments of 1 cmH_2O as tolerated by the child. The goals of therapy include exhaled tidal volume of around 6–7 mL/kg, a normal respiratory rate for age, and oxygen saturation of at least 90%.[4]

In several randomized trials, HFNC and CPAP have fared identically in terms of treatment failure.[2] A recent systematic review on infants up to 24 months of age with bronchiolitis showed that HFNC was superior to standard oxygen therapy via prongs or masks.[5] Thus, both HFNC and CPAP continue to be used based on the clinical scenario, availability, and preference of the treating team.

Bi-level Positive Airway Pressure

Bi-level positive airway pressure (BiPAP) provides both inspiratory peak airway pressure (IPAP) and expiratory peak airway pressure (EPAP) for every breath, the level of pressure support being equal to the difference between the IPAP and EPAP. The IPAP set varies from 4 to 24 cmH_2O, and EPAP from 2 to 20 cmH_2O. Generally, the initial settings for BiPAP are 8–10 cmH_2O IPAP and 2–4 cmH_2O EPAP.[4] Cycling between the two pressures decreases the stress on the diaphragm and accessory muscles by increasing the tidal volume and minute ventilation, opening obstructed alveoli, and reducing the frequency of obstructive apnea and hypopnea.[6]

Bi-level positive airway pressure has traditionally been used for children with chronic lung disease, neuromuscular disorders, and obstructive airways. It has been mostly used in children with a weight above 20 kg due to the concern that smaller children may not initiate supported breaths on BiPAP; however, recent literature supports its use in acute asthma exacerbations in children of all ages.[6]

CPAP and BiPAP have been studied in adult patients. Application in children involves several challenges like limited compliance and cooperation of infants and young children to tolerate the interface, familiarity and experience of the physicians and nurses with usage of the equipment and consumables, and availability of the right size interface. Sedation can compromise respiratory drive and is better avoided in young children. The introduction of dexmedetomidine, an α2-adrenergic receptor agonist that causes sedation without any respiratory depression, has provided an alternative to traditional sedation.

Contraindications of Noninvasive Ventilation

These include:[2]

- Unstable airway (lower cranial nerve palsies and coma/unresponsive patients)
- Bradypnea or poor respiratory efforts (risk of hypoventilation)
- Recent head/neck/esophagus surgery or trauma (tight interface can cause injury or air leak)
- Copious airway secretions (risk of aspiration)
- Uncooperative children (sedation can be tried)
- Pneumothorax or pneumomediastinum (use with caution)

The most important principles that determine the success of NIV are selecting the right patient and having clear targets, failing which the decision for endotracheal intubation and invasive ventilation will be taken in a timely manner.

Endotracheal Intubation

The decision to intubate a child in respiratory failure should be based on clinical assessment without the necessity of blood gas or other investigations. Timely intubation requires the identification of clinical signs that even precede the signs of impending respiratory collapse, listed in **Box 20.7.3**, which appear late on the verge of respiratory/cardiac arrest.

Endotracheal intubation is mostly a clinical decision and must be determined on a case-by-case basis. Adequate preparation and appropriate backup are the key to a successful intubation. The seniormost or the most experienced person in the team should lead the procedure.

A simple mnemonic to be remembered is "SOAP-ME" (suction, oxygenation, airway, positioning, monitors and medications, and equipment and $ETCO_2$ if available).

A secure intravenous (IV) access is mandatory, and in case of an emergency, intraosseous access is important. Nasogastric tube insertion is essential to relieve gastric distension, reduce airway pressures, and also to prevent aspiration.

Emergency drugs should be prepared in advance in the correct dose based on the age or weight of the child. A normal saline bolus and adrenaline (epinephrine) infusion must be kept ready, especially if the child is hemodynamically compromised.

The priority is supporting oxygenation and hemodynamic stability whilst securing the airway. Preoxygenation of the lungs is invaluable, especially in infants and young children, where the length of apnea time tolerated before desaturation is low.

The decision to perform a *rapid sequence induction* (RSI) or a modified RSI should be taken on a case-by-case basis, but neuromuscular blockade should be employed selectively with backup of a pediatric intensive care unit (PICU) facility and an experienced intensivist, preferably along with anesthetist.

Midazolam and morphine are commonly used in combination with either vecuronium or atracurium. Fentanyl and ketamine are suitable alternatives. Propofol is avoided in several centers, except in short-term sedation, because of the risk of *propofol-related infusion syndrome*. Ketamine confers the benefits of bronchodilatation and relative cardiovascular stability. Neuromuscular block will provide

BOX 20.7.3: Signs of impending respiratory collapse.

- *Exhaustion:* Evidenced by listlessness or decreased respiratory effort
- Cyanosis
- Impairment of consciousness
- SpO_2 <92% despite supplemental oxygen FiO_2 0.6
- Recurrent apnea
- Worsening hypercarbia

BOX 20.7.4: Formulae for size and length of tracheal tube (TT).

Sizes for cuffed TT:
- *>3 kg up to 1 year:* Start with size 3.0 mm
- *1–2 years:* Start with size 3.5 mm
- *>2 years:* (age/4) + 3.5 mm

Size for uncuffed TT:
- *<1 year up to 1 kg:* Size 2.5 mm
- *2 kg:* Size 3.0 mm
- *>3 kg:* Size 3.5 mm
- *>1 year:* (age/4) + 4 mm

Depth: (Age/2) + 12 cm or internal diameter of ETT × 3

(ETT: endotracheal tube)

optimal intubating conditions in most cases: Rocuronium, vecuronium, or atracurium is used. The choice of agent depends on the clinical scenario, availability, and experience of the team. Atracurium can precipitate histamine release and may, therefore, worsen bronchoconstriction. Straight laryngoscope blades are generally used in babies up to 6 months and curved blades thereafter. Tracheal tube (TT) size and length should be calculated using the standard formulae given in **Box 20.7.4**[7] A cuffed TT is preferable to an uncuffed TT.

SPECIFIC MANAGEMENT

Physiological stabilization as detailed earlier is paramount and should precede definitive management. Definitive management depends on likely diagnosis and may include antibiotics for pneumonia, hypertonic saline nebulization for bronchiolitis, and inhaled bronchodilators and corticosteroids for acute asthma.

CONCLUSION

Respiratory failure is one of the most common emergencies in children and a common cause of child mortality. Recognition and management decisions are largely based on clinical assessment. A systematic assessment and a focused history and examination are essential to recognize respiratory failure and to categorize the type and severity. Physiological stabilization is more important in the ER and is the initial priority before investigations, diagnosis, and definitive management.

REFERENCES

1. Perin J, Mulick A, Yeung D, Villavicencio F, Lopez G, Strong KL, et al. Global, regional, and national causes of under-5 mortality in 2000-19: An updated systematic analysis with implications for the Sustainable Development Goals. Lancet Child Adolesc Health. 2022;6(2):106-15.
2. Jose D, Parameswaran N. Advances in management of respiratory failure in children. Indian J Pediatr. 2023;90(5): 470-80.
3. Slain KN, Shein SL, Rotta AT. The use of high-flow nasal cannula in the pediatric emergency department. J Pediatr (Rio J). 2017;93(Suppl 1):36-45.
4. Stewart C. Noninvasive airway management techniques: How and when to use them. Emerg Med Pract. 2001;3(7).
5. Dafydd C, Saunders BJ, Kotecha SJ, Edwards MO. Efficacy and safety of high flow nasal oxygen for children with bronchiolitis: Systematic review and meta-analysis. BMJ Open Respir Res. 2021;8(1):e000844.
6. Williams AM, Abramo TJ, Shah MV, Miller R, Burney-Jones C, Rooks S, et al. Safety and clinical findings of BiPAP utilization in children 20 kg or less for asthma exacerbations. Intensive Care Med. 2011;37(8):1338-43.
7. Challands J, Brooks K. Paediatric respiratory distress. BJA Educ. 2019;19(11):350-6.

20.8 Fluid, Electrolytes, and Acid–Base Imbalances

Sasidaran Kandasamy, Divya Selvaraj

INTRODUCTION

Fluids and electrolytes are pivotal in ensuring cellular function, energy metabolism, and overall homeostasis. This chapter explores the body's water compartments, electrolyte composition, and mechanisms regulating osmolality and acid–base balance. It also examines conditions such as dehydration, electrolyte imbalances, and acid–base disturbances, providing detailed insights into their clinical presentation, assessment, and management. The focus on evidence-based strategies highlights their relevance in intensive care, emphasizing timely intervention and precise monitoring to optimize outcomes.

FLUID AND ELECTROLYTES

Fluid Compartments

The regulation of water and electrolytes is crucial for maintaining stability in the body. At birth, total body water (TBW) constitutes about 75% of body weight, decreasing to

TABLE 20.8.1: Electrolyte composition of body fluids.

Electrolytes	ICF	ECF	Interstitial fluid
Cations (mEq/L)			
Na^+	9.0	140	147
K^+	158	4.5	4.0
Ca^{2+}	3.0	5.0	2.5
Mg^{2+}	30	2.0	1.0
Anions (mEq/L)			
Cl^-	4.0	103	114
HCO^-_3	10.0	25	30
Proteins	65	15	0
Phosphates	95	2.0	2.0
Organic acids	4.0	6.0	7.5
Sulfates	22	–	1.0

(ECF: extracellular fluid; ICF: intracellular fluid)

around 65% by 1 year of age, primarily due to a reduction in extracellular water (ECW). After infancy, the ratio between the two main water compartments, intracellular water (ICW) and ECW, stabilizes at 2:1. The extracellular fluid (ECF) is divided into interstitial and intravascular spaces, with the intravascular space comprising roughly 1/12th of the TBW.

Electrolyte Composition

The body fluids differ in their electrolyte composition, with sodium and chloride being predominant in the ECF, while potassium and phosphate dominate within the intracellular fluid (ICF) **(Table 20.8.1)**. Despite some differences, plasma's electrolyte concentration is distinct from that of the interstitial fluid.

Osmolality and Water Balance

Water shifts between compartments are driven by osmolality differences, with water moving from lower to higher osmolality areas. Plasma osmolality is calculated as:[1]

$$\text{Plasma osmolality} = 2 \times (\text{serum Na}^+ \text{ in mEq/L}) + \text{glucose (mg/dL)}/18 + \text{blood urea nitrogen (BUN) (mg/dL)}/2.8$$

Regulation

Plasma osmolality is tightly regulated at 285–295 mOsm/kg. When ECF loses 2% water, thirst is triggered to prevent dehydration. The kidneys regulate water balance and osmolality by controlling solute and water excretion, influenced by antidiuretic hormone (ADH) and natriuretic peptides. ADH secretion increases during hypovolemia or hyperosmolality.

TABLE 20.8.2: Physiological losses.

Source	Losses per 100 kcal metabolized energy		
	Water (mL)	Na^+ (mEq)	K^+ (mEq)
Insensible losses			
Lungs	–15	0	0
Skin	–30	0.1	0.2
Stool losses	–10	0.1	0.2
Urinary losses	–55	3.0	2.0
Water for oxidation	+15		
Total for maintenance	100 mL	3.2 mEq	2.4 mEq

TABLE 20.8.3: Daily maintenance requirement (Holliday and Segar).

Requirements	By body weight	By surface area
Water		
Up to 10 kg	100 mL/kg	1,500 mL/m² (range 1,200–1,800 mL)
• 11–20 kg • >20 kg	• 1000 mL + 50 mL/kg for extra weight above 10 kg • 1500 mL + 20 mL/kg for extra weight above 20 kg	
Sodium	3–4 mEq/kg/day	40–60 mEq/m²
Potassium	2–3 mEq/kg/day	30–40 mEq/m²
Chloride	3–4 mEq/kg/day	–

TABLE 20.8.4: Insensible water loss (ISWL).

Conditions that increase ISWL	Conditions that reduce ISWL
Prematurity	Enclosed incubator
Radiant warmer	Humidified air
Phototherapy	Sedation
Hyperventilation	Decreased activity
Increased activity	Hypothermia
Hyperthermia	

Requirements

Water and electrolyte needs depend on replacing urinary and insensible water losses (ISWLs), as well as water for metabolic processes **(Tables 20.8.2 to 20.8.4)**. A child requires about 110–115 mL of water, 3 mEq of sodium, and 2.5 mEq of potassium per 100 kcal of energy metabolized. Additionally, 10–15 mL of water is produced during the oxidation of carbohydrates, proteins, and fats. Practically, 100 mL of water suffices for 100 kcal metabolism.[2]

Daily fluid and electrolyte maintenance in children is based on body weight **(Table 20.8.3)**. Adjustments are made for factors affecting ISWL **(Table 20.8.4)**. Isotonic fluids, such

TABLE 20.8.5: Neonatal fluid requirements (mL/kg/day).

Birth weight	Day 1	Day 2	Day 3	Day 4	Day 5
<1,000 g	80–100	Advance fluids as per hydration status			
1,000–1,500 g	80	100	120	140	150
>1500 g	60	80	100	120	140

as 0.9% saline with 5% dextrose and added potassium, are the preferred initial choice for maintenance therapy in children.

Neonatal Period

In the neonatal period, fluid requirements are lower during the first few days of life **(Table 20.8.5)**. About 70% of typical maintenance fluid containing dextrose is given in the first two days, increasing to 100% by day 4 or 5. Low-birth-weight infants may need more fluids. Sodium supplementation begins after a newborn loses 6% of birth weight. Potassium is usually supplemented from day 3, based on levels. Low-birth-weight or sick neonates often require calcium supplementation (36–72 mg/kg/day as 10% calcium gluconate 4–8 mL/kg/day) from day 1.

Dehydration

Dehydration, the most common fluid imbalance in infants and children, results from a net loss of body water due to diarrhea, vomiting, or excessive urinary loss. It can be isotonic (equal water and solute loss), hypotonic (greater sodium loss than water), or hypertonic (greater water loss than sodium), leading to intracellular dehydration.

Management of Dehydration

It involves the following several key steps:[3]

- *Estimation of the degree of dehydration* based on clinical history and physical examination **(Table 20.8.6)**, whether mild, moderate, or severe. In malnourished children with reduced subcutaneous tissue, dehydration is often overestimated, while in well-nourished children with more fat reserves, it is underestimated. Thirst, dry mucosa, urine flow, metabolic acidosis, and circulatory status are more reliable indicators. Tachycardia, decreased skin turgor, sunken eyes, fontanel, lethargy, and oliguria suggest over 10% weight loss, though their reliability is debated. Shock symptoms are more pronounced in hypotonic dehydration, while central nervous system (CNS) signs dominate in hypertonic dehydration. Lab tests like blood urea, creatinine, sodium, and osmolality help guide fluid therapy.
- *Rapid restoration of intravascular volume:* To restore perfusion, administer 20–40 mL/kg of 0.9% saline or Ringer's lactate for over 1 hour. If circulation is not restored, an additional 20–40 mL/kg may be given.

TABLE 20.8.6: Severity of dehydration assessment.

Characteristics			
Infants	Mild 1–5%	Moderate 6–9%	Severe ≥10% (>15% shock)
Children	Mild 1–3%	Moderate 4–6%	Severe ≥7% (>9% shock)
Pulse	Normal	Tachycardia	Tachycardia and weak pulse
Systolic BP	Normal	Normal-low	Orthostatic to shock
Urine output	Decreased	Decreased	Oliguria
Buccal mucosa	Slightly dry	Dry	Parched
Anterior fontanel	Normal	Sunken	Markedly sunken
Eyes	Normal	Sunken	Markedly sunken
Skin turgor/ capillary refill	Normal	Decreased	Markedly decreased
Skin (<12 months age)	Normal	Cool	Cool, mottling, and acrocyanosis

- *Rehydration therapy* follows rapid volume restoration. The 24-hour fluid requirement includes maintenance (as previously discussed) and deficit fluids,[4] with the deficit calculated based on the percentage of dehydration. For example, a 10 kg child with 10% dehydration has a 1-liter fluid deficit. After subtracting isotonic fluids used in initial resuscitation, the remaining fluid is replaced over 24 hours with 5% dextrose normal saline (NS) and 20 mEq/l KCl for isonatremic or hyponatremic dehydration. Hypernatremia dehydration requires slower correction to avoid reducing serum sodium by >10 mEq/L per day, using 5% dextrose with 1/2 NS to prevent cerebral edema. Oral rehydration therapy may begin if dehydration is isotonic, and the child has urinated and can drink.
- *Ongoing losses from diarrhea must be replaced* with volumes based on stool output, approximately 50 mL per stool for infants under 6 months, 100 mL for those over 6 months, and 200 mL for older children.
- *Monitoring:* The initial treatment plan is approximate. Continuous monitoring of vital signs, intake/output, weight, volume status, and electrolytes is essential to adjust therapy based on the patient's clinical condition.

ELECTROLYTE DISTURBANCES

Hyponatremia, hypernatremia, hypokalemia, hyperkalemia, hypocalcemia, and hypomagnesemia are important electrolyte disorders in sick children.

TABLE 20.8.7: Syndrome of inappropriate antidiuretic hormone secretion (SIADH) vs. cerebral salt wasting syndrome (CSWS).

Feature	SIADH	CSWS
Sodium	Low	Low
Body water	Increased	Decreased
Serum osmolality	<280 mOsm/L	Decreased
Urine osmolality	>500 mOsm/L	Increased
Urine output	Low	High
Urine Na concentration	Increased	Increased

Hyponatremia

Hyponatremia is defined as a serum sodium level below 135 mEq/L and can result from water retention, sodium loss, or redistribution of sodium and water, particularly in conditions like hyperglycemia or hyperlipidemia. Pseudohyponatremia occurs when high plasma volume falsely lowers sodium levels, with serum sodium decreasing about 1.6 mEq/L for each 100 mg/dL increase in glucose above 100 mg/dL. This condition is common in hospitalized children, often linked to acute diarrhea, pneumonia, meningitis, sepsis, heart failure, or liver and renal diseases, and is associated with severe illness and worse outcomes.[5]

Types

Hyponatremia is of the following types:

- *Hyponatremia with dehydration or hypovolemia*: It results from significant TBW and sodium loss due to diarrhea, vomiting, or renal sodium loss (e.g., from diuretics). In renal sodium loss, urinary sodium exceeds 20 mEq/L.
- *Hypervolemic hyponatremia:* Occurs in conditions like congestive heart failure, nephrotic syndrome, or liver failure, where TBW disproportionately increases compared to sodium. Urinary sodium levels are generally below 5 mEq/L.
- *Euvolemic hyponatremia:* Occurs due to excess of TBW and a slight decrease in total body sodium. Syndrome of inappropriate antidiuretic hormone (SIADH) and water intoxication are important causes. SIADH is seen in CNS disorders such as infections, trauma, or hypoxic-ischemic encephalopathy. Differentiating SIADH from cerebral salt wasting syndrome (CSWS) **(Table 20.8.7)** is essential for treatment.

Clinical Features

They are primarily CNS manifestations due to the movement of water into cells, triggered by extracellular hypoosmolality as the brain is constrained by the rigid skull. It includes nausea, confusion, lethargy, agitation, headache, seizures, and, in severe cases, brainstem herniation. Acute hyponatremia (rapid drop in sodium) is more symptomatic than chronic hyponatremia, which allows for better brain adaptation.

Management

In acute symptomatic hyponatremia, particularly with sodium below 120 mEq/L, immediate treatment with intravenous 3% saline (5–10 mL/kg at 1 mL/min) is necessary to raise sodium by about 5 mEq/L initially. For asymptomatic patients, correction should occur over 48–72 hours. The sodium deficit can be calculated using:

$$\text{Sodium deficit} = 0.6 \times \text{body weight (kg)} \times (135 - \text{observed serum Na})$$

For SIADH, address the underlying cause and restrict fluids, and severe cases may require 3% saline with diuretics like furosemide. In CSWS, high-dose fludrocortisone (0.2–0.4 mg/day) may help manage hyponatremia and volume contraction.

Hypernatremia

Hypernatremia is defined as a serum sodium concentration greater than 145 mEq/L, resulting from a relative water deficit. It can arise from net water loss (e.g., diarrhea, vomiting, diuresis, and burns) or excessive sodium intake. This condition can occur in various hydration states: Dehydration, overhydration, or normal hydration. In dehydration, it is often linked to acute diarrheal diseases, where water loss exceeds electrolyte loss. Diabetes insipidus, hyperventilation, fever, and inadequate water intake are additional causes, while iatrogenic hypernatremia may result from excessive sodium administration in fluids.

Clinical Features

In hypernatremia, signs of dehydration may be minimal due to preserved ECF. Skin turgor may remain, though the skin may feel doughy. Intracellular dehydration can lead to severe hyperosmolality and cerebral damage, resulting in complications like cerebral hemorrhages, thrombosis, or subdural effusion. CNS symptoms are prominent,[6] including hyperirritability and a high-pitched cry with possible seizures. In severe cases, CNS depression, coma, metabolic acidosis, and deep, rapid breathing may develop.

Management

For shock or severe dehydration, rapid intravenous administration of Ringer's lactate or 0.9% saline is crucial. Address the underlying cause of hypernatremia. For acute cases, a safe correction rate is 1 mEq/L/h. For chronic hypernatremia, a slower correction of 0.5 mEq/L/h is recommended, targeting a reduction of 10 mEq/L/d to reach 145 mEq/L. Peritoneal dialysis is indicated when serum sodium exceeds 180 mEq/L. If convulsions occur, 3–5 mL/kg of 3% saline or 20% mannitol may be administered to manage water intoxication or cerebral edema.

Hypokalemia

Hypokalemia is defined as a serum potassium level below 3.6 mEq/L. It can result from gastrointestinal (GI) losses (vomiting, diarrhea, and gastric aspiration), urinary losses (such as with prolonged use of diuretics, renal tubular acidosis, hyperaldosteronism, and steroid therapy), hypomagnesemia, or an intracellular potassium shift caused by conditions like alkalosis, therapy with β-agonists, insulin, or diabetic ketoacidosis (DKA). Other contributing factors include protein–energy malnutrition, carbenicillin therapy, and those who are critically ill.

Clinical Features

Potassium plays a key role in bioelectric processes, such as muscle contraction, nerve conduction, and cardiac pacing. Thus, hypokalemia leads to muscle weakness, hypotonia, diminished reflexes, and paralytic ileus.

Cardiac manifestations include arrhythmias and electrocardiograph (ECG) changes of prominent U-wave, prolonged QTc interval (>0.425 seconds), T-wave inversion, flattening or ST-segment depression, prolonged PR interval, sinoatrial block, and ventricular extrasystoles at levels below 2.5 mEq/L. These changes do not always correlate with the serum potassium level.

Long-term hypokalemia can impair the kidneys' ability to concentrate urine, leading to hypokalemic nephropathy. In severe cases, respiratory paralysis may also occur.

Management

It is essential to address the root cause of hypokalemia, such as GI losses or diuretic therapy. Potassium supplementation at 1–2 mEq/kg/d as oral potassium chloride syrup (Potklor: 15 mL = 20 mEq/L) can be used for mild cases. Intravenous potassium chloride (Injection KCl 1 mL = 2 mEq) is used when oral administration is not possible. The concentration of potassium in IV fluids should not exceed 60 mEq/L.

Rapid correction is indicated if serum potassium is <2.5 mEq/L, the patient is symptomatic, or there are ECG changes. The dose for rapid correction is 0.5–1 mEq/kg given over 1 hour. Potassium should only be administered when urinary flow is established to avoid the risk of potassium buildup, which can lead to hyperkalemia.

If magnesium deficiency is present, it must be corrected alongside potassium replacement. Potassium-sparing diuretics can be added to the treatment regimen to help maintain potassium levels.

Hyperkalemia

Hyperkalemia is defined as a serum potassium level above 5 mEq/L. It most commonly arises due to impaired renal excretion seen in conditions such as oliguria, acute renal failure, adrenal insufficiency, and chronic renal failure. Hyperkalemia can occur due to transcellular shifts such as metabolic acidosis, sepsis, acute hemolysis, acute rhabdomyolysis, tumor lysis syndrome, or tissue necrosis.

Clinical Features

Mild hyperkalemia is often asymptomatic. Severe hyperkalemia affects the cardiac and skeletal muscles, leading to muscle weakness, paresthesia, shock, bradycardia, or cardiac arrhythmias. Early ECG changes include prolonged PR interval, tall T waves, shortened QT interval, and wide QRS complexes with reduced amplitude. In severe cases, absent P waves, first-degree heart block, sine wave patterns, ventricular fibrillation, and cardiac arrest occur.

Management

Managing hyperkalemia involves multiple steps depending on the severity and the presence of ECG changes. The general treatment strategy includes discontinuing any oral or intravenous potassium supplements and identifying and stopping any medications that could precipitate hyperkalemia, like potassium-sparing diuretics or ACE inhibitors. The root cause of hyperkalemia should be treated. If hyperkalemia is accompanied by ECG abnormalities, it is a medical emergency and immediate acute reduction is required.

- *Treatment options for acute reduction in serum potassium:* Injection of calcium gluconate 10% at 100 mg/kg/dose (1 mL/kg/dose) IV over 5–10 minutes acts as a cardiac cell stabilizer.
- *Measures to shift potassium into cells:*[7]
  - Injection of $NaHCO_3$ at 1–2 mEq/kg/dose IV over 5–10 minutes
  - Glucose + insulin at 0.5 g/kg (2 mL/kg of 25% D) 0.1 U/kg regular insulin IV over 1 hour
  - *Nebulized salbutamol:* 2.5 mg for <25 kg, 5 mg for >25 kg
  - *Sodium polystyrene resins:* 0.5–1 g/kg orally/rectally
  - *Furosemide (restricted usage):* 1–2 mg/kg IV/IM

Dialysis is recommended if the above interventions fail to reduce serum potassium levels.

Hypocalcemia

Hypocalcemia occurs when serum calcium levels fall below the normal range of 8.5–10.2 mg/dL (total calcium) or 4.8–7.2 mg/dL (ionized calcium). It is often detected through lab tests, as symptoms may be subtle or absent.

Clinical Features

Symptoms include muscle spasms, fasciculations, Chvostek's and Trousseau's signs, tetany, seizures, bronchospasm, arrhythmias, blood pressure fluctuations, and heart failure. Neurological and cardiovascular symptoms are more pronounced in severe cases (ionized calcium <0.8 mmol/L). Sepsis is commonly associated with hypocalcemia.

Management

Treatment is necessary if the patient is symptomatic or if ionized calcium is below 0.8 mmol/L. Calcium gluconate (10%) is given as 0.5–1.0 mL/kg over 5–10 minutes, followed by continuous infusion of 0.1–0.2 mL/kg/h (equivalent to 0.5–2 mg/kg/h) over the next 2–4 hours. Subsequently, elemental calcium is administered at a rate of 0.3–0.5 mg/kg/h. Calcium chloride (10%) contains 1.36 mEq/mL, while calcium gluconate (10%) contains 0.45 mEq/mL of elemental calcium.

Hypomagnesemia and Hypermagnesemia

Magnesium plays a crucial role in maintaining various cellular functions, particularly through its involvement in the activation of adenosine triphosphate (ATP). Normal serum magnesium (Mg^{2+}) levels range between 1.5 and 2.3 mg/dL.

Hypomagnesemia (<1.5 mEq/L) occurs in a variety of clinical conditions, including protein-energy malnutrition, malabsorption, hypoalbuminemia, sepsis, prolonged GI suctioning, diarrhea, blood transfusions, aminoglycoside therapy, osmotic diuresis, and the use of diuretics. Hypermagnesemia (>2.6 mg/dL) is less common.

Clinical Features

Hypomagnesemia is associated with prolonged PR intervals, widened QRS complexes, ST-segment depression, and low-amplitude T waves on ECG. It can exacerbate dysrhythmias, especially in the presence of hypocalcemia or digitalis toxicity. Refractory hypokalemia unresponsive to treatment is a hallmark of hypomagnesemia and often indicates the need to address the magnesium deficiency.

Hypermagnesemia presents tall, peaked T-waves, and narrow QRS complexes on ECG.

Management

For symptomatic magnesium depletion with normal renal function, the magnesium deficit is 1–2 mEq/kg. Replace with 1 mEq/kg over 24 hours, followed by 0.5 mEq/kg/d for 3–5 days.

FLUID THERAPY IN SPECIAL SITUATIONS

Parenteral Fluid Therapy

Parenteral fluid therapy is essential in certain clinical scenarios, such as:

- *Maintenance fluids:* For comatose or ill children unable to take fluids orally.
- *Adjusted maintenance fluids:* To avoid overhydration or electrolyte imbalances in cases like oliguria/anuria, severe pneumonia, SIADH, raised intracranial pressure (ICP), postoperative care, cardiac failure, or edema.

TABLE 20.8.8: Average electrolyte contents of various gastrointestinal (GI) fluids (mmol/L).

GI fluids	H^+	Na^+	K^+	Cl^-	HCO_3^-
Gastric	80	40	20	150	0
Small bowel	0	130	20	120	30
Pancreatic	0	135	15	100	50

- *Maintenance plus deficit replacement:* For ongoing fluid losses due to vomiting, diarrhea, nasogastric drainage, burns, DKA, salicylate intoxication, or pyloric stenosis.

Gastrointestinal Losses

Fluids lost via nasogastric tubes, ileostomies, or pancreatic fistulas require electrolyte replacement. Gastric fluids are high in hydrogen and chloride, while small-bowel fluids contain more sodium and bicarbonate. **Table 20.8.8** shows the electrolyte composition of various GI fluids.

Increased Intracranial Pressure

In children with increased ICP, it is critical to avoid overhydration. However, fluid restriction, previously recommended, can sometimes be harmful. Instead, close monitoring is essential, especially when osmotic diuretics like mannitol are being used.

Diabetic Ketoacidosis

Diabetic ketoacidosis in children typically presents with an 8–10% fluid deficit, low sodium, normal potassium, and phosphate depletion. Hypokalemia often develops after insulin therapy begins. In shock, fluid resuscitation is the priority over insulin, with a 10–20 mL/kg bolus of normal saline or Ringer's lactate administered over 1 hour. Subsequent fluid rates are calculated based on the fluid deficit[8] (either 5% or 10% dehydration depending on whether the patient has mild, moderate, or severe DKA), and the initial fluid bolus is given along with the maintenance for the next 48 hours (based on Holliday-Segar formula) given as follows:

$$\text{Hourly fluid rate} = [(\text{Deficit} - \text{Initial Bolus})/48 \text{ hour}] + \text{maintenance per hour}$$

Initial choice of fluid is 0.9% saline with 40 mEq/L KCl, which can be changed to 0.45% saline with or without dextrose (5–10%) depending on the monitored sugar and electrolyte values. When the blood glucose level drops to 250 mg/dL, glucose is added to the fluid regimen.

Oliguria and Anuria

In children with oliguria or anuria, fluid therapy should be limited to 300–400 mL/m^2 per day (15–20 mL/kg or 30–40 mL/100 kcal). Urinary water loss is replaced every

4–6 hours, and nonurinary losses are replaced with 10% glucose. Electrolytes are only given for ongoing losses and both hyperkalemia and hypokalemia should be managed by protocols. Renal supportive therapy may be required in cases of acute volume overload.

Fluid Overload

Fluid overload (FO) is common in critically ill children, impairing organ function, especially lung oxygenation, due to excess fluid administration. The Holliday-Segar formula often overestimates fluid needs during acute illness as fluid requirements decrease due to reduced ISWL and altered neurohormonal responses. A persistent positive fluid balance after stabilization harms vital organs, especially the lungs and kidneys, leading to prolonged mechanical ventilation and increased mortality. FO is measured as a percentage using the given formula:[9]

$$FO\ (\%) = \text{Total fluid intake (L)} - \text{total fluid output (L)} / \text{admission weight (kg)} \times 100$$

Management

If fluid overload exceeds 10%, controlled diuresis with low-dose furosemide (0.1–0.4 mg/kg/h) is recommended to achieve a net negative fluid balance. If unresponsive to diuresis or if fluid overload exceeds 20%, early renal replacement therapy (RRT) should be initiated. Fluid balance and clinical indicators should be monitored every 6–12 hours to ensure safe fluid management.

Near-drowning

Patients with poor peripheral perfusion require rapid volume expansion with saline or Ringer's lactate. Central venous pressure and acid-base values must be monitored, and further fluid and electrolyte therapy depends on serum electrolyte levels and complications like cerebral edema.

ACID–BASE BALANCE

Physiology

Maintaining acid-base balance is vital for normal physiological function with a normal blood pH of 7.40 (range 7.35–7.45).[10] Disturbances can arise from respiratory or metabolic imbalances, affecting pH, bicarbonate (HCO^-_3), and partial pressure of carbon dioxide ($PaCO_2$). Acid is a substance that tends to dissociate or give a hydrogen ion (proton donor), whereas base is a substance that tends to bind or associate with a hydrogen ion (proton acceptor).

Acidosis is a blood pH below 7.35, caused by increased $PaCO_2$ (respiratory) or decreased bicarbonate (HCO^-_3) (metabolic).

Alkalosis is a blood pH above 7.45, caused by decreased $PaCO_2$ (respiratory) or increased HCO^-_3 (metabolic).

The body compensates by adjusting $PaCO_2$ and HCO^-_3 levels. For instance, in metabolic acidosis, hyperventilation reduces $PaCO_2$, while in respiratory acidosis, the kidneys retain HCO^-_3. As a rule of thumb, 1 mm Hg increase in $PaCO_2$ decreases pH by 0.01 and 1 mEq/L decrease in HCO^-_3 decreases pH by 0.02. Identifying the primary disturbance and compensation is key for diagnosis and treatment.

Assessment and Identification of Acid–Base Disorders

Comprehensive history and clinical examination focusing on the patient's immediate environment, including fraction of inspired oxygen (FiO_2), barometric pressure, patient's respiratory rate, vital signs, respiratory effort, mental status, and tissue perfusion during the physical examination is done. Laboratory data like previous arterial blood gas (ABG) reports, electrolytes, blood sugar, BUN, hemoglobin, hematocrit, chest X-rays, or pulmonary function tests are important.

Identifying the acid-base disturbance:

- Assess pH:
  - *Low pH (<7.38):* Acidemia
  - *High pH (>7.42):* Alkalemia
- *Determine primary disorder:* Use HCO^-_3 and $PaCO_2$ levels to classify the disturbance **(Table 20.8.9)**.
- *Calculate compensation:* Evaluating compensatory mechanisms is given in **Table 20.8.10**.
- *Calculate the anion gap (discussed under metabolic acidosis):*

$$\text{Anion gap} = Na^+ - (Cl^- + HCO^-_3).$$

A normal range is 8–16 mEq/L, with values >16 indicating high anion gap metabolic acidosis.

TABLE 20.8.9: Identification of primary disturbance.

Primary disorder	***pH***	***HCO^-_3***	***$PaCO_2$***	***Compensation***
Metabolic acidosis	Low	Low	Normal/ low	Fall in $PaCO_2$ and acidic urine
Metabolic alkalosis	High	High	Normal/ high	Rise in $PaCO_2$ and alkaline urine
Respiratory acidosis	Low	Normal/ low	High	Acidic urine
Respiratory alkalosis	High	Normal/ high	Low	Alkaline urine

Example 1: pH 7.3, HCO^-_3 14 = Metabolic acidosis
Example 2: pH 7.57, HCO^-_3 42, and $PaCO_2$ 47 = Metabolic alkalosis
Example 3: pH 7.57, HCO^-_3 18, $PaCO_2$ 18 = Respiratory alkalosis
Example 4: pH 7.2, HCO^-_3 28, and $PaCO_2$ 58 = Respiratory acidosis

TABLE 20.8.10: Compensatory changes for acidosis and alkalosis.

Primary disorder	Compensatory change	Expected compensation
Metabolic acidosis	Fall in HCO^-_3	*Fall in $PaCO_2$:* $\Delta PaCO_2 = 1.2 \times \Delta HCO^-_3$
Metabolic alkalosis	Rise in HCO^-_3	*Rise in $PaCO_2$:* $\Delta PaCO_2 = 0.7 \times \Delta HCO^-_3$
Respiratory acidosis	Rise in $PaCO_2$	• *Acute:* $\Delta HCO^-_3 = 0.1 \times \Delta PaCO_2$ • *Chronic:* $\Delta HCO^-_3 = 0.3 \times \Delta PaCO_2$
Respiratory alkalosis	Fall in $PaCO_2$	• *Acute:* $\Delta HCO^-_3 = 0.2 \times \Delta PaCO_2$ • *Chronic:* $\Delta HCO^-_3 = 0.5 \times \Delta PaCO_2$

This streamlined approach helps accurately diagnose and manage acid-base disturbances.

Metabolic Acidosis

Metabolic acidosis occurs when plasma bicarbonate decreases, leading to compensatory hyperventilation and reduced $PaCO_2$. This results from acid accumulation or bicarbonate loss, disrupting the body's acid-base balance.

Anion gap (AG) results from unmeasured anions like sulfate, phosphate, and organic anions. Normal AG is 8–16 mEq/L. Elevated AG indicates organic acid accumulation, signaling acidosis, even if pH is normal. Elevated AG metabolic acidosis is caused by nonvolatile acids (e.g., lactic acid and ketones), while normal AG metabolic acidosis involves bicarbonate loss and increased chloride. Metabolic acidosis is categorized by whether the AG is elevated or not, depending on the cause.

Causes

Causes of metabolic acidosis are as follows:

- *Normal anion gap acidosis:* Seen in diarrhea, renal tubular acidosis, ureterosigmoidostomy, and early acute renal failure.
- *Increased anion gap acidosis:* Common in DKA, lactic acidosis, inborn metabolic disorders, salicylate or methanol poisoning, uremia, and prolonged starvation.

Clinical Features

The clinical features include:

- *Mild:* Lethargy, fatigue, and Kussmaul breathing.
- *Severe:* Hypotension, stupor, coma, and arrhythmias (pH <7.2)
- *Chronic:* Osteopenia, muscle wasting, and growth retardation in children

Management

Management of metabolic acidosis is done as follows:

- *Emergency measures:* Maintain airway, oxygenation, and perfusion to prevent further H^+ production.
- *Treat underlying causes,* for example, insulin for DKA and antidotes for poisonings.
- *Bicarbonate therapy:* Administer cautiously if pH <7.2 or $HCO^-_3 \leq 5$ mEq/L, with the goal of raising pH to 7.2. Dose = 0.3 × body weight (kg) × base deficit. Dilute for intravenous infusion.
  - *Risks:* Hyperosmolality, hypokalemia, decreased ionized calcium, intracellular acidosis, and worsened tissue hypoxia.
- *Dialysis* is required in severe cases, especially with renal failure or poisoning.

Metabolic Alkalosis

Metabolic alkalosis is marked by elevated bicarbonate (HCO^-_3 >28–30 mEq/L) and a pH above 7.45, typically resulting from excess bicarbonate or acid loss.

Clinical Features

The clinical features include:

- *Mild (HCO^-_3 <36 mEq/L):* Often asymptomatic, discovered through lab tests
- *Moderate (HCO^-_3 36–42 mEq/L):* Symptoms include paresthesia, muscle weakness, orthostatic hypotension, fatigue, muscle cramps, and hyporeflexia.
- *Severe (HCO^-_3 >45–50 mEq/L):* May present with cardiac arrhythmias, tetany, seizures, delirium, hypoventilation, hypoxemia, and difficulty weaning from a ventilator

Management

Management of metabolic alkalosis is done as follows:

- *Chloride-responsive metabolic alkalosis:*
  - *Treat underlying cause:* Address dehydration or vomiting.
  - *Hydration:* Rehydration with 0.9% saline (10 mL/kg over 10–30 minutes)
  - *Potassium supplementation:* Correct hypokalemia with potassium chloride.
  - *Diuretic-induced:* Stop loop diuretics and consider potassium-sparing alternatives.
- *Chloride-resistant metabolic alkalosis:*
  - *Treat underlying condition:* Manage causes like mineralocorticoid excess.
  - *Potassium supplementation:* Replace potassium orally or intravenously.
  - *Potassium-sparing diuretics:* Help retain potassium and correct electrolyte imbalance.

Respiratory Acidosis

Respiratory acidosis occurs when inadequate ventilation leads to CO_2 accumulation, raising $PaCO_2$ above 45 mm Hg and lowering blood pH. Acute cases last up to 12 hours, while chronic cases persist beyond that.

Clinical Features

The clinical features include:

- *Hypercapnia:* Causes headache, irritability, and increased intracranial pressure
- *Severe symptoms:* Drowsiness, coma, muscular tremors, tachycardia, flushed skin, sweating, low blood pressure, and shock
- *Cardiac risk:* Ventricular fibrillation, a life-threatening arrhythmia, may develop.

Management

The management of respiratory acidosis is done as follows:

- *Improve ventilation:* Mechanical or noninvasive ventilation enhances CO_2 elimination.
- *Oxygen therapy:* High-flow oxygen helps reduce CO_2 but must be carefully monitored to avoid respiratory suppression.
- *Sodium bicarbonate:* Administered in cases of hyperkalemia or ventricular fibrillation after ventilation is established to prevent further acid-base imbalance.

Respiratory Alkalosis

It typically results from hyperventilation, either psychogenic or neurogenic, and may signal early sepsis. Acute cases last 6–12 hours, with HCO^-_3 consumption as compensation. Chronic cases involve renal suppression of H^+ excretion and chloride retention.

Clinical Features

Hyperventilation with tetany is due to low ionized calcium caused by alkalosis.

Treatment

Closed-circuit breathing increases CO_2. Treat the underlying cause, sodium bicarbonate is not recommended.

Mixed Acid–Base Disorders

Mixed acid–base disorders occur when two or more primary acid–base disturbances are present simultaneously. These disturbances complicate the body's ability to regulate pH because multiple systems are affected. The most encountered mixed acid–base disorders **(Table 20.8.11)** include:

- Respiratory acidosis + metabolic acidosis
- Respiratory acidosis + metabolic alkalosis
- Respiratory alkalosis + metabolic acidosis
- Respiratory alkalosis + metabolic alkalosis

TABLE 20.8.11: Recognition of mixed acid–base disturbances.

$PaCO_2$ (mm Hg)	*HCO_3^- (mEq/L)*	*Interpretation*
>45	<21	Combined metabolic acidosis + respiratory acidosis
	21–26	Respiratory acidosis
	>6	Mixed metabolic + respiratory acidosis
35–45	<21	Metabolic acidosis
	Normal	Metabolic alkalosis
<35	<21	Mixed metabolic acidosis + respiratory alkalosis
	21–26	Respiratory alkalosis
	>26	Combined respiratory alkalosis + metabolic alkalosis

The most severe forms of mixed acid–base disorders are those where both the respiratory and metabolic components cause a shift in pH in the same direction, either toward acidosis or alkalosis. In such cases, the body's compensatory mechanisms are overwhelmed, leading to a more pronounced deviation in pH.

pH interpretation: The pH helps determine which disorder is primary and which is compensatory, as compensation for mixed acid–base disorders is never complete. Therefore, the pH value will reflect the dominant disturbance.

MONITORING FLUID AND ELECTROLYTE THERAPY

During the early resuscitation phase (first 0–2 hours) of intravenous infusion, it is essential to continuously monitor the pulse, blood pressure, capillary refill time, and sensorium. Urine output should be checked hourly. After this, detailed records of fluid intake, output, and body weight should be kept to detect fluid imbalances. This helps assess renal compensatory mechanisms and adjust therapy accordingly. Parameters should be reviewed every 6 hours, with lab tests (e.g., electrolytes) every 12–24 hours. For infants, the aim is to maintain urine osmolality between 300 and 400 mOsm/L to avoid stressing renal function. Keeping a chart to track all data regularly is valuable.

CONCLUSION

Maintaining fluid, electrolyte, and acid–base homeostasis is essential for managing any critically ill child. Appropriate parenteral fluid therapy is used primarily to correct fluid deficits, to provide maintenance fluids, and to replace ongoing fluid losses. This should be achieved through timely clinical and laboratory parameter monitoring. Understanding physiological mechanisms, promptly identifying acid–base disturbances, and implementing targeted interventions to restore homeostasis ensure optimal patient outcomes and prevent complications in critical care settings.

REFERENCES

1. Greenbaum LA. Fluid and electrolyte disorders. In: Kliegman RM, St. Geme JW, Blum NJ, Shah SS, Tasker RC, Wilson KM (Eds). Nelson Textbook of Pediatrics, 22nd edition. Philadelphia: Elsevier; 2020. pp. 485-532.
2. Holliday MA, Segar WE. The maintenance need for water in parenteral fluid therapy. Pediatrics. 1957;19(5):823-32.
3. National Institute for Health and Care Excellence (NICE). (2020). Intravenous fluid therapy in children and young people in hospital (NICE guideline NG29). [online] Available from https://www.nice.org.uk/guidance/ng29 [Last accessed December, 2024].
4. Ghosh S. Fluid management in paediatric patients. In: Malbrain ML, Wong A, Nasa P, Ghosh S (Eds). Rational Use of Intravenous Fluids in Critically Ill Patients. Cham: Springer; 2024. pp. 395-410.
5. Singhi S. Hyponatremia in hospitalized critically ill children: Current concepts. Indian J Pediatr. 2004;71(9):803-7.
6. Zieg J. Diagnosis and management of hypernatraemia in children. Acta Paediatr. 2022;111(3):505-10. [online] Available from https://doi.org/10.1111/apa.16170 [Last accessed February, 2025].
7. Zieg J, Ghose S, Raina R. Electrolyte disorders related emergencies in children. BMC Nephrol. 2024;25(1):282.
8. British Society for Paediatric Endocrinology and Diabetes. (2021). BSPED guideline for the management of children and young people under the age of 18 years with diabetic keto-acidosis. [online] Available from https://www.bsped.org.uk/media/1798/dka-guideline.pdf [Last accessed December, 2024].
9. El-Nawawy A, Moustafa AA, Antonios MAM, Atta MM. Clinical outcomes associated with fluid overload in critically ill pediatric patients. J Trop Pediatr. 2020;66(2):152-62.
10. Khadra EA. Disorders of the acid base status. Pediatric nephrology in ICU. 2009;19-31.

20.9 Basics of Mechanical Ventilation

Dhiren Gupta, S Ram Sundar, Anil Sachdev

INTRODUCTION

Mechanical ventilation is a crucial tool in the pediatric critical care management. Depending on the underlying disease process, mechanical ventilation support can be full or partial. *Positive pressure ventilation* was first administered in 1880 with the use of a foot bellow; however, most of the information came from the widespread use of *negative pressure ventilation* during the polio epidemic, also referred as the "iron lung". There are now new generation ventilators that operate on partial or total feedback and rely on artificial intelligence, thanks to the numerous advancements made in recent times. In this chapter, we will cover the following topics:[1]

- Physiology
- Indications and approach to mechanical ventilation
- Components of a ventilator
- Modes of ventilation
- Setting up the ventilator

PHYSIOLOGY

Alveolar ventilation is the term used to describe the exchange of gases in the lungs. Alveolar ventilation, calculated as [tidal volume (Vt) – dead space (DS) × respiratory rate (RR)], determines the amount of carbon dioxide (CO_2) eliminated; DS is the anatomical dead space (larger airways) volume.[2]

Ventilation in Dead Space

Alveolar DS is often very little in normal condition but can increase due to inadequate ventilation of perfused alveoli (e.g., pulmonary embolism) or inadequate ventilation of nonperfused alveoli (obstructive airway illnesses such as asthma and bronchitis). Alveolar DS can account for 80–90% of Vt in diseased situations. The typical ratio of DS to Vt is 0.3. Vt or RR can be raised to enhance alveolar ventilation. A rapid increase in Vt can lower CO_2, but at the cost of volutrauma, hyperinflation, a mismatch in ventilation to perfusion (V/Q) ratio and undesired CO_2 retention causing positive end-expiratory pressure (auto-PEEP).

Physiology and Dynamics of Ventilation and Oxygenation

For better understanding of the mechanics of breathing, imagine the respiratory system as a single balloon that represents the lung and chest wall connected to a single tube that represents the airways.[1]

Resistance (R)

The resistance of the lungs and chest wall, as well as the airway resistance (80%), make up resistance. Resistance, R = Pressure (cmH_2O)/Flow(s); this formula describes the resistance to air flow in a long, narrow tube. It is inversely proportional to the fourth power of radius and directly proportional to tube length. The glottis and larynx account for less than 10% of total upper airway resistance, with the trachea and the first five generations contributing the remaining 50%. Nasal airway resistance makes up two-thirds of the total resistance of the respiratory system.

Compliance (C)

Compliance refers to the ease of inflation, which depends on the respiratory system's elastic characteristics (chest wall and lungs). Compliance, C = Volume (V)/Pressure (P), can be derived from the slope between two locations on a pressure-volume curve. The PV curve has a steeper slope during inspiration. Functional residual capacity (FRC) determines compliance, which rises with height and age. In healthy youngsters, specific compliance (also known as compliance/FRC) varies from 35 to 45 mL/cmH_2O and is a better predictor of lung elastic characteristics.

Static and Dynamic Compliance

When there is no airflow, static compliance is assessed, and when air is passing through the lungs, dynamic compliance is measured. The relative compliance of the patient and the circuit, and to a lesser extent the resistance determine the proportion of gas exchange volume. In addition to airway resistance, dynamic compliance indicates stiffness in the chest wall and lungs. Both are low in a stiff lung (pulmonary edema, consolidation, etc.). The airway is occluded if only the dynamic compliance has diminished, which could indicate bronchospasm or endotracheal tube (ETT) occlusion. When choosing PEEP for a patient on mechanical ventilation, we use the static compliance curve. The majority of the collapsed alveoli open at the lower inflection point, while overdistension happens beyond the upper inflection point. There is maximum efficiency in ventilation in the linear compliance area. The lowest inflection point is above the PEEP setting. Then, beyond the upper inflection point, peak pressures and maximal Vt can be identified.

Time Constant (TC)

The time constant of a single lung unit is the rate at which it fills. The lung fills (or empties) entirely over a period of five-times constants. R (cmH_2O/s) × C (cmH_2O) equals Tc(s); time constant is the product of compliance and resistance. An insufficient delivery of Vt may result from a very short inspiratory time (Ti). Inadvertent intrinsic or auto-PEEP may result from insufficient expiratory time (Te).

Pulmonary Pressure Gradients

To understand the pressure settings on ventilator, we need to understand the pressure and pressure gradients. Changes in lung volume occur in response to pressure gradients created by thoracic expansion and contraction. There are four different thoracic pressures involved in breathing (**Fig. 20.9.1**).

- Pm = pressure at the mouth
- Palv = pressure in the alveoli (intrapulmonary pressure)
- Ppl = pressure in the pleural space (intrapleural pressure)
- Pbs = pressure at the body surface

In this context, pulmonary pressures will be expressed relative to atmospheric pressure, which is 760 mm Hg or 1 atmosphere. The mouth pressure (Pm) remains at zero unless there is an application of positive pressure to the airway. The pressure at the body surface (Pbs) is consistently 0, except when the patient is undergoing ventilation using a negative pressure ventilator.

Alveolar pressure (Palv) fluctuates during the respiratory cycle. Pleural pressure (Ppl), typically negative during calm respiration, also fluctuates during the respiratory cycle.

Pressure gradients refer to the variations in pressure between different pressures. The mechanics of breathing require three essential pressure gradients: The transairway/transrespiratory transpulmonary, and transthoracic gradients.[1]

1. *Transairway/transrespiratory pressure gradient* refers to the difference in pressure between the atmosphere (Pm) and the alveoli. This gradient is responsible for the movement of gas into and out of the alveoli during breathing.

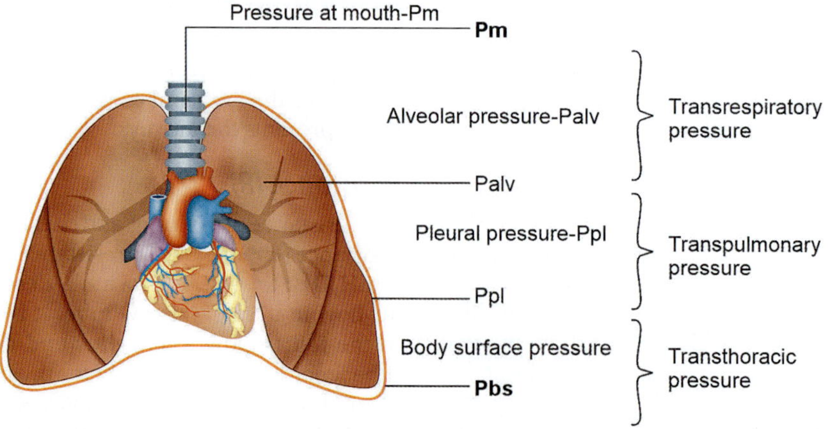

Fig. 20.9.1: Pressure gradient across the respiratory system.

2. *The transpulmonary pressure gradient* refers to the disparity in pressure between the alveoli and the pleural space. This gradient is crucial for sustaining the inflation of the alveoli.
3. *Transthoracic pressure gradient* refers to the pressure gradient between the pressure within the pleural space and the pressure at the body surface. It signifies the overall pressure needed to either expand or contract the lungs and chest wall.

Conceptualize the thorax as a dual compartment system consisting of the airway and the lung. The airway primarily presents resistance, while the lung and chest wall exert elastic forces, which is the inverse of compliance. Air flows through the airway, encountering resistance and subsequently expands the lungs and chest wall, counteracting elastic forces. This pertains to two types of pressures: (1) Transairway or transrespiratory pressure and (2) transthoracic pressure. In volume control positive pressure ventilation, the peak airway pressure indicates changes in the transairway pressure plus transthoracic pressures. Once flows are halted, the only pressure left needed is to inflate the chest wall and maintain lung expansion. This can be demonstrated by an inspiratory hold and the pressure obtained is referred to as plateau pressure. The chest wall often lacks substantial elastic forces in a normal physiological condition, unless there is the presence of edema or elevated abdominal pressure or in other words chest wall is usually highly compliant. Plateau pressure is the result of two opposing forces: The force exerted by the chest wall and the force exerted by the lungs. In order to distinguish between the two, it is necessary to quantify pleural pressure and subsequently transpulmonary pressure.[1]

INDICATIONS AND APPROACH TO MECHANICAL VENTILATION

Respiratory failure is the main reason for using assisted ventilation. Apnea, also known as respiratory arrest, is a severe type of respiratory failure and becomes an absolute indication for mechanical ventilation. Respiratory failure is typically characterized by insufficient oxygenation, insufficient ventilation, or a combination of both. It is advisable to initiate mechanical ventilation prior to the occurrence of respiratory arrest. The common indications are:[3]

- *Hypoxemia (type 1 respiratory failure)*: It is defined as a $PaO_2 \leq 60$ mm Hg ($SaO_2 < 90\%$), e.g., pneumonia and acute respiratory distress syndrome (ARDS).[4]
- *Acute hypoventilation (type 2 respiratory failure)*: It is defined as acute respiratory acidosis [partial pressure of carbon dioxide in arterial blood ($PaCO_2$) > 50–55 mm Hg] with pH <7.25 when ventilatory pump (diaphragm/chest wall muscles) mechanism/their neural control fails. Frequently, respiratory failure is a combination of both hypoxemic and hypercapnic failure.
- *Apnea*: It can be central (absence of respiratory efforts), obstructive (absence of airflow in spite of central drive), or mixed.
- *To reduce the work of breathing (WOB):* Mechanical ventilation decreases the O_2 consumption and relieves discomfort allowing time for the primary disease process to improve, e.g., pneumonia.
- *Anesthesia (secure airway)*: In patients with depressed sensorium, head injury, poor airway reflexes, and in those recovering from anesthesia and during transport of a sick patient. All these patients cannot maintain an intact airway due to tongue fall back, secretions, and poor tone of the laryngeal muscles.
- *To decrease systemic or myocardial O_2 consumption*: Septic and cardiogenic shock
- *To reduce intracranial pressure (ICP):* Controlled hyperventilation causes cerebral vasoconstriction and decreases the ICP.
- *To stabilize the chest wall:* As in flail chest

WHAT IS THE MECHANISM BEHIND THE FUNCTIONING OF A VENTILATOR?

A ventilator primarily facilitates the movement of gas into and out of the lungs. The ventilator receives compressed air and oxygen from the wall through a blender, which can be adjusted to deliver a specific fraction of inspired oxygen (FiO_2). Prior to being delivered to the patient through the breathing circuit, the air-oxygen combination is moistened using a humidifier. When the exhalation valve is closed, it triggers a mechanical breath with positive pressure. Upon reaching the conclusion of the Ti, the exhalation valve is activated, allowing the newborn to release air by exhaling. If there is partial blockage at this end during exhalation, it creates a positive PEEP in the section of the system that is closer to the blockage [or continuous positive airway pressure (CPAP) if the baby is breathing on its own]. Positive pressure breaths can be administered either invasively, through an endotracheal or tracheostomy tube, or noninvasively, through a face mask.[3]

COMPONENTS OF A VENTILATOR[5,6]

Compressor

Compressor is a device that obtains compressed air from the atmosphere and delivers it at a specific pressure (50 PSI) to provide positive pressure ventilation.

Dashboard

Dashboard is an adjustable display monitor with knobs:

- FiO_2
- Peak inspiratory pressure (PIP) (in pressure-controlled mode)

- Tidal volume/minute volume (in volume-controlled mode)
- PEEP
- Measurement of the number of breaths per minute—the RR
- Duration of inhalation (Ti)
- Flow rates

Other parameters measured include mean airway pressure (MAP), I:E ratio (the ratio of Ti to Te), and the expired Vt. Additionally, ventilators visually present wave forms that depict lung function.

Humidifier

The ETT circumvents the normal process of humidification, filtration, and warming in the upper airway. As a result, it is necessary to warm and humidify the inspired gases to avoid hypothermia, thickening of secretions, and damage to the airway lining. Types of humidifiers available are:

- *Basic humidifier:* It adds moisture to the inhaled gas without using a servo control system. An unfavorable aspect is the occurrence of excessive condensation in the tubing, resulting in a decrease in humidity and cooling of the gases by the time they reach the patient.
- *A humidifier with a servo control system* and a heated wire in the tubing. This avoids the build-up of condensation. This system ensures optimal humidification at a temperature of 36-37°C and a relative humidity of 70% at 37°C.

Respiratory Circuit

It is advisable to utilize single-use circuits for each individual. There are specialized pediatric circuits with water traps that can be found in the market.

MODES OF MECHANICAL VENTILATION

There are four basic modes of ventilation **(Flowchart 20.9.1)**.[5,6]

1. *Mandatory or controlled ventilation or continuous mandatory ventilation* (CMV). The clinician sets a minimum rate per minute. Entire breath is machine delivered.
2. *Synchronized intermittent mandatory ventilation (SIMV)*: In SIMV, a set number of mandatory breaths per minute are synchronized with the patient-initiated breaths. Ventilator senses patient's efforts over a brief time period (synchronization window) prior to time of set breath. For example, at a set RR of 30 breaths/min, ventilator will sense patient's effort every 2 seconds during the synchronization window; if patient effort is not detected, ventilator delivers mandatory breath. So, if patient breathes at RR lower than set rate, ventilator provides time-triggered breaths to ensure adequate breaths are delivered. If the patient breathes above the set rate, the extra breaths are allowed and can be supported.
3. *Assist/control ventilation (A/C)*: In this mode, all spontaneous breaths that exceed the trigger sensitivity result in the delivery of a mechanical breath (assist) synchronous to the patient's inspiratory effort. If the patient is apneic, a control breath will be provided at the desired interval.
4. *Supported ventilation*: The breaths are triggered and cycled by the patient but limited by the ventilator, e.g., pressure support ventilation (PSV).

Table 20.9.1 lists the types of breath on a mechanical ventilator.

Flowchart 20.9.1: Modes of mechanical ventilation.

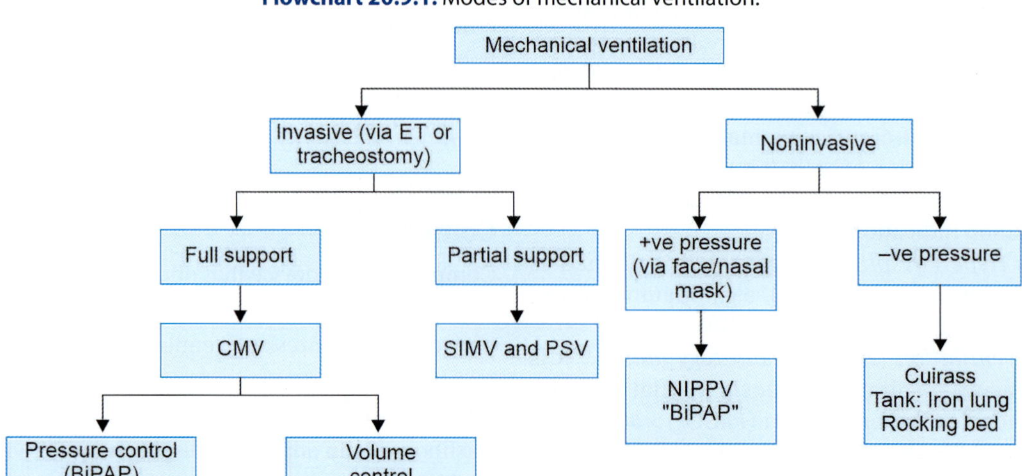

(BiPAP: bilevel positive airway pressure; CMV: continuous mandatory ventilation; ET: endotracheal; NIPPV: noninvasive positive pressure ventilation; PSV: pressure support ventilation; SIMV: synchronized intermittent mandatory ventilation)

TABLE 20.9.1: Types of breath on a mechanical ventilator.

Breath type	Trigger	Phase variable/cycle	Limit
Mandatory	Machine	Machine	Machine
Assisted	Patient	Machine	Machine
Supported	Patient	Patient	Machine
Spontaneous	Patient	Patient	Patient

PHASES OF A VENTILATOR BREATH

A phase variable begins, sustains, and ends one of the four phases of a breath. These four phases are **(Flowchart 20.9.2)**:[7]

1. Change from exhalation to inspiration (trigger variable; time, flow, pressure, and volume triggering)
2. Inspiration (limiting variable; time, pressure, volume, and flow limiting)
3. Change from inspiration to exhalation (cycling variable; volume, time, flow, and pressure cycling)
4. Exhalation (passive process due to elastic recoil of lungs; PEEP is applicable)

Flowchart. 20.9.2: Phases of mechanical ventilation.

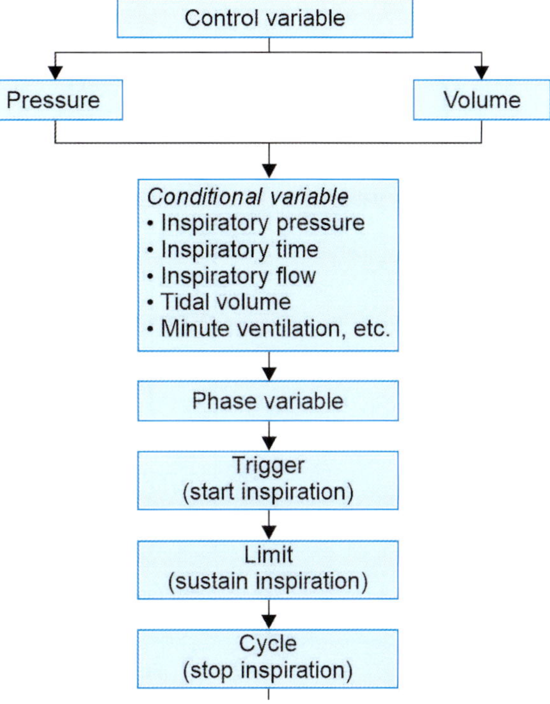

(FRC: functional residual capacity)

Volume-controlled Ventilation

Volume-controlled ventilation (VCV) is a kind of mechanical ventilation where the volume of air delivered to the patient's lungs is controlled. Volume-targeted ventilation or VCV **(Fig. 20.9.2)** is a ventilation mode that seeks to consistently supply a specific Vt. During inspiration, the pressure gradually rises until it reaches the desired Vt. The PIP needed to deliver the desired Vt depends on the lung mechanics, specifically compliance and resistance. The advantages of VCV include the reliable delivery of Vt, reduced risk of lung injury due to excessive Vt (volutrauma), minimized risk of lung collapse due to insufficient Vt (atelectotrauma), and improved stability of arterial CO_2 levels. VCV also provides automatic weaning; pressure support (PIP) needed to achieve the desired Vt gradually drops as the lung compliance improves. In the presence of significant leaks, the volume of air provided (expiratory Vt) may be significantly insufficient, resulting in hypoventilation. Young children have tiny vital capacity and are particularly vulnerable to loss of Vt even with little leaks. Therefore, it is advisable to use cuffed ETTs to minimize air leakage while ventilating children on volume control mode.

Pressure-controlled Ventilation (Fig. 20.9.3)

Pressure-controlled ventilation (PCV) involves regulating the pressure applied to the patient's airway during the breathing cycle.

During positive PCV, the pressure is maintained at a consistent level during the inspiration phase. The movement of gases in the lungs is determined by the pressure difference (PIP - PEEP) and the mechanical properties of the respiratory system. The volume of gas delivered (Vt) is directly related to this pressure difference. When the compliance drops and the resistance increases, the Vt decreases for the same Delta P (pressure difference). The PCV ventilators are configured with the following parameters: Inspiratory duration, RR, PIP, PEEP, and FiO_2. The benefits include a relatively simple design, resistance to major ETT leaks, improved distribution of gas inside the lungs due to the decelerating gas flow pattern, and reduced risk of barotrauma thanks to pressure limitation. One drawback is that the Vt might vary as lung compliance changes, which can result in unintentional hyperventilation and lung injury due to volutrauma.[3]

Table 20.9.2 provides a comparison of pressure- vs. volume-controlled ventilation.

Table 20.9.3 lists the terminologies frequently used during mechanical ventilation.

Trigger Sensitivity

Its objective is to attain synchronization between the patient and the ventilator. The trigger may be activated by either pressure or flow. Traditionally, the majority of ventilators utilized a pressure trigger. The pressure trigger detects a decrease in pressure below the PEEP when the patient breathes naturally. The ventilator maintains a constant flow in the circuit, even when the patient is not actively breathing. During a flow trigger, the ventilator detects any fall in flow

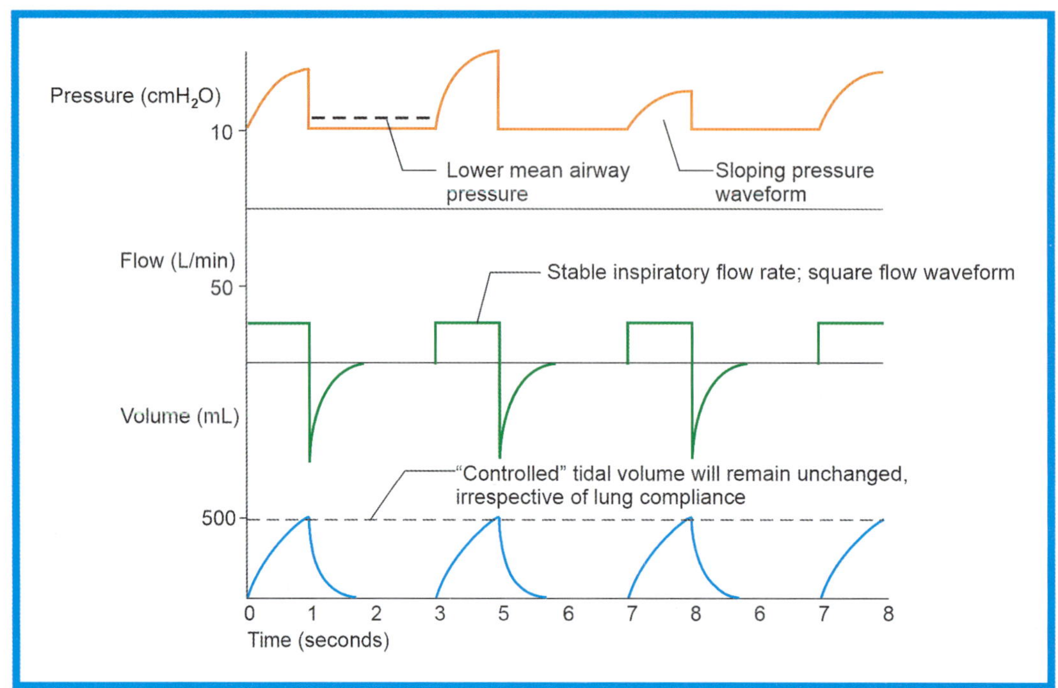

Fig. 20.9.2: Volume-controlled ventilation (PCV).

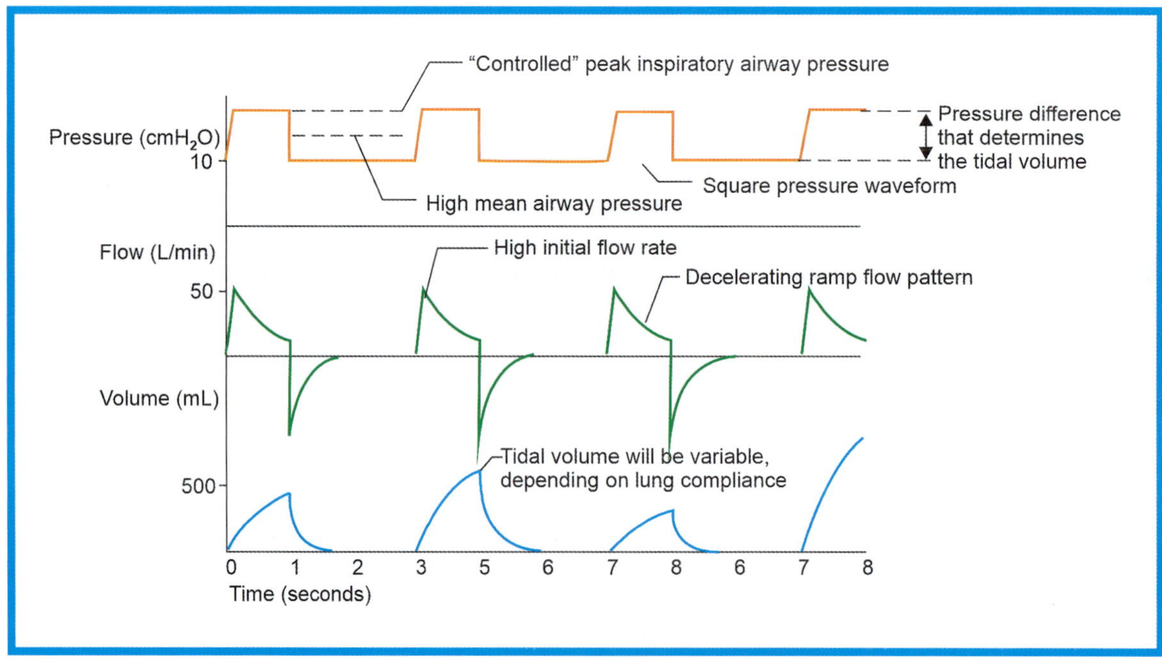

Fig. 20.9.3: Pressure-controlled ventilation (VCV).

below the predetermined bias flow using the expiratory flow sensor, which is interpreted as patient effort. The flow trigger is often chosen over the pressure trigger in most contexts due to its association with reduced WOB. Generally, heightened sensitivity allows the patient to conserve energy when activating the ventilator, resulting in improved patient–ventilator synchronization. Autotriggering refers to the activation of the ventilator due to changes in the airway, such

TABLE 20.9.2: Comparison of pressure- vs. volume-controlled ventilation.

Volume- and pressure-controlled ventilation: Advantages and disadvantages		
	Pressure-controlled ventilation	***Volume-controlled ventilation***
Advantages	• Reduction of peak pressure and risk of barotrauma • Improved gas exchange due to decelerating flow • A more homogeneous ventlation in cases of distribution disorders • Compensation for leaks	• Maintains constant tidal volume • Precise control of $PaCO_2$
Disadvantages	Hypoventilation secondary to changes in lung compliance and resistance	• Potential for high airway pressures and acute lung injury • Inability to compensate for leaks

($PaCO_2$: partial pressure of carbon dioxide in arterial blood)

TABLE 20.9.3: Terminologies frequently used during mechanical ventilation.

• Peak inspiratory pressure (PIP)	• Highest pressure recorded at end of inspiration
• Plateau pressure	• Pressure at end of inspiration and before next expiration by using inspiratory hold knob
• Positive end-expiratory pressure (PEEP)	• Positive distending pressure at the end of expiration
• Mean airway pressure (Paw)	• Average pressure recorded in airways during respiratory cycle
• Inspiratory time (Ti)	• Time of respiratory cycle given for inspiration
• Expiratory time (Te)	• Time of respiratory cycle given for expiration
• Tidal volume (Vt)	• Volume of air delivered with each breath
• Frequency (f)	• Rate of ventilation
• Minute volume	• Vt times frequency

as the presence of water in the circuit, even when there is no real triggering by the patient.

Ventilator Modifications

The clinical state and blood gas levels of the patient are used to decide the ventilator settings. It is recommended that the ventilator settings be adjusted gradually, with modest, accurate steps. It is possible to modify the FiO_2 in increments of 0.05 (5%), the RR in increments of two breaths per minute, the Ti in increments of 0.05 seconds, and the PIP and PEEP values in increments of 1.0 cmH_2O. After a major modification, blood gas analysis can be carried out 20–30 minutes later.[7,8]

Monitoring of a Patient Receiving Mechanical Ventilation

Monitoring is done to reduce side effects such oxygen toxicity, air leakage, ventilator-induced lung damage, and nosocomial infections, and to maximize respiratory assistance.

Signs that there is Enough Ventilation[7,9]

Clinical Characteristics

- Appropriate chest expansion
- Both lungs have satisfactory air entry
- No indications of a retracted chest
- The color pink
- The typical range for capillary filling time (2–3 seconds)
- Ideal blood pressure

Pulse Oximeter

Over 92% oxygen saturation is the ideal level.

Blood Gasses in the Arterial System

- There is a 50–80 mm Hg range in the partial pressure of oxygen in arterial blood (PaO_2).
- The range of $PaCO_2$ is 40–50 mm Hg, with permissive hypercapnia allowing for a maximum of 60 mm Hg.
- There is a 7.35–7.45 pH range.

Assessing the Body's Oxygen Saturation Level

The arterial blood gas (ABG) measures the percentage of oxyhemoglobin saturation and instantaneously measures the blood's PaO_2.[9] A simple, noninvasive device used to measure SpO_2 at the bedside is the pulse oximeter. An accurate way to measure arterial oxygen saturation is with pulse oximetry, especially when the SaO_2 level is higher than 60%. However, it is unable to identify hyperoxia. Furthermore, under circumstances of circulatory shock or local edema, it understates the saturation of arterial oxygen (SaO_2). Moreover, the precision of the test is affected in the presence of other forms of hemoglobin, such as metHb or COHb. For children, an oxygen saturation level (SpO_2) of >92% is ideal. However, a target SaO_2 of 70–75% is deemed appropriate for kids with cyanotic congenital heart disease, provided that other tissue oxygenation markers, like mixed venous oxygen saturation (MvO_2) above 60% and lactate levels below 2, stay within normal bounds.[7]

Keeping an Eye on Ventilation

The $PaCO_2$ readings show how well ventilation is working. Since peripheral venous samples may contain errors in pH and $PaCO_2$ measurements, arterial samples are the better option. Capnography measures end-tidal CO_2 levels (quantitative $ETCO_2$) and can also measure DS, breathing rate and rhythm, ETT location, displacement or obstruction, and asynchrony between the patient and ventilator. Transcutaneous CO_2 detectors and capnography are the two noninvasive techniques for determining CO_2 concentrations.[8,9]

Radiography

A chest radiograph is employed to verify the positioning of central lines, umbilical catheters, and ETTs. In adolescents, the optimal location for an ETT is often one to one and a half inches above the carina. However, the ideal arrangement might be different for younger kids. It can also show abnormalities in the shape of the heart and lung capacity, such as atelectasis or overexpansion. The lungs extend to the 10th rib when the diaphragm flattens, indicating excessive expansion and an increased risk of pulmonary air leaks and lung damage.

VENTILATOR TROUBLESHOOTING

A child on ventilation may experience abrupt deterioration for the following main reasons:[8]

- D: Tube displacement
- O: Blockage in the tube
- P: Pneumothorax
- E: Equipment malfunction

Corrective interventions are necessary for respiratory distress, as previously described (DOPE). The most feared complication in a ventilator is pneumothorax, which requires thoracentesis or immediate needle aspiration of the second intercostal space, followed by the placement of an intercostal drainage (ICD) tube into the fourth or fifth intercostal space for continuous drainage.

When high PEEP is employed, hypotension can occur as a result of diminished venous return. Pneumonia related with ventilators: Develops following 48 hours of mechanical breathing. The use of contaminated equipment or aerosolized drugs, colonization of the aerodigestive tract, recurrent micro aspiration of oropharyngeal secretions, and the use of an ETT or tracheostomy tube are the risk factors for ventilator-associated pneumonia (VAP).

The damage caused to the lungs by mechanical ventilation is known as ventilator induced lung injury. Among the mechanisms of ventilator-induced lung injury (VILI) are:

- *Trauma to the lungs*—damage brought on by excessive lung distension
- *Barotrauma*—high pressure that can harm the epithelium of the airways and disturb the alveoli
- *Atelectotrauma*—harm brought on by recurrent cycles of alveolar recruitment and derecruitment
- *Biotrauma*—harmful effects on the lungs caused by inflammation, infection, and oxidative damage
- *Rheotrauma*—damage brought on by an improper airflow.

REFERENCES

1. Shaffner DH, McCloskey JJ, Huny EA, Tasker RC (Eds). Roger's Textbook of Pediatric Intensive Care, 6th edition. Philadelphia: Wolters Kluwer; 2024.
2. Lands LC. Applying physiology to conventional mechanical ventilation. Paediatr Respir Rev. 2006;7 Suppl 1:S33-6.
3. Khilnani P (Ed). Practical Approach to Pediatric Intensive Care. New Delhi: Jaypee Brothers Medical Publishers Pvt. Ltd.; 2020.
4. Emeriaud G, López-Fernández YM, Iyer NP, Bembea MM, Agulnik A, Barbaro RP, et al.; Second Pediatric Acute Lung Injury Consensus Conference (PALICC-2) Group on behalf of the Pediatric Acute Lung Injury and Sepsis Investigators (PALISI) Network. Executive Summary of the Second International Guidelines for the Diagnosis and Management of Pediatric Acute Respiratory Distress Syndrome (PALICC-2). Pediatr Crit Care Med. 2023;24(2):143-68.
5. Chatburn RL. Understanding mechanical ventilators. Expert Rev Respir Med. 2010;4(6):809-19.
6. Chatburn AL. Classification of mechanical ventilators. Respir Care. 1992;37(9):1009-25.
7. Jubran A, Tobin MJ. Monitoring during mechanical ventilation. Clin Chest Med. 1996;17(3):453-73.
8. Cairo JM, Hinski ST (Eds). Workbook For Pilbeam's Mechanical Ventilation: Physiological And Clinical Applications, 8th edition. Elsevier; 2023.
9. Kliegman RM, Stanton BF, Geme III JWS, Schor NF, Behrman RE (Eds). Nelson Textbook of Pediatrics, 21st edition. Philadelphia: Elsevier; 2020.

20.10 Neurological Emergencies: Clinical Recognition and Management

Namita Ravikumar, Arun Bansal

INTRODUCTION

Neuroemergencies in children are not only associated with high mortality but also lead to significant life-long morbidity due to neurosequelae. Neurological injury is due to both primary and secondary insults, which can occur due to delay in identification, stabilization, and/or inadequate management of the primary pathology or as a result of complications.

Broad categorization of the neurological emergencies include traumatic brain injury (TBI) and nontraumatic brain injury (NTBI), both of which present with common clinical manifestations, namely encephalopathy, seizures, and features of raised intracranial pressure (ICP). The mechanism of brain injury in trauma is a sudden, profound insult, whereas there is a wide variation in NTBI based on whether the etiology is infectious, inflammatory, vascular, or neoplastic.[1]

There are certain differences between pediatric and adult nervous system—higher plasticity of central nervous system (CNS) in children can help recover better than in adult but damage incurred during critical stages of brain development in infancy could be more detrimental. Most of the management protocols in pediatric neurocritical care are extrapolated from adult studies, especially in TBI.[1]

TRAUMATIC BRAIN INJURY

The mechanical forces during trauma like contact force and acceleration/deceleration forces lead to primary insult. Secondary insult could be attributed to hypoxic-ischemic injury, edema, seizures, hyperthermia, hypo- or hypertension, and metabolic derangements. Most common causes of TBI include road traffic accidents and fall from height. TBI has been classified as mild, moderate, and severe. Although mild TBI is most common (75%), it may lead to secondary insult if not managed adequately. The prevalence rate for severe TBI is about 5.4 per 100,000 population per year.[1]

Head Injury Patterns

- Blunt injury
- Sharp injury
- Compression injury
- Penetrating/blast injury

Types of Intracranial Injury

- *Focal cortical gray matter*:
  - Hemorrhagic
  - Nonhemorrhagic
- Diffuse axonal injury
- *Secondary injury*:
  - Edema
  - Hemorrhage

NONTRAUMATIC BRAIN INJURY

Nontraumatic coma in childhood is a common pediatric emergency. The incidence of nontraumatic coma is 30/100,000 children per year. Altered consciousness is the most common presentation followed by seizures and raised ICP. Altered consciousness varies in spectrum from lethargy, obtundation, and stupor to coma. This needs to be differentiated from persistent vegetative state, locked-in state, and akinetic mutism. The most common cause of nontraumatic coma in developing countries is infection, which includes tubercular meningitis (TBM) (19%), encephalitis (18%), and bacterial meningitis (16%). Other causes are toxic-metabolic encephalopathies (19%), status epilepticus (10%), intracranial bleed (7%), and others (4%).[2]

CONCEPT OF INTRACRANIAL PRESSURE AND CEREBRAL PERFUSION PRESSURE

Cranial cavity in children with fused sutures and anterior fontanelle is a closed compartment. According to the Monro–Kellie hypothesis, the brain, blood spaces, and cerebrospinal fluid (CSF) form a closed compartment, and increase in volume of any one compartment compromises the blood flow to the brain **(Fig. 20.10.1)**. Hence, cerebral edema or blockage of CSF drainage can increase the ICP. Cerebral vasodilation can also increase the ICP by increasing the volume of the blood compartment in the skull. Normal ICP in infants is about 10 mm Hg. ICP >20 mm Hg is detrimental and can cause secondary brain injury. Cerebral perfusion pressure (CPP) is the difference between mean arterial pressure (MAP) and ICP. Maintaining the CPP >55 mm Hg in children and >65 mm Hg in adults have been found to have better outcomes than merely targeting ICP lower than 20 mm Hg. Fluid bolus and vasoactive therapy are used to increase the MAP to target the CPP.[1]

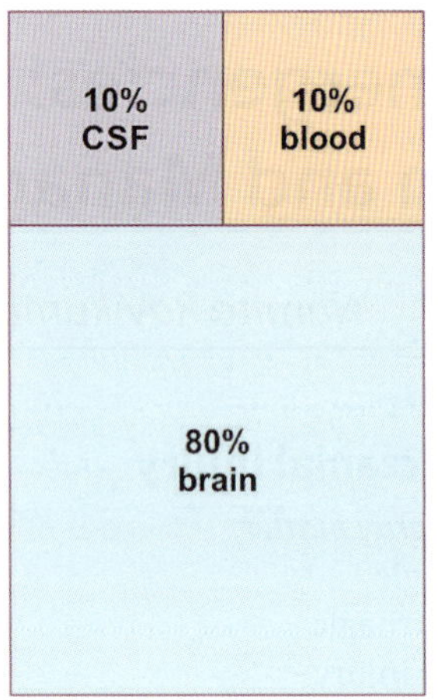

Fig. 20.10.1: The closed cranial compartment depicting brain, blood, and cerebrospinal fluid (CSF) spaces as per Monro–Kellie hypothesis.

Factors Determining Cerebral Perfusion Pressure, Clinical Monitoring, and Targets

- *Blood pressure (BP):* As MAP has a direct effect on CPP, MAP should be maintained between 50th and 90th centile to target CPP >55 mm Hg in children on invasive ICP monitoring.
- *Temperature:* Rise in core body temperature by 1°C can increase cerebral metabolism and increase ICP. Cerebral blood flow (CBF) increases by 7% with every 1°C rise in core body temperature.
- *Hypoxemia:* Hypoxemia causes vasoconstriction and reduced cerebral perfusion. Therefore, SpO_2 to be targeted >92%.
- *Hypercarbia/hypocarbia:* CO_2 is a potent cerebral vasodilator and can cause increase in ICP. Low CO_2 decreases cerebral perfusion by vasoconstriction. Therefore pCO_2 needs to be maintained in the narrow range of 35–40 mm Hg. A change of 11–15 mL/100 g/min in CBF occurs for every 7 mm Hg change in paCO2.
- *Position of head:* Ensure optimal cerebral venous drainage by elevation of head to 30º, thereby preventing kinking of neck veins. Elevation of head beyond 45º decreases the CBF and if less than 15–20º cerebral venous drainage is reduced.
- *Analgesia:* Any painful stimulus can increase ICP and needs to be controlled with adequate analgesia by targeting sedation and pain scores.
- *Seizure:* Seizure leads to increase in oxygen consumption, hypoxia, and rebound increase in ICP. Hence, seizure needs to be controlled by appropriate antiepileptic drugs. Nonconvulsive status epilepticus (NCSE) is also very common in intensive care unit (ICU), which can be detected by continuous electroencephalogram (EEG) monitoring and requires adequate treatment.

CLINICAL PRESENTATION

Traumatic brain injury presents with altered consciousness, seizures, ear, nose, and throat (ENT) bleeds and focal neurological deficits. NTBI can vary in presentation depending on the etiology, but the most common presentations include fever, encephalopathy, seizures, focal neurological deficits, and shock.[1]

INITIAL STABILIZATION

Assessing ABCDE forms the foremost part of the management of both TBI and NTBI.

Airway

Airway can be open and stable, maintainable or obstructed. Simple maneuvers like positioning and suctioning can clear the airway, while some may require advanced airway in the form of endotracheal intubation. In TBI, associated cervical spine injuries are commonly seen which requires cervical spine stabilization with cervical collar. Head-tilt chin left maneuver needs to be avoided and jaw thrust should be performed to keep airway open. Intubation in suspected raised ICP should be done by rapid sequence intubation with lignocaine and adequate sedaoanalgesia to prevent ICP spikes.

Breathing

Disordered control of breathing in neurological diseases can lead to apnea/bradypnea, irregular jerky breathing, or hyperventilation. Ventilatory support may be required in cases of abnormal breathing for controlled ventilation.

Circulation

Children may present in cardiorespiratory arrest or shock. Hypertension and bradycardia along with abnormal respiration form a part of Cushing triad, suggestive of late stage of raised ICP. Fluid boluses with vasoactive support may be required to maintain MAP >50th centile to ensure CPP.

Disability

Consciousness can be assessed using the modified Glasgow Coma Scale (GCS) or AVPU (alert, voice, pain, and unresponsive) scale. Symmetry of movements, posturing, seizures, pupillary size, and reaction are noted. Asymmetry of limb movements suggest paresis, and raised ICP can present with decerebrate posturing. Unequal pupils suggest uncal herniation. Blood glucose level needs to be checked and corrected if hypoglycemia is found.

Exposure

Whole body needs to be examined for presence of external injuries and fractures in case of trauma. The presence of rash, bleeding points, fever, or hypothermia is noted to give a clue in etiology.

EVALUATION

History

A good history can provide a clue into the etiology, neurodeficits, and complications.

- In TBI, history should focus on the details of the injury, force causing the injury, and the site of impact. Important details postinjury include change in consciousness including lucid interval, ENT bleeds, seizures, and features of raised ICP.
- In NTBI, duration of illness can guide us as to the acute, subacute, or chronic nature of illness. Detailed history can help identify the etiology including infectious, inflammatory, vascular, or neoplastic.
- Focality of symptoms such as cranial nerve palsies, and asymmetry of limb movements help in localization of lesion.
- History of chronic illness, any ingestions, clues to metabolic encephalopathy like sibling loss, consanguinity, and history of travel to endemic areas assist in establishing the etiology.

Examination

Vitals

Heart rate (HR)

- *Tachycardia (HR > mean + 2 SD for age)*: Fever, shock, seizure (convulsive or nonconvulsive), and sympathetic toxidrome increase the HR. Nonconvulsive status can present with unexplained tachycardia in a child with altered sensorium.
- *Bradycardia (HR <mean – 2 SD for age)*: It is seen with raised ICP, late stages of shock, electrolyte abnormalities, and hypothermia. It is a late sign of raised ICP and in association with hypertension and altered respiration forms part of Cushing triad. It may also be seen in toxin ingestions like sedatives.

Blood pressure

- *Hypertension (BP >95th centile)*: Increase in BP due to raised ICP occurs to maintain CPP and should not be chased to decrease, as it can precipitate fall in CPP. Hypertensive emergency can also present with encephalopathy, and targeting the MAP to 95th centile is the principal management. Hypertension can also be a part of sympathetic toxidrome.

TABLE 20.10.1: Types of breathing patterns in neurological cases.

Type	*Description*	*Causes*
Tachypnea	Increased RR	Fever and shock
Bradypnea	Decreased RR	Metabolic, sedative drugs, and decreased CNS drive
Apnea	Cessation of breathing	Metabolic, sedative drugs, and decreased CNS drive
Cheyne–Stokes	Gradual increase and decrease in breathing with periods of apnea	Raised ICP and brain stem injury
Biots	Rapid deep respiration with short pauses	TBI and other CNS causes
Kussmaul	Tachypnea with hyperpnea	Metabolic acidosis
Apneustic	Prolonged inspiration with short expiration	Brain stem lesion

(CNS: central nervous system; ICP: intracranial pressure; TBI: traumatic brain injury; RR: respiratory rate)

- *Hypotension (BP <5th centile)*: It may be seen due to neurogenic shock or sedative overdose. This can cause cerebral hypoperfusion and lead to watershed area infarcts.

Respiration: Based on the anatomical location of lesion, various breathing patterns can be seen like Cheyne-Stokes and Apneustic and Biots breathing **(Table 20.10.1)**.

Temperature:

- *Hyperthermia (core body temperature >38.5°C)*: It is seen in infectious causes. Hyperpyrexia (core body temperature >41.5°C with reset of hypothalamic set point) is known in significant CNS damage involving pontine and hypothalamic areas. It may also be a part of anticholinergic toxidrome.
- *Hypothermia (<36°C):* It is seen in infants with infections and may be missed if not looked for.

General Examination

Head to toe examination is done to look for presence of other injuries in TBI. Fractures, abdominal, thoracic, and pelvic injuries need to be ruled out as they can cause occult bleeding and lead to shock. Head size by occipitofrontal circumference, facial dysmorphology, and neurocutaneous markers are points in favor of genetic disorders. Rash, conjunctival congestion, anemia, and jaundice may point toward tropical infections.

Systemic Examination

CNS: Higher mental functions including consciousness, speech, and memory are examined to the extent that is

TABLE 20.10.2: Types of pupil with localization.

Pupil appearance	Etiology/Localization
Small, reactive	Metabolic, hypothalamic
Large, nonreactive, hippus	Tectal
Pinpoint	Pontine, opiate intoxication
Mid-position fixed	Midbrain
Ipsilateral dilated, fixed	Oculomotor nerve, uncal herniation
Bilateral dilated, fixed	Severe hypoxic-ischemic encephalopathy
Dilated and fixed	Anticholinergic poisoning

possible. Cranial nerve examination includes assessment of smell, vision, extraocular movements, pupils, facial symmetry, gag reflex, and neck, shoulder, and jaw movements. Pupil can act as a window to the brain and help in localization **(Table 20.10.2)**. Asymmetry of limb movements suggest focal defects leading to paresis. Muscle wasting suggests lower motor neuron involvement. Deep tendon reflexes (DTR) may be brisk suggesting corticospinal tract involvement and raised ICP. Extensor response of plantars may again suggest upper motor neuron involvement. Sensory examination and cerebellar signs elicited as feasible. Signs of meningeal irritation are present in case of meningitis. Examination of the spine is an important component in both TBI and NTBI.

Other systemic examination: Presence of hepatosplenomegaly helps in diagnosing tropical infections. Respiratory examination for differential air entry is essential to rule out hemo-/pneumothorax in cases of trauma. Similarly muffling of heart sounds may suggest cardiac tamponade.

BEDSIDE NEUROMONITORING TOOLS

Various tools have been developed over the years for bedside monitoring of neurological status.

Noninvasive Tools

Electroencephalogram

Electroencephalogram is a record of brain electrical activity by placing scalp electrodes. This electrical activity is mainly due to the neurons of the outermost layer of the cortex. Different types include conventional EEG, compressed spectral array, and amplitude integrated EEG. It can be done continuously bedside or intermittent detailed EEG. Continuous EEG bedside is a noninvasive monitoring of electrical seizures. It can identify NCSE and location of pathology when there are focal seizures. In deeply sedated and paralyzed children, continuous EEG monitoring becomes essential as they may not show convulsive movement. It is also used to assess response to therapy for NCSE or electrical silence for refractory raised ICP in the form of burst suppression. The characteristic triphasic waves in EEG are seen in hepatic encephalopathy. It can provide information to assess the severity of encephalopathy and in prognostication based on the evoked potentials. Bedside EEG requires separate earthing to avoid interference with other devices in the pediatric intensive care unit (PICU).

Near-infrared Spectroscopy

Near-infrared spectroscopy (NIRS) works on the principle of Beer-Lambert law similar to pulse oximetry and measures regional cerebral oxygen saturation (rSO_2). A continuous-wave spectrometer is most commonly used in clinical devices. Some devices measure "time of flight", which can accurately measure the path length of light. Phase-resolved spectroscopy emits light that is modulated at a known frequency and assesses the phase shift of the transmitted light to derive the path length. Although normative values are yet to be established, it is around 68 ± 10% in healthy children. It differs from pulse oximetry as it does not require pulsatile blood flow. There is no gold standard to compare rSO_2, but it is found to correlate with jugular venous saturation ($SjVO_2$).

Transcranial Doppler

Transcranial Doppler (TCD) is used to assess regional CBF in cerebral arteries and identify perfusion abnormalities in anterior, middle, and posterior circulations. It has been used most commonly for the middle cerebral artery (MCA). In the PICU, its utility lies in measuring blood flow velocities due to vasopressor-induced changes, assessing intactness of cerebral autoregulation, and detecting cerebral vasospasm. In children with sickle cell anemia, TCD is used to assess risk of stroke based on time-averaged mean maximum (TAMM) blood-flow velocity in internal carotid and middle cerebral arteries. TAMM >200 cm/sec is at risk for cerebrovascular accident.

Ocular Ultrasonography for Optic Nerve Sheath Diameter

Optic nerve sheath diameter (ONSD) has been used to detect early raised ICP due to edema. Ultrasonographic examination is performed in both the eyes to measure the ONSD 3 mm behind the globe. Various studies have found the upper limit of normal as 4.5 mm in >1 year of age and 4 mm for <1 year of age. Interobserver variation of 0.1 mm has been found.

Invasive Monitoring

Intracranial Pressure Monitoring

Invasive monitoring of ICP can be done by placing invasive catheters, which are intraparenchymal, subdural, or intraventricular. In comatose children (GCS <8), it gives an objective assessment and can help titrate therapy for raised ICP. Invasive ICP monitoring guides in therapy by giving real-time values. ICP catheter with fiber sensor requires zero calibration prior to insertion and a reference code obtained during insertion. Targeting CPP (MAP-ICP) against ICP-targeted therapy has shown better outcomes both in TBI and in NTBI. Intraventricular catheters can help drain CSF to relieve pressure in addition to monitoring ICP.

Regional Brain Tissue Oxygen Monitoring

Intracranial tissue monitoring is placed alongside ICP catheter in frontal cortex to measure regional partial pressure tissue oxygen and cerebral microdialysis. Here, fluorescent dye is used, which responds to oxygen. Partial pressure of oxygen can also be measured using Clark electrode. Normal values of brain tissue oxygen ($PbtO_2$) are found to be around 25–30 mm Hg, which correlates with normal CPP and ICP.

- Threshold of 20 mm Hg—considered as margin of safety to prevent hypoxia
- <15 mm Hg—significant risk of hypoxia
- <10 mm Hg—ongoing ischemia

The limitation includes that it detects regional rather than global changes.

Brain Tissue Microdialysis

Microdialysis catheter is inserted into the brain, and a perfusion fluid is delivered through a microdialysis pump. This fluid equilibrates with extracellular brain fluid, and samples collected from catheter can be analyzed by an analyzer. Levels of glucose, pyruvate, lactate, glutamate, and other amino acids can be measured.

RADIOLOGICAL INVESTIGATIONS AND MONITORING

Noncontrast Computed Tomography of Brain

Noncontrast computed tomography (NCCT) of brain is the investigation of choice in trauma to diagnose bony injury, intracranial bleed, and obstructive hydrocephalus. CT images of the spine are done to rule out spine fractures. In NTBI, NCCT can reveal edema, infarcts, neoplasms, and inflammatory lesions in the form of hypodense areas, which further require characterization by contrast imaging. Repeat imaging may be required in TBI to see progression of bleed, especially if GCS is worsening. CT brain may help in prognostication by using validated scores—Traumatic Coma Databank (TCDB) CT classification and the Rotterdam CT score, which have correlation with Glasgow Outcome Score. CT takes less time, can be done without requiring much cooperation from the child and lesser sedation.

Contrast Computed Tomography of Brain

Contrast computed tomography of brain helps identify meningeal enhancement in meningitis and intracranial space-occupying lesions (ICSOL) like tumors, brain abscess, tuberculoma, and neurocysticercosis, which show perilesional contrast enhancement. Basal exudates in TBM are well appreciated in contrast images.

Magnetic Resonance Imaging of Brain

Magnetic resonance imaging (MRI) is essential for detailed assessment of gray and white matter and for posterior fossa structures. In trauma, MRI is the imaging modality of choice to look for spinal cord injury. Acute ischemia is best differentiated by diffusion-weighted and susceptibility-weighted MRI. MR angiography/venography are best for visualizing vascular structures of the brain. Spectroscopic imaging analyses signals generated by certain metabolites useful in inborn errors of metabolism. The major disadvantages of MRI are longer duration needed for imaging; requires procedural sedation, and is contraindicated in the presence of metallic implants.

LABORATORY INVESTIGATIONS

Blood Investigations

- Total and differential counts for suspected neuroinfections
- Hemoglobin, platelet count, and coagulogram in trauma and nontraumatic bleed
- Renal function, liver function, electrolytes, blood glucose, and ammonia to rule out metabolic causes of encephalopathy
- Blood culture for suspected sepsis
- Toxicology screen for suspected poisoning

Cerebrospinal Fluid

- Cytology—for meningitis and encephalitis
- Biochemistry—glucose and protein
- Microbiology—Gram stain, cultures, and viral serology

TREATMENT

Management of Raised Intracranial Pressure—Tiers of Treatment[3]

First-line Measures

- Head end elevation up to 30° to facilitate easy venous drainage from head and neck
- Midline position to avoid compression of jugular veins
- *Osmotherapy:*
  - 3% saline bolus of 5–10 mL/kg followed by infusion at 0.1–1 mL/kg/h and can be titrated to target serum Na 145–150 mEq/L

TABLE 20.10.3: Antimicrobial therapy for central nervous system (CNS) infections.

Diagnosis	Drug	Dose	Duration
Pyogenic meningitis	Intravenous (IV) ceftriaxone	100 mg/kg/day in two divided doses	7–10 days
Herpes encephalitis	IV acyclovir	60 mg/kg/day in three divided doses (dilution minimum of 5 mg/mL given over 1 hour)	14–21 days
Cerebral malaria	IV artesunate	2.4 mg/kg at 0, 12, and 24 hours and then OD	Total 7 doses
Scrub typhus	IV/oral doxycycline	5 mg/kg in two divided doses	5–7 days

  - Mannitol 20% for raised ICP has raised concerns, as it can lead to fall in BP and consequently CPP. Persistent spikes of ICP and impending herniation can be treated with mannitol 0.25–0.5 g/kg with cautious BP and urine output monitoring.
- Sedation and analgesia in intubated children to avoid unnecessary stimulus leading to increase in ICP
- Maintaining normothermia (35.5–36.5°C), normocarbia (35–40 mm Hg), normoxemia (>92% saturation), and normoglycemia (80–140 mg/dL)

Second-line Measures

Surgical therapy for mass lesions or obstructive hydrocephalus is needed. Decompressive craniotomy in refractory raised ICP, especially in TBI, has improved mortality but is residual morbidity remains high.

Third-line Measures

Barbiturate coma, hypothermia, and hyperventilation are the last tiers in the management of raised ICP.

Specific Therapy

Traumatic Brain Injury

Mild TBI and moderate TBI with negative CT may only require close observation. Mild neurological deficits and small hemorrhages also need monitoring and observation. Urgent evacuation is necessary for acute bleeds associated with midline shift, those causing significant worsening in GCS, and that which increases over time. Timely compressive craniotomy for TBI has shown improvement in mortality.

Nontraumatic Brain Injury

The treatment depends on the cause and includes antibacterial and antiviral therapies for infections (**Table 20.10.3**), immunomodulatory drugs for inflammatory lesions, and chemo-/radiotherapy for neoplastic lesions.

Supportive Therapy

Seizures are controlled using benzodiazepine (BZD) as initial antiepileptic followed by phenytoin, levetiracetam, valproate, or phenobarbitone if not responding to BZD. Status epilepticus is managed as per protocol. Mechanical ventilation to achieve targets of oxygenation and ventilation may be needed. Shock is managed as per protocol.[4]

PROGNOSIS

Prognosis depends on the etiology, degree, and extent of injury in both TBI and NTBI. Deep coma (GCS <6), abnormal respiration pattern, hypothermia, hypotensive shock, and abnormal tone (flaccidity) have been associated with poor prognosis. The functional status can be assessed on follow up using the Pediatric Overall Performance Category and Pediatric Cerebral Performance Category (POPC/PCPC) scales.

REFERENCES

1. Chapters 57 and 58. In: Nichols DG, Shaffner DH (Ed). Roger's Textbook of Pediatric Intensive Care, 5th edition. Philadelphia: ©Wolters Kluwer; 2016.
2. Jindal A, Singhi SC, Singhi P. Non-Traumatic Coma and Altered Mental Status. Indian J Pediatr. 2012;79(3):367-75.
3. Kumar RR, Singhi SC, Singhi P. Raised Intracranial Pressure (ICP): Management in Emergency Department. Indian J Pediatr. 2012;79(4):518-24.
4. Sasidaran K, Singhi SC, Singhi P. Management of Acute Seizure and Status Epilepticus in Pediatric Emergency. Indian J Pediatr. 2012;79(4):510-7.

20.11 Intrahospital and Interhospital Transport of Critically Ill Child

Jyothi Jayaram, Banani Poddar

INTRODUCTION

Transporting a critically ill child is a complex and high-risk process which requires meticulous planning, necessary equipment and skilled personnel. This is to ensure safe and effective care during transit, minimizing adverse events and optimizing patient outcomes. In this chapter, we discuss the importance of intrahospital and interhospital transport of critically ill children, the types of transport policies, modes of transport, physiological changes during transport, adverse events, risks versus benefits, and the key components of a successful transport process.

WHY IS THE TRANSPORT OF CRITICALLY ILL CHILDREN IMPORTANT?

Transporting critically ill children within a hospital (intrahospital transport) or between different hospitals (interhospital transport) is a complex and potentially risky process that requires careful planning, specialized equipment, and a skilled healthcare team. The critically ill child may deteriorate further during transport if adequate preparation is not done. At the same time, certain diagnostic and therapeutic procedures cannot be done at the bedside or at all levels of healthcare, and hence, intrahospital and interhospital transport become essential.

During any intra- or interhospital transport, the team should try to maintain the same level of care as is provided for a critically ill child in the pediatric intensive care unit (PICU). This includes transport to a diagnostic department, operating room, or specialized care unit in the same hospital or to another hospital. For interhospital transport, this is accomplished by shifting the patient to the nearest facility providing the best level of specialized care. Patient continuity of care should be the goal of both the receiving and the transferring facility. Patient morbidity and death can be considerably increased by an ill-planned and hasty patient transfer.

TYPES OF TRANSPORT[1]

- *Intrahospital transport:* Within the hospital from one place to another.
- *Interhospital transport:* Between different hospitals.
- *Scene run:* From a nonmedical location to the nearest available or designated hospitals.

Intrahospital Transfer

The rationale for transferring a sick child from one site (e.g., ward or emergency) to another (PICU) within the same facility is the need for additional care, including experience and specialized technology that is not accessible at the current location. This also covers the transfer of patients from PICU to operating rooms or to facilities for imaging and radiodiagnosis.

Interhospital Transport

The general indications for transporting a critically ill child from one facility to another are:

- A scarcity of resources and experience to manage the seriously-ill child after initial stabilization.
- A multidisciplinary team approach and care that could be necessary due to the child's serious illness or ailment.
- Involving specialists in subspecialties that are employed by tertiary or quaternary educational institutions.

TYPES OF TRANSPORT POLICIES[1]

There are two types of transport policies:

1. *"Stand and Play"*
    - Transporting the patient only after stabilizing.
    - This is the policy that is followed most, especially during long transport.
2. *"Scoop and Run"*
    - Transporting the patient without wasting much time at the scene.
    - This policy is followed in trauma and bleeding situations or where facilities for stabilization are limited or not available.
    - Even in these situations, stabilization of the airway and fluid resuscitation, if possible, should be done.

MODE OF TRANSPORT[1]

The choice of the mode of transport is determined by several factors, including:

- Severity of illness or injury
- Distance to the referring hospital
- Weather and traffic conditions

Patient transfers occur primarily via two modes: (1) Ground transport, which includes ambulances, and mobile intensive care units (MICUs), and (2) air transport, which includes helicopter or plane. During air transport, the patient has to be moved to the helipad or airport by ground transport, and hence ends up in multiple transports. The relative advantages of each of the modes of transports are listed in **Table 20.11.1**. In the case of intrahospital transfer, patients are typically moved through hospital corridors using a bed or a stretcher.

PHYSIOLOGICAL CHANGES DURING TRANSPORT

During transport, there can be accelerating and decelerating changes due to movement which can lead to significant hemodynamic, respiratory, and neurological changes in the patient. Also, changes in environment, temperature, noise, and equipment can further add to hemodynamic changes. These should be addressed to prevent adverse events during transport.[2]

ADVERSE EVENTS DURING TRANSPORT

Around 68% of adverse events (AEs) during transport are of any severity, whereas 4.2% to 8.9% of AEs are serious.[2,3] Bergman et al. discovered that equipment was a contributor in about 34% of AE.[4] Human errors also contribute to AEs mainly due to patient mix up and poor communication **(Fig. 20.11.1)**.

RISKS VERSUS BENEFITS[1]

Transporting critically unwell children increases their risk of morbidity and death since they have labile physiological factors. The advantages of the transfer must exceed the risks associated with the child's existing clinical status. It is important for the referring physician to wait until they are certain that the child's condition is optimal before transferring the child to the referring hospital.

KEY COMPONENTS OF TRANSPORT

The steps in planning and executing an interhospital transport are shown in **Table 20.11.2**.

Decision to Transfer and Communication

The decision to transfer the child is crucial since it exposes the child and the staff to extra risk as well as additional expenditure for the relatives and the hospital. A senior consultant-level physician makes the choice to transfer the patient after carefully discussing the advantages and disadvantages with the patient's family. Prior to the transfer, the patient's relatives must provide their written, informed consent for the transfer. Direct communication between the transferring and receiving facilities should be initiated, with the sharing of complete information in a written document with respect to patient's clinical status, treatment being administered, reasons for transfer, mode of transfer, and timeline of transfer.

Planning

A standardized transfer plan is created and evaluated on a regular basis as part of a quality improvement process.

Preparation

Before transfer, the patient should be well prepared and stabilized to avoid any adverse events or deterioration in the patient's clinical status. Without unnecessary delay, it is imperative to provide the patient with optimal care and stabilization. Patient's airway, breathing, circulation, and disability, should be assessed during the process of preparation, and any related preventable problems should be fixed. In this situation, using a pretransfer checklist is helpful.[6,7]

- *Is the airway patent and sustainable?* If not, it needs to be secured before the patient is moved. Once intubated, check for end-tidal CO_2 and document the depth of the endotracheal tube placement on chest X-ray. Ensure that the endotracheal tube is securely attached, and that suction is available to maintain the patency of the endotracheal tube.

TABLE 20.11.1: Comparison of modes of transport.[9]

	Ground ambulance	***Fixed-wing aircraft***	***Helicopter***
Availability	Easy availability (most common)	Rare	Rare
Safety	Good	Good	Good
Cabin environment (Space, noise, vibration)	Fair-Good (depends on the road/traffic)	Good	Poor
Transport time	Slow	Rare in India	Excellent
Range	<160 km (typically)	322–3,218 km	160–240 km
Special issues	Road and weather conditions	Need for multiple transfers	Weather conditions

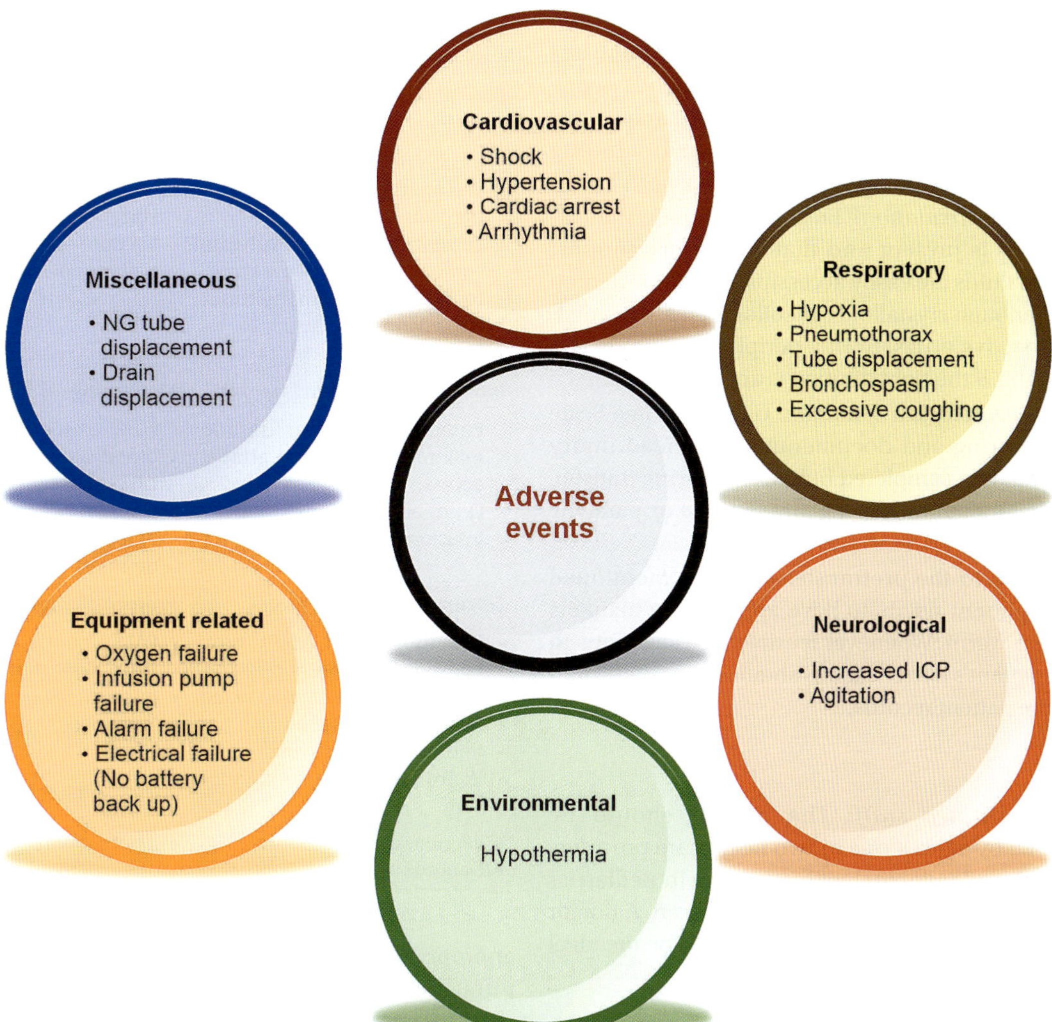

Fig. 20.11.1: Common adverse events during transport. (NG: nasogastric)
Source: Fanara B, Manzon C, Barbot O, Desmettre T, Capellier G. Recommendations for the intra-hospital transport of critically ill patients. Crit Care Lond Engl. 2010;14(3):R87.[5]

TABLE 20.11.2: Steps in the interhospital transport of sick child.[10]

For the receiving hospital: • On receiving the phone call for retrieval, collect patient details and ascertain need for retrieval • Discuss with the pediatric intensive care unit (PICU) consultant about the transport • Inform the transport team and confirm the transport **For the transport team:** • Once everything is ready, call the referring hospital when you start • Once you reach, get detailed hand over • Examine and stabilize the patient • Communicate with parents and complete consent formalities • Monitor the patient continuously during transport and enter all details in the transport/retrieval form	**For the referring hospital:** • Call the receiving hospital and discuss the referral • Confirm bed and treatment availability. Inform parents and get consent • Prepare summary and complete other paperwork • Inform the transport team and confirm the transport • Call the receiving hospital contact person when the transport team starts **For the transport team (after transport):** • Give thorough hand over to the PICU/ER team at the receiving hospital

- *Is the patient's breathing pattern adequate to maintain oxygenation and ventilation during transportation?* It is important to confirm bilateral equal breath sounds to rule out pneumothorax. If breathing is inadequate, maneuvers to increase oxygenation and ventilation (including intubation) should be performed before transport.
- *Is there a stable circulation?* Ensure that a patent intravenous access is present and that circulatory support medications/fluids are easily accessible. It is important to administer enough crystalloids or colloids and, if needed, to start vasoactive drugs. Even a peripheral cannula can be used for this if the right dilution is applied.
- *Disability or neurological condition:* Glasgow Coma Scale (GCS) monitoring and documentation in head injury patients should be completed before and during transfer, as well as before administering any sedative or paralytic medication.

In addition to the pretransfer checklist mentioned earlier, the patient needs to have appropriate blankets to keep them warm. Whenever feasible, investigations to reflect the patient's current status should be repeated and sent with the patient records.

Personnel

- *Adequately trained staff:* The patient should be accompanied by at least one or two healthcare providers (e.g., a nurse and a doctor) with expertise in pediatrics and in the management of critically ill children. A doctor with expertise in managing the airway would be the ideal candidate for one of these roles.
- *Identify a team leader*
- *Clearly define roles*
- *Adequate knowledge about the patient, transport plan, and anticipated problems.*

Teamwork

A multidisciplinary team of doctors (intensive care fellows), nurses, critical care therapists, administrators, and local paramedics is ideal in the ambulance service.

Equipment and Medications

This depends on the age and size of the patient and the clinical status. There should be a checklist for equipment functionality, backup for vital equipment, and battery backup for the journey with additional time in reserve in case of unanticipated delays. The team should know about the functionality of the equipment. Medications for life threatening emergencies that can be drawn up or are readily accessible should be carried along. Stand by drugs and check for adequacy of medications stock prior to the journey. An appropriate supply of equipment and drugs must be available throughout the transfer.

TABLE 20.11.3: List of possible equipment required for patient transport.[10]

Patient movement	***Airway management***
• Trolley • Incubator for children <5 kg. • Restraints to secure patient in transfer. • *Equipment bags:* Multiple compartments to allow access to individual items without unpacking • Drug boxes	• Equipment to establish and maintain a secure airway • Portable mechanical ventilator • Portable oxygen supply • Suction—portable, battery-powered
Intravenous infusions	***Monitoring***
• Equipment to establish and maintain venous and arterial access • Drugs and infusions • Infusion pumps	• ECG, oximetry, noninvasive blood pressure, temperature, capnography, blood gas • Invasive channels (preferably 2) for CVP and invasive BP on monitor
Document folder	***Protocols/algorithms***
• Recording chart, audit form, consent form infusion charts, and crash drug charts—filled in prior to transfer • Information for parents • Warm protective clothing for staff	• PALS algorithms • NALS algorithms • Institutional guidelines • Formulary

(CVP: central venous pressure; ECG: electrocardiogram; PALS: Pediatric Advanced Life Support; NALS: Neonatal Resuscitation)

A comprehensive list of the required equipment has been summarized in **Table 20.11.3**.

Monitoring and Documentation

Ideally, every patient transported should be under the same level of observation as that in an ICU. It is necessary to continuously record electrocardiogram (ECGs) and pulse oximeter readings and to regularly monitor blood pressure, respiratory rate, and pulse rate.

Ensuring proper documentation throughout the entire procedure, including obtaining parental approval, is crucial. Any undesirable incident and its management, as well as the timing, should be well documented in the patient's health record. A detailed handover should be given to the receiving unit to ensure the patient's continuing treatment.

Standard Protocols for Adverse Events

To enhance patient safety and comfort during transportation, a uniform set of protocols is necessary. This will shorten the emergency management team's response time in the event

Appendix 1: Checklist for intrahospital transport.

1. Communication
   a. Patient's relative
   b. Destination department
   c. Supporting staff
2. Timing
   a. Appointment time
   b. Transport
   c. Minimum waiting time
   d. Procedure time
3. Central nervous system (CNS)
   a. Glasgow Coma Scale (GCS) >8 (stable)—yes/no
      If no—
   b. Intracranial pressure raised yes/no
      i. if yes—head end of the bed elevated—yes/no
      ii. Intracranial pressure reducing medication ready—yes/no
   c. On sedation—yes/no
      i. If yes—syringe loaded for entire duration
      ii. Drug loaded for bolus doses
4. Respiration
   a. Airway protected
   b. TT/Endotracheal tube (ETT)—suctioned before transport
   c. Well secured
5. Cardiovascular
   a. Hemodynamically stable—yes/no
   b. Vasopressors—preloaded for entire duration
   c. Unnecessary infusions detached
   d. Intravenous cannula—placed, working
6. Gastrointestinal (GI)
   a. Pretransport random blood sugar checked—yes/no
   b. Abdomen distended—yes/no
   c. Head end of bed elevated—yes/no
   d. Nasogastric tube aspirated
7. Renal
   a. Urinary bag empty and capped
8. Other
   a. Drains—well secured, functioning
   b. Minimum investigations for the procedure—ready
   c. Pretransport ABG checked
9. Drugs
   a. Emergency drugs
   b. Sedatives/relaxants (for bolus also)
10. Equipment
    a. Laryngoscope/ET ready
    b. Ambu bag/Bain's circuit ready
    c. Transport ventilator checked
    d. Oxygen cylinder full
    e. Infusion pumps (battery charged)
11. Monitor—(battery charged)
    a. Pulse oximetry
    b. Intra-arterial BP (preferred if patient is on vasopressors)
    c. Electrocardiogram (ECG)
    d. *Optional:* $EtCO_2$
12. Transport personnel
    a. Trained in managing airway
    b. Knowledgeable about resuscitation guidelines
    c. Knowledgeable about inotropes/vasopressors
13. Drugs that must be available
    a. Adrenaline—10 mg/10 mL
    b. Atropine—0.6 mg/mL
    c. Midazolam—1 mg/mL
    d. Fentanyl—50 µg/mL
    e. Drugs (noradrenaline, $NaHCO_3$) in continuous infusion loaded for full duration
14. Minimum equipment
    a. Laryngoscope—working
    b. Endotracheal tube—proper size
    c. Stylette
    d. Suction catheter—(proper size)
    e. AMBU bag
    f. Mask—appropriate size
    g. Bain's circuit
    h. MRI—minimum 4 pressure monitoring (PM) lines for syringe pump attached, 4 oxygen source connector tube attached

of a transport-related incident. As stated by Beckmann, the transport team members' uncertainty and haste were caused by insufficient protocols.[8] As a result, in order to prevent adverse events, each institute should develop its own procedures based on the resources at its disposal and closely follow them.

Final Checklist

Human error cannot be eliminated due to immense work pressure. Therefore, it is recommended to double-check using a checklist prior to, during, and following the transport. It will assist in following the recommendations and enhance the standard of patient care. A typical check list is available in the **Appendix 1**.

The possible complications and the risk factors for the same are shown in **Boxes 20.11.1 and 20.11.2**, respectively.

BOX 20.11.1: Complications during patient transfer.[11]

- *Pulmonary:* Atelectasis, hypoxemia, pulmonary embolism, bronchospasm, pneumothorax
- *Cardiovascular:* Hypertension, hypotension, arrhythmia, cardiac arrest
- *Endocrine:* Hypoglycemia, hyperglycemia
- *Infectious:* Ventilator-associated pneumonia, infection risk for patient and for personnel
- *Acid-base disorders:* Metabolic acidosis, metabolic alkalosis, respiratory alkalosis, respiratory acidosis
- *Miscellaneous:* Dislodgement of monitoring equipment, interruption of therapy

WHAT IS POSSIBLE IN INDIAN PEDIATRIC INTENSIVE CARE UNIT?

Sparing precious personnel for the intrahospital transport of a critically ill child is difficult. However, depending on the

BOX 20.11.1: Risk factors for the development of complications during transport.[12]

Patient-related
- High positive end-expiratory pressure (>6 cmH_2O)
- History of coronary artery disease
- Postoperative patients
- Severe trauma patients
- Patients on complex medications and/or infusion regimens

Staff-related
- Inexperienced staff
- Unfamiliarity with monitoring equipment/insufficient preparation of the patient
- Poor communication with the receiving facility/inadequate resuscitation
- Lack of checklists
- Failure to prepare monitors before transport: Interruption in therapy.

acuity of illness of the child and the support being given, the following is mandatory for transport.

- *Personnel:* A doctor trained in airway management should accompany the patient along with another paramedical person who can administer drugs, if required.
- *Equipment:* The minimum monitoring required is continuous heart rate and pulse oximetry (for which a portable pulse oximeter would suffice). However, a four channel multiparameter monitor is desirable so that respiratory rate and one invasive/noninvasive pressure monitoring is possible. Battery operated syringe infusion pump (at least one) would definitely be required in case of ongoing vasoactive agent therapy.
- *Dedicated bed/stretcher:* A bed or stretcher that is dedicated for transport would allow easy attachment of oxygen cylinder, monitor, and any other equipment that is required.
- *An indigenously designed transport "bag":* It is wise to be prepared for any eventuality. Hence, carrying the emergency drugs, spare airway supplies, venous cannulae, and intravenous fluids in a designated "bag" enhances the safety of the transport.

CONCLUSION

To conclude, transport of the critically ill child becomes necessary for various reasons; however, the benefits of the transport should outweigh the risks. These children may worsen during the transport if adequate preparation and planning is not undertaken. The level of care required for these children is equivalent to that being provided in a PICU and should follow a protocol which is unique to that particular Institution or organization.

TAKE HOME MESSAGES

- A risk-benefit analysis should be done before deciding whether to transport the patient.
- The transport process should begin after the patient has been stabilized as much as possible.
- To guarantee patient safety during transport, trained staff members and equipment that is convenient for transportation are needed.
- A collaborative and well-communicated strategy within and between teams is required.
- Transport related adverse events can be reduced with the use of standard, individually tailored guidelines, and checklists by each institute.

REFERENCES

1. Pragathesh P, James EJ. Chapter 106. Transport of the Critically Ill Child. In: IAP Textbook of Pediatric ICU Protocols. [online] Available from https://beta-jaypeedigital-com.eu1.proxy.openathens.net/book/9789352709694 [Last accessed December, 2024].
2. Stevenson VW, Haas CF, Wahl WL. Intrahospital transport of the adult mechanically ventilated patient. Respir Care Clin N Am. 2002;8(1):1-35.
3. Papson JPN, Russell KL, Taylor DM. Unexpected events during the intrahospital transport of critically ill patients. Acad Emerg Med. 2007;14(6):574-7.
4. Bergman LM, Pettersson ME, Chaboyer WP, Carlström ED, Ringdal ML. Safety Hazards During Intrahospital Transport: A Prospective Observational Study. Crit Care Med. 2017;45(10):e1043-9.
5. Fanara B, Manzon C, Barbot O, Desmettre T, Capellier G. Recommendations for the intra-hospital transport of critically ill patients. Crit Care. 2010;14(3):R87.
6. Dunn MJG, Gwinnutt CL, Gray AJ. Critical care in the emergency department: patient transfer. Emerg Med J. 2007;24(1):40-4.
7. Martin T. Handbook of Patient Transportation. Oxford: Cambridge University Press; 2001. p. 212.
8. Beckmann U, Gillies DM, Berenholtz SM, Wu AW, Pronovost P. Incidents relating to the intra-hospital transfer of critically ill patients. An analysis of the reports submitted to the Australian Incident Monitoring Study in Intensive Care. Intensive Care Med. 2004;30(8):1579-85.
9. Broman LM, Frenckner B. Transportation of critically ill patients on extracorporeal membrane oxygenation. Front Pediatr. 2016;4:63.
10. IAP Presidential program 2021. Transport of sick children-task module instructor manual first edition. [online] Available from https://iapindia.org/pdf/child-india/2021/CHILD-INDIA-MAY-2021.pdf [Last accessed December, 2024].
11. Damm C, Vandelet P, Petit J, Richard JC, Veber B, Bonmarchand G, et al. Complications during the intrahospital transport in critically ill patients. Ann Fr Anesth Reanim. 2005;24(1):24-30.
12. Knight PH, Maheshwari N, Hussain J, Scholl M, Hughes M, Papadimos TJ, et al. Complications during intrahospital transport of critically ill patients: Focus on risk identification and prevention. Int J Crit Illn Inj Sci. 2015;5(4):256-64.

SECTION

21 Pediatric Subspecialties

Section Editor: Ramachandran Padmanabhan

21.1 Common Behavioral Problems

Manju Mehta

INTRODUCTION

Parents often complain to the pediatrician that their child is very stubborn, does not listen to their commands, and is very demanding and aggressive. School authorities may refer the child for recurrent abdominal pain. These are some examples of behavioral problems. It is important to identify these problems in the initial stages as they can be managed optimally to help the child grow normally and have balanced mental health.

DEFINITION

Behavioral problems in children are reported by parents and school teachers in the developmental period. These children are also termed maladjusted or having emotional disturbance. They may manifest behaviors that deviate from normal behavior expected from a child of the same age. These problems are related to inappropriate behaviors and feelings, unsatisfactory interpersonal relationships, school learning problem, unhappiness, physical symptoms, or fears related to school or personal problems. They range from mild, short-lived periods of unacceptable behavior to more severe problems such as hyperactivity, conduct disorders, and refusal to go to school. Behavioral problems may occasionally occur in any child but require to be managed by the specialist when they become frequent and disrupt school and/or family life. Children who are not able to process their behavior or lack problem-solving skills can have trouble adjusting to a normal life and require medical and educational intervention.

PREVALENCE

Behavioral problems are very common in children, but serious disorders have been reported between 10 and 15% in different studies. With the changing sociocultural scenario, behavioral and emotional problems are on increase. These problems are seen in both genders, but certain problems such as attention deficit hyperactivity disorder (ADHD) are more commonly seen in boys.

BEHAVIORAL AND EMOTIONAL PROBLEMS: CLASSIFICATION

Behavioral problems have a wide spectrum ranging from normal behavior and maladjustment to serious behavioral and emotional disorders. Some behavioral problems that occur during the development period are transient and resolve on their own, whereas some become more complicated and need professional intervention. The criteria to label a child to be having a problem are discussed in the following text.

Age

Certain behaviors are normal for an age; for example, thumb sucking or enuresis in a 2-year-old child is normal but abnormal for a 10-year-old child.

Frequency

If a behavior occurs occasionally it is normal, but if it occurs very often, it is a matter of concern, e.g., a child has abdominal pain every morning before going to school.

Severity

Even a single episode of high intensity or severity requires professional attention, e.g., violent behavior, fainting, and muteness.

Effect on Development

Some behavior is persistent and has negative impact on the growth of the child; for example, poor concentration or hyperactivity causes decline in academic performance. One way to identify a problem in a child is if her/his behavior does not match the expectations within the family. If that behavior inhibits her/his ability to work in the classroom or interact with peers, or if she/he is constantly talking and disrupting other classmates and not focusing on her/his work, then you have an issue.

Behavioral problems can be global as well as culturally specific and ever-evolving. This affects their acceptance in the family as well as society further influencing treatment-seeking behavior; for example, self-injury may warrant acceptance as abnormal behavior but not shyness.

Although International Classification of Diseases and Related Health Problems (10th edition) (ICD-10) and Diagnostic and Statistical Manual of Mental Disorders (5th edition) (DSM-5) are used for classification of mental disorders in children, behavioral problems are classified as externalizing and internalizing.[1] Externalizing behavioral problems include problems related to acting out such as conduct problems, antisocial behavior, aggressiveness, inattention, hyperactivity, impulsiveness, and addiction problems—both drugs and internet and phone. Internalizing disorders include problems such as anxiety, phobia, depression, somatic complaints, somatoform disorders, and obsessive and compulsive disorders (OCDs). Autism spectrum disorders and childhood-onset psychosis are not included under behavioral problems; they are mental disorders.[2]

Behavioral and emotional problems can also manifest as comorbidity with chronic physical problems such as epilepsy, diabetes, and nephrotic syndrome. They also manifest with developmental problems such as intellectual retardation, speech disorders, and specific learning disability.

BEHAVIORAL PROBLEMS

Habit Disorders

In childhood, some habits are very persistent and cause concern to parents. These are tension-discharging phenomena such as head banging, body rocking, temper tantrums, breath holding spells, thumb sucking, nail-biting, teeth grinding (bruxism), and tics. The details are given in **Table 21.1.1**.

TABLE 21.1.1: Habit disorders.

Problem behavior	*Meaning*	*Reason*	*Treatment*
Head banging	Rhythmic rocking and head banging in early life	Sensory stimulation or pleasure for the child who is otherwise uncared for or deprived of human touch or interaction	• Environment should be created in a way that the child cannot get injured • Activities should be provided to the child, which can be comprehended by him and can engage him • Provide emotional security
Temper tantrum	• Disobedient, attention-attracting behavior on part of a child to get demands met, especially in social situations • Breath-holding spells	• The problem increases when the child is recovering from an illness and fatigue or when the child is hungry. This occurs in children when parents fail to discipline a child or get manipulated by the child • Iron deficiency	• Firm, consistent parenting, early social skill training and professional intervention when severe • Role of iron supplementation
Thumb sucking	• Normal in infancy • Abnormal in preschool and above years	May start later after birth of a sibling or when in stress	• Record situation when thumb sucking is done • Occupy child in activity engaging his/her hands • Anxiety management skills • Behavioral reinforcement
Nail-biting	Common in girls and boys in middle and late childhood	It is often associated with anxiety and nervousness	Keeping the child busy and teaching anxiety management
Tics	• Repetitive movement of muscle groups that have no apparent useful function • Mostly muscles of face, neck, shoulders, trunk and hands are involved, e.g., lip smacking and grimacing, tongue thrusting, eye blinking, throat clearing • Unaccompanied by loss of consciousness • Not seen during sleep and can be controlled voluntarily for short periods of time	• Represent discharges of tension originating in emotional and physical states • Must be differentiated from involuntary movements	Combination of pharmacological and nonpharmacological treatment is effective
Teeth grinding or bruxism	• Voluntary grinding of teeth • It may create problems in dental occlusion	• Calcium deficiency • Stress mannerism • Release of tension originating in unexpressed anger or resentment	Helping the child to find ways to express that resentment may relieve the problem

Conduct Disorder

Conduct disorder is defined by DSM-5 as severe repeated acts of aggression that can cause physical harms to themselves and others and violate the basic rights of others or major age-appropriate societal norms or rules are violated. The persistent antisocial behavior of children and adolescents significantly impairs their ability to function in the social or academic area. Such children are arrested as they get in conflict with law such as theft, attempt to murder, and sexual offences. The milder forms are telling lies, running away from school, or stealing. The rate is much higher among boys than girls.

There is evidence for two clusters of symptoms in conduct disorder:

1. Aggressiveness
2. Delinquency

Aggression may be directed toward people (e.g., peers) or animals (cruelty toward animals) or objects (destruction of property). Delinquency, on the other hand, includes antisocial behaviors such as lying, stealing, running away, and truancy that do not primarily involve physical attack on others. The onset of these symptoms may be preceded by the presence of a difficult temperament and a high level of physical aggression in preschool years.

While evaluating a child for conduct disorder, one must consider whether the reported behavior is appropriate developmentally for the age of presentation. Defiance and temper tantrums are often used by children between 1.5 and 3 years of age when frustrated. This often resolves with time. Similarly, 2–4 years old often use lying as a method of playing with language. By observing the reactions of parents and caregivers, preschoolers learn about expectations for honesty in communication. Almost all children steal something at some point in their lives. It becomes a problem when it happens more than once or twice. Thus, certain behaviors become a symptom only when they occur at a greater frequency or persist beyond a developmentally appropriate age. Unlike the previous behaviors, however, truancy, runaway behavior, destruction of property (e.g., through fire-setting), and repeated aggression against animals or others are never developmentally appropriate.

Factors contributing to the development of conduct disorders are as follows:

- Parents who had conduct disorder, antisocial personality disorder, or substance abuse disorders
- High testosterone levels
- Abusive, chaotic, and neglectful family environments
- Exposure to marital conflict and physical aggression, maternal depression, large family size combined with lower socioeconomic status, and early loss of either parent due to divorce

Children with conduct disorders are often school dropouts and have specific learning disability. They may be abusing illegal substances.

Management of a child with conduct disorder is described below:[3]

- *Pharmacological management for reducing aggression:* these include individual therapy based on alliance building and behavioral principles.
- Family therapy designed to improve communication among family members and to elicit underlying conflicts is somewhat effective.
- Correctional schools can address the educational needs of juvenile delinquents.

Childhood conduct disorder often persists into adolescence and predicts antisocial behavior and alcohol or substance abuse in adulthood. In general, risk factors for poor prognosis are childhood onset (<10 years of age), high-level aggression, low intelligence, early court involvement, and peer rejection.

Bullying

Bullying is an intentional and unprovoked abuse of power by one or more adolescents.[4] It causes mental distress and physical pain to the victim. Bullying is a serious problem plaguing school-going adolescents; incidents of bullying among students in recent years have increased and newer methods of bullying are used. Bully victims have a higher risk for conduct problems and hyperactivity and are the most likely to have academic difficulties. Longitudinal studies have shown that adult violent criminals frequently have school records of bullying and other forms of aggressive behavior. When students are victimized, it may negatively affect their feelings of safety at school, reduce their willingness to attend school, and thereby lower their academic achievement. Even minor forms of victimizations, such as minor theft and being bullied, have been linked to these consequences and the effects of bullying may persist into adulthood and produce long-term negative outcomes such as antisocial behavior, drug use and abuse, and criminal behavior. Consequences of bullying victimization can be categorized into four types:

1. Low psychological well-being
2. Poor social adjustment
3. Psychological distress
4. Physical unwellness

Adolescents who do not get emotional support at home may try to attract attention toward themselves in the classroom through bullying. In some cases, a child who is bullied sometimes ends up bullying others. Other factors such as a teacher's indifference to the victims and poor disciplining by parents of bullies can also cause bullying. Some adolescents learn from their homes as their parents may encourage aggressive behaviors.

Oppositional Defiant Disorder

Oppositional defiant disorder is characterized by extreme demanding and aggressive behavior. Adolescent-appropriate behaviors like increased peer group interaction, striving for independence, and experimentation with risky behavior become exaggerated, severe, and disruptive.

Oppositional defiant disorder is seen more often in boys. It involves temper tantrums, continuous arguing, defiance of rules, continual blaming of others, and frequent use of obscene language. An adolescent has a very good relationship with peers outside his immediate family. Treatment approaches are commonly employed including behavior therapy, family therapy, and parent management training.[3]

Substance Abuse

Substance abuse and alcohol are increasing like an epidemic in children and adolescents. The substances abused are inhalants—thinner, white fluid, cough syrups, smokeless tobacco (*pan masala*, *gutka*), opioids, *charas*, and *ganja*. 20% of children and adolescents start experimenting with alcohol and drugs by 11 years of age. Internet and phone addiction is also increasing these days. There are other psychosocial factors, which lead to addiction, namely change in lifestyle, low frustration, tolerance, easy availability of drugs, and peer pressure. The clinical manifestation of substance use in children includes decline in academic performance, change in behavior, irritability, decreased interaction with family members, lying and stealing, and changes in eating and sleeping behavior. These children can be assessed on detailed case history, mental status examination, tobacco, and standardized psychological rating scales such as cut down, annoyed, guilty, and eye opener (CAGE), teen addiction severity index, and Fagerstrom test for nicotine dependence. Cognitive behavior therapy (CBT) and family therapy can help to control the craving and develop coping strategies.[5,6] Parent training can be useful in phone addiction.

Enuresis

Enuresis (bed-wetting) is a very common problem in both boys and girls in the developmental period. It is the involuntary voiding of urine not occasioned by a physical condition. The severity is determined by frequency of urination, and the quantity is not a diagnostic consideration. The child should have a mental age or chronological age of at least 5 years (DSM-5). The diagnosis of enuresis is made when urine is voided twice a week for at least 3 consecutive months or the bed-wetting causes significant distress to the child. While most patients have nocturnal bed-wetting, a diurnal (but during sleep) variety and a combined variety have also been described.

Enuresis is classified as persistent (primary) and regressive (secondary). In primary, the child has never been dry at night. About 75% belong to this category and is probably the result of inadequate or inappropriate toilet training (e.g., parents do not want to wake up the child in the middle of the sleep). The regressive type is often precipitated by stressful environmental events, such as birth of a sibling, marital conflict in parents, or death of a family member. Bed-wetting in this case is transitory and prognosis is better. Methods to control enuresis are given in **Box 21.1.1**.

BOX 21.1.1: Methods to control enuresis.

- Reward the child for dry night
- Once bed-wetting occurs, older children should be asked to wash their own clothes and soiled bedsheets
- Children should not be given any fluids after dinner
- Waking the child 1–2 hours after sleep to void urine again may help
- Punishment and humiliation by parents or siblings should be discouraged
- Stress and anxiety management for the child
- Tricyclic antidepressants

Encopresis (Soiling)

Encopresis refers to a condition of overt psychogenic soiling at inappropriate places at any age when bowel control should have been established. It is very embarrassing for the child as it leads to rejection by peer group; it also indicates a more serious emotional disturbance than enuresis. This condition was less common (around 1% of school age children), but now the problem is on increase due to early morning school timings. Some children try to postpone going to the toilet due to laziness, and then control is lost at the wrong place. Management is primarily with behavioral techniques.

Masturbation

Masturbation in children is a type of self-abuse. Children resort to this type of abuse as a means of self-pleasure. When children are lonely and insecure, they seek pleasure by self-stimulation. Though this is a common problem in older children, sometimes a mother of a 2-3-year-old boy may report that the child rubs his genitalia against the bed repeatedly. Some children engage in this activity even in classroom. Masturbation can be one of the most embarrassing aspects of growing up, and parents feel very disturbed. Parents need to be counseled that masturbation has no physical or mental side effects until taken to an extreme. But the child goes through the fear of being caught with his pants down and brought to shame. This fear leads to an extreme state of anxiety that would require proper counseling and therapy.

Gender Identity Disorder

Gender identity disorder (GID) manifests through a presence of strong and persistent cross-gender identification manifested by a desire to be of other sex, wearing clothes of other gender, e.g., girls dressing in boys' clothes, showing preference in games and play of other sex. There is discomfort in one's own gender role. Both biological (hormones) and psychological factors can precipitate this behavior. In this problem, families with girl children may reinforce a younger child to behave like a boy. In assessment, normal cross dressing in young age should be differentiated with persistent maladaptive behavior. In case family and child insist in corrective sex change operation, comprehensive psychological assessment is required.[7]

Child Sexual Abuse

Victims of child sexual abuse can present with many problems such as shock, mutism, fearfulness, and depressed mood. At times, some victims show high sexual arousal after once being sexually abused. Such sexually aroused children become problematic for their family members as they look at their younger siblings as a source of gratification of their increased sexual arousal. As a result, the problem of incest is commonly reported. For the management of such children, the same therapeutic approach is applied as in the post-traumatic stress disorder. Psychoeducational medical programs of both short-term and long-term types effectively help the individual and the family members.[3]

Pica

This disorder involves repeated or chronic ingestion of non-nutrient substances—plaster, charcoal, clay, toothpaste, paint, and mud; the age of onset is usually 1–2 years. Although tasting or mouthing of objects is normal in infants and toddlers, pica after the second year of life needs investigation. It is associated with mental retardation, iron deficiency, high frequency of maternal and paternal deprivation, family disorganization, poor supervision, and low socioeconomic status. Children with pica are at an increased risk for lead poisoning and parasitic infestations. Pica can be treated with a combination of education and guidance, family counseling, and behavior modification and oral iron where appropriate.

Rumination Disorder

The main characteristic of this disorder is weight loss or failure to gain at the expected level because of repeated regurgitation of food without nausea or associated gastrointestinal illness. This rare condition occurs more commonly in boys and usually appears between 3 and 14 months of age. It is potentially fatal in up to one-fourth of affected children. Behavioral treatment is directed toward positively reinforcing correct eating behavior and negatively reinforcing rumination. Parent counseling and family therapy are often necessary.

Sleep Disorders

A substantial portion of children struggles around bedtime due to difficulty in falling asleep. Many use special methods to help them fall asleep. Infants who show difficulty in establishing regular night-time sleep patterns may also show general fussiness and irritability. In some household, night time is very hectic due to socializing, which causes lack of interest to sleep in children. Sleep difficulty may reflect parental strife or underlying anxiety disorder such as separation anxiety disorder. If there is conflict in parents, alcoholism, or too many demands from parents on the child to excel, it can also lead to sleep problems. Children with ADHD also are reported to have sleep problems like difficulty in falling asleep, restless leg syndrome, and parasomnias. Different types of parasomnias have also been described:

- Nightmares are common phenomena, occurring in the rapid eye movement (REM) phase of sleep. These occur more often in girls with affective or anxiety disorders.
- Night terrors occur in the stage 4 of non-REM sleep. The child usually wakes up with a scream, is confused, shows signs of intense autonomic activity (labored breathing, dilated pupils, sweating, tachycardia), and appears frightened. The patient often does not recall the incident on waking up the next morning. They may be related to a specific developmental conflict or to a precipitating event.
- Sleepwalking or somnambulism occurs in stage 3 or 4 of non-REM sleep. There may be an associated history of enuresis or family history of sleepwalking. It is usually benign, but temporal lobe epilepsy should be ruled out.
- Narcolepsy is characterized by frequent daytime naps, cataplexy, sleep paralysis, and/or hypnagogic hallucinations. Polysomnographic studies, showing early onset of REM sleep following sleep onset, are required for definite diagnosis.

Some children talk in sleep about the things that happened during the day. This is considered normal if it occurs occasionally and does not have an impact on the child's functional ability during the daytime. There are standardized rating scales to assess sleep disorders. For management, the underlying cause should be assessed. Both pharmacotherapy and psychological interventions can be given.[3]

EMOTIONAL DISORDERS

Anxiety Disorders

Anxiety, fearfulness, and worrying are regularly experienced as a part of normal development. When they become disabling to the point that they negatively affect social interactions and development, they are pathologic and warrant intervention. Separation anxiety disorder, social anxiety, overanxious (generalized anxiety) disorder, OCD, phobias, and post-traumatic stress disorder are all defined by occurrence of either diffuse or specific anxiety related to predictable situations. Of these, the former two are more specific in their onset at any age. The prevalence of anxiety disorders has been reported to be 6.8%. About one-third of these children were overanxious, and another third had specific fears or phobias.

Separation Anxiety Disorder

The main characteristic of a child with separation anxiety disorder is excessive anxiety concerning separation from home or a primary caretaker. The antecedents of developmentally normal anxiety initially present at 7–8 months of age as infants begin to differentiate from their primary caregivers.

The prevalence of this disorder has been estimated to be between 3 and 4%. There is a female predominance of 3:1. Children with separation anxiety disorder show intense anxiety to the point of panic when they are separated from their primary caretaker. They can have difficulties playing outside of home, staying with babysitters, going to school, or even being alone in a part of their home. Physical symptoms (e.g., headache, abdominal pain) can occur when separation is about to occur (e.g., when going to school). Sleep disruption can occur with the child, requiring someone to stay with them till they fall asleep. They may also refuse to sleep alone. Children can worry about getting lost and never being reunited with parents. Fears about harm to the family may become exaggerated (e.g., fears of kidnappers/monsters coming into house).

Mothers of children with separation anxiety disorder very commonly have a history of psychiatric illness, especially an anxiety or a depressive disorder. Then, children can be managed by behavior therapy and family therapy.

Social Anxiety

Many teachers report the problem of excessive shyness and social anxiety among the primary school children. Children with social anxiety disorder display an excessive fear in interacting with strangers. They are overly concerned with the fear that they may do something embarrassing or humiliating, or others will think badly of them. These children constantly feel that they are being judged by others, which can lead to a great deal of self-consciousness. These children do not participate in classroom activities, which results in difficulties in integrating them into classroom environment. The management is primarily nonpharmacological. The children are given social skill training and anxiety management.

Overanxious Disorder

Children with this disorder have unrealistic worries about future events, the appropriateness of past behavior, and concerns about competence. They frequently present with somatic complaints (e.g., sweating, palpitation, chest pain, difficulty in breathing, nausea), are markedly self-conscious, need large amounts of reassurance, and have trouble relaxing. These children may be managed with self-control measures like relaxation techniques—yoga and biofeedback.

Examination Anxiety

Many children before examination experience feeling of apprehension and anxiety. The anxiety begins with preparation period and becomes intense near examination. Children with this type of anxiety develop poor appetites, recurring abdominal pain, and headache and sleep disturbance. Mild cases of examination anxiety can be managed by psychological intervention. In severe cases, pharmacological treatment is required.

Phobias

Children with phobias are anxious only under specific conditions. They try to avoid specific objects or situations that automatically lead to anxiety (e.g., animals, closed or open spaces, heights). School phobias are commonly seen in children; in this, the child develops irrational fear to some aspects of school situations. The child is not able to attend school despite deep interest in studies. Although anxiety is prominent, some children also have depressive feelings. Other complaints may be abdominal pain, vomiting, anorexia, headache, and giddiness. The symptoms are usually intense or present during the school-going hours. Generally, the cause of school phobias is disturbed family relationships. The first step of treatment is to help the child to attend school. Behavioral techniques (like graded exposure) are very effective in the management of school phobias. Parents should be given insight into the mechanism involved. Drugs may be considered when anxiety and depression are severe.

Somatoform Disorder

Somatoform disorder or conversion disorder is the most common disorder seen in child psychiatric clinics. It is the disturbance of voluntary motor or sensory system. Often, the symptoms are means to get primary and secondary gains. These patients commonly seek first consultation with the pediatrician as the symptoms are primarily physical such as pseudoseizures, aches and pains, hyperventilation, headache, vomiting, and paralysis. The symptoms are variable and fluctuating and usually do not follow any organic pathway. It occurs in both boys and girls, generally above the age of 8 years.

A variety of methods have been recommended for symptom removal such as reassurance, suggestions, behavioral modification (operant conditioning and aversive therapy), hypnosis, use of placebo, and use of sedatives. Parent counseling is very important to decrease anxiety in parents and to modify their reinforcing behavior. A simple antecedent-behavior-consequence (ABC) chart may be maintained by the parents to understand the cause of the symptoms.

Recurrent Abdominal Pain

Among somatic complaints, recurrent abdominal pain is very common in young children; 80% of these have a nonorganic cause for pain. The pain can occur before going to school before examination or under other stressors. These children are generally anxious, have poor coping skills, and may have unrealistic high expectation in school performance. Parents also are very anxious and reinforce illness behavior in the child. Behavioral assessment helps in understanding cause, and parent's anxiety can be reduced.

Obsessive–Compulsive Disorder

Children with OCD present with repetitive thoughts (obsessions) or repetitive rituals or movements (compulsions). Obsessions have been defined as intrusive thoughts, fears, or images, which become imposed on the conscious mind repeatedly. The fear that some bad event might happen causes anxiety in the child. Compulsions are concerned with fears of contamination. The most common compulsions are "hand-washing", continuous checking of school words, mathematics, or writing and repeated touching. The other fears are death of parent, sexual fears, and moral worries about doing the right thing. This condition is treated with specialized behavioral techniques, e.g., thought stopping, graded exposure, and response prevention. Often, drug treatment and behavior therapy are combined.

Depression

Depression has been on rise in children and adolescents; it presents with sadness and mood disturbance in children. It affects the child's ability to participate in a relationship with parents and peers. The child is not able to enjoy activities, which he/she did earlier. It has an impact on school performance also. Depressed school-aged children present with sad facial expressions, easy tears, irritability, social withdrawal, vegetative symptoms, anxiety, and behavioral disturbances. They have lack of interest in activities liked earlier; there is decline in school performance and decrease in interaction with family members and friends. Delusions are uncommon in psychotically depressed prepubertal children. There is a 2–4% increase in the prevalence of depression with age. The prevalence of depressive disorders in childhood has been estimated to be 0.15–2.0%. Girls report significantly more depressive symptoms than boys. Depressive symptoms vary according to the age and developmental level.

CAUSES OF CHILDHOOD AND ADOLESCENT DISORDERS

Why a child behaves in an abnormal way will depend upon his/her biological and environmental factors, which include family, school, and society in which he/she lives. Some behavioral problems can occur, whatever the family or home situation is. In some cases, however, stressful external events, such as moving home or divorce, may produce periods of behavioral problems. **Table 21.1.2** summarizes these factors.

TABLE 21.1.2: Causes of behavioral and emotional problems.

	Psychosocial		
Biological	***Family***	***School***	***Culture***
• Genetic disposition • Fragile-X syndrome • Down syndrome • Brain damage • Intelligence • Temperament • Illness • Physical handicap • Fatigue • Malnutrition	• Attitudes of parents • Overprotection • Rejection • Child abuse • Discipline • Anxiety • Role model • Expectation • Time spent with child • Conflict • Parents • Family members • Alcoholism	• Stress • Self-esteem • Achievement • Peer group • Discipline • Social skills • Antisocial	• Media • Terrorism • Violence • Neighbor-hood • Ethnicity

Assessment for behavioral problems is carried out in the following steps.

ASSESSMENT OF BEHAVIORAL AND EMOTIONAL DISORDERS

Examination of the child consists of interviewing the child as well as his/her family. Often, a child's understanding of what troubles him/her may be at variance with the reports of his/her parents and teachers. Also, many behavioral problems are situation-specific. For example, a child may have severe temper tantrums only when he/she is with his/her mother or a child who is obedient at school may be destructive at home. Therefore, as a rule, information should be gathered from multiple sources (e.g., parents, peers, teachers). A child's behavior and cooperation may vary from time to time. A child may have his/her good days and bad days. A comprehensive assessment would therefore require observing the child serially over several sessions.

Case History and Mental Status Examination

A detailed case history is taken from the time of conception to the present. This includes beginning of behavioral problem, development of the child, family history, family environment, child's temperament, school performance, and interpersonal relationship.

The mental status examination refers to a child's current abilities to understand his/her actions and interaction with the environment. The child is observed in a structured situation and standard questions are asked to assess his/her feelings and thoughts. Both case history and mental status examination are important in making diagnosis of the child.

Cognitive Assessment

On a standardized objective test, a child's cognitive abilities are assessed. These include attention, concentration, verbal and performance intelligence, social maturity, adaptive behavior, and memory. Attention and concentration can be assessed on digit span test and color/letter cancellation test. Verbal and performance tests of intelligence, Wechsler Intelligence Scale for Children (WISC), and Malin's Intelligence Scale for Indian Children (MISIC) should be used to assess intelligence. In children less than 5 years of age, social maturity level, referred to as social quotient (SQ), can be assessed using Vineland Social Maturity Scale. Mental subnormality, specific learning disorders, and developmental language disorders can be diagnosed based on these tests.

Projective Technique

Projective tests are unstructured stimulus material on which a child's unconscious conflicts and thoughts are elicited. These tests are very useful in understanding the psychodynamic aspect of a child's behavior and his/her interactions with family members. Some of the examples of these types of tests are Draw-a-Person Test and House-Tree-Person Test, in which a child is asked to draw a plain sheet of paper with his/her imagination.[7] In Children's Apperception Test, the child must make a story on the pictures given to him/her. They are very useful in understanding the psychopathology and planning treatment.

Rating Scales and Questionnaires

Rating scales and questionnaires are objective methods to assess psychopathology and personality of the child. Parents or teachers rate the rating scales. Self-rating scales are used for adolescents. The well-known checklists for children are:

- Child Behavior Checklist (CBCL)
- Conner's Rating Scale for assessment of ADHD, parent and teacher versions[8]

Examples of self-report instruments are:

- Child Depression Inventory (CDI)
- Strength and Difficulty Questionnaire (SDQ)
- Perceived Competence Scale (PCS).[9]

There are Indian standardized rating scales and norms available for the assessment. One example of the Indian rating scales is Developmental Psychopathology Checklist for Children.[3]

Behavioral Assessment of a Child

A child's behavior is systematically observed and recorded, according to antecedents (situations), feeling, thought, behavior, and consequences. The parent can be involved in this recording. Older children can do this on their own.

PREVENTION

Majority of behavioral problems in a child arise from a complex interaction between the child and environmental characteristics, related to situational family stresses. Psychoeducation to parents and members of extended family if staying together can help in reducing anxiety in the child and to modify family environment. A pediatrician can help parents cope with troublesome behaviors through education and brief intervention techniques such as behavior modification. In addition, the pediatrician can help to promote "competence" by teaching parents how to interact with their children in more affectionately and cognitively stimulating ways. By providing parenting skills, high expectations from the child can be lowered and his/her needs and uniqueness can be appreciated. In this current situation, parents want the child to be perfect, strong, smart, and quick. He/she may be humiliated for not living up to the expectations of the parents. Thus, parents should create an environment in the family to make the child comfortable and anxiety free. Providing parents with knowledge and helping the child to develop emotional regulation will help in preventing behavioral problems. Parents' own anxiety should be under control. The expectations from the child should be proportionate to the child's cognitive and physical ability.

PRACTICE GUIDELINES

The National Institute for Health and Clinical Excellence (NICE), World Health Organization (WHO), American Academy of Child and Adolescent Psychiatry, and Indian Psychiatric Society (Child Psychiatry Section) have developed detailed practice guidelines. Details can be seen on www.iacap.org. According to these guidelines, the ultimate judgment regarding treatment must be made by the clinician, depending on the clinical evidence provided by the patient and his/her parents. The treatment will be carried out, according to the options and resources available. They have developed pocket cards for each disorder, which include key points, diagnosis and evaluation procedure, criteria for diagnosis, and treatment algorithm.

PRACTICE POINTS/TIPS

Management should begin with an explanation to the parents of the diagnosis, its probable cause, the way in which the child can be helped, and the likely outcome. It is important to reassure parents, as they play an important role in the management of their children. Coping strategies and skill building can be done in a play manner. As much as possible, a sick role should not be given to the child.

Certain elements of standard pharmacological treatment require modification when treating disorders in the context of the developing body and brain. The potential for long-term adverse effects in children of psychotropic drugs on the development of brain and body is of critical concern. Indeed, there are at least two instances of age-related effects of drugs on biological development:

1. Slowing of body growth by psychostimulants (like methylphenidate)
2. Hepatotoxicity induced by valproate

Due to these fears, the clinician will need to carefully consider if pharmacological treatments are required at all.

CONCLUSION

Availability of parents in developing years of the child, consistent discipline style, understanding uniqueness of the child, and ability in parent to control their negative emotions will help the child to have positive mental health.

REFERENCES

1. American Psychiatric Association. Diagnostic and Statistical Manual of Mental Disorders, 5th edition – Text Revision (DSM-V-TR). Washington: American Psychiatric Publishing Inc.; 2022.
2. Bailey A, Philips W, Rutter M. Autism: towards an integration of clinical, genetic, neuropsychological, and neurobiological perspectives. J Child Psychol Psychiatry. 1996;37(1):89-126.
3. Kapur M. Psychological management of childhood problems. In: Kapur M (Ed). Mental Health of Indian Children. New Delhi: Sage Publications; 1995.
4. Mehta M, Pilania VM. Bullying in Indian School Going Adolescents. Indian J Pediatr. 2014;81(11):1143-4.
5. Dhalla S, Kopec JA. The CAGE questionnaire for alcohol misuse: a review of reliability and validity studies. Clin Invest Med. 2007;30(1):33-41.
6. Kaminer Y. The Teen Addiction Severity Index around the Globe: The Tower of Babel revisited. Subst Abus. 2008;29(3):89-94.
7. Machover K. Drawing of the human figure: a method of personality investigation. In: Anderson HH, Anderson GL (Eds). An Introduction to Projective Techniques. New York: Prentice Hall; 1951.
8. Conners CK. Conner's Rating Scales—revised technical manual. Toronto: Multi Health Systems; 1997.
9. Harter S. The perceived competence scale for children. Child Dev. 1982;53(1):87-97.

21.2 Common Surgical Problems

Ketan Parikh

INTRODUCTION

Surgical problems in children are not uncommon. Most often they are brought to the primary pediatrician initially. Parents expect appropriate guidance and information from them. With easy information availability on the internet, parents are likely to cross-check the advice given to them. An obviously improper advice/ guidance can harm the child, spoil the image of the pediatrician and also expose them to unnecessary medico-legal vulnerability.

Early identification, judicious initial assessment, timely primary management and appropriate guidance for referral can significantly enhance child health.

INGUINAL HERNIA AND HYDROCELE

It is the persistence of patency of the processus vaginalis through which the abdominal contents descend into the inguino-scrotal region.

Embryology

During the process of testicular descent antenatally, a tongue of peritoneal fold, the "processus vaginalis" envelops the testis traversing through the inguinal canal. Normally, its communication with the peritoneal cavity should seal off by birth. The persistence of this communication in a variable portion of its extent is termed "patent processus vaginalis" (PPV) **(Fig. 21.2.1)** and may lead to hernia/hydrocele or an encysted hydrocele of the cord.

INGUINAL HERNIA

Clinical Presentation

- *Incidence:* 3–4% of male children are affected but the incidence rises to 25% in premature babies.[1]
- Less common in girls, male:female ratio—6:1.

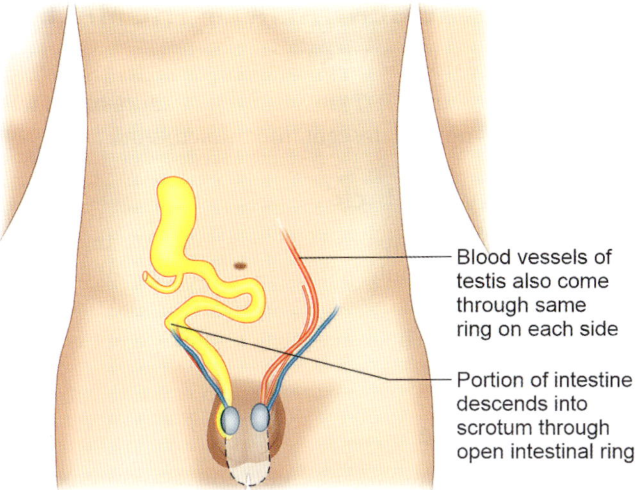

Fig. 21.2.1: Diagrammatic representation of intestines (yellow) passing through patent processus vaginalis.

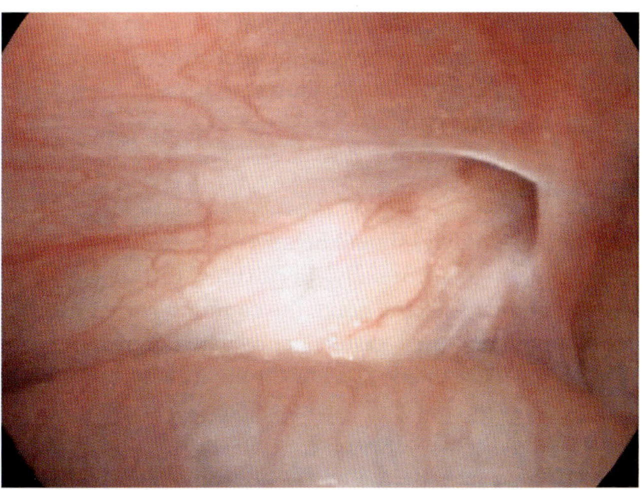

Fig. 21.2.2: A patent processus vaginalis as seen during laparoscopy.

- *Presentation:* Any time after birth but most commonly around the age of 1 year and thus the term "congenital" is a misnomer in most cases.[2]
- *A swelling in the groin or the scrotum:*
  - Bilateral in a small number of cases
  - Often a history of increase in the size of swelling on crying or any activity which increases intra-abdominal pressure.
  - The swelling is reducible unless incarcerated or strangulated.
- *Palpation* of the root of the scrotum after reduction gives a characteristic "silk glove" feeling.
- *Investigations:* No diagnostic investigations are routinely recommended.
- *Ultrasonography (USG) of inguinal region:* USG may help to differentiate from a hydrocele; however, an intermittent hernia may be missed during imaging, especially in a sedated child.
- *Diagnostic laparoscopy to identify a PPV:* Recommended only in select situations **(Fig. 21.2.2)**.
- *Complications:* An inguinal hernia has a high chance of complications in the form of irreducibility (12–17%), obstruction and strangulation.[1]
- Higher chance of complication in premature babies, (as high as 30% in the first 3 months); hence, they should be operated early.[1]
- On strangulation, the edematous and congested sac presses onto the testicular vessels causing a variable degree of testicular ischemia although very few cases develop testicular atrophy.[1]
- In most children, the contents of a hernia are bowel or ovary (in females) and thus strangulation can lead to intestinal gangrene and potentially fatal peritonitis or ovarian gangrene **(Figs. 21.2.3 and 21.2.4)**.

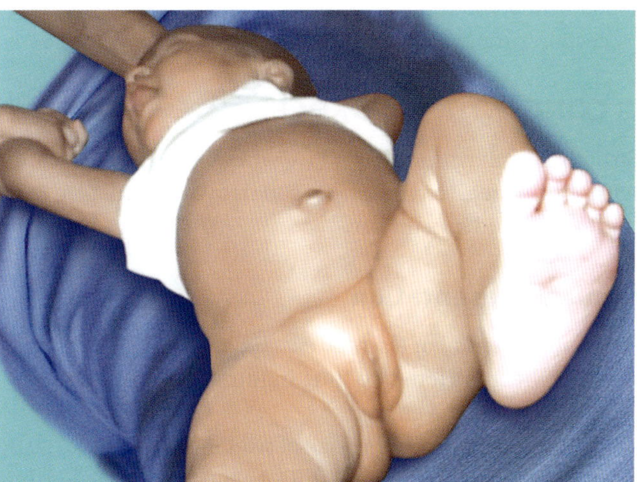

Fig. 21.2.3: Acute right groin swelling in a female child—strangulated hernia.

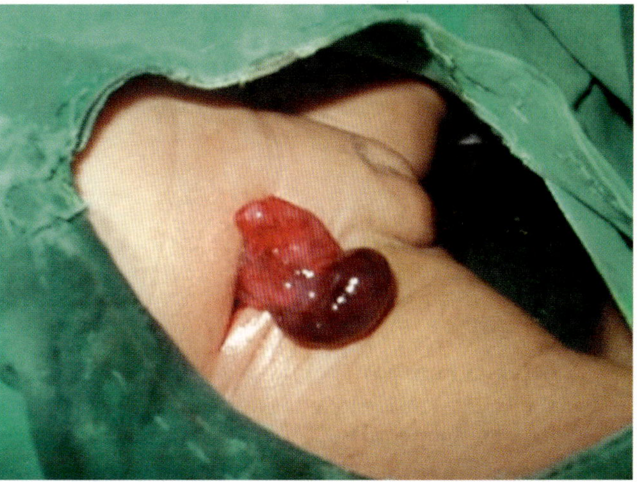

Fig. 21.2.4: Gangrenous ovary in a strangulated hernia.

- The overall surgical complication rate of an obstructed hernia is 10 times more than an unobstructed hernia.
- *Apneic spells:* Premature babies with hernia are known to suffer apneic spells.

Treatment

Surgery (herniotomy) should be advised as soon as a hernia is diagnosed. Traditionally, performed through a small incision in the ipsilateral groin, the communication with the peritoneum is exposed, divided, and ligated. In recent years, herniotomy is also being done by the laparoscopic approach. This modality offers significant magnification and enables the dissection of the vas and vessels from the sac in a relatively easier area (where there are less adhesions). Laparoscopy can also detect a contralateral PPV, which can be tackled simultaneously. It therefore avoids the ad-hoc exploration of the contralateral groin which has often been recommended by certain surgical schools.

CONGENITAL HYDROCELE

Structurally, a hydrocele is a PPV where the communication with peritoneal cavity is very narrow, permitting only peritoneal fluid into the sac.

Clinical Presentation

An inguino-scrotal or a scrotal swelling:
- May be restricted to the inguinal region (encysted hydrocele of the cord)
- Diurnal variation in the size of swelling possible.
- Usually, not easily reducible because of inverted ink-bottle effect.
- Unlike an inguinal hernia, a hydrocele has a high chance of resolution in the first 6 months of life. Since the contents are only fluid, a hydrocele is not prone to complications and thus surgery can be deferred till after infancy. However, in the event of a hernia, an early surgery is advised.

Treatment

Herniotomy

Key Messages

- An inguinal hernia in a child needs to be operated at whichever age it is identified with minimal delay to avoid preventable complications.
- The parents must be warned to identify complications when first consulted for a swelling in the groin.

EXTERNAL GENITALIA OF THE MALE

UNDESCENDED TESTES

Undescended testes (UDT) results from a failure of the testis to complete its normal descent into the scrotum.

Embryology and Incidence

Although the incidence of UDT is almost 3% in the term neonate, it drops to only 0.8% at about the age of 6 months. Most of this postnatal descent is complete by the first month in a term neonate. The exact cause of nondescent is usually not known.

Clinical Features

The ipsilateral scrotum will be empty and less developed than the contralateral normal side and the testis is not palpable within it. The testis may be palpable in the inguinal region.

Various locations of UDT have been described, but clinically the most relevant is to differentiate a palpable gonad from an impalpable one. Careful clinical examination can identify an extra-abdominal gonad in most cases. Inability to palpate the testis along the path of descent would indicate either of these possibilities:
- *Retractile testis:* After a normal descent, the testis may get pulled up due to the hyperactive cremasteric reflex and may temporarily become intra-inguinal. It may become palpable by examining the child in a squatting position or by milking the testis down the inguinal canal. The scrotum is well-formed, and the testis can definitely be located in the scrotum in sleep. An ultrasound examination may misdiagnose these cases as UDT. In most cases, this condition does not require any medical/surgical treatment and only counseling of parents is required.
- An *ectopic testis* is one, which has got diverted from the normal path of descent. Such a testis may be palpable in the superficial inguinal pouch, prepubic, or perineal locations. All these cases need surgical repositioning into the scrotal sac.

A nonpalpable testis could be:
- A high intra-abdominal UDT
- An atrophied testis due to a vascular accident such as torsion
- *Disorder of sex development (DSD)* wherein the nonpalpable gonad is either dysgenetic or a streak gonad or ovotestis/ovary.
- True nondevelopment of ipsilateral testis (rare).

Investigations

Imaging: USG, computed tomography (CT), magnetic resonance imaging (MRI), or radioisotope scanning where they may pick up testicular tissue, but the sensitivity and specificity do not justify their routine use.[2]

Diagnostic laparoscopy: It is the only reliable investigation in UDT. It enables identification of the site of the gonad, its gross structural configuration and also gives a clue to the need for a single or 2-stage orchidopexy.

Complications of an Untreated Undescended Testes

- *Prone to infertility:* Intra-abdominal temperature, which is higher than the scrotal temperature, affects germ cell maturation and the fertility potential of the UDT. Ultramicroscopic changes in the seminiferous tubules have been conclusively documented beyond the age of 1 year in an UDT.
- *Prone to trauma:* In the inguinal region, the testis can get damaged due to blunt trauma.
- *Prone to torsion:* The UDT is significantly more prone to torsion and may present as an acute abdomen or as an enlarged tender mass in the groin.
- *Prone to tumor:* UDT are approximately 50 times more prone to malignant change. The propensity may be decreased by early orchidopexy.
- *An accompanying inguinal hernia* on the ipsilateral side could develop its own complications as discussed earlier.

Treatment

- The testis is extremely unlikely to descend after 6 months of age.
- Efficacy of hormonal treatment has not been proved.
- Only surgical treatment has withstood the test of time universally.
- Desirable to complete therapy by the age of 1 year. Since there may be a need for a two-staged procedure in selected cases, a patient with UDT should undergo his first pediatric surgical assessment by 6 months of age and surgery between the ages of 6 months and 1 year.
- Earlier surgery is indicated in case of:
  - *Presence of an ipsilateral hernia:* Since the hernia needs surgery as early as possible, the orchidopexy should be combined with this surgery, may be done before 6 months of age in such cases.
  - *Any other complication:* Since UDT has a high chance of undergoing torsion, the parents of a child with UDT need to be warned (during the period of observation before 6 months age) that in the event of an acute inflammation in the inguinal region, an urgent surgery may be warranted to derotate the torsion and bring the testis down into the scrotum.

Procedure

Surgery for UDT involves locating the testis, releasing the vascular pedicle from the retroperitoneal tissues to mobilize the testis up to the scrotum and securing the same in the ipsilateral scrotum.

In a nonpalpable testis, *laparoscopy* has emerged as an important modality to locate the testis or confirm its atrophy or absence. It can also be used to mobilize the retroperitoneal vessels in UDT. Additionally, it helps effectively to stage the procedure in case of a high intra-abdominal testis with a short vascular supply.

- A patient with UDT should get his first pediatric surgical assessment latest by the age of 6 months.
- The testis should be brought down into the scrotum by the age of 1 year.
- In case of an ipsilateral hernia, an earlier surgery is necessary.

TESTICULAR TORSION

Testicular torsion signifies a twist of vascular pedicle of the testis. It can occur at any age including the neonatal age.

Clinical Features

- A history of sudden onset of pain in the scrotum with redness and swelling on that side.
- The testis itself is tender and swollen **(Fig. 21.2.5)**.
- In case of neonatal torsion, symptoms are much milder.

Differential Diagnosis

Cellulitis, epididymo-orchitis.

Dictum

An acute scrotum is a surgical emergency. It should be considered testicular torsion unless proved otherwise. This is

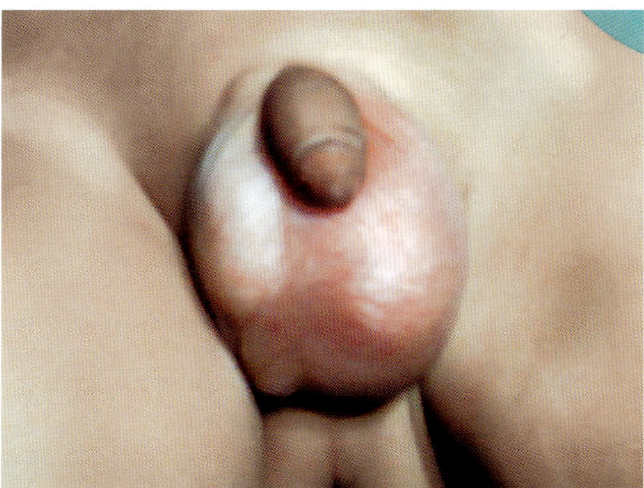

Fig. 21.2.5: Left testicular torsion.

because the resultant ipsilateral testicular hypoxia may lead to the production of autoantibodies to the proteins in the seminiferous tubules and thus, affect the functioning of the contralateral testis even before the affected testis will undergo necrosis.

Investigation

Doppler examination of the scrotal region or a radionuclide scan to see the blood flow to the scrotum is recommended but does not have adequate sensitivity or specificity and delay for surgery is not justifiable for the same.

Treatment

An acute scrotum is one of the most urgent situations in pediatric surgery because of the possibility of vascular damage to the affected testis and the possible immunological effects on the functioning of the contralateral testis. Thus, urgent scrotal exploration is advised in any acute scrotum when torsion cannot be excluded. On exploration, the torsion is corrected if possible and the testis fixed to the scrotum to prevent further episodes of torsion. If the testis has already undergone necrosis **(Fig. 21.2.6)**, orchidectomy should be done to minimize the immune-mediated damage to the contralateral testis. In either case, the contralateral testis should also be exposed and fixed to prevent torsion on that side.

PHIMOSIS

Phimosis is the inability to retract the preputial skin over the glans.

- *Physiological phimosis* (seen in infants) is due to the inadequate separation of the inner preputial skin from the glans penis and does not warrant any active treatment (not even massage). Forceful retraction or massage may lead to tears on the prepuce, which heal with fibrosis and convert the physiological phimosis to pathological.
- *Pathological phimosis* is due to a fibrotic cicatrix of the preputial aperture and thus requires treatment **(Fig. 21.2.7)**.

Symptomatology

Poor stream, straining at micturition, burning micturition, or recurrent attacks of balanoposthitis can be the manifestations. Paraphimosis is an emergency, which occurs due to the forceful retraction of the phimotic prepuce over the coronal sulcus, which then cannot be repositioned leading to edema of the preputial skin and in prolonged cases may also lead to vascular compromise of the prepuce or even the glans penis.

Recent Advances

The earlier aggressive advocacy for circumcision in infants has been diluted by the American Association of Pediatricians.

Circumcision (which involves amputation of a significant portion of the preputial skin) has been the traditional surgical treatment of phimosis. In recent years, *preputioplasty,* a reconstructive surgery of the preputial opening permitting easy retractability **(Figs. 21.2.8A to D)** but preserves the preputial covering, is rapidly becoming popular.[3] Since this procedure preserves the preputial cover of the glans, it enables preservation of its cutaneous sensitivity.

Treatment

In infancy, application of a mild topical steroid with gentle retraction of the prepuce may help in mild phimosis. In case of definite pathological phimosis, surgical treatment (circumcision or preputioplasty) is usually indicated.

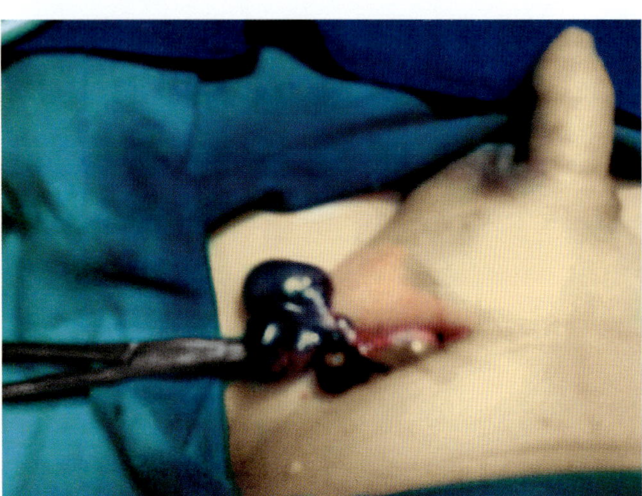

Fig. 21.2.6: Testicular gangrene following a torsion of the testis.

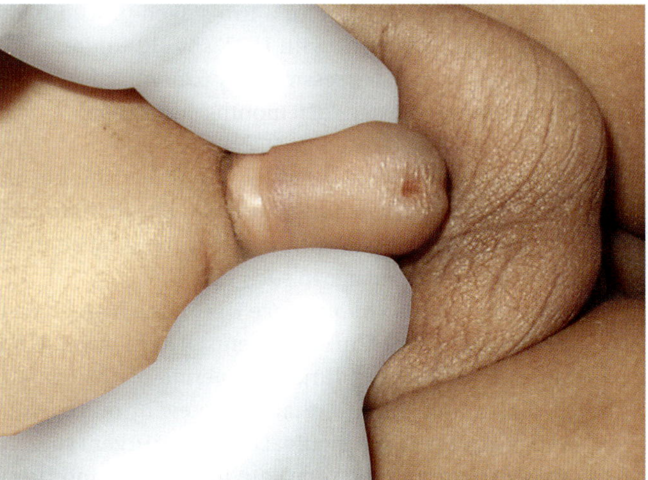

Fig. 21.2.7: Pathological phimosis—fibrotic cicatrix at the tip.

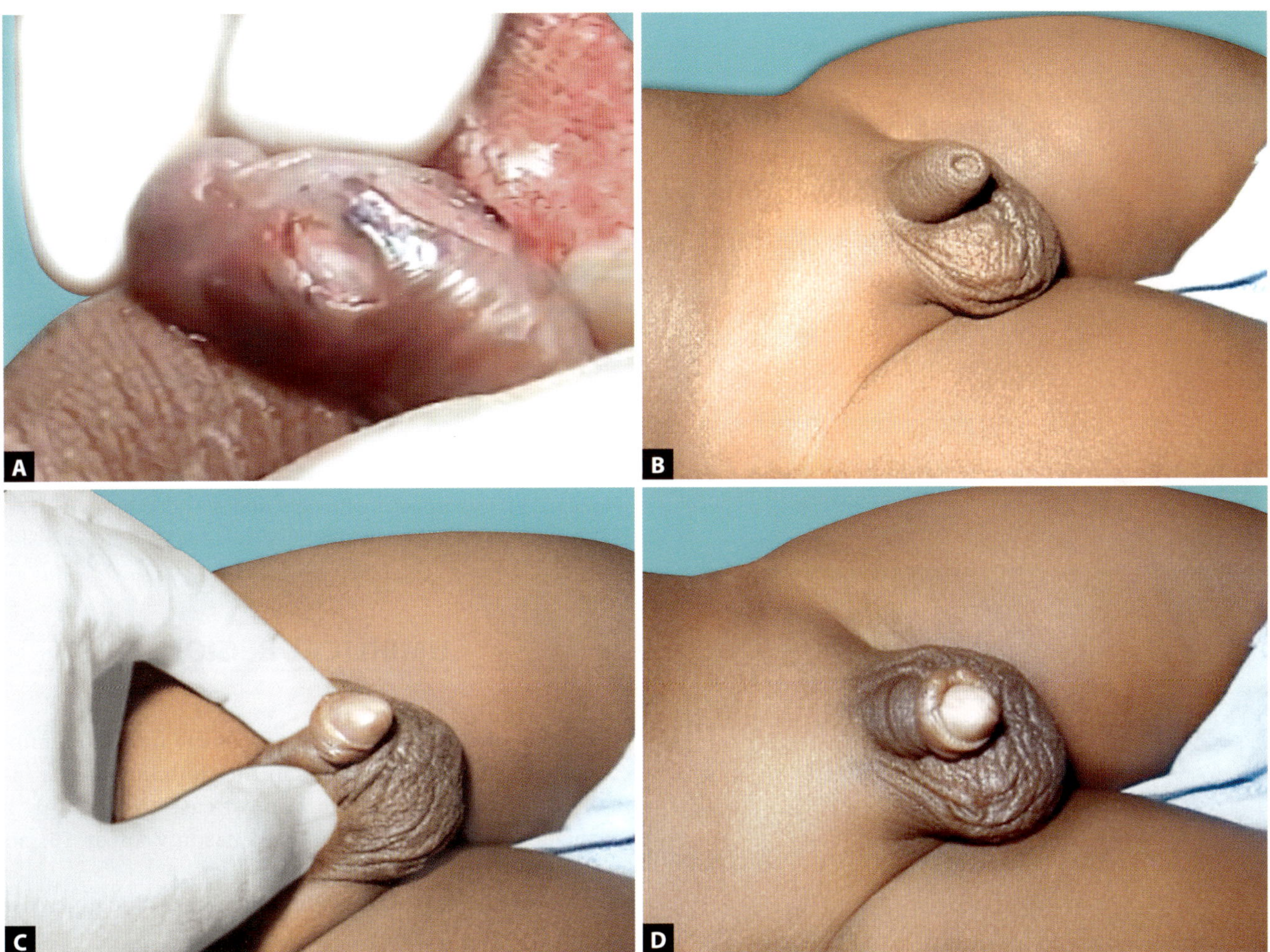

Figs. 21.2.8A to D: Preputioplasty—an alternative surgery for phimosis, which preserves the preputial cover of glans and ensures free retractability; (A) Radial cuts of preputioplasty; (B to D) The postoperative result ensuring easy retractability with an intact preputial covering.

Circumcision done in the neonatal age may cause ammoniacal dermatitis of the glans.

Key Messages

- Phimosis is physiological in most infants.
- Forceful retraction or massage of prepuce can convert a physiological phimosis into pathological phimosis.
- Preputioplasty as an alternative surgery for phimosis is gaining wider acceptance all over the world.

HYPOSPADIAS

Definition

Hypospadias is a condition wherein the urinary opening is abnormally placed on the ventral aspect of the penis. Its classification depends on the position of the urinary opening **(Fig. 21.2.9)**. A multifactorial genetic inheritance pattern has been documented in a few cases.

Associated Anomalies

- *Dorsal hood (common):* A deficiency of the prepuce ventrally with concentration on the dorsum of the penis forming a cape like hood.
- *Chordee (common):* An accompanying ventral curvature of the penis **(Fig. 21.2.10)**.
- Meatal stenosis (common) leading to a very thin (needle point) stream of urine and straining penile shortening occasional)
- A bifid scrotum (uncommon)
- Disorders of sex development (uncommon)**(Fig. 21.2.11)**.

Principles of Management

Meatal stenosis, if present, should be corrected at the earliest, to avoid the harmful effects of obstructive uropathy.

- Distal hypospadias without chordee is compatible with a normal urinary and sexual function. Treatment in these

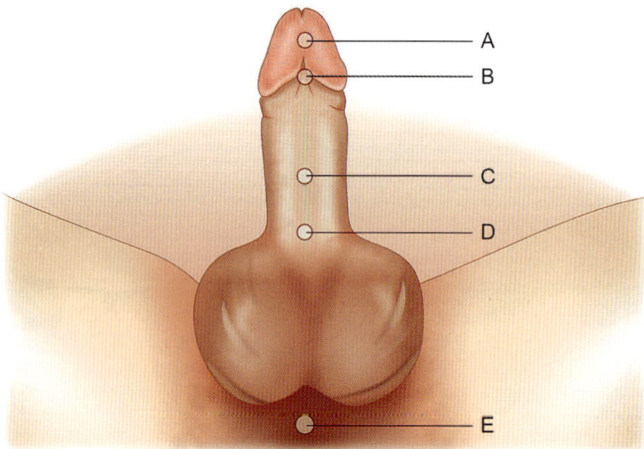

Fig. 21.2.9: Diagrammatic representation of hypospadiac meatus. (A) Glanular; (B) Coronal; (C) Penile; (D) Penoscrotal; (E) Perineal.

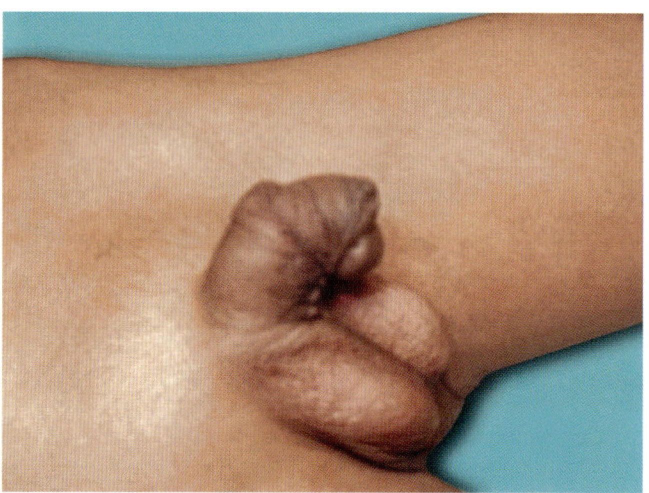

Fig. 21.2.10: Chordee in case of hypospadias.

cases is predominantly for cosmetic and psychological satisfaction.

- Proximal hypospadias may affect fertility.
- Correction of chordee must precede the urethroplasty either in two stages or as a combined single surgery.
- Tissue used for the urethral reconstruction should be hair-free skin or nonmucus secreting mucosa.
- *Timing of the repair:* All the stages of repair should be completed before the child is school-going. Generally speaking, surgery for proximal hypospadias between 9 months and 1 year, and the more severe varieties between 12 months and 24 months.
- *Epispadias:* In this much rare condition, the urethral opening is situated dorsally on the penis.
- The more proximal variety is associated with urinary incontinence.

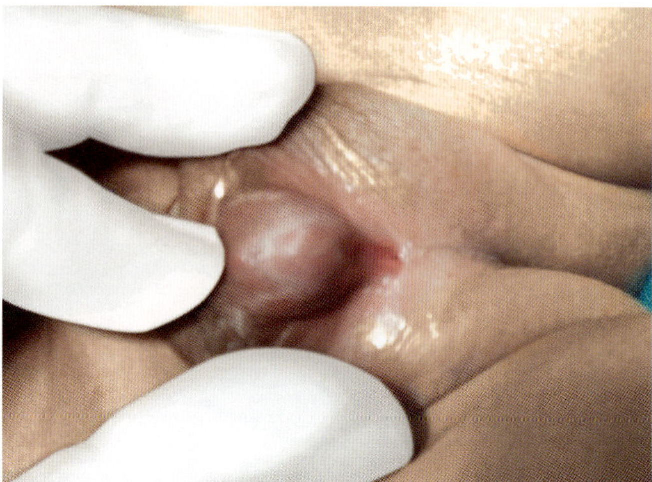

Fig. 21.2.11: Hypospadias with right undescended testes (UDT)—a case of disorder of sex development (DSD) with ovotesticular dysgenesis.

UMBILICAL REGION

HERNIA

Umbilical hernia is the protrusion of the intra-abdominal contents through a weakness in the umbilical fascia into a skin-lined sac. Idiopathic in most cases, may rarely be associated with hypothyroidism, trisomy 13 or 18, and Beckwith-Wiedemann syndrome.

- A variable protrusion of the umbilicus, which increases on crying or straining.
- Palpable defect in the umbilical ring.
- *Outcome:* Most hernias close spontaneously by the age of 2–3 years.
- *Surgery* is indicated for persistent hernia or in case of complications.
- *Complications*: Irreducibility, strangulation, or fear of strangulation.

EXOMPHALOS OR OMPHALOCELE

It is the herniation of the abdominal contents through open umbilical ring into the base of umbilical cord. The contents are not covered by skin but a thin, translucent, and avascular membrane consisting of peritoneum and amniotic membrane sandwiching a thin layer of Wharton's jelly. This sac, translucent at birth, gradually opacifies after a few hours.

The contents range from a small length of bowel to almost the entire bowel, stomach, liver, spleen, pancreas, and bladder. **Table 21.2.1** lists the difference between an exomphalos major and an exomphalos minor **(Fig. 21.2.12)**, as they are of prognostic significance.

TABLE 21.2.1: Difference between exomphalos major and minor.

Exomphalos major	*Exomphalos minor*
Defect is >5 cm in diameter	Defect is <5 cm in diameter
Cord is attached to the base of sac	Cord is attached to the tip of sac
It may contain liver, stomach, etc.	It contains only bowel
Primary closure may not be possible	Primary repair is easy

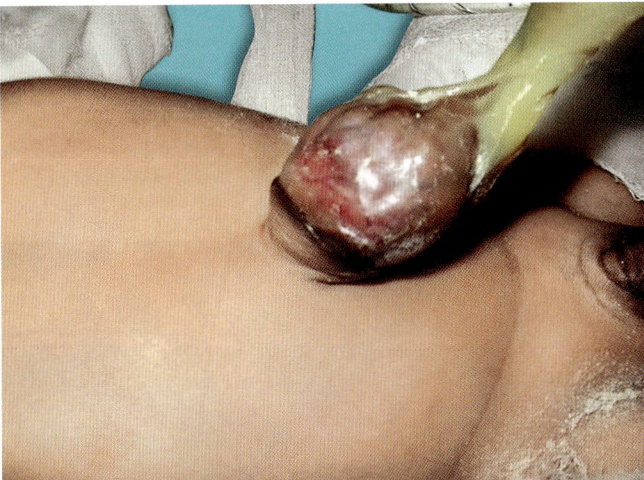

Fig. 21.2.12: Exomphalos minor.

Clinical Features

- Prenatal USG diagnosis, desirable and termination of pregnancy an option.
- *Incidence:* 1:6,000 births
- Associated with many chromosomal defects and syndromes like exomphalos-macroglossia-gigantism (EMG) syndrome.
- Multiorgan defects are common.
- *Complications:* If left untreated—septicemia.

Treatment

- Primary—prevent heat loss and infection.
- Attempt primary closure under general anesthesia (GA).
- If not possible—staged closure or silo method.

ORAL CAVITY

CLEFT LIP AND PALATE

Embryology

The mouth and the lips are formed by a fusion of five processes of mesenchyme. Cleft lip and cleft palate result due to a variable failure of this fusion process **(Fig. 21.2.13)**. In 12% of the cases, the condition is familial.

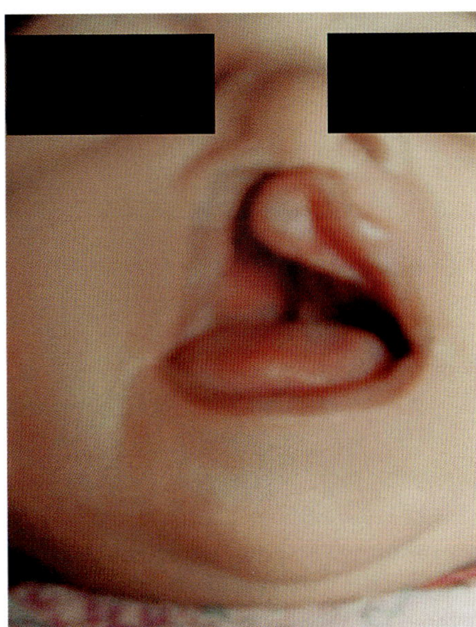

Fig. 21.2.13: Complete cleft of the lip and palate—unilateral.

Cleft Palate

- *Feeding:* Problems with sucking are dealt with by special teats or spoon feeding. However, in most cases, the Indian mother learns to place nipple to the side of mouth and the child manages to suck on the breast.
- *Speech:* Nasal twang is often seen even after successful repair.
- *Breathing:* A special mention must be made of the child with a cleft palate and a short mandible—Pierre-Robin syndrome—these babies have a tendency of tongue fall and choking.
- *Infections:* Recurrent upper respiratory tract infection (URTI) and middle ear infection due to the free communication between the oral and nasal cavities.

Treatment

- Surgical correction of the lip—often advised early to protect parents from psychological trauma. Early repair also allows proper moulding of the alveolus for better long-term results.
- Classically—at 10 weeks, 10 lbs. weight and hemoglobin (Hb) of 10 g/dL; however, some centers repair the lip at birth.
- Repair of the palate between 9 and 12 months.

NECK AND THORAX

BRANCHIAL FISTULA OR SINUS

Remnants or anomalies of the branchial apparatus lead to congenital anomalies, e.g., branchial fistula, sinus, or cyst in that order of frequency **(Fig. 21.2.14)**. Usually, the external

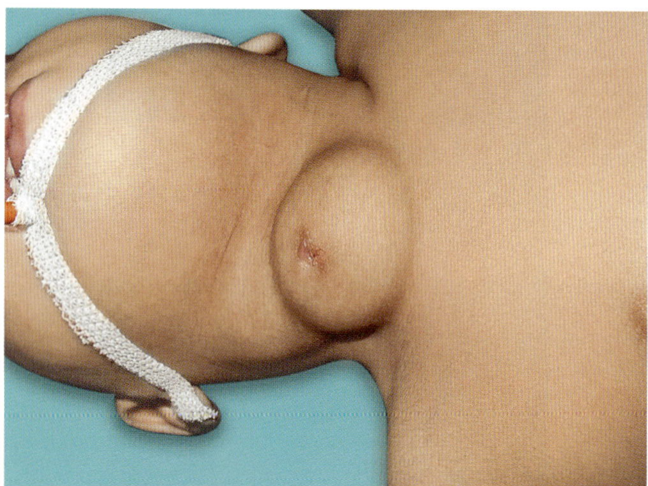

Fig. 21.2.14: Obstructed branchial sinus—the blocked opening is seen in the center of the swelling.

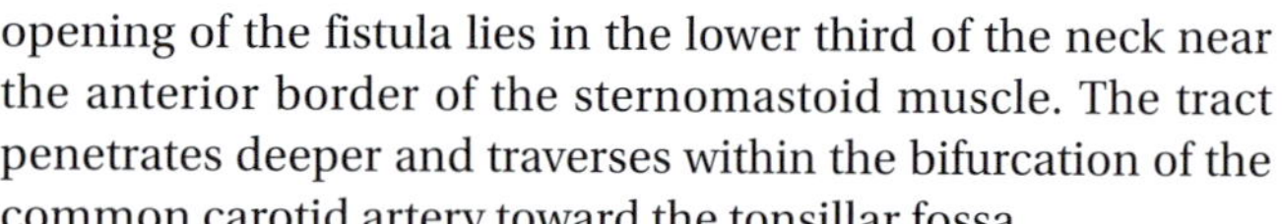

opening of the fistula lies in the lower third of the neck near the anterior border of the sternomastoid muscle. The tract penetrates deeper and traverses within the bifurcation of the common carotid artery toward the tonsillar fossa.

- The opening is often seen later in infancy—intermittent small quantities of mucoid discharge.
- There may be a small skin tag or a tiny cartilaginous tag near the opening.
- Secondary infection may lead to abscess formation. Fistulogram is routinely not recommended.

Complications

There is a high chance of secondary infection. In late cases, malignant transformation of the lining is also known.

Treatment

- If infected, antibiotics and surgical excision in the noninflamed stage.
- Surgery—dissection of the entire tract through the carotid bifurcation up to the tonsillar fossa.

THYROGLOSSAL CYST

The thyroid gland develops from the base of the tongue where it descends to take its formal position. During its course of descent, small groups of cells may get sequestrated, which gradually form a cyst—thyroglossal cyst.

Epidemiology, Clinical Features, and Diagnosis

- About three times more common than branchial remnants in childhood.
- Asymptomatic mass in the midline of neck **(Fig. 21.2.15)**.
- Smooth, round, elastic, and opaque.

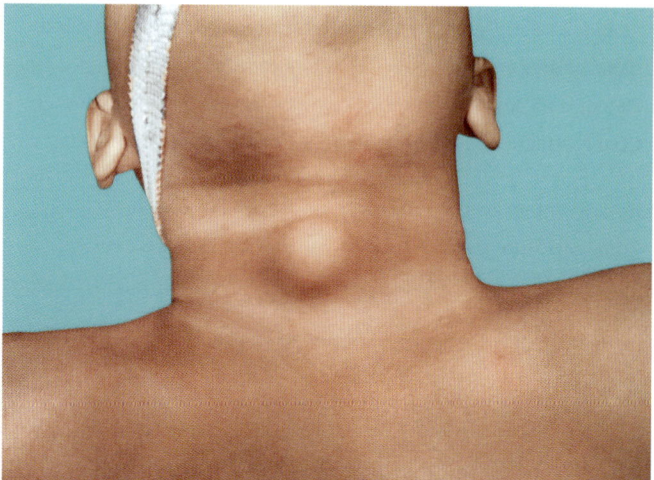

Fig. 21.2.15: Thyroglossal cyst—swelling in the midline of neck.

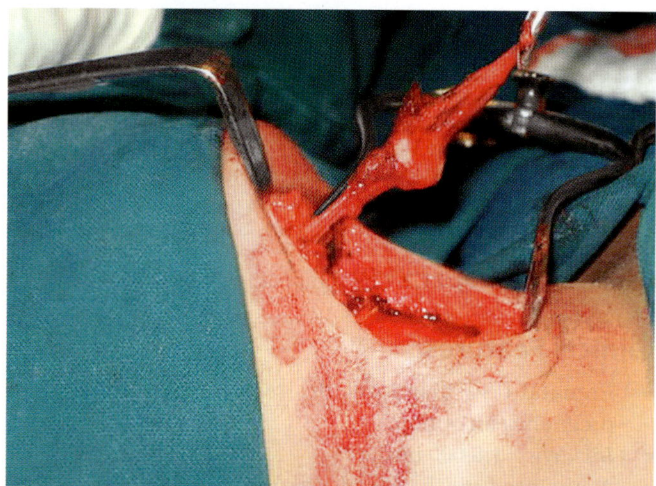

Fig. 21.2.16: Sistrunk's surgery for thyroglossal cyst. Note the excised hyoid bone along with the entire tract till the base of the tongue.

- Moves with deglutition and protrusion of tongue.
- If infected—red and tender and if drained—may form sinus.
- USG may be used for diagnosis.

Treatment

Surgery—excision of the entire tract up till the foramen cecum of the tongue, with body of hyoid bone (Sistrunk's operation) **(Fig. 21.2.16)**.

TRACHEOESOPHAGEAL FISTULA

The trachea and esophagus are formed by splitting of the primitive foregut around the 4th week of intrauterine life. An abnormality during this process causes this anomaly.

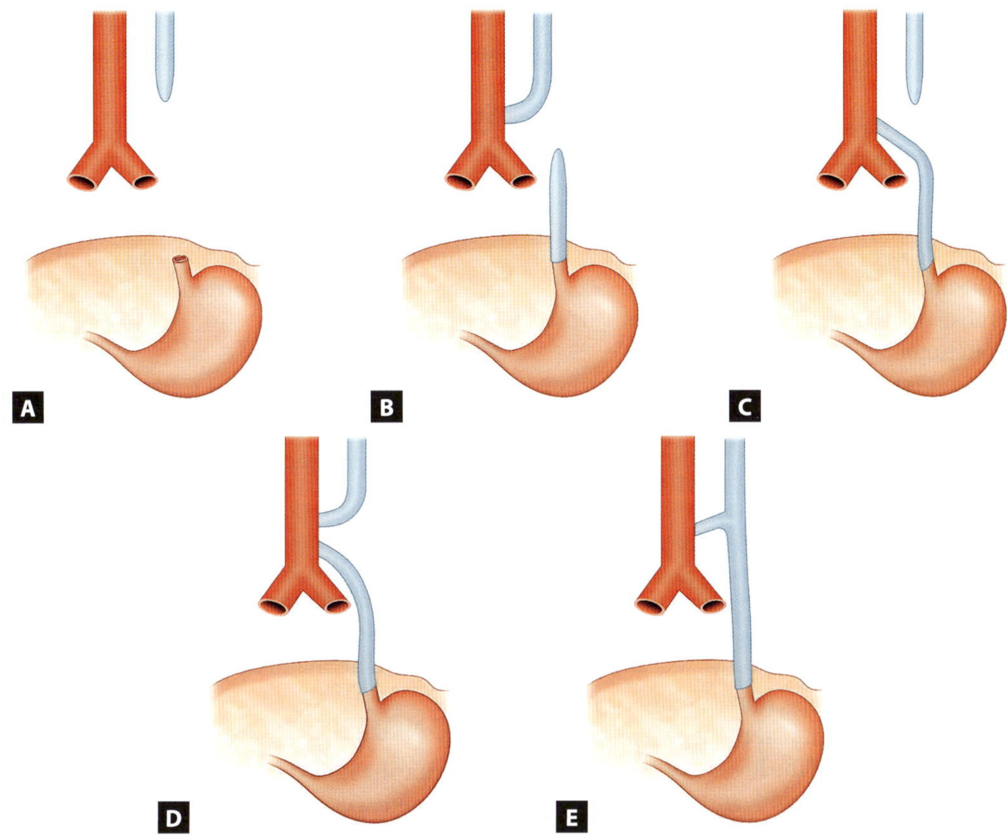

Figs. 21.2.17A to E: Different types of esophageal atresia. (A) Esophageal atresia without tracheoesophageal fistula; (B) Esophageal atresia with an upper pouch fistula; (C) Esophageal atresia with lower end fistula (the most common); (D) Esophageal atresia with fistula at both ends of the esophagus; and (E) H-type tracheoesophageal fistula.

Etiology

Whereas, the exact etiology is unknown, associated anomalies occur as a part of the vertebral, anorectal, tracheoesophageal, and renal anomalies known as VATER association and vertebral, anorectal, cardiac, tracheoesophageal, renal, and limb known as VACTERL association. Incidence ranges from 1:3,000 to 1:4,500 live births. Five types of anomalies are recognizable **(Figs. 21.2.17A to E)**:

1. Esophageal atresia without tracheoesophageal fistula (TEF)
2. Esophageal atresia with an upper pouch fistula
3. Esophageal atresia with lower end fistula (the most common)
4. Esophageal atresia with fistula at both ends of the esophagus

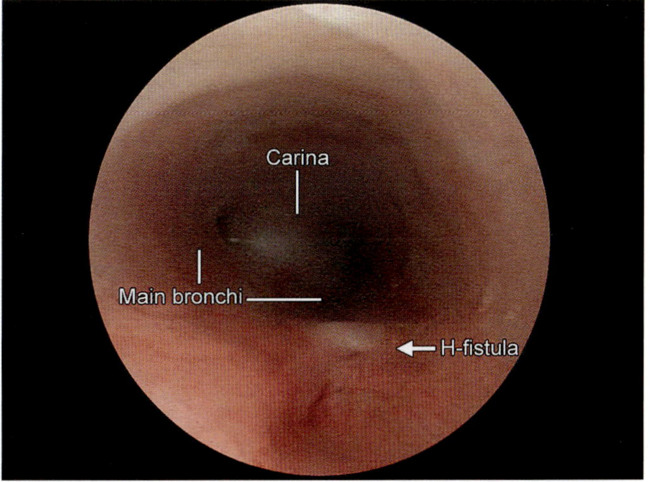

Fig. 21.2.18: Bronchoscopic view of H-type tracheoesophageal fistula (TEF).

H-type Tracheoesophageal Fistula (Fig. 21.2.18)

In the most common variety **(Figs. 21.2.17C and 21.2.19)**, saliva collects in the upper pouch and may spill over in the trachea leading to aspiration pneumonia. Inspired air is partly shunted into the stomach through the fistula causing gaseous distension of the stomach which leads to reflux of the acidic contents of the stomach through the fistula into the trachea and lungs causing chemical pneumonia.

Clinical Features

- *Antenatally:* There may be hydramnios, especially in pure atresia without fistula.
- *Frothing of saliva* is the most characteristic feature due to air bubbling through the collected salivary secretions in the pharynx.
- *Vomiting*—only if baby is inadvertently fed
- *Abdominal distension* is a prominent feature except in type-A where the abdomen is scaphoid.
- *Cyanosis*: Cyanosis may be due to concomitant cardiac anomalies or pneumonia.
- *Associated anomalies:* Vertebral, anorectal, cardiac, tracheoesophageal, renal, and limb defects.
- A baby with an H-fistula usually presents late, with choking during feeds, excessive vomiting, gross aerophagia, and recurrent pneumonia.
- *Diagnostic clinical test in all except the H-type fistula:* A stiff no. 10/12 rubber catheter or Ryle's tube is passed into the pharynx of the baby through mouth, and a characteristic resistance is felt as the catheter gets arrested in the atretic "upper pouch". A soft feeding tube or catheter may coil in the dilated upper pouch and miss the diagnosis. A lateral chest X-ray with the catheter in place will give an idea of the gap between the upper and the lower pouches.
- An H-fistula can be diagnosed only on detailed investigations.

Treatment

On suspicion of a TEF, the prime aim is to prevent pneumonia from aspiration of upper pouch secretions and refluxing gastric contents from the fistula.[4] The therapy for esophageal atresia must consider the maturity and weight of the baby besides the presence if any of the lung infection and associated anomalies. Waterston's criteria are a guide to treatment.

Surgical Priorities

- Disconnection of fistula
- Prevention of salivary pooling
- Establish esophageal continuity

Surgery is performed through a right thoracotomy. In selected cases, a staged approach is adopted.

Recent Advances

The surgery is being done by the thoracoscopic approach, which minimizes the morbidity of an open thoracotomy and facilitates earlier recovery.

Prognosis

Depends on the weight, associated anomalies, and the time elapsed before treatment can be started. If all factors are favorable, survival rates of over 80% can be achieved. Advances in neonatal care have greatly enhanced survival.

CONGENITAL DIAPHRAGMATIC HERNIA

The diaphragm is formed from different embryonal components, viz.:

- The septum transversum
- The pleuroperitoneal membranes
- The dorsal esophageal mesentery and the body wall

Failure of fusion of any one of these components can result in a defect in the diaphragm in approximately 1:3,000 live births,[5] which allows the abdominal viscera to herniate into the chest cavity **(Fig. 21.2.20)**. The most common variety

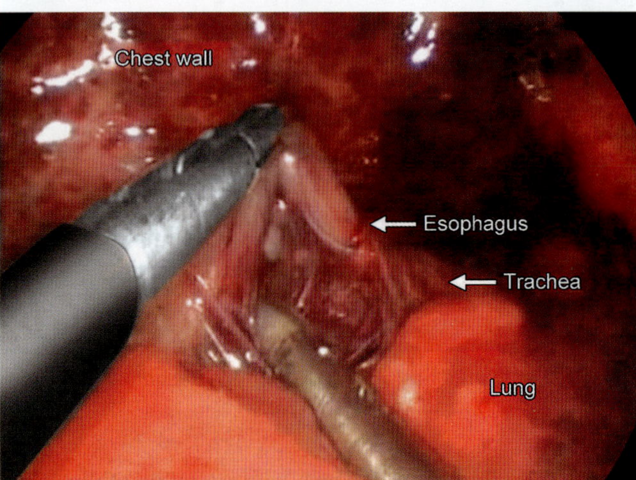

Fig. 21.2.19: Thoracoscopic view of lower esophagus arising from trachea in type "C" esophageal atresia case.

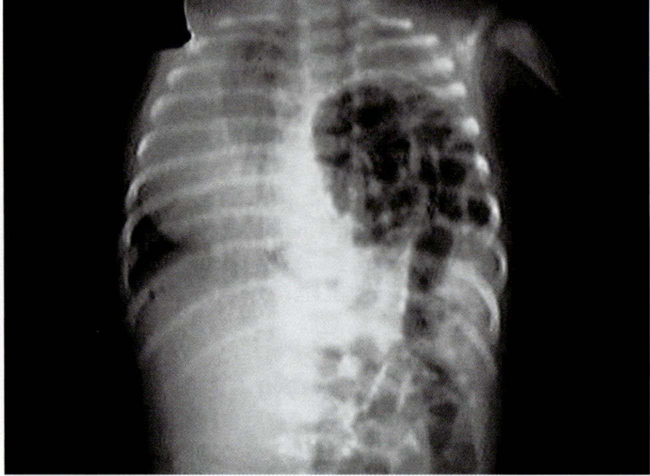

Fig. 21.2.20: Left-sided diaphragmatic hernia with marked mediastinal shift.

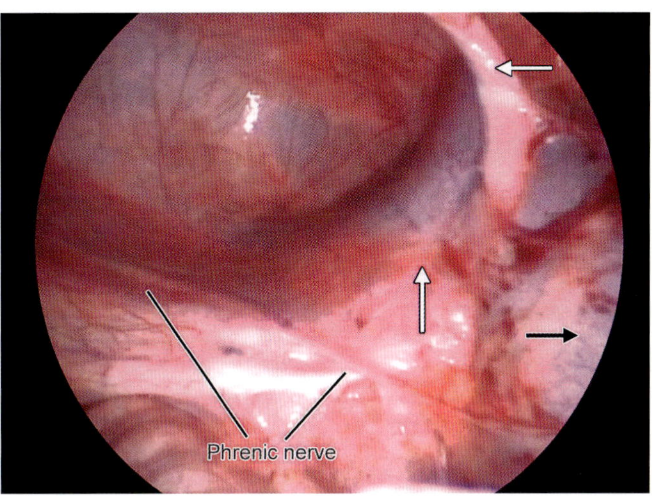

Fig. 21.2.21: Thoracoscopic view of diaphragmatic defect (white arrows) in a case of congenital diaphragmatic hernia (CDH). Black arrow shows the heart.

is the "Bochdalek hernia", which involves the posterolateral part of the diaphragm. It is more common (85%) on the left side **(Fig. 21.2.21)**.[5,6]

Pathophysiology

Pathophysiological events leading to respiratory distress in congenital diaphragmatic hernia (CDH):

- The shift of mediastinum during the antenatal period causes pressure on the contralateral developing lung affecting its development also. This pulmonary hypoplasia limits the gaseous exchange in the available lung tissue.
- Pulmonary hypoplasia also affects the vascular component of the lung. Thus, there is an increased resistance in the pulmonary vasculature resulting in pulmonary hypertension. This may further lead to a persistent fetal circulation.
- The presence of abdominal contents in the chest causes pressure on the lung—this restricts lung expansion, which can be compounded by the gaseous distension of the bowel in a crying baby.
- The hypoplastic lung may not be able to handle normal inspiratory pressures and the resultant alveolar rupture may result in pneumothorax on the affected side or even on the other side.

The severity of symptoms and signs depends mainly on the status of lung development. A severely hypoplastic lung may not be compatible with life, whereas at the other extreme, some cases of CDH may be relatively asymptomatic for years and may present much later in childhood due to repeated chest infections.[6]

Clinical Features

If antenatally diagnosed, these patients must preferably be antenatally transported for birthing in hospitals with adequate facilities for immediate, advanced neonatal care, and neonatal surgical facilities.

Postnatally, in the severely affected baby, there is respiratory distress and cyanosis. The ipsilateral chest appears prominent with evidence of mediastinal shift. Breath sounds on the involved side are absent, occasionally peristaltic sounds can be heard due to displacement of viscera to the chest. In most cases, the abdomen is scaphoid. Heart sounds and apical impulse are on the right side.

Occasionally, patients present late with only recurrent lower respiratory tract infection (LRTI).

Investigations

- A chest X-ray is diagnostic. It shows loops of bowel in the chest cavity. There may be significant mediastinal shift or an associated pneumothorax. In right-sided Bochdalek hernia, liver is the main constituent of the chest cavity.
- In doubtful cases, an abdominal USG or computed tomography (CT) scan of the chest is useful.
- Hypoxia and acidosis should be estimated by arterial blood gas analysis.

Treatment

Primary Management

- Essential to realize that CDH is a physiological emergency rather than a surgical emergency.[5,6]
- A nasogastric tube (NGT) passed immediately to deflate the stomach and reduce aerophagia.
- Intubation with an endotracheal tube at the earliest for a breathless child. Bag and mask ventilation is avoided for fear of increasing aerophagia.
- Ventilation ideally with a high frequency ventilator. However in many cases a pressure-cycle ventilator with high rates may suffice.[5,6]
- Acidosis correction and maintaining mild alkalosis.[5,6]
- In case of severe pulmonary hypertension, drugs to cause pulmonary vasodilatation along with systemic vasopressors are used.[5,6]

Surgery

- Surgery is performed only after stabilizing the baby's condition as much as possible.
- Through a laparotomy, the defect in the diaphragm is identified, the herniated viscera are reposited in the abdomen. The abdominal wall may need to be stretched for accommodating the same. The defect is then repaired.

- Thoracoscopic surgery is being deployed in an increasing number of patients who are stable enough to tolerate the same.
- Very rarely, extracorporeal membrane oxygenation (ECMO) may be indicated in these patients.

Key Messages

- Antenatally diagnosed CDH patients should be delivered in a center with advanced neonatal care.
- Clinically, a strong suspicion should be made on seeing a breathless child with a scaphoid abdomen since other causes of breathlessness cause abdominal distension due to aerophagia.

GASTROINTESTINAL TRACT

INFANTILE HYPERTROPHIC PYLORIC STENOSIS

Incidence

- 1:300 children (Western literature); approximately 1:3,500 for Indian children.[7]
- Mostly sporadic but few cases may run in families.
- The ratio of male:female is 5:1, especially first-born males.[7]

Pathology

Musculature of the pyloric antrum is significantly hypertrophied; thus the pylorus is thickened; pyloric canal is lengthened and narrowed. The olive-shaped pylorus becomes hard to feel when contracted. This hypertrophied pylorus is clinically palpable as a "pyloric tumor" **(Fig. 21.2.22)**. The stomach proximal to the obstruction is dilated and hypertrophied. Gastric mucosa in infancy produces a potent lipase, which hydrolyses milk to free fatty acids. The rancidity of the curdled milk gradually causes progressive mucosal edema and precipitates complete obstruction **(Fig. 21.2.23)**, and thus symptoms often delayed till 3–6 weeks.[7]

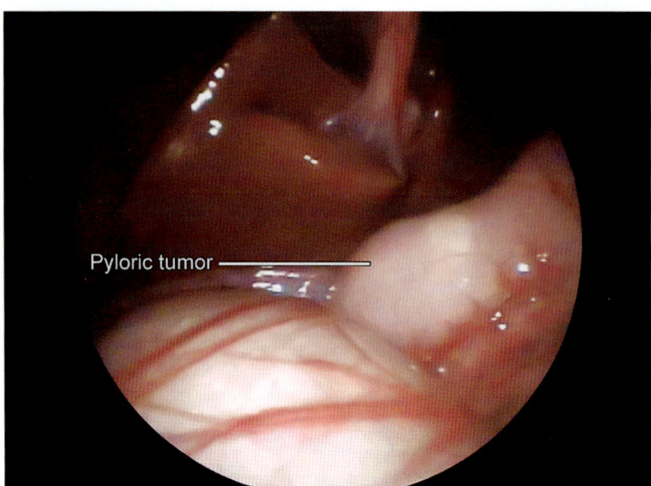

Fig. 21.2.22: Laparoscopic view of the hypertrophied pylorus in a case of infantile hypertrophic pyloric stenosis (IHPS).

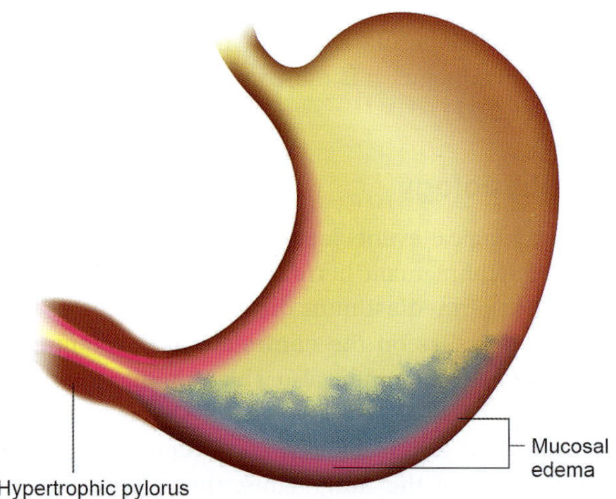

Fig. 21.2.23: Diagrammatic representation of the hypertrophy of the pylorus along with the mucosal edema precipitating the complete obstruction of the pyloric outlet.

Clinical Features

Usually, child is seen between 3 and 6 weeks or any time between 1 week and 4 months.

- Vomiting is the most important presenting symptom—progressive, forcible, projectile, and nonbilious, may come from nose. In most cases, the baby is hungry again after the vomit. There may be altered blood.
- Constipation due to poor intake.
- Weight loss or failure to gain weight.
- Jaundice—occasionally seen due to nutritional deficiencies.
- Facies is characteristic—alert, anxious, and hungry look. Unlike a toxic or septicemic baby, these babies have a slow and shallow breathing due to alkalosis.
- Visible peristalsis on inspection (left to right). Examination must be done with the child comfortably placed in the mother's lap and in good light.
- Palpation of the "tumor" (palpable in 70% cases) is the diagnostic sign. It should be looked for with the left hand, sitting on the patients' left palpating below the right costal margin, underneath the liver border.[7]

Specific Investigations

- *Serum electrolytes:* Hypokalemic, hypochloremic alkalosis
- Ultrasonography shows the "tumor"

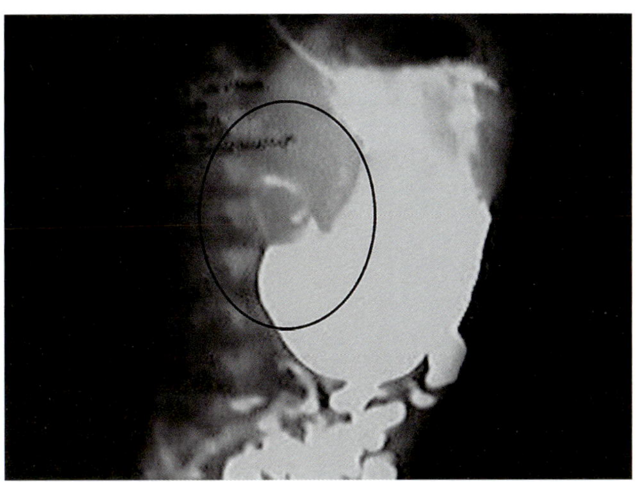

Fig. 21.2.24: String sign seen on barium (Ba) meal examination in case of infantile hypertrophic pyloric stenosis (IHPS).

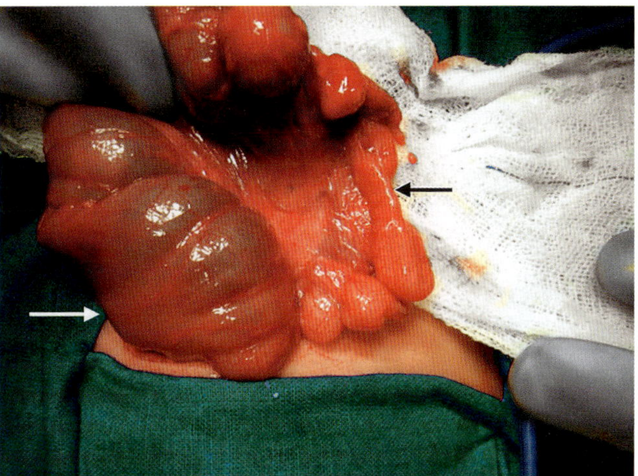

Fig. 21.2.25: Atresia showing complete block of the intestine.

- Contrast studies with barium only if necessary—"string sign", large stomach, delayed emptying, and gastritis **(Fig. 21.2.24)**.

Differential diagnosis includes almost any condition leading to nonbilious vomiting in children, especially gastroenteritis, septicemia, meningitis, and gastroesophageal reflux (GFR).

Treatment

- *Nonsurgical treatment with prokinetics:* To be used only in case of strong contraindication to surgery as the treatment has erratic results and is too prolonged.
- *Surgical treatment:* Treatment of choice.[7]
- *Preoperative:* Correct dehydration and electrolyte imbalance by:
    - *Nasogastric* aspiration and stomach wash with normal saline.
    - Administer 1/3 or 1/2 strength saline through NGT or intravenous (IV).
- *Operation:* Fredet-Ramstedt's pyloromyotomy—laparoscopic surgery possible.
- *Results:* In experienced hands, results are excellent.

INTESTINAL ATRESIA

Intestinal atresia is an obstruction of the intestine due to a complete occlusion of the lumen **(Fig. 21.2.25)**.

Clinical Features and Diagnosis

These are dependent on the site of atresia.

Investigations:

- *Double-bubble sign:* Duodenal atresia **(Fig. 21.2.26)**
- *Multiple fluid levels:* Jejunal or ileal atresia **(Fig. 21.2.27)**

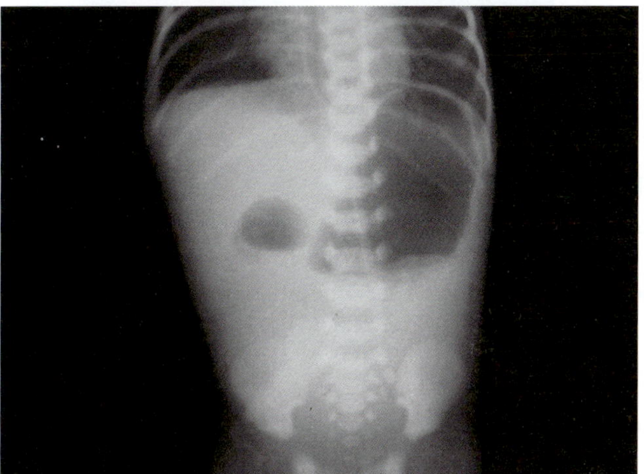

Fig. 21.2.26: An erect plain X-ray showing a double-bubble sign of a duodenal atresia.

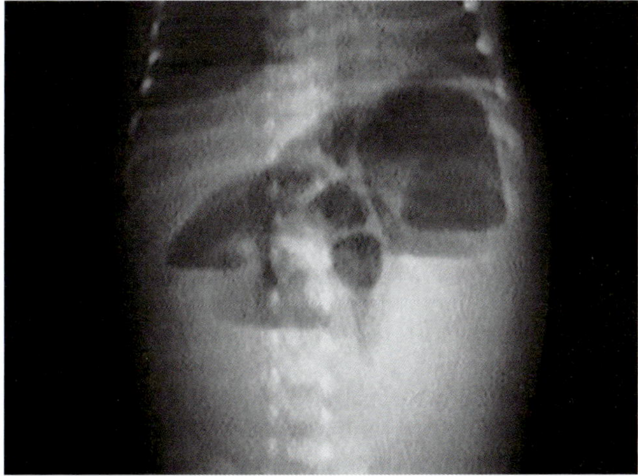

Fig. 21.2.27: An erect X-ray of abdomen showing fluid levels in the upper abdomen with a gasless lower abdomen suggesting a jejunal atresia.

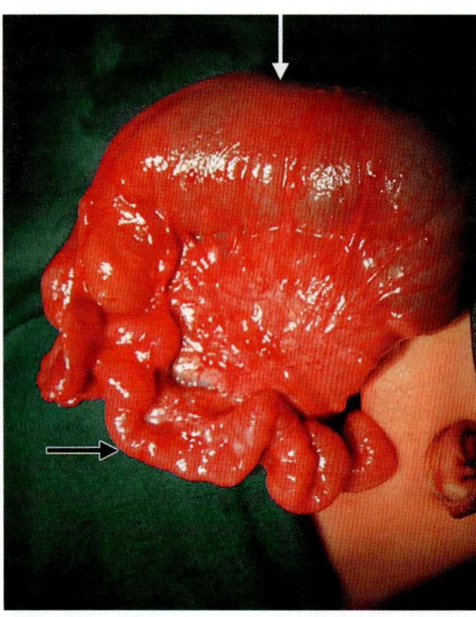

Fig. 21.2.28: Jejunal atresia—massively dilated jejunal loops (white arrow) and collapsed and small caliber distal small bowel (black arrow).

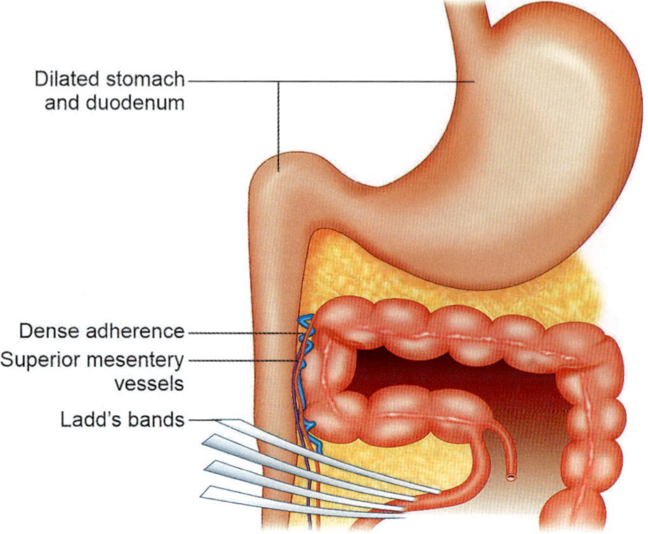

Fig. 21.2.29: Diagrammatic representation of the pathological anatomy in a malrotation—ileocecal region to the left with Ladd's bands crossing from the right abdominal wall toward the ileocecal region compressing the duodenum (which is entirely on right side). Note the narrow root of mesentery—a cause for midgut volvulus.

Treatment

- Early surgery, after at least partial correction of dehydration
- *On laparotomy:* Resection and anastomosis or bypass of atretic segment **(Fig. 21.2.28)**

Prognosis

- Fairly good in uncomplicated cases.
- Deteriorates, if treated late, low birth weight, or premature, or presence of sepsis and other anomalies.
- Poor if multiple atresias or there is a large section of the bowel, which does not have a proper vascular supply (apple peel atresia).

INTESTINAL MALROTATION

If the process of intestinal rotation is incomplete, then malrotation is said to have taken place.

Pathological Anatomy

- The duodenojejunal flexure is to the right of the midline and cecum adjacent on its left, and thus significantly narrowing the root of the mesentery; the ascending and transverse colon are mobile. Together these anomalies can lead to twisting of the intestine (volvulus neonatorum).
- Abnormal peritoneal bands [Ladd's bands **(Fig. 21.2.29)**] run from right peritoneal wall to the cecum over the third part of the duodenum compressing the duodenum.
- In case of volvulus neonatorum, the vascularity of entire midgut can suffer, leading to gangrene, if not corrected early.

Clinical Features

There is a sudden development of upper intestinal obstruction in an apparently normal child, who may have passed normal meconium earlier. If volvulus neonatorum sets in duodenal atresia with gangrene of the midgut [bleeding per rectum (PR)], there is progressive deterioration in the general condition with septicemia.

Diagnosis

- *An erect X-ray of abdomen:* A large stomach bubble or a double-bubble and may show few distal gas shadows. Multiple fluid levels are not seen in this variety of intestinal obstruction.
- *Barium studies:* Duodenum lies to the right of midline; alternatively, a barium enema would show the entire colon to the left of midline.
- Ultrasonography with Doppler can identify the abnormal lie of the superior mesenteric artery and bowel ischemia if any.

Treatment

- Resuscitation as required (high fluid requirement).
- *Exploratory laparotomy:* Ladd's bands released, and root of the mesentery widened to prevent further episodes of volvulus (Ladd's procedure).
- *Gangrenous bowel, if any:* Resection or exteriorization.

Prognosis

Good, if surgery done before gangrene sets in.

INTUSSUSCEPTION

Intussusception indicates the telescoping of one part of the intestine into another—common around 8–10 months of age **(Fig. 21.2.30)**.

Pathology

- The most common site—ileocecal region **(Fig. 21.2.31)**.
- The most common lead point—a hypertrophied Peyer's patch following a change in the bacterial flora during weaning or gastrointestinal infection or due to ingestion of infected respiratory secretions.
- Compression of the mesentery and venous congestion within the innermost layer of intussusception causes secretion of blood and mucus, characteristically labeled as red currant jelly stool. Further, vascular compromise may lead to gangrene of a portion of the bowel.

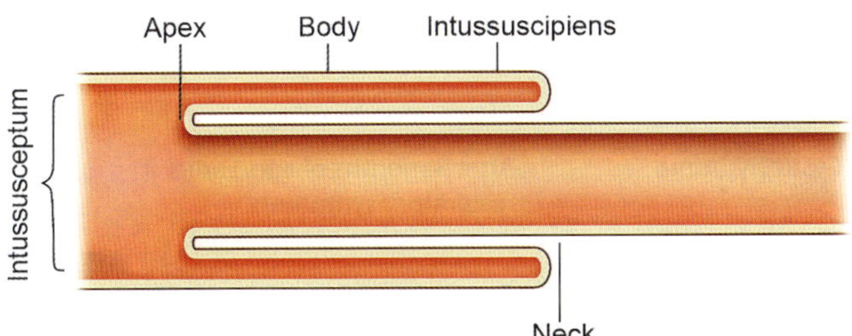

Fig. 21.2.30: Diagrammatic representation of intussusception and its parts.

Clinical Features

- Classically a healthy, well-nourished child, and <1 year of age.
- There may be a prior history of a URTI/URI.
- Colic pain occurs in short bursts with intermittent periods of remission.
- Vomiting—bilious only in late cases.
- Red currant jelly stools—usually with no fecal matter after one to two times (a differentiating feature from dysentery) **(Fig. 21.2.32)**.
- On abdominal palpation—intussusception may be felt as banana-shaped mass with its concavity toward the umbilicus. Occasionally, it can be felt PR.
- In late cases—features of septicemia and peritonitis.

Investigations

- Ultrasound of the abdomen can be diagnostic.
- Alternatively, a barium enema—the coiled spring sign or the claw sign **(Fig. 21.2.33)**.

Treatment

- If diagnosed within 24 hours of attack, hydrostatic reduction attempted by a pediatric surgeon (under USG or radiological control) with facilities for immediate surgery in case of complications.
- *If hydrostatic reduction fails or is contraindicated—exploratory laparotomy:* Operative reduction or if necessary, resection and anastomosis.
- The commonly seen pediatric surgical conditions and the treatment plan are summarized in **Table 21.2.2**.

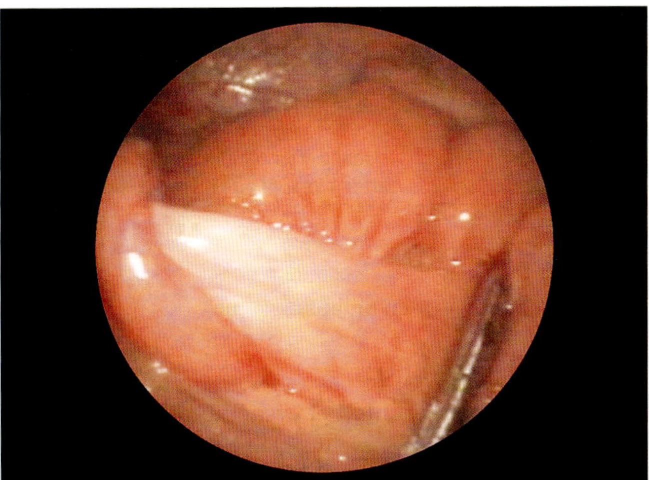

Fig. 21.2.31: Laparoscopic view of an intussusception.

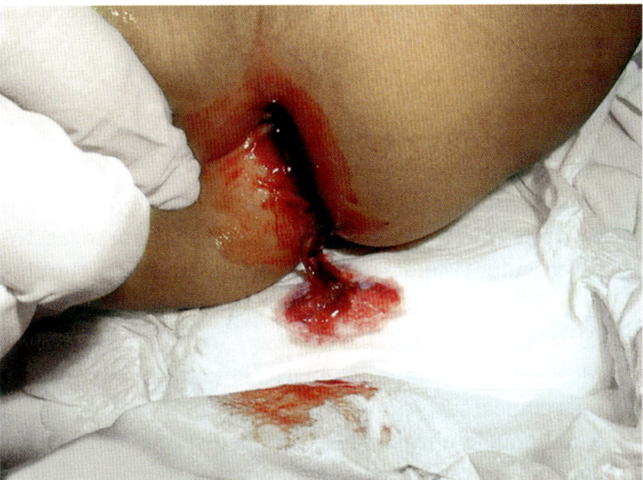

Fig. 21.2.32: Red currant jelly stools.
Courtesy: Dr A Vaidya.

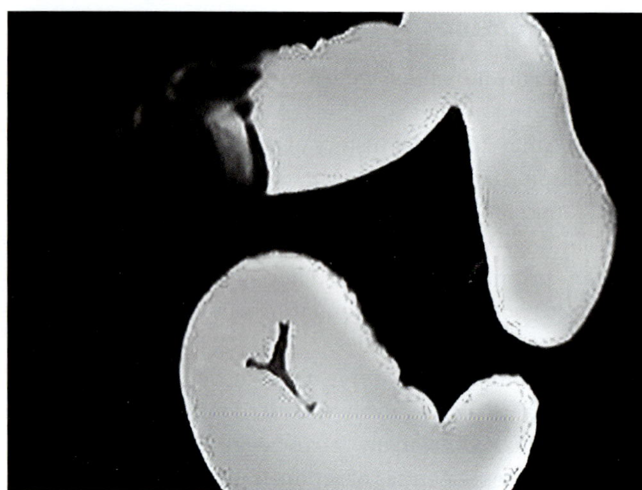

Fig. 21.2.33: Coil spring picture in a barium (Ba) enema for intussusception.

MECKEL'S DIVERTICULUM

This is the persistent proximal part of the vitellointestinal duct. The diverticulum is present on the antimesenteric border of the terminal ileum **(Fig. 21.2.34)**.

The Rule of two: Meckel's diverticulum is present in 2% of the population that is situated 2 feet from the ileocecal junction, is 2-inch-long and is usually symptomatic before the age of 2 years.

Complications

Meckel's diverticulum is symptomatic only if complications arise. These could be:

- *Bleeding:* It is usually painless and profuse. It is due to peptic ulceration in the surrounding ileal mucosa due to acid secretion from heterotopic gastric mucosa seen in some cases.
- Intestinal obstruction:
  - As a lead point of an intussusception.
  - A band from the diverticulum to the umbilicus may cause internal herniation or volvulus.
- *Diverticulitis:* It produces symptoms and signs identical to appendicitis, but the prognosis is worse as the diverticulum is more prone to perforation and peritonitis.

Diagnosis

- Most commonly at abdominal exploration or laparoscopy on a clinical suspicion.
- A radionuclide scan may show the diverticulum as a hot spot only in case there is ectopic gastric mucosa—may be missed during active bleeding.
- Barium study—rarely beneficial.

TABLE 21.2.2: Common pediatric surgical conditions and their basic management plan.

Conditions	*Management plan*
Congenital inguinal hernia	• Operate early even at 1 week of age, if necessary • Fear of strangulation is the highest in newborn period
Tunica vaginal hydrocele/encysted hydrocele of cord	No need for of urgency. Operate after 6 months of age but preferably before 2 years of age unless seen later
Phimosis	Usually after 2 years of age, rarely before 6 months of age. Preputioplasty—an alternative surgery
Paraphimosis	• Reduce as soon as possible (ASAP), plan early surgery • Emergency surgery if not reduced manually
Undescended testis	After 6 months of age and preferably before 1 year of age Earlier, if accompanied with hernia
Cleft lip	Usually around 3 months of age
Cleft palate	Usually between 9 months and 12 months of age
Tongue-tie	Preferably before 1 year of age
Branchial cyst and sinus	After 6 months of age
Cystic hygroma	After 3 months of age. Earlier if respiratory symptoms
Thyroglossal cyst and sinus	Usually after 6 months of age
Torticollis	After 1 year of age
Umbilical hernia	Usually after 2 years of age, any time earlier if history of recurrent irreducibility. Emergency in case of obstruction
Omphalocele	Primary or delayed primary depending on the size
Gastroschisis	At birth
Hypospadias	Usually after 6 months of age, may be after 1 year of age if severe chordee

Treatment

Diverticulectomy—open or laparoscopic.

MECONIUM ILEUS

The neonatal manifestation of cystic fibrosis—a condition affecting all the mucus secreting glands of the body, causing excessive viscidity of the mucus secretion. It is an autosomal recessive disease, which is common in Western countries. In recent years, incidence is increasing in India.

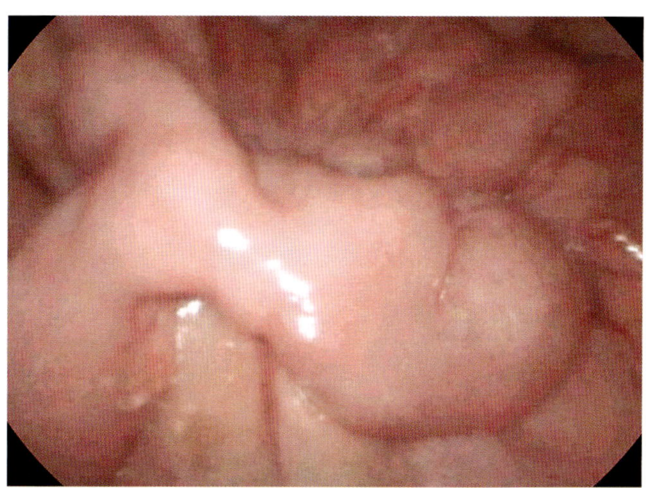

Fig. 21.2.34: Laparoscopic view of a Meckel's diverticulum.

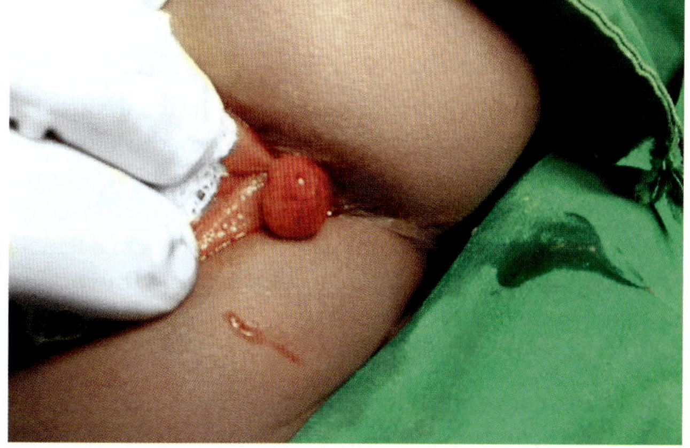

Fig. 21.2.35: Rectal polyp.

Pathology

The mucus secreted in the intestine is extremely sticky, like plasticine, leading to adherence of meconium to the intestinal mucosa, and thus choking up the lumen of the distal intestine, not allowing any contents to pass through.

Clinical Features

- Midintestinal obstruction
- Baby may pass some white chalky meconium
- Viscid meconium may be palpable as a doughy substance in the lower abdomen.

Diagnosis

- *Plain X-ray of the abdomen:* Dilated bowel but no fluid levels.
- *Gastrograffin or (conray/urograffin) enema:* Microcolon (a thin narrow segment of distal relatively unused bowel).

Treatment

The very high osmolarity of conray or gastrograffin enema causes dissolution of the inspissated mucus and may be curative. In case, the obstruction does not resolve after the use of conray, surgery will be required to relieve the obstruction.

RECTAL POLYP

Rectal polyp is a benign adenomatous polyp, usually single. Common in the age group of 3–6 years.

Clinically presents as:

- Bleeding PR—fresh blood in drops at the time of defecation.
- Something coming out PR **(Fig. 21.2.35)**.
  Polyp may be felt on digital examination. It needs to be removed surgically.

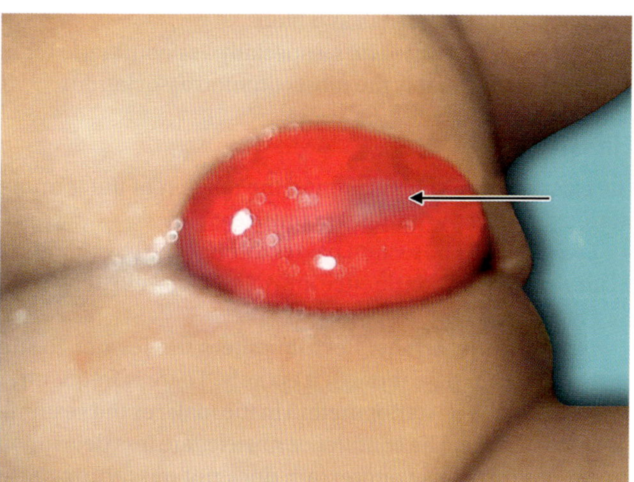

Fig. 21.2.36: Prolapse of rectum—arrow points to the lumen in the center of the prolapse to differentiate from a prolapsed polyp.

RECTAL PROLAPSE

Something coming out PR **(Fig. 21.2.36)**

- Bleeding may be associated.
- *Predisposing factors*: Constipation, diarrhea, and severe cough.

Treatment

- Treatment of the predisposing factors.
- Submucosal sclerosant injections—usually curative.
- Per-rectal/abdominal or laparoscopic surgery required in very rare cases.

ANORECTAL ANOMALIES

Anorectal anomalies are a wide spectrum of anomalies that affect the opening of the terminal anorectum and adjacent perineal structures.

Incidence

Roughly 1 in 5,000 live births.

Pathological Anatomy

The anus does not open normally at the usual site. The opening may be severely stenotic or absent. In the latter case, the rectum ends as a blind pouch. There may be a fistulous communication from the rectal pouch to perineum or the urinary tract in the male or the genital structures in a female. The usual muscles of continence are present in the normal positions but since the terminal gastrointestinal tract (GIT) may not pass through them, they may be poorly developed.

Associated anomalies with these groups:

- *VATER association:* Vertebral, anorectal, tracheo-esophageal, and renal.
- *VACTERL association:* Vertebral, anorectal, cardiac, tracheoesophageal, renal, and limb.
- *Genitourinary anomalies,* especially vesicoureteric reflux (VUR) are probably the most common association.

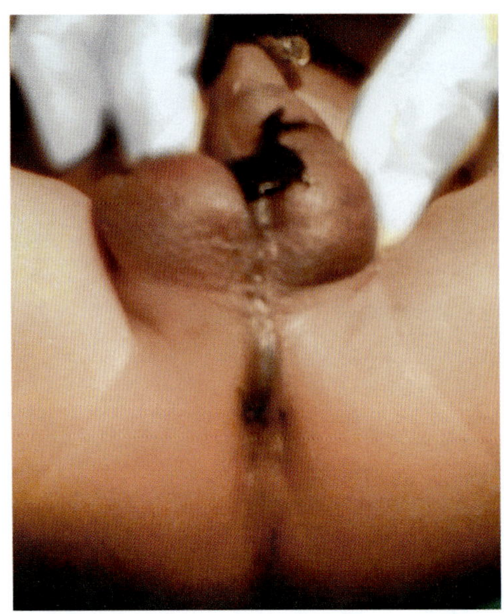

Fig. 21.2.37: Anorectal malformations (ARM)—cutaneous fistula opening on scrotal raphe (low variety).

Classification

The classification centers around the relation of the terminal anorectum with the levator ani muscle.

- *Low variety:* The rectum passes through the levator funnel entirely. The continence muscles are well-developed **(Fig. 21.2.37)**.
- *Intermediate variety:* Rectum enters the levator funnel but does not pass through it entirely. There is frequently a fistula to the posterior urethra in the male, or the vestibule in the female. The continence muscles are less developed.
- *High variety:* The anorectum does not pass through the levator, which is poorly developed—externally manifested as a flat perineum **(Fig. 21.2.38)**, and the fistula is to the urethra or bladder in male and there may be a cloacal anomaly in the female.

Clinically, most varieties of ARM should be identified at birth itself or may present as low-intestinal obstruction. In those with a wide external fistula, the presentation may be of recurrent constipation.

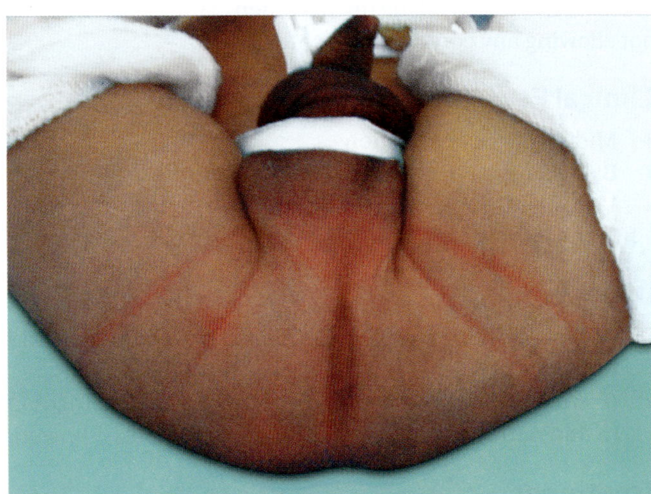

Fig. 21.2.38: Flat perineum as seen in a baby of high anorectal malformations (ARM).

Investigations

Mainly directed at ascertaining the relationship of the anorectum with levator ani and the identification of a fistula if any.

Invertogram or a Prone Lateral Film (Fig. 21.2.39)

It assesses the level of air shadow in the blind rectal pouch with respect to bony landmarks. Since the swallowed air can take 24 hours to reach the rectum, this assessment is likely to be fallacious if done earlier. In patients with an open fistula, the same relationship can be ascertained by dye studies through the fistula.

Treatment

- *Low anomalies:* Since the rectum has already descended through the levator muscles, treated by a surgical exploration of the perineum at birth.
- *Intermediate or high anomaly:* An initial colostomy to relieve the intestinal obstruction. At a later stage, a definitive surgery—the most common being posterior sagittal anorectoplasty (PSARP). The colostomy is closed as the third stage of surgery.

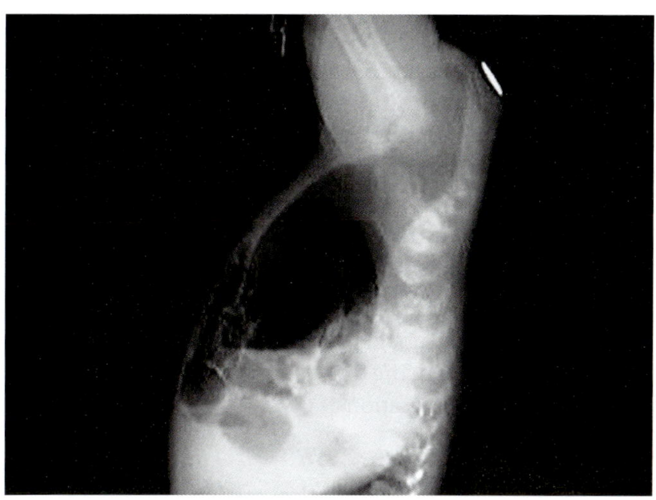

Fig. 21.2.39: Invertogram in case of low anorectal malformations (ARM).

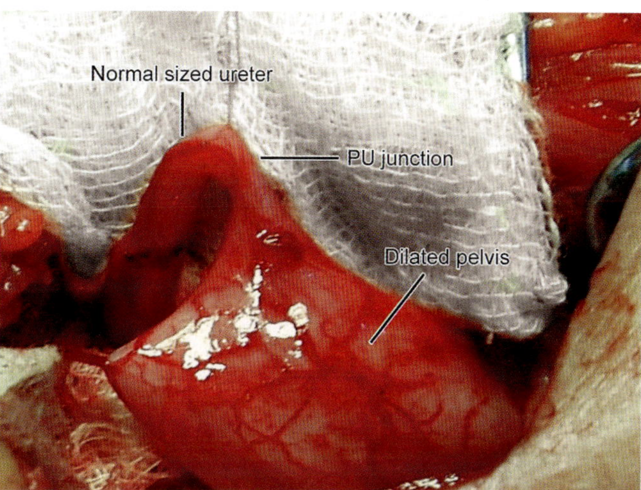

Fig. 21.2.40: Dilated pelvis of a hydronephrotic kidney. (PU: pelviureteric)

KIDNEY AND THE UROGENITAL TRACT

OBSTRUCTIVE UROPATHIES

Obstructive uropathy is a set of condition causing chronic, partial obstruction to the flow of urine anywhere distal to the renal calyces. Obstruction to the flow of urine could lead to:

- Ballooning of calyces and thinning of the renal parenchyma. The renal function gradually deteriorates. High pressures in the antenatal period could cause renal dysplasia.
- Infection further deteriorates renal function.

Common Sites of Obstruction

- Pelviureteric junction **(Fig. 21.2.40)**.
- *Ureteric obstruction:* Usually acquired due to calculus or external compression. Rarely ureteric valves (congenital).
- Vesicoureteric junction.
- *Urethra:* Posterior and anterior urethral valves.

Clinical Features

- Antenatal detection
- Pain in the abdomen
- Recurrent urinary tract infection (UTI)
- Lump in the abdomen—kidney or palpable bladder
- Rarely hematuria
- Gastrointestinal symptoms such as nausea, vomiting, and anorexia, especially in an infant.
- Nonspecific symptoms such as failure to thrive, weakness, and lethargy.
- Poor urinary stream/straining at micturition/retention of urine in case of urethral valves.

Diagnostic and Evaluative Imaging

- *Abdominal ultrasonography:* It identifies the extent of pelvic and ureteric dilatation, bladder hypertrophy, urethral dilatation, and postvoid residue besides any other anomalies.
- *Intravenous pyelography (IVP)—replaced by CT urography or MR urography:* Detailed anatomical delineation.
- A *micturating cystourethrogram (MCUG)* to look for vesicoureteric reflux (VUR) or urethral obstruction, which may mimic or present as a pelviureteric obstruction **(Fig. 21.2.41)**.
- *Isotope renogram:* To assess differential 1 function and scarring (preferably done with an open indwelling bladder catheter).

Complications

- Deterioration of renal function due to progressive renal dilatation.
- Pyonephrosis and septicemia in case of infection.

Pelviureteric Junction Obstruction

- *Pathology:* The obstruction is either due to an adynamic segment or an external compression by an aberrant renal artery. The partial obstruction gets exacerbated during any diuretic period.
- Management principles
    - *Antenatally:* Urgent antenatal consultation required, if there is oligohydramnios. In unilateral isolated hydronephrosis, an expectant line of management is usually followed.
    - *Postnatal management:* Based on the differential renal function, size, and progress of hydronephrosis.
- Spontaneous resolution known in infancy.
- Definite indications for surgery—deteriorating renal function/pain/infection/palpable mass—Anderson-Hynes pyeloplasty (open or laparoscopic).

VESICOURETERIC REFLUX

Vesicoureteric reflux is due to the failure of the normal valvular action at the vesicoureteric junction, which thus permits a variable quantity of urine to reflux back into the ureter and at times even in the renal pelvicalyceal system. Vesicoureteric reflux may be either primary or secondary to high pressures in the bladder either in case of distal outflow obstruction or certain variants of neurogenic bladder.

Pathology

- Features of obstructive uropathy.
- Renal damage could be significant in presence of active infection.

Management Principles

- Prevent and control infection
- Monitor renal function
- Minor degrees of VUR can be self-limiting
- Treat primary cause of VUR, if possible, e.g., posterior urethral valves (PUV) or neurogenic bladder.
- *Surgery (definitive treatment):*
  - *Subureteral-transurethral injection (STING) procedure:* Endoscopic injection of dextranomer hyaluronic acid (Deflux)® at the vesicoureteric junction.
  - *Ureteric reimplantation:*
    - Transvesical
    - Extravesical
    - Laparoscopic

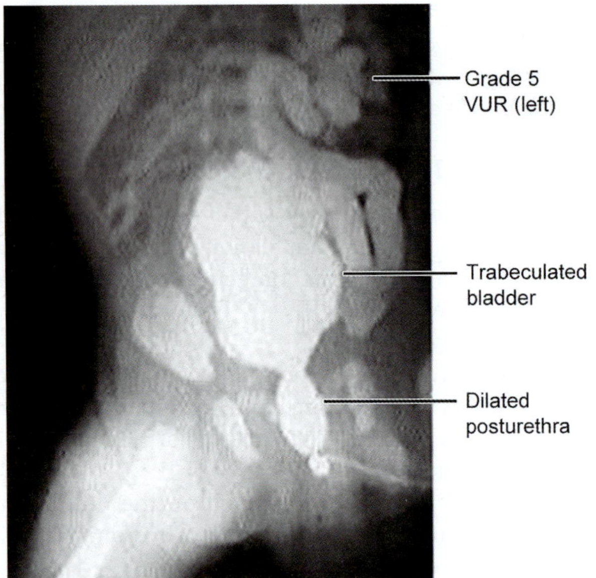

Fig. 21.2.41: Micturating cystourethrogram (MCU) showing grade 5 vesicoureteric reflux (VUR) on left side with trabeculated bladder, dilated posterior urethra with normal caliber distal urethra.

POSTERIOR URETHRAL VALVES

They are the most common cause of end-stage renal disease in children.[3] They are thin curtain like membranes in the posterior urethra causing a partial obstruction to the flow of urine **(Fig. 21.2.42)**. Poor urine stream in a male child should make one suspect PUV.

Management Principles

- Essential to reduce back-pressure on bladder at the earliest.
- Aggressive treatment of azotemia or sepsis, if present.
- Strict asepsis during all urinary tract interventions including catheterizations.

Surgical Options

- Primary urethroscopic fulguration of valves.
- *Diversion of urine: Vesicostomy/ureterostomy/pyelostomy.* Long-term follow up is essential to identify and treat renal malfunction.

Prognosis

- Poor in case of antenatal oligohydramnios
- Guarded in case of early uremia/sepsis
- Cautious in case of significant dilatation of ureters/pelvis
- Good in others.

Key Messages

- Obstructive uropathy or UTI may have insidious presentations.
- Need to identify the patients who will require urgent aggressive treatment.
- Obstruction may resolve or may be progressive.
- Long-term follow-up is essential.

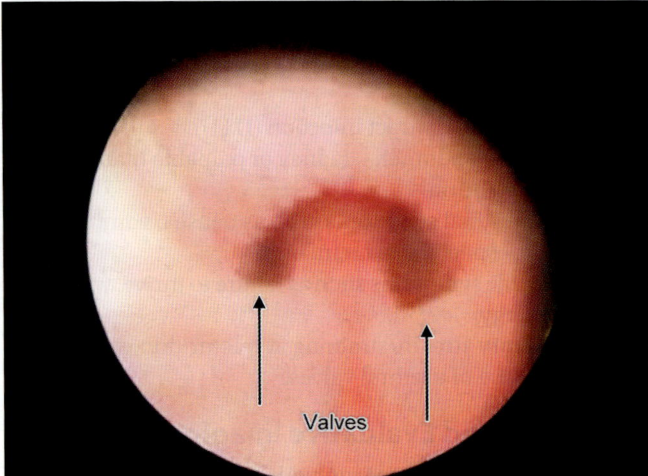

Fig. 21.2.42: Urethroscopic view of posterior urethral valve.

NEONATAL SURGERY

NEONATAL SURGICAL EMERGENCIES

General Principles of Management

- *Nil by mouth (NBM):* When in doubt, keep the baby nil orally.
- Keep baby warm—in the hospital and during transport.
- Cover open wounds, e.g., exomphalos, meningomyelocele, etc.
- *Pass nasogastric tube (NGT) and always keep it open:* (No. 6 or higher), especially in case of vomiting or breathless child (pass NGT minimizes aerophagia and aspiration).
- Transport preferably in prone position.
- Recording passage of urine and meconium with its color and informing surgeon.
- *Supportive:* Antibiotics, intravenous (IV) fluids, and monitoring of vitals.

NEONATAL EMERGENCIES: SPECIFIC CONDITIONS

Intestinal Obstruction

Intestinal obstruction is the failure of aboral progression of intestinal contents.

- *Dynamic obstruction:* It is due to a physical occlusion of a portion of bowel, which may arise either:
  - From outside the wall of the bowel as in compression due to bands, etc.
  - From within the wall, e.g., atresia, etc.
  - From within the lumen like inspissated meconium, etc.
- *Adynamic obstruction:* It is due to absence of peristalsis in the whole or a segment of the bowel.

  Clinically, the presentation is dependent on the level of obstruction, the severity of obstruction, the acuteness of obstruction, and the possibility of vascular compromise, if any.
- *Upper intestinal obstruction:* Early onset of vomiting and failure to tolerate feeds. Abdominal distension, if present, is confined to the upper abdomen. The baby may pass some normal colored meconium or pale colored meconium. Dehydration occurs early and is severe:
  - *Duodenal atresia:* The vomitus may be bilious or nonbilious.
  - Antenatal hydramnios
  - Malrotation with midgut volvulus
- *Small intestinal obstruction:* It is characterized by abdominal distension, failure to pass meconium, and later vomiting (invariably bilious):
  - Jejunal or ileal atresia
  - Meconium ileus
- *Large intestinal obstruction:* The earliest symptom is failure to pass meconium; other symptoms of intestinal obstruction follow. Abdominal distension is gross and generalized:
  - Hirschsprung disease
  - Anorectal malformations (ARM)
  - Meconium plug syndrome
  - Colonic atresias

Key Messages

- Bilious vomiting or bilious gastric aspirate in a newborn is considered pathognomonic of intestinal obstruction.
- Higher the obstruction, more the dehydration.

CONCLUSION

Pediatric surgical conditions can often mimic general symptomatology in children. An alert pediatrician can contribute by timely diagnosis and judicious preliminary assessment.

Successful long-term outcomes of pediatric surgical conditions necessitates effective peri-surgical management, astute but delicate handling of pediatric tissues technically, combined with an empathic approach to the aggrieved child and family. Co-ordinated team management between the primary pediatrician and a well-trained pediatric surgeons can successfully achieve remarkable outcomes.

REFERENCES

1. Bhagwat S, Ramadwar R. Inguinal Hernia and Hydrocoele: In: Redkar R, Agarwal P, Raveenthiran V (Eds). IAPS TB of Pediatric Surgery. New Delhi: Jaypee Brothers; 2020. pp. 795-802.
2. Shah RS, Redddy S, Joshi NM. Undescended Testis. In: Redkar R, Agarwal P, Raveenthiran V (Eds). IAPS TB of Pediatric Surgery. New Delhi: Jaypee Brothers; 2020. pp. 803-11.
3. Sambandan K. Phimosis and Related disorders of the Prepuce. In: Redkar R, Agarwal P, Raveenthiran V, Agarwal P (Eds). IAPS TB of Pediatric Surgery. New Delhi: Jaypee Brothers; 2020. pp. 789-94.
4. Harmon CM, Coran AG. Congenital anomalies of the esophagus. In: Grosfeld JL, O'Neill JA, Fonkalsrud EW, Caldamone AA. Pediatric Surgery. Philadelphia: Mosby Elsevier; 2006. pp. 1051-81.
5. Parelkar S, Sanghvi B, Gupta R. Congenital diaphragmatic hernia. In: Redkar R, Agarwal P, Raveenthiran V (Eds). IAPS Textbook of Pediatric Surgery. New Delhi: Jaypee Brothers; 2020. pp. 305-15.
6. Stolar CJH, Dilon PW. Congenital Diaphragmatic Hernia and Eventeration. In: Grosfeld JL, O'Neill J A, Fonkalsrud EW, Caldamone AA (Eds). Pediatric Surgery. Philadelphia: Mosby Elsevier; 2006. pp. 931-54.
7. Kulkarni S, Kulkarni M. Infantile Hypertrophic Pyloric stenosis. In: Redkar R, Agarwal P, Raveenthiran V (Eds). IAPS Textbook of Pediatric Surgery. New Delhi: Jaypee Brothers; 2020. pp. 369-80.

21.3 Common Pediatric Orthopedic Conditions

Vijay Sriram, Kailash Sarathy

DEVELOPMENTAL DYSPLASIA OF HIP

The term developmental dysplasia of hip (DDH) is preferred to congenital dislocation of hip (CDH) as in many children the hip is not dislocated at birth but there is a spectrum of presentation **(Fig. 21.3.1A)** from dysplasia, subluxation to dislocation. Its significance lies in its early diagnosis because a delay in detection and treatment can yield less than optimum outcome.[1]

Diagnosis

Risk factors include girl child, first born, breech presentation, and positive family history. Clinical tests that may be useful include Barlow and Ortolani tests **(Figs. 21.3.1B and C)**. Ultrasound (USG) is a very important screening tool in neonate. Radiographs are done in older children. Magnetic resonance imaging (MRI) is very rarely indicated.

Treatment

The treatment depends upon the age of the patient. The prognosis is better when treated early. Reduction can be achieved by Pavlik Harness **(Fig. 21.3.2)**; closed reduction under general anesthesia and hip spica cast application **(Figs. 21.3.3A and B)**; open reduction of the hip. Additional surgical procedures may be required to reconstruct a shallow acetabulum or to correct excessive ante version of the femoral neck, especially in older children.

CONGENITAL TALIPES EQUINOVARUS

Clubfoot or congenital talipes equinovarus (CTEV) is the most common congenital anomaly. It is either idiopathic or sometimes associated with other conditions such as spina bifida, arthrogryposis, or limb deficiencies, etc. The deformity consists of equinus (plantar flexion) at the ankle

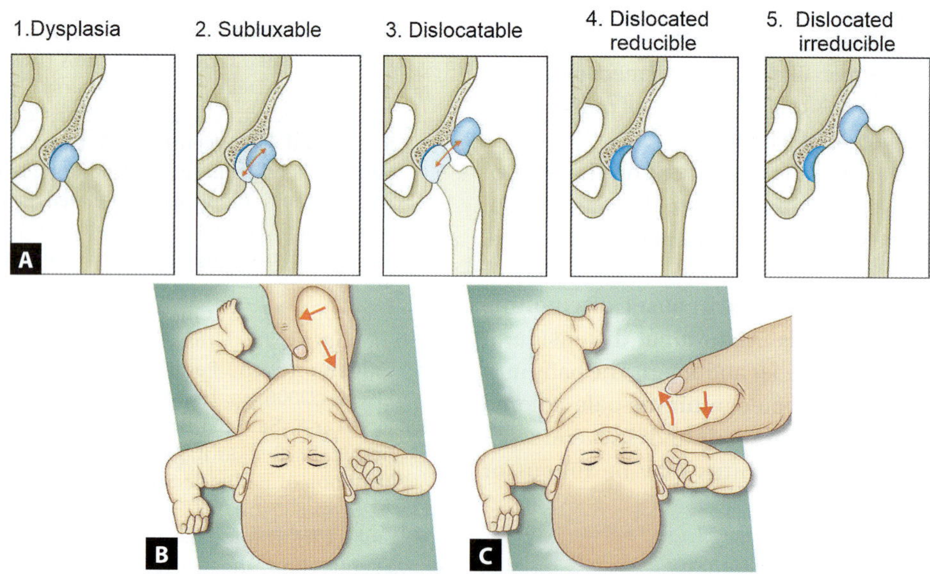

Figs. 21.3.1A to C: (A) The spectrum of developmental dysplasia of hip (DDH)—1. Dysplasia, 2. Subluxable, 3. Dislocatable, 4. Dislocated reducible, and 5. Dislocated and irreducible; (B) Barlow test: The physician grasps the infant's thigh near the hip and with gentle posterior/lateral pressure, attempts to dislocate the femoral head from the acetabulum. Normally, there is no motion in this direction. A distinct "clunk" is felt as the femoral heads pops out of joint indicating that hip can be dislocated; (C) Ortolani test: The hip is abducted and gentle pressure is applied to the proximal thigh from behind. Here, the physician attempts to relocate an already dislocated femoral head back into the acetabulum. A palpable "clunk" is noticed as the head slides back into place, if the joint is dislocated.

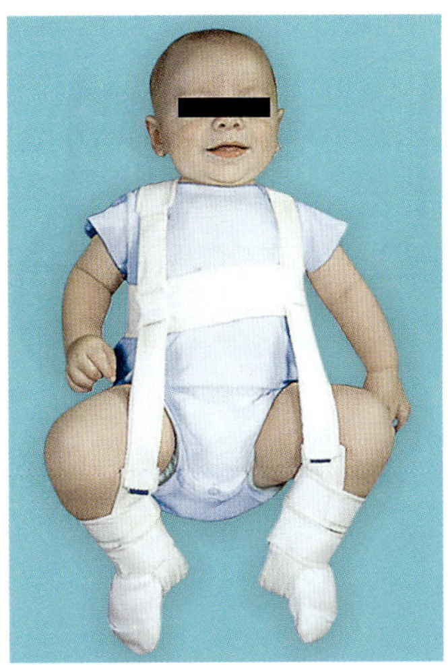

Fig. 21.3.2: Pavlik harness.

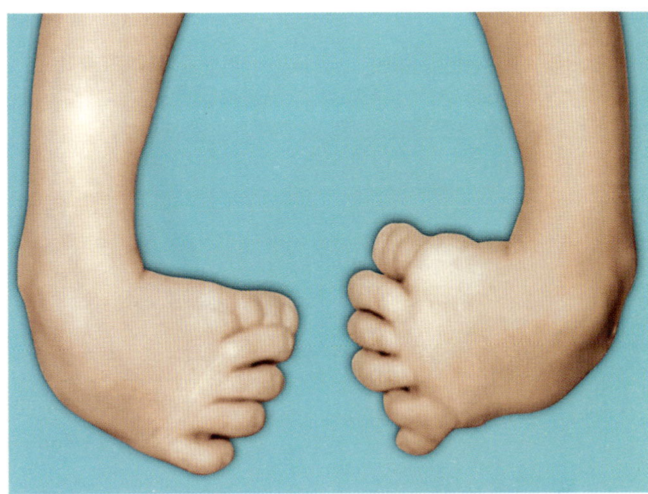

Fig. 21.3.4: An 8-year-old boy with deformity due to clubfoot recurrence.

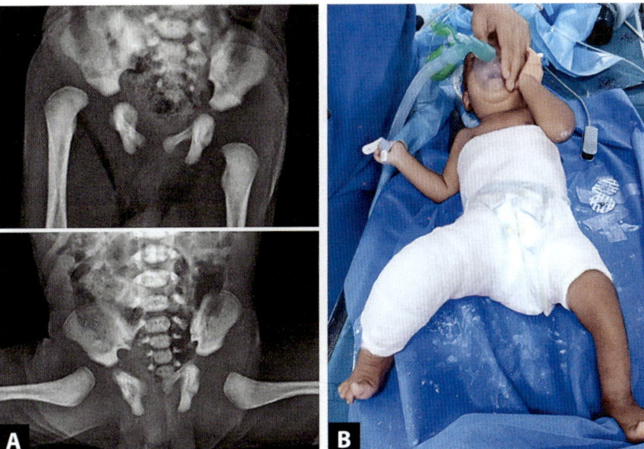

Figs. 21.3.3A and B: (A) X-rays of 8-month-old child with right-sided developmental dysplasia of hip (DDH); (B) Closed reduction and hip spica cast was applied.

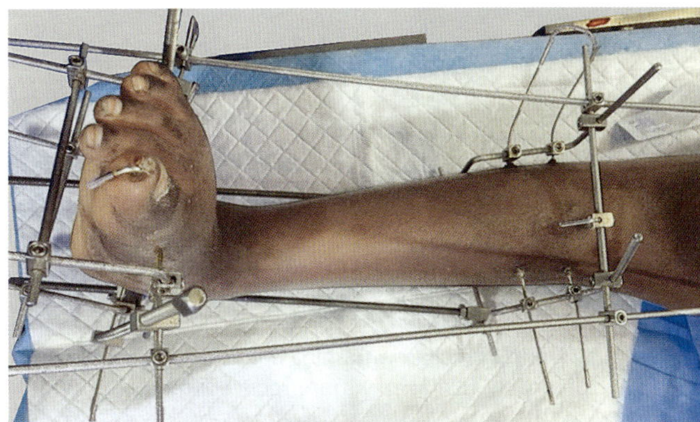

Fig. 21.3.5: Treatment by external fixator application [Joshi external stabilization system (JESS)].

joint, inversion of the foot at the subtalar joint and adduction of the forefoot at the midtarsal joint. There is internal rotation (torsion) of the tibia.[2] It may be unilateral or bilateral. The involved foot, calf, and heel are smaller in size. The deformity cannot be passively corrected due to tightness of the soft tissues, particularly "tendo-Achilles".

In neglected clubfoot, callosities develop over the lateral border or the dorsum of the foot, as the child walks on the lateral border **(Fig. 21.3.4)**.

Management

The treatment is initiated at birth. It involves:

- *Manipulation and casting (Ponseti method)*
- *Surgical methods:* In cases of recurrence post-treatment, neglected deformities, surgical treatment may be necessary.
- In case of naïve feet that are flexible, single stage correction is done by soft tissue releases or soft tissue release combined with bony procedures.
- In children with stiff foot and scarring due to previous surgical procedures, external fixator assisted **(Fig. 21.3.5)** correction is carried out.

SPINA BIFIDA

In spina bifida, defective fusion of the posterior vertebral arch creates a neural tube defect resulting into protrusion of the contents of the spinal canal.[3] It may present merely as a tuft of hair overlying the defect (spina bifida occulta) or as meningocele/myelomeningocele (cystica) **(Fig. 21.3.6)**.

Orthopedic problems are primarily due to muscle weakness and/or muscle imbalance which results in complex deformities in bone and joints (spine, hip, knee, foot, and ankle).

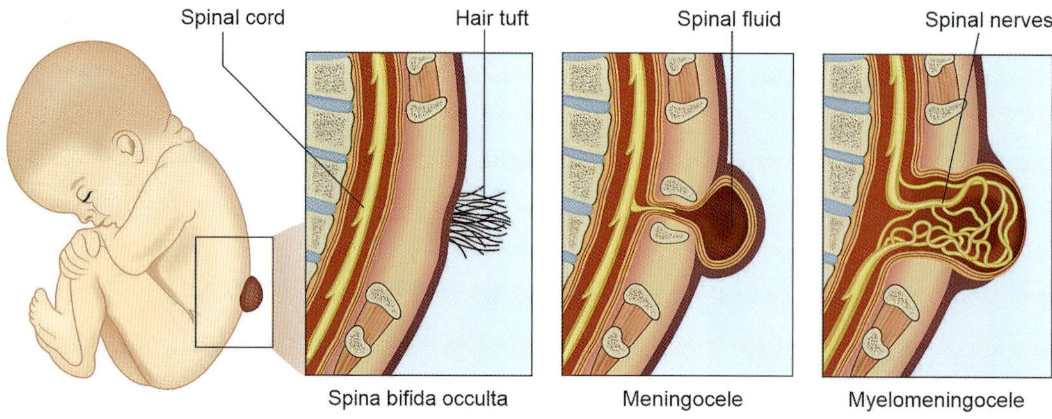

Fig. 21.3.6: Types of spina bifida.

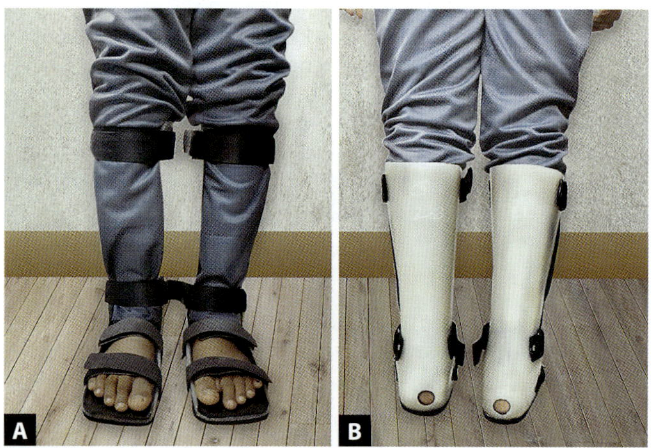

Figs. 21.3.7A and B: A child with spina bifida having flexible foot deformity, managed with corrective orthosis.

Treatment

Orthopedic management includes bracing (to prevent the progression of deformities), surgical (soft tissue and/or bony surgeries). Long-term bracing **(Figs. 21.3.7A and B)** is needed to prevent recurrence.

CONGENITAL PSEUDARTHROSIS OF TIBIA

Congenital pseudarthrosis of the tibia (CPT) is a rare disorder affecting 1 in 140,000 children and about a half of them have underlying neurofibromatosis. CPT is one of the most difficult orthopedic disorders to treat due to significant difficulty in achieving union.[4] The child presents either with a deformity **(Fig. 21.3.8)** or a fracture leading on to nonunion. The problems include deformity, nonunion **(Fig. 21.3.9)**, refractures, and limb length inequality.

Treatment

Treatment ranges from a simple bracing to a more complex reconstruction surgery **(Figs. 21.3.10A and B)**. Aim is to

Fig. 21.3.8: X-ray of a 2-year-old boy with congenital pseudoarthrosis of tibia and fibula.

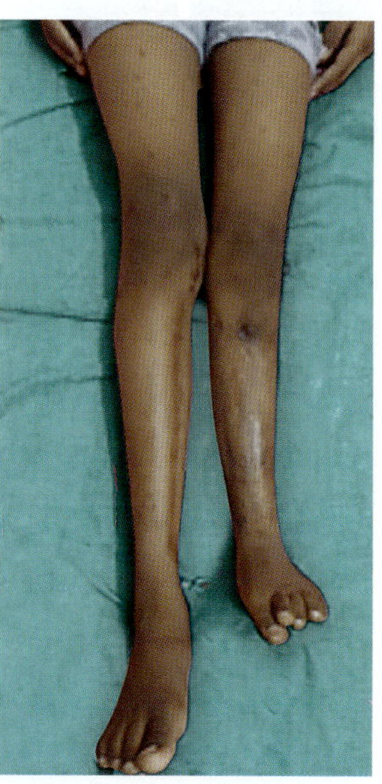

Fig. 21.3.9: An 8-year-old boy with left congenital pseudarthrosis of the tibia (CPT), previously operated multiple times.

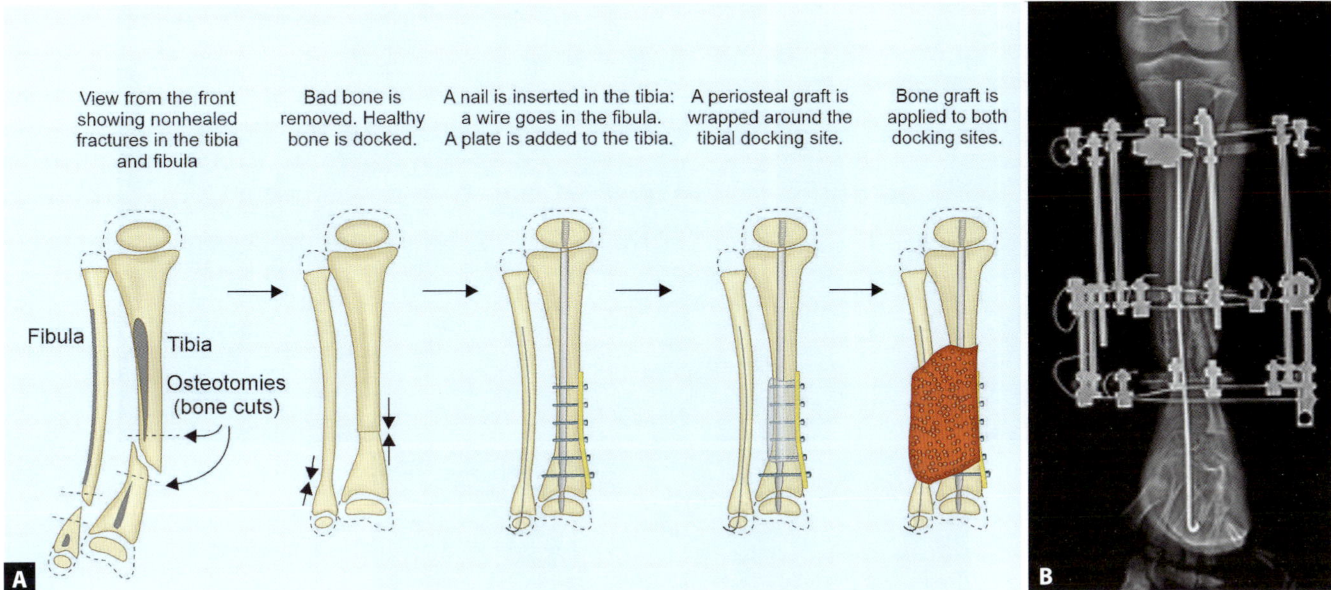

Figs. 21.3.10A and B: Cross-union surgical treatment for congenital pseudarthrosis of the tibia. (A) Surgical treatment for congenital pseudarthrosis of right tibia; (B) Anteroposterior view.

achieve a sound primary union and to maintain it preferably till skeletal maturity. Long-term bracing is also very important to prevent refractures.

ACUTE OSTEOMYELITIS

It is an acute infection of the bone marrow. Most common organism is *Staphylococcus aureus*. Most commonly involves metaphyseal **(Fig. 21.3.11)** region. In places where the metaphysis is intracapsular, septic arthritis can result. Early diagnosis and a high index of clinical suspicion will yield optimum outcomes.[5]

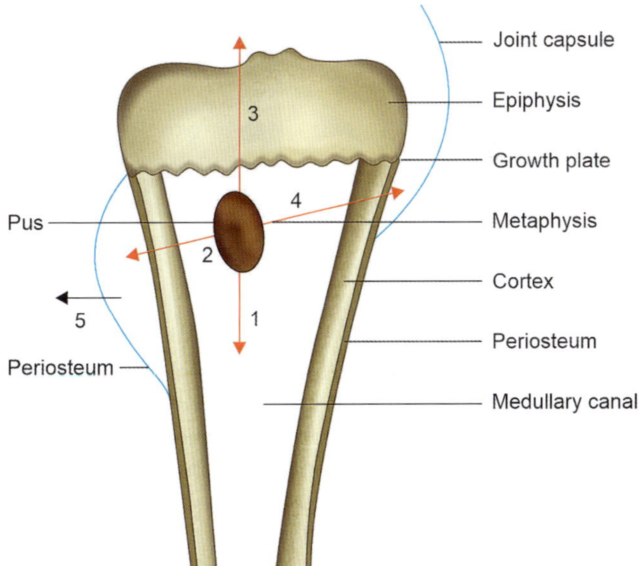

Fig. 21.3.11: Hematogenous (acute) osteomyelitis. Pathogenesis and spread of pus from metaphysis to other areas.

Diagnosis

Most important factor that predicts good outcomes is early diagnosis. Changes in the plain X-rays may not be seen in the first week **(Fig. 21.3.12A)**. MRI can detect even subtle osteomyelitis changes very early **(Figs. 21.3.12B and C)**. The first step is to admit the child and evaluate with monitoring. Antibiotics are the mainstay of treatment, but surgical drainage is indicated when there is a subperiosteal or intraosseous abscess, or when there is a need to identify the organism.

ACUTE SEPTIC ARTHRITIS OF INFANCY (TOM SMITH ARTHRITIS)

Nearly 40% of the neonatal septic arthritis are multifocal. The causative organisms are *Staphylococcus aureus* (methicillin sensitive), gram-negative organisms, or methicillin-resistant (MRSA). Most of the infections are hospital-acquired due to ventilators and catheters. The neonates may be afebrile and inflammatory markers may be negative. The only physical finding may be *pseudoparalysis*. Aspiration from the joints or from infected tissues will show counts exceeding 40,000 cells/mm^3. Many a time, the cultures from aspirates do not yield growth. Concurrent infection of septic arthritis and osteomyelitis is common.

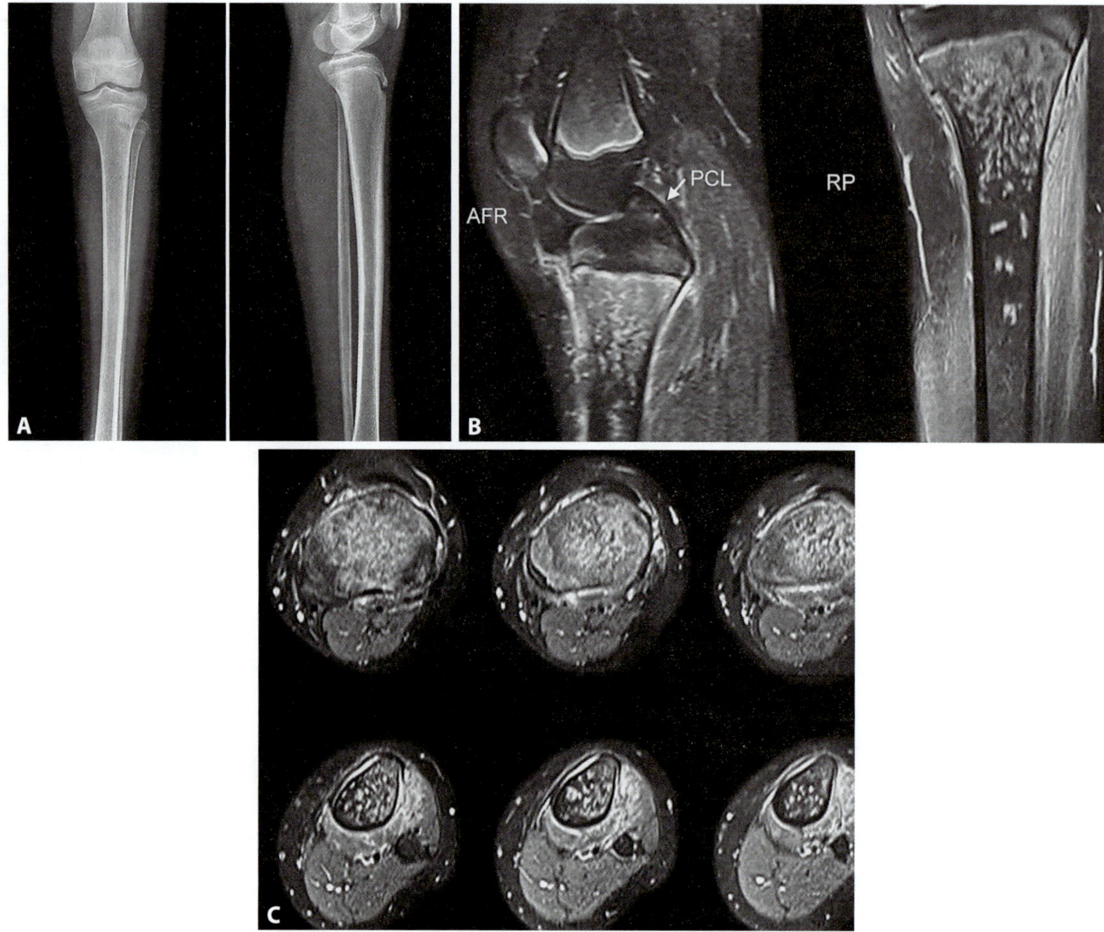

Figs. 21.3.12A to C: (A) A 9-year-old girl with limb pain and suspected bone infection but no significant changes in X-rays; (B and C) MRI shows changes of acute metaphyseal osteomyelitis. (MRI: magnetic resonance imaging)

Management

In septic arthritis of hip **(Fig. 21.3.13A)**, if one side is clinically involved, it is better to do USG screening of all major joints to exclude infection. If the neonate is in septicemia, it is better to do whole body MRI to identify all the areas of infection. The treatment consists of supportive measures, appropriate antibiotics, and immediate arthrotomy of affected joints. If the neonate does not improve in 3–4 days, repeat the MRI to rule out adjacent osteomyelitis or pyomyositis.[5] It is very important to detect septic arthritis early and initiate appropriate treatment. A delay in diagnosis and management may result in long-term sequelae, especially in hip and knee joints **(Figs. 21.3.13B and C)**.

TUBERCULOSIS OF THE SPINE (POTT'S SPINE)

Tuberculosis commonly affects the thoracolumbar spine; however, it is also seen in the other regions of the spine. Pain or discomfort over the back is one of the main and earliest symptoms, which is commonly missed more often.

Deformity of the spine, kyphosis, results from destruction and collapse of the affected vertebra. It is called a *"cold abscess"* because it presents away from the site of activity of the disease, and therefore, does not present with the usual signs of inflammation over it.[6]

Paraplegia/paraparesis is often an important presenting symptom **(Figs. 21.3.14A to C)** in patients with tuberculosis of the dorsal or dorso-lumbar spine. Bowel and bladder function must be analyzed in detail.

Management

Antituberculous drugs are given for a total period of 1 year.

Rest to the affected part is given by means of a POP jacket or a thoracal lumbar sacral orthosis (TLSOR) brace.

A cold abscess may require aspiration or drainage. The cord compression is relieved by various procedures such as costotransversectomy, anterolateral decompression, radical

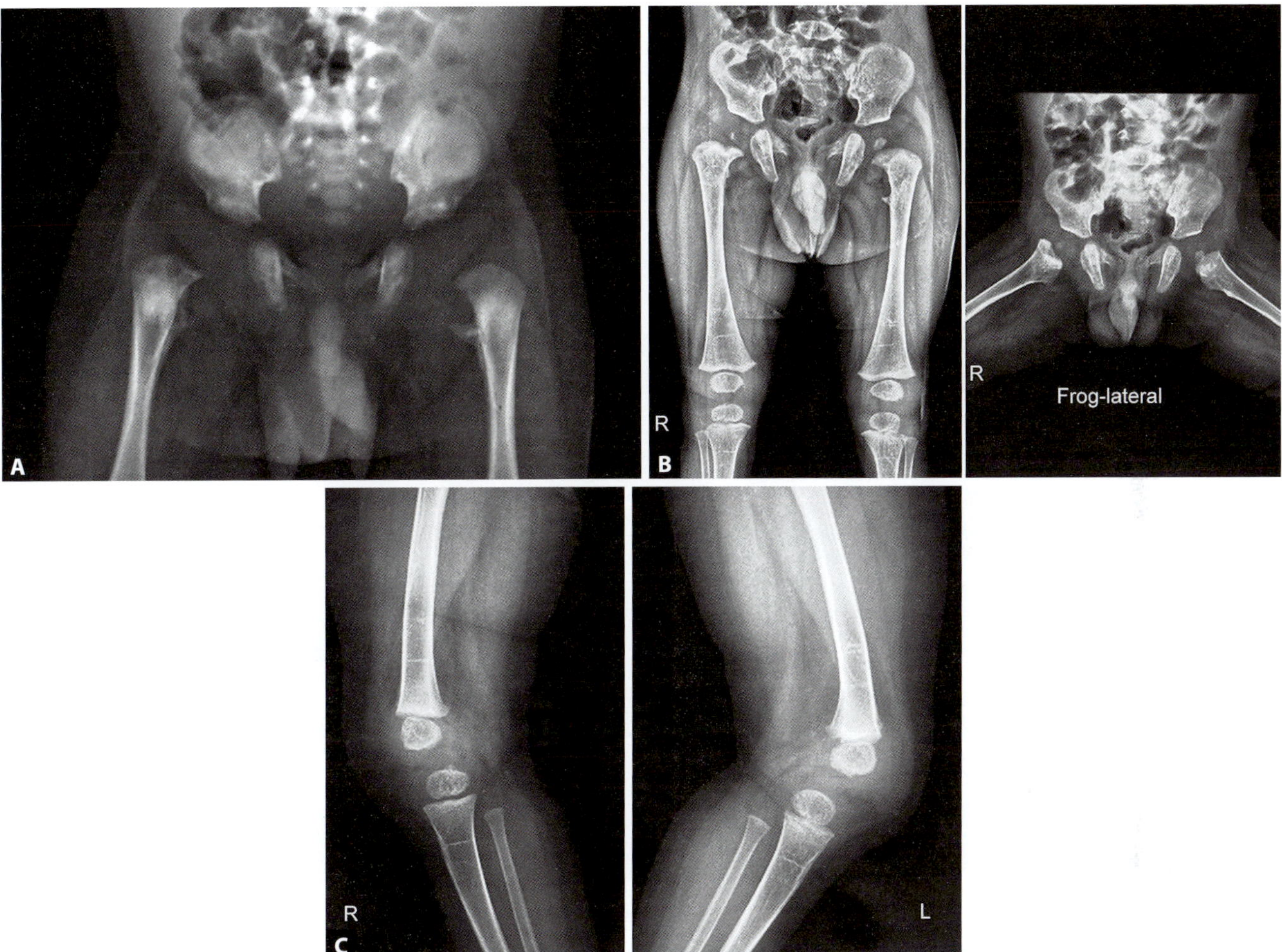

Figs. 21.3.13A to C: (A) Bilateral septic arthritis of hips. Soft tissue swelling and dislocated hips. Neonate had bilateral septic knees as well; (B) 6 months after treatment: Ossific nuclei have appeared in both hips; (C) Knees have normal appearance.

operation, or laminectomy followed by stabilization if <2 levels are involved.

PERTHES DISEASE (LEGG–CALVÉ–PERTHES DISEASE)

Perthes disease, also known as coxa plana, is an avascular necrosis (AVN) of the head of femur **(Fig. 21.3.15)** resulting from interference with its blood supply. The femoral head subsequently revascularizes and may result in deformation.[7] It occurs between the ages of 3 and 10 years, with 80% male preponderance. Usually unilateral but may be bilateral (10%).

Though the classical presentation is that of a painless limp, the child may present with a history of periodic attacks of limping with pain in the hip or referred pain to the knee. In early stages, there is limitation of movement with muscle spasm.

Plain X-ray clinches the diagnosis; however, MRI may be required occasionally.

Treatment

The aim of treatment is prevention of deformity of the femoral head by ensuring containment of the head within the acetabulum by surgical or nonsurgical methods. In the early stage, the child is treated by *skin traction or abduction cast (petri cast* **Fig. 21.3.16**) to relieve pain and muscle spasm. When the muscle spasm is relieved, the child is allowed to walk with a weight-relieving caliper.

Surgery may be required to improve containment of the femoral head within the acetabulum.

PEDIATRIC BONE TUMORS

Osteosarcoma

Osteosarcoma is a highly malignant primary bone tumor that occurs between 10 and 20 years of age. It is commonly seen in males, in the metaphysis of distal end of femur **(Fig. 21.3.17)**, proximal end of tibia and the proximal end of humerus.[8]

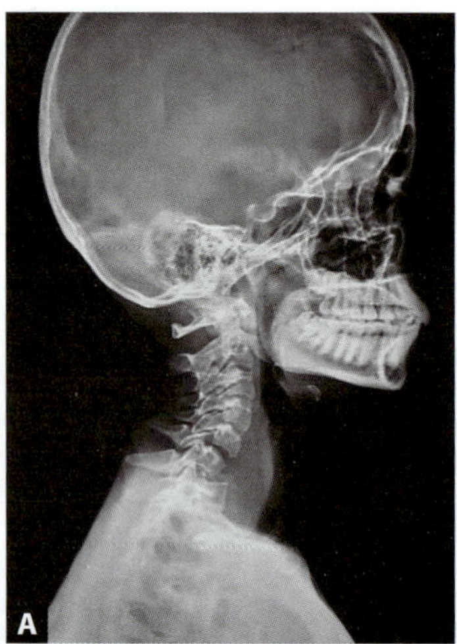

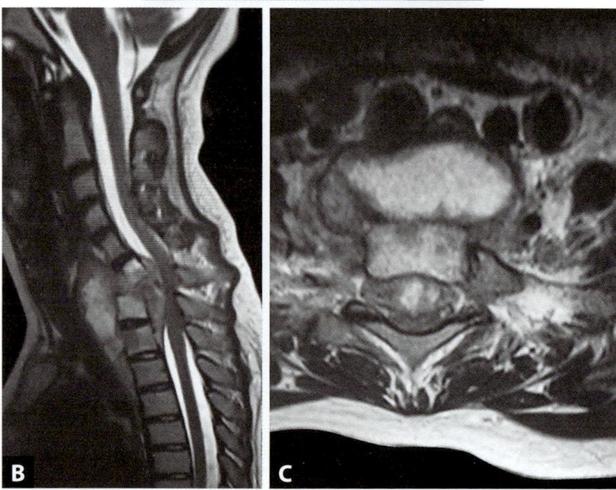

Figs. 21.3.14A to C: (A) A 13-year-old girl presented with acute onset quadriparesis and neck pain; X-ray showing abnormality at the C6–C7 level; (B) Sagittal MRI picture showing abscess and spinal cord compression at C6–C7 level; (C) Axial section at C6 level showing spinal canal compromise due to tuberculosis (TB) cold abscess.

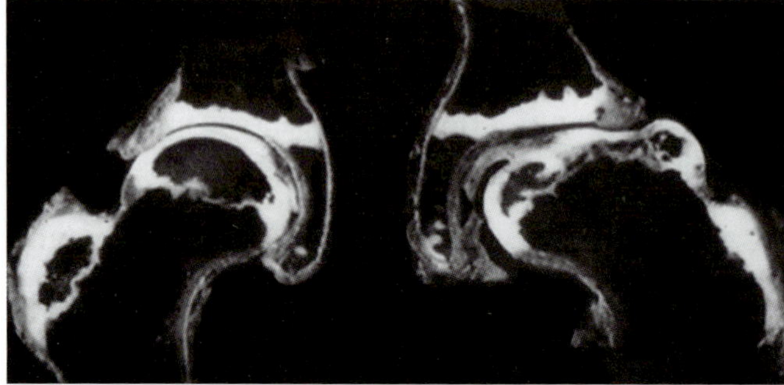

Fig. 21.3.15: Magnetic resonance imaging (MRI) picture of a normal femoral head compared to Perthes' disease.

Clinical Features

Pain is the initial and dominating symptom. After some weeks, a progressively increasing bone swelling appears.

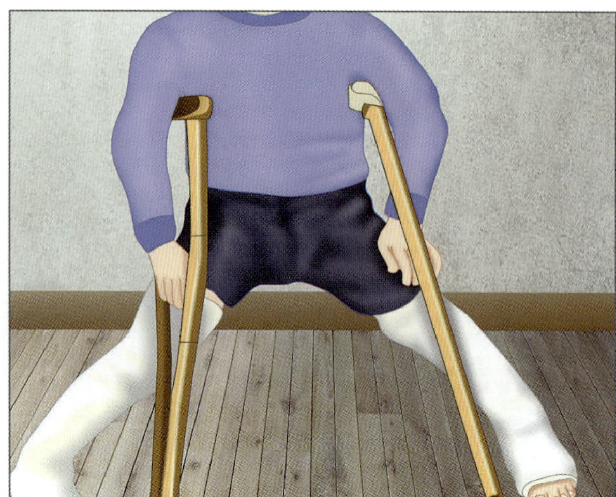

Fig. 21.3.16: A young child with abduction cast/Petri cast, a common method of containment in Perthes disease.

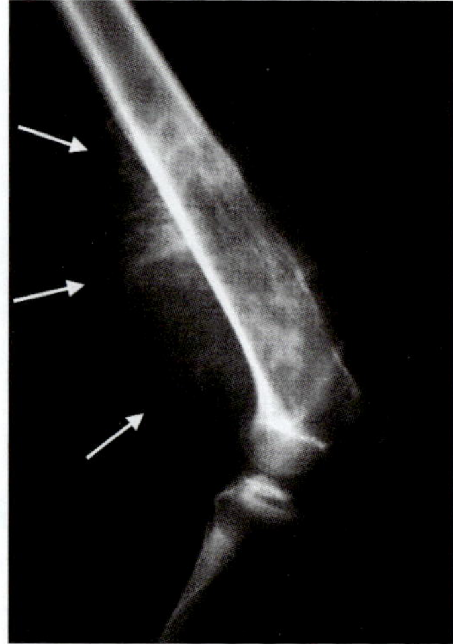

Fig. 21.3.17: Osteosarcoma of lower end of femur.

On examination, the swelling is fusiform; the overlying skin is stretched and shiny with prominent veins. The swelling is warm to touch, and has a variegated consistency. The patient's general health deteriorates with anemia, loss of weight, and cachexia. Biopsy is mandatory to establish the diagnosis.

Treatment

Broadly speaking, the treatment of osteosarcoma is usually a combination of the following:

- *Surgery:* A limb saving surgery is done, after neoadjuvant chemotherapy, if the lesion is small. Amputation is indicated, if limb salvage is not feasible.
- *Radiotherapy and chemotherapy* are indicated for local control of the disease after incomplete surgical removal of the tumor and to control micrometastasis.

A regular follow-up every 3 months is mandatory to detect any recurrence or spread of the tumor.

Ewing Sarcoma

It is an uncommon type of highly malignant bone tumor occurring commonly in males, in the age group of 10–20 years. It affects the diaphysis of long bones such as femur, tibia, and humerus **(Fig. 21.3.18)**. It also occurs in flat bones like pelvis.

Clinical Features

The patient presents with gradually increasing pain, followed by swelling. The swelling is firm to soft in consistency with indefinite margins. There is usually fever, anemia, and leukocytosis, and therefore, the condition often simulates subacute osteomyelitis. The swelling rapidly increases in size with involvement of soft tissues and the general condition deteriorates.

Treatment

Ewing sarcoma is radiosensitive and is best treated by local resection combined with pre- and postoperative chemo- and radiotherapy. This regimen has increased the survival rate from 5 to 50%. Amputation is indicated in locally advanced cases.

MISCELLANEOUS PROBLEMS

Transient Synovitis of the Hip

It is otherwise known as *observation hip*. It is a sterile inflammation and effusion, of unknown etiology, of the hip joint affecting children between 4 and 8 years of age. The importance of this condition lies in the fact that it may precede or be mistaken for other conditions such as septic arthritis of hip or Perthes disease.

The child presents with pain in the groin, limp **(Fig. 21.3.19A)**, or refusal to move the limb or walk. There is usually no fever. The movements of the hip are restricted, especially internal rotation.[9] However, the child is otherwise comfortable when resting in bed.

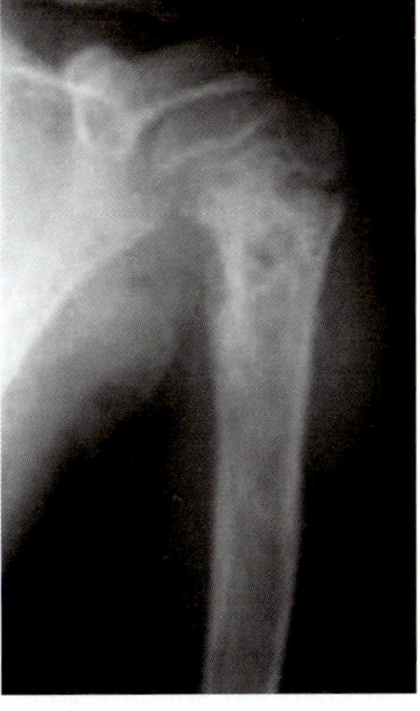

Fig. 21.3.18: Ewing sarcoma.

Management

The child is admitted for observation. Immobilization by skin traction **(Fig. 21.3.19B)** to the limb may relieve muscle spasm and pain. The condition resolves spontaneously within a week's time. Further workup may be needed including blood tests, USG, MRI, etc. if the clinical condition does not resolve.

Bow Legs (Genu Varum) and Knock-Knees (Genu Valgum)

Genu Valgum

Genu valgum or *"knock-knees"* denotes a malalignment in the frontal (coronal) plane, in which the part distal to the site of deformity deviates away from the midline **(Fig. 21.3.20)**. Unilateral genu valgum may be caused by disturbance in the

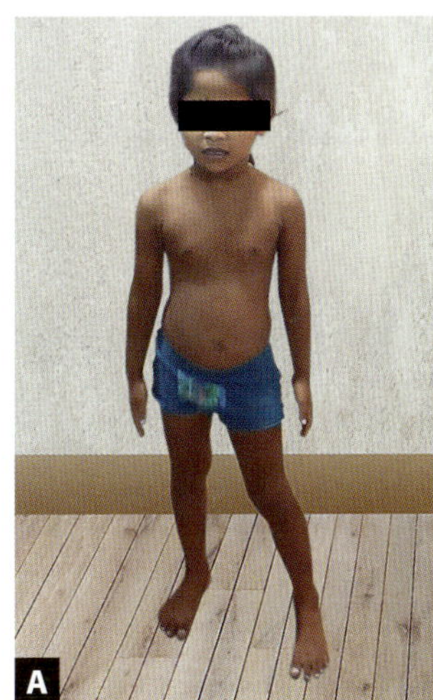

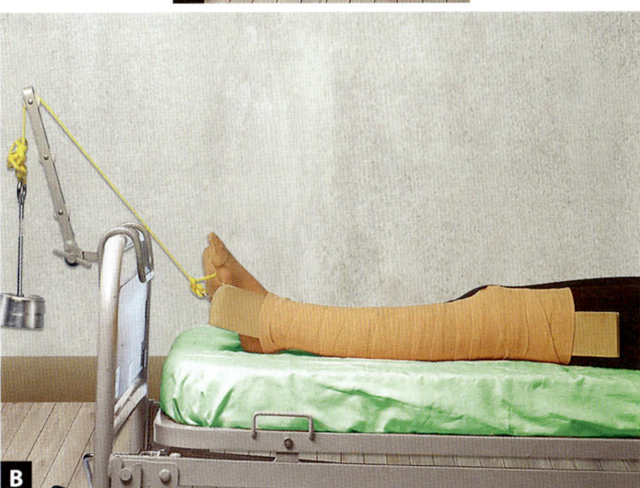

Figs. 21.3.19A and B: (A) A 4-year-old girl with synovitis of left hip, showing apparently longer left lower limb and a significant pelvic tilt; (B) A skin traction is used to relieve spasm and improve symptoms, in older children.

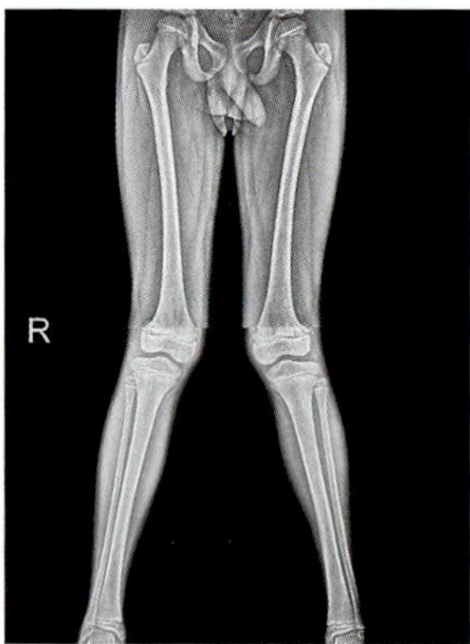

Fig. 21.3.20: Genu valgum.

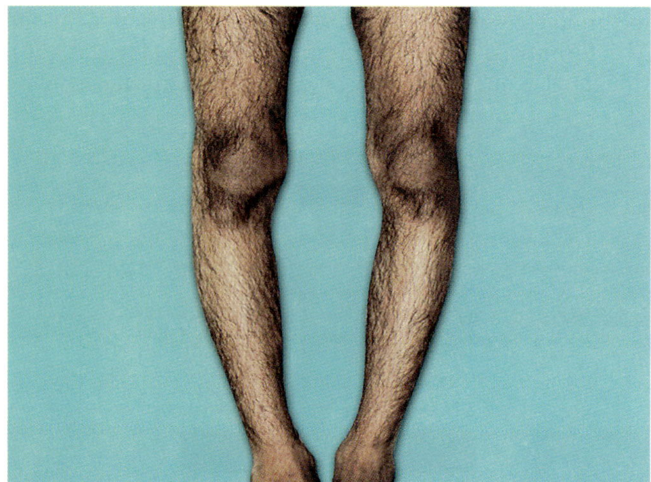

Fig. 21.3.21: Clinical photograph of genu varum of both knee joints.

epiphyseal growth at the lower femur or upper tibia due to trauma or osteomyelitis. Bilateral genu valgum can be caused by endocrine or metabolic disorders, rickets and epiphyseal dysplasia or can be idiopathic.

Treatment: Genu valgum deformity can be ignored in the toddlers as it may get corrected spontaneously. However, if the distance between the two medial malleoli (intermalleolar distance) is >10 cm at the age of 10 years, it will need surgical correction.

Genu Varum

Genu varum or *"bow legs"* is the lateral curvature of leg involving either the tibia or femur or both **(Fig. 21.3.21)**. Mild genu varum is physiological up to 3 years of age and will get corrected spontaneously in the majority. The other causes are rickets, posttraumatic or infective and idiopathic.

Treatment: A mild deformity can be treated by modifications in the shoes. Moderate-to-severe deformity needs surgical correction.

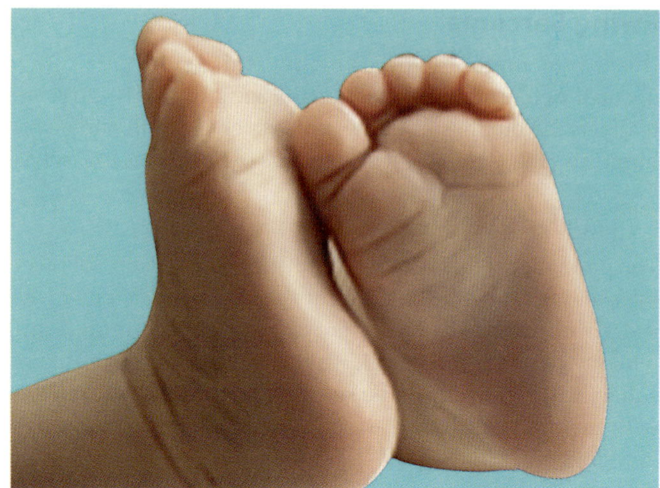

Fig. 21.3.22: Normal arch of the foot.

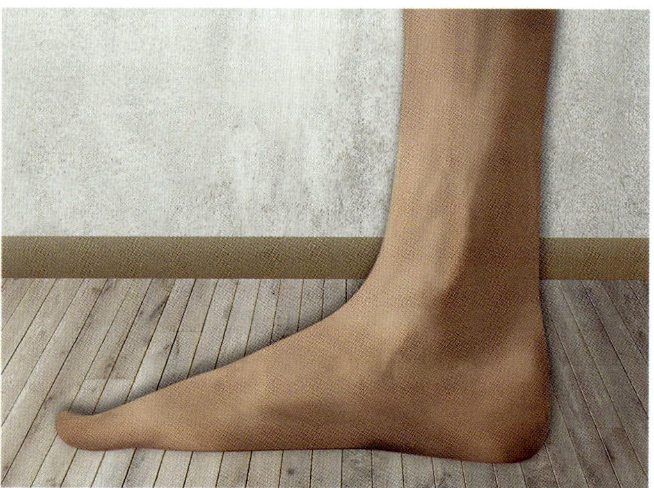

Fig. 21.3.23: Flat foot.

Flat Foot

Normally, the foot has longitudinal and transverse arches. The normal longitudinal arch is visible on the medial side of the foot **(Fig. 21.3.22)**. When this arch is less developed,[10] it is called as flat foot **(Fig. 21.3.23)**.

Causes and types of flat foot

Congenital vertical talus: The talus bone is placed vertically in the foot, instead of being horizontal, which is normal. A radiograph will confirm the diagnosis. The treatment is difficult. Manipulation and serial plaster casts may be indicated in mild cases, whereas severe cases need surgery **(Fig. 21.3.24)**.

Physiological or infantile flat foot: This is the most common type, in which the child has flat feet when he or she starts walking. But gradually, the arch develops within the next 2–3 years. In such a case, no specific treatment is required. However, an arch support inside the shoe and slight

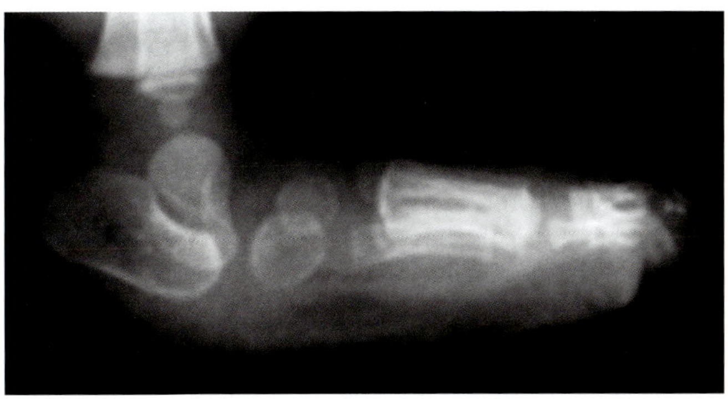

Fig. 21.3.24: Congenital vertical talus.

modification in the sole of the foot may be prescribed. In an older child, exercises for the intrinsic muscles of foot may be taught.

In severe cases, triple arthrodesis, i.e., fusion of the selected tarsal joints is indicated after skeletal maturity.

REFERENCES

1. Vitale MG, Skaggs DL. Developmental dysplasia of the hip from six months to four years of age. J Am Acad Orthop Surg. 2001;9(6):401-11.
2. Dimeglio A. Classification of talipes equinovarus. In: Simons GW (Ed). The Clubfoot: The Present and a View of the Future. New York, NY: Springer-Verlag; 1994. pp. 92-3.
3. Rampersaud E, Melvin EC, Speer MC. In: Wyszynski DF (Ed). Neural Tube Defects: From Origin to Treatment. Oxford University Press; 2006. pp. 165-75.
4. Paley D, Catagni M, Argnani F, Prevot J, Bell D, Armstrong P. Treatment of congenital pseudoarthrosis of the tibia using the Ilizarov technique. Clin Orthop Relat Res. 1992;280:81-93.
5. Doshi C, Sarathy K, Aroojis A. Acute Osteomyelitis and Septic Arthritis in Children - Current Concepts In Diagnosis And Management. J Clin Orthopaed. 2017;2(2):16-24.
6. Jain AK, Dhammi IK. Tuberculosis of the spine: a review. Clin Orthop Relat Res. 2007;460:39-49.
7. Stulberg SD, Cooperman DR, Wallenstein R. The natural history of Legg-Calve-Perthes disease. J Bone Joint Surg Am. 1981;63(7):1095-108.
8. Pilavaki P, Gahanbani Ardakani A, Gikas P, Constantinidou A. Osteosarcoma: Current Concepts and Evolutions in Management Principles. J Clin Med. 2023;12(8):2785.
9. Nouri A, Walmsley D, Pruszczynski B, Synder M. Transient synovitis of the hip: a comprehensive review. J Pediatr Orthop B. 2014;23(1):32-6.
10. Halabchi F, Mazaheri R, Mirshahi M, Abbasian L. Pediatric flexible flatfoot; clinical aspects and algorithmic approach. Iran J Pediatr. 2013;23(3):247-60.

21.4 Common Eye Problems

Payal Gupta

INTRODUCTION

Eye development is critical in the first few months of life; processes that interfere with development may seriously impact vision. It is recommended that children receive their first eye screening at birth, followed by an assessment at 6 months, and thereafter, at every well child visit to the pediatrician **(Table 21.4.1)**, annually between 3 and 6 years and once in 3 years thereafter.

TABLE 21.4.1: Important milestones in the development of the pediatric eye.

	At birth	*1 month*	*2–3 months*	*6 months*	*1 year*	*3 years*
Visual acuity				6/12	6/9	6/6
Fixation reflex		Normal optokinetic nystagmus		Well developed		
Convergence reflex		Starts		Well developed		
Binocularity			Starts	Well developed		
Pupillary reflex	Sluggish	Well developed				
Color vision	Black and white, and shades of gray				Full color	
Menace reflex		Present				

The following children should be referred for ophthalmic evaluation as early as possible:

- Abnormal history (does not make eye contact or focus on and follow objects by 3 months of age, or reach for objects by 6 months of age)
- Abnormal appearance (redness of eyes or eyelids, watery or purulent discharge, white cornea, white pupil, asymmetric pupil size, swelling or drooping of eyelids, and squint)
- Evidence of discomfort (excessive rubbing of eyes, avoids bright light, or keeps one or both eyes closed most of the time).

VISUAL PROBLEMS

Refractive Errors

A refractive error is an optical defect in the eye that prevents light rays from focusing on the macula, thus preventing clear vision. Most children are hypermetropic at birth with enlargement of eyeball over time to attain emmetropia; if the process of enlargement continues, older children will be myopic.[1]

Longer axial length, steeper corneal curvature and higher index causes rays of parallel light to focus nearer, in front of the retina, producing myopia. The reverse situation will cause hypermetropia where rays of parallel light are brought to focus farther behind the retina. Accommodation (increasing the curvature of the lens) shifts the focus anteriorly so that a clear image is formed on the retina. Constant accommodation in hypermetropes causes headaches, eye strain, and excessive convergence (convergent squint). Astigmatism results when the refractive power of the eye is different in different meridia and different foci are formed on the retina.

One should suspect refractive errors when children report difficulty in reading off the blackboard, eyestrain on near work and holding books close to the eyes. Check vision using Snellen chart; repeat using a pinhole. In refractive errors, vision improves with the pinhole since it prevents spherical aberrations by cutting off peripheral rays. Refractive errors are commonly treated using corrective lenses in spectacles or contact lenses.

Amblyopia

Amblyopia (lazy eye) is a partial decrease of vision in the absence of anatomical/structural abnormality. It results when there is inadequate foveal stimulation and/or abnormal binocular interaction (different visual input from the two foveae) during the first few years of life when the visual system is still developing. When there is a difference in the quality of the image recorded by each eye, the brain disregards the blurred image; resulting in the visual system developing more slowly for that eye.[2]

Amblyopia may be due to uncorrected refractive errors, strabismus or due to visual deprivation (ptosis, surgical lid closure, bandaging, corneal opacity, or cataract). In preverbal children, suspect poor vision in one eye when the child protests covering of one eye (the eye with better vision), shows fixation preference for one eye, and has unilateral squint or eccentric fixation.

Management of amblyopia is a slow and tedious process requiring high patience level on the part of parents as well as the doctor. Hence, it is important to counsel parents accordingly. Treatment options include spectacle correction, occlusion therapy, visual exercises, and surgical intervention in cases of cataract and squint.

Color Vision Deficiency

Photosensitive pigments in the cones allow us to see colors. There are three types of cones, each containing a different pigment—red (erythrolabe), green (chlorolabe), or blue (cyanolabe). Genes contain the coding instructions for the three pigments; if the instructions are wrong, the wrong pigments are produced, and the abnormal cones will be sensitive to a different wavelength. All children, especially boys, should have a routine color vision check once during a school health checkup.

Color blindness is most common for red and green colors. Inherited as an X-linked recessive genetic defect, it is seen in 10% of males and 0.4% of females. Blue color blindness, due to defect on chromosome-7, is seen in 5% of people. Color blindness may also be acquired in conditions that involve the cones or the visual pathway (chorioretinitis, diabetic retinopathy, optic neuritis, partial optic atrophy, migraine, stroke, and cerebral trauma). Unlike congenital color blindness, the acquired forms may be unilateral, progressive, or transient, and show no gender predisposition.

Screening tests (Ishihara pseudoisochromatic plates) are used to detect color vision defect. More sophisticated tests (Farnsworth-Munsell 100-Hue test or Lantern test) are required if the objective is to exactly classify the type and degree of defect. Persons with abnormal color vision cannot take up jobs dealing with public safety, and the driving of commercial vehicles, train engines, or airplanes; children should be aware of this when they are considering future careers. There is no treatment for congenital color vision deficiency, although the use of filters can help to differentiate colors in some instances.

Xerophthalmia

Xerophthalmia is a bilateral, dry, lusterless condition of the conjunctiva and cornea due to vitamin A deficiency. It occurs in malnourished children and may be precipitated by exanthematous febrile illness or persistent diarrhea. There

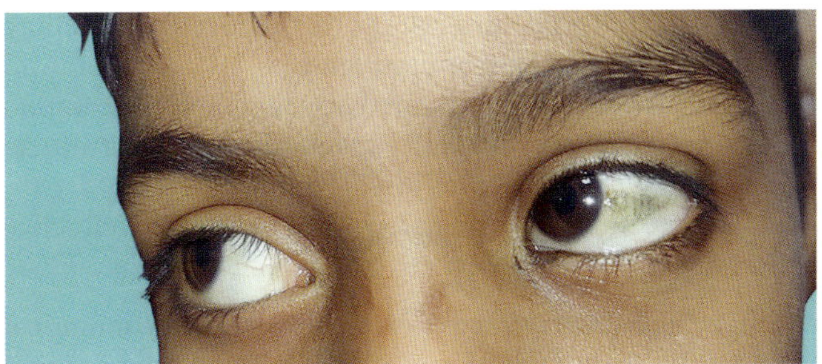

Fig. 21.4.1: Bitot's spot.

may be presence of Bitot's spots **(Fig. 21.4.1)**, conjunctival and corneal xerosis, night blindness, corneal melting (keratomalacia) or corneal scarring.

The child should be referred to an ophthalmologist. Treatment comprises replacement of vitamin A, treatment of the precipitating condition, and taking care of the general health of the child and of the ocular condition. Keratomalacia requires emergency management to prevent corneal perforation. Corneal transplantation is the only treatment once corneal scars form.

INFECTIONS

Infective Conjunctivitis

Etiology

- *Bacterial: Staphylococcus* spp., *Haemophilus* spp., *Neisseria* spp., *Streptococcus* spp., etc.
- *Viral:* Adenovirus, picornavirus, and herpes simplex virus (HSV)
- *Fungal: Aspergillus, Candida,* etc.

Clinical Features

- Redness, itching, and foreign body sensation
- Swollen lids
- Rarely, reduced vision (due to corneal involvement)
- Eye discharge helps in differentiating between viral (watery) and bacterial conjunctivitis (mucopurulent).
- Preauricular lymphadenopathy in viral conjunctivitis due to adenovirus or picornavirus

Management

Etiological diagnosis is usually not necessary. Adenoviral conjunctivitis is very common and is highly contagious (epidemic keratoconjunctivitis). The pediatrician should advise frequent handwashing, separate towels, handkerchiefs, etc. to reduce the risk of spreading infection. There is no specific treatment; however, symptoms can be reduced with instillation of artificial tears, topical antihistamines, or applying cold compresses. Bacterial conjunctivitis resolves spontaneously without specific treatment; however, topical and empirical antibacterial therapy results in earlier microbiological remission.

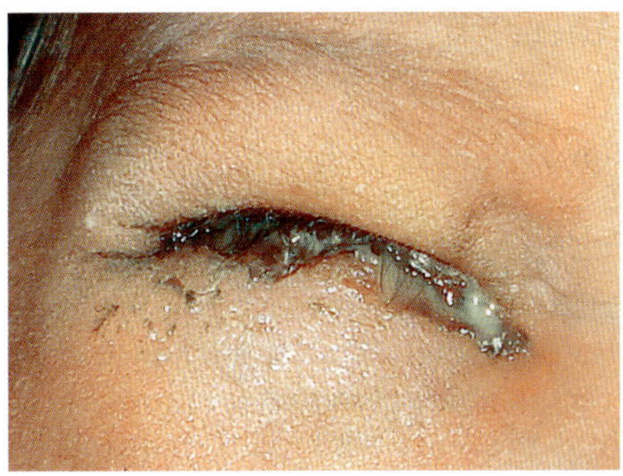

Fig. 21.4.2: Purulent conjunctivitis in a neonate (Ophthalmia neonatorum).

Ophthalmia Neonatorum

Etiology

The infection may be chlamydial, gonococcal, or due to HSV. Conjunctivitis occurs due to infection acquired from the birth canal.

Clinical Features

- Watering and purulent discharge from both eyes in the first few days of life **(Fig. 21.4.2)**.
- There may be an associated keratitis or uveitis.
- In gonococcal infection, the local symptoms and signs are severe; there are also systemic features such as fever, urethritis, arthritis, endocarditis, meningitis, and septicemia.

Management

A conjunctival swab will help to identify the organism, but treatment should begin at once. Wash eyes copiously with saline water frequently. Apply atropine eye ointment, if there is associated keratitis or uveitis (common in gonorrhea).

If the discharge is copious and purulent, treat as for gonorrheal infection: ciprofloxacin eye drops every few minutes till discharge reduces, then 2-hourly. Give parenteral ceftriaxone immediately. In chlamydial infection (the most common), instill tetracycline/erythromycin eye ointment and give oral erythromycin. Infection with HSV may present as keratoconjunctivitis along with skin and mouth lesions. Intravenous acyclovir to limit the spread of the infection along with topical therapy with trifluridine, iododeoxyuridine, or vidarabine is used.

Pregnant women with suspected vaginal infections should be treated well before delivery. If infected women present in labor, instill 2% povidone-iodine or tetracycline or erythromycin ointment into their baby's eyes soon after birth.

Corneal Ulcer

Etiology

Bacterial, fungal, viral, or protozoal.

Clinical Features

- There may be a history of injury with vegetative material (plant leaf, twig, and animal tail in fungal ulcer), fever (in viral ulcer), or abuse of steroid eye drops.
- The child presents with pain, redness of eye, and blepharospasm.
- Diminished vision due to corneal involvement or associated intraocular infection (endophthalmitis)
- The corneal epithelium is abraded and there may be slough resulting in loss of transparency.
- There is mucopurulent (bacterial or fungal ulcer) or watery discharge (viral ulcer).

Management

When a corneal ulcer is suspected, refer urgently to an ophthalmologist. It is best to apply a sterile eye pad during the transfer, although one does not usually patch an eye with an infective ulcer unless it is very deep and could perforate.

Eyelid Infections

Acute Infections

Etiology: Usually caused by *Staphylococcus* species and includes blepharitis, hordeolum externum (stye; due to blockage of the duct of glands associated with an eyelash follicle, i.e., Zeis gland; **Fig. 21.4.3**) and hordeolum internum (suppurative inflammation due to blockage of the duct of a meibomian gland).

Clinical Features

- In stye, there would be painful swelling with a pus point at the base of eyelash follicle (externum); **(Fig. 21.4.3)** whereas in hordeolum internum, the localized swelling will be along the meibomian glands.
- Blepharitis results in inflamed lid margin with ulceration and yellow crusts (ulcerative blepharitis) or dandruff-like flakes (squamous blepharitis).
- May be recurrent, if associated with uncorrected refractive errors or reduced immunity.

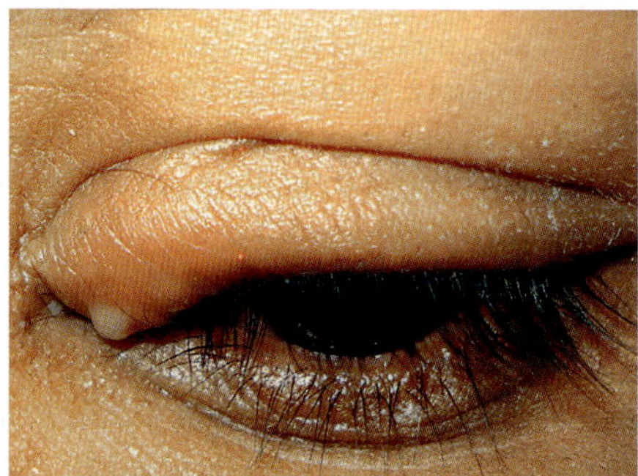

Fig. 21.4.3: Infective swelling in the upper eyelid in the region of the eyelashes (hordeolum externum/stye).

Management: Treat refractive errors and prescribe empirical local antibiotics. If a lid abscess forms, it must be drained under cover of systemic and topical antibiotics.

Chronic Inflammation (Chalazion)

Etiology: Blockage of the duct of a meibomian gland results in a granulomatous reaction to lipid content of the gland.

Clinical features:

- Painless mass in eyelid **(Fig. 21.4.4)**, better felt than seen.
- Free from skin; visible as a bluish discoloration on the conjunctival side.

Management: Chalazion may resolve on its own with hot fomentation and mild topical anti-inflammatory agent. If it is large or does not resolve, intralesional steroid injection may help or it may be incised, and its contents curetted under local anesthesia.

Orbital Cellulitis

Etiology

This is a serious condition; infection of the soft tissue of the orbit usually derives from the adjacent ethmoidal sinus, or from preseptal (eyelid) cellulitis.

Clinical Features

- Painful proptosis
- Lid edema
- Restricted ocular movements
- The cornea may develop exposure keratitis.
- Optic nerve function may be compromised due to increased orbital pressure.
- Signs of regional infection
- There may be systemic signs suggestive of septicemia.

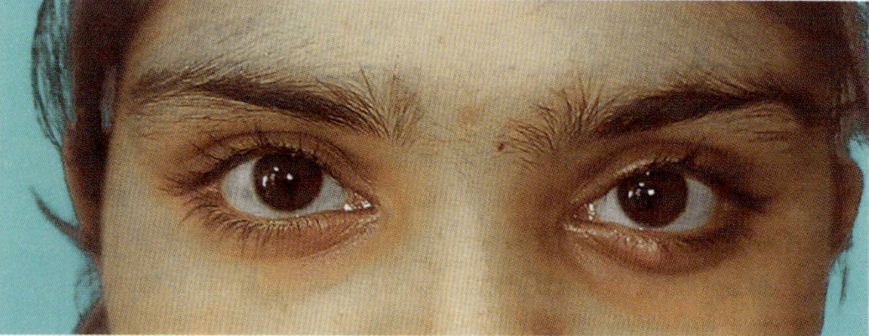

Fig. 21.4.4: Left lower lid chalazion.

Management

The condition mandates an urgent ophthalmic consult, admission, and immediate local and systemic broad-spectrum antibiotic therapy. If an orbital abscess forms, it must be surgically drained.

ALLERGIC AND INFLAMMATORY CONDITIONS

Phlyctenular Keratoconjunctivitis

Etiology

An allergic response to protein from endogenous infections (*Staphylococcus,* mycobacteria, HSV, and helminthiasis).

Clinical Features

- Itching, foreign body sensation, and redness of eye
- One or more phlyctens (blisters) on the bulbar or palpebral conjunctiva, limbus, or cornea
- The blisters ulcerate and heal by scarring, and are recurrent unless the endogenous infection is treated.
- Corneal lesions cause pain, photophobia, and may affect vision.

Management

Topical steroids are recommended. Investigate and treat for any co-existing systemic infections. When there is local staphylococcal infection (conjunctivitis or blepharitis), give topical antibiotics followed later by topical steroids, if required.

Spring Catarrh

Etiology

An allergic conjunctivitis due to exogenous allergens such as pollen, animal hair, etc.

Clinical Features

- It is seen mainly in the 1st decade of life, more often in boys.
- It has seasonal recurrence (in the warm months, subsiding in winter); it usually subsides by puberty.
- The child has itching and ropy mucoid discharge in both eyes.
- In the bulbar form, there are gelatinous papillae around the limbus.
- In the palpebral form, there are large papillae in the palpebral conjunctiva, giving a cobblestone appearance.
- The two forms may coexist; the cornea may be involved too.

Management

The allergen if identified, should be avoided. Topical antihistamines, mast cell stabilizers, steroids under antibiotic cover, immunosuppressants (cyclosporine A), and lubricating drops are given in combination depending on the severity of presentation. Cold compressions give symptomatic relief.

Anterior Uveitis

Etiology

Anterior uveitis in children is seen in a variety of systemic conditions; hence, the pediatrician may be the first to see these patients. Infectious causes include tuberculosis, HSV, *herpes zoster,* and mumps. *Noninfectious* causes are more common; the strongest association is with juvenile idiopathic arthritis (JIA). Other noninfectious causes are spondyloarthropathies and sarcoidosis.

Clinical Features

- Asymptomatic
- Redness of eye from deep ciliary congestion (circumcorneal)
- Pain in the eye
- Blurred vision
- Associated systemic features depending on etiology

Management

A general medical history, physical examination, and specific laboratory tests may elicit cause. Children with these conditions should be seen by an ophthalmologist, even if they have no ocular complaints.

A complete examination of the eye and ocular adnexa is essential, including the cornea (HSV keratitis), uvea (granulomatous or nongranulomatous uveitis), lacrimal glands, and regional lymph nodes (sarcoidosis). A fundus examination is mandatory to detect cystoid macular edema in eyes with chronic uveitis and to rule out posterior uveitis. Topical cycloplegics and topical corticosteroids are the mainstay of treatment.

DISORDERS OF NERVES AND MUSCLES

Squint

Squint (strabismus) is the condition when the axes of the two eyes are misaligned relative to each other. The misalignment may be horizontal or vertical resulting in esotropia **(Fig. 21.4.5)** (one eye is relatively convergent), exotropia **(Fig. 21.4.6)** (one eye is relatively divergent), or hypertropia (one eye is directed upward relative to the other). In addition, deviations may be concomitant (do not vary with direction of gaze) or incomitant (variation of angle of deviation due to paralysis of an extraocular muscle).

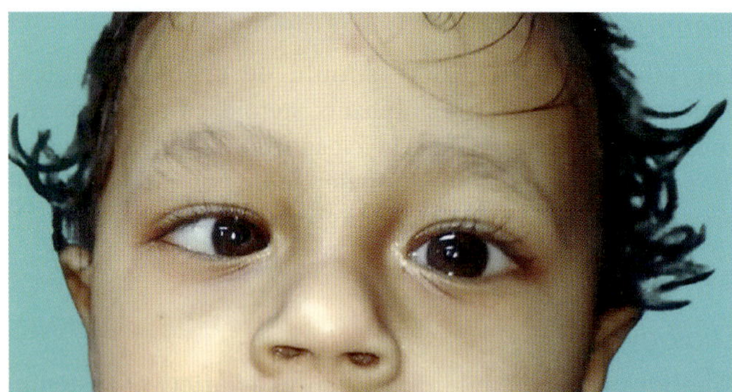

Fig. 21.4.5: Right eye esotropia.

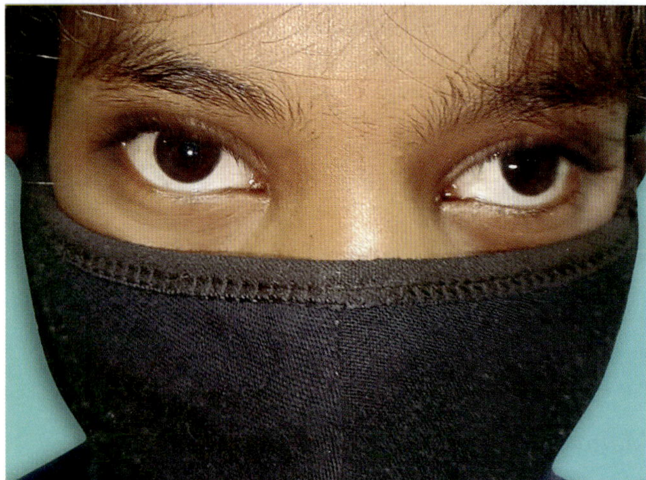

Fig. 21.4.6: Left eye exodeviation.

Squint may be constant, being present throughout the day, or it may appear intermittently.

Etiology

Most squints develop sometime in the first 3 years of life. Newborn babies may squint occasionally, until their binocular reflexes develop; thus, any squint that presents or persists after the age of 3 months must be investigated.

In many cases, the cause is not known. In some, there is a strong family history (infantile esotropia). Squint may occur in uncorrected hypermetropia (excessive accommodation to see clearly causes excessive convergence, producing convergent squint); due to poor vision in one eye; or due to cerebral palsy, hydrocephalus, or brain injury.

Clinical Features

- Misalignment of the visual axes relative to each other
- The fovea of each eye is focusing on a different object; thus, two different images reach the brain leading to confusion. The brain ignores the image coming from the deviated eye, leading eventually to strabismic amblyopia in that eye.
- Binocular vision cannot develop so the child loses depth perception.

Management

Intermittent squint permits each fovea to receive adequate stimulation some of the time; hence treatment, though mandatory, is not emergent. Constant squint, however, needs early and aggressive treatment. If a refractive error is present, children should wear the spectacles constantly. If any squint remains despite spectacle correction, it can be corrected by muscle surgery to straighten the alignment. After surgery, it is usually necessary to continue spectacles, occlusion, and exercise as advised by the ophthalmologist.

A false impression of squint (pseudostrabismus) may result from a flat, wide bridge of nose, or due to epicanthal folds so that the eyes look closer together than they really are. This appearance gradually disappears as the baby's nose bridge grows.

TUMOR AND TUMOR-LIKE CONDITIONS

Dermoid Cysts

Etiology

They represent surface ectoderm that got entrapped during bony fusion; thus, they overlie bony sutures.

Clinical Features

- These are painless, cystic masses usually found around the orbit at birth, near the medial or lateral part of the eyebrow.
- They may have hair.
- They may leak after trauma with sebaceous material causing pain.

Management

While periorbital dermoids are superficial, and thus simpler to remove surgically, orbital ones require an orbital approach.

Retinoblastoma

Retinoblastoma is the most common primary ocular malignancy of childhood. It has been already discussed in Chapter 15.9.

WATERING FROM THE EYES

Congenital Dacryocystitis

Etiology

This is a result of incomplete canalization of the nasolacrimal duct, usually due to epithelial debris, membranes, or valves in the duct.

Clinical Features

- Excessive unilateral or bilateral watering soon after birth
- The lacrimal sac may distend with accumulated secretions to form a palpable, cystic mass below the medial canthal tendon (mucocele).
- *Regurgitation test:* Pressure over the sac area (medial canthus) causes mucopus to regurgitate through the puncta into the conjunctival sac.

Management

The condition is amenable to conservative treatment with lacrimal sac massage several times a day for a few months, to push debris into the nose. Sustained pressure should be applied directly over the lacrimal sac, just under the medial canthal tendon, with the small finger of the parent's hand. The parent should be advised to ensure closure of the eyelids so that the puncta are always occluded during massage. In this way, the lacrimal sac does not empty into the conjunctival sac during massage, ensuring an adequate hydrostatic pressure to push debris into the nose. Empirical antibiotic eye drops are prescribed to prevent infection. If there is no relief after the age of 9 months, syringing and probing (under general anesthesia) should be planned, and may be repeated two or three times if required. Surgery in the form of dacryocystorhinostomy is indicated if obstruction persists after 4 years of age.

Acute Dacryocystitis

Etiology

Bacterial overgrowth in congenital dacryocystitis may produce an acute condition.

Clinical Features

- Painful and erythematous swelling of the lacrimal sac
- The inflamed sac may rupture through the overlying skin resulting in fistula formation.
- Infection may spread beyond the sac to produce preseptal cellulitis, or into the orbit (orbital cellulitis).
- More serious complications (cavernous sinus thrombosis, blindness, and death) may supervene in immunocompromised individuals.

Management

The discharge should be cultured, and immediate broad-spectrum systemic antimicrobial therapy started. If an abscess forms, it should be drained. The condition should be reassessed 2–3 weeks after the acute condition subsides. Scarring from the acute event may prevent successful syringing and probing; dacryocystorhinostomy is usually indicated.

CATARACT AND GLAUCOMA

Pediatric Cataract

Cataract is a visually disabling opacity in the lens. It can occur at birth or develop later. Pediatricians play a vital role in diagnosing cataract since they are able to screen children for ocular abnormalities.

Etiology

Though idiopathic in 50%, a quarter shows autosomal-dominant inheritance. Rest of the cataracts can be due to infection during pregnancy (rubella, chickenpox, cytomegalovirus, herpes, syphilis, and toxoplasmosis), galactosemia, diabetes, hypoglycemia, hypocalcemia, drugs (corticosteroids), trisomy, myotonic dystrophy, ocular abnormalities such as posterior lenticonus and persistent hyperplastic primary vitreous.[3] Acquired cataract can be secondary to uveitis, retinoblastoma, systemic steroids, or ocular trauma **(Fig. 21.4.7)**.

Clinical Features

- White reflex in pupil **(Fig. 21.4.8)**
- Poor response to visual stimulus
- Squint
- Nystagmus

Management

All children with white reflex should be urgently referred to an ophthalmologist. Visually insignificant cataracts need only observation and refractive correction. Surgery is indicated, if the cataract is located centrally, or is large enough to block vision, and must be performed as soon as possible to prevent amblyopia.

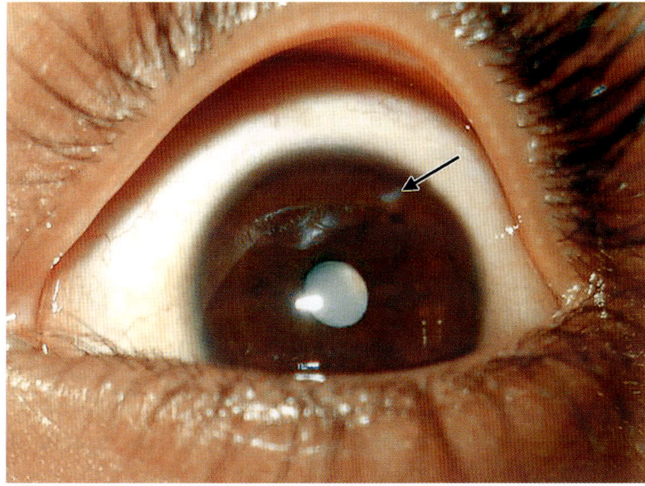

Fig. 21.4.7: Corneal opacity (arrow) and cataract after injury with bow and arrow.

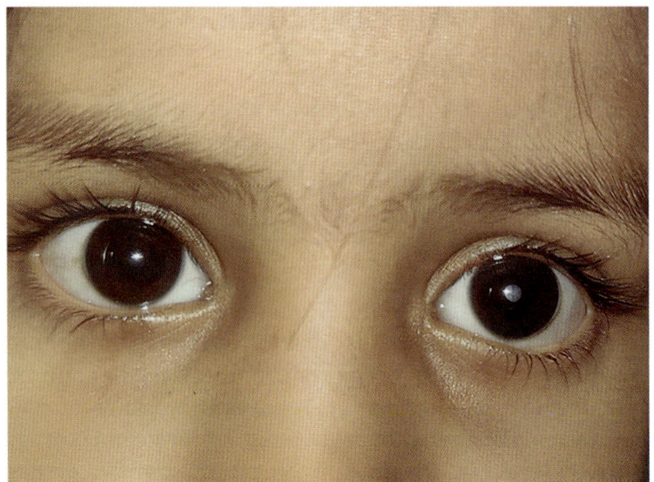

Fig. 21.4.8: White reflex in a unilateral developmental cataract left eye.

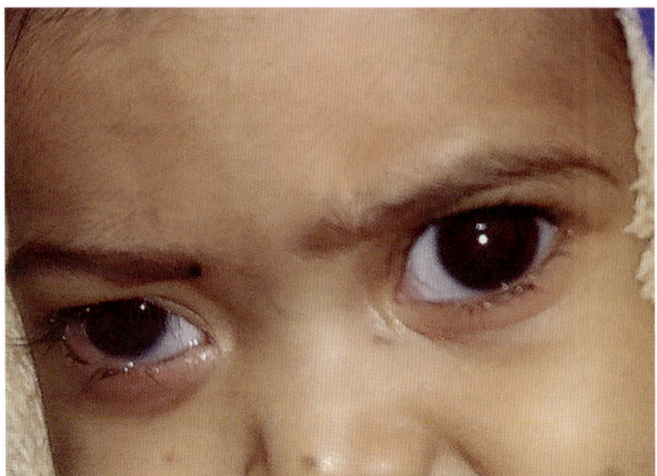

Fig. 21.4.9: Buphthalmos.

Cataract surgery with intraocular lens implantation is recommended under general anesthesia. Postoperatively, long and intensive follow-up is needed to manage refractive changes, amblyopia, squint, and possible complications of surgery.[4] In familial cases, all siblings and offsprings must be screened regularly.

Congenital Glaucoma

Primary developmental glaucoma (congenital glaucoma) results when elevated intraocular pressure occurs in the first 3 years of life. It is rare, its incidence being between 1:10,000 and 30,000 live births.[5] It is bilateral in 75% of cases.

Etiology

The principal defect is a failure in cleavage of the anterior chamber angle during embryogenesis causing aqueous humor to accumulate in the eye.

Clinical Features

- The characteristic clinical picture is enlargement of the eyeball; the infant sclera is more elastic than the adult and stretches in response to elevated intraocular pressure. The enlarged eye resembles that of the ox, and the condition is called "buphthalmos" **(Fig. 21.4.9)**.
- The presenting triad is watering, photophobia, and blepharospasm.
- A horizontal corneal diameter is >12 mm.
- Optic disk cupping
- May be secondary to ocular developmental disorders such as aniridia (congenital absence of iris), or ectopia lentis (subluxation of lens). It may also be associated with systemic syndromes (Sturge-Weber syndrome and neurofibromatosis).

Management

Examination under anesthesia is mandatory to rule out other conditions that mimic congenital glaucoma (megalocornea, keratitis, ophthalmia neonatorum, and mucopolysaccharidosis). The mainstay of treatment is surgical. Pressure must be medically controlled before surgery. Even after successful control of glaucoma, long-term follow-up is needed.

TRAUMA

Ocular injuries are the major cause of morbidity in children.

Etiology

Most injuries occur due to unsupervised play and are preventable. Usual modes of injury in children include stick, bow, and arrow **(Fig. 21.4.7)**, ball, stone, fist, *gilli-danda*, fireworks, scissors, knives, needles, and other sharps.

Clinical Features

- *Superficial foreign body (Particles of sand, wood, metal, or wing cases of insects, or plant seeds):* Watering, redness, and foreign body sensation aggravated by eye movement or blinking.
- *Chemical injury:* Chemosis, redness, pain, and photophobia
- *Blunt injury:* Asymptomatic, blurry vision, pain, and redness.
- *Lacerating injury:* Protrusion of iris tissue through entry wound, pain, and marked loss of vision **(Fig. 21.4.10)**.
- The eyelids, orbits, or eyeball may be involved **(Figs. 21.4.11 to 21.4.13)**.

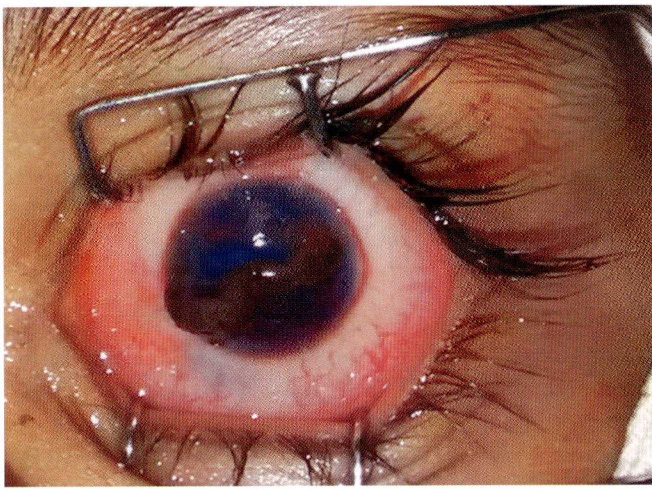

Fig. 21.4.10: Corneal perforation with iris prolapse following firecracker injury.

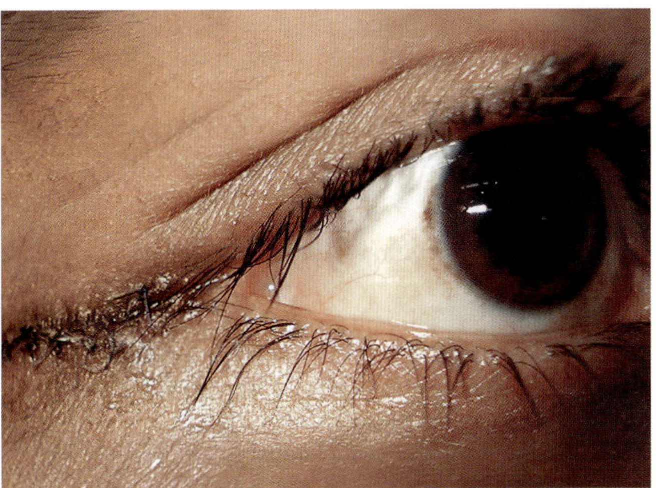

Fig. 21.4.11: Sutured laceration at lateral canthus after injury with a stick.

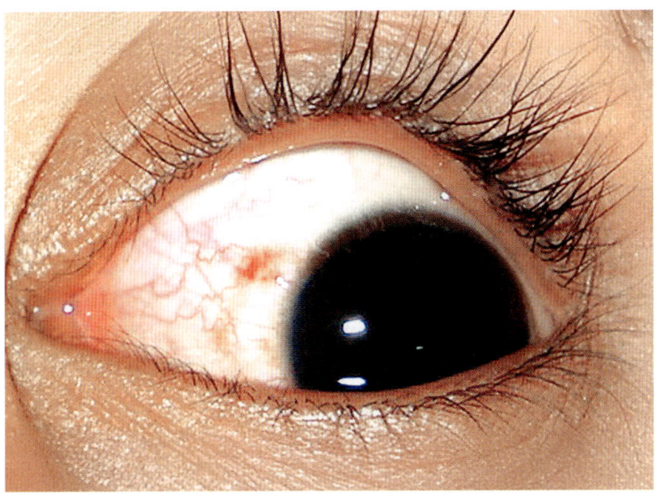

Fig. 21.4.12: Subconjunctival hemorrhage after injury with a pencil.

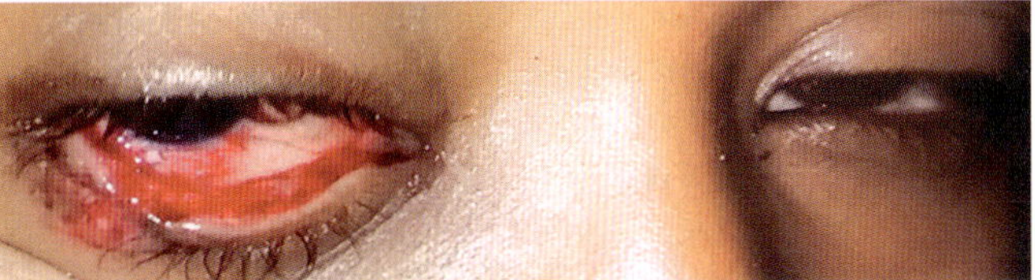

Fig. 21.4.13: Lid laceration with singeing of eyelashes after firecracker injury.

Management

Corneal foreign bodies, if not dislodged by irrigation, need removal under topical anesthesia and high magnification using a sterile cotton swab stick or 26-gauze needle by an ophthalmologist. Chemical injuries must be urgently managed at first presentation by thoroughly washing out all chemicals using any available inert solution; tap water, saline, or Ringer's lactate. Particulate material should be mechanically removed, and washing should continue for 30 minutes, before referral to an ophthalmologist. In mechanical trauma too, the child should be referred; however, if there is bleeding from the eyelid or eyeball, apply a sterile plastic shield before transport. Avoid applying a tight patch and bandage or use of any ointments in cases of lacerating injuries.

RETINAL AND OPTIC NERVE DISORDERS

Papilledema

Papilledema is swelling of the optic nerve head due to elevated intracranial pressure that raises the pressure in the subarachnoid space around the optic nerve, causing stasis of axoplasmic flow and build-up of toxic material.

Etiology

Causes of papilledema include malignant hypertension, central nervous system (CNS) space-occupying lesions, head injury, meningitis, encephalitis, venous sinus thrombosis, hydrocephalus, craniosynostosis, and use of drugs such as tetracycline and corticosteroids.

Clinical Features

- It is usually bilateral and may develop over hours or weeks.
- Elevation of intracranial pressure in infancy, before the fontanels close, may not result in manifest papilledema.
- Symptoms specific to papilledema include transient obscurations of vision, constriction of visual field, and decreased color perception.
- Fundus examination shows blurred disk margins with vascular changes.

Management

Investigative modalities include neuroimaging (CT scan and MRI), perimetry, and fluorescein angiography to establish the diagnosis. Early detection, identification of cause, and its appropriate treatment may be lifesaving.

Retinitis Pigmentosa

Etiology

Retinitis pigmentosa is a group of inherited disorders characterized by retinal pigment dystrophy. The worldwide prevalence is approximately 1 in 5,000.[6] It can be associated with all types of inheritance, with autosomal dominant being the most common. It may also be associated with systemic disease, i.e., hearing loss (Usher syndrome).

Clinical Features

- Progressive night blindness (nyctalopia)
- Loss of peripheral vision (tunnel vision)
- Progression, sometimes up to complete blindness
- It can present at infancy and up to the 3rd or 4th decade of life.
- The characteristic triad seen in the retina includes bony spicules in the midperipheral retina, waxy optic disk pallor, and retinal arteriolar attenuation.
- Some patients develop cystoid macular edema, which reduces central vision as well.

Management

There are very few treatment options available; vitamin A, vitamin E, docosahexaenoic acid, acetazolamide (for macular edema), and lutein/zeaxanthin have been tried. Refraction and low-vision aids may help. Siblings and children of the affected individual should be screened.

Retinopathy of Prematurity

Etiology

Retinopathy of prematurity (ROP) is a fibrovascular proliferation in the retina of premature infants. Vascularization of the fetal retina reaches the periphery by 32–40 weeks of gestation. Thus, eyes of premature babies may have avascular peripheral retina. In response to hyperoxic conditions in the nursery, vasoconstriction occurs to protect the immature retina. When babies are removed from oxygen-rich environments, the resultant relative hypoxia triggers angiogenic factors, which promote neovascularization. All babies <2,000 g birthweight or <34 weeks of gestational age at birth are at risk; other risk factors include hypoxic episodes, supplemental oxygen, sepsis, respiratory distress, hypercarbia, and concurrent illness.[7]

Clinical Features

- Neovascularization at the junction of vascular and avascular retina presenting as demarcation line, fibrovascular ridge, or retinal detachment (RD).
- Complications may include myopia, astigmatism, cataract, glaucoma, amblyopia, strabismus, and phthisis bulbi (shrinking of severely affected eyes).

Management

All high-risk babies should have retinal screening examinations to detect ROP. The first eye examination should be performed at discharge or by 30 days of life, whichever is sooner. Follow-up examinations should continue till the retina is fully vascularized. If ROP signs develop, treatment is initiated in the form of laser, cryotherapy, intravitreal antivascular endothelial growth factor (VEGF) injections or retinal surgery depending on the stage of ROP. Once RD develops, the prognosis is grave and thus treatment must begin early to save sight.

Optic Atrophy

Etiology

Optic atrophy is the endpoint of any disease process that causes retinal ganglion cell axons to degenerate.

In children, it can be hereditary (Leber–optic atrophy) or induced by retinal degeneration (retinitis pigmentosa and ROP), orbital (compression by tumor or inflammation, traumatic neuropathy), or intracranial conditions (optic neuritis in meningitis or encephalitis).

Clinical Features

- Grossly decreased visual acuity
- A relative afferent pupillary defect may be the only objective sign of optic atrophy.
- Visual field defects on field testing

Management

Investigations that may assist in the diagnosis of cause include fundus examination, cranial nerves assessment, ultrasound of orbit, CT or MRI of orbit and brain, visual-evoked response, visual fields, and color vision. Since there is no treatment for the atrophy, it is important to detect and treat the underlying cause before atrophy sets in.

REFERENCES

1. Braverman R. Diagnosis and treatment of refractive errors in the pediatric population. Curr Opin Ophthalmol. 2007;18(5):379-83.
2. von Noorden GK. Amblyopia: a multidisciplinary approach. Proctor lecture. Invest Ophthalmol Vis Sci. 1985;26(12):1704-16.
3. Khokhar SK, Pillay G, Dhull C, Agarwal E, Mahabir M, Aggarwal P. Pediatric cataract. Indian J Ophthalmol. 2017;65(12):1340-9.
4. VanderVeen DK, Drews-Botsch CD, Nizam A, Bothun ED, Wilson LB, Wilson ME, et al.; for the Infant Aphakia Treatment Study. Outcomes of secondary intraocular lens implantation in the Infant Aphakia Treatment Study. J Cataract Refract Surg. 2021;47(2):172-7.
5. Tamçelik N, Atalay E, Bolukbasi S, Çapar O, Ozkok A. Demographic features of subjects with congenital glaucoma. Indian J Ophthalmol. 2014;62(5):565-9.
6. O'Neal TB, Luther EE. Retinitis Pigmentosa. [Updated 2024 Feb 12]. In: StatPearls [Internet]. Treasure Island (FL): StatPearls Publishing; 2024.
7. Shukla R, Murthy GVS, Gilbert C, Vidyadhar B, Mukpalkar S. Operational guidelines for ROP in India: A summary. Indian J Ophthalmol. 2020;68(Suppl 1):S108-S114.

21.5 Common Problems of Ear, Nose, and Throat

Divya Prabhat

HEARING TESTS

Hearing tests are mandatory for the newborn in certain countries. As development of natural speech is all but over by the age of 3–5 years, the earlier an auditory disease is diagnosed, the better are the chances of helping a child to overcome hearing handicap and have a natural speech.

Reflex Tests

- *At birth:* Moro or startle reflex
- *3 months:* Blinking on response to sound
- *5 months:* Eyes turn toward sound
- *6 months:* Head turns toward sound

Behavioral Tests

- *7–18 months:* Distraction tests are performed. The child may be distracted from behind by various sounds.
- *18–30 months:* Child's cooperation is sought. The child is given simple tasks to perform in response to certain sounds.

Performance Tests

These are done between the ages of 2 and 5 years, where the child is asked verbally to perform tasks. Beyond 5 years, pure-tone audiometry is done, which requires the child's response to different sounds.

Subjective Tests

- *Visual reinforcement audiometry (VRA):* Here, a young child is conditioned to press a button when a sound is heard.
- *Conditioned audiometry:* The child is taught to build a tower of bricks each time he or she hears the (test) sound.

Objective Tests

- *Otoacoustic emission (OAE) tests:* It tests the outer hair cells function of the cochlea and can be performed in the neonate.
- *Impedance audiometry:* Here a low frequency sound is introduced into a sealed external canal. The impedance to sound would be much greater, if the tympanic membrane is stiff (e.g., middle ear fluid) than when compliant. Various graphs obtained help us to diagnose Eustachian tube block, serous otitis media, ossicular discontinuity, otosclerosis, etc.
- *Brainstem auditory evoked responses (BERA):* Electrical signals are picked-up by surface electrodes resulting from acoustic signs passing from the cochlear nerve to the brainstem.

DEAFNESS

Depending upon the site of diseases, the hearing loss or deafness is classified as follows:

- *Conductive deafness:* The disease affects the external or middle ear, i.e., involving the sound conducting mechanism of the ear, which is correctable.
- *Sensorineural deafness:* The disease affects the perceiving apparatus, i.e., cochlear or VIII nerve or any area up to the brainstem.

Causes of deafness in children are listed in **Box 21.5.1.**

BOX 21.5.1: Etiology of deafness.

- *Prenatal*
  - *Genetic:*
    - Waardenburg syndrome
    - Klippel–Feil syndrome
    - Pendred syndrome
  - *Nongenetic:*
    - Diseases during pregnancy
    - Toxemia
    - Diabetes mellitus
    - Nephritis
    - Measles and other viral infections
  - *Drugs taken during pregnancy:*
    - Streptomycin
    - Quinine
    - Salicylates
- *Perinatal*
  - *Birth trauma—anoxia/hypoxia*
  - *Hemolytic disease—kernicterus*
  - *Prematurity*
- *Postnatal*
  - *Genetic:*
    - Otosclerosis
    - Familial perceptive deafness
  - *Nongenetic:*
    - Infectious diseases, e.g., measles, mumps, etc.
    - Trauma
    - Otitis media
    - Ototoxic drugs

Management

Conductive deafness is fully corrected by either medical or surgical treatment. Sensorineural deafness is managed by using a hearing aid, which amplifies the basic sound. Children with sensorineural loss not benefitting with a hearing aid are candidates for a cochlear implant, which is done as early as 10 months of age.

FOREIGN BODY IN THE EAR

The types of foreign bodies that are found in the external canal may be living (e.g., maggots or insects) or nonliving (e.g., stones, beads or hygroscopic foreign bodies such as pea, bean, etc.). Symptoms include pain, irritation, discharge, noise, and cough.

Management

- Living foreign bodies are killed by borospirit drops and then syringed out.
- Nonliving foreign bodies are removed with wax hook.
- Forceps *should never be used* for removal as they push the foreign body dangerously further in.
- Impacted hygroscopic foreign bodies may be removed after using glycerin drops, which would shrink the foreign body.
- General anesthesia may be required for the above procedure in a noncooperative child or for impacted foreign bodies.

ACUTE SUPPURATIVE OTITIS MEDIA

Acute suppurative otitis media (ASOM) is nearly always a sequel to an upper respiratory tract infection, which is seen commonly during childhood.[1] In infants, the Eustachian tube is relatively short, wide and horizontal, thus allowing easy access of milk and vomitus in the middle ear. Thus, feeding while lying down, vomiting or forcible nose blowing in older children may lead to acute otitis media.

Etiology

Organisms reach the middle ear:

- Via the Eustachian tube following nasopharyngitis, rhinitis, sinusitis, pharyngitis, etc.
- Through a perforated tympanic membrane due to a previous disease, trauma, or tympanotomy.
- Rarely by blood-borne infections.
- The most common bacterial organisms causing otitis media are *Streptococcus pneumoniae*, nontypeable *Haemophilus influenzae* (NTHi) and *Moraxella catarrhalis*.

Investigations

- Ear discharge for culture and antibiotic sensitivity.[1,2]
- X-ray mastoid to detect the destruction of the mastoid air cells.
- Hearing test to detect the hearing loss.

Treatment

Local

- *Aural toilet* is maintained by sucking out the ear discharge.
- *Borospirit* eardrops are used only after a perforation occurs. Eardrops are not recommended before a perforation as they are unable to disinfect the middle ear, and they may obscure the otoscopic picture.[1,2]

Systemic[2]

- Antibiotic therapy is the most important form of treatment and must be used in all stages of the disease. Commonly used antibiotics are amoxicillin or amoxyclav for 7–10 days.[2-6]
- Nasal decongestant drops are used to improve drainage of the exudate via the Eustachian tube.
- Antihistamines are given to decongest the middle ear, Eustachian tube, and paranasal sinus mucosa.
- Analgesics to relieve pain.

Surgical[2]

Myringotomy may be done only in cases of severe earache with a bulging drum or when impending intracranial complications are present with an inadequate drainage.

CHRONIC OTITIS MEDIA

Types

- *Tubotympanic disease (safe type)* occurs as a residual effect of ASOM.
- *Atticoantral disease (unsafe type)* is associated with a cholesteatoma, which is a three-dimensional epidermal and connective tissue structure in the form of a sac that has the capacity for progressive and independent growth at the expense of the underlying bone **(Fig. 21.5.1)**.
  The characteristic of each type is given in **Table 21.5.1**.

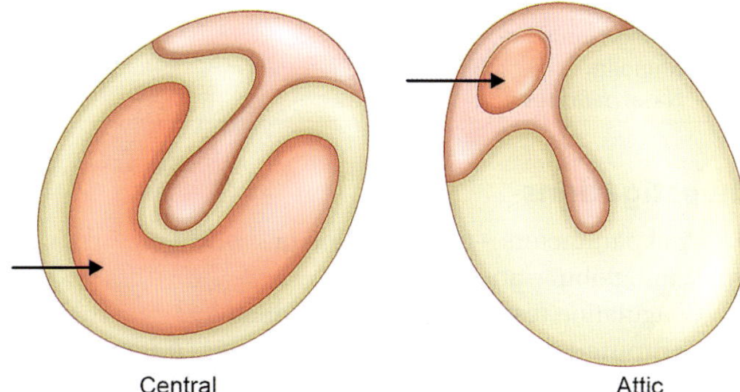

Fig. 21.5.1: Different types of perforation (shaded).

SEROUS OTITIS MEDIA

Serous otitis media is characterized by the presence of nonpurulent fluid in the middle ear, also known as "glue ear".

Etiology

Malfunction of the Eustachian tube is the underlying cause.

Clinical Features

- Deafness—which is of mild conductive type.
- Fullness—with sensation of fluid moving in the ear.
- Air-bubbles or fluid may be seen on otoscopic examination.

Treatment[2]

- Valsalva's inflation to improve Eustachian tube function.
- Local decongestant nasal drops as well as antihistamines for the same
- Myringotomy may be required, if no response to medical line of treatment
- Grommet insertion when recurrence is seen after a myringotomy.

TABLE 21.5.1: Clinical features of chronic otitis media.

Clinical features	***Safe ear***	***Unsafe ear***
Type of disease	Tubotympanic	Atticoantral
Perforation site	Central	Attic
Granulations	Absent	Common
Discharge	Copious, mucoid, and non-foul smelling	Scanty, purulent, and foul smelling
Bleeding	Never	Sometimes
Respiratory tract infection	Increase in the amount of discharge	Not affected
Audiogram	Conductive hearing loss	Mixed hearing loss
X-ray mastoid	Sclerotic	Sclerotic with destruction
Complications	Nil	Common
Treatment	Tympanoplasty	Mastoidectomy

Grommet

Grommet is a hollow tube of inert material, which is placed as a ventilating tube for the middle ear spaces on either side of the eardrum.

NASAL OBSTRUCTION

Causes

Unilateral

- Sinusitis
- Foreign body
- Antrochoanal polyp
- Deviated nasal septum
- Rhinolith
- Unilateral choanal atresia
- Meningocele/encephalocele
- Rhinosporidiosis

Bilateral

- Allergic rhinitis
- Ethmoidal polyp
- Adenoids
- Sinusitis
- Angiofibroma
- Septal abscess
- Atrophic rhinitis

NASAL POLYPS

Nasal polyp is prolapsed edematous respiratory mucosa **(Fig. 21.5.2)**.

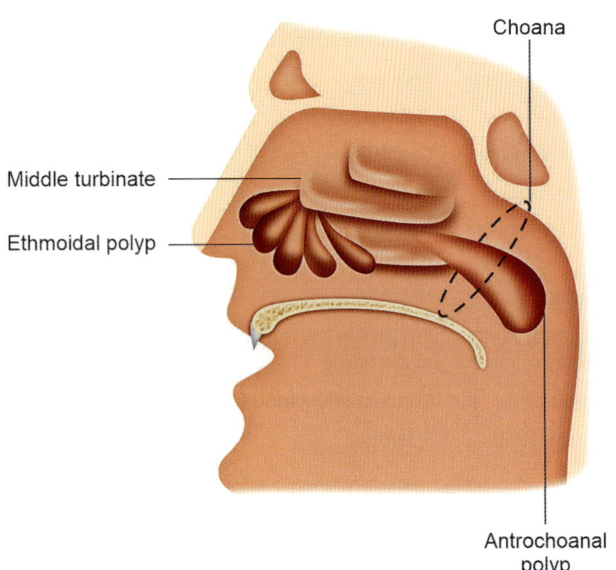

Fig. 21.5.2: Nasal polyps.

TABLE 21.5.2: Clinical features of nasal polyps.

	Antrochoanal	*Ethmoidal*
Number	Single	Multiple
Side	Unilateral	Bilateral
Etiology	Infective/allergy	Allergic
Source	Maxillary sinus	Ethmoid sinus
Age	Small children	Young adults
Type	Triradiate polyp	Single attachment
Direction	Grow toward posterior choanae	Toward anterior choanae
Recurrence	Rare	Common
Operation	Polypectomy with FESS	Polypectomy with FESS

(FESS: functional endoscopic sinus surgery)

Types

Antrochoanal polyp: Antrochoanal polyp arises from the maxillary sinus, enters the nasal cavity through the natural ostia of the sinus and also passes backward into the posterior choanae.

Ethmoidal polyp: Ethmoidal polyp arises from the mucosa of the ethmoidal sinuses and by the effect of gravity occupies the anterior choanae.

Clinical features of nasal polyps are given in **Table 21.5.2.**

EPISTAXIS

Epistaxis is bleeding from the nose.[7] Causes of epistaxis are listed in **Table 21.5.3**.

TABLE 21.5.3: Etiology of epistaxis.

Local	*Systemic*
• *Congenital:* – Osler–Weber–Rendu disease (hereditary hemorrhagic telangiectasia)	• *Cardiovascular system:* – Rheumatic heart disease – Pulmonary hypertension – Infective endocarditis
• *Traumatic:* – *Breach in mucosal continuity:* – Fractures of nose – Operations, e.g., submucosal resection (SMR), polypectomy, etc. – Nose picking	• *Blood disorders:* – Christmas disease – Hemophilia – Purpura – Aplastic anemia
• *Barotrauma:* – Nose blowing – High altitudes	• *Drugs:* – Salicylates – Quinine
• *Inflammatory:* – *Acute:* - Nonspecific rhinitis, e.g., coryza - Specific rhinitis, e.g. diphtheria, adenoiditis, sinusitis, etc. – *Chronic:* - Nonspecific, e.g., atrophic rhinitis - Specific, e.g., scleroma, rhinosporidiosis, chronic sinusitis, etc. - Midline nasal granuloma	• *Renal failure* • *Hepatic failure* • *Septicemia.*
• *Neoplastic:* – *Benign:* - Angiomatous polyp - Papilloma - Nasopharyngeal angiofibroma – *Malignant:* - Carcinoma - Sarcoma of the sinuses/ nasopharynx	
• *Miscellaneous:* – Foreign body – Rhinolith – Nasal parasites	

Investigations

- Vital parameters—for evaluation of shock
- Hemoglobin—anemia
- Coagulation tests—bleeding disorders
- Computed tomography scan—sinusitis, fractures, and tumors
- Biopsy—malignancy

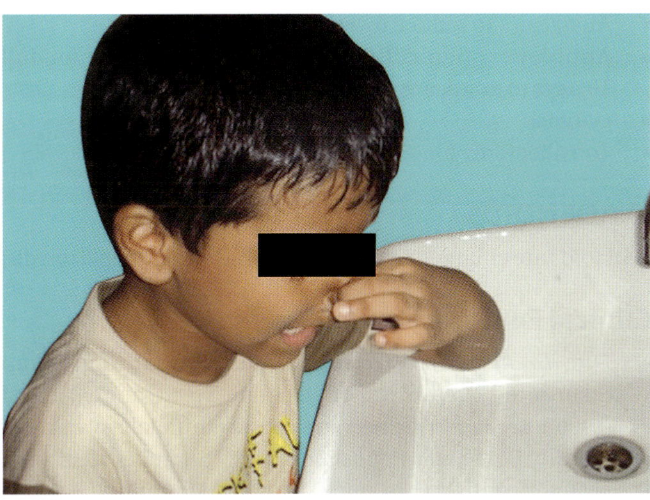

Fig. 21.5.3: Pinching the nostrils.

Management[7]

- *Immediate:*[8]
  - Pressure—by compression of the nose between the thumb and the first two fingers **(Fig. 21.5.3)**
  - Ice cold packs—applied on the bridge of the nose, which may stop the bleeding by reflex vasoconstriction
  - Trotter's method, where the child is made to sit upright and incline forward with mouth open and pinched (self) nostrils, then asked to breathe out quietly spitting out all the blood from pharynx.
  - Assessment of blood loss and vital parameters checked. Treatment of shock and hypovolemia
- *Measures to control bleeding:*
  - Cautery (chemical or electro)
  - Anterior nasal packing
  - Posterior nasal packing
  - Foley's catheter (postnasal)
  - Surgical ligation of the vessels (last resort)
- *General measures:*
  - *Sedation:* This reduces restlessness of the patient and allays anxiety.
  - Hematinics and multivitamins to improve the hemoglobin.
  - Antibiotics are required along with packing to prevent infections.[6]

SINUSITIS

Etiology

- *Age:* It affects children above 5 years of age, but infants are liable to suffer from acute ethmoiditis.
- *Sex:* It affects both equally.
- Acute rhinitis causes spread of infection to the sinuses via their natural ostia from the nasal cavities.
- Pharyngeal infections, especially tonsillitis, act as a focus of infection.
- Dental infections.
- Swimming and diving lead to water penetrating into the sinuses.

Symptoms

- Headache, malaise, and fever
- Loss of normal vocal resonance
- Pain around the various sinuses
- Referred pain in the ear
- Nasal discharge
- Nose block

Signs

- Flushing of the cheek with swelling in case of maxillary sinusitis and involving the upper eyelid in frontal or ethmoid sinusitis.
- Tenderness is elicited at the canine fossa in maxillary sinusitis and above the medial canthus in frontal sinusitis.
- Anterior rhinoscopy reveals redness and mucosal congestion. Pus may be seen trickling from the middle meatus area.

Investigations

- Bacteriological examination is required, if sinusitis does not respond to antibiotic treatment.
- *Radiology:* Water's and Caldwell's view/computed tomography (CT) scan of paranasal sinuses (PNS).
  - Mucosal thickening
  - Opacity of sinuses
  - An air-fluid level
- Nasal sinus endoscopy

Treatment

- Prevention by improving general condition of the child. Lowering of resistance affects the mucosal blanket integrity as well as the ciliary action.
- *Medical:*
  - *Antibiotics:* Appropriate for the infectious agent.[4-6]
  - Local decongestants are used.
  - Analgesics and anti-inflammatory drugs
  - Antihistamines
  - *Steam inhalation:* For clearing out the secretions
- *Surgical:*
  - After the acute phase is over.
  - Correction of a deviated septum—septoplasty
  - Antral puncture (rarely done nowadays)
  - Functional endoscopic sinus surgery (FESS) to restore the normal physiological mucociliary clearance of the sinuses via its natural ostia.

ACUTE TONSILLITIS

It is a triad of sore throat, fever, and malaise lasting for a period of 5 days and usually responds to treatment dramatically.[9]

Etiology

- *Age:* More common between 2 and 5 years.
- *Sex:* Both are equally affected.
- *Organisms:* Bacteria such as group A beta-hemolytic streptococci and viruses such as adenovirus, rhinovirus, and *Enterovirus.*
- *Predisposing factors:*
    - Ingestion of cold foods
    - Contact with infected children
    - Polluted and ill-ventilated environment
        - Preexisting viral upper respiratory tract infection
        - Sinusitis
        - Lowered general resistance

Symptoms

- Throat pain
- Fever
- Malaise and headache
- Neck swelling
- Earache (referred)
- Minimal or absent cough.

Signs

- Tachycardia and fever
- Tonsils are enlarged and congested with exudates
- Pharynx is often inflamed
- Tender and enlarged jugulodigastric lymph nodes (bilateral)

Complications

Local

- Chronic tonsillitis
- Quinsy (peritonsillar abscess)
- Parapharyngeal abscess
- Suppurative cervical lymphadenitis
- Acute otitis media

Systemic

- Rheumatic fever
- Acute glomerulonephritis
- Sydenham's chorea

Treatment[9]

- Bed rest
- Plenty of fluids and soft solid foods
- Analgesics to reduce fever and throat pain
- Antibiotics; penicillin is preferred and given for full 10 days to eradicate the bacteria[4-6]
- Gargles
- Tonsillectomy for chronic tonsillitis

ADENOIDS

Adenoids are enlarged hypertrophied nasopharyngeal tonsils.

Clinical Features

- *Due to nasal obstruction:* Mouth breathing, sleep disordered breathing, obstructive sleep apnea, nasal discharge, and voice becomes nasal (rhinolalia clausa).
- *Due to Eustachian tube blockage:* Earache, deafness, secretory otitis media, and later chronic suppurative otitis media (CSOM).
- *Due to mouth breathing:* Dribbling of saliva, noisy breathing at night, high arched palate, and chronic pharyngitis.
- *General:* Daytime sleepiness, attention deficit hyperactivity disorder, mental backwardness, and lethargy.

Diagnosis

- *Adenoid facies* **(Fig. 21.5.4)**
- Open mouth
- Pinched nostrils
- Nasal discharge
- Narrow maxillary arch
- Crowded protruding teeth
- Vacant facial expression
- X-ray lateral skull reveals the enlarged adenoids
- Nasal endoscopy to visualize the adenoids
- Examination under general anesthesia to visualize or palpate adenoids

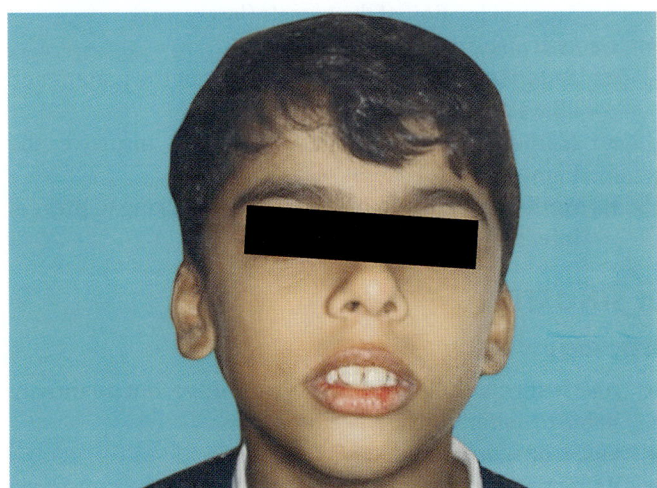

Fig. 21.5.4: Adenoid facies.

Management

Medical

- Antibiotics[5,6]
- Antihistamines
- Local steroid nasal sprays
- Improvement of general condition

Surgical

- Adenoidectomy
- Grommet insertion for treatment of deafness due to serous otitis media
- Nasal sinus endoscopy for sinusitis

TRACHEOBRONCHIAL FOREIGN BODIES

These foreign bodies may lead to a life-threatening situation due to obstruction in the respiratory passage. The absence of a definite history of foreign body aspiration, and the changing clinical signs as the disease evolves, may mimic various other clinical conditions thus making the diagnosis a difficult challenge in children.

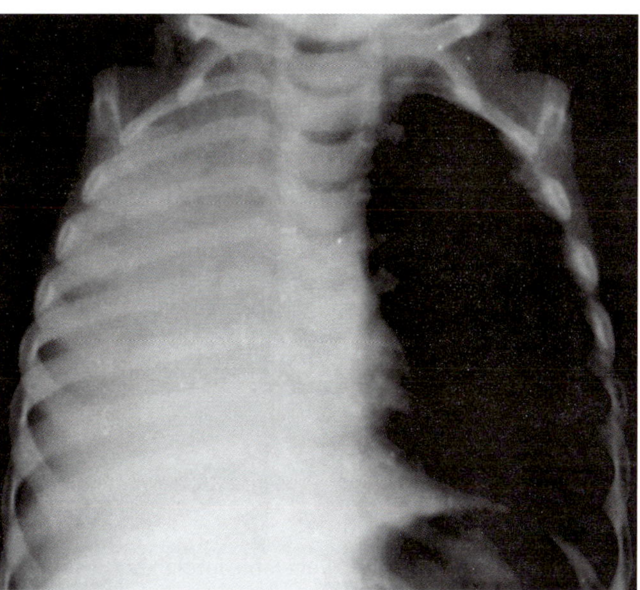

Fig. 21.5.5: Complete collapse of the lung (R) with mediastinal shift and emphysema of the lung (L). Foreign body (*supari*) was removed from the main bronchus (R).

Symptoms

- Sudden onset of cough, choking
- Fever
- Breathlessness
- Stridor

Signs

- Tachycardia
- Tachypnea
- Indrawing of the chest
- Cyanosis
- Unilateral wheeze or decreased/absent breath sounds

Investigations

- Radiograph of chest shows either obstructive emphysema or collapse or mediastinal shift or the foreign body itself (opaque like metallic) or may even be normal **(Figs. 21.5.5 and 21.5.6)**.
- Virtual bronchoscopy scan may be required in some cases.

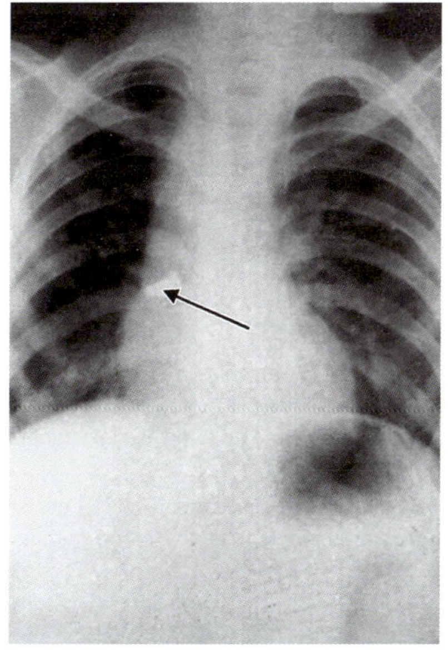

Fig. 21.5.6: Radiopaque foreign body seen in the (R) bronchus (arrow).

Types

Foreign bodies are divided into various types, according to the airflow pattern:

- *Bypass of air:* Foreign bodies such as a button, ring, or bead, which have an opening within itself, allow passage of air to either side **(Fig. 21.5.7)**. Therefore, the child is never breathless, and the radiograph shows no abnormal findings other than the foreign body (if radiopaque).
- *One-way airway obstruction:* Metallic and other nonorganic foreign bodies lead to a unidirectional obstruction in the airway. Inspiration leads to passage of air distal to the foreign body. However, on expiration, it leads to entrapment of air distal to the foreign body. This airway pattern leads to obstructive emphysema as, the radiographic finding and the child clinically presents with breathlessness **(Fig. 21.5.7)**.

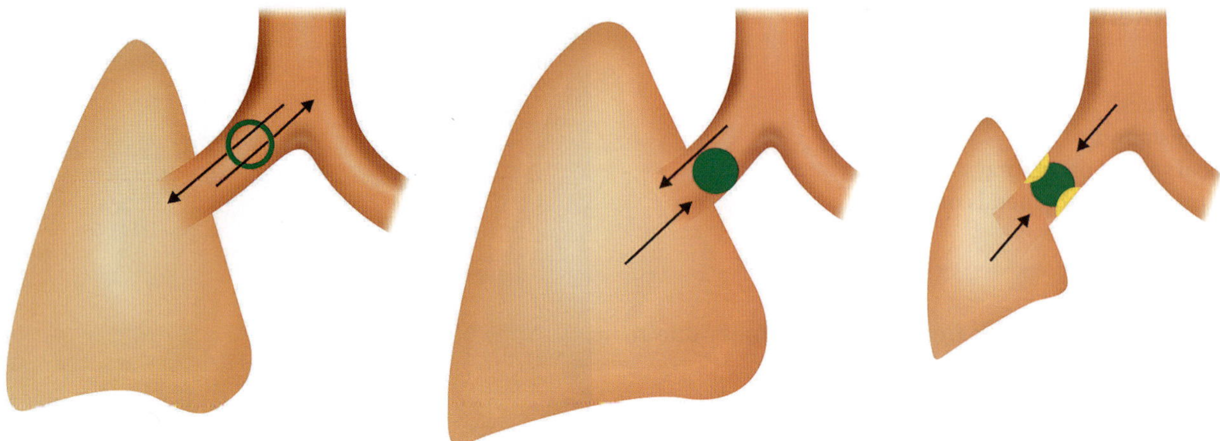

Fig. 21.5.7: X-ray findings with different types of foreign bodies.

- *Total airway obstruction:* Vegetable foreign bodies such as a pea or groundnut swell up in the bronchus due to their hygroscopic nature. The increase in size of foreign body causes impaction of the foreign body onto the bronchial wall. This leads to a collapse of the lung segment/lobe distal to the foreign body **(Fig. 21.5.7)**.and compensatory emphysema of the other segment/lobe.

Management

- Bronchoscopy (rigid or flexible) for removal of the foreign body.
- Tracheostomy (very rare), only as an absolute emergency.

REFERENCES

1. Blanc F, Ayache D, Calmels MN, Deguine O, Francois M, Leboulanger N, et al. Management of otitis media with effusion in children. Eur Ann Otorhinolaryngol Head Neck Dis. 2018:135(4):269-73.
2. Simon F, Haggard M, Rosenfeld RM, Jia H, Peer S, Calmels M-N, et al. International consensus (ICON) on management of otitis media with effusion in children. Eur Ann Otorhinolaryngol Head Neck Dis. 2018;135(1S):S33-9.
3. Choffor-Nchinda E, Atanga LC, Nansseu JR, Djomou F. Effectiveness of amoxicillin alone in the treatment of uncomplicated acute otitis media: A systematic review protocol. BMJ Open. 2018;8(6):e021133.
4. Ivanovska V, Hek K, Mantel-Teeuwisse AK, Leufkens HGM, van Djik L. Age-specific antibiotic prescribing and adherence to guidelines in pediatric patients in primary care. Pediatr Infect Dis J. 2018;37(3):218-23.
5. McCullough AR, Pollack AJ, Hansen MP, Glasziou PP, Locke DF, Britt HC, et al. Antibiotics for acute respiratory infections in general practice: comparison of prescribing rates with guideline recommendations. Med J Aust. 2017;207(2):65-9.
6. Piltcher OB, Kosugi EM, Sakano E, Mion O, Gesta JRG, Romano FR, et al. How to avoid the inappropriate use of antibiotics in upper respiratory tract infections? A position statement from an expert panel. Braz J Otorhinolaryngol. 2018;84(3):265-79.
7. Record S. Practice Guideline: Epistaxis in Children. J Pediatr Health Care. 2015;29(5):484-8.
8. Tanner R, Harney MS. The initial management of epistaxis. Ir Med J. 2015;108(4):123-4.
9. Isaacson G. Pediatric tonsillectomy: An evidence-based approach. Otolaryngol Clin North Am. 2014;47(5):673-90.

21.6 Common Skin Diseases

Parimalam Kumar, Jayakar Thomas

INTRODUCTION

Dermatological problems are seen by pediatricians every day and comprise around one-quarter of a busy outpatient clinic. Most children and adolescents present with skin disorders that can be easily diagnosed and treated. This chapter presents a brief account of the commonly seen skin conditions.

PARASITIC INFESTATIONS

Scabies

Definition/Description: Scabies is a contagious skin infestation.

Epidemiology/Etiology: The primary incubation period is 14 days.[1] It is caused by *Sarcoptes scabiei*, commonly by skin contact.

Clinical evaluation: It is characterized by nocturnal pruritus, burrows, papules, papulopustules, excoriations, vesicles, and urticarial lesions over interdigital spaces, ulnar border of wrist, anterior axillary fold, posterior aspect of elbow, nipple, around umbilicus, inner thighs, and genitals in male children, and gluteal cleft. The face and palms are usually spared, except in infants. Secondary pyogenic infection may complicate neglected scabies **(Fig. 21.6.1)**.

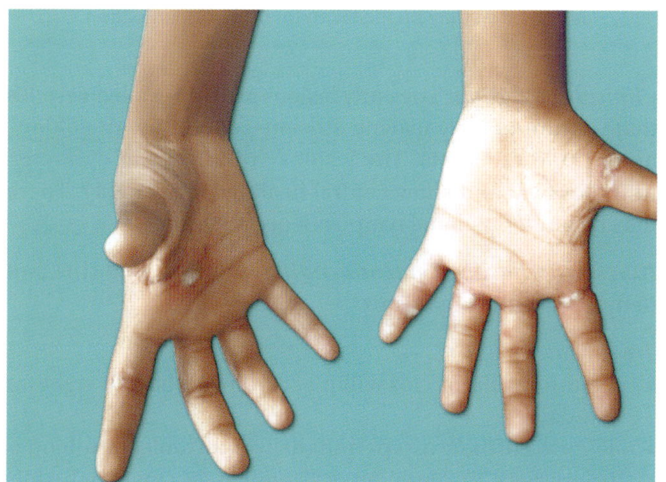

Fig. 21.6.1: Infected scabies of the hands. Note the vesicular lesions with pustules.

Investigations/Dermatopathology: Demonstration of the mite or its products under the microscope, from scraping.

Treatment: All contacts should be treated simultaneously. Clothes should be laundered. Any of the following may be applied from neck to toes after a scrub bath:

- Permethrin 2.5–5%—washed off after 8–12 hours which can be repeated after a week.
- Sulfur precipitate ointment 3–5%—daily for three to four successive nights
- Gamma benzene hexachloride—the same clothing is retained for 48 hours and then washed after shower. Avoided in infants and children with history of seizures.
- Benzyl benzoate emulsion 25–33%—for three successive nights
- Crotamiton 10%—has an antipruritic effect for 2 days.
- Oral ivermectin 3–6 mg, once
- Antihistamine for itching
- Systemic antibiotics—if there is secondary infection.

Pediculosis Capitis

Definition/Description: Pediculosis capitis is an infestation of the scalp.

Epidemiology/Etiology: Pediculus humanus var capitis is the causative agent. Transmission occurs via shared fomites.

Clinical evaluation: Nits appear firmly cemented to the hair shaft. Secondary can mask impetiginization the presence of lice and nits **(Fig. 21.6.2)**. In extreme cases, hair becomes matted (plica polonica). Papular urticaria may be seen on the neck as a reaction to louse bites. The occipital and postauricular lymphadenopathy is commonly associated.

Treatment:

- One of the following preparations may be used:
  - Permethrin 1%—rinse (a synthetic pyrethroid) washed off after 10 minutes
  - Gamma benzene hexachloride—left for 12 hours, followed by shampooing
  - Oral cotrimoxazole
  - Ivermectol 3–12 mg, once
- Nits must be removed using a fine-tooth comb.
- Retreatment may be necessary if lice are found or eggs are observed at the hair-skin junction.

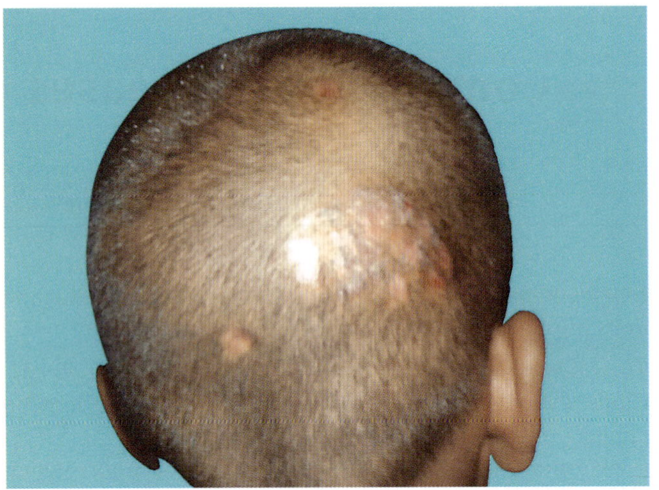

Fig. 21.6.2: Infected pediculosis capitis. Note lymph node behind the right ear.

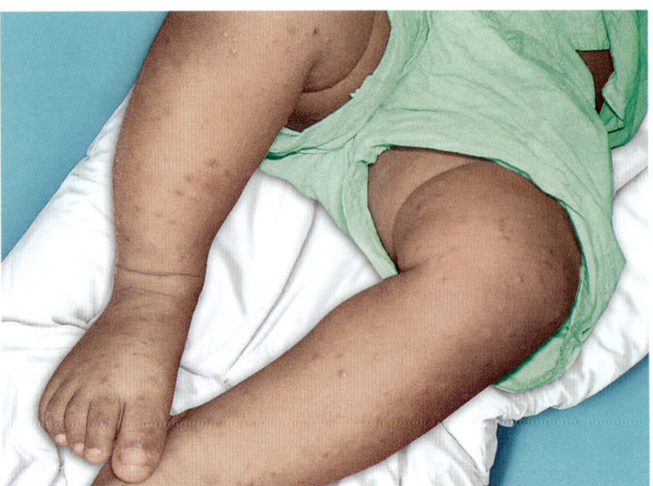

Fig. 21.6.3: Papular urticaria—lesions over legs of the infant.

- Affected family members and contacts should be simultaneously treated.
- Combs and brushes should be washed.
- Secondary bacterial infection should be treated with appropriate systemic antibiotics.

PAPULAR URTICARIA

Definition/Description: Papular urticaria "insect bite allergy" is a reaction pattern to insect bites, most commonly mosquitoes. Quite often, there exists an atopic background.

Clinical evaluation: The lesions are itchy erythematous weals, papules, seen on the legs and forearms relatively sparing the covered areas. Sometimes one new spot provokes all the old ones to come up again and itch intensely **(Fig. 21.6.3)**. Secondary impetiginization and postinflammatory pigmentation are the common sequelae. Recurrence is the hallmark.

Treatment: This is directed essentially toward counseling and prevention. Topical antipruritics (crotamiton), oral antihistamines, and antibiotics if needed can be given.

BACTERIAL INFECTIONS

Impetigo Contagiosa

Definition/Description: Impetigo is a superficial skin infection caused by *Staphylococcus aureus*, and or Group A β-hemolytic streptococci.[2]

Epidemiology/Etiology: Predisposing factors include crowded living conditions, poor hygiene, and neglected minor trauma. Secondary impetiginization of eczema, scabies, and pediculosis capitis are common.

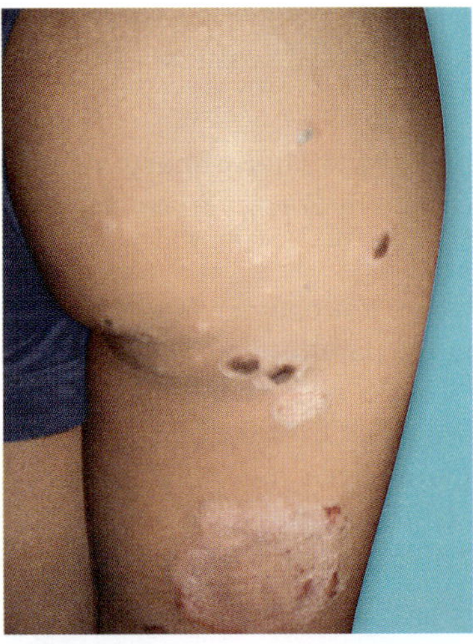

Fig. 21.6.4: Impetigo over the back of right thigh. Note circinate lesions that may be mistaken for ringworm infection.

Clinical evaluation: The early lesions are thin-walled vesicles that rupture quickly leaving erosions, covered with golden/honey-colored crusts. The lesions are 1–3 cm in diameter, round or oval and show central healing **(Fig. 21.6.4)**. There may be tender regional lymph adenopathy.

Investigations/Dermatopathology: Gram's stain can demonstrate the organisms.

Treatment:

- Erythromycin or cloxacillin according to body weight for 5–7 days
- Removal of the crusts permits delivery of topical antibiotics (mupirocin 2% ointment or sisomicin 1% cream or fusidic acid 2% cream or gentamicin 0.1% cream), applied three to four times daily after wash.

Bullous Impetigo

Definition/Description: Bullous impetigo occurs as scattered thin-walled bullae arising in normal skin and containing turbid fluid.

Epidemiology/Etiology: May occur in epidemic form in infant nurseries. Phage Group II staphylococci, the causative agent, can also cause staphylococcal-scalded skin syndrome (SSSS) which is life-endangering if untreated.

Clinical evaluation: Thin-roofed, flaccid bullae with turbid fluid, followed by erosions and brownish crusts. Central healing and peripheral extension may give rise to circinate lesions **(Fig. 21.6.5)**.

Investigations/Dermatopathology:

- Gram's stain of early vesicle shows Gram-positive cocci
- Culture grows *S. aureus*.

Treatment:

- Sparkling cleanliness is the hallmark of management.
- Mupirocin or fusidic acid 2% ointment applied to the lesions and nostrils.
- *Systemic antibiotic:* Erythromycin or cloxacillin according to bodyweight for 7–10 days.

Cellulitis

Definition/Description: It is an acute, spreading infection of dermal and subcutaneous tissues, characterized by red, hot, and tender area of skin, often at the site of bacterial entry.

Epidemiology/Etiology: In children, the cheek, periorbital area, head, and neck are the most common sites, and *H. influenzae* is usually the causative organism. On the extremities, cellulitis is usually caused by *S. aureus* and Group A streptococci. Immunocompromised patients are susceptible to infection with bacteria of low pathogenicity.

Clinical evaluation: A prodrome with higher fever (38.5°C) and chills are usually associated with streptococci; lower fever (37.5°C) with staphylococci. The typical lesion presents as red, hot, edematous, very tender, and elevated area of skin with poorly defined borders. Bluish-purple color is seen with *H. influenzae* **(Fig. 21.6.6)**. Vesicles, bullae, erosions, abscesses, hemorrhage, and necrosis may develop. Lymphangitis may occur. The regional lymph nodes can be enlarged and tender.

Investigations/Dermatopathology:

- *Blood:* White blood cell counts and erythrocyte sedimentation rate (ESR) may be elevated.
- *Blood cultures:* These are positive in only one quarter of cases.
- Fungal and mycobacterial cultures are indicated in atypical cases.

Treatment:

- Supportive measures include rest, immobilization, elevation, moist heat, and analgesics.
- *Mild early cellulitis:* Cloxacillin 0.5–1 g or erythromycin 0.5 g every 6 hours.
- *More severe infections:* Penicillin 100,000–200,000 units/kg bodyweight + cloxacillin 25–50 mg/kg tid IV. Ampicillin 25 mg/kg IV every 4 hours, and vancomycin 10–15 mg/kg tid IV in penicillin-allergic patients may be used. Subsequently, antibiotic is used according to antibiogram.

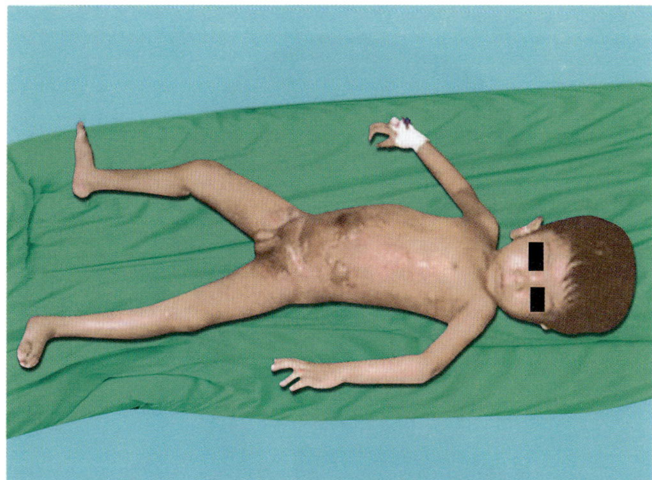

Fig. 21.6.5: Bullous impetigo of staphylococcal origin. Early diagnosis will prevent the development of "staphylococcal-scalded skin syndrome."

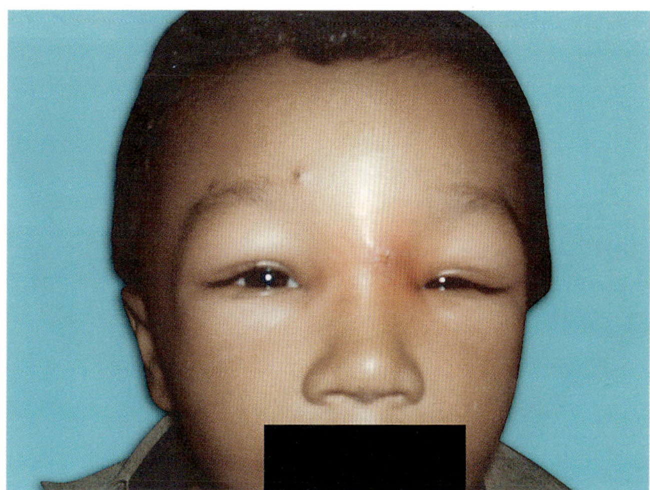

Fig. 21.6.6: Cellulitis following furuncles on the forehead. Note ill-defined borders.

Erysipelas

Definition/Description: A superficial cellulitis with marked lymphatic vessel involvement caused by bacteria.

Epidemiology/Etiology: Etiological agent is Group A or rarely Group C or G β-hemolytic streptococci.

Clinical evaluation: The legs are the most frequent anatomic location. The lesion is well-demarcated, shiny, red, edematous, indurated, and tender; vesicles and bullae sometimes develop **(Fig. 21.6.7)**. Regional lymphadenopathy occasionally occurs. High fever, chills, and malaise are common. Recurrent erysipelas may result in chronic lymphedema. Erysipelas of the face must be differentiated from herpes zoster, angioneurotic edema, and contact dermatitis. Diagnosis is usually clinical.

Investigations/Dermatopathology: The causative organism is difficult to culture from the lesion but may be cultured from blood.

Treatment: Mild cases respond to oral penicillin, cephalosporins, or erythromycin. Severe cases require hospitalization and IV antibiotics. Bed rest, limb elevation, cold packs, and analgesics add to the child's comfort and speed resolution of the illness. Long-term administration of oral penicillin may be warranted to prevent recurrences in selected cases.

Table 21.6.1 lists down the difference between cellulitis and erysipelas as they are of prognostic significance.

Furuncles and Carbuncles

Definition/Description: It is an acute, deep-seated, red, hot, and tender nodule that evolves from a staphylococcal folliculitis. A carbuncle is a conglomerate of multiple coalescing furuncles.

Epidemiology/Etiology: Furuncles are more common in boys. Predisposing factors include chronic staphylococcal nasal carrier state, friction, obesity, excessive sweating, bactericidal defects like hyperimmunoglobulin E (IgE) syndrome, and malnutrition.

Clinical evaluation: Furuncle can be single or multiple, appears as a bright-red, tender, indurated, round, and follicular nodule evolving into a fluctuant abscess with central suppuration and necrotic plug **(Fig. 21.6.8)**. The abscess may rupture forming an ulcer that heals with scar. A carbuncle is a conglomerate of multiple coalescing furuncles with separate "heads," and can leave a deep ulcer with a purulent floor.

TABLE 21.6.1: Cellulitis versus erysipelas.

	Cellulitis	*Erysipelas*
Etiology	Group A β-hemolytic streptococci, *Staphylococcus aureus,* and *Haemophilus influenzae*	Group A (C or G) β-hemolytic streptococci
Fever	Low/high	High
Margin	Poorly-defined	Defined
Blister	In the plaque	Advancing margin
Lymphatic	Usually involved	Markedly involved
Recurrence	Less frequent	More frequent
Treatment	May need surgical intervention (if associated with abscess)	Appropriate medical
Long-term penicillin	No need	In selected cases

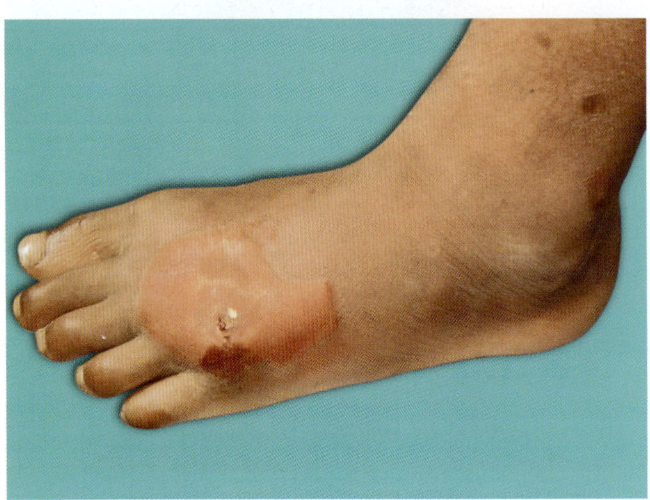

Fig. 21.6.7: Erysipelas with blistering on the dorsum of left foot. Note the well-defined border.

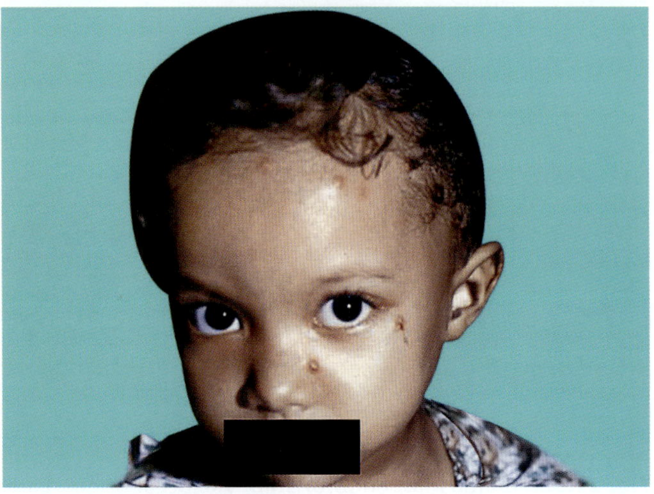

Fig. 21.6.8: Multiple furunculosis.

TABLE 21.6.2: Furuncles versus carbuncles.

Furuncles	*Carbuncles*
Single deep follicle	Multiple coalescing furuncles
Children and adolescents	Middle old age
Bright-red, tender, indurated, round, and follicular nodule	Conglomerate of multiple coalescing furuncles, with separate "heads"
Diabetes less common	Diabetes more common

Investigations/Dermatopathology: Gram stain from the pus and blood culture will help to confirm the diagnosis.

Treatment: Warm compresses and systemic antibiotics such as cloxacillin, erythromycin, or a cephalosporin. Fluctuating lesions should be incised and drained. On the upper lip and nose, great care must be exercised, and incision avoided, because of the dangers of sinus thrombosis. In recurrent furunculosis, mupirocin ointment should be applied daily to the inside of the nares.

The difference between furuncles and carbuncles are described in **Table 21.6.2**.

VIRAL INFECTIONS

Herpes Simplex virus

Etiology: Herpes labialis, gingivostomatitis, whitlow, keratoconjunctivitis and herpes simplex virus (HSV) encephalitis are caused by HSV-1 whereas herpes progenitalis, herpetic vulvovaginitis, and neonatal HSV infection are caused by HSV-2. Recurrence occurs when the virus subsequently migrates along the peripheral sensory nerve. Lifelong latency and periodic recurrences are hallmarks of the disease.

Incubation period: 3–7 days.

Clinical evaluation: Characterized by grouped vesicles on erythematous-base followed by erosions and hypopigmentation **(Fig. 21.6.9)**. Lymphadenopathy and systemic complaints are common during primary infection. Tender submandibular or cervical adenopathy are features of primary infection. Neonatal sepsis and aphthosis should be differentiated.

Investigations: Tzanck smear will show multinucleated giant cells. PCR test is confirmatory. Serology is required in disseminated lesions.

Treatment: Acyclovir oral or parenteral according to severity. Kaposi varicelliform eruption is managed as a dermatological emergency.

Pityriasis Rosea

Definition/Description: Pityriasis rosea is a benign, self-limited, exanthematous, maculopapular, red, and scaling eruption.

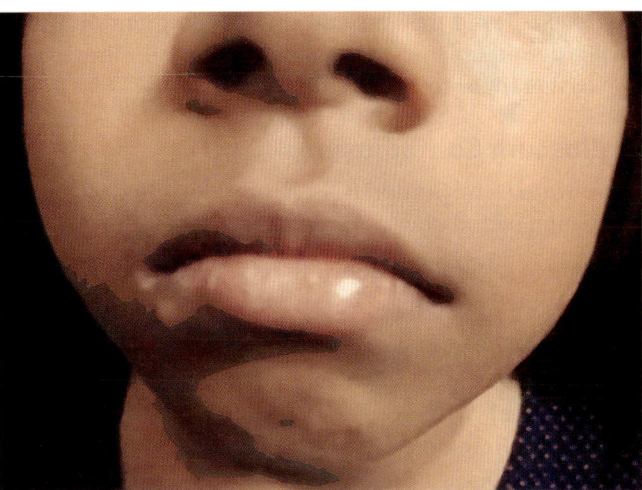

Fig. 21.6.9: Herpes labialis over angle of mouth (right) healed with hypopigmentation.

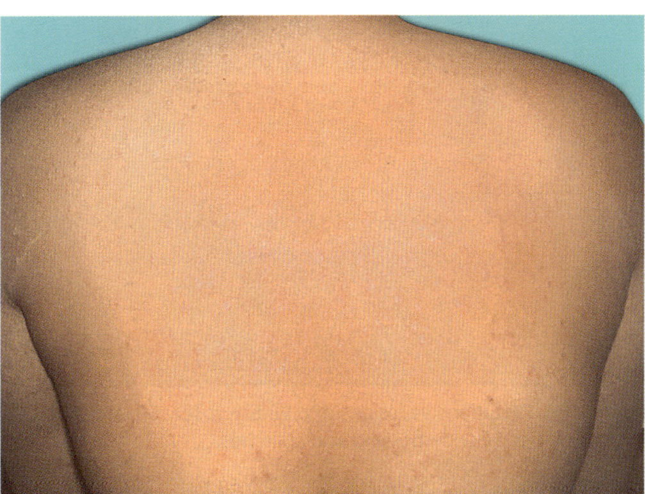

Fig. 21.6.10: Erythematous rash over the back consisting of scaly papules—pityriasis rosea.

Epidemiology/Etiology: It affects 2% of dermatological outpatients and is proposed to be of viral etiology.

Clinical evaluation:

- *Herald patch* seen as erythematous oval patch (2–5 cm) with fine collarette of scaling. In abortive pityriasis rosea, the condition is limited to the herald patch and does not proceed beyond **(Figs. 21.6.10 and 21.6.11)**.
- *Exanthem:* Fine and dull-pink macules with typical marginal collarette of thin with long axes of the lesions following the lines of cleavage in a "Christmas tree" distribution develops following the herald patch. The course lasts for about 6 weeks.

Treatment: Avoid irritants and use an emollient or a mild corticosteroid cream. Oral antihistamine and ultraviolet-B (UV-B) therapy in case of itching.

Molluscum Contagiosum

Definition/Description: It is caused by poxvirus. The incubation period ranges from 14 days to 6 months.

Epidemiology/Etiology: Infection may be acquired through direct contact, or fomites.

Clinical evaluation: Characterized by sessile dome-shaped papules of size 2–10 mm with umbilicated center **(Fig. 21.6.12)**. On squeezing of molluscum body can be expressed. Ultimately, the lesions involute spontaneously and heal without scarring.

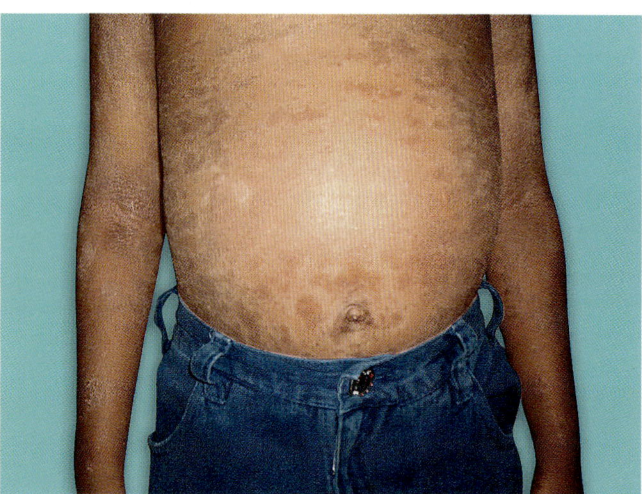

Fig. 21.6.11: Extensive lesions of pityriasis rosea—front of trunk showing scaly patches.

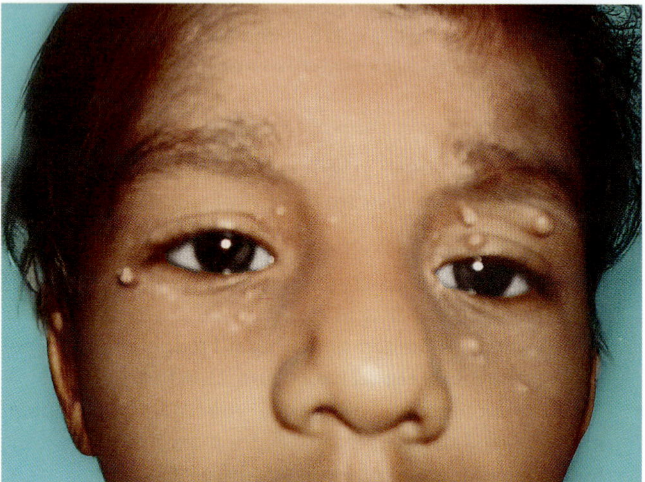

Fig. 21.6.12: Molluscum contagiosum. Note the pearly dome-shaped papules with central umbilication.

The sites of predilection include the face and eyelids, neck, forearms, trunk, anogenital area, and thighs (suspect child abuse).

Investigations/Dermatopathology: Direct microscopic examination of Giemsa-stained central semisolid core reveals "molluscum bodies" (inclusion bodies).

Treatment:

- Simple expression of the contents
- Cryotherapy using liquid nitrogen (10–15 seconds)
- Light electrocautery

Viral Warts

Definition/Description: Viral warts are common, contagious, epithelial tumors caused by at least 60 types of human papillomavirus (HPV).

Epidemiology/Etiology: It may be single or multiple and may develop by autoinoculation with variable course. Complete regression is usual but may persist for years and recur in about 35% of children.

Clinical evaluation: Common warts (verrucae vulgaris) are rough-surfaced, firm papules 2–10 mm in diameter. Periungual and plantar warts are also common. Plantar warts may be exquisitely tender and can be distinguished from corns and calluses by their tendency to pinpoint bleeding when the surface is pared away. Mosaic warts are plaques formed by the coalescence of myriad smaller, closely set plantar warts. Wart involving scalp may present with history of bleeding on combing and may be easily missed over a hairy scalp. **Figure 21.6.13** shows a tiny wart on the scalp.

Treatment: Most common warts disappear spontaneously within 2 years. Any one of the following modalities is effective:

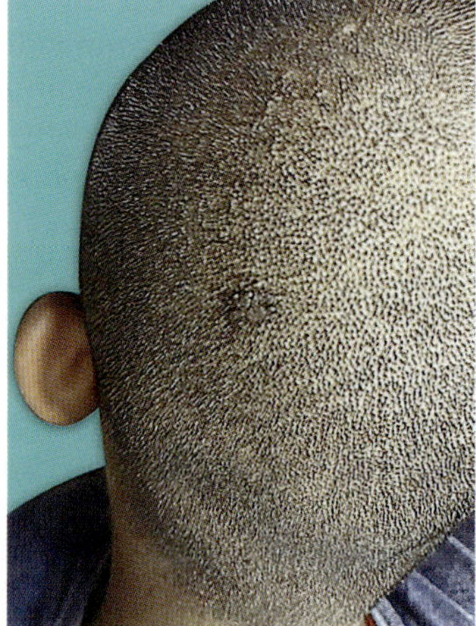

Fig. 21.6.13: Wart over the scalp seen as a small rough, irregular, and firm brown-gray papule.

flexible collodion solution containing 17% salicylic acid and 17% lactic acid, liquid nitrogen freeze; electrodesiccation or laser therapy (care must be taken to avoid scarring).

FUNGAL INFECTIONS

Tinea Capitis

Definition/Description: Tinea capitis is a dermatophyte infection of the scalp.

Epidemiology/Etiology: The causative organisms include epidermophyton, trichophyton, and microsporum.

*Clinical evaluation: Duration ranges from w*eeks to months. Usually, asymptomatic. Pain and tenderness are seen in inflammatory type (kerion).

Types: "Gray patch" and "Black dot" are noninflammatory types while kerion and favus are inflammatory.

- Kerion presents as painful boggy, elevated, and inflamed plaques draining seropus **(Fig. 21.6.14)**.
- Favus is characterized by scutula. These are dry, yellowish, saucer-shaped, and adherent crusts surrounding the openings of hair follicles. Both kerion and favus heal with scarring.
- Regional lymphadenopathy may be present.

Investigations/Dermatopathology:

- Wood's lamp examination reveals bright-green fluorescence in some cases.
- *Direct microscopic examination with 10% potassium hydroxide (KOH):* Endo or ectothrix spores can be seen.
- *Culture* in Sabouraud dextrose agar will confirm the organism.

Treatment: Clipping away of the hair will reduce the infectivity.

- *Oral griseofulvin (ultramicrosize):* 10–12.5 mg/kg bodyweight/day after meals.
- *"Black dot" ringworm:* Treatment continued for 2 weeks after Wood's lamp, KOH examination is done, and cultures are negative.
- *Kerion:* Griseofulvin 250 mg bid for 1–2 months; careful removal of crusts is important. *In kerion favus:* Griseofulvin for 10 weeks.
- Itraconazole may be used instead of griseofulvin for treating certain resistant infections.
- Ketoconazole shampoo can be used to prevent spread in the early phases of therapy.
- Antibiotics may be needed if there is accompanying bacterial infection.

Pityriasis Versicolor

Definition/Description: It is a chronic, asymptomatic, noncontagious, and superficial fungus infection of the skin.

Epidemiology/Etiology: It is caused by *Malassezia furfur,* the pathogenic mycelial phase of the normal flora *Pityrosporum orbiculare*. The disease is common in temperate climates.

Clinical evaluation: Characterized by sharply-marginated, round, or oval hypo- or hyperpigmented macules, with fine branny scaling measuring 1–30 cm **(Figs. 21.6.15 and 21.6.16)**.

Sites of predilection: Upper trunk, upper arms, neck, and abdomen. The face is rarely affected.

Investigations/Dermatopathology: KOH or Parker Quink ink technique reveals short hyphae and round spore, commonly

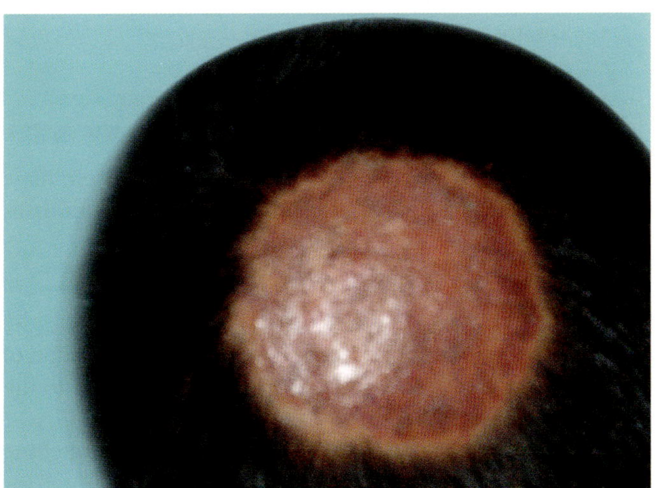

Fig. 21.6.14: Inflammatory type of tinea capitis—kerion.

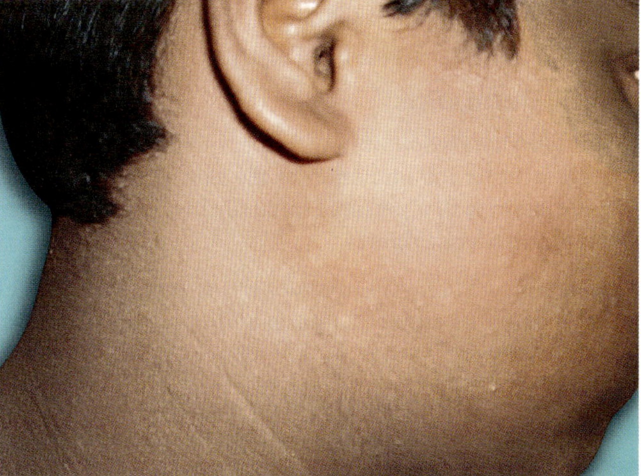

Fig. 21.6.15: Scaly hypopigmented patches of pityriasis versicolor over the sides of the neck.

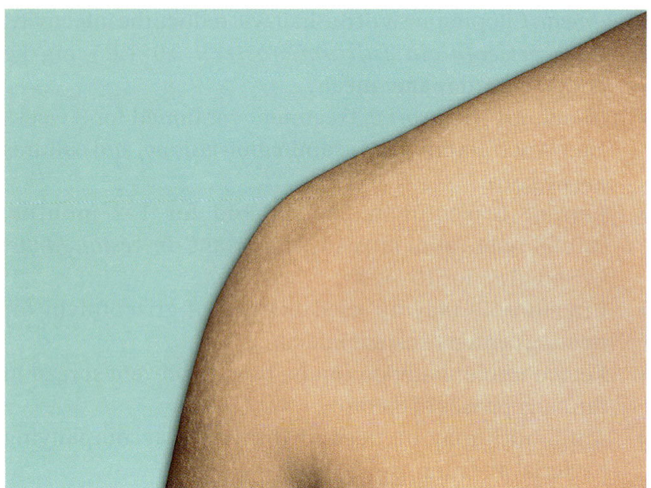

Fig. 21.6.16: Confetti-like patches of pityriasis versicolor over the back.

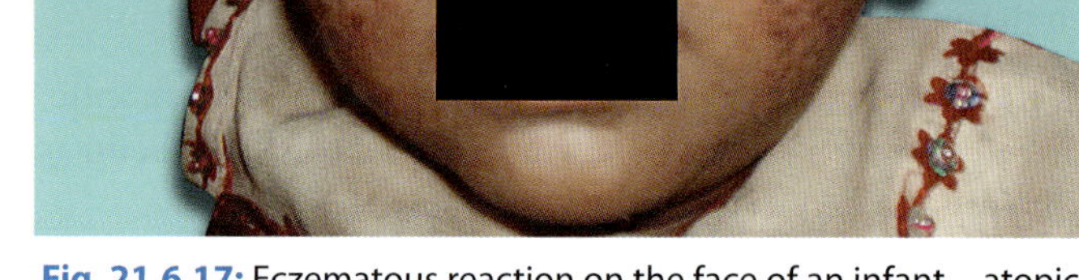

Fig. 21.6.17: Eczematous reaction on the face of an infant—atopic dermatitis.

referred to as "spaghetti and meatballs". Wood's lamp examination shows faint-yellow fluorescence.

Treatment:

- *Topical agents:*
  - Selenium sulfide (2.5%, to be washed off in 30 minutes) for 12 nights. Repeat every 2 weeks.
  - Sodium thiosulfate (25%) solution in water applied once or twice daily
  - Miconazole cream (2%) applied at night
  - Topical ketoconazole (2%) either as shampoo or cream
- *Systemic therapy:* Fluconazole 300 mg orally once a week for 2–4 weeks or itraconazole 200 mg daily for 5–7 days.
- Patients should be warned about the hypopigmentation that may persist after treatment.

DERMATITIS AND ECZEMAS

Atopic Dermatitis

Definition/Description: It is an acute, subacute, but usually chronic pruritic inflammation of the skin, often occurring in association with a personal or family history of hay fever, asthma, and allergic rhinitis.[3]

Epidemiology/Etiology: Over two-thirds have personal or family history of atopic diathesis and in some, related to emotional stress.

Clinical evaluation: Starts after first 2 months of life. Dry skin is the hallmark. Skin lesions include confluent and ill-defined erythema, papules, scaling, excoriations, and crusting. Lichenification occurs with time. Atopic dermatitis passes in three different phases:

1. *Infantile phase:* Age—2 months to 2 years; affects the cheeks and may extend to the forehead. There is no lichenification **(Fig. 21.6.17)**.
2. *Childhood phase (Besnier's prurigo—age: 5–12 years):* The flexural surfaces of the limbs and neck are affected. The lesions consist of itchy papules and lichenified plaques.
3. *Adulthood phase* is marked by disseminated neurodermatitis. Special features include:
   - Generalized infections, especially herpes simplex virus
   - Superimposed staphylococcal infection is also frequent.
   - White dermographism
   - Bilateral cataracts
   - Ichthyosis vulgaris
   - Keratosis pilaris
   - Periorbital pigmentation
   - Infraorbital fold in eyelids (Dennie–Morgan sign)
   - Loss of lateral portions of eyebrows (Hertoghe's sign)

Investigations/Dermatopathology: Some children have elevated IgE levels. Histology shows spongiosis, acanthosis, and dermal perivascular infiltration.

Treatment:

General:

- The most important aspect is sympathetic explanation of the nature of the condition and the complications to the parents.
- Education of the patient to avoid rubbing and scratching is most important.
- Topical antipruritic (menthol/camphor) lotions are helpful in controlling the pruritus.

- Warn parents of the special problems with herpes simplex and frequency of superimposed staphylococcal infection, for which oral erythromycin or cloxacillin is indicated. Acyclovir is indicated if HSV is suspected.

Specific:
- H1-antihistamines are probably useful in reducing itching.
- Hydration (oiled baths) followed by application of unscented emollients (e.g., hydrated petrolatum) is a basic daily treatment needed to prevent xerosis. Soap showers are permissible to wash the body folds, but soap should not be used on the other parts of the skin surface.
- Topical corticosteroids when used judiciously are effective.
- Systemic corticosteroids should be avoided, except in rare instances for only short courses.

Seborrheic Dermatitis

Definition/Description: It is a very common chronic dermatosis characterized by greasy scales.

Epidemiology/Etiology: It is more common in males and affected age groups include infancy and around puberty.

Clinical evaluation: Skin patches are itchy, cause discomfort when it is exudative and affects the major flexures with a tendency to chronicity and recurrence. The morphological variants include:

Infantile variants **(Fig. 21.6.18)**:
- Cradle cap (scalp)
- Lesions on the trunk (including flexures and napkin area)
- *Leiner's disease (nonfamilial and familial C5 dysfunction):* Erythroderma appearing during the 1st few weeks of life, failure to thrive, and diarrhea.

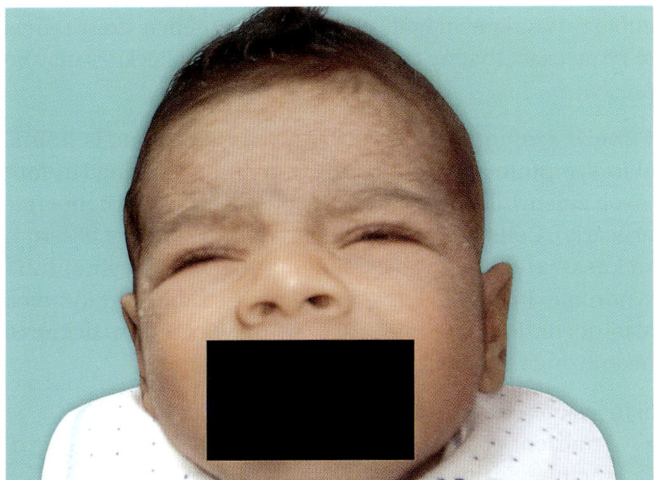

Fig. 21.6.18: Diffuse scaling over the scalp, forehead, and face of an infant—seborrheic dermatitis.

- Dandruff is the earliest manifestation on the scalp in chronic cases, there may be some degree of hair loss.
- Crusted fissure behind the ear in the fold, otitis externa, and blepharitis may occur alone.
- Medial aspect of the eyebrows, glabella, and nasolabial folds are common sites in the face.
- In the flexures, it can manifest as intertrigo. Genitalia may be involved with minimal erythema and scaling to severe crusted dermatitis which may later become psoriasiform.

Investigations/Dermatopathology: The histopathology shows features of both psoriasis and chronic dermatitis.

Treatment: Topical therapy:
- Removal of crusts with 2–3 and salicylic acid in olive oil
- Selenium sulfide/zinc pyrithione/tar/ketoconazole containing shampoos
- Topical vioform-hydrocortisone lotion or betamethasone lotion can be carefully used for severe cases.

Face: This is a difficult therapeutic problem.
- Hydrocortisone acetate cream, 1% or 2.5% bid with or without vioform, is useful.
- Tacrolimus 0.03–0.1% and pimecrolimus 1% are effective.

Napkin Dermatitis

Definition/Description: It is an inflammatory disorder affecting the napkin or diaper area of infants.

Epidemiology/Etiology: There is individual variation to proneness of developing napkin dermatitis, but all children grow out of it when they stop wearing nappies. Factors associated with the etiology include:
- Irritant contact dermatitis due to urine and feces
- Infection with bacteria and *Candida* yeasts
- *Other skin disorders:* Psoriasis, seborrhea, and atopic dermatitis

Clinical evaluation: The disease is characterized by the development of erythema followed by vesicles that rupture to ooze serous discharge over the convexities. The classical "tide mark dermatitis" refers to the erythematous border sparing the depths of the flexures **(Fig. 21.6.19)**. Rarely violaceous nodules may be a presentation—the infantile gluteal granuloma—suggesting candidal reaction.

Treatment: Topical antibiotics, antifungals, and mild steroids, alone or in combination are found to be useful. Avoid wet or dirty nappy.
- Wash and moisturize dry skin at every nappy change. Dimethicone (silicone) barrier creams can also help.
- Apply prescription creams according to directions. Strong steroid creams should be avoided.

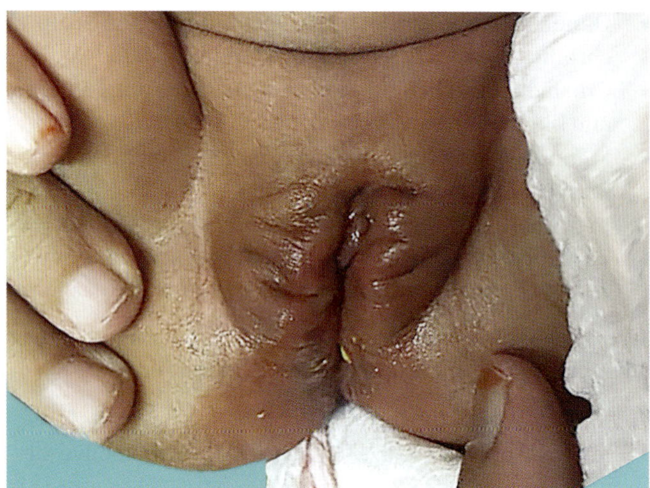

Fig. 21.6.19: Erythema over the convexities and classically sparing the depth of the intertriginous areas—a case of Napkin's dermatitis.

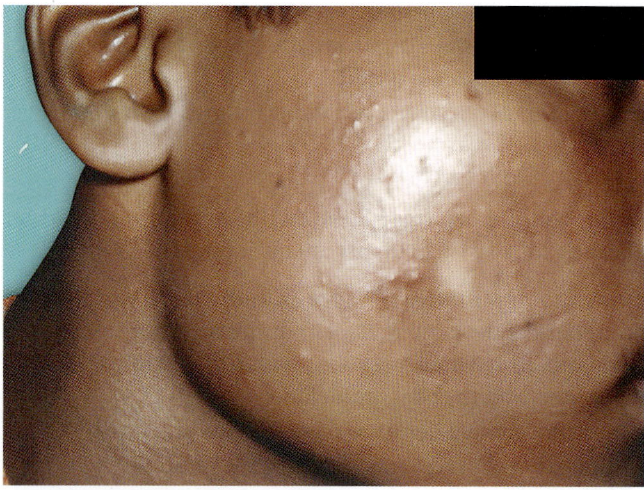

Fig. 21.6.20: Early acne vulgaris with comedones and papules.

Acne Vulgaris

Definition/Description: It is a common chronic inflammation of the pilosebaceous units often followed by scars.[4]

Epidemiology/Etiology: Acne starts at the age of 10–17 years in females and 14–19 years in males and is more severe in males. Multifactorial including genetic, drugs (lithium, hydantoin, and corticosteroids), endocrine (androgens), and emotional stress. Acne is exacerbated by iodine-containing products.[5]

Clinical evaluation: Skin lesions include comedones **(Fig. 21.6.20)**, papules, pustules, nodules, and scars. Seborrhea of the face and scalp is often present. The sites of predilection include the face, upper arms, and trunk.

Treatment: For mild acne—

- Benzoyl peroxide gels (2–5%)
- *Topical retinoids:* Start with tretinoin 0.01% gel and increase after 1 month to 0.025%, applied nightly after washing with a mild soap.

For moderate to severe acne: In adolescents and children above 9 years, topical clascoterone 1% cream, a novel androgen receptor inhibitor is found to be safe and effective.

For severe forms:

- Oral tetracyclines added to the above—minocycline, 50–100 mg bid, tapered to 50 mg/day.
- In females, severe acne can be controlled with careful use of oral estrogens combined with progesterone.

Oral 13-cis-retinoic acid is highly effective for cystic acne and should be used with precaution at 0.5–1 mg/kg/day dose with meals for a 15–20 week course. Careful monitoring is necessary especially in patients with elevated serum triglycerides before therapy is begun.

Urticaria and Angioedema

Definition/Description: Urticaria is characterized by itchy transient weals, and in angioedema, there is involvement of subcutaneous tissue. Urticaria and/or angioedema may be acute or chronic recurrent. In hereditary angioedema, urticarial weals are rarely present.

Epidemiology/Etiology: Angioedema and urticaria can be classified as IgE-mediated, hypocomplementemic, or related to physical stimuli (water, cold, sunlight, and pressure) or idiosyncratic. The syndrome, angioedema-urticaria-eosinophilia syndrome, is related to action of the eosinophil major basic protein. General types include acute urticaria (<6 weeks), often IgE-dependent with atopic background and chronic urticaria (>6 weeks), rarely IgE-dependent; the etiology is unknown in 80–90%; often emotional stress seems to be an exacerbating factor. Intolerance to salicylates may be present.

Clinical evaluation: The duration of the lesions is hours. Skin symptoms include pruritus, pain on walking (in foot involvement), flushing, burning, and wheezing (in cholinergic urticaria). Constitutional symptoms may be present in serum sickness and in the angioedema-urticaria-eosinophilia syndrome. In angioedema, hoarseness, stridor, and dyspnea also occur. Patients may have arthralgia (serum sickness, necrotizing vasculitis, and hepatitis).

Skin lesions consist of:

- Transient pruritic, popular, or weals of 1–8 cm. Weals of cholinergic urticaria measure 1–2 mm.
- *Angioedema:* Skin-colored enlargement of portion of the face (eyelids, lips, and tongue) or extremity **(Fig. 21.6.21)**.

Investigations/Dermatopathology: Diagnosis is mostly clinical. IgE levels and other investigations are done to find the cause.

Serologic tests:

- *Search for hepatitis-associated antigen:* Assessment of the complement system

Hematologic tests:

- Erythrocyte sedimentation rate is often elevated in persistent urticaria (necrotizing vasculitis)
- Hypocomplementemia (necrotizing vasculitis)
- Transient eosinophilia is observed in urticaria from reactions to foods and drugs.
- High levels of eosinophilia are present in the angioedema-urticaria-eosinophilia syndrome.
- Screening for functional C1 esterase inhibitor

Ultrasonography to rule out edema of the bowel.

Treatment: Elimination of etiologic factors is the mainstay.

- Antihistamines H1 blockers, e.g., hydroxyzine, cetirizine, levocetirizine; and if they fail, H1 and H2 blockers (e.g., doxepin).
- Prednisolone is indicated for angioedema-urticaria-eosinophilia syndrome.
- Danazol is indicated as long-term therapy for hereditary angioedema.
- Whole plasma or C1 esterase inhibitor may be used in the acute attack.
- Cyclosporine can be tried with caution in resistant cases of chronic spontaneous urticaria in children above 9 years of age.[6]

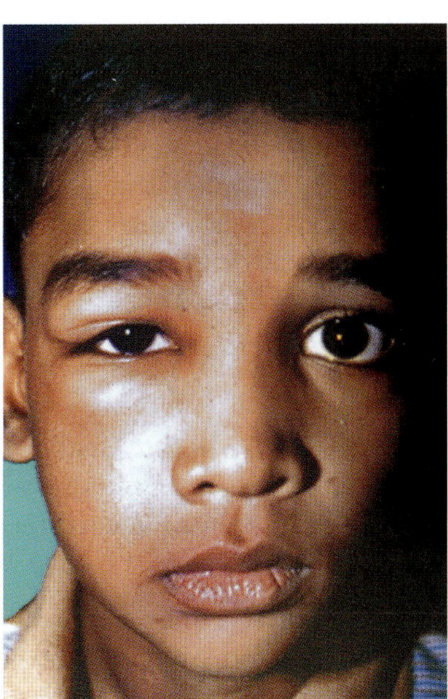

Fig. 21.6.21: A case of angioedema.

- Emergency treatment should start with injection of adrenaline subcutaneously.
- Hydrocortisone IV should follow but not before adrenaline.

Erythema Multiforme

Definition/Description: Erythema multiforme is a reaction of the skin to different causes including viral infections.

Epidemiology/Etiology: Common causes—

- *Drugs:* Sulfonamides, phenytoin, barbiturates, phenylbutazone, and penicillin
- *Infection:* Especially following herpes simplex, mycoplasma
- *Idiopathic:* In >50% of cases, no cause can be detected.

Clinical evaluation: The duration of lesions is several days; lesions develop over 10 days or more. Patients may have a history of prior episode of erythema multiforme. Skin lesions may be pruritic or painful. Mouth lesions are painful and tender and follow constitutional symptoms.

Skin lesions consist of:

- Macules
- Vesicles and bullae (in the center of papule forming the so-called iris or target lesions)
- Lesions may be localized to the hands or generalized **(Fig. 21.6.22)**. They are often symmetrical. The sites of predilection include the dorsa of hands, palms, soles, forearms, feet, elbows, and knees; the penis (50%) and vulva may be also involved.

Mucous membranes: Lesions may occur in the mouth and on the lips (99%) **(Fig. 21.6.23)**.

Other organs: Pulmonary manifestations may be present; the eyes may be affected with corneal ulcers and anterior uveitis.

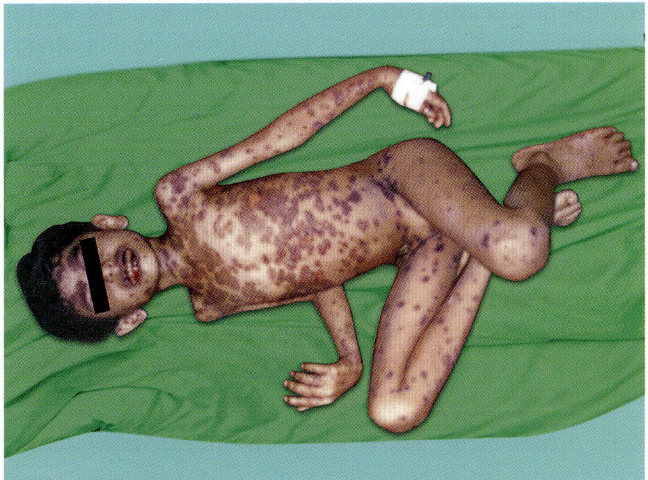

Fig. 21.6.22: Acutely ill child with erythema multiforme.

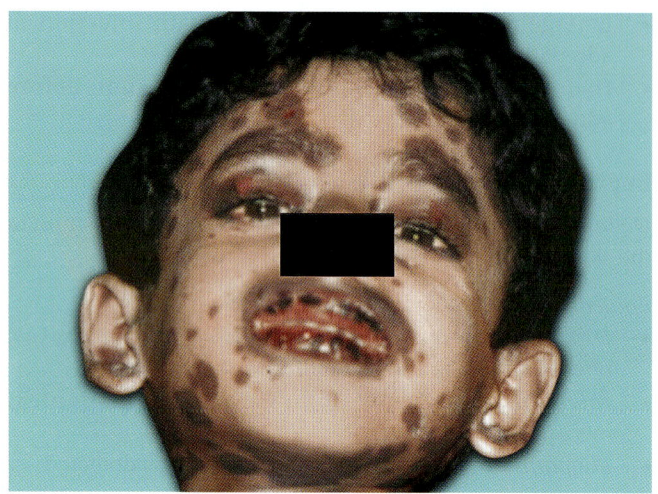

Fig. 21.6.23: Involvement of oral and conjunctival mucosae in erythema multiforme.

Investigations/Dermatopathology: Histology shows eosinophilic keratinocyte necrosis, upper dermal edema, perivascular infiltrate, and subepidermal bulla in some. All attempts must be made to rule out occult infections.

Treatment: In severely ill patients, systemic corticosteroids like prednisolone 50–80 mg daily in divided doses which is quickly tapered, but their effectiveness has not been established by controlled studies. Control of herpes simplex using oral acyclovir may prevent development of recurrent erythema multiforme. Involvement of oral mucosa in a sick dehydrated child warrants inpatient care and meticulous follow-up.[7]

Toxic Epidermal Necrolysis

Synonym: Lyell's syndrome.

Definition/Description: Toxic epidermal necrolysis (TEN) is a life-threatening cutaneous drug-induced or idiopathic reaction pattern characterized by tenderness and erythema of skin and mucosa, followed by extensive exfoliation with multisystem involvement.

Epidemiology/Etiology: Rare in children. Often follows drug intake.

Clinical evaluation: TEN occurs within days of ingestion of the offending drug. Prodrome is associated with mild-to-moderate skin tenderness. Patients are mentally alert but are in distress due to severe pain. Acute renal failure and erosions in lower respiratory tract and gut may complicate the condition.

Skin involvement: Starts as morbilliform or erythema multiforme—such as rash, tender erythema, and small vesicles/bullae becoming irregularly confluent. The necrotic epidermis shears off in large sheets. Epidermal sloughing may result in large and denuded areas resembling a second-degree thermal burn. Denudation is most pronounced over pressure points. Scalp, palms, and soles may be less severely involved or spared, but nails may be shed. Nikolsky's sign is usually positive **(Figs. 21.6.24 and 21.6.25)**.

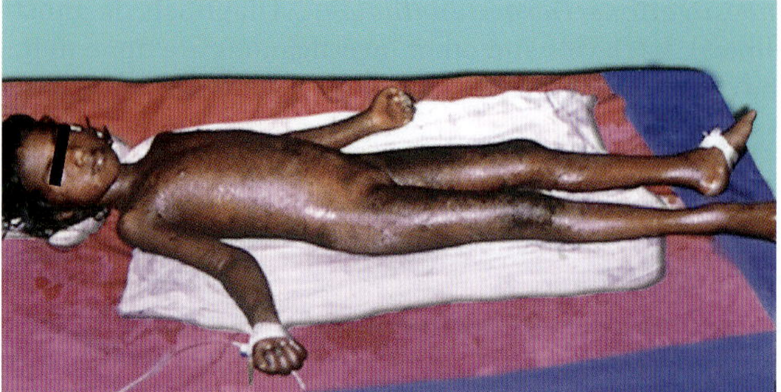

Fig. 21.6.24: Toxic epidermal necrolysis—note positive Nikolsky's sign.

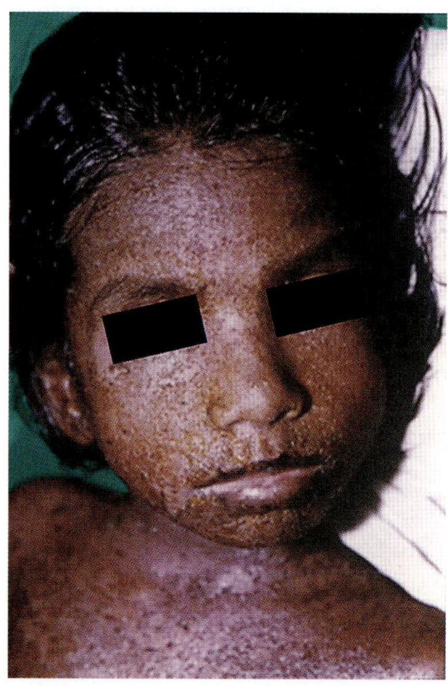

Fig. 21.6.25: The child seen in Figure 21.6.24 with peeling of skin over face and neck.

Mucosal involvement: Oral, ocular, and anogenital mucosae may be severely affected and slough off.

Investigations/Dermatopathology: Histology shows widespread epidermal necrosis, apoptotic keratinocytes, subepidermal split with little or no inflammatory infiltrate.

Treatment:

- Admitted and treated as a thermal burn patient. Silver sulfadiazine to be used with caution for fear of absorption and resultant neutropenia. There is general agreement that corticosteroids should not be used in TEN involving

>20% body surface area (BSA), but it is still unproven whether they will arrest the progression of TEN if given in the first 24–48 hours.

- *Intravenous replacement:* Water, electrolytes, albumin, and plasma.
- *Debridement:* Remove only frankly necrotic tissue.
- Watch for signs of sepsis (fever, hypotension, and change in mental status)
- Eyecare
- Frequent suctioning is needed in oropharyngeal involvement to prevent aspiration pneumonitis.
- Avoid re-exposure to offending drug.

PAPULOSQUAMOUS DISORDERS

Acrodermatitis Enteropathica

Definition/Description: It is a genetic disorder of zinc absorption, presenting in infancy.

Epidemiology/Etiology: In infants bottle-fed with bovine milk, it occurs days to few weeks and in breastfed infants, soon after weaning, and acquired zinc deficiency in older children.

Etiology:

- *Genetic:* Autosomal recessive trait resulting in failure to absorb zinc.
- *Acquired zinc deficiency:* Secondary to reduced dietary intake of zinc, malabsorption, increased urinary loss, and prolonged parenteral nutrition without supplemental zinc.

Clinical evaluation: Characterized by a triad of acral dermatitis (face, hands, feet, and anogenital), alopecia, and diarrhea. Involves skin, mucous membrane, and hair. The skin lesions often become secondarily infected with *Candida albicans* and *S. aureus*. The skin is initially pink, and later, brightly erythematous involving perioral and anogenital area. Scalp, hands and feet, flexural regions, and trunk are also involved. There is impaired wound healing. Children are irritable with depressed mood and have growth failure **(Figs. 21.6.26 and 21.6.27)**.

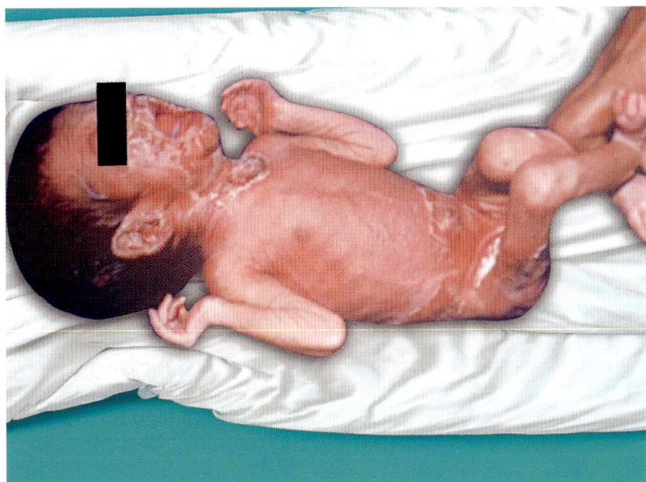

Fig. 21.6.26: Acrodermatitis enteropathica. Note acral lesions and scanty hair.

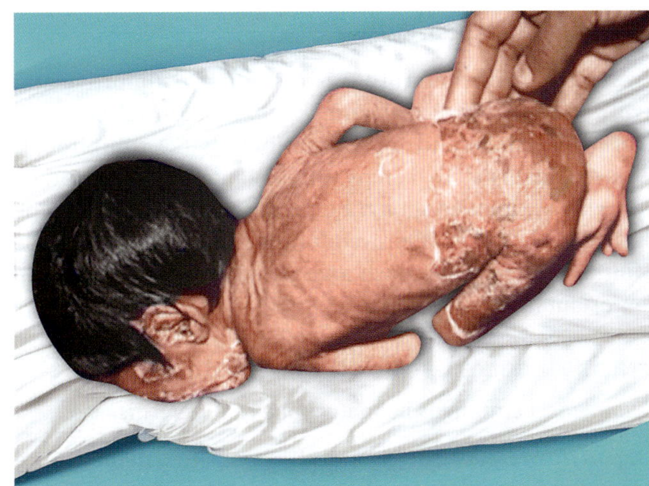

Fig. 21.6.27: Posterior aspect of child is seen in the figure.

Investigations/Dermatopathology:

- *Complete blood count:* Reveals anemia.
- *Biochemistry:* Serum/plasma zinc levels are low.
- *Urine:* Urinary zinc excretion is reduced.
- *Dermatopathology:* Intraepidermal clefts and blisters are observed with acantholysis.

Treatment: Dietary or IV supplementation with zinc salts two to three times, the recommended daily allowances restore normal zinc status in days to weeks. Oral 10 mg/kg of elemental zinc is as effective as parenteral administration and needs to be continued for at least 6 months.

BULLOUS DISORDERS

Epidermolysis Bullosa

Synonym: Mechanobullous disorder

Definition/Description: Epidermolysis bullosa (EB) are a group of dermatoses characterized by easy bullae formation on mild mechanical pressure, leading to erosion, bleeding, infection, and scarring.

Epidemiology/Etiology: EB is genetic and present at birth. Most babies have impaired quality of life due to the psychological effects of easy blistering and scarring.

Clinical evaluation: Several clinical types and subtypes have been described, the major being epidermal, junctional, and dystrophic. **Figure 21.6.28** shows an infant with blistering

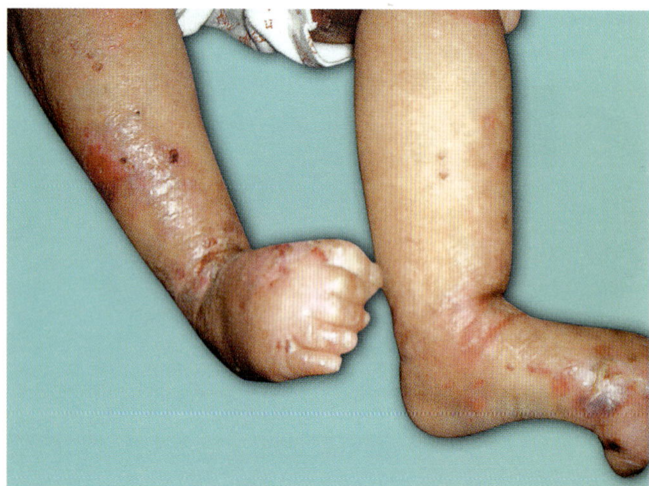

Fig. 21.6.28: Epidermolysis bullosa in an infant. Note the blistering and scarring over the lower limbs.

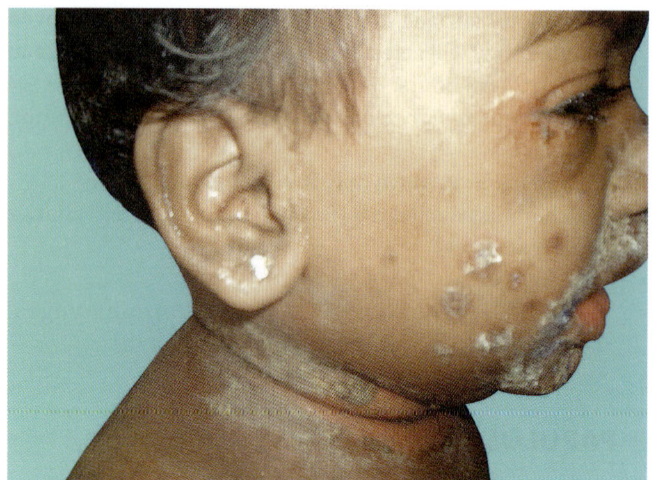

Fig. 21.6.29: Staphylococcal-scalded skin syndrome (SSSS)—exfoliation and erythema over face and neck.

and scarring over the lower limbs. Genetic testing will help in confirming the type of disease.[8]

Treatment: Treatment of EB is essentially supportive and avoidance of physical trauma and nutritional support. Sterile dressings and topical antibiotics (2% mupirocin) form the mainstay of therapy. In resistant cases, appropriate systemic antibiotics should be prescribed. Birch triterpene topical gel has been approved for the treatment of wounds.[9] Multidisciplinary approach and genetic counseling play an important role.

Staphylococcal-scalded Skin Syndrome

Synonyms: Pemphigus neonatorum and Ritter's disease.

Definition/Description: SSSS is a toxin-mediated epidermolytic disease characterized by erythema and widespread detachment of the superficial layers of the epidermis, resembling the effects of scalding. It occurs mainly in newborns and infants under 2 years of age. Severity ranges from a localized form, bullous impetigo, to a generalized form with extensive epidermolysis and desquamation.[1]

Epidemiology/Etiology:

Age: SSSS occurs mainly in infants and young children. Adults with immunosuppression or renal insufficiency are predisposed to SSSS.

Etiology: S. aureus of phase Group II, mostly Type 71.

Clinical evaluation:

- A low-grade fever may be present. The child is irritable, with very tender, ill-defined erythema of the skin, on the face (periorificially), neck, axillae, and groins, becoming more widespread in 24–48 hours followed by sloughing of the epidermis.
- *Scarlatiniform syndrome:* Presentation is like scarlet fever but without pharyngitis, tonsillitis, and strawberry tongue. Nikolsky's sign (gentle lateral pressure causes shearing off superficial epidermis) is positive **(Fig. 21.6.29)**.
- *Mucous membranes:* Usually uninvolved.

Investigations/Dermatopathology: Gram's stain and Culture—*S. aureus* is only present in colonized sites of infection, i.e., umbilical stump, conjunctiva, or external ear canal; culture of sloughing skin or bullae usually yields no pathogens.

Treatment: For a newborn, hospitalization and treatment with IV cloxacillin, 200 mg/kg bodyweight/day in divided every 4 hours, are preferable. Topical care includes baths or compresses, and mupirocin or bacitracin, or silver sulfadiazine/ointment. Surgical intervention of the wound and debridement in children with SSSS is better discouraged.[10]

CONCLUSION

This chapter is not all-encompassing. The reader is requested to refer to the title 'Clinical Pediatric Dermatology' by the same authors.

REFERENCES

1. Gowrishankar NC, Lakshmi S, Ravikumar T, Vijaykumar M (Eds). Management Update for Common Pediatric Problems, 1st edition. New Delhi: Jaypee Brothers Medical Publishers (P) Ltd.; 2004.
2. Parthasarathy A (Ed). Partha's Fundamentals of Pediatrics, 1st edition. New Delhi: Jaypee Brothers Medical Publishers (P) Ltd.; 2007.
3. Thomas J. Atopic dermatitis. In: Thomas J (Ed). Pediatric Dermatology Ward Rounds, 1st edition. New Delhi: Jaypee Brothers Medical Publishers (P) Ltd.; 2007. pp. 17-9.
4. Bhave SY (Ed). Adolescent Health: Case Scenarios, 1st edition. New Delhi: Byword Books Private Limited; 2011.

5. Bhave SY (Ed). Bhave's Textbook of Adolescent Medicine, 1st edition. New Delhi: Jaypee Brothers Medical Publishers (P) Ltd.; 2006.
6. Chang J, Cattelan L, Ben-Shoshan M, Le M, Netchiporouk E. Management of Pediatric Chronic Spontaneous Urticaria: A Review of Current Evidence and Guidelines. J Asthma Allergy. 2021;14:187-99.
7. Goldman RD. Erythema multiforme in children. Can Fam Physician. 2022;68(7):507-8.
8. Hon KL, Chu S, Leung AKC. Epidermolysis Bullosa: Pediatric Perspectives. Curr Pediatr Rev. 2022;18(3):182-90.
9. Pradilla MT, Álvarez E, Novoa M, Lozano I, Trujillo M. Oleogel-S10 in Dystrophic Epidermolysis Bullosa: A Case Series Evaluating the Impact on Wound Burden Over Two Years. Adv Ther. 2024;41(2):867-77.
10. Liy-Wong C, Pope E, Weinstein M, Lara-Corrales I. Staphylococcal scalded skin syndrome: An epidemiological and clinical review of 84 cases. Pediatr Dermatol. 2021;38(1):149-53.

21.7 Understanding Common Oral Health Problems

Akila Ganesh

INTRODUCTION

Knowledge about the human dentition and common oral problems to a pediatrician can pave the way for early diagnosis of common neglected oral diseases. The dentition of a human being is in various stages of development from as early as 14 weeks in utero up to 18–25 years of age. The first tooth to erupt in the oral cavity is the primary lower incisor tooth, with the first evidence of calcification beginning at 14 weeks in utero. The last tooth to erupt in the oral cavity is the permanent third molar which usually erupts between 18 and 25 years of age. During these developmental stages, the gingiva may show physiological signs of pre-eruption, like inflammation.[1]

TYPES OF DENTITIONS

The human dentition comprises of two sets of dentitions. The primary dentition is the first set of teeth to erupt in the mouth. It begins to form prenatally as early as 14 weeks in utero to final root completion at around 3 years of age. The eruption of the primary dentition is between 6 and 8 months of age to about 30–36 months of age. This is followed by the permanent dentition, whose first evidence of calcification begins at birth and the root completion of the third molars ends between 18 and 25 years of age. The eruption phases for the various teeth ranges from 6 to 7 years up to 21 years of age **(Tables 21.7.1 and 21.7.2)**. Between these phases is the mixed dentition period in which there is a mixture of primary and permanent teeth. This period is difficult for the child to handle because of habits, missing teeth, teeth of different color and hues, and crowding of teeth and malposed teeth. A recent meta-analysis reported that primary tooth eruption was earlier in the left quadrant than the right but the role of gender was insignificant while permanent tooth eruption was reported to be earlier in females and in the mandible.[2,3]

TABLE 21.7.1: Chronology of primary teeth.

Tooth	First evidence of calcification (weeks in utero)	Crown completed (months)	Mean age of eruption (months)	Root completed (years)
Maxillary teeth				
Central incisor	14	1½	10	1½
Lateral incisor	16	2½	11	2
Canine	17	9	19	3¼
First molar	15	6	16	2½
Second molar	19	11	29	3
Mandibular teeth				
Central incisor	14	2½	8	1½
Lateral incisor	16	3	13	1½
Canine	17	9	20	3¼
First molar	15½	5½	16	2½
Second molar	18	10	27	3

TYPES OF TEETH

The primary and permanent dentitions have distinct morphological characteristics, which identify them as incisors, canines, and molars. The primary dentition comprises a total of 20 teeth, including two central incisors, two lateral incisors, two canines and four molars in each jaw **(Fig. 21.7.1)**.

TABLE 21.7.2: Chronology of permanent teeth.

Tooth	*First evidence of calcification*	*Crown completed (years)*	*Emergence (eruption) (years)*	*Root completed (years)*
Maxillary teeth				
Central incisor	3–4 months	4–5	7–8	10
Lateral incisor	10–12 months	4 5	8–9	11
Canine	4–5 months	6–7	11–12	13–15
First premolar	1½–1¾ years	5–6	10–11	12–13
Second premolar	2–2½ years	6–7	10–12	12–14
First molar	At birth	2½–3	6–7	9–10
Second molar	2 ½–3 years	7–8	12–13	14–16
Third molar	7–9 years	12–16	17–21	18–25
Mandibular teeth				
Central incisor	3–4 months	4–5	6–7	9
Lateral incisor	3–4 months	4–5	7–8	10
Canine	4–5 months	6–7	9–10	12–14
First premolar	1¼–2 years	5–6	10–12	12–13
Second premolar	2¼–2½ years	6–7	11–12	13–14
First molar	At birth	2½–3	6–7	9–10
Second molar	2 ½–3 years	7–8	11–13	14–15
Third molar	8–10 years	12–16	17–21	18–25

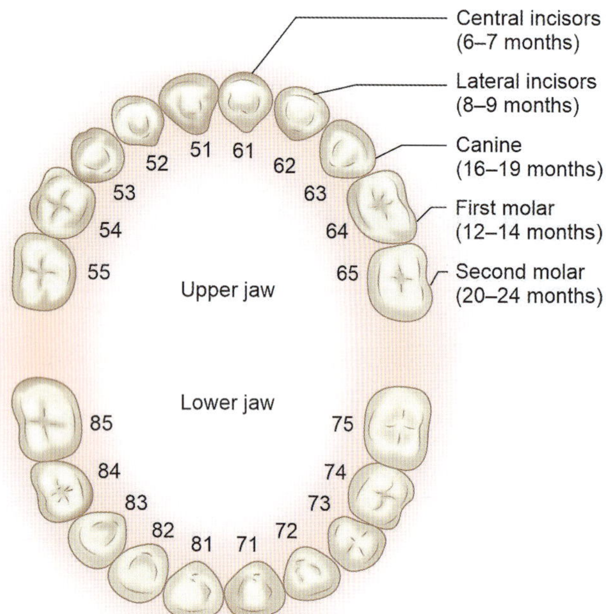

Fig. 21.7.1: Eruption sequence—primary dentition.

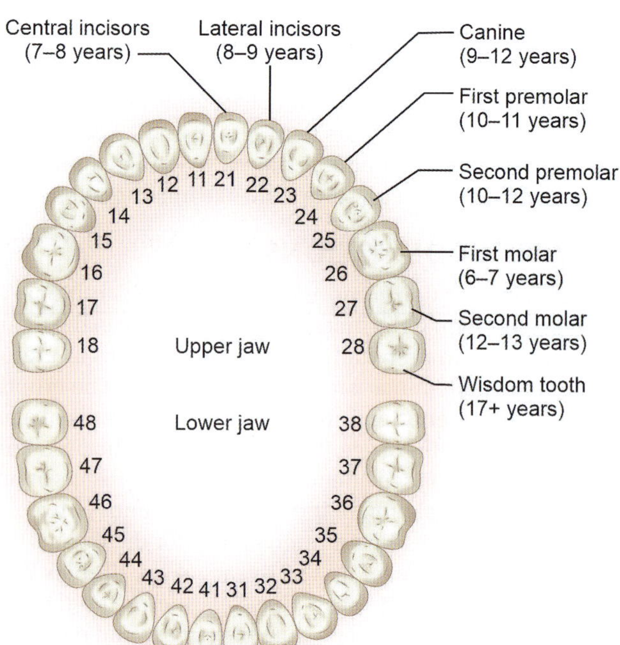

Fig. 21.7.2: Eruption sequence—permanent dentition.

The permanent dentition comprises a total of 32 teeth, including two central incisors, two lateral incisors, two canines, four premolars, and six molars in each jaw **(Fig. 21.7.2)**.

FUNCTIONS OF PRIMARY DENTITION

The primary dentition needs special till its care and should be preserved anticipated exfoliation. The main functions are:

- Mastication
- Esthetics
- Speech
- Psychology of having teeth
- Stimulation of growth of the jaw through mastication
- Prevention of malocclusion through maintaining arch length. Premature loss of primary molar leads to more severe malocclusion.
- Guides occlusion.

DENTAL PROBLEMS

The most common dental diseases are dental caries and periodontal diseases. However, the most common dental disease among children is dental caries, commonly termed "early childhood caries (ECC)".

Early Childhood Caries

Dental caries is a multifactorial infectious disease characterized by demineralization of the inorganic and destruction of the organic substances of the tooth. ECC is dental caries occurring in children below 6 years of age. Earlier there were various terminologies for ECC, including "baby bottle tooth decay", "nursing caries", "night bottle mouth", etc. ECC remains a serious public health challenge globally, especially in the developing countries, with high prevalence among infants, toddlers, and preschoolers around the world, as stated by the American Dental Association (ADA). ECC is one of the commonly neglected diseases among children in India and hence is the most common reason for early loss of primary teeth.

The most commonly affected teeth are the maxillary incisors, from where it can spread rapidly to multiple teeth in a very short span of time **(Figs. 21.7.3.A and B)**. The most common signs and symptoms of ECC include pain, sensitivity associated with thermal changes, difficulty in brushing and chewing, holding the food in the mouth for a long time, teeth abscesses along with fever and even common cold or cough.[4]

The consequences of untreated ECC include prolonged poor food intake, leading to poor general health, caries affecting the newly erupted permanent teeth, loss of school days, poor esthetics, and self-esteem. A healthy permanent dentition, a healthy diet and esthetics depend on the primary dentition; hence the importance of its loss cannot be underestimated.

Prevalence

Ther ECC affects infants and toddlers worldwide. Its prevalence varies from population to population. A recent systematic review has reported an average global prevalence of ECC as 48%,[5] and an Indian prevalence of 49.6%.[6] The greatest prevalence and severity have been reported in Far East Asia, where the prevalence in 3-year-olds ranges from 36 to 85%. An ECC prevalence of 44% has been reported in India among 8- to 48-month-olds. Several studies have reported the skewed distribution of socioeconomic status with ECC. It has been reported that 68.8% of the Indian population live in rural areas. In most cases, detection of the disease is the most crucial factor for control of the oral condition by preventive and therapeutic regimes.

Risk Factors

The epidemiological triad of ECC constitutes of a susceptible tooth (host), cariogenic microorganisms (agent) and fermentable carbohydrates, predominantly free sugars (environment) over a period of time.

There are a few unique risk factors present in young children, which poses them at more risk to caries. These include:

- Oral microbial flora and host defense mechanisms are in the developing stage.
- Newly erupted tooth surfaces have hypoplastic defects which are more susceptible to caries.
- They undergo a transition of feeding practices from liquids to solids and from breastfeeding, bottle-feeding to other possible modes of feeding.

Several studies have evaluated and categorized the risk factors of ECC, such as sociodemographic factors, dietary factors, oral hygiene factors, and factors related to oral bacterial flora and breast-feeding/bottle-feeding. However, the degree to which different risk factors are associated with ECC remains unclear.[7]

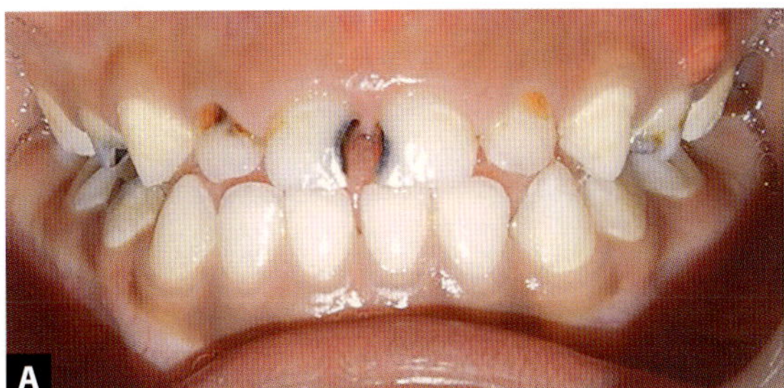

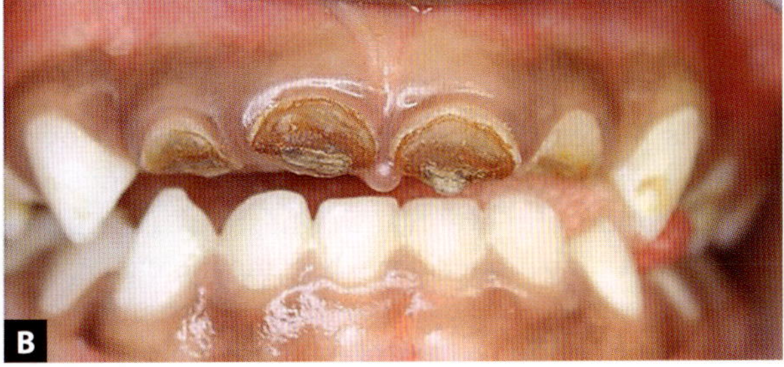

Figs. 21.7.3A and B: Early childhood caries.

A recent systematic review and an umbrella review reported that the most influential risk factor associated with ECC was the presence of enamel defects as a result of improper feeding habits, followed by dentinal caries and high levels of mutans streptococci, increased consumption of soda, daily intake of sugary snacks, and obesity.[8] However, the accumulation of milk or other liquids or food substances on tooth surfaces throughout sleep time might be a substantial causative factor in the occurrence of ECC.

Sleep Time Feeding Practices and ECC

The mode (bottle, sipper, etc.), frequency, duration, and time (daytime, night-time, both) of each feed, and content (in case of bottle and other modes—type of milk, sweetener, or additive) have been reported as risk factors for ECC. During sleep, there is a diminished flow of saliva and lack of tongue movements. Moreover, prolonged contact time of milk on tooth surface during sleep can facilitate continuous, prolonged acid production leading to demineralization, without in-between phases of remineralization, resulting in ECC. In the presence of continuous acid production, the porous enamel of hypoplastic teeth could potentially dissolve rapidly leading to breakdown and ECC. In addition, the child sleeps with the nipple or bottle in the mouth during night-time, early morning hours, and daytime naps.[9]

Role of Medication

One of the important factors that deserves special mention is sugar-containing liquid oral medicines. Some of these pharmaceutical preparations have been reported to have mean sugar content of 55% to make them more palatable and mask the unpleasant taste of drugs, especially for children. Sucrose also acts as a preservative, solvent, and a bulking agent. Further diminution of salivation and mastication during night increases the cariogenic potential of medicines. Some sedatives, anticonvulsants and antihistaminics also lower the salivary flow, which further enhances the cariogenic process. Today, the most widely used caloric sweeteners are xylitol and sorbitol, replacing sucrose in tablets, chewing gums, and pharmaceutical preparations. Xylitol has gained special attention, because it cannot be metabolized by oral microflora and practically no acid is formed.

Feeding Practices

A critical role is played by feeding practices adopted by parents in the development of children's taste preferences, eating habits, nutrition, and eventual weight status. Parents, teachers, and health practitioners have become increasingly concerned about a range of negative outcomes surrounding the eating habits of children. The transition from infancy to toddlerhood has been identified as a critical period for establishing dietary patterns, eating habits, and food preferences. A complete understanding of parental feeding practices is critically important to determining individual differences in eating habits.

Diagnosis

A sharp probe can be used to examine the tooth under good illumination to detect the presence of dental caries. There may not be any pain even when dental caries has involved enamel. The enamel caries can be there for several months but when the caries extents into the dentine, it spreads very fast and reaches the pulp, which becomes very painful. Hence, periodical dental check up with proper illumination with a sharp explorer and mouth mirror will help to detect dental caries, which can be filled with metal or any other restorative resins.

It must also be understood that the enamel is incapable of regeneration. Hence, there is a need for a foreign material to repair the decayed enamel. However, remineralization in the enamel has been found to be possible with topical fluorides and suitable diet rich in calcium and phosphorus **(Figs. 21.7.4A to D)**.

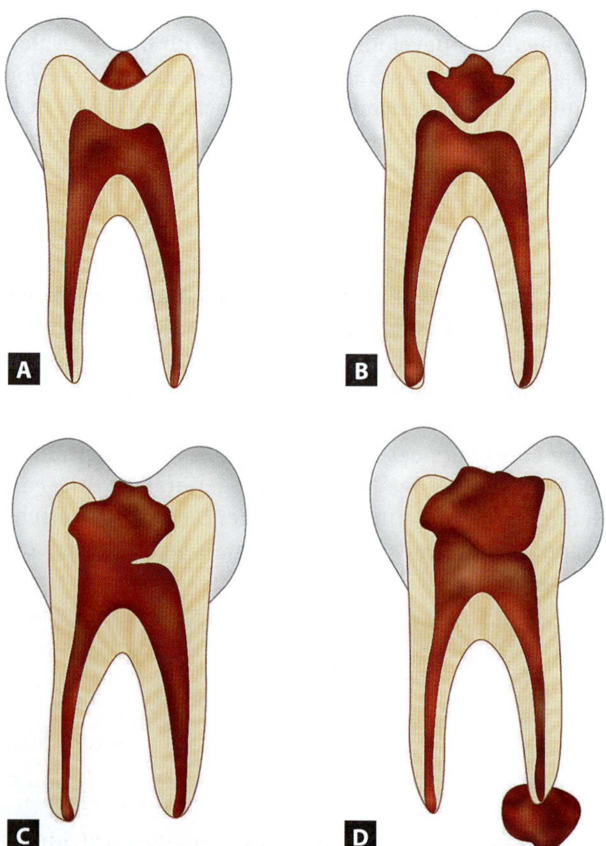

Figs. 21.7.4A to D: (A) Dental caries of enamel; (B) Dental caries of dentin; (C) Pulpitis; (D) Root abscess.

Management of Dental Caries

- Children under 3 years of age with multiple carious lesions may require full mouth rehabilitation under general anesthesia. Older children who are cooperative can be rehabilitated through multiple chairside appointments. These children may mostly require fillings, crowns, multiple root canal treatments, or extraction of teeth.
- *Restoration of the decayed tooth:* The first step is to prevent further progression of the lesion. Gross superficial excavation of the caries and filling the cavity with zinc oxide—eugenol will temporarily arrest the caries process and prevent its rapid progression to the deeper tissues. These cavities can be later filled by permanent filling material.
- *Atraumatic restorative technique (ART):* ART is a procedure based on removing carious tooth structure using hand instrument alone and restoring the cavity with an adhesive restorative material. At present, the restorative material of choice is glass ionomer cement.

Prevention of Dental Caries

- *Pit and fissure sealants:* This is a very important treatment procedure, which protects susceptible surfaces. With improved utilization of this underutilized preventive measure, significant economic and health benefit can be realized.
- *Topical fluorides:* Topical fluoride application can help to prevent caries.
- *Systemic fluorides-water fluoridation:* It is important to understand that fluoride incorporation is beneficial only at the time of calcification of the tooth. There is evidence pointing to considerable tooth decay inhibition when the community water supply having fluoride in the drinking water is approximately 1 ppm, marked inhibition of dental caries without producing significant mottling of the enamel is seen.
- *Reduced intake of fermentable carbohydrates:* Frequency of eating and eating between meals has a direct bearing on the incidence of dental caries, particularly in children. The incidence is more when there is more sugar intake.
- *Detergents diet:* Any food that sticks to the teeth favors caries activity. Hence, such foods should be avoided. Detergent diets play a useful role in the prevention of dental caries. It serves two functions—(1) the fibrous content helps in better blood circulation in the gingiva and (2) it removes all the food debris and plaque between teeth and gums and leaves the mouth clean. It has been observed that cheese and peanuts inhibit caries activity. Almonds and groundnuts are rich source of calcium and phosphorus. Among dry fruits, apricots, figs, and dates also provide rich source of calcium and phosphorus.
- *Sleep time feeding:* Feeding during sleep should be discouraged. During sleep, salivary flow is diminished, and swallowing reflex is absent. Hence, stagnation of milk is possible. The clearance of milk can be encouraged by intake of water.
- *Plaque control:* This can be achieved by tooth brushing, flossing, scaling, and antiseptic mouthwashes.

GINGIVAL DISEASES

Eruption Hematoma

Very rarely a bluish, purple elevated area of gingival tissue, commonly called "eruption hematoma" develops a few weeks before the eruption of a primary or a permanent tooth. The blood-filled "cyst" is most frequently seen in primary second molar to first permanent molar regions. This condition develops because of trauma, which usually subsides within a few days when tooth erupts through the tissue and the hematoma subsides.

Acute Herpetic Gingivostomatitis

Acute herpetic gingivostomatitis is an infection of the oral cavity caused by *Herpes simplex* virus (HSV). The condition usually occurs during and immediately after an episode of febrile disease such as pneumonia, influenza, or typhoid. It also tends to occur during periods of anxiety, strain or exhaustion, and during menstruation.

Clinical Features

This condition appears as a diffuse, erythematous, shiny involvement of the gingiva, and the adjacent oral mucosa with edema and gingival bleeding. In the initial stage, it is characterized by the presence of discrete spherical gray vesicles, which rupture after 24 hours and form painful small ulcers with a red, elevated halo-like margin and a depressed yellowish-gray white central portion. In infants, the disease is marked by irritability and refusal to take food. Cervical adenitis, fever as high as 101°F, and generalized malaise are common. Treatment is only supportive and symptomatic. Antibiotic therapy is of considerable aid in the prevention of secondary infection.

Acute Necrotizing Ulcerative Gingivitis

Acute necrotizing ulcerative gingivitis (ANUG) is an inflammatory destructive disease of the gingiva commonly known as Vincent infection. Spirochetal organism and fusiform bacilli termed *Borrelia* are always found in the disease.

Clinical Features

A well-defined punched-out, crater-like depressions at the crest of the interdental papillae is always seen. This gingival crater is covered by grayish, pseudomembranous slough, demarcated from the remainder of the gingival mucosa by a pronounced linear erythema. The other salient features are constant radiating, gnawing pain that is intensified by eating spicy or hot foods, metallic taste, pasty saliva, and hypersalivation.

Halitosis is always present much to the annoyance of the child and others. Local lymphadenopathy and a slight elevation in temperature are common. However, in severe cases, high fever, increased pulse rate, leukocytosis, loss of appetite, and general lassitude are also seen.

Management

- *Local treatment* for alleviation of the acute inflammation should be started immediately.
- *Systemic:* Appropriate supportive treatment to correct malnutrition and suitable antibiotics.

CANDIDIASIS

Candidiasis is a disease caused by infection with a yeast-like fungus, *Candida albicans*; although, other species may also be involved. This disease is said to be the most opportunistic infection in the world. Acute pseudomembranous candidiasis is one of the more common forms of the disease. It may occur at any age but is especially prone to occur in the debilitated or the chronically ill, or in infants. The oral lesions are characterized by the appearance of soft, white slightly elevated plaques which can be wiped away with a gauze leaving a normal appearing mucosa or an erythematous area.

Treatment

Application of specific antifungal agents such as nystatin or clotrimazole has been beneficial in the treatment. Suspensions of nystatin, held in contact with the oral lesion, have been successfully used in even chronic or severe cases of the disease. Painting the lesion with gentian violet is an older but effective treatment.

MALOCCLUSION

While dental caries has been regarded as the major dental disease throughout the world affecting the child, malocclusion is only next. Malocclusion may involve the teeth, bones, muscle, and nerves. The teeth are irregular, jaw relationship may be good and muscle and nerve function normal. Teeth may be regular in their alignment, but an abnormal jaw relationship may exist so that the teeth do not meet properly during function **(Figs. 21.7.5A and B)**.

Impact of Pediatric Oral Habits

Oral habits can manifest in variety of activities, which may or may not be a concern to the child or parents. They include digit sucking, mentalis habits, lip wetting, lip sucking, abnormal swallowing, tongue thrusting, posture habits, and self-mutilation. Assessment of such habits should be identified immediately to avoid long-term effect on the craniofacial complex and dentition.

Role of Pacifiers

Pacifiers can cause malocclusion of the anterior teeth and posterior cross bites, depending on the frequency, strength, and duration of the pacifier use. Anterior open bite is often seen with pacifier use.

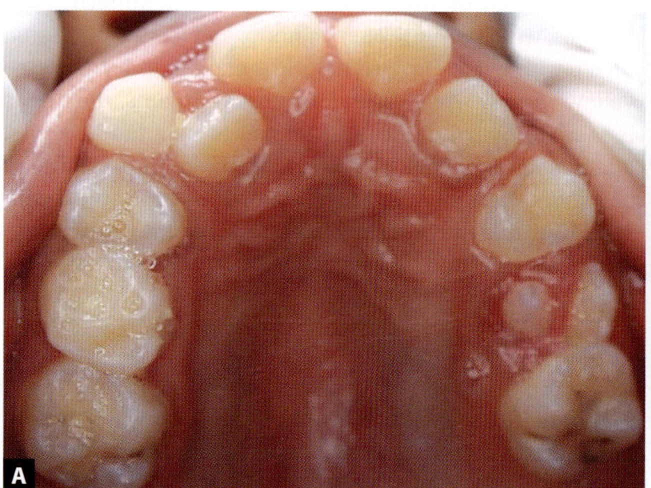

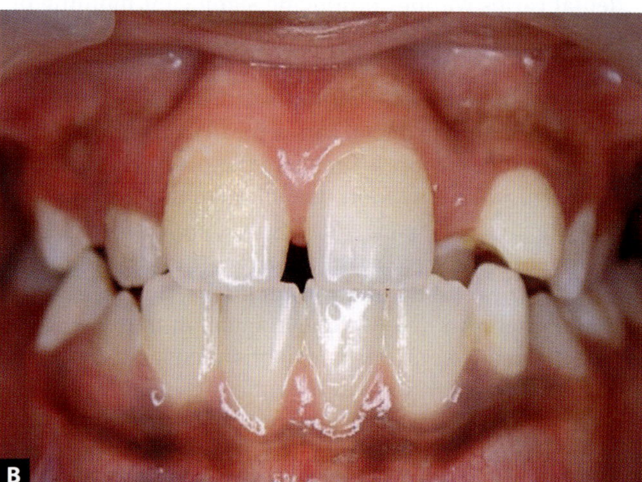

Figs. 21.7.5A and B: Malocclusion.

Epidemiology

The most prevalent type of malocclusion in the primary dentition is anterior open bite, secondary to pernicious habits. In the mixed dentitions, crowding is the most common type of malocclusion. There is no difference in the incidence of malocclusions according to sex. It is interesting to note that the primary dentition usually has good occlusal relationship, particularly in breastfed children. Malocclusion may develop later when the primary teeth are shed, and permanent teeth erupt.

Treatment

Treatment planning is based on a thorough case history, clinical examination, plaster study casts, radiographs, and facial photographs. Treatment should also include:

- Correction of abnormal pressure habits, if any
- Extraction of retained primary teeth
- Extraction of supernumerary teeth, depending on the merits of each patient.

The cause of malocclusion should be identified, and wherever possible, should be eradicated before starting the treatment. This is particularly more relevant when there is a pernicious habit existing. The treatment for malocclusion is usually simple when treatment is given in time. Most malocclusion responds well to removable appliances. However, fixed appliance gives more effective result for severe malocclusion.

RICKETS

Oral examination revealed open-bite, high arched palate, V-shaped maxillary arch, retardation of the teeth eruption, malpositioning of the teeth, gingival abscess, and severe enamel hypoplasia of both the maxillary and mandibular teeth. The disease is responsible for a defect in teeth mineralization, which causes a poorly mineralized and dysplastic dentin, with a noncalcified matrix which is called globular dentin. In these cases, there is also presence of tubular defects which can reach the dentin-enamel junction.

DENTAL EMERGENCIES

It is a dental problem that can happen at virtually any time. Kids playing sports, roughhousing with siblings, or falling while riding a bike are all scenarios in which a dental-related accident can happen. These accidents can result in teeth chipping, breaking, or cracking. In more severe circumstances, a permanent tooth may be knocked out completely.

If the child's permanent tooth does fall out, the dentist must be immediately approached and the tooth should be retrieved. The tooth must be placed in a glass of milk, saline solution, or clean water. The dentist may be able to place the permanent tooth back into the socket, allowing it to reattach with the help of a retainer.

CONCLUSION

Dental diseases affecting children may or may not be symptomatic. Further, certain physiological changes such as eruption of a tooth may be associated with inflammation. Pediatricians should equip themselves to differentiate the physiological changes from pathological lesions. Involving the parents in the prevention, treatment, and recurrence is particularly important in pediatric practice. Prevention of dental diseases should start from educating the pregnant mother.

The recommended age for the first dental visit as per international societies is 6–12 months or at the time of first tooth eruption. This allows the dentist to examine the child and educate his/her parents about effective preventive dental care, diet, injury prevention, fluoride needs, etc.[10] The pediatrician should be aware that teeth and jaws are in the formative stages. They should guide the parents not only in the prevention of dental diseases, but also in ensuring ideal and optimal growth of the dentition.

REFERENCES

1. Nelson SJ. Development and eruption of the teeth. Wheeler's Dental Anatomy, Physiology and Occlusion, 11th Edition. New Delhi: Elsevier Publications; 2020. pp. 20-39.
2. Vandana S, Muthu MS, Akila G, Anusha M, Kandaswamy D, Aswath Narayanan MB. Global variations in eruption chronology of permanent teeth: A systematic review and meta-analysis. Am J Hum Biol. 2024;36(8):e24060.
3. Muthu MS, Vandana S, Akila G, Anusha M, Kandaswamy D, Aswath Narayanan MB. Global variations in eruption chronology of primary teeth: A systematic review and meta-analysis. Arch Oral Biol. 2024;158:105857.
4. Anil S, Anand PS. Early childhood caries: Prevalence, risk factors, and prevention. Front Pediatr. 2017;5:157.
5. Uribe SE, Innes N, Maldupa I. The global prevalence of early childhood caries: A systematic review with meta-analysis using the WHO diagnostic criteria. Int J Paediatr Dent. 2021;31(6):817-30.
6. Ganesh A, Muthu MS, Mohan A, Kirubakaran R. Prevalence of early childhood caries in India - a systematic review. Indian J Pediatr. 2019;86(3):276-86.
7. Harris R, Nicoll AD, Adair PM, Pine CM. Risk factors for dental caries in young children: a systematic review of the literature. Community Dent Health. 2004;21(1 Suppl):71-85.
8. Thang Le VN, Kim JG, Yang YM, Lee DW. Risk Factors for Early Childhood Caries: An Umbrella Review. Pediatr Dent. 2021;43(3):176-94.
9. Ganesh A, Muthu MS, Padmanabhan R, Nuvvula S. Association of sleep time feeding Practices with Early Childhood Caries. Caries Res. 2022;56(4):399-406.
10. American Academy of Pediatric Dentistry. Policy on early childhood caries (ECC): Consequences and preventive strategies. The Reference Manual of Pediatric Dentistry. Chicago, Ill.: American Academy of Pediatric Dentistry; 2023. pp. 88-91.

21.8 Pediatric Radiology

Manisha Jana, Arun Kumar Gupta

INTRODUCTION

Over the last several decades, pediatric radiology has not only emerged in the forefront but also established itself as a definite subspecialty. A pediatric radiologist should not only have knowledge of general radiology, embryology, and basic pediatrics, but also be acutely aware of the indications and technicalities of various procedures and should be radiation conscious. Although a problem-oriented approach is ideal, in this chapter, an organ-oriented approach is used to present the essentials.[1,2]

IMAGING TECHNIQUES

Chest radiograph remains the most commonly performed investigation. Other conventional imaging techniques such as contrast studies of the gastrointestinal tract (GIT) and the lower urinary tract constitute a significant part of pediatric imaging. Ultrasound (USG) is another major relevant imaging modality. Additionally, with the advent of fast multidetector row computed tomography (CT) scanners, and faster sequences in magnetic resonance imaging (MRI), the diagnostic algorithm in several diseases has changed dramatically. The role of important imaging modalities is discussed under each organ system.[1,2]

CHEST

Imaging Techniques

Conventional radiographs are still the most frequently carried out procedures. Proper immobilization is essential. Radiograph is taken in supine anteroposterior (AP) position for children less than 3 years of age and in erect posteroanterior (PA) position for older children. CT is the next best cost-effective imaging technique for complete chest evaluation.[3] MRI and magnetic resonance angiography (MRA) are now increasingly used for assessing the relationship of mediastinal vessels to mediastinal masses or for primary vascular diseases such as aortoarteritis and coarctation. Rapid lung MRI is a promising tool in characterizing pulmonary pathologies in select situations. Sonography has been used for pleural diseases, for mediastinal or pulmonary lesions abutting the chest wall, and for cardiac and major vessel evaluation for a long time. Recent addition of lung USG has opened another dimension to the use of sonography in pediatric radiology, especially in critical care settings. It also bears the advantage of being a quick and easy technique, which can be carried out even at bedside.[1,2]

Normal Chest X-ray

Usually, only a frontal chest radiograph (AP or PA) is taken. If any abnormality is detected or in patients with a high index of suspicion, an appropriate lateral radiograph is also taken.

Interpretation[1,2]

Patient rotation and quality of exposure are first checked because improper patient position or exposure can be disastrous. Next, the image is read either from out-to-in or vice versa. Carefully examine in a sequence, always comparing with the opposite side for soft tissues, bones under review (ribs, clavicles, scapulae, humeri, etc.); aeration of each lung in the upper, mid and lower-thirds as well as medial-mid and outer-thirds; vascularity in each of these zones; tracheal position, diaphragm position and shape; costophrenic angles; mediastinal silhouette on each side; cardiac size and shape; retrocardiac space; position, size, and density of each hilum; and last but not the least, look under the diaphragms for free air and dilated loops.

Lateral radiograph is usually taken to localize a lesion already detected on the frontal films, for evaluation of the hilar nodes and for assessing the position of diaphragm. Its utility is limited, owing to the advent of other cross-sectional imaging modalities.

In a case with suspected free pleural effusion, a lateral decubitus view film is required with the affected side lower and closer to the film cassette.

- *Normal thymus:* An anterior mediastinal soft-tissue "mass" is a common finding on a conventional chest radiograph **(Figs. 21.8.1A and B)** in normal children up to the age of 3 years and is due to normal thymus. Several radiographic signs are helpful to identify it as normal thymus, e.g., *wave sign*, *sail sign*, a change in shape during respiration, and shrinking under the stress of steroid therapy (which reverts to the original size on stoppage of steroid).

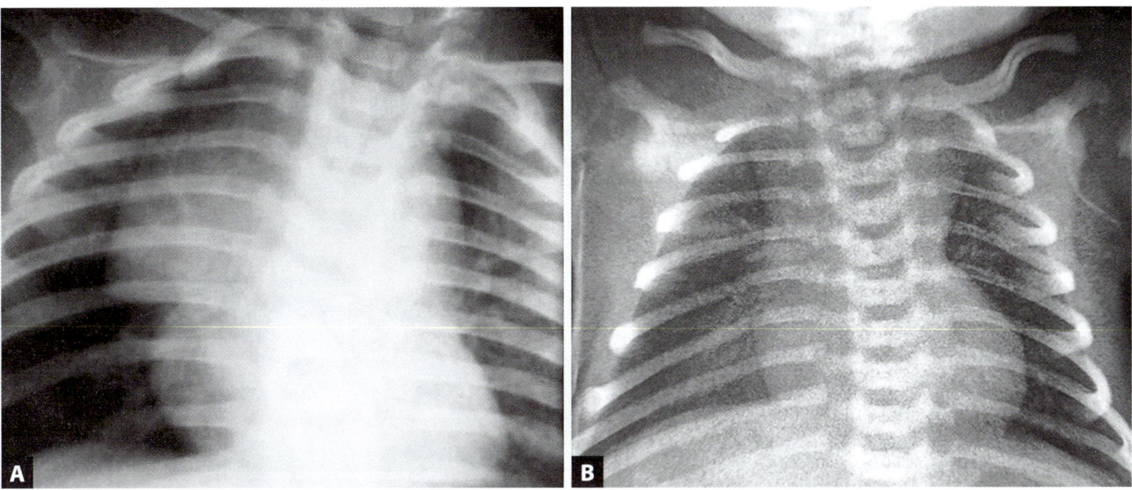

Figs. 21.8.1A and B: Normal thymus in two infants. Note a large right anterior "mediastinal mass" due to normal thymus (sail sign). Correlation with ultrasound and clinical information is mandatory before assigning a pathological label.

Pathological Conditions

Discussions on important neonatal chest conditions such as hyaline membrane disease (HMD), transient tachypnea of the newborn (TTN), and meconium aspiration are beyond the scope of this chapter.

Developmental Anomalies

- *Agenesis of a lung* is an extremely uncommon clinical entity. Completely opaque hemithorax on a frontal chest radiograph and absent pulmonary artery or main bronchus on the pulmonary angiogram or bronchogram, respectively, confirms the diagnosis **(Figs. 21.8.2A to C)**.
- *Congenital diaphragmatic hernia* is seen as air-filled bowel loops in the thoracic cavity, with contralateral mediastinal shift. Clinically, the baby presents with respiratory distress.

Foreign Body Inhalation

One of the most important, noninfective causes of acute respiratory distress in children is inhalation of foreign body, which could be either radiolucent (in about 90%) or radiopaque (in 10%)**(Figs. 21.8.3A and B)**. Radiographic findings depend upon several factors. Collapse, hyperlucent enlarged lobe (or lung) due to ball valve type of block or consolidation may be seen. In a suspected case of radiolucent foreign body inhalation and with equivocal chest radiographic findings, deep expiratory film may be very useful for the correct diagnosis.

Bacterial Pneumonia

Bacterial pneumonia is most commonly caused by *Streptococcus pneumonia, Haemophilus influenzae,* and *Staphylococcus aureus.*

- About 50% of staphylococcal pneumonia cases are complicated by *pneumatoceles* **(Fig. 21.8.4)**.
- Staphylococcal or pneumococcal pneumonia may produce a round-shaped pneumonia termed *round pneumonia*, which may mimic a hydatid cyst or metastatic lesion.
- Abscess **(Fig. 21.8.5)** is not an uncommon complication.
- *Empyema* is another important complication necessitating imaging and many times surgical intervention.

Viral Infection

Unlike bacterial infections, which result in airspace disease, viral infections tend to affect predominantly the airways. The resultant radiologic picture is bilateral hyperinflation with perihilar striations **(Fig. 21.8.6)**, the latter due to peribronchial thickening (cuffing). Radiograph may even appear normal. The pathologic-cum-clinical term used to describe this condition is bronchiolitis or "bronchitis". Thus, in a child presenting with acute respiratory distress but with very subtle radiologic changes, one should suspect this clinical entity.

Pulmonary Tuberculosis

Pulmonary tuberculosis is one of the most commonly seen chest conditions in India. A wide spectrum of radiologic findings is observed in these children:[4,5]

- *Extrapulmonary tuberculosis* can manifest as enlarged mediastinal and hilar nodes. Right paratracheal nodes are most commonly affected **(Figs. 21.8.7A and B)**. Other extrapulmonary sites include pleural or chest wall tuberculosis.
- Pulmonary tuberculosis can present as lobar or segmental consolidation, pneumonic consolidation with

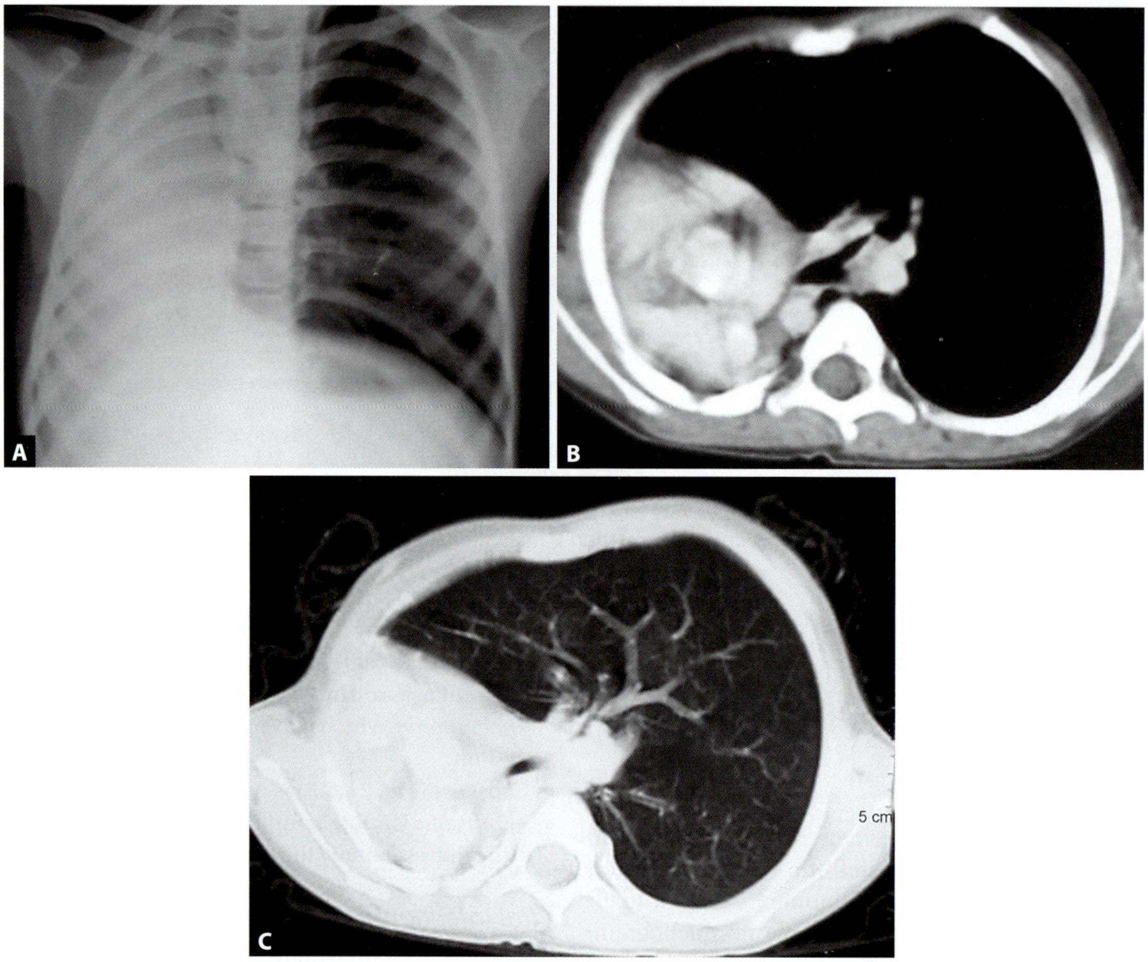

Figs. 21.8.2A to C: Right pulmonary agenesis. The radiographic features include complete opaque hemithorax (A) with ipsilateral mediastinal shift. CT mediastinal window shows no pulmonary artery and parenchyma (B); lung window image shows no right main bronchus (C).

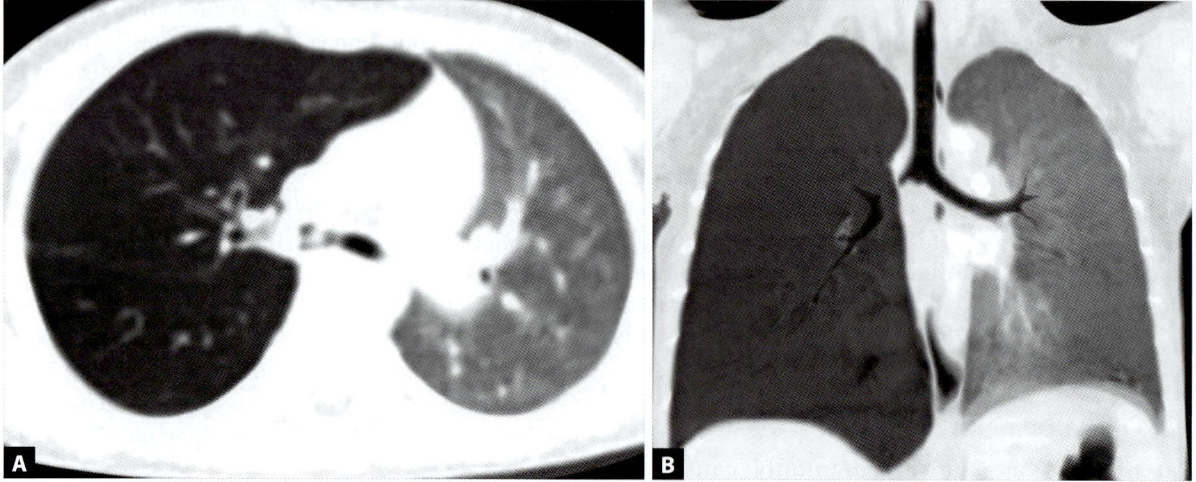

Figs. 21.8.3A and B: Foreign body inhalation. (A) Axial and (B) Coronal minimum intensity projection (MIP) images showing lucent hyperinflated right lung and intraluminal foreign body in the right main bronchus.

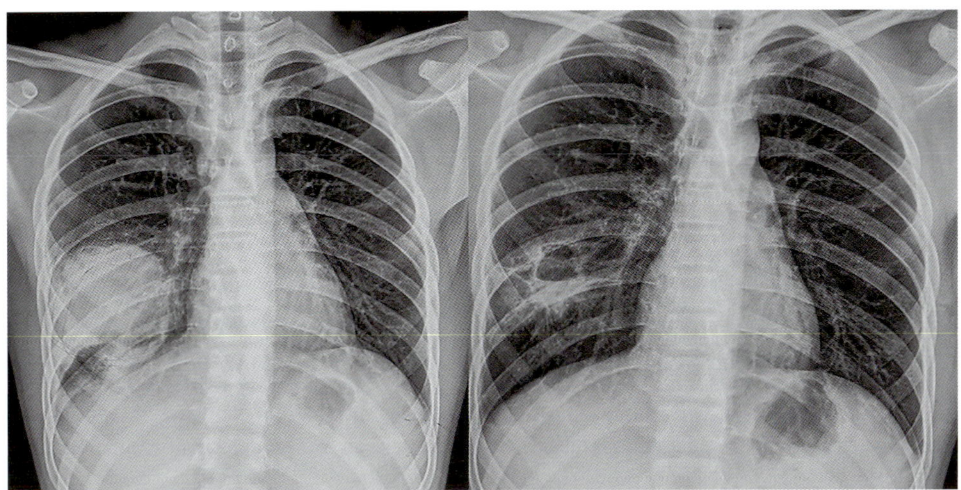

Fig. 21.8.4: Staphylococcal pneumonia with pneumatoceles. Radiograph in the initial phase shows a round pneumonia pattern, which is subsequently replaced by thin-walled cyst/pneumatoceles.

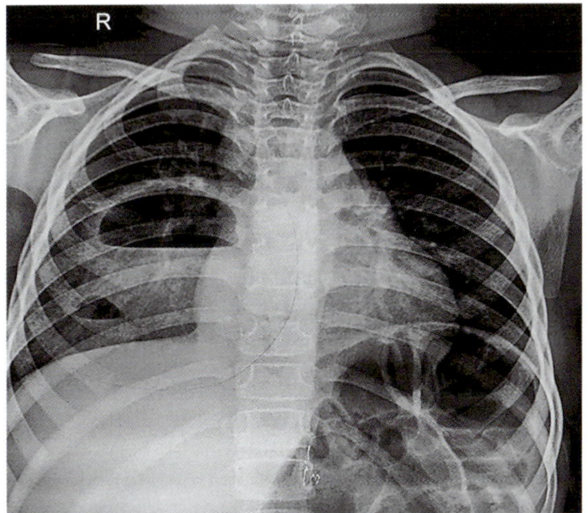

Fig. 21.8.5: Lung abscess in the right lower lobe with air fluid levels.

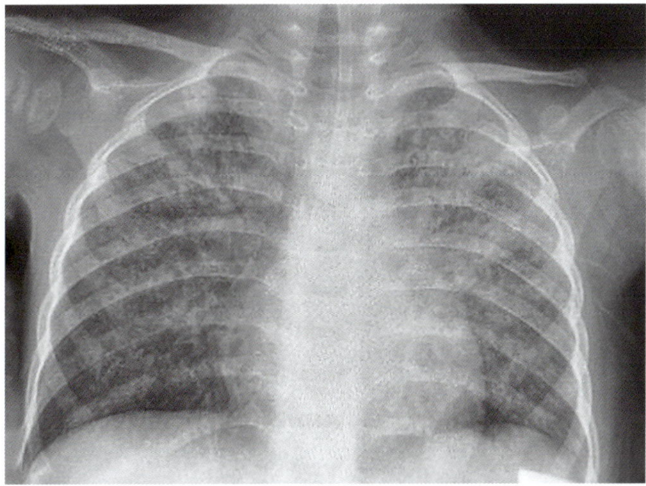

Fig. 21.8.6: Viral pneumonia, bilateral reticular opacities with peribronchial thickening.

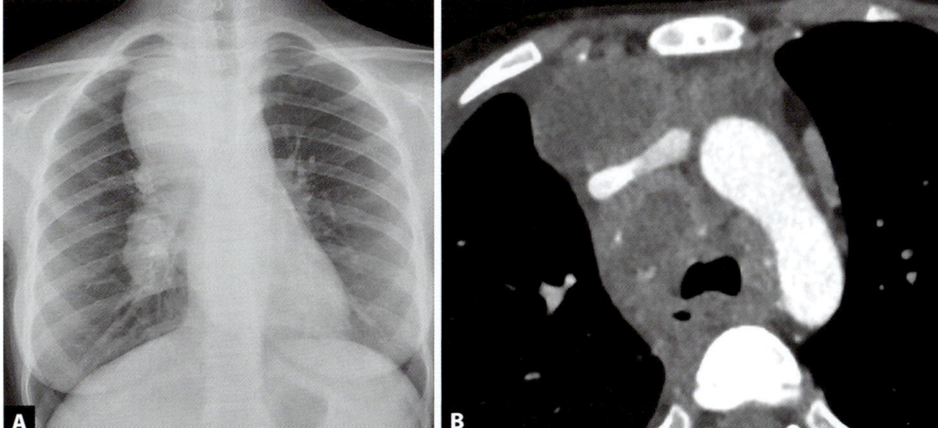

Figs. 21.8.7A and B: Tubercular lymphadenopathy. Right paratracheal lymphadenopathy manifested as widening of the paratracheal stripe. Right hilar lymphadenopathy, manifested as hilar enlargement. CECT chest shows the necrotic nature of nodes, seen as central hypodensity and peripheral rim enhancement.

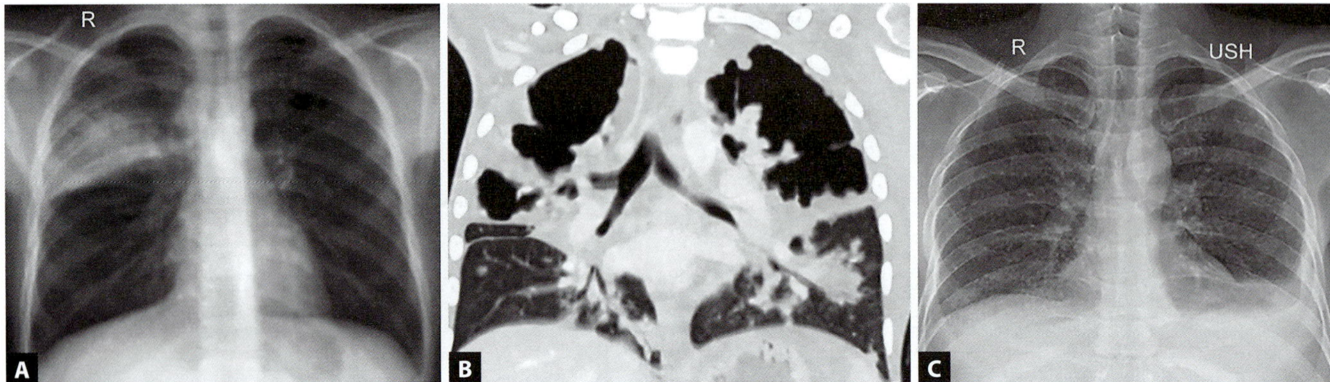

Figs. 21.8.8A to C: Pulmonary tuberculosis. (A) Radiograph showing right upper lobe consolidation; (B) CT coronal reformatted image showing bilateral upper lobe cavitation; (C) Miliary tuberculosis showing small random nodules with concomitant left-sided free pleural effusion.

air bronchogram **(Figs. 21.8.8A and B)**, and pulmonary cavitations.

- Lymphatic or venous seeding in lungs produces miliary tuberculosis **(Fig. 21.8.8C)**.
- Following healing, by chemotherapy or by development of body immunity, chest radiograph may become either completely normal or residual changes like calcified nodes, pulmonary scar, pleural thickening, or loss of volume may be seen.

Bronchiectasis

Bronchiectasis is another common clinical problem, which usually follows infection by tuberculosis, viral, or bacterial pneumonias. After the chest radiographs, thin section, high-resolution CT is the imaging modality of choice to detect subtle bronchiectasis.[3] Bronchograms are rarely, if ever, used nowadays.

Primary Lung Tumors

Primary lung tumors are rare in children. Metastatic lung disease is much more common and is usually from a Wilms tumor.

Mediastinum

Mediastinum is divided into three compartments: (1) Anterior, (2) middle, and (3) posterior. It is important to remember that the radiological division of the mediastinum is different from the anatomical division. Masses can arise from any one of the structures normally present in these compartments:

- Germ cell tumor is an anterior mediastinal malignant tumor.
- Lymph nodes, bronchogenic cyst, pericardial tumors, and hiatus hernia are important masses of middle mediastinum.
- Neurogenic tumors predominate in the posterior mediastinum.

SKELETAL SYSTEM

Imaging Techniques[6]

Conventional radiographs still remain the mainstay for the evaluation of musculoskeletal diseases. CT and MRI provide detailed soft tissue and articular and bony imaging, and are thus helpful, especially for examination of masses regarding their content, extent, and degree of vascular and marrow involvement. MRI is superior to CT due to its better soft-tissue resolution and multiplanar capability. Sonography has a role in the evaluation of congenital dislocation of hip, various causes of joint effusion and synovitis, and soft-tissue masses. USG-guided interventions including joint aspiration/biopsy and intra-articular corticosteroid injection are another additional advantage. Scintigraphy is the primary modality in the detection of metastatic disease and osteomyelitis.[2]

Pathological Conditions[6]

Before interpreting abnormality, one must have knowledge about the normal development of bone, parts of different areas of skeletal system, and several normal variants, which may mimic abnormalities:

- *Rickets* is still a relatively common clinical problem in India. Vitamin D deficiency results in failure of normal mineralization of the growing cartilage into bone. Classic radiographic findings are found in the most rapidly growing ends of bone and include generalized osteopenia, disappearance of zone of provisional calcification, cupping with fraying and irregularity of the metaphyseal ends, and perpendicular striations extending from the metaphyseal end toward epiphysis **(Figs. 21.8.9A and B)**. Enlargement of the anterior ends of ribs (rachitic rosary) and lower ends of radius and ulna may also be noted.

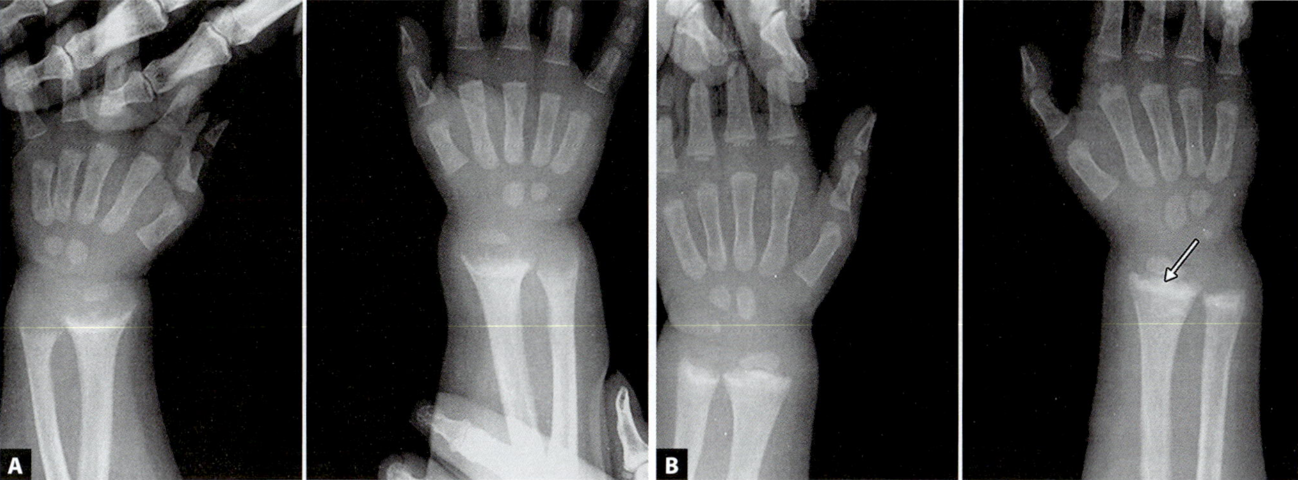

Figs. 21.8.9A and B: Rickets—primarily a metaphyseal disease. Note cupping of metaphyseal ends of both radius and ulna, widened physis, perpendicular striations extending from metaphysis into physis toward the epiphysis. (A) Generalized osteopenia is seen in the background; (B) Post-treatment radiographs show healing.

- *Thalassemia major (homozygous form):* Radiographic changes are at times dramatic **(Figs. 21.8.10A to C)** and are the result of marrow hyperplasia.
- *Congenital syphilis* is caused by transplacental spread. Bony lesions may appear even up to 2 months later. The hallmark of this condition is metaphysitis **(Figs. 21.8.11A to C)**, i.e., a metaphyseal lucent band located directly beneath a dense band in the subphyseal region. Focal destructive bony lesions in diaphysis, periostitis, and pathological fracture may also occur.
- *Skeletal tuberculosis* is still prevalent in India. Tuberculosis may affect any part of the skeletal system. In the spine, it typically affects the vertebral body. Partial collapse produces para- (and/or pre-) vertebral abscess and short angle gibbus. Long bone tuberculosis may be isolated or affect an adjacent joint. A high index of suspicion, chest radiograph, biochemical and hematological findings, family history, and positive tuberculin test all help in establishing the diagnosis in an equivocal case.[4]
- *Developmental dysplasia of hip (congenital dislocation of hip)* is a common clinical problem. Following a thorough clinical examination, USG is usually the first screening modality to confirm the diagnosis. On plain radiographs, several lines have been described to identify cases with subtle dislocation. Nowadays, three-dimensional CT (3D CT) and 3D MRI have shown promising results for in-depth evaluation of this entity.
- *Osteogenic sarcoma* is the most common primary malignant bone tumor between 10 and 25 years of age and is usually located in the metaphysis of a long bone, especially around the knee. Typically, the tumor matrix is ossified and its metastases to lungs may also be ossified.
- *Metastatic disease affecting the skeletal system* is common in the pediatric age group. Commonly, it is due to a round cell tumor—acute lymphoblastic leukemia, neuroblastoma, lymphoma, rhabdomyosarcoma, or Ewing sarcoma. Skeletal survey shows generalized demineralization, "moth-eaten" osteolytic lesions diffusely involving all the bones, metaphyseal lucent bands, and periosteal new bone formation with loss of focal areas of cortical line due to tumor invasion.

Assessment of Skeletal Maturity

Radiology of the skeletal system would be incomplete without a few words on the methodology for skeletal maturity assessment or bone age assessment. The earlier method of observing the appearance and fusion of ossification centers is an obsolete technique; even though in India, it is still the only method used in most hospitals. More accurate methods are by using an atlas either by Greulich–Pyle or by Tanner–Whitehouse 3 (TW3) method. The latter is, at present, the most accurate method for assessment of skeletal maturity in a child. Automated bone age assessment is another new advancement in this regard, which is quick and accurate **(Fig. 21.8.12)**.

GASTROINTESTINAL TRACT

Imaging Techniques

Once again, plain radiograph coupled with contrast examination (barium studies) plays a major role in many GIT disorders. Sonography, CT, and MRI provide valuable information, especially in cases of masses, mesenteric vascular and nodal status, retroperitoneal anatomy, trauma,

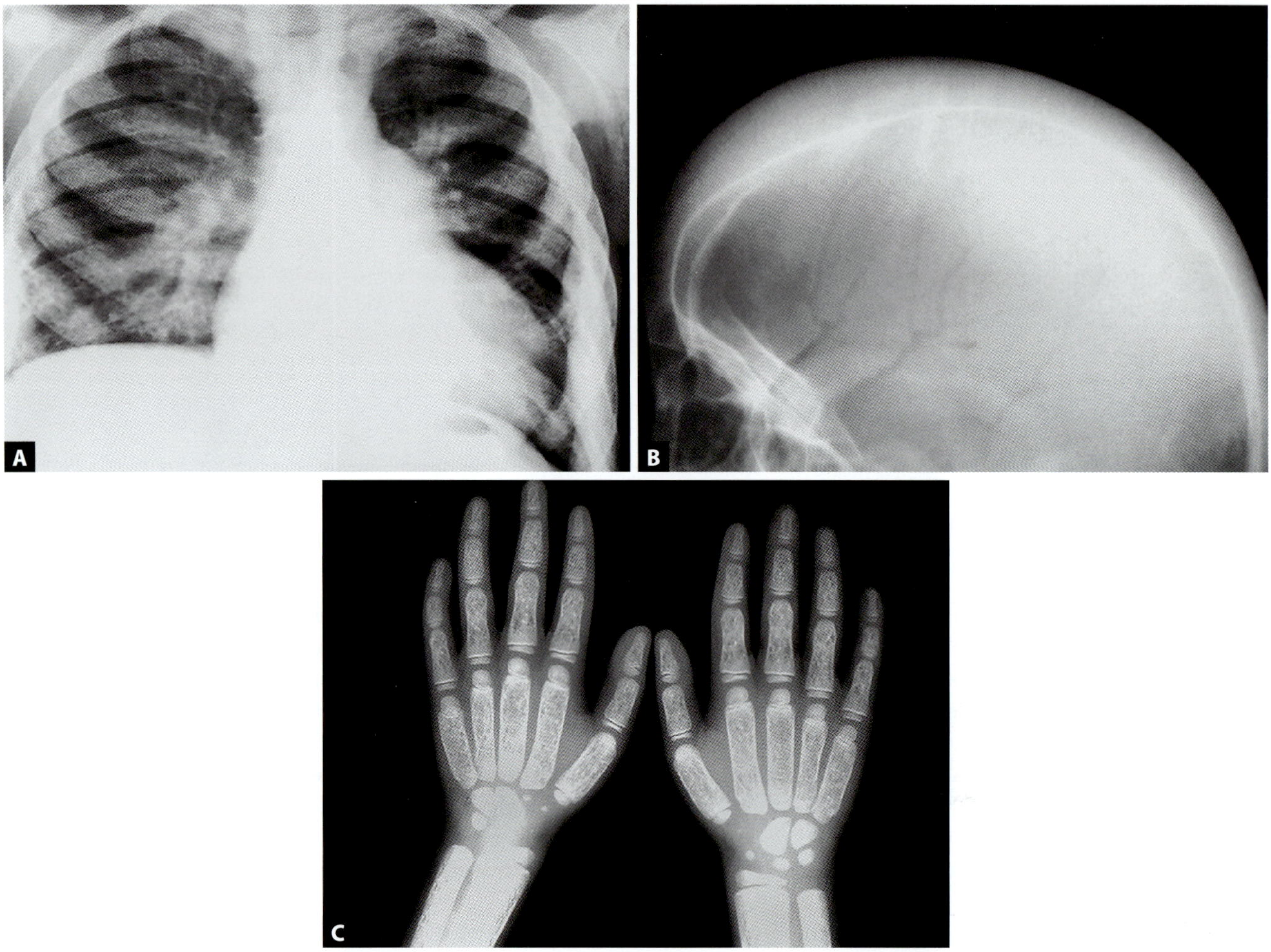

Figs. 21.8.10A to C: Thalassemia major—chest X-ray (CXR) showing marked expansion of the ribs. (A) Striking "hair-on-end" appearance in the skull; (B) Osteoporosis, widening of medullary spaces of all the bones of hands with coarse trabecular pattern, loss of lateral concavity of small bones of hand, and molding abnormality of distal ends of long bones; (C) Radiographic changes reflect a marked degree of marrow proliferation.

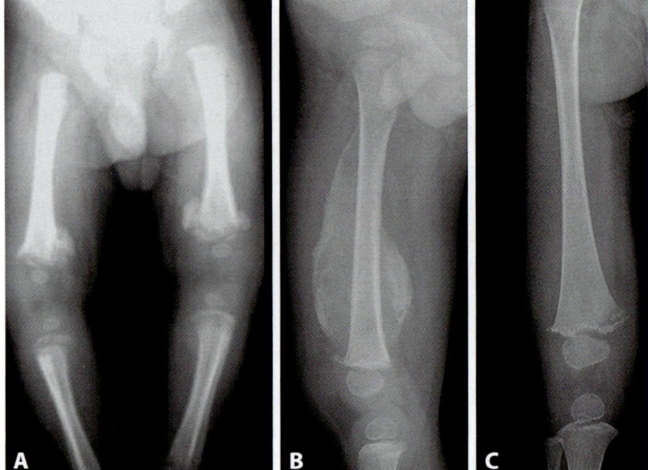

Figs. 21.8.11A to C: Congenital syphilis. Anteroposterior (AP) view of both lower limbs. (A) Characteristic metaphyseal changes (metaphysitis) and periostitis seen in all the long bones. Epiphysis is normal; (B and C) Important differential diagnosis (D/D) is scurvy, which is characterized by osteopenia with subperiosteal hemorrhage lifting the periosteum and metaphyseal changes.

and abscess or other fluid collections. CT enterography and MR enterography are two other important investigations in the evaluation of the GIT, which have the added advantage of detection of luminal as well as extraluminal pathologies.

Pathological Conditions

Erect plain abdominal radiographs are usually adequate in intestinal obstruction **(Figs. 21.8.13A and B)**. Perforation with free air **(Fig. 21.8.14)** or necrotizing enterocolitis (NEC) with classical intramural air **(Fig. 21.8.15)**, calcified mesenteric or retroperitoneal nodes, diseases of the spine (e.g., tuberculosis), and a host of other conditions are also readily diagnosed on plain radiographs.

However, *contrast examination with barium* is required for the diagnosis of mucosal diseases, e.g., polyps or ulcer, and intestinal muscular wall diseases, e.g., congenital hypertrophic pyloric stenosis **(Fig. 21.8.16)** and stricture, obstruction, and Hirschsprung disease. GIT-related masses require a cross-sectional imaging modality, i.e., sonography, CT or MRI, with or without intravenous contrast. Esophageal atresia is diagnosed on day 1 of life, usually with negative contrast, i.e., air only, but positive contrast (i.e., barium or nonionic isotonic contrast) may also be used. Midgut volvulus is another condition which can be diagnosed on contrast study alone **(Figs. 21.8.17A and B)**. Thus, for GIT-related conditions, a radiologist can choose a specific imaging modality in a particular case to derive maximum information with minimum cost and harm (radiation and invasive technique) to the patient.

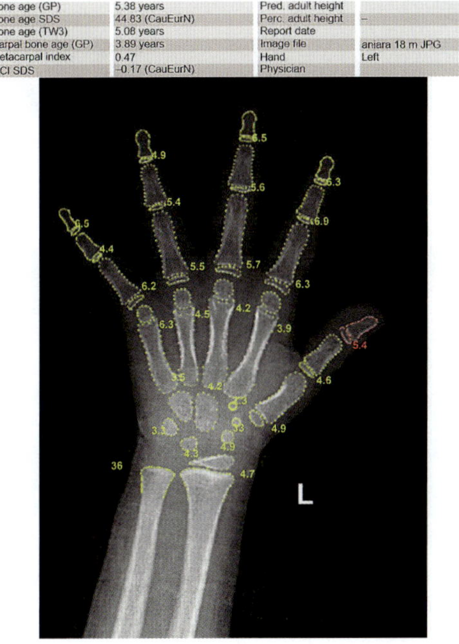

Fig. 21.8.12: Report generated by automated bone age estimation software.

HEPATOBILIARY SYSTEM

Imaging Technique

Nowadays, USG is usually the first imaging modality for evaluating diseases of the hepatobiliary system. In the presence of a tumor, contrast-enhanced CT (CECT) tailored for the suspected pathology is usually adequate. However, magnetic resonance cholangiopancreatography (MRCP) remains the investigation of choice in suspected biliary pathologies.[7] Triple-phase contrast-enhanced MRI with a hepatobiliary specific contrast agent is preferred for hepatic mass characterization. The drawback/hindrance of using MRI in children is the need for general anesthesia or sedation.

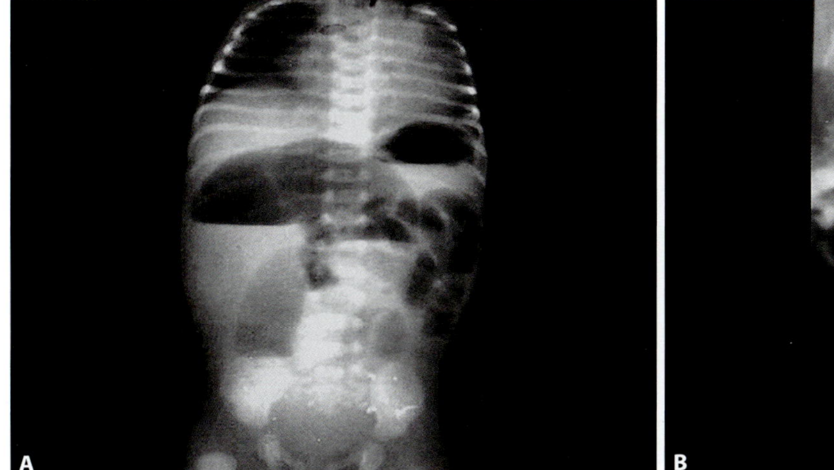

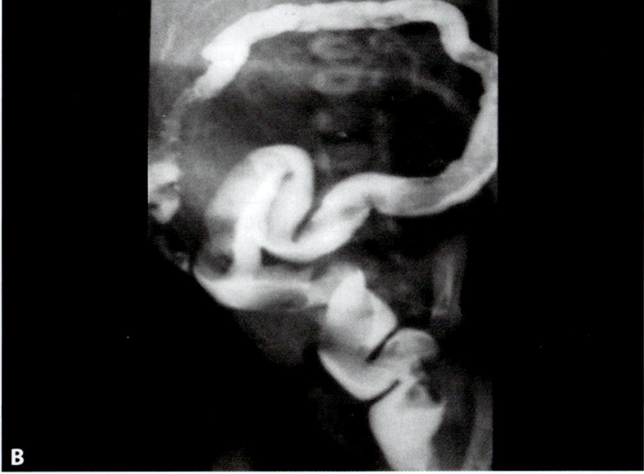

Figs. 21.8.13A and B: Abdomen. Anteroposterior (AP) erect view in a newborn with vomiting and abdominal distention. (A) Multiple, small, air-fluid levels predominantly in the central abdomen. Absent gas in the colon and rectum; a case of ileal atresia. Number, type, and distribution of bowel loops and air-fluid levels help in localizing the level of obstruction; (B) Barium enema revealed microcolon.

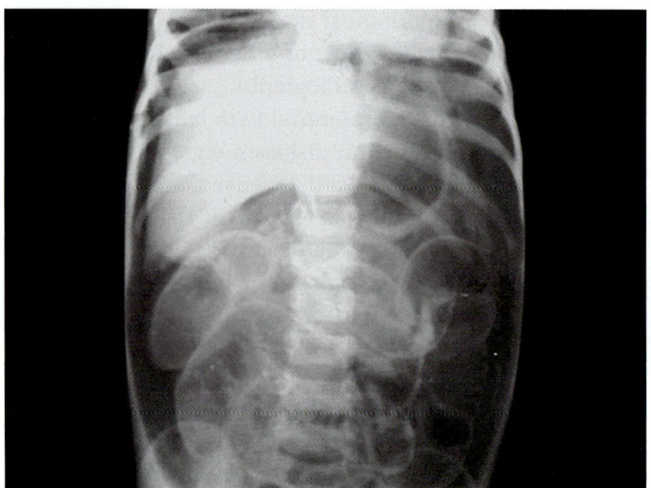

Fig. 21.8.14: Perforation of gastrointestinal tract (GIT) with free peritoneal air seen between the right diaphragm and liver. Both sides of the intestinal walls are visible, another sign of presence of free peritoneal air.

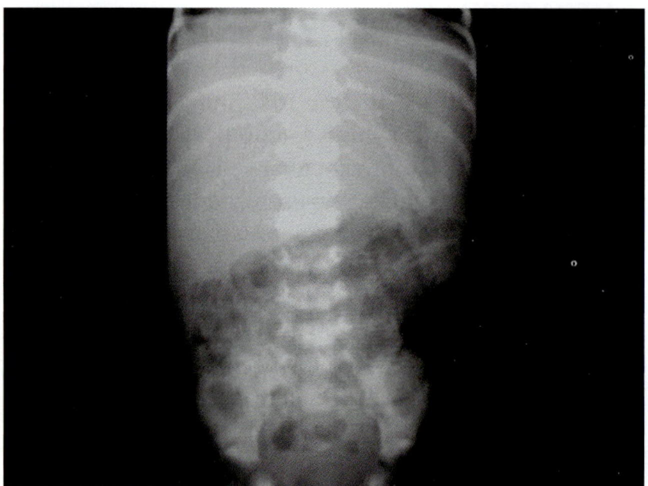

Fig. 21.8.15: Necrotizing enterocolitis in a newborn—classical linear gas shadows due to intramural gas (pneumatosis intestinalis) and bubbly appearance.

Angiography is rarely required either for preoperative arterial roadmap in cases of tumor or for diagnosing primary vascular diseases, e.g., aneurysm, arteritis, etc. Plain radiographs have very limited role, if any.

Pathological Conditions

The most common clinical problem is to differentiate medical from surgical type of jaundice. This differentiation is made by observing the presence or absence of dilatation of biliary channels. Sonography can readily identify dilatation of intra- and/or extrahepatic biliary channels, level of obstruction,

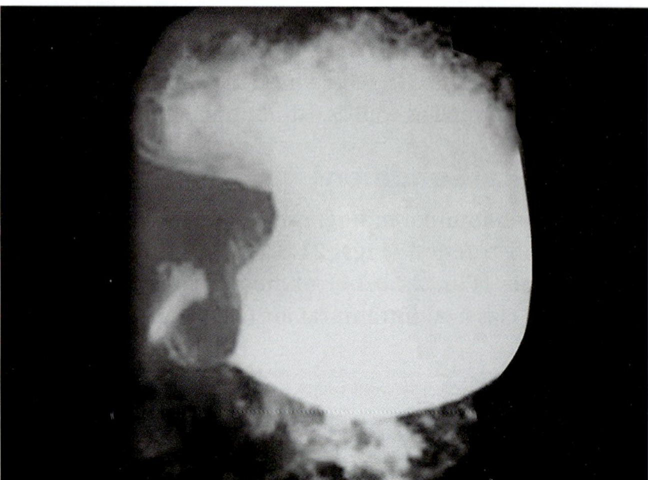

Fig. 21.8.16: Congenital hypertrophic pyloric stenosis.

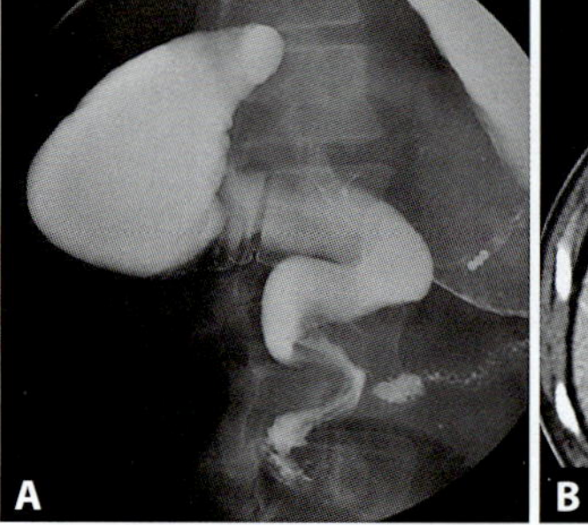

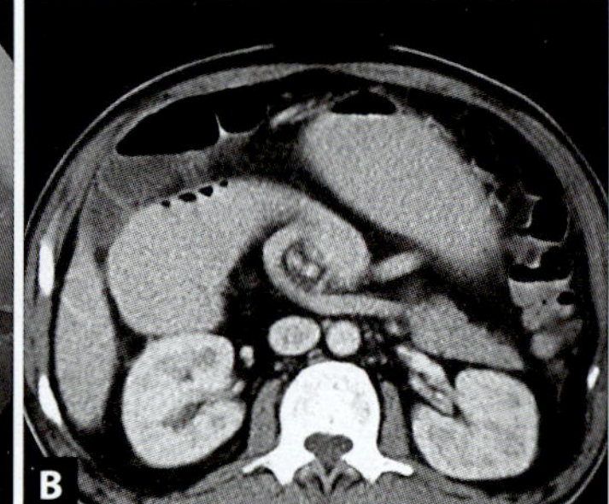

Figs. 21.8.17A and B: Midgut volvulus in a child. (A) Contrast study shows a "corkscrew" pattern; (B) Axial CECT shows a swirling of mesenteric vessels (whirlpool sign).

and many a times, even the cause, e.g., calculus, pancreatic head tumor, or choledochal cyst.

In neonatal age, extrahepatic biliary atresia is an important cause of surgical obstructive jaundice. The sonographic features are a small gall bladder with poor contractility or irregular outline, echogenic "triangular cord" sign, and nonvisualized common bile duct **(Figs. 21.8.18A and B)**. Sometimes, the entire gall bladder may be replaced by a fibrotic echogenic cord-like area, with occasional cystic structure at porta.

Choledochal cysts are congenital ectatic dilatation of biliary channels, either totally extrahepatic, intrahepatic, or a combination of the two. Sonography is usually adequate for its diagnosis **(Fig. 21.8.19A)**, but endoscopic retrograde cholangiopancreatography (ERCP) **(Fig. 21.8.19B)** or MRCP may also be done to demonstrate it preoperatively **(Fig. 21.8.19C)**. Biliary atresia, an important D/D of neonatal jaundice requires ultrasonography (US) coupled with nuclear scan for diagnosis. Nowadays, MRCP is the first and usually

Figs. 21.8.18A and B: Cystic extrahepatic biliary atresia in an infant. Ultrasound image (A) shows a small irregular gallbladder, not showing the normal trilaminar pattern. There is a small cyst at the porta hepatis (B) which is different from a choledochal cyst.

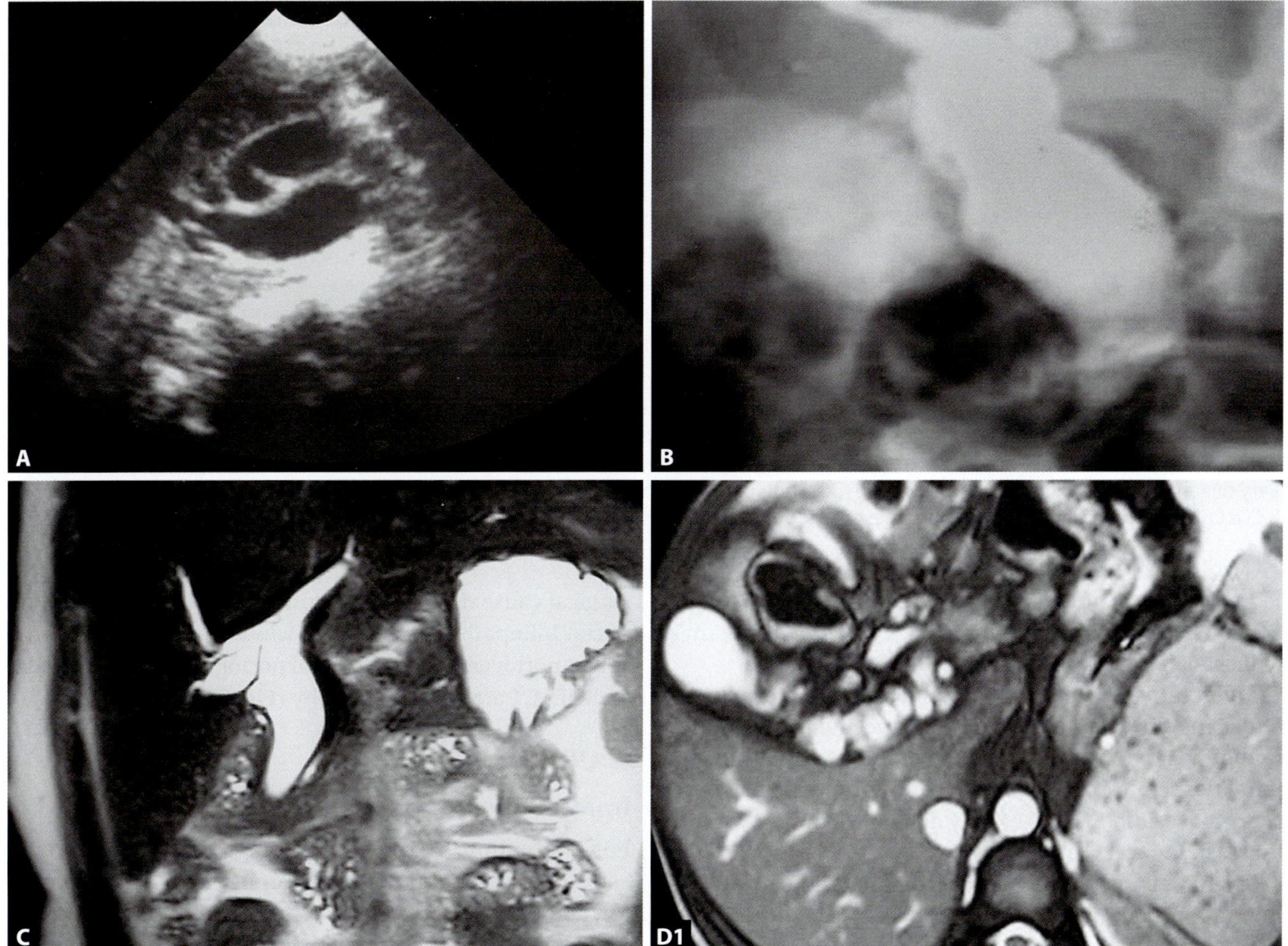

Figs. 21.8.19A to D1

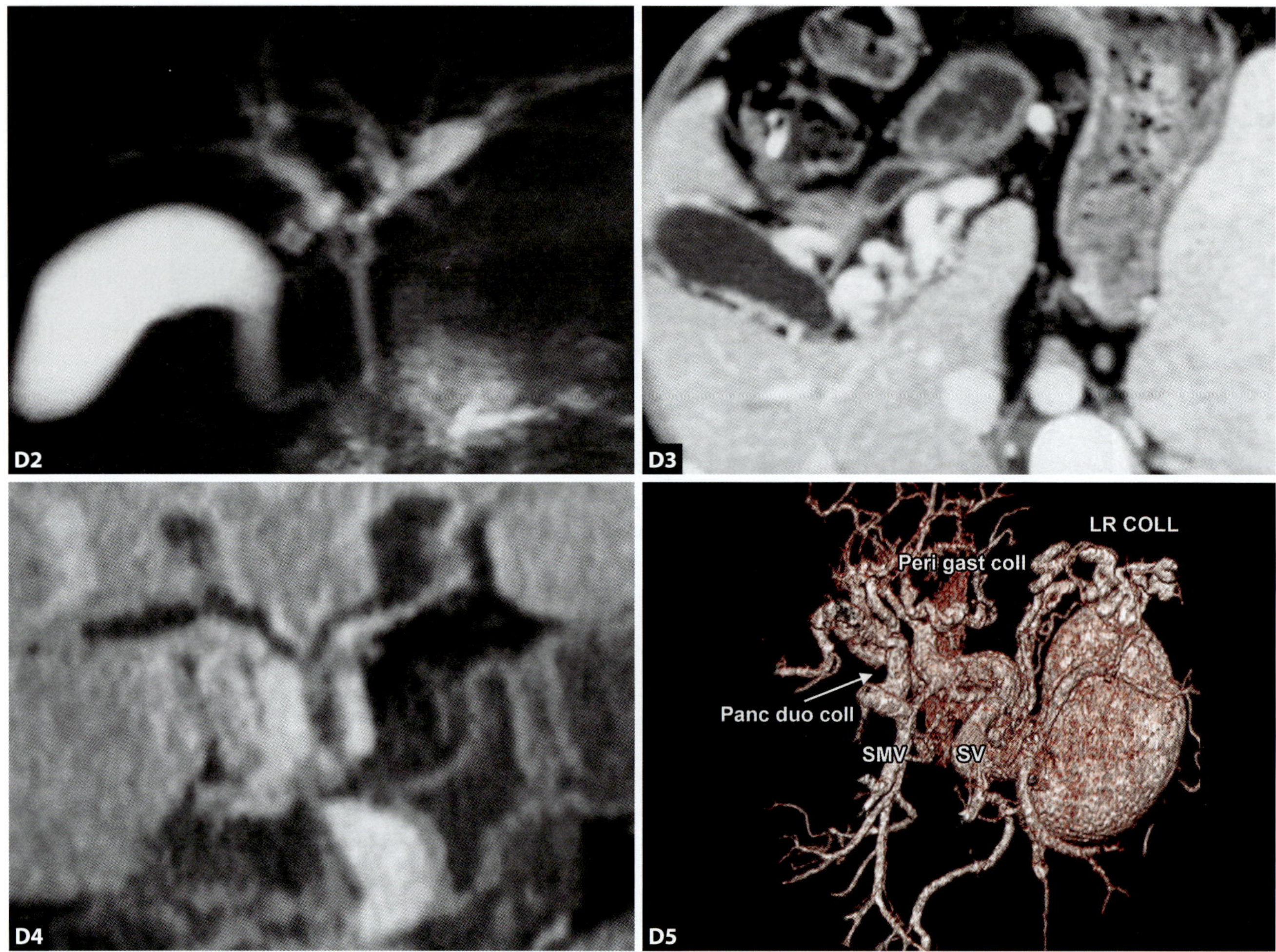

Figs. 21.8.19D2 to D5

Figs. 21.8.19A to D: (A and B) Huge, extrahepatic, cystic choledochal cyst on ultrasound and on ERCP. Note the slightly dilated right main bile duct entering the cyst on ultrasound. Gallbladder should be documented separate from the cyst. (C and D) Magnetic resonance cholangiopancreatography (MRCP) images elegantly documenting the choledochal cyst portal biliopathy: Magnetic resonance imaging (MRI) axial (D1) and coronal (D2), and computed tomography (CT) axial (D3) and coronal (D4) images showing portal cavernoma causing biliary dilatation. Three-dimensional CT (3D CT) (D5) showing exquisite detail of the portosplenic axis and the collaterals developed.
(LR COLL: lienorenal collateral; SMV: super mesenteric vein; SV: splenic vein)

the only imaging modality required to differentiate it from neonatal hepatitis. However, intraoperative cholangiogram is the most definitive investigation for its diagnosis.

Liver tumors are common and of these, malignant neoplasms (hepatoblastoma or hepatocellular carcinoma) are the most common. Any of the cross-sectional imaging modalities can diagnose and stage it. A cystic liver space-occupying lesion (SOL) is usually due to hydatid cyst or liver abscess in India.

Splenic enlargement is another common clinical problem. Malaria and kala-azar are two important medical causes while portal hypertension, usually secondary to extrahepatic block in the splenoportal axis, is the most important surgical cause. Initial evaluation of portal hypertension and portal biliopathy is with USG, which can be confirmed by splenoportovenography, arterial portography, and nowadays with 3D-CT arterial portography **(Fig. 21.8.19D)**.

URINARY SYSTEM

Imaging Techniques

For evaluation of the upper renal tracts, sonography, especially color duplex sonography, is usually adequate for anatomical assessment. High-resolution sonography performed using high-frequency transducers is essential to assess parenchymal renal disease. However, it needs to be

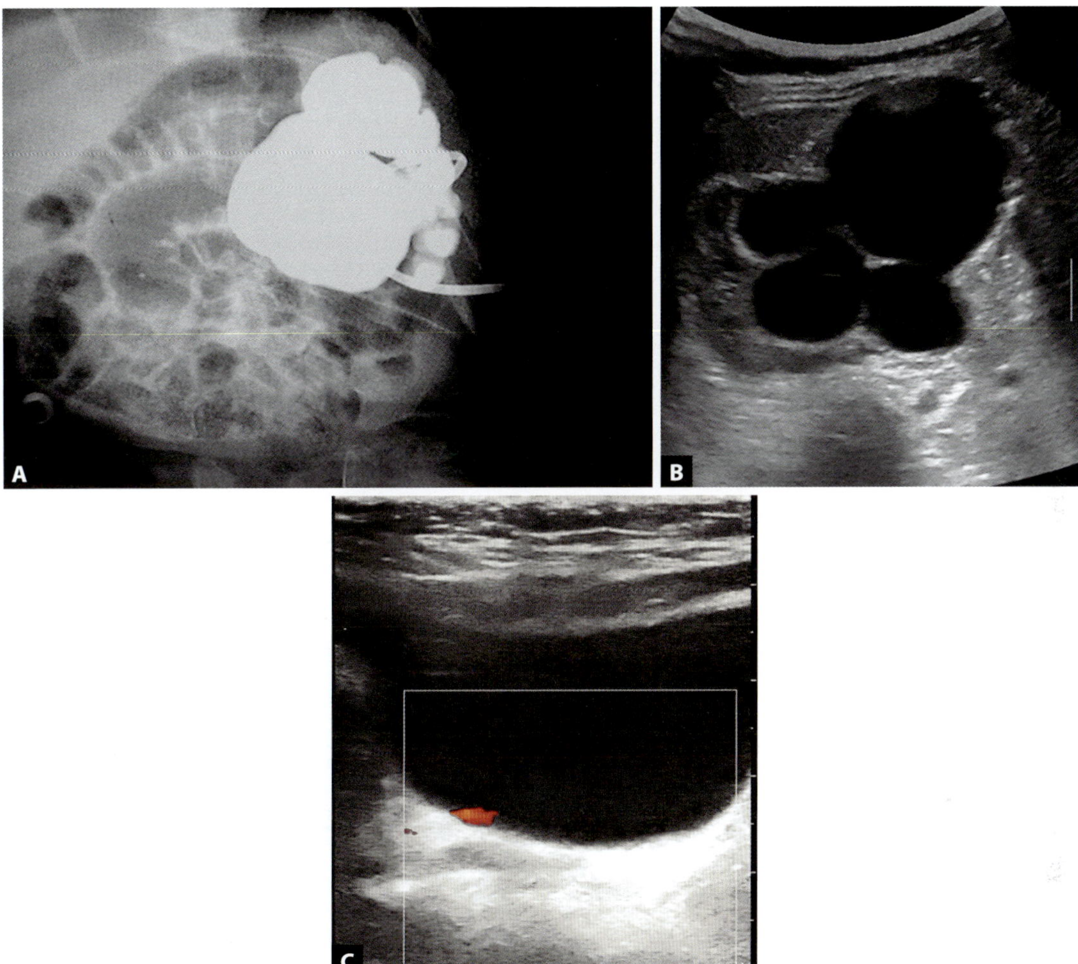

Figs. 21.8.20A to C: Left PUJ obstruction. Nephrostogram of left kidney (A) shows dilated, rounded renal pelvis with caliectasis, a case of pelviureteric junction (PUJ) obstruction. Ureter is not opacified even on delayed images. Ultrasound shows gross hydronephrosis and ballooned-out renal pelvis (B). Color Doppler evaluation of the bladder shows an absent left ureteric jet (C) whereas right-sided jet is visible.

supplemented by a functional study. Excretory urography is required in limited clinical indications, when complex anatomical details need to be clarified or in patients with ureteric disease. CT or MRI is added in the workup of a case of tumor or trauma. For examination of the lower urinary tract, sonography for bladder and contrast examination for urethral evaluation are usually adequate.[7]

Pathological Conditions

Hydronephrosis is one of the most important and common problems encountered in pediatric practice. Sonography and contrast study not only diagnose it reliably, but also provide a clue to its possible cause, e.g., pelviureteric junction (PUJ) obstruction **(Figs. 21.8.20A to C)**, calculus, etc. and it can also delineate an associated hydroureter, if present.

Several congenital anomalies can be seen, e.g., horseshoe kidney, crossed ectopia, low lying kidney, etc.

Of the solid renal masses, Wilms tumor is the most common. On cross-sectional imaging, it is seen as a solid tumor with variegated enhancement due to areas of necrosis. In 10%, it may be bilateral. For staging purposes, CT or MRI may be done in addition to sonography.

Bladder tumors are relatively rare in children, and of these, a malignant tumor, rhabdomyosarcoma, is the most common. On the cystogram phase of a contrast study, characteristic lobulated filling defects are seen from the bladder base. This appearance gives it the name of "sarcoma botryoides".

Vesicoureteric reflex (VUR) is one of the most important causes for urinary tract infection. Voiding cystourethrography (VCUG), using either contrast or an isotope, is required to diagnose it **(Figs. 21.8.21A and B)**. The latter is reported to be more accurate. Nowadays, even sonocystography is used in certain clinical situations to diagnose VUR with the added advantage of lack of ionizing radiation.

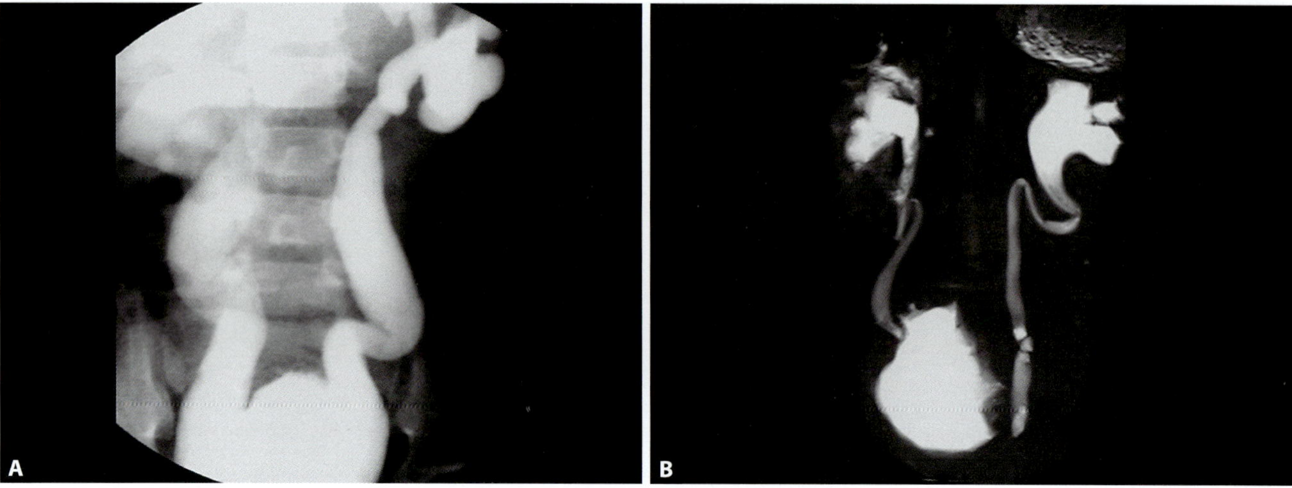

Figs. 21.8.21A and B: (A) Micturating cystourethrography (MCU). Vesicoureteric reflux (VUR) on both sides. Urinary bladder shows trabeculation and sacculations due to neurogenic dysfunction (neurogenic bladder); (B) Same information could be seen on magnetic resonance (MR) urography.

The most common cause for urinary outflow obstruction in a male child is posterior urethral valve (PUV). Micturating cystourethrography (MCU) is mandatory for its diagnosis **(Fig. 21.8.22)**. Backpressure changes in the bladder and associated VUR are common. Magnetic resonance urography has been tried to be useful for demonstrating VUR. Moreover, it is free of radiation.

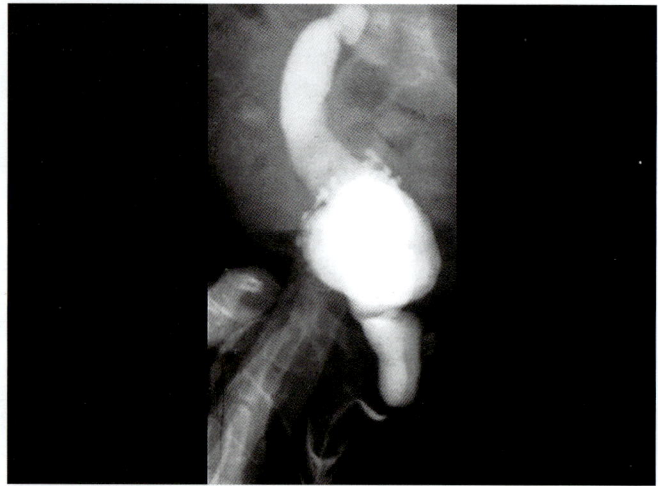

Fig. 21.8.22: Micturating cystourethrography (MCU) shows marked dilatation of posterior urethra, thin urinary stream, and narrowing at the junction of posterior and anterior urethra due to posterior urethral valves. Also, note gross vesicoureteric reflux (VUR) on the right side.

CRANIAL AND SPINAL IMAGING[8]

Imaging Techniques

Conventional radiographs of the skull should include at least frontal and lateral views. Depending upon the suspected clinical disease, more views can be taken, e.g., for sinuses, atlantoaxial junction, pituitary fossa, etc. Plain X-rays of the spine are often the preliminary investigation in the evaluation of back pain and are also done as a part of the skeletal survey.

Transfontanelle cranial US has a role to play, only if the anterior fontanel is open. Diagnosis of hydrocephalus, intracranial bleed, congenital malformations, and tumors of the brain can be made. In neonatal age, transcranial US is a very useful modality in the evaluation of germinal matrix hemorrhage, periventricular leukomalacia, hydrocephalus, and other congenital anomalies. CT is the preferred imaging modality for evaluation of intracranial bleed or calcification.[7] MRI remains the "problem-solving" tool in most intracranial pathologies including tumor, infection, vasculitis, etc. For the evaluation of the spine and its contents, MRI is the modality of choice. However, in infants, US can be used as an excellent alternative, as the posterior elements of the vertebral bodies remain unossified.

Pathological Conditions

The term craniosynostosis denotes premature fusion of cranial sutures. Depending upon the pattern of sutural closure, the shape of the head varies, and different names are used to describe them, e.g., brachycephaly (fused coronal sutures) and scaphocephaly (sagittal sutures fusion). Besides the plain radiographs, CT and nowadays 3D CT is the investigation of choice to assess the sutural status. Growing fracture at times may mimic a widened suture **(Fig. 21.8.23)**.

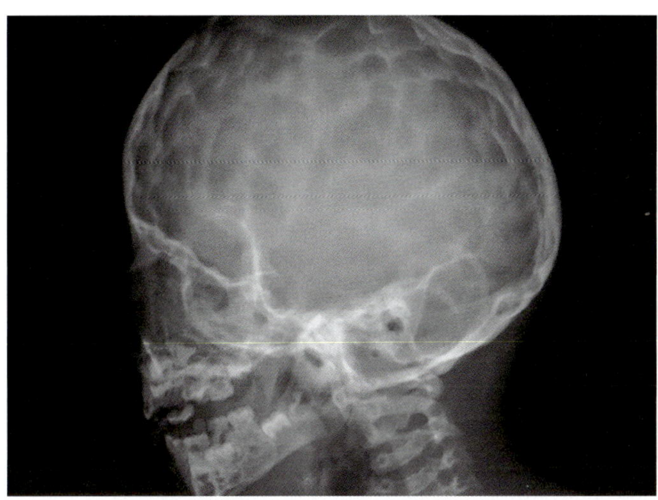

Fig. 21.8.23: Multiple sutural craniosynostosis. Lateral skull radiograph shows "copper beaten" appearance.

Intracranial calcification **(Figs. 21.8.24A to C)** could be seen in postinfectious states, e.g., cytomegalovirus (CMV), toxoplasma infection, and tuberculous meningitis; in brain tumors; hypoparathyroidism; and/or in dysplastic brain tissue. CMV produces periventricular calcifications (a "calcified mold of the ventricles") whereas toxoplasmosis produces diffuse cerebral calcification. In a child with stroke-like presentation and bilateral basal ganglia calcification, mineralizing microangiopathy is a diagnostic possibility. CT is essential for anatomical localization.

Skull vault may be affected in several diseases, e.g., histiocytosis **(Fig. 21.8.25)**, neuroblastoma metastases **(Figs. 21.8.26A and B)**, hematological and metabolic diseases, and various skeletal dysplasias.

Infectious conditions, like brain abscess **(Fig. 21.8.27)**, tuberculomas, and neurocysticercosis (NCC) **(Figs. 21.8.28A and B)**, are readily diagnosed with CT and

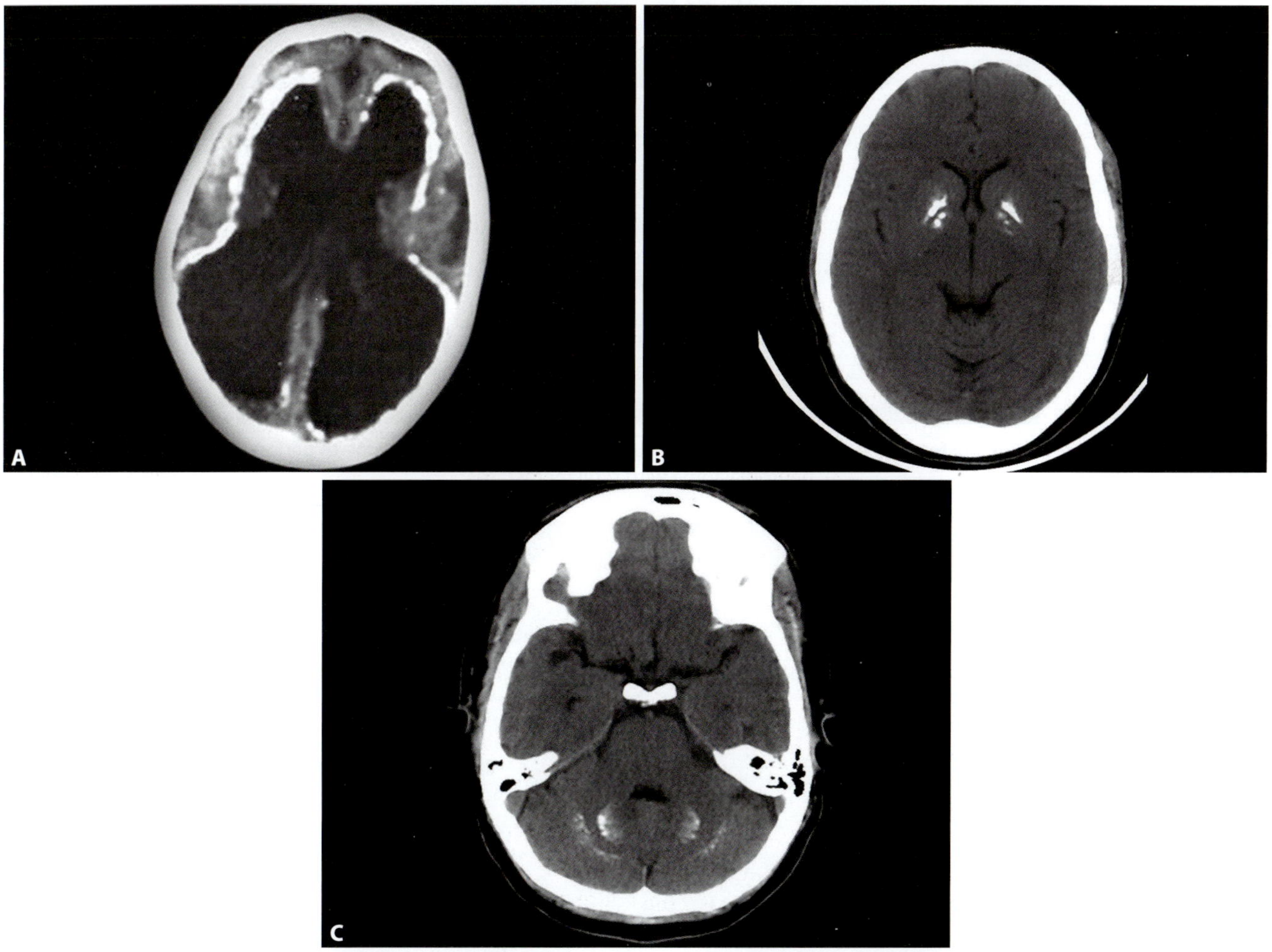

Figs. 21.8.24A to C: Intracranial calcification. (A) Noncontrast computed tomography (NCCT) axial sections showing periventricular calcification in congenital cytomegalovirus (CMV) infection; (B and C) Axial NCCT images showing intracranial calcifications in the bilateral basal ganglias and cerebellar hemispheres—typical presentation of calcification in hypoparathyroidism.

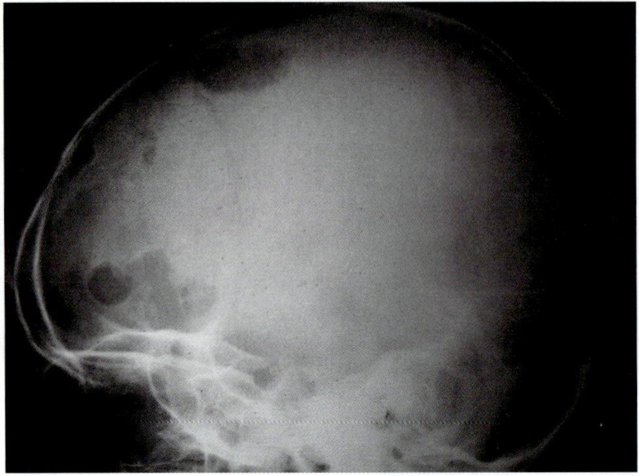

Fig. 21.8.25: Skull X-rays—multiple, large "geographic" type bone destruction, characteristic of histiocytosis. These types of bone lesions indicate relatively slow-growing pathology.

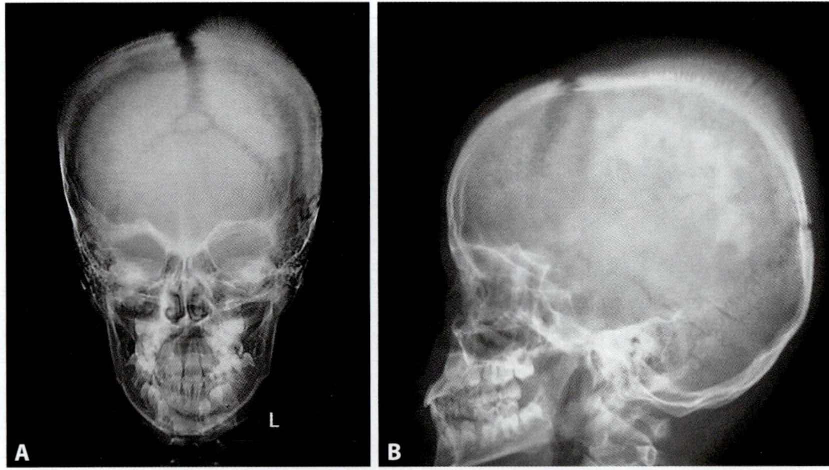

Figs. 21.8.26A and B: Skull posteroanterior and lateral views—sutural diastasis with sunray type of periosteal reaction in a case of neuroblastoma with skull metastases.

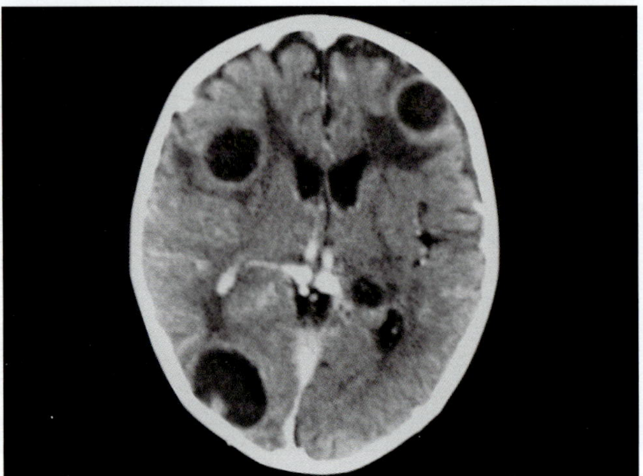

Fig. 21.8.27: Brain abscess—axial computed tomography (CT) showing multiple ring-enhancing lesions in bilateral frontal and right occipital lobes with perilesional edema.

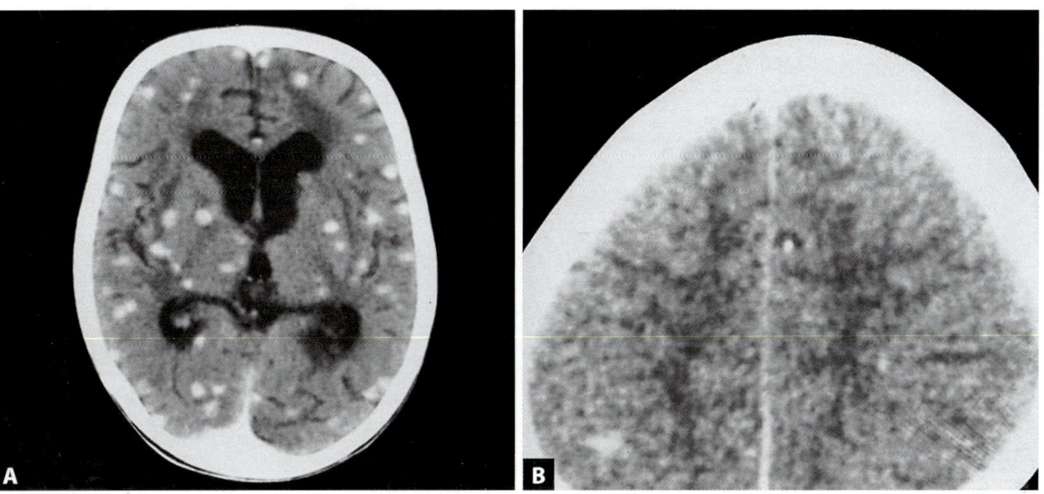

Figs. 21.8.28A and B: Neurocysticercosis (NCC). Multiple hyperdense lesions in brain suggestive of NCC; note the eccentric scolex.

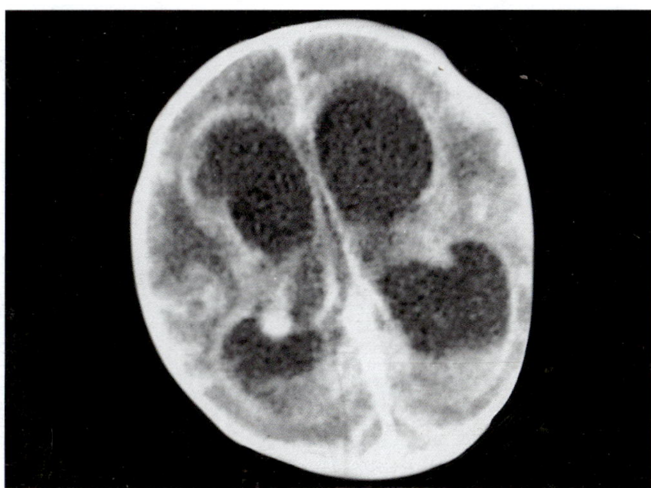

Fig. 21.8.29: Hydrocephalus with ventriculitis—axial CT showing dilated ventricles with enhancing ventricular margin and periventricular ooze.

MRI. Hydrocephalus, one of the most common causes of a large head in children, is readily diagnosed on any one of the cross-sectional imaging modalities **(Fig. 21.8.29)**. Similarly, other intracranial pathologic lesions can be imaged.

Cranial USG is a very useful imaging modality in neonates and early infants. Coronal and sagittal planes of imaging through the anterior fontanel are useful. Ventricular dimension, periventricular white matter changes, and extra-axial pathologies can be visualized with great anatomic detail **(Figs. 21.8.30A and B)**. Color Doppler imaging can be coupled with it to evaluate the resistive index (RI) in the intracranial vessels, which has proven utility in follow-up imaging in hydrocephalus.

Spinal dysraphism is the most common congenital abnormality affecting the spine. It is a complex disorder. Information required by the surgeon regarding the level of spinal involvement, contents of the sac, presence or absence of diastematomyelia (transfixion of the spinal cord by a bony spur congenitally), demyelinating changes in the cord, and associated hydrocephalus and Arnold-Chiari malformations can all be, nowadays, reliably, noninvasively delineated by MRI **(Figs. 21.8.31A to C)**. US of the spine is an accurate and versatile imaging modality which can be performed at the bedside or in the intensive care units (ICUs), and provide great anatomic detail **(Fig. 21.8.32)** without any need of sedation or general anesthesia.

CONCLUSION

Radiographs and USG remain the key imaging modalities in pediatric radiology, especially in the neonatal age group

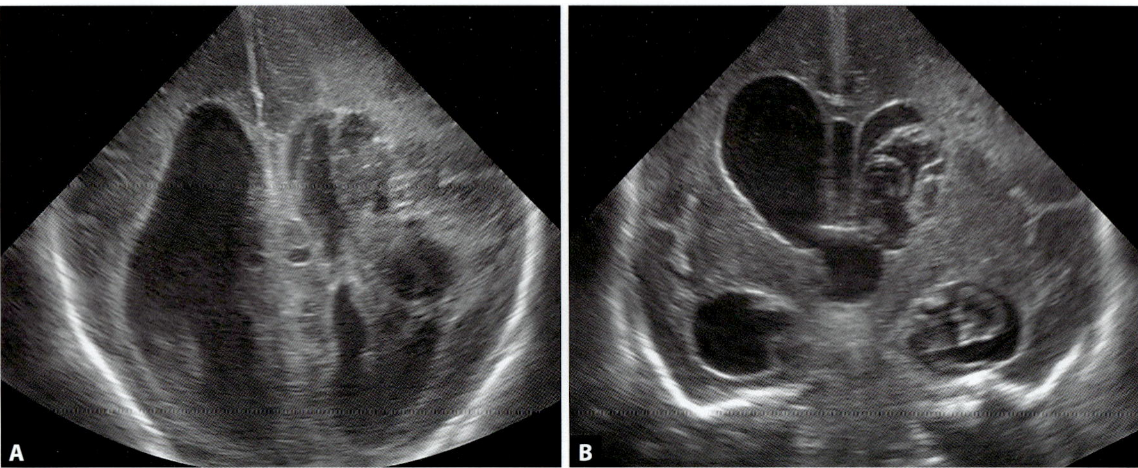

Figs. 21.8.30A and B: Grade IV germinal matrix hemorrhage [periventricular hemorrhagic infarction (PVHI)]. Coronal cranial US showing ventriculomegaly and intraventricular echogenic clots, along with periventricular white matter echogenicity.

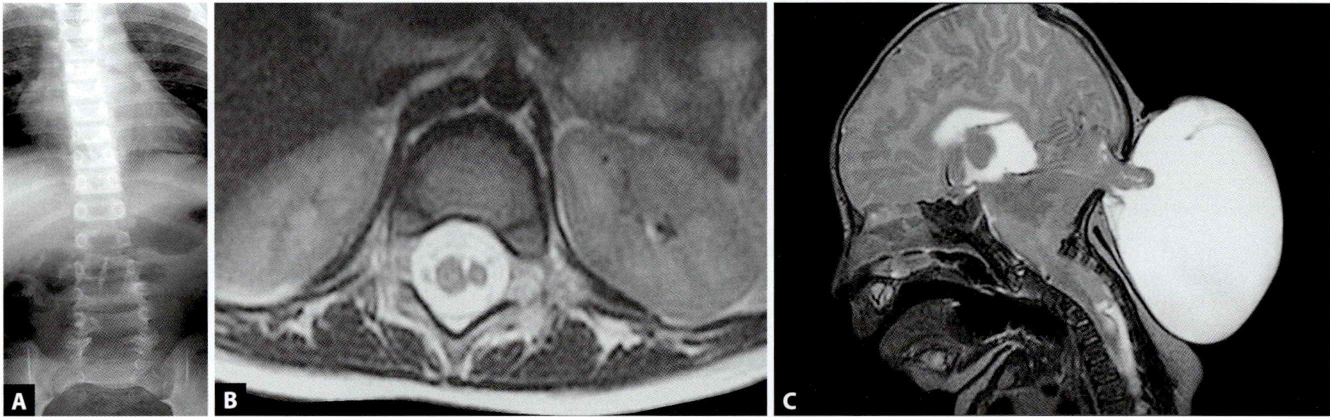

Figs. 21.8.31A to C: Diastematomyelia—radiograph showing bony septum in the spinal canal at L2 level with spina bifida from L3 onward (A) T2-weighted (T2W) axial magnetic resonance imaging (MRI) images; (B) Splitting of the cord into two; (C) Chiari III malformation—sagittal T2W MRI showing herniation of tonsil and brainstem (Chiari II) with occipital meningoencephalocele.

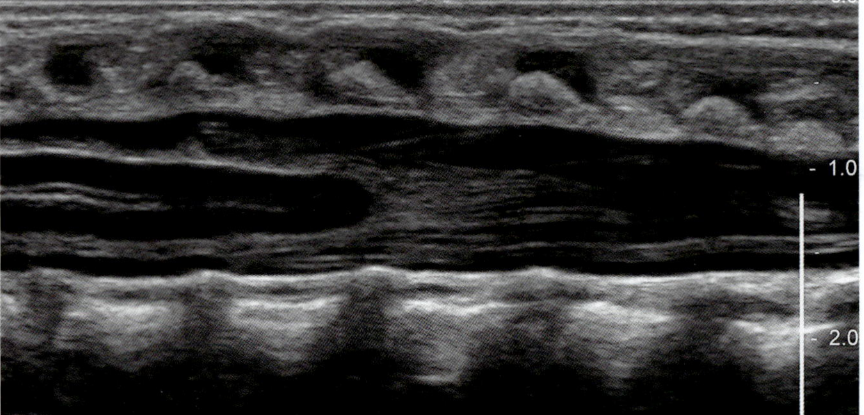

Fig. 21.8.32: Sagittal plane spinal sonography in caudal regression syndrome. The conus medullaris is seen as a club-shaped structure ending abruptly, without showing the normal tapering.

and the critical care scenario. MRI is a versatile imaging technique, with the main drawback of requirement of sedation/general anesthesia. CT scan is the workhorse of pediatric chest and oncologic imaging. Newer imaging techniques such as contrast-enhanced USG, rapid lung MRI, and advanced body MRI have added newer dimensions of pediatric imaging. The choice of imaging modality must be based on critical evaluation of the indication, limitations of the specific modality, and radiation burden.[9]

REFERENCES

1. Gupta AK, Garg A, Sandhu MS (Eds). Pediatric imaging. In: AIIMS-MAMC-PGI Imaging Series: Diagnostic radiology: Pediatric Imaging, 4th edition. New Delhi: Jaypee Brothers Medical Publishers (P) Ltd; 2020.
2. Coley BD (Ed). Caffey's Pediatric Diagnostic Imaging, 13th edition. St Louis: Mosby; 2019.
3. Gräfe D, Anders R, Prenzel F, Sorge I, Roth C, Benkert T, et al. Pediatric MR lung imaging with 3D ultrashort-TE in free breathing: Are we past the conventional T2 sequence? Pediatr Pulmonol. 2021;56(12):3899-907.
4. Mukhopadhyay S, Gupta AK. Imaging in Childhood Tuberculosis. In: Seth V (Ed). Essentials of Tuberculosis in Children. New Delhi: Jaypee Brothers Medical Publishers (P) Ltd.; 1997. pp. 240-63.
5. Sodhi KS, Kritsaneepaiboon S, Jana M, Bhatia A. Ultrasound and magnetic resonance imaging in thoracic tuberculosis in the pediatric population: moving beyond conventional radiology. Pediatr Radiol. 2023;53(12):2552-67.
6. Swischuk LE. Skeletal system and soft tissues. In: Swischuk LE (Ed). Imaging of the Newborn, Infant and Young Child, 4th edition. Philadelphia: Williams and Wilkins; 1997. pp. 678-892.
7. Tiidermann M, Pihlakas T, Saaring J, Märs J, Aasmäe J, Langemets K, et al. Improvement in paediatric CT use and justification: a single-centre experience. BJR Open. 2024;6(1):tzae020.
8. Barkovich AJ, Raybaud C. Pediatric Neuroimaging, 5th edition. Philadelphia: Lippincott Williams and Wilkins; 2011. pp. 367-568.
9. Furlow B. Radiation protection in pediatric imaging. Radiol Technol. 2011;82(5):421-39.

21.9 Environment and Child Health

Ramesh Bajania, D Balachandar

INTRODUCTION

Environmental hazards are among the top health concerns many parents have for their children. There is a felt need to provide more specific training about environmental hazards and parental concerns to medical professionals. The manner in which a child's body handles environmental toxic substances is dependent on the developmental age and genetic programming of the child.[1,2]

TYPES OF POLLUTION

Physical Environment

Anything that comes in contact with the body constitutes the physical environment, for example, air that is in contact with skin and lungs throughout day. It consists of the large geographical macroenvironment made up of smaller units (microenvironment). It differs for every child depending on his/her place of residence, whether the bedroom or kitchen in the house or the surrounding areas like school or road.

The microenvironment differs between children and adults. Mercury vapor is heavier than air and is not evenly dispersed in a room where air is contaminated with mercury. Higher concentration is present near the floor where an infant or child would be more active than an adult who is standing. The exposure and the amount of toxicants also differ for children of same age with different health effects. Preterm babies enduring longer periods of stay in neonatal intensive care units (NICUs) have higher exposure to light, noise, compressed gases, and diagnostic radiation, compared to healthy term babies. Thus, physical location, breathing zones, food consumption, and development of the child, all have a role to play.[1,2]

Added to these, nearly 352 million children between the ages of 5 and 12 years engage in economic activities. Around 50% of these children work in hazardous occupations with poor hygienic conditions, which adversely affect their growth and development, safety, and future health. Nearly 30% of global burden of disease can be attributed to environmental factors. Nearly, 36% of the overall disease burden is due to modifiable environmental risk factors in the age group of 0–4 years and 34% among children of 0–14 years.

Biological Environment

Absorption of pollutants may occur through transplacental, percutaneous, respiratory, and gastrointestinal (GI) routes.

- *Transplacental:* Fat-soluble pollutants and those with low molecular weight [e.g., carbon monoxide (CO)] and some elements (e.g., calcium and lead) can cross placenta.
- *Percutaneous:* Newborns and infants have a relatively large body surface area to body mass. The skin of the preterm newborn has a poor epidermal barrier with few cornified layers leading to increased permeability to exogenous chemicals. Thus, iodine present in povidone-iodine scrub solution may lead to hypothyroidism in a newborn. Hyperbilirubinemia can result from phenolic disinfectants used to clean hospital equipment.
- *Respiratory:* Lungs play a major role in exposure in children. Lungs develop by proliferation of alveoli up to the age of 8 years and later by alveolar expansion. Infants and young children are vulnerable to air pollution, which is associated with decrease in forced expiratory volume in 1 second (FEV_1).
- *Gastrointestinal (GI):* Newborns and infants have relatively less gastric acid secretion, which has an effect on absorption of chemicals. Low acidity also impairs normal bacterial overgrowth in gastrointestinal tract (GIT) resulting in abnormal absorption of some chemicals. The intestines of a child absorb more calcium from food than adults. Lead may be absorbed in place of calcium.

Metabolism

Metabolism results in activation or deactivation. These processes are dependent on developmental age and genetic susceptibility of the individual. These differences may either harm or protect a child from the environmental hazards.[1] **Table 21.9.1** highlights some of the special environmental health risks by stage of child development.

Social Environment

The vulnerability of children to environmental pollution begins with exposure to toxins and/or toxicants in intrauterine period—drugs, tobacco, lead, etc. (The term "toxicant" refers to a chemical agent whereas "toxin" refers to a biological agent.) Epidemiological studies have shown the causal relationship between prenatal and childhood exposure to environmental toxins and toxicants and adverse health effects in fetuses and children.[1] Children are at higher risk as they breathe more air and drink more water. The dosage of air pollutants and water contaminants that a child receives is much more compared with an adult living in the same environment.[1] The diversity and quantity of the food that children consume is another important factor.

TABLE 21.9.1: Special environmental health risks by developmental stage.

Developmental stage	*Time period*	*Health risks related to environmental exposure*
Embryonic period	8 days to 9 weeks of pregnancy	Thalidomide and phocomelia (day 34–50)
Fetal period	9 weeks of pregnancy to birth	In-utero radiation exposure and microcephaly and intellectual deficits (weeks 8–15)
Infancy	Birth to 12 months	• Mercury vapor and acrodynia • Nitrates and methemoglobinemia • Passive smoking and lung disease • Toxigenic molds and pulmonary hemorrhage
Young toddlers	1–2 years	Radiation and thyroid cancer
Older toddlers	2–3 years	Radiation and thyroid cancer
Preschoolers	3–5 years	Radiation and thyroid cancer
School-going children	5–12 years	Nicotine and addiction
Adolescents	12–18 years	Soot exposure and cancer of scrotum

Developing Body Systems

Most body systems in a child are in various stages of development, especially central nervous system (CNS), immunity, GIT, and reproductive system. There are certain windows during which environmental agents can induce irreversible damage. Moreover, unlike adults, children do not have control over their environment; they are explorative by nature, are often unaware of the risks and hazards, and are not in a position to make healthy informed choices on their own.

ENVIRONMENTAL ISSUES

The key environmental pollution problems that affect our children's health are listed in **Box 21.9.1**. The windows and timing of exposure to pollutants during fetal life have different impact as shown in **Table 21.9.2**.

BOX 21.9.1: Key environmental problems faced by children.

- *Air pollution:*
  - Outdoor air pollution
  - Indoor air pollution
- *Water pollution:*
  - Surface water pollution
  - Groundwater pollution
- *Chemical pollution:* Persistent organic pollutants (POPs)
- Noise pollution
- Exposure to radiation

TABLE 21.9.2: Timing and impact of pollutants during fetal period.

Timing	*Impact*
<2 weeks of gestation	Prenatal death and less prone to teratogenic effect
3–8 weeks of gestation	Major morphological abnormalities
After 8 weeks of gestation (fetal period)	Minor morphological abnormalities

AIR POLLUTION

Air pollutants produce ill effects on all systems of human body including behavioral changes. The lungs, being an organ with the largest surface area, receive the brunt of air pollution. Air pollution, outdoor or indoor, is responsible for respiratory infections, pneumonia, respiratory allergy, chronic pulmonary disease, and chronic cough.

Suspended particulate matter (PM) of 2.5 μm and tobacco smoke are the most dangerous pollutants, as they cross lung interstitium to bloodstream causing increase in cardiovascular disease, coagulopathy, insulin-resistant diabetes mellitus, dementia, autism, memory loss, and possible sudden infant death syndrome.[3] International Agency for Research on Cancer (IARC) classified air pollution as a carcinogen in 2013.[1] Air pollution not only triggers allergic airway diseases but also changes the genetic patterns.[3,4]

Outdoor Air Pollution

Outdoor air pollution consists of a complex mixture of pollutants found in ambient air that affects the health of individuals in all age groups. The detrimental effects begin at the preconception stage manifesting in newborn period and childhood and continue into adulthood. The common examples include asthma and respiratory disorders, but it can affect other body systems and even cause malignancy.[1] The potential health risks depend on composition of the pollutant, duration of exposure, age and health status of the child, and genetic makeup.[1]

The main sources of outdoor air pollution are:

- Emissions from automobile exhausts and highway vehicles
- Power-plant emissions
- Industrial emissions
- Open burning of solid wastes, especially in farming
- Construction-related activities
- Accumulated loose soil on the road-side
- Pollen, which is seasonal, or fungi in the atmosphere

Urban air pollution is largely caused by the combustion of fossil fuels for transport and automobile exhausts that are categorized into:

- *Substances that mainly affect the airways:* Oxides of nitrogen (NO_2), sulfur dioxide (SO_2), ozone (O_3), suspended particulate matter, and photochemical oxidants
- *Substances that produce a toxic effect:* CO and lead (Pb)
- *Substances with carcinogenic effect:* Polycyclic aromatic hydrocarbons and aldehydes

The US Environmental Protection Agency (EPA) categorizes air pollution into three major groups:[1]

1. *Criteria air pollutants* (ground-level ozone, respirable PM, SO_2, CO, NO_2, and lead). They are associated with low birthweight, prematurity, stillbirths, respiratory disorders, cardiovascular disorders, and immunological abnormalities.
2. *Toxic chemicals or hazardous air pollutants* released by motor vehicles, industrial facilities, wood combustion, agricultural activities, forest fires, volcanic eruptions, and other sources. They cause neoplasia and reproductive health issues including birth defects and exacerbate respiratory diseases.
3. *Greenhouse gases (GHG) or heat-trapping gases* released into atmosphere generated from burning of fossil fuels and other activities lead to climate change. They lead to bronchitis, asthma, stroke due to heatwave, and lung cancer.

The US EPA has established national ambient air quality standards (NAAQS) for criteria pollutants including O_3, respirable PM, lead, SO_2, CO, and NO_2 based on their effects on human health and environment.[1]

Ozone

Ozone (O_3) is the principal component of urban smog and is a secondary pollutant formed in the atmosphere from a photochemical reaction between volatile organic compounds and nitrogen oxides in the presence of sunlight **(Fig. 21.9.1)**. The primary sources of precursor chemicals include motor vehicle exhaust and emissions from power plants. Hydrocarbon emissions from chemical plants and refineries and evaporative emissions from gasoline and natural sources

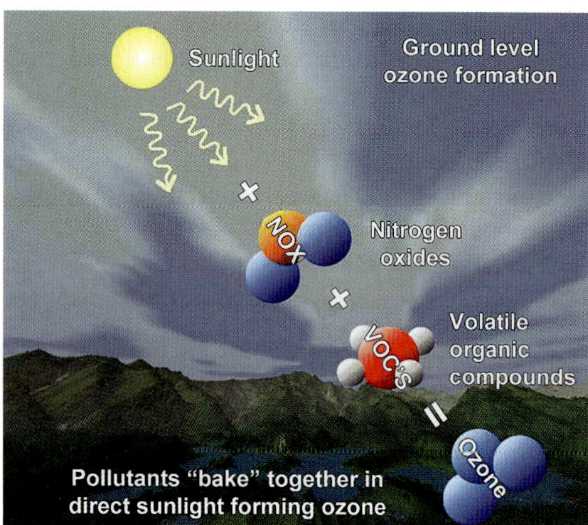

Fig. 21.9.1: Formation of ozone in the environment.

also may contribute to their formation. O_3 concentrations are high in hot dry stagnant summer days with an increase to maximum in the late afternoon. O_3 is an extreme irritant to respiratory tract. Recent observations from India showed an increase in prevalence of asthma, possibly due to production of O_3 from emission of slow-moving traffic in bright sunlight with oxygen.

Particulate Matter

Particulate matter refers to airborne mixture of solid particles and liquid droplets of varying composition and physical properties. Particle size is the primary determinant of whether the PM will be deposited in the lower respiratory tract. Particles <10 μm in aerodynamic diameter is known as PM10. PM2.5 results from combustion of fuels, power plants, combustion of organic material, and wooden stoves. Particles between PM2.5 and PM10 are termed coarse particles and particles below PM2.5 as fine particles, which remain suspended in the air for longer periods, with stronger respiratory effects in children.[5]

Lead

Leaded gasoline is an important source of lead exposure in children even though paints and soil continue to be generally more common sources. It can also come from ferrous and nonferrous melters and battery manufacturing units.[6]

Sulfur Compounds

Sulfur compounds include SO_2, sulfuric acid (H_2SO_4) aerosol, and sulfur particles. In addition to its adverse effects on respiratory system, they contribute to the formation of acid rain.

Carbon Monoxide and Nitrogen Dioxide

Carbon monoxide and NO_2 come usually from motor vehicle emissions and fuel combustion from power plants. NO_2 contributes to the formation of O_3 and nitrogen-bearing particles (nitrate and nitric acid).[1]

Toxic Air Pollutants

Toxic air pollutants represent a large group of substances including volatile organic compounds, metals (mercury), solvents, and combustion byproducts (dioxin). Currently, 187 substances that pose major health threats in urban areas are included in the list of hazardous air pollutants subject to emission regulations under the Clean Air Act, Section 30. Some compounds such as benzene, 1,4-butadiene, and diesel exhaust are emitted primarily from mobile vehicles. Other toxic air pollutants come from large stationary industrial facilities and contribute only to a small proportion of total toxic air exposure.[1]

Greenhouse Gases

Greenhouse gases or heat-trapping gases are released into atmosphere mainly from burning of fossil fuels and to a lesser extent from industrial activities, deforestation, and some agricultural practices. The production of many GHGs such as CO_2, methane, NO_2, hydrocarbons, perfluorocarbons, sulfur hexafluoride, and nitrogen trifluoride is regulated as they endanger public health.[1]

Indoor Air Pollution

Infants and young children spend a major part of their time (80–90%) indoors. The major sources of indoor air pollution include tobacco smoke, gas stoves, wood stoves, pets and pests, molds and other biologicals, furnishings, and construction materials.[7,8] Pediatricians evaluating children with respiratory and allergic disorders should consider exposure to an indoor pollutant as a possible etiology.[1]

Aerobiologicals

These include dust mites, fungi, molds, cockroaches, pollen, pets, and bacteria. Dust mites are microscopic organisms found in the dust that measure 0.1–0.5 mm in size. They are present in places with high humidity, on carpets, upholstered furniture, stuffed toys, woolen blankets, and mattresses. It takes about 100 dust mites/g of dust to develop sensitivity and 500 dust mites/g of dust to develop wheezing. Dust mite concentration varies inversely with altitude. Around 50% of persistent asthma is caused by dust mite allergy.[7,8] About 25% of persistent asthmatics are sensitive to cockroaches. Asthma episodes increase during festivals like *Diwali* by 100%

due to increase of SO_2 in the atmosphere due to burning of crackers.[3,4,7,8]

Pollen and fungi produce allergy in 7.5% of children. Pollen concentration will increase in the atmosphere when the temperature is high, humidity is low, and the wind speed is 1 km/h. The tree pollen is found between April and June, grass pollen between July and November, and weed pollen between November and January.[7]

Only 5% of urban and 7.5% of rural children own pets; of these, 80% are dogs and they are not a major cause of allergy in India. Cat's urine and saliva are more allergic.

Irritants

The source and effects of various irritants are described in **Table 21.9.3**. Children coming from urban ill-ventilated homes, exposed to tobacco smoke, and dirty fuel usage for cooking have more prevalence of asthma.[3,4,7]

Combustion Pollutants

These are released at home from gas ranges and gas heat (when they malfunction or are used as space heaters), or improperly vented wood stoves and fireplaces. Combustion leads to emission of NO_2 and CO. Levels increase usually in winter months with the indoor concentrations reaching double of that in summer. Cooking or heating with wood leads to emission of suspended droplets, suspended particles, and gases such as NO_2 and SO_2. The aerosol mixture of this "smoke" contains particles <10 μm in diameter.[1]

TABLE 21.9.3: Source and effect of irritants.

Irritant	*Source*	*Effect on newborns and children*
Tobacco smoke (major indoor pollutant)[3,4,7,8]	Prenatal maternal exposure (active or passive smoking)	• Low birth weight • Increased infant mortality • Decreased lung function • Increased wheeze • Decreased resistance to respiratory infections
	Postnatal parental smoking	• Improper lung development • Decreased forced expiratory volume at 1 second (FEV_1) • Increased lung hyperreactivity • Persistent wheeze • Asthma exacerbation • Otitis media
Formaldehyde (colorless gas)	Plywood, furniture, tobacco smoke, poorly vented wood, and gas stoves	• Headache • Respiratory tract irritation • Pneumonia • Pulmonary edema
Combustion byproducts (particles, carbon monoxide, carbon dioxide, nitric oxide, nitrogen dioxide, and partially oxidized organic substances)	Combustion of gases, wood-burning stoves, tobacco smoke, poorly ventilated fire places, heaters, and automobile exhausts	• Blurred vision • Drowsiness • Emphysema • Respiratory infection • Asthma • Decreased lung capacity • Death from carbon monoxide poisoning
Cleaning agents and aerosol	Hair sprays, fabric softeners, paints, perfumes, and deodorants	• Irritation of mucous membranes of respiratory tract and eyes • Headache • Mental confusion • Abdominal pain • Triggering of asthma

Air Quality Index

Most metropolitan areas regularly monitor air quality for one or more of the NAAQS. The air quality index (AQI) converts the concentration of 5 specific pollutants (O_3, CO, NO_2, SO_2, and particulate matter) into a number scale from 0 to 500. The AQI is graded as follows:

- *0–50:* Good
- *51–100:* Moderate
- *101–150:* Unhealthy for sensitive groups
- *151–200:* Unhealthy
- *201–300:* Very unhealthy
- *301–500:* Hazardous.

Other Air Pollutants

Traffic-related Air Pollutants and Diesel Exhaust

Traffic emissions are usually complex mixtures and contain numerous respiratory irritants and carcinogens. Traffic pollution induces airway and systemic inflammation and increased airway responsiveness. Studies from USA and Europe have shown the association of an increase in respiratory symptoms and asthma (symptoms and hospitalizations) in areas with high traffic density. Epidemiological studies have confirmed the harm induced by diesel fumes in children leading to development of new allergies and allergic asthma.[1]

Odors

Odors negatively affect the quality of life and exacerbate health problems. Hydrogen sulfide (H_2S), a common air pollutant is emitted as a part of industrial processes. Other sources of odorous air pollution include sewage treatment plants, landfills, composts, livestock feeding lots, tanneries, and geothermal plants.[1]

Occupational Lung Diseases

Children who are exposed to various minerals and chemicals such as silica, asbestos, coal dust, cement, chalk, mica, and iron oxide for long periods of time because of their parent's occupation may suffer from pneumoconiosis, interstitial fibrosis, etc.

Preventive Measures for Air Pollution[2]

The preventive measures for air pollution are as follows:

- Control of automobile emissions by using more public transport and better-quality fuels
- Control of outdoor and indoor pollution
- Use of clean fuel for cooking
- Construction of houses with good cross-ventilation
- Avoid tobacco smoke—most dangerous pollutant
- Drying of mattresses, pillows, and blankets in the sunshine once a week
- Use indoor plants, expose them to sunlight once a week and remove water from trays
- Control of cockroaches and better garbage disposal
- Long-term urban transport planning, certification of in-use vehicles, car-pooling, better traffic management
- Monitoring of hot spots in the city, air quality index (AQI) checks, and avoiding overcrowded places
- Coordination of various municipal and utility services
- Use of better technology to reduce emissions
- Alternatives for fossil fuels
- Education of children, society, and policymakers on the adverse effects of air pollution

WATER POLLUTION

Although 70% of the earth is covered by water, only 3% of the earth's water is fresh. Of that two-thirds is frozen in glaciers and ice caps, leaving only 1% available for human use. Fresh water is classified as either groundwater (0.7%) or surface water such as lakes and rivers (0.3%).[5]

Sources of Surface Water Pollution

Water pollution results from sources of contamination termed either point or nonpoint. Point sources of pollution are municipal wastewater treatment plant discharges and industrial wastewater discharges into the surface. Nonpoint sources are more difficult to identify and control, which include agricultural runoff, urban runoff, soil contamination, and atmospheric deposition.[5] Other sources of contamination include:

- Human and animal wastes
- Sewage
- Storm water runoff
- Industrial discharges
- Cross-media contamination, movement of pollution
- From air to water
- Pesticides and fertilizers drifting during the rainy season

Sources of Groundwater Pollution

They are categorized as biological agents, chemicals, and radionuclides, for example, radon.[5] They include industrial waste pits, discharge of effluents on land, septic tanks, oil wells, and chemicals in groundwater.

Health Hazards of Water Pollution

Several constituents of groundwater contamination due to industrial clusters are caused by electroplating units, tanneries, dyeing, printing units, distilleries, and paper mills. The heavy metal and toxic compounds present in the effluent may pose considerable health risks to the population using such contaminated water. Unfortunately, about 69% of people equate visual cleanliness with safe water.

- *Waterborne diseases:* Water contaminated by fecal matter and urine may produce gastroenteritis, dysentery, amebiasis, cholera, typhoid, paratyphoid, and viral hepatitis. Gastroenteritis is the second biggest killer of the children under the age of 5 years. India displays a high rate of open defecation practices (16%) compared with both the regional average (12%) and the global average (6%). Even today, around 80% of the rural population and 60% of the urban slum population practice open defecation.
- *Water-related vector-borne disease:* Examples of diseases transmitted by the bite of mosquitoes are malaria, dengue fever, Japanese encephalitis, and filarial disease.
- *Water-based disease:* Examples of diseases transmitted by aquatic invertebrate animals and stagnant water contaminated by rat urine are leptospirosis, guinea-worm, and schistosomiasis. The incidence of leptospirosis is increasing in urban slum areas, especially during the rainy season.
- *Water-based chemical diseases:* The major chemicals that enter and contaminate the water are fluoride, arsenic, nitrites, mercury, and lead. Their effects are described in **Table 21.9.4**.

The fetus may be exposed to pollutants when a pregnant mother ingests foods of aquatic food chain in which methyl mercury and polychlorinated biphenyls (PCB) accumulate and are not readily excreted.[5]

Waterborne diseases spread more rapidly in urban communities, where the density of population is higher with no or poor access to water. The World Health Organization (WHO) guidelines for good potable water is the *Escherichia coli* count which should be <10 microbes/100 mL (still low risk) and a higher count always indicates fecal contamination.

Public Health Education to Prevent Water Pollution

Public health education to prevent water pollution include:

- Education of public about use of safe drinking water and toilet hygiene
- Use of water filters
- Prevention of waste production and pollution

TABLE 21.9.4: Chemicals contaminating water and their effects.[5,6]

Chemical	*Mechanism*	*Ill effects*
Fluoride (F)	Affects 6 million children <14 years	Dental fluorosis
	Drinking water with >0.7 mg fluoride/L (US EPA)	• Skeletal fluorosis • Nonskeletal fluorosis
Arsenic (As)	Ingesting water with arsenic content >0.01 mg/L over a period of 5–15 years	• Skin rashes and hyperkeratosis • Cancer of lungs, bladder, and kidneys
Mercury (Hg)	All mercury in India is imported, and used in equipment, batteries, and thermometers	*Major health effects:* Psychological, GIT cramps, and colitis
	Poisoning occurs by ingestion and inhalation	• Persistent cough, emphysema, asthma, and sinusitis • Excessive perspiration • Alzheimer disease and Parkinson's disease • Autism also reported
Nitrites	Seepage from septic tanks, pit latrines, and organic manures into groundwater	• Ingestion of water with >45 mg/L of nitrites—"blue-baby syndrome" and methemoglobinemia • Chronic ingestion and cancer
Lead (Pb)[6]	Ingestion of water from lead pipes, soil, solder, food containers, paint, and insecticides	*Lead level >10 µg/dL in blood:* Progressive GIT, hematologic, peripheral, and central nervous system involvement
	Inhalation of polluted air from leaded petrol, battery storage, crystal glass, ceramic glazes, enamel jewelry, plastic and rubber stabilizers, *surma*, and vermilion	• Anorexia, abdominal pain, and vomiting • Anemia and blue line in gums • Headache, seizures, and altered sensorium • Peripheral neuropathy • Behavioral disturbances • Lower IQ and poor school performance

(GIT: gastrointestinal tract; IQ: intelligence quotient)

- Prevention of waste from various sources entering water and protecting the source of water
- Water storage at home should be covered.
- Avoid using dirty hands or implements to fetch water.
- Drinking water can be purified by chlorination, boiling, slow sand filters, and solar disinfection.
- To reduce hazards from fish consumption, eat small and pan fish rather than predator fish like sharks or tuna. Fatty fishes like mackerel and catfish, which accumulate high levels of chemical pollutants, should be consumed in less amounts. Trim skin and fatty areas where contaminants accumulate but with no effect on removing methyl mercury.

CHEMICAL POLLUTION

Persistent Organic Pollutants

Persistent organic pollutants (POPs) are man-made organic pollutants and are the most dangerous and hazardous compounds to be synthesized. They include pesticides, industrial chemicals, chemicals used in consumer products, and byproducts of certain manufacturing and combustion processes. They have long half-lives, and hence persist in the environment for years or decades. They bioaccumulate and penetrate the food chain thus, polluting and exposing all living things.

They disperse universally and travel in air, water currents, and in living organisms. Most POPs are lipophilic and remain in fat tissue, not well-metabolized or excreted; even small doses ingested daily accumulate to measurable amounts over time. They are endocrine disruptors, mimic, modify, or block the actions of naturally occurring hormones as listed in **Table 21.9.5**. Prenatal exposuret of pesticides negatively affects fetal

TABLE 21.9.5: Reported signs and symptoms by age from chemicals.

Prenatal exposure to low levels of PCB	*Ill effects*
Newborns and infants	Decrease in birth weight, motor delay, and defects in visual recognition memory
4-year-olds	Defects in short-term memory
9–12-year-olds	Lower IQs and delay in cognition
Prenatal exposure to high levels of PCB, PCDF, and DDT	***Ill effects***
Newborns and infants	Low birth weight, conjunctivitis, natal teeth, pigmentation, behavioral disorders, and increased risk of bronchitis
Puberty	Small size penis, growth delay

(DDT: dichlorodiphenyltrichloroethane; IQ: intelligence quotient; PCBs: polychlorinated biphenyls; PCDF: polychlorinated dibenzofurans)

growth in the form of smaller head circumference and shorter birth length.

The major sources of human exposure are food, soil, indoor environment, toys and other objects, air, and leaching from medical products. Infants and children are more heavily exposed than adults. Ingestion is the principal route of exposure to POPs as children eat more food/kg body weight than adults. POPs cross placenta and maternal consumption of foods with high POPs even before pregnancy can result in exposure in utero. Human milk is, therefore, a source of exposure for infants. Infant formula is free of POPs because the lipid in formula comes from coconuts. Workers who apply the pesticides and residents of sprayed houses can have high exposures.[9,10]

The important organic chlorine pesticides developed after dichlorodiphenyltrichloroethane (DDT) and widely used after World War II include aldrin, dieldrin, endrin, chlordane, heptachlor, indane, and pentachlorophenol. They helped a great deal in agriculture, which helped the world economy. Once adverse effects due to their persistence and accumulation in the environment became known, most were discontinued. The "dirty dozen", 12 widespread, highly toxic POPs include aldrin, chlordane, DDT, dieldrin, endrin, heptachlor, hexachlorobenzene, mirex, polychlorinated biphenyls (PCB), polychlorinated dibenzodioxins (PCDD), polychlorinated dibenzofurans (PCDF), and toxaphene. Recent additions include chlordecone, beta-hexachlorocyclohexane, hexabromobiphenyl, lindane, pentachlorobenzene, tetra and pentabromodiphenyl ether, perfluorooctanoic acid (PFOA) and perfluoro octane sulfonic acid (PFOS).[9,10]

PLASTICS AND POLLUTION

Plastics are the most used material in our day-to-day life. They are light, thermo- and chemical resistant, of low cost, strong, and tough. Annual usage of plastic bags in the world is 500 trillion tons. Asia contributes 80% of total plastic leakage to ocean and 4 lakh marine mammals perish annually.

Plastics are made of two compounds:

1. *Polymers or resins (bulk of plastic):*
   a. Polyvinyl chloride (PVC)
   b. Polycarbonate (PC)
   c. High-density polyethylene (HDPE)
   d. Polypropylene (PP)
2. *Plasticizers (additive):*
   a. Phthalates for more flexibility
   b. Bisphenol A (BPA) for more rigidity

Table 21.9.6 lists the sources of phthalates and bisphenols and their effects on the environment.

TABLE 21.9.6: Impact of plasticizers.

Phthalates	***Bisphenols A (BPA)***
• They migrate to the surface of plastics • They either evaporate or leach into the surroundings • They are the most abundant industrial pollutants of the environment	• They are used for production of polycarbonate hand plastic and to make resins to line the metal and beverage cans • With heat, they leach from the source to adjacent materials—water and food from the lining of the cans
Source: Food packaging, food contamination, plastic toys, medical tubings, wall coverings, tablecloths, upholstery, deodorants, insecticides, nail polish, and adhesives	*Source:* Food and beverage cans, gel capsules, cosmetics, flame retardants
Route of exposure: Phthalate leaches out from the above products in high concentration when they are heated	*Route of exposure:* • By inhalation • Ingestion • Skin absorption • Blood through intravenous route by tubings • Transplacental, from maternal bisphenol A

Diseases from Plastics

The following diseases are caused by the plastics:

- *Endocrine-disrupting chemicals with effects in fetal and early postnatal development of male reproductive tract:* Abnormalities such as undescended testes and hypospadias and decreased fertility
- Changes in immune system and inflammatory changes
- Acts as thyroid hormone antagonist
- Behavioral changes
- Early puberty
- Adult-onset diabetes mellitus
- Cancer

Safety Measures for Plastic Use

Figure 21.9.2 shows the safety codes for use of plastic in industry. Safety testing of new chemicals before they are put into market seems ideal, but the long-term hazards of new chemicals until after they have been released into the environment, will not be known. **Table 21.9.7** lists the dos and don'ts of plastics.

NOISE POLLUTION

Unpleasant sounds are called "noise" which affects 800 million people globally. India has the largest deaf population in the world and noise pollution is known to be one of the

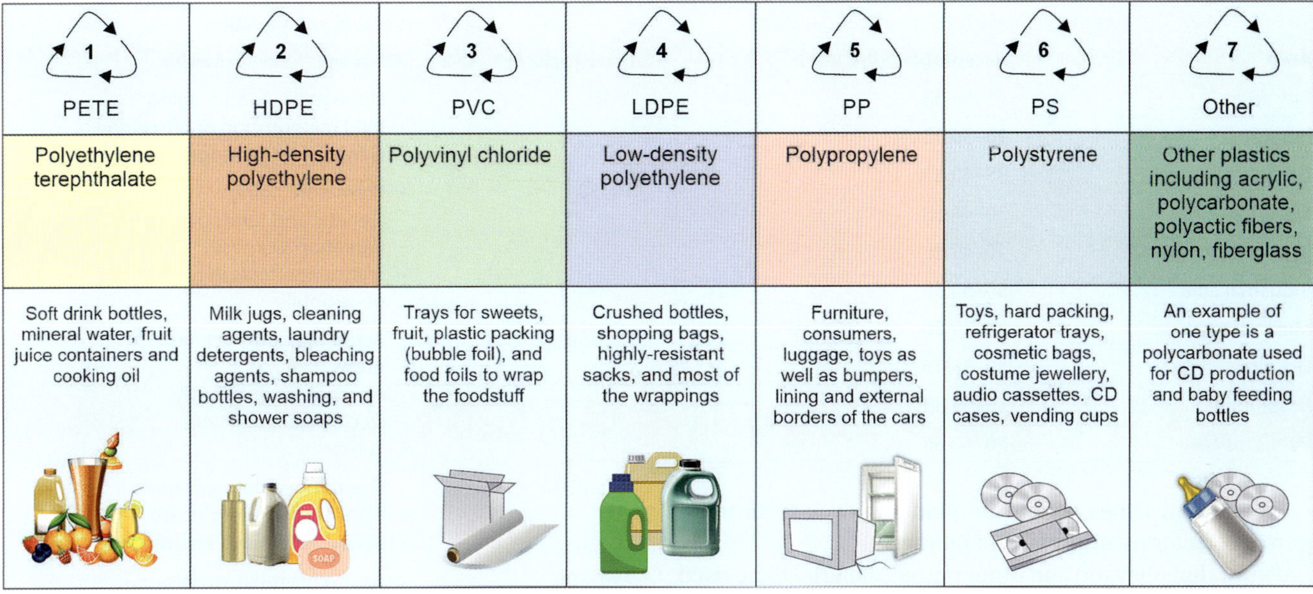

Fig. 21.9.2: Safety codes for use of plastics.

TABLE 21.9.7: Do's and don'ts of plastics.

Do's	*Don'ts*
• Look at recycling code on the bottom of the product to find out the plastic type • Use plastic code 1, 2, 4, and 5, which are considered as safer • Use No. 7 also if it is labeled as "Bio-based or greenware" • Use alternatives—glass and steel cups • Buy phthalate-free toys • Wooden furniture is always better	• Avoid plastic codes 3, 6, and 7 (bisphenol A) • Avoid microwaving the food and drinks in plastics • Avoid dishwashers • Avoid clear plastic bottles • Avoid boiling plastic bottles

significant causes. Environmental noise is one of the many stresses experienced by infants admitted to NICU. American Academy of Pediatrics (AAP) suggests an upper limit of 45 decibels for NICUs and PICUs.[11] The major chronic effect of noise-induced hearing loss depends on the cumulative effect of the magnitude of sound and the duration of exposure.

Noise may be broadly classified as:

- *Industrial noise:* This includes noise from machines in factories, industries, and mills. Significant among them are noise from mechanical saws and pneumatic drills.
- *Transport noise:* This includes road, railway, and air traffic noise.
- *Community noise:* This includes noise from musical instruments, indiscriminate use of amplifiers, and other gadgets in commercial establishments.

TABLE 21.9.8: Psychological and physical effects of different decibel (dB) levels.

Noise level	*Effects*
135 dB	Painful
110 dB	Discomfort
88 dB	Hearing impairment on prolonged exposure
80 dB	Annoying
65 dB	Intrusive

Psychological and physical effects of different decibel levels are given in **Table 21.9.8**.

The acceptable noise level in residential areas is given in **Table 21.9.9.**

The background noise level has increased over the last few decades. The noise level appears to double every decade. An audiological evaluation (pure tone audiometry) should be performed in those with history of excessive environmental noise exposure, poor school performance, short attention span, sensation of ringing in the ears, and speech delay, even if there is no history of acute suppurative otitis media (ASOM) or serous otitis media.[11]

Remedial Measures

The remedial measures include:

- Effective noise control programs in industries and use of protective aids.
- Plantation of trees near schools, hospitals, public offices, and libraries to reduce noise by 6–10 dB

TABLE 21.9.9: The acceptable noise level in residential areas.

Area	*Acceptable noise level*
City area	45–55 dB
Rural area	25–30 dB
Urban residential	35–40 dB
Suburban areas	30–40 dB
Urban business	40–45 dB
Industrial area	50–60 dB
Music theater	30–35 dB
Hospitals	30–35 dB
Restaurants	50–55 dB
Public offices	50–60 dB

- Residential zones should be planned away from main roads, factories, airports, and railways.
- Perforated plywood and other porous material to be used for office floors or ceilings.
- Implementation of noise control regulation on automobiles, social and religious functions, and prayer halls.

RADIATION HAZARDS

Radiation is the emission of energy (as electromagnetic waves) or particle matter from unstable atoms. Some types of radiation are harmful to life while others such as heat energy are beneficial.

Source of Radioactive Substances

Natural sources of ionizing radiation are the most common and include cosmic rays from space and radioactive minerals. In source areas, the gas radon found in soil, rocks, building materials, and granite stone is highly radioactive. Artificial sources of ionizing radiation are external sources including X-ray machines, radioactive isotopes used in diagnosis, and treatment of illnesses, and nuclear reactors. Internal sources include radioactive fallout (ingested in contaminated milk/vegetables) or dermally contaminating or medical radioisotopes (injected or implanted). Risk of cancer associated with most diagnostic radiation is low.[12]

Systemic Effects

Acute radiation syndrome (ARS) is an acute illness resulting from a substantial exposure (>70 rads) to the body. Gastrointestinal syndrome manifests as nausea, vomiting, diarrhea, and anorexia, which occur within minutes to days following exposure. This may progress to mucositis, parotitis, weight loss, infection, dehydration, and electrolyte imbalance. Hemopoietic syndrome manifests within a few hours with reduced lymphocyte and platelet counts.

TABLE 21.9.10: Ill effects of ionizing radiation.

Dose exposure (REM)	*Adverse effects on health*
0–10	• None to premature aging • Mild malnutrition of offspring • Genetic and teratogenic effects
10–50	• Premature aging • Genetic and teratogenic effects • Radiation sickness • Transient effects in lymphocytes and neutrophils
50–150	• Acute radiation sickness • Burns • Abortion and stillbirths • Decreased leukocytes • Tumors
150–250	• Gastrointestinal symptoms • Fetal or embryonic death • Serious infections and death
250–600	• Gastrointestinal symptoms • Loss of hair • Bleeding from gastrointestinal, renal, and nasal sites • Marked destruction of bone marrow leading to death
600–1,000	• Destruction of GI system • Respiratory, hemopoietic, endocrine spleen, and genital problems • Bleeding diathesis and death
>2000	Circulatory system and CNS

(CNS: central nervous system; GI: gastrointestinal; REM: radiation equivalent of mean)

Cutaneous syndrome results from damage of the basal layer of skin with inflammation, erythema, dry or moist desquamation, and epilation over a period of time.[12] The ill effects of ionizing radiation depending on the amount of exposure are summarized in **Table 21.9.10**.

REFERENCES

1. American Academy of Pediatrics Council on Environmental Health. Children's unique vulnerabilities to environmental hazards. In: Etzel RA (Ed). Pediatric Environmental Health, 4th Edition. Itasca, IL: American Academy of Pediatrics; 2019. pp. 8-36.
2. Ratageri VH, Paramesh H. Environmental health of children: Time to translate knowledge into action. Indian J Pediatr. 2018;85(4):282-3.
3. Paramesh H. Asthma and the environment. Indian J Pediatr. 2006;73 (Suppl):S51-5.
4. Paramesh H. Epidemiology of asthma in India. Indian J Pediatr. 2002;69(4):309-12.
5. American Academy of Pediatrics Council on Environmental Health. Drinking Water. In: Etzel RA (Ed). Pediatric Environmental Health, 4th Edition; Itasca, IL: American Academy of Pediatrics; 2019. pp. 277-95.

6. World Health Organization. (2010). Childhood Lead Poisoning. [online] Available from https://iris.who.int/bitstream/handle/10665/136571/9789241500333_eng.pdf [last accessed December, 2024].
7. Paramesh H. Asthma in children: Seasonal Variation. Int J Environ Health. 2008;2(3/4):410-6.
8. Paramesh H. Air pollution and allergic airway diseases: Social determinants and sustainability in the control and prevention. Indian J Pediatr. 2018;85(4):284-94.
9. American Academy of Pediatrics Council on Environmental Health. Persistent organic pollutants. In: Etzel RA (Ed). Pediatric Environmental Health, 4th Edition; Itasca, IL: American Academy of Pediatrics; 2019. pp. 656-62.
10. World Health Organization. (2010). Persistent Organic Pollutants: Impact on Child Health. Geneva. [online] Available from https://www.who.int/publications/i/item/persistent-organic-pollutants-impact-on-child-health [Last accessed December, 2024].
11. American Academy of Pediatrics Council on Environmental Health. Noise. In: Etzel RA, ed. Pediatric Environmental Health, 4th Edition; Itasca, IL: American Academy of Pediatrics; 2019. p. 611.
12. American Academy of Pediatrics Council on Environmental Health. Ionizing Radiation. In: Etzel RA, ed. Pediatric Environmental Health, 4th Edition; Itasca, IL: American Academy of Pediatrics; 2019. p. 533.

SECTION

Community Pediatrics

Section Editor: Alok Gupta

22.1 Vital Statistics

Joseph L Mathew

INTRODUCTION

The term "vital statistics" refers to "systemically collected and compiled data about vital events of life particularly birth and death". Sometimes these include information about additional important events such as marriage, divorce, and adoption. In many ways, these sociodemographic data directly and indirectly reflect the health profile of a community. They can also reflect the adequacy of health services such as family planning, maternal and reproductive health, and immunization programs in a community. The data are also the basis for projections on population growth and time trends. They are also used for the construction of life tables.

A vital statistics system is formally defined as the process of:

- Collection of information on the occurrence of specified and defined vital events, characteristics of the events, and the person(s) concerned
- Compilation, processing, analysis, and evaluation of the data in conventional statistical formats

The vital statistics data collected are represented as indicators that convert the absolute numbers to rates. These are useful for comparing data from different areas and time frames. **Table 22.1.1** summarizes the key vital statistics indicators and the calculation for these.[1-6]

Vital statistics are usually collected and compiled by government agencies, which record the births and deaths

TABLE 22.1.1: Key vital statistics indicators.[1-6]

Vital statistics indicator	*Calculation*
Crude birth rate (CBR)	(Number of live births during the year/mid-year population) × 1,000
Crude death rate (CDR)	(Number of deaths during the year/mid-year population) × 1,000
Age-specific mortality rate (ASMR)	(Number of deaths in a particular age-group/mid-year population of the same age-group) × 1,000
Under-five mortality rate	The probability that a child born in a specific year or period will die before reaching the age of 5 years, subject to current ASMRs
Infant mortality rate (IMR)	(Number of infant deaths during the year/number of live births during the year) × 1,000
Neonatal mortality rate (NMR)	(Number of infant deaths of <28 days during the year/number of live births during the year) × 1,000
Early neonatal mortality rate	(Number of infant deaths of <7 days during the year/number of live births during the year) × 1,000
Late neonatal mortality rate	(Number of infant deaths of 7 days to <28 days during the year/number of live births during the year) × 1,000
Post-neonatal mortality rate (PNMR)	(Number of infant deaths between 28 days and 1 year during the year/number of live births during the year) × 1,000
Perinatal mortality rate (PMR)	(Number of stillbirths and infant deaths of <7 days during the year/number of live births and stillbirths during the year) × 1,000
Stillbirth rate	(Number of stillbirths during the year/number of live births and stillbirths during the year) × 1,000
General fertility rate (GFR)	(Number of live births in a year/mid-year female population in the age-group 15–49 years) × 1,000
Age-specific fertility rate (ASFR)	(Number of live births in a particular age-group/mid-year female population of the same age-group) × 1,000
Total fertility rate (TFR)	5 × (Sum of ASFR for the age-groups, 15–19, 20–24, 25–29 etc.)/1,000. The average number of children a woman would have when she passed through her reproductive years bearing children at the same rates as the women now in each age-group. It is calculated by summing the age specific fertility rates for all ages. If 5 years age-groups are used, then ASFR is multiplied by 5
Age-specific marital fertility rate (ASMFR)	(Number of live births in a particular age-group)/(mid-year married female population of the same age-group) × 1,000

Contd...

Contd...

Vital statistics indicator	***Calculation***
General marital fertility rate (GMFR)	(Number of live births in a year)/(mid-year married female population in the age-group 15–49 years) × 1,000
Total marital fertility rate (TMFR)	5 × (sum of ASMFR for the age-groups 15–19, 20–24, 25–29, etc.)/1,000
Maternal mortality ratio (MMR)	MMR is the ratio of the number of maternal deaths during a given period per 100,000 live births during the same time period. A maternal death refers to a female death from any cause related to or aggravated by pregnancy or its management (excluding accidental or incidental causes) during pregnancy and childbirth or within 42 days of termination of pregnancy, irrespective of the duration, and site of the pregnancy
Maternal mortality rate	Total number of maternal deaths as a proportion of the women in the age-group 15–49, expressed per 100,000 women in that age-group
Lifetime risk	The probability that at least one woman of reproductive age (15–49 years) will die due to childbirth or puerperium assuming that chance of death is uniformly distributed across the entire reproductive span 1– [1– (maternal mortality rate/100,000)]

within a given jurisdiction. In India, the main sources for vital statistics data are from:
- The population census
- Civil Registration System (CRS) records of vital events
- Sample Registration System (SRS)
- Demographic surveys conducted by the National Sample Surveys Organization (NSSO)
- Health surveys such as the National Family Health Survey (NFHS) and District Level Household and Facility Surveys (DLHS)

CIVIL REGISTRATION SYSTEM

The CRS is often referred to as the birth and death registration system. Registration of births, deaths, and stillbirths, within 21 days of the event, is mandatory under the provisions of the Registration of Births and Deaths Act, 1969.[1]

For births and deaths occurring at home, the onus of timely registration rests on the head of the household or nearest relative [in the absence of such person(s), the oldest male person present is responsible]. However, there are additional prescribed notifiers such as Anganwadi workers, auxiliary nurse midwife (ANMs), accredited social health activists (ASHAs), and others. For events occurring in health-care facilities (hospital, health center, or other such institutions), the medical officer in-charge or any person authorized by him/her is responsible. Additional persons responsible for reporting deaths include caretakers of crematoria and burial grounds. Thus, the goal is to ensure that no event is missed from being recorded. Although the CRS is primarily designed for legal purposes, it serves as an important resource for epidemiological and statistical data also.

The most recent vital statistics of India based on the CRS was published in May 2022, and included data till the year 2020.[1,2] Analysis of the total number of births and deaths

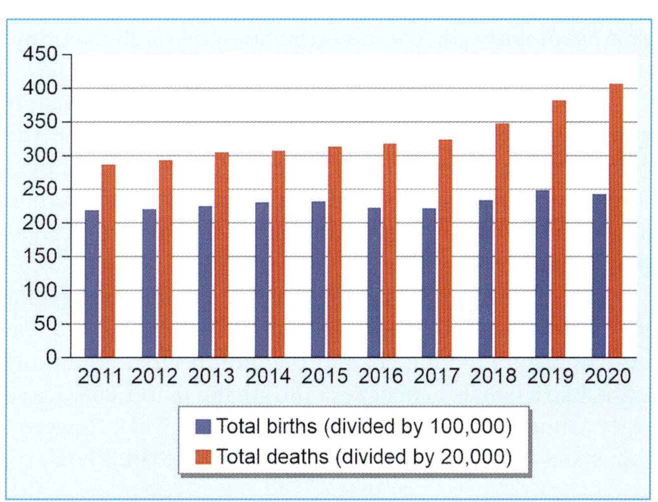

Fig. 22.1.1: The trend of total births and total deaths registered in India during the recent decade (2011–2020). Please note that the total births have been divided by 100,000 and the total deaths by 20,000 for ease of visualization.

over a decade (2011–2020) reveals a steady increase in births during 2011–2015, followed by decline during 2016 and 2017, and then an increase during 2018 and 2019. However, it again declined in 2020. In contrast, the number of deaths rose steadily during the decade from 2011 to 2020. The trends are shown in **Figure 22.1.1**.

The difference in the trends of birth and death can be better appreciated by comparing the change from the previous year, for both the vital statistics. This is shown in **Figure 22.1.2** wherein each vertical bar represents the percentage change over the preceding year. The data suggest a year-on-year increase in the total registered deaths, but no clearly discernible trend in births.

On the one hand, these data can be regarded as robust since they are collected from almost 300,000 registration units across the country. Further, the national level of reporting is greater than 95% in both rural as well as urban areas. On the other hand, state-wise analysis of the reporting presents a somewhat different picture. Only 15 states/union territories had a birth registration rate (within the prescribed 21 days period) of greater than 90%. Eleven states/union territories showed a registration rate between 50 and 90%, and seven had a registration rate of 50% or lower. Nagaland and Arunachal Pradesh had birth registration rates in single-digit figures. This makes it difficult to determine whether the published data are truly representative of the overall vital statistics of the country.

Further, among the registered births, the proportion of male births is significantly higher than female births (52% vs. 48%). Among the registered deaths, the proportion of males was 1.5 times higher than females (60.2% vs. 39.8%). This again raises the question whether the overall data truly represent the national vital statistics.

Among the deaths that occurred in the year 2020, infants contributed to 1.8% of the total. However, here also the completeness of reporting is called into question, as over three quarters of the registered infant deaths were from urban areas. This indirectly suggests that infant deaths in rural areas may be underreported.

The 2022 report did not provide the national average for the "sex ratio at birth". However, state-wise data showed that only one state among 28, and one union territory among eight, had a female to male sex ratio greater than 1,000. These were Arunachal Pradesh and Ladakh, respectively. However, four states did not contribute data. These were Uttar Pradesh, Delhi, Maharashtra, and Sikkim. The absence of data from states with large populations and large birth cohorts, make it difficult to calculate a national average.

SAMPLE REGISTRATION SYSTEM

Despite the mandatory provisions to register births, deaths, and stillbirths through the CRS, the need for reliable data led to the initiation of the SRS, almost six decades back. The SRS relies on two sources of data. The first is the "field investigation" wherein births and deaths are counted in a sample of villages/urban blocks by an enumerator. The second is an independent 6-monthly retrospective survey by a supervisor. The data obtained through these two sources are matched; and nonmatching data are verified. The sampling frame for the SRS is revised every 10 years.[3] The current frame is in use since 2014 and is based on the national census of 2011. **Figure 22.1.3** shows the progressively enlarging sampling frame for the SRS since its inception to the current time.

The SRS in India is widely recognized as the world's single largest demographic survey. It covered nearly 1.5 million households with a total population over 7 million, spread over almost all districts in India. **Table 22.1.2** summarizes the main components of SRS in India.

The data from the SRS are also used to compile "life tables". Currently, the tables for the period 2016–2020 are available. Life expectancy at birth is estimated at 70.0 years for the country as a whole. However, there is an almost 5 years' difference between the expectancy is rural areas (68.6 years) compared to urban areas (73.2 years). The life expectancy at birth is lower for males (68.6 years) compared to females (71.4 years). The life tables also provide life expectancy at different ages, and also by state, gender, and residence.[4]

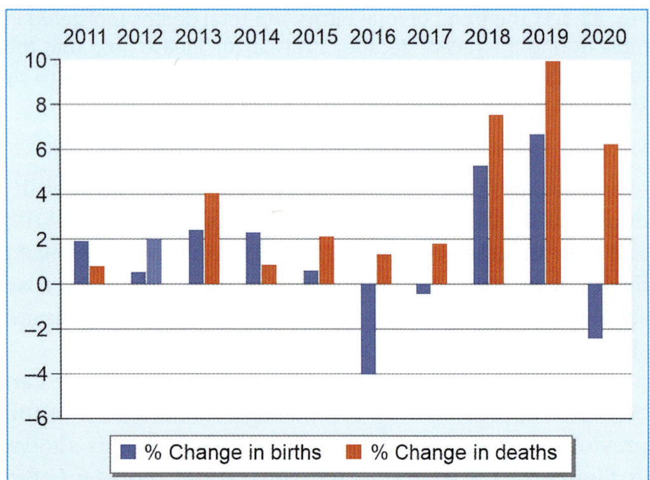

Fig. 22.1.2: The trend of total births and total deaths registered in India during the recent decade (2011–2020) presented as a percentage change from the preceding year.

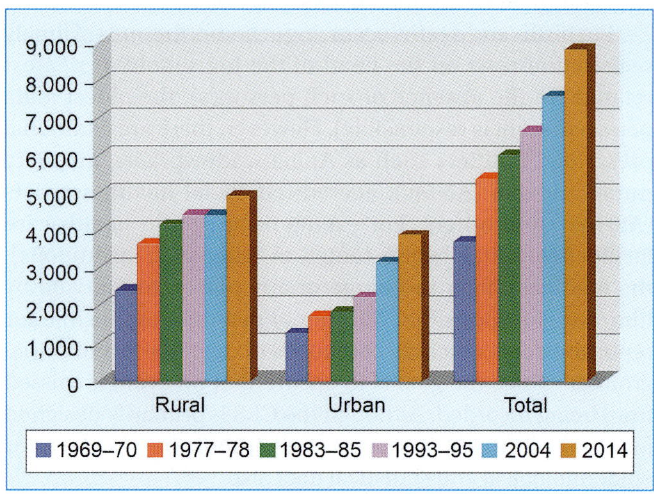

Fig. 22.1.3: Sample sets used for sample registration system (SRS) data collection since its inception.

TABLE 22.1.2: Steps of the sample registration system (SRS) data collection and compilation process.

SRS step	Purpose
Baseline survey of sample units	To assess the resident population of the sample areas
Continuous (longitudinal) enumeration of vital events by an enumerator	To collect the primary data for the sample
Independent retrospective half-yearly surveys for recording births and deaths by a supervisor	To update house lists, household schedule, and list of women in the reproductive age-group (and pregnancy status)
Matching of events recorded during prospective continuous enumeration and retrospective half-yearly survey	Quality control measures to check reliability of data
Field verification of unmatched and partially matched events	To ensure completeness of data
Filling of verbal autopsy forms for finalized deaths	To assign causes of death

Since 1999, the SRS also includes the "survey of causes of deaths (rural)". This uses the "post-death verbal autopsy" technique to estimate the most probable cause of death.[5] The process used to determine the cause of death in the SRS is given the acronym "RHIME" for "Representative, Re-sampled, Routine Household Interview of Mortality with Medical Evaluation method". In this system, every household in the SRS sample frame wherein a death occurs, is visited, to collect the details about signs and symptoms to identify the underlying causes of death. These "verbal autopsy" data are examined to establish the cause of death. In order to maintain quality and ensure reliability, the personnel are trained extensively, and assignment of the cause of death is done centrally by two physicians working independently.

The data for the most recent period (2016–18) showed that noncommunicable diseases (NCD) contributed to 56.0% of the deaths. In contrast, communicable diseases, together with maternal, perinatal, and nutritional, conditions contributed 21.5%. Among the NCD, cardiovascular disease alone accounted for almost 30%, followed by ill-defined conditions, respiratory diseases, malignancy, fever of unknown origin, digestive diseases, and others.

Among the communicable diseases, tuberculosis was the leading cause of death, followed by malaria.

Overall, children under 14 years accounted for 8.7% of the total deaths examined. The age-wise breakup was as follows: 0–1 years: 6.4%, 1–4 years: 1.1%, and 5–14 years: 1.2%. **Figure 22.1.4** summarizes the important causes of death in neonates during the period 2017–19, and **Figure 22.1.5** shows similar data for the age-group of infants <1 year old.

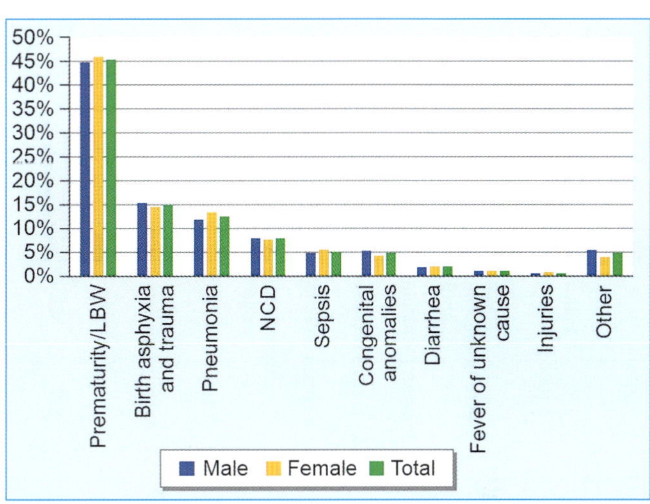

Fig. 22.1.4: Major causes of death in the neonatal age-group (2017–19). (LBW: low birth weight; NCD: noncommunicable disease)

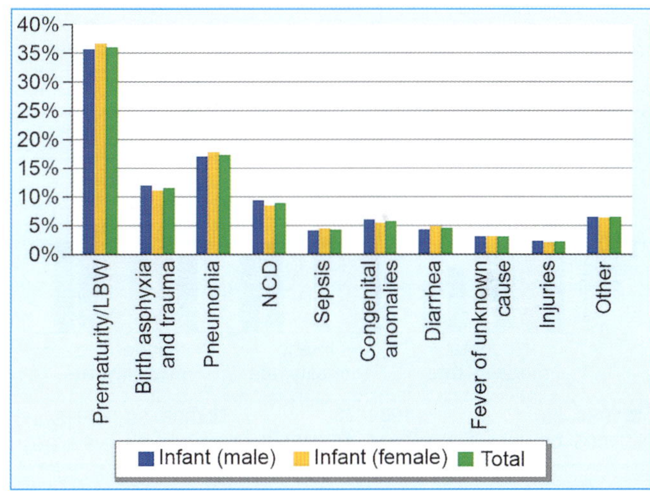

Fig. 22.1.5: Major causes of death in the age-group of 0–1 year (2017–19). (LBW: low birth weight; NCD: noncommunicable disease)

Among children in the age-group of 4–14 years, the pattern of the causes is quite different (as expected). More important, there is a clear gender variation in some of the causes. This is appreciable in **Figure 22.1.6**.

HEALTH SURVEYS

During the recent three decades, additional important sources of vital statistics in our country include the periodic NFHS and the DLHS. The DLHS data reflect various indicators on child health, reproductive health, and health service quality. Five NFHS surveys have been conducted in 1992–93, 1998–99, 2005–06, 2015–16, and 2019–21.[7-11] In recent years, the NFHS data have been regarded as scientifically robust, accurate, and reliable. The first three surveys provided data at the country level and for each of the states and union territories. The most

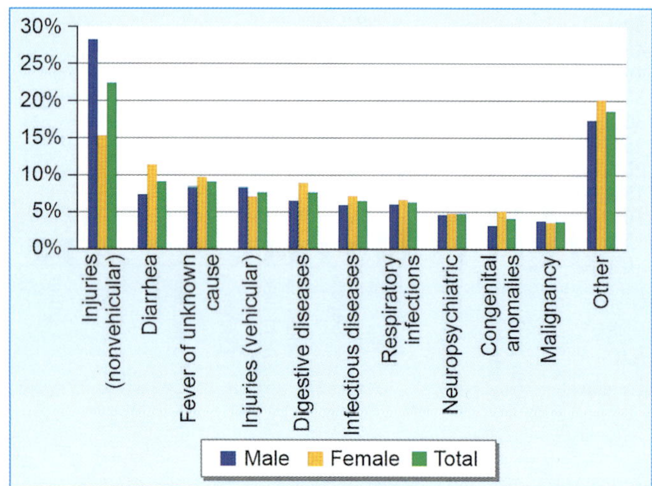

Fig. 22.1.6: Major causes of death in the age-group of 1–14 years (2017–19).

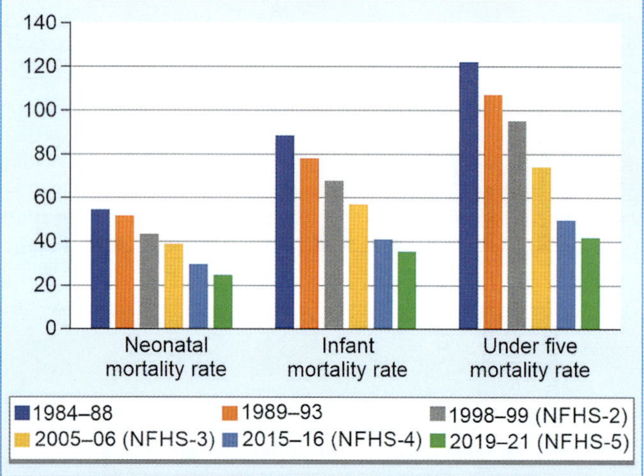

Fig. 22.1.7: Trend of neonatal, infant, and under-five mortality rates in India.

recent surveys (NFHS-4 and NFHS-5) have been expanded to record data at the district level also. In addition to the important vital statistics parameters, the latest survey also added data on blood pressure measurement, blood glucose estimation, etc. Thus, the NFHS surveys provide a wealth of data on vital statistics parameters as well as a wide range of other (direct and indirect) indicators of health. **Figure 22.1.7** shows the impressive decline in neonatal, infant, and under-five mortality over the past three decades.

However, it is interesting that the NFHS data do not match with the SRS data for the same period. For example, the NFHS-5 reported an infant mortality rate (IMR) of 35.2 for 2019–21, whereas the SRS reported 30 for 2019 and 28 for 2020. The respective data from United Nations Children's Fund (UNICEF) published in the Annual State of the World's Children report is 25 for 2021.

Further, the national level data represent an average of the data from various states and districts. Therefore, the range of values may provide a better impression than only the average values.

REFERENCES

1. Office of The Registrar General, India. (2020). Vital Statistics of India Based on the Civil Registration System 2020. [online] Available from https://crsorgi.gov.in/web/uploads/download/CRS_report_2020.pdf [Last accessed December 2024].
2. Office of the Registrar General and Census Commissioner, India. (2021). Vital Statistics Division. [online] Available from https://censusindia.gov.in/census.website/node/180# [Last accessed December 2024].
3. Office of the Registrar General and Census Commissioner, India. (2022). Sample Registration System (SRS): Statistical Report 2020. [online] Available from https://censusindia.gov.in/census.website/data/SRSSTAT [Last accessed December 2024].
4. Office of the Registrar General and Census Commissioner, India. (2022). SRS Based Abridged Life Tables 2016–20. [online] Available from: https://censusindia.gov.in/census.website/data/SRSALT [Last accessed December 2024].
5. Office of the Registrar General and Census Commissioner, India. (2023). Causes of death: Statistics 2017–2019. [online] Available from https://censusindia.gov.in/census.website/data/SRSCOD [Last accessed December 2024].
6. Registrar General India. (2021). Compendium of India's Fertility and Mortality Indicators 1971–2013. [online] Available from https://censusindia.gov.in/census.website/data/SRSCOMP [Last accessed December 2024].
7. International Institute for Population Sciences. (1995). National Family Health Survey (MCH and family planning), India 1992–93 summary report. [online] Available from https://dhsprogram.com/pubs/pdf/SR162/SR162.pdf [Last accessed December 2024].
8. International Institute for Population Sciences; ORC Macro. (2000). National Family Health Survey (NFHS-2), 1998–99: India. [online] Available from https://www.dhsprogram.com/pubs/pdf/FRIND2/FRIND2.pdf [Last accessed December 2024].
9. International Institute for Population Sciences (IIPS); Macro International. (2007). National Family Health Survey, (NFHS-3) 2005–06: India: volume I. [online] Available from https://dhsprogram.com/pubs/pdf/frind3/frind3-vol1andvol2.pdf [Last accessed December 2024].
10. International Institute for Population Sciences; ICF. (2017). National Family Health Survey (NFHS-4) 2015–16: India. [online] Available from https://dhsprogram.com/pubs/pdf/FR339/FR339.pdf [Last accessed December 2024].
11. International Institute for Population Sciences; ICF. (2021). National Family Health Survey (NFHS-5) 2019–21. [online] Available from https://dhsprogram.com/pubs/pdf/FR375/FR375.pdf [Last accessed December 2024].

22.2 Indicators of Child Health

Anupama Singh, Piyush Gupta

INTRODUCTION

Health indicators are statistical measures or instruments used to assess the health of an individual or a defined group. They are variables or measures that can be used to track changes in the level of achievement of health targets, as well as partial or indirect measures of complex situations. There are two types of indicators—qualitative (the presence or absence of an event) and quantitative (ratios, proportions, or rates). They can be classified as socioeconomic factors, demographic pointers, indicators of health status, indicators of health systems, and indicators of health policy, among others.[1]

Mortality indicators related to child health are defined in **Box 22.2.1**. Perinatal mortality and neonatal mortality reflect the health and care of women during pregnancy and the perinatal period, whereas infant mortality is one of the most sensitive indicators of a population's health and quality of life.

UNDER-5 MORTALITY RATE

The under-5 mortality rate (U-5MR) refers to the probability a newborn would die before reaching 5 years of age, expressed per 1,000 live births. It is influenced by the prevalence of disease and malnutrition among under-5 (U-5) children, income and education of their parents, efficacy of health services available, and health status of women. U-5MR is useful for evaluating the effectiveness of public health interventions in a country. It is an indicator for Sustainable Development Goal (SDG) 3: "Ensure healthy lives and promote well-being for all at all ages". It is calculated as:

$$\text{U-5MR} = \frac{\text{Number of deaths in children aged 0–5 years during a year}}{\text{Total number of children born live in the year}} \times 1{,}000$$

Under-5 mortality rate has decreased globally from 146/1,000 in 1970 to 38/1,000 in 2021. Sub-Saharan Africa and Southern Asia contributed 53% of global live births in 2020, but over 80% of the 5 million U-5 deaths. More than 50% of these deaths occurred in six countries: Nigeria, India, Pakistan, China, Ethiopia, and the Democratic Republic of the Congo.[2] **Figure 22.2.1** depicts the distribution of all deaths before the age of 5.[3] In addition to micronutrient deficiency and inadequate breastfeeding, undernutrition is the leading risk factor, accounting for nearly half of all deaths. **Table 22.2.1** shows the U-5MR per 1,000 population in selected countries.[4]

BOX 22.2.1: Mortality indicators of child health.

- *Under-5 mortality rate:* Number of deaths in children aged 0–5 years during a year per 1,000 live births in a given year
- *Neonatal mortality rate:* Number of deaths during the first 28 completed days of life per 1,000 live births in a given year or another period
- *Early neonatal mortality rate:* Number of deaths of a neonate within first 7 days of life expressed as per 1,000 live births in that year or specified duration
- *Late neonatal mortality rate:* Number of deaths of neonates occurring after the 7th day but before 28th day of life per 1,000 live births in that year
- *Post-neonatal mortality rate:* Number of deaths of infants beyond 28th day of life to less than a year of age per 1,000 live births in that year
- *Perinatal mortality rate:* Number of fetuses dying after 28 completed weeks of gestation plus the number of early neonatal deaths per 1,000 total births in that year
- *Infant mortality rate:* Infant mortality rate is the probability of a child born in a specific year or period dying before reaching the age of 1, if subject to age-specific mortality rates of that period
- *Stillbirth rate:* Number of babies born with no signs of life at 28 weeks or more of gestation per 1,000 total births

INFANT MORTALITY RATE

Infant mortality rate (IMR) is the probability of a child born in a specific year or period dying before reaching the age of one, subject to age-specific mortality rates of that period.

$$\text{IMR} = \frac{\text{Number of deaths in children <1 year of age during a year}}{\text{Total number of live birth in the same year}} \times 1000$$

According to United Nations (UN) estimates, the global IMR has dropped from 87 per 1,000 live births between 1975 and 1980 to <28 per 1,000 live births today. **Table 22.2.1** compares IMR in various parts of the world. India had an IMR of >200 per 1,000 live births at the turn of the century (204 in 1911–1915). In India, the current IMR is 28 per 1,000 live births.[5] **Figure 22.2.2** depicts the state-by-state IMR according to Sample Registration Scheme (SRS) in 2020.[6]

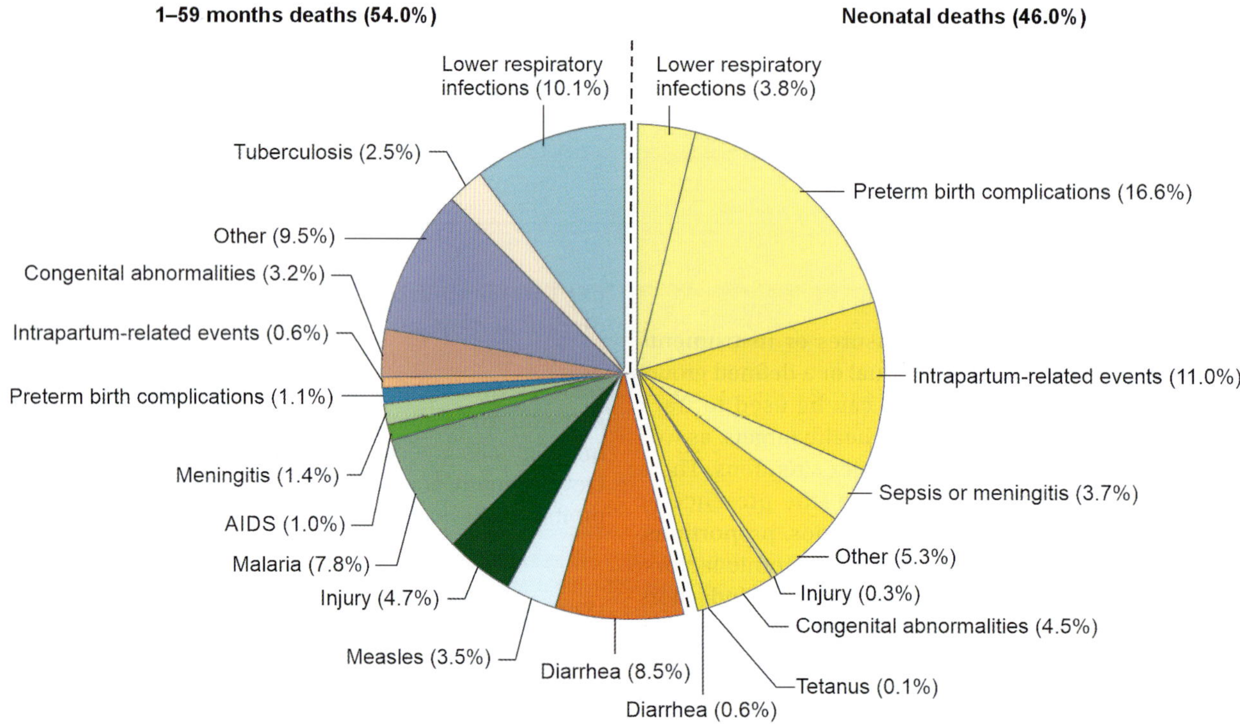

Fig. 22.2.1: Global distribution of causes of death among children aged under-5, by cause 2019.[3] (AIDS: acquired immunodeficiency syndrome)

TABLE 22.2.1: A comparison of under-5, neonatal and infant mortality rate in a few parts of the world.[4]

Country	Under-5 mortality rate	Neonatal (0–27 days) mortality rate	Infant (0–1 year) mortality rate
Afghanistan	56	35	43
Australia	4	2.3	3
Bangladesh	27	17	23
Bhutan	27	15	22
Brazil	14	9	13
China	7	3	5
Egypt	19	10	16
Ethiopia	47	27	34
Finland	2	1	2
France	4	2	3
Germany	4	2	3
India	31	20	25
Indonesia	22	12	19
Japan	2	0.8	2
Malaysia	8	4.2	6
Mali	97	34	62
Nepal	27	17	23
Niger	115	34	60
Pakistan	63	40	53
Singapore	2	0.8	2
Sri Lanka	9	3.9	6
Sweden	7	1.3	2
UK	4	2.8	4
USA	6	3.3	5
Zambia	58	25	40

Causes

The prime causes of infant mortality differ between the neonatal and postnatal periods. A large part of neonatal deaths occur as a result of infections, low birth weight, birth asphyxia, and congenital anomalies, whereas chief causes for post-neonatal mortality are malnutrition and infections (such as diarrhea, respiratory infections, malaria, measles, and other vaccine preventable diseases).

Maternal malnutrition, decreased spacing between births, large family size, and a high fertility rate are the primary causes of low birth weight (2,500 g). Noncompliance with immunization due to illiteracy, ignorance, cultural, and social beliefs, as well as non-practice of exclusive breastfeeding, are major risk factors for infant deaths. Finally, poverty, low living standards, lack of safe water for drinking, and proper sanitary environment are exacerbating factors for the abovementioned issues.

PREVENTION

Preventive measures aim to improve the health status of the mother by providing facilities such as essential antenatal care, safe delivery, essential newborn care, promotion of breastfeeding, immunization, early detection and management of illness, family planning, efficient services for reproductive and child health, improving adolescent health, providing safe drinking water and proper sanitation, and improving the socioeconomic conditions of the population.

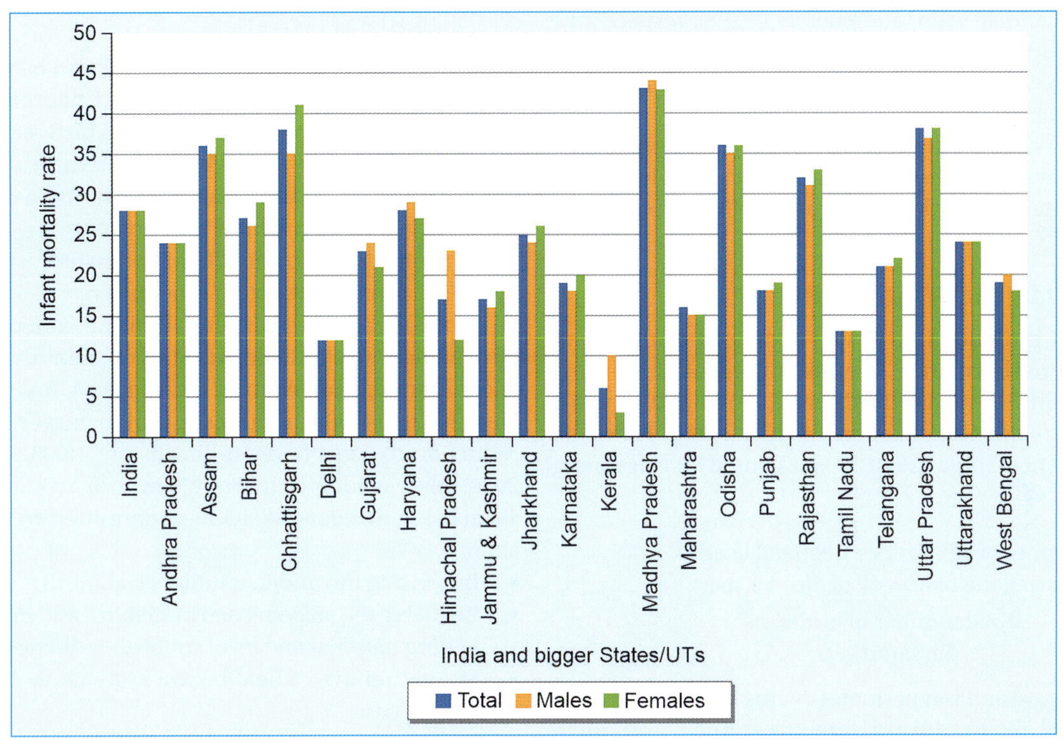

Fig. 22.2.2: Infant mortality rates in India and bigger states/union territories (UTs), 2020.[6]

The National Plan of Action for Children (2019) must be implemented politically, and with a sincere commitment to children's rights. The government must work hard to put policies in place that promote exclusive breastfeeding, use of oral rehydration salt (ORS), universal immunization coverage, and 100% female literacy. Simultaneously, various health programs require ongoing reinforcements with the participation of nongovernmental organizations (NGOs) and the non-health sector.

NEONATAL MORTALITY RATE

Neonatal mortality rate (NMR) is the number of neonatal deaths occurring per 1,000 live births per year.

$$\text{NMR} = \frac{\text{Number of deaths in neonates aged <28 days in a year}}{\text{Total number of live births in the same year}} \times 1{,}000$$

Stillbirth rate (SBR) is the number of stillborn infants (after 28 weeks of gestation) related to total number of births (both live and stillborn) during the same period.

$$\text{SBR} = \frac{\text{Number of stillborn infants in a year}}{\text{Total number of births in the same year}} \times 1{,}000$$

India accounts for 17% of global births (23.1 million) and 18% (13 million) of global newborn deaths. In India, IMR and NMR have decreased significantly over the last few decades. The IMR has fallen from 140 per 1,000 since the early 1970s.

Globally, 3.86 million infant deaths occur annually, out of these 2.4 million occur in the neonatal period; developing countries account for 98% of these deaths. Nearly 65% of these neonatal deaths occur in the first 7 days of life. Neonatal deaths account for 46% of all childhood deaths and >50% of infant mortality. As a result, perinatal and neonatal mortality should be prioritized to reduce infant mortality.

India accounts for 17% of global births (23.1 million) and 18% (13 million) of global newborn deaths. In India, IMR and NMR have decreased significantly over the last few years. The IMR has reduced from 140 to 28 per 1,000 live births since the early 1970s. There has been a reduction in NMR from 72 per 1,000 live births in 1972 to 20 in 2020.[5]

The decrease in NMR is most likely due to three factors:

1. There has been a significant reduction in neonatal tetanus due to the success of tetanus toxoid immunization program for mothers.
2. There has been a steady rise in institutional deliveries and deliveries conducted by skilled birth attendants.
3. Birth spacing

However, the rate of decline in NMR has gradually slowed in recent years. The leading causes of neonatal deaths worldwide are infections, asphyxia, and prematurity. A similar pattern can be found in India, where they account for 13%, 15%, and 45.5% of all neonatal deaths, respectively. It is worth noting that most of these community-level deaths can be avoided by improving maternal and newborn care standards at health facilities.

The NMR varies greatly from as low as 4 in Kerala to as high as 31 in Madhya Pradesh. Other states with a high burden of neonatal mortality include Uttar Pradesh, Uttarakhand, and Rajasthan.

PERINATAL MORTALITY RATE

The perinatal mortality rate (PMR) is defined as the death of a fetus or newborn after 22 weeks of pregnancy, during birth, or within 7 days after birth per 1,000 total births in a year [World Health Organization (WHO), 2006].[7] However, the Government of India uses a 28-week cutoff for calculating PMR in India.

$$\text{PMR} = \frac{\text{Number of stillbirths + neonatal deaths during the first week of life in a year}}{\text{Total number of births in the same year}} \times 1{,}000$$

Every year, >5 million perinatal deaths occur worldwide; half of these occur during late pregnancy and birth (stillbirths), while the other half die within the first week of life (early neonatal mortality).

Perinatal deaths are more common in developing countries than in developed countries, where only 2% of estimated perinatal deaths occur. Africa has the highest PMR, accounting for nearly 25% of all births. Perinatal mortality in these areas is caused by women's poor nutritional status, inadequate pregnancy-related complications prevention, and even unsupervised deliveries. Some of these causes are rooted in society's social, cultural, and economic structure. **Table 22.2.2** summarizes mortality indicators related to child health in India.[6]

STILLBIRTH RATE

For a total of an estimated 2 million stillborn babies each year, WHO and United Nations International Children's Emergency Fund (UNICEF) estimates that one stillbirth occurs every 16 seconds. Stillbirth is a global problem, three quarters of all global stillbirths occur in Sub-Saharan Africa and Southern Asia. High-quality prenatal and postpartum care can help prevent >40% of stillbirths. 20 million babies will be stillborn by 2030 if appropriate action is not taken.

World Health Organization, UNICEF, and other partners have pledged to eliminate preventable stillbirths by 2030. The Global Strategy for Women's, Children's, and Adolescents' Health 2016–2030 includes a global target for stillbirth reduction to 12 or fewer stillbirths per 1,000 total births by 2030, this was adopted in Every Newborn Action Plan (ENAP). To achieve this goal, WHO has committed to the following actions.

- Increasing the understanding of stillbirth
- Reducing the taboo related to stillbirth and misconceptions
- Setting national and local stillbirth reduction targets
- Strengthening of health care systems to provide high-quality care

Working toward the ENAP stillbirth targets is essential, the equity gap within countries can be closed by better ENAP coverage, meeting antenatal and intrapartum quality care targets, reaching agreement on bereavement care and materials, and taking global action to reduce the stigma associated with stillbirth will be required.[8]

WHAT IS RMNCH+A APPROACH?

India has reaffirmed its commitment to make sincere efforts to achieve Millennium Development Goal (MDG) 4 and 5 on a global scale. To reach the desired targets rapidly, a balanced approach to managing child and maternal

TABLE 22.2.2: Comparative rural/urban mortality indicators, 2020, India.[6]

Indicator	*Combined*	*Rural*	*Urban*	*Maximum*	*Minimum*
Crude death rate (2020)	6.0	6.4	5.1	7.7 (Odisha)	4 (Delhi)
Infant mortality rate (2020)	28	31	19	4 (MP)	6 (Kerala)
Percentage of infant deaths/total deaths	9.1	10.3	6	16 (MP)	1.4 (Kerala)
Percentage of neonatal deaths/infant deaths	71.9	74.1	62.4	79.1 (Uttarakhand)	53.4 (Assam)
Percentage of early neonatal/infant deaths	53.3	54.7	44.8	62.9 (Uttarakhand)	40.5 (Kerala)
Neonatal mortality rate	25	27.5	18	29 (MP)	3.4 (Kerala)
Early neonatal mortality rate (NMR)	15	17	9	31 (MP)	4 (Kerala)
Late NMR	5	6	3	–	–
Perinatal mortality rate	32	34	25	43 (Bihar)	6.2 (Kerala)
Stillbirth rate	3	4	3	10 (Odisha)	0 (Delhi)

(MP: Madhya Pradesh)

health care issues is required. It has been recognized that interventions to improve the health of women and children must be done at all levels of the health system, from the home to the community level, and through all health facilities. The RMNCH+A (reproductive, maternal, neonatal, child health plus adolescent) approach was launched to provide state as well as national health secretaries, mission directors, and program managers with a clear vision and understanding of India's comprehensive approach to improving child survival and safe motherhood, as well as achieving MDG 4 and 5. The main concept is "continuum of care" to this approach, which extends from adolescent girls to pregnant women and child health care. This strategy aims to address the leading causes of death among women and children, as well as delays in accessing and utilizing health care and services. The health of an adolescent girl influences pregnancy, whereas the health of a pregnant woman influences the health of the child.

The "plus" in the strategic approach denotes:

- The including adolescence as a distinct stage of life
- The linkage of maternal and child health to reproductive health and other components such as family planning, adolescent health, human immunodeficiency virus (HIV) infection, gender, and preconception and prenatal diagnostic techniques (PC and PNDT)
- The linkage of community and facility-based care, as well as referrals between various levels of health care system

The mode of implementation of RMNCH+A is shown in **Table 22.2.3**.[9]

Key Features of RMNCH+A Strategy

The RMNCH+A strategy approaches include:

- Health systems strengthening (HSS) focusing on infrastructure, human resources, supply chain management, and referral transport measures

TABLE 22.2.3: Mode of implementation of RMNCH+A approach.[9]

Reproductive care	***Pregnancy and childbirth care***	***Newborn and childcare***	
Clinical			
• Comprehensive abortion care • Reproductive tract infections (RTI)/sexually transmitted infections (STIs) case management • Postpartum intrauterine contraceptive device (IUCD) and sterilization; interval IUCD procedures • Adolescent friendly health services	• Skilled obstetric care and immediate newborn care and resuscitation • Preventing parent to child transmission (PPTCT) of human immunodeficiency virus (HIV) • Emergency obstetric care • Postpartum sterilization	• Essential newborn care • Care of sick newborn [special newborn care units (SNCU), newborn stabilization units (NBSU)] • Facility-based care of childhood illnesses (IMNCI) • Care of children with severe acute malnutrition (NRC) • Immunization	
Reproductive health care	*Antenatal care*	*Postnatal care*	*Child health care*
Outreach/subcenter			
• Family planning (including IUCD insertion, oral contraceptive pill, and condoms) • Prevention and management of STIs • Preconception folic acid supplementation	Full antenatal care package PPTCT	• Early detection and treatment of illnesses in mother and newborn • Immunization	• First-level evaluation and treatment of newborn and childhood illnesses • Immunization • Micronutrient supplementation
Family and community			
• Weekly supplementation of iron and folic acid (IFA) • Information and counseling on sexual reproductive health and family planning • Community-based promotion and delivery of contraceptives • Menstrual hygiene	• Counseling and preparation for newborn care, breastfeeding, birth preparedness • Demand generation for pregnancy care and institutional delivery *Janani Suraksha Yojana* (JSY), *Janani Shishu Suraksha Yojana* (JSSY)	• Home-based newborn care (HBNC) and prompt referral HBNC scheme • Antibiotic for suspected case of newborn sepsis • Infant and young child feeding (IYCE), including exclusive breastfeeding and complementary feeding • Child health screening and early intervention services (0–18 years) • Early childhood development (ECD) • Danger sign recognition and care-seeking for illness • Use of oral rehydration salts and zinc in case of diarrhea	
Intersectoral: Water, sanitation, hygiene, nutrition, education, empowerment			

Adolescence/prepregnancy → Pregnancy → Birth → Newborn/postnatal → Childhood

(RMNCH+A: reproductive, maternal, neonatal child health plus adolescent)

TABLE 22.2.4: Current status of key RMNCH+A/RCH indicators.[6]

Indicator	Current status	National Health Policy Target	SDG 2030 Target
Maternal mortality ratio	122	100 by 2020	<70
Neonatal Mortality rate	23	16 by 2025	<12
Under-5 Mortality Rate	37	23 by 2025	≤25

(SRS: Sample Registration System; SDG: Sustainable Development Goal)

- Prioritization of high-impact interventions for various lifecycle stages
- Increasing effectiveness of investments by prioritizing geographical areas based on evidence
- Integrated monitoring and accountability through good governance, use of available data sets, community involvement, and steps to address grievance
- Broad-based collaboration and partnerships with ministries, departments, development partners, civil society, and other stakeholders

The RMNCH+A strategy provides a strong platform for delivery of services across the entire continuum of care, ranging from community to various level of health care system. The current status is depicted in **Table 22.2.4**.[6]

CONCLUSION

The indicators of child health measure the overall health and well-being of children. These indicators are essential for identifying health disparities, planning interventions, and tracking the progress of child health in the community. They reflect the efficiency and penetration of healthcare services in the country and can be compared across the globe. Infant mortality rate is the key indicator that reflects the quality of health services, maternal health and socio-economic conditions of a nation.

REFERENCES

1. Paunović K. Health indicators. In: Kirch W (Eds). Encyclopedia of Public Health. Dordrecht: Springer; 2008.
2. United Nations Children's Fund. (2023). The State of the World's Children 2023: For Every Child, Vaccination. [online] Available from https://www.unicef.org/reports/state-worlds-children-2023 [Last accessed December 2024].
3. United Nations Children's Fund. (2024). Levels and Trends in Child Mortality. United Nations Inter-Agency Group for Child Mortality Estimation (UN IGME), Report 2023. [online] Available from https://data.unicef.org/resources/levels-and-trends-in-child-mortality-2024/ [Last accessed December 2024].
4. United Nations Children's Fund. (2021). Levels and Trends in Child Mortality. United Nations Inter-Agency Group for Child Mortality Estimation (UN IGME), Report, 2021. [online] Available from https://data.unicef.org/resources/levels-and-trends-in-child-mortality-2021/ [Last accessed December 2024].
5. Office of the Registrar General & Census Commissioner, India. (2022). Sample Registration System (SRS)—Bulletin 2020, volume 55-I. [online] Available from https://censusindia.gov.in/nada/index.php/catalog/42687 [Last accessed December 2024].
6. Office of the Registrar General & Census Commissioner, India. (2020). Sample Registration System, Statistical Report 2020. [online] Available from https://new.census.gov.in/nada/index.php/catalog/42634/download/46328/SRS_STAT_2020.pdf [Last accessed December 2024].
7. World Health Organization. (2006). Neonatal and perinatal mortality. https://iris.who.int/bitstream/handle/10665/43444/9241563206_eng.pdf.
8. World Health Organization. Every Newborn Progress Report 2019. Geneva: World Health Organization; United Nations Children's Fund; 2020.
9. Ministry of Health & Family Welfare, Government of India. (2013). A Strategic Approach to Reproductive, Maternal, Newborn, Child, and Adolescent Health (RMNCH+A) in India. [online] Available from https://nhm.gov.in/images/pdf/RMNCH+A/RMNCH+A_Strategy.pdf [Last accessed December 2024].

22.3 National Health Mission

Gnanamurthy Narasimha, Sumitha Nayak

INTRODUCTION

The National Health Mission (NHM) is India's flagship program to revitalize rural and urban health sectors. It envisages universal access to equitable, affordable, and quality healthcare services that are accountable and responsive to people's needs. The main components include strengthening of health system in rural and urban areas, reproductive, maternal, newborn, child, and adolescent health (RMNCH+A) services, and control of communicable and noncommunicable diseases. NHM, comprises the National Rural Health Mission (NRHM) and the National Urban Health Mission (NUHM).[1,2]

Launched in April 2005, the NRHM addresses the health needs of the underserved rural population, especially women, children, and vulnerable sections of the society, providing affordable, accessible, and quality health care. Under the NRHM, the empowered action group states (Bihar, Chhattisgarh, Jharkhand, Madhya Pradesh, Odisha, Rajasthan, Uttarakhand, and Uttar Pradesh), northeastern states, Jammu and Kashmir, and Himachal Pradesh have special focus.[3]

National Urban Health Mission was launched in May 2013 to improve the health status of the urban poor and other vulnerable sections by facilitating their access to quality primary healthcare.[4] NUHM covers all areas with a population of 50,000 and above (as per census 2011) in a phased manner. Cities and towns with population below 50,000 are covered under NRHM.

VISION AND OBJECTIVES

Vision

The vision of NHM is "attainment of universal access to equitable, affordable, and quality healthcare services, accountable and responsive to people's needs, with effective inter-sectoral convergent action to address the wider social determinants of health."

Objectives

The objectives of the NHM are listed in **Box 22.3.1**.[5]

KEY FEATURES

The key features include: To build an integrated network of primary, secondary, and a substantial part of tertiary care, providing a continuum from community level to the district hospital, with robust referral linkages. To address issues of access and continuum of care, to prioritize the creation and upgradation of a set of interconnected facilities based on "time to care and caseloads", ensuring the availability of primary care within 30 minutes and secondary services within 2 hours of any habitation, with an assured referral transport system connecting the two.

Steps include providing free maternal and child health services, including newborn care, immunization, adolescent health, and family planning, and free diagnostic and treatment services to all. District hospitals are being upgraded to superspecialty units to reduce referral load and treatment lag at the tertiary care centers.

Health outcome indicators from various states and districts show uneven progress across the country. Populations in certain geographical locations (e.g., hilly and remote places, tribal areas, and deserts) and the socially and economically disadvantaged (e.g., scheduled castes and tribes and poor) need special focus to ensure they receive the benefits from these investments.

Shortages of skilled workers in remote, rural areas, and other underserved pockets are addressed through appropriate monetary and nonmonetary incentives.

BOX 22.3.1: Objectives of national health mission.

- Reduce MMR to 1/1,000 livebirths
- Reduce IMR to 25/1,000 livebirths
- Reduce TFR to 2.1
- Prevention and reduction of anemia in women aged 15–49 years
- Prevent and reduce mortality and morbidity from communicable and noncommunicable injuries and emerging diseases
- Reduce household out-of-pocket expenditure on total healthcare expenditure
- Reduce annual incidence and mortality from tuberculosis by half
- Reduce the prevalence of leprosy to <1/1,000 population and incidence to zero in all districts
- Annual malaria incidence to be <1/1,000
- Less than 1% microfilaria prevalence in all districts
- Kala-azar elimination by 2015, <1 case per 10,000 population in all block

(IMR: infant mortality rate; MMR: maternal mortality rate; TFR: total fertility rate)

INSTITUTIONAL MECHANISMS

National Level

A Mission Steering Group (MSG) under the chairmanship of Union Minister of Health and Family Welfare directs NHM. An Empowered Program Committee (EPC) headed by Secretary, Department of Health and Family Welfare, scrutinizes all financial proposals before approval by MSG.

The NHM is headed by a Mission Director of Additional Secretary rank, with joint secretaries for the administrative affairs, planning, implementing, and monitoring activities of the mission.

State Level

The State Health Society has a Mission Director and the State Program Management Unit (SPMU).

District Level

The District Health Mission (DHM)/City Health Mission (CHM) with District Health Society (DHS) has the District Collector/ District Magistrate as the Chairperson. The Chief Medical Officer is the Chief Executive Officer (CEO) and is responsible for planning and managing programs in the district.

PROGRAMS UNDER NATIONAL HEALTH MISSION

The key programs under NHM are RMNCH+A services, prevention of communicable diseases, and disease control programs. These programs are elaborated in **Tables 22.3.1 and 22.3.2**, respectively.[1,2,6]

TABLE 22.3.1: Reproductive, maternal, newborn, child, and adolescent health (RMNCH+A) services.

Domain	Key provisions
RMNCH+A services	
Maternal health	Increase coverage and quality of antenatal and postnatal care, access to skilled birth attendance, institutional delivery; basic and comprehensive emergency obstetric care
Access to safe abortion services	Access to comprehensive abortion care, postabortion contraceptive counseling; expanded facilities providing medical termination of pregnancy (MTP) services
Newborn care	Home-based newborn care through Accredited Social Health Activists (ASHAs); essential newborn care, resuscitation at all delivery points. Facility-based care for sick newborns through the newborn stabilization units (NBSU), special newborn care units (SNCU) at first referral units (FRU) and DH
Childcare	Community care for respiratory infections, diarrhea, fevers; institutional care for sick children, severely malnourished children at nutrition rehabilitation centers (NRC); promotion of infant and young child feeding (IYCF) and micronutrient supplementation
Universal immunization	Achieving over 80% routine immunization in districts; introduction of new vaccines; improved cold chain management; adequate number of vaccination sessions and sites, logistics to access remote areas
Child health screening and early intervention services	*Early detection of 4Ds:* Birth defects, diseases, deficiencies, and development delays including disability; providing comprehensive care at appropriate health facilities
Adolescent health	Iron and folic acid (IFA) supplementation, adolescent health services, health promotion activities, information, counseling on sexual and reproductive health (including menstrual hygiene), substance abuse, mental health, noncommunicable diseases, injuries, violence including domestic violence
Family planning	Postpartum and postabortion contraception; spacing methods, especially intrauterine contraceptive devices (IUCDs); doorstep distribution of contraceptives through ASHAs, promotion of healthy spacing after marriage and between the births
Addressing the declining sex ratio	Enforcement of preconception and prenatal diagnostic techniques (PCPNDT) act, monitoring, sensitization of the medical community, proactive support for girl children through the ASHA and anganwadi system

TABLE 22.3.2: Disease control program under National Health Mission.

Program	Key provisions
Control of communicable diseases	
National Vector Borne Diseases Control Program (NVBDCP)	Prevention and control of vector borne diseases: Malaria, Japanese encephalitis (JE), dengue, chikungunya, kala-azar, and filariasis
National Tuberculosis Elimination Program (NTEP)	Revised in January 2020 to NTEP, National Strategic Plan (2017–2025) of Tuberculosis to achieve a TB-free India
National Leprosy Elimination Program (NLEP)	Diagnosis and treatment [multidrug treatment (MDT)] of patients
Integrated Disease Surveillance Program (IDSP)	Prevention and control of outbreaks of communicable diseases
Control of noncommunicable diseases	
National Program for Prevention and Control of Non-Communicable Diseases (NP-NCD)	Prevention of NCDs, screening, early diagnosis, management, referral, and follow up of common NCDs
National Program for the Control of Blindness and Visual Impairment (NPCB&VI)	Screening for detection and management of diabetic retinopathy, refractory defects, and glaucoma
National Mental Health Program (NMHP)	Early detection, treatment of mental illness
National Program for the Health Care of the Elderly (NPHCE)	Specialized healthcare for elderly
National Program for the Prevention and Control of Deafness (NPPCD)	Prevent avoidable hearing loss; early detection/treatment of ear problems
National Tobacco Control and Drug Addiction Treatment Program (NPTCDAT)	Awareness and better implementation of tobacco control
National Oral Health Program (NOHP)	Promotive and preventive oral health care
National Program for Prevention and Control of Fluorosis (NPPCF)	Surveillance, management, health education for prevention, and control of fluorosis
National Iodine Deficiency Disorders Control Program (NIDDCP)	Iodine deficiency-related problems
National Organ Transplant Program (NOTP)	Organ donation from deceased persons, retrieval, storage, and transplantation
National Program for Prevention and Management of Trauma and Burn Injuries (NPPMTBI)	Prevention/treatment of trauma and burn injuries
National Program for Palliative Care (NPPC)	Palliative care for terminal disease

REPRODUCTIVE, MATERNAL, NEWBORN, CHILD, AND ADOLESCENT HEALTH SERVICES

Reproductive, Maternal, Newborn, Child, and Adolescent Health services launched in 2013 address the major causes of mortality among women and children; delays in accessing and utilizing healthcare services. The approach provides "continuum of care" ensuring equal focus on various life stages, including adolescence that is recognized as a distinct "life stage". All the referral linkages between community and the various levels of health system (primary, secondary, and tertiary) are strengthened.

Key RMNCH+A Initiatives

Janani Suraksha Yojana

Janani Suraksha Yojana (JSY) was launched in April 2005 to reduce maternal mortality among pregnant women, encouraging them to deliver in government health facilities. Cash assistance is provided to eligible pregnant women for delivering at government facilities.

Janani Shishu Suraksha Karyakram (JSSK)

Since June 2011, this program entitles all pregnant women to deliver in public health institutions free of charge. This provides with free drugs, consumables, diagnostics, and diet during inpatient stay, provision of blood, transport between home to health institution, and in case of referrals, between health institutions. Similar entitlements available for all sick infants (up to 1 year of age) accessing public health institutions.

Pradhanmantri Surakshit Matritva Abhiyan (PMSMA)

On the 9th of every month, pregnant women are given free health check-up. Private sector gynecologists are encouraged to voluntarily provide antenatal check-ups (ANC) in these health facilities.

Facility-based Newborn Care

It is a continuum of newborn care with home-based and facility-based. Newborn care components ensure essential care from birth and first 48 hours at the health facility, subsequently at home during the initial 42 days. Newborn Care Corners (NBCCs) at delivery points provide essential newborn care at birth; Special Newborn Care Units (SNCUs) at district hospital/medical college, and Newborn Stabilization Units (NBSUs) at first referral units (FRUs) for sick newborns.

Mother and Child Tracking System

Mother and child tracking system is a web-based, name-based tracking system, designed to capture information on and track all pregnant women and children (0–5 years).

Mother and Child Health Wings

Mother and Child Health Wings (MCH wings) are 100/50/30-bedded buildings sanctioned in public health facilities (district hospitals, district women's hospitals, subdistrict hospitals, or community health centers) to overcome the constraints of increasing caseloads and institutional deliveries envisaged to provide advanced, optimal quality obstetric, and newborn care.

National Iron Plus Initiative

National Iron Plus Initiative is a program to prevent and control iron deficiency anemia. Pregnant and lactating women, children, adolescents, and women in reproductive age are provided with iron and folic acid (IFA). Weekly iron and folic acid supplementation (WIFS) for adolescents is an important strategy.

Mission Indradhanush

Mission Indradhanush is a program to strengthen and invigorate the Universal Immunization Program (UIP) and achieve full immunization coverage for all children rapidly. This was launched in December 2014 and ensures immunization to all children below 2 years and pregnant women.

Kayakalp

Kayakalp program promotes cleanliness, hygiene, and infection control practices in public health facilities. Public healthcare facilities are appraised routinely. Those that show exemplary performance of cleanliness, hygiene, and infection control receive awards and commendations.

Free Drugs and Free Diagnostic Services

Extremely high expenditure due to costly drugs and diagnostics are obstacles in provision of accessible and affordable health care for all. Under the NHM, states provide free essential drugs and/or diagnostics to all patients accessing public health facilities, create a robust procurement, logistics and supply chain system, have essential drug list/diagnostic list depending, standard treatment guidelines, and audit prescriptions.

National Ambulance Services (NAS)

States/UTs have provided the facility for people to dial 108 or 102 to call an ambulance. Dial 108 is an emergency response system, designed to attend to patients of critical care, trauma, and accident victims, etc. Dial 102 services consist of basic patient transport.

Daksh Skill Labs

Daksh Skill Labs was established for competency-based training and skill enhancement of healthcare providers for RMNCH+A services. They provide training through repetitive skills practice, simulation of clinical scenarios, and training under the supervision of a trainer.

Dakshata Program

Dakshata Program is a capacity building program for service providers in labor room covering best practices during labor, delivery, and postpartum.

Rashtriya Bal Swasthya Karyakram

Rashtriya Bal Swasthya Karyakram (RBSK) program was launched in February 2013; this enables child health screening and early intervention through early detection and management of 4 Ds, i.e., defects at birth, diseases, deficiencies, and development delays including disability in the age group of 0–18 years. Children diagnosed with any of the 30 specified illnesses would receive follow-up referral support and treatment including surgical interventions at tertiary level free-of-cost.

Rashtriya Kishor Swasthya Karyakram

Rashtriya Kishor Swasthya Karyakram (RKSK) program was launched in January 2014 to reach 253 million adolescents in India. The focus of this program goes beyond reproductive and sexual health and includes life skills, nutrition, injuries, and violence (including gender-based), noncommunicable diseases, mental health, and substance misuse.

National Quality Assurance Framework for Health Facilities

To improve quality of healthcare in over 31,000 public health facilities and provide a clear roadmap to states, quality standards for district hospitals (DHs), CHCs, and PHCs this program was rolled out in November 2014.

Kilkari

Kilkari is an interactive voice response (IVR)-based mobile service, delivering 72 appropriate audio messages weekly, directly to families' mobile phone from second trimester of pregnancy until the child is 1 year of age.

Mobile Academy

Mobile academy is a free audio training course. This will expand and refresh the knowledge of Accredited Social Health Activists (ASHAs) and improve their communication skills.

Comprehensive Primary Health Care

Comprehensive primary health care aims toward primary health care in India, strengthening and expanding the subcenters to provide comprehensive primary health care, and position them as health and wellness centers as first point of care. A mid-level provider (a nurse or an AYUSH provider) will be trained in a 6-month bridge course to provide services.

National Disease Control Program (Table 22.3.2)

Community Process in the National Rural Health Mission

To achieve the goal of active subject involvement in public health, community processes are embedded as described further.

Accredited Social Health Activists

Over 9.43 lakh community health volunteers called ASHAs are engaged, to work as a link between the community and the public health system. ASHA's are the first call for any health-related demands of deprived sections, especially women and children, ASHAs have successfully brought people back to public health system, with increased utilization of hospital facilities, institutional deliveries, and inpatient care.

Rogi Kalyan Samiti (Patient Welfare Committee)

Rogi Kalyan Samiti (RKS) is a registered society with members as trustees managing the hospital affairs. RKS is responsible for upkeep of the facilities, ensuring provision of better facilities to the patients in the hospital. Financial assistance is provided through untied funds.

Village Health Sanitation and Nutrition Committee

Village Health Sanitation and Nutrition Committee (VHSNC) is an important tool of community empowerment and participation at the grassroots level. They take collective action on health issues and its social determinants at the village level. Untied grants of ₹10,000 are provided annually to each VHSNC, which are utilized through involvement of Panchayati Raj representatives and other community members.

GOALS OF NATIONAL HEALTH MISSION

The NHM has several indicators toward which the various programs are geared. **Figure 22.3.1** mentions some of the goals of the NHM.[7]

NATIONAL URBAN HEALTH MISSION

As per Census 2011, urban population comprises 31% of the total population. The access to health services of urban poor is severely restricted due to being "crowded out" of the

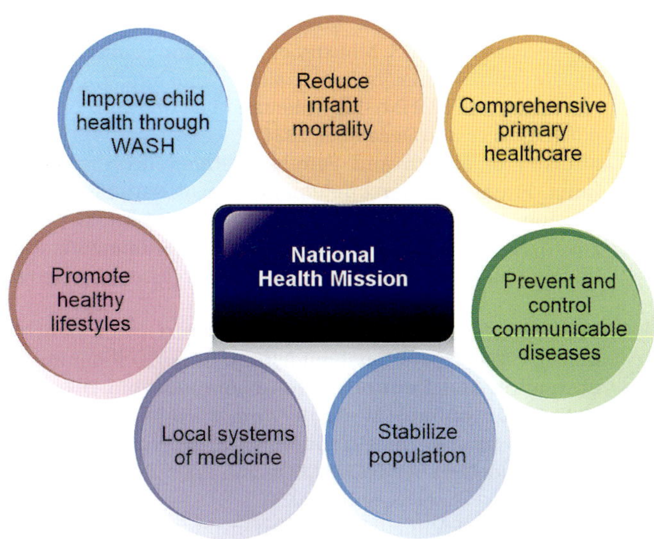

Fig. 22.3.1: Goals of National Health Mission (NHM). (WASH: water, sanitation, and hygiene)

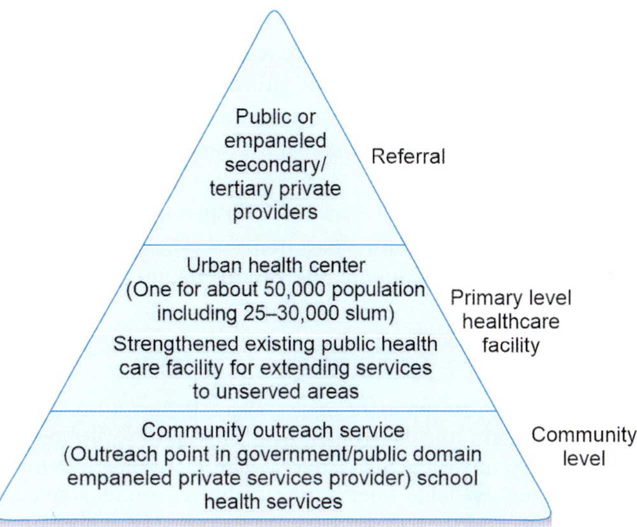

Fig. 22.3.2: Urban Healthcare Delivery Model.[8]

inadequate urban public health system, nonaffordability in private hospitals, social exclusion, lack of referral mechanisms, and information and assistance at the secondary and tertiary hospitals.

To meet this lacuna, the NUHM as a submission of NHM was approved by the cabinet and launched on 20th January 2014.

National Urban Health Mission covers all state capitals, district headquarters, and cities/towns with a population of over 50,000. Support is provided to the states/UTs for strengthening and upgradation of existing infrastructure and human resource augmentation for providing comprehensive primary healthcare services.

Service Delivery Infrastructure under National Urban Health Mission

National Urban Health Mission envisages setting up service delivery infrastructure **(Fig. 22.3.2)**, which is largely absent in cities/towns to address the needs of urban poor.

Urban-Primary Health Center

New Urban-Primary Health Centers (U-PHCs) are established for approximately 50,000 urban population, located within or near a slum for providing preventive, promotive and OPD (consultation), basic laboratory diagnosis, drug/contraceptive dispensing services, and counseling for all communicable and noncommunicable diseases.

Urban-Community Health Center and Referral Hospitals

Around 30–50 bedded Urban-Community Health Centers (U-CHCs) provide inpatient care in cities with a population of above 5 lakhs.

Outreach Services

National Urban Health Mission supports engagement of auxiliary nurse midwives (ANMs) for conducting outreach services to targeted groups particularly slum dwellers, vulnerable populations for providing preventive and promotive healthcare services at the household and community level.

Community Process under National Urban Health Mission

Mahila Arogya Samiti (MAS)

One Samiti covers 250–1,000 beneficiaries and 50–100 households as a community-based peer education group in slums.

ASHA/Link Worker

Frontline community worker (ASHA) serves as an effective and demand-generating link between the health facility and the urban slum population. Each link worker/ASHA has a well-defined service area of about 1,000–2,500 beneficiaries or 200–500 households on geography.

CONCLUSION

1. The National Health Mission is India's flagship program aimed at vitalizing the rural and urban health sectors.
2. While the National Rural Health Mission addresses the health needs of the rural poor, the National Urban Health Mission was envisaged to improve the health status of the urban poor.

3. Several key indicators have been developed to help improve the health of these communities.
4. It consists of programs that address the communicable and noncommunicable diseases, as well as address the reproductive, maternal, newborn and adolescent health services.
5. A National Quality Assurance Framework for health facilities provides the road map for the standards that need to be maintained at the various health setups in the country.

REFERENCES

1. Ministry of Health and Family Welfare, India. (2016). Annual report 2015–16, Department of Health and Family Welfare, Ministry of Health and Family Welfare, Government of India. [online] Available from https://mohfw.gov.in/sites/default/files/56987532145632566578.pdf. [Last accessed December, 2024].
2. Ministry of Health and Family Welfare, India. (2017). Annual report 2016–17, Department of Health and Family Welfare, Ministry of Health and Family Welfare, Government of India. [online] Available from https://mohfw.gov.in/annual-report-department-health-and-family-welfare--2016-17. [Last accessed December, 2024].
3. National Rural Health Mission. (2012). Meeting people's health needs in rural areas: Framework for implementation 2005-2012. Ministry of Health and Family Welfare, Government of India. [online] Available from http://nhm.gov.in/images/pdf/about-nrhm/nrhm-framework-implementation/nrhm-framework-latest.pdf [Last accessed December, 2024].
4. National Urban Health Mission. (2013). Framework for implementation, 2013. Ministry of Health and Family Welfare, Government of India. [online] Available from http://nrhm.gov.in/images/pdf/NUHM/Implementation_Framework_NUHM.pdf. [Last accessed December, 2024].
5. Ministry of Health and Family Welfare, Government of India. Framework for implementation of National Health Mission 2012-2017. [online] Available from https://nhm.gov.in/New_Updates_2018/NHM/NHM_Framework_for_Implementation__08-01-2014.pdf. [Last accessed December, 2024].
6. Ministry of Health and Family Welfare, Government of India. (2023). Operational guidelines. National Program for Prevention and Control of Non-communicable Diseases. 2023-2030. [online] Available from chrome-extension://efaidnbmnnnibpcajpcglclefindmkaj/https://mohfw.gov.in/sites/default/files/NP-NCD%20Operational%20Guidelines_0.pdf [Last accessed December, 2024].
7. Niti Aayog, IIM Ahmedabad, Indian Institute of Public Health, Gandhinagar. National Health Mission. Impact and Learnings for the future - Draft report 2021. [online] Available from https://www.niti.gov.in/sites/default/files/2023-03/Impact%20of%20NHM%20on%20Health%20Systems%20Governance%20%26%20Human%20Resources.pdf. [Last accessed December, 2024].
8. Jagadish B. National Urban Health Mission: Providing adequate urban public health delivery system for the urban poor. [online] Available from https://www.semanticscholar.org/paper/NATIONAL-URBAN-HEALTH-MISSION%3A-PROVIDING-ADEQUATE-Jagadish/26a553ce37f039084391672f518206c0411f15d0. [Last accessed December, 2024].

22.4 National Health Programs Related to Child Health

Pukhraj Bafna, Alok Gupta

INTRODUCTION

The National Health Mission (NHM) of Government of India (GoI) in collaboration with the Ministry of Health and Family Welfare (MoHFW), Ministry of Women and Child Development (MoWCD), and others strives to provide quality health care to all citizens of the country in an equitable manner.

India witnessed a higher decline in maternal and child mortality compared to global average since the inception of NHM. With the National Health Policy (2017) in place, there is an unprecedented opportunity to build upon the gains made in the last 10 years and achieve *Sustainable Development Goals (SDGs)*. Various health programs are in place in all States and Union Territories (UTs) across India implemented with local governments. The State and UT governments are bound to follow these programs funded mostly by the Central Government.

CHILD HEALTH PROGRAMS

Important Child Health Programs in place are:[1]

- Facility-based Newborn and Child Care (FBNC)
- Mother Newborn Care Units
- Janani Shishu Suraksha Karyakram (JSSK)
- Facility-based Integrated Management of Neonatal and Childhood Illness (F-IMNCI)
- Integrated Management of Neonatal and Childhood Illnesses (IMNCI)
- Home-based Newborn Care (HBNC)

- Home-based Care for Young Child (HBYC)
- Strengthening Facility-based Pediatric Care
- Family Participatory Care (FPC)
- Navjat Shishu Suraksha Karyakram (NSSK)
- Reduction in Morbidity and Mortality due to Acute Respiratory Infections (ARI) and Diarrheal Diseases
- Rastriya Bal Swasthya Karyakram (RBSK)
- Pediatric Care
- National Newborn Week
- MusQan
- India Newborn Action Plan (INAP)
- Child Death Review Mechanism
- Intensified Diarrhea Control Fortnight (IDCF)
- Social Awareness and Actions to Neutralize Pneumonia Successfully (SAANS)
- Universal Immunization Program (Mission Indradhanush)

FACILITY-BASED NEWBORN AND CHILD CARE

Neonatal mortality being the major contributor (66%) to the infant mortality, addressing higher neonatal and early neonatal mortality, facility-based newborn care health services have been emphasized upon. Setting up of facilities for care of sick newborn such as Special Newborn Care Units (SNCUs), New Born Stabilization Units (NBSUs), and New Born Care Corners (NBCCs) at different levels is a thrust area under NHM.

- *Special Newborn Care Units* at least one in each district consisting of 12–20 beds, 4 trained doctors, and 10–12 nurses for round-the-clock services. SNCU complex need to have:
  - *Waiting area* in front of SNCU with simple amenities such as comfortable sitting space, safe drinking water, audiovisual (AV) system, tea/coffee vending machine, and a washroom for the parent or attendants
  - *Entry area*—space for gowning, hand washing, shoe rack, etc.
  - *Follow-up area* with AV facilities and adequate space for daily counseling, during discharge and imparting FPC training
  - *Reception area* for receiving the cases and assess under triage area
  - *Newborn care area (SNCU area* for cases admitted as per admission criteria for SNCU)—to accommodate at least 20 radiant warmers with additional clear, designated area as *isolation ward* for the infectious cases such as varicella and diarrhea, and area for procedures (desirable). Separate out-born and inborn units may not be required if strict asepsis protocols like that of an operation theater (OT) are followed.
  - *Additional handwashing facility* within the SNCU, mother's area, and feeding room (human milk storage room) will help in ensuring handwashing before handling of newborn.
  - *Doctor's and sister's duty room* with washrooms, *storage rooms, and Janitors/sluice room*
- *Newborn Stabilization units* of four beds with trained doctors and nurses at community health centers (CHCs)/ first referral units (FRUs) for stabilization of sick newborns
- *Newborn Care Corners* of one bed, attached to the labor room and OT for provision of essential newborn care at each facility where deliveries are taking place.

A comprehensive "Facility-Based Newborn Care Operational Guide-2011, a guideline for Planning and Implementation" have been published and disseminated by Child Health Division, MoHFW, GoI as a reference tool for the states to take necessary steps in implementation of same.

MOTHER NEWBORN CARE UNITS

A separate step-down/Kangaroo mother care (KMC) unit which is existing in many units as per the existing guidelines can now be upgraded and named as "mother newborn care unit (MNCU)", which will be an ideal space to keep the mother–baby dyad together to fulfil the following objectives:

- Decongesting SNCU of newborns who do not require intensive care but need observational care for their medical conditions.
- Making provisions (bed, diet, and treatment) for the mothers of SNCU admissions
- The admission criteria of SNCU as per FBNC Operational Guidelines will continue to be followed.
- No newborn deserving admission in SNCU will be shifted to the MNCU.
- Stepdown/KMC unit may be amalgamated as MNCU to have provisions for both mother and baby.
- MNCU will be jointly owned by both Department/ Unit of Pediatrics and Obstetrics and Gynecology for management of common conditions of both the mother and baby and the designated doctors and nurses will monitor them daily.

JANANI SHISHU SURAKSHA KARYAKRAM (JSSK)

This is discussed in Chapter 22.3.

FACILITY-BASED INTEGRATED MANAGEMENT OF NEONATAL AND CHILDHOOD ILLNESS (F-IMNCI)

This is discussed in Chapter 22.8.

INTEGRATED MANAGEMENT OF NEONATAL AND CHILDHOOD ILLNESSES (IMNCI)

This is discussed in Chapter 22.8.

HOME-BASED NEWBORN CARE

Home-based Newborn Care program, revised in 2014, was launched for accelerated reduction of neonatal mortality and morbidity rates especially in rural, remote areas where access to care is largely unavailable or located faraway. Under this program, Accredited Social Health Activist (ASHA) will make visits to all newborns according to a specified schedule up to the first 42 days of life. This includes six visits in case of institutional deliveries on 3rd, 7th, 14th, 21st, 28th and 42nd days after birth and one additional visit within 24 hours of delivery in case of home deliveries. Additional visits for babies who are preterm, low birth weight (LBW) or ill, and SNCU discharged babies will be conducted.

During the visit, ASHA will do the following activities:

- Information and skills to the mother and family on how to do better care of newborn, on special care for LBW babies, on how to identify danger signs and promote exclusive breastfeeding and immunization.
- Examining every newborn for prematurity and LBW, identification of illness, anything unusual in baby, provision of appropriate care at home, refer to auxiliary nurse and midwife (ANM) or nearest health facilities as defined in the protocols.
- Follow-up for sick newborns after they are discharged from facilities.
- Counseling the mother on postpartum care, recognition of postpartum complications and enabling referral.
- Counseling the mother for adoption of an appropriate family planning method.

Accredited Social Health Activists are being paid incentive of Rs. 250/- per newborn after completion of scheduled home visits at one time after 45 days of delivery, subject to the following:

- Recording of weight of the newborn in MCP card
- Ensuring BCG, first dose of OPV and hepatitis B (HBV) vaccination
- Both the mother and the newborn are safe till 45 days of the delivery, and
- Registration of birth has been done.

A comprehensive "Home-based Newborn Care Operational Guideline–2014 (revised)" has been developed, published, and disseminated by Child Health Division, MoHFW, GoI.

HOME-BASED CARE FOR YOUNG CHILD

Malnutrition continues to be the underlying cause of death for 35% of under-5 mortality reported in India. The interaction between undernutrition and infection can create a vicious cycle of worsening illness and deteriorating nutritional status. Interventions promoting infant and young child feeding (IYCF) are known to improve child survival, growth, and intellectual development. Numerous gaps and barriers are observed in the delivery and practice of IYCF recommendations. Research points to the benefits of integrated delivery platforms, notably combining nutrition interventions with support for parents in promoting play-based learning.

Under NHM, Child Health division, MoHFW, GoI has rolled out "Home Based Care for Young Child (HBYC) Program" in 2018, as an extension of the HBNC program to promote evidence-based interventions delivered in four key domains, namely nutrition, health, early childhood development, and WASH (water, sanitation, and hygiene). An operational guideline for HBYC program was released on 14th April 2018 in Chhattisgarh.

Under HBYC program, the additional five home visits will be carried out by ASHA with support from Anganwadi workers. ASHA will provide home visits on 3rd, 6th, 9th, 12th and 15th months to promote early initiation of breastfeeding, exclusive breastfeeding till 6 months, and continued breastfeeding till 2nd year of life along with adequate complementary feeding, prevention of childhood pneumonia and diarrhea, and to ensure age-appropriate immunization and early childhood development.

Accredited Social Health Activists will be provided incentive of ₹ 250/- for completion of five home visits under HBYC for each young child (₹ 50/- per visit) as per the recommended schedule and additional commodities, namely oral rehydration salt (ORS) packet and iron and folic acid syrup will be provided in the kit. National Deworming Day, Newborn Care, IYCF, and IDCF material, reports, information, education, and communication (IEC) material will be shifted from old website to new website under Child Health section.

STRENGTHENING FACILITY-BASED PEDIATRIC CARE

Facility-based care is complementary to community level interventions in bringing down childhood morbidity and mortality. Newborns and children referred from communities and primary health care (PHC) facilities are often seriously ill and at high risk of dying. Those reaching health facilities need to be managed appropriately and without delay in instituting care. This objective can be achieved by establishing a well-organized unit, adequate human resources, drugs, equipment, and other logistics that provides functional quality of care consistent with clinical standards.

The vision for pediatric care at District Hospital is to set up a comprehensive unit comprising of the following subunits:

- Pediatric outpatient facility (including immunization and counselling services)
- Emergency triage assessment and treatment (ETAT) facility

- Pediatric inpatient facility
- High-dependency unit
- Pediatric ward
- Diarrhea treatment unit
- Isolation room
- Ancillary (e.g., laboratory, imaging, and pharmacy) and auxiliary facilities (e.g., play area and hospital kitchen)

The general pediatric care facility will function in close coordination with specialized units that already have approved guidelines for operationalization and include the following:

- Newborn care facilities (NBCC, NBSU, and SNCU)
- Nutrition rehabilitation center
- District early intervention center

FAMILY PARTICIPATORY CARE

Parents if trained during their stay in the hospital to provide essential care to their sick and small newborns and explained what to do at the time of crises will not only help in improving survival of the babies after discharge from newborn care units but also help in the overall growth and development of the baby. In this regard Child Health division MoHFW, released "Operational Guidelines on Family Participatory Care (FPC)", which essentially provides a setting in which family is empowered, encouraged, and supported as the constant care-provider, in addition to available nursing staff, to complement care of their sick newborn in nursery, from admission until discharge and continue it in home settings. However, the primary responsibility of care continues to rest with the conventional healthcare provider, namely the nurse and doctor. Under FPC capacities of parents-attendants is built in essential newborn care through a structured training program (AV module and a training guide).

The staff at newborn care unit provides continuous supervision and support. Provisions for infrastructure and logistics strengthening required for implementing FPC are ensured in the annual state PIP. States like Madhya Pradesh, Odisha, Rajasthan, and Bihar have already implemented in SNCU across the state [with technical support from National Iron Plus Initiative (NIPI)-Newborn Project]. Parents-attendants are involved in a limited way for maintaining hygiene, cleaning the soiled baby, positioning of babies, and alerting the staff if they notice anything unusual with the baby.

NAVJAT SHISHU SURAKSHA KARYAKRAM

Navjat Shishu Suraksha Karyakram (NSSK) is a program started in 2009 aimed to train health personnel in basic newborn care and resuscitation to address care-at-birth issues, viz.:

- Prevention of hypothermia
- Prevention of infection
- Early initiation of breastfeeding
- Basic newborn resuscitation

With advances in critical care and based on the evidence, the NSSK training package has now been revised with updated algorithm and improved training methodology. The training package is 2 days classroom and hands-on training. It includes a resource manual and flip chart. NSSK aims to train all health workers and doctors involved in delivery and newborn care.

The training package emphasizes the skill imparting techniques by the facilitators and ensures uniform messaging across all the levels. This package is an enabling tool and helps healthcare providers to improve their clinical skills and practices and contribute to newborn survival and health in the country. It is expected to reduce neonatal mortality significantly in the country.

REDUCTION IN MORBIDITY AND MORTALITY DUE TO ACUTE RESPIRATORY INFECTIONS AND DIARRHEAL DISEASES

Childhood Diarrhea

- To control diarrheal diseases, GoI has adopted the World Health Organization (WHO) guidelines on diarrhea management.
- India introduced the low osmolarity Oral Rehydration Solution (ORS), as recommended by WHO for the management of diarrhea.
- Zinc has been approved as an adjunct to ORS for the management of diarrhea. Addition of Zinc would result in reduction of the number and severity of episodes and the duration of diarrhea.
- New guidelines on management of diarrhea have been modified based on the latest available scientific evidence.

Acute Respiratory Infections

- Acute respiratory infections form 19% of all under-5 mortalities in India (WHO 2007 report) and along with diarrhea are two major killers of under-5 children.
- India leads the world in the number of pneumonia cases with nearly 4400,000 cases yearly. Early diagnosis and appropriate case management by rational use of antibiotics remains one of the most effective interventions to prevent deaths due to pneumonia.
- The ARI guidelines are being revised with the inclusion of the latest available global evidence.

RASHTRIYA BAL SWASTHYA KARYAKRAM (RBSK)

This is discussed in Chapters 22.3 and 22.7.

PEDIATRIC CARE (IMNCI AND F-IMNCI)

This is discussed in Chapter 22.8.

NATIONAL NEWBORN WEEK

National Newborn Week is being observed by the MoHFW, GoI from 15th through 21st November to reinforce the importance of newborn health as a key priority area and reiterates its commitment steered at the highest level.

MUSQAN

The key strategy of MusQan is to:

- Strengthen clinical protocols and management process
- Children and parent attendant friendly ambience and infrastructure
- Strengthen referral and follow-up services
- Provision of respectful and dignified care

Through "MusQan", the country aims to make newborn and childcare services friendly, for which the targeted facilities will undertake following rapid improvement cycles. Each cycle will be of two months, and its progress will be rigorously supervised by the states and district level teams.

INDIA NEWBORN ACTION PLAN

India Newborn Action Plan (INAP) was launched in 2014 to make concerted efforts toward attainment of the goals of "Single Digit Neonatal Mortality Rate" and "Single Digit Stillbirth Rate", by 2030.

CHILD DEATH REVIEW MECHANISM

Child Death Review (CDR) strategy implemented with the objectives of:

- To establish a framework to assess the burden of neonatal and child deaths, including trends in numbers and causes of death.
- To generate information about modifiable factors contributing and to use the information to guide actions to prevent similar deaths in the future.
- To use the findings of the child mortality review to formulate appropriate actions to address modifiable factors, thereby preventing future neonatal and child deaths.
- To provide accountability for results and compel decision-makers to pay due attention and respond to the problem.

Child Death Review is of two types:

1. Community-based Child Death Review (CBCDR)
2. Facility-based Child Death Review (FBCDR)

Online portal of Maternal, Perinatal, Child Death Surveillance and Review (MPCDSR) was released on 17th September 2021. This portal will enable real-time recording of all neonatal and child deaths, review causes, and need-based action can be taken based on the report on timely manner.

INTENSIFIED DIARRHEA CONTROL FORTNIGHT

To increase awareness about use of ORS and zinc in diarrhea, an IDCF is being observed during pre-monsoon/monsoon season, with the aim of "zero child deaths due to childhood diarrhea" since 2014. During the fortnight, health workers visit the households of under-5 children, conduct community level awareness generation activities, and distribute ORS packets to the families with children under-5 years of age.

SOCIAL AWARENESS AND ACTIONS TO NEUTRALIZE PNEUMONIA SUCCESSFULLY

Social Awareness and Actions to Neutralize Pneumonia Successfully initiative was launched on 16th November 2019 to accelerate action to reduce deaths due to childhood pneumonia. SAANS Campaign is rolled out in the States/UTs every year with the aim of accelerating action against childhood pneumonia by generating awareness around protect, prevent, and treatment aspects of childhood pneumonia and to enhance early identification and care-seeking behaviors among parents and caregivers.

UNIVERSAL IMMUNIZATION PROGRAM

The goal of Universal Immunization Program (UIP) is to provide every child and pregnant women protection from vaccine-preventable diseases. National Immunization Schedule is available for infants, children, and pregnant women. India's UIP is a part of the Reproductive and Child Health (RCH) Program under NHM. It is one of the largest public health programs in the world under which vaccination is being provided free of cost to all pregnant women and children. Vaccinations are provided against 11 nationally against hepatitis B, poliomyelitis, severe form of tuberculosis, diphtheria, pertussis, tetanus, meningitis, and pneumonia caused by *Haemophilus* type B and pneumococci, rotavirus diarrhea, measles, rubella, and subnationally against Japanese encephalitis in endemic districts.

U-WIN platform captures each and every vaccination event of all pregnant women and children under UIP.

CONCLUSION

India is relatively a country of young people. Nearly 33% of the Indian population is below the age of 18 years, 50% between the age of 18 and 60 years and 13% aged 60 years and above.

To improve the health of children of India in totality, all the 17 SDG goals of UN need to be addressed and met on time.

The most important 20 National Health Programs related to Child Health, as discussed above will help India in becoming 'Fit & Healthy India'.

REFERENCE

1. Child Health Programs, National Health Mission, Ministry of Health and Family Welfare, Government of India. [online] Available from https://nhm.gov.in/index1.php?lang=1&level=3&sublinkid=1179&lid=363 [Last accessed December, 2024].

22.5 Art of Parenting

S Yamuna

INTRODUCTION

India is not only a country of physical, political, linguistic, cultural, and religious multiplicity but also a country with diversity in health needs and distribution. On the one hand, we have been losing many children <5 years in large numbers to infectious diseases and other fatal illnesses of childhood, on the other hand, we are also seeing many children and adolescents with high-risk behaviors that are detrimental not only to their personal growth but also a deterrent to the generation of a healthy human capital for our nation. India would continue to be young till 2050; pediatricians have a window of opportunity and a duty to invest on the holistic health of the children and adolescents to build a wholesome nation.

Studies from many parts of the world have documented that family connectedness, school connectedness, presence of trustworthy adult, and spiritual beliefs as the protective factors associated with healthy adolescence free from high-risk health behaviors such as violence, substance use including smoking, drunken driving, suicide, and high-risk sexual behaviors.

Establishment of family connectedness is dependent on the two-way communicative relationship between parents and the children. Temperament of the child, attachment pattern established during early childhood, parenting styles and practices, and emotional regulation in the family context are some of the determinants of creation of strong family connectedness during adolescence.[1,2]

IS PARENTING AN ART OR SCIENCE?

Parenting practices and styles influence the inculcation of habits, behavior, and personality of the children. All along we have had no formal training on parenting as parenting has been considered an art that is learnt from the previous generation by observation. With rapid economic progress, India has quick urbanization, migration with increase in nuclear families, liberalization, and globalization with the associated confusion about traditionality versus futuristic approach to upbringing of children. In view of this, the science behind parenting is tapped based on evidence to help the knowledge-thirsty educated parents of India to see their children grow with appropriate inputs.

PARENT-CHILD BOND

Parent-child bond is determined by:
- Temperament of the child
- Attachment pattern established during early childhood
- Parenting style
- Communication style of parents

Temperament of the Child

Temperament or innate nature of a child is the trait with which a baby is born in this world. When the parental expectation and the temperamental trait of the child match, the bonding is better because the positive cues given by the parent to the child and the cheerful responses received by the parent from the child are pleasurable and promote attachment.[2]

Activity level, rhythmicity, approach and withdrawal, adaptability, threshold of responsiveness, intensity of reaction, quality of mood, distractibility, attention span, and persistence are temperamental traits. Thus, a child who is active, rhythmic, quick to warm up, with immediate response to cues, easily accommodative, with cheerfulness, with sustained attention, and perseverance would be able to win the hearts of the parents and parental figures more easily than a child who is lethargic, chaotic, slow to warm up, who withdraws at approach, and stays grumpy, whining, with decreased attention span and increased distractibility.

Attachment Pattern Established During Early Childhood

Continuous and consistent reception of warmth, love, care, attention, compassion, and encouragement from parents makes children feel secure with parents even before they turn two. This security is expressed at reunion with parents after a span of separation. Securely attached child is confident of a happy reunion with parents while a child who has received inconsistent responsiveness and attention from parents may either develop an insecure avoidant attachment pattern or insecure ambivalent attachment pattern with expression of avoidance and clinginess respectively. Some children might have received resentment or neglect from parents, who are either preoccupied or ignorant about their role as parent, where the child develops a disorganized attachment pattern. The kind of attachment established during early childhood not only enhances the parent child bonding but also determines the relationships the child would enjoy with friends and marital relationships in future.

Parenting Style

Depending on the parental demandingness and responsiveness to their children, Diana Baumrind classified parenting styles into four types:[1,3]

1. *Authoritarian:* Highly demanding and less responsive
2. *Permissive/indulgent:* Highly responsive and not demanding, but overindulging
3. *Authoritative:* Highly demanding and highly responsive with role modeling
4. *Neglectful:* Not demanding and not responsive and not available

Table 22.5.1 highlights the additional characteristics of each of the parenting style.[3]

TABLE 22.5.1: Characteristic feature of the four parenting styles.[3]

Feature/parenting style	*Authoritarian*	*Permissive/indulgent*	*Authoritative*	*Neglectful*
Demandingness	High	Nil	High	Nil
Responsiveness	Less	High	High	Nil
Style of communication	Aggressive	Passive/submissive	Assertive	Poor/limited to few words
Expression of love	Care is considered as love	Well-expressed	Well-expressed	Rarely expressed
Demonstrative love	Not expressed	Well-expressed	Well-expressed	Nil
Time spent with children	Less	High	High	Minimal
Value inculcation	Through instruction, "do as I say," and not "do as I do"	Left to child as "whatever you do is right for you!"	"We are value loaded and follow what we practice:" Explanations are provided for each expectation	No attempt at value inculcation is made
Insistence on discipline	High with psychological control such as blackmailing, name calling, and sometimes physical abuse	Nil	Firm and high with explanation and negotiation and differential reinforcement such as encouragement for positive behaviors and ignoring negative behaviors	Nil
Role modeling	Minimal	Nil, entire household is child-centered	Very high	Nil
Compassion	Nil	Moderate because the child's best interest is not the priority of the parents	Very high	Nil
Freedom of speech and expression	Nil	Total freedom: Child will not know how to make use of the freedom, gets confused, and anxious	Freedom of expression is given, with a lot of inputs from parents on the right and the wrong. Guidance on modification is offered with compassion	As there is not much of contact, expression is determined by the children who feel not guided
Moralistic	Highly moralistic	Willing to relax all moral values to see happiness in children	High, but not judgmental. Guidance is offered always	Not applicable
Opinionated	Yes	Nil	Not opinionated but explains possible opinions that can be formed by certain behaviors	Not applicable
Care of children	Care is complete, all acts of service done in a methodical but in an impersonal manner. Attempt to self-care is not encouraged. Dependency is seen as obedience and subordination	Very good with personal attention to begin with to the level of not allowing the child to self-learn skills; later years with scare that the child might scold the parents for lapses	Very good with personal attention, involving children in inculcation of habits of self-care very early in life, generation of independence, and preparation of the children to survive without the support of parents is practiced	Care is not adequate and children usually fend for themselves with breach in self-care and hygiene

Contd...

Contd...

Feature/parenting style	*Authoritarian*	*Permissive/indulgent*	*Authoritative*	*Neglectful*
Appreciation and encouragement	Rarely offered	Offered more than necessary as the parents are scared at consequences if not offered	Offered in right doses at right occasions	Not offered as the parents are rarely aware of accomplishments
Criticism	Liberal and frequent	Nil	Yes, but with explanations and ways to rectify	Rarely take note of deviance in behaviors or actions
Outcome in children	Submissive or rebellious, lack of self-control and self-esteem, and self-confidence as they have been controlled always. Performance anxiety is high and accomplishments are less	Self-driven, anxious at outcomes as they have not been exposed to challenges appropriately with guidance from parents; Self-esteem low with reduced confidence at new activities	Self-motivated, self-disciplined, self-confident, children with high self-esteem, and frequent success in many tasks	Feel that they lack direction or may latch on to people to receive direction, which may be right or wrong
Children's perception about the parents	Strict, controlling parents who gave no space for growth	Ineffective parents who offered no guidance and direction	Excellent parents who were available always but at the same time encouraged independence	Nonavailable parents who were totally away in mind, body, and actions

Communication Style of Parents

Parents may use any of the below three styles of communication between themselves with children and with others:

1. Aggressive style communicates authority with minimal empathy and is used by authoritarian parents.
2. Passive style of communication is practiced by permissive parents who are meek, submissive, and are usually not capable of taking decisions.
3. Assertive style of communication is by far the best style used by authoritative parents who express their intent with firmness. This style entertains mutual respect and helps in effective parenting.

ROLE OF THE FAMILY CONTEXT IN THE DEVELOPMENT OF EMOTION REGULATION

Emotion regulation consists of internal and external processes involved in initiating, maintaining, and modulating the occurrence, intensity, and expression of emotions. Emotional regulation helps in the socialization process that happens from infancy to adulthood by modulating one's expression of emotions by understanding the actual emotions, with respect to tone, intensity, and dynamics such as duration of the emotional experience **(Flowchart 22.5.1)**.[4,5]

- *Internal processes* would be child-specific factors such as temperament of the child, child's responsiveness or reactivity to external cues, stage of development, individual thoughts about emotions, and the associated physiological responses to each of the emotion.
- *External processes* would depend on the emotional climate of the family and on the specific characteristics of the parents and the parent figures. Emotional climate of the family is further determined by the status of the marital relationship, parenting styles practiced, attachment patterns established, emotional coaching by parents like "when you are angry take a deep breath, etc.," emotional expressivity of parents, social referencing like adapting the responses of significant others at similar situation, parental role modeling, the predominant emotional state in the family, etc.

INFLUENCE OF PARENTING STYLES

Parent-specific factors are related to the mental health of the parents and the kind of emotional regulation they have imbibed from their parents. With increasing age, the dependency on parents for emotional regulation comes down but the influence of peer group intensifies.[6]

Influence of parenting styles and parenting practices on certain aspects of growth and development in children and adolescents are being studied extensively. The previous endorsement of authoritarian parenting to inculcate certain qualities and habits in children is being replaced by new understandings that are encouraging parents to practice authoritative parenting styles.

Eating Practices

In a study on the influence of parenting styles and the consumption of fruits and vegetables by preschoolers,

Flowchart 22.5.1: Factors determining the emotional regulation of the children in the family context.

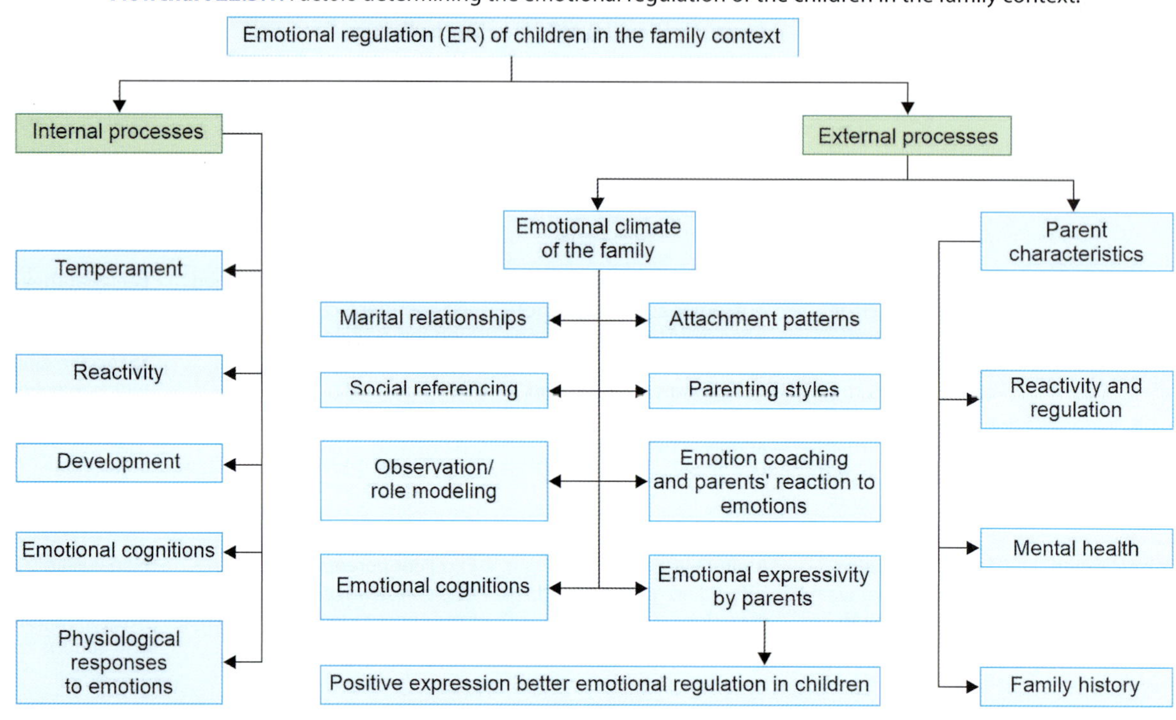

authoritative parenting style emerged as a better style in ensuring cooperation. This has been attributed to the utilization of teachable moments by parents to give information on the benefits of consumption of fruits and vegetables, practical methods such as role modeling by both parents, firmness in maintaining discipline with respect to eating schedules, restriction of availability of junk foods within the household, and limiting accessibility to the same outside the home, and enhancement in the availability of fruits and vegetables at all times of the day.[1,3,7]

Similarly, children with overweight and obesity are less common in families with authoritative parents.

Physical Activity

Though studies on the influence of parenting style on physical activity are not many, the knowledge gained has been quite different. Children's participation in sports, acquisition of skills in a game, and excelling in tournaments has been more commonly associated with permissive style of parenting. Logistic support to continue sports activities is higher in households with permissive parents.[3]

Externalizing Behaviors

Externalizing behaviors like usage of aggression and violence is more common in families with authoritarian style as the children learn by observing parents. It is also widely seen in children brought up by permissive parents because the parents might have failed to establish their role in disciplining between 2 and 6 years when the externalizing behaviors begin and reduce, respectively. Authoritative parents are quite clear about establishing their role and achieving cooperation from children as they practice methods of differential reinforcement, which reduces the negative behaviors.[3,4,6]

MINDFUL PARENTING

Being mindful as a parent means that the parent should have the knowledge of:

- Who are they?
- What is their expectation from the child?
- Is the expectation age and developmentally appropriate for the child?
- Where does this expectation come from?
- Is it from what they received as a kid from their own parents?
- What is the deep-seated emotion surrounding these expectations?
- Is it fear, sadness, worry, anxiety, or pain about being incapable of teaching the child the best?
- Is the underlying emotion disappointment with the child which gets expressed as anger?
- What is the need of the child at that moment?
- Is the need *physical* such as sleep or hunger, *emotional* such as being sad or frustrated at lack of skills, or *social*

such as wanting a hug of appreciation and kiss of nurturance?

- What is the predominant emotion of the child?
- Is the child doing something due to ignorance?
- What can be the ways used to help the child?
- What words to use to convey the same to the child in a way the child feels helped and not judged or ridiculed or criticized?
- When is the best time to explain to the child?
- Willful expression of love and compassion in a manner that is needed and understood by the child.

Mindfulness in all actions that an adult carries out would help the adult to respond to any situation keeping in mind their deep-seated emotion and not react with emotions that surface. Imparting this to parents at every meeting with the pediatrician is likely to help parents inculcate empathy for the child and feel fulfilled as being an effective parent.[8]

PARENTING PROGRAMS

Inculcation of authoritative parenting skills in parents is gradually being adapted in the developing world based on the evidence generated by the developed world. Indian Academy of Pediatrics (IAP) has also created the "Happy Parenting Program" in 2010 where a self-training module titled, "Stepping Stones: Pediatricians' Recipe for Happy Parenting" along with a CD containing slides for introspective learning have been posted to all its members who are now equipped to train the parents.[8,9]

RESEARCH OPTIONS IN THE INDIAN CONTEXT

As of now the parenting styles practiced in India are diverse and in multiple combinations as the parenting responsibility is not limited to biological parents only. The recent generations of parents who are evolving from a collectivistic society to individualistic practices are usually not consistent with the parenting style. Hence, knowledge about the parenting received and the styles being practiced can be accessed from various groups of urban, semiurban, and rural parents by using qualitative research methods and then arrive at new hypotheses for further research.

CONCLUSION

Parenting is a science that is based on human development, temperament, and interpersonal relationships. Use of warm, responsive, firm authoritative parenting style with mindfulness helps in bringing up children as healthy, self-confident, self-reliant, and independent adults. Pediatricians can start introducing parenting principles during well baby visits when parents are usually receptive. Parenting programs can be included as a primary prevention activity to prevent behavior disorders in children.[10]

REFERENCES

1. Berge JM, Wall M, Neumark-Sztainer D, Larson N, Story M. Parenting style and family meals: Cross-sectional and 5-year longitudinal associations. J Am Diet Assoc. 2010;110(7): 1036-42.
2. Lahey BB, Van Hulle CA, Keenan K, Rathouz PJ, D'Onofrio BM, Rodgers JL, et al. Temperament and parenting during the first year of life predict future child conduct problems. J Abnorm Child Psychol. 2008;36(8):1139-58.
3. Darling N. Parenting style and its correlates. ERIC Digest. Illinois: ERIC Clearinghouse on Elementary and Early Childhood Education; 1999.
4. Chang L, Schwartz D, Dodge KA, McBride-Chang C. Harsh parenting in relation to child emotion regulation and aggression. J Fam Psychol. 2003;17:598-606.
5. Morris AS, Silk JS, Steinberg L, Myers JS, Robinson LR. The role of the family context in the development of emotion regulation. Soc Dev. 2007;16:361-88.
6. Buschgens CJ, van Aken MA, Swinkels SH, Ormel J, Verhulst FC, Buitelaar JK. Externalizing behaviors in preadolescents: Familial risk to externalizing behaviors and perceived parenting styles. Eur Child Adolesc Psychiatry. 2010;19(7): 567-75.
7. O'Connor TM, Hughes SO, Watson KB, Baranowski T, Nicklas TA, Fisher JO, et al. Parenting practices are associated with fruit and vegetable consumption in pre-school children. Public Health Nutr. 2010;13(1):91-101.
8. Ugra D, Yamuna S. Stepping Stones: Paediatricians' Recipe for Happy Parenting. Mumbai: Indian Academy of Pediatrics; 2010.
9. Spijkers W, Jansen DE, de Meer G, Reijneveld SA. Effectiveness of a parenting programme in a public health setting: A randomized controlled trial of the positive parenting programme (Triple P) level 3 versus care as usual provided by the preventive child healthcare (PCH). BMC Public Health. 2010;10:131.
10. National Academies of Sciences, Engineering, and Medicine; Division of Behavioral and Social Sciences and Education; Board on Children, Youth, and Families; Committee on Supporting the Parents of Young Children; Breiner H, Ford M, (Eds). Parenting Matters: Supporting Parents of Children Ages 0-8. Washington (DC): National Academies Press (US); 2016.

22.6 Prevention and Control of Injuries

K Nedunchelian

INTRODUCTION

Injuries are important cause of preventable morbidity and mortality among children and adolescents globally. The World Health Organization (WHO) and United Nations Children's Fund (UNICEF) Report (2008) draws global attention to the five leading causes of death related to child injury—road traffic injuries, drowning, poisoning, burns, and fall and set out what could be done to prevent these injuries. Yet there is not much focus on the issue of childhood and adolescent injuries and its prevention, especially in underdeveloped and developing countries.

DEFINITION AND CLASSIFICATION

The term "accident" represents an incident occurring by chance that cannot be predicted and prevented, whereas "injury" represents an event occurring in predictable circumstances among individuals who are at high risk. The term "injury" is preferable in the sense that it promotes awareness program as it leads to proper planning of prevention and possibility of injury control.

Injury control comprises "primary prevention" attempting to prevent injuries, as well as "secondary" and "tertiary" prevention, representing trauma care and rehabilitation, respectively. Instead of just trying to attribute it to accident proneness of children, physical and social environment of children in which injury occurs are to be considered. Injuries can be "unintentional" (road traffic injuries, falls, burns, poisoning, and drowning) or "intentional" (interpersonal violence or homicide, self-inflicted injury or suicide, and war). Injuries are also classified based on the place of injury as "domestic" injuries, injuries at public places, and the settings of injuries as "recreational" injuries and "occupational" injuries (including industrial and agricultural injuries).[1] Our focus here is mainly on the prevention and control of injuries arising out of accidents due to unnatural causes and not those due to natural disasters.

INCIDENCE AND MORTALITY

In the year 2020, the number of road accidents reported was 3,66,138 leading to 3,48,279 injuries. In 2021, it was on the rise with 4,12,432 accidents and 3,84,448 injuries, revealing increase of 12.64% and 10.39%, respectively. In 2022 there were 4,61,000 road accidents across India.[2,3]

RISK FACTORS

Age

Injuries occur at a particular age when a child or an adolescent encounters a new task or hazard against which they may not have the skills to handle. In view of exploratory nature of toddlers, they are at high risk for injuries especially burns, drowning, and falls. They do not know that medications can be poisonous or some houseplants are not to be consumed. Many parents expect young school-aged children to walk home from school, the playground, or the local store, a task for which most children are not developmentally ready. Young school-aged children are at-risk for pedestrian injuries, bicycle-related injuries, motor vehicle occupant injuries, burns, and drowning. The lack of skills and experience leads to motor vehicle injuries, drowning, burns, and risk of intentional trauma among teenagers. Alcohol and other drugs often add to these limitations. Work-related injuries are associated with child labor.[1]

Age also determines the severity of injury and long-term disability. For example, outcome of head injuries among young children is poor when compared to adolescents or adults.

Sex

Males have higher rates of injury than females. Variation in exposure to risk and greater risk-taking behavior, combined with greater frequency of alcohol use, may lead to the disproportionately high rate of motor vehicle crashes among teenage males and not due to developmental differences between the sexes. Children with psychiatric problems, especially those with attention-deficit hyperactivity disorder (ADHD) are at higher risk for injuries.[1]

Ethnicity

Risk for injury is related to poverty, educational status, and presence of hazardous environments, rather than race alone.

Socioeconomic Status and Environment

Mortality from fire, motor vehicle crashes, and drowning are higher among poor children. Other factors are single-parent families, teenage mothers, multiple care providers, family stress, and multiple siblings, which are primarily due to poverty rather than independent risk factors. Poor children are exposed to more hazards in their living environments, in the form of poor housing, which is less likely to be protected by smoke detectors, etc. The roads are more likely to be major thoroughfares. Those with poor environment, experience higher levels of violence, and they are more likely to be victims of assault.

Rural versus Urban Status

Unplanned urbanization with slums and informal urban settlements lead to high risks of injury for children, especially in developing world. Injury rates are higher in rural and homicide rates are higher in urban areas. Case fatality from injury is generally twice as high in rural areas than in urban areas, due to increased severity of some injuries (such as motor vehicle crashes occurring at higher speeds) and poor access to emergency medical and definitive trauma care services. Agricultural injuries are mostly confined to rural areas.

Those prone to injury are more likely to be unsupervised, having families in disharmony, and hazardous environments conducive for injuries.

STRATEGIES TO PREVENT AND CONTROL INJURIES

Children have the right to have a safe environment and protection from injuries. Many developed nations have been able to bring down child deaths related to injuries drastically over the decades by adopting multisectoral, multipronged approaches to child injury prevention.[4] The approach should aim to reduce the:

- Risk of new injuries
- Severity of injuries that occurred
- Frequency and severity of injury-related disability

Following are the strategies suggested in general:[4]

- *Promotion of awareness:* "Passive intervention" is for entire population, irrespective of individual's involvement, whereas "active intervention" requires behavior change of parents and children. Community education is an active intervention, whereas product and environment modification are passive interventions.
- *Education to parents:* Behavior modification is the most important step toward injury control. Focus should be specific, for example, use of car seat restraints, helmets, use of smoke detectors, etc. This will be more successful than vague general instructions.
- *Modification of product designs:* These are more useful than repeated attempts of behavior change among the parents or children. Lowering the water heater temperature, installing smoke detectors, and using child-resistant caps for containers with medicines and household products are examples of effective product modifications. Many interventions require both active and passive measures. Seat belts provide passive protection when used but behavior change is required to use it regularly.
- *Modification of the social and physical environment:* Greater effort is required for this when compared to individual product modification but it is very effective in controlling injuries. Safe roadway traffic and speed limits are examples of such interventions. Changes in the social environment through legislation are needed sometimes, such as laws mandating child seat restraint and use of seat belts, bicycle helmets, and streamlining motor vehicle licensing laws, etc.

Campaigns combining two or more of these approaches have been particularly effective in controlling injuries. All these can be achieved in the following ways:[4]

- Health-promoting initiatives in schools can incorporate injury prevention and safety promotion.
- Child-injury prevention can be taken up by "healthy cities" programs.
- Community-based approaches to child injury prevention can work well.
- Education, skills development, and behavior change, etc. directed toward child injury prevention needs to be integrated with other health promotion campaigns designed to change child and adolescent behavior as well as public in general. An intersectoral approach to injury prevention and control has been suggested by the WHO **(Fig. 22.6.1)**.[4]

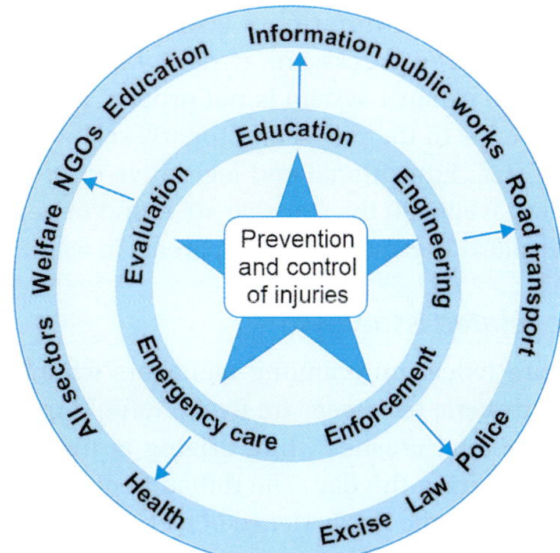

Fig. 22.6.1: An intersectoral approach to injury prevention and control.

Source: WHO. (2002). Strategic Plan for Injury Prevention and Control in South-East Asia. [online] Available from https://iris.who.int/bitstream/handle/10665/206403/B1470.pdf?sequence=1&isAllowed=y [Last accessed December, 2024].

INDIVIDUAL TYPES OF INJURIES AND THEIR PREVENTION

Falls

Falls account for most of the injuries among children. Mostly, falls are from vehicles, walkers, staircases, and while on play, etc. Prevention is by redesigning the furniture and other products, raising the level of railing of staircase, and carpeted, window guards, and playground with energy-absorbent materials like sand, rubberized surfaces, or coir mats. Safety gates can be used, children should never be left unattended, and discourage climbing unreachable heights.

Road Traffic Injuries

Traffic accidents are the major contributors to accidental deaths of unnatural cause and constitute the leading cause of serious and fatal injuries among all age groups. Injury can be to the occupant, driver, or both.

Occupant-related Issues

Injuries to passenger vehicle occupants are the predominant cause of motor vehicle death among children and adolescents, except for the 5–9-year-old group, in whom pedestrian injuries are common. Teach children to always use age- and size-appropriate restraints. Children <13 years should ride in the back seat of the vehicle.

Infants or children weighing <10 kg should be placed in the rear seat facing backward. Toddlers and children can be placed in the rear seat in a forward-facing toddler seat. Children in the back of uncovered vehicles, face the possibility of being thrown out leading to head injury and those in covered trucks are at risk of carbon monoxide poisoning if exhaust system is not proper. The safest place for children is in the rear seat, properly restrained for their age and size. Educational and legislative interventions for children traveling in the rear seat are found to be successful. Audiovisual aids can be shown to parents in waiting rooms.

Driver-related Issue

These are twice more among teenagers when compared to elder drivers; teenagers are five to tenfold more likely to encounter fatal crashes while driving at night compared to driving during the day. The difficulty of driving at night combined with the inexperience of teenagers appear to be a deadly combination. The inexperience in driving and driving in a drunken state is more dangerous.

Pedestrian Injuries

Mostly, injuries occur during the day, with a peak in the after-school period. Risk is more with factors like heavy traffic, high speed, absence of play space near home, household crowding, and low socioeconomic status.

Young children are more prone because of their poor ability to judge distance and speed of vehicles and being easily distracted by playmates or environmental factors. Other factors are poor socioeconomic status, low educational status, living in mobile homes, etc.

Bicycle Injuries

Head trauma is the leading cause of mortality. Educational programs should be organized by physicians and service organizations to promote the use of bicycle helmets in children. Separate bicycle path is an ideal option. Bicycles are to be checked periodically for proper functioning and loose parts.

Prevention of road traffic injuries is by multifaceted approach: Younger children should never cross streets alone until 10 years of age. Select streets with little traffic. Following legislation and police enforcement will be useful:

- Measures to slow the speed of traffic, especially around schools, residential areas, and play areas
- To route traffic away from schools and residential areas
- Networks of "one-way streets"
- Proper placement of transit or school bus stops, sidewalks in urban and suburban areas
- Edge stripping in rural areas to delineate the edge of the road
- Strictly implementing parking rules.

Burns

Flame burns resulting from ignition of clothing are common followed by household fire injuries, especially among small children. Using nonflammable fabrics will minimize this. Scalds from hot liquids and foods are most common in children <5 years. Avoiding taking hot drinks, smoking while holding an infant; keeping children away from pots, and cooking stove; and use of child-resistant lighters are few steps to avoid scalds and burns. Children and parents can undergo mock exercises on coping with a fire accident. A fire extinguisher can be advocated.

Fireworks-related injuries are usually seasonal, where supervision by adults while children use fireworks is mandatory. Smoking constitutes half of the household fires. The combination of smoking and alcohol use will increase risk of injury and mortality. Burns following exposure to corrosives, especially acids and electric shock should be kept in mind. Enforce laws on smoke alarms. Smoke detectors are inexpensive and at the same time, effective methods of preventing majority of these deaths. Sometimes, burns result from setting fire (exploratory play) by children or adolescents.

To treat patients with burns and scalds, a greater number of dedicated burns centers are to be established to have the best outcome for these patients.

Drowning

Drowning is common among older children and adolescents during swimming or boating. It is common among children <5 years of age, as they do not know the consequence of getting into the water and do not call for help, therefore they are more prone to submersion injury. Four-sided fencing of pools, personal flotation devices, and not allowing toddlers unattended in swimming pool or bathtub will prevent drowning. When intoxicated with alcohol, risk increases manyfold. Ensure immediate resuscitation in case of submersion injuries and adults can be trained in cardiopulmonary resuscitation. Feasibility of teaching swimming at least by 4 years of age and practice of wearing life jackets while boating can reduce the morbidity and mortality due to drowning.

Suffocation

Suffocation is more common in infants and toddlers due to food, nuts, parts of toys, etc. getting aspirated into the airway or smothering accidentally by pillow, bed sheet, and strangulation while playing with swings. Prevention of suffocation can be done by making the infants sleep on their backs and using well-fit bedsheets, and children should sleep in the same room as caregivers.

Poisoning

Poisoning with common household substances is a subject by itself (Please refer to *Chapter 20.2: Poisoning and Envenomation in Children* for a detailed description). The prevention can be done by keeping the poisonous substances out of reach of children, stored in proper containers with child-resistant caps, packaging drugs in nonlethal quantities with appropriate labels, etc. Legislation for child-resistant packaging of medicines and poisons is needed. Establish poison control centers to guide, supervise, and manage poisoning-related issues.

Sports

The health benefits of physical activity cannot be underestimated. Children, especially adolescents, who participate in sports and recreational activities are exposed to various injury risks.

Homicide

Homicide may be observed in "infantile" and "adolescent" groups. The earlier group may be subjected to "child abuse" by caretakers and the latter to firearm injuries from peers or otherwise. Firearms should be stored unloaded and kept safely.

MANAGEMENT

Management consists of preventing further injury, transport, maintenance of vitals, and advanced management of the injury. Emergency treatment may need to be instituted immediately in case of respiratory or cardiovascular compromise. Following transfer to a trauma care center, accurate evaluation of the injuries and appropriate management are essential. "Post-traumatic stress disorder" among parents and children who survived near-fatal injuries is yet another important issue, which should be addressed.

CONCLUSION

Since the injuries related to accidents are important cause of preventable morbidity and mortality, it is essential that apart from the prevention, control and management of injuries due to accidents, exposure of the public to various awareness programs prevention and control is equally important.

REFERENCES

1. Chapman JI, Walker DM. Emergency medical services applicable for children/Principles applicable to the developing world–Injuries. In: Kliegman RM, Stanton BF, St. Geme III JW, Schor NF, Behrman RE (Eds). Nelson's Textbook of Pediatrics, First South Asia Edition. New Delhi: Elsevier India; 2016. pp. 385-6.
2. The National Crime Records Bureau (NCRB). Accidental deaths and suicides in India 2015. New Delhi: Ministry of Home Affairs, Government of India; 2016.
3. Ministry of Road Transport and Highways, Government of India. (2022). Road Accidents in India. 2021. [online] Available from https://morth.nic.in/sites/default/files/RA_2022_30_Oct.pdf [Last accessed December, 2024].
4. Harvey A, Towner E, Peden M, Soori H, Bartolomeos K. Injury prevention and the attainment of child and adolescent health. Bull World Health Organ. 2009;87(5):390-4.

22.7 School Health Programs

Swati Ghate

INTRODUCTION

The school-going children constitute a major chunk of our population. In India, the "Right to Education Act" mandates the government to impart schooling to every child between 6 and 14 years. Nearly 80% of this target is achieved and Indian schools cater to over 26.52 crore students (2021–22 data). This huge number is in itself enough to understand the importance of health of school children. Their health status and outcomes obviously, directly reflect on to the current as well as the future health parameters of the community and the country.[1]

WHY "SCHOOL HEALTH"?

School-going children and adolescents are in their peak phase of growth and development. Though this period is regarded as relatively healthy, the school children have their own set of health concerns like physical growth issues, nutritional problems, infections and infestations, mental health problems, etc., for which they need an easily available, affordable, accessible and empathetic medical support system. It is desirable that they are given information, training, monitoring, prevention and treatment services and referral guidance from this system, on various health related issues. Schools, naturally, become the best platforms to offer such services consistently over the entire period of 10–12 schooling years.

Health and learning, including the formal education, are intricately linked. For better academic gains, students need to be healthy, fit and fine. Health and schooling are inseparable and investing in school health programs pays triple dividend, by positively impacting the lives of school children and adolescents today, their adulthood, and their next generation.

Thus, clubbing health with schooling ensures a wide reach and is convenient, cost-effective, time-saving, consistently and easily available over long years and enhances educational outcomes.

HOW IT STARTED?

School health came on priority as the concept of public health gained importance and physical health nutrition, routine health check-ups and health education became an integral part of school health programs. In 1995, World Health Organization (WHO) launched Global School Health Initiative, to mobilize and strengthen health promotion and education activities at the local, national, regional, and global levels. It aimed at improving the health of students, school personnel, families, and other members of the community through schools. The "Health Promoting School" (HPS) concept was initiated. It is a school that constantly strengthens its capacity to become a healthy setting for living, learning, and working. In 2000, WHO, United Nations Children's Fund (UNICEF), and other international organizations working for children started the "Focusing Resources on Effective School Health" (FRESH) Initiative. Its components included health-related school policies, safe learning environment, skill-based health education, and school-based health and nutrition services. The FRESH framework emphasized the need for amalgamation of various sectors like education, healthcare, water, sanitation, agriculture, etc. for the common cause of investing in school health.[2]

COMPONENTS OF SCHOOL HEALTH PROGRAMS

A school health program typically comprises some or all of the following eight domains **(Flowchart 22.7.1)**:[3]

1. *Health education*: Planned, curriculum that addresses the physical, mental, emotional, and social dimensions of health.
2. *Physical education*: Training and promoting physical fitness activities that are enjoyable and pursuable beyond school years.
3. *Health services*: Periodic growth monitoring, daily hygiene check-ups, preventive services, early identification and intervention of health issues, emergency care, primary care, access and referral to community healthcare providers, assisting in managing chronic health conditions like asthma or attention-deficit hyperactivity disorder (ADHD), by providing regular medicines, etc. on time during the school hours.
4. *Nutrition services*: Midday meal and other nutritional supplements like iron, teaching balanced diet, hygienic habits, mindful eating, healthy food choices in school canteen
5. *Psychosocial support*: School environment that promotes positive mental health, empowerment on life skills,

Flowchart 22.7.1: Possible components of school health program.

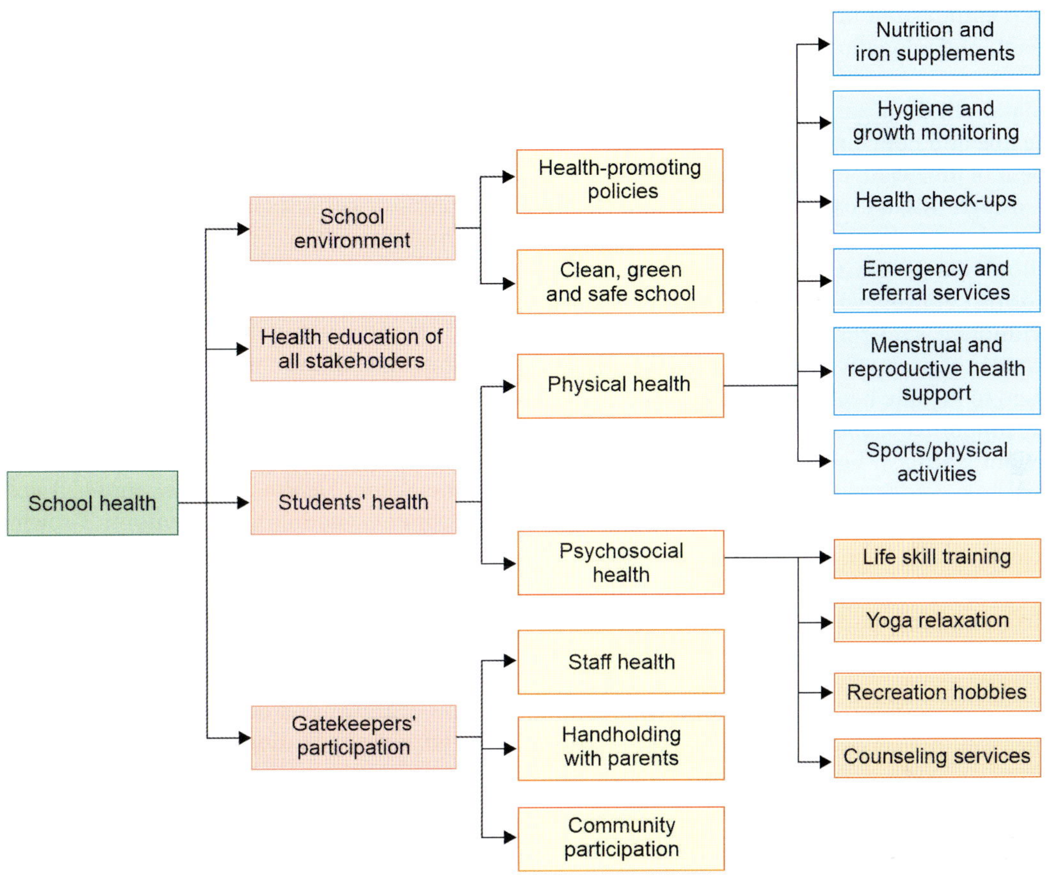

stress management and mental health issues, early identification of red flag signs, counseling services, partnering with family, and timely referrals to mental health professionals. Inclusive schooling including remedial teaching, social service assistance to children like certification/concessions by educational boards [e.g., for learning disability (LD)/autism spectrum disorders (ASDs)], for benefits through the National Trust and other government schemes for children with special needs.

6. *Health promotion for staff*: Arranging routine health check-ups, health education, and fitness activities for the staff members, thereby promoting their health, making them more committed for students' health, and encouraging them to be good role models
7. *Healthy school environment*: Ensuring a nurturing milieu in the school that promotes physical and as well as psychosocial health of all its members
8. *Parent and community involvement*: Encouraging school connectedness of the parents and the civil society members, in ways suitable to them

IMPORTANT GOVERNMENT SCHOOL HEALTH PROGRAMS IN INDIA[4,5]

In India, the first school health activity was done in 1909, in Baroda where school children were medically examined. But the major thrust in this direction came only in 1960s when Tamil Nadu started offering nutritional support to children through schools. In late nineties, cooked meals were served throughout the country to primary school students through *National Program of Nutritional Support to Primary Education (NP-NSPE)*, which provided 300 (now 450) calories and 12 g of protein. In 2001, the Supreme Court of India ordered all the state governments to supply cooked meals to children studying in government-supported primary schools. Students up to up to 8th standard are now distributed 700 calories and 20 g of proteins per day in cooked meals or dry ration form, for 300 days in a year. Earlier named as *National Program of Midday Meals in Schools*, since 2021, this scheme is run by the name *PM-POSHAN (Pradhan Mantri Poshan Shakti Nirman) Abhiyaan*, and serves more than 10 crore students across country.[6]

In 2005, the *National Health Mission (NHM)* was launched, which emphasized on the convergence of varied sectors like health and education to streamline the skewed health indicators. Its main components include reproductive–maternal–neonatal–child and adolescent health (RMNCH+A) and communicable and noncommunicable diseases, which are very pertinent to the health of school-going children and adolescents. Through this, a Comprehensive School Health Program was promoted to integrate health-related activities within the school setup. Apart from the nutritional and growth monitoring services, which were already existent, preventive, promotive, and rehabilitative health services were incorporated in the schools. Formal academic curricula were readdressed to include health education. Additionally, promoting safe, supportive school environment and capacity building of school staff also became a part of the School Health Program.

In 2013, *Rashtriya Bal Swasthya Karyakram (RBSK)* was launched by Government of India to detect and treat the 0–18 age-group problems of developmental delays, disabilities, birth defects, and nutritional deficiencies. For children >6 years of age, the plan got implemented through schools.

India is witnessing a decline in mortality and morbidity due to infectious diseases and an upsurge of noncommunicable diseases, behavioral and mental health issues, substance abuse, accidents, injuries, and climate-related diseases in young population. The National Mental Health Survey in 2016 reported a 7.3% prevalence rate for mental illness in adolescents aged between 13 and 17 years.[7]

Envisioning these trends, the *Rashtriya Kishore Swasthya Karyakram (RKSK)* was launched in 2014 to reach to the adolescents with expansion in services to include injuries and violence (including gender-based violence), noncommunicable diseases, mental health, and substance misuse. The program aims at reaching adolescents in their own environment, making outreach services in schools its important integral part. With its focus on community empowerment, it addresses knowledge building of the gate-keepers of adolescent health, thus multiplying its benefits.

In 2018, through *Ayushman Bharat Scheme,* Government of India established Health and Community Wellness Centers that are directed to promote health-based activities through the schools.

School Health and Wellness Program is being implemented in government and government aided schools since February, 2020. Here, two teachers, preferably one male and one female, from every school, who are called "Health and Wellness Ambassadors" are trained to empower school children on 11 important health-related topics like injuries, violence, substance abuse, risky sexual behaviors, and psychological and emotional disorders. These specially trained teachers then carry out interesting interactive activities, scheduled 1 hour per week for promotion of healthy habits and behaviors. Thus, disease prevention is encouraged among the school-going children. The program, which is a joint initiative of the Department of School Education, Ministry of Human Resource Development, and Ministry of Health and Family Welfare, Government of India, also targets to improve access to health services in an integrated manner at the school level.

Through *Weekly Iron and Folic acid Supplementation (WIFS),* which is Anemia Eradication Program by Government of India, biannually deworming with albendazole 400 g and weekly iron (100 mg elemental) and folic acid (500 µg) is distributed to all the students of classes 6–12 in government and basic screening for anemia and SOS referral is ensured along with empowerment on hygienic measures to prevent worm infestation and dietary measures for better iron intake.

The *School Health Program*, under *Ayushman Bharat,* incorporates a module for students on "Growing up Healthy". It contains information on physical challenges during adolescence and puberty. National Council of Educational Research and Training (NCERT) implements the *Adolescence Education Program* as part of the National Population Education Project where the students are made aware of the process of growing up during adolescence. The aim is to allay their anxieties regarding their growing bodies and inculcate in them a positive attitude regarding the same.

Department of School Education and Literacy (DoSEL), Ministry of Education implements a centrally sponsored Integrated Scheme for School Education *"Samagra Shiksha"* since 2018–19. Under this scheme, the *Swachhta Action Plan* is run and supported financially by the Government of India. This plan is to ensure maintenance of water, sanitation, and hygiene (WASH) in schools, that is, safe drinking water, sanitation" and hygiene (including toilets). In addition, under the "Promotion of Menstrual Hygiene among Adolescent Girls" (10–19 years) program, menstrual hygiene is taught to girls 10–19 years of age. In rural areas, sanitary pads are distributed to them at subsidiary rates by the government in schools or by accredited social health activists (ASHAs).

Schools become the best platforms for mass vaccination campaigns run by the governments. For example, the mumps rubella (MR) vaccine campaign was run across the country and involved most of the schools in 2017.

ROLE OF INDIAN ACADEMY OF PEDIATRICS IN PROMOTING SCHOOL HEALTH

The Indian Academy of Pediatrics (IAP) has long back recognized the need to join hands with government authorities, other organizations like WHO, UNICEF, etc., and other social bodies working in the field of child health. It has worked extensively in guiding the policymakers to ensure healthy childhood and adolescence, and ultimately, a healthful future of the country. It has launched several systematically designed scientific programs and initiatives and empowered thousands of pediatricians, teachers, students, and parents.

The *Child Friendly School Initiative (CFSI)* is to promote schools to follow the following criteria, which are very basic essentials for health of school children:[8]

- No physical punishment
- Bag weight not >10% of child's weight
- Safe and comfortable transportation to school
- Hygienic drinking water
- Clean kitchen or a place where children can bring and eat house food
- Minimum 4 hours for games or physical activity every week
- Properly ventilated, illuminated, well equipped class rooms with not >40 students per class
- Periodic health check-ups and health-related lectures
- Facility for first aid in emergency
- Adequate number of clean toilets, separate for girls and boys.

The IAP programs like Mission Uday, Mission Kishor Uday, Adolescent and Young Adult (AYA) module, Suicide Prevention Module, Mission School Uday, Co-WIN module, Nanhi Kali Program, and many others have components on empowerment of school teachers and students, in which trained pediatricians deliver in the schools lectures and activities.

With a target on holistic well-being of children, they address various issues like growth and development monitoring, reduction in physical health problems including non-communicable diseases, mental health issues, gender biases, etc. The latest Sankalp Sampurn Swasthya focuses on promotion of physical activities and mindful eating using various skill building activities including reading food labels. It also empowers students on judicious media use, sleep hygiene, and mental and environmental health.

During coronavirus disease 2019 (COVID-19) pandemic, IAP came out with a series of advisories and guidelines on "School Reopening, Remote Learning, and Curriculum in and After the COVID-19 Pandemic", which proved useful to the governments, the education sector, and the schools on important issues of physical and psychological health as well as learning during the pandemic.

Medical Emergency Management in Schools (MEMS) is another program run by IAP where teachers and staff are trained on prevention of accidents in school premises and on delivering basic medical support for common health emergencies in school children. Basic life support (BLS) training camps are also conducted in schools.

An online self-learning module for teachers "Nurturing Adolescents in Schools" is freely available on the IAP website. The website also shares 105 guidelines for parents on various topics related to health and schooling concerns of children.

HEALTH PROMOTING SCHOOLS[9]

In the wake of the COVID-19 pandemic and its multi-dimensional aftereffects on children, on October 12th, 2021, WHO, in its Call for Action for Health Promoting Schools, advised its member countries to make health promotion an integral part of every school. The slogan given is "Make Every School a Health Promoting School". This initiative not only focuses on scaling up of health programs for students but also for the school staff, thus compounding the effectiveness. India is signatory to this strategy, which is designed in collaboration with agencies like United Nations (UN), United Nations Educational, Scientific and Cultural Organization (UNESCO), and UNICEF. The target areas suggested are sanitation and hygiene, potable water, nutrition, assessment and management of health conditions, sexual health, and psychosocial support.

Following six key areas are identified for school to work and make it an HPS:

1. Healthy school policies (like health and learning together, institutional capacity building)
2. Physical school environment (like safe playgrounds, potable water, safe clean gender separate latrines)
3. Social school environment (antibullying environment, equity)
4. Health skills and education (like life skills education, promoting healthy eating)
5. Links with parents and community (community involvement, parent–teacher association meetings)
6. Access to health services (school-based health service, school nurse, counselor, tie-up with government or private hospitals)

Aims of Health Promoting School Initiative

An HPS empowers on caring for oneself and others, by creating overall environment and conditions that are conducive to health. It teaches making healthy decisions and being responsible for one's life events. It aims at reducing morbidity and mortality through prevention of leading causes of death, disease and disability: Helminths, tobacco use, human immunodeficiency virus (HIV) and acquired immunodeficiency syndrome (AIDS), sexually transmitted diseases (STD), sedentary lifestyle, drugs and alcohol, violence and injuries, and unhealthy nutrition. There is a capacity building of all the concerned individuals on health-related domains of knowledge, beliefs, skills, attitudes, and values. The ultimate aim is boosting peace, shelter, education, food, income, a stable ecosystem, equity, social justice, and reaching the sustainable developmental goals (SDGs). The important SDGs targeted are related to reduction in violence, tobacco/alcohol use, obesity, suicide, road traffic accident injuries, and HIV infection.

Health Promoting School Strategies

The HPS strategies include the following:

- They promote health and education using all available means like lectures, posters, activities, health camps, etc.
- They bring on one page all the stakeholders like health and education officials, teachers, students, parents, health workers, and community leaders to make the school a healthy place.
- They make all efforts for a healthy environment through physical infrastructure like healthy classrooms, recreation places, healthy eating places, provision of nutritional supplementation, etc. They appoint nurses for physical concerns and counselors for offering psychosocial support. They encourage community participation and outreach projects.
- They take care to respect every individual's well-being and dignity, provide varied opportunities, ways and means to attain their full potentials, and appreciate their honest efforts, intentions, and achievements.
- They work for promotion of health of students, staff, their families and community members. Such schools make efforts to make community leaders understand the importance of joining hands with the schools for a positive health trajectory of the community.

BARRIERS IN IMPLEMENTING SCHOOL HEALTH PROGRAMS

The barriers in the implementation of school health programs include the following:

- Lack of clear-cut policy guidelines for practical implementation of programs
- Inadequate intersectoral coordination (like education and health)
- Insufficient advocacy and awareness among stakeholders
- Tight and demanding academic schedules for the students
- Budget and resource crunch at the government and school level
- Shortage of trainings and skill building of personnel
- Cultural barriers (like resistance for reproductive health education)
- Lack of scientific studies to evaluate evidences of program outcomes.

ROLE OF PEDIATRICIAN IN SCHOOL HEALTH

Pediatrician's care is an integral part of children's growth and development. Many schools voluntarily involve the pediatricians in the school policy-making and take their services for growth monitoring, regular check-ups, special camps, and empowerment of students, teachers, and parents. They also tie up with pediatricians for emergency and referral services. Pediatricians play a vital role as primary healthcare provider for basic health issues. He/she can easily liaison with other specialties, the family and the school for the best outcome of chronic diseases, neurodevelopmental disorders, and psychological issues.

Pediatricians can empower the school students and their caretakers on a variety of topics like nutrition, health and hygiene, growth and development, psychosocial issues, learning problems, study skills, life skills, etc. through interactive engaging activities. Sensitive topics like reproductive health, sexuality, substance abuse, romantic relationships, etc. are best dealt by the pediatricians as they are the most trusted experts for the children and their families.

Such associations of schools and pediatricians are mutually beneficial. Most pediatricians find it very rewarding and take pride in helping the community through the school setting. It adds to not only their esteem but also to their practice. A pediatrician who is attached to the child's school is considered to be more trustworthy by the parents. This positively reflects on the compliance and the ultimate health outcomes.

REFERENCES

1. National Health Mission; Department of Health & Family Welfare, Government of India. (2024). Adolescent Health. [online] Available from https://nhm.gov.in/index1.php?lang=1&level=2&sublinkid=818&lid=221 [Last accessed December 2024].
2. Joerger C, Hoffmann AM. (2002). FRESH: a comprehensive school health approach to achieve EFA (ED-2002/WS/8 REV). [online] Available from https://unesdoc.unesco.org/ark:/48223/pf0000125537 [Last accessed December 2024].
3. World Health Organization. Health Promoting Schools. [online] Available from https://www.who.int/health-topics/health-promoting-schools#tab=tab_2 [Last accessed December 2024].
4. Ministry of Health & Family Welfare; Ministry of Human Resource & Development, Government of India. (2018). Operational Guidelines on School Health Programme Under Ayushman Bharat: Health and Wellness Ambassadors Partnering to Build a Stronger Future. [online] Available from https://nhm.gov.in/New_Updates_2018/NHM_Components/RMNCHA/AH/guidelines/Operational_guidelines_on_School_Health_Programme_under_Ayushman_Bharat.pdf [Last accessed December 2024].
5. Jain YK, Joshi NK, Bhardwaj P, Suthar P. Health-promoting school in India: Approaches and challenges. J Family Med Prim Care. 2019;8(10):3114-9.
6. Department of School Education and Literacy. PM POshan SHAkti Nirman (PM-POSHAN). [online] Available from https://dsel.education.gov.in/scheme/pm-poshan-scheme [Last accessed December 2024].
7. Murthy RS. National Mental Health Survey of India 2015-2016. Indian J Psychiatry. 2017;59(1):21-26.
8. Sukumaran TU. Child friendly school initiative program (CFSI) under IAP Action Plan 2011. Indian Pediatr. 2011;48(3):179-80.
9. Harish R, Pande D. Health Promoting Schools in India: The time has come! Indian Pediatr. 2022;59(12):955-6.

22.8 Integrated Management of Neonatal and Childhood Illnesses

Shashi N Vani

INTRODUCTION

Despite introducing several effective healthcare interventions for past three decades and more, every year nearly 11 million children die globally before reaching age of 5 years. Majority of them die due to a few common illnesses for which we have the knowledge and the capability to prevent or treat. These children, mostly from poor and deprived families, are denied these benefits and unnecessarily succumb to death.

In response to this challenge, the World Health Organization (WHO) and United Nations Children's Fund (UNICEF) designed a fresh strategy named *Integrated Management of Neonatal and Childhood Illness (IMNCI)* in the early 1990s for the developing countries of the world to provide effective and affordable interventions to reduce childhood morbidity and mortality and to improve child health and development. Both preventive and curative healthcare interventions have been included in IMNCI.

BACKGROUND

Nearly 70% of deaths in under-5 (U-5) years children are caused due to a very few common illnesses such as acute respiratory infections (ARIs) (mostly bacterial pneumonia), diarrhea, measles, malaria, and malnutrition or a combination of these conditions. Malnutrition and anemia may not be the direct cause of death, but these are compounding factors with other common childhood illnesses and worsen the condition. Everyday millions of parents seek healthcare for their children, majority of whom suffer because of these few common childhood illnesses. They visit various hospitals, health centers, dispensarics, private practitioners, and traditional healers adding to the burden of the healthcare providers who are not trained to assess, classify, and decide the further approach of management rationally and start early treatment appropriately. They do not have adequate diagnostic and therapeutic facilities, adequate supply of basic but essential drugs or the training for offering quality care. Very often lack of time and awareness regarding parent counseling and preventive and promotive healthcare services such as nutrition advice and immunization are lacking.

Many sick children never reach a healthcare facility due to lack of awareness of the parents or nonavailability of services nearer their homes or sheer poverty. There are many inequities in the health care of these children from deprived families.

During the past three decades or so many successful interventions such as oral rehydration salts (ORS) for diarrheal disease, rational use of antibiotics for pneumonia and other ARIs, early use of antimalarials, immunizations under Expanded Program on Immunization or Universal Immunization Program (EPI/UIP), Anemia Control Program, Vitamin A Supplement Program, etc., have been incorporated in national health programs as vertical programs and have helped in bringing down the childhood mortality to some extent. But, for further reduction of infant and U-5 mortality, a different strategy was needed and with this background, WHO and UNICEF conceived IMNCI approach. It is not a new program. It is an effective strategy or a different approach integrating all the vertical healthcare programs aiming for the holistic care of the young children up to 5 years of age, a care not dependent on sophisticated technology or costly equipment or drugs.[1,2]

ADAPTATIONS OF INTEGRATED MANAGEMENT OF NEONATAL AND CHILDHOOD ILLNESS

Integrated Management of Neonatal and Childhood Illness strategy has been introduced in >100 developing countries all over the world. In the beginning, IMNCI did not include the care of newborns in first week after birth as it was linked with the care of mothers.

In India, the neonatal mortality constitutes almost 50% of under-five mortality rate (U5MR) or 70–80% of infant mortality. Majority of neonatal deaths occur in the first week of life. Hence, neonatal care has been included and the modified strategy of IMNCI has been adopted. Now, many other countries have included neonatal care in their IMNCI. Some African countries have included human immunodeficiency virus/acquired immunodeficiency syndrome (HIV/AIDS) control program in their IMNCI. Many such adaptations have been made depending on the local needs.[2,3]

Main Components of Integrated Management of Neonatal and Childhood Illness

- To improve case management skills of healthcare providers

- To strengthen the health system supports for better child health services delivery
- To improve family and community practices related to childcare

Integrated Management of Neonatal and Childhood Illness Approach[2,4]

Integrated Management of Neonatal and Childhood Illness guidelines are targeted for two groups:

1. Newborns and young infants from birth to 2 months of age. Many deaths occur beyond neonatal age of first 4 weeks. Hence, this group includes infants up to 2 months of age.
2. The second group includes young children >2 months up to 5 years of age.

The clinical guidelines have been developed and they represent evidence-based syndromic approach to case management. That includes rational, effective, and affordable use of drugs and simple diagnostic tools. The clinical decisions based on intuitions, empirical considerations, and without the support of solid evidence are discouraged. The standardized clinical guidelines may not lead to specific diagnosis of a disease, but helps the health worker to classify the condition requiring:

- Emergency management and immediate referral
- Treatment at the outpatient health facility with available resources, or
- Advice for home management

Color-coded standard management charts are provided to help in assessment, classification, and planning further line of management.

- *Pink classification:* Child needs referral and inpatient care.
- *Yellow classification:* Child need specific treatment, provide it at home [e.g., antibiotics, antimalarials, oral dehydration therapy (ORT)]
- *Green classification:* Child needs no medication, home care advice.

Integrated Management of Neonatal and Childhood Illness provides adjustments of interventions to the capacity of the health system and active involvement of family and the community in the healthcare process.[4]

Care of Newborn and Young Infant (Infants Under 2 Months of Age)

- Keep the infant warm
- Initiate breastfeeding immediately after birth and continue exclusive breastfeeding
- Counseling for early and exclusive breastfeeding
- Cord, skin, and eye care
- Recognition of illness in newborn and management and/or referral
- Immunization
- Home visits in the postnatal period

Care of Infant and Children (2 Months Up to 5 Years of Age)

- Management of diarrhea, ARIs (pneumonia), malaria, measles, acute ear infection, malnutrition, and anemia
- Recognition of illness and at-risk conditions and management
- Prevention and management of iron and vitamin A deficiency
- Counseling on feeding of all children below 2 years of age
- Counseling of feeding for malnutrition child between 2 months and 5 years of age[2,4]

FACILITY-BASED INTEGRATED MANAGEMENT OF NEONATAL AND CHILDHOOD ILLNESS

This is yet another adaptation of IMNCI approach in India started since November 2009. Following were a few important considerations for initiating facility-based IMNCI (F-IMNCI) in India for the first time.

Facility-based care for severely ill children is complementary to primary care for providing continuum of care for severely ill children. Good quality inpatient care is required to enhance the impact of primary care and better outcome. There is acute shortage of specialists (pediatricians) at facilities. Thus, it becomes important to build the skill of medical officers and staff nurses at these facilities to manage referred sick infants and children and bridge the gap of specialists to some extent **(Box 22.8.1)**.

Facility-based IMNCI is an integration of existing IMNCI package and the facility-based package with certain added components such as asphyxia management and care of newborns. Critical element of F-IMNCI is again evidence-based integrated approach with a focus on severely ill newborns and children. Salient features of training modules of F-IMNCI are stated in **Box 22.8.1**.

Flowchart 22.8.1 and Table 22.8.1 illustrate the approach in F-IMNCI.

MAJOR ADAPTATIONS OF IMNCI IN INDIA[5,7]

- The entire 0–5 years period is covered including first week of life
- Almost 50% of training time is allotted for management of young infant up to 2 months
- The order of training is reversed; now begins with management of young infant
- Reduced duration of training (8 days)

BOX 22.8.1: Salient features of training modules of facility-based Integrated Management of Neonatal and Childhood Illness (F-IMNCI).

- *Module 1 emergency triage assessment and treatment (ETAT):* Maintain temperature, check, and treat hypoglycemia, airway, and breathing, give oxygen; circulation; coma and convulsions; dehydration.
- *Module 2 facility-based care of sick young infant:* Care at birth including neonatal resuscitation; care of newborn in postnatal wards; management of sick newborn; management of low birth-weight babies; neonatal transport.
- *Module 3 facility-based care of sick children:* Case management of children presenting with cough or difficult breathing, case management of children presenting with fever, case management of children with diarrhea, case management of children with ear problems, case management of children with severe anemia, case management of children with severe malnutrition, effective implementation with proper supplies, and supervision are required for good results from F-IMNCI

Flowchart 22.8.1: Steps in the management of sick young infant and children admitted to hospital.

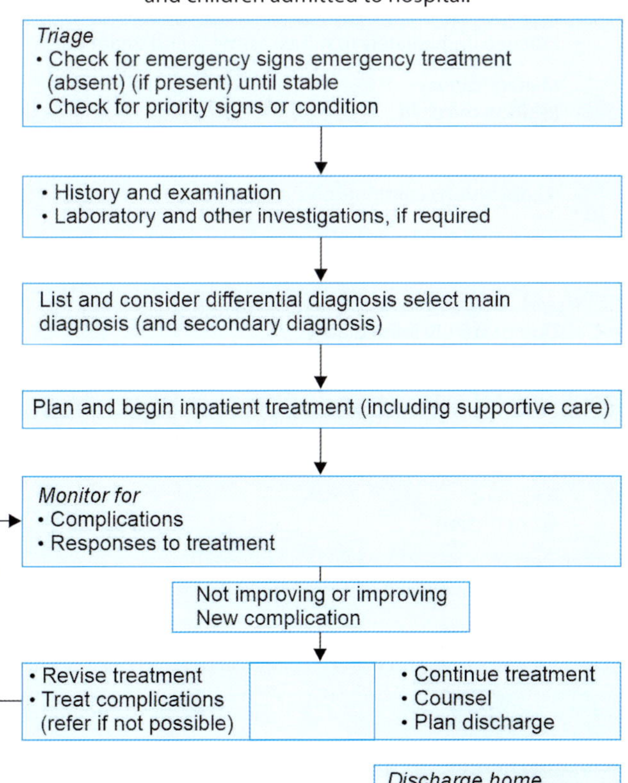

- Separate training material for physicians and other health workers
- Management now consistent with the policies of Ministry of Health and Family Welfare (MOHFW), Department of Women and Child Development (DWCD), and National Anti-Malaria Program (NAMP)
- Home-based care by health workers has been added.

Home Visits for Young Infants

Objectives

- Promote and support early and exclusive breastfeeding
- Promote early direct skin-to-skin contact for all the babies and kangaroo mother care for stable low birth-weight (LBW) infants
- Teach the mothers to recognize the signs of illness for which to seek care
- Identify illness at visit and facilitate referral
- Advise on cord care and hand washing

Schedule of Home Visits for the Newborns

- *All newborns:* Three visits (first within first 24 hours of birth, second on 3rd or 4th day of birth, and third on 7–10 days after birth)
- *For LBW infant:* Three more visits (14th, 21st, and 28th day of birth).

Missing Areas in Integrated Management of Neonatal and Childhood Illness

- Antenatal care/birth preparedness
- Skilled birth attendance
- Management of important problems such as tuberculosis (TB) and others

Role of Private Practitioners in Integrated Management of Neonatal and Childhood Illness

Depending on the scope of practice, private practitioners can adapt IMNCI approach in their clinic works. It will definitely improve their quality of care and rationalize the use of drugs and investigations. In many areas, the community members prefer to take treatment from family physicians/private practitioners than from public health facilities for several reasons. The community health workers also refer their cases to local private doctors. If the private doctor adopts the same IMNCI approach, there will be definitely a better continuum of care benefiting the patient and community at large. Unlike

TABLE 22.8.1: Triage.[5,6]

Assess for emergency signs (in all cases)			***Treat:*** • ***Check for head/neck trauma before treating child (do not move neck if cervical spine injury possible)*** • ***Give appropriate treatment for +ve emergency signs*** • ***Call for help*** • ***Draw blood for glucose, malaria smear, Hb***
Airway and breathing	• Not breathing or gasping or • Central cyanosis or • Severe respiratory distress	Any sign positive	• Manage airway • Provide baby life support (not breathing/gasping) • Give oxygen • Make sure child is warm
Circulation	*Cold extremities with:* • Capillary refill longer than 3 seconds and • Weak and fast pulse	If positive, check for severe acute malnutrition	• If the child has any bleeding, apply pressure to stop the bleeding. Do not use a tourniquet • Give oxygen • Make sure child is warm* • Insert intravenous (IV) and begin giving fluids rapidly • If not able to insert peripheral IV, insert an umbilical or intraosseous line
			• If severe acute malnutrition (age ≥2 months) • *If lethargic or unconscious:* Insert IV line and give glucose and fluids. *If not lethargic or unconscious:* • Give glucose orally or by nasogastric (NG) tube • Proceed immediately to full assessment and treatment
Coma convulsing	• Coma, or • Convulsing (now)	If coma or convulsing	• Manage airway • Position the child • Check and correct hypoglycemia • If convulsions continue, give IV calcium in young infants • If convulsions continue, give anticonvulsants
Severe dehydration (only in cases with diarrhea)	*Diarrhea plus any two of these:* • Lethargy • Sunken eyes • Very slow skin pinch	Diarrhea plus two signs positive, check for severe acute malnutrition	• Make sure child is warm* • Insert IV line and begin giving fluids rapidly following plan C *If severe acute malnutrition (age ≥2 months):* • Do not start IV immediately • Proceed immediately to full assessment and treatment
If there are no emergency signs look for priority signs, these children need prompt assessment and treatment			
• Tiny baby (<2 months) • Bleeding • Pallor (severe) • Malnutrition; visible severe wasting		• Respiratory distress (RR >60/mm) • Trauma or other urgent surgical condition • Referral (urgent) • Edema of both feet	• Temperature <36.5°C or >38.5°C • Restless, continuously irritable or lethargy • Poisoning • Burns (major)

Nonurgent: Proceed with assessment and further treatment according to child's priority.
Note: If a child has trauma or other surgical problems, get surgical help, or follow surgical guidelines.
*Check temperature, if baby is cold to touch, rewarm.

many other healthcare interventions where training is given to doctors in public service alone, IMNCI training is available for family physicians also.

CONCLUSION

If properly implemented and supported by strengthening the health system assuring quality training to all the functionaries, ensuring regular adequate supplies, good supervision and monitoring, and community-based service such as good counseling, behavior change, and communication, IMNCI in India has a great potential to achieve its main goal of reducing newborn and U-5 mortality in children within a short time and come closer to millennium development goals.[5,8,9]

REFERENCES

1. Patwari A, Raina N. Integrated Management of Neonatal and Childhood Illnesses: A robust strategy. Indian Pediatr. 2002;69(1):41-8.
2. Students Handbook for IMNCI (Integrated Management of Neonatal and Childhood Illnesses). World Health Organization/Department of Child and Adolescent Health and Development and the Ministry of Health and Family Welfare, Government of India; 2003.
3. World Health Organization and NRHM, Ministry of Health and Family Welfare. Integrated Management of Neonatal and Childhood Illness: Introduction. World Health Organization and NRHM, Ministry of Health and Family Welfare, Government of India; 2003.
4. Ministry of Health, Newborn, Childhood and Adolescent Health Unit (NCAHU). Integrated Management of Neonatal and Childhood Illness: A guide for healthcare workers, 2017 edition. Ministry of Health, Newborn, Childhood and Adolescent Health Unit (NCAHU), Government of India; 2017.
5. World Health Organization, Ministry of Health and Family Welfare. Facility Based Integrated Management of Neonatal and Childhood Illnesses (F-IMNCI): IMNCI Chart Booklet 2009. World Health Organization, Ministry of Health and Family Welfare, Government of India and National Rural Health Mission; 2009.
6. National Health Mission, Government of Himachal Pradesh. Integrated Management of Neonatal and Childhood Illness: Training modules 1 to 9. National Health Mission, Government of Himachal Pradesh; 2021-22.
7. World Health Organization, Ministry of Health and Family Welfare. Facility Based Integrated Management of Neonatal and Childhood Illness (F-IMNCI): Participants' Manual 2009. World Health Organization, Ministry of Health and Family Welfare, Government of India; 2009.
8. World Health Organization/Department of Child and Adolescent. Integrated Management of Neonatal and Childhood Illness (IMNCI): A guidebook for private practitioners. World Health Organization/Department of Child and Adolescent Health, 2002.
9. World Health Organization, Ministry of Health and Family Welfare and National Rural Health Mission. IMNCI Training modules 1-9, 2009. World Health Organization, Ministry of Health and Family Welfare and National Rural Health Mission, Government of India; 2009.

22.9 Adoption and Care of Orphans

Ramesh D Potdar, Kusum Kalla

INTRODUCTION

Adoption is a process whereby a person assumes the parenting of another, usually a child, from that person's biological or legal parent or parents. Legal adoptions permanently transfer all rights and responsibilities, along with filiation, from the biological parents to the adoptive parents (World Health Organization).

DEFINITION

According to Indian Academy of Pediatrics (IAP), adoption is the act of lawfully assuming the parental rights and responsibilities of another person, usually a child under the age of 18 years. Adopted children become full members of their adopted family and have the same legal status as biological children. Although most people who adopt are married couples, many single people also adopt. The focus is now moving from "parent-centered" to "child-centered" adoptions, and from the concept of "child for a family" to "family for a child."

Adoption is also an instrument through which one can ensure the following important children's rights accepted by the United Nations (UN) convention of rights of children and the world community at large. These are:

- Inherent right to life survival and development
- Right to name and nationality
- Child's interest being always a primary consideration
- Special protection from physical harm and neglect
- No discrimination through universal brotherhood
- Social security through education, employment, and earning
- Special attention to disabled children

TYPES OF ADOPTION IN INDIA

Considering the above definition and objectives, adoptions could be divided into various types. The different types of adoption available in India are detailed here.

Open Adoption

Here, the adoptive parents and the birth parents remain in contact via letters, emails, phone conversations, and even in-person visits. Typically, access is allowed after the adopted child turns 18 years old (in most countries). Additionally, the prospective parents may be met by the birth mother, who will select which pair her child should go to.

Semi-open Adoption

The birth parents and adopted parents do not have any personal interactions. However, the adoptive parents or the adoption agency the mother is registered with may continue to send her letters or pictures. This could go on until the child reaches adulthood. Semi-adoption can change into either an open or closed adoption at any time.

Closed Adoption

As the name implies, there is no communication between the adoptive parents and the birth parents. The adoptive parents may occasionally be given access to the birth parents' medical records. This might occur when a youngster is saved from an abusive situation or removed from it.

Intrafamily Adoption or Relative Adoption

This sort of adoption takes place within the family. A family member or the step-parents may legally adopt a kid if the child's biological parents pass away, remarry, or are otherwise unable to care for the child.

Domestic Adoption

Domestic adoption occurs when the birth parents and adoptive parents are from the same nation.

International Adoption

In this type of adoption, the adoptive parents are not citizens of the country where the child is being adopted. All countries have distinct rules governing international adoption.

Domestic adoption is given preference in India. Other types are single parent adoptions, adoption of older children, and adoption of disabled or "special needs" children. Parents should be strongly advised not to arrange adoptions secretly through hospitals and medical practitioners directly. Adoption must always be done through an institution, which has been recognized by the central government.[1]

LAWS GOVERNING ADOPTION

There are two laws governing adoption in India—(1) the *Hindu Adoption and* (2) *Maintenance Act, 1956* popularly known as HAMA and the *Juvenile Justice (Care and Protection of Children) Act, 2015* popularly known as the JJ Act. Only a Hindu parent (including Sikhs, Jains and Buddhists and excluding Muslims, Christian, Parsi, or Jew) can adopt a Hindu child up to 15 years of age from another Hindu parent under HAMA. Indian citizens of any faith or religion and foreign citizens can adopt a child up to 18 years of age from the specialized adoption agencies (SAAs) under the JJ Act. All adoptions under the JJ Act are regulated by the Central Adoption Resource Authority (CARA) under the Ministry of Women and Child Development (MoWCD). All international adoptions have must happen through JJ Act, and even nonresident Indian Hindus cannot adopt a child from India under HAMA.[2]

Parents are recommended to seek counseling from a certified and trained adoption counselor in deciding upon the relevant law under which they can adopt.

FUNDAMENTAL PRINCIPLES GOVERNING ADOPTION

The following fundamental principles govern adoptions of children from India:

1. The child's best interests shall be of paramount consideration, while processing any adoption placement.
2. Preference shall be given to place the child in adoption with Indian citizens with due regard to the principle of placement of the child in their own sociocultural environment, as far as possible.
3. All applications for adoptions shall be registered on the Designated Portal and confidentiality of the same shall be maintained by the authority.

Eligibility of a Child for Adoption

The following children shall be eligible for adoption:

1. Any orphan or abandoned or surrendered child, declared legally free for adoption by the Child Welfare Committee
2. A child of a relative
3. Child or children of spouse from earlier marriage, surrendered by the biological parents for adoption by the step-parent.

Eligibility Criteria for Prospective Adoptive Parents

1. The prospective adoptive parents shall be physically, mentally, emotionally, and financially capable; they shall not have any life-threatening medical condition and they should not have been convicted in criminal act of any nature.
2. Any prospective adoptive parent, irrespective of their marital status and whether they have biological son or daughter, can adopt a child subject to the following:
    - The consent of both the spouses for the adoption shall be required, in case of a married couple.
    - A single female can adopt a child of any gender.
    - A single male shall not be eligible to adopt a girl child.

3. No child shall be given in adoption to a couple unless they have at least 2 years of stable marital relationship except in the cases of relative or step-parent adoption.
4. The minimum age difference between the child and either of the prospective adoptive parents shall not be <25 years.
5. In case of a couple, the composite age of the prospective adoptive parents shall be counted.
6. The age criteria for prospective adoptive parents shall not be applicable in case of relative adoptions and adoption by step-parent.
7. Couples with two or more children shall only be considered for special needs children and hard-to-place children unless they are relatives or stepchildren.
8. The prospective adoptive parents must revalidate their home study report after a period of 3 years.
9. The seniority of the prospective adoptive parents who have not received a single referral within 3 years shall be counted from their date of registration except those who have crossed composite years of 110 years.[2-4]

Choosing a Child, Medical Screening, and Certifying the "Fit for Adoption" Report

"Choosing" can imply a bias of an arbitrary selection or rejection. However, in the Indian context, it should be left to the social worker to place a child, who is near compatible to adoptive parents in looks, color of the eyes and complexion, and their specific requests if any. This is likely to ensure better adjustment and integration of the baby in the new family and society.

In medical screening for fitness, the doctor should remember that this baby should be examined and certified fit, normal, or otherwise in the context of the situational background that the baby may have suffered.

Clinical examination consists of identification data, anthropometry, systemic examination, detection of any gross deficiency disorders and overt or covert anomalies and their correctability potential, clinical clues to metabolic disorders if observed, and physical and mental milestones evaluation. Standard investigations which are expected to be done are hemogram, urinalysis, tuberculin test, X-ray chest, stool examination for parasites, tests for venereal disease research laboratory (VDRL), human immunodeficiency virus (HIV), hepatitis B virus (HBV), toxoplasmosis, other infections like rubella, cytomegalovirus, and herpes (TORCH) titers, and any other indicated tests with special reference to hypothyroidism, hemolytic anemia, and chromosomal anomalies and metabolic screening tests for intellectual disability like phenylketonuria, galactosemia, aminoaciduria, etc.

The entire exercise should be a balanced one to ensure welfare and maintain interest of both the baby and the adoptive parents with a benefit of doubt given to child (than adoptive parents) since the child is totally dependent on the caregivers.

ADOPTION CERTIFICATE

The adoption certificate is provided to the child who has been adopted by parents. This certificate works as a proof of identity of the adopted child and can be replaced by the original birth certificate. The adoption certificate represents that the child has been adopted by a family on a particular date from an homage or orphanage based on certain rules as per defined by CARA under Government of India.[5] The format of the adoption certificate can be seen at the website of CARA.[4]

ROLE OF PEDIATRICIAN

Every physician, especially a pediatrician should be conversant with the process of adoption, be able to and should advise any prospective adoptive parents on all aspects of adoption including preadoption counseling and awareness, medical examination and investigations of the child, and postadoption counseling. The physician can help in all of the following standard steps of adoption process always using sympathy and empathy at all stages.

PROCESS OF ADOPTION IN INDIA

The adoption procedure in India involves several steps, including:

- *Registration:* The first step in the adoption process is to register with the CARA, which is the central body responsible for regulating and monitoring adoptions in India.
- *Home study:* After registration, a social worker will conduct a home study to evaluate your suitability as an adoptive parent. The home study includes interviews, home visits, and background checks.
- *Referral:* Once you are deemed eligible to adopt, you will be referred to a child who is legally free for adoption. CARA will provide you information about the child's background, medical history, and other relevant details.
- *Acceptance:* If you are satisfied with the referral, you must accept the child and provide a letter of acceptance to CARA.
- *Legal formalities:* The legal formalities involved in adoption include filing a petition in court and obtaining a court order granting you legal guardianship of the child.
- *Follow-up:* After the adoption is finalized, follow-up visits will be conducted to ensure that the child is adjusting well to their new home. It may continue for 1–2 years.[2]

Documents Required for Adoption in India

- Proof of age
- Marriage certificate (if applicable)
- Divorce certificate/death certificate of spouse (if applicable)
- Two letters of reference from relatives supporting adoption
- Medical fitness certificate
- Income proof
- Police clearance certificate
- Home study report
- Letter of acceptance
- Court order

CHALLENGES IN THE ADOPTION PROCESS

Adoption can be a challenging and emotional process, both for the adoptive parents and the child. Some of the challenges that adoptive parents may face include:

- Dealing with the child's emotional and behavioral issues
- Navigating the legal and bureaucratic process
- Coping with societal stigma and discrimination
- Managing financial and logistical challenges

It is important to be prepared for these challenges and seek support when needed.

ADOPTION COUNSELING

Counseling in adoption contributes significantly in creating a positive bond between adoptive parents and adopted children. Counseling is an integral part of the process of adoption. Adoption involves a spectrum of emotions ranging from intense hurt and grief to immense joy and fulfilment for both child and adoptive parents. Counseling in adoption leads to more successful and enriching parenting experiences as mentioned below.

Counseling Biological Mother/Parents in Case of Surrender

The psychosocial status of biological parent/s or unwed mothers cannot be known when they must surrender a child in an institution. After giving up their child, birth mothers lose all custody rights. Birth parent counseling provides birth parents with the chance to express their thoughts, discuss the reasons behind their decision to give up their child, and learn about all their options, including keeping their child with them.

Preadoption Counseling and Home Study Preparation

The preadoption counseling may help adoptive families to identify their difficulties. It is required to:

- Educate them on meaning of adoption
- Help them to assess their capabilities and limitations as a parent
- Point them to families, agencies, and professionals in adoption who can provide detailed inputs from their respective experiences
- Make an informed decision in accepting a child they can support
- Assist them in registering for adoption for the appropriate category of children

Home study preparation is mandatorily done by the social worker of the agency and consists of social and family background of both parents, current marital and family relationships, attitudes and motivation toward infertility, childlessness and adoption, anxieties regarding child's illegitimacy, and social and genetic background. The purpose of this procedure is to protect the rights of the child to the maximum before the irrevocable adoption takes place.

Postadoption Counseling and Follow-up

Postadoption counseling is for anyone affected by adoption. This can be adopted persons, birth parents who have lost a child to adoption, adoptive parents, and adoptive families. This work includes working with issues of transracial adoption. Postadoption counseling focuses on the following issues:

- Coping with parenthood and change of roles
- Feelings of bonding and attachment
- Acceptance of the child by relatives and friends
- Sharing the fact of adoption with the child why, when, and how
- Issues related to the child's schooling and academic performance[2,4]

Follow-up after adoption is necessary for advice and care in the following crisis situations, which are likely to arise in some of the babies:

- *Sudden change crises,* resulting in different types of reactions such as anxiety, rejection, aggression, or any combinations of these
- *Behavior crisis* may be because of pampering and overprotection (or even a covert rejection) by one or both parents and other family members. Such problems may become worse in adolescence if not tackled earlier.
- *Communication and identity crisis* may come up at any age if the child's sense of security is not well ensured by the parents and immediate family members.
- *Crisis of assimilation* is likely to occur in intercountry adoptions in a small number of cases, where the young adults may face discrimination in getting jobs, married, etc.

MEDICAL CARE OF THE ORPHANS AND ADOPTED BABIES

Vast majority of orphans, who go for adoption after 1 month of age or even later, are highly vulnerable to sepsis, malnutrition, and frequent attacks of acute respiratory, gastrointestinal, and skin infections. By introducing simple inputs such as IV fluids, oxygen therapy, and higher antibiotic therapy in the orphanage itself prior to transferring to a higher center, many such sick babies can be saved.

In postadoption care, in addition to problems of general health and standard immunization schedule, an extra caution should be kept on feeding and sleep patterns, and motor and speech development.

TELLING THE CHILD THAT HE/SHE IS AN ADOPTED CHILD, ENCOURAGING, INSISTING, AND HELPING THE PARENTS

Encouraging, insisting, and helping the parents to tell the child about his/her adoption is the most vital postadoption follow-up action. Every child who is adopted must be told that he/she is adopted by the parents themselves; howsoever, it may appear difficult for them. When a child comes to know the fact from sources other than his parents, it can lead to a severe trauma that it might even ruin relations between the parents and the child. *If done between the ages of 6 and 10 years, most children take it into their stride and future problems can be prevented.*

GOLDEN RULES OF CHILD ADOPTION[5]

- The primary responsibility for providing care and protection to children shall be that of his/her family.
- In keeping with the provisions of the various guidelines for adoption issued from time to time, by the State Government, or CARA and notified by the Central Government, children may be given in adoption by a court after satisfying itself regarding the investigations having been carried out, as are required for giving such children in adoption.
- The State Government shall recognize one or more of its institutions or voluntary organizations in each district as specialized adoption agencies.
- Provided that the children's homes and the institutions run by the State Government or a voluntary organization shall ensure that these children are declared fit for adoption by the committee and be referred to the adoption agency in that district for placement of such children in adoption in accordance with the guidelines notified under subsection (3) till the 2 months period for reconsideration by the parent is over in the case of surrendered children, and without his/her consent in the case of a child who can understand and express his/her consent.
- The court may allow a child to be given in adoption:
    - To a person irrespective of marital status
    - To parents to adopt a child of same sex irrespective of the number of living biological sons or daughters
    - To childless couples

CONCLUSION

Children are a nation's most valuable resource and ensuring their well-being is a cumulative responsibility. Adopting a child is a significant decision that transforms the lives of the adoptive parents and also provides a deserving child a chance to live with love, dignity and stability. Adoption is considered a noble act in our country. Government guidelines empower individuals or couples to navigate the intricate yet rewarding journey of adoption in India. Legal procedures outlined by CARA ensure that the process is carried out with utmost care and consideration. Following the principles of love, care and legal diligence, adoption becomes a meaningful venture that contributes positively to the lives of both parents and children.

REFERENCES

1. Rest the Case. (2022). Types of Adoption in India. [online] Available from https://restthecase.com/knowledge-bank/types-of-adoption-in-india [Last accessed December, 2024].
2. Central Adoption Resource Authority (CARA). [online] Available from https://cara.wcd.gov.in/regulation/cara.html [Last accessed December, 2024].
3. Ministry of Women and Child Development. (2017). Adoption Regulations 2017. [online] Available from https://cara.wcd.gov.in/PDF/Regulation_english.pdf [Last accessed December, 2024].
4. Families of Joy Foundation. [online] Available from https://families of joy.org. [Last accessed December, 2024].
5. AplusTopper. (2024). [online] Available from https://www.aplustopper.com/adoption-certificate/ [Last accessed December, 2024].

22.10 Rights of the Child

Swati Y Bhave, S Narmada Ashok

INTRODUCTION

One-third of the 1.4 crore population of India comprises children below 18 years of age of which 73% of children live in rural areas with limited access to nutrition, healthcare, education and protection. The development index which is a summary measure of human development based on life expectancy at birth, knowledge based on expected years of schooling, and standard of living of a country based on per capita is predominantly based on the welfare of our children. Hence, there is a greater responsibility on part of the state to ensure a proper development of children and provide safe environment for them. The entire community especially the media and various professionals who work with children should be well equipped with the skills and ability to identify and have the authority to respond to child abuse in any form. Understanding the rights of our children helps us to contribute to the same and promote the well-being of our children.[1]

This chapter discusses the child rights and the measures taken in our country for the same.

CHILD RIGHTS IN INDIA

India has made some significant commitments toward ensuring the basic rights of children. Several constitutional provisions protect children in India. Various 5-year plans of India have progressively added more schemes for welfare and protection of child. Despite these laws, policies, and commitments, the actual situation for India's children *vis-à-vis* health, education, early childhood care and protection is still not satisfactory.

The United Nations Convention on the Rights of the Child (UNCRC) is a guiding instrument for implementing rights for all children up to the age of 18 years. The four principles of UNCRC are—nondiscrimination, devotion to the best interests of the child, right to life, survival, and development. India was among the 61 countries who first signed the Child Rights and Protection (CRC) on January 26, 1990, and ratified the same in 1992.

The National Policy for Children states that children are supreme assets of India and provides them with four basic rights:[2,3]

1. Right to survival and protection from abuse and exploitation
2. Right to development
3. Right to good health and education
4. To participate in the decisions that have an impact on their lives

WHO IS A CHILD?

The UNCRC, 1989 (Article 1) defined the child as below 18 years of age. There are various definitions of child in various laws in India:

- *Constitution of India, Article 24:* Any one below the age of 14 years
- For obtaining medical care in a government health facility, a child is defined as one who is <12 years of age
- During the initial census of India, persons below the age of 14 years were defined as children and most of the government programs on children are still targeted for the age-group below 14 years
- The legal definition of child varies from 7 to 18 years of age as evident from the various laws in India, but after the introduction of the Juvenile Justice Care and Protection of Children Act, for all practical purposes, a child is considered as a person below 18 years.[4]

LAWS FOR PROTECTION OF CHILD RIGHTS

- *Criminal Law* [*Indian Penal Code (IPC), 1860*]: Nothing is an offence, which is done by a child under 7 years of age (Section 82). Nothing is an offence, which is done by a child above 7 years of age under 12, who has not attained sufficient maturity of understanding to judge the nature and consequence of his conduct on that occasion (Section 83).
- *Family Law (Child Marriage Restraint Act, 1929)*: "Child" means a person who, if a male, has not completed 21 years of age, and if a female, has not completed 18 years of age.
- *Labor Laws (Apprentice Act, 1951), Factories Act, 1948*: It states that a person shall not be qualified to be engaged as a worker unless he/she is not <14 years of age.
- *Mines (Amendment) Act, 1983*: No person below 18 years of age shall be allowed to work in any mine or part thereof.
- *The Child Labour (Prohibition and Regulation) Act, 1986*: "Child" means a person who has not completed his/her 14 years of age. The Act prohibits employment of children below 14 years in hazardous occupations and processes and also regulating the working conditions of children in other employment. In the last 5 years, the number of hazardous "occupations" listed in the schedule of the act

has increased from 7 to 13 and "processes" from 18 to 57. The notice for prohibiting employment of children as domestic servants and in tea shops and roadside eateries (dhabas), etc. is with effect from October 10th, 2006.

- *Factories Act, 1948:* No child who has not completed his 14 years shall be required or allowed to work in any factory.

SPECIAL PROVISIONS FOR CHILDREN ACCORDING TO THE INDIAN CONSTITUTION

- *Article 21(a)* of the Constitution states that all children between the ages of 6 and 14 years should be provided with free and compulsory education.
- To ensure that children are not abandoned by their parents/guardians, *Section 317 of IPC,* provides imprisonment extending up to 7 years for whoever exposes or leaves their child in any place with the intention of wholly abandoning the child.
- *Section 363 of IPC* provides the punishment extending up to 7 years and fine for the offense of kidnaping any child from India or from lawful guardianship.
- *Section 369 of IPC* provides punishment for up to 7 years for whoever kidnaps or abducts any child under the age of 10 years with the intention of taking dishonestly any movable property.
- *Section 363A of IPC* asserts that disfiguring or kidnapping for purposes of begging is a criminal offense under IPC and the offender is liable to imprisonment of up to 10 years.[5,6]

CORE CHILD PROTECTION LEGISLATION—FOUR MAIN LAWS

Though the above laws and provisions are fairly comprehensive and provide the necessary legal framework for addressing the protection and ensuring equal access to children the core child protection legislation is enshrined in four main laws:

1. The Juvenile Justice (Care and Protection of Children) Act 2000, amended in 2015
2. Prohibition of Child Marriage Act (2006)
3. Protection of Children from Sexual Offences (POCSO) Act (2012), amended in 2019
4. Child Labour (Prohibition and Regulation) Act (1986), amended in 2016.

These are detailed in the following text.

The Juvenile Justice (Care and Protection of Children) Act (2000), Amended in 2015

The Act was enacted in 2000; reforms with more transparency were enforced in January 2016 with an aim to reduce crimes in children below 18 years of age. The Act was initially formulated to protect and support children in conflict with law and children in need of care and protection. Lacunae in the law led to revamp of the law especially after the Nirbhaya case, Delhi gang rape where one of the culprit was a juvenile. In 2015 amendment, special provisions have been made to distinguish children in conflict with law and those in need of basic care. The Act defined "orphaned or abandoned children". It gave definitions for petty, serious, and heinous crimes by children.

The law gives more clarity on the two different boards—Juvenile Justice Board and Child Welfare Committee. The Juvenile Justice Board takes care of children in conflict with law, which would be a child-friendly place and not intimidating to the child. The child welfare committees are formed to take care, protect, treat, develop, and rehabilitate children in need as well as provide basic needs and protection. It also made all child care institutions to be registered for better monitoring.

Prohibition of Child Marriage Act (2006)

The objective of this Act is to prohibit solemnization of marriage where either the groom or the bride is below the marriageable age (18 years for girls and 21 years for boys). This Act protects and provides for maintenance and residence of female. Also, the child begotten of such child marriage are deemed as legitimate children and rights are protected. The bill enables to improve the maternal and infant mortality rate. It also prevents child trafficking in the name of marriage.

Protection of Children from Sexual Offences Act (2012), Amended in 2019

In order to effectively address the crimes of sexual abuse and exploitation of children through stringent and less ambiguous legal provisions, the Ministry of Women and Child Development introduced the POCSO Act, 2012. This was further amended in 2019 to make provisions for enhancements of punishments for various offences to deter the perpetrators and to ensure the safety of children. The act is gender-neutral and keeps the welfare of the child as a matter of paramount importance at every stage. The responsibility of supporting children who have been sexually abused should be embraced by the whole community, but it is the professionals that work in this field who play an important role in enabling the healing process. Please refer to Chapter 22.13: Sexual Abuse and Protection of Children from Sexual Offences Act for details.[2]

Child Labour (Prohibition and Regulation) Act (1986), Amended in 2016

Children below the age of 14 years are prohibited from being employed in any kind of hazardous occupations. It also aims to regulate the hours and working conditions of child laborers. The Act was amended in 2016 and prohibited children to be employed in all occupations and adolescents in hazardous occupations. Under the Act, a broad and specific framework has been given for prevention, prohibition, rescue and rehabilitation of children as well as adolescent workers. There have been clarity of issues related to family enterprises.[5,6]

PROGRAMS AND POLICY MEASURES FOR CHILD WELFARE

National Charter for Children, 2003

The charter ensures the following:

- For every child, its inherent right to be a child and enjoy a healthy, happy childhood
- Protection from economic exploitation and all forms of abuse
- Protection of the girl child
- Care, protection, welfare of children of marginalized, and disadvantaged communities
- Strengthening family and ensuring child-friendly procedures in all matters and procedures relating to children, viz., judicial, administrative, educational or social
- Promoting high standards of health and nutrition
- Assuring basic minimum needs and security—play and leisure
- Early childhood care for survival, growth, and development
- Free and compulsory primary education
- Empowering adolescents, equality, freedom of expression, freedom to seek and receive information, freedom of association and peaceful assembly

National Plan of Action for Children, 2005

This covers all rights to all children up to the age of 18 years and includes:

- System of identification, investigation, reporting, follow-up, and referral of children at risk
- Rehabilitate all children in need of care and protection including beggars and those affected by disasters
- Professional counseling services
- Developmental and protective services to children of sex workers and prisoners
- Prevent children to be used in armed conflict
- Facilitate convergence with related ministries

The guiding principles of the National Plan of Action for Children, 2005 are:

- To regard the child as an asset and a person with human rights
- To address issues of discrimination emanating from biases of gender, class, caste, race, religion, and legal status in order to ensure equality
- To accord utmost priority to the most disadvantaged, poorest of the poor and least served child in all policy and programmatic interventions
- To recognize the diverse stages and settings of childhood, and address the needs of each, providing to all children the entitlements that fulfill their rights and meet their needs in each situation.

National Initiative for Protection of Children

National Initiative for Protection of Children (NICP) is a campaign initiated by Ministry of Social Justice and Empowerment, which aims to place child's rights on every agenda through partnership with allied systems for child protection and promotion of child's rights and implemented trough state governments. The allied systems are police, healthcare system, justice (juvenile) system, education system, transport system, labor department, media, and department of telecommunications, corporate sector, and elected representatives.[7]

The Commissions for Protection of Child Rights Act, 2006

India has a National and State Commissions for Protection of Child Rights (NCPCR) and Child Courts, which ensure speedy trial of offences against children or of violation of child rights and matters connected thereto. The aims of this commission are to spread awareness of child rights; review all the laws and other documents for children; setup a mechanism to hear complaints about violation of child rights; undertake and promote research in the field of child rights; and examine the situation of children. The powers of the commission are similar to a Civil Court under Civil Procedure Code (CPC) and they can forward a matter to a magistrate to be tried under Criminal Procedure Code (CrPC). NCPCR guidelines aid professionals involved in providing services to the child and other affected persons including his/her family, thereby fostering better response coordinated mechanisms so as to result in the evolution of a multisectoral, multidisciplinary approach that will go a long way in achieving the objectives of the NCPCR.[6]

Integrated Child Protection Scheme, 2006

Integrated Child Protection Scheme (ICPS) is a centrally sponsored scheme run by the Ministry of Women and Child Development and is based on the cardinal principles of "protection of child rights" and "best interests of the child". It covers punitive measure against perpetrators of abuse and crimes and rehabilitation for all children in need of care and protection. The target groups are any vulnerable children in need of care and protection and children in conflict or contact with the law.

The ICPS brings together multiple existing child protection schemes of the ministry under one comprehensive umbrella and integrates additional interventions for protecting children and preventing harm by fostering partnership with civil society, actors, and international organizations.

The scheme plans to setup a child protection data management system to formulate and implement effective intervention strategies and monitor their outcomes.[8]

Childline, 2006-07

Childline is a first 24-hour service national helpline for children in distress and operates through a national toll free number 1098. The helpline responds to the urgent and emergency needs of children such as medical assistance, shelter, protection from abuse and exploitation, assistance in child missing cases, repatriation, sponsorship, etc. It was in 1996 as a field action project of Tata Institute of Social Sciences, Mumbai and in 2006–07, Ministry of Women and Child Development granted the exclusive "Nodal mother NGO" (nongovernmental organization) status to CHILDLINE India Foundation to set up the services across the country.

Aims and Objectives

- To have a structured approach to respond appropriately to a child in need of care and protection
- To understand the importance of networking with other organizations working for child protection and child well-being
- To understand the helpline protocol

Right to Free and Compulsory Education, 2010

The 86th Constitutional Amendment Act, 2002 has inserted a new Article 21, which provides for free and compulsory education to children of the age-group of 6–14 years being a right to education.[8] Further, there were additions to the Act, which ensured early childhood care and protection up to 6 years of age as a state responsibility and providing opportunities for education to children between 6 and 14 years as a fundamental duty of parents and guardians. The law also encompassed the disabled children and came into effect in India except in the state of Jammu and Kashmir from April 1st, 2010.

Protection of Abused Children, 2012

Abuse and neglect are forms of maltreatment of a child. Abuse can occur by inflicting harm, or by failing to act to prevent harm. Children may be abused in a family, in an institutional or in a community setting, by those known to them or, more rarely, by a stranger. The POCSO Act, 2012 ensures the same and are discussed in Chapter 22.13.[9,10]

Children with Special Needs, 2016

India faces the challenge of providing education with special needs. Though an Act was enacted to give equal opportunities to children with disabilities in 1995, the Act was replaced in 2016, and defined disability as an evolving concept. Special schools with special educators especially in Delhi area are being formed to provide healthy environment for these children. No child with disability can be denied admission and payment of capitation fees is prohibited.

CONCLUSION

India recognizes and acknowledges children as equals to their adults. It is taking measures to protect and shelter them and also give the basic fundamental rights of citizenship. Various laws have been enacted to safeguard their rights and policies have been brought in place to ensure to protect them from exploitation and violence.

REFERENCES

1. Humanium. Realizing child rights in India. [online] Available from https://www.humanium.org/en/india/ [Last accessed December, 2024].
2. United Nation's Children's Fund. Convention on Rights of the Child. [online] Available from https://www.unicef.org/child-rights-convention#:~:text=The%20Convention%20says%20childhood%20is,develop%20and%20flourish%20with%20dignity [Last accessed December, 2024].
3. United Nation's Children's Fund. Child Protection. [online] Available from https://www.unicef.org/india/what-we-do/child-protection [Last accessed December, 2024].
4. National Commission for Protection of Child Rights; UNICEF India. Resource Book for Commissions for Protection of Child Rights, 1st edition. New Delhi: National Commission for the Protection of Child Rights; 2016.
5. Child related legislation. [online] Available from https://wcd.gov.in/documents/legislations. [Last accessed January, 2025].
6. Child rights and legislation. [online] Available from https://egyankosh.ac.in/bitstream/123456789/46438/1/Unit-11.pdf [Last accessed December, 2024].
7. Agarwal K, Dalwai S, Galagali P, Mishra D, Prasad C, Thadani A; Child Rights And Protection Program (CRPP) of Indian Academy of Pediatrics (IAP). Recommendations on recognition and response to child abuse and neglect in the Indian setting. Indian Pediatr. 2010;47(6):493-504.
8. Ministry of Women and Child Development, Government of India. The Integrated Child Protection Scheme (ICPS). [online] Available from https://wcdhry.gov.in/schemes-for-children/icps/. [Last accessed January, 2025].
9. Resource Book. First National Conference on Child Abuse for Multidisciplinary Professionals (COCAMP 2004). Chennai: Indian Council for Child Welfare, Tamil Nadu; Sri Ramchandra Medical College and Research Institute; 2004.
10. Ministry of Women and Child Development, Government of India. Study on Child Abuse: India 2007. New Delhi: Kriti; 2007.

22.11 Child Abuse and Neglect

Chandrika Rao, Aashika Maria Naidu

The true character of a society is revealed in how it treats its children. —**Nelson Mandela**

INTRODUCTION

According to United Nations Convention on Rights of the Child (UNCRC) and in India according to the Juvenile Justice (Care and Protection of Children) Act 2000, any person below the age of 18 years is considered as a child.

WHAT IS CHILD ABUSE?

Child abuse as defined by World Health Organization (WHO) includes all forms of physical and/or emotional ill treatment, sexual abuse, neglect or negligent treatment or commercial or other exploitation, resulting in actual or potential harm to the child's health, survival, development, or dignity in the context of a relationship of responsibility, trust or power.

Definition by World Health Organization and India

The types of abuse and its respective definitions are given by WHO and the same definitions are adapted in India as our country is yet to define child abuse.

- *Physical abuse* is defined as "harm that results in actual or potential physical harm from an interaction or abuse, or lack of an interaction, which is reasonably within the control of a parent or person in a position of responsibility".[1]
- *Emotional abuse* involves the "failure to provide a developmentally abuse-appropriate supportive environment, including the availability of a primary attachment figure, so that the child can develop a stable and full range of emotional and social competencies".[1]
- *Child sexual abuse* is the "involvement of a child in sexual activity that he or she does not fully comprehend, is unable to give informed consent to, or for which the child is not developmentally prepared and cannot give consent".[1]
- *Neglect* can be defined as "the failure to provide for the development of the child in all spheres: Health, education, emotional development, nutrition, shelter, and safe living conditions".[1]

EPIDEMIOLOGY OF CHILD ABUSE IN WORLD AND INDIA

The global prevalence of child abuse according to WHO Global Status Report on preventing violence against children in 2020, estimated that 50% of the children aged between 2 and 17 years have experienced some form of violence each year. Among children in the age-group of 11–15 years, one-third have been bullied by their peers and 120 million girls below the age of 20 years are estimated to have suffered some form of forced sexual contact.[2]

In India, the Indian National Crimes Records Bureau (NCRB) reports that 53% of children report abuse by a parent, relative, or school teacher. The prevalence of child sexual abuse in India is estimated to be between 4 and 66% for females and 4–57% for males.[3]

RISK FACTORS FOR ABUSE

The risk factors of child abuse are multifactorial **(Fig. 22.11.1)**. Broadly they can be classified as individual factors, family factors, community factors, and social factors. **Table 22.11.1** details some of the features of these factors leading to child abuse and neglect.

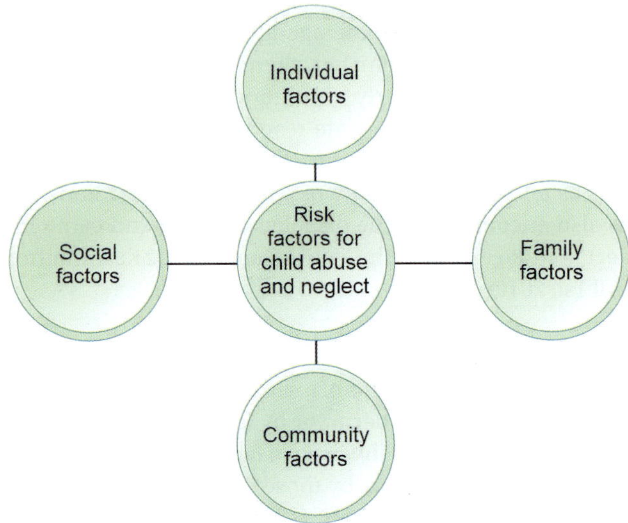

Fig. 22.11.1: The risk factors for child abuse and neglect.

TABLE 22.11.1: The various types of risk factors for child abuse and neglect.

Individual factors	Family factors	Community factors	Social factors
• Age • Gender • Child with disability or mental illness • Adults who were victims of child abuse in their childhood who become perpetrators in their adulthood	• Single parenting • Broken families • Parents with low education • Unemployed parents • Alcohol/drug abuse in the parents • Family conflicts • Partner abuse	• Mistreating female child • Religious practices that prevent the child from being provided with health, food and shelter	• Poverty • Alcohol abuse • Drug abuse • Family stress • School stress • Teenage dating • Bullying

APPROACH TO A CHILD WITH ABUSE

The approach to evaluation of a child with abuse involves a detailed history, good and appropriate clinical examination, selective investigations, and appropriate management **(Table 22.11.2)**.

TABLE 22.11.2: Approach to a child with abuse.

History	• A1: Interview setting • A2: Pattern of interview • A3: Red flag signs of abuse • A4: HEADSSS assessment
Examination	• B1: Anthropometry • B2: Head to toe examination • B3: Examination in cases of sexual abuse
Investigations	• C1: Blood and urine investigations • C2: Radiological investigations • C3: Samples collected during genital examination
Management	• D1: Initial management • D2: Specific management

History

Interview Setting

Interviews should be conducted in a safe and child-friendly environment. The child should be made to feel comfortable by the pediatrician by gaining his/her trust and being nonjudgmental.[5]

Pattern of Interview

- The child should be informed by the pediatrician that the history given by the child will remain confidential and will only be disclosed to parents or concerned authorities only if it is of concern to the child's well-being.
- If the child requests, the pediatrician may consider the presence of a support person to sit during the interview; in such situations the person should be instructed that only the child is allowed to talk *unless* a question is directed to the support person.
- The pediatrician should begin with the interview with general questions such as "Where do you live?", "Which school do you go to?", etc. This helps build rapport with the child.
- Avoid asking the child a direct question as far as possible, such as "Did somebody touch your private parts last week?". Ask open-ended questions such as "I understand something has been bothering you. Please tell me about it."
- During the interview the following points should be clarified:
    - Descriptions of events
    - The identity of the perpetrator(s)
    - If the allegations are single or multiple events
    - The time frame and location/venue
    - The presence and identities of any witnesses
    - Did the child tell anyone about the event(s)
    - If similar events have happened to other children[5]

Red Flag Signs of Abuse

Physical abuse:

- Unexplained injuries
- Unexplained bruises of different ages
- Untreated multiple fractures
- Unexplained burns or scald injuries on an area not likely to come into contact with a hot object or in the shape of an implement (for example, a cigarette tip or iron)
- Repeated, apparent life-threatening events in a child, if the onset is witnessed only by one caregiver and no medical explanation

Sexual abuse:

- Persistent and/or recurrent urinary tract infections
- Unexplained bleeding through vagina or anus
- Evidence of one or more foreign bodies in the vagina or anus that is indicated by offensive vaginal discharge.
- In prepubertal children, presence of sexually transmitted infections
- Pregnancy in a child or young adolescent

Behavioral cues toward child maltreatment:

- Reduced appetite
- Sleeping problems
- Bed wetting
- Social withdrawal

TABLE 22.11.3: HEADSSS assessment in child abuse and neglect.

H *Home*	*E* *Education*	*A* *Activities*	*D* *Drugs and alcohol*	*S* *Sexuality*	*S* *Safety and abuse*	*S* *Self-harm*
Who lives with you?	Are you going to school or college?	What do you do in your spare time?	Have you tried drugs, alcohol, or smoking?	Are you in a relationship?	Do you feel safe at home?	What makes you sad or stressed?
Do you share a room?	Do you have any friends?	Do you exercise?	Do you feel pressurized to do drugs?	Are you sexually active?	Do you feel safe at school/college?	Do you have any thoughts about hurting yourself?
How do you get along with others at home?	Have you experienced bullying at school/college?	Do you share any activity with your friends?	Do you want to continue or stop?	Do you know about contraception?	Does anyone make you feel unsafe?	Have you told anyone about these thoughts?
Who do you talk to when you are upset?	What are your future plans on education?			Do you know about STDs?		

(STDs: sexually transmitted diseases)

- Poor self-regulation
- Regressive behavior compared to what would be expected for the age of the child or adolescent
- Reports or displays of sexualized behavior in a prepubertal child, such as oral-genital contact with another child or a doll; requesting to be touched in the genital area; or inserting or attempting to insert an object, finger, or penis into another child's vagina or anus

HEADSSS Assessment

The HEADSSS assessment is an internationally recognized tool used for structural assessment of an adolescent patient, encompassing *H*ome, *E*ducation, *A*ctivities, *D*rugs and alcohol, *S*exuality, *S*afety and abuse, and *S*elf-harm **(Table 22.11.3)**.[4]

Examination

Anthropometry

- Height, weight, body mass index (BMI)
- Head circumference in children below 2 years of age.

Head-to-toe Examination[5]

These are detailed in **Table 22.11.4** in a descending order.

TABLE 22.11.4: Head-to-toe examination in child with suspected child abuse.

Appearance	General appearance and emotional state of the child
Skin	• The size, shape, color, and location of bruises • Bite marks, abrasions, lacerations, burns
Mouth	• Bruising of lips, buccal mucosa, gums, palate • Mucosal tears or dental trauma
Head	• Infants—anterior fontanelle • Palpate the head for hematomas or fractures
Eyes	• Orbital fracture or globe injury • Fundus examination for retinal hemorrhages
Ears	• Bruising on the pinnae, hemotympanum • Tympanic membrane perforation and cerebrospinal fluid otorrhea
Neck	Ligature or other choke marks
Chest	Costochondral tenderness or chest deformity
Abdomen	• Examine for bruises • Palpate the abdomen for bowel sounds, tenderness, masses
Back	Examine for bruises; palpate for tenderness
Extremities	Limb swelling or fractures

Examination in Cases of Sexual Abuse

Medical examination in a suspected sexual abuse is to be conducted as per the provisions of Section 27 of the Protection of Children against Sexual Offences (POCSO) Act, 2012 and Section 164A of the CrPC, 1973 which states that:

"The examination of the woman with whom rape is alleged or attempted should be by a registered medical practitioner employed in a hospital run by the government or a local authority and in the absence of a such a practitioner, by any other registered medical practitioner, with the consent of such woman or of a person competent to give such consent on her behalf and such woman shall be sent to such registered medical practitioner within 24 hours from the time of receiving the information relating to the commission of such offence."

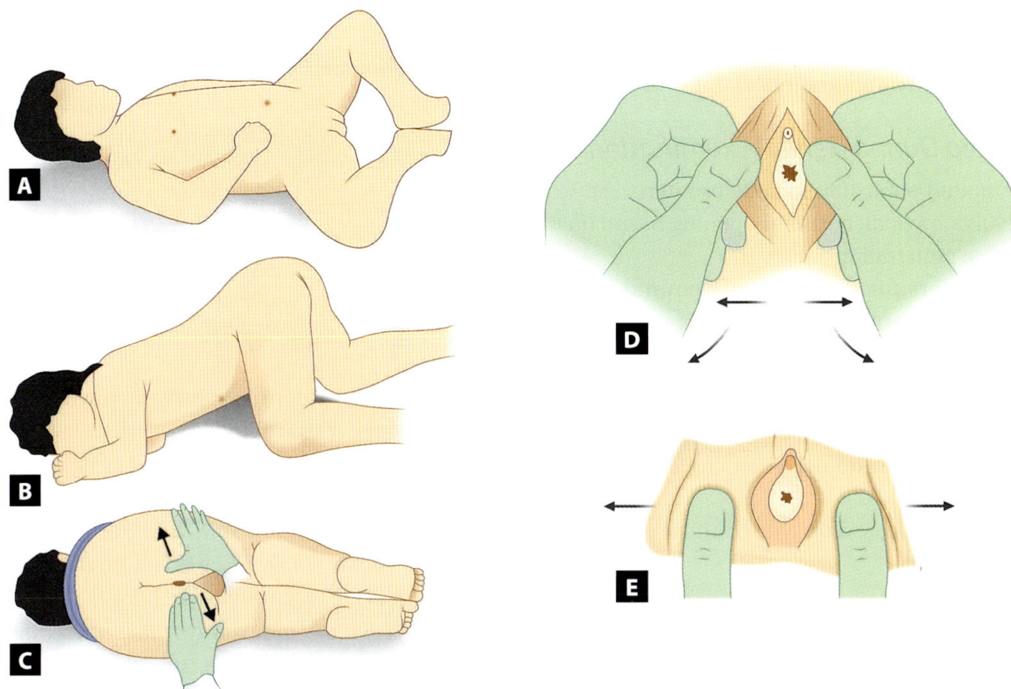

Figs. 22.11.2A to E: The positions for anogenital examination based on the age-group. (A) Supine position; (B) Knee–chest position; (C) Lateral decubitus position; (D) Labial traction; and (E) Labial separation.

In the above legal provision, the term "woman" may be substituted by the term "child", and applied in the context of the POCSO Act, 2012.

Along with the routine head to toe examination done in all cases of abuse, sexual abuse cases require an additional anogenital examination.

Ideally gynecologists who have had specialized training and experience in working with children should conduct genito-anal examinations in children.

Anogenital Examination

The genital examination of the prepubertal child is principally an external visualization. Speculums, anoscopes, and bimanual examinations (two-finger test) of the vagina or rectum of a prepubertal child are not routinely required. The anogenital examination requires special positioning depending on the age of the child as follows **(Figs. 22.11.2A to E)**:

- Young child—on the caregiver's lap
- Prepubertal—supine position
- Pubertal adolescent—lithotomy position
- Anal examination—prone knee-chest position[5]

Figure 22.11.3 shows the normal finding in a genital examination with a semilunar hymen with intravaginally visible longitudinal ridges.

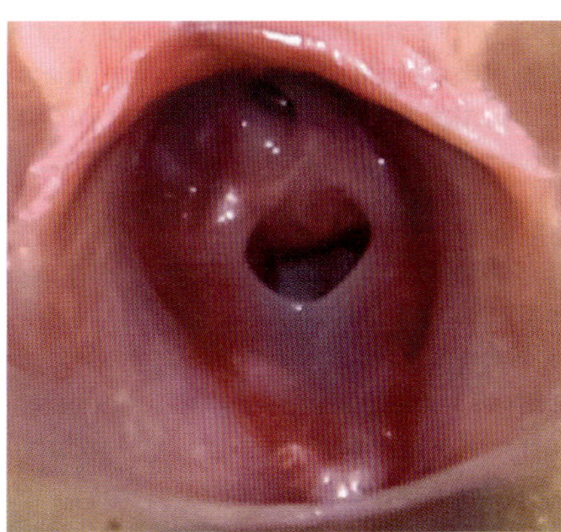

Fig. 22.11.3: Normal finding in genital examination: Semilunar hymen with intravaginally visible longitudinal ridges.

Investigations

- *Blood investigation:* Human immunodeficiency virus (HIV), hepatitis B surface antigen (HbsAg), and venereal disease research laboratory (VDRL) test
- *Urine:* Urine routine for urinary tract infection, urine pregnancy test
- *Radiological investigation*:
  - *X-ray:* Relevant part of the body based on history in case of physical abuse to determine fractures.
  - *Age estimation:* X-ray of left wrist and elbow

- *Ultrasound of the abdomen:* Look for visceral injuries/ hemorrhage.
- *Pregnancy:* Site of implantation, viability of fetus[5]

Samples Collected During Genital Examination

- Clippings of matted pubic hair to detect semen
- Swabs from vulva, vaginal, and anal opening based on the history of orifice penetration
- Two vaginal smears for detection of seminal fluid or examination of spermatozoa[5]

Management—Physical, Emotional, Sexual (Pregnancy and Sexually Transmitted Disease)

Management of child abuse and neglect includes:

- Initial management
- Specific management based on type of abuse

Initial Management

- Stabilize the child and treat the injuries—treatment has to be provided to the child even if FIR is not registered.
- Admit the child if necessary.
- Immediate counseling of the child and parents.

Specific Management

Management of physical abuse: In case a child is in immediate danger, ensure the child's safety. If there are any signs of physical injury, the child should receive prompt medical attention and treat the child's injuries accordingly.

Management of sexual abuse: Management of sexual abuse includes the following:

- Emergency contraception
- HIV prophylaxis
- Prevention of sexually transmitted infections
- Safe abortion in case of pregnancy as per current rules.
  - *Emergency contraception:* Emergency contraception should be offered after informing and counseling regarding the risk of pregnancy in a child abuse victim. Contraception is recommended for girls who are post-monarchial, or those in the initially stages of puberty (Tanner stage 2 or 3) and is recommended for use within 5 days (120 hours) in case of penetrative sex. The contraception provided is one of the following:
    - *Levonorgestrel-only (LNG):* 1.5 mg tablet—single dose
    - *Ulipristal acetate (UPA):* 30 mg tablet—single dose
    - Emergency copper intrauterine device (Cu-IUD)
  - *HIV prophylaxis:* The indications for prophylaxis against HIV include penetrative sexual assault in a child or adolescent especially within 72 hours of assault. The prophylaxis management recommended as per WHO includes:
    - *For children aged 10 years or younger:* Zidovudine (AZT) + Lamivudine (3TC)
    - *For children and adolescents aged 11 years and older (over 30 kg):* Tenofovir disoproxil fumarate (TDF) + Lamivudine (3TC)[6]
  - *Prevention of sexually transmitted infections:*[5]
    - Preferred choice is azithromycin 1 g stat or doxycycline 100 mg bd for 7 days, with metronidazole 400 mg for 7 days.
    - *Hepatitis B immunoglobulin*: Administer 0.06 mL/kg hepatitis B immune globulin immediately up to 72 hours after sexual act.
    - Hepatitis vaccine is recommended as follows:
      - *No, never vaccinated for hepatitis B:* 0, 1, 6 months
      - *Incomplete vaccination:* Complete the schedule as above
      - *Complete vaccination:* No vaccine to be given
  - *Human papillomavirus (HPV) prophylaxis:* For girls aged 9–14 years; while the HPV vaccination is intended for girls before the onset of sexual activity involving vaginal penetration, girls who have been raped may still benefit from the vaccine as they may be infected by a strain not covered in the vaccine or by one of the four strains in the quadrivalent vaccine.[6]

TABLE 22.11.5: Management of emotional abuse in children.

Psychoeducation	*Psychosocial support*
Referral to psychiatrist	• Sleep—Regular bed routines, avoid excessive screen time • Nutrition—Eat regularly, all three meals and some snacks • Physical activity—60 minutes or more of physical activity each day • Social—Participate in school and social activities, spend time with trusted friends and family

Management of emotional abuse: Emotional abuse is managed by psychoeducation and psychosocial support **(Table 22.11.5)**.

PREVENTION OF CHILD ABUSE AND NEGLECT

Methods to Prevent Child Abuse and Neglect

Global Efforts

In May 2021, at the 74th World Health Assembly, member states of WHO adopted the resolution WHA74.17 to end violence against children through health. The strategies put forward were:

- Designate a focal point within ministries of health to ensure coordination.
- Equipment health service providers with the necessary skills to address violence against children.
- Strengthen implementation of legislative frameworks and evidence-based programs consistent with the INSPIRE framework.
  - *I*—Implementation and enforcement of laws
  - *N*—Norms and values
  - *S*—Safe environments
  - *P*—Parent and caregiver support
  - *I*—Income and economic strengthening
  - *R*—Response and support services
  - *E*—Education and life skills[7]
- Prioritize data collection and monitoring.
- Include children, as appropriate, in advocacy, policy development, and action.
- Support, in particular, children in humanitarian settings, children with disabilities, and others who are vulnerable.
- Allocate the necessary budget for national policies and plans.
- Enhance international cooperation.

Indian Scenario

Protection of Children Against Sexual Offences Act

The POCSO Act, 2012 is a law put to force to provide for the protection of children from the offence of sexual assault, sexual harassment, and pornography and to safeguard the interests of the child at every stage of the judicial process.

Child Safety Week

Child Safety Week is a week celebrated by a people-led movement to spread awareness regarding child abuse and encourage collective action toward preventing child abuse in India and addressing the issue of child safety. The entire week from November 14th to 20th is marked for highlighting the relevance of child safety. November 19th is observed as World Day for the Prevention of Child Abuse.

Child Helpline—1098

In India, other than the law enforcement for the protection of children against sexual offences, the nationwide Child Helpline—1098 is available.

At Schools

Children should be taught on how to differentiate between good touch and bad touch. Children should be taught to seek help from parents, friends, teachers, or any trustworthy adult when faced with abuse/neglect. Sex education should be a part of the school curriculum to educate adolescents on sexually transmitted infections.

REFERENCES

1. Runyan D, Wattam C, Ikeda R, Hassan F, Ramiro L. Child abuse and neglect by parents and other caregivers. In: Krug EG, Dahlberg LL, Mercy JA, Zwi AB, Lozano R (Eds). World Report on Violence and Health. Geneva: World Health Organization; 2002. pp. 59-86.
2. World Health Organization. (2020). Global status report on preventing violence against children 2020. [online] Available from unicef.org/media/70731/file/Global-status-report-on-preventing-violence-against-children-2020.pdf [Last accessed December, 2024].
3. National Crime Records Bureau; Ministry of Home Affairs. Crime in India 2020. New Delhi: National Crime Records Bureau; 2021.
4. Katzenellenbogen R. HEADSS: The "Review of Systems" for Adolescents. Virtual Mentor. 2005;7(3):231-3.
5. Ministry of Health and Family Welfare. (2013). Guidelines and Protocols: Medico-legal Care for Survivors/Victims of Sexual Violence. [online] Available from https://mohfw.gov.in/sites/default/files/953522324.pdf [Last accessed December 2024]
6. World Health Organization. Responding to Child Maltreatment: A Clinical Handbook for Health Professionals. Geneva: World Health Organization; 2022.
7. World Health Organization. (2016). INSPIRE: Seven Strategies for Ending Violence Against Children. [online] Available from apps.who.int/iris/bitstream/handle/10665/207717/9789241565356-eng.pdf?sequence=1&isAllowed=y [Last accessed December, 2024]

22.12 Child Labor

Alok Gupta, Kul Bhushan

INTRODUCTION

The problem of child labor continues to pose a major challenge before our nation. The Government of India (GOI) has been taking various proactive measures to tackle this problem. It is essentially a socioeconomic problem inextricably linked to poverty and illiteracy, and requires concerted efforts from all sections of the society to reduce its magnitude and extent.

Child labor in India is a human rights issue as for the entire developed and developing world. It is a serious and extensive problem, with many children compromising their physical, mental, social, and moral health. Being under the age of 14 years working in the carpet-making factories and glass-blowing units and making fireworks with bare little hands make their lives miserable.

Compared with many other countries, child labor is more prevalent in India. According to the Census of India 2011, 10.1 million children are engaged in labor or seeking work. And yet, the National Crime Records Bureau's yearly publication, *Crime in India 2018* reveals that a total of only 464 cases were registered under the Child Labour (Prohibition and Regulation) Amendment Act 2016, (with 810 child victims) across the entire country.[1]

DEFINITION

It is very difficult to define "child work" and "child labor". The problem is compounded by differences in social and cultural perceptions. It is also not easy to draw a distinction between work and labor. The dictionary meaning of "worker" is an employee, especially in manual or industrial work, while a "laborer" is one who for wages does work that requires strength or patience rather than skill or training. In many situations, these two words are synonymous. The word "work" implies full-time commercial work to sustain self or add to the family income. Any child, who is employed in activities to feed self and/or family, is being subjected to "child labor".

Legal Definition

The Government has enacted the Child Labour (Prohibition and Regulation) Act, 1986, which was amended in 2016. The amended act is called the "Child and Adolescent Labour (Prohibition and Regulation) (CALPR) Act, 1986". The act provides for complete prohibition of work or employment of children below 14 years in any occupation and process and adolescents in the age-group of 14–18 years in hazardous occupations and processes.[1]

Child Rights and You Definition

CRY stands for "Child Rights and You". In essence, child labor refers to the exploitation of children through any form of work that deprives them of their childhood, impedes their ability to attend schools, and is detrimental to their physical, mental, social, or moral development.[2]

United Nations Children's Fund Definition

United Nations Children's Fund (UNICEF) has given a comprehensive formulation in its attempt to define child labor as listed below:

- Starting full-time work at too early an age
- Working too long within or outside the family so that the children are unable to attend the school
- Work resulting in excessive physical, social, and psychological strain on the child
- Work and life on the street, which are dangerous and unhealthy
- Inadequate remuneration for working outside the family
- Too much responsibility at too early an age
- Work that does not facilitate the psychological and social developments
- Work that inhibits the child's self-esteem as in bonded labor and prostitution

In conclusion, a simple workable definition of child labor is any work within or outside the family that threatens health and mental development of the child by denying him or her both fundamental as well as nonfundamental rights.[3,4]

CAUSES OF CHILD LABOR

Poverty: Poverty is the single biggest cause of child labor in India. Children from poor families often need to work to support their families financially. They may work in factories, on farms, in industries, or even in streets in restaurants, etc.[5]

Lack of access to quality education: Many children in India do not have access to good schools. When children do not have access to education, they are more likely to work instead of going to school.

Growth of the informal economy: The informal economy is made up of small businesses and self-employed workers. The informal economy often employs them because it is difficult to enforce child labor laws in this sector.

Lack of awareness: Most parents are unaware of the physical, mental, and psychological consequences of this issue.

There are many other factors that contribute to the problem, such as social norms, cultural beliefs, and gender discrimination.[5]

MAJOR FORMS OF CHILD LABOR AND DETERMINANTS OF ITS PATTERN

- *According to duration of work hours:* Two types of workers are classified:
  1. Main workers are those who are engaged in a full-time economic activity
  2. Marginal workers are those who are part-time workers
- *According to work field:* Four types are classified:[2]
  1. Agricultural labor
  2. Domestic labor
  3. Manufacturing and industries
  4. Street and service sector

Many children work in their families as helpers in different household chores including caring for younger siblings. This sort of work discourages school attendance. Rural children are often involved in nondomestic work, which is agricultural in nature and quite a good proportion of them are involved in seasonal work. In cities, on the other hand, children are found to work in marketplaces and almost in every street corner. They are engaged in a variety of working situations such as vendors, waiters in restaurants, helpers in all kinds of shops, private houses, in industries such as carpet weaving, saree-embroidery, brassware, precious stone-polishing, leather tannery, *beedi* (handmade cigarettes) making, bangle manufacturing, glass industry, brick field, matches and fire industries, construction sites, garages, gas stations, fishing, mines, handloom industries, lock industry, and rag-picking.[6]

Girls at an early age are recruited to the profession of *prostitution*. Children involved in gainful employment sometimes are *bonded laborers* in the backward areas of some developing countries. Progenies of *single-parent households* are more likely to join the labor force at an early age. Another factor is the *birth order* of child, the first child having the highest probability of being gainfully employed. Moreover, during the last few decades, in developing societies, the mortality rates have declined markedly, which has resulted in the survival of a larger number of children. The proportion of children under 14 years of age as compared to 15–19 years of age-groups is higher among the poor. Thus, poor families are left with only young children as potential workers.[2]

To summarize, children are engaged in various activities such as visible or invisible, formal or informal, and paid or unpaid. Boys are usually engaged in relatively larger number of occupations than girls. Types of work for urban children are classified here:[7]

- *Within the family:*
  - *Domestic house tasks:* Cooking, childcare, fetching water, cleaning utensils, washing clothes, etc.
  - Handicrafts and cottage industries, weaving, leather work, woodwork, etc.
  - Within the family but outside home, domestic service, construction work, mining, (i.e., quarry mines), informal economy, (i.e., laundry, recycling rubbish)
- *Outside the family:*
  - Bonded labor
  - Apprentices
  - *Skilled traders:* Carpets, embroidery, brassware works, gem polishing, etc.
  - Industries/unskilled occupations, mines, etc.
  - Commercial shops, restaurants, and hotels
  - Begging

CONSEQUENCES OF CHILD LABOR

The child labor leads to harmful effect to the child, society, and the nation as a whole.[6]

Child Consequences

Health risks: This exposes children to hazardous working conditions, physical and mental abuse, and long hours of labor, which can result in injuries, illnesses, and developmental issues.

Education deprivation: Working children are often denied access to education, limiting their future prospects and perpetuating the cycle of poverty.

Stunted development: It disrupts normal childhood development, depriving children of playtime, social interaction, and emotional well-being, hindering their physical, cognitive, and emotional growth.

Antisocial and criminal activities: Working with mature and adult workers leads them to learn bad habits and due to immature thinking, chances of indulgence in criminal activity rises.

Societal Consequences

Undermining human rights: It violates the fundamental rights of children, denying them the right to education, protection, and a safe and healthy environment.

Poverty and inequality: It keeps families trapped in a cycle of poverty, as children's earnings contribute minimally to the household income and hinder their long-term economic prospects.

Social disintegration: It disrupts family and community dynamics as children are forced into work instead of receiving proper care and education. This can lead to a breakdown in social structures and intergenerational poverty.

National Consequences

Economic implications: It deprives children of education, leading to a less skilled workforce, reduced productivity, and limited opportunities for economic advancement.

Human capital loss: It results in the loss of potential human capital as children are denied education and skill development. This diminishes the nation's capacity to compete globally and achieve sustainable development goals.

Social welfare burden: The physical and psychological consequences lead to increased healthcare and social welfare costs for the nation. Governments must allocate resources to address these issues, diverting funds from other critical areas.

Population impact: Since a child laborer starts earning at an early age, marriage takes place early. the need to increase in workforce and better earning motivate them further for early marriage. Due to poor education, they do not understand family planning.

HEALTH HAZARDS FOR WORKING CHILDREN

Chronic starvation and unhealthy environment do contribute to ill health in all children, whether working or otherwise. Also, many children start working at a very early age and do hazardous work for 12–15 hours a day without any holiday. Several occupations may not be hazardous by themselves, but the environment makes them such. These environmental factors include lack of ventilation, presence of dust, gases, fumes and odors, poor lighting, noise, humidity, crowding, and vibrations and ionizing radiations. All the children are in the process of growing and attaining their full physical stature and therefore, their growth is likely to be affected, resulting in stunting. This has been proven in several studies. Children, who started working early in life suffered from deterioration in their nutritional status, but such impact was not seen for those children, who started work after the age of 11 years.

Health effects of labor on children also vary according to the type of work situation. Children, who are engaged in their own household jobs or family-based industries, may have no direct adverse health effects. On the other hand, bonded and wage child workers may have greater effects on health because of the exploitative and unregulated nature of work, in which children are exposed more to health hazards, heavier workload, and physical and mental abuse. Most of the poor child workers go to work without adequate food, clothing, and proper shelter. They ultimately become victims of a wide range of diseases like diarrhea, general weakness, various viral and bacterial infections, and sexually transmitted diseases.[2,3]

Other potential common psychological problems include habit disorders, personality disorders (such as timidity, irritability, sensitiveness, temper tantrums, obstinacy, day-dreaming, negativity, fear, jealousy, inferiority complex), and psychoneurotic disorders (such as nervousness, tremors, headache, pain, hyperventilation syndrome, masturbation, etc.) They are more prone toward developing antisocial behavior such as stealing, sexual offences, premarital sex, psychoses and anxiety neurosis, drug abuse, and psychosexual problems.

OCCUPATIONAL HEALTH HAZARDS

Any occupation which allows the working children to encounter harmful substances like chemicals, as in the balloon and lock industry or fire in glass industry, match and fireworks, or cotton puff and dust as in power loom industry is termed intrinsically hazardous, which may have an adverse effect on physical and psychological development of children.[2,3] Various occupational health hazards are depicted in **Table 22.12.1**.

EXPLOITATION OF CHILD LABOR

Child labor is economically unsound, psychologically disastrous, physically as well as morally harmful and precludes the child's potentialities to unfold completely. It also deprives them of education, training, and skills, which are essential prerequisites of earning power and economic development. Sexual abuse is a common problem faced by girl children who work as a contract labor. The working girls in sleazy B and C grade hotels, lodging houses, restaurants, and in domestic houses are exposed to physical assaults and sexual abuses by their employers and customers.

INITIATIVE AGAINST CHILD LABOR

Child and Adolescent Labour (Prohibition and Regulation) Act

The GOI has enacted the Child Labour (Prohibition and Regulation) Act, 1986, which was amended in 2016. The amended act is called the "Child and Adolescent Labour (Prohibition and Regulation) Act, 1986". The Act provides for complete prohibition of work or employment of children below 14 years in any occupation and process, and

TABLE 22.12.1: Occupational health hazards in children.

Occupation	*Disease/disability*
Balloon factories	Pneumonia, bronchopneumonia, breathlessness, and heart failure
Match and firework	Breathing problems, severe burns, muscle fatigue from lifting heavy loads, deformities due to long hours of work in one position
Lock industry	Tuberculosis and respiratory tract diseases, asthma, acute breathlessness, acid burns, acute headache
Glass industry	Heat strokes, conjunctivitis, tuberculosis (TB) and burns, life span reduced by a third due to heat and dust
Slate industry	Silicosis, TB, pneumoconiosis
Power loom industry	Byssinosis, fibrosis of lung tissue, and TB
Beedi industry/ *gutkha*	*Nicotine poisoning:* Nausea, headache blackouts and muscle fatigue, loss of eyesight Tobacco addiction
Brass industry	Additional burns and TB
Zari industry	Eye diseases, postural deformities and spinal problems
Domestic workers, shop bays, etc.	Overwork, physical and sexual abuse, drug addiction, isolation from society
Carpet industry	Poisoning from coloring agents, lung diseases from fiber dust

Source: Health for the Millions. New Delhi: Voluntary Health Association of India; 1989.

adolescents in the age-group of 14–18 years in hazardous occupations and processes. The amendment also provides for stricter punishment of employers for violation of the act and made the offence as cognizable.[1]

This CALPR Act is enforced by the state government except in railway administration, major ports, mine or oilfield where central government is the appropriate enforcing agency.

The GOI has developed an online portal PENCIL (Platform for Effective Enforcement of No Child Labor) for effective enforcement of CALPR Act. The portal has also a complaint corner for registering the complaint regarding child labor. These complaints are dealt by the respective district nodal officers of the district.[8]

Ministry of Labour and Employment has been implementing National Child Labour Project Scheme (NCLPS) for rehabilitation of child laborers through District Project Societies under the chairmanship of the District Magistrate. Under the NCLPS, the children in the age-group of 9–14 years are rescued or withdrawn from work and enrolled in the NCLP Special Training Centers (STCs), where they are provided with bridge education, vocational training, midday meal, stipend, and healthcare, before being mainstreamed into formal education system. NCLPS has now been subsumed under *Samagara Shiksha Abhiyan (SSA) Scheme* with effect from April 1, 2021.

National Child Labour Project Scheme

Government had initiated the NCLPS in 1988 to rehabilitate working children in 12 child-labor endemic districts of the country.[1,9] This is the major central sector scheme for the rehabilitation of child labor.

- The scheme seeks to adopt a sequential approach with focus on rehabilitation of children working in hazardous occupations and processes in the first instance.
- Under the scheme, survey of child labor engaged in hazardous occupations and processes has been conducted.
- The identified children are to be withdrawn from these occupations and processes and then put into special schools to enable them to be mainstreamed into formal schooling system.
- Project societies at the district level are fully funded for opening of special schools/rehabilitation centers for the rehabilitation of child labor.
- The special schools/rehabilitation centers provide:
    - Nonformal/bridge education
    - Skilled/vocational training
    - Midday meal
    - Stipend @ ₹150/- per child per month.
    - Healthcare facilities through a doctor appointed for a group of 20 schools

The Target Group

The project societies are required to conduct survey to identify children working in hazardous occupations and processes. These children will then form the target group for the project society. Of the children identified, those in the age-group 5–8 years will have to be mainstreamed directly to formal educational system through the SSA scheme. Working children in the age-group of 9–14 years will have to be rehabilitated through NCLP schools established by the Project Society.

Project Implementation

The entire project is required to be implemented through a registered society under the chairmanship of administrative head of the district, namely, District Magistrate/Collector/ Deputy Commissioner of the District. Members of the society may be drawn from concerned government departments, representatives of *Panchayati Raj* Institutions, nongovernmental organizations (NGOs), trade unions, etc.

Funding Pattern

The projects have been taken up in the central sector, the entire funding is done by the Central Government (Ministry of Labour and Employment). Funds are released to the concerned project societies depending upon the progress of project activities.

Present Status of National Child Labour Project Scheme

National Child Labour Project Scheme was approved for implementation up to March 31, 2021 and since then the scheme has been subsumed/merged with the *SSA* scheme of the Ministry of Education. Further, the NCLPS was sanctioned in 324 districts and operational in 59 districts of the country as on March 31, 2021.

The Ministry of Labour and Employment-operated online portal allows government officials, law enforcement agencies, and NGOs to share information and coordinate on child labor cases at the national, state, and local levels to improve enforcement of child labor laws and the implementation of the NCLPS.

The good news is that the incidence of child labor in India has decreased by 2.6 million between 2001 and 2011. Despite the overall numbers trending in the right direction, progress must not stop now.

SOLUTIONS TO THE ISSUE OF CHILD LABOR IN INDIA

Addressing the issue of child labor in India requires a comprehensive approach involving various stakeholders.[9]

- *Strengthening legislative framework:* Enforce and strengthen existing laws, such as the Child Labour (Prohibition and Regulation) Act, to ensure comprehensive protection for children and stricter penalties for offenders. Timely amendments should align with international standards.
- *Access to quality education:* Ensure universal access to free and quality education for all children. Implement and enforce the Right to Education Act, focusing on reducing dropout rates and increasing enrollment in schools.
- *Poverty alleviation:* Tackle the root causes of child labor by implementing poverty alleviation programs, providing economic support to families living in poverty, and promoting livelihood opportunities for parents.
- *Awareness and sensitization:* Conduct widespread awareness campaigns targeting parents, communities, and employers about the detrimental effects of child labor on children's physical, mental, and educational development.
- *Rehabilitation and social protection:* Develop and implement comprehensive rehabilitation programs for rescued child laborers, including access to education, vocational training, healthcare, and psychological support. Establish social protection schemes for vulnerable families to prevent children from entering the labor force.
- *International cooperation:* Collaborate with international organizations, such as the International Labour Organization (ILO) and UNICEF, to access expertise, technical assistance, and financial resources to combat child labor effectively.
- *Empowering local communities:* Involve local communities, including parents, teachers, and community leaders, in preventing child labor. Empower them to identify and report cases of child labor and provide support for rehabilitation and reintegration efforts.

It is important to recognize that addressing child labor is a complex and multifaceted issue that requires sustained efforts, collaboration, and the commitment of all stakeholders to create lasting change.

AREAS TO EXPLORE FOR IMPROVEMENT IN ADOLESCENT WORKERS

Since, we cannot eliminate this problem, we can provide better conditions to adolescent workers.

- *Recreation at workplace:* If healthy environment with some outdoor sports activity is provided to young workers, that will improve their health and keep them away from antisocial company.
- *Separation from adult labor:* Employ them in division where same age-group workers work and keep them away from early exposure to adult habits.
- *Vaccination and regular health check-up:* Vaccination will protect them from many communicable diseases and regular health check-ups are of great help keeping them physically and mentally fit.

CONCLUSION

June 12 was declared by ILO as *World Day Against Child Labor* in 2002 aiming to prevent child labor. We all need to be active and vigilant to make India free of child labor.[3,4]

REFERENCES

1. Ministry of Labour & Employment, Government of India. (2023). About Child Labour. [online] Available from https://labour.gov.in/childlabour/about-child-labour [Last accessed December, 2024].
2. Verma S; iPleaders. (2019). Child Labour Laws in India. [online] Available from https://blog.ipleaders.in/child-labour-laws-in-india [Last accessed December, 2024].
3. International Labour Organization. Child Labour in India. [online] Available from https://www.ilo.org/sites/default/files/wcmsp5/groups/public/@asia/@ro-bangkok/@sro-new_delhi/documents/publication/wcms_557089.pdf [Last accessed December, 2024].

4. International Labour Organization. What is child labour. [online] Available from https://www.ilo.org/international-programme-elimination-child-labour-ipec/what-child-labour [Last accessed December, 2024].
5. Banerjee SR, Bharati P, Vasulu TS, Chakrabarty S, Banerjee P. Whole time domestic child labor in metropolitan city of Kolkata. Indian Pediatr. 2008;45(7):579-82.
6. Kim J, Olsen W. Harmful forms of child labour in India from a time-use perspective. Dev Pract. 2023;33(2):190–204.
7. Kaur N, Byard RW. Prevalence and potential consequences of child labour in India and the possible impact of COVID-19—a contemporary overview. Med Sci Law. 2021;61(3):208-14.
8. PIB Delhi. (2023). PENCIL portal being used for effective enforcement of Child and Adolescent Labour (Prohibition and Regulation) Act. [online] Available from https://pib.gov.in/PressReleseDetail.aspx?PRID=1909997®=3&lang=1 [Last accessed December, 2024].
9. The Borgen Project. (2019). 10 Facts About Child Labor in India. [online] Available from https://borgenproject.org/10-facts-about-child-labor-in-india/ [Last accessed December 2024].

22.13 Sexual Abuse and Protection of Children from Sexual Offences Act

Kiran Aggarwal

INTRODUCTION

World Health Organization (WHO) in 1999 formulated the "Consultation on Child Abuse Prevention", which defined child sexual abuse (CSA) as "the involvement of a child in sexual activity that he or she does not fully comprehend, is unable to give informed consent to, or for which the child is not developmentally prepared and cannot give consent, or that violates laws or social taboos of society".

The CSA is evidenced by the physical, verbal, visual, or online activity between a child and an adult or another child, who by age if the difference is >5 years could be exploitative or who by development is in relationship of responsibility, trust, or power, the activity being intended to gratify or satisfy the needs of the other person but there may be many cases where the offender is a total stranger.[1]

With reference to "Protection of Children from Sexual Offences" (POCSO) Act 2012, a medical professional plays a crucial role in the investigation and handling of cases involving CSA.[2,3]

EPIDEMIOLOGY

The CSA is a universal problem with grave life-long consequences; not a diagnosis or a syndrome with set features or outcomes; but its presentation varies widely based on several factors. The abuser can be of any age, gender, or socioeconomic status, a family member or stranger. Statistics suggest in 80–90% offenders are "known" to the victim. As reported widely, girls even aged 2 and 3 years have been abused by elderly, but even 13- or 14-year-old girls have abused their own classmates and other children. It may not necessarily be penetration but use of force, pain, or may be just touching.

The CSA may take place inside or outside homes, children left by their caregivers for baby-sitting can be the most vulnerable place to be at risk.

Boys are equally abused as girls, as reported worldwide, by an adult or an older child. They usually keep the act to themselves, under a feeling of guilt, may blame self; and as adults they may become abusive husbands, indulge in domestic violence or even may abuse own children to repeat the cycle of abuse.

Children or adolescents sexually abusing a child younger to them to experiment is also considered as CSA. But in such cases the older one (under 18 years) is tried as per Juvenile Justice Act (JJ Act) 2015 that gives complete innocence to a child under 7 years; and for those between 7 and 12 years the court has to assess the mental ability and intention of the child.[4]

Indian Scenario

Results of the National Child Abuse Study in 2007 by Ministry of Women and Child Development (MoWCD) uncovered the earlier total silence maintained on existence of CSA in India. Indian community was too confident of its own culture and joint family system, and thought children were well protected within the four walls of the home.[5] This study included 12,500 children across 13 states. More than half of the children (53%) said they were subjected to one or more forms of abuse

(52.94% were boys and 47.06% girls) indicating one in every two children was sexually abused. Age-wise distribution showed abuse started by 5 years, gained momentum 10 years onward, peaked at 12–15 years. In addition, 9 out of 13 states reported higher percentage of sexual abuse in boys as compared to girls.

The study also noted that children at work faced the highest risk. Of the total children interviewed 20.90% were subjected to severe form of CSA including sexual assault (57.30% were boys and 42.70% girls). It was also disturbing to note that children between 6 and 10 years faced severe form of sexual abuse. Assam, Delhi, Andhra Pradesh, and Bihar reported maximum sexual abuse.

In a self-reported CSA study on a sample of 452 medical students from a medical college in Puducherry, 148 (32.7%) reported one or other form of CSA in both sexes, most were abused at home or at a neighbor's home. Majority (60.1%) did not disclose CSA due to fear of negative consequences or feeling of guilt. Girls and boys equally suffered CSA.[6]

As per the reported data from the National Crime Record Bureau (NCRB) for the year 2022, 38,444 children were raped in the country. Age profile showed that half of them were aged between 16 and 18 years, one-tenth (11%) <12 years, and the rest were aged 12–16 years.[7]

The National Child Abuse Study, 2007 alerted the Government of India (GOI) to act upon and the POCSO Act was brought out as one of the recommendations of the study. Implementation of POCSO Act, 2012 gave courage and confidence to survivors and families for reporting.

ETIOPATHOGENESIS

What may be causing CSA in India?

- *The hesitancy in Indian culture about talking on sexuality:* This is especially true with children and adolescents, even the medical professionals find it difficult to talk about sexuality at ease.
- *Tolerating gender-based violence:* Indian patriarchal society believes firmly that certain things are inevitable to women and children if they cross the limit of moral values and rules applied on them.
- *Indian culture values adults over children:* Children are not viewed as fully developed citizens, their voice is not heard even on issues affecting them, their reasonings are considered disrespectful. If victimized, they may be silenced, and at times the act is considered as the child's fault.

Who may get abused?

Every child is a potential candidate for abuse unless proved otherwise, irrespective of the social, economic, religious, cultural, or educational background. Some children are at more risk than others **(Box 22.13.1)**.

BOX 22.13.1: Who is at higher risk of CSA?

- Special children
- Those questioning sexuality of his/her own being
- Those who come from low socioeconomic status due to lack of supervision
- Those with low self-esteem
- Children of prisoners
- Children who are isolated or have limited friends
- Children who come from broken homes, domestic violence, parent on drug, or alcohol addiction

BOX 22.13.2: Suspecting or warning signs of sexual abuse.

- Disclosure by the child, depending on developmental age
- Detection by pregnancy or sexually transmitted diseases (STDs)
- Sexualized behavior and poor personal hygiene
- Frequent urinary tract infections and injuries to private parts
- Blood-stained nappies in an infant, excessive cries, and feeding difficulties
- Signs and symptoms of isolation, depression, anxiety, and fearfulness
- Sudden onset of bedwetting and unexplained pains or aches
- Avoiding some particular person and place or fear of intimacy or closeness
- Sleep problems and change in eating habits
- Writes, draws, plays and/or dreams of sexual and/or frightening images
- Seems distracted or distant at odd times; suddenly has gifts and/or money
- Suicide attempt, self-harming, drug, and/or alcohol abuse

WARNING SIGNS OF SEXUAL ABUSE

The warning signs of sexual abuse are important as they help to suspect and identify the victims **(Box 22.13.2)**.

IMPORTANT TERMINOLOGIES

- *Incest:* The prohibited sexual relationship between close family members as between parent and child or brother and sister.
- *Commercial sexual exploitation of children (CSEC):* Trafficking of children for sex use, child prostitution, and CSA images
- *Child sex tourism:* Exploitation of children by an individual traveling from their home district/country with sexual intention of using children.
- *Pedophile:* A person with an inclination to exclusive sexual desires for prepubertal children (e.g., they may befriend with a single parent mother but actual target may be her preadolescent daughter).
- *Online sexual abuse/cyber-stalking*: Children feel helpless to exit from online abuse, abuser may contact them any time of day or night, may get sold online for the purpose of live sexual abuse online.

BOX 22.13.3: Why children do not like talking about abuse?

- Children fear that they may not be believed
- They may feel guilty that perhaps it is their fault that the abuse occurred
- Every time they are made to talk about the incident, they have to mentally revisit the situation and hence avoid recalling
- They may fear that the person who groomed/abused them may stop caring or may get into trouble because of them, in cases where the offender is a family member
- The child may have been manipulated to believe it is normal in their relationship, and may not realize being getting abused
- Fear of further abuse may force the child to maintain silence about the incident
- Generally, children are not encouraged to talk about their feelings; if they do so, they may not be listened to or believed
- Lack of verbal skills if the child is too young to communicate, and if abused as play or game, the child may not feel it as abuse

WHY DO CHILDREN NOT DISCLOSE ABUSE?

There can be several reasons why children do not disclose being sexually abused **(Box 22.13.3)**.

Time gap between the abuse and disclosure may vary widely depending on number of factors such as the age, gender, relationship with the abuser, severity of the act, developmental and cognitive abilities, and consequences of disclosure. Hence CSA remains mostly underreported, children may disclose, several years after the incident making the matter difficult to be investigated and dealt with.

HOW THE CHILDHOOD GETS AFFECTED

- *Childhood sexual abuse violates basic child rights:* They are not prepared developmentally for sexual activity, made to believe by grooming to feel it is normal as any other issues in their life
- *Adverse childhood experience (ACE)* disrupts the natural process of physical, sexual, and emotional development.
- *Children may not be ready for overt sexual stimulation.*

PREVENTION

The various levels of prevention include:

- *Primary prevention:* By change in environmental, social, and cultural norms to bring down vulnerability of children and adolescents
- *Secondary prevention:* Early detection/intervention of at risk children
- *Tertiary prevention:* Measures by legal action for treatment of repetition of offence, prevention of intergenerational CSA and restorative justice, and by knowledge, practice, and skills *on* sexuality by all stakeholders that children and adolescents come across during the process of growing up.

Role of Parents

- By providing age-appropriate information on development throughout infancy to adolescent life to children
- Starting educating children from early childhood about right names of private parts, how to keep them clean and safe, and to give child-appropriate expressive skills if inappropriately touched when child is made to learn about body parts.
- They must learn about sexuality. Assist children in growing up by talking at ease to make them learn about safe/unsafe touches, how to say no by life skills, and that "respect" means not "to blindly obey adults".

Role of Schools

- *By creating zero tolerance policy culture on child safety:* In the absence of timely teaching and appropriate knowledge, and also due to myths and ignorance around sexuality, children and adolescents remain uninformed and griped in silence about unsafe sex.
- *Law of the land:* Sex is a crime under 18 years under POCSO Act, adolescents to be warned of their responsibility on consensual sex.
- *At policy level:* Child protection cannot be ensured just by the legislations; formal guidelines are needed by bringing investment plan on child safety intervention in the system.
- *To work on boys:* They need protective shield/life skills/ rehabilitation.
- *Pedophilia awareness:* Keeping in mind prevalence of pedophilia of at least 1% in male population, more research is needed in India. Indicators suggest pedophiles can be reached before acting on their urges.

PROTECTION OF CHILDREN FROM SEXUAL OFFENCES ACT, 2012

The POCSO Act was enacted by GOI introduced by MoWCD and implemented on 14th November 2012 to provide strong legal framework for POCSO, safeguarding the best interest of child or adolescent at every step, by child-friendly mechanisms for reporting, recording of evidence, investigation, and speedy trial of offences through designated special courts. Offenders are brought to justice by giving graded punishment and shifting the burden of proof on accused.

PROVISIONS OF THE ACT

- Applicable to children and adolescents up to 18 years of age
- Gender neutral
- Provides protection from the offences of sexual assault, sexual harassment, and pornography.

- Consensual sexual act under 18 years among children or between a child and an adult is a crime and can be prosecuted irrespective of the consent.
- Mandatory reporting of any information on CSA by all, even by a child under section 19 of POCSO act.
- Police should not refuse first information report (FIR), even if it is a false complaint.
- Police should get medical examination performed within 24 hours of reporting, handover forensic material collection to forensic laboratory at the earliest.
- Police should inform Child Welfare Committee (CWC) within 24 hours of reporting of abuse.
- CWC if asked by police, should decide the place of safety for the survivor within 3 days of reporting to CWC.
- CWC to provide a support person for the child.
- Compensation provided for treatment support to the child at the earliest by the District Child Protection Unit (DCPU) or State Legal Service Authority (SLSA).

CHILD-FRIENDLY PROCEDURES

- Recording of statement of child should be done at the residence of the child, no repeated questioning.
- Recording should be done by a police officer not below rank of subinspector, preferably a lady.
- Police officer should not be in uniform.
- Child should not be detained at the police station in night.
- Child should not be in contact with the accused at any time of trial.
- Defense lawyer cannot directly cross-examine or question the child.

OFFENCES DEFINED UNDER THE ACT

- Penetrative sexual assault (Section 3)
- Aggravated penetrative sexual assault (Section 5)
- Sexual assault (Section 7)
- Aggravated sexual assault (Section 9)
- Sexual harassment of the child (Section 11)
- Use of child for pornographic purposes (Section 13)
- Abetment is treated with same gravity as commission of that offence (Section 16)
- Attempt to commit an offence is penalized, up to half the punishment for that offence (Section 18)

WHY IS THE POCSO ACT IMPORTANT FOR THE MEDICAL PROFESSIONALS?

- *Mandatory reporting* is done as specified under Section 19 of the POCSO Act; Section 21 provides punishment for failure to report or record a CSA.
- *Confidentiality and ethical issues:* While dealing with adolescent's healthcare, the physician may come across several medicolegal issues needing to deal with ethical aspects and confidentiality closely linked with JJ Act 2015 and POCSO Act.
- *Consequences of consensual sex:* Dealing with consensual sex in children <18 years, teen pregnancies and medical termination of pregnancy (MTP) are liable to get punished if not reported to police under POCSO Act 2012. MTP in a teen below 18 years requires signature of parents.
- *No requisition required for medical examination of a rape survivor:* FIR can be lodged after medical examination.
- *Emergency medical treatment not to be refused to any rape survivor:* Even in a case of refusal to medical examination, documentation is a must and it should be signed by the survivor and parent.
- *Consent:* It is an important component in dealing with examination of a rape survivor. Informed consent is separately needed for examination, collection of forensic material, treatment for prophylaxis of sexually transmitted diseases (STDs), human immunodeficiency virus (HIV) and hepatitis B, emergency pregnancy prophylaxis, for photography or any other procedure or examination. A child of 12 years can give consent for examination; below 12 years parent has to give consent. If there is no accompanying person, institutional head should depute a person to give consent.
- *Products of conception from all MTPs of rape survivor* need to go as forensic material collection for deoxyribonucleic acid (DNA) for paternity test.
- *Detailed history* obtained empathetically and in a subjective manner helps to know the extent of medical examination to be performed.
- *Medical examination* should be done in a separate room, in a child friendly manner, keeping dignity of the survivor, giving frequent breaks, and frequent questioning should be avoided. Two finger test not to be performed in a case of child or adolescents (as ruled by the Supreme Court).
- *All cases of sexual assault do not need examination of private parts,* negative findings do not rule out sexual assault.
- Survivors needs to be explained empathetically what is going to be done on them, what is the need for examination? What is expected from them? No instrumentation is to be done in children to examine the private parts and that it is not painful as the fear may be in child's mind.
- *Follow-up of the survivor* is as important as the medical examination and forensic material collection.
- *One stop center scheme:* It was established by MoWCD to provide support to women (and girls) affected by domestic and sexual violence in private and public spaces within the family, community, and workplace to provide medical examination, forensic material collection, and care at one location.

MEDICAL EXAMINATION OF THE SURVIVOR OF SEXUAL ASSAULT

Medical examination is conducted as per the provisions of Section 27 of the POCSO Act, 2012. In case of girl child, it should be done by a lady doctor, in the presence of parents/caregiver; in their absence a female attendant decided by head of the institution should be present. In case a female doctor is not available for the medical examination of a girl, a male doctor (registered medical practitioner) should conduct the examination in the presence of a female attendant.[8] Follow-up of the survivor is as important as the medical examination and forensic material collection.

AGE DETERMINATION

Age determination should be done (by all possible means), if the sexual offender is a person suspected to be under 18 years of age. The child/juvenile will be produced before the Juvenile Justice Board (JJB). JJB will follow all the guidelines given under JJ Act 2015 (revised in 2016).

PUNISHMENT

There is provision of graded punishment under the Act as per the severity of the crime.

IMPORTANT AMENDMENTS IN THE RAPE LAWS

No anticipatory bail can be granted to a person accused of rape of girls of age <16 years.[2,3] Death penalty is prescribed for persons involved in gang rape of a girl of age <12 years.[2,3]

CONCLUSION

Ministry of Health and Family Welfare (MOHFW), GOI in 2014 has brought out special "Guidelines and Protocols, Medico-legal Care for Survivors/Victims of Sexual Violence" with specific POCSO provisions with several clarifications.[8] This describes detailed relevant procedure on interviewing the child, obtaining the consent, medical examination, forensic material collection, prophylaxis, treatment/follow-up, and DOs and DONTs. in a child with suspected CSA.

REFERENCES

1. Seshadri S, Ramaswamy S. Clinical Practice Guidelines for Child Sexual Abuse. Indian J Psychiatry. 2019;61(Suppl 2):317-32.
2. Ministry of Law and Justice. (2019). The Protection of Children from Sexual Offences (Amendment) Act, 2019. [online] Available from https://missionvatsalya.wcd.gov.in/public/pdf/children-related-law/Protection%20of%20Children%20From%20Sexual%20Offences%20(Amendment)%20Act,%202019.pdf [Last accessed December, 2024].
3. The Gazette of India. (2020). The Protection of Children from Sexual Offences Rules, 2020. [online] Available from https://missionvatsalya.wcd.gov.in/public/pdf/children-related-law/POCSO%20Rules%202020.pdf [Last accessed December, 2024].
4. Indian Code. (2015). Juvenile Justice Act 2015 (Amended in 2016). [online] Available from https://www.indiacode.nic.in/handle/123456789/2148#:~:text=An%20Act%20to%20consolidate%20and,friendly%20approach%20in%20the%20adjudication [Last accessed December, 2024].
5. Government of India Ministry of Women and Child Development, 2007, "Study on Child Abuse: India 2007," Working Papers id: 955, eSocialSciences.
6. Rathinam RD, Singh A, Chopra M, Bharathi M, Mathiyalagen P, Bahurupi Y, et al. Spectrum of self-reported childhood sexual abuse among medical students: A single center experience. Indian Pediatr. 2021;58(6):564-67.
7. Government of India, National Crime Records Bureau (NCRB) Report on Crime in India; 2022.
8. Ministry of Health and Family Welfare (MOHFW). (2014). Guidelines & Protocols Medico-legal Care of Survivors/Victims of Sexual Violence. [online] Available from https://mohfw.gov.in/?q=reports/guidelines-and-protocols-medico-legal-care-survivors-victims-sexual-violence [Last accessed December, 2024].

22.14 Urban Slums and Street Children

Rajeev Seth

INTRODUCTION

According to the United Nations agency, UN-HABITAT, a slum is a run-down area of a city characterized by substandard housing, filthy, and lacking in tenure security.[1] The United Nations (UN) has defined slums as regions where individuals living under the same roof lack one or more of the following conditions—access to improved water, access to improved sanitation, sufficient living area, housing durability, and security of tenure. Slums are usually located in urban areas, consisting of densely packed household structures of weak quality. Most slums originate due to rapid rural to urban migration, poverty, high unemployment, informal economy, poor urban resettlement planning, natural disasters, climate change, and results of communal violence, conflict, and wars.[2] World Cities Report 2022—Envisaging the Future of Cities said that the global urban population was back on track post COVID to grow by another 2.2 billion people by 2050.[3] There is a broad consensus that urbanization remains a powerful 21st century mega-trend. Under such a scenario, one of the most important public health concerns is whether our children can inherit an urban future that is more inclusive, safer, and healthier?

The United Nations Convention on the Rights of the Child (UNCRC) is the most widely accepted human rights treaty that recognizes the civil, political, economic, social, and cultural rights of children.[4] In 2017, the UNCRC, via General Comment 21 defined children in street situations (CiSS) as *"children who depend on the streets to live and/or work, whether alone, with peers or with family"* as well as *"a wider population of children who have formed strong connections with public spaces and for whom the street plays a vital role in their everyday lives and identities"*. The UN General Comment 21 provides authoritative guidance to States on developing comprehensive, long-term national strategies on CiSS.[5] The National Commission for Protection of Child Rights (NCPCR), a statutory body of Government of India (GOI) is mandated to ensure that all laws, policies, programs, and administrative mechanisms are in consonance with the child rights perspective, as enshrined in the Constitution of India and also the UNCRC.[6]

Millions of largely invisible children worldwide live in urban slums or work on the streets to escape poverty, domestic abuse, conflict, and trafficking. The issue of street children is a national and global crisis, and far from limited to low-income and middle-income countries (LMICs). It is extremely important to increase the visibility of the issue of street children and develop a rights-based framework for optimizing their health, development, and wellbeing in the medical curriculum.

The *aims and objectives* of this chapter are:

- To understand the health, wellbeing, and rights concerns of street children in Indian slum situations
- To understand how doctors, allied medical professionals, students, and civil society activists can provide access to healthcare, nutrition, development, and protection to the marginalized street children.

EPIDEMIOLOGY

We see street children everywhere, inside railway stations, markets, roadsides, runaways, flower sellers on traffic lights, shoe shiners, tea carriers, rag pickers, and vendors of trinkets and plastic toys. And sometimes we don't see them at all—they are confined to factories, back-room bars, or inside tarpaulin-covered huts. The UN estimates that 150 million children live in street situations worldwide, perhaps 20% of them in India alone, but this estimate remains highly uncertain. Counting CiSS is complicated. Street and working children often do not have a birth certificate to confirm their age or identity. Without legal status, they drop off official statistics. It is also not uncommon for street and working children to avoid legal authorities, frightened of the repercussions.

Many times we pass by these street children in our daily lives, and often we choose to keep them invisible, we look past them, and say nothing. But what if we realize that silence is violence? What if we heed their voices and listen to their stories and see them for the dignified and potential-filled personalities that they are? Despite India being a signatory to the UNCRC in 1992, the life of street children is a violation of basic human rights such as education, health, nutrition, development, and protection.

The Indian Child Abuse Neglect and Child Labour (ICANCL) group of Indian Academy of Pediatrics (IAP) (www.icancl.org) has been working for over 25 years to realize rights and wellbeing of street and working children, which have had poor visibility in healthcare and research. Along with the International Society for Social Pediatrics and Child Health (ISSOP, www.issop.org), the ICANCL group and allied partners formulated a call to action declaration on *"Optimizing the Health, Wellbeing, and Rights of Street and Working Children"* at the International Pediatric association (IPA, www.ipa-world.org) and IAP (www.iapindia.org) PEDICON conference held at Gandhinagar, India in February 2023. Applauding this call, the Lancet Child & Adolescent Health, published an editorial to "Advancing *the rights of street and working children"*. In closing, the Lancet editorial stated that *"we urge governments and international agencies to advance the rights of street and working children, and to engage pediatricians as key partners in this work. Pediatricians must have a seat at the table and hold governments accountable for their obligations to all children.*[7]

ETIOPATHOGENESIS

The etiopathogenesis of health issues in urban slums and among street children is multifaceted and influenced by a variety of interconnected factors:[5]

- *Socioeconomic factors:* Poverty is a fundamental driver of health disparities in the lives of street children.
- *Violence:* Many street children are runaway youths from their families after experiencing intimate partner violence (domestic violence), child physical abuse such as frequent corporal punishment, exploitation as child laborer, sexual exploitation, and emotional abuse.
- *Social determinants of health:* Social factors such as discrimination, social isolation, and lack of community support can adversely affect the mental and emotional well-being of slum dwellers.
- *Mental health challenges:* Street children often face huge adversities and traumatic experiences. Such adverse childhood experiences (ACE) for a long-time lead to toxic stress, epigenetic changes which cause development of adult onset diseases such as hypertension, coronary artery disease (CAD), diabetes mellitus, substance misuse, posttraumatic stress disorder (PTSD), and depression.
- *Limited healthcare access:* Urban slum residents, including street children may have restricted access to healthcare services. They incur huge out of pocket expenditure on healthcare which can exacerbate their poverty. Many street children start smoking; take drugs and alcohol which can exacerbate their health challenges.

CLINICAL FEATURES

The clinical features observed in these populations reflect a combination of infectious, nutritional, and environmental health issues. It is important to have the knowledge of social determinants of health, child protection systems, and experience of working with a multidisciplinary professional approach. Here are some key clinical features specific to the health conditions in street children:

- *Infectious diseases:* Urban slums in India often experience a higher burden of infectious diseases, including respiratory infections (e.g., tuberculosis and pneumonia), waterborne diseases (e.g., cholera and typhoid), and vector-borne diseases (e.g., malaria and dengue).
- *Malnutrition:* Malnutrition is prevalent in urban slums, leading to stunted growth, underweight children, and deficiencies in key micronutrient deficiencies such as iron, vitamin A, and iodine.
- *Maternal and child health issues:* Insufficient prenatal care, inadequate nutrition during pregnancy, and limited access to family planning services contribute to maternal and child health challenges, including low birthweight and neonatal complications.
- *Noncommunicable diseases (NCDs):* As a result of ACEs, including abnormal lifestyles and dietary habits in urban slums, there is an emerging burden of NCDs such as diabetes, hypertension, substance misuse, depression, and PTSD in street children.
- *Respiratory issues:* Poor air quality resulting from industrial pollution, high temperatures, and household cooking practices can contribute to respiratory problems, including chronic obstructive pulmonary disease (COPD), tuberculosis, and asthma.
- *Vector-borne diseases:* Inadequate sanitation and water storage practices in slums create breeding grounds for disease vectors, increasing the risk of diseases such as dengue and malaria.
- *Trauma and injuries:* Overcrowded living conditions and inadequate infrastructure contribute to accidents and injuries, leading to trauma-related health issues.
- *Mental health challenges:* Urban slum residents may face mental health issues due to poverty, social stressors, and limited access to mental health services.
- *Reproductive health issues:* Sexual abuse, including commercial sexual exploitation is common both in boys and girls. Street-based girls may be at risk of sexually transmitted diseases (STDs), early pregnancies, and complications associated with inadequate prenatal care and unsafe childbirth practices.
- *Street children with special needs or neurodisabilities:* Street children with neurodisabilities get further marginalized, and remain most vulnerable, as they need a disability certificate, pension, and are deprived of poor access to multidisciplinary interventions.

DIFFERENTIAL DIAGNOSIS

Children in street situation present in different circumstances. Defining and identifying CiSS appropriately are crucial to provide them with different sets of interventions and services, as per their circumstances and vulnerabilities. For example, those with parents/guardians on the streets will need a different approach and those who have no contact with families or are abandoned or orphans will require a diverse approach and a distinct set of services. The NCPCR SOP 2.0 prescribes various measures/steps to be taken to provide care and protection to the CiSS, there will always be a possibility and need for a customized solution depending on the situation.[8] For proper understanding and need for interventions, the (CiSS) may be categorized under three broad types as follows:

1. *Children without support living on the streets all alone:* These are children without any parental anchor or family support system living on the streets, pavements, or any public places on their own. For them, the street is the home. Examples are missing, runaway, abandoned, and orphan children. They survive on streets by working, begging, selling items/goods, performing on streets, or adopting any other means.
2. *Children stay on the streets in the day and are back home at night with their families who reside in a nearby slum/hutments:* These are children who spend their time on the street, loitering in the daytime. These children may be found simply loitering, begging, picking rags, or selling goods/items.
3. *Children living on the streets with their families:* These are children living with their families on the streets. They are from different parts of the country and have migrated to the city to earn their subsistence. They mostly work in the unorganized sector, such as temporary labor in construction. These families include seasonal as well as permanent migrants.

DIAGNOSIS

In the context of urban slums and street children in India, taking thorough history and understanding the social determinants of health is extremely important in order to differentiate the specific challenges and needs of street children. The medical doctors and allied health professionals need to work through a multidisciplinary approach. Diagnosing health issues in urban slums and among street children in India requires a comprehensive approach that includes clinical assessment, laboratory investigations, and approaches as taught in medical colleges. However, a basic knowledge of child protection systems such as State Commission for the Protection of Child Rights (SCPCR), Child Welfare Committee (CWC), access to local Police station, CHILDLINE 1098, District Child Protection Officers, legal systems, and allied government agencies is needed.

The Juvenile Justice Act (JJ) Act 2015 is the fundamental law dealing with Children in Need & Care & Protection (CNCP). It caters to the needs of CiSS through care, protection, development, treatment, and social reintegration, by adopting a child-friendly approach in the adjudication and disposal of matters in the best interests of children. In the context of Sustainable Development Goals (SDGs), goals like "No Poverty" (SDG No. 1), "Zero Hunger" (SDG No.2), "Good Health and Well Being" (SDG No. 3), "Quality Education" (SDG No. 4), and "Clean Water and Sanitation" (SDG No. 6) have to be addressed. The CiSS is a socioeconomic and legal issue that is getting worse day by day due to lack of appropriate and effective implementation of legal measures and social interventions.[6]

MANAGEMENT

A life on the street constitutes one of the most serious violations of the rights of children—violating their right to education, good health, nutritious food, play, protection, and proper development. The CiSS are a subset of vulnerable and working children. A major category of such children come under children in need of care and protection (CNCP), defined under the Juvenile Justice (Care and Protection of Children) Act, 2015 (hereafter, JJ Act).

The NCPCR "Standard Operating Procedure for Care and Protection of CiSS 2.0" is an endeavor to strengthen the processes and interventions regarding CiSS in the view that there should not be any child in a street situation; rather, they should be with their families. In case the family needs support, it may be provided keeping in mind the best interests of the child. The institutionalization of these children should be assumed as the last resort.[6]

Standard Operating Procedures (SOPs) to be Followed to Ensure Care and Protection of CiSS (Flowchart 22.14.1)

The spirit of the Juvenile Justice Act (JJ Act) is to bring all children needing care and protection into its ambit. The CWC is the focal authority to take decisions on children needing care and protection under the purview of the Act. Therefore, effort should be made to produce all children who need care and protection before the CWC. Once a child is brought into this child protection mechanism, the child can get opportunities to lead a better life.

Production of Child before the Child Welfare Committee

The principle adopted and reflected in JJ Act, 2015, that any child/children who needs care and protection is to be produced before the CWC, is established under Section 27

Flowchart 22.14.1: Possible scenario when a child is produced before the Child Welfare Committee.[6]

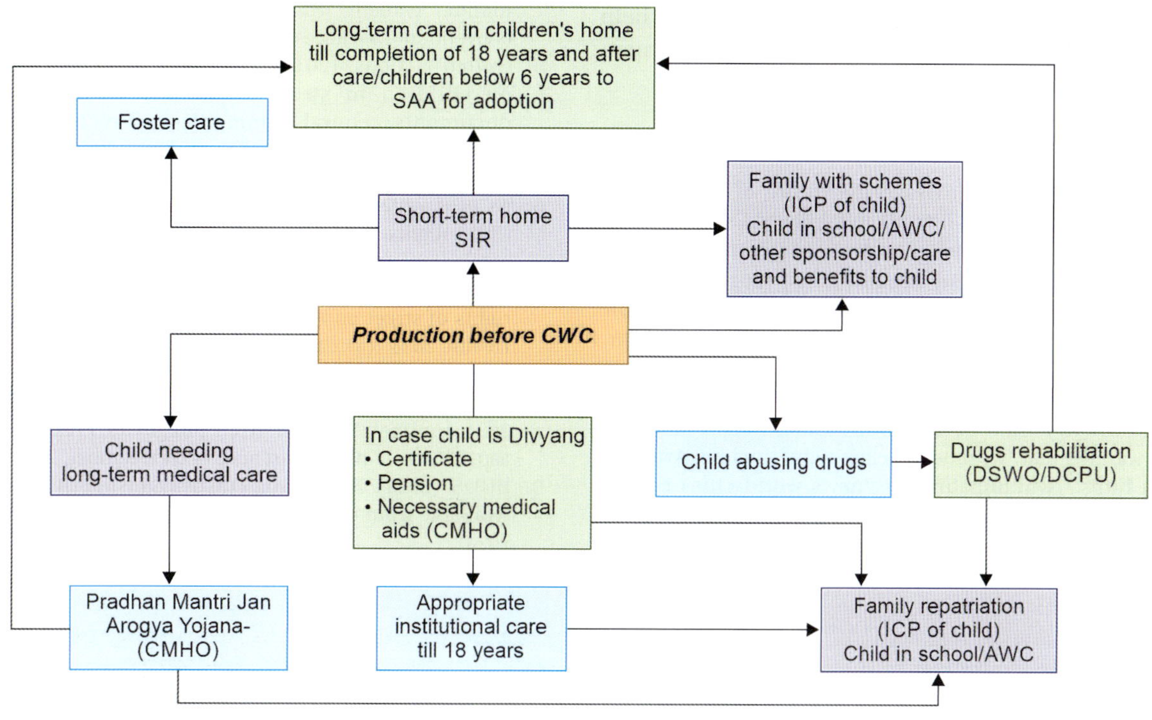

of the Act. It may be noted that under the juvenile justice system, there are two categories of children, namely, children in conflict with law (CICL) and CNCP, to be dealt by the Juvenile Justice Board (JJB) and CWC.[9]

Bal Umang Drishya Sanstha Model

Bal Umang Drishya Sanstha (BUDS) is a nonprofit organization, working with marginalized children and youth. BUDS was established as an Indian Not for Profit Trust 2003, with the country office located in New Delhi, India. Along with a group of pediatricians, doctors, and allied multidisciplinary professionals, BUDS leads *"to provide access to health to street children and marginalized youth through mobile health van (MHV) and drop in center (DIC) model"* to keep children and youth in safe spaces.[9] BUDS currently operates 17 DICs for marginalized children and youth in 4 states of India. DIC offers a safe day care space for children and youth living in urban slums and in marginalized villages, where they are provided free mid-day meals, remedial education, and counseling and health services in a youth friendly environment. The DICs are linked to a dedicated MHV, where the children and youth are provided access to free primary health care and referral services for secondary and tertiary care. BUDS successful strategic initiative of providing access to healthcare, education, development, and comprehensive welfare to marginalized street children in urban slums and rural poor has been included in the youth policy constructed by the GOI, Ministry of Youth Affairs and Sports (MYAS).

CONCLUSION

The state of marginalized street children and youth is a major violation of their human rights and is a huge public health problem. Like any other person, street children and youth from the underprivileged communities have dreams and talents, but they are being left behind. They are discriminated against, stigmatized, and deprived of the most basic rights to health, education, nutrition, play, and protection—in grave violation of the UNCRC. The GOI revised youth policy presented to the G20 nations and has endeavored to address this social injustice.

Pediatricians, doctors, and allied health professionals should obtain experience in this field by volunteering their time with public health institutions, such as ICDS centers *(Anganwadi),* underprivileged schools, childcare institutions (CCI), and local nonprofit organizations. On a local scale, government child protection systems can make a difference by engaging with local NGOs and bringing trauma informed care (TIC) outreach to the marginalized. The MHV clinics and DIC offer an innovative community strategic approach to reach out to provide care to the vulnerable children and youth in street-based situations. The voices and success stories of the youth are truly inspirational case examples, which can help revise and develop regional, state, and national government policies and strengthen their youth welfare systems.

REFERENCES

1. UN Habitat. (2022). Envisage the future of Cities 2022. [online] Available from https://unhabitat.org/sites/default/files/2022/06/wcr_2022.pdf [Last accessed December, 2024].
2. Ministry of Housing and Urban Affairs. (2024). Slums in India. A statistical compendium 2015. [online] Available from http://nbo.gov.in/pdf/SLUMS_IN_INDIA_Slum_Compendium_2015_English.pdf [Last accessed December, 2024].
3. World Urban Forum. (2023). World Cities Report launched with warning that "we must get cities right". [online] Available from https://wuf.unhabitat.org/news/world-cities-report-launched-warning-we-must-get-cities-right [Last accessed December, 2023].
4. UNICEF. (2024). Convention on the Rights of the Child. [online] Available from https://www.unicef.org/child-rights-convention [Last accessed December, 2024].
5. United Nations. (2017). General comment No. 21 (2017) on children in street situations. www.ohchr.org/en/documents/general-comments-and-recommendations/general-comment-no-21-2017-children-street [Last accessed December, 2024].
6. NCPCR. (2024). National Commission for the Protection of Child Rights (NCPCR). [online] Available from www.ncpcr.gov.in [Last accessed December, 2024].
7. The Lancet Child Adolescent Health. Editorial. Advancing the rights of street and working children. Lancet Child Adolesc Health. 2023;7(4):223.
8. Ministry of Women and Child Development. (2021). Juvenile Justice (Care & Protection of Children), Amended Act 2021. [online] Available from pib.gov.in/PressReleasePage.aspx?PRID=1740011 [Last accessed December, 2024].
9. BUDS. (2024). Bal Umang Drishya Sanstha (BUDS). [online] Available from www.budsngo.org [Last accessed December, 2024].

SECTION

23

Pediatric Procedures

Section Editor: Baldev S Prajapati

23.1 Safe Injection Practices

S Sachidananda Kamath, Jaydeep Choudhury

INTRODUCTION

Safe injection practice means that it does no harm to the recipient, does not expose the health worker to any avoidable risks, and does not result in waste that is dangerous to the community.[1] The concept of safe injection has gained much importance in recent years in view of the increased incidence of various blood-borne infections.

According to World Health Organization (WHO), >12 billion injections are administered each year all over the world. Thus, injections are one of the most common healthcare procedures practiced all over the world. Of the vast majority of injections, about 95% are given as curative.[2] Many of these "curative" injections may be unnecessary, ineffective, or inappropriate. Immunization accounts for around 3% of all injections. It is estimated that at least 50% of this are unsafe, posing serious health risks to recipients, health workers, and the public.[1] Reducing unnecessary injections is one way to improve the safety of injections.

Patients sometimes tend to prefer injections because they believe them to be stronger and faster medications. They also nurture a belief that doctors regard injections to be the best treatment. In turn, doctors overprescribe injections. These misconception and misunderstanding can be avoided to a large extent. The doctors have to lead better communication between patients and providers can clarify these issues.

Unsafe injection practices are a powerful engine to transmit blood-borne pathogens, including hepatitis B virus (HBV), hepatitis C virus (HCV), and human immunodeficiency virus (HIV).[3,4] Because infection with these viruses initially presents no symptoms, it is a silent epidemic. However, the consequences of this are increasingly recognized.

- *Hepatitis B virus:* HBV is highly infectious and causes the highest number of infections in developing and transitional countries. About 23.1 million people become infected each year, representing 33% of new HBV infections worldwide.
- *Hepatitis C virus:* Unsafe injections are the most common cause of HCV infection in developing and transitional countries, causing 2 million new infections each year and accounting for 42% of cases.[3,4]
- *Human immunodeficiency virus:* Globally, nearly 2% of all new HIV infections are caused by unsafe injections.

In South Asia, up to 9% of new cases may be caused in this way. Such proportions can no longer be ignored.

Hepatitis B virus, HCV, and HIV cause chronic infections that lead to disease, disability, and death a number of years after the unsafe injection. Those infected with HBV in childhood will typically present with chronic liver disease by the age of 30 years, at the prime of their life. This has a dramatic effect on national economies.

CONDITIONS CAUSING RISK: STEPS RELATED TO INJECTION GIVING

Unsafe injection practices are often viewed as a chronic problem with no easy solution. However, safe and appropriate use of injections can be achieved by adopting a three-part strategy.

Changing Behavior of Healthcare Workers and Patients

30 years into the HIV pandemic, knowledge of HIV among patients and healthcare workers (HCWs) in some countries has driven consumer demand for safe injection equipment and irreversibly improved injection practices. With growing knowledge of HCV and HBV, similar patterns of consumer demand for safe injections should emerge. HIV prevention programs can be expanded to include injection safety components.

Ensuring Availability of Equipment and Supplies

Simply increasing the availability of safe injection equipment can stimulate demand and improve practices. Because the cost of safe disposable syringes is low (about INR 2–5 per unit), patients are usually compliant to pay for safety once they personalize the risks.

Managing Waste Safely and Appropriately

As waste disposal is frequently not an integral part of health planning, unsafe waste management is common. However, when it is appropriately planned, significant results ensue.[5] National healthcare waste management strategies require a national policy to manage healthcare waste, a comprehensive system for implementation, improved awareness, and training of health workers at all levels, as well as the selection of appropriate options for the local solutions.[1]

Specifics of Safe Injection Practices

Medical treatment is intended to save life and improve health, and all health workers have a responsibility to prevent transmission of healthcare-associated infections. Adherence to safe injection practices and related infection control is part of that responsibility—it protects patients and health workers **(Table 23.1.1)**.[1]

Injection is defined as a skin piercing event performed by a syringe and a needle to introduce a vaccine or a curative substance into a patient by various routes such as intravenous (IV), intramuscular (IM), subcutaneous (SC), intradermal (ID), etc.

What is a Safe Injection?

A safe injection, phlebotomy (drawing blood), lancet procedure, or IV device insertion is one that:[6,7]

- Does not harm the recipient.
- Does not expose the provider to any avoidable risk.
- Does not result in any waste that is dangerous for other people.

TABLE 23.1.1: Things to be kept in mind for patients and health workers.

Patients or clients	*Health workers who give injections or collect blood*	*Community or other health workers*
• Unnecessary injections • Reuse of injection equipment • Nonsterile or reprocessed syringes and needles • Poor hand hygiene • Cross-contamination through: – Poor hand hygiene – Medication vials • Improper injection technique or site • Sharps in hospital linen or other unexpected places	• Unnecessary injections • Two-handed recapping of needles • Manipulation of used sharps • Lack of sharps box within arm's reach • Poor positioning of patient • Poor phlebotomy technique • Two-handed transfer of blood • Unsafe transport of blood • Poor hand hygiene • Nonsegregated sharps waste	• Increased waste from unnecessary injections • Unsafe disposal of sharps waste: – Outside safety boxes – Mixed with hospital linen – In nonsecure disposal sites • Lack of protective clothing (boots, gloves, etc.) for waste handlers • Reuse of needles or syringes

Do's and Don'ts of Injection Safety[6,7]

- Do carry out hand hygiene (use soap and water or alcohol rub), and wash carefully, including wrists and spaces between the fingers, for at least 30 seconds.
- Do use one pair of nonsterile gloves per procedure or patient.
- Do use a single-use device for blood sampling and drawing.
- Do disinfect the skin at the venipuncture site.
- Do discard the used device (a needle and syringe is a single unit) immediately into a robust sharps container where recapping of a needle is unavoidable. Do use the one-hand scoop technique.
- Do seal the sharps container with a tamper-proof lid.
- Do place laboratory sample tubes in a sturdy rack before injecting into the rubber stopper.
- Do immediately report any incident or accident linked to a needle or sharp injury, and seek assistance; start postexposure prophylaxis (PEP) as soon as possible, following protocols.
- Do not forget to clean your hands.
- Do not use the same pair of gloves for more than one patient.
- Do not wash gloves for reuse.
- Do not use a syringe, needle, or lancet for more than one patient.
- Do not recap a needle using both hands.
- Do not touch the puncture site after disinfecting it.
- Do not leave an unprotected needle lying outside the sharps container.
- Do not overfill or decant a sharps container.
- Do not inject into a laboratory tube while holding it with the other hand.
- Do not delay PEP after exposure to potentially contaminated material; beyond 72 hours, PEP is not effective.

The essential steps for safe injection practices are:

- Clean workspace for injection preparations (free from any blood contamination).
- Appropriately done hand hygiene (described further). Hand hygiene is a general term that applies to hand washing, antiseptic hand wash, antiseptic hand rub, or surgical hand antisepsis. It is the best and easiest way to prevent the spread of microorganisms.

  Hand hygiene should be carried out as indicated in **Figure 23.1.1**, either with soap and running water (if hands are visibly soiled) or with alcohol rub (if hands appear clean).

Practical Guidance on Hand Hygiene[6,7]

Perform Hand Hygiene Before

- Starting an injection session (i.e., preparing injection material and giving injections)

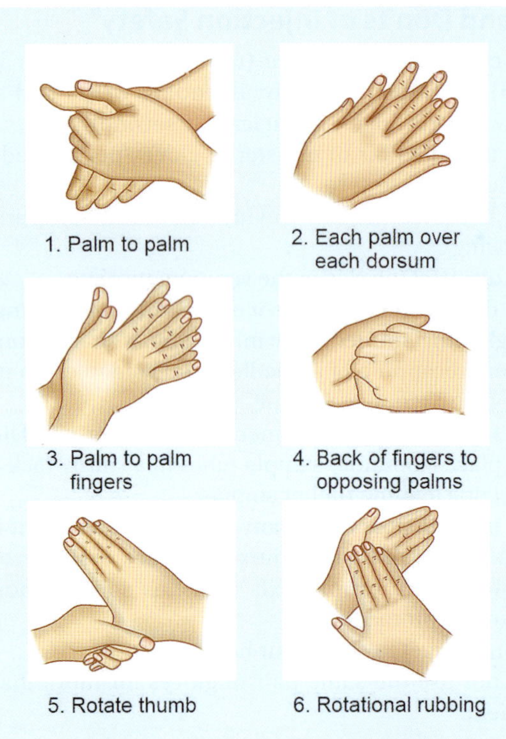

Fig. 23.1.1: Six steps of hand washing.

- Coming into direct contact with patients for healthcare-related procedures
- Putting on gloves (first make sure hands are dry)

Perform Hand Hygiene After

- An injection session
- Any direct contact with patients
- Removing gloves. You may need to perform hand hygiene between injections, depending on the setting and whether there was contact with soil, blood, or body fluids. Avoid giving injections if your skin integrity is compromised by local infection or other skin conditions (e.g., weeping dermatitis, skin lesions, or cuts), and cover any small cuts.

Injection Site Preparation

- Apply a 60–70% alcohol-based solution (isopropyl alcohol or ethanol) on a single-use swab or cotton-wool ball. Do not use methanol or methyl alcohol, as these are not safe for human use.
- Wipe the area from the center of the injection site working outward, without going over the same area.
- Apply the solution for 30 seconds then allow it to dry completely.

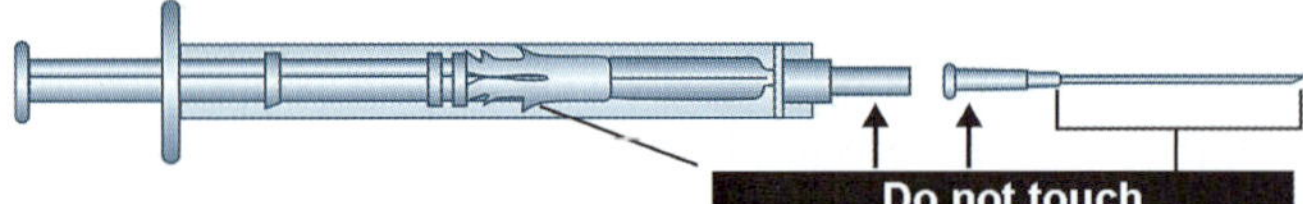

Fig. 23.1.2: Prevention of contamination of injection equipment.

- Do not presoak cotton wool in a container—these become highly contaminated with hand and environmental bacteria.
- Do not use alcohol skin disinfection for administration of vaccinations.

Preventing Injection Equipment from Contamination

- Contamination of injection equipment should be prevented by not touching certain parts as shown in **Figure 23.1.2**.
- The used needles and syringes should be disposed as per biomedical waste management (BWM) rules.

RATIONAL INJECTION THERAPY

People may have different perceptions and meanings regarding the term "rational drug use". However, the conference of experts on the rational use of drugs, convened by the WHO in Nairobi in 1985 defined that "rational use of drugs requires that patients receive medications appropriate to their clinical needs, in doses that meet their own individual requirements for an adequate period of time, at the lowest cost to them and their community".[6,7]

A review of essential drug lists and management guidelines of common illnesses show that injections are recommended only for acute care (emergency setting) and immunization. The reasons given for injection over use are that patients and health workers believe injections are more effective, act fast, and course of management is short.[1]

These are wrong notions. There is need to promote rational injection therapy among all prescribers. It can be achieved through following steps:

- Defining effective and safe protocols
- Promoting minimal essential injection practices
- Promoting rational drug/injection therapy
- Reduction in procurement of injectable drugs at health facilities
- Encouraging prescription auditing at all health facilities, public as well as private sectors
- Continuing medical education for health workers[1]
- Community awareness regarding harmful effects of injections

BEST INJECTION TECHNIQUES[8]

General Principles

- Give injections only when indicated.
- Emergency equipment should be kept ready to use in emergency situations such as anaphylactic reactions—oxygen bag and mask, laryngoscope and endotracheal tubes, as well as emergency drugs such as adrenaline, volume expanders, hydrocortisone, and dopamine should be available. IV cannula, syringes, and needles are also essential.
- Check the appropriate drug or vaccine and its date.
- Make sure that vial or ampoule contains right medication, its appropriate concentration, and doses.
- The drug or vaccine should be kept sterile during the procedure.
- Clean the injection site properly.
- Use disposable or sterile needle and syringe, preferable with reuse prevention feature.
- Do not touch the parts of needle and syringe in which come in contact with injectable drug and body.
- If you accidentally touch these parts, discard the syringe-needle.
- Take care to avoid air bubble in the syringe or bulb.
- While injecting take care to prevent needle stick injury (NSI) (report immediately if you get injured—this is for your own safety).
- Used needles and syringes should be disposed as per standard guidelines.
- Observe the child for 15 minutes, after giving injection.
- Talk to the parents regarding drug or vaccine given by injection, necessary precautions, possible adverse reactions, and necessary remedial measures in case of adverse reactions.
- Guide them to give information to medical person in case of major problems.

Important Points

- Do not allow the needle to touch any contaminated surface.
- Do not reuse a syringe, even if the needle is changed.
- Do not touch the diaphragm after disinfection with the 60–70% alcohol (isopropyl alcohol or ethanol).
- Do not enter several multidose vials with the same needle and syringe.
- Do not re-enter a vial with a needle or syringe used on a patient if that vial will be used to withdraw medication again (whether it is for the same patient or for another patient).
- Do not use bags or bottles of IV solution as a common source of supply for multiple patients (except in pharmacies using laminar flow cabinets).

INTRAMUSCULAR INJECTION

Common Sites

Muscles commonly used for IM injections are:

- Vastus lateralis
- Deltoid
- Gluteus medius

Children do not have well-developed gluteus medius and therefore injections should not be given in gluteal region.

The vastus lateralis (anterolateral aspect of thigh) is preferred site in infants. The specific site in vastus lateralis is the middle third of the area between the greater trochanter and lateral femoral condyle.

In case of deltoid, the site for injection is midway between acromion process and deltoid insertion; it comes to 3–5 cm below the acromion process. This site may be used in children above 5 years and adults. The quantity of drug should be <5 mL. Only watery injections with less viscosity should be injected at deltoid region.

Technique (World Health Organization Technique)

- The site of injection should be exposed well.
- For anterolateral aspect of thigh, the child may be laid supine or be held in mother's lap.
- For deltoid, child may be held in mother's lap or may sit.
- The muscle selected for injection should be relaxed.
- The skin over injection site should be cleaned with spirit. A circular motion of swab is used proceeding from puncture site and extending outward for 5 cm.
- Let the spirit evaporate and skin become dry, otherwise spirit entering into tissues is painful.
- The syringe is filled with the medicine.
- In children, usually 23G needle with 25 mm length is used for IM injections.
- Stretch the skin flat and push the needle down at 90° **(Figs. 23.1.3 and 23.1.4)**
- Aspiration before injecting the vaccine is not required.
- Inject the vaccine at the rate of 1 mL per 10 seconds.
- The needle is withdrawn and injection site is pressed for few seconds.
- Do not rub the injection site.
- Needle should be withdrawn smoothly with steady movement.
- Discard the needle and syringe as per standard guidelines. Alternative to WHO technique, Advisory Committee on Immunization Practices (ACIP) technique may be used. It is also called bunching technique. In this technique, bunch the muscle and direct needle inferiorly along long axis of leg at an angle of 45°. It stabilizes leg and increases the muscle mass.

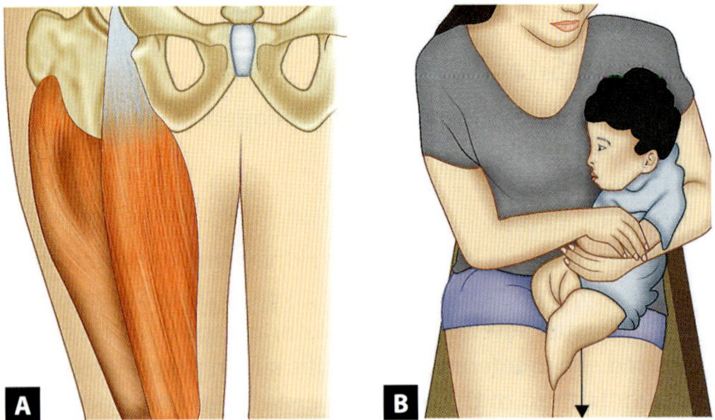

Figs. 23.1.3A and B: Positioning of the child for intramuscular (IM) injection (vastus lateralis).

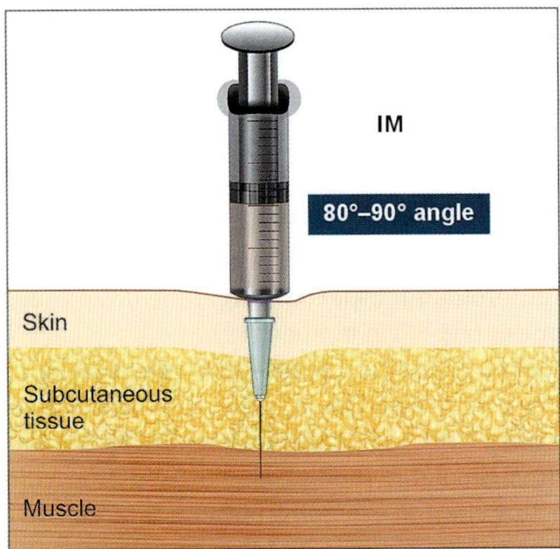

Fig. 23.1.4: Technique for intramuscular (IM) injection.

SUBCUTANEOUS INJECTION

Drugs or vaccines are injected subcutaneously when slow absorption and long duration of action are desired. Another indication of SC route is a coagulopathy, which makes IM injection hazardous, for fear of development of IM hematoma. Insulin and heparin-like drugs as well as measles, varicella, measles, mumps, and rubella (MMR), etc., vaccines are given by SC route.

Technique

- Common sites are arm, thigh, or sometimes anterior abdominal wall. Atrophic and injected areas should be avoided.
- The skin is cleaned and disinfected with spirit.
- 26-G needle with 13-mm length is commonly used for SC injection.

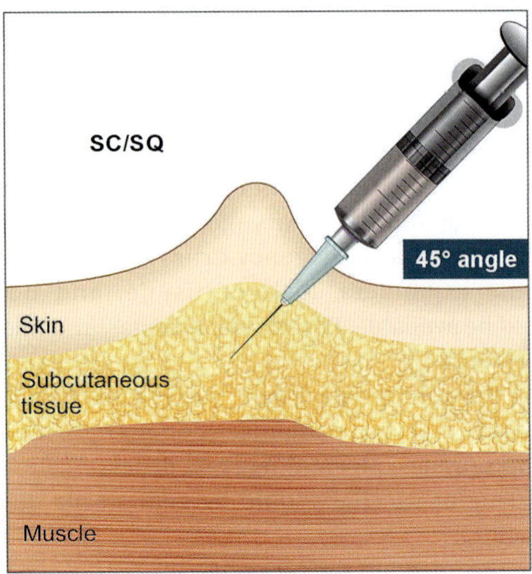

Fig. 23.1.5: Technique for subcutaneous (SC/SQ) injection.

- The skin is raised into a fold with thumb and index finger of the left hand **(Fig. 23.1.5)**.
- The midpoint of the fold is pierced with the needle held at 45° with its surface.
- The tip of the needle is advanced into the SC tissue.
- Aspiration is not required.
- Drugs or vaccine is injected; needle is withdrawn and site is pressed for few minutes.

INTRADERMAL INJECTION

Indications for ID injections are:

- Bacillus Calmette-Guérin (BCG) vaccination
- Rabies vaccine
- Mantoux test
- Skin tests for allergy
- Test for sensitization of certain drugs such as penicillin

Technique

- Ventral (volar) aspect of forearm is commonly used for ID injection.
- Skin is cleaned with spirit or clean water.
- A measured amount of antigen (usually 0.1 mL) is drawn into the syringe.
- 26 or 27-G needle with 1/4–1/2 inch (6.35–12.7 mm) length needle is used for ID injection.
- The skin is held taut between thumb and index finger of the left hand. The syringe is held at an angle of 10–15° with the skin.
- Needle is inserted for about 2 mm, so that entire needle bevel penetrates the skin and the injected solution raises a small bleb of about 5 mm in diameter. The development

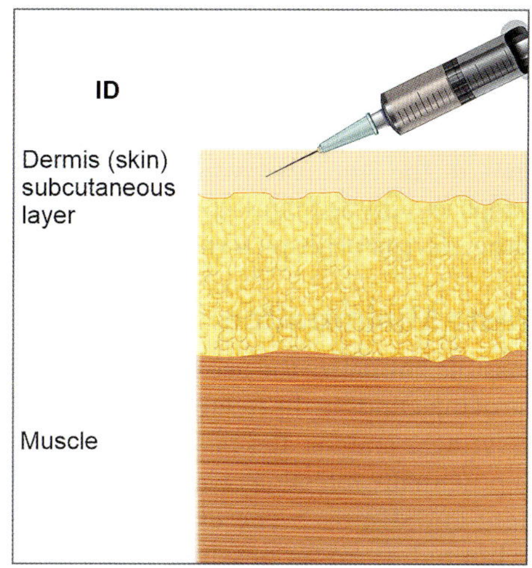

Fig. 23.1.6: Technique for intradermal (ID) injection.

of perifollicular puckering (Peau d'orange) indicates successful ID injection **(Fig. 23.1.6)**.

- The needle is withdrawn.
- The site is circled and it is recorded in patient's chart.
- The reaction is observed in defined time.

NEEDLE STICK INJURY AND POSTEXPOSURE PROPHYLAXIS

Needle Stick Injuries

Needle stick injuries can be defined as an accidental exposure through needles, which may occur before, during, or after the process of injection giving.[9,10] It might place healthcare professional or worker (HCP/HCW) at risk of blood-borne infections such as hepatitis B, hepatitis C, or HIV and many others.[3,4] Globally, NSIs are the most common source of occupational exposures to blood and the primary cause of blood-borne infections of HCWs. The two most common causes of NSIs are two handed recapping and the unsafe collection and disposal of sharps waste.

Determinants of Needle Stick Injuries[9,10]

- Overuse of injections and unnecessary sharps
- *Lack of supplies:* Disposable syringes, safer needle devices, and sharps-disposal containers
- Lack of access to and failure to use sharps containers immediately after injection
- Inadequate or short staffing
- Recapping of needles after use
- Lack of engineering controls such as safer needle devices
- Passing instruments from hand to hand in the operating suite
- Lack of awareness of hazard and lack of training

Flowchart 23.1.1: Management of healthcare professional or worker (HCP/HCW) exposed to hepatitis B injection.

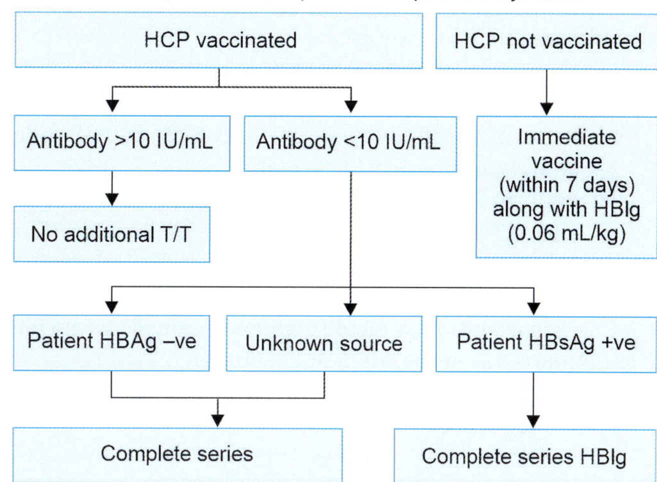

(HBIg: hepatitis B immune globulin; HBsAg: hepatitis B surface antigen; T/T: treatment)

Determinants of Transmission of Infection

The risks of transmission of infection from an infected patient to the HCW following an NSI are hepatitis B, 3–10%; hepatitis C, 3%; and HIV, 0.3%.[3,4]

Immediate Management of Needle Stick Injuries

The exposure site should be cleaned immediately. This is the most important part of PEP. Puncture wounds and other cutaneous injury sites should be copiously washed with soap and water. Exposed oral and nasal mucous membranes should be vigorously flushed with water. Eyes should be irrigated with clean water or saline. There is no evidence that antiseptics for wound care reduce the risk of blood-borne pathogen transmission. The use of bleach or other caustic agents that cause local tissue trauma is not recommended.[9,10]

Postexposure Prophylaxis for Hepatitis B

- If the exposed person is vaccinated and his/her serum antibody titer is >10 IU/mL, no further treatment is required.
- If antibody titer is <10 IU/mL and the exposed person is hepatitis B surface antigen (HbsAg) negative or the source is unknown, then one course of three doses of vaccine is repeated and then antibody titer is rechecked.
- If the exposed person is HbsAg positive, then both, hepatitis B vaccine is repeated and hepatitis B immune globulin (HBIg) is given within hours of exposure.
- If the exposed person is not vaccinated, then vaccination series is started within 7 days.

Flowchart 23.1.1 shows management following exposure to hepatitis B positive patient.

Management of Exposure to Hepatitis C Virus

The following are recommendations for follow-up of occupational HCV exposures:[3]

- For the source, perform anti-HCV
- For the person exposed to HCV positive source:
  - Perform baseline testing for anti-HCV and alanine aminotransferase (ALT) activity.
  - Perform follow-up testing at 4–6 months for anti-HCV and ALT activity.
  - If earlier diagnosis of HCV infection is desired, testing for HCV RNA may be performed at 4–6 weeks.
- Confirm all anti-HCV results reported positive by enzyme immunoassay, using supplement anti-HCV testing.
- Immunoglobulins and antiviral agents are not recommended.

Recommendations for Postexposure Prophylaxis for Human Immunodeficiency Virus

- Indian Academy of Pediatrics (IAP) endorses the National AIDS Control Organization (NACO) guidelines. These should be implemented all over the India.
- If any exposed person reports with NSI to emergency services in a public health facility, it is recommended that immediate care, free testing, and free PEP medicines should be provided.
- A nodal contact person should be in place in all facilities with 24 hours access to deal with immediate management of NSIs/other exposures.
- Healthcare workers should ensure that a startup pack of PEP medication is available in their place of work.

DISPOSAL OF INJECTION WASTE (SYRINGES AND NEEDLES)

Biomedical waste (BMW) management is a process starting from the point of use of a device till its final disposal. It is not only an issue of technology but also requires lot of changes in the way we think. Healthcare waste is hazardous both to the HCP, patients, and public at large.[5]

Government of India under the provision of Environmental Act, 1988 notified the BMW Rules in 1988, which regulates the disposal of all BMW with an objective to ensure safety of health and environment. All healthcare facilities are required to segregate, disinfect, transport, and dispose of the BMW in an environmental-friendly manner. BMW shall not be mixed with other wastes.

As per the Schedule-I, Rule 5 of BMW Rules, sharp wastes are classified in Category 4, which says, sharp wastes means needles, syringes, scalpel blades, glass, etc., that may cause puncture and cuts. This includes both used and unused sharps, which should be treated. As per Schedule-II, color coding of the container for disposal sharps is a must. Blue/white translucent-colored puncture-proof container has to be used and disposed as per the schedule.

Section 4 of the Act has given policy statement. The following steps should be followed—minimization, segregation, handling, storage of hospital waste, and disposal.

Sharp Waste Minimization

As far as possible, minimize the use of sharps. Emphasize the rational use of injections in the treatment of illness. The use of disposable syringes and needles has increased considerably, generating potentially infectious waste with limited options for treatment and disposal. The use of plastic disposables should be limited as far as possible because plastics are nondegradable and more likely to cause reuse.[5]

Segregation of Sharps

Sharps should be segregated at source. The clinical staff is responsible for segregating the waste at source.[5] Blue/white translucent puncture-proof containers should be placed at strategic and easily accessible locations. Needles should not be recapped, removed, and transported by hand. Sharps should be disinfected. Hub-cutters or needle and syringe destroyer should be used at the site of generation to reduce the bulk, to disinfect, and to prevent reusing.

Handling

Sharps containers should be picked-up and carried by the handle provided. They should not be supported at the bottom. Sharp containers should not be carried on back and should not be dropped or thrown. Containers should be labeled. Vehicles used to transport sharp containers should be authorized.

Containers

Sharps decontaminating units (SDUs) for syringes and needles are made of plastic and are puncture-proof; they can be foot operated with an inner-perforated container with secured handles. They should be filled one third with 1% hypochlorite solution (refer to the recent central pollution board guidelines). Sharps in inner containers after treatment with hypochlorite solution should be transferred to puncture-proof containers for shredding. They should be labeled as sharps only.

Mutilation/Destruction/Shredding

Types of waste required to be mutilated are needles, syringes, plastic disposables, etc. Shredders are equipment to cut the waste into small pieces to reduce the volume.[5] They must have safety provisions to prevent contamination. They must be placed in a separate room. Waste must be properly disinfected before feeding into shredder.

Treatment and Disposal

It is necessary to treat certain waste before disposal to prevent hazards to human health and environment. Immediately after use, syringes with needles should be dropped into SDU, so that both parts are completely immersed in disinfectant.[5] When SDU is one-third full, after contact time of 30 minutes the inner perforated container contents are drained into puncture-proof containers for shredding. Heat disinfection, encapsulation, smelting, burial, are incineration are modes for disposal of sharp wastes in mass.

The education and awareness of HCW and public are important. The general public coming to hospital and in the community should know the medical risks of hospital waste so that they keep away from risks and also to demand the proper care, services from the hospital.

NEWER TECHNOLOGIES

Technology plays a supportive role in enhancing the quality of patient care in our day-to-day working. This has over a period of time helped HCPs to deliver services effectively and efficiently. Most of the technological advances have happened as a response to the demands of the healthcare provider. These technologies for ease of understanding can be divided into three different kinds—(1) autodisable (AD) syringes, (2) prefilled AD devices, and (3) HCW safety devices.

Autodisable Syringes

These are disposable syringes that lock once the medication has been injected and hence physically cannot be reused; these syringes prevent reuse and they present the lowest risk of patient-to-patient transmission of blood-borne pathogens. These are available as prefixed 0.5 mL syringes and are presently available for immunization only.

Syringe with different mechanisms are commercially available. These can be broadly divided into two types of AD mechanisms:

1. *Active mechanism:*
    - Requires the user to "actively" disable the syringe/device after use
    - Disadvantage—chances of reuse if mechanism is not activated.
2. *Passive mechanism:*
    - The device is disabled as soon as the drug is fully injected out. The user has no control over the mechanism.
    - No chance of reuse as user has no control over mechanism. WHO-United Nations Children's Fund-United Nations Population Fund joint statement issued in 1999 on the use of AD syringes in immunization services has urged countries to use only AD syringes for immunization after 2003. It is also recommended that in the curative sector also, injection devices with reuse prevention mechanisms should be used **(Fig. 23.1.7)**.

Prefilled Vaccine Devices or Pouch and Needle Devices (Figs. 23.1.8A and B)

Prefilled vaccine devices or pouch and needle devices were also developed by PATH and are used by the pharmaceutical companies and vaccine manufacturers to fill vaccines into them and supply. They combine the benefit of prefilled device with that of AD technologies. Minimally trained volunteers can use them. Several vaccines are now available with this technology.

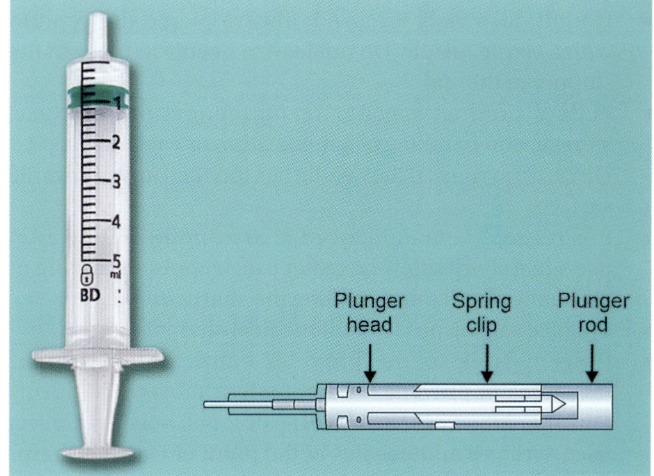

Fig. 23.1.7: Autodisable syringe.

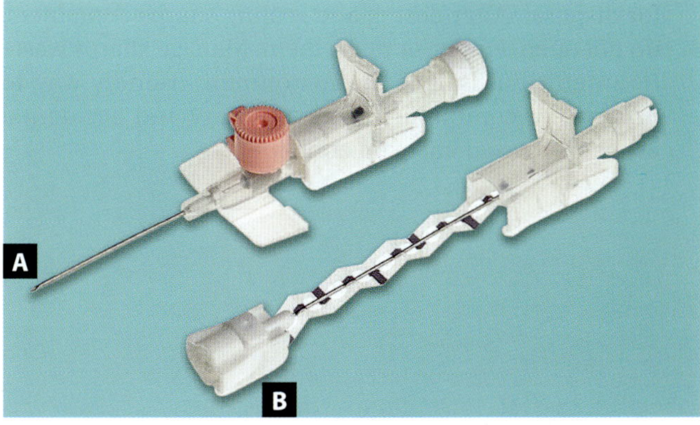

Figs. 23.1.8A and B: Safety cannula and needle shield

Healthcare Worker's Safety Devices

With the identification of the spread of blood-borne pathogens due to NSIs stick injuries and a Needle Stick Safety and Prevention Act passed in the United States in 2000, the trend, globally, is shifting toward use of safety engineered products. Now, a range of products, which help prevent accidental NSIs are available. These products are now widely available in India.

LEARNING POINTS

- Keep hands clean before giving injections.
- Always use "sterile injection equipment". Always use sterile syringe and needle for each injection and to reconstitute each unit of medication.
- Prevent contamination of injection equipment and medicines.
- Prepare each injection in a clean designated area where blood or body fluid contamination is unlikely.
- Clean skin prior to injection with water and wait for it to dry. Do not use cotton balls stored wet in a container.
- If multidose vials are used, always pierce the septum with a sterile needle. Do not leave a needle in place in the stopper of the vial.
- Follow product-specific recommendations for use, storage, and handling of a medication or vaccine.
- Discard a syringe, if the needle has touched any nonsterile surface.
- Ensure safe containment of sharps immediately after use—in a sharp safety box after use, without recapping or manually mutilating/handling the sharps/needles.
- Practice safe disposal for all medical sharps waste.
- Prevent NSIs to the provider—anticipate and take measures to prevent sudden patient movement during and after injection. Do not recap or touch needles. Collect used syringes and needles at the point of use in a sharps container that is puncture-proof and leak-proof. The container should be sealed when three-fourths full.
- Prevent public access to used needles—seal sharps containers before carrying to a secure area in preparation for disposal. After dosing and sealing sharps containers, do not open, empty, or reuse them. Manage sharps waste in an efficient, safe, and environment-friendly way to protect the community from voluntary and accidental exposure to used injection equipment.

REFERENCES

1. World Health Organization (2003). Aide-Memoire for a Strategy to Protect Health Workers from Infection with Bloodborne Viruses. Geneva, Switzerland. [online] Available from: www.who.int/occupational_health/activities/1am_hcw.pdf [Last accessed December, 2024].
2. Hutin YJ, Hauri AM, Armstrong GL. Use of injections in health-care settings worldwide, 2000: literature review and regional estimates. BMJ. 2003;327(7423):1075.
3. Abdel-Aziz F, Habib M, Mohamed MK, Gamil F, Madkour S, Mikhail NN, et al. Hepatitis C virus (HCV) infection in a community in the Nile Delta: population description and HCV prevalence. Hepatology. 2000;32(1):111-5.
4. Frank C, Mohamed MK, Strickland GT, Lavanchy D, Arthur RR, Magder LS, et al. The role of parenteral antischistosomal therapy in the spread of hepatitis C virus in Egypt. Lancet. 2000;355(9207):887-91.
5. World Health Organization. Management of wastes from immunization campaign activities. Practical guidelines for planners and managers. [online] Available from: https://iris.who.int/bitstream/handle/10665/204415/WHO_SDE_WSH_04.11_eng.pdf;jsessionid=041D10A820B0BF1AC0ACE0F6B5040DAC?sequence=1#:~:text=The%20most%20important%20point%20regarding,vaccination%2C%20storage%20or%20disposal%20areas. [Last accessed December, 2024].
6. Kamath SS. IAP workshop on safe injection practices: Recommendations and IAP plan of action. Indian Pediatr. 2005;42(2):155-61.
7. Kamath SS, Bhave S, Shah RC. (2005). IAP Guide Book on Safe Injection Practices. Published by IAP National Task Force on Safe Injection Practices. [online] Available from https://www.indianpediatrics.net/feb2005/155.pdf [Last accessed December, 2024].
8. Royal College of Pediatrics and Child Health (2002). Position Statement in Injection Technique. [online] Available from: www.rcpch.ac.uk/sites/default/files/asset_library/Publications/P/Injections1.pdf [Last accessed December, 2024].
9. Centers for Disease Control and Prevention (1999). National Institute for Occupational Safety and Health (NIOSH) NIOSH Alert: Preventing Needle stick Injuries in Health Care Settings. Publication No. 2000-108. [online] Available from www.cdc.gov/niosh/2000-108.html [Last accessed December, 2024].
10. Prüss-Üstün A, Rapiti E, Hutin Y. Sharps injuries: global burden of disease from sharps injuries to health-care workers. Geneva, Switzerland; WHO; 2003.

23.2 Common Procedures in Pediatric Practice

Baldev S Prajapati

INTRODUCTION

It is very essential for every medical student and practicing pediatrician to learn performing common pediatric procedures. The procedures are best learnt by observation, performing the procedure under supervision and repetitive performances. It should be practical, methodological, and safe for both patients as well as for the individual who performs the procedure.

GENERAL CONSIDERATIONS

Healthcare Counseling

Healthcare counseling (HCC) is a relatively new concept that amalgamates human biology, human psychology, and medical sociology principles, and applies the same in real-time clinical situations. HCC is especially important for the child population as the pediatricians need to partner the parenting responsibilities in different illness care settings covering the period from newborn to adolescence.[1]

Explain to the parents in detail regarding the procedure including its indications, technique of the procedure, possible complications, etc. If the child is older and able to understand, talk to him also in simple language. By this, cooperation is available from parents as well as the child. It decreases the anxiety of all and the procedure can be performed smoothly. An informed consent is a must for all the procedures. In certain procedures such as lumbar puncture, pleural and pericardial tapping, liver biopsy, renal biopsy, exchange transfusion, bone marrow aspiration, and biopsy, it is prudent to get signed consent along with HCC to avoid medicolegal problems.

Procedure Room and Lighting

Separate procedure room is desirable. It should have good daylight and should be well-illuminated and well-equipped. All the equipment and drugs to perform the procedure as well as to manage any emergency if it arises should be made available.

Containers

It is very important to confirm that proper containers are available for collection and transferring the specimens.

Identification of the Patient

It should be a routine to identify the child before performing the procedure. It should be confirmed with hospital staff as well as the parents that you are dealing with the correct child.

Sedation

Children are afraid of procedures and their reactions in the form of crying and struggling and frightened appearance increases the parental anxiety. It affects the performance of the person who is performing the procedure. It results in increased rate of failure and complications related to procedure. In this situation, sedation to the child may help. Promethazine 1 mg/kg/dose or triclofos sodium 20 mg/kg/dose by oral route will suffice in most of the cases. Diazepam, ketamine, and general anesthesia are other options as per indications.

Restraint

Physical restraint of the frightened child may be essential for the successful outcome of any practical procedure. The child may be wrapped with a blanket taking care to prevent aspiration or airway obstruction. The help of the person who is assisting is very crucial in deciding the outcome of the procedure.

Anesthesia

Local anesthesia may be achieved by infiltrating tissues around the site with 0.5–2% lignocaine. The maximum dosage of 1% lignocaine that can be infiltrated is 0.3 mL/kg. An alternative is to apply lignocaine cream to small area of the skin 60 minutes prior to performing the procedure, protected by adhesive dressing. Sedation or general anesthesia may be needed in certain cases.

Asepsis

The physician should scrub hands and forearm using an effective cleaning agent like 4% chlorhexidine or hexachlorophene before undertaking any procedure. Wearing of sterile gloves by the doctor is very important both for his and the patient's safety. The site of the patient's skin is then cleaned with 70% isopropyl alcohol and the surface is allowed to dry, the surface is then again washed three times with 10% povidone-iodine or 0.5% chlorhexidine gluconate in 70% isopropyl alcohol. It should be cleaned in a circular fashion from the center outward.

INTRAMUSCULAR INJECTION

Common Sites

Muscles commonly used for intramuscular (IM) injection are vastus lateralis, deltoid, and gluteus medius. Children do not have well-developed gluteus medius and therefore, it is not the site of preference for IM injections. It has been documented that some vaccines such as hepatitis B and antirabies vaccines administered at gluteal region produce very poor antibody response.

The vastus lateralis (anterolateral aspect of thigh) is the preferred site in infants. The site in vastus lateralis is the middle-third of the area between the greater trochanter and lateral femoral condyle **(Figs. 23.2.1A and B)**.[2]

In case of deltoid, the site for injection is midway between acromion process and deltoid insertion, which is 3–5 cm below the acromion process. This site may be used in children above 5 years and adults. The quantity of drug should be <5 mL. Only watery injections with less viscosity should be injected at deltoid region.

Technique (WHO Technique)

- The site of injection should be exposed well.
- For anterolateral aspect of thigh, the child may be laid supine or be held in mother's lap. For deltoid, child may be held in mother's lap or may sit.
- The muscle selected for injection should be relaxed.
- The skin over injection site should be cleaned with spirit. A circular motion of swab is used, proceeding from puncture site and extending outward for 5 cm. Let the spirit evaporate and skin become dry otherwise spirit entering into tissues is painful.
- The syringe is filled with the medicine.
- In children, usually 23 G needle with 25-mm length are used for IM injections.
- Stretch the skin flat and push the needle down at 90° **(Fig. 23.2.2)**.
- Aspiration before injecting the vaccine is not required.
- Inject the vaccine at the rate of 1 mL per 10 seconds.
- The needle is withdrawn and injection site is pressed for few seconds. Do not rub the injection site.
- Needle should be withdrawn smoothly with steady movement.
- Discard the needle and syringe as per standard guidelines.

Alternative to WHO technique, Advisory Committee on Immunization Practices (ACIP) technique may be used. It is also called *bunching technique*. In this technique, bunch the muscle and direct needle inferiorly along long axis of leg at an angle of 45°. It stabilizes leg and increases the muscle mass.

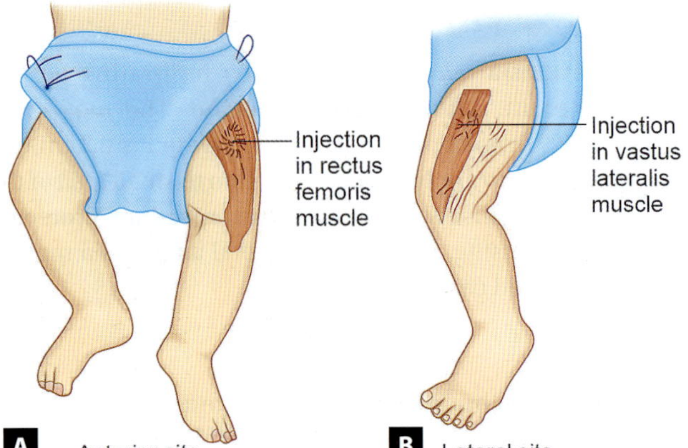

Figs. 23.2.1A and B: Site for intramuscular injections (IM) in an infant.
Source: Prajapati BS. Essential Procedures in Pediatrics, 1st edition. New Delhi: Jaypee Brothers Medical Publishers (P) Ltd; 2003.

SUBCUTANEOUS INJECTION

Drugs or vaccines are injected subcutaneously when slow absorption and long duration of action are desired. Another indication of subcutaneous (SC) injection route is a coagulopathy, which makes IM injection hazardous, for fear of development of IM hematoma. Insulin and heparin such as drugs as well as measles, mumps, and rubella (MMR), varicella vaccines are given by SC route.

Technique

- Common sites are arm, anterior abdominal wall and thigh. Atrophic and infected areas are avoided.

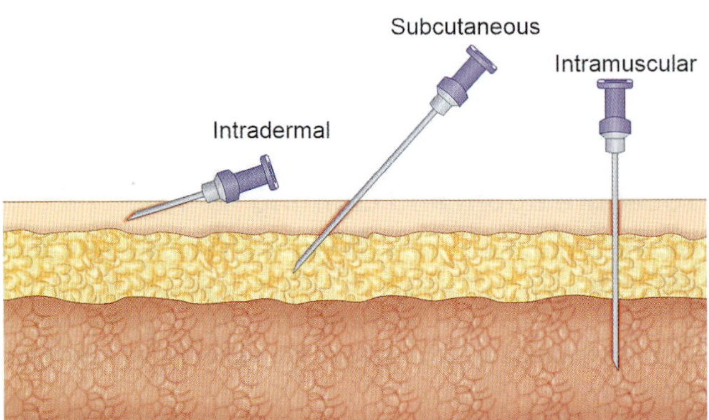

Fig. 23.2.2: The position of the needle during different ways of administering injections.
Source: Wechter EH, Philips J, Holaday B. Nursing Care of Children, 10th edition. Philadelphia: JB Lippincott Co; 1985.

- The skin is cleaned and disinfected with spirit.
- 26 G needle with 13-mm length is commonly used for SC injection.
- The skin is raised into a fold with thumb and index finger of the left hand.
- The midpoint of the fold is pierced with the needle held at 45° with its surface. The tip of the needle is advanced into the SC tissue **(Fig. 23.2.2)**.
- Aspiration is not required.
- Drugs or vaccine is injected, needle is withdrawn and site is pressed for few minutes.

INTRADERMAL INJECTION

Indications for intradermal (ID) injection are bacillus Calmette-Guérin (BCG) vaccination, Mantoux test, skin tests for allergy, and test for sensitization of certain drugs such as penicillin. Antirabies vaccine also can be given by ID route.

Technique

- Ventral (volar) aspect of forearm is commonly used for ID injection.
- Skin is cleaned with sterile water.
- A measured amount of antigen (usually 0.1 mL) is drawn into the syringe.
- 26 G or 27 G needle with 1/4 to 1/2 inch (6.35–12.7 mm) length needle is used for ID injection.
- The skin is held taut between thumb and index finger of the left hand. The syringe is held at an angle of 10–15° with the skin. Needle is inserted for about 2 mm, so that entire needle bevel penetrates the skin and the injected solution raises a small bleb of about 5 mm in diameter. The development of perifollicular puckering (Peau d'orange) indicates successful ID injection **(Fig. 23.2.2)**.
- The needle is withdrawn.
- The site is circled and it is recorded in patient's chart.
- The reaction is observed in defined time.

RECTAL ADMINISTRATION OF DRUGS

It is a safe and easy way of administering drugs. The human rectum represents a body cavity in which drugs can be easily introduced and retained. The absorption of the drugs is well through this route. Rectal administration of drugs is indicated in patients who are not able to take orally due to nausea and vomiting, having convulsions, uncooperative children, before surgery, etc.[2] If the child can understand, it should be explained to him. The child should be relaxed. He is kept in lateral position with knees flexed toward abdomen or in supine position with legs taken upward toward abdomen and the drug is inserted into the rectum through anal orifice, and buttocks are held firmly to prevent expulsion of the drug. Paracetamol, diazepam, midazolam, paraldehyde, glycerine, bisacodyl, diclofenac sodium, steroids, neomycin, artesunate, and many more drugs can be administered through rectal route. When rectal preparations are not available, some liquid preparations such as injection diazepam may be given per rectum. For this purpose, a lubricated tube is inserted into the rectum to a distance of about 5 cm and then the medication is administered through it using a syringe. The buttocks are held together for a couple of minutes. Local irritation and ulcerations in rectum may develop as complication of this procedure, if done repeatedly.

PERIPHERAL INTRAVENOUS ACCESS

Peripheral intravenous (IV) access is one of the mainstays of modern medicine. It allows blood sampling, administration of medicines, fluids, nutrients, blood, and blood products.[3] Intracaths and scalp vein needles are commonly used for this purpose. Various sites for venous access are as follows in order to preference **(Fig. 23.2.3)**:[2,4]

- Veins on dorsum of hand
- Superficial radial vein on radial aspect of wrist
- Superficial veins over volar aspect of forearm
- Basilic vein and median cubital vein over antecubital fossa
- Superficial veins over dorsum of foot and long saphenous vein on medial aspect of leg above the ankle
- Veins of scalp in newborns and infants
- External jugular vein

Straight, large, and easily accessible peripheral veins in healthy SC tissues are ideal for venous access. Veins of the upper extremities are preferred because there are many potential sites and more comfortable to the patient. The distal and superficial veins are preferred as complications are more, following extravasation and thrombophlebitis in proximal and deep veins. When the veins are not visible, they can be palpated at common sites and can be accessed.

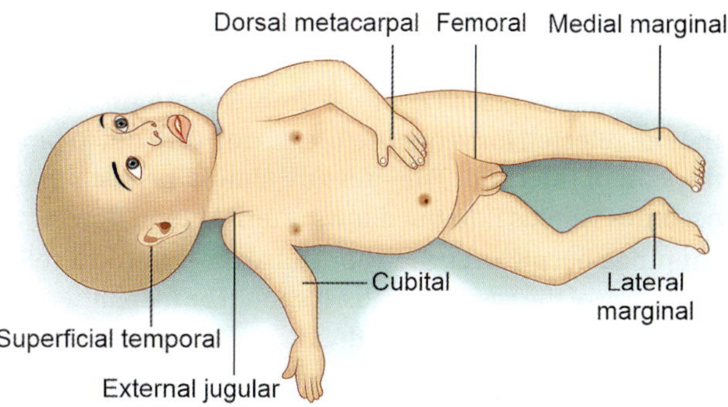

Fig. 23.2.3: Common sites for venipuncture.
Source: Prajapati BS. Essential Procedures in Pediatrics, 1st edition. New Delhi: Jaypee Brothers Medical Publishers (P) Ltd; 2003.

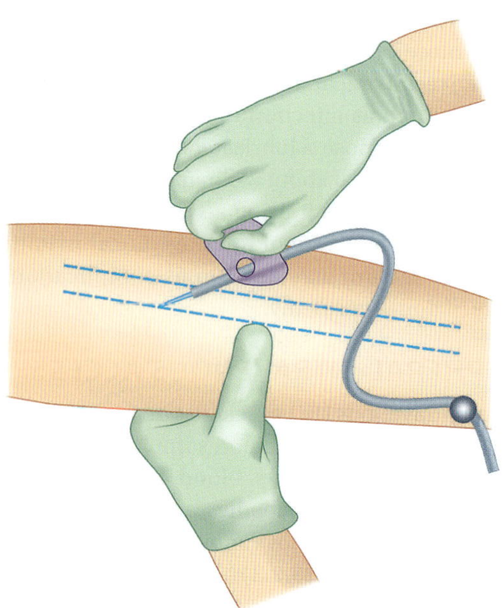

Fig. 23.2.4: Technique of venipuncture with scalp vein needle.
Source: Prajapati BS. Essential Procedures in Pediatrics, 1st edition. New Delhi: Jaypee Brothers Medical Publishers (P) Ltd; 2003.

Scalp vein needle is a hollow needle with butterfly plastic handle, and a plastic tube, at the other end of which, a syringe or infusion set can be attached. It is useful for venous sampling of blood and short-term use of IV route **(Fig. 23.2.4)**.[2] Vein is counter punctured very easily on movement of the limb.

Intracaths are plastic catheters over a hollow metallic needle. The metallic needle just projects beyond the tip of plastic catheter. The metallic needle is to provide stiffness during insertion into the vein, after which it is withdrawn. The plastic catheter is then advanced further gently so that vein is not counter punctured. The plastic catheter is well tolerated. Intracaths and scalp vein needles are available in various sizes from 26 G to 16 G. In children commonly, we use 26 G–21 G depending on age of the child and requirement.[3]

Technique

- A tourniquet is placed over the limb, 3–4 cm proximal to the site selected for venipuncture, taking care not to pinch the skin of the child. The pressure should be such that it occludes venous flow but allows arterial blood flow.
- Tapping sharply over the vein causes mechanical reflex dilatation of the vascular walls. It should be light otherwise pain will cause vasoconstriction.
- Active or passive pumping of extremity enhances blood flow and distends veins.
- A warm moist towel may be applied to the site for several minutes. It causes venous dilatation.
- Aseptic precautions are mandatory.

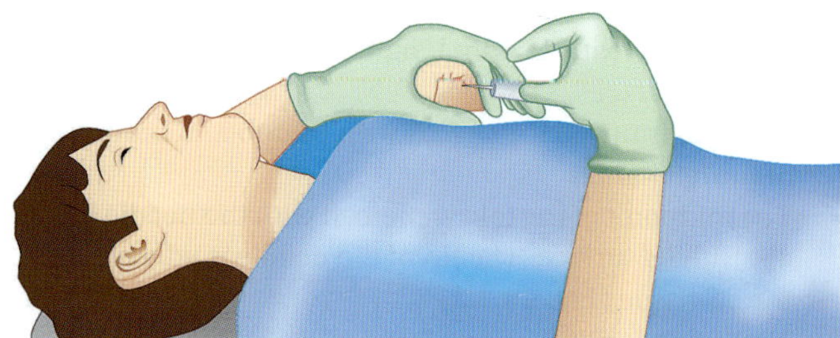

Fig. 23.2.5: For inserting the intravenous (IV) cannula on the dorsum of the hand. The hand may be held flexed at the wrist to occlude venous return and make the veins prominent.

- The methylated spirit is applied over 4–5 cm area at planned site. Let it dry.
- The skin is pulled taut distally to stabilize the vein with a nondominant hand. It is punctured by the needle bevel. up at 15–30° angle parallel to the vein **(Fig. 23.2.5)**. After the entry into the SC tissue, the needle is aligned parallel to the skin surface and along the long axis of the vein. Its tip is depressed a little and is advanced until it penetrates the vein. Then, it is made parallel to the vein again and advanced until it is passed fully into the vein. Blood is collected if indicated and then the IV set is attached to it.
- The tourniquet is removed and the infusion is started by releasing the clamp on the tubing. A hub of the cannula and IV set are secured to the skin with the adhesive plaster.
- For flushing the cannula, normal saline should be used and not the distilled water. Distilled water causes pain at IV site and it also causes hemolysis.
- If venipuncture is performed only for collection of blood, pull the needle gently after collecting the required sample and apply steady pressure at the site with a piece of spirit swab for few minutes.

INTRAOSSEOUS INFUSION

Peripheral percutaneous venous access is the fastest method of obtaining vascular access in children. However, during life-threatening emergencies, rapid access to venous compartment through peripheral or central venous route is occasionally difficult or an impossible procedure for a pediatrician to perform. Small peripheral vessels in children often collapse during shock and efforts at setting up an IV line in a peripheral vein may fail. When IV access cannot be established within three attempts or 90 seconds time, intraosseous route should be used as per the recommendations.[3]

Common Sites

- Anteromedial surface of the proximal tibia, one- or two-finger breadths distal to tibial tuberosity to avoid damage to epiphyseal growth plate

- 2–3 cm above the lateral condyle of the femur in the midline
- Medial surface of the distal tibia proximal to the medial malleolus

Technique (Fig. 23.2.6)

- Specially designed needles, Jamshidi type available for intraosseous infusion should be used, if available. Hypodermic needle can also be used. 20–16 FG needle can be used for children below 18 months of age, and 16–12 FG for older children.[4]
- Identify the site of placement.
- Patient's leg should be restrained, a small sandbag is placed behind the knee.
- The use of local anesthesia is optional, but usually recommended as it may be more painful once the child is resuscitated.
- Aseptic precautions are must.
- Insert the needle perpendicular to the skin and advance to the periosteum and then with a screwing motion penetrate into the marrow. A distinct "give way" sensation indicates that your needle is in marrow. Confirm that the needle is firmly embedded in the bone.
- Insertion of needle to a depth of 1 cm is usually adequate as the distance from skin through the cortex is rarely >1 cm in infants and children.
- The needle should maintain erect posture without support.
- Trocar is removed and correct position is verified by aspiration of marrow and easy flushing with 5–10 mL of normal saline without signs of extravasation.
- The needle should be secured and apply sterile dressing over the site.
- It should be watched for local complications such as extravasation and infection.
- As soon as the peripheral IV route is established, intraosseous needle should be removed.
- Emergency drugs and fluids can be administered via intraosseous route, essentially the same dosage and rates as given by IV route.

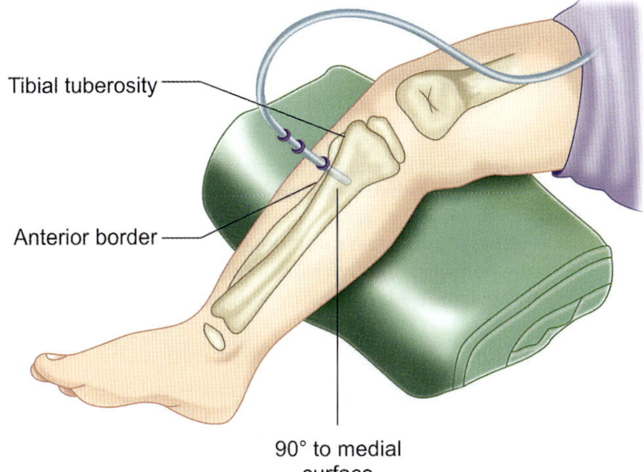

Fig. 23.2.6: Intraosseous cannulation technique.
Source: Chameides L. Textbook of Pediatrics Advanced Life Support. Dallas: American Heart Association—American Academy of Pediatrics; 1988.

VENOUS CUTDOWN (VENESECTION)

Venous cutdown is now rarely resorted to in the present scenario of cannulas and intraosseous access. It is mainly useful when routine IV access has failed in conditions such as shock or when large amounts of fluids have to be given for a long time as in total parenteral nutrition.[3,4]

Sites

- *Lower limb:* Most preferred site is saphenous vein near ankle.
- *Upper limb:* Median cubital or basilic vein in front of elbow
- Cephalic vein at the wrist at anatomical snuff box
- External jugular vein in the neck

Technique (Fig. 23.2.7)[2]

- Get all the instruments ready.
- Prepare the part aseptically. Then it is draped with sterile towels.
- 0.5% Xylocaine is infiltrated subcutaneously at the site of incision. In emergency, local anesthesia can be skipped.
- A 1–2 cm long transverse incision is made 1.5 cm above and in front of medial malleolus over the saphenous vein.

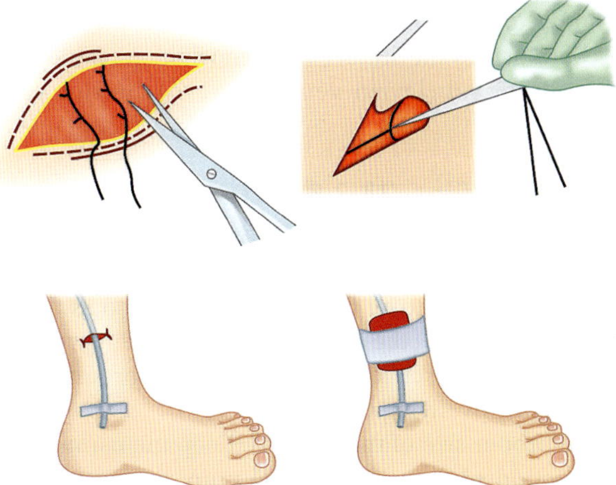

Fig. 23.2.7: Venous cut down.
Source: Prajapati BS. Essential Procedures in Pediatrics, 1st edition. New Delhi: Jaypee Brothers Medical Publishers (P) Ltd.; 2003.

- The vein is exposed by blunt dissection, opening the blades of mosquito forceps parallel to the vein.
- Pass the tip of mosquito artery forceps beneath the vein and elevate at least 1 cm above the vein.
- Pass two silk ligatures under the vein.
- Separate the proximal and distal ligatures for full length of exposed vein.
- Tie the distal ligature and hold the ends with mosquito forceps.
- With venesection scissors put "v"-shaped cut on anterior wall of the vein at middle of the exposed part.
- Introduce polyethylene tube of suitable size proximally through the cut in the vein till the free flow of blood is obtained.
- Cannula is fixed by tying proximal ligature on the vein with cannula in vein.
- Ends of proximal and distal ligatures are trimmed.
- Wound is sutured by silk sutures in a way so that cannula or tube does not get kinked or obstructed.
- Dressing is applied and remaining part of the tube is properly fixed with dressing.
- IV drip is connected to the venesection needle.

Complications

- Wound infections
- Thrombophlebitis
- Deep vein thrombosis
- Air embolism
- Injury to adjacent nerves and vessels.

As alternate route is possible, earliest venesection tube should be removed.

EXTERNAL JUGULAR VEIN PUNCTURE

The external jugular vein is formed below the ear and behind the angle of mandible, passes downward and obliquely backward across the surface of sternocleidomastoid muscle and ends in subclavian vein lateral to anterior scalene muscle.[3,4]

Technique (Figs. 23.2.8 and 23.2.9)

- Place the patient in supine. Both the shoulders should touch the table and head is rotated fully to one side and extended partly over the end of the table so as to extend the vein. Making the child cry makes the vein prominent.[5]
- Restraining the child properly is very important.
- Clean the overlying skin.
- Use proper size of the cannula. Keep the cannula in the direction of the vein with the point aimed toward the same shoulder.
- Make the venipuncture midway between the angle of mandible and midclavicular line.

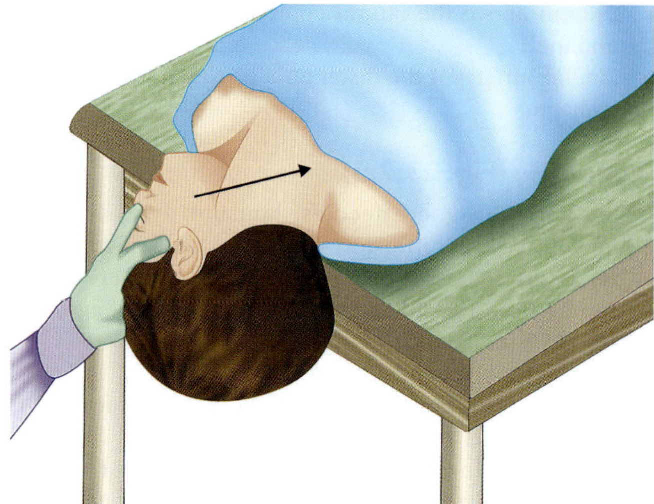

Fig. 23.2.8: Position for jugular vein (both internal and external) puncture. The arrow shows the direction of insertion of the needle for external jugular vein puncture.
Source: Silver HK, Kempe CH, Bruyn HB. Handbook of Pediatrics, 13th edition. Singapore: Lange-Maruzen Asia Publications; 1980.

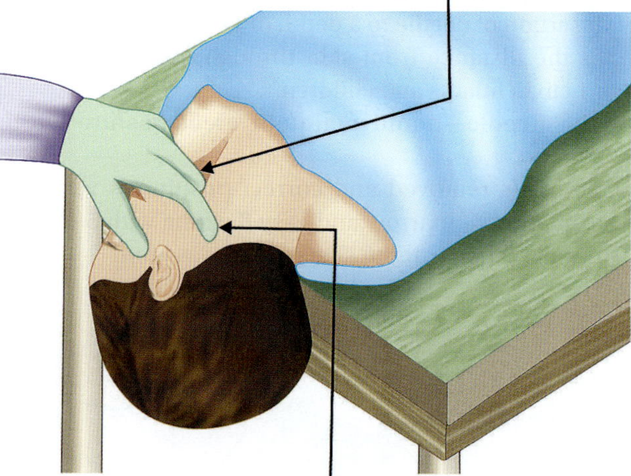

Fig. 23.2.9: Internal jugular vein puncture technique.
Source: Silver HK, Kempe CH, Bruyn HB. Handbook of Pediatrics, 13th edition. Singapore: Lange-Maruzen Asia Publications; 1980.

- Proceed as described for veins of extremities.
- After removing the needle, apply constant pressure at puncture site for 5 minutes while the child is sitting.

FEMORAL VEIN PUNCTURE

In view of the risks of femoral venipuncture, it should be used as a last resort for collection of blood samples in neonates and infants.[3,4]

Technique

- Restraining the infant in frog leg position.
- Clean the inguinal area properly. The part is cleaned properly with spirit—iodine-spirit.
- The femoral artery is located just below the midpoint of inguinal ligament.
- The femoral vein lies medial to the artery.
- Skin is pierced about 1–2 cm as below the inguinal ligament directly over the femoral vein and the needle is advanced at an angle of 30–45° with the skin while maintaining the gentle negative suction. As the vein is punctured, the blood is withdrawn in the syringe.
- If no blood is obtained while needle is inserted, suction should be maintained as the needle is slowly withdrawn. Sometimes needle passes through both the walls of the vein and blood is obtained only when the needle is being withdrawn.
- On removal of needle, apply firm pressure over the site of puncture for at least 3–5 minutes to avoid oozing and hematoma formation.

Precautions

- As far as possible avoid this procedure.
- Strict asepsis is a must as there is potential risk of septic arthritis and osteomyelitis.
- Be careful regarding piercing the femoral artery, which can be identified by bright red color of blood as jet flow of it. If artery is pierced inadvertently, remove the needle and apply pressure for a long time and check the limb periodically for pulsations, color, and warmth.

UMBILICAL VEIN CATHETERIZATION

It is used for exchange transfusion. It may be used for rapid replacement of fluids and blood especially in extreme preterm neonates.[6] Nowadays, exchange transfusion is also preferred by peripheral route.

The umbilical vein spirals through the cord and is at 12 o'clock position at the level of the abdominal wall. Here, it turns cephalad and runs slightly toward right to enter the porta hepatis. It continues with left portal vein, communicates with left hepatic vein and then with inferior vena cava. The umbilical vein is much wider than umbilical arteries.

Technique

- The child should be in supine position with gentle restraining. A padded crucifix splint is used to restrain the baby.
- Sterilize and drape the skin around the umbilical stump.
- The cord is then cut cleanly about 2 cm above the umbilicus and umbilical vein is located at 12 o'clock position. The blood clot in the vein is expressed or pulled out by fine forceps **(Figs. 23.2.10A and B)**.[2]
- Mark the catheter for the correct distance to be inserted, which is about 20% of the crown heel length.

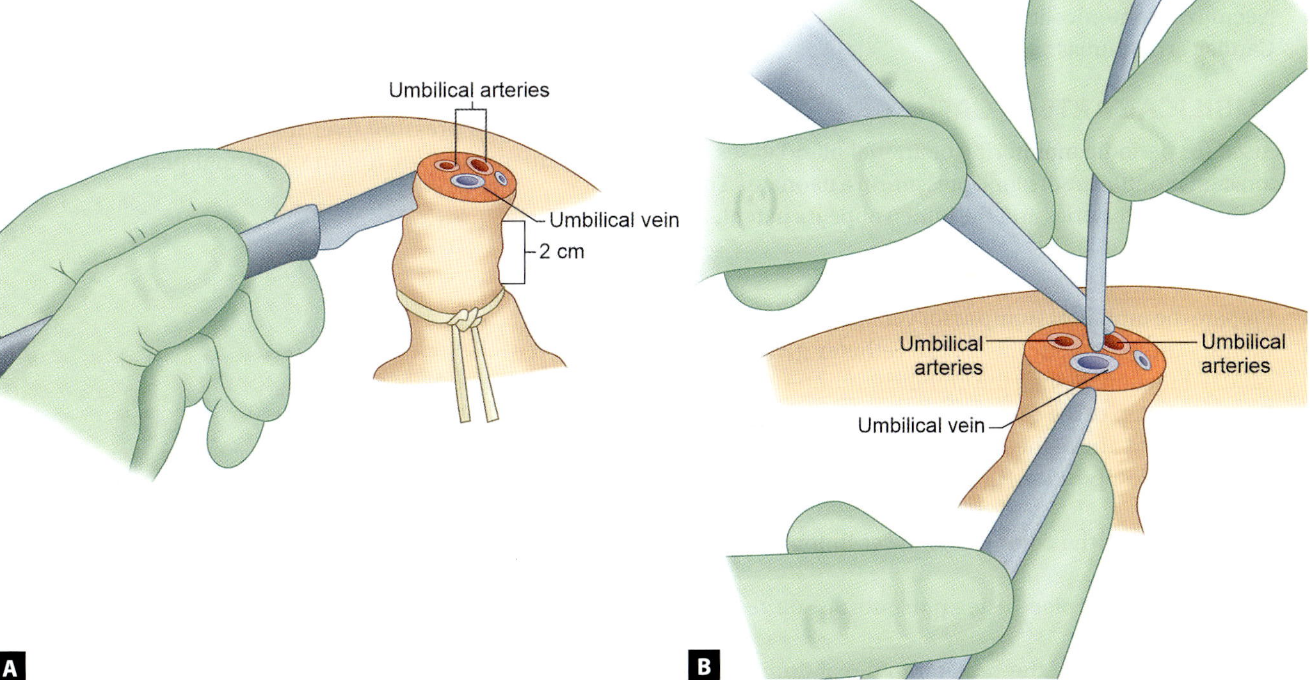

Figs. 23.2.10A and B: (A) Cutting the umbilical cord for vessel catheterization; (B) Insertion of umbilical catheter in umbilical vein.
Source: Prajapati BS. Essential Procedures in Pediatrics, 1st edition. New Delhi: Jaypee Brothers Medical Publishers (P) Ltd; 2003.

- The catheter is passed into the vein slowly and gently, giving caudal traction on the cord stump till free flow of blood is obtained.
- Flush the catheter with heparinized saline.
- The free end of the catheter should be strapped to the abdominal wall.

Special Points

- If the cord is dried up, it can be excised flush with the umbilicus, which can expose the orifice of the umbilical vein at 12 o'clock position. This can be gently dilated with Hagar's dilator and then catheterized.
- If both these methods fail, supraumbilical cut down will become necessary.
- Remove the umbilical vein catheter within 24–48 hours.
- The catheter tip should be advanced up to thoracic portion of the inferior vena cava.
- While passing the catheter, the resistance is felt at the ductus venosus. The catheter should be passed 1–2 cm beyond this point.

Complications

- Infection
- Vessel perforation
- Thrombosis of portal vein and portal hypertension in the future
- Liver infarction
- Liver abscess
- Necrotizing enterocolitis
- Cardiac arrhythmias

UMBILICAL ARTERY CATHETERIZATION

It is used for periodic monitoring of arterial blood gases and for constant monitoring of blood pressure in a neonate.[6] There are two umbilical arteries and the lumen appears patent.

Technique

- Prepare the umbilical stump as for venous catheterization.
- Identify the artery and insert the catheter gently in the caudal direction, pulling the umbilical stump superiorly.
- Position the tip of the catheter at either high (in the lower thoracic aorta above the diaphragm between T4 and T11 vertebre) or low position (in the abdominal aorta opposite L4 vertebra).
- Keep observing the color of the lower limbs during the procedure.
- Fix the catheter in place using purse string sutures at the place.
- Strap the free end of the catheter to the abdominal wall after filling it with heparinized saline and closing the end with a rubber stopper.
- Every time before sampling, remove the heparinized saline in the syringe along with same blood, then collect the sample and reinfuse the previously collected blood to the child.

Complications

- Vessel perforation
- Thromboembolism
- Air embolism
- Hypertension
- Necrotizing enterocolitis
- Infarction of distal extremities
- Renal infarction.

RADIAL ARTERY CATHETERIZATION

It is very useful and frequently used for repeated sampling of arterial blood and for continuous arterial pressure monitoring. The radial artery is easily accessible at the wrist in the groove between the tendon of the flexor carpi radialis medially and the distal radius laterally.[3]

Before puncturing the radial artery, carry out the Allen test to assess the ulnar collateral circulation.

Allen Test (Figs. 23.2.11A to D)[2]

- Make the patient's hands warm to make pulsations easily demonstrable.
- Have the patient open and close the handheld out in front and then clinch the first tightly closed.
- Occlude both radial and ulnar arteries for 30 seconds. Have the patient open the hand. Hand becomes pale due to occlusion of radial and ulnar arteries.
- Release the pressure over the ulnar artery and observe the open hand for return of normal pink color. Return

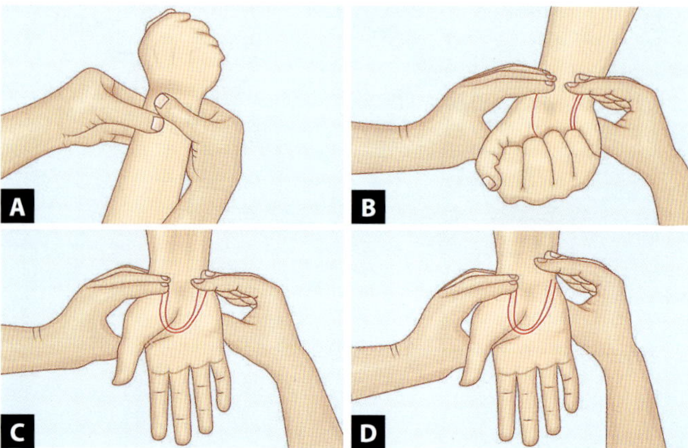

Figs. 23.2.11A to D: Allen test.
Source: Prajapati BS. Essential Procedures in Pediatrics, 1st edition. New Delhi: Jaypee Brothers Medical Publishers (P) Ltd; 2003.

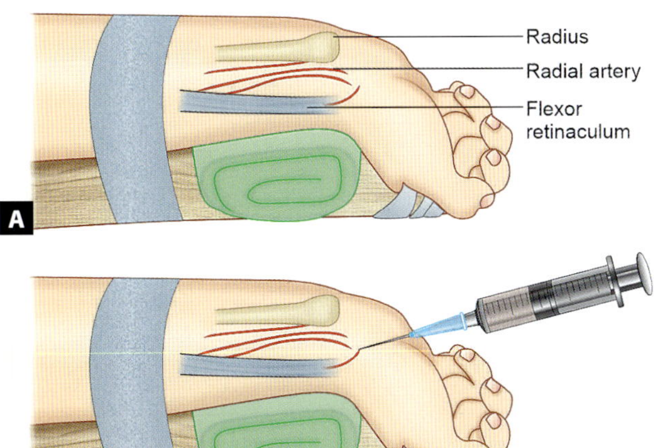

Figs. 23.2.12A and B: Radial artery—(A) Anatomy; (B) Catheterization technique.

of normal color within 6 seconds indicates patency of the ulnar artery and an intact arch with good collateral circulation.

- Delay of appearance of normal color from 10 seconds to 15 seconds indicates slow filling of the ulnar artery and collaterals.
- Persistent blanching for >15 seconds indicates an incomplete arch or poor collaterals.
- Same test can be performed to check patency of radial artery.
- If ulnar collateral circulation is good, radial artery puncture can be performed.

Technique (Figs. 23.2.12A and B)

Patient's hand should be supported and dorsiflexed at the wrist approximately 60° with both hands and lower forearm secured to a board. A roll of gauze behind the wrist will maintain dorsiflexion.

- Locate the radial artery just proximal to head of radius.
- Clean the area and observe the absolutely aseptic precautions.
- Infiltrate the skin with local anesthetic agent.
- Insert the catheter needle at about 30° angle to the surface of the skin and advance the catheter and needle stylet into the artery until blood appears in hub of the needle.
- Remove the needle and attach the hub of the catheter to the connecting tubing.
- Secure the catheter at the place with silk sutures.
- Fix the wrist in a neutral position to the board. It is essential as flexion at wrist can disturb the arterial line.
- Cover the insertion site with sterile dressing.

Special Points

- Do not perform the procedure, if Allen's test is delayed.
- Observe the color of palm periodically after cannulation.
- Before sampling blood, flush the line with 2% normal saline.
- Do not infuse medications and blood products through the arterial line except flushing fluid.

BONE MARROW ASPIRATION

This is a very common ward procedure indicated in children with blood dyscrasias, malignancies and undiagnosed fevers. Needle aspiration, trephine biopsy, and surgical biopsy are three methods available for bone marrow examination. Needle aspiration is commonly practiced in most of the cases in children. It should be done with caution when a defect in clotting mechanism is suspected.[2,7]

Common Sites

- *Iliac crest:* This is the most preferred site in children. It is performed at 1 cm below the posterior iliac crest.
- *Tibia:* At the upper end of tibia, just below tibial tuberosity on its medial aspect.
- *Sternum:* It should be used in children beyond 7–8 years of age. Manubrium sterni can be used 1 cm above sternomanubrial angle, slightly to one side of the midline.
- Rarely, lumbar spinous processes may be used.

Technique

- Atropine should be given as premedication.
- Aseptic and antiseptic precautions are must during the whole procedure.
- Local infiltration of 1% lignocaine from skin to periosteum. In some irritable children, general anesthesia is desirable for successful outcome of the procedure.
- The needle for bone marrow aspiration should be stout and made of hard stainless steel. It is about 7–8 cm long with a well-fitting stylet and an adjustable guard **(Figs. 23.2.13A and B)**.[2] The point of needle and edge of bevel should be sharp. The Sahan and Klima needles are most commonly used needles. Some people prefer to use stout hypodermic needles so that these can be disposed after use and complications of reuse of the needle can be avoided.
- The needle with the guard adjusted 0.5–1 cm from the tip of the needle is introduced into the iliac crest or sternum with screwing or boring movements keeping the needle vertical. The force required varies but needs to be considerable. Sudden giving in of resistance indicates entry of the needle into the bone marrow. Leave the

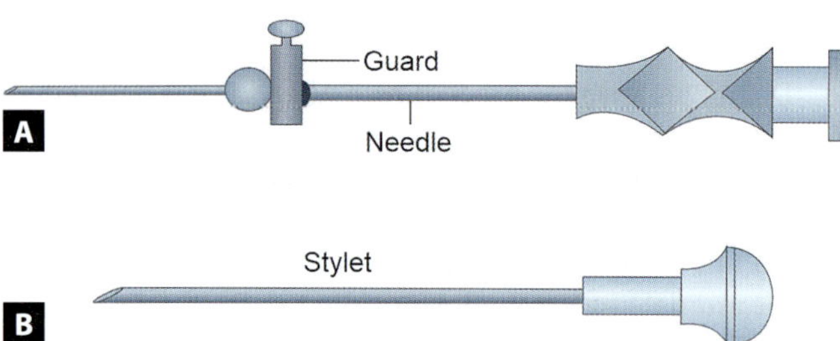

Figs. 23.2.13A and B: Bone marrow aspiration needle.
Source: Prajapati BS. Essential Procedures in Pediatrics, 1st edition. New Delhi: Jaypee Brothers Medical Publishers (P) Ltd; 2003.

needle and if it remains steady, it indicates that the needle is in the bone marrow.

- The stylet is withdrawn and marrow is aspirated with the syringe. About 0.2 mL of marrow is aspirated. This procedure is performed swiftly to obtain only bone marrow particles as slow sluggish aspiration causes dilution of marrow with blood.
- To prevent dilution of marrow with blood, aspirate material only till it appears beyond nozzle of syringe. It is sufficient material for examination. Aspiration beyond it increases the chances of marrow dilution.
- The needle is withdrawn and smear is prepared with marrow. With good material and well-prepared smear marrow, particles can be seen by naked eyes.
- Press the site for 5 minutes. Apply tincture of benzoin seal at puncture site.
- Along with smears of bone marrow, smears from peripheral blood should be prepared and sent for examination.

Complications

- Local pain and hematoma
- Injury to mediastinal structures in case of aspiration at sternum
- Infection
- Dry tap

LUMBAR PUNCTURE

This procedure is performed to obtain cerebrospinal fluid (CSF) sample for analysis in diagnosing infections and other disorders of central nervous system. It is also used for monitoring CSF pressure, intrathecal drug administration, and removing CSF in some cases of hydrocephalus.[2,7]

Contraindications

- Marked raised intracranial pressure (ICP) with closed fontanel because of the risk of herniation of brain substance through foramen magnum. Papilledema is a marker of raised ICP.

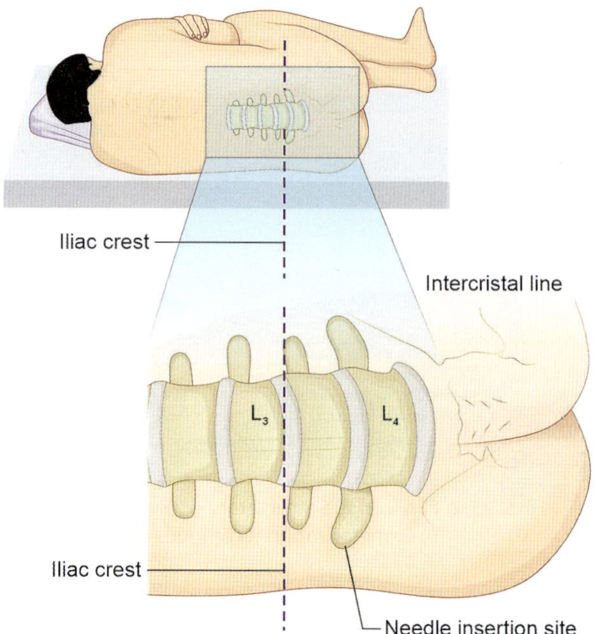

Fig. 23.2.14: Position for lumbar puncture.
Source: Prajapati BS. Essential Procedures in Pediatrics, 1st edition. New Delhi: Jaypee Brothers Medical Publishers (P) Ltd; 2003.

- Local infection
- Cardiovascular and respiratory instability

Technique

- Informed written consent is must.
- The patient is placed on his side at the edge of the table or bed with the knee drawn up toward abdomen and the head flexed to get maximum flexion of the spine **(Fig. 23.2.14)**.[2] If the child is newborn or child has respiratory problem, child should be firmly fixed at shoulders and buttocks only without flexing neck and drawing up knees. In infants, sitting position allows easier identification of the midline. An experienced assistant has a vital role in positioning, restraining, and comforting the patient.
- Aseptic and antiseptic precautions are must.
- Routinely, local anesthesia is not used. But in older children those are irritable; local anesthesia may be useful for performing the procedure smoothly.
- Site of puncture is defined by palpating the iliac crest, which corresponds to L3–L4. Hold the needle between index and middle fingers. In children, instead of lumbar puncture needle with stylet, simple hypodermic needle is commonly used. This should be avoided.
- Gently introduce the needle in midline at above mentioned space, needle being directed toward umbilicus. Entry into the subarachnoid space is indicated by giving the way sensation and free flow of CSF.

- Collect the CSF 0.5 cc in ethylenediaminetetraacetic acid (EDTA) bulb for cell count and 1 cc in plain bulb for biochemistry. It should also be collected in sterile bulb for culture.
- CSF for cell count should be examined at the earliest, usually within 30 minutes.
- Remove the needle and apply firm pressure for few minutes.
- Apply tincture benzoin seal at puncture site.
- In a case of raised ICP, head should be kept little down to prevent herniation of brain through foramen magnum.
- Monitor the patient for some time after the procedure for pulse and respiration.

Complications

- Infection
- Coning
- Headache
- Injury to local structures
- Epidermoid tumor (if hypodermic needles are used instead of lumbar puncture needles)

SUBDURAL TAP

It is indicated for diagnosis of subdural hematoma, effusion, and empyema.[2,7]

Technique

- Before subdural tapping, ultrasonography or CT scan study of cranium is desirable.
- Informed written consent is must.
- Scalp should be shaved, at least 5 cm posterior to the anterior fontanel and 5 cm lateral to midline and anteriorly up to forehead.
- Sedation may be required in irritable infants.
- Child should be in supine position with head at the edge of the table.
- One person should hold the head at the middle position and another person hold the shoulders **(Fig. 23.2.15)**.[2]
- Strict aseptic and antiseptic precautions should be taken.
- Sterilize the area.
- Lateral margins of anterior fontanel are palpated along the coronal sutures and the site is chosen either far lateral as possible or at the area of maximum transillumination.
- It should be at least 2–3 cm from the midline to prevent injury to the underlying sagittal sinus.
- A zig-zag puncture is used to prevent later leakage of subdural fluid.
- A disposable no. 20 G needle is used. The skin is first pulled to one side and then needle is passed perpendicular to the scalp through the suture line and into the subdural space to a depth of approximately 0.3–0.6 cm. A definite pop giving the way is felt on entering the subdural space.

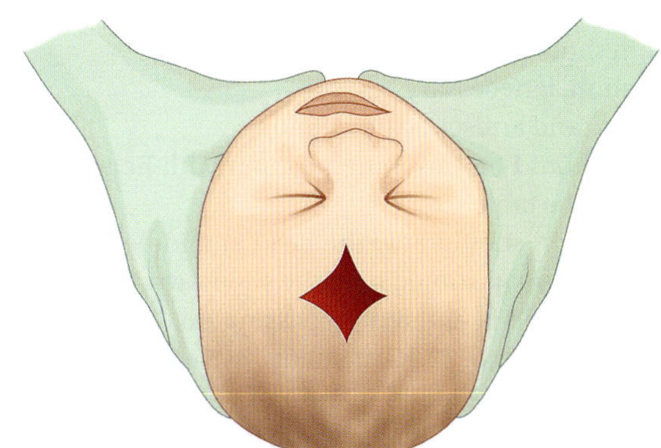

Fig. 23.2.15: Position of head for performing subdural tap.
Source: Prajapati BS. Essential Procedures in Pediatrics, 1st edition. New Delhi: Jaypee Brothers Medical Publishers (P) Ltd; 2003.

The flow of fluid will be there on entering the subdural space. If flow of fluid is not there, slight adjustment or rotation of the needle may be necessary.

- The subdural fluid is allowed to drain spontaneously. The fluid should not be aspirated for fear of drawing pial vessels into the point of needle.
- The subdural fluid is collected in EDTA and plain tubes for examination. Smear for Gram stain should be prepared. It should also be collected for culture.
- The subdural tap must be performed on both the sides. Samples from both the sides should be kept separate and labeled properly indicating right and left side.
- Maximum 10 mL of fluid should be tapped from each side.
- Subdural fluid will be either blood stained or xanthochromic but not clear. If it is clear, it is most likely CSF through ventricular tapping.
- Remove the needle and sterile benzoin seal is done. Dressing should be done tightly with sterile gauze and adhesive tape.

Complications

- Trauma to blood vessels and hematoma formation
- Infection leading to subdural empyema

VENTRICULAR TAP

This procedure is useful in newborns for diagnosis of ventriculitis and intraventricular hemorrhage. It is also performed to relieve the acute rise of ICP in noncommunicating hydrocephalus. In some conditions, it may be done to administer intraventricular drugs.[7]

Technique

- Before ventricular tapping, ultrasonography or computed axial tomography (CAT) scan study of cranium should be done.

- Informed written consent should be taken.
- Scalp should be shaved.
- Sedation, if necessary
- Aseptic and antiseptic precautions
- Child should be in supine position with head at middle edge of the table.
- One person should hold the head at middle position and another person should hold the shoulders.
- The ventricle is entered by passing no. 23 FG needle in neonates and no. 22 FG in infants, 4–5 cm long disposable needle through lateral margin of anterior fontanel and keeping the direction of needle slightly inward toward inner canthus of opposite eye or nasion **(Fig. 23.2.16)**.[2]
- Depending on the degree of ventricular dilatation and size of the patient, the ventricle is reached at the depth of about 2.5 cm.
- Entering the ventricle, gives the way.
- No syringe suction should be applied.
- CSF should be collected in EDTA and plain tubes for examination. Smear should be prepared for Gram stain.
- After removing the needle, press at puncture site for some time.
- Sterile benzoin seal is done. Dressing should be done with sterile gauze and adhesive tape.
- In a case of hydrocephalus, CSF can be drained in large quantity.
- For administering drugs in ventricles, drug should be taken in the syringe and after ventricular puncture, it should be attached with the needle. Let the CSF come in syringe, get the medicine diluted in CSF and then inject back into the ventricle. Drug should not be diluted in any solution.

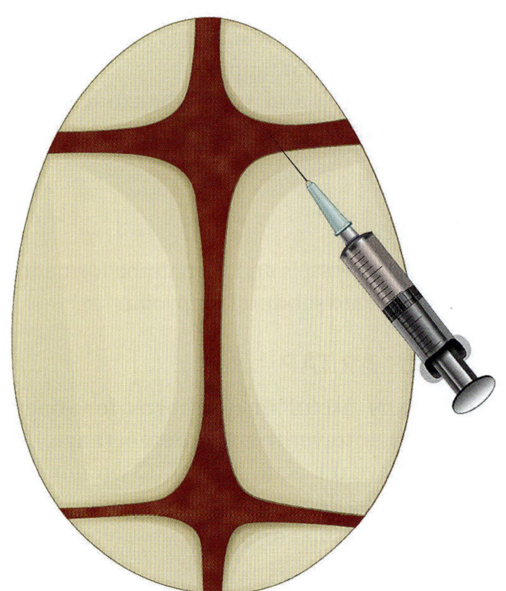

Fig. 23.2.16: Ventricular tapping—the needle should be directed forward and inward toward nasion.
Source: Prajapati BS. Essential Procedures in Pediatrics, 1st edition. New Delhi: Jaypee Brothers Medical Publishers (P) Ltd; 2003.

Complications

- Ventriculitis
- Injury to brain tissues
- Intraventricular hemorrhage

NASOGASTRIC TUBE INSERTION

Nasogastric tube is passed for either aspiration of gastric contents or administration of feeds or therapeutic substances. Nowadays, silastic and polyethylene tubes are being used because they have less tissue reactions.[7]

Indications

Diagnostic

- Gastric aspirate test for diagnosis of neonatal septicemia
- Shake test for lung maturity in preterm babies
- Examination of gastric contents for *Mycobacterium tuberculosis*
- Assessment of upper gastrointestinal (GI) tract bleeding
- Measurement of gastric volume

Therapeutic

- Paralytic ileus
- Intestinal obstruction
- Enteral feeding
- Administration of therapeutic substances

Contraindications

- Esophageal stricture
- Ingestion of alkali—may cause esophageal perforation
- Head and neck injury preventing passage of tube
- Nasal fracture

Technique

- The head is raised in semiupright position.
- The distance from nose to earlobe and from ear lobe to xiphoid process is determined to measure the length of the tube to be passed. The point is marked on the tube **(Figs. 23.2.17A and B)**.
- The more patent nostril is selected for passing the tube.
- The terminal part of the tube is lubricated with a lubricant. It is avoided in newborns to prevent aspiration of an oily substance. In that case, it is wet with water.
- The tube is passed into the nostril, its curve directs downward as it passes along the floor of the nose. In case of difficulty, it is tried in another nostril. Resistance is felt

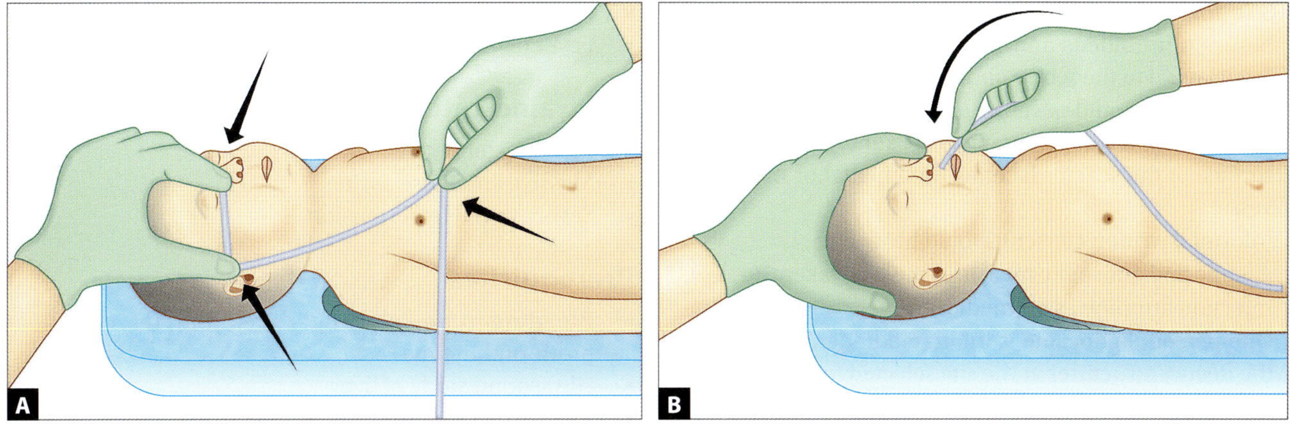

Figs. 23.2.17A and B: Method of inserting a nasogastric tube in a child.
Source: World Health Organization. Management of the child with a serious infection or severe malnutrition: guidelines for care at the first-referral level in Developing Countries Department of Child and Adolescent Health and Development. Geneva: World Health Organization; 2000.

when it reaches the nasopharynx. Getting the patient to sip a little water helps to overcome it.

- With swallowing of the saliva or water by the patients, the tube is advanced into the esophagus.
- If the patient gags or the tube coils up in the mouth, the tube is withdrawn partly and again it is passed.
- The tube is passed up to the mark as measured length of the tube to be passed.
- Confirmation of proper placement is done by the following tests:
    - Aspiration of stomach contents on applying suction at the outer end of the tube with a syringe indicates that the tube lies in the stomach.
    - Air is injected into the tube while epigastric area is auscultated. A sound is heard if the tube is in the stomach.
    - Placing a tube in a glass of water and escape of air bubbles in the water indicate that the tube lies in the trachea.
    - Placement of a radiopaque tube can be assessed by radiography.
- The tube is fixed with a tape in a butterfly fashion around the tube or with vertical tapping over the nose and the tube. The tapping is done in such a way that the tube rests in the middle of the nasal lumen and not directly in contact with mucosa. It is not taped over the forehead as it may cause pressure necrosis of the nose.
- The feed or drug should be allowed to go in the tube by gravity method. It should not be pushed by piston. The tube should be flushed with water periodically.
- While removing the tube, pinch the tube end to prevent spilling of the contents into the trachea.

Complications

- Pulmonary aspiration
- Esophageal perforation
- Gastric perforation
- Nasal necrosis
- Esophageal stricture

Instead of nasogastric tubing, nowadays orogastric tubing is preferred to avoid certain complications.

GASTRIC LAVAGE

It is useful in removing the poisonous substance from the stomach. In corrosives and hydrocarbons ingestion, gastric lavage is contraindicated. In corrosives, passing the tube may cause perforation. Since passing the gastric tube is likely to induce vomiting, it increases the risk of aspiration of hydrocarbons into the trachea and lungs, which causes pneumonia.

After passing the tube in the stomach as described in nasogastric tube insertion, lavage of the stomach using aliquots of normal saline is done in cases of poisoning. It is continued till the color of the lavage is normal.

ABDOMINAL PARACENTESIS

Abdominal paracentesis is performed for diagnostic purpose in case of ascites, peritonitis, and hemorrhage. In huge ascites, it is also done to relieve discomfort and respiratory embarrassment. In some situations, drugs may be instilled in peritoneal cavity such as malignancies.

Technique

- The patient should be placed in supine position. If the patient is not comfortable in supine position, reclining or upright position may be used.

- Site for paracentesis is selected in midline, midway between umbilicus and pubic symphysis or in an iliac fossa lateral to the rectus abdominis.
- The needle should never be advanced through a surgical scar because it can penetrate bowel adherent to the under surface of the scar, or lacerate an omental or mesenteric vessel.
- Informed written consent should be taken.
- Aseptic and antiseptic measures must be taken.
- Injection atropine as premedication
- One percent lignocaine is infiltrated under skin and into the deeper structures at the site selected for paracentesis. Wait for few minutes for full effect of anesthetic agent.
- The hypodermic needle 20 FG is attached to 20 mL syringe. It is passed into the peritoneal cavity perpendicular to the skin. As the needle enters the peritoneal cavity, it gives the way and ascitic fluid starts to drain through the needle.
- In a case of tense ascites, needle should be passed obliquely or skin should be retracted caudally before insertion of the needle to produce a Z-track effect on withdrawing the needle so that needle tract after paracentesis gets sealed properly and persistent drainage can be prevented after removal of the needle.
- After removal of fluid, 10–15 mL for diagnostic purpose, the needle is withdrawn and a seal of tincture benzoin is applied locally.
- If the paracentesis is for therapeutic purpose, the needle should be connected with IV set and regulator of IV set is adjusted in such a way that ascitic fluid is drained slowly. One liter of fluid may be drained over a period of 2–3 hours.
- The patient should be watched following the procedure.

COMPLICATIONS

- Intestinal perforation or laceration
- Peritonitis
- Postparacentesis shock
- Electrolyte imbalance
- Hypoproteinemia
- Perforation of urinary bladder
- Pneumoperitoneum

LIVER BIOPSY

Nowadays, liver biopsy is done under the ultrasound (USG) guidance rather than blind biopsy.[7]

Indications

- Chronic hepatitis
- Undiagnosed hepatomegaly
- Neonatal hepatitis
- Cirrhosis of liver
- Fever of unknown origin

Contraindications

- Bleeding tendency
- Massive and tense ascites
- Severe portal hypertension

Prerequisites

- Bleeding time, clotting time, platelet count, and prothrombin time
- Ultrasound study of liver
- *Premedication:* Atropine 0.01 mg/kg IM 30 minutes before the procedure.

Technique

- Vim–Silverman needle, Menghini's needle, and Tru-cut needles are used for liver biopsy. Tru-cut needle is disposable, easy to operate, and has more success rate, so it is common in use.
- Informed written consent is a must.
- Patient is kept in supine position, near the edge of the bed or table with the right arm under the head and left arm by the side.
- Preparation of the local area
- Aseptic and antiseptic precautions are must.
- 1% lignocaine is infiltrated in the skin, intercostal muscles, and Glisson's capsule. Wait for some time for good effect of the anesthetic agent. Some children may require sedation or general anesthesia.
- The Tru-cut needle is introduced under USG guidance into the liver substance with the inner needle retracted. The latter is then advanced, holding the outer cutting sheath steady. The outer sheath is then advanced to cut the liver in the biopsy notch. The whole apparatus is then withdrawn together quickly. The entire sequence should take only few seconds.
- The Vim–Silverman needle has trocar and bifid needle to cut the liver tissue. In Menghini's needle, the cut piece of liver is sucked into the syringe applied with negative pressure.
- On removal of the needle, the puncture site is sealed with tincture of benzoin.

THORACOCENTESIS (INTERCOSTAL DRAINAGE)

Thoracocentesis refers to temporary insertion of a needle or a catheter into the pleural space for removal of fluid or air from the pleural cavity. The fluid is collected for diagnostic purpose and in some situations, it is done for therapeutic purpose to remove fluid or air, which is in large quantity and causes respiratory embarrassment.[8] Drugs can also be instilled in the pleural cavity by this procedure, if it is indicated, such as in a case of malignancy.

Technique

- Written consent is must.
- *Injection:* Atropine as premedication
- Site of insertion of needle can be decided by chest X-ray, dull note on percussion, and USG study of thorax. Best way to perform the procedure is under USG guidance.
- It should be performed in sitting position of the patient. Patient can lean forward on the table of suitable height with head resting on his forearms **(Fig. 23.2.18)**.
- Strict aseptic and antiseptic measures should be taken.
- 1% lignocaine is infiltrated at the upper border of the rib below the space chosen. Anesthetizing wide area and generous infiltration of local anesthetic agent for good anesthesia help to get good cooperation of the patient, performing the whole procedure comfortably leading to successful performance with minimal chances of complications. Wait for some time for good effect of anesthetic agent.
- A wide-bore needle is connected on one side of the three-way stopcock and opposite to it a syringe is attached. Three-way stopcock is arranged in such a way that there is a single track between the needle, stopcock, and syringe.
- The needle is inserted into the chest in the same manner as for the anesthetic needle, finding the intercostal space and stepping over the lower rib with care, thereby preventing damage to underlying structures **(Fig. 23.2.19)**.[2] Slight suction is applied to the syringe so that the fluid is aspirated in the syringe immediately as the needle enters the pleural space.
- Fluid should be withdrawn slowly and steadily.
- A forceps should be attached to the needle at the skin level, which helps to prevent excessively deep insertion of the needle into the thorax.
- The fluid is aspirated in the syringe and then three-way stopcock is turned to connect the syringe with the outlet, which is attached to IV set.
- Collect the fluid in EDTA and plain tubes. It is also collected for culture. Smear should be prepared for Gram's stain and Ziehl–Neelsen stain.
- The three-way tap is now turned again to connect the syringe with the needle and the pleural space, a further aspiration is carried out. It is expelled into the drainage bag by turning the three-way tap. The drainage bag or bottle should be placed well below the level of the patient's chest.
- As fluid is removed, the lung expands and this often makes the patient to cough.
- The needle is withdrawn and puncture site is covered with a benzoin seal. A sterile gauze is put over it and adhesive tape is applied.

Complications

- Pneumothorax
- Hemothorax
- Infection
- Unilateral pulmonary edema
- Hypoproteinemia

7th intercostal space

Fig. 23.2.18: Another position for doing thoracocentesis.
Source: Johnson KB. The Harriet Lane Handbook—a manual for pediatric house officers, 13th edition. New Delhi: Jaypee Brothers Medical Publishers (P) Ltd; 1993.

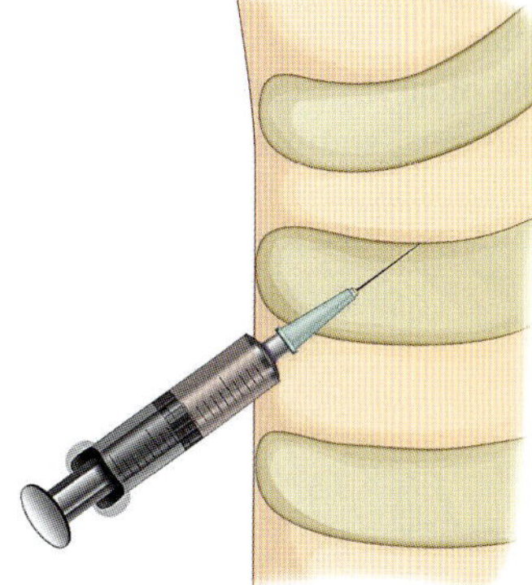

Fig. 23.2.19: Site of needle for pleural fluid aspiration.
Source: Prajapati BS. Essential Procedures in Pediatrics, 1st edition. New Delhi: Jaypee Brothers Medical Publishers (P) Ltd; 2003.

ENDOTRACHEAL INTUBATION

Endotracheal intubation is a procedure, which every pediatrician and one working in intensive care units must be well conversant with.[9] The critically ill patient often requires endotracheal intubation. It secures patent airway. It is a prerequisite for mechanical ventilation. Endotracheal suction can most efficiently be done through an endotracheal tube (ET). It is indicated when bag and mask resuscitation fails in a case of an asphyxiated newborn.

INDICATIONS

- *In neonatal asphyxia:*
  - Bag and mask resuscitation fails.
  - Apparently, stillborn baby after adequate suctioning of upper airways
  - Infants with diaphragmatic hernia
  - Meconium aspiration
- Cardiorespiratory arrest due to any cause
- Central nervous system depression in a case of head injury or comatose child
- Diseases of peripheral nervous system, poliomyelitis, Guillain-Barré syndrome, tetanus, organophosphorus poisoning, etc.
- Administration of general anesthesia

Equipment

- Laryngoscope—with straight blade for neonates
- Endotracheal tubes for various sizes with stylet **(Table 23.2.1)**

Technique

- The patient is placed in a supine position. The operator stands beyond the patient's head. Patient's neck is slightly extended with the head in midline.
- Clear the oropharynx with gentle suctioning.
- Empty the stomach.
- Hold the handle of laryngoscope in left hand with thumb and first three fingers; stabilize the hand with fifth finger resting on patient's cheek. The blade should be pointing away from oneself.
- Open the baby's mouth and push the tongue left with the back of right forefinger and steady the head with the rest of right hand.
- While visualizing insert the blade, midline until the tip is between base of tongue and epiglottis within the vallecula **(Figs. 23.2.20A and B)**.[2]
- If the infant is making respiratory effort, free flow of oxygen with an oxygen tubing held close to the infant's mouth and nose is to be provided during intubation.
- Open the mouth further by pulling on laryngoscope handle, simultaneously tilt the blade tip upward slightly to elevate epiglottis and visualize the glottis. Use base of the tongue as pivot rather than maxilla.

TABLE 23.2.1: Endotracheal tube size according to weight of child.

Weight/age	*Endotracheal tubes size (ID in mm)*
<1,000 g	2.5
1,000–2,000 g	3.0
2,000–3,000 g	3.5
>3,000 g	4.0
1–5 years	4–5
5–12 years	5–6.5

Approximately size of ET, internal diameter (ID) in mm = Age (years) + 16/4.

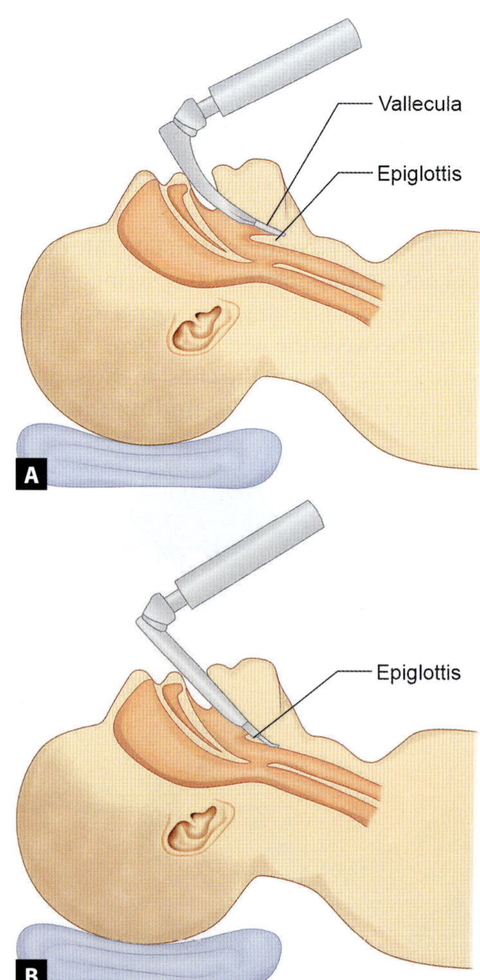

Figs. 23.2.20A and B: Position of laryngoscope blade when using (A) Curved blade, it is in the vallecula; (B) Straight blade, it is over the epiglottis.
Source: Prajapati BS. Essential Procedures in Pediatrics, 1st edition. New Delhi: Jaypee Brothers Medical Publishers (P) Ltd; 2003.

- Suction is needed.
- Have the assistant to palpate suprasternal notch with index finger, applying gentle pressure, if desired.
- Hold the tube with concave curve anterior and pass it down to right side of the mouth, outside the blade, along with maintaining visualization.
- As the patient inspires, pass the tube through cords 2 cm into trachea or until immediately after tip passes under assistant's finger in suprasternal notch.
- The tube is then held firmly at the lips with the right hand, and the laryngoscope and stylet are carefully removed.
- Initially, confirmation of the tube placement is accomplished by attaching a resuscitation bag with the connector and ventilating the infant. With correctly placed tube, the air entry is heard on both sides of the chest, breath sounds are of equal intensity and air is not heard entering the stomach. While listening to the breath sounds, the stethoscope is to be placed at approximately the nipple line.
- Note the centimeter marks on the tube at the level of upper lips and then secure the tube to the infant's face.
- Final confirmation of placement of the tube can be obtained by chest film, if it is needed.
- Attempts to intubate should not exceed 30 seconds. If you are unable to intubate within 30 seconds, abort and continue with bag and mask and then try again after a few minutes. Repeated attempts may cause serious glottic edema and bleeding.
- Intubation is not a matter of prestige. If you are unable to do so, please ask for help.
- ET route is also used for administration of some drugs such as epinephrine, atropine, and naloxone.

Complications

- Hypoxia
- Bradycardia
- Apnea
- Pneumothorax
- Injury and lacerations to tongue, gums, pharynx, epiglottis, trachea, vocal cords, etc.
- Infections
- Postextubation stridor can be managed by nebulized epinephrine or steroids.

Some physicians prefer nasotracheal intubation when long-term ventilation is required.

SUPRAPUBIC BLADDER ASPIRATION

This procedure is performed to collect noncontaminated urine sample in neonates and infants.[6] It is a safe and reliable way of collecting urine samples. It is easy, especially in neonates, as bladder is an intra-abdominal organ in these patients unlike a pelvic organ in older children and adults.

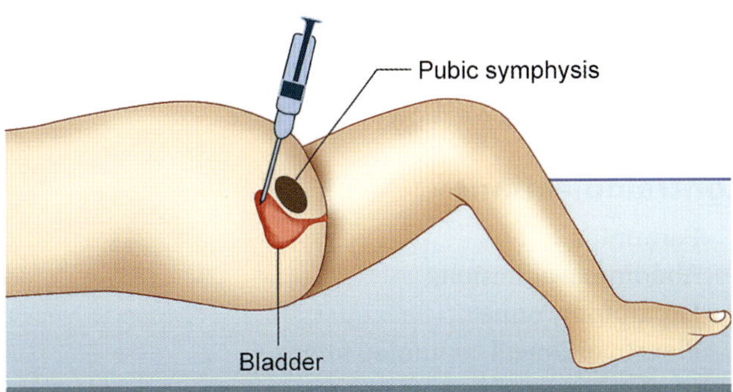

Fig. 23.2.21: Suprapubic bladder puncture technique.
Source: Prajapati BS. Essential Procedures in Pediatrics, 1st edition. New Delhi: Jaypee Brothers Medical Publishers (P) Ltd; 2003.

Technique

- The infant is placed on a flat surface in supine position.
- The assistant stands opposite the operator and immobilizes the infant by grasping the thorax with one hand and thighs and hips with the other.
- Make sure that the bladder is full.
- Local part is cleaned. Aseptic and antiseptic measures are a must.
- A 10 cc disposable syringe with 22 FG, 4–5 cm long needle is taken.
- The pubic symphysis is located with one finger and the needle is inserted 2 cm above the symphysis in the midline with syringe held at 10–20° angles from perpendicular **(Fig. 23.2.21)**.[2]
- With a single steady motion, the needle is inserted until a perceptive change in resistance is felt as the needle enters the bladder.
- Light aspiration is applied to aspirate the urine specimen.
- After removal of needle, a seal of tincture benzoin is applied at puncture site.

PERITONEAL DIALYSIS

Dialysis involves the use of semipermeable membranes that permit the simultaneous passage of smaller molecular weight solutes and water while retarding or inhibiting the movement of large-sized particles. The basic principle controlling the transmembrane movement of solute and water are similar whether the membrane is artificial (hemodialysis) or natural (peritoneal dialysis).[9]

Indications

- Blood urea >300 mg/dL
- Serum hyperkalemia—K^+ >6.5 mEq/L not responding to medical line of treatment
- Severe acidosis

- Pulmonary edema
- Acute left ventricular failure
- Drug intoxications such as barbiturates and salicylates
- Life-threatening electrolyte imbalance

Contraindications

- Peritonitis.
- Abdominal adhesions
- Laparotomy done
- Pleuroperitoneal communication

Technique (Fig. 23.2.22)[2]

- Informed written consent
- Aseptic and antiseptic measures are must.
- Injection atropine 0.01 mg/kg IM 30 minutes before the procedure as the premedication
- Sedation, if required
- Proper restraining
- Bladder is emptied by its own or catheterization, if it is necessary
- Abdominal wall is prepared, painting spirit—betadine spirit. Towel draping
- The catheter is usually placed in the midline few centimeters below the umbilicus.

If midline insertion is not possible, the catheter can be inserted in the flank area, outside the line of inferior epigastric artery.

- The site is anesthetized by injecting 1% lignocaine up to peritoneum.

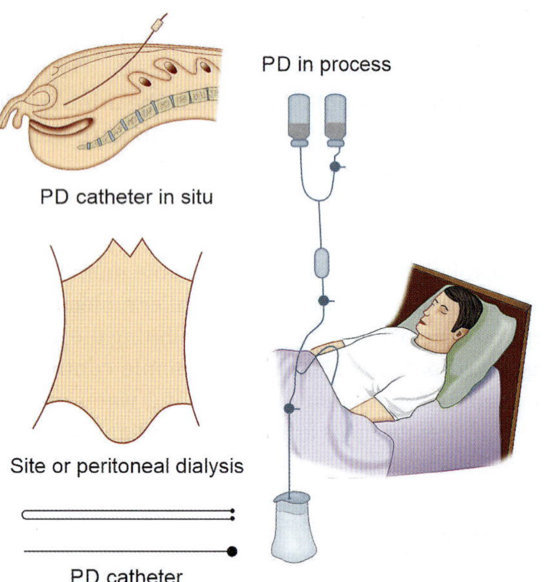

Fig. 23.2.22: Peritoneal dialysis (PD).
Source: Prajapati BS. Essential Procedures in Pediatrics, 1st edition. New Delhi: Jaypee Brothers Medical Publishers (P) Ltd; 2003.

- If there is no ascites, distend the abdomen with 10 mL/kg dialysate solution using 17–20 FG angiocath or needle.
- Needle is withdrawn and a knife blade is used to enlarge the puncture wound in the skin.
- If ascites is present, a very small penetrating incision is made in the skin and the trocar with catheter is stabilized with the fingers of one hand on the skin while the other hand introduces the trocar through the abdominal wall with an alternating drilling motion.
- Penetration up to peritoneum is detected by a definite sensation of giving the way and also by the appearance of fluid in the catheter when trocar is removed.
- On reaching the peritoneal cavity and before removing the trocar, the catheter is gradually advanced in the peritoneal cavity in right or left paracolic gutter and trocar is gradually withdrawn.
- When the catheter is sufficiently introduced in the peritoneal cavity, trocar is removed totally. All the fenestrations on the catheter must be within the peritoneal cavity to avoid SC fluid infiltration in the abdominal wall. In neonates and infants, IV catheters or simple feeding tube can be used.
- The catheter should be stabilized with adhesive plaster.
- The catheter is connected with the administration tubing through small connector, and dialysis fluid is flown.
- Because hyperkalemia is often present, potassium-free fluid is used for the first three–six cycles.
- Time of input of dialysis fluid will be about 10–15 minutes. The fluid is kept in the peritoneal cavity for about 30 minutes. Time for output of dialysis fluid will be about 15–20 minutes. Each cycle will take about an hour. First few cycles should be of half an hour (rapid cycles).
- Record the weight of the patient prior to the procedure and every 12 hours.
- Total duration of dialysis is about 40 hours depending on the clinical and biochemical parameters.
- Warm the dialysate to body temperature.
- Infuse it by gravity flow.
- Each cycle should be of 30–50 mL/kg.
- Blood sugar, blood urea, serum creatinine, serum electrolytes and serum proteins should be checked 12 hourly.
- In the presence of fluid overload, use hypertonic dialysate.
- Tip of the catheter should be sent for culture.
- Close the site of dialysis by sterile bandage
- Peritoneal dialysis-related problems such as pain in abdomen, diarrhea, dyspnea, bleeding, and fluid delivery should be sorted out appropriately.

Complications

- Pain may be due to over distention, peritonitis, etc.
- Bleeding

- Dialysate leak
- Outflow obstruction
- Peritonitis
- Metabolic complications
- Thrombosis
- Pulmonary complications

RENAL BIOPSY

Indications

- Steroid-resistant nephrotic syndrome
- Asymptomatic proteinuria
- Glomerulonephritis associated with conditions such as systemic lupus erythematosus, Henoch-Schönlein purpura, etc.
- Rapidly progressive glomerulonephritis.

Contraindications

- Bleeding diathesis
- Solitary functioning kidney
- Ectopic/horseshoe-shaped kidney
- Severe uncontrolled hypertension

Prerequisites

- Bleeding time, clotting time, partial thromboplastin time (PTT) or activated partial thromboplastin time (APTT), and platelets count
- Blood grouping and cross-matching
- Hypertension and uremia should be controlled.
- Informed written consent is a must.

Technique[10]

- Atropine 0.01 mg/kg IM before 30 minutes of the procedure.
- The patient is placed in the prone position on a firm bed. A pillow is placed under patient's abdomen. This compresses and fixes the kidneys to the posterior abdominal wall, bringing the kidneys closer to the skin and limiting possible ballottement of the kidney by the biopsy needle.
- Ultrasonography is commonly used to mark the location of kidneys and point of entry of the needle into the kidney perpendicular to the skin surface and to obtain depth of tissue from skin surface. Usually, lower pole of left kidney is selected for biopsy.
- The area is prepared and local anesthesia is given. Irritable children may need general anesthesia.
- A 23-gauge exploring lumbar puncture needle is passed downward and obliquely toward the lower pole of the kidney. A needle can be felt going through different structures and renal capsule. Experienced person feels "give-in" feeling up on penetration of capsule of kidney.
- The patient is asked to take slow deep breathings. If the needle is in the kidney, a characteristic pendular movement is seen with respiration, the hub of needle swings through a wide arch, moving toward head during inspiration, and toward buttock during expiration. If the needle is not in the kidney tissue, it is slightly advanced until it penetrates kidneys and moves characteristically on breathing. The depth of the kidney below the skin is measured on the stem of the needle.
- A small nick is made over anesthetized area with a scalpel.
- Franklin modified Vim-Silverman needle and Tru-cut needle are commonly used in the practice. Tru-cut needle is easy to use and having less failure rate. Therefore, Tru-cut needle is preferred nowadays.
- Tru-cut needle is one-piece apparatus with a length of 11.4 cm or 15 cm. The needle with cannula covering the obturator is advanced in the kidney to desired length in a direction perpendicular to skin surface.
- The patient is asked to hold the breath in deep inspiration.
- The obturator is advanced by firm tap on the handle. The specimen is cut by downward movement of cannula over obturator.
- Entire assembly is removed.
- The patient is asked to breathe normally.
- Firm pressure is applied over biopsy site for few minutes and the site is sealed with tincture benzoin. Two good cores of tissue (8–10 mm long) are needed for adequate histological examination. One is immediately fixed in buffered formalin and other in saline (for immunofluorescence study).

Postprocedure Management

- The patient is asked to remain in prone position for 2 hours and in bed for 24 hours.
- Monitoring temperature, pulse, respiratory rate (RR), and blood pressure (BP) 1 hourly for 6 hours and then 4 hourly for 24 hours.
- Urine should be collected in separate bottles during each voiding and should be checked for hematuria.
- Patient is asked to take ample liquids orally.
- Diuretics may be given in case of oliguria to flush any clot in the passage.
- If no frank hematuria and vitals are normal, patient can be discharged after 24 hours with instructions not to do exertion for a week.

Complications

- Hematuria
- Perinephric hematoma
- Arteriovenous (AV) fistula

PERICARDIOCENTESIS

Pericardiocentesis is a procedure for removal of fluid from pericardial cavity for diagnostic purpose or to relieve cardiac tamponade. It is occasionally a life-saving procedure.[9] It is a risky procedure. It should be performed only by skilled person under continuous cardiac monitoring. Echocardiographic diagnosis is must before performing the procedure. It gives idea regarding amount of fluid and also helps to determine the anatomical approach.

Prerequisites

- Echocardiographic diagnosis
- Coagulation profile
- Resuscitation kit including defibrillator
- Cardiac monitor
- IV line
- Premedication with injection atropine 0.01 mg/kg IM 30 minutes before the procedure

Technique

- Informed written consent should be taken.
- Sedation may be required in some patients. If possible, it should be avoided.
- Child should be seated leaning backward at approximately 60° and carefully restrained.
- The best site is xiphocostal angle. The other sites are fourth, fifth, or sixth intercostal spaces 1–2 cm medial to the border of cardiac dullness on percussion.
- Aseptic and antiseptic precautions are must.
- 1% xylocaine is infiltrated in the skin at left xiphocostal angle, 3–4 cm below left costal margin. The needle is advanced initially perpendicular to the skin surface and after traversing the soft tissue under the rib cage, its tip is pointed to the left shoulder. While advancing the needle in the deeper structures, if it reaches to pericardial cavity, the pericardial fluid is withdrawn in the syringe. Local anesthetic agent should not be injected in the pericardial cavity.
- The pericardiocentesis needle is passed along the same path until the fluid is obtained. The distance from skin to the pericardium is <5 cm in a child. A distinct "give" or "pop" is felt when the pericardium is punctured. Pericardial fluid can then be aspirated.
- Getting the fluid confirms the position of needle into the pericardial cavity. Normal saline can be injected under two-dimensional (2D) echo monitoring, which shows bubbles of saline.
- If the blood or bloody fluid is withdrawn, it is vital to determine if cardiac chamber or coronary artery has been punctured. Still uremia and malignant diseases can give rise to hemorrhagic pericardial effusion. Blood obtained from heart or coronary vessel clots immediately.
- Fluid is sent for appropriate examinations.
- The needle is withdrawn and benzoin seal is done at puncture site.
- Postprocedure monitoring of heart rate, RR, and BP should be done. 2D echo may be performed to study postpericardiocentesis condition.

Complications

- Hemopericardium
- Arrhythmias
- Vasovagal reactions
- Infection
- Pneumothorax
- Air embolism
- Perforation of an abdominal viscus, commonly stomach
- Cardiac arrest and death

FINE-NEEDLE ASPIRATION BIOPSY

Fine-needle aspiration biopsy (FNAB) is very useful for cytological and bacteriological evaluation of a mass or a lymph node. It is minimally invasive and requires no sedation. It aids in tissue diagnosis and in determining the course of management.

Requirements

- 1^2 1.5^2 20–25 FG needles. 22 FG 1^2 long is the most commonly used size of needle.
- 10–20 mL plastic disposable syringes
- Clean glass slides
- About 70–90% ethanol for routine wet fixation
- Containers for culture media whenever needed

Technique

- Sterilize the area.
- Anesthesia is usually not required, local anesthetic agent may be used in uncooperative and irritable children.
- Immobilize the lump to be biopsied between your thumb and finger with one hand.
- Hold the syringe in the other hand and insert needle into the assigned area, perpendicular to the skin surface and position the needle within the target tissue.
- Pull the syringe plunger to apply negative pressure.
- While maintaining suction, make several passes through the mass or node.
- Release the negative pressure while needle remains in the target tissue.
- Withdraw the needle.
- Detach the needle, draw 2–3 mL air into the syringe, reattach the needle, and blow the aspirates on to the slide.

- Apply the pressure over the puncture site with cotton swab for 5 minutes.
- Deep biopsies can be done with assistance of radiological imaging techniques such as USG.
- The following situations can give unsatisfactory yield during FNAB:
    - When needle misses the lesion tangentially.
    - When central area is cystic, necrotic, or hemorrhagic and devoid of diagnostic material.
    - When there is a small malignant lesion close to a dominant benign mass.
    - When the target tissue is fibrosclerotic and poor in cells.

REFERENCES

1. Nair MK, Leena ML, Ajithkumar K. Concept of health care counseling for pediatricians. Indian Pediatr. 2016;53(11):961-3.
2. Prajapati BS. Essential Procedures In Pediatrics, 1st edition. New Delhi: Jaypee Brothers Medical Publishers (P) Ltd; 2003.
3. Koebke J, McFarland E, Mein M. Venipuncture Procedures. In: Slockbower JM, Blumenfeld TA (Eds). Collection and Handling of Laboratory Specimens—a Practical Guide. Philadelphia: JB Lippincott Co; 1983. pp. 3-45.
4. Chameides L. Vascular access. In: Textbook of Pediatric Advanced Life Support. USA: American Heart Association American Academy of Pediatrics; 1988. pp. 37-46.
5. Silver HK, Kempe CH, Bruyn HB. Pediatric procedures. In: Handbook of Pediatrics, 13th edition. Singapore: Lange-Maruzen Asia; 1980. pp. 629-44.
6. Singh M. Procedures. In: Singh M (Ed). Care of the Newborn, 4th edition. New Delhi: Sagar Publications. 1991. pp. 340-67.
7. Laing IA, Doyle E. Practical procedures. In: Campbell AGM, Mclntosh N (Eds). Forfar and Arneil's Textbook of Pediatrics, 5th edition. New York: Churchill Livingstone; 1998. pp. 1829-47.
8. Subramanyam L, Thangavelu S, Somu N. Pathophysiology of pleural fluid collection and management of empyema. In: Somu N, Subramanyam L (Eds). Essentials of Pediatric Pulmonology, 2nd edition. Madras: Siva and Co; 1996. pp. 142-9.
9. Singhi S. Procedures in pediatric intensive care. In: Sachdev HPS, Puri RK, Bagga A, Choudhury P (Eds). Principles of Pediatric and Neonatal Emergencies, 1st edition. New Delhi: Jaypee Brothers Medical Publishers (P) Ltd. 1999. pp. 364-72.
10. Prabha S. Renal biopsy in children. In: Nammalwar BR, Vijayakumar M (Eds). Principles and Practice of Pediatric Nephrology, 2nd edition. New Delhi: Jaypee Brothers Medical Publishers (P) Ltd; 1991. pp. 85-9.

23.3 Physiotherapy and Rehabilitation

Somu Sivabalan, Sureshkumar S

INTRODUCTION

Physiotherapy or physical therapy aims to treat and manage any disease or condition physically, enabling people to reach their maximum potential. Physiotherapists or physical therapists are healthcare professionals who diagnose and treat individuals of all ages with illnesses or injuries that limit their ability to mobilize and perform functional activities.

Physical therapy aims to provide treatment techniques that promote mobility, reduce pain, restore function, and prevent disability. In addition, by developing fitness and wellness-oriented programs, it devises strategies to prevent immobility even before it occurs.

REHABILITATION

Rehabilitation means restoring good condition, operability, and capacity to lead a productive life through therapy and education.[1] Pediatric rehabilitation assists in the early detection and management of a variety of injuries, disorders, and diseases that affect the muscles, bones, and joints of infants, children, and adolescents. Optimization of function is brought about by a combination of medications prescribed by the pediatrician and the usage of physical modalities. These include physical training with therapeutic exercise, movement and activity modification, adaptive equipment, chest physiotherapy (to mobilize and bring the secretions out from the airways) and assistive devices, orthotics (braces), and prosthetics, in turn, helping the child to regain independence and in leading a near normal life.

The rehabilitation team consists of physiotherapists, occupational therapists, speech and language pathologists, psychologists, social workers, special educators, prosthetists, and orthotist headed by a physician.

AIMS OF REHABILITATION

The aims of rehabilitation in children include the following:

- To improve the child's gross and fine motor skills
- Maintain balance and coordination
- Improve strength and endurance
- Help in cognitive and sensory processing and integration
- Promote mobility
- Manage pain
- Clearance of secretion clearance and improved expansion of the chest

Goals, Outcome, and Intervention

The goals and outcome as well as the interventions needed to achieve the above aims of rehabilitation are as follows:[2]

- Primary prevention of disability through education and treatment
- Secondary prevention of disabilities such as contractures or deformities, or improvement of the same
- Attain maximum functional goals expected by the child and his/her family
- Improve the lung function and aid in the clearance of secretions
- Help the children lead a near normal life with their disability and to integrate them with the society
- Provide appropriate wheelchairs, orthotics and prosthetics, and modify architectural barriers.

Evaluation

It is the most important component to assess the extent and severity of involvement and also to devise management strategies for a particular patient. The evaluation includes:[3]

- Observation
- Measurement of limb length
- Assessment of muscle power using manual muscle power grading
- Measurement of the active and passive range of motion using goniometer
- Grading spasticity by modified Ashworth scale
- Examination for persistence of abnormal reflexes
- Posture and gait observation
- Chest assessment (physical and radiological)
- Assessment of child's abilities and disabilities

INDICATIONS FOR REHABILITATION

Rehabilitation medicine plays an important role in the following conditions:

- *Neurological conditions*—cerebral palsy, autism, developmental delay, spina bifida, muscular dystrophies, poliomyelitis, infantile hemiplegia, and peripheral nerve lesions
- *Orthopedic conditions*—congenital talipes-equinovarus (CTEV), hip dysplasia, torticollis, and post-traumatic stiffness
- *Genetic diseases*—with motor and sensory involvement
- *Cardiovascular diseases*—mostly involving postoperative care
- *Respiratory disorders*—chronic obstructive pulmonary disease (COPD) which includes bronchial asthma, bronchiectasis, chronic restrictive pulmonary diseases (CRPD), which include chest deformities and neuromuscular disorders
- *Postoperatively*—after an abdominal surgery or urological surgery to train the bladder and bowel muscles
- *Athletes*—for prehabilitation, injury prevention, and rehabilitation of sports injuries

METHODS OF INTERVENTION

To optimize function through the combined use of:

- *Medications*
- *Physical modalities*—warming or cooling the soft tissues
- *Physical training* with therapeutic exercise, movement, and activity modification
- *Respiratory*—Breathing exercises, chest clearance techniques, usage of adjuncts such as incentive spirometer, PEP devices, breath stacking devices such as lung volume recruitment bag, and cough assist devices
- Adaptive equipment and assistive device, orthotics (braces), and prosthesis.

PHYSICAL MODALITIES

There are various methods of warming or cooling the soft tissues.[4]

Warming the Soft Tissues

The sources of heat may be:

- Paraffin wax
- Heat pad
- Moist hot packs
- Interferential therapy (IFT)
- Transcutaneous electrical nerve stimulation (TENS)
- Ultrasound therapy

The modality of choice in an individual depends on the objective of the treatment, the part to be treated, the depth of the lesion, the state of the cutaneous nerve supply, and the underlying pathology.

In pediatric age group, paraffin wax and heating pads are safer. Ultrasound given at the epiphysis end may damage the growth plates. In peripheral nerve lesions such as Erb's palsy and facial palsy, electrical stimulation is indicated and is later followed by tendon transfer surgery.

Ice Therapy or Cooling the Soft Tissues

It is the local or generalized application of cold for therapeutics and prevention. It results in alternating periods of vasoconstriction and vasodilatation, thereby reducing nerve conductivity, and relieving muscle spasm and spasticity. It helps in relieving pain and reducing swelling, spasticity, and hematoma formation.

Cold therapy can be applied by ice cold towels, as an icepack, or by immersion in an ice-filled bath depending upon the comfort of the patient.

Physical Training

Exercises may be in the form of:[5]

- Active/passive exercises
- Stretching
- Strengthening exercises
- Endurance exercises
- Coordination exercises
- Posture correction
- Gait training.

REHABILITATION STRATEGIES IN COMMON DISORDERS

Newborn Babies

Early intervention supports the needs of infants and toddlers with developmental delay and disabilities. Comprehensive care enhances the development of physical, cognitive, communication, social, and emotional development in infants and toddlers. This also encloses the initiation of an adaptive approach among family members, to enhance their capacity to meet the special needs of their children.

Any child at the earliest of age, with obvious developmental delay or who has been found to lag in development as compared to his/her peers requires proper assessment to devise an early and appropriate intervention plan. Physiotherapy and occupational therapy are of prime importance in early intervention. They can act as service coordinators to coordinate with other specialists and therapists for collaborative care.

Assessment of High-risk Children

There are various development assessment scales currently used according to the child's age:[6]

- *Movement assessment of infant (MAI):* From 0 months to 12 months of age
- *Alberta infant motor scale (AIMS):* From 0 months to 18 months of age
- *Test of infant motor performance (TIMP):* From 34 weeks postconception age to 4 months post-term.

At the community level, our own *Trivandrum Developmental Screening Chart (TDSC)* can be utilized.[7] It has been designed in such a way that it takes only around 5 minutes to complete. TDSC (0–6 years) is a simple, reliable, and valid screening tool for use in the community to identify children between 0 and 6 years with developmental delay, enabling early intervention practices.

The BSID-III current version (Bayley Scales of Infant Development) is a standard series of measurements, originally developed by psychologist Nancy Bayley, who used it primarily to assess the motor (fine and gross), language receptive and expressive), and cognitive development of infants and toddlers, <3 years of age.

Physiotherapy helps children achieve meaningful sustained activity. In the initial stages, the aim is to, at the least, take care of their day-to-day needs. The ultimate goal is to achieve normal or near-normal motor skills as their peers.

Physiotherapy also integrates family members and care providers to:[8]

- Understand and meet the child's needs.
- Find resources in their community that are suited to meet their needs.
- Create opportunities for the child to develop motor abilities.
- Provide transition of the child to preschool or other facilities.
- Provide inclusive education in normal schools.
- Help families make decisions on adaptive equipment when and if needed by the child.
- Improve the overall well-being and quality of both the children and their families.

NEUROLOGY AND NEUROMUSCULAR CONDITIONS[9]

Poliomyelitis

- *Acute phase:* Rest and positioning with splint
- *Recovery phase:* Passive exercise, active assisted, and strengthening exercises
- *Residual phase:* Continue exercise and application of orthotics

Cerebral Palsy

A multidisciplinary rehabilitative approach should be initiated at the earliest to get the maximum outcome. The different techniques include neurodevelopment therapy (NDT), sensory integration, and motor relearning theory. The treatment is tailor-made to the child's need and presentation (spastic, hypotonic, athetoid, or mixed type). The aims are:

- Reduce spasticity
- Inhibition of abnormal reflexes

- Sensory integration
- Prevention of deformity/contractures
- Treatment of associated problems such as shearing, visual, and feeding problems

These are achieved by:[10]

- Proper positioning
- Active/passive movements
- Facilitating the development of delayed/missing milestones
- Standing training
- Gait training with or without supports such as ankle-foot orthosis, knee-ankle-foot orthosis, walkers, and crutch
- Stretching and resting splint to relieve spasticity, postbotulinum toxin injection for spastic muscles

Muscular Dystrophy

This is a genetic disorder characterized by progressive muscle weakness. Though many types of dystrophies are reported, Duchenne dystrophy seems quite common. The management includes passive exercise, proper muscular positioning of the weak joints with splints, stretching, chest physiotherapy, and a customized wheelchair to prevent the worsening of the spinal deformity.

Erb's Palsy

This is a nerve injury sustained during birth, affecting the C5–C6 spinal nerves or the whole of the upper trunk of the brachial plexus due to traction injury. The upper extremity is adducted, internally rotated, elbow extended, and forearm pronated. In some babies, nerve recovery occurs on its own. Often, early physiotherapy is required to prevent contractures and regain motor power. However, if the child has not achieved improvement between 6 and 9 months of age nerve graft or nerve decompression is indicated. Sometimes better outcomes are augmented with the physician's choice of Botox injection for stiff muscles.

Spina Bifida

This is a neural tube defect resulting in vertebral and/or spinal cord malformation. Management includes:

- Teaching parents proper positioning and handling of the child
- Educating about the anesthetic skin and potential for sustaining anesthetic ulcers
- Passive stretching exercise to prevent contractures
- Providing appropriate splints

Hypermobile Joints

It is a group of inherited disorders affecting the connective tissues resulting in hypermobility of joints due to lax ligaments and soft tissues. Treatment is directed toward managing symptoms, protecting of muscles and joints with proper exercises, appropriate orthotic supports, and monitoring any complications.

ORTHOPEDIC CONDITIONS

Post-traumatic Muscle Stiffness

The physiotherapy plan is divided into two phases, i.e., during immobilization and mobilization.

1. *During immobilization:*
   - Reduce edema and prevent the formation of adhesions—limb elevation and isometric exercises
   - Avoid undue stress—proper positioning is recommended.
   - Maintain circulation—active movement of extremities
   - Maintain range of joint movements—range of movement (ROM) exercises
   - Maintain function—exercises to unaffected limb and parts
   - Training to use frames, crutches, etc.
2. *During mobilization:*
   - To reduce swelling—limb elevation and active movement
   - Maintain joint range—ROM exercises
   - Strengthen muscles—strengthening exercises and isometric contractions are taught.

Congenital Talipes Equinovarus

It is also known as clubfoot. This deformity is characterized by plantar flexion at the ankle joint, inversion at the subtalar joint, and forefoot adduction. Management includes passive stretching, retaining incorrect positions by adhesive strapping, night splints, gait training, and corrective shoes.

Torticollis

It is commonly known as a twisted neck.[11] The head is typically tilted with a lateral bent to the side of the affected muscle. Birth trauma or intrauterine malpositioning is considered to cause damage to the sternocleidomastoid muscle in the neck. This results in a shortening or excessive contraction of the sternocleidomastoid muscle, often with a limited range of motion in both rotation and lateral bending. The general stretching of the sternocleidomastoid muscle and positioning will help.

Hip Dysplasia

In hip dysplasia or congenital dislocation of the hip, there is dysplasia of the acetabulum and femoral head and dislocation of the femoral head. Management is divided into two phases:

1. *Immobilization phase:*
   - Active movement of all joints of the lower limb including hip

- Splinting
- Isometric exercises

2. *Mobilization phase:*
    - Mobilization exercises
    - Passive adduction
    - Muscle-strengthening exercises
    - Gait training
    - Weight bearing and weight transfers

Dysplasia

This disorder originates from the abnormal organization of cells into tissues leading to abnormal tissue differentiation, e.g., osteogenesis imperfecta. The management includes:

- Instruction to parents about positioning and handling
- Supported sitting in stroller and wheelchairs
- Encourage developmental activities
- Stretching exercises
- Ambulation with assistive orthotic devices

Pediatric Flatfoot

Flatfoot is common in both children and adults.[12] When this deformity occurs in children, it is referred to as pediatric flatfoot. Although there are various forms of flatfoot, they all share one characteristic—partial or total collapse of the arch.

Pediatric flatfoot can be classified as symptomatic or asymptomatic. Symptomatic flatfeet exhibit symptoms, such as pain and limitation of activity, while asymptomatic flat feet show no symptoms. These classifications can assist the foot and ankle surgeon in determining an appropriate treatment plan.

Symptoms

Flatfoot can be apparent at birth or it may not show up until years later. Most children with flatfoot have no symptoms, but some have one or more of the following symptoms:

- Pain, tenderness, or cramping pain in the foot, leg, and knee
- Outward tilting of the heel
- Awkwardness or changes in walking
- Difficulty with shoes
- Reduced energy when participating in physical activities
- Voluntary withdrawal from physical activities

Nonsurgical Treatment

If a child has no symptoms, treatment is often not required. Instead, the condition will be observed and reevaluated periodically by the pediatrician.

- *Activity modifications:* The child needs to temporarily decrease activities that bring pain as well as avoid prolonged walking or standing.
- *Orthotic devices:* The foot and ankle surgeon can provide custom orthotic devices that fit inside the shoe to support the structure of the foot and improve function.
- *Physiotherapy:* Stretching exercises, supervised by the foot and ankle surgeon or a physical therapist, provide relief in some cases of flatfoot.
- *Shoe modifications:* Footwear modifications include in-built medial arches in the shoes to address the navicular drop.

Trigger Finger

A pediatric trigger finger, also known as a congenital trigger finger, is a condition affecting the flexor tendon of the finger or thumb. Symptoms occur when there is a size mismatch between the tendon and the sheath that surrounds the tendon. This causes locking or catching of the finger with attempted bending of the finger with associated pain, which is referred to as "triggering". In pediatric trigger fingers, there is often a nodule (a benign thickening of the tendon) that catches on the overlying sheath, causing the finger or thumb to trigger. This is diagnosed based on history and clinical examination with the finding of triggering of the digit and with a palpable nodule at the base of the finger. Physiotherapy management includes massaging at the A1 pulley level and stretching and/or splinting to keep the finger straight. Trigger thumb is more likely to be successfully treated with surgical techniques.

Sports Injuries

They are increasingly common in pediatrics due to faulty training, musculotendinous imbalance, and anatomical misalignment; including flatfeet, immature structures, improper footwear, and playing surface.[13]

Types of Injuries

- Stress fractures
- Tendonitis and bursitis
- *Joint disorders*:
    - Subluxation
    - Dislocation
    - Ligament injuries

Management

Management in general includes rest, ice compression, strapping/taping, and anti-inflammatory drugs.[14] This has to be followed by muscle-strengthening exercises, proper training, and education for the child as well as the parents. Surgical correction may be required if conservative treatment fails.

PULMONARY DISORDERS

Physiotherapy plays a vital role in the management of obstructive and restrictive pulmonary disorders of the lungs.[15] It plays a role when there is tightness in the bronchial smooth muscles such as bronchial asthma, abnormal secretions in the case of bronchiectasis, cystic fibrosis, or infection such as bronchitis. It is also indicated in restrictive pulmonary disorders such as congenital chest deformities and neuromuscular disorders such as muscular dystrophies.

Physiotherapy also helps in secondary complications in patients who are in intensive care units by proper positioning, Breathing exercises and intensive secretion clearance techniques.

Chest Physiotherapy

It is an airway-clearance technique that combines manual percussion of the chest wall by the caregiver, strategic positioning of the patient for mucus drainage with cough, and breathing techniques. It is useful for individuals with copious mucus or thick secretions, those with weak respiratory mechanics, or those with ineffective cough. Chest physiotherapy consists of various manipulative procedures such as the following:

- *Breathing exercises:* Proper training of diaphragm and intercostal muscles in aiding proper expansion of lungs.
- *Positioning (postural drainage):* Placing the patient in varying positions for optimal gravity drainage of secretions to increase the expansion and prevent occlusion of that individual segment.
- *Percussion (chest percussion, vibration, and thoracic squeezing):* In conjunction with postural drainage; to hasten clearing of secretion from the trachea bronchial tree.
- *Airway clearing technique:* To facilitate clearance of lower airway secretions through the upper airways by cough stimulation, huffing, flutter, cough assist devices, and/or tracheal stimulation.

Breathing Exercises

It is an integral part of chest physiotherapy. It plays a significant role in airway clearance and parenchymal expansion by improving the efficiency of respiratory muscles. Diaphragmatic, costal, and apical breathing techniques are for the different segments of the lungs.

Cough Assist Techniques

They are used to help clear the lungs and airways of secretions. Although limited evidence exists regarding the efficacy of secretion clearance strategies, many patients with impaired airway clearance seem to benefit from the use of secretion clearance devices. Adequate hydration, physical activity, bronchodilators, controlled breathing, and postural drainage in addition help.

"Cough assist device" **(Fig. 23.3.1)** is a handheld device that combines the benefits of both positive expiratory pressure (PEP) therapy (manual) and airway vibrations to mobilize pulmonary secretions. The physiologic rationale is that exhaling against resistance slows down our expiratory phase of breathing. This slower exhalation against resistance or positive pressure generates back pressure, which in turn splints or stents open the more peripheral airways and lessens airway collapse distally. This facilitates the mobilization of secretions from distal or peripheral airways to the larger more central airways. However, the patient or individual must be able to generate adequate airflow to use this device.

Cough Insufflator-insufflator (Mechanical)

A cough assist machine helps to clear secretions in the lungs and bronchioles by using a combination of positive and negative air pressure, by simulating a cough. With correct usage, the device may decrease the risk of chest infections, such as pneumonia due to stagnant secretions that invite a secondary infection.

Single Valve Ambu Bag (Lung Volume Recruitment Bag), PEP Device, and Incentive Spirometer

In restrictive lung disease due to thoracic cage-skeletal anomalies or neuromuscular disease, a single valve Ambu bag, PEP device, and incentive spirometer are useful in removing the secretions **(Figs. 23.3.2A to C)**. "Air/breath stacking method" facilitates breathing in more air, as the bag is squeezed a second time. This should fill the airways further and the patient is asked to hold as long as possible this air,

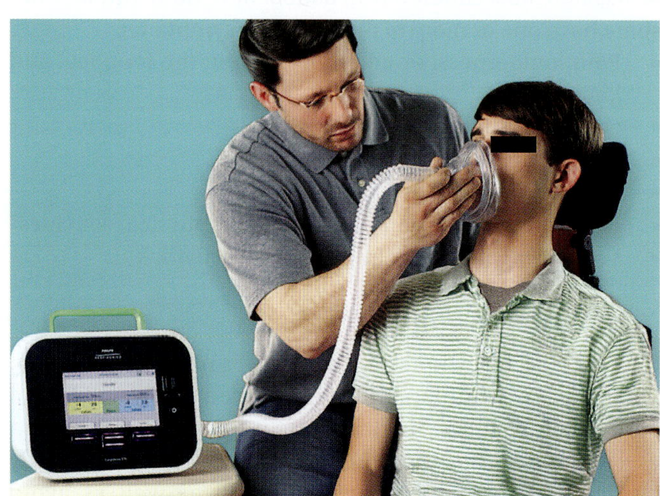

Fig. 23.3.1: Cough assist device.

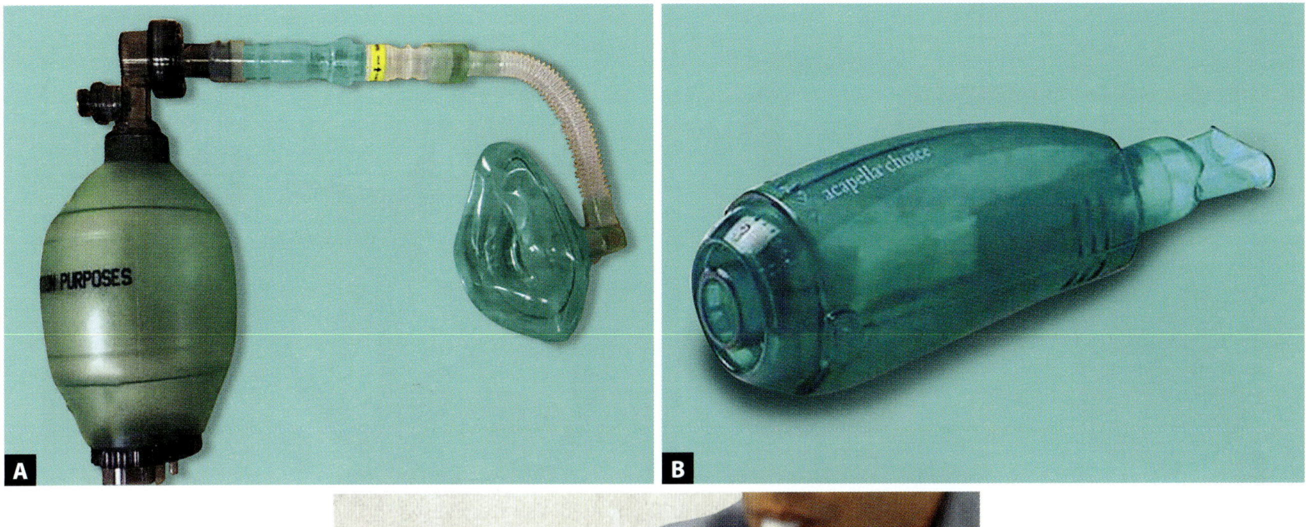

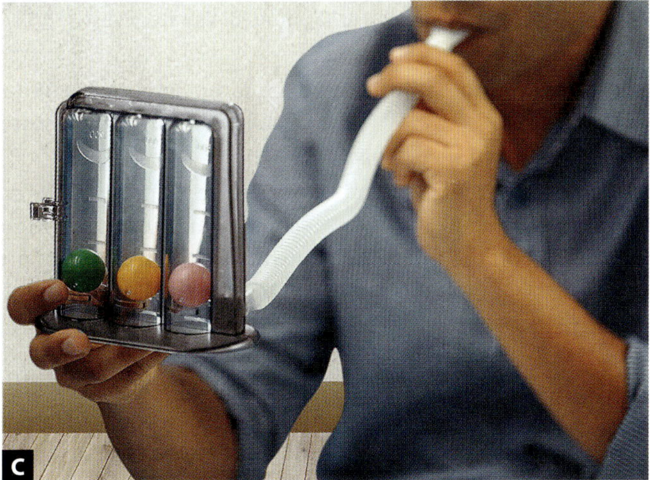

Figs. 23.3.2A to C: (A) Single valve Ambu bag; (B) PEP device; (C) Incentive spirometer.

which then is breathed out as a cough. This helps in removing secretions from the lungs, which further improves ventilation, prevents/clears atelectasis, and assists in coughing.

Vibratory Vest

It is a device used to loosen and thin the mucus by using high-frequency vibration mechanically in the chest walls **(Figs. 23.3.3A and B)**. This promotes airway clearance and improves bronchial drainage. It is one of the main adjuncts used in the management of COPD and most commonly in cystic fibrosis. It is advisable to use the vest for 5 minutes and then cough or huff coughs to clear the mucus. Sessions last about 20–30 minutes.

BURNS

In burns, there is coagulative necrosis of tissue and skin loss. It may be caused due to heat, flame, chemicals, electricity, or radiation. The main aim and treatment line of rehabilitation are to:

- Prevent respiratory complications—chest physiotherapy
- Prevent contractures and deformities—splinting and positioning
- Maintain range of motion and muscle strength—exercises
- Reduce scar contracture—soft tissue release techniques by passive stretching or surgical correction

CARDIOVASCULAR DISORDERS

In older children who are to undergo cardiothoracic surgery, preoperative preparation, and continued postoperative care should be given.

- *Preoperatively,* activities which are to be carried out postoperatively are taught:
  - Breathing exercises with emphasis on deep breathing
  - Incentive spirometry to aid lung expansion

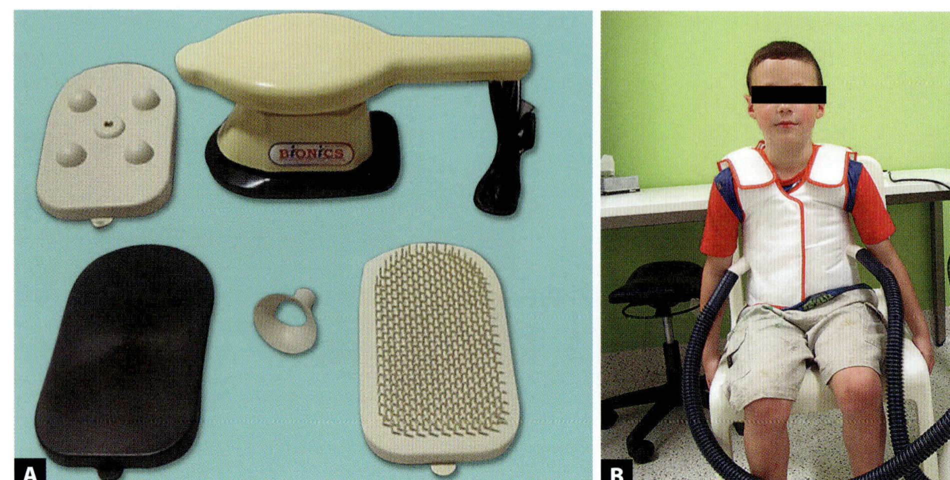

Figs. 23.3.3A and B: (A) Vibrator; (B) Vibratory vest.

- Instructions to effectively cough and splinting techniques
- Postural drainage to remove accumulated secretions
- Lower extremity exercises to maintain circulation and prevent deep vein thrombosis (DVT).

- *On postoperative days,* the emphasis is on the following activities:
  - Promote relaxation and relieve pain
  - Positioning in bed
  - Maintain ventilation through deep breathing exercises and incentive spirometry
  - Assist in secretion removal—begin with deep effective coughing
  - Prevent DVT—lower limb exercises
  - Maintain range of motion—ROM exercises
  - Correct postural defects—positioning and postural training
  - Improve exercise tolerance—graded exercise program.

AUGMENTED BLADDER

Bladder augmentation, also called augmentation cystoplasty, is a surgical procedure used in children who lack adequate bladder capacity or detrusor compliance. Physiotherapy using TENS and exercise to improve the bladder and bowel muscles will help.

POSTURE

Posture is the position in which you hold your body and limbs when standing, sitting, or lying down. Good posture is one that puts the least strain on our back and should be maintained while doing any activity. Poor posture is commonly diagnosed in children and is more frequent in boys. A significant portion of children with poor posture is found between 7 and 11 years of age.

The most frequently detected defects are protruding scapulae and increased lumbar lordosis. Children with poor posture more frequently present with headaches and pain in the cervical and lumbar regions. On average, children spend 4 h/week performing sports activities and >20 h/week watching TV/VCR and playing on mobile phones. Children with limited sports activities have a significantly higher risk of developing poor posture, than children performing sports. Regular exercises such as running, walking, cycling, and playing a variety of sports will help the back to become strong.

Management

This includes maintaining normal spinal curvature and shoulder bracing exercises.

Tips for Proper Posture

- *Standing up:*
  - To have good posture when you are standing, you need to practice. Stand in front of the mirror.
  - Hold your head up and chin in, and look straight ahead
  - Put your shoulders back
  - Tuck your tummy in
  - Keep your knees straight
  - Take a deep breath and relax your shoulders
  - Keep your chest forward
  - Standing for a long time is tiring, so try to rest one foot at a time a bit higher up than the other, like on a step, or a stool

- Slumping sideways into your hip is not good posture and can strain your back muscles. Try to move about rather than standing in one position for too long.

- *Sitting down:*
  - When you sit, try to keep your back straight
  - Put your back against the backrest of the chair
  - Your knees should make a right angle
  - Feet flat on the floor
  - Do not cross your legs.
- *Working on the computer:*
  - If you are working on a computer, then your chair should be moved to fit you.
  - Do not lean forward. Sit back and stretch your arms out to the keyboard.
  - Bring your chair up close to the keyboard so that you can rest your arms on the chair or desk. Keep your shoulders relaxed. Sitting-like this is the least stressful posture for your back.
  - If you are playing computer or video games, be aware that your shoulders may be hunching up as you get more excited.
  - You need to rest and move around every 30 minutes to let your body relax.
  - Try bending back a few times to stretch your muscles and help them relax.
- *Lifting things:*
  - Never lift alone anything that is an awkward shape or is more than a quarter of your body weight.
  - Always bend your knees and straighten your legs as you lift. This way your leg muscles are doing the work and not your back muscles.
  - Use a trolley if you have to move something heavy.
  - To lift something, put your feet apart, hold the object close to your body, and keep your arms bent. This way you are using your arm muscles and not pulling on your shoulder and back muscles.
  - Never lift anything higher than your waist.
  - Bend your legs and hips, tighten your tummy muscles, and use your leg muscles to help you lower the object down again.
- *Lying down:*
  - Even when you are lying down or sleeping, look after your posture by:
  - Keep the natural curves in your back
  - Lie on your side with your knees bent
  - Lie with your head on one soft pillow that your spine is in a natural position.

ASSISTIVE DEVICES

When there is an imbalance in the muscle tissues, assistive devices shall be advised for ambulation and support when there is injury or inflammation.

The following are the different assistive devices:

- Hip-knee-ankle-foot orthosis **(Fig. 23.3.4A)**
- Knee-ankle-foot-orthosis **(Fig. 23.3.4B)**
- Ankle-foot orthosis **(Fig. 23.3.4C)**
- Taylor's brace **(Fig. 23.3.5A)**
- Elbow crutches **(Fig. 23.3.5B)**
- Axillary crutches **(Fig. 23.3.5C)**
- Insoles **(Fig. 23.3.5D)**

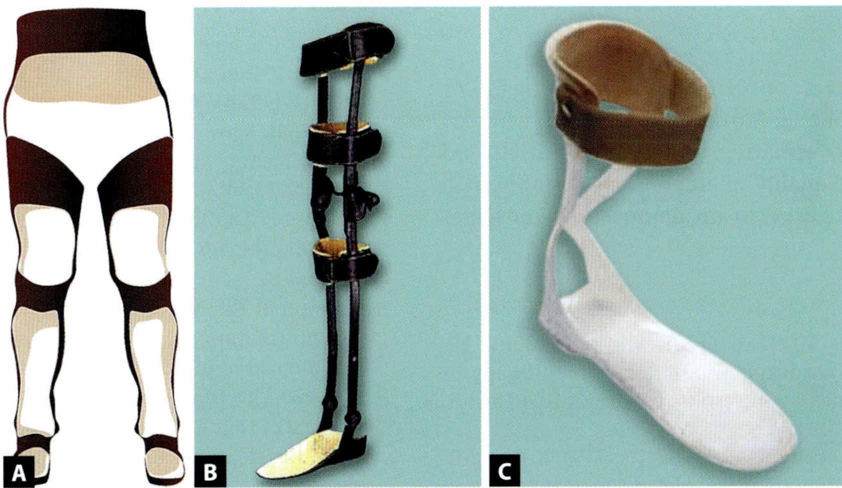

Figs. 23.3.4A to C: (A) Hip-knee-ankle-foot orthosis; (B) Knee-ankle-foot orthosis; (C) Ankle-foot orthosis.

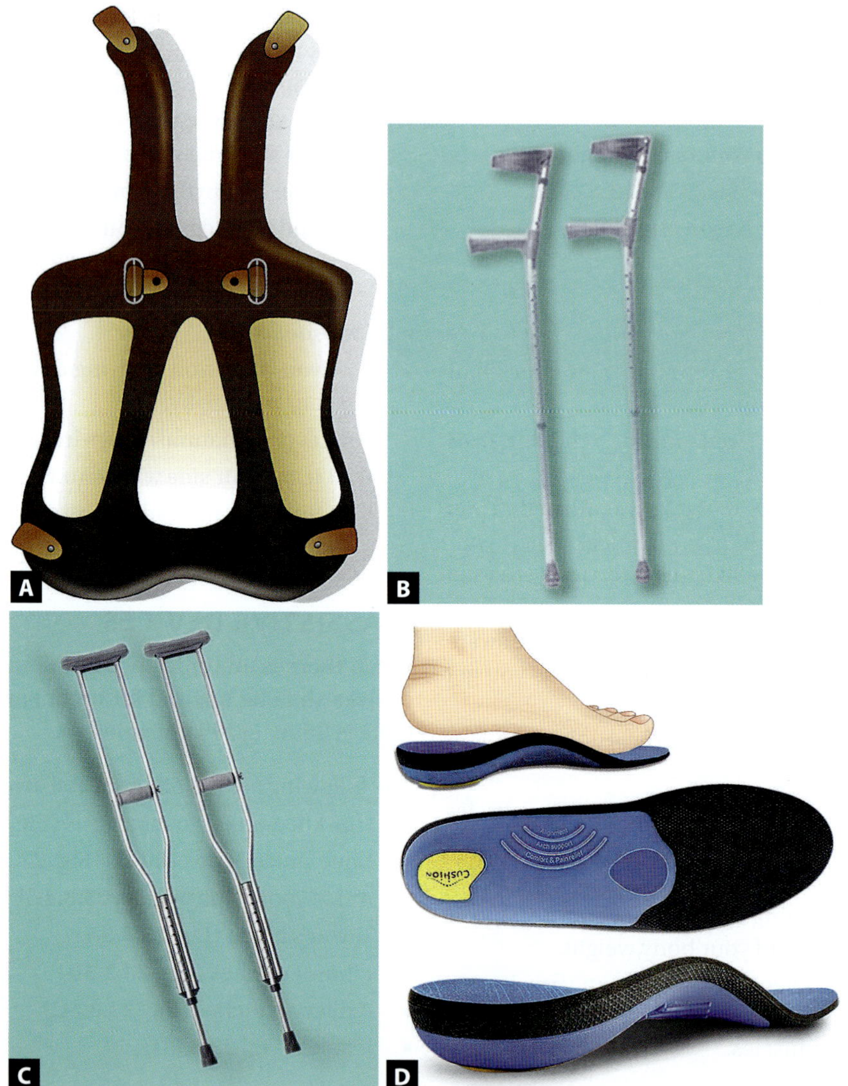

Figs. 23.3.5A to C: (A) Taylor's brace; (B) Elbow crutches; (C) Axillary crutches; and (D) Insoles.

CONCLUSION

Overall, physical therapy is concerned with identifying motor impairment and maximizing movement potential, whereas rehabilitation aims to enhance and restore functional ability and improve the quality of life in those with physical impairments or disabilities due to any neuroskeleto-muscular problems.

REFERENCES

1. Drapeau-Zgoralski V, Beauséjour M, Painchaud AS, Sarda M, Nault ML. Advanced practice physiotherapy in paediatrics: Implementation results. Paediatr Child Health. 2022;27(4):206-12.
2. Pritchard-Wiart L, Thompson-Hodgetts S, McKillop AB. A review of goal setting theories relevant to goal setting in Paediatric Rehabilitation. Clin Rehabil. 2019;33(9):1515-26.
3. Sudhir CS, Sharath HV. A brief overview of recent pediatric physical therapy practices and their importance. Cureus. 2023;15(10):e47863.
4. Casale R, Ferriero G. Physical modalities and pain control in rehabilitation: lights and shadows to dispel. Eur J Phys Rehabil Med. 2022;58(2):280-1.
5. Kisner CC, Colby L. Therapeutic Exercise Foundation and Techniques, 4th edition. Philadelphia: FA Davis Co; 2002. pp. 3, 7, 63-67.
6. Campbell SK, Swanlund A, Smith E, Liao PJ, Zawacki L. Validity of the TIMPSI for estimating concurrent performance on the test of infant motor performance. Pediatr Phys Ther. 2008;20(1):3-10.
7. Nair MK, Nair GS, George B, Suma N, Neethu C, Leena ML, et al. Development and validation of Trivandrum Development Screening Chart for children aged 0-6 years [TDSC (0-6)]. Indian J Pediatr. 2013;80 (Suppl 2):S248-55.

8. Ochandorena-Acha M, Terradas-Monllor M, Sala LL, Cazorla Sánchez ME, Marti MF, Pérez MI, et al. Early Physiotherapy Intervention Program for Preterm Infants and Parents: A Randomized, Single-Blind Clinical Trial. Children (Basel). 2022;9(6):895.
9. Tamburin S, Smania N, Saltuari L, Hoemberg V, Sandrini G. New Advances in Neurorehabilitation. Front Neurol. 2019; 10:1090.
10. Miccinilli S, Santacaterina F, Della Rocca R, Sterzi S, Bressi F, Bravi M. Efficacy of lower limb orthoses in the rehabilitation of children affected by cerebral palsy: A systematic review. Children (Basel). 2024;11(2):212.
11. Kaplan SL, Coulter C, Sargent B. Physical Therapy Management of Congenital Muscular Torticollis: A 2018 Evidence-Based Clinical Practice Guideline From the APTA Academy of Pediatric Physical Therapy. Pediatr Phys Ther. 2018;30(4):240-90.
12. Molina-García C, Banwell G, Rodríguez-Blanque R, Sánchez-García JC, Reinoso-Cobo A, Cortés-Martín J, et al. Efficacy of Plantar Orthoses in Paediatric Flexible Flatfoot: A Five-Year Systematic Review. Children (Basel). 2023;10(2):371.
13. Silva LCE, Teles J, Fragoso I. Sports injuries patterns in children and adolescents according to their sports participation level, age and maturation. BMC Sports Sci Med Rehabil. 2022;14(1):35.
14. Prentice WE. Therapeutic Modalities for Sports Medicine & Athletic Training, 6th ed. New York: Mc Graw Hill; 2009. pp. 17, 33, 104, 123, and 129.
15. Corten L, Morrow BM. Autogenic Drainage in Children With Cystic Fibrosis. Pediatr Phys Ther. 2017;29(2):106-17.

SECTION

24 Pediatric Therapeutics

Section Editor: Jeeson C Unni

24.1 Basics of Pediatric Therapeutics

Sandeep B Bavdekar, Padmaja A Marathe

INTRODUCTION

It is usually believed that every illness should be treated. This principle of therapeutic enthusiasm is clearly appropriate in severe and life-threatening illnesses. It, however, does not apply to all clinical situations. Infants, children, and adolescents have intrinsic recuperative capacities. Therefore, therapeutic intervention may not be required in many conditions. Drug therapy in children differs from that in adults for several reasons. Their abilities to metabolize drugs mature over the years and their capacity to excrete drugs reach adult levels by late infancy. Before initiating drug therapy, the treating doctor should undertake the following steps.[1]

STEPS IN INITIATION OF THERAPY

Reach an Initial Working Diagnosis

Reaching an initial working diagnosis based on history, examination, laboratory findings, and epidemiological considerations is the first step in starting treatment. A critically ill child would require immediate therapy aimed at stabilization of vital signs without waiting for results of investigations. The treatment can be changed subsequently based on results of investigations and response to therapy.

Define Therapeutic Objectives

Once having reached a working diagnosis, the next step is to specify what intends to be achieved through therapy and when. Depending upon the patient's condition and the possible diagnosis, it could include relief of symptoms, prevention of complications, eradication of cause or etiological agents or reversal of metabolic abnormalities, etc. For example, when a patient presents with fever and burning micturition and is diagnosed to have urinary tract infection, therapeutic objectives would include symptomatic relief (relief of pain during micturition and control of fever), eradication of infectious agent (with the help of appropriate antimicrobial therapy), steps to prevent further attacks of urinary tract infection, and preservation of renal function. Defining therapeutic objectives helps the doctor prescribe minimum number of appropriate drugs and provides a benchmark for the assessment of success of therapy.

Assess Effectiveness of Therapies

There is hardly any therapeutic regimen that is completely effective in all cases. Efficacy is dependent on several factors, which include patient's immune status, drug's pharmacokinetic properties, and stage of illness. The treating doctor should be aware of the comparative efficacy of various therapeutic interventions.

Assess Risk to the Patient

Every drug has adverse effects. The risk to patient increases when multiple pharmacological agents are used. The physician should anticipate drug interactions. Complete information regarding adverse effects to newly introduced drugs is not available.

Plan Strategies to Ensure Compliance

A patient will derive benefits from therapy only if the drug is not administered in the correct dose at the right frequency by the correct route for the desired duration. The physician must explain to the parents the importance of administering drug, the symptoms it would help to control or the manifestations that it might ameliorate, by when this is expected to happen and the importance of completing the course. Issues such as taste and smells influence compliance. The sense of smell and taste are well-developed right from the neonatal period. Hence, the doctor should be familiar with the available preparations, their flavors, and unpleasant characteristics.

Consider Costs Involved

For many families, expenses involved including travel expenses, cost of drugs, expenses for diagnostic tests, and professional fees, if any, are some of the important factors determining compliance. Generic drugs are generally less expensive. When time-honored cheaper but effective medications are available, one should not push the parents to buy more expensive drugs.

Enquire About Previous Experience

Another consideration in choosing a drug is to know what has failed with this patient in the past. This includes questions about hypersensitivity, adverse reaction, noncompliance, and noneffectiveness. If a preparation is taken by child with least degree of fuss, it could also mean that the preparation is acceptable to the child in terms of smell, taste, and flavor.

SPECIAL ASPECTS OF PEDIATRIC PHARMACOLOGY[2-7]

Children are not miniature adults, as they differ from adults at every stage of development including physiological and biochemical processes in various organs. Even among children, the rates of drug metabolism, drug excretion as well as pharmacodynamics vary in different age groups. The largest deviation from adult pharmacokinetic profile is observed in infants, when organ functions are developing. Understanding and integrating these developmental changes is crucial while choosing a safe and effective drug therapy. Drug therapy must be individualized on the basis of developmental differences in pharmacokinetics and pharmacodynamics.

Drug Absorption

Gastrointestinal Absorption

Drug absorption in infants and children follows the same principles as in adults. The patient and drug characteristics that affect absorption of a drug from the gastrointestinal tract (GIT) are, in turn, influenced by several factors. These include age of the child, lower secretion of gastric acid, lower concentration of gastrointestinal (GI) enzymes, prolonged gastric emptying, decreased intestinal bile secretion, and slower peristalsis in the first few days of life, which may affect absorption of drugs from the GIT. For example, higher gastric pH in the neonates results in higher bioavailability of ampicillin (a weak basic drug). Similarly the plasma concentration of orally administered paracetamol and phenytoin are lower in infants than those in older children and adults. Delayed development of GI flora results in decreased inactivation of digoxin and increased bioavailability of digoxin in infants. Similarly, decreased bile acid secretion leads to lower concentrations of hydrocortisone in infants as compared to older children.

Parenteral Routes of Absorption

Physiological and physiochemical factors affect the rate and extent of logical drug absorption from parenteral sites. The absorption of the drug administered intramuscularly may be decreased in premature babies with very little muscle mass and in children with diminished perfusion. The factors such as smaller layer of stratum corneum and increased level of hydration of epidermis lead to higher cutaneous perfusion of drugs as compared to adults.

Drug Distribution

Knowledge about drug distribution is important while designing an optimal dosage regimen. The distribution characteristics of drugs differ markedly amongst term infants, premature babies, and children as compared with adults. These differences are a result of much important age-dependent variables. These include the following.

Composition and Size of Body Water Compartments

Neonates have a higher percentage of their body weight in the form of water (70–75%) as compared to adults (50–60%). Similarly, the extracellular water compartment accounts for 40% of the body weight in neonates compared to 20% in adults. The volume of extracellular water compartment is important in determining the concentration of drugs at receptor sites. Thus, water-soluble drugs have a larger volume of distribution in newborns and infants on a per unit body weight basis than in adults. Therefore, neonates require higher doses of gentamicin to achieve equivalent plasma and tissue concentrations. Similarly, infants have a higher proportion of body fat than adults, which may result in larger volumes of distribution per unit body weight for lipid-soluble drugs (e.g., diazepam).

Protein-binding

Albumin and alpha-1-acid glycoprotein, required for binding drugs in the plasma, are present in lower concentrations in neonates and infants. This results in higher free drug concentrations (especially of highly protein-bound drugs) and increased drug distribution to the tissues. This can result in higher toxicity (e.g., phenytoin, salicylates, and ampicillin).

Drug Metabolism

Liver is the primary organ for drug metabolism and different hepatic enzyme systems mature at different ages. The cytochrome P450 monooxygenase system appears to mature rapidly, with adult-like metabolic activity being achieved by 6 months of age. In contrast, glucuronide formation reaches adult values at 3–4 years of life. Although infants are regularly characterized as being slow metabolizers of drugs, some drugs (e.g., theophylline, phenytoin, carbamazepine, and phenobarbitone) are more rapidly metabolized by infants than adults. There are qualitative differences, too. A drug may be preferentially metabolized by one pathway during the neonatal period (e.g., theophylline) as compared to adulthood. All these have practical implications. While determining dosages of drugs that undergo hepatic biotransformation, sequence of maturation of process of drug metabolism must be considered. The drugs (e.g., theophylline) that are metabolized at a rapid rate require higher dose and/or dose frequency.

Drug Excretion

Kidney is the main organ that excretes drugs. The excretion is dependent upon glomerular filtration rate (GFR), renal blood flow (RBF), and rate of active tubular secretion, which, in turn, are dependent on age and maturity. For example, a full-term neonate's GFR and RBF are 30% of the adult values and reach adult values by 8–12 months and 7 months of age, respectively. In preschool children, the tubular secretion capacity can be greater than that in adults. This is the reason for preschool children requiring threefold higher doses of digoxin.

In children, pharmacokinetic rather than pharmacodynamic properties of drugs are studied more extensively. The differences in the pharmacodynamic properties (intensity of response) in adults and children may be secondary to differences in the pathogenesis, receptor levels, receptor-effector mechanisms, target organ sensitivity, and homeostatic feedback mechanisms. For example, children appear to respond differently to antihypertensive drugs and Propofol use leads to prolonged sedation and delayed recovery from general anesthesia. Population pharmacokinetic or pharmacodynamics modeling techniques are statistical methods which predict changes in drug efficacy in relation to drug concentration over time and are used for selecting appropriate dosing regimens for children.

Drug Dosages

Because of the differences in pharmacokinetics in infants and children enumerated earlier, simple proportionate reduction in the adult dose is not adequate to determine a safe and effective pediatric dose. The formulae or rules providing calculations based on age or weight of the child are mere approximations and have been criticized by experts. The most reliable pediatric dose information, wherein the dose is given in terms of weight or surface area, is usually that provided by the manufacturer in the package insert, in the pharmacopoeia, national formulary or textbooks.

METHODS OF DRUG DELIVERY AND PEDIATRIC FORMULATIONS[8]

Oral Administration

Depending on age, various drug forms such as drops, suspensions, dry syrups (powder to be mixed with water before use), dispersible tablets, tablets, and capsules are used for oral administration in children. Suspensions containing sorbitol base or alcohol base provide uniform drug amount even without shaking; but there may be objections on religious or moral grounds for the use of alcohol as a base. Syrupy suspensions contain undissolved particles of drug and these may not be evenly distributed throughout the vehicle. Therefore, the bottle should be shaken prior to administration of each drug dose. Palatability, stability (chemical, physical, or microbiological), dose uniformity, and feasibility of storing may be challenging for liquid formulations. Doses should be prescribed in terms of mL and not in terms of teaspoonful. Use calibrated medicine cups or syringe (without needle) should be encouraged for measuring and administering correct doses. Advent of dispersible tablets has simplified administration of oral medicines. As these tablets can be dissolved in small volume of water, their administration is easier, too. This avoids inaccurate measurement, minimizes spills, and bypasses bad taste. Children over 8–12 years can be taught to take medicines in tablets or capsule form. Safety of excipients used as preservatives, sweeteners, solvents, flavoring or coloring agents is a concern in pediatric formulations. Anecdotal evidence from the past shows that excipient diethylene glycol (an antifreeze agent) used in sulfanilamide elixirs resulted in deaths of children. The safety profile of inactive ingredients needs validation before using them.

Parenteral Administration

This route is resorted to in presence of serious illnesses or when only parenteral form of drug is available. Local application to skin and mucous membranes is mainly used for treating local ailments. Drugs administered by subcutaneous (SC) route are slowly absorbed. The drug behaves as if it is in a reservoir as the SC tissue has limited blood supply. Intramuscular (IM) injections should be administered in the anterolateral aspect of the thigh rather than in the gluteal muscles. This avoids the risk of injury to the sciatic nerve and the possibility of a part of the dose getting injected in the SC fat that is abundant in the buttocks. After 5 years of age, when deltoid mass is generally well-developed that site can be used for IM administration.

Intravenous (IV) administration of drugs to children requires certain special considerations. Some drugs must be administered as IV push so that the drug is placed in the circulation with a minimum delay. This is an important factor when rapid onset of action is essential (e.g., adrenaline for treatment of anaphylaxis and adenosine for managing supraventricular tachycardia). This method should, however, be resorted to only by individuals familiar with acute toxicities of medications. The route carries the risk of sudden cardiac or respiratory collapse, severe anaphylaxis due to sudden antigen-antibody reaction, and local venous thrombosis, if the drug damages the vascular wall (e.g., crystalline penicillin and cloxacillin). Some drugs are required to be administered over a longer period to avoid acute toxicities or vessel wall irritation. Only limited volumes of fluids can be administered to neonates and young infants or to children with renal failure or congestive cardiac failure. Hence, novel methods of IV administration are used in pediatrics. IV piggyback (IVPB) route is used to infuse drugs (e.g., antimicrobial agents) over a period of 1–2 hours.

The dose of medication is injected into volumetric chamber inserted between the IV bag and the device controlling the rate of administration. The method is simple, does not require costly equipment like syringe pump, and as the medication is diluted in existing IV fluid, no extra fluid is administered. The syringe pump method is the gold standard for administration of drugs IV as there is absolute control over drug delivery. The syringe pumps are, however, expensive and entail administration of extra amounts of fluid. The retrograde system is a simpler method mainly used in neonates, as it does not require injection of additional fluids.

There are only limited indications for administration of drugs through sublingual, intrathecal, and intraperitoneal routes. For example, sublingual administration is used for control of severe hypertension with nifedipine, and intrathecal route is used for administering methotrexate in the treatment of childhood leukemia. Antidiuretic hormone (ADH) is administered with the help of a nasal spray for the control of nocturnal enuresis and diabetes insipidus in selected patients. Use of aerosolized drugs has revolutionized the management of childhood asthma. Beta-agonists and steroids are administered through this route. Advantages include almost instantaneous absorption of the drug into the blood through the lungs, avoidance of hepatic first-pass loss, and direct delivery of the drug at the desired site of action and lesser chance of developing systemic toxicity on prolonged use. The cumbersomeness of method of administration that could come in the way of its use in young children has been overcome by using spacer devices or rotahalers. In children aged <5 years, nebulization is a preferred route for pulmonary administration.

Drugs and Breastfeeding[9,10]

When a mother is on medications, drugs may appear in the breast milk. Most drugs are compatible with breastfeeding. However, a physician must consider the pharmacokinetic and safety profile of the drugs, while advising drug therapy to a nursing mother. Detailed information regarding drugs that can be prescribed to nursing mothers can be obtained from drug licensing information, drug formularies, databases like LacMed,[11] and pediatric textbooks.

PRACTICAL HINTS WHILE PRESCRIBING DRUGS FOR CHILDREN

In addition to the usual considerations, it is worthwhile emphasizing the following points that need to be considered while prescribing medications for children:

- Prescribe drugs only when necessary; keeping in mind the risks, benefits, and costs involved. Review therapy as and when additional information becomes available.
- Do not rush to use the latest drug in the market, unless there is a compelling reason to do so.
- Prescribe minimum number of appropriate, inexpensive drugs of good quality, one is familiar with.
- Prescriptions should be legible. They should include the date of prescription, patient details (name, age, and sex), drug details (name, formulation, composition, dose and frequency of administration, and duration for which it needs to be taken), and doctor's details (including name, signature, registration number, and contact details). It is a good practice to write the names of the drugs in capitals and write the generic name of the drugs.
- To ensure compliance, explain to parents the nature of the disease and the likely benefits to be obtained from the therapy. Give clear instruction, preferably in writing to avoid misinterpretation, including the need to complete a given course even if child appears to be asymptomatic. It is important to engage the children old enough to understand in their own care and establish rapport through good communication.
- Prescribe drugs at doses and frequencies as advised in product license, drug formulary, or standard pediatric texts.
- Prescribe appropriate formulations of medicines, e.g., drops for neonates, liquid preparations or dispersible tablets for infants and young children, and tablets and capsules for children older than 8–12 years.
- Direct parents to discard all remaining doses to protect the child from accidental poisoning or improper self-medication later.
- Explain the adverse effects of the drug, if any, to the parents, especially when long-term treatment is suggested. Explain the need for periodical clinical and/or laboratory monitoring when on long-term drug therapy for epilepsy, tuberculosis, renal diseases, etc., to assess the response and prevent serious side effects. Ask the parent to report any worsening, unexplained event, or adverse effect immediately.
- Drug combinations must be used with caution, unless the drugs are in the specified dose requirements. Avoid irrational and inappropriate combinations.
- Interactions can happen between two drugs, if administered simultaneously, e.g., penicillin and aminoglycoside in the same syringe.
- Be conversant with the ongoing developments and progress in the fields of therapeutics and drug development. Base your therapy on quality evidence. Prescribe drugs in a judicious manner to ensure that children do not remain therapeutic orphans and at the same time their safety is not sacrificed while prescribing newer drugs.

CONCLUSION

Prescribing drug therapy to children needs to be done judiciously and the basis should be to provide the 'right drug' in the 'right dose' for the 'right duration' and as per the 'individual child's need'. There is no 'one-size-fits-all' approach as children, especially neonates and infants differ from adults with respect to pharmacokinetics and pharmacodynamics of drugs. Adhering to manufacturer's instructions and/or drug formulary regarding doses to be used is needed rather than relying on formulae based on extrapolation of the adult doses. Educating parents and making them partners in child's therapy ensures satisfactory outcome of the prescribed therapy.

REFERENCES

1. deVaries TPGM, Henning RH, Hogerzeil HV, Fresle DA. Guide to Good Prescribing. Geneva: World Health Organization; 2000.
2. Loebstein R, Vohra S, Koren G. Drug therapy in pediatric patients. In: Carruthers SG, Hoffman BB, Melman KL, Nierenburg DW (Eds). Melmon and Morrelli's Clinical Pharmacology: Basic Principles in Therapeutics, 4th edition. New York: McGraw Hill Medical Publishing Division; 2000. pp. 1143-9.
3. De Cock RFW, Piana C, Krekels EHJ, Danhof M, Allegaert K, Knibbe CAJ. The role of population PK–PD modelling in paediatric clinical research. Eur J Clin Pharmacol. 2011; 67(Suppl 1):5-16.
4. Kearns GL. Abdel-Rahman SM, Alander SW, Blowey DL, Leeder JS, Kauffman RE. Developmental pharmacology—drug disposition, action, and therapy in infants and children. N Engl J Med. 2003;349(12):1157-67.
5. Benjamin Jr DK, Smith PB, Jadhav P, Gobburu JV, Murphy D, Hasselblad V, et al. Pediatric antihypertensive trial failures: analysis of end points and dose range. Hypertension. 2008;51(4):834-40.
6. Mahmood I. Dosing in Children: A Critical Review of the Pharmacokinetic Allometric Scaling and Modelling Approaches in Paediatric Drug Development and Clinical Settings. Clin Pharmacokinet. 2014;53(4):327-46.
7. Batchelor HK, Marriott JF. Paediatric pharmacokinetics: key considerations. Br J Clin Pharmacol. 2015;79(3):395-404.
8. Ivanovska V, Rademaker CM, van Dijk L, Mantel-Teeuwisse AK. Pediatric drug formulations: a review of challenges and progress. Pediatrics. 2014;134(2):361-72.
9. Ito S. Drugs and breastfeeding: the knowledge gap. In: MacLeod S, Hill S, Koren G, Rane A (Eds.). Optimizing Treatment for Children in the Developing World. Switzerland: Springer International; 2015. pp. 71-9.
10. Sachs HC, Committee on Drugs. The transfer of drugs and therapeutics into human breast milk: an update on selected topics. Pediatrics. 2013;132(3):e796-809.
11. National Institute of Child Health and Human Development. (2003). Drugs and Lactation Database (LactMed®). [online] Available from https://www.ncbi.nlm.nih.gov/books/NBK501922/. [Last accessed December, 2024].

24.2 Adverse Drug Reactions, Drug Interactions, and Therapeutic Drug Monitoring

Archana S Kher

ADVERSE DRUG REACTIONS

Introduction

Children constitute a vulnerable group since new drugs get released into the market without adequate trials in children due to ethical reasons, the exceptions being oncology and vaccines. Pharmacokinetics and pharmacodynamics differ in children, neonates, and more so in preterm neonates. Only a careful postmarketing surveillance detects adverse drug reactions (ADRs) occurring in children. Measures should be undertaken to improve detection and reporting of ADRs by all healthcare professionals.

Definitions

Adverse drug reaction generally refers to any unwanted consequence/s of administration of a drug during or following the course of therapy. These unpleasant effects occur at doses intended for therapeutic (prophylactic or diagnostic) effect and necessitate reduction of the dose or withdrawal of the drug or predict a hazard from future administration.

The Joint Commission on the Accreditation of Healthcare Organizations (JCAHO) defines an ADR as "an undesired effect of a medication that either increases toxicity, decreases desired therapeutic effect, or both".

The World Health Organization (WHO) defines ADR as "a response, which is noxious and unintended, and which occurs at doses normally used in humans for the prophylaxis, diagnosis or therapy of disease, or for the modification of physiological function".[1]

Intolerance denotes a low threshold to the normal pharmacological action of a drug.

An *idiosyncratic reaction* is an inherent qualitative abnormal reaction to a drug.

*Harmful reaction*s due to drug overdose (poisoning), drug abuse, and therapeutic errors are excluded from ADRs.[1]

EPIDEMIOLOGY

The ADRs can cause severe morbidity and even death. Incidence rates for ADRs causing hospital admissions ranged from 0.4 to 10.3%, ADRs due to antiepileptics and anti-infectives are common in admitted children. Anti-infectives and nonsteroidal anti-inflammatory drugs (NSAIDs) are the offending drugs among outpatient children. These events result due to a medication poisoning, unsupervised ingestions, mistakes by parents, self-medications, wrong prescriptions, and doses. They are responsible for nearly 7% of admissions and about 60% of reported ADRs could be avoided. ADRs are the seventh most common cause of death. In general, it appears that ADRs are underreported; especially in children and current rates represent only 10–15% of the true rate.[2,3]

Classification

The administration of a drug may result in the development of side effects, untoward effects, toxic effects, or allergic and idiosyncratic effects. ADRs could be either local (irritation, necrosis, and thrombophlebitis) or systemic.[4] They are classified as follows:

- *Type A ADR:* These are also known as augmented, attenuated, or quantitative ADR. They comprise a hyper-response to the main action of the drug, e.g., insulin-induced hypoglycemia. In general, they are dose-dependent and preventable by slow introduction of low dosages. Hypotension by beta-blockers and NSAID-induced gastric ulcers are other examples.
- *Type B ADR:* They are bizarre or qualitative ADRs manifesting as unpredictable or unexpected effects. The exact mechanisms are unclear. They may be serious and often fatal. Examples include halothane-induced hepatitis and chloramphenicol-induced aplastic anemia.
- *Type C ADR:* The effect is time- and dose-related as in analgesic nephropathy. It is often due to continuous drug use, and may be irrevocable, unanticipated, or even unpredictable.
- *Type D ADR:* It is a time-related event as in carcinogenesis. It may be delayed, and may occur even after cessation of treatment, e.g., corneal opacities after thioridazine, ophthalmopathy following chloroquine, retroperitoneal fibrosis following ergot alkaloids, analgesics, and methyldopa.
- *Type E ADR:* These include the end-of-dose or withdrawal reactions. They occur typically with antidepressant drugs. Other examples include seizures on alcohol or benzodiazepine withdrawal.
- *Type F ADR:* These include failure of therapy or ineffective therapy, e.g., augmented hypertension because of inefficient control.

Common Manifestations of Adverse Drug Reactions

The commonly reported ADRs include the following:

- *Dermal reactions:* Erythema multiforme, fixed drug eruptions, and Stevens–Johnson syndrome
- *Gastrointestinal symptoms:* Nausea, vomiting, and diarrhea
- *Hepatic:* Elevated enzymes, liver cell failure, and cholestasis
- *Neurological manifestations:* Tremors, dystonia, and impaired cognitive function
- *Hematological effects:* Neutropenia, aplastic anemia, and thrombocytopenia
- *Anaphylaxis:* Commonly due to penicillin and vaccines

Special Issues Related to Adverse Drug Reaction in Children

Children warrant special attention. Many complaints such as poor attention span and visual impairments may go unnoticed. Their growth potential may get affected with steroids. Children are more vulnerable to dermal reactions. Our pediatric population represents a wide variety of ethnic and sociocultural groups and may therefore react to drugs in a different manner. Infections are widely prevalent in Indian children; therefore it is worth identifying ADRs to drugs used to treat endemic infectious diseases. Over 50% children are malnourished and malnutrition affects drug kinetics. This should be given due consideration while prescribing antitubercular drugs. Very often children are not necessarily treated by pediatricians and irrational multiple drug prescriptions are commonly given. Ayurvedic and homeopathic medicines are additionally prescribed and drug interactions (DIs) may go unnoticed. Ciprofloxacin is not recommended for routine use in children and the reported incidence of ADR is 3.1%, but it is used for resistant enteric fever. Additives, coloring agents, sugars, and flavorings used in medications induce urticaria and asthma; they are often not mentioned on the labels.

Causes of Adverse Drug Reactions

Nondrug Factors

Factors such as age, drug allergy, ethnicity, disease, and genetic predisposition are intrinsic to the patient. Extrinsic factors such as the prescriber and environment influence ADRs. In neonates and infants, the drug distribution is affected by lower proportion of fat and higher proportion of water. The blood–brain barrier is more permeable. The enzyme systems are immature, transporters are not developed, conjugation is impaired and elimination by the kidney is lowered. Drugs such as gentamicin and digoxin have a prolonged half-life. Percutaneous absorption, maternal breast milk, maternal-fetal transmission, impaired metabolism, excipient toxicity, DIs, polypharmacy, and off-label prescribing all play a role. Older children metabolize drugs more rapidly than adults. Heritable conditions such as methemoglobinemia and glucose-6-phosphate dehydrogenase (G6PD) deficiency may precipitate ADRs.

Drug Factors

These factors include the choice of drug and the disease. Side effects of drugs are undesired but are an inevitable part of the pharmacological action of the drug at therapeutic doses, e.g., drowsiness with phenobarbitone. Secondary effects occur due to indirect consequences of a primary drug action, e.g., diuretic-induced hypokalemia leading to digoxin intolerance. A high dose of a drug can cause toxicity, e.g., eighth cranial nerve damage with gentamicin. Incorrect technique of administration of drugs can cause ADRs.

Allergic reactions to drugs result from an interaction of the drug or metabolite with patient and disease and re-exposure may cause severe reactions. Most drugs are simple chemicals and act as incomplete antigens or haptens. Test dose alone at times will be inadequate to rule out any ADR. One must be cautious while using a drug first time, when there is a positive family history of drug allergy. Reactions include rashes, angioedema, serum sickness, anaphylaxis, and asthma.

The reactions can be classified by the time of onset as:

- *Immediate,* which typically begin within 30 minutes of administering the drug.
- *Accelerated,* which are immunoglobulin E (IgE)-mediated and begin in 2–72 hours after the drug use.
- *Late* reactions occur 72 or more hours later, are often unrelated to IgE-mediated mechanisms.

Drugs and the Fetus

Drugs such as thalidomide and anticancer drugs affect cell division, protein synthesis, or deoxyribonucleic acid (DNA) synthesis, and can be teratogenic. Indirect action may result from drugs acting on the placenta or on the uterus (e.g., vasoconstrictors cause fetal anoxia by reducing blood supply). Lipid-soluble drugs easily pass into the fetus; drug metabolites persist due to immature excretory processes.

Pharmacovigilance (PV): Detection and Monitoring of Adverse Drug Reaction

Adverse drug reaction monitoring is generally referred to as pharmacovigilance (PV). The WHO defines PV as the science and activities related to the detection, assessment, understanding, and prevention of ADRs, or any other drug-related problems. Reporting of ADR through periodic safety update is a regulatory requirement. The WHO started the PV programs in 1968. The Uppsala Monitoring Centre (UMC) in Sweden is the WHO collaborating center for this global initiative. The main function of UMC is communication of safety signals recognized through analysis of global data of ADR. Pharmacovigilance Program of India (PvPI) was established in 2010 by the Central Drugs Standard Control Organization (CDSCO) with All India Institute of Medical Sciences (AIIMS), New Delhi as the National Coordination Center.[5,6]

There is a three-tier system with peripheral centers, five regional centers and two zonal centers at KEM Hospital, Mumbai and AIIMS, New Delhi.

The Indian Pharmacopoeia Commission (IPC), functions as the National Coordination Centre (NCC) for the PvPI since April 2011 under the aegis of Ministry of Health and Family Welfare, Government of India. Currently over 250 ADR monitoring centers (AMCs) are functioning in various healthcare institutions.[7]

The major functions of NCC are to collect, collate, and analyze ADRs data as per a standard procedure. The Individual Case Safety Reports (ICSRs) are collected in the standard suspected ADR reporting form, which consists of four sections, i.e., (1) patient's information, (2) suspected adverse reaction, (3) suspected medication(s), and (4) reporter's information. They are analyzed and reported to the NCC to arrive at an inference to recommend regulatory interventions to CDSCO. NCC also communicates risks to healthcare professionals and the public through PvPI newsletters. AMCs have been set up under NCC to collect the ADRs from patients that are rare and not found through clinical trials. Despite all efforts, the underreporting of ADR is a mammoth and daunting challenge for PvPI.[8]

Reporting Adverse Drug Reactions

Suspected ADR reporting forms for healthcare professionals and consumers are available on the website of IPC. The forms are made available in 10 major vernacular languages.

ADRs can be also reported via PvPI helpline number (1-800-180-3024) on weekdays from 9:00 AM to 5:30 PM. The mobile Android application for ADR reporting has also been made available to the public.[5-7]

DRUG INTERACTIONS

Drug interactions refer to the interface of a drug, food, or nutrient in the action of another drug. They result from the use of two or more drugs, this may lead to an enhanced or diminished effect. The effect may be desired or undesired, beneficial, or harmful. They represent 3.5% of all preventable ADRs; also contributes to emergency room visits and hospital admissions. Pediatric patients have immature systems of eliminating drugs, extended half-life of drugs, and therefore behave differently. Analysis of hospital databases revealed that children in intensive care units (ICUs) were exposed to 20 medications during the hospital stay, most common DI being fentanyl and midazolam causing additive effect on respiratory depression.[9] DI is important in the following situations:

- Wrong route of administration and wrong dosages
- Drugs that are enzyme inducers or inhibitors
- Drugs used for the same disorder, e.g., theophylline and salbutamol increase the risk for cardiac arrhythmias, use of beta-blockers, and calcium channel blockers
- Long-term use of any drugs
- Presence of comorbid conditions and multiorgan failure
- Use of multiple drugs.

Drug interactions are of two types: Pharmacokinetic interaction and pharmacodynamic interaction.

Pharmacokinetic Interaction

These are easy to detect and quantify. They are related to the absorption, metabolism, distribution, and excretion of the drug. They can occur outside the body or in the body. Drug incompatibilities may occur before administering when the drugs are mixed, e.g., dopamine with bicarbonate is not compatible, and phenytoin precipitates in dextrose solution. Intravenous solutions must be checked for visible changes such as turbidity, color, and precipitates. Use of correct vehicle and appropriate pH of the infusion is essential. Concomitant administration of aminoglycosides and beta-lactam antibiotics leads to loss of their effectiveness due to chemical inactivation; it is therefore important to monitor serum levels of aminoglycosides and allow an interval of 1–2 hours between the injections. The use of phenobarbitone and valproic acid leads to elevated levels of phenobarbitone and reduced efficacy of valproic acid through enzyme induction. The absorption and protein binding of drugs are different; when drugs are combined, they may be ineffective or their metabolites could be toxic. Few interactions occur through competition at drug transporters.

Pharmacodynamic Interaction

Effects such as synergism and antagonism occur at the action sites of the drugs. They may be mediated through receptors, transport processes, or electrolyte levels, e.g., potassium depletion enhances digoxin effect. Synergism results, when there is summation or addition with two drugs having the same effect. Potentiation also occurs when one drug increases the action of another, e.g., trimethoprim and sulfonamides.

Drugs are metabolized by cytochrome P450 system and many polymorphisms are known in the populations. The differences in the drug metabolism can be genetically determined. In clinical practice, drug-disease and drug-food interactions are evident. Other variables such as gastric pH, gastric emptying, intestinal motility, protein binding, transporter ontogeny, formulations, and changes in CD4 T cells with age, dictate pediatric drug-drug interactions (DDIs). Physiologically based pharmacokinetic (PBPK) models are mathematic models that can be used to predict plasma drug concentrations in pediatric population and acquire greater insight into the influence of age-dependent physiologic differences on drug disposition.

THERAPEUTIC DRUG MONITORING

Therapeutic drug monitoring (TDM) is a domain of clinical laboratory science primarily concerned with monitoring concentration of drugs that have a narrow therapeutic index that is ratio between minimum toxic concentration and minimum effective concentration is defined as therapeutic index. If a drug has a narrow therapeutic range, samples are taken to allow the dose to be adjusted so that the concentration remains between a minimum value for efficacy and a maximum value for safety. This is called "TDM". It has been widely used to adjust dosages of antiepileptic drugs such as phenytoin. Movement of a drug depends upon pharmacokinetic properties—absorption, distribution, metabolism, and elimination.[10]

Monitoring is often advocated as a way of avoiding or mitigating the harm from ADRs. Monitoring for ADRs by repeated laboratory testing probably started with the observation that the antibiotic chloramphenicol could cause bone marrow toxicity of two types, one occurring at high dosage and is reversible, and the other of which could occur at any therapeutic dosage and generally results in fatal aplastic anemia.

The TDM is unlikely to be cost-effective as a monitoring scheme for a rare adverse reaction of little consequence, but very cost-effective to introduce one for a common and serious adverse reaction.

The TDM was introduced in India in late 1980s. It involves tailoring a dose regimen to an individual patient by maintaining plasma or blood concentration within the therapeutic range. Automation has made it possible to develop assays but proper interpretation is required. Genetic variation in metabolism, elimination rates, disease states, pregnancy, nutritional deficiencies, and interactions with other drugs give rise to a wide range of plasma levels in patients administered the same dose.

Ayurvedic, homeopathic, and Unani medicines are often taken together with allopathic medicines. Experimental studies showed that *shankhapushpi* had both pharmacokinetic and pharmacodynamic interactions with phenytoin and phenytoin levels dropped. Drug levels can be altered with a hypoproteinemic state, and conditions such as acquired immune deficiency syndrome (AIDS), which lead to low levels of anti-tuberculosis (TB) drugs. Nutritional deficiencies also affect drug pharmacokinetics. TDM is useful in drugs with a narrow therapeutic index, those that are highly protein-bound or liable to interact or when the metabolites are very toxic.

During estimation of drug level, the actual time that the sample was obtained is important. The levels can be determined anytime during dosing interval for drug with a long half-life, e.g., phenobarbitone. For drugs that have a short half-life, peak, and trough concentrations must be measured at specific times. Concentrations measured during the distribution phase are variable and do not correlate with usual therapeutic range. Ideally, plasma drug samples should be procured after four half-lives of the drug. Peak concentrations are observed within 1–2 hours after oral administration of a drug; to ensure proper absorption levels must be measured before the next dose (trough).

Patients with chronic renal or liver disease, and prolonged therapy with anticonvulsant drugs, need TDM to avoid undertreatment and adverse events. Patients on theophylline can have increased plasma levels and toxicity when given with erythromycin. Cisapride, when given with theophylline can induce cardiac arrhythmias. TDM can help to identify noncompliant patients. Quality of products (drug content and bioavailability) is important especially for drugs with a narrow margin of safety for which TDM is relevant. The TDM service can be used to provide an important early indication of substandard drugs.

The most common indication for TDM of anticonvulsants such as carbamazepine, valproic acid, and phenytoin, has been nonresponse to a standard dose of drug. This allows differentiation between noncompliance, need for a higher dose, and true drug resistance requiring change over to second drug. Other common indications include suspected drug toxicity, dose adjustment in pregnancy, and DIs (especially common with anti-TB drugs). TDM of antimycobacterial drugs offers the clinician a chance to ensure that the patient achieves a serum concentration above the minimum inhibitory concentration (MIC).

Therapeutic drug monitoring can also be used as a useful research tool. In developing countries, TDM is important, where there are spurious poor quality drugs are available, drug legislation is inadequate and self-medication is easily practiced. With good prescribing practices and appropriate use of drug monitoring, therapeutic concentrations can be achieved in over 70% patients. Accuracy of drug assays, laboratory variability in reporting, and poor access to the tests are the limitations. A lot of information in clinical pharmacology and therapeutics is available on the Internet for reference, e.g., www.ascpt.org.

PRACTICE POINTS

- Do not prescribe a drug unless there is a clear indication for its use.
- Ask the child or parents, if he or she had previous allergy or idiosyncrasy to any drug or formulation before prescribing.
- Probe whether the child is already on other drugs including self-medication, health supplements, and alternative therapies as DIs may occur.
- Genetic factors and diseases of liver and kidney may alter the metabolism and excretion of drugs requiring a change in dosage.
- Prescribe as few drugs as possible and avoid polypharmacy.
- Give clear instructions on how to administer the drugs to children.
- Use familiar drugs as far as possible. Be alert to adverse or unexpected effects, whenever a new drug is used.
- Be aware that excipients may be responsible for the ADR. If the ADR is minor, consider prescribing an alternate formulation before altogether abandoning the drug.
- Educate the family that serious ADRs are likely to occur.
- Participate in ADR reporting.

REFERENCES

1. Rieder M. ADR in children: Pediatric pharmacy and drug safety. J Pediatr Pharmacol Ther. 2019;24(1):4-9.
2. Tandon VR, Mahajan V, Khajuria V, Gillani Z. Under-reporting of adverse drug reactions: a challenge for pharmacovigilance in India. Indian J Pharmacol. 2015;47(1):65-71.
3. Smyth RM, Gargon E, Kirkham J, Cresswell L, Golder S, Smyth R, et al. Adverse drug reactions in children—a systematic review. PLoS One. 2012;7(3):e24061.
4. Prakash J, Sachadeva R, Shrivastava TP, Jayachandran CV, Sahu A. Adverse event reporting tools and regulatory measures in India through outcome of pharmacovigilance program of India. Indian J Pharmacol. 2021;50(2):143-52.
5. Amale PN, Deshpande SA, Nakhate YD, Arsod NA. Pharmacovigilance process in India: An overview. J Pharmacovigil. 2018;6(2):259.
6. Kalaiselvan V, Kumar P, Mishra P, Singh GN. System of adverse drug reactions reporting: What, where, how, and whom to report? Indian J Crit Care Med. 2015;19(9):564-6.

7. Mahajan MM, Thatte UM, Gogtay NJ, Deshpande S. An analysis of completeness and quality of adverse drug reaction reports at an adverse drug reaction monitoring centre in Western India. Perspect Clin Res. 2018;9(3):123-6.
8. Singh N, Sharma G, Kumar R, Bhandari V. Pharmacovigilance in India and its impact in patient management. Curr Trends Diagn Treat. 2017;1(1):27-33.
9. Gonzalez D, Sinha J. Potential Drug-Drug Interaction evaluation: Drug, patient population, and methodical considerations. J Clin Pharmacol. 2021;61 Supp 1:S175-87.
10. Simeoli R, Dorlo TPC, Hanff LM, Huitema ADR, Dreesen E. Editorial: Therapeutic Drug Monitoring (TDM): A useful tool in pediatric pharmacology applied to routine clinical practice. Front Pharmacol. 2022:13:931843.

24.3 Rational Drug Therapy in Children

Arun Phatak

INTRODUCTION

Although pediatrics has now firmly established as a specialty in medical practice, it is the family physicians (graduate with or without diploma in pediatrics) who attend to a large majority of children in our country—they are the basic, first-line pediatricians for the families. It is a sick child that is often brought to the family physician and the management likely to involve use of drugs. No drug is 100% safe and it is expected that they are used sensibly based on evidence or reasoning.

EVIDENCE-BASED RATIONAL USE OF DRUG

Rational use of drugs may be defined as effective, safe, and affordable prescribing. A few decades ago, a doctor was considered to be next to God—whatever he/she said or did, was accepted by the patient without any question. The doctor had "clinical freedom" and the treatment was often guided by personal experience. Now the times have changed. Clinical freedom is considered to be "at best, a cloak for ignorance", and at worst, "excuse for quackery". The doctor is now accountable and should be able to justify the treatment he/she gives. The justification (evidence) comes from published and unpublished research papers.

However, one must be cautious in accepting whatever that comes in print or on "net"—one has to learn to assess critically the quality of papers for the robustness of methodology and of the interpretations of the observations **(Box 24.3.1)**. Not everyone is comfortable and competent to do this. But special committees of professional bodies issue practice guidelines that are usually based on evidence from high quality research papers. When high quality evidence is not available, the guidelines express consensus opinion of the experts in the field. As a rule, these guidelines should be followed in clinical practice.

BOX 24.3.1: Order of the quality of different types of research papers.

- Meta-analysis or systemic reviews of randomized clinical trials (RCTs)
- Randomized clinical trials
- Other controlled clinical trials
- Observational studies (cohort and case controlled)
- Case studies, anecdotal, and personal opinion

Evidence from published paper is based on quantifiable patient experiences and adds to the medicine's reliability. However, evidence-based guidelines may not be available or may not applicable because of unavailability of the necessary drugs, equipment, or skill or may be unaffordable or unacceptable to the family. In that case, one tries to do whatever is best with what is available and possible.

One may differ from the standard recommendations. Then the reason for differing along with one's personal observations should be shared with colleagues (clinical meetings of local bodies or as "letter to editor"). A change in current practice is brought about when such lateral thinking is followed by methodical research.

Currently the medical knowledge is almost exploding and new information is quickly available on the net. It should be remembered that current guidelines and recommendations may change as more information and experience becomes available. It is therefore essential to remain updated.

IRRATIONAL DRUG THERAPY—TYPES

Irrational use of drugs has been observed to occur at all levels of clinical practice. Sir William Osler had remarked that "errors in judgment must occur in the practice of an art that largely depends on balancing probabilities". This should be taken not as an excuse but as a warning to be doubly cautious. Irrational use of drugs may occur in three areas—choice of drugs, administration of drugs, and counseling.

Inappropriate Choice of Drugs

Unnecessary Drugs

Medicines may be prescribed when not needed. Use of the so-called "tonics", cough mixtures, and antibiotics are the most common examples of this type of irrationality.

A child with cough-cold and fever is likely to be prescribed an antibiotic and an antipyretic without ascertaining whether it is likely to be viral or bacterial infection or allergy. Such unnecessary use of antibiotics not only carries a risk of adverse reactions in the child but is also likely to lead to antibiotic resistance if misused on a wider scale.

Unnecessary drugs may be inadvertently administered when proprietary medicines are used. Very few of them are single drug preparations. Their composition must be checked to ensure that they do not contain any unwanted drug. For instance, some "cough mixtures" will contain two antihistamines or a cough suppressant with an "expectorant". Tablets and syrup containing both paracetamol and ibuprofen in therapeutic doses are in the market when often only one of them is needed. Single drug preparations should be used whenever possible.

Inappropriate Choice of Indicated Drug

This occurs most frequently while prescribing antibiotics. Before prescribing an antibiotic one should take into consideration the likely pathogen and its known sensitivity and resistance as well as the adverse effects. Moreover one should also take into consideration the route of administration of the selected antibiotic. Since antibiotics are usually given as a "course" of some minimum days, one that can be given both parenterally as well as orally is preferable so that as soon as the acute phase is over, one can shift to the more convenient, comfortable (and cheaper) oral route.

At times one is tempted to prescribe the latest "arrival" without studying its short- and long-term adverse effects. A known familiar drug is always preferable to an unknown newcomer.

Cost of the drug should be another factor considered, especially when the child belongs to low socioeconomic group. Among the group of effective drugs, the cheapest one should be the choice.

Indicated Drug not Used

This is a very rare irrationality that may occur due to ignorance of new developments but more likely to be due to local nonavailability of the drug or nonaffordability by the caretakers.

Inappropriate Administration of Drugs

In children, the dose of drugs varies not only by the weight or surface area of the child but also by the age level—influenced by maturation of various enzyme systems. Moreover, when there is impairment of certain organ system, the dose may need further modification based on the pharmacodynamics and pharmacokinetics of the drug. If one is not sure, it should be checked from the drug formulary. After calculating the required dose, it must be rounded to the nearest measurable weight or volume according to the strength of the available product. Some drugs are marketed in multiple strengths and forms. For instance, paracetamol syrup is available as 125 mg/5 mL and 250 mg/5 mL and paracetamol drops are available as 50 mg, 100 mg, or 125 mg per mL. There is a risk of underdosing or overdosing if the strength is not checked.

Recommendations about frequency of administration of the drug is decided by the timing of attainment and maintenance of optimal blood levels and should be followed meticulously.

Parenteral administration of drug is indicated if rapid effect is needed or if oral route is not possible or not effective. Parenteral administration should be switched to oral as soon as the child stabilizes. It not only reduces the complications of injections and reduces the burden on nursing staff, but also makes the child comfortable and reduces the hospital stay (and cost). In case of antibiotics, if the one being used parenterally cannot be given orally, another belonging to the same group or another reported effective by culture reports can be given.

Inappropriate Prescriptions and Counseling

The trend of giving computerized prescriptions is increasing but still the majority write them with hand. Many drugs have similar syntax and pronunciation. Doctor's handwriting is notorious and serious mistakes have occurred because a wrong medicine was dispensed by the chemist. So, the prescriptions must be written legibly—preferably in capital letters. Moreover, the instructions regarding doses, frequency, and duration are meant for the parents and therefore should be in clear words—not just in symbols—and preferably in a language that the parents understand. The prescription should be written in the standard format **(Box 24.3.2)**.

It is not just enough to write or print the prescription and hand it over to the parents. The parents should be explained

BOX 24.3.2: Standard format for prescriptions.

- Doctor's name, qualification, address, and registration number
- Date of writing prescription
- Patient's name, age, sex, and weight
- Names of the drugs (if necessary the pharmaceutical name) with recommended strengths, forms (drops/liquid/tablet/injection, etc.) and the amount to be bought
- Clear instructions regarding the dose, frequency, and total duration of medication—preferably in a language understood by the parents
- Explanation (at least orally) about common side effects and serious side effects and things to observe and report

verbally how the various drugs are to be administered, how the "dry" syrups are to be made liquid, etc. If the drug has any common side effects or possible adverse reaction, the parents should be counseled about them and informed the symptoms to be watched and reported.

REASONS FOR IRRATIONAL BEHAVIOR

Patient safety demands rational therapy and it is important to know why irrationality creeps into medical practice in spite of 4–6 years of training in the field.

Lack of Conviction and Inappropriate Role Model

The patient profile and the work culture in private practice are different from those in teaching institutions and a doubt prevails in the minds of some practitioners that "what is preached cannot be practiced". The young doctor in the anxiety of "establishing" in private practice, may try to emulate the prescribing behavior of a peer role model, without scrutinizing the rationality.

It is said that it takes about 1,000 days before the new doctor feels comfortable and established in private practice. It is during this waiting period that one should get into the habit keeping updated by regularly reading relevant papers from journal/s devoted to clinical practice and to attending clinical meetings and seminars of the local academic body.

Undue Pressures

With the anxiety of "establishing", the young pediatrician feels that curing the patient quickly will increase the clientele and tries to treat simultaneously every possible cause of the disease (polytherapy). Some parents demand medicines that are not necessary (e.g., antibiotics for minor cold and intravenous (IV) fluids when oral rehydration is possible). The doctor should not succumb to such demands but spend some time counseling the parents about the nature of the disease and its management.

The pharmaceutical industry is a big business with an objective of earning as great a profit as possible. Some of them give rich gifts—sometimes trips abroad, or sponsorship of research or of conferences and seminars. The doctor must be careful not to get enticed into going out of way to favor the company's products. Although doctors claim that such gifts do not influence their prescription-writing, any gift binds the receiver subconsciously to the "gifter" (like the practice of "return gifts" in social functions).

Life Goals

Medical practice is a profession and not a business. While earning to live a decent and comfortable life, our main objective must be the "total care of the patient". In an attempt to earn quick money, some doctors have drifted into malpractice.

Ignorance

As mentioned earlier, the medical science is advancing with leaps and bounds. It is difficult for a busy practitioner to study the original publications to keep up-to-date. An easy way is to become a life member of two or three professional organizations of relevant specialties—in case of pediatric practice the Indian Academy of Pediatrics and its subspecialty groups. One can scan the official journals and select the practice guidelines and other articles relevant to one's clinical practice. One can easily manage to attend the relevant lectures, seminars, workshops, or clinical meetings organized by the local branch.

MEDICAL AUDIT FOR RATIONAL DRUG THERAPY

After the case is closed, the patient's management should be reviewed and audited—checked against the standard recommended practice guideline.

In institutional practice, such medical audits can be done on grouped cases such as how a particular disease was treated, or review of the antibiotics use over the year, or use of cough mixtures or antibiotics in the management of children with upper respiratory infections. The data may be analyzed to compare the performance of different units or individual consultants in charge of the patient management (after concealing the identities of the patients and the consultants) to bring out the disparities. The anonymized results can be published in journals or discussed in clinical meetings. The objective of such studies must always be "improvement in patient care" and not punitive action against those who falter.

It is impossible to learn the whole field of medicine during the 4–5 years at medical college, but during clinical practice, every patient teaches us something. It is possible for the practicing doctor to watch one's own self—self-audit. One way is to review the clinical scenario and its management after the case is closed. Another way is to keep relevant demographic and clinical records in a tabular form ("excel" if the records are digital) and study how various medicines were used in different groups of clinical conditions. Find out places of faltering and try to improve.

ROAD TO RATIONAL USE OF DRUGS

- Know the broad basic aspects of pharmacokinetics and pharmacodynamics of drugs used most commonly in clinical practice and their major side effects, adverse reactions, and drug interactions.

- Keep abreast of the standard practice guidelines issued by the professional bodies.
- Whenever a drug is prescribed think "BRAIN":
  - *B*enefits expected
  - *R*eactions that may occur
  - *A*lternative drugs that may be considered
  - *I*ndividual considerations—availability, acceptability, and affordability
  - *N*ecessary? What will happen if not given?
- Ascertain the dosage and route of administration of the selected drug/s. Write a prescription for the same in the standard format.
- Counsel the child/parents/caretakers on administration of the drug/s and the effects that should be observed and reported.
- Review when the case is closed.
- Practice self-audit for rationalizing use of drugs. Share your experience, if you wish, in local clinical meetings/ medical bulletin.

BIBLIOGRAPHY

1. Feldman W. Evidence-Based Pediatrics. Bengaluru: Panther Publications Private Ltd.; 2001.
2. Greenhalgh T. How to Read a Paper. The Basics of Evidence Based Medicine, 3rd edition. London: Blackwell Publishing Ltd.; 2006.
3. Mathew JL, Singh M. Evidence based child health: fly but with feet on the ground. Indian Pediatr. 2008;45(2):95-8.
4. Raman SK. (2011). The Role of Evidence Based Medicine in Rational Drug Use. [online] Available from https://www.researchgate.net/publication/269997437_The_Role_of_Evidence_-Based_Medicine_in_Rational_Drug_Use. [Last accessed December, 2024].

24.4 What is a Prescription?

Jagdish Chinnappa

INTRODUCTION

A prescription is a fundamental element in the healthcare process, serving as a critical communication tool that embodies the medical authority's judgment for the optimal treatment of a patient's ailment. It is more than just a directive for medication; it is a comprehensive document that reflects a medical practitioner's diagnostic process and therapeutic plan at a particular moment in time.

NOT JUST A PIECE OF PAPER: UNDERSTANDING THE PRESCRIPTION AS A COMMUNICATION TOOL

The prescription bridges three critical points of contact: The doctor, the patient, and the pharmacist.[1-3] For the doctor, it is the culmination of a detailed clinical assessment, encompassing hypothesis formation, diagnosis, and problem identification. For the patient, it is a guide to understanding their health condition and the proposed treatment plan. For the pharmacist, it is a directive for dispensing the appropriate medication and offering additional advice on its proper use.

IMPORTANCE OF PRESCRIPTION IN HEALTHCARE

Prescriptions serve several pivotal roles in healthcare:

- *Medical record:* They act as a vital record of the patient's health condition and the treatment plan, crucial for future consultations and continuity of care.
- *Audit and review:* Prescription audits are essential for evaluating prescribing habits and adherence to evidence-based practices. This retrospective analysis helps in improving healthcare quality and patient safety.
- *Legal and ethical documentation:* Prescriptions are legal documents. They are subject to scrutiny and must adhere to regulatory standards to ensure ethical medical practice.

COMPONENTS OF AN EFFECTIVE PRESCRIPTION

A well-constructed prescription has three major components:[4,5]

1. The header
2. The body
3. The end piece

The Header: Preliminary Steps

1. *Patient details:* This includes the patient's name, age, sex, address, registration number, and contact information like phone number and email. These details are vital for maintaining ongoing communication and personalizing the treatment plan.
2. *Key measurements on which dosage calculations are done:* Key metrics like weight and height are crucial for accurate dosing, particularly in pediatrics and for medications with narrow therapeutic indices.
3. *Healthcare practitioner's information:* The name, qualifications, and registration number and contact details of the prescribing healthcare professional should be clearly mentioned. This ensures accountability and provides a point of reference for any queries or follow-up.
4. *Healthcare facility details:* The address and emergency contact details of the healthcare facility should be included. This is particularly important in case of adverse reactions or the need for urgent follow-up care.
5. *Date of consultation:* The exact date of the consultation provides a timeline for the treatment and is essential for tracking the progression of care.
6. *Diagnosis and allergies:* A clear mention of the diagnosis or problem list, along with any known allergies of the patient, is crucial. This helps in preventing adverse drug reactions and ensures that the prescribed medication is appropriate for the patient's condition.

The Body of the Prescription: Key Considerations

The body of a prescription is where the specific treatment plan is outlined. It is the core of the prescription, detailing the medication regimen designed for the patient's health needs.[1] Precision and clarity in this section are paramount to ensuring the patient's safety and efficacy of the treatment.

1. *Listing medications: The use of generic names*[2,6]
    - *Generic names:* The use of generic names, written in capitals or printed via computer, is emphasized. This practice serves several purposes:
        - *Reduced errors:* Generic names are standardized, reducing confusion caused by multiple brand names.
        - *Cost-effectiveness:* Generic medicines are generally more affordable, making healthcare more accessible.
    - *Supporting local pharmacies:* Encouraging purchases from *Jan Aushadhi Kendras* (People's Medicine Centers) in India supports government initiatives to provide cost-effective medication.
    - *Clear identification:* Each medication should be clearly listed to avoid any confusion during dispensing and administration.
2. *Medication strength*[6]
   Explicit mention: The strength of each medication must be clearly mentioned. This is crucial for ensuring the correct dosage, particularly when a single medication comes in various strengths.
3. *Dosage specificity*[3]
   Precise measurement: Dosages should be specified in precise units (e.g., 2.5 mL) rather than in vague terms like "half a teaspoon". This specificity is vital for:
    - *Accuracy:* Ensuring that the patient receives the correct amount of medication
    - *Safety:* Reducing the risk of underdosing or overdosing, especially in children where dosage accuracy is critical
4. *Frequency and duration of treatment*[2]
    - *Clear frequency:* The prescription must detail how often the medication is to be taken. This could be in hours (e.g., every 6 hours) or as per daily routine (e.g., once every morning).
    - *Duration:* The total length of the treatment course should be explicitly mentioned. This helps in:
        - *Preventing antibiotic resistance:* Particularly important in the case of antibiotics to ensure that the full course is completed
        - *Treatment efficacy:* Ensuring that the treatment is taken for the appropriate duration to be effective
5. *Quantity of medication*
    - *Specific quantities:* The exact number of tablets, capsules, or the volume of liquid medication should be mentioned. This is important for:
        - *Ensuring full treatment course:* The patient should have enough medication to complete the course without interruption.
        - *Preventing waste:* Reducing excess medication which might lead to misuse or be wastefully discarded.

Endpiece of a Prescription: Ensuring Comprehensive Care and Compliance

The endpiece of a prescription plays a pivotal role in ensuring that the patient fully understands and accurately follows the treatment plan.[3-5] It is not merely a formality but a crucial step in the healthcare process, especially in pediatrics, where communication and clarity are paramount.

1. *Language and communication*
    - *Patient's language:* Communicating the prescription details in the patient's language is crucial for clear understanding. This can be achieved through verbal explanation or translation via software applications.
    - *Importance of understanding:* Ensuring that the patient or caregiver comprehends the prescription

BOX 24.4.1: Talking to children about medications.

- *Use age-appropriate language:* Adjust your language to suit the child's age and understanding. Use simple, concrete terms for younger children
- *Explain the purpose:* Describe in simple terms how the medicine will help them feel better or stay healthy
- *Involve them in the process:* For older children, involve them in discussions about their medication. This can empower them and encourage adherence
- *Address fears and concerns:* Children may be afraid of side effects or have misconceptions. Listen to their fears and provide reassurance
- *Demonstrate and practice:* Show them how to take the medicine. For example, with inhalers, demonstrate the technique and let them practice
- *Discuss the importance of adherence:* Explain why it is important to take the medicine exactly as prescribed and what could happen if they do not
- *Use positive reinforcement:* Praise them for taking their medication properly. A reward system for younger children can be effective
- *Be honest about taste and side effects:* Prepare them if the medicine might taste bad or cause mild side effects and discuss ways to cope with these
- *Create a routine:* Establishing a routine can make taking medication a part of their daily schedule, reducing resistance or forgetfulness
- *Use visual aids:* Pictures or stories about how medicine works can be helpful, especially for younger children
- *Ensure understanding:* Ask them to explain back to you what they have understood about their medication to ensure clarity
- *Maintain open communication:* Let them know they can always come to you with questions or problems related to their medication
- *The goal* is to make the child feel comfortable and confident about taking their medicine, understanding its importance in their health and well-being

details reduces the risk of errors and improves adherence to the medication regimen.

- *Talking to children about medications* involves a delicate balance of providing clear information, addressing their concerns, and ensuring that they understand the importance of the medication. **Box 24.4.1** details the salient points to be noted while communicating with children.

2. *Reviewing drug interactions and administration instructions*
    - *Drug interaction check:* A thorough review of potential interactions between prescribed medications is essential to avoid adverse effects.
    - *Minimizing medication quantity:* Limiting the number of medications, whenever possible, simplifies the regimen, especially important in pediatric cases where medication administration can be challenging.
    - *Administration guidelines:* Clear instructions on when to take the medication (before, after, or during meals) and any food interactions should be specified. Medication storage should be emphasized
    - *Side effects and care:* Educating caregivers about common side effects, red flag signs, and care to minimize side effects (like rinsing the mouth after taking certain medications) is vital for patient safety.
3. *Patient education and clarification*
    - *Necessity and administration:* Time should be invested in explaining why the medication is necessary, how to administer it correctly, and addressing any questions or concerns.
    - *Side effects and emergency contact:* Informing about possible side effects, what constitutes an urgent situation, and providing contact details for emergencies are essential aspects of patient education.
    - *Cost transparency:* Discussing the cost of medication can help patients and families plan and understand their financial commitments.
4. *Follow-up and review*
    Scheduling reviews: Advising patients when to return for a follow-up is important for monitoring the effectiveness of the treatment and making necessary adjustments.
5. *Record keeping and transmission*
    - *Prescription copy:* Keeping a copy of the prescription is crucial for future reference and continuity of care. In settings where prescriptions are transmitted directly to pharmacies, a copy should still be provided to the patient.
    - *Importance of records:* Accurate record-keeping facilitates the review of the patient's medication history and aids in the assessment of treatment efficacy.
6. *Special cases: Multiple copies*
    Controlled substances: In the case of controlled medications like morphine, multiple copies of the prescription may be necessary for regulatory compliance and monitoring.
7. *Prescription refills*
    Long-term conditions: Managing a prescription refills for chronic conditions requires as much attention as the initial prescription. This includes ensuring that the patient understands the ongoing nature of the treatment and the process for obtaining refills.
8. *Signature*
    Authentication: The prescription must be authenticated with the signature of the prescribing physician. This is a legal requirement and adds a level of accountability.
9. *Pharmacist's role and verification*
    Pharmacist's stamp and seal: A stamp and seal from the pharmacist, including the date of dispensing, confirm that the medication has been dispensed as per the prescription. This helps in:

BOX 24.4.2: A sample prescription.

Header

Patient's name:	***Physician's Name:*** [Your Name]
Boy/Girl	Dr. ....
Age: ..... Year ..... Months	*Qualifications:* [Your Qualifications] ....
Date: ..(DD)/..(MM)/....(YYYY)	*Registration Number:* [Your Registration Number] ....
Weight: .... Kg	*Clinic/Hospital Address:* [Your Work Address] ....
Parents: Father	*ER* ....
Mother......................	*Contact Number:* [Your Contact Number] Mob. ....
Contact details	
Mobile	

Body

Diagnosis: Fever 1 day
Medication: Paracetamol
Strength: 250 mg/5 mL oral suspension
Dosage: 15 mg/kg/dose
Amount to administer: 150 mg (3 mL) per dose
Frequency: Every 4–6 hours as needed for fever
Duration: Not to exceed 5 days
Route: Oral

End Piece

Instructions: Shake well before use. Administer with or without food. Do not exceed 4 doses in 24 hours. Use the measuring device provided for accurate dosing

Warnings: If fever persists for more than 3 days or if new symptoms appear, consult a physician

Refills: None

Signature: [Your Signature]

- *Preventing misuse:* Ensures that the prescription is used for its intended purpose and timeframe.
- *Duplication prevention:* A stamped and sealed prescription minimizes the risk of duplication and unauthorized reuse.

An example of a complete prescription format is given in **Box 24.4.2**.

Prescription Errors

Some of the common prescription mistakes seen in practice are given in **Box 24.4.3**.

BOX 24.4.3: Common prescription mistakes.

- *Incorrect dosing:* This is particularly critical in pediatrics where doses are often weight-based. Over- or under-dosing can occur due to miscalculation
- *Medication errors:* Prescribing the wrong medication due to similar sounding names (e.g., penicillin vs. penicillamine) or appearance
- *Route of administration errors*: Mistakes in specifying how a drug should be administered (oral, IV, etc.), e.g., Rotavirus vaccine injected!!
- *Frequency mistakes:* Errors in how often the medication should be taken. Patients do not understand OD, QID, etc.
- *Duration errors:* Not specifying or incorrectly specifying the length of time for which the medication should be taken
- *Failing to review allergies:* Overlooking a child's known allergies can lead to serious reactions
- *Neglecting drug interactions:* Not considering other medications the child is taking which could interact with the new prescription
- *Illegible handwriting:* This can lead to misinterpretation of the prescription by pharmacists and caregivers
- *Incomplete instructions:* Failing to provide complete instructions for use, including what to do in case of a missed dose
- *Not tailoring to the patient:* Overlooking patient-specific factors like age, weight, and comorbidities that affect drug choice and dosing

CONCLUSION

The generation of a prescription is a critical component in the patient management process. It ensures that the patient or caregiver is well informed about the treatment, understands how to administer the medication correctly, and is aware of potential side effects and what to do in emergencies. It also serves as a legal document that holds the healthcare provider accountable while providing a reference for the pharmacist. Moreover, it plays a significant role in patient safety and adherence to treatment.

Meticulous attention to these details reflects the commitment of healthcare providers to patient-centered care and the importance of effective communication in the therapeutic process. In sum, the prescription is not just the conclusion of a medical document; it is a comprehensive approach to ensuring that the patient's journey toward recovery is well guided, informed, and safe.

REFERENCES

1. Rajeev M, Bhaskar V. How well are we prescribing medications to our children?. Indian J Child Health. 2014;10(4):47-51.
2. Mandal P, Asad M, Kayal A, Biswas M. Assessment of use of World Health Organization access, watch, reserve antibiotics and core prescribing indicators in pediatric outpatients in a tertiary care teaching hospital in Eastern India. Perspect Clin Res. 2023;14(2):61-7.
3. Maaskant JM, Vermeulen H, Apampa B, Fernando B, Ghaleb MA, Neubert A, et al. Interventions for reducing medication errors in children in hospital. Cochrane Database Syst Rev. 2015;(3):CD006208.
4. Kothari A, Jain AK. Manual of Prescription Writing with Case Scenarios, 2nd edition. New Delhi: CBS Publishers and Distributors Pvt Ltd.; 2023.
5. Sharma S, Sethi GR (Eds). Standard Treatment Guidelines, 6th edition. Delhi Society for Promotion of Rational use of Drugs. Gurgaon: Wolters Kluwer (India) Pvt Ltd.; 2021.
6. Naserifar M, Yousefiabadi SA, Vahdati-Mashhadian N, Ataei M, Hashempour N, Jafari N, et al. Modified Omission of Prescriptions and Inappropriate Prescriptions (POPI) Criteria to Assess the Quality of Prescriptions to Pediatric Patients. Iran J Pediatr. 2023;33(2):e123229.

24.5 Administration of Drugs in Children

Ketan H Shah

INTRODUCTION

Administration of drugs in children is in itself a challenging task. The lack of a suitable preparation, lack of standardization, and lack of knowledge of pharmacokinetics and pharmacodynamics have created a lot of confusion. Standardization and legislation are in operation but not implemented correctly. So many compositions are available in different forms and different concentrations; for example, paracetamol suspension is available in 120 mg/5 mL and 125 mg/5 mL also. Some brands have 250 mg/5 mL and other would have 256 mg/5 mL. In drops, formulations of 100 mg/1 mL and 150 mg/L are also available. These all create prescription errors and will harm children. This chapter highlights common precautions, available modalities of formulations, and a discussion on inert ingredients.

PRECAUTIONS

Before Giving

Every parents should ascertain that medicines are prescribed by a registered medical practitioner. They should avoid taking medicines from any nonmedical person and unlicensed shop. Over-the-counter medicines which do not need prescription should be supervised and carefully selected. Quacks and nonregistered healthcare persons should be identified by parents and should avoid visiting them. Every medicine of any healthcare-related practice can harm the child if given unsupervised. Avoid taking medicines from a person who does not have a license for allopathy practice.

Parents should take help of the doctor and nursing staff for their purchased medicines and should be verified. Sometimes, chemists give wrong medicines or alternate medicines which will have different content and different concentrations. If it is of different concentrations, the dose will be different.

Parents should get knowledge about how to prepare the medicine if it is in powder formulation, e.g., how much water to be added and how to shake and use it. The viability of these reconstituted formulations is usually 7–10 days and they should be discarded afterward. Majority of the antibiotics after reconstitution are kept in refrigeration and the temperature should be maintained. Do not use medicines after their expiry date.

Ready-to-use medicines may contain added sugar as flavor. For a juvenile diabetic patient, they should be avoided.

Some children may have a past history of drug reaction, which may be minor or major like erythema multiforme or Stevens-Johnson syndrome. Some children have glucose-6-phosphate dehydrogenase (G6PD) deficiency, some may have fixed drug eruption as a side effect, and some have renal or hepatic failure. Parents should inform the doctor before giving any medicines. Doses are modified and certain drugs are avoided in certain deficiencies or diseased conditions.

CARE DURING DRUG ADMINISTRATION

Oral Administration

Before giving any oral medicines, parents should check dose, how to prepare the medicine if it is a dry powder preparation, and how to reconstitute. Dropper, measuring cup, or cap and their calibrations should be checked. Overdose and underdose should be avoided. All liquid preparations should be shaken properly to avoid giving supernatant fluid and sometimes precipitations. If a child vomits immediately after taking a medicine, the dose can be repeated. If she/he vomits after sometime, then consult the doctor before repetition of the dose. Certain drugs are given on an empty stomach and a few are given with a fatty meal for better efficacy. Parents should follow the suggestions by the doctor.

Some medicines are bitter in taste and they can be mixed with flavoring liquids like lemon juice, etc. Doses are decided as per pharmacokinetics and dynamics, so "at random" decision should not be taken for the administration of any medicine.

Parenteral Administration

From a pharmacokinetic point of view, parenteral routes can be considered near-ideal ways of administration due to the high bioavailability and rapid onset of action usually obtained. In the case of intravenous (IV) administration, the entire dose reaches the systemic circulation and an immediate physiological response can be achieved. Intramuscular (IM) and subcutaneous (SC) administrations involve an absorption process from the injection site, which leads to a delayed response, since drug molecules have to diffuse in the interstitial space in order to reach the capillaries.[1] All care should be taken before and during parenteral administration of medicines. Dose, dilution, recommendation of dilution, IV cannula for its patency, diluting fluid, etc., should be ascertained. IM injection should be avoided as far as possible. If needed, it is always in thigh and not in gluteal region. SC and intradermal (ID) doses are mainly for vaccination. The SC route is used for administering insulin and growth hormone (GH) in children. Parenteral medications should be either by slow infusion or should be with an infusion pump to avoid rapid push. Certain drugs are given as rapid push like adenosine. In this situation, technique and dilution are important.

The major problem with parenteral administration is the sensation of pain at the injection site resulting in poor patient adherence. The pain is a direct effect of the medicine itself, but several other factors can influence the sensation of the pain like the needle features, injection site, volume of drug injected, speed of injection, and characteristics of the medications like pH and kind of excipients included.[1]

Per Rectal Administration

Few medicines are available in a suppository form like paracetamol, diclofenac, laxative medicines, etc. Due precaution is taken so that the medicine goes in the anorectal area only. Hold the part tight for a few seconds so that the suppository does not come out.

Intramuscular Administration

Except vaccination, IM injections are rarely given in pediatric patients. In small children, the common site for IM injection is always the lateral part of thigh, not the gluteal region. In adolescents, deltoid or gluteal region can be used but safer is the lateral side of thigh. In the gluteal region, chances of sciatic nerve injury are very high (please see *Chapter 23.1: Safe Injection Practices* for more details).

Sublingual Administration

Few medicines are available in sublingual forms like vitamin B_{12}, ondansetron, etc. They are to be kept either on the tongue or below the tongue as instructed. They have an advantage of better absorption.

Inhaled Forms

Intranasal and oral inhalers are available for the management of rhinitis and asthma. The method of administration should be taught to parents.

AFTER GIVING MEDICINES

If any side effect occurs like vomiting, urticarial reaction, tachycardia, respiratory distress, or uneasy feeling, then it should be notified immediately to the healthcare center. Side effects are sometimes idiosyncratic and sometimes related to overdosage. Minor side effects are common for some medications like diarrhea after amoxicillin. Serious side effects should be taken care of. Few medicines like valproic acid (an anticonvulsant) and antitubercular drugs will have slow side effects such as hepatitis, behavioral changes, and neuropathy. Parents have to be informed about these and the patients should be routinely checked and observed. (See *Chapter 24.2: Adverse Drug Reactions, Drug Interactions, and Therapeutic Drug Monitoring* for more details.)

AVAILABLE PREPARATIONS FOR ADMINISTRATION

Various formulations are available for administration.

Oral Preparations

Oral preparations include syrups, suspensions, dispersible tablets, sublingual tablets, powder formulation for reconstitution, tablets which are to be swollen, and slow disintegrating preparations. They release medicines in gut slowly.

Parenteral Preparations

Parenteral preparations include IV, IM, SC, and intradermal preparations.

Per Rectal Preparations

Per rectal preparations include rectal suppositories and rectal solutions.

For a more detailed list of all available preparations of commonly used medicines in children, please refer to *Chapter 24.14: Drugs Licensed for Use in Neonates, Children, and Adolescents.*

EXCIPIENT OR INERT INGREDIENTS

Excipients or inert ingredients are those substances added to pharmacologically active compounds to facilitate dosage form production, enhance drug stability, and improve palatability for the patient.

Common antimicrobial agents include chlorbutol, benzyl alcohol, sodium benzoate, sorbic acid, phenol, thimerosal, parabens, and benzalkonium chloride. Antioxidants used in pharmaceutical products include butylated hydroxytoluene and hydroxyanisole, as well as propyl gallate and sulfites.[2,3] The link between benzyl alcohol and neonatal cardiovascular collapse, "the gasping baby syndrome", is perhaps the most widely publicized adverse reaction related to the use of inert ingredients.

Sweeteners and Flavorings

Saccharin, sucrose, sorbitol, aspartame, and fructose are the most commonly used sweeteners. Lactose is used in the manufacturing of tablet and capsule dosage forms as a diluent or filler, rather than as a sweetener. Diarrhea, abdominal pain, and dental caries are known side effects. Their concentration should be limited in weight/volume (W/V) ratio. The standard guidelines should be followed. Sweeteners will be harmful to patients with diabetes mellitus and those who are on ketogenic diet due to refractory epilepsy treatment. Whenever a cough syrup is prescribed in these patients, sugar-free preparation is preferred.

Dyes and Colorants

There are more than 100 dyes and colorants used in medications to give either color or flavor. This can improve palatability. However, the compositions are sometimes not disclosed and they can cause side effects.

Solvents

Propylene glycol and polyethylene glycol are used as solvents in many dosage formulations as many drugs are not water-soluble. Alcohol derivates (like ethanol) should be restricted in formulation as per standard guidelines.

These inert ingredients can cause many side effects, which may be acute and chronic. The common acute side effects include local side effect like contact dermatitis and systemic side effects like bronchoconstriction, cardiac arrhythmia, sudden anaphylaxis, abdominal pain, and diarrhea. The chronic side effects include dental caries, and some effects may be linked to other systemic chronic diseases.

CONCLUSION

In conclusion, parents should be careful before giving the medicine to their children. Follow the prescription of registered medical doctor only. Check the doses, its content, method of administration and get information of possible side effects.

REFERENCES

1. Sunach I, Martinez R, Festini T, Peris JE. Subcutaneous injection of drugs: Literature review of factors influencing pain sensation at the injection site. Adv Ther. 2019;36(11):2986-96.
2. Golightly LK, Smolinske SS, Bennett ML, Sutherland EW, Rumack BH. Pharmaceutical excipients: Adverse effects associated with 'inactive' ingredients in drug products (Part I). Med Toxicol Adverse Drug Exp. 1988;3(2):128-65.
3. Golightly LK, Smolinske SS, Bennett ML, Sutherland EW, Rumack BH. Pharmaceutical excipients: Adverse effects associated with 'inactive' ingredients in drug products (Part II). Med Toxicol Adverse Drug Exp. 1988;3(3):209-40.

24.6 Antibiotic Stewardship Program

Jeeson C Unni

INTRODUCTION

The commitment of all pediatricians should always be toward evidence-based selection of antibiotics for a given illness; its administration at recommended dose and duration; while ensuring adequate monitoring and audit of usage—and that is the essence of an *Antibiotic Stewardship Program (ASP).*

Therefore, the objectives of the movement are to develop a comprehensive long-term program to maximize antimicrobial benefit, avoid adverse reactions and drug allergies, improve outcomes, reduce cost of treatment of infectious diseases, avoid development of antimicrobial resistance to the extent possible, and create protocols for combating emerging resistance.[1,2] The emergence of drug resistance and the colonization or infection with these organisms is the "collateral damage" that results from the injudicious use of antibiotics.

The World Health Organization (WHO) 2019 Access, Watch, and Reserve (AWaRe) Classification antibiotics database compliance is an indication of optimal use and monitoring of antibiotics in a country. The data published suggests wide country to country differences in use of AWaRe antibiotics in hospitalized neonates and children.[3] India stands 27th in the pediatric and 33rd in the neonatal survey, respectively, among 56 countries.

STRATEGIES FOR IMPLEMENTATION OF ANTIBIOTIC STEWARDSHIP PROGRAM IN AN INSTITUTION

Antimicrobial Stewardship Team

The team, led by a physician, should include an infectious disease physician, a clinical pharmacist with infectious disease training, a clinical microbiologist, and an information system specialist. Support of clinicians and nurses is to be ensured by involving key persons of each group in this committee.

Interventions

Front-end Approach—Formulary Restriction and Preauthorization[4]

Restrictions may be placed on the prescribing of certain antimicrobials on a hospital's formulary. Such restrictions may be based on who can prescribe an antimicrobial (e.g., certain services or expertise), or on acceptable criteria for use of the antimicrobial in the institution. It involves the preapproval of orders before dispensing a drug. Approval is often obtained through consultation between the prescriber and someone responsible for assessing the appropriateness of the request (often an infectious disease specialist and/or infectious disease pharmacist).

This approach is "restrictive" stewardship and may be used in conjunction with "prospective" audit with intervention and feedback to oversee both initial and ongoing use of restricted agents. This strategy has proved to significantly reduce expenditure of the targeted drug but could result in increased use of antimicrobials that are not restricted.

Back-end Approach—Prospective Audit and Feedback[4]

This strategy employs the clinical decisions support software (CDSS) systems to prospectively audit antimicrobial use and send feedback to the prescriber in order to tailor specific antibiotic therapy for a given patient or infection. It would be possible to periodically review certain groups of infections, e.g., extended-spectrum beta-lactamases (ESBLs)—producing urinary tract infection, so that children receive optimal therapy and recommendations for de-escalation may be evolved guided by culture and sensitivity or PCR report; or a group of children, e.g., immunocompromised children, to constitute hospital antibiotic guidelines. This method of stewardship has been shown to decrease antimicrobial use, cost of treatment, and the number of new prescriptions of antimicrobials; in addition to ensuring clinician satisfaction.

Other Strategies that Need to Be in Place

Facility-specific Clinical Practice Guidelines

Periodic dissemination and implementation of evidence-based institutional guidelines on appropriate initiation of oral antibiotics, transition from IV to oral antibiotics, strategies for de-escalation, shortest effective duration of therapy, and changing from broad-spectrum to targeted therapy is an effective way of standardizing prescribing practices based on local epidemiology.[5]

Antimicrobial "Time Out"

A stop order will alert clinicians to revise antimicrobial agents after 72 hours of initiation depending on culture and sensitivity testing results, response to therapy, present condition, and facility needs.[6]

Pharmacy-driven Interventions

Clinical pharmacists play an important role in the development, review, and implementation of ASP guidelines and policies; provide clinical advice, data of audits and feedback to optimize antimicrobial prescribing; and identify medication errors, among other activities.[7] These inputs would aid the primary physician in making appropriate clinical judgment for therapy of a given case.

Educational Interventions

Updates to improve prescriber and patient knowledge of appropriate antibiotic use at regular intervals is an essential component of ASP of an health facility.[8]

Microbiology and Laboratory Inputs

Antibiotic Stewardship Program needs to work with the microbiology to develop stratified antimicrobial susceptibility tests according to the latest Clinical and Laboratory Standard Institute (CLSI) guidelines.[9]

The use of serial procalcitonin (PCT) for intensive care unit (ICU) patients with suspected infection could be recommended by ASP. "Stop Antibiotics on Procalcitonin Guidance Study (SAPS)", the largest PCT trial to date, demonstrated reduction in both antibiotic exposure and mortality in critically ill patients.[10] However, if the institution ICU has a robust ASP, the comparative cost-effectiveness of PCT monitoring needs to be evaluated.

Selective Reporting

It includes a strategy where susceptibilities of broad-spectrum agents and those drugs at risk for overprescription are deliberately withheld; in cascade reporting, antimicrobial agents of each class are ranked based on spectrum of activity, popularity, potential for overprescribing, risk of drug resistance, and cost; and microbiology inputs are used to reduce the use of broad-spectrum, expensive antibiotics, and guide de-escalation without affecting outcome when managing serious infections.[11]

Antimicrobial Measurements

Defined daily dose (DDD), day of therapy (DOT), length of therapy (LOT), antimicrobe-free days, cost of therapy, measures of antimicrobial appropriateness (not developed to the degree that makes them useful and widely applicable), proportion of patients receiving therapy as per facility guideline or algorithm, appropriate use of microbiology inputs, proportion of patients converted to oral therapy, and process measures (documenting an indication for the antimicrobial, filling in an antimicrobial order form, or mandating an infectious diseases consult) are used as measures to monitor antimicrobial therapy.[12] Documentation of all these data should be utilized to revise and update the in-house protocols for ASP.

CONCLUSION

The silent epidemic of antibiotic resistance has made it mandatory that institutions develop guidelines for appropriate use of antimicrobials and create a robust system for monitoring and audit of antibiotic use.

REFERENCES

1. Society for Healthcare Epidemiology of America; Infectious Diseases Society of America; Pediatric Infectious Diseases Society. Policy statement on antimicrobial stewardship by the Society for Healthcare Epidemiology of America (SHEA), the Infectious Diseases Society of America (IDSA), and the Pediatric Infectious Diseases Society (PIDS). Infect Control Hosp Epidemiol. 2012;33(4):322-7.
2. Malani AN, Richards PG, Kapila S, Otto HM, Czerwinski J, Singal B. Clinical and economic outcomes from a community hospital's antimicrobial stewardship program. Am J Infect Control. 2013;41(2):145-8.
3. Hsia Y, Lee BR, Versporten A, Yang Y, Bielicki J, Jackson C, et al.; GARPEC and Global-PPS networks. Use of the WHO Access, Watch, and Reserve classification to define patterns of hospital antibiotic use (AWaRe): an analysis of paediatric survey data from 56 countries. Lancet Glob Health. 2019;7:e861-871.
4. Doron S, Davidson LE. Antimicrobial Stewardship. Mayo Clin Proc. 2011;86(11):1113-23.
5. Bauer KA, West JE, Balada-Llasat JM, Pancholi P, Stevenson KB, Goff DA. An antimicrobial stewardship program's impact with rapid polymerase chain reaction methicillin-resistant Staphylococcus aureus/S. aureus blood culture test in patients with S. aureus bacteremia. Clin Infect Dis. 2010;51(9):1074-80.
6. Barlam TF, Cosgrove SE, Abbo LM, MacDougall C, Schuetz AN, Septimus EJ, et al. Implementing an Antibiotic Stewardship Program: Guidelines by the Infectious Diseases Society of America and the Society for Healthcare Epidemiology of America. Clin Infect Dis. 2016;62(10):e51-77.
7. Unni JC, Chacko M, Jacob J, Warrier A. Randomized control trial on impact of clinical pharmacist led interventions on antibiotic stewardship program in children 0 to 18 years age in a tertiary care hospital in southern India. Am J Infect Control. 2024;52(5):570-4.
8. Gravatt LAH, Patterson JA, Franzese S. Educational Antimicrobial Stewardship Strategies. Curr Treat Options Infect Dis. 2016;8:84-92.
9. Weinstein MP, Lewis JS 2nd. The Clinical and Laboratory Standards Institute Subcommittee on Antimicrobial Susceptibility Testing: Background, Organization, Functions, and Processes. J Clinical Microbiol. 2020;58(3):1-7.
10. de Jong E, van Oers JA, Beishuizen A, Vos P, Vermeijden WJ, Haas LE, et al. Efficacy and safety of procalcitonin guidance in reducing the duration of antibiotic treatment in critically ill patients: a randomised, controlled, open-label trial. Lancet Infect Dis. 2016;16(7):819-27.
11. Wu H, Lutgring JD, McDonald LC, Webb A, Fields V, Blum L, et al. Selective and Cascade Reporting of Antimicrobial Susceptibility Testing Results and Its Impact on Antimicrobial Resistance Surveillance-National Healthcare Safety Network, April 2020 to March 2021. Microbiol Spectr. 2023;11(2):e0164622.
12. Morris AM. Antimicrobial Stewardship Programs: Appropriate Measures and Metrics to Study their Impact. Curr Treat Options Infect Dis. 2014;6(2):101-12.

24.7 Antiviral Agents

Ramachandran Padmanabhan

INTRODUCTION

Viral infections range from subclinical or mild forms with a self-limiting course to life-threatening problems. Compared to antibiotics, antiviral drugs were developed much later. The first antiherpetic drug, idoxuridine was synthesized in 1959.

As the viruses closely integrate with the cellular function, there is a risk of collateral damage to cell function by antiviral agents. The challenge was to develop such molecules which will target the infecting virus without damaging the cells. The other problem encountered in the development of antivirals is the difficulty in confirming viral infections with objective laboratory investigations like culture and sensitivity tests to determine the efficacy of drugs. Advent of molecular diagnostic tests and their availability at affordable cost have helped in choosing appropriate antivirals and also in monitoring the response to treatment. Success of therapy will hinge on collecting appropriate specimens before initiating therapy, assessing the age and the immune status of the child and the function of various organ systems. Drug doses depend on age and suitable modifications may be required depending on renal or liver function. The decision for curative treatment, preventive therapy, and duration is based on whether the child is immunologically competent or not. Immunocompromised children are susceptible to develop severe local or disseminated disease on exposure to common viruses.

MODE OF ACTION OF ANTIVIRAL AGENTS

The commonly targeted sites of action for antiviral agents are at the:

- Viral entry, absorption, penetration, and uncoating (amantadine, rimantadine)
- Transcription or replication of the viral genome (acyclovir, valacyclovir, cidofovir, famciclovir, penciclovir, foscarnet, ganciclovir, valganciclovir, ribavirin, trifluridine)
- Viral protein synthesis [interferons (IFNs)]
- Viral assembly or release (oseltamivir, zanamivir, IFNs)

Antiviral agents exhibit their effect maximally during viral replication inside the cells. They may not eliminate the viruses which are dormant or not replicating actively.

Antiviral resistance is an emerging problem, which can be attributed to high degree of mutation and prolonged and repeated courses of therapy as in immunocompromised children.

CLASSIFICATION OF ANTIVIRAL AGENTS

Nucleoside/Nucleotide Analogs

These agents are structurally similar to the naturally occurring nucleosides/nucleotides. When incorporated into the nucleic acid of the virus, they inhibit viral DNA polymerase and block further addition of nucleotide resulting in chain termination. Their efficacy is based on their selective incorporation into viral nucleic acid in preference to host cell DNA. They are the most effective agents against viruses under the herpes virus family.

Neuraminidase Inhibitors

Neuraminidase inhibitors are drugs which target a viral specific enzyme (neuraminidase) as in influenza virus that helps in the deaggregation as well as prevention of release of newly formed virus from the host cells.

Interferons

Interferons are naturally occurring components of cellular immunity used against viral infections. Currently these are used in conjunction with other antiviral agents for hepatitis B infections.

Antiviral drugs commonly used in practice are against herpes viruses, influenza virus, and hepatitis viruses **(Table 24.7.1)**.[1] Antiviral therapy of human immunodeficiency virus (HIV) is discussed separately.

ANTIVIRAL AGENTS AGAINST HERPES VIRUS INFECTIONS

The important herpes viruses are *herpes simplex virus* (HSV), *varicella zoster virus* (VZV), Epstein-Barr virus (EBV), and cytomegalovirus (CMV). The antivirals effective for herpes viruses predominantly are nucleoside analogs causing inhibition of DNA polymerase of the virus **(Table 24.7.2)**.[1] The important drugs in this group are acyclovir, ganciclovir, valganciclovir, foscarnet, and cidofovir. Some of the prodrugs of these antivirals have better absorption and are orally effective, making them suitable for use in specific situations. For example, valacyclovir is the L-valyl ester of acyclovir and three times more bioavailable than acyclovir.

Acyclovir

Acyclovir is most active against HSV1, HSV2 (twofold less susceptible than for HSV1), and also effective against VZV (requires higher dose). Acyclovir is an analog of guanosine and selectively inhibits HSV and VZV replication. The drug is converted to acyclovir monophosphate by virus-encoded thymidine kinase, a reaction that does not occur

TABLE 24.7.1: Antiviral agents.

Viral infection	*Antivirals*
Herpes [Herpes simplex (HSV), varicella zoster (VZV), cytomegalovirus (CMV)]	Acyclovir, famciclovir, valacyclovir, ganciclovir, valganciclovir, cidofovir, foscarnet
Influenza	Oseltamivir, zanamivir, ribavirin
Respiratory syncytial virus (RSV)	Ribavirin, RSV immune globulin, palivizumab
Hepatitis B	Interferon (IFN), pegylated IFN, entecavir, tenofovir, lamivudine, adefovir, telbivudine
Hepatitis C	Pegylated IFN, ribavirin, sofosbuvir–velpatasvir, ledipasvir–sofosbuvir, glecaprevir–pibrentasvir
Human immunodeficiency virus (HIV)	More than 20 approved drugs

TABLE 24.7.2: Drugs active against herpes viruses.

Drug	*Composition*	*Active component*	*Active against*	*Route of admin*	*Side effects*
Acyclovir	Acyclic nucleoside	Triphosphate	HSV, VZV	Oral, IV, Topical	Renal, neurologic, hematologic
Valacyclovir	Prodrug of acyclovir	Triphosphate	HSV, VZV	Oral	Renal, neurologic, hematologic
Ganciclovir	Acyclic nucleoside	Triphosphate	CMV, HSV, VZV	IV	Hematologic
Valganciclovir	Prodrug—ganciclovir	Triphosphate	CMV	Oral	Hematologic
Foscarnet	Pyrophosphate analog	Drug itself	HSV, CMV (resistant to first-line drugs)	IV	Renal, metabolic
Cidofovir	Nucleotide analog	Diphosphate	CMV, HSV, HPV	IV	Renal, ocular
Trifluridine	Nucleoside analog	Triphosphate	HSV keratitis	Topical	Ocular
Idoxuridine	Nucleoside analog	Triphosphate	HSV keratitis	Topical	Ocular

Note: All of the above inhibit viral DNA polymerase except foscarnet, which inhibits both viral DNA polymerase and reverse transcriptase.
(CMV: cytomegalovirus; HPV: human papillomavirus; HSV: herpes simplex virus; IV: intravenous; VZV: varicella zoster virus)

TABLE 24.7.3: Acyclovir for neonatal herpes simplex virus (HSV) infection.

Clinical situation	*Acyclovir dose*	*Duration of treatment*
Skin, eye, mucous membrane (SEM) disease	IV acyclovir 60 mg/kg/day in 3 divided doses	14 days
Central nervous system (CNS) disease	IV acyclovir 60 mg/kg/day in 3 divided doses	21 days (if HSV PCR positive in CSF at the end of treatment, continue treatment till it becomes negative)
Disseminated disease	IV acyclovir 60 mg/kg/day in 3 divided doses	21 days
Suppressive treatment (in SEM, CNS and disseminated disease)	Oral acyclovir 300 mg/m^2/dose 3 times daily	6 months (monitor neutrophil count)

(CSF: cerebrospinal fluid; IV: intravenous; HSV: herpes simplex virus; PCR: polymerase chain reaction)

to any significant extent in uninfected cells. Subsequent phosphorylation steps are catalyzed by cellular enzymes resulting in high concentrations of acyclovir triphosphate in infected cells. Acyclovir triphosphate inhibits viral DNA synthesis by inactivating viral DNA polymerase resulting in restriction of further DNA chain elongation. Viral DNA polymerase has a much higher affinity for acyclovir triphosphate than does cellular DNA polymerase, resulting in little interference in the function of uninfected cells. This selective antiviral action provides a uniquely high therapeutic index for acyclovir.

Acyclovir does not have an effective action against CMV, EBV, and also RNA viruses like influenza, which lack thymidine kinase, thereby limiting its usefulness in these infections.

Neonatal Herpes Simplex Virus Infection (Table 24.7.3)

In all types of neonatal HSV infections, acyclovir is indicated in parenteral form. This is followed by oral suppressive therapy for 6 months to optimize neurological outcome and to prevent recurrences.[2]

Herpes Simplex Virus Encephalitis

In both suspected or confirmed HSV encephalitis acyclovir is administered intravenously (IV) for 3 weeks followed by confirmation of virological clearance by repeat central nervous system (CNS) examination. Acyclovir therapy in HSV encephalitis and mucocutaneous infection is shown in **Table 24.7.4**.[3]

Varicella Infection

In healthy, immunocompetent children with chickenpox and without any complication, treatment is not routinely recommended as varicella is associated with low rates of morbidity and mortality. For most children, supportive care alone is sufficient. The beneficial clinical effects of acyclovir when administered within 24 hours of onset of rash are:

- Decrease in the number of days in which new lesions appear
- Decrease in the duration of fever by 24 hours
- Decrease in the severity of cutaneous and systemic signs and symptoms
- Decrease in the time to total crusting of lesions by 2 days

Oral acyclovir is well tolerated. Acyclovir therapy is recommended when there is an increased risk of complications as in:

- Adolescents
- Children with chronic skin or respiratory conditions
- Children on steroids
- Secondary cases from household exposure

Oral acyclovir in a dose of 20 mg/kg dose (maximum of 800 mg) four times daily for 5 days is administered. Treatment should be initiated within 72 hours of onset of rash preferably within 24 hours to prevent severe disease. Acyclovir administration does not interfere with the induction of immunity against VZV. An alternative is valacyclovir, approved for use in children >2 years of age, administered in a dose of 20 mg/kg dose thrice daily for 5 days. It is absorbed better than acyclovir **(Table 24.7.5)**.[4]

TABLE 24.7.4: Acyclovir dose for herpes simplex infection in children.

Type of HSV infection	*Acyclovir dose*
HSV encephalitis:	
• >28 days to <3 months	IV acyclovir 20 mg/kg per dose 8 hourly for 21 days
• >3 months to <12 years	IV acyclovir 10–15 mg/kg per dose 8 hourly for 21 days (an increased dose of 20 mg/kg per dose 8 hourly is approved; increased risk of nephrotoxicity and encephalopathy)
• ≥12 years	10 mg/kg per dose IV every 8 hours for 21 days
Mucocutaneous infection (immune-competent)	Acyclovir oral 20 mg/kg per dose 4 times daily for 5–7 days
Mucocutaneous infection (immunocompromised)	Acyclovir IV 5–10 mg/kg per dose 8 hourly for 7 days

TABLE 24.7.5: Acyclovir in varicella zoster virus (VZV) infection.

Clinical situation	*Acyclovir dose and duration*
VZV infection in immunocompetent child	• Oral acyclovir 20 mg/kg/dose 4 times daily for 5 days (maximum 800 mg per dose) • Oral valacyclovir (approved for children >2 years of age) 20 mg/kg/dose 3 times daily for 5 days (maximum 1 g per dose)
VZV infection in immunocompromised child and children with severe varicella (pneumonia, encephalitis, severe thrombocytopenia, severe hepatitis)	10–20 mg/kg/dose IV acyclovir 8 hourly for 7–14 days

Immunocompromised Children and Children with Severe Varicella (Pneumonia, Encephalitis, Severe Thrombocytopenia, Severe Hepatitis)

In these children, IV acyclovir therapy is initiated at the earliest, preferably within 72 hours of onset of rash with the aim of preventing progression and dissemination. It is given in a dose of 20 mg/kg/dose diluted in 5% dextrose as slow IV infusion over 1 hour; given 8 hourly for 7–14 days **(Table 24.7.5)**. Rapid infusion may result in renal damage due to crystalluria. Adequate hydration should be ensured. A switch to oral acyclovir therapy can be considered when the patient is afebrile and new lesion formation has ceased. When feasible, the dosage of immunosuppressive medications should be temporarily reduced. Infection can relapse in immunocompromised children requiring multiple courses of acyclovir therapy.

Resistance to acyclovir is rare, but can occur in children with HIV infection and other immunodeficiency disorders. Such resistant infections may require second-line drugs such as IV foscarnet in a dose of 40 mg/kg/dose 8 hourly for 3 weeks.

Ganciclovir

Cytomegalovirus Infection

Ganciclovir has an uniquely potent action against CMV. It is used for the following indications:[5]

- Infants with symptomatic congenital CMV infection with viral sepsis-like syndrome or at least one end-organ symptom (pneumonitis, myocarditis, severe hepatitis, enterocolitis, severe and refractory thrombocytopenia, sight-threatening retinitis, severe neurologic disease) including isolated CNS involvement
- Preemptive therapy in immunocompromised patients with virologic markers of active infection
- Prophylaxis for high-risk patients, who are CMV seropositive or those who have received transplants from CMV-seropositive donors
- Immunocompromised individuals with invasive CMV disease, including pneumonia, colitis, esophagitis, myocarditis, encephalitis, persistent fever and leukopenia syndrome and viral sepsis syndrome

It is administered in two phases, induction and maintenance **(Table 24.7.6)**. In newborns with congenital CMV infection involving CNS, IV ganciclovir is recommended for 6 weeks. Monitoring has to done for neutropenia. For babies who can take orally, valganciclovir is an alternative.

Valganciclovir

Valganciclovir is a prodrug of ganciclovir and has a similar spectrum of action including potent action against CMV.

TABLE 24.7.6: Treatment of cytomegalovirus (CMV) infection.

Ganciclovir	*Induction:* 5–6 mg/kg/dose IV q 12 h for 2–3 weeks *Maintenance:* 5 mg/kg/dose qd (once daily) 5 days/week (duration individualized depending on the length of immunosuppression) *Newborns with congenital CMV disease of central nervous system (CNS):* 6 mg/kg administered every 12 hours for 6 weeks No maintenance therapy
Valganciclovir	*Induction:* 900 mg PO bid *Maintenance:* 900 mg PO qd *Newborns with congenital CMV disease of CNS:* 15–18 mg/kg/dose every 12 hours PO for 6–12 months

It can be administered orally with a high bioavailability. Treatment of newborns with symptomatic congenital CMV infection can be done with oral valganciclovir (15–18 mg/kg/dose every 12 hours) continued for 6 months. It is as effective as IV ganciclovir, providing improved brain growth and developmental milestones, and reduced risk of hearing loss and progression.

ANTIVIRAL AGENTS FOR VIRAL RESPIRATORY INFECTIONS

Influenza

Neuraminidase Inhibitors (Oseltamivir, Zanamivir, and Peramivir)

Oral oseltamivir and inhaled zanamivir are the drugs used in clinical practice, while IV peramivir is licensed for use in some countries. These inhibit the neuraminidase of influenza A (seasonal H3N2, seasonal H1N1, H1N1pdm2009, and avian influenza viruses, including highly pathogenic H5N1 and H9N2) and influenza B **(Table 24.7.7)**.[6] Oral oseltamivir is available in our country and used in all age-groups.

Indications: As per the revised guidelines of Ministry of Health and Family Welfare (MOHFW), Government of India (GOI) categories B and C of seasonal influenza A H1N1 need treatment with oseltamivir.[7]

Category A: Patients with mild fever plus cough/sore throat with or without body ache, headache, diarrhea, and vomiting will be categorized as Category A. They do not require oseltamivir, and should be treated for the symptoms, confined at home and monitored for their progress. No testing for the virus is required.

Category B: In addition to all the signs and symptoms mentioned under Category A, if the patient has high-grade fever and severe sore throat, he/she may require home isolation and oseltamivir.

TABLE 24.7.7: Antivirals for influenza infection.

Age or weight	***Treatment (dosing for 5 days)***	***Prophylaxis (dosing for 7 days)***
Oseltamivir (oral)		
*<1 year of age**		
0–8 months	3 mg/kg/dose twice daily (3 mg/kg once daily for babies <2 weeks of age)	3 mg/kg once daily from 3 months age
9–11 months	3.5 mg/kg/dose twice daily	3.5 mg/kg/dose once daily
1–12 years of age (based on body weight)		
15 kg or less	30 mg twice daily	30 mg once daily
15.1–23 kg	45 mg twice daily	45 mg once daily
23.1–40 kg	60 mg twice daily	60 mg once daily
40.1 kg or more	75 mg twice daily	75 mg once daily
Zanamivir (inhalation)		
Children ≥7 years	10 mg (two 5 mg inhalations), twice daily	*≥5 years:* 10 mg (two 5 mg inhalations), once daily

*Government of India, Ministry of Health recommendation for oseltamivir: For infants: <3 months 12 mg BD for 5 days; 3–5 months 20 mg BD for 5 days; 6–11 months 25 mg BD for 5 days; preterm infants the dose 1–3 mg/kg/dose BD.[7]

In addition to all the signs and symptoms mentioned under Category A, individuals having one or more of the following high-risk conditions shall be treated with oseltamivir:

- Children with mild illness but with predisposing risk factors
- Patients with lung, heart, liver, or kidney disease, blood disorders, diabetes, neurological disorders, cancer, and HIV/AIDS (acquired immunodeficiency syndrome)
- Patients on long-term corticosteroid therapy

Category C: In addition to the above signs and symptoms of *Category A and B, if the patient has one or more of the following:*

- Breathlessness, chest pain, drowsiness, fall in blood pressure, sputum with blood, cyanosis
- Children with clinical flu-like illness with severe disease as manifested by the red flag signs (somnolence, high and persistent fever, inability to feed well, convulsions, shortness of breath, difficulty in breathing).
- Worsening of underlying chronic conditions

Patients mentioned in Category C require testing, immediate hospitalization, and treatment.

Oseltamivir when administered within 2 days of onset of disease reduces the duration of illness by approximately 1.5 days with a reduction in mortality risk compared with later treatment or no treatment. Treatment also reduces the quantity and duration of viral shedding. Hence, it is also effective in prophylaxis. Reported efficacy in preventing disease in family contacts is up to 90%.

Respiratory Syncytial Virus Infection

Ribavirin

Ribavirin aerosol is licensed for the treatment of respiratory syncytial virus (RSV) bronchiolitis and pneumonia in children. Treatment improves clinical features such as fever, tachypnea, lower respiratory tract signs, and arterial oxygen saturation and also shortens the duration of viral shedding in severely ill patients who receive treatment early in the course of their illness. It is recommended in selected patients with life-threatening RSV infection. There is no documented benefit of treatment in mild cases.

Dose: 6 g of drug reconstituted in a final volume of 300 mL of sterile water (final concentration, 20 mg/mL); a small-particle aerosol generator (SPAG-2 unit) is used to administer the drug continuously during a period of 12–18 hours for 3–7 days. Intermittent high-dose therapy, with drug administered at 60 mg/mL for 2 hours three times daily for 5 days, also appears to be effective and may be better tolerated. It can also be administered through a ventilator.[8]

ANTIVIRAL AGENTS FOR CHRONIC HEPATITIS B AND C INFECTIONS

Perinatal or postnatal hepatitis B and C infections can lead on to chronic hepatitis, liver cirrhosis, and hepatocellular carcinoma. Treatment options with antivirals for the chronic infections due to hepatitis B and C to prevent cirrhosis and hepatocellular carcinoma are available.

Hepatitis B

Diagnosis of chronic hepatitis B is based on a combination of persistent clinical symptoms and laboratory abnormalities, persistence of specific serologic markers such as hepatitis B surface antigen (HBsAg) over a period of at least 6 months and histopathologic characteristics on liver biopsy. The decision to treat chronic hepatitis B is largely based on alanine aminotransferase [ALT or serum glutamic-pyruvic transaminase (SGPT)] level, hepatitis B virus (HBV) viral load and liver histology. Treatment is recommended for those with persistently abnormal ALT (>2 times the upper limit of normal or >60 units/mL) and HBV DNA >20,000 IU/mL or 10^5 copies/mL for at least 4–6 months. Almost all of these children will be hepatitis B e-antigen (HBeAg)-positive.[9]

TABLE 24.7.8: Antivirals for chronic hepatitis B infection.

Drug	Age	Dose	Duration	Advantages	Disadvantages/side effects
Interferon-alpha	≥12 months	5–10 MU/m^2 SC 3 times a week	6 months	Definitive duration, no resistance, immunomodulatory + Antiviral effects	*Parenteral route, side effects:* Flu-like symptoms, anorexia, behavioral problems, lethargy, vomiting, alopecia, rash, neutropenia, arthralgia, thyroid dysfunction
Pegylated interferon-alpha 2-a/b	2–18 years	• 180 µg/1.73 m^2 BSA for a *or* • 1.5 µg/kg weekly for b	6–10 months	Same as above	Same as above
Lamivudine	≥3 years	3 mg/kg/day	≥1 year	Few side effects, oral use, inhibits viral replication	Not a preferred drug due to high rate of resistance
Adefovir	≥12 years	10 mg/day	≥1 year	Oral use	Resistance increases with duration of treatment + Weak antiviral activity
Entecavir	≥3 years	0.5 mg/day (1 mg/day for lamivudine-resistant)	≥1 year	*Preferred nucleos(t)ide analog* Oral use, negligible resistance	Higher resistance in those already exposed to lamivudine
Telbivudine	NA	600 mg/day for adults	≥1 year	Same as above + Renal-sparing effect	Resistance increases with duration of treatment
Tenofovir	12–18 years*	300 mg/day	≥1 year	*Preferred nucleos(t)ide analog* Oral use, high response, no resistance, fewer side effects, useful for patients with lamivudine resistance	Effect on bone mineral density

*Tenofovir disoproxil fumarate (TDF) is licensed for use in children ≥2 years.
(BSA: body surface area; NA: not approved; SC: subcutaneously)

TABLE 24.7.9: Prophylactic agents in viral infections.

Human immunoglobulin	• Prevention of hepatitis A • Treatment of B19 parvovirus infection in immunodeficient individuals
CMV immunoglobulin	• Prophylaxis of CMV in solid organ and hematopoietic stem cell transplant recipients • Treatment of CMV pneumonia in combination with ganciclovir
Hepatitis B immunoglobulin	Prophylaxis of hepatitis B infection especially in newborns born to HBsAg-positive mothers
Rabies immunoglobulin	Post-exposure prophylaxis for rabies
RSV immunoglobulin	Prevention of complications of RSV infection in young infants
Palivizumab (humanized RSV monoclonal antibody with anti-RSV activity)	Prophylactic treatment for prevention of complications of RSV infection in young infants
Varicella zoster immune globulin	Prevention of varicella infection in high risk newborns and Immunocompromised children

(CMV: cytomegalovirus; RSV: respiratory syncytial virus)

Treatment options for chronic HBV in children typically include IFN, or the nucleos(t)ide analogs entecavir or tenofovir. Available drugs are described in **Table 24.7.8.**[10]

Interferon

Interferons are a family of cytokines with immunomodulatory, antiproliferative, and direct antiviral actions. There are three types: α, β, and γ. IFN-α is used in treatment of chronic HBV infection. It acts by inhibiting viral protein synthesis. Combination therapy [e.g., IFN with a nucleos(t)ide analog, or the combination of two nucleos(t)ide analogs] has not been shown to improve clinical outcomes compared with monotherapy.

Hepatitis C

Those who have a detectable hepatitis C virus (HCV) viral level over a period of 6 months should be considered for treatment. Aim of therapy is to achieve a sustained virologic response, defined as being HCV RNA negative 6 months after discontinuation of treatment. Direct-acting antiviral (DAAs) agents currently are the main stay of therapy and can be recommended for all children aged ≥3 years. These agents permit effective, well-tolerated, oral, IFN-free regimens.

The following DAAs are approved for use with a weight based dosing depending on the genotype:

- *For any genotype:* Sofosbuvir–velpatasvir for 12 weeks
- *For any genotype:* Glecaprevir–pibrentasvir for 8 weeks
- *For genotypes 1, 4, 5, and 6:* Ledipasvir–sofosbuvir for 12 weeks[10]

PROPHYLACTIC AGENTS

Besides antivirals, prophylaxis is administered with immunoglobulins and monoclonal antibodies in newborns, immunocompromised children, and for some specific viral exposures. **(Table 24.7.9)**.

CONCLUSION

Antiviral drugs commonly used in practice are the nucleoside/ nucleotide analogs such as acyclovir against herpes viruses, neuraminidase inhibitors such as oseltamivir against influenza virus and interferons against chronic hepatitis B virus infection.

REFERENCES

1. Hammer SM. Antiviral agents. [online] Available from https://www.columbia.edu/itc/hs/medical/pathophys/id/2005/MID40-HammerAntiviralsColor.pdf [Last accessed December 2024].
2. Kimberlin DW, Whitley RJ, Wan W, Powell DA, Storch G, Ahmed A, et al.; National Institute of Allergy and Infectious Diseases Collaborative Antiviral Study Group. Oral acyclovir suppression and neurodevelopment after neonatal herpes. N Engl J Med. 2011;365(4):1284-92.
3. Kimberlin DW. Acyclovir Dosing in the Neonatal Period and Beyond. J Pediatric Infect Dis Soc. 2013;2(2):179-82.
4. American Academy of Pediatrics. Non-HIV antiviral drugs. In: Kimberlin DW, Barnett ED, Lynfield R, Sawyer MH (Eds). Red Book: 2021–2024 Report of the Committee on Infectious Diseases, 32nd edition. Itasca: American Academy of Pediatrics; 2021. p. 930.
5. American Academy of Pediatrics. Cytomegalovirus infection. In: Kimberlin DW, Barnett ED, Lynfield R, Sawyer MH (Eds). Red Book: 2021–2024 Report of the Committee on Infectious Diseases, 32nd edition. Itasca: American Academy of Pediatrics; 2021. p. 294.
6. Committee on Infectious Diseases. Recommendations for Prevention and Control of Influenza in Children, 2023–2024. Pediatrics. 2023;152(4):e2023063772.
7. Directorate General of Health Services; Ministry of Health and Family Welfare, Government of India. Pandemic Influenza A H1N1: Clinical management protocol and infection control guidelines. https://ncdc.mohfw.gov.in/wp-content/uploads/2024/02/72513234671561442053-1.pdf [Accessed December 2024].
8. Hall CB. Respiratory syncytial virus and parainfluenza virus. N Engl J Med. 2001;344(25):1917-28.
9. Sokal EM, Paganelli M, Wirth S, Socha P, Vajro P, Lacaille F, et al.; European Society of Pediatric Gastroenterology, Hepatology and Nutrition. Management of chronic hepatitis B in childhood: ESPGHAN clinical practice guidelines: consensus of an expert panel on behalf of the European Society of Pediatric Gastroenterology, Hepatology and Nutrition. J Hepatol. 2013;59(4):814-29.
10. Ganguly S, Khanna R, Vishwanathan MS. Viral hepatitis. In: Kumar RR, Ratageri VH, Gupta P (Eds). IAP Standard Treatment Guidelines 2022. New Delhi: Jaypee Brothers Medical Publishers; 2023. pp. 639-49.

24.8 Antifungal Therapy

Pooja Dewan, Anjali Tomar

INTRODUCTION

Fungi are nonmotile eukaryotic organisms that include microorganisms such as yeasts and molds. Fungi are characterized by the presence of chitin in their cell walls, which distinguish them from plants and animals. Fungi are ubiquitous in the environment, being found outdoors in soil and on plants and trees as well as on many indoor surfaces and on human skin. Fungi thrive and proliferate well in warm and moist environment. Fungal infections are also more prevalent in warm, moist areas of the body, such as the oral cavity, vaginal, and skin folds. Sweaty clothes and shoes can enhance fungus growth on the skin. Fungi are transmitted from person to person or from objects and surfaces to a person. Also, an individual can transfer fungi to other parts of the body by touching.

RISK FACTORS FOR FUNGAL INFECTIONS

With the widespread use of antibiotics, there has been a steady increase in the incidence of serious secondary fungal infections. Fungi are also dreaded cause of opportunistic infections in immunocompromised hosts [people living with human immunodeficiency virus (PLHIV), acquired and congenital immunodeficiencies], those receiving chemotherapy, those undergoing transplantation, and those receiving immunosuppressive medications and preterm neonates. Children admitted in intensive care set-ups are also predisposed to fungal infections. Older individuals are particularly susceptible to fungal infections. Patients with diabetes are also vulnerable to fungal infections.

FUNGAL INFECTIONS IN HUMANS

Millions of species of fungi have been reported. Most of the fungi are pathogenic in plants. About 400 species of fungi are pathogenic in animals and about 50 species are pathogenic in humans. The infections caused by fungi in animals are called "mycoses". Fungi cause a spectrum of diseases in humans ranging from comparatively innocuous superficial skin diseases to invasive life-threatening infections. The type of fungal disease can be classified depending upon the site of infection, route of acquisition of infection, and virulence of fungal infection.[1]

- *Classification based on site:* Superficial, cutaneous, subcutaneous, or systemic (deep)
- *Classification based on route of acquisition:* Endogenous or exogenous. Endogenous infection involves colonization by a commensal species, or reactivation of a past infection. Exogenous fungi may enter through air or mucocutaneous contact, blood, or gastrointestinal tract
- *Classification based on virulence:* Primary pathogens can establish infections in normal hosts. Opportunistic pathogens cause disease in immunocompromised hosts.

Table 24.8.1 enlists the mycoses encountered in humans with possible fungal etiologic organisms.

CLASSIFICATION OF ANTIFUNGAL DRUGS

With the emergence of invasive fungal illnesses, the market for antifungal drugs has expanded in the recent years. **Table 24.8.2** depicts the antifungal drugs available. However, not all these drugs are approved for use in children and neonates.[1-3]

TABLE 24.8.1: Mycoses encountered in humans.

Type of mycoses	*Disease (etiological agent)*
Superficial	• Black piedra (*Piedraia hortae*) • White piedra (*Trichosporon beigelii*) • Pityriasis versicolor (*Malassezia furfur*) • Tinea nigra (*Phaeoannellomyces werneckii*)
Cutaneous	• *Dermatophytoses: Tinea capitis, Todea barbara, Tinea corporis, Tinea cruris, Tinea unguium, Tinea pedis* (*Epidermophyton, Microsporum,* and *Trichophyton*) • Dermatomycoses (cutaneous infections due to other genera fungi, the most common of which are *Candida* spp.)
Subcutaneous	Chromoblastomycosis (*Fonsecaea pedrosoi, Fonsecaea compacta, Cladosporium carrionii,* and *Phialophora verrucosa*), mycetoma (*Pseudallescheria boydii* and *Nocardia brasiliensis*), and sporotrichosis (*Sporothrix schenckii*)
Systemic (primary infections)	Coccidioidomycosis (*Coccidioides immitis*), histoplasmosis (*Histoplasma capsulatum*), blastomycosis (*Blastomyces dermatitidis*), and *Paracoccidioides brasiliensis*
Systemic (opportunistic infections)	Cryptococcosis (*Cryptococcus neoformans*), candidiasis (*Candida* spp.), Aspergillosis (*Aspergillus* spp.), penicilliosis (*Penicillium marneffei*), zygomucormycosis (*Rhizopus* spp., *Mucor* spp.), trichosporonosis (*Trichosporon beigelii*), and fusariosis (*Fusarium* spp.)

SITE OF ACTION OF ANTIFUNGAL DRUGS

Antifungals can be grouped into various classes based on their site of action **(Fig. 24.8.1)**:[2-4]

- *Interference with fungal cell membrane function:* Polyenes (alter permeability of cell membranes by binding irreversibly)
- *Interference with fungal cell membrane synthesis:* Azoles (inhibit biosynthesis of ergosterol)
- *Interference with cell wall function:* Caspofungin
- *Interference with nucleic acid synthesis:* 5-fluorocytosine
- *Disruption of microtubular function in cells and inhibiting cell division:* Griseofulvin

POLYENE ANTIBIOTICS

Polyene antimycotics are derived from *Streptomyces* bacteria. They bind irreversibly to ergosterol in the fungal cell membrane and alter the permeability of the fungal cell membranes leading to metabolic disruption and cell death.

TABLE 24.8.2: Classes of common antifungal drugs.

Azoles	• *Imidazoles:* Miconazole, ketoconazole, and clotrimazole • *Triazoles:* Fluconazole, itraconazole; voriconazole, ravuconazole, and posaconazole
Echinocandins	• Caspofungin • Micafungin • Anidulafungin • Rezafungin
Polyenes	• Amphotericin B • Nystatin
Allylamine	Terbinafine
Others	• 5-flucytosine • Griseofulvin

Additionally, polyenes act by immune activation leading to oxidation-dependent activation of macrophages.[2,3]

Amphotericin B

The most important polyene antimycotic is amphotericin B (AMB), a heptaene macrolide containing seven conjugated double bonds in the transposition and 3-amino-3,6-dideoxymannose connected to the main ring by a glycosidic bond. The conventional AMB is AMB deoxycholate and is used by intravenous route. The other preparations of AMB with better safety parameters include amphotericin B lipid complex (ABLC), amphotericin B colloidal dispersion (ABCD), and liposomal amphotericin B (LAMB).[5]

Mechanism of Action

Antifungal activity depends upon its binding to a sterol moiety, primarily ergosterol in the membrane of the fungi. This leads to formation of pores in the fungal membrane and increased permeability and leakage of a variety of small molecules.[6]

Pharmacology

The gastrointestinal absorption of AMB is negligible. Pharmacokinetics of AMB differs according to the formulation. LAMB has the highest plasma concentration at therapeutic doses. Conventional AMB is released from its complex with deoxycholate in the blood stream. AMB that remains in the plasma gets bound to B lipoprotein. Concentration of AMB in the fluids from inflamed pleura, peritoneum, synovium, and aqueous humor is approximately two-thirds of the trough concentration in plasma. Penetration into cerebrospinal fluid (CSF), vitreous humor, and normal amniotic fluid is poor. About 60% of AMB gets metabolized in liver. Excretion occurs in urine and bile.[1,4]

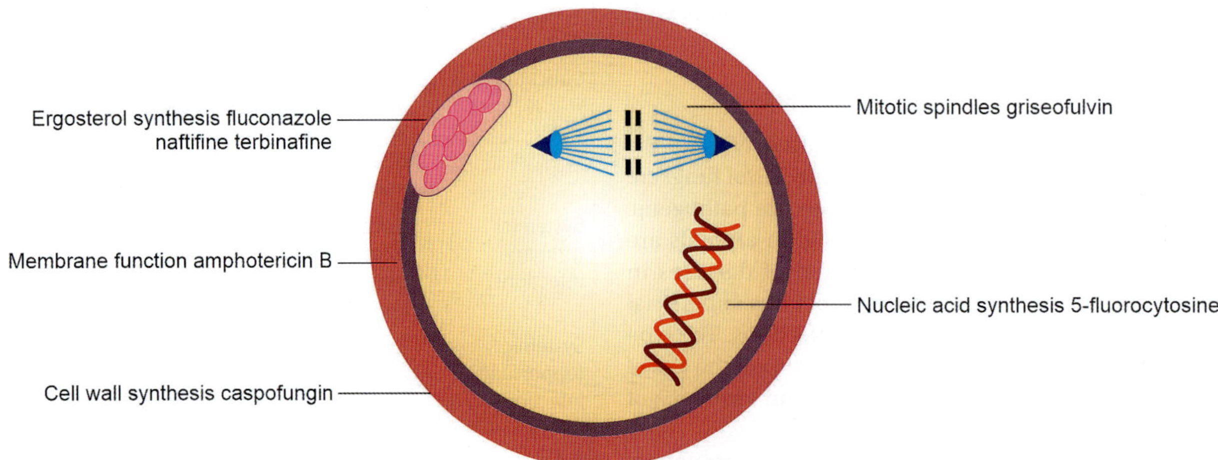

Fig. 24.8.1: Site and mechanism of action of common antifungal drugs.

Antifungal Spectrum

Amphotericin B is a broad-spectrum antifungal active against most invasive fungal infections as well as leishmaniasis and *Naegleria*. It is effective against *Candida* spp., *Cryptococcus neoformans, Blastomyces dermatitidis, Histoplasma capsulatum, Sporothrix schenckii, Aspergillus* spp., *Penicillium marneffei, Paracoccidioides brasiliensis, Coccidioides* spp., *Rhizopus* spp., and *Mucor* spp. AMB is useful for treating children with febrile neutropenia who do not improve with antibacterial therapy and have an underlying risk for invasive fungal infections. AMB is currently the drug of choice for the treatment of systemic infections caused by *Aspergillus* and *Candida* spp.[3]

Dosage and side effects: **Table 24.8.3** shows the recommended dosages for AMB in children and common side effects.

Indications in children: Amphotericin B is useful in invasive fungal infections such as candidiasis and cryptococcal meningitis. It is also recommended in mucormycosis and refractory invasive aspergillosis **(Table 24.8.3)**. AMB can attain good CSF concentration in neonates due to immature blood–brain barrier. Neonates can tolerate AMB better than older children. For cryptococcal meningitis, AMB is given with flucytosine. The duration of therapy is 10–12 weeks after CSF cultures are clear.

AZOLES

Azoles act by inhibiting the cytochrome P450-dependent lanosterol 14α-demethylase (CYP51), which inhibits lanosterol synthesis. This leads to increased cell membrane permeability, impairs membrane-associated oxidative enzymes, and leads to intracellular phospholipid accumulation and cell death. Since azoles act by inhibiting cytochrome P450-dependent enzymes are metabolized by cytochrome P450 isoenzymes, several drugs, which either induce or interact with these cytochrome-dependent enzymes interact with azoles. Astemizole, cisapride, pimozide, quinidine, halofantrine, terfenadine, and ergot alkaloids are contraindicated with azoles as they can lead to azole toxicity. Rifabutin, phenytoin, omeprazole, benzodiazepines, nevirapine, and efavirenz need to monitor as coadministration with azoles can lead to therapeutic failure. Compared to polyenes, azoles take much longer time to begin action. Azoles are effective against many fungal infections, including candidiasis, dermatophytosis, aspergillosis, cryptococcus, and cutaneous sporotrichosis. However, some fungal infections like those due to *Candida krusei* and *C. auris* are resistant to azoles including itraconazole. Azoles are also not useful for treating infections due to rhizopus and mucor.[2,4,5]

Fluconazole

Fluconazole is a first-generation triazole antifungal drug used for treating candidiasis, blastomycosis, coccidioidomycosis, cryptococcosis, histoplasmosis, dermatophytosis, and pityriasis versicolor. Fluconazole is particularly active against *Candida albicans* and *C. neoformans*. It is also used to prevent candidiasis in those who are at high risk such as following organ transplantation, low birth-weight babies, and those with neutropenia. Fluconazole is, however, ineffective against *C. krusei* and *Candida glabrata*.[3,7]

Pharmacokinetics

Fluconazole is almost completely absorbed within 2 hours following oral intake unaffected by gastric acids. It follows zero order kinetics. Only 10% of elimination is due to metabolism, the rest of the drug is excreted in urine and sweat.[1,4]

Dosage and side effects: **Table 24.8.3** shows the recommended dose for fluconazole and the expected side effects with its use.

Itraconazole

Itraconazole is a triazole antifungal drug most active against *Aspergillus* spp. and has greater activity than fluconazole against resistant strains of *Candida* spp. other than *C. albicans*. It is also indicated for the treatment of cryptococcal meningitis, histoplasmosis, nonmeningeal coccidioidomycosis, and infections caused by blastomycosis, *S. schenckii, P. brasiliensis,* and *B. dermatitidis*. Itraconazole is the drug of choice for secondary prophylaxis of histoplasmosis and cryptococcal meningitis in children affected by HIV. The safety of itraconazole in children <18 years and neonates has not been established. Yet, itraconazole is recommended for use in children (not neonates) as salvage or compassionate therapy. Children with cystic fibrosis and allogeneic bone marrow transplant are given itraconazole 2.5–5 mg/kg twice daily for prophylaxis against fungal infections. Gastric acid affects the absorption, and hence therapeutic drug monitoring is recommended with a target trough level of 0.5 μg/mL.[3,7]

Posaconazole

It is a triazole antifungal drug especially active against *Mucor*. Its antifungal spectrum includes *Candida* spp., *Aspergillus* spp., and *Zygomycetes* spp.[8] It is recommended for antifungal prophylaxis (against *Aspergillus* and *Candida* infections) in patients with acute myeloid leukemia, myelodysplastic syndrome, graft-versus-host disease or for patients who have undergone hematopoietic stem cell transplant (HSCT). Oral administration of posaconazole taken with a high-fat meal increases its bioavailability. The safety and efficacy in children <13 years needs to be established.[4]

Voriconazole

It is a triazole antifungal with a structure related to that of fluconazole and a spectrum of activity comparable to that of

TABLE 24.8.3: Therapeutic doses and side effects of common antimycotic drugs.

Antifungal drugs	*Route of administration*	*Dose in neonates*	*Dose in infants*	*Dose in older children*	*Side effects*	*Indications*
Amphotericin B deoxycholate	Intravenous (IV)	0.5–1 mg/kg/day IV infusion q24h; dose in preterm is 0.5 mg/kg/day and in term neonates, the dose is 1 mg/kg/day	0.7–1 mg/kg/day IV infusion q24h	1–1.5 mg/kg/day IV infusion q24h	Anorexia, chills, diarrhea, fever, headache, hypokalemia, hypomagnesemia, hypotension, malaise, pain at injection site, azotemia, renal function abnormalities, vomiting, agranulocytosis, and bone marrow suppression *Renal dose adjustment*: *CrCl <10 mL/min*: 0.5–0.7 mg/kg IV q24–48h	Invasive aspergillosis, cryptococcal meningitis
ABLC	IV	2.5–5 mg/kg/day q24 h	–	5 mg/kg/day q24 h	Less infusion-related toxicity and lesser nephrotoxicity than AMB deoxycholate; rest of side effect profile is similar as AMB deoxycholate	Invasive aspergillosis, cryptococcal meningitis
ABCD	IV	–	3–4 mg/kg/day q24h	3–4 mg/kg/ day q24h	Less infusion-related toxicity and lesser nephrotoxicity than AMB deoxycholate; rest of side effect profile is similar as AMB deoxycholate	Invasive aspergillosis, cryptococcal meningitis
LAMB	IV	3–5 mg/kg/day q24h	3–5 mg/kg/ day q24h	3–5 mg/kg/ day q24h	Less infusion-related toxicity and lesser nephrotoxicity than AMB deoxycholate; rest of side effect profile is similar as AMB deoxycholate	Invasive aspergillosis, cryptococcal meningitis
Fluconazole	IV and oral	25 mg/kg loading dose; 12 mg/kg/day q24h maintenance dose	12 mg/kg/day q24h	6–12 mg/kg/ day q24h	Vomiting, diarrhea, transaminitis, stomachache, chills, and tachycardia	Candidiasis, blastomycosis, coccidioidomycosis, cryptococcosis, histoplasmosis, dermatophytosis, and pityriasis versicolor
Itraconazole	Oral; should be taken with food	–	–	5–10 mg/kg/day q12h	Nausea, vomiting, constipation, headache, dizziness, abnormal liver function tests, swelling, and weight gain	Trichophyton and *Microsporum, T. capitis* infections, and onychomycosis
Posaconazole	IV and oral; should be taken 1 h before meals	–	–	200–400 mg/ dose q6–12h	Fatigue, dry mouth, nausea, diarrhea, vomiting, and hypokalemia	Oral thrush, candidemia, invasive aspergillosis, prophylaxis of invasive *Aspergillus* and *Candida* infections in high-risk, severely immunocompromised patients
Voriconazole	IV and oral; should be taken 20 minutes after a meal	4–6 mg/kg q12h loading dose, 2–3 mg/kg q12h maintenance dose	4–6 mg/kg q12h loading dose, 2–3 mg/kg q12h maintenance dose	7–9 mg/kg q12h loading dose, 5–6 mg/kg q12h maintenance dose	Blurred vision, nausea, vomiting, hepatotoxicity, cardiac arrhythmias, swelling in hands and feet, and photosensitivity	Esophageal candidiasis, invasive aspergillosis, candidemia, scedosporiosis, and fusariosis

Contd...

Antifungal drugs	***Route of administration***	***Dose in neonates***	***Dose in infants***	***Dose in older children***	***Side effects***	***Indications***
Ketoconazole	IV, oral, and topical	–	–	3–6 mg/kg/day	Nausea, vomiting, stomach pain, diarrhea, dizziness, photosensitivity, and QT prolongation on ECG	Blastomycosis, coccidioidomycosis, histoplasmosis, chromomycosis, and paracoccidioidomycosis; not useful for onychomycosis
Caspofungin	IV	25 mg/m^2/day (safety not established)	50 mg/m^2/day	70 mg/m^2/day loading dose; 50 mg/m^2/day maintenance dose	Fever, anaphylaxis, hepatotoxic, diarrhea, vomiting, shivering, rash, and hypokalemia	Candidemia, invasive aspergillosis, empirical therapy for presumed fungal infections in febrile, neutropenic patients
Micafungin	IV	–	2–4 mg/kg/ day	2–4 mg/kg/day (*Prophylax is:* 1 mg/kg/day)	Hepatotoxic, stomachache, nausea, vomiting, weight gain, flushing, and rash	Candidemia, invasive aspergillosis, empirical therapy for presumed fungal infections in febrile, neutropenic patients, prophylaxis of *Candida* infections in HSCT recipients
Anidulafungin	IV	1.5 mg/kg/day	1.5–3 mg/kg/day	1.5–3 mg/kg/day loading dose; 0.75–1.5 mg/kg/day maintenance dose	Flushing, diarrhea, nausea, vomiting, headache, and constipation	Candidemia, esophageal candidiasis
Flucytosine [5-fluorocytosine (5-FC)]	Oral and IV	80–160 mg/kg/day q6h PO	50–150 mg/kg/ day q6h PO	50–150 mg/kg/ day q6h PO	Confusion, headache, dizziness, phototoxicity, sedation, psychosis, bone marrow suppression, nausea, and vomiting	Serious *Candida* infections and cryptococcosis (along with AMB) and chromoblastomycosis
Griseofulvin	Oral; should be given with milk, eggs, and fatty foods	–	–	• *Microsized:* 10–20 mg/kg/ day q12–24h • *Ultramicrosized:* 10–15 mg/kg/ day q12–24h	Headache, nausea, vomiting, diarrhea, photosensitivity, peripheral neuritis, lethargy, mental confusion, and leukopenia	Dermatophytosis, Athlete's foot, and ringworm
Terbinafine	Oral and topical	–	–	• *≥4 years: <25 kg:* 125 mg/day • *25–35 kg:* 187.5 mg/day • *>35 kg:* 250 mg/day	Gastrointestinal distress, headache, hepatotoxicity, severe neutropenia, and Stevens–Johnson syndrome	Dermatophytosis, onychomycosis, pityriasis versicolor, mucosal and cutaneous candidiasis

(ABCD: amphotericin B colloidal dispersion; ABLC: amphotericin B lipid complex; AMB: amphotericin B; HSCT: hematopoietic stem cell transplantation; LAMB: liposomal amphotericin B)

itraconazole. It is effective in treatment of invasive aspergillosis and refractory infections of *Scedosporium apiospermum* and *Fusarium* spp. and empirical therapy in febrile neutropenic patients.[9]

Pharmacokinetics

Voriconazole metabolism follows saturable kinetics. Therefore, increased dosage of voriconazole, a disproportionate increase, is seen in its drug levels. A variable elimination half-life (from 6 to 24 hours) is seen depending on the dosage of voriconazole given. It is well absorbed. However, fatty meal decreases its absorption. Voriconazole is extensively metabolized in the liver. Dose of voriconazole in children is higher than adults as due to higher hepatic clearance and first-pass effect in children.[1,6]

Antifungal Spectrum

Voriconazole has fungicidal action against the various *Aspergillus* spp. most active, especially against *Aspergillus fumigatus*. It is fungistatic against all *Candida* spp. Voriconazole exhibits better potency than fluconazole or itraconazole for most *Candida* isolates studied. Since it can be given orally, it is emerging as a popular choice for empirical antifungal therapy in febrile neutropenic patients when compared to AMB, which must be administered intravenously (IV).[4]

Adverse Effects

Common side effects include visual disturbances, fever, rash, hepatic abnormalities, nausea, vomiting, abdominal pain, and headache.

ECHINOCANDINS

This newer category of antifungal drugs acts by inhibiting the synthesis of glucan in the cell wall. Caspofungin, micafungin, and anidulafungin are semisynthetic echinocandin derivatives with clinical implications.[2,5]

Antifungal Spectrum

Echinocandins are fungicidal against most species of *Candida* (including strains that are fluconazole resistant), but not against *Cryptococcus, Trichosporon,* and *Rhodotorula*. They display synergistic activity with AMB and additive activity with fluconazole against *Candida* spp. Echinocandins are fungistatic against *Aspergillus* and are also partly active against dimorphic fungi (*Blastomyces* and *Histoplasma*). These have some activity against the spores of the fungus *Pneumocystis jirovecii,* formerly known as *Pneumocystis carinii*. Caspofungin is used in the empirical treatment of febrile neutropenia and as salvage therapy for the treatment of invasive aspergillosis, especially refractory invasive aspergillosis is intolerant to other antifungal drugs. Caspofungin is also indicated in invasive candidiasis and the following *Candida* infections: intra-abdominal abscesses, esophageal candidiasis, peritonitis, and pleural space infections. Micafungin is used as prophylaxis against *Candida* infections in HSCT patients. Anidulafungin is a semisynthetic lipopeptide derivative of *Aspergillus nidulans* with a spectrum of activity similar to caspofungin. It has a good activity in vitro against the most commonly pathogenic *Candida* species, with the exception of *Candida parapsilosis* and *Candida guilliermondii,* and has shown to be an effective therapy for invasive candidiasis in animals.[3,7]

Pharmacokinetics

Due to the large molecular weight, echinocandins have poor oral bioavailability and are administered by intravenous infusion. In the plasma, they are 97% bound to albumin. They are metabolized slowly by N-acetylation as well as spontaneous degradation and have a longer half-life in plasma. Due to the larger size, echinocandins are also poorly concentrated in CSF, eyes, and urine.[4,6]

Dosage and side effects: **Table 24.8.3** shows the common side effects and doses for echinocandins.

HETEROCYCLIC BENZOFURAN

Griseofulvin

Griseofulvin is an antifungal agent derived from mold *Penicillium griseofulvum* that is used to treat fungal infection of skin and nails.[5,7]

Mechanism of Action

It causes disruption of the mitotic spindle by interacting with polymerized microtubules. Multinucleated and stunted fungal hyphae result from its action. The effect of the drug is like that of colchicine and vinca alkaloids but its binding sites on the microtubular protein are distinct.[2,6]

Pharmacology

Griseofulvin has very low water solubility, which leads to its irregular absorption from the gastrointestinal tract. To improve its bioavailability, microsized, and ultramicrosized preparations are available. It gets deposited in keratin precursor cells of skin, hair, and nails; it gets concentrated and persists in tinea-infected cells and due to its fungistatic activity, the newly formed keratin is not invaded by the fungus. As the fungus-containing keratin is shed, it is replaced by normal tissue. Griseofulvin is metabolized by methylation and excreted in urine. Its plasma half-life is about 1 day, but it persists for weeks in skin and keratin.[4]

Antifungal Spectrum

It is active against most dermatophytes including *Epidermophyton, Trichophyton, Microsporum,* etc. but not against *Candida* and other fungi-causing deep mycosis.

Dosage and side effects: **Table 24.8.3** shows the recommended dosages in children and the common side effects.

Indications in children: It is mainly used to treat ringworm (*Tinea*) infections. In adolescents and young adults, it is also used to treat athlete's foot (epidermophytosis involving the skin and nails of the foot).

ALLYLAMINES

Terbinafine

Terbinafine is a synthetic allylamine and is a fungistatic agent. It is structurally similar to the topical agent naftifine.[5,7]

Mechanism of Action

It is a noncompetitive inhibitor of squalene epoxidase, which is an early step enzyme in ergosterol biosynthesis by fungi. Accumulation of squalene within the fungal cells is responsible for its action.[6]

Pharmacology

Terbinafine is well absorbed but bioavailability is decreased to about 40% because of first pass metabolism in the liver. It is lipophilic, strongly plasma-protein bound and concentrated in sebum, stratum corneum, and nail plates. It is excreted in urine (80%) and feces (20%).[2]

Antifungal Spectrum

It is used to treat dermatophytosis and onychomycosis and activity is also seen against *Candida* species and *Malassezia furfur*.

Dosage and side effects: **Table 24.8.3** shows the recommended dosages in children and the common side effects.

Indications in children: It is mainly used to treat *Tinea cruris, Tinea corporis, Tinea capitis, and Tinea pedis,* pityriasis versicolor, and onychomycosis. It is less effective against cutaneous and mucosal candidiasis.

FEW IMPORTANT TOPICAL ANTIFUNGALS

Ketoconazole

It is a broad-spectrum antifungal drug, useful in both dermatophytosis and deep mycosis. It is effective in blastomycosis, histoplasmosis, coccidioidomycosis, paracoccidioidomycosis, ringworm, tinea versicolor, chronic mucocutaneous candidiasis, etc.[4,5]

Clotrimazole

It is effective in topical treatment of *Tinea* infections such as ringworm, athlete's foot, otomycosis, oral, cutaneous, and vaginal candidiasis. It is particularly favored for vaginitis because of long-lasting residual effect after once daily application. It is well-tolerated by most patients, but local irritation and stinging and burning sensation occur in some patients.[4,5]

Miconazole

It is used for *Tinea*, pityriasis versicolor, otomycosis, cutaneous, and vulvovaginal candidiasis. It is highly efficacious. Adverse effects from topical application to vagina include burning, itching, irritation and infrequently pelvic cramps headache, and hives.[4,5]

ANTIFUNGALS ON THE HORIZON

Invasive fungal infections can cause severe diseases in humans. During the coronavirus disease 2019 (COVID-19) pandemic, COVID-19 associated fungal infection including the pulmonary aspergillosis and mucormycosis were among the most serious complications. The rapid global spread of the multidrug-resistant yeast *Candida auris* is an example of how fungal infections can challenge health systems and our limited understanding of fungi.[10]

In late 2022, the World Health Organization (WHO) published the first fungal priority pathogens list. The WHO list included newer antifungal agents including rezafungin, ibrexafungerp, olorofim, and fosmanogepix.

Rezafungin

It is a new echinocandin, with a long half-life of around 133 hours and needs less frequent dosing, once every 7 days. On March 22, 2023, the US Food and Drug Administration (FDA) approved rezafungin injection for the treatment of candidemia and invasive candidiasis in patients 18 years of age or older who have limited or no alternative treatment options. It may also be used to treat *Aspergillus* spp. including subsets of echinocandin-resistant *C. auris* and azole-resistant *Aspergillus* isolates.[10]

Ibrexafungerp

It is a triterpenoid antifungal and is the first nonazole agent approved by the US-FDA for the treatment of vaginal yeast infections (*Candida* spp.). The fungicidal action is attributed to inhibition of glucan synthase. It is effective against both *C. albicans* and nonalbicans species such as *C. auris and C. glabrata*. It is an orally used drug and effective as a step-down therapy in outpatient department. Currently, not approved for use in pediatric age.[10]

Olorofim

It is a member of a novel class of antifungal drugs named ortomides. It inhibits an enzyme involved in fungal pyrimidine synthesis. Olorofim has activity against several clinically important groups of fungi, including *Histoplasma* spp., *Aspergillus* spp., and *Scedosporium* spp.[10]

Fosmanogepix

It is a novel drug with a broad-spectrum activity that targets an enzyme in the glycosylphosphatidylinositol anchor biosynthesis pathway. It is currently being tested in a phase 3 trial in which it will be compared with caspofungin plus fluconazole in patients with candidemia and/or invasive candidiasis.[10]

Opelconazole

It is a novel inhaled azole drug which is has been used for treating invasive pulmonary aspergillosis. Currently, having the status of orphan drug and is yet to be approved by FDA.[10]

These new antifungal drugs raise hope that replenishing the arsenal of therapeutic options for invasive fungal infections might be possible. If combined with investments to develop better diagnostic tools and improve surveillance, the availability of new antifungal drugs could open a new page in the fight against pathogenic fungi.

CONCLUSION

Fungal infections are the important cause of hospital stay and mortality especially in high-risk patients like those receiving chemotherapy or immunosuppressive agents, and following solid organ or stem cell transplantation. Amphotericin B is the cornerstone of systemic antifungal therapy. It is a broad-spectrum polyene antifungal agent, active against most invasive fungal infections including aspergillosis. Azole group of antifungal medications include imidazoles (miconazole, ketoconazole) which are commonly used for localized surface infections, and triazoles (itraconazole, fluconazole, voriconazole, posaconazole) which are used for invasive, life-threatening fungal infections including aspergillosis, blastomycosis, candidiasis, cryptococcosis, histoplasmosis, coccidioidomycosis and paracoccidioidomycosis. Fluconazole has fungistatic action and is particularly active against yeast, *Candida albicans* and *C. neoformans*. Voriconazole is also fungistatic against *Candida*, but has fungicidal activity against *Aspergillus*. Most azoles (except ketoconazole) have good penetration in cerebrospinal fluid and are effective in meningitis. Fluconazole is preferred over amphotericin-B for maintenance therapy in cryptococcal meningitis, especially in children living with HIV. In contrast, the echinocandins (micafungin, caspofungin) are fungicidal against *Candida*, including strains that are fluconazole resistant, but fungistatic against *Aspergillus*.

REFERENCES

1. Rang HP, Ritter JM, Flower RJ, Henderson G. Rang and Dale's Pharmacology, 8th edition. London: Elsevier; 2015.
2. Katzung BG. Basic and Clinical Pharmacology, 11th edition. New York: McGraw-Hill; 2015.
3. Bennett JE. Antifungal agents. In: Brunton LL, Hilal-Dandan R (Eds). Goodman and Gilman's Manual of Pharmacology and Therapeutics, 13th edition. New York, NY: McGraw-Hill; 2013.
4. Tripathi KD. Essentials of Medical Pharmacology, 7th edition. New Delhi: Jaypee Brothers Medical Publishers; 2013.
5. Hardman JG, Limbird LE, Gilman AG. Goodman & Gilman's The Pharmacological Basis of Therapeutics, 12th edition. New York: McGraw-Hill; 2011.
6. Ghannoum MA, Rice LB. Antifungal agents: mode of action, mechanisms of resistance, and correlation of these mechanisms with bacterial resistance. Clin Microbiol Rev. 1999;12(4):501-7.
7. Walsh TJ, Dixon DM. Spectrum of Mycoses. In: Baron S (Ed). Medical Microbiology, 4th edition. Galveston, Texas; University of Texas Medical Branch at Galveston, Department of Microbiology and Immunology; 1996.
8. Ribes JA, Vanover-Sams CL, Baker DJ. Zygomycetes in Human Disease. Clin Microbiol Rev. 2000;13(2):236-301.
9. Greer ND. Voriconazole: the newest triazole antifungal agent. Proc (Bayl Univ Med Cent). 2003;16(2):241-8.
10. The Lancet Infectious Diseases. An exciting time for antifungal therapy. Lancet Infect Dis. 2023;23(7):763.

24.9 Biological Agents in Pediatric Therapeutics

Sagar Bhattad, Jyothi Janardhanan

INTRODUCTION

Pediatric rheumatology comprises a spectrum of autoimmune and inflammatory conditions affecting children, often posing unique challenges in diagnosis and management. Over the past few decades, biological therapies have revolutionized the treatment landscape, providing targeted and effective options for many pediatric rheumatic diseases. This chapter explores the role of biologics in pediatric rheumatology, focusing on their mechanisms of action, indications, safety considerations, and future directions.

UNDERSTANDING BIOLOGICS

The term "biologics" refers to a wide range of therapeutic products, including vaccines, blood products, gene and cell therapies, and bioengineered drugs. Often they are used more restrictively to refer to drugs produced through recombinant DNA technology. Biologics or biological disease-modifying antirheumatic drugs (b-DMARDs) differ from nonbiologic or synthetic DMARDs, as biological processes rather than chemical processes produce them. b-DMARDs target specific, well-defined molecules expressed on cells or secreted into the extracellular space.[1]

Biosimilars have been defined by the European Medicines Agency (EMA) as "biological medicine highly similar to another already approved biological medicine (the 'reference medicine')". Biosimilars are approved according to the same standards of pharmaceutical quality, safety, and efficacy that apply to all biological medicines. Biosimilars are different from biocopies, which are biological drugs prepared in other less-resourced countries (e.g., India or China), but which did not pass the high level of scrutiny required by the US Food and Drug Administration (FDA) and EMA and therefore are not available in the US and European markets.

NAMING CONVENTIONS

The International Nonproprietary Name Expert Group (INNEG) of the World Health Organization (WHO) has proposed a standardized nomenclature for monoclonal antibodies (mAbs). This nomenclature comprises a *prefix,* one or two *substems or infixes* (reduced to one substem in the 2017 document), and a *suffix*. The prefix is chosen arbitrarily to ensure a unique and distinct drug name. Substems or infixes convey information about the target (e.g., "ci" for cardiovascular) and the source (host) in which the antibody was originally produced (e.g., "u" for human, "o" for mouse), along with any modifications (e.g., "-xi-" for chimeric, "-zu-" for humanized). The suffix, also referred to as the stem, for mAbs developed between 1990 and 2022 was "mab". However, products named from 2022 onward adopt one of the following suffix options:

- -tug (unmodified immunoglobulin)
- -bart (engineered constant region)
- -mig (bispecific or multispecific)
- -ment (variable region fragment)

Table 24.9.1 provides the commonly used naming conventions using infix and source substems.[2]

TABLE 24.9.1: Naming conventions for biological agents using infix and source substems.

Infix		***Source substem***	
-ci	Cardiovascular	-e	Hamster
-eni	Enzyme inhibition	-i	Primate
-fung	Fungal	-o	Mouse
-gro	Skeletal muscle mass-related growth factors and receptors	-u	Human
-ki	Cytokine and cytokine receptors	-xi	Chimeric
-ler	Allergen	-xizu	Chimeric-humanized
-ne	Neural	-zu	Humanized
-os	Bone		
-pru	Immunosuppressive		
-sto	Immunostimulatory		
-toxa	Toxin		
-ta	Tumor		
-vet	Veterinary use		
-vi	Viral		

Source: Adapted from World Health Organization's International Nonproprietary Names (INN) Scheme for Pharmaceutical Substances, Guidelines on the Use of International Nonproprietary Names (INNs) for Pharmaceutical Substances, and UpToDate.

GENERAL CONSIDERATIONS

The important considerations while prescribing b-DMARDS include:

- b-DMARDS should not be given/started in an active infection.
- Treatment with b-DMARDs is associated with an increased risk of infections.
- Before initiation of a b-DMARD, screening must be done for the presence of tuberculosis and infectious hepatitis.
- Vaccination with live or live-attenuated vaccines is contraindicated in patients on treatment with a b-DMARD.
- All b-DMARDS can be combined with synthetic DMARDs [e.g., methotrexate (MTX), leflunomide, or sulfasalazine].

TUMOR NECROSIS FACTOR-ALPHA INHIBITORS

Tumor necrosis factor (TNF) is an important cytokine implicated in the pathogenesis of juvenile idiopathic arthritis (JIA). Five TNF inhibitors (TNFi) have been approved by the FDA—etanercept, infliximab, adalimumab, golimumab, and certolizumab pegol.[3]

Mechanism of Action

The mechanism of action of TNFi is primarily centered around neutralizing the activity of tumor necrosis factor-alpha (TNF-α), a pro-inflammatory cytokine involved in the immune response. By binding to TNF-α, TNFi prevents the activation of downstream inflammatory pathways. TNF-α normally triggers the release of other inflammatory cytokines, adhesion molecules, and enzymes involved in the inflammatory cascade. Inhibition of TNF-α interrupts this cascade, reducing inflammation.

Etanercept

Etanercept is a recombinant protein made up of an Fc portion of human IgG1 and two human TNF-R2. It was first approved by the FDA for rheumatoid arthritis in 1998.

Dose: 0.4 mg/kg twice weekly or 0.8 mg/kg weekly, subcutaneously (SC); maximum 50 mg/week

Indications:

- Rheumatoid arthritis
- Psoriatic arthritis (PsA)
- Psoriasis
- Ankylosing spondylitis
- JIA (minimum age 2 years)
- Pediatric psoriasis (minimum age 4 years)

Off-label use: Juvenile dermatomyositis

Adalimumab

Adalimumab is a fully human IgGκ mAb to TNF-α. Adalimumab induces strong complement-mediated cytotoxicity and is less immunogenic than infliximab due to the absence of murine variable domains of the immunoglobulin Fab.

Dose:

- *10 kg to <15 kg:* 10 mg every other week SC
- *15 kg to <30 kg:* 20 mg every other week SC
- *≥30 kg:* 40 mg every other week SC

Indications:

- Rheumatoid arthritis
- PsA
- Psoriasis
- Ankylosing spondylitis
- Hidradenitis suppurativa (minimum age 12 years)
- Uveitis (minimum age 2 years)

Off-label use: Sarcoidosis

Infliximab

Infliximab is a chimeric mAb, consisting of murine variable regions and human IgG1 constant regions. It binds both transmembrane and soluble TNF-α with high affinity.

Dose: For JIA 6–10 mg/kg/dose on weeks 0, 2, and 6, then every 4–8 weeks; after that, depending on the course; the dose may be increased further. It is available as 100 mg infliximab/20 mL vial. Premedication with acetaminophen and diphenhydramine is recommended before the infusion.

Indications:

- Crohn's disease and ulcerative colitis
- Rheumatoid arthritis
- PsA
- Psoriasis
- Ankylosing spondylitis

Off-label uses:

- Uveitis
- JIA
- Sarcoidosis
- Pediatric psoriasis
- Kawasaki disease

Adverse Events of Tumor Necrosis Factor Inhibitors

- *Infections:*
    - Reactivation of latent tuberculosis
    - Reactivation of hepatitis B

- *Central nervous system (CNS) involvement:*
  - Headache
  - Behavioral disturbances
  - Serious side effects include Guillain–Barré syndrome, peripheral neuropathies, multiple sclerosis, optic neuritis, and acute transverse myelitis.
- *Drug-induced systemic lupus erythematosus (SLE):* It is mainly seen in patients taking infliximab and, in some cases, after treatment with etanercept and adalimumab.
- *Malignancy:* Few studies have shown an increased risk of non-Hodgkin lymphoma.
- *Antibodies to TNFi:* Serum antibodies to TNFi are called human antichimeric antibodies (HACAs). Concomitant use of MTX is associated with lower incidences of HACA.

B-CELL TARGETED BIOLOGICAL DMARDS

Rituximab

Rituximab is an anti-CD20 mAb that was first approved by the FDA in 1997.

Mechanism of Action

Rituximab is a chimeric mouse and human mAb with binding specificity to CD20.

- The binding of rituximab to CD20 can directly trigger apoptosis through both caspase-dependent and -independent mechanisms.
- Bound rituximab can recruit the C1 complex triggering the classical complement cascade, which leads to the insertion of the membrane attack complex (MAC) and ultimately leads to cell lysis, also known as complement-dependent cytotoxicity (CDC).
- Bound rituximab can recruit natural killer cells *via* recognition by the FcγRIII leading to antibody-dependent cell-mediated cytotoxicity (ADCC). This facilitates the release of perforin, which assembles into membrane-compromising pores in the target cell, and granzyme B, which enters the target cell and triggers apoptosis by cleaving caspases.
- Macrophages recognize CD20-bound rituximab through various Fcγ receptors, which leads to antibody-dependent phagocytosis (ADP) of the target cell.

Dose: 500 mg/m^2 (maximum 1,000 mg) intravenously (IV) on weeks 0 and 2 followed by 375 mg/m^2 weekly for 4 doses.

Indications: Rituximab is licensed to treat B-cell non-Hodgkin lymphoma, adult rheumatoid arthritis, and idiopathic thrombocytopenic purpura.

Off-label uses:

- SLE
- Juvenile dermatomyositis
- Nephrotic syndrome
- Antiphospholipid syndrome
- Antineutrophil cytoplasmic antigens (ANCA)-associated vasculitis
- Sjögren syndrome
- IgA vasculitis
- Uveitis
- Systemic sclerosis
- Pediatric autoimmune encephalitis

Adverse events:

- Serious infusion reactions including anaphylaxis
- Cytopenia
- Hepatitis B reactivation
- Hypogammaglobulinemia
- Infections
- Serum sickness
- Progressive multifocal leukoencephalopathy.

Belimumab

Belimumab is a human mAb to B-lymphocyte stimulator.[4]

Dose: 10 mg/kg IV on weeks 0, 2, 4, then every 4 weeks; 200 mg SC every 1 week

Indications:

- Severe active lupus nephritis
- Severe active CNS system lupus

Adverse events:

- Serious infections including pneumonia, urinary tract infection, cellulitis, bronchitis
- Nausea
- Diarrhea
- Pyrexia
- Injection site reactions
- Others include insomnia, depression, migraine

INTERLEUKIN-6 INHIBITORS

Monoclonal antibodies that block the interleukin-6 receptor (IL-6R) are tocilizumab and sarilumab. Other mAbs target IL-6, however, they are under trial and include sirukumab, olokizumab, clazakizumab, and siltuximab.

Mechanism of Action

Interleukin-6 is a proinflammatory cytokine secreted by macrophages, dendritic cells, and T-cells. IL-6 signaling occurs through its IL-6R. A hexameric complex of IL6R, gp130, and IL-6 is formed, which leads to downstream activation of the JAK-STAT3 pathway and is a major contributor to inflammation. IL-6 activity is inhibited either by blocking IL-6R or by directly blocking IL-6.

Tocilizumab

Dose:

- *Intravenous:*
  - Polyarticular JIA—weight <30 kg: 10 mg/kg; weight >30 kg: 8 mg/kg every 4 weeks
  - Systemic JIA (SJIA)—weight <30 kg: 12 mg/kg; weight >30 kg: 8 mg/kg every 2 weeks; infuse over 1 hour
- *Subcutaneous:*
  - SJIA—weight >30 kg: 162 mg every week; weight <30 kg: 162 mg every 2 weeks
  - Polyarticular JIA—weight >30 kg: 162 mg every 2 weeks; weight <30 kg: 162 mg every 3 weeks

Indications:

- Rheumatoid arthritis
- SJIA

Adverse events:

- Skin and soft-tissue infections
- Transaminitis
- Hypercholesterolemia
- Transient neutropenia

INTERLEUKIN-1 INHIBITOR

Mechanism of Action

Interleukin 1 receptor antagonist (IL-1Ra) is the primary physiological controller of IL-1-induced activity, involving both IL-1-α and IL-1-β. Its pivotal role lies in preventing the interaction between IL-1 and the IL-1 receptor on cell surfaces, thereby averting downstream cell signaling. When there is an imbalance between IL-1 and IL-1Ra, it can result in unregulated inflammation.

In rheumatoid arthritis, IL-1 plays an important role in stimulating synoviocytes and chondrocytes, which produce inflammatory mediators and matrix metalloproteinases (MMP) that lead to cartilage destruction.

Anakinra

Anakinra is a human recombinant form of IL-1Ra.

Dose: 1–2 mg/kg SC daily (maximum 100 mg); safe to use with MTX but should not be combined with TNFi.

Indications:

- Rheumatoid arthritis
- SJIA
- *Autoinflammatory diseases*, e.g., cryopyrin-associated periodic syndrome (CAPS), hyperimmunoglobulin D syndrome (HIDS)
- Macrophage activation syndrome

Adverse events:

- Injection-site reactions
- Increased risk of infections
- Headache
- Gastrointestinal disturbances

Canakinumab

Canakinumab is a fully human IgG1κ mAb specifically targeting IL-1β.

Dose:

- *CAPS:*
  - 40 kg: 150 mg
  - ≥15 kg and ≥40 kg: 2 mg/kg
  - For children 15–40 kg with an inadequate response, the dose can be increased to 3 mg/kg.
  - Administer SC every 8 weeks.
- *SJIA:* ≥7.5 kg: 4 mg/kg (maximum of 300 mg); administer SC every 4 weeks.

Indications:

- CAPS
- SJIA
- Tumor necrosis factor receptor-associated periodic syndrome (TRAPS)
- Familial Mediterranean fever

Adverse events:

- Infections
- Transaminitis
- Neutropenia and thrombocytopenia, usually transient
- Injection-site reactions

INTERLEUKIN-17 AND INTERLEUKIN-23 INHIBITION

Interleukin-17 and interleukin-23 are proinflammatory cytokines and have been implicated in the pathogenesis of psoriasis, PsA, and axial spondyloarthritis (SpA). IL-17 inhibitors include secukinumab, ixekizumab, brodalumab, and bimekizumab. IL-23 inhibitors include guselkumab, tidrakizumab, risankizumab, ustekinumab, and mirikizumab.

Mechanism of Action

Interleukin-17 causes stimulation of osteoclastogenesis, chondrocyte activation, fibrogenesis, angiogenesis, stimulation of proinflammatory cytokines, and MMP production, which leads to inflammation and damage. IL-17 is produced by T helper 17 (Th17) T cells and the differentiation of Th17 T cells is sustained by upstream IL-23. Inhibition of IL-17 and IL-23 is known to be effective in the treatment of psoriasis and PsA. However, in SpA, only IL-17 inhibitors are found to be effective, the exact etiology remains unclear.

Indications:
- Psoriasis
- PsA
- SpA

Adverse events of IL-17 inhibitors:
- Nasopharyngitis
- Diarrhea
- Upper respiratory tract infections

Adverse events of IL-23 inhibitors:
- Nasopharyngitis
- Headache

COSTIMULATORY BLOCKERS

Cytotoxic T-Lymphocyte-associated Antigen-4 Immunoglobulin (Abatacept)

Abatacept was the first CTLA4-Ig (cytotoxic T-lymphocyte-associated antigen-4 immunoglobulin) molecule to be developed.

Mechanism of Action

Resting T cells are activated by the following two signals:
1. The interaction of the T-cell receptor with processed peptide, bound to the appropriate major histocompatibility complex molecule
2. Interaction of CD28 on T cells with CD80/86 on the surface of the antigen-presenting cell

Another high-affinity receptor, CTLA-4, can also bind to CD80/86 with a higher avidity than CD28, thereby preventing the second signal required for T-cell activation.

Abatacept is a fully human, soluble fusion protein comprising the extracellular domain of CTLA-4 and the Fc component of IgG1, which selectively inhibits the costimulatory signal necessary for full T-cell activation. Abatacept inhibits T-cell activation by binding to CD80 and CD86, thereby blocking their interaction with CD28.

Dose:
- *IV:*
  - <75 kg: 10 mg/kg on weeks 0, 2, 4, then every 4 weeks
  - 75–100 kg: 750 mg on weeks 0, 2, 4, then every 4 weeks
  - >100 kg: 1,000 mg on weeks 0, 2, 4, then every 4 weeks
- *SC:*
  - 20 to <25 kg: 50 mg/week
  - 25–50 kg: 87.5 mg/week
  - >50 kg: 125 mg/week

Indications:
- Rheumatoid arthritis
- JIA
- PsA
- Stem cell and renal transplantation

Adverse events:
- Infusion reactions
- Anaphylactoid reactions
- Risk of infections

TABLE 24.9.2: Summary of biologics used in pediatric rheumatology.

Drug	Molecule	Half-life	Laboratory monitoring*†
Etanercept	TNFRII/FcIgG1	4.25 days	CBC, AST, ALT, albumin at baseline and then every 12 weeks
Adalimumab	mAb to TNF	2 weeks	CBC, AST, ALT, and albumin at baseline and then every 12 weeks.
Infliximab	mAb to TNF	8–9.5 days	• CBC, AST, ALT, and albumin at baseline and then every 12 weeks • Test for tuberculosis and infectious hepatitis • Monitor for pregnancy as indicated
Anakinra	IL1-Ra	4–6 hours	• CBC, AST, ALT, and albumin at baseline and then every 12 weeks • Serum lipid monitoring after 2–3 months of therapy
Rituximab	mAb to CD20	32 days	• Examine B-cell numbers before and 1 month after the infusion • Check quantitative immunoglobulins every 3 months • Monitor CBC, AST, and ALT every 4–12 weeks
Tocilizumab	mAb to IL-6 receptor	11–13 days	• AST, ALT, ANC at baseline, second infusion then every 2–4 weeks • Lipid panel 4–8 weeks after start of treatment, then every 6 months
Abatacept	CTLA4-Ig	• IV: 13 days • SC: 14.3 days	CBC, AST, ALT, albumin at baseline and then every 12 weeks

*Withhold for suspected bacterial infection, fungal infection, varicella, or measles.
†All patients should be screened for tuberculosis and hepatitis B before starting biologics.
(ALT: alanine aminotransferase; ANC: absolute neutrophil count; AST: aspartate aminotransferase; CBC: complete blood count; IL-1Ra: interleukin 1 receptor antagonist; IV: intravenous; mAb: monoclonal antibody; SC: subcutaneous; TNF: tumor necrosis factor)

CONCLUSION

Table 24.9.2 summarizes the current use of biologics in pediatric rheumatology.[1,2]

Biologics have revolutionized the treatment of rheumatic diseases by offering targeted therapies that improve disease control, reduce inflammation, and enhance patients' quality of life. However, their use requires careful patient selection and monitoring for potential side effects. Ongoing research continues to refine biologic therapies, with newer agents and biosimilars expanding treatment options.

REFERENCES

1. Brunner HI, Ruperto N. Therapeutics: Biologics and small molecules. In: Petty RE, Laxer RM, Lindsley CB, Wedderburn L, Fuhlbrigge RC, Mellins ED, (Eds). Textbook of Pediatric Rheumatology, 8th edition. Philadelphia: Elsevier; 2021. pp. 174-94.
2. Manis JP. (2024). Overview of therapeutic monoclonal antibodies. [online] Available from https://www.uptodate.com/contents/overview-of-therapeutic-monoclonal-antibodies [Last accessed December 2024].
3. Leone GM, Mangano K, Petralia MC, Nicoletti F, Fagone P. Past, Present and (Foreseeable) Future of Biological Anti-TNF Alpha Therapy. J Clin Med. 2023;12(4):1630.
4. Brunner HI, Abud-Mendoza C, Viola DO, Penades IC, Levy D, Anton J, et al.; Paediatric Rheumatology International Trials Organisation (PRINTO) and the Pediatric Rheumatology Collaborative Study Group (PRCSG). Safety and efficacy of intravenous belimumab in children with systemic lupus erythematosus: results from a randomised, placebo-controlled trial. Ann Rheum Dis. 2020;79(10):1340-8.

24.10 Controlled Drugs and Drug Dependence

Shekhar Seshadri, N Prasanna Kumar

CONTROLLED DRUGS

INTRODUCTION

Drugs that pose a risk of excessive use, leading to misuse and addiction are designated as "controlled drugs". Controlled drugs are prescribed by the doctors for specific ailments that have a recognized therapeutic and medical concern as well as a potential for abuse. "Controlled substances" include both illicit drugs and controlled drugs. These substances carry the risk of misuse and addiction. The government regulates and controls the production, distribution, and possession of these controlled substances.

CONTROLLED MEDICATION AND RISK OF MISUSE AND ADDICTION

The danger of addiction, misuse, and abuse when prescribing controlled medication is very high.[1] Both physical and psychological dependence are possible outcomes. Misuse of controlled drugs is secondary to multifactorial causes. Lack of parental supervision of procuring, storing, and discarding of medications is one of the contributing factors. Preventative measures greatly depend on locating the possible sources from which the teenager/adolescent is obtaining the substance. In majority instances, teenagers get their medication from friends or family members who are already taking it. It is critical to protectively use the controlled substances and dispose them properly.

The Narcotic Drugs and Psychotropic Substances (NDPS) Act in India and the Controlled Substance Act of the US Government **(Table 24.10.1)** both classify controlled medications into distinct schedules.[2] One of the classifications include Schedule one to Schedule five. Schedule one medications have a high risk of misuse and dependence whereas Schedule five medications have the lowest potential for abuse. According to a Central Government of India notification, oxycodone, codeine, hydrocodone, methadone, morphine, and fentanyl were added to the list of essential narcotic substances in India.

VULNERABILITY OF ADOLESCENCE FOR CONTROLLED DRUG ABUSE

Adolescents are particularly susceptible to abusing controlled substances. Adolescents, who are already taking other substances of abuse, have low educational attainment, are truant, and have inadequate parental monitoring are at higher risk. Drugs classified as schedule one narcotics are not prescribed for medical purposes and are not sold in pharmacies.

TABLE 24.10.1: Classification of controlled substances.

Schedule	Potentiality for abuse	Medical use	Drugs
Schedule 1	High	No	Heroin, lysergic acid diethylamide (LSD), 3,4-methylenedioxymethamphetamine (MDMA)
Schedule 2	High	Yes	Cocaine, methadone, oxycodone, methylphenidate
Schedule 3	Moderate	Yes	Ketamine, anabolic steroids
Schedule 4	Low	Yes	Benzodiazepines, tramadol
Schedule 5	Lowest	Yes	Codeine, pregabalin

TABLE 24.10.2: Indications for controlled drugs.

Controlled drugs	Indication
Benzodiazepines	Sleep disorders, anxiety, seizures
Stimulants (methylphenidate)	Attention deficit hyperactivity disorder, sleep disorders
Opioids	Cough, pain
Antiepileptic drugs (AEDs) (pregabalin)	Nerve pain

Controlled medication misuse in adolescents can lead to:

- Risk-taking behaviors, such as reckless driving and unsafe sexual behavior
- Emotional problems that result in suicide attempts
- Abuse of medication in overdose leading to higher rate of hospitalization and mortality

Opioids and stimulants are frequently prescribed controlled substances. The most widely used opioid is codeine and is used for the treatment of pain, persistent diarrhea, and chronic cough **(Table 24.10.2)**. If preventive measures are not taken, adolescents who begin with substance misuse may progress into "substance dependency". Children and adolescents using controlled medication for pain, intractable cough, or stimulants for poor attention must be monitored, and the controlled drugs must be administered by their parents. The transition of medication management may be partially passed to the adolescent with parent supervision and regular monitoring, if the adolescent is maturing and becoming more independent. Adolescents who abuse medication and exhibit signs of addiction attempt to obtain additional pills by visiting several pharmacies and medical professionals, which can result in "prescribers shopping" and, in certain situations, selling the controlled substances to people who abuse them, resulting in "drug diversion".

PRECAUTIONS BY DOCTORS WHILE PRESCRIBING CONTROLLED DRUGS

The prescribing doctor is required to monitor for the possibility of illegitimate use of controlled substances. In order for the pharmacy to accept a prescription for controlled substances, the doctor must adhere to regulations, which include providing a duplicate prescription along with the original. It is imperative that appropriate measures are implemented to ensure that a child or adolescent receiving controlled medication has a suitable caregiver to oversee and administer the medicine. It is necessary to give the family members psychoeducation on the risks of drug abuse, adverse effects, drug interactions, motor impairment, and the precautions they need to take.[3]

Considering Other Alternatives

Prescription of controlled drugs for pain symptoms must be reserved for moderate-to-severe situations, which include cancer-related pain, and only after all other options for pain management have been exhausted. Before administering controlled pain relievers, doctors may first consider nonsteroidal anti-inflammatory drugs (NSAIDs), relaxation techniques including yoga, biofeedback, massage, aerobics, and cognitive behavioral therapy, as well as nerve blocks. If necessary, start with mild opioids like codeine and tramadol before moving on to stronger opioids like morphine. In cases of chronic neuropathic pain, gabapentin, topical lidocaine, tricyclic antidepressants (TCAs), and serotonin and norepinephrine reuptake inhibitors (SNRIs) may be considered. Adolescents who progress to chronic drug usage due to pain symptoms are more susceptible to drug misuse and addiction. If access to controlled drugs is available, self-medication for pain management may result in misuse of drugs. Inappropriate use of controlled drugs occurs when excessive doses are prescribed or when doses are continued in spite of no pain alleviation.[5]

Evaluating Pain

Prescribers must be aware that patients differ in their pain sensitivities and in the ways that the environment, emotions, and behavior impact pain. Before prescribing a controlled substance for pain management, the patient must be thoroughly assessed. Less localized pain with fewer pathological reports are connected with a lower likelihood of addiction than widespread pain symptoms with severe pathology, as well as a history of past substance use. One screening tool available for use of pain assessment is the "Pain Assessment and Documentation Tool (PADT)".

Few adolescents experiencing pain symptoms may also have symptoms of anxiety, restlessness, and persistent fear of pain, a phenomenon known as "pseudoaddiction", and this condition is not associated with physical or psychological dependence.

While prescribing controlled medications, clinicians must evaluate symptoms of intoxication and withdrawal. A clinician must also distinguish between addiction-related abuse and misuse. *Addiction* is defined as a chronic disorder of the reward circuitry in the brain that is linked to cravings, drug tolerance, physical and psychological dependence on a particular substance, and an inability to control or refrain from using drugs despite harmful consequences on the user leading to compulsive drug use. *Misuse* is defined as using the drug for a condition other than what it was prescribed for, as well as for excessive or accidental use.[4]

DRUG ADDICTION

INTRODUCTION

Adolescents are at risk of developing drug addiction. The period of adolescence is characterized by impulsivity. Hormonal changes and brain maturation leads to increased vulnerability to drug addiction. Drug abuse in early ages will have negative outcome compared to late exposure. Centers for Disease Control and Prevention (CDC) reports 15% of high school students ever used illicit drugs. In India, inhalant addiction use among children and adolescents is higher (1.17%) compared to adults. The use of tobacco in adolescents increases as the age of adolescent increases. Tobacco use in adolescents is associated with increased alcohol use.[6] Drug addiction is in the category of *substance use disorders (SUDs)*. SUDs refer to persistent use of psychoactive substances leading to harm and negative consequences to the individual.[7]

ADDICTION BEHAVIOR

Addiction behavior initially starts with curiosity to explore the drug effects and also due to peer pressure. Initially adolescents start the substance as experimental use followed by progress to recreational use and further progress to harmful use and dependence.

Psychosocial stressors including academic difficulties, identity issues, cultural factors, financial difficulties, with past psychiatric illness and physical illness may trigger the addiction behavior. There are high chances of relapse in addiction and complete abstinence can be long-term goal. Delaying the early initiation or first use of substance will help in decreasing the problems with addiction. The early the age of cannabis intake, the higher the chances of being cannabis-dependent.[1]

TABLE 24.10.3: Classification of substance for addiction.

Central nervous system (CNS) action	Drugs
Depressants	Benzodiazepine, alcohol, opioids
Stimulants	Amphetamines, cocaine, caffeine
Hallucinogens	Lysergic acid diethylamide (LSD), 3,4-methylenedioxymethamphetamine (MDMA), ketamine

ADDICTION AND CENTRAL NERVOUS SYSTEM

Addiction is associated with long-term changes in the brain networks. It is associated with changes in gene expression. Reward pathway in the brain circuitry along with changes in neurotransmission of dopamine (DA) potentiates addictive behavior. Brain areas involved include prefrontal cortex, ventral tegmental area, and nucleus accumbens. The existing lower DA activity in reward pathway makes DA-raising substances pleasant. Individuals with low DA function present with low boredom threshold. Increase in DA levels makes more pleasant and reinforcing. Addiction substances are based on the effect on central nervous system **(Table 24.10.3)**.

Determinants of Addiction

The determinants of addiction include:

- *Individual factors:* Genetic predisposition, family history, attention-deficit hyperactivity disorder (ADHD), conduct disorder, academic difficulties, temperament traits and poor life skills
- *Traits:* Impulsivity, increasing boredom, novelty seeking, moody and difficulty in socialization
- *Family-related:* Family conflicts and disturbed families, neglect, abuse, adverse childhood experiences, attachment and poor supervision
- *Social factors:* Peer pressure, poverty, societal norms and laws

Addiction or dependence is considered if the individual has lack of control, tolerance, withdrawal symptoms, craving, is neglecting other pleasures, and is taking substance in spite of harmful effects.

ALCOHOL

Prevalence of alcohol use (10–17 years) is 1.3%.[7] Alcohol dependence is considered as diagnostic category if the individual has:

- Impaired ability to control use of alcohol
- Strong internal drive to use alcohol
- Persistence of use despite harm

- Increasing priority over other activities
- Urge or craving to use alcohol
- Tolerance
- Withdrawal

Alcohol use can lead to harmful use or dependence. Alcohol withdrawal **(Table 24.10.4)** includes *simple withdrawal* characterized by tremors, palpitations, and sweating or *complicated withdrawal* associated with seizures and in some cases with delirium tremens, a medical emergency condition. Withdrawal symptoms can be rated by Clinical Institute Withdrawal Assessment (CIWA). In some individuals, alcohol use can lead to alcohol-induced psychotic disorder characterized by hallucinations, loss of contact with reality, delusions, and disorganized behavior.

Treatment of Alcohol Use Disorder

Detoxification for controlling withdrawal symptoms has to be managed by long-acting benzodiazepines and lorazepam in case of hepatic-compromised individuals. Thiamine supplementation has to be given in alcohol-dependent individuals. The dose of benzodiazepines has to be tapered in 7–10 days based on the withdrawal symptoms. Acamprosate or naltrexone can be considered for managing craving. Acamprosate has to be considered if the individual is motivated for complete abstinence. Reducing the frequency of cues of substance of abuse along with association of coping strategies will help in preventing relapse. Naltrexone has to be considered in case of high levels of craving and to reduce heavy drinking **(Table 24.10.5)**. Educating the individuals for

TABLE 24.10.4: Symptoms of intoxication and withdrawal.

Substance name	***Symptoms of intoxication***	***Symptoms of withdrawal***
Alcohol	Poor coordination, unsteady gait, impaired attention, inappropriate or aggressive behavior, lability of mood, slurred speech, stupor or coma	• Hand tremor, nausea, vomiting, insomnia, autonomic hyperactivity, seizures • Delirium tremens characterized by confusion and disorientation, delusions, and visual, tactile or auditory hallucinations
Cannabis	• Euphoria, perceptual alterations, increased appetite, anxiety, impaired attention, impaired judgment, impaired short-term memory, and sluggishness • Physical signs include red or bloodshot eyes and tachycardia	Insomnia, restlessness, anxiety, dysphoric mood, appetite disturbance, irritability, anger, shakiness, abdominal cramps and muscle aches
Opioids	• Somnolence, impaired judgment, respiratory depression, slurred speech, mood changes, impairment of memory and attention • Pupillary constriction—this sign may be absent when intoxication is due to synthetic opioids	Craving for an opioid, anxiety, nausea or vomiting, abdominal cramps, dysphoric mood, muscle aches, yawning, perspiration, hot and cold flushes, lacrimation, rhinorrhea, hypersomnia or insomnia, diarrhea and piloerection
Sedatives, hypnotics or anxiolytics	Impaired judgment, slurred speech, impaired motor coordination, unsteady gait, somnolence, mood changes, as well as impaired memory, attention and concentration, and nystagmus	Insomnia, increased hand tremor, nausea or vomiting, anxiety, psychomotor agitation, autonomic hyperactivity, seizures and delirium
Cocaine	Euphoria, impaired attention, hypervigilance, psychomotor agitation, anxiety, anger, paranoid ideation, auditory hallucinations, confusion, palpitations, chest pain, elevated blood pressure, and pupillary dilatation	Dysphoric mood, vivid unpleasant dreams, insomnia or hypersomnia, increased appetite, anxiety, psychomotor agitation or retardation, irritability, fatigue, and craving for cocaine
Stimulants including amphetamines, methamphetamine or methcathinone	Anxiety, impaired attention, hypervigilance, psychomotor agitation, anger, paranoid ideation, auditory hallucinations, confusion, tachycardia, elevated blood pressure, pupillary dilatation	Insomnia or (more commonly) hypersomnia, increased appetite, psychomotor agitation or retardation, fatigue
Nicotine	Psychomotor agitation, confusion, burning sensations in the mouth, anxiety, cold sweats, headache, insomnia, and palpitations	Insomnia, irritability, anger, anxiety, difficulty in concentrating, restlessness, bradycardia, increased appetite and weight gain, depressed mood, and craving for tobacco
MDMA-related drugs, including MDA	Anxiety, restlessness, agitation, increased or inappropriate sexual interest and activity, and sweating	Insomnia, depressed mood, anxiety, irritability, fatigue, lethargy, craving, difficulty in concentrating, and appetite disturbance

(MDA: 3,4-methylenedioxyamphetamine; MDMA: 3,4-methylenedioxymethamphetamine)

TABLE 24.10.5: Drug-specific pharmacotherapy for dependance.

Substance name	*Pharmacotherapy in adolescents*
Nicotine	• *Nicotine replacement therapy:* – Nicotine gum, inhaler, lozenge, and nasal spray – *Transdermal patch:* - *<10 cigarettes/day:* 14 mg/day for 6 weeks, then 7 mg/day for 2 weeks, then discontinue - *>10 cigarettes/day:* 21 mg/day for 6 weeks, then 14 mg/day for 2 weeks, then discontinue • *Bupropion:* – *<40 kg:* 150 mg for 12 weeks – *>40 kg:* 150 mg for 3–6 days followed by 150 mg for 12 weeks
Alcohol	• *Naltrexone:* 50 mg/day • *Acamprosate:* 22.2 mg/kg body weight, 666 mg, two times a day • *Benzodiazepines* for alcohol withdrawal
Cannabis	*N-acetylcysteine:* 1,200 mg, two times a day
Opioids	• *Methadone:* (after two documented attempts at short-term detoxification or drug-free treatment) 10–60 mg/day • *Buprenorphine:* Initial dose: 2–8 mg; maximum dose: 24 mg/day

triggers like "hunger, anger, loneliness, and tiredness (HALT)" has to be emphasized.

OPIOIDS

Prevalence of opioid use (10–17 years) is 1.8%.[7] Withdrawal symptoms can be measured with "Clinical Opiate Withdrawal Scale (COWS)". Opioid-induced psychosis or delirium can also be presented in opioid-dependence individuals. Opioid substitution therapy consisting of buprenorphine (sublingual) can be considered for withdrawal and maintenance. Buprenorphine is partial opioid agonist. Clonidine can also be considered for managing withdrawal features of opioids.[8]

INHALANTS

Inhalant abuse is more common in children and adolescents compared to adults. Poor supervision by parents and access to inhalants is one of the predisposing factors. This is associated with significant morbidity and is seen in home settings also. Evaluation of the vulnerable factors and interventions has to be managed accordingly.

ASSESSMENT

Engagement of individual with more open questioning along with reflective listening is needed. CRAFFT (Car, Relax, Alone, Forget, Family, Trouble) is the questionnaire for assessing substance use risk. Michigan Alcohol Screening Test (MAST) is a 25-item questionnaire for evaluation of lifetime alcohol problems **(Table 24.10.6)**.

Assessment should focus on withdrawal symptoms, risk factors, comorbidities, temperament, and motivation. Evaluation has to focus also on individual's strengths and social support. Individual has to be evaluated for the current stage in the stages of motivation, i.e., precontemplation, contemplation, preparation, action, and maintenance followed by relapse.

TABLE 24.10.6: Assessment scales for drugs.

Drug	*Assessment*
Substance use risk	Car, Relax, Alone, Forget, Family, Trouble (CRAFFT)
Alcohol	• Michigan Alcohol Screening Test (MAST) • Clinical Institute Withdrawal Assessment (CIWA)
Opioids	Clinical Opiate Withdrawal Scale (COWS)
Benzodiazepines	Clinical Institute Withdrawal Assessment B (CIWA-B)

GENERAL CONSIDERATIONS IN THE TREATMENT FOR SUBSTANCE USE DISORDERS

Assessment of the amount of the drug along with duration of the drug intake has to be done. Evaluation of other drug intake-associated medical and psychiatric comorbidities has to be noted. Medical and psychological investigations have to be performed. Detoxification and treating medical complications along with management of craving has to be planned. Brief intervention has to be started comprising feedback, personal responsibility, advising, giving menu of strategies and enhancing self-efficacy (FRAMES). For cases of increased craving, intervention focusing on delaying the substance, distracting, discussing, drinking water, and deep breathing has to be discussed. There are chances of relapse even with good treatment. Harm reduction and decreasing the amount of usage of substance has to be emphasized if the patient is resistant and not motivated. Motivation enhancement therapy has to be planned for enhancing motivation to stop substance. Motivational interviewing focus on problem of ambivalence to change on the part of individual. Empathy, giving autonomy fosters motivation. Child strategies to improve family attachment and peer involved interventions are recommended.[4,9]

The vulnerable factors of the individual have to be evaluated and interventions have to be planned accordingly. Individuals with poor life skills or coping skills have to improve by the appropriate interventions. Anxiety and depression have to be managed with cognitive behavioral therapies and medication if needed. Appropriate interventions have to be started if the individual has conduct disorder or ADHD. Medication for ADHD has to be started if needed. Strategies of relapse prevention has to be planned. Family therapy has to be planned for managing family conflicts and dynamics.[4,10]

CONCLUSIONS

- Adolescents are vulnerable to substance abuse based on their brain maturation and environmental factors.
- Evaluation of substance abuse by assessment scales, identification of symptoms of dependence and withdrawal are necessary.
- Detoxification, management of medical complications and relapse prevention are important in treating adolescents with drug addiction.

REFERENCES

1. Singh M, Bala N, Garg PD, Bansal S, Bumrah S, Attri A. Substance abuse in Children and adolescent: A Retrospective Study. Int J Med Res Rev. 2017;5(03):352-6.
2. World Health Organization. (2022). International Classification of Diseases, eleventh revision (BlockL1-6C4). [online] Available from https://www.who.int/standards/classifications/-------------World Health Organization. (2022). International classification [online] Available from https:// icd.who.int/browse/2024-01/mms/en [Last accessed December 2024].
3. Preuss CV, Kalava A, King KC. Prescription of Controlled Substances: Benefits and Risks. In: StatPearls [Internet]. Treasure Island(FL): StatPearls Publishing; 2024.
4. United States Drug Enforcement Administration. Drug Scheduling. [online] Available from https://www.dea.gov/drug-information/drug-scheduling [Last accessed December 2024].
5. Engster SA, Bogen DL, Molina BSG. Adolescent and Parent Management of Controlled Prescription Medications. Subst Use Misuse. 2019;54(14):2264-74.
6. Jaisoorya TS, Beena KV, Beena M, Jose DC, Elangovan K, Thennarasu K. Prevalence & correlates of tobacco use among adolescents in Kerala, India. Indian J Med Res. 2016;144(5):704-11.
7. Ambekar A, Agarwal A, Rao R, Mishra AK, Khandelwal SK, Chadda RK on behalf of the group of investigators for the National Survey on Extent and Pattern of Substance Abuse in India. Magnitude of Substance Use in India. New Delhi: Ministry of Social Justice and Empowerment, Government of India; 2019.
8. Benyamin R, Trescot AM, Datta S, Buenaventura R, Adlaka R, Sehgal N, et al. Opioid complications and side effects. Pain Physician. 2008;11(2 Suppl):S105-20.
9. Ministry of Health & Family Welfare, Government of India. (2021). Training Manual on Mental, Neurological and Substance Use (MNS) Disorders Care for Medical Officer at Ayushman Bharat—Health and Wellness Centres. [online] Available from https://nhsrcindia.org/sites/default/files/2022-05/MNS%20care%20Training%20manual%20for%20CHO.pdf [Last accessed December 2024].
10. Dydyk AM, Sizemore DC, Haddad LM, Lindsay L, Porter BR. NP Safe Prescribing of Controlled Substances While Avoiding Drug Diversion. In: StatPearls [Internet]. Treasure Island (FL): StatPearls Publishing; 2024.

24.11 Antimicrobial Drugs in Renal Impairment

Rehna K Rahman

INTRODUCTION

Renal failure in children creates multiple issues regarding drug administration. Toxicity related to accumulation of the drug or its metabolites is the most common problem. These issues warrant modifying the drug regimen, by reducing the dose or by prescribing alternative drugs. This should be done with caution especially in sick children so that the much needed therapeutic efficacy is not lost. This chapter addresses the optimal use of antimicrobials used among children in a setting of renal impairment.

FACTORS DETERMINING DRUG DOSE MODIFICATION

The degree of renal impairment is the most important factor determining drug dosage.[1] Equally important are the percentage renal elimination of the drug and its toxicity profile. The general rules are as follows:[2]

- If side effects of the medication are minimal or if the predominant metabolism is nonrenal, then dosage alterations may not be needed.
- The glomerular filtration rate (GFR) is used to decide the doses of drugs. Modified Schwartz formula is used to calculate the GFR in a child above 1 year of age and GFR is expressed as mL/min/1.73 m^2. It is calculated using the formula: 0.413*(height in cm)/(serum creatinine in mg/dL)
- Only initial doses are administered for drugs for which plasma drug concentration determines efficacy and toxicity. The latter doses are decided as per plasma levels and treatment response.
- When the renal function is impaired, the renal toxicity of drugs with known nephrotoxicity is exaggerated and hence is better avoided.

ANTIBIOTICS IN RENAL IMPAIRMENT

There are two basic ways of adjusting the dosage—interval adjustment or dose adjustment. These are utilized depending on the characteristics of the antibiotic. Concentration-dependent antibiotics such as aminoglycosides need interval adjustment whereas time-dependent antibiotics such as fluoroquinolones need dose adjustment. Some antibiotics which are less nephrotoxic, e.g., beta-lactams can be either dose- or interval-adjusted, whereas a few antibiotics do not need any dose modification.

Antibiotics Needing no Dose Adjustment

Ceftriaxone, cefotaxime, doxycycline, minocycline, ciprofloxacin, clindamycin, azithromycin, and linezolid are the commonly used antibiotics, which do not need dose modification in renal impairment. Most of these drugs are predominantly metabolized by liver and the metabolites are not toxic in renal failure.

Beta-lactam Antibiotics

Benzylpenicillin

Benzylpenicillin is water-soluble and 60–90% of the dose is excreted by renal elimination. If GFR is >50 mL/min/1.73 m^2, no dose adjustment is needed; if GFR is between 10 and 50 mL/min/1.73 m^2, give normal dose at 8-hourly intervals; and if GFR <10 mL/min/1.73 m^2, give normal dose at 12-hourly intervals.

Ampicillin and Cloxacillin

No dose adjustment is needed for ampicillin if the GFR is above 20 mL/min/1.73 m^2. If GFR is between 10 and 20 mL/min/1.73 m^2, give normal dose 8 hourly; and if below 10 mL/min/1.73 m^2, give 12 hourly. Cloxacillin is not dialyzed and no dose adjustment is needed till GFR is 10 mL/min/1.73 m^2. Below 10 mL/min/1.73 m^2, administer normal dose at 8-hourly intervals.

Amoxiclav

No dose adjustment is required till GFR of 30 mL/min/1.73 m^2. Between 10 and 30 mL/min/1.73 m^2, give normal dose initially followed by 50% of the dose 12 hourly. If GFR is <10 mL/min/1.73 m^2, give normal dose initially followed by 50% of the dose 24 hourly. Regarding oral administration, if GFR is <10 mL/min/1.73 m^2, give 100% of dose at 12-hourly intervals.

Piperacillin–Tazobactam

Piperacillin–tazobactam does not need dose adjustment if GFR is above 50 mL/min/1.73 m^2. Between 30 and 50 mL/min/1.73 m^2 of GFR, administer 50 mg/kg 6 hourly and in GFR <30 mL/min/1.73 m^2, administer 50 mg/kg 8 hourly. Caution is advised when coadministering with vancomycin, because the nephrotoxicity of both the drugs gets potentiated when administered together.[3]

Cephalosporins

The dose adjustments for commonly used cephalosporins are depicted in **Table 24.11.1**.

Cefepime

Cefepime undergoes renal excretion mainly through glomerular filtration. The conventional dose is 50 mg/kg/dose 12 hourly. Between GFR 10 and 50 mL/min/1.73 m^2, give 50 mg/kg 24 hourly and below 10 mL/min/1.73 m^2, give 50 mg/kg 48 hourly. Cefepime is known to cause neurological manifestations including seizures and myoclonus when administered in renal impairment. This is due to concentration-related gamma-aminobutyric acid (GABA) antagonism.

Carbapenems—Meropenem

Meropenem is excreted unchanged in the urine significantly. The regular dosage is 10–20 mg/kg 8 hourly. No dose adjustment needed if GFR is above 50 mL/min/1.73 m^2. In GFR between 20 and 50 mL/min/1.73 m^2, administer normal dose at 12-hourly intervals. In GFR 10–20 mL/min/1.73 m^2, give 50% of dose at 12-hourly intervals. If GFR is <10 mL/min/1.73 m^2, give 50% of the dose 24 hourly.

Macrolide Antibiotics

The dose adjustments of commonly used macrolide antibiotics are given in **Table 24.11.2**.

TABLE 24.11.1: Cephalosporins—dose modification.

Drug	Normal dose	GFR 10–30 mL/min/ 1.73 m²	GFR < 10 mL/min/1.73 m²	HD/PD
Cefazolin (IV)	25 mg/kg/dose q 6 h	25 mg/kg/dose q 12 h	25 mg/kg/dose q 24 h	25 mg/kg q 24 h
Cephalexin (O)	7.5–10 mg/kg/dose q 8 h	5–10 mg/kg /dose q 12 h	5–10 mg/kg/dose q 8 h	5–10 mg/kg q 24 h
Cefadroxil (O)	15 mg/kg/dose q 12 h	15 mg/kg/dose q 24 h	15 mg/kg/dose q 36 h	15 mg/kg q 24 h
	Normal	**GFR 30–50 mL/min/ 1.73 m²**	**GFR 10–30 mL/min/ 1.73 m²**	**GFR <10 mL/min/1.73 m²**
Cefuroxime (IV)	50 mg/kg/dose q 8 h	No dose change	25–50 mg /kg/dose q 12 h	25–50 mg/kg/dose q 24 h
Cefoxitin (IV)	40 mg/kg/dose q 6 h	20–40 mg/kg/dose q 8 h	20–40 mg/kg/dose q 12 h	20–40 mg/kg/dose q 24 h
Ceftazidime (IV)	25–50 mg/kg q 8 h	1st normal dose, then 50 mg/kg q 12 h	1st normal dose, then 50 mg/kg q 24 h	1st normal dose, then 50 mg/kg q 48 h
Cefoperazone (IV)	25–50 mg/kg q 6 h	Same dose q 8 h	Same dose q 12 h	Same dose q 12 h
Cefixime (O)	5 mg/kg/dose q 12 h	No change	No change	4 mg/kg/dose q 12 h

(HD: hemodialysis; IV: intravenous; O: oral; PD: peritoneal dialysis)

TABLE 24.11.2: Dose modification—macrolide antibiotics.

Antibiotic	Regular dose	GFR <30 mL/min/1.73 m²	GFR <10 mL/min/1.73 m²
Erythromycin	10–15 mg/kg q 6 h	No dose adjustment	50–75% q 6 h
Clarithromycin	7.5–15 mg/kg q 12 h	50% dose q 12 h	
Azithromycin	10–15 mg/kg/dose on day 1 7.5 mg/kg/dose q 24 h on day 2–5 orally	No dose adjustment	

(GFR: glomerular filtration rate)

Aminoglycosides

Aminoglycosides are bactericidal antibiotics and possess a narrow range of therapeutic index. Excretion of aminoglycosides is principally via the kidney and accumulation occurs in renal impairment. The different agents exhibit nephrotoxicity and ototoxicity of varying degrees. The toxicity is dependent on the trough levels of the drug and duration of exposure. Since aminoglycosides are concentration-dependent antibiotics, interval between doses must be increased in renal impairment; if the renal impairment is severe, the dose itself should be reduced as well.

Ideally, serum aminoglycoside concentrations must be monitored in patients with renal impairment. Blood samples should be taken just before the next dose is administered ("trough" concentration). If the predose ("trough") concentration is high, the interval between doses must be increased. Dose modifications are given in **Table 24.11.3**.[4]

Tetracyclines

Tetracyclines are bacteriostatic antibiotics, which are used in selective situations. Generally, they are not nephrotoxic except tetracycline. A reversible Fanconi syndrome-like condition is produced by outdated and degraded tetracyclines. Degradation products damage proximal tubules in this setting.

Doxycycline—No adjustment needed; can continue the regular weight-based dosage

Minocycline—No adjustment necessary

Tetracycline—The regular pediatric dose is 25–75 mg/kg intravenous (IV) q 4–6 h (150–300 mg/kg/day). GFR 10–30 mL/min/1.73 m²—same dose q 8 h; GFR < 10 mL/min/1.73 m²—same dose q 12 h

Tigecycline—No adjustment necessary

Fluroquinolones

Fluroquinolones are bactericidal antibiotics and the prototype first-generation quinolone is ciprofloxacin.

Ciprofloxacin

The regular pediatric dosage is 10–20 mg/kg q 12 h orally or 8 hourly IV. No dose adjustment is needed in those with GFR above 30 mL/min/1.73 m². If GFR is between 10 and 30 mL/min/1.73 m², give regular dose at 12-hourly intervals. If GFR is <10 mL/min/1.73 m², give half the dose 12 hourly.

TABLE 24.11.3: Dose modifications—aminoglycoside.[4]

Drug	Regular dose	If drug trough level test available	If drug levels not available
Amikacin	15 mg/kg/day 1 or 2 divided doses	• Give 10 mg/kg IV, take trough level after 24 hours, and hold dose until trough level is available • Afterward, adjust dosage interval according to serum levels, aiming a trough level <10 mg/L	5–7.5 mg/kg q 48 h in GFR <10 mL/min/1.73 m^2 GFR < 50 mL/min/1.73 m^2, same dose is given q 24 h
Tobramycin	2–2.5 mg/kg q 6 h	2.5 mg /kg dose is given and subsequent dosage is determined by blood levels	2.5 mg/kg is given q 24 h
Gentamicin	7–10 mg/kg/day in 1 or 2 divided doses	• Give 2 mg/kg/dose • The target peak levels are 5–10 mg/L and trough level is <1 mg/L	• GFR < 10 mL/min/1.73 m^2, 2–2.5 mg/kg q 48 h • GFR 10–30 mL/min/1.73 m^2, 2–3 mg/kg q 24 h • GFR 30–70 mL/min/1.73 m^2, 3–5 mg/kg q 24 h

(GFR: glomerular filtration rate; IV: intravenous)

TABLE 24.11.4: Vancomycin—dose modification.

GFR (mL/min)	Drug monitoring available	Drug monitoring not available
30–50	Give 10 mg/kg IV, take trough level after 12 hours, give the next dose, and adjust regimen if necessary in order to maintain serum trough level between 5 and 10 mg/L	10 mg/kg/dose q 12 h
10–29	Same as above	10 mg/kg/dose q 24 h
<10	Give 10 mg/kg IV every 24 hours, take trough level after 24 hours and hold dose until the serum trough level is between 5 and 10 mg/L	10 mg/kg/dose q 48 h

Levofloxacin

The regular dosage is 5-10 mg/kg/dose 12 hourly. No dose adjustment is needed above a GFR of 30 mL/min/1.73 m^2. In GFR between 10 and 30 mL/min/1.73 m^2, give same dose 24 hourly. If GFR is <10 mL/min/1.73 m^2, give the same dose at 48-hourly intervals.

Ofloxacin

The regular dosage is 5 mg/kg/dose 8 hourly. If GFR is between 10 and 30 mL/min/1.73 m^2, give 7.5 mg/kg 24 hourly and in those with GFR <10 mL/min/1.73 m^2, give 48 hourly.

Glycopeptide—Vancomycin[4]

Vancomycin is a bactericidal antibiotic active exclusively against resistant gram-positive bacteria. It is partially renally excreted and is known to cause nephrotoxicity, particularly when used in combination with other nephrotoxic drugs like aminoglycosides. The regular dosage is 10-15 mg/kg/dose q 6 hourly. If GFR is >50 mL/min/1.73 m^2, no dose adjustment is recommended, but continue to monitor serum creatinine frequently. The dose modification of vancomycin is given in **Table 24.11.4**.

Clindamycin

Clindamycin is a lincosamide antibiotic, which is predominantly metabolized by liver. The regular pediatric dose is 2.5-10 mg/kg PO q 6-8 h (10-30 mg/kg/day) and IV 6.25-10 mg/kg IV q 6-8 h (25-40 mg/kg/day). No adjustment is required in renal impairment.

Daptomycin

Daptomycin is a lipopeptide antibiotic, which is important in treating resistant staphylococcal infections. The regular dose is 10-12 mg/kg once daily in younger children and 7-9 mg/kg once daily in children above age 6 years. If GFR is <30 mL/min/1.73 m^2, same dose is given IV q 48 h.

Oxazolidinones

Oxazolidinones are linezolid antibiotics and no adjustment is required.

Antitubercular Drugs

- *Isoniazid:* 10-15 mg/kg PO q day; no adjustment is necessary
- *Rifampicin:* 10-20 mg/kg PO/IV q day; if GFR is <10 mL/min/1.73 m^2, 50% PO/IV at same interval
- *Ethambutol:* 15-25 mg/kg PO q day; GFR 10-50 mL/min/1.73 m^2—same dose PO q 24-36 h; GFR <10 mL/min/1.73 m^2—same dose PO q 48 h
- *Pyrazinamide:* 10-40 mg/kg PO q 12-24 h (20-40 mg/kg/day); creatinine clearance (CrCl) <10, 40 mg/kg PO 3 ×/week

Other Antibiotics

- *Chloramphenicol:* Pediatric dose 6.25–25 mg/kg IV q 6 h; no adjustment necessary
- *Colistin:* 2.5–5 mg/kg/day IV in 2–4 doses; GFR 20–50 mL/min/1.73 m^2—75% IV q 12–24 hourly; GFR 10–19 mL/min/1.73 m^2—50% IV q 24 hourly; GFR <10 mL/min/1.73 m^2—25% IV q 36 hourly
- *Metronidazole:* 15–50 mg/kg/day PO/IV q 6–8 h; GFR <10 mL/min/1.73 m^2—50% at same interval
- *Nitrofurantoin:* 1.25–1.75 mg/kg PO QID; GFR <50 mL/min/1.73 m^2—use is not recommended
- *Pyrimethamine:* No adjustment required
- *Trimethoprim/sulfamethoxazole (TMP/SMX):* 4 mg/kg (TMP) PO BD or 15–20 mg/kg/day (TMP) IV divided q 8 h; GFR 15–30 mL/min/1.73 m^2—4 mg/kg mg PO q day; GFR <15 mL/min/1.73 m^2—4 mg/kg PO q 48 h; GFR 15–30 mL/min/1.73 m^2—8–12 mg/kg/day IV divided q 12 h; GFR <15 mL/min/1.73 m^2—8–12 mg/kg IV q 48 h.

ANTIFUNGALS

Systemic antifungals are commonly used in pediatric and neonatal intensive care. Fortunately, most of the antifungals are metabolized through liver and may not need dose modification in renal impairment. Few of them utilize CYP3A4 enzyme system for metabolism and are prone for drug interactions, which has to be kept in mind. Some of the drugs need caution while using in children with hepatic impairment.

Amphotericin B (Liposomal Amphotericin B)

Lipid preparations of amphotericin B are specially designed to be renoprotective. Because of the size of the liposomes, the degree of glomerular filtration and renal elimination is very low and it is not removed by dialysis. Dose of liposomal amphotericin B is 3–5 mg/kg/day 24 hourly. Nephrotoxicity (reduction in GFR) and electrolyte wasting are the major adverse events associated with use. Nephrotoxicity occurs in 15–50% of children and hypokalemia requiring potassium supplementation occurs in up to 40% of children. So frequent laboratory monitoring is warranted. No dose adjustment is needed in renal impairment.

Fluconazole

Fluconazole is a hydrophilic molecule with low protein binding and is well absorbed. It is predominantly renally cleared, with approximately 80% of a dose excreted unchanged in the urine. Fluconazole is used both for prophylaxis and treatment. The dose for prophylaxis is 3 mg/kg (maximum 400 mg) every 24 hours PO/IV and treatment is 6–12 mg/kg 24 hourly PO/IV. In GFR >50 mL/min/1.73 m^2, no dose adjustment needed. In GFR <50 mL/min/1.73 m^2, give one normal dose initially, followed by 50% of the dose subsequently.

Itraconazole

The dose of itraconazole recommended in children is 3–5 mg/kg/day. It is extensively metabolized in liver by CYP3A4 enzymes and are prone for multiple drug interactions. The IV formulation of the drug has a carrier—hydroxypropyl beta cyclodextrin, which accumulates in renal failure and is best avoided in children with GFR <50 mL/min/1.73 m^2.

Voriconazole

Voriconazole is structural analog of fluconazole but with wide spectrum of activity. It is extensively metabolized in the liver and almost all metabolites including the main circulating metabolite, voriconazole N-oxide is renally eliminated. In renal dysfunction, oral preparation does not need dose modification. Regarding IV preparation, there is accumulation of the carrier molecule; once GFR is <50 mL/min/1.73 m^2 and is better avoided.

Echinocandins

Echinocandins have potent fungicidal activity against yeasts, mostly *Candida* species. They are large molecules with poor bioavailability and are only available for parenteral administration. Caspofungin and micafungin are the echinocandins available for pediatric use. They are highly protein bound (92–99%), and have long half-lives in plasma of up to 24–72 hours.

Caspofungin

Caspofungin undergoes spontaneous degradation and further metabolism involves peptide hydrolysis and N-acetylation in the liver. Clearance and volume of distribution of caspofungin are closely related to body surface area (BSA) than weight and dosing is based on BSA.

- *Infants up to 3 months:* 25 mg/m^2 24 hourly
- *3 months to 1 year:* 50 mg/m^2 24 hourly
- *Children 1–18 years:* 70 mg/m^2 as a loading dose followed by 50 mg/m^2 for maintenance 24 hourly
- No dose adjustment is needed in renal failure for both caspofungin and micafungin.

Griseofulvin

Griseofulvin is a fungistatic antifungal with good activity against organisms that cause dermatophyte infections. The dose ranges from 5 to 15 mg/kg/day divided in q 12 hourly doses, not to exceed 750 mg/day. No dose adjustment is needed in renal dysfunction.

TABLE 24.12.5: Dose modification for cidofovir, ganciclovir, valganciclovir, and valacyclovir.

Drug	GFR >55 mL/min/1.73 m^2	GFR 10–55 mL/min/1.73 m^2	GFR <10 mL/min/1.73 m^2
Cidofovir	• 5 mg/kg IV once per week for 2 weeks (induction) • 5 mg/kg IV every 2 weeks (maintenance)	• 1 mg/kg IV 3 times per week for 2 weeks (induction) • 1 mg/kg IV every 2 weeks (maintenance)	• 0.5 mg/kg IV once per week for 2 weeks (induction) • 0.5 mg/kg IV every 2 weeks (maintenance)
	GFR 30–50 mL/min/1.73 m^2	**GFR 10–30 mL/min/1.73 m^2**	**GFR <10 mL/min/1.73 m^2**
Ganciclovir	• IV induction 2.5 mg/kg dose q 24 h • 1.25 mg/kg dose q 24 h (maintenance)	IV induction 1.25 mg/kg dose q 24 h 0.625 mg/kg dose q 24 h (maintenance)	• IV induction 1.25 mg/kg dose 3 ×/week • 0.625 mg/kg dose 3 ×/week (maintenance)
Valganciclovir	20 mg/kg/dose q 8 h	30 mg/kg dose q 12 h	30 mg/kg dose q 24 h
Valacyclovir	1 g every 12 hours	1 g every 24 hours	500 mg every 24 hours

(GFR: glomerular filtration rate; IV: intravenous)

ANTIVIRALS

Oseltamivir

Oseltamivir is predominantly eliminated by kidney after conversion to an active metabolite oseltamivir carboxylate. Dose adjustment is indicated in renal impairment. In GFR 30–60 mL/min/1.73 m^2, give 40% of normal dose twice daily for treatment and once daily for prophylaxis. If GFR is between 10 and 30 mL/min/1.73 m^2, give 40% of normal dose once daily for treatment and 48 hourly for prophylaxis. In GFR <10 mL/min/1.73 m^2, it is better to avoid the use of the drug.

Acyclovir

Acyclovir is cleared by kidneys predominantly. Around 75–80% of acyclovir is excreted unchanged in the urine through glomerular filtration and tubular secretion. If GFR is above 50 mL/min/1.73 m^2, no dose adjustment is needed. If GFR is between 25 and 50 mL/min/1.73 m^2, normal dose IV every 12 hours; if GFR is between 10 and 25 mL/min/1.73 m^2, normal dose IV every 24 hours; and if GFR is <10 mL/min/1.73 m^2, half the normal dose has to be administered every 24 hours.

Cidofovir, Ganciclovir, Valganciclovir, and Valacyclovir[5]

The major route of elimination of cidofovir is renal excretion and dose-dependent nephrotoxicity is the most common adverse effect. Ganciclovir also has nephrotoxicity, but less than cidofovir and myelosuppression is the major adverse effect. It is used both for cytomegalovirus (CMV) prophylaxis and treatment. Valacyclovir is used for treating *herpes* infections. Valganciclovir is the oral prodrug of ganciclovir. The dose for CMV prophylaxis for ganciclovir is calculated by the formula:

$$3 \times BSA \times GFR$$

and for valganciclovir by the formula:

$$7 \times BSA \times GFR$$

The dose is in milligram and has to be given on daily basis. The dose adjustments for above drugs are given in **Table 24.11.5**.

Antiretroviral Drugs

Nevirapine and abacavir do not need any dose modification in renal impairment. Zidovudine does not need modification above GFR of 10 mL/min/1.73 m^2. Half the normal dose is given 8 hourly if GFR is <10 mL/min/1.73 m^2. Lamivudine needs dose modification below GFR of 30 mL/min. If GFR is between 15 and 30 mL/min/1.73 m^2, 150 mg stat dose is given followed by 100 mg/day. If GFR is <15 mL/min/1.73 m^2, 150 mg stat dose is given followed by 50 mg/day.

CONCLUSION

Renal impairment is common among sick children and warrants close monitoring of drug use, both to avoid adverse effects and at the same time to ensure therapeutic efficacy.

REFERENCES

1. British National Formulary for Children 2019-2020. London: BMJ Group; Pharmaceutical Press; 2020. pp 422-3.
2. Phadke KD, Goodyer P, Bitzan M. Manual of Pediatric Nephrology. Heidelberg: Springer; 2014.
3. Blair M, Côté JM, Cotter A, Lynch B, Redahan L, Murray PT. Nephrotoxicity from Vancomycin Combined with Piperacillin-Tazobactam: A Comprehensive Review. Am J Nephrol. 2021;52(2):85-97.
4. Booth R, Patey S. Pediatric Drug Dosage Adjustments in Patients with Renal Impairment or on Renal Replacement Therapies for use on the Intensive Care and Renal Units. London: Great Ormond Street Hospital for Children; NHS Trust; 2014.
5. Jorga K, Reigner B, Chavanne C, Alvaro G, Frey N. Pediatric Dosing of Ganciclovir and Valganciclovir: How Model-Based Simulations Can Prevent Underexposure and Potential Treatment Failure. CPT Pharmacometrics Syst Pharmacol. 2019;8(3):167-76.

24.12 Palliative Care in Children

Lulu Mathews

INTRODUCTION

Pediatric palliative care (PPC) includes the management of distressing symptoms, care at the end of life, and bereavement support. Palliative care (PC) can be introduced at any point throughout a child's life; it is completely individual. PC does not end with the child's death. It neither intentionally hastens nor postpones death. It is all about healing—*"You can't die cured, but you can die healed".* "To die healed" means being able to say or convey: "I love you, Forgive me, I forgive you, Thank you, Good-bye". PC is often said to be "low technology and high touch". It seeks to ensure that compassion and science are both acting side by side in patient care. Accordingly, expensive investigations and treatments are used only when their benefits clearly outweigh any potential burdens.[1]

CASE SCENARIOS

Case 1: Ayub, a 10-year-old boy, presented with pain all over the body and bleeding manifestations. He had undergone several investigations in a tertiary hospital and was diagnosed as acute leukemia. Most of these procedures were very painful which made him very irritable and angry. After the induction of remission for leukemia, he was sent home and was advised to come back regularly for the chemotherapy schedule. But he did not return for his first review. When the family was contacted by the hospital authorities, his mother replied that the family was seeking treatment from a local quack. They decided not to continue treatment because they felt that Ayub had deteriorated following chemotherapy. One month later when they were contacted again, they told us that Ayub was no more.

Case 2: Babu, a 10-year-old boy, was diagnosed with acute leukemia and was referred from another hospital which had a palliative care unit (PCU). As per the advice of PCU, all the investigations were done according to a "procedural pain protocol". Once the diagnosis was confirmed, the patient and family were referred to the hospital PCU, where at a family counseling session, the diagnosis of acute leukemia was broken to the family. The counselor had a session with Babu as well, wherein he also was informed of the diagnosis after confirming that Babu was keen to know the diagnosis. The family continued to get chemotherapy from the oncology unit. He was given treatment for the symptoms which he developed as side effects of drugs used for chemotherapy including nausea, vomiting, and constipation as well as other symptoms due to the disease process like pain, bleeding, and breathlessness. He was given round-the-clock morphine and pain relievers as a result of which his pain was under check. Thus, he was quite comfortable and was also sent home after induction of remission. He was very regular in his follow-up and completed his chemotherapy protocol; investigations were repeated and he was declared as disease-free. Babu continued to visit his treating oncologist at intervals as suggested by the treating team. Meanwhile, the PCU also had a session with his younger siblings. Since the attention of parents was totally on Babu, his youngest sibling had developed sibling rivalry. Babu was linked to the nearest PCU from where he was getting symptomatic treatment for all his needs. Whenever the need arose, he was referred to the treating oncologist at the tertiary center.

After having read these two clinical scenarios, you would note the difference with which both children were treated and the difference in end result. In the first case, the treating team tried their level best to cure his illness, but his felt needs were not considered. His family resorted to further treatment from a quack and he succumbed to the disease within weeks. But in the second case, the investigations were done without inflicting pain, and all his symptoms were managed. The child and his family were properly counseled; he was linked to the nearest PCU, his siblings were taken care of, and most importantly he was declared disease-free.

DEFINITION OF PALLIATIVE CARE

It can be seen that almost all the components of PC have been covered in the care given to Babu when we look at the definition of PPC **(Box 24.12.1)**.[2]

DIFFERENCES FROM CONVENTIONAL TREATMENT

Let us see how PC is different from conventional medical treatment **(Table 24.12.1)**.

STATUS OF PALLIATIVE CARE IN INDIA

In spite of PC offering what is needed for the patient and family, reality regarding its coverage of the population is rather distressing in India but not in Kerala. There are obstacles to

BOX 24.12.1: WHO definition of pediatric palliative care.[2]

- Palliative care for children is the active total care of the child's body, mind, and spirit and also involves giving support to the family
- It begins when illness is diagnosed and continues regardless of whether or not a child receives treatment directed at the disease
- Health providers must evaluate and alleviate a child's physical, psychological, and social distress
- Effective palliative care requires a broad multidisciplinary approach that includes the family and makes use of available community resources; it can be successfully implemented even if resources are limited
- It can be provided in tertiary care facilities, in community health centers, and even in children's homes

TABLE 24.12.1: Differences between conventional and palliative medicine.

Feature	*Conventional medicine*	*Palliative medicine*
Ethos	Military virtue of fighting, not giving up, endurance hardness	• Human dignity as its central value • Solidarity between the patient and the caregiver
Who is in control?	Physician is the "General"	Patient is the "Sovereign"
Power rests with	Physician is all powerful	Physician aware of his/her powerlessness
Aim	Curing	Healing
What is "Disease"?	Disease as a problem to be solved	An experience to be lived
What is "Death"?	A failure of treatment	An inevitable reality
At death	"Don't stand back, just do something"	"Don't just do something, stand back"

the development of PC in India. Though PC is developing in India since the mid-1980s, still only 1–2% of the population have access to PC. In the case of PPC, the coverage is very meagre. The coverage of PC is much better in Kerala where more than 65% get PC. Even now, healthcare professionals equate PC with "terminal care". In the case of parents, they do not want to even think about their child's death. Hence, they are not fond of attending a PCU. Moreover, all the good centers for children's PC are attached to major hospitals like medical colleges or regional cancer centers.

NEED FOR PALLIATIVE CARE FOR CHILDREN

There are several diseases in children where PC is required. Everyone is under the impression that only kids with malignancy need PC, but the truth is that all children with life-limiting illness (LLI) need to come under the umbrella of PC. Some of the chronic illnesses which are common in India, apart from malignancies, are chronic neurological conditions like static and progressive encephalopathy, degenerative neurological diseases, postmeningitic or encephalitic sequelae, chronic hematological diseases like hemolytic diseases, hemophilia, sickle cell disease, operated and inoperable congenital heart diseases, chronic kidney disease, children with HIV/AIDS, diabetes mellitus, congenital surgical conditions like myelomeningocele, and kids with chromosomal anomalies.

Palliative care should be initiated at the diagnosis of a LLI as in the case of Babu in the given scenario. One should not wait till the disease condition reaches a stage when cure is not possible **(Fig. 24.12.1)**. You would have noted that all the symptoms which Babu developed were very well taken care of, thereby improving the quality of his life during the course of treatment. PC does not end with the death of a kid; it extends beyond the death as support to the family members in the form of bereavement care. Unfortunately, people still equate PC with terminal care. Both are not synonymous, but terminal care is a part of PC **(Fig. 24.12.1)**.[1]

Kids can develop several symptoms during the treatment of the LLI, the more common symptoms being pain and gastrointestinal and respiratory symptoms. Pain is the most common symptom to be palliated in any PC clinic. It is quite distressing to note that pain in kids is not evaluated and mostly mismanaged. Hence, very few kids are referred to a PC clinic for pain management.

PAIN MANAGEMENT IN PEDIATRIC PALLIATIVE CARE

Since pain is the most common symptom to be palliated, we shall take a peep into pain management in kids with chronic pain. Pain is a dynamic process and as Margo McCaffery says: "It's whatever the experiencing person says it is, existing whenever and wherever the person says it does."[3] Robert Twycross has made it even simpler, "it is what the patient says hurts him/her."[4] It is an unpleasant sensory and emotional experience associated with actual or potential tissue damage. Just because one cannot see the cause of pain in the child, one should not think that the child has no pain. Pain would be the most unwanted thing in the world as far

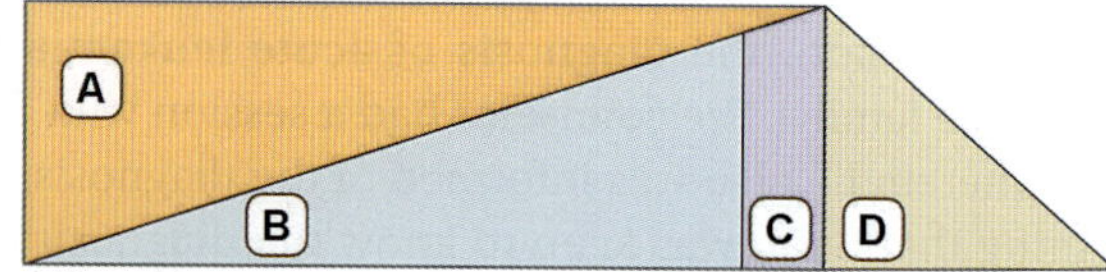

Fig. 24.12.1: Various stages of life-limiting illness. A: Disease-modifying care; B: Palliative care; C: Terminal care; and D: Bereavement care.

as a child is concerned. It is one of the most common and distressing symptoms in cancer patients, occurring in 50–90% of patients with advanced malignancies and 60% of the patients with nonmalignant diseases.[5] We have a duty to treat pain properly **(Box 24.12.2)**.

Concept of Total Pain

Pain is a very subjective phenomenon. Hence, we say pain is what the patient says hurts him/her. So we come to the concept of "total pain" **(Fig. 24.12.2)**.

Case Scenario

Let us go back to our first patient Ayub. He had pain all over the body and also pain inflicted by the various procedures and investigations. This constitutes the *physical component* of pain. He/she is very much depressed by his/her illness is upset emotionally, and refuses to meet his/her friends—this constitutes the *psychological component*. Since the onset of his/her illness, he/she feels that he/she is socially isolated; nobody is open with him/her. This constitutes the *social component*. He/she is an adolescent having doubts like "why has he/she developed such an illness?", "Is he/she being punished by God for not having followed the religious practices regularly?", and "Will he/she be forgiven for his/her misdeeds?". This constitutes the *spiritual component*. The concept of total pain is a way to describe the multidimensional suffering of people with serious illnesses, death, and dying. It was introduced in the early 1960s by Dame Cicely Saunders, an English doctor, nurse, and social worker who founded the modern hospice movement.

BOX 24.12.2: Basic principles of pain management in palliative care.

- Over 80% of the chronic pain can be controlled with inexpensive oral drugs
- Needs proper assessment and systematic use of analgesics
- Access to pain management is a fundamental right!

PRINCIPLES OF MANAGEMENT OF PAIN

Box 24.12.3 describes the basic principles of management of pain.

Start by conveying empathy and with your face and body language, convey, "I care for you". Say what you see: "You seem to be in a lot of pain".

WHO 1986 Guidelines For Pain Management, Revised In 2019[6]

The three main principles of the WHO analgesic ladder are: "By the clock, by the mouth, by the ladder."

1. *By the clock:* Subsequent doses are given before the earlier dose has stopped acting. Persistent pain needs round-the-clock medication. "As and when needed medication" alone is irrational. We should have a good idea regarding the duration of action of common drugs used for pain management **(Table 24.12.2)**.
2. *By the mouth:* The oral route is usually the preferred route for ease of use. However, it may not be possible for all patients (e.g., end-of-life, unconscious, and swallowing issues). When the oral route is not feasible, the least invasive route should be considered (e.g., sublingual or subcutaneous before intravenous). The intramuscular route should never be used.
3. *By the ladder:* When pain occurs, there should be prompt administration of drugs. Drug selection should be appropriate to the severity of the pain **(Fig. 24.12.3)**. The ladder in pediatric pain management has 2 steps.[7] *Step 1* is mild-to-moderate pain and *Step 2* is moderate-to-severe pain. It may be most appropriate with severe

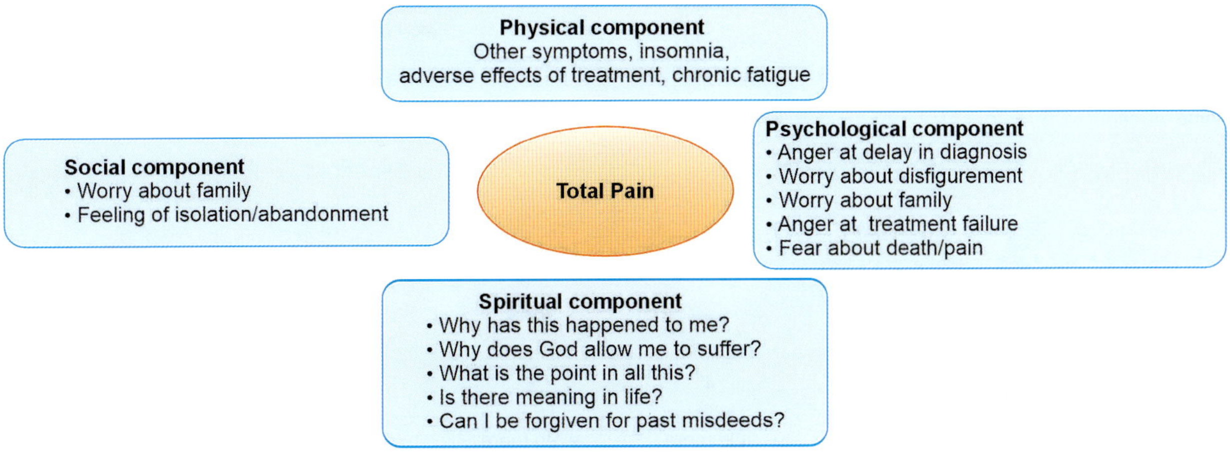

Fig. 24.12.2: Concept of total pain.

pain to begin at the top of the ladder; it is not always necessary to start at *Step 1*. When pain is controlled, the patient should be maintained on the dose that is effective. Along any step in the ladder, additional drugs, "adjuvants", may be used. This two-step approach is inexpensive and 80–90% effective when optimally utilized.

How to Assess Severity of Pain?

There are various tools which can be used in different age groups like FACES Scale, Numeric Rating Scale (NRS), Behavioral Scale, and Visual Analog Scale (VAS). *The Wong-Baker FACES® Pain Rating Scale* **(Fig. 24.12.4)** was created by Donna Wong and Connie Baker in 1983 to help children effectively communicate about their pain. Once practitioners clearly understand the child's pain, they can develop a quality treatment.

BOX 24.12.3: Basic principles of management of pain.

- The earlier the pain is treated, the lesser will be the self-perpetuating changes
- Continuous pain warrants continuous analgesia
- Pain is experienced by people and families and not merely by nerve endings
- Hence need for multimodal and customized therapy in chronic pain
- Importance of proper communication

TABLE 24.12.2: Duration of action, dose, and frequency of common drugs used for pain management.

Drug	*Duration of action (in hours)*	*Dose (mg/kg)*	*Frequency*
Paracetamol	4–6	10–15	4–6 hourly
Ibuprofen	6–8	10	6–8 hourly
Naproxen	8	5	8–12 hourly
Tramadol	6–8	1–2	6–8 hourly
Codeine	4	0.5–1	4 hourly
Morphine	4	0.2	4 hourly

How to Use This Scale?

Explain to the child that each face is for a child who feels happy because he/she has no pain (hurt) or sad because he/she has some or a lot of pain. Face 0 is very happy because he/she does not hurt at all. Face 1 hurts just a little bit. Face 2 hurts a little more and so on. Ask the child to point to the face which belongs to him/her. Here the child internalizes his/her pain and points to a face which gives the numerical value. Once the numerical value is obtained, pain is graded as no pain, mild (1–4), moderate (5–7), and severe (8–10).

If a kid has mild pain, Step 1 drugs are used, i.e., nonopioids [nonsteroidal anti-inflammatory drugs (NSAIDs) and paracetamol]. Use the NSAID you are most comfortable prescribing. *Never prescribe multiple NSAIDs!* Ibuprofen is the most commonly used NSAID in kids for pain management. Paracetamol 1 g qid is equi-analgesic with Diclofenac 50 mg bd. Whenever NSAID is prescribed, one has to start the child on a proton-pump inhibitor (PPI).

If a child has moderate-to-severe pain, he/she should be started on strong opioids, the most commonly used strong opioid being morphine. 60–90% of children with life-limiting or life-threatening diseases undergoing PC receive opioids at the end of life. Morphine remains the gold standard starting opioid for pain relief in PPC.[8]

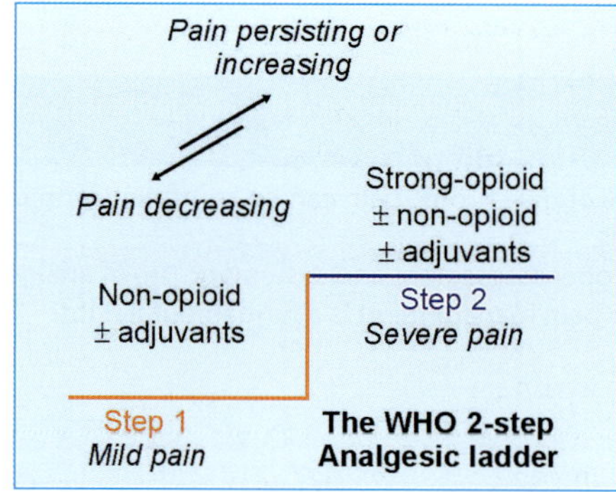

[Non-opioids = acetaminophen (paracetamol); ibuprofen]

Fig. 24.12.3: Drug selection for pain management.

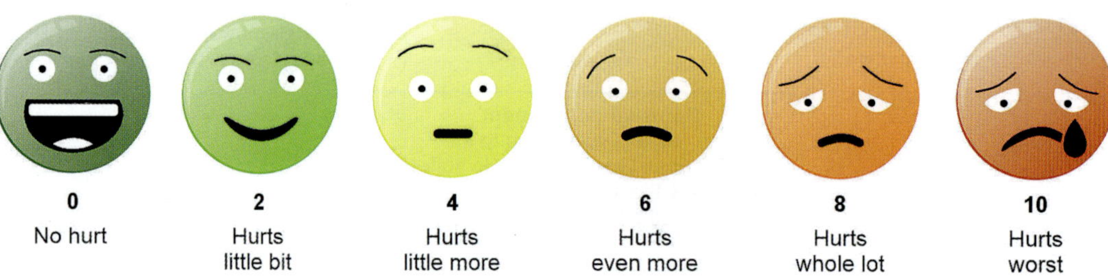

Fig. 24.12.4: Wong-Baker FACES® Pain Rating Scale.

How to Start on Morphine?

- Start with a dose of 0.2 mg/kg Q4h and SOS. 4-hourly dosage, double the dose at bed time. If the child is 10 kg, start on 2 mg Q4h and SOS.
- If the child has breakthrough pain (BTP), i.e., pain in spite of the 4 hourly dose, the same regular, i.e., 2 mg dose, is given as SOS. The dose has to be titrated depending on the degree of pain relief.
- How to follow up on review? On follow-up, the mother tells that the kid had to be given 6 extra doses. So the kid has had a total of 12 doses of 2 mg, i.e., total 24 mg in 24 hours. This should be divided into 6 doses, i.e., 4 mg Q4h and SOS.
- Whenever morphine is started, the child should be started on a stimulant laxative like bisacodyl because morphine induces constipation. The laxative should be continued as long as he/she is on morphine. Another side effect of morphine is emesis, so antiemetic like metoclopramide or haloperidol should be given for the first 2–3 days. After the first 2–3 days, emesis no longer occurs.
- One need not fear to use morphine in kids. There is no maximum dose of morphine
- The dose can be increased depending on the severity of pain. There is no ceiling effect for morphine. *Pain is the physiological antagonist to the central side effects of morphine.*
- Respiratory depression is not a clinical problem because blood level rises slowly on oral therapy. Drowsiness and delirium prevent further intake of drug.
- If used properly in doses adequate for pain relief, chances of addiction are very remote! Initiation of an opioid analgesic should not be delayed by concern over a theoretical likelihood of psychological dependence.[8] There are many myths related to pain and use of morphine in children. It is our duty to dispel these myths and disseminate the facts **(Table 24.12.3)**.
- Morphine and metabolites are excreted by kidneys. So, in renal failure, morphine accumulates and causes toxicity. Depending on the degree of renal failure, the frequency of morphine administration is decreased like Q6h, Q8h, or Q12h.

Why Weak Opioids are not Used in Children?

Commonly used weak opioids in adults are tramadol and codeine. But these are not used in children. Codeine is 1/10th as potent as morphine; that is, 10 mg codeine is converted in the body to 1 mg morphine. But this conversion may not always occur in all children. Moreover, codeine induces severe constipation and hence not used in PPC. Tramadol can lower seizure threshold and is another reason for not commonly using in kids.

TABLE 24.12.3: Myths and facts about pain management with morphine.

Myths	*Facts*
Children and infants do not really feel much pain	Children are more sensitive to pain than adults
Young children have no memory of pain and it has no lasting effect	Pain and distress can endure in even the tiny child's memory
Exposing children to opioid medications will run the risk of drug addiction	Children are at no more risk of becoming addicted to opioids than adults
Children cannot decide their own level of analgesia	Children can indicate how much of morphine they need
If children are in pain, they will tell you and probably overexaggerate	Children are better able to hide their pain than to fake it
We medical professionals are good at assessing childhood pain	Medical professionals consistently and significantly under-rate children's pain

Other Measures in Pain Management

If a child has bone metastases in addition to the above approach, radiotherapy and bisphosphonates may be useful for pain due to bone metastases.[8]

Radiation therapy (RT) is often used as a palliative treatment for children with recurrent malignant disease to ameliorate or prevent symptoms in bone, brain, liver, lung, abdominopelvic and head-and-neck metastases, spinal cord compression, superior vena cava syndrome, and bleeding.[8]

Nonpharmacologic Management

Nonpharmacologic alternatives like ice or heat application, pacifiers, breastfeeding, comforting by parents, bubbles, and videos should be considered the first line for pediatric pain management, especially in the emergency department. These agents are very safe and may act as an effective bridge to pharmacologic treatment options. Nonpharmacologic alternatives can be broken down into two categories: Physical comfort measures and distracting activities. Whereas physical comfort measures are most effective in neonates and younger children, distraction is typically employed in older children and adolescents.[8]

Myths and Facts about Pain Management with Morphine

As a first step to develop CPC, one has to dispel the myths regarding morphine and disseminate the facts **(Table 24.12.3)**. Secondly, believe the children and believe what they have to say.

CONCLUSION

To summarize, PPC is:

- Child-centered rather than disease-focused
- Death-accepting but life-enhancing
- Concerned with healing rather than curing
- Partnership between patient and caregivers

Our aim is to add life to a child's years, not simply add years to a child's life.

REFERENCES

1. Twycross R. Introducing Palliative Care, 3rd edition. 6th Economy Reprint; Part 1. Padstow, Cornwall: TJ International Ltd.; 2003.
2. World Health Organization. Palliative care for children. [online] Available from https://www.who.int/europe/news-room/fact-sheets/item/palliative-care-for-children. [Last accessed December, 2024].
3. Rosdahl CB, Kowalski, MT. Textbook of Basic Nursing, 9th edition. Philadelphia: Lippincott Williams & Wilkins; 2008.
4. Twycross R. Introducing Palliative Care, 3rd edition. Part 3, Symptom management. Padstow, Cornwall: TJ International Ltd.; 2003.
5. Hui D, Abdelghani E, Chen J, Dibaj S, Zhukovsky D, Dev R, et al. Chronic Non-Malignant Pain in Patients with Cancer Seen at a Timely Outpatient Palliative Care Clinic. Cancers (Basel). 2020;12(1):214.
6. World Health Organization. WHO revision of pain management guidelines. [online] Available from https://www.who.int/news/item/27-08-2019-who-revision-of-pain-management-guidelines [Last accessed December, 2024].
7. World Health Organization. Guidelines on the management of chronic pain in children. [online] Available from https://www.who.int/publications/i/item/9789240017870 [Last accessed December, 2024].
8. Unni JC. Pain management in palliative care. Indian J Pract Pediatr. 2022;24(2):212-7.

24.13 Drugs Licensed for Use in Neonates, Children, and Adolescents

Jeeson C Unni, PSN Menon

A

Abacavir

Human immunodeficiency virus (HIV) infection: In combination with at least two other antiretroviral medicines: by mouth (PO), *adolescent:* 300 mg twice daily (bid); *3 months (mo) to 16 years (yr):* 8 mg/kg bid (maximum [max.]. 600 mg daily). For adolescents, the initiation of antiretroviral therapy (ART) is recommended in any patient with a history of an acquired immunodeficiency syndrome (AIDS)-defining infection; with a CD4 count of <350/mm^3; who has HIV-associated nephropathy; or who is being treated for hepatitis B (HBV) infection.

Abciximab

0.25 mg/kg intravenous (IV) bolus, followed by 0.125 µg/kg/min infusion for 12 hours (hr). Platelet counts and coagulation time must be monitored.

Acetazolamide

Epilepsy: as adjunct. Starting dose: *up to 12 yr:* 2.5 mg/kg; *12–18 yr*: 250 mg 2–3 times daily; increase every 4–5 days to maintenance dose of 5–7 mg/kg/dose 2–3 times daily up to 750 mg/day in <12-yr-olds and 1 g/day in 12–18-yr-olds. The IV bolus dose is 6–7 mg/kg 2–3 times daily in <12 yr and 250 mg 2–4 times in 12–18 yr.

Edema: PO or IV starting dose: *up to 12 yr:* 2.5 mg/kg; *12–18 yr:* 250 mg 2–3 times daily.

Raised intracranial pressure (ICP): PO/IV 8 mg/kg thrice daily (tid) and gradually increased.

Hydrocephalus due to communicating intraventricular hemorrhage (IVH): Neonates: 25 mg/kg/24 hr.

Glaucoma: PO/IV 5 mg/kg in *<12 yr;* 250 mg in *12–18 yr*; 2–4 times daily to a max. of 750 mg/day in *<12 yr* and 1 g/day in *12–18 yr.* If creatinine clearance is 10–20 mL/min/1.73 m^2, reduce to bid and if <10 avoid.

Acetylcysteine

Paracetamol poisoning: IV infusion – *Neonate:* initially 150 mg/kg over 1 hr, dose administered in 3 mL/kg glucose 5%; followed by 50 mg/kg over 4 hr, administered in 7 mL/kg glucose 5%; then 100 mg/kg over 16 hr, in 14 mL/kg glucose 5%.

Child (<20 kg): Initially 150 mg/kg over 1 hr, dose administered in 3 mL/kg glucose 5%; followed by 50 mg/kg over 4 hr, in 7 mL/kg glucose 5%; then 100 mg/kg over 16 hr, in 14 mL/kg glucose 5%.

Child (20–39 kg): Initially 150 mg/kg over 1 hr, dose administered in 100 mL glucose 5%; followed by 50 mg/kg over 4 hr, in 250 mL glucose 5%; then 100 mg/kg over 16 hr, in 500 mL glucose 5%.

Child (>40 kg): 150 mg/kg over 1 hr, dose administered in 200 mL glucose 5%; then 50 mg/kg over 4 hr, to be started immediately after completion of first infusion, dose to be administered in 500 mL glucose 5%; then 100 mg/kg over 16 hr, to be started immediately after completion of second infusion, dose to be administered in 1 L glucose 5%.

To avoid excessive dosage in obese patients, a ceiling weight of 110 kg should be used when calculating the dose for paracetamol overdosage.

Meconium ileus: Neonate: 20% injection 200–400 mg up to 3 times a day if required.

Treatment of distal intestinal obstructive syndrome: PO *1 mo to 1 year:* 0.4–3 g as a single dose; *2–6 year:* 2–3 g as a single dose; *7–17 yr:* 4–6 g as a single dose.

Prevention of distal intestinal obstruction syndrome: PO *1 mo to 1 year:* 100–200 mg tid; *2–11 yr:* 200 mg tid; *12–17 yr:* 200–400 mg tid.

Acitretin

Max. duration of continuous treatment is 6 mo. Given PO in *12–18-year-olds* at 500 µg as single dose daily. Occasionally up to 1 mg/kg needed (max. 35 mg daily for short periods).

Activated Charcoal

Dose related more to dose of poison (10 times weight of poison is given) than age/weight of the child. If the amount of toxin is unknown, either give as single dose within 1 hr of ingestion of poison or as multiple doses 4 hrly till toxicity abates or side effects of charcoal become evident—by weight 1 g/kg or by age 25–50 g in 2–12-year-olds.

Acyclovir

Herpes simplex virus 1 (HSV): *Herpes labialis with gingivostomatitis*: PO: *1 mo to 2 yr* 100 mg; 2–18 yr 200 mg 5 times daily for 7 days within 72 hr of onset.

Recurrent herpes labialis with gingivostomatitis: Adolescents: To shorten duration of episode 200–400 mg 5 times daily PO for 5 days.

Long-term prophylaxis for frequent or severe recurrences: 400 mg bid PO.

Herpetic kerato-conjunctivitis: 1 cm acyclovir ointment 5 times daily (continue for at least 3 days after complete healing) - drug of choice.

Prolonged systemic antiviral prophylaxis: For 1 year may help to prevent recurrent herpetic keratitis and amblyopia.

Herpes encephalitis: IV acyclovir infusion, neonate to *3 mo:* 20 mg/kg 8 hrly for 21 days; *3 mo–12 yr:* 250 mg/m^2 tid for 21 days. Double dose in immunocompromised.

Genital herpes: Adolescent: 400 mg tid; *child:* 10–20 mg/kg/dose qid × 7–10 days; extended if healing incomplete (topical - negligible clinical benefit).

Episodic therapy for recurrent genital herpes: Adolescent: 800 mg tid × 2 days (start within the first day of onset or in prodrome)

Herpes simplex prophylaxis in the immunocompromised: PO: *child 1 mo to 2 yr* 100–200 mg 4 times daily; *child 2–18 yr* 200–400 mg qid.

Herpes simplex suppression (suppressive therapy reduces frequency of recurrences by 70–80%): PO: *child 12–18 yr* 400 mg bid or 200 mg qid. Increased to 400 mg tid if recurrences occur on standard suppressive therapy or for suppression of genital herpes during late pregnancy (from 36 wks' gestation). Therapy interrupted every 6–12 mo to reassess recurrence frequency; consider restarting after two or more recurrences.

Chickenpox: Antiviral therapy modifies course in both varicella and Herpes zoster.

Neonates: Regardless of immune status/use of any immunoglobulins - give IV (risk of severe disease). PO not recommended as absorption is variable. *Healthy child: 1 mo to 12 yr:* no treatment. *Adolescent:* Treat within 24 hr.

Immunocompromised and those at special risk (severe CVS/respiratory disease/chronic skin disorder): 10 days with at least 7 days of parenteral treatment. Therapy should start within the first 24 hr.

Herpes zoster: Treatment with the antiviral should be started within 72 hr of the onset of rash and is usually continued for 7–10 days. PO: *1 mo to 2 yr:* 200 mg; *2–6 yr:* 400 mg; *6–12 yr:* 800 mg qid for 5 days; *12–18 yr:* 800 mg 5 times daily for 7 days. In the immunocompromised, continue for 2 days after crusting of lesions. IV infusion: *Neonate to 3 mo:* 10–20 mg/kg 8 hrly for at least 7 days; *3 mo to 12 yr:* 250 mg/m^2; *12–18 yr:* 500 mg/kg 8 hrly for 5 days. At all ages, double dose in encephalitis or immunocompromised (given for 10–14 days in encephalitis, possibly longer if also immunocompromised). To avoid excessive dose in obese, IV dose calculated on the basis of ideal weight for height.

Prophylaxis of chickenpox after delivery: IV infusion: *neonate* 10 mg/kg tid; continued until serological tests confirm absence of virus (VZ IgM).

Attenuation of chickenpox if VZ immunoglobulin not indicated: PO: *1 mo to 18 yr:* 10 mg/kg qid for 7 days starting 1 wk after exposure. IV infusion, reconstitute to 25 mg/mL with water for injection or normal saline (NS), then dilute to concentration of 5 mg/mL with NS or glucose saline and give over 1 hr; or use infusion pump and central line to administer the 25 mg/mL solution over 1 hr.

Dose adjustment in renal impairment: Glomerular filtration rate (GFR) 25–50 mL/min: normal dose IV every 12 hr; GFR 10–25 mL/min: GFR-normal dose IV every 24 hr; GFR < 10 mL/min: GFR-half the normal dose IV every 24 hr.

Dose adjustment on hemodialysis (HD): HD removes approximately 60% of a dose. Give half the normal dose IV every 24 hr after dialysis session.

Dose adjustment in peritoneal dialysis (PD): Not dialyzed. Give half the normal dose IV every 24 hr.

Dose adjustment on continuous veno-venous hemofiltration (CVVH): Filtered. Give normal dose IV every 24 hr. Increase to every 12 hr if severe infection e.g. herpes encephalitis.

Adalimumab
With methotrexate or alone if methotrexate is inappropriate. Subcutaneously (SC) in *child 13–17 yr:* 40 mg alternate week; review treatment if no response in 12 wks.

Adenosine
Up to 12 yr: 0.05 mg/kg IV push and then increase bolus doses by 0.05 mg/kg every 2 min till clinical response occurs or a max. dose of either 0.3 mg/kg or 12 mg. *12–18 yr:* 3 mg IV bolus, increase after 2 min to 6 mg and to 12 mg if supraventricular tachycardia (SVT) is not controlled after another 2 min.

Adrenaline Tartrate (Epinephrine)
Cardiac arrest or profound bradycardia, asystole, ventricular fibrillation, or pulseless electrical activity: IV: 10 µg/kg (0.01 mg/kg); initial dose; intraosseous: 10 µg/kg (0.01 mg/kg); endotracheal: 100 µg/kg (0.10 mg/kg). *Note:* 10 µg/kg = 0.1 mL/kg of 1:10,000 dilution. 100 µg/kg = 0.1 mL/kg of 1:1000 dilution. If administered through an endotracheal tube, follow the dose with saline flush or dilute in isotonic saline flush (1–5 mL) based on patient size. Subsequent doses given every 3–5 min IV: 100 µg/kg (0.1 mg/kg); intraosseous: 100 µg/kg (0.1 mg/kg); endotracheal: 100 µg/kg (0.1 mg/kg). For subsequent doses of epinephrine, a dosage up to 200 µg/kg (0.2 mg/kg) may be given.

Anaphylaxis: SC: 10 g/kg/dose (max. 3 doses); IV: 10 µg/kg/dose: 10 µg/kg = 0.01 mL/kg of 1:1,000 dilution or 0.1 mL/kg of a 1:10,000 dilution. Repeat the SC dose every 20 minutes while attempting IV access. *Note:* Some anaphylactic reactions, e.g. latex allergy, require large doses of epinephrine. A continuous infusion of epinephrine may be required.

Continued shock after volume resuscitation: IV infusion: 0.1–3.0 µg/kg/min. Start at the lowest dose and titrate for desired clinical effect. *Note:* Preparation of infusion solution: 0.6 mg × body weight (kg) diluted to 100 mL. Infuse at 1 mL/h = 0.1 µg/kg/min using a constant infusion pump. Extravasation can result in tissue necrosis injuries.

Status asthmaticus, bronchospasm: SC: 10 µg/kg/dose. 10 µg/kg = 0.01 mL/kg of 1:1,000 dilution. Max. single dose, 300 µg (0.3 mL of 1:1,000 dilution). *Note:* Repeat SC dose every 20 minutes if needed for clinical effect. Total of 3 doses.

Laryngotracheobronchitis: Racemic epinephrine, 2.25% inhalation solution. Dosage: *0–20 kg:* 0.25 mL in 2 mL with normal saline administered by nebulizer; *20–40 kg:* 0.50 mL in 2 mL with normal saline administered by nebulizer; *>40 kg:* 0.75 mL in 2 mL with normal saline administered by nebulizer.

Note: L-Epinephrine: An equal volume of 1% L-epinephrine (1:100) is approximately equivalent in biologic activity to 2.25% racemic epinephrine; one can be substituted for the other in equal volumes for inhalation. Alternatively, 5 mL of 1:1,000 L-epinephrine is equivalent to 0.5 mL of 1:100.

Adrenocorticotropic Hormone (ACTH, Corticotropin)
IM/SC: 1 mo to 18 yr 20–80 units once daily (OD). Duration and frequency of doses depend on the individual child.

Agalsidase Beta
IV: 16–18 yr, 1 mg/kg once in 2 wk.

Albendazole
Whipworm, trichuriasis, pinworm, threadworm, hookworm, roundworm, and ascariasis: <2 yr: 200 mg, *>2 yr:* 400 mg. Single dose. All family members must be treated along with the child and the dose must be repeated after 2–3 wk for all family members and the child for pinworm and threadworm.

Ankylostomiasis: 400 mg single dose.

Strongyloidosis (Strongyloides stercoralis): 2–12 yr: 400 mg OD for 3 days. May repeat after 3 wk if necessary. 400 mg bid for 3 days, repeated after 3 wk. More effective than mebendazole.

Enterobiasis: 100–200 mg single dose, repeated after 4 wk.

Trichinosis: 2–12 yr: 400 mg OD for 5 days. Repeat if necessary.

Tapeworm: 400 mg OD for 3 days.

Neurocysticercosis: Albendazole is used in dose of 15 mg/kg for 3–4 wk. A short course of 8 days is also found to be effective depending upon the location of cyst. 7.5 mg/kg up to max. of 400 mg bid for 14–28 days. Take with food. Repeat if necessary. Under steroid and anticonvulsant and in readiness for shunting for raised ICP.

Hydatid disease, echinococcosis: 15 mg/kg daily for 4 wk. In hydatid disease, a large dose of mebendazole is required

(400–600 mg 3 times a day for 21–30 days). This large dose may cause bone marrow aplasia, and hence albendazole is preferred drug nowadays for hydatid disease. Repeat the dose after 14 days, if required for the next such three doses.

Cutaneous larva migrans: <2 yr: 10 mg/kg bid for 5 days; *2–12 yr:* 400 mg daily once for 5 days.

Toxocariasis: 2–12 yr: 10 mg/kg up to max. of 400 mg; *12–18 yr:* 400 mg bid for 5 days. Steroid cover in symptomatic cases, especially if there is ocular involvement. Albendazole 400 mg bid for 5 days is also used for all the ages. Therapy may be adjunct with corticosteroid if inflammatory symptoms occur with ocular involvement.

Filariasis: It has adjuvant value to DEC or ivermectin in lymphatic filariasis. A single dose in combination has been used in mass programs.

Alemtuzumab
No standard dosage schedules in children are available on pediatric formularies and BNF for children advices to consult local treatment protocols for details. One study used initial infusions with a low dose of 0.06 mg/kg, max. 3 mg; increased over 5 days.

Alendronate
Experience of the use of bisphosphonates in children is limited and expert advice should be sought. 5 mg/day or 35 mg/wk for *<30 kg,* 10 mg/day or 70 mg/wk for *>30 kg;* mean dosage: 0.37 ± 0.069 mg/kg/day.

Alfacalcidol (1 alpha-hydroxycholecalciferol)
Indices of response: Plasma calcium, alkaline phosphatase, parathyroid hormone (PTH), as well as radiological and histological investigations. Monitor carefully for hypercalcemia. In renal bone disease, maintain PTH level at or slightly above the normal range. Oversuppression can result in adynamic bone disease.

Hypophosphatemic rickets: Up to 2 yr and <20 kg: 25–50 ng/kg; *>20 kg* 1 μg IV/PO OD.

Neonatal hypocalcemia: 50–100 ng/kg PO/IV. Up to 2 μg/kg in severe cases. 100 ng/kg/day for prophylaxis in premature.

Prophylaxis of vitamin D deficiency in renal failure: Up to 2 yr and <20 kg: 15–30 ng/kg and *>20 kg* 250–500 ng daily once PO/IV.

Alfentanil
It is used only by a trained anesthetist/interventionist as assisted ventilation is required. Initially 20–50 μg/kg followed by 15 μg/kg both as IV bolus over 30 sec. Alternatively, loading dose 50–100 μg/kg IV over 10 min followed by IV infusion at 500 ng–1 μg/kg/min.

Alginate
Give infants sachets with or after feeds*; <4.5 kg:* sachet; *>4.5 kg* 1 sachet. *>2 yr* give liquid or tablet after meals and at bedtime, *2–12 yr* 1 tab or 5–10 mL liquid and *12–18 yr* 2 tabs or 10–20 mL liquid.

Alglucosidase Alfa
Pompe disease (specialist use only): IV infusion – *Neonate:* 20 mg/kg every 2 wk. *Child:* 20 mg/kg every 2 wk.

Alimemazine Tartrate (Trimeprazine Tartrate)
Urticaria and/or pruritis: PO: *6 mo to 2 yr:* 250 μg/kg (max. 2.5 mg) 3–4 times daily; *2–5 yr:* 2.5 mg 3–4 times daily; *5–12 yr:* 5 mg 3–4 times daily; *12–18 yr:* 10 mg 2–3 times daily, in severe cases up to max. 100 mg daily.

Premedication: PO *2–7 yr:* up to 2 mg/kg 1–2 hr before procedure.

Allopurinol
Hyperuricemia due to tumor lysis syndrome: IV/PO 100 mg/m^2 tid to be commenced 24 hr before starting cytotoxic drugs.

Glycogen storage disease (GSD) and methylmalonic acidemia (MMA): 10–15 mg/kg (max. 400 g) as a single daily dose if serum uric acid > 0.36 mmol/L.

Phosphoribosylpyrophosphate (PRPP) synthetase superactivity and Lesch–Nyhan syndrome: 10–20 mg/kg (max. 400 mg) OD at minimum dose to maintain normal uric acid levels.

Adenine phosphoribosyltransferase (APRT) deficiency: 10 mg/kg (max. 400 mg).

Alprazolam
Anxiety: PO *for 12–18-year-olds:* 200–500 μg tid [max. 4 mg/day in div. (div.) doses] – use minimum effective dose.

Panic disorder: PO *for 12–18-year-olds:* 500 μg tid, increase once in 4 days to max. of 10 mg/day in div. doses.

Aluminum Chloride
Hyperhidrosis: Apply 1–2 mL of aluminum chloride hexahydrate in the affected areas (armpits, palms, and legs) only at night. This can be washed off in the morning. This has to be applied initially for every night in the first week and once the sweating comes down this can be brought down to thrice weekly and then to twice weekly and weekly. Eventually, the patient can be maintained with a weekly dosage.

Bromhidrosis and prevention of tenia pedis: Apply powder to the dry affected skin areas.

Aluminum Hydroxide
Antacid: 4% w/w *6–12 yr:* 5 mL tid; *12–18 yr:* 5–10 mL qid and as required between meals and at bedtime.

Hyperphosphatemia: PO: *1 mo to 1 year:* 2.5–5 mL 3–4 times daily; *1–5 yr:* 5–10 mL 3–4 times daily; *5–12 yr:* 10–20 mL 3–4 times daily; dose may be increased or decreased as required within the ranges given. *12–18 yr:* Tab 840 mg 1–3 tabs 4–5 times daily.

Amikacin

Many dose regimens exist depending on target concentration aimed for and patient groups treated. The doses mentioned are accepted initial doses and dose adjustments done depending on serum levels.

Newborn: Loading dose of 10 mg/kg, then 7.5 mg/kg every 12 hr IV; *<35 wk up to 14 days:* 10 mg/kg OD and *>14 days:* 10 mg/kg loading dose followed by 7.5 mg/kg/dose bid; *>35 wk <14 days:* 15 mg/kg as single dose daily and *>14 days:* 10 mg/kg loading dose followed by 7.5 mg/kg/dose bd. Extended interval dose regimen by slow IV injection or IV infusion: 15 mg/kg every 24 hr.

Children (1 mo to 18 yr): IV/IM 7.5 mg/kg/dose bid up to max. of 500 mg/dose.

Child >12 yr with life-threatening infection: 1.5 g/day in 3 div. doses for up to 10 days may be given. Aim for 1 hr post dose (peak) of 15–30 mg/L.

Once-daily (OD) dose regimen (not for endocarditis or meningitis): Child 1 mo to 18 yr: initially 15 mg/kg and then adjusted according to serum amikacin concentration.

Dose in multidrug-resistant tuberculosis: Single daily dose of 15 mg/kg by IM injection five times weekly.

Dose adjustment in renal impairment/on HD, PD, and continuous veno-venous hemofiltration (CVVH): Give 10 mg/kg IV, take trough level after 24 hr, and hold dose until the trough level is available. Adjust dosage interval according to serum levels - aim to keep trough at <10 mg/L and peak between 20 and 30 mg/L.

Amiloride

Prophylaxis of drug-induced hypokalemia: <12 yr: PO 100–200 μg/kg and *>12 yr:* 5–10 mg bid.

Nephrogenic diabetes insipidus along with hydrochlorothiazide 100 μg/kg tid.

Aminophylline

Bronchial asthma (severe in a theophylline-untreated child) and bronchospasm of anaphylaxis: IV loading dose of 5 mg/kg (max. 500 mg) over 20–30 min if no theophylline is given in prior 24 hr followed by IV infusion at 0.5 mg/kg/hr in *6 wk to 6 mo,* 0.7 mg/kg/hr in *6 mo to 1 yr,* 1 mg/kg/hr in *1–12 yr* and 0.7 mg/kg/hr in *>12 yr.*

Chronic asthma: PO dose of 6 mg/kg for 1 wk and then 12 mg/kg, for *3–12 yr,* 100–200 mg initially and then 200–450 mg in *>12 yr* given bid.

To avoid excessive dosage in obese patients, the dose should be calculated on the basis of ideal weight for height.

Amiodarone Hydrochloride

Loading dose of 5 mg/kg PO (max. 200 mg) 2–3 times daily for 5 days followed by maintenance dose of 5 mg/kg (max. 200 mg) OD. IV loading dose of 5 mg/kg (in rare cases up to max. of 15 mg/kg may be given) slowly over 30 min followed by maintenance continuous infusion at 5–15 μg/kg/min (max. 1.2 g in 24 hr). Central line preferred.

In cardiopulmonary resuscitation (CPR) for shock-resistant ventricular fibrillation and pulseless tachycardia, rapid IV bolus of 5 mg/kg may be given.

Amisulpride

Acute psychotic episode (under specialist supervision): PO: *child 15–18 yr* 200–400 mg bid adjusted according to response; max. 1.2 g daily

Predominantly negative symptoms (under specialist supervision): PO: *child 15–18 yr* 50–300 mg daily

Amitriptyline

Nocturnal enuresis: 6–12 yr 10–25 mg, *12–18 yr* 25–50 mg at bedtime daily for up to 3 mo. Review before deciding on need for further courses.

Depression: >12 yr 25 mg 2–3 times or 50 mg at bedtime, initially at lower dose and increased if tolerated/required. Usual maintenance 50–150 mg/day.

Neuralgic pain: 30 mg bedtime; increased if required/tolerated up to 150 mg/day.

Idiopathic musculoskeletal pain syndromes: 10–50 mg bedtime, starting at lower dose.

Amlodipine

100–200 μg/kg PO daily once, increased if required to max. of 10 mg (*6–15 kg:* 1.25 mg, *16–25 kg:* 2.5 mg, *>25 kg:* 5 mg).

Amodiaquine

Usually taken in combination with another medicine for malaria. PO: The dose is 10 mg/kg/day (range 7.5–15 mg/kg/day). One tablet contains 150 mg amodiaquine base. The dosage should be adjusted in accordance with the patient's age as listed in **Table 24.13.1**.

TABLE 24.13.1: Dosage schedule of amodiaquine.

	Number of tablets/day		
Age	Day 1	Day 2	Day 3
1–6 yr	1	1	1
7–13 yr	2	2	2
>13 yr	4	4	4

Amorolfine

Cream: Apply OD after cleansing in the evening for at least 2–3 wk (up to 6 wk for foot mycosis) continuing for 3–5 days after lesion has healed.

Nail lacquer: Apply to infected nails 1–2 times weekly after filing and cleaning; allow to dry (approx. 3 minutes). Treat fingernails for 6 mo and toe nails for 9–12 mo. Review 3 monthly.

Amoxicillin

20–50 mg/kg/day PO in 2 or 3 div. doses (max. of 500 mg 2–3 times daily).

In uncomplicated gonorrhea: 3 g with 1 g probenecid.

Amphotericin

Amphotericin B Lipid Complex (ABLC): Not licensed for use in children under 1 mo.

Severe invasive candidiasis, severe systemic fungal infections in patients not responding to conventional amphotericin or to other antifungal drugs or where toxicity or renal impairment precludes conventional amphotericin, including invasive aspergillosis, cryptococcal meningitis, and disseminated cryptococcosis in HIV patients – IV infusion – test dose 100 µg/kg (max. dose 1 mg), then 5 mg/kg OD.

Liposomal Amphotericin B (AmBisome): *Severe systemic or deep mycoses* where toxicity (particularly nephrotoxicity) precludes use of conventional amphotericin, suspected or proven infection in febrile neutropenic patients unresponsive to broad-spectrum antibacterials – IV infusion – *Neonate:* 1 mg/kg OD, increased if necessary to 3 mg/kg OD; max. 5 mg/kg/day. *Child:* Test dose 100 µg/kg (max. dose 1 mg), to be given over 10 minutes, then 3 mg/kg OD; max. 5 mg/kg/day.

Visceral leishmaniasis (unresponsive to the antimonial alone): IV infusion: *child:* 1–3 mg/kg daily for 10–21 days to a cumulative dose of 21–30 mg/kg, alternatively 3 mg/kg for 5 consecutive days, followed by 3 mg/kg after 6 days for 1 dose.

Conventional Amphotericin B (Amphotericin B Deoxycholate; Fungizone):

Systemic fungal infections: IV infusion: *Neonate:* 1 mg/kg OD, increased if necessary to 1.5 mg/kg daily for 7 days, then reduced to 1–1.5 mg/kg OD on alternate days if required. *Child:* Test dose 100 µg/kg (max. dose 1 mg), included as part of first dose of 250 µg/kg daily, then increased if tolerated to 1 mg/kg daily, dose is gradually increased over 2–4 days; in severe infection max. 1.5 mg/kg daily or on alternate days. Prolonged treatment usually necessary; if interrupted for longer than 7 days, recommence at 250 µg/kg daily and increase gradually.

Ampicillin

Neonate: 50 mg/kg/dose < 7 days bid, 7–21 days tid, >21 days qid. 100 mg/kg/dose for suspected meningitis and group B streptococcal infection. *Children:* PO: *1 mo to 2 yr* 12.5 mg/kg/dose, *2–12 yr* 250 mg/dose, and *12–18 yr* 500 mg/dose; IV/IM 25 mg/kg/dose (max. 1 g/dose); IV infusion 100 mg/kg/dose (max. 3 g/dose) – all given qid.

Antiscorpion Venom Serum

The usual mode of administration of scorpion antivenin IP is either by IM or by IV route. Generally, 10 mL of the reconstituted scorpion antivenin IP is sufficient for the treatment. However, if the patient continues to show clinical signs of envenomation for more than 3 hr or if the signs aggravate further, 10 mL of the antiserum may be administered by the IV route. In very rare cases, further 10 mL will have to be given.

Antisnake Venom Polyvalent

Prior to administering the snake antivenin, it is obligatory to observe precautions and carry out sensitivity test. The usual mode of administration to snake antivenin is either by IM or by IV route. The actual dose of snake antivenin, to be administered to the patient, varies according to the site of bite, severity of bite, age and physical status, degree of envenomation, involvement of systematic organs, and time factor of initiation of treatment.

A suitable dosage schedule recommended is 100 mL given over 30–60 min by IV route (avoid bolus administration which may rapidly activate the compliment system and result in severe reaction). 50 mL is to be repeated, after 30 min of the initial dose, if active bleeding persists. This may be followed by 100 mL given by slow IV route over 24 hr to counteract the venom absorbed into the circulation from the site of bite which act as a depot. This is specially so for krait, cobra, and Russell's viper bites. Echis carinatus bites require <50 mL of the initial dose.

Some centers use for minimal envenomation: 20–40 mL; moderate envenomation: 50–90 mL; severe envenomation: 100–150 mL; if systemic symptoms increase in severity or new manifestations appear, administer an additional 10–50 mL.

Sea snake and pit viper specific antivenin is not available. However, due to para-specificity of venom and antivenin, the same polyvalent antivenin is recommended. No more test dose is indicated. IM adrenaline is given before administering the antisnake venin as prophylaxis.

Arginine

Carbamoyl phosphate synthetase (CPS) and ornithine transcarbamylase (OCT) deficiency: PO 25–35 mg/kg 3–4 times daily, IV 200 mg once given over 90 min, IV continuous infusion 200 mg/kg/24 hr.

Citrullinemia and argininosuccinic aciduria (ASA): PO 100–175 mg/kg 3–4 times daily up to 700 mg/day, IV 600 mg once given over 90 min, IV continuous infusion 600 mg/kg/24 hr (25 mg/kg/hr).

Growth hormone (GH) stimulation test: IV infusion 500 mg/kg as a single dose over 30 min.

Arginine Vasopressin (AVP, Argipressin, Vasopressin)
A continuous infusion administered when no alternative measures are available and discontinued at earliest. Treatment should not normally continue for more than 72 hr. Monitor carefully. IV over 20–30 min; *birth to 18 yr* 0.3 units/kg. Continuous infusion: 0.3 units/kg/hr or 0.0003–0.006 units/kg/min (max. 1 unit/kg/hr)

Aripiprazole
Schizophrenia: 15–18 yr: PO: 2 mg OD, increased to 5 mg OD after 2 days and then further increased to 10 mg OD after a further 2 days; further increased if necessary in steps of 5 mg to max. 30 mg daily. Start with small doses in severe renal impairment because of increased cerebral sensitivity.

Autism spectrum disorder (ASD): >6 yr age: 2 mg/day, increasing to 5 mg/day, with subsequent increases to 10 or 15 mg/day as needed. Dose adjustments of up to 5 mg/day should occur gradually at intervals of 1 week or greater.

Artesunate + Lumefantrine
Treatment of uncomplicated Plasmodium falciparum and Plasmodium malariae. PO: *Infant or child 5–14 kg:* initially 1 tablet followed by 5 further doses of 1 tablet each at 8, 24, 36, 48, and 60 hr; total 6 tablets over 60 hr. *15–24 kg:* initially 2 tablets followed by 5 further doses of 2 tablets each at 8, 24, 36, 48, and 60 hr (total 12 tablets over 60 hr). *25–34 kg:* initially 3 tablets followed by 5 further doses of 3 tablets each at 8, 24, 36, 48, and 60 hr (total 18 tablets over 60 hr). *Over 34 kg:* initially 4 tablets followed by 5 further doses of 4 tablets each at 8, 24, 36, 48, and 60 hr (total 24 tablets over 60 hr).

Renal impairment: Severe: caution; monitor ECG and plasma potassium.

Hepatic impairment: Severe: caution; monitor ECG and plasma potassium. Nondispersible tablets may be crushed. If the dose is vomited within 1 hr of taking, the dose should be repeated.

Asparaginase
Always consult the current treatment protocol for details of dosage and scheduling. As part of combination therapy: 6,000 units/m^2, 3 times/wk for 3 wk. High-dose IM therapy: 25,000 units/m^2/dose weekly once for doses. IV therapy: 1,000 units/kg/24 hr for 10 days or 200 units/kg/24 hr for 28 days.

Aspirin
Anti-inflammatory, analgesic dose: 80–100 mg/kg/day

Kawasaki disease: 25 mg/kg/dose 4 times daily for 14 days followed by 5 mg/kg OD for 6–8 wk. If there is no evidence of coronary lesions discontinue.

Antiplatelet dose: 3–5 mg/kg/day, given as a single dose (max. 75 mg).

Rheumatic fever: 25 mg/kg/dose for 4 doses/day for 2–3 wks. Then 60 mg/kg/d for a total period of 9–12 wk. Aspirin resistance, as seen in adults is prevalent in children also; 26% in one study.

Atazanavir
PO: With low-dose ritonavir. *6–18 yr 16–20 kg* 150 mg OD; *20–40 kg* 200 mg OD; *>40 kg* 300 mg OD.

Atenolol
Hypertension: PO: *neonate:* 0.5–2 mg/kg OD, dose may be given in 2 div. doses; *1 mo–11 yr:* 0.5–2 mg/kg OD, dose may be given in 2 div. doses, doses higher than 50 mg daily are rarely necessary; *12–17 yr:* 25–50 mg OD, dose may be given in 2 div. doses, higher doses are rarely necessary

Arrhythmias: PO: *neonate:* 0.5–2 mg/kg OD, dose may be given in 2 div. doses; *1 mo to 11 yr*: 0.5–2 mg/kg OD, dose may be given in 2 div. doses; max. 100 mg/day; *12–17 yr:* 50–100 mg OD, dose may be given in 2 div. doses.

Renal failure: No dose adjustment is required in patients with a creatinine clearance (CrCl) > 35 mL/min/1.73 m^2. If CrCl 10–35 mL/min/1.73 m^2 give 50% dose; if <10 mL/min/1.73 m^2, give 30–50% dose and adjust according to response.

In hemodialysis and continuous ambulatory peritoneal dialysis (CAPD), give 30–50% of dose and adjust according to response. 0.5–2 mg/kg OD. Adjust according to pulse and BP. May give 2 times daily up to a max. of 100 mg/24 hr.

Atomoxetine
Children and adolescents may be started at 0.5 mg/kg/day and dose may be increased after a minimum of 3 days to a target dose of 1.2 mg/kg/day, given OD or in 2 div. doses in the morning and late afternoon. No additional benefit is seen in doses more than 1.2 mg/kg/day. Do not exceed 1.4 mg/kg/day or 100 mg/day.

Atorvastatin
Hyperlipidemia including familial hypercholesterolemia. PO – *Child 10–18 yr* initially 10 mg OD, increased if necessary at intervals of at least 4 wk to usual max. 20 mg OD (max. 80 mg OD in homozygous familial hypercholesterolemia.

Atracurium Besylate
Single IV bolus dose: *Neonate:* 300–500 µg/kg; *1 mo to 18 yr* 300–600 µg/kg. Continuous IV infusion: *Neonate* 300–400 µg/kg/hr; *1 mo to 18 yr* 300–600 µg/kg/hr.

Atropine Sulfate
Premedication: Neonates (never give IM) 15 µg/kg; *children:* SC/IM: *1 mo to 12 yr* 20 µg/kg (min 100 µg to max 600 µg); *12–18 yr* 300–600 µg as single dose 45 min before procedure. *<5 kg* 0.2 mg/kg 30 min preoperatively and then 4–6 hrly. *>5 yr* 0.1–0.2 mg/kg 30 min preoperative. IV bolus over 1 min 15 µg/kg; *1 mo to 12 yr* 20 µg/kg (min 100µg to max. 600 g); *12–18 yr* 300–600 µg as a single dose at induction in the un-premedicated patient.

Sinus bradycardia: Neonates (never give IM*) and children:* IV/intratracheal/SC/IM 15 µg/kg may be repeated once 5 min later. *Adolescent:* 0.5–1 mg every 5 min (max. 2 mg).

Organophosphorus poisoning: 0.02–0.05 mg/kg every 10–20 min till atropine effect (mydriasis, tachycardia) and then once in 1–4 hr for at least 24 hr.

Azathioprine
During the first 4 wk of therapy, full blood count (including platelets) should be performed at least weekly and monthly thereafter. More frequent monitoring may be indicated if high dosage is used or in the presence of severe renal or hepatic impairment.

Azelastine
Allergic conjunctivitis: 0.05% soln. *4–18 yr:* Apply 1–2 drops 2 times daily – increase to 4 times if necessary.

Perennial conjunctivitis: 12–18 yr: same dose – max. duration of therapy – 6 wks.

*Rhinitis: >5 yr:*140 µg/nasal spray in each nostril.

Azithromycin
Used in chancroid, legionella infections, atypical pneumonia, pertussis, diphtheria as a second choice to penicillins, multidrug-resistant enteric fever: 6 mo to 12 yr 10 mg/kg/day OD for 3 days up to max. of 200 mg *(3–7 yr)*, 300 mg *(8–11 yr)*, 400 mg *(12–14 yr)*, and 500 mg *(>14 yr)*. Alternatively, 10 mg/kg/day once on first day followed by 5 mg/kg/day OD from day 2 to day 5.

Group A beta-hemolytic streptococcal pharyngitis and tonsillitis (primary prophylaxis of rheumatic fever): 12.5 mg/kg/day – single dose for 5 days. (Not recommended for secondary prophylaxis of rheumatic fever).

Chlamydial infection such as nongonococcal urethritis or cervicitis due to susceptible strains of Chlamydia trachomatis: Adolescents: single dose of 1 g PO.

Bacterial endocarditis prophylaxis: 15 mg/kg (single dose max. 500 mg) 30–60 minutes before procedure in children and adolescents allergic to penicillin.

Treatment and postexposure pertussis prophylaxis [for postexposure prophylaxis, administer to close contacts within 3 wk of exposure, especially in high-risk patients (e.g., infants <12 mo)]: PO dosage: *Infants >6 mo and children*: 10 mg/kg/day (max. 500 mg) on day 1 and then 5 mg/kg/day (max. 250 mg) on days 2–5. *Infants <6 mo:* 10 mg/kg/day for 5 days. Monitor for infantile hypertrophic pyloric stenosis in infants <1 mo old.

Uncomplicated typhoid fever: PO: *Adolescent:* 8–10 mg/kg/day OD for 7 days; 1,000 mg on the first day, followed by 500 mg OD for 6 days. *Children:* 10 mg/kg/day OD for 7 days or 5-day regimen of 20 mg/kg/day. Continued treatment may be needed to prevent relapse in cryptosporidiosis.

Sexually transmitted diseases (STD) caused by C. trachomatis: 12–18 yr 1 g as a single dose.

Diphtheria: Dose is same but to be given for 14 days.

Pertussis: Infants aged <6 mo: 10 mg/kg/day for 5 days. *Infants and children aged >6 mo:* 10 mg/kg (max. 500 mg) on day 1, followed by 5 mg/kg/day (max. 250 mg) on days 2–5.

Multidrug-resistant enteric fever: 10–20 mg/kg/ day for 14 days.

Aztreonam
IV over 3–5 min or IV infusion: <7 days old: 30 mg/kg 12 hrly; rest of neonatal period and *up to 12 yr*: 30 mg/ kg 6–8 hrly.

In severe infection and cystic fibrosis in 2–12-yr-olds: May increase up to 50 mg/kg 6–8 hrly (max. 2 g 6 hrly); *12–18 yr* – 1 g 8 hrly or 2 g 12 hrly (severe infection with *Pseudomonas aeruginosa* or pulmonary infection in cystic fibrosis).

Nebulization for P. aeruginosa pulmonary infection in cystic fibrosis: 6–17 yr: 75 mg 3 times a day for 28 days, doses to be administered at least 4 hr apart.

Renal impairment: CrCl 10–30 mL/min/1.73 m^2 – no change in first dose but subsequent doses to be halved; CrCl < 10 mL/min/1.73 m^2 – no change in the first dose but subsequent doses to be reduced to 1/4th usual dose.

B

Baclofen
Initial dose: 1–12 yr 2.5 mg and *12–18 yr* 5 mg tid and increase gradually every 3 days. Maintenance dose: 5–10 mg *(1–2 yr)*, 10–15 mg *(2–6 yr)*, 15–30 mg *(6–10 yr)* bid, and 10–20 mg *(>10 yr)* tid.

Dosage adjustment in renal impairment: Reduce PO doses by at least 50% (max. dose 5 mg) in patients with impaired renal function and the frequency to tid (mild), bid (moderate), or daily (severe).

Balsalazide Sodium

Treatment of mild-to-moderate ulcerative colitis, acute attack: PO *12–17 yr*: 2.25 g tid until remission occurs or for up to max. of 12 wk.

Maintenance of remission of ulcerative colitis: PO *12–17 yr:* 1.5 g bid (max. dose 3 g), adjusted according to response; max. 6 g/day.

Basiliximab

IV inj. or infusion: *>1 yr and <35 kg*: 10 mg within 2 hr before transplant and 4 day after surgery; *>35 kg*: 20 mg within 2 hr before transplant and 4 day after.

BCG (Bacillus Calmette-Guerin) Vaccine

From birth to 12 mo: 0.05 mL intradermal; *>1 yr*: 0.1 mL intradermal.

Beclomethasone Dipropionate

Aerosol inhaler: 6 mo to 2 yr 50–200 μg and *2–18 yr* 100–400 μg bid as a preventor for regular use. Dry powder inhalers (DPI): *5–18 yr* 100–400 μg bid as a preventor for regular use.

Intranasal for allergic rhinitis: 6–12 yr 50–100 μg (1–2 sprays) into each nostril bid.

Bendroflumethiazide (Bendrofluazide)

PO: 1 mo to 12 yr 50–100 μg/kg; *12–18 yr* 2.5–5 mg OD.

Benzathine Penicillin

Group A streptococcal URI: 25,000–50,000 units/kg as single dose, max. 12 L units/dose or *child < 27 kg*: 3–6 L units as single dose and *>27 kg*: 9 L units as single dose. *Adolescents*: 12 L units as single dose.

Prophylaxis of rheumatic fever: IAP recommends – *Children < 27 kg* 6 L units every 15 days; *≥27 kg* – 1.2 L units every 21 days.

Congenital syphilis: 50,000 units/kg/dose (max. 24 L units) once a week for 3 wk.

Early syphilis in adolescents: 24 L units as single dose in 2 injection sites. If present for >1 yr – 24 L units as single dose in 2 injection sites once weekly for 3 doses.

Benzatropine (Benztropine)

PO: 3–12 yr: 20 μg/kg and *12–18 yr*: 1–2 mg as single dose. Dose can be repeated up to max. of 6 mg/day depending on clinical response. IV/IM *3–12 yr*: 20–100 μg/kg (max. 2 mg), *12–18 yr:* 1–2 mg as single dose – followed, if necessary, with oral treatment.

Benzoyl Peroxide

Topical 2.5% 1–3 times daily sparingly for 15 min. Increase strength and duration of exposure as tolerated. If excessive peeling or redness occurs, decrease to alternate day.

Benzydamine Hydrochloride

>12 yr: Oral rinse of 15 mL every 1½–3 hr as required (diluted with water if stinging occurs) for not more than 7 days; OR as spray onto affected area; *<6 yr:* 1 spray/4 kg up to 4 sprays every 1½–3 hr, *6–12 yr:* 4 sprays every 1½–3 hr, *>12 yr:* 4–8 sprays every 1½–3 hr.

Benzyl Benzoate

Scabies: Apply 25% emulsion to the entire body except head and face after a scrub bath. Wash, rinse, and dry skin well before applying benzyl benzoate. Apply enough medicine to cover the entire skin surface from the neck down, including the soles of your feet, and rub in well. Allow the medicine to remain on the body for 24 hr. Then, thoroughly wash the body with warm water and soap. Rinse thoroughly and dry with a clean towel. Immediately after using benzyl benzoate, wash hands to remove any medicine that may be on them. Treatment may need to be repeated for severe infestation.

Pediculosis: Shampoo, rinse, and dry hair and scalp well before applying benzyl benzoate. Apply enough medicine to thoroughly wet the dry hair and scalp or skin. Allow the medicine to remain on the affected areas for 24 hr. Then, thoroughly wash the affected areas with warm water and soap or regular shampoo. Rinse thoroughly and dry with a clean towel. After rinsing and drying, use a fine-toothed comb (<0.3 mm between the teeth) to remove any remaining nits (eggs) or nit shells from your hair, or, if you have fine hair, you may use a tweezer or your fingernails to pick nits out.

Benzylpenicillin (Penicillin G)

Newborn: 25 mg/kg/dose bid up to 7 days age and tid thereafter. Dose doubled if meningitis diagnosed. *Child:* 25 mg/kg/dose qid. In severe infection and meningitis, 50 mg/kg/dose 6 times daily to max. single dose of 2.4 g and daily dose of 14.4 g/day.

In moderate renal failure (creatinine clearance 10–50 mL/min/1.73 m^2), dosage interval may be increased to 8–12 hr and in severe renal failure (<10 mL/min/1.73 m^2) to every 12 hr.

Beta Carotene

PO OD: 1–4 yr: 60–90 mg, *5–8 yr:* 90–120 mg, *9–12 yr:* 120–150 mg, *13–15 yr:* 150–180 mg, and *>16 yr*: 180–300 mg; protection not total and 2–6 wk treatment should result in yellow discoloration of palms and soles before exposure to sunlight is attempted.

Betaine

PO 50 mg/kg/dose bid; increase according to response – max. 20 g/day. Dosage in renal impairment/liver failure: no information available.

Betamethasone Sodium Phosphate

Ear drops: 2–3 drops into the affected ear (s) 2–3 hrly; reduce frequency when relief obtained.

Nose drops: 2–3 drops into each nostril 2–3 times daily.

Bezafibrate

PO 200 mg/day has been used in adolescents, adjusted according to response to a max. of 200 mg tid but experience in children is limited; refer to an expert.

Biotin

Isolated carboxylase defects: PO/IV bolus: *Neonate:* 5 mg OD, adjusted according to response, maintenance 10–50 mg daily, higher doses may be required. *Child:* 10 mg OD, adjusted according to response; maintenance 10–50 mg daily, increased if necessary up to 100 mg daily.

Defects of biotin metabolism: PO/slow IV injection: *Neonate:* Initially 10 mg OD, adjusted according to response; maintenance 5–20 mg daily, higher doses may be required. *Child:* Initially 10 mg OD, adjusted according to response; maintenance 5–20 mg daily, higher doses may be required.

Bisacodyl

Constipation: PO: *<10 yr:* 5 mg, *>10 yr:* 5–10 mg daily bedtime (max. 15–20 mg). Rectal suppositories *<10 yr:* 5 mg, *>10 yr:* 5–10 mg OD in the morning.

Preparation for surgery or radiological investigation: PO *<10 yr:* 5 mg and *>10 yr*: 5–10 mg at bedtime for 2 days prior to procedure and rectally, if necessary, 1 hr before procedure.

Bleomycin

10–20 units/m^2/dose IV, IM or 0.25–0.50 mg/kg SC 1–2 times/week in combination regimens.

Botulinum A Toxin-Hemagglutinin Complex

Only those who have been trained in its use should administer this drug. It can be an effective tool for reducing muscle tone in the appropriately selected patient. The "ideal" patient is the one who has hypertonia that interferes with function is expected to develop fixed contractures and requires treatment of only a few muscles at any given time. The effect is seen within days–a couple of wk and lasts for 3–8 mo. Use a 23–26 gauge needle and administer on 2 sites of each muscle (used mainly for gastrocnemius muscles) up to a total dose of 4 units/kg. If more than 1 muscle group needs to be injected at the same time, this total dose is div. between these muscles. Dose may be repeated when clinical effect diminishes but not within 2 mo of previous injection.

Blepharospasm: Initially, 1.25–2.5 U injected into the medial and lateral orbicularis oculi of the upper lid and the lateral orbicularis oculi of the lower lid. Subsequently, the dose may be increased up to two-fold. The initial dose should not exceed 25 U per eye. The total dose should not exceed 100 U every 12 wk.

Hemifacial spasm: Treat as for unilateral blepharospasm (as above). Inject other affected facial muscles as needed.

Cervical dystonia: Inject using a 25, 27, or 30 gauge needle (for superficial muscles) or 22 gauge needle (deeper musculature). Tailor dosing to individual patient based on the head and neck position, location of pain, muscle hypertrophy, body weight, and response. Do not inject sternocleidomastoid muscle bilaterally. Max. total dose usually not more than 200 U.

Hyperhidrosis of the axillae: Inject using a 30 gauge needle. Inject 50 U intradermally to each axilla, evenly distributed in multiple sites 1–2 cm apart.

Cerebral palsy: Inject using a 23–26 gauge needle into the medial and lateral heads of the affected gastrocnemius muscle. Recommended total dose: 4 U/kg. Divide dose between two limbs if injected on same occasion. Repeat dose not more frequently than every 2 mo.

Focal spasticity associated with infantile hemiplegia: Inject using a 25, 27, or 30 gauge needle (superficial muscles) or longer needle for deeper musculature. Multiple injection sites may facilitate more uniform contact with the innervation areas of the muscle, especially in larger muscles. Tailor dose and number of sites based on the size, number, and location of muscles involved, the severity of spasticity, and the presence of local muscle weakness.

Brivaracetam

PO, IV, or IV infusion: Child 4–17 yr (up to 50 kg): Initially 0.5–1 mg/kg bid, titrated as required; maintenance dose of 1 mg/kg bid (max. dose 2 mg/kg bid). *If body-weight is >50 kg,* start with a dose of 25–50 mg bid, titrated as required; maintenance dose of 50 mg bid (max. dose 100 mg bid).

Avoid abrupt withdrawal - reduce daily dose in steps of 50 mg at weekly intervals, till a dose of 20 mg daily is arrived at - continue this dose for the final week.

Use cautiously in children with hepatic impairment - if present, an initial dose of 0.5 mg/kg bid, max. maintenance dose of 1.5 mg/kg bid in children weighing < 50 kg and 25 mg bid, max. maintenance dose of 75 mg bid in children weighing >50 kg is suggested.

Budesonide

Prophylaxis and management of BPD: For ventilated babies 400 μg/kg inhaled bid. For nonventilated babies, 500 μg bid inhaled with a nebulizer. May be increased to 1 mg bid in babies >2.5 kg with severe symptoms.

Asthma prophylaxis: Aerosol *1 mo–12 yr:* 50–400 μg, *12–18 yr:* 200–400 μg and turbohaler in *6–18-yr-olds;* 100 μg bid to be used regularly. Can use up to 800 μg/day in severe asthmatics.

Nebulizer in *3 mo to 12 yr:* 250–500 µg and *12–18 yr:* 500 µg to 1 mg bid: Higher doses may be used.

Croup: 1 mo to 18 yr: 2 mg with nebulizer when required.

Bumetanide
PO *1 mo to 12 yr:* 0.015–0.05 mg/kg/dose (max. 2 mg); *12–18 yr:* 1–2 mg 1–4 times daily. IV bolus - *12–18 yr:* 1–2 mg repeated after 20 min if required. IV infusion over 30–60 min: *1 mo to 12 yr:* 0.025–0.050 mg/kg; *12–18 yr:* 1–5 mg.

Bupivacaine Hydrochloride
Caudal block: Children 1–3.7 mg/kg; *adolescen*t 15–30 mL of 0.25% or 0.5%.

Epidural block: Children 1.25 mg/kg/dose; *adolescen*t 10–20 mL of 0.25–0.5%.

Peripheral nerve block: 5 mL of 0.25% (12.5 mg) or 0.5% (25 mg); max. 400 mg/24 hr.

Sympathetic nerve block: 20–50 mL of 0.25% (no epinephrine).

The dosage of bupivacaine will depend upon the site of injection and the procedure used. Expert advice should be obtained. Epidural administration should be carried out by, or under the supervision of, a consultant anesthetist.

Buprenorphine
Moderate-to-severe pain: Sublingual: *Child 16–25 kg:* 100 µg every 6–8 hr; *25–37.5 kg:* 100–200 µg every 6–8 hr; *37.5–50 kg:* 200–300 µg every 6–8 hr; *50 kg and above:* 200–400 µg every 6–8 hr. IM or slow IV: *Child 6 mo to 11 yr:* 3–6 µg/kg every 6–8 hr (max. dose 9 µg/kg); *12–17 yr*: 300–600 µg/every 6–8 hr.

Bupropion
PO 150–300 mg (usually 150 mg) once in the morning.

Buspirone Hydrochloride
PO: 2–12 yr: 5 mg and *12–18 yr:* 5–10 mg 2–3 times daily (max. dose in adolescent 45 mg in div. doses).

C

Caffeine Citrate
Birth to 3 mo: IV/PO loading dose 20 mg/kg followed by maintenance dose 24 hr later at 5–10 mg/kg/day OD or bid.

Calcipotriol
All preparations: Apply to the affected area morning and evening. Do not apply to face. Wash hands after use to avoid inadvertent transfer to other body areas.

Cream/ointment: Weekly max. to be applied: *6–12 yr:* 50 g; adolescents >*12 yr:* 75 g; adults: 100 g.

Scalp solution: Weekly max. to be applied: adults, 60 mL. When used with cream/ointment, weekly max. of total calcipotriol 5 mg.

Calcitonin (Salmon/Salcatonin)
Hypercalcemia: SC/IM injection: *Child:* 2.5–5 units/kg every 12 hr (max. dose 400 units every 6–8 hr), adjusted according to response, no additional benefit with doses over 8 units/kg every 6 hr; IV infusion: *child:* 5–10 units/kg, to be administered by slow IV infusion over at least 6 hr.

Calcitriol (1,25-Dihdroxycholecalciferol)
Premature: 0.05 µg/kg/24 hr IV or 1 µg/24 hr PO; *Children:* 0.01–0.08 µg/kg/24 hr; *Adolescent:* 0.25–1 µg/24 hr.

Calcium (Oral Supplements)
PO: Birth to 4 yr: 0.25 mmol/kg/dose; *5–12 yr:* 0.2 mmol/kg/dose; *12–18 yr:* 10 mmol/dose - qid.

Calcium Carbonate
PO 50–75 mg/kg/day in 2–3 div. doses and adjusted according to plasma phosphate and calcium levels.

Calcium Folinate (Folinic Acid)
IV 15 mg OD. See methotrexate monograph for folate rescue.

Calcium Gluconate
Hypocalcemia: Urgent correction - PO 2 mL/kg of 10% solution, IV bolus over 5–10 min (0.3 mL/kg/dose), followed by PO maintenance. If IV maintenance is desired for a few days, be careful to avoid extravasation and administer 10% solution at 0.1 mL/kg/hr *in neonates,* 0.2 mL/kg/hr *up to 2 yr* and 40 mL/24 hr *in 2–18 yr.*

Cardiopulmonary resuscitation: 0.3 mL/kg of 10% solution as single IV bolus.

Parenteral nutrition regimen: Approximate doses to maintain normal serum calcium - 1 mmol/kg in *neonates,* 0.2–1 mmol/kg up to *2 yr,* 0.2 mmol/kg in *2–12 yr,* and 5–10 mmol/24 hr continuous IV over 12–24 hr.

Hyperkalemia: 1–2 mL/kg IV.

Calcium Polystyrene Sulfonate (Ion Exchange Resin)
Rectally and PO 125–250 mg/kg qid. Not given PO in neonates. Must monitor electrolytes.

Captopril
IAP Working Group on Management of Congenital Heart Disease in India: The starting dose is 0.1 mg/kg/dose. It is gradually increased to 0.5–1 mg/kg/dose tid (increase after every 4–5 doses). Max. dose is 2 mg/kg/dose. BP and renal parameters should be monitored when uptitrating the dose. Captopril is the preferred acetylcholinesterase inhibitor (ACEI) in young infants; requires dosing every 6–8 hr.

Carbamazepine
Children < 6 yr: (use in neonates limited) initially 5 mg/kg/day in 1–2 div. doses; increase by 5 mg/kg/day every 5–7 days till response obtained/toxicity develops/serum levels attained.

6–12 yr: initially 10 mg/kg in 2–4 div. doses; increase by 100 mg or 5 mg/kg/day weekly till effect obtained (usually 800–1,200 mg/24 hr). *12–18 yr:* initially 200 mg bid; increase by 200 mg/day once in a week till effect obtained (usually 1.6–2.4 g/day in 3–4 div. doses).

Carbamylglutamate
PO 12.5–25 mg/kg/dose qid.

Carbaryl
Topical: Gently rub into dry hair and scalp until all the hair is fully soaked. Allow the hair to dry naturally away from heat or sun in a well-ventilated room. After 12 hr, wash in ordinary shampoo and remove dead lice and eggs with comb while the hair is still wet. Repeat after 1 week if lice are still present.

Carbimazole
PO *up to 12 yr:* 250 µg/kg/dose *and 12–18 yr:* 10 mg tid (max. 40 mg). Give until euthyroid and then taper to OD dose barely enough to sustain normal thyroid function.

Carbocisteine
Child 2–4 yr: 62.5–125 mg qid; *5–11 yr:* 250 mg tid; 12–17 yr: Initially 2.25 g daily in div. doses and then reduced to 1.5 g daily in div. doses, as condition improves. *Mucodyne syrup* 250 mg/5 mL has replaced the 125 mg/5 mL formulation – take care to ensure that the appropriate dose is administered.

Carboplatin
Total cumulative doses vary with protocol. An increasing number of protocols employ doses based on GFR (e.g. UKCCSG GC2, MMT 98) or EDTA half-life (e.g. UKCCSF CNS 2000 01).

Solid tumor: 300–600 mg/m^2 IV once in 4 wk.

Brain tumor: 175 mg/m^2 IV once a week for 4 wk. *Adolescent:* 360 mg/m^2 IV once in 4 wk.

Carnitine (Levocarnitine)
Premature: 8–16 mg/kg/24 hr IV infusion; *children:* PO 50–100 mg/kg/24 hr in 2–3 div. doses or IV 50 mg/kg/dose 4–6 hrly (max. 300 mg/kg/24 hr); *adolescent:* 0.33–1 g/dose 2–3 times daily PO.

Carvedilol
PO 0.1 mg/kg/day in 2 div. doses; increase at 1–2 weekly interval to 1 mg/kg/day with a max. of 2 mg/kg/day.

Patients with hepatic impairment: Not recommended for patients with clinically evident hepatic impairment.

Intermittent hemodialysis: Due to its high degree of plasma protein-binding, carvedilol is not likely to be significantly removed by hemodialysis. No supplemental dosage is needed.

Cefaclor
PO: < *1 yr:* 62.5 mg, *1–5 yr:* 125 mg, *6–18 yr:* 250 mg/dose tid. Dose doubled in severe infection with susceptible organisms.

Cefadroxil
Children: PO 30 mg/kg/24 hr in 2 div. doses (max. 2 g/day); *adolescent:* 250–500 mg 8–12 hrly.

Cefazolin
7 days or younger: 25 mg/kg IV or IM 12 hrly; *8–28 days: up to 2 kg:* 25 mg/kg IV or IM 12 hrly, *>2 kg:* 25 mg/kg IV or IM 8 hrly; *1 mo or older: mild-to-moderate infections*: 25–50 mg/kg/day IV or IM in 3 div. doses, max: 3 g/day, *severe infections*: 100–150 mg/kg IV or IM in 3 div. doses, max: 6 g/day.

Treatment of peritonitis: Continuous (the exchange with the loading dose should dwell for 3–6 hr; all subsequent exchanges during therapy should contain the maintenance dose). Loading dose: 500 mg/L intraperitoneally, maintenance dose: 125 mg/L intraperitoneally; intermittent [dose should be applied once a day in the long-dwell (unless otherwise specified)]: 20 mg/kg intraperitoneally once a day.

Peritonitis prophylaxis: Touch contamination (instillation of PD fluid after disconnection of system, disconnection during PD: 125 mg/L intraperitoneally.

Invasive dental procedures while on peritoneal dialysis: 25 mg/kg IV as a single dose 30–60 min before procedure, max: 1 g/dose.

Gastrointestinal (GI) procedures while on peritoneal dialysis: 25 mg/kg IV as a single dose, infused within 60 min before start of surgical procedure, max: 2 g/dose.

Subacute bacterial endocarditis (SBE) prophylaxis: 50 mg/kg IV or IM as single dose 30–60 min before procedure, max: 1 g/dose.

Surgical prophylaxis: Preoperative dose: 30 mg/kg IV as a single dose; max: <120 kg: 2 g/dose, 120 kg: 3 g/dose.

Renal impairment: CrCl 40–70 mL/min: 60% daily dose equally div. 12 hrly; CrCl 20–40 mL/min: 25% daily dose equally div. 12 hrly; CrCl 5–20 mL/min: 10% of usual daily dose one in 24 hr.

Cefdinir
Children: 7 mg/kg/dose bid. *12–18 yr:* 14 mg/kg/day in 2 div. doses or 300 mg/dose bid.

Cefepime
Neonates <14 days: 30 mg/kg/dose bid IV/IM. *Neonates >14 days:* 50 mg/kg/dose bid IV/IM. *Children:* IV 50 mg/kg every 8 hr (max. 2 g/dose). Intraperitoneal 15 mg/kg/dose.

In peritoneal dialysis associated with peritonitis: 1,000 mg/24 hr. However, it is not yet licensed for use in children under 12 yr in UK and US.

Cefixime
8 mg/kg/24 hr in 1–2 div. doses; *adolescent:* 400 mg/24 hr in 1–2 div. doses.

Typhoid: PO cefixime is used in a dose of 15–20 mg/kg/day in 2 div. doses.

Cefoperazone
50–200 mg/kg/day in 2 or more div. doses (max. in adolescent 1–2 g IM/IV 12 hrly).

Cefotaxime
Newborn (severe infections like meningitis): 50 mg/kg/dose <7 *day* bid, 7–21 day tid, *21–30 days* 3–4 times. *1 mo to 12 yr:* 50 mg/kg/dose and *12–18 yr:* 1–3 bid.

Dosage adjustment in renal impairment: Due to extrarenal elimination, it is necessary to reduce dose in severe renal impairment (CrCl <10 mL/min/1.73 m^2). A normal single dose should be given as a loading dose and then the daily dose should be halved without a change in frequency.

Cefpirome
Children 12–18 yr: IV injection or infusion 1g 12 hrly and increased to 2 g 12 hrly in severe infections and infections in immunocompromised children.

Cefpodoxime
9 mg/kg/day in 2 div. doses (max. single dose 200 mg). The dose frequency should be reduced in renal impairment. CrCl 10–40 mL and <10 mL/min/1.73 m^2: Frequency of dosing once in 24 hr and once in 48 hr, respectively.

Ceftazidime
Neonates <7 days and >7 days, <1200 g: 100 mg/kg/24 hr in 2 div doses IV/IM, *>7 days >1200 g:* 150 mg/kg/day div. 8 hrly IM/IV. *Children:* 150 mg/kg/24 hr div. 8 hrly. Max. 6 g/day. Single dose >1 g to be given IV only.

Dose adjustment in renal failure: In mild impairment, give a dose very 12 hr; in moderate impairment (CrCl 10–50 mL/min/1.73 m^2), give a dose OD; and in severe impairment (CrCl <10 mL/min/1.73 m^2), give 50% of dose OD. Levels may be monitored if clinically indicated.

In hemodialysis: Appropriate maintenance dose should be repeated after dialysis.

In peritoneal dialysis: 125–250 mg may be added to 21 of dialysis fluid and given in addition to the IV dose.

Ceftriaxone
Neonates: 50–75 mg/kg OD IM/IV. Infuse over 10–30 min. Avoid in premature, acidotic, or hyperbilirubinemic neonates. *Children:* 50–75 mg/kg OD IV/IM.

Meningitis: Loading dose 75 mg/kg followed by 80–100 mg/kg/24 hr once or div. 12 hrly. Max. 4 g/day.

In *severe renal failure*, reduce dose to a max. of 2 g or 50 mg/kg. No dose adjustment is required in *hepatic impairment*. If there is both hepatic and severe renal impairment, monitor serum concentrations. In patients undergoing dialysis, no supplemental dose is required but serum concentration monitoring advisable.

Cefuroxime
Infections due to sensitive gram-positive and gram-negative bacteria: PO (as cefuroxime axetil): *3 mo to 2 yr:* 10 mg/kg (max. 125 mg) bid; *2–12 yr:* 15 mg/kg (max. 250 mg) bid; *12–18 yr:* 250 mg bid; double the dose for severe lower respiratory tract infections; 125 mg bid in lower urinary tract infection (UTI). IV, IV infusion, IM: *<7 days age:* 25 mg/kg 12 hrly; *7–21 days age:* 25 mg/kg 8 hrly; *21–28 days age:* 25 mg/kg 6 hrly; if severe infection in neonates, give IV at double these doses. *1 mo–18 yr:* 20 mg/kg (max. 750 mg) 8 hrly; increase to 50–60 mg/kg (max. 1.5 g) 6–8 hrly in severe infection and cystic fibrosis.

Lyme disease: PO: *3 mo to 12 yr:* 15 mg/kg (max. 500 mg) BD for 14–21 days (for 28 days in Lyme arthritis); *12–18 yr:* 500 mg BD for 14–21 days (for 28 days in Lyme arthritis).

Surgical prophylaxis: IV: *1 mo to 18 yr:* 50 mg/kg (max. 1.5 g) up to 30 min before procedure; up to 3 more doses of 30 mg/kg (max. 750 mg) may be given IM/IV 8 hrly for high-risk procedures.

Cephalexin
Children: 25–100 mg/kg/24 hr in 3–4 div. doses; *adolescent* 250–500 mg qid (max. 4 g/24 hr).

Reduce dose in severe renal impairment (creatinine clearance < 10 mL/min/1.73 m^2) by reducing dose frequency. If removed by dialysis, an additional dose may be required after dialysis.

Cephalosporins
First-generation cephalosporins: Cephalexin: See above; Cefadroxil: See above.

Second-generation cephalosporins. Cefuroxime: See above; Cefaclor: See above.

Third-generation cephalosporins. Cefixime: See above; Cefpodoxime: See above; Cefdinir: see above.

Fourth-generation cephalosporins. Cefpirome: See above – Cefepime: See above.

Cetirizine
2–6 yr: 5 mg and *6–18 yr:* 10 mg as single or 2 div. doses. In renal impairment, give 50% of the above dose.

Chenodeoxycholic Acid
Cerebrotendinous xanthomatosis: 5 mg/kg/dose tid.

Bile acid synthesis defects: Initially 5 mg/kg/dose tid, then 2.5 mg/kg tid; Others 7 mg/kg/ dose in 1 or div. doses.

Chloral Hydrate

Sedation for procedures: <12 yr: 25–50 mg/kg *12–18 yr:* 1–2 g 45–60 min prior to procedure (max. single dose 100 mg/kg).

Long-term sedation: 20–30 mg/kg/dose qid.

Night sedation: <12 yr: 30–50 mg/kg, *12–18 yr:* 500 mg to 1 g single dose at bedtime.

Chlorambucil

Hodgkin disease and non-Hodgkin lymphoma: Consult the current treatment protocol.

Systemic amyloidosis and severe juvenile idiopathic arthritis (JIA): All ages: 100–120 µg/kg PO OD.

Chloramphenicol

Neonates <14 days: 12.5 mg/kg/dose bid; *>14 days:* 12.5 mg/kg/dose 2–4 times daily – monitor levels. *Children:* 50 mg/kg/day (max. 1 g/day) 4 div. doses – double dose for meningitis, septicemia).

Ear drops: 2–3 drops 2–3 times daily.

Eye drops: 1 drop 4–6 times daily (1–2 hrly in severe infections). In addition, a small amount of ointment may be applied at bedtime.

Eye ointment: Apply 4 times daily (1–2 hrly in severe infections). Continue treatment till 48 hr after the eye is clinically normal. *Eye ointment* may be used in the ear.

Chlorhexidine Gluconate

Dental gel: 1 inch of gel brushed around the teeth and gums once or bid for 1 minute. For gingivitis, apply for 1 mo.

Mouth wash 0.12%: 15 mL for 30 seconds bid. Mouth wash 0.2%: 10 mL for 1 min bid.

Oral spray: Up to 12 actuations to be used bid, morning and night. For the prevention of gingivitis, use for 1 mo. In aphthous ulceration and oral infections, use for 48 hr after the infection has cleared. Postoral surgery/trauma on the advice of the supervising clinician.

Chloroquine

Doses expressed as chloroquine base.

Malaria prophylaxis: 1 mo–12 yr: 5 mg/kg, *12–18 yr:* 300 mg once weekly. Start 1 week before entering and 4 wk after leaving endemic area.

Malaria treatment (Plasmodium vivax, Plasmodium ovale, and sensitive Plasmodium falciparum): PO/IV *1 mo–12 yr:* Initially 10 mg/kg followed by 5 mg/kg 6–8 hr later and then daily once for 2 days. *12–18 yr:* Initially 600 mg followed by 300 mg 6–8 hr later and then daily once for 2 days.

Chlorothiazide

20–40 mg/kg/day in 2 div. doses PO; 2–8 mg/kg twice a day IV.

Chlorpheniramine

PO < *2 yr:* 1 mg 2 times (max. 2 mg), *2–5 yr:* 1–2 mg tid (max. 6 mg), *6–12 yr:* 2–4 mg 3–4 times (max. 12 mg), *12–18 yr:* 4 mg 4–6 times daily (max. 24 mg). IM/IV/SC < *1 yr:* 250 µg/kg; *1–5 yr:* 2.5–5 mg, *6–12 yr:* 5-10 mg, *12–18 yr:* 10–20 mg once. Repeated up to 4 times daily (max. 49 mg in adults).

Chlorpromazine

Withdrawal symptoms in baby born to drug abuser: PO 1 mg/kg/day PO or PO/IV 500–750 µg/kg/ dose 4 times (max. 6 mg/kg/day). Dose doubled if withdrawal is severe.

Children with schizophrenia, violent behavior, agitation: <6 yr: 500 µg/kg/dose qid (max. 40 mg/day); *6–12 yr:* 10 mg/dose (max. 75 mg/day); *and 12–18 yr:* 25 mg/dose qid (max. 300 mg/day).

Intractable hiccup: 6–12 yr: 10 mg/dose 1–3 times daily; *1–18 yr:* 25–50 mg/dose 3–4 times daily.

Nausea and vomiting of terminal illness: 2–12 yr: 500 µg/kg/dose (max. 40 mg/day); *12–18 yr:* 10–25 mg/dose (max. 75 mg/day) qid.

Cholecalciferol (Vitamin D3)

See **Table 24.13.2.**

Colestipol Hydrochloride

PO *12–18 yr* initially 5 g OD. May be increased at intervals of 1 mo to a max. of 30 g daily in 1–2 div. doses.

Cholestyramine

Cholesterol reduction: PO 240 mg/kg/24 hr in 3 div. doses. *12–18 yr* 1 sachet (4 g) start at 1 daily and usually require 4 times daily but up to 9 sachet/day in adults according to cholesterol levels.

Cholestatic pruritus: PO: *<6 yr* half sachet (2 g), *6–12 yr* 1 sachet (4 g) *and 12–18 yr* 1- 2 sachet OD

Diarrhea in ileal resection, Crohn disease, vagotomy, radiation: Same as for cholesterol reduction but alternate treatment to be instituted if no response in 3 days.

TABLE 24.13.2: Cholecalciferol doses (IU) for management of nutritional rickets in children—IAP Consensus Guidelines (2021)

Age	*Daily dose for 12 wk*	*Alternative intermittent dose regimen (if compliance is not good)*	*Maintenance dose (daily)*
<6 mo	2,000	Not recommended	400
6–12 mo	2,000	Equivalent of 2,000 IU/ day may be given on a monthly or weekly basis	400
>12 mo	3,000	60,000 IU fortnightly (after every 2 wk) × 5 doses	600

Choline Salicylate

Children > 4 mo: Apply quarter of an inch of gel to the dried area of the affected oral mucosa, no more frequently than once every 3 hr to a max. of 6 applications in 24 hr. *>12 yr:* Apply half an inch of gel with massage not more often than every 3 hr.

Ciclesonide

Administered OD as MDI in doses of 80–640 µg depending on the clinical severity and response.

Ciclopirox (Topical Antifungal)

Apply once a day with an applicator brush to all affected nails and immediately adjacent skin. Daily applications should be made over the previous coat and removed every 7 days. Up to 48 wk of daily applications, weekly trimming by the patient, and monthly professional removal of the unattached, infected nail, is needed.

Cimetidine

PO/IV < *1 mo:* 5 mg/kg/dose and <*12 yr:* 5–10 mg/kg/dose 4 times daily; *12–18 yr:* 400 mg/dose 2- 4 times/day.

Cinchocaine Hydrochloride + Fluocortolone Caproate + Fluocortolone Pivalate

Hemorrhoids|Pruritus ani: Rectal ointment - *child:* Apply bid for 5–7 days, apply 3–4 times if required, on the first day of treatment, and then apply OD for a few days after symptoms have cleared. As suppository - *child 12–17 yr:* Initially 1 suppository daily for 5–7 days, to be inserted after a bowel movement, and then 1 suppository OD on alternate days for 1 wk.

Hemorrhoids (severe cases), pruritus ani (severe cases): As suppository - *child 12–17 yr:* Initially 1 suppository 2–3 times a day for 5–7 days and then 1 suppository OD on alternate days for 1 wk.

Cinnarizine

Vestibular disorders: PO: *5–12 yr:* 15 mg 3 times daily, *12–18 yr:* 30 mg tid.

Motion sickness: PO: *5–12 yr*: 15 mg 2 hr before travel and then 7.5 mg 8 hrly during journey if necessary; *12–18 yr:* 30 mg 2 hr before travel and then 15 mg 8 hrly during journey if necessary.

Ciprofibrate

PO 2–4 mg/kg (max. 200 mg) has been used in adolescents.

Ciprofloxacin

Fistulating Crohn's disease: PO: *child*: 5 mg/kg bid.

Severe respiratory tract infections and GI infection: PO *Neonate*: 15 mg/kg bid; *Child:* 20 mg/kg bid (max. dose 750 mg); IV infusion: *neonate:* 10 mg/kg 12 hrly, to be given over 60 minutes; *Child:* 10 mg/kg 8 hrly (max. dose 400 mg), to be given over 60 minutes.

Acute exacerbation of bronchiectasis: Child 1–17 yr: 20 mg/kg bid (max. dose 750 mg) for 7–14 days; IV infusion: *child 1–17 yr:* 10 mg/kg 8 hrly (max. dose 400 mg), to be given over 60 min.

Pseudomonal lower respiratory tract infection in cystic fibrosis: PO: *Child:* 20 mg/kg bid (max. dose 750 mg); IV infusion: *child:* 10 mg/kg 8 hrly (max. dose 400 mg), to be given over 60 minutes

Complicated UTI: PO: *neonate:* 10 mg/kg bid; *child:* 10 mg/kg bid, dose to be doubled in severe infection (max. 750 m g bid); IV infusion*: neonate:* 6 mg/kg 12 hrly, to be given over 60 min; *child:* 6 mg/kg 8 hrly; increased to 10 mg/kg 8 hrly (max. dose 400 mg), in severe infection.

Gonorrhea: PO: *child 12–17 yr*: 500 mg for 1 dose.

Anthrax (treatment and postexposure prophylaxis): Child: 15 mg/kg bid (max. dose 500 mg); IV infusion: *child:* 10 mg/kg 12 hrly (max. dose 400 mg).

Prevention of a secondary case of meningococcal meningitis: PO: *Neonate:* 30 mg/kg (max. dose 125 mg) for 1 dose; *Child 1 mo to 4 yr:* 30 mg/kg (max. dose 125 mg) for 1 dose; *Child 5–11 yr:* 250 mg for 1 dose; *Child 12–17 yr*: 500 mg for 1 dose.

Cisapride

PO: Birth to 12 yr 0.15–0.3 mg/kg/dose; *12–18 yr* 10 mg/dose 3–4 times daily. Doses to be given 15–30 min before meals.

Cisplatin

37–75 mg/m^2 once in 3 wk or 50–150 mg/m^2 once in 21–28 days given over 4–6 hr.

Renal failure: CrCl 10–50 mL/min - 75% of dose and if <10 mL/min - 50% of dose.

Citalopram

12–18 yr: 20 mg in the morning and increased to a max. of 60 mg.

Citrulline

Birth to 18 yr: 42.5 mg/kg/dose qid.

Clarithromycin

PO 15 mg/kg/24 hr in 2 div. doses up to a max. of 500 mg bid for 5–10 days.

Helicobacter pylori infection: 1–2 yr: 125 mg, *2–6 yr:* 250 mg, *6–9 yr:* 375 mg, *9–12 yr:* 500 mg, and *12–18 yr:* 1 g/day in 2 div. doses along with amoxycillin and omeprazole or amoxicillin and lansoprazole or metronidazole and omeprazole.

Community-acquired pneumonia (CAP) and pharyngitis in children due to Chlamydophila pneumoniae, Mycoplasma pneumoniae, or Streptococcus pneumoniae: Give for 10 days.

Bacterial endocarditis prophylaxis: 15 mg/kg (single dose max. 500 mg) 3–60 minutes before procedure in children and adolescents allergic to penicillin.

Treatment and postexposure pertussis prophylaxis: For postexposure prophylaxis, administer to close contacts within 3 wk of exposure, especially in high-risk patients (e.g., women in the third trimester, infants < 12 mo). PO dosage*: Infants > 6 mo and children:* 15 mg/kg/day up to a max. of 500 mg bid for 7 days. Not used in neonates.

Patients with renal impairment: CrCl >60 mL/min: no dosage adjustment needed. CrCl 30–60 mL/min: no dosage adjustment needed except in patients receiving concurrent ritonavir. In these patients, reduce the recommended clarithromycin dose by 50%. CrCl <30 mL/min: Reduce the recommended dose by 50%. In patients receiving ritonavir, decrease the recommended clarithromycin dose by 75%.

Clindamycin

Staphylococcal [especially methicillin-resistant Staphylococcus aureus (MRSA)] bone and joint infections such as osteomyelitis, septic arthritis, deep abscess, skin and soft-tissue infection, peritonitis, intra-abdominal sepsis and community-acquired MRSA with Panton-Valentine leukocidin (PVL) toxin-induced necrotizing pneumonia; erysipelas or cellulitis in penicillin-allergic patients (alternative to macrolides): PO *Neonate up to 14 days:* 3–6 mg/kg tid; *14–28 days:* 3–6 mg/kg qid; *>1 mo age*: 3–6 mg/kg qid (max. dose 450 mg). *Child:* 5–7 mg/kg qid; increased if necessary up to 10 mg/kg qid (max. dose 600 mg); IM/IV/IV infusion: *Neonates: <7 days <2,000 g:* 10 mg/kg/day div. 12 hrly IV/IM; *<7 days >2,000 g:* 15 mg/kg/day div. 8 hrly IV/IM; *>7 days <1,200 g:* 10 mg/kg/day div. 12 hrly IV/IM; *1,200–2,000 g:* 15 mg/kg/day div. 8 hrly, *>2,000 g:* 20 mg/kg/day div. 8 hrly IV/IM. *Children:* 10–40 mg/kg/day div. 8 hrly. Doses of 600 mg or more need to be given IV.

Falciparum malaria (alternate therapy) with 20 mg/kg/day for 5 days with quinine, artesunate, or chloroquine.

Acne: Topical clindamycin 1% w/w, available as a foam, a gel, a solution (liquid), a lotion, and a pledget (swab) may be applied as thin film 2 times daily with lotion and once with gel.

Dose adjustment in hepatic failure: Dose reduced and liver function monitored.

Not readily removed by *dialysis or peritoneal dialysis.*

Clobazam

Initially PO: <12 yr: 125 μg/kg/dose, *12–18 yr:* 10 μg/dose bid followed by maintenance of 250 μg/dose (max. 500 μg) in <12 yr *and 10–15 yr:* max. 30 μg /dose in 2 doses.

Clobetasone

Apply a thin layer 2–3 times daily on the affected area for a max. of 2 wk.

Clofazimine

Multibacillary leprosy (in combination with dapsone and rifampicin), PO, *Adolescent:* 50 mg OD and 300 mg once a mo; *Child 10–14 yr:* 50 mg on alternate days and 150 mg once a mo; *Child < 10 yr:* 1 mg/ kg PO OD plus an additional 6 mg/kg PO once per mo in combination with dapsone and rifampin; continue treatment for 12 mo.

Type 2 lepra reaction (erythema nodosum leprosum): PO, *adolescent, and child:* 200–300 mg daily in 2 or 3 div. doses for a max. of 3 mo; 4–6 wk treatment may be required before any effect is seen.

Clomiphene

100 mg daily once: Roughly at the same time each day.

Clomipramine

Start with 25 mg/day and gradually increase up to 250 mg/day according to response usually as single dose at bedtime (may give in div. doses).

Clonazepam

1 mo to 12 yr: Start with 25 μg/kg (0.25 mg: *<5 yr* and 0.5 mg: *6–12 yr*) as a single bedtime dose and increasing every 4 days over 2–4 wk to maintenance of 80 μg/kg/dose (0.1–0.3 mg: <1 yr; 0.3–1 mg: *1–5 yr;* 1–2 mg: *6–12 yr*) 3 times daily. *12–18 yr:* Start with 1 mg bedtime to maintenance of 1–2.5 mg/dose tid.

Clonidine

Hyperactivity and Tourette syndrome: PO initially 0.05 mg/24 hr OD, increase by 0.05 mg once in 5–7 days up to a max. of 0.4 mg/kg/day in 3–4 div. doses.

Hypertension: PO 5–10 μg/kg/day in 2–4 div. doses (max. 0.9 mg/kg/day); IV 2–6 μg/kg as single dose.

Sedation, pain, and narcotic withdrawal: PO initial test dose 1 μg/kg, monitoring for hypotension and escalate in steps of 1-3-5 μg/kg/day if required, tid (max. 5 μg/kg qid).

Growth hormone stimulation test: PO 150 μg/m^2 as single dose.

Clopidogrel

0.2 mg/kg/day is sufficient to achieve a platelet inhibition level similar to that in adults taking the standard dose of 75 mg/day. 80% of children would also be taking aspirin. When appropriate, tablets are rounded to the nearest one-half, one-third, or one-fourth tablet.

Clotrimazole

Apply 2–3 times daily continuing for 14 days after lesions have healed.

Oral thrush: 10–20 drops gently apply to buccal mucosa (covering all lesions) 4 times daily for 5–7 days.

Vaginal candidiasis: Apply 2% vaginal gel 5 g deep into vagina at bedtime for 6 consecutive nights (not to be used during menstruation) or alternatively 100 mg vaginal pessaries for 6 days, 200 mg for 3 days, or 500 mg single dose at bedtime.

Scalp seborrhea: Apply to liquid with selenium to scalp, massage gently, leave for 5 min, and then rinse well with water 2–3 times/wk.

Otomycosis: Instill 4–5 drops in ear 3–4 times daily till 2 wk after infection subsides.

Cloxacillin

Newborn: IV/PO: *<7 days*: 50–100 mg/kg/day in 2 div. doses; *7–21 days:* 75–150 mg/kg/day in 3 div. doses, *>21 days:* 100–200 mg/kg/day in 4 div. doses. May be increased to 100 mg/kg/dose in severe infection (meningitis, cerebral abscess, staph osteitis). PO used only for minor infections.

Children: IV/IM 50–100 mg/kg/day in 4 div. doses (max. single dose 1 g, may be doubled in severe infection). PO: *<1 yr:* 250 mg/day, *1–5 yr:* 500 mg/day, *5–18 yr:* 1 g in 4 div. doses. Doses may be doubled in severe infection.

In renal failure: If CrCl < 10 mL/min/1.73 m^2, increase dosage interval to 8 hrly.

Clozapine

PO: 12–18 yr: Initial dose on 1st day given as inpatient 12.5 mg/dose 1–2 times daily and from 2nd day 25 mg/ dose 1–2 times daily and if tolerated, gradually increase in steps of 25–50 mg over 14–21 day to maintenance dose of 300 mg/day in div. doses (max. 900 mg/day if necessary).

Co-Amoxiclav (Amoxicillin + Clavulanic Acid)

Dose based on amoxycillin content.

Neonates: 30 mg/kg/day in 2 div. doses. *Children:* 20–45 mg/kg in 2–3 div. doses. Higher doses of 80 mg/kg/day may be required in otitis media.

Administration: PO: Give at the start of a meal. Dispersible tablets should be stirred into a little water before taking. IV: Reconstitute a 600 mg vial with 10 mL water for injections (final volume 10.5 mL) and a 1.2 g vial with 20 mL (final volume 20.9 mL). Administer by slow IV injection (over 3–4 minutes, within 20 minutes of reconstitution) or infuse over 30–40 minutes and complete infusion within 4 hr of reconstitution. For infusion, the reconstituted injection can be diluted to 5 times its volume in NaCl 0.9%. Do not infuse in glucose solutions, as co-amoxiclav is less stable in infusions containing glucose.

Co-Careldopa

Metabolic disorders: Start with 250–500 µg/kg/dose of levodopa qid. Increase every 4–5 days to maintenance of 2.5–3 mg/kg/dose of levodopa. Review dose every 3–6 mo in early childhood and adjust if needed according to weight and cerebrospinal fluid (CSF) amine metabolic concentration.

Dystonia: 3 mo–18 yr: start with 250 µg to 1 mg/kg dose of levodopa 2–3 times daily and increase every 2–3 days.

Co-Fluampicil (Ampicillin + Flucloxacillin)

Mixed infections involving beta-lactamase-producing staphylococci: PO: *1 mo–10 yr:* 125/125 mg 6 hrly; *10–18 yr:* 250/250 mg 6 hrly. IM/Slow IV/IV infusion: *1 mo–1 yr:* 62.5/62.5 mg 6 hrly; *2–10 yr:* 125/125 mg 6 hrly; *10–18 yr:* 250/250 mg 6 hrly.

Severe mixed infections involving beta-lactamase producing staphylococci. PO: 1 mo to 10 yr: 250/250 mg 6 hrly; *10–18 yr:* 500/500 mg 6 hrly. IM/ Slow IV/IV infusion: *1 mo–1 yr:* 125/125 mg 6 hrly; *2–10 yr:* 250/250 mg 6 hrly; *10–18 yr*: 500/500 mg 6 hrly. Reduce dose or frequency if GFR is <10 mL/min/1.73 m^2.

Co-Phenotrope (Diphenoxylate + Atropine)

PO: 2–4 yr: ½ tab, *4–12 yr:* 1 tab, *13–16 yr:* 2 tab, *16–18 yr:* initially 4 tab followed by 2 tabs 3–4 times daily. Avoid in treatment of diarrhea in children.

Co-Trimoxazole (Trimethoprim + Sulfamethoxazole)

Gastrointestinal infections and shigella infections: PO: *Children <2 mo of age:* 8 mg/kg of trimethoprim and 40 mg/kg of sulfamethoxazole daily in 2 div. doses every 12 hr. Usual duration is 5 days. IV *Children <2 mo of age:* 8–10 mg/kg of trimethoprim daily (as co-trimoxazole) in 2–4 equally div. doses given for 5 days.

UTI: PO: *Children <2 mo of age:* 8 mg/kg of trimethoprim and 40 mg/kg of sulfamethoxazole daily in 2 div. doses every 12 hr. Usual duration is 10 days. *Severe UTI:* IV *Children <2 mo of age:* 8–10 mg/kg of trimethoprim daily (as co-trimoxazole) in 2–4 equally div. doses given for up to 14 days.

Brucellosis: PO 10 mg/kg daily (up to 480 mg daily) of trimethoprim (as co-trimoxazole) in 2 div. doses for 4–6 wk.

Cholera: PO 4–5 mg/kg of trimethoprim (as co-trimoxazole) bid given for 3 days.

Cyclospora infections: PO 5 mg/kg of trimethoprim and 25 mg/kg of sulfamethoxazole bid given for 7–10 days. HIV-infected patients may require higher dosage and longer treatment.

Granuloma inguinale (donovanosis): PO *Adolescents:* 160 mg of trimethoprim and 800 mg of sulfamethoxazole bid given for 3 wk or until all lesions have healed completely; consider adding IV aminoglycoside (e.g., gentamicin) if improvement is not evident within the first few days of therapy and in HIV-infected patients. Relapse can occur 6–18 mo after apparently effective treatment.

Isosporiasis: PO 5 mg/kg of trimethoprim and 25 mg/kg of sulfamethoxazole bid. Usual duration of treatment is 10 days; higher dosage or more prolonged treatment is necessary in immunocompromised patients.

Pertussis: PO 8 mg/kg of trimethoprim and 40 mg/kg of sulfamethoxazole daily in 2 div. doses. Usual duration is 14 days for treatment or prevention.

Plague postexposure prophylaxis: PO: *Children > 2 mo of age:* 320–640 mg of trimethoprim (as co-trimoxazole) daily in 2 div. doses given for 7 days. Alternatively, 8 mg/kg daily of trimethoprim (as co-trimoxazole) in 2 div. doses given for 7 days.

Pneumocystis jiroveci (P. carinii) pneumonia treatment: PO: *Children >2 mo:* 15–20 mg/kg of trimethoprim and 75–100 mg/kg of sulfamethoxazole daily in 3 or 4 div. doses. Usual duration is 14–21 days. IV: *Children >2 mo:* 15–20 mg/kg of trimethoprim daily (as co-trimoxazole) in 3 or 4 equally div. doses. Usual duration is 14–21 days.

UTI prophylaxis: >3 mo age: 1–2 mg/kg of TMP OD at bedtime. Avoid in infants <3 mo, glucose-6-phosphate dehydrogenase deficiency

HIV prophylaxis in infants and children – primary: PO 150 mg/m^2 of trimethoprim and 750 mg/m^2 of sulfamethoxazole daily in 2 div. doses given on 3 consecutive days each week. Total daily dose should not exceed 320 mg of trimethoprim and 1.6 g of sulfamethoxazole. Alternatively, 150 mg/m^2 of trimethoprim and 750 mg/m^2 of sulfamethoxazole can be administered as a single dose 3 times each week on consecutive days, in 2 div. doses daily 7 days each week, or in 2 div. daily doses given 3 times each week on alternate days.

Prevention of recurrence (secondary prophylaxis) in infants and children: PO 150 mg/m^2 of trimethoprim and 750 mg/m^2 of sulfamethoxazole daily in 2 div. doses given on 3 consecutive days each week. Total daily dose should not exceed 320 mg of trimethoprim and 1.6 g of sulfamethoxazole.

Alternatively, 150 mg/m^2 of trimethoprim and 750 mg/m^2 of sulfamethoxazole can be administered as a single daily dose given for 3 consecutive days each week, in 2 div. doses daily, or in 2 div. daily doses given 3 times a week on alternate days.

Toxoplasmosis – primary prophylaxis in infants and children: PO 150 mg/m^2 of trimethoprim and 750 mg/m^2 of sulfamethoxazole daily in 2 div. doses. The safety of discontinuing toxoplasmosis prophylaxis in HIV-infected children receiving potent ART has not been extensively studied.

Coal Tar

Topical: Bath 60–90 mL of a 5–20% solution or 15–5 mL of 30% solution is added to bath water. Soak for 5–20 min and then pat dry. Use OD to once every 3 days. *Shampoo*: Apply 2 times in a week for 1st 2 wks and then once weekly or more often if needed. *Skin*: Apply to affected areas 1–4 times daily. Decrease frequency to 2–3 times/wk once condition is controlled.

Atopic dermatitis: 2–5% coal tar cream OD or every other day to reduce inflammation.

Scalp psoriasis: Tar oil bath or coal tar solution may be applied sparingly to lesions 3–12 hr before each shampoo.

Psoriasis of body, arms, and legs: Apply at bedtime. If thick scales are present, use a product containing salicylic acid and apply several times during the day.

Codeine Phosphate

Children: Pain: 0.5–1 mg/kg/dose 4–6 hrly (max. 60 mg/dose); *dry cough:* 1–1.5 mg/kg/24 hr div. 4- 6 hrly. *Adolescent: Pain:* 15–60 mg/dose 4–6 hrly and for *cough:* 10–20 mg/dose 4–6 hrly (max. 120 mg/24 hr).

Colchicine

Prophylaxis of Mediterranean fever: Children < 5 yr: 0.5 mg/24 hr and *>5 yr:* 1–1.5 mg/24 hr in 2–3 div. doses.

Colestipol Hydrochloride

PO: 12–18 yr: initially 5 g OD. May be increased at intervals of 1 mo to a max. of 30 g daily in 1–2 div. doses.

Colistin Sulfomethate Sodium

2.6 mg = 1 mg colistin base = 30,000 u. IM, IV over 5min: 40,000 u/kg (adult 2 million units) 8 hrly or 1.25–2.5 mg/of colistin base 12 hrly.

Nebulized along with oral ciprofloxacin for pseudomonas lung infection in cystic fibrosis: <1 yr: 500,000 units, *1–10 yr:* 1 million units, *>10 yr:* 2 million units bid. IV for early pseudomonas infections not cleared by ciprofloxacin and nebulized colistin or moderate-to-severe infection or multiresistant strains along with aminoglycoside where other regimens fail.

Coloxyl

PO: Up to 6 mo: 10 drops tid. *6–18 mo:*15 drops tid.

Copper Histidine

Dosage tailored to individual patient requirements. SC 50–150 µg elemental copper/kg daily once; IM 200 µg elemental copper, increase monthly to max. of 1 g. Daily once.

Crotamiton

Topical: After the patient has a warm bath and dried well, the preparation should be rubbed into the entire body surface excluding face and scalp. The application should be repeated OD preferably in the evening for a total of 3–5 days. Children <3 yr of age should not apply crotamiton more than once a day.

Cyclizine

Children 6–12 yr: PO 25 mg/dose up to 3 times/24 hr as required; *older adolescents:* 50 mg up to 4–6 hrly 30 min before travel (max. 200 mg/24 hr); IM 50 mg 4–6 times.

Cyclopentolate

1–2 drops or as required. Its effect lasts 24 hr.

Cyclophosphamide
Children: Induction: IV 40–50 mg/kg (1.5–1.8 g/m^2) in div. doses over 2–5 days; PO 1–5 mg/kg/24 hr followed by *maintenance* IV 10–15 mg/kg (350–550 mg/m^2) once in 7–10 days or 3–5 mg/kg twice in a week.

Systemic lupus erythematosus (SLE): 500–750 mg/m^2/mo.

Juvenile idiopathic arthritis or vasculitis: IV 10 mg/kg OD in 2 weeks.

Nephrotic syndrome: PO 2–3 mg/kg/24 hr up to 12 wks. In steroid-dependent nephrotic syndrome, use with alternate-day prednisolone. Dose not to exceed 166 mg/kg.

Cycloserine
Tuberculosis: PO 10–20 mg/kg/day in 2 div. doses. Max. 1 g/day. *Adolescent:* 250–500 mg bid for 2 wk and then increased to 500 mg–1 g in div. doses.

Cyclosporin
Juvenile idiopathic arthritis, collagen disease, vasculitis, and uveitis: PO 1–2 mg/kg/dose bid increased gradually up to 3 mg.kg/dose bid.

Organ transplant: PO 5–7 mg/kg/dose bid starting 12 hr before transplant and continued for 1–2 weeks postoperatively gradually reducing to maintenance dose of 1–3 mg/kg/dose. bid.

Cyproheptadine
Pruritus and urticaria: 0.25 mg/kg/day or 8 mg/m^2 body surface area in 2–3 div. doses, or *by age 2–6 yr:* 2 mg PO two to three times a day, not to exceed 12 mg/day; *7–14 yr:* 4 mg PO two to three times a day, not to exceed 16 mg.

Cyproterone acetate
Seek expert advice on use in *McCune-Albright syndrome (MAS) or testotoxicosis.* 1 tablet daily for 21 days starting on the first day of menstrual cycle and repeated after a 7-day interval, usually for several mo.

Cytarabine (Cytosine Arabinoside, Ara-C, Arabinosylcytosine)
Induction: IV 100–200 mg/m^2/24 hr for 5–10 days or until remission followed by maintenance 70–200 mg/m^2/24 hr for 2–5 days/mo. Always consult the current treatment protocols.

 D

Dacarbazine
Solid tumors: 200–470 mg/m^2/24 hr over 5 days once in 21–28 days;

Neuroblastoma: 800–900 mg/m^2 on day 1 of combination therapy once in 3–4 wks.

Hodgkin disease: 375 mg/kg/m^2 on days 1 and 15 of combination therapy and repeat once in 28 days.

Dactinomycin (Actinomycin D)
Children >6 mo age: 15 μg/kg/24 hr or 400–600 μg/m^2/24 hr for 5 days; repeated once in 3–6 wk.

Dalteparin Sodium
Treatment of deep vein thrombosis: SC 200 units/kg/24 hr in 2 div. doses *in <12 yr* and as single dose *in 12–18 yr* not to exceed 18,000 units/24 hr.

Prophylaxis: SC 100 units/kg up to 12 yr and 2,500–5,000 units as a single dose in *12–18 yr.*

Dantrolene
Spasticity: >5 yr: 500 μg/kg/day OD and increase once in 7 days in increments of 500 μg/kg/dose till response achieved; *12–18 yr:* 25 mg daily once and increased gradually till response.

Malignant hyperthermia: IV bolus of 1 mg/kg as a single dose repeated as required at 5–10 min intervals to max. cumulative dose of 10 mg/kg.

Dapsone
Leprosy: PO 1–2 mg/kg/day as a single dose in combination with rifampicin.

Blistering skin conditions: Start at 500 μg/kg/day and increase or decrease as necessary in 12.5 mg increments.

Prophylaxis of P. jiroveci in HIV: >1 mo: 2 mg/kg/day (up to 100 mg) PO OD.

Daunorubicin
Children: Remission induction in ALL (combination therapy) 25–45 mg/m^2 on day 1 of every week for 4 cycles (max: total dose 300 mg/m^2).

Deferasirox
Transfusion-related chronic iron overload in patients with beta-thalassemia major and other anemias who receive frequent blood transfusions (7 mL/kg/mo or more of packed red blood cells): PO *2–17 yr:* Initially 7–21 mg/kg OD, then adjusted in steps of 3.5–7 mg/kg every 3–6 mo, maintenance dose adjusted according to serum-ferritin concentration; max. 28 mg/kg/day; usual max. 21 mg/kg.

Chronic iron overload when desferrioxamine is contraindicated or inadequate in nontransfusion-dependent thalassemia syndromes: PO *10–17 yr:* Initially 7 mg/kg OD, maintenance dose adjusted according to serum-ferritin concentration and liver-iron concentration; max. 7 mg/kg/day.

Deferiprone
PO: >6 yr: 25 mg/kg/dose rounded to the nearest 250 mg dose tid (max. 100 mg/kg/day).

Deflazacort
PO: 1 mo–12 yr: 250 μg–1.5 mg/kg; *12–18 yr:* 2–18 mg OD. Up to 2.4 mg/kg may be used. 2 days dose could be taken as a single dose on alternate days.

Demeclocycline Hydrochloride
PO: Child 12–17 yr: 150 mg qid, alternatively 300 mg bid.

Hepatic impairment: Dose adjustments max. 1 g daily in div. doses.

Renal impairment: May exacerbate renal failure and should not be given to patients with renal impairment.

Desferrioxamine Mesylate
Acute iron poisoning: PO [injection given PO through a nasogastric (NG) tube as very bitter] *1 mo to 12 yr:* 5 g and *12–18 yr:* 5–10 g in 50–100 mL water. IM *1 mo–12 yr:* 1 g, *and 12–18 yr*: 2 g repeated 8 hrly if necessary. IV continuous infusion - initially 15 mg/kg.

Desloratadine
PO: 2–5 yr: 1.25 mg; *6–11 yr:* 2.5 mg; *12–18 yr:* 5 mg OD.

Desmopressin
Nocturnal enuresis: Intranasal in *children > 5 yr* 20 μg once at night; half dose in each nostril for 3 mo and then reassess by stopping for 1 week. Increase if necessary to 40 μg (20 μg in each nostril).

Dexamethasone
Croup: PO 150 μg/kg/dose bid or 600 μg/kg as a single daily dose up to max. of 12 mg/day.

Antiemetic with chemotherapy: IV/PO per dose *<1 yr:* 250 μg–1 mg, *1–5 yr*: 1–2 mg, *6–12 yr:* 2–4 mg and *12–18 yr:* 4 mg tid until 48 hr after chemotherapy.

Headache of increased ICT: IV/PO 250 μg/kg/dose bid for 5 days and then reduce the dose to 62.5–125 μg/kg/dose bid.

Brain tumor edema: IV/PO 125–500 μg/kg/dose bid.

Replacement: IV/PO 250–500 μg/m^2/dose bid

Fetal lung maturation – given to mother: IM 12 mg repeated once after 24 hr and PO 6 mg bid for 4 doses.

Bronchopulmonary dysplasia (BPD): 250 μg/kg IV/PO bid for 3 days, course repeated once every 10 days until the baby is no longer oxygen dependent or 500 μg/kg OD for 3 days and tapered over 6 wk to 100 μg/kg on alternate day during the last week.

Postintubation laryngeal edema: 200 μg/kg IV/PO 8 hrly for 3 doses starting 4 hr before extubation.

Cerebral edema: Initially *<35 kg:* 20 *mg* and *>35 kg:* 24 mg, followed by 1-3rd day 4 mg q3h (<35 kg) and 4 mg q2h (>35 kg), 4th day 4 mg q6h (<35 kg) and 4 mg q4h (>35 kg), 5–8th day 2 mg q6h (<35 kg) and 4 mg q6h (>35 kg), and thereafter taper.

Eye drops: 1 drop 4–6 hrly. In severe conditions, apply hourly till the condition improves and then reduce to 4–6 hrly.

Eye ointment: Small amount into conjunctival sac 3–4 times daily or only at bedtime along with drops during daytime.

Congenital adrenal hyperplasia: 0.25–0.5 mg OD. The drug should be used only after epiphyseal fusion so as to avoid adverse effects on growth.

Dexamphetamine Sulfate
PO: Initially 3–5 yr: 2.5 mg, *>6 yr:* 5–10 mg 1–2 times daily. Increase if required. *<6 yr:* 2.5 mg a day at weekly intervals (max. 20 mg/day); *>6 yr:* 5 mg a day at weekly intervals (max. 40 mg/day). Give maintenance in 2–3 div. doses.

Dextromethorphan
PO 1.25–2 mg/kg/dose qid 15 min before food. PO long-acting suspension 2.5 mg/kg/dose bid.

Diamorphine Hydrochloride (Heroin Hydrochloride)
Acute or chronic pain: PO: *1 mo to 11 yr:* 100–200μg/kg 4 hrly (max. dose 10 mg), adjusted according to response; *12–17 yr:* 5–10 mg 4 hrly, adjusted according to response. IV infusion *1 mo–11 yr:* 12.5–25 μg/kg/hr, adjusted according to response. IV inj.: *1–2 mo:* 20 μg/kg 6 hrly; *3–5 mo:* 25–50 μg/kg 6 hrly; *6–11 mo:* 75 μg/kg 4 hrly; *1–11 yr:* 75–100 μg/kg 4 hrly (max. dose 5 mg); *12–17 yr:* 2.5–5 mg 4 hrly; *at all age groups* – adjust according to response. IM or SC – 12–17 yr: 5 mg 4 hrly, adjusted according to response.

Acute or chronic pain in ventilated neonates: Initially by IV inj.: 50 μg over 30 min, followed by continuous IV infusion at 15 μg/kg/hr, adjusted according to response.

Acute or chronic pain in nonventilated neonates: Continuous IV infusion at 2.5–7 μg/kg/hr, adjusted according to response.

Acute severe pain associated with injury in an emergency setting (specialist supervision in hospital): intranasal *>2 yr – 12–17 kg:* 1.44 mg; *18–23 kg:* 2.16 mg; *24–29 kg:* 2.88 mg; *30–39 kg:* 3.2 mg; *40–50 kg:* 4.8 mg for 1 dose, spray into alternate nostrils.

Hepatic impairment: Dose reduction to be considered. Avoid use or reduce dose in children with renal impairment; opioid effects increased and prolonged; increased cerebral sensitivity.

Diazepam
Sedation: IV slowly 100–200 μg/kg (max. 5 mg *<12 yr* and 10–20 mg *>12 yr.* PO 200–300 μg/kg 45–60 min before procedure. Rectal *1–3 yr:* 5 mg, *3–12 yr:* 5–10 mg, and *12–18 yr* 10 mg.

Premedication: PO *1 mo–1 yr:* 250 µg/kg, *1–5 yr:* 2.5 mg, *5–12 yr:* 5 mg and *12–18 yr:* 10 mg.

Status epilepticus: IV bolus: *Birth to 2 yr:* 300–400 µg/kg; *12–18 yr:* 10–20 mg slowly. Repeat after 10 min if required. Start with the smaller dose and increase to higher dose. IV infusion: *Birth–1 mo:* 50 µg/kg/hr (max. 300 µg/kg/hr), *1 mo–12 yr:* 100 g/kg/hr [max. 125 µg/kg/hr but up to 400 µg/kg/hr have been used in intensive care unit (ICU)], *12–18 yr:* 125 µg/kg/hr. *Rectal birth: 1 mo:* 1.25–2.5 mg, *1 mo–2 yr:* 5 mg, *2–12 yr:* 5–10 mg, *12–18 yr:* 10 mg - repeat if required after 5 min.

Anxiolytic (short term): PO *2–12 yr:* 2–3 mg/dose *and 12–18 yr:* 2–10 mg/dose tid. Not very effective <12 yr.

Suppression of stage IV sleep in parasomnias: PO 2–18 yr: 1.5 mg at bedtime.

Relief of muscle spasm (postoperative, initial dose for tension, and irritability in cerebral spasticity): *<1 yr:* 250 µg/kg, *1–5 yr:* 2.5 mg, *5–12 yr:* 5 mg *and 12–18 yr:* 10 mg (all per dose bid).

Diazoxide
Intractable hypoglycemia: PO 1.7–5 mg/kg/dose tid. Establish response and then gradually increase (max. 15 mg/kg/day up to 20 mg/kg/day used in hyperinsulinemia of infancy). Higher doses are unlikely to be beneficial.

Resistant hypertension: PO 1.7 mg/kg/dose tid (max. 15 mg/kg/day)

Severe hypertension: IV bolus *1 mo–18 yr:* 1–3 mg/kg (max. 150 mg). Repeat after 5–15 min if necessary. Monitor BP. Max. 4 doses/day.

Dichloroacetate
PO 12.5 mg/kg/dose qid (up to 200 mg/kg/day used).

Diclofenac
PO/rectal: >6 mo age: 300 µg–1 mg/kg/dose tid (max. 150 mg/day). IM/IV: *>6 mo age:* 300 µg–1 mg/kg/dose 1–2 times daily (max. 150 mg/day for max. 2 days).

Topical 2–18 yr: Small amount 3–4 times daily.

Dicyclomine Hydrochloride
PO: 6 mo–2 yr: 5–10 mg/dose 3–4 times 15 min before feeds, *2–12 yr:*10 mg/dose; and *12–18 yr:* 10–20 mg/dose tid.

Didanosine (DDI)
PO: >1 mo age: 120 mg/m^2/dose bid and if given with zidovudine 90 mg/m^2/dose bid.

In renal impairment: CrCl (mL/min/1.73 m^2)/dose/frequency: 30–59/60% of normal total dose/2 div. doses, 10–29/40% of normal total dose/OD, <10/30% of normal total dose/OD. Total daily dose may be given OD to improve compliance. Dose reduction is better when reintroducing following discontinuation due to pancreatitis/neuropathy/hepatic impairment.

Diethylcarbamazine
Filariasis and loiasis: PO 300 µg/kg/dose on day 1 and increased over 3 days to 2 mg/kg/dose tid for 3 wk.

Tropical pulmonary eosinophilia: PO 6 mg/kg/day in 3 div. doses for 21 days.

Toxocariasis (visceral larva migrans): PO 160 µg/kg/dose on day 1 and 2 and increased over 3 days to 2 mg/kg/dose 3 times and given for further 7–10 days.

Digoxin
Supraventricular arrhythmia, chronic heart failure: PO: *neonate (<1.5 kg):* initially 25 µg/kg in 3 div. doses for 24 hr, then 4–6 µg/kg daily in 1–2 div. doses; *neonate (1.5–2.5 kg):* initially 30 µg/kg in 3 div. doses for 24 hr, then 4–6 µg/kg daily in 1–2 div. doses; *neonate (>2.6 kg):* initially 45 µg/kg in 3 div. doses for 24 hr, then 10 µg/kg daily in 1–2 div. doses.

1 mo–1 yr: Initially 45 µg/kg in 3 div. doses for 24 hr, then 10 µg/kg daily in 1–2 div. doses.

2–4 yr: Initially 35 µg/kg in 3 div. doses for 24 hr, then 10 µg/kg daily in 1–2 div. doses.

5–9 yr: Initially 25 µg/kg in 3 div. doses (max. per dose 750 µg) for 24 hr, then 6 µg/kg daily in 1–2 div. doses; max. 250 µg/day.

10–17 yr: Initially 0.75–1.5 mg in 3 div. doses for 24 hr, then 62.5–250 µg daily in 1–2 div. doses, higher doses may be necessary.

IV infusion: Neonate (<1.5 kg): initially 20 µg/kg in 3 div. doses for 24 hr, then 4–6 µg/kg daily in 1–2 div. doses; *neonate (1.5–2.5 kg):* initially 30 µg/kg in 3 div. doses for 24 hr, then 4–6 µg/kg daily in 1–2 div. doses; *neonate (>2.6 kg):* initially 35 µg/kg in 3 div. doses for 24 hr, then 10 µg/kg daily in 1–2 div. doses; *1 mo–1 yr:* initially 35 µg/kg in 3 div. doses for 24 hr, then 10 µg/kg daily in 1–2 div. doses; *2–4 yr:* initially 35 µg/kg in 3 div. doses for 24 hr, then 10 µg/kg daily in 1–2 div. doses; *5–9 yr:* initially 25 µg/kg in 3 div. doses (max. per dose 500 µg) for 24 hr, then 6 µg/kg daily in 1–2 div. doses; max. 250 µg/day; *10–17 yr:* initially 0.5–1 mg in 3 div. doses for 24 hr, then 62.5–250 µg daily in 1–2 div. doses, higher doses may be necessary.

Digoxin-Specific Antibody Fragments (Fab)
Each vial will bind to approximately 500 g of digoxin.

Acute ingestion of known quantity: Use the following formula: Dose (number of vials) = total amount ingested (mg) × 0.8/0.5.

Acute ingestion of unknown quantity: <20 kg: clinical judgment; *>20 kg*: start with 10 vials followed by another 10 vials if required.

Toxicity during chronic therapy - steady concentration known: use formula. Dose (number of vials) = serum digoxin conc. (ng/mL) × body wt. (kg)/100.

Toxicity during chronic therapy - steady concentration unknown: <20 kg: 1 vial; *>20 kg:* 6 vials as single dose should reverse toxicity.

Dihydrocodeine Tartrate
Moderate-to-severe pain: PO as immediate release preparation: *1-3 yr:* 500 μg/kg; *4-11 yr:* 0.5-1 mg/kg; *12-17 yr:* 30 mg 4-6 hrly (max. per dose 30 mg). IM or SC: *1-3 yr:* 500 μg/kg; *4-11 yr:* 0.5-1 mg/kg (max. per dose 30 mg); *12-17 yr:* 30 mg 4-6 hrly (max. per dose 50 mg).

Chronic severe pain: PO: modified-release preparations: *12-17 yr:* 60-120 mg 12 hrly.

Severe pain: PO: *12-17 yr:* 40-80 mg tid; max. 240 mg/day.

Hepatic impairment: Dose reduction to be considered.
Avoid use or reduce dose in children with *renal impairment;* opioid effects increased and prolonged; increased cerebral sensitivity.

Diloxanide Furoate
PO: 2-12 yr: 20 mg/kg/day, *12-18 yr:* 1.5 g in 3 div. doses.

Diltiazem
PO: 12-18 yr: 30-60 mg/dose 2-3 times daily.

Dinoprostone (Prostaglandin E2)
PO initially 20-25 μg/kg hrly, doubled if required. If treatment continues for >1 wk, dose/frequency to be reduced. IV infusion initially 5 ng/kg/min increased to 10-20 ng/kg/min in 5 ng/kg/min increments till effect or side effects develop. Monitor heart rate (HR), respiratory rate (RR), blood pressure (BP), and temperature in arms and legs.

Diphenhydramine Hydrochloride
PO: 2-12 yr: 10-25 mg, *12-18 yr:* 25-50 mg once at bedtime.

Diphtheria and Tetanus Vaccine (Adsorbed)
IM: 0.5 mL - Given at 10, 16, and every 10 yr thereafter.

Diphtheria Antitoxin
Differs with site. Half dose in children *<10 yr.*

Nasal: IM 10-20,000 units, *tonsillar*: IM/IV 15-25,000 units, *pharyngeal or laryngeal:* IM/IV 20-40,000 units, *combined types or delayed diagnosis*: IV 40-60,000 units, *severe diphtheria, e.g. with extensive membrane and/or severe edema (bull neck diphtheria)*: IV or part IV and IM 40-100,000 units.

Diphtheria, Tetanus, and Pertussis (Acellular) Vaccine (Adsorbed)
IM 0.5 mL: 3 primary doses at 6, 10, and 14 wk or 2, 3, and 4 mo age followed by boosters at 1½ yr and between 4½ and 5 yr age.

Diphtheria, Tetanus, and Pertussis (Whole Cell) Vaccine (Adsorbed)
IM 0.5 mL; 3 primary doses at 6, 10, and 14 wk or 2, 3, and 4 mo age followed by boosters at 1½ yr and between 4½ and 5 yr age.

Diphtheria, Tetanus, Acellular Pertussis, and Inactivated Poliomyelitis Vaccine (Adsorbed)
IM 0.5 mL: Given at 6, 10, and 14 wk and 1½ and 4½-5 yr boosters.

Diphtheria, Tetanus, Pertussis (Whole Cell), and Hib Vaccine (Adsorbed)
IM 0.5 mL; Given at 6, 10, and 14 wk. If Hib vaccine not given in infancy, it may be given at 1½ yr.

Dipyridamole
Antiplatelet: PO: *1 mo to 12 yr:* 1-2 mg/kg per dose tid; *12-18 yr:* 100-200 mg/dose tid before food (avoid antacids).

Kawasaki disease: PO: *1 mo to 12 yr:* 3 mg/kg in 3 div. doses.

Dithranol
Topical: Apply on a daily basis, leaving on for 20-30 minutes depending on the preparation being used, and then remove by washing off. Always commence treatment with 0.1%, continuing for at least 1 wk, and increasing if necessary to 0.25%, 0.5%, 1%, and 2%. Build up gradually over 4 wk to the highest tolerated strength that gives the best effect. Apply evenly and sparingly to lesions.

Dobutamine Hydrochloride
Continuous IV infusion 5-15 μg/kg/min increased to a max. of 20 μg/kg/min in newborn (side effects more) and rarely up to 40 μg/kg/min in older children if necessary. Correct hypovolemia prior to administration. Adjust the rate of infusion to desired response. Dose may be increased every 10-30 minutes if necessary, up to a max. dose of 40 μg/kg/min. Titrate to discontinue. Infusion should be gradually tapered after 48-72 hr of administration. In cases with low BP, dopamine or noradrenaline infusion may be used concomitantly with dobutamine.

Docusate Sodium
<3 yr: 10-40 mg/24 hr in 1-4 div. doses, *3-6 yr:* 20-60 mg/24 hr in 1-4 div. doses, *6-12 yr:* 40-150 mg/24 hr, *>12 yr:* 50-400 mg/24 hr.

Domperidone
Gastroesophageal reflux and gastric stasis: PO *1 mo-12 yr:* 200-400 μg/kg/dose 3-4 times daily before food and at night. Not often used <2 yr.

Radiotherapy/chemotherapy induced vomiting: PO 1 mo-12 yr: 200-400 μg/kg as a single dose. Could give once in 4-8 hr.

Dopamine Hydrochloride

Continuous low-dose IV infusion for renal effect 2–5 μg/kg/min. *IV infusion in newborn:* Start at 3 μg/kg/min and increase as clinically indicated to max. of 20 μg/kg/min IV infusion; *1 mo–18 yr:* 5–20 g/kg/min.

Dornase Alfa [Phosphorylated Glycosylated Recombinant Human Deoxyribonuclease 1 (rhDNase)]

Inhalation of nebulized solution: Child 5–17 yr: 2,500 units OD, administered by jet nebulizer. Dornase alfa 1,000 units is equivalent to 1 mg.

Dothiepin (Dosulepin Hydrochloride)

PO 12–18 yr: 50–75 mg at bedtime or in div. doses. Increase gradually as needed up to 150 mg/day. In hospital setting, max. 225 mg/day may be used.

Doxapram

IV loading dose 2.5 mg/kg over 5–10 min. IV infusion 300 μg/kg/hr (max. 1.5 mg/kg/hr – side effects if infused for >36 hr). PO 6 mg/kg per dose qid after an IV dose.

Doxorubicin Hydrochloride

Always consult the current treatment protocol for details of dosage and scheduling. *Children:* 35–75 mg/m^2/dose, repeat every 21 days; or 20–30 mg/m^2, repeat every week; or 60–90 mg/m^2, given as continuous infusion over 96 hr once in 3–4 wk.

Hepatic impairment: Reduce dose. If bilirubin 1.2–3 mg reduce by 50% and if bilirubin >3 mg reduce dose by 75%.

Doxycycline

Amebiasis, actinomycosis, brucellosis: >8 yr: 45 kg or less: Initial dose: 4.4 mg/kg IV on the first day, given in 1 or 2 infusions; Maintenance dose: 2.2–4.4 mg/kg IV/day, given in 1 or 2 infusions, depending on the severity of the infection. *>45 kg:* Initial dose: 200 mg IV on the first day, given in 1 or 2 infusions Maintenance dose: 100–200 mg IV/day, depending on the severity of the infection; 200 mg may be given in 1 or 2 infusions PO: *45 kg or less:* Initial dose: 4.4 mg/kg PO on the first day, given in 2 div. doses Maintenance dose: 2.2 mg/kg PO/day, given once a day or in 2 div. doses. More severe infections: Up to 4.4 mg/kg PO/day. *>45 kg:* Initial dose: 200 mg PO on the first day, given in 2 or 4 div. doses; Maintenance dose: 100 mg PO/day, given once a day or in 2 div. doses.

More severe infections: 100 mg PO every 12 hr.

Acne: Initial dose: 100 mg PO bid for 3–6 wk or until improvement occurs. Maintenance dose: 50–150 mg PO OD.

Cholera: Single dose of 4 mg/kg (max. 200 mg).

Multidrug-resistant P. falciparum (resistant to both chloroquine and sulfadoxine-pyrimethamine): With Quinine at 3.5 mg/kg once a day for 7 days.

Malaria prophylaxis – short-term chemoprophylaxis (<6 wk): 100 mg daily in adults and 1.5 mg/kg body weight for children > 8 yr old. The drug should be started 2 days before travel and continued for 4 wk after leaving the malarious area.

Uncomplicated urethral, endocervical, or rectal infections due to C. trachomatis: 8 yr or older: 100 mg PO twice a day for 7 days.

Uncomplicated gonorrhea: 100 mg PO bid for 7 days

Periodontitis: 20 mg PO bid for up to 9 mo.

Plague: 8 yr or older: <45 kg: 2.2 mg/kg IV bid (max. 200 mg/day); *45 kg or more:* 100 mg IV twice a day. *Duration of therapy:* 10 days (or until 2 days after fever subsides).

Mycoplasma pneumonia: 100 mg PO or IV every 12 hr for 10–21 days.

Rocky mountain spotted fever, relapsing fever, or typhus: 100 mg PO or IV twice a day for 7 days

Trachoma: 100 mg PO twice a day for 7 days.

*Tularemia:*100 mg PO or IV twice a day for 14–21 days.

Anthrax postexposure prophylaxis: <45 kg: 2.2 mg/kg PO or IV twice a day; *45 kg or more:* 100 mg PO or IV twice a day. *Total duration of therapy:* 60 days after exposure.

E

Ebastine

6–18 yr: 5–10 mg OD. Both doses significantly reduce the histamine-induced wheal-and-flare areas for up to 28 hr compared with predose values.

Econazole

Apply 2–3 times daily continuing for 14 days after lesions have healed.

Edrophonium Chloride

Myasthenia gravis – for diagnosis: IV: *Birth to 12 yr:* 20 μg/kg followed 30 sec later (if no adverse reaction noted) by remaining dose of 80 μg/kg; *12–18 yr:* 2 mg and then 8 mg.

Cholinergic drug – to differentiate between under- and overdosing: IV given 1 hr after cholinergic. *1 mo–12 yr* 20 μg/kg; *12–18 yr:* 2 mg. In underdosing, muscle strength increases transiently and in overdosing muscle strength decreases transiently.

Nondepolarizing muscular blockade antagonist: IV *1 mo–18 yr:* 500–700 μg/kg slowly over several minutes along with 7 μg/kg of atropine.

Efavirenz

Treatment of HIV infection: PO: *≥3 yr, 32.5–39.9 kg:* 400 mg, *25–32.4 kg:* 350 mg, *20–24.9 kg:* 300 mg, *15–19.9 kg:* 250 mg,

10–14.9 kg: 200 mg, ≥*40 kg:* 600 mg OD at bedtime. For children who can swallow capsules, combine efavirenz with either (1) zidovudine plus lamivudine, emtricitabine, or didanosine or (2) didanosine plus lamivudine or emtricitabine. *Adolescents >40 kg:* 600 mg PO OD at bedtime. Combine efavirenz with either lamivudine or emtricitabine plus either zidovudine or tenofovir.

Enalapril
Neonate: PO 0.1 mg/kg/24 hr in 1–2 doses (max. 0.4 mg/kg/24 hr); IV 5–10 μg/kg/dose every 8–24 hr. *1 mo–12 yr:* PO 0.1–0.5 mg/kg/24 hr in 1–2 doses; IV 5–10 μg/kg/dose every 8–24 hr. *12–18 yr:* PO 2.5–5 mg/24 hr and titrate to max. 40 mg/24 hr in 2 div. doses; IV 0.625–1.25 mg/dose qid (max. 20 mg/24 hr).

Antiproteinuric: Infant and child: 0.1–0.6 mg/kg/24 hr PO, increase p.r.n. over 2 wks, up to 5 mg/24 hr in 2–4 div doses. IV: 0.005–0.01 mg/kg/dose 3–4 times/day, administer over 5 min, up to 5.0 mg 6 hrly may be tolerated for up to 36 hr. Onset of action within 15 min.

Enoxaparin
Prophylaxis: SC *<2 mo:* 1.5 mg/kg/day and *>2 mo:* 1 mg/kg/day in 2 div. doses (max. 40 mg/day).

Treatment: <2 mo: 3 mg/kg/day and *>2 mo:* 2 mg/ kg/day in 2 div. doses.

Ephedrine Hydrochloride
Intranasal 1–2 drops in each nostril 3–4 times daily (15 min before feeds) for max. of 7 days.

Epinephrine
See Adrenaline.

Epoprostenol (Prostacyclin)
Neonate: IV infusion 20 ng/kg/min (max. 40 ng/kg/min) – monitor for systemic hypotension. *Children:* IV infusion 2 ng/kg/min (max. 40 ng/kg/ min) – monitor for systemic hypotension.

Ergocalciferol (Calciferol, Vitamin D2)
Nutritional vitamin-D deficiency rickets: PO: *<6 mo:* 3,000 units daily; dose to be adjusted as necessary; *6 mo–11 yr:* 6,000 units daily, dose to be adjusted as necessary; *12–17 yr:* 10,000 units daily, dose to be adjusted as necessary.

Nutritional or physiological supplement; Prevention of rickets: PO: *neonate:* 400 units daily; *child:* 400–600 units daily.

Vitamin D deficiency in intestinal malabsorption or in chronic liver disease: PO/IM: *1–11 yr:* 10,000–25,000 units daily, dose to be adjusted as necessary; *12–17 yr:* 10,000–40,000 units daily, dose to be adjusted as necessary.

Erythromycin
General indications: Neonates: PO/IV: <7 days age 20 mg/kg/day bid; *>7 days <1,200 g:* 20 mg/kg/day bid; *>7 days >1,200 g:* 30 mg/kg/day 3–4 times daily. *Children:* PO; 30–50 mg/kg/day in 3–4 div. doses max. 250 mg qid may be given. *12–18 yr:* 250–500 mg qid. IV; *1 mo–18 yr:* 12.5 mg/kg/dose qid or as a continuous infusion. Max. dose: 4 g/day. Replace by PO dosage as soon as possible.

Secondary prevention of rheumatic fever: When child is sensitive to penicillin – PO 20 mg/kg/day max. 500 mg bid (contraindicated in liver disorder).

Chlamydia trachomatis pneumonia in infants and neonates: PO 50 mg/kg/day (erythromycin base) in 4 div. doses for 14 days.

Ophthalmia neonatorum caused by C. trachomatis: Neonates: PO 50 mg/kg/day in four div. doses for 14 days. If chlamydial conjunctivitis recurs after discontinuing therapy, the erythromycin dosage regimen should be repeated.

Beta-hemolytic streptococcal (GAS) pharyngitis (primary rheumatic fever prophylaxis as an alternative to penicillin in children allergic to penicillin): 40 mg/kg/day in 4 div. doses × 10 days.

Uncomplicated urethral, endocervical, or rectal gonorrhea, penicillinase-producing Neisseria gonorrhoeae, or for gonorrhea during pregnancy: Adolescent: 500 mg PO qid for 7 days.

Treatment and postexposure pertussis prophylaxis (For postexposure prophylaxis, administer to close contacts within 3 wk of exposure, especially in high-risk patients, e.g., women in 3rd trimester, infants < 12 mo): PO: *infants, children, and adolescents:* 40–50 mg/kg/day (max. 2 g/day) in 4 div. doses for 14 days. *For neonates:* Azithromycin is preferred. If azithromycin is unavailable, erythromycin 40–50 mg/kg/day PO in 4 div. doses may be used. Monitor for infantile hypertrophic pyloric stenosis.

Pneumococcal prophylaxis: 1 mo to 2 yr: 250 mg/day, *2–8 yr:* 500 mg/day, >*9 yr:* 1 g/day in 2 div. doses.

Gastric stasis: PO/IV: *1 mo to 18 yr:* 3 mg/kg qid.

Erythropoietin (Recombinant Human Epoetin)
Start at 50–300 U/kg/dose thrice/week. For children receiving hemodialysis: Up to 450 U/kg/dose 2–3 times/wk. 25–100 units/kg SC/IV 3 times in a week. Monitor the hemoglobin (Hb) at least twice weekly after drug initiation until the Hb stabilizes.

Eslicarbazepine Acetate (ESL)
Adjunctive therapy of focal seizures with or without secondary generalization: PO: *6–17 yr (up to 60 kg):* initially 10 mg/kg OD, then increased in steps of 10 mg/kg daily, every 1–2 wk, and increased, if necessary, up to 30 mg/kg daily (max. per dose 1.2 g); *6–17 yr (60 kg and above):* initially 400 mg OD

for 1–2 wk and then increased to 800 mg OD (max. per dose 1.2 g).

Reduce initial dose in renal impairment to 5 mg/kg OD or 10 mg/kg every other day for 2 wk; then increase to 10 mg/kg OD if CrCl 30–60 mL/min and avoid using if it is <30 mL/min.

Esomeprazole

Nonsteroidal anti-inflammatory drug (NSAID)-associated duodenal ulcer or NSAID-associated gastric ulcer: PO: *Child (weight up to 30 kg):* 0.5–1 mg/kg OD (max. per dose 15 mg OD), doses to be taken in the morning; *Child (weight 30 kg and above):* 15–30 mg OD, doses to be taken in the morning.

Gastroesophageal reflux disease (GERD): PO: *Child (weight up to 30 kg):* 0.5–1 mg/kg OD (max. per dose 15 mg OD), doses to be taken in the morning; *child (weight 30 kg and above):* 15–30 mg OD, doses to be taken in the morning.

Acid-related dyspepsia: PO: *Child (weight up to 30 kg)*: 0.5–1 mg/kg OD (max. per dose 15 mg OD), doses to be taken in the morning; *Child (weight 30 kg and above):* 15–30 mg OD, doses to be taken in the morning.

Fat malabsorption despite pancreatic enzyme replacement therapy in cystic fibrosis: PO: *Child (weight up to 30 kg):* 0.5–1 mg/kg OD (max. per dose 15 mg OD), doses to be taken in the morning; *Child (weight 30 kg and above):* 15–30 mg OD, doses to be taken in the morning.

Patients with hepatic impairment: No dosage adjustment is recommended for mild-to-moderate hepatic impairment. However, in patients with severe hepatic insufficiency, do not exceed 20 mg/day.

Intermittent hemodialysis: No dosage adjustment is necessary. Due to high protein binding, esomeprazole is not expected to be removed by hemodialysis.

Estriol (Topical)

Apply to area of adhesion/fusion (in symptomatic cases) 1–2 times daily for 2–6 wks. Once the adhesions start to separate, the application frequency can be decreased and application of an emollient added.

Etanercept

All patients should have their varicella antibody status measured before commencing treatment. Siblings should be considered for varicella immunization prior to commencement of treatment of the patient.

Ethambutol

20–25 mg/kg/day (max. 1500 mg/day)

Tuberculosis: Daily regimen: 20 mg/kg as a single morning dose (range 15–25 mg/kg; max. dose 1500 mg/day). *Intermittent regimen:* 30 mg/kg (range 25–30 mg/kg).

Ethinyl Estradiol

Induction of puberty: 12–18 yr: 2 μg daily once. Increase every 6 mo – 5, 10, and then 20 μg. Add progestogen after 18–24 mo. Maintenance 20 μg combined with progestogen.

Prevention of tall stature: PO 20–50 μg before 12 yr age.

Priming for GH test in girls with bone age > 10 yr: PO 100 μg, as a single dose for 3 days prior to test (diethylstilbestrol 1 mg twice is alternative for boys and girls).

Ethionamide

Tuberculosis: PO 15–20 mg/kg/day in 2 div. doses. Max. 1 g/day.

Ethosuximide

PO: Start with 5 mg/kg in *2–12 yr old* and 250 mg *in older children.* Increase at 2.5 mg/kg/dose taking 2–3 wk to reach maintenance of 10–20 mg/kg/dose in 2–12 yr old and 500–750 g/dose (max. 1 g) bid.

Etoricoxib

Osteoarthritis: Only for 16–18 yr age: PO 30 mg OD; increased if necessary to 60 mg OD.

Rheumatoid arthritis and ankylosing spondylitis: 90 mg OD.

Acute gout: 120 mg OD for max. 8 days.

Hepatic impairment: Max. 60 mg daily in mild impairment; max. 60 mg on alternate days or 30 mg OD in moderate impairment.

Renal impairment: Avoid if estimated GFR < 30 mL/min/1.73 m^2.

Everolimus

Adjunctive treatment of refractory partial-onset seizures, with or without secondary generalization, associated with tuberous sclerosis complex: *2–17 yr:* dose to be in consultation with experts.

>1 yr of age to treat subependymal giant cell astrocytoma (SEGA) brain tumors and in children older than 2 yr of age to treat partial-onset seizures: The starting dose is 4.5 mg/m^2 OD; max. up to 10 mg.

F

Factor IX

20–25 units/kg dose up to OD. In factor VIII inhibitor patients 75–100 units/kg/dose up to 6 hrly.

Factor VIII

The required dosage may be estimated using the following formula as a guide: Number of factor VIII units required = Body weight (kg) × desired increase (international units) in factor VIII 0.5 (% of normal).

Famotidine

Infants and children: <16 yr: PO/IV.

Peptic ulcer: 0.5 mg/kg/day at bedtime or in 2 div. doses (max. 40 mg/day).

GERD: PO 1 mg/kg/day in 2 div. doses (max. 80 mg/day) or 20 mg bid for up to 6 wks. *16–18 yr:* IV 20 mg 12 hrly.

Duodenal/gastric ulcer: 20 mg/day at bedtime or 10 mg bid for 4–8 wk - max. 40 mg/day.

Hypersecretory conditions: 20 mg 6 hrly and may gradually increase up to 160 mg 6 hrly.

Esophagitis: 20–40 mg bid for up to 12 wks.

Dose adjustment in renal impairment: CrCl 10–50 mL/min: administer normal dose OD or 50% of dose at normal dose interval. CrCl < 10 mL/min; administer normal dose once in 36–48 hr.

Felbamate

Children 2–14 yr with Lennox-Gestaut syndrome: Adjunct therapy - initially 15 mg/kg/day in 3–4 div. doses and increase in 15 mg/kg/day increments at weekly intervals till response is obtained; max. 45 mg/kg/day or 3,600 mg/day whichever is less.

Children > 14 yr: Adjunct therapy: Initially 1,200 mg/day in 3–4 div. doses and increase daily dose by 1,200 mg once every week to max. of 3,600 mg/day.

Conversion to monotherapy: Initially 1,200 mg/day in 3–4 div. doses and from week 2, increase daily dose by 1,200 mg once every week to a max. of 3,600 mg/day. *Decrease dose of other anticonvulsants* by one-third original dose when felbamate is started and at wk 2, when felbamate dose is increased. Continue to reduce other anticonvulsants as clinically indicated.

Fentanyl

For pain relief: Neonates and infants: IV 1–4 µg/kg/dose, repeat every 2–4 hr or continuous infusion 0.5–5 µg/kg/hr. *1–12 yr:* IM/IV 1–3 µg/kg/dose, repeat every 30–60 min or continuous infusion 1–5 µg/kg/hr. *12–18 yr:* 0.5–1 µg/kg/dose, repeat every 30–60 min.

Anesthesia: IV/IM 2–50 µg/kg.

Fexofenadine Hydrochloride

Seasonal allergic rhinitis: PO: *2–11 yr:* 30 mg, *12–18 yr:* 60 mg bid/120 mg OD.

Chronic idiopathic urticaria: PO: *6 mo to 2 yr:* 15 mg, *2–11 yr:* 30 mg bid; *12–18 yr:* 180 mg OD.

For patients with decreased renal function, the recommended starting dose: 2–11 yr: 30 mg OD; 6 mo < *2 yr:* 15 mg OD

Flecainide Acetate

Supraventricular arrhythmias: PO: Modified-release preparation: *child 12–17 yr:* 200 mg daily.

Resistant re-entry supraventricular tachycardia, ventricular ectopic beats or ventricular tachycardia, arrhythmias associated with accessory conduction pathways (e.g., Wolff-Parkinson-White syndrome), paroxysmal atrial fibrillation: PO: *immediate-release preparation, neonate:* 2 mg/kg 2–3 times a day, adjust according to response, also adjust dose according to plasma flecainide concentration. *Child 1 mo to 11 yr:* 2 mg/kg 2–3 times a day, max. 8 mg/kg/day; max. 300 mg/day. *Child 12–17 yr:* Initially 50–100 mg bid; increased if necessary up to 300 mg daily, max. 400 mg daily for ventricular arrhythmias in heavily built children. *Initially by slow IV injection or by IV infusion: Neonate:* initially 1–2 mg/kg, dose to be given over 10–30 minutes, followed by (continuous IV infusion) 100–250 µg/kg/hr if required until arrhythmia is controlled; transfer patient to PO treatment following IV treatment. *Child 1 mo to 11 yr:* Initially 2 mg/kg, dose to be given over 10–30 minutes, followed by (continuous IV infusion) 100–250 µg/kg/hr if required until arrhythmia is controlled, max. cumulative dose of 600 mg in the first 24 hr, transfer patient to PO treatment following IV treatment. *Child 12–17 yr:* Initially 2 mg/kg (max. per dose 150 mg), dose to be given over 10–30 minutes, followed by (continuous IV infusion) 1.5 mg/kg/hr if required for 1 hr, then (by continuous IV infusion) reduced to 100–250 µg/kg/hr until arrhythmia controlled, max. cumulative dose of 600 mg in the first 24 hr, transfer patient to PO treatment following IV treatment.

Drug interactions: Reduce dose by half with concurrent use of amiodarone. Patients stabilized on 200 mg daily immediate-release flecainide may be transferred to modified-release medicines.

Hepatic impairment: Avoid or reduce dose in severe impairment. Monitor plasma-flecainide concentration.

Renal impairment: Reduce dose by 25–50% if estimated GFR <35 mL/min/1.73 m^2. Monitor plasma-flecainide concentration. Monitoring plasma-flecainide concentration for optimal response 200–800 µg/L; blood sample should be taken immediately before the next dose. With IV use, ECG monitoring and resuscitation facilities must be available.

Flucloxacillin

Infections due to beta-lactamase-producing staphylococci including otitis externa, adjunct in pneumonia, impetigo, cellulitis: PO: *Neonate < 7 days:* 25 mg/kg bid; *7–20 days:* 25 mg/kg tid; *21–28 days:* 25 mg/kg qid. *1 mo to 1 yr:* 62.5–125 mg qid; *2–9 yr:* 125–250 mg qid; *10–17 yr:* 250–500 mg qid. *Slow IV/IV infusion: neonate < 7 days:* 25 mg/kg IV 12 hrly; *7–20 days:* 25 mg/kg 8 hrly; *21–28 days:* 25 mg/kg 6 hrly. IM/

IV *child:* 12.5–25 mg/kg 6 hrly (max. IM/dose 500 mg; IV/dose 1 g).

Severe infection: Give IV/IV infusion – double dose for neonates and child (max. IV/dose for child – 2 g).

Endocarditis (in combination with other antibacterial if necessary): Slow IV/IV infusion: *child:* 50 mg/kg 6 hrly (max. IV/dose 2 g).

Osteomyelitis, cerebral abscess, and staphylococcal meningitis: Slow IV/IV infusion: *neonate <7 days:* 50–100 mg/kg IV 12 hrly; *7–20 days:* 50–100 mg/kg 8 hrly; *21–28 days:* 50–100/kg 6 hrly. *Child:* 50 mg/kg 6 hrly (max. IV/dose 2 g).

Staphylococcal lung infection in cystic fibrosis: PO: *child:* 25 mg/kg qid (max. per dose 1 g), alternatively 100 mg/kg daily in 3 div. doses; max. 4 g/day. Slow IV/IV infusion: *child:* 50 mg/kg 6 hrly (max. per dose 2 g).

Prevention of Staphylococcus aureus lung infection in cystic fibrosis-primary prevention: PO: *neonate:* 125 mg bid; *1 mo–3 yr:* 125 mg bid.

Prevention of S. aureus lung infection in cystic fibrosis-secondary prevention: PO: *child:* 50 mg/kg bid (max. per dose 1 g).

Renal failure: With IV use, accumulation of electrolytes can occur in patients with renal failure. Use normal dose every 8 hr if estimated GFR < 10 mL/min/1.73 m^2.

Fluconazole

Newborn: Systemic candidiasis and cryptococcosis: PO/IV: 6–12 mg/kg every 72 hr in <14 day, every 48 hr in 14–28 day, and every 24 hr in >28 day olds.

Mucosal candidiasis: 3 mg/kg in the same intervals. *Children:* PO/IV loading dose 6 mg/kg followed by 3 mg/kg OD for 7–14 days.

Systemic candidiasis and cryptococcosis: 6–12 mg/kg daily once (max. 400 mg). Dose dependent on the severity of infection.

Prophylaxis of fungal infection in immunocompromised: 3–12 mg/kg OD (max. 400 mg); dose dependent on the extent and duration of neutropenia.

Flucytosine

Systemic yeast and fungal infections along with amphotericin in severe systemic candidiasis and other severe or long-standing infections: Newborn: IV/PO 50 mg/kg q12 hr. *Children:* IV/PO 50 mg/kg every 6 hr. Treatment is usually not for >2 wk.

In renal impairment: CrCl in mL/min/1.73 m^2 – 20–40, 50% daily dose in 2 div. doses; 10–20, 25% of daily dose OD; <10, 50 mg/kg as a single dose and adjust dose according to serum levels.

Fludrocortisone Acetate

Adrenal insufficiency: PO *replacement therapy*: 50–200 μg/OD according to potassium and/or plasma renin activity levels. Higher doses are usually required in the neonatal period. (Start with 100 μg OD and increase up to 200 μg daily.)

Sweat test: 3 mg/m^2 single dose on 2 consecutive days prior to sweat test.

Cerebral salt wasting: Start with 100 μg daily and increase up to 200–300 μg according to response.

Flumazenil

IV bolus over 15 sec: *<12 yr:* 10 μg/kg (max. 200 μg) and *>12 yr:* 200 μg as a single dose, repeated every min to max. total dose of 40 μg/kg. IV infusion *<12 yr:* 2–10 μg/kg/hr (max. 400 μg dose/hr) and *>12 yr;* 100–400 μg/kg/hr.

Flunarizine

PO: *3–12 yr:* 5 mg and *>12 yr:* 10 mg daily once. Dose reduction required in liver impairment.

Flunisolide

Intranasal: *5–12 yr:* 1 spray in each nostril up to 3 times daily, *12–18 yr:* 2 sprays in each nostril up to 2–3 times daily.

Fluoride (Sodium Fluoride, Stannous Fluoride)

PO: Drops and tablets (where water fluoride conc. <0.3 ppm/300 μg/L): *6 mo to 3 yr:* 250 μg F/day, *3–6 yr:* 500 μg F/day, *>6 yr:* 1 mg F/day. Doses are expressed as fluoride ion (F). If water fluoride conc. 0.3–0.7 ppm, use ½ dose in *>3-yr-olds* and no fluoride required in *<3-yr-olds.* Gel *(for children > 3-yr-*old): Apply with toothbrush over all surfaces of tooth after normal cleansing with toothpaste. Then gently rub over the tooth surface for 1 min before spitting out excess. No food/drink for 30 min after use for best effect.

Fluoxetine

Depression: PO: *6–18 yr:* 10 mg OD, gradually increase over 3 wk to 20 mg OD.

Bulimia: PO: *12–18 yr:* 60 mg OD.

Obsessive-compulsive disorder (OCD) and anxiety: PO: 6–8 yr 10 mg and *8–18 yr:* 20 mg OD. Gradually increase by 10–20 mg increments once in 2 wk if required (max. 60 mg/day).

Idiopathic musculoskeletal pain: 8–12 yr: 10 mg and *12–18 yr:* 20 mg OD.

Fluticasone Propionate

Inhalation: 2–4 yr: 50–100 μg, *4–16 yr:* 50–200 μg, *>16 yr:* 100 μg – 1 mg bid. *Starting dose* appropriate for severity of disease, adjusted to attain control and then reduced to minimal effective dose according to individual response.

Nebulization: 1 mg bid for *acute exacerbation of asthma.*

Intranasal: 4–12 yr 50 μg (1 spray) in each nostril, 100 μg (2 sprays) in each nostril bid for *allergic rhinitis.*

Treatment of psoriasis: Patients respond preferentially to the 0.005% ointment.

Treatment of eczema: Fluticasone cream 0.05% applied OD is as effective as bid application. *Children and infants 3 mo of age or more:* Fluticasone cream 0.05% applied sparingly to the affected area OD or bid.

Atopic dermatitis: Only fluticasone cream 0.05% has been approved for the treatment of atopic dermatitis in this population. In clinical trials, the 0.05% cream has been applied OD to children for the treatment of atopic dermatitis for up to 4 wk.

Fluticasone/Salmeterol

Aerosol inhaler starting with 125 μg and taper to 50 μg of fluticasone and double dose of DPI.

Fluvoxamine Maleate

PO: *6–18 yr:* 25–50 mg after food bid; *12–18 yr:* 100 mg OD: increasing to max. doses of 300 mg/day needs to be under expert supervision as Indian children tolerate lesser doses than in the West.

Folic Acid

Supplementation in folate deficiency in child; cofactor in metabolic disorders, e.g., homocystinuria: Birth–12 yr: 250 μg/kg; *12–18 yr:* 5–10 mg, OD for 6 mo if cause correctable and lifelong if uncorrectable.

Megaloblastic anemia due to folate deficiency: PO: *newborn:* 1 mg, *<1 yr:* 500 μg/kg, *1–18 yr:* 5 mg daily once for 4 mo.

Hemolytic anemias: PO: *<12 yr:* 2.5 mg; *12–18 yr:* 10 mg OD.

To limit methotrexate-associated side effects when it is used for juvenile idiopathic arthritis: PO: *2–18 yr:* 1 mg OD. Dose may be omitted on the day methotrexate is given. May be given 5 mg weekly or twice weekly.

Preterm babies fed heat-treated human milk may benefit from a 500 μg supplement once a week unless a suitable breastmilk fortifier is used. Supplementation has no impact on the risk of anemia developing in other term or preterm breast or formula-fed babies.

Formaldehyde

Lotion: Apply topically at night as a soak. *Gel:* Apply bid directly to the wart and cover with plaster. Remove the outer dead layers with an emery board or pumice stone as the treatment progresses.

Formoterol Fumarate

Aerosol inhaler/turbohaler > 6 yr: 6–12 μg 1–2 times daily; *DPI:* 12 μg 1–2 times daily. For regular prophylactic use, increase up to 24 μg twice in a day in severe obstruction.

Foscarnet Sodium

Cytomegalovirus (CMV) disease: Retinitis (ganciclovir resistant/immunocompromised patient): IV infusion 1 mo to 8 yr induction 60 mg/kg tid for 2–3 wk and then maintenance 60 mg/kg OD, increased to 90–120 mg/kg if tolerated; if disease progresses on maintenance dose, repeat induction regimen.

Mucocutaneous herpes simplex infection (acyclovir resistant or in immunocompromised patient): IV infusion *1 mo to 18 yr:* 40 mg/kg tid for 2–3 wk or until lesions heal.

Fosphenytoin

Generalized, convulsive status epilepticus or acute tonic-clonic seizures: Adolescents: in patients with unknown, undetectable, or low phenytoin concentrations (i.e., ≤10 μg/mL), the usual loading dose of fosphenytoin is 15–20 mg PE (phenytoin equivalence)/kg IV; not to exceed 150 mg PE/min IV rate.

If seizures are not terminated after the initial loading dose, consider additional anticonvulsants. Some experts give an additional dose of 5–10 mg PE/kg IV if the initial loading dose fails to terminate seizures; max. total loading dose 30 mg PE/kg. The initial maintenance dose is 4–6 mg PE/kg/day IV or IM, div. into 2 or more doses.

Children <12 yr and infants: In patients with unknown, undetectable, or low (i.e. ≤10 μg/mL) phenytoin concentrations, the usual loading dose of fosphenytoin is 15–20 mg PE/kg IV, not to exceed 3 mg PE/kg/min (max: 150 mg PE/ min) IV rate. If seizures are not terminated after the initial loading dose, consider additional anticonvulsants. The initial maintenance dose is 4–6 mg PE/kg/day IV or IM, div. into 2 or more doses.

As a phenytoin substitute when oral phenytoin administration is not possible or when oral phenytoin dosing is inappropriate for the maintenance treatment of tonic-clonic seizures or for partial seizures with complex symptomatology: Adolescents: fosphenytoin, given IV or IM, can be substituted for oral phenytoin sodium at the same total daily dose and frequency. If IV, give no faster than 150 mg PE/min (no faster than 3 mg PE/kg/min - max: 150 mg PE/min in *children < 12 yr*). The daily dose may need to be div. into 2 or more doses to maintain seizure control.

Seizure prophylaxis or for seizure treatment during neurosurgery - Adolescents: The loading dose is 10–20 mg PE/kg IV or IM; if IV give no faster than 150 mg PE/min. The rate of IV administration should not exceed 150 mg PE/min. The initial maintenance dose is 4–6 mg PE/kg/day IV or IM, div. into 2 or more doses. In controlled clinical trials, IM fosphenytoin was administered as a single daily dose using 1 or 2 injection sites, but study was limited to 5 days of treatment. *Children < 12 yr:* The loading dose of fosphenytoin is 10–20 mg PE/kg IV or IM. If IV, give no faster than 3 mg PE/kg/min (max: 150 mg PE/min). The initial maintenance dose is 4–6 mg PE/kg/day IV or IM, div. into 2 or more doses.

Framycetin Sulfate
Eye drops: 1–2 drops 2 hrly and reducing gradually as infection gets controlled to 48 hr after the eye is clinically normal.

Eye ointment: Tid when given alone or at bedtime along with eye drops given during the day.

Cream: Apply 1–3 times daily.

Frusemide
PO: *Newborn:* 1–2 mg/kg/day in 2 div. doses; *1 mo to 12 yr:* 1–2 mg/kg/dose, *12–18 yr*: 20–40 mg/dose 2–3 times daily. IV bolus: *Birth to 12 yr:* 0.5–1 mg/kg; *12–18 yr:* 20–40 mg as a single dose (max: 4 mg/kg). Dose could be repeated every 8 hr. Continuous infusion may be better and safer in acute heart failure and in postoperative setting. The dose does not need to be adjusted in renal or hepatic impairment.

Furazolidone
PO: *1 mo to 12 yr:* 6 mg/kg/day in 4 div. doses; *12–18 yr:* 400 mg/day in 4 div. doses. 7–10 days for giardiasis and for 4–6 days after defervescence in typhoid fever.

G

Granulocyte-Colony Stimulating Factor (G-CSF; Filgrastim)
Prevention of febrile neutropenia: 5 g/kg/day, commencing the day after chemotherapy and finishing after 10–14 days, when the postnadir neutrophil level has reached 10×10^9/L. G-CSF is repeated with each cycle of chemotherapy.

Bone marrow transplantation (BMT): Starting dose of 20–30 µg/kg/day, commencing within 24 hr of the marrow infusion, and tapering the dose according to neutrophil levels during the postnadir neutrophil recovery.

Severe chronic congenital neutropenia: 6 µg/kg SC bid. Titrate dose based on the child's absolute neutrophil count (ANC). The target ANC is 1,500–10,000/mm^3; however, children may experience clinical benefit below this range. Reduce dose if ANC is persistently > 10,000/mm^3. Rarely may require doses ≥100 µg/kg/day.

Severe chronic cyclic neutropenia or idiopathic neutropenia: 5 µg/kg SC OD. Titrate dose based on an individual's ANC. The target ANC is 1,500–10,000/mm^3; however, patients may experience clinical benefit below this range. Reduce dose if the ANC is persistently >10,000/mm^3. Usually, a median dose of 2.1 µg/kg/day is required for cyclic neutropenia and 1.2 µg/kg/day for idiopathic neutropenia.

HIV-induced or drug therapy-induced neutropenia (e.g., ganciclovir-induced neutropenia or zidovudine-induced neutropenia) in patients with HIV disease to decrease the risk of bacterial infections: 5–10 µg/kg/day (300–600 µg/day) SC 1–3 times weekly to maintain ANCs of 2,000–10,000/mm^3 – decreased incidence of severe neutropenia and bacterial infection and allows tolerance of myelosuppressive agents (e.g., ganciclovir or zidovudine).

Gabapentin
PO: *2–12 yr:* 10 mg/kg/dose initially OD, bid on day 2 and tid on day 3 followed by maintenance of 10–20 mg/kg/dose tid. Some children tolerate weekly increments better. *12–18 yr:* Initially 300 mg OD; gradually increase as described to maintenance of 300–800 mg/dose tid.

For renal impairment (CrCl in mL/min/1.73 m^2) adjusted frequency of administration of maintenance doses for <12 yr: 30–40 = bid; 15–30 mL = OD; <15 mL = once on alternate days. On hemodialysis, give a loading dose of 8–12 mg/kg followed by 6–8 mg/kg after every 4 hr dialysis period.

Galsulfase
1 mg/kg of body weight, administered once weekly as an IV infusion over no less than 4 hr.

Gamma Benzene Hexachloride
Scabies: Apply to the whole body surface below neck. Scrub baths after 12–24 hr. If required, one more application may be repeated after a week.

Pediculosis: Massage scalp with emulsion at night and cover with a piece of cloth. The following morning, head bath should be taken ensuring that medication does not enter eyes.

Ganciclovir
Life or sight-threatening CMV infection in immunocompromised and prevention of CMV during immunosuppressive therapy following organ transplantation: IV infusion: *1 mo to 18 yr* initially (induction) 5 mg/kg bid for 14–21 days for treatment or for 7–14 days for prevention; maintenance (for patients at risk of relapse of retinitis), 6 mg/kg daily on 5 days/wk or 5 mg/kg daily until adequate recovery of immunity; if retinitis progresses – repeat initial induction treatment.

CMV infection of the central nervous system (CNS): IV infusion: *neonate:* 6 mg/kg every 12 hr for 6 wk.

Dose in renal impairment: GFR >55 mL/min – normal dose; GFR 10–55 mL/min 1 mg/kg IV 3 times/wk for 2 wk (induction) and then 1 mg/kg IV every 2 wk (maintenance); GFR < 10 mL/min: GFR 0.5 mg/kg IV once/week for 2 wk (induction) and then 0.5 mg/kg IV every 2 wk (maintenance).

Gastrografin
PO or rectal: *<2 yr:* 15–30 mL; *15–25 kg:* 50 mL; *>25 kg:* 100 mL. Dilute well with water. Keep the child well hydrated.

Gelatin
In hypovolemic shock: 10–20 mL/kg bolus as rapidly as possible. Repeat as necessary. In trauma, these requirements

may increase up to 40 mL/kg. At this level, replacement with whole blood should be considered.

Gentamicin

Many dose regimens exist for aminoglycosides depending on target concentration aimed for and patient groups treated. The dose regimens shown here are generally accepted initial doses and dose adjustments should be made in the light of serum concentration measurement.

Neonates: IV/IM: *< 7 days: 1,200–2,000 g:* 2.5 mg/kg once in 12–18 hr; *>2,000 g: 2.5 mg/kg* once in 12 hr; *>7 days: 1,200–2,000 g:* 2.5 mg/kg once in 8–12 hr; *>2,000 g:* 2.5 mg/kg once in 8 hr.

Extended interval dose regimen by slow IV injection or IV infusion: <32 wks gestation: 4–5 mg/kg every 35 hr; *>32 wk gestation:* 4–5 mg/kg every 24 hr. *Children <12 yr:* 7.5 mg/kg/day; *12–18 yr:* 3–6 mg/kg/day in 3 div. doses. Plasma levels done after 3–4 doses to achieve predose level of <2 mg/L and 1 hr post dose peak of 5 mg/L. Alternatively 5–7.5 mg/kg/24 hr IV OD. Plasma levels done 18–24 hr after the 1st dose to achieve a predose level of <1mg/L and 1 hr postdose peak of 16–20 mg/L. *OD dose regimen (not for endocarditis or meningitis) by IV infusion*: *Child 1 mo* to *18 yr:* initially 7 mg/kg and then adjusted according to serum-gentamicin concentration.

Intrathecal/ventricular: Preservative-free preparation: newborn: 1 mg/24 hr; *children:* 1–2 mg/24 hr.

Pseudomonal lung infection in cystic fibrosis: By inhalation of nebulized solution: Child 1 mo to 2 yr: 40 mg bid; *child 2–8 yr:* 80 mg bid; *child 8–18 yr:* 160 mg bid.

0.3% Eye drops: 1–2 drops up to 6 times/day. In severe infections, 1 drop every 15–20 min and gradually decreasing frequency as infection gets controlled till 48 hr after healing. 1.5% eye drops for severe eye infection.

Ear drops: 2–3 drops 3–4 times daily and at night; children and adults.

Gentian violet (1% solution in water)

Candidiasis, oropharyngeal and cutaneous and tenia: Apply qid to bid for 3–7 days.

Glucagon

Hypoglycemia, severe occurring during diabetes treatment: IM/SC/IV bolus: Newborn: 20 µg/kg; *2 yr and up to 25 kg:* 500 µg; *>25 kg:* 500 µg to 1 mg as a single dose. 25% glucose IV if no response in 15 min.

Hyperinsulinemia: IV infusion at 1–10 µg/kg/hr; IM/IV in <2-yr-olds: 1 mg/kg as a single dose. (stimulates insulin release)

Growth hormone testing: >1 mo: 100 µg/kg (max: 1 mg). Eat before discharge to avoid death due to rebound hypoglycemia.

Beta-blocker poisoning: 0.05–0.15 mg/kg IV bolus and then 0.05–0.1 mg/kg/hr infusion.

Glutamine

Child: 250–500 mg/kg/day of L-glutamine have been used. Up to 2 mL/kg can be used in adults; it has been used in children and 2 mL/kg is approximately equivalent to 300 mg/kg L-glutamine.

Glutaraldehyde

Topical: Remove dead skin by gentle rubbing with pumice stone before applying bid. Allow each drop to dry before the next is applied.

Glycerol (Glycerin)

Rectal: <1 yr: 1 g, *1–12 yr:* 2 g; *12–18 yr:* 4 g after moistening as single dose.

Glyceryl Trinitrate (Nitroglycerine)

IV infusion: The initial dose is 0.5 µg//kg/min IV; it is up titrated depending on the response, to a max. of 10 µg/kg/min. Monitor BP and heart rate. Tolerance may develop.

Glycine

50 mg/kg/dose tid. Dose may be increased to 200 mg/kg tid during acute episodes.

Glycopyrrolate

Premedication and intraoperative use: IM/IV: *>1 mo:* 4–8 µg/kg as single dose (max: 200 µg). Larger dose for greater and prolonged antisialogogue effect.

Antagonism of neostigmine muscarinic effect: IV: *>1 mo:* 10 µg/kg as single dose with 50 µg/kg; neostigmine to reverse residual nondepolarizing neuromuscular block.

Controlling upper airway secretions: PO 40–100 µg/kg/dose 3–4 times daily (PO dose is 10 times parenteral dose).

Sialorrhea in cerebral palsy: 0.01–0.09 mg/kg/day in 1–3 div. doses/day.

Glycopyrronium Bromide

Premedication and intraoperative use: IM/IV: *>1 mo:* 4–8 µg/kg as single dose (max: 200 µg). Larger dose for greater and prolonged antisialogogue effect.

Antagonism of neostigmine muscarinic effect: IV: *>1 mo:* 10 µg/kg as single dose with 50 µg/kg; neostigmine to reverse residual nondepolarizing neuromuscular block.

Controlling upper airway secretions: PO 40–100 µg/kg/dose 3–4 times daily (PO dose is 10 times parenteral dose).

Sialorrhea in cerebral palsy: 0.01–0.09 mg/kg/day in 1–3 div. doses/day.

GM-CSF (Molgramostim)

Newborn: Very limited studies: IV infusion over 2 hr 5 μg/kg as single dose.

Cytotoxic chemotherapy: SC 5–10 μg/kg starting 24 hr after the last dose of chemotherapy and continue for 7–10 days.

Bone marrow transplantation: IV infusion over 4–6 hr 10 μg/kg starting 24 hr the day after BMT and continue daily once till ANC is >1 × 10^9/L. Max. duration of therapy is 30 days.

Adjunct to ganciclovir therapy: SC 5 μg/kg daily once. After 5th dose, adjust dose to maintain desirable ANC.

Goserelin

3.6 mg every 4 wk or 10.8 mg every 12 wk. Injections may need to be given more frequently (e.g., every 3 wk or every 10 wk) if patients show signs of failure of hormone suppression.

Granisetron

PO: *1 mo to 12 yr:* 20 μg/kg/dose to a max. of 1 mg; *12–18 yr:* 1 mg administered 1–2 times with the first dose given 1 hr prior to starting chemotherapy. IV: *1 mo to 12 yr:* 40 μg/kg/dose to a max. of 3 mg; *12–18 yr:* 3 mg as a single dose just before administering chemotherapy. 1 more dose may be given within a 24 hr period.

Griseofulvin

1 mo to 12 yr: 10 mg/kg and *12–18 yr:* 500 mg OD.

Growth Hormone (Somatropin)

Chronic renal failure (CRF): 50 μg/kg OD SC.

Growth hormone deficiency: 25–35 μg/kg OD SC.

Intrauterine growth retardation (IUGR): 70 μg/kg OD SC.

Noonan syndrome: 35 μg/kg OD SC.

Prader-Willi syndrome: 70 μg/kg OD SC.

Turner syndrome: 50 μg/kg OD SC.

H

Haemophilus influenzae Type B Vaccine (Hib)

Given at 6–8, 10–12, and 14–16 wk of age. Children 13–48 mo and older children with asplenia who have not received the vaccine need receive only one dose to develop immunity

Haloperidol

Schizophrenia, mania, and tic disorders including Tourette syndrome: 2–12 yr: 25–50 μg/kg/day (max. 10 mg/day); *12–18 yr:* 0.5–30 mg/day (max. 60 mg/day) in 2 div. doses.

Intractable hiccup:12–18 yr 1.5 mg tid. Adjust according to response.

Nausea: 12–18 yr 0.5–2 mg 2–3 times daily.

Halothane

Induction of anesthesia inhaled through calibrated vaporizer: 1 mo to 18 yr: start with 0.5% and increase gradually as required to 2–5% mixed with O_2 or N_2O-O_2. Maintain with 0.5–2% halothane mixed with O_2, O_2–air, or N_2O-O_2.

Heme Arginate (Hematin, Human Hemin)

1 mo to 18 yr: 3 mg/kg OD (max: 250 mg daily) for 4 days. If response is inadequate, repeat 4-day course with close biochemical monitoring. Attacks of porphyria are rare in children but limited experience in tyrosinemia suggests that it is safe to use at this dose.

Heparin [Low Molecular Weight Heparin (LMWH)]

Majority of data in children is with enoxaparin. Other LMWHs are reviparin, dalteparin, and tinzaparin. Dose of enoxaparin is 1.5 mg/kg 12 hrly *for <2 mo (<5 kg)* and 1 mg 12 hrly for *older infants and children.* For preterm babies, a higher dose, up to 1.5–2 mg/kg 12 hrly, may be required.

Heparin (Standard or Unfractionated)

Thromboembolic disease and extracorporeal membrane oxygenation (ECMO): 50 units/kg IV bolus and 15–35 units/kg/hr continuous IV infusion. Maintenance dose - adjust to target activated partial thromboplastin clotting time (aPTT) or heparin level.

Catheter patency: 0.5–1 unit/mL as heparin lock. An IV bolus dose of 75–100 units/kg of heparin.

Hepatitis A and Hepatitis B Vaccines (Combined)

Primary vaccination schedule: This consists of 3 doses, the second being administered 1 mo after the first dose and the third 6 mo after the first dose (a dose in 0.5 mL of the pediatric preparation for children 1–15 yr and 1 mL of the adult preparation for those >16 yr). Once initiated, the primary course of vaccination should be completed with the same preparation.

Booster dose: There is increasing evidence that once a satisfactory serological response had been attained after hepatitis B vaccine, no boosters are necessary. Booster vaccination with the combined vaccine can be recommended from 5 yr after initiation of the primary course. If the monovalent vaccines are used as boosters, they can be administered 5 yr after initiation of the primary course for hepatitis B and 10 yr after initiation of the primary course for hepatitis A.

Hepatitis A Vaccine

Primary vaccination schedule. This consists of 2 doses, the second being administered 6 mo to 1 yr after the first dose. (A dose is 0.5 mL of the pediatric preparation for children aged 1–15 yr. An adult preparation is for those aged >16 yr.) Once initiated, the primary course of vaccination should be completed with the same preparation.

Hepatitis B Immunoglobulin (HBIG)
Baby to be given 200 IU or 40 IU/kg of HBIG immediately after birth. Accelerated course of hepatitis B vaccine to be started on opposite arm: 0.1 mo, 2 mo, and 1 yr doses given.

Hepatitis B Vaccine
This is either given at 6–8, 10–12, and 14–16 wk of age (if HbsAg negativity of mother is certain) or 0, 4–6, and 14 wk or 0, 4–6 wk, and 6 mo. Postexposure prophylaxis might require 4 doses: 0, 1 mo, 2 mo, and 1 yr (accelerated) or 0, 7 and 21 day and 1 yr (superaccelerated).

Human Albumin Solution
In hypovolemic shock: 10–20 mL/kg bolus as rapidly as possible. Repeat as necessary.

In trauma: These requirements may increase up to 40 mL/kg. At this level, replacement with whole blood should be considered.

Nephrotic syndrome: 500 mg to 1 g/kg over 4 hr.

Human Chorionic Gonadotrophin (HCG)
Short stimulation test: IM 1,500–2,000 units daily once for 3 days (testosterone and androgen profile at baseline and on 4th day).

Prolonged simulation test: IM 1,500–2,000 units twice weekly for 3 wk (testosterone and androgen profile at baseline and 4–6 days after the final dose).

Hypogonadotropic hypogonadism: IM 1,000–2,000 units twice weekly in addition to testosterone.

Prepubertal cryptorchidism: 1,000–2,000 units/m^2/dose 3 times a week for 3 wk or 500 units 3 times a week for 4–6 wk.

Human Cytomegalovirus Immunoglobulin
Doses of CMV IgG need to be individualized to suit the patient. *Prophylaxis:* 200 mg/kg *pretransplant;* 100 mg/kg on days 7, 21, 42, and 63.

Treatment: 200 mg/kg on days 1 and 7, given with appropriate antiviral therapy.

Human Normal Immunoglobulin (HNIG)
Measles and polio: IM: *<1 yr:* 250 mg, *1–2 yr:* 500 mg, 3 yr or more: 750 mg

Hepatitis A: <10 yr: 250 mg; *>10 yr:* 500 mg

Rubella in pregnancy: 750 mg.

Human Papillomavirus Vaccine (HPV)
Minimum age: 9 yr

HPV4 (Gardasil®) and HPV2 (Cervarix®) are licensed and available: 2 doses of either of the two HPV vaccines (HPV4 and HPV2) for adolescent/preadolescent girls aged 9–14 yr. The doses are administered in 0–6 mo schedule. For girls 15 yr and older and immunocompromised individuals, 3 doses are recommended. The schedule is HPV4 (0, 2, 6 mo) or HPV2 (0, 1, 6 mo). For a two-dose schedule, the minimum interval between doses should be 5 mo. The minimum acceptable interval, in a 3-dose schedule is 4 wk between dose 1 and dose 2 and 12 wk between dose 2 and dose 3.

Catch-up vaccination: Administer the vaccine series to females (either HPV2 or HPV4) at age 13 through 45 yr if not previously vaccinated.

Hyaluronidase
Infants and children: IV extravasation: SC or intradermal: Reconstitute a 150 unit vial of lyophilized powder in 1 mL NS; dilute 0.1 mL of this soln. With 0.9 mL of NS to prepare a 15 unit/mL soln. - with a 25 or 26 gauge needle, five 0.2 mL injections are made SC or intradermally into the extravasation site at the leading edge, changing the needle after each injection. *In older adolescents,* 150 units of hyaluronidase may be added to the vehicle containing the drug given IM or SC to increase its absorption and dispersion.

Hypodermolysis: SC 15 units added to each 100 mL of IV fluid administered. In premature infants and neonates, the volume of a single clysis should not exceed 25 mL/kg and the rate of administration should not exceed 2 mL/min. In children <3 yr and in >3 yr up to adolescents, the volume of a single clysis should not exceed 200 mL and maintenance IV fluid volume, respectively.

Hydralazine
PO: <12 yr: 0.75 mg/kg/day in 2–3 div. doses; *12–18 yr:* 50 mg in 2 div. doses. Increase if needed to a max. dose of 7.5 mg/kg/day or 200 mg/day.

IV bolus over 20 min: <12 yr: 100–500 µg/kg and *>12 yr:* 5–10 mg as single dose. May be repeated up to 4–6 times daily.

IV infusion: <12 yr: 12.5–50 µg/kg/hr and *>12 yr:* 3–5 mg/hr.

In hepatic and renal impairment, start with small doses or increase interval between doses.

Hydrochlorothiazide
Neonates and infants: PO 2–4 mg/kg/24 hr in 2 div. doses; *>6 mo to 12 yr:* 2 mg/kg/24 hr in 2 div. doses; *12–18 yr:* 12.5–100 mg/24 hr.

Nephrogenic diabetes insipidus: PO: *<2 yr:* 3 mg/kg and *>12 yr:* 37.5–75 mg/day in 3 div. doses.

Hydrocortisone
Acute adrenocortical insufficiency (Addisonian crisis): Initially slow IV infusion. *Neonate:* Initially 10 mg, then (by continuous IV infusion) 100 mg/m^2 daily, alternatively (by IV infusion) 100 mg/m^2 daily in div. doses, to be given every 6–8 hr; adjusted

according to response, when stable reduce over 4–5 days to PO maintenance dose. Slow IV injection or IV infusion: *1 mo to 11 yr:* Initially 2–4 mg/kg and then 2–4 mg/kg every 6 hr, adjusted according to response, when stable reduce over 4–5 days to PO maintenance dose; *12–17 yr:* 100 mg every 6–8 hr.

Congenital adrenal hyperplasia: PO: *Neonates and children:* 9–15 mg/m^2 in 3 div. doses, adjusted according to response.

Adrenal hypoplasia; Addison's disease, chronic maintenance or replacement therapy: PO: *Neonates and children:* 8–10 mg/m^2 daily in 3 div. doses, the larger dose to be given in the morning and the smaller in the evening, higher doses may be needed.

Inflammatory bowel disease – induction of remission: IV: *2–17 yr:* 2.5 mg/kg every 6 hr (max. per dose 100 mg); IV infusion: child *2–17 yr:* 10 mg/kg daily; max. 400 mg/day

Ulcerative colitis, proctitis, proctosigmoiditis: Rectally using rectal foam. *2–17 yr:* Initially 1 metered application 1–2 times a day for 2–3 wk and then reduced to 1 metered application OD on alternate days; to be inserted into the rectum.

Acute hypersensitivity reactions, angioedema: IM/IV: *1–5 mo:* initially 25 mg tid, adjusted according to response; *6 mo to 5 yr:* initially 50 mg tid, adjusted according to response; *6–11 yr:* initially 100 mg tid, adjusted according to response; *12–17 yr:* initially 200 mg tid, adjusted according to response.

Hypotension resistant to inotropic treatment and volume replacement: IV: *Neonate:* Initially 2.5 mg/kg, then 2.5 mg/kg after 4 hr if required, followed by 2.5 mg/kg every 6 hr for 48 hr or until blood pressure recovers, dose to then be reduced gradually over at least 48 hr; *child:* 1 mg/kg every 6 hr (max. per dose 100 mg).

Severe acute asthma, life-threatening acute asthma: IV as sodium succinate: *Child 1 mo to 1 yr:* 4 mg/kg every 6 hr (max. per dose 100 mg), alternatively 25 mg every 6 hr; *2–4 yr:* 4 mg/kg every 6 hr (max. per dose 100 mg), alternatively 50 mg every 6 hr; *5–17 yr:* 4 mg/kg every 6 hr (max. per dose 100 mg), alternatively 100 mg every 6 hr – for all ages, IV doses are given till conversion to PO prednisolone is possible.

Hydrocortisone 1%
Corticosteroid-responsive dermatoses: Topical: nonprescription hydrocortisone preparations should not be used in *children < 2 yr of age* unless directed and supervised by a clinician. *Children > 2 yr of age:* Apply appropriate cream, lotion, ointment, or solution sparingly 1–4 times daily.

Oral lesions: Apply a small amount of paste to the lesion 2 or 3 times daily after meals and at bedtime. If substantial regeneration or repair of oral tissues does not occur after 7 days, further investigate etiology of the lesions.

Ulcerative colitis and anorectal disorders: Retention enema: adjunctive treatment of ulcerative colitis: 100 mg nightly. Some clinicians recommend 100 mg bid followed by 100 mg nightly when improvement occurs. It is usually given for 21 days or until clinical and proctologic remissions are achieved. Lay on left side during and for 30 minutes after administration to distribute drug throughout the left colon. Retain for >1 hr, preferably all night. Symptoms may improve in 3–5 days, followed by proctologic improvement. Discontinue if clinical or proctologic improvement does not occur within 2–3 wk. Proctologic remission may require 2–3 mo of therapy. Following treatment for >21 days, gradually withdraw use; give every other night for 2–3 wk and then discontinue.

Rectal (as foam): Ulcerative proctitis of the distal rectum: 90 mg (1 applicatorful of a 10% aerosol foam suspension) 1 or 2 times daily for 2–3 wk. Then, if necessary, every other day until clinical and proctologic improvement. Symptoms may improve within 5–7 days.

Rectal (as suppository): Adjunctive treatment of ulcerative colitis of the rectum and other inflammatory conditions of the anorectum: 25 mg in the morning and at night for 2 wk. Severe proctitis: 25 mg tid or 50 mg bid.

Hydrocortisone + Gentamicin
Ear: 2–4 drops 3–4 times daily and at night. Alternatively, wicks medicated with the drops may be placed in the ear or mastoid cavity.

Hydrocortisone + Neomycin + Polymyxin
Ear: Place 3 drops into the ear 3–4 times daily.

Hydroxocobalamin (Vitamin B_{12})
Vit B_{12} deficiency: IM 250 µg to 1 mg 3 times weekly for 2 wk followed by 250 µg once weekly till blood counts are normal and then 1 mg once in 2–3 mo as maintenance dose.

Hydroxocobalamin-responsive inborn errors of metabolism: IM initially 1 mg daily for 5 days and assess response. If responsive, continue maintenance at 1 mg once or twice a week. PO up to 10 mg once or twice weekly. PO may be started as soon as response to IM is confirmed, but some patients do not respond to PO administration.

Hydroxychloroquine
PO 5–6.5 mg/kg (max: 400 mg) OD. Adjusted according to plasma levels in severe renal and hepatic impairment.

Hydroxyethyl Starches
Use in children is probably best restricted to an intensive care setting.

IV infusion. <2 yr: 16.9 mL/kg IV daily (up to 50 mL/kg/day); *2–12 yr:* 11 mL/kg IV daily (up to 50 mL/kg/day); *>12 yr:* up to 50 mL/kg IV daily. *Duration of therapy:* Can be administered repetitively over several days. Dosage in children should be adapted to the individual patient colloid needs, considering the disease state, hemodynamic, and hydration status.

Hydroxytryptophan
Given PO at a starting dose of 250–500 µg/kg qid and increased according to patient response, weight, and CSF amine metabolic conc. up to maintenance dose of 2–2.5 mg/kg qid.

Hydroxyurea (Hydroxycarbamide)
Sickle cell disease (to reduce the frequency of painful crises and the need for blood transfusions in children with recurrent moderate-to-severe painful crises): 10–20 mg/kg/day and doses titrated as tolerated. Increase at 5 mg/kg/day every 12 wk according to response (max: 35 mg/kg/day).

Malignant glioma, astrocytoma, medulloblastoma, and primitive neuroectodermal tumors: 1,500–3,000 mg/m^2 PO as a single dose administered every 4–6 wk: given in combination with other chemotherapeutic agents.

Acute myelogenous leukemia (AML): For WBC over 1 L/cumm: 50–75 mg/kg/day PO will cause a rapid decline in the WBC. Once the child is beyond the critical stage, conventional antileukemia therapy may be given. Safety and efficacy have not been established for use in children and adolescents but doses up to 3,000 mg/m^2 have been given PO for malignant glioma (off-label).

Hydroxyzine
Pruritus: PO: *6 mo to 6 yr:* 5–15 mg; *7–12 yr:* 10–15 mg; *12–18 yr:* 25 mg at bedtime. Increase if required to a max. dose of 50 mg/day in *6 mo to 6 yr,* 50–100 mg /day *in 7–12 yr;* 100 mg/day in *12–18 yr* in 3–4 div. doses.

Anxiety: PO: *12–18 yr:* 50–100 mg/dose qid.

In renal impairment, dose needs to be reduced by half.

Hyoscine Butylbromide
PO: *5–12 yr:* 10 mg/dose; *12–18 yr:* 20 mg/dose 3–4 times daily. IM/IV: *<6 yr:* 5 mg/dose; *6–12 yr:* 5–10 mg/dose; *>12 yr:* 20 mg/dose 3–4 tines daily.

Hyoscine Hydrobromide
PO: *2–12 yr:* 10 µg/kg; *12–18 yr:* 300 µg qid.

I

Ibuprofen
Pain/fever: 5–10 mg/kg/dose 3–4 times daily (max. 20 mg/kg/day up to 2.4 g/day).

Juvenile idiopathic arthritis and other rheumatic disorders: 30–50 mg/kg/24 hr in 3–4 div. doses - higher doses in systemic JIA.

Closure of patent ductus arteriosus (PDA) in newborn (IV preparation): Dose as ibuprofen base and given at 24 hr interval: first dose 10 mg/ kg, 2nd and 3rd dose 5 mg/kg. If PDA dose not close 48 hr after the last dose or reopens, a 2nd course of 3 doses may be given.

Idarubicin
Maximal lifetime dose = 137.5 mg/m^2. Lower dose by 25% if severe mucositis develops or if serum bilirubin > 2mg/dL; lower dose by 50% if bilirubin > 2.5 mg/dL; do not give if bilirubin > 5 mg/dL.

Idursulfase
0.5 mg/kg of body weight administered once every week as an IV infusion.

Ifosfamide
Always consult the current treatment protocol for details of dosage and scheduling. *Children:* IV: 1,200–1,800 mg/m^2/24 hr for 5 days every 21–28 days; or 5 g/m^2 as single IV infusion.

Iloprost
12–18 yr: IV infusion start with 0.5 ng/kg/min over 6 hr daily once for 3–5 consecutive days followed by maintenance dose of 1–2 ng/kg/min/day.

Imatinib Mesylate
260 mg and 350 mg/m^2 equivalent to the adult dose of 400 mg *during chronic phase* and 600 mg/day *during accelerated/blast phase crisis* respectively.

Dose adjustment for hepatotoxicity: If elevation in bilirubin >3 times upper limit of normal (ULN) or in liver enzymes >5 times ULN, then stop imatinib. When bilirubin levels have returned to less than 1.5 times ULN and transaminases levels to less than 2.5 times ULN, treatment of imatinib can be continued at a reduced daily dose.

Imiglucerase
Gaucher disease type I: IV infusion: *neonate:* initially 60 units/kg every 2 wk, adjusted according to response, doses as low as 30 units/kg once every 2 wk may be appropriate. *Child:* Initially 60 units/kg every 2 wk, adjusted according to response, doses as low as 30 units/kg once every 2 wk may be appropriate.

Gaucher disease type III: IV infusion: *neonate:* initially 60–120 units/kg every 2 wk, adjusted according to response. *Child:* Initially 60–120 units/kg every 2 wk, adjusted according to response.

Imipenem + Cilastin
Newborn: IV 20 mg/kg/dose in the frequency *<7 days, 7–21 days and >21 days:* at 2, 3, and 4 times daily, respectively. *Children:* IV: <3 mo 80 mg/kg/day, *3 mo to 12 yr:* 60 mg/kg/day, *12–18 yr:* 2 g/day in 4 div. doses. (max. dose *<12 yr:* 500

mg; >*12 yr:* 1 g). *Children:* IV: <3 mo 80 mg/kg/day, *3 mo to 12 yr:* 60 mg/ kg/day, *12–18 yr:* 2 g/day in 4 div. doses. (max. dose < 12 yr: 500 mg; >*12 yr:* 1 g).

Imipramine Hydrochloride

Nocturnal enuresis: 6–12 yr: 25 mg; *12–18 yr:* 25–75 mg ½ hr before bedtime. Max. period of treatment: 3 mo. Review before giving further courses.

Hyperactivity: 6–12 yr: 25–75 mg; *12–17 yr:* 50–75 mg OD. Start at lower doses. Doses >1.5 mg/kg given in 2 div. doses.

Depression: 12–18 yr: 25 mg/dose 1–3 times daily. Increase up to 150–200 mg/day and maintained till improvement noted. Usual maintenance 50–150 mg/day.

Neuropathic pain: Start at 0.2–0.4 mg/kg and gradually increase to 1–3 mg/kg at bedtime.

Immunoglobulin (IV)

Total dose for immunomodulation: 2 g/kg div. over 2–5 days or 1 g/kg for 2 days to be given as IV infusion. May stop if the platelet counts are normal after the 2nd dose. Repeated if symptoms warrant and not according to platelet count. Can be repeated every 3–6 wks.

Indomethacin

Pain/inflammation in rheumatic disease and nephrogenic diabetes insipidus: PO 1–2 mg/kg in 2 div. doses.

Closure of PDA in newborn: IV over 20–30 min 100–200 µg/kg as a single dose followed by 2 doses 100 µg/kg at 24 hr intervals; if residual patency is noted, 100 µg/kg × 3 more doses 24 hrly. Monitor for adequate urine output.

Infliximab

Severe active Crohn's disease: IV infusion *6–17 yr:* initially 5 mg/kg, then 5 mg/kg after 2 wk, then 5 mg/kg after 4 wk, then maintenance 5 mg/kg every 8 wk, interval between maintenance doses adjusted according to response; discontinue if no response within 10 wk of initial dose.

Fistulating Crohn's disease: IV infusion *6–17 yr:* initially 5 mg/kg, then 5 mg/kg after 2 wk, then 5 mg/kg after 4 wk, if the condition has responded, future doses can be given on specialist's recommendation.

Severe active ulcerative colitis: IV infusion *6–17 yr:* initially 5 mg/kg, then 5 mg/kg after 2 wk, then 5 mg/kg after 4 wk, then maintenance 5 mg/kg every 8 wk; discontinue if there is no response within 8 wk of initial dose.

Influenza Vaccine (Inactivated, IIV)

>*6 mo:* 0.5 mL IM. *Those receiving it for the first time between 6 mo and 9 yr:* Will need a 2nd dose after 4 wk. *9 yr and above:* A single dose will suffice. Vaccine is given yearly for those at continuing risk. Quadrivalent IIV is preferred over trivalent IIV.

Insulin

Usual dose of insulin is 0.7 unit/kg/day in prepubertal children and 1.0 unit/kg/day in midpuberty and 1.2 unit/kg/day by the end of puberty.

Insulin regimens: Please refer to Chapter 16.10.

Insulin analogs: Lispro (Humalog: Lilly, Eglucent: Lupin), aspart (Novorapid: Novo), insulin glulisine (Apidra: Sanofi). Insulin analogs begin acting immediately as they exist as monomers. They provide definite peaks at about an hour after injection, last for 2 hr or so, have no overlap and a short tail effect.

Long-acting insulin analogs: Glargine (Lantus: Aventis) and Detemir (Detemir: Novo Nordisk) are long-acting insulin analogs which yield a peakless flat 24 hr profile and produce a near-physiological basal insulin effect. They are used as OD basal insulin as part of a basal bolus regimen.

Tuojeo (U 300 Glargine): Tuojeo has a threefold higher concentration compared to the classical Glargine (U-100). U-300 glargine is peakless and has a longer duration of action (>24 hr) and lesser variability. Currently, it is approved for use above 18 yr of age.

Ultralong-acting insulin: Insulin Degludec (Tresiba: Novo Nordisk) is ultralong-acting peakless insulin. The long half-life (25 hr) and duration of action (42 hr) allows once-a-day dosage of degludec. Its longer course of action provides the opportunity to vary time of injection on different days. It is approved in children above 1 yr of age.

Interferon Alfa

SC: <*12 yr:* 3 million units/m^2; >*12 yr:* 3–10 million units/m^2 usually 3 times/week (daily for hemangioma) for 4–6 mo.

Interferon Gamma-1b (Immune Interferon)

SC surface area <0.5 m^2 1.5 µg/kg/dose and surface area >0.5 m^2 50 µg/kg/dose 3 times in a week. Avoid in children < 6 mo.

Intralipid 10%/Intralipid 20%

The ability to eliminate Intralipid 10%/20% should govern the dosage and infusion rate. 1 g triglycerides correspond to 10 mL Intralipid 10% or 5 mL Intralipid 20%. *Neonates and infants:* 0.5–4 g triglycerides/kg body weight/day. The rate of infusion should not exceed 0.17 g triglycerides/kg body weight/hr (4 g in 24 hr).

Intravenous Immunoglobulin (IVIg)

Total dose for immunomodulation is 2 g/kg div. over 2–5 days or 1 g/kg for 2 days to be given as IV infusion. This may stop if the platelet counts are normal after the 2nd dose. It can be repeated if symptoms warrant and not according to the platelet count. It can be repeated every 3–6 week.

Kawasaki syndrome: IV infusion 2 g/kg given over 8–12 hr period. The treatment should be given within 10 days of the onset of illness, preferably within 7 days (Class I). If active inflammation persists beyond 10 days in the form of persistent fever, raised erythrocyte sedimentation rate (ESR) and C-reactive protein (CRP), or presence of coronary aneurysms, IVIg can be given (Class IIa). IVIg is not indicated in Kawasaki disease after 10 days if there are no signs of ongoing inflammation or coronary aneurysms (Class III). IVIg is also indicated in incomplete Kawasaki disease with echocardiographic demonstration of coronary aneurysms (Class I) or with normal echo (Class IIb). In nonresponders or partial responders, a second course of IVIg may be given after 48 hr.

Immunodeficiency syndrome: IV infusion 400 mg/kg once in 3 wk. Dose depends on severity, infection frequency, and serum IgG.

Intractable epilepsy: IV infusion 400 mg/kg once in 3 wk for 3 doses. If 75% reduction is achieved, continue therapy for 9–12 mo and review.

Juvenile idiopathic arthritis: IV infusion 1 g/kg OD for 2 days. Repeat if clinically needed.

Guillain–Barre syndrome: 400 mg/kg OD for 3–5 days depending on severity and rate to recover.

Myocarditis: 2 g/kg; however, it is generally given over 2 days as the volume of fluid is too much in the presence of ventricular dysfunction.

Iodine

Thyrotoxicosis – neonatal: 1 drop tid.

Thyrotoxicosis (preoperative): 0.1–0.3 mL tid.

Ipratropium Bromide

Inhaled 20–120 g 4 times daily. DPI 40 µg (1 cap) 3–4 times daily.

Nebulized newborn: 25 µg/kg, *<1 yr:* 62.5 µg, *1–5 yr:* 125–250 µg, *5–12 yr:* 250–500 µg, and *12–18 yr:* 500 µg every 20–30 min in the first 2 hr and then tapered according to response.

Iron

All mg doses are expressed as elemental iron.

Newborn infant (birth to 1 mo) for prophylaxis of iron deficiency in low-birth-weight and breast-fed babies: 5–6 mg of elemental iron OD.

Treatment of iron deficiency anemia: 3 mo to 12 yr: 5–6 mg/kg in 2 divided doses. *12–18 yr:* 180 mg of elemental iron in 3 div. doses.

Iron Chloride Injection

1 mL/kg as part of a balanced PN regimen.

Isoniazid (INH)

Treatment and prophylaxis of TB: 10 mg/kg/day. (max: 300 mg/day). Intermittent regimen: 15 mg/kg (range 12–17mg/kg).

INH prophylaxis in doses of 10 mg/kg/day for 6 mo: (1) All asymptomatic contacts (under 6 yr of age) of a smear positive case, after ruling out active disease and irrespective of their BCG, tuberculin skin test (TST), or nutritional status. *(2) All HIV-infected children* who either had a known exposure to an infectious TB case or are TST positive (≥5 mm induration) but have no active TB disease. *(3) All TST-positive children who are receiving immunosuppressive therapy* (e.g., children with nephrotic syndrome, acute leukemia). (4) A child born to a mother who was diagnosed to have TB in pregnancy should receive prophylaxis for 6 mo, provided congenital TB has been ruled out. BCG vaccination can be given at birth even if INH chemoprophylaxis is planned.

Isoproterenol (Isoprenaline)

ECG monitoring required during administration: IV infusion as HCl salt: *newborn:* 20–300 ng/kg/min, *<12 yr:* 20 ng to 1 µg/kg/min, and 12–18 yr: 1–4 µg/min.

Isotretinoin

PO 0.5 mg/kg daily once for 4 wk and if response is good, continue for further 8–12 wk; if response is poor, give up to 1 mg/kg for 8–12 wk. If intolerant, reduce to 0.1–0.2 mg/kg/day.

Topical: Apply 1–2 times daily over affected area.

Ispaghula Husk

Child 2–12 yr: 1 level 5 mL spoonful in water once or bid, preferably at mealtimes. *Child 12–18 yr:* 2 level 5 mL spoonful in water once or bid, preferably at mealtimes.

Itraconazole

PO: *<12 yr:* 3–5 mg/kg and *12–18 yr:* 100 mg OD for 15 days in *tenia corporis, tenia cruris, and oropharyngeal candidiasis* and 30 days for *tenia pedis and tinea manuum.*

Aspergillosis – allergic bronchopulmonary: 3–5 mg/kg in 2 div. doses.

Ivacaftor

Cystic fibrosis PO: *Child 6–17 yr (body-weight 25 kg and above):* 150 mg 12 hrly.

Ivermectin

5–18 yr: 0.15 mg/kg as single dose to repeat every 6–8 mo.

Strongyloidosis: 5–18 yr: 0.2 mg/kg for 2 days as single dose and repeat every 6–12 mo if necessary

Filariasis: Given in a dose of 150 µg/kg once a year for 10 yr. If symptoms recur, then dose is given every 3 mo instead of once a year. Ivermectin is also effective against lymphatic filaria caused by *Wuchereria bancrofti.* In endemic areas, for mass treatments, a single dose of albendazole 400 mg + Ivermectin 200 mg/kg every 12 mo is highly effective in controlling filaria.

Scabies and pediculosis: Recently, a single dose of ivermectin (200 µg/kg) has been found to be highly effective in the treatment of scabies and head lice. Ivermectin is typically helpful in the treatment of crusted scabies found in a patient with immunosuppression (e.g., HIV and leukemia). It is used to prevent and cure the outbreak of scabies in institution.

J

Japanese Encephalitis Vaccine (Inactivated)
Two-dose schedule for those residing in endemic areas:

JEEV: Minimum age: 1 yr. *Primary immunization schedule:* 2 doses of 0.25 mL each administered IM on days 0 and 28 for children between 1 and 3 yr. 2 doses of 0.5 mL for *children > 3 yr and adults aged >18 yr.*

JENVAC: Minimum age: 1 yr. *Primary immunization schedule:* 2 doses of 0.5 mL each administered intramuscularly at 4 wk interval.

Catch-up vaccination: All susceptible children up to 15 yr should be administered during disease outbreak/ahead of anticipated outbreak in campaigns.

Live attenuated, cell culture-derived SA-14-14-2 vaccine: Minimum age: *8 mo;* 2-dose schedule, first dose at 9 mo along with measles vaccine and second at 16–18 mo along with DTP booster. It is used in NIV for all children at 1½ yr age in endemic districts as a single dose.

K

Ketamine
Intermittent IV: <12 yr: 1–2 mg/kg and *12–18 yr:* 1–4.5 mg/kg as induction followed by maintenance as required - usually half induction dose or as IV infusion.

IV infusion induce with 0.5–2 mg/kg followed by maintenance - newborn: 0.5 mg/kg/hr and *1 mo to 18 yr:* 0.6–2.7 mg/kg/hr.

Neuropathic pain for palliative care: 0.1–0.3 mg/kg/hr (max: 1.5 mg/kg/hr) will suffice. IM: 4 mg/kg for diagnostic/pain-causing procedures.

Ketoconazole
Pityriasis versicolor: Use daily for a max. of 5 days.

Seborrheic dermatitis and dandruff: Use twice weekly for 2–4 wk.

Candidiasis, candiduria, or chromomycosis: PO: *Adolescent:* 200 mg PO OD. Serious infection may require 400 mg PO OD. *Children > 2 yr of age:* 3.3–6.6 mg/kg PO OD. *Children < 2 yr of age:* Safety and efficacy have not been established.

Oropharyngeal candidiasis (thrush) in HIV-infected children: PO: *Children:* 3–7 mg/kg/day for 5–49 days till cured.

Vulvovaginal candidiasis: Nonpregnant adolescent females: 200–600 mg PO OD for 3–6 days. *For recurrent vulvovaginal candidiasis*, topical or PO therapy daily for 2 wk and then 6 mo of therapy that could include ketoconazole 100 mg PO every day. It is not recommended in pregnancy.

Tinea capitis, tinea corporis, tinea cruris, tinea pedis, tinea manuum, tinea unguium (onychomycosis) caused by Trichophyton sp., Microsporum sp. or Epidermophyton sp., and tinea versicolor: Adolescent: 200 mg PO OD. Serious infection may require 400 mg PO OD. *Children≥ 2 yr*: 3.3–6.6 mg/kg PO OD.

Ketotifen
Adolescents: 1–2 mg OD with food. Initial treatment is 0.5–1 mg at night. *Children: Over 2 yr:* 1 mg OD with food. Not recommended for children below 2 yr.

L

Labetalol
PO: *1 mo to 12 yr:* 1–2 mg/kg 3–4 times a day; *12–18 yr:* initially 50–100 mg bid increased if required at intervals of 3–14 days to a usual dose of 200–400 mg bid (3–4 div. doses if higher); max. 2.4 g daily. IV: *1 mo to 12 yr:* 250–500 µg/kg as a single dose, max. 20 mg; *12–18 yr:* 50 mg over at least 1 minute, repeated after 5 minutes if necessary, max. total dose 200 mg.

Lactitol Monohydrate
Administer PO OD along with evening meals - the dose may also be given in the morning if that is more convenient.

Constipation: 2–6 yr: 10 mL; *>6 yr:* 10–15 mL.

Prevention of hepatic encephalopathy: 30 mL once in the evening.

Acute phase of hepatic encephalopathy: 45–90 mL div. into 3 doses along with main meals.

Lactulose
Constipation: Initial dose *<1 yr:* 5mL, *1–5 yr*: 10 mL, *5–10 yr:* 20 mL, *>12 yr:* 30 mL in 2 div. doses. Then adjust according to response.

Hepatic encephalopathy: initially 30–50 mL/dose tid. Then adjust to produce 2–3 soft stools/day.

Lamivudine
Dosage: Adolescents (weight ≥ 40 kg): 300 mg/day. Safe and effective use has not been established in adolescent < 40 kg and in children.

Patients with renal impairment: Lamivudine requires dose adjustment in the presence of renal insufficiency.

Lamotrigine

Monotherapy and as an adjunct in focal seizures; primary and secondary generalized tonic-clonic seizures (GTCS); Lennox-Gestaut syndrome: PO along with valproate - *2–12 yr:* initially 50 µg/kg for 2 wks [if *<13 kg:* mg alternate days (A/D) for wks] followed by 300 µg/kg for the next 2 wks; then increase by 300 µg/kg once in 1–2 wks up to 1–5 mg/kg/day in 1–2 div. doses (maintenance) - max: 100 mg/dose. *12–18 yr:* initially 25 mg on A/D for 2 wk followed by 25 mg/day for the next 2 wk; then increase by 25 mg once in 1–2 wk up to 100–200 mg/day in 1–2 div. doses (maintenance).

Adjunct in seizures (with enzyme-inducing drugs) without valproate: 2–12 yr: initially 300 µg/kg/day 2 div. doses for 2 wks followed by 600 µg/kg 2 div. doses for the next 2 wks; then increase by 1.2/kg (max.) every 1–2 wk up to 2.5–5 mg/kg (max: 200 mg/dose) BD. *12–18 yr:* initially 50 mg OD for 2 wk followed by 50 mg BD for the next 2 wk; then increase by max. 100 mg every 1–2 wk up to 100–200 mg BD (maintenance - occasionally up to 700 mg required).

Adjunct in seizures (without enzyme-inducing drugs) without valproate: 2–12 yr: initially 300 µg/kg/d 1–2 div. doses for 2 wk followed by 600 µg/kg 1–2 div. doses for the next 2 wk; then increase by 600 µg/kg (max.) every 1–2 wk up to 1–10 mg/kg/d (max. 200 mg/d) in div doses. *12–18 yr:* initially 25 mg OD for 2 wk followed by 50 mg OD for the next 2 wk; then increase by max. 100 mg every 1–2 wk up to 100–200 mg/day in 1–2 div. doses (maintenance).

Monotherapy of seizures: 12–18 yr: initially 25 mg OD for 2 wk followed by 50 mg OD for the next 2 wk; then increase by max. 100 mg every 1–2 wks up to 100–200 mg/day in 1–2 div. doses (maintenance - occasionally up to 500 mg required).

Monotherapy of atypical absence seizures: 2–12 yr: initially 300 µg/kg/d 2 div. doses for 2 wk followed by 600 µg/kg 2 div. doses for the next 2 wk; then increase by max. 600 µg/kg every 1–2 wk up to 1–10 mg/kg/d in 1–2 div. doses (maintenance - occasionally up to 15 mg/kg/d required).

Note: All dose titrations should be repeated if restarting after an interval of more than 5 days.

Lansoprazole

GERD, acid-related dyspepsia, duodenal and benign gastric ulcer including those following nonsteroidal anti-inflammatory drug (NSAID) therapy: Children < 30 kg: 0.5–1 mg/kg (max: 15 mg) OD; *children > 30 kg:* 15–30 mg OD for 8–12 wk.

Laronidase

Non-neurological manifestations of mucopolysaccharidosis I: IV infusion: *child:* 100 units/kg once weekly.

Leuprorelin Acetate [Leuprolide; Gonadotropin-Releasing Hormone Receptor [GnRHR] Agonist]

3.75 mg every 4 wk or 11.25 mg depot preparation every 12 wk. Injections may need to be given more frequently (e.g., every 3 wk or every 10 wk) if patients show signs of failure of hormone suppression.

Levamisole

Roundworm (ascariasis): <12 yr: 2.5–3 mg/kg, *12–18 yr:* 150 mg as single dose.

Hookworm (ankylostomiasis): <12 yr: 2.5 mg/kg; *12–18 yr:* 150 mg as single dose. Repeat after 7 days if there is severe infection. *Adults:* 300 mg for 1–2 days.

Nephrotic syndrome: 2.5 mg/kg on alternate days for 12–*18 mo.*

Levetiracetam

Monotherapy of focal seizures with or without secondary generalization: PO or IV infusion: *16–17 yr:* Initially 250 mg OD for 1 wk, then increased to 250 mg bid, then increased in steps of 250 mg bid (max. per dose 1.5 g bid), adjusted according to response, dose to be increased every 2 wk.

Adjunctive therapy of focal seizures with or without secondary generalization: PO: *child 1–5 mo:* initially 7 mg/kg OD, then increased in steps of up to 7 mg/kg bid (max. per dose 21 mg/kg bid), dose to be increased every 2 wk. *6 mo to 17 yr (<50 kg):* Initially 10 mg/kg OD, then increased in steps of up to 10 mg/kg bid (max. per dose 30 mg/kg bid), dose to be increased every 2 wk. *12–17 yr (>50 kg):* Initially 250 mg bid, then increased in steps of 500 mg bid (max. per dose 1.5 g bid), dose to be increased every 2–4 wk.

IV infusion: 4–17 yr (< 50 kg): initially 10 mg/kg OD, then increased in steps of up to 10 mg/kg bid (max. per dose 30 mg/kg bid), dose to be increased every 2 wk. *12–17 yr (>50 kg):* Initially 250 mg bid, then increased in steps of 500 mg bid (max. per dose 1.5 g bid), dose to be increased every 2 wk.

Adjunctive therapy of myoclonic seizures and tonic-clonic seizures: PO or IV infusion: *12–17 yr (<50 kg):* Initially 10 mg/kg OD, then increased in steps of up to 10 mg/kg bid (max. per dose 30 mg/kg bid), dose to be increased every 2 wk. *12–17 yr (>50 kg):* Initially 250 mg bid, then increased in steps of 500 mg bid (max. per dose 1.5 g bid), dose to be increased every 2 wk

When levetiracetam is withdrawn, it should be tapered slowly over 2–4 wk to prevent withdrawal seizures.

In adolescents with moderate-to-severe renal impairment, reduce dose by half and give bid.

Hemodialysis removes approximately 50% of a levetiracetam dose in one 4-hr session. Those undergoing hemodialysis should therefore receive a supplemental dose of half their standard maintenance dose after dialysis.

No dosage adjustment is needed in the presence *of hepatic impairment.* But if hepatic impairment is associated with renal impairment with CrCl < 70 mL/min/1.73m^2, half the usual dose is recommended.

Levobupivacaine Hydrochloride
All doses for older adolescent: epidural anesthesia during surgery: 10–20 mL (50–150 mg) of 0.5%–0.75% levobupivacaine as an epidural infusion.

Ophthalmic anesthesia: Regional dosage: 5–15 mL (37.5–112.5 mg) of 0.75% levobupivacaine.

Peripheral nerve block anesthesia including brachial plexus nerve block: Regional dosage: 30 mL (75–150 mg) or 0.4 mL/kg (1–2 mg/kg) of 0.25–0.5% levobupivacaine.

Levocetirizine
PO in the evening as hydrochloride*: 6–11 yr:* 2.5 mg OD (max. dose: >*12 yr:* 5 mg OD) (max. dose: 2.5 mg may suffice in some children).

Levonorgestrel
PO: 30 µg.

Levothyroxine (Thyroxine) Sodium
PO: Initial dose: *newborn:* 10–15 µg/kg, *late neonatal period:* 6–8 µg/kg, *3 mo to 2 yr*: 5–10 µg/kg, *2–12 yr:* 5 µg/kg, *12–18 yr:* 50–100 µg. Adjust dose to correct free thyroxine (FT4) to >20 pmol/L and thyroid-stimulating hormone (TSH) to <1–3 mU/L within 4 wk of therapy. TSH levels take at least 4 wk to show any change following therapy. Monitor thyroid hormone levels 4–6 weekly at onset till target levels are attained and then according to progress. It is ideal to test 6–8 wk after any change in dose and every 3–4 monthly intervals during the second year and biannually or annually as the child grows. It is preferable to monitor TT4 levels to FT4 levels. FT4 is preferred in special circumstances like pregnancy or inappropriately elevated TSH and to cross check central hypothyroidism if the T4 level is borderline as TSH will not be useful.

Lignocaine
Antiarrhythmic: Loading dose IV bolus <*12 yr:* 0.5 mg–1 mg/kg; *12–18 yr:* 50–100 mg (50 mg for thin build or those with severely impaired circulation) followed by maintenance dose IV infusion with ECG monitoring. <*12 yr*: 0.6–3 mg/kg/hr, *12–18 yr:* start with 4 mg/min for 30 min, then 2 mg/kg for 2 hr, and then 1 mg/min for the rest of the day. Lower conc. further if continued beyond 24 hr.

Ventricular fibrillation or pulseless tachycardia: IV: <*12 yr:* 1 mg/kg repeat every 5 min to a max. of 3 mg/kg; *12–18 yr:* 50–100 mg.

Local anesthetic: Local infiltration: <*12 yr:* 3 mg/kg; *12–18 yr:* up to 200 mg – not more frequently than once in 4 hr.

Intraurethral: 3–4 mg/kg prior to catheterization.

Linezolid
IV infusion over 30–120 min: *preterm neonates < 7 days old (gestational age < 34 wk):* 10 mg/kg 12 hrly for 14–28 days and 10 mg/kg 8 hrly in those with a suboptimal clinical response. *Neonates, infants, and children < 12 yr:* 10 mg/kg 8 hrly for 14–28 days. Linezolid is not recommended for empiric treatment of acute CNS infections. ≥*12 yr:* 600 mg 12 hrly for 14–28 days.

PO: Adolescents and children ≥ 12 yr: 600 mg 12 hrly for 10–14 days; *Term neonates, infants, and children < 12 yr:* 10 mg/kg 8 hrly for 10–14 days. *Preterm neonates < 7 days old (gestational age < 34 wk):* 10 mg/kg 12 hrly for 10–14 days; 10 mg/kg 8 hrly in those with a suboptimal clinical response.

Liquid Paraffin
Skin and hair: Topical application as advised in administration section.

Constipation: PO: *3–12 yr*: 0.5–1 mL/kg and *12–18 yr*: 10–30 mL OD.

Lisinopril
Hypertension: PO: *Adolescent:* Initially, 10 mg PO OD. The usual dosage range is 20–40 mg PO OD.

Lower dosage may be necessary in patients *with renal impairment* and in those receiving diuretics. In patients with a CrCl of <30 mL/min, initiate therapy with 5 mg PO OD. Max. daily dose is 80 mg/day. *Children ≥ 6 yr:* Starting dosage is 0.07 mg/kg PO OD (up to 5 mg/day). Adjust dosage based on blood pressure response. Doses > 0.61 mg/kg/day PO or > 40 mg/day have not been studied in pediatric patients.

Renal impairment: Lisinopril is not recommended in children with GFR < 30 mL/min/1.73 m^2. *Children < 6 yr:* Not recommended.

The doses for heart failure in children are not defined.

Lisinopril is removed by *hemodialysis.* For patients receiving dialysis, the initial recommended dosage is 2.5 mg PO OD. Max: 40 mg/day.

Lithium
PO: *12–18 yr:* 200–800 mg/dose tid. Higher dose with citrate—citrate 509 mg = carbonate 200 mg. Maintain plasma level of 0.4–1 mmol/L 12 hr after the last dose. Monitor once in 3 mo.

Loperamide
Chronic diarrhea, e.g., short bowel syndrome: <1 yr: 0.2 mg/kg 30 min before feeds (up to 2 mg/kg/day may be required); *1–12 yr:* 0.1–0.2 mg/kg/dose; *12–18 yr:* 2–4 mg 3–4 times daily.

Acute diarrhea – not recommended in children. 12–18 yr: may be used – start with 4 mg and then give 2 mg after each loose stool up to 6–8 mg/day (max: 16 mg/day). Not given for >5 days.

Loratadine
PO: <*6 yr:* 5 mg; >*6 yr:* 10 mg OD.

Lorazepam
Antiemetic: IV 0.4–0.8 mg/kg/dose 6 hrly as needed.

Anxiety/sedation: Neonates: 0.1–0.4 mg/kg/dose 6 hrly as needed. *Children:* 0.05–0.1 mg/kg/dose 4–8 hrly. *Adolescents:* PO 1–10 mg/24 hr in 2–3 div. doses.

Status epilepticus: Neonates: IV 0.05–0.2 mg/kg/dose over 2–5 min; may repeat in 10–15 min. *Children:* 0.1 mg/kg loading over 2–5 min and if required, another 0.05 mg/kg bolus in 10–15 min. *Adolescent:* 0.07 mg/kg/dose over 2–5 min and may repeat after 10–15 min.

Losartan Potassium
Hypertension: Adolescents: Initially, 50 mg PO OD, unless the patient is volume-depleted. The maintenance dosage range is 25–100 mg/day PO, given in 1–2 div. doses. Maximal effects generally occur within 3–6 wk.

The *addition of a diuretic* has a greater effect on lowering blood pressure than increasing the losartan dosage beyond 50 mg/day. The addition of hydrochlorothiazide 12.5 mg to losartan 50 mg daily results in an additional 50% reduction in diastolic and systolic blood pressure. A modest reduction in blood pressure (up to 3 mm Hg) is achieved by increasing the daily dose of losartan from 50 to 100 mg.

When volume-depletion is suspected (e.g., patients taking diuretics), initiate therapy with 25 mg PO OD. *Children ≥ 6 yr:* The usual recommended starting dose is 0.7 mg/kg PO OD (up to 50 mg/day). *Individualize dosage to attain blood pressure goals.* Doses > 1.4 mg/kg/day (or >100 mg/day) PO have not been studied. Losartan can be prepared extemporaneously as an oral suspension. *Children < 6 yr:* Not recommended.

Chronic congestive cardiac failure: 75–1.4 mg/kg/day.

Other drugs in this group are *Candesartan and Valsartan.* Studies in children are in progress, primarily for treatment of hypertension.

Lumacaftor with Ivacaftor
Cystic fibrosis: PO: *child 6–11 yr:* 200/250 mg every 12 hr; *12–17 yr:* 400/250 mg every 12 hr.

Lymecycline
Susceptible infections (e.g., chlamydia, rickettsia, and mycoplasma): PO: *child 12–17 yr*: 408 mg bid, increased to 1.224–1.632 g daily. *In severe infections:* PO: 408 mg daily for at least 8 wk.

Renal impairment: May exacerbate renal failure.

M

Magnesium Glycerophosphate
PO: <*12 yr:* 0.6 mmol/kg/day; *12–18 yr:* 12–24 mmol/day in 3 div. doses.

Magnesium Salts
5–10 mL at bedtime daily; reduce dose gradually until constipation is relieved.

Magnesium Sulfate
Severe acute asthma; continuing respiratory deterioration in anaphylaxis: IV infusion: *2–17 yr:* 40 mg/kg (max. per dose 2 g), to be given over 20 min.

Persistent pulmonary hypertension of the newborn: Initially by IV infusion: *neonate:* Initially 200 mg/kg, to be given over 0–30 minutes, then (by continuous IV infusion) 20–75 mg/kg/hr for up to 5 days if response occurs after the initial dose (maintain plasma magnesium concentration between 3.5 and 5.5 mmol/L).

Hypomagnesemia: IV infusion: *neonate:* 100 mg/kg every 6–12 hr as required, to be given over at least 10 minutes. *1 mo to 11 yr:* 50 mg/kg every 12 hr as required, to be given over at least 10 minutes. *12–17 yr:* 1 g every 12 hr as required, to be given over at least 10 minutes.

Hypomagnesemia maintenance (e.g., in IV nutrition): IV infusion/IM: *child:* 50–100 mg/kg daily; max: 5 g/day.

Neonatal hypocalcemia: Deep IM/IV infusion: *neonate:* 100 mg/kg every 12 hr for 2–3 doses.

Torsade de pointes: IV infusion: *child:* 25–50 mg/kg (max. per dose 2 g), to be given over 10–15 minutes. Dose may be repeated once if necessary.

Mannitol
Cerebral edema: IV infusion over 30–60 min. *1 mo to 11 yr:* 0.25–1.5 g/kg, repeated if necessary, 1–2 times after 4–8 hr. *12–17 yr:* 0.25–2 g/kg, repeated if necessary, 1–2 times after 4–8 hr.

Peripheral edema and ascites: IV infusion: *child:* 1–2 g/kg, to be given over 2–6 hr.

Mebendazole
Threadworm infections: PO: *6 mo to 17 yr:* 100 mg for 1 dose for all family members – child and all family members to repeat the dose after 2 wks. During treatment and for a few wk afterward, it is also important to follow strict hygiene measures to avoid spreading the threadworm eggs.

Whipworm infections, hookworm infections: PO: *1–17 yr:* 100 mg bid for 3 days.

Roundworm infections: 1 yr: 100 mg bid for 3 days; *2–17 yr:* 100 mg bid for 3 days, alternatively 500 mg for 1 dose.

Hydatid disease: 200–400 mg bid or tid for 3–4 wk, less effective than albendazole.

Reduction in dose for hepatic impairment.

Mebeverine Hydrochloride
PO: *3–4 yr:* 75 mg/day; *4–8 yr:* 150 mg/day, *9–10 yr:* 300 mg/day, *>10 yr:* 450 mg/day in 3 div. doses 10–20 min before meals.

Mebeverine + Ispaghula Husk
PO: *Child 12–17 yr:* 1 sachet bid, in water, morning and evening, 30 minutes before food and 1 sachet daily if required, taken 30 minutes before midday meal.

Mefenamic Acid
Adolescents: 250–500 mg tid, preferably after food. *Children:* 9.5–25 mg/kg/day in div. doses. Except for Still's disease, therapy should not exceed 7 days.

Mefenamic acid should be used with extreme caution in children younger than 14 yr old; safety and effectiveness in these children have not been confirmed.

Mefloquine
Treatment: PO: 15 mg/kg followed by 10 mg/kg 8–12 hr later (max: 1.25 g).

Prophylaxis: PO 1st dose 1 wk before entering malarious area (may be started earlier to make sure drug is tolerated) and given weekly on the same day for 6 wk and continued for 4 wk after return from the malarious area. *3 mo to 3 yr, 6–16 kg:* 62.5 mg (1/4th tab); *4–7 yr 16–25 kg:* 125 mg (1/2 tab); *8–12 yr 25–45 kg:* 187.5 mg (3/4th tab); *>13 yr >45 kg:* 250 mg (1 tab).

Meglumine Antimoniate + Sodium Stibogluconate
Visceral leishmaniasis: Injection of 20 mg of stibogluconate (Sb5+)/kg IM daily for a minimum of 20 days. Treatment should be continued until no parasites are detected in consecutive splenic aspirates taken at 14-day intervals. Patients who relapse following the first course of treatment should be retreated immediately using the same daily dosage.

Cutaneous leishmaniasis except L. aethiopica. Local therapy: Injection of 1–3 mL into the base of the lesion, repeated once or twice if no response is apparent, at intervals of 1–2 days. *Systemic therapy:* 10–20 mg Sb5+/kg IM daily until a few days after clinical cure and slit skin smears are negative. Relapse is unusual.

Leishmania braziliensis therapy: Injection of 20 mg Sb5+/kg IM daily until lesion is healed and for at least 4 wk. Relapse is usually associated with inadequate dosage or interrupted treatment. Should relapse occur following a full course of treatment, pentamidine should be used.

Mucocutaneous leishmaniasis (L. braziliensis): Injection of 20 mg Sb5+/kg daily IM until slit-skin smears are negative and for at least 4 wk. In the event of toxicity or inadequate response, 10–15 mg Sb5+/kg should be administered every 12 hr for the same period. Patients who relapse should be retreated at least twice as long. Those who are unresponsive should receive amphotericin B or pentamidine.

Diffuse cutaneous leishmaniasis (Leishmania amazonensis): Injection of 20 mg Sb 5+/kg daily IM for several mo after clinical improvement occurs. Relapse must be expected until immunity develops.

Melatonin
PO 2–3 mg 20–30 min before bedtime. May be increased to 4–6 mg if the benefit is not achieved in 1–2 wk. Max. of 10 mg tried. If there is still no response in 2 wk, the drug is stopped.

Meloxicam
PO/rectal: *12–18 yr <50 kg:* 7.5 mg; *>50 kg:* 15 mg OD.

In *renal failure*, the dose of 7.5 mg is not to be exceeded.

Melphalan
Always consult the current treatment protocol for details of dosage and scheduling. IV 10–35 mg/m^2/dose once in 21–28 days.

High dose: 140–220 mg/m^2 before BMT. PO 4–20 mg/m^2/day for up to 21 days.

Mepacrine Hydrochloride
PO 100 mg 1–2 times daily.

Mercaptamine (Cysteamine)
PO: Initially: *<12 yr:* 2–3 mg/kg/dose; *>12 yr:* 100 mg qid followed by maintenance of 12.5 mg/kg/dose. *>12 yr:* 500 mg qid.

Eye: 1 drop in each eye 4–6 times daily.

Mercaptopurine
Leukemia/lymphoma/T-non-Hodgkin lymphoma (T-NHL): PO: Induction 2.5–5 mg/kg OD followed by maintenance of 1.5–2.5 mg/kg/day.

Inflammatory bowel disease: 2–18 yr: 1–1.5 mg/kg OD (max. initially 50 mg/day may be increased up to 75 mg/day).

Meropenem
Newborn: 40 mg/kg/day in 2 div. doses <7 days and in 3 div. doses >7 days. Double the dose in meningitis and severe infections.

Children with UTI, gynecological, skin, and soft-tissue infections: 30 mg/kg in 3 div. doses (max. 500 mg/dose).

Pneumonia, peritonitis, neutropenia, septicemia: 60 mg/kg/day in 3 div. doses (max. 1 g/dose).

Meningitis and life-threatening infections: 120 mg/kg/day in 3 div. doses (max. 2 g/dose).

In renal impairment: CrCl (mL/min/1.73m^2) 25–50: give full dose but at 12 hr intervals, 10–25: 50% dose at 12 hr intervals; <10: 50% dose at 24 hr interval.

Dose adjustment in HD/PD: Dialyzed. Give 50% of dose IV every 24 hr, administered after dialysis session.

Dose adjustment on continuous venovenous hemofiltration (CVVH): Give 100% of normal dose every 12 hr or every 8 hr depending upon the severity of infection (e.g., for meningitis).

Mesalazine [5-Aminosalicylic Acid (5-ASA)]
Since other first-line drugs like steroids and azathioprine are more effective, mesalazine is used as an add-on along with these drugs at the stage of remission induction.
ASACOL 400 mg tab

Treatment of mild-to-moderate ulcerative colitis, acute attack: PO: *Child 12–17 yr:* 800 mg tid.

Maintenance of remission of ulcerative colitis and Crohn's ileocolitis: PO: *Child 12–17 yr:* 400–800 mg 2–3 times a day.
ASACOL suppositories

Treatment and maintenance of remission of ulcerative colitis affecting the rectosigmoid region: Rectally: *child 12–17 yr:* 250–500 mg tid, last dose to be administered at bedtime.
PENTASA 500 mg tab

Treatment of mild-to-moderate ulcerative colitis, acute attack: PO: *child 5–17 yr (body-weight up to 40 kg):* 10–20 mg/kg tid; *child 5–17 yr (body-weight 40 kg and above):* 1–2 g bid, total daily dose may alternatively be given in 3 div. doses.

Maintenance of remission of ulcerative colitis: PO: *child 5–17 yr (body-weight up to 40 kg):* 7.5–15 mg/kg bid, total daily dose may alternatively be given in 3 div. doses; *Child 5–17 yr (body-weight 40 kg and above):* 2 g OD.

PENTASA suppositories
Treatment of acute attack, ulcerative proctitis: Rectally: *Child 12–17 yr:* 1 g daily for 2–4 wk.

Maintenance, ulcerative proctitis: Rectally: *Child 12–17 yr:* 1 g daily.
PENTASA retention enema
Treatment of an acute attack of mild-to-moderate ulcerative colitis affecting the rectosigmoid region: Rectally: *Child 12–17 yr:* 1 g OD, dose to be administered at bedtime.
SALOFALK tabs

Treatment of mild-to-moderate ulcerative colitis, acute attack: PO: *child 5–17 yr (body-weight up to 40 kg):* 10–20 mg/kg tid; *child 5–17 yr (body-weight 40 kg and above):* 0.5–1 g tid.

Maintenance of remission of ulcerative colitis: PO: *child 5–17 yr (body-weight up to 40 kg):* 7.5–15 mg/kg bid, total daily dose may alternatively be given in 3 div. doses; *child 5–17 yr (body-weight 40 kg and above):* 500 mg 3 times a day.

SALOFALK enema
Treatment of an acute attack of mild-to-moderate ulcerative colitis or maintenance of remission: Rectally: *Child 12–17 yr:* 2 g OD, dose to be administered at bedtime.

Mesna (Sodium Mercaptoethane Sulfonate)
Uroprotectant: Injection: IV at 20% of dose of cyclophosphamide for 4 doses at 0, 3, 6, 9 hr to protect the bladder. Always consult the current treatment protocols for details of dosage and scheduling.

Mucolytic: Nebule: 3–6 mL of a 20% solution twice.

Metformin Hydrochloride
500 mg/dose 2–3 times daily (max. 1 g/dose 2 times).

Methionine
PO: *<6 yr:* 1 g 4 hrly (max. 4 g/day); *>6 yr:* 2.5 g 4 hrly (max. 10 g/day) started within 8 hr of overdosage. Not effective if given after activated charcoal.

Methotrexate
Severe acute Crohn's disease: SC/IM: *child 7–18 yr:* 15 mg/m^2 (max. 25 mg) once weekly followed by maintenance of remission dose – PO/SC/IM. *Child 7–18 yr:* 15 mg/m^2 (max. 25 mg) once weekly; dose reduced according to response to lowest effective dose.

Juvenile idiopathic arthritis, juvenile dermatomyositis, vasculitis, uveitis, SLE, localized scleroderma, sarcoidosis: PO/SC/IM: *Child 1–18 yr:* 10–15 mg/m^2 (increased to max. 25 mg, if needed) once weekly.

Severe uncontrolled psoriasis unresponsive to conventional therapy: PO: *child 2–18 yr:* initially 200 g/kg (max. 10 mg) once weekly increased according to response to 400 μg/kg (max. 25 mg) once weekly.

Methoxsalen
Psoriasis: PO: *12–18 yr* 600 μg/kg (max. 70 mg) OD – given 2–3 hr before ultraviolet A (UVA) 1–3 times in a week (not to be more frequent than an alternate-day schedule).

Vitiligo: Adolescent – As advised by dermatologist.

Methyldopa
10 mg/kg/day in 2–4 div. doses. Max. 3 g/day.

Methylene Blue
Methemoglobinemia: 1–2 mg/kg or 25–50 mg/m^2; may be repeated after 1 hr if necessary.

NADPH-methemoglobin reductase deficiency: PO: 1–1.5 mg/kg/day (max. 300 mg) given with 5–8 mg/kg/day ascorbic acid.

Methylphenidate Hydrochloride (Controlled Drug)
(0.5–1 mg/kg/day before food). *>6 yr:* 5 mg/dose 1–2 times daily. Increase at weekly increments of 5–10 mg daily. Max. 60 mg/day given in 2–4 div. doses. Avoid dosing in the evenings.

Immediate-release tablets: Duration of action: 4 hr. Initial dose: 5 mg PO bid, preferably 30–45 minutes before breakfast and lunch, and a third dose may be added later between 2 and 4 PM, if necessary. *Maintenance dose:* Doses may be increased weekly in increments of 5–10 mg.

Sustained-release tablets: 18–20 mg; duration of action of approximately 6–8 hr. *Maintenance dose:* increase gradually up to a max. of 60 mg/day.

Extended-release tabs: The recommended starting dose is *6–17 yr:* 18 mg/day; max. dose: *6–12 yr:* 54 mg/day; 13–17 yr: 72 mg/day.

Metoclopramide Hydrochloride
PO, IM, or slow IV: *<12 yr:* 0.3 mg/kg/day (max. 10 g/day) in 3 div. doses. *12–18 yr:* 5–10 mg/dose tid.

Metolazone
2.5–5 mg/day for adolescents, 0.2–0.4 mg/kg/ day in children. Electrolytes must be monitored closely.

Metoprolol
PO: *Children*: 0.2–0.4 mg/kg/day initially; gradually increase to a max. of 1 mg/kg/day in 2 div. doses. A*dolescents:* 100–450 mg/24 hr in 3–4 div. doses. IV 5 mg every 2 min for 3 doses.

Metronidazole
Newborn: IV 15 mg/kg as loading dose followed 24 hr later by 7.5 mg/kg/dose bid.

Anaerobic infections and propionic and methylmalonic acidemia: PO/IV: 7.5 mg/kg/dose (max. 400–500 mg) tid.

Giardiasis: PO 40 mg/kg (max. 2 g) OD for 3 days.

Trichomoniasis: 5 mg/kg/dose (max. 300–499 mg/day) tid daily for 7 days.

Amebiasis (5–10 days) and balantidiasis (5 days): PO 10 mg/kg (max. 400–800 g).

H. pylori infection: PO: *1–6 yr:* 100 mg; *6–12 yr:* 200 mg; *12–18 yr:* 400 mg/dose tid for 14 days with either amoxicillin/omeprazole or clarithromycin/omeprazole.

Renal impairment: Increase dose interval to 12 hr in CrCl < 20 mL/min/1.73 m^2.

Hepatic impairment: Reduce dose and avoid in hepatic encephalopathy.

Miconazole
Topical on skin: Apply on the affected area bid for 10 days after lesions have healed.

Thrush: PO: *<1 mo:* 1.25 mL; *up to 2 yr:* 2.5 mL; *2–12 yr:* 5 mL; *12–18 yr:* 5–10mL 2–4 times daily. Use in the mouth after food and retain as long as possible.

Midazolam
Newborn – sedation: IV infusion 1 µg/kg/min for the 1st 24 hr followed by 0.5 mg/kg/min.

Children – premedication: IM *1–18 yr:* 70–100 µg/kg or PO 500 µg/kg (max. 15 mg) as a single dose 30–60 min before surgery. Monitor from time of administration.

Sedation for procedures: IV: *<12 yr:* 50–100 µg/kg (max. 300 µg/kg); *>12 yr:* 2 mg (if sedation is not adequate, incremental doses of 0.5–1 mg may be given – max. 5 mg); PO 0.5 mg/kg (max. 15 mg); rectal 500–700 µg/kg; intranasal 200–300 µg/kg, half in each nostril.

Sedation in intensive care: 30–300 µg/kg IV bolus over 3–5 min followed by continuous IV infusion of 500 mg or 3.3 µg/kg/min (may not be needed if the child has received morphine or postoperative sedation). Reduce dose in hypovolemia, vasoconstriction, and hypothermia. Lower doses if the child is receiving opiates. Adjust according to response.

Induction of anesthesia: Slow IV bolus: *>7–12 yr:* 150 µg/kg; *12–18 yr:* 200–300 µg/kg as a single dose.

Status epilepticus: IV initial bolus of 0.15–0.2 mg/kg followed by 1 µg/kg/min and increase by 1 µg/kg/min every 15 min until seizures stop (max. 5 µg/kg/min). Buccal/intranasal *<6 mo:* 300 µg/kg, *6 mo to 1 yr:* 2.5 mg; *1–4 yr:* 5 g; *5–9 yr:* 7.5 mg; *>10 yr*: 10 mg as single dose.

Intractable seizures in palliative care: 5 mg/24 hr IV/SC continuous infusion (can be titrated up to 40 mg/24 hr). Dose must be reduced in severe renal impairment and renal failure.

Miglustat
100 mg PO OD.

Milrinone Lactate
IV as 25–50 µg/kg bolus over 10 minutes, followed by infusion at 0.25–0.75 µg/kg/min.

Minocycline
PO: 50 mg/dose bid for minimum of 6 wk.

Paucibacillary leprosy: 50 mg single dose, given as a combination with rifampicin and ofloxacin.

Minoxidil
<12 yr: 0.2 mg/kg (max. 1 mg/kg/day); *12–18 yr:* 5 mg (max. 100 mg/day) – rarely need to give more than 50 mg/day. The dose may be given 1–2 times daily.

Androgenic alopecia: Apply 12 hrly not exceeding 2 mL/day for at least 45 days.

Misoprostol
Prophylaxis of NSAID GI complications: 12–18 yr: 200 µg/dose taken with NSAID along with or after meals qid.

Treatment of NSAID-induced GI complications: 2–12 yr: 5 µg/kg/dose bid; *12–18 yr*: 200 µg/dose 2–4 times daily with breakfast or main meal and at bedtime.

To improve fat absorption in cystic fibrosis: 2–18 yr: 400 µg/day in 4 div. doses.

Mitoxantrone (Mitozantrone)
Acute nonlymphocytic leukemia in children: <2 yr: 0.4 mg/kg/day for 3–5 days; *>2 yr*: 8–12 mg/m^2/day for 5 days.

Solid tumors in children: 18–20 mg/m^2 once in 2–3 wk or 5–8 mg/m^2 weekly.

Mometasone Furoate
Prophylaxis of asthma: DPI *12–17 yr:* Initially 400 µg daily in 1–2 div. doses, single dose to be inhaled in the evening, reduced to 200 µg OD, if control maintained.

Prophylaxis of severe asthma: DPI *12–17 yr:* Increase if necessary up to 400 g bid.

Prophylaxis and treatment of seasonal allergic or perennial rhinitis: Intranasal *3–11 yr:* 50 µg daily, dose to be sprayed into each nostril. *12–17 yr:* 100 µg daily, increased if necessary up to 200 µg daily, dose to be sprayed into each nostril; reduced to 50 µg daily, dose to be reduced when control achieved, dose to be sprayed into each nostril.

Severe inflammatory skin disorders such as eczemas unresponsive to less potent corticosteroids,

Psoriasis: Topical: *child 1 mo to 17 yr:* Apply OD, to be applied thinly (to scalp in case of lotion).

Side effects: Oropharyngeal candidiasis with inhaled mometasone and nasal ulceration with intranasal spray.

Montelukast
PO: *2–5 yr:* 4 mg, *6–14 yr:* 5 mg; *>14 yr:* 10 mg OD in the evening.

Morphine Sulfate (Controlled Drug)
Neonates: IM/IV/SC: *Analgesia:* 0.05–2 mg/kg/dose every 2–4 hr or continuous infusion 0.025–0.05 mg/kg/hr.

Infants and children: IM/IV/SC 0.1–0.2 mg/kg/dose every 2–4 hr. PO 0.2–0.4 mg/kg/dose every 4–6 hr. *Adolescents > 12 yr:* IV 3–4 mg may repeat after 5 min if required.

Mupirocin
Topical cream: Apply to the affected area tid for up to 10 days.

Nasal ointment: Apply to the inner surface of each nostril 2–3 times a day for 5–7 days.

Ointment: Apply to the affected area 2–3 times daily for up to 10 days.

Mycophenolate Mofetil
Prophylaxis of acute rejection in renal transplantation (in combination with a corticosteroid and ciclosporin): PO 600 mg/m^2 bid, max. 2 g/day.

Prophylaxis of acute rejection in renal transplantation (in combination with a corticosteroid and tacrolimus): PO 300 mg/m^2 bid, max. 2 g/day.

Prophylaxis of acute rejection in hepatic transplantation (in combination with a corticosteroid and ciclosporin or tacrolimus): PO 10 mg/kg bid, increased to 20 mg/kg bid, max. 2 g/day.

N

Nalidixic acid
Urinary tract infection due to susceptible organisms: PO: *Adolescents:* 1 g suspension or tablet PO every 6 hr for 1–2 wk. Maintenance dose of 500 mg PO every 6 hr. *Children and infants > 3 mo:* The recommended total daily dosage for initial therapy is 55 mg/ kg/day PO, administered in 4 equally div. doses. For prolonged therapy, the total daily dose may be reduced to 33 mg/kg/day PO.

Urinary tract infection prophylaxis in children: PO: *children and infants > 2 mo to 2 yr:* A dose of 30 mg/kg/day PO in 2 div. doses has been recommended. Max. dosage limits: *Adolescents:* 4 g/day PO. *Children and infants > 3 mo:* 55 mg/kg/day PO. *Infants < 3 mo:* Safe and effective use has not been established.

Patients with hepatic impairment: Exercise caution when using nalidixic acid in patients with liver disease; however, no specific dosage adjustments are indicated.

Patients with renal impairment: Decrease the dose by half in patients with a CrCl ≤ 20 mL/min.

Naloxone
Newborn infant: Do not administer to newborn whose mother is suspected of narcotic abuse as a withdrawal syndrome may be precipitated. Ensure establishment and maintenance of adequate ventilation before administering naloxone. It is specifically indicated for reversal of respiratory depression on newborn of mother who has received narcotics within 4 hr of delivery. IM is preferred because it affords more prolonged effect. 0.1 mg/kg may be repeated after 3–4 min.

In older children with suspected narcotic depression: Same dose (max. 2 mg) may be given IV. Repeat doses to maintain opioid reverse. If no response is seen after 2 doses, diagnosis of opioid toxicity must be reviewed.

Naproxen
PO 10–20 mg/kg in 2 div. doses (max. 1 g/day). In severe cases, up to 15 mg/kg may be used for a few wks.

Nedocromil
Prophylaxis of asthma: Inhalation of aerosol. *5–17 yr:* Initially 4 mg qid; when control is achieved, it may be possible to reduce to bid.

Seasonal and perennial conjunctivitis: Ophthalmic dosage: *6–17 yr:* Apply bid; increased if necessary to qid, max. 12 wk duration of treatment for seasonal allergic conjunctivitis.

Seasonal keratoconjunctivitis: Ophthalmic dosage: *6–17 yr:* Apply 4 times a day.

Neomycin Sulfate

Hepatic coma: *Adolescents:* 0.25–1 g 4 times. *Children:* 12.5 mg/kg/dose PO in diarrhea and 3 g/m^2/day q6h PO.

Eye drops: Superficial eye infection: 1 drop 2–4 times daily, *severe infection* 1 drop every 15–20 min initially and then reducing frequency as infection gets controlled.

Eye ointment: 3–4 times daily. Treatment to continue till 2 days after condition is cured.

Neostigmine

Newborn myasthenia gravis: PO 1–2 mg initially half hr before feed followed by 1–5 mg/dose (adjusted according to response) 6 times daily. IM 0.1 mg initially followed by 0.05–0.25 mg IM or SC (2–3 mg IM/SC is equal to 30 mg PO).

Reversal of nondepolarizing neuromuscular blockade: IV bolus over 1 min – 80 µg/kg with 20 µg/kg of atropine (for drugs other than atracurium) and 50 µg/kg with 20 µg/kg of atropine (for atracurium).

Children: Myasthenia gravis: PO: *1 mo to 5 yr* 7.5 mg/dose, *6–12 yr* 15 mg/dose, and *12–18 yr* 15–30 mg/dose repeated at suitable intervals according to response. IM *1 mo to 12 yr* 0.2–0.5 mg and *12–18 yr* 1–2.5 mg repeated at suitable intervals.

Nesiritide (Hbnp; Human B-Type Natriuretic Peptide)

Infusions starting at 0.01 µg/kg/min and uptitrated to a max. of 0.03 µg/kg/min. Calculate the required bolus volume based on the patient's weight as follows: Bolus volume (in mL) = 0.33 × patient weight (kg). Then withdraw the appropriate bolus volume from the nesiritide infusion bag and inject it over about 60 seconds through an IV port in the tubing. Immediately following the administration of the IV bolus, infuse nesiritide solution at a flow rate of 0.1 mL/kg/hr. The calculation for the infusion flow rate (mL/hr) = 0.1 × patient weight (kg). This will deliver the initial recommended nesiritide maintenance infusion rate of 0.01 µg/kg/min. Nesiritide is generally administered at a fixed IV infusion rate. Due to a long onset and offset of action, nesiritide should be titrated upward no more frequently than every 3 hr. Do not titrate the infusion rate at frequent intervals as is done with other IV agents that have a significantly shorter half-life (e.g., dobutamine, dopamine, nitroglycerin, and nitroprusside).

Netilmicin

Newborn: IV 3 mg/dose 12 hrly. Increase to 8 hrly after *1 week age postnatal.* Monitor after the 3rd dose for 1 hr post dose peak of 8–12 mg/L and a trough of <3 mg/L. Prolong dose interval in PDA, prolonged hypoxia, and indomethacin therapy. *Children*: IV/IM: *<12 yr* 7.5 mg/kg/day and *>12 yr* 6 mg/kg/day in 3 div. doses or *1 mo to 18 yr* 7.5 mg/kg as a single dose daily. Intraperitoneal 7.5–10 mg/L in peritoneal dialysis fluid.

Nevirapine

Treatment of HIV infection in combination with other antiretroviral agents. Neonates ≥ 15 days old, infants, and children: 150 mg/m^2 (not to exceed 400 mg) PO OD for the first 14 days and then 150 mg/m^2 (not to exceed 400 mg) bid. Alternatively, the following volume recommendations per dose of nevirapine 50 mg/5 mL oral suspension, based on body surface area, can be used: *>1.25 m^2:* 20 mL; *1.08–1.25 m^2:* 17.5 mL; *0.92–1.08 m^2:* 15 mL; *0.75–0.92 m^2*: 12.5 mL; *0.58–0.75 m^2:* 10 mL; *0.42–0.58 m^2*: 7.5 mL; *0.25–0.42 m^2:* 5 mL; *0.12–0.25 m^2:* 2.5 mL; and *0.06–0.12 m^2:* 1.25 mL. Same rules as for adolescent in case of rash or appearance of indication for discontinuation of therapy. *Neonates < 15 days old:* Dosing information is unavailable.

HIV prophylaxis – to prevent perinatal transmission of HIV to neonates born to HIV-infected women in labor who have had no prior ART: In patients who are not receiving any ART prior to labor, administer 200 mg PO as a single dose at the onset of labor. *Neonates ≥ 34 wk gestation:* The CDC recommends 2 mg/kg PO as a single dose 48–72 hr after birth. If the mother received nevirapine < 1 hr prior to delivery, the infant should be given 2 mg/kg PO as soon as possible after birth and again at 48–72 hr.

PO dosage (nevirapine and zidovudine combination): Pregnant females – intrapartum: Due to synergistic inhibition of HIV with the combination in vitro, the following regimen has been suggested: nevirapine 200 mg PO as a single dose at the onset of labor plus zidovudine (2 mg/kg IV bolus followed by 1 mg/kg/hr IV continuous infusion until delivery). During or immediately after intrapartum treatment with nevirapine and zidovudine, consider initiation of maternal zidovudine and lamivudine, continuing for 3–7 days, to potentially reduce the development of nevirapine resistance.

Neonates 34 wk gestation: Due to synergistic inhibition of HIV with the combination in vitro, the following regimen has been suggested: nevirapine 2 mg/kg PO as a single PO dose at age 48–72 hr plus zidovudine (2 mg/kg PO every 6 hr for 6 wk). Max. dosage limits: *Adolescents:* 400 mg/day PO. *Children:* 300 mg/m^2.

Niacin (Nicotinic Acid, Vitamin B3)

PO: *Pellagra* – 100–300 mg daily is given in div. doses.
Hartnup disease: 50–200 mg daily.

Nicardipine
Continuous IV infusion initially 500 ng/kg/min followed by maintenance infusion of 1–3 µg/kg/min.

Niclosamide
Tenia solium (pork), Tenia saginata (beef), Diphyllobothrium latum (fish): PO: *<2 yr* 500 mg, *2–6 yr* 1 g, *>7 yr* 2 g OD. Give the dose in 2 div. doses, one before breakfast and the rest 1 hr later.

Hymenolepis nana (dwarf tapeworm): PO single dose on the first day followed by half that dose daily once for the next 6 days. Initial day dose for *<2, 2–6, and 7–18 yr* are 500 mg, 1 g, and 2 g, respectively. No purgative is needed.

Nifedipine
Hypertensive crisis and angina: Sublingual/PO. Pierce the capsule and pour contents sublingually or into mouth 250–500 µg/kg as single dose.

Hypertension and angina: <12 yr 0.2–0.3 mg/kg/dose and *12–18 yr* 5–20 mg/kg/dose tid (max. 100 mg/day).

Raynaud's phenomenon: 2–18 yr 2.5–10 mg 2–4 times daily. Start with low dose at bedtime and gradually increase to avoid postural hypotension.

Nimesulide
5 mg/kg/day in 2 or 3 div. doses. The drug is banned for use in *children below 12 yr* by the Drug Controller General of India (DCGI) after the subcommittee of the government's chief advisory body, the Drug Technical Advisory Board (DTAB), recommended for the same.

Nitazoxanide
Amebiasis, giardiasis, cryptosporidiosis, and helminthiasis: *12–47 mo:* 100 mg 12 hrly for 3 days. *4–11 yr*: 200 mg 12 hrly for 3 days. *Adolescents*: 500 mg 12 hrly for 3 days.

Nitrazepam
PO initially 0.25 mg/kg in 2 div. doses followed by maintenance of 0.5 mg/kg in 2 div. doses (max. 1 mg/kg/day). Total daily dose may be given in 3 div. doses. Achieve target maintenance dose in 2–3 wk.

Renal and hepatic impairment: Dosage reduction is required.

Nitric Oxide
It is delivered along with oxygen through the ventilator circuit in a dose of 5–80 ppm.

>33 wk gestation: Start at 20 ppm. If this produces a raise in postductal pO_2 of at least 3 kPa (while ventilator parameters remain unchanged), reduce the dose after an hr to the lowest dose capable of producing a sustained response.

<33 wk gestation: Start with a dose of 5 ppm and consider increasing in stages to a max. of 40 ppm. If this produces no response, return to 5 ppm and give this for 12 hr. If there is still no response, stop. *Tailing off:* Always try to use the lowest effective dose; failure to do so may result in increasing dependency. Try to reduce the dose further every 12 hr. Drop the concentration by 10% every 3 minutes, but reverse any reduction that causes the arterial saturation to drop by more than 2%.

Nitric oxide should not be used for long term, as it results in methemoglobinemia. BP, pulmonary artery pressure, and arterial oxygen saturation should be monitored during therapy with nitric oxide.

Nitrofurantoin
Contraindicated in infants < 3 mo age.

Urinary tract infection treatment: 3 mo to 12 yr 5–7 mg/kg/day and in *12–18 yr* 200–400 mg/day in 4 div. doses.

Urinary tract infection prophylaxis: 1–2.5 mg/kg/day in at bedtime or in 2 div. doses (max. 100 mg/24 hr).

Nitroglycerine (Glyceryl Trinitrate)
IV infusion: The initial dose is 0.5 µg/kg/min IV; it is uptitrated depending on the response, to a max. of 10 µg/kg/min. Monitor blood pressure and heart rate. Tolerance may develop.

Nitrous Oxide
Inhalation: Nitrous oxide is administered with oxygen to avoid the hypoxia which would otherwise occur. Doses may be self-regulated in most cases by the use of a face-mask connected through a demand valve to the cylinder. The valve is operated by the act of inhalation by the patient and closes when the patient ceases to inhale. This will generally only be possible with children aged about 5 yr and over. It should be administered only by personnel trained in its use. Dose adjustments are not necessary in renal or hepatic disease.

Noradrenaline (Norepinephrine)
IV infusion: 0.3–2 µg/kg/min. Monitor ECG and hemodynamic parameters.

Norethisterone
Induction of sexual maturity: PO: 5 mg OD for the last 7 days of a 28-day cycle. (Norethisterone is added after 1½–2 yr of estrogen therapy or when breakthrough bleeding occurs to regularize menstrual cycles by adding progesterone in the last 7 days of the cycle.)

Postponement of menstruation: PO: 5 mg tid, starting 3 days before the expected onset of menstruation.

Nortriptyline
Nocturnal enuresis: PO: >6 yr 20–25 kg 10 mg; *25–35 kg* 10–20 mg, *>35 kg* 25–35 mg OD (bedtime). Max. duration of treatment is 3 mo. Review before further courses are given.

Depression: PO: *12–18 yr* 30–100 mg OD at night or in div. doses. Use low dose initially and increase if required up to 100 mg.

NTBC [2-(2-nitro-4-trifluoro-methylbenzoyl)-1,3 cyclohexanedione] (nitisinone)
PO 0.5–0.75 mg/kg as single dose initially. May require up to 2 mg/kg/day. Daily dose may be given in 2 div. doses.

Nystatin
Newborn: Treatment and prophylaxis against oral candidiasis: 1 mL 3–4 times daily.

Children: Intestinal and oral candidiasis: 1 mL 3–4 times daily

Oral candidiasis in immunocompromised: 1 mL 4–6 times

Esophageal/intestinal candidiasis: 5 mL or 1 tab 4–6 times daily

 O

Octreotide
Varices: IV infusion 1 µg/kg/hr initially; may be increased to 3 µg/kg/hr till bleeding is controlled. Then taper over 24 hr to avoid rebound bleeding.

Hyperinsulinemia: SC 1 µg/kg 4 hrly initially and increased up to 40 µg/kg/24 hr depending on response.

Renal impairment: No change in dose is required.

Ofloxacin
Eye drops: >1 yr 1 drop 2–4 hrly for the 1st 48 hr and then qid till 2 days after healing is achieved (max. 10 days).

Ear drops: Otitis externa: 1–12 yr 5 drops and *12–18 yr* 10 drops to affected ear(s) bid for 10 days.

Chronic suppurative otitis media (CSOM): >12 yr 10 drops to affected ear(s) bid for 14 days.

Acute otitis media (AOM) with perforation or with tympanostomy tubes: 1–12 yr: 5 drops to affected ear(s) bid for 10 days. IV and PO: 10–15 mg/kg/day in a single dose or div. bid.

Systemic use: It is replaced by levofloxacin which is an S-isomer of ofloxacin and has less side effects.

Olanzapine
12–18 yr: 5–20 mg OD. Usual dose is 10 mg daily.

Olopatadine
Allergic conjunctivitis, including ocular pruritus: Adolescents and children 3 yr: 1 drop in each affected eye two times/day at an interval of 6–8 hr. (This is the max. dosage allowed.) *Children < 3 yr:* Safety and efficacy have not been established.

Renal or hepatic impairment: No dosage adjustment is necessary for ocular administration.

Olsalazine
PO: *Adolescents and children (2–18 yr):* 30 mg/kg/day (not exceeding 3 g/day), in 2 or 3 div. doses. May initiate with 500 mg bid and increase over 1 wk up to a max. of 3 g/day (a single dose not exceeding 1 g). Maintenance dose is 250–500 mg bid.

Patients with hepatic impairment: Specific guidelines for dosage adjustments in hepatic impairment are not available.

Patients with renal impairment: Specific guidelines for dosage adjustments in renal impairment are not available. Olsalazine should be used cautiously in patients with preexisting renal impairment or renal disease due to possibility of renal tubular damage. Monitoring by blood urea nitrogen (BUN), serum creatinine, and urinalysis.

Omeprazole
PO: *<12 yr:* Initially 0.7 mg/kg and increased to 3 mg/kg/day. *12–18 yr:* 20–40 mg initially as single dose and at higher doses in 2 div. doses.

H. pylori infection: PO: *1–12 yr:* 1–2 mg/kg rounded to nearest 10 mg and max. 40 mg. *12–18 yr:* 40 mg as single dose for 14 days with amoxicillin and clarithromycin or amoxicillin and metronidazole or clarithromycin and metronidazole.

Ondansetron
Nausea and vomiting: Chemotherapy induced: IV: *<12 yr:* 5 mg/m^2. *12–18 yr:* 8 mg as single dose just before chemotherapy and repeated 8–12 hrly during therapy and for 24 hr after. PO following initial IV dosing to get control: *<12 yr:* 4 mg. *12–18 yr:* 8 mg 2–3 times daily for up to 5 days after a course of chemotherapy.

Postoperative nausea and vomiting: IV slow infusion *2–12 yr:* 0.1 mg/kg (max. 4 mg). *12–18 yr:* 4 mg.

Pruritus: PO: 2–12 yr 2-4mg/dose and 12–18 yr 4–8 mg/dose bid.

Palliative for nausea/vomiting and pruritus: IV/SC 5 mg/m^2 continuous over 24 hr.

Opioid analgesics
See **Table 24.13.3** for equivalent doses of various opioid analgesics.

Oral Rehydration Salts (ORS)
Fluid and electrolyte loss in diarrhea: PO: *1 mo to 1 yr:* 1–1½ times usual feed volume. *1–12 yr:* 200 mL after every loose motion. *12–18 yr:* 200–400 mL after every loose motion.

Orlistat
PO: *12–18 yr:* 120 mg immediately before, during, or 1 hr after each main meal (max. 3 times/day); specialist advice is

TABLE 24.13.3: Equivalent doses of various opioid analgesics.

An approximate guide: Children should be carefully monitored after any change in medication and dose titration may be required.		
Analgesic	***Route***	***Dose (mg)***
Codeine	PO	100
Diamorphine	IM, IV, SC	3
Dihydrocodeine	PO	2
Morphine	PO	10
Morphine	IM, IV, SC	5
Oxycodone	PO	6.6
Tramadol	PO	100

(IM: intramuscular; IV: intravenous; SC: subcutaneous)

required for treating for more than 12 wk. If meal is missed or if meal contains no fat, the dose may be omitted.

Oseltamivir

Prevention of influenza: PO: *13–18 yr:* 75 mg OD for at least 7 days after exposure or for up to 6 wk during an epidemic.

Treatment of influenza: PO *for children above 1 yr age up to 16 kg:* 30 mg. *16–23 kg:* 45 mg. *23–40 kg:* 60 mg. *>40 kg:* 75 mg – every 12 hr for 5 days.

Oxandrolone

PO 1.25–2.5 mg OD, generally for about 3–6 mo, but has been used occasionally for up to 1 yr; evidence suggests using doses as low as 625 µg for Turner syndrome, in combination with GH - seek expert advice before prescribing

Oxcarbazepine

PO: *6–12 yr:* 8–10 mg/kg/day in 2 div. doses - increase by 5 mg/kg/dose bid weekly till max. of 30 mg/kg/dose for adjunctive therapy and 46 mg/kg/day for monotherapy. *12–18 yr:* 8–10 mg/kg/day (max. initial dose 300 mg/dose) in 2 div. doses. Increase over 2–4 wk to 1,200 mg/24 hr in 2 div. doses (max. 2400 mg/24 hr).

Oxybutynin

PO: *2–5 yr:* 0.2 mg/kg/dose PO q8h. *5–12 yr:* 2.5–5 mg. *12–18 yr:* 5 mg 2–3 times daily (max. in *12–18 yr* 5 mg 4 times daily).

Oxycodone Hydrochloride

Moderate-to-severe pain in palliative care: PO immediate-release preparation: *1 mo to 11 yr:* Initially 200 µg/kg 4–6 hrly (max. per dose 5 mg). *12–17 yr:* Initially 5 mg 4–6 hrly, dose to be increased if necessary, according to the severity of pain.

PO-modified-release preparations: 8–11 yr: initially 5 mg 12 hrly. *12–17 yr:* initially 10 mg 12 hrly, dose to be increased if necessary, according to the severity of pain, use 12-hrly modified-release preparations for this dose; 2 mg PO oxycodone is approximately equivalent to 1 mg parenteral oxycodone.

Severe pain: PO: *12–17 yr:* initially 10 mg every 24 hr, dose to be increased if necessary, according to severity of pain. Some patients may require higher doses than the max. daily dose; max. 400 mg/day.

In mild-to-moderate renal impairment: Max. initial dose 2.5 mg every 6 hr in patients not currently treated with an opioid.

Oxygen

Dependent on condition. In some conditions (e.g., BPD), very low flow rates (e.g., 0.1 L/ min) may maintain oxygen saturation.

Oxymetazoline Hydrochloride

1 drop in each nostril twice daily or when required.

Oxytetracycline

Acne: PO: *12–18 yr:* 250–500 mg/dose 12 hrly.

Infections: 250–500 mg/dose 6 hrly.

P

Paliperidone

Extended-release tablets: *12–17 yr:* Initial dose: 3 mg PO OD; range: 3–12 mg/day; dose increases may be made in increments of 3 mg/day and should occur at intervals of more than 5 days. Max: 12 mg/day.

Palivizumab

15 mg/kg once monthly, starting just prior to the beginning of the respiratory syncytial virus (RSV) season, for a total of 5 doses. Not used in India as of now.

Pamidronate Disodium

Experience of the use of bisphosphonates in children is limited and expert advice should be sought. Their use is only justified when the potential benefits outweigh any risk. *Children:* 1 mg/kg/24 hr for 3 consecutive days once in 3 mo or 10–40 mg/m^2 over 5–8 hr once a mo. Dose adjusted according to serum calcium levels.

Pancreatin

Dose varies widely and should be tailored to each individual patient according to symptoms, stool type, and abdominal findings; should not exceed 10,000 lipase units/kg body weight/day.

Pancuronium Bromide

Newborn: IV loading 0.1 mg/kg followed by maintenance IV 0.05 mg/kg/dose 4–6 times daily as needed. *Children:* IV: *1 mo to 18 yr:* 0.06–0.1 mg/kg initially followed by 0.01–0.02 mg/kg as required.

Pantoprazole
>5 yr old: >15 to <40 kg: 20 mg; *>40 kg:* 40 mg OD × 8 wk.

Zollinger-Ellison syndrome: Adolescents >40 kg: 40 mg bid.

Paracetamol
PO or suppository: *<12 yr:* 15 mg/kg/dose every 4–6 hrly. *12–18 yr:* 325–650 mg every 4–6 hrly. There is no difference between the temperature decrement in patients treated with 15 mg/kg PO acetaminophen and the same or double the dose rectally.

Paraldehyde
Rectal: *<12 yr:* 0.4 mL/kg. *12–18 yr:* 5–10 mL diluted in equal volume of olive or sunflower oil before administration. IM: *Newborn:* 0.2 mL/kg; *1 mo to 12 yr:* 0.1–0.15 mL/kg; *12–18 yr:* 5–10 mL as single dose. Deep IM with Z injection [max. 1 mL (newborn) and 5 mL (older children) per site].

Paromomycin Sulfate
Amebiasis: Asymptomatic cyst passers (intraluminal infections): PO 25–35 mg/kg daily, in 3 div. doses, given for 5–10 days (usually 7 days).

Symptomatic intestinal amebiasis or extraintestinal disease (including amebic liver abscess): PO 25–35 mg/kg daily, in 3 div. doses, given for 5–10 days (usually 7 days). Used as follow-up after initial treatment with a tissue amebicide (PO metronidazole or PO tinidazole).

Cestode (tapeworm) infections – Diphyllobothrium latum (fish tapeworm), Dipylidium caninum (dog and cat tapeworm), T. saginata (beef tapeworm), or T. solium (pork tapeworm) infections: PO 11 mg/kg every 15 min for 4 doses.

Hymenolepis nana (dwarf tapeworm) infections: PO 45 mg/kg daily, given as a single daily dose, for 5–7 days.

Cryptosporidiosis: PO 25–35 mg/kg daily in 2–4 div. doses for HIV-infected children or adolescents. Max. dosage is 500 mg 4 times daily in children.

Dientamoeba fragilis infections: PO 25–35 mg/kg daily, in 3 div. doses, given for 7 days.

Giardiasis: PO 25–35 mg/kg daily, in 3 div. doses, given for 7 days.

Cutaneous leishmaniasis: Topical – apply topically (as a preparation containing paromomycin 15% and methylbenzethonium chloride 12% in white petrolatum) bid for 10–20 days. If effective, clinical healing of lesions usually is complete within several wk to a mo after topical paromomycin treatment is completed. In patients with recurrent disease (leishmaniasis recidivans), more prolonged topical treatment (e.g., bid for about 3 mo) may eliminate the protozoa from cutaneous lesions.

Visceral leishmaniasis (kala-azar): IM 11–20 mg/kg daily for 10–21 days.

Paroxetine
Obsessive-compulsive disorder (OCD): PO: *12–18 yr:* 20 mg (max. 60 mg) OD in the morning. Increase weekly by 10 mg/day to max. dose.

Panic disorder: PO: *12–18 yr:* 12.5 mg/day. Higher doses under supervision of specialist (max. 40 mg) OD in the morning. Increase weekly by 10 mg/day to max. dose.

Idiopathic musculoskeletal pain: PO: *8–12 yr:* 10 mg and *12–18 yr:* 20 mg OD.

Para-amino Salicylic Acid (PAS)
Tuberculosis: PO 150 mg/kg/day in 2–3 div. doses. Max. 12 g/day.

Penicillamine
Complete blood count (CBC), platelet count, and urinalysis should be performed prior to treatment with penicillamine. Urinalysis and CBC should be carried out monthly during treatment. Caution should be exercised in patients with renal insufficiency, and modification of the dosage may be necessary. Renal function should be assessed monthly. An immediate blood count should be carried out if neutropenia or thrombocytopenia is suspected due to symptoms such as a sore throat, glossitis, buccal ulceration, easy bruising, or bleeding. If any abnormal results are found, treatment should be withheld and discussed with the clinician responsible for the child's care. Severe dyspepsia or taste disturbances may necessitate dosage reduction.

Wilson disease: Adjust dose to maintain urinary copper excretion >1 mg/24 hr. PO 20 mg/kg/24hr in 2–4 div. doses (max. 1 g/24 hr).

Lead intoxication: PO 30–40 mg/kg/24 hr in 2–3 div. doses (max. 1.5 g/24 hr).

Juvenile idiopathic arthritis: 3 mg/kg/24 hr in 2 div. doses; increasing once every 3 mo by 3 mg/kg/24 hr up to a max. of 10 mg/kg/24 hr.

Systemic sclerosis: PO: *<12 yr:* 2.5–5 mg/kg/day in 2 div. doses increased 4 weekly to max. of 15–20 mg/kg/day. *12–18 yr:* 125–250 mg/day increased slowly to 250–375 mg in 2 div. doses.

Penicillinase-resistant penicillins (Flucloxacillin/Cloxacillin)
Newborn: IV or PO: <7 days 50–100 mg/ kg/day in 2 div. doses. *7–21 days:* 75–150 mg/kg/day in 3 div. doses. *>21 days:* 100–200 mg/kg/day in 4 div. doses. *Children:* IV/IM 50–100 mg/kg/day in 4 div. doses (max. single dose 1 g – may be doubled in severe infection). PO: *<1 yr:* 250 mg/day. *1–5 yr:* 500 mg/

day. *5–18 yr:* 1 g in 4 div. doses. Doses may be doubled in severe infection.

Penicillins (Benzylpenicillin/Penicillin G)
Given IV. *Newborn:* 25 mg (approx. 40,000 units)/kg/dose bid up to 7 days of age and tid thereafter. Dose is doubled in meningitis. In children, 25 mg/kg/dose qid. Double dose is given in meningitis 6 times daily to a max. single dose of 2.4 g (approx. 40 L units) and a max. daily dose of 14.4 g (approx. 2.3 crore units).

Pentazocine
Adolescents: Inj: 30–60 mg IM or 30 mg IV. May be repeated 3–4 hrly. Doses in excess of 30 mg IV or 60 mg SC or IM not recommended. Max. daily dose: 360 mg. In labor: 30 mg IM or 20 mg IV 2–3 hrly. Max: 2–3 doses. Tab: 25–100 mg repeated when necessary. Max. 600 mg daily. *Children:* Not for children below 12 yr.

Peppermint Oil
Child 15–17 yr: 1–2 capsules tid for up to 3 mo if necessary.

Perampanel [2-(2-oxo-1-phenyl-5-pyridin-2-yl-1,2 dihydropyridin-3-yl benzonitrile hydrate]
Adjunctive treatment of focal seizures with or without secondary generalized seizures: PO: *12–17 yr:* Initially 2 mg OD, before bedtime, then increased, if tolerated, in steps of 2 mg at intervals of at least every 2 wk, and titrated as required; maintenance 4–8 mg OD; max. 12 mg/day.

Adjunctive treatment of primary GTCS: PO: *12–17 yr:* Initially 2 mg OD, before bedtime, then increased, if tolerated, in steps of 2 mg at intervals of at least every 2 wk, and titrated as required, maintenance up to 8 mg OD; max. 12 mg/day.

Monotherapy or adjunctive therapy for generalized and partial-onset seizures with or without secondarily generalization: >4 yr age: start at 2 mg PO at bedtime; increase by 2 mg/day increments in at least weekly intervals to 4–8 mg based on clinical response and tolerability.

Permethrin
Scabies (dermal cream): Single topical application of up to: 1 tube for *children > 12 yr.* Half a tube for *children aged 6–12 yr.* A quarter of a tube for *children aged 1–5 yr.* An eighth of a tube for *children aged 2 mo to 1 yr.* Medical supervision required for children < 2 yr of age. If necessary, a second application may be given not less than 7 days after the initial application. Apply to whole body excluding head. Wash off after 8–12 hr. *Children < 2 yr old* should also have the cream applied to the face, neck, scalp, and ears. If hands or any part are washed, the treatment must be reapplied.

Pediculosis: Head lice (cream rinse): apply to clean damp hair, leave on for 10 minutes, rinse and dry. It is not affected by chlorine in swimming pools.

Pethidine Hydrochloride (Controlled Drug)
SC/IM: *Newborn:* 0.5–1 mg/kg. *<12 yr:* 0.5–2 mg/kg. *12–18 yr:* 25–100 mg as single dose - repeated if required once in 4–6 hr. IV bolus *<12 yr:* 0.5 -1 mg/kg. *12–18 yr*: 25–50 mg repeated if required once in 4–6 hr. IV infusion loading dose of 1 mg/kg followed by 0.1–0.4 mg/kg/hr. Ventilated babies may require higher doses. Newborn and infants are prone to respiratory depression.

Avoid in severe renal impairment, sickle cell crisis, and prolonged infusions as accumulation of metabolite norpethidine can cause seizures. It may precipitate coma in children with liver disease.

Phenobarbitone (Phenobarbital)
Anticonvulsant: Loading dose 15–20 mg/kg PO, IV, or IM; then maintenance. *Newborn:* 3–4 mg/kg/24 hr PO or IV in 2 div. doses or as single daily dose. *Children:* 5–6 mg/kg/24 hr PO or IV in 2 div. doses or as single daily dose. *Adolescents:* 1–3 mg/kg/24 hr PO or IV in 2 div. doses or as single daily dose.

Sedation: Children: 2 mg/kg/dose.

Hyperbilirubinemia: Newborn: 5–8 mg/kg/day PO for 2–7 days. It is not widely used as phototherapy usually suffices.

Phenoxybenzamine Hydrochloride
PO 1–2 mg/kg/24 hr in 2 div. doses. IV infusion 1 mg/kg bolus given IV over 30 min, followed by 0.5–1 mg/kg/day infusion.

Phenoxymethylpenicillin (Penicillin V)
PO 250 mg/day, *1–5 yr*: 500 mg/day. *6–12 yr:* 1 g/day. *12–18 yr:* 2 g/day (severe infection 3 g/day) in 4 div. doses.

Pneumococcal infection prophylaxis: Half the above daily dose in 2 div. doses.

Rheumatic fever prophylaxis: 500 mg/day in 2 div. doses.

Phenytoin
Status epilepticus: Loading dose: *Neonate:* 15–20 mg/kg IV (not to exceed 0.5 mg/kg/min). *Children and adolescents:* 15–18 mg/kg IV (not to exceed 1–3 mg/kg/min).

Antiepileptic: PO/IV: *newborn:* 5 mg/kg/24 hr OD or in 2 div. doses. *<6 yr:* 8–10 mg/kg/24 hr. *7–9 yr*: 6–8 mg/kg/24 hr OD or in 2 div. doses. *10–16 yr:* 6–7 mg/kg/24 hr OD or in 2 div. doses. *>16 yr:* 300–600 mg/24 hr OD or in 2 div. doses.

Arrhythmias: Loading dose 1.25 mg/kg IV once in 5 min until desired effect or total dose 15 mg/kg. *Maintenance: Children:* 8–10 mg/kg/day in 2–3 div. doses; *adolescents:* 250 mg 3–4 times daily.

Pholcodine
PO: *1 mo to 6 yr:* 2 mg/dose. *6–12 yr:* 2.5 mg/dose. *12–18 yr:* 5–10 mg/dose 3–4 times daily.

Phosphates
Hypercalcemia: PO: *newborn*: 1 mmol/kg. *<5 yr:* up to 48 mmol. *>5 yr:* up to 96 mmol.

Hypophosphatemia: PO: *newborn:* 1 mmol/kg. *<5 yr:* up to 36–48 mmol. *>5 yr*: up to 64–96 mmol. May be given in 3 div. doses in hypophosphatemic rickets. IV *newborn:* 1 mmol/kg; *<2 yr:* 0.7 mmol/kg; *>2 yr:* 0.4 mmol/kg.

Phosphocysteamine
PO: *>2 yr:* 6 mg/kg qid. Increase every 2–3 wk by 25 mg/kg/day up to maintenance of 125 mg/kg/day.

Pimozide
Schizophrenia: PO: *12–18 yr:* 1–20 mg usually OD but may be given in div. doses.

Tourette syndrome: PO: *2–12 yr:* 1–4 mg. *12–18 yr:* 2–10 mg usually OD but may be given in div. doses. Do annual ECG to monitor QT interval.

Piperacillin with tazobactam
Hospital-acquired pneumonia, septicemia, complicated infections involving the urinary tract, skin, and soft tissues: IV infusion: *neonate:* 90 mg/kg 8 hrly. *1 mo to 12 yr:* 90 mg/kg 6–8 hrly (max. 4.5 g/dose once in 6 hr). *12–17 yr:* 4.5 g 8 hrly; increased if necessary to 4.5 g 6 hrly.

For acute exacerbation of bronchiectasis used above 1 mo age in the same doses as mentioned.

Infections in a neutropenic child: At 90 mg/kg 6 hrly (max. per dose 4.5 g).

Complicated intra-abdominal infections: IV infusion *2–11 yr:* 112.5 mg/kg 8 hrly (max. per dose 4.5 g). *12–17 yr:* 4.5 g 8 hrly; increased if necessary to 4.5 g 6 hrly.

Note: Piperacillin with tazobactam is not licensed for use in children under 12 yr (except for children 2–12 yr with neutropenia).

Piperazine
Round worm: 4 g OD for 2 days – *children:* 75 g /yr, max. 4 g, because of its capacity to relax worms mainly useful for intestinal obstruction caused by round worms.

Enterobiasis: 50 mg/kg OD for 7 days consecutively or 75 mg/kg single dose.

Piracetam
Learning difficulties: 3 g/day in 3 div. doses for 1 school yr. *Children:* 50 mg/kg in 3 div. doses. Once the desired result has been obtained, reduce the initial dose by half up to 6–8 wk.

Piroxicam
PO: *<15 kg:* 5 mg. *16–25 kg:* 10 mg. *26–45 kg:* 15 mg. *>46 kg:* 20 mg OD.

Pivmecillinam Hydrochloride
PO: *>40 kg:* Initially 400 mg stat and then 200 mg 8 hrly to a total of 10 tablets.

Chronic or recurrent bacteriuria: PO: *>40 kg:* 6–8 hrly

Urinary tract infection: Up to 40 kg: 5–10 mg/kg 6 hrly, alternatively 20–40 mg/kg daily in 3 div. doses. It is not licensed for use in children under 3 mo.

Pizotifen
5–18 yr: Start with 500 µg at night and increase gradually up to 1.5 mg daily in div. doses; max. single dose (at night) – 1 mg.

Pneumococcal Conjugate Vaccine
Deep SC or IM injection: 0.5 mL. The number of doses for a primary course depends on the age of the child. For routine immunization, 3 doses at 1 mo interval from 6 wks of age; if given below 6 mo age, 2 doses at 1 mo interval; if given between 6 mo and 1 yr, 1 dose if given after 1 yr with a booster at 1½ yr age. For these high-risk groups, 3 doses at monthly intervals for children < 2 yr old and 2 doses at a mo apart for those >2 yr. The course should then be followed by a single dose of the plain polysaccharide vaccine to increase the breadth of cover. This should be administered at >2 yr with a minimum interval of 8 wk after the conjugate vaccine.

Pneumococcal Polysaccharide Vaccine
Deep SC or IM: 0.5 mL as single dose. Booster doses of the plain polysaccharide vaccine are not normally recommended and should certainly not take place within 3 yr of the first dose as marked local reactions can occur. As the vaccine could be used in conjunction with the conjugate vaccine in children, one must ensure an 8-week gap between the last conjugate pneumococcal vaccine and the polysaccharide vaccine.

Podophyllum
Topical: Applied twice weekly. Leave on the affected area for not more than 6 hr and then wash off. Protect the surrounding area with soft paraffin. Continue applying till eradication of wart or a max. of 6 wk.

Poliomyelitis Vaccine, Live PO (OPV)
PO: 3 drops (0.135 mL). The primary course is usually given at birth, 8, 12, 16, and 20 wk of age. This is followed by a booster at 1½ and 4½ yr age. It is given on national immunization days to all children < 5 yr age for poliomyelitis eradication.

Polyethylene Glycol 3350
Polyethylene glycol 3350 powder – 1 sachet or 1 heap tablespoon OD – mix with a liquid and give PO once a day as needed for up to 2 wk. It may take 2–4 days for polyethylene glycol 3350 to produce a bowel movement.

Potassium Chloride
Potassium supplementation: PO/IV 0.5–1 mmol/kg bid or 0.5–1 mEq/kg bid.

Acute hypokalemia: 0.08–0.2 mmol/kg/hr or mEq/kg/hr. Check dose carefully as overdose could be fatal. Recheck potassium levels after 3 hr. 1 g KCl = 13.4 mmol or 13.4 mEq.

Potassium Permanganate
Cleansing and deodorizing suppurating eczematous reactions and wounds. For wet dressings or baths, use approx. 0.01% (1 in 10,000) solution OR 1 granule dissolved in 300 mL (2½ glasses) of water.

Povidone-Iodine
Antiseptic paint: Apply bid.

Dry powder: Use for minor wounds and infections.

Ointment: Apply once or bid for up to 14 days.

Shampoo: Use as shampoo twice weekly until improvement is noted followed by once weekly.

Skin cleanser: Retain on infected skin for 3–5 min before rinsing. Repeat bid.

Solutions, tinctures, and scrub: Use undiluted for skin disinfection.

Pralidoxime
Adolescents: Following resuscitation measures, and 2–4 mg atropine inj., 1–2 g IM or IV as 5% soln. over 5–10 min. or infusion in 100 mL sodium chloride over 15–30 min. Repeat therapy if required. *Children:* 20–40 mg/kg OD.

Pravastatin Sodium
PO: *2–12 yr:* 5 mg. *12–18 yr:* 10 mg OD. Increase if needed over 6–12 wk.

Praziquantel
Schistosomiasis hematobium (Schistosoma mansoni): PO: *4–18 yr:* 40 mg/kg/day as single dose or in 2 div. doses with food for 1 day.

Schistosoma japonicum: PO: *4–18 yr:* 60 mg/kg/day in 3 div. doses with food for 1 day.

Liver fluke: PO: *4–18 yr:* 60 mg/kg/day in 2 div. doses with food for 3 days.

Lung fluke (Paragonimus westermani): PO: *4–18 yr:* 75 mg/kg/day in 3 div. doses with food for 3 days.

Intestinal fluke (Fasciolopsis buski): PO: *4–18 yr:* 75 mg/kg/day in 3 div. doses with food for 1 day.

Beef, pork, and fish tapeworm: PO: *4–18 yr:* 10–20 mg/kg/day as single dose with light breakfast for 1 day.

Dwarf tapeworm: PO: *4–18 yr:* 25 mg/kg/day as single dose with light breakfast for 1 day.

Neurocysticercosis: PO: *4–18 yr:* 50 mg/kg/day in 3 div. doses with food for 15–21 days. Give steroids to reduce the severity of adverse reactions.

Echinococcosis: PO: *4–18 yr:* 40 mg/kg/day once in a week with food in combination with albendazole as an adjunct to surgery and for inoperable cysts.

Renal failure and hepatic failure: No dosage adjustment.

Prazosin
Hypertension: PO: *1 mo to 12 yr:* 10–15 μg/kg/dose 2–4 times daily (max. 0.5 mg/kg/day). *12–18 yr:* 0.5 mg/dose 2–3 times daily (max. 20 mg/day).

Congestive cardiac failure: PO: *1 mo–12 yr:* 0.5 μg/kg/dose bid (max. 0.1 mg/kg/day). *12–18 yr:* 0.5 mg/dose 2–4 times daily (max. 20 mg/day).

Prednisolone
Acute asthma: PO 1–2 mg/kg in 2–3 div. doses (max. 40 mg/day) for 1–5 days and stop without tapering if the episode is controlled.

Croup requiring intubation: PO 2 mg/kg/day in 2 div. doses soon after intubation and continued for 24 hr.

Prilocaine Hydrochloride
Children < 10 yr: 1mL; *>10 yr:* 1–2 mL.

Primaquine
PO: *1–12 yr:* 0.25 mg/kg/day. *12–18 yr:* 15 mg OD for 14 days.

For glucose-6-phosphate dehydrogenase (G6PD) deficiency patients: 1–12 yr: 0.5–0.75 mg/kg. *12–18 yr:* 30 mg once in a week for 8 wk.

Primidone
PO: *<2 yr:* initially 125 mg daily at bedtime, increased by 125 mg every 3 days according to response; usual maintenance, 125–250 mg bid. *2–5 yr:* Initially 125 mg daily at bedtime, increased by 125 mg every 3 days according to response; usual maintenance, 250–375 mg bid. *5–9 yr:* Initially 125 mg daily at bedtime, increased by 125 mg every 3 days according to response; usual maintenance, 375–500 mg twice a day. *9–18 yr:* Initially 125 mg daily at bedtime, increased by 125 mg every 3 days to 250 mg bid and then increased.

Hepatic impairment: Reduce dose; may precipitate coma.

Renal impairment: Refer to phenobarbitone (phenobarbital).

Procarbazine
Always consult the current treatment protocol for details of dosage and scheduling.

Hodgkin disease: PO 1.5–3 mg/kg/24 hr (50–100 mg/m^2) OD for 14 days per 28-day cycle.

Bone marrow transplant preparation: 12.5 mg/kg/dose.

Neuroblastoma and medulloblastoma: 100–200 mg/m^2/dose as part of protocol.

Prochlorperazine

PO/rectal: *>1 yr:* 0.1–0.25 mg/kg/dose 2–3 times daily. IM 0.1–0.15 mg/kg/24 hr div. in 2–3 doses.

Procyclidine

PO: *7–12 yr:* 4 mg/kg/day. *12–18 yr:* 7.5 mg/kg/day in 3 div. doses.

Proguanil

PO: *0–12 wk <6 kg:* 25 mg ¼th tab. *12 wk to 11 mo* 6–10 kg: 50 mg ½ tab. *1–3 yr: 10–16 kg:* 75 mg ¾ tab. 4–7 yr: *16–24 kg:* 100 mg 1 tab. *8–12 yr 25–44 kg:* 150 mg. 1½ tab. *>13 yr >45 kg:* 200 mg 2 tab. To be given OD starting 1 week before entering endemic area and continue till 4 wk after return.

Promethazine Hydrochloride

Symptomatic relief of allergy: PO: *<1 yr:* 2.5–5 mg. *1–6 yr:* 5–10 mg. *6–12 yr:* 10–15 mg. *12–18 yr:* 10–20 mg 2–3 times daily.

Vomiting and nausea: PO 1 mg/kg/24 hr in 4 div. doses.

Sedation: PO 1–2 mg/kg as single dose.

Sedation in ICU: Slow IV/PO/deep IM *< 12 yr:* 2–4 mg/kg/day. *>12 yr:* 100–200 mg in 4 div. doses. Start with lower dose and increase gradually depending on response. May use along with chloral hydrate.

Propafenone Hydrochloride

PO 10–20 mg/kg/day in 2 div. doses; starting at lower dose. IV bolus followed by IV infusion 0.2 mg/kg slowly over 10 min repeated every 15 min up to max. 2 mg/kg followed by IV infusion with ECG monitoring of 4 μg/kg/min increasing to 8 μg/kg/min (if required).

Hepatic function is impairment: 20–30% of this total dose.

Propantheline Bromide

PO: *<12 yr:* 0.9–1.2 mg/kg/day in 3–4 div. doses (max. 3 mg/kg/day - larger doses in enuresis). *>12 yr:* 15 mg before meals and 20 mg at bedtime.

Propofol

Sedation: IV 1.5–3 mg/kg/dose over 1–2 min.

Continuous sedation (mechanical ventilation): 5.5 mg/kg for 30 min, increase to 6 mg/kg for 30 min, increase to 8 mg/kg for 1 hr, increase to 10 mg/kg for 1 hr, increase to final infusion rate of 12.5 mg/kg/hr.

Induction of general anesthesia: 1.5–2.5 mg/kg (larger doses in children < 8 yr) and maintain anesthesia with 9–15 mg/kg/hr.

Propranolol

Hypertension: PO: *newborn:* 0.25–0.5 mg/kg. *<12 yr:* 0.25–1 mg/kg tid. *>12 yr:* 80–160 mg bid. Max. in newborn 2 mg/kg/day. In children, increase weekly as required to usual dose 1-5 mg/kg/day.

Migraine prophylaxis and essential tremor: PO: *2–12 yr:* 20 mg/dose. *12–18 yr:* 20–40 mg/dose 2–3 times daily.

Dysarrhythmias: PO: *<12 yr:* 0.25–0.5mg/dose. *>12 yr:* 10–40 mg/dose 3–4 times daily. IV bolus: *<12 yr:* 25–50 μg/kg. *>12 yr:* 1 mg/kg as single dose slowly over 5 min with ECG monitoring. Repeat dose as required up to 4 times daily.

Hyperthyroidism and neonatal thyrotoxicosis: PO: 0.25–0 .75 mg/kg/dose tid. Increase according to response. May require 1 mg/kg/dose tid.

Tetralogy of Fallot: PO: *<12 yr:* 0.25–1 mg/kg/dose bid in newborn and 3–4 times in >1 mo age. IV bolus up to 0.1 mg/kg over 5 min under ECG control bid in newborn and 4 times in >1 mo age.

Hypertrophic obstructive cardiomyopathy: PO: *<12 yr:* 0.25–1 mg/kg/dose. *>12 yr:* 10–40 mg/dose 3–4 times daily (8 mg/kg/day in 4 div. doses).

Propylthiouracil

PO: *<1 yr:* 2.5 mg/kg/dose. *1–4 yr:* 25 mg/dose. *5–12 yr:* 50 mg/dose. *12–18 yr:* 100 mg/dose tid. Dose gradually tapered after child is euthyroid.

Protamine Sulfate

All ages: 1 mg (0.1mL) for each 100 units mucous heparin (or LMWH) or 80 units lung heparin given at last dose. Max. dose 50 mg. Administer within 15 minutes - if the delay is longer, less protamine is required, as heparin is rapidly excreted (after 30 minutes give approximately half dose).

Pseudoephedrine Hydrochloride

PO (not used in newborn): *1 mo–2 yr:* 7.5 mg/dose. *2–12 yr:* 15–30mg/dose. 12–18 yr: 60 mg/dose tid.

Psoralen

Adults: Tab. 0.6–0.7 mg/kg body wt. daily.

Pyrantel Pamoate

11 mg/kg/day as single dose. Repeat after 2 wk (max. 1 g). In heavy hookworm infestation, give for 2 successive days.

Pyrazinamide

PO: *Children:* 30–35 mg/kg/24 hr as single dose or in 2 div. doses (max. 2 g/day) for the first 2 mo of the standard 6 mo regimen. *12–18 yr < 50 kg:* 1.5 g/day and *>50 kg:* 2 g/day as single dose or in 2 div. doses (max. 2 g/day) for the first 2 mo of the standard 6 mo regimen.

Pyridostigmine Bromide
PO initially 1.5 mg/kg/dose (max. *newborn*: 10 mg, *1 mo to 2 yr:* 30 mg; *2–12 yr:* 60 mg; *12–18 yr:* 30– 120 mg). The dose is increased in increments of 25–50% daily till max. improvement is obtained and given in div. doses at suitable intervals. Usual total daily dose in <12 yr is 30–360 mg and >*12 yr* is 300 mg to 1.2 g.

Pyridoxine (Vitamin B6)
Metabolic indications: 50–250 mg/dose 1–2 times daily. Higher doses are given in partially responsive cases and for Wilson disease.

Pyridoxine-dependent seizures: Newborn: PO: Try test dose of 50–100 mg 1–2 times daily for 2 days and if responsive, maintenance of 25–100 mg bid lifelong. Increased dose may be required with intercurrent illness and with growth. IV bolus/IM 50–100 mg as test dose; may give for 2 days and then change to PO. If seizures persist, commence conventional anticonvulsant therapy. *Children*: 20–50 mg 1–2 times daily – up to 500 mg bid may be required. IV bolus – *1 mo to 12 yr:* 25–100 mg as test dose for 2 days and then change to PO.

Pyrimethamine
Toxoplasmosis in pregnancy: If toxoplasma infection is diagnosed in early pregnancy and the fetus is not infected, spiramycin is given (see spiramycin monograph). If the fetus is found to be infected, then pyrimethamine 50 mg OD, sulfadiazine 1 g tid, and calcium folinate (folinic acid) 15 mg 3 times per week are given until delivery.

Toxoplasmosis in infants: Pyrimethamine along with sulfadiazine (50 mg/kg bid) and calcium folinate (folinic acid) (15 mg/kg three times in a week) are given for 12 mo. Pyrimethamine is started with a loading dose of 1 mg/kg/dose bid for 2 days and then 1 mg/kg/dose OD for 6 mo followed by 1 mg/kg/dose thrice in a week for 6 mo. Prednisolone at 0.5/kg/dose bid is also given until signs of CNS inflammation (CSF protein > 10g/L) or active chorioretinitis has settled and then tapered.

Ocular toxoplasmosis, reactivation of toxoplasmosis during HIV infection, and toxoplasmosis in an immunocompromised child with protracted or incapacitating illness: 2 mg/kg loading dose for 2 days followed by 1 mg/kg in <*12 yr* and 25–100 mg in *12– 18 yr olds* for 6 wk to prevent relapse in HIV patients followed by maintenance of a quarter to half of starting dose indefinitely.

Pyrimethamine + Sulfadoxine
PO: *2 mo to 4 yr:* ½ tab; *5–6 yr:* 1 tab; *7–9 yr:* 1½ tab, *10–14 yr:* 2 tab; >*14 yr:* 3 tabs as a single dose after quinine therapy.

Pyritinol
Children: 100–200 mg daily according to age. Continue therapy for several wk. *Infants:* 2.5–5 mL 1–3 times daily.

Q

Quinidine
Adolescents: 200–400 mg 3–4 times daily. Initially give test dose. *Children:* 2 mg/kg test dose to exclude idiosyncrasy. PO: 30 mg/kg/24 hr in div. doses every 4–6 hr.

Quinine
PO: *Birth to 12 yr:* 30 mg/kg/day (sulfate); *12–18 yr:* 1.8 g/day (sulfate) in 3 div. doses for 7 days. IV infusion over 4 hr initial loading dose of 20 mg/kg (max. 1.4 g), then 10 mg/kg (max. 0.7 g) every 12 hr for 48 hr, and then maintenance of 5–7 mg/kg once in 8 hr if IV is needed after 48 hr. As soon as possible, change to PO.

Quinopristin + Dalfopristin
IV into central vein: *1 mo to 18 yr:* 7.5 mg/kg 8 hrly 7 days in *skin and soft-tissue infection,* 10 days in *hospital-acquired pneumonia;* the duration for *Enterococcus faecium* infection depends on the site of infection.

R

Rabies Human Monoclonal Antibodies
Rabishield: The recommended dose is 3.33 IU/kg of body weight.

Twinrab [combination of two murine antirabies mAb, docaravimab (62-71-3) and miromavimab (M777-16-3)]: The recommended dose of Twinrab is 40 IU/kg of body weight.

Rabies Immunoglobulin, Human (HRIG)
20 IU/kg IM and infiltration: Half infiltrated around wound with the rest IM. Give at a different site to the vaccine.

Rabies Vaccine
Pre-exposure: 1 mL on days 0, 7, and 28. 2 doses 4 wk apart may be adequate in those not expecting to handle animals if postexposure treatment will be readily available. In this case, if exposure continues, a further dose after 6–12 mo will be necessary. Boosters may be given every 2–3 yr if there is continuing risk and postexposure treatment is not readily available. After 2–3 boosters, expert advice should be sought before giving more.

Postexposure: When an individual has been exposed via a break in the skin or contamination of a mucosal surface to a potentially rabid animal, consideration should be given to postexposure treatment. Advice should always be sought before starting treatment. *Unimmunized/incompletely immunized (received < 3 doses or had intradermal)*: Low risk: 1 mL on days 0, 3, 7, 14, and 30; high risk: 1 mL on days 0, 3, 7, 14, and 30 plus rabies immunoglobulin. Fully immunized individual: 1 mL on days 0, 3, and 7.

Ramipril

PO: *Children:* 1.5 mg/m^2/24 hr OD. *Adolescents:* 2.5 mg OD. Adjust dosage to achieve proper blood pressure response, up to max. of 20 mg/day. But more studies are required in children before it is used in pediatrics.

Ranitidine

Newborn: PO/IV 1 mg/kg tid (studies with PO treatment in newborn are limited) and IV infusion 30–60 μg/kg/hr (max. 3 mg/kg/day). *Child:* PO: *6 mo to 12 yr:* 2–4 mg/kg/dose (max. 150 mg). *12–18 yr:* 150 mg/dose bid. Up to 9 mg/kg may be used. IV bolus 1 mg/kg 2–4 times daily. IV infusion 125–250 μg/kg/hr.

Severe renal failure: Reduce dose to 50%.

Rasburicase

Chemotherapy-induced hyperuricemia: IV: *Infants and children 1 mo to 17 yr of age:* 0.15 or 0.2 mg/kg OD for 5 days. Safety and efficacy are established only for a single course of treatment. Safety and efficacy of bid dosing, dosing for >5 days, or administration of >1 course of therapy are not established.

Recombinant Human Alpha Glucosidase (Alglucosidase Alfa, Myozyme)

IV infusion of 20 mg/kg body weight given once every 2 wk.

Riboflavin (Vitamin B2)

PO 50 mg OD. May give in frequent smaller doses. Doses up to 300–400 mg/day have been used.

Rifampicin

Rifampicin is to be given in empty stomach.

Tuberculosis in combination with other drugs: PO 10 mg/kg (max. 600 mg/day) as single morning dose.

Meningococcal infection prophylaxis and staphylococcal infections: PO: *<5 yr:* 5 mg/kg/dose; *> 1 yr:* 10 mg/kg/dose (max. 600 mg/dose) bid for 2 days for meningococcal infection prophylaxis and for 10–14 days for staphylococcal infections.

Haemophilus influenzae prophylaxis: PO: *<3 mo:* 10 mg/kg; *>3 mo: 20* mg/kg/dose (max. 600 mg/dose) OD for 4 days.

Cholestasis – pruritis: 5–10 mg/kg (max. 600 mg) OD.

Dose adjustment in liver failure: Avoid altogether or reduce doses for tuberculosis and prophylaxis to 8 mg/kg daily. Prophylaxis of meningococcal and staphylococcal carrier state: *<1 mo:* 5 mg/kg PO or IV every 12 hr for 2 days. *1 mo or older:* 10 mg/kg (not to exceed 600 mg/dose) PO or IV every 12 hr for 2 days.

Risperidone

Aggressive behavior and Tourette syndrome: PO 0.5–2 mg OD or in 2 div. doses.

Schizophrenia: PO 0.5–2 mg OD or in 2 div. doses.

Ritonavir

Low-dose ritonavir to increase the effect of atazanavir: PO: *6–18 yr <20 kg:* 80–100 mg OD; *>20 kg:* 100 mg OD.

Low-dose ritonavir to increase the effect of darunavir: PO: *6–18 yr 20–30 kg:* 50 mg BD; *30–40 kg:* 60 mg BD; *>40 kg:* 100 mg BD.

Rituximab

IV: To check protocols for dosage. 375 mg/m^2 as a 5 hr infusion once weekly for 4–8 wk is a useful guide.

Rotavirus Vaccine

The vaccines may be administered to preterm infants according to their age in wk since birth and infants with controlled GERD. Dose reduction is not necessary in renal or hepatic impairment.

Routine vaccination: Minimum age: 6 wk for all available brands [RV-1 (Rotarix), RV-5 (RotaTeq), RV-116E (Rotavac)] and Rotasil. Only two doses of RV-1 are recommended. If any dose in series was RV-5 or RV-116E or vaccine product is unknown for any dose in the series, a total of 3 doses of RV vaccine should be administered. The max. age of administration of the last dose of any RV vaccine is 32 wk.

Catch-up vaccination: The max. age for the first dose in the series is 14 wk 6 days. Vaccination should not be initiated for infants aged 15 wk 0 day or older. The max. age for the final dose in the series is 8 mo 0 day. However, the upper age limit for administering the 1st dose of Rotavirus vac-cine in the Universal Immunization Program (UIP) is 1 yr.

Roxithromycin

Adolescents: 150 mg bid at least 15 minutes before meals. *Children:* 5–8 mg/kg/day in 2 div. doses for not more than 10 days.

Rubella Vaccine, Live

IM or deep SC: 0.5 mL. Booster doses of single antigen rubella vaccine are not recommended.

Rufinamide

Adjunctive treatment of seizures in Lennox–Gastaut syndrome: PO: *1–3 yr:* Initially 5 mg/kg bid and then increased in steps of up to 5 mg/kg bid (max. per dose 22.5 mg/kg bid), titrated as per clinical status, dose to be increased at intervals of not <3 days to the target dose (max. dose), each dose should be given to the nearest 0.5 mL. *4–17 yr (up to 30 kg):* Initially 100 mg bid, then increased in steps of 100 mg bid (max. per dose 500 mg bid), titrated as per clinical status, dose to be increased at intervals of not <3 days. *4–17 yr (30–50 kg):* Initially 200 mg bid, then increased in steps of 200 mg bid (max. per dose 900 mg bid), titrated as per clinical status, dose to be increased at intervals of not <2 days. *4–17 yr (50–70 kg):* Initially 200 mg bid, then increased in steps of 200 mg bid (max. per dose 1.2

g bid), titrated as per clinical status; dose to be increased at intervals of not <2 days. *4–17 yr (70 kg and above):* Initially 200 mg bid, then increased in steps of 200 mg bid (max. per dose 1.6 g bid), titrated as per clinical status, dose to be increased at intervals of not <2 days.

Adjunctive treatment of seizures in Lennox-Gastaut syndrome with valproate: PO: *1–3 yr:* Same as above except that max. dose is limited to 15 mg/kg per dose bid. *4–17 yr (up to 30 kg):* Same as above except that max. dose is limited to per dose 300 mg bid and dose to be increased at intervals of not <2 days. *4–17 yr (30–50 kg):* Same as above except that max. dose is limited to per dose 600 mg bid. *4–17 yr (50–70 kg):* Same as above except that max. dose is limited to per dose 800 mg bid. *4–17 yr (70 kg and above):* Same as above except that max. dose is limited to per dose 1.1 g bid.

S

Salbutamol
PO: *1 mo to 2 yr:* 0.3–0.4 mg/kg/day. *>2 yr:* 0.3–0 .7 mg/kg/day. *Aerosol inhaler* up to 100–200 µg single dose on demand. *Nebulizer soln.*: 1.25–2.5 mg 1–2 hrly initially and then 4–6 hrly.

Salicylic Acid
Topical: Remove dead skin by gentle rubbing with pumice stone or emery board before applying daily.

Salmeterol
<4 yr: 25 µg; *4–12 yr:* 50 µg; *12–18 yr:* 50–100 µg bid as preventor.

Selenium Sulfide
Seborrheic dermatitis and dandruff: To skin using as shampoo: 5–17 yr: Apply twice weekly for 2 wk, then apply once weekly for 2 wk, and then apply as required.

Pityriasis versicolor: To skin using as shampoo: 5–17 yr: Apply OD for 7 days to the affected area and leave on for 10 minutes before rinsing off. The course may be repeated if necessary. Diluting with a small amount of water prior to application can reduce irritation.

Senna
PO tabs: *6–12 yr:* 1–2 tabs; *12–18 yr:* 2–4 tabs. Liquid: *<2 yr:* 0.5 mg/kg; *2–6 yr:* 2.5–5 mL; *6–12 yr:* 5–10 mL; *12–18 yr:* 10–20mL.

Serratiopeptidase
5–10 mg thrice a day after meals to be swallowed whole without chewing.

Sertraline
Obsessive-compulsive disorder: PO: *6–11 yr:* Initially 25 mg daily for 1 week, then increased to 50 mg daily, then increased in steps of 50 mg at intervals of at least 1 week if required; max. 200 mg/day. *12–17 yr:* Initially 50 mg daily, then increased in steps of 50 mg at intervals of at least 1 week if required; max. 200 mg/day.

Major depression: PO: *12–17 yr*: Initially 50 mg OD, then increased in steps of 50 mg at intervals of at least 1 week if required; max. 200 mg/day.

Sildenafil
Pulmonary arterial hypertension: PO: *neonate to 11 mo:* initially 250–500 g/kg every 4–8 hr, adjusted according to response, start with the lower dose and frequency, especially if used with other vasodilators; max. 30 mg/day. *1–17 yr up to 20 kg:* 10 mg 3 tid, *>20 kg:* 20 mg 3 tid.

Reduce dose with concurrent use of moderate and potent inhibitors of CYP3A4 (avoid with ketoconazole, itraconazole and ritonavir) – no specific recommendation made for children.

Renal and hepatic disease: Dose reduction is required.

Silver Nitrate
Common warts: To the lesion: *child:* apply every 24 hr for up to 3 applications; apply a moistened caustic pencil tip for 1–2 minutes. Ruse by gentle filing and cover with adhesive dressing after application.

Verrucae: To the lesion: *child:* apply every 24 hr for up to 6 applications; apply a moistened caustic pencil tip for 1–2 minutes. Remove dead skin before use by gentle filing and cover with adhesive dressing after application.

Umbilical granuloma: To the granuloma: *child:* apply a moistened caustic pencil tip (usually containing silver nitrate 40%) for 1–2 minutes; protect the surrounding skin with soft paraffin.

Silver Sulfadiazine (Sulfadiazine)
Burns: After cleaning the wound, apply over all affected areas to a depth of 3–5 mm using a sterile gloved hand or sterile spatula. Where necessary, reapply to any area from which it has been removed by patient activity. Reapply at least every 24 hr or more frequently if the volume of exudates is large.

Hand burns: Apply to the burn and enclose the whole hand in a clear plastic bag or glove which is then closed at the wrist. The patient should be encouraged to move the hand and fingers and the dressing should be changed when an excessive amount of exudates has accumulated in the bag.

Leg ulcers/pressure sores: The cavity of the ulcer should be filled with cream to a depth of at least 3–5 mm, followed by application of an absorbent pad or dressing, with further application of pressure bandaging as appropriate. Dressings should be changed daily, but if less exudates every 48 hr may be sufficient.

Finger-tip injuries: Hemostasis of the injury should be achieved prior to the application of a 3–5 mm layer of cream and then the finger should be covered with a finger dressing or the finger of a plastic glove. Dressings should be changed every 2–3 days. In all cases, use the contents of the tube or pot on one person only. Discard 50 g tubes 7 days after opening. Discard 250 and 500 g pots 24 hr after opening.

Silymarin
70–140 mg bid/tid.

Simvastatin
5–10 yr: 5 mg at night increased at 4 wk intervals to 20 mg/night if required. Reduced dose is required with concomitant cyclosporine, danazol, fibrates, amiodarone, diltiazem or verapamil - seek specialized advice.

Sodium Benzoate
Hyperammonemia: PO 250 mg/kg/day in 4 div. doses; IV 250 mg/kg as single infusion over 90 min.

Nonketotic hyperglycinemia: Newborn: 250 mg/kg/day in 4 div. doses; >*1 mo:* 500 mg/kg/day in 4 div. doses.

Sodium Bicarbonate
Renal tubular acidosis: PO: 2 yr: 1–2 mmol/kg/day; >*2 yr*: 70 mmol/m^2/day.

Renal hyperkalemia: IV 1 mmol/kg/day.

Cardiopulmonary resuscitation: 1 mL/kg of 8.4% solution initially followed by 0.5 mL/kg 8.4% if needed.

Sodium Chloride
IV 2–4 mmol/kg/24 hr in continuous IV infusion. PO 2–4 mmol/kg/24 hr in 2–4 div. doses. *Note:* (1) Adjust dose according to clinical requirements for sodium and (2) higher doses may be required in very premature infants because of significant renal loss of electrolytes.

Sodium Chloride Drops
0.9% given as nasal drops or spray may relieve nasal congestion by helping to liquify mucous secretions *in children* with rhinitis. *In infants,* 1–2 drops of sodium chloride 0.9% solution in each nostril before feeds will help relieve congestion and allow more effective suckling.

Sodium Cromoglycate
Inhaler: qid. *Intranasal:* 1 spray 2–4 times daily. PO: <*14 yr:* 100 mg and >*14 yr:* 200 mg/dose qid - increased if required to 40 mg/kg and then reduced according to response.

Sodium Nitrite
3% inj. (30 mg/mL) in water for injection - give IV over 5–20 min. *1 mo to 18 yr:* 4–10 mg/kg (max. 300 mg) or 0.13–0.33 mL/kg (max. 10 mL) followed immediately by 25% inj. (250 mg/mL) sodium thiosulfate in water for injection given 400 mg/kg (max. 12.5g) or 1.6 mL/kg (max. of 50 mL) over 15 min.

Recommended dose of both drugs varies with Hb levels of the child, if the Hb level is known. Sodium nitrite 3% soln. and sodium thiosulfate 25% soln. *Hb 8 g/dL:* Sodium nitrite 6.6 mg/kg (0.22 mL/kg); sodium thiosulfate 1.1 mL/kg. *Hb 10 g/dL:* Sodium nitrite 8.7 mg/kg (0.27 mL/kg); sodium thiosulfate 1.35 mL/kg. *Hb 12 g/dL:* Sodium nitrite 10 mg/kg (0.33 mL/kg); sodium thiosulfate 1.65 mL/kg. *Hb 14g/dL:* Sodium nitrite 11.6 mg/kg (0.39 mL/kg); sodium thiosulfate 1.95 mL/kg. *If Hb is not known:* Sodium nitrite 10 mg/kg (0.33 mL/kg); sodium thiosulfate 1.6 mL/kg - 400 mg/kg IV repeated every 30–60 min to max. of 50 mL.

Sodium Nitroprusside
Hypertensive emergencies: Continuous IV infusion: *neonate:* initially 500 ng/kg/min, then increase in steps of 200 ng/kg/min (max. per dose 8 μg/kg/min) as required, max. 4 μg/kg/min if used for longer than 24 hr. *Child:* Initially 500 ng/kg/min, then increased in steps of 200 ng/kg/min (max. per dose 8 μg/kg/min) as required, max. 4 μg/kg/min if used for longer than 24 hr.

Sodium Phenylbutyrate
PO 250 mg/kg/day in 4 div. doses, IV 250 mg/kg over 50 min, IV infusion 250–600 mg/kg/day as continuous infusion.

Sodium Picosulfate
2–5 yr: 2.5 mL; *5–19 yr:* 2.5–5 mL; >*10 yr:* 5–15 mL as single dose at bedtime.

Sodium Stibogluconate
IV/IM: *1 mo to 18 yr:* 20 mg/kg (max. 850 mg) once daily for 20–30 days. Total daily dose may be given in 2 div. doses 12 hr apart.

Sodium Thiosulfate
25% inj. (250 mg/mL) in water for injection given 400 mg/kg (max. 12.5 g) or 1.6 mL/kg (max. of 50 mL) over 15 min. It is given after IV sodium nitrite. Recommended doses of both drugs vary with Hb levels of the child.

If Hb level is known: Sodium nitrite 3% soln. and sodium thiosulfate 25% solution - *Hb 8 g/dL:* Sodium nitrite 6.6 mg/kg (0.22 mL/kg) + sodium thiosulfate 1.1 mL/kg. *Hb 10 g/dL:* Sodium nitrite 8.7 mg/kg (0.27 mL/kg) + sodium thiosulfate 1.35 mL/kg. *Hb 12 g/dL:* Sodium nitrite 10 mg/kg (0.33 mL/kg) + sodium thiosulfate 1.65 mL/kg. *Hb 14 g/dL:* Sodium nitrite 11.6 mg/kg (0.39 mL/kg) + sodium thiosulfate 1.95 mL/kg. *If Hb is not known:* Sodium nitrite 10 mg/kg (0.33 mL/kg) + sodium thiosulfate 1.6 mL/kg - 400 mg/kg IV repeated every 30–60 min to max. of 50 mL.

Sodium Valproate
PO: Start with 10–15 mg/kg/day in 2 div. doses and maintain at 12.5–15 mg/kg/day. Even doses of 30–40 mg/kg/day have been used in infantile spasms.

Somatropin (Growth Hormone)
Growth hormone deficiency: SC 25–35 μg/kg OD.

Turner syndrome: 50 μg/kg OD.

Chronic renal failure: 50 μg/kg OD.

Prader–Willi syndrome: 70 μg/kg OD.

Noonan syndrome: 35 μg/kg OD.

Intrauterine growth restriction (IUGR): 70 μg/kg OD.

Sotalol
Life-threatening arrhythmias including ventricular tachyarrhythmias: PO: child 12–17 yr: initially 80 mg OD, alternatively initially 40 mg bid, then increased to 80–160 mg bid, dose to be increased gradually at intervals of 2–3 days; higher doses of 480–640 mg daily may be required for life-threatening ventricular arrhythmias (under specialist supervision).

Ventricular arrhythmias, life-threatening ventricular tachyarrhythmia, and supraventricular arrhythmias (initiated under specialist supervision): PO: *neonate:* initially 1 mg/kg bid, increased if necessary up to 4 mg/kg bid, dose to be increased at intervals of 3–4 days.

Atrial flutter, ventricular arrhythmias, life-threatening ventricular tachyarrhythmia, and supraventricular arrhythmias (initiated under specialist supervision): PO: *child 1 mo to 11 yr:* initially 1 mg/kg bid, then increased if necessary up to 4 mg/kg bid (max. per dose 80 mg bid), dose to be increased at intervals of 2–3 days. *Child 12–17 yr:* Initially 80 mg OD, alternatively initially 40 mg bid, increased to 80–160 mg bid, dose to be increased gradually at intervals of 2–3 days.

Renal impairment: Halve normal dose if estimated GFR 30–60 mL/min/1.73 m^2; use one-quarter normal dose if estimated GFR 10–30 mL/min/1.73 m^2. Avoid if estimated GFR < 10 mL/min/1.73 m^2.

Monitoring: Measurement of corrected QT interval and monitoring of ECG and electrolytes required; correct hypokalemia, hypomagnesemia, or other electrolyte disturbances.

Spiramycin
Pregnant women with suspected or confirmed toxoplasma infection: 1.5 g (4.5 million international units) PO bid until term if the fetus is not infected.

Spironolactone
PO 1–3 mg/kg/day in 2 div. doses.

In resistant ascites: Up to 9 mg/kg/day have been given with careful serum potassium monitoring.

Hirsutism: Start with 50 mg in 2 div. doses, gradually increasing to 100 mg; max. up to 200 mg daily can be given.

Stilbestrol
PO 1 mg bid, for 2 days before the test.

Stiripentol (4,4-dimethyl-1-[3,4-(methylene dioxy)-phenyl]-1-penten-3-ol)
Adjunctive therapy of refractory GTCS in patients with severe myoclonic epilepsy in infancy (Dravet syndrome) in combination with clobazam and valproate: PO: *3–5 yr:* initially 20 mg/kg/day for 1 week, then 30 mg/kg/day for 1 week, then 50 mg/kg/day – all in 2–3 div. doses. *6–11 yr:* Initially 20 mg/kg/day for 1 week, then increased in steps of 10 mg/kg/day weekly up to 50 mg/kg/day – all in 2–3 div. doses. *12–17 yr:* Initially 20 mg/kg/day for 1 week, then increased to 30 mg/kg/day for 1 week, then increased in steps of 5 mg/kg/day weekly until the optimum dose is reached based on clinical judgment; max. 50 mg/kg/day.

Streptokinase
Intravascular thrombosis: Initially by IV infusion: *1 mo to 11 yr:* Initially 2,500–4,000 units/kg, dose to be given over 30 minutes, followed by (continuous IV infusion) 500–1,000 units/kg/hr till vascular flow returns or max. of 3 days. 12–17 yr: Initially 2,50,000 units, dose to be given over 30 minutes, followed by (continuous IV infusion) 1,00,000 units/hr till vascular flow returns or max. of 3 days.

Streptomycin
Tuberculosis: IM: Daily regimen – 15 mg/kg as single morning dose (range 15–20 mg/kg; max. dose 1 g/day).

Sucralfate
PO: *<2 yr:* 250 mg; *1–12 yr:* 500 mg; *12–18 yr:* 1 g 4–6 times daily.

Sulfasalazine (Sulphasalazine)
Treatment of an acute attack of mild-to-moderate and severe ulcerative colitis/active Crohn's disease: PO: *child 2–11 yr:* 10–15 mg/kg 4–6 times a day (max. per dose 1 g) until remission occurs; increased if necessary up to 60 mg/kg daily in div. doses. *12–17 yr:* 1–2 g qid until remission occurs. Rectally: *child 5–7 yr:* 500 mg bid; *8–11 yr:* 500 mg, dose to be administered in the morning and 1 g, dose to be administered at night; *12–17 yr:* 0.5–1 g bid.

Maintenance of remission of mild-to-moderate and severe ulcerative colitis: PO: *child 2–11 yr:* 5–7.5 mg/kg qid (max. per dose 500 mg). *12–17 yr:* 500 mg qid. Rectally*: child 5–7 yr:* 500 mg bid. *8–11* yr: 500 mg, dose to be administered in the morning and 1 g, dose to be administered at night. *12–17 yr:* 0.5–1 g bid.

Juvenile idiopathic arthritis: PO: *child 2–11 yr:* initially 5 mg/kg bid for 1 wk, then 10 mg/kg bid for 1 wk, and then 20 mg/kg bid for 1 wk; maintenance 20–25 mg/kg bid; max. 2 g/day. *12–17 yr:* Initially 5 mg/kg bid for 1 wk, then 10 mg/kg bid for

1 wk, and then 20 mg/kg bid for 1 week; maintenance 20–25 mg/kg bid; max. 3 g/day.

Sulfadiazine
<12 yr: 100–200 mg/kg/day; *12–18 yr:* 4–6 g/day in 4 div. doses.

Sumatriptan
PO: *6–10 yr:* 25 mg; *10–12 yr:* 50 mg; *12–18 yr:* 50–100 mg as single dose. May be repeated if migraine recurs (max. 300 mg/day). If there is no response, do not repeat for same attack. SC *>10 yr:* 6 mg single dose. May repeat once not less than 1 hr later for a recurrence (max. 12 mg/day). If there is no response, do not repeat for the same attack.

Surfactants (Natural)
SURVANTA – Treatment of respiratory distress syndrome in preterm neonates, birth-weight over 700 g: Intratracheal: *preterm neonate:* 100 mg/kg, preferably administer within 8 hr of birth; dose may be repeated within 48 hr at intervals of at least 6 hr for up to 4 doses.

Prophylaxis of respiratory distress syndrome in preterm neonates: Intratracheal – *neonate up to 32 wk corrected gestational age:* 100 mg/kg; preferably administer within 15 min of birth; dose may be repeated within 48 hr at intervals of at least 6 hr for up to 4 doses.

Dose equivalence and conversion

Phospholipid 100 mg/kg is equivalent to a volume of 4 mL/kg.

CUROSURF – Treatment of respiratory distress syndrome in neonates, birth weight over 700 g: Intratracheal: *neonate:* 100–200 mg/kg, then 100 mg/kg 12 hrly if required, max. 300–400 mg/kg per course.

Prophylaxis of respiratory distress syndrome: Intratracheal: *neonate 24–31 wk corrected gestational age:* 100–200 mg/kg, administer soon after birth, preferably within 15 minutes, then 100 mg/kg after 6–12 hr if required, then 100 mg/kg after 12 hr if required, and if neonate still intubated. Max. 300–400 mg/kg per course.

Surfactants (Synthetic)
67.5 mg/kg or 5 mL/kg.

Suxamethonium Chloride
Newborn: For 5-10 min muscular paralysis: 2 mg/ kg IV; *for full neuromuscular blockade* 3× mg/kg IV; IM 4×vmg/kg provides 10–30× min muscle paralysis after 2–3 min delay. *Children:* IV: *<12 yr:* 1–2 mg/kg; *12–18 yr:* 1 mg/kg; IM: *<1 yr:* up to 4–5 mg/kg; *>1 yr:* up to 4 mg.

T

Tacalcitol
12–18 yr: Apply sparingly at bedtime.

Tacrolimus
Prophylaxis of graft rejection following liver transplantation, starting 12 hr after transplantation: PO: *Neonates and child:* initially 150 µg/kg bid. IV infusion: *Neonate and child:* initially 50 µg/kg daily for up to 7 days (then transfer to PO therapy) and dose to be administered over 24 hr.

Prophylaxis of graft rejection following kidney transplantation, starting within 24 hr of transplantation: PO: *neonate:* initially 150 µg/kg bid. *Child:* Initially 150 µg/kg bid; a lower initial dose of 100 µg/kg bid has been used in adolescents to prevent very high "trough" concentrations. IV infusion: *Neonate and child:* initially 75–100 µg/kg daily for up to 7 days (then transfer to PO therapy); dose to be administered over 24 hr.

Short-term treatment of moderate-to-severe atopic eczema (including flares) in patients unresponsive to or intolerant of conventional therapy: Topical: *2–15 yr:* apply 0.03% ointment thinly bid for up to 3 wk (consider other treatment if eczema worsens or if no improvement after 2 wk) and then reduce to OD until lesion clears. *16–17 yr:* Apply bid until lesion clears (consider other treatment if eczema worsens or no improvement after 2 wk), initially 0.1% ointment to be applied thinly, reduce frequency to OD or strength of ointment to 0.03% if condition allows.

Prevention of flares in patients with moderate-to-severe atopic eczema and 4 or more flares a yr who have responded to initial treatment with topical tacrolimus: Topical: *2–15 yr:* apply twice weekly, 0.03% ointment to be applied thinly, with an interval of 2–3 days between applications; use short-term treatment regimen during an acute flare; review need for preventative therapy after 1 yr. *16–17 yr:* Apply twice weekly, 0.1% ointment to be applied thinly, with an interval of 2–3 days between applications; use short-term treatment regimen during an acute flare; review need for preventative therapy after 1 yr.

Teicoplanin
Clostridium difficile infection: PO: *children 12–18 yr:* 100–200 mg bid for 7–14 days.

Serious infections caused by gram-positive bacteria (e.g., endocarditis, complicated skin and soft-tissue infections, pneumonia, complicated UTI, bone and joint infections): Initially IV/IV infusion/IM: *neonate:* IV infusion – Initially 16 mg/kg for 1 dose, followed by 8 mg/kg OD, starting 24 hr after first. *Children 2 mo to 11 yr:* Initially 10 mg/kg every 12 hr for 3 doses, followed by 6–10 mg/kg OD. *Children 12–18 yr:* Initially 6 mg/kg every 12 hr for 3 doses and then 6 mg/kg OD.

Streptococcal or enterococcal endocarditis (in combination with another antibacterial) and bone and joint infections: Initially IV/IV infusion: *children 12–18 yr:* 12 mg/kg every 12 hr for 3–5 doses, followed by 12 mg/kg OD.

Peritonitis associated with peritoneal dialysis as intraperitoneal infusion - added to dialysis fluid: Child *12–18 yr:* after a single IV loading dose of 6 mg/kg body weight, 20 mg/L is administered in the bag of the dialysis solution in the first week, 20 mg/L in different bags the second week, and then 20 mg/L in the overnight bag in the third week.

Dose adjustment in renal impairment: GFR 40–60 mL/min: Give normal regimen for the first 3 days and then reduce frequency on day 4 to every 48 hr. GFR < 40 mL/min: Give normal regimen for the first 3 days and then reduce frequency on day 4 to every 72 hr.

Dose adjustment in HD, PD, and CVVH: Not dialyzed. Give normal regimen for the first 3 days and then reduce dose on day 4 to one-third of the dose OD or give 100% of the dose every third day.

Terbinafine
Tinea pedis: Topical: *child:* apply 1–2 times a day for up to 1 week, to be applied thinly. PO: *Child 1–17 yr (10–19 kg):* 62.5 mg; *20–39 kg:* 125 mg; *40 kg and above:* 250 mg OD for 2–6 wk.

Tinea corporis: Topical: *child:* Apply 1–2 times a day for up to 1–2 wk, to be applied thinly, review treatment after 2 wk. PO; *Child 1–17 yr (10–19 kg):* 62.5 mg; *20–39 kg:* 125 mg; *40 kg and above:* 250 mg OD for 4 wk.

Tinea cruris: Topical: *child:* apply 1–2 times a day for up to 1–2 wk, to be applied thinly, review treatment after 2 wk. PO: *Child 1–17 yr (10–19 kg):* 62.5 mg; *20–39 kg:* 125 mg; *40 kg and above:* 250 mg OD for 2-4 wk .

Tinea capitis: PO: *child 1–17 yr (10–19 kg):* 62.5 mg; *20–39 kg:* 125 mg; *40 kg and above:* 250 mg OD for 4 wk.

Dermatophyte infections of the nails: PO: *Child 1–17 yr (10–19 kg):* 62.5 mg; *20–39 kg:* 125 mg; *40 kg and above:* 250 mg OD for 6 wk to 3 mo (occasionally longer in toenail infections).

Cutaneous candidiasis and Pityriasis versicolor: Topical: *child:* Apply 1–2 times a day for up to 1–2 wk, to be applied thinly, review treatment after 2 wk.

Terbutaline
PO: *<7 yr:* 0.25 mg/kg/day in 3 div. doses; *7–12 yr:* 2.5 mg/dose; *12–18 yr:* 2.5–5 mg/dose tid. Aerosol inhaler 250–500 μg/dose 4–6 times daily. Turbohaler 500 μg/dose qid. Nebulized *1 mo to 5 yr:* 2.5–5 mg, *5–12 yr:* 5 mg; *12–18 yr:* 10 mg per dose up to 8 times daily. SC/IM/slow IV: *2–12 yr:* 10 μg/kg/dose (max. 300 μg/dose); *12–18 yr:* 250–500 μg/dose. IV loading dose of 2–4 μg/kg followed by IV infusion of 1–10 μg/kg/hr. IV preparation not available in India.

Testosterone and Esters
Androgen replacement: PO 1 yr: testosterone undecanoate - starting dose 40 mg alternate days, increasing slowly up to 120 mg daily.

Delayed puberty: Dose/dose schedule depends on the product. An example is given but expert advice should be sought from a pediatric endocrinologist. IM injection: 1 mL by deep IM injection every mo for 3 doses.

Priming: IM injection: 1 mL by deep IM injection 3–5 days before the test of GH secretion.

Tetanus Immunoglobulin (Human)
Prevention: A single dose of 250 IU. If there is a risk of heavy contamination or following burns, or more than 24 hr have elapsed since injury, 500 IU should be given.

Treatment of tetanus: 150 IU/kg IM in multiple sites or by IV infusion.

Tetanus Toxoid + Reduced Dose Diphtheria (Td)
Contains tetanus toxoid 5 LF units and 2 LF units of diphtheria toxoid. 0.5 mL deep IM on anterolateral thigh for children above 7 yr age and routinely at 10 and 16 yr (Td to replace TT boosters at 10 and 16 yr).

Tetanus Toxoid, Reduced Diphtheria Toxoid + Acellular Pertussis Vaccine, Adsorbed (Tdap)
Contains tetanus toxoid 5 LF units and 2 LF units of diphtheria toxoid; pertussis Toxoid (PT), Filamentous Hemagglutinin (FHA), Pertactin (PRN). 0.5 mL deep IM on anterolateral thigh for children above 7 yr age and routinely at 10 (Td to replace TT boosters at 10).

Immunization-naïve child: 1 Tdap dose followed by Td vac at 1 and 6 mo. TdaP is preferred to Td for *adolescents aged 11–18 yr* who were vaccinated against tetanus > 5 yr earlier. Require a tetanus toxoid-containing vaccine as part of wound management and have not previously received Tdap. 1 Tdap instead of TT/Td in pregnant women - 27 through 36 wk and repeated in every pregnancy. Catch up to 18 yr and time elapsed since last T or D irrelevant.

Tetanus Vaccine (Adsorbed)
IM/deep SC 0.5 mL.

Tetracosactide (Tetracosactrin)
Diagnosis of adrenocortical insufficiency (diagnostic 30-minute test), standard-dose test: IM/IV: *child:* 145μg/m^2 (max. per dose 250 μg) for 1 dose; *low-dose test*: IM/IV*: child:* 0.3 μg/m^2 for 1 dose.

Infantile spasm: IM depot preparation: *child 1–23 mo:* Initially 500 μg OD on alternate days, adjusted according to response.

Tetracycline
Aphthous ulceration: Local mouth wash with contents of 250 mg cap of tetracycline in water 3–4 times daily for 2–3 min each time (do not swallow) for 3 days.

Susceptible infections (e.g., chlamydia, rickettsia, mycoplasma): PO: *12–17 yr:* 250 mg qid, increased if necessary to 500 mg 3–4 times a day, increased dose used in severe infections.

Acne: PO: *12–17 yr:* 500 mg bid for at least 3 mo, if there is no improvement after the first 3 mo another PO antibacterial should be used, max. improvement usually occurs after 4–6 mo but in more severe cases treatment may need to be continued for 2 yr or longer.

Nongonococcal urethritis: PO: *child 12–17 yr:* 500 mg qid for 7–14 days (21 days if failure or relapse after the first course).

Tetrahydrobiopterin

Monotherapy in tetrahydrobiopterin-sensitive phenylketonuria: PO: *child:* 10 mg/kg bid, adjusted according to response, total daily dose may alternatively be given in 3 div. doses.

In combination with neurotransmitter precursors for tetrahydrobiopterin-sensitive phenylketonuria: PO: *1 mo to 1 yr:* Initially 250–750 µg/kg qid, adjusted according to response, total daily dose may alternatively be given in 3 div. doses; max. 7 mg/kg/day. *2–17 yr:* Initially 250–750 µg/kg qid, adjusted according to response, total daily dose may alternatively be given in 3 div. doses; max. 10 mg/kg/day.

THAM (Trometamol) [Tris (hydroxymethyl) aminomethane]

Dose in mL of 0.3M solution = weight (kg) × base deficit, or 1–2 mEq/kg/dose. Blood gases should be checked before, during, and after administration. Only half the base deficit should be corrected initially. Blood gases should be checked before further correction.

Theophylline

Chronic asthma: PO: modified release preparations: *6 mo to 1 yr:* 12 mg/kg (max. per dose 120 mg); *2–5 yr:* 60–120 mg; *6–11 yr:* 175 mg; *12–17 yr:* 175–350 mg 12 hrly. Dose may be increased in some children with chronic asthma (max. per dose 400 mg), may be appropriate to give larger evening or morning dose to achieve optimum therapeutic effect when symptoms most severe; in patients whose night or daytime symptoms persist despite other therapies, who are not currently receiving theophylline, the total daily requirement may be added as single evening or morning dose.

Thiabendazole

Cutaneous larva migrans: 25 mg/kg (max. 1.5 g), bid for 2 days. Repeat for 2 days if active lesions persist 2 days after completion of the 1st course. 10–15% suspension is applied topically to lesions 4–6 times/day for 2–5 consecutive days.

Dracunculiasis (guinea worm): *1–2 visible worms:* 25 mg/ kg (max. 1.5 g), bid for 1 day. *3–9 visible worms:* 50 mg/kg (max. 1.5 g), 2 times daily for 1 day; *>9 visible worms:* 50 mg/kg (max. 1.5 g), 2 times daily for 1 day, repeat once after 5–8 days.

Trichinosis: 25 mg/kg (max. 1.5 g), 2 times daily for 2–4 days – up to 7 days if required.

Strongyloidiasis: 25 mg/kg (max. 1.5 g), bid for 2 days. *For disseminated infection*: 5–7 day course may be given.

Toxocariasis (visceral larva migrans): Efficacy is limited. A course of 25 mg/kg (max. 1.5 g), bid for 7 days may be tried.

Trichuriasis and hookworm: 25 mg/kg (max. 1.5 g), bid for 2 days. Thiabendazole is not usually first-line therapy for pinworm; other agents are better tolerated and more effective. However, if pinworm infection occurs concurrently with any of the other listed indications for thiabendazole, thiabendazole therapy alone is usually adequate for most patients. May repeat the course after 1 week.

There is limited study of its use in infants and children with weight of <13 kg for any of the indications mentioned.

Patients with renal impairment: Dosage should be modified depending on clinical response and degree of renal impairment, but no quantitative recommendations are available.

Thiamine (Vitamin B1)

Congenital lactic acidosis: PO 100–300 mg OD.

Maple syrup urine disease (MSUD): PO 10–300 mg OD. A trial for 3 wk in newly diagnosed MSUD to determine thiamine responsiveness.

Thiopental (Thiopentone) Sodium

IV bolus 4 mg/kg max. 10 mg/kg (facilities for ventilation must) followed in ventilated babies only with IV infusion 2.5 mg/kg/hr *(newborn)* and 2–8 mg/kg/hr *(1 mo to 18 yr).*

Hepatic disease: Reduce the dose.

Thiotepa

Children: IV 2–65 mg/m^2 every 3–4 wk; high dose 300 mg/m^2/24 hr for 3 doses. Always consult the current treatment protocol for details of dosage and scheduling.

Thyroxine

PO: Initial dose – *newborn:*10–15 µg/kg; *late neonatal period:* 6–8 µg/kg; *3 mo to 2 yr:* 5–10 µg/kg, *2–12 yr:* 5 µg/kg, *12–18 yr:* 50–100 µg. The goal of therapy is to maintain the total thyroxine (TT4) in the upper normal range of 10–15 µg/dL and normalize elevated TSH.

Adjust dose to correct FT4 to >20 pmol/L and TSH to <1–3 mU/L within 4 wk of therapy.

Thyroid-stimulating hormone levels take at least 4 wk to show any change following therapy. Monitor thyroid hormone levels 4–6 weekly at onset till target levels are attained and then according to progress. It is ideal to test 6–8 wk after any change in dose and every 3–4 monthly intervals during the second yr and biannually or annually as the child grows. It is preferable to monitor TT4 levels to FT4 levels. FT4 is preferred in special circumstances like pregnancy or inappropriately elevated TSH, and to cross check central hypothyroidism if the T4 level is borderline as TSH will not be useful.

Tiagabine
Doses are for patients receiving enzyme-induced antiepileptic drugs. Lower doses and slower titration may be required when used in patients not receiving enzyme-induced antiepileptic drugs. Children 12–18 yr: Initially 4 mg OD for 1 week, then 8 mg/day given in 2 div. doses for 1 week, then increase weekly by 4–8 mg/day once (given in 2–4 div. doses, preferably thrice in a day) to a max. of 32 mg/day or till response is obtained. Doses > 32 mg/day have been used in some adolescents for short periods of time.

Ticarcillin + Clavulanic Acid
Infections due to Pseudomonas and Proteus spp: IV infusion: *preterm (<2 kg):* 80 mg/kg 12 hrly. *Preterm (>2 kg):* 80 mg/kg 8 hrly, increased if necessary to 6 hrly. *Term newborn and child up to 40 kg:* 80 mg/kg 8 hrly; increased if necessary to 6 hrly. *Child > 40 kg:* 3.2 g 6–8 hrly, increased to 4 hrly for treating more severe infections.

Renal impairment: In neonates, reduce dose if estimated GFR < 60 mL/min/1.73 m^2. In children aged *1 mo to 18 yr,* use normal dose 8 hrly if GFR is 30–60 mL/min/1.73 m^2; use half normal dose 12 hrly if GFR is <10 mL/min/1.73 m^2.

Tinidazole
Intestinal amoebiasis: PO: *1 mo to 12 yr:* 50–60 mg/kg OD (max. per dose 2 g) for 3 days. *12–17 yr:* 2 g OD for 2–3 days.

Amoebic involvement of liver: PO: *1 mo to 12 yr:* 50–60 mg/kg OD (max. per dose 2 g) for 5 days. *12–17 yr:* 1.5–2 g (max. 2 g per dose) OD for 3–6 days.

Urogenital trichomoniasis and giardiasis: PO: *1 mo to 12 yr:* 50–75 mg/kg OD. *12–17 yr:* 2 g; for 1 single dose, dose may be repeated once if necessary.

Tissue Plasminogen Activator (tPA)
Initiate heparin concurrently to avoid thrombosis and thrombotic emboli. Monitoring: D-dimer, fibrinogen, and bleeding time.

Intravascular thrombosis: IV infusion – *Neonates and child:* 100–500 µg/kg/hr for 3–6 hr, use ultrasound assessment to monitor effect before considering a second course of treatment; max. 100 mg/day.

Tobramycin
Newborn: IV: *<32 wk* 4–5 mg/kg 36 hrly and *>32 wk* 4–5 mg/kg once in 24 hr.

Patent ductus arteriosus, prolonged hypoxia, and indomethacin treatment necessitate increased dose intervals. Extended interval dose regimen by IV injection over 3–5 minutes or by IV infusion: *neonate < 32 wk postmenstrual age:* 4–5 mg/kg every 36 hr; *neonate 32 wk and over postmenstrual age:* 4–5 mg/kg every 24 hr. *Child:* IV/IM 2.5 mg/kg/dose tid or 7 mg/kg as single daily dose. OD dose regimen by IV infusion: *Child 1 mo to 18 yr:* initially 7 mg/kg and then adjusted according to serum tobramycin concentration.

Pseudomonal lung infection in cystic fibrosis: Child 1 mo to 18 yr: 8–10 mg/kg/daily in 3 div. doses. OD dose regimen by IV infusion over 30 minutes. *Child 1 mo to 18 yr*: Initially 10 mg/kg (max. 660 mg) and then adjusted according to serum tobramycin concentration.

Chronic pulmonary P. aeruginosa infection in patients with cystic fibrosis: By inhalation of nebulized solution: *Child 6–18 yr:* 300 mg every 12 hr for 28 days, subsequent courses repeated after a 28-day interval without tobramycin nebulizer solution. Intraventricular: *Newborn* 1 mg/day; *child* 1–2 mg/day; *adolescent* 2–4 mg/day.

Eye drops: 1 drop 2 hrly and then reduce frequency as infection is controlled. To continue till 2 days after healing.

Tolazoline
Correction of pulmonary vasospasm in neonates: IV infusion: *neonate:* initially 1 mg/kg, to be given over 2–5 minutes, followed by (continuous IV infusion); maintenance 200 µg/kg/hr if required. Careful blood pressure monitoring should be carried out; doses above 300 µg/kg/hr are associated with cardiotoxicity and renal failure. Intratracheal: *neonate:* 200 µg/kg.

Tolnaftate
Apply evenly to the affected area and rub gently 2–3 times daily.

Tolterodine
It is usually effective within 4 wk.

Urinary frequency, urinary urgency, and urinary incontinence: PO immediate-release preparations: *2–17 yr:* 1 mg OD, then increased if necessary up to 2 mg bid, adjusted according to response. Modified-release capsules: *2–17 yr:* 4 mg OD.

Nocturnal enuresis associated with overactive bladder incontinence: PO immediate-release preparations: *5–17 yr:* 1 mg OD, dose to be taken at bedtime, then increased if necessary up to 2 mg bid, adjusted according to response.

Dose conversion: Children stabilized on immediate-release tolterodine tartrate 2 mg bid may be transferred to modified-release tolterodine tartrate 4 mg OD.

Topiramate

PO initially 0.5 mg/kg *(1 mo to 12 yr)* and 25 mg *(12–18 yr)* followed by maintenance of 2–4.5 mg/kg *(1 mo to 12 yr)* and 100–200 mg *(12–18 yr)*. Doses up to 6 mg/kg bid have been used. Use starting dose for 2 wk and then increase dose every 2 wk taking at least 6 wk to reach maintenance dose.

Renal impairment: Use with caution in renal failure, titrating dose and intervals between dose adjustments to efficacy and side effects. Supplemental doses required after dialysis.

Migraine prophylaxis: 16–18 yr: initially 25 mg bedtime for 1 wk, increase weekly by 25 mg/day; a dose of 50–100 mg daily in 2 div. doses would suffice (max. 200 mg/day).

Torsemide

On a weight-to-weight basis, torsemide is twice as potent as frusemide and provides a longer duration of action at lower urinary concentrations – allows for a 24-hr dosage interval and avoids the paradoxical antidiuresis seen with frusemide.

Edema associated with congestive heart failure or CRF: PO or IV dosage: *Adolescent:* Initially, 10–20 mg PO or IV OD. If needed, titrate by doubling the dose up to 200 mg PO or IV to achieve a satisfactory diuretic response. The safe use of a single dose ≥ 200 mg has not been evaluated.

Adjunctive treatment of ascites (e.g., due to hepatic cirrhosis) either alone or in combination with spironolactone or amiloride: PO or IV dosage: *adolescent:* Initially, 5–10 mg PO or IV OD. If needed, titrate upward by doubling the dose up to 40 mg PO or IV to achieve a satisfactory diuretic response. Doses ≥ 40 mg have not been evaluated in patients with hepatic cirrhosis. Chronic use in hepatic disease has not been evaluated.

Hypertension: PO dosage: *adolescent:* Initially, 5 mg PO OD. May increase to 10 mg PO OD if the desired reduction in blood pressure is not achieved in 4–6 wk. If this dose is insufficient, an additional antihypertensive agent should be added to the regimen.

Patients with hepatic impairment: No dosage adjustment is needed; see the dosage for the treatment of ascites. Diuretics should be used with caution in patients with hepatic disease since minor alterations of fluid and electrolyte balance may precipitate hepatic coma.

Patients with renal impairment: No dosage adjustment is needed; however, high doses may be effective in patients with end-stage renal disease.

Intermittent hemodialysis: Torsemide is not removed by hemodialysis; no dosage adjustment is needed.

Tranexamic acid

Inhibition of fibrinolysis: PO: *child:* 15–25 mg/kg 2–3 times a day (max. per dose 1.5 g). Slow IV injection: *child:* 10 mg/kg 2–3 times a day (max. per dose 1 g), dose to be given over at least 10 minutes; IV infusion: *child:* 45 mg/kg, dose to be given over 24 hr.

Menorrhagia: PO: *12–17 yr:* 1 g tid for up to 4 days, to be initiated when menstruation starts; max. 4 g/d.

Hereditary angioedema: PO: *child:* 15–25 mg/kg 2–3 times a day (max. per dose 1.5 g), for short-term prophylaxis of hereditary angioedema, tranexamic acid is started several days before planned procedures which may trigger an acute attack of hereditary angioedema (e.g., dental work) and continued for 2–5 days afterward. Slow IV injection*: Child:* 10 mg/kg 2–3 times a day (max. per dose 1 g), dose to be given over at least 10 minutes. IV infusion: *Child:* 45 mg/kg, dose to be given over 24 hr.

Prevention of excessive bleeding after dental procedures (e.g., in hemophilia): IV infusion*: child 6–17 yr:* 10 mg/kg (max. per dose 1.5 g), dose to be given preoperatively. PO: *child 6–17 yr:* 15–25 mg/kg (max. per dose 1.5 g), dose to be given preoperatively, then 15–25 mg/kg 2–3 times a day (max. per dose 1.5 g) for up to 8 days, dose to be given postoperatively.

Prevention of excessive bleeding after dental procedures (e.g., in hemophilia) with mouthwash 5% solution: PO: 6–17 yr: 5–10 mL qid for 2 days, rinse mouth with solution; the solution should not be swallowed.

Tretinoin

Topical: Apply 1–2 times daily thinly. The skin should be thoroughly washed first. Cream is recommended for dry or fair skin and gel for oily or dark skin.

Triamcinolone

Intra-articular: *>1 yr:* 1 mg/kg for large joints (max. 40 mg) and 0.5 mg/kg for small joints (max. 20 mg but max. 10 mg for finger and toe joints).

Triclofos Sodium

PO 30–50 mg/kg as single dose. Doses up to 100 mg/kg used for level 4 sedation required prior to doing procedures. Most used in *children < 12 yr*; chloral hydrate preferred in *children >12 yr.*

Trientine Dihydrochloride

Wilson's disease in patients intolerant of penicillamine: PO: *2–11 yr:* initially 0.6–1.5 g daily; *12–17 yr:* 1.2–2.4 g daily in 2–4 div. doses, adjusted according to response, to be taken before food.

Trifluoperazine
Schizophrenia and severe behavior disorders: 3–5 yr: 1 mg/day in div doses; *6–12 yr:* 2–5 mg in div. doses as required. *12–18 yr:* Start with 5 mg bid and increased by 5 mg/wk up to 15–20 mg/day.

Severe anxiety disorder: PO: *3–5 yr:* up to 1 mg/day; 6–12 yr: up to 4 mg/day; *12–18 yr:* 4 mg/day and increased if required up to 6 mg/day.

Vomiting not responding to other medications: PO: *3–5 yr:* up to 1 mg/day in div doses; up to 4 mg/day in div doses; *12–18 yr:* 2–4 mg/day in div. doses (max. 6 mg).

Trihexyphenidyl (Benzhexol)
Extrapyramidal symptoms and dystonia: 2 mg as single or div. doses.

Antispasmodic: Initial dose of 0.5 mg in <7 yr and 2 mg in >*7 yr* and increased by 0.5–2 mg/day every 10 days till response and given in 3–4 div. doses.

Trimipramine
PO: *6–12 yr:* 50–100 mg and *12–18 yr:* 75—300 mg at bedtime.

Tryptophan (L-Tryptophan)
100 mg/kg in 3 div. doses.

Tuberculin Purified Protein Derivative (PPD)
2 TU 1:1000 solution 0.1 mL intradermal on right forearm.

Typhoid vaccine (polysaccharide)
0.5 mL IM or deep SC.

Typhoid Vi Capsular Polysaccharide Tetanus Toxoid Conjugate Vaccine
Dosage: Single dose 0.5 mL at *9–12 mo age*. Catch-up vaccination is recommended throughout the adolescent period (up to 18 yr).

 U

Urea Cream
Topical: Wash the affected area, rinse off all traces of sap, and apply sparingly bid.

Urokinase
Thromboembolic disease: Loading dose of 4,400 IU/kg in 15 mL solution over 10 min followed by IV infusion 4,400 IU/kg/hr over 6–12 hr.

Blocked arteriovenous shunts, IV cannulas/central lines: 5,000 IU/kg directly into the catheter and clamp off and retain for 2–4 hr. If not cleared, instill 10,000 IU and clamp. Monitor with fibrinogen, thrombin clotting time (TCT), prothrombin time (PT), and aPTT estimations.

Ursodeoxycholic Acid
PO 5–10 mg/kg/dose 2–3 times daily (max. 45 mg/kg/day).

Cystic fibrosis: 10 mg/kg/dose bid.

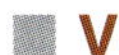 V

Valacyclovir
Heart transplant: 4 mo to 16 yr: total dose (mg) = [7 × BSA × CrCl] PO qid until 100 days post-transplant. Start: Within 10 days of transplant; max. 900 mg/day. Info: Round calculated dose to nearest 25 mg increment; solution preferred, but may use tabs if calculated dose is within 10% of available tab strength; give with food.

Kidney transplant: 4 mo to 16 yr: total dose (mg) = [7 × BSA × CrCl] PO qid until 100 days post-transplant. Start: Within 10 days of transplant; max: 900 mg/day. Info: Round calculated dose to nearest 25 mg increment; solution preferred, but may use tabs if calculated dose is within 10% of available tab strength; give with food.

Renal impairment: Dose adjustment required.

Hepatic dosing: Not defined.

Vancomycin
Clostridium difficile infection: PO: *neonate:* 10 mg/kg every 6 hr for 10 days. *Child 1 mo to 11 yr:* 10 mg/kg every 6 hr for 10 days, tailored to the clinical course of the child; max. 2 g/day. *12–18 yr:* First episode: 125 mg every 6 hr for 10 days; increased if necessary in severe or complicated infection to 500 mg every 6 hr for 10 days and for frequent recurrences - 125 mg every 6 hr for 10 days, followed by either tapering the dose (gradually reducing until 125 mg daily) or a pulse regimen (125–500 mg every 2–3 days for at least 3 wk)

Complicated skin and soft-tissue infections, bone and joint infections, community or hospital-acquired pneumonia including ventilator-associated pneumonia, infective endocarditis, acute bacterial meningitis, septicemia due to MRSA: IV infusion: *neonates up to 29 wk corrected gestational age:* 15 mg/kg OD; *29–35 wk corrected gestational age:* 15 mg/kg 12 hrly; *35 wk corrected gestational age and above:* 15 mg/kg 8 hrly; plasma conc. monitoring to adjust dose in all neonates. *1 mo to 11 yr:* 10–15 mg/kg every 6 hr (max. 60 mg/kg/day). *12–17 yr:* 15–20 mg/kg every 8–12 hr (max. per dose 2 g). Duration should be tailored to type and severity of infection and the individual clinical response. In seriously ill children, a loading dose of 25–30 mg/kg (usual max. 2 g) can be used to facilitate rapid attainment of the target trough serum vancomycin concentration.

Perioperative prophylaxis of bacterial endocarditis (in patients at high risk of developing bacterial endocarditis when undergoing major surgical procedures): IV infusion: *neonate:* 15 mg/kg; *child:* 15 mg/kg, to be given prior to induction of anesthesia, a second dose may be required depending on the duration of surgery. Vancomycin is to be initiated 60–120 minutes prior to incision.

Surgical prophylaxis (when high risk of MRSA): IV infusion: 15 mg/kg IV (max. 2,000 mg/dose) for known MRSA colonization or at high risk for MRSA colonization in the absence of surveillance data (e.g., patients with recent hospitalization, hemodialysis patients)

Central nervous system infection, e.g., ventriculitis: Intraventricular: *neonate:* 10 mg OD; *child*: 10 mg OD, for all children, reduce to 5 mg daily if the ventricular size is reduced or increase to 15–20 mg OD if the ventricular size is increased; adjust dose according to CSF concentration after 3–4 days; aim for pre-dose ("trough") concentration < 10 mg/L. If CSF is not draining freely, reduce dose frequency to once every 2–3 days.

Peritonitis associated with peritoneal dialysis as intraperitoneal infusion – added to dialysis fluid: child: Add to each bag of dialysis fluid to achieve a concentration of 20–25 mg/L.

Eradication of MRSA from the respiratory tract in cystic fibrosis: Nebulization: *child:* 4 mg/kg bid (max. per dose 250 mg) for 5 days, alternatively 4 mg/kg qid (max. per dose 250 mg) for 5 days.

Pseudomembranous colitis: PO vancomycin at 40 mg/kg/day div. q6–8hr for 7–10 days; not to exceed 2 g/day.

Varicella-Zoster Immunoglobulin (VZIG)
Prophylaxis against varicella infection: Deep IM: neonate < 2 kg: 62.5 IU; 2.1–10 kg: 125 IU; >10kg till 5 yr: 250 mg; 6–10 yr: 500 mg, 11–14 yr: 750 mg, 15–17 yr: 1 g – to be administered as soon as possible – not later than 10 days after exposure. Consider a second full dose for high-risk patients who have additional exposures to varicella >3 wk after the initial administration; no evidence that it is effective in severe disease.

Varicella-Zoster Vaccine, Live
All healthy children 12 mo through 12 yr of age should have two doses of chickenpox vaccine, administered at least 3 mo apart. Children who have evidence of immunity to varicella do not need the vaccine.

Vasopressin
By continuous IV infusion (may also be infused directly into superior mesenteric artery: *child 1 mo to 18 yr:* initially 0.3 U/kg (max. 20 U) over 20–30 min and then 0.3 units/kg/hr; adjusted according to response (max. 1 U/kg/hr); if bleeding stops, continue at the same dose for 12 hr and then withdraw gradually over 24–48 hr; max. duration of treatment 72 hr.

Vecuronium Bromide
IV bolus: 80–100 µg/kg as single dose and adjust dose and interval as required. IV infusion: *1 mo to 18 yr*: 50–80 µg/kg/hr.

Velaglucerase Alfa 1 (VPRIV)
Type I Gaucher's disease (specialist use only): IV infusion: *child 4–17 yr:* initially 60 units/kg every 2 wk; adjusted according to response to 15–60 units/kg every 2 wk.

Switching from Imiglucerase to VPRIV: Pediatric patients 4 yr of age and older currently being treated on a stable dosage of imiglucerase for type 1 Gaucher disease may be switched to VPRIV by starting treatment with VPRIV at the previous imiglucerase dosage 2 wk after the last imiglucerase dose.

Verapamil Hydrochloride
PO: *Newborn*: 1–2 mg/kg/dose; *1 mo to 2 yr:* 20 mg/dose; *2–18 yr:* 40–120 mg/dose tid. Slow IV bolus: *Newborn to 1 yr:* 100–200 µg/kg (max. 2 mg); *>1 yr:* 100–300 µg/kg (max. 5 mg) as single dose with ECG monitoring. May repeat after 30 min. Usually, lower doses suffice.

Vigabatrin
PO: *<12 yr:* 15–20 mg/kg/dose. *>12 yr:* 1 g/dose bid as the initial dose followed by maintenance dose of *<12 yr:* 30–40 mg/kg/dose, *>12 yr:* 1–1.5 g/dose bid. Increase to maintenance dose over 2–3 wk except for infantile spasms when the maintenance dose should be reached in 5–7 days.

Impaired renal function: Reduce dose.

Vinblastine Sulfate
Hodgkin disease: IV 2.5–6 mg/m^2/24 hr 1–2/wk for 3–6 wk (max. 12.5 mg/m^2/wk). Always consult the current treatment protocol for details of dosage and scheduling. Max. single dose 10 mg.

Hepatic impairment: A 50% dose reduction has been suggested in patients with serum bilirubin > 50 µmol/L.

Vincristine Sulfate
Children < 10 kg: 0.05 mg/kg once a week, *>10 kg:* 1–2 mg/m^2 once a week. Always consult the current treatment protocol for details of dosage and scheduling. Max. dose in adults is 2 mg weekly. Small infants may be unexpectedly sensitive to vincristine. Dosage reductions may be necessary if toxicity is unacceptable.

Hepatic impairment: An increase in the severity of side effects may be seen in patients with liver disease sufficient to decrease biliary excretion. A 50% dosage reduction is recommended in patients with a serum bilirubin level > 50 µmol/L.

Vitamin A (Retinol)
PO: *<1 yr:* 500 IU; *>1 yr:* 10,000 IU daily.

Prophylaxis of vitamin A deficiency: 1 lakh IU once in 6 mo as in National Program.

Vitamins A + D
Infants 0–6 mo: 2.5 mL of emulsion daily, PO: *6 mo* to *adults:* 5 mL of emulsion of 1 capsule daily.

Vitamin B Complex
Infants: 5 mL daily. *1–12 yr:* 5 mL bid. *12–18 yr:* 5 mL tid.

Therapeutic: Infants: 5 mL tid. *1–12 yr:* 10 mL tid. *12–18 yr:* 10–15 mL tid.

Vitamin C (Ascorbic Acid)
Scurvy: PO initially 500 mg, then 100 mg/day for 1 wk, then 50 mg/day for prophylaxis.

Metabolic indications: 200–400 mg/day.

Transient tyrosinemia: 50–200 mg/day for 1–2 wk.

Hawkinsuria, Tyrosinuria III: Up to 1 g daily for several wk until symptoms subside.

Vitamin E (Alpha Tocopheryl Acetate)
PO: <1 yr: 50 mg, *1–12 yr:* 100 mg; *12–18 yr:* 200 mg OD.

Prophylaxis of vitamin E deficiency in newborn: PO: 0.25 mL (29 mg) daily for all premature infants.

Therapy of symptomatic deficiency/prevention of retrolental fibroplasia (RLF), BPD and IVH: PO: 75–100 mg daily in 3 or 4 div. doses.

Note: (1) 1 mg of d-alpha tocopheryl acetate is equivalent in activity to 1.36 IU of vitamin E. (2) Folic acid status is also important in hemolytic anemia.

Vitamin K
Prophylaxis: In all newborn term babies, 1 mg IM and 0.5 mg IM for *preterm (birth weight < 1,500 g).*

It may be given to patients on *long-term broad-spectrum antibiotics.* PO dose is 5 mg daily.

Another indication for Vitamin K prophylaxis is neonatal cholestasis.

W

Warfarin
Newborn infant (birth to 1 mo): There is very little experience of the use of warfarin in the neonatal period. Always seek expert advice before starting anticoagulation. Initial loading dose is 0.2 mg/kg.

Infants < 1 yr usually need higher maintenance dose compared to older children. The dosage schedule is as per the international normalized ratio (INR) value. Average dose of warfarin in infants and young children is 0.33 mg/kg/day to achieve an INR of 2.0–3.0.

For teenagers, the dose is 0.09 mg/kg/day and *for adults,* 0.04-0.08 mg/kg/day.

Monitoring: Frequent dose adjustments. Warrant close supervision of INR. Vitamin K antagonists have extensive cross-reactivity with several commonly used drugs and dietary agents. Certain point-of-care monitors are commercially available, which are considered reliable and acceptable for checking INR in home setting. These are somewhat similar to glucometers. The INR level is affected by cumulative dose of warfarin taken over the last 5–7 days, so testing INR just after a day of change in dose is not useful.

Dosing of warfarin: Loading dose *(Day 1).* 0.2 mg/kg (max. 10 mg); 0.1 mg/kg in the presence of hepatic dysfunction. *Days 2–4.* INR 1.1–1.3, repeat loading dose. INR 1.4–1.9, give 50% of the initial loading dose. INR 2.0–3.0, give 50% of the initial loading dose. INR 3.1–3.5, give 25% of the initial loading dose. INR >3.5, hold until <3.5, restart at 50% of previous dose.

Maintenance dose (day 5 and beyond). INR 1.1–1.4, increase dose by 20% of previous dose. INR 1.5–1.9, increase dose by 10% of previous dose. INR 2.0–3.0, no change. INR 3.1–3.5, decrease dose by 10% of the previous dose. INR >3.5, hold until <3.5, restart at 20% of previous dose.

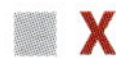

X

Xylometazoline Hydrochloride
Intranasal: *3 mo to 12 yr:* 1–2 drops 1–2 times of 0.05%; *12–18 yr:* 0.1% 2–3 drops or 1 spray 2–3 times daily.

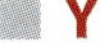

Y

Yellow Fever Vaccine, Live
Deep SC: 0.5 mL repeated every 10 yr while still at risk.

Z

Zafirlukast
5–11 yr: 10 mg PO bid; give 1 hr before or 2 hr after meals; *>12 yr:* 20 mg PO bid; give 1 hr before or 2 hr after meals.

Zidovudine (Azidothymidine, AZT)
Newborn: Prevention of fetomaternal transmission: PO 2 mg/kg/dose qid started within 12 hr of birth and continued for 6 wk. IV 1.5 mg/kg/dose qid. *Child:* PO 180 mg/m^2 bid (max. 250 mg/dose). IV 120 mg/m^2 qid.

Zileuton
Asthma, maintenance >12 yr: 600 mg PO qid; max: 2400 mg/day.

Hepatic impairment: Active hepatic disease/baseline liver function test (LFT) >3 times ULN contraindicated.

Monitoring parameters: ALT at baseline, monthly.

Zinc (Sulfate, Acetate, or Gluconate)

As zinc base. *Acute fluid diarrhea: <6 mo:*10 mg/day as single dose, *>6 mo:* 20 mg/day as single dose for 14 days.

Acrodermatitis enteropathica: PO 0.5–1 mg/kg/dose bid.

Wilson disease: PO *2–12 yr:* 25–37.5 mg/dose; *12–18 yr:* 50 mg/dose 2–4 times daily. Do not give at the same time as penicillamine.

Zinc deficiency: PO: *newborn:* 1 mg/kg OD, *10–30 kg:* 22–25 mg once or bid. *>30 kg:* 45 mg 1–3 times daily. Adjust according to response.

Zinc Sulfate Injection

2–5 μmol/kg depending on age and deficiency state.

Zonisamide

4–8 mg/kg/day. Should be administered once or bid, using 25, 50, or 100 mg capsules. Given PO and can be taken with or without food.

Zopiclone

PO: *12–18 yr:* 3.75 mg OD at bedtime.

Index

Page numbers followed by *b* refer to box, *f* refer to figure, *fc* refer to flowchart, and *t* refer to table.

A

B

C

D

E

F

H

I

J

K

L

M

O

P

T

V

W